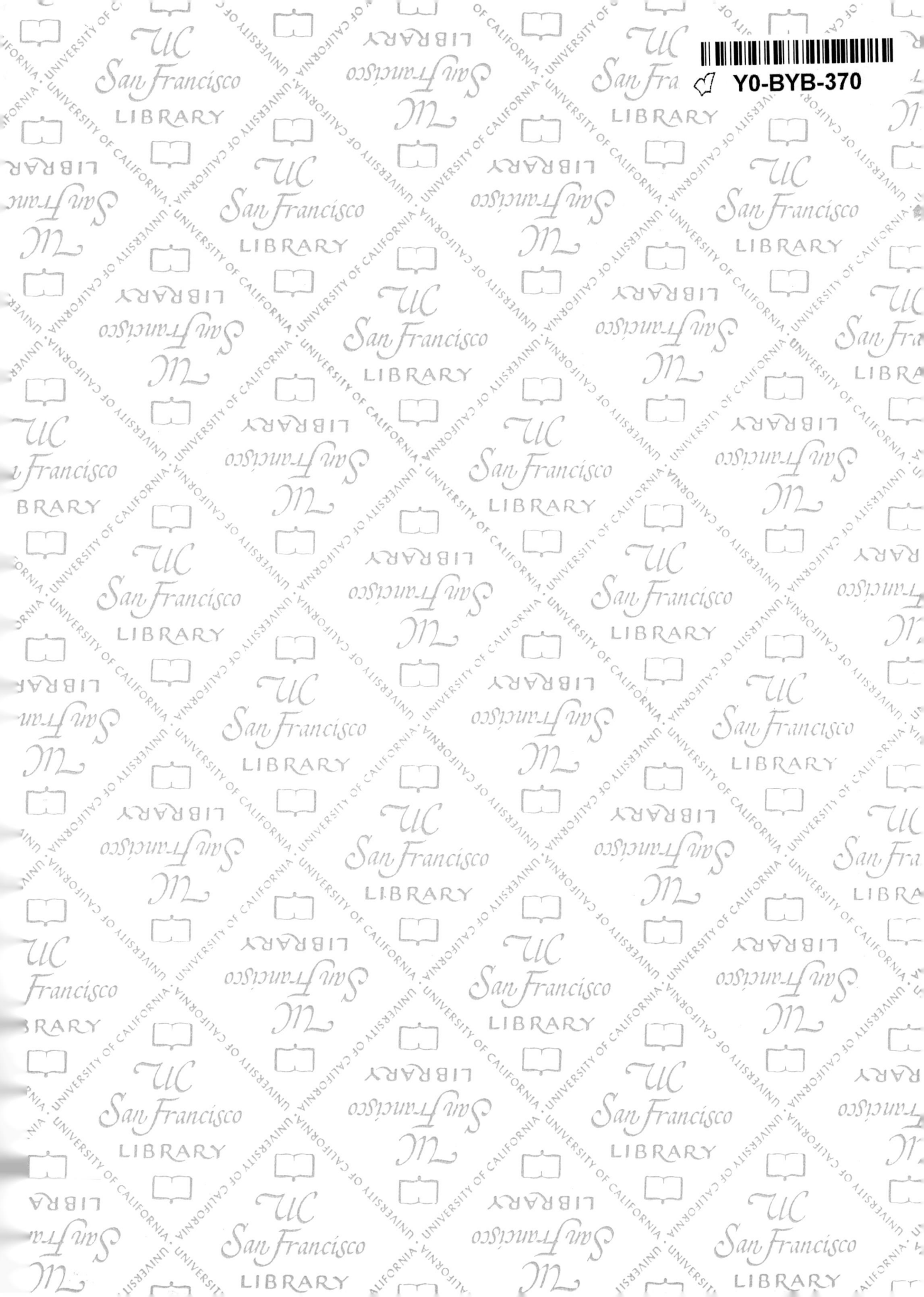

Hospital, Address, Telephone, Administrator, Approval, Facility, and Physician Codes, Health Care System, Network	Classi-fication Codes		Utilization Data					Expense (thousands) of dollars		
★ American Hospital Association (AHA) membership □ Joint Commission on Accreditation of Healthcare Organizations (JCAHO) accreditation + American Osteopathic Hospital Association (AOHA) membership ○ American Osteopathic Association (AOA) accreditation △ Commission on Accreditation of Rehabilitation Facilities (CARF) accreditation Control codes 61, 63, 64, 71, 72 and 73 indicate hospitals listed by AOHA, but not registered by AHA. For definition of numerical codes, see page A4	Control	Service	Beds	Admissions	Census	Outpatient Visits	Births	Total	Payroll	Personnel
ANYTOWN—Universal County ★ COMMUNITY HOSPITAL, First Street and Main Avenue Zip 62835; tel 204/391–2345; Jane Doe, Administrator **A**1 2 3 4 6 9 10 **F**1 2 3 4 5 6 8 9 10 23 24 34; **P**1 2 3 4; **S** Acme HCS **N** ABC	23	10	346	10778	248	75953	1693	20695	9973	796

1 Approval Codes

Reported by the approving bodies specified, as of the dates noted.

1 Accreditation under the hospital program of the Joint Commission on Accreditation of Healthcare Organizations (January 1997).
2 Cancer program approved by American College of Surgeons (January 1997).
3 Approval to participate in residency training, by the Accreditation Council for Graduate Medical Education (January 1997). As of June 30, 1975, internship (formerly code 4) was included under residency, code 3.
5 Medical school affiliation, reported to the American Medical Association (January 1997).

6 Hospital–controlled professional nursing school, reported by National League for Nursing (January 1997).
7 Accreditation by Commission on Accreditation of Rehabilitation Facilities (January 1997).
8 Member of Council of Teaching Hospitals of the Association of American Medical Colleges (January 1997).
9 Hospital contracting or participating in Blue Cross Plan, reported by individual Blue Cross Plans or Blue Cross Association at the time of publication.
10 Certified for participation in the Health Insurance for the Aged (Medicare) Program

by the U.S. Department of Health and Human Services (January 1997).
11 Accreditation by American Osteopathic Association (January 1997).
12 Internship approved by American Osteopathic Association (January 1997).
13 Residency approved by American Osteopathic Association (January 1997).

Nonreporting indicates that the hospital was registered after the mailing of the 1996 Annual Survey, or, that the 1996 Annual Survey questionnaire for the hospital had not been received prior to publication.

2 Facility Codes

Provided directly by the hospital, its health care system, or network, or through a formal arrangement with another provider; for definitions, see page A6.

(Alphabetical/Numerical Order)
1 Adult day care program
2 Alcoholism–drug abuse or dependency inpatient unit
3 Alcoholism–drug abuse or dependency outpatient services
4 Angioplasty
5 Arthritis treatment center
6 Assisted living
7 Birthing room–LDR room–LDRP room
8 Breast cancer screening/mammograms
9 Burn care services
10 Cardiac catheterization laboratory
11 Cardiac intensive care services
12 Case management
13 Children wellness program
14 Community health reporting
15 Community health status assessment
16 Community health status based service planning
17 Community outreach
18 Crisis prevention
19 CT scanner
20 Dental services
21 Diagnostic radioisotope facility

22 Emergency department
23 Extracorporeal shock wave lithotripter (ESWL)
24 Fitness center
25 Freestanding outpatient care center
26 Geriatric services
27 Health facility transportation (to/from)
28 Health fair
29 Health information center
30 Health screenings
31 HIV–AIDS services
32 Home health services
33 Hospice
34 Hospital–based outpatient care center–services
35 Magnetic resonance imaging (MRI)
36 Meals on wheels
37 Medical surgical intensive care services
38 Neonatal intensive care services
39 Nutrition programs
40 Obstetrics services
41 Occupational health services
42 Oncology services
43 Open heart surgery
44 Outpatient surgery
45 Patient education center
46 Patient representative services
47 Pediatric intensive care services
48 Physical rehabilitation inpatient services
49 Physical rehabilitation outpatient services

50 Positron emission tomography scanner (PET)
51 Primary care department
52 Psychiatric acute inpatient services
53 Psychiatric child adolescent services
54 Psychiatric consultation–liaison services
55 Psychiatric education services
56 Psychiatric emergency services
57 Psychiatric geriatric services
58 Psychiatric outpatient services
59 Psychiatric partial hospitalization program
60 Radiation therapy
61 Reproductive health services
62 Retirement housing
63 Single photon emission computerized tomography (SPECT)
64 Skilled nursing or other long–term care services
65 Social work services
66 Sports medicine
67 Support groups
68 Teen outreach services
69 Transplant services
70 Trauma center (certified)
71 Ultrasound
72 Urgent care center
73 Volunteer services department
74 Women's health center/services

3 Physician Codes

Actually available within, and reported by the institution; for definitions, see page A9.

(Alphabetical/Numerical Order)
1 Closed physician–hospital organization (PHO)

2 Equity model
3 Foundation
4 Group practice without walls
5 Independent practice association (IPA)

6 Integrated salary model
7 Management service organization (MSO)
8 Open physician–hospital organization (PHO)

Hospital, Address, Telephone, Administrator, Approval, Facility, and Physician Codes, Health Care System, Network	Classi-fication Codes		Utilization Data					Expense (thousands) of dollars		
	Control	Service	Beds	Admissions	Census	Outpatient Visits	Births	Total	Payroll	Personnel

★ American Hospital Association (AHA) membership
☐ Joint Commission on Accreditation of Healthcare Organizations (JCAHO) accreditation
+ American Osteopathic Hospital Association (AOHA) membership
○ American Osteopathic Association (AOA) accreditation
△ Commission on Accreditation of Rehabilitation Facilities (CARF) accreditation
  Control codes 61, 63, 64, 71, 72 and 73 indicate hospitals listed by AOHA, but not registered by AHA. For definition of numerical codes, see page A4

ANYTOWN—Universal County
★ COMMUNITY HOSPITAL, First Street and Main Avenue Zip 62835; tel 204/391–2345; Jane Doe, Administrator **A**1 2 3 4 6 9 10 **F**1 2 3 4 5 6 8 9 10 23 24 34; **P**1 2 3 4; **S** Acme HCS **N** ABC

	Control	Service	Beds	Admissions	Census	Outpatient Visits	Births	Total	Payroll	Personnel
	23	10	346	10778	248	75953	1693	20695	9973	796

4 **5** **6** **7**

4 Health Care System Code and Name

A code number has been assigned to each health care system headquarters. The inclusion of one of these codes (1) indicates that the hospital belongs to a health care system and (2) identifies the specific system to which the hospital belongs.

5 Network Name

The presence of the letter "N" indicates that the hospital belongs to one or more networks. The name(s) following the "N" identifies the specific network(s) to which the hospital belongs.

6 Classification Codes

Control

Government, nonfederal
12 State
13 County
14 City
15 City–county
16 Hospital district or authority

Nongovernment not–for–profit
21 Church operated
23 Other

Investor–owned (for–profit)
31 Individual
32 Partnership
33 Corporation

Government, federal
41 Air Force
42 Army
43 Navy

44 Public Health Service other than 47
45 Veterans Affairs
46 Federal other than 41–45, 47–48
47 Public Health Service Indian Service
48 Department of Justice

Osteopathic
61 Church operated
63 Other not–for–profit
64 Other
71 Individual for–profit
72 Partnership for–profit
73 Corporation for–profit

Service
10 General medical and surgical
11 Hospital unit of an institution (prison hospital, college infirmary, etc.)
12 Hospital unit within an institution for the mentally retarded
22 Psychiatric

33 Tuberculosis and other respiratory diseases
44 Obstetrics and gynecology
45 Eye, ear, nose, and throat
46 Rehabilitation
47 Orthopedic
48 Chronic disease
49 Other specialty
50 Children's general
51 Children's hospital unit of an institution
52 Children's psychiatric
53 Children's tuberculosis and other respiratory diseases
55 Children's eye, ear, nose, and throat
56 Children's rehabilitation
57 Children's orthopedic
58 Children's chronic disease
59 Children's other specialty
62 Institution for mental retardation
82 Alcoholism and other chemical dependency

* Control codes 61, 63, 64, 71, 72 and 73 indicate hospitals listed by the AOHA but not registered by AHA.

When a hospital restricts its service to a specialty not defined by a specific code, it is coded 49 (59 if a children's hospital) and the specialty is indicated in parentheses following the name of the hospital.

7 Headings

Definitions are based on the American Hospital Association's Hospital Administration Terminology. Where a 12–month period is specified, hospitals were requested to report on the Annual Survey of Hospitals for the 12 months ending September 30, 1996. Hospitals reporting for less than a 12–month period are so designated.

Utilization Data:

Beds–Number of beds regularly maintained (set up and staffed for use) for inpatients as of the close of the reporting period.

Admissions–Number of patients accepted for inpatient service during a 12–month period; does not include newborn.

Census–Average number of inpatients receiving care each day during the 12–month reporting period; does not include newborn.

Outpatient Visits–An outpatient visit is a visit by a patient who is not lodged in the hospital while receiving medical, dental, or other services. Each appearance of an outpatient in each unit constitutes one visit regardless of the number of diagnostic and/or therapeutic treatments that a patient receives.

Births–Number of infants born in the hospital and accepted for service in a newborn infant bassinet during a 12–month period; excludes stillbirths.

Expense: Expense for a 12–month period; both total expense and payroll components are shown. Payroll expenses include all salaries and wages.

Personnel: Includes persons on payroll on September 30, 1996; includes full–time equivalents of part–time personnel. Full–time equivalents were calculated on the basis that two part–time persons equal one full–time person.

AHA Guide to the Health Care Field

1997–98 Edition

Healthcare InfoSource, Inc., a subsidiary
of the American Hospital Association
One North Franklin
Chicago, Illinois 60606-3401

AHA Institutional Members $125
Nonmembers $275
AHA catalog NUMBER C–010097
Telephone ORDERS 1–800–AHA–2626

ISSN 0094–8969
ISBN 0–87258–717–7

Contents

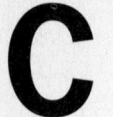

Lists of Health
Organizations,
Agencies and
Providers

Indexes

† List supplied by the Joint Commission on
  Accreditation of Healthcare Organizations

Acknowledgements and Advisements

Acknowledgements

The AHA Guide to the Health Care Field is published annually by Healthcare InfoSource, Inc., a subsidiary of the American Hospital Association. Contributions made by the AHA Communications Group, Computer Application Services, Member Relations, Printing Services Group and Resource Center.

Healthcare InsoSource, Inc. acknowledges the cooperation given by many professional groups and government agencies in the health care field, particularly the following: American College of Surgeons; American Medical Association; American Osteopathic Hospital Association; Blue Cross–Blue Shield Association; Council of Teaching Hospitals of the Association of American Medical Colleges; Joint Commission on Accreditation of Healthcare Organizations; National League for Nursing; Commission on Accreditation of Rehabilitation Facilities; American Osteopathic Association; Health Care Financing Administration; and various offices within the U.S. Department of Health and Human Services.

Advisements

The data published here should be used with the following advisements: The data are based on replies to an annual survey that seeks a variety of information, not all of which is published in this book. The information gathered by the survey includes specific services, but not all of each hospital's services. Therefore, the data do not reflect an exhaustive list of all services offered by all hospitals. For information on the availability of additional data, please contact Healthcare InfoSource, Inc. 312/422–2100.

Healthcare InfoSource, Inc. does not assume responsibility for the accuracy of information voluntarily reported by the individual institutions surveyed. The purpose of this publication is to provide basic data reflecting the delivery of health care in the United States and associated areas, and is not to serve as an official and all inclusive list of services offered by individual hospitals.

Introduction

Each of the three major sections of the AHA Guide begins with its own table of contents and pertinent definitions or explanatory information. Sections B, C and indices have bleed bar tabs for easy identification. The three major sections are:

- Hospitals
- Networks, Health Care Systems and Alliances
- Health Organizations, Agencies and Providers

Please note that many area codes have changed, check before you call.

Hospitals

This section lists:

- AHA–registered and osteopathic hospitals in the U.S. and associated areas, by state within city.
- U.S. government hospitals outside the United States.
- Index of hospitals alphabetically.
- Index of health care professionals.
- AHA Associate members.

AHA member hospitals are identified by a star (★). Hospitals accredited under one of the programs of the Joint Commission on Accreditation of Healthcare Organizations are identified by a hollow box (☐). Preceding the list of hospitals is a statement of the formal requirements for registration by the AHA.

The lists provide a variety of information about each hospital, including the administrator's name; various approvals; selected facilities and services; relationship to a network and/or health care system; classification by control, service; physician arrangement relationships and other selected statistical data from the 1996 AHA Annual Survey.

Also the *AHA Guide* includes state population data from the U.S. Bureau of the Census, *Statistical Abstract of the United States: 1996 (116th edition.) Washington, DC, 1996. They include the following:*

- Total resident population (in thousands)
- Percent of resident population in metro areas
- Birth rate per 1,000 population
- Percent of population 65 years and over
- Percent of persons without health insurance

Some of this information is coded. These include approval, facility and classification codes.

Approval codes refer to approvals held by a hospital; they represent information supplied by various national approving and reporting bodies. For example, code A–1 indicates accreditation under one of the

programs of the Joint Commission on Accreditation of Healthcare Organizations – formal evidence that a hospital meets established standards for quality of patient care.

Physician codes refer to the different types of physician arrangements the hospital participates in.

Health care system names reference specific health care system headquarters. The presence of the system name indicates the hospital belongs to a health care system. Absence of a system name indicates that the hospital does not belong to a health care system.

Network names reference specific network headquarters. The presence of the network name indicates the hospital belongs to a network. Absence of a network name indicates that the hospital does not belong to a network.

Classification codes indicate the type of organization that controls or operates the hospital and type of service. Code numbers in the 10s denote nonfederal (states and local) government hospitals; in the 20s, nongovernment not–for–profit hospitals; in the 40s, federal government hospitals; and in the 60s and 70s, nonregistered osteopathic hospitals.

Among **service codes,** the most common code is 10, indicating a general hospital. Other numbers designate various special services. For example, code 22 indicates psychiatric hospitals and codes in the 50s indicate different types of children's hospitals.

Facility codes refer to facilities and services provided directly by the hospital, it's health care system, or network or through a formal arrangement with another provider.

(For easy reference, there is a alphabetical/numerical list for all of the codes on page A4).

Names of osteopathic hospitals, supplied by the American Osteopathic Hospital Association are interfiled in the list of hospitals. Codes and symbols identifying these institutions are explained on page A4 and in the headnote at the top of each page of the list of hospitals. Also included in this section is an **index of hospitals** in alphabetical order by hospital name, followed by the city and state and the page reference to the hospital's listing in Section A. This section is designated by tabs along the side of the pages. Immediately following this section is an **index of health care professionals** in alphabetical order by name,

followed by the hospital and/or health care system, the city and state and the page reference to the health care professional's listing in section A or B. This section is also designated by tabs along the side of the pages

This section also lists **other AHA institution members** not listed elsewhere in the AHA Guide and **AHA associate members.** The list of AHA institutional members include Canadian hospitals, associated university programs in health administration, hospital schools of nursing, and nonhospital preacute and postacute care facilities. The list of associate members includes ambulatory centers and home care agencies, Blue Cross plans, health maintenance organizations/health care corporations, health system agencies, other inpatient care institutions, shared services organizations and other associate members.

Networks, Health Care Systems and Alliances

Networks

The *AHA Guide* lists the names and addresses of networks including network partners by state, alphabetically by name. Please see page B2 for more information.

Health Care Systems

This is an alphabetical list of health care systems and their hospitals. Data on bed size for each hospital in the system is provided along with an indication of whether the hospital is owned, leased, sponsored or contract– managed.

Following is an index for health care system headquarters geographically by state.

Alliances

Alliances provide information on multistate alliances and their members. Alliances are listed alphabetically by name. Members are listed alphabetically by state, city and then by name.

Health Organizations, Agencies and Providers

There are four major categories in this section.

First is an alphabetical listing of national, international, and regional organizations. Many voluntary organizations that are interested in, or of interest to the health care field are included. Also included is the Healthfinder listing.

The second lists United States government agencies.

The third presents a list of state and local organizations and government agencies. The list for states and provinces include Blue Cross and Blue Shield plans, health systems agencies, hospital associations and councils, hospital licensure agencies, medical and nursing licensure agencies, peer review organizations, state health planning and development agencies, and state and provincial government agencies.

The fourth consists of lists of various health care providers including JCAHO accredited freestanding long–term care organizations, JCAHO accredited freestanding substance abuse organizations, and JCAHO accredited freestanding mental health care organizations, freestanding hospices, freestanding ambulatory surgery centers and health maintenance organizations (HMOs).

Index
This index helps the reader locate specific information quickly. It lists alphabetically the subjects covered in the various sections and where they can be found.

Abbreviations
This is an alphabetical list of all abbreviations used in the *AHA Guide*. In some cases an abbreviation may stand for more than one word or term. In such cases, the meaning will be determined by the context.

We hope you find the *AHA Guide* a valuable resource. If you have any questions or comments, please call Healthcare InfoSource, Inc., at 312/422–2100.

AHA Offices, Officers, and Historical Data

Chicago: One North Franklin, Chicago, IL 60606–3401; tel. 312/422–3000

Washington: 325 Seventh Street, N.W., Suite 700, Washington, DC 20004; tel. 202/638–1100

Speaker of the House of Delegates: Gordon M. Sprenger, Allina Health System, 5601 Smetana Drive, Minneapolis, MN 55440
Chairman of the Board of Trustees: Reginald M. Ballantyne III, PMH Health Resources, Inc., 1201 S. Seventh Avenue, Box 21207, Phoenix, AZ 85036

Chairman–Elect of the Board of Trustees: John G. King, Legacy Health System, 1919 N.W. Lovejoy, Portland, OR 97209
President: Richard J. Davidson, 325 Seventh Street, N.W., Suite 700, Washington, DC 20004; tel. 202/638–1100

Senior Vice President and Secretary: Michael P. Guerin, One North Franklin, Chicago, IL 60606–3401
Vice President, Finance and Assistant Treasurer: Sidney Jacob, One North Franklin, Chicago, IL 60606–3401

Past Presidents/Chairmen†

1899	★James S. Knowles	1931	★Lewis A. Sexton, M.D.	1964	Stanley A. Ferguson
1900	★James S. Knowles	1932	★Paul H. Fesler	1965	Clarence E. Wonnacott
1901	★Charles S. Howell	1933	★George F. Stephens, M.D.	1966	Philip D. Bonnet, M.D.
1902	★J. T. Duryea	1934	★Nathaniel W. Faxon, M.D.	1967	George E. Cartmill
1903	★John Fehrenbatch	1935	★Robert Jolly	1968	★David B. Wilson, M.D.
1904	★Daniel D. Test	1936	★Robin C. Buerki, M.D.	1969	George William Graham, M.D.
1905	★George H. M. Rowe, M.D.	1937	★Claude W. Munger, M.D.	1970	★Mark Berke
1906	★George P. Ludlam	1938	★Robert E. Neff	1971	Jack A. L. Hahn
1907	★Renwick R. Ross, M.D.	1939	★G. Harvey Agnew, M.D.	1972	Stephen M. Morris
1908	★Sigismund S. Goldwater, M.D.	1940	★Fred G. Carter, M.D.	1973	★John W. Kauffman
1909	★John M. Peters, M.D.	1941	★B. W. Black, M.D.	1974	★Horace M. Cardwell
1910	★H. B. Howard, M.D.	1942	★Basil C. MacLean, M.D.	1975	Wade Mountz
1911	★W. L. Babcock, M.D.	1943	★James A. Hamilton	1976	H. Robert Cathcart
1912	★Henry M. Hurd, M.D.	1944	★Frank J. Walter	1977	John M. Stagl
1913	★F. A. Washburn, M.D.	1945	★Donald C. Smelzer, M.D.	1978	★Samuel J. Tibbitts
1914	★Thomas Howell, M.D.	1946	★Peter D. Ward, M.D.	1979	W. Daniel Barker
1915	★William O. Mann, M.D.	1947	★John H. Hayes	1980	Sister Irene Kraus
1916	★Winford H. Smith, M.D.	1948	★Graham L. Davis	1981	Bernard J. Lachner
1917	★Robert J. Wilson, M.D.	1949	★Joseph G. Norby	1982	Stanley R. Nelson
1918	★A. B. Ancker, M.D.	1950	★John H. Hatfield	1983	Elbert E. Gilbertson
1919	★A. R. Warner, M.D.	1951	★Charles F. Wilinsky, M.D.	1984	Thomas R. Matherlee
1920	★Joseph B. Howland, M.D.	1952	★Anthony J. J. Rourke, M.D.	1985	Jack A. Skarupa
1921	★Louis B. Baldwin, M.D.	1953	★Edwin L. Crosby, M.D.	1986	Scott S. Parker
1922	★George O'Hanlon, M.D.	1954	★Ritz E. Heerman	1987	Donald C. Wegmiller
1923	★Asa S. Bacon	1955	★Frank R. Bradley	1988	Eugene W. Arnett
1924	★Malcolm T. MacEachern, M.D.	1956	★Ray E. Brown	1989	Edward J. Connors
1925	★E. S. Gilmore	1957	★Albert W. Snoke, M.D.	1990	David A. Reed
1926	★Arthur C. Bachmeyer, M.D.	1958	★Tol Terrell	1991	C. Thomas Smith
1927	★R. G. Brodrick, M.D.	1959	★Ray Amberg	1992	D. Kirk Oglesby, Jr.
1928	★Joseph C. Doane, M.D.	1960	Russell A. Nelson, M.D.	1993	Larry L. Mathis
1929	★Louis H. Burlingham, M.D.	1961	★Frank S. Groner	1994	Carolyn C. Roberts
1930	★Christopher G. Parnall, M.D.	1962	★Jack Masur, M.D.	1995	Gail L. Warden
		1963	T. Stewart Hamilton, M.D.	1996	Gordon M. Sprenger

Chief Executive Officers

1917–18	★William H. Walsh, M.D.	1943–54	★George Bugbee	1986–91	Carol M. McCarthy, Ph.D., J.D.
1919–24	★Andrew Robert Warner, M.D.	1954–72	★Edwin L. Crosby, M.D.	1991	Jack W. Owen (acting)
1925–27	★William H. Walsh, M.D.	1972	★Madison B. Brown, M.D. (acting)	1991	Richard J. Davidson
1928–42	★Bert W. Caldwell, M.D.	1972–86	J. Alexander McMahon		

Distinguished Service Award

1934	★Matthew O. Foley	1958	★John N. Hatfield	1980	Donald W. Cordes
1939	★Malcolm T. MacEachern, M.D.	1959	★Edwin L. Crosby, M.D.	1981	★Sister Mary Brigh Cassidy
1940	★Sigismund S. Goldwater, M.D.	1960	★Oliver G. Pratt	1982	R. Zach Thomas, Jr.
1941	★Frederic A. Washburn, M.D.	1961	★E. M. Bluestone, M.D.	1983	H. Robert Cathcart
1942	★Winford H. Smith, M.D.	1962	Mother Loretto Bernard, S.C., R.N.	1984	Matthew F. McNulty, Jr., Sc.D.
1943	★Arthur C. Bachmeyer, M.D.	1963	★Ray E. Brown	1985	J. Alexander McMahon
1944	★Rt. Rev. Msgr. Maurice F. Griffin, LL.D.	1964	Russell A. Nelson, M.D.	1986	Sister Irene Kraus
1945	★Asa S. Bacon	1965	★Albert W. Snoke, M.D.	1987	W. Daniel Barker
1946	★George F. Stephens, M.D.	1966	★Frank S. Groner	1988	Elbert E. Gilbertson
1947	★Robin C. Buerki, M.D.	1967	★Rev. John J. Flanagan, S.J.	1989	Donald G. Shropshire
1948	★James A. Hamilton	1968	Stanley W. Martin	1990	John W. Colloton
1949	★Claude W. Munger, M.D.	1969	T. Stewart Hamilton, M.D.	1991	Carol M. McCarthy, Ph.D., J.D.
1950	★Nathaniel W. Faxon, M.D.	1970	★Charles Patteson Cladwell, Jr.	1992	David H. Hitt
1951	★Bert W. Caldwell, M.D.	1971	★Mark Berke	1993	Edward J. Connors
1952	★Fred G. Carter, M.D.	1972	Stanley A. Ferguson		Jack W. Owen
1953	★asil C. MacLean, M.D.	1973	Jack A. L. Hahn	1994	George Adams
1954	★George Bugbee	1974	George William Graham, M.D.	1995	Scott S. Parker
1955	★Joseph G. Norby	1975	George E. Cartmill	1996	John A. Russell
1956	★Charles F. Wilinsky, M.D.	1976	D. O. McClusky, Jr.	1997	D. Kirk Oglesby, Jr.
1957	★John H. Hayes	1977	★Boone Powell		
		1978	★Richard J. Stull		
		1979	★Horace M. Cardwell		

★Deceased

†On June 3, 1972, the House of Delegates changed the title of the chief elected officer to chairman of the Board of Trustees, and the title of president was conferred on the chief executive officer of the Association.

Award of Honor

1966	★Senator Lister Hill	1991	★Haynes Rice			John K. Springer
1967	★Emory W. Morris, D.D.S.	1992	Donald W. Dunn	1996	★Stephen J. Hegarty
1971	Special Committee on Provision of Health		Ira M. Lane, Jr.			Mothers Against Drunk Driving (MADD)
	Services (staff also)	1993	Elliott C. Roberts, Sr.	1997	Paul B. Batalden, M.D.
1982	Walter J. McNemey		William A. Spencer, M.D.			Habitat for Humanity International
1989	Ruth M. Rothstein	1994	Robert A. Derzon			
1990	Joyce C. Clifford, R.N.	1995	Russell G. Mawby, Ph.D.			

Justin Ford Kimball Innovators Award

1958	★E. A. van Steenwyk	1971	★H. Charles Abbott	1984	Joseph F. Duplinsky
1959	George A. Newbury	1972	★John R. Mannix	1985	David W. Stewart
1960	★C. Rufus Rorem, Ph.D.	1973	Herman M. Somers	1988	★Ernest W. Saward, M.D.
1961	★James E. Stuart	1974	William H. Ford, Ph.D.	1990	James A. Vohs
1962	Frank Van Dyk	1975	Earl H. Kammer	1993	John C. Lewin, M.D.
1963	★William S. McNary	1976	J. Ed McConnell	1994	Donald A. Brennan
1964	★Frank S. Groner	1978	Edwin R. Werner	1995	E. George Middleton, Jr.
1965	★J. Douglas Colman	1979	★Robert M. Cunningham, Jr.			Glenn R. Mitchell
1967	Walter J. McNemey	1981	★Maurice J. Norby	1997	Harvey Pettry
1968	★John W. Paynter	1982	Robert E. Rinehimer			D. David Sniff
1970	★Edwin L. Crosby, M.D.	1983	John B. Morgan, Jr.			

Trustees Award

1959	★Joseph V. Friel		Edmond J. Lanigan	1985	★James E. Ferguson
	★John H. Hayes	1974	★James E. Hague			Cleveland Rodgers
1960	Duncan D. Sutphen, Jr.		Sister Marybelle	1986	Rex N. Olsen
1963	Eleanor C. Lambertsen, R.N., Ed.D.	1975	Helen T. Yast	1987	Michael Lesparre
1964	★John R. Mannix	1976	Boynton P. Livingston	1988	Barbara A. Donaho, R.N.
1965	Albert G. Hahn		James Ludlam	1989	Walter H. MacDonald
	★Maurice J. Norby		★Helen McGuire			Donald R. Newkirk
1966	Madison B. Brown, M.D.	1979	★Newton J. Jacobson	1990	William T. Robinson
	Kenneth Williamson		Edward W. Weimer	1992	Jack C. Bills
1967	★Alanson W. Wilcox	1980	★Robert B. Hunter, M.D.			Anne Hall Davis
1968	★E. Dwight Barnett, M.D.		★Samuel J. Tibbitts	1993	Theodore C. Eickhoff, M.D.
1969	★Vane M. Hoge, M.D.	1981	Vernon A. Knutson			Stephen W. Gamble
	Joseph H. McNinch, M.D.		John E. Sullivan			Yoshi Honkawa
1972	David F. Drake, Ph.D.	1982	John Bigelow	1994	Roger M. Busfield, Jr., Ph.D.
	Paul W. Earle		Robert W. O'Leary	1995	Stephen E. Dorn
	Michael Lesparre		Jack W. Owen			William L. Yates
	Andrew Pattullo	1984	Howard J. Berman	1996	Leigh E. Morris
1973	Tilden Cummings		O. Ray Hurst			John Quigley
			James R. Neely			

Citation for Meritorious Service

1968	★F. R. Knautz		Gordon McLachlan	1983	★David M. Kinzer
	Sister Conrad Mary, R.N.	1977	Theodore Cooper, M.D.	1984	Donald L. Custis, M.D.
1971	Hospital Council of Southern California	1979	Norman D. Burkett	1985	John A. D. Cooper, M.D.
1972	College of Misericordia, Dallas, PA		John L. Quigley			Imperial Council of the Ancient Arabic
1973	Madison B. Brown, M.D.		★William M. Whelan			Order of the Nobles of the Mystic Shrine
	★Samuel J. Tibbitts	1980	★Sister Grace Marie Hiltz			for North America
1975	★Kenneth B. Babcock, M.D.		Leo J. Gehrig, M.D.	1986	Howard F. Cook
	Sister Mary Maurita Sengelaube	1981	Richard Davi	1987	David H. Hitt
1976	Chaiker Abbis		Pearl S. Fryar			★Lucile Packard
	★Susan Jenkins	1982	Jorge Brull Nater			

This citation is no longer awarded

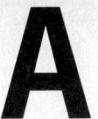
*AHA–registered hospitals in the United States and associated areas are approved for registration by the Executive Committee of the Board of Trustees of the American Hospital Association. This list of registered hospitals is complete as of April 1997. The list of osteopathic hospitals, integrated in this section is supplied by the American Osteopathic Hospital Association.

Registration Requirements for Hospitals

This directory includes hospitals registered by the American Hospital Association and osteopathic hospitals listed by the American Osteopathic Association. Identification codes for both types of hospitals are explained fully on pages A4–5. For the reader's convenience, the codes for osteopathic hospitals are also summarized in the notes at the top of each page of this section. Beginning in November 1970, osteopathic hospitals became eligible to apply for registration with the American Hospital Association. Registered osteopathic hospitals carry the same codes as all other hospitals registered by the American Hospital Association.

The following requirements were approved by the Executive Committee of the Board of Trustees, May 13, 1986.

AHA–Registered Hospitals

Any institution that can be classified as a hospital according to the requirements may be registered if it so desires. Membership in the American Hospital Association is not a prerequisite.

The American Hospital Association may, at the sole discretion of the Executive Committee of the Board of Trustees, grant, deny, or withdraw the registration of an institution.

An Institution may be registered by the American Hospital Association as a hospital if it is accredited as a hospital by the Joint Commission on Accreditation of Healthcare Organizations or is certified as a provider of acute services under Title 18 of the Social Security Act and has provided the Association with documents verifying the accreditation or certification.

In lieu of the preceding accreditation or certification, an institution licensed as a hospital by the appropriate state agency may be registered by AHA as a hospital by meeting the following alternative requirements:

Function: The primary function of the institution is to provide patient services, diagnostic and therapeutic, for particular or general medical conditions.

1. The institution shall maintain at lease six inpatient beds, which shall be continuously available for the care of patients who are nonrelated and who stay on the average in excess of 24 hours per admission.
2. The institution shall be constructed, equipped, and maintained to ensure the health and safety of patients and to provide uncrowded, sanitary facilities for the treatment of patients.
3. There shall be an identifiable governing authority legally and morally responsible for the conduct of the hospital.
4. There shall be a chief executive to whom the governing authority delegates the continuous responsibility for the operation of the hospital in accordance with established policy.
5. There shall be an organized medical staff of fully licensed physicians* that may include other licensed individuals permitted by law and by the hospital to provide patient care services independently in the hospital. The medical staff shall be accountable to the governing authority for maintaining proper standards of medical care, and it shall be governed by bylaws adopted by said staff and approved by the governing authority.
6. Each patient shall be admitted on the authority of a member of the medical staff who has been granted the privilege to admit patients to inpatient services in accordance with state law and criteria for standards of medical care established by the individual medical staff. Each patient's general medical condition is the responsibility of a qualified physician member of the medical staff. When nonphysician members of the medical staff are granted privileges to admit patients, provision is made for prompt medical evaluation of these patients by a qualified physician. Any graduate of a foreign medical school who is permitted to assume responsibilities for patient care shall possess a valid license to practice medicine, or shall be certified by the Educational Commission for Foreign Medical Graduates, or shall have qualified for and have successfully completed an academic year of supervised clinical training under the direction of a medical school approved by the Liaison Committee onGAT Medical Education.
7. Registered nurse supervision and other nursing services are continuous.
8. A current and complete+ medical record shall be maintained by the institution for each patient and shall be available for reference.
9. Pharmacy service shall be maintained in the institution and shall be supervised by a registered pharmacist.
10. The institution shall provide patients with food service that meets their nutritional and therapeutic requirements; special diets shall also be available.

*Physician–Term used to describe an individual with an M.D. or D.O. degree who is fully licensed to practice medicine in all its phases.

‡The completed records in general shall contain at least the following: the patient's identifying data and consent forms, medical history, record of physical examination, physicians' progress notes, operative notes, nurses' notes, routine x–ray and laboratory reports, doctors' orders, and final diagnosis.

Types of Hospitals

In addition to meeting these 10 general registration requirements, hospitals are registered as one of four types of hospitals: general, special, rehabilitation and chronic disease, or psychiatric. The following definitions of function by type of hospital and special requirements for registration are employed:

General

The primary function of the institution is to provide patient services, diagnostic and therapeutic, for a variety of medical conditions. A general hospital also shall provide:
- diagnostic x–ray services with facilities and staff for a variety of procedures
- clinical laboratory service with facilities and staff for a variety of procedures and with anatomical pathology services regularly and conveniently available
- operating room service with facilities and staff.

Special

The primary function of the institution is to provide diagnostic and treatment services for patients who have specified medical conditions, both surgical and nonsurgical. A special hospital also shall provide:
- such diagnostic and treatment services as may be determined by the Executive Committee of the Board of Trustees of the American Hospital Association to be appropriate for the specified medical conditions for which medical services are provided shall be maintained in the institution with suitable facilities and staff. If such conditions do not normally require diagnostic x–ray service, laboratory service, or operating room service, and if any such services are therefore not maintained in the institution, there shall be written arrangements to make them available to patients requiring them.
- clinical laboratory services capable of providing tissue diagnosis when offering pregancy termination services.

Rehabilitation and Chronic Disease

The primary function of the institution is to provide diagnostic and treatment services to handicapped or disabled individuals requiring restorative and adjustive services. A rehabilitation and chronic disease hospital also shall provide:
- arrangements for diagnostic x–ray services, as required, on a regular and conveniently available basis
- arrangements for clinical laboratory service, as required on a regular and conveniently available basis
- arrangements for operating room service, as required, on a regular and conveniently available basis
- a physical therapy service with suitable facilities and staff in the institution
- an occupational therapy service with suitable facilities and staff in the institution
- arrangements for psychological and social work services on a regular and conveniently available basis
- arrangements for educational and vocational services on a regular and conveniently available basis

- written arrangements with a general hospital for the transfer of patients who require medical, obstetrical, or surgical services not available in the institution.

Psychiatric

The primary function of the institution is to provide diagnostic and treatment services for patients who have psychiatric–related illnesses. A psychiatric hospital also shall provide:
- arrangements for clinical laboratory service, as required, on a regular and conveniently available basis
- arrangements for diagnostic x–ray services, as required on a regular and conveniently available basis
- psychiatric, psychological, and social work service with facilities and staff in the institution
- arrangements for electroencephalograph services, as required, on a regular and conveniently available basis.
- written arrangements with a general hospital for the transfer of patients who require medical, obstetrical, or surgical services not available in the institution.

The American Hospital Association may, at the sole discretion of the Executive Committee of the Board of Trustees, grant, deny, or withdraw the registration of an institution.

AOHA–Listed Hospitals

The list of osteopathic hospitals includes both members and nonmembers of the American Osteopathic Hospital Association.

*Physician–Term used to describe an individual with an M.D. or D.O. degree who is fully licensed to practice medicine in all its phases.

‡The completed records in general shall contain at least the following: the patient's identifying data and consent forms, medical history, record of physical examination, physicians' progress notes, operative notes, nurses' notes, routine x–ray and laboratory reports, doctors' orders, and final diagnosis.

Explanation of Hospital Listings

Hospital, Address, Telephone, Administrator, Approval, Facility, and Physician Codes, Health Care System, Network	Classi- fication Codes		Utilization Data						Expense (thousands) of dollars		
	Control	Service	Beds	Admissions	Census	Outpatient Visits	Births	Total	Payroll	Personnel

★ American Hospital Association (AHA) membership
□ Joint Commission on Accreditation of Healthcare Organizations (JCAHO) accreditation
+ American Osteopathic Hospital Association (AOHA) membership
○ American Osteopathic Association (AOA) accreditation
△ Commission on Accreditation of Rehabilitation Facilities (CARF) accreditation
Control codes 61, 63, 64, 71, 72 and 73 indicate hospitals listed by AOHA, but not registered by AHA. For definition of numerical codes, see page A4

ANYTOWN—Universal County
★ COMMUNITY HOSPITAL, First Street and Main Avenue Zip 62835; tel 204/391–2345; Jane Doe, Administrator **A**1 2 3 4 6 9 10 **F**1 2 3 4 5 6 8 9 10 23 24 34; **P**1 2 3 4; **S** Acme HCS **N** ABC

23	10	346	10778	248	75953	1693	20695	9973	796

1   2   3

1 Approval Codes

Reported by the approving bodies specified, as of the dates noted.

1 Accreditation under the hospital program of the Joint Commission on Accreditation of Healthcare Organizations (January 1997).

2 Cancer program approved by American College of Surgeons (January 1997).

3 Approval to participate in residency training, by the Accreditation Council for Graduate Medical Education (January 1997). As of June 30, 1975, internship (formerly code 4) was included under residency, code 3.

5 Medical school affiliation, reported to the American Medical Association (January 1997).

6 Hospital–controlled professional nursing school, reported by National League for Nursing (January 1997).

7 Accreditation by Commission on Accreditation of Rehabilitation Facilities (January 1997).

8 Member of Council of Teaching Hospitals of the Association of American Medical Colleges (January 1997).

9 Hospital contracting or participating in Blue Cross Plan, reported by individual Blue Cross Plans or Blue Cross Association at the time of publication.

10 Certified for participation in the Health Insurance for the Aged (Medicare) Program

by the U.S. Department of Health and Human Services (January 1997).

11 Accreditation by American Osteopathic Association (January 1997).

12 Internship approved by American Osteopathic Association (January 1997).

13 Residency approved by American Osteopathic Association (January 1997).

Nonreporting indicates that the hospital was registered after the mailing of the 1996 Annual Survey, or, that the 1996 Annual Survey questionnaire for the hospital had not been received prior to publication.

2 Facility Codes

Provided directly by the hospital, its health care system, or network, or through a formal arrangement with another provider; for definitions, see page A6.

(Alphabetical/Numerical Order)

1 Adult day care program
2 Alcoholism–drug abuse or dependency inpatient unit
3 Alcoholism–drug abuse or dependency outpatient services
4 Angioplasty
5 Arthritis treatment center
6 Assisted living
7 Birthing room–LDR room–LDRP room
8 Breast cancer screening/mammograms
9 Burn care services
10 Cardiac catheterization laboratory
11 Cardiac intensive care services
12 Case management
13 Children wellness program
14 Community health reporting
15 Community health status assessment
16 Community health status based service planning
17 Community outreach
18 Crisis prevention
19 CT scanner
20 Dental services
21 Diagnostic radioisotope facility

22 Emergency department
23 Extracorporeal shock wave lithotripter (ESWL)
24 Fitness center
25 Freestanding outpatient care center
26 Geriatric services
27 Health facility transportation (to/from)
28 Health fair
29 Health information center
30 Health screenings
31 HIV–AIDS services
32 Home health services
33 Hospice
34 Hospital–based outpatient care center–services
35 Magnetic resonance imaging (MRI)
36 Meals on wheels
37 Medical surgical intensive care services
38 Neonatal intensive care services
39 Nutrition programs
40 Obstetrics services
41 Occupational health services
42 Oncology services
43 Open heart surgery
44 Outpatient surgery
45 Patient education center
46 Patient representative services
47 Pediatric intensive care services
48 Physical rehabilitation inpatient services
49 Physical rehabilitation outpatient services

50 Positron emission tomography scanner (PET)
51 Primary care department
52 Psychiatric acute inpatient services
53 Psychiatric child adolescent services
54 Psychiatric consultation–liaison services
55 Psychiatric education services
56 Psychiatric emergency services
57 Psychiatric geriatric services
58 Psychiatric outpatient services
59 Psychiatric partial hospitalization program
60 Radiation therapy
61 Reproductive health services
62 Retirement housing
63 Single photon emission computerized tomography (SPECT)
64 Skilled nursing or other long–term care services
65 Social work services
66 Sports medicine
67 Support groups
68 Teen outreach services
69 Transplant services
70 Trauma center (certified)
71 Ultrasound
72 Urgent care center
73 Volunteer services department
74 Women's health center/services

3 Physician Codes

Actually available within, and reported by the institution; for definitions, see page A9.

(Alphabetical/Numerical Order)

1 Closed physician–hospital organization (PHO)

2 Equity model
3 Foundation
4 Group practice without walls
5 Independent practice association (IPA)

6 Integrated salary model
7 Management service organization (MSO)
8 Open physician–hospital organization (PHO)

© 1997 AHA Guide

Hospital, Address, Telephone, Administrator, Approval, Facility, and Physician Codes, Health Care System, Network	Classi-fication Codes		Utilization Data						Expense (thousands) of dollars		
★ American Hospital Association (AHA) membership □ Joint Commission on Accreditation of Healthcare Organizations (JCAHO) accreditation + American Osteopathic Hospital Association (AOHA) membership ○ American Osteopathic Association (AOA) accreditation △ Commission on Accreditation of Rehabilitation Facilities (CARF) accreditation Control codes 61, 63, 64, 71, 72 and 73 indicate hospitals listed by AOHA, but not registered by AHA. For definition of numerical codes, see page A4	Control	Service	Beds	Admissions	Census	Outpatient Visits	Births	Total	Payroll	Personnel
ANYTOWN—Universal County ★ COMMUNITY HOSPITAL, First Street and Main Avenue Zip 62835; tel 204/391–2345; Jane Doe, Administrator **A**1 2 3 4 6 9 10 **F**1 2 3 4 5 6 8 9 10 23 24 34; **P**1 2 3 4; **S** Acme HCS **N** ABC	23	10	346	10778	248	75953	1693	20695	9973	796

Below the table, brackets label: **4**, **5**, **6**, **7**

4 Health Care System Code and Name

A code number has been assigned to each health care system headquarters. The inclusion *of one of these codes (1) indicates that the hospital belongs to a health care system and* *(2) identifies the specific system to which the hospital belongs.*

5 Network Name

The presence of the letter "N" indicates that the hospital belongs to one or more networks. The *name(s) following the "N" identifies the specific network(s) to which the hospital belongs.*

6 Classification Codes

Control

Government, nonfederal
12 State
13 County
14 City
15 City–county
16 Hospital district or authority

Nongovernment not–for–profit
21 Church operated
23 Other

Investor–owned (for–profit)
31 Individual
32 Partnership
33 Corporation

Government, federal
41 Air Force
42 Army
43 Navy

44 Public Health Service other than 47
45 Veterans Affairs
46 Federal other than 41–45, 47–48
47 Public Health Service Indian Service
48 Department of Justice

Osteopathic
61 Church operated
63 Other not–for–profit
64 Other
71 Individual for–profit
72 Partnership for–profit
73 Corporation for–profit

Service
10 General medical and surgical
11 Hospital unit of an institution (prison hospital, college infirmary, etc.)
12 Hospital unit within an institution for the mentally retarded
22 Psychiatric

33 Tuberculosis and other respiratory diseases
44 Obstetrics and gynecology
45 Eye, ear, nose, and throat
46 Rehabilitation
47 Orthopedic
48 Chronic disease
49 Other specialty
50 Children's general
51 Children's hospital unit of an institution
52 Children's psychiatric
53 Children's tuberculosis and other respiratory diseases
55 Children's eye, ear, nose, and throat
56 Children's rehabilitation
57 Children's orthopedic
58 Children's chronic disease
59 Children's other specialty
62 Institution for mental retardation
82 Alcoholism and other chemical dependency

* Control codes 61, 63, 64, 71, 72 and 73 indicate hospitals listed by the AOHA but not registered by AHA.

When a hospital restricts its service to a specialty not defined by a specific code, it is coded 49 (59 if a children's hospital) and the specialty is indicated in parentheses following the name of the hospital.

7 Headings

Definitions are based on the American Hospital Association's Hospital Administration Terminology. Where a 12–month period is specified, hospitals were requested to report on the Annual Survey of Hospitals for the 12 months ending September 30, 1996. Hospitals reporting for less than a 12–month period are so designated.

Utilization Data:

Beds–Number of beds regularly maintained (set up and staffed for use) for inpatients as of the close of the reporting period.

Admissions–Number of patients accepted for inpatient service during a 12–month period; does not include newborn.

Census–Average number of inpatients receiving care each day during the 12–month reporting period; does not include newborn.

Outpatient Visits–An outpatient visit is a visit by a patient who is not lodged in the hospital while receiving medical, dental, or other services. Each appearance of an outpatient in each unit constitutes one visit regardless of the number of diagnostic and/or therapeutic treatments that a patient receives.

Births–Number of infants born in the hospital and accepted for service in a newborn infant bassinet during a 12–month period; excludes stillbirths.

Expense: Expense for a 12–month period; both total expense and payroll components are shown. Payroll expenses include all salaries and wages.

Personnel: Includes persons on payroll on September 30, 1996; includes full–time equivalents of part–time personnel. Full–time equivalents were calculated on the basis that two part–time persons equal one full–time person.

Annual Survey

Each year, an annual survey of hospitals is conducted by Healthcare InfoSource, Inc., a subsidiary of the American Hospital Association (AHA).

Until the 1981 edition, this publication included a copy of both the Annual Survey and instructions and definitions that accompanied the survey instrument. However, because of their size, the questionnaire and associated definitions are no longer reproduced. The definitions of facility codes are presented instead.

The facilities and services found below are either provided by the hospital, its health care system, or network or through a formal arrangement with another provider.

The AHA Guide to the Health Care Field does not include all data collected from the 1996 Annual Survey. Requests for purchasing other Annual Survey data should be directed to Healthcare InfoSource, Inc., One North Franklin, Chicago, IL 60606–3401, 312/422–2100.

Definitions of Facility Codes

1. **Adult day care program** Program providing supervision, medical and psychological care, and social activities for older adults who live at home or in another family setting, but cannot be alone or prefer to be with others during the day. May include intake assessment, health monitoring, occupational therapy, personal care, noon meal, and transportation services.

2. **Alcoholism–drug abuse or dependency inpatient services** Provides, diagnosis and therapeutic services to patients with alcoholism or other drug dependencies. Includes care for inpatient/residential treatment for patients whose course of treatment involves more intensive care than provided in an outpatient setting or where patient requires supervised withdrawal.

3. **Alcoholism–drug abuse or dependency outpatient services** Organized hospital services that provide medical care and/or rehabilitative treatment services to outpatients for whom the primary diagnosis is alcoholism or other chemical dependency.

4. **Angioplasty** The reconstruction of restructuring of a blood vessel by operative means or by nonsurgical techniques such as balloon dilation or laser.

5. **Arthritis treatment center** Specifically equipped and staffed center for the diagnosis and treatment of arthritis and other joint disorders.

6. **Assisted living** A special combination of housing, supportive services, personalized assistance and health care designed to respond to the individual needs of those who need help in activities of daily living and instrumental activities of daily living. Supportive services are available, 24 hours a day, to meet scheduled and unscheduled needs, in a way that promotes maximum independence and dignity for each resident and encourages the involvement of a resident's family, neighbor and friends.

7. **Birthing room–LDR room–LDRP room** A single room–type of maternity care with a more homelike setting for families than the traditional three–room unit (labor/delivery/recovery) with a separate postpartum area. A birthing room combines labor and delivery in one room. An LDR room accommodates three stages in the birthing process—labor, delivery, and recovery. An LDRP room accommodates all four stages of the birth process—labor, delivery, recovery and postpartum.

8. **Breast cancer screening/mammograms** Mammography screening The use of breast x–ray to detect unsuspected breast cancer in asymptomatic women. Diagnostic mammography The x–ray imaging of breast tissue in symptomatic women who are considered to have a substantial likelihood of having breast cancer already.

9. **Burn care services** Provides care to severely burned patients. Severely burned patients are those with any of the following: 1. Second–degree burns of more than 25% total body surface area for adults or 20% total body surface area for children; 2. Third–degree burns of more than 10% total body surface area; 3. Any severe burns of the hands, face, eyes, ears or feet or; 4. All inhalation injuries, electrical burns, complicated burn injuries involving fractures and other major traumas, and all other poor risk factors.

10. **Cardiac catheterization laboratory** Facilities offering special diagnostic procedures for cardiac patients. Available procedures must include, but need not be limited to, introduction of a catheter into the interior of the heart by way of a vein or artery or by direct needle puncture. Procedures must be performed in a laboratory or a special procedure room.

11. **Cardiac intensive care services** Provides patient care of a more specialized nature than the usual medical and surgical care, on the basis of physicians' orders and approved nursing care plans. The unit is staffed with specially trained nursing personnel and contains monitoring and specialized support or treatment equipment for patients who, because of heart seizure, open–heart surgery, or other life–threatening conditions, require intensified, comprehensive observation and care. May include myocardial infarction, pulmonary care, and heart transplant units.

12. **Case management** A system of assessment, treatment planning, referral and follow–up that ensures the provision of comprehensive and continuous services and the coordination of payment and reimbursement for care.

13. **Children wellness program** A program that encourages improved health status and a healthful lifestyle of children through health education, exercise, nutrition and health promotion.

14. **Community health reporting** Does your hospital either by itself or in conjunction with others disseminate

reports to the community on the quality and costs of health care services?

15. **Community health status assessment** Does your hospital work with other providers, public agencies, or community representatives to conduct a health status assessment of the community?

16. **Community health status based service planning** Does your hospital use health status indicators (such as rates of health problems or surveys of self–reported health) for defined populations to design new services or modify existing services?

17. **Community outreach** A program that systematically interacts with the community to identify those in need of services, alerting persons and their families to the availability of services, locating needed services, and enabling persons to enter the service delivery system.

18. **Crisis prevention** Services provided in order to promote physical and mental well being and the early identification of disease and ill health prior to the onset and recognition of symptoms so as to permit early treatment.

19. **CT scanner** Computed tomographic scanner for head or whole body scans.

20. **Dental services** An organized dental service, not necessarily involving special facilities, that provides dental or oral services to inpatients or outpatients.

21. **Diagnostic radioisotope facility** The use of radioactive isotopes (Radiopharmaceutical) as tracers or indicators to detect an abnormal condition or disease.

22. **Emergency department** Hospital facilities for the provision of unscheduled outpatient services to patients whose conditions require immediate care. Must be staffed 24 hours a day.

23. **Extracorporeal shock wave lithotripter (ESWL)** A medical device used for treating stones in the kidney or ureter. The device disintegrates kidney stones noninvasively through the transmission of acoustic shock waves directed at the stones.

24. **Fitness center** Provides exercise, testing, or evaluation programs and fitness activities to the community and hospital employees.

25. **Freestanding outpatient care center** A facility owned and operated by the hospital, but physically separate from the hospital, that provides various medical treatments on an outpatient basis only. In addition to treating minor illnesses or injuries, the center will stabilize seriously ill or injured patients before transporting them to a hospital. Laboratory and radiology services are usually available.

26. **Geriatric services** The branch of medicine dealing with the physiology of aging and the diagnosis and treatment of disease affecting the aged. Services could include: Adult day care program; Alzheimer's diagnostic–assessment services; Comprehensive geriatric assessment; Emergency response system; Geriatric acute care unit; and/or Geriatric clinics.

27. **Health facility transportation (to/from)** A long–term care support service designed to assist the mobility of the elderly. Some programs offer improved financial access by offering reduced rates and barrier–free buses or vans with ramps and lifts to assist the elderly or handicapped; others offer subsidies for public transport systems or operate mini–bus services exclusively for use by senior citizens.

28. **Health fair** Community health education events that focus on the prevention of disease and promotion of health through such activities as audiovisual exhibits and free diagnostic services.

29. **Health information center** Education which is directed at increasing the information of individuals and populations. It is intended to increase the ability to make informed personal, family and community health decision by providing consumers with informed choices about health matters with the objective of improving health status.

30. **Health screenings** A preliminary procedure, such as a test or examination to detect the most characteristic sign or signs of a disorder that may require further investigation.

31. **HIV–AIDS services** Services may include one or more of the following: HIV–AIDS unit (special unit or team designated and equipped specifically for diagnosis, treatment, continuing care planning, and counseling services for HIV–AIDS patients and their families.), General inpatient care for HIV–AIDS (inpatient diagnosis and treatment for human immunodeficiency virus and acquired immunodeficiency syndrome patients, but dedicated unit is not available.) Specialized outpatient program for HIV–AIDS (special outpatient program providing diagnostic, treatment, continuing care planning, and counseling for HIV–AIDS patients and their families.)

32. **Home health services** Service providing nursing, therapy, and health–related homemaker or social services in the patient's home.

33. **Hospice** A program providing palliative care, chiefly medical relief of pain and supportive services, addressing the emotional, social, financial, and legal needs of terminally ill patients and their families. Care can be provided in a variety of settings, both inpatient and at home.

34. **Hospital–based outpatient care center–services** Organized hospital health care services offered by appointment on an ambulatory basis. Services may include outpatient surgery, examination, diagnosis, and treatment of a variety of medical conditions on a nonemergency basis, and laboratory and other diagnostic testing as ordered by staff or outside physician referral.

35. **Magnetic resonance imaging (MRI)** The use of a uniform magnetic field and radio frequencies to study tissue and structure of the body. This procedure enables the visualization of biochemical activity of the cell in vivo without the use of ionizing radiation, radioisotopic substances, or high–frequency sound.

36. **Meals on wheels** A hospital sponsored program which delivers meals to people, usually the elderly, who are unable to prepare their own meals. Low cost, nutritional meals are delivered to individuals' homes on a regular basis.

37. **Medical surgical intensive care services** Provides patient care of a more intensive nature than the usual medical and surgical care, on the basis of physicians' orders and approved nursing care plans. These units are staffed with specially trained nursing personnel and contain monitoring and specialized support equipment of patients who, because of shock, trauma, or other life–threatening conditions, require intensified,

comprehensive observation and care. Includes mixed intensive care units.

38. **Neonatal intensive care services** A unit that must be separate from the newborn nursery providing intensive care to all sick infants including those with the very lowest birth weights (less that 1500 grams). NICU has potential for providing mechanical ventilation, neonatal surgery, and special care for the sickest infants born in the hospital or transferred from another institution. A full–time neonatologist serves as director of the NICU.

39. **Nutrition programs** Those services within a health care facility which are designed to provide inexpensive, nutritionally sound meals to patients.

40. **Obstetrics services** Levels should be designated: (1) unit provides services for uncomplicated maternity and newborn cases; (2) unit provides services for uncomplicated cases, the majority of complicated problems, and special neonatal services; and (3) unit provides services for all serious illnesses and abnormalities and is supervised by a full–time maternal/fetal specialist.

41. **Occupational health services** Includes services designed to protect the safety of employees from hazards in the work environment.

42. **Oncology services** An organized program for the treatment of cancer by the use of drugs or chemicals.

43. **Open heart surgery** Heart surgery where the chest has been opened and the blood recirculated and oxygenated with the proper equipment and the necessary staff to perform the surgery.

44. **Outpatient surgery** Scheduled surgical services provided to patients who do not remain in the hospital overnight. The surgery may be performed in operating suites also used for inpatient surgery, specially designated surgical suites for outpatient surgery, or procedure rooms within an outpatient care facility.

45. **Patient education center** Written goals and objectives for the patient and/or family related to therapeutic regimens, medical procedures, and self care.

46. **Patient representative services** Organized hospital services providing personnel through whom patients and staff can seek solutions to institutional

problems affecting the delivery of high–quality care and services.

47. **Pediatric intensive care services** Provides care to pediatric patients that is of a more intensive nature than that usually provided to pediatric patients. The unit is staffed with specially trained personnel and contains monitoring and specialized support equipment for treatment of patients who, because of shock, trauma, or other life–threatening conditions, require intensified, comprehensive observation and care.

48. **Physical rehabilitation inpatient services** Provides care encompassing a comprehensive array of restoration services for the disabled and all support services necessary to help patients attain their maximum functional capacity.

49. **Physical rehabilitation outpatient services** Outpatient program providing medical, health–related, therapy, social, and/or vocational services to help disabled persons attain or retain their maximum functional capacity.

50. **Positron emission tomography scanner (PET)** is a nuclear medicine imaging technology which uses radioactive (positron emitting) isotopes created in a cyclotron or generator and computers to produce composite pictures of the brain and heart at work. PET scanning produces sectional images depicting metabolic activity or blood flow rather than anatomy.

51. **Primary care department** A unit of clinic within the hospital that provides primary care services (e.g. general pediatric care, general internal medicine, family practice and gynecology) through hospital–salaried medical and or nursing staff, focusing on evaluating and diagnosing medical problems and providing medical treatment on an outpatient basis.

52. **Psychiatric acute inpatient services** Provides acute or long–term care to emotionally disturbed patients, including patients admitted for diagnosis and those admitted for treatment of psychiatric problems, on the basis of physicians' orders and approved nursing care plans. Long–term care may include intensive supervision to the chronically mentally ill, mentally disordered, or other mentally incompetent persons.

53. **Psychiatric child adolescent services** Provides care to emotionally disturbed

children and adolescents, including those admitted for diagnosis and those admitted for treatment.

54. **Psychiatric consultation–liaison services** Provides organized psychiatric consultation/liaison services to nonpsychiatric hospital staff and/or department on psychological aspects of medical care that may be generic or specific to individual patients.

55. **Psychiatric education services** Provides psychiatric educational services to community agencies and workers such as schools, police, courts, public health nurses, welfare agencies, clergy and so forth. The purpose is to expand the mental health knowledge and competence of personnel not working in the mental health field and to promote good mental health through improved understanding, attitudes, and behavioral patterns.

56. **Psychiatric emergency services** Services or facilities available on a 24–hour basis to provide immediate unscheduled outpatient care, diagnosis, evaluation, crisis intervention, and assistance to persons suffering acute emotional or mental distress.

57. **Psychiatric geriatric services** Provides care to emotionally disturbed elderly patients, including those admitted for diagnosis and those admitted for treatment.

58. **Psychiatric outpatient services** Provides medical care, including diagnosis and treatment of psychiatric outpatients.

59. **Psychiatric partial hospitalization program** Organized hospital services of intensive day/evening outpatient services of three hours or more duration, distinguished from other outpatient visits of one hour.

60. **Radiation therapy** The branch of medicine concerned with radioactive substances and using various techniques of visualization, with the diagnosis and treatment of disease using any of the various sources of radiant energy. Services could include: megavoltage radiation therapy; radioactive implants; stereotactic radiosurgery; therapeutic radioisotope facility; X–ray radiation therapy.

61. **Reproductive health services** Services that include any or all of the following:

Fertility counseling A service that counsels and educates on infertility problems and includes laboratory and surgical workup and management for individuals having problems conceiving children.

In vitro fertilization Program providing for the induction of fertilization of a surgically removed ovum by donated sperm in a culture medium followed by a short incubation period. The embryo is then reimplanted in the womb.

62. **Retirement housing** A facility which provides social activities to senior citizens, usually retired persons, who do not require health care but some short–term skilled nursing care may be provided. A retirement center may furnish housing and may also have acute hospital and long–term care facilities, or it may arrange for acute and long term care through affiliated institutions.

63. **Single photon emission computerized tomography (SPECT)** is a nuclear medicine imaging technology that combines existing technology of gamma camera imaging with computed tomographic imaging technology to provide a more precise and clear image.

64. **Skilled nursing or other long–term care services** Provides non–acute medical and skilled nursing care services, therapy, and social services under the supervision of a licensed registered nurse on a 24–hour basis.

65. **Social work services** Services may include one or more of the following: Organized social work services (services that are properly directed and sufficiently staffed by qualified individuals who provide assistance and counseling to patients and their families in dealing with social, emotional, and environmental problems associated with illness or disability, often in the context of financial or discharge planning coordination.), Outpatient social work services (social work services provided in ambulatory care areas.) Emergency department social work services (social work services provided to emergency department patients by social workers dedicated to the emergency department or on call.)

66. **Sports medicine** Provision of diagnostic screening and assessment and clinical and rehabilitation services for the prevention and treatment of sports–related injuries.

67. **Support groups** A hospital sponsored program which allows a group of individuals with the same or similar problems who meet periodically to share experiences, problems, and solutions, in order to support each other.

68. **Teen outreach services** A program focusing on the teenager which encourages an improved health status and a healthful lifestyle including physical, emotional, mental, social, spiritual and economic through health education, exercise, nutrition and health promotion.

69. **Transplant services** The branch of medicine that transfers an organ or tissue from one person to another or from one body part to another to replace a diseased structure or to restore function or to change appearance. Services could includes: Bone marrow transplant program; kidney transplant; organ transplant (other than kidney); tissue transplant.

70. **Trauma center (certified)** A facility certified to provide emergency and specialized intensive care to critically ill and injured patients.

71. **Ultrasound** The use of acoustic waves above the range of 20,000 cycles per second to visualize internal body structures.

72. **Urgent care center** A facility that provides care and treatment for problems that are not life–threatening but require attention over the short term. These units function like emergency rooms but are separate from hospitals with which they may have backup affiliation arrangements.

73. **Volunteer services department** An organized hospital department responsible for coordinating the services of volunteers working within the institution.

74. **Women's health center/services** An area set aside for coordinated education and treatment services specifically for and promoted by women as provided by this special unit. Services may or may not include obstetrics but include a range of services other than OB.

Definitions of Physician Codes

1. **Closed physician–hospital organization (PHO)** A PHO that restricts physician membership to those practitioners who meet criteria for cost effectiveness and/or high quality.

2. **Equity model** Allows established practitioners to become shareholders in a professional corporation in exchange for tangible and intangible assets of their existing practices.

3. **Foundation** A corporation, organized either as a hospital affiliate or subsidiary, which purchases both the tangible and intangible assets of one or more medical group practices. Physicians remain in a separate corporate entity but sign a professional services agreement with the foundation.

4. **Group practice without walls** Hospital sponsors the formation of, or provides capital to physicians to establish, a 'quasi' group to share administrative expenses while remaining independent practitioners.

5. **Independent practice association (IPA)** An IPA is a legal entity that hold managed care contracts. The IPA then contracts with physicians, usually in solo practice, to provide care either on a fee–for–services or capitated basis. The purpose of an IPA is to assist solo physicians in obtaining managed care contracts.

6. **Integrated salary model** Physicians are salaried by the hospital or another entity of a health system to provide medical services for primary care and specialty care.

7. **Management services organization (MSO)** A corporation, owned by the hospital or a physician/hospital joint venture, that provides management services to one or more medical group practices. The MSO purchases the tangible assets of the practices and leases them back as part of a full–service management agreement, under which the MSO employs all non–physician staff and provides all supplies/administrative systems for a fee.

8. **Open physician–hospital organization (PHO)** A joint venture between the hospital and all members of the medical staff who wish to participate. The PHO can act as a unified agent in managed care contracting, own a managed care plan, own and operate ambulatory care centers or ancillary services projects, or provide administrative services to physician members.

ALABAMA

Resident population 4,253 (in thousands)
Resident population in metro areas 67.5%
Birth rate per 1,000 population 14.8
65 years and over 13.0%
Percent of persons without health insurance 19.2%

Hospital, Address, Telephone, Administrator, Approval, Facility, and Physician Codes, Health Care System, Network	Classi-fication Codes		Utilization Data					Expense (thousands) of dollars		
	Control	Service	Beds	Admissions	Census	Outpatient Visits	Births	Total	Payroll	Personnel

★ American Hospital Association (AHA) membership
□ Joint Commission on Accreditation of Healthcare Organizations (JCAHO) accreditation
+ American Osteopathic Hospital Association (AOHA) membership
○ American Osteopathic Association (AOA) accreditation
△ Commission on Accreditation of Rehabilitation Facilities (CARF) accreditation
Control codes 61, 63, 64, 71, 72 and 73 indicate hospitals listed by AOHA, but not registered by AHA. For definition of numerical codes, see page A4

Hospital	Control	Service	Beds	Admissions	Census	Outpatient Visits	Births	Total	Payroll	Personnel
ALABASTER—Shelby County										
✠ SHELBY BAPTIST MEDICAL CENTER, 1000 First Street North, Zip 35007–0488; Mailing Address: Box 488, Zip 35007–0488; tel. 205/620–8100; Charles C. Colvert, President (Total facility includes 18 beds in nursing home–type unit) (Nonreporting) **A**1 2 9 10 **S** Baptist Health System, Birmingham, AL **N** Baptist Health System, Birmingham, AL	13	10	228	—	—	—	—	—	—	—
ALEXANDER CITY—Tallapoosa County										
✠ RUSSELL HOSPITAL, U.S. 280 By–Pass, Zip 35010, Mailing Address: P.O. Box 939, Zip 35011–0939; tel. 205/329–7100; Frank W. Harris, President and Chief Executive Officer (Nonreporting) **A**1 9 10	23	10	75	—	—	—	—	—	—	—
ANDALUSIA—Covington County										
✠ COLUMBIA ANDALUSIA HOSPITAL, 849 South Three Notch Street, Zip 36420–0760, Mailing Address: Box 760, Zip 36420; tel. 334/222–8466; James L. Sample, Chief Executive Officer (Nonreporting) **A**1 9 10 **S** Columbia/HCA Healthcare Corporation, Nashville, TN	33	10	101	—	—	—	—	—	—	—
ANNISTON—Calhoun County										
✠ NORTHEAST ALABAMA REGIONAL MEDICAL CENTER, 400 East Tenth Street, Zip 36207, Mailing Address: Box 2208, Zip 36202; tel. 205/235–5121; Allen P. Fletcher, President **A**1 2 9 10 **F**7 8 10 14 15 16 19 21 22 30 31 32 34 35 37 40 41 42 44 46 49 52 54 55 56 57 59 60 65 66 70 71 73	16	10	259	14482	181	110273	1520	79664	34464	1198
□ STRINGFELLOW MEMORIAL HOSPITAL, 301 East 18th Street, Zip 36207; tel. 205/235–8900; Michael E. Cassidy, Administrator **A**1 9 10 **F**1 2 6 8 10 12 15 19 20 21 22 28 30 32 33 35 36 37 39 40 41 42 44 45 46 49 52 60 63 65 66 67 71 73 **P**3 **S** Health Management Associates, Naples, FL	23	10	66	2297	26	15810	0	—	—	269
ASHLAND—Clay County										
□ CLAY COUNTY HOSPITAL, 544 East First Avenue, Zip 36251, Mailing Address: P.O. Box 1270, Zip 36251–1277; tel. 205/354–2131; Linda U. Jordan, Administrator (Total facility includes 63 beds in nursing home–type unit) (Nonreporting) **A**1 9 10	13	10	116	—	—	—	—	—	—	—
ATHENS—Limestone County										
✠ ATHENS–LIMESTONE HOSPITAL, 700 West Market Street, Zip 35611, Mailing Address: Box 999, Zip 35611; tel. 205/233–9292; Philip E. Dotson, Administrator and Chief Executive Officer **A**1 9 10 **F**7 8 12 15 16 19 21 22 26 28 30 32 37 39 40 44 45 49 65 71 74 **P**6 **N** HealthGroup of Alabama, L.L.C., Madison, AL	16	10	101	4286	49	46635	385	33536	14859	477
ATMORE—Escambia County										
□ ATMORE COMMUNITY HOSPITAL, 401 Medical Park Drive, Zip 36502; tel. 334/368–2500; Lavon Henley, Administrator (Nonreporting) **A**1 9 10 **S** Escambia County Health Care Authority, Brewton, AL	13	10	51	—	—	—	—	—	—	—
BAY MINETTE—Baldwin County										
✠ NORTH BALDWIN HOSPITAL, 1815 Hand Avenue, Zip 36507, Mailing Address: P.O. Box 1409, Zip 36507; tel. 334/937–5521; Gary W. Farrow, Administrator (Nonreporting) **A**1 9 10	13	10	55	—	—	—	—	—	—	—
BESSEMER—Jefferson County										
✠ BESSEMER CARRAWAY MEDICAL CENTER, 995 Ninth Avenue S.W., Zip 35023, Mailing Address: Box 847, Zip 35021–0847; tel. 205/481–7000; Dan M. Eagar, Jr., Administrator **A**1 2 9 10 **F**2 3 7 8 10 11 12 14 19 21 22 27 28 33 37 39 41 42 44 48 49 52 54 55 56 57 65 67 70 71 73 74 **P**4	23	10	210	7005	107	77456	391	51491	20810	780
BIRMINGHAM—Jefferson County										
✠ BIRMINGHAM BAPTIST MEDICAL CENTER–MONTCLAIR CAMPUS, 800 Montclair Road, Zip 35213; tel. 205/592–1000; Dana S. Hensley, President (Total facility includes 112 beds in nursing home–type unit) **A**1 2 3 5 8 9 10 **F**2 3 4 6 7 8 10 11 12 14 15 16 17 19 21 22 24 26 29 31 32 33 34 35 37 38 40 41 42 43 44 45 46 48 49 52 53 54 55 56 57 58 59 60 61 62 63 64 65 70 71 73 74 **P**6 7 **S** Baptist Health System, Birmingham, AL **N** National Cardiovascular Network, Atlanta, GA; Baptist Health System, Birmingham, AL	21	10	1023	32302	440	304063	1687	247972	102938	3415
✠ BIRMINGHAM BAPTIST MEDICAL CENTER–PRINCETON, 701 Princeton Avenue S.W., Zip 35211–1305; tel. 205/783–3000; Dana S. Hensley, President and Chief Executive Officer (Nonreporting) **A**1 2 3 5 8 9 10 **S** Baptist Health System, Birmingham, AL **N** Baptist Health System, Birmingham, AL	21	10	1033	—	—	—	—	—	—	—
BRADFORD HEALTH SERVICES AT BIRMINGHAM, 1221 Alton Drive, Zip 35210, Mailing Address: P.O. Box 129, Warrior, Zip 35180; tel. 205/833–4000; W. Clay Simmons, Executive Director (Nonreporting) **A**9	33	82	90	—	—	—	—	—	—	—
□ BROOKWOOD MEDICAL CENTER, 2010 Brookwood Medical Center Drive, Zip 35209; tel. 205/877–1000; Gregory H. Burfitt, President and Chief Executive Officer (Nonreporting) **A**1 2 9 10 **S** TENET Healthcare Corporation, Santa Barbara, CA **N** Alabama Health Services, Birmingham, AL	33	10	515	—	—	—	—	—	—	—

Hospital, Address, Telephone, Administrator, Approval, Facility, and Physician Codes, Health Care System, Network	Classi-fication Codes		Utilization Data					Expense (thousands) of dollars		
	Control	Service	Beds	Admissions	Census	Outpatient Visits	Births	Total	Payroll	Personnel

★ American Hospital Association (AHA) membership
☐ Joint Commission on Accreditation of Healthcare Organizations (JCAHO) accreditation
+ American Osteopathic Hospital Association (AOHA) membership
◯ American Osteopathic Association (AOA) accreditation
△ Commission on Accreditation of Rehabilitation Facilities (CARF) accreditation
Control codes 61, 63, 64, 71, 72 and 73 indicate hospitals listed by AOHA, but not registered by AHA. For definition of numerical codes, see page A4

Hospital	Control	Service	Beds	Admissions	Census	Outpatient Visits	Births	Total	Payroll	Personnel
★ △ CARRAWAY METHODIST MEDICAL CENTER, 1600 Carraway Boulevard, Zip 35234–1990; tel. 205/502–6000; Warren E. Callaway, FACHE, Administrator **A**1 2 3 5 7 8 9 10 **F**2 4 7 8 10 11 12 14 15 16 17 19 20 22 23 24 25 26 28 30 31 32 33 34 35 37 39 40 41 42 43 44 45 46 48 49 51 52 53 54 55 56 57 58 60 65 67 70 71 73 **P**6 8	23	10	383	13449	217	206826	543	139163	54050	1726
★ CHILDREN'S HOSPITAL OF ALABAMA, 1600 Seventh Avenue South, Zip 35233–1785; tel. 205/939–9100; Jim Dearth, M.D., Chief Executive Officer **A**1 3 5 9 10 **F**9 12 13 14 15 16 17 19 20 21 22 25 29 30 31 34 35 38 39 41 42 44 45 46 47 49 51 52 53 54 56 58 65 66 67 70 71 72 73 **P**1 2 3 5 7	23	50	218	10727	154	283204	0	111828	62728	1883
☐ COOPER GREEN HOSPITAL, 1515 Sixth Avenue South, Zip 35233; tel. 205/930–3600; Max Michael, M.D., Chief Executive Officer and Medical Director **A**1 3 5 9 10 **F**4 7 8 10 12 15 16 17 19 21 22 23 28 30 31 32 34 35 37 39 40 41 42 43 44 47 48 49 60 65 71 73 74 **P**3 5	13	10	130	5950	77	105985	1412	58485	22356	698
★ EYE FOUNDATION HOSPITAL, 1720 University Boulevard, Zip 35233–1816; tel. 205/325–8100; Gordon L. Smith, Administrator **A**1 3 5 9 10 **F**15 16 17 19 22 30 34 35 41 44 65 71 73	23	45	23	1292	5	16171	0	12833	4846	157
★ △ HEALTHSOUTH LAKESHORE REHABILITATION HOSPITAL, 3800 Ridgeway Drive, Zip 35209; tel. 205/868–2000; Terry Brown, Administrator and Chief Executive Officer **A**1 7 9 10 **F**6 12 15 19 25 34 35 39 41 48 49 54 65 67 71 73 **S** HEALTHSOUTH Corporation, Birmingham, AL	33	46	100	1786	81	8714	0	—	—	267
★ HEALTHSOUTH MEDICAL CENTER, 1201 11th Avenue South, Zip 35205; tel. 205/930–7000; Frank R. Gannon, Administrator and Chief Executive Officer **A**1 9 10 **F**8 10 12 14 19 21 22 34 35 37 42 44 48 49 64 65 66 71 73 **S** HEALTHSOUTH Corporation, Birmingham, AL	33	10	201	6678	91	—	0	66057	22953	654
☐ HILL CREST BEHAVIORAL HEALTH SERVICES, 6869 Fifth Avenue South, Zip 35212; tel. 205/833–9000; Steve McCabe, Chief Executive Officer (Nonreporting) **A**1 9 10 **S** Ramsay Health Care, Inc., Coral Gobles, FL	32	22	100							
★ △ MEDICAL CENTER EAST, 50 Medical Park East Drive, Zip 35235–9987; tel. 205/838–3000; David E. Crawford, FACHE, Executive Vice President and Chief Operating Officer **A**1 2 3 5 7 9 10 **F**1 2 3 4 6 7 8 9 10 11 12 14 15 16 17 19 21 22 23 24 25 27 28 29 30 31 32 33 34 35 37 38 39 40 41 42 43 44 45 46 47 48 49 51 52 53 54 55 56 57 58 59 60 61 62 64 65 67 69 70 71 72 73 74 **P**5 6 7 **S** Eastern Health System, Inc., Birmingham, AL **N** Alabama Health Services, Birmingham, AL	23	10	282	11999	154	104220	853	107952	47115	984
★ ST. VINCENT'S HOSPITAL, 810 St. Vincent's Drive, Zip 35205, Mailing Address: P.O. Box 12407, Zip 35202–2407; tel. 205/939–7000; Vincent C. Caponi, President and Chief Executive Officer **A**1 2 3 5 9 10 **F**4 5 7 8 10 11 12 15 16 17 18 19 21 22 24 25 26 27 28 29 30 31 32 33 34 35 36 37 38 39 40 41 42 43 44 45 46 49 51 52 54 55 56 57 60 63 65 67 71 73 **P**5 **S** Daughters of Charity National Health System, Saint Louis, MO	23	10	338	15161	198	109980	2326	116438	51662	1618
★ UNIVERSITY OF ALABAMA HOSPITAL, 619 South 19th Street, Zip 35233–6505; tel. 205/934–4011; Kevin E. Lofton, Executive Director and Chief Executive Officer (Total facility includes 36 beds in nursing home–type unit) **A**1 2 3 5 8 9 10 12 **F**3 4 5 7 8 9 10 11 12 14 15 16 17 19 21 22 23 24 25 26 28 31 32 33 34 35 37 40 41 42 43 44 46 48 49 51 52 53 54 55 57 60 61 65 67 69 70 71 **P**1 **N** University of Alabama Hospital/UAB Health System, Birmingham, AL	12	10	828	37978	642	—	3088	404441	159071	5123
★ VETERANS AFFAIRS MEDICAL CENTER, 700 South 19th Street, Zip 35233–1996; tel. 205/933–8101; Y. C. Parris, Director **A**1 2 3 5 8 9 **F**3 4 5 8 10 11 16 17 19 20 21 22 24 25 26 27 28 29 30 31 32 33 34 37 39 41 42 43 44 46 49 51 54 56 58 59 61 65 67 69 71 72 73 74 **P**6 **S** Department of Veterans Affairs, Washington, DC	45	10	317	6200	146	183470	0	112376	57096	1683
BOAZ—Marshall County										
★ BOAZ–ALBERTVILLE MEDICAL CENTER, U.S. Highway 431 North, Zip 35957–0999, Mailing Address: Drawer Z, Zip 35957–0999; tel. 205/593–8310; Marlin Hanson, Administrator **A**1 9 10 **F**7 8 15 16 17 19 21 22 28 30 34 35 37 40 42 44 49 54 60 63 65 66 71 73 74 **S** Marshall County Health Care Authority, Guntersville, AL	13	10	102	4782	66	145340	401	34655	16203	569
BREWTON—Escambia County										
★ D. W. MCMILLAN MEMORIAL HOSPITAL, 1301 Belleville Avenue, Zip 36426, Mailing Address: Box 908, Zip 36427; tel. 334/867–8061; Phillip L. Parker, Administrator (Nonreporting) **A**1 9 10 **S** Escambia County Health Care Authority, Brewton, AL	23	10	83	—	—	—	—	—	—	—
BRIDGEPORT—Jackson County										
☐ NORTH JACKSON HOSPITAL, Mailing Address: 47005 U.S. Highway 72, Zip 35740; tel. 205/437–2101; Rodney C. Watford, Administrator (Total facility includes 60 beds in nursing home–type unit) (Nonreporting) **A**1 9 10	16	10	109							
CAMDEN—Wilcox County										
J. PAUL JONES HOSPITAL, 317 McWilliams Avenue, Zip 36726; tel. 205/682–4131; Arden Chesnut, Administrator **A**9 10 **F**15 19 22 32 71	15	10	20	476	5	18397	0	2414	1249	54
CARROLLTON—Pickens County										
☐ PICKENS COUNTY MEDICAL CENTER, Route 2, Zip 35447, Mailing Address: P.O. Box 478, Zip 35447–0478; tel. 205/367–8111; Tunisia Lavender, R.N., Interim Chief Operating Officer (Nonreporting) **A**1 9 10	13	10	45	—	—	—	—	—	—	—
CENTRE—Cherokee County										
★ CHEROKEE BAPTIST MEDICAL CENTER, 400 Northwood Drive, Zip 35960–1023; tel. 205/927–5531; Barry S. Cochran, President **A**1 9 10 **F**8 11 12 14 16 17 19 21 22 27 28 29 30 32 33 44 45 51 71 73 74 **S** Baptist Health System, Birmingham, AL **N** The Medical Resource Network, L.L.C., Atlanta, GA; Baptist Health System, Birmingham, AL	23	10	45	1332	14	71153	0	8676	3500	155

Hospital, Address, Telephone, Administrator, Approval, Facility, and Physician Codes, Health Care System, Network	Classi-fication Codes		Utilization Data					Expense (thousands) of dollars		
★ American Hospital Association (AHA) membership ☐ Joint Commission on Accreditation of Healthcare Organizations (JCAHO) accreditation + American Osteopathic Hospital Association (AOHA) membership ○ American Osteopathic Association (AOA) accreditation △ Commission on Accreditation of Rehabilitation Facilities (CARF) accreditation Control codes 61, 63, 64, 71, 72 and 73 indicate hospitals listed by AOHA, but not registered by AHA. For definition of numerical codes, see page A4	Control	Service	Beds	Admissions	Census	Outpatient Visits	Births	Total	Payroll	Personnel

CENTREVILLE—Bibb County

BIBB MEDICAL CENTER, 164 Pierson Avenue, Zip 35042; tel. 205/926–4881; Terry J. Smith, Administrator (Total facility includes 113 beds in nursing home–type unit) **A**9 10 **F**7 19 22 32 40 44 49 62 64 71 | 13 | 10 | 138 | 770 | 107 | 17787 | 63 | 6725 | — | 212

CHATOM—Washington County

WASHINGTON COUNTY INFIRMARY AND NURSING HOME, St. Stephens Avenue, Zip 36518, Mailing Address: Box 597, Zip 36518–0597; tel. 334/847–2223; Howard C. Holcomb, Administrator (Total facility includes 73 beds in nursing home–type unit) (Nonreporting) **A**9 10 **S** Infirmary Health System, Inc., Mobile, AL | 13 | 10 | 88 | — | — | — | — | — | — | —

CLANTON—Chilton County

☐ VAUGHAN CHILTON MEDICAL CENTER, 1010 Lay Dam Road, Zip 35045; tel. 205/755–2500; Jeffrey Potts, Administrator (Nonreporting) **A**1 9 10 **S** Healthcorp of Tennessee, Inc., Chattanooga, TN | 23 | 10 | 45 | — | — | — | — | — | — | —

CULLMAN—Cullman County

☒ CULLMAN REGIONAL MEDICAL CENTER, 1912 Alabama Highway 157, Zip 35055, Mailing Address: P.O. Box 1108, Zip 35056–1108; tel. 205/737–2000; Jesse O. Weatherly, Administrator **A**1 2 9 10 **F**4 7 8 10 12 14 15 16 17 19 21 22 24 28 30 32 33 35 37 40 41 42 44 46 49 60 65 66 67 71 73 74 **P**3 **S** Baptist Health System, Birmingham, AL **N** Baptist Health System, Birmingham, AL | 23 | 10 | 115 | 6152 | 66 | 137549 | 611 | 39894 | 14510 | 605

☐ WOODLAND COMMUNITY HOSPITAL, 1910 Cherokee Avenue S.E., Zip 35055; tel. 205/739–3500; Lowell Benton, Executive Director (Nonreporting) **A**1 9 10 **S** Community Health Systems, Inc., Brentwood, TN | 33 | 10 | 67 | — | — | — | — | — | — | —

DADEVILLE—Tallapoosa County

★ LAKESHORE COMMUNITY HOSPITAL, 201 Mariarden Road, Zip 36853, Mailing Address: P.O. Box 248, Zip 36853; tel. 205/825–7821; Mavis B. Halko, Administrator (Nonreporting) **A**9 10 **S** Healthcorp of Tennessee, Inc., Chattanooga, TN | 23 | 10 | 27 | — | — | — | — | — | — | —

DAPHNE—Baldwin County

☒ MERCY MEDICAL, 101 Villa Drive, Zip 36526, Mailing Address: P.O. Box 1090, Zip 36526; tel. 334/626–2694; Sister Mary Eileen Wilhelm, President and Chief Executive Officer (Total facility includes 132 beds in nursing home–type unit) **A**1 9 10 **F**6 12 15 16 17 20 26 31 32 33 34 36 39 42 49 62 64 65 67 73 **S** Eastern Mercy Health System, Radnor, PA | 21 | 46 | 157 | 1512 | 130 | 191876 | 0 | 26644 | 13674 | 662

DECATUR—Morgan County

☒ DECATUR GENERAL HOSPITAL, 1201 Seventh Street S.E., Zip 35601, Mailing Address: Box 2239, Zip 35609–2239; tel. 205/341–2000; Robert L. Smith, President and Chief Executive Officer **A**1 2 9 10 **F**4 7 8 10 11 15 16 19 21 22 28 29 32 34 35 37 39 40 42 44 45 46 52 53 54 55 56 57 58 59 60 63 65 71 73 **N** HealthGroup of Alabama, L.L.C., Madison, AL | 16 | 10 | 256 | 8956 | 120 | 106603 | 1895 | 68664 | 29663 | 976

☐ DECATUR GENERAL HOSPITAL–WEST, 2205 Beltline Road S.W., Zip 35602, Mailing Address: P.O. Box 2240, Zip 35609–2240; tel. 205/350–1450; Dennis Griffin, Vice President (Nonreporting) **A**1 9 **N** HealthGroup of Alabama, L.L.C., Madison, AL | 33 | 22 | 64 | — | — | — | — | — | — | —

☐ NORTH ALABAMA REGIONAL HOSPITAL, Highway 31 South, Zip 35609, Mailing Address: P.O. Box 2221, Zip 35609; tel. 205/353–9433; Kay Greenwood, R.N., MS, Facility Director **A**1 10 **F**14 15 16 46 49 52 56 65 73 | 12 | 22 | 74 | 473 | 111 | 0 | 0 | 7667 | 4825 | 166

☐ PARKWAY MEDICAL CENTER HOSPITAL, 1874 Beltline Road S.W., Zip 35601, Mailing Address: P.O. Box 2211, Zip 35609; tel. 205/350–2211; Philip J. Mazzuca, Executive Director (Nonreporting) **A**1 9 10 **S** Community Health Systems, Inc., Brentwood, TN | 33 | 10 | 94 | — | — | — | — | — | — | —

DEMOPOLIS—Marengo County

☒ BRYAN W. WHITFIELD MEMORIAL HOSPITAL, Highway 80 West, Zip 36732, Mailing Address: Box 890, Zip 36732; tel. 334/289–4000; Charles E. Nabors, Chief Executive Officer and Administrator **A**1 9 10 **F**1 8 12 14 15 16 17 19 21 22 24 28 30 32 37 39 40 42 44 45 63 65 71 73 **P**5 **N** Provider of Rural Health Network, Montgomery, AL | 14 | 10 | 99 | 3727 | 48 | 19659 | 479 | 17487 | 8081 | 341

DOTHAN—Houston County

☒ FLOWERS HOSPITAL, 4370 West Main Street, Zip 36301, Mailing Address: Box 6907, Zip 36302–6907; tel. 334/793–5000; Keith Granger, President and Chief Executive Officer (Nonreporting) **A**1 2 9 10 **S** Quorum Health Group/Quorum Health Resources, Inc., Brentwood, TN | 33 | 10 | 215 | — | — | — | — | — | — | —

☐ SOUTHEAST ALABAMA MEDICAL CENTER, 1108 Ross Clark Circle, Zip 36301, Mailing Address: P.O. Box 6987, Zip 36302; tel. 334/793–8111; James R. Blackmon, Chief Executive Officer (Nonreporting) **A**1 2 9 10 **N** Principal Health Care of Georgia, Atlanta, GA | 16 | 10 | 347 | — | — | — | — | — | — | —

ELBA—Coffee County

ELBA GENERAL HOSPITAL, 987 Drayton Street, Zip 36323; tel. 334/897–2257; Ellen Briley, Administrator and Chief Executive Officer (Total facility includes 101 beds in nursing home–type unit) **A**9 10 **F**19 22 34 50 64 71 **P**6 | 16 | 10 | 121 | 1480 | 106 | 7503 | 0 | — | — | 166

ENTERPRISE—Coffee County

☒ MEDICAL CENTER ENTERPRISE, 400 North Edwards Street, Zip 36330–9981; tel. 334/347–0584; John L. Robertson, Chief Executive Officer (Nonreporting) **A**1 9 10 **S** Quorum Health Group/Quorum Health Resources, Inc., Brentwood, TN | 33 | 10 | 113 | — | — | — | — | — | — | —

EUFAULA—Barbour County

☐ LAKEVIEW COMMUNITY HOSPITAL, 820 West Washington Street, Zip 36027; tel. 205/687–5761; Carl D. Brown, Administrator (Nonreporting) **A**1 9 10 **S** Healthcorp of Tennessee, Inc., Chattanooga, TN | 33 | 10 | 74 | — | — | — | — | — | — | —

Hospital, Address, Telephone, Administrator, Approval, Facility, and Physician Codes, Health Care System, Network	Classi-fication Codes		Utilization Data					Expense (thousands) of dollars		
	Control	Service	Beds	Admissions	Census	Outpatient Visits	Births	Total	Payroll	Personnel

★ American Hospital Association (AHA) membership
□ Joint Commission on Accreditation of Healthcare Organizations (JCAHO) accreditation
+ American Osteopathic Hospital Association (AOHA) membership
○ American Osteopathic Association (AOA) accreditation
△ Commission on Accreditation of Rehabilitation Facilities (CARF) accreditation
Control codes 61, 63, 64, 71, 72 and 73 indicate hospitals listed by AOHA, but not registered by AHA. For definition of numerical codes, see page A4

EUTAW—Greene County

Hospital	Control	Service	Beds	Admissions	Census	Outpatient Visits	Births	Total	Payroll	Personnel
GREENE COUNTY HOSPITAL, 509 Wilson Avenue, Zip 35462; tel. 205/372–3388; Robert J. Coker, Jr., Administrator (Nonreporting) **A**9 10	13	10	72	—	—	—	—	—	—	—

FAIRFIELD—Jefferson County

Hospital	Control	Service	Beds	Admissions	Census	Outpatient Visits	Births	Total	Payroll	Personnel
☒ LLOYD NOLAND HOSPITAL AND HEALTH SYSTEM, 701 Lloyd Noland Parkway, Zip 35064–2699; tel. 205/783–5106; Gary M. Glasscock, Administrator (Nonreporting) **A**1 2 3 5 9 10 **S** TENET Healthcare Corporation, Santa Barbara, CA **N** Alabama Health Services, Birmingham, AL	23	10	222	—	—	—	—	—	—	—

FAIRHOPE—Baldwin County

Hospital	Control	Service	Beds	Admissions	Census	Outpatient Visits	Births	Total	Payroll	Personnel
☒ THOMAS HOSPITAL, 750 Morphy Avenue, Zip 36532–1812, Mailing Address: Drawer 929, Zip 36533–0929; tel. 334/928–2375; Owen Bailey, Administrator **A**1 5 9 10 **F**7 8 17 19 21 22 24 25 28 29 30 35 37 40 41 44 45 46 49 52 54 56 57 58 65 67 71 73 **P**1 3 7	16	10	108	5086	52	245486	643	31483	11685	510

FAYETTE—Fayette County

Hospital	Control	Service	Beds	Admissions	Census	Outpatient Visits	Births	Total	Payroll	Personnel
☒ FAYETTE MEDICAL CENTER, (Formerly Fayette County Hospital and Home), 1653 Temple Avenue North, Zip 35555, Mailing Address: P.O. Drawer 878, Zip 35555; tel. 205/932–5966; Harold Reed, Administrator (Total facility includes 122 beds in nursing home–type unit) **A**1 9 10 **F**4 8 19 21 28 30 32 33 34 35 39 40 42 44 45 49 63 64 65 71 73 **S** DCH Healthcare Authority, Tuscaloosa, AL	13	10	162	1642	142	37257	0	15066	8024	287

FLORALA—Covington County

Hospital	Control	Service	Beds	Admissions	Census	Outpatient Visits	Births	Total	Payroll	Personnel
FLORALA MEMORIAL HOSPITAL, 515 East Fifth Avenue, Zip 36442–0189, Mailing Address: P.O. Box 189, Zip 36442–0189; tel. 334/858–3287; Blair W. Henson, Administrator (Nonreporting) **A**9 10 **S** United Hospital Corporation, Memphis, TN	33	10	23	—	—	—	—	—	—	—

FLORENCE—Lauderdale County

Hospital	Control	Service	Beds	Admissions	Census	Outpatient Visits	Births	Total	Payroll	Personnel
☒ COLUMBIA FLORENCE HOSPITAL, 2111 Cloyd Boulevard, Zip 35630, Mailing Address: Box 2010, Zip 35631; tel. 205/767–8700; Glen M. Jones, Chief Executive Officer (Nonreporting) **A**1 9 10 **S** Columbia/HCA Healthcare Corporation, Nashville, TN	33	10	155	—	—	—	—	—	—	—
☒ ELIZA COFFEE MEMORIAL HOSPITAL, (Includes Mitchell–Hollingsworth Annex), 205 Marengo Street, Zip 35630, Mailing Address: Box 818, Zip 35631; tel. 205/767–9191; Richard H. Peck, Administrator (Total facility includes 214 beds in nursing home–type unit) **A**1 9 10 **F**4 7 8 10 11 19 21 22 26 28 31 34 35 37 40 42 43 44 45 46 49 52 53 54 55 56 57 64 65 67 71 73 **N** HealthGroup of Alabama, L.L.C., Madison, AL	16	10	457	11243	370	61280	1204	78067	32393	1553

FOLEY—Baldwin County

Hospital	Control	Service	Beds	Admissions	Census	Outpatient Visits	Births	Total	Payroll	Personnel
☒ SOUTH BALDWIN HOSPITAL, 1613 North McKenzie Street, Zip 36535; tel. 334/952–3400; Robert F. Jernigan, Jr., Administrator **A**1 9 10 **F**7 8 12 14 15 16 19 22 32 35 37 39 40 41 42 44 45 46 65 67 70 71 73 **P**3	16	10	76	4334	46	59623	306	21234	9624	379

FORT PAYNE—DeKalb County

Hospital	Control	Service	Beds	Admissions	Census	Outpatient Visits	Births	Total	Payroll	Personnel
☒ DEKALB BAPTIST MEDICAL CENTER, 200 Medical Center Drive, Zip 35967, Mailing Address: P.O. Box 778, Zip 35967–0778; tel. 205/845–3150; Barry S. Cochran, President **A**1 9 10 **F**7 8 12 14 15 16 19 21 22 24 26 27 30 31 32 33 35 37 40 41 42 44 46 62 65 66 68 70 71 73 74 **P**3 5 7 **S** Baptist Health System, Birmingham, AL **N** Baptist Health System, Birmingham, AL	21	10	91	3942	45	49003	555	26622	9841	349

FORT RUCKER—Coffee County

Hospital	Control	Service	Beds	Admissions	Census	Outpatient Visits	Births	Total	Payroll	Personnel
☒ LYSTER U. S. ARMY COMMUNITY HOSPITAL, U.S. Army Aeromedical Center, Zip 36362–5333; tel. 334/255–7360; Lieutenant Colonel Melvin Leggett, Jr., Deputy Commander, Administration **A**1 9 **F**1 2 3 4 5 6 7 8 9 10 11 12 13 14 15 16 17 18 19 20 21 22 23 24 25 26 27 28 29 30 31 32 33 34 35 36 37 38 39 40 41 42 43 44 45 46 47 48 49 50 51 52 53 54 55 56 57 58 59 60 61 62 63 64 65 66 67 68 69 71 72 73 74 **S** Department of the Army, Office of the Surgeon General, Falls Church, VA	42	10	42	2820	17	191209	0	31111	18340	504

GADSDEN—Etowah County

Hospital	Control	Service	Beds	Admissions	Census	Outpatient Visits	Births	Total	Payroll	Personnel
☒ GADSDEN REGIONAL MEDICAL CENTER, 1007 Goodyear Avenue, Zip 35999; tel. 205/494–4000; William Russell Spray, Chief Executive Officer **A**1 2 9 10 **F**4 7 8 10 11 12 14 16 19 21 22 23 30 32 33 35 37 40 42 43 44 46 49 52 56 57 60 65 70 71 74 **P**5 **S** Quorum Health Group/Quorum Health Resources, Inc., Brentwood, TN	33	10	257	11315	163	122215	1196	76296	29047	1110
□ MOUNTAIN VIEW HOSPITAL, 3001 Scenic Highway, Zip 35901–9956, Mailing Address: P.O. Box 8406, Zip 35902–8406; tel. 205/546–9265; Jon Orr, Administrator **A**1 9 10 **F**1 2 3 4 5 6 7 8 10 11 12 13 14 16 17 18 19 20 21 22 25 26 27 29 30 31 32 33 34 35 36 37 39 40 41 42 43 44 45 46 48 49 50 51 52 53 54 55 56 57 58 59 60 61 62 63 64 65 66 67 68 71 72 74 **P**4 8	33	22	68	1277	42	12600	0	—	—	127
□ RIVERVIEW REGIONAL MEDICAL CENTER, 600 South Third Street, Zip 35901, Mailing Address: P.O. Box 268, Zip 35999–0268; tel. 205/543–5200; David A. McClellan, Executive Director **A**1 9 10 **F**4 7 8 10 11 12 16 17 19 21 22 26 28 29 30 32 34 35 36 37 39 40 41 42 43 44 45 46 49 60 63 65 66 70 71 72 73 74 **P**5 **S** Health Management Associates, Naples, FL	33	10	281	7237	110	54159	222	—	—	624

GENEVA—Geneva County

Hospital	Control	Service	Beds	Admissions	Census	Outpatient Visits	Births	Total	Payroll	Personnel
☒ WIREGRASS HOSPITAL, 1200 West Maple Avenue, Zip 36340; tel. 334/684–3655; H. Randolph Smith, Administrator (Total facility includes 86 beds in nursing home–type unit) (Nonreporting) **A**1 9 10 **S** Quorum Health Group/Quorum Health Resources, Inc., Brentwood, TN	13	10	151	—	—	—	—	—	—	—

GEORGIANA—Butler County

Hospital	Control	Service	Beds	Admissions	Census	Outpatient Visits	Births	Total	Payroll	Personnel
GEORGIANA DOCTORS HOSPITAL, 515 Miranda Street, Zip 36033, Mailing Address: Box 548, Zip 36033; tel. 334/376–2205; David Paris, Administrator **A**9 10 **F**11 22 32 37 44 71	33	10	22	969	11	15828	0	2942	1554	73

© 1997 AHA Guide

Hospital, Address, Telephone, Administrator, Approval, Facility, and Physician Codes, Health Care System, Network	Classi- fication Codes		Utilization Data					Expense (thousands) of dollars		
★ American Hospital Association (AHA) membership ☐ Joint Commission on Accreditation of Healthcare Organizations (JCAHO) accreditation + American Osteopathic Hospital Association (AOHA) membership ○ American Osteopathic Association (AOA) accreditation △ Commission on Accreditation of Rehabilitation Facilities (CARF) accreditation Control codes 61, 63, 64, 71, 72 and 73 indicate hospitals listed by AOHA, but not registered by AHA. For definition of numerical codes, see page A4	Control	Service	Beds	Admissions	Census	Outpatient Visits	Births	Total	Payroll	Personnel

GRAYSVILLE—Jefferson County

LONGVIEW GENERAL HOSPITAL, 1100 Bankhead Highway S.W., Zip 35073; tel. 205/674–9422; Dianne Cantrell, Acting Administrator (Nonreporting) **A**9 10	33	10	25	—	—	—	—	—	—	—

GREENSBORO—Hale County

HALE COUNTY HOSPITAL, 508 Green Street, Zip 36744; tel. 334/624–3024; Richard M. McGill, Administrator (Nonreporting) **A**9 10	13	10	30							

GREENVILLE—Butler County

L. V. STABLER MEMORIAL HOSPITAL, Highway 10 West, Zip 36037–0915, Mailing Address: Box 1000, Zip 36037–0915; tel. 334/382–2676; Dwayne Moss, Administrator (Nonreporting) **A**9 10 **S** Community Health Systems, Inc., Brentwood, TN	33	10	74							

GROVE HILL—Clarke County

☐ GROVE HILL MEMORIAL HOSPITAL, 295 South Jackson Street, Zip 36451, Mailing Address: P.O. Box 935, Zip 36451; tel. 334/275–3191; Floyd N. Price, Administrator **A**1 9 10 **F**7 8 19 22 32 40 44 48 49 71 **S** Infirmary Health System, Inc., Mobile, AL	14	10	46	972	8	17423	200	4282	1884	104

GUNTERSVILLE—Marshall County

⊞ GUNTERSVILLE–ARAB MEDICAL CENTER, 8000 Alabama Highway 69, Zip 35976; tel. 205/753–8000; Gary R. Gore, Administrator (Nonreporting) **A**1 9 10 **S** Marshall County Health Care Authority, Guntersville, AL	16	10	90	—	—	—	—	—	—	—

HALEYVILLE—Winston County

⊞ CARRAWAY BURDICK WEST MEDICAL CENTER, (Formerly Burdick–West Memorial Hospital), Highway 195 East, Zip 35565, Mailing Address: Box 780, Zip 35565–0780; tel. 205/486–5213; Ronald L. Sparkman, Administrator **A**1 9 10 **F**8 16 19 20 21 22 28 30 32 33 35 37 44 45 46 51 65 71	23	10	36	1658	19	22003	0	5802	—	140

HAMILTON—Marion County

⊞ MARION BAPTIST MEDICAL CENTER, 1315 Military Street South, Zip 35570; tel. 205/921–7861; Evan S. Dillard, President (Total facility includes 69 beds in nursing home–type unit) **A**1 9 10 **F**8 12 14 15 16 19 22 25 27 28 30 32 34 35 37 42 44 45 46 49 51 54 63 64 65 66 71 73 74 **P**2 4 **S** Baptist Health System, Birmingham, AL **N** Baptist Health System, Birmingham, AL	33	10	112	1453	87	17350	0	10599	4816	139

HARTSELLE—Morgan County

☐ HARTSELLE MEDICAL CENTER, 201 Pine Street N.W., Zip 35640, Mailing Address: P.O. Box 969, Zip 35640; tel. 205/773–6511; Mike H. McNair, Chief Executive Officer (Nonreporting) **A**1 9 10 **S** Community Health Systems, Inc., Brentwood, TN	33	10	150							

HUNTSVILLE—Madison County

⊞ COLUMBIA MEDICAL CENTER OF HUNTSVILLE, (Formerly Columbia Hospital of Huntsville), One Hospital Drive, Zip 35801–3403; tel. 205/882–3100; Thomas M. Weiss, Chief Executive Officer (Nonreporting) **A**1 9 10 **S** Columbia/HCA Healthcare Corporation, Nashville, TN	33	10	120	—	—	—	—	—	—	—
☐ △ HEALTHSOUTH REHABILITATION HOSPITAL OF NORTH ALABAMA, (Formerly North Alabama Rehabilitation Hospital), 107 Governors Drive, Zip 35801; tel. 205/535–2300; Rod Moss, Chief Executive Officer **A**1 7 9 10 **F**12 14 15 16 19 21 25 35 48 49 66 67 71 **S** HEALTHSOUTH Corporation, Birmingham, AL	33	46	50	1104	49	25728	0	9161	5710	162
⊞ HUNTSVILLE HOSPITAL, 101 Sivley Road, Zip 35801–9990; tel. 205/517–8123; Ronald S. Owen, Chief Executive Officer **A**1 2 3 5 9 10 **F**4 7 8 10 11 12 14 15 16 17 19 21 22 23 24 25 28 29 30 32 34 35 37 38 39 40 41 42 43 44 45 46 47 49 52 55 56 57 58 59 60 65 71 73 74 **P**7 **S** Huntsville Hospital System, Huntsville, AL **N** HealthGroup of Alabama, L.L.C., Madison, AL	16	10	558	26940	369	195432	3517	188558	89243	2577
☐ HUNTSVILLE HOSPITAL EAST, 911 Big Cove Road S.E., Zip 35801–3784; tel. 205/517–8020; L. Joe Austin, Chief Executive Officer **A**1 9 10 **F**4 7 8 10 11 12 14 15 16 19 21 22 23 24 25 27 28 32 34 35 37 38 39 40 41 42 43 44 46 47 49 52 55 56 57 58 59 60 65 71 73 74 **P**7 **S** Huntsville Hospital System, Huntsville, AL **N** HealthGroup of Alabama, L.L.C., Madison, AL	16	10	223	6280	76	51217	1099	45147	17493	444
NORTH ALABAMA REHABILITATION HOSPITAL See Healthsouth Rehabilitation Hospital of North Alabama										

JACKSON—Clarke County

VAUGHN JACKSON MEDICAL CENTER, 220 Hospital Drive, Zip 36545, Mailing Address: Box 428, Zip 36545; tel. 205/246–9021; Teresa F. Grimes, Administrator (Nonreporting) **A**9 10	33	10	35	—	—	—	—	—	—	—

JACKSONVILLE—Calhoun County

⊞ JACKSONVILLE HOSPITAL, 1701 Pelham Road South, Zip 36265, Mailing Address: P.O. Box 999, Zip 36265; tel. 205/435–4970; Richard L. McConahy, Chief Executive Officer **A**1 9 10 **F**8 19 22 25 31 35 36 37 40 41 44 49 61 71 73 **P**1 **S** Quorum Health Group/Quorum Health Resources, Inc., Brentwood, TN	33	10	56	1955	17	26732	269	13022	5671	165

JASPER—Walker County

⊞ WALKER BAPTIST MEDICAL CENTER, 3400 Highway 78 East, Zip 35501, Mailing Address: Box 3547, Zip 35502–3547; tel. 205/387–4000; Jeff Brewer, President (Nonreporting) **A**1 9 10 **S** Baptist Health System, Birmingham, AL **N** Baptist Health System, Birmingham, AL	21	10	267	—	—	—	—	—	—	—

LUVERNE—Crenshaw County

CRENSHAW BAPTIST HOSPITAL, 1625 South Forrest Avenue, Zip 36049, Mailing Address: Box 432, Zip 36049; tel. 334/335–3374; Wayne Sasser, Administrator **A**9 10 **F**2 7 12 14 15 16 17 19 22 25 32 34 41 44 49 56 57 58 65 71 73	23	10	52	1080	22	7618	166	—	—	120

MADISON—Madison County

BRADFORD HEALTH SERVICES AT HUNTSVILLE, 1600 Browns Ferry Road, Zip 35758, Mailing Address: P.O. Box 176, Zip 35758–0176; tel. 205/461–7272; Bob Hinds, Executive Director (Nonreporting) **A**9 **S** Bradford Health Services, Birmingham, AL	33	82	84	—	—	—	—	—	—	—

Hospital, Address, Telephone, Administrator, Approval, Facility, and Physician Codes, Health Care System, Network	Classi- fication Codes		Utilization Data					Expense (thousands) of dollars		
	Control	Service	Beds	Admissions	Census	Outpatient Visits	Births	Total	Payroll	Personnel

★ American Hospital Association (AHA) membership
□ Joint Commission on Accreditation of Healthcare Organizations (JCAHO) accreditation
+ American Osteopathic Hospital Association (AOHA) membership
○ American Osteopathic Association (AOA) accreditation
△ Commission on Accreditation of Rehabilitation Facilities (CARF) accreditation
Control codes 61, 63, 64, 71, 72 and 73 indicate hospitals listed by AOHA, but not registered by AHA. For definition of numerical codes, see page A4

MARION—Perry County

Hospital	Control	Service	Beds	Admissions	Census	Outpatient Visits	Births	Total	Payroll	Personnel
VAUGHAN PERRY HOSPITAL, 505 East Lafayette Street, Zip 36756–0149, Mailing Address: P.O. Box 149, Zip 36756–0149; tel. 334/683–9696; Hugh Nichols, Administrator (Total facility includes 61 beds in nursing home–type unit) **A**9 10 **F**9 11 15 22 32 37 38 40 44 47 48	23	10	76	540	62	9489	0	—	—	64

MOBILE—Mobile County

Hospital	Control	Service	Beds	Admissions	Census	Outpatient Visits	Births	Total	Payroll	Personnel
□ CHARTER BEHAVIORAL HEALTH SYSTEM, (Formerly Charter Hospital of Mobile), 5800 Southland Drive, Zip 36693, Mailing Address: P.O. Box 991800, Zip 36691; tel. 334/661–3001; Keith Cox, CHE, Chief Executive Officer **A**1 5 9 10 **F**2 3 15 17 52 53 54 55 56 57 58 59 64 **S** Magellan Health Services, Atlanta, GA	33	22	94	1514	52	0	0	—	—	72
★ MOBILE INFIRMARY MEDICAL CENTER, (Includes Rotary Rehabilitation Hospital), 5 Mobile Infirmary Drive North, Zip 36604, Mailing Address: P.O. Box 2144, Zip 36652–2144; tel. 334/431–4700; E. Chandler Bramlett, Jr., President and Chief Executive Officer **A**1 2 5 9 10 **F**4 5 7 8 10 11 12 14 15 19 21 22 24 25 27 28 29 31 32 34 35 37 40 41 42 43 44 45 46 47 48 49 52 53 54 55 57 60 61 63 64 65 66 67 71 73 74 **P**3 4 6 8 **S** Infirmary Health System, Inc., Mobile, AL	23	10	550	22096	372	214973	836	154609	59442	2350
★ PROVIDENCE HOSPITAL, 6801 Airport Boulevard, Zip 36608, Mailing Address: P.O. Box 850429, Zip 36685; tel. 334/633–1000; John R. Roeder, President **A**1 2 9 10 **F**4 7 8 10 11 12 15 16 17 19 21 22 23 24 25 30 31 32 33 34 35 37 40 42 43 44 46 49 60 65 66 67 71 73 **P**5 6 7 **S** Daughters of Charity National Health System, Saint Louis, MO	21	10	349	16715	233	161180	1031	107411	43893	1518
ROTARY REHABILITATION HOSPITAL See Mobile Infirmary Medical Center										
□ SPRINGHILL MEMORIAL HOSPITAL, 3719 Dauphin Street, Zip 36608–1798, Mailing Address: Box 8246, Zip 36608; tel. 205/344–9630; Bill A. Mason, President **A**1 9 10 **F**8 19 21 22 24 31 34 40 44 45 46 60 65 71 74	31	10	218	8945	115	60347	1358	—	—	1146
UNIVERSITY OF SOUTH ALABAMA HOSPITAL See USA Doctors Hospital										
□ UNIVERSITY OF SOUTH ALABAMA KNOLLWOOD PARK HOSPITAL, 5600 Girby Road, Zip 36693–3398; tel. 334/660–5120; Stanley K. Hammack, Administrator (Nonreporting) **A**1 3 5 9 10 **S** University of South Alabama Hospitals, Mobile, AL	12	10	150							
□ UNIVERSITY OF SOUTH ALABAMA MEDICAL CENTER, 2451 Fillingim Street, Zip 36617; tel. 334/471–7000; Stephen H. Simmons, Administrator (Nonreporting) **A**1 2 3 5 8 9 10 **S** University of South Alabama Hospitals, Mobile, AL	12	10	316							
□ USA DOCTORS HOSPITAL, (Formerly University of South Alabama Hospital), 1700 Center Street, Zip 36604–3391; tel. 334/415–1000; Thomas J. Gibson, Administrator (Nonreporting) **A**1 3 5 9 10 **S** University of South Alabama Hospitals, Mobile, AL	12	10	131							

MONROEVILLE—Monroe County

Hospital	Control	Service	Beds	Admissions	Census	Outpatient Visits	Births	Total	Payroll	Personnel
□ MONROE COUNTY HOSPITAL, 1901 South Alabama Avenue, Zip 36460, Mailing Address: P.O. Box 886, Zip 36461–0886; tel. 334/575–3111; Joe Zager, Chief Executive Officer (Nonreporting) **A**1 9 10 **S** Quorum Health Group/Quorum Health Resources, Inc., Brentwood, TN	13	10	59							

MONTGOMERY—Montgomery County

Hospital	Control	Service	Beds	Admissions	Census	Outpatient Visits	Births	Total	Payroll	Personnel
★ BAPTIST MEDICAL CENTER, 2105 East South Boulevard, Zip 36116–2498, Mailing Address: Box 11010, Zip 36111–1101; tel. 334/288–2100; Michael D. DeBoer, President and Chief Executive Officer **A**1 3 5 9 10 **F**2 3 4 7 8 10 11 12 13 14 15 16 17 19 21 22 23 24 25 28 29 30 31 32 33 34 35 37 38 39 40 41 42 43 44 45 46 48 49 51 52 55 56 58 59 62 63 65 67 71 72 73 74 **P**2 6 7	23	10	357	16936	224	88781	2358	110405	41932	1859
★ COLUMBIA EAST MONTGOMERY MEDICAL CENTER, 400 Taylor Road, Zip 36117, Mailing Address: P.O. Box 241267, Zip 36124–1267; tel. 334/277–8330; John W. Melton, Chief Executive Officer (Nonreporting) **A**1 5 9 10 **S** Columbia/HCA Healthcare Corporation, Nashville, TN	33	10	150							
★ COLUMBIA REGIONAL MEDICAL CENTER, (Formerly Columbia Montgomery Medical Center), 301 South Ripley Street, Zip 36104–4495; tel. 334/269–8000; Ron MacLaren, Chief Executive Officer (Nonreporting) **A**1 3 5 9 10 **S** Columbia/HCA Healthcare Corporation, Nashville, TN	33	10	250							
□ △ HEALTHSOUTH REHABILITATION HOSPITAL OF MONTGOMERY, 4465 Narrow Lane Road, Zip 36116; tel. 334/284–7700; Arnold F. McRae, Administrator and Chief Executive Officer (Nonreporting) **A**1 7 9 10 **S** HEALTHSOUTH Corporation, Birmingham, AL	33	46	80							
★ JACKSON HOSPITAL AND CLINIC, 1235 Forest Avenue, Zip 36106–1125; tel. 334/293–8000; Donald M. Ball, President **A**1 2 9 10 **F**7 10 11 15 19 22 23 30 33 34 35 37 39 40 41 42 44 46 49 52 54 56 60 65 66 71 73 **P**6	23	10	264	11894	166	66527	840	74351	32704	1227
★ MAXWELL HOSPITAL, 330 Kirkpatrick Avenue East, Zip 36112–6219; tel. 334/953–7801; Colonel Herman R. Greenberg, Administrator **A**1 9 **F**7 8 12 13 17 18 19 20 22 28 29 30 31 32 35 39 40 41 44 45 46 47 51 54 55 56 57 58 61 65 71 73 **S** Department of the Air Force, Washington, DC	41	10	30	1228	6	196905	301	—	—	598
★ VETERANS AFFAIRS MEDICAL CENTER, 215 Perry Hill Road, Zip 36109–3798; tel. 334/272–4670; John R. Rowan, Director **A**1 9 **F**14 15 16 19 20 22 33 34 35 37 39 41 49 51 54 58 65 71 73 74 **P**6 **S** Department of Veterans Affairs, Washington, DC	45	10	124	1770	73	51272	0	41550	18906	510

MOULTON—Lawrence County

Hospital	Control	Service	Beds	Admissions	Census	Outpatient Visits	Births	Total	Payroll	Personnel
★ LAWRENCE BAPTIST MEDICAL CENTER, 202 Hospital Street, Zip 35650–0039, Mailing Address: P.O. Box 39, Zip 35650–0039; tel. 205/974–2200; Cheryl Hays, Administrator (Nonreporting) **A**1 9 10 **S** Baptist Health System, Birmingham, AL **N** Baptist Health System, Birmingham, AL	13	10	30							

Hospital, Address, Telephone, Administrator, Approval, Facility, and Physician Codes, Health Care System, Network	Classi-fication Codes		Utilization Data					Expense (thousands) of dollars		
★ American Hospital Association (AHA) membership □ Joint Commission on Accreditation of Healthcare Organizations (JCAHO) accreditation + American Osteopathic Hospital Association (AOHA) membership ○ American Osteopathic Association (AOA) accreditation △ Commission on Accreditation of Rehabilitation Facilities (CARF) accreditation Control codes 61, 63, 64, 71, 72 and 73 indicate hospitals listed by AOHA, but not registered by AHA. For definition of numerical codes, see page A4	Control	Service	Beds	Admissions	Census	Outpatient Visits	Births	Total	Payroll	Personnel

MOUNT VERNON—Mobile County

□ SEARCY HOSPITAL, Mailing Address: P.O. Box 1001, Zip 36560–1001; tel. 334/829–9411; John T. Bartlett, Director (Nonreporting) **A**1 3 5 10

| | 12 | 52 | 530 | — | — | — | — | — | — | — |

MUSCLE SHOALS—Colbert County

⊠ MEDICAL CENTER SHOALS, 201 Avalon Avenue, Zip 35661, Mailing Address: P.O. Box 3359, Zip 35662; tel. 205/386–1600; Connie Hawthorne, Chief Executive Officer (Nonreporting) **A**1 9 10 **S** Columbia/HCA Healthcare Corporation, Nashville, TN

| | 33 | 10 | 128 | — | — | — | — | — | — | — |

NORTHPORT—Tuscaloosa County

⊠ NORTHPORT HOSPITAL–DCH, 2700 Hospital Drive, Zip 35476; tel. 205/333–4500; Charles L. Stewart, Administrator **A**1 9 10 **F**2 4 7 8 10 11 12 14 15 16 17 18 19 21 22 23 24 25 26 28 29 30 31 32 34 35 37 38 39 40 41 42 43 44 45 46 47 48 49 52 54 55 56 57 60 65 66 67 70 71 73 74 **P**7 **S** DCH Healthcare Authority, Tuscaloosa, AL

| | 16 | 10 | 132 | 4506 | 62 | 54089 | 682 | 33644 | 13290 | 446 |

ONEONTA—Blount County

★ BLOUNT MEMORIAL HOSPITAL, 1000 Lincoln Avenue, Zip 35121, Mailing Address: P.O. Box 220, Zip 35121; tel. 205/625–3511; George McGowan, Chief Executive Officer **A**9 10 **F**8 13 14 15 16 19 21 22 28 29 30 32 34 37 39 44 46 49 65 71 73 **S** Eastern Health System, Inc., Birmingham, AL **N** Alabama Health Services, Birmingham, AL

| | 13 | 10 | 57 | 1906 | 23 | 35999 | 0 | 13342 | 5855 | 224 |

OPELIKA—Lee County

⊠ EAST ALABAMA MEDICAL CENTER, 2000 Pepperell Parkway, Zip 36802–3201; tel. 334/749–3411; Terry W. Andrus, President (Total facility includes 24 beds in nursing home–type unit) **A**1 2 9 10 **F**2 4 7 8 10 11 12 14 19 21 22 26 31 32 33 34 35 37 39 40 42 43 44 45 49 52 53 56 57 60 64 65 70 71 73 **P**7 8

| | 16 | 10 | 279 | 13565 | 202 | — | 1533 | 88587 | 38781 | 1342 |

OPP—Covington County

★ MIZELL MEMORIAL HOSPITAL, 702 Main Street, Zip 36467–1626, Mailing Address: P.O. Box 1010, Zip 36467–1010; tel. 334/493–3541; Allen Foster, Administrator **A**9 10 **F**7 8 11 12 15 16 17 19 21 22 28 31 32 35 40 41 44 45 49 65 66 71 73 74 **S** Baptist Health Care Corporation, Pensacola, FL **N** Baptist Health Care, Inc., Pensacola, FL

| | 23 | 10 | 57 | 1695 | 22 | 18514 | 91 | 6501 | 3598 | 175 |

OZARK—Dale County

□ DALE MEDICAL CENTER, 100 Hospital Avenue, Zip 36360; tel. 334/774–2601; Robert F. Bigley, Administrator **A**1 9 10 **F**7 8 10 19 21 22 25 30 32 37 40 42 44 45 46 49 65 66 71 73 **P**5

| | 15 | 10 | 85 | 3000 | 37 | 29601 | 330 | 14498 | 7347 | 305 |

PELHAM—Shelby County

BRADFORD HEALTH SERVICES AT OAK MOUNTAIN, 2280 Highway 35, Zip 35124; tel. 205/664–3460; Jerry Caltrider, Administrator (Nonreporting) **A**9 **S** Bradford Health Services, Birmingham, AL

| | 33 | 52 | 84 | — | — | — | — | — | — | — |

PELL CITY—St. Clair County

★ ST. CLAIR REGIONAL HOSPITAL, 2805 Hospital Drive, Zip 35125; tel. 205/338–3301; George McGowan, Chief Executive Officer (Nonreporting) **A**9 10 **S** Eastern Health System, Inc., Birmingham, AL **N** Alabama Health Services, Birmingham, AL

| | 13 | 10 | 51 | — | — | — | — | — | — | — |

PHENIX CITY—Russell County

⊠ PHENIX REGIONAL HOSPITAL, 1707 21st Avenue, Zip 36867, Mailing Address: Box 190, Zip 36868–0190; tel. 334/291–8502; Lance B. Duke, FACHE, President and Chief Executive Officer (Nonreporting) **A**1 9 10 **N** Columbus Regional HealthCare System, Inc., Columbus, GA; Principal Health Care of Georgia, Atlanta, GA; The Medical Resource Network, L.L.C., Atlanta, GA

| | 23 | 10 | 140 | — | — | — | — | — | — | — |

PRATTVILLE—Autauga County

⊠ COLUMBIA NORTHRIDGE MEDICAL CENTER, 124 South Memorial Drive, Zip 36067; tel. 334/365–0651; Duane Brookhart, Ph.D., President and Chief Executive Officer (Nonreporting) **A**1 9 10 **S** Columbia/HCA Healthcare Corporation, Nashville, TN

| | 33 | 10 | 50 | — | — | — | — | — | — | — |

RED BAY—Franklin County

RED BAY HOSPITAL, 211 Hospital Road, Zip 35582, Mailing Address: Box 490, Zip 35582; tel. 205/356–9532; Ralph J. Wilson, Administrator **A**9 10 **F**8 14 19 32 44 71 **P**5

| | 13 | 10 | 33 | 1075 | 12 | 17384 | 0 | 4891 | 1777 | 83 |

REDSTONE ARSENAL—Madison County

⊠ FOX ARMY COMMUNITY HOSPITAL, Zip 35809–7000; tel. 205/876–4147; Major Mark A. Miller, Deputy Commander **A**1 9 **F**2 3 4 5 6 7 8 9 10 11 12 13 17 18 19 20 21 22 24 26 27 28 29 30 31 32 33 34 35 36 37 38 39 40 41 42 43 44 45 46 47 48 49 50 51 52 53 54 55 56 57 58 59 60 61 63 64 65 66 67 68 69 70 71 72 73 74 **S** Department of the Army, Office of the Surgeon General, Falls Church, VA

| | 42 | 10 | 29 | 1265 | 7 | 129255 | 0 | — | — | 312 |

ROANOKE—Randolph County

★ RANDOLPH COUNTY HOSPITAL, 1000 Wadley Highway, Zip 36274, Mailing Address: Box 670, Zip 36274; tel. 334/863–4111; Moultrie D. Plowden, CHE, Administrator **A**9 10 **F**2 7 8 15 19 21 22 28 32 34 35 37 40 44 49 65 71 73

| | 13 | 10 | 66 | 1504 | 25 | 19279 | 95 | 9098 | 3775 | 171 |

RUSSELLVILLE—Franklin County

⊠ NORTHWEST MEDICAL CENTER, Highway 43 By-Pass, Zip 35653, Mailing Address: P.O. Box 1089, Zip 35653; tel. 205/332–1611; Christine R. Stewart, President and Chief Executive Officer (Nonreporting) **A**1 9 10 **S** Columbia/HCA Healthcare Corporation, Nashville, TN

| | 33 | 10 | 100 | — | — | — | — | — | — | — |

SCOTTSBORO—Jackson County

□ JACKSON COUNTY HOSPITAL, 380 Woods Cove Road, Zip 35768, Mailing Address: Box 1050, Zip 35768; tel. 205/259–4444; James K. Mason, Administrator (Total facility includes 50 beds in nursing home–type unit) **A**1 9 10 **F**7 11 14 15 16 19 22 32 35 40 44 64 65 71 73

| | 13 | 10 | 142 | 4254 | 102 | 86825 | 356 | 23336 | 10013 | 318 |

Hospital, Address, Telephone, Administrator, Approval, Facility, and Physician Codes, Health Care System, Network	Classi-fication Codes		Utilization Data					Expense (thousands) of dollars		
	Control	Service	Beds	Admissions	Census	Outpatient Visits	Births	Total	Payroll	Personnel

★ American Hospital Association (AHA) membership
□ Joint Commission on Accreditation of Healthcare Organizations (JCAHO) accreditation
+ American Osteopathic Hospital Association (AOHA) membership
○ American Osteopathic Association (AOA) accreditation
△ Commission on Accreditation of Rehabilitation Facilities (CARF) accreditation
Control codes 61, 63, 64, 71, 72 and 73 indicate hospitals listed by AOHA, but not registered by AHA. For definition of numerical codes, see page A4

SELMA—Dallas County

Hospital	Control	Service	Beds	Admissions	Census	Outpatient Visits	Births	Total	Payroll	Personnel
⊞ COLUMBIA FOUR RIVERS MEDICAL CENTER, 1015 Medical Center Parkway, Zip 36701; tel. 334/872–8461; Robert F. Bigley, Chief Executive Officer (Nonreporting) **A**1 2 3 5 9 10 **S** Columbia/HCA Healthcare Corporation, Nashville, TN	33	10	150	—	—	—	—	—	—	—
⊞ VAUGHAN REGIONAL MEDICAL CENTER, 1050 West Dallas Avenue, Zip 36701; Mailing Address: Box 328, Zip 36702–0328; tel. 334/418–6000; Donald J. Jones, Administrator **A**1 3 5 9 10 **F**7 8 12 16 17 19 21 22 24 28 29 30 32 35 40 44 46 63 65 67 71 73 **P**3 5 7	23	10	114	5598	66	43377	971	25464	12380	556

SHEFFIELD—Colbert County

Hospital	Control	Service	Beds	Admissions	Census	Outpatient Visits	Births	Total	Payroll	Personnel
⊞ HELEN KELLER HOSPITAL, 1300 South Montgomery Avenue, Zip 35660, Mailing Address: Box 610, Zip 35660; tel. 205/386–4556; Ralph Clark, Jr., President **A**1 9 10 **F**2 3 7 8 10 11 16 19 21 22 23 26 27 34 35 37 40 41 44 46 49 52 60 63 65 66 71 73 74 **P**6	16	10	152	5904	88	62999	712	36477	14379	690

SYLACAUGA—Talladega County

Hospital	Control	Service	Beds	Admissions	Census	Outpatient Visits	Births	Total	Payroll	Personnel
⊞ COOSA VALLEY BAPTIST MEDICAL CENTER, 315 West Hickory Street, Zip 35150–2996; tel. 205/249–5000; Steven M. Johnson, President (Total facility includes 75 beds in nursing home–type unit) **A**1 9 10 **F**7 12 15 16 17 19 21 22 24 28 30 32 34 35 37 39 40 42 44 49 54 60 64 65 66 67 71 73 74 **P**5 **S** Baptist Health System, Birmingham, AL **N** Baptist Health System, Birmingham, AL	21	10	176	5789	126	86789	519	24258	10704	691

TALLADEGA—Talladega County

Hospital	Control	Service	Beds	Admissions	Census	Outpatient Visits	Births	Total	Payroll	Personnel
⊞ CITIZENS BAPTIST MEDICAL CENTER, 604 Stone Avenue, Zip 35160, Mailing Address: P.O. Box 978, Zip 35161; tel. 205/362–8111; Steven M. Johnson, President (Nonreporting) **A**1 9 10 **S** Baptist Health System, Birmingham, AL **N** Baptist Health System, Birmingham, AL	23	10	97	—	—	—	—	—	—	—

TALLASSEE—Elmore County

Hospital	Control	Service	Beds	Admissions	Census	Outpatient Visits	Births	Total	Payroll	Personnel
□ COMMUNITY HOSPITAL, 805 Friendship Road, Zip 36078, Mailing Address: Box 707, Zip 36078–0707; tel. 205/283–6541; Jennie Rhinehart, Administrator (Nonreporting) **A**1 9 10	23	10	69	—	—	—	—	—	—	—

THOMASVILLE—Clarke County

Hospital	Control	Service	Beds	Admissions	Census	Outpatient Visits	Births	Total	Payroll	Personnel
□ VAUGHN THOMASVILLE MEDICAL CENTER, 1440 Highway 43 North, Zip 36784, Mailing Address: P.O. Box 429, Zip 36784; tel. 334/636–4431; Wendy Ackerman, Administrator (Nonreporting) **A**1 9 10	33	10	37	—	—	—	—	—	—	—

TROY—Pike County

Hospital	Control	Service	Beds	Admissions	Census	Outpatient Visits	Births	Total	Payroll	Personnel
⊞ EDGE REGIONAL MEDICAL CENTER, 1330 Highway 231 South, Zip 36081–1224; tel. 334/670–5000; David E. Loving, Chief Executive Officer (Nonreporting) **A**1 9 10 **S** Community Health Systems, Inc., Brentwood, TN	14	10	87	—	—	—	—	—	—	—

TUSCALOOSA—Tuscaloosa County

Hospital	Control	Service	Beds	Admissions	Census	Outpatient Visits	Births	Total	Payroll	Personnel
□ BRYCE HOSPITAL, 200 University Boulevard, Zip 35401; tel. 205/759–0799; James F. Reddoch, Jr., Director (Total facility includes 354 beds in nursing home–type unit) **A**1 10 **F**8 15 16 19 20 21 31 35 37 41 44 49 52 53 54 55 56 57 58 59 64 65 67 71 73 **P**6	12	22	870	739	849	0	0	53499	34325	1211
⊞ DCH REGIONAL MEDICAL CENTER, 809 University Boulevard East, Zip 35401–9961; tel. 205/759–7111; Bryan N. Kindred, Chief Executive Officer **A**1 2 3 5 9 10 **F**4 7 8 10 11 12 14 16 17 18 19 21 22 23 24 25 28 30 31 32 33 34 35 37 38 39 40 41 42 43 44 45 46 47 48 49 52 54 55 56 57 60 63 64 65 66 67 70 71 73 74 **P**7 **S** DCH Healthcare Authority, Tuscaloosa, AL	23	10	476	21777	363	212535	1971	154273	69615	2324
⊞ VETERANS AFFAIRS MEDICAL CENTER, 3701 Loop Road, Zip 35404–9983; tel. 205/554–2000; W. Kenneth Ruyle, Director (Total facility includes 195 beds in nursing home–type unit) **A**1 9 **F**3 11 15 16 17 20 22 24 26 27 28 29 30 31 32 35 39 41 42 46 48 49 51 52 55 56 57 58 64 65 73 74 **P**8 **S** Department of Veterans Affairs, Washington, DC	45	22	307	2987	268	85798	0	—	—	999

TUSKEGEE—Macon County

Hospital	Control	Service	Beds	Admissions	Census	Outpatient Visits	Births	Total	Payroll	Personnel
⊞ VETERANS AFFAIRS MEDICAL CENTER, 2400 Hospital Road, Zip 36083–5001; tel. 334/727–0550; Jim Clay, Director (Total facility includes 152 beds in nursing home–type unit) **A**1 3 5 9 **F**2 3 11 12 17 19 20 21 22 25 26 27 31 32 34 37 41 44 45 46 48 49 52 54 55 56 57 58 63 64 65 67 71 73 74 **S** Department of Veterans Affairs, Washington, DC	45	10	679	4735	560	91037	0	76961	48944	1242

UNION SPRINGS—Bullock County

Hospital	Control	Service	Beds	Admissions	Census	Outpatient Visits	Births	Total	Payroll	Personnel
BULLOCK COUNTY HOSPITAL, 102 West Conecuh Avenue, Zip 36089; tel. 334/738–2140; Diane S. Hall, Administrator **A**9 10 **F**14 16 18 19 22 28 32 44 71	33	10	30	1177	11	7835	5	—	—	96

VALLEY—Chambers County

Hospital	Control	Service	Beds	Admissions	Census	Outpatient Visits	Births	Total	Payroll	Personnel
□ GEORGE H. LANIER MEMORIAL HOSPITAL AND HEALTH SERVICES, 4800 48th Street, Zip 36854–3666; tel. 334/756–3111; Robert J. Humphrey, Administrator (Total facility includes 93 beds in nursing home–type unit) **A**1 9 10 **F**4 7 8 14 16 19 20 21 22 23 26 28 29 30 31 32 33 34 35 37 39 40 42 44 45 46 64 65 67 71 73	23	10	175	4059	135	42852	373	21921	10173	351

WEDOWEE—Randolph County

Hospital	Control	Service	Beds	Admissions	Census	Outpatient Visits	Births	Total	Payroll	Personnel
WEDOWEE HOSPITAL, 290 North Main Street, Zip 36278, Mailing Address: Box 307, Zip 36278; tel. 205/357–2111; Kerlene Mitchell, Administrator (Nonreporting) **A**9 10	23	10	34	—	—	—	—	—	—	—

WETUMPKA—Elmore County

Hospital	Control	Service	Beds	Admissions	Census	Outpatient Visits	Births	Total	Payroll	Personnel
★ ELMORE COMMUNITY HOSPITAL, 500 Hospital Drive, Zip 36092, Mailing Address: P.O. Box 120, Zip 36092–0120; tel. 334/567–4311; Tommy R. McDougal, Jr., Administrator **A**9 10 **F**2 3 8 15 16 19 21 22 28 30 32 33 34 37 39 44 46 49 63 65 66 67 71 73	15	10	46	1622	23	19121	0	8068	3162	152

Hospital, Address, Telephone, Administrator, Approval, Facility, and Physician Codes, Health Care System, Network	Classi-fication Codes		Utilization Data					Expense (thousands) of dollars		
★ American Hospital Association (AHA) membership ☐ Joint Commission on Accreditation of Healthcare Organizations (JCAHO) accreditation + American Osteopathic Hospital Association (AOHA) membership ○ American Osteopathic Association (AOA) accreditation △ Commission on Accreditation of Rehabilitation Facilities (CARF) accreditation Control codes 61, 63, 64, 71, 72 and 73 indicate hospitals listed by AOHA, but not registered by AHA. For definition of numerical codes, see page A4	Control	Service	Beds	Admissions	Census	Outpatient Visits	Births	Total	Payroll	Personnel

WINFIELD—Marion County

☒ CARRAWAY NORTHWEST MEDICAL CENTER, Highway 78 West, Zip 35594, Mailing Address: Box 130, Zip 35594–0130; tel. 205/487–4234; Robert E. Henger, Administrator **A**1 9 10 **F**7 8 12 14 15 16 17 19 21 22 28 29 30 32 34 37 39 40 41 42 44 45 46 49 51 59 61 63 65 66 71 73 74 **P**1 5

	21	10	63	2212	26	33758	255	11581	4748	238

ALASKA

Resident population 604 (in thousands)
Resident population in metro areas 41.8%
Birth rate per 1,000 population 18.5
65 years and over 4.9%
Percent of persons without health insurance 13.3%

★ American Hospital Association (AHA) membership
□ Joint Commission on Accreditation of Healthcare Organizations (JCAHO) accreditation
+ American Osteopathic Hospital Association (AOHA) membership
◯ American Osteopathic Association (AOA) accreditation
△ Commission on Accreditation of Rehabilitation Facilities (CARF) accreditation
Control codes 61, 63, 64, 71, 72 and 73 indicate hospitals listed by AOHA, but not
registered by AHA. For definition of numerical codes, see page A4

Hospital, Address, Telephone, Administrator, Approval, Facility, and Physician Codes, Health Care System, Network	Control	Service	Beds	Admissions	Census	Outpatient Visits	Births	Total	Payroll	Personnel
ANCHORAGE—2nd Judicial Division										
□ ALASKA PSYCHIATRIC HOSPITAL, 2900 Providence Drive, Zip 99508–4677; tel. 907/269–7100; Randall Burns, Director (Nonreporting) **A**1 9 10	12	22	79	—	—	—	—	—	—	—
□ CHARTER NORTH STAR BEHAVIORAL HEALTH SYSTEM, 2530 Debarr Road, Zip 99508; tel. 907/258–7575; Kathleen Cronen, Administrator (Nonreporting) **A**1 9 10 **S** Magellan Health Services, Atlanta, GA	33	22	80	—	—	—	—	—	—	—
⊞ COLUMBIA ALASKA REGIONAL HOSPITAL, 2801 Debarr Road, Zip 99508, Mailing Address: P.O. Box 143889, Zip 99514–3889; tel. 907/276–1131; Ernie Meier, President and Chief Executive Officer (Nonreporting) **A**1 9 10 **S** Columbia/HCA Healthcare Corporation, Nashville, TN	33	10	238	—	—	—	—	—	—	—
□ NORTH STAR HOSPITAL AND COUNSELING CENTER, 1650 South Bragaw, Zip 99508–3467; tel. 907/277–1522; Bob Marshall, Administrator (Nonreporting) **A**1 10 **N** Ketchikan General Hospital, Ketchikan, AK	33	22	34	—	—	—	—	—	—	—
⊞ PROVIDENCE ALASKA MEDICAL CENTER, 3200 Providence Drive, Zip 99508, Mailing Address: P.O. Box 196604, Zip 99519–6604; tel. 907/562–2211; Douglas A. Bruce, Chief Executive Alaska Service Area (Nonreporting) **A**1 9 10 **S** Sisters of Providence Health System, Seattle, WA	21	10	341	—	—	—	—	—	—	—
⊞ U. S. PUBLIC HEALTH SERVICE ALASKA NATIVE MEDICAL CENTER, 255 Gambell Street, Zip 99501, Mailing Address: P.O. Box 107741, Zip 99510; tel. 907/279–6661; Richard Mandsager, M.D., Director (Nonreporting) **A**1 5 10 **S** U. S. Public Health Service Indian Health Service, Rockville, MD	47	10	140	—	—	—	—	—	—	—
BARROW—4th Judicial Division										
⊞ SAMUEL SIMMONDS MEMORIAL HOSPITAL, (Formerly U. S. Public Health Service Alaska Native Hospital), Zip 99723; tel. 907/852–4611; John Morrow, Administrator (Nonreporting) **A**1 10 **S** U. S. Public Health Service Indian Health Service, Rockville, MD	47	10	15	—	—	—	—	—	—	—
BETHEL—1st Judicial Division										
⊞ YUKON–KUSKOKWIM DELTA REGIONAL HOSPITAL, P.O. Box 528, Zip 99559–3000; tel. 907/543–6300; Edwin L. Hansen, Vice President (Nonreporting) **A**1 10 **S** U. S. Public Health Service Indian Health Service, Rockville, MD	47	10	50	—	—	—	—	—	—	—
CORDOVA—2nd Judicial Division										
★ CORDOVA COMMUNITY MEDICAL CENTER, 602 Chase Avenue, Zip 99574, Mailing Address: Box 160, Zip 99574; tel. 907/424–8000; Greg Porter, Administrator and Chief Executive Officer (Total facility includes 13 beds in nursing home–type unit) (Nonreporting) **A**9 10	14	10	23	—	—	—	—	—	—	—
DILLINGHAM—1st Judicial Division										
⊞ KANAKANAK HOSPITAL, Mailing Address: P.O. Box 130, Zip 99576; tel. 907/842–5201; Darrel C. Richardson, Chief Operating Officer (Nonreporting) **A**1 9 10 **S** U. S. Public Health Service Indian Health Service, Rockville, MD	47	10	16	—	—	—	—	—	—	—
ELMENDORF AFB—2nd Judicial Division										
⊞ U. S. AIR FORCE REGIONAL HOSPITAL, 24800 Hospital Drive, Zip 99506–3700; tel. 907/552–4033; Colonel Larry J. Sutterer, MSC, USAF, Administrator **A**1 5 **F**2 3 7 8 12 14 15 16 17 19 20 21 22 24 27 28 29 30 31 34 35 37 39 40 41 42 44 46 48 49 51 52 53 54 55 56 58 61 63 65 68 71 74 **S** Department of the Air Force, Washington, DC	41	10	64	4674	31	267439	785	58912	34423	870
FAIRBANKS—1st Judicial Division										
⊞ FAIRBANKS MEMORIAL HOSPITAL, 1650 Cowles Street, Zip 99701; tel. 907/452–8181; Michael K. Powers, Administrator (Total facility includes 92 beds in nursing home–type unit) **A**1 2 9 10 **F**3 4 7 8 12 13 14 17 19 21 22 27 28 32 34 35 36 37 39 40 41 44 49 52 55 56 58 63 64 65 66 67 70 71 73 **S** Lutheran Health Systems, Fargo, ND	23	10	200	5897	141	181801	972	77151	32899	751
FORT WAINWRIGHT—1st Judicial Division										
⊞ BASSETT ARMY COMMUNITY HOSPITAL, Fort Wainwright, Zip 99703–7400; tel. 907/353–5108; Lieutenant Colonel Gordon Lewis, Deputy Commander for Administration **A**1 **F**3 7 8 12 13 14 15 17 18 19 20 22 24 25 28 29 30 31 34 39 40 44 46 49 51 54 55 56 58 61 65 66 67 71 72 74 **P**1 **S** Department of the Army, Office of the Surgeon General, Falls Church, VA	42	10	43	2493	16	152282	620	—	—	495
HOMER—3rd Judicial Division										
★ SOUTH PENINSULA HOSPITAL, 4300 Bartlett Street, Zip 99603; tel. 907/235–8101; Charles C. Franz, Chief Executive Officer (Total facility includes 20 beds in nursing home–type unit) **A**9 10 **F**7 8 11 12 15 19 21 22 28 32 37 40 44 49 64 65 71	16	10	40	845	28	14480	136	12993	5937	176
JUNEAU—3rd Judicial Division										
⊞ BARTLETT REGIONAL HOSPITAL, (Formerly Bartlett Memorial Hospital), 3260 Hospital Drive, Zip 99801; tel. 907/586–2611; Robert F. Valliant, Administrator (Nonreporting) **A**1 9 10 **S** Quorum Health Group/Quorum Health Resources, Inc., Brentwood, TN	15	10	64	—	—	—	—	—	—	—

Hospital, Address, Telephone, Administrator, Approval, Facility, and Physician Codes, Health Care System, Network	Classi-fication Codes		Utilization Data					Expense (thousands) of dollars		
★ American Hospital Association (AHA) membership □ Joint Commission on Accreditation of Healthcare Organizations (JCAHO) accreditation + American Osteopathic Hospital Association (AOHA) membership ○ American Osteopathic Association (AOA) accreditation △ Commission on Accreditation of Rehabilitation Facilities (CARF) accreditation Control codes 61, 63, 64, 71, 72 and 73 indicate hospitals listed by AOHA, but not registered by AHA. For definition of numerical codes, see page A4	Control	Service	Beds	Admissions	Census	Outpatient Visits	Births	Total	Payroll	Personnel

KETCHIKAN—3rd Judicial Division

▣ KETCHIKAN GENERAL HOSPITAL, 3100 Tongass Avenue, Zip 99901–5746; tel. 907/225–5171; Edward F. Mahn, Chief Executive Officer (Total facility includes 26 beds in nursing home–type unit) **A**1 9 10 **F**2 3 7 8 11 14 16 19 21 22 29 31 34 37 40 41 44 45 49 52 56 63 64 65 70 71 73 **S** PeaceHealth, Bellevue, WA **N** PeaceHealth, Bellevue, WA; Ketchikan General Hospital, Ketchikan, AK
— 21 10 53 1851 34 45124 350 22995 12031 228

KODIAK—2nd Judicial Division

★ PROVIDENCE KODIAK ISLAND HOSPITAL AND MEDICAL CENTER, (Formerly Kodiak Island Hospital and Care Center), 1915 East Rezanof Drive, Zip 99615; tel. 907/486–3281; Phillip E. Cline, Administrator (Total facility includes 19 beds in nursing home–type unit) (Nonreporting) **A**9 10 **S** Lutheran Health Systems, Fargo, ND
— 13 10 44 — — — — — — —

KOTZEBUE—2nd Judicial Division

▣ MANIILAQ HEALTH CENTER, Zip 99752–0043; tel. 907/442–3321; Jan Harris, Vice President **A**1 10 **F**2 7 8 13 14 15 16 17 20 22 25 26 27 28 29 30 31 32 33 34 36 39 40 45 46 51 54 56 58 61 64 65 67 71 74 **P**6 **S** U. S. Public Health Service Indian Health Service, Rockville, MD
— 47 10 17 903 9 — 88 — — 192

NOME—2nd Judicial Division

▣ NORTON SOUND REGIONAL HOSPITAL, Bering Street, Zip 99762, Mailing Address: Box 966, Zip 99762; tel. 907/443–3311; Charles Fagerstrom, Vice President (Total facility includes 15 beds in nursing home–type unit) (Nonreporting) **A**1 9 10 **S** U. S. Public Health Service Indian Health Service, Rockville, MD **N** Norton Sound Regional Hospital, Nome, AK
— 23 10 34 — — — — — — —

PALMER—2nd Judicial Division

▣ VALLEY HOSPITAL, 515 East Dahlia Street, Zip 99645, Mailing Address: P.O. Box 1687, Zip 99645; tel. 907/352–2860; Cliff Orme, Executive Director **A**1 9 10 **F**7 8 12 15 16 17 19 21 22 32 33 34 35 37 40 44 45 46 49 65 71 72 **P**7 8
— 23 10 36 2224 20 32625 404 26337 11761 323

PETERSBURG—3rd Judicial Division

PETERSBURG MEDICAL CENTER, 103 Fram Street, Zip 99833, Mailing Address: Box 589, Zip 99833–0589; tel. 907/772–4291; Gary W. Grandy, Administrator (Total facility includes 14 beds in nursing home–type unit) **A**9 10 **F**2 7 8 11 15 16 22 25 30 31 32 34 40 42 44 49 52 56 64 66 71 **P**6
— 14 10 25 195 15 13140 21 3890 2173 57

SEWARD—2nd Judicial Division

★ PROVIDENCE SEWARD MEDICAL CENTER, 417 First Avenue, Zip 99664, Mailing Address: P.O. Box 365, Zip 99664–0365; tel. 907/224–5205; Colleen Bridge, Administrator (Nonreporting) **A**9 10
— 14 10 20 — — — — — — —

SITKA—3rd Judicial Division

▣ SEARHC MT. EDGECUMBE HOSPITAL, 222 Tongass Drive, Zip 99835–9416; tel. 907/966–2411; Arthur C. Willman, Vice President Operations **A**1 10 **F**2 7 8 12 15 16 20 22 24 27 28 34 40 44 52 53 54 56 57 58 65 67 68 71 74 **S** U. S. Public Health Service Indian Health Service, Rockville, MD
— 23 10 72 1664 25 31234 68 — — 273

▣ SITKA COMMUNITY HOSPITAL, 209 Moller Avenue, Zip 99835–7145; tel. 907/747–3241; Grant Asay, Chief Executive Officer (Total facility includes 5 beds in nursing home–type unit) **A**1 9 10 **F**7 8 19 22 32 34 44 49 64 65 71 73 **P**6
— 15 10 22 484 9 16875 79 6963 3188 78

SOLDOTNA—3rd Judicial Division

▣ CENTRAL PENINSULA GENERAL HOSPITAL, 250 Hospital Place, Zip 99669; tel. 907/262–4404; Rulon J. Barlow, Administrator **A**1 9 10 **F**2 3 7 8 11 12 15 16 17 19 22 26 28 30 31 34 37 39 40 41 42 44 46 49 52 56 65 67 70 71 73 **P**5 **S** Lutheran Health Systems, Fargo, ND
— 23 10 58 2164 21 31539 429 20884 9648 227

VALDEZ—3rd Judicial Division

★ VALDEZ COMMUNITY HOSPITAL, 911 Meals Avenue, Zip 99686–0550, Mailing Address: Box 550, Zip 99686–0550; tel. 907/835–2249; James R. Culley, Administrator **A**9 10 **F**7 8 14 15 22 28 32 40 44 64 71 **P**4
— 14 10 7 136 2 4913 45 2392 1223 28

WRANGELL—3rd Judicial Division

★ WRANGELL GENERAL HOSPITAL AND LONG TERM CARE FACILITY, First Avenue & Bennett Street, Zip 99929, Mailing Address: P.O. Box 1081, Zip 99929; tel. 907/874–7000; Brian D. Gilbert, Administrator (Total facility includes 14 beds in nursing home–type unit) **A**9 10 **F**7 8 11 15 16 22 28 29 34 40 44 64 71
— 14 10 21 197 15 10435 16 3799 1825 44

ARIZONA

Resident population 4,218 (in thousands)
Resident population in metro areas 87.3%
Birth rate per 1,000 population 17.5
65 years and over 13.3%
Percent of persons without health insurance 20.2%

Hospital, Address, Telephone, Administrator, Approval, Facility, and Physician Codes, Health Care System, Network	Classi-fication Codes		Utilization Data					Expense (thousands) of dollars		
	Control	Service	Beds	Admissions	Census	Outpatient Visits	Births	Total	Payroll	Personnel

★ American Hospital Association (AHA) membership
□ Joint Commission on Accreditation of Healthcare Organizations (JCAHO) accreditation
+ American Osteopathic Hospital Association (AOHA) membership
○ American Osteopathic Association (AOA) accreditation
△ Commission on Accreditation of Rehabilitation Facilities (CARF) accreditation
Control codes 61, 63, 64, 71, 72 and 73 indicate hospitals listed by AOHA, but not registered by AHA. For definition of numerical codes, see page A4

BENSON—Cochise County

□ BENSON HOSPITAL, 450 South Ocotillo Street, Zip 85602, Mailing Address: P.O. Box 2290, Zip 85602–2290; tel. 520/586–2261; Ronald A. McKinnon, Administrator (Nonreporting) **A**1 9 10 — Control 16, Service 10, Beds 22

BISBEE—Cochise County

□ COPPER QUEEN COMMUNITY HOSPITAL, 101 Cole Avenue, Zip 85603–1399; tel. 520/432–5383; Jim Tavary, Chief Executive Officer and Administrator (Total facility includes 21 beds in nursing home–type unit) **A**1 9 10 **F**7 8 14 15 16 17 20 22 28 32 33 34 40 41 44 49 51 56 64 65 66 67 71 73 **P**5 — Control 23, Service 10, Beds 49, Admissions 529, Census 26, Outpatient Visits 12247, Births 39, Total 5602, Payroll 2911, Personnel 168

BULLHEAD CITY—Mohave County

⊠ BULLHEAD COMMUNITY HOSPITAL, 2735 Silver Creek Road, Zip 86442; tel. 520/763–2273; Ronald W. Tenbarge, Executive Vice President and Chief Executive Officer (Total facility includes 120 beds in nursing home–type unit) **A**1 9 10 **F**3 8 10 12 14 15 16 19 21 22 23 24 28 29 32 33 35 37 40 41 42 44 45 49 53 54 55 56 57 58 64 65 67 71 73 **P**1 3 7 **S** Baptist Hospitals and Health Systems, Inc., Phoenix, AZ **N** Baptist Hospitals and Health Systems, Phoenix, AZ — Control 23, Service 10, Beds 182, Admissions 4347, Census 155, Outpatient Visits 48828, Births 617, Total 31130, Payroll 11411, Personnel 329

★ MOHAVE VALLEY HOSPITAL AND MEDICAL CENTER, 1225 East Hancock Road, Zip 86442; tel. 520/758–3931; Stan Lentz, Administrator and Chief Executive Officer **A**9 10 **F**12 14 15 16 19 22 26 30 31 34 35 42 44 50 51 60 63 71 72 73 **P**1 — Control 33, Service 10, Beds 12, Admissions 583, Census 5, Outpatient Visits 28210, Births 0, Total 11345, Payroll 3513, Personnel 78

CASA GRANDE—Pinal County

⊠ CASA GRANDE REGIONAL MEDICAL CENTER, 1800 East Florence Boulevard, Zip 85222; tel. 520/426–6300; J. Stephen Hockins, Administrator (Total facility includes 128 beds in nursing home–type unit) **A**1 9 10 **F**7 8 12 13 14 15 16 19 21 22 27 28 29 30 34 35 37 39 40 41 44 45 49 64 65 67 70 71 72 73 74 **P**5 8 **N** Arizona Voluntary Hospital Federation, Tempe, AZ — Control 23, Service 10, Beds 244, Admissions 6222, Census 193, Outpatient Visits 54659, Births 756, Total 43671, Payroll 17325, Personnel 520

CHANDLER—Maricopa County

⊠ CHANDLER REGIONAL HOSPITAL, 475 South Dobson Road, Zip 85224–4230; tel. 602/963–4561; Kaylor E. Shemberger, President and Chief Executive Officer **A**1 9 10 **F**7 8 12 15 16 17 19 21 22 25 28 30 31 32 34 35 37 39 40 41 42 44 46 49 65 67 70 71 72 73 74 **P**1 5 **N** Arizona Voluntary Hospital Federation, Tempe, AZ — Control 23, Service 10, Beds 120, Admissions 9545, Census 80, Outpatient Visits 78235, Births 2749, Total 64800, Payroll 25430, Personnel 839

□ CHARTER BEHAVIORAL HEALTH SYSTEM–EAST VALLEY, 2190 North Grace Boulevard, Zip 85224; tel. 602/899–8989; James Plummer, Chief Executive Officer **A**1 9 10 **F**2 3 15 16 52 53 54 55 56 57 58 59 **S** Magellan Health Services, Atlanta, GA — Control 33, Service 22, Beds 80, Admissions 1444, Census 47, Outpatient Visits 2274, Births 0

CHINLE—Apache County

⊠ CHINLE COMPREHENSIVE HEALTH CARE FACILITY, Highway 191, Zip 86503, Mailing Address: P.O. Drawer PH, Zip 86503; tel. 520/674–5281; Ronald Tso, Chief Executive Officer **A**1 10 **F**3 7 13 14 15 16 17 20 22 25 27 30 34 37 39 40 44 45 46 49 51 54 55 58 61 65 67 68 71 74 **P**6 **S** U. S. Public Health Service Indian Health Service, Rockville, MD — Control 47, Service 10, Beds 60, Admissions 2827, Census 29, Outpatient Visits 129930, Births 593, Personnel 458

CLAYPOOL—Gila County

⊠ COBRE VALLEY COMMUNITY HOSPITAL, One Hospital Drive, Zip 85532, Mailing Address: P.O. Box 3261, Zip 85532–3261; tel. 520/425–3261; John L. Hoopes, Administrator and Chief Executive Officer **A**1 9 10 **F**11 15 16 19 22 28 35 40 44 65 67 71 73 74 **P**3 **S** Brim, Inc., Portland, OR — Control 23, Service 10, Beds 38, Admissions 1977, Census 17, Outpatient Visits 58367, Births 411, Total 14378, Payroll 5519, Personnel 257

COTTONWOOD—Yavapai County

⊠ MARCUS J. LAWRENCE MEDICAL CENTER, 202 South Willard Street, Zip 86326; tel. 520/634–2251; Rita M. Poindexter, President and Chief Operating Officer **A**1 9 10 **F**7 8 12 14 15 16 17 19 21 22 23 28 29 30 32 33 34 35 37 39 40 41 42 44 45 49 51 60 63 65 67 71 73 **P**1 4 5 **N** Northern Arizona Healthcare, Flagstaff, AZ — Control 23, Service 10, Beds 64, Admissions 3731, Census 36, Outpatient Visits 44128, Births 514, Total 28367, Payroll 10971, Personnel 357

DAVIS–MONTHAN AFB—Pima County

⊠ U. S. AIR FORCE HOSPITAL, 4175 South Alamo Avenue, Zip 85707–4405; tel. 520/228–2930; Colonel Stanley F. Uchman, Commander **A**1 **F**15 16 19 22 35 39 41 44 45 46 49 51 53 54 55 56 57 58 71 74 **S** Department of the Air Force, Washington, DC — Control 41, Service 10, Beds 20, Admissions 2269, Census 12, Outpatient Visits 169188, Births 250, Total 39659, Payroll 21135, Personnel 535

DOUGLAS—Cochise County

□ SOUTHEAST ARIZONA MEDICAL CENTER, Route 1, Box 30, Zip 85607; tel. 520/364–7931; Robert C. Benjamin, Chief Executive Officer (Total facility includes 43 beds in nursing home–type unit) **A**1 9 10 **F**1 14 17 19 22 24 26 27 30 31 32 37 40 41 42 44 46 49 64 65 71 — Control 23, Service 10, Beds 75, Admissions 1503, Census 41, Outpatient Visits 56684, Births 365, Total 10887, Payroll 5209, Personnel 210

FLAGSTAFF—Coconino County

ASPEN HILL HOSPITAL See BHC Aspen Hill Hospital

⊠ BHC ASPEN HILL HOSPITAL, (Formerly Aspen Hill Hospital), 305 West Forest Avenue, Zip 86001–1464; tel. 520/773–1060; Alan G. Chapman, Administrator and Chief Executive Officer **A**1 9 10 **F**3 14 15 16 52 53 54 55 56 57 58 59 **P**4 6 **S** Behavioral Healthcare Corporation, Nashville, TN — Control 33, Service 22, Beds 26, Admissions 387, Census 15, Births 0, Total 2430, Payroll 1138, Personnel 56

Hospital, Address, Telephone, Administrator, Approval, Facility, and Physician Codes, Health Care System, Network	Classi-fication Codes		Utilization Data					Expense (thousands) of dollars		
★ American Hospital Association (AHA) membership □ Joint Commission on Accreditation of Healthcare Organizations (JCAHO) accreditation + American Osteopathic Hospital Association (AOHA) membership ○ American Osteopathic Association (AOA) accreditation △ Commission on Accreditation of Rehabilitation Facilities (CARF) accreditation Control codes 61, 63, 64, 71, 72 and 73 indicate hospitals listed by AOHA, but not registered by AHA. For definition of numerical codes, see page A4	Control	Service	Beds	Admissions	Census	Outpatient Visits	Births	Total	Payroll	Personnel

Hospital	Control	Service	Beds	Admissions	Census	Outpatient Visits	Births	Total	Payroll	Personnel
⊠ △ FLAGSTAFF MEDICAL CENTER, 1200 North Beaver Street, Zip 86001; tel. 602/779–3366; Stephen G. Carlson, President and Chief Operating Officer (Total facility includes 18 beds in nursing home–type unit) (Nonreporting) **A**1 7 9 10 **N** Northern Arizona Healthcare, Flagstaff, AZ; Arizona Voluntary Hospital Federation, Tempe, AZ	23	10	128	—	—	—	—	—	—	—
FLORENCE—Pinal County										
□ CENTRAL ARIZONA MEDICAL CENTER, Adamsville Road, Zip 85232, Mailing Address: Box 2080, Zip 85232; tel. 520/868–2003; Darrold Bertsch, Administrator (Total facility includes 27 beds in nursing home–type unit) (Nonreporting) **A**1 9 10	23	10	77	—	—	—	—	—	—	—
FORT DEFIANCE—Apache County										
⊠ U. S. PUBLIC HEALTH SERVICE FORT DEFIANCE INDIAN HEALTH SERVICE HOSPITAL, Mailing Address: P.O. Box 649, Zip 86504; tel. 520/729–3223; Franklin Freeland, Ed.D., Chief Executive Officer **A**1 10 **F**3 7 13 14 15 16 20 22 27 28 30 34 39 40 44 46 49 51 58 60 65 71 72 **P**6 **S** U. S. Public Health Service Indian Health Service, Rockville, MD	47	10	49	1712	16	94835	344	—	—	297
FORT HUACHUCA—Cochise County										
⊠ RAYMOND W. BLISS ARMY COMMUNITY HOSPITAL, Zip 85613–7040; tel. 520/533–2350; Lieutenant Colonel Michael H. Kennedy, Deputy Commander **A**1 **F**3 7 8 12 15 17 18 19 20 24 25 27 28 29 30 34 35 37 39 40 44 45 46 49 51 54 55 56 58 65 73 74 **S** Department of the Army, Office of the Surgeon General, Falls Church, VA	42	10	30	1515	8	192083	0	45801	20040	448
GANADO—Apache County										
□ SAGE MEMORIAL HOSPITAL, Highway 264, Zip 86505, Mailing Address: P.O. Box 457, Zip 86505; tel. 520/755–3411; Liz Johnson, Chief Executive Officer (Nonreporting) **A**1 10	23	10	25	—	—	—	—	—	—	—
GLENDALE—Maricopa County										
⊠ ARROWHEAD COMMUNITY HOSPITAL AND MEDICAL CENTER, 18701 North 67th Avenue, Zip 85308–5722; tel. 602/561–1000; Richard S. Alley, Executive Vice President and Chief Executive Officer **A**1 9 10 **F**3 4 7 8 10 11 12 16 19 21 22 28 29 30 32 33 35 37 38 40 43 44 47 49 62 64 65 67 70 71 73 74 **P**1 5 **S** Baptist Hospitals and Health Systems, Inc., Phoenix, AZ **N** Baptist Hospitals and Health Systems, Phoenix, AZ	23	10	80	4877	44	43282	1508	20401	12651	354
□ CHARTER BEHAVIORAL HEALTH SYSTEM–GLENDALE, 6015 West Peoria Avenue, Zip 85302; tel. 602/878–7878; Kim Hall, Chief Executive Officer **A**1 9 10 **F**2 3 15 16 52 53 54 55 56 57 58 59 **S** Magellan Health Services, Atlanta, GA	33	22	90	2034	65	12604	0	—	—	—
□ △ HEALTHSOUTH VALLEY OF THE SUN REHABILITATION HOSPITAL, 13460 North 67th Avenue, Zip 85304; tel. 602/878–8800; Michael S. Wallace, Administrator and Chief Executive Officer (Total facility includes 18 beds in nursing home–type unit) **A**1 7 10 **F**12 15 16 28 29 34 45 46 48 49 64 65 66 67 73 **S** HEALTHSOUTH Corporation, Birmingham, AL	33	46	42	862	40	—	0	11593	4322	154
SAMARITAN BEHAVIORAL HEALTH CENTER–THUNDERBIRD SAMARITAN CAMPUS See Thunderbird Samaritan Medical Center										
⊠ THUNDERBIRD SAMARITAN MEDICAL CENTER, (Includes Samaritan Behavioral Health Center–Thunderbird Samaritan Campus), 5555 West Thunderbird Road, Zip 85306; tel. 602/588–5555; Robert H. Curry, Senior Vice President and Chief Executive Officer **A**1 9 10 **F**1 3 4 7 8 10 12 14 15 16 17 18 19 21 22 23 25 26 27 28 30 31 32 33 34 35 39 40 41 42 43 44 46 50 51 52 53 54 55 56 57 58 59 60 61 63 65 67 68 69 71 72 73 74 **P**5 7 **S** Samaritan Health System, Phoenix, AZ **N** Samaritan Health Services, Phoenix, AZ	23	10	227	13871	138	75566	4065	93907	34651	1012
⊠ U. S. AIR FORCE HOSPITAL LUKE, Luke AFB, Zip 85309–1525; tel. 602/856–7501; Colonel Robert P. Edwards, Administrator **A**1 **F**7 8 12 13 14 15 16 17 18 19 20 21 22 24 27 29 30 34 37 39 40 44 45 46 49 51 54 58 65 71 73 74 **S** Department of the Air Force, Washington, DC	41	10	23	2873	14	203944	540	25458	—	711
KEAMS CANYON—Navajo County										
⊠ U. S. PUBLIC HEALTH SERVICES INDIAN HOSPITAL, Mailing Address: P.O. Box 98, Zip 86034; tel. 520/738–2211; Taylor Satala, Service Unit Director **A**1 10 **F**2 3 4 5 7 8 9 10 11 12 13 14 15 16 17 19 20 21 22 25 26 27 28 30 31 34 35 37 38 40 43 44 45 47 48 49 50 51 52 53 54 55 56 57 58 59 60 63 64 65 68 71 **S** U. S. Public Health Service Indian Health Service, Rockville, MD	47	10	17	438	3	36107	71	6400	3601	157
KINGMAN—Mohave County										
⊠ KINGMAN REGIONAL MEDICAL CENTER, 3269 Stockton Hill Road, Zip 86401; tel. 520/757–0602; Brian Turney, Chief Executive Officer (Total facility includes 14 beds in nursing home–type unit) **A**1 9 10 **F**7 8 10 14 19 21 22 32 33 34 35 37 39 40 41 42 44 45 46 49 63 64 65 70 71 73 **P**2 5 8 **N** Arizona Voluntary Hospital Federation, Tempe, AZ	23	10	124	6118	76	55324	592	32377	13507	500
LAKE HAVASU CITY—Mohave County										
⊠ HAVASU SAMARITAN REGIONAL HOSPITAL, 101 Civic Center Lane, Zip 86403; tel. 520/855–8185; Kevin P. Poorten, Vice President and Chief Executive Officer (Total facility includes 20 beds in nursing home–type unit) **A**1 9 10 **F**7 8 12 15 16 19 22 31 32 34 37 40 41 42 44 46 49 54 56 58 64 65 71 73 **P**3 5 7 **S** Samaritan Health System, Phoenix, AZ **N** Samaritan Health Services, Phoenix, AZ	23	10	118	4104	53	37373	553	34904	11995	401
MESA—Maricopa County										
⊠ DESERT SAMARITAN MEDICAL CENTER, (Includes Samaritan Behavioral Health Center–Desert Samaritan Medical Center, 2225 West Southern Avenue, Zip 85202; tel. 602/464–4000), 1400 South Dobson Road, Zip 85202–9879; tel. 602/835–3000; Bruce E. Pearson, Vice President and Chief Executive Officer **A**1 2 9 10 **F**1 3 4 5 7 8 10 11 14 15 16 19 21 22 25 29 31 32 33 34 35 39 40 41 42 43 44 49 50 52 53 54 55 58 59 61 63 64 65 69 70 71 73 **P**3 5 7 **S** Samaritan Health System, Phoenix, AZ **N** Samaritan Health Services, Phoenix, AZ	23	10	511	22483	359	79219	5797	164178	56801	1748

Hospital, Address, Telephone, Administrator, Approval, Facility, and Physician Codes, Health Care System, Network	Classi-fication Codes		Utilization Data					Expense (thousands) of dollars		
	Control	Service	Beds	Admissions	Census	Outpatient Visits	Births	Total	Payroll	Personnel

★ American Hospital Association (AHA) membership
□ Joint Commission on Accreditation of Healthcare Organizations (JCAHO) accreditation
+ American Osteopathic Hospital Association (AOHA) membership
○ American Osteopathic Association (AOA) accreditation
△ Commission on Accreditation of Rehabilitation Facilities (CARF) accreditation
Control codes 61, 63, 64, 71, 72 and 73 indicate hospitals listed by AOHA, but not registered by AHA. For definition of numerical codes, see page A4

Hospital	Control	Service	Beds	Admissions	Census	Outpatient Visits	Births	Total	Payroll	Personnel
□ DESERT VISTA BEHAVIORAL HEALTH SERVICES, 570 West Brown Road, Zip 85201; tel. 602/962–3900; Allen S. Nohre, Chief Executive Officer (Total facility includes 19 beds in nursing home–type unit) **A**1 9 10 **F**1 2 3 12 17 18 26 29 30 41 45 52 53 54 55 56 57 58 59 64 65 67 **S** Ramsay Health Care, Inc., Coral Gobles, FL	33	22	119	1371	62	12798	0	7870	3977	192
□ ○ MESA GENERAL HOSPITAL MEDICAL CENTER, 515 North Mesa Drive, Zip 85201; tel. 602/969–9111 (Total facility includes 13 beds in nursing home–type unit) **A**1 9 10 11 12 13 **F**1 3 4 7 8 10 12 14 15 16 19 21 22 25 26 28 30 31 32 33 34 35 37 38 39 40 41 42 43 44 45 48 49 50 53 54 55 56 57 58 59 63 64 65 71 73 74 **P**5 7 8 **S** TENET Healthcare Corporation, Santa Barbara, CA	33	10	125	9337	53	67787	1034	34719	15400	479
⊞ △ MESA LUTHERAN HOSPITAL, 525 West Brown Road, Zip 85201–3299; tel. 602/834–1211; Don Evans, Chief Executive Officer (Total facility includes 60 beds in nursing home–type unit) **A**1 2 7 9 10 **F**4 7 8 10 12 15 16 17 18 19 20 21 22 23 26 27 28 29 30 32 33 34 35 36 37 39 40 41 42 43 44 45 48 49 52 57 59 60 64 65 67 70 71 73 74 **P**5 7 8 **S** Lutheran Health Systems, Fargo, ND **N** Lutheran Healthcare Network, Mesa, AZ	23	10	278	11348	118	61672	2292	85753	36522	1064
SAMARITAN BEHAVIORAL HEALTH CENTER–DESERT SAMARITAN MEDICAL CENTER See Desert Samaritan Medical Center										
⊞ VALLEY LUTHERAN HOSPITAL, 6644 Baywood Avenue, Zip 85206; tel. 602/981–4100; Don Evans, Chief Executive Officer (Nonreporting) **A**1 9 10 **S** Lutheran Health Systems, Fargo, ND **N** Lutheran Healthcare Network, Mesa, AZ	23	10	172	—	—	—	—	—	—	—
NOGALES—Santa Cruz County										
⊞ CARONDOLET HOLY CROSS HOSPITAL, 1171 Target Range Road, Zip 85621; tel. 520/287–2771; Carol Field, Administrator (Total facility includes 49 beds in nursing home–type unit) (Nonreporting) **A**1 9 10 **S** Carondelet Health System, Saint Louis, MO **N** Carondelet Health Network, Inc., Tucson, AZ	21	10	80	—	—	—	—	—	—	—
PAGE—Coconino County										
⊞ PAGE HOSPITAL, North Navajo Drive and Vista Avenue, Zip 86040, Mailing Address: P.O. Box 1447, Zip 86040; tel. 520/645–2424; Preston M. Simmons, Administrator **A**1 9 10 **F**1 7 8 12 15 16 17 19 22 28 30 31 32 34 40 41 42 44 46 49 65 71 73 **P**3 5 7 **S** Samaritan Health System, Phoenix, AZ	23	10	25	529	4	13746	210	5867	2753	86
PARKER—La Paz County										
★ ○ PARKER COMMUNITY HOSPITAL, 1200 Mohave Road, Zip 85344, Mailing Address: Box 1149, Zip 85344; tel. 520/669–9201; William G. Coe, Administrator and Chief Executive Officer (Nonreporting) **A**9 10 11	23	10	39	—	—	—	—	—	—	—
⊞ U. S. PUBLIC HEALTH SERVICE INDIAN HOSPITAL, Mailing Address: Route 1, Box 12, Zip 85344; tel. 520/669–2137; Gary Davis, Service Unit Director (Nonreporting) **A**1 10 **S** U. S. Public Health Service Indian Health Service, Rockville, MD	47	10	18	—	—	—	—	—	—	—
PAYSON—Gila County										
⊞ PAYSON REGIONAL MEDICAL CENTER, 807 South Ponderosa Street, Zip 85541; tel. 520/474–3222; Duane H. Anderson, President and Chief Executive Officer **A**1 9 10 **F**7 8 14 15 16 19 21 22 28 30 32 34 35 37 40 44 46 49 65 66 67 68 70 71 73 **N** Arizona Voluntary Hospital Federation, Tempe, AZ	23	10	34	1671	16	20959	158	14693	6395	251
PHOENIX—Maricopa County										
□ ARIZONA STATE HOSPITAL, 2500 East Van Buren Street, Zip 85008; tel. 602/244–1331; John R. Migliaro, Ph.D., Chief Executive Officer **A**1 10 **F**1 3 4 5 6 7 8 10 12 14 15 16 17 18 19 20 21 22 23 26 27 28 29 30 31 32 33 34 35 37 39 41 42 43 44 45 46 49 50 51 52 53 54 55 56 57 58 59 60 61 62 63 65 66 67 68 69 70 71 72 73 74	12	22	372	477	422	0	0	40478	17512	508
⊞ CARL T. HAYDEN VETERANS AFFAIRS MEDICAL CENTER, 650 East Indian School Road, Zip 85012–1894; tel. 602/277–5551; John R. Fears, Director (Total facility includes 120 beds in nursing home–type unit) **A**1 2 3 5 **F**1 2 3 4 8 9 10 11 12 14 16 17 18 19 20 21 22 23 24 25 26 27 28 30 31 32 34 35 37 39 40 41 42 43 44 46 48 49 50 51 52 54 56 57 58 59 60 63 64 65 67 69 71 72 73 74 **P**6 **S** Department of Veterans Affairs, Washington, DC	45	10	422	10725	322	304013	0	126520	65838	1580
⊞ COLUMBIA MEDICAL CENTER PHOENIX, 1947 East Thomas Road, Zip 85016; tel. 602/650–7600; Denny W. Powell, Chief Executive Officer (Total facility includes 13 beds in nursing home–type unit) (Nonreporting) **A**1 10 **S** Columbia/HCA Healthcare Corporation, Nashville, TN **N** National Cardiovascular Network, Atlanta, GA	33	10	295	—	—	—	—	—	—	—
⊞ COLUMBIA PARADISE VALLEY HOSPITAL, 3929 East Bell Road, Zip 85032; tel. 602/867–1881; Rebecca C. Kuhn, R.N., President and Chief Executive Officer (Nonreporting) **A**1 2 9 10 **S** Columbia/HCA Healthcare Corporation, Nashville, TN	33	10	140	—	—	—	—	—	—	—
□ ○ COMMUNITY HOSPITAL MEDICAL CENTER, 6501 North 19th Avenue, Zip 85015; tel. 602/249–3434; Randall Hempling, Chief Executive Officer (Nonreporting) **A**1 10 11 12 13 **S** TENET Healthcare Corporation, Santa Barbara, CA	33	10	59	—	—	—	—	—	—	—
⊞ △ GOOD SAMARITAN REGIONAL MEDICAL CENTER, 1111 East McDowell Road, Zip 85006, Mailing Address: Box 2989, Zip 85062; tel. 602/239–2000; Steven L. Seiler, Senior Vice President and Chief Executive Officer (Total facility includes 30 beds in nursing home–type unit) **A**1 2 3 5 7 8 9 10 **F**1 3 4 5 7 8 9 10 11 15 16 19 21 22 23 26 29 31 32 33 34 35 37 39 40 41 42 43 44 48 49 50 52 53 54 55 57 58 59 60 61 63 64 65 69 70 71 73 74 **P**3 5 7 **S** Samaritan Health System, Phoenix, AZ **N** Samaritan Health Services, Phoenix, AZ	23	10	714	27669	459	192644	6993	283452	103256	3224

Hospital, Address, Telephone, Administrator, Approval, Facility, and Physician Codes, Health Care System, Network	Control	Service	Beds	Admissions	Census	Outpatient Visits	Births	Total	Payroll	Personnel

Classification Codes / Utilization Data / Expense (thousands) of dollars

★ American Hospital Association (AHA) membership
□ Joint Commission on Accreditation of Healthcare Organizations (JCAHO) accreditation
+ American Osteopathic Hospital Association (AOHA) membership
○ American Osteopathic Association (AOA) accreditation
△ Commission on Accreditation of Rehabilitation Facilities (CARF) accreditation
Control codes 61, 63, 64, 71, 72 and 73 indicate hospitals listed by AOHA, but not registered by AHA. For definition of numerical codes, see page A4

Hospital	Control	Service	Beds	Admissions	Census	Outpatient Visits	Births	Total	Payroll	Personnel
✪ JOHN C. LINCOLN HEALTH NETWORK, (Formerly John C. Lincoln Hospital and Health Center), 250 East Dunlap Avenue, Zip 85020–2446; tel. 602/943–2381; Dan C. Coleman, President and Chief Executive Officer (Total facility includes 22 beds in nursing home–type unit) **A**1 9 10 **F**1 4 7 8 10 11 12 13 15 17 19 20 21 22 24 27 28 29 30 32 33 34 35 37 40 42 43 44 45 49 54 60 62 63 64 65 66 67 68 70 71 73 74 **P**1 5 6	23	10	223	10279	127	96781	930	85495	37941	1444
JOHN C. LINCOLN HOSPITAL AND HEALTH CENTER See John C. Lincoln Health Network										
✪ MARICOPA MEDICAL CENTER, 2601 East Roosevelt Street, Zip 85008, Mailing Address: P.O. Box 5099, Zip 85010; tel. 602/267–5011; Frank D. Alvarez, Chief Executive Officer **A**1 2 3 5 8 9 10 **F**4 7 8 9 11 12 13 14 15 16 17 18 19 20 21 22 23 25 26 27 28 29 30 31 32 33 34 35 37 38 39 40 42 43 44 45 46 47 49 51 52 53 54 55 56 57 58 59 60 61 63 65 69 70 71 72 73 74 **P**1 **S** Quorum Health Group/Quorum Health Resources, Inc., Brentwood, TN **N** Maricopa Integrated Health System, Phoenix, AZ	13	10	481	18461	287	392822	3610	197420	85609	2664
✪ MARYVALE SAMARITAN MEDICAL CENTER, 5102 West Campbell Avenue, Zip 85031; tel. 602/848–5101; Robert H. Curry, Senior Vice President and Chief Executive Officer (Total facility includes 26 beds in nursing home–type unit) **A**1 2 9 10 **F**1 3 4 7 8 10 14 15 16 19 21 22 31 32 33 34 35 40 42 44 45 46 49 50 60 63 64 65 69 70 71 73 **P**3 5 7 **S** Samaritan Health System, Phoenix, AZ **N** Samaritan Health Services, Phoenix, AZ	23	10	213	10452	94	64115	2612	68249	25356	708
✪ PHOENIX BAPTIST HOSPITAL AND MEDICAL CENTER, 6025 North 20th Avenue, Zip 85015; tel. 602/249–0212; Richard S. Alley, Chief Executive Officer (Nonreporting) **A**1 2 3 5 9 10 **S** Baptist Hospitals and Health Systems, Inc., Phoenix, AZ **N** Baptist Hospitals and Health Systems, Phoenix, AZ	23	10	222	—	—	—	—	—	—	—
✪ PHOENIX CHILDREN'S HOSPITAL, 1111 East McDowell Road, Zip 85006, Mailing Address: 1300 North 12th Street, Suite 404, Zip 85006; tel. 602/239–5920; Leland G. Clabots, President and Chief Executive Officer **A**1 3 5 9 **F**10 15 16 17 19 20 21 22 25 27 28 29 30 31 32 34 35 38 39 41 42 43 44 45 46 47 49 50 52 53 54 55 56 58 60 65 67 70 71 73	23	50	205	8139	152	38036	0	84737	32171	598
★ ○ PHOENIX GENERAL HOSPITAL AND MEDICAL CENTER, 19829 North 27th Avenue, Zip 85027–4002; tel. 602/879–6100; H. Douglas Garner, Chief Executive Officer (Total facility includes 23 beds in nursing home–type unit) **A**9 10 11 **F**4 7 8 10 11 12 13 15 17 19 20 21 22 28 29 30 31 33 34 35 37 39 40 41 42 43 44 45 46 48 49 54 56 57 58 64 65 71 73 74 **P**5 8 **S** Quorum Health Group/Quorum Health Resources, Inc., Brentwood, TN	23	10	97	2530	33	—	250	33507	10966	292
✪ PMH HEALTH SERVICES NETWORK, 1201 South Seventh Avenue, Zip 85007–3995; tel. 602/258–5111; Jeffrey Norman, Chief Executive Officer (Total facility includes 28 beds in nursing home–type unit) **A**1 2 10 **F**1 2 3 4 5 6 7 8 9 10 11 12 13 14 15 16 17 18 19 20 21 22 23 24 25 26 27 28 29 30 31 32 33 34 35 36 37 39 40 41 42 43 44 45 46 47 48 49 50 51 52 53 54 55 56 57 58 59 60 61 62 63 65 66 67 68 69 70 71 72 73 74 **P**1 4 5 6 7 8 **S** PMH Health Resources, Inc., Phoenix, AZ **N** Arizona Voluntary Hospital Federation, Tempe, AZ	23	10	211	12712	124	208564	1620	106294	32957	947
★ SAMARITAN–WENDY PAINE O'BRIEN TREATMENT CENTER, 5055 North 34th Street, Zip 85018; tel. 602/955–6200; Mike Todd, Chief Executive Officer (Nonreporting) **A**10 **S** Samaritan Health System, Phoenix, AZ **N** Samaritan Health Services, Phoenix, AZ	23	22	23	—	—	—	—	—	—	—
✪ △ ST. JOSEPH'S HOSPITAL AND MEDICAL CENTER, 350 West Thomas Road, Zip 85013, Mailing Address: Box 2071, Zip 85001–2071; tel. 602/406–3100; Mary G. Yarbrough, President and Chief Executive Officer **A**1 2 3 5 7 8 9 10 **F**1 4 7 8 10 11 12 13 14 15 16 17 18 19 20 21 22 23 24 25 26 27 28 29 30 31 32 33 34 35 37 38 39 40 41 42 43 44 45 46 47 48 49 50 51 52 54 55 58 59 60 61 63 65 66 67 68 69 70 71 73 74 **P**1 6 **S** Catholic Healthcare West, San Francisco, CA **N** Catholic HealthCare West (CHW), San Francisco, CA	21	10	514	24064	339	352230	4643	280297	115705	3201
□ ST. LUKE'S BEHAVIORAL HEALTH CENTER, 1800 East Van Buren, Zip 85006–3742; tel. 602/251–8484; Patrick D. Waugh, Chief Executive Officer **A**1 9 10 **F**1 2 3 7 8 10 12 13 14 15 16 17 19 22 25 26 28 29 30 32 34 35 41 42 44 45 46 49 52 53 54 55 56 57 58 59 60 66 73 74 **N** Saint Lukes Health System, Phoenix, AZ	33	22	86	1936	33	—	0	—	—	121
□ ST. LUKE'S MEDICAL CENTER, 1800 East Van Buren Street, Zip 85006–3742; tel. 602/251–8100; Mary Starmann–Harrison, FACHE, Chief Executive Officer (Total facility includes 55 beds in nursing home–type unit) (Nonreporting) **A**1 9 10 **S** TENET Healthcare Corporation, Santa Barbara, CA **N** Saint Lukes Health System, Phoenix, AZ	33	10	296	—	—	—	—	—	—	—
✪ U. S. PUBLIC HEALTH SERVICE PHOENIX INDIAN MEDICAL CENTER, 4212 North 16th Street, Zip 85016–5389; tel. 602/263–1200; Anna Albert, Chief Executive Officer **A**1 5 10 **F**7 8 10 12 14 15 16 19 20 21 22 34 35 37 40 42 44 45 46 49 51 53 54 56 58 61 65 71 73 74 **P**6 **S** U. S. Public Health Service Indian Health Service, Rockville, MD	44	10	137	5226	76	175422	703	—	—	699
□ VENCOR HOSPITAL–PHOENIX, 40 East Indianola, Zip 85012; tel. 602/280–7000; John L. Harrington, Jr., FACHE, Administrator **A**1 10 **F**12 15 16 19 20 21 22 27 29 31 35 37 39 42 45 46 50 63 65 71 73 **P**7 **S** Vencor, Incorporated, Louisville, KY	33	10	58	467	44	0	0	11600	5579	156
WESTBRIDGE TREATMENT CENTER, 1830 East Roosevelt, Zip 85006; tel. 602/254–0884; Mike Perry, Chief Executive Officer **A**10 **F**52 53 58 59 **P**8 **S** Century Healthcare Corporation, Tulsa, OK	33	52	78	137	93	0	0	8532	4733	116

Hospital, Address, Telephone, Administrator, Approval, Facility, and Physician Codes, Health Care System, Network	Classification Codes		Utilization Data					Expense (thousands) of dollars		
	Control	Service	Beds	Admissions	Census	Outpatient Visits	Births	Total	Payroll	Personnel

★ American Hospital Association (AHA) membership
□ Joint Commission on Accreditation of Healthcare Organizations (JCAHO) accreditation
+ American Osteopathic Hospital Association (AOHA) membership
○ American Osteopathic Association (AOA) accreditation
△ Commission on Accreditation of Rehabilitation Facilities (CARF) accreditation
Control codes 61, 63, 64, 71, 72 and 73 indicate hospitals listed by AOHA, but not registered by AHA. For definition of numerical codes, see page A4.

PRESCOTT—Yavapai County

★ VETERANS AFFAIRS MEDICAL CENTER, 500 Highway 89 North, Zip 86313; tel. 520/445–4860; Patricia A. McKlem, Medical Center Director (Total facility includes 70 beds in nursing home–type unit) **A**1 **F**1 2 6 8 15 16 17 19 22 26 30 31 32 33 35 37 39 42 44 45 46 48 49 51 52 54 56 57 58 60 64 65 67 70 71 72 73 74 **P**6 **S** Department of Veterans Affairs, Washington, DC — 45 10 287 2836 240 77705 0 37351 21534 539

□ YAVAPAI REGIONAL MEDICAL CENTER, 1003 Willow Creek Road, Zip 86301; tel. 520/445–2700; Timothy Barnett, Chief Executive Officer **A**1 9 10 **F**7 8 11 14 15 16 17 19 21 22 24 25 28 30 32 33 34 35 40 41 42 44 46 48 49 56 63 64 65 67 71 73 **P**1 **N** Arizona Voluntary Hospital Federation, Tempe, AZ — 23 10 84 5768 54 54065 788 39785 17673 529

SACATON—Pinal County

★ HUHUKAM MEMORIAL HOSPITAL, Seed Farm Road, Zip 85247–0038, Mailing Address: P.O. Box 38, Zip 85247; tel. 602/562–3321; Viola L. Johnson, Chief Executive Officer (Nonreporting) **A**1 10 **S** U. S. Public Health Service Indian Health Service, Rockville, MD — 47 10 10 — — — — — — — —

SAFFORD—Graham County

★ MOUNT GRAHAM COMMUNITY HOSPITAL, 1600 20th Avenue, Zip 85546; tel. 520/348–4000; Karl E. Johnson, Chief Executive Officer **A**1 9 10 **F**7 8 11 14 15 19 22 24 28 30 32 33 34 35 37 40 41 44 46 49 65 71 73 **P**1 — 16 10 40 2630 20 48104 545 12500 5739 232

SAN CARLOS—Middlesex County

★ U. S. PUBLIC HEALTH SERVICE INDIAN HOSPITAL, Mailing Address: P.O. Box 208, Zip 85550; tel. 520/562–3382; Viola L. Johnson, Service Unit Director (Nonreporting) **A**1 10 **S** U. S. Public Health Service Indian Health Service, Rockville, MD — 47 10 28 — — — — — — — —

SCOTTSDALE—Maricopa County

□ △ HEALTHSOUTH MERIDIAN POINT REHABILITATION HOSPITAL, 11250 North 92nd Street, Zip 85260–6148; tel. 602/860–0671; Warren Kyle West, Administrator and Chief Executive Officer (Nonreporting) **A**1 7 10 **S** HEALTHSOUTH Corporation, Birmingham, AL — 33 46 43 — — — — — — — —

★ SAMARITAN BEHAVIORAL HEALTH CENTER–SCOTTSDALE, 7575 East Earll Drive, Zip 85251–6998; tel. 602/941–7500; Robert F. Meyer, M.D., Chief Executive Officer **A**1 **F**1 2 3 4 5 8 10 11 12 13 14 19 21 22 25 26 28 29 30 31 32 33 34 35 37 38 40 41 42 43 44 45 46 47 48 49 51 52 53 54 55 56 57 58 59 60 61 64 65 66 67 69 70 71 72 73 74 **P**5 7 **S** Samaritan Health System, Phoenix, AZ **N** Samaritan Health Services, Phoenix, AZ — 23 22 60 1914 39 5843 0 7954 4284 117

★ SCOTTSDALE MEMORIAL HOSPITAL–NORTH, 9003 East Shea Boulevard, Zip 85260; tel. 602/860–3000; Thomas J. Sadvary, FACHE, Senior Vice President and Administrator **A**1 2 3 5 9 10 **F**1 2 3 4 5 6 7 8 9 10 11 12 13 14 15 16 17 18 19 20 21 22 23 24 25 26 27 28 29 30 31 32 33 34 35 36 37 38 39 40 41 42 43 44 45 46 47 48 49 51 52 56 60 61 63 64 65 67 68 69 70 71 72 73 74 **P**1 3 7 **S** Scottsdale Memorial Health Systems, Inc., Scottsdale, AZ — 23 10 242 15046 161 56758 2032 117933 41862 1498

★ △ SCOTTSDALE MEMORIAL HOSPITAL–OSBORN, 7400 East Osborn Road, Zip 85251; tel. 602/481–4000; David R. Carpenter, FACHE, Senior Vice President and Administrator (Total facility includes 60 beds in nursing home–type unit) **A**1 2 3 5 7 9 10 **F**1 4 7 8 10 11 12 13 14 15 16 17 19 21 22 24 25 26 27 28 29 30 32 33 34 35 36 37 39 40 41 42 43 44 45 46 48 49 51 54 56 60 61 63 64 65 67 70 71 72 73 **P**1 3 7 **S** Scottsdale Memorial Health Systems, Inc., Scottsdale, AZ — 23 10 258 13817 200 69427 1151 136875 57719 2076

SELLS—Pima County

★ U. S. PUBLIC HEALTH SERVICE INDIAN HOSPITAL, Mailing Address: P.O. Box 548, Zip 85634; tel. 520/383–7251; Darrell Rumley, Service Unit Director (Nonreporting) **A**1 10 **S** U. S. Public Health Service Indian Health Service, Rockville, MD — 47 10 34 — — — — — — — —

SHOW LOW—Navajo County

★ NAVAPACHE REGIONAL MEDICAL CENTER, 2200 Show Low Lake Road, Zip 85901; tel. 520/537–4375; Leigh Cox, Chief Executive Officer **A**1 9 10 **F**7 8 11 12 15 16 17 19 21 22 24 29 30 32 35 39 40 44 45 49 63 65 67 70 71 73 **P**3 **S** Brim, Inc., Portland, OR — 23 10 54 3205 25 33623 678 20471 9689 289

SIERRA VISTA—Cochise County

★ SIERRA VISTA COMMUNITY HOSPITAL, 300 El Camino Real, Zip 85635; tel. 520/458–4641; Dale A. Decker, Chief Executive Officer **A**1 9 10 **F**7 8 19 21 22 25 28 29 30 32 33 34 35 37 40 42 44 49 63 65 71 — 23 10 60 3742 31 — 1105 25627 11644 363

SPRINGERVILLE—Apache County

★ WHITE MOUNTAIN COMMUNITIES HOSPITAL, 118 South Mountain Avenue, Zip 85938, Mailing Address: Box 880, Zip 85938–0471; tel. 520/333–4368; David J. Ross, Administrator (Total facility includes 64 beds in nursing home–type unit) **A**1 9 10 **F**7 8 12 14 15 19 21 22 28 31 34 40 44 48 49 64 70 71 73 **N** Samaritan Health Services, Phoenix, AZ — 23 10 89 1105 67 13585 54 5102 1915 104

SUN CITY—Maricopa County

★ WALTER O. BOSWELL MEMORIAL HOSPITAL, 10401 West Thunderbird Boulevard, Zip 85351, Mailing Address: Box 1690, Zip 85372; tel. 602/977–7211; George Perez, Executive Vice President and Chief Operating Officer (Total facility includes 40 beds in nursing home–type unit) **A**1 2 9 10 **F**1 4 8 10 11 12 15 16 17 19 21 24 27 28 29 30 32 33 34 35 36 39 41 42 43 44 45 48 49 52 54 55 56 57 58 59 64 67 70 71 72 73 **P**1 3 5 **S** Sun Health Corporation, Sun City, AZ **N** Sun Health Corporation, Sun City, AZ — 23 10 297 14058 216 52999 0 100327 35533 1191

Hospital, Address, Telephone, Administrator, Approval, Facility, and Physician Codes, Health Care System, Network	Classi-fication Codes		Utilization Data					Expense (thousands) of dollars		
★ American Hospital Association (AHA) membership □ Joint Commission on Accreditation of Healthcare Organizations (JCAHO) accreditation + American Osteopathic Hospital Association (AOHA) membership ◯ American Osteopathic Association (AOA) accreditation △ Commission on Accreditation of Rehabilitation Facilities (CARF) accreditation Control codes 61, 63, 64, 71, 72 and 73 indicate hospitals listed by AOHA, but not registered by AHA. For definition of numerical codes, see page A4	Control	Service	Beds	Admissions	Census	Outpatient Visits	Births	Total	Payroll	Personnel

SUN CITY WEST—Maricopa County

▣ DEL E. WEBB MEMORIAL HOSPITAL, 14502 West Meeker Boulevard, Zip 85375, Mailing Address: P.O. Box 5169, Zip 85375; tel. 602/214–4000; Thomas C. Dickson, Executive Vice President and Chief Operating Officer (Total facility includes 40 beds in nursing home–type unit) **A**1 9 10 **F**1 3 4 8 10 11 12 15 16 17 19 21 22 26 27 28 29 30 31 32 33 34 35 36 39 41 42 43 44 45 46 48 49 52 54 55 56 57 58 59 60 64 65 67 70 71 73 **P**1 5 **S** Sun Health Corporation, Sun City, AZ **N** Sun Health Corporation, Sun City, AZ	23	10	181	5075	90	39684	0	37688	14126	395

TEMPE—Maricopa County

▣ TEMPE ST. LUKE'S HOSPITAL, 1500 South Mill Avenue, Zip 85281–6699; tel. 602/784–5501; Thomas A. Salerno, Chief Executive Officer **A**1 9 10 12 13 **F**1 2 3 4 5 7 8 9 10 11 12 13 15 17 18 19 20 21 22 23 24 25 26 27 28 29 30 31 32 33 34 35 36 37 38 39 40 41 42 43 44 45 46 47 48 49 50 51 52 53 54 55 56 57 58 59 60 61 63 64 65 66 67 68 69 70 71 72 73 74 **P**2 4 5 6 7 **S** TENET Healthcare Corporation, Santa Barbara, CA **N** Saint Lukes Health System, Phoenix, AZ	33	10	110	3846	32	28817	603	20682	8596	274

TUBA CITY—Coconino County

▣ TUBA CITY INDIAN MEDICAL CENTER, Main Street, Zip 86045–6211, Mailing Address: P.O. Box 600, Zip 86045–6211; tel. 520/283–2827; Susie John, M.D., Chief Executive Officer (Nonreporting) **A**1 10 **S** U. S. Public Health Service Indian Health Service, Rockville, MD	47	10	69	—	—	—	—	—	—	—

TUCSON—Pima County

▣ △ CARONDELET ST. JOSEPH'S HOSPITAL, 350 North Wilmot Road, Zip 85711; tel. 520/296–3211; Sister St. Joan Willert, President and Chief Executive Officer **A**1 7 9 10 **F**3 4 7 8 10 11 12 14 15 16 17 19 21 22 28 29 30 31 32 33 34 35 37 39 40 44 46 48 49 52 53 54 55 56 57 58 59 63 65 67 71 72 73 74 **P**1 2 6 7 **S** Carondelet Health System, Saint Louis, MO **N** Carondelet Health Network, Inc., Tucson, AZ	21	10	287	12257	150	68369	1786	83540	38233	1208
▣ △ CARONDELET ST. MARY'S HOSPITAL, 1601 West St. Mary's Road, Zip 85745–2682; tel. 602/622–5833; Sister St. Joan Willert, President and Chief Executive Officer **A**1 5 7 9 10 **F**4 7 8 9 10 11 12 14 15 16 17 19 21 22 26 28 29 30 31 32 33 34 35 36 37 40 41 42 43 44 46 48 49 52 53 54 55 56 57 58 59 63 65 67 71 72 73 74 **P**1 2 6 7 **S** Carondelet Health System, Saint Louis, MO **N** Carondelet Health Network, Inc., Tucson, AZ	21	10	345	16288	207	69877	619	118407	54863	1744
▣ △ COLUMBIA EL DORADO HOSPITAL, 1400 North Wilmot, Zip 85712, Mailing Address: Box 13070, Zip 85732; tel. 520/886–6361; Rhonda Dean, Chief Executive Officer (Total facility includes 31 beds in nursing home–type unit) **A**1 7 9 10 **F**4 8 10 11 12 15 16 19 22 26 28 32 34 35 36 37 39 41 43 44 48 49 52 57 64 65 70 71 73 **P**2 5 6 7 **S** Columbia/HCA Healthcare Corporation, Nashville, TN	33	10	166	4651	72	—	0	32910	14812	565
□ DESERT HILLS CENTER FOR YOUTH AND FAMILIES, 2797 North Introspect Drive, Zip 85745; tel. 602/622–5437; Boyd Dover, Executive Director **A**1 3 **F**3 12 13 16 34 39 41 52 53 54 55 56 58 59 **P**8	33	52	140	624	94	4396	0	12552	6290	232
□ △ HEALTHSOUTH REHABILITATION INSTITUTE OF TUCSON, 2650 North Wyatt Drive, Zip 85712; tel. 520/325–1300; Joni K. Raneri, Administrator (Nonreporting) **A**1 7 10 **S** HEALTHSOUTH Corporation, Birmingham, AL	33	46	80	—	—	—	—	—	—	—
□ KINO COMMUNITY HOSPITAL, 2800 East Ajo Way, Zip 85713; tel. 520/294–4471; Richard Carmona, M.D., Chief Executive Officer (Total facility includes 20 beds in nursing home–type unit) **A**1 3 5 9 10 **F**3 6 7 8 12 13 17 18 19 20 22 26 28 29 30 31 32 34 36 37 39 40 41 42 44 46 49 51 52 56 61 64 65 71 72 73 74	13	10	114	4690	76	110136	704	49983	20400	790
▣ NORTHWEST HOSPITAL, 6200 North La Cholla Boulevard, Zip 85741; tel. 520/742–9000; Sharon Gregoire, Chief Operating Officer (Total facility includes 16 beds in nursing home–type unit) (Nonreporting) **A**1 2 9 10 **S** Columbia/HCA Healthcare Corporation, Nashville, TN	33	10	152	—	—	—	—	—	—	—
★ PALO VERDE MENTAL HEALTH SERVICES, (Formerly Palo Verde Hospital), 2695 North Craycroft, Zip 85712, Mailing Address: P.O. Box 40030, Zip 85717–0030; tel. 520/324–5438; Rodrigo A. Pascualy, Administrator (Nonreporting) **A**9 **N** Health Partners of Southern Arizona, Tucson, AZ	23	22	62	—	—	—	—	—	—	—
SIERRA TUCSON, (BEHAVIORAL/ ALCH), 16500 North Lago Del Oro Parkway, Zip 85739; tel. 520/624–4000; Terry A. Stephens, Executive Director **F**1 2 3 4 5 6 7 8 10 12 13 14 16 17 18 19 20 21 22 23 24 25 26 27 28 29 30 31 32 33 34 35 36 39 41 42 43 44 45 46 49 50 51 52 53 54 55 56 57 58 59 60 61 62 63 65 66 67 68 69 70 71 72 73 74 **P**1	33	49	70	738	43	0	0	8620	4550	123
□ ◯ TUCSON GENERAL HOSPITAL, 3838 North Campbell Avenue, Zip 85719; tel. 520/318–6300; William C. Behnke, Jr., Chief Executive Officer **A**1 9 10 11 12 13 **F**2 3 7 8 10 12 14 15 16 19 21 22 26 28 29 30 34 35 36 37 40 42 44 46 49 52 57 64 65 71 73 **P**2 5 6 7 8 **S** TENET Healthcare Corporation, Santa Barbara, CA	33	10	80	2969	36	24810	442	20026	9234	313
▣ TUCSON MEDICAL CENTER, 5301 East Grant Road, Zip 85712–2874, Mailing Address: Box 42195, Zip 85733–2195; tel. 520/324–5438; Rodrigo A. Pascualy, Administrator (Total facility includes 50 beds in nursing home–type unit) **A**1 2 3 5 9 10 **F**2 3 4 6 7 8 10 11 12 13 14 15 16 17 18 19 21 22 23 24 25 26 27 28 29 30 31 32 33 34 35 37 38 39 40 41 42 43 44 45 46 47 48 49 51 52 53 54 55 56 57 58 59 60 61 63 64 65 67 70 71 72 73 74 **P**3 4 5 6 8 **N** Health Partners of Southern Arizona, Tucson, AZ	23	10	432	24550	265	133688	3727	156471	64913	2186

Hospital, Address, Telephone, Administrator, Approval, Facility, and Physician Codes, Health Care System, Network	Classi-fication Codes		Utilization Data					Expense (thousands) of dollars		
	Control	Service	Beds	Admissions	Census	Outpatient Visits	Births	Total	Payroll	Personnel

★ American Hospital Association (AHA) membership
□ Joint Commission on Accreditation of Healthcare Organizations (JCAHO) accreditation
+ American Osteopathic Hospital Association (AOHA) membership
○ American Osteopathic Association (AOA) accreditation
△ Commission on Accreditation of Rehabilitation Facilities (CARF) accreditation
  Control codes 61, 63, 64, 71, 72 and 73 indicate hospitals listed by AOHA, but not registered by AHA. For definition of numerical codes, see page A4.

✠ UNIVERSITY MEDICAL CENTER, 1501 North Campbell Avenue, Zip 85724; tel. 602/694-0111; Gregory A. Pivirotto, President and Chief Executive Officer **A**1 2 3 5 8 9 10 **F**4 7 8 10 11 12 14 15 16 17 19 21 22 23 26 28 30 31 32 34 35 36 37 38 39 40 41 42 43 44 46 47 49 50 52 53 54 55 56 57 58 60 61 65 67 69 70 71 73 74 **P**5 **N** Arizona Voluntary Hospital Federation, Tempe, AZ	23	10	322	18102	240	371240	3243	191957	78204	2267
□ VENCOR HOSPITAL–TUCSON, 355 North Wilmot Road, Zip 85711; tel. 520/747-8200; Charles E. Bill, Administrator and Chief Executive Officer (Nonreporting) **A**1	33	49	51	—	—	—	—	—	—	—
✠ VETERANS AFFAIRS MEDICAL CENTER, 3601 South 6th Avenue, Zip 85723; tel. 520/792-1450; Jonathan H. Gardner, Chief Executive Officer (Total facility includes 88 beds in nursing home–type unit) **A**1 3 5 8 **F**2 3 4 5 6 8 10 11 17 19 20 21 23 25 26 27 28 29 30 31 32 33 34 35 37 39 41 42 43 44 45 46 48 49 51 52 54 55 56 57 58 60 63 64 65 66 67 69 71 72 73 74 **P**6 **S** Department of Veterans Affairs, Washington, DC	45	10	288	6820	218	223045	0	106229	53014	1330

WHITERIVER—Navajo County

✠ U. S. PUBLIC HEALTH SERVICE INDIAN HOSPITAL, State Route 73, Box 860, Zip 85941-0860; tel. 520/338-4911; Carla Alchesay-Nachu, Service Unit Director (Nonreporting) **A**1 **S** U. S. Public Health Service Indian Health Service, Rockville, MD	47	10	45	—	—	—	—	—	—	—

WICKENBURG—Maricopa County

✠ WICKENBURG REGIONAL HOSPITAL, 520 Rose Lane, Zip 85390; tel. 520/684-5421; Carol Schmoyer, Administrator (Total facility includes 57 beds in nursing home–type unit) **A**1 9 10 **F**8 14 15 19 22 26 28 29 32 33 34 39 44 49 64 65 68 71 72 73 **P**3	23	10	80	748	58	9112	3	6515	3020	134

WILLCOX—Cochise County

✠ NORTHERN COCHISE COMMUNITY HOSPITAL, 901 West Rex Allen Drive, Zip 85643; tel. 520/384-3541; Chris Cronberg, Chief Executive Officer (Total facility includes 24 beds in nursing home–type unit) **A**1 9 10 **F**7 8 12 15 16 19 22 26 28 33 34 39 44 46 49 51 64 65 71 73 **S** Brim, Inc., Portland, OR	16	10	48	582	34	11192	55	5292	2439	96

WINSLOW—Navajo County

★ WINSLOW MEMORIAL HOSPITAL, 1501 Williamson Avenue, Zip 86047; tel. 520/289-4691; Michael King, Administrator **A**9 10 **F**3 7 8 14 15 16 19 20 22 26 28 30 31 32 33 34 39 40 44 46 65 71 73 74	33	10	34	1196	10	17978	251	7657	3445	138

YUMA—Imperial County

U. S. PUBLIC HEALTH SERVICE INDIAN HOSPITAL See Winterhaven, CA										
✠ YUMA REGIONAL MEDICAL CENTER, 2400 Avenue A, Zip 85364-7170; tel. 520/344-2000; Robert T. Olsen, Chief Executive Officer (Total facility includes 20 beds in nursing home–type unit) **A**1 9 10 **F**4 7 8 10 11 12 15 16 19 20 21 22 23 24 26 28 30 31 32 34 35 37 39 40 41 42 44 56 60 64 65 67 70 71 73 **P**5 8 **N** Arizona Voluntary Hospital Federation, Tempe, AZ	23	10	238	13547	151	79252	2871	76345	32861	919

ARKANSAS

Resident population 2,484 (in thousands)
Resident population in metro areas 45.0%
Birth rate per 1,000 population 14.1
65 years and over 14.5%
Percent of persons without health insurance 17.4%

Hospital, Address, Telephone, Administrator, Approval, Facility, and Physician Codes, Health Care System, Network	Classi-fication Codes		Utilization Data					Expense (thousands) of dollars		
	Control	Service	Beds	Admissions	Census	Outpatient Visits	Births	Total	Payroll	Personnel

★ American Hospital Association (AHA) membership
□ Joint Commission on Accreditation of Healthcare Organizations (JCAHO) accreditation
+ American Osteopathic Hospital Association (AOHA) membership
○ American Osteopathic Association (AOA) accreditation
△ Commission on Accreditation of Rehabilitation Facilities (CARF) accreditation
Control codes 61, 63, 64, 71, 72 and 73 indicate hospitals listed by AOHA, but not registered by AHA. For definition of numerical codes, see page A4

Hospital	Control	Service	Beds	Admissions	Census	Outpatient Visits	Births	Total	Payroll	Personnel
ARKADELPHIA—Clark County										
✠ BAPTIST MEDICAL CENTER ARKADELPHIA, 3050 Twin Rivers Drive, Zip 71923; tel. 501/245–1100; Dan Gathright, Senior Vice President and Administrator **A**1 9 10 **F**7 8 12 15 16 19 21 22 27 30 31 32 33 35 36 37 40 41 42 44 49 65 71 73 **P**1 5 6 7 **S** Baptist Health, Little Rock, AR **N** Arkansas' FirstSource, Little Rock, AR; Baptist Health, Little Rock, AR	23	10	57	1487	15	19587	280	12940	4981	226
ASHDOWN—Little River County										
LITTLE RIVER MEMORIAL HOSPITAL, Fifth and Locke Streets, Zip 71822–0577, Mailing Address: Box 577, Zip 71822; tel. 501/898–5011; Judy Adams, Administrator **A**10 **F**8 11 15 16 19 22 32 44 49 63 71 **P**5 **N** Arkansas' FirstSource, Little Rock, AR	13	10	33	817	10	9450	0	4331	2156	124
BATESVILLE—Independence County										
✠ WHITE RIVER MEDICAL CENTER, 1710 Harrison Street, Zip 72501, Mailing Address: P.O. Box 2197, Zip 72503–2197; tel. 501/793–1200; Gary Bebow, Administrator and Chief Executive Officer **A**1 9 10 **F**7 8 10 11 12 14 15 16 19 22 23 25 28 30 31 32 34 35 37 40 41 42 44 46 49 52 57 64 65 66 71 73 **P**3 8 **N** Arkansas' FirstSource, Little Rock, AR	23	10	146	7935	108	77182	252	41170	16419	727
BENTON—Saline County										
□ RIVENDELL PSYCHIATRIC CENTER, 100 Rivendell Drive, Zip 72015; tel. 501/794–1255; Mark E. Schneider, Chief Executive Officer (Nonreporting) **A**1 9 10 **S** Vendell Heralthcare, Inc., Nashville, TN	33	52	77	—	—	—	—	—	—	—
✠ SALINE MEMORIAL HOSPITAL, 1 Medical Park Drive, Zip 72015; tel. 501/776–6000; Roger D. Feldt, FACHE, President and Chief Executive Officer (Total facility includes 12 beds in nursing home–type unit) **A**1 9 10 **F**7 8 12 19 21 22 32 33 34 35 37 40 44 52 57 64 65 71 73 **P**8 **S** Quorum Health Group/Quorum Health Resources, Inc., Brentwood, TN **N** Arkansas' FirstSource, Little Rock, AR; Arkansas Network, North Little Rock, AR	23	10	141	4324	64	34669	348	27398	11222	490
BENTONVILLE—Benton County										
BATES MEDICAL CENTER See Northwest Medical Center, Springdale										
BERRYVILLE—Carroll County										
★ CARROLL REGIONAL MEDICAL CENTER, 214 Carter Street, Zip 72616, Mailing Address: P.O. Box 387, Zip 72616; tel. 501/423–5230; J. Rudy Darling, President and Chief Executive Officer **A**9 10 **F**7 12 19 28 30 31 32 33 35 37 39 40 41 42 44 45 46 49 51 61 66 67 71 73 **P**3 8 **S** Sisters of Mercy Health System–St. Louis, Saint Louis, MO **N** Arkansas' FirstSource, Little Rock, AR	23	10	39	1932	16	14104	261	10975	5095	201
BLYTHEVILLE—Mississippi County										
✠ BAPTIST MEMORIAL HOSPITAL–BLYTHEVILLE, 1520 North Division Street, Zip 72315, Mailing Address: P.O. Box 108, Zip 72316–0108; tel. 501/762–3300; Randy King, Administrator (Total facility includes 70 beds in nursing home–type unit) **A**1 9 10 **F**8 11 12 13 14 15 16 17 19 21 22 24 28 29 30 31 32 33 35 37 39 40 41 44 45 46 49 52 57 64 65 67 71 73 **P**3 7 **S** Baptist Memorial Health Care Corporation, Memphis, TN **N** Arkansas' FirstSource, Little Rock, AR	21	10	210	3472	112	29423	734	16869	6192	292
BOONEVILLE—Logan County										
★ BOONEVILLE COMMUNITY HOSPITAL, 880 West Main, Zip 72927, Mailing Address: P.O. Box 290, Zip 72927; tel. 501/675–2800; Robert R. Bash, Administrator **A**9 10 **F**8 19 22 28 30 32 34 44 49 65 71 73 **P**1 **N** Arkansas' FirstSource, Little Rock, AR	23	10	26	564	8	17428	0	3194	1471	70
CALICO ROCK—Izard County										
MEDICAL CENTER OF CALICO ROCK, 103 Grasse Street, Zip 72519; tel. 501/297–3726; Terry L. Amstutz, CHE, Chief Executive Officer and Administrator (Nonreporting) **A**10 **N** Arkansas' FirstSource, Little Rock, AR	23	10	26	—	—	—	—	—	—	—
CAMDEN—Ouachita County										
✠ OUACHITA MEDICAL CENTER, 638 California Street, Zip 71701, Mailing Address: Box 797, Zip 71701; tel. 501/836–1000; C. C. McAllister, President and Chief Executive Officer **A**1 5 9 10 **F**1 2 3 7 8 12 15 16 17 19 21 22 26 27 28 30 32 33 34 37 40 42 44 45 46 49 51 52 57 63 65 67 71 73 **P**1 **N** Arkansas' FirstSource, Little Rock, AR; Arkansas Network, North Little Rock, AR	23	10	118	3020	42	21840	394	18013	9045	515
CHEROKEE VILLAGE—Sharp County										
✠ EASTERN OZARKS REGIONAL HEALTH SYSTEM, 122 South Allegheny Drive, Zip 72529; tel. 501/257–4101; Norman Steinig, Administrator (Nonreporting) **A**1 9 10 **N** Arkansas' FirstSource, Little Rock, AR	33	10	40	—	—	—	—	—	—	—
CLARKSVILLE—Johnson County										
★ JOHNSON REGIONAL MEDICAL CENTER, 1100 East Poplar Street, Zip 72830, Mailing Address: P.O. Box 738, Zip 72830–0738; tel. 501/754–5454; Kenneth R. Wood, Administrator **A**10 **F**7 8 14 15 19 20 21 27 28 30 32 35 37 39 40 41 44 45 46 49 53 54 56 61 65 71 73 **P**3 8 **N** Arkansas' FirstSource, Little Rock, AR	23	10	58	2179	24	25677	276	10732	4881	230
CLINTON—Van Buren County										
VAN BUREN COUNTY MEMORIAL HOSPITAL, Highway 65 South, Zip 72031, Mailing Address: Box 206, Zip 72031; tel. 501/745–2401; Alan Finley, Administrator (Total facility includes 120 beds in nursing home–type unit) **A**9 10 **F**8 12 15 16 22 26 27 28 29 30 34 44 45 49 64 65 71 **P**8 **S** United Hospital Corporation, Memphis, TN **N** Arkansas' FirstSource, Little Rock, AR	23	10	144	570	124	10990	2	5421	2638	160

Hospital, Address, Telephone, Administrator, Approval, Facility, and Physician Codes, Health Care System, Network	Classi-fication Codes		Utilization Data					Expense (thousands) of dollars		
	Control	Service	Beds	Admissions	Census	Outpatient Visits	Births	Total	Payroll	Personnel

★ American Hospital Association (AHA) membership
□ Joint Commission on Accreditation of Healthcare Organizations (JCAHO) accreditation
+ American Osteopathic Hospital Association (AOHA) membership
○ American Osteopathic Association (AOA) accreditation
△ Commission on Accreditation of Rehabilitation Facilities (CARF) accreditation
Control codes 61, 63, 64, 71, 72 and 73 indicate hospitals listed by AOHA, but not registered by AHA. For definition of numerical codes, see page A4

CONWAY—Faulkner County

⊞ CONWAY REGIONAL MEDICAL CENTER, 2302 College Avenue, Zip 72032–6297; tel. 501/329–3831; James A. Summersett, III, FACHE, President and Chief Executive Officer **A**1 9 10 **F**7 8 10 11 12 15 19 20 21 22 23 24 28 32 33 34 35 37 40 41 42 44 46 49 52 57 60 64 65 66 67 71 73 **P**3 8 **N** Arkansas' FirstSource, Little Rock, AR	23	10	116	5774	63	53119	1112	46813	17869	666

CROSSETT—Ashley County

★ ASHLEY MEMORIAL HOSPITAL, 400 Main Street, Zip 71635, Mailing Address: Box 400, Zip 71635; tel. 501/364–4111; Ernie Helin, Interim Administrator **A**9 10 **F**8 12 16 19 22 24 32 35 37 44 52 57 65 71	23	10	44	1408	12	18225	6	8213	3964	135

DANVILLE—Yell County

CHAMBERS MEMORIAL HOSPITAL, Highway 10 at Detroit, Zip 72833, Mailing Address: P.O. Box 639, Zip 72833–0639; tel. 501/495–2241; Scott Peek, Administrator **A**10 **F**17 19 22 28 32 40 41 44 49 64 65 71 **N** Arkansas' FirstSource, Little Rock, AR	15	10	36	1068	10	20405	79	6100	2287	115

DARDANELLE—Yell County

DARDANELLE HOSPITAL, 200 North Third Street, Zip 72834, Mailing Address: Box 578, Zip 72834; tel. 501/229–4677; Shawn Cathey, Administrator **A**9 10 **F**8 15 16 19 22 26 28 32 44 49 52 57 65 71 73 74	13	10	44	847	8	11269	0	3639	1296	79

DE QUEEN—Sevier County

★ COLUMBIA DE QUEEN REGIONAL MEDICAL CENTER, 1306 Collin Raye Drive, Zip 71832–2198; tel. 501/584–4111; Charles H. Long, Chief Executive Officer **A**9 10 **F**7 8 12 16 19 20 21 22 23 28 29 30 32 33 34 35 37 38 39 40 44 49 65 69 71 73 74 **P**2 7 **S** Columbia/HCA Healthcare Corporation, Nashville, TN **N** Arkansas' FirstSource, Little Rock, AR	33	10	75	1817	19	50525	234	11813	4116	180

DE WITT—Arkansas County

DEWITT CITY HOSPITAL, Highway 1 and Madison Street, Zip 72042, Mailing Address: Box 32, Zip 72042; tel. 501/946–3571; Joe E. Smith, Administrator and Chief Executive Officer (Total facility includes 54 beds in nursing home–type unit) (Nonreporting) **A**9 10 **N** Arkansas' FirstSource, Little Rock, AR	14	10	88	—	—	—	—	—	—	—

DUMAS—Desha County

★ DELTA MEMORIAL HOSPITAL, 300 East Pickens Street, Zip 71639, Mailing Address: Box 887, Zip 71639–0887; tel. 501/382–4303; Rodney McPherson, Administrator **A**9 10 **F**1 12 15 17 19 22 26 27 28 30 32 34 41 44 49 52 57 59 63 65 71 **P**8 **S** Quorum Health Group/Quorum Health Resources, Inc., Brentwood, TN **N** Arkansas' FirstSource, Little Rock, AR; Arkansas Network, North Little Rock, AR	23	10	35	1429	12	51156	107	7087	3117	149

EL DORADO—Union County

⊞ MEDICAL CENTER OF SOUTH ARKANSAS, (Includes Union Medical Center, 700 West Grove Street, Warner Brown Hospital, 460 West Oak Street, tel. 501/863–2000), 700 West Grove, Zip 71730, Mailing Address: P.O. Box 1998, Zip 71731–1998; tel. 501/864–3200; Luther J. Lewis, Chief Executive Officer **A**1 3 5 10 **F**3 7 8 10 12 14 15 16 17 19 21 22 23 26 28 29 30 31 32 33 34 35 37 38 39 40 41 42 44 45 46 48 49 52 54 55 56 57 58 59 60 63 64 65 66 67 68 71 73 74 **P**3 8 **S** Columbia/HCA Healthcare Corporation, Nashville, TN **N** Arkansas' FirstSource, Little Rock, AR	32	10	195	6420	93	34977	813	33098	13028	637
UNION MEDICAL CENTER See Medical Center of South Arkansas										
WARNER BROWN HOSPITAL See Medical Center of South Arkansas										

EUREKA SPRINGS—Carroll County

★ EUREKA SPRINGS HOSPITAL, 24 Norris Street, Zip 72632; tel. 501/253–7400; Joe Hammond, Administrator **A**9 10 **F**8 14 15 22 28 32 33 34 44 48 49 51 64 65 67 71 73 **P**1 3 5 **N** Arkansas' FirstSource, Little Rock, AR	23	10	16	502	7	5121	0	3024	1699	80

FAYETTEVILLE—Washington County

□ CHARTER BEHAVIORAL HEALTH SYSTEM OF NORTHWEST ARKANSAS, (Formerly Charter Vista Hospital), 4253 Crossover Road, Zip 72702; tel. 501/521–5731; Lucinda DeBruce, Administrator **A**1 9 10 **F**3 14 18 25 34 52 53 54 55 56 57 58 59 65 **S** Magellan Health Services, Atlanta, GA	33	22	49	804	39	1874	0	—	—	68
FAYETTEVILLE CITY HOSPITAL, 221 South School Street, Zip 72701; tel. 501/442–5100; Michael A. McLean, R.N., Administrator (Total facility includes 138 beds in nursing home–type unit) (Nonreporting) **A**5 9	23	10	144	—	—	—	—	—	—	—
□ △ NORTHWEST ARKANSAS REHABILITATION HOSPITAL, 153 Monte Painter Drive, Zip 72703; tel. 501/444–2200; Dennis R. Shelby, Chief Executive Officer **A**1 7 9 10 **F**5 12 15 17 25 27 28 30 34 41 48 49 64 65 66 67 73 **S** Continental Medical Systems, Inc., Mechanicsburg, PA	33	46	60	1066	50	14960	0	12016	5075	168
⊞ VETERANS AFFAIRS MEDICAL CENTER, 1100 North College Avenue, Zip 72703–6995; tel. 501/443–4301; Richard F. Robinson, Director **A**1 5 9 **F**3 12 15 16 19 20 26 27 29 30 32 34 37 44 45 46 49 51 52 56 58 60 64 65 71 72 73 74 **S** Department of Veterans Affairs, Washington, DC	45	10	94	2992	57	91475	0	36581	19514	469
⊞ WASHINGTON REGIONAL MEDICAL CENTER, 1125 North College Avenue, Zip 72703; tel. 501/442–1000; Patrick D. Flynn, President and Chief Executive Officer (Total facility includes 12 beds in nursing home–type unit) **A**1 2 3 5 9 10 **F**4 6 7 8 10 11 12 13 14 15 16 17 19 20 21 22 23 24 26 27 28 29 30 31 32 33 35 37 39 40 41 42 43 44 49 52 57 63 64 65 67 71 73 74 **P**4 8 **N** Arkansas' FirstSource, Little Rock, AR	23	10	203	10662	122	114559	2014	81254	35147	1156

FORDYCE—Dallas County

DALLAS COUNTY HOSPITAL, 201 Clifton Street, Zip 71742; tel. 501/352–3155; Greg R. McNeil, Administrator **A**9 10 **F**8 19 22 27 32 49 65 71 **S** Healthcorp of Tennessee, Inc., Chattanooga, TN	33	10	32	1060	12	—	0	9556	4358	250

Hospital, Address, Telephone, Administrator, Approval, Facility, and Physician Codes, Health Care System, Network	Classi- fication Codes		Utilization Data					Expense (thousands) of dollars		
★ American Hospital Association (AHA) membership □ Joint Commission on Accreditation of Healthcare Organizations (JCAHO) accreditation + American Osteopathic Hospital Association (AOHA) membership ○ American Osteopathic Association (AOA) accreditation △ Commission on Accreditation of Rehabilitation Facilities (CARF) accreditation Control codes 61, 63, 64, 71, 72 and 73 indicate hospitals listed by AOHA, but not registered by AHA. For definition of numerical codes, see page A4	Control	Service	Beds	Admissions	Census	Outpatient Visits	Births	Total	Payroll	Personnel

FORREST CITY—St. Francis County

⊞ BAPTIST MEMORIAL HOSPITAL–FORREST CITY, 1601 Newcastle Road, Zip 72335, Mailing Address: P.O. Box 667, Zip 72336–0667; tel. 501/633–2020; George S. Fray, Administrator **A**1 9 10 **F**7 8 15 16 17 19 21 22 26 30 32 33 35 38 40 44 46 49 52 55 57 65 69 71 73 **S** Baptist Memorial Health Care Corporation, Memphis, TN **N** Arkansas' FirstSource, Little Rock, AR	23	10	86	2177	31	31057	542	12665	4367	241

FORT SMITH—Sebastian County

HARBOR VIEW MERCY HOSPITAL, 10301 Mayo Road, Zip 72903, Mailing Address: P.O. Box 17000, Zip 72917–7000; tel. 501/484–5550; Sister Judith Marie Keith, President and Chief Executive Officer **A**10 **F**2 3 15 16 19 22 26 32 34 35 52 53 54 55 56 57 58 59 65 67 71 73 **P**1 **S** Sisters of Mercy Health System–St. Louis, Saint Louis, MO **N** Saint Edward Mercy Medical Center, Fort Smith, AR; Arkansas' FirstSource, Little Rock, AR	21	22	80	1077	44	25545	0	—	—	113
□ HEALTHSOUTH REHABILITATION HOSPITAL OF FORT SMITH, 1401 South J Street, Zip 72901; tel. 501/785–3300; Claudia A. Eisenmann, Director Operations (Nonreporting) **A**1 10 **S** HEALTHSOUTH Corporation, Birmingham, AL	33	46	80	—	—	—	—	—	—	—
⊞ SPARKS REGIONAL MEDICAL CENTER, 1311 South I Street, Zip 72901–4995, Mailing Address: P.O. Box 17006, Zip 72917–7006; tel. 501/441–4000; Charles R. Shuffield, President **A**1 2 3 5 9 10 **F**3 4 7 8 10 11 12 16 17 19 21 22 23 24 25 26 27 28 29 30 31 32 34 35 37 38 39 40 42 43 44 45 47 48 49 52 53 55 56 57 58 63 64 65 67 71 73 **P**1	23	10	439	17035	291	86197	1906	99411	41058	1529
⊞ ST. EDWARD MERCY MEDICAL CENTER, 7301 Rogers Avenue, Zip 72903, Mailing Address: P.O. Box 17000, Zip 72917–7000; tel. 501/484–6000; Sister Judith Marie Keith, President and Chief Executive Officer **A**1 2 5 9 10 **F**1 3 4 7 8 10 14 15 16 19 20 21 22 24 25 26 29 31 32 33 34 35 37 40 41 42 43 44 49 52 53 54 55 56 57 58 59 60 63 64 65 67 69 71 72 73 **P**6 8 **S** Sisters of Mercy Health System–St. Louis, Saint Louis, MO **N** Saint Edward Mercy Medical Center, Fort Smith, AR; Arkansas' FirstSource, Little Rock, AR	21	10	260	13118	202	89582	1520	80997	32587	1179

GRAVETTE—Benton County

GRAVETTE MEDICAL CENTER HOSPITAL, 1101 Jackson Street S.W., Zip 72736–0470, Mailing Address: P.O. Box 470, Zip 72736–0470; tel. 501/787–5291; John F. Phillips, Administrator **A**9 10 **F**8 11 14 17 19 21 22 28 34 40 44 46 65 71 73 **N** Arkansas' FirstSource, Little Rock, AR	23	10	58	2003	22	—	387	6508	3602	177

HARRISON—Boone County

★ NORTH ARKANSAS MEDICAL CENTER, 620 North Willow Street, Zip 72601; tel. 501/365–2000; Brian L. Clemens, Chief Executive Officer (Total facility includes 14 beds in nursing home–type unit) **A**9 10 **F**7 8 10 12 14 15 16 17 19 21 22 23 28 30 32 33 34 35 41 42 44 45 46 49 60 64 65 67 71 73 74 **N** Arkansas' FirstSource, Little Rock, AR	13	10	125	4749	54	242882	452	27473	13584	582

HEBER SPRINGS—Cleburne County

⊞ BAPTIST MEDICAL CENTER HEBER SPRINGS, (Formerly Cleburne Memorial Hospital), Highway 110 West, Zip 72543–1087, Mailing Address: P.O. Box 1087, Zip 72543–1087; tel. 501/362–3121; Harrell E. Clendenin, Vice President and Administrator **A**1 9 10 **F**8 14 15 16 19 22 28 30 32 34 44 71 **S** Baptist Health, Little Rock, AR **N** Arkansas' FirstSource, Little Rock, AR	23	10	22	425	5	12397	0	4986	2377	99

HELENA—Phillips County

⊞ HELENA REGIONAL MEDICAL CENTER, 155 Newman Drive, Zip 72342, Mailing Address: Box 788, Zip 72342–0788; tel. 501/338–5800; Steve Reeder, Chief Executive Officer **A**1 10 **F**7 19 21 22 27 28 32 37 40 41 44 48 49 54 56 61 65 67 71 73 **P**1 **S** Quorum Health Group/Quorum Health Resources, Inc., Brentwood, TN **N** Arkansas' FirstSource, Little Rock, AR	23	10	125	3210	43	28344	600	17419	8003	322

HOPE—Hempstead County

⊞ MEDICAL PARK HOSPITAL, 2001 South Main Street, Zip 71801; tel. 501/777–2323; Jimmy Leopard, Chief Executive Officer **A**1 9 10 **F**8 12 14 15 16 19 22 26 27 28 30 32 34 35 37 38 39 40 44 46 49 52 57 61 65 67 71 73 74 **P**7 8 **S** Columbia/HCA Healthcare Corporation, Nashville, TN **N** Arkansas' FirstSource, Little Rock, AR	33	10	75	3237	42	145854	300	27785	10945	328

HOT SPRINGS—Garland County

□ NATIONAL PARK MEDICAL CENTER, 1910 Malvern Avenue, Zip 71901; tel. 501/321–1000; Jerry D. Mabry, Executive Director **A**1 9 10 **F**4 7 8 10 12 16 19 21 22 23 27 28 29 32 34 35 37 39 40 42 43 44 46 48 49 52 55 56 57 59 63 64 65 71 73 74 **P**1 2 4 5 6 7 8 **S** TENET Healthcare Corporation, Santa Barbara, CA	33	10	166	5868	108	147820	583	42832	14972	812
⊞ ST. JOSEPH'S REGIONAL HEALTH CENTER, 300 Werner Street, Zip 71913; tel. 501/622–1000; Randall J. Fale, President and Chief Executive Officer (Total facility includes 48 beds in nursing home–type unit) **A**1 2 9 10 **F**4 7 8 10 11 12 15 16 17 19 21 26 27 28 29 30 32 34 35 36 37 39 40 42 43 44 46 48 49 51 60 64 65 66 67 70 71 73 74 **P**7 **S** Sisters of Mercy Health System–St. Louis, Saint Louis, MO **N** Arkansas' FirstSource, Little Rock, AR	21	10	274	11832	198	204945	835	95490	36813	1377

HOT SPRINGS NATIONAL PARK—Garland County

⊞ LEVI HOSPITAL, 300 Prospect Avenue, Zip 71901, Mailing Address: P.O. Box 850, Zip 71902; tel. 501/624–1281; Patrick McCabe, Jr., Executive Director **A**1 10 **F**5 15 16 19 21 26 27 28 29 32 33 34 35 48 49 52 54 56 57 58 59 65 67 71 **P**3	23	46	25	284	6	—	0	5210	3188	140

JACKSONVILLE—Pulaski County

⊞ △ REBSAMEN REGIONAL MEDICAL CENTER, 1400 West Braden Street, Zip 72076; tel. 501/985–7000; Thomas R. Siemers, Chief Executive Officer **A**1 7 9 10 **F**7 8 10 11 12 17 19 21 22 26 28 30 32 34 35 37 39 40 42 48 49 51 52 57 65 66 67 71 73 74 **P**7 8 **S** Quorum Health Group/Quorum Health Resources, Inc., Brentwood, TN **N** Arkansas' FirstSource, Little Rock, AR; Arkansas Network, North Little Rock, AR	23	10	113	3667	54	42611	384	26518	11000	474

Hospital, Address, Telephone, Administrator, Approval, Facility, and Physician Codes, Health Care System, Network	Classification Codes		Utilization Data					Expense (thousands) of dollars		
	Control	Service	Beds	Admissions	Census	Outpatient Visits	Births	Total	Payroll	Personnel

★ American Hospital Association (AHA) membership
□ Joint Commission on Accreditation of Healthcare Organizations (JCAHO) accreditation
+ American Osteopathic Hospital Association (AOHA) membership
○ American Osteopathic Association (AOA) accreditation
△ Commission on Accreditation of Rehabilitation Facilities (CARF) accreditation
Control codes 61, 63, 64, 71, 72 and 73 indicate hospitals listed by AOHA, but not registered by AHA. For definition of numerical codes, see page A4

Hospital	Control	Service	Beds	Admissions	Census	Outpatient Visits	Births	Total	Payroll	Personnel
⊠ U. S. AIR FORCE HOSPITAL LITTLE ROCK, Little Rock AFB, Zip 72099–5057; tel. 501/988–7411; Colonel Norman L. Sims, MSC, USAF, Commander A1 9 F13 14 15 16 20 24 30 39 51 58 61 S Department of the Air Force, Washington, DC	41	10	12	599	5	120000	0	—	—	348

JONESBORO—Craighead County

Hospital	Control	Service	Beds	Admissions	Census	Outpatient Visits	Births	Total	Payroll	Personnel
□ GREENLEAF CENTER, 2712 East Johnson, Zip 72401; tel. 501/932–2800; John S. Hart, Administrator A1 10 F1 2 3 4 5 6 7 8 9 10 11 12 13 14 15 16 17 18 19 20 21 22 23 24 25 26 27 28 29 30 31 32 33 34 35 36 37 38 39 40 41 42 43 44 45 46 47 48 49 50 51 52 53 54 55 56 57 58 59 60 61 62 63 64 65 66 67 68 69 70 71 72 73 74 S Greenleaf Health Systems, Inc., Chattanooga, TN N Arkansas' FirstSource, Little Rock, AR	33	22	40	1018	39	5327	0	5723	3654	116
⊠ METHODIST HOSPITAL OF JONESBORO, 3024 Stadium Boulevard, Zip 72401; tel. 501/972–7000; Philip H. Walkley, Jr., Chief Executive Officer A1 5 9 10 F2 4 7 8 10 11 12 17 19 20 21 22 23 26 28 29 30 31 32 33 34 35 37 38 39 40 41 42 43 44 45 46 47 48 49 53 54 56 58 59 63 65 66 67 69 71 73 74 P8 S TENET Healthcare Corporation, Santa Barbara, CA	33	10	104	3865	42	110877	942	22445	9378	380
⊠ △ NORTHEAST ARKANSAS REHABILITATION HOSPITAL, 1201 Fleming Avenue, Zip 72401, Mailing Address: P.O. Box 1680, Zip 72403–1680; tel. 501/932–0440; Wayne E. Sensor, Chief Executive Officer A1 7 9 10 F12 15 16 17 19 25 27 28 30 34 48 49 65 66 67 71 P8 N Arkansas' FirstSource, Little Rock, AR	33	46	60	878	57	13830	0	11826	6101	178
⊠ ST. BERNARDS REGIONAL MEDICAL CENTER, 224 East Matthews Street, Zip 72401, Mailing Address: P.O. Box 9320, Zip 72403–9320; tel. 501/972–4100; Ben E. Owens, President A1 2 3 5 9 10 F4 7 8 10 11 12 13 14 15 19 20 21 22 23 28 30 31 32 33 34 35 37 39 40 41 42 43 44 45 46 49 60 64 65 66 67 71 73 74 P2 3 7 8 N Arkansas' FirstSource, Little Rock, AR	21	10	319	16553	227	58251	1427	102520	33265	1109

LAKE VILLAGE—Chicot County

Hospital	Control	Service	Beds	Admissions	Census	Outpatient Visits	Births	Total	Payroll	Personnel
★ CHICOT COUNTY MEMORIAL HOSPITAL, 2729 Highway 65 and 82 South, Zip 71653–0000, Mailing Address: Box 512, Zip 71653–0441; tel. 501/265–5351; Robert R. Reddish, Administrator and Chief Executive Officer A9 10 F8 11 14 19 22 28 30 32 33 34 37 40 44 45 53 56 57 65 67 71 73 P3 S Quorum Health Group/Quorum Health Resources, Inc., Brentwood, TN N Arkansas' FirstSource, Little Rock, AR; Arkansas Network, North Little Rock, AR	13	10	35	2206	23	49701	197	8308	4349	204

LITTLE ROCK—Pulaski County

Hospital	Control	Service	Beds	Admissions	Census	Outpatient Visits	Births	Total	Payroll	Personnel
⊠ △ ARKANSAS CHILDREN'S HOSPITAL, 800 Marshall Street, Zip 72202–3591; tel. 501/320–8000; Jonathan R. Bates, M.D., President and Chief Executive Officer A1 3 5 7 8 9 10 F3 4 5 9 10 11 12 13 15 16 17 19 20 22 23 27 28 30 31 34 35 38 39 42 43 44 46 47 48 49 51 52 53 54 56 58 59 60 63 65 66 67 69 71 73 P7 8 N Arkansas' FirstSource, Little Rock, AR	23	50	266	9506	192	260379	0	154392	70795	2332
⊠ ARKANSAS STATE HOSPITAL, 4313 West Markham Street, Zip 72205–4096; tel. 501/686–9000; Glenn R. Sago, Administrator (Nonreporting) A1 3 5 9 10	12	22	206	—	—	—	—	—	—	—
⊠ BAPTIST MEDICAL CENTER, 9601 Interstate 630, Exit 7, Zip 72205–7299; tel. 501/202–2000; Steven B. Lampkin, Senior Vice President and Administrator A1 3 5 6 9 10 F2 3 4 6 7 8 10 11 12 13 15 16 17 18 19 20 21 22 23 24 25 26 27 28 29 30 31 32 33 34 35 37 38 39 40 41 42 43 44 45 46 48 49 52 53 54 55 56 57 59 60 61 62 63 64 65 66 67 68 69 70 71 72 73 74 P1 3 5 6 7 S Baptist Health, Little Rock, AR N Arkansas' FirstSource, Little Rock, AR; Baptist Health, Little Rock, AR	23	10	635	26770	436	261852	2089	231654	84450	2611
⊠ △ BAPTIST REHABILITATION INSTITUTE OF ARKANSAS, 9601 Interstate 630, Exit 7, Zip 72205–7249; tel. 501/202–7000; Steven Douglas Weeks, Vice President and Administrator A1 3 5 7 9 10 F2 3 4 6 7 8 10 11 12 13 15 16 17 18 19 20 21 22 23 24 25 27 28 29 30 31 32 33 34 35 36 37 38 39 40 41 42 43 44 45 46 48 49 51 52 53 54 55 56 57 58 59 60 62 63 64 65 66 67 68 69 70 71 72 73 74 P1 3 5 6 7 S Baptist Health, Little Rock, AR N Arkansas' FirstSource, Little Rock, AR; Baptist Health, Little Rock, AR	23	46	100	1600	69	29448	0	16770	8104	218
□ BHC PINNACLE POINTE HOSPITAL, (Formerly CPC Pinnacle Pointe Hospital), 11501 Financial Center Parkway, Zip 72211–3715; tel. 501/223–3322; Joseph Fischer, Chief Executive Officer A1 9 10 F3 12 14 15 16 52 53 54 55 56 57 58 59 65 67 S Behavioral Healthcare Corporation, Nashville, TN	33	22	98	1038	74	0	0	7686	4419	115
⊠ COLUMBIA DOCTORS HOSPITAL, 6101 West Capitol, Zip 72205–5331; tel. 501/661–4000; Maura Walsh, President and Chief Executive Officer A1 9 10 F4 7 8 10 11 12 14 15 16 19 21 22 29 34 37 38 40 41 42 43 44 45 46 48 51 52 57 58 59 63 64 65 71 73 74 P6 7 S Columbia/HCA Healthcare Corporation, Nashville, TN	33	10	308	7688	99	27621	2612	—	—	579
CPC PINNACLE POINTE HOSPITAL See BHC Pinnacle Pointe Hospital										
⊠ SOUTHWEST HOSPITAL, 11401 Interstate 30, Zip 72209; tel. 501/455–7100; Timothy E. Hill, President and Chief Executive Officer A1 9 10 F8 10 15 16 19 21 22 26 27 30 35 41 44 49 51 52 57 64 65 71 73 74 P6 S Quorum Health Group/Quorum Health Resources, Inc., Brentwood, TN	23	10	125	1936	38	11990	0	21686	7310	256
⊠ ST. VINCENT INFIRMARY MEDICAL CENTER, Two St. Vincent Circle, Zip 72205–5499; tel. 501/660–3000; Diana T. Hueter, President and Chief Executive Officer (Total facility includes 52 beds in nursing home–type unit) A1 2 3 5 9 10 F1 2 3 4 7 8 10 11 12 13 14 15 16 17 19 20 21 22 23 26 27 28 29 30 31 32 33 34 35 36 37 38 39 40 41 42 43 44 45 46 47 49 50 52 54 55 56 57 58 59 63 64 65 66 70 71 73 74 P2 4 7 8 S Sisters of Charity of Nazareth Health System, Nazareth, KY N National Cardiovascular Network, Atlanta, GA; Arkansas Network, North Little Rock, AR	21	10	570	19709	348	149729	826	185271	77797	2245

Hospital, Address, Telephone, Administrator, Approval, Facility, and Physician Codes, Health Care System, Network	Classi-fication Codes		Utilization Data					Expense (thousands) of dollars		
★ American Hospital Association (AHA) membership ☐ Joint Commission on Accreditation of Healthcare Organizations (JCAHO) accreditation + American Osteopathic Hospital Association (AOHA) membership ○ American Osteopathic Association (AOA) accreditation △ Commission on Accreditation of Rehabilitation Facilities (CARF) accreditation Control codes 61, 63, 64, 71, 72 and 73 indicate hospitals listed by AOHA, but not registered by AHA. For definition of numerical codes, see page A4	Control	Service	Beds	Admissions	Census	Outpatient Visits	Births	Total	Payroll	Personnel

⊠ UNIVERSITY HOSPITAL OF ARKANSAS, 4301 West Markham Street, Zip 72205; tel. 501/686–7000; Richard Pierson, Executive Director, Clinical Programs **A**1 2 3 5 8 9 10 **F**4 5 7 8 10 11 12 16 19 20 21 22 26 27 28 30 31 32 34 35 37 38 39 40 41 42 43 44 45 46 49 51 61 63 65 66 69 70 71 72 73 74	12	10	291	12088	220	230974	2010	161142	64502	2244
⊠ VETERANS AFFAIRS MEDICAL CENTER, (Includes North Little Rock Division, North Little Rock), 4300 West Seventh Street, Zip 72205–5484; tel. 501/661–1202; George H. Gray, Jr., Director (Total facility includes 176 beds in nursing home–type unit) **A**1 2 3 5 8 9 **F**1 2 3 4 5 6 8 10 11 12 17 19 20 21 22 24 26 28 30 31 32 33 34 37 39 41 42 43 44 45 46 48 49 50 51 52 54 55 56 57 58 59 63 64 65 67 71 73 74 **P**6 **S** Department of Veterans Affairs, Washington, DC	45	10	830	13949	613	317556	0	207247	108279	3025
MAGNOLIA—Columbia County										
⊠ MAGNOLIA HOSPITAL, 101 Hospital Drive, Zip 71753–2416, Mailing Address: Box 629, Zip 71753–0629; tel. 501/235–3000; William D. Hedden, Administrator **A**1 10 **F**19 22 32 34 37 39 40 44 45 65 71 73 **S** Sisters of Charity of the Incarnate Word Healthcare System, Houston, TX **N** Arkansas' FirstSource, Little Rock, AR	14	10	65	1930	30	26205	201	11320	5866	282
MALVERN—Hot Spring County										
★ H.S.C. MEDICAL CENTER, 1001 Schneider Drive, Zip 72104; tel. 501/337–4911; Jeff Curtis, President and Chief Executive Officer **A**10 **F**7 8 11 14 15 19 21 22 24 28 32 37 40 44 51 52 54 56 57 71 73 **P**8 **N** Arkansas' FirstSource, Little Rock, AR	23	10	77	2790	39	22776	130	12442	7606	379
MAUMELLE—Pulaski County										
☐ CHARTER BEHAVIORAL HEALTH SYSTEM OF LITTLE ROCK, 1601 Murphy Drive, Zip 72113; tel. 501/851–8700; Rose K. Gantner, Chief Executive Officer **A**1 9 10 **F**1 2 3 12 14 15 16 17 18 52 53 54 55 56 57 58 59 **P**5 **S** Magellan Health Services, Atlanta, GA	33	22	60	967	35	851	0	5088	2329	71
MCGEHEE—Desha County										
MCGEHEE–DESHA COUNTY HOSPITAL, 900 South Third, Zip 71654–0351, Mailing Address: Box 351, Zip 71654–0351; tel. 501/222–5600; William A. Conway, Administrator (Nonreporting) **A**10 **N** Arkansas' FirstSource, Little Rock, AR	13	10	34	—	—	—	—	—	—	—
MENA—Polk County										
MENA MEDICAL CENTER, 311 North Morrow Street, Zip 71953; tel. 501/394–6100; Albert Pilkington, III, Administrator and Chief Executive Officer **A**10 **F**7 8 11 14 15 16 19 22 32 33 34 35 40 41 44 52 57 64 71 **P**8 **S** Quorum Health Group/Quorum Health Resources, Inc., Brentwood, TN **N** Arkansas' FirstSource, Little Rock, AR; Arkansas Network, North Little Rock, AR	14	10	42	1647	19	59704	252	9813	4817	220
MONTICELLO—Drew County										
★ DREW MEMORIAL HOSPITAL, 778 Scogin Drive, Zip 71655–5728; tel. 501/367–2411; Darren Caldwell, Chief Executive Officer **A**9 10 **F**8 12 14 15 16 19 21 22 28 30 32 34 35 37 39 40 41 42 44 45 46 49 65 71 **P**1 **N** Arkansas' FirstSource, Little Rock, AR	13	10	50	3187	30	17709	327	9593	4269	185
MORRILTON—Conway County										
★ CONWAY COUNTY HOSPITAL, 4 Hospital Drive, Zip 72110–4510; tel. 501/354–3512; Johnson L. Smith, Chief Executive Officer and Administrator **A**9 10 **F**1 7 8 11 12 16 17 19 21 22 26 32 33 35 37 40 41 44 46 49 52 56 57 64 65 66 67 71 73 **P**8 **N** Arkansas' FirstSource, Little Rock, AR	21	10	69	1713	29	18011	97	10535	5039	237
MOUNTAIN HOME—Baxter County										
⊠ BAXTER COUNTY REGIONAL HOSPITAL, 624 Hospital Drive, Zip 72653; tel. 501/424–1000; H. William Anderson, Administrator (Total facility includes 35 beds in nursing home–type unit) **A**1 2 5 9 10 **F**7 8 10 11 12 15 16 19 20 21 22 23 27 28 30 32 33 34 35 37 38 39 40 41 42 44 45 46 48 49 60 64 65 66 67 71 73 74 **P**3 8 **N** Arkansas' FirstSource, Little Rock, AR	23	10	194	9138	123	62389	700	52316	23864	952
MOUNTAIN VIEW—Stone County										
STONE COUNTY MEDICAL CENTER, Highway 14 East, Zip 72560–0510, Mailing Address: P.O. Box 510, Zip 72560; tel. 501/269–4361; Stanley Townsend, Administrator (Nonreporting) **A**5 9 10 **N** Arkansas' FirstSource, Little Rock, AR	33	10	48	—	—	—	—	—	—	—
MURFREESBORO—Pike County										
PIKE COUNTY MEMORIAL HOSPITAL, 315 East 13th Street, Zip 71958; tel. 501/285–3182; Rosemary Fritts, Administrator **A**9 10 **F**19 22 32 34 71 **P**5 **N** Arkansas' FirstSource, Little Rock, AR	13	10	32	454	5	6496	0	1530	841	51
NASHVILLE—Howard County										
★ HOWARD MEMORIAL HOSPITAL, 800 West Leslie Street, Zip 71852–0381, Mailing Address: Box 381, Zip 71852–0381; tel. 501/845–4400; Lynn Crowell, Chief Executive Officer **A**10 **F**8 14 15 16 19 21 22 26 28 29 30 32 37 44 46 49 52 57 64 67 71 **P**3 8 **S** Quorum Health Group/Quorum Health Resources, Inc., Brentwood, TN **N** Arkansas' FirstSource, Little Rock, AR; Arkansas Network, North Little Rock, AR	23	10	50	1098	16	40976	0	8308	3676	183
NEWPORT—Jackson County										
☐ HARRIS HOSPITAL, 1205 McLain Street, Zip 72112; tel. 501/523–8911; Timothy E. Schmidt, Interim Chief Executive Officer **A**1 10 **F**7 8 10 11 12 14 15 16 17 19 20 21 22 26 28 30 32 33 35 39 40 41 42 44 46 49 52 57 61 65 71 73 74 **P**1 **S** Community Health Systems, Inc., Brentwood, TN **N** Arkansas' FirstSource, Little Rock, AR	33	10	88	3261	44	18932	505	11758	5153	222
★ NEWPORT HOSPITAL AND CLINIC, 2000 McLain, Zip 72112; tel. 501/523–6721; Eugene Zuber, Administrator **A**9 10 **F**8 10 11 17 19 21 22 28 30 31 32 34 40 42 44 71 73 **N** Arkansas' FirstSource, Little Rock, AR	33	10	86	2974	37	15921	161	9842	4289	201

Hospital, Address, Telephone, Administrator, Approval, Facility, and Physician Codes, Health Care System, Network	Classi-fication Codes		Utilization Data					Expense (thousands) of dollars		
★ American Hospital Association (AHA) membership □ Joint Commission on Accreditation of Healthcare Organizations (JCAHO) accreditation + American Osteopathic Hospital Association (AOHA) membership ○ American Osteopathic Association (AOA) accreditation △ Commission on Accreditation of Rehabilitation Facilities (CARF) accreditation Control codes 61, 63, 64, 71, 72 and 73 indicate hospitals listed by AOHA, but not registered by AHA. For definition of numerical codes, see page A4	Control	Service	Beds	Admissions	Census	Outpatient Visits	Births	Total	Payroll	Personnel

NORTH LITTLE ROCK—Pulaski County

☒ BAPTIST MEMORIAL MEDICAL CENTER, One Pershing Circle, Zip 72114–1899; tel. 501/202–3000; Harrison M. Dean, Senior Vice President and Administrator **A**1 9 10 **F**4 7 8 10 11 12 13 14 16 17 19 21 22 27 28 29 30 34 35 37 39 40 41 42 44 45 46 48 49 52 54 55 56 58 59 60 62 63 65 67 71 73 74 **P**1 3 5 7 **S** Baptist Health, Little Rock, AR **N** Arkansas' FirstSource, Little Rock, AR; Baptist Health, Little Rock, AR

| 23 | 10 | 200 | 7313 | 91 | 68190 | 572 | 52589 | 21288 | 794 |

□ BRIDGEWAY, 21 Bridgeway Road, Zip 72113; tel. 501/771–1500; Barry Pipkin, Chief Executive Officer (Nonreporting) **A**1 9 10 **S** Universal Health Services, Inc., King of Prussia, PA

| 33 | 22 | 70 | — | — | — | — | — | — | — |

NORTH LITTLE ROCK DIVISION See Veterans Affairs Medical Center, Little Rock

OSCEOLA—Mississippi County

☒ BAPTIST MEMORIAL HOSPITAL–OSCEOLA, 611 West Lee Avenue, Zip 72370, Mailing Address: Box 607, Zip 72370–0607; tel. 501/563–7000; Al Sypniewski, Administrator **A**1 9 10 **F**2 7 12 14 15 16 19 22 28 29 30 32 33 37 44 45 46 49 52 65 71 **P**3 7 **S** Baptist Memorial Health Care Corporation, Memphis, TN **N** Arkansas' FirstSource, Little Rock, AR

| 21 | 10 | 59 | 2030 | 23 | 15105 | 0 | 7355 | 3023 | 114 |

OZARK—Franklin County

★ MERCY HOSPITAL–TURNER MEMORIAL, 801 West River, Zip 72949; tel. 501/667–4138; Sister Mary Werner Keith, Administrator (Nonreporting) **A**9 10 **S** Sisters of Mercy Health System–St. Louis, Saint Louis, MO **N** Saint Edward Mercy Medical Center, Fort Smith, AR; Arkansas' FirstSource, Little Rock, AR

| 21 | 10 | 39 | — | — | — | — | — | — | — |

PARAGOULD—Greene County

☒ ARKANSAS METHODIST HOSPITAL, 900 West Kingshighway, Zip 72450, Mailing Address: Box 339, Zip 72450; tel. 501/239–7000; Ronald K. Rooney, President **A**1 9 10 **F**7 8 10 12 14 16 19 22 23 28 30 32 34 35 37 39 40 44 45 46 49 65 71 73 **P**5 8 **N** Arkansas' FirstSource, Little Rock, AR

| 23 | 10 | 129 | 4117 | 50 | — | 389 | 19162 | 8247 | 384 |

PARIS—Logan County

★ NORTH LOGAN MERCY HOSPITAL, 500 East Academy, Zip 72855–4099; tel. 501/963–6101; Jim L. Maddox, Chief Administrative Officer **A**9 10 **F**2 3 4 7 8 9 10 11 14 15 16 19 20 21 22 24 25 28 30 31 32 33 34 35 37 38 39 40 41 42 43 44 47 50 52 53 54 55 56 57 58 59 60 62 65 66 67 69 71 73 **P**1 **S** Sisters of Mercy Health System–St. Louis, Saint Louis, MO **N** Saint Edward Mercy Medical Center, Fort Smith, AR; Arkansas' FirstSource, Little Rock, AR

| 21 | 10 | 16 | 266 | 3 | 8350 | 0 | 2766 | 1189 | 49 |

PIGGOTT—Clay County

★ PIGGOTT COMMUNITY HOSPITAL, 1206 Gordon Duckworth Drive, Zip 72454; tel. 501/598–3881; Betty J. Reams, Executive Director (Nonreporting) **A**9 10 **N** Arkansas' FirstSource, Little Rock, AR

| 14 | 10 | 35 | — | — | — | — | — | — | — |

PINE BLUFF—Jefferson County

☒ JEFFERSON REGIONAL MEDICAL CENTER, 1515 West 42nd Avenue, Zip 71603–7089; tel. 501/541–7100; Robert P. Atkinson, President and Chief Executive Officer (Total facility includes 112 beds in nursing home–type unit) **A**1 2 3 5 6 10 **F**3 4 7 8 10 11 12 14 15 16 18 19 21 22 23 24 25 27 28 29 30 31 32 33 34 35 37 38 39 40 41 42 43 44 45 46 48 49 51 52 54 55 56 57 58 59 60 63 64 65 66 67 68 70 71 72 73 74 **P**7 **N** Arkansas' FirstSource, Little Rock, AR

| 23 | 10 | 487 | 12992 | 323 | 84571 | 1646 | 102212 | 40198 | 1563 |

POCAHONTAS—Randolph County

□ RANDOLPH COUNTY MEDICAL CENTER, 2801 Medical Center Drive, Zip 72455; tel. 501/892–4511; Brad S. Morse, Executive Director (Nonreporting) **A**1 9 10 **S** Community Health Systems, Inc., Brentwood, TN **N** Arkansas' FirstSource, Little Rock, AR

| 33 | 10 | 50 | — | — | — | — | — | — | — |

ROGERS—Benton County

★ ST. MARY–ROGERS MEMORIAL HOSPITAL, 1200 West Walnut Street, Zip 72756–3599; tel. 501/636–0200; Michael J. Packnett, President and Chief Executive Officer **A**2 5 9 10 **F**1 7 8 10 11 12 14 15 16 19 21 22 24 28 30 32 33 34 35 36 38 39 40 41 42 44 49 63 64 65 66 67 71 73 **P**3 5 **S** Sisters of Mercy Health System–St. Louis, Saint Louis, MO **N** Arkansas' FirstSource, Little Rock, AR

| 21 | 10 | 110 | 6357 | 70 | 44223 | 1138 | 36672 | 18744 | 644 |

RUSSELLVILLE—Pope County

□ △ SAINT MARY'S REGIONAL MEDICAL CENTER, 1808 West Main Street, Zip 72801; tel. 501/968–2841; Mike McCoy, Chief Executive Officer **A**1 7 9 10 **F**7 8 10 12 15 16 19 21 22 23 24 25 28 29 30 32 34 35 37 39 40 41 42 44 46 48 49 60 63 64 65 71 73 74 **S** TENET Healthcare Corporation, Santa Barbara, CA **N** Arkansas' FirstSource, Little Rock, AR

| 33 | 10 | 152 | 5160 | 69 | 39505 | 1006 | 30166 | 10350 | 477 |

SALEM—Fulton County

FULTON COUNTY HOSPITAL, Highway 9, Zip 72576, Mailing Address: P.O. Box 517, Zip 72576; tel. 501/895–2691; Franklin E. Wise, Administrator **A**9 10 **F**19 22 32 34 40 44 71 **N** Arkansas' FirstSource, Little Rock, AR

| 13 | 10 | 30 | 883 | 10 | 18385 | 41 | 3720 | 1990 | 105 |

SEARCY—White County

□ △ CENTRAL ARKANSAS HOSPITAL, 1200 South Main, Zip 72143; tel. 501/278–3131; David C. Laffoon, Executive Director **A**1 2 7 9 10 **F**7 10 11 12 14 15 16 19 22 24 32 35 37 38 40 42 44 48 52 54 56 57 58 59 65 71 74 **P**6 7 8 **S** TENET Healthcare Corporation, Santa Barbara, CA

| 33 | 10 | 173 | 5984 | 88 | 74574 | 833 | 25710 | 10876 | 409 |

☒ WHITE COUNTY MEDICAL CENTER, 3214 East Race, Zip 72143–4847; tel. 501/268–6121; Raymond W. Montgomery, II, President and Chief Executive Officer **A**1 2 9 10 **F**7 10 11 12 13 15 16 19 20 21 22 23 24 28 30 31 32 33 34 35 37 38 40 41 42 44 45 46 49 65 66 68 71 73 74 **P**3 **N** Arkansas' FirstSource, Little Rock, AR

| 23 | 10 | 104 | 4360 | 54 | 25213 | 342 | 21776 | 9531 | 444 |

Hospital, Address, Telephone, Administrator, Approval, Facility, and Physician Codes, Health Care System, Network	Classi- fication Codes		Utilization Data					Expense (thousands) of dollars		
★ American Hospital Association (AHA) membership □ Joint Commission on Accreditation of Healthcare Organizations (JCAHO) accreditation + American Osteopathic Hospital Association (AOHA) membership ○ American Osteopathic Association (AOA) accreditation △ Commission on Accreditation of Rehabilitation Facilities (CARF) accreditation Control codes 61, 63, 64, 71, 72 and 73 indicate hospitals listed by AOHA, but not registered by AHA. For definition of numerical codes, see page A4	Control	Service	Beds	Admissions	Census	Outpatient Visits	Births	Total	Payroll	Personnel

SHERWOOD—Pulaski County

□ △ ST. VINCENT–NORTH REHABILITATION HOSPITAL, (Formerly Central Arkansas Rehabilitation Hospital), 2201 Wildwood Avenue, Zip 72120–5074, Mailing Address: P.O. Box 6930, Zip 72124–6930; tel. 501/834–1800; Douglas W. Parker, Chief Executive Officer (Total facility includes 10 beds in nursing home–type unit) **A**1 7 9 10 **F**5 12 14 16 27 34 41 46 48 49 64 65 73 **S** Continental Medical Systems, Inc., Mechanicsburg, PA

| | 32 | 46 | 60 | 874 | 48 | 9305 | 0 | 11791 | 5374 | 146 |

SILOAM SPRINGS—Benton County

★ SILOAM SPRING MEMORIAL HOSPITAL, 205 East Jefferson Street, Zip 72761; tel. 501/524–4141; Donald E. Patterson, Administrator **A**9 10 **F**7 12 16 19 21 22 28 30 32 34 37 39 40 41 44 46 64 65 67 71 **S** Quorum Health Group/Quorum Health Resources, Inc., Brentwood, TN **N** Arkansas' FirstSource, Little Rock, AR; Arkansas Network, North Little Rock, AR

| | 14 | 10 | 52 | 2294 | 32 | 18255 | 148 | 11172 | 5421 | 242 |

SPRINGDALE—Washington County

⊠ NORTHWEST MEDICAL CENTER, (Includes Bates Medical Center, 602 North Walton Boulevard, Bentonville, Zip 72712; tel. 501/273–2481; Thomas P. O'Neal, Executive Vice President and Chief Operating Officer), 609 West Maple Avenue, Zip 72764, Mailing Address: P.O. Box 47, Zip 72765; tel. 501/751–5711; Russ D. Sword, President and Chief Executive Officer (Total facility includes 22 beds in nursing home–type unit) **A**1 2 5 9 10 **F**3 4 7 8 10 11 12 13 14 15 16 17 18 19 20 21 22 24 25 26 27 28 29 30 31 32 33 34 35 37 38 39 40 41 42 43 44 45 46 49 51 52 53 54 55 56 57 58 59 60 63 64 65 66 67 71 72 73 74 **P**2 5 6 8 **N** Arkansas Network, North Little Rock, AR

| | 23 | 10 | 222 | 10831 | 134 | 92547 | 713 | 82366 | 35919 | 1708 |

STUTTGART—Arkansas County

★ STUTTGART REGIONAL MEDICAL CENTER, North Buerkle Road, Zip 72160, Mailing Address: Box 1905, Zip 72160; tel. 501/673–3511; Jim E. Bushmaier, Administrator and Chief Executive Officer (Nonreporting) **A**9 10 **N** Arkansas' FirstSource, Little Rock, AR

| | 23 | 10 | 89 | — | — | — | — | — | — | — |

VAN BUREN—Crawford County

□ CRAWFORD MEMORIAL HOSPITAL, East Main & South 20th Streets, Zip 72956, Mailing Address: Box 409, Zip 72956; tel. 501/474–3401; Richard Boone, Executive Director **A**1 9 10 **F**8 12 15 19 21 22 23 32 34 35 37 39 42 44 49 65 71 73 **S** Health Management Associates, Naples, FL **N** Arkansas' FirstSource, Little Rock, AR

| | 33 | 10 | 103 | 3109 | 37 | 28507 | 0 | 17487 | 7085 | 356 |

WALDRON—Scott County

★ MERCY HOSPITAL OF SCOTT COUNTY, Highways 71 and 80, Zip 72958–9984, Mailing Address: Box 2230, Zip 72958–2230; tel. 501/637–4135; Sister Mary Alvera Simon, Administrator (Total facility includes 105 beds in nursing home–type unit) **A**10 **F**6 15 19 22 30 31 32 33 34 44 49 64 65 71 **P**1 4 7 **S** Sisters of Mercy Health System–St. Louis, Saint Louis, MO **N** Saint Edward Mercy Medical Center, Fort Smith, AR; Arkansas' FirstSource, Little Rock, AR

| | 21 | 10 | 127 | 483 | 106 | 13142 | 0 | 4844 | 2532 | 119 |

WALNUT RIDGE—Lawrence County

LAWRENCE MEMORIAL HOSPITAL, (Includes Lawrence Hall Nursing Home), 1309 West Main, Zip 72476–0839, Mailing Address: Box 839, Zip 72476; tel. 501/886–1200; Larry Morse, Administrator (Total facility includes 189 beds in nursing home–type unit) **A**10 **F**8 13 15 16 19 22 28 30 32 34 36 42 44 64 65 67 71 73 **P**5 6 8 **N** Arkansas' FirstSource, Little Rock, AR

| | 13 | 10 | 201 | 883 | 180 | 8020 | 0 | 7779 | 3907 | 240 |

WARREN—Bradley County

★ BRADLEY COUNTY MEMORIAL HOSPITAL, 404 South Bradley Street, Zip 71671; tel. 501/226–3731; Harry H. Stevens, Administrator **A**9 10 **F**1 6 7 8 11 12 13 15 16 17 18 19 20 21 22 24 26 27 28 29 30 31 32 33 34 36 39 41 44 46 49 51 53 54 55 56 57 58 59 63 65 67 71 73 **P**1 3 **N** Arkansas' FirstSource, Little Rock, AR

| | 13 | 10 | 60 | 1358 | 21 | 16409 | 130 | 9836 | 4322 | 205 |

WEST MEMPHIS—Crittenden County

□ △ CRITTENDEN MEMORIAL HOSPITAL, 200 Tyler Street, Zip 72301, Mailing Address: Box 2248, Zip 72303–2248; tel. 501/735–1500; Ross Hooper, Chief Executive Officer **A**1 7 9 10 **F**7 8 11 15 17 19 20 21 22 24 28 30 32 33 34 35 37 40 42 44 46 48 49 65 71 73 **N** Arkansas' FirstSource, Little Rock, AR

| | 23 | 10 | 95 | 4859 | 81 | 54940 | 525 | 31278 | 13794 | 544 |

WYNNE—Cross County

★ CROSS COUNTY HOSPITAL, 310 South Falls Boulevard, Zip 72396, Mailing Address: P.O. Box 590, Zip 72396; tel. 501/238–3300; Harry M. Baker, Chief Executive Officer **A**9 10 **F**11 15 19 22 32 40 44 65 71 **N** Arkansas' FirstSource, Little Rock, AR

| | 13 | 10 | 53 | 1537 | 19 | 20943 | 140 | 5777 | 2996 | 148 |

CALIFORNIA

Resident population 31,589 (in thousands)
Resident population in metro areas 96.7%
Birth rate per 1,000 population 18.8
65 years and over 11.0%
Percent of persons without health insurance 21.1%

Hospital, Address, Telephone, Administrator, Approval, Facility, and Physician Codes, Health Care System, Network	Classi-fication Codes		Utilization Data					Expense (thousands) of dollars		
	Control	Service	Beds	Admissions	Census	Outpatient Visits	Births	Total	Payroll	Personnel

★ American Hospital Association (AHA) membership
□ Joint Commission on Accreditation of Healthcare Organizations (JCAHO) accreditation
+ American Osteopathic Hospital Association (AOHA) membership
○ American Osteopathic Association (AOA) accreditation
△ Commission on Accreditation of Rehabilitation Facilities (CARF) accreditation
Control codes 61, 63, 64, 71, 72 and 73 indicate hospitals listed by AOHA, but not registered by AHA. For definition of numerical codes, see page A4

ALAMEDA—Alameda County

✸ ALAMEDA HOSPITAL, 2070 Clinton Avenue, Zip 94501; tel. 510/522–3700; William J. Dal Cielo, Chief Executive Officer (Total facility includes 23 beds in nursing home–type unit) **A**1 9 10 **F**7 8 16 19 21 22 26 28 29 32 33 34 35 37 39 40 41 42 44 45 49 52 57 63 64 71 73 **P**1 4 5 6 7 **N** East Bay Medical Network, Emeryville, CA	23	10	120	4311	63	35567	555	31675	20707	384

ALHAMBRA—Los Angeles County

□ △ ALHAMBRA HOSPITAL, 100 South Raymond Avenue, Zip 91801, Mailing Address: Box 510, Zip 91802–0510; tel. 818/570–1606; Timothy McGlew, Chief Executive Officer (Total facility includes 42 beds in nursing home–type unit) **A**1 2 7 9 10 **F**8 11 12 14 15 16 19 21 22 27 28 29 30 34 37 39 41 42 44 46 48 49 60 63 64 65 71 73 **P**5	32	10	144	2594	67	18324	0	29306	11410	194

ALTURAS—Modoc County

★ MODOC MEDICAL CENTER, 228 McDowell Street, Zip 96101; tel. 916/233–5131; Woody J. Laughnan, Chief Executive Officer (Total facility includes 71 beds in nursing home–type unit) **A**9 10 **F**7 8 15 16 17 20 22 28 32 34 40 44 45 49 64 65 71 73 74 **N** InterMountain Healthcare Network, Alturas, CA	13	10	87	324	62	10243	58	6473	2927	116

ANAHEIM—Orange County

□ ANAHEIM GENERAL HOSPITAL, 3350 West Ball Road, Zip 92804–9998; tel. 714/827–6700; Timothy L. Carda, Chief Executive Officer **A**1 9 10 **F**4 8 12 15 19 22 27 28 29 31 32 34 35 37 39 40 41 42 44 49 61 65 71 74 **P**5 **S** Pacific Health Corporation, Long Beach, CA	32	10	88	3220	38	25565	738	—	—	307
□ ANAHEIM MEMORIAL HOSPITAL, 1111 West La Palma Avenue, Zip 92801, Mailing Address: Box 3005, Zip 92803; tel. 714/774–1450; Chris D. Van Gorder, President and Chief Executive Officer **A**1 2 5 9 10 **F**4 7 8 10 11 12 14 15 16 17 19 21 22 24 25 26 27 28 29 30 32 34 35 37 38 39 40 41 42 43 44 45 46 47 48 49 51 61 64 65 66 67 69 70 71 72 73 74 **P**4 5 7 **S** Memorial Health Services, Long Beach, CA	23	10	192	7390	99	41022	754	63822	22174	636
✸ COLUMBIA WEST ANAHEIM MEDICAL CENTER, 3033 West Orange Avenue, Zip 92804–3184; tel. 714/827–3000; David Culberson, Chief Executive Officer (Total facility includes 22 beds in nursing home–type unit) (Nonreporting) **A**1 2 5 9 10 **S** Columbia/HCA Healthcare Corporation, Nashville, TN	33	10	219	—	—	—	—	—	—	—
✸ KAISER FOUNDATION HOSPITAL, 441 North Lakeview Avenue, Zip 92807; tel. 714/279–4100; Gerald A. McCall, Administrator **A**1 2 3 10 **F**2 3 4 7 8 10 11 12 13 14 15 16 17 18 19 21 22 23 28 29 30 31 32 33 35 37 38 39 40 41 42 43 44 45 46 48 49 51 52 53 54 55 57 58 59 60 61 63 64 65 66 67 68 69 71 72 73 **P**4 **S** Kaiser Foundation Hospitals, Oakland, CA	23	10	131	8075	79	—	2511	—	—	690
✸ MARTIN LUTHER HOSPITAL–ANAHEIM, 1830 West Romneya Drive, Zip 92801–1854; tel. 714/491–5200; Stephen E. Dixon, President and Chief Executive Officer (Total facility includes 22 beds in nursing home–type unit) **A**1 2 9 10 **F**1 3 4 7 8 9 10 11 12 13 14 15 16 17 19 20 21 22 23 27 28 29 30 32 33 35 37 38 39 40 41 43 44 45 46 49 51 53 54 55 56 57 58 59 60 61 64 65 66 67 68 69 70 71 72 73 74 **P**3 5 7 **S** UniHealth, Burbank, CA **N** UniHealth, Burbank, CA	23	10	205	6652	84	49775	2119	49981	20814	483
✸ WESTERN MEDICAL CENTER HOSPITAL ANAHEIM, 1025 South Anaheim Boulevard, Zip 92805; tel. 714/533–6220; Doug Norris, Chief Operating Officer (Nonreporting) **A**1 9 10 **S** TENET Healthcare Corporation, Santa Barbara, CA	23	10	171	—	—	—	—	—	—	—

ANTIOCH—Contra Costa County

✸ SUTTER DELTA MEDICAL CENTER, (Formerly Delta Memorial Hospital), 3901 Lone Tree Way, Zip 94509; tel. 510/779–7200; Linda Horn, Administrator (Nonreporting) **A**1 9 10 **S** Sutter Health, Sacramento, CA **N** East Bay Medical Network, Emeryville, CA; Sutter\CHS, Sacramento, CA	23	10	111	—	—	—	—	—	—	—

APPLE VALLEY—San Bernardino County

✸ ST. MARY REGIONAL MEDICAL CENTER, 18300 Highway 18, Zip 92307–0725; Mailing Address: Box 7025, Zip 92307–0725; tel. 619/242–2311; Catherine M. Pelley, President and Chief Executive Officer (Nonreporting) **A**1 2 9 10 **S** St. Joseph Health System, Orange, CA **N** Saint Joseph Health System, Orange, CA	21	10	137	—	—	—	—	—	—	—

ARCADIA—Los Angeles County

✸ METHODIST HOSPITAL OF SOUTHERN CALIFORNIA, 300 West Huntington Drive, Zip 91007, Mailing Address: P.O. Box 60016, Zip 91066–6016; tel. 818/445–4441; Dennis M. Lee, President (Total facility includes 26 beds in nursing home–type unit) **A**1 2 9 10 **F**4 7 8 10 11 12 17 19 21 22 28 30 32 33 34 36 37 38 39 40 41 42 43 44 45 48 49 52 54 55 56 57 58 59 60 64 65 66 67 70 71 73 **P**1 3 5 7 **S** Southern California Healthcare System, Pasadena, CA **N** Southern California Healthcare Systems, Pasadena, CA	23	10	304	11564	165	56094	1265	87517	38746	979

ARCATA—Humboldt County

□ MAD RIVER COMMUNITY HOSPITAL, 3800 Janes Road, Zip 95521, Mailing Address: P.O. Box 1115, Zip 95521–1115; tel. 707/822–3621; Michael Young, Administrator (Nonreporting) **A**1 9 10	33	10	78	—	—	—	—	—	—	—

Hospital, Address, Telephone, Administrator, Approval, Facility, and Physician Codes, Health Care System, Network	Classi-fication Codes		Utilization Data					Expense (thousands) of dollars		
	Control	Service	Beds	Admissions	Census	Outpatient Visits	Births	Total	Payroll	Personnel

★ American Hospital Association (AHA) membership
☐ Joint Commission on Accreditation of Healthcare Organizations (JCAHO) accreditation
+ American Osteopathic Hospital Association (AOHA) membership
○ American Osteopathic Association (AOA) accreditation
△ Commission on Accreditation of Rehabilitation Facilities (CARF) accreditation
Control codes 61, 63, 64, 71, 72 and 73 indicate hospitals listed by AOHA, but not registered by AHA. For definition of numerical codes, see page A4

ARROYO GRANDE—San Luis Obispo County

☐ ARROYO GRANDE COMMUNITY HOSPITAL, 345 South Halcyon Road, Zip 93420; tel. 805/489–4261; Richard N. Woolslayer, Chief Executive Officer **A**1 9 10 **F**4 8 15 16 19 21 22 23 26 28 31 32 34 35 37 41 42 44 49 66 71 72 — 23 10 35 2380 25 59679 0 18029 6444 209

ARTESIA—Los Angeles County

☐ PIONEER HOSPITAL, 17831 South Pioneer Boulevard, Zip 90701; tel. 310/865–6291; Sharon L. Jose, MS, R.N., Vice President, Hospital Operations **A**1 9 10 **F**2 4 7 8 10 14 15 16 17 18 19 20 21 22 26 29 30 31 32 34 35 37 38 39 40 41 42 43 44 45 46 47 48 49 50 52 53 54 56 57 60 64 65 72 73 74 **P**5 7 — 33 10 99 5232 52 18194 1812 — — 294

ATASCADERO—San Luis Obispo County

☐ ATASCADERO STATE HOSPITAL, 10333 El Camino Real, Zip 93422–7001, Mailing Address: P.O. Box 7001, Zip 93423–7001; tel. 805/461–2000; Jon Demorales, Executive Director **A**1 3 5 **F**14 15 20 31 41 45 46 52 65 73 **P**6 — 12 22 981 1356 935 0 0 95659 61535 1576

ATWATER—Merced County

BLOSS MEMORIAL HOSPITAL DISTRICT, 1691 Third Street, Zip 95301; tel. 209/358–8201; L. Ned Miller, CHE, Administrator and Chief Executive Officer **A**9 10 **F**22 34 51 65 67 71 73 **P**3 — 16 10 23 321 4 41116 0 5335 — 99

AUBURN—Placer County

✶ SUTTER AUBURN FAITH HOSPITAL, 11815 Education Street, Zip 95604, Mailing Address: Box 8992, Zip 95604–8992; tel. 916/888–4518; Joel E. Grey, Chief Executive Officer (Total facility includes 12 beds in nursing home–type unit) **A**1 9 **F**7 8 11 12 14 15 16 19 21 22 23 27 28 32 33 34 35 37 39 40 41 42 44 46 48 49 50 63 64 65 71 73 **S** Sutter Health, Sacramento, CA **N** Sutter\CHS, Sacramento, CA — 23 10 105 5636 66 41073 620 43551 20362 493

AVALON—Los Angeles County

AVALON MUNICIPAL HOSPITAL AND CLINIC, 100 Falls Canyon Road, Zip 90704, Mailing Address: Box 1563, Zip 90704–1563; tel. 310/510–0700; Karla Parsons, R.N., Administrator (Total facility includes 4 beds in nursing home–type unit) (Nonreporting) **A**9 10 — 23 10 12 — — — — — — —

BAKERSFIELD—Kern County

✶ BAKERSFIELD MEMORIAL HOSPITAL, 420 34th Street, Zip 93301, Mailing Address: Box 1888, Zip 93303–1888; tel. 805/327–1792; C. Larry Carr, President (Total facility includes 24 beds in nursing home–type unit) **A**1 2 9 10 **F**2 3 4 7 8 10 11 12 15 16 17 18 19 21 22 23 27 28 30 32 35 37 38 40 41 42 43 44 49 52 53 54 58 59 60 64 65 71 72 73 74 **P**1 3 4 5 7 **S** Catholic Healthcare West, San Francisco, CA **N** Catholic HealthCare West (CHW), San Francisco, CA — 23 10 379 11279 196 42963 1675 100921 39602 1072

☐ COLUMBIA GOOD SAMARITAN HOSPITAL, 901 Olive Drive, Zip 93308–4137; tel. 805/399–4461; Jim Bennett, Administrator **A**1 10 **F**8 11 12 13 14 15 17 18 19 20 25 26 27 29 30 31 32 33 34 35 37 39 41 44 46 49 52 54 55 57 58 59 60 63 65 67 71 72 **P**5 6 7 **S** Columbia/HCA Healthcare Corporation, Nashville, TN — 32 10 64 1692 30 21672 0 10549 4500 161

☐ HEALTHSOUTH BAKERSFIELD REHABILITATION HOSPITAL, 5001 Commerce Drive, Zip 93309; tel. 805/323–5500; Jo Ann Bennett, Chief Operating Officer (Nonreporting) **A**1 10 **S** HEALTHSOUTH Corporation, Birmingham, AL — 33 46 60 — — — — — — —

☐ KERN MEDICAL CENTER, 1830 Flower Street, Zip 93305–4197; tel. 805/326–2000; Gerald A. Starr, Chief Executive Officer **A**1 2 3 5 8 9 10 **F**1 3 4 7 8 10 11 14 15 16 17 18 19 21 22 24 25 26 28 29 30 31 34 35 36 37 38 39 40 41 42 43 44 45 46 49 51 52 53 54 56 60 61 65 71 73 **P**6 — 13 10 198 14794 176 203028 3698 106878 54161 1448

☐ MEMORIAL CENTER, 5201 White Lane, Zip 93309; tel. 805/398–1800; Deirdre Terleski, Chief Executive Officer **A**1 9 10 **F**1 2 3 12 14 15 16 32 52 53 54 55 56 57 58 59 67 **P**5 — 23 22 37 1000 14 20235 0 7451 3263 99

✶ MERCY HEALTHCARE–BAKERSFIELD, (Formerly Mercy Hospital), (Includes Mercy Southwest Hospital, 400 Old River Road, Zip 93311; tel. 805/663–6000), 2215 Truxtun Avenue, Zip 93301, Mailing Address: Box 119, Zip 93302; tel. 805/632–5000; Bernard J. Herman, President and Chief Executive Officer (Total facility includes 50 beds in nursing home–type unit) **A**1 2 9 10 **F**7 8 10 15 16 17 19 22 23 30 32 34 35 37 38 39 40 42 44 45 46 49 60 64 65 67 71 72 73 74 **P**2 3 5 7 **S** Catholic Healthcare West, San Francisco, CA **N** Catholic HealthCare West (CHW), San Francisco, CA — 21 10 261 11144 168 144188 1729 85325 37741 1309

MERCY SOUTHWEST HOSPITAL See Mercy Healthcare–Bakersfield

✶ SAN JOAQUIN COMMUNITY HOSPITAL, 2615 Eye Street, Zip 93301, Mailing Address: Box 2615, Zip 93303–2615; tel. 805/395–3000; Fred Manchur, President (Nonreporting) **A**1 9 10 **S** Adventist Health, Roseville, CA — 23 10 178 — — — — — — —

BANNING—Riverside County

✶ SAN GORGONIO MEMORIAL HOSPITAL, 600 North Highland Springs Avenue, Zip 92220; tel. 909/845–1121; Kay Lang, Chief Executive Officer **A**1 9 10 **F**8 13 14 15 17 18 19 21 22 26 27 28 29 30 32 33 34 37 39 40 41 42 44 45 46 49 51 54 58 59 65 67 68 71 73 **S** Brim, Inc., Portland, OR — 23 10 68 2587 27 30583 343 14529 7209 197

BARSTOW—San Bernardino County

☐ BARSTOW COMMUNITY HOSPITAL, 555 South Seventh Avenue, Zip 92311; tel. 619/256–1761; Russell V. Judd, Chief Executive Officer **A**1 2 9 10 **F**7 8 11 14 15 16 19 21 22 28 35 37 40 41 44 71 73 **P**7 **S** Community Health Systems, Inc., Brentwood, TN — 33 10 56 2966 27 27441 495 15964 6446 195

BEALE AFB—Yuba County

✶ U. S. AIR FORCE HOSPITAL, 15301 Warren Shingle Road, Zip 95903–1907; tel. 916/634–4838; Lieutenant Colonel Robert G. Quinn, MSC, USAF, FACHE, Administrator **A**1 **F**3 8 12 13 20 27 29 30 34 39 44 46 49 51 65 71 **S** Department of the Air Force, Washington, DC — 41 10 6 136 1 60560 0 — — 362

Hospital, Address, Telephone, Administrator, Approval, Facility, and Physician Codes, Health Care System, Network	Classi-fication Codes		Utilization Data					Expense (thousands) of dollars		
★ American Hospital Association (AHA) membership □ Joint Commission on Accreditation of Healthcare Organizations (JCAHO) accreditation + American Osteopathic Hospital Association (AOHA) membership ○ American Osteopathic Association (AOA) accreditation △ Commission on Accreditation of Rehabilitation Facilities (CARF) accreditation Control codes 61, 63, 64, 71, 72 and 73 indicate hospitals listed by AOHA, but not registered by AHA. For definition of numerical codes, see page A4	Control	Service	Beds	Admissions	Census	Outpatient Visits	Births	Total	Payroll	Personnel

BELLFLOWER—Los Angeles County

Hospital	Control	Service	Beds	Admissions	Census	Outpatient Visits	Births	Total	Payroll	Personnel
□ BELLFLOWER MEDICAL CENTER, 9542 East Artesia Boulevard, Zip 90706; tel. 310/925–8355; Stanley Otake, Chief Executive Officer **A**1 9 10 **F**8 19 21 22 27 35 37 39 40 44 48 49 52 58 65 71 73 **P**5 **S** Pacific Health Corporation, Long Beach, CA	33	10	145	4335	59	6506	794	22556	9425	305
□ BELLWOOD GENERAL HOSPITAL, 10250 East Artesia Boulevard, Zip 90706; tel. 562/866–9028; Joseph Sharp, Administrator **A**1 9 10 **F**15 17 19 22 27 28 30 34 35 37 40 44 49 51 61 65 71 73 74 **P**5 **S** Paracelsus Healthcare Corporation, Houston, TX	33	10	65	2752	38	20532	584	23573	8336	240
⊠ KAISER FOUNDATION HOSPITAL, (Includes Kaiser Foundation Hospital, Norwalk, 12500 South Hoxie, Norwalk, Zip 90650), 9400 East Rosecrans Avenue, Zip 90706–2246; tel. 310/461–3000; Timothy A. Reed, Administrator (Nonreporting) **A**1 2 10 **S** Kaiser Foundation Hospitals, Oakland, CA	23	10	248	—	—	—	—	—	—	—

BELMONT—San Mateo County

Hospital	Control	Service	Beds	Admissions	Census	Outpatient Visits	Births	Total	Payroll	Personnel
□ BHC BELMONT HILLS HOSPITAL, (Formerly CPC Belmont Hills Hospital), 1301 Ralston Avenue, Zip 94002; tel. 415/593–2143; Harold G. Marohn, Acting Chief Executive Officer (Nonreporting) **A**1 9 10 **S** Behavioral Healthcare Corporation, Nashville, TN	33	22	53	—	—	—	—	—	—	—

BERKELEY—Alameda County

Hospital	Control	Service	Beds	Admissions	Census	Outpatient Visits	Births	Total	Payroll	Personnel
⊠ △ ALTA BATES MEDICAL CENTER–ASHBY CAMPUS, (Includes Alta Bates Medical Center–Herrick Campus, 2001 Dwight Way, Zip 94704; tel. 510/204–4444), 2450 Ashby Avenue, Zip 94705; tel. 510/204–4444; Albert Lawrence Greene, President and Chief Executive Officer (Total facility includes 63 beds in nursing home–type unit) (Nonreporting) **A**1 2 7 9 10 **S** Sutter Health, Sacramento, CA **N** East Bay Medical Network, Emeryville, CA; Sutter\CHS, Sacramento, CA	23	10	453	—	—	—	—	—	—	—

BIG BEAR LAKE—San Bernardino County

Hospital	Control	Service	Beds	Admissions	Census	Outpatient Visits	Births	Total	Payroll	Personnel
⊠ BEAR VALLEY COMMUNITY HOSPITAL, 41870 Garstin Road, Zip 92315, Mailing Address: P.O. Box 1649, Zip 92315–1649; tel. 909/866–6501; Jim Sato, Chief Executive Officer (Total facility includes 15 beds in nursing home–type unit) (Nonreporting) **A**1 9 10 **S** Brim, Inc., Portland, OR	16	10	30	—	—	—	—	—	—	—

BISHOP—Inyo County

Hospital	Control	Service	Beds	Admissions	Census	Outpatient Visits	Births	Total	Payroll	Personnel
⊠ NORTHERN INYO HOSPITAL, 150 Pioneer Lane, Zip 93514–2599; tel. 760/873–5811; Herman J. Spencer, Administrator **A**1 9 10 **F**7 15 19 22 33 34 37 40 44 49 65 71	16	10	30	1366	10	21403	333	16748	8588	217

BLYTHE—Riverside County

Hospital	Control	Service	Beds	Admissions	Census	Outpatient Visits	Births	Total	Payroll	Personnel
★ PALO VERDE HOSPITAL, 250 North First Street, Zip 92225, Mailing Address: P.O. Drawer Z, Zip 92226; tel. 619/922–4115; M. Victoria Clark, Administrator **A**9 10 **F**7 8 12 13 14 16 17 19 22 28 29 30 32 35 37 40 44 46 49 61 65 71	33	10	40	1877	14	18891	365	11069	3779	158

BRAWLEY—Imperial County

Hospital	Control	Service	Beds	Admissions	Census	Outpatient Visits	Births	Total	Payroll	Personnel
⊠ PIONEERS MEMORIAL HEALTHCARE DISTRICT, 207 West Legion Road, Zip 92227–9699; tel. 619/351–3333; William W. Daniel, Administrator and Chief Executive Officer **A**1 9 10 **F**7 8 14 15 16 19 20 22 28 30 34 35 37 38 40 41 44 46 65 67 71 73 **P**4 5 7 **S** Brim, Inc., Portland, OR	16	10	80	3803	38	45045	1020	30053	13051	442

BREA—Orange County

Hospital	Control	Service	Beds	Admissions	Census	Outpatient Visits	Births	Total	Payroll	Personnel
□ BREA COMMUNITY HOSPITAL, 380 West Central Avenue, Zip 92621; tel. 714/529–0211; Dave Yeager, Chief Executive Officer (Nonreporting) **A**1 9 10	33	10	60	—	—	—	—	—	—	—
□ THC–ORANGE COUNTY, 875 Brea Boulevard, Zip 92821; tel. 714/529–6842; Donna Hoover, Chief Executive Officer (Nonreporting) **A**1 10 **S** Transitional Hospitals Corporation, Las Vegas, NV	33	10	48	—	—	—	—	—	—	—

BUENA PARK—Orange County

Hospital	Control	Service	Beds	Admissions	Census	Outpatient Visits	Births	Total	Payroll	Personnel
□ BUENA PARK MEDICAL CENTER, (Formerly Buena Park Doctors Medical Center), 5742 Beach Boulevard, Zip 90621; tel. 714/521–4770; Timothy L. Carda, Administrator and Chief Executive Officer (Nonreporting) **A**1 9 **S** Pacific Health Corporation, Long Beach, CA	33	10	58	—	—	—	—	—	—	—
□ ORANGE COUNTY COMMUNITY HOSPITAL OF BUENA PARK, 6850 Lincoln Avenue, Zip 90620–5703; tel. 562/827–1161; Joseph Sharp, Acting Administrator **A**1 9 10 **F**1 12 41 44 52 58 59 65 **P**5 **S** Paracelsus Healthcare Corporation, Houston, TX	33	22	55	695	15	20744	0	10187	3377	132

BURBANK—Los Angeles County

Hospital	Control	Service	Beds	Admissions	Census	Outpatient Visits	Births	Total	Payroll	Personnel
⊠ PROVIDENCE SAINT JOSEPH MEDICAL CENTER, 501 South Buena Vista Street, Zip 91505–4866; tel. 818/843–5111; Michael J. Madden, Chief Executive Los Angeles Service Area (Total facility includes 121 beds in nursing home–type unit) **A**1 2 9 10 **F**4 7 8 10 11 12 13 14 15 16 17 19 20 21 22 23 24 26 28 29 30 31 32 33 34 35 37 38 39 40 41 42 43 44 45 46 48 49 60 64 65 67 68 71 72 73 74 **P**5 **S** Sisters of Providence Health System, Seattle, WA **N** Providence Health System in California, Burbank, CA	21	10	423	18441	294	320117	2739	169123	69202	1778
□ THOMPSON MEMORIAL MEDICAL CENTER, 466 East Olive Avenue, Zip 91501; tel. 818/953–6500; Jerry Gillman, President and Chief Executive Officer **A**1 9 10 **F**11 12 15 16 17 19 22 30 31 32 35 42 44 59 65 71 73	33	10	56	1964	24	—	0	19884	7481	225

BURLINGAME—San Mateo County

Hospital	Control	Service	Beds	Admissions	Census	Outpatient Visits	Births	Total	Payroll	Personnel
⊠ △ MILLS–PENINSULA HEALTH SERVICES, (Formerly Mills–Peninsula Hospitals), (Includes Mills Hospital, 100 South San Mateo Drive, San Mateo, Zip 94401; tel. 415/696–4400; Peninsula Hospital, 1783 El Camino Real, tel. 415/696–5400), 1783 El Camino Real, Zip 94010–3205; tel. 415/696–5400; Robert W. Merwin, Chief Executive Officer (Total facility includes 55 beds in nursing home–type unit) **A**1 2 7 9 10 **F**1 2 3 4 5 7 8 10 11 12 14 15 16 17 19 21 22 23 24 25 26 30 32 33 34 35 37 38 39 40 41 42 43 44 45 46 48 49 52 53 54 55 56 57 58 59 60 63 64 65 67 71 73 **P**5 7 **S** Sutter Health, Sacramento, CA **N** Sutter\CHS, Sacramento, CA	23	10	414	16253	251	389222	2337	175587	87894	1258
PENINSULA HOSPITAL See Mills–Peninsula Health Services										

Hospital, Address, Telephone, Administrator, Approval, Facility, and Physician Codes, Health Care System, Network	Classi-fication Codes		Utilization Data					Expense (thousands) of dollars		
★ American Hospital Association (AHA) membership □ Joint Commission on Accreditation of Healthcare Organizations (JCAHO) accreditation + American Osteopathic Hospital Association (AOHA) membership ○ American Osteopathic Association (AOA) accreditation △ Commission on Accreditation of Rehabilitation Facilities (CARF) accreditation Control codes 61, 63, 64, 71, 72 and 73 indicate hospitals listed by AOHA, but not registered by AHA. For definition of numerical codes, see page A4	Control	Service	Beds	Admissions	Census	Outpatient Visits	Births	Total	Payroll	Personnel

CALEXICO—Imperial County
CALEXICO HOSPITAL, 450 Birch Street, Zip 92231; tel. 619/357–1191; Randolph R. Smith, Administrator (Nonreporting) **A**9 — 16 10 34 — — — — — — —

CAMARILLO—Ventura County
□ CAMARILLO STATE HOSPITAL AND DEVELOPMENTAL CENTER, 1878 South Lewis Road, Zip 93012, Mailing Address: P.O. Box 6022, Zip 93011–6022; tel. 805/484–3661; Norm Kramer, Administrator (Nonreporting) **A**1 9 10 — 12 22 1119 — — — — — — —

★ ST. JOHN'S PLEASANT VALLEY HOSPITAL, 2309 Antonio Avenue, Zip 93010–1459; tel. 805/389–5800; Daniel R. Herlinger, President and Chief Executive Officer (Total facility includes 99 beds in nursing home–type unit) **A**1 9 10 **F**7 8 11 15 16 17 19 21 22 23 28 29 30 32 35 37 40 44 45 46 49 60 63 64 65 67 71 73 **P**3 5 7 **S** Catholic Healthcare West, San Francisco, CA **N** Catholic HealthCare West (CHW), San Francisco, CA — 23 10 153 3799 121 40164 636 32087 14395 369

CAMP PENDLETON—San Diego County
★ NAVAL HOSPITAL, Mailing Address: Box 555191, Zip 92055–5191; tel. 619/725–1288; Captain B. B. Potter, Commanding Officer **A**1 3 5 **F**1 2 3 4 5 6 7 8 9 10 11 12 13 16 17 18 19 20 21 22 23 24 25 26 27 28 29 30 31 32 33 34 35 36 37 38 39 40 41 42 43 44 45 46 47 48 49 50 51 52 53 54 55 56 57 58 59 60 61 63 64 65 66 67 68 69 70 71 72 73 74 **P**6 **S** Department of Navy, Washington, DC — 43 10 209 7234 73 644240 1119 — — —

CAMPBELL—Santa Clara County
CHEMICAL DEPENDENCY INSTITUTE OF NORTHERN CALIFORNIA, 3333 South Bascom Avenue, Zip 95008; tel. 408/559–2000; Roy R. Shelden, Administrator and Chief Executive Officer (Nonreporting) — 33 82 40 — — — — — — —

CANOGA PARK—Los Angeles County, See Los Angeles

CARMICHAEL—Sacramento County
★ MERCY AMERICAN RIVER/MERCY SAN JUAN HOSPITAL, (Formerly Mercy Healthcare Sacramento), (Includes Mercy American River Hospital, Mercy San Juan Hospital), 6501 Coyle Avenue, Zip 95608, Mailing Address: P.O. Box 479, Zip 95608; tel. 916/537–5000; Sister Bridget McCarthy, President **A**1 9 10 **F**4 6 7 10 12 16 19 22 23 25 28 30 32 33 35 39 41 42 43 44 49 50 64 65 71 72 73 74 **P**3 5 **S** Catholic Healthcare West, San Francisco, CA **N** Catholic HealthCare West (CHW), San Francisco, CA — 21 10 352 17063 221 140200 2683 — — 1516

CASTRO VALLEY—Alameda County
□ EDEN HOSPITAL MEDICAL CENTER, 20103 Lake Chabot Road, Zip 94546; tel. 510/537–1234; Edward Schreck, President and Chief Executive Officer (Total facility includes 67 beds in nursing home–type unit) **A**1 2 9 10 **F**6 7 8 10 11 12 14 15 17 19 21 22 26 27 29 30 32 35 37 38 39 40 41 42 44 46 48 49 52 57 58 59 60 62 64 65 67 70 71 73 74 **P**5 **N** Sutter\CHS, Sacramento, CA — 16 10 258 9399 148 111060 1116 71047 28957 640

CATHEDRAL CITY—Riverside County
□ CHARTER BEHAVIORAL HEALTH SYSTEM–PALM SPRINGS, 69–696 Ramon Road, Zip 92234; tel. 619/321–2000; Robert Deney, Chief Executive Officer (Nonreporting) **A**1 10 **S** Magellan Health Services, Atlanta, GA — 33 22 80 — — — — — — —

CEDARVILLE—Modoc County
SURPRISE VALLEY COMMUNITY HOSPITAL, Main and Washington Streets, Zip 96104, Mailing Address: P.O. Box 246, Zip 96104–0246; tel. 916/279–6111; Joyce Gysin, Administrator (Total facility includes 19 beds in nursing home–type unit) **A**9 10 **F**14 15 20 22 26 28 30 32 34 36 39 64 71 73 **P**6 **N** InterMountain Healthcare Network, Alturas, CA — 16 10 26 118 22 2159 10 2261 — 64

CERES—Stanislaus County
MEMORIAL HOSPITALS–CERES See Memorial Hospitals Association, Modesto

CERRITOS—Los Angeles County
□ COLLEGE HOSPITAL, 10802 College Place, Zip 90703–1579; tel. 562/924–9581; Stephen Witt, Chief Executive Officer **A**1 3 9 10 **F**1 14 15 19 21 27 35 46 50 52 53 54 55 56 57 58 59 63 65 71 **P**5 **S** College Health Enterprises, Huntington Beach, CA — 33 22 125 3761 71 15326 0 13912 6656 241

CHESTER—Plumas County
SENECA DISTRICT HOSPITAL, 130 Brentwood Drive, Zip 96020, Mailing Address: Box 737, Zip 96020; tel. 916/258–2151; Bernard G. Hietpas, Administrator (Total facility includes 16 beds in nursing home–type unit) **A**9 10 **F**7 8 14 22 28 31 33 34 40 44 64 65 71 73 — 16 10 26 380 20 11624 52 5839 2892 92

CHICO—Butte County
□ △ CHICO COMMUNITY HOSPITAL, 560 Cohasset Road, Zip 95926; tel. 916/896–5000; Fredrick W. Hodges, Chief Executive Officer (Total facility includes 21 beds in nursing home–type unit) **A**1 7 9 10 **F**14 15 16 19 21 22 27 35 44 49 56 57 65 67 71 73 **P**5 **S** Paracelsus Healthcare Corporation, Houston, TX — 33 10 105 2627 48 26575 0 28135 10542 329

★ N. T. ENLOE MEMORIAL HOSPITAL, West Fifth Avenue and Esplanade, Zip 95926–3386; tel. 916/891–7300; Philip R. Wolfe, Executive Director **A**1 2 9 10 **F**4 7 8 10 11 14 15 17 19 21 22 25 28 30 31 32 33 35 36 37 38 39 40 41 42 43 44 45 51 60 65 67 70 71 72 73 **P**7 — 23 10 208 10623 136 168270 1749 106840 49651 1441

CHINO—San Bernardino County
□ BHC CANYON RIDGE HOSPITAL, (Formerly Canyon Ridge Hospital), 5353 G Street, Zip 91710; tel. 909/590–3700; Diana L. Goulet, Chief Executive Officer **A**1 9 10 **F**1 3 16 27 52 53 54 55 56 57 58 59 65 67 68 **S** Behavioral Healthcare Corporation, Nashville, TN — 33 22 59 2127 36 3254 0 6220 3457 149
CANYON RIDGE HOSPITAL See BHC Canyon Ridge Hospital

Hospital, Address, Telephone, Administrator, Approval, Facility, and Physician Codes, Health Care System, Network	Classi-fication Codes		Utilization Data					Expense (thousands) of dollars		
	Control	Service	Beds	Admissions	Census	Outpatient Visits	Births	Total	Payroll	Personnel

★ American Hospital Association (AHA) membership
□ Joint Commission on Accreditation of Healthcare Organizations (JCAHO) accreditation
+ American Osteopathic Hospital Association (AOHA) membership
○ American Osteopathic Association (AOA) accreditation
△ Commission on Accreditation of Rehabilitation Facilities (CARF) accreditation
Control codes 61, 63, 64, 71, 72 and 73 indicate hospitals listed by AOHA, but not registered by AHA. For definition of numerical codes, see page A4

Hospital	Control	Service	Beds	Admissions	Census	Outpatient Visits	Births	Total	Payroll	Personnel
✶ COLUMBIA CHINO VALLEY MEDICAL CENTER, 5451 Walnut Avenue, Zip 91710; tel. 909/464–8600; Anthony A. Armada, Chief Executive Officer (Total facility includes 14 beds in nursing home–type unit) **A**1 9 10 **F**7 8 16 17 19 21 22 28 30 32 33 35 37 39 40 44 49 64 65 66 67 71 73 **P**2 5 7 **S** Columbia/HCA Healthcare Corporation, Nashville, TN	33	10	104	6015	60	—	1188	32220	14589	402
HOSPITAL OF THE CALIFORNIA INSTITUTION FOR MEN, 14901 Central Avenue, Zip 91710, Mailing Address: Box 128, Zip 91710; tel. 909/597–1821; Pat Garleb, Administrator **F**1 2 3 4 5 6 9 10 11 12 18 19 20 21 22 25 27 29 30 31 33 34 35 37 39 41 42 43 44 45 46 48 49 50 51 52 54 55 56 57 58 59 60 63 64 65 67 69 70 71 72	12	11	80	1192	62	58187	0	—	—	280
CHOWCHILLA—Madera County										
CHOWCHILLA DISTRICT MEMORIAL HOSPITAL, 1104 Ventura Avenue, Zip 93610, Mailing Address: Box 1027, Zip 93610; tel. 209/665–3781; Julia Kiil, Administrator (Nonreporting) **A**9 10	16	10	23	—	—	—	—	—	—	—
CHULA VISTA—San Diego County										
□ BAYVIEW HOSPITAL AND MENTAL HEALTH SYSTEM, (Formerly Bayview Hospital), 330 Moss Street, Zip 91911–2005; tel. 619/426–6310; Roy Rodriguez, Chief Executive Officer **A**1 9 **F**1 2 12 15 16 17 18 41 52 53 54 55 56 57 58 59 65 67	33	22	64	999	25	9811	0	5990	2802	155
✶ SCRIPPS MEMORIAL HOSPITAL–CHULA VISTA, 435 H Street, Zip 91912–1537, Mailing Address: Box 1537, Zip 91910–1537; tel. 619/691–7000; Thomas A. Gammiere, Vice President and Administrator **A**1 9 10 **F**1 2 3 4 6 7 8 10 11 12 14 15 16 17 19 21 22 23 24 25 26 27 28 29 30 31 32 33 34 35 36 37 38 39 40 41 42 43 44 45 46 48 49 50 52 53 54 55 56 57 58 59 60 63 64 65 67 68 69 70 71 72 73 74 **P**3 4 5 7 **S** Scripps Health, San Diego, CA **N** ScrippsHealth, San Diego, CA	23	10	159	8034	101	61048	2032	53173	25100	527
□ SHARP CHULA VISTA MEDICAL CENTER, 751 Medical Center Court, Zip 91911, Mailing Address: Box 1297, Zip 91912; tel. 619/482–5800; Britt Berrett, Chief Executive Officer (Total facility includes 133 beds in nursing home–type unit) (Nonreporting) **A**1 2 3 9 10 **S** Sharp Healthcare, San Diego, CA **N** Sharp Healthcare, San Diego, CA	23	10	306	—	—	—	—	—	—	—
CLEARLAKE—Lake County										
✶ REDBUD COMMUNITY HOSPITAL, 18th Avenue and Highway 53, Zip 95422, Mailing Address: Box 6720, Zip 95422; tel. 707/994–6486; Michael Schultz, Chief Executive Officer **A**1 9 10 **F**7 8 12 15 16 17 19 21 22 27 28 30 32 34 35 37 39 40 41 44 45 46 49 51 65 71 73 74 **P**3 6 **S** Adventist Health, Roseville, CA	16	10	34	1376	13	55054	297	17769	8994	194
CLOVIS—Fresno County										
□ CLOVIS COMMUNITY HOSPITAL, 2755 Herndon Avenue, Zip 93611; tel. 209/323–4060; Mike Barber, Facility Service Integrator (Nonreporting) **A**1 9 10 **S** Community Hospitals of Central California, Fresno, CA	23	10	143	—	—	—	—	—	—	—
COALINGA—Fresno County										
COALINGA REGIONAL MEDICAL CENTER, 1191 Phelps Avenue, Zip 93210; tel. 209/935–6562; James J. Dickson, Administrator and Chief Executive Officer (Total facility includes 54 beds in nursing home–type unit) **A**9 10 **F**19 35 40 44 49 51 64 66 71 72 73 74	16	10	78	1007	46	36511	112	15790	4719	163
COLUSA—Colusa County										
□ COLUSA COMMUNITY HOSPITAL, 199 East Webster Street, Zip 95932, Mailing Address: P.O. Box 331, Zip 95932–0331; tel. 916/458–5821; Edward C. Bland, Chief Executive Officer **A**1 9 10 **F**7 8 11 12 15 16 17 19 21 22 25 28 30 32 34 37 40 41 44 49 64 65 67 71 73	23	10	36	1045	12	19454	246	9792	3949	119
CONCORD—Contra Costa County										
✶ MOUNT DIABLO MEDICAL CENTER, 2540 East Street, Zip 94520, Mailing Address: P.O. Box 4110, Zip 94524–4110; tel. 510/682–8200; Michael L. Wall, President and Chief Executive Officer **A**1 2 9 10 **F**2 3 4 5 7 8 10 11 12 15 16 19 20 21 22 23 24 26 27 28 29 30 31 32 34 35 37 38 39 40 41 42 43 44 45 46 48 49 52 54 55 56 57 58 59 60 61 63 64 65 66 67 71 73 74 **P**4 5 **N** East Bay Medical Network, Emeryville, CA	16	10	209	8310	98	220361	787	108654	46298	837
CORCORAN—Kings County										
CORCORAN DISTRICT HOSPITAL, 1310 Hanna Avenue, Zip 93212, Mailing Address: Box 758, Zip 93212; tel. 209/992–5051; Jimmy M. Knight, Administrator and Chief Executive Officer **A**9 10 **F**12 14 19 22 28 34 44 64 71 73 **P**4	16	10	32	1164	15	—	1	11131	2385	104
CORONA—Riverside County										
□ CHARTER BEHAVIORAL HEALTH SYSTEM OF SOUTHERN CALIFORNIA–CORONA, 2055 Kellogg Avenue, Zip 91719; tel. 909/735–2910; Diana C. Hanyak, Chief Executive Officer (Nonreporting) **A**1 9 10 **S** Magellan Health Services, Atlanta, GA	33	22	92	—	—	—	—	—	—	—
□ △ CORONA REGIONAL MEDICAL CENTER, (Includes Corona Regional Medical Center–Rehabilitation, 730 Magnolia Avenue, Zip 91719; tel. 909/736–7200), 800 South Main Street, Zip 91720; tel. 909/736–6240; Marlene Woodworth, Chief Executive Officer (Total facility includes 30 beds in nursing home–type unit) **A**1 2 7 9 10 **F**4 7 8 12 15 16 17 19 21 22 26 27 28 29 30 32 33 35 37 39 40 41 42 43 44 45 46 48 49 52 54 57 58 59 60 64 65 67 69 71 73 74 **P**5	23	10	228	8219	104	84079	1659	62471	20593	554
CORONADO—San Diego County										
□ SHARP CORONADO HOSPITAL, 250 Prospect Place, Zip 92118; tel. 619/522–3600; Marcia K. Hall, Chief Executive Officer (Total facility includes 149 beds in nursing home–type unit) (Nonreporting) **A**1 9 10 **S** Sharp Healthcare, San Diego, CA	23	10	195	—	—	—	—	—	—	—

Hospital, Address, Telephone, Administrator, Approval, Facility, and Physician Codes, Health Care System, Network	Classi- fication Codes		Utilization Data					Expense (thousands) of dollars		
★ American Hospital Association (AHA) membership □ Joint Commission on Accreditation of Healthcare Organizations (JCAHO) accreditation + American Osteopathic Hospital Association (AOHA) membership ○ American Osteopathic Association (AOA) accreditation △ Commission on Accreditation of Rehabilitation Facilities (CARF) accreditation Control codes 61, 63, 64, 71, 72 and 73 indicate hospitals listed by AOHA, but not registered by AHA. For definition of numerical codes, see page A4	Control	Service	Beds	Admissions	Census	Outpatient Visits	Births	Total	Payroll	Personnel

COSTA MESA—Orange County

□ COLLEGE HOSPITAL COSTA MESA, 301 Victoria Street, Zip 92627; tel. 714/642–2607; Eric Rabjohns, Chief Executive Officer **A**1 9 10 **F**3 12 17 18 19 25 26 27 35 37 39 44 49 52 53 54 56 57 58 59 65 67 71 73 **S** College Health Enterprises, Huntington Beach, CA	33	22	119	4372	76	—	0	20852	9195	256

COVINA—Los Angeles County

⊡ CHARTER BEHAVIORAL HEALTH SYSTEM OF SOUTHERN CALIFORNIA–CHARTER OAK, 1161 East Covina Boulevard, Zip 91724–1161; tel. 818/966–1632; Todd A. Smith, Chief Executive Officer **A**1 9 10 **F**3 15 52 53 57 59 65 **P**5 7 8 **S** Magellan Health Services, Atlanta, GA	33	22	95	2848	48	0	0	—	—	97
□ CITRUS VALLEY MEDICAL CENTER INTER–COMMUNITY CAMPUS, 210 West San Bernardino Road, Zip 91723–1901; tel. 818/331–7331; Warren J. Kirk, Administrator **A**1 2 9 10 **F**4 7 8 10 11 12 14 15 16 17 19 21 22 28 29 30 32 33 34 35 36 37 38 39 40 41 42 43 44 45 46 48 49 52 60 63 64 65 66 67 71 73 74 **P**1 5 7 **S** Citrus Valley Health Partners, Covina, CA	23	10	252	10004	144	54302	836	72885	28747	725

CRESCENT CITY—Del Norte County

⊡ SUTTER COAST HOSPITAL, 800 East Washington Boulevard, Zip 95531; tel. 707/464–8511; John E. Menaugh, Chief Executive Officer **A**1 9 10 **F**7 8 13 16 17 19 22 23 28 29 30 31 32 33 34 35 37 40 41 44 45 49 65 71 72 73 74 **P**3 5 7 **S** Sutter Health, Sacramento, CA **N** Sutter\CHS, Sacramento, CA	23	10	47	2531	30	102701	319	25987	9824	339

CULVER CITY—Los Angeles County

□ BROTMAN MEDICAL CENTER, 3828 Delmas Terrace, Zip 90231–2459, Mailing Address: Box 2459, Zip 90231–2459; tel. 310/836–7000; John V. Fenton, Chief Executive Officer (Total facility includes 21 beds in nursing home–type unit) (Nonreporting) **A**1 9 10 **S** TENET Healthcare Corporation, Santa Barbara, CA	33	10	240	—	—	—	—	—	—	—
□ WASHINGTON MEDICAL CENTER, 12101 West Washington Boulevard, Zip 90231, Mailing Address: Box 2787, Zip 90231; tel. 310/391–0601; Peter Friedman, Administrator (Nonreporting) **A**1 9 10	33	10	99	—	—	—	—	—	—	—

DALY CITY—San Mateo County

⊡ SETON MEDICAL CENTER, 1900 Sullivan Avenue, Zip 94015–2229; tel. 415/992–4000; Bernadette Smith, Chief Operating Officer (Total facility includes 66 beds in nursing home–type unit) (Nonreporting) **A**1 2 3 5 9 10 **S** Catholic Healthcare West, San Francisco, CA **N** Catholic HealthCare West (CHW), San Francisco, CA	21	10	279	—	—	—	—	—	—	—

DANA POINT—Orange County

□ CAPISTRANO BY THE SEA HOSPITAL, 34000 Capistrano by the Sea Drive, Zip 92629–2104, Mailing Address: Box 398, Zip 92629–2104; tel. 714/496–5702; Barbara Messer, R.N., Administrator (Nonreporting) **A**1 9 10	33	22	82	—	—	—	—	—	—	—

DAVIS—Yolo County

⊡ SUTTER DAVIS HOSPITAL, 2000 Sutter Place, Zip 95616, Mailing Address: P.O. Box 1617, Zip 95617; tel. 916/756–6440; Lawrence A. Maas, Administrator **A**1 9 10 **F**7 12 13 15 16 17 19 20 22 23 28 32 35 37 40 41 42 44 65 68 71 73 **P**3 **S** Sutter Health, Sacramento, CA **N** Sutter\CHS, Sacramento, CA	23	10	48	3012	20	68966	1097	27927	10238	230

DEER PARK—Napa County

⊡ ST. HELENA HOSPITAL, 650 Sanitarium Road, Zip 94576, Mailing Address: P.O. Box 250, Zip 94576; tel. 707/963–3611; JoAline Olson, R.N., President and Chief Executive Officer (Total facility includes 23 beds in nursing home–type unit) (Nonreporting) **A**1 9 10 **S** Adventist Health, Roseville, CA **N** Adventist Health–Northern California, Deer Park, CA	21	10	168	—	—	—	—	—	—	—

DELANO—Kern County

□ DELANO REGIONAL MEDICAL CENTER, 1401 Garces Highway, Zip 93215, Mailing Address: Box 460, Zip 93216; tel. 805/725–4800; Bryan M. Ballard, Executive Director (Total facility includes 45 beds in nursing home–type unit) **A**1 9 10 **F**7 8 10 12 14 15 16 17 19 20 21 22 27 28 30 31 32 35 39 40 44 45 46 49 59 64 65 71 73 **P**5	23	10	156	3777	79	22582	1092	21815	9795	496

DINUBA—Tulare County

★ ALTA DISTRICT HOSPITAL, 500 Adelaide Way, Zip 93618–1698; tel. 209/591–4171; Robert M. Montion, Administrator (Total facility includes 18 beds in nursing home–type unit) **A**9 10 **F**15 19 20 22 34 35 36 44 64 65 71 73	16	10	50	1322	19	39947	0	9431	3396	119

DOS PALOS—Merced County

□ DOS PALOS MEMORIAL HOSPITAL, 2118 Marguerite Street, Zip 93620; tel. 209/392–6106; Darryl E. Henley, Administrator (Nonreporting) **A**9 10	23	10	15	—	—	—	—	—	—	—

DOWNEY—Los Angeles County

□ DOWNEY COMMUNITY HOSPITAL FOUNDATION, (Includes Downey Community Hospital, 11500 Brookshire Avenue, Mailing Address: P.O. Box 7010, Zip 90241–7010; tel. 310/904–5000; Rio Hondo Memorial Hospital, 8300 East Telegraph Road, Zip 90240; tel. 310/806–1821), 11500 Brookshire Avenue, Zip 90241–4990; tel. 310/904–5000; Allen R. Korneff, President and Chief Executive Officer (Total facility includes 20 beds in nursing home–type unit) **A**1 9 10 12 **F**4 7 8 10 11 12 19 21 22 23 26 27 28 30 32 35 36 37 38 40 41 42 43 44 45 48 49 60 63 64 65 67 71 73 **P**7	23	10	222	11639	140	149211	1883	89451	38006	1087
⊡ △ LAC–RANCHO LOS AMIGOS MEDICAL CENTER, 7601 East Imperial Highway, Zip 90242; tel. 562/401–7022; Consuelo C. Diaz, Chief Executive Officer **A**1 3 5 7 9 10 **F**1 2 4 5 7 9 10 11 12 13 14 15 16 17 19 20 21 22 23 25 26 27 28 29 30 31 32 34 35 37 38 39 40 41 42 43 44 45 46 47 48 49 50 51 52 53 54 55 56 57 58 59 60 61 63 64 65 66 68 69 70 71 72 73 74 **P**3 5 6 **S** Los Angeles County–Department of Health Services, Los Angeles, CA RIO HONDO MEMORIAL HOSPITAL See Downey Community Hospital Foundation	13	46	300	3819	304	68584	0	236462	79395	1927

Hospital, Address, Telephone, Administrator, Approval, Facility, and Physician Codes, Health Care System, Network	Classi-fication Codes		Utilization Data					Expense (thousands) of dollars		
★ American Hospital Association (AHA) membership □ Joint Commission on Accreditation of Healthcare Organizations (JCAHO) accreditation + American Osteopathic Hospital Association (AOHA) membership ○ American Osteopathic Association (AOA) accreditation △ Commission on Accreditation of Rehabilitation Facilities (CARF) accreditation Control codes 61, 63, 64, 71, 72 and 73 indicate hospitals listed by AOHA, but not registered by AHA. For definition of numerical codes, see page A4	Control	Service	Beds	Admissions	Census	Outpatient Visits	Births	Total	Payroll	Personnel

DUARTE—Los Angeles County

✸ CITY OF HOPE NATIONAL MEDICAL CENTER, (CANCER), 1500 East Duarte Road, Zip 91010–3000; tel. 818/359–8111; Charles M. Balch, M.D., President and Chief Executive Officer **A**1 2 3 5 9 10 **F**8 12 15 16 17 19 20 21 30 32 34 35 37 41 42 44 45 46 49 50 60 65 69 71 73 **P**6	23	49	145	4139	109	102406	0	171252	75343	1905
□ SANTA TERESITA HOSPITAL, 819 Buena Vista Street, Zip 91010–1703; tel. 818/359–3243; Michael J. Costello, Jr., Chief Executive Officer (Total facility includes 133 beds in nursing home–type unit) (Nonreporting) **A**1 2 9 10	21	10	283	—	—	—	—	—	—	—

EDWARDS AFB—Kern County

✸ U. S. AIR FORCE HOSPITAL, 30 Hospital Road, Building 5500, Zip 93524–1730; tel. 805/277–2010; Major Greg Allen, MSC, USAF, Commander **A**1 **F**1 2 3 4 5 6 7 8 9 10 11 12 13 14 15 16 17 18 19 20 21 22 23 24 25 26 27 28 29 30 31 32 33 34 35 36 37 38 39 40 41 42 43 44 45 46 47 48 49 50 51 52 53 54 55 56 57 58 59 60 61 62 63 64 65 66 67 68 69 71 72 73 74 **S** Department of the Air Force, Washington, DC	41	10	10	1002	5	96654	256	—	—	378

EL CAJON—San Diego County

KAISER FOUNDATION HOSPITAL See Kaiser Foundation Hospital, San Diego

✸ SCRIPPS HOSPITAL–EAST COUNTY, 1688 East Main Street, Zip 92021; tel. 619/593–5600; Robin B. Brown, Vice President and Administrator (Total facility includes 35 beds in nursing home–type unit) **A**1 9 10 **F**4 7 8 10 11 12 13 17 19 22 27 28 31 32 34 35 36 37 38 40 41 42 44 45 46 48 49 52 56 57 59 64 65 69 70 71 73 74 **P**1 3 5 7 8 **S** Scripps Health, San Diego, CA **N** ScrippsHealth, San Diego, CA	23	10	105	3271	42	35513	0	37830	11121	246

EL CENTRO—Imperial County

✸ EL CENTRO REGIONAL MEDICAL CENTER, 1415 Ross Avenue, Zip 92243; tel. 619/339–7100; Ted Fox, Administrator and Chief Executive Officer **A**1 9 10 **F**8 16 17 19 21 22 23 25 28 30 34 35 37 38 40 41 44 45 46 54 56 60 63 65 67 71 73 **P**4 5	14	10	107	6412	60	55149	1424	37560	14782	504

ELDRIDGE—Sonoma County

SONOMA DEVELOPMENTAL CENTER, 15000 Arnold Drive, Zip 95431; tel. 707/938–6000; Timothy L. Meeker, Executive Director **A**9 10 **F**1 2 3 4 5 8 9 10 11 12 16 17 18 19 20 21 22 23 24 25 26 27 28 29 30 31 32 33 34 35 37 38 39 41 42 43 44 45 46 47 48 49 50 51 52 53 54 55 56 57 58 59 60 61 62 63 64 65 66 67 68 69 70 71 72 73 74 **P**6	12	62	996	18	1038	0	0	110618	63762	1661

ENCINITAS—San Diego County

□ BHC SAN LUIS REY HOSPITAL, (Formerly CPC San Luis Rey Hospital), 335 Saxony Road, Zip 92024–2723; tel. 619/753–1245; William T. Sparrow, Chief Executive Officer (Nonreporting) **A**1 9 10 **S** Behavioral Healthcare Corporation, Nashville, TN	33	22	117	—	—	—	—	—	—	—
✸ △ SCRIPPS MEMORIAL HOSPITAL–ENCINITAS, 354 Santa Fe Drive, Zip 92024, Mailing Address: P.O. Box 817, Zip 92023; tel. 619/753–6501; Gerald E. Bracht, Vice President and Administrator (Nonreporting) **A**1 2 7 9 10 **S** Scripps Health, San Diego, CA **N** ScrippsHealth, San Diego, CA	23	10	145	—	—	—	—	—	—	—

ENCINO—Los Angeles County, See Los Angeles

ESCONDIDO—San Diego County

✸ PALOMAR MEDICAL CENTER, 555 East Valley Parkway, Zip 92025–3084; tel. 619/739–3000; Victoria M. Penland, Administrator and Chief Operating Officer (Total facility includes 96 beds in nursing home–type unit) **A**1 2 9 10 **F**3 4 7 8 10 17 19 21 22 23 25 27 28 29 30 31 32 33 34 35 37 38 39 40 41 42 43 44 45 46 49 51 52 54 55 56 57 58 59 60 61 63 64 65 66 70 71 73 **P**6 7 **S** Palomar Pomerado Health System, San Diego, CA **N** Health First Network, San Diego, CA	16	10	395	15074	239	180417	2971	124628	47494	1297

EUREKA—Humboldt County

✸ △ GENERAL HOSPITAL, 2200 Harrison Avenue, Zip 95501; tel. 707/445–5111; David S. Wanger, Chief Executive Officer **A**1 7 9 10 **F**7 8 12 16 19 20 21 22 23 25 28 31 32 33 34 35 37 38 40 41 44 48 49 51 56 61 63 65 71 72 73	33	10	65	3233	40	34893	629	28138	11867	306
✸ SAINT JOSEPH HOSPITAL, 2700 Dolbeer Street, Zip 95501; tel. 707/445–8121; Paul J. Chodkowski, President and Chief Executive Officer **A**1 2 9 10 **F**3 7 8 9 10 11 14 15 16 17 19 20 21 22 27 28 29 30 31 32 33 34 35 37 40 41 42 44 45 46 49 60 65 67 71 73 74 **P**3 5 6 7 **S** St. Joseph Health System, Orange, CA **N** Saint Joseph Health System, Orange, CA	21	10	62	3474	43	126732	0	35725	12271	375

EXETER—Tulare County

□ MEMORIAL HOSPITAL AT EXETER, 215 Crespi Avenue, Zip 93221–1399; tel. 209/592–2151; Sally Brewer, Chief Executive Officer (Total facility includes 62 beds in nursing home–type unit) **A**1 9 10 **F**8 13 16 17 19 21 22 26 28 30 34 41 44 64 65 71 72 74 **P**5	23	10	80	221	65	21413	0	8872	4080	165

FAIRFIELD—Solano County

✸ NORTHBAY MEDICAL CENTER, 1200 B. Gale Wilson Boulevard, Zip 94533–3587; tel. 707/429–3600; Deborah Sugiyama, President (Total facility includes 11 beds in nursing home–type unit) **A**1 2 9 10 **F**7 8 10 12 13 14 15 16 17 19 21 22 23 28 30 32 33 35 36 37 39 40 41 42 44 49 60 64 65 67 71 73 73 **P**3 5 **S** NorthBay Healthcare System, Fairfield, CA **N** NorthBay Healthcare System, Fairfield, CA	23	10	92	5196	49	73848	1636	53273	22318	340

FALL RIVER MILLS—Shasta County

MAYERS MEMORIAL HOSPITAL DISTRICT, Highway 299 East, Zip 96028, Mailing Address: Box 459, Zip 96028; tel. 916/336–5511; Everett L. Beck, Administrator (Total facility includes 50 beds in nursing home–type unit) (Nonreporting) **A**9 10 **N** InterMountain Healthcare Network, Alturas, CA	16	10	72	—	—	—	—	—	—	—

Hospital, Address, Telephone, Administrator, Approval, Facility, and Physician Codes, Health Care System, Network	Classi-fication Codes		Utilization Data					Expense (thousands) of dollars		
★ American Hospital Association (AHA) membership □ Joint Commission on Accreditation of Healthcare Organizations (JCAHO) accreditation + American Osteopathic Hospital Association (AOHA) membership ○ American Osteopathic Association (AOA) accreditation △ Commission on Accreditation of Rehabilitation Facilities (CARF) accreditation Control codes 61, 63, 64, 71, 72 and 73 indicate hospitals listed by AOHA, but not registered by AHA. For definition of numerical codes, see page A4	Control	Service	Beds	Admissions	Census	Outpatient Visits	Births	Total	Payroll	Personnel

FALLBROOK—San Diego County

✠ FALLBROOK HOSPITAL DISTRICT, 624 East Elder Street, Zip 92028; tel. 619/728–1191; Corey A. Seale, Chief Executive Officer (Total facility includes 95 beds in nursing home–type unit) **A**1 9 10 **F**7 8 11 12 14 15 19 21 22 25 27 30 32 33 34 35 37 40 42 44 49 51 54 64 65 67 71 **P**4

| 16 | 10 | 142 | 2324 | 96 | — | 537 | 20410 | 11046 | 337 |

FOLSOM—Sacramento County

✠ MERCY HOSPITAL OF FOLSOM, 1650 Creekside Drive, Zip 95630–3405; tel. 916/983–7400; Donald C. Hudson, Vice President and Chief Operating Officer **A**1 9 10 **F**4 7 8 9 10 11 12 14 15 17 19 22 25 26 28 30 31 32 33 35 37 38 40 41 42 43 44 46 47 48 49 50 60 62 64 65 67 71 72 73 74 **P**3 5 **S** Catholic Healthcare West, San Francisco, CA **N** Catholic HealthCare West (CHW), San Francisco, CA

| 21 | 10 | 95 | 3429 | 31 | 28147 | 721 | 22668 | 9869 | 318 |

□ VENCOR HOSPITAL–SACRAMENTO, 223 Fargo Way, Zip 95630; tel. 916/351–9151; Meredith Taylor, Administrator (Nonreporting) **A**1 9 10 **S** Vencor, Incorporated, Louisville, KY

| 33 | 10 | 32 | — | — | — | — | — | — | — |

FONTANA—San Bernardino County

✠ KAISER FOUNDATION HOSPITAL, 9961 Sierra Avenue, Zip 92335–6794; tel. 909/427–5000; Patricia Siegel, Senior Vice President, Health Plan, Hospitals and Inland Empire Area Manager **A**1 2 3 5 10 **F**2 3 4 7 8 10 11 12 14 15 16 19 21 22 23 25 28 29 30 32 33 35 37 38 41 42 43 44 45 46 48 49 51 53 54 55 56 58 59 60 61 63 65 66 67 68 69 71 73 **S** Kaiser Foundation Hospitals, Oakland, CA

| 23 | 10 | 287 | 17158 | 173 | 62997 | 3249 | — | — | 811 |

FORT BRAGG—Mendocino County

□ MENDOCINO COAST DISTRICT HOSPITAL, 700 River Drive, Zip 95437; tel. 707/961–1234; Elizabeth MacGard, Chief Executive Officer **A**1 9 10 **F**7 8 11 12 14 15 16 17 19 21 22 26 28 29 30 31 32 33 34 35 36 37 39 40 41 42 44 45 46 49 60 63 65 67 68 71 73 **P**3

| 16 | 10 | 54 | 1983 | 23 | 53946 | 231 | 19653 | 9048 | 242 |

FORT IRWIN—San Bernardino County

✠ WEED ARMY COMMUNITY HOSPITAL, Zip 92310–5065; tel. 619/380–3108; Colonel James Beson, Commander **A**1 **F**2 3 8 11 12 14 15 16 17 19 20 21 22 25 28 29 30 31 34 35 37 38 39 40 41 45 46 47 51 52 54 56 58 61 65 70 71 73 **P**5 **S** Department of the Army, Office of the Surgeon General, Falls Church, VA

| 42 | 10 | 27 | 1707 | 11 | 121357 | 289 | 23070 | — | 314 |

FORTUNA—Humboldt County

✠ REDWOOD MEMORIAL HOSPITAL, 3300 Renner Drive, Zip 95540; tel. 707/725–3361; Paul J. Chodkowski, President and Chief Executive Officer (Nonreporting) **A**1 2 9 10 **S** St. Joseph Health System, Orange, CA **N** Saint Joseph Health System, Orange, CA

| 21 | 10 | 35 | — | — | — | — | — | — | — |

FOUNTAIN VALLEY—Orange County

□ FOUNTAIN VALLEY REGIONAL HOSPITAL AND MEDICAL CENTER, 17100 Euclid at Warner, Zip 92708; tel. 714/966–7200; Richard E. Butler, Chief Executive Officer (Total facility includes 80 beds in nursing home–type unit) **A**1 2 5 9 10 **F**1 4 7 8 10 11 12 14 15 16 17 19 21 22 27 28 29 30 31 32 34 35 37 38 39 40 41 42 43 44 45 46 47 49 52 57 59 60 63 64 65 67 71 73 74 **P**5 7 **S** TENET Healthcare Corporation, Santa Barbara, CA

| 33 | 10 | 413 | 14854 | 191 | 67063 | 3955 | 106043 | 47027 | 1286 |

□ ORANGE COAST MEMORIAL MEDICAL CENTER, 9920 Talbert Avenue, Zip 92708; tel. 714/378–7000; Barry Arbuckle, Ph.D., Chief Operating Officer **A**1 3 10 **F**2 3 4 7 8 9 10 11 12 13 16 17 19 21 22 23 25 26 27 28 30 32 33 34 35 37 38 39 40 41 42 43 44 45 46 47 48 49 50 51 52 53 54 55 56 57 58 59 60 61 63 64 65 67 69 71 72 73 74 **P**1 2 3 5 6 7 **S** Memorial Health Services, Long Beach, CA

| 23 | 10 | 230 | 8241 | 86 | 27184 | 1166 | — | — | 585 |

FREMONT—Alameda County

□ BHC FREMONT HOSPITAL, (Formerly Fremont Hospital), 39001 Sundale Drive, Zip 94538; tel. 510/796–1100; Terry Johnson, Chief Executive Officer **A**1 9 10 **F**2 3 12 15 16 22 52 53 55 56 57 58 59 65 67 **S** Behavioral Healthcare Corporation, Nashville, TN

| 33 | 22 | 78 | 1529 | 35 | 4858 | 0 | — | — | 83 |

✠ WASHINGTON TOWNSHIP HEALTH CARE DISTRICT, 2000 Mowry Avenue, Zip 94538–1716; tel. 510/797–1111; Nancy D. Farber, Chief Executive Officer (Nonreporting) **A**1 2 9 10 **N** East Bay Medical Network, Emeryville, CA

| 16 | 10 | 202 | — | — | — | — | — | — | — |

FRENCH CAMP—San Joaquin County

□ △ SAN JOAQUIN GENERAL HOSPITAL, 500 West Hospital Road, Zip 95231, Mailing Address: P.O. Box 1020, Stockton, Zip 95201; tel. 209/468–6600; Michael N. Smith, Director Healthcare Services **A**1 3 5 7 9 10 **F**2 3 4 7 8 10 11 12 15 16 17 18 19 20 21 22 23 25 26 27 28 31 32 33 34 35 37 38 39 40 42 43 44 46 48 49 51 52 53 54 55 56 57 58 60 63 65 67 68 69 71 72 73 **P**6

| 13 | 10 | 195 | 8142 | 129 | 197675 | 1842 | 91690 | 40215 | 1340 |

FRESNO—Fresno County

□ BHC CEDAR VISTA HOSPITAL, (Formerly Cedar Vista Hospital Comprehensive Psychiatric Services), 7171 North Cedar Avenue, Zip 93720; tel. 209/449–8000; Arthur M. Ginsberg, Chief Executive Officer **A**1 9 10 **F**2 3 12 14 15 52 53 55 56 57 58 59 65 **S** Behavioral Healthcare Corporation, Nashville, TN
CEDAR VISTA HOSPITAL COMPREHENSIVE PSYCHIATRIC SERVICES See BHC Cedar Vista Hospital

| 33 | 22 | 61 | 1671 | 31 | 2529 | 0 | 5906 | 3287 | 105 |

✠ △ FRESNO COMMUNITY HOSPITAL AND MEDICAL CENTER, Fresno and R Streets, Zip 93721, Mailing Address: Box 1232, Zip 93715; tel. 209/442–6000; J. Philip Hinton, M.D., Chief Executive Officer **A**1 2 7 9 10 **F**1 2 3 4 7 8 10 11 14 15 16 17 19 21 22 23 25 26 28 29 30 31 32 33 34 35 37 38 39 40 41 42 43 44 45 46 48 49 50 52 53 54 55 56 57 58 59 60 61 63 64 65 69 71 73 74 **P**5 7 8 **S** Community Hospitals of Central California, Fresno, CA

| 23 | 10 | 375 | 17356 | 236 | 204035 | 4816 | 150924 | 66566 | 1827 |

Hospital, Address, Telephone, Administrator, Approval, Facility, and Physician Codes, Health Care System, Network	Classi-fication Codes		Utilization Data					Expense (thousands) of dollars		
★ American Hospital Association (AHA) membership □ Joint Commission on Accreditation of Healthcare Organizations (JCAHO) accreditation + American Osteopathic Hospital Association (AOHA) membership ○ American Osteopathic Association (AOA) accreditation △ Commission on Accreditation of Rehabilitation Facilities (CARF) accreditation Control codes 61, 63, 64, 71, 72 and 73 indicate hospitals listed by AOHA, but not registered by AHA. For definition of numerical codes, see page A4	Control	Service	Beds	Admissions	Census	Outpatient Visits	Births	Total	Payroll	Personnel

FRESNO SURGERY CENTER–THE HOSPITAL FOR SURGERY, (SURGICAL), 6125 North Fresno Street, Zip 93710; tel. 209/431–8000; Alan H. Pierrot, M.D., Chief Executive Officer **A**10 **F**6 8 14 15 23 28 34 44	32	49	20	1703	9	4355	0	15056	6331	152
✠ KAISER FOUNDATION HOSPITAL, 7300 North Fresno Street, Zip 93720; tel. 209/448–4500; Edward S. Glavis, Administrator **A**1 10 **F**2 3 4 7 8 9 10 11 12 13 14 15 16 17 18 19 21 22 23 25 26 27 28 29 30 31 32 33 34 35 37 38 39 40 41 42 43 44 45 46 47 48 49 50 51 52 53 54 55 56 57 58 59 60 61 63 64 65 66 67 68 69 70 71 72 73 74 **P**6 **S** Kaiser Foundation Hospitals, Oakland, CA	23	10	89	4375	41	—	1257	—	—	—
✠ SAINT AGNES MEDICAL CENTER, 1303 East Herndon Avenue, Zip 93720–3397; tel. 209/449–3000; Sister Ruth Marie Nickerson, President and Chief Executive Officer **A**1 2 9 10 **F**1 3 4 6 7 8 10 11 12 15 16 19 22 25 26 28 29 30 31 32 33 34 35 37 38 39 40 41 42 43 44 45 49 53 54 55 56 57 58 59 60 62 65 66 67 68 70 71 72 73 74 **P**1 5 7 **S** Holy Cross Health System Corporation, South Bend, IN	21	10	326	20475	232	297171	3247	190009	74270	1986
□ △ SAN JOAQUIN VALLEY REHABILITATION HOSPITAL, 7173 North Sharon Avenue, Zip 93720; tel. 209/436–3600; W. David Smiley, Chief Executive Officer (Nonreporting) **A**1 7 10	33	46	62							
□ △ VALLEY CHILDREN'S HOSPITAL, 3151 North Millbrook, Zip 93703; tel. 209/225–3000; James D. Northway, M.D., President and Chief Executive Officer **A**1 3 5 7 9 10 **F**10 13 14 15 16 17 19 21 22 25 28 30 32 34 35 38 41 42 43 44 45 46 47 48 49 51 58 60 65 67 71 72 73 **P**1 5	23	50	201	9064	145	137127	0	110795	53519	1687
□ VALLEY MEDICAL CENTER OF FRESNO, 445 South Cedar Avenue, Zip 93702–2907; tel. 209/453–4000; Terry Henry, Interim Administrator (Nonreporting) **A**1 2 3 5 8 9 10	13	10	257							
✠ VETERANS AFFAIRS MEDICAL CENTER, 2615 East Clinton Avenue, Zip 93703; tel. 209/225–6100; James C. DeNiro, Director (Total facility includes 60 beds in nursing home–type unit) **A**1 2 3 5 **F**1 2 3 4 6 8 10 14 15 16 19 20 21 22 26 27 28 29 30 31 32 33 34 35 37 39 41 42 44 45 46 49 51 52 54 56 57 58 60 64 65 67 71 73 74 **P**6 **S** Department of Veterans Affairs, Washington, DC	45	10	220	4326	144	134981	0	63039	42795	774
FULLERTON—Orange County										
✠ △ ST. JUDE MEDICAL CENTER, 101 East Valencia Mesa Drive, Zip 92635; tel. 714/992–3000; Robert J. Fraschetti, President and Chief Executive Officer **A**1 2 7 9 10 **F**2 3 4 7 8 10 11 12 13 14 15 16 17 18 19 21 22 23 26 27 28 29 30 31 32 33 34 35 36 37 38 39 40 41 42 43 44 46 48 49 51 52 54 55 56 57 58 59 60 63 64 65 67 68 71 73 74 **P**3 5 7 **S** St. Joseph Health System, Orange, CA **N** Friendly Hills HealthCare Network, LaHabra, CA; Saint Joseph Health System, Orange, CA	21	10	347	13819	197	175001	2269	120662	46781	1455
GARBERVILLE—Humboldt County										
SOUTHERN HUMBOLDT COMMUNITY HEALTHCARE DISTRICT, 733 Cedar Street, Zip 95542–3292; tel. 707/923–3921; Michael E. Helroid, Administrator and Chief Executive Officer (Total facility includes 8 beds in nursing home–type unit) **A**9 10 **F**3 6 7 8 11 12 13 14 15 16 17 22 27 28 29 30 31 32 33 34 36 39 40 41 45 46 49 51 61 64 65 66 67 68 71 **P**3	16	10	18	358	12	17640	34	3584	1824	73
GARDEN GROVE—Orange County										
□ GARDEN GROVE HOSPITAL AND MEDICAL CENTER, 12601 Garden Grove Boulevard, Zip 92843–1959; tel. 714/741–2700; Timothy Smith, President and Chief Executive Officer (Total facility includes 12 beds in nursing home–type unit) **A**1 9 10 **F**7 12 16 19 21 22 23 26 27 28 30 31 32 33 34 35 37 38 40 41 42 44 49 63 64 65 71 73 **P**5 7 **S** TENET Healthcare Corporation, Santa Barbara, CA **N** Tenet Healthcare Corporation, Santa Barbara, CA	33	10	167	8417	84	45739	2763	40052	19893	509
GARDENA—Los Angeles County										
□ COMMUNITY HOSPITAL OF GARDENA, 1246 West 155th Street, Zip 90247–4062; tel. 310/323–5330; Raymond N. Smith, Chief Executive Officer (Total facility includes 20 beds in nursing home–type unit) **A**1 9 10 **F**8 15 19 21 22 25 28 33 34 35 37 41 44 49 50 51 60 63 64 65 71 72 **P**5	33	10	58	640	12	3238	0	—	—	—
□ MEMORIAL HOSPITAL OF GARDENA, 1145 West Redondo Beach Boulevard, Zip 90247; tel. 310/532–4200; Frank Katsuda, Administrator (Nonreporting) **A**1 9 10	33	10	107	—	—	—	—	—	—	—
GILROY—Santa Clara County										
✠ COLUMBIA SOUTH VALLEY HOSPITAL, (Formerly South Valley Hospital), 9400 No Name Uno, Zip 95020–2368; tel. 408/848–2000; Beverly Gilmore, Chief Executive Officer (Total facility includes 21 beds in nursing home–type unit) (Nonreporting) **A**1 9 10 **S** Columbia/HCA Healthcare Corporation, Nashville, TN	33	10	93	—	—	—	—	—	—	—
GLENDALE—Los Angeles County										
✠ □ GLENDALE ADVENTIST MEDICAL CENTER, 1509 Wilson Terrace, Zip 91206–4007; tel. 818/409–8000; David Nelson, Chief Operating Officer **A**1 2 3 5 7 9 10 **F**3 4 5 6 7 8 10 11 12 15 16 17 18 19 21 22 23 24 27 28 29 30 32 34 35 37 38 40 41 42 43 44 48 49 52 53 54 55 56 57 58 59 60 64 65 67 68 69 71 72 73 74 **P**3 5 **S** Adventist Health, Roseville, CA **N** Adventist Health–Southern California, Glendale, CA	21	10	396	13982	226	240952	2876	117477	51706	1521
✠ GLENDALE MEMORIAL HOSPITAL AND HEALTH CENTER, 1420 South Central Avenue, Zip 91204–2594; tel. 818/502–1900; Roger E. Seaver, President and Chief Executive Officer (Total facility includes 30 beds in nursing home–type unit) **A**1 2 9 10 **F**3 4 7 8 10 11 12 16 17 18 19 21 22 24 27 28 29 30 32 34 36 37 39 40 41 42 43 44 45 48 49 52 54 56 59 60 63 64 65 67 71 73 **P**3 4 5 7 **S** UniHealth, Burbank, CA **N** UniHealth, Burbank, CA	23	10	273	12448	174	116119	1762	89671	42754	1020

Hospital, Address, Telephone, Administrator, Approval, Facility, and Physician Codes, Health Care System, Network	Classi-fication Codes		Utilization Data					Expense (thousands) of dollars		
	Control	Service	Beds	Admissions	Census	Outpatient Visits	Births	Total	Payroll	Personnel

★ American Hospital Association (AHA) membership
□ Joint Commission on Accreditation of Healthcare Organizations (JCAHO) accreditation
+ American Osteopathic Hospital Association (AOHA) membership
○ American Osteopathic Association (AOA) accreditation
△ Commission on Accreditation of Rehabilitation Facilities (CARF) accreditation
Control codes 61, 63, 64, 71, 72 and 73 indicate hospitals listed by AOHA, but not registered by AHA. For definition of numerical codes, see page A4

Hospital	Control	Service	Beds	Admissions	Census	Outpatient Visits	Births	Total	Payroll	Personnel
⊠ VERDUGO HILLS HOSPITAL, 1812 Verdugo Boulevard, Zip 91208, Mailing Address: P.O. Box 1431, Zip 91209–1431; tel. 818/790–7100; Bernard Glossy, President (Total facility includes 18 beds in nursing home–type unit) **A**1 2 9 10 **F**7 8 11 12 13 14 15 16 19 20 21 22 24 26 28 29 32 35 37 40 42 44 45 49 52 57 59 63 64 65 66 67 71 73 **P**5 7 **S** Southern California Healthcare System, Pasadena, CA **N** Southern California Healthcare Systems, Pasadena, CA	23	10	134	5081	49	37877	1106	41399	17526	438
GLENDORA—Los Angeles County										
⊠ FOOTHILL PRESBYTERIAN HOSPITAL–MORRIS L. JOHNSTON MEMORIAL, 250 South Grand Avenue, Zip 91741; tel. 818/857–3235; Bryan R. Rogers, President and Chief Executive Officer **A**1 2 9 10 **F**4 7 8 10 11 12 14 15 16 17 19 21 22 28 29 30 32 33 34 35 36 37 39 40 41 42 43 44 45 46 49 60 63 65 66 67 71 73 74 **P**1 3 5 7 **S** Citrus Valley Health Partners, Covina, CA	23	10	106	5164	50	67327	1180	33263	14656	536
⊠ HUNTINGTON EAST VALLEY HOSPITAL, 150 West Alosta Avenue, Zip 91740–4398; tel. 818/335–0231; James W. Maki, Chief Executive Officer **A**1 9 10 **F**7 8 14 15 16 17 19 21 22 26 28 30 37 40 44 52 57 59 65 71 73 74 **P**3 4 5 7 **S** Southern California Healthcare System, Pasadena, CA **N** Southern California Healthcare Systems, Pasadena, CA	23	10	128	2663	30	11138	1134	17171	8014	269
GRANADA HILLS—Los Angeles County, See Los Angeles										
GRASS VALLEY—Nevada County										
⊠ SIERRA NEVADA MEMORIAL HOSPITAL, 155 Glasson Way, Zip 95945–5792, Mailing Address: Box 1029, Zip 95945–5792; tel. 916/274–6000; C. Thomas Collier, President and Chief Executive Officer (Total facility includes 17 beds in nursing home–type unit) **A**1 9 10 **F**7 8 11 12 14 15 16 19 22 34 35 37 39 40 42 44 45 49 60 64 71 **S** Catholic Healthcare West, San Francisco, CA **N** Catholic HealthCare West (CHW), San Francisco, CA	23	10	111	5676	66	96147	550	44967	17380	526
GREENBRAE—Marin County										
⊠ MARIN GENERAL HOSPITAL, 250 Bon Air Road, Zip 94904, Mailing Address: Box 8010, San Rafael, Zip 94912–8010; tel. 415/925–7000; Henry J. Buhrmann, President and Chief Executive Officer **A**1 2 9 10 **F**4 7 8 10 11 12 14 15 16 19 21 22 23 24 28 29 30 31 32 34 35 37 38 40 41 42 43 44 45 46 49 52 53 54 55 56 57 58 59 60 65 71 73 74 **P**1 3 7 **S** Sutter Health, Sacramento, CA **N** Sutter\CHS, Sacramento, CA	23	10	108	9836	97	81047	1621	99117	40200	957
GREENVILLE—Plumas County										
INDIAN VALLEY HOSPITAL DISTRICT, 174 Hot Springs Road, Zip 95947; tel. 916/284–7191; Lynn Seaberg, Administrator and Chief Executive Officer (Total facility includes 19 beds in nursing home–type unit) **A**9 10 **F**15 16 22 28 44 64 71 **P**5 **N** InterMountain Healthcare Network, Alturas, CA	16	10	26	296	21	11836	11	4023	2031	79
GRIDLEY—Butte County										
BIGGS–GRIDLEY MEMORIAL HOSPITAL, 240 Spruce Street, Zip 95948, Mailing Address: Box 97, Zip 95948; tel. 916/846–5671; Charles R. Norton, Administrator (Nonreporting) **A**9 10	23	10	55	—						
HANFORD—Kings County										
□ CENTRAL VALLEY GENERAL HOSPITAL, 1025 North Douty Street, Zip 93230, Mailing Address: Box 480, Zip 93232; tel. 209/583–2100; Gary K. Wiggins, Chief Executive Officer **A**1 9 10 **F**16 19 21 22 25 30 34 37 39 40 44 51 71 73 74 **P**7	33	10	40	2639	22	66723	1127	17027	6292	250
⊠ HANFORD COMMUNITY MEDICAL CENTER, 450 Greenfield Avenue, Zip 93230–0240, Mailing Address: Box 240, Zip 93232–0240; tel. 209/582–9000; Stan B. Berry, FACHE, President **A**1 9 10 **F**7 8 10 12 14 15 16 19 20 22 23 25 28 30 32 33 34 35 37 39 40 41 42 44 45 46 51 60 65 70 71 72 73 74 **P**3 **S** Adventist Health, Roseville, CA	21	10	59	4976	47	161781	1138	46937	16891	650
HARBOR CITY—Los Angeles County, See Los Angeles										
HAWTHORNE—Los Angeles County										
□ HAWTHORNE HOSPITAL, 13300 South Hawthorne Boulevard, Zip 90250; tel. 310/679–3321; Marvin Herschberg, Chief Executive Officer (Nonreporting) **A**1 9 10 **S** Pacific Health Corporation, Long Beach, CA	33	10	73	—	—	—	—	—	—	—
⊠ ROBERT F. KENNEDY MEDICAL CENTER, 4500 West 116th Street, Zip 90250; tel. 310/973–1711; Peter P. Aprato, Administrator and Chief Operating Officer (Total facility includes 34 beds in nursing home–type unit) **A**1 9 10 **F**8 11 12 15 16 17 19 21 22 27 28 30 31 37 41 42 44 45 46 49 52 56 59 63 64 65 67 71 73 **P**5 **S** Catholic Healthcare West, San Francisco, CA **N** Catholic HealthCare West (CHW), San Francisco, CA; Essential HealthCare Network, Monterey Park, CA	23	10	195	5324	109	34975	0	46693	21928	522
HAYWARD—Alameda County										
⊠ KAISER FOUNDATION HOSPITAL, 27400 Hesperian Boulevard, Zip 94545–4297; tel. 510/784–4313; Lisa Koltun, Administrator (Nonreporting) **A**1 10 **S** Kaiser Foundation Hospitals, Oakland, CA **N** Kaiser Foundation Health Plan of Northern California, Oakland, CA	23	10	190	—	—	—	—	—	—	—
□ ST. ROSE HOSPITAL, 27200 Calaroga Avenue, Zip 94545–4383; tel. 510/264–4000; Michael P. Mahoney, President and Chief Executive Officer (Total facility includes 46 beds in nursing home–type unit) (Nonreporting) **A**1 2 9 10 **S** Via Christi Health System, Wichita, KS	21	10	175	—	—	—	—	—	—	—
HEALDSBURG—Sonoma County										
⊠ HEALDSBURG GENERAL HOSPITAL, 1375 University Avenue, Zip 95448; tel. 707/431–6500; Kenneth Madfes, Chief Executive Officer **A**1 9 10 **F**1 11 19 22 31 32 37 40 41 44 49 57 64 71 73 **S** Columbia/HCA Healthcare Corporation, Nashville, TN	33	10	49	2008	23	18573	209	17270	8379	250

Hospital, Address, Telephone, Administrator, Approval, Facility, and Physician Codes, Health Care System, Network	Classi-fication Codes		Utilization Data					Expense (thousands) of dollars		
★ American Hospital Association (AHA) membership □ Joint Commission on Accreditation of Healthcare Organizations (JCAHO) accreditation + American Osteopathic Hospital Association (AOHA) membership ○ American Osteopathic Association (AOA) accreditation △ Commission on Accreditation of Rehabilitation Facilities (CARF) accreditation Control codes 61, 63, 64, 71, 72 and 73 indicate hospitals listed by AOHA, but not registered by AHA. For definition of numerical codes, see page A4	Control	Service	Beds	Admissions	Census	Outpatient Visits	Births	Total	Payroll	Personnel

HEMET—Riverside County

□ HEMET VALLEY MEDICAL CENTER, 1117 East Devonshire Avenue, Zip 92543; tel. 909/652–2811; John Ruffner, Administrator (Nonreporting) A1 9 10 S Valley Health System, Hemet, CA — 16 10 285 — — — — — — —

HOLLISTER—San Benito County

□ HAZEL HAWKINS MEMORIAL HOSPITAL, (Includes Hazel Hawkins Convalescent Hospital–Southside, 3110 Southside Road, Zip 95023; tel. 408/637–5711), 911 Sunset Drive, Zip 95023–5695; tel. 408/637–5711; Louis D. Kraml, Administrator (Total facility includes 52 beds in nursing home–type unit) (Nonreporting) A1 9 10 S Brim, Inc., Portland, OR — 16 10 86 — — — — — — —

HOLLYWOOD—Los Angeles County, See Los Angeles

HUNTINGTON BEACH—Orange County

⊞ COLUMBIA HUNTINGTON BEACH HOSPITAL AND MEDICAL CENTER, 17772 Beach Boulevard, Zip 92647–9932; tel. 714/842–1473; Carol B. Freeman, Chief Executive Officer (Total facility includes 12 beds in nursing home–type unit) A1 9 10 F4 8 11 12 15 16 17 18 19 21 22 23 27 28 32 35 37 39 41 42 44 49 52 55 59 64 65 71 73 P5 S Columbia/HCA Healthcare Corporation, Nashville, TN — 33 10 135 3398 50 59849 163 34843 13406 355

□ PACIFICA HOSPITAL, 18800 Delaware Street, Zip 92648; tel. 714/596–8000; Barbara J. Foster, President and Chief Executive Officer A1 9 10 F1 2 3 4 5 6 7 8 9 10 12 13 15 17 18 19 20 21 22 23 24 25 26 27 28 29 30 31 32 33 34 35 36 38 39 40 41 42 43 44 45 46 47 48 49 50 51 53 54 55 56 57 58 59 60 61 62 63 65 66 67 68 69 70 71 72 73 74 P4 5 7 — 33 10 83 1561 46 32867 0 26639 8138 199

HUNTINGTON PARK—Los Angeles County

□ COMMUNITY HOSPITAL OF HUNTINGTON PARK, (Formerly Community and Mission Hospitals of Huntington), (Includes Mission Hospital of Huntington Park, 3111 East Florence Avenue, tel. 213/582–8261), 2623 East Slauson Avenue, Zip 90255; tel. 213/583–1931; Charles Martinez, Ph.D., Chief Executive Officer (Nonreporting) A1 9 10 S TENET Healthcare Corporation, Santa Barbara, CA N Essential HealthCare Network, Monterey Park, CA — 33 10 226 — — — — — — —

MISSION HOSPITAL OF HUNTINGTON PARK See Community Hospital of Huntington Park

INDIO—Riverside County

□ JOHN F. KENNEDY MEMORIAL HOSPITAL, 47–111 Monroe Street, Zip 92201, Mailing Address: P.O. Drawer LLLL, Zip 92202–2558; tel. 619/347–6191; Michael A. Rembis, Chief Executive Officer A1 9 10 F7 8 10 12 15 16 17 19 22 28 29 30 34 35 36 37 39 40 41 42 44 45 46 49 65 67 71 73 74 P1 2 3 4 5 6 7 8 S TENET Healthcare Corporation, Santa Barbara, CA N Tenet Healthcare Corporation, Santa Barbara, CA — 33 10 130 7732 75 49259 2178 40746 17471 485

INGLEWOOD—Los Angeles County

□ △ CENTINELA HOSPITAL MEDICAL CENTER, 555 East Hardy Street, Zip 90301–4073, Mailing Address: Box 720, Zip 90307–0720; tel. 310/673–4660; John Smithhisler, CHE, Chief Executive Officer (Total facility includes 24 beds in nursing home–type unit) A1 2 3 7 9 10 F4 5 8 10 12 14 15 16 17 19 21 22 23 24 25 27 28 29 30 31 32 34 35 37 38 40 41 42 43 44 45 46 48 49 51 60 61 63 64 65 66 71 72 73 74 P5 7 S TENET Healthcare Corporation, Santa Barbara, CA — 33 10 375 13606 203 161950 2388 125740 58273 1438

⊞ △ DANIEL FREEMAN MEMORIAL HOSPITAL, 333 North Prairie Avenue, Zip 90301–4514; tel. 310/674–7050; Joseph W. Dunn, Ph.D., Chief Executive Officer (Total facility includes 29 beds in nursing home–type unit) A1 2 5 7 9 10 F4 7 10 11 12 17 19 21 22 24 27 28 30 32 34 35 37 38 39 40 41 42 43 44 45 46 48 49 51 53 61 63 64 65 66 67 71 72 73 74 S Carondelet Health System, Saint Louis, MO — 21 10 365 14275 224 53164 0 128163 57609 —

IRVINE—Orange County

□ IRVINE MEDICAL CENTER, 16200 Sand Canyon Avenue, Zip 92618–3714; tel. 714/753–2000; Richard H. Robinson, Chief Executive Officer (Total facility includes 35 beds in nursing home–type unit) A1 10 F1 4 7 8 10 11 12 15 16 17 19 20 21 22 23 24 25 27 28 29 30 31 32 33 34 35 37 38 39 40 41 42 43 44 45 49 56 59 60 64 65 66 67 70 71 72 73 74 P4 5 7 S TENET Healthcare Corporation, Santa Barbara, CA N Tenet Healthcare Corporation, Santa Barbara, CA — 33 10 153 5646 78 — 1523 55284 18611 384

JACKSON—Amador County

⊞ SUTTER AMADOR HOSPITAL, 810 Court Street, Zip 95642–2379; tel. 209/223–7500; Scott Stenberg, Chief Executive Officer (Total facility includes 44 beds in nursing home–type unit) A1 9 10 F7 8 15 19 21 22 25 26 28 29 30 31 35 37 40 42 44 63 64 65 71 73 P3 5 S Sutter Health, Sacramento, CA N Sutter\CHS, Sacramento, CA — 23 10 85 2601 54 47001 285 20504 9135 231

JOSHUA TREE—San Bernardino County

⊞ HI–DESERT MEDICAL CENTER, 6601 White Feather Road, Zip 92252–6601; tel. 619/366–3711; James R. Larson, President and Chief Executive Officer (Total facility includes 85 beds in nursing home–type unit) A1 9 10 F8 15 16 17 19 20 21 22 25 26 28 30 31 32 33 34 35 37 39 41 44 45 46 49 64 65 67 71 73 P1 — 16 10 115 2944 115 56603 0 30287 11074 471

KENTFIELD—Marin County

□ BHC ROSS HOSPITAL, (Formerly Ross Hospital), 1111 Sir Francis Drake Boulevard, Zip 94904; tel. 415/258–6900; Judy G. House, Chief Executive Officer (Nonreporting) A1 9 10 S Behavioral Healthcare Corporation, Nashville, TN — 33 22 56 — — — — — — —

Hospital, Address, Telephone, Administrator, Approval, Facility, and Physician Codes, Health Care System, Network	Classi-fication Codes		Utilization Data					Expense (thousands) of dollars		
★ American Hospital Association (AHA) membership □ Joint Commission on Accreditation of Healthcare Organizations (JCAHO) accreditation + American Osteopathic Hospital Association (AOHA) membership ○ American Osteopathic Association (AOA) accreditation △ Commission on Accreditation of Rehabilitation Facilities (CARF) accreditation Control codes 61, 63, 64, 71, 72 and 73 indicate hospitals listed by AOHA, but not registered by AHA. For definition of numerical codes, see page A4	Control	Service	Beds	Admissions	Census	Outpatient Visits	Births	Total	Payroll	Personnel

Hospital	Control	Service	Beds	Admissions	Census	Outpatient Visits	Births	Total	Payroll	Personnel
★ △ KENTFIELD REHABILITATION HOSPITAL, 1125 Sir Francis Drake Boulevard, Zip 94904, Mailing Address: P.O. Box 338, Zip 94914–0338; tel. 415/456–9680; John Behrmann, Administrator and Chief Executive Officer (Total facility includes 12 beds in nursing home–type unit) (Nonreporting) A1 7 9 10 S Continental Medical Systems, Inc., Mechanicsburg, PA	33	46	60	—	—	—	—	—	—	—
KING CITY—Monterey County										
□ GEORGE L. MEE MEMORIAL HOSPITAL, 300 Canal Street, Zip 93930–3410; tel. 408/385–6000; Walter Beck, Chief Executive Officer (Nonreporting) A1 9 10	23	10	42	—	—	—	—	—	—	—
KINGSBURG—Fresno County										
KINGSBURG DISTRICT HOSPITAL, 1200 Smith Street, Zip 93631; tel. 209/897–5841; Rod Holt, Administrator (Total facility includes 20 beds in nursing home–type unit) (Nonreporting) A9 10	16	10	35	—	—	—	—	—	—	—
LA HABRA—Orange County										
★ FRIENDLY HILLS REGIONAL MEDICAL CENTER, 1251 West Lambert Road, Zip 90631; tel. 310/694–3838; Gloria Mayer, Executive Director (Nonreporting) A1 2 9 10 N Friendly Hills HealthCare Network, LaHabra, CA	33	10	140	—	—	—	—	—	—	—
LA JOLLA—San Diego County										
★ GREEN HOSPITAL OF SCRIPPS CLINIC, 10666 North Torrey Pines Road, Zip 92037–1093; tel. 619/455–9100; Glenn W. Chong, Senior Vice President and Administrator A1 2 3 5 8 9 10 F1 2 3 4 7 8 10 12 14 15 16 17 19 20 21 22 24 25 26 27 28 29 30 31 32 34 35 36 37 39 40 41 42 43 44 45 48 51 52 53 54 55 56 57 58 59 60 61 63 64 65 66 67 69 70 71 72 73 74 P3 5 7 S Scripps Health, San Diego, CA N ScrippsHealth, San Diego, CA	23	10	165	8095	88	112170	0	96195	33310	698
★ SCRIPPS MEMORIAL HOSPITAL–LA JOLLA, 9888 Genesee Avenue, Zip 92037–1276, Mailing Address: Box 28, Zip 92038–0028; tel. 619/626–4123; Glenn W. Chong, Senior Vice President and Administrator (Total facility includes 29 beds in nursing home–type unit) A1 2 3 9 10 F1 2 3 4 7 8 10 11 12 14 15 16 19 21 22 23 24 25 26 27 33 35 36 37 38 40 41 42 43 44 45 46 49 50 52 53 54 55 56 57 58 59 60 61 63 64 65 66 67 69 70 71 72 73 74 P5 7 S Scripps Health, San Diego, CA N ScrippsHealth, San Diego, CA	23	10	431	13560	185	—	2850	137847	50182	843
LA MESA—San Diego County										
□ △ GROSSMONT HOSPITAL, 5555 Grossmont Center Drive, Zip 91942, Mailing Address: Box 158, Zip 91944–0158; tel. 619/465–0711; Michele T. Tarbet, R.N., Chief Executive Officer (Nonreporting) A1 2 3 7 9 10 12 S Sharp Healthcare, San Diego, CA N Sharp Healthcare, San Diego, CA	23	10	377	—	—	—	—	—	—	—
LA PALMA—Orange County										
★ △ LA PALMA INTERCOMMUNITY HOSPITAL, 7901 Walker Street, Zip 90623–5850, Mailing Address: P.O. Box 5850, Buena Park, Zip 90622; tel. 714/670–7400; Stephen E. Dixon, President and Chief Executive Officer A1 2 7 9 10 F3 7 12 14 15 16 17 19 22 27 28 31 35 39 41 44 49 57 58 59 65 71 73 74 P5 7 S UniHealth, Burbank, CA N UniHealth, Burbank, CA	23	10	139	4070	50	46847	926	40102	14084	383
LAGUNA HILLS—Orange County										
□ △ SADDLEBACK MEMORIAL MEDICAL CENTER, 24451 Health Center Drive, Zip 92653; tel. 714/837–4500; Nolan Draney, Executive Vice President (Total facility includes 18 beds in nursing home–type unit) A1 2 5 7 9 10 F4 5 6 7 8 10 12 14 15 16 17 18 19 21 22 25 26 28 29 30 31 32 33 34 35 36 37 38 39 40 41 42 43 44 45 46 48 49 51 59 60 61 64 65 70 71 72 73 74 P3 5 7 S Memorial Health Services, Long Beach, CA	23	10	220	10281	118	140875	2076	86715	33452	916
LAKE ARROWHEAD—San Bernardino County										
□ SAN BERNARDINO MOUNTAINS COMMUNITY HOSPITAL DISTRICT, (Formerly Mountains Community Hospital), 29101 Hospital Road, Zip 92352, Mailing Address: Box 70, Zip 92352; tel. 909/336–3651; John J. McCormick, Chief Executive Officer (Total facility includes 18 beds in nursing home–type unit) A1 9 10 F7 8 17 18 19 22 25 26 30 31 32 34 36 39 41 44 49 51 64 65 67 71 72 73 P3 8	16	10	36	1001	22	18619	148	10761	4661	140
LAKE ISABELLA—Kern County										
□ KERN VALLEY HOSPITAL DISTRICT, 6412 Laurel Avenue, Zip 93240, Mailing Address: P.O. Box 1628, Zip 93240; tel. 619/379–2681; Ronald E. Dahlgren, Chief Executive Officer (Total facility includes 74 beds in nursing home–type unit) A1 9 10 F12 15 16 17 19 22 28 32 34 37 41 44 46 49 51 64 65 71 73 P3	16	10	101	1206	76	14925	0	14076	4931	216
LAKEPORT—Lake County										
★ SUTTER LAKESIDE HOSPITAL, 5176 Hill Road East, Zip 95453–6111; tel. 707/262–5001; Paul J. Hensler, Chief Executive Officer (Nonreporting) A1 9 10 S Sutter Health, Sacramento, CA N Sutter\CHS, Sacramento, CA	23	10	54	—	—	—	—	—	—	—
LAKEWOOD—Los Angeles County										
DOCTORS HOSPITAL OF LAKEWOOD See Lakewood Regional Medical Center										
□ LAKEWOOD REGIONAL MEDICAL CENTER, (Includes Doctors Hospital of Lakewood, 3700 East South Street, New Beginnings Doctors Hospital of Lakewood–Clark, 5300 Clark Avenue, tel. 213/866–9711), 3700 East South Street, Zip 90712; tel. 310/531–2550; Gustavo A. Valdespino, Chief Executive Officer A1 2 3 9 10 F3 4 7 8 10 11 12 15 16 19 21 22 26 27 28 30 32 33 34 35 37 39 40 41 42 43 44 46 48 49 52 57 58 59 65 70 71 73 74 P5 7 S TENET Healthcare Corporation, Santa Barbara, CA N Tenet Healthcare Corporation, Santa Barbara, CA NEW BEGINNINGS DOCTORS HOSPITAL OF LAKEWOOD–CLARK See Lakewood Regional Medical Center	33	10	148	5900	79	50662	691	43085	17729	522

Hospital, Address, Telephone, Administrator, Approval, Facility, and Physician Codes, Health Care System, Network	Classification Codes		Utilization Data					Expense (thousands) of dollars		
	Control	Service	Beds	Admissions	Census	Outpatient Visits	Births	Total	Payroll	Personnel

★ American Hospital Association (AHA) membership
□ Joint Commission on Accreditation of Healthcare Organizations (JCAHO) accreditation
+ American Osteopathic Hospital Association (AOHA) membership
○ American Osteopathic Association (AOA) accreditation
△ Commission on Accreditation of Rehabilitation Facilities (CARF) accreditation
Control codes 61, 63, 64, 71, 72 and 73 indicate hospitals listed by AOHA, but not registered by AHA. For definition of numerical codes, see page A4

LANCASTER—Los Angeles County

✠ ANTELOPE VALLEY HOSPITAL, 1600 West Avenue J, Zip 93534–2894; tel. 805/949–5000; Robert J. Harenski, Chief Executive Officer (Total facility includes 32 beds in nursing home–type unit) **A**1 9 10 **F**4 7 8 10 11 14 15 16 17 19 21 22 23 30 31 32 33 34 35 37 38 39 40 41 43 44 46 49 52 53 54 56 58 60 61 64 65 67 71 72 73 74	16	10	281	16731	188	135044	4878	95732	46449	1211
✠ LAC–HIGH DESERT HOSPITAL, 44900 North 60th Street West, Zip 93536; tel. 805/945–8461; Mel Grussing, Administrator (Total facility includes 50 beds in nursing home–type unit) **A**1 9 10 **F**2 8 11 12 13 15 16 17 19 20 21 25 28 30 31 32 33 34 35 37 41 42 43 44 46 48 49 51 60 63 64 65 71 73 **P**6 **S** Los Angeles County–Department of Health Services, Los Angeles, CA	13	10	76	1350	74	60039	0	56588	21260	572
□ LANCASTER COMMUNITY HOSPITAL, 43830 North Tenth Street West, Zip 93534; tel. 805/948–4781; Steve Schmidt, Administrator and Chief Executive Officer (Total facility includes 22 beds in nursing home–type unit) **A**1 9 10 **F**4 10 11 12 14 15 16 19 21 22 23 27 32 33 34 35 37 41 42 43 44 45 46 64 71 73 **P**5 **S** Paracelsus Healthcare Corporation, Houston, TX	33	10	123	5688	69	44984	0	35351	15197	417

LEMOORE—Kings County

✠ NAVAL HOSPITAL, 930 Franklin Avenue, Zip 93246–5000; tel. 209/998–4201; Captain Jerry W. Brickeen, MSC, USN, Commanding Officer **A**1 **F**2 3 4 7 8 11 12 13 15 16 17 18 19 20 21 22 27 32 35 37 38 39 40 41 42 43 44 45 46 47 48 49 51 52 53 55 56 58 59 60 61 65 67 69 71 73 74 **P**5 8 **S** Department of Navy, Washington, DC	43	10	25	1052	5	206408	338	21142	6115	—

LINDSAY—Tulare County

✠ LINDSAY DISTRICT HOSPITAL, 740 North Sequoia Avenue, Zip 93247, Mailing Address: Box 40, Zip 93247; tel. 209/562–4955; David S. Wanger, Chief Executive Officer (Total facility includes 53 beds in nursing home–type unit) **A**1 9 10 **F**7 22 37 40 41 44 45 64 70 71 73 **P**5 **N** UniHealth, Burbank, CA	16	10	106	1765	57	24659	578	9335	3987	211

LIVERMORE—Alameda County

VALLEY MEMORIAL HOSPITAL, 1111 East Stanley Boulevard, Zip 94550; tel. 510/447–7000; Richard E. Herington, President and Chief Executive Officer (Total facility includes 14 beds in nursing home–type unit) (Nonreporting) **A**2 9 10 **S** ValleyCare Health System, Pleasanton, CA	23	10	110							
VETERANS AFFAIRS MEDICAL CENTER See Veterans Affairs Palo Alto Health Care System, Palo Alto										

LODI—San Joaquin County

✠ △ LODI MEMORIAL HOSPITAL, (Includes Lodi Memorial Hospital West, 800 South Lower Sacramento Road, Zip 95242; tel. 209/333–0211), 975 South Fairmont Avenue, Zip 95240–5179, Mailing Address: P.O. Box 3004, Zip 95241–1908; tel. 209/334–3411; Joseph P. Harrington, Chief Executive Officer (Total facility includes 43 beds in nursing home–type unit) **A**1 7 9 10 **F**1 2 3 4 5 7 8 9 10 11 12 13 14 15 16 17 19 20 21 22 23 24 25 27 28 29 30 32 34 35 37 38 39 40 41 42 43 44 45 46 47 48 49 51 52 53 54 55 56 57 58 59 60 61 63 64 65 66 67 69 71 72 73 **P**5 7	23	10	166	6146	96	106935	1198	53565	26600	792

LOMA LINDA—San Bernardino County

✠ JERRY L. PETTIS MEMORIAL VETERANS MEDICAL CENTER, 11201 Benton Street, Zip 92357; tel. 909/825–7084; Dean R. Stordahl, Director (Total facility includes 108 beds in nursing home–type unit) **A**1 3 5 8 **F**2 3 4 5 8 10 11 12 14 18 19 20 21 22 23 26 27 28 30 31 32 33 34 35 37 39 41 42 43 44 45 46 48 49 51 52 54 55 56 57 58 59 60 61 63 64 65 67 69 71 72 73 74 **P**1 **S** Department of Veterans Affairs, Washington, DC	45	10	315	6534	246	230373	0	108919	53724	1282
✠ △ LOMA LINDA UNIVERSITY MEDICAL CENTER, (Includes Loma Linda University Community Medical Center, 25333 Barton Road, Zip 92354–3053; tel. 909/796–0167), 11234 Anderson Street, Zip 92354–2870, Mailing Address: P.O. Box 2000, Zip 92354–0200; tel. 909/824–0800; J. David Moorhead, M.D., President (Nonreporting) **A**1 2 3 5 7 8 9 10 **S** Adventist Health System–Loma Linda, Loma Linda, CA **N** Adventist Health System–Loma Linda, Loma Linda, CA	21	10	729	—	—	—	—	—	—	—

LOMPOC—Santa Barbara County

□ LOMPOC DISTRICT HOSPITAL, 508 East Hickory Street, Zip 93436, Mailing Address: Box 1058, Zip 93438; tel. 805/737–3300; Scott Rhine, Administrator and Chief Executive Officer (Total facility includes 110 beds in nursing home–type unit) (Nonreporting) **A**1 9 10	16	10	170							

LONE PINE—Inyo County

SOUTHERN INYO HEALTHCARE DISTRICT, 501 East Locust Street, Zip 93545, Mailing Address: Box 1009, Zip 93545; tel. 619/876–5501; Raye Burhardt, Acting Administrator (Nonreporting) **A**9 10	16	10	37	—	—	—	—	—	—	—

LONG BEACH—Los Angeles County

✠ LONG BEACH COMMUNITY MEDICAL CENTER, 1720 Termino Avenue, Zip 90804; tel. 310/498–1000; Makoto Nakayama, Interim President and Chief Executive Officer (Total facility includes 27 beds in nursing home–type unit) **A**1 2 9 10 **F**1 4 7 8 10 11 12 14 15 16 17 19 21 22 26 27 28 29 30 31 34 35 37 38 39 40 41 42 43 44 45 46 47 49 51 52 54 55 56 57 58 59 60 63 64 65 67 71 72 73 74 **P**1 2 4 5 7 **S** UniHealth, Burbank, CA **N** UniHealth, Burbank, CA	23	10	290	11258	140	66190	2920	91887	33105	945
□ LONG BEACH DOCTORS HOSPITAL, 1725 Pacific Avenue, Zip 90813–1798; tel. 310/599–3551; Manuel Anel, M.D., Administrator and Chief Executive Officer (Nonreporting) **A**1 9 10	32	10	43	—	—	—	—	—	—	—
□ △ LONG BEACH MEMORIAL MEDICAL CENTER, 2801 Atlantic Avenue, Zip 90806, Mailing Address: Box 1428, Zip 90801–1428; tel. 562/933–2000; Thomas J. Collins, President and Chief Executive Officer (Total facility includes 62 beds in nursing home–type unit) **A**1 2 3 5 7 8 9 10 13 **F**4 5 6 7 8 10 11 12 14 15 16 17 19 20 21 22 23 25 26 28 29 30 31 32 33 34 35 37 38 39 40 41 42 43 44 45 46 47 48 49 50 51 60 61 63 64 65 66 67 70 71 72 73 74 **P**3 5 7 **S** Memorial Health Services, Long Beach, CA	23	10	726	27311	403	—	4814	269277	115946	2720

Hospital, Address, Telephone, Administrator, Approval, Facility, and Physician Codes, Health Care System, Network	Classi-fication Codes		Utilization Data					Expense (thousands) of dollars		
	Control	Service	Beds	Admissions	Census	Outpatient Visits	Births	Total	Payroll	Personnel

★ American Hospital Association (AHA) membership
□ Joint Commission on Accreditation of Healthcare Organizations (JCAHO) accreditation
+ American Osteopathic Hospital Association (AOHA) membership
○ American Osteopathic Association (AOA) accreditation
△ Commission on Accreditation of Rehabilitation Facilities (CARF) accreditation
Control codes 61, 63, 64, 71, 72 and 73 indicate hospitals listed by AOHA, but not registered by AHA. For definition of numerical codes, see page A4

□ ○ PACIFIC HOSPITAL OF LONG BEACH, 2776 Pacific Avenue, Zip 90806–2699, Mailing Address: P.O. Box 1268, Zip 90801; tel. 562/595–1911; Gerald S. Goldberg, Administrator and Chief Executive Officer (Total facility includes 27 beds in nursing home–type unit) **A**1 5 9 10 11 12 13 **F**8 11 12 15 16 17 19 20 21 22 26 27 28 30 31 32 33 34 35 37 40 41 42 44 49 51 52 56 57 58 59 61 64 65 71 73 **P**5	23	10	179	3459	70	49438	651	27138	11672	378
REDGATE MEMORIAL HOSPITAL, 1775 Chestnut Avenue, Zip 90813; tel. 310/599–8444; Robert Worrell, Chief Executive Officer (Nonreporting)	23	82	63	—	—	—	—	—	—	—
★ SAINT MARY MEDICAL CENTER, 1050 Linden Avenue, Zip 90801, Mailing Address: P.O. Box 887, Zip 90801; tel. 310/491–9000; Tammie McMann Brailsford, Administrator (Total facility includes 80 beds in nursing home–type unit) **A**1 2 3 5 9 10 **F**4 6 7 8 10 12 15 16 17 19 21 22 24 25 26 30 31 32 33 34 35 37 38 40 41 42 43 44 46 47 48 49 50 51 52 57 58 59 60 63 64 65 69 70 71 72 73 **P**5 7 **S** Catholic Healthcare West, San Francisco, CA **N** Catholic HealthCare West (CHW), San Francisco, CA	23	10	479	12163	214	254033	2112	121190	50004	1641
★ VETERANS AFFAIRS MEDICAL CENTER, 5901 East Seventh Street, Zip 90822–5201; tel. 562/494–5400; Jerry B. Boyd, Director (Total facility includes 266 beds in nursing home–type unit) (Nonreporting) **A**1 2 3 5 8 **S** Department of Veterans Affairs, Washington, DC	45	10	1131	—	—	—	—	—	—	—
□ WOODRUFF COMMUNITY HOSPITAL, 3800 Woodruff Avenue, Zip 90808; tel. 310/421–8241; Robert Glass, Executive Director (Nonreporting) **A**1 9 10 **S** TENET Healthcare Corporation, Santa Barbara, CA	33	10	96	—	—	—	—	—	—	—

LOS ALAMITOS—Orange County

□ LOS ALAMITOS MEDICAL CENTER, 3751 Katella Avenue, Zip 90720; tel. 310/598–1311; Gustavo A. Valdespino, Chief Executive Officer (Total facility includes 20 beds in nursing home–type unit) (Nonreporting) **A**1 2 9 10 **S** TENET Healthcare Corporation, Santa Barbara, CA	33	10	173	—	—	—	—	—	—	—

LOS ANGELES—Los Angeles County
(Mailing Addresses - Canoga Park, Encino, Granada Hills, Harbor City, Hollywood, Mission Hills, North Hollywood, Northridge, Panorama City, San Pedro, Sepulveda, Sherman Oaks, Sun Valley, Sylmar, Tarzana, Van Nuys, West Hills, West Los Angeles, Woodland Hills)

★ BARLOW RESPIRATORY HOSPITAL, 2000 Stadium Way, Zip 90026–2696; tel. 213/250–4200; Margaret W. Crane, Chief Executive Officer **A**1 3 5 9 10 **F**12 14 15 16 17 34 37 45 49 65 67	23	33	49	271	32	714	0	14857	7328	214
★ BAY HARBOR HOSPITAL, 1437 West Lomita Boulevard, Harbor City, Zip 90710–2097; tel. 310/325–1221; Jack W. Weiblen, FACHE, Chief Executive Officer (Total facility includes 212 beds in nursing home–type unit) **A**1 2 9 10 **F**2 4 8 9 10 11 12 15 17 19 22 27 28 32 33 34 35 37 38 40 41 42 43 44 45 47 48 49 51 52 53 54 58 60 64 65 71 73 **P**3	23	10	346	5651	194	33693	531	57498	23115	780
★ CALIFORNIA HOSPITAL MEDICAL CENTER, 1401 South Grand Avenue, Zip 90015; tel. 213/748–2411; Melinda D. Beswick, President and Chief Executive Officer (Total facility includes 19 beds in nursing home–type unit) **A**1 2 3 5 9 10 **F**1 4 7 8 10 11 12 13 15 17 18 19 21 22 25 26 27 28 30 32 34 37 38 40 41 42 43 44 45 46 47 49 52 54 55 56 57 58 59 60 61 64 65 67 68 69 71 72 73 74 **P**5 **S** UniHealth, Burbank, CA **N** UniHealth, Burbank, CA	23	10	309	13401	155	107373	5248	99446	43184	1047
★ CEDARS–SINAI MEDICAL CENTER, 8700 Beverly Boulevard, Zip 90048–0750, Mailing Address: Box 48750, Zip 90048–0750; tel. 310/855–5000; Thomas M. Priselac, President and Chief Executive Officer **A**1 2 3 5 8 9 10 **F**3 4 5 7 8 10 11 12 13 14 15 16 17 18 19 20 21 22 23 26 27 28 29 30 31 32 33 34 35 36 37 38 39 40 41 42 43 44 45 46 47 48 49 50 51 52 53 54 55 56 57 58 59 60 61 63 64 65 66 67 68 69 70 71 73 74 **P**3 5 7 8 **N** National Cardiovascular Network, Atlanta, GA; Cedars–Sinai Health System, Los Angeles, CA	23	10	754	35903	576	—	6848	561767	225735	5285
□ CENTURY CITY HOSPITAL, 2070 Century Park East, Zip 90067; tel. 310/553–6211; John R. Nickens, III, Chief Executive Officer (Nonreporting) **A**1 9 10 **S** TENET Healthcare Corporation, Santa Barbara, CA **N** Tenet Healthcare Corporation, Santa Barbara, CA	33	10	135	—	—	—	—	—	—	—
★ CHILDRENS HOSPITAL OF LOS ANGELES, 4650 Sunset Boulevard, Zip 90027–6089, Mailing Address: Box 54700, Zip 90054–0700; tel. 213/660–2450; Walter W. Noce, Jr., President and Chief Executive Officer **A**1 2 3 5 9 10 **F**4 5 10 12 13 14 15 16 17 18 19 20 21 22 27 28 30 31 32 34 35 38 39 41 42 43 44 45 46 47 48 49 51 53 54 55 56 58 60 65 66 67 68 69 70 71 72 73 **P**4 5 6	23	50	302	11113	216	193194	0	215084	97385	2263
★ COLUMBIA WEST HILLS MEDICAL CENTER, 7300 Medical Center Drive, West Hills, Zip 91307, Mailing Address: P.O. Box 7937, Zip 91309–7937; tel. 818/712–4110; Howard H. Levine, President and Chief Executive Officer **A**1 10 **F**4 7 8 10 11 12 14 19 20 21 22 24 26 27 28 30 31 32 33 34 35 37 38 39 40 41 42 43 44 46 49 51 54 60 61 64 65 66 67 71 73 74 **P**4 5 7 **S** Columbia/HCA Healthcare Corporation, Nashville, TN	33	10	236	8114	107	30397	1404	62302	29409	757
□ EAST LOS ANGELES DOCTORS HOSPITAL, 4060 Whittier Boulevard, Zip 90023; tel. 213/268–5514; Frank Kutsuda, Administrator and Chief Executive Officer (Total facility includes 25 beds in nursing home–type unit) (Nonreporting) **A**1 9 10	33	10	127	—	—	—	—	—	—	—
□ EDGEMONT HOSPITAL, 4841 Hollywood Boulevard, Zip 90027; tel. 213/913–9000; Lynn Ordway, Administrator **A**1 9 10 **F**52 56 57 58 59	33	22	61	1478	55	0	0	8647	4518	125
□ ENCINO–TARZANA REGIONAL MEDICAL CENTER, (Includes Encino–Tarzana Regional Medical Center, 16237 Ventura Boulevard, Encino, Zip 91436–2201; tel. 818/995–5000), 18321 Clark Street, Tarzana, Zip 91356; tel. 818/881–0800; Arnold R. Schaffer, Chief Executive Officer (Nonreporting) **A**1 3 9 10 **S** TENET Healthcare Corporation, Santa Barbara, CA **N** Tenet Healthcare Corporation, Santa Barbara, CA	33	10	382	—	—	—	—	—	—	—

Hospital, Address, Telephone, Administrator, Approval, Facility, and Physician Codes, Health Care System, Network	Classi-fication Codes		Utilization Data					Expense (thousands) of dollars		
★ American Hospital Association (AHA) membership □ Joint Commission on Accreditation of Healthcare Organizations (JCAHO) accreditation + American Osteopathic Hospital Association (AOHA) membership ○ American Osteopathic Association (AOA) accreditation △ Commission on Accreditation of Rehabilitation Facilities (CARF) accreditation Control codes 61, 63, 64, 71, 72 and 73 indicate hospitals listed by AOHA, but not registered by AHA. For definition of numerical codes, see page A4	Control	Service	Beds	Admissions	Census	Outpatient Visits	Births	Total	Payroll	Personnel

Hospital	Control	Service	Beds	Admissions	Census	Outpatient Visits	Births	Total	Payroll	Personnel
□ GATEWAYS HOSPITAL AND MENTAL HEALTH CENTER, 1891 Effie Street, Zip 90026–1711; tel. 213/644–2000; Saul Goldfarb, Chief Executive Officer **A**1 9 10 **F**14 15 16 26 52 53 55 57 58 59	23	22	55	565	28	—	0	12421	8641	197
✸ GRANADA HILLS COMMUNITY HOSPITAL, 10445 Balboa Boulevard, Granada Hills, Zip 91394–9400; tel. 818/360–1021; Dennis E. Coleman, President and Chief Executive Officer (Total facility includes 23 beds in nursing home–type unit) **A**1 9 10 **F**4 8 10 11 12 15 16 17 19 20 21 22 24 26 27 28 29 30 34 35 39 40 41 42 43 44 49 56 61 63 64 65 67 71 72 73 74 **P**5 7	23	10	139	5439	65	24492	1631	35680	15385	445
□ HOLLYWOOD COMMUNITY HOSPITAL OF HOLLYWOOD, (Includes Hollywood Community Hospital of Van Nuys, 14433 Emelita Street, Zip 91401; tel. 818/787–1511; Sandra Allen, Administrator), 6245 De Longpre Avenue, Zip 90028; tel. 213/462–2271; Steven Courtier, Chief Executive Officer (Nonreporting) **A**1 9 10 **S** Paracelsus Healthcare Corporation, Houston, TX HOLLYWOOD COMMUNITY HOSPITAL OF VAN NUYS See Hollywood Community Hospital of Hollywood	33	10	160	—	—	—	—	—	—	—
□ △ HOSPITAL OF THE GOOD SAMARITAN, 616 South Witmer Street, Zip 90017–2395; tel. 213/977–2121; Andrew B. Leeka, Chief Executive Officer **A**1 2 5 7 8 9 10 **F**4 7 8 10 11 12 15 17 19 21 22 23 24 27 28 29 30 32 35 37 38 40 41 42 43 44 45 46 47 48 49 56 58 60 63 64 65 66 67 70 71 73 74 **P**5	23	10	318	13843	230	65658	2271	162415	68796	1940
✸ KAISER FOUNDATION HOSPITAL, (Includes Kaiser Foundation Mental Health Center, 765 West College Street, Zip 90012; tel. 213/580–7200), 4747 Sunset Boulevard, Zip 90027; tel. 213/783–4011; Joseph Wm Hummel, Senior Vice President and Area Manager (Nonreporting) **A**1 2 3 5 10 **S** Kaiser Foundation Hospitals, Oakland, CA	23	10	311	—	—	—	—	—	—	—
✸ KAISER FOUNDATION HOSPITAL, 25825 South Vermont Avenue, Harbor City, Zip 90710; tel. 310/325–5111; Mary Ann Barnes, Administrator **A**1 2 10 **F**2 3 4 7 8 10 11 12 14 15 16 19 21 22 23 25 26 28 29 30 31 32 33 34 35 39 40 41 42 43 44 45 46 49 51 53 54 55 56 57 58 59 60 61 63 65 67 68 69 71 72 73 **S** Kaiser Foundation Hospitals, Oakland, CA	23	10	179	8151	91	—	1660	—	—	—
✸ KAISER FOUNDATION HOSPITAL, 13652 Cantara Street, Panorama City, Zip 91402; tel. 818/375–2000; Dev Mahadevan, Administrator **A**1 2 5 10 **F**3 4 7 8 10 11 12 13 14 15 16 17 18 19 21 22 26 27 28 29 30 31 32 33 34 35 37 38 40 41 42 43 44 45 46 49 50 51 53 54 55 56 57 58 59 60 61 63 65 66 67 68 69 71 72 73 **P**4 **S** Kaiser Foundation Hospitals, Oakland, CA	23	10	269	8617	88	—	1802	—	—	—
✸ KAISER FOUNDATION HOSPITAL, 5601 DeSoto Avenue, Woodland Hills, Zip 91365–4084; tel. 818/719–2000; James L. Breeden, Administrator **A**1 3 5 10 **F**2 3 4 7 8 10 11 12 13 15 16 17 18 19 21 22 26 27 28 29 30 31 32 33 35 37 38 39 40 41 42 43 44 45 48 49 50 51 52 53 54 55 56 58 59 60 61 63 64 65 66 67 68 69 71 72 73 74 **S** Kaiser Foundation Hospitals, Oakland, CA	23	10	139	8003	80	—	1851	—	—	653
✸ KAISER FOUNDATION HOSPITAL–WEST LOS ANGELES, 6041 Cadillac Avenue, Zip 90034; tel. 213/857–2201; Ivette Estrada, Administrator (Nonreporting) **A**1 2 3 5 10 **S** Kaiser Foundation Hospitals, Oakland, CA	23	10	161	—	—	—	—	—	—	—
✸ LAC–KING–DREW MEDICAL CENTER, 12021 South Wilmington Avenue, Zip 90059; tel. 310/668–4321; Foster Randall, Administrator and Chief Executive Officer **A**1 2 3 5 8 9 10 **F**1 4 7 8 9 10 11 12 13 15 16 17 18 19 20 21 22 23 25 26 27 28 30 31 32 34 35 37 38 40 41 42 44 45 47 48 49 50 51 52 53 54 55 56 57 58 59 60 61 63 64 65 69 70 71 72 73 74 **P**3 5 **S** Los Angeles County–Department of Health Services, Los Angeles, CA	13	10	264	17973	264	246666	3060	345895	133332	3127
✸ LAC–UNIVERSITY OF SOUTHERN CALIFORNIA MEDICAL CENTER, (Includes General Hospital, 1200 North State Street, Zip 90033; Women's and Children's Hospital, 1240 North Mission Road, Zip 90033), 1200 North State Street, Zip 90033–1084; tel. 213/226–2622; Douglas D. Bagley, Executive Director **A**1 2 3 5 8 9 10 **F**1 2 3 4 5 6 7 8 9 10 11 12 13 14 15 16 17 18 19 20 21 22 23 25 26 27 28 29 30 31 32 34 35 37 38 39 40 41 42 43 44 45 46 47 48 49 51 52 53 54 55 56 57 58 59 60 61 63 64 65 66 67 68 69 70 71 72 73 74 **P**1 3 6 8 **S** Los Angeles County–Department of Health Services, Los Angeles, CA	13	10	1157	51551	852	795861	4906	1054467	308153	7228
□ LINCOLN HOSPITAL MEDICAL CENTER, 443 South Soto Street, Zip 90033; tel. 213/261–1181; Tim Kollars, Administrator (Nonreporting) **A**1 9 10	33	10	61	—	—	—	—	—	—	—
□ LOS ANGELES COMMUNITY HOSPITAL, (Includes Los Angeles Community Hospital of Norwalk, 13222 Bloomfield Avenue, Zip 90650; tel. 310/863–4763), 4081 East Olympic Boulevard, Zip 90023; tel. 213/267–0477; Thomas McClintock, Chief Executive Officer (Nonreporting) **A**1 9 10 **S** Paracelsus Healthcare Corporation, Houston, TX	33	10	186	—	—	—	—	—	—	—
LOS ANGELES COUNTY CENTRAL JAIL HOSPITAL, 441 Bauchet Street, Zip 90012; tel. 213/974–5045; Tom Flaherty, Assistant Administrator (Nonreporting)	13	11	190	—	—	—	—	—	—	—
□ LOS ANGELES METROPOLITAN MEDICAL CENTER, 2231 South Western Avenue, Zip 90018–1399; tel. 213/737–7372; Marc A. Furstman, Chief Executive Officer **A**1 9 10 **F**2 4 8 11 12 14 15 16 17 19 27 28 30 41 44 48 52 54 55 56 58 65 **S** Pacific Health Corporation, Long Beach, CA	33	10	115	1643	32	5284	0	9979	4606	199
□ MIDWAY HOSPITAL MEDICAL CENTER, 5925 San Vicente Boulevard, Zip 90019; tel. 213/938–3161; John V. Fenton, Chief Executive Officer (Nonreporting) **A**1 9 10 **S** TENET Healthcare Corporation, Santa Barbara, CA MISSION COMMUNITY HOSPITAL–PANORAMA CITY CAMPUS See Mission Community Hospital–San Fernando Campus, San Fernando	33	10	291	—	—	—	—	—	—	—

Hospital, Address, Telephone, Administrator, Approval, Facility, and Physician Codes, Health Care System, Network	Classi-fication Codes		Utilization Data					Expense (thousands) of dollars		
	Control	Service	Beds	Admissions	Census	Outpatient Visits	Births	Total	Payroll	Personnel

Hospital, Address, Telephone, Administrator, Approval, Facility, and Physician Codes, Health Care System, Network	Control	Service	Beds	Admissions	Census	Outpatient Visits	Births	Total	Payroll	Personnel
✠ MOTION PICTURE AND TELEVISION FUND HOSPITAL AND RESIDENTIAL SERVICES, 23388 Mulholland Drive, Woodland Hills, Zip 91364–2792; tel. 818/876–1888; William F. Haug, FACHE, President and Chief Executive Officer (Total facility includes 165 beds in nursing home–type unit) (Nonreporting) **A**1 9 10	23	10	218	—	—	—	—	—	—	—
□ NORTH HOLLYWOOD MEDICAL CENTER, 12629 Riverside Drive, North Hollywood, Zip 91607–3495; tel. 818/980–9200; Dale Surowitz, President and Chief Executive Officer **A**1 9 10 **F**1 4 5 7 8 10 11 12 13 16 17 19 21 22 26 28 29 30 31 32 34 35 37 38 40 41 42 43 44 45 46 47 48 49 51 52 56 57 58 59 61 63 64 65 71 73 74 **P**2 5 6 7 **S** TENET Healthcare Corporation, Santa Barbara, CA **N** Tenet Healthcare Corporation, Santa Barbara, CA	33	10	150	4775	70	—	1002	33820	14389	—
✠ NORTHRIDGE HOSPITAL AND MEDICAL CENTER, SHERMAN WAY CAMPUS, 14500 Sherman Circle, Van Nuys, Zip 91405; tel. 818/997–0101; Richard D. Lyons, President and Chief Administrative Officer (Total facility includes 38 beds in nursing home–type unit) **A**1 10 **F**1 3 4 7 8 10 11 12 15 16 17 18 19 21 22 23 24 26 27 28 30 31 32 33 34 35 37 38 39 40 41 42 43 44 45 46 47 48 49 51 52 53 54 55 56 57 58 59 60 61 63 64 65 66 67 68 70 71 73 74 **P**3 5 7 **S** UniHealth, Burbank, CA **N** UniHealth, Burbank, CA	23	10	195	6070	84	45325	1000	39773	18719	408
✠ △ NORTHRIDGE HOSPITAL MEDICAL CENTER–ROSCOE BOULEVARD CAMPUS, 18300 Roscoe Boulevard, Northridge, Zip 91328; tel. 818/885–8500; Roger E. Seaver, President and Chief Executive Officer (Total facility includes 30 beds in nursing home–type unit) **A**1 5 7 10 **F**1 3 4 7 8 10 11 12 15 17 18 19 21 22 24 26 28 30 31 32 34 35 37 38 39 40 41 42 43 44 45 46 47 48 49 52 53 54 55 56 57 58 59 60 63 64 65 67 68 70 71 73 74 **P**3 5 **S** UniHealth, Burbank, CA **N** UniHealth, Burbank, CA	23	10	368	15349	256	149189	2585	165291	65296	1404
✠ OLIVE VIEW–UCLA MEDICAL CENTER, 14445 Olive View Drive, Sylmar, Zip 91342–1495; tel. 818/364–1555; Melinda Anderson, Administrator **A**1 3 5 9 10 **F**3 4 7 8 10 11 12 13 17 19 20 21 22 25 26 27 28 29 30 31 32 33 34 35 37 38 39 40 41 42 43 44 45 46 49 50 51 52 53 54 56 57 58 59 60 61 63 65 67 68 69 70 71 72 73 74 **P**6 8 **S** Los Angeles County–Department of Health Services, Los Angeles, CA	13	10	241	13563	213	195054	3052	242398	81529	1842
□ ORTHOPAEDIC HOSPITAL, 2400 South Flower Street, Zip 90007, Mailing Address: Box 60132, Terminal Annex, Zip 90060; tel. 213/742–1000; James V. Luck, Jr., M.D., Chief Executive Officer and Medical Director (Nonreporting) **A**1 2 3 5 9 10	23	47	152	—	—	—	—	—	—	—
✠ PACIFIC ALLIANCE MEDICAL CENTER, 531 West College Street, Zip 90012; tel. 213/624–8411; John R. Edwards, Chief Executive Officer (Nonreporting) **A**1 10 **N** Essential HealthCare Network, Monterey Park, CA	32	10	89	—	—	—	—	—	—	—
□ PACIFICA HOSPITAL OF THE VALLEY, 9449 San Fernando Road, Sun Valley, Zip 91352; tel. 818/252–2380; Trude Williams, R.N., Administrator (Total facility includes 64 beds in nursing home–type unit) **A**1 9 10 **F**8 10 11 12 14 15 16 19 22 29 32 35 38 40 44 47 49 52 56 59 64 65 67 71 73 **P**5	32	10	236	5874	114	—	816	37339	16273	395
✠ △ PROVIDENCE HOLY CROSS MEDICAL CENTER, 15031 Rinaldi Street, Mission Hills, Zip 91345–1285; tel. 818/365–8051; Michael J. Madden, Chief Executive Los Angeles Service Area (Total facility includes 48 beds in nursing home–type unit) **A**1 7 10 **F**4 7 8 10 11 12 14 15 16 17 19 20 21 22 23 28 29 30 32 33 34 35 37 40 41 42 43 44 45 46 48 49 60 64 65 67 70 71 72 73 74 **P**5 **S** Sisters of Providence Health System, Seattle, WA **N** Providence Health System in California, Burbank, CA	21	10	257	10086	137	69070	1417	84581	35215	937
□ QUEEN OF ANGELS–HOLLYWOOD PRESBYTERIAN MEDICAL CENTER, 1300 North Vermont Avenue, Zip 90027–0069; tel. 213/413–3000; Sylvester Graff, President and Chief Executive Officer (Total facility includes 89 beds in nursing home–type unit) **A**1 2 9 10 **F**4 7 8 11 15 16 17 19 21 22 27 28 30 31 32 33 34 35 37 38 40 41 42 43 44 45 46 48 49 60 64 65 71 73 74 **P**3 5 7 **N** Essential HealthCare Network, Monterey Park, CA	23	10	409	19010	287	120064	6120	113312	48464	1381
✠ △ SAN PEDRO PENINSULA HOSPITAL, 1300 West Seventh Street, San Pedro, Zip 90732; tel. 310/832–3311; John M. Wilson, President (Total facility includes 128 beds in nursing home–type unit) **A**1 7 9 10 **F**2 3 7 8 10 11 12 14 19 21 22 23 25 26 27 31 32 33 34 35 37 38 40 41 42 43 44 48 49 52 54 57 59 60 64 65 71 73 **P**3 5 7 **N** Little Company of Mary Health Services, Torrance, CA	23	10	309	6666	210	145214	646	70607	32291	724
□ SAN VICENTE HOSPITAL, 6000 San Vicente Boulevard, Zip 90036; tel. 213/937–2504; R. Wayne Ives, Administrator (Nonreporting) **A**1 9	33	44	17	—	—	—	—	—	—	—
✠ SANTA MARTA HOSPITAL, 319 North Humphreys Avenue, Zip 90022; tel. 213/266–6500; James G. Ovieda, President and Chief Executive Officer **A**1 10 **F**8 11 15 17 19 22 27 35 37 38 40 44 45 46 47 65 71 72 73 74 **P**5 **S** Carondelet Health System, Saint Louis, MO **N** Essential HealthCare Network, Monterey Park, CA	21	10	110	5110	45	—	1338	27675	11133	370
□ SHERMAN OAKS HOSPITAL AND HEALTH CENTER, 4929 Van Nuys Boulevard, Sherman Oaks, Zip 91403; tel. 818/981–7111; David Levinsonn, Chief Executive Officer (Total facility includes 18 beds in nursing home–type unit) **A**1 9 10 **F**1 8 9 11 12 17 19 21 22 23 28 30 31 32 35 37 39 41 42 44 45 46 49 50 59 63 64 65 66 67 71 73 **P**5	23	50	156	3470	55	18507	0	32119	13711	398
✠ SHRINERS HOSPITALS FOR CHILDREN, LOS ANGELES, 3160 Geneva Street, Zip 90020–1199; tel. 213/388–3151; Paul D. Hargis, Administrator **A**1 3 5 **F**15 17 19 21 22 27 34 35 41 47 48 51 56 65 70 71 73 **P**6 **S** Shriners Hospitals for Children, Tampa, FL	23	57	50	1651	37	11934	0	—	—	227

Hospital, Address, Telephone, Administrator, Approval, Facility, and Physician Codes, Health Care System, Network	Classi-fication Codes		Utilization Data					Expense (thousands) of dollars		
★ American Hospital Association (AHA) membership □ Joint Commission on Accreditation of Healthcare Organizations (JCAHO) accreditation + American Osteopathic Hospital Association (AOHA) membership ○ American Osteopathic Association (AOA) accreditation △ Commission on Accreditation of Rehabilitation Facilities (CARF) accreditation Control codes 61, 63, 64, 71, 72 and 73 indicate hospitals listed by AOHA, but not registered by AHA. For definition of numerical codes, see page A4	Control	Service	Beds	Admissions	Census	Outpatient Visits	Births	Total	Payroll	Personnel

	Control	Service	Beds	Admissions	Census	Outpatient Visits	Births	Total	Payroll	Personnel
✠ ST. VINCENT MEDICAL CENTER, 2131 West Third Street, Zip 90057–0992, Mailing Address: P.O. Box 57992, Zip 90057; tel. 213/484–7111; Vincent F. Guinan, President and Chief Executive Officer (Total facility includes 27 beds in nursing home–type unit) **A**1 3 5 9 10 **F**4 8 10 11 12 15 16 17 19 21 25 26 27 29 30 31 32 33 34 35 36 37 39 41 42 43 44 45 46 49 60 63 64 65 66 67 68 69 71 72 73 **P**5 7 8 **S** Catholic Healthcare West, San Francisco, CA **N** Catholic HealthCare West (CHW), San Francisco, CA	21	10	350	10141	168	40109	0	114510	39810	1143
□ TEMPLE COMMUNITY HOSPITAL, 235 North Hoover Street, Zip 90004; tel. 213/382–7252; Herbert G. Needman, Administrator and Chief Executive Officer (Total facility includes 11 beds in nursing home–type unit) **A**1 9 10 **F**8 11 19 20 21 31 35 37 44 45 60 63 64 71 73 **P**5	33	10	130	3595	70	—	0	28049	8852	287
✠ UNIVERSITY OF CALIFORNIA LOS ANGELES MEDICAL CENTER, 10833 Le Conte Avenue, Zip 90095–1730; tel. 310/825–9111; Michael Karpf, M.D., Vice Provost Hospital System and Director Medical Center **A**1 2 3 5 8 9 10 **F**4 5 7 8 10 11 12 13 17 19 20 21 22 23 25 26 27 28 29 30 31 32 34 35 37 38 40 41 42 43 44 45 46 47 48 49 50 51 60 61 63 65 67 69 70 71 72 73 74 **P**6 **S** University of California–Systemwide Administration, Oakland, CA	23	10	610	23634	392	491090	1450	460457	197940	6016
✠ UNIVERSITY OF CALIFORNIA LOS ANGELES NEUROPSYCHIATRIC HOSPITAL, 760 Westwood Plaza, Zip 90024–1759; tel. 310/825–9548; G. Michael Arnold, Interim Director **A**1 3 5 9 10 **F**12 15 52 53 54 55 56 57 58 59 **S** University of California–Systemwide Administration, Oakland, CA	12	22	117	1642	52	32867	0	26798	15643	555
✠ UNIVERSITY OF SOUTHERN CALIFORNIA–KENNETH NORRIS JR. CANCER HOSPITAL, (ACUTE CANCER CARE), 1441 Eastlake Avenue, Zip 90033–0804, Mailing Address: P.O. Box 33804, Zip 90033; tel. 213/764–3000; G. Peter Shostak, Administrator **A**1 2 3 5 9 10 **F**8 14 15 16 17 19 21 23 29 30 31 32 34 35 37 42 44 45 50 54 60 63 65 67 69 71 73 74 **P**4 5 6	23	49	60	2024	35	35028	0	47405	12768	316
✠ VALLEY PRESBYTERIAN HOSPITAL, 15107 Vanowen Street, Van Nuys, Zip 91405; tel. 818/782–6600; Robert C. Bills, President and Vice Chairman (Total facility includes 32 beds in nursing home–type unit) (Nonreporting) **A**1 2 9 10	23	10	315	—	—	—	—	—	—	—
□ VALUEMARK PINE GROVE BEHAVIORAL HEALTHCARE SYSTEM, 7011 Shoup Avenue, Canoga Park, Zip 91307; tel. 818/348–0500; Diane Sharpe, Chief Executive Officer (Nonreporting) **A**1 9 10 **S** ValueMark Healthcare Systems, Inc., Atlanta, GA	33	22	62	—	—	—	—	—	—	—
□ VAN NUYS HOSPITAL, 15220 Vanowen Street, Van Nuys, Zip 91405; tel. 818/787–0123; Brent Lamb, Administrator (Nonreporting) **A**1 9 10	33	22	41	—	—	—	—	—	—	—
□ VENCOR HOSPITAL–LOS ANGELES, 5525 West Slauson Avenue, Zip 90056; tel. 310/642–0325; Billie Anne Schoppman, R.N., Administrator (Nonreporting) **A**1 9 10 **S** Vencor, Incorporated, Louisville, KY	33	49	81	—	—	—	—	—	—	—
✠ VETERANS AFFAIRS MEDICAL CENTER–WEST LOS ANGELES, 11301 Wilshire Boulevard, Zip 90073–0275; tel. 310/268–3132; Kenneth J. Clark, Executive Director and Chief Executive Officer (Total facility includes 240 beds in nursing home–type unit) **A**1 3 5 8 **F**1 2 3 4 5 6 8 10 11 12 14 15 16 17 18 19 20 21 22 23 24 25 26 27 28 29 30 31 32 34 35 37 39 41 42 43 44 45 46 48 49 50 51 52 54 55 56 57 58 59 60 61 63 64 65 67 71 73 74 **S** Department of Veterans Affairs, Washington, DC	45	10	1327	13139	956	458762	0	302688	206268	3626
✠ △ WHITE MEMORIAL MEDICAL CENTER, 1720 Cesar E Chavez Avenue, Zip 90033–2481; tel. 213/268–5000; Beth D. Zachary, Chief Operating Officer (Total facility includes 41 beds in nursing home–type unit) (Nonreporting) **A**1 3 5 7 9 10 **S** Adventist Health, Roseville, CA **N** Adventist Health–Southern California, Glendale, CA	21	10	354	—	—	—	—	—	—	—
LOS BANOS—Merced County										
□ MEMORIAL HOSPITAL LOS BANOS, 520 West I Street, Zip 93635; tel. 209/826–0591; Gil Silbernagel, Administrator (Nonreporting) **A**1 9 10 **N** Sutter\CHS, Sacramento, CA	23	10	48	—	—	—	—	—	—	—
LOS GATOS—Santa Clara County										
□ △ COMMUNITY HOSPITAL OF LOS GATOS, 815 Pollard Road, Zip 95030; tel. 408/378–6131; Truman L. Gates, Chief Executive Officer (Nonreporting) **A**1 7 9 10 **S** TENET Healthcare Corporation, Santa Barbara, CA **N** Tenet Healthcare Corporation, Santa Barbara, CA	33	10	209	—	—	—	—	—	—	—
LOYALTON—Sierra County										
SIERRA VALLEY DISTRICT HOSPITAL, 700 Third Street, Zip 96118, Mailing Address: Box 178, Zip 96118; tel. 916/993–1225; Billie Weatherson, Administrator (Total facility includes 34 beds in nursing home–type unit) (Nonreporting) **A**9 10	16	10	40	—	—	—	—	—	—	—
LYNWOOD—Los Angeles County										
✠ ST. FRANCIS MEDICAL CENTER, 3630 East Imperial Highway, Zip 90262; tel. 310/603–6000; Gerald T. Kozai, Administrator and Chief Operating Officer (Total facility includes 30 beds in nursing home–type unit) **A**1 6 9 10 **F**4 7 8 10 12 14 15 16 17 19 20 27 28 29 32 33 34 35 37 38 40 41 42 43 44 45 46 49 52 59 64 65 67 70 71 72 73 74 **P**2 3 4 5 7 **S** Catholic Healthcare West, San Francisco, CA **N** Catholic HealthCare West (CHW), San Francisco, CA; Essential HealthCare Network, Monterey Park, CA	21	10	414	29476	255	219948	5292	126251	56510	1487
MADERA—Madera County										
□ MADERA COMMUNITY HOSPITAL, 1250 East Almond Avenue, Zip 93637–5696, Mailing Address: Box 1328, Zip 93639–1328; tel. 209/675–5501; Robert C. Kelley, President and Chief Executive Officer **A**1 9 10 **F**7 8 11 15 16 19 21 22 25 29 32 37 40 41 44 46 47 49 65 71 73	23	10	100	4051	42	97837	1333	26493	12552	410

Hospital, Address, Telephone, Administrator, Approval, Facility, and Physician Codes, Health Care System, Network	Classi-fication Codes		Utilization Data					Expense (thousands) of dollars		
★ American Hospital Association (AHA) membership □ Joint Commission on Accreditation of Healthcare Organizations (JCAHO) accreditation + American Osteopathic Hospital Association (AOHA) membership ○ American Osteopathic Association (AOA) accreditation △ Commission on Accreditation of Rehabilitation Facilities (CARF) accreditation Control codes 61, 63, 64, 71, 72 and 73 indicate hospitals listed by AOHA, but not registered by AHA. For definition of numerical codes, see page A4	Control	Service	Beds	Admissions	Census	Outpatient Visits	Births	Total	Payroll	Personnel

MAMMOTH LAKES—Mono County

□ MAMMOTH HOSPITAL, 85 Sierra Park Road, Zip 93546, Mailing Address: P.O. Box 660, Zip 93546; tel. 619/934–3311; Gary Myers, Administrator (Nonreporting) **A**1 9 10	23	10	15	—	—	—	—	—	—	—

MANTECA—San Joaquin County

□ DOCTORS HOSPITAL OF MANTECA, 1205 East North Street, Zip 95336, Mailing Address: Box 191, Zip 95336; tel. 209/823–3111; Patrick W. Rufferty, Chief Executive Officer **A**1 9 10 **F**2 3 4 7 8 9 10 11 12 15 16 19 21 22 24 25 26 27 28 29 30 32 33 34 35 36 37 38 40 41 42 43 44 45 46 47 48 49 51 52 54 55 56 58 59 60 61 64 65 66 67 70 71 72 73 74 **P**1 5 7 8 **S** TENET Healthcare Corporation, Santa Barbara, CA **N** Tenet Healthcare Corporation, Santa Barbara, CA	33	10	73	2794	31	43950	562	23010	9873	278
★ ST. DOMINIC'S HOSPITAL, 1777 West Yosemite Avenue, Zip 95337; tel. 209/825–3500; Richard Aldred, Chief Administrative Officer **A**9 10 **F**3 4 6 7 8 10 11 12 13 14 15 16 17 19 21 22 28 29 30 32 33 35 37 38 40 41 42 43 44 45 46 49 51 54 55 56 57 58 59 60 62 63 65 67 71 72 73 74 **P**7 **S** Catholic Healthcare West, San Francisco, CA **N** Catholic HealthCare West (CHW), San Francisco, CA	21	10	40	1694	29	22291	412	16626	5827	211

MARINA DEL REY—Los Angeles County

⊞ DANIEL FREEMAN MARINA HOSPITAL, 4650 Lincoln Boulevard, Zip 90292–6360; tel. 310/823–8911; Joseph W. Dunn, Ph.D., Chief Executive Officer (Nonreporting) **A**1 9 10 **S** Carondelet Health System, Saint Louis, MO	21	10	180	—	—	—	—	—	—	—

MARIPOSA—Mariposa County

JOHN C. FREMONT HEALTHCARE DISTRICT, 5189 Hospital Road, Zip 95338, Mailing Address: Box 216, Zip 95338; tel. 209/966–3631; Claire Kuczkowski, Administrator (Total facility includes 10 beds in nursing home–type unit) (Nonreporting) **A**9 10	16	10	34	—	—	—	—	—	—	—

MARTINEZ—Contra Costa County

KAISER FOUNDATION HOSPITAL See Kaiser Foundation Hospital, Walnut Creek										
□ MERRITHEW MEMORIAL HOSPITAL, 2500 Alhambra Avenue, Zip 94553; tel. 510/370–5000; Frank J. Puglisi, Jr., Executive Director **A**1 2 3 5 10 **F**1 3 4 8 10 12 13 15 16 17 18 19 20 21 22 23 26 27 28 29 30 31 32 33 34 35 36 37 39 40 41 42 43 44 45 46 49 51 52 53 54 55 56 57 58 60 61 64 65 67 68 70 71 72 73 74 **P**6	13	10	104	7325	120	321171	1323	133097	69790	978

MARYSVILLE—Yuba County

RIDEOUT MEMORIAL HOSPITAL, 726 Fourth Street, Zip 95901–2128, Mailing Address: Box 2128, Zip 95901–2128; tel. 916/749–4300; Thomas P. Hayes, Chief Executive Officer (Total facility includes 11 beds in nursing home–type unit) **A**9 10 **F**7 8 10 14 15 16 17 19 22 25 26 28 32 33 34 35 37 41 44 45 60 64 71 72 **P**5 **S** Fremont–Rideout Health Group, Yuba City, CA **N** Fremont–Rideout Health Group, Yuba City, CA	23	10	97	4791	85	58395	0	43937	17542	545

MATHER AFB—Sacramento County

□ U. S. AIR FORCE HOSPITAL, 10535 Hospital Way, Zip 95655–1200; tel. 916/643–7166; Richard Davis, Foreman Biomedical Equipment Maintenance (Nonreporting) **A**1	41	10	40	—	—	—	—	—	—	—

MENLO PARK—San Mateo County

□ RECOVERY INN OF MENLO PARK, 570 Willow Road, Zip 94025; tel. 415/324–8500; Ann Klein, Executive Director (Nonreporting) **A**1 10	33	10	16	—	—	—	—	—	—	—

MERCED—Merced County

MERCED COMMUNITY MEDICAL CENTER See Sutter Merced Medical Center										
⊞ MERCY HOSPITAL AND HEALTH SERVICES, 2740 M Street, Zip 95340–2880; tel. 209/384–6444; Kelly C. Morgan, President and Chief Executive Officer **A**1 9 10 **F**8 11 14 15 16 17 19 22 23 25 26 32 34 35 40 42 44 49 65 71 73 **S** Catholic Healthcare West, San Francisco, CA **N** Catholic HealthCare West (CHW), San Francisco, CA	21	10	101	5115	60	37020	947	33617	15150	468
⊞ SUTTER MERCED MEDICAL CENTER, (Formerly Merced Community Medical Center), 301 East 13th Street, Zip 95340–6211, Mailing Address: Box 231, Zip 95341–0231; tel. 209/385–7000; Brian S. Bentley, Administrator **A**1 3 5 9 10 **F**7 8 10 11 12 14 15 16 17 19 22 23 25 30 32 37 39 40 41 44 46 49 51 63 65 71 73 **S** Sutter Health, Sacramento, CA **N** Sutter\CHS, Sacramento, CA	13	10	158	6182	65	84975	1781	47275	23346	632

MISSION HILLS—Los Angeles County, See Los Angeles

MISSION VIEJO—Orange County

□ CHARTER BEHAVIORAL HEALTH SYSTEM OF SOUTHERN CALIFORNIA/MISSION VIEJO, 23228 Madero, Zip 92691; tel. 714/830–4800; James S. Plummer, Chief Executive Officer (Nonreporting) **A**1 10 **S** Magellan Health Services, Atlanta, GA	33	22	80	—	—	—	—	—	—	—
⊞ MISSION HOSPITAL REGIONAL MEDICAL CENTER, 27700 Medical Center Road, Zip 92691; tel. 714/364–1400; Peter F. Bastone, President and Chief Executive Officer **A**1 2 5 9 10 **F**2 4 7 8 10 11 12 13 14 15 16 17 19 21 22 23 24 25 26 28 29 30 32 33 34 35 37 38 39 40 41 42 43 44 46 47 48 49 60 63 65 67 70 71 73 74 **P**3 5 7 **S** St. Joseph Health System, Orange, CA	21	10	208	11679	127	100341	2859	102259	36877	987

MODESTO—Stanislaus County

□ △ DOCTORS MEDICAL CENTER, 1441 Florida Avenue, Zip 95350–4418, Mailing Address: P.O. Box 4138, Zip 95352–4138; tel. 209/578–1211; Chris DiCicco, Chief Executive Officer **A**1 2 7 9 10 **F**1 4 7 10 11 12 14 15 16 17 19 21 22 23 25 27 32 33 34 35 37 38 39 40 41 42 43 44 45 46 49 54 60 61 63 65 67 69 71 72 73 **P**5 6 **S** TENET Healthcare Corporation, Santa Barbara, CA **N** Tenet Healthcare Corporation, Santa Barbara, CA	33	10	289	15890	211	62428	4095	140963	60837	1568

Hospital, Address, Telephone, Administrator, Approval, Facility, and Physician Codes, Health Care System, Network	Classi-fication Codes		Utilization Data					Expense (thousands) of dollars		
★ American Hospital Association (AHA) membership □ Joint Commission on Accreditation of Healthcare Organizations (JCAHO) accreditation + American Osteopathic Hospital Association (AOHA) membership ○ American Osteopathic Association (AOA) accreditation △ Commission on Accreditation of Rehabilitation Facilities (CARF) accreditation Control codes 61, 63, 64, 71, 72 and 73 indicate hospitals listed by AOHA, but not registered by AHA. For definition of numerical codes, see page A4	Control	Service	Beds	Admissions	Census	Outpatient Visits	Births	Total	Payroll	Personnel
✠ MEMORIAL HOSPITALS ASSOCIATION, (Includes Memorial Hospitals–Ceres, 1905 Memorial Drive, Ceres, Zip 95307; Memorial Medical Center, 1700 Coffee Road, Zip 95355; Mailing Address: P.O. Box 942, Zip 95353; tel. 209/526–4500; David P. Benn, President and Chief Executive Officer (Total facility includes 48 beds in nursing home–type unit) (Nonreporting) **A**1 2 9 10 **S** Sutter Health, Sacramento, CA **N** Sutter\CHS, Sacramento, CA	23	10	373	—	—	—	—	—	—	—
STANISLAUS BEHAVIORAL HEALTH CENTER, 1501 Claus Road, Zip 95355; tel. 209/524–4888; Larry B. Poaster, Ph.D., Director **F**14 52 53 54 55 56 57 58 59 60	13	22	46	2064	45	0	0	9002	4332	103
□ STANISLAUS MEDICAL CENTER, 830 Scenic Drive, Zip 95350, Mailing Address: Box 3271, Zip 95353; tel. 209/558–7000; Beverly M. Finley, Chief Executive Officer (Nonreporting) **A**1 3 5 9 10	13	10	84	—	—	—	—	—	—	—
MONROVIA—Los Angeles County										
□ MONROVIA COMMUNITY HOSPITAL, 323 South Heliotrope Avenue, Zip 91016, Mailing Address: Box 707, Zip 91017–0707; tel. 818/359–8341; Steve Courtier, Administrator **A**1 9 10 **F**19 21 22 26 32 34 35 36 37 44 49 65 71 **S** Paracelsus Healthcare Corporation, Houston, TX	32	10	49	2127	29	4039	0	10212	4359	132
MONTCLAIR—San Bernardino County										
□ U.S. FAMILYCARE MEDICAL CENTER, 5000 San Bernardino Street, Zip 91763; tel. 909/625–5411; Ronald W. Porter, Chief Executive Officer (Nonreporting) **A**1 9 10 12 13	33	10	102	—	—	—	—	—	—	—
MONTEBELLO—Los Angeles County										
✠ BEVERLY HOSPITAL, 309 West Beverly Boulevard, Zip 90640; tel. 213/726–1222; Matthew S. Gerlach, Chief Executive Officer and Administrator **A**1 2 9 10 **F**4 7 8 10 11 19 20 21 22 27 28 30 32 35 37 38 40 43 44 45 49 60 63 65 67 71 73 **P**4 5 7 8 **S** Southern California Healthcare System, Pasadena, CA **N** Southern California Healthcare Systems, Pasadena, CA	23	10	120	9993	116	52434	2445	—	—	—
MONTEREY—Monterey County										
✠ COMMUNITY HOSPITAL OF THE MONTEREY PENINSULA, 23625 Holman Highway, Zip 93940, Mailing Address: Box 'HH', Zip 93942–1085; tel. 408/624–5311; Jay Hudson, President and Chief Executive Officer **A**1 2 9 10 **F**1 3 7 8 14 15 16 19 21 22 23 28 31 32 34 35 37 40 41 42 44 52 53 54 56 57 58 59 60 63 65 67 71 73 **P**7	23	10	174	10736	124	169253	1712	124452	52349	1093
MONTEREY PARK—Los Angeles County										
□ △ GARFIELD MEDICAL CENTER, 525 North Garfield Avenue, Zip 91754; tel. 818/573–2222; Philip A. Cohen, Chief Executive Officer **A**1 2 7 9 10 **F**4 7 8 10 11 12 16 17 19 21 22 27 28 29 30 32 34 35 37 38 39 40 41 42 43 44 46 48 49 60 64 65 71 73 **P**5 **S** TENET Healthcare Corporation, Santa Barbara, CA **N** Tenet Healthcare Corporation, Santa Barbara, CA; Essential HealthCare Network, Monterey Park, CA	33	10	207	11209	214	32598	3655	64982	31323	992
□ MONTEREY PARK HOSPITAL, 900 South Atlantic Boulevard, Zip 91754; tel. 818/570–9000; Dan F. Ausman, Chief Executive Officer (Nonreporting) **A**1 2 10 **S** TENET Healthcare Corporation, Santa Barbara, CA	33	10	95	—	—	—	—	—	—	—
MORENO VALLEY—Riverside County										
□ MORENO VALLEY COMMUNITY HOSPITAL, 27300 Iris Avenue, Zip 92555; tel. 909/243–0811; Janice Ziomek, Administrator (Nonreporting) **A**1 10 **S** Valley Health System, Hemet, CA	16	10	66	—	—	—	—	—	—	—
MORGAN HILL—Santa Clara County										
✠ SAINT LOUISE HOSPITAL, 18500 Saint Louise Drive, Zip 95037; tel. 408/779–1500; William C. Finlayson, President and Chief Executive Officer (Total facility includes 19 beds in nursing home–type unit) **A**1 9 10 **F**1 2 3 4 7 8 10 11 12 14 15 16 17 18 19 20 21 22 23 24 25 26 27 28 29 30 31 32 33 35 37 38 39 40 41 42 43 44 45 46 47 49 52 53 54 55 56 57 58 59 60 63 64 65 66 67 68 69 71 73 74 **P**2 3 5 6 7 **S** Catholic Healthcare West, San Francisco, CA **N** Catholic HealthCare West (CHW), San Francisco, CA	21	10	40	2008	29	23019	381	19534	6438	141
MOSS BEACH—San Mateo County										
✠ SETON MEDICAL CENTER COASTSIDE, (GEN ACUTE CARE WITH DIST SKIL), 600 Marine Boulevard, Zip 94038; tel. 415/728–5521; Deborah E. Stebbins, FACHE, President and Chief Executive Officer (Total facility includes 116 beds in nursing home–type unit) **A**1 9 10 **F**1 2 3 4 5 6 7 8 9 10 11 12 14 16 17 18 19 21 22 23 24 25 26 27 28 29 30 31 32 33 34 35 36 37 38 39 40 41 42 43 44 45 46 47 48 49 51 52 53 54 55 56 57 58 59 60 63 64 65 66 67 68 71 72 73 74 **P**2 3 5 7 **S** Catholic Healthcare West, San Francisco, CA **N** Catholic HealthCare West (CHW), San Francisco, CA	21	49	121	179	109	10847	0	7455	4057	90
MOUNT SHASTA—Siskiyou County										
✠ MERCY MEDICAL CENTER MOUNT SHASTA, 914 Pine Street, Zip 96067, Mailing Address: P.O. Box 239, Zip 96067–0239; tel. 916/926–6111; James R. Hoss, President and Chief Executive Officer (Total facility includes 47 beds in nursing home–type unit) **A**1 9 10 **F**7 8 15 17 19 22 24 25 26 28 31 32 33 35 37 39 40 41 44 56 64 65 66 70 71 73 **P**5 **S** Catholic Healthcare West, San Francisco, CA **N** Catholic HealthCare West (CHW), San Francisco, CA	23	10	80	1641	55	30560	150	16988	7113	272
MOUNTAIN VIEW—Santa Clara County										
✠ CAMINO HEALTHCARE, 2500 Grant Road, Zip 94040, Mailing Address: P.O. Box 7025, Zip 94039; tel. 415/940–7000; Joann Zimmerman, Vice President Patient Services and Chief Operating Officer (Nonreporting) **A**1 9 10	16	10	290	—	—	—	—	—	—	—
MURRIETA—Riverside County										
SHARP HEALTHCARE MURRIETA, 25500 Medical Center Drive, Zip 92562–5966; tel. 909/696–6000; Juanice Lovett, Chief Executive Officer (Total facility includes 42 beds in nursing home–type unit) (Nonreporting) **A**9 10 **S** Sharp Healthcare, San Diego, CA **N** Sharp Healthcare, San Diego, CA	23	10	91	—	—	—	—	—	—	—

Hospital, Address, Telephone, Administrator, Approval, Facility, and Physician Codes, Health Care System, Network	Classi-fication Codes		Utilization Data					Expense (thousands) of dollars		
★ American Hospital Association (AHA) membership □ Joint Commission on Accreditation of Healthcare Organizations (JCAHO) accreditation + American Osteopathic Hospital Association (AOHA) membership ○ American Osteopathic Association (AOA) accreditation △ Commission on Accreditation of Rehabilitation Facilities (CARF) accreditation Control codes 61, 63, 64, 71, 72 and 73 indicate hospitals listed by AOHA, but not registered by AHA. For definition of numerical codes, see page A4	Control	Service	Beds	Admissions	Census	Outpatient Visits	Births	Total	Payroll	Personnel

NAPA—Napa County

□ NAPA STATE HOSPITAL, 2100 Napa–Vallejo Highway, Zip 94558; tel. 707/253–5454; Frank Turley, Ph.D., Executive Director **A**1 3 9 10 **F**1 19 20 22 26 29 31 35 37 41 45 52 53 57 58 59 64 65 71 73	12	22	1110	511	829	—	0	105010	64489	1644
⊞ QUEEN OF THE VALLEY HOSPITAL, 1000 Trancas Street, Zip 94558, Mailing Address: Box 2340, Zip 94558; tel. 707/252–4411; Howard Levant, President and Chief Executive Officer (Total facility includes 24 beds in nursing home–type unit) (Nonreporting) **A**1 2 9 10 **S** St. Joseph Health System, Orange, CA **N** Saint Joseph Health System, Orange, CA	21	10	176	—	—	—	—	—	—	—

NATIONAL CITY—San Diego County

⊞ △ PARADISE VALLEY HOSPITAL, 2400 East Fourth Street, Zip 91950; tel. 619/470–4321; Fred M. Harder, President and Chief Executive Officer (Total facility includes 12 beds in nursing home–type unit) (Nonreporting) **A**1 7 9 10 **S** Adventist Health, Roseville, CA	21	10	130	—	—	—	—	—	—	—

NEEDLES—San Bernardino County

⊞ NEEDLES–DESERT COMMUNITIES HOSPITAL, 1401 Bailey Avenue, Zip 92363; tel. 619/326–4531; Donna Beane, Administrator **A**1 9 10 **F**7 8 12 15 16 19 22 24 28 34 36 37 40 44 49 65 71 **P**5 **S** Brim, Inc., Portland, OR **N** Samaritan Health Services, Phoenix, AZ	14	10	39	1558	14	12118	101	—	—	165

NEWHALL—Los Angeles County

NEWHALL COMMUNITY HOSPITAL, 22607 6th Street, Zip 91322–1328, Mailing Address: Box 221328, Zip 91321–1328; tel. 805/259–4555; Bienvenido Tan, M.D., Chief Executive Officer (Nonreporting) **A**9 10	12	10	13	—	—	—	—	—	—	—

NEWPORT BEACH—Orange County

⊞ HOAG MEMORIAL HOSPITAL PRESBYTERIAN, One Hoag Drive, Zip 92663–4120, Mailing Address: Box 6100, Zip 92658–6100; tel. 714/645–8600; Michael D. Stephens, President and Chief Executive Officer **A**1 2 5 9 10 **F**2 3 4 7 8 10 11 12 15 16 17 19 22 23 25 28 30 31 32 34 35 37 38 39 40 41 42 43 44 46 48 49 60 65 69 71 72 74 **P**1 5	23	10	355	20085	222	192113	4064	226478	73540	2362

NORTH HOLLYWOOD—Los Angeles County, See Los Angeles
NORTHRIDGE—Los Angeles County, See Los Angeles
NORWALK—Los Angeles County

□ COAST PLAZA DOCTORS HOSPITAL, 13100 Studebaker Road, Zip 90650; tel. 310/868–3751; Gerald J. Garner, Chairman of the Board (Total facility includes 12 beds in nursing home–type unit) **A**1 9 10 12 **F**11 12 15 16 17 19 21 22 26 28 34 35 37 44 46 49 58 59 60 64 66 71 73 **P**5	32	10	68	2940	32	7450	2	14717	—	236
KAISER FOUNDATION HOSPITAL, NORWALK See Kaiser Foundation Hospital, Bellflower										
LOS ANGELES COMMUNITY HOSPITAL OF NORWALK See Los Angeles Community Hospital, Los Angeles										
□ METROPOLITAN STATE HOSPITAL, 11400 Norwalk Boulevard, Zip 90650; tel. 310/863–7011; William G. Silva, Administrator **A**1 5 9 10 **F**20 22 24 30 39 41 45 46 52 55 59 65 67 73	12	22	600	854	514	0	0	75239	48693	1281

NOVATO—Marin County

⊞ NOVATO COMMUNITY HOSPITAL, 1625 Hill Road, Zip 94947, Mailing Address: P.O. Box 1108, Zip 94948; tel. 415/897–3111; Anne Hosfeld, Chief Administrative Officer **A**1 9 10 **F**4 7 8 10 11 12 14 15 16 19 21 22 23 24 27 28 29 30 31 32 33 34 35 37 38 40 41 42 43 44 45 46 47 48 49 52 53 54 55 56 57 58 59 60 65 71 73 **P**1 3 4 7 **S** Sutter Health, Sacramento, CA **N** Sutter\CHS, Sacramento, CA	23	10	30	2110	23	37460	191	20870	9715	261

OAKDALE—Stanislaus County

⊞ OAK VALLEY DISTRICT HOSPITAL, 350 South Oak Street, Zip 95361; tel. 209/847–3011; Gary D. Rapaport, Administrator and Chief Executive Officer (Total facility includes 108 beds in nursing home–type unit) **A**1 9 10 **F**7 8 11 15 16 17 19 20 21 22 30 34 35 37 40 41 44 46 49 64 65 67 71 72 73 74 **P**5 **N** Sutter\CHS, Sacramento, CA	16	10	141	2155	116	54612	361	19043	8078	348

OAKLAND—Alameda County

□ ALAMEDA COUNTY MEDICAL CENTER–HIGHLAND CAMPUS, 1411 East 31st Street, Zip 94602; tel. 510/437–5081; Michael Smart, Chief Executive Officer (Nonreporting) **A**1 3 5 10 12 **S** Alameda County Health Care Services Agency, San Leandro, CA	13	10	247	—	—	—	—	—	—	—
□ CHILDREN'S HOSPITAL OAKLAND, 747 52nd Street, Zip 94609; tel. 510/428–3000; Antonie H. Paap, President and Chief Executive Officer **A**1 3 5 9 10 **F**4 9 10 12 13 14 15 16 17 19 20 21 22 25 28 29 30 31 32 33 34 35 38 39 42 43 44 45 47 48 49 51 53 54 55 56 58 65 66 67 68 70 71 72 73 **P**5 8	23	50	193	8918	146	160118	0	144928	70327	1230
⊞ KAISER FOUNDATION HOSPITAL, 280 West MacArthur Boulevard, Zip 94611; tel. 510/596–1000; Donald Oxley, Vice President, Area Manager and Chief Executive Officer (Nonreporting) **A**1 3 5 10 **S** Kaiser Foundation Hospitals, Oakland, CA **N** Kaiser Foundation Health Plan of Northern California, Oakland, CA	23	10	263	—	—	—	—	—	—	—
□ SUMMIT MEDICAL CENTER, 350 Hawthorne Avenue, Zip 94609; tel. 510/655–4000; Irwin C. Hansen, President and Chief Executive Officer (Total facility includes 48 beds in nursing home–type unit) (Nonreporting) **A**1 2 9 10	23	10	420	—	—	—	—	—	—	—

OCEANSIDE—San Diego County

⊞ TRI–CITY MEDICAL CENTER, 4002 Vista Way, Zip 92056–4593; tel. 619/724–8411; John P. Lauri, President and Chief Executive Officer (Nonreporting) **A**1 2 9 10	16	10	371	—	—	—	—	—	—	—

Hospital, Address, Telephone, Administrator, Approval, Facility, and Physician Codes, Health Care System, Network	Classi-fication Codes		Utilization Data					Expense (thousands) of dollars		
★ American Hospital Association (AHA) membership □ Joint Commission on Accreditation of Healthcare Organizations (JCAHO) accreditation + American Osteopathic Hospital Association (AOHA) membership ○ American Osteopathic Association (AOA) accreditation △ Commission on Accreditation of Rehabilitation Facilities (CARF) accreditation Control codes 61, 63, 64, 71, 72 and 73 indicate hospitals listed by AOHA, but not registered by AHA. For definition of numerical codes, see page A4	Control	Service	Beds	Admissions	Census	Outpatient Visits	Births	Total	Payroll	Personnel

OJAI—Ventura County

☒ OJAI VALLEY COMMUNITY HOSPITAL, 1306 Maricopa Highway, Zip 93023–3180; tel. 805/646–1401; William E. Price, Interim Chief Executive Officer (Total facility includes 45 beds in nursing home–type unit) (Nonreporting) **A**1 9 10 **S** Principal Hospital Group, Brentwood, TN

| | 33 | 10 | 116 | — | — | — | — | — | — | — |

ONTARIO—San Bernardino County

□ VENCOR HOSPITAL–ONTARIO, 550 North Monterey, Zip 91764; tel. 909/391–0333; Virgis Narbutas, Administrator (Nonreporting) **A**1 5 **S** Vencor, Incorporated, Louisville, KY

| | 33 | 10 | 100 | — | — | — | — | — | — | — |

ORANGE—Orange County

□ CHAPMAN MEDICAL CENTER, 2601 East Chapman Avenue, Zip 92869; tel. 714/633–0011; Maxine T. Cooper, Chief Executive Officer **A**1 9 10 **F**2 3 4 5 6 7 8 9 10 11 12 13 16 17 18 19 20 21 22 23 24 25 26 27 28 29 30 31 32 33 34 35 37 38 39 40 41 42 43 44 45 46 47 48 49 50 51 52 53 54 55 56 57 58 60 61 62 63 64 65 66 67 68 69 70 71 72 73 74 **P**1 2 4 5 7 8 **S** TENET Healthcare Corporation, Santa Barbara, CA

| | 33 | 10 | 135 | 2672 | 27 | 17704 | 613 | — | — | 233 |

☒ CHILDREN'S HOSPITAL OF ORANGE COUNTY, 455 South Main Street, Zip 92868–3874; tel. 714/997–3000; Kimberly C. Cripe, Acting Chief Executive Officer **A**1 2 3 5 9 10 **F**12 13 14 15 16 17 27 31 32 34 38 39 42 44 47 49 53 54 58 65 67 69 72 73 **P**3 4 5 7 8

| | 23 | 50 | 192 | 6065 | 89 | 122856 | 0 | 112601 | 40734 | 1002 |

☒ ST. JOSEPH HOSPITAL, 1100 West Stewart Drive, Zip 92668, Mailing Address: P.O. Box 5600, Zip 92613–5600; tel. 714/633–9111; Larry K. Ainsworth, President and Chief Executive Officer (Total facility includes 34 beds in nursing home–type unit) **A**1 2 3 5 9 10 **F**2 3 4 7 8 10 11 12 14 15 16 17 18 19 20 21 22 23 24 25 26 28 30 32 33 34 35 36 37 38 39 40 41 42 43 44 47 48 49 52 56 58 59 60 64 65 67 69 71 73 74 **P**2 3 4 5 7 **S** St. Joseph Health System, Orange, CA **N** Saint Joseph Health System, Orange, CA

| | 21 | 10 | 367 | 19148 | 226 | 194333 | 5354 | 196180 | 72226 | 1924 |

☒ UNIVERSITY OF CALIFORNIA, IRVINE MEDICAL CENTER, 101 The City Drive, Zip 92668–3298; tel. 714/456–7890; Mark R. Laret, Executive Director **A**1 2 3 5 8 9 10 **F**4 5 8 9 10 11 12 13 14 15 16 17 18 19 21 22 25 26 28 29 30 31 34 35 37 38 39 40 41 42 43 44 45 46 47 48 49 51 52 53 54 55 56 57 58 59 60 65 66 67 68 69 70 71 72 73 74 **P**5 6 **S** University of California–Systemwide Administration, Oakland, CA

| | 23 | 10 | 383 | 13269 | 238 | 184417 | 1954 | 196888 | 84577 | 2149 |

OROVILLE—Butte County

□ OROVILLE HOSPITAL, 2767 Olive Highway, Zip 95966–6185; tel. 916/533–8500; Robert J. Wentz, President and Chief Executive Officer (Total facility includes 20 beds in nursing home–type unit) **A**1 9 10 **F**7 8 12 13 15 16 17 19 20 21 22 25 28 30 31 32 34 35 37 39 40 41 44 45 46 49 51 61 63 64 65 67 70 71 72 73 74 **P**8

| | 23 | 10 | 120 | 5307 | 68 | — | 654 | 49603 | 22784 | 674 |

OXNARD—Ventura County

☒ △ ST. JOHN'S REGIONAL MEDICAL CENTER, 1600 North Rose Avenue, Zip 93030; tel. 805/988–2500; Daniel R. Herlinger, President and Chief Executive Officer **A**1 7 9 10 **F**4 7 8 10 11 15 16 17 19 21 22 23 28 29 30 32 34 35 37 38 40 41 42 43 44 45 46 48 49 60 63 65 67 71 73 **P**3 5 7 **S** Catholic Healthcare West, San Francisco, CA **N** Catholic HealthCare West (CHW), San Francisco, CA

| | 23 | 10 | 230 | 11637 | 151 | 98000 | 1964 | 79639 | 36328 | 980 |

PALM SPRINGS—Riverside County

□ DESERT HOSPITAL, 1150 North Indian Canyon Drive, Zip 92262, Mailing Address: Box 2739, Zip 92263; tel. 619/323–6511; Robert A. Minkin, CHE, President and Chief Executive Officer (Nonreporting) **A**1 2 9 10

| | 23 | 10 | 348 | — | — | — | — | — | — | — |

PALO ALTO—Santa Clara County

□ LUCILE SALTER PACKARD CHILDREN'S HOSPITAL AT STANFORD, 725 Welch Road, Zip 94304; tel. 415/497–8000; Peter Van Etten, President **A**1 3 5 9 10 **F**4 5 8 10 12 13 15 16 17 18 19 21 22 23 29 30 31 32 34 35 38 39 41 42 43 44 45 46 47 49 50 51 53 54 55 56 58 59 60 65 67 68 69 70 73

| | 23 | 50 | 162 | 5908 | 124 | 57566 | 0 | 132620 | 53725 | 980 |

VETERANS AFFAIRS MEDICAL CENTER See Veterans Affairs Palo Alto Health Care System

☒ VETERANS AFFAIRS PALO ALTO HEALTH CARE SYSTEM, (Includes Veterans Affairs Medical Center, 4951 Arroyo Road, Livermore, Zip 94550; tel. 510/447–2560; Clarence H. Nixon, Director; Veterans Affairs Medical Center, 3801 Miranda Avenue, tel. 415/493–5000), 3801 Miranda Avenue, Zip 94304–1207; tel. 415/493–5000; James A. Goff, FACHE, Director (Total facility includes 379 beds in nursing home–type unit) **A**1 2 3 5 8 **F**1 2 3 4 5 6 8 10 11 12 14 15 16 17 18 19 20 21 22 23 25 26 27 28 30 31 32 33 34 35 37 39 41 42 43 44 45 46 48 49 50 51 52 54 55 56 57 58 59 60 61 63 64 65 67 69 71 72 73 74 **P**6 **S** Department of Veterans Affairs, Washington, DC

| | 45 | 10 | 1028 | 8176 | 519 | 342998 | 0 | 325916 | 160784 | 3424 |

PANORAMA CITY—Los Angeles County, See Los Angeles

PARADISE—Butte County

☒ FEATHER RIVER HOSPITAL, 5974 Pentz Road, Zip 95969–5593; tel. 916/877–9361; George Pifer, President (Total facility includes 21 beds in nursing home–type unit) **A**1 9 10 **F**7 8 10 11 12 15 17 19 22 25 27 28 29 30 31 32 34 35 36 37 40 41 44 46 49 64 65 67 71 73 74 **P**3 4 5 **S** Adventist Health, Roseville, CA **N** Adventist Health–Northern California, Deer Park, CA

| | 21 | 10 | 122 | 4659 | 59 | 89849 | 504 | 36851 | 17782 | 565 |

PARAMOUNT—Los Angeles County

□ SUBURBAN MEDICAL CENTER, 16453 South Colorado Avenue, Zip 90723; tel. 310/531–3110; Michael D. Kerr, Chief Executive Officer **A**1 9 10 **F**10 11 12 16 19 21 22 27 37 40 44 64 71 73 **P**5 7 **S** TENET Healthcare Corporation, Santa Barbara, CA **N** Essential HealthCare Network, Monterey Park, CA

| | 33 | 10 | 130 | 6616 | 67 | 67449 | 3415 | 30318 | 13722 | 432 |

Hospital, Address, Telephone, Administrator, Approval, Facility, and Physician Codes, Health Care System, Network	Classi-fication Codes		Utilization Data					Expense (thousands) of dollars		
★ American Hospital Association (AHA) membership □ Joint Commission on Accreditation of Healthcare Organizations (JCAHO) accreditation + American Osteopathic Hospital Association (AOHA) membership ○ American Osteopathic Association (AOA) accreditation △ Commission on Accreditation of Rehabilitation Facilities (CARF) accreditation Control codes 61, 63, 64, 71, 72 and 73 indicate hospitals listed by AOHA, but not registered by AHA. For definition of numerical codes, see page A4	Control	Service	Beds	Admissions	Census	Outpatient Visits	Births	Total	Payroll	Personnel

PASADENA—Los Angeles County

★ COLUMBIA LAS ENCINAS HOSPITAL, 2900 East Del Mar Boulevard, Zip 91107–4375; tel. 818/795–9901; Roland Metivier, Chief Executive Officer **A**1 9 10 **F**1 2 3 12 17 18 26 27 28 34 46 52 53 54 55 56 57 58 59 64 65 67 68 73 **P**7 **S** Columbia/HCA Healthcare Corporation, Nashville, TN | 33 | 22 | 138 | 1913 | 60 | 6670 | 0 | — | — | 228

★ HUNTINGTON MEMORIAL HOSPITAL, 100 West California Boulevard, Zip 91105, Mailing Address: P.O. Box 7013, Zip 91109–7013; tel. 818/397–5000; Stephen A. Ralph, President and Chief Executive Officer (Total facility includes 75 beds in nursing home–type unit) **A**1 3 5 8 9 10 **F**4 7 8 10 12 15 16 17 19 21 22 23 26 28 29 30 31 32 34 35 37 38 40 41 42 44 47 48 49 51 52 54 55 56 57 58 59 60 61 64 65 70 71 73 **P**3 5 **S** Southern California Healthcare System, Pasadena, CA **N** Southern California Healthcare Systems, Pasadena, CA | 23 | 10 | 472 | 23419 | 397 | 211013 | 4196 | 207129 | 93152 | 2463

IMPACT DRUG AND ALCOHOL TREATMENT CENTER, 1680 North Fair Oaks Avenue, Zip 91103; tel. 818/681–2575; James M. Stillwell, Director (Nonreporting) | 23 | 82 | 130 | — | — | — | — | — | — | —

□ ST. LUKE MEDICAL CENTER, 2632 East Washington Boulevard, Zip 91107–1994; tel. 818/797–1141; Mark Uffer, Chief Executive Officer (Total facility includes 18 beds in nursing home–type unit) (Nonreporting) **A**1 2 9 10 **S** TENET Healthcare Corporation, Santa Barbara, CA | 33 | 10 | 120 | — | — | — | — | — | — | —

PATTERSON—Stanislaus County

DEL PUERTO HOSPITAL, South Ninth Street, Zip 95363–0187, Mailing Address: Box 187, Zip 95363–0187; tel. 209/892–8781; Michael Petrie, Chief Executive Officer (Total facility includes 23 beds in nursing home–type unit) (Nonreporting) **A**9 10 | 16 | 10 | 30 | — | — | — | — | — | — | —

PATTON—San Bernardino County

□ PATTON STATE HOSPITAL, 3102 East Highland Avenue, Zip 92369; tel. 909/425–7000; William L. Summers, Executive Director **A**1 9 **F**8 9 10 11 12 14 16 19 20 21 22 23 26 28 30 31 34 35 37 39 40 41 42 46 47 50 52 54 55 56 57 63 64 65 67 70 71 73 **N** East Bay Medical Network, Emeryville, CA | 12 | 22 | 1133 | 1122 | 1130 | 0 | 0 | 93518 | 61711 | 1602

PETALUMA—Sonoma County

□ PETALUMA VALLEY HOSPITAL, 400 North McDowell Boulevard, Zip 94954–2339; tel. 707/778–1111; Neil Martin, President and Chief Executive Officer (Total facility includes 14 beds in nursing home–type unit) (Nonreporting) **A**1 2 9 10 **S** St. Joseph Health System, Orange, CA | 16 | 10 | 84 | — | — | — | — | — | — | —

PINOLE—Contra Costa County

□ DOCTORS HOSPITAL OF PINOLE, 2151 Appian Way, Zip 94564; tel. 510/724–5000; Gary Sloan, Chief Executive Officer (Total facility includes 40 beds in nursing home–type unit) **A**1 9 10 **F**2 3 4 7 8 10 11 12 14 15 16 17 19 21 22 28 29 31 32 33 34 35 37 39 42 43 44 46 49 50 53 57 58 60 63 64 65 67 69 71 73 74 **P**5 7 **S** TENET Healthcare Corporation, Santa Barbara, CA **N** Tenet Healthcare Corporation, Santa Barbara, CA | 33 | 10 | 137 | 4102 | 85 | 28529 | 0 | 41841 | 20194 | 296

PLACENTIA—Orange County

□ PLACENTIA–LINDA HOSPITAL, 1301 Rose Drive, Zip 92870; tel. 714/993–2000; Maxine T. Cooper, Chief Executive Officer **A**1 9 10 **F**7 8 11 14 15 16 17 19 21 22 28 30 31 32 34 35 36 37 39 40 41 42 44 46 49 54 56 61 63 65 66 67 71 73 **P**5 7 8 **S** TENET Healthcare Corporation, Santa Barbara, CA **N** Tenet Healthcare Corporation, Santa Barbara, CA | 33 | 10 | 114 | 2110 | 19 | 20204 | 437 | 18614 | 7723 | 217

PLACERVILLE—El Dorado County

★ MARSHALL HOSPITAL, Marshall Way, Zip 95667–3439; tel. 916/622–1441; Frank Nachtman, Administrator (Nonreporting) **A**1 9 10 | 23 | 10 | 107 | — | — | — | — | — | — | —

PLEASANTON—San Benito County

VALLEYCARE MEDICAL CENTER, 5555 West Los Positas Boulevard, Zip 94588; tel. 510/847–3000 (Nonreporting) **A**9 10 **S** ValleyCare Health System, Pleasanton, CA | 23 | 10 | 68 | — | — | — | — | — | — | —

POMONA—Los Angeles County

★ △ CASA COLINA HOSPITAL FOR REHABILITATIVE MEDICINE, 255 East Bonita Avenue, Zip 91767–9966, Mailing Address: P.O. Box 6001, Zip 91769–6001; tel. 909/593–7521; Dale E. Eazell, Ph.D., President and Chief Executive Officer (Total facility includes 11 beds in nursing home–type unit) **A**1 7 9 10 **F**1 12 14 17 24 25 26 32 34 41 45 48 49 64 65 67 73 | 23 | 46 | 38 | 490 | 31 | 9160 | 0 | 8061 | 3860 | 129

LANTERMAN DEVELOPMENTAL CENTER, 3530 Pomona Boulevard, Zip 91768, Mailing Address: P.O. Box 100, Zip 91769; tel. 909/595–1221; Ruth Maples, Executive Director **A**10 **F**2 3 4 5 6 7 8 9 10 11 12 13 17 18 19 20 21 22 23 24 25 26 27 28 29 30 31 32 33 34 35 36 37 38 39 40 41 42 43 44 45 46 47 48 49 50 51 52 53 54 55 56 57 58 59 60 61 62 63 64 65 66 67 68 69 70 71 72 73 74 **P**1 | 12 | 62 | 771 | 597 | 806 | 0 | 0 | 79000 | 47200 | 1204

★ POMONA VALLEY HOSPITAL MEDICAL CENTER, 1798 North Garey Avenue, Zip 91767–2918; tel. 909/865–9500; Richard E. Yochum, President (Total facility includes 38 beds in nursing home–type unit) **A**1 2 3 9 10 **F**4 7 8 10 11 12 14 15 16 17 19 20 21 22 23 24 25 28 29 30 31 34 35 36 37 38 39 40 41 42 43 44 45 46 47 60 64 65 66 67 71 72 73 74 **P**5 | 23 | 10 | 381 | 17759 | 221 | 362652 | 4814 | 165833 | 73573 | 1483

PORT HUENEME—Ventura County

□ ANACAPA HOSPITAL, 307 East Clara Street, Zip 93041; tel. 805/488–3661; John J. Megara, Administrator **A**1 9 10 **F**1 12 19 21 35 52 53 54 55 56 58 59 65 67 68 71 **P**8 | 33 | 22 | 40 | 660 | 27 | | 0 | 8268 | 2328 | —

PORTERVILLE—Tulare County

PORTERVILLE DEVELOPMENTAL CENTER, 26501 Avenue 140, Zip 93257–9430, Mailing Address: Box 2000, Zip 93258–2000; tel. 209/782–2222; Harold Pitchford, Executive Director **A**9 10 **F**6 7 12 16 17 18 19 20 21 24 26 27 28 29 30 31 32 35 41 44 46 50 53 54 57 60 64 65 67 73 **P**6 | 12 | 62 | 808 | 68 | 739 | 0 | 0 | — | — | 1397

Hospital, Address, Telephone, Administrator, Approval, Facility, and Physician Codes, Health Care System, Network	Classi-fication Codes		Utilization Data					Expense (thousands) of dollars		
	Control	Service	Beds	Admissions	Census	Outpatient Visits	Births	Total	Payroll	Personnel

★ American Hospital Association (AHA) membership
□ Joint Commission on Accreditation of Healthcare Organizations (JCAHO) accreditation
+ American Osteopathic Hospital Association (AOHA) membership
○ American Osteopathic Association (AOA) accreditation
△ Commission on Accreditation of Rehabilitation Facilities (CARF) accreditation
Control codes 61, 63, 64, 71, 72 and 73 indicate hospitals listed by AOHA, but not registered by AHA. For definition of numerical codes, see page A4

Hospital	Control	Service	Beds	Admissions	Census	Outpatient Visits	Births	Total	Payroll	Personnel
SIERRA VIEW DISTRICT HOSPITAL, 465 West Putnam Avenue, Zip 93257–3320; tel. 209/784–1110; Edwin L. Ermshar, President and Chief Executive Officer **A**9 10 **F**7 8 17 19 21 22 28 29 30 32 34 35 37 40 41 44 45 51 60 65 71 72 73 74 **P**5 8	16	10	93	5337	56	72279	1146	40451	15136	504
PORTOLA—Plumas County										
EASTERN PLUMAS DISTRICT HOSPITAL, 500 First Avenue, Zip 96122; tel. 916/832–4277; Charles Guenther, Administrator (Total facility includes 14 beds in nursing home–type unit) **A**9 10 **F**7 8 13 14 15 16 17 22 32 34 40 41 44 45 46 64 71 72 73 74 **P**6	16	10	24	493	20	18760	40	5903	2354	152
POWAY—San Diego County										
★ POMERADO HOSPITAL, 15615 Pomerado Road, Zip 92064; tel. 619/485–4600; Marvin W. Levenson, M.D., Administrator and Chief Operating Officer (Total facility includes 149 beds in nursing home–type unit) **A**1 2 9 10 **F**3 4 7 8 10 12 14 15 16 17 19 21 22 25 27 28 29 30 31 32 33 34 35 36 37 38 40 41 42 43 44 45 46 49 52 56 57 59 60 61 63 64 65 67 71 72 73 74 **P**3 5 6 7 **S** Palomar Pomerado Health System, San Diego, CA **N** Health First Network, San Diego, CA	16	10	258	5637	188	72582	1504	48670	19874	578
QUINCY—Plumas County										
□ PLUMAS DISTRICT HOSPITAL, 1065 Bucks Lake Road, Zip 95971–9599; tel. 916/283–2121; R. Michael Barry, Administrator (Nonreporting) **A**1 9 10	16	10	32	—	—	—	—	—	—	—
RANCHO MIRAGE—Riverside County										
★ EISENHOWER MEMORIAL HOSPITAL AND BETTY FORD CENTER AT EISENHOWER, 39000 Bob Hope Drive, Zip 92270; tel. 619/340–3911; Andrew W. Deems, President and Chief Executive Officer **A**1 2 5 9 10 **F**1 4 5 7 8 10 11 12 15 19 21 22 24 25 29 32 33 34 35 37 38 39 40 41 42 43 44 45 46 49 60 65 66 67 71 72 73 74 **P**5	23	10	261	13075	161	214941	1628	139634	47612	1149
RED BLUFF—Tehama County										
★ ST. ELIZABETH COMMUNITY HOSPITAL, 2550 Sister Mary Columba Drive, Zip 96080–4397; tel. 916/529–8005; Thomas F. Grimes, III, Executive Vice President and Chief Operating Officer **A**1 9 10 **F**7 11 12 15 16 17 19 22 28 32 33 34 35 40 44 49 65 68 71 73 **S** Catholic Healthcare West, San Francisco, CA **N** Catholic HealthCare West (CHW), San Francisco, CA	21	10	53	3231	34	—	617	30894	12624	394
REDDING—Shasta County										
★ MERCY MEDICAL CENTER, 2175 Rosaline Avenue, Zip 96001, Mailing Address: Box 496009, Zip 96049–6009; tel. 916/225–6000; George A. Govier, President and Chief Executive Officer **A**1 2 3 5 9 10 **F**4 7 8 10 11 15 16 19 21 22 23 24 25 27 29 30 31 32 33 34 36 37 38 39 40 41 42 43 44 49 60 63 64 65 67 70 71 72 73 74 **P**3 5 **S** Catholic Healthcare West, San Francisco, CA **N** Catholic HealthCare West (CHW), San Francisco, CA	21	10	220	11026	120	102739	1606	104295	41366	1085
□ REDDING MEDICAL CENTER, 1100 Butte Street, Zip 96001–0853, Mailing Address: Box 496072, Zip 96049–6072; tel. 916/244–5454; Jeff Koury, Chief Executive Officer **A**1 9 10 **F**2 3 4 5 7 8 9 10 11 12 14 15 16 17 18 19 20 22 27 28 30 32 33 34 35 36 37 38 39 40 41 42 43 44 47 48 49 52 53 54 57 58 59 60 61 63 64 65 67 69 70 71 72 73 74 **P**4 5 7 **S** TENET Healthcare Corporation, Santa Barbara, CA **N** Tenet Healthcare Corporation, Santa Barbara, CA; Kaiser Foundation Health Plan of Northern California, Oakland, CA	33	10	162	7457	110	110688	397	82165	31670	882
REDLANDS—San Bernardino County										
□ LOMA LINDA UNIVERSITY BEHAVIORAL MEDICINE CENTER, 1710 Barton Road, Zip 92373; tel. 909/793–9333; Nolan Kerr, Administrator (Nonreporting) **A**1 5 9 10 **S** Adventist Health System–Loma Linda, Loma Linda, CA **N** Adventist Health System–Loma Linda, Loma Linda, CA	21	22	89	—	—	—	—	—	—	—
□ REDLANDS COMMUNITY HOSPITAL, 350 Terracina Boulevard, Zip 92373, Mailing Address: Box 3391, Zip 92373–0742; tel. 909/335–5500; James R. Holmes, President (Nonreporting) **A**1 9 10	23	10	194	—	—	—	—	—	—	—
REDONDO BEACH—Los Angeles County										
□ SOUTH BAY MEDICAL CENTER, 514 North Prospect Avenue, Zip 90277; tel. 310/376–9474; Jerald R. Happel, Executive Director (Total facility includes 30 beds in nursing home–type unit) **A**1 9 **F**7 8 11 12 15 17 19 22 24 28 30 34 35 36 38 39 41 44 46 52 64 65 67 71 73 **P**7 **S** TENET Healthcare Corporation, Santa Barbara, CA **N** Tenet Healthcare Corporation, Santa Barbara, CA	33	10	149	2575	35	14328	707	28429	10834	287
REDWOOD CITY—San Mateo County										
★ KAISER FOUNDATION HOSPITAL, 1150 Veterans Boulevard, Zip 94063–2087; tel. 415/299–2000; Carol Kiecker, Chief Executive Officer, Vice President and Area Manager **A**1 3 5 10 **F**2 3 4 5 7 8 9 10 11 12 13 14 16 18 19 21 22 23 25 26 28 29 30 31 32 33 34 35 37 38 39 40 41 42 43 44 45 46 47 48 49 50 51 52 53 54 55 56 57 58 59 60 61 63 64 65 66 67 69 71 72 73 **P**3 **S** Kaiser Foundation Hospitals, Oakland, CA **N** Kaiser Foundation Health Plan of Northern California, Oakland, CA	23	10	144	6729	72	518352	1601	—	—	591
★ SEQUOIA HOSPITAL, 170 Alameda De Las Pulgas, Zip 94062–2799; tel. 415/367–5561; Glenna L. Vaskelis, Administrator (Total facility includes 72 beds in nursing home–type unit) **A**1 9 10 **F**1 2 4 7 8 10 11 12 15 17 18 19 21 22 28 29 30 31 32 33 34 35 37 38 39 40 41 42 43 44 45 46 48 49 52 53 56 59 60 64 65 66 67 71 73 **P**5 **S** Catholic Healthcare West, San Francisco, CA **N** Catholic HealthCare West (CHW), San Francisco, CA	16	10	249	10606	140	95474	1289	124946	48363	919
REEDLEY—Fresno County										
★ SIERRA–KINGS DISTRICT HOSPITAL, 372 West Cypress Avenue, Zip 93654; tel. 209/638–8155; Daniel DeSantis, Administrator **A**1 9 10 **F**7 8 12 13 14 15 16 17 19 22 24 28 34 39 40 44 45 49 65 71 73	16	10	36	1380	9	37427	693	9122	3667	157

Hospital, Address, Telephone, Administrator, Approval, Facility, and Physician Codes, Health Care System, Network	Control	Service	Beds	Admissions	Census	Outpatient Visits	Births	Total	Payroll	Personnel

RICHMOND—Contra Costa County

☐ EAST BAY HOSPITAL, 820 23rd Street, Zip 94804–1397; tel. 510/234–2525; Lois K. Patsey, Administrator and Chief Executive Officer **A**1 9 10 **F**41 44 52 55 59 65 73 — Control 33, Service 10, Beds 87, Admissions 1682, Census 62, Outpatient Visits 5166, Births 0, Total —, Payroll —, Personnel 83

RIDGECREST—Kern County

✠ RIDGECREST COMMUNITY HOSPITAL, 1081 North China Lake Boulevard, Zip 93555; tel. 619/446–3551; David A. Mechtenberg, Chief Executive Officer **A**1 9 10 **F**7 11 15 16 19 22 28 32 35 36 37 40 41 44 45 46 49 65 71 73 **P**8 — Control 23, Service 10, Beds 80, Admissions 2360, Census 24, Outpatient Visits 42031, Births 491, Total 19763, Payroll 8563, Personnel 250

RIVERSIDE—Riverside County

✠ KAISER FOUNDATION HOSPITAL–RIVERSIDE, 10800 Magnolia Avenue, Zip 92505–3000; tel. 909/353–4600; Robert S. Lund, Administrator **A**1 2 3 10 **F**3 4 7 8 10 12 14 15 16 21 22 31 32 33 35 37 38 40 41 42 43 45 46 53 54 55 56 58 63 65 69 71 72 73 74 **S** Kaiser Foundation Hospitals, Oakland, CA — Control 23, Service 10, Beds 121, Admissions 8073, Census 78, Outpatient Visits 32120, Births 2123, Total —, Payroll —, Personnel 641

☐ PARKVIEW COMMUNITY HOSPITAL MEDICAL CENTER, 3865 Jackson Street, Zip 92503; tel. 909/688–2211; Norm Martin, President and Chief Executive Officer **A**1 2 9 10 **F**7 8 10 11 12 15 16 17 19 21 22 28 30 35 36 37 38 40 41 42 43 44 46 49 65 68 71 72 73 — Control 23, Service 10, Beds 193, Admissions 11999, Census 113, Outpatient Visits 130155, Births 4189, Total 71020, Payroll 28018, Personnel 975

☐ RIVERSIDE COMMUNITY HOSPITAL, 4445 Magnolia Avenue, Zip 92501–1669, Mailing Address: Box 1669, Zip 92502–1669; tel. 909/788–3000; Nancy J. Bitting, President and Chief Executive Officer (Nonreporting) **A**1 9 10 — Control 23, Service 10, Beds 254

☐ RIVERSIDE GENERAL HOSPITAL–UNIVERSITY MEDICAL CENTER, 9851 Magnolia Avenue, Zip 92503; tel. 909/358–7811; Tomi Hadfield, Administrator **A**1 3 5 9 10 **F**4 7 8 12 14 15 16 17 18 19 20 21 22 27 28 29 30 31 34 35 37 38 39 40 41 42 43 44 47 49 53 54 55 56 57 58 59 61 65 67 70 71 72 73 74 **P**6 — Control 13, Service 10, Beds 239, Admissions 10657, Census 139, Outpatient Visits 164217, Births 1501, Total 118743, Payroll 45161, Personnel 1258

ROSEMEAD—Los Angeles County

☐ BHC ALHAMBRA HOSPITAL, 4619 North Rosemead Boulevard, Zip 91770–1498, Mailing Address: P.O. Box 369, Zip 91770; tel. 818/286–1191; Peggy Minnick, Administrator (Nonreporting) **A**1 9 10 **S** Behavioral Healthcare Corporation, Nashville, TN — Control 33, Service 22, Beds 98

ROSEVILLE—Placer County

✠ SUTTER ROSEVILLE MEDICAL CENTER, One Medical Plaza, Zip 95661–3477; tel. 916/781–1000; Joel E. Grey, Chief Executive Officer (Total facility includes 14 beds in nursing home–type unit) **A**1 2 9 10 **F**4 7 10 11 12 13 15 16 17 19 20 21 22 26 28 29 30 31 32 33 37 39 40 41 42 44 45 46 49 60 63 64 65 66 67 70 71 73 **P**3 5 7 **S** Sutter Health, Sacramento, CA **N** Sutter\CHS, Sacramento, CA — Control 23, Service 10, Beds 183, Admissions 10856, Census 119, Outpatient Visits 166736, Births 1575, Total 90206, Payroll 39166, Personnel 742

SACRAMENTO—Sacramento County

✠ BHC HERITAGE OAKS HOSPITAL, 4250 Auburn Boulevard, Zip 95841; tel. 916/489–3336; Ingrid L. Whipple, Chief Executive Officer (Nonreporting) **A**1 9 10 **S** Behavioral Healthcare Corporation, Nashville, TN — Control 33, Service 22, Beds 76

☐ BHC SIERRA VISTA HOSPITAL, (Formerly CPC Sierra Vista Hospital), 8001 Bruceville Road, Zip 95823; tel. 916/423–2000; Kenneth A. Meibert, Chief Executive Officer (Nonreporting) **A**1 9 10 **S** Behavioral Healthcare Corporation, Nashville, TN — Control 33, Service 22, Beds 72

CPC SIERRA VISTA HOSPITAL See BHC Sierra Vista Hospital

✠ KAISER FOUNDATION HOSPITAL, 2025 Morse Avenue, Zip 95825–2115; tel. 916/978–1710; Sarah Krevans, Administrator (Nonreporting) **A**1 3 5 10 **S** Kaiser Foundation Hospitals, Oakland, CA — Control 23, Service 10, Beds 304

✠ KAISER FOUNDATION HOSPITAL, 6600 Bruceville Road, Zip 95823; tel. 916/688–2430; Sarah Krevans, Area Manager (Nonreporting) **A**1 3 10 **S** Kaiser Foundation Hospitals, Oakland, CA **N** Kaiser Foundation Health Plan of Northern California, Oakland, CA — Control 23, Service 10, Beds 221

✠ MERCY GENERAL HOSPITAL, 4001 J Street, Zip 95819; tel. 916/453–4950; Thomas A. Petersen, Vice President and Chief Operating Officer (Total facility includes 117 beds in nursing home–type unit) **A**1 2 5 9 10 **F**4 7 8 10 11 12 15 17 18 19 21 22 23 25 26 28 29 30 31 32 33 34 35 37 38 39 40 41 42 43 44 46 48 49 50 53 54 55 56 57 58 59 60 61 64 65 66 67 68 71 72 73 74 **P**3 5 **S** Catholic Healthcare West, San Francisco, CA **N** National Cardiovascular Network, Atlanta, GA; Catholic HealthCare West (CHW), San Francisco, CA — Control 21, Service 10, Beds 405, Admissions 18403, Census 275, Births 3779, Total 147989, Payroll 59979, Personnel 1367

☐ METHODIST HOSPITAL, 7500 Hospital Drive, Zip 95823–5477; tel. 916/423–3000; Stanley C. Oppegard, Vice President and Chief Operating Officer (Total facility includes 142 beds in nursing home–type unit) **A**1 3 9 10 **F**4 5 7 8 10 12 14 15 16 17 19 20 21 22 23 24 25 26 27 28 29 30 31 32 33 34 35 37 39 40 41 42 43 44 45 46 49 50 51 53 54 55 56 57 58 59 60 63 64 65 66 67 69 70 71 72 73 74 **P**3 5 **S** Catholic Healthcare West, San Francisco, CA **N** Catholic HealthCare West (CHW), San Francisco, CA — Control 23, Service 10, Beds 303, Admissions 6034, Census 187, Outpatient Visits 48996, Births 670, Total 50100, Payroll 24001, Personnel 661

★ SUTTER CENTER FOR PSYCHIATRY, 7700 Folsom Boulevard, Zip 95826–2608; tel. 916/386–3000; Diane Gail Stewart, Administrator **A**9 10 **F**2 3 4 7 8 10 11 12 13 15 16 17 19 21 22 26 28 29 30 31 32 33 34 35 37 38 39 40 41 42 43 44 45 46 47 48 49 50 51 52 53 54 55 57 58 59 60 61 63 65 66 67 68 69 71 72 73 74 **P**3 5 **S** Sutter Health, Sacramento, CA **N** Sutter\CHS, Sacramento, CA — Control 23, Service 22, Beds 69, Admissions 1735, Census 38, Births 0, Total 8770, Payroll 4615, Personnel 176

✠ SUTTER COMMUNITY HOSPITALS, (Includes Sutter General Hospital, 2801 L Street, Zip 95816; tel. 916/454–2222; Sutter Memorial Hospital, 5151 F Street), 5151 F Street, Zip 95819–3295; tel. 916/454–3333; Lou Lazatin, Chief Executive Officer (Total facility includes 198 beds in nursing home–type unit) **A**1 2 3 5 9 10 **F**1 2 3 4 5 7 8 10 11 12 14 15 16 17 18 19 20 21 22 23 25 26 27 28 29 30 31 32 33 34 35 36 37 38 40 41 42 43 44 45 46 47 49 50 52 53 54 55 56 57 58 59 60 61 62 63 64 65 67 68 69 70 71 72 73 74 **P**3 5 **S** Sutter Health, Sacramento, CA **N** Sutter\CHS, Sacramento, CA — Control 23, Service 10, Beds 499, Admissions 26745, Census 307, Outpatient Visits 260569, Births 5697, Total 254912, Payroll 107383, Personnel 2808

Hospital, Address, Telephone, Administrator, Approval, Facility, and Physician Codes, Health Care System, Network	Classi-fication Codes		Utilization Data					Expense (thousands) of dollars		
	Control	Service	Beds	Admissions	Census	Outpatient Visits	Births	Total	Payroll	Personnel

★ American Hospital Association (AHA) membership
□ Joint Commission on Accreditation of Healthcare Organizations (JCAHO) accreditation
+ American Osteopathic Hospital Association (AOHA) membership
○ American Osteopathic Association (AOA) accreditation
△ Commission on Accreditation of Rehabilitation Facilities (CARF) accreditation
Control codes 61, 63, 64, 71, 72 and 73 indicate hospitals listed by AOHA, but not registered by AHA. For definition of numerical codes, see page A4

Hospital	Control	Service	Beds	Admissions	Census	Outpatient Visits	Births	Total	Payroll	Personnel
★ UNIVERSITY OF CALIFORNIA, DAVIS MEDICAL CENTER, 2315 Stockton Boulevard, Zip 95817–2282; tel. 916/734–2011; Frank J. Loge, Director **A**1 2 3 5 8 9 10 **F**4 7 8 9 10 11 12 13 14 15 16 17 18 19 20 21 22 23 25 26 28 29 30 31 32 33 34 35 37 38 39 40 41 42 43 44 45 46 47 48 49 50 51 53 54 55 56 57 58 60 61 63 65 66 67 68 69 70 71 72 73 74 **P**6 **S** University of California–Systemwide Administration, Oakland, CA	12	10	448	21901	337	499618	1200	395246	185425	4682
SALINAS—Monterey County										
★ NATIVIDAD MEDICAL CENTER, 1330 Natividad Road, Zip 93906, Mailing Address: Box 81611, Zip 93912–1611; tel. 408/755–4111; Howard H. Classen, Chief Executive Officer (Total facility includes 52 beds in nursing home–type unit) (Nonreporting) **A**1 3 5 10	13	10	181	—	—	—	—	—	—	—
★ SALINAS VALLEY MEMORIAL HOSPITAL, 450 East Romie Lane, Zip 93901–4098; tel. 408/757–4333; Samuel W. Downing, Chief Executive Officer **A**1 2 9 10 **F**4 7 8 10 11 12 13 14 15 16 17 19 20 21 22 24 25 27 28 29 30 32 33 34 35 36 37 39 40 41 42 43 44 45 46 48 49 60 63 64 65 67 71 72 73 74 **P**3 5 7 8	16	10	177	11077	114	75401	2594	128312	60332	1085
SAN ANDREAS—Calaveras County										
★ MARK TWAIN ST. JOSEPH'S HOSPITAL, 768 Mountain Ranch Road, Zip 95249–9710; tel. 209/754–3521; Kathy Yarbrough, Administrator (Nonreporting) **A**1 9 10 **S** Catholic Healthcare West, San Francisco, CA **N** Catholic HealthCare West (CHW), San Francisco, CA	23	10	33	—	—	—	—	—	—	—
SAN BERNARDINO—San Bernardino County										
□ COMMMUNITY HOSPITAL OF SAN BERNARDINO, 1805 Medical Center Drive, Zip 92411; tel. 909/887–6333; Bruce G. Satzger, Administrator and Chief Executive Officer (Total facility includes 99 beds in nursing home–type unit) **A**1 9 10 **F**1 7 8 10 12 15 16 19 20 21 22 27 28 29 31 32 34 35 36 37 38 39 40 41 42 44 45 46 48 49 52 53 54 56 57 58 61 64 65 67 71 73 74 **P**5 7	23	10	380	10783	241	116566	2365	72330	34201	1244
★ ○ SAN BERNARDINO COUNTY MEDICAL CENTER, 780 East Gilbert Street, Zip 92415–0935; tel. 909/387–8188; Charles R. Jervis, Director **A**1 2 3 5 9 10 11 12 13 **F**3 4 7 9 10 12 14 15 16 19 20 21 22 26 29 31 32 35 37 38 40 41 42 44 45 51 52 53 56 57 58 59 60 61 63 65 69 70 71 72 73 **P**5	13	10	293	14959	201	194734	1759	141322	62427	1555
★ ST. BERNARDINE MEDICAL CENTER, 2101 North Waterman Avenue, Zip 92404; tel. 909/883–8711; Maureen O'Connor, Interim Administrator and Chief Operating Officer (Total facility includes 29 beds in nursing home–type unit) (Nonreporting) **A**1 2 9 10 **S** Catholic Healthcare West, San Francisco, CA **N** Catholic HealthCare West (CHW), San Francisco, CA	23	10	447	—	—	—	—	—	—	—
SAN CLEMENTE—Orange County										
★ COLUMBIA SAN CLEMENTE HOSPITAL AND MEDICAL CENTER, 654 Camino De Los Mares, Zip 92673; tel. 714/496–1122; Tony Struthers, Chief Executive Officer (Nonreporting) **A**1 9 10 **S** Samaritan Health System, Phoenix, AZ **N** Samaritan Health Services, Phoenix, AZ	23	10	86	—	—	—	—	—	—	—
SAN DIEGO—San Diego County										
□ ALVARADO HOSPITAL MEDICAL CENTER, 6655 Alvarado Road, Zip 92120–5298; tel. 619/229–3100; Barry G. Weinbaum, Chief Executive Officer **A**1 2 3 9 10 **F**4 7 8 10 11 12 15 16 17 19 22 23 30 32 34 35 37 38 39 40 42 43 44 45 46 49 61 63 65 67 71 73 **S** TENET Healthcare Corporation, Santa Barbara, CA **N** Tenet Healthcare Corporation, Santa Barbara, CA	33	10	144	7888	91	—	986	—	—	860
□ CHARTER BEHAVIORAL HEALTH SYSTEM OF SAN DIEGO, 11878 Avenue of Industry, Zip 92128; tel. 619/487–3200; Jerry Greene, Chief Executive Officer **A**1 9 10 **F**1 2 3 12 34 52 53 54 55 56 57 58 59 65 73 **S** Magellan Health Services, Atlanta, GA	33	22	80	1236	35	5229	0	8035	—	88
□ △ CHILDREN'S HOSPITAL AND HEALTH CENTER, 3020 Children's Way, Zip 92123–4282; tel. 619/576–1700; Blair L. Sadler, President (Total facility includes 59 beds in nursing home–type unit) **A**1 2 3 5 7 9 10 **F**5 10 13 15 16 17 19 20 21 22 28 31 32 33 34 35 38 41 42 43 44 46 47 48 49 53 54 58 64 65 69 70 71 72 73 **P**5	23	50	283	10636	187	197606	0	148063	63360	1608
★ COLUMBIA MISSION BAY HOSPITAL, 3030 Bunker Hill Street, Zip 92109–5780; tel. 619/274–7721; Deborah Brehe, Chief Executive Officer (Total facility includes 26 beds in nursing home–type unit) **A**1 9 10 **F**8 11 12 14 16 17 19 22 26 28 30 32 35 37 44 46 52 57 64 65 71 73 **P**5 7 **S** Columbia/HCA Healthcare Corporation, Nashville, TN	33	10	117	2362	36	67086	0	26112	11131	294
□ HARBOR VIEW MEDICAL CENTER, 120 Elm Street, Zip 92101; tel. 619/232–4331; Steve Hall, Chief Executive Officer **A**1 9 10 **F**1 2 3 4 5 6 7 8 9 10 11 12 13 16 17 18 19 20 21 22 23 24 25 26 27 28 29 30 31 32 33 34 35 36 37 38 39 40 41 42 43 44 45 46 47 48 49 50 52 53 54 55 56 57 58 59 60 61 62 63 64 65 66 67 68 69 70 71 72 73 74 **P**5 7 **S** TENET Healthcare Corporation, Santa Barbara, CA	33	10	146	5355	117	38083	0	26777	11131	282
★ KAISER FOUNDATION HOSPITAL, (Includes Kaiser Foundation Hospital, 203 Travelodge Drive, El Cajon, Zip 92020; tel. 619/528–5000), 4647 Zion Avenue, Zip 92120; tel. 619/528–5000; Kenneth F. Colling, Administrator **A**1 2 3 5 10 **F**2 3 4 7 8 10 11 12 13 14 15 16 17 18 19 21 22 23 25 26 28 29 30 31 32 33 34 35 37 38 39 40 41 42 43 44 45 46 51 52 53 56 58 59 60 61 63 64 65 67 69 71 72 73 74 **S** Kaiser Foundation Hospitals, Oakland, CA MERCY HEALTHCARE–SAN DIEGO See Scripps Mercy Medical Center	23	10	277	20341	201	—	4444	—	—	—
★ NAVAL MEDICAL CENTER, 34800 Bob Wilson Drive, Zip 92134–5000; tel. 619/532–6400; Rear Admiral R. A. Nelson, MC, USN, Commander (Nonreporting) **A**1 2 3 5 **S** Department of Navy, Washington, DC	43	10	386	—	—	—	—	—	—	—

Hospital, Address, Telephone, Administrator, Approval, Facility, and Physician Codes, Health Care System, Network	Classi-fication Codes		Utilization Data					Expense (thousands) of dollars		
★ American Hospital Association (AHA) membership □ Joint Commission on Accreditation of Healthcare Organizations (JCAHO) accreditation + American Osteopathic Hospital Association (AOHA) membership ○ American Osteopathic Association (AOA) accreditation △ Commission on Accreditation of Rehabilitation Facilities (CARF) accreditation Control codes 61, 63, 64, 71, 72 and 73 indicate hospitals listed by AOHA, but not registered by AHA. For definition of numerical codes, see page A4	Control	Service	Beds	Admissions	Census	Outpatient Visits	Births	Total	Payroll	Personnel

□ SAN DIEGO COUNTY PSYCHIATRIC HOSPITAL, 3851 Rosecrans Street, Zip 92110, Mailing Address: P.O. Box 85524, Zip 92138–5524; tel. 619/692–8211; Karen C. Hogan, Administrator and Chief Executive Officer (Nonreporting) A1 9 10	13	22	109	—	—	—	—	—	—	—
★ SAN DIEGO HOSPICE, (SPECIALITY), 4311 Third Avenue, Zip 92103; tel. 619/688–1600; Janet E. Cetti, President and Chief Executive Officer A10 F14 15 16 67	23	49	24	345	17	0	0	4543	1798	—
⊠ SCRIPPS MERCY MEDICAL CENTER, (Formerly Mercy Healthcare–San Diego), 4077 Fifth Avenue, Zip 92103–2180; tel. 619/260–7101; Nancy Wilson, Senior Vice President and Regional Administrator (Nonreporting) A1 2 3 5 9 10 S Scripps Health, San Diego, CA N ScrippsHealth, San Diego, CA	21	10	417	—	—	—	—	—	—	—
□ SHARP CABRILLO HOSPITAL, 3475 Kenyon Street, Zip 92110–5067; tel. 619/221–3400; Randi Larsson, Senior Vice President and Administrator (Total facility includes 79 beds in nursing home–type unit) (Nonreporting) A1 9 10 S Sharp Healthcare, San Diego, CA N Sharp Healthcare, San Diego, CA	23	10	227	—	—	—	—	—	—	—
□ △ SHARP MEMORIAL HOSPITAL, 7901 Frost Street, Zip 92123–2788; tel. 619/541–3400; Dan Gross, Chief Executive Officer (Nonreporting) A1 2 3 7 9 10 S Sharp Healthcare, San Diego, CA N Sharp Healthcare, San Diego, CA	23	10	488	—	—	—	—	—	—	—
⊠ UNIVERSITY OF CALIFORNIA SAN DIEGO MEDICAL CENTER, 200 West Arbor Drive, Zip 92103–8970; tel. 619/543–6222; David B. Coats, President (Nonreporting) A1 2 3 5 8 9 10 S University of California–Systemwide Administration, Oakland, CA	12	10	412	—	—	—	—	—	—	—
□ VENCOR HOSPITAL–SAN DIEGO, 1940 El Cajon Boulevard, Zip 92104; tel. 619/543–4500; Michael D. Cress, Administrator A1 10 F14 16 19 21 22 34 35 37 46 50 63 65 71 P5 S Vencor, Incorporated, Louisville, KY	33	10	70	435	31	2528	0	10838	5382	123
⊠ VETERANS AFFAIRS MEDICAL CENTER, 3350 LaJolla Village Drive, Zip 92161; tel. 619/552–8585; Thomas B. Arnold, Chief Operating Officer (Total facility includes 44 beds in nursing home–type unit) A1 2 3 5 8 F1 2 3 4 5 8 10 11 12 14 15 17 18 19 20 21 22 23 24 25 26 27 28 29 31 32 33 34 35 37 39 41 42 43 44 45 46 48 49 51 52 54 56 57 58 59 60 64 65 67 69 71 72 73 74 P6 S Department of Veterans Affairs, Washington, DC	45	10	269	7224	190	287056	0	141429	71641	1865
□ VILLAVIEW COMMUNITY HOSPITAL, 5550 University Avenue, Zip 92105, Mailing Address: P.O. Box 5587, Zip 92105; tel. 619/582–3516; Stuart A. Jed, Administrator (Nonreporting) A1 9 10	23	10	100	—	—	—	—	—	—	—
SAN DIMAS—Los Angeles County										
□ SAN DIMAS COMMUNITY HOSPITAL, 1350 West Covina Boulevard, Zip 91773–0308; tel. 909/599–6811; Larry Peterson, Chief Executive Officer (Nonreporting) A1 2 9 10 S TENET Healthcare Corporation, Santa Barbara, CA N Tenet Healthcare Corporation, Santa Barbara, CA	33	10	93	—	—	—	—	—	—	—
SAN FERNANDO—Los Angeles County										
⊠ MISSION COMMUNITY HOSPITAL–SAN FERNANDO CAMPUS, (Includes Mission Community Hospital–Panorama City Campus, 14850 Roscoe Boulevard, Panorama City, Zip 91402–4618; tel. 818/787–2222), 700 Chatsworth Drive, Zip 91340–4299; tel. 818/361–7331; Cathy Fickes, R.N., Chief Executive Officer (Nonreporting) A1 9	23	10	152	—	—	—	—	—	—	—
SAN FRANCISCO—San Francisco County										
⊠ △ CALIFORNIA PACIFIC MEDICAL CENTER, Clay at Buchanan Street, Zip 94115, Mailing Address: P.O. Box 7999, Zip 94120; tel. 415/563–4321; Martin Brotman, M.D., President and Chief Executive Officer (Total facility includes 95 beds in nursing home–type unit) A1 2 3 5 7 8 9 10 F2 3 4 7 8 9 10 11 12 13 14 15 16 17 19 20 21 22 23 26 28 29 30 31 32 33 34 35 37 38 40 41 42 43 44 45 46 47 48 49 50 51 52 53 54 56 57 58 59 60 61 64 65 66 67 69 71 72 73 74 P3 5 7 S Sutter Health, Sacramento, CA N Sutter\CHS, Sacramento, CA	23	10	520	21209	319	364604	4263	281086	125697	2748
⊠ CHINESE HOSPITAL, 845 Jackson Street, Zip 94133–4899; tel. 415/982–2400; Thomas M. Harlan, Chief Executive Officer A1 9 10 F4 7 8 9 10 14 15 16 17 19 21 22 28 29 30 32 33 35 37 38 39 40 41 42 43 44 45 46 47 48 50 52 60 63 64 65 67 69 71 73 P5 7	23	10	47	2392	33	39203	213	22413	8933	198
⊠ DAVIES MEDICAL CENTER, Castro and Duboce Streets, Zip 94114; tel. 415/565–6000; Greg Monardo, President (Total facility includes 51 beds in nursing home–type unit) A1 3 5 9 10 F8 11 12 14 15 16 17 19 20 21 22 26 28 31 32 33 34 35 39 41 42 44 46 48 49 51 52 54 55 57 60 64 65 66 67 71 72 73 74 P5	23	10	205	3507	90	76070	0	60165	27882	651
⊠ KAISER FOUNDATION HOSPITAL, 2425 Geary Boulevard, Zip 94115; tel. 415/202–2000; Rosemary Fox, Acting Administrator (Nonreporting) A1 3 5 10 S Kaiser Foundation Hospitals, Oakland, CA N Kaiser Foundation Health Plan of Northern California, Oakland, CA	23	10	210	—	—	—	—	—	—	—
★ LAGUNA HONDA HOSPITAL AND REHABILITATION CENTER, 375 Laguna Honda Boulevard, Zip 94116–1499; tel. 415/664–1580; Anthony G. Wagner, Executive Administrator (Total facility includes 1145 beds in nursing home–type unit) (Nonreporting) A10	15	48	1203	—	—	—	—	—	—	—
□ PACIFIC COAST HOSPITAL, 1210 Scott Street, Zip 94115–4000; tel. 415/563–3444; Robert C. Hughes, Healthcare and Hospital Administrator (Nonreporting) A1 9 10	23	49	28	—	—	—	—	—	—	—
⊠ SAINT FRANCIS MEMORIAL HOSPITAL, 900 Hyde Street, Zip 94109, Mailing Address: Box 7726, Zip 94120–7726; tel. 415/353–6000; John G. Williams, President and Chief Executive Officer (Total facility includes 34 beds in nursing home–type unit) A1 2 3 9 10 F8 9 10 11 12 14 15 16 17 19 21 22 30 31 32 34 35 37 41 42 44 48 49 52 54 56 57 60 64 65 66 67 71 73 P3 5 7 S Catholic Healthcare West, San Francisco, CA N Catholic HealthCare West (CHW), San Francisco, CA	23	10	190	5965	109	157249	0	70313	32793	679

Hospital, Address, Telephone, Administrator, Approval, Facility, and Physician Codes, Health Care System, Network	Classi-fication Codes		Utilization Data					Expense (thousands) of dollars		
	Control	Service	Beds	Admissions	Census	Outpatient Visits	Births	Total	Payroll	Personnel

★ American Hospital Association (AHA) membership
□ Joint Commission on Accreditation of Healthcare Organizations (JCAHO) accreditation
+ American Osteopathic Hospital Association (AOHA) membership
○ American Osteopathic Association (AOA) accreditation
△ Commission on Accreditation of Rehabilitation Facilities (CARF) accreditation
Control codes 61, 63, 64, 71, 72 and 73 indicate hospitals listed by AOHA, but not registered by AHA. For definition of numerical codes, see page A4

Hospital	Control	Service	Beds	Admissions	Census	Outpatient Visits	Births	Total	Payroll	Personnel
□ SAN FRANCISCO GENERAL HOSPITAL MEDICAL CENTER, 1001 Potrero Avenue, Zip 94110; tel. 415/206–8000; Richard Cordova, Executive Director **A**1 2 3 5 9 10 **F**3 4 7 8 10 11 15 16 17 18 19 20 22 29 31 34 35 37 38 39 40 41 42 44 45 46 49 51 52 54 56 61 63 65 66 67 70 71 73 74 **P**1 6	15	10	357	17613	273	337829	1581	298948	126482	3747
✖ SHRINERS HOSPITALS FOR CHILDREN, SAN FRANCISCO, 1701 19th Avenue, Zip 94122–4599; tel. 415/665–1100; Margaret Bryan–Williams, Administrator (Nonreporting) **A**1 3 5 **S** Shriners Hospitals for Children, Tampa, FL	23	57	48	—	—	—	—	—	—	—
□ ST. LUKE'S HOSPITAL, 3555 Cesar Chavez Street, Zip 94110; tel. 415/647–8600; Jack Fries, President (Total facility includes 39 beds in nursing home–type unit) (Nonreporting) **A**1 9 10	23	10	242	—	—	—	—	—	—	—
✖ ST. MARY'S MEDICAL CENTER, 450 Stanyan Street, Zip 94117–1079; tel. 415/668–1000; John G. Williams, President (Total facility includes 48 beds in nursing home–type unit) **A**1 2 3 5 8 9 10 **F**1 3 4 8 10 12 15 16 17 19 21 22 26 27 30 31 32 35 37 42 43 44 46 48 49 52 53 54 55 56 57 58 59 60 64 65 66 67 71 73 74 **P**3 5 7 **S** Catholic Healthcare West, San Francisco, CA **N** Catholic HealthCare West (CHW), San Francisco, CA	21	10	256	8844	189	117613	0	108076	55837	1025
✖ UNIVERSITY OF CALIFORNIA SAN FRANCISCO MEDICAL CENTER, (Includes Langley Porter Psychiatric Hospital, 401 Parnassus Avenue, Zip 94143–0984, Mailing Address: Box F–0984, Zip 94143–0984; tel. 415/476–7347; University of California–San Francisco Mount Zion Medical Center, 1600 Divisadero Street, Zip 94143–1601; tel. 415/567–6600), 500 Parnassus, Zip 94143–0296; tel. 415/476–1000; William B. Kerr, Director (Total facility includes 31 beds in nursing home–type unit) **A**1 2 3 5 8 9 10 **F**1 3 4 5 7 8 10 11 12 13 14 17 18 19 20 21 22 23 24 25 26 27 30 31 32 34 35 37 38 39 40 41 42 43 44 45 46 47 48 49 50 51 53 54 55 56 57 58 59 60 61 63 64 65 66 67 68 69 70 71 72 73 74 **P**1 4 5 6 **S** University of California–Systemwide Administration, Oakland, CA	23	10	663	24774	409	479461	1638	446328	199210	4901
UNIVERSITY OF CALIFORNIA–SAN FRANCISCO MOUNT ZION MEDICAL CENTER See University of California San Francisco Medical Center										
✖ VETERANS AFFAIRS MEDICAL CENTER, 4150 Clement Street, Zip 94121–1598; tel. 415/750–2041; Lawrence C. Stewart, Director (Total facility includes 120 beds in nursing home–type unit) **A**1 3 5 8 **F**3 4 10 11 16 19 20 21 22 25 26 28 31 32 33 34 35 37 39 41 42 43 44 45 46 48 49 51 52 54 56 58 63 64 65 71 73 74 **P**6 **S** Department of Veterans Affairs, Washington, DC	45	10	372	7179	272	273626	0	164897	83022	1774

SAN GABRIEL—Los Angeles County

Hospital	Control	Service	Beds	Admissions	Census	Outpatient Visits	Births	Total	Payroll	Personnel
✖ SAN GABRIEL VALLEY MEDICAL CENTER, 218 South Santa Anita Street, Zip 91776, Mailing Address: P.O. Box 1507, Zip 91778–1507; tel. 818/289–5454; Makoto Nakayama, President and Chief Executive Officer (Total facility includes 46 beds in nursing home–type unit) **A**1 9 10 **F**1 7 8 10 12 14 15 17 19 21 22 23 27 32 34 35 37 38 39 40 41 42 43 44 46 49 52 53 57 59 60 61 63 64 65 69 71 73 74 **P**3 5 7 **S** UniHealth, Burbank, CA **N** UniHealth, Burbank, CA	23	10	271	9091	152	49572	1671	69113	27335	641

SAN JOSE—Santa Clara County

Hospital	Control	Service	Beds	Admissions	Census	Outpatient Visits	Births	Total	Payroll	Personnel
□ ALEXIAN BROTHERS HOSPITAL, 225 North Jackson Avenue, Zip 95116–1691; tel. 408/259–5000; Steven R. Barron, Chief Executive Officer (Nonreporting) **A**1 9 10 **S** Alexian Brothers Health System, Inc., Elk Grove Village, IL	21	10	192	—	—	—	—	—	—	—
✖ COLUMBIA GOOD SAMARITAN HOSPITAL, 2425 Samaritan Drive, Zip 95124, Mailing Address: P.O. Box 240002, Zip 95154–2402; tel. 408/559–2011; Joan C. White, Chief Executive Officer (Nonreporting) **A**1 9 10 **S** Columbia/HCA Healthcare Corporation, Nashville, TN	33	10	348	—	—	—	—	—	—	—
✖ COLUMBIA SAN JOSE MEDICAL CENTER, (Formerly San Jose Medical Center), 675 East Santa Clara Street, Zip 95112, Mailing Address: P.O. Box 240003, Zip 95154–2403; tel. 408/998–3212; Mary Schwind, R.N., MS, Chief Executive Officer (Total facility includes 26 beds in nursing home–type unit) (Nonreporting) **A**1 2 3 5 9 10 **S** Columbia/HCA Healthcare Corporation, Nashville, TN	33	10	327	—	—	—	—	—	—	—
✖ O'CONNOR HOSPITAL, 2105 Forest Avenue, Zip 95128–1471; tel. 408/947–2500; William C. Finlayson, President and Chief Executive Officer (Total facility includes 24 beds in nursing home–type unit) **A**1 2 9 10 **F**2 3 4 7 8 10 12 14 15 16 17 19 21 22 23 24 25 27 28 30 31 32 33 34 35 37 38 39 40 41 42 43 44 45 46 47 48 49 50 51 52 54 56 57 58 59 60 61 63 64 65 66 67 68 69 70 71 73 74 **P**2 3 5 6 7 **S** Catholic Healthcare West, San Francisco, CA **N** Catholic HealthCare West (CHW), San Francisco, CA	21	10	141	8299	128	209703	3371	99270	30921	806
SAN JOSE MEDICAL CENTER See Columbia San Jose Medical Center										
□ △ SANTA CLARA VALLEY MEDICAL CENTER, 751 South Bascom Avenue, Zip 95128; tel. 408/885–5000; Robert Sillen, Executive Director (Nonreporting) **A**1 2 3 5 7 10	13	10	377	—	—	—	—	—	—	—
✖ SANTA TERESA COMMUNITY HOSPITAL, 250 Hospital Parkway, Zip 95119; tel. 408/972–7000 **A**1 3 10 **F**2 3 4 7 8 9 10 11 12 13 14 15 16 17 19 21 22 23 24 25 26 28 29 30 31 32 33 35 37 38 39 40 41 42 43 44 45 46 47 48 49 50 51 52 53 54 55 56 58 59 60 61 63 64 65 66 67 68 69 71 72 73 74 **P**5 **S** Kaiser Foundation Hospitals, Oakland, CA	23	10	178	8518	86	—	2460	—	—	531

SAN LEANDRO—Alameda County

Hospital	Control	Service	Beds	Admissions	Census	Outpatient Visits	Births	Total	Payroll	Personnel
ALAMEDA COUNTY MEDICAL CENTER, (Formerly Fairmont Hospital), 15400 Foothill Boulevard, Zip 94578–1091; tel. 510/667–7920; Michael G. Smart, Chief Executive Officer (Total facility includes 119 beds in nursing home–type unit) (Nonreporting) **A**9 **S** Alameda County Health Care Services Agency, San Leandro, CA	13	49	193							

Hospital, Address, Telephone, Administrator, Approval, Facility, and Physician Codes, Health Care System, Network	Classi-fication Codes		Utilization Data					Expense (thousands) of dollars		
	Control	Service	Beds	Admissions	Census	Outpatient Visits	Births	Total	Payroll	Personnel

★ American Hospital Association (AHA) membership
☐ Joint Commission on Accreditation of Healthcare Organizations (JCAHO) accreditation
+ American Osteopathic Hospital Association (AOHA) membership
○ American Osteopathic Association (AOA) accreditation
△ Commission on Accreditation of Rehabilitation Facilities (CARF) accreditation
Control codes 61, 63, 64, 71, 72 and 73 indicate hospitals listed by AOHA, but not registered by AHA. For definition of numerical codes, see page A4

Hospital	Control	Service	Beds	Admissions	Census	Outpatient Visits	Births	Total	Payroll	Personnel
⊠ COLUMBIA SAN LEANDRO HOSPITAL, (Formerly San Leandro Hospital), 13855 East 14th Street, Zip 94578–0398; tel. 510/667–4510; Kelly Mather, Executive Director (Nonreporting) **A**1 9 10 **S** Columbia/HCA Healthcare Corporation, Nashville, TN **N** East Bay Medical Network, Emeryville, CA	33	10	136	—	—	—	—	—	—	—
FAIRMONT HOSPITAL See Alameda County Medical Center										
SAN LEANDRO HOSPITAL See Columbia San Leandro Hospital										
☐ VENCOR HOSPITAL–SAN LEANDRO, 2800 Benedict Drive, Zip 94577; tel. 510/357–8300; Wayne M. Lingenfelter, Ed.D., Administrator and Chief Executive Officer (Nonreporting) **A**1 9 10 **S** Vencor, Incorporated, Louisville, KY	33	10	42	—	—	—	—	—	—	—
SAN LUIS OBISPO—San Luis Obispo County										
CALIFORNIA MENS COLONY HOSPITAL, Highway 1, Zip 93409–8101, Mailing Address: P.O. Box 8101, Zip 93409–8101; tel. 805/547–7913; Galen Kirn, Administrator (Nonreporting)	12	11	39							
☐ FRENCH HOSPITAL MEDICAL CENTER, 1911 Johnson Avenue, Zip 93401; tel. 805/543–5353; William L. Gilbert, Chief Executive Officer (Nonreporting) **A**1 9 10 **S** TENET Healthcare Corporation, Santa Barbara, CA	33	10	124	—	—	—	—	—	—	—
☐ SAN LUIS OBISPO GENERAL HOSPITAL, 2180 Johnson Avenue, Zip 93401, Mailing Address: Box 8113, Zip 93403–8113; tel. 805/781–4800; Susan G. Zepeda, Ph.D., Administrator **A**1 9 10 **F**7 14 15 16 19 22 25 26 27 31 34 35 36 37 40 44 45 46 49 51 65 71 72 73 **P**6	13	10	46	1767	16	51417	800	25735	10827	276
☐ △ SIERRA VISTA REGIONAL MEDICAL CENTER, 1010 Murray Street, Zip 93405, Mailing Address: Box 1367, Zip 93406–1367; tel. 805/546–7600; Harold E. Chilton, Chief Executive Officer **A**1 7 9 10 **F**7 8 10 11 12 15 16 19 21 22 23 34 35 38 39 40 41 42 44 46 48 49 60 63 65 69 71 73 **S** TENET Healthcare Corporation, Santa Barbara, CA **N** Tenet Healthcare Corporation, Santa Barbara, CA	33	10	117	5733	73	41729	1098	37704	14754	451
SAN MATEO—San Mateo County										
MILLS HOSPITAL See Mills–Peninsula Health Services, Burlingame										
☐ SAN MATEO COUNTY GENERAL HOSPITAL, 222 West 39th Avenue, Zip 94403–4398; tel. 415/573–2222; Timothy B. McMurdo, Chief Executive Officer (Total facility includes 124 beds in nursing home–type unit) **A**1 3 5 10 **F**8 12 14 15 16 17 19 20 21 22 25 26 27 28 29 30 31 32 34 36 37 39 42 44 45 46 49 51 52 54 56 57 58 60 61 64 65 71 73 74 **P**4 6	13	10	240	3951	189	144760	2	80911	32597	—
SAN PABLO—Contra Costa County										
☐ BROOKSIDE HOSPITAL, 2000 Vale Road, Zip 94806; tel. 510/235–7000; Michael P. Lawson, President and Chief Executive Officer (Total facility includes 106 beds in nursing home–type unit) **A**1 2 9 10 **F**4 7 8 9 10 11 12 14 15 16 17 19 22 25 26 28 30 31 32 34 37 38 39 40 41 42 43 44 46 49 51 52 57 60 64 65 67 71 73 74 **P**4 5 **S** TENET Healthcare Corporation, Santa Barbara, CA	16	10	286	7086	157	142040	870	78131	31571	717
SAN PEDRO—Los Angeles County, See Los Angeles										
SAN RAFAEL—Marin County										
⊠ KAISER FOUNDATION HOSPITAL, 99 Montecillo Road, Zip 94903–3397; tel. 415/444–2000; Richard R. Pettingill, Chief Executive Officer **A**1 10 **F**4 8 9 10 14 19 21 22 23 29 31 32 33 34 35 37 38 39 40 41 42 43 44 45 46 47 48 49 52 53 54 63 64 65 69 70 71 73 **S** Kaiser Foundation Hospitals, Oakland, CA **N** Kaiser Foundation Health Plan of Northern California, Oakland, CA	23	10	119	3745	42	379407	0	—	—	267
SAN RAMON—Contra Costa County										
☐ △ SAN RAMON REGIONAL MEDICAL CENTER, 6001 Norris Canyon Road, Zip 94583; tel. 510/275–9200; Philip P. Gustafson, Chief Executive Officer **A**1 7 9 10 **F**2 3 7 8 10 11 12 15 16 17 19 21 22 30 35 37 38 39 40 41 42 44 48 49 61 64 65 67 71 73 74 **P**5 7 **S** TENET Healthcare Corporation, Santa Barbara, CA **N** Tenet Healthcare Corporation, Santa Barbara, CA	33	10	103	3638	38	37779	795	—	17306	267
SANGER—Fresno County										
☐ SANGER GENERAL HOSPITAL, 2558 Jensen Avenue, Zip 93657–2296; tel. 209/875–6571; Lynda Bisseger, Chief Executive Officer (Nonreporting) **A**1 9 10	32	10	25	—	—	—	—	—	—	—
SANTA ANA—Orange County										
☐ COASTAL COMMUNITIES HOSPITAL, 2701 South Bristol Street, Zip 92704–9911, Mailing Address: P.O. Box 5240, Zip 92704–0240; tel. 714/754–5454; Mark Meyers, Chief Executive Officer (Total facility includes 46 beds in nursing home–type unit) **A**1 9 10 **F**8 12 15 16 19 20 21 22 34 35 37 39 40 41 44 46 51 52 57 60 63 64 65 71 73 74 **P**2 5 7 **S** TENET Healthcare Corporation, Santa Barbara, CA	32	10	177	4739	75	21284	2053	—	—	266
DOCTORS HOSPITAL OF SANTA ANA, 1901 North College Avenue, Zip 92706; tel. 714/547–2565; R. Michael Hartman, Chief Executive Officer (Nonreporting) **A**9	33	10	54	—	—	—	—	—	—	—
☐ SANTA ANA HOSPITAL MEDICAL CENTER, 1901 North Fairview Street, Zip 92706; tel. 714/554–1653; Michael H. Sussman, Acting Chief Executive Officer (Nonreporting) **A**1 9 10 **S** TENET Healthcare Corporation, Santa Barbara, CA	33	10	90	—	—	—	—	—	—	—
☐ WESTERN MEDICAL CENTER–SANTA ANA, 1001 North Tustin Avenue, Zip 92705–3502; tel. 714/835–3555; Richard E. Butler, Chief Executive Officer (Nonreporting) **A**1 2 3 5 9 10 **S** TENET Healthcare Corporation, Santa Barbara, CA	23	10	288	—	—	—	—	—	—	—
SANTA BARBARA—Santa Barbara County										
☐ GOLETA VALLEY COTTAGE HOSPITAL, (Formerly Goleta Valley Community Hospital), 351 South Patterson Avenue, Zip 93111, Mailing Address: Box 6306, Zip 93160; tel. 805/967–3411; Diane Wisby, Vice President (Nonreporting) **A**1 9 10 **S** Cottage Health System, Santa Barbara, CA	23	10	79	—	—	—	—	—	—	—

Hospital, Address, Telephone, Administrator, Approval, Facility, and Physician Codes, Health Care System, Network	Classi-fication Codes		Utilization Data					Expense (thousands) of dollars		
★ American Hospital Association (AHA) membership □ Joint Commission on Accreditation of Healthcare Organizations (JCAHO) accreditation + American Osteopathic Hospital Association (AOHA) membership ○ American Osteopathic Association (AOA) accreditation △ Commission on Accreditation of Rehabilitation Facilities (CARF) accreditation Control codes 61, 63, 64, 71, 72 and 73 indicate hospitals listed by AOHA, but not registered by AHA. For definition of numerical codes, see page A4	Control	Service	Beds	Admissions	Census	Outpatient Visits	Births	Total	Payroll	Personnel
□ △ REHABILITATION INSTITUTE AT SANTA BARBARA, 427 Camino Del Remedio, Zip 93110; tel. 805/683–3788; Rusty Pollock, President and Chief Executive Officer (Nonreporting) **A**1 7 9 10	23	46	40	—	—	—	—	—	—	—
□ SANTA BARBARA COTTAGE HOSPITAL, (Includes Santa Barbara Cottage Care Center), Pueblo at Bath Streets, Zip 93105, Mailing Address: Box 689, Zip 93102; tel. 805/682–7111; James L. Ash, President and Chief Executive Officer (Nonreporting) **A**1 2 3 5 9 10 **S** Cottage Health System, Santa Barbara, CA	23	10	307	—	—	—	—	—	—	—
□ ST. FRANCIS MEDICAL CENTER OF SANTA BARBARA, 601 East Micheltorena Street, Zip 93103; tel. 805/962–7661; Ron Biscaro, Administrator (Total facility includes 34 beds in nursing home–type unit) **A**1 9 10 **F**7 8 10 11 13 14 15 16 19 22 28 30 35 37 39 40 41 44 49 64 65 67 71 73 **P**5	21	10	96	3361	42	19226	326	26377	11713	273
SANTA CLARA—Santa Clara County										
⊞ KAISER FOUNDATION HOSPITAL, 900 Kiely Boulevard, Zip 95051–5386; tel. 408/236–6400 **A**1 3 5 10 **F**2 3 4 7 8 9 11 12 13 14 15 16 19 21 22 25 26 28 29 30 31 32 33 34 35 37 38 39 40 41 42 44 45 46 47 48 49 50 51 52 53 54 55 56 57 58 59 60 61 63 64 65 66 67 68 69 71 72 73 74 **P**6 **S** Kaiser Foundation Hospitals, Oakland, CA **N** Kaiser Foundation Health Plan of Northern California, Oakland, CA	23	10	249	12038	123	—	2986	—	—	482
SANTA CRUZ—Santa Cruz County										
⊞ DOMINICAN SANTA CRUZ HOSPITAL, 1555 Soquel Drive, Zip 95065–1794; tel. 408/462–7700; Sister Julie Hyer, President and Chief Executive Officer (Total facility includes 36 beds in nursing home–type unit) **A**1 9 10 **F**4 6 7 8 10 12 13 14 15 16 17 19 22 25 30 32 34 35 37 38 40 41 42 43 44 45 46 48 49 52 54 56 59 60 62 64 65 66 67 71 72 73 74 **P**3 5 7 8 **S** Catholic Healthcare West, San Francisco, CA **N** Catholic HealthCare West (CHW), San Francisco, CA	21	10	284	12309	176	105806	1712	105683	47011	889
SANTA MARIA—Santa Barbara County										
⊞ MARIAN MEDICAL CENTER, 1400 East Church Street, Zip 93454, Mailing Address: Box 1238, Zip 93456; tel. 805/739–3000; Charles J. Cova, Executive Vice President (Total facility includes 95 beds in nursing home–type unit) **A**1 9 10 **F**4 7 8 10 11 12 14 15 16 17 19 20 21 22 26 28 29 30 31 32 33 34 35 39 40 41 42 43 44 45 46 49 54 56 60 64 65 67 70 71 73 74 **P**7	21	10	225	7435	143	91679	1571	55601	22187	625
□ VALLEY COMMUNITY HOSPITAL, 505 East Plaza Drive, Zip 93454–9943; tel. 805/925–0935; William C. Rasmussen, Chief Executive Officer (Nonreporting) **A**1 9 10 **S** TENET Healthcare Corporation, Santa Barbara, CA	33	10	70	—	—	—	—	—	—	—
SANTA MONICA—Los Angeles County										
⊞ SAINT JOHN'S HOSPITAL AND HEALTH CENTER, 1328 22nd Street, Zip 90404; tel. 310/829–5511; Sister Marie Madeleine Shonka, President **A**1 2 9 10 **F**2 3 4 7 8 10 11 12 14 15 16 17 19 21 22 28 29 30 32 33 34 35 36 37 38 39 40 41 42 43 44 45 49 50 52 54 55 56 57 58 59 60 64 65 71 73 74 **P**1 4 5 7 **S** Sisters of Charity of Leavenworth Health Services Corporation, Leavenworth, KS	21	10	234	10716	162	161282	1061	126155	52983	939
⊞ SANTA MONICA–UCLA MEDICAL CENTER, 1250 16th Street, Zip 90404–1200; tel. 310/319–4000; William D. Parente, Director and Chief Executive Officer **A**1 2 3 5 9 10 **F**4 7 8 10 12 15 17 18 19 20 21 22 24 28 30 31 34 37 38 40 41 42 43 44 49 61 64 65 71 73 **P**3 5 7 **S** University of California–Systemwide Administration, Oakland, CA **N** UniHealth, Burbank, CA	12	10	221	10036	151	10497	2249	86727	32196	—
SANTA PAULA—Ventura County										
□ SANTA PAULA MEMORIAL HOSPITAL, 825 North Tenth Street, Zip 93060–0270, Mailing Address: P.O. Box 270, Zip 93060–0270; tel. 805/525–7171; William M. Greene, FACHE, President (Nonreporting) **A**1 9 10 **S** Quorum Health Group/Quorum Health Resources, Inc., Brentwood, TN	23	10	54	—	—	—	—	—	—	—
SANTA ROSA—Sonoma County										
⊞ COMMUNITY HOSPITAL, 3325 Chanate Road, Zip 95404; tel. 707/576–4000; Cliff Coates, Chief Executive Officer (Total facility includes 16 beds in nursing home–type unit) **A**1 3 5 9 10 **F**4 7 8 10 12 13 14 15 16 19 21 22 26 31 34 35 37 38 39 40 41 44 49 51 52 54 56 58 64 65 67 71 72 73 74 **P**1 **S** Sutter Health, Sacramento, CA **N** Sutter\CHS, Sacramento, CA	23	10	128	5021	85	76388	1529	57677	23393	396
⊞ KAISER FOUNDATION HOSPITAL, 401 Bicentennial Way, Zip 95403; tel. 707/571–4000; Richard R. Pettingill, President and Chief Executive Officer (Nonreporting) **A**1 10 **S** Kaiser Foundation Hospitals, Oakland, CA	23	10	117	—	—	—	—	—	—	—
□ NORTH COAST HEALTH CARE CENTERS–EAST CAMPUS, (Formerly North Coast Rehabilitation Center), 151 Sotoyome Street, Zip 95405; tel. 707/543–2500; Pamela J. McFadden, President and Chief Executive Officer **A**1 9 10 **F**5 12 15 16 22 24 25 26 31 32 34 39 41 42 48 49 52 57 59 64 65	33	10	119	2023	76	47919	0	17391	9056	293
⊞ SANTA ROSA MEMORIAL HOSPITAL, 1165 Montgomery Drive, Zip 95405, Mailing Address: Box 522, Zip 95402; tel. 707/546–3210; Robert H. Fish, President and Chief Executive Officer **A**1 2 9 10 **F**4 7 8 9 10 11 12 14 15 16 17 19 20 22 30 31 32 34 35 37 38 40 41 42 43 44 46 48 49 60 65 67 69 70 71 72 73 **P**7 **S** St. Joseph Health System, Orange, CA **N** Saint Joseph Health System, Orange, CA	21	10	225	12872	157	40715	1550	96709	41484	814
□ WARRACK MEDICAL CENTER HOSPITAL, 2449 Summerfield Road, Zip 95405; tel. 707/542–9030; Dale E. Iversen, President and Chief Executive Officer (Nonreporting) **A**1 9 10	33	10	79	—	—	—	—	—	—	—
SEBASTOPOL—Sonoma County										
⊞ COLUMBIA PALM DRIVE HOSPITAL, 501 Petaluma Avenue, Zip 95472; tel. 707/823–8511; Jeff Frandsen, Chief Executive Officer (Total facility includes 10 beds in nursing home–type unit) (Nonreporting) **A**1 9 10 **S** Columbia/HCA Healthcare Corporation, Nashville, TN	33	10	48	—	—	—	—	—	—	—

Hospital, Address, Telephone, Administrator, Approval, Facility, and Physician Codes, Health Care System, Network	Classi-fication Codes		Utilization Data					Expense (thousands) of dollars		
★ American Hospital Association (AHA) membership □ Joint Commission on Accreditation of Healthcare Organizations (JCAHO) accreditation + American Osteopathic Hospital Association (AOHA) membership ○ American Osteopathic Association (AOA) accreditation △ Commission on Accreditation of Rehabilitation Facilities (CARF) accreditation Control codes 61, 63, 64, 71, 72 and 73 indicate hospitals listed by AOHA, but not registered by AHA. For definition of numerical codes, see page A4	Control	Service	Beds	Admissions	Census	Outpatient Visits	Births	Total	Payroll	Personnel

SELMA—Fresno County

□ SELMA DISTRICT HOSPITAL, 1141 Rose Avenue, Zip 93662–3293; tel. 209/891–2201; Terrence A. Curley, Executive Director (Total facility includes 14 beds in nursing home–type unit) **A**1 5 9 10 **F**7 8 14 15 16 19 21 22 35 40 44 64 65 71 **P**3

| 16 | 10 | 57 | 2365 | 22 | 52801 | 569 | 13376 | 4521 | 202 |

SEPULVEDA—Los Angeles County, See Los Angeles

SHERMAN OAKS—Los Angeles County, See Los Angeles

SIMI VALLEY—Ventura County

⊞ SIMI VALLEY HOSPITAL AND HEALTH CARE SERVICES, (Includes Simi Valley Hospital and Health Care Services–South Campus, 1850 Heywood Street, Zip 93065; tel. 805/582–5050), 2975 North Sycamore Drive, Zip 93065–1277; tel. 805/527–2462; Alan J. Rice, President (Total facility includes 74 beds in nursing home–type unit) **A**1 2 9 10 **F**2 3 4 7 8 9 10 11 12 13 14 15 16 17 18 19 21 22 25 26 27 28 29 30 31 32 33 34 35 37 38 39 40 41 42 43 44 45 46 47 48 49 52 54 55 56 57 58 59 60 62 63 64 65 66 69 71 73 74 **P**1 3 4 5 6 7 8 **S** Adventist Health, Roseville, CA **N** Adventist Health–Southern California, Glendale, CA

| 21 | 10 | 225 | 6647 | 137 | 99799 | 907 | 58532 | 25121 | 652 |

SOLVANG—Santa Barbara County

□ SANTA YNEZ VALLEY COTTAGE HOSPITAL, (Formerly Santa Ynez Valley Hospital), 700 Alamo Pintado Road, Zip 93463; tel. 805/688–6431; Bobbie Kline, R.N., Vice President (Nonreporting) **A**1 9 10 **S** Cottage Health System, Santa Barbara, CA

| 23 | 10 | 20 | — | — | — | — | — | — | — |

SONOMA—Sonoma County

□ SONOMA VALLEY HOSPITAL, 347 Andrieux Street, Zip 95476–6811, Mailing Address: Box 600, Zip 95476–0600; tel. 707/935–5000; Dennis R. Burns, Administrator and Chief Executive Officer (Nonreporting) **A**1 9 10

| 16 | 10 | 86 | — | — | — | — | — | — | — |

SONORA—Tuolumne County

⊞ SONORA COMMUNITY HOSPITAL, 1 South Forest Road, Zip 95370; tel. 209/532–3161; Lary Davis, President (Total facility includes 63 beds in nursing home–type unit) **A**1 9 10 **F**7 8 11 12 15 16 17 19 22 25 26 28 30 32 34 35 37 39 40 41 44 46 49 51 64 65 67 71 72 73 **S** Adventist Health, Roseville, CA

| 21 | 10 | 113 | 3592 | 96 | 140232 | 543 | 40682 | 17029 | 529 |

□ TUOLUMNE GENERAL HOSPITAL, 101 Hospital Road, Zip 95370; tel. 209/533–7100; Joseph K. Mitchell, Administrator (Total facility includes 32 beds in nursing home–type unit) (Nonreporting) **A**1 9 10

| 13 | 10 | 77 | — | — | — | — | — | — | — |

SOUTH EL MONTE—Los Angeles County

□ GREATER EL MONTE COMMUNITY HOSPITAL, 1701 South Santa Anita Avenue, Zip 91733–9918; tel. 818/579–7777; Elizabeth A. Primeaux, Chief Executive Officer (Total facility includes 13 beds in nursing home–type unit) **A**1 9 10 **F**2 3 4 5 7 8 10 11 12 13 15 16 17 18 19 20 21 22 23 24 25 26 27 28 29 30 31 32 33 34 35 36 37 38 39 40 41 42 43 44 45 46 47 48 49 50 51 52 53 54 55 56 57 58 59 60 61 62 63 64 65 66 67 68 69 70 71 72 73 74 **P**1 2 3 4 5 6 7 8 **S** TENET Healthcare Corporation, Santa Barbara, CA **N** Essential HealthCare Network, Monterey Park, CA

| 33 | 10 | 113 | 4622 | 53 | 23242 | 1495 | 24129 | 12076 | 253 |

SOUTH LAGUNA—Orange County

⊞ SOUTH COAST MEDICAL CENTER, 31872 Coast Highway, Zip 92677; tel. 714/499–1311; T. Michael Murray, President (Total facility includes 29 beds in nursing home–type unit) **A**1 9 10 **F**2 3 7 8 11 12 15 16 17 19 21 22 25 27 28 29 30 31 32 34 35 36 37 39 40 41 42 44 45 46 49 52 56 57 58 59 60 64 65 67 71 73 74 **P**4 5 7

| 23 | 10 | 155 | 4752 | 63 | 39096 | 603 | 37050 | 16967 | 478 |

SOUTH LAKE TAHOE—El Dorado County

□ BARTON MEMORIAL HOSPITAL, 2170 South Avenue, Zip 96158, Mailing Address: Box 9578, Zip 96158; tel. 916/541–3420; William G. Gordon, Chief Executive Officer (Nonreporting) **A**1 9 10

| 23 | 10 | 81 | — | — | — | — | — | — | — |

SOUTH SAN FRANCISCO—San Mateo County

⊞ KAISER FOUNDATION HOSPITAL, 1200 El Camino Real, Zip 94080–3299; tel. 415/742–2547; Rosemary Fox, Coutinuing Care Leader **A**1 10 **F**1 2 3 4 7 8 9 10 11 12 13 14 15 16 17 19 21 22 25 26 28 29 30 31 32 33 34 35 36 37 38 39 40 41 42 43 44 45 46 47 48 49 51 52 53 56 57 58 59 60 63 64 65 67 68 69 70 71 72 73 **P**7 **S** Kaiser Foundation Hospitals, Oakland, CA **N** Kaiser Foundation Health Plan of Northern California, Oakland, CA

| 23 | 10 | 79 | 4714 | 49 | 658918 | 1 | 41839 | 19922 | 877 |

STANFORD—Santa Clara County

⊞ STANFORD UNIVERSITY HOSPITAL, 300 Pasteur Drive, Zip 94305–5584; tel. 415/723–4000; Peter Van Etten, President and Chief Executive Officer (Total facility includes 22 beds in nursing home–type unit) **A**1 3 5 8 9 10 **F**3 4 5 7 8 10 11 12 15 16 17 19 21 22 27 29 30 31 34 35 37 40 42 43 44 45 46 48 49 50 51 52 53 54 55 56 57 58 59 60 61 63 64 65 66 67 69 70 71 72 73 74 **P**1 3 5 6 7

| 23 | 10 | 479 | 23765 | 318 | 599142 | 4220 | 539225 | 194167 | 4770 |

STOCKTON—San Joaquin County

□ DAMERON HOSPITAL, 525 West Acacia Street, Zip 95203; tel. 209/944–5550; Luis Arismendi, M.D., Administrator (Nonreporting) **A**1 9 10 **N** Sutter\CHS, Sacramento, CA

| 23 | 10 | 211 | — | — | — | — | — | — | — |

⊞ ST. JOSEPH'S BEHAVIORAL HEALTH CENTER, 2510 North California Street, Zip 95204–5568; tel. 209/948–2100; James Sondecker, Administrator **A**1 9 10 **F**2 3 14 15 16 26 32 52 53 54 55 56 57 58 59 65 **P**5 **S** Catholic Healthcare West, San Francisco, CA **N** Catholic HealthCare West (CHW), San Francisco, CA

| 23 | 22 | 35 | 1360 | 26 | 4542 | 0 | — | — | 74 |

Hospital, Address, Telephone, Administrator, Approval, Facility, and Physician Codes, Health Care System, Network	Control	Service	Beds	Admissions	Census	Outpatient Visits	Births	Total	Payroll	Personnel

★ American Hospital Association (AHA) membership
□ Joint Commission on Accreditation of Healthcare Organizations (JCAHO) accreditation
+ American Osteopathic Hospital Association (AOHA) membership
○ American Osteopathic Association (AOA) accreditation
△ Commission on Accreditation of Rehabilitation Facilities (CARF) accreditation
Control codes 61, 63, 64, 71, 72 and 73 indicate hospitals listed by AOHA, but not registered by AHA. For definition of numerical codes, see page A4

Hospital	Control	Service	Beds	Admissions	Census	Outpatient Visits	Births	Total	Payroll	Personnel
✣ ST. JOSEPH'S MEDICAL CENTER, 1800 North California Street, Zip 95204–6088, Mailing Address: P.O. Box 213008, Zip 95213–9008; tel. 209/943–2000; Edward G. Schroeder, President and Chief Executive Officer (Total facility includes 43 beds in nursing home–type unit) **A**1 2 9 10 **F**2 3 4 6 7 8 10 11 12 13 14 15 16 17 18 19 20 21 22 23 25 26 27 28 29 30 31 32 33 34 35 37 38 39 40 41 42 43 44 45 46 49 51 52 53 54 55 56 57 58 59 60 62 64 65 66 67 68 69 71 72 73 74 **P**3 4 5 7 **S** Catholic Healthcare West, San Francisco, CA **N** Catholic HealthCare West (CHW), San Francisco, CA	21	10	312	15390	194	314171	1992	139899	60039	1591
SUN CITY—Riverside County										
□ MENIFEE VALLEY MEDICAL CENTER, 28400 McCall Boulevard, Zip 92585–9537; tel. 909/679–8888; Susan Ballard, Administrator (Nonreporting) **A**1 10 **S** Valley Health System, Hemet, CA	16	10	84							
SUN VALLEY—Los Angeles County, See Los Angeles										
SUSANVILLE—Lassen County										
□ LASSEN COMMUNITY HOSPITAL, 560 Hospital Lane, Zip 96130–4809; tel. 916/257–5325; David S. Anderson, FACHE, Administrator (Total facility includes 31 beds in nursing home–type unit) **A**1 9 10 **F**7 8 12 15 16 20 22 26 28 30 32 35 40 44 51 64 65 71 73 **S** Lutheran Health Systems, Fargo, ND	21	10	59	1115	30	19187	258	9803	4218	141
SYLMAR—Los Angeles County, See Los Angeles										
TAFT—Kern County										
WEST SIDE DISTRICT HOSPITAL, 110 East North Street, Zip 93268; tel. 805/763–4211; Margo Arnold, Administrator (Total facility includes 52 beds in nursing home–type unit) (Nonreporting) **A**9 10	16	10	72							
TEHACHAPI—Kern County										
TEHACHAPI HOSPITAL, 115 West E Street, Zip 93561, Mailing Address: Box 648, Zip 93581; tel. 805/822–3241; David P. Jacobsen, Chief Executive Officer **A**9 10 **F**8 15 22 28 34 44 51 67 73	16	10	28	158	17	29596	2	5878	2366	86
TEMPLETON—San Luis Obispo County										
□ TWIN CITIES COMMUNITY HOSPITAL, 1100 Las Tablas Road, Zip 93465; tel. 805/434–3500; Harold E. Chilton, Chief Executive Officer **A**1 9 10 **F**8 10 12 15 19 22 25 28 30 34 35 37 40 41 42 44 46 49 65 71 73 **S** TENET Healthcare Corporation, Santa Barbara, CA **N** Tenet Healthcare Corporation, Santa Barbara, CA	33	10	84	4072	44	75176	296	—	—	374
THOUSAND OAKS—Los Angeles County										
✣ COLUMBIA LOS ROBLES HOSPITAL AND MEDICAL CENTER, 215 West Janss Road, Zip 91360–1899; tel. 805/497–2727; Ronald C. Phelps, Chief Executive Officer (Total facility includes 18 beds in nursing home–type unit) **A**1 2 9 10 **F**4 7 8 10 11 14 15 16 17 19 21 22 26 29 30 31 32 34 35 36 37 38 39 40 41 42 44 45 49 60 63 64 65 67 71 73 74 **P**5 **S** Columbia/HCA Healthcare Corporation, Nashville, TN	33	10	185	9668	119	65896	2010	69314	32407	872
TORRANCE—Los Angeles County										
□ DEL AMO HOSPITAL, 23700 Camino Del Sol, Zip 90505; tel. 310/530–1151; E. Daniel Thomas, Administrator and Chief Executive Officer (Nonreporting) **A**1 9 10 **S** Universal Health Services, Inc., King of Prussia, PA	33	22	166	—	—	—	—	—	—	—
✣ LAC–HARBOR–UNIVERSITY OF CALIFORNIA AT LOS ANGELES MEDICAL CENTER, 1000 West Carson Street, Zip 90509; tel. 310/222–2101; Tecla A. Mickoseff, Administrator **A**1 2 3 5 9 10 **F**4 8 10 11 16 19 21 22 23 29 31 34 35 37 38 40 41 42 43 44 45 47 52 54 56 58 60 61 63 65 66 69 70 71 72 73 74 **P**6 **S** Los Angeles County–Department of Health Services, Los Angeles, CA	13	10	455	23192	350	328727	2366	427717	136963	2877
✣ LITTLE COMPANY OF MARY HOSPITAL, 4101 Torrance Boulevard, Zip 90503–4698; tel. 310/540–7676; Mark Costa, President (Total facility includes 121 beds in nursing home–type unit) **A**1 2 9 10 **F**3 4 5 7 8 10 11 12 17 19 21 22 23 25 27 29 32 33 34 35 37 38 40 41 42 43 44 46 49 51 54 56 57 59 60 63 64 65 67 71 72 73 74 **P**3 5 7 **S** Little Company of Mary Sisters Healthcare System, Evergreen Park, IL **N** Little Company of Mary Health Services, Torrance, CA	23	10	335	13794	242	123697	2671	105263	41666	1121
✣ TORRANCE MEMORIAL MEDICAL CENTER, 3330 Lomita Boulevard, Zip 90505–5073; tel. 310/325–9110; George W. Graham, President **A**1 2 9 10 **F**3 4 7 8 9 10 17 19 21 22 23 25 26 27 28 29 30 31 32 33 34 35 37 38 40 41 42 43 44 45 46 49 51 52 54 55 56 57 58 59 60 65 67 71 72 73 74 **P**5	23	10	360	21131	236	116769	4774	137829	57648	1569
TRACY—San Joaquin County										
✣ TRACY COMMUNITY MEMORIAL HOSPITAL, 1420 North Tracy Boulevard, Zip 95376–3497; tel. 209/835–1500; Larry L. Meyer, Vice President and Administrator (Total facility includes 11 beds in nursing home–type unit) **A**1 9 10 **F**7 8 11 15 16 17 19 21 22 28 29 30 32 33 34 35 37 39 40 41 44 49 50 63 64 67 71 73 **P**3 5 8 **S** Sutter Health, Sacramento, CA **N** Sutter\CHS, Sacramento, CA	23	10	63	2664	29	72309	445	24051	9859	276
TRAVIS AFB—Solano County										
✣ DAVID GRANT MEDICAL CENTER, 101 Bodin Circle, Zip 94535–1800; tel. 707/423–7300; Colonel D. Creager Brown, MSC, USAF, Administrator **A**1 2 3 5 **F**2 3 4 7 8 10 11 12 14 15 16 17 18 19 20 21 22 28 29 30 34 35 37 38 39 40 41 42 44 45 46 49 51 52 53 54 55 56 57 58 59 60 63 65 67 68 71 73 **S** Department of the Air Force, Washington, DC	41	10	185	11838	146	414183	776	—	—	2046
TRUCKEE—Nevada County										
□ TAHOE FOREST HOSPITAL DISTRICT, 10121 Pine Avenue, Zip 96161, Mailing Address: Box 759, Zip 96160; tel. 916/582–3481; Lawrence C. Long, Chief Executive Officer (Total facility includes 30 beds in nursing home–type unit) **A**1 9 10 **F**3 7 8 12 15 16 17 19 22 23 28 29 30 32 33 34 35 37 40 41 42 44 46 49 64 65 66 67 71 72 73 **P**3 5 7 8	16	10	72	1921	48	61434	359	27671	10183	326

Hospital, Address, Telephone, Administrator, Approval, Facility, and Physician Codes, Health Care System, Network	Classification Codes		Utilization Data					Expense (thousands) of dollars		
★ American Hospital Association (AHA) membership □ Joint Commission on Accreditation of Healthcare Organizations (JCAHO) accreditation + American Osteopathic Hospital Association (AOHA) membership ○ American Osteopathic Association (AOA) accreditation △ Commission on Accreditation of Rehabilitation Facilities (CARF) accreditation Control codes 61, 63, 64, 71, 72 and 73 indicate hospitals listed by AOHA, but not registered by AHA. For definition of numerical codes, see page A4	Control	Service	Beds	Admissions	Census	Outpatient Visits	Births	Total	Payroll	Personnel

TULARE—Tulare County

☒ TULARE DISTRICT HOSPITAL, 869 Cherry Street, Zip 93274–2287; tel. 209/688–0821; Jerry W. Boyter, Administrator **A**1 9 10 **F**7 8 12 14 15 19 22 30 32 34 35 37 40 42 44 46 65 71 73 **P**1 5

| | | 16 | 10 | 88 | 3811 | 41 | 57050 | 972 | 31693 | 13518 | 450 |

TURLOCK—Stanislaus County

☒ EMANUEL MEDICAL CENTER, 825 Delbon Avenue, Zip 95382, Mailing Address: Box 2120, Zip 95381–2120; tel. 209/667–4200; Robert A. Moen, President and Chief Executive Officer (Total facility includes 145 beds in nursing home–type unit) **A**1 9 10 **F**3 6 7 8 12 15 16 17 19 21 22 23 25 26 28 29 30 31 32 33 34 35 36 37 38 40 41 42 44 45 46 49 60 62 64 65 67 71 72 73 74 **P**1

| | | 21 | 10 | 334 | 7379 | 247 | 73631 | 1719 | 51943 | 21440 | 883 |

TUSTIN—Orange County

□ TUSTIN HOSPITAL, 14662 Newport Avenue, Zip 92680; tel. 714/838–9600 (Total facility includes 24 beds in nursing home–type unit) (Nonreporting) **A**1

| | | 33 | 10 | 117 | — | — | — | — | — | — | — |

□ △ TUSTIN REHABILITATION HOSPITAL, 14851 Yorba Street, Zip 92680; tel. 714/832–9200; Page Van Hoy, Chief Executive Officer (Nonreporting) **A**1 7 10

| | | 33 | 46 | 117 | — | — | — | — | — | — | — |

TWENTYNINE PALMS—San Bernardino County

☒ NAVAL HOSPITAL, Mailing Address: Box 788250, MCAGCC, Zip 92278–8250; tel. 619/830–2492; Captain R. S. Kayler, MSC, USN, Commanding Officer (Nonreporting) **A**1 **S** Department of Navy, Washington, DC

| | | 43 | 10 | 29 | — | — | — | — | — | — | — |

UKIAH—Mendocino County

☒ UKIAH VALLEY MEDICAL CENTER, (Includes Ukiah Valley Medical Center–Dora Street, 1120 South Dora Street, Ukiah Valley Medical Center–Hospital Drive), 275 Hospital Drive, Zip 95482; tel. 707/462–3111; ValGene Devitt, President and Chief Executive Officer (Nonreporting) **A**1 9 10 **S** Adventist Health, Roseville, CA **N** Adventist Health–Northern California, Deer Park, CA

| | | 21 | 10 | 101 | — | — | — | — | — | — | — |

UPLAND—San Bernardino County

☒ SAN ANTONIO COMMUNITY HOSPITAL, 999 San Bernardino Road, Zip 91786–4920, Mailing Address: Box 5001, Zip 91785; tel. 909/985–2811; George A. Kuykendall, President **A**1 2 9 10 **F**2 3 4 7 8 10 11 12 14 15 19 21 22 25 28 29 30 32 34 35 37 38 40 41 43 44 46 49 52 58 59 60 61 63 65 67 71 72 73 **P**5 7

| | | 23 | 10 | 308 | 17117 | 176 | 254499 | 3867 | 129960 | 55792 | 1510 |

VACAVILLE—Solano County

CALIFORNIA MEDICAL FACILITY, 1600 California Drive, Zip 95687–2000; tel. 707/448–6841; Velma Alcorn, Administrator **F**1 3 4 10 11 19 20 21 22 27 30 31 33 35 41 42 43 44 49 52 54 56 58 60 65 69 70 71

| | | 12 | 11 | 215 | 877 | 51 | 92260 | 0 | — | — | 435 |

★ VACAVALLEY HOSPITAL, 1000 Nut Tree Road, Zip 95687; tel. 707/446–5716; Deborah Sugiyama, President **A**9 10 **F**7 8 10 12 13 14 15 16 17 19 21 22 23 28 30 32 33 35 36 37 38 39 40 41 42 44 49 60 64 65 67 71 72 73 **P**3 5 **S** NorthBay Healthcare System, Fairfield, CA **N** NorthBay Healthcare System, Fairfield, CA

| | | 23 | 10 | 35 | 1556 | 14 | 19955 | 0 | — | — | 102 |

VALENCIA—Los Angeles County

□ △ HENRY MAYO NEWHALL MEMORIAL HOSPITAL, 23845 McBean Parkway, Zip 91355; tel. 805/253–8000; Duffy Watson, President and Chief Executive Officer (Total facility includes 62 beds in nursing home–type unit) **A**1 2 7 9 10 **F**1 7 8 11 12 14 15 16 17 18 19 20 21 22 25 26 27 28 29 30 31 32 33 35 37 40 41 42 44 45 46 48 49 52 56 57 58 59 63 64 65 67 70 71 73

| | | 23 | 10 | 227 | 8262 | 125 | 53776 | 1542 | 69034 | 24413 | 534 |

VALLEJO—Solano County

□ FIRST HOSPITAL VALLEJO, 525 Oregon Street, Zip 94590; tel. 707/648–2200; John E. Wiley, Chief Executive Officer and Administrator **A**1 10 **F**19 21 22 27 35 50 52 53 54 55 56 58 59 63 65 67 71 **P**7 **S** First Hospital Corporation, Norfolk, VA

| | | 33 | 22 | 61 | 1404 | 34 | — | 0 | — | — | 83 |

☒ KAISER FOUNDATION HOSPITAL AND REHABILITATION CENTER, 975 Sereno Drive, Zip 94589; tel. 707/648–6230; Vivian M. Rittenhouse, Vice President and Market Leader **A**1 10 **F**2 3 7 8 9 11 12 13 14 15 16 17 19 22 25 29 30 32 33 35 37 38 40 41 45 46 47 48 49 51 52 54 58 60 64 65 67 71 72 73 **P**1 **S** Kaiser Foundation Hospitals, Oakland, CA **N** Kaiser Foundation Health Plan of Northern California, Oakland, CA

| | | 23 | 10 | 219 | 11859 | 118 | 734863 | 2291 | — | — | 881 |

☒ SUTTER SOLANO MEDICAL CENTER, 300 Hospital Drive, Zip 94589–2517, Mailing Address: P.O. Box 3189, Zip 94589; tel. 707/554–4444; Patrick R. Brady, Administrator (Total facility includes 9 beds in nursing home–type unit) **A**1 9 10 **F**7 8 10 11 12 14 15 16 19 21 22 28 30 32 34 35 36 39 41 42 44 49 63 64 65 71 73 74 **S** Sutter Health, Sacramento, CA **N** Sutter\CHS, Sacramento, CA

| | | 23 | 10 | 63 | 5246 | 53 | — | 837 | 41773 | 18382 | 444 |

VAN NUYS—Los Angeles County, See Los Angeles

VANDENBERG AFB—Santa Barbara County

☒ U. S. AIR FORCE HOSPITAL, 338 South Dakota, Zip 93437–6307; tel. 805/734–8232; Colonel John A. Reyburn, Jr., Commander **A**1 **F**8 12 13 15 20 22 24 28 29 30 34 39 44 45 46 49 51 53 56 58 65 71 73 **P**4 **S** Department of the Air Force, Washington, DC

| | | 41 | 10 | 8 | 1116 | 6 | 110585 | 0 | — | — | 344 |

VENTURA—Ventura County

BHC VISTA DEL MAR HOSPITAL, (Formerly CPC Vista Del Mar Hospital), 801 Seneca Street, Zip 93001; tel. 805/653–6434; Jerry Conway, Chief Executive Officer (Nonreporting) **A**9 **S** Behavioral Healthcare Corporation, Nashville, TN

| | | 33 | 22 | 87 | — | — | — | — | — | — | — |

☒ COMMUNITY MEMORIAL HOSPITAL OF SAN BUENAVENTURA, Loma Vista Road at Brent, Zip 93003–2854; tel. 805/652–5011; Michael D. Bakst, Ph.D., Executive Director **A**1 9 10 **F**4 7 8 10 11 15 16 17 19 21 22 23 24 25 28 29 30 35 37 38 40 41 43 44 63 64 65 67 71 73 **P**5

| | | 23 | 10 | 217 | 11280 | 138 | 89776 | 2620 | 76360 | 33581 | 991 |

CPC VISTA DEL MAR HOSPITAL See BHC Vista Del Mar Hospital

Hospital, Address, Telephone, Administrator, Approval, Facility, and Physician Codes, Health Care System, Network	Classi-fication Codes		Utilization Data					Expense (thousands) of dollars		
★ American Hospital Association (AHA) membership □ Joint Commission on Accreditation of Healthcare Organizations (JCAHO) accreditation + American Osteopathic Hospital Association (AOHA) membership ○ American Osteopathic Association (AOA) accreditation △ Commission on Accreditation of Rehabilitation Facilities (CARF) accreditation Control codes 61, 63, 64, 71, 72 and 73 indicate hospitals listed by AOHA, but not registered by AHA. For definition of numerical codes, see page A4	Control	Service	Beds	Admissions	Census	Outpatient Visits	Births	Total	Payroll	Personnel
□ VENTURA COUNTY MEDICAL CENTER, 3291 Loma Vista Road, Zip 93003; tel. 805/652–6058; Samuel Edwards, Administrator **A**1 3 9 10 **F**3 4 8 10 11 12 15 16 17 18 19 21 22 25 27 28 29 30 31 34 35 36 37 38 39 41 42 43 44 45 46 49 51 52 53 54 55 56 57 58 59 61 65 67 68 71 72 73 74 **P**6	13	10	162	8794	130	527483	2015	146285	52041	279
VICTORVILLE—San Bernardino County										
★ DESERT VALLEY HOSPITAL, 16850 Bear Valley Road, Zip 92392; tel. 619/241–8000; Sidney Ono, Administrator **A**1 10 **F**8 10 11 12 19 21 22 23 27 28 30 32 33 34 35 36 39 40 41 42 43 44 45 46 50 51 54 60 61 65 67 69 71 72 73 74 **P**3 5 6	31	10	83	5355	39	—	907	68137	10544	318
□ VICTOR VALLEY COMMUNITY HOSPITAL, 15248 11th Street, Zip 92392; tel. 619/245–8691; Ralph L. Parks, Administrator and Chief Executive Officer (Nonreporting) **A**1 9 10	23	10	119							
VISALIA—Tulare County										
★ KAWEAH DELTA HEALTHCARE DISTRICT, (Includes Community Health Center, 1633 South Court Street, Zip 93277, Mailing Address: Box 911, Zip 93277; tel. 209/625–7221; Lindsay K. Mann, Senior Vice President), 400 West Mineral King Avenue, Zip 93291; tel. 209/625–2211; Thomas M. Johnson, Chief Executive Officer (Total facility includes 63 beds in nursing home–type unit) **A**1 2 9 10 **F**3 4 7 8 10 12 14 15 16 17 19 21 22 23 24 28 29 30 32 34 35 37 40 42 43 44 45 46 48 49 52 57 60 64 65 67 71 72 73	16	10	298	13290	157	—	3556	120785	57098	1737
WALNUT CREEK—Contra Costa County										
□ BHC WALNUT CREEK HOSPITAL, 175 La Casa Via, Zip 94598; tel. 510/933–7990; Jay R. Kellison, Chief Executive Officer (Nonreporting) **A**1 9 10 **S** Behavioral Healthcare Corporation, Nashville, TN	33	22	108	—	—					
★ JOHN MUIR MEDICAL CENTER, 1601 Ygnacio Valley Road, Zip 94598–3194; tel. 510/939–3000; J. Kendall Anderson, President and Chief Executive Officer (Total facility includes 29 beds in nursing home–type unit) (Nonreporting) **A**1 2 9 10	23	10	256							
★ KAISER FOUNDATION HOSPITAL, (Includes Kaiser Foundation Hospital, 200 Muir Road, Martinez, Zip 94553–4696; tel. 510/372–1000), 1425 South Main Street, Zip 94596; tel. 510/295–4000; Anna Robinson, Administrator (Nonreporting) **A**1 5 10 **S** Kaiser Foundation Hospitals, Oakland, CA **N** Kaiser Foundation Health Plan of Northern California, Oakland, CA	23	10	268							
WATSONVILLE—Santa Cruz County										
□ WATSONVILLE COMMUNITY HOSPITAL, 298 Green Valley Road, Zip 95076; tel. 408/724–4741; John P. Friel, President and Chief Executive Officer (Total facility includes 13 beds in nursing home–type unit) **A**1 9 10 **F**2 3 7 8 10 11 15 16 17 19 21 22 24 25 27 28 30 31 32 34 35 37 38 39 40 41 42 44 46 64 65 66 67 68 71 72 73 **P**4 5	23	10	130	5466	76	185350	1658	50609	25970	566
WEAVERVILLE—Trinity County										
TRINITY HOSPITAL, 410 North Taylor Street, Zip 96093, Mailing Address: P.O. Box 1229, Zip 96093–1229; tel. 916/623–5541; Bob Robertson, Administrator (Total facility includes 42 beds in nursing home–type unit) (Nonreporting) **A**9 10	13	10	65	—	—	—	—	—	—	—
WEST COVINA—Los Angeles County										
□ CITRUS VALLEY MEDICAL CENTER–QUEEN OF THE VALLEY CAMPUS, (Formerly Queen of the Valley Hospital), 1115 South Sunset Avenue, Zip 91790, Mailing Address: Box 1980, Zip 91793; tel. 818/962–4011; Warren J. Kirk, Administrator and Chief Operating Officer **A**1 2 9 10 **F**4 7 8 10 11 12 13 14 15 16 17 19 21 22 23 28 29 30 31 32 33 34 35 36 37 38 39 40 41 42 43 44 45 46 48 49 60 63 64 65 66 67 68 71 72 73 74 **P**1 5 7 **S** Citrus Valley Health Partners, Covina, CA	23	10	263	18045	208	103438	4292	91698	37674	1105
□ COVINA VALLEY COMMUNITY HOSPITAL, 845 North Lark Ellen Avenue, Zip 91791; tel. 818/339–5451; John Hogue, Administrator (Nonreporting) **A**1 9 10	32	10	76	—	—					
□ DOCTORS HOSPITAL OF WEST COVINA, 725 South Orange Avenue, Zip 91790–2614; tel. 818/338–8481; Gerald H. Wallman, Administrator (Total facility includes 24 beds in nursing home–type unit) **A**1 9 10 **F**3 19 35 37 40 44 49 58 59 64 65 71 **P**5	33	10	51	987	17	—	437	—	—	—
QUEEN OF THE VALLEY HOSPITAL See Citrus Valley Medical Center–Queen of the Valley Campus										
WEST HILLS—Los Angeles County, See Los Angeles										
WEST LOS ANGELES—Los Angeles County, See Los Angeles										
WESTLAKE VILLAGE—Los Angeles County										
★ WESTLAKE MEDICAL CENTER, 4415 South Lakeview Canyon Road, Zip 91361; tel. 818/706–8000; Ronald C. Phelps, Chief Executive Officer (Nonreporting) **A**1 9 10 **S** Columbia/HCA Healthcare Corporation, Nashville, TN	33	10	60	—	—					
WHITTIER—Los Angeles County										
★ PRESBYTERIAN INTERCOMMUNITY HOSPITAL, 12401 Washington Boulevard, Zip 90602–1099; tel. 562/698–0811; Daniel F. Adams, President and Chief Executive Officer (Nonreporting) **A**1 2 3 5 9 10	23	10	312	—	—	—	—	—	—	—
□ WHITTIER HOSPITAL MEDICAL CENTER, 15151 Janine Drive, Zip 90605; tel. 562/907–1541; Sandra M. Chester, Chief Executive Officer (Total facility includes 39 beds in nursing home–type unit) **A**1 9 10 **F**7 8 11 12 14 15 16 17 19 21 22 26 27 28 30 32 34 35 37 39 40 41 44 46 49 61 64 65 71 73 74 **P**2 5 7 **S** TENET Healthcare Corporation, Santa Barbara, CA	33	10	159	4876	76	36951	1838	33563	16092	371
WILDOMAR—Riverside County										
□ INLAND VALLEY REGIONAL MEDICAL CENTER, 36485 Inland Valley Drive, Zip 92595; tel. 909/677–1111; B. Ann Kuss, Chief Executive Officer and Managing Director **A**1 10 **F**7 8 10 12 14 15 19 21 22 27 28 29 30 32 35 37 39 40 41 44 46 49 67 70 71 73 74 **S** Universal Health Services, Inc., King of Prussia, PA	33	10	80	5095	40	31847	876	26123	13337	359

Hospital, Address, Telephone, Administrator, Approval, Facility, and Physician Codes, Health Care System, Network	Classi-fication Codes		Utilization Data					Expense (thousands) of dollars		
	Control	Service	Beds	Admissions	Census	Outpatient Visits	Births	Total	Payroll	Personnel
WILLITS—Mendocino County ☒ FRANK R. HOWARD MEMORIAL HOSPITAL, 1 Madrone Street, Zip 95490; tel. 707/459–6801; Robert J. Walker, President **A**1 9 10 **F**8 12 15 16 17 19 22 28 32 33 35 37 39 41 44 45 48 49 71 72 73 **P**3 **S** Adventist Health, Roseville, CA **N** Adventist Health–Northern California, Deer Park, CA	23	10	28	896	9	10717	6	10131	4030	122
WILLOWS—Glenn County GLENN MEDICAL CENTER, 1133 West Sycamore Street, Zip 95988; tel. 916/934–1800; Bernard G. Hietpas, Chief Executive Officer **A**9 10 **F**8 12 13 22 25 27 30 34 39 44 51 71 72 73	23	10	27	282	2	27559	0	4923	2025	80
WINTERHAVEN—Imperial County ☒ U. S. PUBLIC HEALTH SERVICE INDIAN HOSPITAL, Mailing Address: P.O. Box 1368, Yuma, AZ, Zip 85366–8368; tel. 619/572–0217; Hortense Miguel, R.N., Acting Service Unit Director (Nonreporting) **A**1 9 10 **S** U. S. Public Health Service Indian Health Service, Rockville, MD	47	10	17	—	—	—	—	—	—	—
WOODLAND—Yolo County ☒ WOODLAND MEMORIAL HOSPITAL, 1325 Cottonwood Street, Zip 95695–5199; tel. 916/662–3961; D. Scott Ideson, Interim Chief Executive Officer (Nonreporting) **A**1 9 10 **S** Catholic Healthcare West, San Francisco, CA **N** Catholic HealthCare West (CHW), San Francisco, CA	23	10	103	—	—	—	—	—	—	—
WOODLAND HILLS—Los Angeles County, See Los Angeles										
YOUNTVILLE—Napa County ★ VETERANS HOME OF CALIFORNIA, 100 California Drive, Zip 94599–1413; tel. 707/944–4500; James D. Helzer, Administrator (Total facility includes 514 beds in nursing home–type unit) (Nonreporting) **A**10	12	10	540	—	—	—	—	—	—	—
YREKA—Siskiyou County ☐ SISKIYOU GENERAL HOSPITAL, 818 South Main Street, Zip 96097; tel. 916/842–4121; Kenneth E. Monfore, Jr., Administrator (Nonreporting) **A**1 9 10	23	10	48	—	—	—	—	—	—	—
YUBA CITY—Sutter County ☐ FREMONT MEDICAL CENTER, 970 Plumas Street, Zip 95991; tel. 916/751–4000; Thomas P. Hayes, Chief Executive Officer **A**1 10 **F**7 8 10 14 15 16 17 19 22 25 26 28 32 33 34 35 37 38 40 44 45 49 60 71 **P**5 **S** Fremont–Rideout Health Group, Yuba City, CA **N** Fremont–Rideout Health Group, Yuba City, CA	23	10	92	7938	78	37977	2261	38281	15617	458

COLORADO

Resident population 3,747 (in thousands)
Resident population in metro areas 84.4%
Birth rate per 1,000 population 15.2
65 years and over 10.0%
Percent of persons without health insurance 12.4%

Hospital, Address, Telephone, Administrator, Approval, Facility, and Physician Codes, Health Care System, Network	Classi-fication Codes		Utilization Data					Expense (thousands) of dollars		
★ American Hospital Association (AHA) membership □ Joint Commission on Accreditation of Healthcare Organizations (JCAHO) accreditation + American Osteopathic Hospital Association (AOHA) membership ○ American Osteopathic Association (AOA) accreditation △ Commission on Accreditation of Rehabilitation Facilities (CARF) accreditation Control codes 61, 63, 64, 71, 72 and 73 indicate hospitals listed by AOHA, but not registered by AHA. For definition of numerical codes, see page A4	Control	Service	Beds	Admissions	Census	Outpatient Visits	Births	Total	Payroll	Personnel

ALAMOSA—Alamosa County
★ SAN LUIS VALLEY REGIONAL MEDICAL CENTER, 106 Blanca Avenue, Zip 81101–2393; tel. 719/589–2511; Paul Herman, Administrator (Nonreporting) **A**1 9 10 — 21 10 85 — — — — — — — —

ASPEN—Pitkin County
★ ASPEN VALLEY HOSPITAL DISTRICT, 0401 Castle Creek Road, Zip 81611; tel. 970/925–1120; Randy Middlebrook, Chief Executive Officer (Nonreporting) **A**1 9 10 — 16 10 41 — — — — — — — —

AURORA—Adams County
AURORA PRESBYTERIAN HOSPITAL See North Campus and Columbia Aurora Presbyterian Transitional Care Center
AURORA REGIONAL MEDICAL CENTER See Columbia Regional Medical Center–South Campus
★ COLUMBIA MEDICAL CENTER OF AURORA, (Includes Columbia Regional Medical Center–South Campus, 1501 South Potomac, North Campus and Columbia Aurora Presbyterian Transitional Care Center, 700 Potomac Street, Zip 80011–6792; tel. 303/363–7200), 1501 South Potomac Street, Zip 80012; tel. 303/695–2600; Louis O. Garcia, President and Chief Executive Officer (Nonreporting) **A**1 2 9 10 **S** Columbia/HCA Healthcare Corporation, Nashville, TN **N** Columbia – Health One, Englewood, CO — 33 10 334 — — — — — — — —
★ △ SPALDING REHABILITATION HOSPITAL, 900 Potomac Street, Zip 80011; tel. 303/367–1166; Russell W. York, President and Chief Executive Officer (Nonreporting) **A**1 5 7 9 10 **S** Columbia/HCA Healthcare Corporation, Nashville, TN — 33 46 176 — — — — — — — —

BOULDER—Boulder County
★ △ BOULDER COMMUNITY HOSPITAL, 1100 Balsam, Zip 80304–3496, Mailing Address: P.O. Box 9019, Zip 80301–9019; tel. 303/440–2273; David P. Gehant, President **A**1 2 7 9 10 **F**2 3 4 5 7 8 10 11 12 13 14 15 19 21 22 24 25 26 29 30 31 32 33 34 35 37 40 41 42 43 44 45 46 48 49 51 52 53 54 55 56 57 58 59 60 63 65 66 67 68 70 71 72 73 74 **P**4 7 8 — 23 10 197 9138 105 148845 1671 99966 43395 1202

BRIGHTON—Adams County
★ PLATTE VALLEY MEDICAL CENTER, 1850 Egbert Street, Zip 80601, Mailing Address: P.O. Box 98, Zip 80601; tel. 303/659–1531; John R. Hicks, Administrator **A**1 9 10 **F**7 8 11 13 14 15 16 17 19 21 22 24 27 28 30 32 33 34 35 36 37 39 40 41 42 44 46 49 51 64 65 66 67 69 71 73 **P**3 4 5 8 — 21 10 40 1678 14 23651 635 15182 6954 219

BRUSH—Morgan County
★ EAST MORGAN COUNTY HOSPITAL, 2400 West Edison, Zip 80723; tel. 970/842–5151; Anne Platt, Administrator (Nonreporting) **A**1 9 10 **S** Lutheran Health Systems, Fargo, ND **N** High Plains Rural Health Network, Fort Morgan, CO — 23 10 29 — — — — — — — —

BURLINGTON—Kit Carson County
KIT CARSON COUNTY MEMORIAL HOSPITAL, 286 16th Street, Zip 80807–1697; tel. 719/346–5311; DeAnn K. Cure, Chief Executive Officer (Nonreporting) **A**9 10 **N** High Plains Rural Health Network, Fort Morgan, CO — 13 10 24 — — — — — — — —

CANON CITY—Fremont County
★ ST. THOMAS MORE HOSPITAL AND PROGRESSIVE CARE CENTER, 1338 Phay Avenue, Zip 81212–2221; tel. 719/269–2000; C. Ray Honker, Administrator and Senior Vice President (Total facility includes 163 beds in nursing home–type unit) (Nonreporting) **A**1 9 10 **S** Catholic Health Initiatives, Denver, CO — 21 10 218 — — — — — — — —

CHEYENNE WELLS—Cheyenne County
★ KEEFE MEMORIAL HOSPITAL, 602 North Sixth Street West, Zip 80810, Mailing Address: P.O. Box 578, Zip 80810; tel. 719/767–5661; Linda Roth, Administrator **A**1 9 10 **F**8 13 14 15 16 19 20 22 26 28 30 32 33 35 36 39 42 44 45 46 49 65 71 73 74 **N** High Plains Rural Health Network, Fort Morgan, CO — 13 10 14 145 2 9839 0 2605 1166 58

COLORADO SPRINGS—El Paso County
□ CEDAR SPRINGS PSYCHIATRIC HOSPITAL, 2135 Southgate Road, Zip 80906–2693; tel. 719/633–4114; Connie Mull, Chief Executive Officer **A**1 10 **F**1 2 3 12 15 18 26 46 52 53 54 55 56 57 58 59 65 67 **S** Healthcare America, Inc., Austin, TX — 33 22 101 898 63 6691 0 — — 127
★ MEMORIAL HOSPITAL, 1400 East Boulder Street, Zip 80909–5599, Mailing Address: Box 1326, Zip 80901; tel. 719/475–5000; J. Robert Peters, Executive Director **A**1 2 9 10 **F**4 7 8 9 10 11 12 14 15 16 17 19 21 22 26 28 29 30 31 32 34 35 37 38 39 40 41 42 43 44 45 46 47 49 51 60 63 65 67 70 71 72 73 74 **P**5 7 **N** Health & Medical Network of Colorado, Colorado Springs, CO — 14 10 340 14941 205 185767 2418 — — 2321
PENROSE HOSPITAL See Penrose–St. Francis Health Services
★ PENROSE–ST. FRANCIS HEALTH SERVICES, (Formerly Penrose–St Francis Health System), (Includes Penrose Hospital, 2215 North Cascade Avenue, Mailing Address: P.O. Box 7021, Zip 80933–7021; tel. 719/776–5000; St Francis Health Center, 825 East Pikes Peak Avenue, Zip 80903; tel. 719/776–8800), 2215 North Cascade Avenue, Zip 80907; tel. 719/776–5000; Donna L. Bertram, R.N., Administrator (Total facility includes 64 beds in nursing home–type unit) (Nonreporting) **A**1 2 3 5 9 10 **S** Catholic Health Initiatives, Denver, CO **N** Centura Penrose–St Francis Health Services, Colorado Springs, CO — 21 10 522 — — — — — — — —
ST FRANCIS HEALTH CENTER See Penrose–St. Francis Health Services

Hospital, Address, Telephone, Administrator, Approval, Facility, and Physician Codes, Health Care System, Network	Classi-fication Codes		Utilization Data					Expense (thousands) of dollars		
★ American Hospital Association (AHA) membership □ Joint Commission on Accreditation of Healthcare Organizations (JCAHO) accreditation + American Osteopathic Hospital Association (AOHA) membership ○ American Osteopathic Association (AOA) accreditation △ Commission on Accreditation of Rehabilitation Facilities (CARF) accreditation Control codes 61, 63, 64, 71, 72 and 73 indicate hospitals listed by AOHA, but not registered by AHA. For definition of numerical codes, see page A4	Control	Service	Beds	Admissions	Census	Outpatient Visits	Births	Total	Payroll	Personnel

CORTEZ—Montezuma County

★ SOUTHWEST MEMORIAL HOSPITAL, 1311 North Mildred Road, Zip 81321; tel. 970/565–6666; Stephen R. Selzer, Administrator **A**1 9 10 **F**7 8 12 14 15 16 17 19 20 22 27 30 31 33 35 36 37 39 40 41 44 45 46 49 65 67 71 73 **P**3 8 **S** Quorum Health Group/Quorum Health Resources, Inc., Brentwood, TN — 23 10 56 2448 20 20397 245 17829 7365 280

CRAIG—Moffat County

★ MEMORIAL HOSPITAL, 785 Russell Street, Zip 81625–9906; tel. 970/824–9411; M. Randell Phelps, Administrator (Nonreporting) **A**1 9 10 **S** Quorum Health Group/Quorum Health Resources, Inc., Brentwood, TN — 13 10 27 — — — — — — —

DELTA—Delta County

★ DELTA COUNTY MEMORIAL HOSPITAL, 100 Stafford Lane, Zip 81416–2297, Mailing Address: P.O. Box 10100, Zip 81416–5003; tel. 970/874–7681; Edwin E. Hurysz, Administrator **A**1 9 10 **F**8 14 19 21 22 28 32 37 40 41 44 49 65 71 73 **P**5 **S** Presbyterian Healthcare Services, Albuquerque, NM — 16 10 44 2241 21 28577 233 13607 6640 247

DENVER—Denver, Adams and Arapahoe Counties

□ CENTURA SPECIAL CARE HOSPITAL, (Formerly Provenant Acute Long Stay Hospital), 1601 North Lowell, Zip 80204; tel. 303/899–5170; Silas M. Weir, Chief Executive Officer (Nonreporting) **A**1 10 — 23 10 24 — — — — — — —

★ CHILDREN'S HOSPITAL, 1056 East 19th Avenue, Zip 80218–1088; tel. 303/861–8888; Lua R. Blankenship, Jr., President and Chief Executive Officer **A**1 3 5 9 10 **F**4 5 9 10 12 13 14 15 16 17 18 19 20 21 22 25 28 29 30 31 32 34 35 38 39 41 42 43 44 45 46 47 49 51 52 53 54 55 56 58 59 60 65 67 68 69 70 71 72 73 **P**4 7 **N** The Children's Hospital, Denver, CO — 23 50 199 6939 124 242921 0 139874 63176 1873

□ COLORADO MENTAL HEALTH INSTITUTE AT FORT LOGAN, 3520 West Oxford Avenue, Zip 80236; tel. 303/761–0220; Allan Brock Willett, M.D., Director **A**1 9 10 **F**1 2 3 4 5 6 7 8 9 10 11 12 13 14 15 16 17 18 19 20 21 22 23 24 25 26 27 28 29 30 31 32 33 34 35 36 37 38 39 40 41 42 43 44 45 46 47 48 49 50 51 52 53 54 55 56 57 58 59 60 61 62 63 64 65 66 67 68 69 70 71 72 73 74 **P**4 6 — 12 22 315 782 302 — 0 29762 18110 475

★ COLUMBIA HEALTHONE–BEHAVIORAL HEALTH SERVICES, 4400 East Iliff Avenue, Zip 80222; tel. 303/758–1514; William Kent, Ph.D., Vice President Behavioral Health **A**1 9 10 **F**1 2 3 4 5 6 7 8 9 10 11 12 13 14 15 16 17 18 19 20 21 22 23 24 25 26 27 28 29 30 31 32 33 34 35 36 37 38 39 40 41 42 43 44 45 46 47 48 49 50 52 53 54 55 56 57 58 59 60 61 62 63 64 65 66 67 68 69 70 71 72 73 74 **P**1 8 **S** Columbia/HCA Healthcare Corporation, Nashville, TN — 33 22 86 117 2 14384 0 6519 4417 —

★ COLUMBIA PRESBYTERIAN–ST. LUKE'S MEDICAL CENTER, (Formerly Presbyterian–St. Luke's Medical Center), (Includes Presbyterian–Denver Hospital, 1719 East 19th Avenue, Zip 80218–1124; tel. 303/839–6565), 1719 East 19th Avenue, Zip 80218; tel. 303/839–6000; William K. Atkinson, Ph.D., Chief Executive Officer **A**1 2 3 5 9 10 12 13 **F**1 2 3 4 5 6 7 8 10 12 14 15 16 17 19 20 21 22 23 24 25 26 27 28 29 30 32 33 34 35 36 37 38 39 40 41 42 43 44 45 46 47 48 49 51 53 54 55 56 57 59 60 61 62 63 64 65 66 67 68 69 70 71 72 73 74 **P**5 6 7 **S** Columbia/HCA Healthcare Corporation, Nashville, TN **N** Columbia – Health One, Englewood, CO — 23 10 479 15842 280 79891 1716 125511 59850 1590

★ COLUMBIA ROSE MEDICAL CENTER, 4567 East Ninth Avenue, Zip 80220; tel. 303/320–2101; Kenneth H. Feiler, Chief Executive Officer **A**1 2 3 5 9 10 **F**1 2 3 4 5 7 8 9 10 11 12 14 15 16 17 19 20 21 22 23 25 26 27 28 29 30 31 32 33 34 35 37 38 39 40 41 42 43 44 45 46 47 48 49 51 52 53 54 55 56 57 58 59 61 63 64 65 66 67 69 70 71 72 73 74 **P**4 5 7 **S** Columbia/HCA Healthcare Corporation, Nashville, TN **N** Columbia – Health One, Englewood, CO — 33 10 250 13853 156 152882 3921 110311 41281 1335

□ DENVER HEALTH MEDICAL CENTER, (Formerly Denver Health and Hospitals), 777 Bannock Street, Zip 80204–4507; tel. 303/436–6000; Patricia A. Gabow, M.D., Chief Executive Officer and Medical Director (Nonreporting) **A**1 3 5 9 10 — 15 10 312 — — — — — — —

★ NATIONAL JEWISH MEDICAL AND RESEARCH CENTER, (Formerly National Jewish Center for Immunology and Respiratory Medicine), 1400 Jackson Street, Zip 80206–2762; tel. 303/388–4461; Lynn M. Taussig, M.D., President and Chief Executive Officer (Nonreporting) **A**1 3 5 9 10 — 23 49 75 — — — — — — —

★ PORTER CARE HOSPITAL, 2525 South Downing Street, Zip 80210–5876; tel. 303/778–1955; Ruthita J. Fike, Administrator (Total facility includes 34 beds in nursing home–type unit) **A**1 2 3 5 9 10 **F**3 4 6 7 8 10 11 12 13 14 15 16 17 18 19 21 22 24 25 26 27 28 29 30 31 32 33 34 35 37 38 39 40 41 42 43 44 45 46 48 49 51 52 53 54 55 56 57 58 59 60 61 62 63 64 65 66 67 68 70 71 72 73 74 **P**1 4 5 7 — 21 10 339 12437 178 102290 912 122639 49849 2458

PRESBYTERIAN–ST. LUKE'S MEDICAL CENTER See Columbia Presbyterian–St. Luke's Medical Center

PROVENANT ACUTE LONG STAY HOSPITAL See Centura Special Care Hospital

PROVENANT ST. ANTHONY HOSPITAL CENTRAL See St. Anthony Hospital Central

★ SAINT JOSEPH HOSPITAL, 1835 Franklin Street, Zip 80218; tel. 303/837–7111; Sister Marianna Bauder, President and Chief Executive Officer **A**1 2 3 9 10 **F**3 4 7 8 10 11 14 15 16 17 19 21 22 23 26 29 30 31 34 35 37 38 39 40 41 42 43 44 45 46 49 51 52 54 55 56 57 58 59 60 63 65 66 67 68 71 72 73 74 **P**1 6 **S** Sisters of Charity of Leavenworth Health Services Corporation, Leavenworth, KS **N** Primera Health Care, Denver, CO — 21 10 394 23293 264 254360 5282 157250 73161 1685

★ ST. ANTHONY HOSPITAL CENTRAL, (Formerly Provenant St. Anthony Hospital Central), 4231 West 16th Avenue, Zip 80204–4098; tel. 303/629–3511; Michael H. Erne, Senior Vice President and Administrator **A**1 2 3 5 10 **F**1 4 8 10 11 12 15 19 21 22 24 26 28 32 33 34 35 37 40 42 43 44 45 46 48 49 51 52 57 60 64 65 70 71 73 74 **P**3 7 **S** Catholic Health Initiatives, Denver, CO — 21 10 238 15778 170 105632 1389 — — —

Hospital, Address, Telephone, Administrator, Approval, Facility, and Physician Codes, Health Care System, Network	Classi-fication Codes		Utilization Data					Expense (thousands) of dollars		
★ American Hospital Association (AHA) membership □ Joint Commission on Accreditation of Healthcare Organizations (JCAHO) accreditation + American Osteopathic Hospital Association (AOHA) membership ○ American Osteopathic Association (AOA) accreditation △ Commission on Accreditation of Rehabilitation Facilities (CARF) accreditation Control codes 61, 63, 64, 71, 72 and 73 indicate hospitals listed by AOHA, but not registered by AHA. For definition of numerical codes, see page A4	Control	Service	Beds	Admissions	Census	Outpatient Visits	Births	Total	Payroll	Personnel
⊞ UNIVERSITY OF COLORADO HOSPITAL, 4200 East Ninth Avenue, Zip 80262; tel. 303/399–1211; Dennis C. Brimhall, President A1 2 5 8 9 10 F4 5 7 8 9 10 12 14 15 16 17 18 19 20 21 22 24 25 26 29 30 31 32 34 35 37 38 39 40 41 42 43 44 45 46 48 49 51 52 53 54 56 58 59 60 61 63 65 66 67 68 69 70 71 72 73 74	16	10	318	14025	203	285644	2057	269405	77005	1992
⊞ VETERANS AFFAIRS MEDICAL CENTER, 1055 Clermont Street, Zip 80220–3877; tel. 303/399–8020; Ed Thorsland, Jr., Director (Total facility includes 60 beds in nursing home–type unit) A1 2 3 5 8 F2 3 4 8 10 14 15 16 17 19 20 21 22 23 26 27 28 31 32 33 34 35 37 39 41 42 43 44 45 46 48 49 51 52 54 55 56 58 59 60 64 65 69 71 73 74 P6 S Department of Veterans Affairs, Washington, DC	45	10	336	7063	249	253060	0	122251	61351	1882
DURANGO—La Plata County										
MERCY BEHAVIORAL HEALTH, 3801 North Main Avenue, Zip 81301; tel. 970/382–2400; Jerry Brown, Manager (Nonreporting) A9	16	22	20	—	—	—	—	—	—	—
⊞ MERCY MEDICAL CENTER, 375 East Park Avenue, Zip 81301; tel. 970/247–4311; Renato V. Baciarelli, Administrator A1 9 10 F3 4 7 8 10 12 14 15 16 17 19 20 21 22 23 24 25 28 29 30 31 32 33 34 35 36 37 38 39 40 41 42 44 46 49 51 52 53 56 58 64 65 66 67 70 71 72 73 74 P1 4 5 6 7 8 S Catholic Health Initiatives, Denver, CO	21	10	92	3686	37	302029	656	57061	27051	581
EADS—Kiowa County										
★ WEISBROD MEMORIAL HOSPITAL, 1208 Luther Street, Zip 81036, Mailing Address: P.O. Box 817, Zip 81036–0817; tel. 719/438–5401; Marvin O. Bishop, Administrator (Total facility includes 34 beds in nursing home–type unit) (Nonreporting) A9 10	16	10	42	—	—	—	—	—	—	—
ENGLEWOOD—Arapahoe County										
⊞ COLUMBIA SWEDISH MEDICAL CENTER, (Formerly Swedish Medical Center), 501 East Hampden Avenue, Zip 80110–0101, Mailing Address: P.O. Box 2901, Zip 80150–0101; tel. 303/788–5000; Mary M. White, President and Chief Executive Officer (Nonreporting) A1 2 3 5 9 10 S Columbia/HCA Healthcare Corporation, Nashville, TN N Columbia – Health One, Englewood, CO	23	10	328	—	—	—	—	—	—	—
⊞ △ CRAIG HOSPITAL, 3425 South Clarkson, Zip 80110; tel. 303/789–8000; Dennis O'Malley, President A1 7 9 10 F12 14 16 17 19 20 21 22 23 24 32 34 35 39 41 44 45 46 48 49 50 60 63 65 67 70 71 73	23	46	70	502	62	5846	0	27998	12598	350
SWEDISH MEDICAL CENTER See Columbia Swedish Medical Center										
ESTES PARK—Larimer County										
★ ESTES PARK MEDICAL CENTER, 555 Prospect, Zip 80517, Mailing Address: P.O. Box 2740, Zip 80517–2740; tel. 970/586–2317; Andrew Wills, Chief Executive Officer (Total facility includes 60 beds in nursing home–type unit) A9 10 F7 14 15 16 21 22 26 28 32 33 34 41 42 44 45 46 49 51 62 64 65 69 71 73 P7 8 N High Plains Rural Health Network, Fort Morgan, CO	16	10	74	474	49	31486	40	7700	3525	173
FORT CARSON—El Paso County										
⊞ EVANS U. S. ARMY COMMUNITY HOSPITAL, Zip 80913–5101; tel. 719/526–7200; Colonel Kenneth W. Leisher, Deputy Commander, Administration A1 2 F3 7 8 12 13 14 15 16 17 18 19 20 21 22 24 25 28 29 30 31 32 34 37 39 40 41 42 44 45 46 49 51 52 53 54 56 58 59 65 66 67 71 73 74 P6 S Department of the Army, Office of the Surgeon General, Falls Church, VA	42	10	103	7565	51	432687	1430	61837	22139	—
FORT COLLINS—Larimer County										
□ MOUNTAIN CREST HOSPITAL, 4601 Corbett Drive, Zip 80525; tel. 970/225–9191; Kathleen Mechler, Chief Executive Officer A1 10 F1 2 3 12 14 15 16 17 18 26 28 29 30 31 45 46 52 53 54 55 56 57 58 59 67 68	33	22	44	792	21	0	0	5619	2024	76
⊞ POUDRE VALLEY HOSPITAL, 1024 Lemay Avenue, Zip 80524–3998; tel. 970/495–7000; Rulon F. Stacey, President A1 2 3 9 10 F3 4 7 8 10 12 15 16 19 20 21 22 24 25 29 30 32 33 34 35 36 37 40 41 42 43 44 45 46 47 48 49 51 52 53 54 55 56 57 58 59 60 63 65 67 71 73 P5	23	10	222	13181	134	284458	2066	114662	50898	1331
FORT LYON—Bent County										
⊞ VETERANS AFFAIRS MEDICAL CENTER, Zip 81038; tel. 719/456–1260; W. David Smith, Director (Total facility includes 209 beds in nursing home–type unit) A1 F14 16 19 20 22 26 29 30 31 34 39 41 44 45 46 49 51 52 54 58 64 65 67 71 73 74 P6 S Department of Veterans Affairs, Washington, DC	45	22	299	779	294	40540	0	34428	11988	522
FORT MORGAN—Morgan County										
⊞ COLORADO PLAINS MEDICAL CENTER, 1000 Lincoln Street, Zip 80701; tel. 970/867–3391; Keith Mesmer, Administrator and Chief Executive Officer A1 9 10 F7 8 11 14 15 16 19 22 28 29 30 32 34 35 37 40 41 42 44 45 46 47 49 65 66 67 70 71 73 P8 S Principal Hospital Group, Brentwood, TN N High Plains Rural Health Network, Fort Morgan, CO	33	10	40	2144	22	74755	391	14735	6344	206
FRUITA—Mesa County										
FAMILY HEALTH WEST, 228 North Cherry Street, Zip 81521, Mailing Address: Box 130, Zip 81521–0130; tel. 303/858–9871; Dennis E. Ficklin, Executive Director (Total facility includes 352 beds in nursing home–type unit) (Nonreporting) A9 10	23	10	358	—	—	—	—	—	—	—
GLENWOOD SPRINGS—Garfield County										
⊞ VALLEY VIEW HOSPITAL, 1906 Blake Avenue, Zip 81601, Mailing Address: Box 1970, Zip 81602; tel. 970/945–6535; Norman L. McBride, Chief Executive Officer A1 9 10 F2 7 8 15 16 19 22 23 32 34 35 36 37 39 40 41 42 44 46 49 63 65 66 71 73 P5 S Quorum Health Group/Quorum Health Resources, Inc., Brentwood, TN	23	10	61	2832	30	—	533	27715	12454	338

Hospital, Address, Telephone, Administrator, Approval, Facility, and Physician Codes, Health Care System, Network	Classi-fication Codes		Utilization Data					Expense (thousands) of dollars		
★ American Hospital Association (AHA) membership □ Joint Commission on Accreditation of Healthcare Organizations (JCAHO) accreditation + American Osteopathic Hospital Association (AOHA) membership ○ American Osteopathic Association (AOA) accreditation △ Commission on Accreditation of Rehabilitation Facilities (CARF) accreditation Control codes 61, 63, 64, 71, 72 and 73 indicate hospitals listed by AOHA, but not registered by AHA. For definition of numerical codes, see page A4	Control	Service	Beds	Admissions	Census	Outpatient Visits	Births	Total	Payroll	Personnel

GRAND JUNCTION—Mesa County

□ + ○ COMMUNITY HOSPITAL, 2021 North 12th Street, Zip 81501; tel. 970/242–0920; Roger C. Zumwalt, Executive Director (Nonreporting) **A**1 9 10 11 **N** Community Health Providers Organization, Grand Junction, CO — 23 10 51 — — — — — — —

COMMUNITY HOSPITAL	23	10	51	—		—		—	—	—
ST. MARY'S HOSPITAL AND MEDICAL CENTER	21	10	273	12196	132	280953	1315	108637	47841	1409
VETERANS AFFAIRS MEDICAL CENTER	45	10	116	1905	69	51129	0	23480	12646	315
NORTH COLORADO MEDICAL CENTER	23	10	262	12862	156	233196	1796	115530	50236	1505
GUNNISON VALLEY HOSPITAL	13	10	24	587	5	19268	114	4932	2426	72
HAXTUN HOSPITAL DISTRICT	16	10	48	—		—		—	—	—
MELISSA MEMORIAL HOSPITAL	16	10	18	297	5	9417	22	3017	1598	64
LINCOLN COMMUNITY HOSPITAL AND NURSING HOME	13	10	56	513	34	9742	41	3952	1742	92
SEDGWICK COUNTY MEMORIAL HOSPITAL	13	10	58	240	34	5955	23	2575	1224	63
KREMMLING MEMORIAL HOSPITAL	16	10	19	277	10	14988	0	3253	1243	63
CONEJOS COUNTY HOSPITAL	16	10	49	1076	34	—	36	4424	2261	—
ARKANSAS VALLEY REGIONAL MEDICAL CENTER	21	10	187	2801	158	44268	315	18892	9049	372
PROWERS MEDICAL CENTER	16	10	40	1509	13	24853	256	9561	4226	149
ST. VINCENT GENERAL HOSPITAL	16	10	31	—	—	—	—	—	—	—
PORTER CARE HOSPITAL–LITTLETON	21	10	106	7091	62	—	2028	46699	18366	492

⊞ ST. MARY'S HOSPITAL AND MEDICAL CENTER, 2635 North 7th Street, Zip 81501–1628, Mailing Address: P.O. Box 1628, Zip 81502; tel. 970/244–2273; Sister Lynn Casey, President and Chief Executive Officer **A**1 2 3 9 10 **F**1 3 4 5 6 7 8 9 10 11 12 13 14 15 16 17 18 19 20 21 22 23 24 26 27 28 29 30 31 32 33 34 35 36 37 38 39 40 41 42 43 44 45 46 48 49 51 52 53 54 55 56 57 58 59 60 61 63 64 65 66 67 68 70 71 72 73 74 **P**3 5 6 7 **S** Sisters of Charity of Leavenworth Health Services Corporation, Leavenworth, KS

⊞ VETERANS AFFAIRS MEDICAL CENTER, 2121 North Avenue, Zip 81501–6499; tel. 970/242–0731; Robert R. Rhyne, D.D.S., Director (Total facility includes 30 beds in nursing home–type unit) **A**1 **F**2 3 4 10 14 15 16 17 19 20 21 22 23 26 30 31 32 33 34 35 37 39 41 42 43 44 45 46 49 51 52 54 58 59 60 64 65 67 71 73 74 **P**6 **S** Department of Veterans Affairs, Washington, DC

GREELEY—Weld County

⊞ NORTH COLORADO MEDICAL CENTER, 1801 16th Street, Zip 80631–5199; tel. 970/350–6000; Karl B. Gills, Administrator **A**1 2 3 9 10 **F**2 3 4 7 8 9 10 12 14 15 16 17 19 21 22 23 25 26 27 29 30 31 32 33 34 35 37 39 40 41 42 43 44 45 46 48 49 51 52 53 54 55 56 57 58 59 60 63 64 65 66 67 70 71 73 74 **P**5 7 8 **S** Lutheran Health Systems, Fargo, ND **N** High Plains Rural Health Network, Fort Morgan, CO

GUNNISON—Gunnison County

GUNNISON VALLEY HOSPITAL, 214 East Denver Avenue, Zip 81230; tel. 970/641–1456; Robert S. Austin, President **A**9 10 **F**7 8 11 14 15 19 20 22 28 29 32 35 37 40 41 44 47 49 65 66 71 73

HAXTUN—Phillips County

★ HAXTUN HOSPITAL DISTRICT, 235 West Fletcher Street, Zip 80731–0308, Mailing Address: Box 308, Zip 80731–0308; tel. 970/774–6123; James E. Brundige, Administrator (Total facility includes 32 beds in nursing home–type unit) (Nonreporting) **A**9 10 **N** High Plains Rural Health Network, Fort Morgan, CO

HOLYOKE—Phillips County

★ MELISSA MEMORIAL HOSPITAL, 505 South Baxter Avenue, Zip 80734–1496; tel. 970/854–2241; Geo V. Larson, II, Administrator **A**9 10 **F**7 8 14 15 17 19 20 22 24 27 28 30 32 34 40 41 44 45 49 71 73 **P**3 6 **N** High Plains Rural Health Network, Fort Morgan, CO

HUGO—Lincoln County

★ LINCOLN COMMUNITY HOSPITAL AND NURSING HOME, 111 Sixth Street, Zip 80821, Mailing Address: Box 248, Zip 80821; tel. 719/743–2421; Mary L. Thompson, Administrator (Total facility includes 35 beds in nursing home–type unit) **A**9 10 **F**7 8 14 15 16 19 32 34 35 40 41 44 49 64 65 71 **N** High Plains Rural Health Network, Fort Morgan, CO

JULESBURG—Sedgwick County

SEDGWICK COUNTY MEMORIAL HOSPITAL, 900 Cedar Street, Zip 80737; tel. 970/474–3323; Bill Patten, Administrator (Total facility includes 32 beds in nursing home–type unit) **A**9 10 **F**1 7 8 11 14 15 16 19 20 24 27 28 29 30 32 34 35 37 39 40 41 42 44 45 46 49 51 64 65 66 71 **P**7

KREMMLING—Grand County

KREMMLING MEMORIAL HOSPITAL, Fourth and Grand Avenue, Zip 80459, Mailing Address: Box 399, Zip 80459–0399; tel. 970/724–3442 **A**9 10 **F**8 14 15 16 17 24 28 39 44 49 51 71 73 **P**6

LA JARA—Conejos County

□ CONEJOS COUNTY HOSPITAL, Mailing Address: Box 639, Zip 81140–0639; tel. 719/274–5121; Monica Morris, Administrator (Total facility includes 34 beds in nursing home–type unit) **A**1 9 10 **F**7 13 14 15 22 28 30 33 40 41 43 44 46 49 57 64 65 71 73

LA JUNTA—Otero County

⊞ ARKANSAS VALLEY REGIONAL MEDICAL CENTER, 1100 Carson Avenue, Zip 81050; tel. 719/384–5412; Dale D. Stoll, Chief Executive Officer (Total facility includes 120 beds in nursing home–type unit) **A**1 9 10 **F**7 8 10 15 17 19 22 23 28 30 32 34 35 37 40 42 44 46 49 64 65 67 71 **P**5

LAMAR—Prowers County

⊞ PROWERS MEDICAL CENTER, 401 Kendall Drive, Zip 81052–3993; tel. 719/336–4343; Earl J. Steinhoff, Chief Executive Officer **A**1 9 10 **F**1 2 3 4 5 7 8 9 10 11 14 15 16 17 19 20 21 22 23 25 26 27 28 29 30 32 33 34 35 36 37 38 39 40 41 42 43 44 45 46 47 48 49 50 51 52 53 54 55 56 57 58 59 60 61 63 64 65 66 67 69 70 71 73 74 **S** Quorum Health Group/Quorum Health Resources, Inc., Brentwood, TN **N** High Plains Rural Health Network, Fort Morgan, CO

LEADVILLE—Lake County

ST. VINCENT GENERAL HOSPITAL, 822 West Fourth Street, Zip 80461–3897; tel. 719/486–0230; Sam Radke, Interim Chief Executive Officer (Nonreporting) **A**9 10

LITTLETON—Arapahoe County

⊞ PORTER CARE HOSPITAL–LITTLETON, 7700 South Broadway, Zip 80122; tel. 303/730–8900; Ruthita J. Fike, Administrator **A**1 9 **F**3 7 8 11 12 13 14 15 16 17 18 19 21 22 24 25 26 27 28 29 30 31 32 33 34 35 37 38 39 40 41 44 45 46 48 49 51 52 53 54 55 56 57 58 59 60 61 62 63 64 65 66 67 68 69 70 71 72 73 74 **P**1 4 5 7

Hospital, Address, Telephone, Administrator, Approval, Facility, and Physician Codes, Health Care System, Network	Classi-fication Codes		Utilization Data						Expense (thousands) of dollars		
★ American Hospital Association (AHA) membership □ Joint Commission on Accreditation of Healthcare Organizations (JCAHO) accreditation + American Osteopathic Hospital Association (AOHA) membership ○ American Osteopathic Association (AOA) accreditation △ Commission on Accreditation of Rehabilitation Facilities (CARF) accreditation Control codes 61, 63, 64, 71, 72 and 73 indicate hospitals listed by AOHA, but not registered by AHA. For definition of numerical codes, see page A4	Control	Service	Beds	Admissions	Census	Outpatient Visits	Births	Total	Payroll	Personnel

LONGMONT—Boulder County

✸ LONGMONT UNITED HOSPITAL, 1950 West Mountain View Avenue, Zip 80501–3162, Mailing Address: Box 1659, Zip 80502–1659; tel. 303/651–5111; Kenneth R. Huey, President and Chief Executive Officer (Total facility includes 15 beds in nursing home–type unit) **A**1 2 9 10 **F**1 3 7 8 12 14 16 17 19 20 21 22 24 25 26 27 28 29 30 31 32 33 34 35 37 39 40 41 42 44 45 46 48 49 52 53 54 55 56 57 58 59 60 64 65 66 67 68 69 70 71 73 **P**8	23	10	122	5483	65	153015	820	46349	20499	721

LOUISVILLE—Boulder County

□ CHARTER CENTENNIAL PEAKS HEALTH SYSTEM, 2255 South 88th Street, Zip 80027; tel. 303/673–9990; Sharon Worsham, Administrator (Nonreporting) **A**1 9 10 **S** Magellan Health Services, Atlanta, GA	33	22	72	—	—	—	—	—	—	—
✸ PORTERCARE HOSPITAL–AVISTA, 100 Health Park Drive, Zip 80027–9583; tel. 303/673–1000; John Sackett, Administrator **A**1 3 9 10 **F**7 8 10 12 13 14 15 16 17 19 21 22 25 26 28 29 30 32 33 34 35 37 39 40 41 42 44 46 49 61 65 66 67 71 73 **P**3 5	21	10	58	3719	29	41481	1432	28258	11422	351

LOVELAND—Larimer County

✸ MCKEE MEDICAL CENTER, 2000 Boise Avenue, Zip 80538–4281; tel. 970/669–4640; Charles F. Harms, Administrator **A**1 9 10 **F**1 7 8 12 14 15 16 17 18 19 21 22 23 28 30 31 32 33 34 35 39 41 44 45 46 49 55 60 63 64 65 70 71 73 **P**7 8 **S** Lutheran Health Systems, Fargo, ND	23	10	109	5059	54	51546	647	38594	17048	616

MEEKER—Rio Blanco County

★ PIONEERS HOSPITAL OF RIO BLANCO COUNTY, (Includes Walbridge Memorial Convalescent Wing), 345 Cleveland Street, Zip 81641–0000; tel. 970/878–5047; Jim Murphy, Administrator (Total facility includes 29 beds in nursing home–type unit) **A**9 10 **F**1 8 14 15 20 22 24 25 26 27 28 32 36 39 41 44 49 64 71 72 73 74 **P**1 **S** Quorum Health Group/Quorum Health Resources, Inc., Brentwood, TN **N** Quorum Health Network of Colorado, Boulder, CO	15	10	41	264	29	8420	1	4628	2087	94

MONTROSE—Montrose County

✸ MONTROSE MEMORIAL HOSPITAL, 800 South Third Street, Zip 81401–4291; tel. 970/249–2211; Tyler Erickson, Administrator **A**1 9 10 **F**2 3 7 8 11 12 14 15 16 17 19 20 21 22 23 24 26 28 29 30 33 34 35 37 39 40 41 42 44 45 46 47 48 49 52 53 54 55 56 57 58 63 65 66 67 68 71 73 74 **P**5 8 **S** Quorum Health Group/Quorum Health Resources, Inc., Brentwood, TN	13	10	60	2813	30	58525	456	24286	10699	324

PUEBLO—Pueblo County

□ COLORADO MENTAL HEALTH INSTITUTE AT PUEBLO, 1600 West 24th Street, Zip 81003–1499; tel. 719/546–4000; Robert L. Hawkins, Superintendent (Nonreporting) **A**1 9 10	12	22	605	—	—	—	—	—	—	—
✸ PARKVIEW EPISCOPAL MEDICAL CENTER, 400 West 16th Street, Zip 81003; tel. 719/584–4000; C. W. Smith, President (Total facility includes 6 beds in nursing home–type unit) **A**1 9 10 **F**1 2 3 4 7 8 10 12 14 15 16 17 18 19 22 23 26 28 30 31 32 35 37 39 40 41 42 43 44 45 46 48 49 52 53 54 55 56 57 58 59 64 65 66 70 71 73 **P**7 8 **S** Quorum Health Group/Quorum Health Resources, Inc., Brentwood, TN	23	10	259	8792	134	96799	887	69945	31584	1296
✸ ST. MARY–CORWIN REGIONAL MEDICAL CENTER, 1008 Minnequa Avenue, Zip 81004–3798; tel. 719/560–4000; Walter Sackett, Senior Vice President and Administrator (Total facility includes 16 beds in nursing home–type unit) (Nonreporting) **A**1 2 3 9 10 **S** Catholic Health Initiatives, Denver, CO	21	10	261	—	—	—	—	—	—	—

RANGELY—Rio Blanco County

★ RANGELY DISTRICT HOSPITAL, 511 South White Avenue, Zip 81648–2104; tel. 970/675–5011; Kent Harmon, Interim Chief Executive Officer **A**9 10 **F**8 15 22 28 30 32 34 44 46 49 51 64 71 **P**6	16	10	25	82	13	9776	0	3171	1744	62

RIFLE—Garfield County

★ GRAND RIVER HOSPITAL DISTRICT, 701 East Fifth Street, Zip 81650–2970, Mailing Address: P.O. Box 912, Zip 81650–0912; tel. 970/625–1510; Edwin A. Gast, Administrator (Total facility includes 57 beds in nursing home–type unit) (Nonreporting) **A**9 10 **S** Quorum Health Group/Quorum Health Resources, Inc., Brentwood, TN **N** Quorum Health Network of Colorado, Boulder, CO	16	10	75	—	—	—	—	—	—	—

SALIDA—Chaffee County

★ HEART OF THE ROCKIES REGIONAL MEDICAL CENTER, 448 East First Street, Zip 81201–0429, Mailing Address: P.O. Box 429, Zip 81201–0429; tel. 719/539–6661; Howard D. Turner, Administrator and Chief Executive Officer (Nonreporting) **A**9 10 **S** Quorum Health Group/Quorum Health Resources, Inc., Brentwood, TN	16	10	38	—	—	—	—	—	—	—

SPRINGFIELD—Baca County

★ SOUTHEAST COLORADO HOSPITAL AND LONG TERM CARE, 373 East Tenth Avenue, Zip 81073; tel. 719/523–4501; Annie L. Dukes, JD, Chief Executive Officer (Total facility includes 56 beds in nursing home–type unit) **A**9 10 **F**11 13 14 15 16 17 19 22 26 27 28 29 30 31 32 33 34 42 44 45 46 49 51 60 64 65 67 71 73 **P**5 6	23	10	81	402	49	27463	0	—	—	144

STEAMBOAT SPRINGS—Routt County

✸ ROUTT MEMORIAL HOSPITAL, 80 Park Avenue, Zip 80487–5010; tel. 970/879–1322; Margaret D. Sabin, Chief Executive Officer (Total facility includes 50 beds in nursing home–type unit) **A**1 9 10 **F**3 7 8 14 15 19 21 22 26 28 34 35 37 40 41 42 44 49 53 54 55 56 57 58 63 64 65 66 70 71 74	23	10	74	907	49	—	176	11888	5386	194

Hospital, Address, Telephone, Administrator, Approval, Facility, and Physician Codes, Health Care System, Network	Classi-fication Codes		Utilization Data					Expense (thousands) of dollars		
★ American Hospital Association (AHA) membership □ Joint Commission on Accreditation of Healthcare Organizations (JCAHO) accreditation + American Osteopathic Hospital Association (AOHA) membership ○ American Osteopathic Association (AOA) accreditation △ Commission on Accreditation of Rehabilitation Facilities (CARF) accreditation Control codes 61, 63, 64, 71, 72 and 73 indicate hospitals listed by AOHA, but not registered by AHA. For definition of numerical codes, see page A4	Control	Service	Beds	Admissions	Census	Outpatient Visits	Births	Total	Payroll	Personnel

STERLING—Logan County

★ STERLING REGIONAL MEDCENTER, 615 Fairhurst, Zip 80751–0500, Mailing Address: Box 3500, Zip 80751; tel. 970/522–0122; James O. Pernau, Administrator **A**1 9 10 **F**7 8 11 12 13 15 16 17 19 21 22 23 24 26 28 29 30 32 33 35 36 37 39 40 41 42 44 45 46 48 49 50 63 64 65 66 67 71 73 **P**4 5 7 8 **S** Lutheran Health Systems, Fargo, ND **N** High Plains Rural Health Network, Fort Morgan, CO — 23 10 36 1880 21 82615 248 21609 9181 297

THORNTON—Adams County

□ △ MEDIPLEX REHABILITATION–DENVER, 8451 Pearl Street, Zip 80229; tel. 303/288–3000; Harvey Ross, Executive Director and Chief Executive Officer (Total facility includes 50 beds in nursing home–type unit) **A**1 5 7 9 10 **F**14 15 16 19 21 25 27 35 48 49 50 52 59 63 64 71 73 — 33 46 117 1073 5 0 0 — — 189

★ NORTH SUBURBAN MEDICAL CENTER, 9191 Grant Street, Zip 80229; tel. 303/451–7800; Jay S. Weinstein, Chief Executive Officer (Total facility includes 15 beds in nursing home–type unit) **A**1 9 10 **F**1 2 3 4 5 6 7 8 9 10 11 12 13 14 15 16 17 18 19 20 21 22 23 24 25 26 27 28 29 30 31 32 33 34 35 36 37 38 39 40 41 42 43 44 45 46 47 48 49 50 51 52 53 54 55 56 57 58 59 60 61 62 63 64 65 66 67 68 69 70 71 72 73 74 **P**7 **S** Columbia/HCA Healthcare Corporation, Nashville, TN **N** Columbia – Health One, Englewood, CO — 33 10 125 5095 66 46089 877 33336 15725 558

TRINIDAD—Las Animas County

★ MOUNT SAN RAFAEL HOSPITAL, 410 Benedicta Avenue, Zip 81082–2093; tel. 719/846–9213; James P. D'Agostino, Chief Executive Officer **A**1 9 10 **F**7 19 21 22 32 35 37 40 44 46 51 71 **P**8 **S** Quorum Health Group/Quorum Health Resources, Inc., Brentwood, TN — 23 10 31 1179 14 34008 119 8085 3610 148

USAF ACADEMY—El Paso County

★ U. S. AIR FORCE ACADEMY HOSPITAL, 4102 Pinion Drive, Zip 80840–4000; tel. 719/333–5111; Colonel David L. Hammer, USAF, MC, Commander **A**1 **F**7 8 12 14 15 16 19 20 21 22 24 25 28 29 30 34 35 37 39 40 41 44 45 46 48 49 51 53 54 55 56 57 58 59 61 65 66 67 71 73 74 **S** Department of the Air Force, Washington, DC — 41 10 46 5127 29 263573 633 — — 721

VAIL—Eagle County

★ VAIL VALLEY MEDICAL CENTER, 181 West Meadow Drive, Zip 81657; tel. 970/476–2451; Howard C. Andersen, Chief Executive Officer **A**1 3 9 10 **F**4 7 8 10 12 17 19 21 22 24 28 30 31 32 33 35 39 41 44 46 49 65 66 67 68 70 71 73 74 **P**5 7 — 23 10 49 2169 16 38034 505 37470 15780 502

WALSENBURG—Huerfano County

★ HUERFANO MEDICAL CENTER, 23500 U.S. Highway 160, Zip 81089; tel. 719/738–5100; Vonnie Maier, President and Chief Executive Officer **A**9 10 **F**3 5 8 15 16 17 19 20 22 26 27 28 29 30 31 32 33 34 35 39 41 44 45 46 49 65 66 71 73 74 — 16 10 24 819 18 21610 0 6139 2159 173

WESTMINSTER—Jefferson County

★ CLEO WALLACE CENTER HOSPITAL, 8405 West 100th Avenue, Zip 80021; tel. 303/466–7391; James M. Cole, President and Chief Executive Officer (Nonreporting) **A**1 9 10 — 23 52 61 — — — — — —

PROVENANT ST. ANTHONY HOSPITAL NORTH See St. Anthony Hospital North

★ ST. ANTHONY HOSPITAL NORTH, (Formerly Provenant St. Anthony Hospital North), 2551 West 84th Avenue, Zip 80030; tel. 303/426–2151; Michael H. Erne, Senior Vice President and Administrator **A**10 **F**1 4 8 10 11 12 15 19 22 24 26 28 32 33 34 35 37 40 42 43 44 45 46 48 49 51 52 57 60 64 65 70 71 73 74 **P**3 7 **S** Catholic Health Initiatives, Denver, CO — 21 10 110 7469 63 60982 954 — — —

WHEAT RIDGE—Jefferson County

★ LUTHERAN MEDICAL CENTER, (Includes West Pines at Lutheran Medical Center, 3400 Lutheran Parkway, Zip 80033; tel. 303/467–4001; Edward A. Ross, Director Mental Health), 8300 West 38th Avenue, Zip 80033–6005; tel. 303/425–4500; Kay R. Phillips, President and Chief Executive Officer (Total facility includes 18 beds in nursing home–type unit) **A**1 2 9 10 **F**2 3 4 5 6 7 8 9 10 11 12 13 14 15 16 17 19 21 22 24 26 27 29 30 31 32 33 34 35 36 37 39 40 41 42 43 44 45 46 47 48 49 51 52 53 54 55 56 57 58 59 60 61 62 64 65 66 67 68 70 71 72 73 74 **P**5 6 7 **N** Primera Health Care, Denver, CO — 23 10 335 14128 167 157286 1886 131607 66823 1884

WEST PINES AT LUTHERAN MEDICAL CENTER See Lutheran Medical Center

WRAY—Yuma County

WRAY COMMUNITY DISTRICT HOSPITAL, 1017 West 7th Street, Zip 80758–1420; tel. 970/332–4811; Daniel Dennis, Administrator (Nonreporting) **A**3 9 10 **N** High Plains Rural Health Network, Fort Morgan, CO — 16 10 25 — — — — — — —

YUMA—Yuma County

★ YUMA DISTRICT HOSPITAL, 910 South Main Street, Zip 80759–3098, Mailing Address: P.O. Box 306, Zip 80759–0306; tel. 970/848–5405; Michael G. Clark, Administrator **A**9 10 **F**7 8 14 15 22 28 31 32 39 40 44 49 71 73 **N** High Plains Rural Health Network, Fort Morgan, CO — 16 10 11 210 2 15527 21 2306 1195 64

CONNECTICUT

Resident population 3,275 (in thousands)
Resident population in metro areas 95.7%
Birth rate per 1,000 population 14.2
65 years and over 14.3%
Percent of persons without health insurance 10.4%

Hospital, Address, Telephone, Administrator, Approval, Facility, and Physician Codes, Health Care System, Network	Classi-fication Codes		Utilization Data					Expense (thousands) of dollars		
★ American Hospital Association (AHA) membership □ Joint Commission on Accreditation of Healthcare Organizations (JCAHO) accreditation + American Osteopathic Hospital Association (AOHA) membership ○ American Osteopathic Association (AOA) accreditation △ Commission on Accreditation of Rehabilitation Facilities (CARF) accreditation Control codes 61, 63, 64, 71, 72 and 73 indicate hospitals listed by AOHA, but not registered by AHA. For definition of numerical codes, see page A4	Control	Service	Beds	Admissions	Census	Outpatient Visits	Births	Total	Payroll	Personnel

BETHLEHEM—Litchfield County

★ WELLSPRING FOUNDATION, 21 Arch Bridge Road, Zip 06751–0370, Mailing Address: P.O. Box 370, Zip 06751–0370; tel. 203/266–7235; Herbert L. Hall, Chief Executive Officer **F**2 9 11 12 18 20 22 27 29 30 31 37 39 40 44 45 47 48 49 51 52 53 54 55 56 58 59 65 67 70 **P**6

	23	22	36	82	20	—	0	2953	1951	62

BRANFORD—New Haven County

□ THE CONNECTICUT HOSPICE, INC., 61 Burban Drive, Zip 06405–4003; tel. 203/481–6231; Rosemary Johnson Hurzeler, President and Chief Executive Officer (Nonreporting) **A**1 10

	33	49	52	—	—	—	—	—	—	—

BRIDGEPORT—Fairfield County

⊠ BRIDGEPORT HOSPITAL, 267 Grant Street, Zip 06610–2875, Mailing Address: P.O. Box 5000, Zip 06610–0120; tel. 203/384–3000; Robert J. Trefry, President and Chief Executive Officer **A**1 2 3 5 6 8 9 10 **F**2 4 7 8 9 10 11 12 13 14 15 16 17 19 21 22 25 27 28 29 30 31 32 33 34 35 36 37 38 39 40 41 42 43 44 45 46 47 48 49 51 52 53 54 55 56 57 58 59 60 61 65 66 67 68 69 70 71 72 73 74 **P**1 3 5 7 8

	23	10	335	17232	263	130506	2118	170281	71595	1654

GREATER BRIDGEPORT COMMUNITY MENTAL HEALTH CENTER, 1635 Central Avenue, Zip 06610–0902, Mailing Address: Box 5117, Zip 06610; tel. 203/579–6646; James M. Lehane, III, Director **A**10 **F**2 6 12 14 15 16 17 18 39 45 52 54 55 56 57 58 59 65 67 **S** Connecticut State Department of Mental Health, Hartford, CT

	12	22	62	1153	35	122117	0	18057	15624	395

⊠ ST. VINCENT'S MEDICAL CENTER, 2800 Main Street, Zip 06606–4292; tel. 203/576–6000; William J. Riordan, President and Chief Executive Officer **A**1 2 3 5 8 9 10 **F**1 2 3 4 7 8 10 11 12 14 15 16 17 19 21 22 25 26 28 29 30 31 32 34 35 37 39 40 41 42 43 44 46 49 51 52 53 54 55 56 57 58 59 60 65 67 68 70 71 72 73 **P**2 6 7 **S** Daughters of Charity National Health System, Saint Louis, MO

	21	10	289	15313	261	81495	1873	134239	66124	1413

BRISTOL—Hartford County

⊠ BRISTOL HOSPITAL, P.O. Box 977, Brewster Road, Zip 06011–0977; tel. 860/585–3000; Thomas D. Kennedy, III, President and Chief Executive Officer **A**1 2 5 9 10 **F**3 7 8 12 13 17 18 19 21 22 29 30 32 33 34 35 37 39 40 41 42 44 46 49 51 52 54 58 59 63 65 71 73 74 **P**1 7

	23	10	160	7053	86	175071	936	70587	35128	782

DANBURY—Fairfield County

⊠ DANBURY HOSPITAL, 24 Hospital Avenue, Zip 06810–6099; tel. 203/797–7000; Frank J. Kelly, President and Chief Executive Officer **A**1 2 3 5 8 9 10 **F**3 4 5 7 8 10 11 12 13 14 15 16 17 18 19 20 21 22 24 26 28 29 30 31 32 33 34 35 37 38 39 40 41 42 44 45 46 48 49 51 52 53 54 56 58 59 60 61 63 65 67 68 70 71 73 74 **P**1 7

	23	10	250	14055	212	201748	2427	173240	80209	1830

DERBY—New Haven County

⊠ GRIFFIN HOSPITAL, 130 Division Street, Zip 06418; tel. 203/735–7421; John Bustelos, Jr., President **A**1 2 3 5 9 10 **F**1 3 7 8 14 15 16 19 20 21 22 28 29 30 35 37 38 41 42 44 49 51 52 53 56 58 59 61 71 72 73 74 **P**5

	23	10	160	5464	95	88920	605	61495	29174	693

FARMINGTON—Hartford County

⊠ UNIVERSITY OF CONNECTICUT HEALTH CENTER, JOHN DEMPSEY HOSPITAL, 263 Farmington Avenue, Zip 06030–1956; tel. 860/679–2000; Andria Martin, MS, Director **A**1 2 3 5 8 9 10 **F**2 3 4 5 7 8 10 12 14 15 19 20 21 22 23 26 28 30 34 35 36 37 38 39 40 41 42 43 44 45 46 49 51 52 54 55 56 58 59 60 61 65 66 67 71 73 74 **P**5

	12	10	201	7122	146	426182	553	121951	47622	983

GREENWICH—Fairfield County

⊠ GREENWICH HOSPITAL, 5 Perryridge Road, Zip 06830–4697; tel. 203/863–3901; Frank A. Corvino, President and Chief Executive Officer **A**1 2 3 5 9 10 **F**2 3 4 7 8 10 11 12 13 14 15 16 17 18 19 20 21 22 24 25 26 28 29 30 31 32 33 34 35 37 38 39 40 41 42 44 45 46 49 51 53 54 55 56 58 60 61 63 64 65 67 68 71 73 **P**5 7

	23	10	167	7275	115	218032	1356	93028	48128	1141

GROTON—New London County

⊠ NAVAL HOSPITAL, 1 Wahoo Drive, Box 600, Zip 06349–5600; tel. 860/449–3261; Captain R. B. Hall, II, Commanding Officer **A**1 5 9 **F**8 12 14 15 16 18 19 20 22 24 28 29 30 36 37 39 41 44 45 46 49 54 56 58 65 67 71 72 73 **S** Department of Navy, Washington, DC

	43	10	25	2067	11	208862	0	—	—	—

HARTFORD—Hartford County

⊠ CONNECTICUT CHILDREN'S MEDICAL CENTER, 282 Washington Street, Zip 06106–3316; tel. 860/545–8551; Larry M. Gold, President and Chief Executive Officer (Nonreporting) **A**1 3 5 9 10

	23	50	76	—	—	—	—	—	—	—

⊠ HARTFORD HOSPITAL, (Includes Institute of Living, 400 Washington Street, Zip 06106–3392; tel. 860/545–7000), 80 Seymour Street, Zip 06102–5037, Mailing Address: P.O. Box 5037, Zip 06102–5037; tel. 860/545–5555; John J. Meehan, President and Chief Executive Officer (Total facility includes 104 beds in nursing home–type unit) **A**1 2 3 5 8 9 10 **F**1 3 4 7 8 10 11 14 15 16 19 20 21 22 26 30 31 32 33 34 35 36 37 38 40 41 42 43 44 45 46 47 48 49 50 51 52 53 54 55 56 57 58 59 60 61 64 65 66 67 69 70 71 72 73 74 **P**4 5 8

	23	10	879	34515	646	155842	4682	355525	196021	5404

Hospital, Address, Telephone, Administrator, Approval, Facility, and Physician Codes, Health Care System, Network	Classi-fication Codes		Utilization Data					Expense (thousands) of dollars		
★ American Hospital Association (AHA) membership □ Joint Commission on Accreditation of Healthcare Organizations (JCAHO) accreditation + American Osteopathic Hospital Association (AOHA) membership ○ American Osteopathic Association (AOA) accreditation △ Commission on Accreditation of Rehabilitation Facilities (CARF) accreditation Control codes 61, 63, 64, 71, 72 and 73 indicate hospitals listed by AOHA, but not registered by AHA. For definition of numerical codes, see page A4	Control	Service	Beds	Admissions	Census	Outpatient Visits	Births	Total	Payroll	Personnel
✶ SAINT FRANCIS HOSPITAL AND MEDICAL CENTER, 114 Woodland Street, Zip 06105–1299; tel. 860/714–4000; David D'Eramo, President and Chief Executive Officer **A**1 2 3 5 6 8 9 10 **F**3 4 7 8 10 11 12 13 14 15 16 17 19 20 21 22 25 26 28 29 30 31 32 33 34 35 37 38 40 41 42 43 44 45 46 49 51 52 53 54 55 56 57 58 59 60 61 63 65 66 67 68 70 71 72 73 74 **P**1 4 7 **N** Saint Francis Physician Hospital Organization, Hartford, CT	21	10	525	25195	391	284966	2942	302859	143772	3439
MANCHESTER—Hartford County										
✶ MANCHESTER MEMORIAL HOSPITAL, 71 Haynes Street, Zip 06040–4188; tel. 860/646–1222; Barry G. Beeman, Chief Executive Officer **A**1 9 10 **F**7 8 11 12 13 15 16 17 18 19 20 21 22 26 28 29 30 31 32 33 34 35 36 37 39 40 41 42 44 45 46 48 49 52 53 54 55 56 57 58 59 63 64 65 66 67 68 71 72 73 74 **P**4 5 6 8 **N** Eastern Connecticut Health Network, Manchester, CT	23	10	178	8071	101	156597	1146	83415	43679	950
MANSFIELD CENTER—Tolland County										
□ NATCHAUG HOSPITAL, 189 Storrs Road, Zip 06250–1638; tel. 860/456–1311; Stephen W. Larcen, Ph.D., Chief Executive Officer **A**1 9 10 **F**2 3 15 16 52 53 54 55 56 57 58 59 **P**1 6	23	22	58	1110	41	30372	0	12925	7030	190
MERIDEN—New Haven County										
✶ VETERANS MEMORIAL MEDICAL CENTER, (Includes East Campus, 883 Paddock Avenue, Zip 06450–7094; tel. 203/238–8200), One King Place, Zip 06450–1009, Mailing Address: P.O. Box 1009, Zip 06450–1009; tel. 203/238–8200; Theodore H. Horwitz, FACHE, President **A**1 2 9 10 **F**1 3 7 8 15 16 17 18 19 21 22 24 26 28 30 31 32 33 34 35 37 40 41 42 44 46 52 53 54 55 56 57 58 59 60 63 65 67 68 71 72 73 74 **P**1 5 8	23	10	107	7530	92	113044	1110	91508	46829	1089
MIDDLETOWN—Middlesex County										
□ CONNECTICUT VALLEY HOSPITAL, (Includes Whiting Forensic Division of Connecticut Valley Hospital, O'Brien Drive, Zip 06457, Mailing Address: Box 70, Zip 06457–3942; tel. 203/344–2541), Eastern Drive, Zip 06457–7023, Mailing Address: P.O. Box 351, Zip 06457–7023; Garrell S. Mullaney, Superintendent (Nonreporting) **A**1 3 5 9 10 **S** Connecticut State Department of Mental Health, Hartford, CT	12	22	418	—	—	—	—	—	—	—
✶ MIDDLESEX HOSPITAL, 28 Crescent Street, Zip 06457–3650; tel. 860/344–6000; Robert Gerard Kiely, President and Chief Executive Officer **A**1 2 3 5 9 10 **F**3 7 8 11 12 13 14 15 16 17 18 19 20 21 22 25 26 27 28 29 30 31 32 33 34 35 37 39 40 41 42 44 45 49 51 52 53 54 55 56 57 58 59 60 61 63 64 65 66 67 68 71 72 73 **P**5 6 7	23	10	109	9073	102	457594	1212	105661	53323	1243
RIVERVIEW HOSPITAL FOR CHILDREN, River Road, Zip 06457, Mailing Address: Box 621, Zip 06457; tel. 203/344–2700; Richard J. Wiseman, Ph.D., Superintendent (Nonreporting) **A**3 9	12	52	55	—	—	—	—	—	—	—
WHITING FORENSIC DIVISION OF CONNECTICUT VALLEY HOSPITAL See Connecticut Valley Hospital										
MILFORD—New Haven County										
✶ MILFORD HOSPITAL, 2047 Bridgeport Avenue, Zip 06460–4606; tel. 203/876–4000; Paul E. Moss, President **A**1 2 9 10 **F**7 12 14 19 21 22 28 30 32 35 36 37 39 40 42 44 46 63 65 67 71 73 **P**5	23	10	72	3857	51	44463	529	33885	18883	390
NEW BRITAIN—Hartford County										
✶ △ HOSPITAL FOR SPECIAL CARE, (CHRONIC DISEASE & REHAB), 2150 Corbin Avenue, Zip 06053–2263; tel. 860/827–4761; Katherine C. III, M.D., President **A**1 7 9 10 **F**12 20 24 25 26 34 39 41 48 49 54 63 65 67 71 73 **P**6	23	49	199	530	171	16000	0	48434	27576	656
✶ NEW BRITAIN GENERAL HOSPITAL, 100 Grand Street, Zip 06052–2000, Mailing Address: P.O. Box 100, Zip 06050–0100; tel. 860/224–5011; Laurence A. Tanner, President and Chief Executive Officer **A**1 2 3 5 8 9 10 **F**1 2 3 4 7 8 10 11 12 14 15 16 17 18 19 21 22 23 24 25 26 30 31 32 33 34 35 37 38 39 40 41 42 43 44 46 48 49 51 52 53 54 55 56 57 58 59 60 61 63 65 66 67 71 73 74 **P**5 8	23	10	263	13073	184	126419	2065	140528	80812	1910
NEW CANAAN—Fairfield County										
✶ SILVER HILL HOSPITAL, 208 Valley Road, Zip 06840–3899; tel. 203/966–3561; Richard J. Frances, M.D., President and Medical Director **A**1 **F**3 52 53 54 55 56 57 58 59	23	22	61	1037	41	7184	0	15742	9269	221
NEW HAVEN—New Haven County										
□ CONNECTICUT MENTAL HEALTH CENTER, 34 Park Street, Zip 06519, Mailing Address: Box 1842, Zip 06508–1842; tel. 203/789–7290; Selby Jacobs, M.D., M.P.H., Director **A**1 3 5 9 10 **F**3 12 17 18 19 20 21 22 35 39 46 52 53 55 56 58 59 65 67 71 **S** Connecticut State Department of Mental Health, Hartford, CT	12	22	49	743	38	81966	0	—	—	—
✶ HOSPITAL OF SAINT RAPHAEL, 1450 Chapel Street, Zip 06511–1450; tel. 203/789–3000; James J. Cullen, President (Total facility includes 125 beds in nursing home–type unit) **A**1 2 3 5 8 9 10 **F**3 4 7 8 10 11 12 13 14 15 16 17 18 19 20 21 22 26 27 28 29 30 31 32 34 35 37 39 40 41 42 43 44 46 48 49 51 52 53 54 55 56 57 58 59 60 61 63 64 65 67 68 70 71 72 73 74 **P**2 7 8 **N** Connecticut Health System, Inc., Hartford, CT	21	10	511	21265	361	158865	1275	243328	114667	2652
□ YALE PSYCHIATRIC INSTITUTE, 184 Liberty Street, Zip 06519, Mailing Address: Box 208038, Zip 06520; tel. 203/785–7200; Thomas H. McGlashan, M.D., Director (Nonreporting) **A**1 3 5 9 10	23	22	55	—	—	—	—	—	—	—
✶ YALE–NEW HAVEN HOSPITAL, 20 York Street, Zip 06504; tel. 203/785–4242; Joseph A. Zaccagnino, President and Chief Executive Officer **A**1 2 3 5 8 9 10 **F**3 4 7 8 10 11 12 13 14 15 16 17 18 19 20 21 22 23 24 25 26 29 30 31 32 34 35 37 38 39 40 42 43 44 45 46 47 48 49 50 51 52 53 54 55 56 57 58 59 60 61 63 65 66 67 68 69 70 71 72 73 74 **P**5 7 8	23	10	764	34793	533	347594	4814	422167	199662	4979

Hospital, Address, Telephone, Administrator, Approval, Facility, and Physician Codes, Health Care System, Network	Classi-fication Codes		Utilization Data					Expense (thousands) of dollars		
	Control	Service	Beds	Admissions	Census	Outpatient Visits	Births	Total	Payroll	Personnel

★ American Hospital Association (AHA) membership
□ Joint Commission on Accreditation of Healthcare Organizations (JCAHO) accreditation
+ American Osteopathic Hospital Association (AOHA) membership
○ American Osteopathic Association (AOA) accreditation
△ Commission on Accreditation of Rehabilitation Facilities (CARF) accreditation
Control codes 61, 63, 64, 71, 72 and 73 indicate hospitals listed by AOHA, but not registered by AHA. For definition of numerical codes, see page A4

NEW LONDON—New London County

☒ LAWRENCE AND MEMORIAL HOSPITAL, 365 Montauk Avenue, Zip 06320–4769; tel. 860/442–0711; William T. Christopher, President and Chief Executive Officer **A**1 9 10 **F**3 8 10 11 12 13 14 15 16 19 21 22 25 30 31 32 33 34 35 37 38 39 40 41 42 44 45 46 48 49 51 52 53 54 55 56 58 59 60 61 65 71 72 73 **P**4 5 6 | 23 | 10 | 223 | 12135 | 172 | 95604 | 1807 | 119172 | 60461 | 1154

NEW MILFORD—Litchfield County

☒ NEW MILFORD HOSPITAL, 21 Elm Street, Zip 06776–2993; tel. 860/355–2611; Richard E. Pugh, President and Chief Executive Officer (Nonreporting) **A**1 9 10 **N** Columbia Presbyterian Regional Network, New York, NY | 23 | 10 | 63 | — | — | — | — | — | — | —

NEWINGTON—Hartford County

□ CEDARCREST REGIONAL HOSPITAL, 525 Russell Road, Zip 06111–1595; tel. 203/666–4613; David E. K. Hunter, Ph.D., Superintendent **A**1 9 10 **F**1 2 3 4 5 6 9 10 11 12 14 16 17 18 19 20 21 22 23 24 25 26 27 28 29 30 31 32 33 34 35 36 37 38 39 40 41 42 43 44 45 46 48 49 50 51 52 53 54 55 56 57 58 59 60 61 62 63 64 65 66 67 69 70 71 72 73 74 **P**1 **S** Connecticut State Department of Mental Health, Hartford, CT | 12 | 22 | 146 | 2850 | 154 | — | 0 | 30761 | 18226 | 376

VETERANS AFFAIRS MEDICAL CENTER, NEWINGTON CAMPUS See Veterans Affairs Connecticut Healthcare System, West Haven

NORWALK—Fairfield County

☒ △ NORWALK HOSPITAL, Maple Street, Zip 06856–5050; tel. 203/852–2000; David W. Osborne, President and Chief Executive Officer **A**1 2 3 5 7 9 10 **F**2 3 7 8 10 11 12 13 15 16 17 18 19 20 21 22 25 26 28 29 30 31 32 33 34 35 37 38 39 40 41 42 44 45 48 49 51 52 53 54 55 56 57 58 59 60 61 65 67 68 71 73 74 **P**5 8 | 23 | 10 | 220 | 14109 | 212 | 202091 | 2018 | 143949 | 77999 | 1537

NORWICH—New London County

☒ WILLIAM W. BACKUS HOSPITAL, 326 Washington Street, Zip 06360–2742; tel. 860/889–8331; Thomas P. Pipicelli, President and Chief Executive Officer **A**1 3 9 10 **F**7 8 10 12 14 15 16 19 21 22 28 29 30 31 32 33 34 35 37 38 39 40 41 42 44 45 49 52 54 56 58 59 60 65 67 68 71 72 73 | 23 | 10 | 159 | 9312 | 119 | 595391 | 1209 | 81621 | 40662 | 938

PORTLAND—Middlesex County

□ ELMCREST PSYCHIATRIC INSTITUTE, 25 Marlborough Street, Zip 06480–1829; tel. 860/342–0480; Lane Ameen, M.D., Chief Executive Officer **A**1 9 10 **F**2 3 12 17 29 34 39 41 45 46 52 53 54 55 56 57 58 59 67 68 74 **P**1 **S** Magellan Health Services, Atlanta, GA | 32 | 22 | 92 | 2286 | 76 | 42380 | 0 | 21239 | 12651 | 389

PUTNAM—Windham County

☒ DAY KIMBALL HOSPITAL, 320 Pomfret Street, Zip 06260, Mailing Address: P.O. Box 6001, Zip 06260–9417; tel. 860/928–6541; Charles F. Schneider, President **A**1 5 9 10 **F**3 7 8 12 13 15 16 17 18 19 21 22 25 26 27 28 29 30 32 33 34 35 37 39 40 41 42 44 45 46 49 52 54 55 56 57 58 59 61 63 65 66 67 68 71 72 73 74 **P**8 | 23 | 10 | 102 | 4524 | 52 | 209221 | 592 | 42324 | 22809 | 464

ROCKY HILL—Hartford County

□ VETERANS HOME AND HOSPITAL, 287 West Street, Zip 06067–3501; tel. 860/529–2571; Sharon R. Wood, Administrator (Nonreporting) **A**1 10 | 12 | 48 | 296 | — | — | — | — | — | — | —

SHARON—Litchfield County

☒ SHARON HOSPITAL, 50 Hospital Hill Road, Zip 06069–0789, Mailing Address: P.O. Box 789, Zip 06069–0789; tel. 203/364–4141; James E. Sok, President **A**1 2 9 10 **F**7 8 14 15 16 17 19 21 22 29 30 33 34 35 37 39 40 41 42 44 46 49 63 65 67 71 72 73 **P**5 7 | 23 | 10 | 78 | 2837 | 40 | — | 349 | 30445 | 12466 | 372

SOMERS—Tolland County

CONNECTICUT DEPARTMENT OF CORRECTION'S HOSPITAL, Mailing Address: Box 100, Zip 06071; tel. 203/749–8391; Edward A. Blanchette, M.D., Director (Nonreporting) | 12 | 11 | 29 | — | — | — | — | — | — | —

SOUTHINGTON—Hartford County

☒ BRADLEY MEMORIAL HOSPITAL AND HEALTH CENTER, 81 Meriden Avenue, Zip 06489–3297; tel. 203/276–5000; Clarence J. Silvia, President **A**1 9 10 **F**8 11 12 14 15 17 19 22 26 28 29 30 33 34 35 37 39 41 42 44 45 49 55 56 63 65 67 71 73 74 **P**8 | 23 | 10 | 74 | 2392 | 36 | 34067 | 0 | 25450 | 12319 | 277

STAFFORD SPRINGS—Tolland County

□ JOHNSON MEMORIAL HOSPITAL, 201 Chestnut Hill Road, Zip 06076–0860, Mailing Address: P.O. Box 860, Zip 06076–0860; tel. 860/684–4251; Alfred A. Lerz, President and Chief Executive Officer **A**1 9 10 **F**3 7 8 12 13 14 15 16 17 18 19 21 22 24 25 26 28 29 30 31 32 33 34 35 37 39 40 41 42 44 45 46 49 51 52 53 54 55 56 57 58 59 65 67 68 71 73 74 **P**5 | 23 | 10 | 89 | 3779 | 52 | 52723 | 273 | 32642 | 18207 | 418

STAMFORD—Fairfield County

☒ ST. JOSEPH MEDICAL CENTER, 128 Strawberry Hill Avenue, Zip 06904–1222, Mailing Address: P.O. Box 1222, Zip 06904–1222; tel. 203/353–2000; William J. Riordan, President and Chief Executive Officer **A**1 3 5 9 10 **F**7 8 10 12 15 16 17 18 19 21 22 26 28 29 30 33 34 35 37 39 40 44 45 46 48 49 56 65 67 68 71 73 74 **P**6 7 | 21 | 10 | 147 | 4279 | 86 | 67914 | 472 | 53245 | 23362 | 553

☒ STAMFORD HOSPITAL, Shelburne Road and West Broad Street, Zip 06902, Mailing Address: P.O. Box 9317, Zip 06904–9317; tel. 203/325–7000; Philip D. Cusano, President and Chief Executive Officer **A**1 2 3 5 8 9 10 **F**3 7 8 10 12 14 15 16 17 19 21 22 24 25 26 28 29 30 31 32 33 34 35 37 38 39 40 41 42 44 45 46 49 51 52 53 54 55 56 57 58 59 60 61 63 65 67 69 70 71 72 73 74 **P**5 7 8 **N** Westchester Health Services Network, Mt Kisco, NY | 23 | 10 | 241 | 11036 | 163 | 122794 | 2127 | 107369 | 52775 | 1106

Hospital, Address, Telephone, Administrator, Approval, Facility, and Physician Codes, Health Care System, Network	Classi-fication Codes		Utilization Data					Expense (thousands) of dollars		
★ American Hospital Association (AHA) membership □ Joint Commission on Accreditation of Healthcare Organizations (JCAHO) accreditation + American Osteopathic Hospital Association (AOHA) membership ○ American Osteopathic Association (AOA) accreditation △ Commission on Accreditation of Rehabilitation Facilities (CARF) accreditation Control codes 61, 63, 64, 71, 72 and 73 indicate hospitals listed by AOHA, but not registered by AHA. For definition of numerical codes, see page A4	Control	Service	Beds	Admissions	Census	Outpatient Visits	Births	Total	Payroll	Personnel

TORRINGTON—Litchfield County

□ CHARLOTTE HUNGERFORD HOSPITAL, 540 Litchfield Street, Zip 06790, Mailing Address: Box 988, Zip 06790–0988; tel. 860/496–6666; David R. Newton, President and Executive Director **A**1 2 9 10 **F**7 8 11 12 13 14 15 16 17 18 19 20 21 22 25 28 29 30 31 32 33 34 35 37 39 40 41 42 44 45 46 49 52 53 54 56 58 59 60 63 65 66 67 70 71 72 73 **P**1 — 23, 10, 109, 5088, 72, 159648, 572, 58503, 27712, 692

VERNON ROCKVILLE—Hartford County

✠ ROCKVILLE GENERAL HOSPITAL, 31 Union Street, Zip 06066–3160; tel. 860/872–0501; Barry G. Beeman, Chief Executive Officer (Nonreporting) **A**1 9 10 **N** Eastern Connecticut Health Network, Manchester, CT — 23, 10, 95, —, —, —, —, —, —, —

WALLINGFORD—New Haven County

✠ △ GAYLORD HOSPITAL, Gaylord Farm Road, Zip 06492–7049, Mailing Address: P.O. Box 400, Zip 06492–0400; tel. 203/284–2801; Paul H. Johnson, President and Chief Executive Officer **A**1 5 7 9 10 **F**2 3 12 14 25 26 28 34 41 45 46 48 49 54 65 66 67 71 73 **P**6 **N** Connecticut Health System, Inc., Hartford, CT — 23, 46, 88, 1116, 76, 49364, 0, 34052, 19658, 465

✠ MASONIC GERIATRIC HEALTHCARE CENTER, (GENERAL GERIATRIC MEDICAL), 22 Masonic Avenue, Zip 06492–3048, Mailing Address: P.O. Box 70, Zip 06492–7002; tel. 203/284–3900; Ronald L. Waack, President (Total facility includes 468 beds in nursing home–type unit) **A**1 9 10 **F**1 6 8 12 16 17 19 20 21 22 26 27 28 29 30 32 33 34 35 39 41 44 45 46 49 51 52 54 55 57 58 59 62 64 65 67 71 73 **P**6 — 23, 49, 503, 1207, 460, 13026, 0, 39771, 21236, 608

WATERBURY—New Haven County

✠ ST. MARY'S HOSPITAL, 56 Franklin Street, Zip 06706–1200; tel. 203/574–6000; Sister Marguerite Waite, President and Chief Executive Officer **A**1 2 3 5 9 10 **F**3 5 7 8 10 11 12 13 14 15 16 17 18 19 20 21 22 25 26 28 29 30 31 32 33 34 35 36 37 39 40 41 42 44 45 46 49 51 52 54 55 56 58 59 60 63 65 67 70 71 72 73 **P**7 8 **N** Saint Mary's Hospital, Waterbury, CT — 21, 10, 223, 10674, 137, 169030, 1327, 115406, 58913, 1313

✠ WATERBURY HOSPITAL, 64 Robbins Street, Zip 06721, Mailing Address: P.O. Box 1589, Zip 06721–1589; tel. 203/573–6000; John H. Tobin, President **A**1 2 3 5 9 10 **F**5 7 8 10 11 12 14 15 16 17 18 19 20 21 22 24 27 28 29 30 31 32 33 34 35 37 38 39 40 41 42 44 49 51 52 53 54 55 56 57 58 59 60 65 67 69 70 71 72 73 74 **P**1 7 — 23, 10, 223, 11861, 172, 724322, 1378, 124112, 61028, 1339

WEST HARTFORD—Hartford County

★ HEBREW HOME AND HOSPITAL, (COMPREHENSIVE GERIATRIC HEALTH), 1 Abrahms Boulevard, Zip 06117–1525; tel. 203/523–3800; Irving Kronenberg, President and Executive Director (Total facility includes 293 beds in nursing home–type unit) **A**5 9 10 **F**1 12 17 18 19 20 21 26 27 29 30 32 33 34 35 36 39 41 42 45 46 49 51 54 55 56 57 58 63 64 65 67 69 73 **P**6 — 23, 49, 334, 676, 329, —, 0, —, —, 376

WEST HAVEN—New Haven County

✠ VETERANS AFFAIRS CONNECTICUT HEALTHCARE SYSTEM, (Includes Veterans Affairs Medical Center, Newington Campus, 555 Willard Avenue, Newington, Zip 06111–2600; tel. 860/666–6951; Veterans Affairs Medical Center, West Haven Campus, 950 Campbell Avenue, Zip 06516–2700; tel. 203/932–5711), 950 Campbell Avenue, Zip 06516; tel. 203/932–5711; Vincent Ng, Director (Total facility includes 74 beds in nursing home–type unit) **A**1 2 3 5 8 9 **F**1 2 3 4 6 8 10 11 12 15 17 18 19 20 21 22 26 27 28 29 30 31 32 33 34 35 37 39 41 42 43 44 45 46 49 50 51 52 54 55 56 57 58 59 60 61 64 65 67 69 70 71 73 74 **S** Department of Veterans Affairs, Washington, DC — 45, 10, 343, 7110, 335, 324879, 0, 175718, 115266, 1910

WESTPORT—Fairfield County

✠ HALL–BROOKE HOSPITAL, A DIVISION OF HALL–BROOKE FOUNDATION, 47 Long Lots Road, Zip 06880–3800; tel. 203/227–1251; Seth Berman, Executive Director **A**1 9 10 **F**1 2 3 14 15 16 26 34 52 53 54 56 57 58 59 73 **P**1 — 23, 22, 52, 650, 33, 22670, 0, 8850, 5428, 168

WILLIMANTIC—Windham County

□ WINDHAM COMMUNITY MEMORIAL HOSPITAL, 112 Mansfield Avenue, Zip 06226–2082; tel. 860/456–9116; Duane A. Carlberg, President **A**1 9 10 **F**3 7 8 12 13 15 17 18 19 21 22 25 28 30 31 33 34 35 37 39 40 41 42 44 45 49 53 54 56 58 59 63 65 67 68 71 73 **P**8 — 23, 10, 94, 4158, 52, 89154, 506, 44160, 18121, 469

DELAWARE

Resident population 717 (in thousands)
Resident population in metro areas 82.7%
Birth rate per 1,000 population 15.1
65 years and over 12.6%
Percent of persons without health insurance 13.5%

★ American Hospital Association (AHA) membership
□ Joint Commission on Accreditation of Healthcare Organizations (JCAHO) accreditation
+ American Osteopathic Hospital Association (AOHA) membership
○ American Osteopathic Association (AOA) accreditation
△ Commission on Accreditation of Rehabilitation Facilities (CARF) accreditation
Control codes 61, 63, 64, 71, 72 and 73 indicate hospitals listed by AOHA, but not registered by AHA. For definition of numerical codes, see page A4

			Classification Codes		Utilization Data					Expense (thousands) of dollars		
			Control	Service	Beds	Admissions	Census	Outpatient Visits	Births	Total	Payroll	Personnel

DOVER—Kent County
★ KENT GENERAL HOSPITAL, 640 South State Street, Zip 19901–3597; tel. 302/674–4700; Dennis E. Klima, President and Chief Executive Officer **A**1 2 9 10 **F**1 3 11 13 15 16 17 19 21 22 23 24 25 28 29 30 31 32 34 35 37 38 39 40 41 42 44 45 46 49 51 52 53 54 55 56 57 58 59 60 61 63 64 65 66 70 71 72 73 74 **P**8 **S** Bayhealth Medical Center, Dover, DE — 23 10 193 9965 135 154244 1223 80818 36800 1055

DOVER AFB—Kent County
★ U. S. AIR FORCE HOSPITAL DOVER, 307 Tuskegee Boulevard, Zip 19902–7307; tel. 302/677–2525; Major David M. Allen, MSC, Administrator **A**1 **F**7 8 12 13 14 15 16 17 18 20 24 27 28 29 30 34 40 41 44 45 46 49 51 56 58 65 67 68 71 72 73 74 **S** Department of the Air Force, Washington, DC — 41 10 16 1184 5 131874 336 9615 — 380

LEWES—Sussex County
★ BEEBE MEDICAL CENTER, 424 Savannah Road, Zip 19958–0226; tel. 302/645–3300; Jeffrey M. Fried, FACHE, President and Chief Executive Officer (Total facility includes 89 beds in nursing home–type unit) **A**1 2 6 9 10 **F**1 3 4 7 8 12 15 16 17 19 21 22 23 25 27 30 31 32 34 35 37 39 40 41 42 44 49 51 52 53 54 55 56 57 58 59 60 63 64 65 67 71 72 73 74 **P**8 — 23 10 214 6617 164 109524 607 54709 25165 817

MILFORD—Sussex County
★ △ BAYHEALTH MEDICAL CENTER, MILFORD MEMORIAL CAMPUS, (Formerly Milford Memorial Hospital), 21 West Clarke Avenue, Zip 19963, Mailing Address: P.O. Box 199, Zip 19963–0199; tel. 302/424–5613; Joseph K. Whiting, Executive Vice President and Chief Operating Officer **A**1 2 7 9 10 **F**7 8 12 15 17 19 21 22 24 25 28 29 30 32 33 34 35 37 39 40 41 42 44 45 46 48 49 63 64 65 66 67 71 73 74 **P**6 **S** Bayhealth Medical Center, Dover, DE — 23 10 130 4919 86 128755 360 41652 18633 576

NEW CASTLE—New Castle County
□ DELAWARE PSYCHIATRIC CENTER, Dupont Highway, Zip 19720–1199; tel. 302/577–4381; Jiro R. Shimono, Director (Total facility includes 59 beds in nursing home–type unit) **A**1 3 9 10 **F**2 12 14 18 19 20 21 22 26 29 35 39 45 46 49 50 52 56 57 58 63 65 67 71 73 **P**6 — 12 22 336 1194 337 0 0 30973 17942 686
□ MEADOW WOOD BEHAVIORAL HEALTH SYSTEM, 575 South Dupont Highway, Zip 19720; tel. 302/328–3330; Joseph Pyle, Administrator (Nonreporting) **A**1 9 10 **S** Hospital Group of America, Wayne, PA — 33 52 50 — — — — — — —

NEWARK—New Castle County
★ ROCKFORD CENTER, 100 Rockford Drive, Zip 19713; tel. 302/996–5480; Walter J. Yokobosky, Jr., Chief Executive Officer (Nonreporting) **A**1 9 10 **S** Columbia/HCA Healthcare Corporation, Nashville, TN — 33 22 70 — — — — — — —

SEAFORD—Sussex County
★ NANTICOKE MEMORIAL HOSPITAL, 801 Middleford Road, Zip 19973–3698; tel. 302/629–6611; Edward H. Hancock, President (Total facility includes 90 beds in nursing home–type unit) **A**1 9 10 **F**2 3 4 7 8 10 12 14 15 16 17 19 22 24 28 30 35 37 39 40 41 42 44 45 46 49 52 56 57 58 59 64 65 66 67 71 73 74 **P**1 5 6 7 8 **N** Nanticoke Health Services, Seaford, DE — 23 10 199 6492 153 44518 737 46044 20700 830

WILMINGTON—New Castle County
ALFRED I. DUPONT INSTITUTE See duPont Hospital for Children
CHRISTIANA HOSPITAL See Medical Center of Delaware
★ △ DUPONT HOSPITAL FOR CHILDREN, (Formerly Alfred I. duPont Institute), 1600 Rockland Road, Zip 19803–3616, Mailing Address: Box 269, Zip 19899–0269; tel. 302/651–4000; Thomas P. Ferry, Administrator and Chief Executive (Nonreporting) **A**1 3 5 7 9 10 — 23 52 128 — — — — — — —
EUGENE DUPONT MEMORIAL HOSPITAL See Medical Center of Delaware
★ + MEDICAL CENTER OF DELAWARE, (Includes Christiana Hospital, Eugene Dupont Memorial Hospital, Riverside Hospital, Wilmington Hospital), 501 West 14th Street, Zip 19801, Mailing Address: P.O. Box 1668, Zip 19899–1668; tel. 302/733–1000; Charles M. Smith, M.D., President and Chief Executive Officer **A**1 2 3 5 8 9 10 12 13 **F**4 7 8 10 11 15 16 17 19 20 21 22 23 25 29 30 31 32 34 35 37 38 39 40 41 42 43 44 45 46 47 48 49 51 53 54 56 58 59 60 61 63 64 65 67 68 69 70 71 73 74 **P**8 **N** Medical Center of Delaware Foundation, Wilmington, DE — 23 10 603 35734 569 467588 6105 427326 209407 4449
RIVERSIDE HOSPITAL See Medical Center of Delaware
★ ST. FRANCIS HOSPITAL, Seventh and Clayton Streets, Zip 19805–0500, Mailing Address: P.O. Box 2500, Zip 19805–0500; tel. 302/421–4100; Steven C. Bjelich, President and Chief Executive Officer **A**1 2 3 5 9 10 **F**4 5 7 8 10 12 13 14 15 16 17 19 20 21 22 23 25 26 28 29 30 31 32 34 35 39 41 42 44 45 46 49 51 54 55 56 57 58 59 63 65 66 67 68 71 72 73 74 **P**6 **S** Catholic Health Initiatives, Denver, CO — 21 10 277 10307 165 294075 1150 109664 51617 1342
★ VETERANS AFFAIRS MEDICAL CENTER, 1601 Kirkwood Highway, Zip 19805–4989; tel. 302/633–5201; Dexter D. Dix, Director (Total facility includes 60 beds in nursing home–type unit) (Nonreporting) **A**1 3 5 8 9 **S** Department of Veterans Affairs, Washington, DC — 45 10 210 — — — — — — —
WILMINGTON HOSPITAL See Medical Center of Delaware

DISTRICT OF COLUMBIA

Resident population 554 (in thousands)
Resident population in metro areas 100%
Birth rate per 1,000 population 18.4
65 years and over 13.9%
Percent of persons without health insurance 16.4%

Hospital, Address, Telephone, Administrator, Approval, Facility, and Physician Codes, Health Care System, Network	Classi-fication Codes		Utilization Data					Expense (thousands) of dollars		
★ American Hospital Association (AHA) membership □ Joint Commission on Accreditation of Healthcare Organizations (JCAHO) accreditation + American Osteopathic Hospital Association (AOHA) membership ○ American Osteopathic Association (AOA) accreditation △ Commission on Accreditation of Rehabilitation Facilities (CARF) accreditation Control codes 61, 63, 64, 71, 72 and 73 indicate hospitals listed by AOHA, but not registered by AHA. For definition of numerical codes, see page A4	Control	Service	Beds	Admissions	Census	Outpatient Visits	Births	Total	Payroll	Personnel

WASHINGTON—District of Columbia County

★ CHILDREN'S NATIONAL MEDICAL CENTER, 111 Michigan Avenue N.W., Zip 20010–2970; tel. 202/884–5000; Edwin K. Zechman, Jr., President and Chief Executive Officer **A**1 3 5 8 9 10 **F**4 5 9 10 12 14 15 16 17 19 20 21 22 25 27 28 29 30 31 32 33 34 35 38 39 41 42 43 44 45 46 47 49 51 52 53 54 55 56 58 59 63 65 67 68 69 70 71 73 **P**6	23	50	167	10074	164	188109	0	169215	78202	1791
★ COLUMBIA HOSPITAL FOR WOMEN MEDICAL CENTER, 2425 L Street N.W., Zip 20037–1433; tel. 202/293–6500; Susan M. Hansen, President and Chief Executive Officer **A**1 9 10 **F**7 8 14 15 16 17 21 28 29 30 37 38 39 40 42 44 45 46 51 60 61 65 67 68 71 73 74 **P**3 6	23	44	75	11299	77	71647	4301	63960	27714	673
★ DISTRICT OF COLUMBIA GENERAL HOSPITAL, 19th Street & Massachusetts Avenue S.E., Zip 20003; tel. 202/675–5000; John A. Fairman, Executive Director **A**1 3 5 9 10 **F**2 7 8 10 11 13 14 15 16 17 19 20 21 22 27 29 30 31 34 37 38 40 41 42 44 46 49 54 56 60 61 65 70 71 73 **P**6	14	10	250	10510	187	137410	837	114014	61576	1607
★ GEORGE WASHINGTON UNIVERSITY HOSPITAL, 901 23rd Street N.W., Zip 20037; tel. 202/994–1000; Phillip S. Schaengold, JD, Chief Executive Officer **A**1 2 3 5 8 9 10 **F**4 7 10 11 12 14 15 16 17 19 21 22 23 31 34 35 37 38 40 41 42 43 44 46 49 52 53 54 55 56 57 58 59 60 61 63 65 70 71 73	23	10	295	14790	228	—	1377	159195	72179	1677
□ GEORGETOWN UNIVERSITY HOSPITAL, 3800 Reservoir Road N.W., Zip 20007–2197; tel. 202/784–3000; Janice M. Feldman, Interim Administrator **A**1 2 3 5 8 9 10 **F**3 4 5 8 10 12 13 17 18 19 20 21 22 23 25 26 28 29 30 31 34 35 37 38 39 40 41 42 43 44 45 46 47 49 51 52 53 54 55 56 57 58 59 60 61 63 65 66 67 68 69 70 71 72 73 74 **P**6	23	10	404	15266	289	189503	1350	220970	95347	2297
★ GREATER SOUTHEAST COMMUNITY HOSPITAL, 1310 Southern Avenue S.E., Zip 20032–4699; tel. 202/574–6000; Robert C. Winfrey, President and Chief Operating Officer (Total facility includes 24 beds in nursing home–type unit) **A**1 2 3 5 9 10 **F**1 8 10 11 12 14 15 16 17 19 21 22 26 28 30 31 32 34 36 37 38 39 40 41 42 44 45 46 48 49 51 52 53 54 60 61 62 64 65 71 73 74 **P**1 5 **S** Greater Southeast Healthcare System, Washington, DC	23	10	305	12520	271	76240	1287	110624	54490	1367
□ HADLEY MEMORIAL HOSPITAL, 4601 Martin Luther King Jr. Avenue S.W., Zip 20032; tel. 202/574–5700; Ana Raley, Administrator (Total facility includes 39 beds in nursing home–type unit) **A**1 9 10 **F**8 15 19 21 28 37 44 64 65 **P**5 7	16	10	109	2386	115	15295	0	26115	10695	354
★ △ HOSPITAL FOR SICK CHILDREN, 1731 Bunker Hill Road N.E., Zip 20017; tel. 202/635–6125; Robert J. Moylan, CHE, Chief Executive Officer **A**1 5 7 9 **F**12 14 15 17 20 27 28 31 34 41 42 45 46 54 65 67 68 73 **P**6	23	56	114	305	90	3505	0	32365	16326	343
★ HOWARD UNIVERSITY HOSPITAL, 2041 Georgia Avenue N.W., Zip 20060; tel. 202/865–6100; Sherman P. McCoy, Executive Director and Chief Executive Officer **A**1 2 3 5 8 9 10 **F**7 8 10 11 12 14 15 16 17 19 20 21 22 25 28 29 30 31 34 35 37 38 40 41 42 44 45 46 49 50 52 53 54 56 57 58 60 61 63 65 66 69 70 71 73 74 **P**8	23	10	355	11029	233	113608	794	182374	91161	2258
MALCOLM GROW MEDICAL CENTER See Andrews AFB, MD										
★ △ NATIONAL REHABILITATION HOSPITAL, 102 Irving Street N.W., Zip 20010–2949; tel. 202/877–1000; Edward A. Eckenhoff, President and Chief Executive Officer **A**1 3 5 7 9 10 **F**3 4 5 8 10 12 13 14 16 17 19 20 21 22 25 26 27 28 29 30 31 32 33 34 35 39 41 42 43 44 45 46 48 49 50 51 53 54 55 56 57 58 59 60 61 64 65 66 67 69 70 71 72 73 74 **P**3 6 8 **S** Medlantic Healthcare Group, Washington, DC **N** Medlantic Healthcare Group, Washington, DC	23	46	160	1629	108	75870	0	52534	28505	684
★ PROVIDENCE HOSPITAL, 1150 Varnum Street N.E., Zip 20017–2180; tel. 202/269–7000; Sister Carol Keehan, President (Total facility includes 240 beds in nursing home–type unit) **A**1 3 5 9 10 **F**2 3 7 8 9 10 11 14 15 16 17 18 19 22 24 25 26 27 28 29 30 33 34 35 36 37 38 39 40 41 42 44 45 47 48 49 51 52 54 55 56 57 58 59 61 64 65 67 71 72 73 74 **S** Daughters of Charity National Health System, Saint Louis, MO	21	10	556	13001	387	71001	1675	115658	59088	1676
□ PSYCHIATRIC INSTITUTE OF WASHINGTON, 4228 Wisconsin Avenue N.W., Zip 20016; tel. 202/965–8550; Kenneth F. Courage, Jr., Chief Executive Officer (Nonreporting) **A**1 5 9 10	33	22	99	—	—	—	—	—	—	—
★ SIBLEY MEMORIAL HOSPITAL, 5255 Loughboro Road N.W., Zip 20016; tel. 202/537–4000; Robert L. Sloan, Chief Executive Officer (Total facility includes 18 beds in nursing home–type unit) **A**1 2 3 5 9 10 **F**7 8 10 11 12 16 17 19 21 22 26 30 31 32 34 35 37 39 40 41 42 44 45 46 49 52 53 55 56 57 58 60 61 64 65 66 67 71 73 74 **P**8	23	10	252	12062	188	75002	924	93576	46207	1046
★ ST. ELIZABETHS HOSPITAL, 2700 Martin Luther King Jr. Avenue S.E., Zip 20032; tel. 202/373–7166; Sam Fantasia, Director, Division of Administration and Financial Services (Nonreporting) **A**1 5 10	14	22	1024	—	—	—	—	—	—	—
★ VETERANS AFFAIRS MEDICAL CENTER, 50 Irving Street N.W., Zip 20422; tel. 202/745–8100; Sanford M. Garfunkel, Medical Center Director (Total facility includes 112 beds in nursing home–type unit) **A**1 2 3 5 8 9 **F**1 3 4 8 10 14 15 16 18 19 20 21 22 23 26 28 29 30 31 32 35 37 39 41 42 43 44 45 46 49 51 52 54 55 56 57 58 59 60 64 65 67 71 73 74 **S** Department of Veterans Affairs, Washington, DC	45	10	451	8022	373	305207	0	166192	112294	1909

Hospital, Address, Telephone, Administrator, Approval, Facility, and Physician Codes, Health Care System, Network	Classi-fication Codes		Utilization Data					Expense (thousands) of dollars		
★ American Hospital Association (AHA) membership □ Joint Commission on Accreditation of Healthcare Organizations (JCAHO) accreditation + American Osteopathic Hospital Association (AOHA) membership ○ American Osteopathic Association (AOA) accreditation △ Commission on Accreditation of Rehabilitation Facilities (CARF) accreditation Control codes 61, 63, 64, 71, 72 and 73 indicate hospitals listed by AOHA, but not registered by AHA. For definition of numerical codes, see page A4	Control	Service	Beds	Admissions	Census	Outpatient Visits	Births	Total	Payroll	Personnel
✵ WALTER REED HEALTH CARE SYSTEM, Zip 20307–5001; tel. 202/782–6393; Colonel Robert James Heckert, Jr., MSC, Chief of Staff **A**1 2 3 5 **F**2 3 4 5 7 8 10 11 12 13 14 15 17 18 19 20 21 22 23 24 25 27 28 29 30 31 34 35 37 38 39 40 41 42 43 44 45 46 47 48 49 51 52 53 54 55 56 57 58 59 60 61 63 64 65 66 67 69 71 73 **S** Department of the Army, Office of the Surgeon General, Falls Church, VA	42	10	474	21454	450	640553	0	—	—	3453
✵ WASHINGTON HOSPITAL CENTER, 110 Irving Street N.W., Zip 20010–2975; tel. 202/877–7000; Kenneth A. Samet, President **A**1 2 3 5 8 9 10 **F**2 3 4 5 7 8 9 10 11 12 16 17 18 19 20 21 22 26 27 28 29 30 31 32 33 34 35 37 38 39 40 41 42 43 44 45 46 48 49 51 52 54 56 57 58 60 61 64 65 66 67 68 69 70 71 73 **P**1 6 **S** Medlantic Healthcare Group, Washington, DC **N** Medlantic Healthcare Group, Washington, DC; National Cardiovascular Network, Atlanta, GA	23	10	772	31844	551	222610	2669	414815	203813	4148

FLORIDA

Resident population 14,166 (in thousands)
Resident population in metro areas 93.0%
Birth rate per 1,000 population 14.0
65 years and over 18.6%
Percent of persons without health insurance 17.2%

Hospital, Address, Telephone, Administrator, Approval, Facility, and Physician Codes, Health Care System, Network	Control	Service	Beds	Admissions	Census	Outpatient Visits	Births	Total	Payroll	Personnel

★ American Hospital Association (AHA) membership
□ Joint Commission on Accreditation of Healthcare Organizations (JCAHO) accreditation
+ American Osteopathic Hospital Association (AOHA) membership
○ American Osteopathic Association (AOA) accreditation
△ Commission on Accreditation of Rehabilitation Facilities (CARF) accreditation
Control codes 61, 63, 64, 71, 72 and 73 indicate hospitals listed by AOHA, but not registered by AHA. For definition of numerical codes, see page A4

ALTAMONTE SPRINGS—Seminole County
FLORIDA HOSPITAL–ALTAMONTE See Florida Hospital, Orlando

APALACHICOLA—Franklin County
EMERALD COAST HOSPITAL, One Washington Square, Zip 32320, Mailing Address: P.O. Box 610, Zip 32329; tel. 904/653–8853; Kenneth E. Dykes, Sr., Administrator (Nonreporting) **A**9 10 — 33 10 29

APOPKA—Orange County
FLORIDA HOSPITAL–APOPKA See Florida Hospital, Orlando

ARCADIA—De Soto County
✠ DESOTO MEMORIAL HOSPITAL, 900 North Robert Avenue, Zip 34265, Mailing Address: P.O. Box 2180, Zip 34265–2180; tel. 941/494–3535; Gary M. Moore, President and Chief Executive Officer **A**1 5 9 10 **F**8 12 13 15 16 17 19 21 22 26 27 28 30 32 33 34 35 37 39 40 41 44 49 50 51 63 65 67 71 72 **P**6 **S** Quorum Health Group/Quorum Health Resources, Inc., Brentwood, TN — 23 10 62 1991 19 — 465 17851 7709 64

G. PIERCE WOOD MEMORIAL HOSPITAL, 5847 S.E. Highway 31, Zip 33821–9627; tel. 813/494–3323; Richard J. Bradley, Administrator **A**5 10 **F**26 46 52 57 65 73 **P**6 — 12 22 450 316 398 0 0 40925 23851 1121

ATLANTIS—Palm Beach County
✠ COLUMBIA J. F. K. MEDICAL CENTER, (Formerly JFK Medical Center), 5301 South Congress Avenue, Zip 33462; tel. 561/965–7300; Phillip D. Robinson, Chief Executive Officer (Total facility includes 20 beds in nursing home–type unit) **A**1 2 9 10 **F**3 4 7 8 10 11 12 14 15 16 17 19 21 22 23 25 28 30 31 32 34 35 37 39 41 42 43 44 46 49 51 52 53 54 55 56 57 58 59 60 64 65 67 71 72 73 74 **P**6 7 **S** Columbia/HCA Healthcare Corporation, Nashville, TN **N** Lake Okeechobee Rural Health Network, Belle Glade, FL — 33 10 363 18394 255 125813 0 147438 52508 1414

AVON PARK—Highlands County
FLORIDA CENTER FOR ADDICTIONS AND DUAL DISORDERS, 100 West College Drive, Zip 33825; tel. 941/452–3858; Arthur J. Cox, Sr., Director (Nonreporting) — 23 82 50
✠ FLORIDA HOSPITAL–WALKER, 2501 U.S. Highway 27 North, Zip 33825–1200, Mailing Address: P.O. Box 1200, Zip 33826–1200; tel. 941/453–7511; Samuel Leonor, President (Nonreporting) **A**1 9 10 **S** Adventist Health System Sunbelt Health Care Corporation, Winter Park, FL **N** Adventist Health System, Winter Park, FL — 21 10 151

BARTOW—Polk County
✠ COLUMBIA BARTOW MEMORIAL HOSPITAL, (Formerly Bartow Memorial Hospital), 1239 East Main Street, Zip 33830–5005, Mailing Address: Box 1050, Zip 33830–1050; tel. 941/533–8111; Thomas C. Mathews, Administrator **A**1 9 10 **F**1 3 4 7 8 10 12 16 17 19 20 21 22 23 24 26 27 28 29 30 31 32 33 34 35 36 37 39 40 41 42 43 44 45 46 49 50 51 53 54 55 56 57 58 59 60 61 63 64 65 69 70 71 72 73 **P**5 **S** Columbia/HCA Healthcare Corporation, Nashville, TN — 32 10 88 2778 28 34573 587 16736 6522 204

BAY PINES—Pinellas County
✠ VETERANS AFFAIRS MEDICAL CENTER, 10000 Bay Pines Boulevard, Zip 33744, Mailing Address: P.O. Box 5005, Zip 33744; tel. 813/398–6661; Thomas H. Weaver, FACHE, Director (Total facility includes 168 beds in nursing home–type unit) **A**1 2 3 5 **F**2 3 6 8 11 12 15 17 19 20 21 22 24 25 26 27 28 29 30 31 32 33 34 35 37 39 41 42 44 45 46 48 49 52 54 55 56 57 58 61 64 65 67 71 72 73 74 **S** Department of Veterans Affairs, Washington, DC — 45 10 773 10277 609 280025 0 157864 82430 1944

BELLE GLADE—Palm Beach County
✠ GLADES GENERAL HOSPITAL, 1201 South Main Street, Zip 33430; tel. 561/996–6571; Michael G. Layfield, Chief Executive Officer **A**1 9 10 **F**7 8 12 15 17 19 22 24 26 28 29 30 31 33 34 35 37 40 44 45 48 49 65 68 71 73 74 **P**7 **S** Quorum Health Group/Quorum Health Resources, Inc., Brentwood, TN **N** Lake Okeechobee Rural Health Network, Belle Glade, FL — 16 10 47 2150 20 24390 374 14712 5962 125

BLOUNTSTOWN—Calhoun County
CALHOUN–LIBERTY HOSPITAL, 424 Burns Avenue, Zip 32424–1097; tel. 904/674–5411; Josh Plummer, Administrator **A**9 10 **F**22 32 **N** Panhandle Area Health Network, Marianna, FL — 23 10 30 445 4 11131 1 8400 2500 170

BOCA RATON—Palm Beach County
✠ BOCA RATON COMMUNITY HOSPITAL, 800 Meadows Road, Zip 33486–2368; tel. 561/395–7100; Randolph J. Pierce, President and Chief Executive Officer **A**1 2 9 10 **F**7 8 10 11 14 15 16 19 21 22 23 24 26 27 28 29 30 31 32 34 35 37 39 40 41 42 44 45 46 49 51 60 61 65 67 71 72 73 74 **P**3 8 **N** Florida Health Choice, Del Ray Beach, FL — 23 10 331 16117 235 — 732 135492 55748 1393

□ WEST BOCA MEDICAL CENTER, 21644 State Road 7, Zip 33428–1899; tel. 407/488–8000; Richard Gold, Chief Executive Officer **A**1 9 10 **F**4 7 8 10 11 12 13 14 15 16 17 19 21 22 23 27 28 29 30 32 35 37 38 40 41 44 45 46 47 49 64 65 66 67 70 71 73 74 **P**5 7 **S** TENET Healthcare Corporation, Santa Barbara, CA **N** Tenet South Florida Health System Network, Fort Lauderdale, FL — 33 10 150 8035 85 80972 1885 27328 18497 400

Hospital, Address, Telephone, Administrator, Approval, Facility, and Physician Codes, Health Care System, Network	Classi-fication Codes		Utilization Data					Expense (thousands) of dollars		
★ American Hospital Association (AHA) membership □ Joint Commission on Accreditation of Healthcare Organizations (JCAHO) accreditation + American Osteopathic Hospital Association (AOHA) membership ○ American Osteopathic Association (AOA) accreditation △ Commission on Accreditation of Rehabilitation Facilities (CARF) accreditation Control codes 61, 63, 64, 71, 72 and 73 indicate hospitals listed by AOHA, but not registered by AHA. For definition of numerical codes, see page A4	Control	Service	Beds	Admissions	Census	Outpatient Visits	Births	Total	Payroll	Personnel

BONIFAY—Holmes County

□ DOCTORS MEMORIAL HOSPITAL, 401 East Byrd Avenue, Zip 32425, Mailing Address: Box 188, Zip 32425; tel. 904/547–1120; Dale Larson, Executive Director (Nonreporting) **A**1 9 10 **S** Community Health Systems, Inc., Brentwood, TN **N** Panhandle Area Health Network, Marianna, FL

| | 33 | 10 | 34 | — | — | — | — | — | — | — |

BOYNTON BEACH—Palm Beach County

✠ BETHESDA MEMORIAL HOSPITAL, 2815 South Seacrest Boulevard, Zip 33435; tel. 561/737–7733; Robert B. Hill, President **A**1 2 9 10 **F**1 7 8 10 11 17 19 22 23 24 25 26 27 28 30 32 33 34 35 37 38 39 40 42 44 49 52 54 55 57 58 59 60 63 65 66 67 71 73 74 **P**1 7

| | 23 | 10 | 362 | 13060 | 169 | 105664 | 2387 | 101794 | 39444 | 1639 |

BRADENTON—Manatee County

✠ △ COLUMBIA BLAKE MEDICAL CENTER, 2020 59th Street West, Zip 34209, Mailing Address: P.O. Box 25004, Zip 34206–5004; tel. 941/792–6611; Lindell W. Orr, Chief Executive Officer (Total facility includes 23 beds in nursing home–type unit) **A**1 2 7 9 10 **F**4 7 8 10 11 12 13 14 15 16 17 19 21 22 23 24 25 26 28 30 32 33 34 35 37 39 40 41 42 43 44 45 46 48 49 60 64 65 67 71 72 73 74 **S** Columbia/HCA Healthcare Corporation, Nashville, TN **N** Columbia/HCA Tampa Bay Division, Tampa, FL; The Health Advantage Network, Winter Park, FL

| | 33 | 10 | 284 | 11842 | 182 | 76200 | 540 | 85837 | 38456 | 1086 |

□ MANATEE MEMORIAL HOSPITAL, 206 Second Street East, Zip 34208; tel. 941/745–7373; Michael Marquez, Chief Executive Officer **A**1 2 9 10 **F**2 3 4 7 8 10 11 12 14 15 16 17 19 21 22 24 25 28 30 32 34 37 38 40 41 42 43 44 45 46 49 52 53 58 59 61 65 67 72 73 74 **P**8 **S** Universal Health Services, Inc., King of Prussia, PA **N** BayCare Health Network, Inc., Clearwater, FL

| | 33 | 10 | 512 | 13984 | 187 | 80014 | 1766 | 100055 | 35441 | — |

BRANDON—Hillsborough County

✠ COLUMBIA BRANDON REGIONAL MEDICAL CENTER, 119 Oakfield Drive, Zip 33511–5799; tel. 813/681–5551; H. Rex Etheredge, President and Chief Executive Officer **A**1 5 9 10 **F**7 8 10 11 12 14 16 19 21 22 27 28 30 32 35 37 38 40 42 44 45 47 49 59 63 64 65 67 71 73 **P**5 7 8 **S** Columbia/HCA Healthcare Corporation, Nashville, TN **N** Columbia/HCA Tampa Bay Division, Tampa, FL; The Health Advantage Network, Winter Park, FL

| | 33 | 10 | 225 | 13470 | 151 | 90291 | 2752 | — | — | — |

BROOKSVILLE—Hernando County

✠ BROOKSVILLE REGIONAL HOSPITAL, 55 Ponce De Leon Boulevard, Zip 34601–0037, Mailing Address: Box 37, Zip 34605–0037; tel. 352/796–5111; Robert Foreman, Associate Administrator (Nonreporting) **A**1 9 10 **S** Quorum Health Group/Quorum Health Resources, Inc., Brentwood, TN **N** BayCare Health Network, Inc., Clearwater, FL

| | 23 | 10 | 91 | — | — | — | — | — | — | — |

□ GREENBRIER HOSPITAL, 7007 Grove Road, Zip 34609; tel. 352/596–4306; James E. O'Shea, Administrator **A**1 10 **F**2 3 12 14 15 16 17 19 20 21 27 32 35 48 50 52 54 55 56 57 58 59 63 65 71 **P**8

| | 33 | 22 | 36 | 1162 | 34 | — | 0 | — | — | 97 |

BUNNELL—Flagler County

★ MEMORIAL HOSPITAL–FLAGLER, Moody Boulevard, Zip 32110, Mailing Address: HCR1, Box 2, Zip 32110; tel. 904/437–2211; Clark P. Christianson, Senior Vice President and Administrator (Total facility includes 8 beds in nursing home–type unit) **A**9 10 **F**8 12 14 15 16 17 19 20 21 22 25 26 28 29 30 31 32 33 34 37 39 41 42 44 45 46 49 64 65 66 67 71 73 74 **P**1 2 6 8 **S** Memorial Health Systems, Ormond Beach, FL

| | 23 | 10 | 81 | 1718 | 24 | 28957 | 0 | 16435 | 7583 | 202 |

CAPE CORAL—Lee County

□ CAPE CORAL HOSPITAL, 636 Del Prado Boulevard, Zip 33990; tel. 941/574–2323; Earl Tamar, Executive Director and System Vice President (Nonreporting) **A**1 2 9 10

| | 23 | 10 | 201 | — | — | — | — | — | — | — |

CHATTAHOOCHEE—Gadsden County

FLORIDA STATE HOSPITAL, U.S. Highway 90 East, Zip 32324–1000, Mailing Address: P.O. Box 1000, Zip 32324–1000; tel. 904/663–7536; Robert B. Williams, Administrator (Total facility includes 111 beds in nursing home–type unit) **A**5 10 **F**4 8 10 11 12 17 19 20 21 22 23 26 28 29 30 31 35 37 39 40 41 42 44 50 52 54 55 57 60 63 64 65 67 70 71 73 74 **P**6

| | 12 | 22 | 1001 | 668 | 914 | 0 | 0 | 92569 | 57180 | 2606 |

CHIPLEY—Washington County

✠ NORTHWEST FLORIDA COMMUNITY HOSPITAL, 1360 Brickyard Road, Zip 32428–5010, Mailing Address: P.O. Box 889, Zip 32428; tel. 904/638–1610; Stephen D. Mason, Administrator **A**1 9 10 **F**8 11 15 19 22 24 27 28 30 32 33 34 41 44 49 54 65 71 73 **N** Panhandle Area Health Network, Marianna, FL

| | 13 | 10 | 45 | 1517 | 24 | 123951 | 0 | 13523 | 6218 | 283 |

CLEARWATER—Pinellas County

✠ COLUMBIA CLEARWATER COMMUNITY HOSPITAL, 1521 Druid Road East, Zip 34616–6193, Mailing Address: P.O. Box 9068, Zip 34618–9068; tel. 813/447–4571; Thomas L. Herron, FACHE, Chief Executive Officer (Total facility includes 20 beds in nursing home–type unit) (Nonreporting) **A**1 10 **S** Columbia/HCA Healthcare Corporation, Nashville, TN **N** Columbia/HCA Tampa Bay Division, Tampa, FL; The Health Advantage Network, Winter Park, FL

HORIZON HOSPITAL See Psychiatric Hospital of Florida

| | 32 | 10 | 133 | — | — | — | — | — | — | — |

□ MORTON PLANT HOSPITAL, 323 Jeffords Street, Zip 34616–3892, Mailing Address: Box 210, Zip 34617–0210; tel. 813/462–7000; Frank V. Murphy, III, President and Chief Executive Officer (Total facility includes 126 beds in nursing home–type unit) (Nonreporting) **A**1 2 5 9 10 **N** Morton Plant Mease Health Care, Dunedin, FL; BayCare Health Network, Inc., Clearwater, FL

| | 23 | 10 | 742 | — | — | — | — | — | — | — |

Hospital, Address, Telephone, Administrator, Approval, Facility, and Physician Codes, Health Care System, Network	Classi-fication Codes		Utilization Data					Expense (thousands) of dollars		Personnel
	Control	Service	Beds	Admissions	Census	Outpatient Visits	Births	Total	Payroll	

★ American Hospital Association (AHA) membership
□ Joint Commission on Accreditation of Healthcare Organizations (JCAHO) accreditation
+ American Osteopathic Hospital Association (AOHA) membership
○ American Osteopathic Association (AOA) accreditation
△ Commission on Accreditation of Rehabilitation Facilities (CARF) accreditation
Control codes 61, 63, 64, 71, 72 and 73 indicate hospitals listed by AOHA, but not registered by AHA. For definition of numerical codes, see page A4

□ PSYCHIATRIC HOSPITAL OF FLORIDA, (Formerly Horizon Hospital), 11300 U.S. 19 North, Zip 34624; tel. 813/541–2646; C. William Brett, Ph.D., Chief Executive Officer **A**1 10 **F**2 26 27 28 52 54 55 56 57 58 59 65 67	33	22	50	909	37	5938	0	—	—	93
CLERMONT—Lake County										
⊞ SOUTH LAKE HOSPITAL, 847 Eighth Street, Zip 34711; tel. 352/394–4071; P. Shannon Elswick, Administrator and Chief Executive Officer **A**1 9 10 **F**8 12 14 15 16 19 21 22 29 30 32 34 35 37 41 44 45 49 65 71 73 **S** Orlando Regional Healthcare System, Orlando, FL **N** Orlando Regional Healthcare System, Orlando, FL	16	10	68	2038	27	20786	0	12734	6339	176
CLEWISTON—Hendry County										
⊞ HENDRY REGIONAL MEDICAL CENTER, 500 West Sugarland Highway, Zip 33440; tel. 941/983–9121; J. Rudy Reinhardt, Administrator **A**1 9 10 **F**3 8 12 13 15 16 17 18 19 20 21 22 26 28 29 30 31 33 34 35 37 39 41 44 45 49 51 53 54 55 56 57 58 63 65 69 71 73 **P**6 **S** Quorum Health Group/Quorum Health Resources, Inc., Brentwood, TN **N** Lake Okeechobee Rural Health Network, Belle Glade, FL	16	10	45	1065	14	22494	0	10371	4315	165
COCOA BEACH—Brevard County										
⊞ HEALTH FIRST/CAPE CANAVERAL HOSPITAL, 701 West Cocoa Beach Causeway, Zip 32931, Mailing Address: P.O. Box 320069, Zip 32932–0069; tel. 407/799–7111; Christopher S. Kennedy, President and Chief Operating Officer **A**1 9 10 **F**4 7 8 10 11 12 14 16 17 19 21 22 23 24 27 28 29 30 32 33 34 35 37 38 40 41 42 43 44 45 46 49 50 60 63 64 65 67 71 72 74 **P**6 7	23	10	128	6089	67	—	824	53575	22750	585
CORAL GABLES—Dade County										
□ CORAL GABLES HOSPITAL, 3100 Douglas Road, Zip 33134–6990; tel. 305/445–8461; Martha Garcia, Chief Executive Officer (Nonreporting) **A**1 10 **S** TENET Healthcare Corporation, Santa Barbara, CA	33	10	205	—	—	—	—	—	—	—
□ HEALTHSOUTH DOCTORS' HOSPITAL, 5000 University Drive, Zip 33146–2094; tel. 305/666–2111; Lincoln S. Mendez, Chief Executive Officer (Total facility includes 29 beds in nursing home–type unit) **A**1 3 9 10 **F**5 7 8 10 12 14 15 16 19 21 22 24 27 30 31 32 34 35 37 39 40 41 42 44 45 46 49 64 65 66 67 71 73 **S** HEALTHSOUTH Corporation, Birmingham, AL	33	10	157	5928	80	65376	1056	55661	21446	658
□ VENCOR HOSPITAL–CORAL GABLES, 5190 S.W. Eighth Street, Zip 33134; tel. 305/445–1364; Theodore Welding, Chief Executive Officer (Nonreporting) **A**1 10 **S** Vencor, Incorporated, Louisville, KY	33	10	53	—	—	—	—	—	—	—
CORAL SPRINGS—Broward County										
⊞ CORAL SPRINGS MEDICAL CENTER, 3000 Coral Hills Drive, Zip 33065; tel. 954/344–3000; A. Gary Muller, FACHE, Regional Vice President Administration **A**1 9 10 **F**4 5 7 8 10 11 12 14 15 16 17 19 21 22 23 24 25 27 28 29 30 31 32 33 34 35 37 38 39 40 41 42 43 44 45 49 50 51 54 56 57 60 63 65 66 67 70 71 72 73 74 **P**6 8 **S** North Broward Hospital District, Fort Lauderdale, FL **N** Community Health Network of South Florida, Ft Lauderdale, FL	16	10	167	9380	102	80157	2142	59672	24262	658
CRESTVIEW—Okaloosa County										
□ NORTH OKALOOSA MEDICAL CENTER, 151 Redstone Avenue S.E., Zip 32539–6026; tel. 904/689–8100; Roger L. Hall, Chief Executive Officer (Total facility includes 10 beds in nursing home–type unit) **A**1 9 10 **F**7 8 12 14 15 16 17 19 22 24 28 29 30 32 33 34 35 37 40 41 44 45 46 49 51 63 64 65 67 71 72 73 74 **P**1 5 7 **S** Community Health Systems, Inc., Brentwood, TN **N** Columbia/HCA North & NorthEast Florida Division, Jacksonville, FL; The Health Advantage Network, Winter Park, FL	33	10	91	3829	47	57600	495	24451	10030	466
CRYSTAL RIVER—Citrus County										
□ + SEVEN RIVERS COMMUNITY HOSPITAL, 6201 North Suncoast Boulevard, Zip 34428; tel. 904/795–6560; Michael L. Collins, Chief Executive Officer **A**1 9 10 **F**7 8 10 11 12 14 16 17 19 21 22 23 24 28 29 30 34 35 37 39 40 41 42 44 45 49 52 54 55 56 57 59 60 63 65 67 71 73 74 **S** TENET Healthcare Corporation, Santa Barbara, CA	33	10	128	5818	75	43895	257	32628	12692	453
DADE CITY—Pasco County										
⊞ COLUMBIA DADE CITY HOSPITAL, 13100 Fort King Road, Zip 33525–5294; tel. 904/521–1100; Robert Meade, Chief Executive Officer (Nonreporting) **A**1 10 **S** Columbia/HCA Healthcare Corporation, Nashville, TN **N** Columbia/HCA Tampa Bay Division, Tampa, FL; The Health Advantage Network, Winter Park, FL	33	10	120	—	—	—	—	—	—	—
DAYTONA BEACH—Volusia County										
⊞ COLUMBIA MEDICAL CENTER–DAYTONA, 400 North Clyde Morris Boulevard, Zip 32114, Mailing Address: Box 9000, Zip 32120; tel. 904/239–5000; Thomas R. Pentz, Chief Executive Officer (Nonreporting) **A**1 10 **S** Columbia/HCA Healthcare Corporation, Nashville, TN **N** Columbia/HCA Central Florida Division, Winter Park, FL; The Health Advantage Network, Winter Park, FL	33	10	214	—	—	—	—	—	—	—
⊞ HALIFAX COMMUNITY HEALTH SYSTEM, (Formerly Halifax Medical Center), (Includes Halifax Behavioral Center, 841 Jimmy Ann Drive, Zip 32117–4599; tel. 904/274–5333), 303 North Clyde Morris Boulevard, Zip 32114; tel. 904/254–4065; Ron R. Rees, Administrator **A**1 2 3 5 9 10 **F**1 7 8 10 12 13 15 16 17 18 19 21 22 23 24 25 26 27 28 29 30 31 32 33 34 35 37 38 39 40 41 42 44 45 46 49 51 52 53 54 55 56 57 58 59 60 61 63 64 65 66 67 68 69 70 71 72 73 74 **P**5 6	16	10	491	18987	250	—	2322	179665	64153	2001
DE FUNIAK SPRINGS—Walton County										
WALTON REGIONAL HOSPITAL, 336 College Avenue, Zip 32433; tel. 904/892–5171; Jon Hufstedler, Administrator **A**9 10 **F**8 14 15 19 32 34 35 37 44 46 70 71 73 **P**5	33	10	34	1000	11	19711	0	7219	3137	167

Hospital, Address, Telephone, Administrator, Approval, Facility, and Physician Codes, Health Care System, Network	Classi-fication Codes		Utilization Data					Expense (thousands) of dollars		
	Control	Service	Beds	Admissions	Census	Outpatient Visits	Births	Total	Payroll	Personnel

★ American Hospital Association (AHA) membership
☐ Joint Commission on Accreditation of Healthcare Organizations (JCAHO) accreditation
+ American Osteopathic Hospital Association (AOHA) membership
◯ American Osteopathic Association (AOA) accreditation
△ Commission on Accreditation of Rehabilitation Facilities (CARF) accreditation
    Control codes 61, 63, 64, 71, 72 and 73 indicate hospitals listed by AOHA, but not
    registered by AHA. For definition of numerical codes, see page A4.

DELAND—Union County

✠ MEMORIAL HOSPITAL–WEST VOLUSIA, 701 West Plymouth Avenue, Zip 32720, Mailing Address: Box 509, Zip 32721–0509; tel. 904/734–3320; Johnette L. Vodenicker, Senior Vice President and Administrator **A**1 9 10 **F**2 4 7 8 10 11 12 13 14 15 16 17 19 21 22 23 24 28 29 30 32 33 34 35 37 39 40 41 42 43 44 45 49 52 60 63 64 65 66 67 71 72 73 74 **P**1 2 6 8 **S** Memorial Health Systems, Ormond Beach, FL	23	10	156	5976	80	80170	832	46422	18166	561

DELRAY—Palm Beach County

☐ △ PINECREST REHABILITATION HOSPITAL, 5360 Linton Boulevard, Zip 33484; tel. 407/495–0400; Paul D. Echelard, Administrator (Nonreporting) **A**1 7 10	33	46	90	—	—	—	—	—	—	—

DELRAY BEACH—Palm Beach County

☐ DELRAY COMMUNITY HOSPITAL, 5352 Linton Boulevard, Zip 33484; tel. 407/498–4440; Mitchell S. Feldman, Chief Executive Officer **A**1 9 10 **F**1 2 3 4 8 10 11 12 16 17 18 19 20 21 22 25 27 28 30 31 32 34 35 37 38 39 40 41 42 43 44 45 46 47 48 49 52 53 54 55 56 57 58 59 60 64 65 70 71 73 **P**5 7 **S** TENET Healthcare Corporation, Santa Barbara, CA **N** Tenet South Florida Health System Network, Fort Lauderdale, FL	33	10	211	11602	185	92707	0	98476	29953	1327
☐ FAIR OAKS HOSPITAL, 5440 Linton Boulevard, Zip 33484; tel. 561/495–1000; Michael B. Gittelman, Chief Executive Officer **A**1 10 **F**1 2 3 26 32 52 54 55 56 57 58 59	33	22	102	1617	40	2241	0	—	—	88

DUNEDIN—Pinellas County

☐ MEASE HOSPITAL DUNEDIN, 601 Main Street, Zip 34698, Mailing Address: P.O. Box 760, Zip 34697–0760; tel. 813/733–1111; Philip K. Beauchamp, FACHE, President and Chief Executive Officer (Total facility includes 20 beds in nursing home–type unit) (Nonreporting) **A**1 9 10 **S** Mease Health Care, Palm Harbor, FL **N** Morton Plant Mease Health Care, Dunedin, FL; BayCare Health Network, Inc., Clearwater, FL	23	10	258	—	—	—	—	—	—	—

EGLIN AFB—Okaloosa County

✠ U. S. AIR FORCE REGIONAL HOSPITAL, 307 Boatner Road, Suite 114, Zip 32542–1282; tel. 904/883–8221; Colonel William C. Head, MSC, USAF, Administrator **A**1 3 5 **F**2 3 4 6 7 8 9 10 11 12 13 17 18 19 20 21 22 24 25 26 27 28 29 30 31 32 33 34 35 36 37 38 39 40 41 42 43 44 45 46 47 48 49 50 51 52 53 54 55 56 57 58 59 60 61 62 63 64 65 66 67 68 69 70 71 72 73 74 **P**6 **S** Department of the Air Force, Washington, DC	41	10	85	6710	51	277718	1002	—	—	—

ENGLEWOOD—Sarasota County

✠ COLUMBIA ENGLEWOOD COMMUNITY HOSPITAL, 700 Medical Boulevard, Zip 34223; tel. 941/475–6571; Terry L. Moore, Chief Executive Officer **A**1 10 **F**8 10 12 14 15 16 17 19 20 21 22 25 26 28 29 30 32 34 35 37 41 42 44 46 49 51 59 64 65 66 71 73 **P**6 **S** Columbia/HCA Healthcare Corporation, Nashville, TN **N** Columbia/HCA SouthWest Florida Division, Fort Myers, FL; The Health Advantage Network, Winter Park, FL	33	10	100	3930	57	—	0	35316	16568	—

EUSTIS—Lake County

✠ FLORIDA HOSPITAL WATERMAN, 201 North Eustis Street, Zip 32726, Mailing Address: P.O. Box B, Zip 32727–0377; tel. 352/589–3333; Royce C. Thompson, President (Total facility includes 29 beds in nursing home–type unit) **A**1 2 10 **F**7 8 10 12 14 15 16 17 19 21 22 23 24 25 27 28 30 31 32 33 34 35 37 39 40 42 44 45 46 49 63 64 65 66 67 68 71 73 74 **P**1 5 6 7 **S** Adventist Health System Sunbelt Health Care Corporation, Winter Park, FL **N** Adventist Health System, Winter Park, FL; Florida Hospital Health Network, Orlando, FL	21	10	182	7839	125	—	609	74353	32510	1140

FERNANDINA BEACH—Nassau County

☐ BAPTIST MEDICAL CENTER–NASSAU, 1250 South 18th Street, Zip 32034; tel. 904/321–3501; Jim L. Mayo, Administrator **A**1 9 10 **F**2 3 4 7 8 10 11 12 14 15 16 17 18 19 20 21 22 23 24 25 26 28 29 30 31 32 34 35 37 38 39 40 41 42 43 44 45 46 47 48 49 50 51 52 53 54 55 56 57 58 59 60 61 63 64 65 66 67 71 72 73 74 **P**1 **N** Baptist/St. Vincent's Health System, Jacksonville, FL	23	10	48	1656	16	28321	383	13340	6103	231

FORT LAUDERDALE—Broward County

☐ BHC FORT LAUDERDALE HOSPITAL, (Formerly CPC Fort Lauderdale Hospital), 1601 East Las Olas Boulevard, Zip 33301–2393; tel. 954/463–4321; Andrew Fuhrman, Chief Executive Officer (Nonreporting) **A**1 10 **S** Behavioral Healthcare Corporation, Nashville, TN	33	22	100	—	—	—	—	—	—	—
✠ BROWARD GENERAL MEDICAL CENTER, 1600 South Andrews Avenue, Zip 33316–2510; tel. 954/355–4400; Ruth A. Eldridge, R.N., Regional Vice President, Administration (Total facility includes 20 beds in nursing home–type unit) **A**1 2 9 10 **F**4 7 8 10 11 12 15 16 17 19 21 22 23 24 25 27 28 29 30 31 32 33 34 35 37 38 39 40 41 42 43 44 45 46 47 48 49 50 51 52 54 56 57 58 60 63 64 65 66 67 70 71 72 73 74 **P**1 6 **S** North Broward Hospital District, Fort Lauderdale, FL **N** Community Health Network of South Florida, Ft Lauderdale, FL	16	10	548	20798	370	180158	3180	171418	70894	2070
☐ CLEVELAND CLINIC HOSPITAL, 2835 North Ocean Boulevard, Zip 33308; tel. 954/568–1000; Margaret S. McRae, Site Administrator **A**1 3 9 10 **F**8 10 12 14 15 16 17 19 21 22 24 26 27 29 30 31 32 33 34 35 37 39 41 42 43 44 45 46 49 51 60 65 66 67 71 73 74 **P**3 5	23	10	120	5087	72	31789	0	46685	15080	411
☐ CORAL RIDGE PSYCHIATRIC HOSPITAL, 4545 North Federal Highway, Zip 33308; tel. 954/771–2711; Michael J. Held, Administrator **A**1 10 **F**2 15 52 53 54 55 57 58 59 65 67 68	31	22	86	1004	45	0	0	—	—	124
CPC FORT LAUDERDALE HOSPITAL See BHC Fort Lauderdale Hospital										

Hospital, Address, Telephone, Administrator, Approval, Facility, and Physician Codes, Health Care System, Network	Classi-fication Codes		Utilization Data					Expense (thousands) of dollars		
★ American Hospital Association (AHA) membership □ Joint Commission on Accreditation of Healthcare Organizations (JCAHO) accreditation + American Osteopathic Hospital Association (AOHA) membership ○ American Osteopathic Association (AOA) accreditation △ Commission on Accreditation of Rehabilitation Facilities (CARF) accreditation Control codes 61, 63, 64, 71, 72 and 73 indicate hospitals listed by AOHA, but not registered by AHA. For definition of numerical codes, see page A4	Control	Service	Beds	Admissions	Census	Outpatient Visits	Births	Total	Payroll	Personnel
□ FLORIDA MEDICAL CENTER HOSPITAL, 5000 West Oakland Park Boulevard, Zip 33313–1585; tel. 305/735–6000; Denny De Narvaez, Chief Executive Officer A1 9 10 F1 4 7 8 10 11 12 14 15 16 19 21 22 23 26 27 32 33 35 37 41 42 43 44 45 46 49 52 53 55 56 57 58 60 61 63 64 65 66 67 71 73 P8 S TENET Healthcare Corporation, Santa Barbara, CA N Med Connect, Ft Lauderdale, FL	32	10	459	13602	235	135732	0	113146	39608	1263
□ △ HEALTHSOUTH SUNRISE REHABILITATION HOSPITAL, 4399 Nob Hill Road, Zip 33351–5899; tel. 305/749–0300; Kevin R. Conn, Administrator A1 7 10 F12 17 25 26 27 34 41 46 48 49 65 66 67 73 S HEALTHSOUTH Corporation, Birmingham, AL	33	46	108	2008	102	30551	0	27609	11081	271
□ △ HOLY CROSS HOSPITAL, 4725 North Federal Highway, Zip 33308, Mailing Address: Box 23460, Zip 33307; tel. 305/771–8000; Ray Budrys, President and Chief Executive Officer (Nonreporting) A1 7 9 10 S Eastern Mercy Health System, Radnor, PA N Community Health Network of South Florida, Ft Lauderdale, FL	21	10	437	—	—	—	—	—	—	—
☒ IMPERIAL POINT MEDICAL CENTER, 6401 North Federal Highway, Zip 33308–1495; tel. 954/776–8500; Dorothy J. Mancini, R.N., Regional Vice President Administration A1 9 10 F4 5 7 8 10 12 14 15 16 17 19 22 23 24 26 28 30 31 32 33 34 35 37 39 41 42 43 44 49 51 52 56 57 58 59 60 65 66 70 71 73 P6 S North Broward Hospital District, Fort Lauderdale, FL N Community Health Network of South Florida, Ft Lauderdale, FL	16	10	154	4900	94	54081	0	45100	18410	521
NORTH RIDGE MEDICAL CENTER, 5757 North Dixie Highway, Zip 33334; tel. 305/776–6000; Emil P. Miller, Chief Executive Officer A9 10 F4 7 8 10 11 12 14 15 16 19 21 22 25 26 27 28 30 31 32 35 37 39 40 42 43 44 46 49 51 61 64 65 67 71 73 74 P4 5 8 S TENET Healthcare Corporation, Santa Barbara, CA N National Cardiovascular Network, Atlanta, GA; Med Connect, Ft Lauderdale, FL	33	10	391	7883	138	87635	175	69733	25471	—
□ VENCOR HOSPITAL–FORT LAUDERDALE, 1516 East Las Olas Boulevard, Zip 33301–2399; tel. 954/764–8900; Lewis A. Ransdell, Administrator A1 10 F12 14 15 16 19 20 22 26 27 32 35 37 41 54 65 71 73 S Vencor, Incorporated, Louisville, KY	33	10	64	248	57	0	0	—	—	287
FORT MYERS—Lee County										
□ CHARTER GLADE BEHAVIORAL HEALTH SYSTEM, 3550 Colonial Boulevard, Zip 33912, Mailing Address: P.O. Box 60120, Zip 33906; tel. 813/939–0403; Vickie Lewis, Chief Executive Officer (Nonreporting) A1 10 S Magellan Health Services, Atlanta, GA	33	22	104	—	—	—	—	—	—	—
☒ ○ COLUMBIA GULF COAST HOSPITAL, 13681 Doctors Way, Zip 33912; tel. 941/768–5000; Valerie A. Jackson, Chief Executive Officer (Nonreporting) A1 10 11 S Columbia/HCA Healthcare Corporation, Nashville, TN N Columbia/HCA SouthWest Florida Division, Fort Myers, FL; The Health Advantage Network, Winter Park, FL	33	10	120	—	—	—	—	—	—	—
☒ COLUMBIA REGIONAL MEDICAL CENTER OF SOUTHWEST FLORIDA, 2727 Winkler Avenue, Zip 33901–9396; tel. 941/939–1147; Nick Carbone, Chief Executive Officer (Nonreporting) A1 2 10 S Columbia/HCA Healthcare Corporation, Nashville, TN N Columbia/HCA SouthWest Florida Division, Fort Myers, FL; The Health Advantage Network, Winter Park, FL	33	10	400	—	—	—	—	—	—	—
☒ △ LEE MEMORIAL HEALTH SYSTEM, 2776 Cleveland Avenue, Zip 33901, Mailing Address: P.O. Box 2218, Zip 33902; tel. 941/332–1111; James R. Nathan, President (Total facility includes 90 beds in nursing home–type unit) A1 2 7 9 10 F4 7 8 10 11 12 14 15 17 19 21 22 24 26 29 30 31 32 34 35 37 38 39 40 41 42 43 44 45 47 48 49 60 61 63 64 65 66 67 69 70 71 73 P6 8	16	10	659	22811	409	143886	2823	193037	80488	3322
FORT PIERCE—St. Lucie County										
☒ COLUMBIA LAWNWOOD REGIONAL MEDICAL CENTER, (Includes Lawnwood Pavilion, 1860 North Lawnwood Circle, Zip 34950, Mailing Address: P.O. Box 1540, Zip 34954–1540; tel. 407/466–1500), 1700 South 23rd Street, Zip 34950–0188; tel. 561/461–4000; Gary Cantrell, President and Chief Executive Officer (Total facility includes 33 beds in nursing home–type unit) A1 9 10 F3 4 7 8 10 11 12 13 14 15 16 17 19 20 22 23 24 25 28 29 30 31 32 33 34 35 36 37 38 39 40 41 42 44 45 46 49 52 53 55 58 59 60 64 65 66 71 73 74 S Columbia/HCA Healthcare Corporation, Nashville, TN N Columbia/HCA Central Florida Division, Winter Park, FL; The Health Advantage Network, Winter Park, FL	33	10	363	12124	217	75153	1346	81480	38367	1102
LAWNWOOD PAVILION See Columbia Lawnwood Regional Medical Center										
FORT WALTON BEACH—Okaloosa County										
☒ COLUMBIA FORT WALTON BEACH MEDICAL CENTER, 1000 Mar–Walt Drive, Zip 32547–6708; tel. 904/862–1111; Wayne Campbell, Chief Executive Officer A1 9 10 F4 7 8 10 11 12 14 15 16 17 19 21 22 31 32 34 37 40 41 42 44 45 48 49 52 54 55 56 57 59 63 64 66 71 73 74 S Columbia/HCA Healthcare Corporation, Nashville, TN N Columbia/HCA North & NorthEast Florida Division, Jacksonville, FL; The Health Advantage Network, Winter Park, FL	33	10	247	8616	126	70106	1006	45114	20830	657
GULF COAST TREATMENT CENTER, (Formerly Rivendell Psychiatric Hospital), 1015 Mar–Walt Drive, Zip 32547; tel. 904/863–4160; Raul D. Ruelas, M.D., Administrator (Nonreporting) A10 S Ramsay Health Care, Inc., Coral Gobles, FL	33	52	79	—	—	—	—	—	—	—

Hospital, Address, Telephone, Administrator, Approval, Facility, and Physician Codes, Health Care System, Network	Classi-fication Codes		Utilization Data					Expense (thousands) of dollars		
★ American Hospital Association (AHA) membership □ Joint Commission on Accreditation of Healthcare Organizations (JCAHO) accreditation + American Osteopathic Hospital Association (AOHA) membership ○ American Osteopathic Association (AOA) accreditation △ Commission on Accreditation of Rehabilitation Facilities (CARF) accreditation Control codes 61, 63, 64, 71, 72 and 73 indicate hospitals listed by AOHA, but not registered by AHA. For definition of numerical codes, see page A4	Control	Service	Beds	Admissions	Census	Outpatient Visits	Births	Total	Payroll	Personnel

GAINESVILLE—Alachua County

ALACHUA GENERAL HOSPITAL See Shands at AGH

★ COLUMBIA NORTH FLORIDA REGIONAL MEDICAL CENTER, 6500 Newberry Road, Zip 32605–4392, Mailing Address: P.O. Box 147006, Zip 32614–7006; tel. 352/333–4000; Brian C. Robinson, Chief Executive Officer (Total facility includes 24 beds in nursing home–type unit) **A**1 9 10 **F**4 7 8 10 11 12 14 15 16 19 22 23 24 25 28 30 32 34 35 37 39 40 41 42 43 44 46 49 51 60 64 65 66 67 71 72 73 74 **P**8 **S** Columbia/HCA Healthcare Corporation, Nashville, TN **N** Columbia/HCA North & NorthEast Florida Division, Jacksonville, FL; The Health Advantage Network, Winter Park, FL	33	10	278	13923	178	215246	1673	90065	40356	1411
★ SHANDS AT AGH, (Formerly Alachua General Hospital), 801 S.W. Second Avenue, Zip 32601; tel. 352/372–4321; Robert B. Williams, Administrator (Total facility includes 30 beds in nursing home–type unit) **A**1 2 3 5 9 10 **F**1 2 3 4 7 8 10 11 14 15 16 19 21 22 23 28 29 30 31 32 34 35 36 37 38 40 41 42 43 44 45 46 48 49 52 53 54 55 56 57 58 59 60 63 64 65 67 71 **S** Shands Health System, University of Florida Health Science Center, Gainesville, FL	23	10	269	4664	172	171841	372	32007	14701	1135
★ SHANDS AT THE UNIVERSITY OF FLORIDA, 1600 S.W. Archer Road, Zip 32610–0326, Mailing Address: P.O. Box 100326, Zip 32610–0326; tel. 352/395–0111; J. Richard Gaintner, M.D., Chief Executive Officer **A**1 2 3 5 8 9 10 **F**2 3 4 7 8 9 10 11 12 14 16 17 18 19 20 21 22 23 25 26 28 29 30 31 32 34 35 36 37 38 39 40 41 42 43 44 45 46 47 48 49 50 51 52 53 54 55 56 57 58 59 60 61 63 64 65 66 67 69 71 73 74 **P**6 **S** Shands Health System, University of Florida Health Science Center, Gainesville, FL	23	10	564	24725	428	284910	2497	357772	140895	4980
★ △ UPREACH REHABILITATION HOSPITAL, 8900 N.W. 39th Avenue, Zip 32606–5625; tel. 352/338–0091; Cynthia M. Toth, Administrator **A**1 7 10 **F**2 3 4 7 8 9 10 11 12 14 15 16 17 18 19 21 22 23 25 28 29 30 31 32 34 35 36 37 38 39 40 41 42 43 44 45 46 47 48 49 50 52 53 54 58 59 60 63 64 65 66 67 69 71 73 74 **P**6 **S** Shands Health System, University of Florida Health Science Center, Gainesville, FL	23	46	40	484	27	1722	0	4261	2367	108
★ VETERANS AFFAIRS MEDICAL CENTER, 1601 S.W. Archer Road, Zip 32608–1197; tel. 352/376–1611; Malcom Randall, Director (Total facility includes 90 beds in nursing home–type unit) **A**1 3 5 8 **F**1 2 3 4 8 10 15 16 17 18 19 20 21 23 25 26 27 28 29 30 31 32 33 34 35 37 39 41 42 43 44 46 49 51 52 54 55 56 57 58 59 60 63 64 65 67 71 73 74 **P**1 **S** Department of Veterans Affairs, Washington, DC	45	10	384	7291	269	268583	0	145459	66362	1632

GRACEVILLE—Jackson County

CAMPBELLTON GRACEVILLE HOSPITAL, 5429 College Drive, Zip 32440; tel. 904/263–4431; Neil Whipkey, Administrator **A**9 10 **F**8 14 15 16 19 22 30 32 33 37 40 44 64 65 71 **P**5 8 **N** Panhandle Area Health Network, Marianna, FL	16	10	35	563	7	6777	0	3520	1783	78

GREEN COVE SPRINGS—Clay County

□ VENCOR–NORTH FLORIDA, 801 Oak Street, Zip 32043; tel. 904/284–9230; Tim Simpson, Administrator (Nonreporting) **A**1 10 **S** Vencor, Incorporated, Louisville, KY	33	49	48							

GULF BREEZE—Santa Rosa County

□ GULF BREEZE HOSPITAL, 1110 Gulf Breeze Parkway, Zip 32561–1110, Mailing Address: P.O. Box 159, Zip 32562–0159; tel. 904/934–2000; Richard C. Fulford, Administrator **A**1 9 10 **F**2 3 4 7 8 9 10 11 12 13 14 15 16 19 21 22 23 26 27 28 31 32 33 35 37 39 40 41 42 43 44 45 46 48 49 51 52 53 54 55 56 57 58 59 60 61 62 63 64 65 66 67 70 71 72 73 74 **P**4 5 7 **S** Baptist Health Care Corporation, Pensacola, FL **N** Baptist Health Care, Inc., Pensacola, FL	23	10	45	1984	23	31749	0	16281	5319	181
THE FRIARY OF BAPTIST HEALTH CENTER, 4400 Hickory Shores Boulevard, Zip 32561; tel. 904/932–9375; Leo J. Donnelly, Executive Director (Nonreporting)	23	82	30	—	—	—	—	—	—	—

HAINES CITY—Polk County

□ HEART OF FLORIDA HOSPITAL, Tenth Street and Wood Avenue, Zip 33844, Mailing Address: Box 67, Zip 33844; tel. 813/422–4971; Robert Mahaffey, Administrator (Nonreporting) **A**1 9 10 **S** Health Management Associates, Naples, FL	33	10	51							

HIALEAH—Dade County

★ HIALEAH HOSPITAL, 651 East 25th Street, Zip 33013–3878; tel. 305/693–6100; Clifford J. Bauer, Chief Executive Officer (Nonreporting) **A**1 9 10 **S** TENET Healthcare Corporation, Santa Barbara, CA **N** Tenet South Florida Health System Network, Fort Lauderdale, FL	33	10	411							
□ PALM SPRINGS GENERAL HOSPITAL, 1475 West 49th Street, Zip 33012, Mailing Address: Box 2804, Zip 33012; tel. 305/558–2500; Carlos Milanes, Executive Vice President and Administrator **A**1 10 **F**11 19 22 26 30 34 35 37 44 45 46 49 65 67 71 73 **P**5	33	10	190	8227	133	24514	0	—	—	600
□ PALMETTO GENERAL HOSPITAL, 2001 West 68th Street, Zip 33016; tel. 305/823–5000; John C. Johnson, Chief Executive Officer (Nonreporting) **A**1 9 10 12 13 **S** TENET Healthcare Corporation, Santa Barbara, CA **N** Tenet South Florida Health System Network, Fort Lauderdale, FL	33	10	360							
□ ○ SOUTHERN WINDS HOSPITAL, 4225 West 20th Street, Zip 33012; tel. 305/558–9700; Michael J. Gerber, Chief Executive Officer (Nonreporting) **A**1 10 11	33	22	60							

HOLLYWOOD—Broward County

□ △ HOLLYWOOD MEDICAL CENTER, 3600 Washington Street, Zip 33021; tel. 954/966–4500; Holly Lerner, Chief Executive Officer (Nonreporting) **A**1 7 10 **S** TENET Healthcare Corporation, Santa Barbara, CA **N** Tenet South Florida Health System Network, Fort Lauderdale, FL	33	10	238							

Hospital, Address, Telephone, Administrator, Approval, Facility, and Physician Codes, Health Care System, Network	Classi-fication Codes		Utilization Data					Expense (thousands) of dollars		
★ American Hospital Association (AHA) membership ☐ Joint Commission on Accreditation of Healthcare Organizations (JCAHO) accreditation + American Osteopathic Hospital Association (AOHA) membership ◯ American Osteopathic Association (AOA) accreditation △ Commission on Accreditation of Rehabilitation Facilities (CARF) accreditation Control codes 61, 63, 64, 71, 72 and 73 indicate hospitals listed by AOHA, but not registered by AHA. For definition of numerical codes, see page A4	Control	Service	Beds	Admissions	Census	Outpatient Visits	Births	Total	Payroll	Personnel
☐ HOLLYWOOD PAVILION, 1201 North 37th Avenue, Zip 33021; tel. 954/962–1355; Karen Kallen–Zury, Chief Executive Officer (Nonreporting) **A**1 10	33	22	46	—	—	—	—	—	—	—
★ △ MEMORIAL REGIONAL HOSPITAL, 3501 Johnson Street, Zip 33021–5421; tel. 954/987–2000; Patricia A. Flury, Administrator (Total facility includes 120 beds in nursing home–type unit) **A**1 2 3 7 9 10 **F**1 2 3 4 5 7 8 9 10 11 12 14 15 16 17 18 19 20 21 22 23 24 25 26 27 28 29 30 31 32 33 34 35 37 38 39 40 41 42 43 44 47 48 49 51 52 56 57 58 59 60 61 64 65 66 67 69 70 71 72 73 74 **P**1 3 4 5 7 8 **S** Memorial Healthcare System, Hollywood, FL **N** Memorial Healthcare System, Hollywood, FL	16	10	792	26506	537	366638	3193	241061	101983	3510
HOMESTEAD—Dade County										
☐ HOMESTEAD HOSPITAL, 160 N.W. 13th Street, Zip 33030–4299; tel. 305/248–3232; Bo Boulenger, Chief Executive Officer **A**1 9 10 **F**2 3 4 5 7 8 10 11 12 14 15 16 17 18 19 20 21 22 23 24 25 26 27 28 29 30 31 32 33 34 35 37 38 39 40 41 42 43 44 45 46 47 48 49 50 51 52 60 61 63 64 65 66 67 68 71 72 73 74 **P**1 3 5 6 7 8 **N** Dimensions Health/Baptist Health Systems, Miami, FL	23	10	100	5094	58	42141	827	29988	12299	474
HUDSON—Pasco County										
★ COLUMBIA REGIONAL MEDICAL CENTER AT BAYONET POINT, 14000 Fivay Road, Zip 34667–7199; tel. 813/863–2411; J. Daniel Miller, President and Chief Executive Officer **A**1 9 10 **F**2 3 4 5 7 8 10 11 12 13 14 15 16 17 18 19 21 22 23 24 25 26 28 29 30 32 34 35 37 38 40 41 42 43 44 45 46 48 49 50 51 52 60 64 65 66 67 71 72 73 74 **P**1 **S** Columbia/HCA Healthcare Corporation, Nashville, TN **N** Columbia/HCA Tampa Bay Division, Tampa, FL; The Health Advantage Network, Winter Park, FL	33	10	256	12000	158	60000	0	—	—	1054
INVERNESS—Citrus County										
★ CITRUS MEMORIAL HOSPITAL, 502 Highland Boulevard, Zip 34452–4754; tel. 904/726–1551; Charles A. Blasband, Chief Executive Officer **A**1 9 10 **F**7 8 10 12 14 15 19 21 22 25 28 30 32 34 35 36 37 39 40 44 49 51 65 67 71 72 73 **P**7	23	10	171	8165	104	143322	519	60956	21143	790
JACKSONVILLE—Duval County										
★ BAPTIST MEDICAL CENTER, 800 Prudential Drive, Zip 32207–8203; tel. 904/202–2000; William C. Mason, Chief Executive Officer **A**1 2 3 5 9 10 **F**2 3 4 7 8 10 11 12 13 14 15 16 17 18 19 20 21 22 23 24 25 26 27 28 29 30 31 32 33 34 35 36 37 38 39 40 41 42 43 44 45 46 47 49 51 52 53 54 55 56 57 58 59 60 61 64 65 66 67 68 69 71 72 73 74 **P**1 2 5 6 8 **N** Baptist/St. Vincent's Health System, Jacksonville, FL	23	10	501	22501	300	378425	4196	201879	79132	3460
☐ BHC ST. JOHNS RIVER HOSPITAL, (formerly CPC St. Johns River Hospital), 6300 Beach Boulevard, Zip 32216; tel. 904/724–9202; Patricia Vandergrift, Administrator **A**1 10 **F**2 3 14 15 16 19 21 22 27 35 52 53 54 55 56 57 58 59 65 67 **S** Behavioral Healthcare Corporation, Nashville, TN	33	22	60	1728	37	7474	0	5569	2980	89
★ COLUMBIA MEMORIAL HOSPITAL JACKSONVILLE, 3625 University Boulevard South, Zip 32216, Mailing Address: Box 16325, Zip 32216; tel. 904/399–6111; Winston Rushing, President **A**1 2 9 10 **F**1 3 4 7 8 10 11 12 14 16 17 18 19 21 22 23 24 25 27 28 29 30 32 33 34 35 37 38 39 40 41 42 43 44 45 46 47 48 49 50 51 52 53 54 55 56 58 59 61 64 65 67 70 71 73 74 **P**1 3 7 **S** Columbia/HCA Healthcare Corporation, Nashville, TN **N** Columbia/HCA North & NorthEast Florida Division, Jacksonville, FL; The Health Advantage Network, Winter Park, FL	32	10	310	16618	220	128092	2437	113859	45027	1377
★ COLUMBIA SPECIALTY HOSPITAL JACKSONVILLE, (LONG TERM ACUTE CARE), 4901 Richard Street, Zip 32207; tel. 904/737–3120; W. Raymond C. Ford, Administrator and Chief Executive Officer **A**1 10 **F**3 4 7 8 9 10 11 12 14 16 17 19 21 22 23 24 25 26 27 28 29 30 31 32 33 34 35 37 39 40 41 42 43 44 45 46 48 49 50 51 54 55 56 57 58 59 60 61 65 66 67 71 73 74 **P**7 8 **S** Columbia/HCA Healthcare Corporation, Nashville, TN **N** Columbia/HCA North & NorthEast Florida Division, Jacksonville, FL; The Health Advantage Network, Winter Park, FL	33	49	61	611	48	0	0	18109	6970	155
CPC ST. JOHNS RIVER HOSPITAL See BHC St. Johns River Hospital										
★ △ GENESIS REHABILITATION HOSPITAL, 3599 University Boulevard South, Zip 32216–4211, Mailing Address: P.O. Box 16406, Zip 32245–6406; tel. 904/858–7600; Stephen K. Wilson, President **A**1 7 10 **F**3 4 5 7 8 9 10 11 12 14 15 16 17 19 21 22 23 24 25 26 27 28 29 30 31 32 33 34 35 37 38 39 40 41 42 43 44 45 46 47 48 49 50 51 60 61 64 65 66 67 69 71 72 73 74 **P**5 8 **N** Genesis Health, Inc., Jacksonville, FL	23	46	110	1471	106	—	0	24152	12940	331
★ METHODIST MEDICAL CENTER, 580 West Eighth Street, Zip 32209–6553; tel. 904/798–8000; Marcus E. Drewa, President **A**1 5 9 **F**4 8 10 11 12 14 15 16 17 19 22 26 28 29 30 31 32 33 34 35 37 39 41 44 45 49 51 65 67 69 71 73 74 **P**7 **S** Methodist Health System, Jacksonville, FL **N** Methodist Health Systems, Jacksonville, FL	23	10	160	7046	118	42677	0	67783	22434	744
METHODIST PATHWAY CENTER, 580 West Eighth Street, Zip 32209–6553; tel. 904/798–8250; Marcus E. Drewa, President (Nonreporting) **A**10 **S** Methodist Health System, Jacksonville, FL **N** Methodist Health Systems, Jacksonville, FL	23	82	25	—	—	—	—	—	—	—
★ NAVAL HOSPITAL, 2080 Child Street, Zip 32214–5000; tel. 904/777–7300; Captain M. J. Benson, MSC, USN, Commanding Officer (Nonreporting) **A**1 3 5 **S** Department of Navy, Washington, DC	43	10	96	—	—	—	—	—	—	—
★ ST. LUKE'S HOSPITAL, 4201 Belfort Road, Zip 32216; tel. 904/296–3700; J. Larry Read, President (Total facility includes 17 beds in nursing home–type unit) **A**1 2 3 5 8 9 10 **F**4 8 9 10 11 12 19 21 22 23 25 28 30 32 34 35 37 39 41 42 43 44 49 51 60 63 64 65 66 67 69 71 73 **P**3 6 **S** Mayo Foundation, Rochester, MN	23	10	220	7365	115	51114	0	95545	35754	1336

Hospital, Address, Telephone, Administrator, Approval, Facility, and Physician Codes, Health Care System, Network	Classification Codes		Utilization Data					Expense (thousands) of dollars		
	Control	Service	Beds	Admissions	Census	Outpatient Visits	Births	Total	Payroll	Personnel

★ = American Hospital Association (AHA) membership
□ = Joint Commission on Accreditation of Healthcare Organizations (JCAHO) accreditation
+ = American Osteopathic Hospital Association (AOHA) membership
○ = American Osteopathic Association (AOA) accreditation
△ = Commission on Accreditation of Rehabilitation Facilities (CARF) accreditation
Control codes 61, 63, 64, 71, 72 and 73 indicate hospitals listed by AOHA, but not registered by AHA. For definition of numerical codes, see page A4

Hospital	Control	Service	Beds	Admissions	Census	Outpatient Visits	Births	Total	Payroll	Personnel
☒ ST. VINCENT'S MEDICAL CENTER, 1800 Barrs Street, Zip 32204, Mailing Address: P.O. Box 2982, Zip 32203–2982; tel. 904/308–7300; John W. Logue, Executive Vice President and Chief Operating Officer (Total facility includes 240 beds in nursing home–type unit) **A**1 2 3 5 9 10 **F**2 4 7 8 10 11 12 14 15 16 17 18 19 21 22 23 24 25 26 27 28 29 30 31 32 34 35 37 38 39 40 41 42 43 44 45 46 47 49 51 52 53 54 56 57 59 60 61 64 65 66 67 71 73 74 **P**5 **S** Daughters of Charity National Health System, Saint Louis, MO **N** Baptist/St. Vincent's Health System, Jacksonville, FL	21	10	756	22747	559	254229	2082	206755	83897	2702
□ UNIVERSITY MEDICAL CENTER, 655 West Eighth Street, Zip 32209; tel. 904/549–5000; W. A. McGriff, III, President and Chief Executive Officer **A**1 2 3 5 8 9 10 **F**1 4 7 8 10 11 12 14 15 16 17 18 19 20 21 22 28 30 31 34 35 37 38 40 41 42 43 44 45 46 47 49 51 52 53 54 55 56 58 60 61 63 65 69 70 71 73 74	23	10	518	18719	275	292711	2931	208283	68068	2248
JACKSONVILLE BEACH—Duval County										
□ BAPTIST MEDICAL CENTER–BEACHES, 1350 13th Avenue South, Zip 32250–3205; tel. 904/247–2900; Jerry L. Miller, Administrator **A**1 9 10 **F**4 7 8 10 11 12 19 21 22 24 28 30 32 33 35 37 40 41 42 43 44 45 46 47 49 52 54 56 59 60 63 65 71 73 **P**5 **N** Baptist/St. Vincent's Health System, Jacksonville, FL	23	10	76	3054	40	52789	0	26231	10428	464
JASPER—Hamilton County										
★ COLUMBIA HAMILTON MEDICAL CENTER, 506 N.W. Fourth Street, Zip 32052; tel. 904/792–7200; Amelia Tuten, R.N., Administrator (Nonreporting) **A**9 10 **S** Columbia/HCA Healthcare Corporation, Nashville, TN **N** Columbia/HCA North & NorthEast Florida Division, Jacksonville, FL; The Health Advantage Network, Winter Park, FL	33	10	42							
JAY—Santa Rosa County										
JAY HOSPITAL, 221 South Alabama Street, Zip 32565, Mailing Address: P.O. Box 397, Zip 32565; tel. 904/675–8000; H. D. Cannington, Administrator **A**9 10 **F**8 12 15 17 19 21 22 27 28 30 32 33 34 35 39 44 49 63 64 65 71 73 **P**4 5 7 **S** Baptist Health Care Corporation, Pensacola, FL **N** Baptist Health Care, Inc., Pensacola, FL	23	10	47	1543	28	22820	—	8225	3325	133
JUPITER—Palm Beach County										
☒ JUPITER MEDICAL CENTER, 1210 South Old Dixie Highway, Zip 33458; tel. 407/747–2234; Donald A. Mayer, Chief Executive Officer (Total facility includes 120 beds in nursing home–type unit) **A**1 2 9 10 **F**8 19 21 22 31 32 34 35 37 44 64 65 71 73 **P**7 **S** Quorum Health Group/Quorum Health Resources, Inc., Brentwood, TN	23	10	276	6472	190	55740	0	68609	27750	783
KEY WEST—Monroe County										
DE POO HOSPITAL See Lower Florida Keys Health System										
FLORIDA KEYS MEMORIAL HOSPITAL See Lower Florida Keys Health System										
☒ LOWER FLORIDA KEYS HEALTH SYSTEM, (Includes De Poo Hospital, 1200 Kennedy Drive, Zip 33041; tel. 305/294–4692; Florida Keys Memorial Hospital, 5900 College Road, tel. 305/294–5531), 5900 College Road, Zip 33040, Mailing Address: P.O. Box 9107, Zip 33041–9107; tel. 305/294–5531; James K. Simon, President and Chief Executive Officer (Nonreporting) **A**1 9 10	23	10	169	—						
KISSIMMEE—Osceola County										
□ CHARTER HOSPITAL ORLANDO SOUTH, 206 Park Place Drive, Zip 34741; tel. 407/846–0444; Daniel Kearney, Chief Executive Officer **A**1 10 **F**2 3 14 22 26 29 30 34 45 52 53 54 55 56 57 58 59 65 67 **P**6 **S** Magellan Health Services, Atlanta, GA	33	22	60	1254	38	5090	0	8036	2869	74
☒ COLUMBIA MEDICAL CENTER–OSCEOLA, (Formerly Columbia Osceola Regional Hospital), 700 West Oak Street, Zip 34741, Mailing Address: P.O. Box 422589, Zip 34742–2589; tel. 407/846–2266; E. Tim Cook, Chief Executive Officer (Nonreporting) **A**1 9 10 **S** Columbia/HCA Healthcare Corporation, Nashville, TN **N** Columbia/HCA Central Florida Division, Winter Park, FL; The Health Advantage Network, Winter Park, FL	33	10	156							
COLUMBIA OSCEOLA REGIONAL HOSPITAL See Columbia Medical Center–Osceola										
FLORIDA HOSPITAL KISSIMMEE See Florida Hospital, Orlando										
LAKE BUTLER—Union County										
NORTH FLORIDA RECEPTION CENTER HOSPITAL, Mailing Address: P.O. Box 628, Zip 32054–0628; tel. 904/496–6111; Bob Torrescano, Administrator **F**19 21 35 44 50 52 56 58 60 63 65 71 72	12	11	153	1843	95	37812	0	—	—	288
LAKE CITY—Columbia County										
☒ COLUMBIA LAKE CITY MEDICAL CENTER, 1701 West U.S. Highway 90, Zip 32055; tel. 904/752–2922; David P. Steitz, Chief Executive Officer (Total facility includes 5 beds in nursing home–type unit) **A**1 9 10 **F**8 12 14 15 16 17 19 21 22 23 26 28 31 32 33 34 35 37 39 41 44 45 49 52 54 55 56 57 58 59 63 64 65 66 71 73 **P**7 **S** Columbia/HCA Healthcare Corporation, Nashville, TN **N** Columbia/HCA North & NorthEast Florida Division, Jacksonville, FL; The Health Advantage Network, Winter Park, FL	33	10	75	3260	49	184620	0	27217	12870	439
LAKE SHORE HOSPITAL See Shands at Lake Shore										
☒ SHANDS AT LAKE SHORE, (Formerly Lake Shore Hospital), 560 East Franklin Street, Zip 32055, Mailing Address: Box 1989, Zip 32056–1989; tel. 904/755–3200; Linda A. McKnew, R.N., Chief Operating Officer **A**1 9 10 **F**1 2 3 4 5 7 8 9 10 11 12 14 15 16 17 18 19 20 21 22 23 24 26 28 29 30 31 32 34 35 36 37 38 39 40 41 42 43 44 46 47 48 49 51 52 53 56 57 59 60 61 64 65 66 67 69 71 73 **S** Shands Health System, University of Florida Health Science Center, Gainesville, FL	23	10	128	1522	41	28762	173	7585	3381	269

Hospital, Address, Telephone, Administrator, Approval, Facility, and Physician Codes, Health Care System, Network	Classi- fication Codes		Utilization Data					Expense (thousands) of dollars		
★ American Hospital Association (AHA) membership □ Joint Commission on Accreditation of Healthcare Organizations (JCAHO) accreditation + American Osteopathic Hospital Association (AOHA) membership ○ American Osteopathic Association (AOA) accreditation △ Commission on Accreditation of Rehabilitation Facilities (CARF) accreditation Control codes 61, 63, 64, 71, 72 and 73 indicate hospitals listed by AOHA, but not registered by AHA. For definition of numerical codes, see page A4	Control	Service	Beds	Admissions	Census	Outpatient Visits	Births	Total	Payroll	Personnel

✦ VETERANS AFFAIRS MEDICAL CENTER, 801 South Marion Street, Zip 32025–5898; tel. 904/755–3016; Alline L. Norman, Director (Total facility includes 180 beds in nursing home–type unit) **A**1 3 5 **F**2 3 11 15 16 19 20 21 22 25 26 28 32 33 34 37 39 41 44 45 46 48 49 51 52 54 55 56 58 64 65 67 71 73 74 **S** Department of Veterans Affairs, Washington, DC	45	10	360	5256	333	72889	0	65397	44098	942
LAKE WALES—Polk County										
✦ LAKE WALES MEDICAL CENTERS, 410 South 11th Street, Zip 33853, Mailing Address: P.O. Box 3460, Zip 33859–3460; tel. 941/676–1433; Joe M. Connell, Chief Executive Officer (Total facility includes 177 beds in nursing home–type unit) **A**1 9 10 **F**2 3 7 8 10 11 13 14 17 19 21 22 23 24 26 28 29 30 32 33 35 36 37 38 39 40 41 42 43 44 45 46 47 48 49 51 52 53 54 55 56 57 58 59 60 63 64 65 67 71 72 73 74 **P**6 **N** Mid–Florida Medical Services, Inc., Winter Haven, FL	23	10	264	2821	195	42693	280	25778	15392	510
LAKELAND—Polk County										
□ HEART OF FLORIDA BEHAVIORAL CENTER, 2510 North Florida Avenue, Zip 33805; tel. 941/682–6105; David M. Polunas, Administrator and Chief Executive Officer (Nonreporting) **A**1 10 **S** Health Management Associates, Naples, FL	33	22	66	—	—	—	—	—	—	—
✦ LAKELAND REGIONAL MEDICAL CENTER, 1324 Lakeland Hills Boulevard, Zip 33805–4543, Mailing Address: P.O. Box 95448, Zip 33804–5448; tel. 941/687–1100; Jack T. Stephens, Jr., President and Chief Executive Officer **A**1 2 5 9 10 **F**2 3 4 7 10 11 14 15 16 17 19 21 22 23 26 27 28 29 30 34 37 38 39 40 42 43 44 47 52 53 54 55 56 57 58 59 60 65 67 71 72 73 74	23	10	649	24599	354	129887	2502	206776	89606	2210
LANTANA—Palm Beach County										
A. G. HOLLEY STATE HOSPITAL, 1199 West Lantana Road, Zip 33462, Mailing Address: Box 3084, Zip 33465–3084; tel. 407/582–5666; David Ashkin, M.D., Medical Executive Director (Nonreporting) **A**10	12	33	50	—	—	—	—	—	—	—
LARGO—Pinellas County										
□ CHARTER BEHAVIORAL HEALTH SYSTEM AT MEDFIELD, 12891 Seminole Boulevard, Zip 34648–2300; tel. 813/587–6000; Jim Hill, Chief Executive Officer (Nonreporting) **A**1 10 **S** Magellan Health Services, Atlanta, GA	33	22	64	—	—	—	—	—	—	—
✦ COLUMBIA LARGO MEDICAL CENTER, 201 14th Street S.W., Zip 33770, Mailing Address: P.O. Box 2905, Zip 33779; tel. 813/586–1411; Thomas L. Herron, FACHE, President and Chief Executive Officer (Total facility includes 13 beds in nursing home–type unit) **A**1 2 9 10 **F**4 8 10 11 12 14 15 16 17 19 21 22 23 27 28 29 30 32 33 34 35 37 38 39 40 41 42 43 44 45 49 51 60 61 64 65 67 70 71 72 73 74 **P**1 2 7 **S** Columbia/HCA Healthcare Corporation, Nashville, TN **N** Columbia/HCA Tampa Bay Division, Tampa, FL; The Health Advantage Network, Winter Park, FL	33	10	243	9529	127	51466	0	—	—	731
□ △ HEALTHSOUTH REHABILITATION HOSPITAL, 901 North Clearwater–Largo Road, Zip 34640–1955; tel. 813/586–2999; Vincent O. Nico, Regional Vice President (Nonreporting) **A**1 7 10 **S** HEALTHSOUTH Corporation, Birmingham, AL	33	46	60	—	—	—	—	—	—	—
✦ + ○ SUN COAST HOSPITAL, 2025 Indian Rocks Road, Zip 34644, Mailing Address: Box 2025, Zip 34649–2025; tel. 813/581–9474; Jeffrey A. Collins, Chief Executive Officer (Total facility includes 14 beds in nursing home–type unit) (Nonreporting) **A**1 10 11 12 13 **S** Quorum Health Group/Quorum Health Resources, Inc., Brentwood, TN	23	10	241	—	—	—	—	—	—	—
LECANTO—Citrus County										
□ HERITAGE BEVERLY HILLS HOSPITAL, 2804 West Marc Knighton Court, Zip 34461; tel. 352/746–9000; Charles Visalli, Administrator **A**1 10 **F**15 16 52 53 54 55 56 57 58 59 **P**1 5	33	22	88	1125	48	0	0	5016	2882	104
LEESBURG—Lake County										
✦ △ LEESBURG REGIONAL MEDICAL CENTER, 600 East Dixie Avenue, Zip 34748; tel. 352/323–5000; Joe D. DePew, President and Chief Executive Officer (Total facility includes 120 beds in nursing home–type unit) **A**1 7 9 10 **F**7 8 10 12 14 15 19 21 22 23 24 25 26 28 30 32 37 40 41 42 44 46 48 49 63 64 65 71 72 73 **S** Quorum Health Group/Quorum Health Resources, Inc., Brentwood, TN	23	10	414	10856	137	68735	1065	75311	29098	1008
LEHIGH ACRES—Lee County										
✦ COLUMBIA EAST POINTE HOSPITAL, 1500 Lee Boulevard, Zip 33936; tel. 941/369–2101; Valerie A. Jackson, Chief Executive Officer (Total facility includes 13 beds in nursing home–type unit) **A**1 9 10 **F**4 6 7 8 10 11 12 13 14 15 16 17 18 19 20 21 22 23 26 27 28 29 30 31 32 33 34 35 36 37 39 40 41 42 43 44 45 46 47 48 49 55 56 57 59 60 61 63 64 65 66 67 68 69 70 71 72 73 74 **P**7 8 **S** Columbia/HCA Healthcare Corporation, Nashville, TN **N** Columbia/HCA SouthWest Florida Division, Fort Myers, FL; The Health Advantage Network, Winter Park, FL	33	10	88	2516	36	27820	210	20981	9313	242
LIVE OAK—Suwannee County										
✦ SHANDS AT LIVE OAK, (Formerly Suwannee Hospital), 1100 S.W. 11th Avenue, Zip 32060, Mailing Address: P.O. Drawer X, Zip 32060; tel. 904/362–1413; Rhonda Sherrod, Administrator (Nonreporting) **A**1 9 10 **S** Shands Health System, University of Florida Health Science Center, Gainesville, FL	23	10	16	—	—	—	—	—	—	—
LONGWOOD—Seminole County										
✦ SOUTH SEMINOLE HOSPITAL, (Formerly Columbia South Seminole Hospital), 555 West State Road 434, Zip 32750; tel. 407/767–1200; Sue Whelan–Williams, Site Administrator **A**1 9 10 **F**2 3 4 7 8 9 10 11 12 13 14 15 19 21 22 23 24 26 27 28 29 30 31 32 33 34 35 37 38 40 42 43 44 46 47 48 49 52 53 54 55 56 57 58 59 60 63 64 65 70 71 73 74 **S** Orlando Regional Healthcare System, Orlando, FL **N** Orlando Regional Healthcare System, Orlando, FL; Columbia/HCA Central Florida Division, Winter Park, FL; The Health Advantage Network, Winter Park, FL	32	10	206	5659	73	81965	827	34682	15012	382

Hospital, Address, Telephone, Administrator, Approval, Facility, and Physician Codes, Health Care System, Network	Classification Codes		Utilization Data					Expense (thousands) of dollars		
	Control	Service	Beds	Admissions	Census	Outpatient Visits	Births	Total	Payroll	Personnel

★ American Hospital Association (AHA) membership
□ Joint Commission on Accreditation of Healthcare Organizations (JCAHO) accreditation
+ American Osteopathic Hospital Association (AOHA) membership
○ American Osteopathic Association (AOA) accreditation
△ Commission on Accreditation of Rehabilitation Facilities (CARF) accreditation
Control codes 61, 63, 64, 71, 72 and 73 indicate hospitals listed by AOHA, but not registered by AHA. For definition of numerical codes, see page A4

LOXAHATCHEE—Palm Beach County

| ⊞ COLUMBIA PALMS WEST HOSPITAL, 13001 Southern Boulevard, Zip 33470–1150; tel. 407/798–3300; Alex M. Marceline, Chief Executive Officer (Nonreporting) **A**1 9 10 **S** Columbia/HCA Healthcare Corporation, Nashville, TN **N** Med Connect, Ft Lauderdale, FL; Columbia/HCA South Florida Division, Miami Lakes, FL; The Health Advantage Network, Winter Park, FL | 33 | 10 | 117 | — | — | — | — | — | — | — |

LUTZ—Hillsborough County

| □ CHARTER HOSPITAL OF PASCO, 21808 State Road 54, Zip 33549; tel. 813/948–2441; Miriam K. Williams, Administrator **A**1 10 **F**2 3 15 52 54 55 56 57 58 59 65 67 **S** Magellan Health Services, Atlanta, GA | 33 | 22 | 72 | 1321 | 36 | 0 | 0 | — | — | 69 |

MACCLENNY—Baker County

| ED FRASER MEMORIAL HOSPITAL, 159 North Third Street, Zip 32063–0484; tel. 904/259–3151; Dennis R. Markos, Chief Executive Officer (Total facility includes 62 beds in nursing home–type unit) (Nonreporting) **A**9 10 | 23 | 10 | 68 | — | — | — | — | — | — | — |

MACDILL AFB—Hillsborough County

| ⊞ U. S. AIR FORCE HOSPITAL, 8415 Bayshore Boulevard, Zip 33621–1607; tel. 813/828–3258; Colonel Roger H. Bower, MC, USAF, Commander (Nonreporting) **A**1 **S** Department of the Air Force, Washington, DC | 41 | 10 | 50 | — | — | — | — | — | — | — |

MADISON—Madison County

| MADISON COUNTY MEMORIAL HOSPITAL, 201 East Marion Street, Zip 32340; tel. 904/973–2271; Miriam Ross, Acting Administrator **A**9 10 **F**8 11 15 20 26 27 28 30 32 36 39 44 49 51 65 67 68 71 74 **P**5 | 23 | 10 | 26 | 364 | 6 | 10356 | 0 | 4223 | 2437 | 102 |

MARATHON—Monroe County

| □ FISHERMEN'S HOSPITAL, 3301 Overseas Highway, Zip 33050–0068; tel. 305/743–5533; Patrice L. Tavernier, Administrator (Nonreporting) **A**1 9 10 **S** Health Management Associates, Naples, FL | 33 | 10 | 58 | — | — | — | — | — | — | — |

MARGATE—Broward County

| ⊞ COLUMBIA NORTHWEST MEDICAL CENTER, 2801 North State Road 7, Zip 33063, Mailing Address: P.O. Box 639002, Zip 33063–9002; tel. 305/978–4000; Gina Becker, Acting Chief Executive Officer **A**1 9 10 **F**2 7 8 9 12 15 17 19 22 24 27 28 29 30 32 33 34 35 37 38 39 40 44 46 47 48 49 52 61 64 66 67 71 73 74 **S** Columbia/HCA Healthcare Corporation, Nashville, TN **N** Columbia/HCA South Florida Division, Miami Lakes, FL; The Health Advantage Network, Winter Park, FL | 33 | 10 | 150 | 6617 | 78 | 44156 | 775 | 38162 | 16883 | 477 |

MARIANNA—Jackson County

| ⊞ JACKSON HOSPITAL, 4250 Hospital Drive, Zip 32446, Mailing Address: P.O. Box 1608, Zip 32447–1608; tel. 904/526–2200; Richard L. Wooten, Administrator **A**1 9 10 **F**7 8 12 15 16 17 19 21 22 23 24 28 30 31 34 35 37 40 44 45 46 49 65 66 71 73 **P**5 **S** Quorum Health Group/Quorum Health Resources, Inc., Brentwood, TN **N** Panhandle Area Health Network, Marianna, FL | 16 | 10 | 84 | 3490 | 44 | 41783 | 682 | 21424 | 8645 | 326 |

MELBOURNE—Brevard County

□ CIRCLES OF CARE, 400 East Sheridan Road, Zip 32901–3184; tel. 407/722–5200; James B. Whitaker, President (Nonreporting) **A**1 10	23	22	72	—	—	—	—	—	—	—
DEVEREUX HOSPITAL AND CHILDREN'S CENTER OF FLORIDA, 8000 Devereux Drive, Zip 32940–7907; tel. 407/242–9100; James E. Colvin, Executive Director **F**52 53 **P**6 **S** Devereux Foundation, Devon, PA	23	52	100	92	99	0	0	9972	5175	219
□ △ HEALTHSOUTH SEA PINES REHABILITATION HOSPITAL, 101 East Florida Avenue, Zip 32901–9966; tel. 407/984–4600; Henry J. Cranston, Chief Operating Officer (Nonreporting) **A**1 7 10 **S** HEALTHSOUTH Corporation, Birmingham, AL	33	46	80	—	—	—	—	—	—	—
⊞ HOLMES REGIONAL MEDICAL CENTER, 1350 South Hickory Street, Zip 32901; tel. 407/727–7000; Stephen P. Bunker, President and Chief Operating Officer (Total facility includes 30 beds in nursing home–type unit) **A**1 2 9 10 **F**4 7 8 10 11 12 13 15 16 17 19 21 22 23 24 25 27 28 29 30 32 33 34 35 37 38 39 40 41 42 43 44 45 46 49 51 54 56 60 61 63 64 65 66 67 71 72 73 74 **P**6 7	23	10	528	23643	308	194501	2117	181387	73431	3067

MIAMI—Dade County

⊞ △ BAPTIST HOSPITAL OF MIAMI, 8900 North Kendall Drive, Zip 33176–2197; tel. 305/596–6503; Fred M. Messing, Chief Executive Officer **A**1 2 3 7 9 10 **F**2 3 4 5 7 8 10 12 14 15 16 17 19 21 22 24 25 26 27 28 29 30 31 32 33 34 35 37 38 40 41 42 43 44 45 46 47 49 50 60 61 63 64 65 66 67 71 72 73 74 **P**1 5 6 7 **N** Dimensions Health/Baptist Health Systems, Miami, FL	23	10	392	23790	334	—	3692	219076	91804	2874
⊞ BASCOM PALMER EYE INSTITUTE–ANNE BATES LEACH EYE HOSPITAL, 900 N.W. 17th Street, Zip 33136–1199, Mailing Address: Box 016880, Zip 33101–6880; tel. 305/326–6000; David Bixler, Administrator **A**1 3 5 9 10 **F**22 27 30 34 39 41 44 45 46 60 65 69 71 73 **P**6 **S** Quorum Health Group/Quorum Health Resources, Inc., Brentwood, TN	23	45	35	1052	5	128853	0	28778	12915	419
CHARTER HOSPITAL OF MIAMI See Columbia Behavioral Health Center										
⊞ COLUMBIA AVENTURA HOSPITAL AND MEDICAL CENTER, 20900 Biscayne Boulevard, Zip 33180–1407; tel. 305/682–7100; Davide M. Carbone, Chief Executive Officer **A**1 9 10 **F**1 2 3 4 5 7 8 10 11 12 13 14 15 16 17 18 19 20 21 22 23 25 26 27 28 29 30 31 32 33 34 35 37 38 39 40 42 43 44 45 46 47 49 51 52 53 54 55 56 57 58 59 60 61 63 64 65 67 71 72 73 74 **P**5 7 **S** Columbia/HCA Healthcare Corporation, Nashville, TN **N** Columbia/HCA South Florida Division, Miami Lakes, FL; The Health Advantage Network, Winter Park, FL	33	10	407	12245	168	57187	604	76412	28234	850
□ COLUMBIA BEHAVIORAL HEALTH CENTER, (Formerly Charter Hospital of Miami), 11100 N.W. 27th Street, Zip 33172; tel. 305/591–3230; Cheryl Siegwald–Mays, Administrator **A**1 10 **F**1 3 4 5 7 8 11 12 14 15 16 17 18 19 21 22 26 27 28 30 31 32 34 35 37 42 43 44 45 49 52 53 54 55 56 57 58 59 60 61 63 65 67 71 72 73 74 **S** Columbia/HCA Healthcare Corporation, Nashville, TN	33	22	88	806	17	164	0	2979	1244	86

Hospital, Address, Telephone, Administrator, Approval, Facility, and Physician Codes, Health Care System, Network	Classi-fication Codes		Utilization Data					Expense (thousands) of dollars		
	Control	Service	Beds	Admissions	Census	Outpatient Visits	Births	Total	Payroll	Personnel

★ American Hospital Association (AHA) membership
□ Joint Commission on Accreditation of Healthcare Organizations (JCAHO) accreditation
+ American Osteopathic Hospital Association (AOHA) membership
○ American Osteopathic Association (AOA) accreditation
△ Commission on Accreditation of Rehabilitation Facilities (CARF) accreditation
Control codes 61, 63, 64, 71, 72 and 73 indicate hospitals listed by AOHA, but not registered by AHA. For definition of numerical codes, see page A4

✠ COLUMBIA CEDARS MEDICAL CENTER, (Includes Victoria Pavilion, 955 N.W. Third Street, Zip 33128, Mailing Address: Box 016216, Flagler Station, Zip 33101; tel. 305/545–8050), 1400 N.W. 12th Avenue, Zip 33136–1003; tel. 305/325–5511; Ralph A. Aleman, Chief Executive Officer **A**1 2 3 5 10 **F**1 2 3 4 5 8 10 11 12 14 15 16 17 19 21 22 23 25 26 27 28 30 31 32 34 35 37 39 40 41 42 43 44 45 46 49 52 53 54 55 56 57 58 59 60 63 64 65 67 71 73 74 **P**3 6 7 **S** Columbia/HCA Healthcare Corporation, Nashville, TN **N** Columbia/HCA South Florida Division, Miami Lakes, FL; The Health Advantage Network, Winter Park, FL	32	10	500	19620	336	77467	0	133490	56048	1567
✠ COLUMBIA DEERING HOSPITAL, 9333 S.W. 152nd Street, Zip 33157; tel. 305/256–5100; Anthony M. Degina, Jr., Chief Executive Officer (Nonreporting) **A**1 9 10 **S** Columbia/HCA Healthcare Corporation, Nashville, TN **N** Columbia/HCA South Florida Division, Miami Lakes, FL; The Health Advantage Network, Winter Park, FL	33	10	233							
✠ COLUMBIA KENDALL MEDICAL CENTER, (Formerly Columbia Kendall Regional Medical Center), 11750 Bird Road, Zip 33175–3530; tel. 305/223–3000; Victor Maya, Chief Executive Officer **A**1 9 10 **F**1 2 3 4 5 7 8 10 11 12 14 15 16 19 20 21 22 23 26 27 28 30 31 32 33 34 35 37 39 40 41 42 43 44 45 46 48 49 52 53 54 55 56 57 58 59 60 63 65 67 68 69 71 72 73 **P**2 3 4 5 **S** Columbia/HCA Healthcare Corporation, Nashville, TN **N** Columbia/HCA South Florida Division, Miami Lakes, FL; The Health Advantage Network, Winter Park, FL GOLDEN GLADES REGIONAL MEDICAL CENTER See Parkway Regional Medical Center–West	32	10	235	10599	157	134604	560	79466	29022	746
□ HARBOR VIEW, 1861 N.W. South River Drive, Zip 33125; tel. 305/642–3555; Nelson Rodney, Administrator **A**1 10 **F**16 52 54 55	33	22	94	1146	57	0	0	7252	3515	126
□ HEALTHSOUTH REHABILITATION HOSPITAL, 20601 Old Cutler Road, Zip 33189; tel. 305/251–3800; Jude Torchia, Chief Executive Officer (Nonreporting) **A**1 10 **S** HEALTHSOUTH Corporation, Birmingham, AL HIGHLAND PARK HOSPITAL See Jackson Memorial Hospital	33	46	45							
✠ △ JACKSON MEMORIAL HOSPITAL, (Includes Highland Park Hospital, 1660 N.W. Seventh Court, Zip 33136; tel. 305/324–8111; Stuart Podolnick, Administrator), 1611 N.W. 12th Avenue, Zip 33136–1094; tel. 305/585–6754; Ira C. Clark, President **A**1 2 3 5 6 7 8 9 10 **F**1 2 3 4 5 7 8 9 10 11 12 13 14 15 16 17 18 19 20 21 22 23 24 25 26 27 28 29 30 31 32 34 35 37 38 39 40 41 42 43 44 45 46 47 48 49 51 52 53 54 55 56 57 58 59 60 61 63 64 65 66 67 68 69 70 71 72 73 74 **P**6	13	10	1376	49223	967	485683	5957	666149	288937	8053
✠ △ MERCY HOSPITAL, 3663 South Miami Avenue, Zip 33133–4237; tel. 305/854–4400; Edward J. Rosasco, Jr., President **A**1 2 6 7 9 10 **F**3 4 5 7 8 10 11 12 14 15 16 17 18 19 21 22 23 25 26 27 28 29 30 31 32 33 34 35 37 38 39 40 41 42 43 44 45 46 48 49 50 51 52 54 55 57 58 59 60 61 63 64 65 66 67 68 69 71 72 73 74 **P**4 5 8	21	10	365	15444	259	131549	1968	137247	60466	1735
✠ MIAMI CHILDREN'S HOSPITAL, 3100 S.W. 62nd Avenue, Zip 33155–3009; tel. 305/666–6511; William A. McDonald, President and Chief Executive Officer **A**1 3 5 9 10 **F**2 3 4 5 6 7 8 10 11 12 13 14 17 18 19 20 21 22 23 24 25 26 27 28 29 30 31 32 33 34 35 37 38 39 41 42 43 44 45 46 47 49 51 52 53 54 55 56 57 58 59 60 61 64 65 66 67 68 69 70 71 72 73 74 **P**1 7	23	50	268	8399	161	186859	0	171765	82277	2250
✠ MIAMI HEART INSTITUTE, (Includes Miami Heart Institute–South, 250 63rd Street, Zip 33141; tel. 305/672–1111), 4701 Meridian Avenue, Zip 33140–2910; tel. 305/674–3114; Tim Parker, Chief Executive Officer (Total facility includes 10 beds in nursing home–type unit) **A**1 9 10 **F**1 4 7 8 10 11 12 14 15 16 19 21 22 29 31 32 33 35 37 39 41 42 43 44 46 49 52 57 58 59 64 65 71 72 73 **P**7 **S** Columbia/HCA Healthcare Corporation, Nashville, TN **N** Columbia/HCA South Florida Division, Miami Lakes, FL; The Health Advantage Network, Winter Park, FL	32	10	278	9418	169	48571	282	104173	30147	1164
✠ MIAMI JEWISH HOME AND HOSPITAL FOR AGED, 5200 N.E. Second Avenue, Zip 33137–2706; tel. 305/751–8626; Terry Goodman, Executive Director **A**1 3 10 **F**1 3 6 12 15 16 17 20 25 26 27 28 29 30 34 39 49 55 56 57 58 59 65 67 71 73	23	10	32	424	13	14500	0	3729	1601	74
□ NORTH SHORE MEDICAL CENTER, 1100 N.W. 95th Street, Zip 33150–2098; tel. 305/835–6000; Steven M. Klein, President and Chief Executive Officer **A**1 2 9 10 **F**1 8 11 14 16 19 21 22 28 29 30 31 32 34 35 37 38 40 41 42 44 45 49 52 55 56 57 58 59 60 65 71 73 74 **P**1 **S** TENET Healthcare Corporation, Santa Barbara, CA	23	10	286	11161	168	89705	2112	86120	37782	1183
✠ PAN AMERICAN HOSPITAL, 5959 N.W. Seventh Street, Zip 33126–3198; tel. 305/264–1000; Carolina Calderin, Chief Executive Officer **A**1 10 **F**1 8 11 12 14 15 17 19 21 22 26 27 29 30 32 34 35 37 44 45 49 51 60 65 67 71 73 74 **P**7 8	23	10	144	6426	118	83939	0	57248	22607	725
□ PARKWAY REGIONAL MEDICAL CENTER–WEST, (Formerly Golden Glades Regional Medical Center), 17300 N.W. Seventh Avenue, Zip 33169; tel. 305/652–4200; Stephen M. Patz, Chief Executive Officer (Nonreporting) **A**1 10	33	10	127	—	—	—	—	—	—	—
□ SOUTH FLORIDA EVALUTATION AND TREATMENT CENTER, 2200 N.W. 7th Avenue, Zip 33127; tel. 305/637–2500; Cheryl Y. Brantley, Administrator **A**1 **F**14 15 16 52 53 54 55 56 57 58 59	12	22	200	191	190	0	0	—	—	420
□ △ SOUTH MIAMI HOSPITAL, 6200 S.W. 73rd Street, Zip 33143–9990; tel. 305/661–4611; D. Wayne Brackin, Chief Executive Officer (Nonreporting) **A**1 2 7 9 10 **N** Dimensions Health/Baptist Health Systems, Miami, FL	23	10	397	—	—	—	—	—	—	—

Hospital, Address, Telephone, Administrator, Approval, Facility, and Physician Codes, Health Care System, Network	Classification Codes		Utilization Data					Expense (thousands) of dollars		
	Control	Service	Beds	Admissions	Census	Outpatient Visits	Births	Total	Payroll	Personnel

★ American Hospital Association (AHA) membership
☐ Joint Commission on Accreditation of Healthcare Organizations (JCAHO) accreditation
+ American Osteopathic Hospital Association (AOHA) membership
○ American Osteopathic Association (AOA) accreditation
△ Commission on Accreditation of Rehabilitation Facilities (CARF) accreditation
Control codes 61, 63, 64, 71, 72 and 73 indicate hospitals listed by AOHA, but not registered by AHA. For definition of numerical codes, see page A4

	Control	Service	Beds	Admissions	Census	Outpatient Visits	Births	Total	Payroll	Personnel
✠ UNIVERSITY OF MIAMI HOSPITAL AND CLINICS, 1475 N.W. 12th Avenue, Zip 33136–1002; tel. 305/243–6418; John Rossfeld, Administrator **A**1 2 3 5 9 10 **F**8 12 14 15 16 17 19 20 21 22 27 29 30 31 34 35 42 44 45 46 51 54 58 60 63 65 67 71 73 **P**1 **S** Quorum Health Group/Quorum Health Resources, Inc., Brentwood, TN	23	10	40	852	17	137728	0	52236	13889	400
✠ VETERANS AFFAIRS MEDICAL CENTER, 1201 N.W. 16th Street, Zip 33125–1624; tel. 305/324–4455; Thomas C. Doherty, Medical Center Director (Total facility includes 240 beds in nursing home–type unit) **A**1 3 5 8 **F**1 3 4 5 8 10 11 12 14 15 16 18 19 20 21 22 23 25 26 27 28 29 30 31 32 33 34 35 37 39 41 42 43 44 45 46 48 49 51 52 54 55 56 57 58 59 60 63 64 65 67 69 71 73 74 **S** Department of Veterans Affairs, Washington, DC	45	10	669	8445	536	364035	0	185707	98070	2691
VICTORIA PAVILION See Columbia Cedars Medical Center										
+ ○ WESTCHESTER GENERAL HOSPITAL, 2500 S.W. 75th Avenue, Zip 33155–9947; tel. 305/264–5252; Gilda Baldwin, Chief Administrative Officer and Chief Operating Officer (Nonreporting) **A**10 11 12 13	33	10	110	—	—	—	—	—	—	—

MIAMI BEACH—Dade County

	Control	Service	Beds	Admissions	Census	Outpatient Visits	Births	Total	Payroll	Personnel
☐ △ MOUNT SINAI MEDICAL CENTER, 4300 Alton Road, Zip 33140–2800; tel. 305/674–2121; Fred D. Hirt, President and Chief Executive Officer (Total facility includes 150 beds in nursing home–type unit) **A**1 2 3 5 7 8 9 10 **F**2 3 4 7 8 10 12 14 15 16 17 19 20 21 22 23 25 26 28 29 30 31 32 33 34 35 37 40 41 42 43 44 45 46 48 49 51 52 54 57 58 59 60 63 64 65 67 71 73 74 **P**1 4 6 7	23	10	721	20997	533	144963	1665	229319	107108	3084
✠ △ SOUTH SHORE HOSPITAL AND MEDICAL CENTER, (GERIATRICS), 630 Alton Road, Zip 33139; tel. 305/672–2100; William Zubkoff, Ph.D., Chief Executive Officer **A**1 7 10 **F**1 12 14 15 16 17 19 21 22 26 27 31 32 33 34 37 41 44 45 46 49 52 57 59 65 71 72 73 **P**5	23	49	178	4586	142	21879	0	37424	17015	662

MILTON—Santa Rosa County

	Control	Service	Beds	Admissions	Census	Outpatient Visits	Births	Total	Payroll	Personnel
✠ SANTA ROSA MEDICAL CENTER, 1450 Berryhill Road, Zip 32570, Mailing Address: P.O. Box 648, Zip 32572; tel. 904/626–7762; Barbara H. Thames, Chief Executive Officer (Total facility includes 10 beds in nursing home–type unit) **A**1 9 10 **F**1 3 4 7 8 10 11 12 14 15 16 17 19 21 22 26 28 29 30 33 35 36 37 39 40 41 42 44 46 49 51 54 56 64 65 67 71 73 74 **P**8 **S** Paracelsus Healthcare Corporation, Houston, TX **N** Columbia/HCA North & NorthEast Florida Division, Jacksonville, FL; The Health Advantage Network, Winter Park, FL	33	10	129	3375	42	50078	461	22564	9418	306

NAPLES—Collier County

	Control	Service	Beds	Admissions	Census	Outpatient Visits	Births	Total	Payroll	Personnel
✠ △ NAPLES COMMUNITY HOSPITAL, 350 Seventh Street North, Zip 34102–3029, Mailing Address: P.O. Box 413029, Zip 34101–3029; tel. 941/436–5000; William G. Crone, President and Chief Executive Officer **A**1 2 7 9 10 **F**2 3 4 7 8 9 10 11 12 13 14 15 16 17 19 21 22 23 24 25 26 28 29 30 32 33 34 35 37 38 39 40 41 42 43 44 45 46 47 48 49 51 52 56 57 59 60 64 65 66 67 70 71 72 73 74 **P**8	23	10	434	21447	282	161483	2189	153918	69250	2066
WILLOUGH AT NAPLES, 9001 Tamiami Trail East, Zip 34113–3316; tel. 941/775–4500; Gary Centafanti, Vice President and Executive Director **A**10 **F**2 3 15 16 17 18 25 27 29 52 53 54 55 56 57 58 59 67 73 **P**6	33	22	64	1158	43	0	0	7866	3310	99

NEW PORT RICHEY—Pasco County

	Control	Service	Beds	Admissions	Census	Outpatient Visits	Births	Total	Payroll	Personnel
✠ COLUMBIA NEW PORT RICHEY HOSPITAL, 5637 Marine Parkway, Zip 34652, Mailing Address: Box 996, Zip 34656–0996; tel. 813/848–1733; Andrew Oravec, Jr., Administrator (Nonreporting) **A**1 9 10 **S** Columbia/HCA Healthcare Corporation, Nashville, TN **N** Columbia/HCA Tampa Bay Division, Tampa, FL; The Health Advantage Network, Winter Park, FL	33	10	414	—	—	—	—	—	—	—
☐ NORTH BAY MEDICAL CENTER, 6600 Madison Street, Zip 34652; tel. 813/842–8468; Dennis A. Taylor, Administrator (Nonreporting) **A**1 9 10 **S** TENET Healthcare Corporation, Santa Barbara, CA **N** BayCare Health Network, Inc., Clearwater, FL	33	10	122	—	—	—	—	—	—	—

NEW SMYRNA BEACH—Volusia County

	Control	Service	Beds	Admissions	Census	Outpatient Visits	Births	Total	Payroll	Personnel
✠ BERT FISH MEDICAL CENTER, 401 Palmetto Street, Zip 32168; tel. 904/424–5000; James R. Foster, President and Chief Executive Officer (Nonreporting) **A**1 9 10 **S** Quorum Health Group/Quorum Health Resources, Inc., Brentwood, TN	16	10	82	—	—	—	—	—	—	—

NICEVILLE—Okaloosa County

	Control	Service	Beds	Admissions	Census	Outpatient Visits	Births	Total	Payroll	Personnel
✠ COLUMBIA TWIN CITIES HOSPITAL, 2190 Highway 85 North, Zip 32578; tel. 904/678–4131; David Whalen, Chief Executive Officer **A**1 9 10 **F**8 12 14 15 16 17 19 21 22 25 28 29 30 32 33 37 44 45 49 51 63 71 **S** Columbia/HCA Healthcare Corporation, Nashville, TN **N** Columbia/HCA North & NorthEast Florida Division, Jacksonville, FL; The Health Advantage Network, Winter Park, FL	33	10	60	2221	28	26366	0	13833	6230	285

NORTH MIAMI—Dade County

	Control	Service	Beds	Admissions	Census	Outpatient Visits	Births	Total	Payroll	Personnel
✠ △ VILLA MARIA HOSPITAL, 1050 N.E. 125th Street, Zip 33161; tel. 305/891–8850; Jack Rutenberg, Administrator (Total facility includes 212 beds in nursing home–type unit) **A**1 7 **F**1 6 19 20 21 26 27 32 33 34 35 39 48 49 50 54 64 65 67 71 73	21	46	272	1043	212	2217	0	16999	5252	234

NORTH MIAMI BEACH—Dade County

	Control	Service	Beds	Admissions	Census	Outpatient Visits	Births	Total	Payroll	Personnel
☐ △ PARKWAY REGIONAL MEDICAL CENTER, 160 N.W. 170th Street, Zip 33169; tel. 305/654–5050; Stephen M. Patz, Chief Executive Officer **A**1 7 9 **F**5 7 8 10 11 12 15 16 17 19 22 25 26 27 28 30 31 32 33 34 35 37 38 39 40 41 42 44 45 46 47 48 49 51 52 56 57 58 59 60 64 65 66 67 71 73 74 **P**1 7 **S** TENET Healthcare Corporation, Santa Barbara, CA	33	10	392	19729	168	184645	2193	—	—	—

Hospital, Address, Telephone, Administrator, Approval, Facility, and Physician Codes, Health Care System, Network	Classi-fication Codes		Utilization Data					Expense (thousands) of dollars		
	Control	Service	Beds	Admissions	Census	Outpatient Visits	Births	Total	Payroll	Personnel

★ American Hospital Association (AHA) membership
□ Joint Commission on Accreditation of Healthcare Organizations (JCAHO) accreditation
+ American Osteopathic Hospital Association (AOHA) membership
○ American Osteopathic Association (AOA) accreditation
△ Commission on Accreditation of Rehabilitation Facilities (CARF) accreditation
Control codes 61, 63, 64, 71, 72 and 73 indicate hospitals listed by AOHA, but not registered by AHA. For definition of numerical codes, see page A4

OCALA—Marion County

Hospital	Control	Service	Beds	Admissions	Census	Outpatient Visits	Births	Total	Payroll	Personnel
□ CHARTER SPRINGS HOSPITAL, 3130 S.W. 27th Avenue, Zip 34474, Mailing Address: P.O. Box 3338, Zip 34478; tel. 352/237–7293; James Duff, Administrator **A**1 10 **F**1 2 3 12 14 15 17 18 19 26 35 44 45 49 52 53 54 55 58 59 60 65 67 72 **S** Magellan Health Services, Atlanta, GA	33	22	92	1244	37	3409	0	—	—	112
✣ COLUMBIA OCALA REGIONAL MEDICAL CENTER, 1431 S.W. First Avenue, Zip 34474, Mailing Address: Box 2200, Zip 34478–2200; tel. 352/401–1000; Terry Upton, Chief Executive Officer **A**1 2 9 10 **F**4 7 8 10 12 14 19 21 22 32 33 34 35 39 41 42 43 44 45 46 49 60 63 65 66 71 73 **P**8 **S** Columbia/HCA Healthcare Corporation, Nashville, TN **N** Columbia/HCA North & NorthEast Florida Division, Jacksonville, FL; The Health Advantage Network, Winter Park, FL	33	10	216	10963	147	59345	908	73137	32625	1013
✣ MUNROE REGIONAL MEDICAL CENTER, 131 S.W. 15th Street, Zip 34474, Mailing Address: Box 6000, Zip 34478; tel. 904/351–7200; Dyer T. Michell, President **A**1 5 9 10 **F**4 7 8 10 11 14 15 16 19 21 22 23 24 26 28 29 30 31 32 34 37 39 40 41 43 44 45 46 49 51 65 66 71 72 73 74 **P**6 7 8	23	10	319	14044	189	92558	1285	117791	44493	1380

OCOEE—Orange County

Hospital	Control	Service	Beds	Admissions	Census	Outpatient Visits	Births	Total	Payroll	Personnel
✣ HEALTH CENTRAL, 10000 West Colonial Drive, Zip 34761, Mailing Address: P.O. Box 614007, Orlando, Zip 32861–4007; tel. 407/296–1000; Richard M. Irwin, Jr., President and Chief Executive Officer (Total facility includes 228 beds in nursing home–type unit) **A**1 9 10 **F**1 4 7 8 10 11 12 14 15 17 19 20 21 22 23 27 28 30 31 32 33 34 35 37 39 40 41 42 44 45 46 49 64 65 66 67 69 70 71 72 73 74 **P**3	16	10	338	4326	264	—	519	43152	15541	503

OKEECHOBEE—Okeechobee County

Hospital	Control	Service	Beds	Admissions	Census	Outpatient Visits	Births	Total	Payroll	Personnel
✣ COLUMBIA RAULERSON HOSPITAL, 1796 Highway 441 North, Zip 34972, Mailing Address: Box 1307, Zip 34973–1307; tel. 941/763–2151; Frank Irby, Chief Executive Officer **A**1 9 10 **F**11 12 16 19 22 23 28 30 32 33 34 35 37 42 44 46 58 60 64 71 73 **P**5 **S** Columbia/HCA Healthcare Corporation, Nashville, TN **N** Columbia/HCA Central Florida Division, Winter Park, FL; The Health Advantage Network, Winter Park, FL	33	10	101	3902	61	45104	0	22517	11303	327

ORANGE PARK—Clay County

Hospital	Control	Service	Beds	Admissions	Census	Outpatient Visits	Births	Total	Payroll	Personnel
✣ COLUMBIA ORANGE PARK MEDICAL CENTER, 2001 Kingsley Avenue, Zip 32073–5156; tel. 904/276–8500; Robert M. Krieger, Chief Executive Officer (Nonreporting) **A**1 9 10 **S** Columbia/HCA Healthcare Corporation, Nashville, TN **N** Columbia/HCA North & NorthEast Florida Division, Jacksonville, FL; The Health Advantage Network, Winter Park, FL	33	10	196	—	—	—	—	—	—	—

ORLANDO—Orange County

Hospital	Control	Service	Beds	Admissions	Census	Outpatient Visits	Births	Total	Payroll	Personnel
✣ △ COLUMBIA PARK MEDICAL CENTER, 818 South Main Lane, Zip 32801; tel. 407/649–6111; Rick O'Connell, Chief Executive Officer (Total facility includes 20 beds in nursing home–type unit) **A**1 7 9 10 **F**1 3 4 7 8 10 11 12 15 16 17 19 20 21 22 23 24 25 26 27 28 29 30 31 32 33 34 35 36 37 39 40 41 42 43 44 46 48 49 51 53 54 55 56 57 58 59 61 63 64 65 66 67 71 72 73 74 **P**1 **S** Columbia/HCA Healthcare Corporation, Nashville, TN **N** Columbia/HCA Central Florida Division, Winter Park, FL; The Health Advantage Network, Winter Park, FL	33	10	267	9218	137	38906	751	69058	27266	1067
✣ ○ △ FLORIDA HOSPITAL, (Includes Florida Hospital East Orlando, 7727 Lake Underhill Drive, Zip 32822; tel. 407/277–8110; Florida Hospital Kissimmee, 200 Hilda Street, Kissimmee, Zip 34741–2301; tel. 407/846–4343; Florida Hospital–Altamonte, 601 East Altamonte Drive, Altamonte Springs, Zip 32701; tel. 407/830–4321; Florida Hospital–Apopka, 201 North Park Avenue, Apopka, Zip 32703; tel. 407/889–2566), 601 East Rollins Street, Zip 32803–1489; tel. 407/896–6611; Thomas L. Werner, President (Nonreporting) **A**1 2 3 5 7 9 10 11 12 13 **S** Adventist Health System Sunbelt Health Care Corporation, Winter Park, FL **N** National Cardiovascular Network, Atlanta, GA; Adventist Health System, Winter Park, FL; Florida Hospital Health Network, Orlando, FL	21	10	1406	—	—	—	—	—	—	—
✣ △ ORLANDO REGIONAL MEDICAL CENTER, (Includes Arnold Palmer Hospital for Children and Women; M. D. Anderson Cancer Center; and Sand Lake Hospital), 1414 Kuhl Avenue, Zip 32806–2093; tel. 407/841–5111; John Hillenmeyer, President **A**1 2 3 5 7 8 9 10 **F**2 3 4 7 8 9 10 11 12 13 14 15 16 17 18 19 21 22 23 24 25 26 27 28 29 30 31 32 34 35 37 38 39 40 41 42 43 44 45 46 47 48 49 51 52 53 54 55 56 57 58 59 60 61 62 63 64 65 66 67 68 69 70 71 72 73 74 **P**3 4 5 6 7 **S** Orlando Regional Healthcare System, Orlando, FL **N** Orlando Regional Healthcare System, Orlando, FL	23	10	807	40958	539	456534	6199	391303	188520	7075
□ PRINCETON HOSPITAL, 1800 Mercy Drive, Zip 32808; tel. 407/295–5151; Randall Phillips, President and Chief Executive Officer **A**1 10 **F**7 8 10 11 12 14 15 16 19 21 22 23 26 27 28 30 31 32 34 35 37 39 40 41 42 44 45 46 49 52 54 56 57 61 65 67 71 73 74 **P**8	23	10	150	3539	43	32000	350	32399	10926	407
□ UNIVERSITY BEHAVIORAL CENTER, 2500 Discovery Drive, Zip 32826; tel. 407/281–7000; Gregory P. Roth, Executive Director (Nonreporting) **A**1 10 **S** Health Management Associates, Naples, FL	33	22	100	—	—	—	—	—	—	—
□ VALUEMARK BEHAVIORAL HEALTHCARE OF FLORIDA, (Formerly ValueMark–Laurel Oaks Behavioral Healthcare System), 6601 Central Florida Parkway, Zip 32821; tel. 407/345–5000; Marni Berger, Chief Executive Officer **A**1 **F**1 3 12 15 16 17 26 30 52 53 55 56 57 58 59 65 67 **P**6 **S** ValueMark Healthcare Systems, Inc., Atlanta, GA	31	52	52	104	29	0	0	—	—	—

ORMOND BEACH—Volusia County

Hospital	Control	Service	Beds	Admissions	Census	Outpatient Visits	Births	Total	Payroll	Personnel
□ ○ COLUMBIA MEDICAL CENTER PENINSULA, (Formerly Peninsula Medical Center), 264 South Atlantic Avenue, Zip 32176–8192; tel. 904/672–4161; Thomas R. Pentz, Chief Executive Officer **A**1 10 11 12 13 **F**8 12 14 15 16 19 20 21 22 27 28 30 32 35 37 39 41 44 48 49 63 65 71 73 **P**5 **S** Columbia/HCA Healthcare Corporation, Nashville, TN	33	10	119	2873	56	25250	0	—	—	310

Hospital, Address, Telephone, Administrator, Approval, Facility, and Physician Codes, Health Care System, Network	Classi-fication Codes		Utilization Data					Expense (thousands) of dollars		
	Control	Service	Beds	Admissions	Census	Outpatient Visits	Births	Total	Payroll	Personnel

American Hospital Association (AHA) membership
☐ Joint Commission on Accreditation of Healthcare Organizations (JCAHO) accreditation
+ American Osteopathic Hospital Association (AOHA) membership
○ American Osteopathic Association (AOA) accreditation
△ Commission on Accreditation of Rehabilitation Facilities (CARF) accreditation
Control codes 61, 63, 64, 71, 72 and 73 indicate hospitals listed by AOHA, but not registered by AHA. For definition of numerical codes, see page A4

✶ △ MEMORIAL HOSPITAL–ORMOND BEACH, 875 Sterthaus Avenue, Zip 32174–5197; tel. 904/676–6000; Clark P. Christianson, Senior Vice President and Administrator (Total facility includes 17 beds in nursing home–type unit) **A**1 7 9 10 **F**4 7 8 10 11 12 14 15 16 17 19 20 21 22 23 24 25 26 28 29 30 31 32 33 34 35 37 39 40 41 42 43 44 45 46 49 60 61 64 65 66 67 71 73 74 **P**1 2 6 8 **S** Memorial Health Systems, Ormond Beach, FL	23	10	205	7657	122	51465	500	78105	30926	874

PENINSULA MEDICAL CENTER See Columbia Medical Center Peninsula

PAHOKEE—Palm Beach County

☐ EVERGLADES REGIONAL MEDICAL CENTER, 200 South Barfield Highway, Zip 33476–1897; tel. 407/924–5200; Donald A. Anderson, President and Chief Executive Officer **A**1 9 10 **F**8 10 15 19 21 22 25 35 37 40 44 46 49 65 71 **P**5 7 8	23	10	63	2867	31	15060	541	18032	8025	321

PALATKA—Putnam County

✶ COLUMBIA PUTNAM MEDICAL CENTER, Highway 20 West, Zip 32177, Mailing Address: P.O. Box 778, Zip 32178–0778; tel. 904/328–5711; David Whalen, President and Chief Executive Officer **A**1 9 10 **F**7 8 14 15 16 17 19 21 22 26 27 28 29 30 31 32 33 34 35 37 39 40 41 42 44 45 46 49 51 52 54 55 56 57 59 60 63 64 65 66 67 71 72 73 74 **P**4 5 7 8 **S** Columbia/HCA Healthcare Corporation, Nashville, TN **N** Columbia/HCA North & NorthEast Florida Division, Jacksonville, FL; The Health Advantage Network, Winter Park, FL	33	10	161	6333	87	81612	497	—	—	477

PALM BEACH GARDENS—Palm Beach County

☐ PALM BEACH GARDENS MEDICAL CENTER, 3360 Burns Road, Zip 33410–4304; tel. 407/622–1411 (Nonreporting) **A**1 9 10 **S** TENET Healthcare Corporation, Santa Barbara, CA **N** Tenet South Florida Health System Network, Fort Lauderdale, FL; Med Connect, Ft Lauderdale, FL	33	10	204	—	—	—	—	—	—	—

PANAMA CITY—Bay County

✶ BAY MEDICAL CENTER, 615 North Bonita Avenue, Zip 32401–2515, Mailing Address: P.O. Box 2515, Zip 32402; tel. 904/769–1511; Ronald V. Wolff, President and Chief Executive Officer **A**1 9 10 **F**4 7 8 10 14 15 16 17 19 21 22 25 27 28 30 31 32 33 34 35 37 40 41 42 43 44 46 49 52 59 60 63 65 71 73 74 **P**5	16	10	315	12285	182	92638	685	98151	40034	1429
✶ COLUMBIA GULF COAST MEDICAL CENTER, (Formerly Columbia Gulf Coast Hospital), 449 West 23rd Street, Zip 32405, Mailing Address: P.O. Box 15309, Zip 32406–5309; tel. 904/769–8341; Donald E. Butts, Chief Executive Officer **A**1 2 9 10 **F**7 8 10 11 12 17 19 21 22 23 24 25 28 29 32 34 35 37 39 40 41 42 44 46 49 60 63 65 66 71 72 73 74 **P**1 7 **S** Columbia/HCA Healthcare Corporation, Nashville, TN **N** Columbia/HCA North & NorthEast Florida Division, Jacksonville, FL; The Health Advantage Network, Winter Park, FL	33	10	176	7471	85	93393	1321	—	—	629
✶ U. S. AIR FORCE HOSPITAL, Tyndall AFB, Zip 32403–5300; tel. 904/283–7515; Colonel Jay Sprenger, Commander (Nonreporting) **A**1 **S** Department of the Air Force, Washington, DC	41	10	25	—	—	—	—	—	—	—

PATRICK AFB—Brevard County

★ U. S. AIR FORCE HOSPITAL, 1381 South Patrick Drive, Zip 32925–3606; tel. 407/494–8102; Colonel William Trent, MSC, USAF, Commanding Officer **F**2 3 4 5 7 8 9 10 11 12 13 15 16 17 18 19 20 21 22 23 24 25 26 27 28 29 30 31 32 34 35 37 38 39 41 42 43 44 45 46 47 48 49 50 51 52 53 54 55 56 57 58 59 60 61 63 64 65 67 71 73 **S** Department of the Air Force, Washington, DC	41	10	15	753	4	129325	0	19348	—	—

PEMBROKE PINES—Broward County

✶ MEMORIAL HOSPITAL PEMBROKE, 2301 University Drive, Zip 33024; tel. 954/962–9650; J. E. Piriz, Administrator (Nonreporting) **A**1 9 10 **S** Memorial Healthcare System, Hollywood, FL **N** Memorial Healthcare System, Hollywood, FL; Columbia/HCA South Florida Division, Miami Lakes, FL; The Health Advantage Network, Winter Park, FL	16	10	301	—	—	—	—	—	—	—
✶ MEMORIAL HOSPITAL WEST, 703 North Flamingo Road, Zip 33028; tel. 954/436–5000; Zeff Ross, Administrator **A**1 10 **F**1 2 3 4 5 7 8 10 11 12 13 14 15 16 17 18 19 20 21 22 23 24 25 26 27 28 29 30 31 32 33 34 35 36 37 38 39 40 41 42 43 44 46 47 48 49 51 52 53 54 55 56 57 58 59 60 61 63 64 65 66 67 68 69 70 71 72 73 74 **P**1 3 7 **S** Memorial Healthcare System, Hollywood, FL **N** Memorial Healthcare System, Hollywood, FL; Community Health Network of South Florida, Ft Lauderdale, FL	16	10	110	8379	86	121064	2828	57337	22671	537
SOUTH FLORIDA STATE HOSPITAL, 1000 S.W. 84th Avenue, Zip 33025; tel. 954/967–7000; Thomas S. Gramley, Administrator (Nonreporting) **A**10	12	22	355	—	—	—	—	—	—	—

PENSACOLA—Escambia County

✶ BAPTIST HOSPITAL, 1000 West Moreno, Zip 32501–2393, Mailing Address: P.O. Box 17500, Zip 32522–7500; tel. 904/469–2313; Quinton Studer, President (Total facility includes 57 beds in nursing home–type unit) **A**1 2 9 10 **F**3 4 7 8 10 11 12 14 15 16 17 18 19 21 22 23 24 25 26 27 28 29 30 31 32 34 35 37 40 41 42 44 45 46 48 49 51 52 53 54 55 56 57 58 59 60 61 62 63 64 65 66 67 68 70 71 72 73 74 **P**4 5 7 **S** Baptist Health Care Corporation, Pensacola, FL **N** Baptist Health Care, Inc., Pensacola, FL	23	10	521	13165	260	123836	1027	103980	38716	1517
✶ △ COLUMBIA WEST FLORIDA REGIONAL MEDICAL CENTER, (Includes Rehabilitation Institute of West Florida, tel. 904/494–6000; The Pavilion, tel. 904/494–5000; West Florida Hospital, tel. 904/494–4000), 8383 North Davis Highway, Zip 32514, Mailing Address: P.O. Box 18900, Zip 32523–8900; tel. 904/494–4000; Stephen Brandt, Chief Executive Officer (Total facility includes 40 beds in nursing home–type unit) **A**1 2 7 9 10 **F**2 3 4 7 8 10 11 12 14 17 19 21 23 24 26 27 29 30 32 35 36 37 39 40 41 42 43 44 45 48 49 52 53 54 56 57 58 59 60 63 64 65 66 67 70 71 73 74 **S** Columbia/HCA Healthcare Corporation, Nashville, TN **N** Columbia/HCA North & NorthEast Florida Division, Jacksonville, FL; The Health Advantage Network, Winter Park, FL	33	10	531	13123	229	131679	770	106716	40196	1956

Hospital, Address, Telephone, Administrator, Approval, Facility, and Physician Codes, Health Care System, Network	Classi-fication Codes		Utilization Data					Expense (thousands) of dollars		
★ American Hospital Association (AHA) membership □ Joint Commission on Accreditation of Healthcare Organizations (JCAHO) accreditation + American Osteopathic Hospital Association (AOHA) membership ○ American Osteopathic Association (AOA) accreditation △ Commission on Accreditation of Rehabilitation Facilities (CARF) accreditation Control codes 61, 63, 64, 71, 72 and 73 indicate hospitals listed by AOHA, but not registered by AHA. For definition of numerical codes, see page A4	Control	Service	Beds	Admissions	Census	Outpatient Visits	Births	Total	Payroll	Personnel
☒ NAVAL HOSPITAL, 6000 West Highway 98, Zip 32512–0003; tel. 904/452–6413; Commander H. M. Chinnery, Director, Administration (Nonreporting) **A**1 3 5 **S** Department of Navy, Washington, DC	43	10	104	—	—	—	—	—	—	—
REHABILITATION INSTITUTE OF WEST FLORIDA See Columbia West Florida Regional Medical Center										
☒ SACRED HEART HOSPITAL OF PENSACOLA, 5151 North Ninth Avenue, Zip 32504, Mailing Address: P.O. Box 2700, Zip 32513–2700; tel. 904/416–7000; Patrick J. Madden, President and Chief Executive Officer (Total facility includes 89 beds in nursing home–type unit) **A**1 2 3 5 9 10 **F**4 7 8 10 11 12 13 14 15 16 17 19 21 22 23 24 25 28 29 30 32 33 34 35 37 38 39 40 41 42 43 44 45 46 47 49 56 60 61 63 64 65 66 67 68 70 71 72 73 74 **P**4 7 **S** Daughters of Charity National Health System, Saint Louis, MO	21	10	520	20298	349	238420	2664	144518	60117	2157
THE PAVILION See Columbia West Florida Regional Medical Center										
WEST FLORIDA HOSPITAL See Columbia West Florida Regional Medical Center										
PERRY—Taylor County										
☒ DOCTOR'S MEMORIAL HOSPITAL, 407 East Ash Street, Zip 32347, Mailing Address: P.O. Box 1847, Zip 32347–1847; tel. 904/584–0800; Thomas O. Logue, Jr., Ph.D., Administrator and Chief Executive Officer **A**9 10 **F**8 12 15 19 22 28 32 34 37 44 45 49 51 71 73 **P**8	23	10	28	858	10	35891	4	9398	4668	166
PLANT CITY—Hillsborough County										
☒ SOUTH FLORIDA BAPTIST HOSPITAL, 301 North Alexander Street, Zip 33566–9058, Mailing Address: Drawer H, Zip 33564–9058; tel. 813/757–1200; William H. Anderson, Administrator and Chief Executive Officer (Total facility includes 15 beds in nursing home–type unit) **A**1 9 10 **F**7 8 12 14 15 19 21 22 25 27 28 32 35 37 40 42 44 49 63 64 65 67 71 72 73 74 **N** BayCare Health Network, Inc., Clearwater, FL	23	10	100	4263	55	58217	514	35762	14493	501
PLANTATION—Broward County										
☒ COLUMBIA PLANTATION GENERAL HOSPITAL, 401 N.W. 42nd Avenue, Zip 33317–2882; tel. 954/587–5010; Anthony M. Degina, Jr., Chief Executive Officer **A**1 9 10 **F**4 7 8 10 11 12 14 15 16 17 19 21 22 23 28 29 30 33 34 35 37 38 39 40 41 44 45 46 47 49 61 65 67 71 73 74 **P**5 7 **S** Columbia/HCA Healthcare Corporation, Nashville, TN **N** Med Connect, Ft Lauderdale, FL; Columbia/HCA South Florida Division, Miami Lakes, FL; The Health Advantage Network, Winter Park, FL	33	10	264	9675	116	60976	3497	57611	21902	659
☒ COLUMBIA WESTSIDE REGIONAL MEDICAL CENTER, 8201 West Broward Boulevard, Zip 33324–9937; tel. 954/473–6600; Michael G. Joseph, Chief Executive Officer **A**1 9 10 **F**2 3 4 5 7 8 10 11 12 13 15 16 17 19 20 21 22 23 25 26 27 28 29 30 31 32 33 34 35 37 38 39 40 41 42 44 45 46 47 48 49 51 52 53 54 55 56 57 61 64 65 66 67 68 71 72 73 74 **P**5 7 **S** Columbia/HCA Healthcare Corporation, Nashville, TN **N** Columbia/HCA South Florida Division, Miami Lakes, FL; The Health Advantage Network, Winter Park, FL	33	10	204	8817	104	40575	661	56499	21122	649
□ ○ FLORIDA MEDICAL CENTER SOUTH, 6701 West Sunrise Boulevard, Zip 33313; tel. 954/581–7800; Denny DeNaruaez, Chief Executive Officer (Nonreporting) **A**1 10 11 12 13 **S** TENET Healthcare Corporation, Santa Barbara, CA	33	10	127	—	—	—	—	—	—	—
POMPANO BEACH—Broward County										
☒ COLUMBIA POMPANO BEACH MEDICAL CENTER, 600 S.W. Third Street, Zip 33060–6979; tel. 954/782–2000; Heather J. Rohan, Chief Executive Officer **A**1 9 10 **F**4 7 8 10 11 12 14 15 16 17 18 19 22 23 25 27 28 30 31 32 33 34 35 37 41 42 43 44 49 53 54 55 57 58 59 60 65 66 67 71 73 74 **P**5 8 **S** Columbia/HCA Healthcare Corporation, Nashville, TN **N** Columbia/HCA South Florida Division, Miami Lakes, FL; The Health Advantage Network, Winter Park, FL	33	10	80	4678	51	—	0	31936	12677	377
☒ △ NORTH BROWARD MEDICAL CENTER, 201 Sample Road, Zip 33064–3502; tel. 954/941–8300; James R. Chromik, Regional Vice President, Administration (Total facility includes 18 beds in nursing home–type unit) **A**1 2 7 9 10 **F**3 4 7 8 10 11 12 13 14 15 16 17 18 19 21 22 23 24 26 27 28 29 30 31 32 33 34 35 37 38 39 40 41 42 43 44 45 46 47 48 49 50 51 52 53 54 55 56 57 58 59 60 61 63 64 65 66 67 68 70 71 72 73 **P**6 7 **S** North Broward Hospital District, Fort Lauderdale, FL **N** Community Health Network of South Florida, Ft Lauderdale, FL	16	10	334	12329	213	—	0	95686	38857	1103
PORT CHARLOTTE—Charlotte County										
☒ BON SECOURS–ST. JOSEPH HOSPITAL, 2500 Harbor Boulevard, Zip 33952–5396; tel. 941/625–4122; Michael L. Harrington, Executive Vice President and Administrator (Total facility includes 101 beds in nursing home–type unit) **A**1 5 9 10 **F**1 8 10 12 14 15 16 17 18 19 22 24 25 26 27 28 29 30 32 33 34 35 37 39 40 41 42 44 45 46 49 60 61 64 65 66 67 71 72 73 74 **P**5 8 **S** Bon Secours Health System, Inc., Marriottsville, MD	21	10	313	8403	192	51278	977	60735	19168	962
☒ △ COLUMBIA FAWCETT MEMORIAL HOSPITAL, 21298 Olean Boulevard, Zip 33952–6765, Mailing Address: P.O. Box 4028, Punta Gorda, Zip 33949–4028; tel. 941/629–1181; Steve Dobbs, Chief Executive Officer (Total facility includes 15 beds in nursing home–type unit) **A**1 7 10 **F**5 8 10 12 14 15 16 19 21 22 23 25 26 27 28 29 30 32 33 34 35 37 39 41 42 44 45 46 48 49 57 59 64 65 66 67 71 73 **P**7 8 **S** Columbia/HCA Healthcare Corporation, Nashville, TN **N** Columbia/HCA SouthWest Florida Division, Fort Myers, FL; The Health Advantage Network, Winter Park, FL	33	10	249	7648	119	213383	0	69583	32245	941
PORT ST. JOE—Gulf County										
GULF PINES HOSPITAL, 102 20th Street, Zip 32456, Mailing Address: P.O. Box 70, Zip 32456; tel. 904/227–1121; Brian Upton, Administrator and Chief Executive Officer (Nonreporting) **A**9 10	33	10	45	—	—	—	—	—	—	—

Hospital, Address, Telephone, Administrator, Approval, Facility, and Physician Codes, Health Care System, Network	Classi-fication Codes		Utilization Data					Expense (thousands) of dollars		
	Control	Service	Beds	Admissions	Census	Outpatient Visits	Births	Total	Payroll	Personnel

★ American Hospital Association (AHA) membership
☐ Joint Commission on Accreditation of Healthcare Organizations (JCAHO) accreditation
+ American Osteopathic Hospital Association (AOHA) membership
○ American Osteopathic Association (AOA) accreditation
△ Commission on Accreditation of Rehabilitation Facilities (CARF) accreditation
 Control codes 61, 63, 64, 71, 72 and 73 indicate hospitals listed by AOHA, but not registered by AHA. For definition of numerical codes, see page A4

PORT ST. LUCIE—St. Lucie County

Hospital	Control	Service	Beds	Admissions	Census	Outpatient Visits	Births	Total	Payroll	Personnel
✲ COLUMBIA MEDICAL CENTER–PORT ST. LUCIE, 1800 S.E. Tiffany Avenue, Zip 34952–7580; tel. 407/335–4000; Michael P. Joyce, President and Chief Executive Officer (Total facility includes 24 beds in nursing home–type unit) **A**1 9 10 **F**2 3 4 7 8 10 11 12 14 15 16 17 19 21 22 23 25 26 28 29 30 32 34 35 37 38 39 40 41 42 44 45 46 49 51 52 53 54 55 56 57 58 60 64 65 67 68 71 72 73 74 **S** Columbia/HCA Healthcare Corporation, Nashville, TN **N** Columbia/HCA Central Florida Division, Winter Park, FL; The Health Advantage Network, Winter Park, FL	33	10	150	6979	90	54808	584	41120	17618	1208
☐ SAVANNAS HOSPITAL, 2550 S.E. Walton Road, Zip 34952; tel. 407/335–0400; Patricia W. Brown, Executive Director (Nonreporting) **A**1 10	33	22	70	—	—	—	—	—	—	—

PUNTA GORDA—Charlotte County

Hospital	Control	Service	Beds	Admissions	Census	Outpatient Visits	Births	Total	Payroll	Personnel
☐ CHARLOTTE REGIONAL MEDICAL CENTER, 809 East Marion Avenue, Zip 33950–3898; tel. 941/637–3128; Donald B. McElroy, Executive Director (Nonreporting) **A**1 9 10 **S** Health Management Associates, Naples, FL	21	10	148	—	—	—	—	—	—	—

QUINCY—Gadsden County

Hospital	Control	Service	Beds	Admissions	Census	Outpatient Visits	Births	Total	Payroll	Personnel
GADSDEN COMMUNITY HOSPITAL, U.S. Highway 90 East, Zip 32353, Mailing Address: P.O. Box 1979, Zip 32353–1979; tel. 904/875–1100; Donna Gatch, Administrator (Nonreporting) **A**9 10	23	10	51	—	—	—	—	—	—	—

ROCKLEDGE—Brevard County

Hospital	Control	Service	Beds	Admissions	Census	Outpatient Visits	Births	Total	Payroll	Personnel
☐ WUESTHOFF HOSPITAL, 110 Longwood Avenue, Zip 32955, Mailing Address: P.O. Box 565002, Mail Stop 1, Zip 32956–5002; tel. 407/636–2211; Robert O. Carman, President **A**1 2 10 **F**3 4 7 8 10 11 12 14 15 17 19 21 22 23 24 26 28 29 30 31 32 33 34 35 37 38 39 40 41 42 43 44 45 46 49 52 53 54 55 57 58 59 63 65 66 67 71 73 74 **P**5 7 8	23	10	235	10963	135	129560	934	89293	39380	1282

SAFETY HARBOR—Pinellas County

Hospital	Control	Service	Beds	Admissions	Census	Outpatient Visits	Births	Total	Payroll	Personnel
MEASE COUNTRYSIDE HOSPITAL, 3231 McMullen–Booth Road, Zip 34695–1098, Mailing Address: P.O. 1098, Zip 34695–1098; tel. 813/725–6111; James A. Pfeiffer, Chief Administrative Officer (Nonreporting) **A**9 10 **S** Mease Health Care, Palm Harbor, FL **N** Morton Plant Mease Health Care, Dunedin, FL; BayCare Health Network, Inc., Clearwater, FL	23	10	100	—	—	—	—	—	—	—

SAINT AUGUSTINE—St. Johns County

Hospital	Control	Service	Beds	Admissions	Census	Outpatient Visits	Births	Total	Payroll	Personnel
✲ FLAGLER HOSPITAL, (Includes Flagler Hospital Psychiatric Center, 200 River Haven Way, tel. 904/824–9800; Brian Trella, Program Director; Flagler Hospital–West, 1955 U.S. 1 South, tel. 904/826–4700), 400 Health Park Boulevard, Zip 32086; tel. 904/829–5155; James D. Conzemius, President **A**1 9 10 **F**7 8 10 15 16 19 21 22 28 32 34 35 37 40 44 49 52 56 65 71 73 74	23	10	254	7990	128	90080	817	58836	24049	833

SAINT CLOUD—Lowndes County

Hospital	Control	Service	Beds	Admissions	Census	Outpatient Visits	Births	Total	Payroll	Personnel
✲ ST. CLOUD HOSPITAL, A DIVISION OF ORLANDO REGIONAL HEALTHCARE SYSTEM, 2906 17th Street, Zip 34769–6099; tel. 407/892–2135; Jim Norris, Executive Director (Nonreporting) **A**1 9 **S** Orlando Regional Healthcare System, Orlando, FL **N** Orlando Regional Healthcare System, Orlando, FL	23	10	68	—	—	—	—	—	—	—

SAINT PETERSBURG—Pinellas County

Hospital	Control	Service	Beds	Admissions	Census	Outpatient Visits	Births	Total	Payroll	Personnel
✲ ALL CHILDREN'S HOSPITAL, (PEDIATRIC SPECIALTY), 801 Sixth Street South, Zip 33701–4899; tel. 813/898–7451; J. Dennis Sexton, President **A**1 3 5 8 9 10 **F**4 10 12 13 14 15 17 19 20 22 24 25 27 28 30 31 34 35 37 38 39 41 42 43 44 45 49 51 53 65 67 69 71 73 **P**1 **N** BayCare Health Network, Inc., Clearwater, FL	23	59	168	6566	129	77287	0	129354	58854	1664
✲ △ BAYFRONT MEDICAL CENTER, 701 Sixth Street South, Zip 33701–4891; tel. 813/823–1234; Sue G. Brody, President **A**1 2 3 5 7 9 10 **F**4 7 8 10 11 12 13 14 15 16 17 19 21 24 25 26 27 28 29 30 31 32 34 35 37 38 39 40 41 42 43 44 45 46 48 49 50 51 60 61 63 64 65 66 67 70 71 72 73 74 **P**3 8 **N** BayCare Health Network, Inc., Clearwater, FL	23	10	268	15943	232	162655	3139	137205	55857	1848
✲ COLUMBIA EDWARD WHITE HOSPITAL, 2323 Ninth Avenue North, Zip 33713, Mailing Address: P.O. Box 12018, Zip 33733–2018; tel. 813/323–1111; Barry S. Stokes, Chief Executive Officer (Total facility includes 10 beds in nursing home–type unit) **A**1 10 **F**4 7 8 10 11 12 14 17 19 20 21 22 23 24 25 26 28 29 30 31 32 33 34 35 37 40 41 42 43 44 46 49 51 59 63 64 65 66 67 71 73 74 **P**7 8 **S** Columbia/HCA Healthcare Corporation, Nashville, TN **N** Columbia/HCA Tampa Bay Division, Tampa, FL; The Health Advantage Network, Winter Park, FL	33	10	134	3172	50	56473	0	28655	12005	305
✲ COLUMBIA NORTHSIDE MEDICAL CENTER, 6000 49th Street North, Zip 33709; tel. 813/521–4411; Bradley K. Grover, Sr., Chief Executive Officer **A**1 9 10 **F**3 4 7 8 10 11 12 13 14 15 16 17 18 19 20 21 22 23 26 27 28 29 30 32 33 34 35 37 38 39 40 41 42 43 44 45 46 49 51 57 58 59 61 64 65 66 67 71 73 74 **P**1 7 **S** Columbia/HCA Healthcare Corporation, Nashville, TN **N** Columbia/HCA Tampa Bay Division, Tampa, FL; The Health Advantage Network, Winter Park, FL	33	10	301	7432	114	47720	0	—	—	829
✲ COLUMBIA ST. PETERSBURG MEDICAL CENTER, 6500 38th Avenue North, Zip 33710; tel. 813/384–1414; Bradley K. Grover, Sr., President and Chief Executive Officer (Total facility includes 20 beds in nursing home–type unit) **A**1 9 10 **F**3 4 7 8 10 12 13 14 15 16 17 19 20 21 22 23 24 25 26 27 28 29 30 31 32 33 34 35 37 39 40 41 42 43 44 45 46 49 51 59 61 64 65 66 67 71 73 74 **P**5 7 8 **S** Columbia/HCA Healthcare Corporation, Nashville, TN **N** Columbia/HCA Tampa Bay Division, Tampa, FL; The Health Advantage Network, Winter Park, FL	33	10	199	7129	69	59475	1085	40225	15684	536
☐ PALMS OF PASADENA HOSPITAL, 1501 Pasadena Avenue South, Zip 33707; tel. 813/381–1000; John D. Bartlett, Chief Executive Officer **A**1 2 10 **F**8 10 11 12 15 19 22 25 27 32 35 37 42 44 60 65 66 71 73 **P**5 **S** TENET Healthcare Corporation, Santa Barbara, CA **N** Tenet South Florida Health System Network, Fort Lauderdale, FL	33	10	267	7079	118	122812	0	—	—	663

Hospital, Address, Telephone, Administrator, Approval, Facility, and Physician Codes, Health Care System, Network	Classification Codes		Utilization Data					Expense (thousands) of dollars		
	Control	Service	Beds	Admissions	Census	Outpatient Visits	Births	Total	Payroll	Personnel

★ American Hospital Association (AHA) membership
□ Joint Commission on Accreditation of Healthcare Organizations (JCAHO) accreditation
+ American Osteopathic Hospital Association (AOHA) membership
○ American Osteopathic Association (AOA) accreditation
△ Commission on Accreditation of Rehabilitation Facilities (CARF) accreditation
Control codes 61, 63, 64, 71, 72 and 73 indicate hospitals listed by AOHA, but not registered by AHA. For definition of numerical codes, see page A4

✦ ST. ANTHONY'S HOSPITAL, 1200 Seventh Avenue North, Zip 33705, Mailing Address: P.O. Box 12588, Zip 33733; tel. 813/825–1100; Revonda L. Shumaker, R.N., President (Total facility includes 30 beds in nursing home–type unit) **A**1 2 9 10 **F**2 4 7 8 10 11 15 16 17 19 21 22 24 25 26 27 28 29 30 31 32 33 34 35 37 39 40 41 42 43 44 45 46 49 52 54 55 56 57 59 60 64 65 66 67 71 73 74 **P**5 7 8 **S** Allegany Health System, Tampa, FL **N** BayCare Health Network, Inc., Clearwater, FL; Allegany Health System, Tampa, FL	23	10	329	11246	207	166176	418	82309	29299	1061
□ VENCOR HOSPITAL–ST PETERSBURG, 3030 Sixth Street South, Zip 33705; tel. 813/894–8719; Pamela M. Riter, R.N., Administrator (Nonreporting) **A**1 10 **S** Vencor, Incorporated, Louisville, KY	33	49	60	—	—	—	—	—	—	—
SANFORD—Seminole County										
✦ COLUMBIA MEDICAL CENTER SANFORD, 1401 West Seminole Boulevard, Zip 32771–6764; tel. 407/321–4500; Doug Sills, President and Chief Executive Officer (Nonreporting) **A**1 9 10 **S** Columbia/HCA Healthcare Corporation, Nashville, TN **N** Columbia/HCA Central Florida Division, Winter Park, FL; The Health Advantage Network, Winter Park, FL	33	10	226	—	—	—	—	—	—	—
SARASOTA—Sarasota County										
✦ COLUMBIA DOCTORS HOSPITAL OF SARASOTA, 5731 Bee Ridge Road, Zip 34233; tel. 941/342–1100; William C. Lievense, President and Chief Executive Officer **A**1 9 10 **F**3 4 7 8 10 12 14 15 16 19 21 22 26 27 30 32 35 37 40 41 42 44 46 49 57 63 71 73 74 **P**1 **S** Columbia/HCA Healthcare Corporation, Nashville, TN **N** Columbia/HCA SouthWest Florida Division, Fort Myers, FL; The Health Advantage Network, Winter Park, FL	12	10	147	6637	82	29322	548	48375	18567	641
□ △ HEALTHSOUTH REHABILITATION HOSPITAL OF SARASOTA, 3251 Proctor Road, Zip 34231–8538; tel. 941/921–8600; Jeff Garber, Administrator and Chief Executive Officer (Nonreporting) **A**1 7 10 **S** HEALTHSOUTH Corporation, Birmingham, AL	33	46	60	—	—	—	—	—	—	—
✦ △ SARASOTA MEMORIAL HOSPITAL, 1700 South Tamiami Trail, Zip 34239–3555; tel. 941/917–9000; Michael H. Covert, FACHE, President and Chief Executive Officer **A**1 2 5 7 9 10 **F**2 3 4 7 8 10 11 12 14 15 16 17 19 21 22 23 25 26 28 29 30 32 34 35 37 38 39 40 42 43 44 45 46 48 49 50 51 52 53 54 55 56 58 59 63 64 65 66 67 71 72 73 74	16	10	543	24269	388	290829	2264	240147	86778	2345
SEBASTIAN—Indian River County										
□ SEBASTIAN RIVER MEDICAL CENTER, 13695 North U.S. Highway 1, Zip 32958, Mailing Address: Box 780838, Zip 32978; tel. 561/589–3186; Stephen L. Midkiff, Executive Director (Nonreporting) **A**1 9 10 **S** Health Management Associates, Naples, FL	33	10	133	—	—	—	—	—	—	—
SEBRING—Highlands County										
□ HIGHLANDS REGIONAL MEDICAL CENTER, 3600 South Highlands Avenue, Zip 33870–5495, Mailing Address: Drawer 2066, Zip 33871–2066; tel. 941/385–6101; Kevin Dilallo, Executive Director (Nonreporting) **A**1 9 10 **S** Health Management Associates, Naples, FL	33	10	126	—	—	—	—	—	—	—
SEMINOLE—Pasco County										
□ ○ COLUMBIA UNIVERSITY GENERAL HOSPITAL, 10200 Seminole Boulevard, Zip 34642–0005, Mailing Address: P.O. Box 4005, Zip 34642–0005; tel. 813/397–5511; Barry S. Stokes, Chief Operating Officer (Nonreporting) **A**1 10 11 12 13 **S** Columbia/HCA Healthcare Corporation, Nashville, TN	33	10	152	—	—	—	—	—	—	—
SOUTH MIAMI—Dade County										
□ LARKIN HOSPITAL, (Formerly Healthsouth Larkin Hospital), 7031 S.W. 62nd Avenue, Zip 33143; tel. 305/284–7500; Mel D. Deutsch, Administrator (Nonreporting) **A**1 9 10	33	10	112	—	—	—	—	—	—	—
SPRING HILL—Hernando County										
✦ COLUMBIA REGIONAL MEDICAL CENTER, 11375 Cortez Boulevard, Zip 34613, Mailing Address: P.O. Box 5300, Zip 34606; tel. 904/596–6632; John R. Finnegan, Administrator and Chief Operating Officer **A**1 9 10 **F**4 7 8 10 12 15 16 17 19 20 21 22 25 28 30 32 34 37 40 41 42 44 46 49 63 65 71 73 **P**1 **S** Columbia/HCA Healthcare Corporation, Nashville, TN **N** Columbia/HCA Tampa Bay Division, Tampa, FL; The Health Advantage Network, Winter Park, FL	16	10	204	9428	121	62032	424	—	—	805
✦ SPRING HILL REGIONAL HOSPITAL, 10461 Quality Drive, Zip 34609; tel. 904/688–3053; Sonia I. Gonzalez, R.N., Chief Operating Officer **A**1 9 10 **F**7 8 10 16 19 21 22 25 35 37 40 44 49 71 73 74 **S** Quorum Health Group/Quorum Health Resources, Inc., Brentwood, TN **N** BayCare Health Network, Inc., Clearwater, FL	23	10	75	3370	37	27653	610	20302	6428	216
STARKE—Bradford County										
✦ SHANDS AT STARKE, (Formerly Bradford Hospital), 922 East Call Street, Zip 32091, Mailing Address: P.O. Box 1210, Zip 32091–1210; tel. 904/964–6000; Jeannie Baker, Chief Operating Officer **A**1 9 10 **F**8 14 19 22 28 30 34 41 44 49 51 71 73 **S** Shands Health System, University of Florida Health Science Center, Gainesville, FL	23	10	23	290	9	16800	0	—	—	112
STUART—Martin County										
✦ MARTIN MEMORIAL HEALTH SYSTEM, (Includes Martin Memorial Hospital South, 2100 S.E. Salerno Road, Zip 34997; tel. 407/223–2300), 300 S.E. Hospital Drive, Zip 34994, Mailing Address: P.O. Box 9010, Zip 34995–9010; tel. 561/223–5945; Richmond M. Harman, President and Chief Executive Officer **A**1 2 9 10 **F**5 7 8 10 12 14 15 16 17 19 21 22 23 24 25 26 27 28 29 30 31 32 33 34 35 36 37 39 40 41 42 44 45 46 49 51 54 60 63 65 66 67 71 72 73 74 **P**1 3 **N** Lake Okeechobee Rural Health Network, Belle Glade, FL	23	10	260	13371	178	166867	1216	117218	51013	1467

Hospital, Address, Telephone, Administrator, Approval, Facility, and Physician Codes, Health Care System, Network	Classi-fication Codes		Utilization Data					Expense (thousands) of dollars		
★ American Hospital Association (AHA) membership □ Joint Commission on Accreditation of Healthcare Organizations (JCAHO) accreditation + American Osteopathic Hospital Association (AOHA) membership ○ American Osteopathic Association (AOA) accreditation △ Commission on Accreditation of Rehabilitation Facilities (CARF) accreditation Control codes 61, 63, 64, 71, 72 and 73 indicate hospitals listed by AOHA, but not registered by AHA. For definition of numerical codes, see page A4	Control	Service	Beds	Admissions	Census	Outpatient Visits	Births	Total	Payroll	Personnel

SUN CITY CENTER—Hillsborough County

⊞ COLUMBIA SOUTH BAY HOSPITAL, 4016 State Road 674, Zip 33573–5298; tel. 813/634–3301; Marcia Easley, Chief Operating Officer **A**1 9 10 **F**8 11 12 14 16 22 26 28 32 35 37 42 44 45 49 59 64 65 67 71 73 **S** Columbia/HCA Healthcare Corporation, Nashville, TN **N** Columbia/HCA Tampa Bay Division, Tampa, FL; The Health Advantage Network, Winter Park, FL

	33	10	112	4188	71	34856	0	—	—	550

SUNRISE—Broward County

□ THE RETREAT, 555 S.W. 148th Avenue, Zip 33325; tel. 954/370–0200; Maryann J. Greenwell, Executive Director (Nonreporting) **A**1 10

	33	22	100	—	—	—	—	—	—	—

TALLAHASSEE—Leon County

⊞ COLUMBIA TALLAHASSEE COMMUNITY HOSPITAL, 2626 Capital Medical Boulevard, Zip 32308; tel. 904/656–5000; Gary L. Brewer, Chief Executive Officer **A**1 9 10 **F**2 4 7 8 11 12 19 21 22 24 32 35 37 38 40 42 43 44 47 49 60 71 73 **S** Columbia/HCA Healthcare Corporation, Nashville, TN **N** Columbia/HCA North & NorthEast Florida Division, Jacksonville, FL; The Health Advantage Network, Winter Park, FL

	33	10	180	6533	77	61281	857	43900	19353	535

□ △ HEALTHSOUTH REHABILITATION HOSPITAL OF TALLAHASSEE, 1675 Riggins Road, Zip 32308–5315; tel. 904/656–4800; Mike Marshall, Chief Executive Officer **A**1 7 10 **F**1 5 12 14 16 17 24 26 28 29 30 39 41 42 45 48 49 53 54 55 57 58 59 65 66 67 73 **S** HEALTHSOUTH Corporation, Birmingham, AL

	33	46	70	1110	57	10913	0	—	—	271

⊞ TALLAHASSEE MEMORIAL REGIONAL MEDICAL CENTER, 1300 Miccosukee Road, Zip 32308–5093; tel. 904/681–1155; Duncan Moore, President and Chief Executive Officer (Total facility includes 110 beds in nursing home–type unit) **A**1 2 3 5 9 10 **F**4 7 8 10 11 14 15 16 17 19 21 22 23 24 25 26 27 28 29 30 31 32 34 35 37 38 39 40 41 42 43 44 45 46 47 49 51 52 53 54 55 56 57 58 59 60 61 63 64 65 66 67 69 71 73 74 **P**6

	23	10	587	23179	431	212631	3577	184171	84818	2745

TAMARAC—Broward County

⊞ COLUMBIA UNIVERSITY HOSPITAL AND MEDICAL CENTER, (Includes University Pavilion, 7425 North University Drive, Zip 33328; tel. 305/722–9933), 7201 North University Drive, Zip 33321; tel. 305/721–2200; James A. Cruickshank, Chief Executive Officer (Nonreporting) **A**1 9 10 **S** Columbia/HCA Healthcare Corporation, Nashville, TN **N** Columbia/HCA South Florida Division, Miami Lakes, FL; The Health Advantage Network, Winter Park, FL

	33	10	211	—	—	—	—	—	—	—

TAMPA—Hillsborough County

□ CHARTER BEHAVIORAL HEALTH SYSTEM OF TAMPA BAY, 4004 North Riverside Drive, Zip 33603; tel. 813/238–8671; James C. Hill, Chief Executive Officer (Nonreporting) **A**1 10 **S** Magellan Health Services, Atlanta, GA

	33	22	146	—	—	—	—	—	—	—

⊞ H. LEE MOFFITT CANCER CENTER AND RESEARCH INSTITUTE, (CANCER), 12902 Magnolia Drive, Zip 33612–9497; tel. 813/972–4673; John C. Ruckdeschel, M.D., Director and Chief Executive Officer **A**1 2 3 5 8 9 10 **F**8 14 16 17 19 20 21 26 30 31 33 34 37 39 42 44 45 46 49 54 55 58 60 65 67 69 71 73 74

	23	49	115	4148	82	66199	0	98831	38487	1072

⊞ JAMES A. HALEY VETERANS HOSPITAL, 13000 Bruce B. Downs Boulevard, Zip 33612–4798; tel. 813/972–2000; Richard A. Silver, Director (Total facility includes 209 beds in nursing home–type unit) **A**1 3 5 8 **F**1 3 4 5 8 10 11 12 14 15 16 17 18 20 22 23 24 26 28 29 30 31 32 33 34 37 39 41 42 43 48 52 64 **P**6 **S** Department of Veterans Affairs, Washington, DC

	45	10	640	10447	474	450187	0	181418	—	2627

□ MEMORIAL HOSPITAL OF TAMPA, 2901 Swann Avenue, Zip 33609–4057; tel. 813/873–6400; Stephen Mahan, Chief Executive Officer **A**1 5 9 10 **F**1 2 3 4 8 10 11 12 16 17 18 19 21 22 24 26 28 29 30 31 32 33 35 37 38 39 41 42 44 45 47 48 49 51 52 56 57 58 59 63 64 65 71 73 74 **P**5 7 8 **S** TENET Healthcare Corporation, Santa Barbara, CA **N** Tenet South Florida Health System Network, Fort Lauderdale, FL

	32	10	174	4529	81	30893	0	31680	12045	388

⊞ SHRINERS HOSPITALS FOR CHILDREN, TAMPA, 12502 North Pine Drive, Zip 33612–9499; tel. 813/972–2250; John Holtz, Administrator (Nonreporting) **A**1 3 5 **S** Shriners Hospitals for Children, Tampa, FL **N** Tenet South Florida Health System Network, Fort Lauderdale, FL

	23	57	60	—	—	—	—	—	—	—

⊞ ST. JOSEPH'S HOSPITAL, (Includes Tampa Children's Hospital at St. Joseph's, St. Joseph's Women's Hospital – Tampa, 3030 West Dr. Martin L. King Boulevard, Zip 33607–6394; tel. 813/879–4730), 3001 West Martin Luther King Boulevard, Zip 33607–6387, Mailing Address: P.O. Box 4227, Zip 33677–4227; tel. 813/870–4000; Charles Francis Scott, President (Total facility includes 19 beds in nursing home–type unit) **A**1 2 5 9 10 **F**4 6 7 8 10 11 16 17 19 21 22 24 26 29 30 31 32 34 35 37 38 40 41 42 43 44 46 47 49 52 54 55 56 58 59 60 63 64 65 67 70 71 73 74 **P**1 5 6 7 8 **S** Allegany Health System, Tampa, FL **N** BayCare Health Network, Inc., Clearwater, FL; Allegany Health System, Tampa, FL

	21	10	883	33761	501	—	5965	263682	98461	3834

⊞ △ TAMPA GENERAL HEALTHCARE, (Includes TGH–University Psychiatry Center, 3515 East Fletcher Avenue, Zip 33613–4788; tel. 813/972–3000), Davis Islands, Zip 33606, Mailing Address: P.O. Box 1289, Zip 33601; tel. 813/251–7000; Bruce Siegel, M.D., M.P.H., President and Chief Executive Officer (Total facility includes 24 beds in nursing home–type unit) **A**1 3 5 7 8 9 10 **F**3 4 5 7 8 9 10 11 12 13 14 15 16 17 18 19 21 22 23 24 25 26 28 29 30 31 32 34 35 37 38 40 41 42 43 44 45 46 47 48 49 51 52 53 54 55 56 57 58 59 60 61 64 65 66 67 68 69 70 71 72 73 74 **P**4 7
TGH–UNIVERSITY PSYCHIATRY CENTER See Tampa General Healthcare

	16	10	829	22991	446	275952	3134	306027	108977	2951

□ TOWN AND COUNTRY HOSPITAL, 6001 Webb Road, Zip 33615–3291; tel. 813/885–6666; Stephen Mahan, Chief Executive Officer **A**1 5 9 10 **F**2 3 5 8 10 12 14 16 19 21 22 24 28 30 31 32 34 35 41 42 44 45 46 49 51 54 55 56 57 58 59 63 64 65 66 67 71 73 **P**7 8 **S** TENET Healthcare Corporation, Santa Barbara, CA **N** Tenet South Florida Health System Network, Fort Lauderdale, FL

	32	10	148	4423	70	37956	76	27603	11455	363

Hospital, Address, Telephone, Administrator, Approval, Facility, and Physician Codes, Health Care System, Network	Classi-fication Codes		Utilization Data					Expense (thousands) of dollars		
★ American Hospital Association (AHA) membership □ Joint Commission on Accreditation of Healthcare Organizations (JCAHO) accreditation + American Osteopathic Hospital Association (AOHA) membership ○ American Osteopathic Association (AOA) accreditation △ Commission on Accreditation of Rehabilitation Facilities (CARF) accreditation Control codes 61, 63, 64, 71, 72 and 73 indicate hospitals listed by AOHA, but not registered by AHA. For definition of numerical codes, see page A4	Control	Service	Beds	Admissions	Census	Outpatient Visits	Births	Total	Payroll	Personnel
□ TRANSITIONAL HOSPITAL OF TAMPA, 4801 North Howard Avenue, Zip 33603; tel. 813/874–7575; Robert N. Helms, Jr., Divisional Vice President, Operations (Nonreporting) **A**1 5 10 **S** Transitional Hospitals Corporation, Las Vegas, NV	33	49	102	—	—	—	—	—	—	—
□ UNIVERSITY COMMUNITY HOSPITAL, 3100 East Fletcher Avenue, Zip 33613–4688; tel. 813/971–6000; Norman V. Stein, President (Total facility includes 20 beds in nursing home–type unit) **A**1 2 9 10 **F**4 7 8 10 11 12 14 15 16 17 19 20 21 22 23 24 26 27 28 29 30 31 32 34 35 37 38 39 40 41 42 43 44 45 46 47 48 49 60 61 63 64 65 67 71 72 73 74 **P**5 **N** BayCare Health Network, Inc., Clearwater, FL	23	10	424	16384	246	—	1992	143213	66658	1849
□ ○ UNIVERSITY COMMUNITY HOSPITAL–CARROLLWOOD, 7171 North Dale Mabry Highway, Zip 33614–2699; tel. 813/558–8001; Larry J. Archbell, Vice President Operations **A**1 10 11 12 13 **F**4 7 8 10 11 12 14 15 16 17 19 20 21 22 23 24 26 27 28 29 30 31 32 34 35 37 38 39 40 41 42 43 44 45 46 47 48 49 60 61 63 64 65 67 71 72 73 74 **P**5 **N** BayCare Health Network, Inc., Clearwater, FL	23	10	120	3415	44	25416	0	22284	11167	391
□ VENCOR HOSPITAL–TAMPA, (LONG TERM ACUTE CARE), 4555 South Manhattan Avenue, Zip 33611; tel. 813/839–6341; Theresa Hunkins, Administrator **A**1 3 5 10 **F**12 15 16 17 19 20 22 26 27 35 37 39 41 42 46 65 67 71 73 **P**8 **S** Vencor, Incorporated, Louisville, KY	33	49	73	389	60	0	0	—	—	181
TARPON SPRINGS—Pinellas County										
★ HELEN ELLIS MEMORIAL HOSPITAL, 1395 South Pinellas Avenue, Zip 34689–3721, Mailing Address: P.O. Box 1487, Zip 34688–1487; tel. 813/942–5000; Joseph N. Kiefer, Administrator (Total facility includes 18 beds in nursing home–type unit) **A**1 5 9 10 **F**7 8 10 11 12 16 17 19 21 22 25 26 28 29 30 34 35 37 39 40 41 42 44 45 46 49 64 65 67 71 72 73 **P**8	23	10	168	7010	107	64996	456	52151	19351	649
★ NORTHPOINTE BEHAVIORAL HEALTH SYSTEM, (Formerly The Manors), 1527 Riverside Drive, Zip 34689–2023; tel. 813/937–4211; Trish Mitchell, Chief Executive Officer (Total facility includes 16 beds in nursing home–type unit) (Nonreporting) **A**1 10 THE MANORS See Northpointe Behavioral Health System	32	22	130	—	—	—	—	—	—	—
TAVERNIER—Monroe County										
★ MARINERS HOSPITAL, 50 High Point Road, Zip 33070; tel. 305/852–4418; Robert H. Luse, Chief Executive Officer **A**1 9 10 **F**8 15 16 17 19 21 22 28 32 33 34 35 37 44 49 63 65 71 73 **P**1 **N** Dimensions Health/Baptist Health Systems, Miami, FL	23	10	35	1188	14	14956	1	10310	4460	134
TEQUESTA—Martin County										
□ SANDYPINES, 11301 S.E. Tequesta Terrace, Zip 33469; tel. 407/744–0211; David L. Beardsley, Administrator (Nonreporting) **A**1 **S** Health Management Associates, Naples, FL	33	52	60	—	—	—	—	—	—	—
TITUSVILLE—Brevard County										
□ PARRISH MEDICAL CENTER, 951 North Washington Avenue, Zip 32796–2194; tel. 407/268–6111; Rod L. Baker, President and Chief Executive Officer **A**1 2 9 10 **F**7 8 10 12 14 15 16 19 20 21 22 23 24 25 27 28 30 32 33 34 35 37 39 40 41 42 44 45 46 49 51 53 56 58 60 63 65 67 68 71 73 **P**8	16	10	210	8254	104	100489	579	51486	22749	735
VENICE—Sarasota County										
★ BON SECOURS–VENICE HOSPITAL, 540 The Rialto, Zip 34285; tel. 941/485–7711; Roy Hess, Executive Vice President and Administrator (Total facility includes 120 beds in nursing home–type unit) (Nonreporting) **A**1 2 9 10 **S** Bon Secours Health System, Inc., Marriottsville, MD	21	10	390	—	—	—	—	—	—	—
VERO BEACH—Indian River County										
□ △ HEALTHSOUTH TREASURE COAST REHABILITATION HOSPITAL, 1600 37th Street, Zip 32960–6549; tel. 407/778–2100; Denise B. McGrath, Chief Executive Officer (Nonreporting) **A**1 7 10 **S** HEALTHSOUTH Corporation, Birmingham, AL	33	46	70	—	—	—	—	—	—	—
★ INDIAN RIVER MEMORIAL HOSPITAL, 1000 36th Street, Zip 32960–6592; tel. 407/567–4311; Michael J. O'Grady, Jr., President and Chief Executive Officer **A**1 2 9 10 **F**3 7 8 10 11 12 14 15 16 17 19 21 22 23 27 28 29 30 31 32 33 34 35 37 39 40 41 42 44 45 46 49 51 52 53 54 55 56 57 58 59 60 63 65 66 67 71 73 74 **P**8 **N** Community Health Network of Indian River County, Vero Beach, FL	23	10	300	10475	170	60872	835	93046	37073	1089
WEST PALM BEACH—Palm Beach County										
45TH STREET MENTAL HEALTH CENTER, 1041 45th Street, Zip 33407; tel. 407/844–9741; Terry H. Allen, Executive Director (Nonreporting) **A**10	23	22	44	—	—	—	—	—	—	—
★ ○ COLUMBIA HOSPITAL, 2201 45th Street, Zip 33407–2069; tel. 561/842–6141; Michael M. Fencel, Chief Executive Officer (Nonreporting) **A**1 9 10 11 12 **S** Columbia/HCA Healthcare Corporation, Nashville, TN	33	10	250	—	—	—	—	—	—	—
★ GOOD SAMARITAN MEDICAL CENTER, Flagler Drive at Palm Beach Lakes Boulevard, Zip 33401; tel. 561/655–5511; Phillip C. Dutcher, Interim President **A**1 2 10 **F**1 3 7 8 10 12 13 15 16 17 19 21 22 23 24 26 28 30 31 32 33 34 35 37 38 40 42 44 49 51 53 54 55 56 57 58 59 60 65 70 71 73 **P**1 3 4 5 7 **S** Allegany Health System, Tampa, FL **N** Med Connect, Ft Lauderdale, FL	23	10	341	10460	152	67275	2301	103612	30619	—
HOSPICE OF PALM BEACH COUNTY, 5300 East Avenue, Zip 33407–2352; tel. 407/848–5200; Deborah S. Dailey, President and Chief Executive Officer (Nonreporting)	23	49	24	—	—	—	—	—	—	—
★ △ ST. MARY'S HOSPITAL, 901 45th Street, Zip 33407–2495, Mailing Address: P.O. Box 24620, Zip 33416–4620; tel. 561/844–6300; Phillip C. Dutcher, Interim President and Chief Executive Officer **A**1 7 9 10 **F**1 4 7 8 10 11 12 14 15 16 19 21 22 24 26 28 30 31 32 35 37 38 40 41 42 44 48 49 51 52 56 57 58 59 60 65 66 67 70 71 72 73 74 **P**1 3 5 7 **S** Allegany Health System, Tampa, FL **N** The Mount Sinai Health System, New York, NY; Med Connect, Ft Lauderdale, FL; Allegany Health System, Tampa, FL	23	10	433	16355	260	95033	3637	156018	53990	2259

Hospital, Address, Telephone, Administrator, Approval, Facility, and Physician Codes, Health Care System, Network	Classi-fication Codes		Utilization Data					Expense (thousands) of dollars		
★ American Hospital Association (AHA) membership □ Joint Commission on Accreditation of Healthcare Organizations (JCAHO) accreditation + American Osteopathic Hospital Association (AOHA) membership ○ American Osteopathic Association (AOA) accreditation △ Commission on Accreditation of Rehabilitation Facilities (CARF) accreditation Control codes 61, 63, 64, 71, 72 and 73 indicate hospitals listed by AOHA, but not registered by AHA. For definition of numerical codes, see page A4	Control	Service	Beds	Admissions	Census	Outpatient Visits	Births	Total	Payroll	Personnel

	Control	Service	Beds	Admissions	Census	Outpatient Visits	Births	Total	Payroll	Personnel
★ VETERANS AFFAIRS MEDICAL CENTER, 7305 North Military Trail, Zip 33410–6400; tel. 561/882–8262; Richard D. Isaac, Administrator (Total facility includes 90 beds in nursing home–type unit) **F**1 2 3 4 8 10 11 12 14 15 16 17 18 19 20 21 22 23 25 26 27 28 29 30 31 32 33 34 35 37 39 42 43 44 45 46 48 49 50 51 52 54 55 56 57 58 59 60 61 64 65 67 69 71 72 73 74 **P**6 **S** Department of Veterans Affairs, Washington, DC	45	10	242	1380	103	245000	0	—	—	1436
□ ○ WELLINGTON REGIONAL MEDICAL CENTER, 10101 Forest Hill Boulevard, Zip 33414; tel. 561/798–8500; Gregory E. Boyer, Chief Executive Officer (Nonreporting) **A**1 2 9 10 11 12 13 **S** Universal Health Services, Inc., King of Prussia, PA	33	10	93	—	—	—	—	—	—	—
WILLISTON—Levy County										
□ NATURE COAST REGIONAL HEALTH NETWORK, (Formerly Nature Coast Regional Hospital), 125 S.W. Seventh Street, Zip 32696, Mailing Address: P.O. Drawer 550, Zip 32696; tel. 352/528–2801; Chris Wearmouth, Administrator **A**1 9 10 **F**15 19 21 22 26 27 28 30 32 33 34 37 41 44 46 48 49 51 64 65 71 73 **P**6	33	10	40	838	10	16499	0	7749	3785	149
WINTER GARDEN—Orange County										
HEALTH CENTRAL See Ocoee										
WINTER HAVEN—Polk County										
✠ △ WINTER HAVEN HOSPITAL, 200 Avenue F N.E., Zip 33881; tel. 941/297–1899; Lance W. Anastasio, President (Total facility includes 47 beds in nursing home–type unit) **A**1 7 9 10 **F**7 8 10 11 13 14 15 16 17 18 19 20 21 22 23 24 28 29 30 32 33 34 35 37 38 39 40 41 42 44 45 48 49 51 52 53 54 55 56 57 58 59 60 64 65 67 71 72 73 74 **N** Mid–Florida Medical Services, Inc., Winter Haven, FL	23	10	435	18016	256	203293	2140	130615	63701	2184
WINTER PARK—Orange County										
✠ WINTER PARK MEMORIAL HOSPITAL, (Formerly Columbia Winter Park Memorial Hospital), (Includes Winter Park Psychiatric Care Center, 1600 Dodd Road, Zip 32792; tel. 407/677–6842), 200 North Lakemont Avenue, Zip 32792–3273; tel. 407/646–7000; Douglas P. DeGraaf, Chief Executive Officer (Nonreporting) **A**1 9 10 **S** Columbia/HCA Healthcare Corporation, Nashville, TN **N** Columbia/HCA Central Florida Division, Winter Park, FL; The Health Advantage Network, Winter Park, FL	33	10	339	—	—	—	—	—	—	—
ZEPHYRHILLS—Pasco County										
✠ EAST PASCO MEDICAL CENTER, 7050 Gall Boulevard, Zip 33541–1399; tel. 813/788–0411; Bob A. Dodd, President (Total facility includes 11 beds in nursing home–type unit) (Nonreporting) **A**1 9 10 **S** Adventist Health System Sunbelt Health Care Corporation, Winter Park, FL **N** BayCare Health Network, Inc., Clearwater, FL; Adventist Health System, Winter Park, FL	21	10	120	—	—	—	—	—	—	—

GEORGIA

Resident population 7,201 (in thousands)
Resident population in metro areas 68.1%
Birth rate per 1,000 population 16.0
65 years and over 10.0%
Percent of persons without health insurance 16.2%

Hospital, Address, Telephone, Administrator, Approval, Facility, and Physician Codes, Health Care System, Network	Classi-fication Codes		Utilization Data					Expense (thousands) of dollars		
★ American Hospital Association (AHA) membership □ Joint Commission on Accreditation of Healthcare Organizations (JCAHO) accreditation + American Osteopathic Hospital Association (AOHA) membership ○ American Osteopathic Association (AOA) accreditation △ Commission on Accreditation of Rehabilitation Facilities (CARF) accreditation Control codes 61, 63, 64, 71, 72 and 73 indicate hospitals listed by AOHA, but not registered by AHA. For definition of numerical codes, see page A4	Control	Service	Beds	Admissions	Census	Outpatient Visits	Births	Total	Payroll	Personnel

ADEL—Cook County

MEMORIAL HOSPITAL OF ADEL, 706 North Parrish Avenue, Zip 31620–0677, Mailing Address: Box 677, Zip 31620–0677; tel. 912/896–2251; Wade E. Keck, Chief Executive Officer (Total facility includes 95 beds in nursing home–type unit) **A**10 **F**7 14 15 16 17 19 22 32 37 40 44 46 49 64 71 73 **S** Memorial Health Services, Adel, GA — 33 10 155 2474 119 — 190 15869 6495 287

ALBANY—Dougherty County

COLUMBIA PALMYRA MEDICAL CENTERS, 2000 Palmyra Road, Zip 31701, Mailing Address: Box 1908, Zip 31702–1908; tel. 912/434–2000; Allen Golson, Chief Executive Officer **A**1 10 **F**8 11 12 14 15 16 19 21 22 23 24 26 28 30 31 34 35 37 39 41 42 44 45 46 48 49 57 66 67 70 71 72 73 **P**1 2 3 4 5 6 7 8 **S** Columbia/HCA Healthcare Corporation, Nashville, TN **N** Principal Health Care of Georgia, Atlanta, GA; Georgia 1st, Inc., Decatur, GA — 33 10 156 4768 92 50840 0 40137 14779 514

PHOEBE PUTNEY MEMORIAL HOSPITAL, 417 Third Avenue, Zip 31701–1828, Mailing Address: P.O. Box 1828, Zip 31703–1828; tel. 912/883–1800; Joel Wernick, President and Chief Executive Officer (Nonreporting) **A**1 2 3 5 9 10 **N** The Medical Resource Network, L.L.C., Atlanta, GA — 23 10 418 — — — — — — —

ALMA—Bacon County

BACON COUNTY HOSPITAL, 302 South Wayne Street, Zip 31510, Mailing Address: P.O. Drawer 1987, Zip 31510; tel. 912/632–8961; Patsy Busbin, Acting Chief Executive Officer (Total facility includes 88 beds in nursing home–type unit) **A**1 9 10 **F**7 8 14 15 16 19 22 26 30 31 35 37 40 41 44 45 46 49 57 61 64 65 71 73 74 **P**8 — 16 10 126 1668 105 14519 50 11348 4959 215

AMERICUS—Sumter County

SUMTER REGIONAL HOSPITAL, 100 Wheatley Drive, Zip 31709; tel. 912/924–6011; Jerry W. Adams, President (Total facility includes 100 beds in nursing home–type unit) **A**1 9 10 **F**4 7 8 10 11 15 16 17 19 21 22 23 26 27 28 29 30 32 33 34 35 37 39 40 42 43 44 45 46 48 49 51 52 56 57 64 65 67 69 70 71 73 **P**8 **N** Principal Health Care of Georgia, Atlanta, GA; Georgia 1st, Inc., Decatur, GA — 16 10 252 5250 171 39116 886 32984 14075 601

ARLINGTON—Calhoun County

CALHOUN MEMORIAL HOSPITAL, 209 Academy & Carswell Streets, Zip 31713, Mailing Address: Drawer R, Zip 31713; tel. 912/725–4272; Peggy Pierce, Administrator (Nonreporting) **A**10 **N** The Medical Resource Network, L.L.C., Atlanta, GA — 16 10 24 — — — — — — —

ATHENS—Clarke County

ATHENS REGIONAL MEDICAL CENTER, 1199 Prince Avenue, Zip 30606–2793; tel. 706/549–9977; John A. Drew, President and Chief Executive Officer **A**1 9 10 **F**2 3 4 7 8 10 11 15 16 17 19 21 22 23 25 30 31 32 33 35 37 38 40 41 42 43 44 46 49 52 53 54 55 56 57 61 65 66 67 71 73 **N** Georgia 1st, Inc., Decatur, GA; The Medical Resource Network, L.L.C., Atlanta, GA — 16 10 315 14810 209 96623 1514 124120 51178 1654

CHARTER WINDS HOSPITAL, 240 Mitchell Bridge Road, Zip 30606; tel. 706/546–7277; Susan Lister, Chief Executive Officer (Nonreporting) **A**1 10 **S** Magellan Health Services, Atlanta, GA — 33 22 80 — — — — — — —

ST. MARY'S HEALTH CARE SYSTEM, 1230 Baxter Street, Zip 30606–3791; tel. 706/548–7581; Edward J. Fechtel, Jr., President and Chief Executive Officer (Total facility includes 120 beds in nursing home–type unit) **A**1 9 10 **F**7 8 10 12 14 15 16 17 19 21 22 24 26 27 28 29 30 31 32 33 34 35 37 38 39 40 41 42 44 45 46 49 60 64 65 66 67 71 73 **P**6 7 8 **N** Principal Health Care of Georgia, Atlanta, GA — 23 10 290 7163 209 73627 1068 74279 36897 1021

ATLANTA—Fulton and De Kalb Counties County

★ ANCHOR HOSPITAL, 5454 Yorktowne Drive, Zip 30349–5305; tel. 770/991–6044; Benjamin H. Underwood, CHE, FAAMA, President and Chief Executive Officer **A**9 10 **F**2 3 14 15 16 17 27 34 45 46 52 53 54 55 56 57 58 59 65 67 73 **P**6 — 33 82 84 2380 37 8975 0 5166 2289 151

CHARTER BEHAVIORAL HEALTH SYSTEM OF ATLANTA, 811 Juniper Street N.E., Zip 30308; tel. 404/881–5800; Dennis Workman, M.D., Medical Director (Nonreporting) **A**1 10 **S** Magellan Health Services, Atlanta, GA — 33 22 40 — — — — — — —

CHARTER BEHAVIORAL HEALTH SYSTEM OF ATLANTA AT PEACHFORD, 2151 Peachford Road, Zip 30338; tel. 770/455–3200; Aleen S. Davis, Chief Executive Officer (Nonreporting) **A**1 10 **S** Magellan Health Services, Atlanta, GA — 33 22 224 — — — — — — —

COLUMBIA DUNWOODY MEDICAL CENTER, 4575 North Shallowford Road, Zip 30338; tel. 770/454–2000; Thomas D. Gilbert, President and Chief Executive Officer **A**1 10 **F**7 8 10 12 14 15 16 17 18 19 21 22 23 25 27 28 29 30 32 34 35 37 38 39 40 41 44 45 46 49 61 63 65 66 67 70 71 72 73 74 **P**1 2 4 8 **S** Columbia/HCA Healthcare Corporation, Nashville, TN — 33 10 122 4187 43 27704 1026 34915 13749 410

COLUMBIA METROPOLITAN HOSPITAL, 3223 Howell Mill Road N.W., Zip 30327; tel. 404/351–0500; Neil Heatherly, Chief Executive Officer (Nonreporting) **A**1 10 **S** Columbia/HCA Healthcare Corporation, Nashville, TN — 33 49 64 — — — — — — —

Hospital, Address, Telephone, Administrator, Approval, Facility, and Physician Codes, Health Care System, Network	Classification Codes		Utilization Data					Expense (thousands) of dollars		
★ American Hospital Association (AHA) membership □ Joint Commission on Accreditation of Healthcare Organizations (JCAHO) accreditation + American Osteopathic Hospital Association (AOHA) membership ○ American Osteopathic Association (AOA) accreditation △ Commission on Accreditation of Rehabilitation Facilities (CARF) accreditation Control codes 61, 63, 64, 71, 72 and 73 indicate hospitals listed by AOHA, but not registered by AHA. For definition of numerical codes, see page A4.	Control	Service	Beds	Admissions	Census	Outpatient Visits	Births	Total	Payroll	Personnel
★ + ○ COLUMBIA NORTHLAKE REGIONAL MEDICAL CENTER, 1455 Montreal Road, Zip 30084, Mailing Address: P.O. Box 450000, Zip 31145; tel. 770/270–3000; Michael R. Burroughs, President and Chief Executive Officer A1 2 10 11 F7 8 12 14 17 19 21 22 27 28 32 35 37 38 39 40 41 42 44 48 49 65 71 73 P5 7 S Columbia/HCA Healthcare Corporation, Nashville, TN	33	10	120	2526	36	25422	510	—	—	377
★ COLUMBIA WEST PACES MEDICAL CENTER, 3200 Howell Mill Road N.W., Zip 30327–4101; tel. 404/351–0351; Thomas E. Anderson, President and Chief Executive Officer (Nonreporting) A1 2 3 10 S Columbia/HCA Healthcare Corporation, Nashville, TN	33	10	294	—	—	—	—	—	—	—
★ CRAWFORD LONG HOSPITAL OF EMORY UNIVERSITY, 550 Peachtree Street N.E., Zip 30365–2225; tel. 404/686–4411; John Dunklin Henry, Sr., Chief Executive Officer (Nonreporting) A1 2 3 5 8 9 10 N Georgia 1st, Inc., Decatur, GA	23	10	419	—	—	—	—	—	—	—
★ △ EGLESTON CHILDREN'S HOSPITAL AT EMORY UNIVERSITY, 1405 Clifton Road N.E., Zip 30322–1101; tel. 404/325–6000; Alan J. Gayer, President (Nonreporting) A1 3 5 7 8 9 10 N Principal Health Care of Georgia, Atlanta, GA; Georgia 1st, Inc., Decatur, GA; The Medical Resource Network, L.L.C., Atlanta, GA	23	50	196	—	—	—	—	—	—	—
★ △ EMORY UNIVERSITY HOSPITAL, 1364 Clifton Road N.E., Zip 30322–1102; tel. 404/727–7021; John Dunklin Henry, Sr., Chief Executive Officer (Nonreporting) A1 2 3 5 7 8 9 10 N Candler Health System, Savannah, GA; National Cardiovascular Network, Atlanta, GA; Georgia 1st, Inc., Decatur, GA	23	10	523	—	—	—	—	—	—	—
★ △ GEORGIA BAPTIST HEALTH CARE SYSTEM, 303 Parkway Drive N.E., Zip 30312; tel. 404/265–4000; David E. Harrell, President and Chief Executive Officer (Total facility includes 72 beds in nursing home–type unit) A1 2 3 5 7 8 10 F4 6 7 8 10 11 12 13 14 16 17 18 19 21 22 23 24 25 26 27 28 29 30 31 32 33 34 35 37 38 39 40 41 42 43 44 45 46 48 49 51 52 54 55 56 57 58 59 60 61 62 63 64 65 67 71 72 73 74 P6 7	21	10	450	15195	271	113453	2614	161828	66623	2298
□ GEORGIA MENTAL HEALTH INSTITUTE, 1256 Briarcliff Road N.E., Zip 30306; tel. 404/894–5911; B. C. Robbins, Superintendent A1 3 5 10 F2 14 15 22 45 52 53 54 55 56 65 73 P6	12	22	222	4126	174	—	0	27050	17198	496
★ GRADY MEMORIAL HOSPITAL, 80 Butler Street S.E., Zip 30335–3801, Mailing Address: P.O. Box 26189, Zip 30335–3801; tel. 404/616–4252; Edward J. Renford, President and Chief Executive Officer (Total facility includes 354 beds in nursing home–type unit) (Nonreporting) A1 2 3 5 8 10 N Grady Health System, Atlanta, GA	16	10	1200	—	—	—	—	—	—	—
★ HILLSIDE HOSPITAL, 690 Courtney Drive N.E., Zip 30306–0206, Mailing Address: P.O. Box 8247, Zip 31106–0247; tel. 404/875–4551; Teresa Stoker, Executive Director F14 15 16 52 53 55 56 59 65 67	23	52	61	33	61	0	0	7892	3939	159
★ NORTHSIDE HOSPITAL, 1000 Johnson Ferry Road N.E., Zip 30342–1611; tel. 404/851–8000; Sidney Kirschner, President and Chief Executive Officer (Nonreporting) A1 2 9 10 N Principal Health Care of Georgia, Atlanta, GA; Georgia 1st, Inc., Decatur, GA; The Medical Resource Network, L.L.C., Atlanta, GA	23	44	352	—	—	—	—	—	—	—
★ PIEDMONT HOSPITAL, 1968 Peachtree Road N.W., Zip 30309–1231; tel. 404/605–5000; Richard B. Hubbard, III, President and Chief Executive Officer (Total facility includes 37 beds in nursing home–type unit) (Nonreporting) A1 2 3 5 9 10 N Promina Health System, Inc., Atlanta, GA; Principal Health Care of Georgia, Atlanta, GA; The Medical Resource Network, L.L.C., Atlanta, GA	23	10	444	—	—	—	—	—	—	—
★ SAINT JOSEPH'S HOSPITAL OF ATLANTA, 5665 Peachtree Dunwoody Road N.E., Zip 30342–1764; tel. 404/851–7001; Brue Chandler, President and Chief Executive Officer (Nonreporting) A1 2 9 10 S Eastern Mercy Health System, Radnor, PA N Saint Joseph's Hospital of Atlanta, Atlanta, GA	23	10	346	—	—	—	—	—	—	—
★ △ SCOTTISH RITE CHILDREN'S MEDICAL CENTER, 1001 Johnson Ferry Road N.E., Zip 30342; tel. 404/256–5252; James E. Tally, Ph.D., President and Chief Executive Officer A1 3 5 7 9 F12 13 15 16 17 19 20 21 22 29 30 34 35 38 39 41 42 44 45 46 47 48 49 51 54 60 65 66 67 70 71 72 73 P1 N Principal Health Care of Georgia, Atlanta, GA	23	50	165	7476	103	139605	0	121424	53509	1341
★ △ SHEPHERD CENTER, 2020 Peachtree Road N.W., Zip 30309–1465; tel. 404/352–2020; Gary R. Ulicny, Ph.D., President and Chief Executive Officer A1 5 7 9 10 F12 14 15 17 19 20 22 24 27 34 35 37 39 45 46 48 49 53 54 58 61 65 67 70 71 73 P6 7 N Principal Health Care of Georgia, Atlanta, GA; The Medical Resource Network, L.L.C., Atlanta, GA	23	46	100	752	69	15513	0	37479	18811	519
□ SOUTHWEST HOSPITAL AND MEDICAL CENTER, 501 Fairburn Road S.W., Zip 30331–2099; tel. 404/699–1111; Marie Cameron, FACHE, President and Chief Executive Officer (Nonreporting) A1 3 5 9 10	23	10	80	—	—	—	—	—	—	—
□ VENCOR HOSPITAL–ATLANTA, 705 Juniper Street N.E., Zip 30365; tel. 404/873–2871; Skip Wright, Administrator (Nonreporting) A1 10 S Vencor, Incorporated, Louisville, KY	33	49	66	—	—	—	—	—	—	—
★ WESLEY WOODS GERIATRIC HOSPITAL, 1821 Clifton Road N.E., Zip 30329–5102; tel. 404/728–6200; William L. Minnix, Chief Executive Officer A1 3 5 10 F3 4 6 8 10 11 12 17 19 20 21 22 25 26 27 28 29 30 33 34 35 37 39 41 42 43 44 45 46 48 49 50 51 52 54 55 56 57 58 59 60 62 63 64 65 67 69 70 71 73 74 P6 N Emory University System of Healthcare Affiliate Network, Atlanta, GA	23	22	91	1792	66	24766	0	24557	9944	328

AUGUSTA—Richmond County

★ COLUMBIA AUGUSTA MEDICAL CENTER, (Formerly Columbia Augusta Regional Medical Center), 3651 Wheeler Road, Zip 30909–6426; tel. 706/651–3232; Michael K. Kerner, President and Chief Executive Officer A1 9 10 F2 3 7 8 9 10 12 16 19 21 22 25 28 30 32 35 37 40 41 42 44 48 49 51 52 53 58 59 60 65 67 73 P1 S Columbia/HCA Healthcare Corporation, Nashville, TN	33	10	284	8643	126	75511	1139	63072	26997	864

Hospital, Address, Telephone, Administrator, Approval, Facility, and Physician Codes, Health Care System, Network	Classi-fication Codes		Utilization Data					Expense (thousands) of dollars		
	Control	Service	Beds	Admissions	Census	Outpatient Visits	Births	Total	Payroll	Personnel

★ American Hospital Association (AHA) membership
□ Joint Commission on Accreditation of Healthcare Organizations (JCAHO) accreditation
+ American Osteopathic Hospital Association (AOHA) membership
○ American Osteopathic Association (AOA) accreditation
△ Commission on Accreditation of Rehabilitation Facilities (CARF) accreditation
Control codes 61, 63, 64, 71, 72 and 73 indicate hospitals listed by AOHA, but not registered by AHA. For definition of numerical codes, see page A4

Hospital	Control	Service	Beds	Admissions	Census	Outpatient Visits	Births	Total	Payroll	Personnel
□ GEORGIA REGIONAL HOSPITAL AT AUGUSTA, 3405 Mike Padgett Highway, Zip 30906; tel. 706/792–7019; Benjamin H. Walker, Acting Superintendent **A**1 3 10 **F**1 2 3 4 5 6 7 8 9 10 11 12 13 14 17 18 19 20 21 22 23 24 25 26 27 28 29 30 31 32 33 34 35 36 37 38 39 40 41 42 43 44 45 46 47 48 49 50 51 52 53 54 55 56 57 58 59 60 61 62 63 64 65 66 67 68 69 70 71 72 73 74 **P**3 6	12	22	262	3214	213	0	0	22667	14258	520
⊠ MEDICAL COLLEGE OF GEORGIA HOSPITAL AND CLINICS, 1120 15th Street, Zip 30912–5000; tel. 706/721–0211; Patricia Sodomka, Executive Director **A**1 2 3 5 8 9 10 12 **F**4 7 8 9 10 11 12 13 15 16 17 19 20 21 22 23 26 27 28 29 30 31 34 35 37 38 39 40 41 42 43 44 46 47 49 51 52 53 54 55 56 57 58 59 60 61 63 65 66 67 69 70 71 73 74 **P**6 **N** Georgia 1st, Inc., Decatur, GA	12	10	459	16381	300	439873	1734	233314	116158	3263
⊠ ST. JOSEPH HOSPITAL, 2260 Wrightsboro Road, Zip 30904–4726; tel. 706/481–7000; J. William Paugh, President and Chief Executive Officer **A**1 9 10 **F**7 8 10 12 14 15 16 17 19 22 23 25 26 28 29 30 32 33 34 35 37 38 39 40 42 44 45 49 51 62 65 67 71 73 74 **P**8 **S** Carondelet Health System, Saint Louis, MO	21	10	145	5818	83	443015	1228	72941	33422	1126
⊠ UNIVERSITY HOSPITAL, 1350 Walton Way, Zip 30901–2629; tel. 706/722–9011; Donald C. Bray, President and Chief Executive Officer **A**1 2 3 5 9 10 **F**1 2 3 4 6 7 8 10 11 12 14 15 16 17 18 20 21 22 23 24 25 28 29 30 31 32 34 35 37 38 39 40 41 42 43 44 45 46 47 48 49 51 52 54 55 56 57 58 59 61 63 64 65 66 67 68 71 72 73 74 **P**1 2 5 7 **N** Principal Health Care of Georgia, Atlanta, GA; The Medical Resource Network, L.L.C., Atlanta, GA; University Health, Inc., Augusta, GA	23	10	528	21713	337	297683	2483	233651	86176	3121
⊠ VETERANS AFFAIRS MEDICAL CENTER, 1 Freedom Way, Zip 30904–6285; tel. 706/733–0188; David Whatley, Director (Total facility includes 60 beds in nursing home–type unit) **A**1 2 3 5 8 **F**1 2 3 4 8 10 11 12 14 15 16 17 19 20 21 22 24 26 27 31 32 33 34 35 37 39 41 42 43 44 45 46 48 49 51 52 54 56 57 58 59 60 63 64 65 67 71 73 74 **S** Department of Veterans Affairs, Washington, DC	45	10	587	8313	490	104356	0	145652	78375	2171
⊠ △ WALTON REHABILITATION HOSPITAL, 1355 Independence Drive, Zip 30901–1037; tel. 706/823–8505; Dennis B. Skelley, President and Chief Executive Officer **A**1 7 9 10 **F**1 2 3 4 5 6 7 8 9 10 11 12 13 14 15 16 17 18 19 20 21 22 23 24 25 26 27 28 29 30 31 32 33 34 35 36 37 38 39 40 41 42 43 44 45 46 47 48 49 50 51 52 53 54 55 56 57 58 59 60 61 62 63 64 65 66 67 68 69 70 71 72 73 74 **S** Carondelet Health System, Saint Louis, MO **N** Principal Health Care of Georgia, Atlanta, GA	23	46	58	914	43	20117	0	16917	7365	231
AUSTELL—Cobb County										
⊠ △ PROMINA COBB HOSPITAL, 3950 Austell Road, Zip 30001–1121; tel. 770/732–4000; Betty Whisenant, Site Manager **A**1 2 7 9 10 **F**2 3 6 7 8 10 11 12 13 14 15 16 17 18 19 20 21 22 24 25 26 28 29 30 31 32 33 34 35 37 38 39 40 41 42 44 45 46 48 49 50 51 52 53 54 55 56 57 58 59 60 61 62 64 65 66 67 68 70 71 72 73 74 **P**1 3 7 **S** Promina Northwest Health System, Austell, GA **N** Promina Health System, Inc., Atlanta, GA; Principal Health Care of Georgia, Atlanta, GA; The Medical Resource Network, L.L.C., Atlanta, GA	23	10	311	14039	176	128089	2825	99891	43355	1251
BAINBRIDGE—Decatur County										
⊠ MEMORIAL HOSPITAL AND MANOR, 1500 East Shotwell Street, Zip 31717; tel. 912/246–3500; James G. Peak, Director (Total facility includes 107 beds in nursing home–type unit) (Nonreporting) **A**1 9 10 **N** Principal Health Care of Georgia, Atlanta, GA	16	10	187	—	—	—	—	—	—	—
BAXLEY—Appling County										
□ APPLING HEALTHCARE SYSTEM, 301 East Tollison Street, Zip 31513; tel. 912/367–9841; Luther E. Reeves, Chief Executive Officer (Total facility includes 101 beds in nursing home–type unit) (Nonreporting) **A**1 10 **N** Candler Health System, Savannah, GA; Principal Health Care of Georgia, Atlanta, GA; Georgia 1st, Inc., Decatur, GA; The Medical Resource Network, L.L.C., Atlanta, GA	16	10	141	—	—	—	—	—	—	—
BLAIRSVILLE—Union County										
★ UNION GENERAL HOSPITAL, 214 Hospital Drive, Zip 30512; tel. 706/745–2111, Rebecca T. Dyer, Administrator (Total facility includes 105 beds in nursing home–type unit) **A**9 10 **F**7 8 15 16 19 20 21 22 28 30 34 37 40 44 64 65 71 73	16	10	150	2091	123	24980	215	12027	5730	241
BLAKELY—Early County										
□ EARLY MEMORIAL HOSPITAL, 630 Columbia Street, Zip 31723; tel. 912/723–4241 (Total facility includes 127 beds in nursing home–type unit) (Nonreporting) **A**1 9 10 **S** Archbold Medical Center, Thomasville, GA **N** Georgia 1st, Inc., Decatur, GA; The Medical Resource Network, L.L.C., Atlanta, GA	16	10	176	—	—	—	—	—	—	—
BLUE RIDGE—Fannin County										
□ FANNIN REGIONAL HOSPITAL, Highway 5 North, Zip 30513, Mailing Address: Box 1549, Zip 30513; tel. 706/632–3711; Kent W. McMackin, Chief Executive Officer (Nonreporting) **A**1 9 10 **S** Community Health Systems, Inc., Brentwood, TN	33	10	46	—	—	—	—	—	—	—
BOWDON—Carroll County										
BOWDON AREA HOSPITAL, 501 Mitchell Avenue, Zip 30108; tel. 770/258–7207; Yvonne Willis, Administrator **A**9 10 **F**8 15 19 22 28 33 35 39 41 44 48 49 65 67 71 73 **S** Bowdon Corporate Offices, Atlanta, GA	33	10	41	850	16	5124	0	4324	1441	63
BREMEN—Haralson County										
★ HIGGINS GENERAL HOSPITAL, 200 Allen Memorial Drive, Zip 30110, Mailing Address: Box 655, Zip 30110; tel. 770/537–5851; Robbie Smith, Administrator **A**9 10 **F**8 14 15 16 19 22 28 30 37 44 45 46 49 65 71 **P**8 **N** Principal Health Care of Georgia, Atlanta, GA; Georgia 1st, Inc., Decatur, GA; The Medical Resource Network, L.L.C., Atlanta, GA	15	10	39	847	13	15313	0	7593	3128	134

Hospital, Address, Telephone, Administrator, Approval, Facility, and Physician Codes, Health Care System, Network	Classi-fication Codes		Utilization Data						Expense (thousands) of dollars		
★ American Hospital Association (AHA) membership □ Joint Commission on Accreditation of Healthcare Organizations (JCAHO) accreditation + American Osteopathic Hospital Association (AOHA) membership ○ American Osteopathic Association (AOA) accreditation △ Commission on Accreditation of Rehabilitation Facilities (CARF) accreditation Control codes 61, 63, 64, 71, 72 and 73 indicate hospitals listed by AOHA, but not registered by AHA. For definition of numerical codes, see page A4	Control	Service	Beds	Admissions	Census	Outpatient Visits	Births	Total	Payroll	Personnel

BRUNSWICK—Glynn County											
✠ SOUTHEAST GEORGIA REGIONAL MEDICAL CENTER, 3100 Kemble Avenue, Zip 31520, Mailing Address: Box 1518, Zip 31521; tel. 912/264–7000; E. Berton Whitaker, President and Chief Executive Officer **A**1 10 **F**7 8 10 11 14 15 16 19 21 22 28 29 30 31 33 34 35 37 40 41 42 44 45 46 49 52 56 58 59 60 65 67 71 73 **P**1 3 **S** Quorum Health Group/Quorum Health Resources, Inc., Brentwood, TN **N** Principal Health Care of Georgia, Atlanta, GA; Georgia 1st, Inc., Decatur, GA	16	10	337	12514	186	98385	1151	98861	42259	1326
CAIRO—Grady County											
□ GRADY GENERAL HOSPITAL, 1155 Fifth Street S.E., Zip 31728, Mailing Address: P.O. Box 360, Zip 31728; tel. 912/377–1150; Glen C. Davis, Administrator (Nonreporting) **A**1 9 10 **S** Archbold Medical Center, Thomasville, GA **N** Georgia 1st, Inc., Decatur, GA; The Medical Resource Network, L.L.C., Atlanta, GA	23	10	45	—	—	—	—	—	—	—
CALHOUN—Gordon County											
✠ GORDON HOSPITAL, 1035 Red Bud Road, Zip 30701, Mailing Address: P.O. Box 12938, Zip 30703–7013; tel. 706/629–2895; Dennis Kiley, President **A**1 9 10 **F**8 10 12 15 17 19 21 22 26 28 30 32 34 35 37 40 44 45 49 50 57 63 65 67 71 72 73 **P**1 **S** Adventist Health System Sunbelt Health Care Corporation, Winter Park, FL **N** Principal Health Care of Georgia, Atlanta, GA; The Medical Resource Network, L.L.C., Atlanta, GA	21	10	50	2767	28	92556	354	22953	9193	338
CAMILLA—Mitchell County											
□ MITCHELL COUNTY HOSPITAL, 90 Stephens Street, Zip 31730, Mailing Address: P.O. Box 639, Zip 31730; tel. 912/336–5284; Ronald M. Gilliard, FACHE, Administrator (Total facility includes 156 beds in nursing home–type unit) (Nonreporting) **A**1 9 10 **S** Archbold Medical Center, Thomasville, GA **N** Georgia 1st, Inc., Decatur, GA; The Medical Resource Network, L.L.C., Atlanta, GA	23	10	182	—	—	—	—	—	—	—
CANTON—Cherokee County											
✠ R. T. JONES HOSPITAL, 201 Hospital Road, Zip 30114, Mailing Address: P.O. Box 906, Zip 30114; tel. 770/720–5100; Douglas M. Parker, Chief Executive Officer **A**1 9 10 **F**7 8 15 16 19 21 22 28 29 31 35 37 39 40 42 44 45 49 67 70 71 73 **N** Principal Health Care of Georgia, Atlanta, GA	16	10	84	2670	33	28493	233	19036	8103	254
CARROLLTON—Carroll County											
✠ TANNER MEDICAL CENTER, 705 Dixie Street, Zip 30117–3818; tel. 770/836–9666; Loy M. Howard, Chief Executive Officer **A**1 9 10 **F**7 8 10 12 15 17 18 19 20 21 22 23 28 30 34 35 37 40 41 42 44 46 48 52 59 60 63 64 65 71 73 74 **P**7 8 **S** Quorum Health Group/Quorum Health Resources, Inc., Brentwood, TN **N** Principal Health Care of Georgia, Atlanta, GA; Georgia 1st, Inc., Decatur, GA	23	10	183	7588	95	81665	1057	50090	21481	788
CARTERSVILLE—Bartow County											
✠ COLUMBIA CARTERSVILLE MEDICAL CENTER, 960 Joe Frank Harris Parkway, Zip 30120, Mailing Address: P.O. Box 200008, Zip 30120–9001; tel. 770/382–1530; Keith Sandlin, Chief Executive Officer (Nonreporting) **A**1 9 10 **S** Columbia/HCA Healthcare Corporation, Nashville, TN **N** Principal Health Care of Georgia, Atlanta, GA	33	10	80	—	—	—	—	—	—	—
CEDARTOWN—Polk County											
✠ COLUMBIA POLK GENERAL HOSPITAL, (Formerly Polk General Hospital), 424 North Main Street, Zip 30125; tel. 770/748–2500; Mark Nichols, Chief Executive Officer (Nonreporting) **A**1 9 10	16	10	35	—	—	—	—	—	—	—
CHATSWORTH—Murray County											
✠ COLUMBIA MURRAY MEDICAL CENTER, 707 Old Ellijay Road, Zip 30705, Mailing Address: P.O. Box 1406, Zip 30705; tel. 706/695–4564; Richard Cook, Administrator (Nonreporting) **A**1 9 10 **S** Columbia/HCA Healthcare Corporation, Nashville, TN **N** NorthWest Georgia Healthcare Partnership, Dalton, GA	33	10	42	—	—	—	—	—	—	—
CLAXTON—Evans County											
□ EVANS MEMORIAL HOSPITAL, 200 North River Street, Zip 30417, Mailing Address: Box 518, Zip 30417; tel. 912/739–5000; Eston Price, Jr., Administrator **A**1 9 10 **F**6 8 14 15 16 19 22 39 40 41 44 46 49 65 71 **P**3	16	10	32	1320	14	12516	93	7212	3524	157
CLAYTON—Rabun County											
★ RABUN COUNTY MEMORIAL HOSPITAL, South Main Street, Zip 30525, Mailing Address: Box 705, Zip 30525–0705; tel. 706/782–4233; Richard B. Wallace, Chief Executive Officer (Nonreporting) **A**10	16	10	26	—	—	—	—	—	—	—
✠ RIDGECREST HOSPITAL, 393 Ridgecrest Circle, Zip 30525; tel. 706/782–4297; Gerald E. Knepp, Chief Executive Officer **A**1 10 **F**2 3 8 18 19 22 26 27 28 30 32 33 34 39 44 49 51 52 54 55 56 57 58 59 64 65 67 71 72 73 **P**5 6 7 8 **S** Quorum Health Group/Quorum Health Resources, Inc., Brentwood, TN **N** Principal Health Care of Georgia, Atlanta, GA	23	10	45	1532	16	10012	0	9724	4270	171
✠ WOODRIDGE HOSPITAL, 394 Ridgecrest Circle, Zip 30525; tel. 706/782–3100; Gerald E. Knepp, Chief Executive Officer **A**1 10 **F**2 3 8 12 13 18 19 22 26 27 28 30 32 33 34 39 44 49 51 52 54 55 56 57 58 59 64 65 71 73 **P**5 6 7 8 **S** Quorum Health Group/Quorum Health Resources, Inc., Brentwood, TN	23	22	32	506	13	—	0	5552	2241	55
COCHRAN—Bleckley County											
BLECKLEY MEMORIAL HOSPITAL, 408 Peacock Street, Zip 31014–1559, Mailing Address: Box 536, Zip 31014–0536; tel. 912/934–6211; Henry T. Gibbs, Administrator **A**10 **F**15 16 19 20 22 28 30 34 37 44 46 65 67 69 71 73 **P**5 **S** Memorial Health Services, Adel, GA	16	10	45	1051	10	9770	2	3884	1772	88
COLQUITT—Miller County											
MILLER COUNTY HOSPITAL, 209 North Cuthbert Street, Zip 31737, Mailing Address: P.O. Box 7, Zip 31737; tel. 912/758–3385; Colleen B. Houston, Administrator (Total facility includes 97 beds in nursing home–type unit) **A**10 **F**15 16 19 22 34 40 44 64 71	16	10	135	485	100	4924	40	4294	2314	134

Hospital, Address, Telephone, Administrator, Approval, Facility, and Physician Codes, Health Care System, Network	Classi-fication Codes		Utilization Data					Expense (thousands) of dollars		
★ American Hospital Association (AHA) membership □ Joint Commission on Accreditation of Healthcare Organizations (JCAHO) accreditation + American Osteopathic Hospital Association (AOHA) membership ○ American Osteopathic Association (AOA) accreditation △ Commission on Accreditation of Rehabilitation Facilities (CARF) accreditation Control codes 61, 63, 64, 71, 72 and 73 indicate hospitals listed by AOHA, but not registered by AHA. For definition of numerical codes, see page A4	Control	Service	Beds	Admissions	Census	Outpatient Visits	Births	Total	Payroll	Personnel

COLUMBUS—Muscogee County

BRADLEY CENTER OF ST. FRANCIS See St. Francis Hospital

⊞ COLUMBIA DOCTORS HOSPITAL, 616 19th Street, Zip 31901–1528, Mailing Address: P.O. Box 2188, Zip 31902–2188; tel. 706/571–4262; Hugh D. Wilson, Chief Executive Officer (Nonreporting) **A**1 2 10 **S** Columbia/HCA Healthcare Corporation, Nashville, TN **N** Principal Health Care of Georgia, Atlanta, GA	33	10	219	—	—	—	—	—	—	—
⊞ COLUMBIA HUGHSTON SPORTS MEDICINE HOSPITAL, 100 Frist Court, Zip 31908–7188, Mailing Address: P.O. Box 7188, Zip 31908–7188; tel. 706/576–2100; Hugh D. Wilson, Chief Executive Officer **A**1 3 5 10 **F**2 3 4 7 8 10 11 12 15 16 17 19 21 22 26 28 30 34 35 37 40 42 43 44 45 46 48 49 52 60 65 66 71 73 74 **P**2 3 4 5 **S** Columbia/HCA Healthcare Corporation, Nashville, TN	33	47	100	3613	38	8808	0	24577	7508	300
⊞ ST. FRANCIS HOSPITAL, (Includes Bradley Center of St. Francis, 2000 16th Avenue, Zip 31906–0308; tel. 706/649–6450), 2122 Manchester Expressway, Zip 31904–6878, Mailing Address: Box 7000, Zip 31908–7000; tel. 706/596–4000; Michael E. Garrigan, President and Chief Executive Officer (Nonreporting) **A**1 10 **S** SSM Health Care System, Saint Louis, MO	23	10	281	—	—	—	—	—	—	—
⊞ THE MEDICAL CENTER, 710 Center Street, Zip 31902, Mailing Address: Box 951, Zip 31902; tel. 706/571–1000; Lance B. Duke, FACHE, President and Chief Executive Officer (Total facility includes 150 beds in nursing home–type unit) **A**1 2 3 5 9 10 12 **F**2 3 6 7 8 10 12 14 15 16 17 18 19 21 22 23 26 27 28 29 30 31 34 35 37 38 40 41 42 44 45 46 47 48 49 51 52 54 55 56 59 60 63 64 65 67 68 70 71 72 73 74 **P**8 **N** Community Healthcare Network, Columbus, GA; Columbus Regional HealthCare System, Inc., Columbus, GA; Principal Health Care of Georgia, Atlanta, GA; Georgia 1st, Inc., Decatur, GA; The Medical Resource Network, L.L.C., Atlanta, GA	23	10	559	13634	314	104184	3104	107196	46823	1320

COMMERCE—Jackson County

⊞ BJC MEDICAL CENTER, 70 Medical Center Drive, Zip 30529–9989; tel. 706/335–1000; J. David Lawrence, Jr., Chief Executive Officer (Total facility includes 167 beds in nursing home–type unit) **A**1 9 10 **F**8 11 15 16 19 21 22 28 30 33 34 37 40 41 44 46 49 64 65 71 73	16	10	257	1833	184	20708	89	10273	5792	222

CONYERS—Rockdale County

⊞ ROCKDALE HOSPITAL, 1412 Milstead Avenue N.E., Zip 30207–9990; tel. 770/918–3000; Nelson Toebbe, Chief Executive Officer (Nonreporting) **A**1 2 9 10 **N** Principal Health Care of Georgia, Atlanta, GA	23	10	107	—	—	—	—	—	—	—

CORDELE—Crisp County

□ CRISP REGIONAL HOSPITAL, 902 North Seventh Street, Zip 31015–5007; tel. 912/276–3100; D. Wayne Martin, Administrator and Chief Executive Officer **A**1 9 10 **F**7 15 19 22 23 27 32 35 37 40 44 60 65 71 73 74 **N** Georgia 1st, Inc., Decatur, GA; The Medical Resource Network, L.L.C., Atlanta, GA	16	10	65	2931	33	62878	340	—	—	408

COVINGTON—Newton County

⊞ NEWTON GENERAL HOSPITAL, 5126 Hospital Drive, Zip 30209; tel. 770/786–7053; James F. Weadick, Administrator and Chief Executive Officer **A**1 9 10 **F**7 8 15 17 19 22 23 28 29 30 32 33 34 35 37 40 41 44 45 56 63 65 67 69 71 73 **P**8 **N** Principal Health Care of Georgia, Atlanta, GA; Georgia 1st, Inc., Decatur, GA	23	10	90	3571	37	70108	406	24118	12671	394

CUMMING—Forsyth County

□ BAPTIST NORTH HOSPITAL, 133 Samaritan Drive, Zip 30130, Mailing Address: Box 768, Zip 30130; tel. 770/887–2355; John M. Herron, Administrator **A**1 10 **F**4 6 7 8 10 11 12 13 15 16 17 18 19 21 22 23 24 25 26 27 28 29 30 31 32 33 34 35 37 38 39 40 41 42 43 44 45 46 48 49 51 52 54 55 56 57 58 59 60 61 62 63 64 65 67 71 72 73 74 **P**6 7	21	10	30	1543	19	26419	0	12860	4704	183

CUTHBERT—Randolph County

★ SOUTHWEST GEORGIA REGIONAL MEDICAL CENTER, 109 Randolph Street, Zip 31740–1338; tel. 912/732–2181; Earnest E. Benton, Chief Executive Officer (Total facility includes 80 beds in nursing home–type unit) **A**9 10 **F**8 19 22 34 40 42 44 46 64 71 73 **N** Community Healthcare Network, Columbus, GA; The Medical Resource Network, L.L.C., Atlanta, GA	16	10	120	810	91	9359	101	6391	2243	176

DAHLONEGA—Lumpkin County

⊞ CHESTATEE REGIONAL HOSPITAL, 1111 Mountain Drive, Zip 30533; tel. 706/864–6136; Stephen G. Widener, President and Chief Executive Officer (Nonreporting) **A**1 10 **S** NetCare Health Systems, Inc., Nashville, TN	21	10	52	—	—	—	—	—	—	—

DALLAS—Paulding County

⊞ PROMINA PAULDING MEMORIAL MEDICAL CENTER, 600 West Memorial Drive, Zip 30132–1335; tel. 770/445–4411; T. Mark Haney, Administrator (Total facility includes 169 beds in nursing home–type unit) **A**1 10 **F**2 3 6 7 8 10 11 12 13 14 15 16 17 18 19 20 21 22 24 25 26 28 29 30 31 32 33 34 35 37 38 39 40 41 42 44 45 46 48 49 50 51 52 53 54 55 56 57 58 59 60 61 62 65 66 67 68 70 71 72 73 74 **P**1 3 7 **S** Promina Northwest Health System, Austell, GA **N** Principal Health Care of Georgia, Atlanta, GA; The Medical Resource Network, L.L.C., Atlanta, GA	23	10	208	1304	176	30837	0	16028	7427	284

DALTON—Whitfield County

⊞ HAMILTON MEDICAL CENTER, 1200 Memorial Drive, Zip 30720, Mailing Address: P.O. Box 1168, Zip 30722–1168; tel. 706/272–6000; Ned B. Wilford, President and Chief Executive Officer **A**1 2 10 **F**3 6 7 8 10 15 16 17 18 19 21 22 23 24 27 28 30 31 32 33 34 35 37 39 40 41 42 44 45 46 49 52 53 54 55 56 57 58 59 60 62 65 67 70 71 72 73 **P**8 **N** NorthWest Georgia Healthcare Partnership, Dalton, GA; The Medical Resource Network, L.L.C., Atlanta, GA	23	10	282	11157	132	198514	2214	85590	39063	1160

Hospital, Address, Telephone, Administrator, Approval, Facility, and Physician Codes, Health Care System, Network	Classi-fication Codes		Utilization Data					Expense (thousands) of dollars		
★ American Hospital Association (AHA) membership □ Joint Commission on Accreditation of Healthcare Organizations (JCAHO) accreditation + American Osteopathic Hospital Association (AOHA) membership ○ American Osteopathic Association (AOA) accreditation △ Commission on Accreditation of Rehabilitation Facilities (CARF) accreditation Control codes 61, 63, 64, 71, 72 and 73 indicate hospitals listed by AOHA, but not registered by AHA. For definition of numerical codes, see page A4	Control	Service	Beds	Admissions	Census	Outpatient Visits	Births	Total	Payroll	Personnel

DECATUR—De Kalb County

☒ DECATUR HOSPITAL, 450 North Candler Street, Zip 30030, Mailing Address: Box 40, Zip 30031; tel. 404/377–0221; Richard T. Schmidt, Executive Director (Nonreporting) **A**1 10 **N** Promina Health System, Inc., Atlanta, GA; Principal Health Care of Georgia, Atlanta, GA; The Medical Resource Network, L.L.C., Atlanta, GA
23 | 10 | 120 | — | — | — | — | — | — | —

☒ △ DEKALB MEDICAL CENTER, 2701 North Decatur Road, Zip 30033; tel. 404/501–1000; John R. Gerlach, Chief Executive Officer/Administrator (Total facility includes 48 beds in nursing home–type unit) **A**1 2 7 9 10 **F**2 3 5 7 8 10 11 12 15 17 19 20 21 22 23 24 25 26 27 28 29 30 31 32 33 34 35 37 38 39 40 41 42 44 45 46 48 49 51 52 54 55 56 57 58 59 60 61 63 64 65 66 67 68 70 71 72 73 74 **P**1 4 5 6 7 **N** Promina Health System, Inc., Atlanta, GA; Principal Health Care of Georgia, Atlanta, GA; The Medical Resource Network, L.L.C., Atlanta, GA
23 | 10 | 397 | 19272 | 251 | 180121 | 4285 | 165652 | 73590 | 2386

□ GEORGIA REGIONAL HOSPITAL AT ATLANTA, 3073 Panthersville Road, Zip 30034–3828; tel. 404/243–2100; Ronald C. Hogan, Superintendent (Total facility includes 43 beds in nursing home–type unit) **A**1 3 5 10 **F**1 3 4 5 6 7 8 10 12 13 14 15 17 18 19 20 21 22 23 24 25 27 28 29 30 31 32 33 34 35 36 39 41 42 43 44 45 46 49 50 51 52 53 54 55 56 57 58 59 60 61 63 64 65 66 67 68 69 70 71 72 73 74 **P**6
12 | 22 | 273 | 6353 | 224 | — | 0 | 30859 | 18497 | 638

☒ VETERANS AFFAIRS MEDICAL CENTER, 1670 Clairmont Road, Zip 30033–4098; tel. 404/728–7600; Robert A. Perreault, Director (Total facility includes 110 beds in nursing home–type unit) **A**1 3 5 8 **F**1 2 3 4 5 8 10 11 12 19 20 21 22 23 26 27 30 31 32 33 34 35 37 39 41 42 43 44 45 46 48 49 50 51 52 54 55 56 57 58 59 60 63 64 65 67 70 71 73 74 **S** Department of Veterans Affairs, Washington, DC
45 | 10 | 378 | 6748 | 329 | 251892 | 0 | 142656 | 68795 | 1825

DEMOREST—Habersham County

☒ HABERSHAM COUNTY MEDICAL CENTER, Highway 441, Zip 30535, Mailing Address: Box 37, Zip 30535; tel. 706/754–2161; C. Richard Dwozan, President (Total facility includes 84 beds in nursing home–type unit) (Nonreporting) **A**1 9 10 **S** Quorum Health Group/Quorum Health Resources, Inc., Brentwood, TN **N** Georgia 1st, Inc., Decatur, GA
16 | 10 | 140 | — | — | — | — | — | — | —

DONALSONVILLE—Seminole County

□ DONALSONVILLE HOSPITAL, Hospital Circle, Zip 31745, Mailing Address: Box 677, Zip 31745; tel. 912/524–5217; Charles H. Orrick, Administrator (Total facility includes 75 beds in nursing home–type unit) **A**1 10 **F**14 15 16 19 21 44 64 71 **N** The Medical Resource Network, L.L.C., Atlanta, GA
23 | 10 | 140 | 2151 | 80 | 17055 | 0 | 10245 | 3908 | 148

DOUGLAS—Coffee County

☒ COFFEE REGIONAL MEDICAL CENTER, 1101 Ocilla Road, Zip 31533–1248, Mailing Address: P.O. Box 1248, Zip 31533; tel. 912/384–1900; George L. Heck, III, President and Chief Executive Officer **A**1 10 **F**7 8 12 13 14 15 16 17 18 19 21 22 27 28 29 30 31 37 40 44 49 51 63 65 67 68 71 73
16 | 10 | 108 | 5391 | 51 | 72832 | 943 | 36329 | 16467 | 540

DOUGLASVILLE—Douglas County

INNER HARBOUR HOSPITALS, 4685 Dorsett Shoals Road, Zip 30135; tel. 770/942–2391; Ron Scroggy, Interim Group Administrator **F**15 16 20 22 39 46 52 53 54 55 59 65 67 73 **P**6
23 | 52 | 132 | 239 | 122 | 0 | 0 | 11546 | 6381 | 257

☒ PROMINA DOUGLAS HOSPITAL, 8954 Hospital Drive, Zip 30134–2282; tel. 770/949–1500; Tom Hill, Chief Executive Officer **A**1 9 10 **F**2 3 6 7 8 10 11 12 13 14 15 16 17 18 19 20 21 22 24 25 26 28 29 30 31 32 33 34 35 36 37 38 39 40 41 42 44 45 46 48 49 50 51 52 53 54 55 56 57 58 59 60 61 62 64 65 66 67 68 70 71 72 73 74 **P**1 3 7 **S** Promina Northwest Health System, Austell, GA **N** Principal Health Care of Georgia, Atlanta, GA; The Medical Resource Network, L.L.C., Atlanta, GA
23 | 10 | 98 | 3149 | 31 | 47916 | 169 | 22685 | 9630 | 298

DUBLIN—Laurens County

☒ COLUMBIA FAIRVIEW PARK HOSPITAL, 200 Industrial Boulevard, Zip 31021, Mailing Address: Box 1408, Zip 31040; tel. 912/275–2000; Jeffrey T. Whiteborn, Chief Executive Officer (Nonreporting) **A**1 2 9 10 **S** Columbia/HCA Healthcare Corporation, Nashville, TN **N** Principal Health Care of Georgia, Atlanta, GA; Georgia 1st, Inc., Decatur, GA; Emory University System of Healthcare Affiliate Network, Atlanta, GA
33 | 10 | 190 | — | — | — | — | — | — | —

☒ VETERANS AFFAIRS MEDICAL CENTER, 1826 Veterans Boulevard, Zip 31021; tel. 912/277–2701; William O. Edgar, Director (Total facility includes 112 beds in nursing home–type unit) **A**1 3 **F**3 6 12 14 15 16 17 18 19 20 21 22 24 26 27 29 30 31 32 33 34 37 39 41 44 45 46 48 49 51 52 54 55 56 58 64 65 67 71 72 73 74 **P**1 **S** Department of Veterans Affairs, Washington, DC
45 | 10 | 253 | 3463 | 241 | 87284 | 0 | 57194 | 30537 | 817

DULUTH—Gwinnett County

JOAN GLANCY MEMORIAL HOSPITAL See Promina Gwinnett Hospital System, Lawrenceville

EAST POINT—Fulton County

☒ SOUTH FULTON MEDICAL CENTER, 1170 Cleveland Avenue, Zip 30344; tel. 404/305–3500; H. Neil Copelan, President and Chief Executive Officer (Total facility includes 36 beds in nursing home–type unit) **A**1 2 9 10 **F**7 8 10 11 12 16 17 19 21 22 24 28 29 30 32 35 37 39 40 41 42 44 46 48 49 51 60 63 64 65 67 68 71 73 74 **P**8 **N** Principal Health Care of Georgia, Atlanta, GA; The Medical Resource Network, L.L.C., Atlanta, GA
23 | 10 | 369 | 11537 | 180 | 71053 | 1990 | 96382 | 44191 | 1396

EASTMAN—Dodge County

□ DODGE COUNTY HOSPITAL, 715 Griffin Street, Zip 31023, Mailing Address: Box 4309, Zip 31023; tel. 912/374–4000; Meredith H. Smith, Administrator **A**1 9 10 **F**8 15 17 19 21 22 30 36 37 40 44 45 46 49 52 57 67 71 73 **N** Principal Health Care of Georgia, Atlanta, GA; The Medical Resource Network, L.L.C., Atlanta, GA
16 | 10 | 87 | 2720 | 45 | 20903 | 135 | 14072 | 6826 | 318

Hospital, Address, Telephone, Administrator, Approval, Facility, and Physician Codes, Health Care System, Network	Classi-fication Codes		Utilization Data					Expense (thousands) of dollars		
★ American Hospital Association (AHA) membership □ Joint Commission on Accreditation of Healthcare Organizations (JCAHO) accreditation + American Osteopathic Hospital Association (AOHA) membership ○ American Osteopathic Association (AOA) accreditation △ Commission on Accreditation of Rehabilitation Facilities (CARF) accreditation Control codes 61, 63, 64, 71, 72 and 73 indicate hospitals listed by AOHA, but not registered by AHA. For definition of numerical codes, see page A4	Control	Service	Beds	Admissions	Census	Outpatient Visits	Births	Total	Payroll	Personnel

EATONTON—Putnam County

□ PUTNAM GENERAL HOSPITAL, Lake Oconee Parkway, Zip 31024–4330, Mailing Address: Box 4330, Zip 31024–4330; tel. 706/485–2711; Darrell M. Oglesby, Administrator **A**1 10 **F**8 11 14 16 17 19 20 22 28 29 30 31 33 34 36 37 39 41 43 44 45 46 48 49 65 71 73 **N** Principal Health Care of Georgia, Atlanta, GA; The Medical Resource Network, L.L.C., Atlanta, GA	16	10	50	977	10	13382	0	6525	2947	124

ELBERTON—Elbert County

★ ELBERT MEMORIAL HOSPITAL, 4 Medical Drive, Zip 30635–1897; tel. 706/283–3151; Tim Merritt, Administrator **A**1 9 10 **F**7 8 14 15 16 19 21 22 23 24 28 34 37 40 44 45 46 49 65 66 67 71 73 **P**5 **S** Quorum Health Group/Quorum Health Resources, Inc., Brentwood, TN **N** Georgia 1st, Inc., Decatur, GA	16	10	52	2245	29	9456	118	12324	5762	218

ELLIJAY—Gilmer County

□ NORTH GEORGIA MEDICAL CENTER AND GILMER NURSING HOME, Jasper Road, Zip 30540–0346, Mailing Address: Box 346, Zip 30540–0346; tel. 706/276–4741; Mickey M. Rabuka, Administrator (Total facility includes 100 beds in nursing home–type unit) **A**1 9 10 **F**15 19 20 21 22 27 28 30 33 34 35 37 39 41 42 44 46 49 63 64 65 66 71 **P**1 **S** NetCare Health Systems, Inc., Nashville, TN **N** Principal Health Care of Georgia, Atlanta, GA	33	10	150	2186	121	17416	0	15435	5584	205

FITZGERALD—Ben Hill County

★ DORMINY MEDICAL CENTER, Perry House Road, Zip 31750, Mailing Address: Drawer 1447, Zip 31750–1447; tel. 912/424–7100; Steve Barber, Administrator **A**1 9 10 **F**7 8 14 19 21 22 28 33 34 35 37 40 44 49 50 63 65 71 73	16	10	60	2009	26	23234	183	12774	5940	277

FOLKSTON—Charlton County

CHARLTON MEMORIAL HOSPITAL, 1203 Third Street, Zip 31537, Mailing Address: Box 188, Zip 31537; tel. 912/496–2531; James L. Leis, Jr., Administrator and Chief Executive Officer **A**9 10 **F**8 14 15 16 19 21 22 26 27 29 34 37 44 45 46 49 51 65 71 73 **P**6	16	10	35	879	11	16828	0	3640	2527	99

FORSYTH—Monroe County

□ MONROE COUNTY HOSPITAL, 88 Martin Luther King Jr. Drive, Zip 31029, Mailing Address: Box 1068, Zip 31029–1068; tel. 912/994–2521; Gale V. Tanner, Administrator **A**1 9 10 **F**8 19 22 31 34 35 42 44 48 59 65 71 73 **N** The Medical Resource Network, L.L.C., Atlanta, GA	16	10	37	993	10	18707	0	5775	—	94

FORT BENNING—Muscogee County

★ MARTIN ARMY COMMUNITY HOSPITAL, Zip 31905–6100; tel. 706/544–2041; Colonel Stephen L. Markelz, Deputy Commander, Administration (Nonreporting) **A**1 2 3 **S** Department of the Army, Office of the Surgeon General, Falls Church, VA	42	10	126	—	—	—	—	—	—	—

FORT GORDON—Richmond County

★ DWIGHT DAVID EISENHOWER ARMY MEDICAL CENTER, Zip 30905–5650; tel. 706/787–8192; Colonel Ronald J. Dunn, Deputy Commander for Administration (Nonreporting) **A**1 2 3 5 **S** Department of the Army, Office of the Surgeon General, Falls Church, VA	42	10	313	—	—	—	—	—	—	—

FORT OGLETHORPE—Catoosa County

□ GREENLEAF CENTER, 500 Greenleaf Circle, Zip 30742; tel. 706/861–4357; Richard A. Waxler, Administrator (Nonreporting) **A**1 9 10 **S** Greenleaf Health Systems, Inc., Chattanooga, TN	33	22	90	—	—	—	—	—	—	—
★ HUTCHESON MEDICAL CENTER, 100 Gross Crescent Circle, Zip 30742; tel. 706/858–2000; Robert T. Jones, M.D., President and Chief Executive Officer (Total facility includes 109 beds in nursing home–type unit) **A**1 9 10 **F**1 2 3 7 8 10 11 12 14 15 16 19 21 22 28 29 30 32 33 35 37 38 40 41 42 44 49 52 53 54 55 56 57 58 64 65 66 70 71 73 74 **P**3 **N** Principal Health Care of Georgia, Atlanta, GA	16	10	297	7880	208	70383	1196	69947	34566	1283

FORT STEWART—Liberty County

★ WINN ARMY COMMUNITY HOSPITAL, Zip 31314–5300; tel. 912/370–6001; Lieutenant Colonel Jimmy Sanders, Administrator **A**1 5 **F**3 8 12 13 14 17 18 19 20 22 27 28 30 31 37 39 41 44 46 51 52 53 54 56 58 65 67 **S** Department of the Army, Office of the Surgeon General, Falls Church, VA	42	10	100	5839	49	432188	1527	—	—	839

FORT VALLEY—Peach County

□ PEACH REGIONAL MEDICAL CENTER, (Formerly Peach County Hospital), 601 North Camellia Boulevard, Zip 31030–4599; tel. 912/825–8691; Nancy Peed, Administrator **A**1 9 10 **F**8 11 12 14 15 16 17 18 19 22 24 28 29 30 39 41 44 45 46 48 49 65 71 73 **N** The Medical Resource Network, L.L.C., Atlanta, GA	16	10	41	695	7	21398	0	6018	2425	95

GAINESVILLE—Hall County

★ COLUMBIA LANIER PARK HOSPITAL, 675 White Sulphur Road, Zip 30505, Mailing Address: P.O. Box 1354, Zip 30503; tel. 770/503–3000; Jerry Fulks, Chief Executive Officer (Nonreporting) **A**1 10 **S** Columbia/HCA Healthcare Corporation, Nashville, TN **N** Chattahoochee Health Network, Gainesville, GA	33	10	124	—	—	—	—	—	—	—
★ △ NORTHEAST GEORGIA MEDICAL CENTER, 743 Spring Street N.E., Zip 30501–3899; tel. 770/535–3553; Henry Rigdon, Executive Vice President (Total facility includes 15 beds in nursing home–type unit) (Nonreporting) **A**1 2 7 9 10 **N** Principal Health Care of Georgia, Atlanta, GA; Georgia 1st, Inc., Decatur, GA; The Medical Resource Network, L.L.C., Atlanta, GA	23	10	338	—	—	—	—	—	—	—

GLENWOOD—Wheeler County

WHEELER COUNTY HOSPITAL, Third Street, Zip 30428, Mailing Address: P.O. Box 398, Zip 30428; tel. 912/523–5113; Charles M. Mayo, Administrator (Nonreporting) **A**10 **S** Accord Health Care Corporation, Clearwater, FL	33	10	30	—	—	—	—	—	—	—

Hospital, Address, Telephone, Administrator, Approval, Facility, and Physician Codes, Health Care System, Network	Control	Service	Beds	Admissions	Census	Outpatient Visits	Births	Total	Payroll	Personnel

★ American Hospital Association (AHA) membership
□ Joint Commission on Accreditation of Healthcare Organizations (JCAHO) accreditation
+ American Osteopathic Hospital Association (AOHA) membership
○ American Osteopathic Association (AOA) accreditation
△ Commission on Accreditation of Rehabilitation Facilities (CARF) accreditation
Control codes 61, 63, 64, 71, 72 and 73 indicate hospitals listed by AOHA, but not registered by AHA. For definition of numerical codes, see page A4

GRACEWOOD—Richmond County
GRACEWOOD STATE SCHOOL AND HOSPITAL, Zip 30812; tel. 706/790–2030; Joanne P. Miklas, Ph.D., Superintendent (Total facility includes 56 beds in nursing home–type unit) (Nonreporting) A10 — 12 12 71 — — — — — — —

GREENSBORO—Greene County
□ MINNIE G. BOSWELL MEMORIAL HOSPITAL, 1201 Siloam Highway, Zip 30642, Mailing Address: P.O. Box 329, Zip 30642; tel. 706/453–7331; Larry W. Anderson, Administrator (Total facility includes 29 beds in nursing home–type unit) A1 9 10 F7 8 14 15 16 19 22 28 33 34 39 40 41 44 64 65 66 71 73 P5 N The Medical Resource Network, L.L.C., Atlanta, GA; University Health, Inc., Augusta, GA — 16 10 58 1167 43 14632 209 7314 3647 169

GRIFFIN—Spalding County
□ SPALDING REGIONAL HOSPITAL, 601 South Eighth Street, Zip 30224, Mailing Address: P.O. Drawer V, Zip 30224–1168; tel. 770/228–2721; Phil Shaw, Executive Director A1 9 10 F7 8 10 12 14 15 16 17 19 20 21 22 23 25 26 28 30 31 32 35 37 39 40 41 42 44 49 65 66 67 71 72 73 74 P6 7 8 S TENET Healthcare Corporation, Santa Barbara, CA N Principal Health Care of Georgia, Atlanta, GA; Georgia 1st, Inc., Decatur, GA — 33 10 160 6518 78 111661 844 40976 14644 616

HAHIRA—Lowndes County
SMITH HOSPITAL, 117 East Main Street, Zip 31632, Mailing Address: P.O. Box 337, Zip 31632; tel. 912/794–2502; Amanda M. Hall, Administrator (Nonreporting) A9 10 S Memorial Health Services, Adel, GA — 33 10 71 — — — — — — —

HARTWELL—Hart County
⊞ HART COUNTY HOSPITAL, Gibson and Cade Streets, Zip 30643–0280, Mailing Address: P.O. Box 280, Zip 30643–0280; tel. 706/856–6100; Samuel A. Strickland, Administrator (Nonreporting) A1 9 10 N Principal Health Care of Georgia, Atlanta, GA — 13 10 65 — — — — — — —

HAWKINSVILLE—Pulaski County
⊞ TAYLOR REGIONAL HOSPITAL, Macon Highway, Zip 31036; tel. 912/783–0200; Dan S. Maddock, President A1 9 10 F7 8 10 14 15 17 19 21 22 23 27 28 30 32 34 35 37 44 45 46 49 63 65 66 71 73 P3 6 N Principal Health Care of Georgia, Atlanta, GA; The Medical Resource Network, L.L.C., Atlanta, GA — 23 10 55 2335 22 33719 377 20218 7494 293

HAZLEHURST—Jeff Davis County
JEFF DAVIS HOSPITAL, 1215 South Tallahassee Street, Zip 31539, Mailing Address: Box 1200, Zip 31539; tel. 912/375–7781; Oreta Williams, Administrator (Nonreporting) A10 — 16 10 50 — — — — — — —

HIAWASSEE—Towns County
□ CHATUGE REGIONAL HOSPITAL AND NURSING HOME, 110 Main Street, Zip 30546, Mailing Address: Box 509, Zip 30546–0509; tel. 706/896–2222; Thomas I. Edwards, President and Chief Executive Officer (Total facility includes 76 beds in nursing home–type unit) (Nonreporting) A1 10 S NetCare Health Systems, Inc., Nashville, TN — 33 10 116 — — — — — — —

HINESVILLE—Liberty County
□ LIBERTY REGIONAL MEDICAL CENTER, 112 East Oglethorpe Boulevard, Zip 31313, Mailing Address: Box 919, Zip 31313; tel. 912/369–9400; H. Scott Kroell, Jr., Chief Executive Officer A1 9 10 F7 14 15 16 19 22 32 35 40 44 45 49 66 71 73 N Candler Health System, Savannah, GA; Principal Health Care of Georgia, Atlanta, GA; Georgia 1st, Inc., Decatur, GA; The Medical Resource Network, L.L.C., Atlanta, GA — 16 10 41 1454 11 29513 224 9931 4206 185

HOMERVILLE—Clinch County
★ CLINCH MEMORIAL HOSPITAL, 524 Carswell Street, Zip 31634, Mailing Address: P.O. Box 516, Zip 31634; tel. 912/487–5211; Randy Sauls, Interim Administrator A10 F8 15 16 19 20 22 34 44 46 49 65 71 73 — 13 10 36 1100 12 22386 0 4688 2527 100

JACKSON—Butts County
SYLVAN GROVE HOSPITAL, 1050 McDonough Road, Zip 30233; tel. 404/775–7861; Jack F. Frayer, Administrator (Nonreporting) A10 S Healthcare Management Group, Inc., Macon, GA — 16 10 28 — — — — — — —

JESUP—Wayne County
⊞ WAYNE MEMORIAL HOSPITAL, 865 South First Street, Zip 31598, Mailing Address: Box 408, Zip 31598; tel. 912/427–6811; Charles R. Morgan, Administrator A1 10 F7 8 12 15 19 22 28 29 30 34 35 37 39 40 41 44 45 46 49 65 71 73 S Quorum Health Group/Quorum Health Resources, Inc., Brentwood, TN N Principal Health Care of Georgia, Atlanta, GA — 16 10 110 3905 55 — 341 22155 10683 403

KENNESAW—Cobb County
DEVEREUX CENTER–GEORGIA, 1291 Stanley Road, Zip 30152; tel. 770/427–0147; Ralph L. Comerford, Director F14 15 16 22 52 53 55 P6 S Devereux Foundation, Devon, PA — 23 52 115 77 108 0 0 11630 6878 281

LA GRANGE—Troup County
⊞ WEST GEORGIA HEALTH SYSTEM, (Formerly West Georgia Medical Center), 1514 Vernon Road, Zip 30240–4199; tel. 706/882–1411; Charles L. Foster, Jr., FACHE, President and Chief Executive Officer (Total facility includes 150 beds in nursing home–type unit) A1 2 10 F2 3 4 7 8 10 11 12 13 14 15 17 18 19 21 22 26 27 28 29 30 32 33 34 35 37 39 40 41 42 44 46 49 50 51 52 53 54 55 57 58 59 60 63 64 65 67 68 70 71 73 74 P7 8 N Community Healthcare Network, Columbus, GA; Georgia 1st, Inc., Decatur, GA — 15 10 363 8886 280 330054 1061 69204 32070 1283

LAKELAND—Lanier County
⊞ LOUIS SMITH MEMORIAL HOSPITAL, 852 West Thigpen Avenue, Zip 31635–1099; tel. 912/482–3110; Randy Sauls, Administrator (Total facility includes 62 beds in nursing home–type unit) A1 10 F7 8 14 15 16 22 27 28 33 34 40 44 46 49 64 65 71 73 P3 N Principal Health Care of Georgia, Atlanta, GA; Georgia 1st, Inc., Decatur, GA — 23 10 102 788 74 7370 47 6075 3000 180

Hospital, Address, Telephone, Administrator, Approval, Facility, and Physician Codes, Health Care System, Network	Classi-fication Codes		Utilization Data					Expense (thousands) of dollars		
★ American Hospital Association (AHA) membership □ Joint Commission on Accreditation of Healthcare Organizations (JCAHO) accreditation + American Osteopathic Hospital Association (AOHA) membership ○ American Osteopathic Association (AOA) accreditation △ Commission on Accreditation of Rehabilitation Facilities (CARF) accreditation Control codes 61, 63, 64, 71, 72 and 73 indicate hospitals listed by AOHA, but not registered by AHA. For definition of numerical codes, see page A4	Control	Service	Beds	Admissions	Census	Outpatient Visits	Births	Total	Payroll	Personnel

LAWRENCEVILLE—Gwinnett County

✠ PROMINA GWINNETT HOSPITAL SYSTEM, (Includes Gwinnett Medical Center, 1000 Medical Center Boulevard, Zip 30245; Joan Glancy Memorial Hospital, McClure Bridge Road, Duluth, Zip 30136; tel. 770/497–4800), Mailing Address: Box 348, Zip 30246–0348; tel. 770/995–4321; Franklin M. Rinker, President and Chief Executive Officer (Nonreporting) **A**1 2 9 10 **N** Promina Health System, Inc., Atlanta, GA; Principal Health Care of Georgia, Atlanta, GA	16	10	390	—	—	—	—	—	—	—

LITHIA SPRINGS—Douglas County

✠ COLUMBIA PARKWAY MEDICAL CENTER, 1000 Thornton Road, Zip 30057; Mailing Address: P.O. Box 570, Zip 30057; tel. 770/732–7777; Deborah S. Guthrie, Chief Executive Officer **A**1 2 10 **F**2 3 7 8 10 12 14 15 16 17 18 19 21 22 23 24 25 26 27 28 30 31 32 34 35 37 39 40 41 42 44 46 48 49 52 53 54 55 56 57 58 59 60 61 64 65 67 71 73 74 **P**5 7 **S** Columbia/HCA Healthcare Corporation, Nashville, TN	33	10	233	4729	82	36006	830	35829	12259	407

LOUISVILLE—Jefferson County

□ JEFFERSON HOSPITAL, 1067 Peachtree Street, Zip 30434; tel. 912/625–7000; Rita Culvern, Administrator (Nonreporting) **A**1 9 10 **N** Principal Health Care of Georgia, Atlanta, GA; The Medical Resource Network, L.L.C., Atlanta, GA; University Health, Inc., Augusta, GA	16	10	37	—	—	—	—	—	—	—

MACON—Bibb County

□ CHARTER BEHAVIORAL HEALTH SYSTEM/CENTRAL GEORGIA, 3500 Riverside Drive, Zip 31210; tel. 912/474–6200; Blair R. Johanson, Administrator (Nonreporting) **A**1 10 **S** Magellan Health Services, Atlanta, GA	33	22	118	—	—	—	—	—	—	—
✠ COLUMBIA COLISEUM MEDICAL CENTERS, 350 Hospital Drive, Zip 31213; tel. 912/765–7000; Michael S. Boggs, Chief Executive Officer **A**1 9 10 **F**3 7 8 10 12 13 16 19 21 22 23 25 27 28 29 30 33 34 35 37 40 41 42 44 45 46 47 48 49 51 52 53 54 55 56 58 59 60 61 65 67 71 72 73 74 **P**1 7 **S** Columbia/HCA Healthcare Corporation, Nashville, TN **N** Principal Health Care of Georgia, Atlanta, GA	33	10	188	7961	113	55346	1215	—	—	847
✠ COLUMBIA COLISEUM PSYCHIATRIC HOSPITAL, 340 Hospital Drive, Zip 31201–8002; tel. 912/741–1355; Edward W. Ruffin, Administrator **A**1 9 10 **F**2 3 7 8 11 12 15 16 17 18 19 22 23 25 28 29 30 34 35 37 38 39 40 41 44 45 46 48 49 51 52 53 54 55 56 57 58 59 65 67 71 72 73 74 **P**1 6 7 **S** Columbia/HCA Healthcare Corporation, Nashville, TN	33	22	92	1133	30	12260	—	—	—	82
□ △ HEALTHSOUTH CENTRAL GEORGIA REHABILITATION HOSPITAL, 3351 Northside Drive, Zip 31210; tel. 912/471–3536; Elbert T. McQueen, Chief Executive Officer (Nonreporting) **A**1 7 10 **S** HEALTHSOUTH Corporation, Birmingham, AL **N** The Medical Resource Network, L.L.C., Atlanta, GA	33	46	50	—	—	—	—	—	—	—
✠ MACON NORTHSIDE HOSPITAL, 400 Charter Boulevard, Zip 31210, Mailing Address: P.O. Box 4627, Zip 31208; tel. 912/757–8200; Richard Gaston, Administrator **A**1 10 **F**2 3 7 8 10 12 19 21 22 25 28 29 30 34 35 37 38 39 40 41 44 45 46 49 51 52 53 54 55 56 58 59 60 63 65 71 72 73 74 **S** Quorum Health Group/Quorum Health Resources, Inc., Brentwood, TN	33	10	103	2536	32	27432	0	31689	11034	344
✠ MEDICAL CENTER OF CENTRAL GEORGIA, 777 Hemlock Street, Zip 31201, Mailing Address: Box 6000, Zip 31208; tel. 912/633–1000; A. Donald Faulk, FACHE, President (Nonreporting) **A**1 2 3 5 8 9 10 **N** Georgia 1st, Inc., Decatur, GA; The Medical Resource Network, L.L.C., Atlanta, GA	16	10	518	—	—	—	—	—	—	—
✠ MIDDLE GEORGIA HOSPITAL, 888 Pine Street, Zip 31201, Mailing Address: Box 6278, Zip 31208–6278; tel. 912/751–1111; William W. Fox, III, Chief Executive Officer (Nonreporting) **A**1 10 **S** Quorum Health Group/Quorum Health Resources, Inc., Brentwood, TN	33	10	119	—	—	—	—	—	—	—

MADISON—Morgan County

MORGAN MEMORIAL HOSPITAL, Canterbury Park, Zip 30650, Mailing Address: Box 860, Zip 30650; tel. 706/342–1667; Patrick Green, Administrator **A**10 **F**22 28 30 44 49 71 73 **S** Healthcare Management Group, Inc., Macon, GA	16	10	26	280	3	6102	0	1797	892	61

MARIETTA—Cobb County

✠ △ KENNESTONE HOSPITAL, 677 Church Street, Zip 30060; tel. 770/793–5000; Thomas E. Hill, Chief Executive Officer **A**1 2 7 9 10 **F**2 3 6 / 8 10 11 12 13 14 15 16 17 18 19 20 21 22 24 25 26 28 29 30 31 32 33 34 35 37 38 39 40 41 42 44 45 46 48 49 50 51 52 53 54 55 56 57 58 59 60 61 62 63 64 65 66 67 68 70 71 72 73 74 **P**1 3 7 **S** Promina Northwest Health System, Austell, GA **N** Promina Health System, Inc., Atlanta, GA; The Medical Resource Network, L.L.C., Atlanta, GA	23	10	439	23892	285	235578	4514	172098	73464	2023
✠ △ PROMINA WINDY HILL HOSPITAL, 2540 Windy Hill Road, Zip 30067; tel. 770/644–1000; T. Mark Haney, Administrator **A**1 7 9 10 **F**2 3 6 7 8 10 11 12 13 14 15 16 17 18 19 20 21 22 24 25 26 28 29 30 31 32 33 34 35 37 38 39 40 41 42 43 44 45 46 48 49 50 51 52 53 54 55 56 57 58 59 60 61 62 64 65 66 67 68 70 71 72 73 74 **P**1 3 7 **S** Promina Northwest Health System, Austell, GA **N** Principal Health Care of Georgia, Atlanta, GA; The Medical Resource Network, L.L.C., Atlanta, GA	23	10	100	1503	17	57613	0	26987	10254	248

MCRAE—Telfair County

TELFAIR COUNTY HOSPITAL, U.S. 341 South, Zip 31055, Mailing Address: P.O. Box 150, Zip 31055; tel. 912/868–5621; Gail B. Norris, Administrator (Nonreporting) **A**9 10 **S** Memorial Health Services, Adel, GA	33	10	52	—	—	—	—	—	—	—

METTER—Candler County

★ CANDLER COUNTY HOSPITAL, Cedar Road, Zip 30439, Mailing Address: Box 597, Zip 30439–0597; tel. 912/685–5741; Charles Balkcom, President **A**9 10 **F**15 16 22 26 28 30 33 37 39 44 45 46 49 71 **N** Candler Health System, Savannah, GA; Georgia 1st, Inc., Decatur, GA; The Medical Resource Network, L.L.C., Atlanta, GA	16	10	47	1513	21	24375	0	8147	3603	141

Hospital, Address, Telephone, Administrator, Approval, Facility, and Physician Codes, Health Care System, Network	Classi-fication Codes		Utilization Data					Expense (thousands) of dollars		
★ American Hospital Association (AHA) membership □ Joint Commission on Accreditation of Healthcare Organizations (JCAHO) accreditation + American Osteopathic Hospital Association (AOHA) membership ○ American Osteopathic Association (AOA) accreditation △ Commission on Accreditation of Rehabilitation Facilities (CARF) accreditation Control codes 61, 63, 64, 71, 72 and 73 indicate hospitals listed by AOHA, but not registered by AHA. For definition of numerical codes, see page A4	Control	Service	Beds	Admissions	Census	Outpatient Visits	Births	Total	Payroll	Personnel

MILLEDGEVILLE—Baldwin County

□ CENTRAL STATE HOSPITAL, (MENTAL HEALTH/RETARDATION), Zip 31062; tel. 912/453–4128; Britton B. Dennis, Sr., Superintendent (Total facility includes 1751 beds in nursing home–type unit) **A**1 3 10 **F**1 2 3 6 8 12 17 18 20 21 22 28 30 31 34 37 39 41 44 45 46 51 52 53 54 55 56 57 58 64 65 67 68 71 73 **P**6 | 12 | 49 | 1898 | 3289 | 1775 | 55537 | 0 | 144287 | 86183 | 3478

✠ OCONEE REGIONAL MEDICAL CENTER, 821 North Cobb Street, Zip 31061, Mailing Address: Box 690, Zip 31061; tel. 912/454–3500; Brian L. Riddle, Chief Executive Officer **A**1 9 10 **F**7 8 12 14 15 16 17 19 21 22 23 24 27 28 29 30 34 35 36 37 39 40 42 44 45 46 49 60 65 66 67 70 71 72 73 74 **S** Quorum Health Group/Quorum Health Resources, Inc., Brentwood, TN **N** Principal Health Care of Georgia, Atlanta, GA; Georgia 1st, Inc., Decatur, GA; The Medical Resource Network, L.L.C., Atlanta, GA | 16 | 10 | 145 | 4785 | 54 | 55688 | 618 | 35920 | 15595 | 532

MILLEN—Jenkins County

★ JENKINS COUNTY HOSPITAL, 515 East Winthrope Avenue, Zip 30442; tel. 912/982–4221; Watson W. Rocker, President and Chief Executive Officer (Nonreporting) **A**9 10 | 16 | 10 | 35 | — | — | — | — | — | — | —

MONROE—Walton County

✠ WALTON MEDICAL CENTER, 330 Alcovy Street, Zip 30655, Mailing Address: Box 1346, Zip 30655; tel. 770/267–8461; Edgar L. Belcher, Administrator (Total facility includes 58 beds in nursing home–type unit) **A**1 9 10 **F**7 8 16 19 20 21 22 23 24 28 30 34 35 37 40 42 44 49 64 65 67 71 73 74 **S** Quorum Health Group/Quorum Health Resources, Inc., Brentwood, TN **N** Georgia 1st, Inc., Decatur, GA | 16 | 10 | 115 | 2153 | 80 | 43432 | 188 | 19373 | 8617 | 320

MONTEZUMA—Macon County

★ FLINT RIVER COMMUNITY HOSPITAL, 509 Sumter Street, Zip 31063–0770, Mailing Address: P.O. Box 770, Zip 31063–0770; tel. 912/472–3100; Michael Clark, Chief Executive Officer **A**10 **F**8 14 15 16 19 21 22 31 32 34 35 44 70 71 **S** Paracelsus Healthcare Corporation, Houston, TX | 33 | 10 | 50 | 1171 | 11 | 18209 | 0 | 7318 | 3638 | 121

MONTICELLO—Jasper County

JASPER MEMORIAL HOSPITAL, 898 College Street, Zip 31064; tel. 706/468–6411; Donna Holman, Administrator (Total facility includes 44 beds in nursing home–type unit) **A**10 **F**11 14 15 16 17 19 22 27 29 30 31 32 34 35 41 49 64 65 71 73 **P**5 | 16 | 10 | 72 | 281 | 46 | 5316 | 0 | 2709 | 1192 | 82

MOODY AFB—Lowndes County

✠ U. S. AIR FORCE HOSPITAL MOODY, 3278 Mitchell Boulevard, Zip 31699–1500; tel. 912/257–3772; Colonel Stephan A. Giesecke, USAF, MSC, Commander **A**1 **F**7 15 16 24 27 29 30 40 44 45 46 49 51 55 56 58 64 65 67 72 73 **S** Department of the Air Force, Washington, DC | 41 | 10 | 16 | 665 | 4 | 112780 | 232 | — | — | 281

MOULTRIE—Colquitt County

✠ COLQUITT REGIONAL MEDICAL CENTER, 3131 South Main Street, Zip 31768–6701, Mailing Address: P.O. Box 40, Zip 31776–0040; tel. 912/985–3420; James R. Lowry, FACHE, Chief Executive Officer **A**1 9 10 **F**7 8 10 11 14 15 16 17 19 20 21 22 23 26 27 28 29 30 31 32 33 34 35 37 39 40 42 44 45 46 49 51 58 61 63 65 67 71 73 74 **P**3 8 | 16 | 10 | 155 | 3874 | 49 | 96295 | 533 | 31166 | 14266 | 663

TURNING POINT HOSPITAL, 319 East By–Pass, Zip 31776, Mailing Address: P.O. Box 1177, Zip 31768; tel. 912/985–4815; Ben Marion, Chief Executive Officer **A**10 **F**2 3 14 15 16 **P**1 **S** Universal Health Services, Inc., King of Prussia, PA | 33 | 82 | 59 | 562 | 9 | 6842 | 0 | 3078 | 1771 | 64

NASHVILLE—Berrien County

□ BERRIEN COUNTY HOSPITAL, 1221 East McPherson Street, Zip 31639, Mailing Address: P.O. Box 665, Zip 31639; tel. 912/686–7471; James P. Seward, Jr., Executive Director (Total facility includes 108 beds in nursing home–type unit) (Nonreporting) **A**1 10 **S** Community Health Systems, Inc., Brentwood, TN **N** Principal Health Care of Georgia, Atlanta, GA; The Medical Resource Network, L.L.C., Atlanta, GA | 33 | 10 | 155 | — | — | — | — | — | — | —

NEWNAN—Coweta County

✠ COLUMBIA PEACHTREE REGIONAL HOSPITAL, 60 Hospital Road, Zip 30264, Mailing Address: Box 2228, Zip 30264; tel. 770/253–1912; Linda Jubinsky, Chief Executive Officer (Nonreporting) **A**1 10 **S** Columbia/HCA Healthcare Corporation, Nashville, TN **N** Principal Health Care of Georgia, Atlanta, GA | 33 | 10 | 144 | — | — | — | — | — | — | —

✠ NEWNAN HOSPITAL, 80 Jackson Street, Zip 30263–1941, Mailing Address: Box 997, Zip 30264–0997; tel. 770/253–2330; Glenn M. Flake, Executive Director (Total facility includes 143 beds in nursing home–type unit) **A**1 9 10 **F**8 10 17 19 21 22 23 24 30 33 35 37 44 46 49 64 65 71 73 | 23 | 10 | 253 | 4243 | 198 | 46472 | 0 | 40055 | 14596 | 572

OCILLA—Irwin County

IRWIN COUNTY HOSPITAL, 710 North Irwin Avenue, Zip 31774; tel. 912/468–7411; Sue Spivey, Administrator (Total facility includes 30 beds in nursing home–type unit) **A**10 **F**14 19 22 44 64 71 **P**6 | 16 | 10 | 64 | 938 | 40 | 4800 | 28 | 4782 | 2552 | 124

PERRY—Houston County

✠ PERRY HOSPITAL, 1120 Morningside Drive, Zip 31069, Mailing Address: Drawer 1004, Zip 31069–1004; tel. 912/987–3600; Nadine L. Weems, Administrator **A**1 9 10 **F**2 3 7 8 10 12 13 14 15 16 17 18 19 20 22 26 27 28 29 30 31 32 33 34 35 36 37 39 40 44 45 46 49 51 52 54 56 65 66 67 68 71 72 73 **P**7 **N** The Medical Resource Network, L.L.C., Atlanta, GA | 16 | 10 | 45 | 1917 | 20 | 29968 | 289 | 12450 | 7020 | 210

QUITMAN—Brooks County

□ BROOKS COUNTY HOSPITAL, 903 North Court Street, Zip 31643, Mailing Address: P.O. Box 5000, Zip 31643; tel. 912/263–4171; Ken Brooker, Interim Administrator (Nonreporting) **A**1 9 10 **S** Archbold Medical Center, Thomasville, GA **N** Georgia 1st, Inc., Decatur, GA; The Medical Resource Network, L.L.C., Atlanta, GA | 23 | 10 | 35 | — | — | — | — | — | — | —

© 1997 AHA Guide

Hospital, Address, Telephone, Administrator, Approval, Facility, and Physician Codes, Health Care System, Network	Classi-fication Codes		Utilization Data					Expense (thousands) of dollars		
★ American Hospital Association (AHA) membership □ Joint Commission on Accreditation of Healthcare Organizations (JCAHO) accreditation + American Osteopathic Hospital Association (AOHA) membership ○ American Osteopathic Association (AOA) accreditation △ Commission on Accreditation of Rehabilitation Facilities (CARF) accreditation Control codes 61, 63, 64, 71, 72 and 73 indicate hospitals listed by AOHA, but not registered by AHA. For definition of numerical codes, see page A4	Control	Service	Beds	Admissions	Census	Outpatient Visits	Births	Total	Payroll	Personnel

REIDSVILLE—Tattnall County

TATTNALL MEMORIAL HOSPITAL, Highway 121 South, Zip 30453, Mailing Address: Route 1, Box 261, Zip 30453; tel. 912/557–4731; Ken Ford, Administrator **A**9 10 **F**7 8 15 16 19 22 40 44 49 71
| | | 16 | 10 | 40 | 897 | 9 | 14334 | 52 | 4084 | 1735 | 81 |

RICHLAND—Stewart County

STEWART–WEBSTER HOSPITAL, 300 Alston Street, Zip 31825, Mailing Address: Box 190, Zip 31825; tel. 912/887–3366; Jerry R. Wise, Administrator (Nonreporting) **A**9 10 **S** Accord Health Care Corporation, Clearwater, FL
| | | 33 | 10 | 25 | — | — | — | — | — | — | — |

RIVERDALE—Clayton County

⊞ SOUTHERN REGIONAL MEDICAL CENTER, 11 Upper Riverdale Road S.W., Zip 30274–2600; tel. 770/991–8000; Donald B. Logan, President and Chief Executive Officer (Nonreporting) **A**1 2 9 10 **N** Promina Health System, Inc., Atlanta, GA; Principal Health Care of Georgia, Atlanta, GA; Georgia 1st, Inc., Decatur, GA
| | | 23 | 10 | 324 | — | — | — | — | — | — | — |

ROBINS AFB—Houston County

⊞ U. S. AIR FORCE HOSPITAL ROBINS, Zip 31098–2227; tel. 912/926–9381; Lieutenant Colonel Ronald M. Gilliard, MSC, USAF, FACHE, Administrator (Nonreporting) **A**1 **S** Department of the Air Force, Washington, DC
| | | 41 | 10 | 32 | | | | | | | |

ROME—Floyd County

⊞ COLUMBIA REDMOND REGIONAL MEDICAL CENTER, 501 Redmond Road, Zip 30165–7001, Mailing Address: Box 107001, Zip 30164–7001; tel. 706/291–0291; James R. Thomas, Chief Executive Officer **A**1 2 9 10 **F**4 8 10 11 12 14 16 19 21 22 23 25 28 32 34 35 37 41 42 43 44 45 46 49 63 65 67 71 72 73 74 **P**7 **S** Columbia/HCA Healthcare Corporation, Nashville, TN
| | | 33 | 10 | 188 | 9289 | 124 | 64835 | 0 | 57298 | 22684 | 887 |

⊞ △ FLOYD MEDICAL CENTER, 304 Turner McCall Boulevard, Zip 30165, Mailing Address: Box 233, Zip 30162–0233; tel. 706/802–2000; Kurt Stuenkel, FACHE, President and Chief Executive Officer **A**1 2 3 5 7 9 10 **F**2 3 7 8 10 11 12 14 16 18 19 21 22 23 26 27 28 29 30 32 33 34 35 37 38 40 41 42 44 45 46 48 49 51 52 54 55 56 57 58 59 60 61 63 65 66 67 68 70 71 72 73 74 **P**6 8 **N** Principal Health Care of Georgia, Atlanta, GA; Georgia 1st, Inc., Decatur, GA; The Medical Resource Network, L.L.C., Atlanta, GA
| | | 16 | 10 | 234 | 10549 | 127 | 161237 | 2049 | 85583 | 31534 | 1225 |

□ NORTHWEST GEORGIA REGIONAL HOSPITAL, 1305 Redmond Circle, Zip 30161; tel. 706/295–6246; Jean W. Morgan, Superintendent **A**1 10 **F**14 52 53 56 57 65 73
| | | 12 | 22 | 340 | 2444 | 306 | 0 | 0 | 28330 | 17905 | 690 |

ROSWELL—Fulton County

□ NORTH FULTON REGIONAL HOSPITAL, 3000 Hospital Boulevard, Zip 30076–9930; tel. 404/751–2500; Frederick R. Bailey, Chief Executive Officer (Nonreporting) **A**1 10 **S** TENET Healthcare Corporation, Santa Barbara, CA **N** Georgia 1st, Inc., Decatur, GA
| | | 33 | 10 | 168 | — | — | — | — | — | — | — |

ROYSTON—Franklin County

⊞ COBB MEMORIAL HOSPITAL, (Includes Brown Memorial Convalescent Center, Cobb Health Care Center and Cobb Terrace Personal Care Center), 577 Franklin Springs Street, Zip 30662, Mailing Address: Box 589, Zip 30662–0589; tel. 706/245–5034; H. Thomas Brown, Administrator (Total facility includes 260 beds in nursing home–type unit) **A**1 9 10 **F**6 7 12 13 14 15 16 17 19 21 22 28 32 33 36 37 39 40 41 44 46 49 62 64 65 71 73 **N** Principal Health Care of Georgia, Atlanta, GA
| | | 23 | 10 | 331 | 2579 | 295 | 32881 | 203 | 21584 | 10311 | 399 |

SAINT MARYS—Camden County

⊞ CAMDEN MEDICAL CENTER, 2000 Dan Proctor Drive, Zip 31558–0805, Mailing Address: Box 805, Zip 31558–0805; tel. 912/576–4200; Warren Manley, Administrator (Nonreporting) **A**1 9 10 **S** Quorum Health Group/Quorum Health Resources, Inc., Brentwood, TN **N** Georgia 1st, Inc., Decatur, GA
| | | 23 | 10 | 40 | — | — | — | — | — | — | — |

SAINT SIMONS ISLAND—Glynn County

□ CHARTER BY–THE–SEA BEHAVIORAL HEALTH SYSTEM, 2927 Demere Road, Zip 31522–1620; tel. 912/638–1999; Wes Robbins, Chief Executive Officer (Nonreporting) **A**1 9 10 **S** Magellan Health Services, Atlanta, GA
| | | 33 | 22 | 101 | | | | | | | |

SANDERSVILLE—Washington County

⊞ WASHINGTON COUNTY REGIONAL HOSPITAL, (Formerly Memorial Hospital of Washington County), 610 Sparta Highway, Zip 31082, Mailing Address: Box 636, Zip 31082; tel. 912/552–3901; Shirley R. Roberts, Administrator (Total facility includes 60 beds in nursing home–type unit) **A**1 10 **F**3 7 8 11 15 16 17 19 21 22 24 27 28 29 30 35 37 39 40 42 44 45 49 53 54 57 58 64 65 66 67 71 73 74 **N** Principal Health Care of Georgia, Atlanta, GA
| | | 16 | 10 | 116 | 1910 | 79 | 25125 | 43 | 15252 | 7362 | 389 |

SAVANNAH—Chatham County

⊞ △ CANDLER HOSPITAL, 5353 Reynolds Street, Zip 31405, Mailing Address: Box 9787, Zip 31412–9787; tel. 912/692–6000; Paul P. Hinchey, President and Chief Executive Officer (Nonreporting) **A**1 7 10 **N** Candler Health System, Savannah, GA; Principal Health Care of Georgia, Atlanta, GA; Georgia 1st, Inc., Decatur, GA; The Medical Resource Network, L.L.C., Atlanta, GA
| | | 23 | 10 | 335 | — | — | — | — | — | — | — |

□ CHARTER SAVANNAH BEHAVIORAL HEALTH SYSTEM, 1150 Cornell Avenue, Zip 31406; tel. 912/354–3911; Ron Fincher, Chief Executive Officer (Nonreporting) **A**1 9 10 **S** Magellan Health Services, Atlanta, GA
| | | 33 | 22 | 112 | — | — | — | — | — | — | — |

□ GEORGIA REGIONAL HOSPITAL AT SAVANNAH, Eisenhower Drive at Varnedoe, Zip 31406, Mailing Address: Box 13607, Zip 31416–0607; tel. 912/356–2011; Doug Osborne, Interim Superintendent **A**1 10 **F**15 16 20 26 27 31 45 46 52 53 54 55 56 57 65 73
| | | 12 | 22 | 232 | 1833 | 200 | 0 | 0 | 19845 | — | 451 |

Hospital, Address, Telephone, Administrator, Approval, Facility, and Physician Codes, Health Care System, Network	Classi-fication Codes		Utilization Data					Expense (thousands) of dollars		
★ American Hospital Association (AHA) membership ☐ Joint Commission on Accreditation of Healthcare Organizations (JCAHO) accreditation + American Osteopathic Hospital Association (AOHA) membership ○ American Osteopathic Association (AOA) accreditation △ Commission on Accreditation of Rehabilitation Facilities (CARF) accreditation Control codes 61, 63, 64, 71, 72 and 73 indicate hospitals listed by AOHA, but not registered by AHA. For definition of numerical codes, see page A4	Control	Service	Beds	Admissions	Census	Outpatient Visits	Births	Total	Payroll	Personnel

⊠ △ MEMORIAL MEDICAL CENTER, 4700 Waters Avenue, Zip 31404, Mailing Address: Box 23089, Zip 31403–3089; tel. 912/350–8000; Robert A. Colvin, President and Chief Executive Officer **A**1 2 3 5 7 8 10 **F**3 4 7 8 10 11 12 15 16 17 18 19 21 22 23 26 27 28 29 30 31 32 34 35 37 38 39 40 41 42 43 44 46 47 48 49 51 52 53 54 55 56 57 58 59 60 61 63 65 67 70 71 73 74 **P**7 **S** Quorum Health Group/Quorum Health Resources, Inc., Brentwood, TN **N** Principal Health Care of Georgia, Atlanta, GA	16	10	373	20517	310	211761	2488	207456	80815	3056
⊠ △ ST. JOSEPH'S HOSPITAL, 11705 Mercy Boulevard, Zip 31419–1791; tel. 912/927–5404; Paul P. Hinchey, President and Chief Executive Officer (Nonreporting) **A**1 2 7 9 10 **S** Sisters of Mercy of the Americas–Regional Community of Baltimore, Baltimore, MD **N** Premier Health Systems, Inc., Columbia, SC	21	10	305	—	—	—	—	—	—	—
SMYRNA—Cobb County										
⊠ EMORY–ADVENTIST HOSPITAL, 3949 South Cobb Drive, Zip 30080; tel. 770/434–0710; Larry D. Luce, President (Total facility includes 12 beds in nursing home–type unit) **A**1 10 **F**1 8 10 15 19 21 22 23 35 37 41 44 46 51 63 64 65 71 72 73 **S** Adventist Health System Sunbelt Health Care Corporation, Winter Park, FL **N** Georgia 1st, Inc., Decatur, GA	23	10	54	1333	23	27011	0	18426	6603	—
⊠ RIDGEVIEW INSTITUTE, 3995 South Cobb Drive, Zip 30080; tel. 770/434–4567; John E. Gronewald, Chief Operating Officer **A**1 3 5 9 10 **F**2 3 12 15 16 19 52 53 54 55 56 57 58 59 65 74	23	22	124	1871	42	19785	0	13953	6372	256
☐ VALUEMARK–BRAWNER BEHAVIORAL HEALTHCARE SYSTEM–NORTH, 3180 Atlanta Street S.E., Zip 30080; tel. 404/436–0081; John J. Cascone, Chief Executive Officer (Nonreporting) **A**1 3 10 **S** ValueMark Healthcare Systems, Inc., Atlanta, GA	33	22	108	—	—	—	—	—	—	—
SNELLVILLE—Gwinnett County										
⊠ COLUMBIA EASTSIDE MEDICAL CENTER, 1700 Medical Way, Zip 30278, Mailing Address: P.O. Box 587, Zip 30278; tel. 770/979–0200; Les Beard, Chief Executive Officer (Nonreporting) **A**1 9 10 **S** Columbia/HCA Healthcare Corporation, Nashville, TN **N** Georgia 1st, Inc., Decatur, GA	33	10	114	—	—	—	—	—	—	—
SPARTA—Hancock County										
★ HANCOCK MEMORIAL HOSPITAL, 453 Boland Street, Zip 31087, Mailing Address: P.O. Box 490, Zip 31087; tel. 706/444–7006; Daniel D. Holtz, FACHE, Administrator and Chief Executive Officer **A**9 10 **F**8 14 19 22 28 44 48 71 **S** Quorum Health Group/Quorum Health Resources, Inc., Brentwood, TN **N** Emory University System of Healthcare Affiliate Network, Atlanta, GA	23	10	35	1465	16	8227	6	7072	3265	163
SPRINGFIELD—Effingham County										
⊠ EFFINGHAM HOSPITAL, 459 Highway 119 South, Zip 31329, Mailing Address: Box 386, Zip 31329–0386; tel. 912/754–6451; W. Scott Burnette, Chief Executive Officer (Total facility includes 105 beds in nursing home–type unit) **A**1 10 **F**8 12 15 16 19 22 24 25 28 33 44 45 46 49 51 64 65 71 72 73 **N** Candler Health System, Savannah, GA; Principal Health Care of Georgia, Atlanta, GA; Georgia 1st, Inc., Decatur, GA; The Medical Resource Network, L.L.C., Atlanta, GA	16	10	146	574	109	19585	0	9356	4471	189
STATESBORO—Bulloch County										
⊠ BULLOCH MEMORIAL HOSPITAL, 500 East Grady Street, Zip 30458, Mailing Address: P.O. Box 1048, Zip 30459–1048; tel. 912/764–6671; C. Scott Campbell, Executive Director **A**1 2 10 **F**7 8 11 12 17 19 20 21 22 23 26 28 29 30 32 33 34 35 37 39 40 44 45 49 63 65 66 70 71 73 **S** Health Management Associates, Naples, FL **N** Principal Health Care of Georgia, Atlanta, GA	33	10	158	5770	66	52185	1113	32884	13681	460
⊠ WILLINGWAY HOSPITAL, 311 Jones Mill Road, Zip 30458; tel. 912/764–6236; Jimmy Mooney, Chief Executive Officer **A**1 10 **F**2 3 **N** Premier Health Systems, Inc., Columbia, SC; Candler Health System, Savannah, GA; The Medical Resource Network, L.L.C., Atlanta, GA	33	82	40	474	23	4385	0	4156	2493	104
STOCKBRIDGE—Henry County										
⊠ HENRY MEDICAL CENTER, 1133 Eagle's Landing Parkway, Zip 30281–5099; tel. 770/389–2200; Joseph G. Brum, President and Chief Executive Officer **A**1 9 10 **F**7 8 10 11 14 15 16 17 19 21 22 28 29 30 34 35 37 38 39 40 44 45 60 63 65 67 68 70 71 72 73 74	16	10	118	6328	73	52397	1302	58154	21444	678
SUMMERVILLE—Chattooga County										
CHATTOOGA COUNTY HOSPITAL, 1010 Highland Avenue, Zip 30747, Mailing Address: Box 449, Zip 30747–0449; tel. 706/857–4761; Stephen W. Johnson, Executive Director (Total facility includes 151 beds in nursing home–type unit) **A**9 10 **F**32 34 64 71 **N** The Medical Resource Network, L.L.C., Atlanta, GA	16	10	182	925	152	7262	0	6950	3603	197
SWAINSBORO—Emanuel County										
⊠ EMANUEL COUNTY HOSPITAL, 117 Kite Road, Zip 30401, Mailing Address: P.O. Box 879, Zip 30401; tel. 912/237–9911; Richard W. Clarke, Chief Executive Officer (Total facility includes 49 beds in nursing home–type unit) (Nonreporting) **A**1 10 **S** Quorum Health Group/Quorum Health Resources, Inc., Brentwood, TN **N** Principal Health Care of Georgia, Atlanta, GA; The Medical Resource Network, L.L.C., Atlanta, GA; University Health, Inc., Augusta, GA	16	10	119	—	—	—	—	—	—	—
SYLVANIA—Screven County										
★ SCREVEN COUNTY HOSPITAL, 215 Mims Road, Zip 30467; tel. 912/564–7426; Michael T. Hutchins, Chief Executive Officer **A**10 **F**8 19 22 34 41 44 49 65 71 73	16	10	40	792	10	11933	2	4798	1776	89
SYLVESTER—Worth County										
⊠ WORTH COUNTY HOSPITAL, 807 South Isabella Street, Zip 31791–0545, Mailing Address: Box 545, Zip 31791–0545; tel. 912/776–6961; Loron H. Coxwell, Administrator **A**1 10 **F**15 17 19 22 30 40 44 46 65 71 73	33	10	50	1005	11	12221	59	4351	1981	85

Hospital, Address, Telephone, Administrator, Approval, Facility, and Physician Codes, Health Care System, Network	Classi-fication Codes		Utilization Data					Expense (thousands) of dollars		
★ American Hospital Association (AHA) membership □ Joint Commission on Accreditation of Healthcare Organizations (JCAHO) accreditation + American Osteopathic Hospital Association (AOHA) membership ○ American Osteopathic Association (AOA) accreditation △ Commission on Accreditation of Rehabilitation Facilities (CARF) accreditation Control codes 61, 63, 64, 71, 72 and 73 indicate hospitals listed by AOHA, but not registered by AHA. For definition of numerical codes, see page A4	Control	Service	Beds	Admissions	Census	Outpatient Visits	Births	Total	Payroll	Personnel

THOMASTON—Upson County
✠ UPSON REGIONAL MEDICAL CENTER, 801 West Gordon Street, Zip 30286–2831, Mailing Address: Box 1059, Zip 30286; tel. 706/647–8111; Samuel S. Gregory, Administrator (Nonreporting) **A**1 9 10 **S** Quorum Health Group/Quorum Health Resources, Inc., Brentwood, TN **N** Principal Health Care of Georgia, Atlanta, GA; Georgia 1st, Inc., Decatur, GA; The Medical Resource Network, L.L.C., Atlanta, GA	23	10	115	—	—	—	—	—	—	—

THOMASVILLE—Thomas County
✠ JOHN D. ARCHBOLD MEMORIAL HOSPITAL, 910 South Broad Street, Zip 31792, Mailing Address: P.O. Box 1018, Zip 31799; tel. 912/228–2000; Jason H. Moore, President and Chief Executive Officer (Total facility includes 64 beds in nursing home–type unit) **A**1 2 9 10 **F**1 2 3 4 7 8 10 11 12 14 15 16 17 18 19 20 21 22 23 25 26 27 28 29 30 31 32 33 34 35 37 39 40 41 42 44 45 46 48 49 50 51 52 53 54 55 56 57 58 59 60 61 63 64 65 66 67 69 70 71 72 73 **P**8 **S** Archbold Medical Center, Thomasville, GA **N** Georgia 1st, Inc., Decatur, GA; The Medical Resource Network, L.L.C., Atlanta, GA	23	10	328	10175	221	141214	922	76852	35322	1376

THOMSON—McDuffie County
✠ MCDUFFIE COUNTY HOSPITAL, 521 Hill Street S.W., Zip 30824; tel. 706/595–1411; Douglas C. Keir, Chief Executive Officer **A**1 9 10 **F**11 14 16 17 19 22 24 28 29 30 33 34 37 39 44 45 48 49 65 66 67 71 73 **S** Quorum Health Group/Quorum Health Resources, Inc., Brentwood, TN **N** Principal Health Care of Georgia, Atlanta, GA; The Medical Resource Network, L.L.C., Atlanta, GA; University Health, Inc., Augusta, GA	16	10	47	1633	19	24685	4	9570	4536	186

TIFTON—Tift County
✠ TIFT GENERAL HOSPITAL, 901 East 18th Street, Zip 31794, Mailing Address: Drawer 747, Zip 31793; tel. 912/382–7120; William T. Richardson, President and Chief Executive Officer **A**1 9 10 **F**7 8 10 12 14 17 19 21 22 23 28 33 35 37 39 40 41 42 44 45 46 48 49 61 65 71 73 74 **P**7 8 **N** Georgia 1st, Inc., Decatur, GA; Emory University System of Healthcare Affiliate Network, Atlanta, GA	16	10	181	7613	95	69918	1097	50396	18195	712

TOCCOA—Stephens County
✠ STEPHENS COUNTY HOSPITAL, 2003 Falls Road, Zip 30577; tel. 706/886–6841; Edward C. Gambrell, Jr., Administrator (Total facility includes 82 beds in nursing home–type unit) **A**1 10 **F**6 7 8 14 15 16 17 19 22 23 28 30 35 37 40 41 44 45 49 62 63 64 65 69 71 73 **N** Principal Health Care of Georgia, Atlanta, GA	16	10	178	3833	111	30383	388	24226	11683	394

VALDOSTA—Lowndes County
□ GREENLEAF CENTER, 2209 Pineview Drive, Zip 31602; tel. 912/247–4357; Michael Lane, Administrator and Chief Executive Officer (Nonreporting) **A**1 10 **S** Greenleaf Health Systems, Inc., Chattanooga, TN	33	22	70	—	—	—	—	—	—	—
✠ SOUTH GEORGIA MEDICAL CENTER, 2501 North Patterson Street, Zip 31602, Mailing Address: Box 1727, Zip 31603–1727; tel. 912/333–1000; John S. Bowling, President and Chief Executive Officer **A**1 2 10 **F**1 2 4 6 7 8 10 11 12 13 15 16 17 19 20 21 22 23 25 26 27 28 29 30 33 34 35 37 38 39 40 41 42 44 45 46 48 49 51 52 53 54 55 56 57 60 62 63 65 66 67 70 71 72 73 74 **P**8 **N** Principal Health Care of Georgia, Atlanta, GA; Georgia 1st, Inc., Decatur, GA; The Medical Resource Network, L.L.C., Atlanta, GA	16	10	288	12386	171	127612	1484	89204	38331	1437

VIDALIA—Toombs County
★ MEADOWS REGIONAL MEDICAL CENTER, 1703 Meadows Lane, Zip 30475, Mailing Address: P.O. Box 1048, Zip 30474; tel. 912/537–8921; Barry Michael, Chief Executive Officer (Total facility includes 35 beds in nursing home–type unit) **A**10 **F**7 8 10 14 15 16 17 19 21 22 23 25 28 30 31 34 35 37 39 40 41 44 45 46 49 63 64 65 67 71 72 73 **P**3 **N** Candler Health System, Savannah, GA; Principal Health Care of Georgia, Atlanta, GA	16	10	122	4143	77	35192	602	25157	11245	352

VIENNA—Dooly County
□ DOOLY MEDICAL CENTER, 1300 Union Street, Zip 31092, Mailing Address: Box 278, Zip 31092; tel. 912/268–4141; Kevin Paul, Administrator **A**1 10 **F**8 15 19 21 22 23 28 30 32 33 37 40 44 48 49 65 70 71 73 **P**8 **N** Principal Health Care of Georgia, Atlanta, GA; The Medical Resource Network, L.L.C., Atlanta, GA	16	10	38	659	7	3309	0	4017	—	89

VILLA RICA—Carroll County
✠ TANNER MEDICAL CENTER–VILLA RICA, 601 Dallas Road, Zip 30180, Mailing Address: Box 638, Zip 30180; tel. 770/459–7100; Larry N. Steed, Administrator **A**1 9 10 **F**8 11 15 16 19 21 22 23 30 33 40 44 63 65 71 73 **P**8 **S** Quorum Health Group/Quorum Health Resources, Inc., Brentwood, TN **N** Principal Health Care of Georgia, Atlanta, GA; Georgia 1st, Inc., Decatur, GA	16	10	45	1455	13	16204	162	9209	4134	124

WARM SPRINGS—Meriwether County
MERIWETHER REGIONAL HOSPITAL, Mailing Address: P.O. Box 8, Zip 31830; tel. 706/655–3331; William E. Daniel, Administrator (Total facility includes 79 beds in nursing home–type unit) **A**10 **F**14 15 16 19 22 32 33 40 44 49 64 65 71 **N** Community Healthcare Network, Columbus, GA	21	10	105	741	27	7474	27	—	—	143
□ ROOSEVELT WARM SPRINGS INSTITUTE FOR REHABILITATION, Mailing Address: P.O. Box 1000, Zip 31830–0268; tel. 706/655–5001; Frank C. Ruzycki, Executive Director; Paul E. Peach, Medical Director **A**1 10 **F**15 48 49	12	46	78	755	49	5817	0	16635	5679	495

WARNER ROBINS—Houston County
✠ HOUSTON MEDICAL CENTER, 1601 Watson Boulevard, Zip 31093–3431, Mailing Address: Box 2886, Zip 31099–2886; tel. 912/922–4281; Arthur P. Christie, Administrator **A**1 9 10 **F**7 8 10 12 14 15 16 19 20 21 22 23 25 28 33 34 35 36 37 38 39 40 42 44 45 46 49 52 54 55 56 57 58 59 65 66 67 71 72 73 **P**7 **N** Georgia 1st, Inc., Decatur, GA; The Medical Resource Network, L.L.C., Atlanta, GA	16	10	186	10309	107	77345	894	53371	23192	938

Hospital, Address, Telephone, Administrator, Approval, Facility, and Physician Codes, Health Care System, Network	Classi-fication Codes		Utilization Data					Expense (thousands) of dollars		
★ American Hospital Association (AHA) membership □ Joint Commission on Accreditation of Healthcare Organizations (JCAHO) accreditation + American Osteopathic Hospital Association (AOHA) membership ○ American Osteopathic Association (AOA) accreditation △ Commission on Accreditation of Rehabilitation Facilities (CARF) accreditation Control codes 61, 63, 64, 71, 72 and 73 indicate hospitals listed by AOHA, but not registered by AHA. For definition of numerical codes, see page A4	Control	Service	Beds	Admissions	Census	Outpatient Visits	Births	Total	Payroll	Personnel

WASHINGTON—Wilkes County

WILLS MEMORIAL HOSPITAL, 120 Gordon Street, Zip 30673, Mailing Address: Box 370, Zip 30673-0370; tel. 706/678-2151; Vincent DiFranco, Chief Executive Officer (Nonreporting) **A**9 10 **S** Quorum Health Group/Quorum Health Resources, Inc., Brentwood, TN **N** University Health, Inc., Augusta, GA

	16	10	50	—	—	—	—	—	—	—

WAYCROSS—Ware County

✠ SATILLA REGIONAL MEDICAL CENTER, 410 Darling Avenue, Zip 31501, Mailing Address: P.O. Box 139, Zip 31502-0139; tel. 912/283-3030; Eugene Johnson, President and Chief Executive Officer **A**1 9 10 **F**8 11 16 19 20 22 23 32 33 35 37 38 40 41 42 44 46 49 54 55 57 58 59 60 65 71 73 **P**8 **N** Principal Health Care of Georgia, Atlanta, GA

	23	10	116	6716	82	118882	712	35942	17467	683

WAYNESBORO—Burke County

□ BURKE COUNTY HOSPITAL, 351 Liberty Street, Zip 30830; tel. 706/554-4435; Gloria Cochran, Administrator **A**1 9 10 **F**7 8 15 16 17 19 22 28 30 37 40 44 45 46 49 65 67 71 73 **N** Principal Health Care of Georgia, Atlanta, GA; The Medical Resource Network, L.L.C., Atlanta, GA; University Health, Inc., Augusta, GA

	13	10	40	1571	16	8448	176	7303	2612	113

WILDWOOD—Dade County

WILDWOOD LIFESTYLE CENTER AND HOSPITAL, Lifestyle Lane, Zip 30757; tel. 706/820-1493; Larry E. Clements, Administrator (Nonreporting)

	23	10	13	—	—	—	—	—	—	—

WINDER—Barrow County

✠ COLUMBIA BARROW MEDICAL CENTER, 316 North Broad Street, Zip 30680, Mailing Address: Box 768, Zip 30680; tel. 770/867-3400; Joe T. Hutchins, Chief Executive Officer (Total facility includes 4 beds in nursing home-type unit) **A**1 9 10 **F**7 8 12 15 16 19 21 22 27 32 34 35 37 39 40 44 49 63 64 65 71 73 **P**2 3 7 8 **S** Columbia/HCA Healthcare Corporation, Nashville, TN

	33	10	60	1831	20	29675	266	18000	6149	221

HAWAII

Resident population 1,187 (in thousands)
Resident population in metro areas 74.2%
Birth rate per 1,000 population 16.8
65 years and over 12.6%
Percent of persons without health insurance 9.2%

Hospital, Address, Telephone, Administrator, Approval, Facility, and Physician Codes, Health Care System, Network	Classi-fication Codes		Utilization Data					Expense (thousands) of dollars		
★ American Hospital Association (AHA) membership □ Joint Commission on Accreditation of Healthcare Organizations (JCAHO) accreditation + American Osteopathic Hospital Association (AOHA) membership ○ American Osteopathic Association (AOA) accreditation △ Commission on Accreditation of Rehabilitation Facilities (CARF) accreditation Control codes 61, 63, 64, 71, 72 and 73 indicate hospitals listed by AOHA, but not registered by AHA. For definition of numerical codes, see page A4	Control	Service	Beds	Admissions	Census	Outpatient Visits	Births	Total	Payroll	Personnel

EWA BEACH—Honolulu County

☒ KAHI MOHALA, 91-2301 Fort Weaver Road, Zip 96706; tel. 808/671-8511; Margi Drue, Administrator (Nonreporting) **A**1 3 10 **S** Sutter Health, Sacramento, CA — 33 22 88 — — — — — — — —

☒ ST. FRANCIS MEDICAL CENTER—WEST, 91-2141 Fort Weaver Road, Zip 96706; tel. 808/678-7000; Sister Gretchen Gilroy, President and Chief Executive Officer **A**1 5 10 **F**4 7 8 10 11 12 15 16 17 19 20 21 22 28 29 30 31 32 33 34 35 37 40 41 42 43 44 45 46 49 60 65 68 69 71 73 **P**3 **S** Sisters of the 3rd Franciscan Order, Syracuse, NY — 21 10 87 3380 70 — 577 35629 18344 491

HILO—Hawaii County

☒ HILO MEDICAL CENTER, 1190 Waianuenue Avenue, Zip 96720-2095; tel. 808/974-4743; William Carnett, D.O., Acting Administrator (Total facility includes 108 beds in nursing home–type unit) **A**1 5 9 10 **F**7 8 11 14 15 16 19 20 21 22 25 26 29 31 32 33 35 37 40 41 42 44 45 49 52 54 55 56 57 59 60 64 65 71 73 **P**5 **S** State of Hawaii, Department of Health, Honolulu, HI — 12 10 274 8102 241 — 1246 59287 25364 731

HONOKAA—Hawaii County

★ HONOKAA HOSPITAL, Mailing Address: P.O. Box 237, Zip 96727-0237; tel. 808/775-7211; Romel de la Cruz, Administrator **A**9 10 **F**15 16 20 22 44 51 64 65 67 73 **S** State of Hawaii, Department of Health, Honolulu, HI — 12 10 50 455 29 2807 0 6303 2578 85

HONOLULU—Honolulu County

☒ KAISER FOUNDATION HOSPITAL, 3288 Moanalua Road, Zip 96819; tel. 808/834-5333; Bruce Behnke, Administrator (Total facility includes 55 beds in nursing home–type unit) **A**1 2 3 5 10 **F**3 4 7 8 10 11 12 13 14 16 17 19 20 21 22 23 25 26 27 28 30 31 32 33 34 35 37 38 39 40 41 42 43 44 45 46 49 51 53 54 55 57 58 59 60 61 63 64 65 67 68 69 70 71 72 73 74 **P**4 **S** Kaiser Foundation Hospitals, Oakland, CA — 23 10 198 10555 147 1154069 2108 — — 938

☒ KAPIOLANI MEDICAL CENTER FOR WOMEN AND CHILDREN, 1319 Punahou Street, Zip 96826-1032; tel. 808/973-8511; Frances A. Hallonquist, Chief Executive Officer **A**1 3 5 10 **F**5 7 8 10 12 13 14 15 16 17 18 19 21 22 25 27 28 30 31 32 34 38 39 40 41 42 43 44 45 46 47 49 51 53 54 55 56 58 60 61 65 66 67 68 70 /1 72 73 74 **P**2 5 7 — 23 44 276 12201 155 147200 5467 120136 46800 1193

☒ KUAKINI MEDICAL CENTER, 347 North Kuakini Street, Zip 96817-2381; tel. 808/536-2236; Gary K. Kajiwara, President and Chief Executive Officer **A**1 2 3 5 9 10 **F**1 4 8 10 11 12 14 15 16 19 21 22 23 25 26 28 29 30 32 33 34 35 37 39 41 42 43 44 45 46 49 60 63 64 65 66 67 71 73 **P**8 **N** Pacific Health Care, Honolulu, HI — 23 10 189 6015 125 35199 0 88776 44876 1120

★ LEAHI HOSPITAL, 3675 Kilauea Avenue, Zip 96816; tel. 808/733-8000; Fred D. Horwitz, Administrator (Total facility includes 179 beds in nursing home–type unit) **A**3 5 9 10 **F**1 16 19 20 21 34 35 41 50 57 63 64 65 71 **P**6 **S** State of Hawaii, Department of Health, Honolulu, HI — 12 33 192 98 158 — 0 16610 8639 —

☒ QUEEN'S MEDICAL CENTER, 1301 Punchbowl Street, Zip 96813; tel. 808/538-9011; Arthur A. Ushijima, President and Chief Executive Officer (Total facility includes 30 beds in nursing home–type unit) **A**1 2 3 5 8 9 10 **F**3 4 6 7 8 10 11 14 15 16 17 18 19 20 21 22 23 25 26 27 28 29 30 31 32 33 34 35 36 37 39 40 41 42 44 45 46 52 53 54 55 56 57 58 59 60 61 63 64 65 67 69 70 71 72 73 74 **P**5 7 **S** Queen's Health Systems, Honolulu, HI **N** Queens Health Systems, Honolulu, HI — 23 10 496 19737 454 205829 2095 305905 138625 3047

☒ △ REHABILITATION HOSPITAL OF THE PACIFIC, 226 North Kuakini Street, Zip 96817-9881; tel. 808/531-3511; William D. O'Connor, President and Chief Executive Officer **A**1 7 9 10 **F**12 14 15 16 19 21 25 27 32 34 35 36 39 41 46 48 49 54 57 58 65 66 67 71 73 **P**2 — 23 46 86 1472 71 46500 0 28000 16800 354

☒ SHRINERS HOSPITALS FOR CHILDREN, HONOLULU, (Formerly Shriners Hospitals for Crippled Children), 1310 Punahou Street, Zip 96826-1099; tel. 808/941-4466; James B. Brasel, Administrator (Nonreporting) **A**1 3 5 **S** Shriners Hospitals for Children, Tampa, FL — 23 57 40 — — — — — — —

☒ ST. FRANCIS MEDICAL CENTER, 2230 Liliha Street, Zip 96817-9979, Mailing Address: P.O. Box 30100, Zip 96820-0100; tel. 808/547-6011; Cynthia Okinaka, Administrator (Total facility includes 46 beds in nursing home–type unit) **A**1 2 3 5 9 10 **F**2 3 4 7 8 10 14 15 16 17 18 19 20 21 22 26 28 30 32 33 34 35 37 39 41 42 43 44 45 46 49 51 54 60 63 64 65 67 68 69 70 71 73 **P**7 8 **S** Sisters of the 3rd Franciscan Order, Syracuse, NY **N** Pacific Health Care, Honolulu, HI — 21 10 221 4962 202 340862 0 127575 55744 1566

□ STRAUB CLINIC AND HOSPITAL, 888 South King Street, Zip 96813; tel. 808/522-4000; Blake E. Waterhouse, M.D., President and Chief Executive Officer **A**1 2 3 5 9 10 **F**3 4 8 9 10 14 15 19 21 22 25 26 28 30 31 32 34 35 36 37 39 41 42 43 44 45 46 48 49 51 53 54 55 56 57 58 60 61 63 65 66 67 71 72 73 74 **P**3 — 33 10 139 6036 106 — 0 199465 98310 1720

☒ TRIPLER ARMY MEDICAL CENTER, Zip 96859-5000; tel. 808/433-6661; Brigadier General Warren A. Todd, Jr., MSC, Commander **A**1 2 3 5 **F**2 3 4 7 8 10 12 13 14 15 16 17 18 19 20 21 22 24 25 28 29 30 31 34 35 37 38 39 40 41 42 43 44 45 46 47 49 50 51 52 53 54 55 56 57 58 59 60 61 63 65 66 67 68 70 71 72 73 74 **P**5 6 **S** Department of the Army, Office of the Surgeon General, Falls Church, VA — 42 10 354 17112 246 593859 2905 152653 43529 2787

Hospital, Address, Telephone, Administrator, Approval, Facility, and Physician Codes, Health Care System, Network	Classi-fication Codes		Utilization Data					Expense (thousands) of dollars		
★ American Hospital Association (AHA) membership □ Joint Commission on Accreditation of Healthcare Organizations (JCAHO) accreditation + American Osteopathic Hospital Association (AOHA) membership ○ American Osteopathic Association (AOA) accreditation △ Commission on Accreditation of Rehabilitation Facilities (CARF) accreditation Control codes 61, 63, 64, 71, 72 and 73 indicate hospitals listed by AOHA, but not registered by AHA. For definition of numerical codes, see page A4	Control	Service	Beds	Admissions	Census	Outpatient Visits	Births	Total	Payroll	Personnel

KAHUKU—Honolulu County

☒ KAHUKU HOSPITAL, Mailing Address: P.O. Box 219, Zip 96731; tel. 808/293–9221; Keith R. Ridley, Chief Executive Officer (Nonreporting) **A**1 9 10

| | 23 | 10 | 24 | — | — | — | — | — | — | — |

KAILUA—Honolulu County

☒ CASTLE MEDICAL CENTER, 640 Ulukahiki Street, Zip 96734–4498; tel. 808/263–5500; Kenneth A. Finch, President and Administrator (Total facility includes 10 beds in nursing home–type unit) **A**1 9 10 **F**2 3 7 8 10 14 15 16 17 19 21 22 28 29 30 32 35 37 40 41 42 44 46 49 52 53 58 59 64 65 67 71 73 74 **P**5 8 **S** Adventist Health, Roseville, CA

| | 21 | 10 | 150 | 6029 | 93 | 55944 | 542 | 56011 | 27126 | 618 |

KANEOHE—Honolulu County

□ HAWAII STATE HOSPITAL, 45–710 Keaahala Road, Zip 96744–3597; tel. 808/236–8237; Marvin O. St. Clair, Administrator **A**1 3 5 **F**15 19 20 21 26 27 31 35 41 42 46 48 49 52 54 55 57 59 60 63 64 65 67 71 73

| | 12 | 22 | 167 | 89 | 170 | 0 | 0 | 38488 | 19603 | 557 |

KAPAA—Kauai County

★ SAMUEL MAHELONA MEMORIAL HOSPITAL, (SNF/ ACUTE PSYCHIATRIC), 4800 Kawaihau Road, Zip 96746–1998; tel. 808/822–4961; Neva M. Olson, Administrator (Total facility includes 61 beds in nursing home–type unit) **A**9 10 **F**14 15 16 26 33 41 49 52 64 65 73 **S** State of Hawaii, Department of Health, Honolulu, HI

| | 12 | 49 | 82 | 136 | 65 | | 0 | 7428 | 4248 | 133 |

KAUNAKAKAI—Maui County

☒ MOLOKAI GENERAL HOSPITAL, Mailing Address: P.O. Box 408, Zip 96748–0408; tel. 808/553–5331; Calvin M. Ichinose, Administrator (Total facility includes 16 beds in nursing home–type unit) **A**1 9 10 **F**1 2 3 4 5 6 7 8 9 10 11 13 14 15 16 17 18 19 20 21 22 23 24 25 26 27 28 29 30 31 32 33 34 36 37 38 39 41 42 43 44 45 46 47 48 49 51 52 53 54 55 56 57 58 59 60 61 62 64 65 66 67 68 69 70 71 73 **P**4 5 7 **S** Queen's Health Systems, Honolulu, HI **N** Queens Health Systems, Honolulu, HI

| | 23 | 10 | 30 | 154 | 15 | 7137 | 47 | 6002 | 2456 | 81 |

KEALAKEKUA—Hawaii County

☒ KONA COMMUNITY HOSPITAL, Mailing Address: P.O. Box 69, Zip 96750–0069; tel. 808/322–4429; David W. Patton, Chief Executive Officer (Total facility includes 22 beds in nursing home–type unit) **A**1 9 10 **F**1 7 14 15 16 19 20 22 36 37 40 41 42 44 49 56 59 64 65 71 73 **S** State of Hawaii, Department of Health, Honolulu, HI

| | 12 | 10 | 75 | 3355 | 61 | 13211 | 616 | 25061 | 11791 | 314 |

KOHALA—Hawaii County

★ KOHALA HOSPITAL, Mailing Address: P.O. Box 10, Kapaau, Zip 96755–0010; tel. 808/889–6211; Manuel Anduha, Administrator **A**9 10 **F**1 2 3 4 5 6 7 8 9 10 11 12 13 15 16 17 18 19 20 21 22 23 24 25 26 27 28 29 30 31 32 33 34 35 36 37 38 39 40 41 42 43 44 45 46·47 48 49 50 51 52 53 54 55 56 57 58 59 60 61 62 63 64 65 66 67 68 69 70 71 72 73 74 **P**1 2 3 4 5 6 7 8 **S** State of Hawaii, Department of Health, Honolulu, HI

| | 12 | 10 | 26 | 45 | 24 | 1807 | 0 | — | — | 43 |

KULA—Maui County

★ KULA HOSPITAL, (NURSING FACILITY), 204 Kula Highway, Zip 96790–9499; tel. 808/878–1221; Michael P. Gagne, Administrator (Total facility includes 103 beds in nursing home–type unit) **A**9 10 **F**14 15 16 34 64 **P**6 **S** State of Hawaii, Department of Health, Honolulu, HI

| | 12 | 49 | 105 | 34 | 99 | 322 | 0 | 10513 | 5379 | 185 |

LANAI CITY—Maui County

★ LANAI COMMUNITY HOSPITAL, 628 Seventh Street, Zip 96763–0797, Mailing Address: P.O. Box 797, Zip 96763–0797; tel. 808/565–6411; Herbert K. Yim, Administrator **A**9 10 **F**22 **P**5 **S** State of Hawaii, Department of Health, Honolulu, HI

| | 12 | 10 | 14 | 21 | 8 | 2861 | 0 | 2029 | 1049 | 28 |

LIHUE—Kauai County

☒ WILCOX MEMORIAL HOSPITAL, 3420 Kuhio Highway, Zip 96766; tel. 808/245–1100; Larry K. Mangold, Interim President and Chief Executive Officer (Total facility includes 110 beds in nursing home–type unit) **A**1 2 9 10 **F**1 7 8 15 16 19 20 21 22 25 26 27 28 29 30 31 32 33 34 37 39 40 41 42 44 45 49 51 61 63 64 65 68 71 72 73 **P**5 6

| | 23 | 10 | 177 | 4416 | 158 | 39923 | 733 | 42520 | 20322 | 559 |

PAHALA—Hawaii County

★ KAU HOSPITAL, Mailing Address: P.O. Box 40, Zip 96777; tel. 808/928–8331; Dawn S. Pung, Administrator (Total facility includes 19 beds in nursing home–type unit) **A**9 10 **F**1 22 64 **S** State of Hawaii, Department of Health, Honolulu, HI

| | 12 | 10 | 21 | 10 | 13 | 3147 | 0 | 2480 | 1228 | 32 |

WAHIAWA—Honolulu County

☒ WAHIAWA GENERAL HOSPITAL, 128 Lehua Street, Zip 96786, Mailing Address: P.O. Box 580, Zip 96786–0580; tel. 808/621–8411; David L. Hill, President and Chief Executive Officer (Total facility includes 93 beds in nursing home–type unit) (Nonreporting) **A**1 3 5 9 10

| | 23 | 10 | 162 | — | — | — | — | — | — | — |

WAILUKU—Maui County

☒ MAUI MEMORIAL HOSPITAL, 221 Mahalani Street, Zip 96793–2581; tel. 808/244–9056; Alan G. Lee, Administrator (Nonreporting) **A**1 2 9 10 **S** State of Hawaii, Department of Health, Honolulu, HI

| | 12 | 10 | 180 | — | — | — | — | — | — | — |

WAIMEA—Kauai County

☒ KAUAI VETERANS MEMORIAL HOSPITAL, Waimea Canyon Road, Zip 96796, Mailing Address: P.O. Box 337, Zip 96796–0337; tel. 808/338–9431; Orianna A. Skomoroch, Administrator (Total facility includes 20 beds in nursing home–type unit) **A**1 9 10 **F**7 8 11 12 14 15 16 22 28 33 39 40 44 46 49 64 65 71 **S** State of Hawaii, Department of Health, Honolulu, HI

| | 12 | 10 | 49 | 762 | 30 | 4897 | 13 | 9711 | 4929 | 140 |

IDAHO

Resident population 1,163 (in thousands)
Resident population in metro areas 30.7%
Birth rate per 1,000 population 15.8
65 years and over 11.4%
Percent of persons without health insurance 14.0%

Hospital, Address, Telephone, Administrator, Approval, Facility, and Physician Codes, Health Care System, Network	Classi-fication Codes		Utilization Data					Expense (thousands) of dollars		
	Control	Service	Beds	Admissions	Census	Outpatient Visits	Births	Total	Payroll	Personnel

★ American Hospital Association (AHA) membership
□ Joint Commission on Accreditation of Healthcare Organizations (JCAHO) accreditation
+ American Osteopathic Hospital Association (AOHA) membership
○ American Osteopathic Association (AOA) accreditation
△ Commission on Accreditation of Rehabilitation Facilities (CARF) accreditation
Control codes 61, 63, 64, 71, 72 and 73 indicate hospitals listed by AOHA, but not registered by AHA. For definition of numerical codes, see page A4

AMERICAN FALLS—Power County

★ HARMS MEMORIAL HOSPITAL DISTRICT, 510 Roosevelt, Zip 83211–0420, Mailing Address: P.O. Box 420, Zip 83211–0420; tel. 208/226–2327; Dale E. Polla, Administrator (Total facility includes 31 beds in nursing home–type unit) **A**9 10 **F**1 3 7 8 11 15 17 20 21 22 26 28 32 34 41 46 49 64 65 73 **P**5 — 16 10 41 161 32 9501 10 3490 1668 77

ARCO—Butte County

★ LOST RIVERS DISTRICT HOSPITAL, 551 Highland Drive, Zip 83213, Mailing Address: P.O. Box 145, Zip 83213; tel. 208/527–3616; Cindy Charyulu, Chief Executive Officer (Total facility includes 33 beds in nursing home–type unit) (Nonreporting) **A**9 10 — 16 10 41 — — — — — — —

BLACKFOOT—Bingham County

✠ BINGHAM MEMORIAL HOSPITAL, 98 Poplar Street, Zip 83221–1799; tel. 208/785–4100; Robert M. Peterson, Administrator (Total facility includes 75 beds in nursing home–type unit) **A**1 9 10 **F**7 8 14 15 16 17 19 21 22 28 29 30 35 37 39 40 41 44 45 46 49 64 65 67 71 73 **P**8 **S** Quorum Health Group/Quorum Health Resources, Inc., Brentwood, TN — 13 10 115 1500 77 30015 354 12413 4544 194

STATE HOSPITAL SOUTH, 700 East Alice Street, Zip 83221–0400, Mailing Address: Box 400, Zip 83221–0400; tel. 208/785–1200; Ray Laible, Administrative Director (Total facility includes 30 beds in nursing home–type unit) **F**52 53 54 55 56 57 64 **P**6 — 12 22 136 335 108 0 0 15720 8315 245

BOISE—Ada County

□ BHC INTERMOUNTAIN HOSPITAL, (Formerly CPC Intermountain Hospital), 303 North Allumbaugh Street, Zip 83704–9266; tel. 208/377–8400; Vernon G. Garrett, Chief Executive Officer (Nonreporting) **A**1 9 10 **S** Behavioral Healthcare Corporation, Nashville, TN — 33 22 75 — — — — — — —

★ △ IDAHO ELKS REHABILITATION HOSPITAL, 204 Fort Place, Zip 83702–4597, Mailing Address: Box 1100, Zip 83701–1100; tel. 208/343–2583; Joseph P. Caroselli, Administrator (Total facility includes 10 beds in nursing home–type unit) **A**7 10 **F**12 24 27 39 41 46 48 49 53 64 65 66 67 73 — 23 46 62 1292 46 33782 0 12690 7483 300

✠ △ SAINT ALPHONSUS REGIONAL MEDICAL CENTER, 1055 North Curtis Road, Zip 83706–1370; tel. 208/378–2121; Sandra B. Bruce, President and Chief Executive Officer (Total facility includes 11 beds in nursing home–type unit) **A**1 2 3 5 7 9 10 **F**3 4 8 10 11 12 15 16 17 18 19 21 22 23 25 26 27 28 29 30 31 32 33 34 35 37 39 41 42 43 44 45 46 48 49 51 52 53 54 55 56 57 58 60 64 65 67 69 70 71 72 73 **P**5 6 7 8 **S** Holy Cross Health System Corporation, South Bend, IN — 21 10 287 14788 178 243222 0 133570 50676 1671

✠ ST. LUKE'S REGIONAL MEDICAL CENTER, 190 East Bannock Street, Zip 83712–6298; tel. 208/381–2222; Edwin E. Dahlberg, President **A**1 2 3 5 9 10 **F**4 7 8 10 11 12 13 14 15 16 17 19 20 21 22 23 24 25 26 28 29 30 31 32 33 34 35 36 37 38 39 40 41 42 43 44 45 46 47 49 51 53 54 56 57 58 60 63 65 67 68 69 71 72 73 74 **P**6 — 23 10 312 20286 187 312987 4578 158703 66746 2063

✠ VETERANS AFFAIRS MEDICAL CENTER, 500 West Fort Street, Zip 83702–4598; tel. 208/422–1000; Wayne C. Tippets, Director (Total facility includes 40 beds in nursing home–type unit) **A**1 3 5 **F**2 3 10 12 14 17 19 20 21 22 26 27 28 30 31 32 33 34 37 39 42 44 45 46 49 51 52 54 56 57 58 59 60 64 65 67 71 73 74 **S** Department of Veterans Affairs, Washington, DC — 45 10 176 3316 90 96241 — — — 592

BONNERS FERRY—Boundary County

★ BOUNDARY COMMUNITY HOSPITAL, (Includes Boundary County Nursing Home), 6640 Kaniksu Street, Zip 83805, Mailing Address: HCR 61, Box 61A, Zip 83805; tel. 208/267–3141; William T. McClintock, FACHE, Chief Executive Officer (Total facility includes 52 beds in nursing home–type unit) **A**9 10 **F**1 12 14 15 17 22 26 27 28 30 32 33 34 39 41 44 49 51 56 57 64 65 67 72 73 **P**8 **N** North Idaho Rural Health Consortium, Coeur d'Alene, ID — 13 10 62 474 52 10269 0 4564 2744 136

BURLEY—Cassia County

✠ CASSIA REGIONAL MEDICAL CENTER, 1501 Hiland Avenue, Zip 83318; tel. 208/678–4444; Richard Packer, Administrator (Total facility includes 34 beds in nursing home–type unit) (Nonreporting) **A**1 2 9 10 **S** Intermountain Health Care, Inc., Salt Lake City, UT **N** Intermountain HealthCare/Amerinet, Salt Lake City, UT — 23 10 87 — — — — — — —

CALDWELL—Canyon County

✠ COLUMBIA WEST VALLEY MEDICAL CENTER, 1717 Arlington, Zip 83605–4864; tel. 208/459–4641; Mark Adams, Chief Executive Officer (Total facility includes 16 beds in nursing home–type unit) (Nonreporting) **A**1 9 10 **S** Columbia/HCA Healthcare Corporation, Nashville, TN — 33 10 122 — — — — — — —

CASCADE—Valley County

★ CASCADE MEDICAL CENTER, 402 Old State Highway, Zip 83611, Mailing Address: P.O. Box 151, Zip 83611; tel. 208/382–4242; Richard Holm, Administrator (Nonreporting) **A**9 10 **S** Holy Cross Health System Corporation, South Bend, IN — 13 10 10 — — — — — — —

COEUR D'ALENE—Kootenai County

□ INLAND BEHAVIORAL HEALTH INSTITUTE, (Formerly Pine Crest Hospital), 2301 North Ironwood Place, Zip 83814; tel. 208/765–4800; Albert J. Gale, Chief Executive Officer **A**1 10 **F**2 3 12 15 16 52 53 54 56 57 58 65 — 33 22 48 644 26 177 0 3986 2031 111

Hospital, Address, Telephone, Administrator, Approval, Facility, and Physician Codes, Health Care System, Network	Classi-fication Codes		Utilization Data					Expense (thousands) of dollars		
★ American Hospital Association (AHA) membership □ Joint Commission on Accreditation of Healthcare Organizations (JCAHO) accreditation + American Osteopathic Hospital Association (AOHA) membership ○ American Osteopathic Association (AOA) accreditation △ Commission on Accreditation of Rehabilitation Facilities (CARF) accreditation Control codes 61, 63, 64, 71, 72 and 73 indicate hospitals listed by AOHA, but not registered by AHA. For definition of numerical codes, see page A4	Control	Service	Beds	Admissions	Census	Outpatient Visits	Births	Total	Payroll	Personnel

	Control	Service	Beds	Admissions	Census	Outpatient Visits	Births	Total	Payroll	Personnel
⊠ KOOTENAI MEDICAL CENTER, 2003 Lincoln Way, Zip 83814; tel. 208/666–2000; Joe Morris, Chief Executive Officer (Total facility includes 25 beds in nursing home–type unit) **A**1 2 9 10 **F**1 4 7 8 10 11 15 16 17 18 19 21 22 23 25 27 28 29 30 31 32 34 35 37 39 40 41 42 44 45 46 48 49 52 54 55 56 57 58 59 60 64 65 66 67 70 71 72 73 **P**8 **N** North Idaho Rural Health Consortium, Coeur d'Alene, ID	16	10	212	9890	93	73841	1213	54586	25766	762
PINE CREST HOSPITAL See Inland Behavioral Health Institute										
COTTONWOOD—Idaho County										
★ ST. MARY'S HOSPITAL, Lewiston and North Streets, Zip 83522, Mailing Address: P.O. Box 137, Zip 83522–0137; tel. 208/962–3251; Casey Uhling, Administrator (Total facility includes 10 beds in nursing home–type unit) (Nonreporting) **A**9 10 **S** Benedictine Health System, Duluth, MN	21	10	28	—	—	—	—	—	—	—
COUNCIL—Adams County										
COUNCIL COMMUNITY HOSPITAL AND NURSING HOME, 205 North Berkley Street, Zip 83612; tel. 208/253–4242; Sandy Niehm, Administrator (Total facility includes 20 beds in nursing home–type unit) **A**9 10 **F**22 32 33 64 **P**5	13	10	26	219	20	0	0	1755	830	36
DRIGGS—Teton County										
★ TETON VALLEY HOSPITAL, 283 North First East, Zip 83422–0728, Mailing Address: P.O. Box 728, Zip 83422–0728; tel. 208/354–2383; Susan Kunz, Administrator **A**9 10 **F**7 8 14 15 17 22 28 29 32 33 40 41 42 44 46 49 51 65 71 73 **P**3	13	10	13	335	3	21962	47	3255	1664	71
EMMETT—Gem County										
WALTER KNOX MEMORIAL HOSPITAL, 1202 East Locust Street, Zip 83617; tel. 208/365–3561; Max Long, Chief Executive Officer (Nonreporting) **A**9 10	13	10	24	—	—	—	—	—	—	—
GOODING—Gooding County										
GOODING COUNTY MEMORIAL HOSPITAL, 1120 Montana Street, Zip 83330; tel. 208/934–4433; Kenneth W. Archer, Administrator (Total facility includes 13 beds in nursing home–type unit) (Nonreporting) **A**9 10 **N** South Central Health Network, Twin Falls, ID	16	10	27	—	—	—	—	—	—	—
GRANGEVILLE—Idaho County										
SYRINGA GENERAL HOSPITAL, 607 West Main Street, Zip 83530–1396; tel. 208/983–1700; Jess Hawley, Administrator **A**9 10 **F**7 8 11 12 19 22 32 34 37 40 44 71 **P**5	16	10	16	434	3	9966	39	2954	1530	63
HAILEY—Blaine County										
BLAINE COUNTY MEDICAL CENTER See Wood River Medical Center, Sun Valley										
IDAHO FALLS—Bonneville County										
⊠ COLUMBIA EASTERN IDAHO REGIONAL MEDICAL CENTER, (Formerly Eastern Idaho Regional Medical Center), 3100 Channing Way, Zip 83404, Mailing Address: P.O. Box 2077, Zip 83403–2077; tel. 208/529–6111; Ronald G. Butler, Chief Executive Officer **A**1 9 10 **F**4 5 7 8 10 12 14 15 16 17 18 19 21 22 24 25 28 30 32 35 37 38 39 40 41 42 43 44 45 48 49 52 53 54 56 57 58 61 63 64 65 66 67 70 71 72 73 74 **P**8 **S** Columbia/HCA Healthcare Corporation, Nashville, TN	33	10	286	11020	157	162230	1709	74177	31153	1099
★ IDAHO FALLS RECOVERY CENTER, 1957 East 17th Street, Zip 83404; tel. 208/529–5285; Jackie Street, President **A**10 **F**3 15 16	23	10	10	650	3	0	0	—	—	18
JEROME—Jerome County										
★ ST. BENEDICTS FAMILY MEDICAL CENTER, 709 North Lincoln Avenue, Zip 83338, Mailing Address: Box 586, Zip 83338–0586; tel. 208/324–4301; David Farnes, Administrator (Total facility includes 40 beds in nursing home–type unit) **A**9 10 **F**7 8 13 14 15 16 17 19 21 22 25 28 30 32 34 35 37 39 40 44 46 49 51 64 71 72 73 **P**6 8 **S** Holy Cross Health System Corporation, South Bend, IN **N** South Central Health Network, Twin Falls, ID	21	10	65	1045	40	20148	295	10146	3987	176
KELLOGG—Shoshone County										
⊠ SHOSHONE MEDICAL CENTER, 3 Jacobs Gulch, Zip 83837–2096; tel. 208/784–1221; Robert A. Morasko, Chief Executive Officer (Total facility includes 20 beds in nursing home–type unit) (Nonreporting) **A**1 9 10 **N** North Idaho Rural Health Consortium, Coeur d'Alene, ID	16	10	46	—	—	—	—	—	—	—
LEWISTON—Nez Perce County										
⊠ ST. JOSEPH REGIONAL MEDICAL CENTER, 415 Sixth Street, Zip 83501–0816; tel. 208/743–2511; Howard A. Hayes, President and Chief Executive Officer (Total facility includes 16 beds in nursing home–type unit) **A**1 2 9 10 **F**7 8 13 14 15 16 17 18 19 20 21 23 24 25 26 27 28 29 30 31 32 33 34 35 36 37 39 40 41 42 44 45 46 49 52 54 55 56 57 58 59 60 63 64 65 66 67 69 70 71 73 74 **S** Carondelet Health System, Saint Louis, MO	21	10	156	6536	82	107429	749	49215	22017	570
MALAD CITY—Oneida County										
ONEIDA COUNTY HOSPITAL, 150 North 200 West, Zip 83252–0126, Mailing Address: Box 126, Zip 83252–0126; tel. 208/766–2231; Robert O. Kent, Administrator and Chief Executive Officer (Total facility includes 41 beds in nursing home–type unit) **A**9 10 **F**1 7 14 22 26 28 32 34 40 44 64 65 **P**3 5	13	10	52	259	35	5239	14	3277	1392	87
MCCALL—Valley County										
★ MCCALL MEMORIAL HOSPITAL, 1000 State Street, Zip 83638, Mailing Address: P.O. Box 906, Zip 83638; tel. 208/634–2221; Karen J. Kellie, President **A**9 10 **F**7 8 14 15 19 22 28 32 33 37 39 40 41 44 45 49 65 71 73 **P**3 **S** Holy Cross Health System Corporation, South Bend, IN	16	10	12	593	4	13804	90	4967	2125	73
MONTPELIER—Bear Lake County										
★ BEAR LAKE MEMORIAL HOSPITAL, 164 South Fifth Street, Zip 83254; tel. 208/847–1630; Rod Jacobson, Administrator (Total facility includes 37 beds in nursing home–type unit) **A**9 10 **F**14 15 16 19 22 28 30 32 33 37 44 46 49 64 65 71 73	13	10	58	544	42	13127	72	4601	2369	126

Hospital, Address, Telephone, Administrator, Approval, Facility, and Physician Codes, Health Care System, Network	Classi-fication Codes		Utilization Data					Expense (thousands) of dollars		
	Control	Service	Beds	Admissions	Census	Outpatient Visits	Births	Total	Payroll	Personnel
MOSCOW—Latah County										
★ GRITMAN MEDICAL CENTER, 710 South Washington Street, Zip 83843; tel. 208/882–4511; Daniel R. Smigelski, Chief Executive Officer A1 9 10 F7 8 11 12 15 16 17 19 21 22 23 27 28 29 30 32 33 34 35 37 39 40 41 42 44 45 46 49 64 65 66 67 70 71 73 P5 8 S Quorum Health Group/Quorum Health Resources, Inc., Brentwood, TN	23	10	35	1953	17	41075	438	15529	6683	236
MOUNTAIN HOME—Elmore County										
★ ELMORE MEDICAL CENTER, 895 North Sixth East Street, Zip 83647, Mailing Address: P.O. Box 1270, Zip 83647–0348; tel. 208/587–8401; Gregory L. Maurer, Administrator (Total facility includes 55 beds in nursing home–type unit) A9 10 F7 8 14 15 19 22 28 40 44 49 64 71 S Holy Cross Health System Corporation, South Bend, IN	16	10	78	1073	56	18847	64	6500	3310	98
MOUNTAIN HOME AFB—Elmore County										
★ U. S. AIR FORCE HOSPITAL MOUNTAIN HOME, Zip 83648–5300; tel. 208/828–7600; Lieutenant Colonel Randall E. Fellman, MC, USAF, Commanding Officer (Nonreporting) A1 S Department of the Air Force, Washington, DC	41	10	29	—	—	—	—	—	—	—
NAMPA—Canyon County										
★ △ MERCY MEDICAL CENTER, 1512 12th Avenue Road, Zip 83686–6008; tel. 208/467–1171; Joseph Messmer, President and Chief Executive Officer A1 7 9 10 F2 3 4 7 8 10 14 15 16 19 22 27 32 33 35 36 37 40 41 44 49 64 65 66 71 73 S Catholic Health Initiatives, Denver, CO	21	10	144	6061	73	108161	1388	38847	17237	566
OROFINO—Clearwater County										
★ CLEARWATER VALLEY HOSPITAL, 301 Cedar, Zip 83544–9029; tel. 208/476–4555; James E. Robertson, Jr., Chief Executive Officer A9 10 F7 8 14 16 19 22 30 32 33 34 44 49 71 P6 S Brim, Inc., Portland, OR	13	10	23	679	8	48530	78	6468	3374	100
STATE HOSPITAL NORTH, 300 Hospital Drive, Zip 83544; tel. 208/476–4511; Gerald L. Hart, Chief Executive Officer F2 14 15 16 52 54 65	12	22	60	375	50	0	0	5193	3131	104
POCATELLO—Bannock County										
★ BANNOCK REGIONAL MEDICAL CENTER, 651 Memorial Drive, Zip 83201; tel. 208/239–1000; Fred R. Eaton, Administrator (Total facility includes 118 beds in nursing home–type unit) A1 2 3 9 10 F7 8 12 13 14 15 16 17 19 21 22 23 25 26 28 29 30 31 32 33 34 35 37 38 39 40 41 42 44 45 46 47 49 60 63 64 65 66 67 69 70 71 72 73 74 P5	13	10	241	5291	159	131022	1286	44396	16967	592
★ △ POCATELLO REGIONAL MEDICAL CENTER, 777 Hospital Way, Zip 83201; tel. 208/234–0777; Earl L. Christison, Administrator (Total facility includes 9 beds in nursing home–type unit) A1 3 7 9 10 F4 7 8 10 11 12 14 15 16 17 19 21 22 28 29 30 32 34 35 39 40 41 44 46 48 49 51 63 64 65 67 71 73 74 P3 S Intermountain Health Care, Inc., Salt Lake City, UT N Intermountain HealthCare/Amerinet, Salt Lake City, UT	23	10	87	2672	33	72345	193	27541	12483	386
PRESTON—Franklin County										
★ FRANKLIN COUNTY MEDICAL CENTER, 44 North First East Street, Zip 83263; tel. 208/852–0137; Michael G. Andrus, Administrator and Chief Executive Officer (Total facility includes 45 beds in nursing home–type unit) A9 10 F7 8 20 21 22 26 28 32 33 34 44 49 64 65 71	13	10	65	545	49	—	145	4633	2276	89
REXBURG—Madison County										
★ MADISON MEMORIAL HOSPITAL, 450 East Main, Zip 83440, Mailing Address: Box 310, Zip 83440–0310; tel. 208/356–3691; Keith M. Steiner, Chief Executive Officer A9 10 F8 11 15 17 18 19 20 21 22 28 29 31 32 37 39 40 41 44 45 46 49 58 65 66 71 73 P1	13	10	52	2628	18	28499	809	11259	5042	210
RUPERT—Minidoka County										
★ MINIDOKA MEMORIAL HOSPITAL AND EXTENDED CARE FACILITY, 1224 Eighth Street, Zip 83350; tel. 208/436–0481; Randall G. Holom, Administrator (Total facility includes 78 beds in nursing home–type unit) A9 10 F8 15 16 19 21 22 26 28 30 31 32 34 35 37 40 41 44 46 51 64 65 71 73 P5 N South Central Health Network, Twin Falls, ID	13	10	101	1227	76	21360	160	13612	4776	178
SAINT MARIES—Benewah County										
★ BENEWAH COMMUNITY HOSPITAL, 229 South Seventh Street, Zip 83861; tel. 208/245–5551; Camille Scott, Administrator A9 10 F7 8 12 14 15 16 17 19 22 27 28 30 32 33 37 39 40 41 44 49 51 64 65 71 74 P7 8 N North Idaho Rural Health Consortium, Coeur d'Alene, ID	13	10	25	723	5	10526	71	6000	2637	97
SALMON—Lemhi County										
★ STEELE MEMORIAL HOSPITAL, Main and Daisy Streets, Zip 83467, Mailing Address: Box 700, Zip 83467; tel. 208/756–4291; Kay H. Springer, Administrator A9 10 F7 8 22 34 37 40 44 46 56 71	13	10	28	609	5	11732	81	3059	1729	52
SANDPOINT—Bonner County										
★ BONNER GENERAL HOSPITAL, 520 North Third Avenue, Zip 83864–0877, Mailing Address: Box 1448, Zip 83864–0877; tel. 208/263–1441; Gene Tomt, FACHE, Chief Executive Officer A1 9 10 F7 8 11 17 19 22 28 30 31 32 33 34 39 40 41 44 46 49 56 65 71 73 P3 8 N North Idaho Rural Health Consortium, Coeur d'Alene, ID	23	10	62	2286	16	24634	482	12528	6410	206
SODA SPRINGS—Caribou County										
★ CARIBOU MEMORIAL HOSPITAL AND NURSING HOME, 300 South Third West Street, Zip 83276; tel. 208/547–3341; Arthur J. Phillips, Administrator (Total facility includes 43 beds in nursing home–type unit) (Nonreporting) A9 10	13	10	65	—	—	—	—	—	—	—

Hospital, Address, Telephone, Administrator, Approval, Facility, and Physician Codes, Health Care System, Network	Classi-fication Codes		Utilization Data					Expense (thousands) of dollars		
	Control	Service	Beds	Admissions	Census	Outpatient Visits	Births	Total	Payroll	Personnel
SUN VALLEY—Blaine County										
★ WOOD RIVER MEDICAL CENTER, (Includes Blaine County Medical Center, 706 South Main Street, Hailey, Zip 83333, Mailing Address: Box 927, Zip 83333; tel. 208/788–2222; Moritz Community Hospital, Mailing Address: P.O. Box 86, Zip 83353; tel. 208/622–3333), Sun Valley Road, Zip 83353, Mailing Address: P.O. Box 86, Zip 83353; tel. 208/622–3333; Alan Stevenson, Administrator (Total facility includes 25 beds in nursing home–type unit) **A**9 10 **F**7 8 15 17 19 20 21 22 24 34 35 37 40 41 44 49 56 64 65 66 68 71 73 74 **N** South Central Health Network, Twin Falls, ID	15	10	64	1744	37	21291	209	13829	6231	199
TWIN FALLS—Twin Falls County										
⊠ MAGIC VALLEY REGIONAL MEDICAL CENTER, 650 Addison Avenue West, Zip 83301, Mailing Address: Box 409, Zip 83303–0409; tel. 208/737–2000; John Bingham, Administrator (Total facility includes 20 beds in nursing home–type unit) **A**1 2 9 10 **F**7 8 15 16 19 21 22 26 28 30 32 33 35 37 38 40 41 42 44 46 47 49 60 64 65 67 70 71 73 **P**5 **N** South Central Health Network, Twin Falls, ID	13	10	146	5212	64	76630	1097	43272	17099	586
TWIN FALLS CLINIC HOSPITAL, 666 Shoshone Street East, Zip 83301, Mailing Address: Box 1233, Zip 83301; tel. 208/733–3700; Marley D. Jackman, Administrator (Nonreporting) **A**9 10 **N** South Central Health Network, Twin Falls, ID	33	10	40	—	—	—	—	—	—	—
WEISER—Washington County										
★ MEMORIAL HOSPITAL, 645 East Fifth Street, Zip 83672, Mailing Address: Box 550, Zip 83672; tel. 208/549–0370; Philip Krueger, M.D., Ph.D., Administrator **A**9 10 **F**7 8 14 15 16 22 32 34 44 71 73	16	10	18	509	3	15611	68	3175	1400	65

ILLINOIS

Resident population 11,830 (in thousands)
Resident population in metro areas 84.1%
Birth rate per 1,000 population 16.3
65 years and over 12.5%
Percent of persons without health insurance 11.4%

Hospital, Address, Telephone, Administrator, Approval, Facility, and Physician Codes, Health Care System, Network	Classi-fication Codes		Utilization Data					Expense (thousands) of dollars		
★ American Hospital Association (AHA) membership □ Joint Commission on Accreditation of Healthcare Organizations (JCAHO) accreditation + American Osteopathic Hospital Association (AOHA) membership ○ American Osteopathic Association (AOA) accreditation △ Commission on Accreditation of Rehabilitation Facilities (CARF) accreditation Control codes 61, 63, 64, 71, 72 and 73 indicate hospitals listed by AOHA, but not registered by AHA. For definition of numerical codes, see page A4	Control	Service	Beds	Admissions	Census	Outpatient Visits	Births	Total	Payroll	Personnel

ALEDO—Mercer County

★ MERCER COUNTY HOSPITAL, 409 N.W. Ninth Avenue, Zip 61231; tel. 309/582–5301; Bruce D. Peterson, Administrator (Total facility includes 18 beds in nursing home–type unit) **A**9 10 **F**8 15 19 22 30 31 32 34 36 37 40 41 44 48 51 58 64 65 69 71 73 **P**3 **N** Mercer County Community Care Network, Aledo, IL
13 10 45 791 27 20473 44 8092 4180 218

ALTON—Madison County

✠ ALTON MEMORIAL HOSPITAL, One Memorial Drive, Zip 62002–6722; tel. 618/463–7311; Ronald B. McMullen, President (Total facility includes 64 beds in nursing home–type unit) **A**1 2 9 10 **F**7 8 10 12 15 16 17 19 21 22 28 30 31 32 33 34 35 36 37 40 41 42 44 46 60 63 64 65 67 71 73 **P**2 4 5 6 7 8 **S** BJC Health System, Saint Louis, MO **N** BJC Health System, St. Louis, MO
23 10 224 5524 135 70408 614 49579 21590 675

□ ALTON MENTAL HEALTH CENTER, 4500 College Avenue, Zip 62002–5099; tel. 618/465–5593; Karl Kruckeberg, Director **A**1 10 **F**1 20 48 52 55 65
12 22 194 465 164 0 0 18129 — 423

✠ SAINT ANTHONY'S HEALTH CENTER, (Includes Saint Clare's Hospital, 915 East Fifth Street, Zip 62002–6434; tel. 618/463–5151), Saint Anthony's Way, Zip 62002, Mailing Address: P.O. Box 340, Zip 62002–0340; tel. 618/465–2571; William E. Kessler, President (Total facility includes 38 beds in nursing home–type unit) **A**1 2 9 10 **F**1 2 3 4 7 8 9 10 12 13 14 15 16 17 18 19 20 21 22 23 24 26 27 28 29 30 31 32 33 34 35 36 37 38 39 40 41 42 43 44 45 47 48 49 51 52 53 54 55 56 57 58 59 60 61 63 64 65 66 67 68 69 71 72 73 74 **P**3 7 8 **N** Unity Health System, St. Louis, MO
SAINT CLARE'S HOSPITAL See Saint Anthony's Health Center
23 10 254 6404 95 136302 690 61989 24867 785

ANNA—Union County

□ CHOATE MENTAL HEALTH AND DEVELOPMENTAL CENTER, 1000 North Main Street, Zip 62906–1699; tel. 618/833–5161; Tom Richards, Facility Director **A**1 5 **F**1 2 3 14 15 19 21 22 31 35 50 52 53 54 55 56 57 58 59 63 64 71
12 22 488 569 339 0 0 25940 20710 578

✠ UNION COUNTY HOSPITAL DISTRICT, 517 North Main Street, Zip 62906–1696; tel. 618/833–1511; Carol L. Goodman, Administrator (Total facility includes 10 beds in nursing home–type unit) **A**1 9 10 **F**8 14 15 16 17 19 21 22 32 34 44 45 46 49 51 64 71 73
16 10 46 1152 19 27976 0 8859 4642 203

ARLINGTON HEIGHTS—Cook County

✠ NORTHWEST COMMUNITY HOSPITAL, 800 West Central Road, Zip 60005–2392; tel. 847/618–1000; Bruce K. Crowther, President and Chief Executive Officer **A**1 2 9 10 **F**1 4 7 8 10 11 12 14 15 16 17 19 21 22 23 24 26 27 28 29 30 32 33 35 37 39 40 41 42 43 44 45 46 49 52 53 54 55 56 57 58 59 60 63 64 65 66 67 70 71 72 73 74 **P**1 **N** Northwestern Health Care Network, Chicago, IL
23 10 401 18739 219 376418 2640 160201 74884 2005

AURORA—Du Page and Kane Counties County

✠ △ COPLEY MEMORIAL HOSPITAL, 2000 Ogden Avenue, Zip 60504–4206; tel. 630/978–6200; D. Chet McKee, President **A**1 2 3 5 7 9 10 **F**1 2 3 4 5 6 7 8 9 10 11 12 13 14 15 16 17 18 19 20 21 22 23 24 25 26 27 28 29 30 31 32 33 34 35 36 37 38 39 40 41 42 43 44 45 46 47 48 49 50 51 52 53 54 55 56 57 58 59 60 61 62 63 64 65 66 67 68 69 70 71 72 73 74 **P**5 7 8 **S** Rush–Presbyterian–St. Luke's Medical Center, Chicago, IL **N** Rush System for Health, Chicago, IL
23 10 140 6404 82 68630 1216 61089 25379 556

□ MERCY CENTER FOR HEALTH CARE SERVICES, 1325 North Highland Avenue, Zip 60506; tel. 630/859–2222; John K. Barto, Jr., President and Chief Executive Officer (Total facility includes 15 beds in nursing home–type unit) **A**1 2 9 10 **F**2 3 4 7 8 10 14 15 16 19 22 28 30 34 35 36 37 39 40 41 42 43 44 45 46 49 52 53 57 58 59 64 65 67 70 71 73 **S** Mercy–Chicago Region Healthcare System, Naperville, IL
21 10 193 9570 120 56157 1520 62824 27414 820

BARRINGTON—Lake County

✠ GOOD SHEPHERD HOSPITAL, 450 West Highway 22, Zip 60010–1999; tel. 847/381–9600; Russell E. Feurer, Chief Executive **A**1 2 9 10 **F**7 8 12 15 16 17 18 19 21 22 23 27 28 30 32 33 34 35 36 37 39 40 41 42 44 46 49 52 53 54 55 56 57 58 60 63 65 66 67 70 71 73 **P**5 7 8 **S** Advocate Health Care, Oakbrook, IL **N** Advocate Health Care, Oak Brook, IL; MEDACOM Tri–State, Oakbrook, IL
21 10 154 7688 80 80973 1966 63943 24566 —

BELLEVILLE—St. Clair County

✠ MEMORIAL HOSPITAL, 4500 Memorial Drive, Zip 62226–5399; tel. 618/233–7750; Harry R. Maier, President (Total facility includes 108 beds in nursing home–type unit) **A**1 2 9 10 **F**3 4 7 8 10 16 19 21 22 23 24 28 30 32 33 34 35 37 40 41 42 43 44 45 46 49 52 56 58 60 63 64 65 66 67 71 73 **P**8
23 10 449 14754 277 189461 1430 104069 44981 1736

✠ △ ST. ELIZABETH'S HOSPITAL, 211 South Third Street, Zip 62222–0694; tel. 618/234–2120; Gerald M. Harman, Chief Executive Officer and Executive Vice President **A**1 2 3 7 9 10 **F**1 2 3 4 7 8 10 12 13 14 15 16 17 18 19 20 21 22 23 24 25 26 28 29 30 31 32 33 34 35 36 37 38 39 40 41 42 43 44 45 46 47 48 49 52 54 55 56 57 58 59 60 64 65 66 67 68 70 71 73 **P**5 8 **S** Hospital Sisters Health System, Springfield, IL **N** Unity Health System, St. Louis, MO
21 10 379 12048 213 95545 548 93218 36818 1302

Hospital, Address, Telephone, Administrator, Approval, Facility, and Physician Codes, Health Care System, Network	Classi-fication Codes		Utilization Data					Expense (thousands) of dollars		
★ American Hospital Association (AHA) membership □ Joint Commission on Accreditation of Healthcare Organizations (JCAHO) accreditation + American Osteopathic Hospital Association (AOHA) membership ○ American Osteopathic Association (AOA) accreditation △ Commission on Accreditation of Rehabilitation Facilities (CARF) accreditation Control codes 61, 63, 64, 71, 72 and 73 indicate hospitals listed by AOHA, but not registered by AHA. For definition of numerical codes, see page A4	Control	Service	Beds	Admissions	Census	Outpatient Visits	Births	Total	Payroll	Personnel

BELVIDERE—Boone County

□ HIGHLAND COMMUNITY HOSPITAL, 1625 South State Street, Zip 61008; tel. 815/547–5441; Joan Elliott, MSN, R.N., Chief Operating Officer (Nonreporting) **A**1 9 10

	23	10	69	—	—	—	—	—	—	—

✠ SAINT JOSEPH HOSPITAL, 1005 Julien Street, Zip 61008–9932; tel. 815/544–3411; David A. Schertz, Administrator (Total facility includes 34 beds in nursing home–type unit) **A**1 9 10 **F**19 22 32 36 44 64 71 72 73 **P**6 **S** OSF Healthcare System, Peoria, IL

	21	10	58	1565	37	21903	0	13034	5739	189

BENTON—Franklin County

✠ FRANKLIN HOSPITAL AND SKILLED NURSING CARE UNIT, 201 Bailey Lane, Zip 62812; tel. 618/439–3161; Ron Slaviero, Administrator (Total facility includes 83 beds in nursing home–type unit) **A**1 9 10 **F**8 14 15 16 19 21 22 26 30 32 33 34 36 37 39 44 45 49 51 64 65 71 **P**3 **S** Southern Illinois Hospital Services, Carbondale, IL

	16	10	117	1246	89	34044	0	9010	4175	212

BERWYN—Cook County

✠ MACNEAL HOSPITAL, 3249 South Oak Park Avenue, Zip 60402; tel. 708/795–9100; Brian J. Lemon, President (Total facility includes 40 beds in nursing home–type unit) **A**1 2 3 5 8 9 10 **F**2 3 4 7 8 10 12 14 15 16 17 18 19 20 21 22 23 25 26 27 28 29 30 31 32 33 34 35 36 37 39 40 41 42 44 45 49 51 52 53 54 55 56 57 58 59 60 61 63 65 66 67 68 70 71 73 74 **P**5 6 7 8

	23	10	297	17251	228	94593	2329	136052	67618	2065

BLOOMINGTON—McLean County

BROMENN LIFECARE CENTER See BroMenn Healthcare, Normal

✠ OSF ST. JOSEPH MEDICAL CENTER, (Formerly St. Joseph Medical Center), 2200 East Washington Street, Zip 61701–4364; tel. 309/662–3311; Kenneth J. Natzke, Administrator (Total facility includes 13 beds in nursing home–type unit) (Nonreporting) **A**1 2 9 10 **S** OSF Healthcare System, Peoria, IL

	21	10	152	—	—	—	—	—	—	—

BLUE ISLAND—Cook County

✠ ST. FRANCIS HOSPITAL AND HEALTH CENTER, 12935 South Gregory Street, Zip 60406–2470; tel. 708/597–2000; Jay E. Kreuzer, President **A**1 2 9 10 **F**4 7 8 10 12 14 16 17 18 19 21 22 24 25 28 29 30 31 32 33 34 35 36 37 39 40 41 42 43 44 49 54 60 63 65 67 71 72 73 74 **P**6 8 **S** SSM Health Care System, Saint Louis, MO **N** MEDACOM Tri–State, Oakbrook, IL

	21	10	258	12522	166	—	1270	112332	49149	1271

BREESE—Clinton County

✠ ST. JOSEPH'S HOSPITAL, 9515 Holy Cross Lane, Zip 62230–0099, Mailing Address: P.O. Box 99, Zip 62230–0099; tel. 618/526–4511; Jacolyn M. Schlautman, Executive Vice President and Administrator **A**1 9 10 **F**7 8 14 15 16 19 21 22 28 30 32 33 34 35 37 40 44 49 65 71 73 **S** Hospital Sisters Health System, Springfield, IL

	21	10	57	2074	21	38833	466	14394	6395	219

CANTON—Fulton County

✠ GRAHAM HOSPITAL, 210 West Walnut Street, Zip 61520; tel. 309/647–5240; D. Ray Slaubaugh, President (Total facility includes 54 beds in nursing home–type unit) **A**1 6 9 10 **F**7 8 12 14 15 16 17 19 21 22 28 30 32 33 35 37 40 42 44 46 64 65 67 71 73

	23	10	124	2800	75	46145	291	24297	11036	448

CARBONDALE—Jackson County

✠ MEMORIAL HOSPITAL OF CARBONDALE, 405 West Jackson Street, Zip 62902, Mailing Address: P.O. Box 10000, Zip 62902–9000; tel. 618/549–0721; George Maroney, Administrator **A**1 2 3 5 9 10 **F**7 8 10 15 16 17 19 21 22 23 28 30 32 33 35 37 38 40 42 44 45 49 60 63 65 66 67 71 73 **P**8 **S** Southern Illinois Hospital Services, Carbondale, IL

	23	10	132	11230	73	110182	2117	49187	20683	612

CARLINVILLE—Macoupin County

✠ CARLINVILLE AREA HOSPITAL, 1001 East Morgan Street, Zip 62626–1499; tel. 217/854–3141; Robert W. Porteus, President and Chief Executive Officer (Nonreporting) **A**1 9 10

	23	10	31	—	—	—	—	—	—	—

CARMI—White County

✠ CARMI TOWNSHIP HOSPITAL, (Formerly White County Hospital), 400 Plum Street, Zip 62821–1799; tel. 618/382–4171; Joe E. Gamble, Chief Executive Officer (Total facility includes 98 beds in nursing home–type unit) **A**1 9 10 **F**8 12 19 21 22 28 30 32 33 34 37 39 41 44 49 64 65 71 **S** Quorum Health Group/Quorum Health Resources, Inc., Brentwood, TN

	16	10	126	498	96	27741	0	7835	3084	139

CARROLLTON—Greene County

★ THOMAS H. BOYD MEMORIAL HOSPITAL, (Includes Reisch Memorial Nursing Home), 800 School Street, Zip 62016–1498; tel. 217/942–6946; Deborah Campbell, Administrator (Total facility includes 38 beds in nursing home–type unit) **A**9 10 **F**8 14 15 16 22 24 28 44 49 64 67 71 **S** Quorum Health Group/Quorum Health Resources, Inc., Brentwood, TN

	23	10	60	291	41	14826	0	3666	1959	112

CARTHAGE—Hancock County

✠ MEMORIAL HOSPITAL, South Adams Street, Zip 62321, Mailing Address: P.O. Box 160, Zip 62321; tel. 217/357–3131; Keith E. Heuser, Chief Executive Officer **A**1 9 10 **F**7 8 12 19 21 22 28 29 34 35 40 41 44 45 49 65 67 71 73 **S** Quorum Health Group/Quorum Health Resources, Inc., Brentwood, TN

	23	10	59	1258	12	14989	63	8864	4189	139

CENTRALIA—Marion County

✠ ST. MARY'S HOSPITAL, 400 North Pleasant Avenue, Zip 62801–3091; tel. 618/532–6731; James W. McDowell, President and Chief Executive Officer **A**1 2 9 10 **F**1 2 3 7 8 12 14 15 16 17 18 19 21 22 26 27 30 31 32 33 34 35 37 39 40 41 42 44 45 46 49 51 52 53 54 55 56 57 58 59 60 63 65 66 67 69 71 73 74 **P**6 **N** Felician Health Care, Inc., Chicago, IL

	21	10	276	8302	130	116996	554	57395	22180	905

Hospital, Address, Telephone, Administrator, Approval, Facility, and Physician Codes, Health Care System, Network	Classi-fication Codes		Utilization Data					Expense (thousands) of dollars		
	Control	Service	Beds	Admissions	Census	Outpatient Visits	Births	Total	Payroll	Personnel

★ American Hospital Association (AHA) membership
☐ Joint Commission on Accreditation of Healthcare Organizations (JCAHO) accreditation
+ American Osteopathic Hospital Association (AOHA) membership
○ American Osteopathic Association (AOA) accreditation
△ Commission on Accreditation of Rehabilitation Facilities (CARF) accreditation
Control codes 61, 63, 64, 71, 72 and 73 indicate hospitals listed by AOHA, but not registered by AHA. For definition of numerical codes, see page A4

CENTREVILLE—St. Clair County

Hospital	Control	Service	Beds	Admissions	Census	Outpatient Visits	Births	Total	Payroll	Personnel
★ TOUCHETTE REGIONAL HOSPITAL, 5900 Bond Avenue, Zip 62207; tel. 618/332–3060; Mark S. Brodeur, President **A**1 9 10 **F**7 8 12 13 14 15 16 17 19 21 22 27 28 30 31 33 34 35 37 38 40 44 49 65 71 72 73 74 **P**8	23	10	104	2326	27	26185	940	18930	9543	311

CHAMPAIGN—Champaign County

Hospital	Control	Service	Beds	Admissions	Census	Outpatient Visits	Births	Total	Payroll	Personnel
BURNHAM HOSPITAL See Covenant Medical Center, Urbana										
☐ THE PAVILION, 809 West Church Street, Zip 61820; tel. 217/373–1700; Nina W. Eisner, Chief Executive Officer (Nonreporting) **A**1 9 10 **S** Universal Health Services, Inc., King of Prussia, PA **N** The Carle Foundation, Urbana, IL	33	22	38	—						

CHESTER—Randolph County

Hospital	Control	Service	Beds	Admissions	Census	Outpatient Visits	Births	Total	Payroll	Personnel
☐ CHESTER MENTAL HEALTH CENTER, Chester Road, Zip 62233–0031, Mailing Address: Box 31, Zip 62233–0031; tel. 618/826–4571; Stephen L. Hardy, Ph.D., Facility Director (Nonreporting) **A**1	12	22	314							
☐ MEMORIAL HOSPITAL, 1900 State Street, Zip 62233–0609, Mailing Address: Box 609, Zip 62233; tel. 618/826–4581; Eric Freeburg, Administrator **A**1 9 10 **F**3 7 8 11 15 16 17 18 19 21 22 23 27 28 30 33 35 36 37 39 40 42 44 49 58 65 66 67 71 72 73 **S** Quorum Health Group/Quorum Health Resources, Inc., Brentwood, TN **N** BJC Health System, St. Louis, MO	16	10	50	1216	16	48626	102	9980	4505	191

CHICAGO—Cook County

Hospital	Control	Service	Beds	Admissions	Census	Outpatient Visits	Births	Total	Payroll	Personnel
BERNARD MITCHELL HOSPITAL See University of Chicago Hospitals										
★ BETHANY HOSPITAL, 3435 West Van Buren, Zip 60624; tel. 773/265–7700; Lena L. Shields, Chief Executive **A**1 9 10 **F**2 3 7 8 12 13 14 15 16 17 18 19 21 22 25 26 27 28 29 30 32 33 34 35 37 39 40 41 42 44 49 51 52 54 59 60 61 65 71 73 **P**6 8 **S** Advocate Health Care, Oakbrook, IL **N** Advocate Health Care, Oak Brook, IL; MEDACOM Tri–State, Oakbrook, IL	23	10	120	5904	70	68909	1108	42408	17363	463
CHICAGO LYING–IN HOSPITAL See University of Chicago Hospitals										
CHICAGO–READ MENTAL HEALTH CENTER, 4200 North Oak Park Avenue, Zip 60634; tel. 773/794–4000; Thomas Simpatico, M.D., Facility Director and Network System Manager **A**10 **F**1 3 11 12 14 15 16 20 26 37 52 53 56 57 58 65 73	12	22	281	1941	245	0	0	31321	25131	600
★ CHILDREN'S MEMORIAL HOSPITAL, 2300 Children's Plaza, Zip 60614; tel. 773/880–4000; Jan R. Jennings, President and Chief Executive Officer **A**1 2 3 5 8 9 10 **F**4 5 10 12 13 15 16 17 19 20 21 22 25 28 29 30 31 32 34 35 38 39 42 43 44 45 46 47 49 51 52 53 54 55 56 58 59 63 65 67 69 70 71 72 73 **P**7 8 **N** Northwestern Health Care Network, Chicago, IL	23	50	237	9824	164	240360	0	199717	86571	—
★ COLUMBIA CHICAGO LAKESHORE HOSPITAL, 4840 North Marine Drive, Zip 60640; tel. 773/907–4601; Marcia S. Shapiro, Administrator and Chief Executive Officer **A**1 3 5 9 10 **F**2 3 14 15 17 18 19 21 27 32 34 35 52 53 54 55 56 57 58 59 67 **S** Columbia/HCA Healthcare Corporation, Nashville, TN	33	22	102	2086	69	9277	0	—	—	173
★ △ COLUMBIA GRANT HOSPITAL, 550 West Webster Avenue, Zip 60614–9980; tel. 773/883–2000; Nancy R. Hellyer, R.N., Chief Executive Officer (Total facility includes 33 beds in nursing home–type unit) **A**1 3 7 9 10 **F**2 3 4 8 10 12 14 16 17 19 20 21 22 26 28 29 30 31 32 34 35 37 39 41 42 43 44 48 49 51 52 53 54 55 56 57 58 59 60 64 65 67 68 71 73 **P**2 5 7 **S** Columbia/HCA Healthcare Corporation, Nashville, TN	33	10	213	6048	115	—	0	44791	20846	620
★ △ COLUMBIA MICHAEL REESE HOSPITAL AND MEDICAL CENTER, 2929 South Ellis Avenue, Zip 60616; tel. 312/791–2000; F. Scott Winslow, President and Chief Executive Officer (Nonreporting) **A**1 2 3 5 7 8 9 10 **S** Columbia/HCA Healthcare Corporation, Nashville, TN	33	10	523	—	—	—	—	—	—	—
★ COLUMBUS HOSPITAL, 2520 North Lakeview Avenue, Zip 60614; tel. 773/883–7300; Sister Theresa Peck, President and Chief Executive Officer **A**1 2 3 5 9 10 **F**2 3 4 5 6 7 8 10 12 16 17 19 22 25 26 27 28 30 31 32 33 34 35 37 38 40 41 42 43 44 46 48 49 52 54 55 56 57 58 59 60 63 64 65 66 67 68 71 73 74 **P**4 5 6 8 **S** Catholic Health Partners, Chicago, IL **N** Family Health Network, Inc., Chicago, IL; Catholic Health Partners, Chicago, IL	21	10	291	10058	158	73402	1292	112973	45732	1243
★ COOK COUNTY HOSPITAL, 1835 West Harrison Street, Zip 60612; tel. 312/633–6000; Ruth M. Rothstein, Hospital Director **A**1 2 3 5 8 9 10 **F**3 4 5 8 9 10 11 12 13 14 15 16 17 18 19 20 21 22 23 25 27 28 29 30 31 32 33 34 35 37 38 39 40 41 42 43 44 45 46 47 49 51 53 54 55 56 60 61 65 67 68 70 71 72 73 74 **P**6 **S** Cook County Bureau of Health Services, Chicago, IL	13	10	770	27808	474	662137	2696	360748	288029	—
☐ DOCTORS HOSPITAL OF HYDE PARK, 5800 South Stony Island Avenue, Zip 60637–2099; tel. 773/643–9200; Stephen M. Weinstein, President and Chief Executive Officer (Nonreporting) **A**1 9 10	31	10	200							
★ EDGEWATER MEDICAL CENTER, 5700 North Ashland Avenue, Zip 60660–4086; tel. 773/878–6000; Peter G. Rogan, Chief Executive Officer **A**1 2 3 9 10 **F**2 3 4 8 10 14 17 19 21 22 26 27 28 30 31 32 33 34 37 42 43 44 49 54 56 60 65 71 **P**5	23	10	215	8280	147	27339	0	56255	21893	653
☐ HARTGROVE HOSPITAL, 520 North Ridgeway Avenue, Zip 60624; tel. 773/722–3113; Karen E. Johnson, Administrator **A**1 9 10 **F**1 3 52 53 54 55 56 57 58 59 65 **S** Hospital Group of America, Wayne, PA	33	22	119	2259	91	5346	0	—	—	171
★ △ HOLY CROSS HOSPITAL, 2701 West 68th Street, Zip 60629–1882; tel. 773/471–8000; Mark C. Clement, President and Chief Executive Officer (Total facility includes 37 beds in nursing home–type unit) **A**1 2 7 9 10 **F**4 7 8 10 11 12 13 14 15 16 17 19 21 22 25 27 28 29 30 32 33 34 35 37 39 40 42 44 46 48 49 51 63 64 65 66 71 72 73 74 **P**3 4 5 7 8	23	10	299	12794	211	123837	923	95850	53124	1389
★ ILLINOIS MASONIC MEDICAL CENTER, 836 West Wellington Avenue, Zip 60657–5193; tel. 773/975–1600; Bruce C. Campbell, President (Total facility includes 220 beds in nursing home–type unit) **A**1 2 3 5 8 9 10 **F**1 3 4 7 8 10 11 12 13 14 15 16 17 18 19 20 21 22 25 26 27 28 29 30 31 32 33 34 35 37 38 39 40 41 42 43 44 45 46 47 49 51 52 53 54 55 56 57 58 59 60 61 63 64 65 66 67 69 70 71 73 74 **P**5 6 8 **N** Rush System for Health, Chicago, IL	23	10	582	14403	563	257750	2737	178880	90902	3124

Hospital, Address, Telephone, Administrator, Approval, Facility, and Physician Codes, Health Care System, Network	Classi-fication Codes		Utilization Data					Expense (thousands) of dollars		
	Control	Service	Beds	Admissions	Census	Outpatient Visits	Births	Total	Payroll	Personnel

★ American Hospital Association (AHA) membership
☐ Joint Commission on Accreditation of Healthcare Organizations (JCAHO) accreditation
+ American Osteopathic Hospital Association (AOHA) membership
○ American Osteopathic Association (AOA) accreditation
△ Commission on Accreditation of Rehabilitation Facilities (CARF) accreditation
Control codes 61, 63, 64, 71, 72 and 73 indicate hospitals listed by AOHA, but not registered by AHA. For definition of numerical codes, see page A4

Hospital	Control	Service	Beds	Admissions	Census	Outpatient Visits	Births	Total	Payroll	Personnel
☐ JACKSON PARK HOSPITAL, 7531 Stony Island Avenue, Zip 60649–3993; tel. 773/947–7500; Peter E. Friedell, M.D., President **A**1 2 3 9 10 **F**2 3 5 8 12 14 15 16 17 18 19 20 21 22 26 28 29 30 31 32 33 40 41 42 44 45 46 49 51 52 54 56 57 58 60 65 66 71 73	23	10	254	13098	165	67567	505	—	—	663
JOHNSTON R. BOWMAN HEALTH CENTER See Rush–Presbyterian–St. Luke's Medical Center										
⊠ LARABIDA CHILDREN'S HOSPITAL AND RESEARCH CENTER, (PEDIATRIC–CHRONIC DISEASE), East 65th Street at Lake Michigan, Zip 60649–1395; tel. 773/363–6700; Paula Jaudes, M.D., Interim Director **A**1 5 9 10 **F**12 15 16 22 34 45 49 65 73 **P**6	23	59	62	1470	40	24095	0	27867	13968	472
☐ LORETTO HOSPITAL, 645 South Central Avenue, Zip 60644–9987; tel. 773/626–4300; Steven C. Drucker, President **A**1 9 10 **F**2 3 8 14 15 16 18 19 22 28 30 34 37 39 41 44 49 51 52 56 58 65 67 71 73 **P**5	23	10	120	4930	116	35743	0	32699	15834	494
⊠ LOUIS A. WEISS MEMORIAL HOSPITAL, 4646 North Marine Drive, Zip 60640–1501; tel. 773/878–8700; Gregory A. Cierlik, President and Chief Executive Officer **A**1 2 3 5 9 10 **F**2 3 4 7 8 9 10 12 15 16 17 19 21 22 27 28 30 31 33 34 35 37 38 39 40 41 42 43 44 45 47 48 49 52 60 65 66 67 69 70 71 73 **P**3 5 6 7 8 **S** Louis A Weiss Memorial Hospital/University of Chicago Hospitals, Chicago, IL **N** University of Chicago Hospitals & Health System, Chicago, IL	23	10	200	8004	132	119136	420	83043	34675	982
⊠ MERCY HOSPITAL AND MEDICAL CENTER, Stevenson Expressway at King Drive, Zip 60616–2477; tel. 312/567–2006; Winkle Lee, Chief Executive Officer (Total facility includes 28 beds in nursing home–type unit) **A**1 2 3 5 8 9 10 **F**1 2 3 4 5 7 8 10 11 12 13 16 17 19 20 21 22 25 26 28 29 30 31 32 33 35 37 38 39 40 41 42 43 44 45 46 48 49 51 52 53 54 55 56 57 58 59 60 63 64 65 66 67 68 71 73 74 **P**5 7 8 **S** Mercy–Chicago Region Healthcare System, Naperville, IL	21	10	392	15983	232	275068	2529	158437	77845	1956
☐ METHODIST HOSPITAL OF CHICAGO, 5025 North Paulina Street, Zip 60640–2797; tel. 773/271–9040; Steven H. Friedman, Ph.D., Executive Vice President (Total facility includes 17 beds in nursing home–type unit) (Nonreporting) **A**1 2 9 10	23	10	189	—	—	—	—	—	—	—
METROPOLITAN CHILDREN AND ADOLESCENT INSTITUTE, 1601 Taylor Street, Zip 60612; tel. 312/433–8300; James T. Barter, M.D., Director **F**15 16 52 53 **P**6	12	22	83	324	62	0	0	11753	—	227
⊠ MOUNT SINAI HOSPITAL MEDICAL CENTER OF CHICAGO, California Avenue and 15th Street, Zip 60608–1610; tel. 312/542–2000; Benn Greenspan, President and Chief Executive Officer **A**1 2 3 5 8 9 10 **F**1 2 3 4 7 8 10 11 12 13 14 15 16 17 18 19 20 21 22 23 26 27 28 29 30 31 32 34 35 37 38 39 40 41 42 43 44 45 46 47 48 49 51 52 53 54 55 56 57 58 59 60 61 65 66 67 68 69 70 71 72 73 74 **P**6 **N** Family Health Network, Inc., Chicago, IL	23	10	315	13854	232	262674	2957	129842	66301	1734
NORMAN AND IDA STONE INSTITUTE OF PSYCHIATRY See Northwestern Memorial Hospital										
⊠ NORTHWESTERN MEMORIAL HOSPITAL, (Includes Norman and Ida Stone Institute of Psychiatry, 320 East Huron Street, Zip 60611; Passavant Pavilion, 303 East Superior Street, Zip 60611; tel. 312/908–2000; Prentice Women's Hospital, 333 East Superior Street, Zip 60611; tel. 312/908–2000; Wesley Pavilion, 250 East Superior Street, Zip 60611; tel. 312/908–2000), Superior Street and Fairbanks Court, Zip 60611–2950; tel. 312/908–2000; Gary A. Mecklenburg, President and Chief Executive Officer **A**1 2 3 5 8 9 10 **F**3 4 5 7 8 10 12 13 14 15 16 17 18 19 20 21 22 23 24 26 27 28 29 30 31 32 33 34 35 37 38 39 40 41 42 43 44 45 46 47 49 51 52 53 54 55 56 57 58 59 60 61 63 64 65 66 67 68 69 70 71 73 74 **P**4 5 7 8 **N** Northwestern Health Care Network, Chicago, IL	23	10	730	34718	413	215594	5806	385600	165717	3824
⊠ NORWEGIAN–AMERICAN HOSPITAL, 1044 North Francisco Avenue, Zip 60622; tel. 773/292–8200; Clarence A. Nagelvoort, President and Chief Executive Officer (Nonreporting) **A**1 9 10 **N** Family Health Network, Inc., Chicago, IL	23	10	230	—	—	—	—	—	—	—
⊠ OUR LADY OF THE RESURRECTION MEDICAL CENTER, 5645 West Addison Street, Zip 60634–4455; tel. 312/282–7000; John Sullivan, Chief Executive Officer (Total facility includes 56 beds in nursing home–type unit) **A**1 9 10 **F**3 4 6 7 8 10 15 17 18 19 20 21 22 24 25 27 28 29 30 32 33 34 35 37 39 41 42 43 44 45 46 49 51 60 61 62 63 64 65 67 71 72 73 74 **P**5 6 **N** Unified Health Care Network, Maywood, IL	21	10	293	10857	227	105597	0	79141	33568	1059
PASSAVANT PAVILION See Northwestern Memorial Hospital										
PRENTICE WOMEN'S HOSPITAL See Northwestern Memorial Hospital										
⊠ PROVIDENT HOSPITAL OF COOK COUNTY, 500 East 51st Street, Zip 60615; tel. 773/572–1200; Shirley Bomar–Cole, Chief Operating Officer **A**1 10 **F**2 3 4 5 7 8 9 10 12 13 14 15 16 17 18 19 20 21 22 23 25 26 28 29 30 31 34 35 37 38 39 40 41 42 43 44 45 46 47 49 51 52 63 64 65 66 67 68 69 70 71 72 73 74 **P**6 **S** Cook County Bureau of Health Services, Chicago, IL	13	10	100	4822	67	96933	929	66507	28233	726
⊠ △ RAVENSWOOD HOSPITAL MEDICAL CENTER, 4550 North Winchester Avenue, Zip 60640–5205; tel. 773/878–4300; John E. Blair, President **A**1 2 3 5 6 7 9 10 **F**2 3 4 5 7 8 10 11 12 13 14 15 16 17 18 19 20 21 22 24 25 26 27 28 29 30 31 32 33 34 35 37 39 40 41 43 44 45 46 49 52 53 54 56 57 58 59 60 61 63 64 65 66 67 68 71 72 73 74 **P**1 3 5 6 7 **S** Advocate Health Care, Oakbrook, IL **N** Advocate Health Care, Oak Brook, IL	23	10	301	11258	172	212442	1856	103259	53792	1617
⊠ △ REHABILITATION INSTITUTE OF CHICAGO, 345 East Superior Street, Zip 60611–4496; tel. 312/908–6017; Wayne M. Lerner, Dr.PH, President and Chief Executive Officer (Nonreporting) **A**1 3 5 7 9 10	23	46	176	—	—	—	—	—	—	—

Hospital, Address, Telephone, Administrator, Approval, Facility, and Physician Codes, Health Care System, Network	Classi-fication Codes		Utilization Data					Expense (thousands) of dollars		
★ American Hospital Association (AHA) membership □ Joint Commission on Accreditation of Healthcare Organizations (JCAHO) accreditation + American Osteopathic Hospital Association (AOHA) membership ○ American Osteopathic Association (AOA) accreditation △ Commission on Accreditation of Rehabilitation Facilities (CARF) accreditation Control codes 61, 63, 64, 71, 72 and 73 indicate hospitals listed by AOHA, but not registered by AHA. For definition of numerical codes, see page A4	Control	Service	Beds	Admissions	Census	Outpatient Visits	Births	Total	Payroll	Personnel

Hospital	Control	Service	Beds	Admissions	Census	Outpatient Visits	Births	Total	Payroll	Personnel
★ △ RESURRECTION MEDICAL CENTER, 7435 West Talcott Avenue, Zip 60631–3746; tel. 773/774–8000; Sister Donna Marie, Chief Executive Officer (Total facility includes 298 beds in nursing home–type unit) **A**1 2 3 5 7 9 10 **F**3 4 7 8 10 15 16 17 19 21 22 24 29 31 32 34 35 37 38 40 41 42 43 44 45 48 49 53 54 55 56 57 58 59 60 64 65 66 67 71 73 74 **P**1 5 6 7 **N** Unified Health Care Network, Maywood, IL	21	10	658	16859	553	198357	1231	149776	61959	2671
★ ROSELAND COMMUNITY HOSPITAL, 45 West 111th Street, Zip 60628; tel. 773/995–3000; Denise R. Williams, President **A**1 9 10 **F**2 14 15 16 19 22 25 34 35 37 39 40 44 46 65 71 73 **P**1	23	10	131	4905	71	34453	859	31716	14380	600
★ △ RUSH–PRESBYTERIAN–ST. LUKE'S MEDICAL CENTER, (Includes Johnston R. Bowman Health Center, 700 South Paulina, Zip 60612; tel. 312/942–7000; James T. Frankenbach, President), 1653 West Congress Parkway, Zip 60612–3833; tel. 312/942–5000; Leo M. Henikoff, President and Chief Executive Officer (Total facility includes 44 beds in nursing home–type unit) **A**1 2 3 5 7 8 9 10 **F**1 2 3 4 5 6 7 8 10 11 14 15 16 17 19 20 21 22 23 26 28 30 31 32 33 34 35 36 37 38 40 41 42 43 44 46 47 48 49 50 51 52 53 54 55 56 57 58 59 60 61 63 64 65 66 67 69 71 73 74 **P**5 6 7 8 **S** Rush–Presbyterian–St. Luke's Medical Center, Chicago, IL **N** Rush System for Health, Chicago, IL	23	10	783	26814	549	429195	2367	609897	302763	7214
□ SACRED HEART HOSPITAL, 3240 West Franklin Boulevard, Zip 60624–1599; tel. 773/722–3020; Edward Novak, President and Chief Executive Officer (Nonreporting) **A**1 9 10	33	10	96	—	—	—	—	—	—	—
★ SAINT ANTHONY HOSPITAL, 2875 West 19th Street, Zip 60623; tel. 773/521–1710; Sister Theresa Peck, President and Chief Executive Officer **A**1 9 10 **F**2 3 4 5 6 7 8 10 12 16 17 19 22 25 26 27 28 30 31 32 33 34 35 37 38 40 41 42 43 44 46 48 49 52 54 55 56 57 58 59 60 63 64 65 66 67 68 71 73 74 **P**4 5 6 8 **S** Catholic Health Partners, Chicago, IL **N** Family Health Network, Inc., Chicago, IL; Catholic Health Partners, Chicago, IL	21	10	186	8946	136	46530	2340	59395	27032	688
★ SAINT MARY OF NAZARETH HOSPITAL CENTER, 2233 West Division Street, Zip 60622–3086; tel. 312/770–2000; Sister Stella Louise, President and Chief Executive Officer **A**1 2 3 9 10 **F**4 8 10 11 15 16 17 19 21 22 26 27 28 30 31 32 33 34 35 37 39 40 41 42 43 44 45 48 49 52 53 54 55 56 57 58 59 60 61 65 67 71 73 74 **P**5 8 **S** Sisters of the Holy Family of Nazareth–Sacred Heart Province, Des Plaines, IL **N** Unified Health Care Network, Maywood, IL	21	10	305	12656	221	179931	—	104660	52525	1425
★ △ SCHWAB REHABILITATION HOSPITAL AND CARE NETWORK, 1401 South California Boulevard, Zip 60608–1612; tcl. 773/522–2010; Kathleen C. Yosko, President and Chief Executive Officer **A**1 3 7 9 10 **F**3 8 11 14 17 19 20 21 26 27 32 34 35 37 38 40 41 42 43 44 46 47 48 49 51 52 54 56 58 59 60 61 65 67 70 71 72 73 **P**6 **N** Family Health Network, Inc., Chicago, IL	23	46	85	1162	76	49844	0	25796	15854	373
★ SHRINERS HOSPITALS FOR CHILDREN–CHICAGO, (Formerly Shriners Hospitals for Crippled Children, Chicago Unit), 2211 North Oak Park Avenue, Zip 60607–3392; tel. 773/622–5400; A. James Spang, Administrator **A**1 3 5 **F**5 12 13 15 16 17 19 20 21 27 34 35 39 41 44 45 49 53 54 65 66 67 68 71 73 **P**6 **S** Shriners Hospitals for Children, Tampa, FL	23	57	60	1538	26	14788	0	—	—	229
★ SOUTH SHORE HOSPITAL, 8012 South Crandon Avenue, Zip 60617–1199; tel. 773/768–0810; John D. Harper, Administrator **A**1 9 10 **F**12 14 15 17 19 20 21 22 26 28 29 30 33 34 35 37 39 44 45 46 51 65 71 73 **P**5 8	23	10	125	3717	61	27833	0	27974	14432	443
□ ST. BERNARD HOSPITAL AND HEALTH CARE CENTER, 64th & Dan Ryan Expressway, Zip 60621; tel. 773/962–3900; Sister Elizabeth Van Straten, President and Chief Executive Officer (Nonreporting) **A**1 9 10 **N** Family Health Network, Inc., Chicago, IL; Unified Health Care Network, Maywood, IL	21	10	194	—	—	—	—	—	—	—
★ ST. ELIZABETH'S HOSPITAL, 1431 North Claremont Avenue, Zip 60622; tel. 773/278–2000; JoAnn Birdzell, President and Chief Executive Officer (Total facility includes 27 beds in nursing home–type unit) **A**1 2 3 9 10 **F**2 3 5 8 10 12 13 14 15 16 17 18 19 22 23 25 26 27 28 29 30 31 32 33 34 35 36 37 39 41 42 44 45 46 49 51 52 54 55 56 57 58 59 64 65 67 71 72 73 **P**3 5 6 7 8 **S** Ancilla Systems Inc., Hobart, IN **N** Midwest Health Net, LLC., Fort Wayne, IN; Family Health Network, Inc., Chicago, IL	21	10	240	10279	182	142224	0	70683	31878	841
★ ST. JOSEPH HOSPITAL, (Formerly St. Joseph Health Centers and Hospital), 2900 North Lake Shore Drive, Zip 60657–6274; tel. 773/665–3000; Sister Theresa Peck, President and Chief Executive Officer **A**1 2 3 5 9 10 **F**2 3 4 5 6 7 8 10 11 12 16 17 19 22 25 26 27 28 30 31 32 33 34 35 37 38 39 40 41 42 43 44 46 49 52 54 55 56 57 58 59 60 61 63 64 65 66 67 68 71 73 74 **P**4 5 6 8 **S** Catholic Health Partners, Chicago, IL **N** Family Health Network, Inc., Chicago, IL; Catholic Health Partners, Chicago, IL	21	10	347	10882	203	86834	1750	109716	51311	1580
★ SWEDISH COVENANT HOSPITAL, 5145 North California Avenue, Zip 60625–3688; tel. 773/878–8200; Edward A. Cucci, President **A**1 2 3 5 9 10 **F**4 7 8 10 12 13 14 15 16 17 19 20 21 22 23 24 26 27 28 29 30 31 32 33 35 36 37 38 39 40 41 42 43 44 45 46 47 48 49 51 52 55 56 57 58 60 62 63 64 65 66 67 69 70 71 72 73 74 **P**1 5 7 **N** Northwestern Health Care Network, Chicago, IL	21	10	280	11134	203	144475	1122	93524	46443	1337
THC–CHICAGO See Transitional Hospital of Chicago										
★ THOREK HOSPITAL AND MEDICAL CENTER, 850 West Irving Park Road, Zip 60613; tel. 773/525–6780; Frank A. Solare, President and Chief Executive Officer **A**1 3 5 9 10 **F**8 14 15 19 21 22 27 28 30 31 33 36 37 41 42 44 46 49 51 60 65 66 67 71 73 **P**5 6	23	10	142	5363	94	111283	0	46878	20192	506

Hospital, Address, Telephone, Administrator, Approval, Facility, and Physician Codes, Health Care System, Network	Classi-fication Codes		Utilization Data					Expense (thousands) of dollars		
	Control	Service	Beds	Admissions	Census	Outpatient Visits	Births	Total	Payroll	Personnel

Codes legend:

★ American Hospital Association (AHA) membership
☐ Joint Commission on Accreditation of Healthcare Organizations (JCAHO) accreditation
+ American Osteopathic Hospital Association (AOHA) membership
○ American Osteopathic Association (AOA) accreditation
△ Commission on Accreditation of Rehabilitation Facilities (CARF) accreditation
Control codes 61, 63, 64, 71, 72 and 73 indicate hospitals listed by AOHA, but not registered by AHA. For definition of numerical codes, see page A4.

	Control	Service	Beds	Admissions	Census	Outpatient Visits	Births	Total	Payroll	Personnel
☐ TRANSITIONAL HOSPITAL OF CHICAGO, (Formerly THC–Chicago), 4058 West Melrose Street, Zip 60641; tel. 773/736–7000; Darryl L. Duncan, Chief Executive Officer **A**1 9 10 **F**12 15 19 21 35 39 44 45 64 71 **P**5 **S** Transitional Hospitals Corporation, Las Vegas, NV	33	10	81	423	60	300	0	18107	7413	293
✠ TRINITY HOSPITAL, 2320 East 93rd Street, Zip 60617; tel. 773/978–2000; John N. Schwartz, Chief Executive Officer **A**1 5 10 **F**2 3 7 8 10 12 15 16 17 19 20 21 22 27 28 29 30 32 34 35 37 39 40 41 42 44 45 46 49 51 54 58 62 65 67 68 71 73 74 **P**1 2 6 7 8 **S** Advocate Health Care, Oakbrook, IL **N** MEDACOM Tri–State, Oakbrook, IL	21	10	218	9794	129	84930	1650	73169	30211	791
☐ UNIVERSITY HOSPITAL, 1116 North Kedzie Avenue, Zip 60651; tel. 773/276–5200; Michael F. Huber, Administrator and Chief Executive Officer **A**1 9 10 **F**15 16 27 52 53 54 55 56 57 58 59 65 67	33	22	85	1952	56	—	0	—	—	162
✠ UNIVERSITY OF CHICAGO HOSPITALS, (Includes Bernard Mitchell Hospital, Chicago Lying–in Hospital, Wyler Children's Hospital, tel. 312/702–6168), 5841 South Maryland, Zip 60637–1470; tel. 773/702–1000; Ralph W. Muller, President **A**1 2 3 5 8 9 10 **F**4 5 7 8 9 10 11 12 13 16 17 19 20 21 22 23 24 26 27 28 30 32 34 35 36 37 38 39 40 41 42 43 44 45 47 49 50 51 52 53 54 55 56 57 58 59 60 61 63 65 67 69 70 71 73 74 **P**6 **S** Louis A Weiss Memorial Hospital/University of Chicago Hospitals, Chicago, IL **N** University of Chicago Hospitals & Health System, Chicago, IL	23	10	526	23407	418	454614	2860	416690	193756	4586
✠ △ UNIVERSITY OF ILLINOIS AT CHICAGO MEDICAL CENTER, 1740 West Taylor Street, Zip 60612–4348; tel. 312/996–3900; Sidney E. Mitchell, Executive Director **A**1 2 3 5 7 8 9 10 **F**3 4 5 7 8 10 11 14 15 16 19 20 22 25 26 27 28 29 30 31 34 35 37 38 40 41 42 43 44 45 46 47 48 49 51 52 53 54 55 56 57 58 59 60 61 64 65 66 67 68 69 70 71 73 74 **P**4 6	12	10	430	18125	301	359249	3035	202494	127979	3200
✠ VA CHICAGO HEALTH CARE SYSTEM–LAKESIDE DIVISION, (Formerly Veterans Affairs Lakeside Medical Center), 333 East Huron Street, Zip 60611–3004; tel. 312/640–2100; Joseph L. Moore, Director **A**1 3 5 8 **F**2 3 4 5 6 8 10 11 12 14 15 16 17 18 19 20 21 22 23 25 26 27 28 29 30 31 32 33 34 35 37 39 41 42 43 44 45 48 49 51 52 54 55 56 57 58 59 60 65 67 69 71 73 74 **S** Department of Veterans Affairs, Washington, DC	45	10	252	6607	187	205200	0	91105	54872	1248
✠ VA CHICAGO HEALTH CARE SYSTEM–WEST SIDE DIVISION, (Formerly Veteran Affairs West Side Medical Center), 820 South Damen Avenue, Zip 60612, Mailing Address: Box 8195, Zip 60680; tel. 312/666–6500; Joseph L. Moore, Director (Nonreporting) **A**1 2 3 5 8 **S** Department of Veterans Affairs, Washington, DC	45	10	323	—	—	—	—	—	—	—
VENCOR HOSPITAL–CHICAGO NORTH, (LONG TERM ACUTE CARE), 2544 West Montrose Avenue, Zip 60618; tel. 773/267–2622; Steven A. Matarelli, Administrator **F**16 19 22 37 52 56 65 71 **S** Vencor, Incorporated, Louisville, KY	33	49	111	1133	92	0	0	20933	9883	240
WESLEY PAVILION See Northwestern Memorial Hospital										
WYLER CHILDREN'S HOSPITAL See University of Chicago Hospitals										
CHICAGO HEIGHTS—Cook County										
✠ ST. JAMES HOSPITAL AND HEALTH CENTERS, 1423 Chicago Road, Zip 60411–9934; tel. 708/756–1000; Peter J. Murphy, President and Chief Executive Officer (Total facility includes 101 beds in nursing home–type unit) **A**1 2 9 10 **F**7 8 10 11 14 15 16 17 19 21 22 26 27 28 29 30 32 33 34 35 36 37 40 41 42 44 45 46 51 60 64 65 66 67 68 71 73 74 **P**5 6 8 **S** Sisters of St. Francis Health Services, Inc., Mishawaka, IN **N** MEDACOM Tri–State, Oakbrook, IL	21	10	332	11699	228	74681	1285	92891	42215	1104
CLIFTON—Iroquois County										
✠ CENTRAL COMMUNITY HOSPITAL, 335 East Fifth Avenue, Zip 60927, Mailing Address: Box 68, Zip 60927; tel. 815/694–2392; Steve Wilder, President and Chief Executive Officer **A**1 9 10 **F**19 20 21 22 25 26 28 30 33 34 36 39 44 45 51 65 71 **P**6 **S** ServantCor, Kankakee, IL **N** Servantcor, Clifton, IL	23	10	33	423	4	6176	0	3613	958	38
CLINTON—Dewitt County										
★ DR. JOHN WARNER HOSPITAL, 422 West White Street, Zip 61727–2199; tel. 217/935–9571; Sally Waite, Acting Administrator (Total facility includes 9 beds in nursing home–type unit) **A**9 10 **F**8 11 15 19 20 22 32 34 42 44 45 49 54 64 65 66 71	14	10	37	1201	15	35578	0	8565	3809	138
DANVILLE—Vermilion County										
✠ UNITED SAMARITANS MEDICAL CENTER, (Includes United Samaritans Medical Center, 600 Sager Avenue, Zip 61832; tel. 217/442–6300), 812 North Logan, Zip 61832–3788; tel. 217/442–6300; Dennis J. Doran, President and Chief Executive Officer (Total facility includes 49 beds in nursing home–type unit) **A**1 2 9 10 **F**2 3 7 8 12 15 16 19 22 26 28 29 30 32 33 34 35 36 37 39 40 41 42 44 45 46 49 52 55 57 58 60 64 65 67 70 71 73 **P**6 8 **S** Franciscan Sisters Health Care Corporation, Frankfort, IL **N** MEDACOM Tri–State, Oakbrook, IL	21	10	308	10751	161	244753	968	82917	35184	1365
✠ VETERANS AFFAIRS MEDICAL CENTER, 1900 East Main Street, Zip 61832; tel. 217/442–8000; James S. Jones, Director (Total facility includes 175 beds in nursing home–type unit) **A**1 3 5 **F**1 3 6 12 14 15 16 17 18 19 20 21 22 26 27 28 29 30 31 32 34 37 39 41 44 45 46 48 49 51 52 54 55 57 58 63 64 65 67 71 73 74 **P**6 **S** Department of Veterans Affairs, Washington, DC	45	10	531	5241	373	140897	0	83032	47862	1298
DE KALB—De Kalb County										
✠ KISHWAUKEE COMMUNITY HOSPITAL, 626 Bethany Road, Zip 60115, Mailing Address: Box 707, Zip 60115; tel. 815/756–1521; Robert S. Thebeau, President **A**1 2 9 10 **F**3 7 8 14 15 16 19 21 22 26 28 29 30 31 35 37 40 41 44 46 49 52 53 54 55 56 57 58 59 60 61 65 66 67 71 73 74 **P**5	23	10	114	4335	40	135719	846	30944	12439	426
DECATUR—Macon County										
✠ DECATUR MEMORIAL HOSPITAL, 2300 North Edward Street, Zip 62526; tel. 217/876–8121; Kenneth L. Smithmier, President and Chief Executive Officer (Total facility includes 59 beds in nursing home–type unit) **A**1 2 3 5 9 10 **F**7 8 10 11 12 14 15 16 17 19 21 22 26 27 28 29 30 31 32 33 35 37 39 40 41 42 44 45 47 49 60 61 64 65 66 67 71 72 73 74 **P**3 6 8	23	10	247	9128	122	185621	906	80742	34143	1254

Hospital, Address, Telephone, Administrator, Approval, Facility, and Physician Codes, Health Care System, Network	Classi-fication Codes		Utilization Data					Expense (thousands) of dollars		
	Control	Service	Beds	Admissions	Census	Outpatient Visits	Births	Total	Payroll	Personnel

American Hospital Association (AHA) membership

★
□ Joint Commission on Accreditation of Healthcare Organizations (JCAHO) accreditation
+ American Osteopathic Hospital Association (AOHA) membership
○ American Osteopathic Association (AOA) accreditation
△ Commission on Accreditation of Rehabilitation Facilities (CARF) accreditation
Control codes 61, 63, 64, 71, 72 and 73 indicate hospitals listed by AOHA, but not registered by AHA. For definition of numerical codes, see page A4

Hospital	Control	Service	Beds	Admissions	Census	Outpatient Visits	Births	Total	Payroll	Personnel
⊞ ST. MARY'S HOSPITAL, 1800 East Lake Shore Drive, Zip 62521–3883; tel. 217/464–2966; Keith L. Callahan, Executive Vice President and Administrator (Total facility includes 45 beds in nursing home–type unit) **A**1 2 3 5 9 10 **F**1 3 7 8 14 15 16 17 18 19 21 22 23 26 27 28 29 30 33 34 35 36 37 39 40 41 42 44 45 47 49 52 53 54 55 56 57 58 59 60 64 65 67 71 72 73 **P**3 7 **S** Hospital Sisters Health System, Springfield, IL	21	10	205	7662	130	213989	947	61325	26175	960
DES PLAINES—Cook County										
□ FOREST HOSPITAL, 555 Wilson Lane, Zip 60016–4794; tel. 847/635–4100; Richard Michael Ackley, Administrator and Chief Executive Officer (Nonreporting) **A**1 9 10	31	22	80	—	—	—	—	—	—	—
□ HOLY FAMILY MEDICAL CENTER, 100 North River Road, Zip 60016; tel. 847/297–1800; Sister Patricia Ann Koschalke, President and Chief Executive Officer (Nonreporting) **A**1 2 5 9 10 **S** Sisters of the Holy Family of Nazareth–Sacred Heart Province, Des Plaines, IL **N** Rush System for Health, Chicago, IL	23	10	183	—	—	—	—	—	—	—
DIXON—Lee County										
⊞ KATHERINE SHAW BETHEA HOSPITAL, 403 East First Street, Zip 61021; tel. 815/288–5531; Darryl L. Vandervort, President and Chief Executive Officer (Total facility includes 15 beds in nursing home–type unit) **A**1 2 9 10 **F**7 8 11 12 14 15 16 17 19 20 21 22 24 26 27 28 29 30 32 33 34 35 36 37 39 40 41 42 44 45 46 49 51 52 53 54 55 56 57 58 59 60 63 64 65 66 67 71 73 **P**4 6	23	10	101	3388	43	67475	319	33006	13958	475
DOWNERS GROVE—Du Page County										
⊞ GOOD SAMARITAN HOSPITAL, 3815 Highland Avenue, Zip 60515; tel. 630/275–5900; David M. McConkey, Chief Executive (Total facility includes 20 beds in nursing home–type unit) **A**1 2 9 10 **F**1 4 7 8 10 11 12 15 16 17 19 21 22 23 24 25 26 27 28 29 30 31 32 33 34 37 38 39 40 41 42 43 44 45 49 51 52 53 54 55 56 57 58 59 61 62 63 64 65 66 67 70 71 72 73 74 **P**1 2 3 4 5 6 7 **S** Advocate Health Care, Oakbrook, IL **N** National Cardiovascular Network, Atlanta, GA; Advocate Health Care, Oak Brook, IL; MEDACOM Tri–State, Oakbrook, IL	21	10	259	14173	188	163274	2341	145087	53451	1973
DU QUOIN—Perry County										
⊞ MARSHALL BROWNING HOSPITAL, 900 North Washington Street, Zip 62832, Mailing Address: Box 192, Zip 62832–0192; tel. 618/542–2146; William J. Huff, Chief Executive Officer **A**1 9 10 **F**7 8 14 15 16 19 21 22 30 32 34 36 40 44 49 65 71	23	10	33	1090	13	77520	138	7870	3214	144
EAST ST. LOUIS—St. Clair County										
⊞ ST. MARY'S HOSPITAL, 129 North Eighth Street, Zip 62201–2999; tel. 618/274–1900; Richard J. Mark, President and Chief Executive Officer **A**1 9 10 **F**8 14 15 16 17 18 19 22 27 28 29 30 32 37 39 44 45 46 49 51 52 58 59 65 66 67 70 71 72 73 **P**4 **S** Ancilla Systems Inc., Hobart, IN **N** Midwest Health Net, LLC., Fort Wayne, IN; Saint Louis Health Care Network, St. Louis, MO	21	10	119	4246	88	95326	0	31672	14140	503
EFFINGHAM—Effingham County										
⊞ ST. ANTHONY'S MEMORIAL HOSPITAL, 503 North Maple Street, Zip 62401–2099; tel. 217/347–1495; Anthony D. Pfitzer, Administrator **A**1 2 9 10 **F**7 8 14 15 16 19 21 22 23 33 34 35 36 37 39 40 42 44 49 60 63 65 67 71 73 **S** Hospital Sisters Health System, Springfield, IL	21	10	131	6062	70	148213	734	38023	14898	455
ELDORADO—Saline County										
★ FERRELL HOSPITAL, 1201 Pine Street, Zip 62930; tel. 618/273–3361; E. T. Seely, Acting Administrator and Chief Financial Officer (Nonreporting) **A**9 10 **S** Southern Illinois Hospital Services, Carbondale, IL	33	10	51	—	—	—	—	—	—	—
ELGIN—Kane County										
□ ELGIN MENTAL HEALTH CENTER, 750 South State Street, Zip 60123–7692; tel. 847/742–1040; Nancy Staples, MS, Administrator **A**1 **F**12 14 16 52 54 55 56 57 58 59 65 67 73 **P**6	12	22	708	1412	640	0	0	53995	43370	1178
⊞ SAINT JOSEPH HOSPITAL, 77 North Airlite Street, Zip 60123–4912; tel. 847/695–3200; Larry Narum, President and Chief Executive Officer **A**1 2 9 10 **F**3 7 8 10 12 15 16 17 18 19 21 22 25 26 27 28 29 30 31 32 33 34 35 36 37 39 40 41 42 44 45 46 48 49 52 53 54 55 56 57 58 59 60 64 65 66 67 70 71 72 73 74 **P**3 5 8 **S** Franciscan Sisters Health Care Corporation, Frankfort, IL **N** MEDACOM Tri–State, Oakbrook, IL	23	10	202	5955	88	234669	671	63561	27421	799
⊞ SHERMAN HOSPITAL, 934 Center Street, Zip 60120–2198; tel. 847/742–9800; John A. Graham, President and Chief Executive Officer **A**1 2 9 10 **F**3 4 7 8 10 11 12 13 15 16 17 19 21 22 23 25 27 28 29 30 31 32 33 34 35 36 37 38 39 40 41 42 43 44 45 49 55 63 64 65 67 70 71 72 73 74 **P**7 8	23	10	252	11407	137	137643	2456	112515	40559	1627
ELK GROVE VILLAGE—Cook County										
⊞ △ ALEXIAN BROTHERS MEDICAL CENTER, 800 Biesterfield Road, Zip 60007–3397; tel. 847/437–5500; Brother Philip Kennedy, President and Chief Executive Officer **A**1 2 5 7 9 10 **F**2 3 4 7 8 10 11 12 13 14 15 16 17 18 19 20 21 22 25 26 27 28 29 30 31 32 33 35 36 37 39 40 41 42 43 44 45 46 48 49 51 52 53 54 55 56 57 58 59 60 61 64 65 66 67 68 69 70 71 72 73 74 **P**1 5 6 7 **S** Alexian Brothers Health System, Inc., Elk Grove Village, IL **N** Alexian Brothers Health System, Inc., Elk Grove Village, IL	21	10	391	17864	252	182794	3405	142376	64877	2059
ELMHURST—Du Page County										
⊞ ELMHURST MEMORIAL HOSPITAL, 200 Berteau Avenue, Zip 60126–2989; tel. 630/833–1400; Leo F. Fronza, Jr., President and Chief Executive Officer (Total facility includes 28 beds in nursing home–type unit) **A**1 2 9 10 **F**3 4 7 8 10 11 14 15 16 19 21 22 23 24 26 28 29 30 31 32 33 34 35 37 38 39 40 41 42 43 44 45 46 49 52 54 55 56 57 58 59 60 61 63 64 65 67 69 70 71 73 74 **P**1 5 6 7 8	23	10	305	15796	194	132605	1943	144127	67330	1967

Hospital, Address, Telephone, Administrator, Approval, Facility, and Physician Codes, Health Care System, Network	Classi-fication Codes		Utilization Data					Expense (thousands) of dollars		
★ American Hospital Association (AHA) membership ☐ Joint Commission on Accreditation of Healthcare Organizations (JCAHO) accreditation + American Osteopathic Hospital Association (AOHA) membership ○ American Osteopathic Association (AOA) accreditation △ Commission on Accreditation of Rehabilitation Facilities (CARF) accreditation Control codes 61, 63, 64, 71, 72 and 73 indicate hospitals listed by AOHA, but not registered by AHA. For definition of numerical codes, see page A4	Control	Service	Beds	Admissions	Census	Outpatient Visits	Births	Total	Payroll	Personnel

EUREKA—Woodford County

EUREKA COMMUNITY HOSPITAL See BroMenn Healthcare, Normal

EVANSTON—Cook County

✶ △ EVANSTON HOSPITAL, (Includes Glenbrook Hospital, 2100 Pfingsten Road, Glenview, Zip 60025; tel. 847/657–5800), 2650 Ridge Avenue, Zip 60201; tel. 847/570–2000; Mark R. Neaman, President and Chief Executive Officer (Total facility includes 26 beds in nursing home–type unit) **A**1 2 3 5 7 8 9 10 **F**1 2 3 4 5 7 8 9 10 11 12 14 15 16 17 18 19 20 21 22 23 24 25 26 28 29 30 31 32 33 34 35 36 37 38 39 40 41 42 43 44 45 46 48 49 51 52 53 54 55 56 57 58 59 60 61 63 64 65 66 67 68 69 70 71 73 74 **P**1 5 6 7 **N** Northwestern Health Care Network, Chicago, IL | 23 | 10 | 466 | 26424 | 346 | 760671 | 3799 | 247742 | 105013 | 3128

✶ ST. FRANCIS HOSPITAL OF EVANSTON, 355 Ridge Avenue, Zip 60202–3399; tel. 847/316–4000; James C. Gizzi, President and Chief Executive Officer (Total facility includes 105 beds in nursing home–type unit) **A**1 2 3 5 6 9 10 **F**3 4 5 7 8 10 11 12 14 15 16 17 18 19 21 22 25 27 28 29 30 32 33 34 35 36 37 40 41 42 43 44 45 46 49 51 52 53 54 56 57 58 59 60 63 64 66 67 70 71 72 73 74 **P**5 7 **S** Sisters of St. Francis Health Services, Inc., Mishawaka, IN **N** National Cardiovascular Network, Atlanta, GA | 21 | 10 | 440 | 14008 | 304 | 144490 | 1335 | 144981 | 62739 | 1700

EVERGREEN PARK—Cook County

☐ LITTLE COMPANY OF MARY HOSPITAL AND HEALTH CARE CENTERS, 2800 West 95th Street, Zip 60805–2795; tel. 708/422–6200; Sister Kathleen McIntyre, President **A**1 2 3 5 9 10 **F**1 2 3 7 8 10 11 12 15 16 17 18 19 21 22 25 26 28 29 30 31 32 33 34 35 37 38 39 40 41 42 44 45 46 47 49 51 52 53 54 55 56 57 58 59 60 63 65 67 71 72 73 74 **P**1 7 **S** Little Company of Mary Sisters Healthcare System, Evergreen Park, IL | 21 | 10 | 372 | 17562 | 227 | 126933 | 2020 | 123683 | 56875 | 1377

FAIRFIELD—Wayne County

✶ FAIRFIELD MEMORIAL HOSPITAL, 303 N.W. 11th Street, Zip 62837; tel. 618/842–2611; Albert Ban, Jr., Chief Executive Officer (Total facility includes 104 beds in nursing home–type unit) **A**1 9 10 **F**7 8 15 16 19 22 26 28 32 34 35 36 37 40 42 44 49 64 65 71 73 **S** Alliant Health System, Louisville, KY | 23 | 10 | 185 | 1412 | 117 | 16261 | 166 | 9941 | 4416 | 238

FLORA—Clay County

✶ CLAY COUNTY HOSPITAL, 700 North Mill Street, Zip 62839, Mailing Address: P.O. Box 280, Zip 62839; tel. 618/662–2131; John E. Monnahan, President and Senior Executive Officer **A**1 9 10 **F**7 8 15 16 17 19 22 28 30 33 34 36 39 40 44 49 65 71 73 **S** BJC Health System, Saint Louis, MO **N** BJC Health System, St. Louis, MO | 13 | 10 | 31 | 985 | 11 | 21072 | 55 | 5787 | 2465 | 138

FOREST PARK—Cook County

✶ COLUMBIA RIVEREDGE HOSPITAL, 8311 West Roosevelt Road, Zip 60130–2500; tel. 708/771–7000; Mary Palmer, President and Chief Executive Officer **A**1 5 9 10 **F**2 15 16 19 35 52 53 55 56 57 58 59 65 67 71 **S** Columbia/HCA Healthcare Corporation, Nashville, TN | 33 | 22 | 120 | 1526 | 82 | 6800 | 0 | 14556 | 6086 | 175

FREEPORT—Stephenson County

✶ FREEPORT MEMORIAL HOSPITAL, 1045 West Stephenson Street, Zip 61032; tel. 815/235–4131; Joseph E. Bonnett, Executive Vice President and Chief Executive Officer (Total facility includes 43 beds in nursing home–type unit) **A**1 2 9 10 **F**1 3 7 8 10 12 13 14 15 16 17 19 21 22 23 24 26 27 28 29 30 31 32 33 35 36 39 40 41 42 44 45 49 51 53 54 55 56 57 58 60 64 65 66 67 68 70 71 72 73 74 **P**3 5 6 8 **N** Freeport Regional Health Plan, Freeport, IL | 23 | 10 | 174 | 6175 | 96 | 112308 | 685 | 41123 | 16272 | 636

GALENA—Jo Daviess County

★ GALENA–STAUSS HOSPITAL, 215 Summit Street, Zip 61036–1697; tel. 815/777–1340; Roger D. Hervey, Administrator (Total facility includes 60 beds in nursing home–type unit) **A**9 10 **F**1 15 19 22 24 28 30 44 49 64 65 71 | 16 | 10 | 85 | 425 | 62 | 17705 | 0 | 4242 | 1951 | 109

GALESBURG—Knox County

✶ GALESBURG COTTAGE HOSPITAL, 695 North Kellogg Street, Zip 61401; tel. 309/343–8131; Steven J. West, President and Chief Executive Officer **A**1 9 10 **F**2 3 7 8 11 15 19 21 22 30 32 33 35 36 37 40 42 44 49 52 54 55 56 58 63 64 65 70 71 73 **P**6 | 23 | 10 | 189 | 5394 | 77 | 49544 | 429 | 39186 | 17101 | 529

✶ ST. MARY MEDICAL CENTER, 3333 North Seminary Street, Zip 61401–1299; tel. 309/344–3161; Richard S. Kowalski, Administrator and Chief Executive Officer (Total facility includes 14 beds in nursing home–type unit) **A**1 2 9 10 **F**2 3 7 8 10 11 12 13 15 16 17 18 19 21 22 23 28 30 32 35 36 37 39 40 41 42 44 46 48 49 52 60 64 65 66 67 70 71 73 74 **P**6 **S** OSF Healthcare System, Peoria, IL | 21 | 10 | 156 | 4093 | 53 | 60598 | 455 | 33920 | 15527 | 444

GENESEO—Henry County

✶ HAMMOND–HENRY HOSPITAL, 210 West Elk Street, Zip 61254–1099; tel. 309/944–6431; Nathan C. Olson, President and Chief Executive Officer (Total facility includes 57 beds in nursing home–type unit) **A**1 9 10 **F**7 8 11 14 16 19 22 32 34 35 40 44 64 65 71 73 **S** Brim, Inc., Portland, OR | 16 | 10 | 105 | 1057 | 52 | 36754 | 143 | 11200 | 4383 | 187

GENEVA—Kane County

✶ DELNOR–COMMUNITY HOSPITAL, 300 Randall Road, Zip 60134–4200; tel. 630/208–3000; Craig A. Livermore, President and Chief Executive Officer **A**1 2 9 10 **F**7 8 10 12 14 15 16 17 19 20 21 22 24 28 29 30 32 33 37 39 40 41 42 44 45 46 49 53 63 65 66 67 70 71 73 74 **P**5 7 **N** MEDACOM Tri–State, Oakbrook, IL | 23 | 10 | 118 | 6507 | 67 | 72121 | 1453 | 53521 | 22184 | 643

GIBSON CITY—Ford County

✶ GIBSON COMMUNITY HOSPITAL, (Includes Gibson Community Hospital Annex), 1120 North Melvin Street, Zip 60936, Mailing Address: P.O. Box 429, Zip 60936–0429; tel. 217/784–4251; Craig A. Jesiolowski, Chief Executive Officer (Total facility includes 42 beds in nursing home–type unit) (Nonreporting) **A**1 9 10 **S** Quorum Health Group/Quorum Health Resources, Inc., Brentwood, TN | 23 | 10 | 82 | — | — | — | — | — | — | —

Hospital, Address, Telephone, Administrator, Approval, Facility, and Physician Codes, Health Care System, Network	Classi-fication Codes		Utilization Data					Expense (thousands) of dollars		
	Control	Service	Beds	Admissions	Census	Outpatient Visits	Births	Total	Payroll	Personnel

★ American Hospital Association (AHA) membership
☐ Joint Commission on Accreditation of Healthcare Organizations (JCAHO) accreditation
+ American Osteopathic Hospital Association (AOHA) membership
○ American Osteopathic Association (AOA) accreditation
△ Commission on Accreditation of Rehabilitation Facilities (CARF) accreditation
Control codes 61, 63, 64, 71, 72 and 73 indicate hospitals listed by AOHA, but not registered by AHA. For definition of numerical codes, see page A4

GLENDALE HEIGHTS—Du Page County

★ GLENOAKS HOSPITAL AND MEDICAL CENTER, 701 Winthrop Avenue, Zip 60139; tel. 630/545–8000; Jorge A. Heyde, Administrator **A**1 9 10 **F**1 2 3 4 7 8 10 11 12 15 16 17 18 19 21 22 25 27 28 29 30 31 32 33 34 35 37 39 40 41 42 43 44 46 47 48 49 52 53 54 55 56 58 59 60 61 63 65 66 67 68 69 70 71 73 **P**5 7 8 — 21 10 115 3559 47 49872 703 39739 13241 465

GLENVIEW—Cook County

GLENBROOK HOSPITAL See Evanston Hospital, Evanston

GRANITE CITY—Madison County

★ ST. ELIZABETH MEDICAL CENTER, 2100 Madison Avenue, Zip 62040; tel. 618/798–3000; Ted Eilerman, President **A**1 2 3 9 10 **F**2 3 7 8 10 12 13 14 15 16 17 18 19 21 22 24 28 29 30 32 33 34 35 36 37 39 40 41 42 44 45 46 49 51 52 53 54 55 56 57 58 59 63 64 65 66 67 68 71 73 74 **P**4 6 **N** Unity Health System, St. Louis, MO — 21 10 276 7028 123 154632 451 63781 25257 946

GREAT LAKES—Lake County

★ NAVAL HOSPITAL, Zip 60088–5230; tel. 847/688–4560; Captain R. William Holden, MC, USN, Commanding Officer (Nonreporting) **A**1 2 **S** Department of Navy, Washington, DC — 43 10 136 — — — — — — —

GREENVILLE—Bond County

★ EDWARD A. UTLAUT MEMORIAL HOSPITAL, (Includes Fair Oaks), 200 Health Care Drive, Zip 62246; tel. 618/664–1230; Charles Bouis, President and Chief Executive Officer (Total facility includes 160 beds in nursing home–type unit) **A**1 9 10 **F**7 8 19 22 28 29 34 35 40 44 45 49 64 65 67 71 73 — 23 10 192 1082 122 43507 153 11117 5100 158

HARRISBURG—Saline County

★ HARRISBURG MEDICAL CENTER, 100 Hospital Drive, Zip 62946–0017, Mailing Address: P.O. Box 428, Zip 62946–0428; tel. 618/253–7671; Claude Chatterton, Chief Executive Officer **A**1 10 **F**8 14 15 17 19 21 22 26 30 31 32 34 35 37 39 41 42 44 45 48 49 52 54 56 57 58 59 60 63 65 66 67 71 73 **P**7 — 23 10 78 2389 37 49121 0 14716 5993 291

HARVARD—McHenry County

★ HARVARD MEMORIAL HOSPITAL, 901 Grant Street, Zip 60033–1898; tel. 815/943–5431; Dan Colby, Administrator (Total facility includes 45 beds in nursing home–type unit) (Nonreporting) **A**1 9 10 — 16 10 81 — — — — — — —

HARVEY—Cook County

★ △ INGALLS MEMORIAL HOSPITAL, One Ingalls Drive, Zip 60426–3591; tel. 708/333–2300; Robert L. Harris, President and Chief Executive Officer (Total facility includes 39 beds in nursing home–type unit) **A**1 2 7 9 10 **F**2 3 4 7 8 10 11 15 16 17 18 19 20 21 22 24 25 26 27 28 29 30 31 32 33 34 35 37 39 40 41 42 43 44 45 46 48 49 51 52 54 55 56 57 58 59 60 61 64 65 66 67 71 72 73 74 **P**1 3 4 7 **N** Northwestern Health Care Network, Chicago, IL — 23 10 424 19042 281 256034 2268 148346 66541 1794

HAVANA—Mason County

★ MASON DISTRICT HOSPITAL, 520 East Franklin Street, Zip 62644–0530, Mailing Address: Box 530, Zip 62644–0530; tel. 309/543–4431; Harry Wolin, Administrator and Chief Executive Officer **A**1 9 10 **F**8 14 15 16 19 22 28 32 35 36 37 41 44 49 64 65 71 72 73 — 16 10 36 598 8 31149 0 7585 3453 145

HAZEL CREST—Cook County

★ SOUTH SUBURBAN HOSPITAL, 17800 South Kedzie Avenue, Zip 60429; tel. 708/799–8000; Robert Rutkowski, Chief Executive (Total facility includes 41 beds in nursing home–type unit) **A**1 2 9 10 **F**7 8 10 12 14 15 16 17 19 21 22 25 28 30 32 33 34 35 37 40 41 42 44 49 60 63 64 67 71 73 **P**1 7 **S** Advocate Health Care, Oakbrook, IL **N** Advocate Health Care, Oak Brook, IL; MEDACOM Tri–State, Oakbrook, IL — 23 10 216 10513 156 85180 1260 81197 36674 876

HERRIN—Williamson County

★ HERRIN HOSPITAL, 201 South 14th Street, Zip 62948; tel. 618/942–2171; Virgil Hannig, Administrator (Total facility includes 13 beds in nursing home–type unit) **A**1 9 10 **F**8 10 11 15 17 19 21 22 28 29 30 31 32 33 34 35 37 38 40 44 45 46 47 49 61 64 65 66 67 71 73 74 **P**8 **S** Southern Illinois Hospital Services, Carbondale, IL — 23 10 84 3062 51 58502 0 22406 8427 293

HIGHLAND—Madison County

★ ST. JOSEPH'S HOSPITAL, 1515 Main Street, Zip 62249–1656; tel. 618/654–7421; Anthony G. Mastrangelo, Executive Vice President and Chief Executive Officer (Total facility includes 30 beds in nursing home–type unit) **A**1 9 10 **F**8 14 15 16 17 19 21 22 27 28 29 30 31 32 33 34 35 36 37 41 42 44 46 49 51 63 64 65 66 67 69 71 73 **P**8 **S** Hospital Sisters Health System, Springfield, IL **N** Unity Health System, St. Louis, MO — 21 10 76 1404 40 39419 0 12189 5438 216

HIGHLAND PARK—Lake County

★ HIGHLAND PARK HOSPITAL, 718 Glenview Avenue, Zip 60035–2497; tel. 847/432–8000; Ronald G. Spaeth, President and Chief Executive Officer (Total facility includes 28 beds in nursing home–type unit) **A**1 2 9 10 **F**1 3 4 7 8 10 11 12 14 15 16 17 19 20 21 22 23 26 28 29 30 32 33 34 35 36 37 39 40 41 42 43 44 45 46 49 52 53 54 55 56 57 58 59 60 61 63 64 65 66 67 70 71 73 74 **P**5 7 8 **N** Northwestern Health Care Network, Chicago, IL — 23 10 219 8275 101 192091 1903 89161 35603 1013

HILLSBORO—Montgomery County

☐ HILLSBORO AREA HOSPITAL, 1200 East Tremont Street, Zip 62049; tel. 217/532–6111; Rex H. Brown, President (Total facility includes 40 beds in nursing home–type unit) **A**1 9 10 **F**7 8 12 14 15 16 17 19 20 21 22 26 27 28 30 32 33 34 35 37 39 40 42 44 45 49 64 65 66 67 70 71 73 **S** Brim, Inc., Portland, OR — 23 10 95 1674 39 21315 111 9091 4033 179

Hospital, Address, Telephone, Administrator, Approval, Facility, and Physician Codes, Health Care System, Network	Classi-fication Codes		Utilization Data					Expense (thousands) of dollars		
	Control	Service	Beds	Admissions	Census	Outpatient Visits	Births	Total	Payroll	Personnel

★ American Hospital Association (AHA) membership
□ Joint Commission on Accreditation of Healthcare Organizations (JCAHO) accreditation
+ American Osteopathic Hospital Association (AOHA) membership
○ American Osteopathic Association (AOA) accreditation
△ Commission on Accreditation of Rehabilitation Facilities (CARF) accreditation
Control codes 61, 63, 64, 71, 72 and 73 indicate hospitals listed by AOHA, but not registered by AHA. For definition of numerical codes, see page A4

HINES—Cook County

□ JOHN J. MADDEN MENTAL HEALTH CENTER, 1200 South First Avenue, Zip 60141; tel. 708/338-7202; Ugo Formigoni, Metro-West Network Manager **A**1 5 10 **F**14 15 52 56

| | 12 | 22 | 185 | 1764 | 175 | 0 | 0 | 21604 | 17184 | 412 |

★ VETERANS AFFAIRS EDWARD HINES, JR. HOSPITAL, Fifth Avenue & Roosevelt Road, Zip 60141-5000, Mailing Address: P.O. Box 5000, Zip 60141-5000; tel. 708/343-7200; John J. DeNardo, Director (Total facility includes 240 beds in nursing home-type unit) (Nonreporting) **A**1 3 5 8 9 **S** Department of Veterans Affairs, Washington, DC

| | 45 | 10 | 896 | — | — | — | — | — | — | — |

HINSDALE—Du Page County

★ △ HINSDALE HOSPITAL, 120 North Oak Street, Zip 60521; tel. 630/856-9000; Ronald Sackett, President **A**1 2 3 5 7 9 10 **F**1 2 3 4 7 8 10 11 12 13 14 17 18 19 20 21 22 23 24 25 26 27 28 29 30 31 32 33 34 35 36 37 39 40 41 42 43 44 45 46 47 48 49 51 52 53 54 55 56 57 58 59 60 61 63 64 65 66 67 68 69 70 71 72 73 74 **P**3 5 7

| | 21 | 10 | 371 | 14026 | 163 | 1073426 | 2952 | 164477 | 62735 | 1644 |

□ SUBURBAN HOSPITAL, 55th Street & County Line Road, Zip 60521-8900; tel. 708/323-5800; James Richard Prister, Chief Operating Officer (Nonreporting) **A**1 9 10

| | 16 | 10 | 81 | — | — | — | — | — | — | — |

HOFFMAN ESTATES—Cook County

★ COLUMBIA ESTATES MEDICAL CENTER, 1555 North Barrington Road, Zip 60194; tel. 847/843-2000; Edward Goldberg, President and Chief Executive Officer (Total facility includes 23 beds in nursing home-type unit) **A**1 2 9 10 **F**1 2 3 4 7 8 10 11 12 14 15 16 17 19 21 22 27 30 32 34 35 36 37 39 40 41 42 44 45 46 49 51 52 53 54 55 56 57 61 63 64 65 67 70 71 73 74 **P**1 5 7 8 **S** Columbia/HCA Healthcare Corporation, Nashville, TN

| | 33 | 10 | 195 | 10536 | 121 | 51925 | 2422 | — | — | 790 |

★ COLUMBIA WOODLAND HOSPITAL, 1650 Moon Lake Boulevard, Zip 60194-5000; tel. 847/882-1600; John F. Buckley, Chief Executive Officer (Nonreporting) **A**1 9 10 **S** Columbia/HCA Healthcare Corporation, Nashville, TN

| | 33 | 22 | 94 | — | — | — | — | — | — | — |

HOOPESTON—Vermilion County

★ HOOPESTON COMMUNITY MEMORIAL HOSPITAL, 701 East Orange Street, Zip 60942-1896; tel. 217/283-5531; Darryl Wahler, Administrator (Total facility includes 75 beds in nursing home-type unit) **A**1 9 10 **F**6 19 22 34 41 44 46 49 64 65 67 71 72

| | 23 | 10 | 97 | 415 | 63 | 8520 | 0 | 5427 | 2729 | 137 |

HOPEDALE—Tazewell County

HOPEDALE MEDICAL COMPLEX, 107 Tremont Street, Zip 61747; tel. 309/449-3321; L. J. Rossi, M.D., Chief Executive Officer (Total facility includes 95 beds in nursing home-type unit) (Nonreporting) **A**9 10

| | 23 | 10 | 119 | — | — | — | — | — | — | — |

JACKSONVILLE—Morgan County

★ PASSAVANT AREA HOSPITAL, 1600 West Walnut Street, Zip 62650; tel. 217/245-9541; Chester A. Wynn, President and Chief Executive Officer **A**1 2 9 10 **F**4 7 8 15 16 17 19 20 21 22 28 29 30 31 33 35 36 37 39 40 42 44 45 46 49 51 53 57 59 63 65 66 67 70 71 72 73 **P**8

| | 23 | 10 | 115 | 4192 | 56 | 69672 | 374 | 34137 | 14973 | 595 |

JERSEYVILLE—Jersey County

□ JERSEY COMMUNITY HOSPITAL, 400 Maple Summit Road, Zip 62052, Mailing Address: P.O. Box 426, Zip 62052; tel. 618/498-6402; Lawrence P. Bear, Administrator **A**1 9 10 **F**3 7 8 10 14 15 16 17 19 21 22 27 28 30 31 33 35 36 37 39 40 41 42 43 44 45 46 49 53 54 58 60 65 66 67 71 73

| | 16 | 10 | 67 | 1828 | 15 | 28274 | 339 | 11597 | 5047 | 180 |

JOLIET—Will County

★ △ SAINT JOSEPH MEDICAL CENTER, 333 North Madison Street, Zip 60435-6595; tel. 815/741-7236; David W. Benfer, President and Chief Executive Officer (Total facility includes 35 beds in nursing home-type unit) **A**1 2 5 7 9 10 **F**3 4 7 8 10 11 12 14 15 16 17 18 19 20 21 22 24 25 26 27 28 29 30 31 32 33 34 35 37 40 41 42 43 44 45 46 47 48 49 51 52 53 54 55 56 57 58 59 60 63 64 65 66 67 70 71 73 74 **P**1 5 7 **S** Franciscan Sisters Health Care Corporation, Frankfort, IL **N** MEDACOM Tri-State, Oakbrook, IL

| | 21 | 10 | 505 | 15421 | 243 | 350196 | 1647 | 145283 | 64255 | 1616 |

★ SILVER CROSS HOSPITAL, 1200 Maple Road, Zip 60432; tel. 815/740-1100; Paul Pawlak, President **A**1 2 9 10 **F**1 2 3 4 5 6 7 8 9 10 11 12 15 16 17 18 19 20 21 22 23 24 25 26 27 28 29 30 32 33 34 35 36 37 38 39 40 41 42 43 44 45 46 47 48 49 50 52 53 54 55 56 57 58 59 60 61 62 63 64 65 66 67 68 69 70 71 73 **P**3 6 7 8 **N** Northwestern Health Care Network, Chicago, IL

| | 23 | 10 | 228 | 10957 | 138 | 97822 | 1612 | 87226 | 36366 | 1034 |

KANKAKEE—Kankakee County

★ △ RIVERSIDE HEALTHCARE, (Formerly Riverside Medical Center), 350 North Wall Street, Zip 60901-0749; tel. 815/933-1671; Dennis C. Millirons, President and Chief Executive Officer (Total facility includes 100 beds in nursing home-type unit) **A**1 2 7 9 10 **F**2 3 6 7 8 10 11 12 13 14 15 16 17 18 19 20 21 22 23 26 27 28 29 30 31 32 33 34 35 36 37 39 40 41 42 44 45 46 48 49 52 53 54 55 56 57 58 59 60 61 62 63 64 65 66 67 68 69 70 71 73 74 **P**5 6 8 **N** Rush System for Health, Chicago, IL

| | 23 | 10 | 381 | 8665 | 210 | 165745 | 1086 | 79619 | 33869 | 1220 |

★ ST. MARY'S HOSPITAL, 500 West Court Street, Zip 60901; tel. 815/937-2400; Allan C. Sonduck, President and Chief Executive Officer (Total facility includes 24 beds in nursing home-type unit) **A**1 2 9 10 **F**1 4 5 7 8 10 12 15 16 17 19 21 22 23 26 27 28 29 30 31 32 33 35 37 39 40 41 42 43 44 45 46 49 50 51 52 53 54 55 56 57 58 59 60 61 63 64 65 66 69 70 71 73 74 **P**8 **S** ServantCor, Kankakee, IL **N** Servantcor, Clifton, IL

| | 21 | 10 | 209 | 7813 | 112 | 126905 | 609 | 61046 | 23424 | 951 |

KEWANEE—Henry County

★ KEWANEE HOSPITAL, 719 Elliott Street, Zip 61443-2711, Mailing Address: P.O. Box 747, Zip 61443-0747; tel. 309/853-3361; Roger L. Holloway, Chief Executive Officer (Total facility includes 14 beds in nursing home-type unit) **A**1 9 10 **F**7 8 11 15 16 19 22 30 32 33 34 35 36 37 40 42 44 49 64 65 66 67 71 73 74 **P**6 8

| | 23 | 10 | 63 | 2171 | 29 | 48335 | 195 | 22232 | 10317 | 362 |

Hospital, Address, Telephone, Administrator, Approval, Facility, and Physician Codes, Health Care System, Network	Classi-fication Codes		Utilization Data					Expense (thousands) of dollars		
★ American Hospital Association (AHA) membership □ Joint Commission on Accreditation of Healthcare Organizations (JCAHO) accreditation + American Osteopathic Hospital Association (AOHA) membership ○ American Osteopathic Association (AOA) accreditation △ Commission on Accreditation of Rehabilitation Facilities (CARF) accreditation Control codes 61, 63, 64, 71, 72 and 73 indicate hospitals listed by AOHA, but not registered by AHA. For definition of numerical codes, see page A4	Control	Service	Beds	Admissions	Census	Outpatient Visits	Births	Total	Payroll	Personnel

LA GRANGE—Cook County

☒ COLUMBIA LA GRANGE MEMORIAL HOSPITAL, 5101 South Willow Springs Road, Zip 60525–2680; tel. 708/352–1200; Cathleen D. Biga, President and Chief Executive Officer (Total facility includes 47 beds in nursing home–type unit) **A**1 2 3 5 9 10 **F**4 7 8 10 11 15 16 17 19 21 22 26 27 28 29 30 31 32 33 34 35 37 39 40 41 42 43 44 45 46 49 60 63 64 65 66 67 70 71 73 74 **P**8 **S** Columbia/HCA Healthcare Corporation, Nashville, TN **N** MEDACOM Tri–State, Oakbrook, IL

| | 33 | 10 | 231 | 9562 | 141 | 108721 | 926 | 99420 | 36459 | 989 |

LAKE FOREST—Lake County

☒ △ LAKE FOREST HOSPITAL, 660 North Westmoreland Road, Zip 60045–1696; tel. 847/234–5600; William G. Ries, President (Total facility includes 88 beds in nursing home–type unit) **A**1 2 7 9 10 **F**1 3 5 7 8 12 14 15 17 19 21 22 24 25 26 28 30 31 32 33 34 35 36 37 39 40 41 42 44 45 46 49 51 54 56 60 61 63 64 65 66 67 70 71 73 74 **P**1 6 7 **N** Rush System for Health, Chicago, IL

| | 23 | 10 | 199 | 6538 | 146 | 199522 | 1912 | 91315 | 41755 | 910 |

LAWRENCEVILLE—Lawrence County

★ LAWRENCE COUNTY MEMORIAL HOSPITAL, West State Street, Zip 62439; tel. 618/943–1000; Gerald E. Waldroup, Administrator **A**9 10 **F**7 8 11 14 15 17 19 22 29 33 34 35 37 39 40 44 46 49 52 53 54 55 56 57 59 63 65 67 71 73 **P**5

| | 13 | 10 | 59 | 1297 | 19 | 27345 | 52 | 7716 | 3780 | 173 |

LEMONT—Du Page County

□ THE ROCK CREEK CENTER, 40 Timberline Drive, Zip 60439; tel. 630/257–3636; Wendy Mamoon, Chief Operating Officer **A**1 9 10 **F**3 14 15 16 52 53 54 55 56 57 58 59

| | 32 | 22 | 60 | 814 | 33 | 24873 | 0 | 16989 | 7738 | 227 |

LIBERTYVILLE—Lake County

☒ CONDELL MEDICAL CENTER, 801 South Milwaukee Avenue, Zip 60048–3199; tel. 847/362–2900; Eugene Pritchard, President **A**1 2 9 10 **F**1 3 7 8 15 16 19 21 22 24 25 32 33 34 35 37 40 42 44 46 49 52 57 58 59 60 63 65 66 67 70 71 72 73 **P**1 5

| | 23 | 10 | 175 | 9154 | 89 | 231943 | 1476 | 71251 | 31381 | 1095 |

LINCOLN—Logan County

☒ ABRAHAM LINCOLN MEMORIAL HOSPITAL, 315 8th Street, Zip 62656–2698; tel. 217/732–2161; Forrest G. Hester, President and Chief Executive Officer **A**1 9 10 **F**1 3 8 12 15 16 18 19 21 22 27 33 34 35 37 39 40 42 44 46 49 65 71 72 73 **P**4 **S** Memorial Health System, Springfield, IL

| | 23 | 10 | 47 | 2100 | 24 | 35886 | 232 | 16872 | 7537 | 229 |

LINCOLN DEVELOPMENTAL CENTER, 861 South State Street, Zip 62656–2599; tel. 217/735–2361; Martin Downs, Facility Director **F**20 53 54 55 56 57 58 59 60 65 73 **P**1

| | 12 | 62 | 450 | 24 | 446 | 0 | 0 | 25427 | 21024 | 697 |

LITCHFIELD—Montgomery County

☒ ST. FRANCIS HOSPITAL, 1215 East Union Avenue, Zip 62056–1215, Mailing Address: P.O. Box 1215, Zip 62056–1215; tel. 217/324–2191; Michael Sipkoski, Executive Vice President and Chief Executive Officer (Total facility includes 35 beds in nursing home–type unit) **A**1 9 10 **F**7 8 11 14 15 16 19 22 30 32 33 35 37 39 40 41 44 45 63 64 65 67 71 **S** Hospital Sisters Health System, Springfield, IL

| | 21 | 10 | 97 | 2924 | 42 | 56481 | 371 | 18442 | 8334 | 288 |

MACOMB—McDonough County

☒ MCDONOUGH DISTRICT HOSPITAL, 525 East Grant Street, Zip 61455; tel. 309/833–4101; Stephen R. Hopper, President and Chief Executive Officer (Total facility includes 16 beds in nursing home–type unit) **A**1 2 9 10 **F**1 3 7 8 14 15 16 19 21 22 23 26 29 30 32 33 35 37 39 40 41 42 44 46 53 56 57 58 64 65 67 71 73 74 **P**6 7 8

| | 16 | 10 | 144 | 3925 | 57 | 37204 | 310 | 29859 | 14437 | 488 |

MARION—Williamson County

☒ MARION MEMORIAL HOSPITAL, 917 West Main Street, Zip 62959; tel. 618/997–5341; Edward Cunningham, Interim Administrator **A**1 9 10 **F**7 8 12 15 16 17 19 20 21 22 26 28 29 30 31 32 33 34 36 37 38 39 40 41 42 44 45 46 47 49 51 56 63 64 65 66 67 68 71 73 **P**5 6 **S** Community Health Systems, Inc., Brentwood, TN

| | 14 | 10 | 84 | 2997 | 40 | 61413 | 265 | 22197 | 9854 | 370 |

☒ VETERANS AFFAIRS MEDICAL CENTER, 2401 West Main Street, Zip 62959–1194; tel. 618/997–5311; Linda Kurz, Director (Total facility includes 60 beds in nursing home–type unit) **A**1 5 **F**3 8 16 19 20 21 22 25 26 27 31 32 33 34 35 37 41 42 44 46 49 51 54 58 64 65 67 71 73 74 **S** Department of Veterans Affairs, Washington, DC

| | 45 | 10 | 162 | 3603 | 65 | 122761 | 0 | 41575 | 26508 | 520 |

MARYVILLE—Madison County

☒ ANDERSON HOSPITAL, 6800 State Route 162, Zip 62062, Mailing Address: P.O. Box 1000, Zip 62062; tel. 618/288–5711; R. Coert Shepard, President **A**1 9 10 **F**4 7 8 10 14 16 17 19 21 22 26 28 30 32 33 35 36 37 40 44 45 46 56 65 71 73

| | 23 | 10 | 110 | 4680 | 46 | 60279 | 785 | 28178 | 12562 | 456 |

MATTOON—Coles County

☒ SARAH BUSH LINCOLN HEALTH SYSTEM, 1000 Health Center Drive, Zip 61938–0372, Mailing Address: P.O. Box 372, Zip 61938; tel. 217/258–2525; Eugene A. Leblond, FACHE, President and Chief Executive Officer (Total facility includes 23 beds in nursing home–type unit) **A**1 2 9 10 **F**7 8 11 12 14 19 20 21 22 23 24 26 28 30 31 32 34 35 37 39 40 41 42 44 45 46 49 52 53 54 55 56 57 58 59 60 63 64 65 66 67 70 71 73 74 **P**4 5 6 7

| | 23 | 10 | 174 | 6598 | 78 | 185216 | 882 | 59040 | 24852 | 759 |

MAYWOOD—Cook County

☒ LOYOLA UNIVERSITY MEDICAL CENTER, 2160 South First Avenue, Zip 60153–5585; tel. 708/216–9000; Anthony L. Barbato, M.D., President and Chief Executive Officer **A**1 5 8 9 10 **F**3 4 5 7 8 9 10 11 12 13 14 15 16 17 18 19 20 21 22 23 24 25 26 27 28 29 30 31 32 33 34 35 37 38 39 40 41 42 43 44 45 46 47 49 51 52 53 54 55 56 57 58 59 60 61 63 64 65 66 67 68 69 70 71 72 73 74 **P**3 7 8 **N** Unified Health Care Network, Maywood, IL; MEDACOM Tri–State, Oakbrook, IL

| | 23 | 10 | 536 | 18618 | 337 | 321337 | 1241 | 367361 | 149095 | 4023 |

Hospital, Address, Telephone, Administrator, Approval, Facility, and Physician Codes, Health Care System, Network	Classi-fication Codes		Utilization Data					Expense (thousands) of dollars		
★ American Hospital Association (AHA) membership ☐ Joint Commission on Accreditation of Healthcare Organizations (JCAHO) accreditation + American Osteopathic Hospital Association (AOHA) membership ○ American Osteopathic Association (AOA) accreditation △ Commission on Accreditation of Rehabilitation Facilities (CARF) accreditation Control codes 61, 63, 64, 71, 72 and 73 indicate hospitals listed by AOHA, but not registered by AHA. For definition of numerical codes, see page A4	Control	Service	Beds	Admissions	Census	Outpatient Visits	Births	Total	Payroll	Personnel

MCHENRY—McHenry County

☒ △ NORTHERN ILLINOIS MEDICAL CENTER, 4201 Medical Center Drive, Zip 60050–9506; tel. 815/344–5000; Jim D. Redding, Chief Executive Officer (Total facility includes 12 beds in nursing home–type unit) **A**1 2 7 9 10 **F**2 3 4 7 8 10 12 14 15 16 17 18 19 20 22 24 25 26 27 28 29 30 32 33 34 35 36 37 39 40 41 42 44 46 48 49 52 53 54 55 56 57 58 59 60 64 65 67 70 71 73 74 **P**4 5 6 7 **N** Centegra Health System, McHenry, IL — 23 10 160 7395 96 162524 907 72239 28690 876

MCLEANSBORO—Hamilton County

☒ HAMILTON MEMORIAL HOSPITAL DISTRICT, 611 South Marshall Avenue, Zip 62859; tel. 618/643–2361; James M. Hayes, Administrator (Total facility includes 60 beds in nursing home–type unit) **A**1 9 10 **F**15 16 19 21 22 28 30 34 44 45 46 49 64 65 71 — 16 10 91 1204 73 14985 0 6793 3680 137

MELROSE PARK—Cook County

☒ GOTTLIEB MEMORIAL HOSPITAL, 701 West North Avenue, Zip 60160–1692; tel. 708/681–3200; John Morgan, President (Total facility includes 32 beds in nursing home–type unit) **A**1 5 9 10 **F**4 5 7 8 10 11 12 15 16 17 18 19 21 22 26 27 28 29 30 31 32 33 34 35 37 39 40 41 42 43 44 45 49 63 64 65 66 67 70 71 73 74 **P**8 — 23 10 212 9178 124 114537 1087 81111 37219 1089

☒ △ WESTLAKE COMMUNITY HOSPITAL, 1225 Lake Street, Zip 60160; tel. 708/681–3000; David R. Hey, Chief Operating Officer (Total facility includes 17 beds in nursing home–type unit) (Nonreporting) **A**1 2 3 5 7 9 10 **N** Rush System for Health, Chicago, IL; Synergon Health System, Oak Park, IL — 23 10 239 — — — — — — —

MENDOTA—La Salle County

☒ MENDOTA COMMUNITY HOSPITAL, 1315 Memorial Drive, Zip 61342; tel. 815/539–7461; Susan Urso, Administrator **A**1 9 10 **F**3 7 8 19 21 22 30 32 36 37 39 40 41 42 44 46 65 67 71 73 — 23 10 68 1696 18 49056 103 10765 5570 172

METROPOLIS—Massac County

☒ MASSAC MEMORIAL HOSPITAL, 28 Chick Street, Zip 62960–2481, Mailing Address: P.O. Box 850, Zip 62960–0850; tel. 618/524–2176; James Marshall, Chief Executive Officer **A**1 9 10 **F**19 21 22 32 33 37 44 51 71 **S** Alliant Health System, Louisville, KY — 16 10 31 1320 15 22003 0 8261 3527 162

MOLINE—Rock Island County

TRINITY MEDICAL CENTER–EAST CAMPUS See Trinity Medical Center–West Campus, Rock Island

MONMOUTH—Warren County

COMMUNITY MEMORIAL HOSPITAL, 1000 West Harlem Avenue, Zip 61462–1099; tel. 309/734–3141; Donald G. Brown, Chief Executive Officer (Total facility includes 34 beds in nursing home–type unit) **A**9 10 **F**8 11 14 15 16 17 18 19 20 21 22 26 28 30 32 33 37 39 41 44 45 49 51 63 64 65 67 69 70 71 73 — 14 10 68 1302 38 19684 0 8337 3681 122

MONTICELLO—Piatt County

☒ JOHN AND MARY KIRBY HOSPITAL, 1111 North State Street, Zip 61856; tel. 217/762–2115; Thomas D. Dixon, Administrator **A**1 9 10 **F**8 14 15 16 22 28 32 33 34 41 44 45 46 49 51 53 54 55 56 57 58 59 65 67 69 71 73 — 23 10 16 414 6 21276 0 4294 1876 83

MORRIS—Grundy County

☒ MORRIS HOSPITAL, 150 West High Street, Zip 60450; tel. 815/942–2932; Clifford L. Corbett, President and Chief Executive Officer **A**1 2 9 10 **F**8 15 16 19 21 22 26 28 29 30 33 34 35 36 37 39 40 41 42 44 46 49 54 56 58 65 70 71 73 — 23 10 82 3273 33 45645 277 36492 16480 386

MORRISON—Whiteside County

★ MORRISON COMMUNITY HOSPITAL, 303 North Jackson Street, Zip 61270–3042; tel. 815/772–4003; Mark F. Fedyk, Administrator (Total facility includes 38 beds in nursing home–type unit) (Nonreporting) **A**9 10 **S** Mercy Health Services, Farmington Hills, MI — 16 10 114 — — — — — — —

MOUNT CARMEL—Wabash County

☒ WABASH GENERAL HOSPITAL DISTRICT, 1418 College Drive, Zip 62863; tel. 618/262–8621; James R. Farris, CHE, Chief Executive Officer **A**1 9 10 **F**8 12 15 16 19 22 28 30 32 33 35 37 42 44 46 49 65 71 73 **S** Alliant Health System, Louisville, KY — 16 10 56 1190 16 12583 0 9360 3649 161

MOUNT VERNON—Jefferson County

CROSSROADS COMMUNITY HOSPITAL, 8 Doctors Park Road, Zip 62864; tel. 618/244–5500; Edward Cunningham, Executive Director (Nonreporting) **A**9 10 **S** Community Health Systems, Inc., Brentwood, TN — 33 10 49 — — — — — — —

☒ GOOD SAMARITAN REGIONAL HEALTH CENTER, 605 North 12th Street, Zip 62864; tel. 618/242–4600; Leo F. Childers, Jr., FACHE, President **A**1 2 9 10 **F**4 7 8 10 12 14 15 16 17 18 19 20 21 22 23 24 25 28 29 30 31 32 33 34 35 37 39 40 42 44 45 46 48 49 57 58 60 65 67 71 73 **P**2 3 4 5 6 7 8 **S** SSM Health Care System, Saint Louis, MO **N** MEDACOM Tri-State, Oakbrook, IL — 21 10 152 5298 78 58881 598 55384 24255 833

MURPHYSBORO—Jackson County

☒ ST. JOSEPH MEMORIAL HOSPITAL, 2 South Hospital Drive, Zip 62966; tel. 618/684–3156; Betty Gaffney, Administrator (Nonreporting) **A**1 9 10 **S** Southern Illinois Hospital Services, Carbondale, IL — 23 10 59 — — — — — — —

NAPERVILLE—Du Page County

☒ EDWARD HOSPITAL, 801 South Washington Street, Zip 60566–7060; tel. 708/355–0450; Pamela Meyer Davis, President and Chief Executive Officer (Total facility includes 14 beds in nursing home–type unit) **A**1 2 9 10 **F**3 4 7 8 10 12 13 14 15 16 17 18 19 20 22 24 25 28 29 30 32 34 35 37 39 40 41 42 43 44 45 46 49 51 53 54 55 56 57 58 59 61 64 65 67 70 71 72 73 74 **P**8 — 23 10 155 9457 99 132874 2358 100348 37433 968

Hospital, Address, Telephone, Administrator, Approval, Facility, and Physician Codes, Health Care System, Network	Classi-fication Codes		Utilization Data					Expense (thousands) of dollars		
★ American Hospital Association (AHA) membership □ Joint Commission on Accreditation of Healthcare Organizations (JCAHO) accreditation + American Osteopathic Hospital Association (AOHA) membership ○ American Osteopathic Association (AOA) accreditation △ Commission on Accreditation of Rehabilitation Facilities (CARF) accreditation Control codes 61, 63, 64, 71, 72 and 73 indicate hospitals listed by AOHA, but not registered by AHA. For definition of numerical codes, see page A4	Control	Service	Beds	Admissions	Census	Outpatient Visits	Births	Total	Payroll	Personnel

NASHVILLE—Washington County

☒ WASHINGTON COUNTY HOSPITAL, 705 South Grand Street, Zip 62263–1532; tel. 618/327–8236; Michael P. Ellermann, President (Total facility includes 27 beds in nursing home–type unit) **A**1 9 10 **F**3 4 5 7 8 9 10 11 12 13 14 17 18 19 21 22 25 27 28 29 30 31 32 33 34 35 37 38 39 40 41 42 43 44 45 47 49 51 52 53 54 55 56 57 58 59 60 61 63 64 65 66 67 69 70 71 72 73 74 **P**1 6 7 **S** SSM Health Care System, Saint Louis, MO **N** Saint Louis Health Care Network, St. Louis, MO
→ 16 | 10 | 53 | 792 | 29 | 25152 | 64 | 5866 | 2486 | 113

NORMAL—McLean County

☒ BROMENN HEALTHCARE, (Includes Bromenn Lifecare Center, 807 North Main Street, Bloomington, Zip 61701; tel. 309/454–1400; Bromenn Regional Medical Center, tel. 309/454–1400; Eureka Community Hospital, 101 South Major Street, Eureka, Zip 61530, Mailing Address: P.O. Box 203, Zip 61530; tel. 309/467–2371; Virginia and Franklin Streets, Zip 61761, Mailing Address: P.O. Box 2850, Bloomington, Zip 61702–2850; tel. 309/454–0700; Dale S. Strassheim, President (Total facility includes 146 beds in nursing home–type unit) **A**1 2 9 10 **F**1 2 3 7 8 10 12 13 15 16 17 18 19 21 22 24 25 26 27 28 29 30 31 32 33 34 35 37 38 39 40 41 42 44 46 48 49 51 52 53 54 55 56 57 58 59 61 63 64 65 67 68 70 71 72 73 **P**6 7 8
→ 21 | 10 | 327 | 8886 | 230 | 92526 | 1426 | 104000 | 45426 | 1524

BROMENN REGIONAL MEDICAL CENTER See BroMenn Healthcare

NORTH CHICAGO—Lake County

☒ VETERANS AFFAIRS MEDICAL CENTER, 3001 Green Bay Road, Zip 60064; tel. 847/688–1900; Alfred S. Pate, Director (Total facility includes 373 beds in nursing home–type unit) (Nonreporting) **A**1 3 5 9 **S** Department of Veterans Affairs, Washington, DC
→ 45 | 49 | 836 | — | — | — | — | — | — | —

OAK FOREST—Cook County

☒ △ OAK FOREST HOSPITAL OF COOK COUNTY, (LONG TERM ACUTE CARE), 15900 South Cicero Avenue, Zip 60452; tel. 708/687–7200; Cynthia T. Henderson, M.D., M.P.H., Interim Hospital Director (Total facility includes 526 beds in nursing home–type unit) **A**1 3 5 7 9 10 **F**3 8 10 12 13 14 15 16 17 20 22 25 26 27 28 29 30 31 33 34 36 37 39 41 42 44 45 46 48 49 51 54 57 58 64 65 67 71 73 **P**6 **S** Cook County Bureau of Health Services, Chicago, IL
→ 15 | 49 | 627 | 2316 | 584 | 60541 | 0 | 102708 | 62897 | 1821

OAK LAWN—Cook County

☒ △ CHRIST HOSPITAL AND MEDICAL CENTER, 4440 West 95th Street, Zip 60453–2699; tel. 708/425–8000; Carol Schneider, Chief Executive (Nonreporting) **A**1 2 3 5 7 9 10 **S** Advocate Health Care, Oakbrook, IL **N** Advocate Health Care, Oak Brook, IL; MEDACOM Tri–State, Oakbrook, IL
→ 21 | 10 | 800 | — | — | — | — | — | — | —

OAK PARK—Cook County

☒ △ OAK PARK HOSPITAL, 520 South Maple Avenue, Zip 60304–1097; tel. 708/383–9300; Leonard J. Muller, President (Total facility includes 47 beds in nursing home–type unit) (Nonreporting) **A**1 2 5 7 9 10 **S** Wheaton Franciscan Services, Inc., Wheaton, IL **N** Rush System for Health, Chicago, IL; Synergon Health System, Oak Park, IL
→ 23 | 10 | 176 | — | — | — | — | — | — | —

☒ WEST SUBURBAN HOSPITAL MEDICAL CENTER, Erie at Austin Boulevard, Zip 60302–2599; tel. 708/383–6200; David M. Cecero, President and Chief Executive Officer (Total facility includes 20 beds in nursing home–type unit) (Nonreporting) **A**1 2 3 5 9 10
→ 23 | 10 | 273 | — | — | — | — | — | — | —

OLNEY—Richland County

☒ RICHLAND MEMORIAL HOSPITAL, 800 East Locust Street, Zip 62450–2598; tel. 618/395–2131; Harvey H. Pettry, Administrator (Total facility includes 28 beds in nursing home–type unit) **A**1 2 9 10 **F**7 8 12 14 15 16 19 20 21 27 28 29 30 31 32 33 34 35 36 37 39 40 41 42 44 45 46 49 52 54 56 59 63 64 65 66 67 71 73
→ 13 | 10 | 97 | 3077 | 55 | 67463 | 324 | 19806 | 8662 | 369

OLYMPIA FIELDS—Cook County

★ ○ COLUMBIA OLYMPIA FIELDS OSTEOPATHIC HOSPITAL AND MEDICAL CENTER, 20201 Crawford Avenue, Zip 60461–1080; tel. 708/747–4000; Barry S. Schneider, President and Chief Executive Officer **A**9 11 12 13 **F**4 5 7 8 10 11 12 13 14 16 17 19 21 22 25 26 28 29 30 32 34 35 37 38 39 40 41 42 43 44 45 46 48 49 51 52 54 55 56 57 60 61 64 65 66 67 70 71 72 73 74 **P**5 7 **S** Columbia/HCA Healthcare Corporation, Nashville, TN
→ 33 | 10 | 174 | 6792 | 90 | 132087 | 606 | 87113 | 26999 | 678

OTTAWA—La Salle County

☒ + COMMUNITY HOSPITAL OF OTTAWA, 1100 East Norris Drive, Zip 61350; tel. 815/433–3100; Robert Schmelter, President **A**1 9 10 **F**1 2 3 4 6 7 8 11 15 19 20 21 22 26 27 28 29 30 32 33 36 39 40 42 44 45 46 49 52 53 54 56 57 58 65 67 70 71 73 **P**3 8
→ 23 | 10 | 113 | 3917 | 51 | 53242 | 399 | 27214 | 12285 | 430

PALOS HEIGHTS—Cook County

☒ PALOS COMMUNITY HOSPITAL, 12251 South 80th Avenue, Zip 60463–0930; tel. 708/923–4000; Sister Margaret Wright, President **A**1 2 9 10 **F**2 3 7 8 10 11 16 19 21 22 25 31 32 34 35 36 37 39 40 41 42 44 45 49 52 53 54 56 57 58 59 63 65 66 67 71 72 73
→ 23 | 10 | 337 | 16204 | 210 | 168693 | 2166 | 154203 | 76695 | 1703

PANA—Christian County

☒ PANA COMMUNITY HOSPITAL, 101 East Ninth Street, Zip 62557; tel. 217/562–2131; Michael J. Laird, Administrator and Chief Executive Officer **A**1 9 10 **F**8 12 14 15 16 19 21 22 29 31 32 33 34 36 37 42 44 45 46 49 51 54 65 71
→ 23 | 10 | 44 | 641 | 6 | 15676 | 0 | 6280 | 2924 | 123

PARIS—Edgar County

☒ PARIS COMMUNITY HOSPITAL, 721 East Court Street, Zip 61944–2420; tel. 217/465–4141; John M. Dillon, Chief Executive Officer **A**1 9 10 **F**8 15 19 21 22 30 33 34 36 37 41 42 44 48 49 64 65 67 71 73 **P**6 **S** Alliant Health System, Louisville, KY
→ 23 | 10 | 49 | 957 | 16 | 14172 | 0 | 7699 | 3430 | 145

Hospital, Address, Telephone, Administrator, Approval, Facility, and Physician Codes, Health Care System, Network	Classi- fication Codes		Utilization Data					Expense (thousands) of dollars		
	Control	Service	Beds	Admissions	Census	Outpatient Visits	Births	Total	Payroll	Personnel

★ American Hospital Association (AHA) membership
□ Joint Commission on Accreditation of Healthcare Organizations (JCAHO) accreditation
+ American Osteopathic Hospital Association (AOHA) membership
○ American Osteopathic Association (AOA) accreditation
△ Commission on Accreditation of Rehabilitation Facilities (CARF) accreditation
　　Control codes 61, 63, 64, 71, 72 and 73 indicate hospitals listed by AOHA, but not registered by AHA. For definition of numerical codes, see page A4

PARK RIDGE—Cook County

✠ △ LUTHERAN GENERAL HOSPITAL, 1775 Dempster Street, Zip 60068–1174; tel. 847/723–2210; Kenneth J. Rojek, Chief Executive **A**1 2 3 5 7 8 9 10 **F**1 2 3 4 5 6 7 8 10 11 12 14 15 16 17 19 21 22 23 24 26 27 28 29 30 31 32 33 34 35 36 37 38 39 40 41 42 43 44 46 47 48 49 51 52 53 54 55 56 57 58 59 60 61 62 64 65 66 67 68 69 70 71 73 74 **P**1 2 3 4 5 6 7 8 **S** Advocate Health Care, Oakbrook, IL **N** Advocate Health Care, Oak Brook, IL | 21 | 10 | 559 | 25148 | 376 | 190252 | 4343 | 324701 | 119755 | 3514

PEKIN—Tazewell County

✠ PEKIN HOSPITAL, 600 South 13th Street, Zip 61554–5098; tel. 309/347–1151; Robert J. Moore, CHE, Chief Executive Officer (Total facility includes 20 beds in nursing home–type unit) **A**1 9 10 **F**2 3 4 7 8 10 12 14 15 16 17 18 19 20 21 22 24 26 28 29 30 31 32 34 35 37 38 39 40 41 42 43 44 45 46 47 49 51 52 53 54 55 56 57 58 59 60 61 63 64 65 66 67 68 69 70 71 72 73 74 **P**1 5 7 | 23 | 10 | 125 | 4276 | 59 | 65760 | 470 | 34506 | 14309 | 533

PEORIA—Peoria County

□ GEORGE A. ZELLER MENTAL HEALTH CENTER, 5407 North University Street, Zip 61614–4785; tel. 309/693–5228; Robert W. Vyverberg, Ed.D., Director (Nonreporting) **A**1 10 | 12 | 22 | 154 | — | — | — | — | — | — | —

✠ △ METHODIST MEDICAL CENTER OF ILLINOIS, 221 N.E. Glen Oak Avenue, Zip 61636; tel. 309/672–5522; James K. Knoble, President **A**1 2 3 5 6 7 9 10 **F**1 2 3 4 7 8 10 11 12 13 14 16 18 19 21 22 23 24 25 26 27 28 29 30 32 33 35 37 39 40 41 42 43 44 45 46 48 49 50 51 52 53 54 55 56 57 58 59 60 61 63 64 65 67 69 71 72 73 74 **P**1 6 7 | 23 | 10 | 315 | 13213 | 213 | 285132 | 1760 | — | — | 2236

✠ PROCTOR HOSPITAL, 5409 North Knoxville Avenue, Zip 61614–5094; tel. 309/691–1000; Norman H. LaConte, President and Chief Executive Officer (Total facility includes 30 beds in nursing home–type unit) **A**1 9 10 **F**2 3 4 7 8 10 12 13 14 15 16 19 21 22 24 28 29 30 34 35 36 37 39 40 41 43 44 46 49 63 64 65 70 71 73 **P**1 6 | 23 | 10 | 185 | 5969 | 105 | 140859 | 623 | 55716 | 22747 | 821

✠ △ SAINT FRANCIS MEDICAL CENTER, 530 N.E. Glen Oak Avenue, Zip 61637; tel. 309/655–2000; Sister M. Canisia, Administrator **A**1 2 3 5 7 9 10 **F**1 3 4 5 6 7 8 10 11 12 13 14 15 16 17 18 19 20 21 22 23 24 25 26 27 28 29 30 31 32 33 34 35 36 37 38 39 40 41 42 43 44 45 46 47 48 49 50 51 52 53 54 55 56 57 58 59 60 61 62 63 64 65 66 67 68 69 70 71 72 73 74 **P**1 4 5 **S** OSF Healthcare System, Peoria, IL **N** Unified Health Care Network, Maywood, IL | 21 | 10 | 534 | 21277 | 354 | 440297 | 2281 | 265658 | 121194 | 3541

PERU—La Salle County

✠ ILLINOIS VALLEY COMMUNITY HOSPITAL, 925 West Street, Zip 61354–2799; tel. 815/223–3300; Ralph B. Berkley, Administrator (Total facility includes 12 beds in nursing home–type unit) **A**1 9 10 **F**1 7 8 10 15 16 19 21 22 23 26 28 29 30 31 32 33 35 36 37 39 40 41 42 44 45 46 49 52 53 54 55 56 57 58 59 64 65 66 67 71 73 74 **P**8 | 23 | 10 | 104 | 3641 | 57 | 70489 | 378 | 29780 | 12275 | 426

PINCKNEYVILLE—Perry County

★ PINCKNEYVILLE COMMUNITY HOSPITAL, 101 North Walnut Street, Zip 62274; tel. 618/357–2187; John D. Schubert, Administrator and Chief Executive Officer (Total facility includes 50 beds in nursing home–type unit) (Nonreporting) **A**9 10 **N** BJC Health System, St. Louis, MO | 16 | 10 | 92 | — | — | — | — | — | — | —

PITTSFIELD—Pike County

✠ ILLINI COMMUNITY HOSPITAL, 640 West Washington Street, Zip 62363; tel. 217/285–2113; Jete Edmisson, President and Chief Executive Officer **A**1 9 10 **F**8 11 15 16 19 20 22 24 26 28 29 30 32 33 36 37 39 40 41 44 46 49 51 65 71 73 **P**6 **S** Quorum Health Group/Quorum Health Resources, Inc., Brentwood, TN | 23 | 10 | 45 | 937 | 10 | 30669 | 67 | 9690 | 4384 | 178

PONTIAC—Livingston County

✠ SAINT JAMES HOSPITAL, 610 East Water Street, Zip 61764; tel. 815/842–2828; David Ochs, Administrator (Total facility includes 16 beds in nursing home–type unit) **A**1 9 10 **F**7 8 12 14 15 16 17 19 21 22 24 28 29 30 32 33 34 35 36 37 39 40 41 42 44 45 49 64 65 66 67 71 74 **P**4 6 7 **S** OSF Healthcare System, Peoria, IL **N** Unified Health Care Network, Maywood, IL | 21 | 10 | 81 | 2602 | 31 | 57896 | 317 | 23380 | 11626 | 286

PRINCETON—Bureau County

✠ PERRY MEMORIAL HOSPITAL, 530 Park Avenue East, Zip 61356–2598; tel. 815/875–2811; William H. Spitler, III, President (Total facility includes 15 beds in nursing home–type unit) **A**1 9 10 **F**7 8 15 16 17 19 21 22 28 29 30 34 35 37 40 41 44 49 64 65 67 71 **P**3 8 | 14 | 10 | 87 | 2599 | 34 | 41453 | 198 | 19019 | 8184 | 259

QUINCY—Adams County

✠ BLESSING HOSPITAL, (Includes Blessing Hospital, Broadway & 14th Street, Mailing Address: P.O. Box 7005, Zip 62305–7005; tel. 217/223–1200), Broadway at 11th Street, Zip 62301, Mailing Address: P.O. Box 7005, Zip 62305–7005; tel. 217/223–5811; Lawrence L. Swearingen, President (Total facility includes 44 beds in nursing home–type unit) **A**1 2 3 5 9 10 **F**1 2 5 7 8 10 12 13 14 15 16 17 19 20 21 22 23 24 26 27 28 29 30 31 32 33 34 35 36 37 39 40 41 42 44 45 46 48 49 52 53 56 60 63 64 65 67 70 71 72 73 74 **P**8 | 23 | 10 | 323 | 11261 | 194 | 253381 | 1271 | 73146 | 36838 | 1319

RED BUD—Randolph County

✠ ST. CLEMENT HEALTH SERVICES, One St. Clement Boulevard, Zip 62278–1194; tel. 618/282–3831; Michael Thomas McManus, President (Total facility includes 40 beds in nursing home–type unit) **A**1 9 10 **F**7 8 15 16 17 18 19 21 22 24 28 29 30 32 33 34 35 37 40 42 44 49 63 64 65 66 67 71 74 **S** Sisters of Mercy Health System–St. Louis, Saint Louis, MO **N** Unity Health System, St. Louis, MO; BJC Health System, St. Louis, MO | 21 | 10 | 105 | 1506 | 47 | 50113 | 138 | 15681 | 7136 | 228

Hospital, Address, Telephone, Administrator, Approval, Facility, and Physician Codes, Health Care System, Network	Classi-fication Codes		Utilization Data					Expense (thousands) of dollars		
	Control	Service	Beds	Admissions	Census	Outpatient Visits	Births	Total	Payroll	Personnel

★ American Hospital Association (AHA) membership
□ Joint Commission on Accreditation of Healthcare Organizations (JCAHO) accreditation
+ American Osteopathic Hospital Association (AOHA) membership
○ American Osteopathic Association (AOA) accreditation
△ Commission on Accreditation of Rehabilitation Facilities (CARF) accreditation
Control codes 61, 63, 64, 71, 72 and 73 indicate hospitals listed by AOHA, but not registered by AHA. For definition of numerical codes, see page A4

ROBINSON—Crawford County

✠ CRAWFORD MEMORIAL HOSPITAL, 1000 North Allen Street, Zip 62454, Mailing Address: P.O. Box 151, Zip 62454; tel. 618/544–3131; William E. Schirmer, FACHE, Interim Chief Executive Officer (Total facility includes 48 beds in nursing home–type unit) **A**1 9 10 **F**7 8 13 14 15 16 18 19 22 27 28 30 32 33 34 35 36 37 39 40 41 42 44 46 49 51 64 65 67 71 **P**6 8 **S** Quorum Health Group/Quorum Health Resources, Inc., Brentwood, TN	16	10	102	1948	60	30427	282	15124	6307	251

ROCHELLE—Ogle County

✠ ROCHELLE COMMUNITY HOSPITAL, 900 North Second Street, Zip 61068–0330; tel. 815/562–2181; Peter Jennings, Interim Administrator **A**1 9 10 **F**7 8 12 15 16 19 21 22 24 30 31 32 37 40 44 49 51 65 67 71 72 **P**5 8	23	10	43	1089	12	48011	74	8079	3831	104

ROCK ISLAND—Rock Island County

✠ △ TRINITY MEDICAL CENTER–WEST CAMPUS, (Includes Trinity Medical Center–East Campus, 501 Tenth Avenue, Moline, Zip 61265; tel. 309/757–3131), 2701 17th Street, Zip 61201; tel. 309/757–3822; Eric Crowell, President and Chief Executive Officer (Total facility includes 29 beds in nursing home–type unit) **A**1 7 9 10 **F**2 3 7 8 9 10 11 12 13 14 15 16 17 18 19 21 22 23 24 25 26 27 28 29 30 31 32 33 34 35 37 38 39 40 41 42 44 45 46 48 49 52 53 54 55 56 57 58 59 60 61 63 64 65 66 67 70 71 72 73 74 **P**4 8 **N** Advocate Health Care, Oak Brook, IL	23	10	369	14216	207	250014	1464	109040	49129	1442

ROCKFORD—Winnebago County

□ H. DOUGLAS SINGER MENTAL HEALTH AND DEVELOPMENTAL CENTER, 4402 North Main Street, Zip 61103–1278; tel. 815/987–7096; Robert Vyverberger, Acting Facility Director and Network Manager **A**1 10 **F**2 4 7 8 9 10 11 15 19 20 21 22 31 35 37 38 40 42 43 44 47 48 49 50 52 53 56 60 63 64 65 71 73 **P**6	12	22	162	654	146	0	0	13500	10097	200
✠ △ ROCKFORD MEMORIAL HOSPITAL, 2400 North Rockton Avenue, Zip 61103–3692; tel. 815/971–5000; Thomas David DeFauw, President and Chief Executive Officer **A**1 2 5 7 9 10 **F**2 3 4 5 7 8 10 11 14 15 16 17 19 21 22 26 28 29 30 31 32 34 35 36 37 38 39 40 41 42 43 44 45 46 47 48 49 51 53 54 55 56 57 58 59 60 61 65 67 70 71 73 74 **P**1 3 4 8	23	10	408	14270	244	281096	2182	179198	74258	2148
✠ SAINT ANTHONY MEDICAL CENTER, 5666 East State Street, Zip 61108–2472; tel. 815/226–2000; David A. Schertz, Administrator **A**1 2 3 5 9 10 **F**4 7 8 9 10 11 12 14 15 16 17 19 21 22 23 24 26 27 28 29 30 31 32 34 35 36 37 39 40 41 42 43 44 46 48 49 51 60 63 64 65 66 67 70 71 72 73 **P**4 5 6 7 8 **S** OSF Healthcare System, Peoria, IL	21	10	210	8216	115	131369	816	104007	45218	1325
✠ SWEDISHAMERICAN HOSPITAL, 1400 Charles Street, Zip 61104–2298; tel. 815/968–4400; Robert B. Klint, M.D., President **A**1 2 3 5 9 10 **F**2 3 4 7 8 10 11 12 14 16 17 18 19 21 26 28 29 30 31 32 33 34 35 37 39 40 41 42 43 44 45 46 47 48 49 51 52 53 54 55 56 57 58 59 60 63 64 65 67 70 71 73 74 **P**4 6 7 **N** SwedishAmerican Health System, Rockford, IL; MEDACOM Tri-State, Oakbrook, IL	23	10	296	11047	144	—	1782	102338	45596	1294

ROSICLARE—Hardin County

✠ HARDIN COUNTY GENERAL HOSPITAL, Ferrell Road, Zip 62982; tel. 618/285–6634; Roby D. Williams, Administrator (Nonreporting) **A**1 9 10	23	10	48	—	—	—	—	—	—	—

RUSHVILLE—Schuyler County

★ SARAH D. CULBERTSON MEMORIAL HOSPITAL, 238 South Congress Street, Zip 62681, Mailing Address: P.O. Box 440, Zip 62681; tel. 217/322–4321; Michael C. O'Brien, Administrator (Total facility includes 25 beds in nursing home–type unit) **A**9 10 **F**8 14 17 19 22 28 30 34 36 40 42 44 49 64 71 72 73 **P**6	16	10	53	794	32	19322	141	5851	2220	113

SALEM—Marion County

✠ PUBLIC HOSPITAL OF THE TOWN OF SALEM, 1201 Ricker Drive, Zip 62881–6250, Mailing Address: P.O. Box 1250, Zip 62881–1250; tel. 618/548–3194; Clarence E. Lay, Chief Executive Officer **A**1 9 10 **F**8 14 15 16 17 19 22 28 30 32 33 36 37 39 41 44 65 69 71 73 **N** BJC Health System, St. Louis, MO	14	10	33	1722	22	36088	0	11715	5095	203

SANDWICH—De Kalb County

★ SANDWICH COMMUNITY HOSPITAL, 11 East Pleasant Avenue, Zip 60548–0901; tel. 815/786–8484; Roland R. Carlson, Administrator **A**9 10 **F**7 8 19 21 22 28 30 34 35 37 39 40 41 44 45 49 65 71 73 **S** Quorum Health Group/Quorum Health Resources, Inc., Brentwood, TN	23	10	50	1065	10	21346	81	9203	3583	121

SCOTT AFB—St. Clair County

✠ SCOTT MEDICAL CENTER, Zip 62225–5252; tel. 618/256–7012; Colonel Stephen J. Pribyl, MSC, USAF, Administrator **A**1 2 3 5 **F**3 7 8 10 12 13 15 16 17 18 19 20 22 24 25 28 29 30 34 35 39 40 41 42 44 45 46 49 51 52 53 54 55 56 58 61 65 67 68 69 71 73 74 **P**5 8 **S** Department of the Air Force, Washington, DC	41	10	59	5284	34	323252	561	33000	—	1257

SHELBYVILLE—Shelby County

✠ SHELBY MEMORIAL HOSPITAL, 200 South Cedar Street, Zip 62565–1899; tel. 217/774–3961; John Bennett, President and Chief Executive Officer (Total facility includes 15 beds in nursing home–type unit) **A**1 9 10 **F**8 11 14 15 16 19 21 22 31 32 35 37 41 42 44 49 63 64 65 66 71	23	10	60	1726	32	30150	0	8270	3564	145

SILVIS—Rock Island County

✠ ILLINI HOSPITAL, 801 Hospital Road, Zip 61282; tel. 309/792–9363; Gary E. Larson, Chief Executive Officer **A**1 9 10 **F**6 7 8 19 21 22 24 25 26 28 29 30 32 35 37 40 41 44 45 62 63 65 71 72 73 **P**6 7 8 **N** Genesis Health System, Davenport, IA	23	10	133	4506	45	68934	627	31300	13336	480

Hospital, Address, Telephone, Administrator, Approval, Facility, and Physician Codes, Health Care System, Network	Classi-fication Codes		Utilization Data					Expense (thousands) of dollars		
	Control	Service	Beds	Admissions	Census	Outpatient Visits	Births	Total	Payroll	Personnel

★ American Hospital Association (AHA) membership
☐ Joint Commission on Accreditation of Healthcare Organizations (JCAHO) accreditation
+ American Osteopathic Hospital Association (AOHA) membership
○ American Osteopathic Association (AOA) accreditation
△ Commission on Accreditation of Rehabilitation Facilities (CARF) accreditation
Control codes 61, 63, 64, 71, 72 and 73 indicate hospitals listed by AOHA, but not registered by AHA. For definition of numerical codes, see page A4

SKOKIE—Cook County

⊠ RUSH NORTH SHORE MEDICAL CENTER, 9600 Gross Point Road, Zip 60076–1257; tel. 847/677–9600; John S. Frigo, President **A**1 2 3 5 9 10 **F**4 7 8 10 14 15 16 17 19 21 22 26 28 29 34 35 36 39 40 41 42 43 44 46 49 52 54 55 56 57 58 59 60 63 65 70 71 73 74 **P**8 **S** Rush–Presbyterian–St. Luke's Medical Center, Chicago, IL **N** Rush System for Health, Chicago, IL | 23 | 10 | 229 | 9443 | 153 | 197037 | 652 | 89083 | 40089 | 1196

SPARTA—Randolph County

★ SPARTA COMMUNITY HOSPITAL, 818 East Broadway Street, Zip 62286–0297, Mailing Address: P.O. Box 297, Zip 62286–0297; tel. 618/443–2177; Joann Emge, Chief Executive Officer **A**9 10 **F**1 7 8 12 14 15 16 17 19 22 25 28 30 32 33 34 40 41 42 44 46 49 51 65 67 71 73 74 **P**6 **S** Brim, Inc., Portland, OR | 16 | 10 | 39 | 809 | 8 | 27739 | 131 | 8468 | 4153 | 135

SPRING VALLEY—Bureau County

⊠ ST. MARGARET'S HOSPITAL, 600 East First Street, Zip 61362–2034; tel. 815/664–5311; Timothy Muntz, President (Total facility includes 33 beds in nursing home–type unit) **A**1 2 9 10 **F**1 7 8 10 14 15 16 19 21 22 23 24 27 30 32 33 35 37 39 40 41 42 44 48 49 60 62 64 65 66 67 71 73 74 **P**6 **S** Sisters of Mary of the Presentation Health Corporation, Fargo, ND | 21 | 10 | 127 | 2968 | 53 | 86611 | 399 | 25242 | 10417 | 335

SPRINGFIELD—Sangamon County

☐ ANDREW MCFARLAND MENTAL HEALTH CENTER, 901 Southwind Road, Zip 62703; tel. 217/786–6994; Nieves Tan–Lachica, M.D., Superintendent (Nonreporting) **A**1 | 12 | 22 | 146 | — | — | — | — | — | — | —

☐ DOCTORS HOSPITAL, 5230 South Sixth Street, Zip 62703, Mailing Address: P.O. Box 19254, Zip 62794–9254; tel. 217/529–7151; Jim Bohl, President and Chief Executive Officer (Nonreporting) **A**1 9 10 | 33 | 10 | 150 | — | — | — | — | — | — | —

⊠ △ MEMORIAL MEDICAL CENTER, 800 North Rutledge Street, Zip 62781–0001; tel. 217/788–3000; Robert T. Clarke, President and Chief Executive Officer **A**1 2 3 5 7 8 9 10 **F**3 4 6 7 8 9 10 11 12 15 17 18 19 21 22 23 25 29 30 32 33 34 35 36 37 39 40 41 42 43 44 45 46 48 49 51 52 53 54 55 56 57 58 59 60 65 66 67 69 70 71 72 73 **P**3 4 5 7 **S** Memorial Health System, Springfield, IL | 23 | 10 | 455 | 17900 | 304 | 344774 | 1897 | 204162 | 84228 | 2441

⊠ ST. JOHN'S HOSPITAL, 800 East Carpenter Street, Zip 62769; tel. 217/544–6464; Allison C. Laabs, Executive Vice President and Administrator (Total facility includes 53 beds in nursing home–type unit) **A**1 2 3 5 8 9 10 **F**1 3 4 8 10 12 14 15 16 19 21 22 26 28 30 32 33 35 36 37 38 39 40 41 42 43 44 46 47 49 52 57 58 59 60 64 65 69 70 71 73 **S** Hospital Sisters Health System, Springfield, IL **N** National Cardiovascular Network, Atlanta, GA | 21 | 10 | 580 | 22136 | 375 | 177273 | 1803 | 222312 | 91722 | 2987

STAUNTON—Macoupin County

⊠ COMMUNITY MEMORIAL HOSPITAL, 400 Caldwell Street, Zip 62088–1499; tel. 618/635–2200; Patrick B. Heise, Chief Executive Officer **A**1 9 10 **F**8 19 22 32 44 65 71 73 **P**3 **S** Quorum Health Group/Quorum Health Resources, Inc., Brentwood, TN **N** Unity Health System, St. Louis, MO | 23 | 10 | 57 | 843 | 9 | 16094 | 0 | 7151 | 3301 | 144

STERLING—Whiteside County

⊠ CGH MEDICAL CENTER, 100 East LeFevre Road, Zip 61081–1279; tel. 815/625–0400; Edward Andersen, President and Chief Executive Officer **A**1 2 9 10 **F**7 8 12 14 15 16 17 19 21 22 23 27 28 29 30 31 32 33 35 37 39 40 41 42 44 46 48 49 60 63 64 65 66 67 69 70 71 73 **P**4 7 | 14 | 10 | 147 | 6116 | 66 | 75926 | 767 | 42386 | 18391 | 641

STREAMWOOD—Cook County

☐ BHC STREAMWOOD HOSPITAL, (Formerly CPC Streamwood Hospital), 1400 East Irving Park Road, Zip 60107; tel. 630/837–9000; Jeff Bergren, Chief Operating Officer and Administrator **A**1 9 10 **F**2 9 11 37 38 40 41 47 52 53 54 55 56 57 58 59 65 **S** Behavioral Healthcare Corporation, Nashville, TN | 33 | 22 | 100 | 233 | 17 | 3314 | 0 | — | — | 120

STREATOR—La Salle County

⊠ ST. MARY'S HOSPITAL, 111 East Spring Street, Zip 61364; tel. 815/673–2311; James F. Dover, Administrator and Executive Vice President (Total facility includes 30 beds in nursing home–type unit) **A**1 9 10 **F**1 3 7 8 14 15 16 17 19 20 21 22 24 26 27 28 29 30 32 33 34 35 37 38 39 40 41 42 44 45 49 60 63 64 65 67 69 71 73 **P**8 **S** Hospital Sisters Health System, Springfield, IL | 21 | 10 | 170 | 4198 | 70 | 36264 | 302 | 26110 | 12526 | 392

SYCAMORE—De Kalb County

☐ VENCOR HOSPITAL–SYCAMORE, 225 Edward Street, Zip 60178; tel. 815/895–2144; Donald Van Voorhis, Administrator (Nonreporting) **A**1 9 10 **S** Vencor, Incorporated, Louisville, KY | 14 | 10 | 50 | — | — | — | — | — | — | —

TAYLORVILLE—Christian County

⊠ ST. VINCENT MEMORIAL HOSPITAL, 201 East Pleasant Street, Zip 62568–1597; tel. 217/824–3331; Daniel J. Raab, President and Chief Executive Officer (Total facility includes 50 beds in nursing home–type unit) **A**1 9 10 **F**7 8 12 13 14 15 16 17 19 21 22 26 28 29 31 32 33 34 35 36 37 39 40 42 44 45 46 49 51 54 64 65 67 71 72 73 74 **P**5 **S** Memorial Health System, Springfield, IL | 21 | 10 | 149 | 2424 | 70 | 58281 | 196 | 17673 | 8322 | 347

TINLEY PARK—Cook County

☐ TINLEY PARK MENTAL HEALTH CENTER, 7400 West 183rd Street, Zip 60477–3695; tel. 708/614–4000; Delores Newman, MS, Network Manager, Metro South Network (Nonreporting) **A**1 5 10 | 12 | 22 | 280 | — | — | — | — | — | — | —

URBANA—Champaign County

⊠ △ CARLE FOUNDATION HOSPITAL, 611 West Park Street, Zip 61801–2595; tel. 217/383–3311; Michael H. Fritz, President (Total facility includes 240 beds in nursing home–type unit) **A**1 2 3 5 7 9 10 **F**2 4 6 7 8 10 12 13 14 15 16 17 19 22 23 25 26 27 28 29 30 31 32 33 38 39 40 41 42 43 44 45 46 48 49 62 64 65 67 70 71 72 73 **P**5 **N** The Carle Foundation, Urbana, IL | 23 | 10 | 540 | 12276 | 326 | 44076 | 1526 | 110738 | 43747 | 1189

Hospital, Address, Telephone, Administrator, Approval, Facility, and Physician Codes, Health Care System, Network	Classi-fication Codes		Utilization Data					Expense (thousands) of dollars		
	Control	Service	Beds	Admissions	Census	Outpatient Visits	Births	Total	Payroll	Personnel

★ American Hospital Association (AHA) membership
□ Joint Commission on Accreditation of Healthcare Organizations (JCAHO) accreditation
+ American Osteopathic Hospital Association (AOHA) membership
○ American Osteopathic Association (AOA) accreditation
△ Commission on Accreditation of Rehabilitation Facilities (CARF) accreditation
Control codes 61, 63, 64, 71, 72 and 73 indicate hospitals listed by AOHA, but not registered by AHA. For definition of numerical codes, see page A4

✶ △ COVENANT MEDICAL CENTER, (Includes Burnham Hospital, 407 South Fourth Street, Champaign, Zip 61820; tel. 217/337–2500; Mercy Hospital), 1400 West Park Street, Zip 61801; tel. 217/337–2000; Joseph W. Beard, President and Chief Executive Officer **A**1 2 3 5 7 9 10 **F**4 7 10 12 16 17 19 21 22 23 24 26 30 32 33 34 35 37 38 39 40 41 42 43 44 48 49 52 54 55 56 58 59 60 63 64 65 67 71 73 **P**4 **S** ServantCor, Kankakee, IL **N** Servantcor, Clifton, IL MERCY HOSPITAL See Covenant Medical Center	21	10	268	10886	137	136837	1563	88575	36339	1192
VANDALIA—Fayette County										
✶ FAYETTE COUNTY HOSPITAL AND LONG TERM CARE, Seventh and Taylor Streets, Zip 62471–1296; tel. 618/283–1231; Daniel L. Gantz, President (Total facility includes 92 beds in nursing home–type unit) **A**1 9 10 **F**8 14 15 16 17 19 20 21 22 28 30 32 33 35 36 41 42 44 45 46 49 50 58 64 65 71 72 73 **P**1 5 6 7 8 **S** BJC Health System, Saint Louis, MO **N** BJC Health System, St. Louis, MO	16	10	133	1486	95	25652	0	10170	4681	228
WATSEKA—Iroquois County										
✶ IROQUOIS MEMORIAL HOSPITAL AND RESIDENT HOME, 200 Fairman Avenue, Zip 60970–1644; tel. 815/432–5841; Melvin H. Fahs, President (Total facility includes 46 beds in nursing home–type unit) **A**1 9 10 **F**7 8 14 15 16 17 19 20 21 22 28 30 32 33 34 36 37 38 40 42 44 45 49 58 63 64 65 67 71 73 **P**5	23	10	112	2029	66	27884	192	16997	7756	247
WAUKEGAN—Lake County										
✶ △ SAINT THERESE MEDICAL CENTER, 2615 Washington Street, Zip 60085–4988; tel. 847/249–3900; Timothy P. Selz, President (Total facility includes 25 beds in nursing home–type unit) **A**1 2 7 9 10 **F**3 4 7 8 10 11 12 13 14 15 16 17 18 19 20 21 22 23 24 25 26 27 28 29 30 31 32 33 34 35 39 40 41 42 44 45 46 48 49 51 52 53 54 55 56 58 59 63 64 65 66 67 68 70 71 72 73 74 **P**3 5 7 8 **S** Franciscan Sisters Health Care Corporation, Frankfort, IL **N** MEDACOM Tri–State, Oakbrook, IL	21	10	254	8289	112	224190	1263	67062	30030	832
✶ VICTORY MEMORIAL HOSPITAL, 1324 North Sheridan Road, Zip 60085–2181; tel. 847/360–3000; Timothy Harrington, President **A**1 2 9 10 **F**1 2 3 4 7 8 10 12 14 15 16 18 19 21 22 24 25 26 28 29 30 32 33 34 35 37 39 40 41 42 44 45 46 49 52 54 55 56 57 58 59 60 63 64 65 67 71 73 **P**1 7	23	10	171	7630	91	87015	1321	63462	26605	780
WEST FRANKFORT—Franklin County										
★ UNITED MINE WORKERS OF AMERICA UNION HOSPITAL, 507 West St. Louis Street, Zip 62896–1999; tel. 618/932–2155; Ronald Slaviero, Administrator **A**9 10 **F**19 32 44 70 71 73 **S** Southern Illinois Hospital Services, Carbondale, IL	23	10	32	361	4	—	0	4688	2042	—
WHEATON—Du Page County										
✶ △ MARIANJOY REHABILITATION HOSPITAL AND CLINICS, 26 West 171 Roosevelt Road, Zip 60187, Mailing Address: P.O. Box 795, Zip 60189–0795; tel. 630/462–4000; Bruce A. Schurman, President **A**1 3 5 7 9 10 **F**5 17 19 21 22 25 27 29 32 34 35 41 45 46 48 49 50 54 62 63 65 66 67 71 73 **P**1 **S** Wheaton Franciscan Services, Inc., Wheaton, IL	21	46	107	1610	94	17234	0	38969	17966	431
WINFIELD—Du Page County										
ALCOHOLISM TREATMENT CENTER, 27 West 350 High Lake Road, Zip 60190; tel. 708/653–4000; David Fox, President (Nonreporting)	23	82	52	—	—	—	—	—	—	—
✶ CENTRAL DUPAGE HOSPITAL, 25 North Winfield Road, Zip 60190; tel. 630/682–1600; George G. Holzhauer, President **A**1 2 9 10 **F**2 3 4 7 8 10 11 12 15 16 17 19 20 21 22 23 25 28 29 30 32 33 34 35 37 38 40 41 42 43 44 45 46 47 49 51 52 53 54 56 57 58 59 62 64 65 67 70 71 72 73 **P**6	23	10	326	13185	143	216624	3141	140231	54453	1308
WOOD RIVER—Madison County										
✶ WOOD RIVER TOWNSHIP HOSPITAL, 101 East Edwardsville Road, Zip 62095–1332; tel. 618/254–3821; Max L. Ludeke, FACHE, Interim Chief Executive Officer (Total facility includes 15 beds in nursing home–type unit) **A**1 9 10 **F**3 7 8 10 12 13 14 15 16 17 18 19 21 22 26 27 28 29 30 31 32 33 34 35 36 37 38 39 40 41 44 45 46 47 48 49 51 52 54 55 56 57 58 60 64 65 66 67 68 71 73 74 **S** Brim, Inc., Portland, OR	16	10	128	1816	35	16164	229	18953	7849	288
WOODSTOCK—McHenry County										
✶ MEMORIAL MEDICAL CENTER, Highway 14 and Doty Road, Zip 60098–3797, Mailing Address: P.O. Box 1990, Zip 60098; tel. 815/338–2500; Jim D. Redding, Chief Executive Officer (Total facility includes 20 beds in nursing home–type unit) **A**1 2 9 10 **F**2 3 4 7 8 10 12 14 15 16 17 18 19 20 22 24 26 27 28 29 30 32 33 34 35 36 37 39 40 41 42 44 45 46 48 49 52 53 54 55 56 57 58 59 60 64 65 66 67 68 70 71 73 74 **P**4 5 6 7 **N** Centegra Health System, McHenry, IL	23	10	128	4662	65	48522	553	47071	18726	520
ZION—Lake County										
□ MIDWESTERN REGIONAL MEDICAL CENTER, 2501 Emmaus Avenue, Zip 60099–2587; tel. 847/872–4561; Roger C. Cary, President and Chief Executive Officer **A**1 2 9 10 **F**8 12 14 15 16 17 19 21 22 27 28 29 30 31 33 34 35 37 39 41 42 44 45 46 49 51 54 60 65 66 68 69 71 73 **S** Cancer Treatment Centers of America, Arlington Heights, IL	33	10	70	2103	30	81500	0	51885	12129	372

INDIANA

Resident population 5,803 (in thousands)
Resident population in metro areas 71.7%
Birth rate per 1,000 population 14.7
65 years and over 12.5%
Percent of persons without health insurance 10.5%

Hospital, Address, Telephone, Administrator, Approval, Facility, and Physician Codes, Health Care System, Network

★ American Hospital Association (AHA) membership
□ Joint Commission on Accreditation of Healthcare Organizations (JCAHO) accreditation
\+ American Osteopathic Hospital Association (AOHA) membership
○ American Osteopathic Association (AOA) accreditation
△ Commission on Accreditation of Rehabilitation Facilities (CARF) accreditation
Control codes 61, 63, 64, 71, 72 and 73 indicate hospitals listed by AOHA, but not registered by AHA. For definition of numerical codes, see page A4

Hospital	Classification Codes		Utilization Data					Expense (thousands) of dollars		
	Control	Service	Beds	Admissions	Census	Outpatient Visits	Births	Total	Payroll	Personnel
ANDERSON—Madison County										
★□ COMMUNITY HOSPITAL OF ANDERSON AND MADISON COUNTY, 1515 North Madison Avenue, Zip 46011–3453; tel. 765/642–8011; William C. Vanness, II, M.D., Chief Executive Officer (Total facility includes 30 beds in nursing home–type unit) (Nonreporting) **A**1 2 9 10 **N** Midwest Health Net, LLC., Fort Wayne, IN	23	10	177	—	—	—	—	—	—	—
★□ SAINT JOHN'S HEALTH SYSTEM, 2015 Jackson Street, Zip 46016–4339; tel. 765/649–2511; James H. Stephens, President and Chief Executive Officer (Total facility includes 29 beds in nursing home–type unit) **A**1 2 9 10 **F**1 2 3 4 7 8 10 12 14 15 16 17 18 19 20 21 22 23 25 26 27 28 29 30 31 32 33 34 35 37 39 40 41 42 44 45 48 49 52 53 54 55 56 57 58 59 60 63 64 65 66 67 68 71 72 73 74 **P**8 **S** Holy Cross Health System Corporation, South Bend, IN **N** Sagamore Health Network, Inc., Carmel, IN; Holy Cross Health System, South Bend, IN	21	10	371	8131	139	247701	461	90836	34809	1278
ANGOLA—Steuben County										
★ CAMERON MEMORIAL COMMUNITY HOSPITAL, 416 East Maumee Street, Zip 46703; tel. 219/665–2141; Dennis L. Knapp, President **A**9 10 **F**3 7 8 14 15 19 22 29 30 32 33 34 35 36 37 39 40 44 46 49 58 65 67 71 73 **N** LutheranPreferred Network, Fort Wayne, IN; Midwest Health Net, LLC., Fort Wayne, IN; Sagamore Health Network, Inc., Carmel, IN	23	10	30	1245	9	65561	352	13779	6877	239
AUBURN—De Kalb County										
★□ DEKALB MEMORIAL HOSPITAL, 1316 East Seventh Street, Zip 46706–0542, Mailing Address: P.O. Box 542, Zip 46706; tel. 219/925–4600; Jack M. Corey, President **A**1 9 10 **F**7 8 11 12 14 15 16 17 19 21 22 24 26 28 29 30 32 33 34 37 39 40 41 42 44 45 46 49 51 65 67 71 72 73 **P**4 6 7 **N** LutheranPreferred Network, Fort Wayne, IN; Midwest Health Net, LLC., Fort Wayne, IN	23	10	47	2040	18	43617	458	21116	9846	311
BATESVILLE—Franklin County										
★□ MARGARET MARY COMMUNITY HOSPITAL, 321 Mitchell Avenue, Zip 47006–8953, Mailing Address: P.O. Box 226, Zip 47006–0226; tel. 812/934–6624; James L. Amos, President (Total facility includes 35 beds in nursing home–type unit) **A**1 9 10 **F**7 8 15 19 20 21 22 26 28 30 32 33 34 35 36 37 40 41 42 44 49 63 64 65 67 71 73	23	10	94	2202	49	88482	394	17603	8215	261
BEDFORD—Lawrence County										
★□ BEDFORD REGIONAL MEDICAL CENTER, 2900 West 16th Street, Zip 47421; tel. 812/275–1200; John R. Birdzell, FACHE, Chief Executive Officer **A**1 2 9 10 **F**7 8 10 14 15 17 19 20 21 22 27 28 30 32 33 34 35 37 39 40 42 44 45 46 49 51 63 65 71 72 73 **P**6 **N** Midwest Health Net, LLC., Fort Wayne, IN	23	10	60	2917	23	164274	408	32324	13200	378
★□ DUNN MEMORIAL HOSPITAL, 1600 23rd Street, Zip 47421–4704; tel. 812/275–3331; Richard W. Hahn, Executive Director **A**1 9 10 **F**1 7 8 10 11 13 17 19 22 27 28 29 30 31 32 33 34 37 39 40 42 44 45 46 49 51 65 71 73 74 **P**3 **N** Sagamore Health Network, Inc., Carmel, IN	13	10	96	2963	34	40172	285	25212	12168	455
BEECH GROVE—Marion County										
★□ ST. FRANCIS HOSPITAL AND HEALTH CENTERS, 1600 Albany Street, Zip 46107–1593; tel. 317/787–3311; Robert J. Brody, President and Chief Executive Officer (Nonreporting) **A**1 2 3 5 9 10 **S** Sisters of St. Francis Health Services, Inc., Mishawaka, IN **N** Sagamore Health Network, Inc., Carmel, IN	21	10	396	—	—	—	—	—	—	—
BLOOMINGTON—Monroe County										
★□ BLOOMINGTON HOSPITAL, 601 West Second Street, Zip 47403–2317, Mailing Address: Box 1149, Zip 47402–1149; tel. 812/336–6821; Nancy S. Carlstedt, President (Total facility includes 362 beds in nursing home–type unit) **A**1 9 10 **F**1 2 4 6 7 8 10 11 12 14 15 16 17 19 21 22 23 25 26 27 29 30 31 32 33 34 35 36 37 40 41 42 43 44 45 46 48 49 52 53 54 55 56 57 59 60 64 65 66 67 70 71 73 74 **P**8	23	10	617	13723	306	242258	1792	109173	49885	1541
BLUFFTON—Wells County										
★□ CAYLOR–NICKEL MEDICAL CENTER, One Caylor–Nickel Square, Zip 46714; tel. 219/824–3500; William F. Brockmann, President and Chief Executive Officer (Total facility includes 19 beds in nursing home–type unit) **A**1 2 9 10 **F**3 5 7 8 10 11 12 14 15 16 17 19 20 21 22 24 25 26 30 32 33 34 35 37 39 40 41 42 44 45 46 49 51 52 53 54 56 57 58 60 64 65 67 71 73 **P**1 7 **N** LutheranPreferred Network, Fort Wayne, IN; Health Quest, Bluffton, IN; Midwest Health Net, LLC., Fort Wayne, IN	23	10	99	3225	40	72960	278	27308	11450	460
★□ WELLS COMMUNITY HOSPITAL, 1100 South Main Street, Zip 46714; tel. 219/824–3210; Martin P. Braaksma, Executive Director (Nonreporting) **A**1 9 10 **N** LutheranPreferred Network, Fort Wayne, IN; Midwest Health Net, LLC., Fort Wayne, IN; Sagamore Health Network, Inc., Carmel, IN	13	10	38	—	—	—	—	—	—	—
BOONVILLE—Warrick County										
★□ ST. MARY'S HOSPITAL WARRICK, (Formerly Warrick Hospital), 1116 Millis Avenue, Zip 47601–0629, Mailing Address: Box 629, Zip 47601–0629; tel. 812/897–4800; John D. O'Neil, Executive Vice President and Administrator **A**1 9 10 **F**8 14 15 16 17 19 20 22 28 31 32 37 41 44 49 64 65 71 73 **S** Daughters of Charity National Health System, Saint Louis, MO **N** Sagamore Health Network, Inc., Carmel, IN	23	10	36	1294	14	10840	0	9931	5235	257

Hospital, Address, Telephone, Administrator, Approval, Facility, and Physician Codes, Health Care System, Network	Classification Codes		Utilization Data					Expense (thousands) of dollars		
	Control	Service	Beds	Admissions	Census	Outpatient Visits	Births	Total	Payroll	Personnel

★ American Hospital Association (AHA) membership
□ Joint Commission on Accreditation of Healthcare Organizations (JCAHO) accreditation
+ American Osteopathic Hospital Association (AOHA) membership
○ American Osteopathic Association (AOA) accreditation
△ Commission on Accreditation of Rehabilitation Facilities (CARF) accreditation
Control codes 61, 63, 64, 71, 72 and 73 indicate hospitals listed by AOHA, but not registered by AHA. For definition of numerical codes, see page A4

BRAZIL—Clay County

✠ CLAY COUNTY HOSPITAL, 1206 East National Avenue, Zip 47834–2797; tel. 812/448–2675; Jay P. Jolly, Administrator and Chief Executive Officer **A**1 9 10 **F**7 8 19 20 21 22 30 34 35 37 40 42 44 45 51 65 67 71 73 **N** Sagamore Health Network, Inc., Carmel, IN — 13 10 58 1102 12 23450 93 8453 3507 164

BREMEN—Marshall County

★ COMMUNITY HOSPITAL OF BREMEN, 411 South Whitlock Street, Zip 46506–1699; tel. 219/546–2211; Scott R. Graybill, Administrator and Chief Executive Officer **A**9 10 **F**8 12 15 17 19 22 26 27 32 33 34 41 44 45 49 51 53 54 55 56 57 58 59 64 65 66 71 73 **P**1 3 **S** Ancilla Systems Inc., Hobart, IN **N** Ancilla Systems, Inc., Hobart, IN; Sagamore Health Network, Inc., Carmel, IN — 23 10 28 474 4 30123 79 5625 2334 95

CARMEL—Hamilton County

ST. VINCENT CARMEL HOSPITAL See St. Vincent Hospitals and Health Services, Indianapolis

CHARLESTOWN—Clark County

□ MEDICAL CENTER OF SOUTHERN INDIANA, 2200 Market Street, Zip 47111–0069, Mailing Address: P.O. Box 69, Zip 47111–0069; tel. 812/256–3301; Kevin J. Miller, Chief Executive Officer **A**1 10 **F**4 6 7 8 9 12 13 14 15 16 19 20 21 22 23 25 26 28 29 30 31 32 34 35 37 38 39 40 41 42 43 44 45 46 47 48 49 50 51 52 57 58 59 60 63 64 65 66 67 69 70 71 72 73 74 **P**5 7 **N** Sagamore Health Network, Inc., Carmel, IN — 23 10 80 1916 42 27816 0 13423 7588 274

CLINTON—Vermillion County

□ WEST CENTRAL COMMUNITY HOSPITAL, (Formerly Vermillion County Hospital), 801 South Main Street, Zip 47842–0349; tel. 317/832–2451; Marilyn J. Custer-Mitchell, Chief Executive Officer **A**1 9 10 **F**7 8 12 19 21 22 24 25 28 34 37 39 40 42 44 46 49 65 67 71 73 — 13 10 23 1167 16 32036 70 9947 3795 178

COLUMBIA CITY—Whitley County

□ WHITLEY MEMORIAL HOSPITAL, (Formerly Whitley County Memorial Hospital), 353 North Oak Street, Zip 46725; tel. 219/244–6191; John M. Hatcher, President (Total facility includes 82 beds in nursing home–type unit) (Nonreporting) **A**1 9 10 **N** Parkview Health System, Fort Wayne, IN; Midwest Health Net, LLC., Fort Wayne, IN; Sagamore Health Network, Inc., Carmel, IN — 13 10 130 — — — — — — —

COLUMBUS—Bartholomew County

✠ △ COLUMBUS REGIONAL HOSPITAL, 2400 East 17th Street, Zip 47201–5360; tel. 812/379–4441; John C. McGinty, Jr., President and Chief Executive Officer (Total facility includes 20 beds in nursing home–type unit) **A**1 2 7 9 10 **F**7 8 10 12 14 15 16 17 18 19 21 22 23 27 28 29 30 32 33 34 35 36 37 39 40 41 42 44 45 46 48 49 51 52 53 54 55 56 57 58 59 60 63 64 65 66 67 71 72 73 74 **P**3 5 6 7 8 — 13 10 237 9569 113 111840 1343 91330 38501 1152

□ KOALA BEHAVIORAL HEALTH–COLUMBUS CAMPUS, 2223 Poshard Drive, Zip 47203; tel. 812/376–1711; Thomas N. Theroult, Administrator **A**1 9 10 **F**2 3 12 16 18 27 34 46 52 53 54 55 56 57 58 59 65 68 **S** Sterling Healthcare Corporation, Bellevue, WA — 33 22 60 816 30 3500 0 4182 2538 83

CONNERSVILLE—Fayette County

✠ FAYETTE MEMORIAL HOSPITAL, 1941 Virginia Avenue, Zip 47331–9990; tel. 765/825–5131; David Brandon, Chief Executive Officer **A**1 9 10 **F**3 7 8 12 14 15 16 19 21 22 24 26 27 28 29 30 31 32 33 34 37 39 40 41 44 45 49 52 53 54 55 56 58 59 65 66 67 71 72 73 **P**1 3 4 6 — 23 10 111 2880 38 57561 260 25522 11436 485

CORYDON—Harrison County

✠ HARRISON COUNTY HOSPITAL, 245 Atwood Street, Zip 47112–1774; tel. 812/738–4251; Steven L. Taylor, Chief Executive Officer **A**1 9 10 **F**7 8 14 15 16 19 21 22 28 30 32 33 34 35 37 40 41 42 44 46 49 51 63 65 66 71 **P**6 7 **S** Alliant Health System, Louisville, KY — 13 10 46 1507 16 28398 135 13240 5816 255

CRAWFORDSVILLE—Montgomery County

□ CULVER UNION HOSPITAL, 1710 Lafayette Road, Zip 47933; tel. 765/362–2800; Gregory D. Starnes, Chief Executive Officer (Total facility includes 17 beds in nursing home–type unit) **A**1 9 10 **F**7 8 11 12 14 15 16 19 22 28 32 34 35 36 37 39 40 41 42 44 48 49 52 54 56 57 64 66 67 71 72 73 74 **P**2 4 5 6 7 8 **S** TENET Healthcare Corporation, Santa Barbara, CA — 33 10 98 3926 48 50485 387 23244 8087 346

CROWN POINT—Lake County

✠ ST. ANTHONY MEDICAL CENTER, 1201 South Main Street, Zip 46307–8483; tel. 219/738–2100; Stephen O. Leurck, President **A**1 2 6 9 10 **F**1 4 6 7 8 10 11 12 13 15 16 17 18 19 21 22 24 25 28 30 32 33 34 35 36 39 40 41 42 43 44 45 48 49 50 51 54 55 56 57 60 63 64 65 67 71 72 73 **P**3 4 6 7 **N** Sagamore Health Network, Inc., Carmel, IN — 21 10 248 8360 127 72278 849 92450 39224 854

DANVILLE—Hendricks County

✠ HENDRICKS COMMUNITY HOSPITAL, 1000 East Main Street, Zip 46122–0409, Mailing Address: P.O. Box 409, Zip 46122–0409; tel. 317/745–4451; Dennis W. Dawes, President **A**1 9 10 **F**2 7 8 12 14 15 16 19 20 21 22 24 28 29 30 31 32 34 35 36 37 39 40 41 42 44 45 49 51 52 54 55 56 57 65 66 67 71 72 73 74 **P**6 7 8 **N** Sagamore Health Network, Inc., Carmel, IN; Suburban Health Organization, Indianapolis, IN — 13 10 127 5446 56 163313 795 42222 19614 555

DECATUR—Adams County

★ ADAMS COUNTY MEMORIAL HOSPITAL, 805 High Street, Zip 46733, Mailing Address: P.O. Box 151, Zip 46733; tel. 219/724–2145; Marvin L. Baird, Executive Director (Total facility includes 22 beds in nursing home–type unit) **A**9 10 **F**1 7 8 30 11 14 15 16 19 21 22 26 27 28 30 32 35 40 41 42 44 46 49 51 52 53 56 57 58 59 62 64 65 71 72 73 74 **N** LutheranPreferred Network, Fort Wayne, IN; Sagamore Health Network, Inc., Carmel, IN — 13 10 87 2315 41 55454 242 17851 8169 279

Hospital, Address, Telephone, Administrator, Approval, Facility, and Physician Codes, Health Care System, Network	Classi-fication Codes		Utilization Data					Expense (thousands) of dollars		
	Control	Service	Beds	Admissions	Census	Outpatient Visits	Births	Total	Payroll	Personnel

★ American Hospital Association (AHA) membership
□ Joint Commission on Accreditation of Healthcare Organizations (JCAHO) accreditation
+ American Osteopathic Hospital Association (AOHA) membership
○ American Osteopathic Association (AOA) accreditation
△ Commission on Accreditation of Rehabilitation Facilities (CARF) accreditation
   Control codes 61, 63, 64, 71, 72 and 73 indicate hospitals listed by AOHA, but not registered by AHA. For definition of numerical codes, see page A4

DYER—Lake County

SAINT MARGARET MERCY HEALTHCARE CENTERS–SOUTH CAMPUS See Saint Margaret Mercy Healthcare Centers, Hammond

EAST CHICAGO—Lake County

| ST. CATHERINE HOSPITAL, 4321 Fir Street, Zip 46312; tel. 219/392–7000; JoAnn Birdzell, President and Chief Executive Officer **A**1 9 10 **F**4 7 8 10 12 14 15 16 17 19 21 22 23 24 25 28 29 30 31 32 33 34 35 39 40 41 42 43 44 45 46 50 52 56 60 63 64 65 71 73 74 **P**2 3 6 7 8 **S** Ancilla Systems Inc., Hobart, IN **N** Ancilla Systems, Inc., Hobart, IN; Midwest Health Net, LLC., Fort Wayne, IN; Sagamore Health Network, Inc., Carmel, IN | 21 | 10 | 204 | 6800 | 115 | 41153 | 492 | 61399 | 22412 | 670 |

ELKHART—Elkhart County

| ELKHART GENERAL HOSPITAL, 600 East Boulevard, Zip 46514, Mailing Address: Box 1329, Zip 46515; tel. 219/294–2621; Gregory W. Lintjer, President (Total facility includes 42 beds in nursing home–type unit) **A**1 9 10 **F**3 7 8 10 11 12 15 16 17 19 21 22 23 30 31 32 35 37 38 39 40 41 43 44 49 52 53 54 55 56 58 59 60 64 65 67 71 73 **P**5 8 **N** Memorial Health System, Inc., South Bend, IN | 23 | 10 | 308 | 11623 | 170 | 98323 | 1599 | 91640 | 39094 | 1289 |

ELWOOD—Madison County

| ST. VINCENT MERCY HOSPITAL, 1331 South A Street, Zip 46036–1942; tel. 765/552–4600; Ann C. Parsons, Interim Administrator **A**1 9 10 **F**7 8 11 15 17 19 20 22 31 33 35 37 40 41 42 44 49 51 61 64 65 66 67 71 73 **P**3 5 8 **N** Sagamore Health Network, Inc., Carmel, IN; Saint Vincent Hospitals and Health Services, Inc., Indianapolis, IN | 21 | 10 | 40 | 1762 | 21 | 26429 | 124 | 9909 | 4492 | — |

EVANSVILLE—Vanderburgh County

△ DEACONESS HOSPITAL, 600 Mary Street, Zip 47747–0001; tel. 812/426–3000; Thomas H. Kramer, President (Total facility includes 48 beds in nursing home–type unit) **A**1 2 3 5 7 9 10 **F**2 4 7 8 10 11 14 15 16 17 19 21 22 23 24 26 27 28 29 30 31 32 33 34 35 36 37 39 40 41 42 43 44 46 47 49 51 54 56 60 61 62 63 64 65 67 70 71 73 74 **P**1 6 7 8	23	10	388	16757	249	101237	1330	140029	62905	1898
EVANSVILLE STATE HOSPITAL, 3400 Lincoln Avenue, Zip 47714–0146; tel. 812/473–2100; Ralph Nichols, Superintendent **A**1 9 **F**14 20 41 49 52 57 65 73	12	22	330	73	282	0	0	21182	11733	522
△ HEALTHSOUTH TRI–STATE REHABILITATION HOSPITAL, 4100 Covert Avenue, Zip 47714, Mailing Address: P.O. Box 5349, Zip 47716–5349; tel. 812/476–9983; Gerald F. Vozel, Administrator and Chief Executive Officer **A**1 7 9 10 **F**12 15 16 19 27 32 34 35 48 49 65 67 71 73 **S** HEALTHSOUTH Corporation, Birmingham, AL	33	46	80	772	47	6150	0	12633	6033	190
ST. MARY'S MEDICAL CENTER OF EVANSVILLE, 3700 Washington Avenue, Zip 47750; tel. 812/485–4000; Richard C. Breon, President and Chief Executive Officer (Total facility includes 128 beds in nursing home–type unit) **A**1 2 3 5 9 10 **F**3 4 7 8 10 11 12 14 15 16 17 19 21 22 23 24 25 28 30 32 34 35 37 38 40 41 42 43 44 47 49 52 54 55 56 57 58 59 60 61 64 65 66 67 68 71 72 73 74 **P**7 8 **S** Daughters of Charity National Health System, Saint Louis, MO **N** Ancilla Systems, Inc., Hobart, IN; Sagamore Health Network, Inc., Carmel, IN	21	10	549	12160	310	220504	2006	123139	54024	1740
△ WELBORN MEMORIAL BAPTIST HOSPITAL, 401 Southeast Sixth Street, Zip 47713–1299; tel. 812/426–8000; Marjorie Z. Soyugenc, President and Chief Executive Officer (Total facility includes 19 beds in nursing home–type unit) **A**1 2 7 9 10 **F**2 3 4 7 8 10 11 12 14 15 16 19 21 22 23 24 26 28 29 30 31 32 33 35 36 37 38 39 40 41 42 43 44 45 46 48 49 51 52 53 54 55 56 58 59 60 61 63 64 65 67 69 71 73 **P**1 5 6 7	23	10	296	10217	156	—	1037	84210	41437	1244

FORT WAYNE—Allen County

CHARTER BEACON, 1720 Beacon Street, Zip 46805; tel. 219/423–3651; Robert Hails, Chief Executive Officer **A**1 9 10 **F**3 14 15 16 17 18 25 26 52 53 54 55 56 57 58 59 **S** Magellan Health Services, Atlanta, GA	33	22	97	1105	46	0	0	—	—	118
LUTHERAN HOSPITAL OF INDIANA, 7950 West Jefferson Boulevard, Zip 46804–1677; tel. 219/435–7001; William L. Anderson, Chief Executive Officer **A**1 3 5 9 10 **F**3 4 7 8 10 11 14 15 16 18 19 20 21 22 23 26 28 29 30 31 32 33 34 35 36 37 38 39 40 41 42 43 44 47 49 52 54 55 56 57 58 59 60 61 63 64 65 66 69 71 72 73 74 **P**5 7 **S** Quorum Health Group/Quorum Health Resources, Inc., Brentwood, TN **N** LutheranPreferred Network, Fort Wayne, IN; Memorial Health System, Inc., South Bend, IN	33	10	342	12979	175	129214	1537	—	—	1292
△ PARKVIEW MEMORIAL HOSPITAL, 2200 Randallia Drive, Zip 46805; tel. 219/484–6636; Frank D. Byrne, M.D., President (Total facility includes 28 beds in nursing home–type unit) **A**1 3 5 7 9 10 **F**2 3 4 7 8 10 11 12 14 15 16 17 18 19 21 22 24 25 27 28 30 32 33 34 36 37 38 39 40 41 42 43 44 45 46 47 48 49 51 52 53 54 55 56 57 58 59 60 64 65 67 68 71 72 73 74 **P**6 7 8 **N** Parkview Health System, Fort Wayne, IN; Midwest Health Net, LLC., Fort Wayne, IN; Sagamore Health Network, Inc., Carmel, IN	23	10	493	22200	310	130572	3733	222757	105974	2980
△ ST. JOSEPH MEDICAL CENTER OF FORT WAYNE, 700 Broadway, Zip 46802; tel. 219/425–3000; John T. Farrell, Sr., President and Chief Executive Officer **A**1 3 5 7 9 10 **F**2 4 7 8 10 11 12 13 14 15 16 17 19 21 22 24 26 27 28 30 31 32 34 35 36 37 39 40 41 43 44 46 48 49 52 64 65 71 72 73 **P**3 6 7 8 **S** Ancilla Systems Inc., Hobart, IN **N** Ancilla Systems, Inc., Hobart, IN; Midwest Health Net, LLC., Fort Wayne, IN; Sagamore Health Network, Inc., Carmel, IN	21	10	194	7050	112	118317	723	66237	24409	748
VETERANS AFFAIRS NORTHERN INDIANA HEALTH CARE SYSTEM–FORT WAYNE DIVISION, 2121 Lake Avenue, Zip 46805–5347; tel. 219/426–5431; Michael W. Murphy, Ph.D., Director (Total facility includes 123 beds in nursing home–type unit) **A**1 9 **F**1 2 3 8 17 19 20 21 22 26 27 30 31 32 33 34 35 37 39 42 44 46 48 49 51 52 54 55 56 57 58 59 60 64 65 67 71 73 74 **P**1 **S** Department of Veterans Affairs, Washington, DC	45	22	568	3658	479	102564	0	97219	60820	1243

Hospital, Address, Telephone, Administrator, Approval, Facility, and Physician Codes, Health Care System, Network	Classi-fication Codes		Utilization Data					Expense (thousands) of dollars		
	Control	Service	Beds	Admissions	Census	Outpatient Visits	Births	Total	Payroll	Personnel

★ American Hospital Association (AHA) membership
☐ Joint Commission on Accreditation of Healthcare Organizations (JCAHO) accreditation
+ American Osteopathic Hospital Association (AOHA) membership
○ American Osteopathic Association (AOA) accreditation
△ Commission on Accreditation of Rehabilitation Facilities (CARF) accreditation
Control codes 61, 63, 64, 71, 72 and 73 indicate hospitals listed by AOHA, but not registered by AHA. For definition of numerical codes, see page A4

FRANKFORT—Clinton County

✠ CLINTON COUNTY HOSPITAL, 1300 South Jackson Street, Zip 46041–3394, Mailing Address: P.O. Box 669, Zip 46041–0669; tel. 765/659–4731; Brian R. Zeh, Executive Director **A**1 9 10 **F**7 8 14 19 21 22 24 26 27 28 29 30 31 32 34 35 37 39 40 41 42 44 45 46 49 54 63 65 66 71 73 74 **P**1 6 **N** Midwest Health Net, LLC., Fort Wayne, IN; Sagamore Health Network, Inc., Carmel, IN; Suburban Health Organization, Indianapolis, IN	13	10	53	1554	13	39253	321	14311	6539	178

FRANKLIN—Johnson County

✠ JOHNSON MEMORIAL HOSPITAL, 1125 West Jefferson Street, Zip 46131–2140, Mailing Address: P.O. Box 549, Zip 46131–0549; tel. 317/736–3300; Gregg A. Bechtold, President and Chief Executive Officer (Total facility includes 87 beds in nursing home–type unit) **A**1 9 10 **F**1 7 8 12 14 15 16 17 19 21 22 26 28 29 30 34 35 37 39 40 41 42 44 45 46 49 51 64 65 67 71 73 **P**6 8 **N** Midwest Health Net, LLC., Fort Wayne, IN; Sagamore Health Network, Inc., Carmel, IN; Suburban Health Organization, Indianapolis, IN	13	10	160	4030	104	66850	543	31779	13293	438

GARY—Lake County

✠ △ METHODIST HOSPITALS, (Includes Northlake Campus, Southlake Campus, 8701 Broadway, Merrillville, Zip 46410; tel. 219/738–5500), 600 Grant Street, Zip 46402; tel. 219/886–4000; John H. Betjemann, President (Total facility includes 26 beds in nursing home–type unit) **A**1 2 3 5 7 9 10 **F**1 2 3 4 5 7 8 10 11 15 19 21 22 23 26 28 29 30 34 35 37 38 39 40 41 42 43 44 48 49 51 52 53 54 55 57 58 60 61 63 64 65 67 71 72 73 74 **P**5 6 7	23	10	639	23003	391	240661	2405	198540	88575	2540

GOSHEN—Elkhart County

✠ GOSHEN GENERAL HOSPITAL, 200 High Park Avenue, Zip 46526, Mailing Address: P.O. Box 139, Zip 46527; tel. 219/533–2141; James O. Dague, President (Nonreporting) **A**1 9 10	23	10	90	—	—	—	—	—	—	—
☐ OAKLAWN PSYCHIATRIC CENTER, INC., 330 Lakeview Drive, Zip 46526–9365, Mailing Address: P.O. Box 809, Zip 46527–0809; tel. 219/533–1234; Harold C. Loewen, President **A**1 9 10 **F**1 3 12 15 16 17 18 26 27 31 52 53 54 55 56 57 58 59 65 73 **P**3 6 **N** Sagamore Health Network, Inc., Carmel, IN	23	22	40	1085	27	70125	0	17570	8943	386

GREENCASTLE—Putnam County

☐ PUTNAM COUNTY HOSPITAL, 1542 Bloomington Street, Zip 46135; tel. 765/653–5121; John D. Fajt, Executive Director **A**1 2 9 10 **F**7 8 14 15 16 17 19 20 21 22 26 28 30 32 35 37 39 40 41 42 44 46 48 49 56 65 67 71 **P**8 **N** Sagamore Health Network, Inc., Carmel, IN; Suburban Health Organization, Indianapolis, IN	13	10	85	1814	26	44560	239	12831	5961	242

GREENFIELD—Hancock County

✠ HANCOCK MEMORIAL HOSPITAL AND HEALTH SERVICES, 801 North State Street, Zip 46140–2537, Mailing Address: Box 827, Zip 46140; tel. 317/462–5544; Robert C. Keen, Ph.D., President and Chief Executive Officer (Total facility includes 21 beds in nursing home–type unit) **A**1 9 10 **F**3 7 8 10 11 14 15 16 17 19 21 22 24 28 30 31 32 33 34 35 36 37 39 40 41 42 44 45 46 49 52 57 60 64 65 66 67 68 71 72 73 74 **P**1 7 **N** Midwest Health Net, LLC., Fort Wayne, IN; Sagamore Health Network, Inc., Carmel, IN; Suburban Health Organization, Indianapolis, IN	13	10	102	3478	47	148294	511	38272	17295	489

GREENSBURG—Decatur County

✠ DECATUR COUNTY MEMORIAL HOSPITAL, 720 North Lincoln Street, Zip 47240–1398; tel. 812/663–4331; Charles Duffy, President **A**1 9 10 **F**1 7 8 16 19 20 21 22 23 27 28 30 32 33 34 35 36 37 40 41 42 44 45 46 49 63 65 67 71 73 **P**3 **S** Alliant Health System, Louisville, KY **N** Midwest Health Net, LLC., Fort Wayne, IN	13	10	75	1685	29	55595	253	14766	6450	227

GREENWOOD—Johnson County

☐ BHC VALLE VISTA HOSPITAL, (Formerly CPC Valle Vista Hospital), 898 East Main Street, Zip 46143; tel. 317/887–1348; Sheila Mishler, Chief Executive Officer (Nonreporting) **A**1 9 10 **S** Behavioral Healthcare Corporation, Nashville, TN	33	22	96	—	—	—	—	—	—	—

HAMMOND—Lake County

✠ SAINT MARGARET MERCY HEALTHCARE CENTERS, (Includes Saint Margaret Mercy Healthcare Centers–North Campus, Saint Margaret Mercy Healthcare Centers–South Campus, 24 Joliet Street, Dyer, Zip 46311–1799; tel. 219/865–2141), 5454 Hohman Avenue, Zip 46320; tel. 219/933–2074; Eugene C. Diamond, President and Chief Executive Officer (Total facility includes 67 beds in nursing home–type unit) **A**1 2 3 9 10 **F**2 3 4 7 8 10 11 12 13 14 15 16 17 19 20 21 22 27 28 29 30 32 34 35 36 37 38 39 40 42 43 44 45 46 47 48 49 51 52 53 54 55 56 57 58 59 60 64 65 67 68 71 73 74 **P**7 8 **S** Sisters of St. Francis Health Services, Inc., Mishawaka, IN **N** Sagamore Health Network, Inc., Carmel, IN	21	10	624	21241	359	117672	1549	171105	74197	2348

HARTFORD CITY—Blackford County

✠ BLACKFORD COUNTY HOSPITAL, 503 East Van Cleve Street, Zip 47348; tel. 765/348–0300; Mark A. Edwards, Chief Executive Officer **A**1 9 10 **F**14 15 16 19 22 28 30 32 33 34 35 40 44 45 49 63 65 70 71 72 **S** Alliant Health System, Louisville, KY **N** LutheranPreferred Network, Fort Wayne, IN	13	10	36	887	12	19736	66	6508	2824	130

HOBART—Lake County

☐ CHARTER BEHAVIORAL HEALTH SYSTEM OF NORTHWEST INDIANA, 101 West 61st Avenue and State Road 51, Zip 46342; tel. 219/947–4464; Michael J. Brown, Jr., Chief Executive Officer **A**1 9 10 **F**1 2 3 12 15 16 17 18 19 20 21 22 23 24 25 26 27 28 29 30 31 32 33 34 35 36 37 38 39 41 42 43 44 45 46 47 48 49 50 51 52 53 54 55 56 57 58 59 60 61 62 63 64 65 66 67 68 69 70 71 72 73 74 **S** Magellan Health Services, Atlanta, GA	33	22	60	1126	33	3722	0	—	—	61

Hospital, Address, Telephone, Administrator, Approval, Facility, and Physician Codes, Health Care System, Network	Classi-fication Codes		Utilization Data					Expense (thousands) of dollars		
	Control	Service	Beds	Admissions	Census	Outpatient Visits	Births	Total	Payroll	Personnel

★ American Hospital Association (AHA) membership
□ Joint Commission on Accreditation of Healthcare Organizations (JCAHO) accreditation
+ American Osteopathic Hospital Association (AOHA) membership
○ American Osteopathic Association (AOA) accreditation
△ Commission on Accreditation of Rehabilitation Facilities (CARF) accreditation
Control codes 61, 63, 64, 71, 72 and 73 indicate hospitals listed by AOHA, but not registered by AHA. For definition of numerical codes, see page A4

✖ ST. MARY MEDICAL CENTER, 1500 South Lake Park Avenue, Zip 46342; tel. 219/942–0551; Milton Triana, President and Chief Executive Officer (Nonreporting) **A**1 10 **S** Ancilla Systems Inc., Hobart, IN **N** Midwest Health Net, LLC., Fort Wayne, IN; Sagamore Health Network, Inc., Carmel, IN	21	10	102	—	—	—	—	—	—	—

HUNTINGBURG—Dubois County

□ ST. JOSEPH'S HOSPITAL, 1900 Medical Arts Drive, Zip 47542–9521, Mailing Address: P.O. Box 148, Zip 47542–0148; tel. 812/683–2121; Dale R. Mulder, President and Chief Executive Officer (Nonreporting) **A**1 9 10	23	10	76	—	—	—	—	—	—	—

HUNTINGTON—Huntington County

✖ HUNTINGTON MEMORIAL HOSPITAL, 1215 Etna Avenue, Zip 46750–3696; tel. 219/356–3000; L. Kent McCoy, President **A**1 9 10 **F**2 3 7 8 11 15 16 17 19 22 24 27 28 29 30 32 33 34 35 36 37 40 41 42 44 46 48 67 71 73 **P**1 3 5 7 **N** Parkview Health System, Fort Wayne, IN; LutheranPreferred Network, Fort Wayne, IN; Midwest Health Net, LLC., Fort Wayne, IN; Sagamore Health Network, Inc., Carmel, IN	23	10	37	1888	20	43484	249	17041	8068	269

INDIANAPOLIS—Marion County

□ CHARTER INDIANAPOLIS BEHAVIORAL HEALTH SYSTEM, 5602 Caito Drive, Zip 46226; tel. 317/545–2111; Marina Cecchini, Chief Executive Officer **A**1 9 10 **F**2 3 14 15 16 52 53 54 55 56 57 58 59 65 **P**8 **S** Magellan Health Services, Atlanta, GA	33	22	80	1441	53	33040	0	—	—	127
✖ COLUMBIA WOMEN'S HOSPITAL–INDIANAPOLIS, 8111 Township Line Road, Zip 46260–8043; tel. 317/875–5994; Steven B. Reed, President and Chief Executive Officer **A**1 9 10 **F**7 8 19 26 28 30 38 40 44 45 46 52 57 59 61 65 71 73 74 **S** Columbia/HCA Healthcare Corporation, Nashville, TN	33	10	132	3890	39	—	2411	20410	8938	297
□ △ COMMUNITY HOSPITALS INDIANAPOLIS, (Includes Community Hospital North; Community Hospital South, 1402 East County Line Road South, Zip 46227; tel. 317/887–7000), 1500 North Ritter Avenue, Zip 46219–3095; tel. 317/355–1411; William E. Corley, President (Nonreporting) **A**1 2 3 5 7 9 10	23	10	822	—	—	—	—	—	—	—
FAIRBANKS HOSPITAL, 8102 Clearvista Parkway, Zip 46256–4698; tel. 317/849–8222; Timothy J. Kelly, M.D., President (Nonreporting) **A**9 10 **N** Sagamore Health Network, Inc., Carmel, IN	23	82	96	—	—	—	—	—	—	—
✖ INDIANA UNIVERSITY MEDICAL CENTER, (Includes Riley Hospital, University Hospital and Outpatient Center), 550 North University Boulevard, Zip 46202–5262; tel. 317/274–5000; David J. Handel, Director **A**1 2 3 5 8 9 10 **F**2 4 5 7 8 9 10 11 12 13 14 15 16 17 19 20 21 22 23 30 31 32 34 35 37 38 39 40 41 42 43 44 46 47 49 50 51 53 54 55 56 57 58 60 61 63 65 68 69 71 73 74 **P**1 **N** LutheranPreferred Network, Fort Wayne, IN; Sagamore Health Network, Inc., Carmel, IN	12	10	552	20236	376	386005	1144	329477	127453	3700
□ LARUE D. CARTER MEMORIAL HOSPITAL, 2601 Cold Spring Road, Zip 46222; tel. 317/941–4000; Diana Haugh, MS, Superintendent **A**1 3 5 9 10 **F**12 16 27 29 30 31 34 45 46 50 52 53 54 55 56 58 65 67 73 **P**1	12	22	146	263	149	2328	0	16286	9326	366
✖ METHODIST HOSPITAL OF INDIANA, 1701 North Senate Boulevard, Zip 46202, Mailing Address: I. 65 at 21st Street, P.O. Box 1367, Zip 46206–1367; tel. 317/929–2000; William J. Loveday, President and Chief Executive Officer (Total facility includes 60 beds in nursing home–type unit) **A**1 2 3 5 8 9 10 **F**2 3 4 5 7 8 10 11 12 13 14 15 16 17 18 19 20 21 22 23 25 26 28 29 30 31 32 33 34 35 36 37 38 39 40 41 42 43 44 45 46 47 48 49 51 52 53 54 55 56 57 58 59 60 61 63 64 65 66 67 68 69 70 71 72 73 74 **P**1 4 5 7 **N** Midwest Health Net, LLC., Fort Wayne, IN; Sagamore Health Network, Inc., Carmel, IN; Methodist Hospital of Indiana, Indianapolis, IN	23	10	779	43375	570	420095	3737	401537	175590	4777
✖ △ REHABILITATION HOSPITAL OF INDIANA, 4141 Shore Drive, Zip 46254–2607; tel. 317/329–2000; Kim D. Eicher, Administrator and Chief Executive Officer (Nonreporting) **A**1 7 10 **N** Sagamore Health Network, Inc., Carmel, IN; Methodist Hospital of Indiana, Indianapolis, IN	23	46	80	—	—	—	—	—	—	—
✖ RICHARD L. ROUDEBUSH VETERANS AFFAIRS MEDICAL CENTER, 1481 West Tenth Street, Zip 46202; tel. 317/635–7401; Alice Wood, Director (Total facility includes 35 beds in nursing home–type unit) **A**1 3 5 8 9 **F**1 3 4 5 8 10 11 12 14 15 16 17 18 19 20 21 22 23 26 27 28 29 30 31 32 34 35 37 39 41 42 43 44 45 46 48 49 50 51 52 54 55 56 57 58 59 60 64 65 67 69 71 73 74 **P**6 **S** Department of Veterans Affairs, Washington, DC	45	10	197	6207	171	271698	0	145091	67576	1562
RILEY HOSPITAL See Indiana University Medical Center										
✖ ST. VINCENT HOSPITALS AND HEALTH SERVICES, (Formerly St. Vincent Hospital and Health Center), (Includes St. Vincent Carmel Hospital, 13500 North Meridian Street, Carmel, Zip 46032; tel. 317/582–7000; St. Vincent Stress Center, 8401 Harcourt Road, Mailing Address: P.O. Box 80160, Zip 46280; tel. 317/338–4600; Anita J. Harden, Administrator), 2001 West 86th Street, Zip 46260, Mailing Address: Box 40970, Zip 46240–0970; tel. 317/338–2345; Douglas D. French, President and Chief Executive Officer **A**1 2 3 5 9 10 **F**2 3 4 6 7 8 10 11 12 13 14 15 16 17 18 19 20 21 22 23 24 25 26 27 28 29 30 31 32 33 34 35 37 38 39 40 41 42 43 44 45 46 49 51 52 53 54 55 56 57 58 59 60 63 65 66 67 68 69 70 71 72 73 74 **P**5 6 7 8 **S** Daughters of Charity National Health System, Saint Louis, MO **N** National Cardiovascular Network, Atlanta, GA; Sagamore Health Network, Inc., Carmel, IN	21	10	427	30829	444	841512	3953	392997	168401	4754
ST. VINCENT STRESS CENTER See St. Vincent Hospitals and Health Services										
UNIVERSITY HOSPITAL AND OUTPATIENT CENTER See Indiana University Medical Center										

Hospital, Address, Telephone, Administrator, Approval, Facility, and Physician Codes, Health Care System, Network	Classi-fication Codes		Utilization Data					Expense (thousands) of dollars		
★ American Hospital Association (AHA) membership □ Joint Commission on Accreditation of Healthcare Organizations (JCAHO) accreditation + American Osteopathic Hospital Association (AOHA) membership ○ American Osteopathic Association (AOA) accreditation △ Commission on Accreditation of Rehabilitation Facilities (CARF) accreditation Control codes 61, 63, 64, 71, 72 and 73 indicate hospitals listed by AOHA, but not registered by AHA. For definition of numerical codes, see page A4	Control	Service	Beds	Admissions	Census	Outpatient Visits	Births	Total	Payroll	Personnel
+ ○ WESTVIEW HOSPITAL, 3630 Guion Road, Zip 46222–1699; tel. 317/924–6661; David C. Dyar, President and Administrator (Total facility includes 18 beds in nursing home–type unit) (Nonreporting) **A**9 10 11 12 13 **N** Midwest Health Net, LLC., Fort Wayne, IN; Sagamore Health Network, Inc., Carmel, IN; Suburban Health Organization, Indianapolis, IN	23	10	67	—	—	—	—	—	—	—
□ WINONA MEMORIAL HOSPITAL, 3232 North Meridian Street, Zip 46208–4693; tel. 317/924–3392; Keith R. King, Chief Executive Officer (Total facility includes 28 beds in nursing home–type unit) **A**1 10 **F**2 3 4 8 10 12 14 15 16 19 21 22 26 28 30 31 32 34 35 37 39 41 42 44 45 46 48 49 51 52 54 56 57 58 59 64 65 67 71 72 73 **P**5 7 **S** TENET Healthcare Corporation, Santa Barbara, CA	33	10	159	3281	70	72079	0	37701	20409	524
★ WISHARD HEALTH SERVICES, (Formerly William N. Wishard Memorial Hospital), 1001 West 10th Street, Zip 46202–2879; tel. 317/630–7356; John F. Williams, Jr., M.D., Director (Total facility includes 240 beds in nursing home–type unit) **A**1 3 5 8 9 10 **F**1 3 4 7 8 9 10 12 14 15 16 17 18 19 20 21 22 23 25 26 27 28 30 31 32 34 35 36 37 38 39 40 41 42 43 44 46 49 50 51 52 53 54 55 56 57 58 59 60 61 63 64 65 66 67 68 69 70 71 72 73 74 **P**3 5 8	16	10	531	14195	395	612763	2460	185716	81968	2906
JASPER—Dubois County										
★ MEMORIAL HOSPITAL AND HEALTH CARE CENTER, 800 West Ninth Street, Zip 47546–2516; tel. 812/482–2345; Sister M. Adrian Davis, Ph.D., President and Chief Executive Officer (Total facility includes 24 beds in nursing home–type unit) **A**1 2 9 10 **F**7 8 10 14 15 16 18 19 21 22 26 28 29 30 32 33 34 35 37 39 40 41 42 44 45 46 49 52 53 54 55 56 57 58 63 64 65 66 67 71 73 **S** Little Company of Mary Sisters Healthcare System, Evergreen Park, IL	21	10	125	4755	78	95370	516	39136	19557	562
JEFFERSONVILLE—Clark County										
□ CHARTER BEHAVIORAL HEALTH SYSTEM OF INDIANA AT JEFFERSON, 2700 River City Park Road, Zip 47130; tel. 812/284–3400; Michael D. Coppol, Chief Executive Officer (Nonreporting) **A**1 10 **S** Magellan Health Services, Atlanta, GA	33	22	100							
★ CLARK MEMORIAL HOSPITAL, 1220 Missouri Avenue, Zip 47130–3743, Mailing Address: Box 69, Zip 47131–0069; tel. 812/282–6631; Merle E. Stepp, President and Chief Executive Officer (Total facility includes 52 beds in nursing home–type unit) **A**1 9 10 **F**3 7 8 10 11 16 17 19 21 22 23 28 29 30 31 32 33 34 35 39 40 41 42 44 45 46 49 52 53 54 55 56 57 58 59 60 63 64 65 71 73 74 **S** Jewish Hospital Healthcare Services, Louisville, KY **N** Jewish Hospital Healthcare Services, Louisville, KY	13	10	265	9093	170	95947	1120	68110	33475	1163
KENDALLVILLE—Noble County										
★ MCCRAY MEMORIAL HOSPITAL, 951 East Hospital Drive, Zip 46755, Mailing Address: P.O. Box 249, Zip 46755; tel. 219/347–1100; Peter A. Marotti, Chief Executive Officer **A**1 9 10 **F**3 7 8 16 17 19 20 21 22 24 25 27 28 30 32 33 34 35 37 40 41 42 44 46 49 52 54 55 56 57 58 63 65 71 72 73 **P**7 **S** Continuum, Kendallville, IN **N** LutheranPreferred Network, Fort Wayne, IN; Midwest Health Net, LLC., Fort Wayne, IN; Sagamore Health Network, Inc., Carmel, IN	15	10	51	1602	21	77441	211	17755	6881	147
KNOX—Starke County										
★ STARKE MEMORIAL HOSPITAL, 102 East Culver Road, Zip 46534–2299; tel. 219/772–6231; Kathryn J. Norem, Executive Director (Nonreporting) **A**1 9 10 **N** Sagamore Health Network, Inc., Carmel, IN	13	10	35	—	—	—	—	—	—	—
KOKOMO—Howard County										
★ HOWARD COMMUNITY HOSPITAL, 3500 South La Fountain Street, Zip 46904–9011; tel. 765/453–0702; James C. Bigogno, FACHE, President and Chief Executive Officer (Total facility includes 18 beds in nursing home–type unit) **A**1 2 9 10 **F**3 7 8 10 12 13 14 15 16 19 21 22 23 24 26 29 30 32 34 35 37 39 40 42 44 45 49 52 53 54 55 56 57 58 59 60 61 64 65 67 68 71 73 74 **P**2 8 **N** Midwest Health Net, LLC., Fort Wayne, IN	13	10	115	4479	66	140553	263	41994	20659	724
□ KOKOMO REHABILITATION HOSPITAL, 829 North Dixon Road, Zip 46901; tel. 765/452–6700; Paul V. Peiffer, Chief Executive Officer (Nonreporting) **A**1 9 10	33	46	60							
★ SAINT JOSEPH HOSPITAL & HEALTH CENTER, 1907 West Sycamore Street, Zip 46904–9010; tel. 765/456–5300; Kathleen Korbelak, President and Chief Executive Officer (Total facility includes 20 beds in nursing home–type unit) **A**1 9 10 **F**2 3 7 8 10 12 14 15 16 17 19 21 22 23 25 26 27 28 30 31 32 33 34 35 36 37 39 40 41 42 44 45 46 49 51 53 54 55 56 58 59 60 63 64 65 66 67 68 71 73 74 **P**8 **S** Daughters of Charity National Health System, Saint Louis, MO **N** Saint Vincent Hospitals and Health Services, Inc., Indianapolis, IN	21	10	157	6479	85	—	1155	50896	22185	818
LA PORTE—La Porte County										
★ LA PORTE HOSPITAL, State and Madison Streets, Zip 46350–0250, Mailing Address: P.O. Box 250, Zip 46352–0250; tel. 219/326–1234; Leigh E. Morris, President (Total facility includes 55 beds in nursing home–type unit) (Nonreporting) **A**1 2 9 10 **N** Sagamore Health Network, Inc., Carmel, IN; Memorial Health System, Inc., South Bend, IN	23	10	227							
LAFAYETTE—Tippecanoe County										
□ CHARTER BEHAVIORAL HEALTH SYSTEMS, 3700 Rome Drive, Zip 47905, Mailing Address: P.O. Box 5969, Zip 47903; tel. 765/448–6999; Stewart Graham, Administrator **A**1 9 10 **F**3 14 15 16 52 53 54 55 56 57 58 59 **S** Magellan Health Services, Atlanta, GA	33	22	64	1065	25	—	0	4476	—	77
★ LAFAYETTE HOME HOSPITAL, 2400 South Street, Zip 47904; tel. 765/447–6811; John R. Walling, President and Chief Executive Officer (Total facility includes 21 beds in nursing home–type unit) **A**1 9 10 **F**6 7 8 10 12 15 16 19 20 21 22 23 24 26 28 29 30 31 32 34 35 36 37 38 39 40 41 42 44 45 46 48 49 52 54 56 57 58 61 62 63 64 65 66 67 71 73 74 **P**6	23	10	276	9546	141	87072	2189	77454	34540	1175

Hospital, Address, Telephone, Administrator, Approval, Facility, and Physician Codes, Health Care System, Network	Classi-fication Codes		Utilization Data					Expense (thousands) of dollars		
★ American Hospital Association (AHA) membership □ Joint Commission on Accreditation of Healthcare Organizations (JCAHO) accreditation + American Osteopathic Hospital Association (AOHA) membership ○ American Osteopathic Association (AOA) accreditation △ Commission on Accreditation of Rehabilitation Facilities (CARF) accreditation Control codes 61, 63, 64, 71, 72 and 73 indicate hospitals listed by AOHA, but not registered by AHA. For definition of numerical codes, see page A4	Control	Service	Beds	Admissions	Census	Outpatient Visits	Births	Total	Payroll	Personnel

Hospital	Control	Service	Beds	Admissions	Census	Outpatient Visits	Births	Total	Payroll	Personnel
✠ ST. ELIZABETH MEDICAL CENTER, 1501 Hartford Street, Zip 47904–2126, Mailing Address: Box 7501, Zip 47903–7501; tel. 765/423–6011; Douglas W. Eberle, President and Chief Executive Officer (Total facility includes 43 beds in nursing home–type unit) **A**1 2 6 9 10 **F**4 7 8 10 11 14 15 16 17 19 21 22 23 25 26 28 30 31 32 33 34 35 37 39 40 41 42 43 44 45 49 56 60 63 64 65 66 67 71 72 73 74 **S** Sisters of St. Francis Health Services, Inc., Mishawaka, IN	21	10	205	6284	108	128000	428	70893	30269	988
LAGRANGE—LaGrange County										
□ VENCOR HOSPITAL–LAGRANGE, 207 North Townline Road, Zip 46761; tel. 219/463–2143; Joe Murrell, Administrator **A**1 9 10 **F**7 8 12 14 15 16 19 21 22 30 31 34 35 37 39 40 41 42 44 48 49 65 71 73 **S** Vencor, Incorporated, Louisville, KY	33	10	57	1372	20	20455	438	9199	4718	192
LAWRENCEBURG—Dearborn County										
✠ DEARBORN COUNTY HOSPITAL, 600 Wilson Creek Road, Zip 47025–1199; tel. 812/537–1010; Peter V. Resnick, Executive Director (Total facility includes 15 beds in nursing home–type unit) **A**1 9 10 **F**7 8 10 15 16 19 21 22 23 28 30 32 33 35 37 40 41 42 44 49 60 63 64 65 66 67 71 73 **P**3	13	10	88	2748	31	103468	354	—	—	397
LEBANON—Boone County										
□ WITHAM MEMORIAL HOSPITAL, 1124 North Lebanon Street, Zip 46052–1776, Mailing Address: P.O. Box 1200, Zip 46052–3005; tel. 317/482–2700; Stephen J. White, FACHE, President and Chief Executive Officer (Nonreporting) **A**1 9 10 **N** Midwest Health Net, LLC., Fort Wayne, IN; Sagamore Health Network, Inc., Carmel, IN; Suburban Health Organization, Indianapolis, IN	13	10	60	—	—	—	—	—	—	—
LINTON—Greene County										
✠ GREENE COUNTY GENERAL HOSPITAL, Rural Route 1, Box 1000, Zip 47441–9457; tel. 812/847–2281; Jonas S. Uland, Executive Director **A**1 9 10 **F**8 14 15 16 19 20 22 28 29 30 32 34 37 40 42 44 49 54 56 71 73 **P**3 **N** Midwest Health Net, LLC., Fort Wayne, IN; Sagamore Health Network, Inc., Carmel, IN	13	10	56	1557	19	—	91	11924	5717	221
LOGANSPORT—Cass County										
□ LOGANSPORT STATE HOSPITAL, 1098 South State Road 25, Zip 46947–9699; tel. 219/722–4141; Jeffrey H. Smith, Ph.D., Superintendent **A**1 9 **F**9 11 20 26 37 45 48 52 64 73	12	22	438	159	393	0	0	30130	18446	765
✠ MEMORIAL HOSPITAL, 1101 Michigan Avenue, Zip 46947–1596, Mailing Address: P.O. Box 7013, Zip 46947–7013; tel. 219/753–7541; George W. Poor, President and Chief Executive Officer **A**1 9 10 **F**3 7 8 14 15 16 19 21 22 28 30 32 33 35 36 37 39 40 42 44 46 49 52 53 56 57 58 59 63 65 67 71 73 **N** Sagamore Health Network, Inc., Carmel, IN	13	10	104	3262	34	43242	559	25551	11500	415
MADISON—Jefferson County										
✠ KING'S DAUGHTERS' HOSPITAL, One King's Daughters' Drive, Zip 47250, Mailing Address: Box 447, Zip 47250; tel. 812/265–5211; Roger J. Allman, Chief Executive Officer (Total facility includes 29 beds in nursing home–type unit) **A**1 9 10 **F**7 8 10 11 14 15 16 17 19 21 22 23 25 27 28 30 32 33 34 35 39 40 41 42 44 49 60 64 65 66 67 71 73 **P**6	23	10	115	5153	78	47185	463	34549	16071	557
□ MADISON STATE HOSPITAL, 711 Green Road, Zip 47250; tel. 812/265–2611; Steven Covington, Superintendent **A**1 9 10 **F**2 15 16 20 52 53 57 65 73 **P**6	12	22	335	208	304	0	0	21515	12959	556
MARION—Grant County										
✠ MARION GENERAL HOSPITAL, 441 North Wabash Avenue, Zip 46952–2690; tel. 765/662–1441; Albert C. Knauss, President and Chief Executive Officer (Total facility includes 21 beds in nursing home–type unit) **A**1 9 10 **F**7 8 10 11 15 16 19 21 22 28 30 32 33 34 35 36 37 39 40 41 42 44 46 49 63 64 65 66 67 68 71 73 74 **P**6 7	23	10	212	8519	116	220518	717	64985	30977	1001
✠ VETERANS AFFAIRS NORTHERN INDIANA HEALTH CARE SYSTEM–MARION CAMPUS, 1700 East 38th Street, Zip 46953–4589; tel. 765/674–3351; Michael W. Murphy, Ph.D., Director (Total facility includes 69 beds in nursing home–type unit) (Nonreporting) **A**1 9 **S** Department of Veterans Affairs, Washington, DC	45	22	580	—	—	—	—	—	—	—
MARTINSVILLE—Morgan County										
★ MORGAN COUNTY MEMORIAL HOSPITAL, 2209 John R. Wooden Drive, Zip 46151, Mailing Address: P.O. Box 1717, Zip 46151; tel. 765/349–6501; S. Dean Melton, President and Chief Executive Officer **A**9 10 **F**7 8 14 15 16 19 21 22 28 29 30 32 34 35 36 37 39 40 41 42 44 45 49 51 65 71 73 **P**6 8 **N** Midwest Health Net, LLC., Fort Wayne, IN; Sagamore Health Network, Inc., Carmel, IN; Suburban Health Organization, Indianapolis, IN	13	10	86	1965	25	80991	180	29794	8297	292
MERRILLVILLE—Lake County										
SOUTHLAKE CAMPUS See Methodist Hospitals, Gary										
MICHIGAN CITY—La Porte County										
✠ MEMORIAL HOSPITAL OF MICHIGAN CITY, 515 Pine Street, Zip 46360–3370; tel. 219/879–0202; Norman D. Steider, President **A**1 9 10 **F**2 3 4 7 8 12 14 15 16 17 18 19 20 21 22 28 29 30 31 32 33 34 35 36 37 39 40 41 42 44 45 46 48 49 52 53 54 55 56 57 59 60 63 65 66 67 68 71 73	23	10	120	2707	44	16368	265	21183	7497	226
✠ △ SAINT ANTHONY HOSPITAL AND HEALTH CENTERS, 301 West Homer Street, Zip 46360–4358; tel. 219/879–8511; Bruce E. Rampage, President and Chief Executive Officer (Total facility includes 19 beds in nursing home–type unit) **A**1 7 9 10 **F**4 7 8 10 11 12 17 19 21 22 23 26 28 29 30 32 33 34 35 36 37 39 40 41 42 44 45 46 48 49 51 60 63 64 65 67 71 73 **S** Sisters of St. Francis Health Services, Inc., Mishawaka, IN **N** Sagamore Health Network, Inc., Carmel, IN	21	10	190	6280	95	241346	492	48680	19542	699

Hospital, Address, Telephone, Administrator, Approval, Facility, and Physician Codes, Health Care System, Network	Classi-fication Codes		Utilization Data					Expense (thousands) of dollars		
	Control	Service	Beds	Admissions	Census	Outpatient Visits	Births	Total	Payroll	Personnel

★ American Hospital Association (AHA) membership
☐ Joint Commission on Accreditation of Healthcare Organizations (JCAHO) accreditation
+ American Osteopathic Hospital Association (AOHA) membership
◯ American Osteopathic Association (AOA) accreditation
△ Commission on Accreditation of Rehabilitation Facilities (CARF) accreditation
Control codes 61, 63, 64, 71, 72 and 73 indicate hospitals listed by AOHA, but not registered by AHA. For definition of numerical codes, see page A4

MISHAWAKA—St. Joseph County

✸ ST. JOSEPH COMMUNITY HOSPITAL, 215 West Fourth Street, Zip 46544; tel. 219/259–2431; Stephen L. Crain, President and Chief Executive Officer **A**1 9 10 **F**3 4 7 8 10 12 13 14 15 16 17 18 19 21 22 23 25 26 28 30 32 34 35 37 39 40 41 42 44 45 46 48 49 51 52 53 54 56 63 65 66 67 71 72 73 **P**3 4 6 7 8 **S** Ancilla Systems Inc., Hobart, IN **N** Ancilla Systems, Inc., Hobart, IN; Midwest Health Net, LLC., Fort Wayne, IN; Sagamore Health Network, Inc., Carmel, IN; Memorial Health System, Inc., South Bend, IN	21	10	187	5952	77	79908	1149	64189	24813	709

MONTICELLO—White County

✸ WHITE COUNTY MEMORIAL HOSPITAL, 1101 O'Connor Boulevard, Zip 47960; tel. 219/583–7111; John M. Avers, Chief Executive Officer (Nonreporting) **A**1 9 10 **N** Midwest Health Net, LLC., Fort Wayne, IN; Sagamore Health Network, Inc., Carmel, IN	15	10	59	—	—	—	—	—	—	—

MOORESVILLE—Morgan County

☐ KENDRICK MEMORIAL HOSPITAL, 1201 Hadley Road N.W., Zip 46158–1789; tel. 317/831–1160; Charles D. Swisher, Executive Director (Nonreporting) **A**1 9 10 **N** Sagamore Health Network, Inc., Carmel, IN	23	10	60	—	—	—	—	—	—	—

MUNCIE—Delaware County

✸ △ BALL MEMORIAL HOSPITAL, 2401 University Avenue, Zip 47303–3499; tel. 765/747–3111; Mitchell C. Carson, President (Total facility includes 30 beds in nursing home–type unit) **A**1 3 5 7 9 10 **F**2 3 4 7 8 10 11 14 15 16 17 19 20 21 22 23 24 26 28 29 30 31 32 33 34 35 36 37 38 39 40 41 42 43 44 45 46 48 49 51 52 54 55 56 57 60 61 63 64 65 66 67 71 73 74 **P**7 8	23	10	430	17428	268	157178	1748	146598	61419	1937

MUNSTER—Lake County

☐ COMMUNITY HOSPITAL, 901 MacArthur Boulevard, Zip 46321–2959; tel. 219/836–1600; Edward P. Robinson, Administrator (Nonreporting) **A**1 2 9 10	23	10	292	—	—	—	—	—	—	—

NEW ALBANY—Floyd County

✸ FLOYD MEMORIAL HOSPITAL AND HEALTH SERVICES, 1850 State Street, Zip 47150; tel. 812/949–5500; Bryant R. Hanson, President **A**1 2 9 10 **F**7 8 10 11 12 14 15 19 21 22 23 32 35 37 40 41 42 44 46 49 60 63 65 67 70 71 72 73 74 **P**1 **N** Sagamore Health Network, Inc., Carmel, IN	13	10	215	8174	101	140753	877	66391	30150	890
✸ △ SOUTHERN INDIANA REHABILITATION HOSPITAL, 3104 Blackiston Boulevard, Zip 47150; tel. 812/941–8300; Randy L. Napier, President **A**1 7 10 **F**1 4 8 9 10 11 12 14 15 16 19 20 21 22 25 28 29 30 32 34 35 37 38 39 40 41 42 43 44 46 47 48 49 51 52 64 65 66 67 69 71 72 73 74 **S** Jewish Hospital Healthcare Services, Louisville, KY	32	46	60	668	46	5168	0	—	—	138

NEW CASTLE—Henry County

✸ HENRY COUNTY MEMORIAL HOSPITAL, 1000 North 16th Street, Zip 47362–4319, Mailing Address: Box 490, Zip 47362–0490; tel. 765/521–0890; Jack Basler, President **A**1 9 10 **F**7 8 14 15 16 17 19 21 22 32 34 35 42 44 46 65 66 67 71 73 74 **P**8 **N** Midwest Health Net, LLC., Fort Wayne, IN; Sagamore Health Network, Inc., Carmel, IN; Suburban Health Organization, Indianapolis, IN	13	10	107	3551	39	45854	441	27501	12472	510

NOBLESVILLE—Hamilton County

✸ RIVERVIEW HOSPITAL, 395 Westfield Road, Zip 46060–1425, Mailing Address: P.O. Box 220, Zip 46061–0220; tel. 317/773–0760; Seward Horner, President (Nonreporting) **A**1 9 10 **N** Midwest Health Net, LLC., Fort Wayne, IN; Sagamore Health Network, Inc., Carmel, IN; Suburban Health Organization, Indianapolis, IN	13	10	111	—	—	—	—	—	—	—

NORTH VERNON—Jennings County

★ JENNINGS COMMUNITY HOSPITAL, 301 Henry Street, Zip 47265; tel. 812/346–6200; Dale P. Wernke, Chief Executive Officer **A**9 10 **F**8 15 19 22 28 30 34 39 41 44 51 64 71 72 73 **N** Saint Vincent Hospitals and Health Services, Inc., Indianapolis, IN	23	10	34	537	15	16415	0	7825	3236	131

OAKLAND CITY—Gibson County

★ + WIRTH REGIONAL HOSPITAL, Highway 64 West, Zip 47660–9379, Mailing Address: Rural Route 3, Box 14A, Zip 47660–9379; tel. 812/749–6111; Ralph Paulding, Administrator **A**9 10 **F**15 19 22 40 41 44 49 65 71 **S** Brim, Inc., Portland, OR	23	10	11	444	5	12672	17	3555	1550	58

PAOLI—Orange County

★ ORANGE COUNTY HOSPITAL, 642 West Hospital Road, Zip 47454–0499, Mailing Address: P.O. Box 499, Zip 47454–0499; tel. 812/723–2811; James W. Pope, Chief Executive Officer **A**9 10 **F**7 8 11 12 14 15 16 17 19 22 28 29 30 32 33 34 37 40 41 42 44 49 67 71 72 **N** Sagamore Health Network, Inc., Carmel, IN	13	10	37	1092	10	27940	170	9174	4376	183

PERU—Miami County

✸ DUKES MEMORIAL HOSPITAL, Grant and Boulevard, Zip 46970–1698; tel. 765/473–6621; R. Joe Johnston, President and Chief Executive Officer (Total facility includes 35 beds in nursing home–type unit) **A**1 9 10 **F**7 8 11 14 15 16 17 19 21 22 24 26 28 30 32 33 34 35 36 39 40 41 42 44 45 46 49 63 64 65 67 68 71 73 **P**6 **N** LutheranPreferred Network, Fort Wayne, IN; Midwest Health Net, LLC., Fort Wayne, IN; Sagamore Health Network, Inc., Carmel, IN	15	10	140	1795	45	51867	396	17850	7871	306

PLYMOUTH—Marshall County

☐ KOALA HOSPITAL AND COUNSELING CENTER, 1800 North Oak Road, Zip 46563; tel. 219/936–3784; Wayne T. Miller, Administrator (Nonreporting) **A**1 10 **S** Sterling Healthcare Corporation, Bellevue, WA	33	22	80	—	—	—	—	—	—	—
✸ ST. JOSEPH'S HOSPITAL OF MARSHALL COUNTY, 1915 Lake Avenue, Zip 46563–9905, Mailing Address: P.O. Box 670, Zip 46563–9905; tel. 219/936–3181; Brian E. Dietz, President **A**1 9 10 **F**1 4 6 7 8 10 12 14 15 16 19 21 22 23 24 26 27 28 31 33 35 36 37 40 41 42 43 44 47 48 49 60 64 65 70 71 73 74 **P**7 8 **S** Holy Cross Health System Corporation, South Bend, IN **N** Sagamore Health Network, Inc., Carmel, IN; Holy Cross Health System, South Bend, IN	21	10	58	2130	21	44894	311	16085	5485	204

Hospital, Address, Telephone, Administrator, Approval, Facility, and Physician Codes, Health Care System, Network	Classi-fication Codes		Utilization Data					Expense (thousands) of dollars		
	Control	Service	Beds	Admissions	Census	Outpatient Visits	Births	Total	Payroll	Personnel

★ American Hospital Association (AHA) membership
□ Joint Commission on Accreditation of Healthcare Organizations (JCAHO) accreditation
+ American Osteopathic Hospital Association (AOHA) membership
○ American Osteopathic Association (AOA) accreditation
△ Commission on Accreditation of Rehabilitation Facilities (CARF) accreditation
Control codes 61, 63, 64, 71, 72 and 73 indicate hospitals listed by AOHA, but not registered by AHA. For definition of numerical codes, see page A4

PORTLAND—Jay County

⊠ JAY COUNTY HOSPITAL, 500 West Votaw Street, Zip 47371–1322; tel. 219/726–7131; Thomas J. Valerius, Chief Executive Officer **A**1 9 10 **F**7 8 15 19 21 22 28 30 32 33 34 35 37 40 41 42 44 46 49 67 71 73 74 **P**3 8 **S** Alliant Health System, Louisville, KY **N** LutheranPreferred Network, Fort Wayne, IN; Health Quest, Bluffton, IN	13	10	55	1664	17	27472	175	10936	4436	160

PRINCETON—Gibson County

⊠ GIBSON GENERAL HOSPITAL, 1808 Sherman Drive, Zip 47670–1043; tel. 812/385–3401; Michael J. Budnick, Administrator and Chief Executive Officer (Total facility includes 45 beds in nursing home–type unit) **A**1 9 10 **F**3 6 7 8 12 14 15 16 17 18 19 20 22 26 28 29 30 32 33 34 35 37 39 40 41 42 44 49 52 53 54 55 56 57 58 60 63 64 65 66 71 73 74 **P**5 **S** Alliant Health System, Louisville, KY **N** Sagamore Health Network, Inc., Carmel, IN	23	10	109	1879	62	27120	128	11631	5662	254

RENSSELAER—Jasper County

★ JASPER COUNTY HOSPITAL, 1104 East Grace Street, Zip 47978–3296; tel. 219/866–5141; Timothy M. Schreeg, President and Chief Executive Officer (Total facility includes 21 beds in nursing home–type unit) **A**9 10 **F**7 8 11 14 17 19 20 21 22 23 24 26 27 28 29 30 31 32 33 34 35 36 37 39 40 41 42 44 45 46 49 53 54 55 56 57 58 59 64 65 66 67 71 73 **P**6	13	10	69	1733	38	40767	176	14492	7634	292

RICHMOND—Wayne County

⊠ REID HOSPITAL AND HEALTH CARE SERVICES, 1401 Chester Boulevard, Zip 47374; tel. 765/983–3000; Barry S. MacDowell, President **A**1 2 9 10 **F**2 3 7 8 10 11 14 15 16 17 19 21 22 23 28 30 32 33 35 37 40 41 42 44 46 49 50 52 54 56 60 63 65 67 71 73 **P**1 3	23	10	199	11216	139	112491	943	71705	32251	913
□ RICHMOND STATE HOSPITAL, 498 N.W. 18th Street, Zip 47374–2898; tel. 765/966–0511; James McCormick, Superintendent **A**1 9 10 **F**2 12 17 20 26 28 29 30 31 39 41 45 46 52 53 54 55 57 64 65 67 73	12	22	339	288	310	0	0	27195	15384	652

ROCHESTER—Fulton County

★ WOODLAWN HOSPITAL, 1400 East Ninth Street, Zip 46975–8937; tel. 219/224–1173; Michael L. Gordon, President (Nonreporting) **A**9 10	13	10	49	—	—	—	—	—	—	—

RUSHVILLE—Rush County

★ RUSH MEMORIAL HOSPITAL, 1300 North Main Street, Zip 46173–1198; tel. 765/932–4111; H. William Hartley, Chief Executive Officer **A**9 10 **F**8 15 16 17 19 22 30 32 34 35 37 39 42 44 46 49 71 73 **S** Alliant Health System, Louisville, KY **N** Sagamore Health Network, Inc., Carmel, IN	13	10	52	984	27	67700	0	8943	4224	176

SALEM—Washington County

⊠ WASHINGTON COUNTY MEMORIAL HOSPITAL, 911 North Shelby Street, Zip 47167; tel. 812/883–5881; Rodney M. Coats, Executive Director **A**1 9 10 **F**2 6 7 8 11 14 15 17 18 19 20 22 27 28 29 30 32 33 34 37 39 40 42 44 49 52 54 55 56 57 64 67 71 73 **P**6 **S** Jewish Hospital Healthcare Services, Louisville, KY **N** Jewish Hospital Healthcare Services, Louisville, KY	13	10	50	1598	22	25030	142	11422	4761	248

SCOTTSBURG—Scott County

⊠ SCOTT MEMORIAL HOSPITAL, 1415 North Gardner Street, Zip 47170–0456, Mailing Address: Box 430, Zip 47170–0430; tel. 812/752–8500; Clifford D. Nay, Executive Director **A**1 9 10 **F**7 8 11 12 14 15 16 17 19 22 28 30 32 34 35 37 39 40 41 42 44 49 65 67 71 73 **S** Jewish Hospital Healthcare Services, Louisville, KY **N** Jewish Hospital Healthcare Services, Louisville, KY	13	10	40	1047	12	15374	137	8955	4566	150

SEYMOUR—Jackson County

⊠ MEMORIAL HOSPITAL, 411 West Tipton Street, Zip 47274–5000, Mailing Address: P.O. Box 2349, Zip 47274; tel. 812/522–2349; George H. James, Jr., President and Chief Executive Officer **A**1 2 9 10 **F**7 8 14 15 16 19 21 22 28 30 32 33 34 35 36 37 40 42 44 45 46 49 63 65 67 71 73	13	10	107	4172	47	108915	654	31636	13772	471

SHELBYVILLE—Shelby County

⊠ MAJOR HOSPITAL, 150 West Washington Street, Zip 46176–1236; tel. 317/392–3211; Anthony B. Lennen, President and Chief Executive Officer **A**1 9 10 **F**7 8 12 14 15 16 17 19 21 22 28 30 32 34 35 36 37 39 40 41 42 44 45 49 63 65 66 71 73 74 **P**7 8	15	10	51	2260	25	78433	274	19677	8998	305

SOUTH BEND—St. Joseph County

⊠ △ MEMORIAL HOSPITAL OF SOUTH BEND, 615 North Michigan Street, Zip 46601–9986; tel. 219/234–9041; Philip A. Newbold, President and Chief Executive Officer **A**1 2 3 5 7 9 10 **F**2 3 4 7 8 10 11 13 14 15 16 17 18 19 20 21 22 23 24 25 26 27 28 29 30 31 32 34 35 37 38 39 40 41 42 43 44 46 47 48 49 50 51 52 53 54 55 56 57 58 59 60 61 63 64 65 66 67 70 71 72 73 74 **P**1 6	23	10	340	14941	203	105404	2667	151733	60166	1691
⊠ △ ST. JOSEPH'S MEDICAL CENTER, 801 East LaSalle, Zip 46617, Mailing Address: Box 1935, Zip 46634; tel. 219/237–7111; Brian E. Dietz, Interim Chief Executive Officer **A**1 2 3 5 7 9 10 **F**1 4 6 7 8 10 11 12 13 14 15 16 17 19 21 22 23 24 26 27 28 29 30 31 32 34 35 37 38 40 41 42 43 44 45 47 48 49 51 60 62 64 65 66 67 68 71 73 74 **P**1 6 7 **S** Holy Cross Health System Corporation, South Bend, IN **N** Select Health Network, South Bend, IN; Sagamore Health Network, Inc., Carmel, IN; Holy Cross Health System, South Bend, IN	21	10	289	11074	164	126604	971	125795	47180	1340
★ + ○ ST. MARY COMMUNITY HOSPITAL, 2515 East Jefferson Boulevard, Zip 46615–2691; tel. 219/288–8311; Stephen L. Crain, President (Nonreporting) **A**9 10 11 12 13 **S** Ancilla Systems Inc., Hobart, IN **N** Ancilla Systems, Inc., Hobart, IN; Midwest Health Net, LLC., Fort Wayne, IN; Sagamore Health Network, Inc., Carmel, IN	23	10	70	—	—	—	—	—	—	—

Hospital, Address, Telephone, Administrator, Approval, Facility, and Physician Codes, Health Care System, Network	Classi-fication Codes		Utilization Data					Expense (thousands) of dollars		
	Control	Service	Beds	Admissions	Census	Outpatient Visits	Births	Total	Payroll	Personnel

★ American Hospital Association (AHA) membership
□ Joint Commission on Accreditation of Healthcare Organizations (JCAHO) accreditation
+ American Osteopathic Hospital Association (AOHA) membership
○ American Osteopathic Association (AOA) accreditation
△ Commission on Accreditation of Rehabilitation Facilities (CARF) accreditation
Control codes 61, 63, 64, 71, 72 and 73 indicate hospitals listed by AOHA, but not registered by AHA. For definition of numerical codes, see page A4.

Hospital	Control	Service	Beds	Admissions	Census	Outpatient Visits	Births	Total	Payroll	Personnel
SULLIVAN—Sullivan County										
⊞ MARY SHERMAN HOSPITAL, 320 North Section Street, Zip 47882, Mailing Address: P.O. Box 10, Zip 47882–0010; tel. 812/268–4311; Thomas J. Hudgins, Administrator **A**1 9 10 **F**7 8 12 13 14 15 16 17 19 20 21 22 26 28 29 30 31 32 35 37 39 40 41 42 44 45 49 53 54 55 56 57 58 63 65 66 67 68 71 73 74 **S** Quorum Health Group/Quorum Health Resources, Inc., Brentwood, TN **N** Sagamore Health Network, Inc., Carmel, IN	13	10	53	1709	25	42033	155	10454	4295	190
TELL CITY—Perry County										
⊞ PERRY COUNTY MEMORIAL HOSPITAL, 1 Hospital Road, Zip 47586–0362; tel. 812/547–7011; Bradford W. Dykes, Chief Executive Officer **A**1 9 10 **F**7 8 12 17 19 21 22 26 28 29 30 32 33 34 35 37 39 40 42 44 45 46 49 58 63 64 65 67 71 73 **S** Alliant Health System, Louisville, KY	13	10	38	1211	12	48664	69	9901	4060	168
TERRE HAUTE—Vigo County										
⊞ COLUMBIA TERRE HAUTE REGIONAL HOSPITAL, 3901 South Seventh Street, Zip 47802–4299; tel. 812/232–0021; Jerry Dooley, Chief Executive Officer (Total facility includes 25 beds in nursing home–type unit) **A**1 9 10 **F**2 3 4 7 8 10 11 12 14 16 17 19 21 22 26 28 30 32 34 36 37 39 40 41 42 43 44 46 50 52 54 55 56 57 58 59 60 61 64 65 66 67 71 72 73 74 **P**3 7 8 **S** Columbia/HCA Healthcare Corporation, Nashville, TN	33	10	236	7033	108	97915	849	34370	16418	784
HAMILTON CENTER, 620 Eighth Avenue, Zip 47804–0323; tel. 812/231–8323; Galen Goode, Chief Executive Officer (Nonreporting) **A**9 10	23	22	45	—	—	—	—	—	—	—
⊞ △ UNION HOSPITAL, 1606 North Seventh Street, Zip 47804–2780; tel. 812/238–7000; Frank Shelton, President **A**1 2 3 5 7 9 10 **F**3 4 5 7 8 10 11 12 14 15 16 17 19 20 21 22 23 24 25 28 29 30 31 32 33 34 35 37 38 39 40 41 42 43 44 45 46 47 48 49 51 52 53 56 58 59 60 61 64 65 66 67 71 72 73 74 **P**5 6 **N** Sagamore Health Network, Inc., Carmel, IN	23	10	295	13016	210	581014	1529	131145	56687	1846
TIPTON—Tipton County										
⊞ TIPTON COUNTY MEMORIAL HOSPITAL, 1000 South Main Street, Zip 46072–9799; tel. 317/675–8500; Alfonso W. Gatmaitan, Chief Executive Officer (Total facility includes 50 beds in nursing home–type unit) **A**1 2 9 10 **F**7 8 12 19 21 22 28 30 32 35 36 37 39 40 41 42 44 45 46 49 50 63 64 65 66 71 73 74 **P**8 **N** Midwest Health Net, LLC., Fort Wayne, IN; Sagamore Health Network, Inc., Carmel, IN; Suburban Health Organization, Indianapolis, IN	13	10	100	1986	53	34283	154	16664	7524	289
VALPARAISO—Porter County										
⊞ △ PORTER MEMORIAL HOSPITAL, 814 La Porte Avenue, Zip 46383–5898; tel. 219/465–4600; Wiley N. Carr, President and Chief Executive Officer **A**1 7 9 10 **F**3 4 7 8 10 14 15 16 17 18 19 21 22 23 28 32 34 35 37 38 40 41 42 43 44 45 48 49 52 53 54 55 56 57 58 59 60 61 63 65 68 70 71 72 73 74 **P**3 8	13	10	364	12605	203	285041	1300	107523	45099	1418
VINCENNES—Knox County										
⊞ GOOD SAMARITAN HOSPITAL, 520 South Seventh Street, Zip 47591–1098; tel. 812/882–5220; A. John Hidde, President and Chief Executive Officer (Total facility includes 26 beds in nursing home–type unit) **A**1 2 9 10 **F**3 4 7 8 10 11 13 14 15 16 19 20 21 22 23 24 28 29 30 32 33 34 35 37 39 40 41 42 43 44 45 46 52 53 54 55 56 57 58 59 60 63 64 65 67 71 72 73 74 **P**8	13	10	254	10322	164	204626	502	80704	37837	1350
WABASH—Wabash County										
⊞ WABASH COUNTY HOSPITAL, 710 North East Street, Zip 46992, Mailing Address: Box 548, Zip 46992–0548; tel. 219/563–3131; David C. Hunter, Chief Executive Officer (Total facility includes 25 beds in nursing home–type unit) **A**1 2 9 10 **F**7 8 12 13 17 19 21 22 24 28 29 30 32 33 34 35 36 37 39 40 41 42 44 45 46 64 67 71 73 **S** Alliant Health System, Louisville, KY **N** LutheranPreferred Network, Fort Wayne, IN; Midwest Health Net, LLC., Fort Wayne, IN; Sagamore Health Network, Inc., Carmel, IN	13	10	75	1932	31	184553	238	21467	9046	295
WARSAW—Kosciusko County										
⊞ KOSCIUSKO COMMUNITY HOSPITAL, 2101 East Dubois Drive, Zip 46580; tel. 219/267–3200; Wayne Hendrix, President (Total facility includes 89 beds in nursing home–type unit) **A**1 9 10 **F**3 7 8 12 13 14 15 16 17 19 21 22 26 27 28 29 30 32 33 34 35 36 37 39 40 41 42 44 45 49 51 64 65 66 67 71 72 73 **P**1 3 4 **N** LutheranPreferred Network, Fort Wayne, IN; Midwest Health Net, LLC., Fort Wayne, IN; Sagamore Health Network, Inc., Carmel, IN	23	10	161	3440	107	143408	666	35182	16090	568
WASHINGTON—Daviess County										
⊞ DAVIESS COUNTY HOSPITAL, 1314 Grand Avenue, Zip 47501–2198, Mailing Address: P.O. Box 760, Zip 47501–0760; tel. 812/254–2760; Marc Chircop, Chief Executive Officer (Total facility includes 29 beds in nursing home–type unit) **A**1 9 10 **F**7 8 11 12 15 16 17 19 21 22 32 33 34 35 36 37 39 40 41 42 44 45 49 53 55 56 58 59 63 64 65 66 67 71 73 **P**3 7 8 **S** Quorum Health Group/Quorum Health Resources, Inc., Brentwood, TN	13	10	85	2492	46	52985	364	18757	8137	286
WEST LAFAYETTE—Tippecanoe County										
□ WABASH VALLEY HOSPITAL, 2900 North River Road, Zip 47906–3766; tel. 317/463–2555; R. Craig Lysinger, Administrator (Nonreporting) **A**1 9 10	23	22	70	—	—	—	—	—	—	—
WILLIAMSPORT—Warren County										
★ ST. VINCENT WILLIAMSPORT HOSPITAL, (Formerly Community Hospital), 412 North Monroe Street, Zip 47993–0215; tel. 765/762–2496; Jane Craigin, Chief Executive Officer (Nonreporting) **A**9 10 **N** Saint Vincent Hospitals and Health Services, Inc., Indianapolis, IN	23	10	22	—	—	—	—	—	—	—
WINAMAC—Pulaski County										
⊞ PULASKI MEMORIAL HOSPITAL, 616 East 13th Street, Zip 46996–1117; tel. 219/946–6131; Richard H. Mynark, Administrator **A**1 9 10 **F**7 8 14 15 19 21 22 26 29 30 32 33 35 37 39 40 41 42 44 45 49 58 65 67 71 73 **N** Sagamore Health Network, Inc., Carmel, IN	13	10	24	1157	12	34805	106	9140	4941	168

Hospital, Address, Telephone, Administrator, Approval, Facility, and Physician Codes, Health Care System, Network	Classi-fication Codes		Utilization Data					Expense (thousands) of dollars		
★ American Hospital Association (AHA) membership □ Joint Commission on Accreditation of Healthcare Organizations (JCAHO) accreditation + American Osteopathic Hospital Association (AOHA) membership ○ American Osteopathic Association (AOA) accreditation △ Commission on Accreditation of Rehabilitation Facilities (CARF) accreditation Control codes 61, 63, 64, 71, 72 and 73 indicate hospitals listed by AOHA, but not registered by AHA. For definition of numerical codes, see page A4	Control	Service	Beds	Admissions	Census	Outpatient Visits	Births	Total	Payroll	Personnel

WINCHESTER—Randolph County

★ RANDOLPH COUNTY HOSPITAL, 325 South Oak Street, Zip 47394, Mailing Address: P.O. Box 407, Zip 47394; tel. 765/584–9001; James M. Full, Chief Executive Officer **A**9 10 **F**7 8 13 15 16 17 19 21 22 25 26 28 30 32 33 34 35 37 40 41 42 44 46 49 61 65 66 71 73 74 **P**3 **S** Alliant Health System, Louisville, KY **N** Health Quest, Bluffton, IN; Midwest Health Net, LLC., Fort Wayne, IN; Sagamore Health Network, Inc., Carmel, IN

13	10	27	984	10	94744	123	9947	3831	155

IOWA

Resident population 2,842 (in thousands)
Resident population in metro areas 44.0%
Birth rate per 1,000 population 13.4
65 years and over 15.2%
Percent of persons without health insurance 9.7%

Hospital, Address, Telephone, Administrator, Approval, Facility, and Physician Codes, Health Care System, Network	Classi-fication Codes		Utilization Data					Expense (thousands) of dollars		
★ American Hospital Association (AHA) membership □ Joint Commission on Accreditation of Healthcare Organizations (JCAHO) accreditation + American Osteopathic Hospital Association (AOHA) membership ○ American Osteopathic Association (AOA) accreditation △ Commission on Accreditation of Rehabilitation Facilities (CARF) accreditation Control codes 61, 63, 64, 71, 72 and 73 indicate hospitals listed by AOHA, but not registered by AHA. For definition of numerical codes, see page A4	Control	Service	Beds	Admissions	Census	Outpatient Visits	Births	Total	Payroll	Personnel

ALBIA—Monroe County

MONROE COUNTY HOSPITAL, RR 3, Box 311–11, Zip 52531; tel. 515/932–2134; Gregory A. Paris, Administrator **A**9 10 **F**8 15 16 17 19 22 28 30 32 33 34 35 36 42 44 49 54 65 67 71 73 **P**3 **N** Mercy Network of Health Services, Des Moines, IA — 13 10 46 494 23 — 0 4651 1807 101

ALGONA—Kossuth County

★ KOSSUTH REGIONAL HEALTH CENTER, 1515 South Phillips Street, Zip 50511; tel. 515/295–2451; James G. Fitzpatrick, Administrator **A**9 10 **F**7 8 12 14 15 16 17 19 22 26 28 30 31 32 33 34 35 36 37 39 40 41 42 44 45 48 49 58 64 65 66 67 71 73 **P**6 **S** Mercy Health Services, Farmington Hills, MI **N** North Iowa Mercy Health Network, Mason City, IA — 13 10 29 630 8 14900 92 7091 2464 93

AMES—Story County

⊞ MARY GREELEY MEDICAL CENTER, 1111 Duff Avenue, Zip 50010; tel. 515/239–2011; Kimberly A. Russel, President and Chief Executive Officer (Total facility includes 20 beds in nursing home–type unit) **A**1 2 9 10 **F**6 7 8 10 14 15 16 17 18 19 21 22 26 28 29 30 31 32 33 34 35 36 37 38 39 40 41 42 44 45 48 49 52 53 54 55 56 57 58 59 60 61 63 64 65 66 67 71 73 — 14 10 216 8867 118 133418 1153 60642 28218 996

ANAMOSA—Jones County

⊞ ANAMOSA COMMUNITY HOSPITAL, 104 Broadway Place, Zip 52205; tel. 319/462–6131; Margaret Robinson, Administrator **A**1 9 10 **F**1 7 8 12 13 15 16 17 19 22 26 30 32 33 34 39 41 44 45 46 49 65 71 73 **P**1 5 **S** Iowa Health System, Des Moines, IA — 23 10 18 347 5 13814 6 3743 1462 88

ATLANTIC—Cass County

★ CASS COUNTY MEMORIAL HOSPITAL, 1501 East Tenth Street, Zip 50022–1997; tel. 712/243–3250; Patricia Markham, Administrator **A**9 10 **F**1 7 8 15 16 19 21 22 28 30 32 33 34 35 36 37 39 40 41 42 44 52 53 55 56 57 58 59 63 65 67 71 **P**7 8 — 13 10 72 1664 27 33276 185 13171 6597 257

AUDUBON—Audubon County

AUDUBON COUNTY MEMORIAL HOSPITAL, 515 Pacific Street, Zip 50025–1099; tel. 712/563–2611; David G. Couser, Administrator **A**9 10 **F**8 14 15 19 22 30 33 34 35 40 42 44 49 63 71 **P**1 3 **N** Mercy Network of Health Services, Des Moines, IA — 13 10 29 517 5 13707 30 3319 1477 60

BELMOND—Wright County

★ BELMOND COMMUNITY HOSPITAL, 403 First Street S.E., Zip 50421–0326, Mailing Address: P.O. Box 326, Zip 50421; tel. 515/444–3223; Allan Atkinson, Administrator **A**9 10 **F**3 8 14 15 16 17 19 22 28 30 31 32 33 36 39 44 49 53 54 55 58 71 73 **P**1 2 3 4 5 6 7 8 **S** Mercy Health Services, Farmington Hills, MI **N** North Iowa Mercy Health Network, Mason City, IA — 14 10 22 310 7 6996 0 2490 1223 50

BLOOMFIELD—Davis County

DAVIS COUNTY HOSPITAL, 507 North Madison Street, Zip 52537–1299; tel. 515/664–2145; Randy Simmons, Administrator (Total facility includes 32 beds in nursing home–type unit) **A**9 10 **F**7 13 14 15 16 19 20 22 24 28 30 31 32 34 35 36 37 39 40 42 44 45 49 64 67 71 73 **P**6 **N** Mercy Network of Health Services, Des Moines, IA — 13 10 80 1032 45 11853 66 7873 3434 170

BOONE—Boone County

⊞ BOONE COUNTY HOSPITAL, 1015 Union Street, Zip 50036–4898; tel. 515/432–3140; Joseph S. Smith, Chief Executive Officer **A**1 9 10 **F**7 8 11 15 19 22 24 28 30 32 35 36 39 40 41 44 48 49 64 71 73 **P**3 **S** Quorum Health Group/Quorum Health Resources, Inc., Brentwood, TN — 13 10 57 1593 22 33343 128 13211 5874 214

BRITT—Hancock County

★ HANCOCK COUNTY MEMORIAL HOSPITAL, 531 Second Street N.W., Zip 50423, Mailing Address: Box 68, Zip 50423–0068; tel. 515/843–3801; Harriet Thompson, Administrator **A**9 10 **F**1 8 14 15 17 22 27 30 33 34 36 40 41 44 46 64 65 67 71 **P**6 **S** Mercy Health Services, Farmington Hills, MI **N** North Iowa Mercy Health Network, Mason City, IA — 13 10 26 472 7 13120 3 3699 1702 56

BURLINGTON—Des Moines County

⊞ BURLINGTON MEDICAL CENTER, (Includes Burlington Medical Center Klein Unit, 2910 Madison Road, Zip 52601; tel. 319/753–3500), 602 North Third Street, Zip 52601–5088; tel. 319/753–3011; Mark D. Richardson, President and Chief Executive Officer (Total facility includes 167 beds in nursing home–type unit) **A**1 9 10 **F**2 3 4 8 10 12 13 14 15 16 17 18 19 21 22 23 24 28 29 30 32 34 35 36 37 38 39 40 41 42 44 45 46 48 49 52 53 54 55 56 57 58 60 63 64 65 66 67 70 71 73 — 23 10 388 7427 230 180192 748 55048 24250 798

CARROLL—Carroll County

⊞ ST. ANTHONY REGIONAL HOSPITAL, South Clark Street, Zip 51401; tel. 712/792–8231; Gary P. Riedmann, President and Chief Executive Officer (Total facility includes 79 beds in nursing home–type unit) **A**1 9 10 **F**1 7 8 12 14 15 16 17 19 20 21 22 26 28 29 30 31 32 33 34 35 36 37 39 40 41 42 44 45 46 49 51 52 53 54 55 56 57 58 59 60 62 63 64 65 66 67 68 71 73 **P**6 **N** Mercy Network of Health Services, Des Moines, IA — 21 10 142 2318 108 43746 234 16931 7202 286

Hospital, Address, Telephone, Administrator, Approval, Facility, and Physician Codes, Health Care System, Network	Classi-fication Codes		Utilization Data					Expense (thousands) of dollars		
	Control	Service	Beds	Admissions	Census	Outpatient Visits	Births	Total	Payroll	Personnel

★ American Hospital Association (AHA) membership
□ Joint Commission on Accreditation of Healthcare Organizations (JCAHO) accreditation
+ American Osteopathic Hospital Association (AOHA) membership
○ American Osteopathic Association (AOA) accreditation
△ Commission on Accreditation of Rehabilitation Facilities (CARF) accreditation
  Control codes 61, 63, 64, 71, 72 and 73 indicate hospitals listed by AOHA, but not registered by AHA. For definition of numerical codes, see page A4

CEDAR FALLS—Black Hawk County

✴ SARTORI MEMORIAL HOSPITAL, 515 College Street, Zip 50613–2599; tel. 319/266–3584; Verna M. Klinkenborg, President (Total facility includes 18 beds in nursing home–type unit) **A**1 9 10 **F**8 12 17 19 20 22 24 30 32 33 34 35 36 37 39 41 44 49 51 64 65 66 67 71 73	14	10	101	1757	22	67713	0	17559	8105	247

CEDAR RAPIDS—Linn County

✴ MERCY MEDICAL CENTER, 701 Tenth Street S.E., Zip 52403; tel. 319/398–6011; A. James Tinker, President and Chief Executive Officer (Total facility includes 90 beds in nursing home–type unit) **A**1 2 3 9 10 **F**2 3 4 7 8 10 11 12 14 15 16 19 20 21 22 24 26 28 29 30 31 32 33 34 35 37 40 41 42 44 45 46 47 48 49 52 54 55 56 57 58 59 60 63 64 65 67 69 70 71 73 74 **P**1 5	21	10	406	9747	200	106222	977	83982	37180	1309
✴ △ ST. LUKE'S HOSPITAL, 1026 A Avenue N.E., Zip 52402–3026, Mailing Address: P.O. Box 3026, Zip 52406–3026; tel. 319/369–7211; Stephen E. Vanourny, M.D., President (Total facility includes 28 beds in nursing home–type unit) **A**1 3 7 9 10 **F**3 4 7 8 10 11 12 14 15 16 17 19 20 21 22 24 25 26 27 28 29 30 31 32 33 34 35 36 37 38 39 40 41 42 43 44 45 46 47 48 49 51 52 53 54 55 56 57 58 59 61 64 65 66 67 68 70 71 72 73 74 **P**3 7 8 **S** Iowa Health System, Des Moines, IA	23	10	406	13921	213	186019	2146	127061	57285	1726

CENTERVILLE—Appanoose County

✴ ST. JOSEPH'S MERCY HOSPITAL, 1 St. Joseph's Drive, Zip 52544; tel. 515/437–3411; William C. Assell, President and Chief Executive Officer (Total facility includes 24 beds in nursing home–type unit) **A**1 9 10 **F**7 8 14 15 16 19 21 22 26 28 29 30 32 33 34 35 36 37 39 40 44 45 51 64 65 66 67 71 73 **S** Catholic Health Initiatives, Denver, CO **N** Mercy Network of Health Services, Des Moines, IA	21	10	58	1096	43	40615	71	7760	3703	167

CHARITON—Lucas County

★ LUCAS COUNTY HEALTH CENTER, 1200 North Seventh Street, Zip 50049; tel. 515/774–3000; Cathy Stotts, Chief Executive Officer **A**9 10 **F**1 3 6 7 8 15 16 19 21 22 27 28 30 32 34 35 44 49 51 53 54 55 56 57 58 59 61 62 65 66 67 70 71 72 73 **P**7	13	10	56	579	7	12546	102	8726	3496	154

CHARLES CITY—Floyd County

FLOYD COUNTY MEMORIAL HOSPITAL, 800 Eleventh Street, Zip 50616–3499; tel. 515/228–6830; Bill D. Faust, Administrator **A**9 10 **F**7 8 11 14 15 16 19 22 28 29 30 32 33 34 36 37 39 40 41 42 44 49 51 53 57 58 65 66 67 71 73 **S** Mayo Foundation, Rochester, MN	13	10	29	1311	16	38861	107	9209	3850	151

CHEROKEE—Cherokee County

□ MENTAL HEALTH INSTITUTE, 1200 West Cedar Street, Zip 51012; tel. 712/225–2594; Tom Deiker, Ph.D., Superintendent **A**1 10 13 **F**1 14 15 16 27 45 52 53 54 55 56 58 59 65	12	22	174	927	79	2896	0	14452	9855	259
★ SIOUX VALLEY MEMORIAL HOSPITAL, 300 Sioux Valley Drive, Zip 51012; tel. 712/225–5101; John M. Comstock, Chief Executive Officer **A**9 10 **F**7 8 11 12 14 15 17 19 22 24 26 28 29 30 31 32 33 34 35 36 39 40 41 42 44 45 46 49 51 53 54 55 56 57 58 64 65 66 67 71 73 **P**4 6	23	10	40	1202	14	20956	118	8957	4488	165

CLARINDA—Page County

★ CLARINDA REGIONAL HEALTH CENTER, (Formerly Clarinda Municipal Hospital), 17th and Wells Streets, Zip 51632, Mailing Address: P.O. Box 217, Zip 51632–0217; tel. 712/542–2176; Rudy Snedigar, Administrator **A**9 10 **F**8 14 15 16 19 21 22 24 26 28 30 32 34 35 36 39 42 44 46 49 58 65 67 71 73	14	10	26	626	12	30202	79	4978	2257	126
MENTAL HEALTH INSTITUTE, Mailing Address: Box 338, Zip 51632–0338; tel. 712/542–2161; Mark Lund, Superintendent (Total facility includes 63 beds in nursing home–type unit) **F**4 11 14 15 16 19 20 21 25 26 35 37 40 41 44 48 50 52 54 55 56 57 58 60 63 64 65 71 73	12	22	83	201	69	0	0	—	—	135

CLARION—Wright County

★ COMMUNITY MEMORIAL HOSPITAL, 1316 South Main Street, Zip 50525–0429; tel. 515/532–2811; Steve J. Simonin, Chief Executive Officer **A**9 10 **F**7 8 14 17 19 20 22 30 32 33 34 35 36 39 40 41 42 44 49 62 65 67 71 73 **P**7 8 **S** Iowa Health System, Des Moines, IA	14	10	33	566	14	21769	89	4744	1926	85

CLINTON—Clinton County

✴ SAMARITAN HEALTH SYSTEM, (Includes Samaritan Hospital North, 1410 North Fourth Street, tel. 319/244–5555; Samaritan Services for Aging, 600 14th Avenue North, tel. 319/244–3888), 1410 North Fourth Street, Zip 52732, Mailing Address: P.O. Box 2960, Zip 52733–2960; tel. 319/244–5555; Thomas J. Hesselmann, President and Chief Executive Officer (Total facility includes 189 beds in nursing home–type unit) **A**1 9 10 **F**1 3 7 8 10 11 12 15 16 17 18 19 20 21 22 23 26 27 28 29 30 32 33 34 35 36 40 41 42 44 46 49 52 53 54 55 56 57 58 59 60 62 63 64 65 67 71 73 74 **P**8 **S** Mercy Health Services, Farmington Hills, MI	21	10	360	6428	259	43530	479	40467	17259	751

CORNING—Adams County

✴ ALEGENT HEALTH MERCY HOSPITAL, (Formerly Mercy Hospital), Rosary Drive, Zip 50841, Mailing Address: Box 368, Zip 50841; tel. 515/322–3121; James C. Ruppert, Regional Administrator **A**1 9 10 **F**8 12 15 16 19 22 28 29 30 32 33 34 35 36 39 40 41 42 44 49 58 63 65 67 71 73 **P**6 **S** Catholic Health Initiatives, Denver, CO **N** Alegent Health, Omaha, NE	21	10	24	524	8	39503	47	4886	2162	114

CORYDON—Wayne County

★ WAYNE COUNTY HOSPITAL, 417 South East Street, Zip 50060, Mailing Address: Box 305, Zip 50060; tel. 515/872–2260; Bill D. Wilson, Administrator **A**9 10 **F**7 8 12 13 14 15 17 19 20 22 28 30 32 33 34 36 37 39 40 44 45 49 51 64 65 70 71 73 **P**8 **N** Mercy Network of Health Services, Des Moines, IA	13	10	20	991	14	11226	79	4063	1870	87

Hospital, Address, Telephone, Administrator, Approval, Facility, and Physician Codes, Health Care System, Network	Classi-fication Codes		Utilization Data					Expense (thousands) of dollars		
	Control	Service	Beds	Admissions	Census	Outpatient Visits	Births	Total	Payroll	Personnel

★ American Hospital Association (AHA) membership
☐ Joint Commission on Accreditation of Healthcare Organizations (JCAHO) accreditation
+ American Osteopathic Hospital Association (AOHA) membership
○ American Osteopathic Association (AOA) accreditation
△ Commission on Accreditation of Rehabilitation Facilities (CARF) accreditation
Control codes 61, 63, 64, 71, 72 and 73 indicate hospitals listed by AOHA, but not registered by AHA. For definition of numerical codes, see page A4

COUNCIL BLUFFS—Pottawattamie County

✸ ALEGENT HEALTH MERCY HOSPITAL, (Formerly Mercy Hospital), 800 Mercy Drive, Zip 51503, Mailing Address: Box 1C, Zip 51502; tel. 712/328–5000; Charles J. Marr, Chief Executive Officer (Total facility includes 24 beds in nursing home–type unit) **A**1 9 10 **F**1 2 3 4 7 8 10 11 12 15 16 17 18 19 20 21 22 23 24 25 26 27 28 29 30 31 32 33 34 35 36 37 38 39 40 41 42 43 44 45 46 48 49 50 51 52 53 54 55 56 57 58 59 60 61 62 63 64 65 66 67 68 71 72 73 74 **P**8 **S** Catholic Health Initiatives, Denver, CO **N** Alegent Health, Omaha, NE	21	10	194	5565	79	51163	444	43942	18174	656
✸ JENNIE EDMUNDSON MEMORIAL HOSPITAL, 933 East Pierce Street, Zip 51503–4652, Mailing Address: P.O. Box 2C, Zip 51502–3002; tel. 712/328–6000; David M. Holcomb, President and Chief Executive Officer (Total facility includes 17 beds in nursing home–type unit) **A**1 5 6 9 10 **F**3 7 8 10 12 15 17 19 21 22 23 28 29 30 31 32 33 35 36 37 39 40 41 42 44 46 49 52 53 54 55 56 57 58 59 60 63 64 65 66 67 71 73 **P**3 8	23	10	108	5742	94	63542	638	47364	21631	659
MERCY HOSPITAL See Alegent Health Mercy Hospital										

CRESCO—Howard County

★ HOWARD COUNTY HOSPITAL, 235 Eighth Avenue West, Zip 52136–1098; tel. 319/547–2101; Elizabeth A. Doty, Administrator **A**9 10 **F**7 8 15 19 22 30 33 39 40 44 49 71 73 **P**3 4 5 8 **S** Mercy Health Services, Farmington Hills, MI **N** North Iowa Mercy Health Network, Mason City, IA	13	10	32	418	4	14324	94	4113	1870	76

CRESTON—Union County

★ GREATER COMMUNITY HOSPITAL, 1700 West Townline, Zip 50801–1099; tel. 515/782–7091; Marlys Scherlin, Administrator **A**9 10 **F**7 8 12 14 15 16 19 20 22 24 27 28 29 30 31 32 33 34 35 36 37 39 40 41 42 44 49 50 54 56 58 59 60 63 65 67 69 71 73 **P**3	15	10	53	1451	19	26675	204	10068	4651	188

DAVENPORT—Scott County

☐ ○ DAVENPORT MEDICAL CENTER, 1111 West Kimberly Road, Zip 52806; tel. 319/391–2020; Richard A. Seidler, Chief Executive Officer **A**1 9 10 11 12 13 **F**7 8 12 14 15 16 19 20 22 26 30 32 34 37 39 40 41 42 44 45 46 61 63 64 65 67 71 72 73 74 **P**1 2 5 **S** TENET Healthcare Corporation, Santa Barbara, CA	33	10	106	1559	19	35529	241	19622	7612	239
✸ △ GENESIS MEDICAL CENTER, (Includes Genesis Medical Center–East Campus, Genesis Medical Center–West Campus, 1401 West Central Park, Zip 52804–1769; tel. 319/383–1000), 1227 East Rusholme Street, Zip 52803; tel. 319/421–6000; Leo A. Bressanelli, President and Chief Executive Officer (Total facility includes 41 beds in nursing home–type unit) **A**1 2 3 5 7 9 10 **F**2 3 4 5 7 8 10 11 12 15 16 17 18 19 20 21 22 23 25 27 29 30 31 32 33 34 35 36 37 38 39 40 41 42 43 44 46 48 49 51 52 53 54 56 57 60 63 64 65 67 71 72 73 **P**6 7 8 **N** MEDACOM Tri–State, Oakbrook, IL; Genesis Health System, Davenport, IA	23	10	466	18660	321	162246	2278	166179	66274	3388

DE WITT—Clinton County

✸ DEWITT COMMUNITY HOSPITAL, 1118 11th Street, Zip 52742; tel. 319/659–3241; C. James Christensen, Chief Executive Officer (Total facility includes 77 beds in nursing home–type unit) **A**1 9 10 **F**8 9 12 14 15 16 17 19 20 22 26 27 28 29 30 33 36 38 39 44 45 46 49 51 64 65 66 67 71 72 73 **P**1 5 8 **N** Genesis Health System, Davenport, IA	23	10	101	461	82	19536	0	5660	2517	142

DECORAH—Winneshiek County

✸ WINNESHIEK COUNTY MEMORIAL HOSPITAL, 901 Montgomery Street, Zip 52101; tel. 319/382–2911; Paul J. Anderson, Administrator **A**1 9 10 **F**7 8 11 12 14 15 17 19 21 22 28 30 31 32 33 34 36 37 39 40 41 42 44 45 46 49 65 66 67 71 73	13	10	83	1179	12	33910	256	8459	4374	172

DENISON—Crawford County

CRAWFORD COUNTY MEMORIAL HOSPITAL, 2020 First Avenue South, Zip 51442; tel. 712/263–5021; Gary L. Petersen, Administrator **A**9 10 **F**3 7 8 14 15 16 17 18 19 20 21 22 24 26 27 28 29 30 31 32 33 34 35 37 39 40 41 42 44 45 46 49 51 53 54 55 56 57 58 59 62 65 66 67 68 71 72 73 74 **P**1 3	13	10	72	895	12	19276	122	4892	3085	121

DES MOINES—Polk County

✸ BROADLAWNS MEDICAL CENTER, 1801 Hickman Road, Zip 50314–1597; tel. 515/282–2200; Willis F. Fry, Executive Director **A**1 3 5 9 10 **F**1 2 3 7 8 12 14 15 16 17 18 19 20 21 22 27 28 31 33 34 35 37 38 39 40 41 43 44 46 49 51 52 53 54 55 56 58 59 65 67 71 72 73 **P**6	13	10	107	5031	59	200129	579	55949	27655	839
✸ + ○ DES MOINES GENERAL HOSPITAL, 603 East 12th Street, Zip 50309–5515; tel. 515/263–4200; Roy W. Wright, Chief Executive Officer (Total facility includes 15 beds in nursing home–type unit) (Nonreporting) **A**1 9 10 11 12 13 **S** Quorum Health Group/Quorum Health Resources, Inc., Brentwood, TN	23	10	112	—	—	—	—	—	—	—
✸ IOWA LUTHERAN HOSPITAL, 700 East University Avenue, Zip 50316–2392; tel. 515/263–5612; James H. Skogsbergh, President (Total facility includes 16 beds in nursing home–type unit) **A**1 3 5 9 10 **F**1 2 3 4 7 8 9 10 11 12 13 14 15 16 17 18 19 21 22 24 25 26 27 28 29 30 31 32 33 34 35 37 39 40 41 42 43 44 45 46 47 48 49 51 52 53 54 55 56 57 58 59 60 61 63 64 65 66 67 68 69 70 71 72 73 **P**1 2 3 6 7 **S** Iowa Health System, Des Moines, IA	23	10	243	9010	139	308638	1262	—	—	—
✸ IOWA METHODIST MEDICAL CENTER, (Includes Powell Convalescent Center, Raymond Blank Memorial Hospital for Children, Younker Memorial Rehabilitation Center), 1200 Pleasant Street, Zip 50309–9976; tel. 515/241–6212; James H. Skogsbergh, President **A**1 2 3 5 6 9 10 **F**1 2 3 4 7 8 9 10 11 12 14 15 16 17 18 19 21 22 24 25 26 27 28 29 30 31 32 33 34 35 37 39 40 41 42 43 44 45 46 47 48 49 51 52 53 54 55 56 57 58 59 60 61 63 64 65 66 67 68 69 70 71 72 73 **P**1 3 6 7 **S** Iowa Health System, Des Moines, IA **N** St Lukes/Iowa Health System, Des Moines, IA	23	10	557	19549	312	248552	2020	—	— 4277

Hospital, Address, Telephone, Administrator, Approval, Facility, and Physician Codes, Health Care System, Network	Classi-fication Codes		Utilization Data					Expense (thousands) of dollars		
	Control	Service	Beds	Admissions	Census	Outpatient Visits	Births	Total	Payroll	Personnel

✠ MERCY HOSPITAL MEDICAL CENTER, (Includes Mercy Franklin Center, 1818 48th Street, Zip 50310; tel. 515/271–6000), 400 University Avenue, Zip 50314; tel. 515/247–4278; Thomas A. Reitinger, President and Chief Executive Officer (Total facility includes 35 beds in nursing home–type unit) **A**1 2 3 6 9 10 **F**1 3 4 5 6 7 8 10 11 12 14 15 16 17 18 19 20 21 22 23 24 25 26 28 30 31 32 33 34 35 37 38 39 40 41 42 43 44 47 49 51 52 53 54 55 56 57 58 59 60 62 64 65 66 67 69 70 71 72 73 74 **P**1 **S** Catholic Health Initiatives, Denver, CO **N** Mercy Network of Health Services, Des Moines, IA	21	10	584	25970	401	179393	3161	266858	99087	3068
✠ VETERANS AFFAIRS MEDICAL CENTER, 3600 30th Street, Zip 50310–5774; tel. 515/255–2173; Ellen DeGeorge–Smith, Director **A**1 2 3 5 **F**2 3 4 8 9 10 11 12 18 19 20 21 22 23 26 27 29 30 31 32 33 35 37 39 41 42 43 44 46 49 51 52 54 55 56 57 58 59 60 63 64 65 67 69 70 71 73 74 **P**6 **S** Department of Veterans Affairs, Washington, DC	45	10	99	3604	77	100964	0	45503	27625	666

DUBUQUE—Dubuque County

✠ FINLEY HOSPITAL, 350 North Grandview Avenue, Zip 52001–6392; tel. 319/582–1881; Kevin L. Rogols, President and Chief Executive Officer (Total facility includes 17 beds in nursing home–type unit) **A**1 2 9 10 **F**4 7 8 12 14 15 16 17 19 21 22 23 24 26 27 28 29 30 31 32 33 34 35 36 37 39 40 41 42 44 45 46 49 60 61 63 64 65 66 67 70 71 72 73 74 **P**1 5 7	23	10	143	5194	71	42721	550	44285	18013	680
✠ △ MERCY HEALTH CENTER, (Includes Mercy Health Center–St. Mary's Unit, 1111 Third Street S.W., Dyersville, Zip 52040; tel. 319/875–7101), 250 Mercy Drive, Zip 52001–7360; tel. 319/589–8000; Sister Helen Huewe, President (Total facility includes 69 beds in nursing home–type unit) **A**1 7 9 10 **F**1 2 3 4 7 8 10 12 13 15 16 17 19 20 21 22 23 24 26 27 28 29 30 31 32 34 35 37 38 39 40 41 42 43 44 45 48 49 52 53 54 55 56 57 58 59 60 63 64 65 66 67 68 69 70 71 72 73 74 **P**8 **S** Mercy Health Services, Farmington Hills, MI	21	10	385	9815	123	47470	980	71744	31404	1098

DYERSVILLE—Dubuque County

MERCY HEALTH CENTER–ST. MARY'S UNIT See Mercy Health Center, Dubuque

ELDORA—Hardin County

★ ELDORA REGIONAL MEDICAL CENTER, 2413 Edgington Avenue, Zip 50627–1541; tel. 515/858–5416; Greg Reed, Administrator **A**9 10 **F**8 15 16 19 21 22 28 30 33 34 41 42 44 46 49 70 71 73 **P**6 **S** Mercy Health Services, Farmington Hills, MI **N** North Iowa Mercy Health Network, Mason City, IA	14	10	18	310	3	11488	2	3109	1634	48

ELKADER—Clayton County

★ CENTRAL COMMUNITY HOSPITAL, 901 Davidson Street, Zip 52043–9799; tel. 319/245–2250; Lisa Manson, Administrator **A**9 10 **F**7 8 11 12 15 16 17 18 19 22 24 26 28 29 30 31 32 33 34 37 39 40 41 42 44 45 46 48 49 58 64 66 67 71 73 74 **P**3 **S** Lutheran Health Systems, Fargo, ND	23	10	29	319	4	8458	27	2742	949	67

EMMETSBURG—Palo Alto County

PALO ALTO COUNTY HOSPITAL, 3201 First Street, Zip 50536; tel. 712/852–2434; Darrell E. Vondrak, Administrator (Total facility includes 22 beds in nursing home–type unit) **A**9 10 **F**7 8 14 15 16 19 21 22 26 27 29 30 32 33 34 35 36 37 39 40 41 42 44 49 64 65 67 71 **P**7 **S** Mercy Health Services, Farmington Hills, MI	13	10	54	791	30	20036	71	5223	2720	128

ESTHERVILLE—Emmet County

✠ HOLY FAMILY HEALTH SERVICES, (Formerly Holy Family Hospital), 826 North Eighth Street, Zip 51334–1598; tel. 712/362–2631; Thomas Nordwick, President and Chief Executive Officer **A**1 9 10 **F**1 3 7 8 12 13 15 17 18 19 22 26 27 30 31 32 33 34 35 36 37 39 40 42 44 49 58 65 67 71 **S** Presentation Health System, Yankton, SD	21	10	36	1016	14	29151	74	8002	3822	188

FAIRFIELD—Jefferson County

★ JEFFERSON COUNTY HOSPITAL, 400 Highland Avenue, Zip 52556, Mailing Address: Box 588, Zip 52556; tel. 515/472–4111; Walter W. Brownlee, President (Total facility includes 36 beds in nursing home–type unit) **A**9 10 **F**7 8 14 15 16 19 22 30 32 34 35 37 39 40 41 42 44 49 52 53 54 56 58 59 64 65 71	13	10	83	1791	52	26121	98	10221	4417	179

FORT DODGE—Webster County

✠ TRINITY REGIONAL HOSPITAL, 802 Kenyon Road, Zip 50501; tel. 515/573–3101; Tom Tibbitts, President (Total facility includes 12 beds in nursing home–type unit) **A**1 9 10 **F**2 3 7 8 12 14 15 16 17 19 21 22 23 27 29 30 31 32 33 34 35 37 39 40 41 44 46 48 49 52 53 54 55 56 57 58 59 61 63 64 65 66 67 68 71 73 **P**7	23	10	184	6259	83	103826	503	46543	20748	706

FORT MADISON—Lee County

✠ FORT MADISON COMMUNITY HOSPITAL, Highway 61 West, Zip 52627–0174, Mailing Address: Highway 61 West, Box 174, Zip 52627–0174; tel. 319/372–6530; C. James Platt, Administrator **A**1 9 10 **F**8 12 14 15 16 19 22 24 27 28 30 35 37 40 41 42 44 45 46 48 49 60 64 65 71 73 74 **S** Quorum Health Group/Quorum Health Resources, Inc., Brentwood, TN	23	10	50	1997	23	31553	167	15132	6074	207

GLENWOOD—Mills County

GLENWOOD STATE HOSPITAL SCHOOL, Zip 51534; tel. 712/527–4811; William E. Campbell, Ph.D., Superintendent **F**6 12 14 15 16 17 18 20 24 48 52 53 54 65 73 **P**6	12	62	437	30	401	0	0	36692	25198	840

GREENFIELD—Adair County

ADAIR COUNTY MEMORIAL HOSPITAL, 609 S.E. Kent Street, Zip 50849; tel. 515/743–2123; Myrna Erb, Administrator **A**9 10 **F**7 8 14 15 19 22 26 30 32 34 35 36 39 42 44 49 71 **N** Mercy Network of Health Services, Des Moines, IA	13	10	31	447	6	6655	19	2631	1188	77

Hospital, Address, Telephone, Administrator, Approval, Facility, and Physician Codes, Health Care System, Network	Classi-fication Codes		Utilization Data					Expense (thousands) of dollars		
★ American Hospital Association (AHA) membership □ Joint Commission on Accreditation of Healthcare Organizations (JCAHO) accreditation + American Osteopathic Hospital Association (AOHA) membership ○ American Osteopathic Association (AOA) accreditation △ Commission on Accreditation of Rehabilitation Facilities (CARF) accreditation Control codes 61, 63, 64, 71, 72 and 73 indicate hospitals listed by AOHA, but not registered by AHA. For definition of numerical codes, see page A4	Control	Service	Beds	Admissions	Census	Outpatient Visits	Births	Total	Payroll	Personnel

GRINNELL—Poweshiek County

⊞ GRINNELL REGIONAL MEDICAL CENTER, 210 Fourth Avenue, Zip 50112–1833; tel. 515/236–7511; Todd C. Linden, President and Chief Executive Officer **A**1 9 10 **F**1 12 13 14 15 16 17 19 20 22 24 27 29 30 31 32 33 35 36 37 39 40 41 42 44 45 46 49 51 58 62 63 65 67 70 71 73 **P**3 7	23	10	46	2323	25	33953	190	17916	—	211

GRUNDY CENTER—Grundy County

GRUNDY COUNTY MEMORIAL HOSPITAL, 201 East J Avenue, Zip 50638–2096; tel. 319/824–5421; James A. Faulwell, Administrator (Total facility includes 55 beds in nursing home–type unit) **A**9 10 **F**8 12 14 15 16 17 19 22 26 28 30 33 39 41 44 45 46 49 64 65 67 71 72 **P**3	13	10	73	389	61	41081	4	3565	1818	119

GUTHRIE CENTER—Guthrie County

★ GUTHRIE COUNTY HOSPITAL, 710 North 12th Street, Zip 50115; tel. 515/747–2201; Stuart Bell, Administrator **A**9 10 **F**7 8 11 12 15 17 19 20 21 22 33 34 35 36 39 40 41 42 44 49 58 65 70 71 73	13	10	26	478	6	7014	16	3016	1200	56

GUTTENBERG—Clayton County

★ GUTTENBERG MUNICIPAL HOSPITAL, Second and Main Street, Zip 52052–0550, Mailing Address: Box 550, Zip 52052–0550; tel. 319/252–1121; Timothy J. Wick, Chief Executive Officer **A**9 10 **F**7 8 19 21 22 26 28 30 32 33 36 37 39 40 42 44 64 66 71 **P**5 **S** Brim, Inc., Portland, OR	14	10	29	480	6	13011	45	3671	1490	82

HAMBURG—Fremont County

GRAPE COMMUNITY HOSPITAL, Highway 275 North, Zip 51640, Mailing Address: P.O. Box 246, Zip 51640–0246; tel. 712/382–1515; Carolyn K. Hess, Administrator **A**9 10 **F**7 8 15 19 22 30 32 34 35 36 37 39 40 42 44 45 49 71 73	23	10	49	611	21	12236	15	4709	2252	103

HAMPTON—Franklin County

★ FRANKLIN GENERAL HOSPITAL, 1720 Central Avenue East, Zip 50441–1859; tel. 515/456–4721; Laura Olander, Chief Executive Officer (Total facility includes 52 beds in nursing home–type unit) **A**9 10 **F**3 4 5 7 8 10 11 12 14 15 16 18 19 20 22 26 27 29 30 31 32 33 34 35 37 39 40 41 42 43 44 45 49 56 58 60 62 64 65 66 67 71 72 73 74 **P**2 6 8 **S** Mercy Health Services, Farmington Hills, MI **N** North Iowa Mercy Health Network, Mason City, IA	13	10	82	527	60	21206	0	4734	2378	116

HARLAN—Shelby County

★ SHELBY COUNTY MYRTUE MEMORIAL HOSPITAL, 1213 Garfield Avenue, Zip 51537; tel. 712/755–5161; Stephen L. Goeser, Administrator **A**9 10 **F**7 8 12 13 14 15 16 17 18 19 21 22 24 28 30 32 33 34 35 36 37 40 41 42 44 49 51 53 54 56 58 63 67 68 71 73 **P**6 8	13	10	52	1208	18	21477	72	8489	3437	161

HAWARDEN—Sioux County

HAWARDEN COMMUNITY HOSPITAL, 1111 11th Street, Zip 51023; tel. 712/552–3100; Stuart A. Katz, FACHE, Chief Executive Officer **A**9 10 **F**8 12 15 16 17 19 21 22 27 28 30 32 33 34 35 42 44 46 49 51 54 58 67 68 71 73 **P**1 **S** Mercy Health Services, Farmington Hills, MI	14	10	19	199	5	12162	0	1594	717	35

HUMBOLDT—Humboldt County

HUMBOLDT COUNTY MEMORIAL HOSPITAL, 1000 North 15th Street, Zip 50548; tel. 515/332–4200; Kari L. Engholm, Administrator **A**9 10 **F**7 8 15 17 19 21 22 30 33 34 35 39 40 41 44 49 65 71 **P**3	13	10	49	567	28	22290	57	4556	2211	105

IDA GROVE—Ida County

★ HORN MEMORIAL HOSPITAL, 701 East Second Street, Zip 51445; tel. 712/364–3311; Dan Ellis, Administrator **A**9 10 **F**8 14 15 16 19 22 32 33 34 36 37 40 41 42 44 51 54 64 71 73	23	10	36	698	10	21056	100	3830	1972	70

INDEPENDENCE—Buchanan County

□ MENTAL HEALTH INSTITUTE, 2277 Iowa Avenue, Zip 50644, Mailing Address: Box 111, Zip 50644; tel. 319/334–2583; B. J. Dave, M.D., Superintendent **A**1 10 **F**14 15 16 20 22 27 45 46 51 52 53 54 55 56 58 65 67 73 **P**6	12	22	213	1052	153	13	0	18224	12993	374
★ PEOPLE'S MEMORIAL HOSPITAL OF BUCHANAN COUNTY, 1600 First Street East, Zip 50644–3155; tel. 319/334–6071; Robert J. Richard, Administrator (Total facility includes 59 beds in nursing home–type unit) **A**9 10 **F**7 8 14 15 16 19 22 28 30 31 32 33 36 40 41 44 49 64 65 71 **P**4	13	10	109	478	63	25552	42	6172	3110	144

IOWA CITY—Johnson County

⊞ MERCY HOSPITAL, 500 East Market Street, Zip 52245; tel. 319/339–0300; Ronald R. Reed, President and Chief Executive Officer (Total facility includes 12 beds in nursing home–type unit) **A**1 2 3 5 9 10 **F**4 7 8 10 14 15 16 17 19 22 23 26 28 29 30 32 33 35 37 38 39 40 41 42 43 44 45 49 52 60 63 64 66 67 71 73 **P**8 **S** Mercy–Chicago Region Healthcare System, Naperville, IL	21	10	240	8932	134	199167	1250	62700	28236	783
STATE PSYCHIATRIC HOSPITAL See University of Iowa Hospitals and Clinics										
⊞ UNIVERSITY OF IOWA HOSPITALS AND CLINICS, (Includes Chemical Dependency Center, Oakdale, tel. 319/335–4165; State Psychiatric Hospital, tel. 319/356–4658; University Hospital School, tel. 319/353–6456), 200 Hawkins Drive, Zip 52242–1009; tel. 319/356–1616; R. Edward Howell, Director and Chief Executive Officer **A**1 2 3 5 8 9 10 **F**2 3 4 5 7 8 9 10 11 12 13 14 15 16 17 19 20 21 22 23 25 26 27 28 29 30 31 33 34 35 37 38 39 40 41 42 43 44 45 46 47 48 49 50 51 52 53 54 55 56 57 58 59 60 61 63 65 66 67 69 70 71 72 73 74 **P**1	12	10	840	39042	631	632138	1352	399565	170315	5251
⊞ VETERANS AFFAIRS MEDICAL CENTER, Highway 6 West, Zip 52246–2208; tel. 319/338–0581; Gary L. Wilkinson, Director **A**1 3 5 8 **F**1 3 4 8 10 12 16 19 20 21 22 23 26 27 28 30 31 32 33 34 35 37 39 41 42 43 44 45 46 49 50 51 52 54 56 58 60 63 65 67 69 71 73 74 **S** Department of Veterans Affairs, Washington, DC	45	10	159	5621	113	121069	0	71533	41096	1044

Hospital, Address, Telephone, Administrator, Approval, Facility, and Physician Codes, Health Care System, Network	Classi-fication Codes		Utilization Data					Expense (thousands) of dollars		
★ American Hospital Association (AHA) membership □ Joint Commission on Accreditation of Healthcare Organizations (JCAHO) accreditation + American Osteopathic Hospital Association (AOHA) membership ○ American Osteopathic Association (AOA) accreditation △ Commission on Accreditation of Rehabilitation Facilities (CARF) accreditation Control codes 61, 63, 64, 71, 72 and 73 indicate hospitals listed by AOHA, but not registered by AHA. For definition of numerical codes, see page A4	Control	Service	Beds	Admissions	Census	Outpatient Visits	Births	Total	Payroll	Personnel

IOWA FALLS—Hardin County

⊞ ELLSWORTH MUNICIPAL HOSPITAL, 110 Rocksylvania Avenue, Zip 50126–2431; tel. 515/648–4631; John O'Brien, Administrator **A**1 2 9 10 **F**1 3 7 8 11 12 13 14 15 16 19 22 24 27 28 29 30 31 33 35 37 39 40 41 42 44 45 49 52 53 54 55 56 57 58 59 61 65 67 71 72 73 **P**3 5 8 **S** Mercy Health Services, Farmington Hills, MI | 14 | 10 | 40 | 1337 | 17 | 13133 | 166 | 8438 | 4743 | 154 |

JEFFERSON—Greene County

⊞ GREENE COUNTY MEDICAL CENTER, 1000 West Lincolnway, Zip 50129–1697; tel. 515/386–2114; Karen L. Bossard, Administrator (Total facility includes 62 beds in nursing home–type unit) **A**1 9 10 **F**1 7 8 11 12 13 14 15 16 17 18 19 21 22 26 28 29 30 31 32 33 34 35 39 40 41 42 44 45 49 62 64 65 66 67 68 71 73 74 **P**5 | 13 | 10 | 115 | 1012 | 92 | 22932 | 102 | 8840 | 4519 | 208 |

KEOKUK—Lee County

⊞ KEOKUK AREA HOSPITAL, 1600 Morgan Street, Zip 52632; tel. 319/524–7150; Allan Zastrow, FACHE, Chief Executive Officer (Total facility includes 20 beds in nursing home–type unit) **A**1 9 10 **F**3 7 8 11 14 15 16 17 19 21 22 23 28 29 30 32 33 34 35 40 44 45 46 49 52 53 54 55 56 61 64 65 66 67 71 73 **N** BJC Health System, St. Louis, MO | 23 | 10 | 113 | 4282 | 65 | 41951 | 314 | 20810 | 9682 | 395 |

KEOSAUQUA—Van Buren County

★ VAN BUREN COUNTY HOSPITAL, Highway 1 North, Zip 52565, Mailing Address: Box 70, Zip 52565; tel. 319/293–3171; Lisa Wagner Schnedler, Administrator **A**9 10 **F**1 7 8 12 14 15 16 17 19 22 26 28 30 34 35 39 40 41 42 45 44 45 46 49 53 54 55 56 57 58 59 64 65 71 73 74 **P**6 **S** Sisters of Mary of the Presentation Health Corporation, Fargo, ND | 13 | 10 | 40 | 569 | 17 | 11154 | 60 | 3868 | 1819 | 78 |

KNOXVILLE—Marion County

⊞ KNOXVILLE AREA COMMUNITY HOSPITAL, 1002 South Lincoln Street, Zip 50138–3121; tel. 515/842–2151; Daryl Mackender, Chief Executive Officer (Total facility includes 14 beds in nursing home–type unit) **A**1 9 10 **F**7 8 11 15 16 19 21 22 28 30 33 34 35 37 40 41 44 45 49 56 63 64 65 66 67 71 73 **P**8 **S** Quorum Health Group/Quorum Health Resources, Inc., Brentwood, TN | 23 | 10 | 52 | 1434 | 26 | 14142 | 111 | 7897 | 3026 | 137 |

⊞ VETERANS AFFAIRS MEDICAL CENTER, 1515 West Pleasant, Zip 50138–3399; tel. 515/842–3101; Ellen DeGeorge–Smith, Acting Director (Total facility includes 260 beds in nursing home–type unit) **A**1 **F**2 3 15 22 26 30 31 32 34 35 41 44 46 48 49 51 52 54 55 56 57 58 64 65 71 73 74 **S** Department of Veterans Affairs, Washington, DC | 45 | 22 | 565 | 2672 | 479 | 64070 | 0 | 49766 | 38657 | 853 |

LAKE CITY—Calhoun County

★ STEWART MEMORIAL COMMUNITY HOSPITAL, 1301 West Main, Zip 51449–1585; tel. 712/464–3171; Jon L. Jensen, Interim Administrator **A**9 10 **F**7 8 14 19 22 29 30 32 33 34 35 36 37 40 41 42 44 45 49 56 65 71 **P**5 6 | 23 | 10 | 49 | 1997 | 32 | 43674 | 174 | 8829 | 4235 | 168 |

LE MARS—Plymouth County

FLOYD VALLEY HOSPITAL, Highway 3 East, Zip 51031, Mailing Address: P.O. Box 10, Zip 51031; tel. 712/546–7871; G. Frank LaBonte, FACHE, Chief Executive Officer **A**9 10 **F**3 7 8 11 13 15 16 17 18 19 22 24 28 29 30 32 33 34 35 36 39 40 41 42 44 45 46 48 49 56 65 66 67 71 73 **P**5 **S** St. Luke's Health System, Inc., Sioux City, IA | 14 | 10 | 44 | 1325 | 18 | 32689 | 134 | 8182 | 3466 | 126 |

LEON—Decatur County

⊞ DECATUR COUNTY HOSPITAL, 1405 N.W. Church Street, Zip 50144–1299; tel. 515/446–4871; Neil Davenport, Administrator **A**1 9 10 **F**8 14 15 16 19 22 34 37 39 40 41 42 44 45 46 49 53 54 55 56 57 58 59 67 71 73 | 13 | 10 | 49 | 583 | 13 | 45000 | 87 | 4458 | 2011 | 97 |

MANCHESTER—Delaware County

DELAWARE COUNTY MEMORIAL HOSPITAL, 709 West Main Street, Zip 52057–0359; tel. 319/927–3232; Lon D. Butikofer, R.N., Ph.D., Administrator and Chief Executive Officer (Total facility includes 12 beds in nursing home–type unit) **A**9 10 **F**7 8 12 13 14 15 16 17 18 19 22 24 26 27 28 29 30 31 32 33 34 37 39 40 41 42 44 45 46 49 51 54 55 56 58 64 66 67 71 73 **P**3 5 | 13 | 10 | 49 | 841 | 33 | 49331 | 183 | 9803 | 5236 | 169 |

MANNING—Carroll County

MANNING GENERAL HOSPITAL, 410 Main Street, Zip 51455; tel. 712/653–2072; Mitchel S. Ketcham, Administrator (Total facility includes 12 beds in nursing home–type unit) **A**9 10 **F**1 2 3 7 8 14 18 19 21 22 26 29 30 31 32 34 35 40 41 44 45 46 51 54 56 64 65 67 71 73 **P**3 **N** Mercy Network of Health Services, Des Moines, IA | 23 | 10 | 41 | 453 | 14 | 8725 | 49 | 2865 | 1361 | 78 |

MAQUOKETA—Jackson County

⊞ JACKSON COUNTY PUBLIC HOSPITAL, 700 West Grove Street, Zip 52060–0910; tel. 319/652–2474; Harold S. Geller, Administrator (Total facility includes 18 beds in nursing home–type unit) **A**1 9 10 **F**7 8 19 21 22 24 30 32 34 36 37 39 40 44 45 46 49 63 64 65 71 73 | 13 | 10 | 61 | 1156 | 27 | 17521 | 121 | 8196 | 4014 | 175 |

MARENGO—Iowa County

MARENGO MEMORIAL HOSPITAL, 300 West May Street, Zip 52301, Mailing Address: Box 228, Zip 52301; tel. 319/642–5543; James H. Ragland, Administrator **A**9 10 **F**16 19 22 27 28 30 33 36 39 44 49 65 71 73 **P**6 **N** St Lukes/Iowa Health System, Des Moines, IA | 14 | 10 | 44 | 221 | 33 | 9967 | 0 | 3449 | 1612 | 93 |

MARSHALLTOWN—Marshall County

⊞ MARSHALLTOWN MEDICAL AND SURGICAL CENTER, 3 South Fourth Avenue, Zip 50158; tel. 515/754–5151; Robert Cooper, Chief Executive Officer (Total facility includes 26 beds in nursing home–type unit) **A**1 9 10 **F**7 8 12 14 15 16 17 19 21 22 25 26 27 28 29 30 32 34 35 36 37 39 40 41 42 44 45 46 49 51 64 65 66 67 68 70 71 73 74 **P**7 | 23 | 10 | 111 | 3818 | 54 | 142433 | 396 | 31520 | 15497 | 503 |

Hospital, Address, Telephone, Administrator, Approval, Facility, and Physician Codes, Health Care System, Network	Classi-fication Codes		Utilization Data					Expense (thousands) of dollars		
★ American Hospital Association (AHA) membership □ Joint Commission on Accreditation of Healthcare Organizations (JCAHO) accreditation + American Osteopathic Hospital Association (AOHA) membership ○ American Osteopathic Association (AOA) accreditation △ Commission on Accreditation of Rehabilitation Facilities (CARF) accreditation Control codes 61, 63, 64, 71, 72 and 73 indicate hospitals listed by AOHA, but not registered by AHA. For definition of numerical codes, see page A4	Control	Service	Beds	Admissions	Census	Outpatient Visits	Births	Total	Payroll	Personnel

MASON CITY—Cerro Gordo County

☒ NORTH IOWA MERCY HEALTH CENTER, 1000 Fourth Street S.W., Zip 50401; tel. 515/422–7000; David H. Vellinga, President and Chief Executive Officer (Total facility includes 30 beds in nursing home–type unit) **A**1 2 3 5 9 10 **F**1 3 4 7 8 10 12 13 14 15 16 17 18 19 20 21 22 23 26 27 28 29 30 31 32 33 34 35 36 37 38 39 40 41 42 43 44 45 46 49 51 52 53 54 55 56 57 58 59 60 62 64 65 66 67 68 71 73 74 **P**1 6 7 **S** Mercy Health Services, Farmington Hills, MI **N** North Iowa Mercy Health Network, Mason City, IA | 21 | 10 | 285 | 11316 | 149 | 536539 | 1236 | 120142 | 53986 | 1579

MISSOURI VALLEY—Harrison County

☒ ALEGENT HEALTH COMMUNITY MEMORIAL HOSPITAL, 631 North Eighth Street, Zip 51555–1199; tel. 712/642–2784; James A. Seymour, Regional Administrator **A**1 10 **F**8 12 15 16 19 22 28 29 30 32 33 34 39 41 42 44 49 53 56 58 65 66 67 71 **P**8 **N** Alegent Health, Omaha, NE | 23 | 10 | 35 | 701 | 8 | 20466 | 0 | 4792 | 2374 | 77

MOUNT AYR—Ringgold County

RINGGOLD COUNTY HOSPITAL, 211 Shellway Drive, Zip 50854; tel. 515/464–3226; Gordon W. Winkler, Administrator **A**9 10 **F**2 3 8 22 27 30 33 40 41 42 44 71 **P**6 **N** Mercy Network of Health Services, Des Moines, IA | 13 | 10 | 36 | 382 | 6 | 14348 | 2 | 3912 | 1770 | 78

MOUNT PLEASANT—Henry County

★ HENRY COUNTY HEALTH CENTER, Saunders Park, Zip 52641–2299; tel. 319/385–3141; Robert Miller, Chief Executive Officer (Total facility includes 49 beds in nursing home–type unit) **A**9 10 **F**7 8 11 12 13 14 15 16 17 18 19 20 21 22 26 27 28 29 30 32 34 35 37 39 40 41 42 44 45 49 51 52 54 56 61 64 65 66 67 71 73 74 **P**5 8 | 13 | 10 | 81 | 1411 | 63 | 40464 | 151 | 13104 | 5804 | 258

MENTAL HEALTH INSTITUTE, 1200 East Washington Street, Zip 52641; tel. 319/385–7231; David J. Scurr, Superintendent **A**10 **F**2 3 20 45 52 65 73 | 12 | 82 | 80 | 996 | 70 | 57 | 0 | 4876 | 3269 | 74

MUSCATINE—Muscatine County

□ MUSCATINE GENERAL HOSPITAL, 1518 Mulberry Avenue, Zip 52761–3499; tel. 319/264–9100; Jonathan R. Goble, Chief Executive Officer (Total facility includes 8 beds in nursing home–type unit) **A**1 9 10 **F**3 7 8 14 17 19 21 22 26 30 33 35 36 37 39 40 42 44 49 64 65 71 | 13 | 10 | 58 | 2348 | 23 | 30287 | 433 | 19009 | 8282 | 233

NEVADA—Story County

★ STORY COUNTY HOSPITAL AND LONG TERM CARE FACILITY, 630 Sixth Street, Zip 50201; tel. 515/382–2111; Todd Willert, Administrator (Total facility includes 80 beds in nursing home–type unit) **A**9 10 **F**19 20 22 24 26 27 28 30 32 33 34 36 37 39 41 42 44 48 49 57 64 65 66 67 71 73 **P**3 6 7 **N** Mercy Network of Health Services, Des Moines, IA | 13 | 10 | 122 | 326 | 85 | 16445 | 0 | 5990 | 2489 | 134

NEW HAMPTON—Chickasaw County

☒ SAINT JOSEPH COMMUNITY HOSPITAL, 308 North Maple Avenue, Zip 50659; tel. 515/394–4121; Thomas Thompson, President (Total facility includes 35 beds in nursing home–type unit) **A**1 9 10 **F**1 7 8 12 14 15 16 17 18 19 22 26 27 28 29 30 32 33 34 39 40 41 44 45 46 49 58 64 65 66 67 71 73 74 **P**6 7 8 **S** Mercy Health Services, Farmington Hills, MI | 21 | 10 | 55 | 870 | 39 | 18196 | 74 | 5936 | 2731 | —

NEWTON—Jasper County

☒ SKIFF MEDICAL CENTER, 204 North Fourth Avenue East, Zip 50208; tel. 515/792–1273; Eric L. Lothe, Chief Executive Officer **A**1 9 10 **F**7 8 13 15 16 19 22 32 33 34 35 37 39 40 41 44 49 52 53 54 55 56 57 59 63 67 71 | 14 | 10 | 68 | 2193 | 25 | 54514 | 165 | 16089 | 7966 | 282

OAKDALE—Johnson County

IOWA MEDICAL AND CLASSIFICATION CENTER, Zip 52319; tel. 319/626–2391; R. E. Rogerson, Warden **F**2 3 4 5 7 8 9 10 11 12 19 20 21 22 23 25 26 29 30 31 35 37 39 40 41 42 43 44 45 46 48 49 50 51 52 54 55 56 57 58 60 61 63 64 65 66 67 69 70 71 72 73 74 | 12 | 22 | 23 | 170 | 22 | 0 | 0 | 2701 | — | 26

OELWEIN—Fayette County

☒ MERCY HOSPITAL OF FRANCISCAN SISTERS, 201 Eighth Avenue S.E., Zip 50662; tel. 319/283–6000; Richard Schrupp, President and Chief Executive Officer (Total facility includes 39 beds in nursing home–type unit) **A**1 9 10 **F**3 7 8 14 15 16 17 19 22 26 27 28 29 30 32 33 34 36 37 39 40 41 44 45 46 49 63 64 65 66 67 68 71 **P**6 **S** Wheaton Franciscan Services, Inc., Wheaton, IL | 21 | 10 | 64 | 946 | 48 | 43354 | 64 | 8250 | 3708 | 158

ONAWA—Monona County

☒ BURGESS MEMORIAL HOSPITAL, 1600 Diamond Street, Zip 51040–1548; tel. 712/423–2311; Francis Tramp, President **A**1 9 10 **F**7 8 14 15 16 17 19 21 22 24 28 30 32 33 34 40 42 44 49 65 67 71 73 74 | 23 | 10 | 48 | 1453 | 18 | 31213 | 90 | 8712 | 3986 | 154

ORANGE CITY—Sioux County

ORANGE CITY MUNICIPAL HOSPITAL, 400 Central Avenue N.W., Zip 51041–1398; tel. 712/737–4984; Martin W. Guthmiller, Administrator (Total facility includes 83 beds in nursing home–type unit) **A**9 10 **F**7 8 13 14 15 16 17 18 19 20 21 22 29 30 32 33 35 36 37 39 40 41 42 44 45 46 58 64 65 66 67 71 73 74 **P**6 **S** St. Luke's Health System, Inc., Sioux City, IA | 14 | 10 | 113 | 1113 | 97 | 28767 | 175 | 10219 | 3798 | 225

OSAGE—Mitchell County

★ MITCHELL COUNTY REGIONAL HEALTH CENTER, 616 North Eighth Street, Zip 50461–1498; tel. 515/732–3781; Richard C. Hamilton, Chief Executive Officer **A**9 10 **F**7 8 15 16 19 22 39 42 44 65 71 **P**1 **S** Mercy Health Services, Farmington Hills, MI **N** North Iowa Mercy Health Network, Mason City, IA | 13 | 10 | 40 | 985 | 9 | 50432 | 79 | 7904 | 2422 | 86

OSCEOLA—Clarke County

★ CLARKE COUNTY HOSPITAL, 800 South Fillmore Street, Zip 50213–0427, Mailing Address: P.O. Box 427, Zip 50213–0427; tel. 515/342–2184; Kris Baumgart, Administrator **A**9 10 **F**8 14 15 16 19 21 22 24 30 33 36 37 42 44 49 71 **S** Iowa Health System, Des Moines, IA | 13 | 10 | 48 | 662 | 36 | 13110 | 1 | 4044 | 1690 | 98

Hospital, Address, Telephone, Administrator, Approval, Facility, and Physician Codes, Health Care System, Network	Classi-fication Codes		Utilization Data					Expense (thousands) of dollars		
	Control	Service	Beds	Admissions	Census	Outpatient Visits	Births	Total	Payroll	Personnel

Approval codes key:

★ American Hospital Association (AHA) membership
□ Joint Commission on Accreditation of Healthcare Organizations (JCAHO) accreditation
+ American Osteopathic Hospital Association (AOHA) membership
○ American Osteopathic Association (AOA) accreditation
△ Commission on Accreditation of Rehabilitation Facilities (CARF) accreditation
Control codes 61, 63, 64, 71, 72 and 73 indicate hospitals listed by AOHA, but not registered by AHA. For definition of numerical codes, see page A4

	Control	Service	Beds	Admissions	Census	Outpatient Visits	Births	Total	Payroll	Personnel
OSKALOOSA—Mahaska County										
✠ MAHASKA COUNTY HOSPITAL, 1229 C Avenue East, Zip 52577; tel. 515/672-3100; David E. Rutter, Administrator **A**1 9 10 **F**3 4 7 8 10 11 12 13 14 15 16 17 18 19 20 21 22 23 25 26 27 28 29 30 31 32 33 34 35 36 39 40 41 42 43 44 45 46 49 50 51 53 54 55 56 57 58 59 60 61 63 64 65 66 67 68 69 70 71 72 **P**1 **S** Iowa Health System, Des Moines, IA	13	10	53	1701	15	57045	213	11495	5108	204
OTTUMWA—Wapello County										
✠ OTTUMWA REGIONAL HEALTH CENTER, 1001 Pennsylvania Avenue, Zip 52501-2186; tel. 515/684-2300; Clarence Cory, President (Total facility includes 13 beds in nursing home–type unit) **A**1 2 9 10 **F**1 2 3 7 8 14 15 19 21 22 23 24 28 29 30 32 33 34 35 36 37 39 40 41 42 44 46 49 52 55 56 57 58 59 60 62 63 64 65 67 71 73 **P**6 8	23	10	90	6104	87	127063	769	45077	19688	711
PELLA—Marion County										
✠ PELLA REGIONAL HEALTH CENTER, (Formerly Pella Community Hospital), 404 Jefferson Street, Zip 50219; tel. 515/628-3150; Robert D. Kroese, Chief Executive Officer (Total facility includes 109 beds in nursing home–type unit) **A**1 9 10 **F**1 7 8 11 14 15 16 17 19 22 28 29 30 32 33 34 35 39 40 41 42 44 45 46 49 64 65 67 71 73 **P**1 5 6	23	10	156	1466	136	66799	203	14635	6750	342
PERRY—Dallas County										
★ DALLAS COUNTY HOSPITAL, 610 10th Street, Zip 50220, Mailing Address: P.O. Box 608, Zip 50220; tel. 515/465-3547; Vernette Riley, Administrator and Chief Executive Officer **A**9 10 **F**1 17 19 22 26 30 33 34 42 44 49 67 70 71 72 73	13	10	42	631	9	20654	1	5970	2468	100
POCAHONTAS—Pocahontas County										
★ POCAHONTAS COMMUNITY HOSPITAL, 606 N.W. Seventh, Zip 50574; tel. 712/335-3501; Jay Christensen, Administrator **A**9 10 **F**8 11 19 22 28 30 32 33 34 37 41 44 49 65 67 71 **P**6	14	10	25	421	5	20475	1	2738	1256	65
PRIMGHAR—Obrien County										
★ BAUM HARMON MEMORIAL HOSPITAL, 255 North Welch Avenue, Zip 51245, Mailing Address: P.O. Box 528, Zip 51245; tel. 712/757-3905; Ronald Bender, Administrator **A**9 10 **F**8 12 14 15 16 19 22 24 28 30 32 33 34 35 36 37 40 41 42 44 49 65 66 67 71 **P**6 8 **S** Mercy Health Services, Farmington Hills, MI	14	10	19	366	3	10365	18	2326	822	42
RED OAK—Montgomery County										
★ MONTGOMERY COUNTY MEMORIAL HOSPITAL, 2301 Eastern Avenue, Zip 51566; tel. 712/623-7000; Allen E. Pohren, Administrator **A**9 10 **F**7 8 12 14 15 16 17 19 22 23 30 32 33 34 35 36 37 39 40 41 42 44 49 58 63 65 71 73	13	10	40	1722	26	35948	7	11478	4803	192
ROCK RAPIDS—Lyon County										
★ MERRILL PIONEER COMMUNITY HOSPITAL, 801 South Greene Street, Zip 51246-1998; tel. 712/472-2591; Gordon Smith, Administrator **A**9 10 **F**7 8 19 22 28 33 40 44 49 71 **P**6 7 **S** Sioux Valley Health System, Sioux Falls, SD **N** Sioux Valley Health System, Sioux Falls, SD	23	10	30	395	4	6667	39	2171	1011	52
ROCK VALLEY—Sioux County										
★ HEGG MEMORIAL HEALTH CENTER, 1202 21st Avenue, Zip 51247-1497; tel. 712/476-5305; Daniel L. Drees, Administrator and Chief Executive Officer (Total facility includes 95 beds in nursing home–type unit) **A**9 10 **F**6 7 8 12 15 16 17 19 20 22 24 28 29 30 32 33 34 36 37 39 40 44 49 62 64 65 71 73 **S** Presentation Health System, Yankton, SD	23	10	123	294	93	10904	27	4381	2519	143
SAC CITY—Sac County										
★ LORING HOSPITAL, Highland Avenue, Zip 50583-0217; tel. 712/662-7105; Greg Miner, Administrator (Total facility includes 21 beds in nursing home–type unit) **A**9 10 **F**3 4 5 7 8 10 11 13 14 15 16 17 19 22 23 26 28 29 30 31 32 33 34 35 39 40 42 43 44 45 46 49 51 53 54 55 56 57 58 59 60 64 65 67 69 71 73 **S** Iowa Health System, Des Moines, IA	23	10	54	818	30	9076	37	3738	2106	99
SHELDON—Obrien County										
★ NORTHWEST IOWA HEALTH CENTER, 118 North Seventh Avenue, Zip 51201; tel. 712/324-5041; Charles R. Miller, Chief Executive Officer (Total facility includes 70 beds in nursing home–type unit) **A**9 10 **F**1 3 8 15 16 17 18 19 20 22 26 28 30 32 33 34 35 36 39 40 41 42 44 45 46 49 53 54 55 56 57 58 59 64 65 66 67 71 73 **P**6 **S** Sioux Valley Health System, Sioux Falls, SD **N** Sioux Valley Health System, Sioux Falls, SD	23	10	95	918	78	23293	93	6446	2881	167
SHENANDOAH—Page County										
★ SHENANDOAH MEMORIAL HOSPITAL, 300 Pershing Avenue, Zip 51601; tel. 712/246-1230; Charles L. Millburg, CHE, Chief Executive Officer (Total facility includes 62 beds in nursing home–type unit) **A**9 10 **F**7 8 21 22 24 30 34 36 37 40 44 45 46 49 64 65 71 73	23	10	106	908	67	6766	75	8592	3474	199
SIBLEY—Osceola County										
★ OSCEOLA COMMUNITY HOSPITAL, Ninth Avenue North, Zip 51249-0258, Mailing Address: P.O. Box 258, Zip 51249-0258; tel. 712/754-2574; Janet Dykstra, Chief Executive Officer **A**9 10 **F**2 3 7 8 11 13 14 15 16 17 19 20 21 22 26 27 28 29 30 31 32 33 34 35 36 39 40 41 42 44 45 46 48 49 51 53 54 55 56 57 58 60 62 64 65 66 67 68 69 71 73 74	23	10	32	572	7	14696	88	3567	1543	75
SIGOURNEY—Keokuk County										
KEOKUK COUNTY HEALTH CENTER, 1312 South Stuart Street, Zip 52591-0286, Mailing Address: P.O. Box 286, Zip 52591-0286; tel. 515/622-2720; Douglas A. Sheetz, Chief Executive Officer **A**9 10 **F**14 19 21 22 30 33 35 39 41 44 50 63 65 69 71	13	10	26	162	14	7302	0	1897	964	52
SIOUX CENTER—Sioux County										
SIOUX CENTER COMMUNITY HOSPITAL AND HEALTH CENTER, 605 South Main Avenue, Zip 51250; tel. 712/722-1271; Marla Toering, Administrator (Total facility includes 69 beds in nursing home–type unit) **A**9 10 **F**7 8 15 16 19 21 22 28 30 32 33 34 35 39 41 44 49 64 65 66 67 71 74 **S** Presentation Health System, Yankton, SD	23	10	90	752	76	26995	188	7507	3248	161

Hospital, Address, Telephone, Administrator, Approval, Facility, and Physician Codes, Health Care System, Network	Classi-fication Codes		Utilization Data					Expense (thousands) of dollars		
★ American Hospital Association (AHA) membership □ Joint Commission on Accreditation of Healthcare Organizations (JCAHO) accreditation + American Osteopathic Hospital Association (AOHA) membership ○ American Osteopathic Association (AOA) accreditation △ Commission on Accreditation of Rehabilitation Facilities (CARF) accreditation Control codes 61, 63, 64, 71, 72 and 73 indicate hospitals listed by AOHA, but not registered by AHA. For definition of numerical codes, see page A4	Control	Service	Beds	Admissions	Census	Outpatient Visits	Births	Total	Payroll	Personnel

SIOUX CITY—Woodbury County

☒ △ MARIAN HEALTH CENTER, (Includes Marian Behavioral Health Center, 4301 Sergeant Road, Zip 51106; tel. 712/279–2446; St. Vincent Hospital, 624 Jones Street, Zip 51105, Mailing Address: Box 3168, Zip 51102), 801 Fifth Street, Zip 51102, Mailing Address: Box 3168, Zip 51102; tel. 712/279–2010 **A**1 2 3 5 7 9 10 **F**1 2 3 4 7 8 10 11 12 13 14 15 16 17 19 21 22 25 26 27 28 29 30 31 32 33 34 35 36 37 39 40 41 42 43 44 45 46 48 49 51 52 53 54 55 56 57 58 59 60 65 67 70 71 72 73 **P**5 6 7 8 **S** Mercy Health Services, Farmington Hills, MI ... 21 10 267 10982 172 255175 882 121182 44532 1582

☒ ST. LUKE'S REGIONAL MEDICAL CENTER, 2720 Stone Park Boulevard, Zip 51104–2000; tel. 712/279–3500; John D. Daniels, President and Chief Executive Officer (Total facility includes 20 beds in nursing home–type unit) **A**1 2 3 5 6 9 10 **F**3 4 6 7 8 9 10 11 12 16 19 20 21 22 23 24 26 27 29 30 32 33 34 35 36 37 38 39 40 41 42 44 45 46 47 49 52 53 56 60 62 63 64 65 67 70 71 72 73 **P**1 **S** Iowa Health System, Des Moines, IA ... 23 10 192 10153 121 90392 1615 77093 31016 1168

SPENCER—Clay County

★ SPENCER MUNICIPAL HOSPITAL, 1200 First Avenue East, Zip 51301–4321; tel. 712/264–6111; James L. Striepe, Administrator (Total facility includes 14 beds in nursing home–type unit) **A**9 10 **F**3 7 8 12 14 15 16 17 19 20 21 22 26 27 28 30 31 32 33 34 36 37 39 40 41 42 44 45 46 49 52 54 55 56 57 58 59 63 64 65 66 67 71 73 ... 14 10 86 2964 36 23790 260 19518 8909 339

SPIRIT LAKE—Dickinson County

□ DICKINSON COUNTY MEMORIAL HOSPITAL, Highway 71 South, Zip 51360, Mailing Address: Box AB, Zip 51360; tel. 712/336–1230; Richard C. Kielman, President and Chief Executive Officer **A**1 9 10 **F**7 8 14 16 19 22 27 28 30 35 36 37 40 42 44 65 66 67 71 73 **P**5 ... 13 10 49 1671 20 28234 170 10058 4542 185

STORM LAKE—Buena Vista County

☒ BUENA VISTA COUNTY HOSPITAL, 1525 West Fifth Street, Zip 50588–0309; tel. 712/732–4030; James O. Nelson, Administrator **A**1 9 10 **F**1 3 7 8 11 12 14 15 16 19 21 22 24 27 29 30 32 33 34 35 36 37 39 40 41 42 44 45 49 65 67 71 73 **P**3 ... 13 10 30 1731 16 56097 279 11146 5498 223

SUMNER—Bremer County

COMMUNITY MEMORIAL HOSPITAL, 909 West First Street, Zip 50674, Mailing Address: Box 148, Zip 50674–0148; tel. 319/578–3275; Scott Knode, Co–Administrator **A**9 10 **F**3 7 8 14 19 22 30 32 33 34 36 39 41 44 49 65 71 73 ... 23 10 29 381 5 12638 15 3060 1400 57

VINTON—Benton County

★ VIRGINIA GAY HOSPITAL, 502 North Ninth Avenue, Zip 52349; tel. 319/472–2348; Michael J. Riege, Administrator (Total facility includes 58 beds in nursing home–type unit) **A**9 10 **F**8 10 13 14 15 16 17 19 20 22 26 27 28 29 30 31 32 33 34 35 39 41 42 44 45 49 51 53 54 55 56 57 58 59 60 64 65 67 71 73 **S** Iowa Health System, Des Moines, IA **N** St Lukes/Iowa Health System, Des Moines, IA ... 23 10 97 333 64 12178 0 5052 2479 107

WASHINGTON—Washington County

★ WASHINGTON COUNTY HOSPITAL, 400 East Polk Street, Zip 52353, Mailing Address: P.O. Box 909, Zip 52353; tel. 319/653–5481; Ronald D. Davis, Chief Executive Officer (Total facility includes 43 beds in nursing home–type unit) **A**9 10 **F**7 8 11 15 19 22 28 30 32 33 36 40 44 45 49 64 65 71 73 **S** Quorum Health Group/Quorum Health Resources, Inc., Brentwood, TN ... 13 10 83 1405 58 36907 125 9562 4130 161

WATERLOO—Black Hawk County

☒ ALLEN MEMORIAL HOSPITAL, 1825 Logan Avenue, Zip 50703; tel. 319/235–3941; Larry W. Pugh, President and Chief Executive Officer (Total facility includes 20 beds in nursing home–type unit) **A**1 3 5 6 9 10 **F**3 4 7 8 10 12 14 15 16 17 19 20 21 22 23 24 25 28 29 30 31 32 33 34 35 37 39 40 41 42 43 44 45 46 49 51 52 53 54 55 56 57 58 59 60 64 65 67 68 71 73 74 **P**3 4 7 8 **S** Iowa Health System, Des Moines, IA ... 23 10 176 8291 117 183920 767 61087 26680 839

☒ △ COVENANT MEDICAL CENTER, (Includes Kimball–Ridge Center, 2101 Kimball Avenue, Zip 50702), 3421 West Ninth Street, Zip 50702–5499; tel. 319/272–8000; Raymond F. Burfeind, President (Total facility includes 44 beds in nursing home–type unit) **A**1 2 3 5 7 9 10 **F**2 3 4 6 7 8 12 15 16 17 18 19 20 21 22 23 24 26 27 28 29 30 31 32 33 34 35 37 39 40 41 42 44 45 48 49 51 52 53 54 55 56 57 58 59 60 63 64 65 66 67 70 71 73 74 **P**6 7 **S** Wheaton Franciscan Services, Inc., Wheaton, IL ... 21 10 293 11066 167 404950 1419 99262 46520 1460

KIMBALL–RIDGE CENTER See Covenant Medical Center

WAUKON—Allamakee County

VETERANS MEMORIAL HOSPITAL, 40 First Street S.E., Zip 52172–2099; tel. 319/568–3411; Daniel J. Woods, Administrator **A**9 10 **F**3 7 8 14 15 16 17 19 22 24 28 29 30 32 33 34 39 40 41 42 44 49 58 65 66 67 68 71 72 ... 14 10 25 767 8 28099 64 4124 2101 100

WAVERLY—Bremer County

☒ WAVERLY MUNICIPAL HOSPITAL, 312 Ninth Street S.W., Zip 50677; tel. 319/352–4120; Arnold Flessner, Administrator **A**1 9 10 **F**7 8 14 15 19 22 24 29 31 34 35 39 40 41 44 45 46 49 51 65 66 67 70 71 73 **P**3 ... 14 10 38 916 10 17519 105 6874 3098 128

WEBSTER CITY—Hamilton County

□ HAMILTON COUNTY PUBLIC HOSPITAL, 800 Ohio Street, Zip 50595; tel. 515/832–9400; Roger W. Lenz, Administrator **A**1 9 10 **F**7 8 15 16 19 22 28 30 35 36 39 40 41 44 49 63 65 71 73 **P**3 **N** Mercy Network of Health Services, Des Moines, IA ... 13 10 40 2317 25 15720 166 10838 5178 170

Hospital, Address, Telephone, Administrator, Approval, Facility, and Physician Codes, Health Care System, Network	Classi-fication Codes		Utilization Data					Expense (thousands) of dollars		
★ American Hospital Association (AHA) membership □ Joint Commission on Accreditation of Healthcare Organizations (JCAHO) accreditation + American Osteopathic Hospital Association (AOHA) membership ○ American Osteopathic Association (AOA) accreditation △ Commission on Accreditation of Rehabilitation Facilities (CARF) accreditation Control codes 61, 63, 64, 71, 72 and 73 indicate hospitals listed by AOHA, but not registered by AHA. For definition of numerical codes, see page A4	Control	Service	Beds	Admissions	Census	Outpatient Visits	Births	Total	Payroll	Personnel

WEST UNION—Fayette County

★ PALMER LUTHERAN HEALTH CENTER, 112 Jefferson Street, Zip 52175; tel. 319/422–3811; Jeanine Matt, President **A**9 10 **F**7 8 15 16 19 22 26 29 30 31 32 33 34 41 42 44 49 52 57 58 65 67 68 71 73

	23	10	30	852	9	51335	128	7142	3101	179

WINTERSET—Madison County

MADISON COUNTY MEMORIAL HOSPITAL, 300 Hutchings Street, Zip 50273–2199; tel. 515/462–2373; James Anderson, Interim Administrator **A**9 10 **F**3 8 12 17 19 22 26 30 31 32 33 34 35 37 39 41 42 44 45 48 49 51 53 54 57 58 65 66 67 68 71 73

	13	10	31	692	11	37094	0	5809	2183	94

WOODWARD—Boone County

WOODWARD STATE HOSPITAL–SCHOOL, Zip 50276–9999; tel. 515/438–2600; Michael J. Davis, Ph.D., Superintendent **F**4 5 8 9 10 11 19 20 21 22 23 27 31 35 37 42 43 44 47 50 52 53 54 55 56 57 58 60 63 65 70 71 73

	12	62	284	29	277	0	0	29841	20804	647

KANSAS

Resident population 2,565 (in thousands)
Resident population in metro areas 54.9%
Birth rate per 1,000 population 14.8
65 years and over 13.7%
Percent of persons without health insurance 12.9%

Hospital, Address, Telephone, Administrator, Approval, Facility, and Physician Codes, Health Care System, Network	Classi-fication Codes		Utilization Data					Expense (thousands) of dollars		
★ American Hospital Association (AHA) membership □ Joint Commission on Accreditation of Healthcare Organizations (JCAHO) accreditation + American Osteopathic Hospital Association (AOHA) membership ○ American Osteopathic Association (AOA) accreditation △ Commission on Accreditation of Rehabilitation Facilities (CARF) accreditation Control codes 61, 63, 64, 71, 72 and 73 indicate hospitals listed by AOHA, but not registered by AHA. For definition of numerical codes, see page A4	Control	Service	Beds	Admissions	Census	Outpatient Visits	Births	Total	Payroll	Personnel

ABILENE—Dickinson County

★ MEMORIAL HOSPITAL, 511 N.E. Tenth Street, Zip 67410, Mailing Address: P.O. Box 219, Zip 67410–0219; tel. 913/263–2100; Leon J. Boor, Chief Executive Officer **A**9 10 **F**7 8 15 19 22 24 30 32 33 34 36 39 40 42 44 49 64 65 67 71 73 **P**8 **N** Sunflower Health Network, Inc., Salina, KS ... 16 10 30 718 7 13489 88 5892 2885 121

ANTHONY—Harper County

HOSPITAL DISTRICT NUMBER SIX OF HARPER COUNTY, 1101 East Spring Street, Zip 67003; tel. 316/842–5111; Cindy M. McCray, Chief Executive Officer **A**9 10 **F**8 15 19 22 42 44 51 61 64 65 71 **P**6 ... 16 10 30 314 21 18715 0 3219 1958 72

ARKANSAS CITY—Cowley County

✠ SOUTH CENTRAL KANSAS REGIONAL MEDICAL CENTER, (Formerly Arkansas City Memorial Hospital), 216 West Birch Avenue, Zip 67005, Mailing Address: P.O. Box 1107, Zip 67005; tel. 316/442–2500; Webster T. Russell, Chief Executive Officer (Total facility includes 10 beds in nursing home–type unit) **A**1 9 10 **F**7 8 11 12 14 15 16 17 19 22 32 34 35 36 39 40 42 44 46 64 71 73 ... 14 10 85 1251 16 74242 145 7428 3416 152

ASHLAND—Clark County

★ ASHLAND HEALTH CENTER, 709 Oak Street, Zip 67831, Mailing Address: P.O. Box 188, Zip 67831; tel. 316/635–2241; Bryan Stacey, Administrator (Total facility includes 36 beds in nursing home–type unit) **A**9 10 **F**1 8 20 24 27 29 30 32 33 34 41 44 46 49 54 56 58 64 65 71 **S** Great Plains Health Alliance, Inc., Phillipsburg, KS **N** Great Plains Health Alliance, Phillipsburg, KS ... 16 10 48 103 33 — 0 1956 1116 58

ATCHISON—Atchison County

✠ ATCHISON HOSPITAL, 1301 North Second Street, Zip 66002; tel. 913/367–2131; W. David Drew, President and Chief Executive Officer (Total facility includes 43 beds in nursing home–type unit) **A**1 9 10 **F**7 8 14 15 16 17 19 21 22 23 27 28 30 32 33 34 35 37 40 44 46 48 49 51 52 54 57 64 65 66 67 71 73 **P**4 7 ... 23 10 95 2164 59 20794 193 14279 7378 274

ATWOOD—Rawlins County

RAWLINS COUNTY HOSPITAL, 707 Grant Street, Zip 67730–4700, Mailing Address: Box 47, Zip 67730–4700; tel. 913/626–3211; Donald J. Kessen, Administrator **A**9 10 **F**3 7 8 14 15 16 17 19 20 22 26 30 31 32 34 35 39 42 44 49 62 63 65 71 **S** Great Plains Health Alliance, Inc., Phillipsburg, KS **N** Great Plains Health Alliance, Phillipsburg, KS; Hays Medical Center, Hays, KS; High Plains Rural Health Network, Fort Morgan, CO ... 13 10 24 137 2 5696 13 1983 1170 44

AUGUSTA—Butler County

AUGUSTA MEDICAL COMPLEX, 2101 Dearborn Street, Zip 67010–0430, Mailing Address: Box 430, Zip 67010–0430; tel. 316/775–5421; Larry D. Wilkerson, Chief Executive Officer (Total facility includes 107 beds in nursing home–type unit) **A**9 10 **F**2 3 8 14 19 21 22 27 28 30 32 33 41 42 44 49 64 65 67 71 ... 23 10 147 434 105 12728 0 6486 3054 164

BELLEVILLE—Republic County

✠ REPUBLIC COUNTY HOSPITAL, 2420 G Street, Zip 66935; tel. 913/527–2255; Charles A. Westin, FACHE, Administrator (Total facility includes 38 beds in nursing home–type unit) **A**1 9 10 **F**7 8 12 14 15 17 19 20 21 22 26 28 33 34 39 41 42 44 45 46 49 64 65 66 71 **P**8 **S** Great Plains Health Alliance, Inc., Phillipsburg, KS **N** Sunflower Health Network, Inc., Salina, KS; Great Plains Health Alliance, Phillipsburg, KS ... 23 10 86 1180 51 6225 67 5654 2631 128

BELOIT—Mitchell County

✠ MITCHELL COUNTY HOSPITAL, 400 West Eighth, Zip 67420, Mailing Address: P.O. Box 399, Zip 67420; tel. 913/738–2266; John M. Osse, Administrator (Total facility includes 40 beds in nursing home–type unit) **A**1 9 10 **F**7 8 17 19 20 22 26 32 33 34 35 36 41 42 44 45 49 64 65 71 **S** Great Plains Health Alliance, Inc., Phillipsburg, KS **N** Sunflower Health Network, Inc., Salina, KS; Great Plains Health Alliance, Phillipsburg, KS ... 23 10 89 1538 59 12858 101 8581 4118 166

BURLINGTON—Coffey County

COFFEY COUNTY HOSPITAL, 801 North Fourth Street, Zip 66839, Mailing Address: Box 189, Zip 66839–0189; tel. 316/364–2121; Dennis L. George, Administrator **A**9 10 **F**7 8 11 15 19 22 25 28 32 34 37 40 41 44 62 71 73 **P**6 ... 13 10 20 738 7 10496 64 8566 3906 148

CALDWELL—Sumner County

SUMNER COUNTY HOSPITAL DISTRICT ONE, 601 South Osage Street, Zip 67022; tel. 316/845–6492; Virgil Watson, Administrator **A**9 10 **F**1 14 15 17 28 30 32 33 34 39 42 44 48 49 64 70 71 73 ... 16 10 27 245 3 5196 1 1614 834 35

CEDAR VALE—Chautauqua County

CEDAR VALE COMMUNITY HOSPITAL, (Formerly Cedar Vale Regional Hospital), 501 Cedar Street, Zip 67024, Mailing Address: Box 398, Zip 67024; tel. 316/758–2266; William A. Lybarger, Administrator **A**9 10 **F**15 21 27 28 32 51 65 71 **P**5 ... 23 10 16 190 13 — 0 1181 — 40

CHANUTE—Neosho County

✠ NEOSHO MEMORIAL REGIONAL MEDICAL CENTER, 629 South Plummer, Zip 66720; tel. 316/431–4000; Murray L. Brown, Administrator **A**1 9 10 **F**7 8 15 19 20 22 23 27 28 32 33 35 37 40 41 44 49 65 71 73 **S** Quorum Health Group/Quorum Health Resources, Inc., Brentwood, TN **N** SouthEast Kansas Network, Coffeyville, KS ... 13 10 60 2492 30 15471 319 13709 5621 231

Hospital, Address, Telephone, Administrator, Approval, Facility, and Physician Codes, Health Care System, Network	Classi-fication Codes		Utilization Data					Expense (thousands) of dollars		
★ American Hospital Association (AHA) membership □ Joint Commission on Accreditation of Healthcare Organizations (JCAHO) accreditation + American Osteopathic Hospital Association (AOHA) membership ○ American Osteopathic Association (AOA) accreditation △ Commission on Accreditation of Rehabilitation Facilities (CARF) accreditation Control codes 61, 63, 64, 71, 72 and 73 indicate hospitals listed by AOHA, but not registered by AHA. For definition of numerical codes, see page A4	Control	Service	Beds	Admissions	Census	Outpatient Visits	Births	Total	Payroll	Personnel

CLAY CENTER—Clay County

★ CLAY COUNTY HOSPITAL, 617 Liberty Street, Zip 67432; tel. 913/632–2144; John F. Wiebe, Chief Executive Officer **A**9 10 **F**7 8 15 19 22 28 33 39 44 45 49 65 67 71 **P**3 8 **N** Sunflower Health Network, Inc., Salina, KS	13	10	35	972	12	17728	70	5561	2461	117

COFFEYVILLE—Montgomery County

⊠ COFFEYVILLE REGIONAL MEDICAL CENTER, 1400 West Fourth, Zip 67337–3306; tel. 316/251–1200; Gerald Joseph Marquette, Jr., Administrator (Total facility includes 33 beds in nursing home–type unit) **A**1 2 9 10 **F**3 7 8 14 15 16 19 21 22 27 28 30 31 32 33 37 40 42 44 49 52 53 57 58 60 64 65 71 73 74 **P**8 **S** Quorum Health Group/Quorum Health Resources, Inc., Brentwood, TN **N** SouthEast Kansas Network, Coffeyville, KS	14	10	123	3688	67	17719	241	19644	8812	356

COLBY—Thomas County

□ CITIZENS MEDICAL CENTER, 100 East College Drive, Zip 67701–3799; tel. 913/462–7511; Richard B. Gamel, Chief Executive Officer **A**1 9 10 **F**7 8 11 15 19 21 22 29 32 33 34 36 37 40 42 44 45 46 49 51 65 67 71 73 **N** MED–OP, Oakley, KS	23	10	40	1163	12	9394	142	6693	2797	110

COLDWATER—Comanche County

COMANCHE COUNTY HOSPITAL, Second and Frisco Streets, Zip 67029, Mailing Address: HC 65, Box 8A, Zip 67029; tel. 316/582–2144; Nancy Zimmerman, Administrator **A**9 10 **F**8 15 20 22 24 30 31 32 33 36 39 40 41 42 44 49 56 64 70 71 **P**6	13	10	14	198	3	3763	6	—	—	36

COLUMBUS—Cherokee County

MAUDE NORTON MEMORIAL CITY HOSPITAL, 220 North Pennsylvania Street, Zip 66725–1197; tel. 316/429–2545; Cindy Neely, Administrator and Chief Executive Officer (Nonreporting) **A**9 **N** SouthEast Kansas Network, Coffeyville, KS	14	10	30	—	—	—	—	—	—	—

CONCORDIA—Cloud County

★ CLOUD COUNTY HEALTH CENTER, 1100 Highland Drive, Zip 66901–3997; tel. 913/243–1234; Daniel R. Bartz, Chief Executive Officer **A**9 10 **F**8 15 16 17 19 20 21 22 26 27 28 30 33 34 35 36 37 39 41 44 45 46 49 50 51 53 54 55 56 57 58 59 64 65 67 70 71 73 **N** Via Christi Health System, Wichita, KS; Sunflower Health Network, Inc., Salina, KS	23	10	57	1163	18	45414	0	6929	3480	148

COUNCIL GROVE—Morris County

MORRIS COUNTY HOSPITAL, 600 North Washington Street, Zip 66846, Mailing Address: P.O. Box 275, Zip 66846; tel. 316/767–6811; Jim Reagan, M.D., Administrator **A**9 10 **F**7 8 14 15 16 17 19 22 25 28 30 32 33 34 37 39 40 41 42 44 46 49 65 67 71 73 **P**3 **N** Community Health Alliance, Winchester, KS	13	10	28	698	9	14871	67	3848	1783	83

DIGHTON—Lane County

★ LANE COUNTY HOSPITAL, 243 South Second, Zip 67839, Mailing Address: Box 969, Zip 67839; tel. 316/397–5321; Donna McGowan, R.N., Administrator (Total facility includes 21 beds in nursing home–type unit) **A**9 10 **F**1 8 15 19 22 26 28 32 34 35 41 49 51 64 65 66 71 **S** Great Plains Health Alliance, Inc., Phillipsburg, KS **N** Great Plains Health Alliance, Phillipsburg, KS	13	10	31	200	21	4759	0	2056	1095	52

DODGE CITY—Ford County

⊠ COLUMBIA WESTERN PLAINS REGIONAL HOSPITAL, 3001 Avenue A, Zip 67801, Mailing Address: Box 1478, Zip 67801; tel. 316/225–8401; Ken Hutchenrider, President and Chief Executive Officer (Total facility includes 5 beds in nursing home–type unit) **A**1 9 10 **F**8 12 14 15 16 17 19 20 21 22 23 28 30 32 35 37 39 40 41 44 45 46 48 49 63 64 65 66 67 73 **S** Columbia/HCA Healthcare Corporation, Nashville, TN	33	10	85	2791	40	—	677	—	—	291

EL DORADO—Butler County

⊠ SUSAN B. ALLEN MEMORIAL HOSPITAL, 720 West Central Avenue, Zip 67042–2144; tel. 316/321–3300; Jim Wilson, President and Chief Executive Officer (Total facility includes 21 beds in nursing home–type unit) **A**1 9 10 **F**7 19 21 22 24 26 28 32 35 36 37 39 40 44 52 57 64 65 71 73	23	10	85	1982	30	40874	172	15575	7589	261

ELKHART—Morton County

★ MORTON COUNTY HEALTH SYSTEM, (Formerly Morton County Hospital), 445 Hilltop Street, Zip 67950–0937, Mailing Address: Box 937, Zip 67950–0937; tel. 316/697–2141; Glen A. Wood, Chief Executive Officer (Total facility includes 60 beds in nursing home–type unit) (Nonreporting) **A**9 10	13	10	100	—	—	—	—	—	—	—

ELLINWOOD—Barton County

★ ELLINWOOD DISTRICT HOSPITAL, 605 North Main Street, Zip 67526; tel. 316/564–2548; Marge Conell, R.N., Administrator **A**9 **F**8 19 20 22 34 35 36 49 65 69 71 **S** Great Plains Health Alliance, Inc., Phillipsburg, KS **N** Great Plains Health Alliance, Phillipsburg, KS	23	10	12	178	3	3959	0	1474	705	30

ELLSWORTH—Ellsworth County

ELLSWORTH COUNTY HOSPITAL, 300 Kingsley Street, Zip 67439, Mailing Address: Drawer 87, Zip 67439; tel. 913/472–3111; Roger W. Pearson, Administrator **A**9 10 **F**15 19 21 28 41 48 49 64 71 73 **P**8 **N** Sunflower Health Network, Inc., Salina, KS	13	10	19	603	9	8255	0	2532	1100	52

EMPORIA—Lyon County

⊠ NEWMAN MEMORIAL COUNTY HOSPITAL, (Formerly Newman Memorial Hospital), 1201 West 12th Avenue, Zip 66801–2597; tel. 316/343–6800; Terry R. Lambert, Chief Executive Officer (Total facility includes 18 beds in nursing home–type unit) **A**1 9 10 **F**3 7 8 15 19 21 22 23 28 30 31 32 33 34 35 36 37 40 41 42 44 45 46 49 56 64 65 67 71 **S** Quorum Health Group/Quorum Health Resources, Inc., Brentwood, TN	13	10	110	3720	55	57416	523	25718	11880	391

Hospital, Address, Telephone, Administrator, Approval, Facility, and Physician Codes, Health Care System, Network	Classi- fication Codes		Utilization Data					Expense (thousands) of dollars		
	Control	Service	Beds	Admissions	Census	Outpatient Visits	Births	Total	Payroll	Personnel

★ American Hospital Association (AHA) membership
□ Joint Commission on Accreditation of Healthcare Organizations (JCAHO) accreditation
+ American Osteopathic Hospital Association (AOHA) membership
○ American Osteopathic Association (AOA) accreditation
△ Commission on Accreditation of Rehabilitation Facilities (CARF) accreditation
Control codes 61, 63, 64, 71, 72 and 73 indicate hospitals listed by AOHA, but not registered by AHA. For definition of numerical codes, see page A4

EUREKA—Greenwood County

★ GREENWOOD COUNTY HOSPITAL, 100 West 16th Street, Zip 67045; tel. 316/583–7451; Emmett Schuster, Administrator and Chief Executive Officer **A**9 10 **F**3 7 8 12 15 16 17 19 20 22 26 30 31 32 33 34 35 39 44 46 49 53 54 56 57 58 65 71 73 **P**1 7 8

| 13 | 10 | 46 | 923 | 15 | 4733 | 0 | 5223 | 1946 | 119 |

FORT LEAVENWORTH—Leavenworth County

⊞ MUNSON ARMY COMMUNITY HOSPITAL, 550 Pope Avenue, Zip 66027–2332; tel. 913/684–6420; Colonel Cloyd B. Gatrell, Commander **A**1 9 **F**2 3 4 8 9 11 15 16 19 20 21 22 24 28 30 33 35 37 38 39 40 41 42 43 44 45 46 47 49 50 51 52 53 54 55 56 58 59 60 61 63 65 71 72 73 74 **P**6 **S** Department of the Army, Office of the Surgeon General, Falls Church, VA

| 42 | 10 | 20 | 1306 | 6 | 159183 | 0 | 40100 | 14100 | 328 |

FORT RILEY—Geary County

⊞ IRWIN ARMY COMMUNITY HOSPITAL, Building 600, Zip 66442; tel. 913/239–7100; Colonel J. Thomas Hardy, Commanding Officer **A**1 2 9 **F**3 8 12 14 15 16 18 19 20 21 22 28 29 30 31 34 35 37 39 40 41 42 44 45 46 49 51 65 67 70 71 73 74 **S** Department of the Army, Office of the Surgeon General, Falls Church, VA

| 42 | 10 | 56 | 4291 | 24 | 325836 | 906 | 51814 | 33581 | 692 |

FORT SCOTT—Bourbon County

⊞ MERCY HEALTH SYSTEM OF KANSAS, (Formerly Mercy Hospitals of Kansas), 821 Burke Street, Zip 66701; tel. 316/223–2200; Susan Barrett, President and Chief Executive Officer (Total facility includes 23 beds in nursing home–type unit) **A**1 9 10 **F**7 8 12 14 15 16 17 19 21 22 23 24 27 28 30 32 33 35 37 38 39 40 41 44 48 49 51 64 65 67 71 73 **P**6 **S** Sisters of Mercy Health System–St. Louis, Saint Louis, MO **N** SouthEast Kansas Network, Coffeyville, KS

| 21 | 10 | 105 | 4081 | 54 | 44698 | 247 | 19731 | 9666 | 464 |

FREDONIA—Wilson County

★ FREDONIA REGIONAL HOSPITAL, 1527 Madison Street, Zip 66736, Mailing Address: Box 579, Zip 66736; tel. 316/378–2121; Terry Deschaine, Administrator **A**9 10 **F**8 14 15 19 22 32 44 49 58 62 65 71 **S** Great Plains Health Alliance, Inc., Phillipsburg, KS **N** Great Plains Health Alliance, Phillipsburg, KS; SouthEast Kansas Network, Coffeyville, KS

| 14 | 10 | 42 | 450 | 7 | 14035 | 0 | 3614 | 1600 | 76 |

GARDEN CITY—Finney County

⊞ ST. CATHERINE HOSPITAL, 410 East Walnut, Zip 67846–5672; tel. 316/272–2222; Gary L. Rowe, President and Chief Executive Officer **A**1 5 9 10 **F**7 8 14 15 16 17 19 20 21 23 26 28 30 31 33 35 36 37 38 39 40 41 42 44 46 49 52 54 55 56 57 58 60 65 69 71 73 **S** Catholic Health Initiatives, Denver, CO

| 21 | 10 | 99 | 4869 | 59 | 37885 | 1050 | 33667 | 13868 | 499 |

GARDNER—Johnson County

△ MEADOWBROOK HOSPITAL, 427 West Main Street, Zip 66030; tel. 913/884–8711; Anita Macke, Administrator (Total facility includes 21 beds in nursing home–type unit) (Nonreporting) **A**7 9 10

| 33 | 46 | 84 | — | — | — | — | — | — | — |

GARNETT—Anderson County

ANDERSON COUNTY HOSPITAL, 421 South Maple, Zip 66032, Mailing Address: Box 309, Zip 66032; tel. 913/448–3131; James K. Johnson, Administrator (Total facility includes 32 beds in nursing home–type unit) **A**9 10 **F**8 11 14 15 16 19 22 26 32 33 35 39 41 44 49 54 57 58 64 65 71 **P**8 **S** Saint Luke's Shawnee Mission Health System, Kansas City, MO **N** Jayhawk Health Alliance, Olathe, KS

| 13 | 10 | 66 | 642 | 40 | 17137 | 0 | 4867 | 2355 | 114 |

GIRARD—Crawford County

★ CRAWFORD COUNTY HOSPITAL DISTRICT ONE, 302 North Hospital Drive, Zip 66743–2000; tel. 316/724–8291; Jerry Hanson, Administrator **A**9 10 **F**7 8 11 15 19 21 22 32 33 35 36 37 40 41 42 44 45 49 54 56 58 63 66 71 73

| 16 | 10 | 38 | 1409 | 15 | 22690 | 95 | 6410 | 3292 | 144 |

GOODLAND—Sherman County

GOODLAND REGIONAL MEDICAL CENTER, 220 West Second Street, Zip 67735–1602; tel. 913/899–3625; Jim Chaddic, Chief Executive Officer **A**9 10 **F**3 8 10 11 14 15 16 19 20 21 22 26 28 31 33 34 35 36 37 39 40 42 44 45 46 48 49 58 63 64 65 67 70 71 73 **N** MED–OP, Oakley, KS

| 13 | 10 | 49 | 938 | 16 | 34240 | 58 | 6059 | 2597 | 114 |

GREAT BEND—Barton County

⊞ CENTRAL KANSAS MEDICAL CENTER, (Includes Central Kansas Medical Center–St. Joseph Campus, 923 Carroll Avenue, Larned, Zip 67550; tel. 316/285–3161), 3515 Broadway Street, Zip 67530; tel. 316/792–2511; Gary L. Barnett, President and Chief Executive Officer (Total facility includes 79 beds in nursing home–type unit) **A**1 9 10 **F**3 7 8 15 16 19 21 22 23 28 30 32 33 34 35 36 37 39 40 41 42 44 45 49 51 60 64 65 66 67 71 73 **P**1 **S** Catholic Health Initiatives, Denver, CO

| 21 | 10 | 175 | 3211 | 74 | 171776 | 400 | 32407 | 15369 | 583 |

GREENSBURG—Kiowa County

KIOWA COUNTY MEMORIAL HOSPITAL, 501 South Walnut Street, Zip 67054; tel. 316/723–3341; Ronald J. Baker, Administrator **A**9 10 **F**8 15 22 24 28 30 32 34 36 39 44 49 65 71 **P**6 **S** Great Plains Health Alliance, Inc., Phillipsburg, KS **N** Great Plains Health Alliance, Phillipsburg, KS

| 13 | 10 | 38 | 323 | 9 | 5533 | 22 | 3912 | — | 85 |

HALSTEAD—Harvey County

⊞ COLUMBIA HALSTEAD HOSPITAL, 328 Poplar Street, Zip 67056–2099; tel. 316/835–2651; David Nevill, President and Chief Executive Officer (Total facility includes 17 beds in nursing home–type unit) **A**1 9 10 **F**3 4 8 10 11 12 14 15 16 17 19 20 21 22 23 24 26 27 28 29 30 32 33 34 35 36 37 39 41 42 43 44 45 46 49 51 52 53 54 55 56 57 58 60 61 63 64 65 67 71 72 73 **P**5 **S** Columbia/HCA Healthcare Corporation, Nashville, TN

| 33 | 10 | 137 | 3038 | 50 | 18636 | 0 | 24669 | 9639 | 340 |

HANOVER—Washington County

HANOVER HOSPITAL, 205 South Hanover, Zip 66945, Mailing Address: Box 38, Zip 66945; tel. 913/337–2214; Roger D. Warren, M.D., Administrator (Total facility includes 32 beds in nursing home–type unit) **A**9 10 **F**11 14 15 26 32 36 37 40 44 48 49 64 71

| 16 | 10 | 50 | 408 | 28 | 1209 | 14 | 2213 | 1217 | 39 |

Hospital, Address, Telephone, Administrator, Approval, Facility, and Physician Codes, Health Care System, Network	Classi-fication Codes		Utilization Data					Expense (thousands) of dollars		
★ American Hospital Association (AHA) membership □ Joint Commission on Accreditation of Healthcare Organizations (JCAHO) accreditation + American Osteopathic Hospital Association (AOHA) membership ○ American Osteopathic Association (AOA) accreditation △ Commission on Accreditation of Rehabilitation Facilities (CARF) accreditation Control codes 61, 63, 64, 71, 72 and 73 indicate hospitals listed by AOHA, but not registered by AHA. For definition of numerical codes, see page A4	Control	Service	Beds	Admissions	Census	Outpatient Visits	Births	Total	Payroll	Personnel

HARPER—Harper County

★ HOSPITAL DISTRICT NUMBER FIVE OF HARPER COUNTY, 1204 Maple, Zip 67058–1438; tel. 316/896–7324; Vernon Minnis, Chief Executive Officer **A**9 10 **F**1 8 12 14 19 22 28 30 32 33 34 35 36 44 49 51 64 65 71 73 **P**6

| | 16 | 10 | 38 | 483 | 15 | 5330 | 0 | — | — | 97 |

HAYS—Ellis County

⊞ △ HAYS MEDICAL CENTER, (Includes Hadley Campus, 201 East Seventh Street, Zip 67601–4198; St. Anthony Campus, 2220 Canterbury Drive, Zip 67601–2342, Mailing Address: P.O. Box 8100, Zip 67601), 2220 Canterbury Road, Zip 67601–2323, Mailing Address: P.O. Box 8100, Zip 67601; tel. 913/623–5407; Stephen F. Ronstrom, President and Chief Executive Officer **A**1 2 5 7 9 10 **F**7 8 10 11 12 13 15 16 17 18 19 21 23 26 27 28 29 30 32 33 34 35 36 37 38 39 40 41 42 44 45 46 48 49 51 52 54 55 56 57 58 60 63 64 65 67 71 73 74 **P**6 **N** MED–OP, Oakley, KS; High Plains Rural Health Network, Fort Morgan, CO
ST. ANTHONY CAMPUS See Hays Medical Center

| | 23 | 10 | 161 | 5411 | 86 | 120000 | 539 | 53066 | 22741 | 746 |

HERINGTON—Dickinson County

HERINGTON MUNICIPAL HOSPITAL, 100 East Helen Street, Zip 67449; tel. 913/258–2207; William D. Peterson, Administrator (Total facility includes 18 beds in nursing home–type unit) **A**9 **F**7 8 11 14 15 16 19 20 22 26 28 32 33 35 40 41 44 64 71 **P**5 **N** Sunflower Health Network, Inc., Salina, KS

| | 14 | 10 | 38 | 596 | 13 | 17165 | 31 | — | — | — |

HIAWATHA—Brown County

⊞ HIAWATHA COMMUNITY HOSPITAL, 300 Utah Street, Zip 66434; tel. 913/742–2131; John Moore, Administrator **A**1 9 10 **F**3 7 8 14 19 20 22 28 30 32 34 35 36 37 39 40 41 44 48 49 55 64 65 71 73 74 **P**8

| | 23 | 10 | 29 | 928 | 13 | 24083 | 79 | 6293 | 2653 | 123 |

HILL CITY—Graham County

★ GRAHAM COUNTY HOSPITAL, 304 West Prout Street, Zip 67642, Mailing Address: P.O. Box 339, Zip 67642; tel. 913/421–2121; Fred J. Meis, Administrator **A**9 10 **F**1 7 8 12 15 16 19 22 28 32 33 34 36 39 44 71 **N** MED–OP, Oakley, KS

| | 13 | 10 | 26 | 869 | 12 | 11603 | 13 | 3531 | 1814 | 79 |

HILLSBORO—Marion County

SALEM HOSPITAL, 701 South Main Street, Zip 67063–9981; tel. 316/947–3114; Robert G. Senneff, Chief Executive Officer (Total facility includes 60 beds in nursing home–type unit) **A**9 10 **F**1 7 8 12 14 15 16 17 19 22 26 28 30 32 33 34 35 40 44 49 57 62 64 65 67 71 **P**5 **S** Great Plains Health Alliance, Inc., Phillipsburg, KS **N** Great Plains Health Alliance, Phillipsburg, KS

| | 21 | 10 | 86 | 480 | 54 | 5672 | 22 | 4293 | 2384 | 124 |

HOISINGTON—Barton County

CLARA BARTON HOSPTIAL, 250 West Ninth Street, Zip 67544; tel. 316/653–2114; James Turnbull, Administrator and Chief Executive Officer (Total facility includes 12 beds in nursing home–type unit) **A**9 10 **F**2 3 7 8 15 19 20 22 24 34 35 36 37 40 44 49 64 71 73

| | 23 | 10 | 48 | 488 | 11 | 12166 | 60 | 3167 | 1677 | 115 |

HOLTON—Jackson County

HOLTON COMMUNITY HOSPITAL, 510 Kansas Avenue, Zip 66436; tel. 913/364–2116; Diane S. Gross, Administrator **A**9 10 **F**1 7 8 11 12 13 15 16 17 19 22 27 29 30 32 33 34 36 39 40 41 44 45 46 49 64 65 66 67 68 71 73 74 **P**8 **N** Community Health Alliance, Winchester, KS

| | 14 | 10 | 13 | 400 | 5 | 23228 | 32 | 2650 | 1391 | 69 |

HORTON—Brown County

HORTON HEALTH FOUNDATION, (Formerly Horton Community Hospital), 240 West 18th Street, Zip 66439; tel. 913/486–2642 **A**9 10 **F**3 8 12 15 16 19 28 30 32 36 41 44 65 71 **P**8 **N** Community Health Alliance, Winchester, KS

| | 23 | 10 | 35 | 520 | 6 | 30269 | 0 | 3940 | 1825 | 84 |

HOXIE—Sheridan County

SHERIDAN COUNTY HOSPITAL, 826 18th Street, Zip 67740–0167, Mailing Address: P.O. Box 167, Zip 67740–0167; tel. 913/675–3281; Joy Bretz, Administrator (Total facility includes 48 beds in nursing home–type unit) **A**9 10 **F**1 6 8 14 15 16 19 22 28 32 33 36 40 44 58 64 65 71 **N** MED–OP, Oakley, KS

| | 13 | 10 | 66 | 315 | 48 | 6811 | 7 | 3468 | 1755 | 75 |

HUGOTON—Stevens County

STEVENS COUNTY HOSPITAL, 1006 South Jackson Street, Zip 67951, Mailing Address: Box 10, Zip 67951; tel. 316/544–8511; Ted Strote, Administrator **A**9 10 **F**8 12 15 19 22 24 28 30 32 34 39 41 44 45 49 65 67 71 73 **N** Allina Health System, Minnetonka, MN

| | 13 | 10 | 17 | 437 | 6 | 16884 | 0 | 4165 | 2103 | 85 |

HUTCHINSON—Reno County

⊞ HUTCHINSON HOSPITAL CORPORATION, 1701 East 23rd Street, Zip 67502–1191; tel. 316/665–2000; Gene E. Schmidt, President (Total facility includes 18 beds in nursing home–type unit) **A**1 9 10 **F**3 6 7 10 15 16 18 19 21 22 23 28 32 33 34 37 40 41 42 44 46 48 49 51 52 53 54 55 56 57 58 59 60 62 64 65 67 68 71 73

| | 23 | 10 | 149 | 6886 | 114 | 171029 | 648 | 43086 | 18544 | 701 |

INDEPENDENCE—Montgomery County

⊞ MERCY HOSPITALS OF KANSAS, 800 West Myrtle Street, Zip 67301, Mailing Address: Box 388, Zip 67301–0388; tel. 316/331–2200; Susan Barrett, President and Chief Executive Officer (Total facility includes 18 beds in nursing home–type unit) **A**1 9 10 **F**7 8 12 15 16 17 19 21 22 27 28 30 32 34 35 41 44 49 64 65 71 73 **P**1 **S** Sisters of Mercy Health System–St. Louis, Saint Louis, MO

| | 21 | 10 | 58 | 2023 | 28 | 62013 | 152 | 13846 | 5726 | 229 |

IOLA—Allen County

⊞ ALLEN COUNTY HOSPITAL, 101 South First Street, Zip 66749, Mailing Address: P.O. Box 540, Zip 66749–0540; tel. 316/365–3131; Franklin K. Wilson, Administrator **A**1 9 10 **F**19 21 22 23 28 30 31 32 33 35 37 40 42 44 65 71 72 73 **S** Health Midwest, Kansas City, MO **N** Health Midwest, Kansas City, MO; SouthEast Kansas Network, Coffeyville, KS

| | 23 | 10 | 41 | 1408 | 18 | 20083 | 79 | 8542 | 3433 | 135 |

Hospital, Address, Telephone, Administrator, Approval, Facility, and Physician Codes, Health Care System, Network	Classi-fication Codes		Utilization Data					Expense (thousands) of dollars		
	Control	Service	Beds	Admissions	Census	Outpatient Visits	Births	Total	Payroll	Personnel

★ American Hospital Association (AHA) membership
□ Joint Commission on Accreditation of Healthcare Organizations (JCAHO) accreditation
+ American Osteopathic Hospital Association (AOHA) membership
○ American Osteopathic Association (AOA) accreditation
△ Commission on Accreditation of Rehabilitation Facilities (CARF) accreditation
Control codes 61, 63, 64, 71, 72 and 73 indicate hospitals listed by AOHA, but not registered by AHA. For definition of numerical codes, see page A4

JETMORE—Hodgeman County

★ HODGEMAN COUNTY HEALTH CENTER, 809 Bramley, Zip 67854, Mailing Address: P.O. Box 367, Zip 67854; tel. 316/357-8361; Roger Salisbury, Administrator (Total facility includes 36 beds in nursing home–type unit) **A**9 10 **F**7 8 12 14 15 19 20 22 26 27 32 35 40 44 45 49 51 64 65 71

| | 13 | 10 | 52 | 386 | 37 | 3904 | 7 | 3100 | 1548 | 77 |

JOHNSON—Stanton County

★ STANTON COUNTY HEALTH CARE FACILITY, (Formerly Stanton County Hospital and Long–Term Care Unit), 404 North Chestnut Street, Zip 67855-0779, Mailing Address: Box 779, Zip 67855-0779; tel. 316/492-6250; Ed Finley, Administrator (Total facility includes 28 beds in nursing home–type unit) **A**9 10 **F**1 7 8 14 15 16 22 26 28 30 32 34 39 49 64 71 73

| | 15 | 10 | 40 | 194 | 26 | 2293 | 90 | 2149 | 1215 | 62 |

JUNCTION CITY—Geary County

⊞ GEARY COMMUNITY HOSPITAL, Ash and St. Mary's Road, Zip 66441, Mailing Address: Box 490, Zip 66441-0490; tel. 913/238-4131; David K. Bradley, Chief Executive Officer **A**1 5 9 10 **F**3 8 15 16 19 20 21 22 23 31 32 33 34 35 37 39 40 42 44 45 46 49 51 65 67 71 **N** Community Health Alliance, Winchester, KS

| | 13 | 10 | 49 | 1570 | 19 | 91946 | 72 | 11680 | 5826 | 257 |

KANSAS CITY—Wyandotte County

⊞ △ BETHANY MEDICAL CENTER, 51 North 12th Street, Zip 66102-9990; tel. 913/281-8400; John L. Millard, President and Chief Executive Officer (Total facility includes 51 beds in nursing home–type unit) **A**1 2 3 5 7 9 10 **F**2 3 4 7 8 10 12 14 15 16 17 19 20 21 22 23 26 28 29 30 32 33 34 35 37 39 40 41 42 43 44 45 46 48 49 51 52 53 54 55 56 58 60 64 65 67 69 71 73 **P**1 2 4 7

| | 23 | 10 | 251 | 8908 | 157 | 66247 | 721 | 66222 | 28447 | 912 |

⊞ PROVIDENCE MEDICAL CENTER, 8929 Parallel Parkway, Zip 66112-0430; tel. 913/596-4000; Francis V. Creeden, Jr., President (Total facility includes 36 beds in nursing home–type unit) **A**1 2 10 **F**4 7 8 10 12 15 16 17 18 19 20 21 22 26 27 28 29 30 31 32 33 34 35 37 39 40 41 42 43 44 45 46 49 52 53 54 55 56 57 58 59 60 63 64 65 66 67 71 73 74 **P**1 4 5 6 7 8 **S** Sisters of Charity of Leavenworth Health Services Corporation, Leavenworth, KS **N** Jayhawk Health Alliance, Olathe, KS

| | 21 | 10 | 219 | 8036 | 125 | 40593 | 991 | 61420 | 26369 | 839 |

⊞ △ UNIVERSITY OF KANSAS HOSPITAL, 3901 Rainbow Boulevard, Zip 66160-7200; tel. 913/588-5000; Irene M. Cumming, Chief Executive Officer **A**1 2 3 5 7 8 10 **F**3 4 5 7 8 9 10 11 15 16 18 19 21 22 23 24 25 26 28 29 30 31 34 35 37 38 39 40 41 42 43 44 46 47 48 49 51 52 53 54 55 56 57 58 60 61 63 65 66 67 69 71 73 74 **P**1 3 **N** Jayhawk Health Alliance, Olathe, KS

| | 12 | 10 | 456 | 13016 | 247 | 386995 | 1009 | 165032 | 62699 | 2101 |

KINGMAN—Kingman County

★ KINGMAN COMMUNITY HOSPITAL, 750 Avenue D West, Zip 67068; tel. 316/532-3147; Gary L. Tiller, Administrator **A**9 10 **F**7 8 14 15 16 17 19 22 28 29 30 32 34 35 36 40 41 42 44 46 48 49 58 64 65 67 71 73 **P**3 6 7

| | 23 | 10 | 35 | 643 | 9 | 15670 | 62 | 5166 | 2597 | 111 |

KIOWA—Barber County

★ KIOWA DISTRICT HOSPITAL, 810 Drumm Street, Zip 67070; tel. 316/825-4131; Buck McKinney, Jr., Chief Executive Officer **A**9 10 **F**8 12 14 15 16 19 22 28 33 44 51 65 71

| | 16 | 10 | 24 | 251 | 3 | 3775 | 1 | 1280 | 761 | 36 |

LA CROSSE—Rush County

★ RUSH COUNTY MEMORIAL HOSPITAL, Eighth and Locust Streets, Zip 67548, Mailing Address: P.O. Box 520, Zip 67548-0520; tel. 913/222-2545; Donna L. Myers, Administrator and Chief Executive Officer (Total facility includes 26 beds in nursing home–type unit) **A**9 10 **F**7 14 15 19 22 28 32 33 35 40 44 49 64 71 **P**5 **N** MED–OP, Oakley, KS

| | 13 | 10 | 50 | 425 | 34 | 9956 | 16 | 1690 | 824 | 52 |

LAKIN—Kearny County

KEARNY COUNTY HOSPITAL, 500 Thorpe Street, Zip 67860, Mailing Address: Box 744, Zip 67860; tel. 316/355-7111; Steven S. Reiner, Administrator **A**9 10 **F**1 3 7 8 13 14 15 16 17 19 20 22 27 28 30 31 32 34 36 37 40 44 49 51 62 65 67 71 **P**6

| | 13 | 10 | 20 | 161 | 5 | 3312 | 9 | 2689 | 1337 | 49 |

LARNED—Pawnee County

□ LARNED STATE HOSPITAL, Mailing Address: Rural Route 3, P.O. Box 89, Zip 67550-9365; tel. 316/285-2131; Mani Lee, Ph.D., Superintendent **A**1 10 **F**2 7 8 11 19 20 21 23 31 35 37 39 40 41 42 44 45 46 47 52 53 56 57 60 65 67 71 72 73 **P**6

| | 12 | 22 | 362 | 1417 | 333 | 0 | 0 | 29950 | 20376 | 797 |

LAWRENCE—Douglas County

□ LAWRENCE MEMORIAL HOSPITAL, 325 Maine, Zip 66044-1393; tel. 913/749-6100; Robert B. Ohlen, President and Chief Executive Officer (Total facility includes 14 beds in nursing home–type unit) **A**1 5 9 10 **F**7 8 10 14 15 16 19 20 21 22 28 31 32 33 35 36 37 39 40 41 44 46 49 52 64 65 71 73 **N** Jayhawk Health Alliance, Olathe, KS

| | 14 | 10 | 80 | 5723 | 80 | 69480 | 849 | 42230 | 19590 | 654 |

LEAVENWORTH—Leavenworth County

□ CUSHING MEMORIAL HOSPITAL, 711 Marshall Street, Zip 66048; tel. 913/684-1100; Charles L. Rogers, President (Nonreporting) **A**1 9 10

| | 23 | 10 | 77 | — | — | — | — | — | — | — |

⊞ DWIGHT D. EISENHOWER VETERANS AFFAIRS MEDICAL CENTER, 4101 South Fourth Street Trafficway, Zip 66048-5055; tel. 913/682-2000; Carole Bishop Smith, Center Director (Total facility includes 99 beds in nursing home–type unit) **A**1 3 5 9 **F**1 3 4 6 8 10 15 16 19 20 21 23 26 30 31 32 33 34 35 37 41 42 43 44 45 46 48 49 50 51 52 54 56 57 58 60 63 64 65 67 69 70 71 73 74 **S** Department of Veterans Affairs, Washington, DC **N** Hays Medical Center, Hays, KS

| | 45 | 10 | 122 | 2942 | 109 | 106848 | 0 | 60095 | 36216 | 919 |

Hospital, Address, Telephone, Administrator, Approval, Facility, and Physician Codes, Health Care System, Network	Classification Codes		Utilization Data					Expense (thousands) of dollars		
	Control	Service	Beds	Admissions	Census	Outpatient Visits	Births	Total	Payroll	Personnel

★ American Hospital Association (AHA) membership
□ Joint Commission on Accreditation of Healthcare Organizations (JCAHO) accreditation
+ American Osteopathic Hospital Association (AOHA) membership
○ American Osteopathic Association (AOA) accreditation
△ Commission on Accreditation of Rehabilitation Facilities (CARF) accreditation
Control codes 61, 63, 64, 71, 72 and 73 indicate hospitals listed by AOHA, but not registered by AHA. For definition of numerical codes, see page A4

Hospital	Control	Service	Beds	Admissions	Census	Outpatient Visits	Births	Total	Payroll	Personnel
✠ SAINT JOHN HOSPITAL, 3500 South Fourth Street, Zip 66048–5092; tel. 913/680–6000; Francis V. Creeden, Jr., President (Total facility includes 6 beds in nursing home–type unit) **A**1 9 10 **F**7 8 15 16 17 19 22 26 28 30 31 32 33 34 37 40 41 42 44 49 63 64 65 67 71 73 74 **P**1 4 5 6 7 8 **S** Sisters of Charity of Leavenworth Health Services Corporation, Leavenworth, KS **N** Jayhawk Health Alliance, Olathe, KS	21	10	36	1858	19	40952	293	13813	6553	224
LENEXA—Johnson County										
□ BHC COLLEGE MEADOWS HOSPITAL, (Formerly CPC College Meadows Hospital), 14425 College Boulevard, Zip 66215; tel. 913/469–1100; Lisa Redmond, Chief Executive Officer (Nonreporting) **A**1 9 10 **S** Behavioral Healthcare Corporation, Nashville, TN	33	22	120	—	—	—	—	—	—	—
LEOTI—Wichita County										
★ WICHITA COUNTY HOSPITAL, (Includes Wichita County Hospital Long Term Care, Mailing Address: P.O. Box 968, Zip 67861), 211 East Earl, Zip 67861–0968, Mailing Address: RR2, Box 38, Zip 67861–0968; tel. 316/375–2233; Julie Diehl, Administrator (Total facility includes 30 beds in nursing home–type unit) (Nonreporting) **A**9 10	23	10	51							
LIBERAL—Seward County										
✠ SOUTHWEST MEDICAL CENTER, 315 West 15th Street, Zip 67901–1340, Mailing Address: Box 1340, Zip 67905–1340; tel. 316/624–1651; Dave Kindel, President and Chief Executive Officer (Total facility includes 18 beds in nursing home–type unit) **A**1 9 10 **F**7 8 14 15 16 17 19 21 22 23 24 28 32 33 35 37 39 40 44 49 52 57 64 65 67 71 73	13	10	87	3106	33	33086	813	—	—	402
LINCOLN—Lincoln County										
LINCOLN COUNTY HOSPITAL, 624 North Second Street, Zip 67455, Mailing Address: P.O. Box 406, Zip 67455; tel. 913/524–4403; Jolene Yager, R.N., Administrator (Total facility includes 20 beds in nursing home–type unit) **A**9 10 **F**15 22 32 33 34 36 41 44 64 65 71 **S** Great Plains Health Alliance, Inc., Phillipsburg, KS **N** Sunflower Health Network, Inc., Salina, KS; Great Plains Health Alliance, Phillipsburg, KS	13	10	34	424	23	5065	0	2873	—	68
LINDSBORG—McPherson County										
★ LINDSBORG COMMUNITY HOSPITAL, 605 West Lincoln Street, Zip 67456–2399; tel. 913/227–3308; Greg Lundstrom, Interim Administrator **A**9 10 **F**15 24 28 32 34 36 39 42 44 49 64 71 **P**3 **N** Sunflower Health Network, Inc., Salina, KS	23	10	12	542	4	31239	0	3408	1491	69
LYONS—Rice County										
★ RICE COUNTY HOSPITAL DISTRICT NUMBER ONE, 619 South Clark Street, Zip 67554, Mailing Address: P.O. Box 828, Zip 67554; tel. 316/257–5173; Robert L. Mullen, Administrator **A**9 10 **F**6 7 8 12 14 15 16 17 20 26 28 30 32 33 36 39 40 44 46 49 62 65 71 **N** SouthEast Kansas Network, Coffeyville, KS	16	10	44	636	18	5515	142	3298	1575	73
MANHATTAN—Riley County										
MEMORIAL HOSPITAL See Mercy Health Center of Manhattan										
✠ MERCY HEALTH CENTER OF MANHATTAN, (Includes Memorial Hospital, 1105 Sunset Avenue, Zip 66502, Mailing Address: Box 1208, Zip 66502; tel. 913/776–3300; Saint Mary Hospital, 1823 College Avenue, Zip 66502, Mailing Address: Box 1047, Zip 66502–0041), Mailing Address: 1823 College Avenue, Zip 66502; E. Michael Nunamaker, President and Chief Executive Officer **A**1 9 10 **F**7 8 12 15 16 17 19 21 22 23 24 28 29 30 31 32 34 35 36 39 40 41 42 44 46 47 48 49 52 53 54 55 56 58 59 60 61 63 65 67 71 73 74 **S** Via Christi Health System, Wichita, KS **N** Community Health Alliance, Winchester, KS; Via Christi Health System, Wichita, KS	21	10	178	4288	51	64159	900	30925	13348	628
MANKATO—Jewell County										
JEWELL COUNTY HOSPITAL, 100 Crestvue, Zip 66956, Mailing Address: Box 327, Zip 66956–0327; tel. 913/378–3137; Rodney Brockelman, Administrator (Total facility includes 43 beds in nursing home–type unit) **A**9 **F**15 22 28 33 49 62 64 **P**5 **N** Sunflower Health Network, Inc., Salina, KS	13	10	49	75	40	806	0	1775	1191	57
MARION—Marion County										
★ ST. LUKE HOSPITAL, 1014 East Melvin, Zip 66861; tel. 316/382–2179; Craig Hanson, Administrator (Total facility includes 32 beds in nursing home–type unit) **A**9 10 **F**7 8 11 12 14 15 17 19 20 21 22 26 29 30 32 33 34 36 37 39 40 41 42 44 45 46 49 51 64 65 71 73 74 **S** Lutheran Health Systems, Fargo, ND	23	10	54	604	38	18265	50	4589	2351	107
MARYSVILLE—Marshall County										
★ COMMUNITY MEMORIAL HOSPITAL, 708 North 18th Street, Zip 66508–1399; tel. 913/562–2311; Harley B. Appel, Chief Executive Officer (Total facility includes 77 beds in nursing home–type unit) **A**9 10 **F**1 3 7 8 12 14 15 16 19 21 22 24 26 28 32 33 34 35 36 40 41 42 44 46 53 54 55 56 57 58 59 63 64 65 67 71 73 **P**3 7 **N** Community Health Alliance, Winchester, KS	23	10	132	1283	52	20368	82	8057	2655	138
MCPHERSON—McPherson County										
★ MEMORIAL HOSPITAL, 1000 Hospital Drive, Zip 67460–2321; tel. 316/241–2250; Stan Regehr, President and Chief Executive Officer **A**9 10 **F**7 8 14 15 16 17 19 21 22 24 28 31 32 33 35 36 37 39 40 41 42 44 45 46 49 65 71 73 **N** Sunflower Health Network, Inc., Salina, KS	23	10	41	1540	20	61333	179	10656	4956	202
MEADE—Meade County										
MEADE DISTRICT HOSPITAL, 510 East Carthage Street, Zip 67864–0680, Mailing Address: P.O. Box 680, Zip 67864–0680; tel. 316/873–2141; Michael P. Thomas, Administrator (Nonreporting) **A**9 10	16	10	20	—	—	—	—	—	—	—
MEDICINE LODGE—Barber County										
★ MEDICINE LODGE MEMORIAL HOSPITAL, 710 North Walnut Street, Zip 67104, Mailing Address: P.O. Drawer C, Zip 67104; tel. 316/886–3771; Kevin A. White, Administrator **A**9 10 **F**8 15 16 20 22 26 34 44 49 71 **S** Great Plains Health Alliance, Inc., Phillipsburg, KS **N** Great Plains Health Alliance, Phillipsburg, KS	16	10	42	729	16	7688	0	4318	2109	88

Hospital, Address, Telephone, Administrator, Approval, Facility, and Physician Codes, Health Care System, Network	Classi-fication Codes		Utilization Data					Expense (thousands) of dollars		
★ American Hospital Association (AHA) membership □ Joint Commission on Accreditation of Healthcare Organizations (JCAHO) accreditation + American Osteopathic Hospital Association (AOHA) membership ○ American Osteopathic Association (AOA) accreditation △ Commission on Accreditation of Rehabilitation Facilities (CARF) accreditation Control codes 61, 63, 64, 71, 72 and 73 indicate hospitals listed by AOHA, but not registered by AHA. For definition of numerical codes, see page A4	Control	Service	Beds	Admissions	Census	Outpatient Visits	Births	Total	Payroll	Personnel

MINNEAPOLIS—Ottawa County

★ OTTAWA COUNTY HOSPITAL, 215 East Eighth, Zip 67467, Mailing Address: Box 209, Zip 67467; tel. 913/392–2122; Joy Reed, R.N., Administrator (Total facility includes 23 beds in nursing home–type unit) **A**9 10 **F**1 14 15 16 17 20 21 22 24 26 27 32 34 36 45 49 58 64 65 71 **S** Great Plains Health Alliance, Inc., Phillipsburg, KS **N** Sunflower Health Network, Inc., Salina, KS; Great Plains Health Alliance, Phillipsburg, KS

| 23 | 10 | 53 | 452 | 48 | — | 0 | 2968 | 1670 | 90 |

MINNEOLA—Clark County

★ MINNEOLA DISTRICT HOSPITAL, 212 Main Street, Zip 67865; tel. 316/885–4264; Blaine K. Miller, Administrator **A**9 10 **F**8 16 22 28 33 34 41 44 49 56 62 65 71 **S** Great Plains Health Alliance, Inc., Phillipsburg, KS **N** Great Plains Health Alliance, Phillipsburg, KS

| 16 | 10 | 15 | 617 | 8 | 5254 | 52 | 2392 | 887 | 40 |

MOUNDRIDGE—McPherson County

★ MERCY HOSPITAL, 218 East Pack Street, Zip 67107, Mailing Address: Box 180, Zip 67107; tel. 316/345–6391; Doyle K. Johnson, Administrator (Total facility includes 6 beds in nursing home–type unit) **A**9 10 **F**15 22 26 40 44 49 64

| 21 | 10 | 22 | 269 | 3 | 4771 | 28 | 1038 | 544 | 31 |

NEODESHA—Wilson County

★ WILSON COUNTY HOSPITAL, 205 Mill Street, Zip 66757, Mailing Address: Box 360, Zip 66757; tel. 316/325–2611; Deanna Pittman, Administrator **A**9 10 **F**1 7 15 16 17 19 22 26 30 31 32 33 39 40 41 44 52 57 65 67 71 73 **S** Quorum Health Group/Quorum Health Resources, Inc., Brentwood, TN **N** SouthEast Kansas Network, Coffeyville, KS

| 13 | 10 | 38 | 573 | 11 | 5995 | 54 | 4036 | 1925 | 88 |

NESS CITY—Ness County

★ NESS COUNTY HOSPITAL NUMBER TWO, 312 East Custer Street, Zip 67560; tel. 913/798–2291; Clyde T. McCracken, Administrator (Total facility includes 27 beds in nursing home–type unit) **A**9 10 **F**15 17 19 22 28 30 32 35 39 44 48 49 64 65 67 71 **P**6 **N** MED–OP, Oakley, KS

| 16 | 10 | 52 | 375 | 34 | 3474 | 3 | 3066 | 1577 | 97 |

NEWTON—Harvey County

⊞ NEWTON MEDICAL CENTER, Mailing Address: P.O. Box 308, Zip 67114–0308; tel. 316/283–2700; W. Charles Waters, President (Total facility includes 11 beds in nursing home–type unit) **A**1 9 10 **F**7 14 15 19 21 22 23 26 28 29 30 31 32 33 34 35 37 40 41 44 49 56 64 65 71

| 23 | 10 | 72 | 2837 | 38 | 26429 | 433 | 17145 | 8473 | 315 |

□ PRAIRIE VIEW, 1901 East First Street, Zip 67114, Mailing Address: Box 467, Zip 67114–0467; tel. 316/283–2400; Melvin Goering, Chief Executive Officer **A**1 10 **F**3 12 14 15 16 17 18 22 27 28 30 32 52 53 54 55 56 57 58 59 65 67 73 **P**6

| 23 | 22 | 30 | 1081 | 23 | — | 0 | 14565 | 9273 | 247 |

NORTON—Norton County

★ NORTON COUNTY HOSPITAL, 102 East Holme, Zip 67654–0250, Mailing Address: P.O. Box 250, Zip 67654–0250; tel. 913/877–3351; Richard Miller, Administrator **A**9 10 **F**7 8 15 16 19 20 21 22 26 28 30 32 33 34 36 39 40 42 44 45 46 48 49 51 53 54 55 56 57 58 64 65 71 73 **P**4 **N** MED–OP, Oakley, KS

| 13 | 10 | 22 | 566 | 14 | 20413 | 20 | 4262 | 2166 | 84 |

OAKLEY—Logan County

LOGAN COUNTY HOSPITAL, 211 Cherry Street, Zip 67748; tel. 913/672–3211; Rodney Bates, Administrator (Total facility includes 30 beds in nursing home–type unit) **A**9 10 **F**6 7 15 22 27 28 32 33 34 36 37 40 42 44 49 62 64 65 71 **N** MED–OP, Oakley, KS

| 13 | 10 | 51 | 453 | 34 | 10299 | 23 | 2553 | 1443 | 71 |

OBERLIN—Decatur County

★ DECATUR COUNTY HOSPITAL, 810 West Columbia, Zip 67749, Mailing Address: P.O. Box 268, Zip 67749; tel. 913/475–2208; R. Kim Hardman, Administrator (Total facility includes 50 beds in nursing home–type unit) **A**9 10 **F**7 8 12 14 15 16 19 22 26 28 30 32 34 35 36 37 42 44 46 49 64 65 71 **S** Lutheran Health Systems, Fargo, ND **N** MED–OP, Oakley, KS

| 23 | 10 | 74 | 623 | 55 | 10832 | 57 | 4305 | 2178 | 96 |

OLATHE—Johnson County

⊞ OLATHE MEDICAL CENTER, 20333 West 151st Street, Zip 66061–5352; tel. 913/791–4200; Frank H. Devocelle, President and Chief Executive Officer **A**1 2 5 9 10 **F**4 7 8 10 12 14 15 16 17 19 21 22 28 30 31 32 33 34 35 37 40 44 46 49 65 67 71 72 73 **P**6 **N** Jayhawk Health Alliance, Olathe, KS

| 23 | 10 | 130 | 7424 | 78 | 100075 | 941 | 47953 | 22299 | 651 |

ONAGA—Pottawatomie County

COMMUNITY HOSPITAL ONAGA, 120 West Eighth Street, Zip 66521–0120; tel. 913/889–4272; Joseph T. Engelken, Chief Executive Officer (Total facility includes 42 beds in nursing home–type unit) **A**9 10 **F**1 2 3 4 5 6 7 8 9 10 11 12 13 14 15 16 17 19 20 21 22 23 24 25 26 27 28 29 30 31 32 33 34 35 37 38 39 40 41 42 43 44 45 46 47 48 49 50 51 52 53 54 55 56 57 58 59 60 61 62 63 64 65 66 67 68 69 70 71 72 73 74 **P**1 4 **N** Community Health Alliance, Winchester, KS

| 23 | 10 | 67 | 856 | 54 | 32957 | 129 | 9164 | 5108 | 232 |

OSAWATOMIE—Miami County

□ OSAWATOMIE STATE HOSPITAL, 500 State Hospital Drive, Zip 66064–9757, Mailing Address: P.O. Box 500, Zip 66064–9757; tel. 913/755–3151; Stephen H. Feinstein, Ph.D., Superintendent **A**1 10 **F**2 8 19 20 21 22 26 42 44 45 46 50 51 52 53 57 60 65 70 73 **P**6

| 12 | 22 | 275 | 1196 | 198 | 0 | 0 | 28414 | 14590 | 515 |

OSBORNE—Osborne County

★ OSBORNE COUNTY MEMORIAL HOSPITAL, 424 West New Hampshire Street, Zip 67473–0070, Mailing Address: P.O. Box 70, Zip 67473–0070; tel. 913/346–2121; Patricia Bernard, R.N., Administrator **A**9 10 **F**7 8 19 20 22 33 34 36 44 71 **S** Great Plains Health Alliance, Inc., Phillipsburg, KS **N** Sunflower Health Network, Inc., Salina, KS; Great Plains Health Alliance, Phillipsburg, KS

| 13 | 10 | 29 | 407 | 4 | 6950 | 22 | 2256 | 1070 | 60 |

Hospital, Address, Telephone, Administrator, Approval, Facility, and Physician Codes, Health Care System, Network	Classi-fication Codes		Utilization Data					Expense (thousands) of dollars		
	Control	Service	Beds	Admissions	Census	Outpatient Visits	Births	Total	Payroll	Personnel

★   American Hospital Association (AHA) membership
□   Joint Commission on Accreditation of Healthcare Organizations (JCAHO) accreditation
+   American Osteopathic Hospital Association (AOHA) membership
○   American Osteopathic Association (AOA) accreditation
△   Commission on Accreditation of Rehabilitation Facilities (CARF) accreditation
    Control codes 61, 63, 64, 71, 72 and 73 indicate hospitals listed by AOHA, but not registered by AHA. For definition of numerical codes, see page A4

OTTAWA—Franklin County

✠ RANSOM MEMORIAL HOSPITAL, 1301 South Main Street, Zip 66067–3598; tel. 913/242–3344; Robert E. Bregant, Jr., Administrator **A**1 9 10 **F**7 8 15 17 19 21 22 26 27 28 30 32 33 34 35 37 39 40 41 42 44 45 46 49 56 63 65 67 68 71 73	13	10	45	1908	25	34997	181	12114	6235	277

OVERLAND PARK—Johnson County

✠ COLUMBIA OVERLAND PARK REGIONAL MEDICAL CENTER, 10500 Quivira Road, Zip 66215–2373, Mailing Address: P.O. Box 15959, Zip 66215; tel. 913/541–5000; Kevin J. Hicks, President and Chief Executive Officer (Total facility includes 17 beds in nursing home–type unit) **A**1 9 10 **F**4 7 8 10 11 12 14 15 16 17 19 26 27 28 29 30 31 32 33 34 35 37 38 39 40 41 42 43 44 45 46 47 49 51 52 53 54 55 56 57 58 59 60 61 64 65 66 67 68 70 71 72 73 74 **S** Columbia/HCA Healthcare Corporation, Nashville, TN	33	10	287	9681	125	77901	2067	70167	27677	835
★ MENORAH MEDICAL CENTER, 5721 West 119th Street, Zip 66209; tel. 913/498–6000; Steven D. Wilkinson, Chief Executive Officer **A**2 9 10 **F**1 2 3 4 5 7 8 10 11 12 14 15 16 17 18 19 20 21 22 23 24 25 26 27 28 29 30 31 32 33 34 35 37 38 39 40 41 42 43 44 45 46 48 49 51 52 53 54 55 56 57 58 59 60 61 63 65 66 67 68 69 70 71 72 73 74 **P**1 5 6 7 8 **S** Health Midwest, Kansas City, MO	23	10	70	1267	15	27091	396	29699	10224	556
✠ △ MID–AMERICA REHABILITATION HOSPITAL, 5701 West 110th Street, Zip 66211; tel. 913/491–2400; Richard L. Allen, Chief Executive Officer (Total facility includes 15 beds in nursing home–type unit) **A**1 7 9 10 **F**12 14 15 16 17 19 20 21 25 27 34 35 41 46 48 49 60 64 65 66 67 71 73 **P**5 7	33	46	80	799	57	18742	0	18435	8670	170

PAOLA—Miami County

★ MIAMI COUNTY MEDICAL CENTER, 2100 Baptiste, Zip 66071–0365, Mailing Address: P.O. Box 365, Zip 66071–0365; tel. 913/294–2327; Gerald Wiesner, Vice President and Chief Operating Officer **A**9 10 **F**8 13 16 19 21 22 28 30 31 32 33 34 39 41 42 44 46 48 49 51 56 65 66 71 73 **N** Jayhawk Health Alliance, Olathe, KS	23	10	18	541	6	20565	0	7041	2890	124

PARSONS—Labette County

✠ + LABETTE COUNTY MEDICAL CENTER, 1902 South U.S. Highway 59, Zip 67357, Mailing Address: P.O. Box 956, Zip 67357; tel. 316/421–4880; Richard A. Nye, Chief Executive Officer (Total facility includes 12 beds in nursing home–type unit) **A**1 9 10 **F**7 8 10 14 15 17 19 21 22 23 28 29 30 32 34 35 36 37 39 40 41 42 44 46 49 64 65 67 71 73 **N** SouthEast Kansas Network, Coffeyville, KS	13	10	81	2953	42	38500	289	25848	10667	390
PARSONS STATE HOSPITAL AND TRAINING CENTER, 2601 Gabriel Street, Zip 67357–0738, Mailing Address: Box 738, Zip 67357–0738; tel. 316/421–6550; Gary J. Daniels, Ph.D., Superintendent (Nonreporting)	12	62	222	—	—	—	—	—	—	—

PHILLIPSBURG—Phillips County

★ PHILLIPS COUNTY HOSPITAL, 1150 State Street, Zip 67661, Mailing Address: Box 607, Zip 67661; tel. 913/543–5226; James L. Giedd, Administrator (Total facility includes 33 beds in nursing home–type unit) **A**9 10 **F**1 7 8 15 19 20 22 28 34 35 42 44 46 49 64 65 71 73 **S** Great Plains Health Alliance, Inc., Phillipsburg, KS **N** Great Plains Health Alliance, Phillipsburg, KS; Hays Medical Center, Hays, KS	23	10	62	938	41	9646	37	5477	2516	113

PITTSBURG—Crawford County

✠ + MOUNT CARMEL MEDICAL CENTER, Centennial and Rouse Streets, Zip 66762–6686; tel. 316/231–6100; John Daniel Lingor, President and Chief Executive Officer (Total facility includes 20 beds in nursing home–type unit) **A**1 2 9 10 **F**1 7 8 12 15 16 19 21 22 23 27 28 29 30 32 35 36 37 39 40 41 42 44 45 46 49 51 52 54 55 56 59 60 63 64 65 66 67 71 73 **P**1 2 3 4 5 6 7 8 **S** Via Christi Health System, Wichita, KS **N** Via Christi Health System, Wichita, KS; SouthEast Kansas Network, Coffeyville, KS	23	10	119	4450	58	66119	300	29386	13144	488

PLAINVILLE—Rooks County

PLAINVILLE RURAL HOSPITAL DISTRICT NUMBER ONE, 304 South Colorado Avenue, Zip 67663; tel. 913/434–4553; Leonard Hernandez, Administrator **A**9 10 **F**1 3 4 5 6 7 8 10 12 13 14 15 16 17 18 19 20 21 22 23 24 25 26 27 28 29 30 31 32 33 34 35 36 39 41 42 43 44 45 49 51 53 54 55 56 57 58 59 60 62 65 66 67 68 69 70 71 72 73 74 **P**5 **N** MED–OP, Oakley, KS	15	10	27	322	7	2525	9	2287	1027	61

PRATT—Pratt County

✠ PRATT REGIONAL MEDICAL CENTER, 200 Commodore Street, Zip 67124–3099; tel. 316/672–7451; Susan M. Page, President and Chief Executive Officer (Total facility includes 15 beds in nursing home–type unit) **A**1 9 10 **F**7 8 13 15 16 19 21 22 23 24 25 26 28 29 30 31 32 33 34 35 36 37 39 40 42 44 45 46 49 61 64 65 66 67 71 73 **P**7	23	10	84	1799	26	25466	167	14962	6574	229

QUINTER—Gove County

GOVE COUNTY MEDICAL CENTER, Fifth and Garfield Streets, Zip 67752; tel. 913/754–3341; Paul Davis, Administrator **A**9 10 **F**6 7 8 19 22 27 28 32 33 34 44 49 64 65 71 **N** MED–OP, Oakley, KS	13	10	80	820	11	8056	60	4601	2303	120

RANSOM—Ness County

★ GRISELL MEMORIAL HOSPITAL DISTRICT ONE, 210 South Vermont, Zip 67572–0268, Mailing Address: P.O. Box 268, Zip 67572–0268; tel. 913/731–2231; Kristine Ochs, R.N., Administrator (Total facility includes 34 beds in nursing home–type unit) **A**9 10 **F**7 8 19 20 22 26 32 33 35 36 41 44 49 51 56 64 65 71 **S** Great Plains Health Alliance, Inc., Phillipsburg, KS **N** Great Plains Health Alliance, Phillipsburg, KS; Hays Medical Center, Hays, KS	16	10	46	156	35	7991	3	2402	1335	62

Hospital, Address, Telephone, Administrator, Approval, Facility, and Physician Codes, Health Care System, Network	Classi-fication Codes		Utilization Data					Expense (thousands) of dollars		
★ American Hospital Association (AHA) membership □ Joint Commission on Accreditation of Healthcare Organizations (JCAHO) accreditation + American Osteopathic Hospital Association (AOHA) membership ○ American Osteopathic Association (AOA) accreditation △ Commission on Accreditation of Rehabilitation Facilities (CARF) accreditation Control codes 61, 63, 64, 71, 72 and 73 indicate hospitals listed by AOHA, but not registered by AHA. For definition of numerical codes, see page A4	Control	Service	Beds	Admissions	Census	Outpatient Visits	Births	Total	Payroll	Personnel

RUSSELL—Russell County

✠ RUSSELL REGIONAL HOSPITAL, 200 South Main Street, Zip 67665; tel. 913/483–3131; Talton L. Francis, FACHE, President and Chief Executive Officer (Total facility includes 23 beds in nursing home–type unit) **A**1 9 10 **F**14 15 16 19 21 22 27 28 29 30 32 34 36 37 40 44 45 48 49 51 64 65 67 71 73 **N** Sunflower Health Network, Inc., Salina, KS
13 10 · 57 · 797 · 31 · 16356 · 29 · 5650 · 2987 · 123

SABETHA—Nemaha County

★ SABETHA COMMUNITY HOSPITAL, 14th and Oregon Streets, Zip 66534, Mailing Address: P.O. Box 229, Zip 66534; tel. 913/284–2121; Rita K. Buurman, Administrator **A**9 10 **F**1 7 8 15 16 17 19 20 22 26 28 30 32 34 35 41 42 44 45 49 54 56 58 65 71 **P**6 **S** Great Plains Health Alliance, Inc., Phillipsburg, KS **N** Great Plains Health Alliance, Phillipsburg, KS
23 10 · 27 · 541 · 8 · 15881 · 48 · 3861 · 1983 · 64

SAINT FRANCIS—Maricopa County

★ CHEYENNE COUNTY HOSPITAL, 210 West First Street, Zip 67756, Mailing Address: P.O. Box 547, Zip 67756–0547; tel. 913/332–2104; Leslie Lacy, Administrator **A**9 10 **F**7 8 15 16 19 22 35 42 44 49 51 65 71 **S** Great Plains Health Alliance, Inc., Phillipsburg, KS **N** Great Plains Health Alliance, Phillipsburg, KS; Hays Medical Center, Hays, KS; High Plains Rural Health Network, Fort Morgan, CO
23 10 · 23 · 202 · 3 · 8875 · 0 · 1807 · 681 · 40

SALINA—Saline County

✠ △ SALINA REGIONAL HEALTH CENTER, (Includes Salina Regional Health Center–Penn Campus, 139 North Penn Street, Salina Regional Health Center–Santa Fe Campus), 400 South Santa Fe Avenue, Zip 67401, Mailing Address: P.O. Box 5080, Zip 67401; tel. 913/452–7000; Clay D. Edmands, President (Total facility includes 31 beds in nursing home–type unit) **A**1 2 3 7 9 10 **F**4 7 8 10 15 16 17 19 20 21 22 23 24 26 27 28 29 30 31 32 33 34 35 36 37 38 39 40 41 42 44 45 46 48 49 52 54 55 56 57 58 60 63 64 65 66 68 71 73 74 **P**3 8 **N** Via Christi Health System, Wichita, KS; Sunflower Health Network, Inc., Salina, KS
23 10 · 229 · 9366 · 143 · 114452 · 1075 · 70123 · 29778 · 1086

★ ST. FRANCIS AT SALINA, 5097 Cloud Street, Zip 67401, Mailing Address: 509 East Elm, Zip 67401; tel. 913/825–0563; Reverend Phillip J. Rapp, President and Chief Executive Officer (Nonreporting) **A**9
23 22 · 26 · — · — · — · — · — · — · —

SATANTA—Haskell County

★ SATANTA DISTRICT HOSPITAL, 401 South Cheyenne Street, Zip 67870, Mailing Address: P.O. Box 159, Zip 67870–0159; tel. 316/649–2761; T. G. Lee, Administrator (Total facility includes 29 beds in nursing home–type unit) **A**9 10 **F**7 8 15 17 19 22 32 34 35 39 41 44 45 49 64 65 71 **P**4 **S** Great Plains Health Alliance, Inc., Phillipsburg, KS **N** Pioneer Network, Santana, KS; Great Plains Health Alliance, Phillipsburg, KS; Hays Medical Center, Hays, KS
16 10 · 42 · 314 · 28 · 4836 · 0 · 3566 · 1745 · 95

SCOTT CITY—Scott County

★ SCOTT COUNTY HOSPITAL, 310 East Third Street, Zip 67871; tel. 316/872–5811; Greg Unruh, Chief Executive Officer **A**9 10 **F**7 15 19 22 28 36 39 42 44 65 71 73 **N** MED-OP, Oakley, KS
13 10 · 27 · 812 · 11 · 8120 · 77 · — · — · 96

SEDAN—Chautauqua County

SEDAN CITY HOSPITAL, 300 North Street, Zip 67361, Mailing Address: Box C, Zip 67361; tel. 316/725–3115; Janice Shippy, R.N., Administrator **A**9 10 **F**8 14 15 16 22 28 32 33 51 57 64 71 **P**6
14 10 · 30 · 128 · 8 · 6609 · 0 · 2795 · 1303 · 59

SENECA—Nemaha County

NEMAHA VALLEY COMMUNITY HOSPITAL, 1600 Community Drive, Zip 66538; tel. 913/336–6181; Michael J. Ryan, President and Chief Executive Officer **A**9 10 **F**7 8 15 19 22 26 28 30 32 34 35 40 41 44 49 65 67 70 71 **N** Community Health Alliance, Winchester, KS
23 10 · 24 · 473 · 6 · 9081 · 50 · 3644 · 1468 · 66

SHAWNEE MISSION—Johnson County

MENORAH MEDICAL CENTER See Overland Park

✠ SHAWNEE MISSION MEDICAL CENTER, 9100 West 74th Street, Zip 66204–4019, Mailing Address: Box 2923, Zip 66201–1323; tel. 913/676–2000; William G. Robertson, Senior Executive Officer **A**1 2 5 9 10 **F**2 3 4 7 8 10 11 12 13 15 16 17 19 21 22 23 24 28 29 30 31 32 33 34 35 37 38 39 40 41 42 43 44 45 46 49 52 53 54 55 56 57 58 59 61 64 65 66 67 68 69 71 72 73 74 **P**5 6 7 8 **S** Saint Luke's Shawnee Mission Health System, Kansas City, MO
21 10 · 333 · 16964 · 195 · 216054 · 3108 · 133356 · 60280 · 1721

SMITH CENTER—Smith County

★ SMITH COUNTY MEMORIAL HOSPITAL, 614 South Main Street, Zip 66967–0349, Mailing Address: P.O. Box 349, Zip 66967–0349; tel. 913/282–6845; John Terrill, Administrator (Total facility includes 28 beds in nursing home–type unit) **A**9 10 **F**1 7 8 19 22 34 35 44 49 64 71 **S** Great Plains Health Alliance, Inc., Phillipsburg, KS **N** Sunflower Health Network, Inc., Salina, KS; Great Plains Health Alliance, Phillipsburg, KS
23 10 · 54 · 658 · 34 · 9455 · 50 · 3604 · 1743 · 96

STAFFORD—Stafford County

STAFFORD DISTRICT HOSPITAL, 502 South Buckeye Street, Zip 67578, Mailing Address: Box 190, Zip 67578; tel. 316/234–5221; Douglas Newman, Administrator **A**9 10 **F**8 11 12 13 15 16 17 19 20 21 22 25 26 28 29 30 31 32 33 34 35 36 39 42 44 45 46 49 51 56 63 64 65 66 71 73 74 **P**6
16 10 · 25 · 387 · 6 · 3739 · 0 · — · — · 43

SYRACUSE—Hamilton County

HAMILTON COUNTY HOSPITAL, East Avenue G and Huser Street, Zip 67878–0909, Mailing Address: Box 909, Zip 67878–0909; tel. 316/384–7461; Arthur R. Smith, Chief Executive Officer and Administrator (Total facility includes 44 beds in nursing home–type unit) **A**9 10 **F**6 7 8 15 17 19 22 26 27 28 32 34 35 36 39 44 49 51 62 64 65 71 72 **P**4
13 10 · 73 · 283 · 43 · — · 6 · 3637 · 1793 · 94

Hospital, Address, Telephone, Administrator, Approval, Facility, and Physician Codes, Health Care System, Network	Classi-fication Codes		Utilization Data					Expense (thousands) of dollars		
★ American Hospital Association (AHA) membership □ Joint Commission on Accreditation of Healthcare Organizations (JCAHO) accreditation + American Osteopathic Hospital Association (AOHA) membership ○ American Osteopathic Association (AOA) accreditation △ Commission on Accreditation of Rehabilitation Facilities (CARF) accreditation Control codes 61, 63, 64, 71, 72 and 73 indicate hospitals listed by AOHA, but not registered by AHA. For definition of numerical codes, see page A4	Control	Service	Beds	Admissions	Census	Outpatient Visits	Births	Total	Payroll	Personnel

TOPEKA—Shawnee County

☒ C. F. MENNINGER MEMORIAL HOSPITAL, (Includes Child and Adolescent Services of the Menninger Clinic, 5800 S.W. Sixth Avenue, Mailing Address: Box 829, Zip 66601; tel. 913/350–5000), 5800 West Sixth Avenue, Zip 66606, Mailing Address: Box 829, Zip 66601–0829; tel. 913/350–5000; W. Pearl Washington, MSN, Administrator **A**1 3 9 10 **F**1 2 3 4 7 8 9 10 11 14 15 16 19 21 22 23 31 32 33 34 35 37 40 42 43 44 47 52 53 55 56 57 58 59 60 65 71 74 **P**1

| | 23 | 22 | 143 | 1436 | 105 | 72297 | 0 | 33111 | 20079 | 528 |

CHILD AND ADOLESCENT SERVICES OF THE MENNINGER CLINIC See C. F. Menninger Memorial Hospital

☒ COLMERY–O'NEIL VETERANS AFFAIRS MEDICAL CENTER, 2200 Gage Boulevard, Zip 66622; tel. 913/350–3111; Edgar Tucker, Director (Total facility includes 129 beds in nursing home–type unit) **A**1 3 9 **F**1 2 3 6 8 10 11 12 14 15 16 17 18 19 20 21 22 24 26 27 28 29 30 31 32 34 35 37 39 41 42 44 45 46 48 49 51 52 54 55 56 57 58 59 63 64 65 67 71 72 73 74 **S** Department of Veterans Affairs, Washington, DC

| | 45 | 10 | 437 | 3762 | 279 | 163355 | 0 | 73116 | 43696 | 1071 |

KANSAS NEUROLOGICAL INSTITUTE, 3107 West 21st Street, Zip 66604–3298; tel. 913/296–5301; Robert Day, Ph.D., Superintendent **F**20 39 73 **P**6

| | 12 | 62 | 251 | 0 | 242 | 0 | 0 | 24758 | 16355 | 697 |

□ △ KANSAS REHABILITATION HOSPITAL, 1504 S.W. Eighth, Zip 66606–2714; tel. 913/235–6600; Julie De Jean, Administrator (Total facility includes 17 beds in nursing home–type unit) **A**1 7 9 10 **F**10 14 15 41 48 49 64 65 67 73 74

| | 46 | 46 | 79 | 690 | 38 | 18582 | 0 | 10576 | 5450 | 161 |

□ PARKVIEW HOSPITAL OF TOPEKA, 3707 S.W. Sixth Street, Zip 66606; tel. 913/295–3000; Thomas G. Smith, Administrator **A**1 9 10 **F**2 3 14 15 16 52 53 54 55 56 57 58 59 65 67 **P**5 7 **S** Health Management Associates, Naples, FL

| | 33 | 22 | 60 | 669 | 16 | 9134 | 0 | 4235 | 2142 | 93 |

☒ △ ST. FRANCIS HOSPITAL AND MEDICAL CENTER, 1700 West Seventh Street, Zip 66606–1690; tel. 913/295–8000; Sister Loretto Marie Colwell, President **A**1 2 3 5 7 9 10 **F**2 3 4 7 8 10 11 12 15 19 20 21 22 24 27 28 30 31 32 34 35 37 40 41 42 43 44 45 46 48 49 51 56 60 63 65 67 71 73 **P**8 **S** Sisters of Charity of Leavenworth Health Services Corporation, Leavenworth, KS **N** Community Health Alliance, Winchester, KS; Heart of America Network, Wichita, KS

| | 21 | 10 | 308 | 10023 | 142 | 217388 | 1141 | 93697 | 42315 | 1301 |

☒ STORMONT–VAIL HEALTHCARE, (Formerly Stormont–Vail Regional Medical Center), 1500 S.W. Tenth Street, Zip 66604–1353; tel. 913/354–6000; Maynard F. Oliverius, President and Chief Executive Officer **A**1 3 5 9 10 **F**4 7 8 10 11 12 14 15 16 17 19 21 22 23 24 26 27 28 29 30 31 32 33 34 35 36 37 38 39 40 41 42 43 44 45 46 47 49 52 53 55 56 57 58 60 65 67 71 73 74 **P**6 **S** Stormont–Vail HealthCare, Topeka, KS

| | 23 | 10 | 313 | 10227 | 155 | 86272 | 1841 | 151006 | 75838 | 2041 |

TRIBUNE—Greeley County

★ GREELEY COUNTY HOSPITAL, 506 Third Street, Zip 67879, Mailing Address: Box 338, Zip 67879; tel. 316/376–4221; Cynthia K. Schneider, Administrator (Total facility includes 31 beds in nursing home–type unit) **A**9 10 **F**7 8 15 16 19 20 22 27 32 36 39 44 46 49 56 57 64 67 71 **S** Great Plains Health Alliance, Inc., Phillipsburg, KS **N** Great Plains Health Alliance, Phillipsburg, KS

| | 23 | 10 | 49 | 440 | 33 | 6272 | 51 | 2934 | 1418 | 71 |

ULYSSES—Grant County

★ BOB WILSON MEMORIAL GRANT COUNTY HOSPITAL, 415 North Main Street, Zip 67880; tel. 316/356–1266; Bruce K. Birchell, Administrator **A**9 10 **F**8 15 19 21 22 28 29 32 34 35 37 44 45 49 65 71 73 **P**5 **S** Quorum Health Group/Quorum Health Resources, Inc., Brentwood, TN

| | 13 | 10 | 39 | 733 | 9 | 15674 | 23 | 7587 | 2894 | 130 |

WAKEENEY—Trego County

★ TREGO COUNTY–LEMKE MEMORIAL HOSPITAL, 320 13th Street, Zip 67672–2099; tel. 913/743–2182; James Wahlmeier, Administrator (Total facility includes 45 beds in nursing home–type unit) **A**9 10 **F**3 7 8 15 16 17 19 20 22 32 33 34 44 45 49 64 65 71 **S** Great Plains Health Alliance, Inc., Phillipsburg, KS **N** Great Plains Health Alliance, Phillipsburg, KS; Hays Medical Center, Hays, KS

| | 13 | 10 | 73 | 672 | 52 | 6987 | 1 | 4502 | 2034 | 103 |

WAMEGO—Pottawatomie County

WAMEGO CITY HOSPITAL, 711 Genn Drive, Zip 66547; tel. 913/456–2295; Lisa J. Freeborn, Administrator **A**9 10 **F**15 16 19 22 28 32 44 49 64 65 71 **S** Stormont–Vail HealthCare, Topeka, KS

| | 14 | 10 | 26 | 560 | 7 | 12269 | 0 | 4225 | 2411 | 105 |

WASHINGTON—Washington County

WASHINGTON COUNTY HOSPITAL, 304 East Third Street, Zip 66968–2098; tel. 913/325–2211; Everett Lutjemeier, Administrator **A**9 10 **F**1 7 8 9 14 15 22 24 28 30 33 36 37 40 44 49 51 64 65 71 **P**5

| | 13 | 10 | 27 | 269 | 8 | 3546 | 15 | 1605 | 759 | 36 |

WELLINGTON—Sumner County

★ SUMNER REGIONAL MEDICAL CENTER, 1323 North A Street, Zip 67152–1323; tel. 316/326–7453; Raymond Williams, III, President and Chief Executive Officer (Total facility includes 11 beds in nursing home–type unit) **A**9 10 **F**7 14 15 19 22 32 34 36 40 44 64 71 73 **P**8

| | 14 | 10 | 49 | 1174 | 16 | 27079 | 155 | 6151 | 2735 | 111 |

WESTMORELAND—Pottawatomie County

DECHAIRO HOSPITAL, First and North Streets, Zip 66549; tel. 913/457–3311; Paula Lauer, Administrator (Nonreporting) **A**9 10 **S** Stormont–Vail HealthCare, Topeka, KS

| | 33 | 10 | 13 | — | — | — | — | — | — | — |

WICHITA—Sedgwick County

☒ COLUMBIA WESLEY MEDICAL CENTER, 550 North Hillside Avenue, Zip 67214–4976; tel. 316/688–2468; Kevin Gross, Interim President and Chief Executive Officer **A**1 2 3 5 9 10 **F**4 7 8 10 11 12 15 16 18 19 20 21 22 23 24 26 27 28 29 30 31 32 33 34 35 37 38 39 40 41 42 43 44 46 47 49 51 54 56 60 61 64 65 66 67 69 70 71 73 74 **P**6 7 **S** Columbia/HCA Healthcare Corporation, Nashville, TN

| | 33 | 10 | 553 | 22377 | 331 | 186885 | 3634 | 220066 | 87008 | 2434 |

Hospital, Address, Telephone, Administrator, Approval, Facility, and Physician Codes, Health Care System, Network	Classification Codes		Utilization Data					Expense (thousands) of dollars		
	Control	Service	Beds	Admissions	Census	Outpatient Visits	Births	Total	Payroll	Personnel
+ ○ RIVERSIDE HEALTH SYSTEM, 2622 West Central Street, Zip 67203–4999; tel. 316/946–5000; Robert Dixon, President and Chief Executive Officer (Total facility includes 22 beds in nursing home–type unit) **A**9 10 11 12 13 **F**7 8 11 12 13 14 15 16 17 19 20 21 22 26 28 29 30 31 35 37 39 40 41 42 44 45 46 49 54 56 63 64 65 66 67 71 73 **P**3 6 ST. FRANCIS REGIONAL MEDICAL CENTER See Via Christi Regional Medical Center ST. JOSEPH MEDICAL CENTER See Via Christi Regional Medical Center	23	10	117	3158	35	27643	225	34261	15612	518
✦ VETERANS AFFAIRS MEDICAL AND REGIONAL OFFICE CENTER, 5500 East Kellogg, Zip 67218; tel. 316/685–2221; Robert D. Morrel, Associate Director **A**1 3 5 9 **F**3 8 19 20 21 22 26 31 35 39 41 44 45 46 49 51 52 56 57 58 60 65 67 73 **P**6 **S** Department of Veterans Affairs, Washington, DC	45	10	83	3330	71	91412	0	—	—	—
✦ △ VIA CHRISTI REGIONAL MEDICAL CENTER, (Includes Via Christi Regional Medical Center–St. Francis Campus, 929 North St. Francis Street, tel. 316/268–5000; Via Christi Regional Medical Center–St. Joseph Campus, 3600 East Harry Street, Zip 67218–3713; tel. 316/685–1111), 929 North St. Francis Street, Zip 67214–3882; tel. 316/268–5000; Randall G. Nyp, President and Chief Executive Officer (Nonreporting) **A**1 3 5 7 9 10 **S** Via Christi Health System, Wichita, KS **N** Heart of America Network, Wichita, KS; Via Christi Health System, Wichita, KS VIA CHRISTI REGIONAL MEDICAL CENTER–ST. FRANCIS CAMPUS See Via Christi Regional Medical Center VIA CHRISTI REGIONAL MEDICAL CENTER–ST. JOSEPH CAMPUS See Via Christi Regional Medical Center	21	10	1098	—	—	—	—	—	—	—
□ VIA CHRISTI REHABILITATION CENTER, 1151 North Rock Road, Zip 67206–1262; tel. 316/634–3400; Laurie Labarca, Chief Operating Officer (Total facility includes 19 beds in nursing home–type unit) **A**1 10 **F**1 2 3 4 6 7 8 9 10 11 12 13 14 15 16 17 18 19 20 21 22 23 24 25 26 27 28 29 30 31 32 33 34 35 37 38 39 40 41 42 43 44 45 46 47 48 49 50 51 52 53 54 55 56 57 58 59 60 62 63 64 65 66 67 68 69 70 71 72 73 74	21	46	42	441	19	5104	0	8997	4731	150
□ △ WESLEY REHABILITATION HOSPITAL, 8338 West 13th Street North, Zip 67212–2984; tel. 316/729–9999; Joseph F. Pitingolo, Jr., Chief Executive Officer (Total facility includes 15 beds in nursing home–type unit) **A**1 7 9 10 **F**12 14 16 19 21 22 25 27 34 35 45 46 48 49 50 60 63 64 71 73 **P**1 5 **S** Continental Medical Systems, Inc., Mechanicsburg, PA	33	46	65	761	42	15806	0	—	—	149
WINCHESTER—Jefferson County										
JEFFERSON COUNTY MEMORIAL HOSPITAL, 408 Delaware Street, Zip 66097, Mailing Address: Rural Route 1, Box 1, Zip 66097; tel. 913/774–4340; Steven F. Ashcraft, Administrator (Total facility includes 85 beds in nursing home–type unit) **A**9 10 **F**7 8 15 16 19 21 22 26 27 30 33 34 35 36 39 40 44 49 64 65 71 73 **N** Community Health Alliance, Winchester, KS	23	10	113	128	68	5743	9	—	—	98
WINFIELD—Cowley County										
✦ WILLIAM NEWTON MEMORIAL HOSPITAL, 1300 East Fifth Street, Zip 67156–2495; tel. 316/221–2300; Richard H. Vaught, Administrator (Total facility includes 14 beds in nursing home–type unit) **A**1 9 10 **F**7 8 13 16 17 19 21 22 27 28 30 32 36 37 39 40 41 42 44 45 46 49 52 58 64 65 66 67 71 73	14	10	57	1483	16	40571	266	12494	7033	283
WINFIELD STATE HOSPITAL AND TRAINING CENTER, 1320 North McCabe, Zip 67156–9701; tel. 316/221–1200; William P. Brooks, Superintendent **F**6 20 46 48 65 73	12	62	222	0	242	0	0	26500	—	600

KENTUCKY

Resident population 3,860 (in thousands)
Resident population in metro areas 48.3%
Birth rate per 1,000 population 14.0
65 years and over 12.6%
Percent of persons without health insurance 15.2%

Hospital, Address, Telephone, Administrator, Approval, Facility, and Physician Codes, Health Care System, Network	Classi-fication Codes		Utilization Data					Expense (thousands) of dollars		
★ American Hospital Association (AHA) membership □ Joint Commission on Accreditation of Healthcare Organizations (JCAHO) accreditation + American Osteopathic Hospital Association (AOHA) membership ○ American Osteopathic Association (AOA) accreditation △ Commission on Accreditation of Rehabilitation Facilities (CARF) accreditation Control codes 61, 63, 64, 71, 72 and 73 indicate hospitals listed by AOHA, but not registered by AHA. For definition of numerical codes, see page A4	Control	Service	Beds	Admissions	Census	Outpatient Visits	Births	Total	Payroll	Personnel

ALBANY—Clinton County

CLINTON COUNTY HOSPITAL, 723 Burkesville Road, Zip 42602; tel. 606/387–6421; Randel Flowers, Ph.D., Administrator **A**9 10 **F**11 19 22 71 **N** Center Care, Bowling Green, KY	23	10	42	2221	26	11872	0	5789	2885	133

ASHLAND—Boyd County

✠ △ KING'S DAUGHTERS' MEDICAL CENTER, 2201 Lexington Avenue, Zip 41101, Mailing Address: P.O. Box 151, Zip 41105–0151; tel. 606/327–4000; Fred L. Jackson, Chief Executive Officer (Total facility includes 10 beds in nursing home–type unit) **A**1 2 7 9 10 **F**4 7 8 10 12 15 16 17 19 21 22 25 27 28 30 31 32 33 34 35 36 37 38 39 40 41 42 43 44 45 46 48 49 52 53 54 55 56 57 58 60 63 64 65 66 67 71 72 73 74 **P**8	23	10	340	15546	241	119186	1056	119632	46591	1350
✠ OUR LADY OF BELLEFONTE HOSPITAL, St. Christopher Drive, Zip 41105–0789, Mailing Address: P.O. Box 789, Zip 41105–0789; tel. 606/833–3333; Robert J. Maher, President **A**1 9 10 **F**2 3 7 8 12 13 14 15 16 19 20 21 22 24 28 30 31 32 34 35 36 37 39 40 41 42 44 45 46 49 52 54 55 56 58 60 65 66 67 71 73 **P**1 **S** Franciscan Sisters of the Poor Health System, Inc., New York, NY **N** CHA Provider Network, Inc., Lexington, KY	21	10	194	7876	110	124431	59	60682	24598	846

BARBOURVILLE—Knox County

✠ KNOX COUNTY GENERAL HOSPITAL, 321 High Street, Zip 40906, Mailing Address: P.O. Box 160, Zip 40906; tel. 606/546–4175; Craig Morgan, Administrator (Total facility includes 16 beds in nursing home–type unit) **A**1 9 10 **F**7 19 21 22 37 40 44 64 65 71 73 **N** CHA Provider Network, Inc., Lexington, KY; Blue Grass Family Health Plan, Lexington, KY	13	10	58	1954	32	26058	188	7281	4015	194

BARDSTOWN—Nelson County

✠ FLAGET MEMORIAL HOSPITAL, 201 Cathedral Manor, Zip 40004–1299; tel. 502/348–3923; Suzanne Reasbeck, President and Chief Executive Officer (Nonreporting) **A**1 9 10 **S** Sisters of Charity of Nazareth Health System, Nazareth, KY **N** Community Health Delivery System, Inc., Louisville, KY	21	10	36	—	—	—	—	—	—	—

BENTON—Marshall County

✠ MARSHALL COUNTY HOSPITAL, 503 George McClain Drive, Zip 42025, Mailing Address: P.O. Box 630, Zip 42025; tel. 502/527–4800; David G. Fuqua, R.N., Chief Executive Officer (Total facility includes 34 beds in nursing home–type unit) **A**1 9 10 **F**1 8 14 15 19 21 22 26 35 37 44 49 64 65 67 71 **P**3 **S** Quorum Health Group/Quorum Health Resources, Inc., Brentwood, TN	16	10	80	782	47	13444	0	7776	3263	165

BEREA—Madison County

✠ BEREA HOSPITAL, 305 Estill Street, Zip 40403; tel. 606/986–3151; David E. Burgio, FACHE, Administrator and Chief Executive Officer (Total facility includes 62 beds in nursing home–type unit) **A**1 5 9 10 **F**8 12 14 15 16 17 19 20 21 22 26 27 28 30 31 34 37 39 41 44 46 49 64 65 67 71 73 74 **N** CHA Provider Network, Inc., Lexington, KY; Blue Grass Family Health Plan, Lexington, KY	23	10	110	1886	82	38465	0	17094	6827	301

BOWLING GREEN—Warren County

✠ COLUMBIA GREENVIEW HOSPITAL, 1801 Ashley Circle, Zip 42104, Mailing Address: Box 90024, Zip 42102–9024; tel. 502/793–1000; Harry Alvis, Chief Executive Officer **A**1 9 10 **F**4 7 8 10 11 12 14 15 16 17 19 21 22 23 28 29 30 32 33 34 35 37 40 41 42 44 45 46 65 67 71 73 74 **P**5 7 **S** Columbia/HCA Healthcare Corporation, Nashville, TN	33	10	211	6167	87	131952	951	—	—	572
□ MEDIPLEX REHABILITATION HOSPITAL, 1300 Campbell Lane, Zip 42104; tel. 502/782–6900; Jeffrey L. Durham, Chief Executive Officer (Total facility includes 10 beds in nursing home–type unit) **A**1 10 **F**12 14 17 20 25 34 39 41 48 49 57 58 64 65 67 73 **P**5	33	46	55	839	52	10545	0	15752	4293	171
✠ THE MEDICAL CENTER AT BOWLING GREEN, 250 Park Street, Zip 42101, Mailing Address: Box 90010, Zip 42102–9010; tel. 502/745–1000; Laurence C. Hinsdale, Chief Executive Officer **A**1 9 10 **F**2 3 4 7 8 10 11 12 17 18 19 21 22 25 26 27 28 30 31 32 34 35 37 38 40 41 42 43 44 45 46 49 52 54 55 56 57 60 64 65 67 69 71 72 73 74 **P**8 **N** Center Care, Bowling Green, KY	23	10	298	9621	134	32434	872	—	—	1187

BURKESVILLE—Cumberland County

★ CUMBERLAND COUNTY HOSPITAL, Highway 90 West, Zip 42717–0280, Mailing Address: P.O. Box 280, Zip 42717–0280; tel. 502/864–2511; Mark Thompson, Chief Executive Officer **A**9 10 **F**7 8 12 15 19 22 27 34 44 46 49 65 71 **S** Quorum Health Group/Quorum Health Resources, Inc., Brentwood, TN **N** Center Care, Bowling Green, KY	23	10	31	1655	19	15607	20	5198	2202	106

CADIZ—Trigg County

★ TRIGG COUNTY HOSPITAL, Highway 68 East, Zip 42211, Mailing Address: Box 312, Zip 42211; tel. 502/522–3215; Richard Chapman, Administrator **A**9 10 **F**15 16 19 44 49 51 65 71 73 **N** Community Health Delivery System, Inc., Louisville, KY	33	10	30	435	5	8255	0	3620	—	—

CALHOUN—McLean County

MCLEAN COUNTY GENERAL HOSPITAL, 200 Highway 81 North, Zip 42327; tel. 502/273–5252; Mynette Dennis, R.N., Administrator (Nonreporting) **A**9 10	13	10	26	—	—	—	—	—	—	—

Hospital, Address, Telephone, Administrator, Approval, Facility, and Physician Codes, Health Care System, Network	Classification Codes		Utilization Data					Expense (thousands) of dollars		
	Control	Service	Beds	Admissions	Census	Outpatient Visits	Births	Total	Payroll	Personnel

★ American Hospital Association (AHA) membership
□ Joint Commission on Accreditation of Healthcare Organizations (JCAHO) accreditation
+ American Osteopathic Hospital Association (AOHA) membership
○ American Osteopathic Association (AOA) accreditation
△ Commission on Accreditation of Rehabilitation Facilities (CARF) accreditation
Control codes 61, 63, 64, 71, 72 and 73 indicate hospitals listed by AOHA, but not registered by AHA. For definition of numerical codes, see page A4

CAMPBELLSVILLE—Taylor County

⊞ TAYLOR COUNTY HOSPITAL, 1700 Old Lebanon Road, Zip 42718; tel. 502/465–3561; David R. Hayes, President **A**1 2 9 10 **F**7 8 10 14 15 19 21 22 23 24 27 28 29 30 32 33 35 37 39 40 42 44 45 46 49 50 60 63 70 71 73 **S** Jewish Hospital Healthcare Services, Louisville, KY **N** Jewish Hospital Healthcare Services, Louisville, KY

| 16 | 10 | 80 | 3461 | 43 | 41195 | 347 | 25075 | 9217 | 405 |

CARLISLE—Nicholas County

⊞ NICHOLAS COUNTY HOSPITAL, (Includes Johnson–Mathers Nursing Home), 2323 Concrete Road, Zip 40311, Mailing Address: Box 232, Zip 40311; tel. 606/289–7181; James J. Wente, Administrator (Total facility includes 55 beds in nursing home–type unit) **A**1 9 10 **F**8 13 14 15 16 19 22 26 28 32 33 34 36 39 41 44 49 64 65 67 71 73 **P**5 **N** CHA Provider Network, Inc., Lexington, KY

| 23 | 10 | 83 | 716 | 67 | 38995 | 0 | 5773 | 3202 | 124 |

CARROLLTON—Carroll County

★ CARROLL COUNTY MEMORIAL HOSPITAL, 309 11th Street, Zip 41008; tel. 502/732–4321; Roger Williams, Chief Executive Officer (Nonreporting) **A**9 10 **S** Alliant Health System, Louisville, KY **N** Community Health Delivery System, Inc., Louisville, KY

| 13 | 10 | 39 | — | — | — | — | — | — | — |

COLUMBIA—Adair County

□ WESTLAKE REGIONAL HOSPITAL, (Formerly Westlake Cumberland Hospital), Westlake Drive, Zip 42728, Mailing Address: P.O. Box 468, Zip 42728–0468; tel. 502/384–4753; Rex A. Tungate, Administrator (Nonreporting) **A**1 9 10 **N** Center Care, Bowling Green, KY

| 16 | 10 | 80 | | | | | | | |

CORBIN—Whitley County

⊞ BAPTIST REGIONAL MEDICAL CENTER, 1 Trillium Way, Zip 40701–8420; tel. 606/528–1212; John S. Henson, President **A**1 9 10 **F**2 3 7 8 10 12 16 17 18 19 21 22 24 28 30 34 35 40 41 42 44 45 46 48 49 52 53 54 55 56 58 59 65 67 71 72 73 74 **P**7 8 **S** Baptist Healthcare System, Louisville, KY **N** Blue Grass Family Health Plan, Lexington, KY; Community Health Delivery System, Inc., Louisville, KY; Center Care, Bowling Green, KY; Baptist Healthcare System, Louisville, KY

| 23 | 10 | 255 | 9132 | 129 | 80178 | 886 | 50955 | 20105 | 807 |

COVINGTON—Kenton County

□ CHILDREN'S PSYCHIATRIC HOSPITAL OF NORTHERN KENTUCKY, 502 Farrell Drive, Zip 41011, Mailing Address: Box 2680, Zip 41012–2680; tel. 606/578–3200; Gary Goetz, Director **A**1 9 10 **F**14 15 16 52 53 54 56 58

| 23 | 52 | 26 | 319 | 18 | 351 | 0 | 3068 | 1316 | 64 |

⊞ ST. ELIZABETH MEDICAL CENTER–NORTH, (Includes St. Elizabeth Medical Center–South, 1 Medical Village Drive, Edgewood, Zip 41017; tel. 606/344–2000), 401 East 20th Street, Zip 41014; tel. 606/292–4000; Joseph W. Gross, President and Chief Executive Officer (Total facility includes 66 beds in nursing home–type unit) **A**1 2 3 5 9 10 **F**3 4 7 8 10 14 15 16 17 19 21 22 28 29 30 31 32 33 34 35 41 42 43 44 49 55 56 58 59 60 65 66 67 71 73 74 **P**1 5 6 **N** Community Health Delivery System, Inc., Louisville, KY; Center Care, Bowling Green, KY; Saint Elizabeth Medical Center, Covington, KY

| 21 | 10 | 466 | 23520 | 300 | 306186 | 2760 | 177228 | 85159 | 2566 |

CYNTHIANA—Harrison County

⊞ HARRISON MEMORIAL HOSPITAL, Mailing Address: P.O. Box 250, Zip 41031–0250; tel. 606/234–2300; Darwin E. Root, Administrator (Total facility includes 34 beds in nursing home–type unit) **A**1 9 10 **F**7 8 19 21 22 24 26 32 33 34 37 39 40 42 44 49 64 65 71 73 **P**5 **N** CHA Provider Network, Inc., Lexington, KY; Blue Grass Family Health Plan, Lexington, KY

| 23 | 10 | 99 | 1867 | 58 | 27744 | 142 | 12176 | 5443 | 235 |

DANVILLE—Boyle County

⊞ EPHRAIM MCDOWELL REGIONAL MEDICAL CENTER, 217 South Third Street, Zip 40422–9983; tel. 606/239–1000; Thomas W. Smith, President and Chief Executive Officer (Total facility includes 25 beds in nursing home–type unit) **A**1 5 9 10 **F**3 7 8 10 12 14 16 17 19 20 22 24 25 26 28 29 30 33 34 36 37 38 39 40 41 42 44 45 46 49 52 55 56 57 60 64 65 66 67 71 73 74 **P**8

| 23 | 10 | 177 | 6050 | 109 | 66429 | 960 | 42795 | 18816 | 689 |

EDGEWOOD—Kenton County

□ △ HEALTHSOUTH NORTHERN KENTUCKY REHABILITATION HOSPITAL, 201 Medical Village Drive, Zip 41017; tel. 606/341–2044; Ronald L. Bierman, Chief Executive Officer (Nonreporting) **A**1 7 9 10 **S** HEALTHSOUTH Corporation, Birmingham, AL

| 33 | 46 | 40 | — | — | — | — | — | — | — |

ST. ELIZABETH MEDICAL CENTER–SOUTH See St. Elizabeth Medical Center–North, Covington

ELIZABETHTOWN—Hardin County

⊞ HARDIN MEMORIAL HOSPITAL, 913 North Dixie Highway, Zip 42701–2599; tel. 502/737–1212; Gary R. Colberg, President and Chief Executive Officer **A**1 9 10 **F**5 7 8 10 11 12 14 15 17 19 21 22 27 28 34 35 37 40 42 44 46 48 49 52 56 60 63 65 71 72 73 74 **P**3 **S** Jewish Hospital Healthcare Services, Louisville, KY **N** Jewish Hospital Healthcare Services, Louisville, KY

| 13 | 10 | 276 | 11442 | 175 | 119850 | 1189 | 79725 | 34697 | 1094 |

□ △ LAKEVIEW REHABILITATION HOSPITAL, 134 Heartland Drive, Zip 42701; tel. 502/769–3100; James H. Wesp, Administrator **A**1 7 9 10 **F**15 48 49 **N** Center Care, Bowling Green, KY

| 32 | 46 | 40 | 560 | 29 | 11793 | 0 | 8357 | 4208 | 110 |

FLEMINGSBURG—Fleming County

⊞ FLEMING COUNTY HOSPITAL, 920 Elizaville Avenue, Zip 41041, Mailing Address: Box 388, Zip 41041–0388; tel. 606/849–5000; Bobby B. Emmons, Administrator (Nonreporting) **A**1 9 10 **S** Quorum Health Group/Quorum Health Resources, Inc., Brentwood, TN

| 13 | 10 | 52 | — | — | — | — | — | — | — |

Hospital, Address, Telephone, Administrator, Approval, Facility, and Physician Codes, Health Care System, Network	Classi-fication Codes		Utilization Data					Expense (thousands) of dollars		
	Control	Service	Beds	Admissions	Census	Outpatient Visits	Births	Total	Payroll	Personnel

★ American Hospital Association (AHA) membership
□ Joint Commission on Accreditation of Healthcare Organizations (JCAHO) accreditation
+ American Osteopathic Hospital Association (AOHA) membership
○ American Osteopathic Association (AOA) accreditation
△ Commission on Accreditation of Rehabilitation Facilities (CARF) accreditation
Control codes 61, 63, 64, 71, 72 and 73 indicate hospitals listed by AOHA, but not registered by AHA. For definition of numerical codes, see page A4

FLORENCE—Boone County

★ ST. LUKE HOSPITAL WEST, 7380 Turfway Road, Zip 41042; tel. 606/525–5200; John D. Hoyle, Senior Executive Officer (Total facility includes 16 beds in nursing home–type unit) **A**9 10 **F**1 2 3 4 7 8 9 10 11 12 13 14 15 16 17 18 19 20 21 22 24 25 26 27 28 29 30 31 32 33 34 35 36 37 38 39 40 41 42 43 44 45 46 47 48 49 50 51 52 53 54 55 56 57 58 59 60 61 63 64 65 66 67 69 70 71 72 73 74 **P**1 2 6 7 **S** Health Alliance of Greater Cincinnati, Cincinnati, OH **N** The Healthcare Alliance of Greater Cincinnati, Cincinnati, OH; CHA Provider Network, Inc., Lexington, KY	23	10	152	6802	81	126200	747	35921	16307	568

FORT CAMPBELL—Christian County

⊞ COLONEL FLORENCE A. BLANCHFIELD ARMY COMMUNITY HOSPITAL, 650 Joel Drive, Zip 42223–5349; tel. 502/798–8040; Colonel Lester Martinez–Lopez, Director Health Services **A**1 2 **F**3 8 12 13 18 19 20 22 25 29 30 34 35 37 39 40 41 42 44 46 49 51 52 53 54 56 58 65 71 74 **P**6 **S** Department of the Army, Office of the Surgeon General, Falls Church, VA	42	10	107	10489	54	676921	1935	—	—	1150

FORT KNOX—Hardin County

⊞ IRELAND ARMY COMMUNITY HOSPITAL, 851 Ireland Loop, Zip 40121–5520; tel. 502/624–9020; Lieutenant Colonel Robert T. Foster, Deputy Commander for Administrtaion **A**1 5 **F**3 7 8 12 13 17 18 19 20 21 22 25 27 30 34 37 39 40 44 46 49 51 53 54 55 56 58 63 65 66 71 73 74 **P**1 **S** Department of the Army, Office of the Surgeon General, Falls Church, VA	42	10	76	4954	25	365024	587	39940	13026	1002

FORT THOMAS—Campbell County

⊞ ST. LUKE HOSPITAL EAST, 85 North Grand Avenue, Zip 41075–1796; tel. 606/572–3100; Daniel M. Vinson, CPA, Senior Executive Officer (Total facility includes 26 beds in nursing home–type unit) **A**1 2 10 **F**1 2 3 4 7 8 9 10 11 12 13 14 15 16 17 18 19 20 21 22 24 25 26 27 28 29 30 31 32 33 34 35 36 37 38 39 40 41 42 43 44 45 46 47 48 49 50 51 52 53 54 55 56 57 58 59 60 61 63 64 65 66 67 69 70 71 72 73 74 **P**1 2 6 7 **S** Health Alliance of Greater Cincinnati, Cincinnati, OH **N** The Healthcare Alliance of Greater Cincinnati, Cincinnati, OH; CHA Provider Network, Inc., Lexington, KY	23	10	221	8897	121	143691	852	55309	22040	793

FRANKFORT—Franklin County

⊞ COLUMBIA HOSPITAL FRANKFORT, 299 King's Daughters Drive, Zip 40601–4186; tel. 502/875–5240; David P. Steitz, Chief Executive Officer **A**1 9 10 **F**2 3 7 8 10 11 12 14 15 16 19 20 21 22 28 29 32 33 34 35 37 39 40 42 44 46 49 51 52 54 60 63 65 67 71 73 **P**7 **S** Columbia/HCA Healthcare Corporation, Nashville, TN **N** Blue Grass Family Health Plan, Lexington, KY	33	10	147	4541	59	50057	558	28829	11176	466

FRANKLIN—Simpson County

★ FRANKLIN–SIMPSON MEMORIAL HOSPITAL, Brookhaven Road, Zip 42135–2929, Mailing Address: P.O. Box 2929, Zip 42135–2929; tel. 502/586–3253; William P. Macri, Administrator (Total facility includes 6 beds in nursing home–type unit) **A**9 10 **F**8 14 15 16 19 22 28 37 44 46 51 64 71 73 **P**8 **S** Quorum Health Group/Quorum Health Resources, Inc., Brentwood, TN **N** Community Care Network, Henderson, KY; Center Care, Bowling Green, KY	13	10	36	853	11	10484	0	5541	2355	97

FULTON—Fulton County

□ PARKWAY REGIONAL HOSPITAL, 2000 Holiday Lane, Zip 42041; tel. 502/472–2522; Mary Jo Lewis, Chief Executive Officer (Nonreporting) **A**1 9 10 **S** Community Health Systems, Inc., Brentwood, TN	33	10	70	—	—	—	—	—	—	—

GEORGETOWN—Scott County

⊞ COLUMBIA HOSPITAL GEORGETOWN, 1140 Lexington Road, Zip 40324; tel. 502/868–1100; Britt T. Reynolds, Chief Executive Officer (Total facility includes 10 beds in nursing home–type unit) (Nonreporting) **A**1 9 10 **S** Columbia/HCA Healthcare Corporation, Nashville, TN **N** Blue Grass Family Health Plan, Lexington, KY	33	10	61	—	—	—	—	—	—	—

GLASGOW—Barren County

⊞ T. J. SAMSON COMMUNITY HOSPITAL, 1301 North Race Street, Zip 42141–3483; tel. 502/651–4444; H. Glenn Joiner, Chief Executive Officer (Total facility includes 16 beds in nursing home–type unit) **A**1 9 10 **F**4 7 8 10 12 14 15 17 19 21 22 28 30 31 32 33 34 37 38 39 40 41 42 44 45 46 49 51 64 65 67 71 73 **N** Center Care, Bowling Green, KY	23	10	196	7360	103	60912	966	41770	18780	799

GREENSBURG—Green County

★ JANE TODD CRAWFORD MEMORIAL HOSPITAL, 202–206 Milby Street, Zip 42743, Mailing Address: P.O. Box 220, Zip 42743; tel. 502/932–4211; Larry Craig, Chief Executive Officer (Total facility includes 12 beds in nursing home–type unit) **A**9 10 **F**2 8 15 16 19 22 25 28 37 42 44 46 52 53 55 56 57 64 67 71 **N** Community Health Delivery System, Inc., Louisville, KY	13	10	64	1411	36	17608	0	6371	2820	125

GREENVILLE—Muhlenberg County

⊞ MUHLENBERG COMMUNITY HOSPITAL, 440 Hopkinsville Street, Zip 42345, Mailing Address: P.O. Box 387, Zip 42345; tel. 502/338–8000; Charles D. Lovell, Jr., Chief Executive Officer (Total facility includes 45 beds in nursing home–type unit) (Nonreporting) **A**1 9 10 **S** Quorum Health Group/Quorum Health Resources, Inc., Brentwood, TN **N** Community Care Network, Henderson, KY; Center Care, Bowling Green, KY	23	10	135	—	—	—	—	—	—	—

HARDINSBURG—Breckinridge County

★ BRECKINRIDGE MEMORIAL HOSPITAL, 1011 Old Highway 60, Zip 40143–2597; tel. 502/756–7000; George Walz, CHE, Chief Executive Officer (Total facility includes 18 beds in nursing home–type unit) **A**9 10 **F**8 14 19 22 32 33 34 42 44 46 64 71 73 **P**5 **S** Alliant Health System, Louisville, KY **N** Community Health Delivery System, Inc., Louisville, KY	23	10	45	1052	26	38720	0	6207	2775	152

Hospital, Address, Telephone, Administrator, Approval, Facility, and Physician Codes, Health Care System, Network	Classi-fication Codes		Utilization Data					Expense (thousands) of dollars		
★ American Hospital Association (AHA) membership □ Joint Commission on Accreditation of Healthcare Organizations (JCAHO) accreditation + American Osteopathic Hospital Association (AOHA) membership ○ American Osteopathic Association (AOA) accreditation △ Commission on Accreditation of Rehabilitation Facilities (CARF) accreditation Control codes 61, 63, 64, 71, 72 and 73 indicate hospitals listed by AOHA, but not registered by AHA. For definition of numerical codes, see page A4	Control	Service	Beds	Admissions	Census	Outpatient Visits	Births	Total	Payroll	Personnel

HARLAN—Harlan County

□ HARLAN ARH HOSPITAL, 81 Ball Park Road, Zip 40831–1792; tel. 606/573–8100; Daniel Fitzpatrick, Administrator (Nonreporting) **A**1 9 10 **S** Appalachian Regional Healthcare, Lexington, KY **N** CHA Provider Network, Inc., Lexington, KY
| | 23 | 10 | 125 | — | — | — | — | — | — | |

HARRODSBURG—Mercer County

★ THE JAMES B. HAGGIN MEMORIAL HOSPITAL, 464 Linden Avenue, Zip 40330–1862; tel. 606/734–5441; Earl James Motzer, Ph.D., FACHE, Chief Executive Officer (Total facility includes 25 beds in nursing home–type unit) **A**9 10 **F**8 11 14 15 16 17 19 22 28 29 30 33 34 37 39 42 44 49 53 64 65 67 68 71 **P**5 **S** Alliant Health System, Louisville, KY **N** CHA Provider Network, Inc., Lexington, KY; Blue Grass Family Health Plan, Lexington, KY; Center Care, Bowling Green, KY
| | 23 | 10 | 59 | 906 | 40 | 22500 | 0 | 7058 | 3194 | 132 |

HARTFORD—Ohio County

⊞ OHIO COUNTY HOSPITAL, 1211 Main Street, Zip 42347; tel. 502/298–7411; Blaine Pieper, Administrator (Nonreporting) **A**1 9 10 **S** Quorum Health Group/Quorum Health Resources, Inc., Brentwood, TN **N** Center Care, Bowling Green, KY
| | 23 | 10 | 54 | — | — | — | — | — | — | |

HAZARD—Perry County

□ ARH REGIONAL MEDICAL CENTER, 100 Medical Center Drive, Zip 41701–1000; tel. 606/439–6610; David R. Lyon, Administrator **A**1 3 5 9 10 **F**7 8 10 16 19 21 22 28 32 33 34 35 37 40 41 42 44 49 51 52 53 54 55 57 60 65 67 71 72 73 **P**5 8 **S** Appalachian Regional Healthcare, Lexington, KY **N** CHA Provider Network, Inc., Lexington, KY
| | 23 | 10 | 288 | 7844 | 118 | 198341 | 482 | 47558 | 18714 | 736 |

HENDERSON—Henderson County

⊞ COMMUNITY METHODIST HOSPITAL, 1305 North Elm Street, Zip 42420, Mailing Address: Box 48, Zip 42420–0048; tel. 502/827–7700; Bruce D. Begley, Executive Director (Nonreporting) **A**1 9 10 **N** Community Care Network, Henderson, KY
| | 21 | 10 | 213 | — | — | — | — | — | — | |

HOPKINSVILLE—Christian County

□ CUMBERLAND HALL HOSPITAL, 210 West 17th Street, Zip 42240; tel. 502/886–1919; William C. Heard, Administrator and Chief Executive Officer (Nonreporting) **A**1 10
| | 33 | 52 | 50 | — | — | — | — | — | — | |

⊞ JENNIE STUART MEDICAL CENTER, 320 West 18th Street, Zip 42240–6315; tel. 502/887–0100; Lewis T. Peeples, Chief Executive Officer **A**1 9 10 **F**7 8 11 12 14 15 19 21 22 23 28 30 32 35 37 40 42 44 45 46 49 60 65 67 71 73 **P**5 7 **S** Quorum Health Group/Quorum Health Resources, Inc., Brentwood, TN **N** Community Care Network, Henderson, KY
| | 23 | 10 | 139 | 5604 | 68 | 53442 | 619 | 42276 | 15604 | 641 |

□ WESTERN STATE HOSPITAL, Russellville Road, Zip 42241, Mailing Address: Box 2200, Zip 42241; tel. 502/886–4431; Wayne Taylor, Director (Total facility includes 144 beds in nursing home–type unit) **A**1 9 10 **F**20 27 39 41 45 46 52 55 56 57 65 67 73 **P**6
| | 12 | 22 | 355 | 1171 | 215 | 0 | 0 | — | — | 453 |

HORSE CAVE—Hart County

★ CAVERNA MEMORIAL HOSPITAL, 1501 South Dixie Street, Zip 42749; tel. 502/786–2191; James J. Kerins, Sr., Administrator **A**9 10 **F**8 14 15 16 19 22 28 30 34 37 44 64 71 **S** Alliant Health System, Louisville, KY **N** Community Health Delivery System, Inc., Louisville, KY; Center Care, Bowling Green, KY
| | 23 | 10 | 28 | 822 | 8 | 12826 | 84 | 3057 | 1489 | 75 |

HYDEN—Leslie County

MARY BRECKINRIDGE HOSPITAL, Hospital Drive, Zip 41749–0000; tel. 606/672–2901; A. Ray Branaman, Administrator **A**9 10 **F**19 22 32 40 49 51 65 71 **N** CHA Provider Network, Inc., Lexington, KY
| | 23 | 10 | 40 | 1497 | 16 | 40580 | 174 | 11861 | 6887 | 305 |

IRVINE—Estill County

★ MARCUM AND WALLACE MEMORIAL HOSPITAL, 60 Mercy Court, Zip 40336, Mailing Address: P.O. Box 928, Zip 40336; tel. 606/723–2115; Christopher M. Goddard, Administrator **A**9 10 **F**8 15 16 17 19 22 28 34 44 49 71 **P**1 2 4 5 6 7 8 **S** Mercy Health System, Cincinnati, OH **N** CHA Provider Network, Inc., Lexington, KY; Blue Grass Family Health Plan, Lexington, KY
| | 21 | 10 | 16 | 493 | 8 | 34959 | 0 | 3665 | 1679 | 98 |

JACKSON—Madison County

KENTUCKY RIVER MEDICAL CENTER, 540 Jett Drive, Zip 41339–9620; tel. 606/666–4971; O. David Bevins, Chief Executive Officer (Nonreporting) **A**3 9 10 **S** Community Health Systems, Inc., Brentwood, TN
| | 33 | 10 | 55 | — | — | — | — | — | — | |

JENKINS—Letcher County

□ JENKINS COMMUNITY HOSPITAL, Main Street, Zip 41537, Mailing Address: P.O. Box 472, Zip 41537; te!. 606/832–2171; Sherrie Newcomb, Acting Administrator (Nonreporting) **A**1 9 10 **S** First Health, Inc., Batesville, MS **N** CHA Provider Network, Inc., Lexington, KY
| | 33 | 10 | 60 | — | — | — | — | — | — | |

LA GRANGE—Oldham County

⊞ TRI COUNTY BAPTIST HOSPITAL, 1025 New Moody Lane, Zip 40031–0559; tel. 502/222–5388; David L. Gray, Administrator (Total facility includes 30 beds in nursing home–type unit) **A**1 9 10 **F**2 3 4 7 8 10 11 12 13 14 15 16 17 18 19 21 22 26 28 29 30 31 32 34 35 37 38 39 40 41 42 43 44 45 46 48 49 52 53 54 55 56 57 58 59 60 61 63 64 65 67 68 71 72 73 74 **S** Baptist Healthcare System, Louisville, KY **N** Community Health Delivery System, Inc., Louisville, KY; Baptist Healthcare System, Louisville, KY
| | 23 | 10 | 120 | 2500 | 55 | 38160 | 280 | 19350 | 7880 | 218 |

LANCASTER—Garrard County

★ GARRARD COUNTY MEMORIAL HOSPITAL, 308 West Maple Avenue, Zip 40444–1098; tel. 606/792–6844; W. David MacCool, Administrator **A**9 10 **F**8 19 22 35 41 44 49 64 65 71 **N** CHA Provider Network, Inc., Lexington, KY; Blue Grass Family Health Plan, Lexington, KY
| | 13 | 10 | 131 | 534 | 7 | 14119 | 0 | 7154 | 3144 | 102 |

Hospital, Address, Telephone, Administrator, Approval, Facility, and Physician Codes, Health Care System, Network	Classi-fication Codes		Utilization Data					Expense (thousands) of dollars		
★ American Hospital Association (AHA) membership □ Joint Commission on Accreditation of Healthcare Organizations (JCAHO) accreditation + American Osteopathic Hospital Association (AOHA) membership ○ American Osteopathic Association (AOA) accreditation △ Commission on Accreditation of Rehabilitation Facilities (CARF) accreditation Control codes 61, 63, 64, 71, 72 and 73 indicate hospitals listed by AOHA, but not registered by AHA. For definition of numerical codes, see page A4	Control	Service	Beds	Admissions	Census	Outpatient Visits	Births	Total	Payroll	Personnel

LEBANON—Marion County

☒ COLUMBIA SPRING VIEW HOSPITAL, 320 Loretto Road, Zip 40033–0320; tel. 502/692–3161; John D. Brock, Chief Executive Officer (Total facility includes 38 beds in nursing home–type unit) (Nonreporting) **A**1 9 10 **S** Columbia/HCA Healthcare Corporation, Nashville, TN
| | 33 | 10 | 113 | — | — | — | — | — | — | — |

LEITCHFIELD—Grayson County

★ TWIN LAKES REGIONAL MEDICAL CENTER, 910 Wallace Avenue, Zip 42754; tel. 502/259–9400; Stephen L. Meredith, Chief Executive Officer **A**9 10 **F**8 12 14 15 16 19 22 24 32 35 37 40 44 45 46 49 62 65 66 71 73 **P**3 6 **S** Alliant Health System, Louisville, KY **N** Community Health Delivery System, Inc., Louisville, KY; Center Care, Bowling Green, KY
| | 23 | 10 | 75 | 2162 | 29 | 36629 | 302 | 15687 | 6204 | 257 |

LEXINGTON—Fayette County

★ △ CARDINAL HILL REHABILITATION HOSPITAL, 2050 Versailles Road, Zip 40504–1499; tel. 606/254–5701; Kerry G. Gillihan, President and Chief Executive Officer **A**3 5 7 9 10 **F**5 12 14 15 16 17 20 22 25 27 28 30 34 39 41 45 46 48 49 54 64 65 66 67 70 72 73 **P**6 **N** CHA Provider Network, Inc., Lexington, KY
| | 23 | 46 | 90 | 1490 | 70 | 33327 | 0 | 21367 | 12564 | 442 |

☒ CENTRAL BAPTIST HOSPITAL, 1740 Nicholasville Road, Zip 40503; tel. 606/275–6100; William G. Sisson, President (Total facility includes 12 beds in nursing home–type unit) **A**1 2 3 5 9 10 **F**4 7 8 10 11 12 15 16 19 21 22 29 30 32 34 37 38 40 41 42 43 44 45 46 49 60 61 63 65 71 73 74 **P**6 7 **S** Baptist Healthcare System, Louisville, KY **N** Blue Grass Family Health Plan, Lexington, KY; Community Health Delivery System, Inc., Louisville, KY; Center Care, Bowling Green, KY; Baptist Healthcare System, Louisville, KY
| | 23 | 10 | 321 | 15965 | 227 | 110013 | 3121 | 147149 | 53847 | 1721 |

□ CHARTER RIDGE HOSPITAL, 3050 Rio Dosa Drive, Zip 40509–9990; tel. 606/269–2325; Ali A. Elhaj, Chief Executive Officer **A**1 3 5 9 10 **F**2 3 19 20 22 35 52 53 55 58 59 65 67 **S** Magellan Health Services, Atlanta, GA **N** CHA Provider Network, Inc., Lexington, KY
| | 33 | 22 | 110 | 1984 | 58 | 5941 | 0 | — | — | 98 |

☒ COLUMBIA HOSPITAL LEXINGTON, 310 South Limestone Street, Zip 40508–3008; tel. 606/252–6612; Barton A. Hove, Chief Executive Officer (Total facility includes 34 beds in nursing home–type unit) **A**1 2 9 10 **F**3 7 8 10 11 12 14 15 16 19 21 22 26 28 29 30 31 32 34 36 37 39 40 41 42 44 45 46 49 52 53 54 55 56 57 58 59 61 64 65 67 71 73 74 **P**7 8 **S** Columbia/HCA Healthcare Corporation, Nashville, TN
| | 33 | 10 | 219 | 6402 | 92 | 38119 | 235 | — | — | 669 |

□ EASTERN STATE HOSPITAL, 627 West Fourth Street, Zip 40508–9990; tel. 606/246–7000; Daniel J. Luchtefeld, Director **A**1 5 9 10 **F**15 16 20 26 52 55 56 57 65 73
| | 12 | 22 | 197 | 1708 | 137 | 0 | 0 | 26788 | 11903 | 390 |

□ FEDERAL MEDICAL CENTER, 3301 Leestown Road, Zip 40511; tel. 606/255–6812; A. F. Beeler, Warden (Nonreporting) **A**1
| | 33 | 22 | 56 | — | — | — | — | — | — | — |

☒ LEXINGTON HOSPITAL, 150 North Eagle Creek Drive, Zip 40509–1807; tel. 606/268–4800; Rebecca Lewis, President **A**1 5 9 10 **F**4 7 8 10 11 12 17 19 21 22 26 27 30 31 32 33 37 39 40 41 42 43 44 45 46 49 51 63 65 66 71 73 **S** Jewish Hospital Healthcare Services, Louisville, KY **N** Jewish Hospital Healthcare Services, Louisville, KY
| | 33 | 10 | 174 | 5271 | 72 | 33524 | 607 | 37937 | 15449 | 463 |

☒ SHRINERS HOSPITALS FOR CHILDREN–LEXINGTON UNIT, 1900 Richmond Road, Zip 40502; tel. 606/266–2101; Tony Lewgood, Administrator **A**1 3 5 **F**9 15 16 17 45 49 65 71 73 **P**6 **S** Shriners Hospitals for Children, Tampa, FL
| | 23 | 57 | 50 | 1034 | 19 | 12053 | 0 | — | — | 182 |

☒ ST. JOSEPH HOSPITAL, One St. Joseph Drive, Zip 40504; tel. 606/278–3436; Thomas J. Murray, President (Total facility includes 22 beds in nursing home–type unit) **A**1 2 3 5 9 10 **F**2 3 4 8 10 11 12 15 16 17 19 21 22 25 26 28 29 30 31 33 35 37 39 41 42 43 44 45 46 47 49 51 52 53 54 55 56 57 58 59 60 63 64 65 66 67 71 73 74 **P**6 **S** Sisters of Charity of Nazareth Health System, Nazareth, KY **N** Blue Grass Family Health Plan, Lexington, KY; Community Health Delivery System, Inc., Louisville, KY; Center Care, Bowling Green, KY
| | 21 | 10 | 324 | 13672 | 229 | 64007 | 0 | 121824 | 48630 | 1587 |

☒ UNIVERSITY OF KENTUCKY HOSPITAL, 800 Rose Street, Zip 40536–0084; tel. 606/323–5000; Frank Butler, Director **A**1 2 3 5 8 9 10 **F**4 7 8 9 10 11 12 15 16 17 18 19 20 21 22 24 25 26 29 30 31 32 34 35 37 38 39 40 41 42 43 44 45 46 47 49 51 52 53 54 55 56 57 58 59 60 61 65 66 67 69 70 71 73 74 **P**1 7 8 **N** CHA Provider Network, Inc., Lexington, KY
| | 12 | 10 | 421 | 19987 | 336 | 364175 | 2210 | 218025 | 84699 | 2814 |

☒ VETERANS AFFAIRS MEDICAL CENTER–LEXINGTON, 2250 Leestown Pike, Zip 40511–1093; tel. 606/233–4511; Helen K. Cornish, Director (Total facility includes 86 beds in nursing home–type unit) **A**1 2 3 5 8 9 **F**2 3 4 8 10 11 12 16 19 20 21 22 24 26 27 28 29 30 31 32 33 34 35 37 39 41 42 43 44 45 46 48 49 51 52 54 56 57 58 59 60 63 64 65 67 71 73 74 **P**6 **S** Department of Veterans Affairs, Washington, DC
| | 45 | 10 | 613 | 7273 | 526 | 144151 | 0 | 120514 | 70376 | 1765 |

LONDON—Laurel County

☒ MARYMOUNT MEDICAL CENTER, (Formerly Marymount Hospital), 310 East Ninth Street, Zip 40741–1299; tel. 606/878–6520; Lowell Jones, President (Total facility includes 24 beds in nursing home–type unit) (Nonreporting) **A**1 9 10 **S** Sisters of Charity of Nazareth Health System, Nazareth, KY **N** Blue Grass Family Health Plan, Lexington, KY; Community Health Delivery System, Inc., Louisville, KY
| | 21 | 10 | 95 | — | — | — | — | — | — | — |

LOUISA—Lawrence County

□ THREE RIVERS MEDICAL CENTER, Highway 644, Zip 41230, Mailing Address: Box 769, Zip 41230; tel. 606/638–9451; Greg Kiser, Chief Executive Officer **A**1 9 10 **F**11 13 15 16 19 22 23 26 28 29 35 37 40 44 45 46 52 55 56 57 58 59 63 65 71 73 **S** Community Health Systems, Inc., Brentwood, TN **N** CHA Provider Network, Inc., Lexington, KY
| | 33 | 10 | 90 | 2436 | 31 | 22992 | 67 | — | — | 177 |

Hospital, Address, Telephone, Administrator, Approval, Facility, and Physician Codes, Health Care System, Network	Classi-fication Codes		Utilization Data					Expense (thousands) of dollars		
	Control	Service	Beds	Admissions	Census	Outpatient Visits	Births	Total	Payroll	Personnel

★ American Hospital Association (AHA) membership
□ Joint Commission on Accreditation of Healthcare Organizations (JCAHO) accreditation
+ American Osteopathic Hospital Association (AOHA) membership
○ American Osteopathic Association (AOA) accreditation
△ Commission on Accreditation of Rehabilitation Facilities (CARF) accreditation
Control codes 61, 63, 64, 71, 72 and 73 indicate hospitals listed by AOHA, but not registered by AHA. For definition of numerical codes, see page A4

LOUISVILLE—Jefferson County

Hospital	Control	Service	Beds	Admissions	Census	Outpatient Visits	Births	Total	Payroll	Personnel
★ ALLIANT HOSPITALS, (Includes Alliant Medical Pavilion, 315 East Broadway, tel. 502/629–2000; Kosair Children's Hospital, 231 East Gray Street, Mailing Address: P.O. Box 35070, Zip 40232–5070; tel. 502/629–6000; Norton Hospital, 200 East Chestnut, Mailing Address: P.O. Box 35070, Zip 40232–5070; tel. 502/629–8000), 200 East Chestnut Street, Zip 40202, Mailing Address: Box 35070, Zip 40232–5070; tel. 502/629–8000; Shirley B. Powers, Senior Executive Officer (Total facility includes 17 beds in nursing home–type unit) **A**1 2 3 5 9 10 **F**3 4 5 7 8 9 10 11 12 13 14 15 16 17 19 20 21 22 23 24 26 28 29 30 31 32 33 34 35 37 38 40 41 42 43 44 45 46 47 49 52 53 54 55 56 57 58 59 60 61 64 65 67 69 70 71 72 73 74 **P**3 7 **S** Alliant Health System, Louisville, KY **N** Community Health Delivery System, Inc., Louisville, KY; Alliant Health System, Louisville, KY	23	10	709	28824	463	185938	5492	286222	122290	4190
★ △ BAPTIST HOSPITAL EAST, 4000 Kresge Way, Zip 40207–4676; tel. 502/897–8100; Susan Stout Tamme, President **A**1 2 7 9 10 **F**2 3 4 7 8 10 11 12 13 14 15 16 17 18 19 21 22 26 28 29 30 32 34 35 37 40 41 42 43 44 45 46 48 49 52 53 54 55 56 57 58 59 60 64 65 67 68 71 72 73 74 **S** Baptist Healthcare System, Louisville, KY **N** Community Health Delivery System, Inc., Louisville, KY; Center Care, Bowling Green, KY; Baptist Healthcare System, Louisville, KY	23	10	407	18759	295	129665	2881	139775	61274	1992
★ CARITAS MEDICAL CENTER, 1850 Bluegrass Avenue, Zip 40215–1199; tel. 502/361–6000; Peter J. Bernard, President and Chief Executive Officer (Total facility includes 33 beds in nursing home–type unit) **A**1 9 10 **F**2 3 5 6 8 10 11 12 14 15 16 17 19 21 22 24 26 27 28 32 34 35 36 37 39 41 42 44 45 46 49 50 51 52 53 54 55 56 57 58 59 60 63 64 65 66 67 68 71 73 **P**3 7 **S** Sisters of Charity of Nazareth Health System, Nazareth, KY **N** Community Health Delivery System, Inc., Louisville, KY; Baptist Healthcare System, Louisville, KY; Caritas Health Services, Louisville, KY	21	10	177	7628	112	86193	0	72238	30747	892
★ CARITAS PEACE CENTER, 2020 Newburg Road, Zip 40205; tel. 502/451–3330; Peter J. Bernard, President and Chief Executive Officer **A**1 9 10 **F**3 14 15 16 35 52 53 54 55 56 57 58 59 65 67 73 **S** Sisters of Charity of Nazareth Health System, Nazareth, KY **N** Community Health Delivery System, Inc., Louisville, KY; Baptist Healthcare System, Louisville, KY; Caritas Health Services, Louisville, KY	23	22	156	2036	101	39559	0	19530	8385	295
□ CENTRAL STATE HOSPITAL, 10510 LaGrange Road, Zip 40223–1228; tel. 502/245–4121; Paula Tamme, Chief Executive Officer (Nonreporting) **A**1 5 10	12	22	175	—	—	—	—	—	—	—
□ CHARTER LOUISVILLE BEHAVIORAL HEALTH SYSTEM, (Formerly Charter Hospital of Louisville), 1405 Browns Lane, Zip 40207; tel. 502/896–0495; Charles L. Webb, Jr., Administrator **A**1 9 10 **F**3 12 14 15 16 17 18 25 26 28 34 46 52 53 54 55 56 57 58 59 65 **S** Magellan Health Services, Atlanta, GA	33	22	66	1476	49	388	0	—	—	73
★ COLUMBIA AUDUBON HOSPITAL, One Audubon Plaza Drive, Zip 40217–1397, Mailing Address: Box 17550, Zip 40217–0550; tel. 502/636–7111; James E. Rogers, President and Chief Executive Officer (Nonreporting) **A**1 2 5 9 10 **S** Columbia/HCA Healthcare Corporation, Nashville, TN	33	10	480	—	—	—	—	—	—	—
★ COLUMBIA SOUTHWEST HOSPITAL, 9820 Third Street Road, Zip 40272–9984; tel. 502/933–8100; Cathryn A. Hibbs, Chief Executive Officer (Total facility includes 23 beds in nursing home–type unit) (Nonreporting) **A**1 10 **S** Columbia/HCA Healthcare Corporation, Nashville, TN	33	10	150	—	—	—	—	—	—	—
★ COLUMBIA SUBURBAN HOSPITAL, 4001 Dutchmans Lane, Zip 40207; tel. 502/893–1000; Tracy A. Rogers, President and Chief Executive Officer (Total facility includes 37 beds in nursing home–type unit) **A**1 9 10 **F**4 5 6 7 8 10 11 12 14 15 16 19 21 22 23 28 31 32 33 34 35 37 38 39 40 41 42 43 44 45 47 49 51 60 61 64 65 66 67 69 71 73 74 **P**6 **S** Columbia/HCA Healthcare Corporation, Nashville, TN	33	10	380	11587	161	72485	1918	67545	—	1217
★ △ FRAZIER REHABILITATION CENTER, 220 Abraham Flexner Way, Zip 40202–1887; tel. 502/582–7400; Jason Roeback, President **A**1 3 5 7 9 **F**1 3 4 7 8 10 12 15 16 17 18 19 20 22 23 25 26 27 28 29 30 31 32 34 35 37 39 40 41 42 43 44 45 46 48 49 51 53 54 55 56 57 58 59 60 63 64 65 67 69 70 71 73 74 **S** Jewish Hospital Healthcare Services, Louisville, KY **N** Jewish Hospital Healthcare Services, Louisville, KY	23	46	93	1557	84	100409	0	23278	11006	322
★ JEWISH HOSPITAL, 217 East Chestnut Street, Zip 40202–1886; tel. 502/587–4011; Douglas E. Shaw, President **A**1 2 5 8 9 10 **F**1 2 3 4 6 7 8 9 10 11 12 13 14 15 16 17 18 19 20 21 22 24 25 26 27 28 29 30 31 32 33 34 35 36 37 38 39 40 41 42 43 44 45 46 47 48 49 51 52 53 54 55 56 57 58 59 60 61 63 64 65 66 67 68 69 70 71 72 73 74 **S** Jewish Hospital Healthcare Services, Louisville, KY **N** National Cardiovascular Network, Atlanta, GA; Jewish Hospital Healthcare Services, Louisville, KY; Center Care, Bowling Green, KY	23	10	404	19057	340	102773	0	216584	68873	2103
KOSAIR CHILDREN'S HOSPITAL See Alliant Hospitals										
NORTON HOSPITAL See Alliant Hospitals										
□ TEN BROECK HOSPITAL, 8521 Old LaGrange Road, Zip 40242; tel. 502/426–6380; Pat Hammer, Chief Executive Officer **A**1 10 **F**1 2 3 14 15 16 19 21 22 26 27 34 35 48 52 53 54 55 56 57 58 59 65 67 68 71 **S** United Medical Corporation, Windermere, FL	33	22	94	1724	56	4516	0	8263	3713	167
★ UNIVERSITY OF LOUISVILLE HOSPITAL, 530 South Jackson Street, Zip 40202–3611; tel. 502/562–3000; James H. Taylor, President and Chief Executive Officer **A**1 2 3 5 8 9 10 **F**4 8 9 10 11 12 15 16 17 19 21 22 23 28 30 35 37 38 40 41 42 43 44 45 46 49 50 52 54 56 60 63 65 67 70 71 73 **P**4 **S** Jewish Hospital Healthcare Services, Louisville, KY	23	10	269	12019	215	109639	1741	132305	48053	1781

Hospital, Address, Telephone, Administrator, Approval, Facility, and Physician Codes, Health Care System, Network	Classi-fication Codes		Utilization Data					Expense (thousands) of dollars		
	Control	Service	Beds	Admissions	Census	Outpatient Visits	Births	Total	Payroll	Personnel

★ American Hospital Association (AHA) membership
□ Joint Commission on Accreditation of Healthcare Organizations (JCAHO) accreditation
+ American Osteopathic Hospital Association (AOHA) membership
○ American Osteopathic Association (AOA) accreditation
△ Commission on Accreditation of Rehabilitation Facilities (CARF) accreditation
Control codes 61, 63, 64, 71, 72 and 73 indicate hospitals listed by AOHA, but not registered by AHA. For definition of numerical codes, see page A4

Hospital	Control	Service	Beds	Admissions	Census	Outpatient Visits	Births	Total	Payroll	Personnel
⊠ VENCOR HOSPITAL–LOUISVILLE, 1313 St. Anthony Place, Zip 40204; tel. 502/627–1102; James H. Wesp, Administrator (Total facility includes 37 beds in nursing home–type unit) **A**1 9 10 **F**8 16 19 21 34 35 42 44 60 64 65 71 **S** Vencor, Incorporated, Louisville, KY	33	10	156	399	53	10374	0	21173	12436	496
⊠ VETERANS AFFAIRS MEDICAL CENTER–LOUISVILLE, 800 Zorn Avenue, Zip 40206–1499; tel. 502/895–3401; Larry J. Sander, FACHE, Director **A**1 2 3 5 8 9 **F**3 8 10 11 16 19 20 22 25 26 28 31 32 33 34 35 37 39 41 42 43 44 46 49 51 52 54 58 60 64 65 71 73 74 **S** Department of Veterans Affairs, Washington, DC	45	10	229	6873	158	170268	0	94336	49008	1235
MADISONVILLE—Hopkins County										
⊠ REGIONAL MEDICAL CENTER OF HOPKINS COUNTY, 900 Hospital Drive, Zip 42431–1694; tel. 502/825–5100; Bobby H. Dampier, Chief Executive Officer **A**1 2 3 5 9 10 **F**3 4 7 8 10 11 12 15 16 17 19 20 21 22 23 24 28 30 31 32 34 35 37 38 39 40 41 42 43 44 45 46 47 49 52 53 56 57 58 60 63 65 66 67 71 73 **P**1 4 5 **N** Community Care Network, Henderson, KY	23	10	410	10460	148	56652	729	75213	33587	1168
MANCHESTER—Clay County										
⊠ MEMORIAL HOSPITAL, 401 Memorial Drive, Zip 40962–9156; tel. 606/598–5104; T. Henry Scoggins, FACHE, President (Total facility includes 11 beds in nursing home–type unit) **A**1 9 10 **F**7 8 15 16 17 19 20 21 22 24 28 30 32 33 37 39 40 44 45 46 49 51 62 64 65 71 74 **S** Adventist Health System Sunbelt Health Care Corporation, Winter Park, FL **N** CHA Provider Network, Inc., Lexington, KY	21	10	55	2831	36	32143	325	17229	7834	323
MARION—Crittenden County										
⊠ CRITTENDEN COUNTY HOSPITAL, Highway 60 South, Zip 42064–0386, Mailing Address: Box 386, Zip 42064; tel. 502/965–5281; Rick Napper, Chief Executive Officer **A**1 9 10 **F**2 3 15 16 17 52 53 54 55 56 57 58 59 65 73 **S** Quorum Health Group/Quorum Health Resources, Inc., Brentwood, TN **N** Community Care Network, Henderson, KY	33	22	67	671	25	1532	0	5036	2526	92
MARTIN—Floyd County										
⊠ OUR LADY OF THE WAY HOSPITAL, 11022 Main Street, Zip 41649–0910; tel. 606/285–5181; Lowell Jones, Chief Executive Officer (Total facility includes 13 beds in nursing home–type unit) **A**1 9 10 **F**8 15 16 17 19 22 30 39 44 49 64 65 66 67 71 73 **S** Catholic Health Initiatives, Denver, CO **N** CHA Provider Network, Inc., Lexington, KY	21	10	39	1715	24	22278	0	8468	3376	120
MAYFIELD—Graves County										
⊠ + COLUMBIA PINELAKE REGIONAL HOSPITAL, 1099 Medical Center Circle, Zip 42066, Mailing Address: P.O. Box 1099, Zip 42066; tel. 502/251–4100; Don A. Horstkotte, Chief Executive Officer (Total facility includes 14 beds in nursing home–type unit) **A**1 9 10 **F**7 8 10 12 14 15 16 19 21 22 28 29 30 32 35 37 40 41 42 44 45 54 63 64 65 66 67 70 71 74 **P**1 2 3 4 5 6 7 8 **S** Columbia/HCA Healthcare Corporation, Nashville, TN **N** Center Care, Bowling Green, KY	33	10	106	3764	48	58733	470	20277	8414	391
MAYSVILLE—Mason County										
⊠ COLUMBIA HOSPITAL MAYSVILLE, 989 Medical Park Drive, Zip 41056; tel. 606/759–5311; J. Timothy Browne, Chief Executive Officer (Total facility includes 10 beds in nursing home–type unit) **A**1 9 10 **F**7 8 10 12 14 15 16 18 19 21 22 28 30 35 37 38 40 44 46 49 64 65 66 71 73 74 **P**8 **S** Columbia/HCA Healthcare Corporation, Nashville, TN **N** Blue Grass Family Health Plan, Lexington, KY; Center Care, Bowling Green, KY	33	10	90	3204	36	—	440	16629	6986	287
MCDOWELL—Floyd County										
□ MCDOWELL ARH HOSPITAL, Route 122, Zip 41647, Mailing Address: Box 247, Zip 41647; tel. 606/377–3400; Jerry Haynes, Administrator **A**1 9 10 **F**2 3 4 7 8 11 12 14 15 16 17 19 21 22 25 26 28 29 30 32 34 35 36 37 38 39 40 41 42 44 46 47 49 51 52 53 54 55 56 57 58 59 60 64 65 66 67 71 73 74 **P**5 8 **S** Appalachian Regional Healthcare, Lexington, KY **N** CHA Provider Network, Inc., Lexington, KY	23	10	74	1584	21	47503	0	9944	3957	148
MIDDLESBORO—Bell County										
□ MIDDLESBORO APPALACHIAN REGIONAL HOSPITAL, 3600 West Cumberland Avenue, Zip 40965, Mailing Address: Box 340, Zip 40965–0340; tel. 606/242–1101; Paul V. Miles, Administrator **A**1 9 10 **F**7 8 15 16 19 22 28 30 31 32 34 35 37 40 44 49 65 67 71 73 **S** Appalachian Regional Healthcare, Lexington, KY **N** CHA Provider Network, Inc., Lexington, KY	23	10	96	4656	57	71532	233	21991	9082	266
MONTICELLO—Wayne County										
□ WAYNE COUNTY HOSPITAL, 166 Hospital Street, Zip 42633–2416; tel. 606/348–9343; Eddy R. Stockton, Administrator **A**1 9 10 **F**8 15 16 19 21 22 44 46 65 71 73	23	10	30	925	17	22102	0	5475	2121	92
MOREHEAD—Rowan County										
⊠ ST. CLAIRE MEDICAL CENTER, 222 Medical Circle, Zip 40351–1180; tel. 606/783–6500; Mark J. Neff, President and Chief Executive Officer **A**1 5 9 10 **F**3 4 7 8 10 14 15 16 17 18 19 20 21 22 23 24 25 26 28 30 31 32 33 34 35 37 40 41 42 44 45 46 49 51 52 53 54 55 56 57 58 60 63 65 67 70 71 73 74 **P**6 **N** CHA Provider Network, Inc., Lexington, KY	21	10	133	5510	65	316677	516	47644	22987	829
MORGANFIELD—Union County										
□ UNION COUNTY METHODIST HOSPITAL, 4604 Highway 60 West, Zip 42437–9570; tel. 502/389–3030; Patrick Donahue, Administrator (Total facility includes 16 beds in nursing home–type unit) **A**1 9 10 **F**8 12 15 16 19 20 22 26 28 30 32 33 35 37 39 44 49 53 56 57 58 64 65 71 73 **P**8 **N** Community Care Network, Henderson, KY	21	10	54	600	16	16097	0	5169	2206	98

Hospital, Address, Telephone, Administrator, Approval, Facility, and Physician Codes, Health Care System, Network	Classi-fication Codes		Utilization Data					Expense (thousands) of dollars		
★ American Hospital Association (AHA) membership □ Joint Commission on Accreditation of Healthcare Organizations (JCAHO) accreditation + American Osteopathic Hospital Association (AOHA) membership ○ American Osteopathic Association (AOA) accreditation △ Commission on Accreditation of Rehabilitation Facilities (CARF) accreditation Control codes 61, 63, 64, 71, 72 and 73 indicate hospitals listed by AOHA, but not registered by AHA. For definition of numerical codes, see page A4	Control	Service	Beds	Admissions	Census	Outpatient Visits	Births	Total	Payroll	Personnel

MOUNT STERLING—Montgomery County

★ GATEWAY REGIONAL HEALTH SYSTEM, Sterling Avenue, Zip 40353–0007, Mailing Address: P.O. Box 7, Zip 40353; tel. 606/497–7701; Jeffrey L. Buckley, President and Chief Executive Officer (Total facility includes 40 beds in nursing home–type unit) **A**1 9 10 **F**7 8 11 12 14 15 16 17 19 20 21 22 24 28 30 35 37 39 40 41 42 44 46 49 56 63 64 65 71 73 74 **P**6 7 — 23 | 10 | 103 | 2418 | 68 | 68196 | 664 | 18715 | 7486 | 476

MOUNT VERNON—Rockcastle County

ROCKCASTLE HOSPITAL, 145 Newcomb Avenue, Zip 40456, Mailing Address: P.O. Box 1310, Zip 40456; tel. 606/256–2195; Lee D. Keene, Administrator (Total facility includes 60 beds in nursing home–type unit) **A**9 10 **F**8 19 21 22 34 41 44 49 64 65 71 **N** CHA Provider Network, Inc., Lexington, KY — 23 | 10 | 86 | 1153 | 71 | 21783 | 0 | 14440 | 7775 | 303

MURRAY—Calloway County

★ MURRAY–CALLOWAY COUNTY HOSPITAL, 803 Poplar Street, Zip 42071–2432; tel. 502/762–1100; Stuart Poston, President (Total facility includes 214 beds in nursing home–type unit) **A**1 9 10 **F**1 7 8 10 19 21 22 32 33 35 37 40 41 42 44 46 54 55 56 57 58 60 63 64 65 67 70 71 73 74 **N** Community Care Network, Henderson, KY — 15 | 10 | 352 | 5680 | 287 | 97614 | 602 | 43422 | 19350 | 863

OWENSBORO—Daviess County

MERCY HOSPITAL See Owensboro Mercy Health System

★ △ OWENSBORO MERCY HEALTH SYSTEM, (Includes Mercy Hospital, 1006 Ford Avenue, Zip 42301, Mailing Address: P.O. Box 2839, Zip 42302; tel. 502/686–6100; Owensboro–Daviess County Hospital, 811 East Parrish Avenue, Zip 42304), 811 East Parrish Avenue, Zip 42303, Mailing Address: P.O. Box 20007, Zip 42303; tel. 502/688–2000; Greg L. Carlson, President and Chief Executive Officer (Total facility includes 24 beds in nursing home–type unit) **A**1 2 7 9 10 **F**4 7 8 10 11 12 14 15 16 17 19 20 21 22 23 24 25 26 27 28 29 30 31 32 33 34 35 37 39 40 41 42 43 44 45 46 48 49 52 54 55 56 57 58 60 64 65 66 67 70 71 72 73 74 **P**7 **N** Community Care Network, Henderson, KY; Center Care, Bowling Green, KY — 23 | 10 | 380 | 17194 | 240 | 221804 | 1689 | 125975 | 48280 | 1692

OWENSBORO–DAVIESS COUNTY HOSPITAL See Owensboro Mercy Health System

RIVERVALLEY BEHAVIORAL HEALTH HOSPITAL, (Formerly Valley Hospital), 1000 Industrial Drive, Zip 42301–8715; tel. 502/686–8477; William Bach, M.D., Administrator and Medical Director **A**9 10 **F**1 3 12 14 15 16 17 18 25 27 29 45 52 53 54 55 56 58 59 67 73 — 23 | 52 | 75 | 548 | 68 | 0 | 0 | 9797 | 4551 | 182

OWENTON—Owen County

OWEN COUNTY MEMORIAL HOSPITAL, 330 Roland Avenue, Zip 40359; tel. 502/484–3441; Richard D. McLeod, Administrator (Total facility includes 20 beds in nursing home–type unit) **A**9 10 **F**8 11 14 15 19 22 25 30 33 37 41 42 44 49 51 64 65 71 72 **P**1 6 **N** CHA Provider Network, Inc., Lexington, KY; Blue Grass Family Health Plan, Lexington, KY — 33 | 10 | 50 | 948 | 39 | — | 0 | 5071 | 2750 | 126

PADUCAH—McCracken County

□ CHARTER BEHAVIORAL HEALTH SYSTEM OF PADUCAH, 435 Berger Road, Zip 42001, Mailing Address: P.O. Box 7609, Zip 42002–7609; tel. 502/444–0444; Pat Harrod, Chief Executive Officer **A**1 9 10 **F**3 15 16 52 53 54 55 56 57 58 59 **S** Magellan Health Services, Atlanta, GA — 33 | 22 | 56 | 730 | 34 | — | 0 | — | | 62

★ △ LOURDES HOSPITAL, 1530 Lone Oak Road, Zip 42002, Mailing Address: P.O. Box 7100, Zip 42002–7100; tel. 502/444–2444; Douglas Borders, President and Chief Executive Officer (Total facility includes 30 beds in nursing home–type unit) **A**1 7 9 10 **F**1 4 7 8 10 11 12 14 15 16 17 19 20 21 22 23 24 26 28 29 30 31 32 33 34 35 36 37 39 40 41 42 43 44 45 46 48 49 52 55 56 64 65 67 71 73 **P**5 7 **S** Mercy Health System, Cincinnati, OH — 21 | 10 | 290 | 11263 | 178 | 269529 | 302 | 96656 | 39673 | 1481

★ WESTERN BAPTIST HOSPITAL, 2501 Kentucky Avenue, Zip 42003; tel. 502/575–2100; Larry O. Barton, President **A**1 9 10 **F**4 7 8 10 11 12 15 19 21 22 24 28 30 32 35 37 38 39 40 41 42 43 44 49 60 65 67 71 72 73 74 **P**5 8 **S** Baptist Healthcare System, Louisville, KY **N** Community Health Delivery System, Inc., Louisville, KY; Baptist Healthcare System, Louisville, KY — 21 | 10 | 310 | 11777 | 178 | 141812 | 1144 | 96539 | 36251 | 1217

PAINTSVILLE—Johnson County

□ PAUL B. HALL REGIONAL MEDICAL CENTER, 625 James S Trimble Boulevard, Zip 41240, Mailing Address: P.O. Box 1487, Zip 41240; tel. 606/789–3511; Deborah T. Meadows, Administrator (Nonreporting) **A**1 9 10 **S** Health Management Associates, Naples, FL — 33 | 10 | 72 | — | — | — | — | — | — | —

PARIS—Bourbon County

★ COLUMBIA HOSPITAL PARIS, (Formerly Bourbon General Hospital), 9 Linville Drive, Zip 40361; tel. 606/987–1000; John R. Grant, Chief Executive Officer **A**1 9 10 **F**8 10 14 15 16 19 21 22 28 35 37 41 44 46 49 52 53 55 56 58 63 65 66 71 **P**7 **S** Columbia/HCA Healthcare Corporation, Nashville, TN **N** Blue Grass Family Health Plan, Lexington, KY — 33 | 10 | 58 | 1700 | 24 | 22615 | 0 | 9865 | 4093 | 234

PIKEVILLE—Pike County

★ PIKEVILLE UNITED METHODIST HOSPITAL OF KENTUCKY, 911 South Bypass, Zip 41501–1595; tel. 606/437–3500; Martha O'Regan Chill, Administrator and Chief Executive Officer (Nonreporting) **A**1 2 9 10 **N** Center Care, Bowling Green, KY — 23 | 10 | 171 | — | — | — | — | — | — | —

PINEVILLE—Bell County

★ PINEVILLE COMMUNITY HOSPITAL ASSOCIATION, Riverview Avenue, Zip 40977–0850; tel. 606/337–3051; J. Milton Brooks, III, Administrator (Total facility includes 30 beds in nursing home–type unit) **A**1 9 10 **F**7 8 14 19 21 22 26 28 30 32 34 37 40 44 46 64 65 71 73 **P**5 **N** CHA Provider Network, Inc., Lexington, KY — 23 | 10 | 150 | 3986 | 83 | 21885 | 263 | 16562 | 7272 | 332

Hospital, Address, Telephone, Administrator, Approval, Facility, and Physician Codes, Health Care System, Network	Classi-fication Codes		Utilization Data					Expense (thousands) of dollars		
	Control	Service	Beds	Admissions	Census	Outpatient Visits	Births	Total	Payroll	Personnel

★ American Hospital Association (AHA) membership
□ Joint Commission on Accreditation of Healthcare Organizations (JCAHO) accreditation
+ American Osteopathic Hospital Association (AOHA) membership
○ American Osteopathic Association (AOA) accreditation
△ Commission on Accreditation of Rehabilitation Facilities (CARF) accreditation
  Control codes 61, 63, 64, 71, 72 and 73 indicate hospitals listed by AOHA, but not registered by AHA. For definition of numerical codes, see page A4

PRESTONSBURG—Floyd County

	Control	Service	Beds	Admissions	Census	Outpatient Visits	Births	Total	Payroll	Personnel
✚ HIGHLANDS REGIONAL MEDICAL CENTER, 5000 Kentucky Route 321, Zip 41653, Mailing Address: Box 668, Zip 41653-0668; tel. 606/886-8511; Clarence Traum, President and Chief Executive Officer (Nonreporting) **A**1 2 5 9 10 **N** CHA Provider Network, Inc., Lexington, KY	23	10	184	—	—	—	—	—	—	—

PRINCETON—Caldwell County

✚ CALDWELL COUNTY HOSPITAL, 101 Hospital Drive, Zip 42445-0410, Mailing Address: Box 410, Zip 42445-0410; tel. 502/365-0300; John Svoboda, Chief Executive Officer **A**1 9 10 **F**7 8 15 16 19 22 28 30 32 34 39 40 44 45 46 71 72 **P**8 **S** Alliant Health System, Louisville, KY **N** Community Care Network, Henderson, KY; Community Health Delivery System, Inc., Louisville, KY	23	10	15	905	9	25139	116	8862	3928	171

RADCLIFF—Hardin County

✚ LINCOLN TRAIL BEHAVIORAL HEALTH SYSTEM, 3909 South Wilson Road, Zip 40160-9714, Mailing Address: P.O. Box 369, Zip 40159-0369; tel. 502/351-9444; Melvin E. Modderman, Administrator (Nonreporting) **A**1 9 10 **S** Park Healthcare Company, Nashville, TN	33	22	67	—	—	—	—	—	—	—

RICHMOND—Madison County

✚ PATTIE A. CLAY HOSPITAL, EKU By-Pass, Zip 40475, Mailing Address: P.O. Box 1600, Zip 40476-2603; tel. 606/625-3131; Richard M. Thomas, President **A**1 9 10 **F**7 8 10 12 13 17 19 21 22 28 30 31 34 35 37 39 40 41 44 45 46 49 58 60 61 63 65 66 67 68 70 71 72 73 74 **S** Jewish Hospital Healthcare Services, Louisville, KY **N** CHA Provider Network, Inc., Lexington, KY; Jewish Hospital Healthcare Services, Louisville, KY; Blue Grass Family Health Plan, Lexington, KY	23	10	96	4310	51	—	902	—	—	494

RUSSELL SPRINGS—Russell County

RUSSELL COUNTY HOSPITAL, Dowell Road, Zip 42642, Mailing Address: P.O. Box 1610, Zip 42642; tel. 502/866-4141; William J. Hurteau, FACHE, Administrator **A**9 10 **F**14 15 16 19 20 22 28 29 30 32 33 37 44 45 49 65 71 **S** Alliant Health System, Louisville, KY	13	10	45	1142	21	14500	0	7982	3397	159

RUSSELLVILLE—Logan County

✚ COLUMBIA LOGAN MEMORIAL HOSPITAL, 1625 South Nashville Road, Zip 42276-0010, Mailing Address: P.O. Box 10, Zip 42276; tel. 502/726-4011 (Total facility includes 8 beds in nursing home-type unit) **A**1 9 10 **F**7 8 11 12 15 16 17 19 22 28 35 37 39 40 44 49 64 65 71 73 **S** Columbia/HCA Healthcare Corporation, Nashville, TN **N** Center Care, Bowling Green, KY	33	10	64	1734	23	30323	170	—	—	183

SALEM—Livingston County

★ LIVINGSTON HOSPITAL AND HEALTHCARE SERVICES, 131 Hospital Drive, Zip 42078, Mailing Address: Box 138, Zip 42078; tel. 502/988-2299; William C. Smith, Chief Executive Officer **A**9 10 **F**8 14 15 16 17 19 22 28 30 32 33 35 42 44 46 48 71 **N** Community Care Network, Henderson, KY	23	10	26	1208	13	13606	0	8908	3381	140

SCOTTSVILLE—Allen County

★ MEDICAL CENTER AT SCOTTSVILLE, 456 Burnley Road, Zip 42164; tel. 502/622-2800; Connie Smith, Senior Vice President (Nonreporting) **A**9 10 **N** Center Care, Bowling Green, KY	23	10	47	—	—	—	—	—	—	—

SHELBYVILLE—Shelby County

✚ JEWISH HOSPITAL–SHELBYVILLE, 727 Hospital Drive, Zip 40065; tel. 502/647-4301; Timothy L. Jarm, President (Total facility includes 8 beds in nursing home-type unit) **A**1 9 10 **F**2 4 7 8 9 10 11 12 13 14 15 16 17 18 19 21 22 23 24 25 26 27 28 29 30 32 33 34 35 37 39 40 41 42 43 44 45 46 48 49 50 51 52 53 54 55 56 57 58 59 60 62 63 64 65 66 67 69 70 71 73 74 **S** Jewish Hospital Healthcare Services, Louisville, KY **N** Jewish Hospital Healthcare Services, Louisville, KY	21	10	66	2501	32	16531	—	19670	7586	277

SOMERSET—Pulaski County

✚ △ COLUMBIA LAKE CUMBERLAND REGIONAL HOSPITAL, 305 Langdon Street, Zip 42501, Mailing Address: Box 620, Zip 42502-2750; tel. 606/679-7441; Kenneth W. Lukhard, President and Chief Executive Officer **A**1 2 7 9 10 **F**2 3 7 8 10 12 15 16 18 19 21 22 23 28 29 30 32 33 35 37 39 40 41 42 44 46 48 49 52 53 54 55 56 57 58 59 60 64 65 67 71 73 **P**5 7 **S** Columbia/HCA Healthcare Corporation, Nashville, TN	33	10	227	10597	145	37439	1512	40426	17356	722

SOUTH WILLIAMSON—Pike County

□ WILLIAMSON ARH HOSPITAL, 260 Hospital Drive, Zip 41503; tel. 606/237-1700; John A. Grah, Administrator (Total facility includes 50 beds in nursing home-type unit) **A**1 9 10 **F**4 7 8 12 13 15 16 17 19 22 25 28 30 32 33 34 35 37 39 40 42 44 49 52 54 56 57 58 60 63 64 65 71 73 **P**2 3 5 6 **S** Appalachian Regional Healthcare, Lexington, KY **N** Partners in Health Network, Inc., Charleston, WV; CHA Provider Network, Inc., Lexington, KY	23	10	148	4500	130	90409	158	25548	12669	403

STANFORD—Lincoln County

✚ FORT LOGAN HOSPITAL, 124 Portman Avenue, Zip 40484-1200; tel. 606/365-2187; Terry C. Powers, Administrator (Total facility includes 30 beds in nursing home-type unit) **A**1 9 10 **F**7 8 14 15 16 19 20 22 26 30 31 34 40 41 44 46 49 64 65 71 **N** CHA Provider Network, Inc., Lexington, KY; Blue Grass Family Health Plan, Lexington, KY	23	10	73	1175	45	12863	104	8108	3474	166

TOMPKINSVILLE—Monroe County

✚ MONROE COUNTY MEDICAL CENTER, 529 Capp Harlan Road, Zip 42167; tel. 502/487-9231; Carolyn E. Riley, Chief Executive Officer **A**1 9 10 **F**8 15 16 19 22 27 32 34 39 44 45 49 65 70 71 **P**8 **S** Quorum Health Group/Quorum Health Resources, Inc., Brentwood, TN **N** Center Care, Bowling Green, KY	23	10	49	2703	35	23348	0	10057	4675	252

Hospital, Address, Telephone, Administrator, Approval, Facility, and Physician Codes, Health Care System, Network	Classi-fication Codes		Utilization Data					Expense (thousands) of dollars		
	Control	Service	Beds	Admissions	Census	Outpatient Visits	Births	Total	Payroll	Personnel

VERSAILLES—Woodford County

★ WOODFORD HOSPITAL, 360 Amsden Avenue, Zip 40383–1286; tel. 606/873–3111; Nancy Littrell, Chief Executive Officer (Total facility includes 23 beds in nursing home–type unit) **A**9 10 **F**8 10 12 14 15 16 17 19 20 21 22 26 28 29 30 32 33 34 37 39 40 41 44 45 46 49 54 64 65 66 67 71 73 **N** CHA Provider Network, Inc., Lexington, KY; Blue Grass Family Health Plan, Lexington, KY
23 10 73 933 32 9804 0 8515 3408 159

WEST LIBERTY—Morgan County

□ MORGAN COUNTY APPALACHIAN REGIONAL HOSPITAL, 476 Liberty Road, Zip 41472, Mailing Address: Box 579, Zip 41472–0579; tel. 606/743–3186; Dennis R. Chaney, Administrator (Total facility includes 15 beds in nursing home–type unit) **A**1 9 10 **F**8 15 16 19 22 28 29 30 32 33 34 40 45 64 65 71 73 **S** Appalachian Regional Healthcare, Lexington, KY **N** CHA Provider Network, Inc., Lexington, KY
23 10 55 1087 34 35015 0 8253 3887 122

WHITESBURG—Letcher County

□ WHITESBURG APPALACHIAN REGIONAL HOSPITAL, 550 Jenkins Road, Zip 41858; tel. 606/633–3600; Nick Lewis, Administrator **A**1 9 10 **F**7 8 12 14 15 16 19 21 22 23 28 32 34 35 37 40 42 44 46 60 65 71 73 **P**6 **S** Appalachian Regional Healthcare, Lexington, KY **N** CHA Provider Network, Inc., Lexington, KY
23 10 71 3958 48 64480 409 18606 7880 275

WILLIAMSTOWN—Grant County

✠ ST. ELIZABETH MEDICAL CENTER–GRANT COUNTY, 238 Barnes Road, Zip 41097; tel. 606/824–2400; Chris Carle, Administrator **A**1 9 10 **F**2 3 4 8 10 11 14 15 16 19 21 22 27 32 33 35 37 39 40 42 43 44 46 48 49 52 64 65 67 71 73 74 **P**1 5 **N** Community Health Delivery System, Inc., Louisville, KY; Center Care, Bowling Green, KY; Saint Elizabeth Medical Center, Covington, KY
21 10 20 559 5 25626 0 4646 1692 73

WINCHESTER—Clark County

✠ CLARK REGIONAL MEDICAL CENTER, West Lexington Avenue, Zip 40391, Mailing Address: P.O. Box 630, Zip 40392–0630; tel. 606/745–3500; Robert D. Fraraccio, Administrator **A**1 5 9 10 **F**7 8 11 12 19 20 21 22 28 30 31 33 34 37 39 40 41 42 44 49 64 65 67 71 73 74 **N** CHA Provider Network, Inc., Lexington, KY; Blue Grass Family Health Plan, Lexington, KY
23 10 75 2350 29 — 251 16660 6938 244

LOUISIANA

Resident population 4,342 (in thousands)
Resident population in metro areas 75.1%
Birth rate per 1,000 population 16.2
65 years and over 11.4%
Percent of persons without health insurance 19.2%

★ American Hospital Association (AHA) membership
□ Joint Commission on Accreditation of Healthcare Organizations (JCAHO) accreditation
+ American Osteopathic Hospital Association (AOHA) membership
○ American Osteopathic Association (AOA) accreditation
△ Commission on Accreditation of Rehabilitation Facilities (CARF) accreditation
Control codes 61, 63, 64, 71, 72 and 73 indicate hospitals listed by AOHA, but not registered by AHA. For definition of numerical codes, see page A4

Hospital, Address, Telephone, Administrator, Approval, Facility, and Physician Codes, Health Care System, Network	Classi-fication Codes		Utilization Data					Expense (thousands) of dollars		
	Control	Service	Beds	Admissions	Census	Outpatient Visits	Births	Total	Payroll	Personnel

ABBEVILLE—Vermilion Parish

□ ABBEVILLE GENERAL HOSPITAL, 118 North Hospital Drive, Zip 70510, Mailing Address: P.O. Box 580, Zip 70511–0580; tel. 318/893–5466; Ray A. Landry, Administrator **A**1 9 10 **F**8 14 15 16 19 21 22 32 33 34 35 37 39 40 42 44 52 57 58 59 65 71 73

	16	10	121	3748	57	40578	213	17996	8423	300

ABITA SPRINGS—St. Tammany Parish

□ SOUTHEAST LOUISIANA HOSPITAL, Mailing Address: P.O. Box 3850, Mandeville, Zip 70470–3850; tel. 504/626–6300; Joseph C. Vinturella, Chief Executive Officer **A**1 10 **F**15 16 52 53 54 56 57 65 73 **S** Louisiana State Hospitals, New Orleans, LA

	12	22	251	827	237	0	0	28600	18742	669

ALEXANDRIA—Rapides Parish

✠ DEPARTMENT OF VA MEDICAL CENTER–ALEXANDRIA, (Formerly Veterans Affairs Medical Center), Shreveport Highway, Zip 71306–6002; tel. 318/473–0010; Allan S. Goss, Director (Total facility includes 197 beds in nursing home–type unit) **A**1 2 3 5 **F**3 8 16 18 19 20 21 22 25 26 27 28 30 34 35 37 41 42 44 46 49 51 52 54 57 58 60 64 65 67 71 73 74 **P**6 **S** Department of Veterans Affairs, Washington, DC

	45	10	401	3555	347	94453	0	59172	43156	1021

✠ RAPIDES REGIONAL MEDICAL CENTER, 211 Fourth Street, Zip 71301–8421, Mailing Address: Box 30101, Zip 71301–8421; tel. 318/473–3000; Lynn Truelove, President **A**1 2 9 10 **F**1 3 4 5 6 7 8 10 12 13 14 15 17 18 19 20 21 22 23 24 25 26 27 28 29 30 31 32 33 34 35 36 37 39 40 41 42 43 44 45 46 47 49 50 51 52 53 54 55 56 57 58 59 60 61 62 63 64 65 66 67 68 69 70 71 72 73 74 **P**8 **S** Columbia/HCA Healthcare Corporation, Nashville, TN

	23	10	359	13662	180	103649	1577	110252	41489	1516

✠ △ ST. FRANCES CABRINI HOSPITAL, 3330 Masonic Drive, Zip 71301; tel. 318/487–1122; Sister Olive Bordelon, Chief Executive Officer (Total facility includes 19 beds in nursing home–type unit) **A**1 7 9 10 **F**4 7 8 10 11 12 14 15 16 17 19 21 22 24 26 27 28 29 30 32 33 34 35 37 38 39 40 41 42 43 44 45 46 48 49 50 52 53 54 55 56 57 58 59 60 63 64 65 66 67 68 69 70 71 72 73 74 **P**1 4 5 7 8 **S** Sisters of Charity of the Incarnate Word Healthcare System, Houston, TX **N** Ochsner/Sisters of Charity Health Network, New Orleans, LA

	23	10	227	8597	134	106973	568	78750	31827	961

AMITE—Tangipahoa Parish

★ HOOD MEMORIAL HOSPITAL, 301 West Walnut Street, Zip 70422; tel. 504/748–9485; A. D. Richardson, Administrator (Nonreporting) **A**9 10

	16	10	40	—	—	—	—	—	—	—

BASTROP—Morehouse Parish

✠ MOREHOUSE GENERAL HOSPITAL, 323 West Walnut Street, Zip 71220, Mailing Address: Box 1060, Zip 71221–1060; tel. 318/283–3601; William W. Bing, Administrator (Total facility includes 18 beds in nursing home–type unit) **A**1 9 10 **F**1 7 8 11 14 15 16 17 19 20 21 22 26 28 29 30 32 34 35 37 39 40 41 42 44 45 46 49 52 55 57 59 63 64 65 67 68 71 73 **P**1

	16	10	100	3156	50	37025	339	23600	9688	420

BATON ROUGE—East Baton Rouge Parish

★ BATON ROUGE GENERAL HEALTH CENTER, 8585 Picardy Avenue, Zip 70809, Mailing Address: P.O. Box 84330, Zip 70884–4330; tel. 504/763–4000; Linda Lee, Administrator (Nonreporting) **A**9 10 **S** General Health System, Baton Rouge, LA

	23	10	72	—	—	—	—	—	—	—

✠ BATON ROUGE GENERAL MEDICAL CENTER, 3600 Florida Street, Zip 70806, Mailing Address: P.O. Box 2511, Zip 70821–2511; tel. 504/387–7770; Chris W. Barnette, President and Chief Executive Officer (Total facility includes 47 beds in nursing home–type unit) **A**1 2 3 5 6 8 9 10 **F**1 2 3 4 7 8 9 10 11 12 13 15 16 17 18 19 20 21 22 23 24 26 28 29 30 31 32 33 34 35 37 38 39 41 42 43 44 45 46 47 49 52 53 54 55 56 57 58 59 60 61 64 65 66 67 69 71 73 74 **P**3 4 7 **S** General Health System, Baton Rouge, LA

	23	10	355	11365	170	67241	0	113145	48149	1413

□ BHC MEADOW WOOD HOSPITAL, (Formerly CPC Meadow Wood Hospital), 9032 Perkins Road, Zip 70810; tel. 504/766–8553; Ralph J. Waite, III, Chief Executive Officer **A**1 10 **F**2 3 15 16 17 18 34 52 53 54 55 56 57 58 59 65 67 **S** Behavioral Healthcare Corporation, Nashville, TN

	33	22	55	1374	31	3500	0	4074	2408	72

✠ COLUMBIA MEDICAL CENTER, 17000 Medical Center Drive, Zip 70816–3224; tel. 504/755–4800; Joseph R. Dicapo, Chief Executive Officer (Total facility includes 24 beds in nursing home–type unit) (Nonreporting) **A**1 9 10 **S** Columbia/HCA Healthcare Corporation, Nashville, TN **N** Ochsner/Sisters of Charity Health Network, New Orleans, LA

	33	10	183	—	—	—	—	—	—	—

□ CONCORD HOSPITAL, (Formerly Parkland Hospital), 2414 Bunker Hill Drive, Zip 70808; tel. 504/925–1290; Theresa Harris, Clinical Administrator (Nonreporting) **A**1 10

	33	22	170	—	—	—	—	—	—	—

CPC MEADOW WOOD HOSPITAL See BHC Meadow Wood Hospital

□ EARL K. LONG MEDICAL CENTER, 5825 Airline Highway, Zip 70805; tel. 504/358–1000; Margaret Alvis, MSN, R.N., Chief Executive Officer **A**1 3 5 10 **F**7 14 15 16 19 22 31 34 37 38 40 44 47 52 54 60 61 65 71 73 **P**1 6 **S** Louisiana Health Care Authority, Baton Rouge, LA **N** Louisiana Health Care Authority, Baton Rouge, LA

	12	10	204	9583	162	168069	1595	—	—	808

Hospital, Address, Telephone, Administrator, Approval, Facility, and Physician Codes, Health Care System, Network	Classi-fication Codes		Utilization Data					Expense (thousands) of dollars		
★ American Hospital Association (AHA) membership □ Joint Commission on Accreditation of Healthcare Organizations (JCAHO) accreditation + American Osteopathic Hospital Association (AOHA) membership ○ American Osteopathic Association (AOA) accreditation △ Commission on Accreditation of Rehabilitation Facilities (CARF) accreditation Control codes 61, 63, 64, 71, 72 and 73 indicate hospitals listed by AOHA, but not registered by AHA. For definition of numerical codes, see page A4	Control	Service	Beds	Admissions	Census	Outpatient Visits	Births	Total	Payroll	Personnel
□ HEALTHSOUTH REHABILITATION HOSPITAL OF SOUTH LOUISIANA, 4040 North Boulevard, Zip 70806–3829; tel. 504/383–5055; Sharon S. Black, R.N., Chief Operating Officer (Nonreporting) **A**1 10 **S** HEALTHSOUTH Corporation, Birmingham, AL	33	46	40	—	—	—	—	—	—	—
⊠ △ OUR LADY OF THE LAKE REGIONAL MEDICAL CENTER, (Includes Our Lady of the Lake–Assumption, 135 Highway 402, Napoleonville, Zip 70390, Mailing Address: P.O. Drawer 546, Zip 70390; tel. 504/369–3600), 5000 Henessy Boulevard, Zip 70808–4350; tel. 504/765–6565; Robert C. Davidge, President and Chief Executive Officer (Total facility includes 178 beds in nursing home–type unit) **A**1 2 5 7 9 10 **F**1 2 3 4 6 8 10 11 12 14 15 16 17 19 21 22 23 24 26 27 28 29 30 31 32 33 34 35 37 39 41 42 43 44 45 46 47 48 49 50 51 52 53 54 55 56 57 58 59 60 62 63 64 65 66 67 68 69 71 73 **P**1 **S** Franciscan Missionaries of Our Lady Health System, Inc., Baton Rouge, LA **N** Franciscan Missionaries of Our Lady Health Network, Baton Rouge, LA PARKLAND HOSPITAL See Concord Hospital	21	10	660	22291	390	—	0	—	—	2830
⊠ △ REHABILITATION HOSPITAL OF BATON ROUGE, 8595 United Plaza Boulevard, Zip 70809; tel. 504/927–0567; Jeff Henderson, Chief Executive Officer **A**1 7 10 **F**12 14 15 16 32 34 41 48 49 66	33	46	80	653	44	27297	0	16390	—	236
⊠ WOMAN'S HOSPITAL, 9050 Airline Highway, Zip 70815, Mailing Address: Box 95009, Zip 70895–9009; tel. 504/927–1300; Teri G. Fentonot, President and Chief Executive Officer **A**1 2 5 9 10 **F**7 8 12 14 15 16 17 18 19 24 25 28 29 30 32 34 37 38 40 42 44 45 46 49 61 65 67 68 71 73 74	23	44	203	10857	101	89135	6706	79935	37271	1007
BERNICE—Union Parish										
TRI–WARD GENERAL HOSPITAL, 409 First Street, Zip 71222, Mailing Address: P.O. Box 697, Zip 71222–0697; tel. 318/285–9066; Charolette Thompson, Administrator **A**9 10 **F**15 22 70	16	10	11	184	2	987	0	1940	1065	40
BOGALUSA—Washington Parish										
⊠ BOGALUSA COMMUNITY MEDICAL CENTER, 433 Plaza Street, Zip 70429–0940; tel. 504/732–7122; Terry G. Whittington, Chief Executive Officer and Administrator (Nonreporting) **A**1 9 10 **S** Quorum Health Group/Quorum Health Resources, Inc., Brentwood, TN	23	10	102	—	—	—	—	—	—	—
□ WASHINGTON–ST. TAMMANY REGIONAL MEDICAL CENTER, 400 Memphis Street, Zip 70427–0040, Mailing Address: Box 40, Zip 70429–0040; tel. 504/735–1322; Larry R. King, Administrator **A**1 10 **F**14 15 16 19 22 31 34 41 44 45 46 49 52 59 65 67 70 71 73 74 **S** Louisiana Health Care Authority, Baton Rouge, LA **N** Louisiana Health Care Authority, Baton Rouge, LA	12	10	55	1980	31	56513	0	12778	5986	182
BOSSIER CITY—Bossier Parish										
⊠ BOSSIER MEDICAL CENTER, 2105 Airline Drive, Zip 71111; tel. 318/741–6000; Jack F. Houghton, Chief Executive Officer (Total facility includes 20 beds in nursing home–type unit) **A**1 9 10 **F**4 7 8 10 12 15 16 17 19 22 25 26 27 28 29 30 32 33 34 35 37 40 41 42 43 44 45 49 51 52 57 63 64 65 67 71 72 73 **P**5 8	14	10	131	4424	64	121038	334	44035	19334	605
□ SUMMIT HOSPITAL OF NORTHWEST LOUISIANA, 4900 Medical Drive, Zip 71112, Mailing Address: P.O. Box 8450, Zip 71112–8450; tel. 318/747–9500; Louise Wiggins, Administrator (Nonreporting) **A**1 10 **S** Summit Hospital Corporation	33	22	54	—	—	—	—	—	—	—
BREAUX BRIDGE—St. Martin Parish										
GARY MEMORIAL HOSPITAL, 210 Champagne Boulevard, Zip 70517–3852, Mailing Address: Box 357, Zip 70517–0357; tel. 318/332–2178; Burton Dupuis, Administrator (Nonreporting) **A**9 10	16	10	12	—	—	—	—	—	—	—
BUNKIE—Avoyelles Parish										
★ BUNKIE GENERAL HOSPITAL, Evergreen Highway, Zip 71322, Mailing Address: Box 380, Zip 71322–0380; tel. 318/346–6681; Donald L. Kannady, Administrator **A**9 10 **F**15 16 19 21 22 24 26 28 29 32 34 35 44 46 49 52 53 59 71 73 **N** Ochsner/Sisters of Charity Health Network, New Orleans, LA	16	10	48	977	22	25501	0	6613	3097	145
CAMERON—Cameron Parish										
SOUTH CAMERON MEMORIAL HOSPITAL, 5360 West Creole Highway, Zip 70631; tel. 318/542–4111; Joseph L. Soileau, Chief Executive Officer (Nonreporting) **A**9 10	16	10	33	—	—	—	—	—	—	—
CHALMETTE—St. Bernard Parish										
□ CHALMETTE MEDICAL CENTERS, (Includes Chalmette Medical Center, 801 Virtue Street, William E. Price, Managing Director), 9001 Patricia Street, Zip 70043; tel. 504/277–8011; Larry M. Graham, Chief Executive Officer (Nonreporting) **A**1 9 10 **S** Universal Health Services, Inc., King of Prussia, PA	33	10	196	—	—	—	—	—	—	—
CHURCH POINT—Acadia Parish										
ACADIA–ST. LANDRY HOSPITAL, 810 South Broadway Street, Zip 70525; tel. 318/684–5435; Alcus Trahan, Administrator (Nonreporting) **A**9 10	23	10	39	—	—	—	—	—	—	—
COLUMBIA—Caldwell Parish										
CALDWELL MEMORIAL HOSPITAL, 410 Main Street, Zip 71418, Mailing Address: Box 899, Zip 71418; tel. 318/649–6111; Ronnie Wagnon, Administrator (Nonreporting) **A**9 10	33	10	31	—	—	—	—	—	—	—
COUSHATTA—Red River Parish										
L. S. HUCKABAY MD MEMORIAL HOSPITAL, 1635 Marvel Street, Zip 71019, Mailing Address: Box 369, Zip 71019; tel. 318/932–5784; Betty Bell, Team Administrator (Nonreporting) **A**9 10	33	10	74	—	—	—	—	—	—	—
COVINGTON—St. Tammany Parish										
⊠ COLUMBIA LAKEVIEW REGIONAL MEDICAL CENTER, 95 East Fairway Drive, Zip 70433; tel. 504/876–3800; Scott Koenig, Chief Executive Officer **A**1 9 10 **F**4 7 8 10 11 12 14 15 16 17 19 21 22 25 26 27 30 32 34 35 37 38 40 41 42 43 44 49 51 52 57 60 64 65 67 71 72 73 74 **P**1 7 **S** Columbia/HCA Healthcare Corporation, Nashville, TN **N** Columbia Lakeview Regional Medical Center, Covington, LA	33	10	163	5664	68	39530	1156	48805	19551	563

Hospital, Address, Telephone, Administrator, Approval, Facility, and Physician Codes, Health Care System, Network	Classi-fication Codes		Utilization Data					Expense (thousands) of dollars		
	Control	Service	Beds	Admissions	Census	Outpatient Visits	Births	Total	Payroll	Personnel

★ American Hospital Association (AHA) membership
☐ Joint Commission on Accreditation of Healthcare Organizations (JCAHO) accreditation
+ American Osteopathic Hospital Association (AOHA) membership
○ American Osteopathic Association (AOA) accreditation
△ Commission on Accreditation of Rehabilitation Facilities (CARF) accreditation
Control codes 61, 63, 64, 71, 72 and 73 indicate hospitals listed by AOHA, but not registered by AHA. For definition of numerical codes, see page A4

Hospital	Control	Service	Beds	Admissions	Census	Outpatient Visits	Births	Total	Payroll	Personnel
☐ GREENBRIER HOSPITAL, 201 Greenbrier Boulevard, Zip 70433; tel. 504/893–2970; Pam McCullough Broughton, Chief Executive Officer (Nonreporting) **A**1 9 10 **S** Ramsay Health Care, Inc., Coral Gobles, FL	33	22	66	—	—	—	—	—	—	—
⊞ ST. TAMMANY PARISH HOSPITAL, 1202 South Tyler Street, Zip 70433–2394; tel. 504/898–4000; Thomas J. Stone, Administrator **A**1 2 9 10 **F**4 7 8 10 12 14 15 19 21 22 23 25 26 30 31 32 33 34 35 36 37 38 39 40 41 42 43 44 46 49 51 61 63 64 65 71 72 73 74 **P**6	16	10	131	5504	74	95032	857	51249	24471	675
CROWLEY—Acadia Parish										
★ AMERICAN LEGION HOSPITAL, 1305 Crowley Rayne Highway, Zip 70526–9410; tel. 318/783–3222; Leonard J. Spears, Administrator **A**9 10 **F**2 8 15 16 19 21 22 32 37 39 40 44 46 52 57 65 71 **P**2	23	10	178	3294	35	29821	507	20156	8353	343
CUT OFF—Lafourche Parish										
⊞ LADY OF THE SEA GENERAL HOSPITAL, 200 West 134th Place, Zip 70345; tel. 504/632–6401; Lane M. Cheramie, Chief Executive Officer **A**1 9 10 **F**1 8 12 14 15 16 17 19 22 23 25 28 29 30 32 33 34 35 37 39 42 44 45 46 49 51 52 54 55 56 57 58 59 65 67 71 73 **S** Brim, Inc., Portland, OR **N** Ochsner/Sisters of Charity Health Network, New Orleans, LA	16	10	55	1586	26	16467	0	14991	4840	186
DE QUINCY—Calcasieu Parish										
DEQUINCY MEMORIAL HOSPITAL, 110 West Fourth Street, Zip 70633, Mailing Address: Box 1166, Zip 70633; tel. 318/786–1200; Michael E. Daiken, Administrator (Nonreporting) **A**9 10	14	10	41	—	—	—	—	—	—	—
DE RIDDER—Beauregard Parish										
⊞ BEAUREGARD MEMORIAL HOSPITAL, 600 South Pine Street, Zip 70634, Mailing Address: P.O. Box 730, Zip 70634–0730; tel. 318/462–7100; Theodore J. Badger, Jr., Chief Executive Officer (Total facility includes 26 beds in nursing home–type unit) **A**1 9 10 **F**8 10 15 16 19 20 21 22 23 24 28 32 37 42 44 46 63 64 65 71 73 **P**1 7 **N** Ochsner/Sisters of Charity Health Network, New Orleans, LA	16	10	93	3860	50	25451	645	19348	9114	323
DELHI—Richland Parish										
RICHLAND PARISH HOSPITAL–DELHI, 507 Cincinnati Street, Zip 71232; tel. 318/878–5171; Michael W. Carroll, Administrator (Nonreporting) **A**9 10	16	10	42	—	—	—	—	—	—	—
DONALDSONVILLE—Ascension Parish										
⊞ PREVOST MEMORIAL HOSPITAL, 301 Memorial Drive, Zip 70346, Mailing Address: Box 186, Zip 70346; tel. 504/473–7931; Vince A. Cataldo, Administrator (Nonreporting) **A**1 9 10	16	10	35	—	—	—	—	—	—	—
EUNICE—St. Landry Parish										
⊞ MOOSA MEMORIAL HOSPITAL, Moosa Boulevard, Zip 70535, Mailing Address: Box 1026, Zip 70535; tel. 318/457–5244; Craig A. Ortego, Administrator **A**1 9 10 **F**1 8 14 15 16 19 21 22 23 28 32 34 35 37 40 42 44 46 49 52 53 54 55 56 57 58 59 65 67 69 71 73 74 **P**7	16	10	67	1943	31	21870	234	13674	5663	220
FARMERVILLE—Union Parish										
UNION GENERAL HOSPITAL, 901 James Avenue, Zip 71241, Mailing Address: P.O. Box 398, Zip 71241; tel. 318/368–9751; Evalyn Ormond, Administrator **A**9 10 **F**9 15 22 26 28 30 32 34 39 44 48 49 52 57 65 71 73	23	10	35	608	8	27138	0	4538	—	87
FERRIDAY—Concordia Parish										
RIVERLAND MEDICAL CENTER, 1700 North E 'E' Wallace Boulevard, Zip 71334, Mailing Address: Box 111, Zip 71334; tel. 318/757–6551; Vernon R. Stevens, Jr., Administrator (Nonreporting) **A**9 10 **N** Ochsner/Sisters of Charity Health Network, New Orleans, LA	16	10	49	—	—	—	—	—	—	—
FORT POLK—Vernon Parish										
⊞ BAYNE–JONES ARMY COMMUNITY HOSPITAL, Zip 71459–6000; tel. 318/531–3928; Colonel Joe W. Butler, Jr., Deputy Commander and Administrator (Nonreporting) **A**1 **S** Department of the Army, Office of the Surgeon General, Falls Church, VA	42	10	52	—	—	—	—	—	—	—
FRANKLIN—St. Mary Parish										
⊞ FRANKLIN FOUNDATION HOSPITAL, 1501 Hospital Avenue, Zip 70538, Mailing Address: Box 577, Zip 70538–0577; tel. 318/828–0760; A. Dale Morgan, Administrator **A**1 9 10 **F**4 8 19 20 21 22 30 32 37 40 41 44 48 49 65 66 71 **P**2 5 6 7 8 **S** Quorum Health Group/Quorum Health Resources, Inc., Brentwood, TN	16	10	60	1331	16	20287	164	12317	4382	196
FRANKLINTON—Washington Parish										
⊞ RIVERSIDE MEDICAL CENTER, 1900 Main Street, Zip 70438; tel. 504/839–4431; John E. Walker, Chief Executive Officer **A**1 9 10 **F**8 19 22 32 35 37 41 42 44 71	16	10	53	1674	21	13920	0	9010	4025	166
GONZALES—Ascension Parish										
☐ ASCENSION HOSPITAL, 615 East Worthy Road, Zip 70737; tel. 504/647–2891; Michael J. Nolan, Chief Executive Officer (Nonreporting) **A**1 9 10	16	49	118	—	—	—	—	—	—	—
⊞ COLUMBIA RIVERVIEW MEDICAL CENTER, 1125 West Louisiana Highway 30, Zip 70737; tel. 504/647–5000; James W. White, Chief Executive Officer (Total facility includes 15 beds in nursing home–type unit) (Nonreporting) **A**1 9 10 **S** Columbia/HCA Healthcare Corporation, Nashville, TN	33	10	104	—	—	—	—	—	—	—
GREENSBURG—St. Helena Parish										
★ ST. HELENA PARISH HOSPITAL, Highway 43 North, Zip 70441, Mailing Address: Box 337, Zip 70441–0337; tel. 504/222–6111; L. J. Pecot, Administrator (Total facility includes 72 beds in nursing home–type unit) (Nonreporting) **A**9 10	16	10	99	—	—	—	—	—	—	—
GREENWELL SPRINGS—East Baton Rouge Parish										
⊞ GREENWELL SPRINGS HOSPITAL, 23260 Greenwell Springs Road, Zip 70739, Mailing Address: P.O. Box 549, Zip 70739–0549; tel. 504/261–2730; Warren T. Price, Jr., Chief Executive Officer (Nonreporting) **A**1 **S** Louisiana State Hospitals, New Orleans, LA	12	22	104	—	—	—	—	—	—	—

Hospital, Address, Telephone, Administrator, Approval, Facility, and Physician Codes, Health Care System, Network	Classi-fication Codes		Utilization Data					Expense (thousands) of dollars		
★ American Hospital Association (AHA) membership □ Joint Commission on Accreditation of Healthcare Organizations (JCAHO) accreditation + American Osteopathic Hospital Association (AOHA) membership ○ American Osteopathic Association (AOA) accreditation △ Commission on Accreditation of Rehabilitation Facilities (CARF) accreditation Control codes 61, 63, 64, 71, 72 and 73 indicate hospitals listed by AOHA, but not registered by AHA. For definition of numerical codes, see page A4	Control	Service	Beds	Admissions	Census	Outpatient Visits	Births	Total	Payroll	Personnel

GRETNA—Jefferson Parish

□ MEADOWCREST HOSPITAL, 2500 Belle Chase Highway, Zip 70056; tel. 504/392–3131; Jaime A. Wesolowski, Chief Executive Officer (Total facility includes 24 beds in nursing home–type unit) **A**1 3 9 10 **F**1 4 7 8 10 11 12 16 19 20 21 22 23 24 28 30 31 32 35 37 38 39 40 41 42 43 44 45 46 47 48 49 52 53 54 55 56 57 58 59 63 64 65 66 71 72 73 **P**1 5 7 **S** TENET Healthcare Corporation, Santa Barbara, CA **N** Tenet Louisiana Health System Network, Metairie, LA — 33 10 181 6231 77 44386 1771 37649 15147 643

HAMMOND—Tangipahoa Parish

✇ NORTH OAKS MEDICAL CENTER, 15790 Medical Center Drive, Zip 70403, Mailing Address: Box 2668, Zip 70404; tel. 504/345–2700; James E. Cathey, Jr., Chief Executive Officer **A**1 9 10 **F**1 4 7 8 10 12 15 16 19 22 23 26 28 32 33 34 35 37 38 39 41 42 43 44 45 46 48 49 52 56 57 58 64 65 66 67 71 73 74 **S** Quorum Health Group/Quorum Health Resources, Inc., Brentwood, TN **N** Center Care, Bowling Green, KY — 16 10 245 8926 117 105088 1453 79572 42567 1411

HOMER—Claiborne Parish

HOMER MEMORIAL HOSPITAL, 620 East College Street, Zip 71040; tel. 318/927–2024; J. Larry Jordan, Administrator (Nonreporting) **A**3 5 9 10 **N** Ochsner/Sisters of Charity Health Network, New Orleans, LA — 14 10 57

HOUMA—Terrebonne Parish

□ BAYOU OAKS HOSPITAL, 8134 Main Street, Zip 70360, Mailing Address: P.O. Box 4374, Zip 70361–4374; tel. 504/876–2020; George H. Perry, Ph.D., Chief Executive Officer (Nonreporting) **A**1 10 **S** Ramsay Health Care, Inc., Coral Gobles, FL — 33 22 86

□ LEONARD J. CHABERT MEDICAL CENTER, 1978 Industrial Boulevard, Zip 70363; tel. 504/873–2200; William C. Bankston, Acting Administrator **A**1 3 10 **F**8 19 21 22 25 31 37 38 40 41 42 44 45 49 51 52 53 65 70 71 73 74 **S** Louisiana Health Care Authority, Baton Rouge, LA **N** Louisiana Health Care Authority, Baton Rouge, LA — 12 10 151 7041 81 156742 1159 49129 21427 926

✇ TERREBONNE GENERAL MEDICAL CENTER, 936 East Main Street, Zip 70360, Mailing Address: Box 6037, Zip 70361; tel. 504/873–4664; Alex B. Smith, Ph.D., Executive Director (Total facility includes 16 beds in nursing home–type unit) **A**1 9 10 **F**3 4 7 8 10 11 12 13 14 15 16 17 18 19 21 22 26 27 28 29 30 32 33 34 35 37 39 40 41 42 43 44 45 46 48 49 51 60 63 64 65 67 68 71 72 73 74 **P**6 7 — 16 10 261 10269 160 74686 885 83841 40071 1333

INDEPENDENCE—Tagipahoa Parish

□ LALLIE KEMP MEDICAL CENTER, 52579 Highway 51 South, Zip 70443; tel. 504/878–9421; LeVern Meades, Acting Administrator **A**1 10 **F**2 8 12 13 15 16 17 19 20 21 28 29 30 31 32 34 37 39 42 44 45 49 51 65 67 71 72 73 74 **P**1 3 **S** Louisiana Health Care Authority, Baton Rouge, LA **N** Louisiana Health Care Authority, Baton Rouge, LA — 12 10 68 3137 53 125540 0 27581 14197 462

JACKSON—East Feliciana Parish

□ EAST LOUISIANA STATE HOSPITAL, Mailing Address: P.O. Box 498, Zip 70748; tel. 504/634–0100; Warren T. Price, Jr., Chief Executive Officer (Nonreporting) **A**1 10 **S** Louisiana State Hospitals, New Orleans, LA — 12 22 452 — — — — — — —

✇ VILLA FELICIANA CHRONIC DISEASE HOSPITAL AND REHABILITATION CENTER, Mailing Address: P.O. Box 438, Zip 70748; tel. 504/634–4000; Bob L. Wilson, Administrator (Total facility includes 264 beds in nursing home–type unit) **A**1 10 **F**20 26 27 54 57 64 65 73 — 12 48 275 71 258 0 0 15835 9760 437

JEFFERSON—Jefferson Parish

✇ COLUMBIA JEFFERSON MEDICAL CENTER, 1221 South Clearview Parkway, Zip 70121; tel. 504/734–1900; David E. Hoidal, Chief Executive Officer (Nonreporting) **A**1 10 **S** Columbia/HCA Healthcare Corporation, Nashville, TN — 33 10 108 — — — — — — —

JENA—La Salle Parish

★ LA SALLE GENERAL HOSPITAL, Highway 84, Zip 71342–1388, Mailing Address: P.O. Box 1388, Zip 71342; tel. 318/992–8231; Mary M. Denton, Administrator (Total facility includes 10 beds in nursing home–type unit) **A**9 10 **F**19 22 28 30 32 44 49 59 64 71 — 16 10 67 1641 34 11547 0 9327 4201 179

JENNINGS—Jefferson Davis Parish

✇ JENNINGS AMERICAN LEGION HOSPITAL, 1634 Elton Road, Zip 70546; tel. 318/821–4151; Terry J. Terrebonne, Administrator **A**1 9 10 **F**7 8 12 15 16 17 19 21 22 30 32 34 35 37 39 40 42 44 45 46 65 71 73 **N** Ochsner/Sisters of Charity Health Network, New Orleans, LA — 23 10 49 2577 23 16740 342 11681 4285 201

JONESBORO—Jackson Parish

JACKSON PARISH HOSPITAL, 165 Beech Springs Road, Zip 71251; tel. 318/259–4435; Delmar J. Medill, Interim Chief Executive Officer (Nonreporting) **A**9 10 **S** Brim, Inc., Portland, OR — 16 10 59

KAPLAN—Vermilion Parish

ABROM KAPLAN MEMORIAL HOSPITAL, 1310 West Seventh Street, Zip 70548; tel. 318/643–8300; Lyman Trahan, Administrator **A**9 10 **F**8 11 16 19 21 22 28 30 32 33 35 37 39 41 44 52 54 55 56 57 58 59 65 71 73 — 16 10 60 745 18 33870 0 7284 2032 87

KENNER—Jefferson Parish

□ KENNER REGIONAL MEDICAL CENTER, (Formerly St. Jude Medical Center), 180 West Esplanade Avenue, Zip 70065; tel. 504/468–8600; Steven J. Greene, Chief Executive Officer **A**1 9 10 **F**2 3 4 6 7 8 10 12 13 14 15 19 20 21 22 24 25 26 27 28 29 30 31 32 33 34 35 37 38 39 41 42 43 44 45 46 47 48 49 50 52 53 54 55 56 57 58 59 60 61 63 64 65 66 67 68 69 71 72 73 74 **P**1 5 7 **S** TENET Healthcare Corporation, Santa Barbara, CA **N** Tenet Louisiana Health System Network, Metairie, LA — 33 10 213 4105 75 26110 278 31921 13015 423

Hospital, Address, Telephone, Administrator, Approval, Facility, and Physician Codes, Health Care System, Network	Classi-fication Codes		Utilization Data					Expense (thousands) of dollars		
★ American Hospital Association (AHA) membership □ Joint Commission on Accreditation of Healthcare Organizations (JCAHO) accreditation + American Osteopathic Hospital Association (AOHA) membership ○ American Osteopathic Association (AOA) accreditation △ Commission on Accreditation of Rehabilitation Facilities (CARF) accreditation Control codes 61, 63, 64, 71, 72 and 73 indicate hospitals listed by AOHA, but not registered by AHA. For definition of numerical codes, see page A4	Control	Service	Beds	Admissions	Census	Outpatient Visits	Births	Total	Payroll	Personnel

KINDER—Allen Parish

★ ALLEN PARISH HOSPITAL, Mailing Address: P.O. Box 1670, Zip 70648; tel. 318/738–2527; William C. Jeanmard, Chief Executive Officer **A**9 10 **F**2 15 16 19 22 32 34 52 65 71 73 **P**5

| | 16 | 10 | 42 | 906 | 21 | 4612 | 0 | 4318 | 2306 | 81 |

LAFAYETTE—Lafayette Parish

⊠ CHARTER CYPRESS BEHAVIORAL HEALTH SYSTEM, 302 Dulles Drive, Zip 70506; tel. 318/233–9024; Denise Guthrie, Chief Executive Officer (Nonreporting) **A**1 **S** Magellan Health Services, Atlanta, GA

| | 33 | 22 | 70 | — | — | — | — | — | — | — |

⊠ COLUMBIA MEDICAL CENTER OF SOUTHWEST LOUISIANA, 2810 Ambassador Caffery Parkway, Zip 70506; tel. 318/981–2949; Gerald A. Fornoff, Chief Executive Officer **A**1 9 10 **F**4 8 10 12 15 16 19 21 22 30 32 34 35 37 41 43 44 45 46 48 49 63 64 65 71 73 **P**7 8 **S** Columbia/HCA Healthcare Corporation, Nashville, TN **N** Center Care, Bowling Green, KY

| | 33 | 10 | 107 | 3723 | 53 | 99625 | 0 | 31325 | 12053 | 334 |

⊠ COLUMBIA WOMEN'S AND CHILDREN'S HOSPITAL, 4600 Ambassador Caffery Parkway, Zip 70508, Mailing Address: P.O. Box 88030, Zip 70598–8030; tel. 318/981–9100; Madeleine L. Roberson, Chief Executive Officer **A**1 9 10 **F**7 8 11 12 14 15 16 19 20 24 32 34 35 37 38 40 41 43 44 48 49 64 65 71 73 74 **P**1 7 **S** Columbia/HCA Healthcare Corporation, Nashville, TN **N** Center Care, Bowling Green, KY

| | 33 | 44 | 96 | 3558 | 36 | 36876 | 2202 | 15817 | 7220 | 280 |

⊠ △ LAFAYETTE GENERAL MEDICAL CENTER, 1214 Coolidge Avenue, Zip 70503, Mailing Address: Box 52009 OCS, Zip 70505; tel. 318/289–7991; John J. Burdin, Jr., President and Chief Executive Officer (Total facility includes 30 beds in nursing home–type unit) **A**1 2 6 7 9 10 **F**1 2 3 4 7 8 10 11 12 13 14 15 16 17 18 19 20 21 22 24 25 27 28 29 30 32 33 34 35 36 37 38 39 40 41 42 43 44 45 46 47 48 49 50 52 53 54 55 56 57 58 60 61 63 64 65 66 67 68 71 72 73 74 **P**5 7 8

| | 23 | 10 | 320 | 13524 | 179 | — | 1286 | 114887 | 48066 | 1600 |

⊠ △ OUR LADY OF LOURDES REGIONAL MEDICAL CENTER, 611 St. Landry Street, Zip 70506–4697, Mailing Address: Box 4027, Zip 70502–4027; tel. 318/289–2000; Dudley Romero, President and Chief Executive Officer (Total facility includes 25 beds in nursing home–type unit) **A**1 2 7 9 10 **F**4 7 8 10 11 12 13 14 15 16 17 19 21 22 23 24 25 26 28 29 30 31 32 33 34 35 37 39 40 41 42 43 44 45 46 48 49 60 63 64 65 66 67 69 71 73 **P**7 8 **S** Franciscan Missionaries of Our Lady Health System, Inc., Baton Rouge, LA **N** Franciscan Missionaries of Our Lady Health Network, Baton Rouge, LA

| | 21 | 10 | 293 | 10398 | 162 | 67398 | 390 | 94694 | 37343 | 1232 |

□ UNIVERSITY MEDICAL CENTER, 2390 West Congress Street, Zip 70506, Mailing Address: P.O. Box 4016–C, Zip 70502–4016; tel. 318/261–6004; Lawrence T. Dorsey, Administrator **A**1 2 3 5 10 **F**2 8 10 19 21 22 25 31 37 38 39 40 42 44 45 46 49 51 52 56 57 59 60 61 65 67 71 73 74 **P**1 **S** Louisiana Health Care Authority, Baton Rouge, LA **N** Louisiana Health Care Authority, Baton Rouge, LA

| | 12 | 10 | 161 | 8686 | 112 | 152511 | 1182 | 46105 | 23693 | 1004 |

★ VERMILION HOSPITAL, 2520 North University, Zip 70507, Mailing Address: P.O. Box 91526, Zip 70509–1526; tel. 318/234–5614; John P. Patout, Administrator (Nonreporting) **A**10 **S** General Health System, Baton Rouge, LA

| | 23 | 22 | 54 | — | — | — | — | — | — | — |

LAKE CHARLES—Calcasieu Parish

□ CHARTER BEHAVIORAL HEALTH SYSTEM OF LAKE CHARLES, 4250 Fifth Avenue South, Zip 70605–3812; tel. 318/474–6133; Charles P. Whitson, Chief Executive Officer (Nonreporting) **A**1 10 **S** Magellan Health Services, Atlanta, GA
COLUMBIA LAKE AREA MEDICAL CENTER See Columbia Women and Children's Hospital–Lake Charles

| | 33 | 22 | 60 | — | — | — | — | — | — | — |

⊠ COLUMBIA WOMEN AND CHILDREN'S HOSPITAL–LAKE CHARLES, (Formerly Columbia Lake Area Medical Center), 4200 Nelson Road, Zip 70605; tel. 318/474–6370; Alan E. McMillin, Chief Executive Officer **A**1 9 10 **F**7 8 12 19 22 32 37 38 40 44 49 61 65 71 73 74 **P**7 **S** Columbia/HCA Healthcare Corporation, Nashville, TN

| | 33 | 10 | 72 | 2101 | 20 | 19662 | 1154 | 12962 | 5878 | 166 |

□ LAKE CHARLES MEMORIAL HOSPITAL, 1701 Oak Park Boulevard, Zip 70601, Mailing Address: P.O. Drawer M, Zip 70602; tel. 318/494–3000; Elton L. Williams, Jr., CPA, President (Total facility includes 20 beds in nursing home–type unit) (Nonreporting) **A**1 2 3 9 10

| | 16 | 10 | 303 | — | — | — | — | — | — | — |

⊠ △ ST. PATRICK HOSPITAL OF LAKE CHARLES, 524 South Ryan Street, Zip 70601, Mailing Address: P.O. Box 3401, Zip 70602–3401; tel. 318/436–2511; J. William Hankins, President and Chief Executive Officer (Total facility includes 22 beds in nursing home–type unit) **A**1 2 7 9 10 **F**2 3 4 7 8 10 11 12 15 16 17 19 21 22 24 28 29 30 32 33 35 37 39 40 41 42 43 44 46 48 49 51 57 60 64 65 66 67 71 73 74 **P**7 8 **S** Sisters of Charity of the Incarnate Word Healthcare System, Houston, TX **N** Ochsner/Sisters of Charity Health Network, New Orleans, LA

| | 21 | 10 | 298 | 9787 | 163 | 94710 | 405 | 80235 | 31302 | 1128 |

WALTER OLIN MOSS REGIONAL MEDICAL CENTER, 1000 Walters Street, Zip 70605; tel. 318/475–8100; Philip H. Rome, Administrator **A**5 10 **F**8 10 11 13 14 15 16 19 21 22 25 27 30 31 34 35 37 39 42 44 45 46 48 49 51 52 53 54 56 58 60 64 65 71 73 **P**7 **S** Louisiana Health Care Authority, Baton Rouge, LA **N** Louisiana Health Care Authority, Baton Rouge, LA

| | 12 | 10 | 66 | 2566 | 40 | 57233 | 0 | — | — | 459 |

LAKE PROVIDENCE—East Carroll Parish

EAST CARROLL PARISH HOSPITAL, 226 North Hood Street, Zip 71254; tel. 318/559–2441; Ladonna Englerth, Administrator (Nonreporting) **A**9 10

| | 16 | 10 | 29 | — | — | — | — | — | — | — |

LAPLACE—St. John the Baptist Parish

□ RIVER PARISHES HOSPITAL, 500 Rue De Sante, Zip 70068; tel. 504/652–7000; John Lloyd Hummer, Chief Executive Officer and Managing Director **A**1 9 **F**7 8 12 14 15 16 17 19 21 22 27 28 30 32 35 37 40 44 49 54 57 58 59 63 65 66 71 73 **P**1 **S** Universal Health Services, Inc., King of Prussia, PA

| | 33 | 10 | 60 | 2238 | 23 | 30608 | 422 | 22741 | — | 245 |

Hospital, Address, Telephone, Administrator, Approval, Facility, and Physician Codes, Health Care System, Network	Classi-fication Codes		Utilization Data					Expense (thousands) of dollars		
★ American Hospital Association (AHA) membership □ Joint Commission on Accreditation of Healthcare Organizations (JCAHO) accreditation + American Osteopathic Hospital Association (AOHA) membership ○ American Osteopathic Association (AOA) accreditation △ Commission on Accreditation of Rehabilitation Facilities (CARF) accreditation Control codes 61, 63, 64, 71, 72 and 73 indicate hospitals listed by AOHA, but not registered by AHA. For definition of numerical codes, see page A4	Control	Service	Beds	Admissions	Census	Outpatient Visits	Births	Total	Payroll	Personnel

LEESVILLE—Vernon Parish
□ BYRD REGIONAL HOSPITAL, 1020 Fertitta Boulevard, Zip 71446; tel. 318/239–9041; Donald Henderson, Executive Director **A**1 9 10 **F**8 10 12 15 16 19 28 30 35 37 44 57 63 71 **P**7 8 **S** Community Health Systems, Inc., Brentwood, TN **N** Ochsner/Sisters of Charity Health Network, New Orleans, LA	33	10	59	2151	29	18655	0	—	—	229

LULING—St. Charles Parish
□ ST. CHARLES PARISH HOSPITAL, 1057 Paul Maillard Road, Zip 70070, Mailing Address: P.O. Box 87, Zip 70070–0087; tel. 504/785–6242; Fred Martinez, Jr., Administrator **A**1 9 10 **F**8 11 12 14 15 17 19 22 26 28 29 30 32 34 35 37 41 42 44 45 49 52 54 55 56 57 65 66 67 71 73 **P**8	16	10	104	1437	48	16698	7	18425	8300	323

LUTCHER—St. James Parish
✚ ST. JAMES PARISH HOSPITAL, 2471 Louisiana Avenue, Zip 70071; tel. 504/869–5512; Joan Murray, R.N., Administrator **A**1 9 10 **F**8 15 16 17 22 26 28 30 34 36 39 41 44 45 46 49 52 53 54 56 57 58 65 67 71 **P**8	16	10	28	319	4	12778	0	6939	2974	109

MAMOU—Evangeline Parish
✚ SAVOY MEDICAL CENTER, 801 Poinciana Avenue, Zip 70554; tel. 318/468–5261; J. E. Richardson, Chief Executive Officer (Total facility includes 355 beds in nursing home–type unit) **A**1 9 10 **F**1 2 3 7 8 12 15 16 19 21 22 26 28 29 30 31 32 33 34 35 37 40 42 44 45 46 48 49 52 53 57 61 64 65 68 71 73 **P**8 **S** Columbia/HCA Healthcare Corporation, Nashville, TN	33	10	503	3864	319	—	531	48784	20103	787

MANSFIELD—De Soto Parish
★ DE SOTO REGIONAL HEALTH SYSTEM, (Formerly De Soto General Hospital), 207 Jefferson Street, Zip 71052, Mailing Address: P.O. Box 672, Zip 71052; tel. 318/872–4610; William F. Barrow, President and Chief Executive Officer **A**9 10 **F**8 14 15 19 22 28 32 42 44 49 52 57 71 73 **P**3 **N** Ochsner/Sisters of Charity Health Network, New Orleans, LA	23	10	49	1267	20	11335	0	6734	2456	116

MANY—Sabine Parish
□ SABINE MEDICAL CENTER, 240 Highland Drive, Zip 71449–3718; tel. 318/256–5691; Mark Nosacka, Executive Director (Nonreporting) **A**1 9 **S** Community Health Systems, Inc., Brentwood, TN **N** Ochsner/Sisters of Charity Health Network, New Orleans, LA	33	10	68	—	—	—	—	—	—	—

MARKSVILLE—Avoyelles Parish
✚ AVOYELLES HOSPITAL, 4231 Highway 1192, Zip 71351, Mailing Address: Box 255, Zip 71351; tel. 318/253–8611; David M. Mitchel, Chief Executive Officer (Nonreporting) **A**1 9 10 **S** Columbia/HCA Healthcare Corporation, Nashville, TN	33	10	55	—	—	—	—	—	—	—

MARRERO—Jefferson Parish
✚ WEST JEFFERSON MEDICAL CENTER, 1101 Medical Center Boulevard, Zip 70072–3191; tel. 504/347–5511; David M. Smith, FACHE, President and Chief Executive Officer (Total facility includes 30 beds in nursing home–type unit) **A**1 9 10 **F**1 2 4 7 8 10 11 12 14 15 17 19 20 21 22 23 24 28 30 32 35 37 38 40 41 42 43 44 45 46 47 48 49 50 51 52 56 60 63 64 65 66 67 70 71 73 74 **N** Healthcare Advantage, Inc., New Orleans, LA; Ochsner/Sisters of Charity Health Network, New Orleans, LA	16	10	382	13421	190	114382	1277	109560	47154	1692

METAIRIE—Jefferson Parish
✚ COLUMBIA LAKESIDE HOSPITAL, (Formerly Lakeside Hospital), 4700 I–10 Service Road, Zip 70001–1269; tel. 504/885–3333; M. P. Gandy, Jr., President (Nonreporting) **A**1 9 10 **S** Columbia/HCA Healthcare Corporation, Nashville, TN	33	44	99	—	—	—	—	—	—	—
✚ DOCTORS HOSPITAL OF JEFFERSON, 4320 Houma Boulevard, Zip 70006–2973; tel. 504/456–5800; Gerald L. Parton, Chief Executive Officer (Nonreporting) **A**1 9 10 **S** TENET Healthcare Corporation, Santa Barbara, CA **N** Tenet Louisiana Health System Network, Metairie, LA; Healthcare Advantage, Inc., New Orleans, LA	33	10	114	—	—	—	—	—	—	—
✚ △ EAST JEFFERSON GENERAL HOSPITAL, 4200 Houma Boulevard, Zip 70011–9987; tel. 504/454–4000; Peter J. Betts, President and Chief Executive Officer (Total facility includes 71 beds in nursing home–type unit) **A**1 2 3 5 7 9 10 **F**3 4 7 8 10 11 16 19 20 22 27 29 30 32 33 34 35 37 38 39 40 41 42 43 44 48 49 52 58 60 64 65 67 68 71 73 74 **P**6 7 8 **N** Healthcare Advantage, Inc., New Orleans, LA	16	10	447	17843	304	152798	1528	171418	69935	2437
LAKESIDE HOSPITAL See Columbia Lakeside Hospital										

MINDEN—Webster Parish
□ MINDEN MEDICAL CENTER, 1 Medical Plaza, Zip 71055; tel. 318/377–2321; George E. French, III, Chief Executive Officer **A**1 9 10 **F**7 8 12 14 15 16 17 19 22 28 29 32 33 35 37 40 41 42 44 46 49 52 57 65 66 71 73 74 **S** TENET Healthcare Corporation, Santa Barbara, CA **N** Ochsner/Sisters of Charity Health Network, New Orleans, LA	33	10	121	3681	41	76996	672	17713	9438	296

MONROE—Ouachita Parish
✚ △ COLUMBIA NORTH MONROE HOSPITAL, 3421 Medical Park Drive, Zip 71203; tel. 318/388–1946; George E. Miller, Chief Executive Officer (Total facility includes 13 beds in nursing home–type unit) (Nonreporting) **A**1 7 9 **S** Columbia/HCA Healthcare Corporation, Nashville, TN	33	10	210	—	—	—	—	—	—	—
□ E. A. CONWAY MEDICAL CENTER, 4864 Jackson Street, Zip 71202, Mailing Address: P.O. Box 1881, Zip 71210–8005; tel. 318/330–7000; Roy D. Bostick, Director **A**1 3 5 10 **F**8 15 19 22 28 31 35 37 38 40 42 43 44 52 56 60 65 71 73 **P**1 **S** Louisiana Health Care Authority, Baton Rouge, LA **N** Louisiana Health Care Authority, Baton Rouge, LA	12	10	223	7834	129	160514	1648	47198	22865	880
✚ ST. FRANCIS MEDICAL CENTER, 309 Jackson Street, Zip 71201, Mailing Address: Box 1901, Zip 71210–1901; tel. 318/327–4000; H. Gerald Smith, President and Chief Executive Officer **A**1 2 9 10 **F**4 7 8 10 11 16 17 19 20 21 22 24 26 28 29 30 31 32 33 34 35 36 37 38 39 41 42 43 44 46 49 50 52 57 59 60 64 65 71 73 74 **P**8 **S** Franciscan Missionaries of Our Lady Health System, Inc., Baton Rouge, LA **N** Franciscan Missionaries of Our Lady Health Network, Baton Rouge, LA	21	10	385	11266	206	67509	993	109870	40423	1406

Hospital, Address, Telephone, Administrator, Approval, Facility, and Physician Codes, Health Care System, Network	Classification Codes		Utilization Data					Expense (thousands) of dollars		
★ American Hospital Association (AHA) membership □ Joint Commission on Accreditation of Healthcare Organizations (JCAHO) accreditation + American Osteopathic Hospital Association (AOHA) membership ○ American Osteopathic Association (AOA) accreditation △ Commission on Accreditation of Rehabilitation Facilities (CARF) accreditation Control codes 61, 63, 64, 71, 72 and 73 indicate hospitals listed by AOHA, but not registered by AHA. For definition of numerical codes, see page A4	Control	Service	Beds	Admissions	Census	Outpatient Visits	Births	Total	Payroll	Personnel

MORGAN CITY—St. Mary Parish

☒ LAKEWOOD MEDICAL CENTER, (Formerly Lakewood Hospital), 1125 Marguerite Street, Zip 70380, Mailing Address: Drawer 2308, Zip 70381; tel. 504/384–2200; Joyce Grove Hein, Chief Executive Officer (Total facility includes 10 beds in nursing home–type unit) **A**1 9 10 **F**7 8 10 11 14 15 16 17 19 22 23 26 28 30 32 34 35 37 39 40 42 44 45 46 49 52 55 56 57 59 64 65 71 73 74 **S** Quorum Health Group/Quorum Health Resources, Inc., Brentwood, TN ... 16 | 10 | 122 | 2928 | 30 | 38319 | 481 | 21150 | 9261 | 345

NAPOLEONVILLE—Assumption Parish

OUR LADY OF THE LAKE–ASSUMPTION See Our Lady of the Lake Regional Medical Center, Baton Rouge

NATCHITOCHES—Natchitoches Parish

□ NATCHITOCHES PARISH HOSPITAL, 501 Keyser Avenue, Zip 71457, Mailing Address: Box 2009, Zip 71457–2009; tel. 318/352–1200; Eugene Spillman, Executive Director (Total facility includes 112 beds in nursing home–type unit) **A**1 9 10 **F**1 7 8 14 16 19 21 22 23 24 26 30 32 33 34 36 37 40 41 44 46 49 52 57 59 64 65 71 73 **P**5 **N** Ochsner/Sisters of Charity Health Network, New Orleans, LA ... 13 | 10 | 166 | 3024 | 139 | 36773 | 515 | 14796 | 6889 | 212

NEW IBERIA—Iberia Parish

☒ COLUMBIA DAUTERIVE HOSPITAL, 600 North Lewis Street, Zip 70560, Mailing Address: P.O. Box 11210, Zip 70562–1210; tel. 318/365–7311; Kyle J. Viator, Chief Executive Officer (Total facility includes 10 beds in nursing home–type unit) (Nonreporting) **A**1 9 10 **S** Columbia/HCA Healthcare Corporation, Nashville, TN **N** Center Care, Bowling Green, KY ... 33 | 10 | 92

☒ IBERIA GENERAL HOSPITAL AND MEDICAL CENTER, 2315 East Main Street, Zip 70560, Mailing Address: P.O. Box 13338, Zip 70562–3338; tel. 318/364–0441; Robert R. Stanley, Chief Executive Officer (Total facility includes 12 beds in nursing home–type unit) **A**1 9 10 **F**7 8 10 13 14 19 21 22 28 30 32 35 37 40 41 44 49 64 71 73 **P**8 ... 16 | 10 | 75 | 3855 | 48 | 60634 | 510 | 29134 | 11268 | 434

NEW ORLEANS—Orleans Parish

□ BHC EAST LAKE HOSPITAL, (Formerly CPC Metro Behavioral Health Services), 5650 Read Boulevard, Zip 70127–3145; tel. 504/241–0888; Darlene Salvant, Chief Executive Officer (Nonreporting) **A**1 10 **S** Behavioral Healthcare Corporation, Nashville, TN ... 33 | 22 | 72

CHARITY CAMPUS See Medical Center of Louisiana at New Orleans

□ △ CHILDREN'S HOSPITAL, 200 Henry Clay Avenue, Zip 70118–5799; tel. 504/899–9511; Steve Worley, President and Chief Executive Officer **A**1 2 3 5 7 9 10 **F**4 5 10 12 19 20 21 22 28 31 34 35 38 39 42 43 44 46 47 48 49 53 54 56 58 65 66 67 69 71 72 73 **P**8 ... 23 | 50 | 175 | 6246 | 99 | 126308 | 0 | — | — | 1004

COLUMBIA DEPAUL HOSPITAL See DePaul/Tulane Behavioral Health Center

☒ △ COLUMBIA LAKELAND MEDICAL CENTER, (Formerly Lakeland Medical Center), 6000 Bullard Avenue, Zip 70128; tel. 504/241–6335; Trudy Land, Chief Executive Officer **A**1 7 9 10 **F**2 3 4 7 8 10 11 12 15 16 17 18 19 21 22 23 24 25 28 30 31 32 33 34 35 37 38 39 40 42 43 44 45 47 48 49 51 52 53 54 55 56 57 58 59 60 61 63 64 65 67 69 70 71 73 **P**7 8 **S** Columbia/HCA Healthcare Corporation, Nashville, TN ... 33 | 10 | 130 | 5086 | 77 | 31024 | 1002 | 32978 | 14285 | 508

CPC METRO BEHAVIORAL HEALTH SERVICES See BHC East Lake Hospital

☒ DEPAUL/TULANE BEHAVIORAL HEALTH CENTER, (Formerly Columbia DePaul Hospital), 1040 Calhoun Street, Zip 70118; tel. 504/899–8282; David E. Hoidal, Chief Executive Officer (Nonreporting) **A**1 10 **S** Behavioral Healthcare Corporation, Nashville, TN ... 33 | 22 | 102

□ JO ELLEN SMITH MEDICAL CENTER, 4444 General Meyer Avenue, Zip 70131; tel. 504/363–7011; Michael Manning, Chief Executive Officer (Nonreporting) **A**1 3 9 10 **N** Tenet Louisiana Health System Network, Metairie, LA ... 33 | 10 | 186

LAKELAND MEDICAL CENTER See Columbia Lakeland Medical Center

□ MEDICAL CENTER OF LOUISIANA AT NEW ORLEANS, (Includes Charity Campus, 1532 Tulane Avenue, Zip 70140; tel. 504/568–3201; University Campus, 2021 Perdido Street, Mailing Address: Box 61262, Zip 70161–1262), 2021 Perdido Street, Zip 70112–1396; tel. 504/588–3000; Jonathan Roberts, Dr.PH, President and Chief Executive Officer (Nonreporting) **A**1 2 3 5 8 9 10 **N** Tenet Louisiana Health System Network, Metairie, LA; Louisiana Health Care Authority, Baton Rouge, LA ... 12 | 10 | 746

☒ △ MEMORIAL MEDICAL CENTER, (Formerly Mercy Baptist Medical Center), (Includes Eye, Ear, Nose and Throat Hospital, 2626 Napoleon Avenue, tel. 504/896–1100; Memorial Medical Center–Baptist Campus, Memorial Medical Center–Mercy Campus, 301 North Jefferson Davis Parkway, Zip 70119; tel. 504/483–5000), 2700 Napoleon Avenue, Zip 70115; tel. 504/899–9311; Randall L. Hoover, Chief Executive Officer **A**1 2 3 5 7 9 10 **F**1 4 7 8 10 11 12 19 22 24 26 28 30 32 33 35 37 38 40 41 42 43 44 45 46 49 60 64 65 66 67 69 71 72 73 74 **S** TENET Healthcare Corporation, Santa Barbara, CA ... 33 | 10 | 522 | 13806 | 305 | 68540 | 1327 | 118361 | 50753 | 2012

MEMORIAL MEDICAL CENTER–MERCY CAMPUS See Memorial Medical Center
MERCY BAPTIST MEDICAL CENTER See Memorial Medical Center
MERCY HOSPITAL OF NEW ORLEANS See Memorial Medical Center

□ METHODIST BEHAVIORAL RESOURCES, 5610 Read Boulevard, Zip 70127; tel. 504/244–5661; Daniel Aguillard, Chief Executive Officer **A**1 10 **F**1 2 3 14 18 22 25 26 32 34 41 52 53 54 55 56 57 58 59 65 **P**5 ... 32 | 22 | 36 | 1137 | 40 | — | 0 | 7072 | 3164 | 85

Hospital, Address, Telephone, Administrator, Approval, Facility, and Physician Codes, Health Care System, Network	Classi-fication Codes		Utilization Data					Expense (thousands) of dollars		
★ American Hospital Association (AHA) membership □ Joint Commission on Accreditation of Healthcare Organizations (JCAHO) accreditation + American Osteopathic Hospital Association (AOHA) membership ○ American Osteopathic Association (AOA) accreditation △ Commission on Accreditation of Rehabilitation Facilities (CARF) accreditation Control codes 61, 63, 64, 71, 72 and 73 indicate hospitals listed by AOHA, but not registered by AHA. For definition of numerical codes, see page A4	Control	Service	Beds	Admissions	Census	Outpatient Visits	Births	Total	Payroll	Personnel

Hospital	Control	Service	Beds	Admissions	Census	Outpatient Visits	Births	Total	Payroll	Personnel
□ NEW ORLEANS ADOLESCENT HOSPITAL, 210 State Street, Zip 70118; tel. 504/897–3400; Michael E. Teague, Chief Executive Officer (Nonreporting) **A**1 10 **S** Louisiana State Hospitals, New Orleans, LA	12	22	99	—	—	—	—	—	—	—
★ △ OCHSNER FOUNDATION HOSPITAL, 1516 Jefferson Highway, Zip 70121; tel. 504/842–3000; Mary W. Brown, Executive Vice President and Director (Total facility includes 31 beds in nursing home–type unit) (Nonreporting) **A**1 2 3 5 7 8 9 10 **N** Ochsner/Sisters of Charity Health Network, New Orleans, LA	23	10	411	—	—	—	—	—	—	—
★ PENDLETON MEMORIAL METHODIST HOSPITAL, 5620 Read Boulevard, Zip 70127–3154; tel. 504/244–5100; Frederick C. Young, Jr., President (Total facility includes 22 beds in nursing home–type unit) **A**1 9 10 **F**4 10 11 15 17 19 22 23 32 35 37 38 39 40 42 43 44 46 49 60 64 71 73 **N** Healthcare Advantage, Inc., New Orleans, LA; Ochsner/Sisters of Charity Health Network, New Orleans, LA	23	10	163	6746	108	71836	1012	81686	32881	991
□ RIVER OAKS HOSPITAL, 1525 River Oaks Road West, Zip 70123; tel. 504/734–1740; Daryl Sue White, R.N., Managing Director (Nonreporting) **A**1 10 **S** Universal Health Services, Inc., King of Prussia, PA	33	22	94	—	—	—	—	—	—	—
□ ST. CHARLES GENERAL HOSPITAL, 3700 St. Charles Avenue, Zip 70115; tel. 504/899–7441; Lynn C. Orfgen, Chief Executive Officer **A**1 9 10 **F**2 11 14 16 17 19 20 22 27 34 35 37 38 40 41 44 45 46 47 48 49 52 64 65 67 71 73 **P**1 5 7 **S** TENET Healthcare Corporation, Santa Barbara, CA **N** Tenet Louisiana Health System Network, Metairie, LA	33	10	137	3662	62	7518	0	—	—	272
□ ST. CLAUDE MEDICAL CENTER, (Formerly United Medical Center), 3419 St. Claude Avenue, Zip 70117; tel. 504/948–8200; Joseph R. Tucker, President (Nonreporting) **A**1 9 10 **S** United Medical Corporation, Windermere, FL	33	10	136	—	—	—	—	—	—	—
□ THC–NEW ORLEANS, 3601 Coliseum Street, Zip 70115; tel. 504/899–1555; John R. Watkins, Chief Executive Officer (Nonreporting) **A**1 10 **S** Transitional Hospitals Corporation, Las Vegas, NV	33	10	78	—	—	—	—	—	—	—
□ △ TOURO INFIRMARY, 1401 Foucher Street, Zip 70115–3593; tel. 504/897–7011; Gary M. Stein, President and Chief Executive Officer **A**1 2 3 5 7 8 9 10 **F**1 4 7 8 10 11 12 14 15 16 17 18 19 21 22 23 24 25 26 28 29 30 32 34 35 37 38 39 40 41 42 43 44 45 46 48 49 51 52 54 55 56 57 58 59 60 61 63 64 65 66 67 70 71 72 73 74 **P**1 7	23	10	326	8916	181	119625	915	103279	45748	1332
★ TULANE UNIVERSITY HOSPITAL AND CLINIC, 1415 Tulane Avenue, Zip 70112–2632; tel. 504/588–5263; Stephen A. Pickett, President and Chief Executive Officer **A**1 2 3 5 8 9 10 **F**3 4 7 8 10 11 14 16 19 21 22 23 28 30 31 32 34 35 37 38 39 40 41 42 43 44 46 47 49 51 52 53 54 55 56 57 58 59 63 65 69 71 73 74 **P**1 **S** Columbia/HCA Healthcare Corporation, Nashville, TN	33	10	259	9289	165	290564	605	—	—	1558
UNITED MEDICAL CENTER See St. Claude Medical Center										
UNIVERSITY CAMPUS See Medical Center of Louisiana at New Orleans										
UNIVERSITY REHABILITATION HOSPITAL, 3125 Canal Street, Zip 70119; tel. 504/822–8222; Robert A. Leonhard, Jr., Administrator (Nonreporting) **A**10	33	10	40	—	—	—	—	—	—	—
★ VETERANS AFFAIRS MEDICAL CENTER, 1601 Perdido Street, Zip 70146; tel. 504/568–0811; John D. Church, Jr., Director (Total facility includes 60 beds in nursing home–type unit) **A**1 2 3 5 8 **F**2 3 4 8 10 11 12 14 15 16 17 18 19 20 22 26 27 28 29 30 31 32 33 34 35 37 39 42 43 44 45 46 49 51 52 54 55 56 57 58 59 63 64 65 67 71 73 74 **S** Department of Veterans Affairs, Washington, DC	45	10	285	7095	237	277417	0	—	—	1971
NEW ROADS—Pointe Coupee Parish										
★ POINTE COUPEE GENERAL HOSPITAL, 2202 False River Drive, Zip 70760; tel. 504/638–6331; Larry J. Ayres, Administrator and Chief Executive Officer (Nonreporting) **A**9 10	16	10	29	—	—	—	—	—	—	—
OAK GROVE—West Carroll Parish										
WEST CARROLL MEMORIAL HOSPITAL, Ross Street, Zip 71263, Mailing Address: Box 748, Zip 71263; tel. 318/428–3237; Randall R. Morris, Administrator **A**9 10 **F**17 19 22 32 34 35 45 63	23	10	21	997	10	—	0	—	—	148
OAKDALE—Allen Parish										
★ OAKDALE COMMUNITY HOSPITAL, 130 North Hospital Drive, Zip 71463, Mailing Address: Box 629, Zip 71463; tel. 318/335–3700; LaQuita Johnson, Chief Executive Officer (Nonreporting) **A**1 9 10 **S** Columbia/HCA Healthcare Corporation, Nashville, TN	32	10	60	—	—	—	—	—	—	—
OLLA—La Salle Parish										
★ HARDTNER MEDICAL CENTER, Mailing Address: P.O. Box 1218, Zip 71465; tel. 318/495–3131; David Hamner, Administrator **A**9 10 **F**7 19 22 26 40 44 46 49 52 57 65 67 71 73	16	10	31	822	9	10855	118	3850	1777	79
OPELOUSAS—St. Landry Parish										
★ COLUMBIA DOCTORS' HOSPITAL OF OPELOUSAS, 5101 Highway 167 South, Zip 70570; tel. 318/948–2100; Daryl J. Doise, Administrator (Nonreporting) **A**1 9 10 **S** Columbia/HCA Healthcare Corporation, Nashville, TN **N** Center Care, Bowling Green, KY	32	10	105	—	—	—	—	—	—	—
★ OPELOUSAS GENERAL HOSPITAL, 520 Prudhomme Lane, Zip 70570, Mailing Address: Box 1208, Zip 70571–1208; tel. 318/948–3011; Patrick Brian Carrier, Administrator (Total facility includes 13 beds in nursing home–type unit) **A**1 2 9 10 **F**7 10 15 16 17 18 19 21 22 24 28 31 32 35 37 40 42 44 45 46 49 51 60 63 64 65 71 73 74 **P**7 8 **S** Quorum Health Group/Quorum Health Resources, Inc., Brentwood, TN	16	10	126	4604	61	93191	552	34387	13682	511

Hospital, Address, Telephone, Administrator, Approval, Facility, and Physician Codes, Health Care System, Network	Classi-fication Codes		Utilization Data					Expense (thousands) of dollars		
★ American Hospital Association (AHA) membership □ Joint Commission on Accreditation of Healthcare Organizations (JCAHO) accreditation + American Osteopathic Hospital Association (AOHA) membership ○ American Osteopathic Association (AOA) accreditation △ Commission on Accreditation of Rehabilitation Facilities (CARF) accreditation Control codes 61, 63, 64, 71, 72 and 73 indicate hospitals listed by AOHA, but not registered by AHA. For definition of numerical codes, see page A4	Control	Service	Beds	Admissions	Census	Outpatient Visits	Births	Total	Payroll	Personnel

PINEVILLE—Rapides Parish

□ CENTRAL LOUISIANA STATE HOSPITAL, 242 West Shamrock Avenue, Zip 71360, Mailing Address: P.O. Box 5031, Zip 71361–5031; tel. 318/484–6200; Gary S. Grand, Chief Executive Officer **A**1 10 **F**16 20 27 30 39 52 53 65 73 **S** Louisiana State Hospitals, New Orleans, LA

| | | 12 | 22 | 280 | 337 | 243 | 0 | 0 | 24197 | 13046 | 497 |

□ HUEY P. LONG MEDICAL CENTER, 352 Hospital Boulevard, Zip 71360, Mailing Address: Box 5352, Zip 71361–5352; tel. 318/448–0811; James E. Morgan, Director (Nonreporting) **A**1 3 5 10 **S** Louisiana Health Care Authority, Baton Rouge, LA **N** Louisiana Health Care Authority, Baton Rouge, LA

| | | 12 | 10 | 143 | — | — | — | — | — | — | — |

□ RIVERNORTH HOSPITAL, 5505 Shreveport Highway, Zip 71360; tel. 318/640–0222; Daniel W. Johnson, Chief Executive Officer (Nonreporting) **A**1 10 **S** Community Health Systems, Inc., Brentwood, TN **N** Ochsner/Sisters of Charity Health Network, New Orleans, LA

| | | 33 | 22 | 53 | — | — | — | — | — | — | — |

PLAQUEMINE—Iberville Parish

□ RIVER WEST MEDICAL CENTER, 59355 River West Drive, Zip 70764–9543; tel. 504/687–9222; Steve Grimm, Chief Executive Officer (Nonreporting) **A**1 9 10 **S** Community Health Systems, Inc., Brentwood, TN **N** Ochsner/Sisters of Charity Health Network, New Orleans, LA

| | | 32 | 10 | 119 | — | — | — | — | — | — | — |

RACELAND—Lafourche Parish

□ ST. ANNE GENERAL HOSPITAL, Highway 1 and Twin Oaks Drive, Zip 70394, Mailing Address: Box 440, Zip 70394; tel. 504/537–6841; Milton D. Bourgeois, Jr., Administrator (Total facility includes 11 beds in nursing home–type unit) **A**1 9 10 **F**8 10 16 19 21 22 32 35 37 40 42 44 46 52 57 58 64 65 71 73 **N** Ochsner/Sisters of Charity Health Network, New Orleans, LA

| | | 16 | 10 | 78 | 1637 | 16 | 13773 | 348 | 14680 | 5924 | 254 |

RAYVILLE—Richland Parish

RICHARDSON MEDICAL CENTER, Christian Drive at Greer Road, Zip 71269–9985, Mailing Address: P.O. Box 388, Zip 71269–9985; tel. 318/728–4181; David D. Kervin, Administrator (Nonreporting) **A**9 10

| | | 16 | 10 | 60 | — | — | — | — | — | — | — |

RUSTON—Lincoln Parish

⊠ LINCOLN GENERAL HOSPITAL, 401 East Vaughn Street, Zip 71270, Mailing Address: P.O. Drawer 1368, Zip 71273–1368; tel. 318/254–2100; E. Allen Tuten, Administrator (Total facility includes 12 beds in nursing home–type unit) **A**1 9 10 **F**4 7 8 10 11 12 14 19 20 21 22 23 28 32 33 35 37 40 41 44 46 64 65 67 70 71 73

| | | 23 | 10 | 141 | 5744 | 73 | 31150 | 548 | 32428 | 14231 | 477 |

□ △ NORTH LOUISIANA REHABILITATION HOSPITAL, 1401 Ezell Street, Zip 71270, Mailing Address: P.O. Box 490, Zip 71273–0490; tel. 318/251–5354; Alice M. Prophit, Chief Executive Officer (Nonreporting) **A**1 7 10

| | | 33 | 46 | 90 | — | — | — | — | — | — | — |

SAINT FRANCISVILLE—West Feliciana Parish

★ WEST FELICIANA PARISH HOSPITAL, Mailing Address: Box 368, Zip 70775–0368; tel. 504/635–3811; John H. Green, Administrator **A**9 10 **F**8 22 25 28 32 54 56 65 71 **P**5 6

| | | 16 | 10 | 23 | 237 | 3 | — | 0 | 3739 | 1934 | 66 |

SHREVEPORT—Bossier Parish

□ BRENTWOOD BEHAVIORAL HEALTHCARE, 1006 Highland Avenue, Zip 71101; tel. 318/227–2221; Scott F. Blakley, Administrator (Nonreporting) **A**1

| | | 33 | 22 | 200 | — | — | — | — | — | — | — |

□ CHARTER FOREST BEHAVIORAL HEALTH SYSTEM, 9320 Linwood Avenue, Zip 71106, Mailing Address: P.O. Box 18130, Zip 71138–1130; tel. 318/688–3930; Randy J. Watson, Administrator **A**1 3 10 **F**2 3 12 15 16 17 18 19 25 35 39 52 53 55 56 57 58 59 **S** Magellan Health Services, Atlanta, GA

| | | 33 | 22 | 60 | 1489 | 49 | 776 | 0 | 7440 | 3916 | 110 |

⊠ COLUMBIA HIGHLAND HOSPITAL, 1453 East Bert Kouns Industrial Loop, Zip 71105–6050; tel. 318/798–4300; Anthony S. Sala, Jr., Chief Executive Officer (Nonreporting) **A**1 9 10 **S** Columbia/HCA Healthcare Corporation, Nashville, TN

| | | 33 | 10 | 121 | — | — | — | — | — | — | — |

□ △ DOCTORS' HOSPITAL OF SHREVEPORT, 1130 Louisiana Avenue, Zip 71101, Mailing Address: Box 1526, Zip 71165; tel. 318/227–1211; Charles E. Boyd, Administrator (Nonreporting) **A**1 7 9 10 **S** Universal Health Services, Inc., King of Prussia, PA

| | | 33 | 10 | 118 | — | — | — | — | — | — | — |

★ LIFECARE HOSPITALS, (LONG TERM ACUTE CARE), 1128 Louisiana Avenue, Suite A, Zip 71101, Mailing Address: P.O. Box 1680, Zip 71165–1680; tel. 318/222–2273; Kim B. Bird, Administrator **A**10 **F**12 15 17 19 21 22 27 30 35 41 45 46 48 49 64 65 67 71

| | | 33 | 49 | 40 | 240 | 29 | 0 | 0 | — | — | 127 |

□ LSU MEDICAL CENTER–UNIVERSITY HOSPITAL, 1541 Kings Highway, Zip 71130–3932, Mailing Address: Box 33932, Zip 71130; tel. 318/675–5000; Ingo Angermeier, FACHE, Administrator and Chief Executive Officer **A**1 2 3 5 8 9 10 **F**4 5 7 8 9 10 13 16 17 19 20 21 22 23 26 28 30 31 34 35 37 38 39 40 41 42 43 44 47 49 50 51 52 56 57 58 60 61 65 69 70 71 72 73 74 **P**1 5

| | | 12 | 10 | 421 | 19614 | 307 | 420195 | 2095 | 177912 | 103884 | 4231 |

⊠ OVERTON BROOKS VETERANS AFFAIRS MEDICAL CENTER, 510 East Stoner Avenue, Zip 71101–4295; tel. 318/221–8411; Michael E. Hamilton, Director **A**1 2 3 5 8 **F**3 4 8 10 11 15 16 17 19 20 21 22 23 25 26 27 28 30 31 33 34 35 37 39 41 42 43 44 46 49 50 51 52 54 56 57 58 60 65 67 69 71 73 74 **P**6 **S** Department of Veterans Affairs, Washington, DC

| | | 45 | 10 | 197 | 6498 | 145 | 142369 | 0 | 78917 | 40452 | 1080 |

⊠ △ SCHUMPERT MEDICAL CENTER, One St. Mary Place, Zip 71101, Mailing Address: P.O. Box 21976, Zip 71120–1076; tel. 318/681–4500; Arthur A. Gonzalez, Dr.PH, President and Chief Executive Officer (Nonreporting) **A**1 2 3 5 7 9 10 **S** Sisters of Charity of the Incarnate Word Healthcare System, Houston, TX **N** Ochsner/Sisters of Charity Health Network, New Orleans, LA

| | | 21 | 10 | 486 | — | — | — | — | — | — | — |

Hospital, Address, Telephone, Administrator, Approval, Facility, and Physician Codes, Health Care System, Network	Classi-fication Codes		Utilization Data					Expense (thousands) of dollars		
★ American Hospital Association (AHA) membership □ Joint Commission on Accreditation of Healthcare Organizations (JCAHO) accreditation + American Osteopathic Hospital Association (AOHA) membership ○ American Osteopathic Association (AOA) accreditation △ Commission on Accreditation of Rehabilitation Facilities (CARF) accreditation Control codes 61, 63, 64, 71, 72 and 73 indicate hospitals listed by AOHA, but not registered by AHA. For definition of numerical codes, see page A4	Control	Service	Beds	Admissions	Census	Outpatient Visits	Births	Total	Payroll	Personnel

★ SHRINERS HOSPITALS FOR CHILDREN, SHREVEPORT, 3100 Samford Avenue, Zip 71103; tel. 318/222–5704; Thomas R. Schneider, Administrator **A**1 3 5 **F**5 15 16 34 39 49 65 71 73 **S** Shriners Hospitals for Children, Tampa, FL	23	57	45	817	23	9436	0	—	—	151
★ U. S. AIR FORCE HOSPITAL, Barksdale AFB, Zip 71110–5300; tel. 318/456–6004; Colonel Richard Weltzin, MSC, USAF, Administrator **A**1 **F**1 2 3 4 5 6 7 8 9 10 11 12 13 14 15 16 17 18 19 20 21 22 23 24 25 26 27 28 29 30 31 32 33 34 35 36 37 38 39 40 41 42 43 44 45 46 47 48 49 50 51 52 53 54 55 56 57 58 59 60 61 62 63 64 65 66 67 68 69 70 71 72 73 74 **P**1 2 3 4 5 6 7 8 **S** Department of the Air Force, Washington, DC	41	10	25	2006	9	135551	271	—	—	571
★ △ WILLIS–KNIGHTON MEDICAL CENTER, 2600 Greenwood Road, Zip 71103–2600, Mailing Address: P.O. Box 32600, Zip 71130–2600; tel. 318/632–4600; James K. Elrod, President (Nonreporting) **A**1 3 5 7 9 10	23	10	426	—	—	—	—	—	—	—
SLIDELL—St. Tammany Parish										
□ NORTH SHORE PSYCHIATRIC HOSPITAL, 104 Medical Center Drive, Zip 70461; tel. 504/646–5500; Becky Reeves, Administrator **A**1 10 **F**3 15 16 18 26 34 52 53 55 56 57 58 59 **P**5 6 7 8	33	22	58	1007	40	13013	0	6852	3640	94
□ NORTHSHORE REGIONAL MEDICAL CENTER, 100 Medical Center Drive, Zip 70461–8572; tel. 504/649–7070; Charles F. Miller, Chief Executive Officer (Total facility includes 13 beds in nursing home–type unit) (Nonreporting) **A**1 9 10 **S** TENET Healthcare Corporation, Santa Barbara, CA **N** Tenet Louisiana Health System Network, Metairie, LA; Ochsner/Sisters of Charity Health Network, New Orleans, LA	33	10	147	—	—	—	—	—	—	—
★ SLIDELL MEMORIAL HOSPITAL AND MEDICAL CENTER, 1001 Gause Boulevard, Zip 70458–2987; tel. 504/643–2200; Monica P. Gates, Chief Executive Officer **A**1 2 9 10 **F**4 7 8 10 12 14 15 16 17 19 21 22 23 24 27 28 29 30 32 33 34 35 37 38 39 40 41 42 43 44 45 46 48 49 51 60 63 64 65 66 67 71 73 74 **P**1 3 7	16	10	173	7225	102	57552	670	67486	28951	880
SPRINGHILL—Webster Parish										
★ COLUMBIA SPRINGHILL MEDICAL CENTER, 2001 Doctors Drive, Zip 71075, Mailing Address: Box 920, Zip 71075–0920; tel. 318/539–1000; John D. Anderson, Chief Executive Officer (Nonreporting) **A**1 9 10 **S** Columbia/HCA Healthcare Corporation, Nashville, TN	33	10	86	—	—	—	—	—	—	—
STERLINGTON—Ouachita Parish										
STERLINGTON HOSPITAL, Highway 2, Zip 71280, Mailing Address: P.O. Box 567, Zip 71280–0567; tel. 318/665–2526; Evalyn Ormond, Administrator (Nonreporting) **A**9 10	23	10	32	—	—	—	—	—	—	—
SULPHUR—Calcasieu Parish										
★ WEST CALCASIEU CAMERON HOSPITAL, Cypress Street, Zip 70663, Mailing Address: P.O. Box 2509, Zip 70664–2509; tel. 318/527–4240; Wayne A. Swiniarski, FACHE, Chief Executive Officer (Total facility includes 10 beds in nursing home–type unit) **A**1 9 10 **F**8 12 13 16 17 19 22 24 27 28 29 30 32 35 37 39 40 41 44 45 49 63 64 65 66 71 73 **P**5 **N** Ochsner/Sisters of Charity Health Network, New Orleans, LA	16	10	120	3267	35	56279	245	31417	14761	563
TALLULAH—Madison Parish										
MADISON PARISH HOSPITAL, 900 Johnson Street, Zip 71282, Mailing Address: P.O. Box 1559, Zip 71284–1559; tel. 318/574–2374; Elizabeth A. Bullard, Administrator (Nonreporting) **A**9 10	23	10	47	—	—	—	—	—	—	—
THIBODAUX—Lafourche Parish										
★ △ THIBODAUX REGIONAL MEDICAL CENTER, (Formerly Thibodaux Hospital and Health Centers), 602 North Acadia Road, Zip 70301, Mailing Address: Box 1118, Zip 70302–1118; tel. 504/447–5500; Greg K. Stock, Chief Executive Officer (Nonreporting) **A**1 7 9 10 **S** Quorum Health Group/Quorum Health Resources, Inc., Brentwood, TN	16	10	130	—	—	—	—	—	—	—
VILLE PLATTE—Evangeline Parish										
★ VILLE PLATTE MEDICAL CENTER, 800 East Main Street, Zip 70586, Mailing Address: Box 349, Zip 70586; tel. 318/363–5684; Linda Deville, Chief Executive Officer **A**1 9 10 **F**7 8 12 15 16 19 22 30 32 34 35 37 42 44 49 52 57 65 73 **P**8	23	10	116	3150	37	37912	181	13764	6263	218
VIVIAN—Caddo Parish										
★ NORTH CADDO MEDICAL CENTER, (Formerly North Caddo Memorial Hospital), 1000 South Spruce Street, Zip 71082, Mailing Address: Box 792, Zip 71082; tel. 318/375–3235; Patricia S. Wilkins, Administrator **A**1 9 10 **F**11 13 14 15 16 19 22 26 28 30 34 44 57 58 59 65 71	16	10	33	726	8	5273	0	3473	1671	86
WELSH—Jefferson Davis Parish										
WELSH GENERAL HOSPITAL, 410 South Simmons Street, Zip 70591–5000; tel. 318/734–2555; Doug Landreneau, Administrator (Total facility includes 60 beds in nursing home–type unit) (Nonreporting) **A**9 10	14	10	128	—	—	—	—	—	—	—
WEST MONROE—Ouachita Parish										
★ GLENWOOD REGIONAL MEDICAL CENTER, 503 McMillan Road, Zip 71291, Mailing Address: Box 35805, Zip 71294–5805; tel. 318/329–4200; Raymond L. Ford, President and Chief Executive Officer (Total facility includes 12 beds in nursing home–type unit) **A**1 2 9 10 **F**7 8 10 11 12 15 16 17 19 20 21 22 23 24 28 29 30 31 32 33 34 35 36 37 39 40 41 42 44 45 46 47 48 49 60 64 65 66 67 68 71 73 74 **P**8	23	10	184	8598	106	65030	398	59621	20666	743
□ LAKEVIEW REGIONAL HOSPITAL, 6200 Cypress Street, Zip 71291–9012; tel. 318/396–5900; Edward C. Tschopp, Administrator (Nonreporting) **A**1 10 **S** Innovative Healthcare Systems, Inc., Birmingham, AL	33	22	60	—	—	—	—	—	—	—

Hospital, Address, Telephone, Administrator, Approval, Facility, and Physician Codes, Health Care System, Network	Classi-fication Codes		Utilization Data					Expense (thousands) of dollars		
★ American Hospital Association (AHA) membership □ Joint Commission on Accreditation of Healthcare Organizations (JCAHO) accreditation + American Osteopathic Hospital Association (AOHA) membership ○ American Osteopathic Association (AOA) accreditation △ Commission on Accreditation of Rehabilitation Facilities (CARF) accreditation Control codes 61, 63, 64, 71, 72 and 73 indicate hospitals listed by AOHA, but not registered by AHA. For definition of numerical codes, see page A4	Control	Service	Beds	Admissions	Census	Outpatient Visits	Births	Total	Payroll	Personnel

WINNFIELD—Winn Parish

✠ WINN PARISH MEDICAL CENTER, 301 West Boundary Street, Zip 71483, Mailing Address: Box 152, Zip 71483; tel. 318/628–2721; Bobby Jordan, Chief Executive Officer (Nonreporting) **A**1 9 10 **S** Columbia/HCA Healthcare Corporation, Nashville, TN	33	10	103	—	—	—	—	—	—	—

WINNSBORO—Franklin Parish

FRANKLIN MEDICAL CENTER, 2106 Loop Road, Zip 71295; tel. 318/435–9411; Ann Netherland, Chief Executive Officer **A**9 10 **F**14 15 16 17 19 21 22 26 27 28 32 37 44 52 57 65 71 73	16	10	47	2457	28	33337	0	10159	3951	183

ZACHARY—East Baton Rouge Parish

✠ LANE MEMORIAL HOSPITAL, 6300 Main Street, Zip 70791–9990; tel. 504/658–4000; Charlie L. Massey, Administrator (Total facility includes 50 beds in nursing home–type unit) **A**1 9 10 **F**7 8 12 17 19 20 21 22 28 29 30 31 32 34 35 37 39 41 44 45 49 63 64 65 71 73 **P**6 7 **S** Quorum Health Group/Quorum Health Resources, Inc., Brentwood, TN **N** Ochsner/Sisters of Charity Health Network, New Orleans, LA	16	10	136	4572	99	79069	308	30898	14667	510

MAINE

Resident population 1,241 (in thousands)
Resident population in metro areas 35.9%
Birth rate per 1,000 population 12.2
65 years and over 13.9%
Percent of persons without health insurance 13.1%

Hospital, Address, Telephone, Administrator, Approval, Facility, and Physician Codes, Health Care System, Network	Control	Service	Beds	Admissions	Census	Outpatient Visits	Births	Total	Payroll	Personnel

★ American Hospital Association (AHA) membership
□ Joint Commission on Accreditation of Healthcare Organizations (JCAHO) accreditation
+ American Osteopathic Hospital Association (AOHA) membership
○ American Osteopathic Association (AOA) accreditation
△ Commission on Accreditation of Rehabilitation Facilities (CARF) accreditation
Control codes 61, 63, 64, 71, 72 and 73 indicate hospitals listed by AOHA, but not registered by AHA. For definition of numerical codes, see page A4.

AUGUSTA—Kennebec County

Hospital	Control	Service	Beds	Admissions	Census	Outpatient Visits	Births	Total	Payroll	Personnel
□ AUGUSTA MENTAL HEALTH INSTITUTE, Arsenal Street, Zip 04330, Mailing Address: Box 724, Zip 04330; tel. 207/287–7200; Rodney Bouffard, Superintendent **A**1 9 10 **F**14 15 16 52 57	12	22	133	410	125	0	0	27437	14189	351
★ KENNEBEC VALLEY MEDICAL CENTER, 6 East Chestnut Street, Zip 04330–9988; tel. 207/626–1000; Warren C. Kessler, President (Total facility includes 29 beds in nursing home–type unit) **A**1 2 3 5 9 10 **F**1 2 3 7 8 11 12 14 15 16 17 19 20 21 22 24 25 26 28 30 31 32 33 34 35 37 39 40 41 42 44 49 51 52 53 54 55 56 57 58 59 60 64 65 66 67 71 73 **P**4 5 8	23	10	173	6294	97	124936	553	55431	24381	741

BANGOR—Penobscot County

Hospital	Control	Service	Beds	Admissions	Census	Outpatient Visits	Births	Total	Payroll	Personnel
★ ACADIA HOSPITAL, 268 Stillwater Avenue, Zip 04401, Mailing Address: P.O. Box 422, Zip 04402–0422; tel. 207/973–6100; Dennis P. King, President **A**1 9 10 **F**2 3 4 5 6 7 8 10 11 13 16 17 18 19 21 22 24 26 28 29 30 31 32 33 34 37 38 39 40 41 42 43 44 45 46 47 48 49 51 52 53 54 55 56 57 58 59 60 61 63 64 65 66 67 68 71 72 73 74 **P**1 5 6 **S** Eastern Maine Healthcare, Bangor, ME **N** Health Net, Inc., Bangor, ME	23	22	72	1462	68	3018	0	17150	8878	333
□ BANGOR MENTAL HEALTH INSTITUTE, 656 State Street, Zip 04402–0926, Mailing Address: P.O. Box 926, Zip 04402–0926; tel. 207/941–4000; N. Lawrence Ventura, Superintendent **A**1 9 10 **F**1 15 16 19 21 26 27 35 45 50 52 56 57 59 63 65 71 73 **P**6	12	22	188	245	164	1277	0	—	—	459
★ EASTERN MAINE MEDICAL CENTER, (Includes Ross Skilled Nursing Facility), 489 State Street, Zip 04401, Mailing Address: P.O. Box 404, Zip 04402–0404; tel. 207/973–7000; Norman A. Ledwin, President and Chief Executive Officer (Total facility includes 15 beds in nursing home–type unit) **A**1 2 3 5 9 10 12 **F**2 3 4 6 7 8 10 11 12 13 15 17 18 19 21 22 24 26 28 29 30 31 32 33 34 35 37 38 39 40 41 42 43 44 45 46 47 48 49 51 52 53 54 55 56 57 58 59 60 61 63 64 65 66 67 68 71 72 73 74 **P**1 2 4 5 6 **S** Eastern Maine Healthcare, Bangor, ME **N** Health Net, Inc., Bangor, ME	23	10	344	16122	247	269054	1533	182003	77956	2133
★ ST. JOSEPH HOSPITAL, 360 Broadway, Zip 04401–3897, Mailing Address: P.O. Box 403, Zip 04402–0403; tel. 207/262–1100; Sister Mary Norberta Malinowski, President **A**1 9 10 **F**8 12 15 16 17 19 21 22 23 26 30 32 33 35 37 39 41 42 44 45 46 49 63 65 66 67 71 72 73 74 **P**5 7 **N** Synernet, Portland, ME	21	10	72	3038	46	90224	0	37546	14465	565

BAR HARBOR—Hancock County

Hospital	Control	Service	Beds	Admissions	Census	Outpatient Visits	Births	Total	Payroll	Personnel
★ MOUNT DESERT ISLAND HOSPITAL, Wayman Lane, Zip 04609–0008, Mailing Address: P.O. Box 8, Zip 04609–0008; tel. 207/288–5081; Leslie A. Hawkins, Chief Executive Officer **A**1 9 10 **F**3 7 8 15 16 17 19 21 22 28 30 34 37 39 40 41 42 44 49 51 56 65 66 67 71 74 **P**6 **N** Synernet, Portland, ME	23	10	37	1663	20	20398	80	12264	5659	184

BATH—Sagadahoc County

Hospital	Control	Service	Beds	Admissions	Census	Outpatient Visits	Births	Total	Payroll	Personnel
★ MID COAST HOSPITAL, (Includes Bath Memorial Hospital, Mailing Address: 1356 Washington Street, Zip 04530–2897; Regional Memorial Hospital, 58 Baribeau Drive, Brunswick, Zip 04011–3286; tel. 207/729–0181), 1356 Washington Street, Zip 04530–2897; tel. 207/443–5524; Herbert Paris, President (Total facility includes 16 beds in nursing home–type unit) **A**1 9 10 **F**3 6 7 8 10 12 15 16 17 18 19 21 22 26 27 28 29 30 31 32 33 34 35 36 37 39 40 41 42 44 45 46 49 52 53 54 55 56 57 58 59 60 62 63 64 65 67 69 71 72 73 74 **P**1 5 6 **N** Synernet, Portland, ME	23	10	119	4019	63	93641	281	28036	13646	409

BELFAST—Waldo County

Hospital	Control	Service	Beds	Admissions	Census	Outpatient Visits	Births	Total	Payroll	Personnel
□ WALDO COUNTY GENERAL HOSPITAL, Northport Avenue, Zip 04915, Mailing Address: P.O. Box 287, Zip 04915–0287; tel. 207/338–2500; Mark A. Biscone, Executive Director **A**1 9 10 **F**1 3 6 7 8 11 14 15 16 18 19 22 24 28 30 32 33 34 35 37 40 41 42 44 46 49 53 54 55 56 57 58 62 63 65 66 67 71 73 **N** Synernet, Portland, ME	23	10	45	1933	28	71004	173	13335	7044	266

BIDDEFORD—York County

Hospital	Control	Service	Beds	Admissions	Census	Outpatient Visits	Births	Total	Payroll	Personnel
★ SOUTHERN MAINE MEDICAL CENTER, One Medical Center Drive, Zip 04005, Mailing Address: P.O. Box 626, Zip 04005–0626; tel. 207/283–7000; Edward J. McGeachey, President and Chief Executive Officer **A**1 2 9 10 **F**7 8 10 14 15 16 19 21 22 26 28 29 30 31 34 35 37 39 40 41 42 44 45 49 52 53 54 55 56 57 58 59 60 61 65 71 73 74 **N** Synernet, Portland, ME	23	10	112	4810	69	93605	501	39999	19111	654

BLUE HILL—Hancock County

Hospital	Control	Service	Beds	Admissions	Census	Outpatient Visits	Births	Total	Payroll	Personnel
★ BLUE HILL MEMORIAL HOSPITAL, Water Street, Zip 04614–0823, Mailing Address: P.O. Box 823, Zip 04614–0823; tel. 207/374–2836; Bruce D. Cummings, Chief Executive Officer **A**1 9 10 **F**6 7 8 12 15 16 17 19 22 26 28 30 32 33 34 37 40 42 44 49 51 54 58 62 63 65 67 71 72 73 74 **P**1 6 **N** Synernet, Portland, ME; Blue Hill Memorial Hospital Foundation, Blue Hill, ME	23	10	19	886	11	23650	161	9957	4986	175

BOOTHBAY HARBOR—Lincoln County

Hospital	Control	Service	Beds	Admissions	Census	Outpatient Visits	Births	Total	Payroll	Personnel
★ ST. ANDREWS HOSPITAL AND HEALTHCARE CENTER, 3 St. Andrews Lane, Zip 04538, Mailing Address: P.O. Box 417, Zip 04538–0417; tel. 207/633–2121; Margaret G. Pinkham, Administrator (Total facility includes 30 beds in nursing home–type unit) **A**1 9 10 **F**8 15 16 17 22 26 30 32 39 44 49 51 61 64 65 66 67 71 73 74	23	10	50	442	33	13450	7	6577	3443	131

Hospital, Address, Telephone, Administrator, Approval, Facility, and Physician Codes, Health Care System, Network	Classi-fication Codes		Utilization Data					Expense (thousands) of dollars		
★ American Hospital Association (AHA) membership □ Joint Commission on Accreditation of Healthcare Organizations (JCAHO) accreditation + American Osteopathic Hospital Association (AOHA) membership ○ American Osteopathic Association (AOA) accreditation △ Commission on Accreditation of Rehabilitation Facilities (CARF) accreditation Control codes 61, 63, 64, 71, 72 and 73 indicate hospitals listed by AOHA, but not registered by AHA. For definition of numerical codes, see page A4	Control	Service	Beds	Admissions	Census	Outpatient Visits	Births	Total	Payroll	Personnel

BRIDGTON—Cumberland County

☒ NORTHERN CUMBERLAND MEMORIAL HOSPITAL, South High Street, Zip 04009, Mailing Address: P.O. Box 230, Zip 04009–0230; tel. 207/647–8841; John Wiesendanger, President **A**1 9 10 **F**7 8 11 12 15 17 19 21 22 39 40 41 42 44 45 63 65 67 71 73 **P**4 7 8 **N** Synernet, Portland, ME; Central Maine Healthcare Corp, Lewiston, ME

| | 23 | 10 | 40 | 1524 | 17 | 19541 | 81 | 12047 | 5536 | 212 |

BRUNSWICK—Cumberland County

☒ PARKVIEW HOSPITAL, 329 Maine Street, Zip 04011–3398; tel. 207/729–1641; Jon W. Gepford, President and Chief Executive Officer **A**1 9 10 **F**7 8 15 16 17 19 22 26 28 29 30 31 32 33 34 37 39 40 42 44 45 46 49 54 65 67 71 73 74

| | 21 | 10 | 22 | 2008 | 18 | 51248 | 650 | 14745 | 7476 | 207 |

CALAIS—Washington County

☒ CALAIS REGIONAL HOSPITAL, 50 Franklin Street, Zip 04619–1398; tel. 207/454–7521; Ray H. Davis, Jr., Chief Executive Officer (Total facility includes 8 beds in nursing home–type unit) **A**1 9 10 **F**3 7 8 14 16 19 21 22 34 35 37 40 44 49 60 64 65 71 73 **S** Quorum Health Group/Quorum Health Resources, Inc., Brentwood, TN

| | 23 | 10 | 57 | 1273 | 25 | 26098 | 122 | 11153 | 5075 | 176 |

CARIBOU—Aroostook County

☒ CARY MEDICAL CENTER, 37 Van Buren Road, Zip 04736–2599; tel. 207/498–3111; Kris Doody–Chabre, Interim Executive Director (Total facility includes 9 beds in nursing home–type unit) **A**1 9 10 **F**4 7 8 10 11 12 13 15 16 17 18 19 20 21 22 24 25 26 27 28 29 30 31 32 33 34 35 36 37 39 40 41 42 44 45 46 49 51 53 54 55 56 57 58 59 60 63 65 66 67 69 70 71 72 73 74 **P**8 **S** Quorum Health Group/Quorum Health Resources, Inc., Brentwood, TN

| | 14 | 10 | 59 | 2364 | 44 | 64044 | 154 | 22064 | 10203 | 409 |

DAMARISCOTTA—Lincoln County

☒ MILES MEMORIAL HOSPITAL, Bristol Road, Zip 04543, Mailing Address: Rural Route 2, Box 4500, Zip 04543; tel. 207/563–1234; Judith Tarr, Chief Executive Officer **A**1 9 10 **F**1 7 8 11 12 14 15 16 17 18 19 22 24 32 33 37 39 40 44 48 49 62 64 65 68 71 72 74 **P**5 **N** Synernet, Portland, ME

| | 23 | 10 | 30 | 1590 | 16 | 39707 | 148 | 14884 | 6055 | 361 |

DOVER–FOXCROFT—Piscataquis County

☒ MAYO REGIONAL HOSPITAL, 75 West Main Street, Zip 04426; tel. 207/564–8401; George Avery, Interim Chief Executive Officer **A**1 9 10 **F**3 7 8 14 15 16 17 19 22 28 30 33 37 40 42 44 49 65 71 73 **P**7 **S** Quorum Health Group/Quorum Health Resources, Inc., Brentwood, TN

| | 16 | 10 | 46 | 1641 | 18 | 37890 | 142 | 12460 | 5864 | 205 |

ELLSWORTH—Hancock County

☒ MAINE COAST MEMORIAL HOSPITAL, 72 Union Street, Zip 04605–1599; tel. 207/667–5311; Paul Raymond Barrette, President and Chief Executive Officer **A**1 9 10 **F**7 8 12 15 16 17 18 19 21 22 24 25 26 28 29 30 31 33 34 35 37 39 40 41 44 45 46 49 51 53 56 57 58 60 63 65 66 71 72 73 74 **P**6 8 **S** Quorum Health Group/Quorum Health Resources, Inc., Brentwood, TN

| | 23 | 10 | 48 | 2334 | 29 | 30947 | 207 | 19657 | 8530 | 302 |

FARMINGTON—Franklin County

☒ FRANKLIN MEMORIAL HOSPITAL, One Hospital Drive, Zip 04938–9990; tel. 207/778–6031; Richard A. Batt, President and Chief Executive Officer **A**1 9 10 **F**7 8 12 14 15 16 17 19 22 28 30 34 37 39 40 41 42 44 49 51 58 65 66 67 71 73 **P**5 8 **N** Synernet, Portland, ME

| | 23 | 10 | 70 | 2636 | 26 | 78211 | 366 | 21560 | 9411 | 291 |

FORT FAIRFIELD—Aroostook County

COMMUNITY GENERAL HOSPITAL See Aroostook Medical Center, Presque Isle

FORT KENT—Aroostook County

☒ NORTHERN MAINE MEDICAL CENTER, 143 East Main Street, Zip 04743; tel. 207/834–3155; Martin B. Bernstein, Executive Director (Total facility includes 45 beds in nursing home–type unit) **A**1 9 10 **F**7 8 12 14 15 16 19 21 22 28 32 33 34 35 36 37 39 40 41 42 44 45 46 49 52 53 54 55 56 57 58 63 64 65 71 **P**6 **N** Synernet, Portland, ME

| | 23 | 10 | 97 | 1247 | 59 | 29218 | 99 | 14725 | 6459 | 255 |

GREENVILLE—Piscataquis County

CHARLES A. DEAN MEMORIAL HOSPITAL, Pritham Avenue, Zip 04441–1395, Mailing Address: P.O. Box 1129, Zip 04441; tel. 207/695–2223; Andrew Finegan, Administrator (Total facility includes 36 beds in nursing home–type unit) **A**9 10 **F**8 14 15 16 22 24 40 44 64 65 71

| | 23 | 10 | 50 | 566 | 40 | 20582 | 35 | 4345 | 2532 | 103 |

HOULTON—Aroostook County

☒ HOULTON REGIONAL HOSPITAL, 20 Hartford Street, Zip 04730–9998; tel. 207/532–9471; Thomas J. Moakler, Administrator and Chief Executive Officer (Total facility includes 28 beds in nursing home–type unit) (Nonreporting) **A**1 9 10 **S** Quorum Health Group/Quorum Health Resources, Inc., Brentwood, TN

| | 23 | 10 | 69 | — | — | — | — | — | — | — |

LEWISTON—Androscoggin County

☒ CENTRAL MAINE MEDICAL CENTER, 300 Main Street, Zip 04240–0305; tel. 207/795–0111; William W. Young, Jr., President **A**1 2 3 5 9 10 12 **F**7 8 10 11 12 14 15 17 19 21 22 24 25 28 29 30 31 32 35 37 40 41 42 44 45 46 48 49 51 60 63 64 65 67 69 71 73 **P**6 8

| | 23 | 10 | 116 | 8700 | 116 | 143713 | 890 | 71971 | 31087 | 934 |

☒ ST. MARY'S REGIONAL MEDICAL CENTER, 45 Golder Street, Zip 04240, Mailing Address: P.O. Box 291, Zip 04243–0291; tel. 207/777–8100; James E. Cassidy, President and Chief Executive Officer **A**1 2 9 10 **F**2 3 7 8 10 12 14 15 16 17 18 19 20 21 22 24 26 28 29 30 33 34 35 37 39 40 41 42 44 46 49 52 53 54 55 56 57 58 59 63 64 65 67 71 73 74 **P**6 **S** Covenant Health Systems, Inc., Lexington, MA **N** Synernet, Portland, ME

| | 23 | 10 | 173 | 5605 | 101 | 75000 | 363 | 42559 | 14815 | 480 |

LINCOLN—Penobscot County

☒ PENOBSCOT VALLEY HOSPITAL, Transalpine Road, Zip 04457–0368, Mailing Address: P.O. Box 368, Zip 04457–0368; tel. 207/794–3321; Ronald D. Victory, Administrator (Total facility includes 9 beds in nursing home–type unit) **A**1 3 9 10 **F**7 8 15 16 19 21 22 27 28 30 31 34 35 36 37 39 40 41 42 44 45 46 49 64 65 66 71 73 **P**6 **S** Quorum Health Group/Quorum Health Resources, Inc., Brentwood, TN

| | 16 | 10 | 42 | 1335 | 18 | 32845 | 104 | 8857 | 4252 | 169 |

Hospital, Address, Telephone, Administrator, Approval, Facility, and Physician Codes, Health Care System, Network	Classi-fication Codes		Utilization Data					Expense (thousands) of dollars		
	Control	Service	Beds	Admissions	Census	Outpatient Visits	Births	Total	Payroll	Personnel

American Hospital Association (AHA) membership
Joint Commission on Accreditation of Healthcare Organizations (JCAHO) accreditation
American Osteopathic Hospital Association (AOHA) membership
American Osteopathic Association (AOA) accreditation
Commission on Accreditation of Rehabilitation Facilities (CARF) accreditation
Control codes 61, 63, 64, 71, 72 and 73 indicate hospitals listed by AOHA, but not registered by AHA. For definition of numerical codes, see page A4

Hospital	Control	Service	Beds	Admissions	Census	Outpatient Visits	Births	Total	Payroll	Personnel
MACHIAS—Washington County										
★ DOWN EAST COMMUNITY HOSPITAL, Upper Court Street, Zip 04654, Mailing Address: Rural Route 1, Box 11, Zip 04654; tel. 207/255–3356; Richard Hanley, Chief Executive Officer **A**1 9 10 **F**8 13 14 15 16 17 19 21 22 30 40 42 44 49 65 67 71 **S** Quorum Health Group/Quorum Health Resources, Inc., Brentwood, TN	23	10	38	1622	18	—	152	12504	5065	184
MARS HILL—Aroostook County										
AROOSTOOK HEALTH CENTER See Aroostook Medical Center, Presque Isle										
MILLINOCKET—Penobscot County										
★ MILLINOCKET REGIONAL HOSPITAL, 200 Somerset Street, Zip 04462; tel. 207/723–5161; Craig A. Kantos, Chief Executive Officer **A**1 9 10 **F**7 8 17 19 22 24 30 35 37 39 40 41 42 44 46 49 65 71 73 **S** Quorum Health Group/Quorum Health Resources, Inc., Brentwood, TN	23	10	20	1062	15	23771	68	10488	4427	140
NORWAY—Oxford County										
★ STEPHENS MEMORIAL HOSPITAL, 80 Main Street, Zip 04268–1297; tel. 207/743–5933; Timothy A. Churchill, President **A**1 9 10 **F**2 3 7 8 15 16 19 21 22 29 33 35 37 40 41 44 49 64 65 71 **P**6 8 **N** Synernet, Portland, ME; Central Maine Healthcare Corp, Lewiston, ME	23	10	50	2119	27	88919	267	17043	8846	274
PITTSFIELD—Somerset County										
★ SEBASTICOOK VALLEY HOSPITAL, 99 Grove Street, Zip 04967–1199; tel. 207/487–5141; Ann Morrison, R.N., Chief Executive Officer **A**9 10 **F**2 3 8 12 17 19 22 27 28 30 33 34 37 39 41 42 44 46 49 65 67 71 73 **P**8 **N** Synernet, Portland, ME	23	10	28	1394	14	—	0	8842	3747	115
PORTLAND—Cumberland County										
□ + BRIGHTON CAMPUS OF MAINE MEDICAL CENTER, (Formerly Brighton Medical Center), 335 Brighton Avenue, Zip 04102–9735, Mailing Address: P.O. Box 9735, Zip 04102–9735; tel. 207/879–8000; Vincent S. Conti, President (Nonreporting) **A**1 9 10 **N** Synernet, Portland, ME	23	10	110	—	—	—	—	—	—	—
□ △ HEALTHSOUTH REHABILITATION HOSPITAL, (Formerly New England Rehabilitation Hospital), 13 Charles Street, Zip 04102–9924; tel. 207/775–4000; Patricia McMurry, Executive Vice President and Chief Executive Officer (Nonreporting) **A**1 7 9 10 **S** HEALTHSOUTH Corporation, Birmingham, AL	33	46	76	—	—	—	—	—	—	—
★ MAINE MEDICAL CENTER, 22 Bramhall Street, Zip 04102; tel. 207/871–0111; Donald L. McDowell, President and Chief Executive Officer **A**1 2 3 5 8 9 10 **F**4 8 10 11 12 13 14 15 16 17 18 19 20 21 22 23 25 26 27 28 29 30 31 32 34 35 37 38 39 40 41 42 43 44 45 46 48 49 51 52 53 54 55 56 57 58 59 60 61 63 65 67 69 70 71 72 73 74 **P**4 6 7 8 **N** National Cardiovascular Network, Atlanta, GA	23	10	573	24555	421	138527	2252	279935	123532	3760
★ MERCY HOSPITAL PORTLAND, 144 State Street, Zip 04101–3795; tel. 207/879–3000; Howard R. Buckley, President **A**1 3 9 10 **F**2 3 7 8 15 16 17 19 21 22 25 26 27 28 30 31 32 33 34 35 37 39 40 42 44 49 51 54 58 65 67 71 72 73 **P**6 **S** Eastern Mercy Health System, Radnor, PA **N** Synernet, Portland, ME	21	10	159	9388	113	87391	1370	57254	25626	725
NEW ENGLAND REHABILITATION HOSPITAL See HealthSouth Rehabilitation Hospital										
PRESQUE ISLE—Aroostook County										
★ AROOSTOOK MEDICAL CENTER, (Includes Aroostook Health Center, 15 Highland Avenue, Mars Hill, Zip 04758, Mailing Address: P.O. Box 410, Zip 04758; tel. 207/768–4900; Arthur R. Gould Memorial Hospital, Academy Street, Mailing Address: P.O. Box 151, Zip 04769; tel. 207/768–4000; Community General Hospital, 3 Green Street, Fort Fairfield, Zip 04742; tel. 207/768–4700; Washburn Regional Health Center, Washburn, Mailing Address: P.O. Box 510, Zip 04786), Academy Street, Zip 04769, Mailing Address: P.O. Box 151, Zip 04769–0151; tel. 207/768–4000; David A. Peterson, President and Chief Executive Officer (Total facility includes 76 beds in nursing home–type unit) **A**1 9 10 **F**7 8 15 16 19 21 22 25 26 28 30 33 34 35 36 37 39 40 41 42 44 48 49 51 52 53 55 56 58 59 60 64 65 67 71 73 74 **P**2 6	23	10	164	3040	114	73304	333	33187	14843	577
ARTHUR R. GOULD MEMORIAL HOSPITAL See Aroostook Medical Center										
ROCKPORT—Knox County										
★ PENOBSCOT BAY MEDICAL CENTER, 6 Glen Cove Drive, Zip 04856–4241; tel. 207/596–8000; Gary R. Daniels, President (Total facility includes 57 beds in nursing home–type unit) **A**1 2 9 10 **F**2 3 7 8 11 15 16 19 22 27 28 32 33 35 37 40 41 42 44 48 49 52 54 56 59 64 65 67 71 73 74 **P**6 **N** Synernet, Portland, ME	23	10	157	4272	112	79668	395	38358	21571	639
RUMFORD—Oxford County										
★ RUMFORD COMMUNITY HOSPITAL, 420 Franklin Street, Zip 04276, Mailing Address: P.O. Box 619, Zip 04276; tel. 207/364–4581; John H. Welsh, Chief Executive Officer **A**1 2 9 10 **F**2 3 7 8 11 14 16 19 20 21 22 24 28 30 40 44 48 49 65 73 **P**1 **N** Synernet, Portland, ME; Central Maine Healthcare Corp, Lewiston, ME	23	10	27	1154	14	27867	61	12113	4701	143
SANFORD—York County										
★ HENRIETTA D. GOODALL HOSPITAL, 25 June Street, Zip 04073–2645; tel. 207/324–4310; Peter G. Booth, President (Total facility includes 88 beds in nursing home–type unit) **A**1 9 10 **F**6 7 8 13 15 16 17 19 22 28 30 34 35 37 40 41 44 49 64 65 71 73 **N** Synernet, Portland, ME	23	10	156	2174	115	40387	312	24387	10788	311
SKOWHEGAN—Somerset County										
★ REDINGTON–FAIRVIEW GENERAL HOSPITAL, Fairview Avenue, Zip 04976, Mailing Address: P.O. Box 468, Zip 04976; tel. 207/474–5121; Richard Willett, Chief Executive Officer **A**1 2 9 10 **F**7 8 11 12 15 16 17 19 21 22 30 32 33 34 35 40 41 42 44 49 54 56 58 65 66 67 71 73 **N** Synernet, Portland, ME	23	10	65	3107	33	57091	244	21061	9714	331

Hospital, Address, Telephone, Administrator, Approval, Facility, and Physician Codes, Health Care System, Network	Classi-fication Codes		Utilization Data					Expense (thousands) of dollars		
★ American Hospital Association (AHA) membership □ Joint Commission on Accreditation of Healthcare Organizations (JCAHO) accreditation + American Osteopathic Hospital Association (AOHA) membership ○ American Osteopathic Association (AOA) accreditation △ Commission on Accreditation of Rehabilitation Facilities (CARF) accreditation Control codes 61, 63, 64, 71, 72 and 73 indicate hospitals listed by AOHA, but not registered by AHA. For definition of numerical codes, see page A4	Control	Service	Beds	Admissions	Census	Outpatient Visits	Births	Total	Payroll	Personnel

SOUTH PORTLAND—Cumberland County

□ JACKSON BROOK INSTITUTE, 175 Running Hill Road, Zip 04106; tel. 207/761–2200; Vincent Furey, President (Nonreporting) **A**1 3 9 10 **S** Community Care Systems, Inc., Wellesley Hills, MA

| | 33 | 22 | 106 | — | — | — | — | — | — | — |

TOGUS—Kennebec County

✠ VETERANS AFFAIRS MEDICAL CENTER, Zip 04330; tel. 207/623–8411; John H. Sims, Jr., Director (Total facility includes 100 beds in nursing home–type unit) **A**1 2 3 5 **F**1 2 3 12 14 15 16 17 18 19 20 21 25 26 27 30 31 32 33 34 37 39 41 42 44 46 49 51 52 54 56 57 58 59 63 64 65 67 71 72 73 74 **P**6 **S** Department of Veterans Affairs, Washington, DC

| | 45 | 10 | 241 | 3834 | 209 | 146348 | 0 | 53563 | 35669 | 1000 |

WASHBURN—Aroostook County

WASHBURN REGIONAL HEALTH CENTER See Aroostook Medical Center, Presque Isle

WATERVILLE—Kennebec County

★ + ○ INLAND HOSPITAL, Kennedy Memorial Drive, Zip 04901; tel. 207/861–3000; Wilfred J. Addison, Administrator **A**9 10 11 **F**7 8 15 16 19 22 24 28 32 33 34 35 41 42 44 49 51 66 71 73 **P**5 **S** Quorum Health Group/Quorum Health Resources, Inc., Brentwood, TN **N** Synernet, Portland, ME

| | 23 | 10 | 44 | 1536 | 17 | 36810 | 286 | 16009 | 6929 | 210 |

✠ MID–MAINE MEDICAL CENTER, 149 North Street, Zip 04901–4974; tel. 207/872–1000; Scott B. Bullock, President (Total facility includes 18 beds in nursing home–type unit) **A**1 2 3 5 9 10 **F**1 2 3 7 8 11 13 14 15 16 19 21 22 30 34 35 37 39 40 41 42 44 46 48 49 51 52 53 54 55 56 58 59 60 63 64 65 66 67 68 71 73 **P**5 8

| | 23 | 10 | 220 | 7514 | 125 | 302116 | 638 | 67274 | 32668 | 995 |

WESTBROOK—Cumberland County

WESTBROOK COMMUNITY HOSPITAL, 40 Park Road, Zip 04092; tel. 207/854–8464; Joel P. Rogers, Chief Executive Officer (Nonreporting) **A**9 10 **N** Synernet, Portland, ME

| | 23 | 82 | 30 | — | — | — | — | — | — | — |

YORK—York County

✠ YORK HOSPITAL, 15 Hospital Drive, Zip 03909–1099; tel. 207/363–4321; Jud Knox, President (Total facility includes 13 beds in nursing home–type unit) **A**1 9 10 **F**3 4 7 8 10 11 12 15 16 19 21 22 23 24 26 27 30 31 32 33 35 37 39 40 42 44 45 46 49 54 58 64 65 67 68 69 71 73 **P**8 **N** Synernet, Portland, ME

| | 23 | 10 | 79 | 2820 | 35 | 38455 | 291 | 30306 | 13077 | 387 |

MARYLAND

Resident population 5,042 (in thousands)
Resident population in metro areas 92.7%
Birth rate per 1,000 population 15.1
65 years and over 11.3%
Percent of persons without health insurance 12.6%

Hospital, Address, Telephone, Administrator, Approval, Facility, and Physician Codes, Health Care System, Network	Classi-fication Codes		Utilization Data					Expense (thousands) of dollars		
★ American Hospital Association (AHA) membership □ Joint Commission on Accreditation of Healthcare Organizations (JCAHO) accreditation + American Osteopathic Hospital Association (AOHA) membership ○ American Osteopathic Association (AOA) accreditation △ Commission on Accreditation of Rehabilitation Facilities (CARF) accreditation Control codes 61, 63, 64, 71, 72 and 73 indicate hospitals listed by AOHA, but not registered by AHA. For definition of numerical codes, see page A4	Control	Service	Beds	Admissions	Census	Outpatient Visits	Births	Total	Payroll	Personnel

ANDREWS AFB—Kern County

★ MALCOLM GROW MEDICAL CENTER, 1050 West Perimeter, Suite A1–19, Zip 20748, Mailing Address: Andrews AFB, Washington, DC, Zip 20331–6600; tel. 301/981–3002; Colonel James F. Geiger, Administrator (Nonreporting) **A**1 2 3 5 **S** Department of the Air Force, Washington, DC
— 41 10 185 — — — — — — —

ANNAPOLIS—Anne Arundel County

★ ANNE ARUNDEL MEDICAL CENTER, Franklin and Cathedral Streets, Zip 21401–2777; tel. 410/267–1000; Martin L. Doordan, President **A**1 2 9 10 **F**3 7 8 10 11 14 15 16 17 19 21 22 28 29 30 32 33 35 37 40 42 44 45 46 49 56 60 65 67 71 73 74
— 23 10 291 14255 144 140607 3036 108211 51095 1472

BALTIMORE—Baltimore City County

★ BON SECOURS HOSPITAL, 2000 West Baltimore Street, Zip 21223–1597; tel. 410/362–3000; Jane Durney Crowley, Chief Executive Officer (Total facility includes 32 beds in nursing home–type unit) **A**1 9 10 **F**3 8 10 11 12 14 15 16 17 19 20 21 22 25 26 27 28 30 31 32 33 34 35 37 39 41 44 46 49 51 54 58 62 64 65 67 68 71 73 **P**1 5 6 7 **S** Bon Secours Health System, Inc., Marriottsville, MD
— 21 10 148 6274 107 49827 0 59248 23818 646

★ △ CHILDREN'S HOSPITAL AND CENTER FOR RECONSTRUCTIVE SURGERY, 3825 Greenspring Avenue, Zip 21211–1398; tel. 410/462–6800; Robert A. Chrzan, President and Chief Executive Officer **A**1 3 5 7 9 10 **F**12 15 19 20 21 24 28 30 32 34 35 37 39 41 44 45 46 48 49 65 66 73
— 23 47 76 892 9 39816 0 14986 5788 185

★ CHURCH HOSPITAL CORPORATION, 100 North Broadway, Zip 21231–1593; tel. 410/522–8000; James R. Bobb, President (Total facility includes 31 beds in nursing home–type unit) **A**1 9 10 **F**1 2 3 4 5 6 7 8 10 12 13 14 15 16 17 18 19 20 21 22 23 25 26 27 28 29 30 31 32 33 34 35 37 38 39 40 41 42 43 44 45 46 48 49 51 53 54 55 56 57 58 59 60 61 62 63 64 65 66 67 68 71 72 73 74 **P**1 2 5 7 **S** Helix Health, Lutherville, MD **N** Helix Health System, Lutherville, MD
— 23 10 165 5977 105 21579 0 49385 23015 721

★ DEATON SPECIALTY HOSPITAL AND HOME, 611 South Charles Street, Zip 21230–3898; tel. 410/547–8500; Errol G. Newport, President and Chief Executive Officer (Total facility includes 152 beds in nursing home–type unit) **A**1 5 9 10 **F**27 33 41 46 49 54 57 64 65 73 **N** University of Maryland Medical System, Baltimore, MD
— 21 48 275 605 277 0 0 27471 11698 448

★ FRANKLIN SQUARE HOSPITAL CENTER, 9000 Franklin Square Drive, Zip 21237–3998; tel. 410/682–7000; Charles D. Mross, President and Chief Executive Officer **A**1 3 5 8 9 10 **F**2 3 4 7 8 10 11 12 14 16 17 18 19 21 22 23 24 25 26 28 29 30 31 32 33 34 35 37 38 39 40 41 42 43 44 45 46 48 49 51 52 53 54 55 56 57 58 59 60 61 62 63 64 65 66 67 68 71 72 73 74 **P**2 5 7 **S** Helix Health, Lutherville, MD **N** Helix Health System, Lutherville, MD
— 23 10 405 19752 235 135901 2966 139703 70611 2125

★ △ GOOD SAMARITAN HOSPITAL OF MARYLAND, 5601 Loch Raven Boulevard, Zip 21239–2995; tel. 410/532–8000; Lawrence M. Beck, President **A**1 3 5 7 9 10 **F**1 3 4 5 6 7 8 10 11 12 14 15 16 17 18 19 20 21 22 23 24 25 26 28 29 30 31 32 33 34 35 37 38 39 40 41 42 43 44 45 46 47 48 49 51 52 53 54 55 56 57 58 59 60 61 62 63 64 65 66 67 68 69 71 72 73 74 **P**5 7 **S** Helix Health, Lutherville, MD **N** Helix Health System, Lutherville, MD
— 23 10 274 9775 185 110173 0 94006 42186 1240

★ GREATER BALTIMORE MEDICAL CENTER, 6701 North Charles Street, Zip 21204–6892; tel. 410/828–2000; Robert P. Kowal, President **A**1 2 3 5 8 9 10 **F**3 7 8 10 11 12 16 17 19 21 22 26 29 30 32 33 34 35 37 38 40 42 44 45 46 49 51 60 61 65 66 67 68 71 73 74 **P**1 3 5 7 **N** Maryland Health Network, Columbia, MD
— 23 10 304 24227 263 110895 5505 182919 89272 2568

□ GUNDRY–GLASS HOSPITAL, 2 North Wickham Road, Zip 21229, Mailing Address: 1777 Reisterstown Road, Pikesville, Zip 21208; tel. 410/484–2700; Sheldon D. Glass, M.D., President (Nonreporting) **A**1 9 10
— 33 22 84 — — — — — — —

★ HARBOR HOSPITAL CENTER, 3001 South Hanover Street, Zip 21225–1290; tel. 410/347–3200; L. Barney Johnson, President and Chief Executive Officer (Total facility includes 26 beds in nursing home–type unit) **A**1 3 5 9 10 **F**1 7 8 10 12 14 15 16 17 19 21 22 24 26 27 28 30 32 34 35 37 39 40 41 42 44 46 49 51 53 54 58 60 63 64 65 67 68 71 73 74 **P**6 **S** Helix Health, Lutherville, MD
— 23 10 176 11853 172 75222 1718 99555 49647 1414

★ △ JAMES LAWRENCE KERNAN HOSPITAL, (ORTHO/SPECIALITY SURGERY/REHAB), 2200 Kernan Drive, Zip 21207–6697; tel. 410/448–2500; James E. Ross, FACHE, Chief Executive Officer **A**1 3 5 7 9 10 **F**1 2 3 4 7 8 10 11 12 13 17 18 19 20 22 25 26 28 29 30 31 32 33 34 35 37 38 40 42 43 44 46 47 48 49 51 52 53 54 55 56 57 58 59 60 61 64 65 66 67 69 70 71 73 74 **P**1 3 **N** University of Maryland Medical System, Baltimore, MD
— 23 46 152 2694 119 23908 0 41991 18556 473

★ JOHNS HOPKINS BAYVIEW MEDICAL CENTER, 4940 Eastern Avenue, Zip 21224–2780; tel. 410/550–0100; Ronald R. Peterson, President (Total facility includes 304 beds in nursing home–type unit) **A**1 3 5 8 9 10 **F**1 2 3 4 5 7 8 9 10 11 12 13 14 15 16 17 18 19 20 21 22 23 24 25 26 27 28 29 30 31 32 33 34 35 37 38 39 40 41 42 43 44 45 46 47 49 50 51 52 53 54 55 56 57 58 59 60 61 63 64 65 66 67 68 69 70 71 72 73 74 **P**5 6 **S** Johns Hopkins Health System, Baltimore, MD **N** Johns Hopkins Health System, Baltimore, MD
— 23 10 667 18054 521 245338 1018 170548 59497 2521

Hospital, Address, Telephone, Administrator, Approval, Facility, and Physician Codes, Health Care System, Network	Classi-fication Codes		Utilization Data					Expense (thousands) of dollars		
★ American Hospital Association (AHA) membership □ Joint Commission on Accreditation of Healthcare Organizations (JCAHO) accreditation + American Osteopathic Hospital Association (AOHA) membership ○ American Osteopathic Association (AOA) accreditation △ Commission on Accreditation of Rehabilitation Facilities (CARF) accreditation Control codes 61, 63, 64, 71, 72 and 73 indicate hospitals listed by AOHA, but not registered by AHA. For definition of numerical codes, see page A4	Control	Service	Beds	Admissions	Census	Outpatient Visits	Births	Total	Payroll	Personnel

Hospital	Control	Service	Beds	Admissions	Census	Outpatient Visits	Births	Total	Payroll	Personnel
⊠ △ JOHNS HOPKINS HOSPITAL, 600 North Wolfe Street, Zip 21287; tel. 410/955–5000; Ronald R. Peterson, President A1 2 3 5 7 8 9 10 F1 2 3 4 5 7 8 9 10 11 12 13 14 15 16 17 19 20 21 22 23 24 25 26 27 28 29 30 31 32 33 34 35 37 38 39 40 41 42 43 44 45 46 47 48 49 50 51 52 53 54 55 56 57 58 59 60 61 63 64 65 66 67 68 69 70 71 72 73 74 P1 2 5 6 7 8 S Johns Hopkins Health System, Baltimore, MD N Johns Hopkins Health System, Baltimore, MD	23	10	886	39096	706	286437	2055	536824	191734	6158
⊠ △ KENNEDY KRIEGER CHILDREN'S HOSPITAL, (CHILDREN'S–OTHER SPECIALTY), 707 North Broadway, Zip 21205–1890; tel. 410/550–9000; Gary W. Goldstein, M.D., President A1 7 9 10 F6 12 14 15 16 17 19 20 21 22 32 34 35 39 45 46 48 49 50 51 53 54 55 58 63 65 67 70 71 73 P6	23	59	63	426	45	87180	0	44403	21947	1339
⊠ △ LEVINDALE HEBREW GERIATRIC CENTER AND HOSPITAL, (NURSING HOME SPECIALTY HOSP), 2434 West Belvedere Avenue, Zip 21215–5299; tel. 410/466–8700; Stanford A. Alliker, FACHE, President A1 7 9 10 F1 12 15 16 19 20 21 26 31 32 33 35 36 45 48 52 54 57 59 64 65 67 73	23	49	288	1069	254	—	0	28838	13928	470
⊠ LIBERTY MEDICAL CENTER, 2600 Liberty Heights Avenue, Zip 21215; tel. 410/383–4000; Jane Durney Crowley, Chief Executive Officer A1 9 10 F3 8 12 13 14 15 16 17 18 19 20 21 22 27 28 29 30 31 32 33 34 35 37 39 42 44 45 46 49 50 51 52 53 54 55 56 58 59 63 65 67 71 73 74 P3 5 7 8 S Bon Secours Health System, Inc., Marriottsville, MD	23	10	160	6465	111	64515	0	67998	30516	732
⊠ △ MARYLAND GENERAL HOSPITAL, 827 Linden Avenue, Zip 21201–4606; tel. 410/225–8000; James R. Wood, Chairman and Chief Executive Officer A1 2 3 5 7 9 10 F3 7 8 10 11 12 14 17 19 21 22 25 26 27 28 29 30 31 32 34 35 37 39 40 41 42 44 45 48 49 51 52 54 55 56 57 58 59 60 61 65 67 68 71 72 73 74 P8	23	10	225	8972	151	94712	415	79794	43917	1198
⊠ MERCY MEDICAL CENTER, 301 St. Paul Place, Zip 21202–2165; tel. 410/332–9000; Sister Helen Amos, President and Chief Executive Officer A1 3 5 9 10 F2 3 4 7 8 10 11 12 16 17 19 20 21 22 23 25 26 29 30 33 35 37 38 39 40 41 42 44 45 46 49 52 53 56 60 65 67 71 72 73 74 P4 5 S Sisters of Mercy of the Americas–Regional Community of Baltimore, Baltimore, MD	21	10	218	13140	167	103534	2253	131070	57536	1598
⊠ △ MT. WASHINGTON PEDIATRIC HOSPITAL, (PEDIATRIC SPECIALTY & REHAB), 1708 West Rogers Avenue, Zip 21209–4596; tel. 410/578–8600; Francis A. Pommett, Jr., President A1 5 7 9 10 F12 14 15 16 17 20 27 28 31 32 34 39 41 45 46 48 49 53 54 58 65 71 73 P6	23	59	84	359	53	6073	0	18891	7760	315
⊠ SHEPPARD AND ENOCH PRATT HOSPITAL, 6501 North Charles Street, Zip 21285–6815, Mailing Address: P.O. Box 6815, Zip 21285–6815; tel. 410/938–3000; Steven S. Sharfstein, M.D., President, Medical Director and Chief Executive Officer A1 3 5 9 10 F1 3 6 12 14 15 16 17 18 25 26 27 28 29 32 34 45 46 52 53 54 55 57 58 59 65 67 68 72 73 P3 6	23	22	172	3840	146	85571	0	51370	28233	906
⊠ △ SINAI HOSPITAL OF BALTIMORE, 2401 West Belvedere Avenue, Zip 21215–5271; tel. 410/601–9000; Warren A. Green, President and Chief Executive Officer A1 2 3 5 7 8 9 10 F1 2 3 4 5 6 7 8 9 10 11 12 13 15 16 17 18 19 20 21 22 23 24 25 26 27 28 29 30 31 32 33 34 35 36 37 38 39 40 41 42 43 44 45 46 47 48 49 50 51 52 53 54 55 56 57 58 59 60 61 62 63 64 65 66 67 68 69 70 71 72 73 74 P3 5 6 7 N National Cardiovascular Network, Atlanta, GA	23	10	436	21261	311	100236	2657	235865	121407	3068
⊠ ST. AGNES HEALTHCARE, 900 Caton Avenue, Zip 21229–5299; tel. 410/368–6000; Robert E. Pezzoli, President and Chief Executive Officer (Total facility includes 24 beds in nursing home–type unit) A1 2 3 5 9 10 F3 7 8 10 11 12 13 15 16 17 19 21 22 26 28 29 30 32 33 34 35 37 38 39 40 41 42 44 45 46 47 49 51 53 54 55 57 58 60 61 63 64 65 67 68 70 71 73 74 P6 7 8 S Daughters of Charity National Health System, Saint Louis, MO N Maryland Health Network, Columbia, MD	23	10	422	19029	260	196678	2082	172560	84075	2282
⊠ △ UNION MEMORIAL HOSPITAL, 201 East University Parkway, Zip 21218–2391; tel. 410/554–2000; Kenneth R. Buser, President and Chief Executive Officer (Total facility includes 31 beds in nursing home–type unit) A1 3 5 6 7 9 10 F1 3 4 7 8 10 11 12 13 14 15 16 17 19 20 21 22 26 28 30 31 32 33 34 35 37 38 39 40 41 42 43 44 48 49 51 52 54 56 57 58 59 60 61 64 65 66 67 70 71 72 73 74 P1 5 6 7 S Helix Health, Lutherville, MD N Helix Health System, Lutherville, MD	23	10	378	15554	250	124608	907	165340	84838	2180
⊠ UNIVERSITY OF MARYLAND MEDICAL SYSTEM, 22 South Greene Street, Zip 21201–1595; tel. 410/328–8667; Morton I. Rapoport, M.D., President and Chief Executive Officer A1 2 3 5 8 9 10 F3 4 5 7 8 10 11 12 13 14 15 16 17 19 20 21 22 23 25 26 27 28 29 30 31 32 33 34 35 37 38 39 40 41 42 43 44 45 46 47 49 51 52 53 54 55 56 57 58 59 60 61 65 66 67 68 69 70 71 72 73 74 P1 7 N University of Maryland Medical System, Baltimore, MD	23	10	768	26166	496	182132	1748	368902	149626	4462
⊠ VETERANS AFFAIRS MEDICAL CENTER, 10 North Greene Street, Zip 21201–1524; tel. 410/605–7001; Dennis H. Smith, Director (Total facility includes 140 beds in nursing home–type unit) A1 2 3 5 8 9 F1 2 3 4 8 10 11 12 17 19 22 25 26 27 28 30 31 32 33 34 35 37 39 41 42 43 44 46 48 49 51 52 54 56 57 58 60 64 65 67 69 71 72 73 74 S Department of Veterans Affairs, Washington, DC	45	10	897	11999	737	412253	0	220019	123798	3291
BERLIN—Worcester County										
⊠ ATLANTIC GENERAL HOSPITAL, 9733 Healthway Drive, Zip 21811–1151; tel. 410/641–1100; Donald E. Annis, Chief Executive Officer (Total facility includes 24 beds in nursing home–type unit) A1 9 10 F8 15 16 17 19 21 22 28 30 35 37 39 41 44 45 51 64 71 72 P6 S Quorum Health Group/Quorum Health Resources, Inc., Brentwood, TN	23	10	62	2117	32	26672	2	17771	7448	284

Hospital, Address, Telephone, Administrator, Approval, Facility, and Physician Codes, Health Care System, Network	Classi-fication Codes		Utilization Data					Expense (thousands) of dollars		
★ American Hospital Association (AHA) membership □ Joint Commission on Accreditation of Healthcare Organizations (JCAHO) accreditation + American Osteopathic Hospital Association (AOHA) membership ○ American Osteopathic Association (AOA) accreditation △ Commission on Accreditation of Rehabilitation Facilities (CARF) accreditation Control codes 61, 63, 64, 71, 72 and 73 indicate hospitals listed by AOHA, but not registered by AHA. For definition of numerical codes, see page A4	Control	Service	Beds	Admissions	Census	Outpatient Visits	Births	Total	Payroll	Personnel

BETHESDA—Montgomery County

★ NATIONAL NAVAL MEDICAL CENTER, Zip 20889–5600; tel. 301/295–5800; Rear Admiral Richard T. Ridenour, MC, USN, Commander **A**1 2 3 5 **F**4 7 8 10 11 15 16 18 19 20 21 22 24 28 29 30 31 34 35 37 38 39 40 41 42 43 44 45 46 49 51 52 53 54 55 56 57 58 60 61 65 66 67 71 72 73 74 **P**6 **S** Department of Navy, Washington, DC	43	10	217	15703	157	573193	1631	334075	—	1057
★ SUBURBAN HOSPITAL, 8600 Old Georgetown Road, Zip 20814–1497; tel. 301/896–3100; Brian G. Grissler, President and Chief Executive Officer (Total facility includes 26 beds in nursing home–type unit) **A**1 2 3 5 10 **F**2 3 6 8 10 11 12 15 16 17 19 21 22 26 28 30 32 34 35 37 42 44 49 51 52 55 56 57 58 59 60 61 64 65 67 70 71 73 74 **P**1 2 4 5 8	23	10	250	11155	190	84783	0	102850	47187	1272
★ WARREN G. MAGNUSON CLINICAL CENTER, NATIONAL INSTITUTES OF HEALTH, (BIOMEDICAL RESEARCH), 9000 Rockville Pike, Zip 20892–1504; tel. 301/496–4114; John I. Gallin, M.D., Director **A**1 3 5 8 **F**3 4 8 10 19 20 21 24 26 27 31 34 35 37 39 41 42 43 44 46 49 50 52 53 54 55 57 58 59 63 65 71 73 **S** U. S. Public Health Service Indian Health Service, Rockville, MD	44	49	330	6858	160	68346	0	222327	87346	1838

CAMBRIDGE—Dorchester County

★ DORCHESTER GENERAL HOSPITAL, 300 Byrn Street, Zip 21613–1908; tel. 410/228–5511; Kenneth A. Richmond, President and Chief Executive Officer **A**1 2 9 10 **F**7 8 12 15 16 17 19 21 22 28 29 30 31 34 35 37 39 40 41 44 45 49 51 52 53 54 56 58 65 71 73 74 **P**3 6	23	10	66	3648	54	47179	232	24201	11510	375
□ EASTERN SHORE HOSPITAL CENTER, Mailing Address: Box 800, Zip 21613; tel. 410/221–2300; Mary K. Noren, Acting Superintendent **A**1 10 **F**14 15 16 28 37 45 46 48 52 54 55 57 58 65 73 **P**6	12	22	101	200	70	0	0	13854	8725	254

CATONSVILLE—Baltimore County

□ SPRING GROVE HOSPITAL CENTER, Wade Avenue, Zip 21228; tel. 410/455–6000; William B. Landis, Acting Superintendent (Total facility includes 70 beds in nursing home–type unit) (Nonreporting) **A**1 3 5 10	12	22	360	—	—	—	—	—	—	—

CHESTERTOWN—Kent County

★ KENT AND QUEEN ANNE'S HOSPITAL, 100 Brown Street, Zip 21620–1499; tel. 410/778–3300; William R. Kirk, Jr., President and Chief Executive Officer **A**1 9 10 **F**7 8 11 12 14 15 16 17 19 21 22 24 28 30 35 37 39 40 42 44 45 49 56 63 64 65 67 69 71 73	23	10	64	2660	32	38945	194	16448	7824	241
□ UPPER SHORE COMMUNITY MENTAL HEALTH CENTER, Scheeler Road, Zip 21620, Mailing Address: P.O. Box 229, Zip 21620; tel. 410/778–6800; Mary K. Noren, Acting Administrator and Chief Executive Officer **A**1 10 **F**20 52 54 55 56 73	12	22	64	159	50	0	0	6161	3436	105

CHEVERLY—Prince George's County

□ GLADYS SPELLMAN SPECIALTY HOSPITAL AND NURSING CENTER, 2900 Mercy Lane, Zip 20785; tel. 301/618–2010; Hattie Courtney, Administrator (Nonreporting) **A**1	33	48	30	—	—	—	—	—	—	—
★ PRINCE GEORGE'S HOSPITAL CENTER, 3001 Hospital Drive, Zip 20785–1189; tel. 301/618–2000; Allan Earl Atzrott, President **A**1 3 5 10 **F**3 4 7 8 10 11 12 14 15 16 17 18 19 20 21 22 24 25 26 27 28 29 30 31 32 34 35 36 37 39 40 41 42 43 44 45 46 48 49 51 52 53 54 56 58 59 60 63 64 65 67 68 70 71 72 73 **P**1 7 **S** Dimensions Health Corporation, Landover, MD **N** Dimensions HealthCare System, Landover, MD	23	10	370	16328	258	114792	3381	134002	67502	1942

CLINTON—Prince George's County

★ SOUTHERN MARYLAND HOSPITAL, 7503 Surratts Road, Zip 20735–3395; tel. 301/868–8000; Francis P. Chiaramonte, M.D., Chief Executive Officer (Nonreporting) **A**1 2 10	33	10	250	—	—	—	—	—	—	—

COLUMBIA—Howard County

★ HOWARD COUNTY GENERAL HOSPITAL, 5755 Cedar Lane, Zip 21044–2999; tel. 410/740–7890; Victor A. Broccolino, President and Chief Executive Officer **A**1 2 5 9 10 **F**7 8 10 14 15 16 19 21 22 26 28 29 30 32 33 34 35 37 40 42 44 45 46 49 52 56 57 59 60 64 65 67 68 71 73 **P**8	23	10	182	12286	123	54866	3079	75782	31980	808

CRISFIELD—Somerset County

□ EDWARD W. MCCREADY MEMORIAL HOSPITAL, 201 Hall Highway, Zip 21817–1299; tel. 410/968–1200; J. Allan Bickling, Chief Executive Officer **A**1 9 10 **F**8 14 15 16 17 19 22 23 24 26 28 30 32 35 39 41 44 46 49 52 57 65 71 73 **P**5	23	10	45	558	26	11254	0	5794	2505	129

CROWNSVILLE—Anne Arundel County

□ CROWNSVILLE HOSPITAL CENTER, Zip 21032; tel. 410/987–6200; Barry Rudnick, M.D., Acting Clinical Director (Nonreporting) **A**1 10	12	22	248	—	—	—	—	—	—	—

CUMBERLAND—Allegany County

★ △ MEMORIAL HOSPITAL AND MEDICAL CENTER OF CUMBERLAND, 600 Memorial Avenue, Zip 21502–3797; tel. 301/777–4000; Thomas C. Dowdell, Executive Director **A**1 2 7 9 10 **F**1 5 7 8 10 11 14 15 16 17 18 19 20 21 22 23 26 28 29 30 31 32 33 34 36 37 39 40 41 42 44 45 46 48 49 52 54 56 58 60 64 65 66 67 70 71 73 74	23	10	222	8537	133	61906	530	66607	30346	889
★ SACRED HEART HOSPITAL, 900 Seton Drive, Zip 21502–1874; tel. 301/759–4200; Edward M. Dinan, President and Chief Executive Officer (Nonreporting) **A**1 2 9 10 **S** Daughters of Charity National Health System, Saint Louis, MO	23	10	272	—	—	—	—	—	—	—
□ THOMAS B. FINAN CENTER, Country Club Road, Zip 21501, Mailing Address: Box 1722, Zip 21501–1722; tel. 301/777–2240; Archie T. Wallace, Chief Executive Officer (Nonreporting) **A**1 10	12	22	119	—	—	—	—	—	—	—

Hospital, Address, Telephone, Administrator, Approval, Facility, and Physician Codes, Health Care System, Network	Classi-fication Codes		Utilization Data					Expense (thousands) of dollars		
	Control	Service	Beds	Admissions	Census	Outpatient Visits	Births	Total	Payroll	Personnel

★ American Hospital Association (AHA) membership
□ Joint Commission on Accreditation of Healthcare Organizations (JCAHO) accreditation
+ American Osteopathic Hospital Association (AOHA) membership
○ American Osteopathic Association (AOA) accreditation
△ Commission on Accreditation of Rehabilitation Facilities (CARF) accreditation
Control codes 61, 63, 64, 71, 72 and 73 indicate hospitals listed by AOHA, but not registered by AHA. For definition of numerical codes, see page A4.

EAST NEW MARKET—Dorchester County

CHARTER BEHAVIORAL HEALTH SYSTEM AT WARWICK MANOR, 3680 Warwick Road, Zip 21631; tel. 410/943–8108; John S. Lacy, Executive Director (Nonreporting) **A**9 — 33 82 42 — — — — — — — —

EASTON—Talbot County

☒ MEMORIAL HOSPITAL AT EASTON MARYLAND, 219 South Washington Street, Zip 21601–2996; tel. 410/822–1000; Joseph P. Ross, President and Chief Executive Officer (Total facility includes 31 beds in nursing home–type unit) **A**1 2 6 10 **F**3 7 8 10 12 14 15 16 17 19 20 21 22 23 25 26 28 29 30 31 32 34 35 37 39 40 41 42 44 45 49 52 54 56 57 58 59 60 63 64 65 67 70 71 72 73 74 **P**3 — 23 10 188 8202 117 284040 751 61191 26525 945

ELKTON—Cecil County

☒ UNION HOSPITAL, 106 Bow Street, Zip 21921–5596; tel. 410/398–4000; Steve N. Owen, Chief Executive Officer **A**1 9 10 **F**1 7 8 12 14 15 16 17 19 21 22 25 28 29 30 31 34 35 37 40 41 44 45 49 52 54 56 65 66 71 73 **P**5 7 8 — 23 10 105 5862 62 90970 615 40125 17487 516

ELLICOTT CITY—Howard County

□ TAYLOR MANOR HOSPITAL, 4100 College Avenue, Zip 21043, Mailing Address: Box 396, Zip 21041–0396; tel. 410/465–3322; Morris L. Scherr, Executive Vice President **A**1 9 10 **F**14 15 16 19 21 34 35 46 48 50 52 53 55 56 57 58 59 63 65 71 **P**5 — 33 22 110 928 49 — 0 9890 6070 203

EMMITSBURG—Frederick County

MOUNTAIN MANOR TREATMENT CENTER, Route 15, Zip 21727, Mailing Address: Box E, Zip 21727; tel. 301/447–2361; William J. Roby, Executive Vice President (Nonreporting) — 33 82 140 — — — — — — — —

FALLSTON—Harford County

☒ FALLSTON GENERAL HOSPITAL, 200 Milton Avenue, Zip 21047–2777; tel. 410/877–3700; Lyle Ernest Sheldon, Executive Vice President and Chief Operating Officer **A**1 9 10 **F**7 8 10 11 12 14 15 16 17 18 19 21 22 24 25 28 29 30 32 33 35 37 40 41 44 45 46 49 52 54 55 56 57 58 63 65 67 71 72 73 **P**3 7 **S** Upper Chesapeake Health System, Fallston, MD — 23 10 115 6721 80 39397 0 40021 15833 527

FORT GEORGE G MEADE—Anne Arundel County

★ KIMBROUGH ARMY COMMUNITY HOSPITAL, Zip 20755; tel. 301/677–4171; Colonel David W. Roberts, Commanding Officer (Nonreporting) **A**5 **S** Department of the Army, Office of the Surgeon General, Falls Church, VA — 42 10 22 — — — — — — — —

FORT HOWARD—Baltimore County

☒ VETERANS AFFAIRS MEDICAL CENTER, 9600 North Point Road, Zip 21052–9989; tel. 410/477–1800; Dennis H. Smith, Director (Total facility includes 47 beds in nursing home–type unit) (Nonreporting) **A**1 5 9 **S** Department of Veterans Affairs, Washington, DC — 45 49 245 — — — — — — — —

FORT WASHINGTON—Prince George's County

☒ FORT WASHINGTON HOSPITAL, 11711 Livingston Road, Zip 20744–5164; tel. 301/292–7000; Theodore M. Lewis, President and Chief Executive Officer (Nonreporting) **A**1 10 **S** Greater Southeast Healthcare System, Washington, DC — 33 10 33 — — — — — — — —

FREDERICK—Frederick County

☒ FREDERICK MEMORIAL HOSPITAL, 400 West Seventh Street, Zip 21701–4593; tel. 301/698–3300; James K. Kluttz, President and Chief Executive Officer **A**1 2 9 10 **F**7 8 10 12 13 14 15 16 17 18 19 20 21 22 25 28 29 30 31 32 33 34 35 37 39 40 41 42 44 46 48 49 52 53 54 55 56 58 59 60 63 65 66 67 71 73 74 **P**1 5 — 23 10 164 12750 150 245096 2029 93971 44221 1321

GLEN BURNIE—Anne Arundel County

☒ NORTH ARUNDEL HOSPITAL, 301 Hospital Drive, Zip 21061–5899; tel. 410/787–4000; James R. Walker, FACHE, President and Chief Executive Officer **A**1 9 10 **F**6 8 10 11 12 15 16 17 19 21 22 26 27 28 29 30 32 34 37 39 41 42 44 49 51 52 56 57 59 65 66 67 71 72 73 74 **P**2 6 7 — 23 10 230 15246 191 85929 0 103226 46927 1392

HAGERSTOWN—Washington County

□ BROOK LANE PSYCHIATRIC CENTER, 13218 Brook Lane Drive, Zip 21742–1945, Mailing Address: P.O. Box 1945, Zip 21742–1945; tel. 301/733–0330; R. Lynn Rushing, Chief Executive Officer **A**1 9 10 **F**1 3 14 15 16 25 26 34 39 46 52 53 54 55 56 57 58 59 65 **P**5 — 23 22 65 1236 31 18505 0 7975 5133 159

☒ WASHINGTON COUNTY HOSPITAL ASSOCIATION, 251 East Antietam Street, Zip 21740–5771; tel. 301/790–8000; Horace W. Murphy, President (Total facility includes 47 beds in nursing home–type unit) **A**1 2 9 10 **F**3 4 7 8 10 11 14 15 16 17 18 19 21 22 23 25 26 28 29 30 31 32 33 34 35 36 37 39 40 41 42 44 45 46 48 49 51 52 54 55 56 58 59 60 61 63 64 65 66 67 70 71 73 74 **P**6 8 — 23 10 333 16675 226 162684 1619 105335 52475 1388

□ WESTERN MARYLAND CENTER, 1500 Pennsylvania Avenue, Zip 21742–3194; tel. 301/791–4400; Carl A. Fischer, M.D., Director (Total facility includes 60 beds in nursing home–type unit) (Nonreporting) **A**1 9 10 — 12 48 120 — — — — — — — —

HAVRE DE GRACE—Harford County

☒ HARFORD MEMORIAL HOSPITAL, 501 South Union Avenue, Zip 21078–3493; tel. 410/939–2400; Lyle Ernest Sheldon, President and Chief Executive Officer **A**1 9 10 **F**7 8 10 11 12 14 15 16 17 18 19 21 22 25 28 29 30 32 33 35 37 40 44 45 46 49 52 54 55 56 57 58 63 65 67 71 72 73 **P**3 7 **S** Upper Chesapeake Health System, Fallston, MD — 23 10 168 6849 71 47118 777 39397 16884 582

JESSUP—Anne Arundel County

□ CLIFTON T. PERKINS HOSPITAL CENTER, 8450 Dorsey Run Road, Zip 20794, Mailing Address: P.O. Box 1000, Zip 20794–1000; tel. 410/792–4022; M. Richard Fragala, M.D., Superintendent **A**1 5 **F**3 14 16 27 45 52 55 58 65 73 **P**6 — 12 22 200 70 170 0 0 24115 15523 495

Hospital, Address, Telephone, Administrator, Approval, Facility, and Physician Codes, Health Care System, Network	Classi-fication Codes		Utilization Data					Expense (thousands) of dollars		
★ American Hospital Association (AHA) membership □ Joint Commission on Accreditation of Healthcare Organizations (JCAHO) accreditation + American Osteopathic Hospital Association (AOHA) membership ○ American Osteopathic Association (AOA) accreditation △ Commission on Accreditation of Rehabilitation Facilities (CARF) accreditation Control codes 61, 63, 64, 71, 72 and 73 indicate hospitals listed by AOHA, but not registered by AHA. For definition of numerical codes, see page A4	Control	Service	Beds	Admissions	Census	Outpatient Visits	Births	Total	Payroll	Personnel

LA PLATA—Charles County

☒ PHYSICIANS MEMORIAL HOSPITAL, 701 East Charles Street, Zip 20646, Mailing Address: P.O. Box 1070, Zip 20646; tel. 301/609–4000; Susan L. Hunsaker, CHE, President and Chief Executive Officer **A**1 9 10 **F**7 8 12 14 15 16 17 18 19 21 22 25 28 29 30 31 32 35 37 39 40 42 44 49 56 61 65 71 73 74 — 23 10 110 5214 65 46810 572 38023 17675 506

LANHAM—Prince George's County

☒ DOCTORS COMMUNITY HOSPITAL, 8118 Good Luck Road, Zip 20706–3596; tel. 301/552–8118; Philip Down, President **A**1 10 **F**4 8 10 11 12 14 16 17 19 21 22 28 29 30 32 34 37 39 41 42 44 45 49 60 64 65 67 71 73 — 23 10 200 8450 131 67871 0 67428 25787 701

LAUREL—Prince George's County

☒ △ LAUREL REGIONAL HOSPITAL, 7300 Van Dusen Road, Zip 20707–9266; tel. 301/725–4300; Patrick F. Mutch, President **A**1 7 10 **F**2 3 4 5 7 8 10 11 12 15 17 18 19 20 21 22 23 25 26 28 29 30 31 32 33 34 35 36 37 38 39 40 41 42 43 44 45 46 48 49 51 52 53 54 55 56 57 58 59 60 64 65 67 68 69 70 71 72 73 **P**1 6 7 **S** Dimensions Health Corporation, Landover, MD — 23 10 185 6570 102 40971 737 53624 26240 592

LEONARDTOWN—St. Marys County

☒ ST. MARY'S HOSPITAL, 25500 Point Lookout Road, Zip 20650, Mailing Address: P.O. Box 527, Zip 20650; tel. 301/475–6001; Christine R. Wray, Chief Executive Officer **A**1 2 9 10 **F**7 8 12 15 16 17 19 20 22 26 27 28 29 30 32 33 34 35 37 39 40 41 42 44 46 49 52 54 55 56 57 59 65 67 68 71 73 **P**2 — 23 10 107 5646 64 108225 788 33110 15272 509

OAKLAND—Garrett County

☒ GARRETT COUNTY MEMORIAL HOSPITAL, 251 North Fourth Street, Zip 21550–1398; tel. 301/334–2155; Walter P. Donalson, III, President and Chief Executive Officer **A**1 9 10 **F**7 8 11 14 15 16 17 18 19 20 21 22 28 30 33 34 36 37 39 40 44 45 46 49 54 56 63 65 67 71 73 **P**3 8 — 23 10 76 2898 31 59428 315 20422 9910 299

OLNEY—Montgomery County

☒ MONTGOMERY GENERAL HOSPITAL, 18101 Prince Philip Drive, Zip 20832–1512; tel. 301/774–8882; Peter W. Monge, President and Chief Executive Officer **A**1 2 9 10 **F**1 2 3 7 8 11 12 15 17 18 19 21 22 26 27 28 29 32 35 37 40 41 42 44 49 51 52 56 57 58 59 60 63 65 67 68 71 73 74 **P**1 6 7 **N** Maryland Health Network, Columbia, MD — 23 10 164 7830 103 29237 972 56464 27700 783

PATUXENT RIVER—St. Marys County

★ NAVAL HOSPITAL, Zip 20670–5370; tel. 301/342–1418; Captain Paul E. Campbell, MSC, USN, Commanding Officer **F**3 13 16 21 22 25 27 28 29 30 34 44 46 49 51 55 58 64 65 67 71 **S** Department of Navy, Washington, DC — 43 10 5 380 2 71325 0 — — 214

PERRY POINT—Cecil County

☒ VA MARYLAND HEALTH CARE SYSTEM, Circle Drive, Zip 21902; tel. 410/642–2411; Dennis H. Smith, Director (Total facility includes 80 beds in nursing home–type unit) (Nonreporting) **A**1 5 9 **S** Department of Veterans Affairs, Washington, DC — 45 22 526 — — — — — — —

PRINCE FREDERICK—Calvert County

☒ CALVERT MEMORIAL HOSPITAL, 100 Hospital Road, Zip 20678–9675; tel. 410/535–4000; James J. Xinis, President and Chief Executive Officer **A**1 2 9 10 **F**8 13 14 15 16 17 18 19 22 25 28 29 30 32 33 35 36 37 39 40 41 42 44 45 46 49 52 53 54 56 59 65 66 67 71 73 74 **P**8 — 23 10 109 5448 64 58634 661 28572 14046 506

RANDALLSTOWN—Baltimore County

☒ NORTHWEST HOSPITAL CENTER, 5401 Old Court Road, Zip 21133–5185; tel. 410/521–2200; Robert W. Fischer, President **A**1 2 9 10 **F**8 10 11 12 14 15 16 17 19 21 22 28 29 30 31 32 34 35 37 39 41 42 44 45 46 49 51 56 60 65 67 71 73 **P**1 6 7 **N** Maryland Health Network, Columbia, MD — 23 10 198 10998 157 51069 0 80336 37705 1090

ROCKVILLE—Montgomery County

□ CHARTER BEHAVIORAL HEALTH SYSTEM OF POTOMAC RIDGE, 14901 Broschart Road, Zip 20850–3321; tel. 301/251–4500; Craig S. Juengling, Chief Executive Officer (Nonreporting) **A**1 10 **S** Magellan Health Services, Atlanta, GA — 33 22 140 — — — — — — —

☒ CHESTNUT LODGE HOSPITAL, (Formerly CPC Health–Chestnut Lodge Hospital), 500 West Montgomery Avenue, Zip 20850; tel. 301/424–8300; Steven Goldstein, Ph.D., Chief Executive Officer (Nonreporting) **A**1 10 **S** Community Psychiatric Centers — 33 22 50 — — — — — — —

CPC HEALTH–CHESTNUT LODGE HOSPITAL See Chestnut Lodge Hospital

□ SHADY GROVE ADVENTIST HOSPITAL, 9901 Medical Center Drive, Zip 20850–3395; tel. 301/279–6000; Bryan L. Breckenridge, President (Nonreporting) **A**1 10 — 21 10 253 — — — — — — —

SALISBURY—Wicomico County

□ DEER'S HEAD CENTER, Mailing Address: Box 2018, Zip 21802–2018; tel. 410/543–4000; Dorothy A. Bradshaw, Director (Total facility includes 68 beds in nursing home–type unit) **A**1 10 **F**4 8 10 11 14 15 16 19 20 21 22 26 28 29 30 31 33 35 37 42 44 45 46 48 49 52 53 54 55 56 57 58 60 64 65 67 69 71 73 74 **P**6 — 12 48 90 84 74 20367 0 11499 4536 262

□ △ HEALTHSOUTH CHESAPEAKE REHABILITATION HOSPITAL, 220 Tilghman Road, Zip 21804; tel. 410/546–4600; William Rothman, Chief Executive Officer **A**1 7 9 10 **F**14 48 49 **P**6 **S** HEALTHSOUTH Corporation, Birmingham, AL — 33 46 42 421 40 8296 0 3949 1962 127

☒ PENINSULA REGIONAL MEDICAL CENTER, 100 East Carroll Street, Zip 21801–5422; tel. 410/546–6400; Dan H. Akin, President **A**1 2 9 10 **F**4 7 8 10 11 14 15 16 17 19 20 21 22 23 24 25 26 28 29 30 31 32 34 35 37 39 40 41 42 43 44 45 51 52 54 56 57 60 65 67 70 71 72 73 **P**6 — 23 10 377 16756 234 326654 1878 119511 54939 1694

Hospital, Address, Telephone, Administrator, Approval, Facility, and Physician Codes, Health Care System, Network	Classi-fication Codes		Utilization Data					Expense (thousands) of dollars		
★ American Hospital Association (AHA) membership □ Joint Commission on Accreditation of Healthcare Organizations (JCAHO) accreditation + American Osteopathic Hospital Association (AOHA) membership ○ American Osteopathic Association (AOA) accreditation △ Commission on Accreditation of Rehabilitation Facilities (CARF) accreditation Control codes 61, 63, 64, 71, 72 and 73 indicate hospitals listed by AOHA, but not registered by AHA. For definition of numerical codes, see page A4	Control	Service	Beds	Admissions	Census	Outpatient Visits	Births	Total	Payroll	Personnel

SILVER SPRING—Montgomery County

☒ HOLY CROSS HOSPITAL OF SILVER SPRING, 1500 Forest Glen Road, Zip 20910; tel. 301/754–7000; James P. Hamill, President **A**1 3 5 8 10 **F**1 3 4 7 8 9 10 11 12 13 15 16 17 18 19 21 22 25 27 28 29 30 32 33 34 35 36 37 38 39 40 42 43 44 45 46 47 48 49 51 52 53 54 55 56 57 58 59 60 63 64 65 66 67 71 73 74 **P**1 2 3 7 **S** Holy Cross Health System Corporation, South Bend, IN **N** Maryland Health Network, Columbia, MD

	21	10	434	23899	280	188928	6764	150413	61762	1691

★ SAINT LUKE INSTITUTE, 8901 New Hampshire Avenue, Zip 20903; tel. 301/445–7970; Reverend Stephen J. Rossetti, Ph.D., President and Chief Executive Officer (Nonreporting)

	23	22	24	—	—	—	—	—	—	—

SYKESVILLE—Carroll County

□ SPRINGFIELD HOSPITAL CENTER, 6655 Sykesville Road, Zip 21784; tel. 410/795–2100; Paula A. Langmead, Superintendent **A**1 10 **F**14 16 52 55 57 65 73

	12	22	360	380	366	0	0		—	998

TAKOMA PARK—Montgomery County

☒ WASHINGTON ADVENTIST HOSPITAL, 7600 Carroll Avenue, Zip 20912–6392; tel. 301/891–7600; Kiltie Leach, Chief Operating Officer (Nonreporting) **A**1 9 10

	21	10	300	—	—	—	—	—	—	—

TOWSON—Baltimore County

☒ ST. JOSEPH MEDICAL CENTER, 7620 York Road, Zip 21204–7582; tel. 410/337–1000; John S. Prout, President and Chief Executive Officer **A**1 10 **F**4 5 7 8 10 11 12 13 14 15 16 17 18 19 20 21 22 25 26 28 29 30 31 32 33 34 35 37 38 39 40 41 42 43 44 45 46 49 51 52 54 55 56 57 60 65 67 68 71 72 73 74 **P**2 7 **S** Catholic Health Initiatives, Denver, CO

	21	10	460	19604	258	60047	1718	150562	63200	1683

WESTMINSTER—Carroll County

☒ CARROLL COUNTY GENERAL HOSPITAL, 200 Memorial Avenue, Zip 21157–5799; tel. 410/848–3000; John M. Sernulka, President and Chief Executive Officer **A**1 9 10 **F**4 7 8 10 12 15 16 17 19 20 21 22 23 28 30 32 33 35 37 40 42 44 45 46 52 53 54 63 65 67 71 73 74 **P**3 7

	23	10	158	9145	113	71788	887	54283	24937	896

MASSACHUSETTS

Resident population 6,074 (in thousands)
Resident population in metro areas 96.1%
Birth rate per 1,000 population 14.1
65 years and over 14.2%
Percent of persons without health insurance 12.5%

Hospital, Address, Telephone, Administrator, Approval, Facility, and Physician Codes, Health Care System, Network	Classi-fication Codes		Utilization Data					Expense (thousands) of dollars		
	Control	Service	Beds	Admissions	Census	Outpatient Visits	Births	Total	Payroll	Personnel

★   American Hospital Association (AHA) membership
☐   Joint Commission on Accreditation of Healthcare Organizations (JCAHO) accreditation
+   American Osteopathic Hospital Association (AOHA) membership
○   American Osteopathic Association (AOA) accreditation
△   Commission on Accreditation of Rehabilitation Facilities (CARF) accreditation
Control codes 61, 63, 64, 71, 72 and 73 indicate hospitals listed by AOHA, but not registered by AHA. For definition of numerical codes, see page A4

AMHERST—Hampshire County

Hospital	Control	Service	Beds	Admissions	Census	Outpatient Visits	Births	Total	Payroll	Personnel
UNIVERSITY HEALTH SERVICES, University of Massachusetts, Zip 01003–4310; tel. 413/577–5000; Bernette A. Melby, Executive Director **A**3 9 10 **F**15 20 28 29 30 31 45 46 58 66 71 72 74 **P**6	12	11	6	78	1	80310	0	—	—	—

ANDOVER—Essex County

Hospital	Control	Service	Beds	Admissions	Census	Outpatient Visits	Births	Total	Payroll	Personnel
ISHAM HEALTH CENTER, Phillips Academy, Zip 01810; tel. 508/749–4455; Margaret Lankow, Administrator (Nonreporting)	23	59	20	—	—	—	—	—	—	—

ARLINGTON—Middlesex County

Hospital	Control	Service	Beds	Admissions	Census	Outpatient Visits	Births	Total	Payroll	Personnel
☐ SYMMES HOSPITAL AND MEDICAL CENTER, (Formerly Medical Center at Symmes), Hospital Road, Zip 02174–2199; tel. 617/646–1500; Peter D. Goldbach, M.D., Chief Executive Officer (Nonreporting) **A**1 9 10	23	10	88	—	—	—	—	—	—	—

ASHBURNHAM—Worcester County

Hospital	Control	Service	Beds	Admissions	Census	Outpatient Visits	Births	Total	Payroll	Personnel
NAUKEAG HOSPITAL, 216 Lake Road, Zip 01430; tel. 617/827–5115; Geraldine A. McQuoid, Director (Nonreporting) **A**9	33	82	26	—	—	—	—	—	—	—

ATHOL—Worcester County

Hospital	Control	Service	Beds	Admissions	Census	Outpatient Visits	Births	Total	Payroll	Personnel
☐ ATHOL MEMORIAL HOSPITAL, 2033 Main Street, Zip 01331–3598; tel. 508/249–3511; William DiFederico, President **A**1 5 9 10 **F**8 15 16 17 19 20 22 29 30 31 32 33 34 37 39 41 42 44 45 46 49 53 54 58 65 67 71 73 **P**5 8 **N** Fallon Healthcare System, Worcester, MA	23	10	46	1804	22	34869	0	15131	7637	330

ATTLEBORO—Bristol County

Hospital	Control	Service	Beds	Admissions	Census	Outpatient Visits	Births	Total	Payroll	Personnel
✠ STURDY MEMORIAL HOSPITAL, 211 Park Street, Zip 02703, Mailing Address: P.O. Box 2963, Zip 02703; tel. 508/236–8000; Linda Shyavitz, President and Chief Executive Officer **A**1 2 9 10 **F**7 8 12 13 15 16 17 18 19 20 21 22 23 25 26 28 29 30 31 33 34 35 37 39 40 41 42 44 45 46 49 51 54 61 63 65 67 68 71 72 73 74 **P**5	23	10	117	4795	61	162395	791	49994	26728	646

AYER—Middlesex County

Hospital	Control	Service	Beds	Admissions	Census	Outpatient Visits	Births	Total	Payroll	Personnel
✠ DEACONESS–NASHOBA HOSPITAL, 200 Groton Road, Zip 01432; tel. 508/772–0200; Jeffrey R. Kelly, President and Chief Executive Officer **A**1 9 10 **F**1 2 8 9 11 12 14 15 16 17 19 20 21 22 26 28 29 30 31 32 33 34 35 37 38 39 41 42 44 45 47 48 49 56 58 63 64 65 67 70 71 73 74 **P**5 6 8 **S** CareGroup, Boston, MA **N** CareGroup, Boston, MA; Fallon Healthcare System, Worcester, MA	23	10	49	2043	25	77199	0	21687	9512	297

BEDFORD—Middlesex County

Hospital	Control	Service	Beds	Admissions	Census	Outpatient Visits	Births	Total	Payroll	Personnel
✠ EDITH NOURSE ROGERS MEMORIAL VETERANS HOSPITAL, 200 Springs Road, Zip 01730; tel. 617/687–2000; William A. Conte, Director (Total facility includes 265 beds in nursing home–type unit) (Nonreporting) **A**1 3 5 9 **S** Department of Veterans Affairs, Washington, DC	45	22	680	—	—	—	—	—	—	—

BELMONT—Middlesex County

Hospital	Control	Service	Beds	Admissions	Census	Outpatient Visits	Births	Total	Payroll	Personnel
✠ MCLEAN HOSPITAL, 115 Mill Street, Zip 02178–9106; tel. 617/855–2000; Steven M. Mirin, M.D., President and Psychiatrist in Chief (Nonreporting) **A**1 3 5 9 10 **S** Partners HealthCare System, Boston, MA	23	22	201	—	—	—	—	—	—	—

BEVERLY—Essex County

Hospital	Control	Service	Beds	Admissions	Census	Outpatient Visits	Births	Total	Payroll	Personnel
✠ BEVERLY HOSPITAL, (Includes Addison Gilbert Hospital, 298 Washington Street, Gloucester, Zip 01930–4887; tel. 508/283–4000; Robert L. Shafner, President), 85 Herrrick Street, Zip 01915–1777; tel. 508/922–3000; Robert R. Fanning, Jr., Chief Executive Officer **A**1 2 3 9 10 **F**1 2 3 4 5 6 7 8 10 11 12 13 14 15 16 17 18 19 20 22 23 24 25 26 28 29 30 31 32 33 34 35 36 37 39 40 41 42 44 45 46 48 49 51 52 53 54 55 56 57 58 59 60 61 62 64 65 66 67 68 69 71 73 74 **P**1 2 3 4 5 6 8 **N** Northeast Health Systems, Beverly, MA	23	10	360	13609	172	112273	2854	128120	61476	1431

BOSTON—Suffolk County

Hospital	Control	Service	Beds	Admissions	Census	Outpatient Visits	Births	Total	Payroll	Personnel
☐ ARBOUR HOSPITAL, 49 Robinwood Avenue, Zip 02130, Mailing Address: P.O. Box 9, Zip 02130; tel. 617/522–4400; Roy A. Ettlinger, Chief Executive Officer (Nonreporting) **A**1 10 **S** Universal Health Services, Inc., King of Prussia, PA	33	22	118	—	—	—	—	—	—	—
✠ BETH ISRAEL DEACONESS MEDICAL CENTER, 330 Brookline Avenue, Zip 02215; tel. 617/667–2000; David Dolins, President (Total facility includes 48 beds in nursing home–type unit) **A**1 2 3 5 8 9 10 **F**4 5 7 8 10 11 12 14 15 16 17 18 19 20 21 22 23 24 25 26 27 28 29 30 31 32 33 34 35 37 38 39 40 41 42 43 44 45 46 48 49 51 52 53 54 55 56 57 58 59 60 61 63 64 65 66 67 69 70 71 72 73 74 **P**1 2 3 5 6 7 **S** CareGroup, Boston, MA **N** CareGroup, Boston, MA; Fallon Healthcare System, Worcester, MA	23	10	671	34754	506	680541	5264	651140	242450	7644
BOSTON CITY HOSPITAL See Boston Medical Center										
✠ BOSTON MEDICAL CENTER, (Includes Boston City Hospital, 818 Harrison Avenue, Zip 02118; tel. 617/534–5365; Boston University Medical Center–University Hospital, 88 East Newton Street, tel. 617/638–8000), One Boston Medical Ctr Place, Zip 02118–2393; tel. 617/638–8000; Elaine S. Ullian, President and Chief Executive Officer (Total facility includes 24 beds in nursing home–type unit) **A**1 2 3 5 8 9 10 **F**1 2 3 4 5 6 7 8 9 10 11 12 13 14 15 16 17 19 20 21 22 23 24 25 26 27 28 29 30 31 32 34 35 36 37 38 39 40 41 42 44 45 46 47 48 49 51 52 53 54 56 57 58 60 61 62 63 64 65 66 67 68 69 70 71 72 73 74 **P**3 4 5 6 8 **N** New England Health Partnership, Waltham, MA	23	10	489	22955	442	453388	1540	—	—	4329
BOSTON UNIVERSITY MEDICAL CENTER–UNIVERSITY HOSPITAL See Boston Medical Center										

Hospital, Address, Telephone, Administrator, Approval, Facility, and Physician Codes, Health Care System, Network	Classi-fication Codes		Utilization Data					Expense (thousands) of dollars		
	Control	Service	Beds	Admissions	Census	Outpatient Visits	Births	Total	Payroll	Personnel

★ American Hospital Association (AHA) membership
□ Joint Commission on Accreditation of Healthcare Organizations (JCAHO) accreditation
+ American Osteopathic Hospital Association (AOHA) membership
○ American Osteopathic Association (AOA) accreditation
△ Commission on Accreditation of Rehabilitation Facilities (CARF) accreditation
Control codes 61, 63, 64, 71, 72 and 73 indicate hospitals listed by AOHA, but not registered by AHA. For definition of numerical codes, see page A4

Hospital	Control	Service	Beds	Admissions	Census	Outpatient Visits	Births	Total	Payroll	Personnel
✠ BRIGHAM AND WOMEN'S HOSPITAL, 75 Francis Street, Zip 02115–6195; tel. 617/732–5500; Jeffrey Otten, President A1 2 3 5 8 9 10 F2 3 4 5 7 8 9 10 11 12 13 14 15 16 17 18 19 20 21 22 23 24 25 26 28 29 30 31 32 34 35 37 38 39 40 41 42 43 44 45 46 47 48 49 50 51 52 53 54 55 56 57 58 59 60 61 63 64 65 66 67 68 69 70 71 72 73 74 P1 3 5 6 7 8 S Partners HealthCare System, Boston, MA N Fallon Healthcare System, Worcester, MA; Partners HealthCare System, Boston, MA	23	10	617	34901	508	699638	8421	660033	248473	6981
✠ CARNEY HOSPITAL, 2100 Dorchester Avenue, Zip 02124–5666; tel. 617/296–4000; Joyce A. Murphy, President and Chief Executive Officer (Nonreporting) A1 2 3 5 9 10 S Caritas Christi Health Care System, Boston, MA	21	10	194	—	—	—	—	—	—	—
✠ CHILDREN'S HOSPITAL, 300 Longwood Avenue, Zip 02115; tel. 617/355–6000; David Stephen Weiner, President A1 3 5 8 9 10 F10 11 12 13 14 15 16 17 19 21 23 29 30 31 34 35 38 39 41 42 43 44 45 46 47 49 50 51 52 53 54 55 56 58 60 61 63 65 66 67 68 69 70 71 72 73 P5 7 N Fallon Healthcare System, Worcester, MA; Children's Hospital, Boston, MA	23	50	325	18099	234	262667	0	344577	120371	3941
✠ DANA–FARBER CANCER INSTITUTE, (COMPREHENSIVE CANCER CENTER), 44 Binney Street, Zip 02115–6084; tel. 617/632–3000; David G. Nathan, M.D., President A1 3 9 10 F8 15 16 17 19 20 21 22 30 34 35 39 41 42 44 45 46 54 56 60 63 65 67 69 71 73 74 P6 N Fallon Healthcare System, Worcester, MA	23	49	34	1566	30	58978	0	171787	74890	1166
✠ FAULKNER HOSPITAL, Mailing Address: 1153 Centre Sreet, Zip 02130; tel. 617/983–7000; David J. Trull, President and Chief Executive Officer A1 2 3 5 8 9 10 F1 3 4 8 10 11 12 14 15 16 17 19 21 22 25 30 31 33 34 35 37 39 41 42 44 45 46 49 51 52 54 55 56 57 58 59 61 65 67 68 71 72 73 P5	23	10	144	6142	90	156763	0	67318	33916	866
□ △ FRANCISCAN CHILDREN'S HOSPITAL AND REHABILITATION CENTER, Mailing Address: 30 Warren Street, Zip 02135–3680; tel. 617/254–3800; Paul J. Dellarocco, President and Chief Executive Officer (Nonreporting) A1 5 7 9 10	21	56	60	—	—	—	—	—	—	—
★ HEBREW REHABILITATION CENTER FOR AGED, (LTC GERIATRIC), Mailing Address: 1200 Centre Street, Zip 02131–1097; tel. 617/325–8000; Maurice I. May, President A10 F1 6 15 16 17 20 24 26 27 28 30 33 34 36 39 46 49 51 54 57 58 62 64 65 67 73 P6	23	49	725	176	710	169	0	49451	27501	756
✠ JEWISH MEMORIAL HOSPITAL AND REHABILITATION CENTER, (CHRONIC DISEASE & REHAB), 59 Townsend Street, Zip 02119–9918; tel. 617/442–8760; Donald E. Schwarz, President and Chief Executive Officer A1 3 5 9 10 F1 12 15 16 19 20 21 22 26 30 31 32 33 35 36 39 42 45 48 49 52 54 57 65 67 71 73 P6 8	23	49	110	758	99	9800	0	26138	13233	325
✠ LEMUEL SHATTUCK HOSPITAL, 170 Morton Street, Jamaica Plain, Zip 02130–3787; tel. 617/522–8110; Robert D. Wakefield, Jr., Executive Director (Nonreporting) A1 3 5 6 9 10 S Massachusetts Department of Mental Health, Boston, MA	12	10	230	—	—	—	—	—	—	—
□ MASSACHUSETTS EYE AND EAR INFIRMARY, 243 Charles Street, Zip 02114–3096; tel. 617/523–7900; F. Curtis Smith, President (Nonreporting) A1 3 5 9 10	23	45	47	—	—	—	—	—	—	—
✠ MASSACHUSETTS GENERAL HOSPITAL, 55 Fruit Street, Zip 02114; tel. 617/726–2000; James J. Mongan, M.D., President and Chief Operating Officer A1 2 3 5 8 9 10 F2 3 4 5 6 7 8 9 10 11 12 14 15 16 17 19 20 21 22 23 25 26 27 28 29 30 31 32 33 34 35 37 38 39 40 41 42 43 44 45 46 47 48 49 50 51 52 53 54 55 56 57 58 59 60 61 62 63 65 66 67 68 69 70 71 72 73 74 P3 4 8 S Partners HealthCare System, Boston, MA N Fallon Healthcare System, Worcester, MA; Partners HealthCare System, Boston, MA	23	10	794	33899	616	623099	1513	650848	287941	10803
★ MASSACHUSETTS MENTAL HEALTH CENTER, 74 Fenwood Road, Zip 02115; tel. 617/734–1300; Catherine Howard, Chief Executive Officer (Nonreporting) A3 5 9 S Massachusetts Department of Mental Health, Boston, MA	12	22	27	—	—	—	—	—	—	—
✠ NEW ENGLAND BAPTIST HOSPITAL, 125 Parker Hill Avenue, Zip 02120–3297; tel. 617/738–5800; Alan H. Robbins, M.D., President (Total facility includes 20 beds in nursing home–type unit) A1 3 5 6 9 10 F1 4 5 8 10 12 15 16 17 19 20 21 22 23 24 25 26 29 30 32 34 35 37 39 41 42 43 44 45 49 51 54 60 64 65 66 70 71 72 73 P1 5 6 8 S CareGroup, Boston, MA N CareGroup, Boston, MA; Fallon Healthcare System, Worcester, MA	23	10	141	5742	95	72851	0	90313	35695	883
✠ NEW ENGLAND MEDICAL CENTER, 750 Washington Street, Zip 02111–1845; tel. 617/636–5000; Thomas F. O'Donnell, Jr., M.D., FACS, President and Chief Executive Officer (Total facility includes 21 beds in nursing home–type unit) A1 2 3 5 8 9 10 F3 4 5 7 8 9 10 11 12 13 14 15 16 17 18 19 20 21 22 25 26 27 28 29 30 31 34 35 37 38 39 40 41 42 43 44 45 46 49 51 52 53 54 55 57 58 59 60 64 65 66 67 68 69 70 71 73 74 P5 6 N National Cardiovascular Network, Atlanta, GA	23	10	348	15098	272	346292	1239	344248	125456	4854
✠ SHRINERS HOSPITALS FOR CHILDREN, BURNS INSTITUTE BOSTON UNIT, (PEDIATRIC BURNS), 51 Blossom Street, Zip 02114–2699; tel. 617/722–3000; Robert F. Bories, Jr., FACHE, Administrator A1 5 F16 19 21 22 35 45 49 53 65 67 71 73 S Shriners Hospitals for Children, Tampa, FL	23	59	30	649	18	3248	0	—	—	266
✠ △ SPAULDING REHABILITATION HOSPITAL, 125 Nashua Street, Zip 02114; tel. 617/720–6400; Manuel J. Lipson, M.D., President (Total facility includes 37 beds in nursing home–type unit) A1 3 7 9 10 F2 3 12 17 19 20 21 22 25 26 27 28 29 30 32 34 35 39 41 45 46 48 49 53 54 55 56 57 58 60 64 65 66 71 73 S Partners HealthCare System, Boston, MA	23	46	284	3672	253	75841	0	—	—	1246
✠ ST. ELIZABETH'S MEDICAL CENTER OF BOSTON, 736 Cambridge Street, Zip 02135; tel. 617/789–3000; Michael F. Collins, M.D., President A1 2 3 5 6 8 9 10 F1 2 3 4 7 8 10 11 12 14 15 16 17 18 19 20 21 22 23 25 26 28 29 30 31 32 33 34 35 37 38 39 40 41 42 43 44 45 46 49 51 52 54 55 56 57 58 59 60 61 65 66 67 70 71 72 73 74 P5 7 S Caritas Christi Health Care System, Boston, MA N Caritas Christi Health Network, Boston, MA	21	10	256	13433	247	147498	1824	194443	79101	2306

Hospital, Address, Telephone, Administrator, Approval, Facility, and Physician Codes, Health Care System, Network	Classi-fication Codes		Utilization Data					Expense (thousands) of dollars		
	Control	Service	Beds	Admissions	Census	Outpatient Visits	Births	Total	Payroll	Personnel

Approval/membership symbols

★ American Hospital Association (AHA) membership
□ Joint Commission on Accreditation of Healthcare Organizations (JCAHO) accreditation
+ American Osteopathic Hospital Association (AOHA) membership
○ American Osteopathic Association (AOA) accreditation
△ Commission on Accreditation of Rehabilitation Facilities (CARF) accreditation
Control codes 61, 63, 64, 71, 72 and 73 indicate hospitals listed by AOHA, but not registered by AHA. For definition of numerical codes, see page A4

Hospital	Control	Service	Beds	Admissions	Census	Outpatient Visits	Births	Total	Payroll	Personnel
□ VENCOR HOSPITAL–BOSTON, 1515 Commonwealth Avenue, Zip 02135; tel. 617/254–1100; Steven E. Levitsky, Administrator (Nonreporting) **A**1 10	33	49	59	—	—	—	—	—	—	—
✦ VETERANS AFFAIRS MEDICAL CENTER, Mailing Address: 150 South Huntington Avenue, Jamaica Plain Station, Zip 02130–4820; tel. 617/232–9500; Elwood J. Headley, M.D., Director **A**1 2 3 5 8 **F**2 3 5 8 10 11 12 18 19 20 21 22 24 25 27 28 29 30 31 32 33 34 35 37 39 41 42 44 45 46 48 49 51 52 54 55 56 58 60 65 67 69 71 72 73 74 **P**6 **S** Department of Veterans Affairs, Washington, DC	45	10	418	9520	314	362236	0	—	—	1886
BRAINTREE—Norfolk County										
✦ △ BRAINTREE HOSPITAL REHABILITATION NETWORK, 250 Pond Street, Zip 02185; tel. 617/848–5353; Ernest J. Broadbent, President and Chief Executive Officer **A**1 3 7 9 10 **F**1 5 12 13 14 15 16 17 18 19 21 24 25 26 27 28 29 30 32 34 35 41 42 44 45 48 49 50 51 63 64 65 66 67 71 73 74 **P**5 6 **S** Continental Medical Systems, Inc., Mechanicsburg, PA	33	46	187	2747	171	237962	0	64109	39863	1033
✦ MASSACHUSETTS RESPIRATORY HOSPITAL, 2001 Washington Street, Zip 02184; tel. 617/848–2600; Edward F. Kittredge, Chief Executive Officer **A**1 9 10 **F**12 14 15 17 26 28 30 32 34 41 45 46 49 58 59 65 67 73 **P**6 **S** Quorum Health Group/Quorum Health Resources, Inc., Brentwood, TN	13	48	110	625	62	7428	0	17534	9437	243
BRIDGEWATER—Plymouth County										
BRIDGEWATER STATE HOSPITAL, Administration Road, Zip 02324; tel. 617/697–8161; Kenneth W. Nelson, Superintendent (Nonreporting)	12	22	350	—	—	—	—	—	—	—
BRIGHTON—Suffolk County										
✦ ST. JOHN OF GOD HOSPITAL, 296 Allston Street, Zip 02146–1659; tel. 617/277–5750; William K. Brinkert, President **A**1 9 10 **F**1 2 3 4 7 8 10 11 12 17 19 22 26 30 31 32 33 34 35 37 38 40 41 42 43 44 48 49 50 51 52 54 56 57 58 60 61 64 65 66 71 73 74 **P**8 **S** Caritas Christi Health Care System, Boston, MA **N** Caritas Christi Health Network, Boston, MA	21	48	31	342	36	0	0	8304	4570	90
BROCKTON—Plymouth County										
✦ BROCKTON HOSPITAL, 680 Centre Street, Zip 02402–3395; tel. 508/941–7000; Norman B. Goodman, President and Chief Executive Officer **A**1 2 3 5 6 9 10 **F**3 7 8 10 11 12 13 14 15 16 17 18 19 21 22 26 28 29 30 31 34 37 39 40 41 42 44 46 49 50 51 52 54 55 56 57 58 59 60 61 63 65 66 67 71 72 73 74 **P**1 6	23	10	259	9385	132	105216	1081	88622	51987	1154
✦ BROCKTON–WEST ROXBURY VETERANS AFFAIRS MEDICAL CENTER, 940 Belmont Street, Zip 02401; tel. 508/583–4500; Michael E. Lawson, Director (Total facility includes 149 beds in nursing home–type unit) (Nonreporting) **A**1 3 5 8 **S** Department of Veterans Affairs, Washington, DC	45	10	765	—	—	—	—	—	—	—
✦ GOOD SAMARITAN MEDICAL CENTER, (Includes Good Samaritan Medical Center – Cushing Campus, 235 North Pearl Street, Zip 02401–1794; tel. 508/427–3000; Good Samaritan Medical Center – Goddard Campus, 909 Sumner Street, Stoughton, Zip 02072; tel. 617/344–5100), 235 North Pearl Street, Zip 02401; tel. 508/427–3000; Frank J. Larkin, President and Chief Executive Officer **A**1 2 5 9 10 **F**7 8 11 12 15 16 17 19 20 21 22 23 26 28 30 33 35 37 39 40 41 42 44 45 46 49 54 56 65 67 71 72 73 74 **P**5 **S** Caritas Christi Health Care System, Boston, MA **N** Caritas Christi Health Network, Boston, MA	23	10	218	13129	176	141331	1224	91289	39779	957
BROOKLINE—Norfolk County										
□ BOURNEWOOD HOSPITAL, 300 South Street, Zip 02167–3694; tel. 617/469–0300; Nasir A. Khan, M.D., Director (Nonreporting) **A**1 9 10	33	22	76	—	—	—	—	—	—	—
□ H. R. I. HOSPITAL, 227 Babcock Street, Zip 02146; tel. 617/731–3200; Roy A. Ettlinger, Chief Executive Officer **A**1 3 5 9 10 **F**16 26 34 52 53 55 57 58 59 65 74 **S** Universal Health Services, Inc., King of Prussia, PA	33	22	51	942	38	24308	0	10354	4817	64
BURLINGTON—Middlesex County										
✦ LAHEY HITCHCOCK CLINIC, 41 Mall Road, Zip 01805–0001; tel. 617/744–5100; Bruce W. Steinhauer, M.D., Chief Executive Officer (Nonreporting) **A**1 2 3 5 8 9 10 **N** Lahey Network, Burlington, MA; New England Health Partnership, Waltham, MA	23	10	272	—	—	—	—	—	—	—
CAMBRIDGE—Middlesex County										
✦ CAMBRIDGE PUBLIC HEALTH COMMISSION, (Formerly Cambridge Public Health Authority), (Includes Cambridge Hospital, 1493 Cambridge Street, Somerville Hospital, 230 Highland Avenue, Somerville, Zip 02143; tel. 617/666–4400; Carl Zack, President; 1493 Cambridge Street, Zip 02139–1099; tel. 617/498–1000; John G. O'Brien, Chief Executive Officer (Nonreporting) **A**1 3 5 6 9 10	16	10	257	—	—	—	—	—	—	—
□ M. I. T. MEDICAL DEPARTMENT, 77 Massachusetts Avenue, Zip 02139; tel. 617/253–4481; Arnold N. Weinberg, M.D., Director (Nonreporting) **A**1	23	11	18	—	—	—	—	—	—	—
✦ MOUNT AUBURN HOSPITAL, 330 Mount Auburn Street, Zip 02238; tel. 617/492–3500; Francis P. Lynch, President and Chief Executive Officer **A**1 2 3 5 8 9 10 **F**3 4 7 8 10 11 12 14 15 16 17 19 21 22 23 26 28 29 30 31 32 34 35 36 37 39 40 41 42 43 44 45 46 49 51 52 54 55 56 57 58 59 60 61 65 67 68 70 71 72 73 74 **P**3 5 6 7 **S** CareGroup, Boston, MA **N** CareGroup, Boston, MA	23	10	172	9618	135	240116	1160	115590	57618	1813
✦ STILLMAN INFIRMARY, HARVARD UNIVERSITY HEALTH SERVICES, 75 Mount Auburn Street, Zip 02138; tel. 617/495–2010; David S. Rosenthal, M.D., Director (Nonreporting) **A**1 9 10	23	11	18	—	—	—	—	—	—	—
✦ △ YOUVILLE LIFECARE, 1575 Cambridge Street, Zip 02138–4398; tel. 617/876–4344; T. Richard Quigley, President and Chief Executive Officer (Total facility includes 140 beds in nursing home–type unit) **A**1 6 7 9 10 **F**12 15 16 17 26 30 34 42 48 49 51 54 64 65 67 73 **P**6 **S** Covenant Health Systems, Inc., Lexington, MA	21	46	286	2653	204	6768	0	46148	25265	621

Hospital, Address, Telephone, Administrator, Approval, Facility, and Physician Codes, Health Care System, Network	Classi-fication Codes		Utilization Data					Expense (thousands) of dollars		
★ American Hospital Association (AHA) membership □ Joint Commission on Accreditation of Healthcare Organizations (JCAHO) accreditation + American Osteopathic Hospital Association (AOHA) membership ○ American Osteopathic Association (AOA) accreditation △ Commission on Accreditation of Rehabilitation Facilities (CARF) accreditation Control codes 61, 63, 64, 71, 72 and 73 indicate hospitals listed by AOHA, but not registered by AHA. For definition of numerical codes, see page A4	Control	Service	Beds	Admissions	Census	Outpatient Visits	Births	Total	Payroll	Personnel

CANTON—Norfolk County

✠ MASSACHUSETTS HOSPITAL SCHOOL, 3 Randolph Street, Zip 02021–2397; tel. 617/828–2440; John H. Britt, Executive Director **A**1 5 10 **F**12 15 28 45 46 48 49 51 54 65 67 73 **P**6	12	56	110	74	58	1743	0	14289	8223	242

CHELSEA—Suffolk County

✠ LAWRENCE F. QUIGLEY MEMORIAL HOSPITAL, 91 Crest Avenue, Zip 02150–2199; tel. 617/884–5660; William D. Thompson, Commandant (Total facility includes 88 beds in nursing home–type unit) (Nonreporting) **A**1 10	12	49	159	—	—	—	—	—	—	—

CHICOPEE—Hampden County

□ CHARLES RIVER HOSPITAL–WEST, 350 Memorial Drive, Zip 01020–5025; tel. 413/594–2211; Robert W. Spiegel, President and Chief Executive Officer (Nonreporting) **A**1 10 **S** Community Care Systems, Inc., Wellesley Hills, MA	33	22	90	—	—	—	—	—	—	—

CLINTON—Worcester County

□ CLINTON HOSPITAL, 201 Highland Street, Zip 01510; tel. 508/368–3000; Thomas Devins, Chief Executive Officer **A**1 5 9 10 **F**2 3 8 14 15 16 19 22 26 28 30 31 41 44 46 48 49 52 54 55 57 65 71 72 73 **N** Fallon Healthcare System, Worcester, MA	23	10	46	1361	37	18312	0	8037	4208	196

CONCORD—Middlesex County

✠ EMERSON HOSPITAL, 133 Old Road to Nine Acre Corner, Zip 01742–9120; tel. 508/369–1400; Geoffrey F. Cole, President and Chief Executive Officer **A**1 2 5 9 10 **F**3 7 8 11 13 15 16 17 19 21 22 28 29 30 31 32 33 34 35 36 37 39 40 42 44 45 46 49 52 53 54 55 56 57 58 59 60 61 63 65 66 67 68 71 73 **P**5 6 8	23	10	165	7451	92	178351	1526	68791	34525	894

EVERETT—Middlesex County

WHIDDEN MEMORIAL HOSPITAL See UniCare Health System, Melrose

FALL RIVER—Bristol County

CHARLTON MEMORIAL HOSPITAL See Southcoast Hospitals Group

✠ SAINT ANNE'S HOSPITAL, 795 Middle Street, Zip 02721–1798; tel. 508/674–5741; Joseph W. Wilczek, President **A**1 2 9 10 **F**3 8 15 16 19 21 22 28 30 31 33 34 35 37 39 41 42 44 46 49 54 56 58 60 63 65 67 71 73 **P**5 6 7 **S** Caritas Christi Health Care System, Boston, MA **N** Caritas Christi Health Network, Boston, MA	21	10	165	4841	80	—	0	51014	23045	630
✠ △ SOUTHCOAST HOSPITALS GROUP, (Includes Charlton Memorial Hospital, 363 Highland Avenue, Zip 02720–3794; tel. 508/679–7013; St. Luke's Hospital of New Bedford, 101 Page Street, New Bedford, Zip 02740; Mailing Address: P.O. Box H–3000, Zip 02741–3000; tel. 508/997–1515; Tobey Hospital, 43 High Street, Wareham, Zip 02571; tel. 508/295–0880), 363 Highland Avenue, Zip 02720; tel. 508/679–7013; Ronald B. Goodspeed, M.D., President (Total facility includes 20 beds in nursing home–type unit) **A**1 2 7 9 10 **F**3 7 8 10 11 12 13 14 15 16 17 19 20 21 22 23 24 25 26 27 28 29 30 31 32 33 34 35 37 39 40 41 42 44 45 46 48 49 51 52 54 55 56 57 58 59 60 61 63 64 65 66 67 68 71 72 73 74 **P**5 6 7	23	10	685	31674	527	235717	3668	282650	144971	3440

FALMOUTH—Barnstable County

✠ FALMOUTH HOSPITAL, 100 Ter Heun Drive, Zip 02540–2599; tel. 508/457–3500; Roy A. Hitchings, Jr., FACHE, President **A**1 9 10 **F**6 7 10 12 15 16 17 19 22 26 27 28 29 30 32 33 34 35 37 39 40 42 44 46 49 65 67 71 72 73 74 **P**6 8 **N** Cape Cod Healthcare, Inc., Hyannisport, MA	23	10	84	4742	57	126998	630	43166	21289	620

FITCHBURG—Worcester County

HEALTH ALLIANCE–BURBANK HOSPITAL See Health Alliance Hospitals, Leominster

FRAMINGHAM—Middlesex County

✠ COLUMBIA METROWEST MEDICAL CENTER, (Includes Framingham Union Hospital, 115 Lincoln Street, tel. 508/383–1000; Leonard Morse Hospital, 67 Union Street, Natick, Zip 01760; tel. 508/650–7000), 115 Lincoln Street, Zip 01701; tel. 508/383–1000; Lawrence Kaplan, M.D., President and Chief Executive Officer (Nonreporting) **A**1 2 3 5 6 9 10 **S** Columbia/HCA Healthcare Corporation, Nashville, TN	33	10	423	—	—	—	—	—	—	—

GARDNER—Worcester County

□ HEYWOOD HOSPITAL, 242 Green Street, Zip 01440; tel. 508/632–3420; Daniel P. Moen, President and Chief Executive Officer (Total facility includes 19 beds in nursing home–type unit) **A**1 5 9 10 **F**5 7 8 15 16 17 19 21 22 26 30 31 33 34 35 37 40 41 42 44 46 49 51 52 53 57 64 65 67 68 71 73 **P**5 8	23	10	126	4179	71	126033	403	34182	17160	506

GEORGETOWN—Essex County

BALDPATE HOSPITAL, Baldpate Road, Zip 01833; tel. 617/352–2131; Lucille M. Batal, Administrator (Nonreporting) **A**9 10	33	22	59							

GLOUCESTER—Essex County

ADDISON GILBERT HOSPITAL See Beverly Hospital, Beverly

GREAT BARRINGTON—Berkshire County

✠ FAIRVIEW HOSPITAL, 29 Lewis Avenue, Zip 01230–1713; tel. 413/528–0790; Claire L. Bowen, President **A**1 9 10 **F**7 8 10 12 15 16 17 19 20 21 22 25 26 28 29 30 31 32 33 34 35 37 39 40 41 42 44 46 49 54 55 56 61 65 66 67 71 73 74 **S** Berkshire Health Systems, Inc., Pittsfield, MA **N** Berkshire Health System, Pittsfield, MA	23	10	34	1294	15	—	165	15133	6394	166

GREENFIELD—Franklin County

✠ FRANKLIN MEDICAL CENTER, 164 High Street, Zip 01301; tel. 413/773–0211; Harlan J. Smith, President **A**1 2 9 10 **F**1 2 3 7 8 12 13 15 16 17 18 19 21 22 26 27 29 30 31 32 33 34 35 37 39 40 41 42 44 49 51 52 53 54 55 56 57 58 59 63 65 67 68 71 73 **P**3 5 6 7 8 **S** Baystate Health Systems, Inc., Springfield, MA **N** Baystate Health System, Springfield, MA	23	10	105	4908	60	230907	579	56673	27090	668

Hospital, Address, Telephone, Administrator, Approval, Facility, and Physician Codes, Health Care System, Network	Classi-fication Codes		Utilization Data					Expense (thousands) of dollars		
★ American Hospital Association (AHA) membership □ Joint Commission on Accreditation of Healthcare Organizations (JCAHO) accreditation + American Osteopathic Hospital Association (AOHA) membership ○ American Osteopathic Association (AOA) accreditation △ Commission on Accreditation of Rehabilitation Facilities (CARF) accreditation Control codes 61, 63, 64, 71, 72 and 73 indicate hospitals listed by AOHA, but not registered by AHA. For definition of numerical codes, see page A4	Control	Service	Beds	Admissions	Census	Outpatient Visits	Births	Total	Payroll	Personnel

HAVERHILL—Essex County

✠ HALE HOSPITAL, 140 Lincoln Avenue, Zip 01830; tel. 508/374–2000; Jeffrey Doran, Chief Executive Officer **A**1 9 10 **F**7 8 12 14 15 16 17 19 21 22 28 29 30 34 35 37 39 40 41 42 44 45 49 53 54 56 57 58 61 63 65 67 68 71 73 74 **S** Quorum Health Group/Quorum Health Resources, Inc., Brentwood, TN **N** New England Health Partnership, Waltham, MA	14	10	113	4997	69	59462	595	39607	18362	500
✠ △ WHITTIER REHABILITATION HOSPITAL, 76 Summer Street, Zip 01830; tel. 508/372–8000; Alfred Arcidi, M.D., President (Nonreporting) **A**1 7 10	33	46	60	—	—	—	—	—	—	—

HOLYOKE—Hampden County

✠ HOLYOKE HOSPITAL, 575 Beech Street, Zip 01040–2296; tel. 413/534–2500; Hank J. Porten, President **A**1 2 5 9 10 **F**3 6 7 8 11 12 13 14 15 16 17 18 19 21 22 25 26 28 29 30 31 32 33 34 35 37 39 40 41 42 44 45 46 49 51 52 53 54 55 56 57 58 59 60 61 63 64 65 67 68 71 73 74 **P**6 8	23	10	201	6151	99	131718	227	—	—	751
✠ SOLDIERS' HOME IN HOLYOKE, 110 Cherry Street, Zip 01040; tel. 413/532–9475; Rudy Chmura, Superintendent (Total facility includes 238 beds in nursing home–type unit) **A**1 9 10 **F**15 16 20 34 41 49 58 64 65 73 **P**6	12	10	265	251	291	11226	0	15345	9819	285

HYANNIS—Barnstable County

✠ CAPE COD HOSPITAL, 27 Park Street, Zip 02601; tel. 508/771–1800; Roy A. Hitchings, Jr., FACHE, President (Nonreporting) **A**1 2 5 9 10 **N** Cape Cod Healthcare, Inc., Hyannisport, MA	23	10	258	—	—	—	—	—	—	—

LAWRENCE—Essex County

□ LAWRENCE GENERAL HOSPITAL, 1 General Street, Zip 01842–0389, Mailing Address: P.O. Box 189, Zip 01842–0389; tel. 508/683–4000; Joseph S. McManus, President and Chief Executive Officer (Nonreporting) **A**1 2 3 9 10 **N** Fallon Healthcare System, Worcester, MA	23	10	230	—	—	—	—	—	—	—

LEOMINSTER—Worcester County

✠ HEALTH ALLIANCE HOSPITALS, (Formerly Health Alliance Hospital–Leominster), (Includes Health Alliance–Burbank Hospital, 275 Nichols Road, Fitchburg, Zip 01420–8209; tel. 508/343–5000), 60 Hospital Road, Zip 01453–8004; tel. 508/537–4811; Douglas L. Fairfax, President and Chief Executive Officer **A**1 3 5 9 10 **F**1 7 8 10 12 14 15 16 17 19 21 22 26 28 30 31 32 33 34 35 37 40 41 42 44 48 49 51 52 53 54 56 57 58 59 61 64 65 66 67 68 70 71 72 73 74 **P**5 8 **N** Fallon Healthcare System, Worcester, MA	23	10	208	8419	106	198323	1732	74921	33796	685

LOWELL—Middlesex County

H. C. SOLOMON MENTAL HEALTH CENTER, 391 Varnum Avenue, Zip 01854–2199; tel. 508/454–8851; Kathleen Bown, Director **A**10 **F**12 34 52 53 54 55 57 58 65 **P**6	12	22	16	180	14	—	0	—	—	71
✠ LOWELL GENERAL HOSPITAL, 295 Varnum Avenue, Zip 01854–2195; tel. 508/937–6000; Robert A. Donovan, President and Chief Executive Officer (Total facility includes 21 beds in nursing home–type unit) **A**1 2 9 10 **F**1 3 7 8 10 12 14 15 16 19 21 22 26 28 29 30 31 34 35 37 39 40 41 42 44 45 46 49 52 54 55 56 57 58 59 60 64 65 67 70 71 73 74 **P**1 5	23	10	231	9524	126	146605	2357	68753	32820	939
✠ SAINTS MEMORIAL MEDICAL CENTER, (Includes Saints Memorial Medical Center–East Campus, Saints Memorial Medical Center–West Campus, 220 Pawtucket Street, Zip 01854–3071; tel. 508/453–1761), One Hospital Drive, Zip 01852; tel. 508/458–1411; Thomas Clark, President and Chief Executive Officer (Total facility includes 23 beds in nursing home–type unit) (Nonreporting) **A**1 2 9 10 **N** Fallon Healthcare System, Worcester, MA	23	10	242	—	—	—	—	—	—	—

LUDLOW—Hampden County

✠ △ REHABILITATION HOSPITAL OF WESTERN MASSACHUSETTS, (Formerly Rehabilitation Hospital of Western New England), 14 Chestnut Place, Zip 01056; tel. 413/589–7581; Mark D. Kramer, Administrator **A**1 7 9 10 **F**12 15 16 34 41 42 48 49 54 65 66 67 **S** HEALTHSOUTH Corporation, Birmingham, AL	33	46	40	575	30	13365	0	9007	4343	115

LYNN—Essex County

✠ ATLANTICARE MEDICAL CENTER, 500 Lynnfield Street, Zip 01904–1487; tel. 617/581–9200; Andrew J. Riddell, President and Chief Executive Officer (Total facility includes 24 beds in nursing home–type unit) **A**1 2 5 9 10 **F**2 3 8 10 11 12 14 15 16 17 18 19 22 26 28 29 30 31 32 34 35 37 39 42 44 45 46 48 49 52 60 64 65 66 67 68 71 73 **P**3 4 5 **N** Lahey Network, Burlington, MA	23	10	189	6829	119	—	0	69859	29294	697

MALDEN—Middlesex County

✠ MALDEN HOSPITAL, 100 Hospital Road, Zip 02148–3591; tel. 617/322–7560; Stanley W. Krygowski, President (Total facility includes 23 beds in nursing home–type unit) **A**1 3 5 9 10 **F**4 5 7 8 10 12 14 15 16 17 18 19 21 22 26 28 29 30 32 33 34 35 37 39 40 41 42 44 45 49 51 52 54 55 56 57 58 59 60 61 63 64 65 66 67 71 72 73 **P**5 7 **N** New England Health Partnership, Waltham, MA	23	10	176	5357	102	76195	544	54535	24469	708

MARLBOROUGH—Middlesex County

✠ MARLBOROUGH HOSPITAL, 57 Union Street, Zip 01752; tel. 508/481–5000; Anne Burgeois, Interim Chief Executive Officer **A**1 5 9 10 **F**2 3 8 12 15 16 17 18 19 20 22 26 28 30 32 33 34 35 37 39 41 42 44 46 49 52 54 56 57 58 59 65 66 67 68 71 72 73 74 **P**5 7 8 **N** Continuum of Care Network, Marlborough, MA; Fallon Healthcare System, Worcester, MA	23	10	71	3342	47	65281	0	32749	16246	402

MEDFIELD—Norfolk County

✠ MEDFIELD STATE HOSPITAL, 45 Hospital Road, Zip 02052; tel. 508/359–7312; Theodore E. Kirousis, Area Director (Nonreporting) **A**1 9 10 **S** Massachusetts Department of Mental Health, Boston, MA	12	22	212	—	—	—	—	—	—	—

MEDFORD—Middlesex County

✠ LAWRENCE MEMORIAL HOSPITAL OF MEDFORD, 170 Governors Avenue, Zip 02155; tel. 617/306–6000; Charles F. Johnson, President (Total facility includes 19 beds in nursing home–type unit) **A**1 2 5 6 9 10 **F**8 13 14 15 16 17 19 21 22 25 26 27 29 30 32 34 36 37 39 42 44 49 51 52 54 57 58 59 60 63 64 65 67 71 73 74 **P**5 6 8	23	10	169	5686	105	140605	0	52543	28347	873

Hospital, Address, Telephone, Administrator, Approval, Facility, and Physician Codes, Health Care System, Network	Classi-fication Codes		Utilization Data					Expense (thousands) of dollars		
★ American Hospital Association (AHA) membership □ Joint Commission on Accreditation of Healthcare Organizations (JCAHO) accreditation + American Osteopathic Hospital Association (AOHA) membership ○ American Osteopathic Association (AOA) accreditation △ Commission on Accreditation of Rehabilitation Facilities (CARF) accreditation Control codes 61, 63, 64, 71, 72 and 73 indicate hospitals listed by AOHA, but not registered by AHA. For definition of numerical codes, see page A4	Control	Service	Beds	Admissions	Census	Outpatient Visits	Births	Total	Payroll	Personnel

MELROSE—Middlesex County

MELROSE–WAKEFIELD HOSPITAL See UniCare Health System

☒ UNICARE HEALTH SYSTEM, (Includes Melrose–Wakefield Hospital, 585 Lebanon Street, tel. 617/979–3000; Whidden Memorial Hospital, 103 Garland Street, Everett, Zip 02149–5095), 585 Lebanon Street, Zip 02176; tel. 617/979–3000; Richard S. Quinlan, President and Chief Executive Officer (Total facility includes 21 beds in nursing home–type unit) (Nonreporting) **A**1 2 9 10 — 23 10 343

| | 23 | 10 | 343 | | | | | | | |

METHUEN—Essex County

☒ HOLY FAMILY HOSPITAL AND MEDICAL CENTER, 70 East Street, Zip 01844–4597; tel. 508/687–0151; William L. Lane, President **A**1 2 9 10 **F**3 7 8 10 11 12 13 14 15 16 17 18 19 20 21 22 23 25 26 28 29 30 31 32 33 34 35 37 38 39 40 41 42 44 45 46 49 51 52 53 54 55 56 57 58 59 60 63 65 66 67 68 69 71 72 73 74 **P**3 5 6 7 **S** Caritas Christi Health Care System, Boston, MA **N** Caritas Christi Health Network, Boston, MA; Fallon Healthcare System, Worcester, MA

| | 21 | 10 | 247 | 8268 | 138 | 76127 | 968 | 64882 | 32513 | 868 |

MIDDLEBOROUGH—Plymouth County

□ CRANBERRY SPECIALTY HOSPITAL OF PLYMOUTH COUNTY, 52 Oak Street, Zip 02346; tel. 508/947–1000; Edward B. Leary, President (Nonreporting) **A**1 9 10

| | 13 | 46 | 68 | — | — | — | — | — | — | — |

MILFORD—Worcester County

☒ MILFORD–WHITINSVILLE REGIONAL HOSPITAL, (Includes Whitinsville Medical Center, 18 Granite Street, Whitinsville, Zip 01588; tel. 508/234–6311), 14 Prospect Street, Zip 01757; tel. 508/473–1190; Francis M. Saba, President and Chief Executive Officer (Nonreporting) **A**1 5 9 10 **N** Fallon Healthcare System, Worcester, MA

| | 23 | 10 | 125 | | | | | | | |

MILTON—Norfolk County

☒ MILTON HOSPITAL, 92 Highland Street, Zip 02186–3807; tel. 617/696–4600; George A. Geary, President (Nonreporting) **A**1 2 9 10

| | 23 | 10 | 137 | — | — | — | — | — | — | — |

NANTUCKET—Nantucket County

☒ NANTUCKET COTTAGE HOSPITAL, 57 Prospect Street, Zip 02554–2799; tel. 508/228–1200; Lucille C. Giddings, R.N., CHE, President and Chief Executive Officer **A**1 9 10 **F**1 3 7 8 13 14 15 17 19 22 28 30 31 32 33 37 40 41 42 44 49 65 67 71

| | 23 | 10 | 19 | 632 | 8 | 35148 | 66 | 8539 | 4626 | 109 |

NATICK—Middlesex County

LEONARD MORSE HOSPITAL See Columbia MetroWest Medical Center, Framingham

NEEDHAM—Norfolk County

☒ DEACONESS–GLOVER HOSPITAL CORPORATION, 148 Chestnut Street, Zip 02192–2483; tel. 617/444–5600; John Dalton, President and Chief Executive Officer **A**1 2 9 10 **F**2 3 4 7 8 10 11 12 15 16 17 18 19 20 21 22 24 25 26 27 28 29 30 31 32 33 34 35 36 37 39 40 41 42 43 44 45 46 49 50 51 52 53 54 55 56 57 58 59 60 61 63 64 65 66 67 69 71 73 74 **P**5 7 8 **S** CareGroup, Boston, MA **N** CareGroup, Boston, MA; Fallon Healthcare System, Worcester, MA

| | 23 | 10 | 54 | 2190 | 33 | 54678 | 0 | 21602 | 10043 | 274 |

NEW BEDFORD—Bristol County

ST. LUKE'S HOSPITAL OF NEW BEDFORD See Southcoast Hospitals Group, Fall River

NEWBURYPORT—Essex County

☒ ANNA JAQUES HOSPITAL, 25 Highland Avenue, Zip 01950–3894; tel. 508/463–1000; Allan L. DesRosiers, President (Total facility includes 20 beds in nursing home–type unit) **A**1 9 10 **F**7 8 11 12 13 15 16 17 18 19 21 22 28 29 30 31 32 33 34 35 36 37 39 40 41 42 44 45 46 49 52 53 54 56 58 59 63 64 65 66 67 71 73 **P**5

| | 23 | 10 | 145 | 6367 | 92 | 129285 | 813 | 53317 | 23767 | 733 |

NEWTON—Middlesex County

☒ NEWTON–WELLESLEY HOSPITAL, 2014 Washington Street, Zip 02162; tel. 617/243–6000; John P. Bihldorff, President and Chief Executive Officer **A**1 2 3 5 9 10 **F**1 3 7 8 12 13 14 15 16 17 18 19 22 26 30 31 32 34 35 37 38 40 41 42 44 46 49 51 52 53 54 55 56 57 58 59 61 65 66 67 71 73 **P**5 8

| | 23 | 10 | 240 | 13497 | 159 | 96552 | 4163 | 121000 | 60163 | 1447 |

NORFOLK—Norfolk County

☒ SOUTHWOOD COMMUNITY HOSPITAL, 111 Dedham Street, Zip 02056; tel. 508/668–0385; Yolanda Landrau, R.N., Ed.D., President and Chief Executive Officer (Nonreporting) **A**1 2 9 10 **S** Neponset Valley Health System, Norwood, MA

| | 23 | 10 | 182 | — | — | — | — | — | — | — |

NORTH ADAMS—Berkshire County

☒ NORTH ADAMS REGIONAL HOSPITAL, Hospital Avenue, Zip 01247; tel. 413/663–3701; John C. J. Cronin, President and Chief Executive Officer **A**1 2 9 10 **F**4 8 10 12 13 15 16 17 19 22 27 28 30 31 32 33 35 37 39 40 41 42 44 45 46 49 52 54 55 65 67 71 73

| | 23 | 10 | 134 | 5000 | 76 | 66903 | 351 | 32531 | 15274 | 390 |

NORTHAMPTON—Hampshire County

☒ COOLEY DICKINSON HOSPITAL, 30 Locust Street, Zip 01061–5001, Mailing Address: P.O. Box 5001, Zip 01061–5001; tel. 413/582–2000; Craig N. Melin, President and Chief Executive Officer **A**1 2 9 10 **F**3 7 8 12 14 15 16 17 19 20 21 22 27 28 30 31 32 33 34 35 37 39 40 41 42 44 45 46 49 52 54 55 56 57 58 60 63 65 66 67 68 71 72 73 **P**6 8

| | 23 | 10 | 149 | 7018 | 85 | 135940 | 945 | 57645 | 31025 | 630 |

☒ VETERANS AFFAIRS MEDICAL CENTER, Route 9, Zip 01060–1288; tel. 413/584–4040; Bruce A. Gordon, Director (Total facility includes 50 beds in nursing home–type unit) (Nonreporting) **A**1 **S** Department of Veterans Affairs, Washington, DC

| | 45 | 22 | 361 | — | — | — | — | — | — | — |

Hospital, Address, Telephone, Administrator, Approval, Facility, and Physician Codes, Health Care System, Network	Classi-fication Codes		Utilization Data					Expense (thousands) of dollars		
★ American Hospital Association (AHA) membership □ Joint Commission on Accreditation of Healthcare Organizations (JCAHO) accreditation + American Osteopathic Hospital Association (AOHA) membership ○ American Osteopathic Association (AOA) accreditation △ Commission on Accreditation of Rehabilitation Facilities (CARF) accreditation Control codes 61, 63, 64, 71, 72 and 73 indicate hospitals listed by AOHA, but not registered by AHA. For definition of numerical codes, see page A4	Control	Service	Beds	Admissions	Census	Outpatient Visits	Births	Total	Payroll	Personnel

NORWOOD—Norfolk County

⊞ NORWOOD HOSPITAL, 800 Washington Street, Zip 02062; tel. 617/769–4000; Yolanda Landrau, R.N., Ed.D., President and Chief Executive Officer (Nonreporting) **A**1 2 5 9 10 **S** Neponset Valley Health System, Norwood, MA
| | 23 | 10 | 150 | — | — | — | — | — | — | — |

OAK BLUFFS—Dukes County

⊞ MARTHA'S VINEYARD HOSPITAL, Linton Lane, Zip 02557, Mailing Address: P.O. Box 1477, Zip 02557; tel. 508/693–0410; Charles S. Kinney, Chief Executive Officer (Total facility includes 81 beds in nursing home–type unit) (Nonreporting) **A**1 9 10
| | 23 | 10 | 123 | — | — | — | — | — | — | — |

PALMER—Hampden County

⊞ WING MEMORIAL HOSPITAL AND MEDICAL CENTERS, 40 Wright Street, Zip 01069–1138; tel. 413/283–7651; Richard H. Scheffer, President **A**1 2 5 9 10 **F**3 8 12 19 21 22 25 30 32 33 34 37 41 42 44 49 51 52 53 54 55 56 57 58 61 65 66 67 71 72 73 74 **P**6 **N** Lahey Network, Burlington, MA
| | 23 | 10 | 46 | 2088 | 29 | 124678 | — | 27920 | 14909 | 389 |

PEABODY—Essex County

□ THC–BOSTON, 15 King Street, Zip 01960; tel. 508/531–2900; Della Underwood, Chief Executive Officer (Nonreporting) **A**1 9 10 **S** Transitional Hospitals Corporation, Las Vegas, NV
| | 14 | 10 | 59 | — | — | — | — | — | — | — |

PEMBROKE—Plymouth County

□ PEMBROKE HOSPITAL, 199 Oak Street, Zip 02359; tel. 617/826–8161; Michael P. Krupa, Ed.D., Chief Executive Officer (Nonreporting) **A**1 9
| | 33 | 22 | 115 | — | — | — | — | — | — | — |

PITTSFIELD—Berkshire County

⊞ △ BERKSHIRE MEDICAL CENTER, (Includes Hillcrest Hospital, 165 Tor Court, Zip 01201–3099, Mailing Address: Box 1155, Zip 01202–1155; tel. 413/443–4761; Eugene A. Dellea, President and Chief Executive Officer), 725 North Street, Zip 01201; tel. 413/447–2000; Ruth P. Blodgett, Chief Operating Officer **A**1 2 3 5 7 8 9 10 12 **F**2 3 4 6 8 10 11 12 13 15 16 17 18 19 20 21 22 26 28 30 31 32 34 35 37 39 40 41 42 44 45 46 48 49 51 52 53 54 56 57 58 59 60 64 65 66 70 71 72 73 74 **S** Berkshire Health Systems, Inc., Pittsfield, MA **N** Berkshire Health System, Pittsfield, MA
HILLCREST HOSPITAL See Berkshire Medical Center
| | 23 | 10 | 330 | 12884 | 226 | 109706 | 1022 | 131026 | 63405 | 1401 |

PLYMOUTH—Plymouth County

⊞ JORDAN HOSPITAL, 275 Sandwich Street, Zip 02360–2196; tel. 508/746–2001; Alan D. Knight, President and Chief Executive Officer **A**1 2 9 10 **F**1 2 3 4 7 8 11 12 15 16 17 18 19 21 22 23 27 28 29 30 31 32 33 34 35 37 39 40 41 42 43 44 45 46 48 49 52 53 54 56 60 64 65 66 67 68 71 73 **P**4 5 6 7 **S** Quorum Health Group/Quorum Health Resources, Inc., Brentwood, TN
| | 23 | 10 | 123 | 6393 | 82 | 173289 | 848 | 63812 | 28642 | 596 |

POCASSET—Barnstable County

□ BARNSTABLE COUNTY HOSPITAL, 870 County Road, Zip 02559; tel. 508/563–5941; Edward B. Leary, President (Nonreporting) **A**1 9 10
| | 13 | 46 | 39 | — | — | — | — | — | — | — |

QUINCY—Norfolk County

⊞ QUINCY HOSPITAL, 114 Whitwell Street, Zip 02169–1899; tel. 617/773–6100; Ralph DiPisa, Chief Executive Officer (Total facility includes 28 beds in nursing home–type unit) (Nonreporting) **A**1 9 10 **S** Quorum Health Group/Quorum Health Resources, Inc., Brentwood, TN **N** New England Health Partnership, Waltham, MA
| | 14 | 10 | 254 | — | — | — | — | — | — | — |

SALEM—Essex County

⊞ SALEM HOSPITAL, (Includes North Shore Children's Hospital, tel. 508/745–2100), 81 Highland Avenue, Zip 01970; tel. 508/741–1200; Michael J. Geaney, Jr., President **A**1 2 3 5 9 10 **F**2 3 7 8 10 11 12 15 16 19 21 22 23 24 25 26 27 28 29 30 31 32 33 34 35 37 39 40 41 42 44 45 46 49 51 52 53 54 55 56 58 59 60 63 65 66 67 68 71 72 73 74 **P**5 6 8 **S** Partners HealthCare System, Boston, MA **N** Partners HealthCare System, Boston, MA
| | 23 | 10 | 291 | 11810 | 155 | 398776 | 1710 | 130755 | 69902 | 1698 |

⊞ △ SHAUGHNESSY–KAPLAN REHABILITATION HOSPITAL, Dove Avenue, Zip 01970; tel. 508/745–9000; Anthony Sciola, President and Chief Executive Officer (Total facility includes 40 beds in nursing home–type unit) **A**1 7 9 10 **F**2 3 7 8 10 11 12 13 14 15 16 17 18 19 20 21 22 23 26 27 28 29 30 31 32 33 34 35 37 38 40 41 42 44 45 46 47 48 49 51 52 53 54 56 57 58 59 60 61 63 65 66 67 71 72 73 74 **P**6 8 **S** Partners HealthCare System, Boston, MA **N** Partners HealthCare System, Boston, MA
| | 23 | 46 | 160 | 2015 | 117 | 22293 | 0 | 21222 | 10730 | 234 |

SOMERVILLE—Middlesex County

SOMERVILLE HOSPITAL See Cambridge Public Health Commission, Cambridge

SOUTH ATTLEBORO—Bristol County

□ FULLER MEMORIAL HOSPITAL, 200 May Street, Zip 02703–5599; tel. 508/761–8500; Landon Kite, President (Nonreporting) **A**1 9 10 **S** Universal Health Services, Inc., King of Prussia, PA
| | 33 | 22 | 46 | — | — | — | — | — | — | — |

SOUTH WEYMOUTH—Norfolk County

⊞ SOUTH SHORE HOSPITAL, 55 Fogg Road, Zip 02190–2455; tel. 617/340–8000; David T. Hannan, President and Chief Executive Officer (Total facility includes 25 beds in nursing home–type unit) **A**1 2 9 10 **F**7 11 14 16 19 21 22 23 26 28 30 32 33 34 35 37 39 40 41 42 44 45 46 49 54 56 60 61 64 65 67 68 71 **P**1 3 7
| | 23 | 10 | 277 | 14879 | 188 | 438946 | 3069 | 160189 | 79595 | 2110 |

SOUTHBRIDGE—Worcester County

⊞ HARRINGTON MEMORIAL HOSPITAL, 100 South Street, Zip 01550–4045; tel. 508/765–9771; Richard M. Mangion, President and Chief Executive Officer **A**1 5 9 10 **F**1 3 4 5 6 7 8 10 11 12 14 15 16 17 18 19 20 21 22 23 24 25 26 27 28 30 31 32 33 34 35 36 37 39 40 41 42 43 44 45 46 49 50 51 52 53 54 55 56 57 58 59 60 61 62 63 65 66 67 68 69 70 71 73 74 **P**8 **N** Fallon Healthcare System, Worcester, MA
| | 23 | 10 | 113 | 4022 | 52 | 199804 | 383 | 36451 | 20488 | 515 |

Hospital, Address, Telephone, Administrator, Approval, Facility, and Physician Codes, Health Care System, Network	Classi-fication Codes		Utilization Data					Expense (thousands) of dollars		
★ American Hospital Association (AHA) membership □ Joint Commission on Accreditation of Healthcare Organizations (JCAHO) accreditation + American Osteopathic Hospital Association (AOHA) membership ○ American Osteopathic Association (AOA) accreditation △ Commission on Accreditation of Rehabilitation Facilities (CARF) accreditation Control codes 61, 63, 64, 71, 72 and 73 indicate hospitals listed by AOHA, but not registered by AHA. For definition of numerical codes, see page A4	Control	Service	Beds	Admissions	Census	Outpatient Visits	Births	Total	Payroll	Personnel

SPRINGFIELD—Hampden County

★ BAYSTATE MEDICAL CENTER, 759 Chestnut Street, Zip 01199–0001; tel. 413/784–0000; Mark R. Tolosky, Chief Executive Officer **A**1 2 3 5 6 8 9 10 **F**4 7 8 10 11 13 14 15 16 17 19 20 21 22 23 24 25 26 27 28 30 31 32 33 34 35 37 38 39 40 41 42 43 44 45 46 47 49 51 52 53 54 55 56 57 58 59 60 61 63 64 65 67 68 69 70 71 72 73 74 **P**1 3 5 6 **S** Baystate Health Systems, Inc., Springfield, MA **N** Baystate Health System, Springfield, MA | 23 | 10 | 660 | 28178 | 452 | 325417 | 5164 | 332077 | 146103 | 3701 |

★ △ MERCY HOSPITAL, 271 Carew Street, Zip 01104, Mailing Address: P.O. Box 9012, Zip 01102–9012; tel. 413/748–9000; Vincent J. McCorkle, President and Chief Executive Officer **A**1 2 7 9 10 **F**1 3 7 8 10 11 12 14 15 16 17 19 20 21 22 25 26 28 29 30 31 32 34 35 37 39 40 41 42 44 45 46 48 49 51 53 54 55 56 57 58 59 60 63 65 67 68 71 73 74 **S** Sisters of Providence Health System, Springfield, MA **N** Sisters of Providence Health System, Springfield, MA | 21 | 10 | 262 | 8489 | 164 | 97608 | 2 | 82192 | 34887 | 1078 |

□ OLYMPUS SPECIALTY HOSPITAL–SPRINGFIELD, (Formerly Springfield Municipal Hospital), 1400 State Street, Zip 01109–2589; tel. 413/787–6700; Marilyn M. Riddle, Chief Executive Officer (Total facility includes 220 beds in nursing home–type unit) (Nonreporting) **A**1 5 10 | 14 | 49 | 394 | | | | | | | |

★ SHRINERS HOSPITALS FOR CHILDREN, SPRINGFIELD, 516 Carew Street, Zip 01104–2396; tel. 413/787–2000; Mark L. Niederpruem, Administrator (Nonreporting) **A**1 3 5 **S** Shriners Hospitals for Children, Tampa, FL | 23 | 57 | 40 | | | | | | | |

SPRINGFIELD MUNICIPAL HOSPITAL See Olympus Specialty Hospital–Springfield

STOCKBRIDGE—Berkshire County

★ AUSTEN RIGGS CENTER, 25 Main Street, Zip 01262–0962, Mailing Address: P.O. Box 962, Zip 01262–0962; tel. 413/298–5511; Edward R. Shapiro, M.D., Medical Director and Chief Executive Officer (Nonreporting) **A**1 3 | 23 | 22 | 47 | | | | | | | |

STONEHAM—Middlesex County

□ BOSTON REGIONAL MEDICAL CENTER, 5 Woodland Road, Zip 02180, Mailing Address: P.O. Box 9102, Zip 02180–9102; tel. 617/979–7000; Charles S. Ricks, D.D.S., President and Chief Executive Officer (Nonreporting) **A**1 2 3 9 10 **N** Fallon Healthcare System, Worcester, MA | 21 | 10 | 187 | | | | | | | |

STOUGHTON—Plymouth County

GOOD SAMARITAN MEDICAL CENTER See Brockton

GOOD SAMARITAN MEDICAL CENTER – GODDARD CAMPUS See Good Samaritan Medical Center, Brockton

★ △ NEW ENGLAND SINAI HOSPITAL AND REHABILITATION CENTER, (CHRONIC DISEASE & REHAB), 150 York Street, Zip 02072–1881; tel. 617/364–4850; Donald H. Goldberg, President **A**1 3 7 9 10 **F**1 5 12 15 16 20 28 33 34 39 42 48 49 54 65 66 67 71 73 | 23 | 49 | 160 | 1450 | 147 | 26386 | 0 | 37111 | 21277 | 499 |

TAUNTON—Bristol County

★ MORTON HOSPITAL AND MEDICAL CENTER, 88 Washington Street, Zip 02780–2499; tel. 508/828–7000; Thomas C. Porter, President **A**1 2 9 10 **F**7 8 10 12 13 14 15 16 17 19 21 22 23 25 28 30 34 35 37 39 40 41 44 45 46 49 51 60 65 66 67 68 71 72 73 74 **P**6 | 23 | 10 | 178 | 5445 | 84 | 148447 | 634 | 69434 | 32231 | 785 |

□ TAUNTON STATE HOSPITAL, 60 Hodges Avenue Extension, Zip 02780, Mailing Address: P.O. Box 4007, Zip 02780; tel. 508/824–7551; Gary Phillips, Administrator and Chief Operating Officer **A**1 9 10 **F**1 12 15 16 17 18 52 53 54 55 56 57 59 65 73 **S** Massachusetts Department of Mental Health, Boston, MA | 12 | 22 | 185 | 365 | 176 | 0 | | — | — | 423 |

TEWKSBURY—Middlesex County

★ TEWKSBURY HOSPITAL, East Street, Zip 01876–1998; tel. 508/851–7321; Raymond D. Sanzone, Executive Director **A**1 6 10 **F**3 15 16 20 22 27 31 34 42 46 49 52 54 55 65 67 73 **P**6 **S** Massachusetts Department of Mental Health, Boston, MA | 12 | 48 | 527 | 379 | 483 | 0 | 0 | 35096 | — | 712 |

WALTHAM—Middlesex County

★ DEACONESS WALTHAM HOSPITAL, Hope Avenue, Zip 02254–9116; tel. 617/647–6000; Jeanette G. Clough, President and Chief Executive Officer (Total facility includes 21 beds in nursing home–type unit) **A**1 2 5 9 10 **F**2 3 7 8 11 12 13 14 15 16 17 18 19 20 21 22 23 26 27 28 29 30 31 32 33 35 36 37 40 41 42 44 45 46 49 51 52 53 54 55 56 57 58 59 60 61 64 65 66 67 68 70 71 72 73 74 **P**3 4 5 6 8 **S** CareGroup, Boston, MA **N** CareGroup, Boston, MA; Fallon Healthcare System, Worcester, MA | 23 | 10 | 198 | 6678 | 123 | 61211 | 318 | 57893 | 29552 | 786 |

□ MIDDLESEX HOSPITAL, 775 Trapelo Road, Zip 02254, Mailing Address: P.O. Box 9151, Zip 02254–9151; tel. 617/895–7000; Jeanne M. Boyle, R.N., Chief Operating Officer (Nonreporting) **A**1 9 10 | 13 | 48 | 120 | — | — | — | — | — | — | — |

WARE—Hampshire County

★ MARY LANE HOSPITAL, 85 South Street, Zip 01082; tel. 413/967–6211; Christine Shirtcliff, Executive Vice President (Nonreporting) **A**1 9 10 **S** Baystate Health Systems, Inc., Springfield, MA **N** Baystate Health System, Springfield, MA | 23 | 10 | 35 | — | — | — | — | — | — | — |

WAREHAM—Plymouth County

TOBEY HOSPITAL See Southcoast Hospitals Group, Fall River

WEBSTER—Worcester County

★ HUBBARD REGIONAL HOSPITAL, 340 Thompson Road, Zip 01570–0608; tel. 508/943–2600; Gerald J. Barbini, Administrator and Chief Executive Officer **A**1 9 10 **F**8 14 15 19 21 22 27 30 34 37 39 41 42 44 45 46 49 56 58 65 71 72 73 74 **P**3 7 **S** Quorum Health Group/Quorum Health Resources, Inc., Brentwood, TN **N** Fallon Healthcare System, Worcester, MA; New England Health Partnership, Waltham, MA | 23 | 10 | 34 | 1298 | 18 | — | 0 | 14049 | 6525 | 200 |

Hospital, Address, Telephone, Administrator, Approval, Facility, and Physician Codes, Health Care System, Network	Classi-fication Codes		Utilization Data					Expense (thousands) of dollars		
★ American Hospital Association (AHA) membership ☐ Joint Commission on Accreditation of Healthcare Organizations (JCAHO) accreditation + American Osteopathic Hospital Association (AOHA) membership ○ American Osteopathic Association (AOA) accreditation △ Commission on Accreditation of Rehabilitation Facilities (CARF) accreditation Control codes 61, 63, 64, 71, 72 and 73 indicate hospitals listed by AOHA, but not registered by AHA. For definition of numerical codes, see page A4	Control	Service	Beds	Admissions	Census	Outpatient Visits	Births	Total	Payroll	Personnel

WELLESLEY—Norfolk County

☐ CHARLES RIVER HOSPITAL, 203 Grove Street, Zip 02181; tel. 617/235–8400; Juliette Fay, President and Chief Executive Officer **A**1 3 9 10 **F**3 12 14 15 16 26 34 52 53 54 55 56 57 58 59 65 **P**5 **S** Community Care Systems, Inc., Wellesley Hills, MA | 33 | 22 | 62 | 766 | 22 | 809 | 0 | 5375 | 4838 | 183

SIMPSON INFIRMARY, WELLESLEY COLLEGE, Worcester Street, Zip 02181–8277; tel. 617/283–2810; Charlotte K. Sanner, M.D., Director Health Service **A**9 **F**14 15 16 28 29 34 39 45 51 61 66 67 74 | 23 | 11 | 11 | 116 | 1 | 8208 | 0 | — | — | 13

WESTBOROUGH—Worcester County

☐ WESTBOROUGH STATE HOSPITAL, Mailing Address: P.O. Box 288, Zip 01581; tel. 617/727–9830; Theodore E. Kirousis, Area Director (Nonreporting) **A**1 5 9 10 **S** Massachusetts Department of Mental Health, Boston, MA | 12 | 22 | 220 | — | — | — | — | — | — | —

WESTFIELD—Hampden County

☒ NOBLE HOSPITAL, 115 West Silver Street, Zip 01086–1634; tel. 413/572–5040; George J. Koller, President and Chief Executive Officer **A**1 2 5 9 10 **F**8 14 15 16 19 21 22 28 29 30 32 33 35 37 39 41 42 44 45 46 48 49 52 54 55 56 65 67 71 72 73 74 **P**8 | 23 | 10 | 97 | 2924 | 58 | 95971 | 0 | 26478 | 14139 | 359

WESTWOOD—Norfolk County

☐ WESTWOOD LODGE HOSPITAL, 45 Clapboardtree Street, Zip 02090; tel. 617/762–7764; Michael P. Krupa, Ed.D., Chief Executive Officer (Nonreporting) **A**1 9 10 | 33 | 22 | 100 | — | — | — | — | — | — | —

WHITINSVILLE—Worcester County

WHITINSVILLE MEDICAL CENTER See Milford–Whitinsville Regional Hospital, Milford

WINCHESTER—Middlesex County

☒ WINCHESTER HOSPITAL, 41 Highland Avenue, Zip 01890–9920; tel. 617/729–9000; Stephen R. Laverty, President and Chief Executive Officer (Nonreporting) **A**1 2 5 9 10 | 23 | 10 | 156 | — | — | — | — | — | — | —

WOBURN—Middlesex County

★ CHOATE HEALTH SYSTEMS, 23 Warren Avenue, Zip 01801; tel. 617/933–6700; David Fassler, M.D., President (Nonreporting) **A**10 | 33 | 22 | 21 | — | — | — | — | — | — | —

☐ △ HEALTHSOUTH NEW ENGLAND REHABILITATION HOSPITAL, (Formerly New England Rehabilitation Hospital), Two Rehabilitation Way, Zip 01801–6098; tel. 617/935–5050; Guido J. Cubellis, Chief Executive Officer (Nonreporting) **A**1 7 9 10 **S** HEALTHSOUTH Corporation, Birmingham, AL | 33 | 46 | 198 | — | — | — | — | — | — | —

WORCESTER—Worcester County

ADCARE HOSPITAL OF WORCESTER, 107 Lincoln Street, Zip 01605–2499; tel. 508/799–9000; David W. Hillis, President (Nonreporting) **A**9 10 | 33 | 82 | 88 | — | — | — | — | — | — | —

☐ △ FAIRLAWN REHABILITATION HOSPITAL, 189 May Street, Zip 01602–4399; tel. 508/791–6351; Ellen Ferrante, President and Chief Executive Officer **A**1 5 7 9 10 **F**12 15 25 26 34 45 46 48 49 65 73 **S** HEALTHSOUTH Corporation, Birmingham, AL | 33 | 46 | 110 | 1675 | 94 | 19796 | 0 | 21551 | 9981 | 322

MEDICAL CENTER OF CENTRAL MASSACHUSETTS See Memorial Health Care

☒ MEMORIAL HEALTH CARE, (Formerly Medical Center of Central Massachusetts), 119 Belmont Street, Zip 01605–2982; tel. 508/793–6611; Peter H. Levine, M.D., President and Chief Executive Officer (Total facility includes 31 beds in nursing home–type unit) **A**1 2 3 5 8 9 10 12 **F**3 7 8 10 11 12 13 15 16 17 19 21 22 23 25 26 28 29 30 31 32 33 34 35 37 38 40 42 44 45 49 51 52 53 54 55 56 57 58 59 60 61 63 64 65 66 67 68 71 72 73 74 **P**2 8 | 23 | 10 | 377 | 21126 | 259 | 328786 | 3775 | 184425 | 86251 | 2291

☐ SAINT VINCENT HOSPITAL, 25 Winthrop Street, Zip 01604–4593; tel. 508/798–1234; Robert E. Maher, Jr., President and Chief Executive Officer (Nonreporting) **A**1 2 3 5 8 9 10 12 **S** TENET Healthcare Corporation, Santa Barbara, CA **N** Fallon Healthcare System, Worcester, MA | 23 | 10 | 369 | — | — | — | — | — | — | —

☒ UNIVERSITY OF MASSACHUSETTS MEDICAL CENTER, 55 Lake Avenue North, Zip 01655; tel. 508/856–0011; Lin C. Weeks, Dr.PH, R.N., Director (Nonreporting) **A**1 2 3 5 8 9 10 **N** Fallon Healthcare System, Worcester, MA | 12 | 10 | 388 | — | — | — | — | — | — | —

☐ WORCESTER STATE HOSPITAL, 305 Belmont Street, Zip 01604; tel. 508/752–4681; Bernard Kingsley, Chief Operating Officer (Nonreporting) **A**1 5 9 10 **S** Massachusetts Department of Mental Health, Boston, MA | 12 | 22 | 176 | — | — | — | — | — | — | —

MICHIGAN

Resident population 9,549 (in thousands)
Resident population in metro areas 82.5%
Birth rate per 1,000 population 14.8
65 years and over 12.4%
Percent of persons without health insurance 10.8%

Hospital, Address, Telephone, Administrator, Approval, Facility, and Physician Codes, Health Care System, Network	Classi-fication Codes		Utilization Data						Expense (thousands) of dollars		
★ American Hospital Association (AHA) membership □ Joint Commission on Accreditation of Healthcare Organizations (JCAHO) accreditation + American Osteopathic Hospital Association (AOHA) membership ○ American Osteopathic Association (AOA) accreditation △ Commission on Accreditation of Rehabilitation Facilities (CARF) accreditation Control codes 61, 63, 64, 71, 72 and 73 indicate hospitals listed by AOHA, but not registered by AHA. For definition of numerical codes, see page A4	Control	Service	Beds	Admissions	Census	Outpatient Visits	Births	Total	Payroll	Personnel

	Control	Service	Beds	Admissions	Census	Outpatient Visits	Births	Total	Payroll	Personnel
ADDISON—Lenawee County										
□ ADDISON COMMUNITY HOSPITAL, 421 North Steer Street, Zip 49220; tel. 517/547–6151; Trevor J. Dyksterhouse, Administrator (Nonreporting) **A**1 9 10	16	10	24	—	—	—	—	—	—	—
ADRIAN—Lenawee County										
⊞ BIXBY MEDICAL CENTER, 818 Riverside Avenue, Zip 49221; tel. 517/265–0900; John R. Robertstad, President and Chief Executive Officer **A**1 2 9 10 **F**3 7 8 14 15 16 19 20 22 33 34 35 37 40 42 44 46 49 52 54 57 58 60 65 66 67 71 73 **P**8	23	10	103	4368	49	102613	625	37339	18141	580
ALBION—Calhoun County										
□ TRILLIUM HOSPITAL, (Formerly Albion Community Hospital), 809 West Erie Street, Zip 49224–1556; tel. 517/629–2191; Michael G. Boff, President **A**1 9 10 **F**7 8 10 11 12 14 15 16 17 19 20 21 22 26 28 29 30 32 33 34 35 37 39 40 41 42 44 51 53 54 55 56 57 58 59 63 65 71 72 73 **P**1 5 8	23	10	61	1421	13	66376	113	12394	5938	201
ALLEGAN—Allegan County										
⊞ ALLEGAN GENERAL HOSPITAL, 555 Linn Street, Zip 49010–1594; tel. 616/673–8424; James Klun, President (Nonreporting) **A**1 9 10 **S** Quorum Health Group/Quorum Health Resources, Inc., Brentwood, TN **N** Hospital Network Inc., Kalamazoo, MI	23	10	63							
ALMA—Gratiot County										
⊞ GRATIOT COMMUNITY HOSPITAL, 300 South Warwick Drive, Zip 48801; tel. 517/463–1101; Bob M. Baker, President and Chief Executive Officer (Nonreporting) **A**1 9 10	23	10	127	—	—	—	—	—	—	—
ALPENA—Alpena County										
⊞ ALPENA GENERAL HOSPITAL, 1501 West Chisholm Street, Zip 49707–1498; tel. 517/356–7390; John A. McVeety, Chief Executive Officer **A**1 2 9 10 **F**2 3 4 7 8 10 12 15 16 17 19 21 22 27 28 29 30 31 32 33 34 35 36 37 39 40 41 42 43 44 45 46 49 52 53 54 55 56 57 58 63 65 66 67 68 71 72 73 74	13	10	149	5466	69	61447	518	48367	23680	655
ANN ARBOR—Washtenaw County										
⊞ △ ST. JOSEPH MERCY HEALTH SYSTEM, (Formerly Catherine McAuley Health System), (Includes St. Joseph Mercy Hospital), 5301 East Huron River Drive, Zip 48106, Mailing Address: Box 995, Zip 48106–0992; tel. 313/712–3456; Garry C. Faja, President and Chief Executive Officer **A**1 2 3 5 7 8 9 10 **F**1 3 4 7 8 10 11 12 13 14 15 16 17 19 20 21 22 25 26 28 29 30 31 32 33 34 35 37 39 40 41 42 43 44 45 46 48 49 51 52 53 54 55 56 57 58 59 60 63 65 66 67 68 70 71 72 73 74 **P**1 **S** Mercy Health Services, Farmington Hills, MI **N** Mercy Health Services, Farmington Hills, MI	21	10	481	26175	363	439338	3951	316924	127368	3774
□ UNIVERSITY OF MICHIGAN HOSPITALS, 1150 West Medical Center Drive, Zip 48109–0603; tel. 313/936–4000; Larry Warren, Interim Executive Director **A**1 2 3 5 8 9 10 **F**2 3 4 5 7 8 9 10 11 12 13 14 17 18 19 20 21 22 23 24 25 26 28 29 30 31 32 34 35 36 37 38 39 40 41 42 43 44 45 46 47 48 49 50 51 52 53 54 55 56 57 58 60 61 63 65 66 67 69 70 71 72 73 74	23	10	848	33016	657	1016941	2406	882176	324257	8361
⊞ VETERANS AFFAIRS MEDICAL CENTER, 2215 Fuller Road, Zip 48105; tel. 313/769–7100; Edward L. Gamache, Director (Total facility includes 60 beds in nursing home–type unit) **A**1 3 5 8 9 **F**2 3 4 5 8 10 11 14 16 19 20 21 22 23 25 26 27 28 29 30 31 32 33 34 35 37 39 41 42 43 44 45 46 49 50 51 52 54 55 56 57 58 59 60 64 65 67 69 71 72 73 74 **S** Department of Veterans Affairs, Washington, DC	45	10	238	5691	183	295797	0	111904	62993	1722
AUBURN HILLS—Oakland County										
□ HAVENWYCK HOSPITAL, 1525 University Drive, Zip 48326–2675; tel. 810/373–9200; Robert A. Kercorian, Chief Executive Officer (Nonreporting) **A**1 9 10 **S** Ramsay Health Care, Inc., Coral Gobles, FL	33	22	120	—	—	—	—	—	—	—
BAD AXE—Huron County										
⊞ HURON MEMORIAL HOSPITAL, 1100 South Van Dyke Road, Zip 48413–9799; tel. 517/269–9521; James B. Gardner, President **A**1 9 10 **F**7 8 14 15 16 19 21 22 27 28 30 32 33 34 37 39 40 41 42 44 49 63 65 67 71	23	10	64	1707	18	43686	236	17036	7391	253
BATTLE CREEK—Calhoun County										
⊞ BATTLE CREEK HEALTH SYSTEM, (Includes Community Hospital, 183 West Street, Zip 49016; Fieldstone Center, 165 North Washington Avenue, Zip 49016; tel. 616/964–7121; Leila Hospital, 300 North Avenue, Zip 49016), 300 North Avenue, Zip 49016–3396; tel. 616/966–8000; Stephen L. Abbott, President and Chief Executive Officer (Total facility includes 77 beds in nursing home–type unit) **A**1 2 9 10 **F**2 3 7 8 10 12 13 14 15 16 17 18 19 21 22 26 27 28 29 30 34 35 37 39 40 41 42 44 45 48 49 52 53 54 55 56 57 58 59 60 63 64 65 66 67 70 71 72 73 74 **P**1 **S** Mercy Health Services, Farmington Hills, MI **N** Mercy Health Services, Farmington Hills, MI; Battle Creek Health System, Battle Creek, MI	23	10	402	12143	264	128988	1196	113534	46735	1488
FIELDSTONE CENTER See Battle Creek Health System										
★ △ SOUTHWESTERN MICHIGAN REHABILITATION HOSPITAL, 183 West Street, Zip 49017; tel. 616/965–3206; David Mungenast, President **A**7 9 10 **F**15 17 34 48 49 65	23	46	30	379	13	23278	0	5046	1670	51

Hospital, Address, Telephone, Administrator, Approval, Facility, and Physician Codes, Health Care System, Network	Classi-fication Codes		Utilization Data					Expense (thousands) of dollars		
★ American Hospital Association (AHA) membership □ Joint Commission on Accreditation of Healthcare Organizations (JCAHO) accreditation + American Osteopathic Hospital Association (AOHA) membership ○ American Osteopathic Association (AOA) accreditation △ Commission on Accreditation of Rehabilitation Facilities (CARF) accreditation Control codes 61, 63, 64, 71, 72 and 73 indicate hospitals listed by AOHA, but not registered by AHA. For definition of numerical codes, see page A4	Control	Service	Beds	Admissions	Census	Outpatient Visits	Births	Total	Payroll	Personnel

✠ VETERANS AFFAIRS MEDICAL CENTER, 5500 Armstrong Road, Zip 49016; tel. 616/966–5600; Michael K. Wheeler, Director (Total facility includes 191 beds in nursing home–type unit) **A**1 5 9 **F**1 2 3 4 5 6 8 10 12 15 16 17 18 19 20 21 22 23 24 25 26 27 28 29 30 31 32 33 34 35 36 37 39 41 43 44 45 46 48 49 50 51 52 54 55 56 57 58 59 60 63 64 65 67 70 71 72 73 74 **S** Department of Veterans Affairs, Washington, DC	45	22	640	4112	580	151901	0	87370	52479	1403
BAY CITY—Bay County										
✠ △ BAY MEDICAL CENTER, (Includes Bay Medical Center–West Campus, 3250 East Midland Road, Zip 48706; tel. 517/667–6750; Samaritan Health Center, 713 Ninth Street, tel. 517/894–3799), 1900 Columbus Avenue, Zip 48708; tel. 517/894–3000; Anthony W. Armstrong, President **A**1 2 7 9 10 12 **F**2 3 6 7 8 10 12 14 15 16 17 18 19 20 21 22 26 28 29 30 31 32 33 34 35 36 37 39 40 41 42 44 45 46 48 49 52 54 55 56 58 59 60 63 65 66 67 70 71 72 73 74 **P**6 8	23	10	339	15748	224	238984	1163	112593	51357	1716
BAY SPECIAL CARE, (Formerly Bay Special Care Center), 3250 East Midland Road, Suite 1, Zip 48706; tel. 517/667–6802; Cheryl A. Burzynski, President (Nonreporting) **A**10	23	48	20	—	—	—	—	—	—	—
BERRIEN CENTER—Berrien County										
LAKELAND MEDICAL CENTER, BERRIEN CENTER See Lakeland Medical Center–St. Joseph, Saint Joseph										
BIG RAPIDS—Mecosta County										
✠ MECOSTA COUNTY GENERAL HOSPITAL, 405 Winter Avenue, Zip 49307–2099; tel. 616/796–8691; Thomas E. Daugherty, Chief Executive Officer **A**1 9 10 **F**7 8 10 15 16 19 22 33 34 36 37 40 41 42 44 45 48 49 63 65 71 72 73 **P**4 7 **S** Quorum Health Group/Quorum Health Resources, Inc., Brentwood, TN	13	10	74	2351	26	73258	653	18504	7775	258
BRIGHTON—Livingston County										
★ BRIGHTON HOSPITAL, 12851 East Grand River Avenue, Zip 48116–8596; tel. 810/227–1211; Deborah A. Sopo, President **A**9 10 **F**2 3 14 15 16 39	23	82	63	1301	41	9726	0	7063	3026	128
CADILLAC—Wexford County										
✠ MERCY HEALTH SERVICES–NORTH, (Formerly Mercy Hospital), 400 Hobart Street, Zip 49601–9596; tel. 616/876–7200; Dennis J. Renander, President and Chief Executive Officer **A**1 9 10 **F**3 7 8 10 12 14 15 16 17 19 20 21 22 24 28 29 30 31 32 33 34 35 37 39 40 41 42 44 45 46 49 51 52 54 55 56 58 63 65 66 67 71 73 **P**1 2 3 4 5 6 7 8 **S** Mercy Health Services, Farmington Hills, MI **N** Mercy Health Services, Farmington Hills, MI	21	10	89	4835	50	70472	567	37491	14717	572
CARO—Tuscola County										
□ CARO CENTER, 2000 Walk Road, Zip 48723–0153, Mailing Address: Box A, Zip 48723–0153; tel. 517/673–3191; Rose Laskowski, R.N., Facility Director (Nonreporting) **A**1 9 10	12	22	234	—	—	—	—	—	—	—
★ CARO COMMUNITY HOSPITAL, 401 North Hooper Street, Zip 48723, Mailing Address: P.O. Box 71, Zip 48723; tel. 517/673–3141; William P. Miller, President and Chief Executive Officer (Nonreporting) **A**9 10	15	10	19	—	—	—	—	—	—	—
CARSON CITY—Montcalm County										
+ ○ CARSON CITY HOSPITAL, 406 East Elm Street, Zip 48811–0879, Mailing Address: P.O. Box 879, Zip 48811–0879; tel. 517/584–3131; Bruce L. Traverse, President **A**9 10 11 12 13 **F**7 14 15 16 17 19 20 22 28 30 32 34 35 41 42 44 51 52 54 55 56 58 65 67 71 73 74 **P**6 **N** Butterworth Health System, Grand Rapids, MI	23	10	78	2436	27	44798	379	18934	9496	385
CASS CITY—Tuscola County										
✠ HILLS AND DALES GENERAL HOSPITAL, 4675 Hill Street, Zip 48726–1099; tel. 517/872–2121; Dee McKrow, Chief Executive Officer **A**1 9 10 **F**7 8 12 15 16 17 19 21 22 24 28 29 30 31 32 33 34 39 40 41 42 44 45 46 49 51 63 65 66 67 71 73 **P**5	23	10	47	807	9	23442	0	7763	3289	150
CHARLEVOIX—Charlevoix County										
✠ CHARLEVOIX AREA HOSPITAL, 14700 Lake Shore Drive, Zip 49720–1931; tel. 616/547–4024; Richard L. Krueger, President **A**1 9 10 **F**7 8 14 15 16 17 20 22 28 30 37 40 41 44 49 65 66 71 73	23	10	33	1305	12	18793	169	10473	4818	152
CHARLOTTE—Eaton County										
✠ HAYES–GREEN–BEACH MEMORIAL HOSPITAL, 321 East Harris Street, Zip 48813; tel. 517/543–1050; Scott D. Currie, Chief Operating Officer **A**1 9 10 **F**7 8 14 15 16 19 21 22 24 28 29 30 32 34 36 39 40 44 49 65 66 67 71 73	23	10	45	1505	15	90993	175	14260	7840	218
CHEBOYGAN—Cheboygan County										
✠ COMMUNITY MEMORIAL HOSPITAL, 748 South Main Street, Zip 49721–2299, Mailing Address: P.O. Box 419, Zip 49721–0419; tel. 616/627–5601; Howard J. Purcell, Jr., President (Total facility includes 50 beds in nursing home–type unit) **A**1 9 10 **F**8 15 16 19 20 21 22 32 33 34 37 40 44 64 71 73	23	10	92	2343	72	81986	210	19750	9698	359
CHELSEA—Washtenaw County										
□ △ CHELSEA COMMUNITY HOSPITAL, 775 South Main Street, Zip 48118–1399; tel. 313/475–1311; Willard H. Johnson, President **A**1 3 5 7 9 10 **F**3 8 14 15 17 19 21 22 24 25 26 28 29 30 32 34 37 39 41 42 44 45 46 48 49 52 53 54 55 57 58 59 61 65 67 71 72 73 74	23	10	105	3051	60	119358	0	41348	20023	581
CLARE—Clare County										
✠ ○ MIDMICHIGAN REGIONAL MEDICAL CENTER–CLARE, 104 West Sixth Street, Zip 48617–1409; tel. 517/386–9951; Lawrence F. Barco, President **A**1 9 10 11 **F**7 8 15 17 19 21 22 28 30 32 33 35 40 41 42 44 45 49 63 67 71 72 73 74 **P**6 8 **S** MidMichigan Regional Health System, Midland, MI	23	10	64	2642	25	31922	307	17407	8271	259

Hospital, Address, Telephone, Administrator, Approval, Facility, and Physician Codes, Health Care System, Network	Classi-fication Codes		Utilization Data					Expense (thousands) of dollars		
	Control	Service	Beds	Admissions	Census	Outpatient Visits	Births	Total	Payroll	Personnel

★ American Hospital Association (AHA) membership
□ Joint Commission on Accreditation of Healthcare Organizations (JCAHO) accreditation
+ American Osteopathic Hospital Association (AOHA) membership
○ American Osteopathic Association (AOA) accreditation
△ Commission on Accreditation of Rehabilitation Facilities (CARF) accreditation
  Control codes 61, 63, 64, 71, 72 and 73 indicate hospitals listed by AOHA, but not registered by AHA. For definition of numerical codes, see page A4

CLINTON TOWNSHIP—Macomb County

| ☒ ST. JOSEPH'S MERCY HOSPITALS AND HEALTH SERVICES, (Includes St. Joseph's Mercy Hospital–East, 215 North Avenue, Mount Clemens, Zip 48043; tel. 810/466–9300; St. Joseph's Mercy Hospital–West, 15855 19 Mile Road, Zip 48038; tel. 810/263–2300; St. Joseph's Mercy–North, 80650 North Van Dyke, Romeo, Zip 48065; tel. 810/798–3551), Robert L. Beyer, President and Chief Executive Officer **A**1 9 10 **F**3 6 7 8 10 11 12 13 15 16 17 19 21 22 26 27 28 29 30 31 32 33 34 35 36 37 39 40 41 42 44 45 46 48 49 52 54 55 56 57 58 59 61 64 65 67 68 71 72 73 74 **P**6 7 8 **S** Mercy Health Services, Farmington Hills, MI **N** Mercy Health Services, Farmington Hills, MI | 23 | 10 | 380 | 15155 | 236 | 279568 | 1947 | 119156 | 55969 | 2043 |

COLDWATER—Branch County

| ☒ + ○ COMMUNITY HEALTH CENTER OF BRANCH COUNTY, 274 East Chicago Street, Zip 49036–2088; tel. 517/279–5489; Douglas L. Rahn, Chief Executive Officer **A**1 9 10 11 12 **F**3 7 8 10 16 19 21 22 31 35 37 40 41 42 44 49 51 52 54 55 56 57 58 59 63 65 67 70 71 73 **P**6 **S** Quorum Health Group/Quorum Health Resources, Inc., Brentwood, TN | 13 | 10 | 96 | 3739 | 43 | 75875 | 415 | 31015 | 13213 | 444 |

COMMERCE TOWNSHIP—Oakland County

| ☒ HURON VALLEY HOSPITAL, 1601 East Commerce Road, Zip 48382; tel. 810/360–3300; Elliot Joseph, Senior Vice President, Oakland Region **A**1 3 5 10 **F**7 8 10 14 15 19 21 22 27 28 30 31 33 34 37 39 40 42 44 45 46 49 54 65 66 67 71 73 **P**4 6 **S** Detroit Medical Center, Detroit, MI **N** Detroit Medical Center, Detroit, MI | 23 | 10 | 139 | 7932 | 91 | 57816 | 1866 | 65925 | 22548 | 685 |

CRYSTAL FALLS—Iron County

CRYSTAL FALLS COMMUNITY HOSPITAL See Iron County Community Hospital, Iron River

DEARBORN—Wayne County

| ☒ OAKWOOD HOSPITAL AND MEDICAL CENTER–DEARBORN, 18101 Oakwood Boulevard, Zip 48124, Mailing Address: P.O. Box 2500, Zip 48123–2500; tel. 313/593–7000; Gerald D. Fitzgerald, President and Chief Executive Officer **A**1 2 3 5 8 9 10 **F**1 2 3 4 6 7 8 10 11 12 13 14 15 16 17 18 19 20 21 22 23 24 25 26 27 28 29 30 31 32 33 34 35 36 37 38 39 40 41 42 43 44 45 46 48 49 51 52 53 54 55 56 57 58 59 60 61 62 63 64 65 66 67 68 69 71 72 73 74 **P**2 5 6 **S** Oakwood Healthcare System, Dearborn, MI | 23 | 10 | 560 | 27092 | 406 | 627508 | 4535 | 289078 | 149165 | 3331 |

DECKERVILLE—Sanilac County

| ☒ DECKERVILLE COMMUNITY HOSPITAL, 3559 Pine Street, Zip 48427–0126, Mailing Address: P.O. Box 126, Zip 48427–0126; tel. 810/376–2835; Charlotte Williams, Interim Administrator **A**1 9 10 **F**5 8 15 17 19 22 28 30 32 34 41 42 44 45 46 49 65 67 70 71 72 **S** Mercy Health Services, Farmington Hills, MI **N** Mercy Health Services, Farmington Hills, MI | 23 | 10 | 17 | 346 | 3 | 14065 | 0 | 3033 | 1535 | 66 |

DETROIT—Wayne County

□ ○ AURORA HOSPITAL FOR CHILDREN, 3737 Lawton, Zip 48208; tel. 313/361–7600; Patricia Strong, Administrator **A**1 10 11 **F**12 16 18 52 53 54 55 56 59 65 67 **S** Michigan Health Care Corporation, Southfield, MI	23	52	80	1096	47	—	0	18339	6212	241
☒ △ CHILDREN'S HOSPITAL OF MICHIGAN, 3901 Beaubien, Zip 48201–9985; tel. 313/745–0073; Thomas M. Rozek, Senior Vice President **A**1 3 5 7 8 9 10 **F**2 3 4 5 6 7 8 9 10 11 12 13 14 15 16 17 19 20 21 22 24 25 26 27 28 29 30 31 33 34 35 36 37 38 39 40 41 42 43 44 45 46 47 48 49 50 51 52 54 55 56 57 58 60 61 64 65 66 67 69 70 71 72 73 74 **P**2 3 4 5 6 8 **S** Detroit Medical Center, Detroit, MI **N** Detroit Medical Center, Detroit, MI	23	50	245	14127	172	206602	0	182780	66299	1800
☒ DETROIT RECEIVING HOSPITAL AND UNIVERSITY HEALTH CENTER, 4201 St. Antoine Boulevard, Zip 48201–2194; tel. 313/745–3605; Leslie C. Bowman, Regional Administrator, Ancillary Services and Site Administrator **A**1 3 5 8 10 **F**4 7 8 9 10 11 12 17 18 19 21 22 23 27 28 29 30 31 32 34 35 37 39 41 42 43 44 46 49 50 51 52 54 56 57 58 60 65 67 70 71 72 73 **S** Detroit Medical Center, Detroit, MI **N** Detroit Medical Center, Detroit, MI	23	10	290	12180	216	116647	0	163111	58898	1752
☒ ○ DETROIT RIVERVIEW HOSPITAL, 7733 East Jefferson Avenue, Zip 48214; tel. 313/499–3000; Richard T. Young, Administrator (Nonreporting) **A**1 9 10 11 **S** Detroit–Macomb Hospital Corporation, Warren, MI **N** Detroit–Macomb Hospital Corp, Warren, MI	23	10	230	—	—	—	—	—	—	—
☒ GRACE HOSPITAL, 6071 West Outer Drive, Zip 48235; tel. 313/966–3300; Anne M. Regling, Regional Executive **A**1 3 5 8 9 10 12 **F**1 2 3 4 7 8 9 10 11 12 13 17 18 19 20 21 22 23 25 26 27 28 29 30 31 32 33 34 35 37 38 39 40 41 42 43 44 45 46 47 48 49 50 51 52 53 54 55 56 57 58 59 60 61 63 64 65 66 67 68 69 70 71 72 73 74 **P**5 6 7 8 **S** Detroit Medical Center, Detroit, MI **N** Detroit Medical Center, Detroit, MI	23	10	352	17122	259	135949	2893	213548	79321	2039
☒ HARPER HOSPITAL, 3990 John R, Zip 48201–9027; tel. 313/745–8040; Paul L. Broughton, FACHE, Senior Vice President **A**1 2 3 5 8 9 10 **F**2 3 4 7 8 9 10 11 12 13 14 15 16 17 18 19 20 21 22 23 24 25 26 27 28 29 30 31 32 33 34 35 36 37 38 39 40 41 42 43 44 45 46 47 48 49 50 51 52 53 54 55 56 57 58 60 61 63 64 65 66 67 68 69 70 71 72 73 74 **P**2 3 4 5 6 8 **S** Detroit Medical Center, Detroit, MI **N** Detroit Medical Center, Detroit, MI	23	10	427	18609	366	178774	0	309854	102695	2569
☒ HENRY FORD HOSPITAL, 2799 West Grand Boulevard, Zip 48202–2689; tel. 313/876–2600; Stephen H. Velick, Chief Executive Officer **A**1 2 3 5 6 8 9 10 **F**1 2 3 4 5 6 7 8 9 10 11 12 13 14 15 16 17 18 19 20 21 22 23 24 25 26 27 28 29 30 31 32 33 34 35 36 37 38 39 40 41 42 43 44 45 46 47 48 49 51 52 53 54 55 56 57 58 59 60 61 63 64 65 66 67 68 69 70 71 72 73 74 **P**6 **S** Henry Ford Health System, Detroit, MI **N** Henry Ford Health System, Detroit, MI	23	10	605	35141	494	—	2535	332639	127615	5373

Hospital, Address, Telephone, Administrator, Approval, Facility, and Physician Codes, Health Care System, Network	Classi-fication Codes		Utilization Data					Expense (thousands) of dollars		
★ American Hospital Association (AHA) membership □ Joint Commission on Accreditation of Healthcare Organizations (JCAHO) accreditation + American Osteopathic Hospital Association (AOHA) membership ○ American Osteopathic Association (AOA) accreditation △ Commission on Accreditation of Rehabilitation Facilities (CARF) accreditation Control codes 61, 63, 64, 71, 72 and 73 indicate hospitals listed by AOHA, but not registered by AHA. For definition of numerical codes, see page A4	Control	Service	Beds	Admissions	Census	Outpatient Visits	Births	Total	Payroll	Personnel
⊞ HOLY CROSS HOSPITAL, 4777 East Outer Drive, Zip 48234–0401; tel. 313/369–9100; Michael F. Breen, President **A**1 9 10 **F**1 2 3 4 5 6 7 8 9 10 11 12 13 14 15 16 17 18 19 21 22 23 24 25 26 27 28 29 30 31 32 33 34 35 36 37 38 39 40 41 42 43 44 45 46 47 48 49 50 51 52 53 54 55 56 57 58 59 60 61 62 64 65 66 67 70 71 72 73 74 **P**5 8 **S** Sisters of St. Joseph Health System, Ann Arbor, MI **N** Saint John Health System, Detroit, MI	21	10	161	2470	120	22637	0	21123	10605	498
⊞ HUTZEL HOSPITAL, 4707 St. Antoine Boulevard, Zip 48201–0154; tel. 313/745–7555; Susan A. Erickson, Clinical Services Administrator for Women's Services and Site Administrator **A**1 3 5 8 9 10 **F**1 3 4 5 7 8 9 10 11 12 13 14 15 16 17 18 19 20 21 22 23 24 25 26 27 28 29 30 31 32 33 34 35 36 37 38 39 40 41 42 43 44 45 46 47 48 49 50 51 52 53 54 55 56 57 58 59 60 61 63 64 65 66 67 68 69 70 71 72 73 74 **P**2 4 5 7 8 **S** Detroit Medical Center, Detroit, MI **N** Detroit Medical Center, Detroit, MI	23	10	243	12144	120	84919	6493	176969	61845	1651
⊞ MERCY HOSPITAL, 5555 Conner Avenue, Zip 48213–3499; tel. 313/579–4000; Brenita Crawford, President and Chief Executive Officer **A**1 3 10 **F**1 2 3 4 7 8 10 12 13 14 15 16 17 18 19 20 22 23 24 25 26 27 28 30 31 32 33 34 35 37 40 41 42 43 44 49 51 52 53 54 55 56 58 59 60 62 64 65 67 69 71 72 73 74 **P**5 6 8 **S** Mercy Health Services, Farmington Hills, MI **N** Mercy Health Services, Farmington Hills, MI	21	10	248	9345	186	215397	891	98425	42999	1201
+ ○ MICHIGAN HOSPITAL AND MEDICAL CENTER, 2700 Martin Luther King Jr. Boulevard, Zip 48208; tel. 313/361–8112; Barbara J. Clark, Vice President and Chief Operating Officer (Nonreporting) **A**9 10 11 12 13 **S** Michigan Health Care Corporation, Southfield, MI	23	10	416	—	—	—	—	—	—	—
□ NEW CENTER HOSPITAL, 801 Virginia Park, Zip 48202; tel. 313/874–2800; Alfred Moore, Chief Executive Officer (Nonreporting) **A**1 9 10	23	10	145	—	—	—	—	—	—	—
⊞ △ REHABILITATION INSTITUTE OF MICHIGAN, 261 Mack Boulevard, Zip 48201; tel. 313/745–1203; Bruce M. Gans, M.D., Senior Vice President **A**1 3 5 7 9 10 **F**3 4 5 7 8 9 10 11 13 14 16 17 19 20 21 22 23 24 25 26 27 28 29 30 31 32 33 34 35 37 38 39 40 41 42 43 44 45 47 48 49 50 51 52 53 54 55 56 57 58 59 60 61 63 64 65 66 67 69 70 71 72 73 74 **P**4 5 6 **S** Detroit Medical Center, Detroit, MI **N** Detroit Medical Center, Detroit, MI	23	46	96	1781	75	79386	0	46362	21426	541
SARATOGA COMMUNITY HOSPITAL See St. John Health System–Saratoga Campus										
⊞ ○ △ SINAI HOSPITAL, 6767 West Outer Drive, Zip 48235–2899; tel. 313/493–6800 **A**1 3 5 7 8 9 10 11 12 **F**4 5 7 8 10 11 12 14 15 16 17 18 19 20 21 22 24 25 26 27 28 29 30 32 33 34 35 37 38 40 41 42 43 44 45 46 47 48 49 51 52 53 54 55 56 57 58 59 60 61 65 66 67 70 71 72 73 74 **P**6 8 **S** Detroit Medical Center, Detroit, MI	23	10	469	20634	364	269160	3318	282923	147147	3118
⊞ △ ST. JOHN HEALTH SYSTEM–SARATOGA CAMPUS, (Formerly Saratoga Community Hospital), 15000 Gratiot Avenue, Zip 48205–1999; tel. 313/245–1200; Michael F. Breen, President **A**1 7 9 10 **F**8 12 14 15 16 17 19 21 22 25 26 27 28 30 31 34 37 39 42 44 45 48 49 63 64 65 67 71 73 **P**5 8 **S** Sisters of St. Joseph Health System, Ann Arbor, MI **N** Saint John Health System, MI	23	10	170	3999	105	21826	3	34121	15218	617
⊞ ST. JOHN HOSPITAL AND MEDICAL CENTER, 22101 Moross Road, Zip 48236–2172; tel. 313/343–4000; Timothy J. Grajewski, President and Chief Executive Officer **A**1 2 3 5 8 9 10 **F**2 3 4 7 8 10 11 12 13 14 15 16 17 18 19 20 22 23 25 27 28 29 30 31 32 33 35 37 38 39 40 41 42 43 44 46 48 49 51 52 53 56 58 59 60 61 62 64 65 66 67 68 69 70 71 72 73 74 **P**3 5 6 8 **S** Sisters of St. Joseph Health System, Ann Arbor, MI **N** Saint John Health System, Detroit, MI; Port Huron Hospital/Blue Water Health Services, Port Huron, MI	21	10	599	27932	443	245163	3335	316150	149529	3947
⊞ VETERANS AFFAIRS MEDICAL CENTER, 4646 John R Street, Zip 48201; tel. 313/576–1000; Carlos B. Lott, Jr., Director (Total facility includes 90 beds in nursing home–type unit) **A**1 2 3 8 9 **F**2 3 4 5 6 8 10 11 12 14 15 16 17 18 19 20 21 22 23 26 27 28 29 30 31 32 33 34 35 37 39 41 42 43 44 45 46 49 50 51 52 54 55 56 58 59 60 61 63 64 65 67 69 70 71 72 73 74 **P**6 **S** Department of Veterans Affairs, Washington, DC	45	10	432	7774	252	211818	0	131259	71185	1562
DOWAGIAC—Cass County										
⊞ LEE MEMORIAL HOSPITAL, 420 West High Street, Zip 49047–1907; tel. 616/782–8681; Fritz Fahrenbacher, Vice President and Regional Hospital Administrator **A**1 9 10 **F**8 11 14 15 16 19 22 25 28 29 30 33 35 36 39 42 44 45 49 53 54 55 56 57 58 59 65 66 67 71 72 73 **P**6 8 **S** Sisters of St. Joseph Health System, Ann Arbor, MI **N** First Choice Network, Watervliet, MI	21	10	47	1695	20	29069	0	11340	5119	179
EAST CHINA—St. Clair County										
⊞ RIVER DISTRICT HOSPITAL, 4100 South River Road, Zip 48054; tel. 810/329–7111; John E. Knox, President **A**1 9 10 **F**3 7 8 12 15 16 19 21 22 30 32 37 40 41 42 44 46 49 56 58 65 67 71 73 **P**6 8 **S** Sisters of St. Joseph Health System, Ann Arbor, MI **N** Saint John Health System, Detroit, MI; Port Huron Hospital/Blue Water Health Services, Port Huron, MI	23	10	68	2771	25	55004	698	22229	10378	307
EATON RAPIDS—Eaton County										
□ EATON RAPIDS COMMUNITY HOSPITAL, 1500 South Main Street, Zip 48827–0130, Mailing Address: P.O. Box 130, Zip 48827–0130; tel. 517/663–2671; Jack L. Denton, President **A**1 9 10 **F**8 12 14 15 16 19 22 28 30 34 35 36 39 42 44 45 46 51 56 65 71 72 73	23	10	21	716	7	27684	0	6846	3061	127
ESCANABA—Delta County										
⊞ ST. FRANCIS HOSPITAL, 3401 Ludington Street, Zip 49829; tel. 906/786–3311; Roger M. Burgess, Administrator **A**1 5 9 10 **F**7 8 15 16 19 22 28 30 32 33 34 35 37 40 41 42 44 45 49 65 67 69 71 72 73 74 **P**6 **S** OSF Healthcare System, Peoria, IL	23	10	66	3367	45	63524	424	28624	13366	473

Hospital, Address, Telephone, Administrator, Approval, Facility, and Physician Codes, Health Care System, Network	Classi-fication Codes		Utilization Data					Expense (thousands) of dollars		
	Control	Service	Beds	Admissions	Census	Outpatient Visits	Births	Total	Payroll	Personnel

★ American Hospital Association (AHA) membership
□ Joint Commission on Accreditation of Healthcare Organizations (JCAHO) accreditation
+ American Osteopathic Hospital Association (AOHA) membership
○ American Osteopathic Association (AOA) accreditation
△ Commission on Accreditation of Rehabilitation Facilities (CARF) accreditation
Control codes 61, 63, 64, 71, 72 and 73 indicate hospitals listed by AOHA, but not registered by AHA. For definition of numerical codes, see page A4

FARMINGTON HILLS—Oakland County

★ + ○ △ BOTSFORD GENERAL HOSPITAL, 28050 Grand River Avenue, Zip 48336–5933; tel. 248/471–8000; Gerson I. Cooper, President **A**7 9 10 11 12 13 **F**3 5 7 8 10 11 12 14 15 16 17 19 21 22 24 25 26 27 28 29 30 31 32 33 34 35 37 40 41 42 44 45 46 48 49 51 52 54 57 58 62 64 65 66 67 69 71 72 73 74 **P**5 6 7 **N** Great Lakes Health Network, Southfield, MI	23	10	333	12769	220	352726	906	154630	77632	2009

FERNDALE—Oakland County

⊞ KINGSWOOD HOSPITAL, 10300 West Eight Mile Road, Zip 48220; tel. 810/398–3200; Kathleen Emrich, R.N., Ed.D., Assistant Vice President and Chief Operating Officer **A**1 3 9 10 **F**19 21 22 35 52 53 54 55 58 59 65 71 **P**4 **S** Henry Ford Health System, Detroit, MI **N** Henry Ford Health System, Detroit, MI	23	22	64	2801	43	7874	0	8765	5420	157

FLINT—Genesee County

⊞ HURLEY MEDICAL CENTER, One Hurley Plaza, Zip 48503–5993; tel. 810/257–9000; Glenn A. Fosdick, President and Chief Executive Officer **A**1 2 3 5 8 9 10 **F**3 7 8 9 10 11 12 13 14 15 16 17 18 19 20 21 22 24 25 26 27 28 29 30 31 32 33 34 35 37 38 39 40 41 42 44 45 46 47 48 49 51 52 53 54 55 56 59 60 61 63 64 65 66 67 69 70 71 72 73 74 **P**3 5 6 7 8	14	10	495	19749	293	360960	3166	223526	98826	2667
⊞ △ MCLAREN REGIONAL MEDICAL CENTER, 401 South Ballenger Highway, Zip 48532–3685; tel. 810/342–2000; Philip A. Incarnati, President and Chief Executive Officer **A**1 2 3 5 7 8 9 10 **F**1 2 3 4 7 8 10 11 12 13 14 15 16 17 18 19 20 21 22 24 25 26 27 28 29 30 31 32 33 34 35 37 38 39 40 41 42 43 44 45 46 47 48 49 51 52 53 54 55 56 57 58 59 60 61 63 64 65 66 67 69 71 72 73 74 **P**4 6	23	10	436	17361	264	611221	1077	190964	94630	2078

FRANKFORT—Benzie County

⊞ PAUL OLIVER MEMORIAL HOSPITAL, 224 Park Avenue, Zip 49635; tel. 616/352–9621; James D. Austin, CHE, Administrator (Total facility includes 40 beds in nursing home–type unit) **A**1 9 10 **F**8 14 15 16 17 19 21 22 26 28 30 32 33 34 35 44 46 49 64 65 71 73 74 **P**1 3 5 7 **S** Munson Healthcare, Traverse City, MI **N** Munson Healthcare, Traverse City, MI	23	10	48	265	35	23501	0	6107	1928	75

FREMONT—Newaygo County

⊞ GERBER MEMORIAL HOSPITAL, 212 South Sullivan Street, Zip 49412; tel. 616/924–3300; Ned B. Hughes, Jr., President **A**1 9 10 **F**7 8 14 15 16 17 19 22 26 30 32 33 34 37 39 40 41 42 44 45 46 49 52 54 55 56 57 58 65 66 67 71 72 73 74 **N** Butterworth Health System, Grand Rapids, MI	23	10	73	2292	28	64678	343	25505	12841	401

GARDEN CITY—Wayne County

+ ○ GARDEN CITY HOSPITAL, 6245 North Inkster Road, Zip 48135; tel. 313/421–3300; Gary R. Ley, President and Chief Executive Officer **A**9 10 11 12 13 **F**2 3 7 8 10 11 12 14 15 16 17 19 22 27 28 29 33 34 35 37 39 40 41 42 44 46 48 49 51 60 65 66 67 71 72 73 **P**5 8 **N** Great Lakes Health Network, Southfield, MI	23	10	253	10289	182	72736	804	91113	43342	1307

GAYLORD—Otsego County

⊞ OTSEGO MEMORIAL HOSPITAL, (Includes McReynolds Hall), 825 North Center Street, Zip 49735; tel. 517/731–2216; John L. Macleod, Administrator and Chief Executive Officer (Total facility includes 34 beds in nursing home–type unit) **A**1 9 10 **F**7 8 14 15 16 19 22 24 28 30 32 33 34 35 37 40 41 44 49 63 64 65 67 71 72 73 **P**6 8	23	10	73	1870	47	45948	206	13898	6360	229

GLADWIN—Gladwin County

⊞ MIDMICHIGAN REGIONAL MEDICAL CENTER–GLADWIN, 455 South Quarter Street, Zip 48624; tel. 517/426–9286; Mark E. Bush, Executive Vice President **A**1 9 10 **F**14 15 16 17 19 22 28 30 32 34 44 51 71 72 73 **P**1 6 **S** MidMichigan Regional Health System, Midland, MI	23	10	32	1542	18	36951	0	9266	4051	158

GRAND BLANC—Genesee County

⊞ + ○ △ GENESYS REGIONAL MEDICAL CENTER, One Genesys Parkway, Zip 48439–1477; tel. 810/606–6600; Young S. Suh, President and Chief Executive Officer **A**1 2 3 5 7 9 10 11 12 13 **F**1 2 3 4 7 8 10 11 12 13 14 15 16 17 18 19 21 22 23 25 26 27 29 30 31 32 33 34 35 37 39 40 41 42 43 44 45 46 48 49 51 53 54 56 57 58 60 63 64 65 67 68 70 71 72 73 74 **P**1 6 7 **S** Sisters of St. Joseph Health System, Ann Arbor, MI	21	10	599	26808	364	310224	2628	231629	120985	2923

GRAND HAVEN—Ottawa County

⊞ NORTH OTTAWA COMMUNITY HOSPITAL, 1309 Sheldon Road, Zip 49417–2488; tel. 616/842–3600; Jevne Conover, President and Chief Executive Officer **A**1 9 10 **F**3 7 8 14 19 21 22 26 28 30 31 32 33 34 35 36 39 41 42 44 46 49 63 65 66 67 68 71 72 73	16	10	81	2568	27	207848	519	32534	13656	396

GRAND RAPIDS—Kent County

⊞ BLODGETT MEMORIAL MEDICAL CENTER, (Includes Blodgett, Ferguson Campus, 72 Sheldon Boulevard S.E., Zip 49503–4294; tel. 616/356–4000), 1840 Wealthy Street S.E., Zip 49506–2921; tel. 616/774–7444; Terrence Michael O'Rourke, President (Nonreporting) **A**1 2 3 5 8 9 10	23	10	382	—	—	—	—	—	—	—
⊞ BUTTERWORTH HOSPITAL, 100 Michigan Street N.E., Zip 49503–2551; tel. 616/391–1774; Philip H. McCorkle, Jr., Chief Executive Officer **A**1 2 3 5 8 9 10 **F**1 2 3 4 6 7 8 10 11 13 14 15 16 17 19 21 22 23 25 26 28 29 30 31 32 33 34 35 37 38 39 40 41 42 43 44 45 46 47 48 49 51 52 53 54 55 56 57 58 59 60 61 64 65 67 68 69 70 71 72 73 74 **P**1 5 8 **N** Butterworth Health System, Grand Rapids, MI	23	10	529	25849	370	510535	5301	268156	125619	3899
□ FOREST VIEW HOSPITAL, 1055 Medical Park Drive S.E., Zip 49546; tel. 616/942–9610; John F. Kuhn, Chief Executive Officer **A**1 10 **F**17 26 34 41 46 52 53 55 56 57 58 59 65 67 **S** Universal Health Services, Inc., King of Prussia, PA	33	22	62	849	18	7371	0	4848	2397	95

Hospital, Address, Telephone, Administrator, Approval, Facility, and Physician Codes, Health Care System, Network	Classi- fication Codes		Utilization Data					Expense (thousands) of dollars		
★ American Hospital Association (AHA) membership □ Joint Commission on Accreditation of Healthcare Organizations (JCAHO) accreditation + American Osteopathic Hospital Association (AOHA) membership ○ American Osteopathic Association (AOA) accreditation △ Commission on Accreditation of Rehabilitation Facilities (CARF) accreditation Control codes 61, 63, 64, 71, 72 and 73 indicate hospitals listed by AOHA, but not registered by AHA. For definition of numerical codes, see page A4	Control	Service	Beds	Admissions	Census	Outpatient Visits	Births	Total	Payroll	Personnel

	Control	Service	Beds	Admissions	Census	Outpatient Visits	Births	Total	Payroll	Personnel
✠ KENT COMMUNITY HOSPITAL, (LTC CHEM DEPENDENCY), 750 Fuller Avenue N.E., Zip 49503–1995; tel. 616/336–3300; Lori Portfleet, Chief Executive Officer (Total facility includes 338 beds in nursing home–type unit) **A**1 9 10 **F**2 3 14 16 64 65 73	13	49	374	2115	284	—	0	20399	8931	522
✠ △ MARY FREE BED HOSPITAL AND REHABILITATION CENTER, 235 Wealthy S.E., Zip 49503–5299; tel. 616/242–0300; William H. Blessing, President **A**1 7 9 10 **F**15 16 19 21 25 27 32 34 35 39 41 45 48 49 65 67 71 73	23	46	80	772	53	44642	0	23345	14414	454
+ ○ △ METROPOLITAN HOSPITAL, 1919 Boston Street S.E., Zip 49506, Mailing Address: P.O. Box 158, Zip 49501–0158; tel. 616/247–7200; Michael D. Faas, President and Chief Executive Officer **A**7 9 10 11 12 13 **F**1 3 4 7 8 10 12 14 15 16 17 19 21 23 24 25 26 28 29 30 31 32 33 34 35 37 39 40 41 42 44 48 49 51 53 54 55 56 57 58 59 60 61 63 65 66 67 70 71 73 74 **P**3 6 7 8 **N** Butterworth Health System, Grand Rapids, MI	23	10	201	7818	111	145098	1057	74129	36607	921
✠ PINE REST CHRISTIAN MENTAL HEALTH SERVICES, 300 68th Street S.E., Zip 49501–0165, Mailing Address: P.O. Box 165, Zip 49501–0165; tel. 616/455–5000; Daniel L. Holwerda, President and Chief Executive Officer **A**1 3 5 9 10 **F**3 4 7 8 9 10 11 12 13 14 15 16 17 19 21 22 24 25 29 30 32 35 37 38 40 42 43 44 45 46 47 50 52 53 54 55 56 57 58 59 60 61 63 64 65 71 73 74 **N** Butterworth Health System, Grand Rapids, MI	23	22	106	2305	55	70853	0	30591	18346	516
✠ SAINT MARY'S HEALTH SERVICES, 200 Jefferson Avenue S.E., Zip 49503; tel. 616/752–6090; David J. Ameen, President and Chief Executive Officer **A**1 2 3 5 9 10 **F**7 8 10 12 14 15 16 17 19 20 21 22 24 25 26 28 29 30 31 32 34 35 37 39 40 42 44 45 49 52 54 55 59 60 63 64 65 66 67 69 70 71 73 74 **P**3 **S** Mercy Health Services, Farmington Hills, MI **N** Mercy Health Services, Farmington Hills, MI	21	10	287	12158	172	505150	2205	144434	61364	2015
GRAYLING—Crawford County										
✠ MERCY HEALTH SERVICES NORTH–GRAYLING, 1100 Michigan Avenue, Zip 49738–1398; tel. 517/348–5461; Dennis J. Renander, President and Chief Executive Officer (Total facility includes 40 beds in nursing home–type unit) **A**1 9 10 **F**7 8 10 11 15 16 17 19 22 28 29 32 33 34 35 37 39 40 41 44 48 49 64 65 71 73 **P**8 **S** Mercy Health Services, Farmington Hills, MI **N** Mercy Health Services, Farmington Hills, MI	21	10	98	2913	61	65564	253	26006	10953	422
GREENVILLE—Montcalm County										
✠ UNITED MEMORIAL HOSPITAL ASSOCIATION, 615 South Bower Street, Zip 48838–2614, Mailing Address: P.O. Box 430, Zip 48838–0430; tel. 616/754–4691; Larry R. Davis, Chief Executive Officer (Total facility includes 40 beds in nursing home–type unit) **A**1 9 10 **F**7 8 14 15 16 17 19 22 25 28 37 40 41 42 44 46 49 51 61 64 65 71 73 **P**3 **N** Butterworth Health System, Grand Rapids, MI	23	10	100	2638	59	180261	278	24313	8298	374
GROSSE POINTE—Wayne County										
✠ BON SECOURS HOSPITAL, 468 Cadieux Road, Zip 48230; tel. 313/343–1000; Michael Serilla, Acting Executive Vice President and Administrator **A**1 3 5 9 10 **F**3 7 8 10 15 16 17 18 19 21 22 24 25 26 27 28 29 30 31 32 33 35 36 37 39 40 42 44 45 46 49 51 53 63 64 65 67 71 73 74 **P**3 **S** Bon Secours Health System, Inc., Marriottsville, MD	21	10	242	10510	159	121821	1342	97556	51643	1419
GROSSE POINTE FARMS—Wayne County										
✠ HENRY FORD COTTAGE HOSPITAL OF GROSSE POINTE, 159 Kercheval Avenue, Zip 48236–3692; tel. 313/640–1000; Gregory J. Vasse, President and Chief Executive Officer **A**1 3 9 10 **F**1 7 8 14 15 16 18 19 22 27 28 29 30 31 33 34 39 40 42 44 45 46 49 52 54 55 56 57 58 59 63 65 66 67 71 72 73 74 **P**6 **S** Henry Ford Health System, Detroit, MI **N** Henry Ford Health System, Detroit, MI	23	10	144	4768	83	173054	627	57282	29906	833
HANCOCK—Houghton County										
✠ PORTAGE HEALTH SYSTEM, 200 Michigan Avenue, Zip 49930; tel. 906/487–8000; James Bogan, Chief Executive Officer (Total facility includes 30 beds in nursing home–type unit) **A**1 9 10 **F**1 7 8 12 13 14 15 16 17 19 22 26 28 30 31 32 33 34 35 36 37 39 40 41 44 45 49 51 54 56 57 58 61 63 64 65 66 67 71 73 74 **P**6	23	10	74	2170	51	61258	449	20111	11331	281
HARBOR BEACH—Huron County										
★ HARBOR BEACH COMMUNITY HOSPITAL, Broad and First Streets, Zip 48441–1236, Mailing Address: P.O. Box 40, Zip 48441; tel. 517/479–3201; Pauline Siemen–Messing, R.N., President and Chief Executive Officer (Total facility includes 40 beds in nursing home–type unit) **A**9 10 **F**7 8 16 19 22 26 30 34 40 44 49 51 64 65 71 **P**6	23	10	67	502	43	15044	6	5252	2948	148
HARRISON TOWNSHIP—Macomb County										
✠ △ ST. JOHN HOSPITAL–MACOMB CENTER, 26755 Ballard Road, Zip 48045–2458; tel. 810/465–5501; David Sessions, President **A**1 7 10 **F**2 3 4 6 7 8 10 11 12 13 14 15 16 17 18 19 20 21 22 23 25 26 27 28 29 30 31 32 33 34 35 36 37 38 39 40 41 42 43 44 45 46 47 48 49 51 52 54 55 56 57 58 59 60 63 64 65 66 67 69 70 71 72 73 74 **P**5 8 **S** Sisters of St. Joseph Health System, Ann Arbor, MI **N** Saint John Health System, Detroit, MI	21	10	66	1441	32	20337	0	15991	8056	267
HASTINGS—Barry County										
□ PENNOCK HOSPITAL, 1009 West Green Street, Zip 49058–1790; tel. 616/945–3451; Daniel Hamilton, Chief Executive Officer **A**1 9 10 **F**7 8 10 11 12 14 15 16 19 21 22 24 26 28 29 30 32 33 34 35 37 39 40 41 42 44 45 46 49 56 62 63 65 66 67 71 73	23	10	88	2971	39	108313	362	22827	10114	395
HILLSDALE—Hillsdale County										
✠ HILLSDALE COMMUNITY HEALTH CENTER, 168 South Howell Street, Zip 49242–2081; tel. 517/437–4451; Charles A. Bianchi, President (Total facility includes 21 beds in nursing home–type unit) **A**1 9 10 **F**7 8 14 15 16 17 19 22 28 30 34 35 37 39 40 41 44 46 49 51 63 64 65 67 71 72 73	23	10	68	2929	46	82448	352	18535	7253	298

Hospital, Address, Telephone, Administrator, Approval, Facility, and Physician Codes, Health Care System, Network	Classification Codes		Utilization Data					Expense (thousands) of dollars		
	Control	Service	Beds	Admissions	Census	Outpatient Visits	Births	Total	Payroll	Personnel

★ American Hospital Association (AHA) membership
□ Joint Commission on Accreditation of Healthcare Organizations (JCAHO) accreditation
+ American Osteopathic Hospital Association (AOHA) membership
○ American Osteopathic Association (AOA) accreditation
△ Commission on Accreditation of Rehabilitation Facilities (CARF) accreditation
Control codes 61, 63, 64, 71, 72 and 73 indicate hospitals listed by AOHA, but not registered by AHA. For definition of numerical codes, see page A4

HOLLAND—Ottawa County

△ HOLLAND COMMUNITY HOSPITAL, 602 Michigan Avenue, Zip 49423–4999; tel. 616/392–5141; Judeth N. Javorek, R.N., President and Chief Executive Officer **A**1 7 9 10 **F**7 14 15 16 19 21 22 28 32 34 35 36 37 39 40 41 42 44 45 49 52 53 54 55 56 57 58 59 63 65 67 71 72 73 **P**8 — 23 10 163 7897 81 182902 1694 52848 24920 691

HOWELL—Livingston County

MCPHERSON HOSPITAL, 620 Byron Road, Zip 48843–1093; tel. 517/545–6000; C. W. Lauderbach, Jr., Chief Operating Officer **A**1 9 10 **F**1 2 3 4 5 7 8 9 10 11 12 14 15 16 17 19 20 21 22 23 24 25 26 30 31 32 33 34 35 37 38 39 40 41 42 43 44 46 47 48 49 50 51 52 53 54 56 57 58 59 60 61 63 64 65 66 67 68 69 70 71 72 73 74 **P**2 5 7 8 **S** Mercy Health Services, Farmington Hills, MI **N** Mercy Health Services, Farmington Hills, MI — 21 10 63 3423 35 240151 729 42669 20112 556

HUDSON—Lenawee County

★ THORN HOSPITAL, 458 Cross Street, Zip 49247; tel. 517/448–2371; Rodney M. Nelson, President and Chief Executive Officer **A**9 10 **F**2 3 7 8 11 14 15 16 22 24 28 30 32 34 35 37 40 41 42 44 45 46 48 49 51 52 64 67 73 **P**6 — 23 10 22 246 2 7578 0 4627 2281 51

IONIA—Ionia County

IONIA COUNTY MEMORIAL HOSPITAL, 479 Lafayette Street, Zip 48846–1834, Mailing Address: Box 1001, Zip 48846–1899; tel. 616/527–4200; Evonne G. Ulmer, Chief Executive Officer **A**1 9 10 **F**7 8 11 14 15 16 17 19 22 26 28 29 30 32 33 34 37 39 40 41 42 44 49 51 53 54 55 56 57 58 65 66 67 71 72 74 **P**6 — 23 10 55 1333 16 86414 172 9607 4934 167

IRON MOUNTAIN—Dickinson County

DICKINSON COUNTY HEALTHCARE SYSTEM, 1721 South Stephenson Avenue, Zip 49801; tel. 906/774–1313; John Schon, Administrator and Chief Executive Officer **A**1 9 10 **F**7 8 14 16 19 21 22 28 29 32 35 37 39 40 41 42 44 46 49 53 54 58 65 66 67 71 73 **P**3 — 13 10 95 4756 56 103884 592 39239 20320 521

VETERANS AFFAIRS MEDICAL CENTER, 325 East H Street, Zip 49801–4792; tel. 906/774–3300; Glen W. Grippen, Director (Total facility includes 40 beds in nursing home–type unit) **A**1 5 9 **F**2 3 8 12 17 19 20 21 22 26 27 30 31 33 34 37 39 42 44 45 46 49 51 58 64 65 71 72 73 74 **P**6 **S** Department of Veterans Affairs, Washington, DC — 45 10 133 1755 80 52969 0 29253 14571 374

IRON RIVER—Iron County

IRON COUNTY COMMUNITY HOSPITAL, (Includes Crystal Falls Community Hospital, 212 South Third Street, Crystal Falls, Zip 49920, Mailing Address: P.O. Box 60, Zip 49920–0060; tel. 906/875–6661), 1400 West Ice Lake Road, Zip 49935; tel. 906/265–6121; David L. Hoff, Chief Executive Officer (Nonreporting) **A**1 9 10 — 13 10 71 — — — — — — —

IRONWOOD—Gogebic County

GRAND VIEW HOSPITAL, N10561 Grand View Lane, Zip 49938–9622; tel. 906/932–2525; Frederick Geissler, Chief Executive Officer **A**1 9 10 **F**7 11 14 15 16 17 19 21 22 28 32 33 34 39 40 41 42 44 45 49 61 65 66 67 71 73 74 **P**8 **N** Northern Lakes Health Consortium, Duluth, MN — 23 10 54 1871 22 56634 219 15108 6499 191

ISHPEMING—Marquette County

□ BELL MEMORIAL HOSPITAL, 101 South Fourth Street, Zip 49849; tel. 906/486–4431; Kevin P. Calhoun, President and Chief Executive Officer **A**1 9 10 **F**7 11 14 15 16 17 19 22 27 28 30 33 34 39 40 41 44 49 51 58 65 71 72 73 **P**3 6 — 23 10 30 1740 16 46940 226 13070 6345 180

JACKSON—Jackson County

★ + ○ DOCTORS HOSPITAL OF JACKSON, 110 North Elm Avenue, Zip 49202–3595; tel. 517/787–1440; Michael J. Falatko, President and Chief Executive Officer **A**9 10 11 **F**8 11 14 15 17 19 21 22 29 30 34 35 37 41 42 44 46 49 63 65 71 72 73 **N** Midwest Health Net, LLC., Fort Wayne, IN — 23 10 40 1516 16 41796 0 18415 8353 269

DUANE L. WATERS HOSPITAL, 3857 Cooper Street, Zip 49201; tel. 517/780–5600; Gerald De Voss, Acting Administrator **A**1 **F**4 10 18 19 20 21 22 23 24 25 26 30 31 33 34 35 39 42 43 44 49 50 52 54 56 57 58 60 63 64 65 67 71 **P**6 — 12 11 86 1211 69 44697 0 — — 396

□ W. A. FOOTE MEMORIAL HOSPITAL, 205 North East Avenue, Zip 49201–1789; tel. 517/788–4800; Georgia R. Fojtasek, President and Chief Executive Officer **A**1 9 10 **F**2 3 7 8 10 11 12 14 15 16 17 18 19 21 22 24 26 28 29 30 32 33 34 35 36 37 39 40 41 42 44 45 46 49 51 52 53 54 55 56 57 58 59 60 63 65 66 67 71 73 74 **P**1 5 — 23 10 326 16796 169 332857 1930 119401 58098 1806

KALAMAZOO—Kalamazoo County

△ BORGESS MEDICAL CENTER, (Includes Borgess–Pipp Health Center, 411 Naomi Street, Plainwell, Zip 49080–9911; tel. 616/685–6811; Fritz Fahrenbacher, Vice President and Regional Hospital Administrator), 1521 Gull Road, Zip 49001–1640; tel. 616/226–7000; R. Timothy Stack, FACHE, President and Chief Executive Officer (Nonreporting) **A**1 2 3 5 7 9 10 **S** Sisters of St. Joseph Health System, Ann Arbor, MI **N** First Choice Network, Watervliet, MI — 21 10 394 — — — — — — —

BRONSON METHODIST HOSPITAL, 252 East Lovell Street, Zip 49007–5345; tel. 616/341–6000; Frank J. Sardone, President and Chief Executive Officer **A**1 2 3 5 6 9 10 **F**2 3 4 6 7 8 9 10 11 12 13 14 15 16 17 18 19 20 21 22 23 24 25 26 27 28 29 30 31 32 33 34 35 37 38 39 40 41 42 43 44 45 48 49 51 52 53 54 55 56 57 58 59 60 61 62 63 64 65 66 67 68 70 71 72 73 74 **P**2 5 7 8 **S** Bronson Healthcare Group, Inc., Kalamazoo, MI **N** Hospital Network Inc., Kalamazoo, MI; Lakeland Regional Health System, St. Joseph, MI — 23 10 314 15669 208 313917 2803 160079 72124 1725

Hospital, Address, Telephone, Administrator, Approval, Facility, and Physician Codes, Health Care System, Network	Classi-fication Codes		Utilization Data					Expense (thousands) of dollars		
★ American Hospital Association (AHA) membership □ Joint Commission on Accreditation of Healthcare Organizations (JCAHO) accreditation + American Osteopathic Hospital Association (AOHA) membership ○ American Osteopathic Association (AOA) accreditation △ Commission on Accreditation of Rehabilitation Facilities (CARF) accreditation Control codes 61, 63, 64, 71, 72 and 73 indicate hospitals listed by AOHA, but not registered by AHA. For definition of numerical codes, see page A4	Control	Service	Beds	Admissions	Census	Outpatient Visits	Births	Total	Payroll	Personnel

Hospital	Control	Service	Beds	Admissions	Census	Outpatient Visits	Births	Total	Payroll	Personnel
□ KALAMAZOO REGIONAL PSYCHIATRIC HOSPITAL, 1312 Oakland Drive, Zip 49008; tel. 616/337–3000; James Coleman, Director **A**1 9 10 **F**4 5 8 10 14 16 19 20 21 22 23 24 27 29 30 31 33 35 42 43 44 45 46 51 52 53 54 55 56 57 60 61 65 70 71 72 73 74	12	22	220	565	167	0	0	30405	19516	469
KALKASKA—Kalkaska County										
★ KALKASKA MEMORIAL HEALTH CENTER, 419 Coral Street, Zip 49646, Mailing Address: P.O. Box 249, Zip 49646–0249; tel. 616/258–9142; James D. Austin, CHE, Administrator (Total facility includes 68 beds in nursing home–type unit) **A**9 10 **F**8 14 15 16 19 28 32 33 34 49 58 64 65 67 71 74 **S** Munson Healthcare, Traverse City, MI **N** Munson Healthcare, Traverse City, MI	16	10	76	283	67	32900	0	8209	3838	121
L'ANSE—Baraga County										
□ BARAGA COUNTY MEMORIAL HOSPITAL, 770 North Main Street, Zip 49946–1195; tel. 906/524–6166; John P. Tembreull, Administrator (Total facility includes 28 beds in nursing home–type unit) **A**1 9 10 **F**15 16 19 21 22 32 44 58 64 65 67 71	13	10	52	980	37	17365	0	7556	3538	119
LAKEVIEW—Montcalm County										
□ KELSEY MEMORIAL HOSPITAL, 418 Washington Avenue, Zip 48850; tel. 517/352–7211 (Total facility includes 48 beds in nursing home–type unit) **A**1 9 10 **F**8 15 16 19 22 24 28 30 32 33 34 41 44 46 48 49 51 54 64 65 71 72 73 **P**5	23	10	72	844	53	26431	44	10907	5752	183
LANSING—Ingham County										
INGHAM MEDICAL CENTER See Michigan Capital Healthcare										
LANSING GENERAL HOSPITAL See Michigan Capital Healthcare										
✠ ○ △ MICHIGAN CAPITAL HEALTHCARE, (Formerly Michigan Affiliated Health System), (Includes Michigan Capital Medical Center, Greenlawn Campus, tel. 517/334–2121; Michigan Capital Medical Center, Pennsylvania Campus, 2727 South Pennsylvania Avenue, Zip 48910; tel. 517/372–8220), 401 West Greenlawn Avenue, Zip 48910–2819; tel. 517/334–2121; Dennis M. Litos, President and Chief Executive Officer (Total facility includes 28 beds in nursing home–type unit) **A**1 3 5 7 8 10 11 12 13 **F**2 3 4 6 7 8 9 10 11 12 13 14 15 16 17 18 19 20 21 22 23 24 25 26 28 29 30 31 32 33 34 35 36 37 38 39 40 41 42 43 44 45 46 47 48 49 51 52 53 54 55 56 57 58 59 60 61 62 63 64 65 66 67 68 70 71 72 73 74 **P**1 **N** Michigan Capital Healthcare, Lansing, MI	23	10	343	14394	232	—	850	172040	79825	3084
MICHIGAN CAPITAL MEDICAL CENTER, GREENLAWN CAMPUS See Michigan Capital Healthcare										
MICHIGAN CAPITAL MEDICAL CENTER, PENNSYLVANIA CAMPUS See Michigan Capital Healthcare										
✠ △ SPARROW HEALTH SYSTEM, (Includes Edward W. Sparrow Hospital), 1215 East Michigan Avenue, Zip 48912, Mailing Address: P.O. Box 30480, Zip 48909–7980; tel. 517/483–2700; Joseph F. Damore, President and Chief Executive Officer **A**1 2 3 5 7 9 10 12 **F**2 3 4 6 7 8 9 10 11 12 14 15 16 17 18 19 21 22 23 28 29 30 32 33 34 35 36 37 38 39 40 41 42 43 44 46 47 48 49 51 52 53 54 55 56 57 58 59 60 61 63 65 67 68 70 71 72 73 74 **P**1 6	23	10	379	20535	278	—	4293	220518	110401	2993
✠ ○ ST. LAWRENCE HOSPITAL AND HEALTHCARE SERVICES, 1210 West Saginaw Street, Zip 48915–1999; tel. 517/372–3610; Arthur Knueppel, President and Chief Executive Officer (Total facility includes 178 beds in nursing home–type unit) **A**1 2 3 5 9 10 11 12 **F**2 3 5 7 8 11 12 14 15 16 17 18 19 21 22 24 25 26 27 28 30 31 32 33 34 37 40 41 42 44 49 51 52 53 54 55 56 57 58 59 64 65 66 67 71 73 74 **P**4 5 6 8 **S** Mercy Health Services, Farmington Hills, MI **N** Mercy Health Services, Farmington Hills, MI	23	10	375	8160	274	174664	1012	74768	36175	1528
LAPEER—Lapeer County										
□ LAPEER REGIONAL HOSPITAL, 1375 North Main Street, Zip 48446; tel. 810/667–5500; Donald C. Kooy, President and Chief Executive Officer **A**1 9 10 **F**1 2 3 4 7 8 10 11 12 13 14 15 16 17 18 19 20 21 22 24 25 26 27 28 29 30 31 32 33 34 35 37 38 39 40 41 42 43 44 45 46 47 48 49 51 52 53 54 55 56 57 58 59 60 61 63 64 65 67 71 72 73 74 **P**4 6	23	10	203	5606	81	270351	776	55385	28289	764
LAURIUM—Houghton County										
✠ KEWEENAW MEMORIAL MEDICAL CENTER, 205 Osceola Street, Zip 49913–2199; tel. 906/337–3100; Rick Wright, FACHE, CPA, President and Chief Executive Officer **A**1 9 10 **F**7 8 11 12 16 17 19 21 22 31 32 35 37 40 44 46 65 71 74 **P**6	23	10	48	1547	19	29392	66	10401	4935	177
LINCOLN PARK—Wayne County										
✠ OAKWOOD HOSPITAL DOWNRIVER CENTER–LINCOLN PARK, 25750 West Outer Drive, Zip 48146–1574; tel. 313/382–6000; Thomas Kochis, Administrator (Nonreporting) **A**1 9 10 **S** Oakwood Healthcare System, Dearborn, MI	23	10	49	—	—	—	—	—	—	—
□ VENCOR HOSPITAL–DETROIT, 26400 West Outer Drive, Zip 48146; tel. 313/594–6000; Judith A. Curtiss, Administrator **A**1 9 10 **F**16 22 27 37 65 67 73 **P**6 **S** Vencor, Incorporated, Louisville, KY	33	10	112	502	68	0	0	14163	7734	335
LIVONIA—Wayne County										
✠ ST. MARY HOSPITAL, 36475 West Five Mile Road, Zip 48154–1988; tel. 313/655–4800; Sister Mary Modesta Piwowar, President and Chief Executive Officer **A**1 9 10 **F**2 3 4 6 7 8 10 11 12 13 14 15 17 18 19 20 21 22 23 24 26 27 28 29 30 32 33 34 35 37 39 40 41 42 43 44 45 46 49 52 54 55 56 57 58 59 60 63 65 67 69 70 71 72 73 74 **P**4 5 8 **N** William Beaumont Hospital Corp, Royal Oak, MI	21	10	246	9979	160	134223	614	86554	44868	1174
LUDINGTON—Mason County										
✠ MEMORIAL MEDICAL CENTER OF WEST MICHIGAN, One Atkinson Drive, Zip 49431–1999; tel. 616/843–2591; Robert C. Marquardt, FACHE, President **A**1 9 10 **F**7 8 14 15 16 17 19 21 22 30 32 34 35 37 39 40 41 44 49 52 54 55 56 57 63 65 67 71 73 74 **P**6	23	10	80	3089	40	63086	362	24446	11253	390

Hospital, Address, Telephone, Administrator, Approval, Facility, and Physician Codes, Health Care System, Network	Classi-fication Codes		Utilization Data					Expense (thousands) of dollars		
★ American Hospital Association (AHA) membership □ Joint Commission on Accreditation of Healthcare Organizations (JCAHO) accreditation + American Osteopathic Hospital Association (AOHA) membership ○ American Osteopathic Association (AOA) accreditation △ Commission on Accreditation of Rehabilitation Facilities (CARF) accreditation Control codes 61, 63, 64, 71, 72 and 73 indicate hospitals listed by AOHA, but not registered by AHA. For definition of numerical codes, see page A4	Control	Service	Beds	Admissions	Census	Outpatient Visits	Births	Total	Payroll	Personnel

MADISON HEIGHTS—Oakland County

✠ MADISON COMMUNITY HOSPITAL, 30671 Stephenson Highway, Zip 48071; tel. 810/588-8000; Craig J. Yanos, Administrator (Nonreporting) **A**1 9 10

	23	10	56	—	—	—	—	—	—	—

□ + ○ OAKLAND GENERAL HOSPITAL, 27351 Dequindre, Zip 48071; tel. 810/967-7000; Robert Deputat, President **A**1 9 10 11 12 13 **F**1 2 3 4 6 7 8 9 10 11 12 13 14 15 16 17 18 19 20 21 22 23 24 25 26 27 28 29 30 31 32 33 34 35 36 37 38 39 40 41 42 43 44 45 46 47 48 49 50 51 52 53 54 55 56 57 58 59 60 61 62 63 64 65 66 67 68 69 70 71 72 73 74 **P**4 5 6 7 8 **S** Sisters of St. Joseph Health System, Ann Arbor, MI **N** Saint John Health System, Detroit, MI; Great Lakes Health Network, Southfield, MI

	21	10	166	6389	124	38446	0	61699	28427	888

MANISTEE—Manistee County

□ WEST SHORE HOSPITAL, 1465 East Parkdale Avenue, Zip 49660; tel. 616/723-3501; Burton O. Parks, III, Administrator **A**1 9 10 **F**7 8 10 11 12 14 15 16 19 21 22 24 28 30 32 33 34 35 39 40 41 42 44 45 46 49 51 63 65 67 71 73 74 **P**3 8

	13	10	54	1758	21	38801	161	17092	8207	250

MANISTIQUE—Schoolcraft County

✠ SCHOOLCRAFT MEMORIAL HOSPITAL, 500 Main Street, Zip 49854-0000; tel. 906/341-3200; David B. Jahn, Administrator and Chief Financial Officer **A**1 9 10 **F**2 3 4 7 8 9 10 11 15 17 18 19 20 21 22 23 24 26 27 28 29 30 31 32 33 34 35 36 37 38 39 40 41 42 43 44 45 46 47 48 49 51 52 53 54 55 56 57 58 59 60 63 64 65 66 67 70 71 72 73 74 **P**4

	13	10	38	716	6	29974	126	7745	4122	117

MARLETTE—Sanilac County

✠ MARLETTE COMMUNITY HOSPITAL, 2770 Main Street, Zip 48453-0307, Mailing Address: P.O. Box 307, Zip 48453-0307; tel. 517/635-4000; David S. McEwen, Chief Executive Officer (Total facility includes 43 beds in nursing home–type unit) **A**1 9 10 **F**1 14 15 16 19 21 22 26 30 33 36 37 42 44 45 48 62 64 65 71 **S** Quorum Health Group/Quorum Health Resources, Inc., Brentwood, TN

	23	10	91	1101	58	32865	0	14812	6900	274

MARQUETTE—Marquette County

✠ △ MARQUETTE GENERAL HOSPITAL, 420 West Magnetic Street, Zip 49855; tel. 906/228-9440; N. Bruce Clement, Chief Executive Officer **A**1 2 3 5 7 9 10 **F**2 3 4 5 7 8 10 11 12 13 14 15 16 17 19 21 22 23 26 28 29 30 32 33 34 35 37 38 39 40 41 42 43 44 45 46 48 49 51 52 53 54 55 56 57 58 60 65 66 67 70 71 73 74 **P**6

	23	10	320	10206	173	285488	601	139261	68954	1862

MARSHALL—Calhoun County

✠ OAKLAWN HOSPITAL, 200 North Madison Street, Zip 49068; tel. 616/781-4271; Rob Covert, President and Chief Executive Officer **A**1 9 10 **F**3 4 5 7 8 10 12 15 16 17 19 21 22 24 29 30 31 32 33 34 35 36 37 39 40 41 43 44 45 46 49 52 54 55 56 57 58 59 61 63 65 66 67 71 73 **N** Hospital Network Inc., Kalamazoo, MI

	23	10	94	2685	30	62895	559	25333	12560	370

MIDLAND—Midland County

✠ △ MIDMICHIGAN REGIONAL MEDICAL CENTER, 4005 Orchard Drive, Zip 48670; tel. 517/839-3000; David A. Reece, President **A**1 2 3 5 7 9 10 **F**6 7 8 10 11 12 15 19 20 21 22 26 27 28 29 30 31 32 33 34 35 36 37 39 40 41 42 44 45 46 48 49 51 52 54 55 56 57 58 59 60 64 65 66 67 71 72 73 74 **P**1 2 5 6 7 **S** MidMichigan Regional Health System, Midland, MI

	23	10	221	10037	138	178055	1166	114467	50481	1334

MONROE—Monroe County

✠ MERCY MEMORIAL HOSPITAL, 740 North Macomb Street, Zip 48161-9974, Mailing Address: P.O. Box 67, Zip 48161-0067; tel. 313/241-1700; Richard S. Hiltz, President and Chief Executive Officer (Total facility includes 70 beds in nursing home–type unit) **A**1 9 10 **F**1 2 3 4 5 6 7 8 9 10 11 12 13 14 15 16 17 18 19 20 21 22 23 24 25 26 27 28 29 30 31 32 33 34 35 36 37 38 39 40 41 42 43 44 45 46 47 48 49 50 51 52 53 54 55 56 57 58 59 60 62 63 64 65 66 67 68 69 70 71 72 73 74 **N** Lake Erie Health Alliance, Toledo, OH; Midwest Health Net, LLC., Fort Wayne, IN

	23	10	243	269	172	98978	943	65498	32469	887

MORENCI—Lenawee County

□ MORENCI AREA HOSPITAL, 13101 Sims Highway, Zip 49256-1099; tel. 517/458-2236; Rodney M. Nelson, President and Chief Executive Officer **A**1 9 10 **F**15 16 22 28 30 36 37 39 42 44 46 49 64 66 71 73

	14	10	18	170	1	9866	0	2531	—	18

MOUNT CLEMENS—Macomb County

★ + ○ MOUNT CLEMENS GENERAL HOSPITAL, 1000 Harrington Boulevard, Zip 48043-2992; tel. 810/493-8000; Ralph J. La Gro, President and Chief Executive Officer **A**9 10 11 12 13 **F**4 7 8 10 12 13 15 16 17 18 19 20 21 24 25 26 27 28 29 30 31 32 33 34 35 37 39 40 41 42 43 44 45 46 49 51 61 63 65 66 67 68 70 71 72 73 74 **P**4 5 6 7 8 **N** Great Lakes Health Network, Southfield, MI; William Beaumont Hospital Corp, Royal Oak, MI

	23	10	241	11268	153	—	1397	147965	68666	1832

MOUNT PLEASANT—Isabella County

✠ + ○ CENTRAL MICHIGAN COMMUNITY HOSPITAL, 1221 South Drive, Zip 48858-3234; tel. 517/772-6700; Mark A. Cwiek, President and Chief Executive Officer **A**1 9 10 11 **F**8 14 15 16 19 20 21 22 24 25 28 29 30 31 32 34 35 37 39 40 41 42 44 48 52 53 54 55 57 59 63 66 67 71 72 73 74 **P**6 8

	23	10	118	3722	39	138620	460	33738	17979	573

MUNISING—Alger County

□ MUNISING MEMORIAL HOSPITAL, 1500 Sand Point Road, Zip 49862, Mailing Address: Route 1, Box 501, Zip 49862; tel. 906/387-4110; Carl J. Velte, Chief Executive Officer (Nonreporting) **A**1 9 10

	23	10	40	—	—	—	—	—	—	—

MUSKEGON—Muskegon County

✠ HACKLEY HEALTH, 1700 Clinton Street, Zip 49443-3302, Mailing Address: P.O. Box 3302, Zip 49443-3302; tel. 616/726-3511; Gordon A. Mudler, President and Chief Executive Officer **A**1 2 9 10 **F**7 8 10 12 14 15 16 17 19 20 21 22 24 26 27 29 30 32 35 37 39 40 41 42 44 45 46 48 49 51 52 55 56 57 59 60 63 65 66 67 71 72 73 74 **P**5 6 7

	23	10	226	8742	115	353998	1388	84080	39470	1068

Hospital, Address, Telephone, Administrator, Approval, Facility, and Physician Codes, Health Care System, Network	Classification Codes		Utilization Data					Expense (thousands) of dollars		
	Control	Service	Beds	Admissions	Census	Outpatient Visits	Births	Total	Payroll	Personnel

★ American Hospital Association (AHA) membership
☐ Joint Commission on Accreditation of Healthcare Organizations (JCAHO) accreditation
+ American Osteopathic Hospital Association (AOHA) membership
○ American Osteopathic Association (AOA) accreditation
△ Commission on Accreditation of Rehabilitation Facilities (CARF) accreditation
Control codes 61, 63, 64, 71, 72 and 73 indicate hospitals listed by AOHA, but not registered by AHA. For definition of numerical codes, see page A4

Hospital	Control	Service	Beds	Admissions	Census	Outpatient Visits	Births	Total	Payroll	Personnel
+ ○ MERCY GENERAL HEALTH PARTNERS–OAK AVENUE CAMPUS, (Formerly Muskegon General Hospital), 1700 Oak Avenue, Zip 49442; tel. 616/773–3311; Roger Spoelman, Chief Executive Officer (Nonreporting) **A**9 10 11 12 13 **S** Mercy Health Services, Farmington Hills, MI **N** Mercy General Health Partners, Muskegon, MI; Mercy Health Services, Farmington Hills, MI	23	10	127	—	—	—	—	—	—	—
⊞ MERCY GENERAL HEALTH PARTNERS–SHERMAN BOULEVARD CAMPUS, 1500 East Sherman Boulevard, Zip 49443, Mailing Address: P.O. Box 358, Zip 49443–0358; tel. 616/739–9341; Roger Spoelman, Chief Executive Officer (Nonreporting) **A**1 9 10 12 **S** Mercy Health Services, Farmington Hills, MI **N** Mercy General Health Partners, Muskegon, MI	23	10	123	—	—	—	—	—	—	—
MUSKEGON GENERAL HOSPITAL See Mercy General Health Partners–Oak Avenue Campus										
NEW BALTIMORE—Macomb County										
☐ HARBOR OAKS HOSPITAL, 35031 23 Mile Road, Zip 48047; tel. 810/725–5777; Gary J. LaHood, Administrator and Chief Executive Officer (Nonreporting) **A**1 9 10 **S** Pioneer Healthcare, Peabody, MA	32	22	64	—	—	—	—	—	—	—
NEWBERRY—Luce County										
⊞ HELEN NEWBERRY JOY HOSPITAL, (Includes Helen Newberry Joy Hospital Annex), 502 West Harrie Street, Zip 49868–0070; tel. 906/293–9200; Bruce C. Huron, Interim Chief Executive Officer (Total facility includes 48 beds in nursing home–type unit) **A**1 9 10 **F**8 14 15 16 17 19 21 22 28 32 34 35 44 64 71 72	13	10	86	838	56	38247	1	10277	5321	194
NILES—Berrien County										
⊞ LAKELAND MEDICAL CENTER–NILES, 31 North St. Joseph Avenue, Zip 49120–2287; tel. 616/683–5510; Joseph A. Wasserman, President and Chief Executive Officer **A**1 9 10 **F**3 7 8 12 14 15 16 19 21 22 30 32 33 34 35 36 37 40 41 42 44 49 65 67 71 73 **P**8 **S** Lakeland Regional Health System, Inc., Saint Joseph, MI **N** Lakeland Regional Health System, St. Joseph, MI	23	10	106	3644	36	103096	463	27851	13660	418
NORTHPORT—Leelanau County										
⊞ LEELANAU MEMORIAL HEALTH CENTER, 215 South High Street, Zip 49670, Mailing Address: P.O. Box 217, Zip 49670; tel. 616/386–5101; Jayne R. Bull, Administrator (Total facility includes 72 beds in nursing home–type unit) **A**1 10 **F**1 8 13 15 22 24 27 36 41 44 45 51 65 71 73 **P**3 5 6 7 8 **S** Munson Healthcare, Traverse City, MI **N** Munson Healthcare, Traverse City, MI	23	10	91	338	64	10515	0	5462	2806	184
NORTHVILLE—Wayne County										
☐ HAWTHORN CENTER, 18471 Haggerty Road, Zip 48167; tel. 810/349–3000; Neil Wasserman, Director **A**1 3 5 9 **F**20 52 53 55 56 65 **P**6	12	52	118	110	90	0	0	17479	9230	320
☐ NORTHVILLE PSYCHIATRIC HOSPITAL, 41001 West Seven Mile Road, Zip 48167; tel. 810/349–1800; Ed Stovall, Administrative Officer (Nonreporting) **A**1 10	12	22	360	—	—	—	—	—	—	—
ONTONAGON—Ontonagon County										
☐ ONTONAGON MEMORIAL HOSPITAL, 601 Seventh Street, Zip 49953; tel. 906/884–4134; Fred Nelson, Administrator (Total facility includes 46 beds in nursing home–type unit) **A**1 9 10 **F**8 15 16 17 19 20 21 22 25 26 28 29 30 34 39 41 44 49 51 64 65 66 71 **N** Northern Lakes Health Consortium, Duluth, MN	14	10	72	737	57	18926	0	7275	3695	169
OWOSSO—Shiawassee County										
⊞ MEMORIAL HEALTHCARE CENTER, 826 West King Street, Zip 48867–2198; tel. 517/723–5211; Margaret S. Gulick, President and Chief Executive Officer (Total facility includes 16 beds in nursing home–type unit) **A**1 9 10 **F**3 7 8 11 12 14 15 16 17 19 21 22 27 30 32 33 34 35 36 37 39 40 41 42 44 45 46 48 49 51 52 54 55 56 57 58 59 64 65 66 67 71 73 **P**1 7	23	10	138	5030	76	213668	484	45927	23203	778
PAW PAW—Van Buren County										
⊞ LAKEVIEW COMMUNITY HOSPITAL, 408 Hazen Street, Zip 49079, Mailing Address: Box 209, Zip 49079–0209; tel. 616/657–3141; Sue E. Johnson–Phillippe, Chief Executive Officer (Total facility includes 120 beds in nursing home–type unit) **A**1 9 10 **F**7 8 12 14 15 16 17 19 20 22 26 30 32 33 34 35 37 39 40 41 44 45 49 52 54 55 57 59 61 64 65 67 71 72 73 74 **P**3 4 5 **S** Quorum Health Group/Quorum Health Resources, Inc., Brentwood, TN	16	10	168	1703	143	51526	0	19944	10057	391
PETOSKEY—Emmet County										
⊞ NORTHERN MICHIGAN HOSPITAL, 416 Connable Avenue, Zip 49770–2297; tel. 616/348–4000; Jeffrey T. Wendling, President **A**1 2 9 10 **F**1 3 4 6 7 8 10 12 14 15 16 17 19 20 21 22 25 27 28 29 30 31 32 33 34 35 36 37 39 40 41 42 43 44 45 46 49 51 52 53 54 56 58 59 60 61 64 65 66 67 71 72 73 **P**7	23	10	261	9013	127	74496	962	76471	31111	943
PIGEON—Huron County										
⊞ SCHEURER HOSPITAL, 170 North Caseville Road, Zip 48755–9704; tel. 517/453–3223; Dwight Gascho, President and Chief Executive Officer (Total facility includes 19 beds in nursing home–type unit) **A**1 9 10 **F**8 15 16 19 21 22 28 29 30 33 34 36 39 40 41 42 44 45 46 49 51 62 63 64 65 67 71 72 **P**6	23	10	42	696	27	29554	1	9285	4550	151
PLAINWELL—Allegan County										
BORGESS–PIPP HEALTH CENTER See Borgess Medical Center, Kalamazoo										
PONTIAC—Oakland County										
☐ CLINTON VALLEY CENTER, 140 Elizabeth Lake Road, Zip 48341–1000; tel. 810/452–8700; Neil Wasserman, Director **A**1 10 **F**1 2 3 4 6 7 8 9 10 11 12 14 15 16 17 18 19 20 21 22 23 25 26 27 28 30 39 42 43 44 45 46 48 49 50 51 52 53 54 55 56 57 58 59 60 61 63 65 66 67 68 69 70 71 73 74	12	22	275	310	298	0	0	43971	26042	618
⊞ NORTH OAKLAND MEDICAL CENTERS, 461 West Huron Street, Zip 48341–1651; tel. 810/857–7200; Robert L. Davis, President and Chief Executive Officer **A**1 3 5 10 **F**4 7 8 10 12 14 15 16 17 18 19 20 21 22 25 26 28 29 30 31 33 34 37 38 39 40 41 42 44 45 46 48 49 51 52 54 55 56 57 58 60 61 63 65 67 68 71 72 73 **P**3 7 8 **N** William Beaumont Hospital Corp, Royal Oak, MI	23	10	222	9620	134	90333	1685	97604	45633	1222

Hospital, Address, Telephone, Administrator, Approval, Facility, and Physician Codes, Health Care System, Network	Classification Codes		Utilization Data					Expense (thousands) of dollars		
	Control	Service	Beds	Admissions	Census	Outpatient Visits	Births	Total	Payroll	Personnel

★ American Hospital Association (AHA) membership
□ Joint Commission on Accreditation of Healthcare Organizations (JCAHO) accreditation
+ American Osteopathic Hospital Association (AOHA) membership
○ American Osteopathic Association (AOA) accreditation
△ Commission on Accreditation of Rehabilitation Facilities (CARF) accreditation
Control codes 61, 63, 64, 71, 72 and 73 indicate hospitals listed by AOHA, but not registered by AHA. For definition of numerical codes, see page A4

+ ○ PONTIAC OSTEOPATHIC HOSPITAL, 50 North Perry Street, Zip 48342; tel. 810/338–5000; Patrick Lamberti, Chief Executive Officer **A**9 10 11 12 13 **F**3 8 10 12 13 15 16 17 18 19 21 22 24 25 26 28 29 30 31 32 33 34 35 37 39 41 42 44 45 46 49 51 54 61 63 65 66 67 71 72 73 74 **P**4 5 6 8 **N** Great Lakes Health Network, Southfield, MI	23	10	161	6823	93	117944	64	75125	37453	1047
⊠ △ ST. JOSEPH MERCY OAKLAND, 900 Woodward Avenue, Zip 48341–2985; tel. 810/858–3000; Thomas L. Feurig, President and Chief Executive Officer **A**1 3 5 7 9 10 **F**2 3 4 6 7 8 10 11 12 13 14 15 16 17 19 21 22 25 26 28 29 30 31 32 33 34 35 36 37 39 40 41 42 43 44 46 47 48 49 52 53 54 55 56 57 58 59 61 62 64 65 66 67 70 71 72 73 74 **P**2 5 6 8 **S** Mercy Health Services, Farmington Hills, MI **N** Mercy Health Services, Farmington Hills, MI	21	10	417	17923	263	218877	2630	172754	74377	2292
PORT HURON—St. Clair County										
⊠ △ MERCY HOSPITAL, 2601 Electric Avenue, Zip 48061–6518; tel. 810/985–1510; Mary R. Trimmer, President and Chief Executive Officer **A**1 2 7 9 10 **F**4 8 10 12 14 15 16 17 19 21 22 28 30 31 32 33 34 35 37 39 41 42 43 44 45 46 48 49 60 63 65 67 71 73 74 **S** Mercy Health Services, Farmington Hills, MI **N** Mercy Health Services, Farmington Hills, MI	21	10	119	4361	66	57076	0	42255	17012	573
⊠ PORT HURON HOSPITAL, 1221 Pine Grove Avenue, Zip 48061–5011; tel. 810/987–5000; Donald C. Fletcher, President and Chief Executive Officer **A**1 2 9 10 **F**3 4 7 8 10 11 12 14 15 16 17 19 20 21 22 26 29 30 31 33 34 35 37 40 41 42 43 44 45 46 49 52 54 55 56 57 58 59 63 65 66 67 71 73 74 **P**7 **S** Blue Water Health Services Corporation, Port Huron, MI **N** Saint John Health System, Detroit, MI; Port Huron Hospital/Blue Water Health Services, Port Huron, MI	23	10	184	8457	103	156840	1070	67610	30657	764
REED CITY—Osceola County										
⊠ REED CITY HOSPITAL CORPORATION, 7665 Patterson Road, Zip 49677–1122, Mailing Address: P.O. Box 75, Zip 49677; tel. 616/832–3271; David M. Coates, Ph.D., President and Chief Executive Officer (Total facility includes 54 beds in nursing home–type unit) **A**1 9 10 **F**8 10 14 15 16 19 22 26 28 29 30 32 33 34 36 37 39 41 42 44 49 51 64 65 71 73 **P**4 8	23	10	79	1630	68	22292	0	11330	4484	192
ROCHESTER—Oakland County										
⊠ CRITTENTON HOSPITAL, 1101 West University Drive, Zip 48307–1831; tel. 810/652–5000; Dennis P. Markiewicz, Vice President, Hospital Operations **A**1 2 9 10 **F**7 8 10 11 14 15 16 19 21 22 24 28 29 30 32 33 34 35 37 39 40 41 42 44 45 46 48 49 52 54 55 56 57 58 59 60 63 65 66 67 71 73 74	23	10	224	11241	144	149182	1631	96043	43828	1275
ROGERS CITY—Presque Isle County										
△ ROGERS CITY REHABILITATION HOSPITAL, (Formerly Tendercare Rehabilitation Hospital), 555 North Bradley Highway, Zip 49779; tel. 517/734–7545; Darlene Park, Executive Director **A**7 10 **F**48 65	33	46	17	189	9	0	0	3096	809	59
ROYAL OAK—Oakland County										
⊠ △ WILLIAM BEAUMONT HOSPITAL–ROYAL OAK, 3601 West Thirteen Mile Road, Zip 48073–6769; tel. 810/551–5000; John D. Labriola, Vice President and Director **A**1 2 3 5 7 8 9 10 **F**1 4 6 7 8 10 11 12 14 15 16 17 19 21 22 23 24 25 26 28 29 30 31 32 33 34 35 37 38 39 40 42 43 44 45 46 47 48 49 50 51 52 54 55 56 57 59 60 61 63 64 65 66 67 69 71 73 74 **P**5 7 8 **S** William Beaumont Hospital Corporation, Royal Oak, MI **N** National Cardiovascular Network, Atlanta, GA; William Beaumont Hospital Corp, Royal Oak, MI	23	10	856	44677	674	628133	5856	518853	239175	7315
SAGINAW—Saginaw County										
⊠ △ HEALTHSOURCE SAGINAW, (LTC REHAB PSYCH CHEM DEP), 3340 Hospital Road, Zip 48603, Mailing Address: P.O. Box 6280, Zip 48608–6280; tel. 517/790–7700; Lester Heyboer, Jr., President and Chief Executive Officer (Total facility includes 213 beds in nursing home–type unit) **A**1 7 9 10 **F**2 3 15 20 26 39 41 45 46 48 49 52 53 54 55 57 58 64 65 67 73 **P**6	13	49	319	1768	194	14236	0	19479	10327	413
⊠ SAGINAW GENERAL HOSPITAL, 1447 North Harrison Street, Zip 48602; tel. 517/771–4000; William J. Heath, President and Chief Executive Officer **A**1 3 5 9 10 **F**7 8 10 11 12 15 16 19 21 22 25 30 31 32 33 34 35 37 38 39 40 41 42 44 45 46 49 52 56 59 61 65 67 71 73 74 **P**1	23	10	249	12973	165	95291	3203	97502	45661	1239
⊠ △ ST. LUKE'S HOSPITAL, 700 Cooper Avenue, Zip 48602; tel. 517/771–6001; Spencer Maidlow, President **A**1 3 5 7 9 10 **F**4 7 8 10 11 12 15 16 19 22 25 27 28 34 37 40 41 42 43 44 45 46 47 48 49 51 65 66 70 71 72 73 **P**3 6	23	10	273	13553	202	191670	663	128602	59432	1590
⊠ ST. MARY'S MEDICAL CENTER, 830 South Jefferson Avenue, Zip 48601–2594; tel. 517/776–8000; Frederic L. Fraizer, President and Chief Executive Officer **A**1 2 3 5 9 10 **F**4 8 9 10 11 14 15 16 19 21 22 25 27 28 30 34 35 37 39 42 43 44 45 46 49 54 56 60 63 65 70 71 73 **P**6 8 **S** Daughters of Charity National Health System, Saint Louis, MO	21	10	268	11319	190	124709	0	114390	49581	1310
⊠ VETERANS AFFAIRS MEDICAL CENTER, 1500 Weiss Street, Zip 48602; tel. 517/793–2340; Robert H. Sabin, Medical Center Director (Total facility includes 120 beds in nursing home–type unit) **A**1 5 9 **F**3 12 15 16 17 19 20 22 25 26 27 30 31 32 33 34 35 37 39 42 44 46 49 51 54 58 64 65 67 71 72 73 74 **S** Department of Veterans Affairs, Washington, DC	45	10	215	2231	132	62225	0	32963	19487	445
SAINT IGNACE—Mackinac County										
MACKINAC STRAITS HOSPITAL AND HEALTH CENTER, 220 Burdette Street, Zip 49781; tel. 906/643–8585; Mary E. Tamlyn, Administrator (Total facility includes 99 beds in nursing home–type unit) **A**9 10 **F**15 16 22 34 64 65	16	10	107	213	74	15525	0	6433	3558	133
SAINT JOHNS—Clinton County										
⊠ CLINTON MEMORIAL HOSPITAL, 805 South Oakland Street, Zip 48879–0260; tel. 517/224–6881; Paul E. McNamara, President **A**1 9 10 **F**7 8 14 15 16 17 19 22 24 26 29 32 33 35 36 40 41 42 44 48 49 65 66 71 72 73 **P**8	23	10	28	952	9	22543	125	16604	5296	182

Hospital, Address, Telephone, Administrator, Approval, Facility, and Physician Codes, Health Care System, Network	Classi-fication Codes		Utilization Data					Expense (thousands) of dollars		
★ American Hospital Association (AHA) membership □ Joint Commission on Accreditation of Healthcare Organizations (JCAHO) accreditation + American Osteopathic Hospital Association (AOHA) membership ○ American Osteopathic Association (AOA) accreditation △ Commission on Accreditation of Rehabilitation Facilities (CARF) accreditation Control codes 61, 63, 64, 71, 72 and 73 indicate hospitals listed by AOHA, but not registered by AHA. For definition of numerical codes, see page A4	Control	Service	Beds	Admissions	Census	Outpatient Visits	Births	Total	Payroll	Personnel

□ RIVENDELL OF MICHIGAN, 101 West Townsend Road, Zip 48879; tel. 517/224–1177; Michael Talmo, Chief Executive Officer (Nonreporting) **A**1 **S** Vendell Heralthcare, Inc., Nashville, TN	33	22	63	—	—	—	—	—	—	—
SAINT JOSEPH—Berrien County										
✠ △ LAKELAND MEDICAL CENTER-ST. JOSEPH, (Includes Lakeland Medical Center, Berrien Center, 6418 Dean's Hill Road, Berrien Center, Zip 49102–9704; tel. 616/471–7761), 1234 Napier Avenue, Zip 49085; tel. 616/983–8300; Joseph A. Wasserman, President and Chief Executive Officer **A**1 2 7 9 10 **F**3 4 7 8 10 12 15 16 19 21 22 26 28 29 30 31 32 33 34 35 37 40 41 42 43 44 48 49 51 52 56 59 60 63 65 66 67 71 73 74 **P**8 **S** Lakeland Regional Health System, Inc., Saint Joseph, MI **N** Lakeland Regional Health System, St. Joseph, MI	23	10	254	10662	143	227556	1071	102220	43378	1530
SALINE—Washtenaw County										
✠ SALINE COMMUNITY HOSPITAL, 400 West Russell Street, Zip 48176–1101; tel. 313/429–1500; Garry C. Faja, President and Chief Executive Officer **A**1 9 10 **F**2 3 8 12 14 15 17 19 20 21 22 28 30 31 33 34 41 44 49 65 67 71 73 **P**3 **S** Mercy Health Services, Farmington Hills, MI **N** Mercy Health Services, Farmington Hills, MI	21	10	48	1802	23	84069	0	21510	9695	237
SANDUSKY—Sanilac County										
★ MCKENZIE MEMORIAL HOSPITAL, 120 Delaware Street, Zip 48471–1087; tel. 810/648–3770; Joseph W. Weiler, President **A**9 10 **F**3 8 12 15 16 19 21 22 26 28 33 34 37 40 41 42 44 45 46 49 54 56 63 65 69 71 73 **P**6	23	10	25	927	7	17769	94	8645	4058	124
SAULT STE. MARIE—Chippewa County										
✠ CHIPPEWA COUNTY WAR MEMORIAL HOSPITAL, 500 Osborn Boulevard, Zip 49783–4467; tel. 906/635–4460; Daniel Wakeman, Chief Executive Officer (Total facility includes 51 beds in nursing home–type unit) **A**1 9 10 **F**3 7 8 11 12 14 15 16 19 21 22 34 35 37 40 41 42 44 45 46 49 63 64 65 71 72 73 **S** Brim, Inc., Portland, OR	23	10	130	2595	77	47778	418	22824	10022	415
SHELBY—Oceana County										
✠ LAKESHORE COMMUNITY HOSPITAL, 72 South State Street, Zip 49455–1299; tel. 616/861–2156; Martin E. Anderson, Administrator **A**1 9 10 **F**7 8 14 15 16 17 22 28 30 31 34 40 42 44 45 51 71 73	23	10	32	784	7	29419	145	4641	2322	86
SHERIDAN—Montcalm County										
+ ○ SHERIDAN COMMUNITY HOSPITAL, 301 North Main Street, Zip 48884, Mailing Address: P.O. Box 279, Zip 48884–0279; tel. 517/291–3261; Christopher Noland, Chief Executive Officer **A**9 10 11 **F**8 14 15 16 17 19 22 25 28 30 32 33 37 41 42 44 46 49 51 71 73	23	10	19	494	6	22267	0	6282	3463	110
SOUTH HAVEN—Van Buren County										
✠ SOUTH HAVEN COMMUNITY HOSPITAL, 955 South Bailey Avenue, Zip 49090; tel. 616/637–5271; Craig J. Marks, President and Chief Executive Officer **A**1 9 10 **F**1 4 5 7 8 14 15 16 19 21 22 24 26 28 30 31 32 33 35 36 37 39 40 41 42 44 45 48 49 53 54 55 56 57 58 59 60 61 65 66 69 71 72 73 74 **P**4 **N** Lakeland Regional Health System, St. Joseph, MI	16	10	52	1362	10	82374	312	13562	5609	182
SOUTHFIELD—Oakland County										
○ △ GREAT LAKES REHABILITATION HOSPITAL, 22401 Foster Winter Drive, Zip 48075; tel. 810/569–1500; Gerald L. Berger, CPA, Chief Operating Officer (Total facility includes 10 beds in nursing home–type unit) **A**7 9 10 11 **F**12 14 15 16 20 34 39 41 45 46 48 49 54 58 64 65 67 73	33	46	55	723	47	3699	0	10204	6310	196
✠ PROVIDENCE HOSPITAL AND MEDICAL CENTERS, 16001 West Nine Mile Road, Zip 48075–4854, Mailing Address: Box 2043, Zip 48037–2043; tel. 810/424–3000; Brian M. Connolly, President and Chief Executive Officer **A**1 2 3 5 8 9 10 **F**1 3 4 7 8 10 11 12 13 14 15 16 17 19 21 22 25 26 27 28 29 30 31 32 33 34 35 37 38 39 40 41 42 43 44 45 46 48 49 51 52 53 54 55 56 57 58 59 60 65 66 67 70 71 72 73 74 **P**8 **S** Daughters of Charity National Health System, Saint Louis, MO	21	10	351	19236	280	603407	3877	275109	126476	2576
✠ STRAITH HOSPITAL FOR SPECIAL SURGERY, 23901 Lahser Road, Zip 48034–3296; tel. 810/357–3360; Gregory R. Hoose, Chief Executive Officer **A**1 9 10 **F**12 14 15 44 65 69	23	45	23	1030	13	6047	0	10504	4222	123
STANDISH—Arenac County										
□ STANDISH COMMUNITY HOSPITAL, 805 West Cedar Street, Zip 48658, Mailing Address: P.O. Box 579, Zip 48658; tel. 517/846–4521; Thomas G. Westhoff, Chief Executive Officer (Total facility includes 44 beds in nursing home–type unit) **A**1 9 10 **F**8 11 19 22 27 34 37 44 49 63 64 65 67 71 72 73	23	10	72	952	53	26302	0	11937	6380	242
STURGIS—St. Joseph County										
✠ STURGIS HOSPITAL, 916 Myrtle, Zip 49091–2001; tel. 616/659–4400; David James, Chief Executive Officer **A**1 9 10 **F**7 8 11 14 15 16 17 18 19 20 21 22 24 25 28 29 30 32 33 34 35 36 37 39 40 41 42 44 45 46 49 51 63 65 67 71 73 **P**6 **S** Quorum Health Group/Quorum Health Resources, Inc., Brentwood, TN **N** Hospital Network Inc., Kalamazoo, MI	14	10	67	2296	22	70040	390	22982	8508	308
TAWAS CITY—Iosco County										
✠ TAWAS ST. JOSEPH HOSPITAL, 200 Hemlock Street, Zip 48763, Mailing Address: P.O. Box 659, Zip 48764–0659; tel. 517/362–3411; Paul R. Schmidt, President and Chief Executive Officer **A**1 9 10 **F**7 8 14 15 16 17 19 22 25 26 27 29 30 32 33 34 37 39 40 41 42 44 49 63 67 71 73 **P**5 **S** Sisters of St. Joseph Health System, Ann Arbor, MI	23	10	69	2414	25	91778	324	22897	10494	375
TAYLOR—Wayne County										
✠ OAKWOOD HOSPITAL–HERITAGE CENTER, 10000 Telegraph Road, Zip 48180–3349; tel. 313/295–5000; Thomas E. Johnson, Vice President and Administrator **A**1 9 10 **F**1 3 4 7 8 10 11 12 13 14 15 16 17 18 19 20 21 22 25 26 27 28 29 30 31 32 33 34 35 36 37 38 39 40 41 42 43 44 45 46 48 49 50 51 52 53 54 55 56 57 58 59 60 61 62 63 64 65 67 68 70 71 72 73 74 **P**3 4 5 7 **S** Oakwood Healthcare System, Dearborn, MI	23	10	243	7823	169	—	0	66412	30617	655

Hospital, Address, Telephone, Administrator, Approval, Facility, and Physician Codes, Health Care System, Network	Classi- fication Codes		Utilization Data					Expense (thousands) of dollars		
	Control	Service	Beds	Admissions	Census	Outpatient Visits	Births	Total	Payroll	Personnel

Approval codes legend:
★ American Hospital Association (AHA) membership
□ Joint Commission on Accreditation of Healthcare Organizations (JCAHO) accreditation
+ American Osteopathic Hospital Association (AOHA) membership
○ American Osteopathic Association (AOA) accreditation
△ Commission on Accreditation of Rehabilitation Facilities (CARF) accreditation
Control codes 61, 63, 64, 71, 72 and 73 indicate hospitals listed by AOHA, but not registered by AHA. For definition of numerical codes, see page A4

TECUMSEH—Lenawee County

Hospital	Control	Service	Beds	Admissions	Census	Outpatient Visits	Births	Total	Payroll	Personnel
★ ○ HERRICK MEMORIAL HOSPITAL, 500 East Pottawatamie Street, Zip 49286–2097; tel. 517/423–3834; Michael J. Mihora, Chief Operating Officer (Total facility includes 25 beds in nursing home–type unit) A1 9 10 11 F3 7 8 11 15 16 17 19 21 22 24 28 29 30 37 40 41 44 45 46 48 49 52 53 58 59 61 64 65 67 71 72 73 P8	23	10	91	2343	48	59505	267	19677	8678	275

THREE RIVERS—St. Joseph County

Hospital	Control	Service	Beds	Admissions	Census	Outpatient Visits	Births	Total	Payroll	Personnel
★ △ THREE RIVERS AREA HOSPITAL, 1111 West Broadway, Zip 49093–9362; tel. 616/278–1145; Bradley Solberg, President and Chief Executive Officer A1 7 9 10 F7 8 10 12 15 16 17 19 21 22 24 28 30 31 32 34 35 37 39 40 41 42 44 45 48 49 61 65 71 73 74 S Quorum Health Group/Quorum Health Resources, Inc., Brentwood, TN	16	10	60	1634	25	36092	213	18751	7780	269

TRAVERSE CITY—Grand Traverse County

Hospital	Control	Service	Beds	Admissions	Census	Outpatient Visits	Births	Total	Payroll	Personnel
★ △ MUNSON MEDICAL CENTER, 1105 Sixth Street, Zip 49684–2386; tel. 616/935–5000; Ralph J. Cerny, President and Chief Executive Officer A1 2 7 9 10 12 13 F2 3 4 7 8 10 11 12 14 15 16 17 19 20 21 22 23 24 25 26 27 28 29 30 31 32 33 34 35 37 38 39 40 41 42 43 44 45 46 48 49 51 52 54 55 56 57 59 60 61 65 66 67 68 71 72 73 74 P5 7 8 S Munson Healthcare, Traverse City, MI	23	10	368	17075	224	272577	1790	151869	71470	2184

TRENTON—Wayne County

Hospital	Control	Service	Beds	Admissions	Census	Outpatient Visits	Births	Total	Payroll	Personnel
★ OAKWOOD HOSPITAL SEAWAY CENTER, 5450 Fort Street, Zip 48183; tel. 313/671–3800; Edward Freisinger, Vice President and Administration A1 9 10 F2 3 4 6 7 8 10 11 12 14 15 16 17 19 21 22 23 25 26 28 29 30 31 32 33 34 35 36 37 39 40 41 42 43 44 45 46 48 49 52 53 54 55 56 57 58 59 60 61 62 63 64 65 66 67 68 69 71 72 73 74 S Oakwood Healthcare System, Dearborn, MI	23	10	103	3172	40	50787	153	32084	13351	327
+ ○ RIVERSIDE OSTEOPATHIC HOSPITAL, 150 Truax Street, Zip 48183–2151; tel. 313/676–4200; Dennis R. Lemanski, D.O., Vice President and Chief Administrative Officer A9 10 11 12 13 F7 8 10 11 12 14 15 16 17 18 19 21 22 24 26 27 28 29 30 31 32 33 34 35 36 37 39 40 41 42 44 45 46 49 52 54 55 56 57 60 61 63 65 66 67 70 71 73 74 S Henry Ford Health System, Detroit, MI N Great Lakes Health Network, Southfield, MI	23	10	148	5502	81	126022	765	56251	27061	568

TROY—Oakland County

Hospital	Control	Service	Beds	Admissions	Census	Outpatient Visits	Births	Total	Payroll	Personnel
★ WILLIAM BEAUMONT HOSPITAL–TROY, 44201 Dequindre Road, Zip 48098–1198; tel. 810/828–5100; Eugene F. Michalski, Vice President and Hospital Director A1 3 9 10 F1 4 6 7 8 10 11 12 14 15 16 17 19 21 22 23 24 25 26 28 29 30 31 32 33 34 35 37 38 39 40 42 43 44 45 46 47 48 49 50 51 52 54 55 56 57 59 60 61 63 64 65 66 67 69 71 73 74 P5 7 8 S William Beaumont Hospital Corporation, Royal Oak, MI N William Beaumont Hospital Corp, Royal Oak, MI	23	10	189	11755	148	348002	1586	120483	55640	1666

VICKSBURG—Kalamazoo County

Hospital	Control	Service	Beds	Admissions	Census	Outpatient Visits	Births	Total	Payroll	Personnel
★ △ BRONSON VICKSBURG HOSPITAL, 13326 North Boulevard, Zip 49097–1099; tel. 616/649–2321; Frank J. Sardone, President A1 7 9 10 F8 12 14 19 21 22 26 28 30 34 35 41 44 45 48 49 54 65 71 73 S Bronson Healthcare Group, Inc., Kalamazoo, MI N Hospital Network Inc., Kalamazoo, MI	23	46	41	359	12	31296	0	7450	2462	89

WARREN—Macomb County

Hospital	Control	Service	Beds	Admissions	Census	Outpatient Visits	Births	Total	Payroll	Personnel
□ ARBORVIEW HOSPITAL, 6902 Chicago Road, Zip 48092; tel. 810/264–8875; Donald L. Warner, Chief Operating Officer A1 10 F15 16 52 53 54 55 56 57 58 59 P5	33	22	40	1061	13	0	0	4613	2127	87
+ ○ △ BI-COUNTY COMMUNITY HOSPITAL, 13355 East Ten Mile Road, Zip 48089–2065; tel. 810/759–7300; Gary W. Popiel, Vice President and Chief Administrative Officer A7 9 10 11 12 13 F3 7 8 10 12 14 15 16 19 21 22 24 27 28 29 30 31 32 33 34 35 37 39 40 41 42 44 45 46 48 49 51 53 54 55 60 61 63 65 66 71 73 74 P6 S Henry Ford Health System, Detroit, MI N Great Lakes Health Network, Southfield, MI	23	10	152	6162	108	135628	554	68513	32142	527
□ KERN HOSPITAL FOR SPECIAL SURGERY, (PODIATRY), 21230 Dequindre, Zip 48091–2287; tel. 810/759–4520; Irvin Kanat, DPM, Chief Executive Officer A1 9 10 F14 27 44 65	23	49	20	486	9	—	0	4668	3204	86
★ MACOMB HOSPITAL CENTER, 11800 East Twelve Mile Road, Zip 48093; tel. 810/573–5000; Timothy J. Ryan, JD, President and Chief Executive Officer A1 2 9 10 F7 8 10 11 14 15 16 17 19 20 21 22 27 28 29 30 32 33 34 35 37 39 40 42 44 45 46 48 49 51 52 54 55 56 57 58 59 60 63 65 66 67 71 73 P4 5 6 8 S Detroit–Macomb Hospital Corporation, Warren, MI N Detroit–Macomb Hospital Corp, Warren, MI	23	10	297	12006	206	102250	1302	116757	54761	1369

WATERVLIET—Berrien County

Hospital	Control	Service	Beds	Admissions	Census	Outpatient Visits	Births	Total	Payroll	Personnel
★ △ COMMUNITY HOSPITAL, Medical Park Drive, Zip 49098–0158, Mailing Address: Box 158, Zip 49098; tel. 616/463–3111; Dennis Turney, Chief Executive Officer A1 7 9 10 F8 10 12 14 15 16 19 22 26 28 29 30 32 33 34 35 37 39 44 45 46 48 49 54 63 65 67 71 72 73 74 P1 S Quorum Health Group/Quorum Health Resources, Inc., Brentwood, TN N First Choice Network, Watervliet, MI	23	10	54	1835	29	34166	0	14031	6142	226

WAYNE—Wayne County

Hospital	Control	Service	Beds	Admissions	Census	Outpatient Visits	Births	Total	Payroll	Personnel
★ OAKWOOD HOSPITAL ANNAPOLIS CENTER, (Includes Oakwood Hospital Merriman Center–Westland, 2345 Merriman Road, Westland, Zip 48185; tel. 313/467–2300), 33155 Annapolis Road, Zip 48184; tel. 313/467–4000; Mark Anthony, Vice President and Administrator A1 9 10 F1 3 4 6 7 8 10 11 12 13 14 15 16 17 18 19 20 21 22 26 27 28 29 30 32 33 34 35 37 38 39 40 41 42 43 44 45 46 48 49 52 54 55 56 57 58 59 60 61 62 63 64 65 66 67 68 71 72 73 74 P3 6 S Oakwood Healthcare System, Dearborn, MI	23	10	360	11600	196	91155	695	83055	31569	926

Hospital, Address, Telephone, Administrator, Approval, Facility, and Physician Codes, Health Care System, Network	Control	Service	Beds	Admissions	Census	Outpatient Visits	Births	Total	Payroll	Personnel
WEST BRANCH—Ogemaw County										
★ TOLFREE MEMORIAL HOSPITAL, 335 East Houghton Avenue, Zip 48661–1199; tel. 517/345–3660; Douglas E. Pattullo, Chief Executive Officer **A**1 9 10 **F**7 11 15 16 19 22 33 40 42 44 63	14	10	92	3301	38	41626	333	15972	7525	292
WESTLAND—Wayne County										
OAKWOOD HOSPITAL MERRIMAN CENTER–WESTLAND See Oakwood Hospital Annapolis Center, Wayne										
□ WALTER P. REUTHER PSYCHIATRIC HOSPITAL, 30901 Palmer Road, Zip 48185–5389; tel. 313/722–4500; Norma C. Josef, M.D., Director **A**1 10 **F**14 19 20 21 26 35 48 50 52 54 56 57 63 64 65 73 **P**5	12	22	176	171	182	0	0	24771	14322	343
WYANDOTTE—Wayne County										
★ △ HENRY FORD WYANDOTTE HOSPITAL, 2333 Biddle Avenue, Zip 48192; tel. 313/284–2400; William R. Alvin, President **A**1 7 9 10 **F**1 7 8 10 11 14 17 19 22 25 30 33 34 35 37 40 41 42 44 46 48 49 52 53 54 56 57 58 59 60 65 66 67 71 72 73 **P**6 **S** Henry Ford Health System, Detroit, MI **N** Henry Ford Health System, Detroit, MI	23	10	355	13074	235	—	1115	105028	56792	1535
YALE—St. Clair County										
★ YALE COMMUNITY HOSPITAL, 420 North Street, Zip 48097, Mailing Address: P.O. Box 129, Zip 48097–0129; tel. 810/387–3211; Joyce Laupichler, Administrator **A**1 9 10 **F**8 16 28 34 44 49 51 71 72 **P**6 **N** Port Huron Hospital/Blue Water Health Services, Port Huron, MI	23	10	22	142	1	16144	0	2161	1201	47
YPSILANTI—Washtenaw County										
★ OAKWOOD HOSPITAL BEYER CENTER–YPSILANTI, 135 South Prospect Street, Zip 48198–5693; tel. 313/484–2200; Richard Hillbom, Acting Administrator **A**1 9 10 **F**3 7 8 10 14 15 16 17 19 21 22 26 28 30 32 33 34 35 37 40 41 42 44 45 46 49 56 58 63 65 67 71 74 **P**1 4 5 7 **S** Oakwood Healthcare System, Dearborn, MI	23	10	82	3393	48	40064	299	31290	14229	306
ZEELAND—Ottawa County										
★ ZEELAND COMMUNITY HOSPITAL, 100 South Pine Street, Zip 49464; tel. 616/772–4644; Henry A. Veenstra, President **A**1 9 10 **F**7 8 11 14 15 16 17 19 22 28 30 33 36 39 40 41 42 44 45 49 60 71 72 73 74 **P**4 8 **N** Butterworth Health System, Grand Rapids, MI	23	10	55	1811	20	41384	329	16356	7381	235

MINNESOTA

Resident population 4,610 (in thousands)
Resident population in metro areas 69.4%
Birth rate per 1,000 population 14.3
65 years and over 12.4%
Percent of persons without health insurance 9.5%

Hospital, Address, Telephone, Administrator, Approval, Facility, and Physician Codes, Health Care System, Network	Classification Codes		Utilization Data					Expense (thousands) of dollars		
★ American Hospital Association (AHA) membership □ Joint Commission on Accreditation of Healthcare Organizations (JCAHO) accreditation + American Osteopathic Hospital Association (AOHA) membership ○ American Osteopathic Association (AOA) accreditation △ Commission on Accreditation of Rehabilitation Facilities (CARF) accreditation Control codes 61, 63, 64, 71, 72 and 73 indicate hospitals listed by AOHA, but not registered by AHA. For definition of numerical codes, see page A4	Control	Service	Beds	Admissions	Census	Outpatient Visits	Births	Total	Payroll	Personnel

ADA—Norman County

★ BRIDGES MEDICAL SERVICES, (Includes John Wimmer Memorial Home), 405 East Second Avenue, Zip 56510–0233, Mailing Address: P.O. Box 233, Zip 56510–0233; tel. 218/784–5000; Kyle Rasmussen, Administrator (Total facility includes 49 beds in nursing home–type unit) **A**9 10 **F**11 15 19 21 22 27 34 44 49 64 71 **P**6

| | 14 | 10 | 63 | 354 | 46 | 8679 | 0 | 4275 | 2361 | 114 |

ADRIAN—Nobles County

ARNOLD MEMORIAL HEALTH CARE CENTER, 601 Louisiana Avenue, Zip 56110–0279, Mailing Address: Box 279, Zip 56110–0279; tel. 507/483–2668; Gerald E. Carl, Administrator (Total facility includes 41 beds in nursing home–type unit) **A**9 10 **F**6 8 26 28 32 33 34 49 64 71 **S** Sioux Valley Health System, Sioux Falls, SD

| | 15 | 10 | 50 | 92 | 40 | 1561 | 0 | 1873 | 1096 | 50 |

AITKIN—Aitkin County

RIVERWOOD HEALTH CARE CENTER, 301 Minnesota Avenue South, Zip 56431–1626; tel. 218/927–2121; Debra Boardman, Chief Executive Officer (Total facility includes 48 beds in nursing home–type unit) **A**9 10 **F**7 8 11 15 19 22 28 32 33 35 42 44 49 64 65 67 71 73 **P**8 **N** Northern Lakes Health Consortium, Duluth, MN

| | 23 | 10 | 68 | 952 | 58 | 19819 | 48 | 8745 | 3813 | 154 |

ALBANY—Stearns County

★ ALBANY AREA HOSPITAL AND MEDICAL CENTER, 300 Third Avenue, Zip 56307; tel. 320/845–2121; Ben Koppelman, Administrator **A**9 10 **F**7 8 15 16 19 22 30 32 33 40 44 48 58 64 65 71 73 **P**6 **S** Catholic Health Initiatives, Denver, CO

| | 21 | 10 | 13 | 365 | 3 | 4817 | 76 | 3951 | 1295 | 67 |

ALBERT LEA—Freeborn County

⊠ △ NAEVE HOSPITAL, 404 West Fountain Street, Zip 56007–2473; tel. 507/373–2384; Theodore Myers, M.D., Chief Executive Officer (Nonreporting) **A**1 7 9 10 **S** Mayo Foundation, Rochester, MN

| | 23 | 10 | 72 | — | — | — | — | — | — | — |

ALEXANDRIA—Douglas County

⊠ DOUGLAS COUNTY HOSPITAL, 111 17th Avenue East, Zip 56308–3798; tel. 320/762–1511; William G. Flaig, Administrator **A**1 9 10 **F**3 7 8 14 15 19 21 22 23 28 29 31 32 33 34 35 36 37 40 41 42 44 45 49 54 55 56 58 59 63 65 66 67 71 73

| | 13 | 10 | 110 | 3995 | 45 | 45691 | 490 | 28659 | 13290 | 411 |

ANOKA—Anoka County

□ ANOKA–METROPOLITAN REGIONAL TREATMENT CENTER, 3300 Fourth Avenue North, Zip 55303–1119; tel. 612/576–5500; Judith Krohn, Ph.D., Chief Executive Officer **A**1 9 10 **F**14 52 54 55 56 57 58 65 73 **P**6

| | 12 | 22 | 247 | 520 | 256 | — | 0 | 25000 | 16500 | 400 |

APPLETON—Swift County

APPLETON MUNICIPAL HOSPITAL AND NURSING HOME, 30 South Behl Street, Zip 56208–1699; tel. 612/289–2422; Mark E. Paulson, Administrator (Total facility includes 84 beds in nursing home–type unit) **A**9 10 **F**7 14 17 19 22 32 33 34 36 39 41 44 45 49 58 62 63 64 65 71 73 **P**7 **N** Minnesota Rural Health Cooperative, Willmar, MN

| | 14 | 10 | 104 | 354 | 85 | 3577 | 9 | 5356 | 2151 | 103 |

ARLINGTON—Sibley County

□ ARLINGTON MUNICIPAL HOSPITAL, 601 West Chandler Street, Zip 55307; tel. 507/964–2271; Lynette Froehlich, R.N., Administrator **A**1 9 10 **F**1 3 8 15 19 20 22 27 31 32 33 35 42 44 45 46 49 53 62 65 66 67 71 73 **P**7 8

| | 14 | 10 | 17 | 340 | 4 | 4109 | 0 | 2573 | 1293 | 48 |

AURORA—St. Louis County

★ WHITE COMMUNITY HOSPITAL, 5211 Highway 110, Zip 55705; tel. 218/229–2211; Cheryl A. High, Administrator (Total facility includes 69 beds in nursing home–type unit) **A**9 10 **F**7 16 17 22 26 28 30 31 34 36 44 49 60 64 65 66 67 **N** Northern Lakes Health Consortium, Duluth, MN

| | 23 | 10 | 85 | 283 | 70 | 4289 | 0 | 4538 | 2384 | 112 |

AUSTIN—Mower County

□ AUSTIN MEDICAL CENTER, 1000 First Drive N.W., Zip 55912; tel. 507/437–4551; Donald R. Brezicka, Executive Vice President (Nonreporting) **A**1 10 **S** Mayo Foundation, Rochester, MN **N** Mayo Foundation, Rochester, MN

| | 23 | 10 | 108 | — | — | — | — | — | — | — |

BAGLEY—Clearwater County

★ CLEARWATER HEALTH SERVICES, 203 Fourth Street N.W., Zip 56621, Mailing Address: Rural Route 3, Box 46, Zip 56621; tel. 218/694–6501; Larry Laudon, Administrator (Total facility includes 70 beds in nursing home–type unit) **A**9 10 **F**7 8 15 19 22 40 44 49 71

| | 13 | 10 | 92 | 549 | 72 | 9821 | 30 | 5881 | 2652 | 125 |

BAUDETTE—Lake of the Woods County

★ LAKEWOOD HEALTH CENTER, 600 South Main Avenue, Zip 56623, Mailing Address: Route 1, Box 2120, Zip 56623; tel. 218/634–2120; David A. Nelson, President and Chief Executive Officer (Total facility includes 52 beds in nursing home–type unit) **A**9 10 **F**7 8 13 14 15 16 17 19 22 27 28 30 32 35 40 44 63 64 65 71 **S** Catholic Health Initiatives, Denver, CO **N** Northstar Health Consortium, Roseau, MN

| | 21 | 10 | 73 | 421 | 52 | 5071 | 50 | 5081 | 2164 | 103 |

BEMIDJI—Beltrami County

⊠ NORTH COUNTRY REGIONAL HOSPITAL, 1100 West 38th Street, Zip 56601–9972; tel. 218/751–5430; John Skjerven, Interim Chief Executive Officer (Total facility includes 78 beds in nursing home–type unit) **A**1 9 10 **F**4 7 8 12 14 15 16 17 19 21 22 28 29 30 32 33 34 35 37 39 40 41 42 44 45 49 62 64 65 67 71 73 **P**6

| | 23 | 10 | 172 | 5100 | 127 | 33645 | 725 | 34385 | 15289 | 422 |

Hospital, Address, Telephone, Administrator, Approval, Facility, and Physician Codes, Health Care System, Network	Classi- fication Codes		Utilization Data					Expense (thousands) of dollars		
★ American Hospital Association (AHA) membership □ Joint Commission on Accreditation of Healthcare Organizations (JCAHO) accreditation + American Osteopathic Hospital Association (AOHA) membership ○ American Osteopathic Association (AOA) accreditation △ Commission on Accreditation of Rehabilitation Facilities (CARF) accreditation Control codes 61, 63, 64, 71, 72 and 73 indicate hospitals listed by AOHA, but not registered by AHA. For definition of numerical codes, see page A4	Control	Service	Beds	Admissions	Census	Outpatient Visits	Births	Total	Payroll	Personnel

BENSON—Swift County

★ SWIFT COUNTY–BENSON HOSPITAL, 1815 Wisconsin Avenue, Zip 56215–1653; tel. 320/843–4232; John Stindt, Chief Executive Officer **A**9 10 **F**7 8 11 15 16 19 22 28 32 33 34 35 36 37 39 40 41 44 49 54 58 64 65 71 **S** Brim, Inc., Portland, OR **N** Minnesota Rural Health Cooperative, Willmar, MN — 15 | 10 | 31 | 394 | 4 | — | 30 | 3315 | 1455 | 51

BIGFORK—Itasca County

★ NORTHERN ITASCA HEALTH CARE CENTER, 258 Pine Tree Drive, Zip 56628, Mailing Address: P.O. Box 258, Zip 56628–0258; tel. 218/743–3177; Richard M. Ash, Administrator (Total facility includes 40 beds in nursing home–type unit) **A**9 10 **F**1 6 7 8 15 16 19 20 22 26 27 28 32 33 40 42 44 49 64 65 71 **P**5 **N** Northern Lakes Health Consortium, Duluth, MN; Itasca Partnership for Quality Healthcare, Grand Rapids, MN — 16 | 10 | 56 | 357 | 43 | 11827 | 25 | 4486 | 2124 | 97

BLUE EARTH—Faribault County

⊞ UNITED HOSPITAL DISTRICT, 515 South Moore Street, Zip 56013–2158, Mailing Address: P.O. Box 160, Zip 56013–0160; tel. 507/526–3273; Brian Kief, President **A**1 9 10 **F**7 8 15 16 17 19 22 26 27 28 30 31 32 33 34 35 36 37 39 40 41 42 44 45 49 53 54 55 58 65 67 71 **S** Allina Health System, Minneapolis, MN **N** Allina Health System, Minnetonka, MN; Quality Health Alliance, Mankato, MN — 16 | 10 | 43 | 919 | 9 | 26016 | 52 | 7827 | 3160 | 135

BRAINERD—Crow Wing County

□ BRAINERD REGIONAL HUMAN SERVICES CENTER, 1777 Highway 18 East, Zip 56401; tel. 218/828–2201; Harvey G. Caldwell, Administrator and Chief Executive Officer (Nonreporting) **A**1 10 — 12 | 22 | 288 | — | — | — | — | — | — | —

□ ST. JOSEPH'S MEDICAL CENTER, 523 North Third Street, Zip 56401–3098; tel. 218/829–2861; Thomas K. Prusak, President **A**1 9 10 **F**2 3 7 8 11 12 15 16 19 21 22 28 29 30 31 32 33 34 35 36 39 40 41 42 44 46 48 49 52 53 54 55 56 58 59 65 66 67 71 73 **S** Benedictine Health System, Duluth, MN — 21 | 10 | 153 | 6000 | 73 | — | 600 | 42140 | 18399 | 534

BRECKENRIDGE—Wilkin County

⊞ ST. FRANCIS MEDICAL CENTER, 415 Oak Street, Zip 56520; tel. 218/643–3000; Mark C. McNelly, President and Chief Executive Officer (Total facility includes 124 beds in nursing home–type unit) **A**1 5 9 10 **F**1 3 6 7 8 15 16 17 19 20 21 22 26 28 29 30 32 33 35 36 37 39 40 41 44 45 46 49 51 53 54 55 56 57 58 60 64 65 66 67 71 72 73 **S** Catholic Health Initiatives, Denver, CO — 21 | 10 | 171 | 1798 | 139 | 14246 | 272 | 15851 | 6923 | 300

BUFFALO—Wright County

⊞ BUFFALO HOSPITAL, 303 Catlin Street, Zip 55313–1947, Mailing Address: P.O. Box 609, Zip 55313–0609; tel. 612/682–7180; Mary Ellen Wells, President **A**1 9 10 **F**7 8 11 14 15 16 17 19 21 22 27 28 30 32 33 34 35 37 39 40 41 42 44 46 48 49 65 67 71 73 **P**5 6 **S** Allina Health System, Minneapolis, MN **N** Allina Health System, Minnetonka, MN — 23 | 10 | 30 | 1669 | 13 | 16046 | 390 | 12528 | 6212 | 159

BURNSVILLE—Dakota County

⊞ FAIRVIEW RIDGES HOSPITAL, 201 East Nicollet Boulevard, Zip 55337–5799; tel. 612/892–2000; Mark M. Enger, Senior Vice President and Administrator **A**1 9 10 **F**2 3 7 8 15 16 17 19 21 22 32 33 34 35 37 40 41 42 44 45 48 49 54 65 66 67 71 73 74 **S** Fairview Hospital and Healthcare Services, Minneapolis, MN **N** Fairview Health System, Minneapolis, MN — 21 | 10 | 124 | 8350 | 60 | 56026 | 2567 | 48721 | 18587 | 459

CAMBRIDGE—Isanti County

⊞ CAMBRIDGE MEDICAL CENTER, 701 South Dellwood Street, Zip 55008–1920; tel. 612/689–7700; Lowell L. Becker, M.D., President **A**1 9 10 **F**2 3 7 8 11 12 15 16 17 19 20 21 22 24 26 28 29 30 31 32 33 34 35 36 39 40 41 42 44 45 46 49 51 52 54 55 56 57 58 60 62 65 66 67 70 71 72 73 **P**3 8 **S** Allina Health System, Minneapolis, MN **N** Allina Health System, Minnetonka, MN — 23 | 10 | 81 | 3924 | 43 | 23642 | 389 | 31991 | 17028 | 565

CANBY—Yellow Medicine County

★ CANBY COMMUNITY HEALTH SERVICES, (Includes Senior Haven Convalescent Nursing Center), 112 St. Olaf Avenue South, Zip 56220–1433; tel. 507/223–7277; Robert J. Salmon, Chief Executive Officer (Total facility includes 75 beds in nursing home–type unit) **A**9 10 **F**7 8 15 17 19 21 22 26 27 28 29 30 32 33 34 35 37 39 40 41 42 44 49 53 62 64 65 66 67 71 73 **P**6 **S** Sioux Valley Health System, Sioux Falls, SD **N** Minnesota Rural Health Cooperative, Willmar, MN; Southwest Minnesota Health Alliance, Luverne, MN; Sioux Valley Health System, Sioux Falls, SD — 23 | 10 | 99 | 405 | 77 | 5676 | 30 | 5594 | 2211 | —

CANNON FALLS—Goodhue County

★ COMMUNITY HOSPITAL, 1116 West Mill Street, Zip 55009–1898; tel. 507/263–4221; Randy Ulseth, Interim Administrator **A**9 10 **F**1 2 3 4 5 6 7 8 9 10 11 12 13 14 17 18 19 20 21 22 23 24 25 26 27 28 29 30 31 32 33 34 35 36 37 39 40 41 42 43 44 45 46 47 48 49 50 51 52 53 54 55 56 57 58 60 61 62 63 64 65 66 67 68 69 70 71 72 73 74 **P**8 — 16 | 10 | 21 | 410 | 3 | — | 32 | 3444 | 1494 | —

CASS LAKE—Cass County

⊞ U. S. PUBLIC HEALTH SERVICE INDIAN HOSPITAL, 7th Street and Grant Utley Avenue N.W., Zip 56633; tel. 218/335–2293; Luella Brown, Service Unit Director (Nonreporting) **A**1 5 10 **S** U. S. Public Health Service Indian Health Service, Rockville, MD — 47 | 10 | 13 | — | — | — | — | — | — | —

CHISAGO CITY—Chisago County

⊞ CHISAGO HEALTH SERVICES, 11685 Lake Boulevard North, Zip 55013–9540; tel. 612/257–8400; Scott Wordelman, President and Chief Executive Officer (Total facility includes 40 beds in nursing home–type unit) **A**1 9 10 **F**7 8 11 12 15 16 17 19 22 26 32 33 34 35 37 39 40 41 42 44 45 46 49 51 54 64 65 68 71 72 73 74 **P**8 **S** Fairview Hospital and Healthcare Services, Minneapolis, MN **N** Fairview Health System, Minneapolis, MN; I–35 Corridor Health Network, Duluth, MN — 23 | 10 | 89 | 1584 | 46 | 58887 | 272 | 30809 | 14374 | 422

Hospital, Address, Telephone, Administrator, Approval, Facility, and Physician Codes, Health Care System, Network	Classi-fication Codes		Utilization Data					Expense (thousands) of dollars		
★ American Hospital Association (AHA) membership □ Joint Commission on Accreditation of Healthcare Organizations (JCAHO) accreditation + American Osteopathic Hospital Association (AOHA) membership ○ American Osteopathic Association (AOA) accreditation △ Commission on Accreditation of Rehabilitation Facilities (CARF) accreditation Control codes 61, 63, 64, 71, 72 and 73 indicate hospitals listed by AOHA, but not registered by AHA. For definition of numerical codes, see page A4	Control	Service	Beds	Admissions	Census	Outpatient Visits	Births	Total	Payroll	Personnel

CLOQUET—Carlton County

COMMUNITY MEMORIAL HOSPITAL AND CONVALESCENT AND NURSING CARE SECTION, 512 Skyline Boulevard, Zip 55720–1199; tel. 218/879–4641; James J. Carroll, Administrator (Total facility includes 88 beds in nursing home–type unit) **A**9 10 **F**7 8 12 19 22 28 30 32 34 35 36 37 39 40 41 42 44 45 46 49 51 64 65 67 71 72 73 **P**3 8 **N** Northern Lakes Health Consortium, Duluth, MN
23 | 10 | 124 | 1279 | 98 | 22740 | 93 | 12149 | 6119 | 208

COOK—St. Louis County

★ COOK HOSPITAL AND CONVALESCENT NURSING CARE UNIT, 10 South Fifth Street East, Zip 55723; tel. 218/666–5945; Allen J. Vogt, Administrator (Total facility includes 41 beds in nursing home–type unit) **A**9 10 **F**1 8 14 15 16 17 22 26 33 41 49 64 65 71 73 **N** Northern Lakes Health Consortium, Duluth, MN
16 | 10 | 55 | 252 | 42 | 11436 | 0 | 3515 | 1611 | 79

COON RAPIDS—Anoka County

⊞ MERCY HOSPITAL, 4050 Coon Rapids Boulevard, Zip 55433–2586; tel. 612/422–4500 **A**1 9 10 **F**2 3 4 7 8 10 11 12 14 15 16 17 18 19 21 22 23 24 27 28 32 33 35 36 37 39 40 41 42 43 44 45 46 49 52 53 54 55 56 57 58 60 63 65 67 68 70 71 72 73 **P**3 4 5 6 7 **S** Allina Health System, Minneapolis, MN
23 | 10 | 194 | 11752 | 127 | 68998 | 0 | 95843 | 39600 | 1078

CROOKSTON—Polk County

⊞ RIVERVIEW HEALTHCARE ASSOCIATION, 323 South Minnesota Street, Zip 56716–1600; tel. 218/281–9200; Thomas C. Lenertz, President and Chief Executive Officer (Total facility includes 162 beds in nursing home–type unit) **A**1 5 9 10 **F**1 2 3 7 8 15 16 17 19 20 21 22 26 28 29 30 31 32 33 36 37 40 41 44 45 46 49 56 64 65 66 67 70 71 73 **P**5
23 | 10 | 234 | 1731 | 173 | 17097 | 144 | 15224 | 7609 | 320

CROSBY—Crow Wing County

★ CUYUNA REGIONAL MEDICAL CENTER, 320 East Main Street, Zip 56441; tel. 218/546–7000; Thomas F. Reek, Chief Executive Officer (Total facility includes 130 beds in nursing home–type unit) **A**9 10 **F**7 8 15 16 19 22 26 28 30 31 32 33 34 35 37 40 41 42 44 49 64 65 66 71 73 **P**7 8 **N** Northern Lakes Health Consortium, Duluth, MN
16 | 10 | 158 | 1370 | 138 | 16888 | 175 | 15833 | 7085 | 292

DAWSON—Lac Qui Parle County

JOHNSON MEMORIAL HEALTH SERVICES, 1282 Walnut Street, Zip 56232; tel. 612/769–4323; Vern Silvernale, Administrator (Total facility includes 70 beds in nursing home–type unit) **A**9 10 **F**7 8 16 17 19 22 26 32 33 34 36 40 41 44 45 49 64 65 71 73 **P**6 **N** Minnesota Rural Health Cooperative, Willmar, MN
16 | 10 | 94 | 392 | 72 | 2847 | 20 | 5160 | 2266 | 118

DEER RIVER—Itasca County

★ DEER RIVER HEALTHCARE CENTER, 1002 Comstock Drive, Zip 56636; tel. 218/246–2900; Michael Hedrix, Chief Executive Officer (Total facility includes 50 beds in nursing home–type unit) **A**9 10 **F**1 6 7 8 15 16 26 27 28 30 32 39 40 44 49 62 64 65 70 73 **N** Northern Lakes Health Consortium, Duluth, MN; Itasca Partnership for Quality Healthcare, Grand Rapids, MN
23 | 10 | 70 | 516 | 54 | 8654 | 42 | 5935 | 2917 | 130

DETROIT LAKES—Becker County

⊞ ST. MARY'S REGIONAL HEALTH CENTER, 1027 Washington Avenue, Zip 56501–3598; tel. 218/847–5611; John H. Solheim, Chief Executive Officer (Total facility includes 100 beds in nursing home–type unit) **A**1 9 10 **F**2 3 7 8 10 12 15 16 17 19 21 22 28 30 32 33 34 35 37 40 41 42 44 46 49 60 62 64 65 66 67 69 71 73 74 **S** Benedictine Health System, Duluth, MN
21 | 10 | 167 | 2265 | 124 | 11312 | 334 | 14064 | 5936 | —

DULUTH—St. Louis County

⊞ △ MILLER DWAN MEDICAL CENTER, 502 East Second Street, Zip 55805–1982; tel. 218/727–8762; William H. Palmer, President **A**1 5 7 9 10 **F**2 3 6 9 12 14 15 16 17 18 19 21 26 31 34 35 37 39 41 42 44 45 46 48 49 52 53 55 56 57 58 59 60 65 67 71 73 **P**5 **N** Northern Lakes Health Consortium, Duluth, MN
14 | 10 | 152 | 3331 | 74 | 79482 | 0 | 43567 | 20722 | 587

⊞ ST. LUKE'S HOSPITAL, 915 East First Street, Zip 55805–2193; tel. 218/726–5555; John Strange, President and Chief Executive Officer **A**1 2 3 5 9 10 **F**3 4 7 8 10 11 12 14 15 16 19 20 21 22 23 28 30 31 32 33 34 35 37 39 40 41 42 43 44 49 51 52 53 54 55 56 57 58 59 60 63 65 67 70 71 72 73 **P**3 **N** Northern Lakes Health Consortium, Duluth, MN
23 | 10 | 262 | 7001 | 91 | 76927 | 934 | 74304 | 36905 | 927

⊞ ST. MARY'S MEDICAL CENTER, 407 East Third Street, Zip 55805–1984; tel. 218/726–4000; Sister Kathleen Hofer, President **A**1 3 5 9 10 **F**2 3 4 5 6 7 8 9 10 11 14 15 16 17 18 19 20 21 22 23 24 27 29 30 31 32 33 34 35 36 37 38 39 40 41 42 43 44 45 46 47 48 49 51 52 53 54 55 56 57 58 59 60 61 62 63 64 65 66 67 70 71 72 73 **S** Benedictine Health System, Duluth, MN
21 | 10 | 286 | 15778 | 218 | 97791 | 1425 | 131920 | 58501 | 1613

ELBOW LAKE—Grant County

★ GRANT COUNTY HEALTH CENTER, 930 First Street N.E., Zip 56531; tel. 218/685–4461; Larry Rapp, Chief Medical and Executive Officer (Nonreporting) **A**9 10
23 | 10 | 15 | — | — | — | — | — | — | —

ELY—St. Louis County

★ ELY–BLOOMENSON COMMUNITY HOSPITAL, 328 West Conan Street, Zip 55731–1198; tel. 218/365–3271; Larry Ravenberg, Administrator (Total facility includes 99 beds in nursing home–type unit) **A**9 10 **F**1 7 8 11 15 17 19 21 22 32 33 34 35 36 39 40 44 49 64 65 67 71 72 73 **P**6 **N** Northern Lakes Health Consortium, Duluth, MN
23 | 10 | 130 | 586 | 101 | 5564 | 56 | 8126 | 4617 | 171

FAIRMONT—Martin County

⊞ FAIRMONT COMMUNITY HOSPITAL, (Includes Lutz Wing Convalescent and Nursing Care Unit), 835 Johnson Street, Zip 56031–4523, Mailing Address: P.O. Box 835, Zip 56031–0835; tel. 507/238–4254; Gerry Gilbertson, President (Total facility includes 40 beds in nursing home–type unit) **A**1 9 10 **F**6 7 8 14 15 16 19 20 21 22 24 28 29 30 32 33 34 35 37 40 41 42 44 45 46 49 60 61 64 65 66 71 72 73 **S** Allina Health System, Minneapolis, MN **N** Allina Health System, Minnetonka, MN
23 | 10 | 108 | 1836 | 59 | 36046 | 288 | 15449 | 8183 | 229

Hospital, Address, Telephone, Administrator, Approval, Facility, and Physician Codes, Health Care System, Network	Control	Service	Beds	Admissions	Census	Outpatient Visits	Births	Total	Payroll	Personnel

★ American Hospital Association (AHA) membership
□ Joint Commission on Accreditation of Healthcare Organizations (JCAHO) accreditation
+ American Osteopathic Hospital Association (AOHA) membership
○ American Osteopathic Association (AOA) accreditation
△ Commission on Accreditation of Rehabilitation Facilities (CARF) accreditation
Control codes 61, 63, 64, 71, 72 and 73 indicate hospitals listed by AOHA, but not registered by AHA. For definition of numerical codes, see page A4

FARIBAULT—Rice County

	Control	Service	Beds	Admissions	Census	Outpatient Visits	Births	Total	Payroll	Personnel
⊠ DISTRICT ONE HOSPITAL, (Formerly Rice County District One Hospital), 631 S.E. First Street, Zip 55021–6345; tel. 507/334–6451; James N. Wolf, Chief Executive Officer **A**1 10 **F**7 8 10 15 16 19 20 21 22 28 30 32 33 35 36 37 39 40 41 42 44 45 65 67 71 73	16	10	64	2071	19	37653	300	14809	6290	189
FARIBAULT REGIONAL CENTER, 802 Circle Drive, Zip 55021–6399; tel. 507/332–3000; Bridget K. Stroud, Chief Executive Officer (Nonreporting)	12	62	263	—	—	—	—	—	—	—
□ WILSON CENTER PSYCHIATRIC FACILITY FOR CHILDREN AND ADOLESCENTS, 1800 14th Street N.E., Zip 55021, Mailing Address: P.O. Box 917, Zip 55021; tel. 507/334–5561; Kevin J. Mahoney, President (Nonreporting) **A**1 9	33	22	50	—	—	—	—	—	—	—

FARMINGTON—Dakota County

	Control	Service	Beds	Admissions	Census	Outpatient Visits	Births	Total	Payroll	Personnel
⊠ SOUTH SUBURBAN MEDICAL CENTER, 3410–213th Street West, Zip 55024–1197; tel. 612/463–7825; Robert D. Johnson, Chief Executive Officer (Total facility includes 65 beds in nursing home–type unit) **A**1 9 10 **F**6 7 8 15 16 17 19 21 22 26 28 29 32 33 34 35 37 40 41 42 44 45 46 49 51 62 64 65 67 71 72 73 **P**6	23	10	95	430	67	11471	85	8017	3377	114

FERGUS FALLS—Otter Tail County

	Control	Service	Beds	Admissions	Census	Outpatient Visits	Births	Total	Payroll	Personnel
□ FERGUS FALLS REGIONAL TREATMENT CENTER, Fir and Union Avenues, Zip 56537, Mailing Address: Box 157, Zip 56537–0157; tel. 218/739–7200; Michael Ackley, Administrator (Nonreporting) **A**1 10	12	22	281	—	—	—	—	—	—	—
⊠ LAKE REGION HOSPITAL CORPORATION, (Formerly Lake Region Hospital and Nursing Home), 712 South Cascade Street, Zip 56537, Mailing Address: P.O. Box 728, Zip 56538–0728; tel. 218/736–8000; Edward J. Mehl, Chief Executive Officer (Total facility includes 44 beds in nursing home–type unit) **A**1 9 10 **F**7 15 19 21 22 32 34 35 37 40 41 44 49 52 53 54 55 56 57 64 65 66 67 71 73	23	10	136	3435	87	32522	300	28191	12949	433

FOREST LAKE—Washington County

	Control	Service	Beds	Admissions	Census	Outpatient Visits	Births	Total	Payroll	Personnel
⊠ DISTRICT MEMORIAL HOSPITAL, 246 11th Avenue S.E., Zip 55025–1898; tel. 612/464–3341; John F. Lannon, Administrator **A**1 9 10 **F**3 7 8 12 14 18 19 21 22 30 32 33 35 37 40 44 46 49 65 67 71 72 73 **P**5 6 **S** Fairview Hospital and Healthcare Services, Minneapolis, MN	16	10	44	824	7	10837	116	7197	3992	95

FOSSTON—Polk County

	Control	Service	Beds	Admissions	Census	Outpatient Visits	Births	Total	Payroll	Personnel
★ FIRST CARE MEDICAL SERVICES, 900 South Hilligoss Boulevard East, Zip 56542–1599; tel. 218/435–1133; David Hubbard, Chief Executive Officer (Total facility includes 50 beds in nursing home–type unit) **A**9 10 **F**7 8 14 15 16 19 26 27 32 34 35 36 44 49 51 63 64 65 66 67 70 71	23	10	70	595	54	—	65	6629	2949	141

FRIDLEY—Anoka County

	Control	Service	Beds	Admissions	Census	Outpatient Visits	Births	Total	Payroll	Personnel
★ UNITY HOSPITAL, 550 Osborne Road N.E., Zip 55432–2799; tel. 612/422–4500 **A**2 **F**2 3 7 8 10 12 14 15 16 17 18 19 21 22 23 27 28 29 30 32 33 35 36 37 39 40 41 42 43 44 45 46 49 52 53 54 55 56 57 58 59 60 63 65 67 68 70 71 72 73 **P**3 4 5 6 7 8 **S** Allina Health System, Minneapolis, MN	23	10	190	10605	106	88382	1992	82727	37032	984

GLENCOE—McLeod County

	Control	Service	Beds	Admissions	Census	Outpatient Visits	Births	Total	Payroll	Personnel
★ GLENCOE AREA HEALTH CENTER, 705 East 18th Street, Zip 55336–1499; tel. 320/864–3121; Jon D. Braband, Chief Executive Officer (Total facility includes 110 beds in nursing home–type unit) **A**9 10 **F**1 6 7 8 11 15 16 19 22 26 27 28 30 32 33 34 35 37 40 41 42 44 49 58 62 63 64 65 71 73 **S** HealthSystem Minnesota, Saint Louis Park, MN	14	10	149	1210	117	16753	120	13635	6757	232

GLENWOOD—Pope County

	Control	Service	Beds	Admissions	Census	Outpatient Visits	Births	Total	Payroll	Personnel
★ GLACIAL RIDGE HOSPITAL, 10 Fourth Avenue S.E., Zip 56334–1898; tel. 320/634–4521; Douglas J. Reker, Administrator and Chief Executive Officer **A**9 10 **F**7 8 14 15 19 21 22 24 32 33 34 35 37 40 41 44 49 53 54 65 70 71 73 **P**6	16	10	20	500	4	7908	50	5888	2301	110

GOLDEN VALLEY—Hennepin County

	Control	Service	Beds	Admissions	Census	Outpatient Visits	Births	Total	Payroll	Personnel
⊠ TRANSITIONAL HOSPITAL CORPORATION OF MINNEAPOLIS, 4101 Golden Valley Road, Zip 55422; tel. 612/588–2750; Patrick A. Auman, Ph.D., Chief Executive Officer **A**1 9 10 **F**12 19 27 35 65 **P**8 **S** Transitional Hospitals Corporation, Las Vegas, NV	33	10	111	315	43	—	0	—	—	190

GRACEVILLE—Big Stone County

	Control	Service	Beds	Admissions	Census	Outpatient Visits	Births	Total	Payroll	Personnel
GRACEVILLE HEALTH CENTER, 115 West Second Street, Zip 56240–0157, Mailing Address: P.O. Box 157, Zip 56240–0157; tel. 320/748–7223; Carollee Brinkman, Chief Executive Officer (Total facility includes 60 beds in nursing home–type unit) **A**9 10 **F**3 7 8 12 13 17 18 22 26 27 28 29 30 32 33 34 41 44 45 46 49 51 61 64 65 67 73 **N** Minnesota Rural Health Cooperative, Willmar, MN	23	10	92	334	58	7281	15	3280	1485	82

GRAND MARAIS—Cook County

	Control	Service	Beds	Admissions	Census	Outpatient Visits	Births	Total	Payroll	Personnel
COOK COUNTY NORTH SHORE HOSPITAL, Mailing Address: P.O. Box 10, Zip 55604–0010; tel. 218/387–1500; Diane Pearson, Administrator (Total facility includes 47 beds in nursing home–type unit) **A**9 10 **F**7 8 11 17 22 32 33 40 49 64 65 71 73 **N** Northern Lakes Health Consortium, Duluth, MN	16	10	56	192	34	9543	27	3902	2087	75

GRAND RAPIDS—Itasca County

	Control	Service	Beds	Admissions	Census	Outpatient Visits	Births	Total	Payroll	Personnel
⊠ ITASCA MEDICAL CENTER, 126 First Avenue S.E., Zip 55744–3698; tel. 218/326–3401; Tom Papin, Administrator (Total facility includes 35 beds in nursing home–type unit) **A**1 9 10 **F**1 2 7 8 11 12 15 17 19 21 22 26 31 32 34 39 40 41 44 46 48 49 56 57 59 65 66 71 73 74 **N** Benedictine Health System, Duluth, MN; Northern Lakes Health Consortium, Duluth, MN; Itasca Partnership for Quality Healthcare, Grand Rapids, MN	13	10	94	2517	59	24441	338	21421	10541	343

GRANITE FALLS—Yellow Medicine County

	Control	Service	Beds	Admissions	Census	Outpatient Visits	Births	Total	Payroll	Personnel
⊠ GRANITE FALLS MUNICIPAL HOSPITAL AND MANOR, 345 Tenth Avenue, Zip 56241–1499; tel. 320/564–3111; George Gerlach, President (Total facility includes 64 beds in nursing home–type unit) **A**1 9 10 **F**8 14 15 16 17 19 22 28 30 31 32 33 35 36 40 44 46 49 63 64 65 71 **S** Allina Health System, Minneapolis, MN **N** Allina Health System, Minnetonka, MN; Minnesota Rural Health Cooperative, Willmar, MN	14	10	87	516	69	9823	0	6680	3201	132

Hospital, Address, Telephone, Administrator, Approval, Facility, and Physician Codes, Health Care System, Network	Classification Codes		Utilization Data					Expense (thousands) of dollars		
★ American Hospital Association (AHA) membership □ Joint Commission on Accreditation of Healthcare Organizations (JCAHO) accreditation + American Osteopathic Hospital Association (AOHA) membership ○ American Osteopathic Association (AOA) accreditation △ Commission on Accreditation of Rehabilitation Facilities (CARF) accreditation Control codes 61, 63, 64, 71, 72 and 73 indicate hospitals listed by AOHA, but not registered by AHA. For definition of numerical codes, see page A4	Control	Service	Beds	Admissions	Census	Outpatient Visits	Births	Total	Payroll	Personnel
HALLOCK—Kittson County KITTSON MEMORIAL HOSPITAL, 1010 South Birch Street, Zip 56728, Mailing Address: P.O. Box 700, Zip 56728; tel. 218/843–3612; Richard J. Failing, Chief Executive Officer (Total facility includes 95 beds in nursing home–type unit) **A**9 10 **F**8 11 15 16 19 22 28 32 35 39 40 44 49 64 65 71 **P**5 **N** Northstar Health Consortium, Roseau, MN	23	10	115	282	89	7450	9	4723	1768	118
HARMONY—Fillmore County HARMONY COMMUNITY HOSPITAL, 815 South Main Avenue, Zip 55939, Mailing Address: Route 1, Box 173, Zip 55939; tel. 507/886–6544; Greg Braun, Administrator (Total facility includes 45 beds in nursing home–type unit) **A**9 10 **F**1 15 16 17 26 27 28 30 32 33 34 41 54 64 67 72 73 **P**3	23	10	53	175	46	—	0	2536	1253	60
HASTINGS—Dakota County □ REGINA MEDICAL CENTER, 1175 Nininger Road, Zip 55033; tel. 612/437–3121; Lynn W. Olson, Administrator and Chief Executive Officer (Total facility includes 61 beds in nursing home–type unit) (Nonreporting) **A**1 9 10	23	10	130	—	—	—	—	—	—	—
HENDRICKS—Lincoln County ★ HENDRICKS COMMUNITY HOSPITAL, 503 East Lincoln Street, Zip 56136; tel. 507/275–3134; Kirk Stensrud, Administrator (Total facility includes 70 beds in nursing home–type unit) **A**9 10 **F**1 6 7 8 11 12 14 15 16 17 19 20 21 22 24 28 30 31 32 33 34 35 37 40 44 63 64 65 67 71 73 **N** Minnesota Rural Health Cooperative, Willmar, MN	23	10	93	302	71	4619	44	3916	2085	—
HIBBING—St. Louis County ⊞ UNIVERSITY MEDICAL CENTER–MESABI, 750 East 34th Street, Zip 55746; tel. 218/262–4881; Frances J. Gardeski, Chief Executive Officer **A**1 9 10 **F**1 2 3 7 8 12 15 19 20 21 22 28 29 31 32 33 34 35 36 37 39 40 42 44 49 52 53 54 55 56 57 58 59 60 65 66 67 70 71 73 **P**5 **S** Fairview Hospital and Healthcare Services, Minneapolis, MN **N** Northern Lakes Health Consortium, Duluth, MN	23	10	132	3795	55	65014	269	27793	12628	389
HUTCHINSON—McLeod County ⊞ HUTCHINSON AREA HEALTH CARE, 1095 Highway 15 South, Zip 55350–3182; tel. 320/234–5000; Philip G. Graves, President (Total facility includes 127 beds in nursing home–type unit) **A**1 9 10 **F**1 3 7 8 11 15 16 17 18 19 22 26 28 29 30 32 33 34 35 36 39 40 41 42 44 45 49 52 53 54 55 56 57 58 59 64 65 66 67 71 73 74 **S** Allina Health System, Minneapolis, MN **N** Allina Health System, Minnetonka, MN	14	10	187	2422	144	39124	360	24317	10390	358
INTERNATIONAL FALLS—Koochiching County ⊞ FALLS MEMORIAL HOSPITAL, 1400 Highway 71, Zip 56649–2189; tel. 218/283–4481; James F. Hanko, Administrator and Chief Executive Officer **A**1 9 10 **F**7 8 11 14 15 16 17 19 20 21 22 28 30 32 33 35 37 40 42 44 46 48 49 56 64 65 71 73 **S** Quorum Health Group/Quorum Health Resources, Inc., Brentwood, TN **N** Northern Lakes Health Consortium, Duluth, MN	23	10	35	996	9	30972	132	7477	3545	119
IVANHOE—Lincoln County ★ DIVINE PROVIDENCE HEALTH CENTER, 312 East George Street, Zip 56142–0136, Mailing Address: P.O. Box G, Zip 56142–0136; tel. 507/694–1414; James C. Rossow, Administrator (Total facility includes 51 beds in nursing home–type unit) (Nonreporting) **A**9 10 **S** Presentation Health System, Yankton, SD **N** Minnesota Rural Health Cooperative, Willmar, MN	23	10	79	—	—	—	—	—	—	—
JACKSON—Jackson County ★ JACKSON MEDICAL CENTER, 1430 North Highway, Zip 56143–1098; tel. 507/847–2420; Charlotte Heitkamp, Chief Executive Officer (Total facility includes 21 beds in nursing home–type unit) **A**9 10 **F**22 33 44 58 64 **P**6 **S** Sioux Valley Health System, Sioux Falls, SD	14	10	41	286	23	9407	0	3579	1352	71
LAKE CITY—Wabasha County ⊞ LAKE CITY HOSPITAL, 904 South Lakeshore Drive, Zip 55041; tel. 612/345–3321; Mark Rinehardt, Chief Executive Officer (Total facility includes 115 beds in nursing home–type unit) **A**1 9 10 **F**3 8 10 15 17 19 22 26 32 33 40 43 44 46 64 65 71 72 73	14	10	140	609	111	4195	51	7037	3055	165
LE SUEUR—Le Sueur County MINNESOTA VALLEY HEALTH CENTER, (Includes Gardenview Nursing Home), 621 South Fourth Street, Zip 56058–2203; tel. 507/665–3375; Jennifer D. Pfeffer, Administrator and Chief Executive Officer (Total facility includes 85 beds in nursing home–type unit) (Nonreporting) **A**9 10	23	10	103	—	—	—	—	—	—	—
LITCHFIELD—Meeker County ★ MEEKER COUNTY MEMORIAL HOSPITAL, 612 South Sibley Avenue, Zip 55355–3398; tel. 320/693–3242; Ronald E. Johnson, Administrator **A**9 10 **F**7 8 15 19 21 22 26 28 29 30 34 35 37 40 42 44 45 49 63 67 71	13	10	31	1140	11	13940	164	6912	3172	105
LITTLE FALLS—Morrison County ⊞ ST. GABRIEL'S HOSPITAL, 815 Second Street S.E., Zip 56345–3596; tel. 320/632–5441; Larry A. Schulz, President and Chief Executive Officer (Total facility includes 150 beds in nursing home–type unit) (Nonreporting) **A**1 9 10 **S** Catholic Health Initiatives, Denver, CO	21	10	205	—	—	—	—	—	—	—
LONG PRAIRIE—Todd County ⊞ LONG PRAIRIE MEMORIAL HOSPITAL AND HOME, 20 Ninth Street S.E., Zip 56347–1404; tel. 320/732–2141; Clayton R. Peterson, President (Total facility includes 123 beds in nursing home–type unit) **A**1 9 10 **F**1 7 8 11 14 15 16 19 22 27 28 32 33 34 35 36 40 41 44 49 64 65 71 73 **P**3 **S** Allina Health System, Minneapolis, MN **N** Allina Health System, Minnetonka, MN	23	10	141	570	121	10164	70	7928	3468	177

Hospital, Address, Telephone, Administrator, Approval, Facility, and Physician Codes, Health Care System, Network	Classi-fication Codes		Utilization Data					Expense (thousands) of dollars		
★ American Hospital Association (AHA) membership □ Joint Commission on Accreditation of Healthcare Organizations (JCAHO) accreditation + American Osteopathic Hospital Association (AOHA) membership ○ American Osteopathic Association (AOA) accreditation △ Commission on Accreditation of Rehabilitation Facilities (CARF) accreditation Control codes 61, 63, 64, 71, 72 and 73 indicate hospitals listed by AOHA, but not registered by AHA. For definition of numerical codes, see page A4	Control	Service	Beds	Admissions	Census	Outpatient Visits	Births	Total	Payroll	Personnel

LUVERNE—Rock County

LUVERNE COMMUNITY HOSPITAL, 305 East Luverne Street, Zip 56156–2519, Mailing Address: P.O. Box 1019, Zip 56156; tel. 507/283–2321; Gerald E. Carl, Administrator **A**9 10 **F**7 8 15 16 19 22 30 32 33 34 35 39 40 41 42 44 49 64 65 67 71 **P**3 **S** Sioux Valley Health System, Sioux Falls, SD **N** Southwest Minnesota Health Alliance, Luverne, MN

	14	10	38	986	11	9879	153	7260	3178	116

MADELIA—Watonwan County

☒ MADELIA COMMUNITY HOSPITAL, 121 Drew Avenue S.E., Zip 56062; tel. 507/642–3255; Candace Fenske, R.N., Administrator **A**1 9 10 **F**7 14 15 16 17 19 20 21 22 28 29 32 33 34 36 40 41 44 45 49 64 65 71

	23	10	25	350	3	4895	40	2170	1078	43

MADISON—Lac Qui Parle County

★ LAC QUI PARLE HOSPITAL OF MADISON, (Formerly Madison Hospital), 820 Third Avenue, Zip 56256, Mailing Address: P.O. Box 184, Zip 56256; tel. 320/598–7556; John Fossum, Chief Executive Officer (Nonreporting) **A**9 10 **N** Minnesota Rural Health Cooperative, Willmar, MN

	21	10	21	—	—	—	—	—	—	—

MAHNOMEN—Mahnomen County

MAHNOMEN HEALTH CENTER, (Formerly Mahnomen County and Village Hospital, Clinic and Nursing Center), 414 Jefferson Avenue, Zip 56557, Mailing Address: Box 396, Zip 56557–0396; tel. 218/935–2511; Craig Doughty, Chief Executive Officer (Total facility includes 48 beds in nursing home–type unit) **A**9 10 **F**8 11 17 19 22 24 26 28 30 31 33 34 35 39 44 46 48 49 53 64 65 71 **P**6

	23	10	66	221	47	6569	0	2793	1682	84

MANKATO—Blue Earth County

☒ IMMANUEL ST. JOSEPH'S—MAYO HEALTH SYSTEM, (Formerly Immanuel–St. Joseph's Hospital), 1025 Marsh Street, Zip 56001, Mailing Address: P.O. Box 8673, Zip 56002–8673; tel. 507/625–4031; Jerome A. Crest, Executive Vice President **A**1 2 3 5 9 10 **F**2 3 7 8 10 12 15 16 17 19 20 21 22 23 28 29 30 31 32 33 34 35 37 39 40 41 42 44 45 49 52 53 54 55 56 57 58 59 60 63 65 67 71 73 74 **P**8 **S** Mayo Foundation, Rochester, MN
IMMANUEL–ST. JOSEPH'S HOSPITAL See Immanuel St. Joseph's–Mayo Health System

	23	10	147	6861	79	50704	972	46441	20691	670

MAPLEWOOD—Ramsey County

★ HEALTHEAST ST. JOHN'S HOSPITAL, 1575 Beam Avenue, Zip 55109; tel. 612/232–7000; William Knutson, Vice President and Administrator **A**3 5 9 10 **F**2 3 4 7 8 10 11 12 14 15 16 17 19 21 22 25 26 27 29 31 32 33 34 35 36 37 38 39 40 41 42 43 44 45 46 52 60 62 63 64 70 71 73 **P**2 3 4 5 6 7 8 **S** HealthEast, Saint Paul, MN **N** Healtheast, St. Paul, MN

	23	10	150	10268	101	62973	2378	66113	29248	676

MARSHALL—Lyon County

☒ WEINER MEMORIAL MEDICAL CENTER, 300 South Bruce Street, Zip 56258–1934; tel. 507/532–9661; Ronald Jensen, Administrator (Total facility includes 76 beds in nursing home–type unit) **A**1 9 10 **F**1 7 8 14 15 16 17 19 20 22 23 24 26 27 28 29 30 31 32 33 34 35 37 39 40 41 42 44 45 49 56 57 58 62 63 64 65 67 71 73 **P**3 4 **N** Minnesota Rural Health Cooperative, Willmar, MN; Affiliated Community Health Network, Inc., Willmar, MN

	14	10	116	1776	89	15481	441	13758	6865	261

MELROSE—Stearns County

MELROSE HOSPITAL AND PINE VILLA NURSING HOME, 11 North Fifth Avenue West, Zip 56352; tel. 320/256–4231; Joan Jackson, Administrator (Total facility includes 75 beds in nursing home–type unit) **A**9 10 **F**1 7 8 14 15 16 17 19 20 22 26 27 32 33 34 35 36 37 39 40 41 44 49 51 57 58 62 64 65 66 67 71 73 **P**5

	14	10	91	404	78	8810	54	5245	3183	111

MINNEAPOLIS—Hennepin County

☒ △ ABBOTT NORTHWESTERN HOSPITAL, (Includes Sister Kenny Institute), 800 East 28th Street, Zip 55407–3799; tel. 612/863–4203; Robert K. Spinner, President (Total facility includes 18 beds in nursing home–type unit) **A**1 2 3 5 7 9 10 **F**3 4 5 7 8 10 11 12 15 17 19 21 22 23 24 25 26 27 28 29 30 31 32 33 34 35 36 37 39 40 41 42 43 44 45 46 48 49 51 52 53 54 55 56 57 58 59 60 61 63 64 65 67 69 71 72 73 74 **P**5 6 8 **S** Allina Health System, Minneapolis, MN **N** National Cardiovascular Network, Atlanta, GA; Allina Health System, Minnetonka, MN

	23	10	612	28387	430	129536	2643	352862	148354	3564

□ CHILDREN'S HEALTH CARE, MINNEAPOLIS, 2525 Chicago Avenue South, Zip 55404–9976; tel. 612/813–6100; Brock D. Nelson, Chief Executive Officer **A**1 2 3 9 10 **F**4 10 12 13 14 15 16 17 19 20 21 22 23 25 27 29 30 31 32 33 34 35 38 39 41 42 43 44 45 46 47 49 50 51 53 54 55 56 58 60 63 65 67 68 70 71 73 **P**1 3

	23	50	163	6267	111	64691	0	101454	50696	1331

FAIRVIEW RIVERSIDE HOSPITAL See Fairview–University Medical Center

☒ FAIRVIEW SOUTHDALE HOSPITAL, 6401 France Avenue South, Zip 55435–2199; tel. 612/924–5000; Mark M. Enger, Senior Vice President and Administrator (Nonreporting) **A**1 2 9 10 **S** Fairview Hospital and Healthcare Services, Minneapolis, MN **N** Fairview Health System, Minneapolis, MN

	23	10	390	—	—	—	—	—	—	—

☒ FAIRVIEW–UNIVERSITY MEDICAL CENTER, (Includes Fairview Riverside Hospital, 2312 South Sixth Street, Zip 55454; St. Mary's Hospital and Rehabilitation Center, 2414 South Seventh Street, Zip 55454; tel. 612/338–2229; University of Minnesota Hospital and Clinic, 420 S.E. Delaware Street, Box 502, Zip 55455–0392; tel. 612/626–3000), 2450 Riverside Avenue, Zip 55454–1400; tel. 612/672–6300; Peter Rapp, Senior Vice President and Administrator (Total facility includes 115 beds in nursing home–type unit) (Nonreporting) **A**1 2 3 5 6 8 9 10 **S** Fairview Hospital and Healthcare Services, Minneapolis, MN **N** Fairview Health System, Minneapolis, MN; I–35 Corridor Health Network, Duluth, MN; Quality Health Network, Inc., Redwing, MN

	23	10	1362	—	—	—	—	—	—	—

Hospital, Address, Telephone, Administrator, Approval, Facility, and Physician Codes, Health Care System, Network	Classi-fication Codes		Utilization Data					Expense (thousands) of dollars		
	Control	Service	Beds	Admissions	Census	Outpatient Visits	Births	Total	Payroll	Personnel

★ American Hospital Association (AHA) membership
□ Joint Commission on Accreditation of Healthcare Organizations (JCAHO) accreditation
+ American Osteopathic Hospital Association (AOHA) membership
○ American Osteopathic Association (AOA) accreditation
△ Commission on Accreditation of Rehabilitation Facilities (CARF) accreditation
Control codes 61, 63, 64, 71, 72 and 73 indicate hospitals listed by AOHA, but not registered by AHA. For definition of numerical codes, see page A4

	Control	Service	Beds	Admissions	Census	Outpatient Visits	Births	Total	Payroll	Personnel
▣ △ HENNEPIN COUNTY MEDICAL CENTER, 701 Park Avenue South, Zip 55415; tel. 612/347–2121; John W. Bluford, Administrator **A**1 2 3 5 7 8 9 10 **F**3 4 5 7 8 9 10 11 12 13 14 16 17 18 19 20 21 22 23 25 26 27 28 29 30 31 35 37 38 39 40 41 42 43 44 45 46 47 48 49 51 52 53 54 55 56 57 58 59 60 61 65 66 67 69 70 71 72 73 74 **P**1	13	10	462	19797	290	376122	1842	269856	128921	3323
▣ PHILLIPS EYE INSTITUTE, 2215 Park Avenue, Zip 55404–3756; tel. 612/336–6000; Shari E. Levy, President **A**1 10 **F**2 3 4 5 7 8 10 11 12 14 15 16 17 18 19 21 22 24 25 26 27 28 29 30 31 32 33 34 35 37 39 40 41 42 43 44 45 46 47 48 49 51 52 53 54 55 56 57 58 59 60 61 64 65 66 67 69 71 72 73 74 **P**3 4 8 **S** Allina Health System, Minneapolis, MN **N** Allina Health System, Minnetonka, MN	23	45	10	727	2	11118	0	12810	4651	112
▣ SHRINERS HOSPITALS FOR CHILDREN, TWIN CITIES UNIT, 2025 East River Road, Zip 55414–3696; tel. 612/335–5300; Laurence E. Johnson, Administrator **A**1 3 5 **F**15 19 34 35 39 44 45 46 49 53 65 67 71 73 **P**6 **S** Shriners Hospitals for Children, Tampa, FL	23	57	40	830	18	8283	0	—	—	154
ST. MARY'S HOSPITAL AND REHABILITATION CENTER See Fairview–University Medical Center										
▣ VETERANS AFFAIRS MEDICAL CENTER, One Veterans Drive, Zip 55417–2399; tel. 612/725–2000; Charles A. Milbrandt, Director (Total facility includes 110 beds in nursing home–type unit) (Nonreporting) **A**1 2 3 5 8 **S** Department of Veterans Affairs, Washington, DC	45	10	519	—	—	—	—	—	—	—
MONTEVIDEO—Chippewa County										
CHIPPEWA COUNTY MONTEVIDEO HOSPITAL, 824 North 11th Street, Zip 56265; tel. 320/269–8877; Fred Knutson, Administrator (Nonreporting) **A**9 10 **N** Minnesota Rural Health Cooperative, Willmar, MN	15	10	29	—	—	—	—	—	—	—
MONTICELLO—Wright County										
▣ MONTICELLO BIG LAKE HOSPITAL, 1013 Hart Boulevard, Zip 55362; tel. 612/295–2945; Barbara Schwientek, Executive Director (Total facility includes 91 beds in nursing home–type unit) **A**1 9 10 **F**1 3 7 8 14 15 19 22 32 33 34 35 37 40 42 44 58 64 65 66 71	16	10	103	953	96	25382	240	12325	5022	213
MOOSE LAKE—Carlton County										
★ MERCY HOSPITAL AND HEALTH CARE CENTER, 710 South Kenwood Avenue, Zip 55767; tel. 218/485–4481; Dianne Mandernach, Chief Executive Officer (Total facility includes 94 beds in nursing home–type unit) **A**9 10 **F**7 8 12 14 15 16 17 19 22 24 28 30 32 34 37 39 40 41 44 45 46 49 61 64 65 66 67 70 71 73 **P**5 **N** Northern Lakes Health Consortium, Duluth, MN; I–35 Corridor Health Network, Duluth, MN	16	10	119	854	100	7483	96	8860	4629	166
MORA—Kanabec County										
▣ KANABEC HOSPITAL, 300 Clark Street, Zip 55051; tel. 320/679–1212; John A. Kayfes, FACHE, Administrator **A**1 9 10 **F**8 14 16 17 19 21 22 28 30 35 37 40 41 42 44 45 46 49 64 65 71 73 **N** I–35 Corridor Health Network, Duluth, MN	13	10	36	1000	11	10413	175	7360	3676	127
MORRIS—Stevens County										
▣ STEVENS COMMUNITY MEDICAL CENTER, 400 East First Street, Zip 56267–1407, Mailing Address: P.O. Box 660, Zip 56267; tel. 612/589–1313; John Rau, President **A**1 9 10 **F**3 7 8 11 14 15 17 18 19 20 22 27 28 30 31 32 33 34 35 37 40 41 42 44 45 46 49 51 53 54 55 56 57 58 65 67 71 **P**6 **S** Allina Health System, Minneapolis, MN	23	10	37	950	12	—	72	9961	3521	151
NEW PRAGUE—Le Sueur County										
▣ QUEEN OF PEACE HOSPITAL, 301 Second Street N.E., Zip 56071–1799; tel. 612/758–4431; Sister Jean Juenemann, Chief Executive Officer **A**1 9 10 **F**6 7 8 11 13 16 17 19 20 21 22 24 28 30 32 34 35 39 40 41 42 44 45 46 49 51 60 62 64 67 71 72 73	23	10	28	1311	12	—	153	9934	4386	137
NEW ULM—Brown County										
▣ NEW ULM MEDICAL CENTER, 1324 Fifth Street North, Zip 56073–1553, Mailing Address: P.O. Box 577, Zip 56073; tel. 507/354–2111; Rickie L. Ressler, R.N., Interim President **A**1 9 10 **F**2 3 7 8 15 17 18 19 20 21 22 24 27 28 30 32 33 34 35 36 37 39 40 41 42 44 45 46 49 51 52 53 54 56 57 58 65 66 67 71 72 **S** Allina Health System, Minneapolis, MN **N** Allina Health System, Minnetonka, MN; Quality Health Alliance, Mankato, MN	23	10	47	2093	22	49041	388	24048	8537	304
NORTHFIELD—Rice County										
▣ NORTHFIELD HOSPITAL, (Includes H. O. Dilley Skilled Nursing Facility), 801 West First Street, Zip 55057–1697; tel. 507/645–6661; Kendall C. Bank, President (Total facility includes 40 beds in nursing home–type unit) **A**1 9 10 **F**11 14 15 16 19 20 21 22 27 28 30 32 33 34 35 36 39 40 41 42 44 45 46 49 51 64 65 66 67 71 73 **S** Allina Health System, Minneapolis, MN **N** Allina Health System, Minnetonka, MN	14	10	69	1425	47	16996	290	12998	5859	189
OLIVIA—Renville County										
RENVILLE COUNTY HOSPITAL, 611 East Fairview Avenue, Zip 56277–1397; tel. 612/523–1261; Dean G. Slagter, Administrator **A**9 10 **F**1 7 8 11 14 15 17 19 20 21 22 28 30 33 34 35 36 39 40 41 42 44 49 63 71 **N** Minnesota Rural Health Cooperative, Willmar, MN	13	10	30	650	5	5856	51	3584	1570	54
ONAMIA—Mille Lacs County										
▣ MILLE LACS HEALTH SYSTEM, 200 North Elm Street, Zip 56359–7978; tel. 320/532–3154; Frederick W. Haack, President (Total facility includes 80 beds in nursing home–type unit) **A**1 9 10 **F**1 3 7 8 12 15 16 17 19 20 21 22 26 27 28 29 30 32 40 41 42 44 45 49 51 64 65 66 67 71 **P**5 6 **S** Allina Health System, Minneapolis, MN **N** Allina Health System, Minnetonka, MN; Northern Lakes Health Consortium, Duluth, MN	23	10	98	827	85	12474	55	9600	5179	169

Hospital, Address, Telephone, Administrator, Approval, Facility, and Physician Codes, Health Care System, Network	Classi-fication Codes		Utilization Data					Expense (thousands) of dollars		
★ American Hospital Association (AHA) membership □ Joint Commission on Accreditation of Healthcare Organizations (JCAHO) accreditation + American Osteopathic Hospital Association (AOHA) membership ○ American Osteopathic Association (AOA) accreditation △ Commission on Accreditation of Rehabilitation Facilities (CARF) accreditation Control codes 61, 63, 64, 71, 72 and 73 indicate hospitals listed by AOHA, but not registered by AHA. For definition of numerical codes, see page A4	Control	Service	Beds	Admissions	Census	Outpatient Visits	Births	Total	Payroll	Personnel

ORTONVILLE—Big Stone County

★ ORTONVILLE AREA HEALTH SERVICES, 750 Eastvold Avenue, Zip 56278; tel. 320/839–2502; Frederick Peterson, Administrator (Total facility includes 74 beds in nursing home–type unit) (Nonreporting) **A**9 10 **S** Lutheran Health Systems, Fargo, ND **N** Minnesota Rural Health Cooperative, Willmar, MN — 14 10 105 — — — — — — —

OWATONNA—Steele County

⊞ OWATONNA HOSPITAL, 903 Oak Street South, Zip 55060–3234; tel. 507/451–3850; Richard G. Slieter, President **A**1 9 10 **F**7 8 12 15 16 19 21 22 28 30 32 33 35 36 37 40 44 49 52 54 55 56 57 58 65 66 67 71 **S** Allina Health System, Minneapolis, MN **N** Allina Health System, Minnetonka, MN — 23 10 66 1957 21 24357 410 13683 5721 189

PARK RAPIDS—Hubbard County

⊞ ST JOSEPH'S AREA HEALTH SERVICES, 600 Pleasant Avenue, Zip 56470; tel. 218/732–3311; David R. Hove, President and Chief Executive Officer **A**1 9 10 **F**7 8 15 16 17 19 22 30 32 33 35 37 40 44 49 63 65 67 71 **S** Catholic Health Initiatives, Denver, CO — 21 10 42 1600 20 18620 150 13137 6137 217

PAYNESVILLE—Stearns County

★ PAYNESVILLE AREA HEALTH CARE SYSTEM, 200 First Street West, Zip 56362; tel. 320/243–3767; William M. LaCroix, Administrator (Total facility includes 64 beds in nursing home–type unit) **A**9 10 **F**1 7 8 11 14 15 19 21 22 24 26 27 32 34 35 36 39 40 42 44 46 48 52 58 62 64 65 67 71 **P**8 — 16 10 94 631 69 10343 77 9342 4558 162

PERHAM—Otter Tail County

⊞ PERHAM MEMORIAL HOSPITAL AND HOME, 665 Third Street S.W., Zip 56573–1199; tel. 218/346–4500; Chuck Hofius, Administrator (Total facility includes 102 beds in nursing home–type unit) (Nonreporting) **A**1 9 10 — 16 10 130 — — — — — — —

PIPESTONE—Pipestone County

PIPESTONE COUNTY MEDICAL CENTER, 911 Fifth Avenue S.W., Zip 56164, Mailing Address: P.O. Box 370, Zip 56164; tel. 507/825–5811; Carl P. Vaagenes, Administrator (Total facility includes 43 beds in nursing home–type unit) **A**9 10 **F**1 7 8 12 19 21 22 30 32 33 34 35 39 40 41 44 49 63 64 71 73 **S** Presentation Health System, Yankton, SD — 13 10 76 723 49 14055 82 7483 2960 140

PRINCETON—Sherburne County

⊞ FAIRVIEW NORTHLAND REGIONAL HOSPITAL, 911 Northland Drive, Zip 55371; tel. 612/389–1313; Glenn G. Erickson, Vice President and Administrator (Nonreporting) **A**1 9 10 **S** Fairview Hospital and Healthcare Services, Minneapolis, MN **N** Fairview Health System, Minneapolis, MN — 23 10 41 — — — — — — —

RED WING—Goodhue County

⊞ ST. JOHN'S REGIONAL HEALTH CENTER, 1407 West Fourth Street, Zip 55066–2198; tel. 612/388–6721; Craig Stoeckel, Interim Administrator **A**1 9 10 **F**2 3 7 8 11 15 16 17 19 26 28 29 30 31 32 33 34 35 36 37 39 40 41 42 44 45 46 49 51 62 65 67 71 73 **N** Quality Health Network, Inc., Redwing, MN — 23 10 68 2174 27 21082 417 17457 7178 219

REDLAKE—Beltrami County

⊞ U.S. PUBLIC HEALTH SERVICE INDIAN HOSPITAL, Zip 56671; tel. 218/679–3912; Essimae Stevens, Service Unit Director (Nonreporting) **A**1 10 **S** U. S. Public Health Service Indian Health Service, Rockville, MD — 47 10 23 — — — — — — —

REDWOOD FALLS—Redwood County

★ REDWOOD FALLS MUNICIPAL HOSPITAL, 100 Fallwood Road, Zip 56283–1828; tel. 507/637–2907; James E. Schulte, Administrator **A**9 10 **F**1 7 8 11 12 14 15 16 17 19 20 21 22 24 27 28 29 30 32 33 34 35 39 40 42 44 45 46 49 63 65 67 71 73 **N** Minnesota Rural Health Cooperative, Willmar, MN; Affiliated Community Health Network, Inc., Willmar, MN — 14 10 35 900 7 9141 150 — — 87

ROBBINSDALE—Hennepin County

⊞ △ NORTH MEMORIAL HEALTH CARE, 3300 Oakdale Avenue North, Zip 55422–2900; tel. 612/520–5200; Scott R. Anderson, President and Chief Executive Officer **A**1 2 3 5 7 9 10 **F**1 4 7 8 10 11 12 14 15 16 17 19 20 21 22 26 27 28 30 32 33 34 35 36 37 38 39 40 41 42 43 44 46 48 49 51 52 54 55 56 57 61 63 65 67 70 71 72 73 74 **P**1 — 23 10 371 20438 259 — 3328 223097 99581 2651

ROCHESTER—Olmsted County

⊞ OLMSTED MEDICAL CENTER, 210 Ninth Street S.E., Zip 55904–4300; tel. 507/288–3443; Mark W. Jenkins, Chief Administrative Officer **A**1 9 10 **F**7 15 19 22 24 36 37 40 44 71 73 **P**3 — 13 10 49 1954 15 17441 880 13036 6574 182

⊞ ROCHESTER METHODIST HOSPITAL, 201 West Center Street, Zip 55902–3084; tel. 507/266–7180; Stephen C. Waldhoff, Administrator **A**1 3 5 9 10 **F**3 4 5 6 7 8 10 12 13 14 15 16 17 18 19 20 21 22 23 24 25 26 27 28 30 32 33 34 35 37 38 39 40 41 42 43 44 45 46 49 51 53 54 55 56 57 58 59 60 61 62 63 65 66 67 68 69 70 71 72 73 74 **P**6 **S** Mayo Foundation, Rochester, MN **N** Mayo Foundation, Rochester, MN — 23 10 335 14757 215 — 1744 — — —

⊞ △ SAINT MARYS HOSPITAL, 1216 Second Street S.W., Zip 55902–1970; tel. 507/255–5123; John M. Panicek, Administrator **A**1 5 7 8 9 10 **F**2 3 4 5 6 7 8 10 11 12 13 14 15 16 17 18 19 20 21 22 23 24 25 26 27 28 29 30 31 32 33 34 35 37 38 40 41 42 43 44 45 46 47 48 49 51 52 53 54 55 56 57 58 59 60 61 62 63 65 66 67 68 69 70 71 72 73 74 **P**6 **S** Mayo Foundation, Rochester, MN **N** Mayo Foundation, Rochester, MN — 23 10 797 33888 642 — 0 — — —

ROSEAU—Roseau County

⊞ ROSEAU AREA HOSPITAL AND HOMES, 715 Delmore Avenue, Zip 56751; tel. 218/463–2500; David F. Hagen, President and Executive Officer (Total facility includes 124 beds in nursing home–type unit) **A**1 9 10 **F**7 8 10 11 12 13 14 15 16 19 21 22 28 30 32 33 34 35 39 41 42 44 45 49 58 60 63 64 65 67 71 73 **P**5 **N** Northstar Health Consortium, Roseau, MN — 23 10 161 1030 130 16368 270 12386 5393 280

Hospital, Address, Telephone, Administrator, Approval, Facility, and Physician Codes, Health Care System, Network	Classi-fication Codes		Utilization Data					Expense (thousands) of dollars		
	Control	Service	Beds	Admissions	Census	Outpatient Visits	Births	Total	Payroll	Personnel

★ American Hospital Association (AHA) membership
□ Joint Commission on Accreditation of Healthcare Organizations (JCAHO) accreditation
+ American Osteopathic Hospital Association (AOHA) membership
○ American Osteopathic Association (AOA) accreditation
△ Commission on Accreditation of Rehabilitation Facilities (CARF) accreditation
Control codes 61, 63, 64, 71, 72 and 73 indicate hospitals listed by AOHA, but not registered by AHA. For definition of numerical codes, see page A4

RUSH CITY—Chisago County

RUSH CITY HOSPITAL, 760 West Fourt Street, Zip 55069; tel. 612/358–4708; Mark Lunseth, Administrator **A**9 10 **F**8 15 16 17 19 22 28 30 32 33 34 35 41 44 49 71 72 73 **P**6 **N** Northern Lakes Health Consortium, Duluth, MN; I–35 Corridor Health Network, Duluth, MN — 14 10 26 279 2 13818 0 3214 1204 50

SAINT CLOUD—Stearns County

★ ST. CLOUD HOSPITAL, 1406 Sixth Avenue North, Zip 56303–0016; tel. 320/251–2700; John Frobenius, President and Chief Executive Officer **A**1 2 9 10 **F**1 2 3 4 5 6 7 8 10 11 12 13 14 15 16 17 18 19 20 21 22 23 25 26 27 28 29 30 31 32 33 34 35 36 37 38 39 40 41 42 43 44 45 46 48 49 51 52 53 54 55 56 57 58 59 60 61 62 65 66 67 70 71 72 73 74 **P**3 6 — 21 10 332 14467 197 89298 2233 121732 56582 1682

★ VETERANS AFFAIRS MEDICAL CENTER, 4801 Eighth Street North, Zip 56303–2099; tel. 320/252–1670; Barry I. Bahl, Associate Director (Total facility includes 210 beds in nursing home–type unit) **A**1 **F**1 2 3 6 8 12 19 20 22 26 30 33 34 35 39 41 44 46 49 51 52 56 57 58 59 64 65 67 73 74 **P**6 **S** Department of Veterans Affairs, Washington, DC — 45 22 570 2800 500 93700 0 53000 40000 880

SAINT JAMES—Watonwan County

ST. JAMES HEALTH SERVICES, (Formerly Watonwan Memorial Hospital), 1207 Sixth Avenue South, Zip 56081; tel. 507/375–3261; Lee Holter, Chief Executive Officer **A**9 10 **F**7 8 15 16 17 19 20 21 22 28 30 32 33 39 40 44 45 46 49 51 65 67 71 **P**6 **N** Quality Health Alliance, Mankato, MN — 23 10 24 203 2 16382 30 4296 — 54

SAINT LOUIS PARK—Hennepin County

★ △ METHODIST HOSPITAL HEALTHSYSTEM MINNESOTA, 6500 Excelsior Boulevard, Zip 55426–4702, Mailing Address: Box 650, Minneapolis, Zip 55440–0650; tel. 612/993–5000; James Reinertsen, M.D., Chief Executive Officer (Total facility includes 35 beds in nursing home–type unit) **A**1 2 3 5 7 9 10 **F**3 4 5 6 7 8 10 11 12 14 15 17 18 19 20 22 23 24 25 26 28 29 30 31 32 33 34 35 36 37 40 41 42 43 44 45 46 48 49 51 53 54 55 56 57 58 60 61 64 65 66 67 68 69 70 71 72 73 **P**6 **S** HealthSystem Minnesota, Saint Louis Park, MN — 23 10 376 18759 239 187737 3072 139185 64087 1739

SAINT PAUL—Ramsey County

★ CHILDREN'S HEALTH CARE–ST. PAUL, 345 North Smith Avenue, Zip 55102; tel. 612/220–6000; Brock D. Nelson, Chief Executive Officer **A**1 3 5 9 10 **F**2 3 4 7 10 13 14 15 16 17 19 20 21 22 23 24 27 31 32 33 34 35 38 39 41 42 43 44 45 46 47 48 49 51 52 53 54 55 56 58 59 60 61 65 67 68 70 71 73 **P**1 — 23 50 105 5508 74 74902 0 63160 26506 589

□ △ GILLETTE CHILDREN'S SPECIALTY HEALTHCARE, (Formerly Gillette Children's Hospital), (PEDIATRIC SPECIALITY), 200 University Avenue East, Zip 55101; tel. 612/291–2848; Margaret Perryman, Chief Executive Officer **A**1 3 5 7 9 10 **F**5 14 15 16 17 19 20 21 22 34 35 39 41 44 45 46 47 48 49 50 63 65 67 70 71 73 **P**4 7 — 23 59 43 918 15 14248 0 24162 10529 269

★ △ HEALTHEAST BETHESDA LUTHERAN HOSPITAL AND REHABILITATION CENTER, 559 Capitol Boulevard, Zip 55103; tel. 612/232–2133; Scott Batulis, Administrator **A**1 7 9 10 **F**1 2 3 4 5 6 7 8 9 10 11 12 13 14 15 16 17 18 19 20 21 22 23 24 25 26 27 28 29 30 31 32 33 34 35 36 37 38 39 40 41 42 43 44 45 46 47 48 49 50 51 52 53 54 55 56 57 58 59 60 61 62 63 64 65 66 67 68 69 70 71 72 73 74 **P**1 3 4 5 6 8 **S** HealthEast, Saint Paul, MN **N** Healtheast, St. Paul, MN — 23 48 127 887 100 1011 0 31280 16011 465

★ HEALTHEAST ST. JOSEPH'S HOSPITAL, 69 West Exchange Street, Zip 55102; tel. 612/232–3000; William Knutson, Vice President and Administrator (Nonreporting) **A**1 2 3 5 9 10 **S** HealthEast, Saint Paul, MN **N** Healtheast, St. Paul, MN — 23 10 292 — — — — — — —

★ △ ST. PAUL–RAMSEY MEDICAL CENTER, 640 Jackson Street, Zip 55101–2595; tel. 612/221–3456; Terry S. Finzen, President **A**1 2 3 5 7 8 9 10 **F**2 3 4 5 7 8 9 10 11 17 18 19 20 21 22 25 26 29 31 32 33 34 35 37 38 40 41 42 43 44 46 47 48 49 51 52 53 54 56 57 58 61 65 70 71 72 73 74 **P**3 5 8 **N** HealthPartners, Minneapolis, MN — 23 10 409 17597 260 342376 1500 208247 94981 2608

★ UNITED HOSPITAL, 333 North Smith Street, Zip 55102–2389; tel. 612/220–8000; David Jones, President **A**1 2 3 5 9 10 **F**3 4 7 8 10 12 14 15 16 17 19 21 22 23 24 27 28 29 30 31 32 33 34 35 37 39 40 41 42 43 44 45 46 48 49 51 52 53 54 55 58 59 60 61 63 65 67 71 73 **S** Allina Health System, Minneapolis, MN **N** Allina Health System, Minnetonka, MN — 23 10 386 23650 303 137462 4478 207863 88333 2195

SAINT PETER—Nicollet County

COMMUNITY HOSPITAL AND HEALTH CARE CENTER, 618 West Broadway, Zip 56082–1327; tel. 507/931–2200; Jeanne Johnson, Chief Executive Officer (Total facility includes 85 beds in nursing home–type unit) (Nonreporting) **A**10 — 14 10 118 — — — — — — —

MINNESOTA SECURITY HOSPITAL See St. Peter Regional Treatment Center

□ ST. PETER REGIONAL TREATMENT CENTER, (Includes Minnesota Security Hospital, Sheppard Drive, Zip 56082; tel. 507/931–7100), 100 Freeman Drive, Zip 56082–1599; tel. 507/931–7100; William L. Pedersen, Chief Executive Officer **A**1 9 10 **F**2 14 15 16 20 46 52 56 57 65 73 **N** Quality Health Alliance, Mankato, MN — 12 22 560 930 495 — 0 40000 25000 890

SANDSTONE—Pine County

PINE MEDICAL CENTER, 109 Court Avenue South, Zip 55072; tel. 612/245–2212; Vivian Swanson, Interim Administrator (Total facility includes 86 beds in nursing home–type unit) **A**9 10 **F**8 12 15 16 19 22 41 42 44 49 51 64 65 71 **P**6 **N** Northern Lakes Health Consortium, Duluth, MN; I–35 Corridor Health Network, Duluth, MN — 16 10 91 464 85 7912 0 7148 2824 —

Hospital, Address, Telephone, Administrator, Approval, Facility, and Physician Codes, Health Care System, Network	Classi-fication Codes		Utilization Data					Expense (thousands) of dollars		
★ American Hospital Association (AHA) membership □ Joint Commission on Accreditation of Healthcare Organizations (JCAHO) accreditation + American Osteopathic Hospital Association (AOHA) membership ○ American Osteopathic Association (AOA) accreditation △ Commission on Accreditation of Rehabilitation Facilities (CARF) accreditation Control codes 61, 63, 64, 71, 72 and 73 indicate hospitals listed by AOHA, but not registered by AHA. For definition of numerical codes, see page A4	Control	Service	Beds	Admissions	Census	Outpatient Visits	Births	Total	Payroll	Personnel

SAUK CENTRE—Stearns County
★ ST. MICHAEL'S HOSPITAL, 425 North Elm Street, Zip 56378; tel. 320/352–2221; Del Christianson, Administrator **A**9 10 **F**7 8 11 15 16 19 20 22 26 32 33 34 35 36 41 42 44 45 51 62 64 65 67 71 72 73 — 14 10 78 477 63 12031 55 5719 2317 —

SHAKOPEE—Scott County
⊞ ST. FRANCIS REGIONAL MEDICAL CENTER, 1455 St. Francis Avenue, Zip 55379–1228; tel. 612/403–3000; Venetia Kudrle, President (Nonreporting) **A**1 2 9 10 **S** Allina Health System, Minneapolis, MN **N** Benedictine Health System, Duluth, MN; Allina Health System, Minnetonka, MN — 21 10 63 — — — — — — —

SLAYTON—Murray County
MURRAY COUNTY MEMORIAL HOSPITAL, 2042 Juniper Avenue, Zip 56172; tel. 507/836–6111; Jerry Bobeldyk, Administrator **A**9 10 **F**8 15 19 30 33 35 44 60 71 **S** Sioux Valley Health System, Sioux Falls, SD **N** Southwest Minnesota Health Alliance, Luverne, MN; Sioux Valley Health System, Sioux Falls, SD — 13 10 30 570 5 8934 0 3009 1320 50

SLEEPY EYE—Brown County
SLEEPY EYE MUNICIPAL HOSPITAL, 400 Fourth Avenue N.W., Zip 56085; tel. 507/794–3571; Chad Cooper, Administrator **A**9 10 **F**7 8 11 12 15 16 17 19 20 22 24 28 30 33 34 35 36 37 39 40 41 44 49 67 71 **N** Quality Health Alliance, Mankato, MN — 14 10 20 470 4 5697 20 2583 1232 48

SPRING GROVE—Houston County
TWEETEN LUTHERAN HEALTH CARE CENTER, 125 Fifth Avenue S.E., Zip 55974; tel. 507/498–3211; Robert Schmidt, Chief Executive Officer (Total facility includes 79 beds in nursing home–type unit) **A**9 10 **F**3 12 14 15 16 17 20 26 27 28 29 30 32 33 34 36 39 41 44 45 46 48 49 61 62 64 65 66 68 71 73 74 **P**6 — 23 10 89 131 70 4577 0 3448 1812 87

SPRING VALLEY—Fillmore County
COMMUNITY MEMORIAL HOSPITAL AND NURSING HOME, 800 Memorial Drive, Zip 55975; tel. 507/346–7381; David Herder, Administrator (Total facility includes 50 beds in nursing home–type unit) (Nonreporting) **A**9 — 23 10 74 — — — — — — —

SPRINGFIELD—Brown County
□ SPRINGFIELD COMMUNITY HOSPITAL, 625 North Jackson, Zip 56087, Mailing Address: Box 146, Zip 56087; tel. 507/723–6201; Scott Thoreson, Administrator **A**1 9 10 **F**7 8 15 16 19 22 28 30 32 39 40 41 44 49 58 64 65 71 **N** Quality Health Alliance, Mankato, MN — 14 10 24 426 4 6486 40 3634 923 50

STAPLES—Wadena County
GREATER STAPLES HOSPITAL AND CARE CENTER, 401 East Prairie Avenue, Zip 56479–9415; tel. 218/894–1515; Tim Rice, Administrator (Total facility includes 100 beds in nursing home–type unit) **A**9 10 **F**7 8 14 15 16 19 22 26 27 28 30 32 33 35 41 44 45 46 49 64 65 67 71 **P**5 — 16 10 124 1010 107 14743 110 10603 4370 229

STARBUCK—Pope County
★ MINNEWASKA DISTRICT HOSPITAL, 610 West Sixth Street, Zip 56381, Mailing Address: P.O. Box 160, Zip 56381–0610; tel. 320/239–2201; Roxann A. Wellman, Chief Executive Officer **A**9 10 **F**7 8 14 15 19 22 27 28 32 33 34 35 36 37 40 41 44 62 64 65 71 — 16 10 19 387 5 888 15 2074 923 33

STILLWATER—Washington County
⊞ LAKEVIEW HOSPITAL, 927 West Churchill Street, Zip 55082–5930; tel. 612/439–5330; Jeffrey J. Robertson, Administrator **A**1 9 10 **F**7 8 11 15 16 17 19 21 22 28 29 30 32 33 34 35 37 39 40 41 42 44 45 46 49 65 66 67 68 71 73 74 **P**5 — 23 10 48 2354 21 21711 540 22554 9048 278

THIEF RIVER FALLS—Pennington County
⊞ NORTHWEST MEDICAL CENTER, 120 LaBree Avenue South, Zip 56701–2819; tel. 218/681–4240; Richard A. Spyhalski, Chief Executive Officer (Total facility includes 90 beds in nursing home–type unit) **A**1 9 10 **F**7 8 11 15 16 19 21 22 28 29 30 34 35 36 37 39 40 42 44 45 46 49 52 53 54 55 56 57 58 60 64 65 66 67 71 73 74 — 23 10 165 2046 110 13703 213 16738 8933 334

TRACY—Lyon County
★ TRACY MUNICIPAL HOSPITAL, 251 Fifth Street East, Zip 56175–1536; tel. 507/629–3200; Thomas J. Quinlivan, Administrator **A**9 10 **F**6 7 8 11 14 15 16 17 19 22 26 28 29 30 31 32 33 34 35 37 40 41 42 44 45 48 49 51 54 58 62 65 71 74 **P**5 **S** Sioux Valley Health System, Sioux Falls, SD **N** Southwest Minnesota Health Alliance, Luverne, MN; Sioux Valley Health System, Sioux Falls, SD — 14 10 28 424 3 10291 10 2313 1195 45

TWO HARBORS—Lake County
LAKE VIEW MEMORIAL HOSPITAL, 325 11th Avenue, Zip 55616–1298; tel. 218/834–7300; Brian J. Carlson, Administrator (Total facility includes 50 beds in nursing home–type unit) **A**9 10 **F**3 7 14 15 40 44 49 64 65 70 71 73 **N** Northern Lakes Health Consortium, Duluth, MN — 23 10 66 416 52 6924 27 4882 2132 105

TYLER—Lincoln County
★ TYLER HEALTHCARE CENTER, 240 Willow Street, Zip 56178–0280; tel. 507/247–5521; James Rotert, Administrator (Total facility includes 43 beds in nursing home–type unit) **A**10 **F**1 7 8 15 16 19 22 24 26 32 33 35 36 40 44 49 58 64 67 71 **P**6 **S** Presentation Health System, Yankton, SD **N** Minnesota Rural Health Cooperative, Willmar, MN — 23 10 63 214 44 5704 0 3257 1574 85

VIRGINIA—St. Louis County
⊞ △ VIRGINIA REGIONAL MEDICAL CENTER, 901 Ninth Street North, Zip 55792–2398; tel. 218/741–3340; Kyle Hopstad, Administrator (Total facility includes 116 beds in nursing home–type unit) **A**1 7 10 **F**4 7 8 14 15 16 19 21 22 23 26 28 30 32 34 35 37 40 42 44 48 64 65 66 67 71 73 **S** Quorum Health Group/Quorum Health Resources, Inc., Brentwood, TN **N** Northern Lakes Health Consortium, Duluth, MN — 14 10 199 2920 151 13744 265 26421 12097 393

Hospital, Address, Telephone, Administrator, Approval, Facility, and Physician Codes, Health Care System, Network	Classi-fication Codes		Utilization Data					Expense (thousands) of dollars		
★ American Hospital Association (AHA) membership □ Joint Commission on Accreditation of Healthcare Organizations (JCAHO) accreditation + American Osteopathic Hospital Association (AOHA) membership ○ American Osteopathic Association (AOA) accreditation △ Commission on Accreditation of Rehabilitation Facilities (CARF) accreditation Control codes 61, 63, 64, 71, 72 and 73 indicate hospitals listed by AOHA, but not registered by AHA. For definition of numerical codes, see page A4	Control	Service	Beds	Admissions	Census	Outpatient Visits	Births	Total	Payroll	Personnel

WABASHA—Wabasha County

☒ ST. ELIZABETH HOSPITAL, 1200 Fifth Grand Boulevard West, Zip 55981; tel. 612/565–4531; Thomas Crowley, President (Total facility includes 152 beds in nursing home–type unit) **A**1 10 **F**1 2 3 4 5 6 7 8 9 10 11 12 13 14 15 16 17 18 19 20 21 22 23 24 25 26 27 28 29 30 31 32 33 34 35 36 37 38 39 40 41 42 43 44 45 46 47 48 49 50 51 52 53 54 55 56 57 58 59 60 61 62 63 64 65 66 67 68 69 70 71 72 73 74 **P**1 2 3 4 5 6 7 8 **S** Sisters of the Sorrowful Mother United States Health System, Tulsa, OK

| | 21 | 10 | 183 | 550 | 144 | 14423 | 80 | 8947 | 4570 | 204 |

WACONIA—Carver County

☒ RIDGEVIEW MEDICAL CENTER, 500 South Maple Street, Zip 55387; tel. 612/442–2191; Robert Stevens, President and Chief Executive Officer **A**1 10 **F**7 8 11 14 15 17 18 19 20 21 22 28 30 32 33 34 35 37 39 40 41 42 44 45 49 60 63 65 66 67 70 71 72 73 74 **P**4 5

| | 14 | 10 | 102 | 4845 | 44 | 56570 | 928 | 39378 | 18414 | 537 |

WADENA—Wadena County

☒ TRI–COUNTY HOSPITAL, 415 Jefferson Street North, Zip 56482; tel. 218/631–3510; Dennis C. Miley, Administrator **A**1 10 **F**7 8 11 14 15 16 17 19 21 22 26 28 30 32 33 34 35 36 37 39 40 41 42 44 45 49 53 54 58 64 65 66 67 71 73 **P**3

| | 23 | 10 | 23 | 1339 | 16 | 11606 | 180 | 10485 | 4892 | 182 |

WARREN—Marshall County

★ NORTH VALLEY HEALTH CENTER, 109 South Minnesota Street, Zip 56762–1499; tel. 218/745–4211; Everett A. Butler, Administrator **A**9 10 **F**8 11 13 15 16 17 19 22 24 28 29 30 32 33 35 37 39 41 44 45 48 49 66 71 73 **P**4 **N** Northstar Health Consortium, Roseau, MN

| | 23 | 10 | 18 | 400 | 4 | | 0 | 3107 | 1033 | 59 |

WASECA—Waseca County

☒ WASECA AREA MEDICAL CENTER, (Formerly Waseca Area Memorial Hospital), 100 Fifth Avenue N.W., Zip 56093–2422; tel. 507/835–1210; Michael Milbrath, Administrator **A**1 10 **F**3 7 8 11 14 15 16 17 22 24 30 32 36 39 40 41 44 46 48 49 65 66 71 72 **P**1 **N** Quality Health Alliance, Mankato, MN

| | 23 | 10 | 19 | 480 | 3 | — | 75 | 6074 | 1906 | 81 |

WESTBROOK—Cottonwood County

WESTBROOK HEALTH CENTER, (Formerly Schmidt Memorial Hospital), 920 Bell Avenue, Zip 56183, Mailing Address: P.O. Box 188, Zip 56183–0188; tel. 507/274–6121; Judy Lichty, Administrator **A**10 **F**8 17 19 22 28 30 33 35 36 37 42 44 51 64 71 **P**3 5 **S** Sioux Valley Health System, Sioux Falls, SD **N** Sioux Valley Health System, Sioux Falls, SD

| | 23 | 10 | 8 | 153 | 2 | — | 1 | 816 | 401 | 19 |

WHEATON—Traverse County

WHEATON COMMUNITY HOSPITAL, 401 12th Street North, Zip 56296–1099; tel. 612/563–8226; James J. Talley, Administrator **A**10 **F**7 11 12 14 15 16 17 19 20 21 22 24 27 28 29 30 32 33 34 35 37 39 40 41 42 44 46 48 49 52 53 54 55 57 58 63 64 67 71 73 **P**5

| | 14 | 10 | 28 | 514 | 6 | 11528 | 26 | 3042 | 1323 | 53 |

WILLMAR—Kandiyohi County

☒ RICE MEMORIAL HOSPITAL, 301 Becker Avenue S.W., Zip 56201–3395; tel. 320/231–4227; Lawrence J. Massa, Chief Executive Officer (Total facility includes 86 beds in nursing home–type unit) **A**1 2 9 10 **F**7 8 15 19 21 22 23 30 33 34 35 37 40 42 44 45 49 52 54 55 56 57 58 60 63 64 65 67 71 73 **N** Minnesota Rural Health Cooperative, Willmar, MN; Affiliated Community Health Network, Inc., Willmar, MN

| | 14 | 10 | 204 | 5182 | 143 | 27399 | 780 | 44328 | 20982 | 622 |

□ WILLMAR REGIONAL TREATMENT CENTER, North Highway 71, Zip 56201–1128, Mailing Address: Box 1128, Zip 56201–1128; tel. 612/231–5100; Gregory G. Spartz, Chief Executive Officer **A**1 10 **F**1 2 3 6 12 14 15 16 17 18 19 20 21 22 25 26 27 29 32 34 35 41 44 45 46 52 53 54 55 56 57 58 64 65 67 71 73 **P**6 **N** Affiliated Community Health Network, Inc., Willmar, MN

| | 12 | 22 | 375 | 1150 | 303 | — | 0 | 31000 | 21000 | — |

WINDOM—Cottonwood County

WINDOM AREA HOSPITAL, Highways 60 and 71 North, Zip 56101, Mailing Address: P.O. Box 339, Zip 56101; tel. 507/831–2400; J. Stephen Pautler, CHE, Administrator **A**10 **F**7 8 16 17 19 20 22 28 30 33 34 35 40 44 49 64 65 67 71 73 **P**6 **S** Sioux Valley Health System, Sioux Falls, SD **N** Southwest Minnesota Health Alliance, Luverne, MN; Sioux Valley Health System, Sioux Falls, SD

| | 14 | 10 | 17 | 820 | 8 | 12932 | 160 | 4314 | 1591 | 63 |

WINONA—Winona County

☒ COMMUNITY MEMORIAL HOSPITAL AND CONVALESCENT AND REHABILITATION UNIT, 855 Mankato Avenue, Zip 55987–4894, Mailing Address: P.O. Box 5600, Zip 55987–0600; tel. 507/454–3650; Roger L. Metz, President (Total facility includes 104 beds in nursing home–type unit) **A**1 10 **F**1 2 6 7 8 10 11 15 16 17 19 21 22 23 24 26 28 30 32 33 35 37 39 40 41 44 45 46 49 51 52 53 54 55 56 57 60 63 64 65 67 71 73

| | 23 | 10 | 185 | 3296 | 138 | 32792 | 417 | 23862 | 12418 | 448 |

WORTHINGTON—Nobles County

□ WORTHINGTON REGIONAL HOSPITAL, 1018 Sixth Avenue, Zip 56187, Mailing Address: P.O. Box 997, Zip 56187; tel. 507/372–2941; Melvin J. Platt, Administrator **A**1 10 **F**7 15 19 21 22 27 30 32 33 35 36 37 40 41 44 49 52 53 64 65 71 73 **S** Sioux Valley Health System, Sioux Falls, SD **N** Southwest Minnesota Health Alliance, Luverne, MN

| | 14 | 10 | 83 | 2359 | 26 | 26843 | 348 | 12797 | 6233 | 191 |

ZUMBROTA—Goodhue County

☒ ZUMBROTA HEALTH CARE, 383 West Fifth Street, Zip 55992; tel. 507/732–5131; Daniel Will, Administrator (Nonreporting) **A**1 10

| | 23 | 10 | 19 | — | — | — | — | — | — | — |

MISSISSIPPI

Resident population 2,697 (in thousands)
Resident population in metro areas 35.0%
Birth rate per 1,000 population 16.0
65 years and over 12.3%
Percent of persons without health insurance 17.8%

Hospital, Address, Telephone, Administrator, Approval, Facility, and Physician Codes, Health Care System, Network	Classification Codes		Utilization Data					Expense (thousands) of dollars		
★ American Hospital Association (AHA) membership □ Joint Commission on Accreditation of Healthcare Organizations (JCAHO) accreditation + American Osteopathic Hospital Association (AOHA) membership ○ American Osteopathic Association (AOA) accreditation △ Commission on Accreditation of Rehabilitation Facilities (CARF) accreditation Control codes 61, 63, 64, 71, 72 and 73 indicate hospitals listed by AOHA, but not registered by AHA. For definition of numerical codes, see page A4	Control	Service	Beds	Admissions	Census	Outpatient Visits	Births	Total	Payroll	Personnel

ABERDEEN—Monroe County

| ABERDEEN–MONROE COUNTY HOSPITAL, 400 South Chestnut Street, Zip 39730; Mailing Address: Box 747, Zip 39730; tel. 601/369–2455; Frank Harrington, Administrator A9 10 F8 15 19 22 49 71 73 P2 5 | 15 | 10 | 27 | 666 | 10 | 5243 | 0 | — | — | 93 |

ACKERMAN—Choctaw County

| CHOCTAW COUNTY MEDICAL CENTER, 148 West Cherry Street, Zip 39735–0417, Mailing Address: P.O. Box 417, Zip 39735–0417; tel. 601/285–6235; Ouida Loper, Administrator (Total facility includes 66 beds in nursing home–type unit) A9 10 F2 22 64 65 P6 | 13 | 10 | 88 | 315 | 74 | 3361 | 0 | | | 67 |

AMORY—Monroe County

| ✠ GILMORE MEMORIAL HOSPITAL, 1105 Earl Frye Boulevard, Zip 38821, Mailing Address: P.O. Box 459, Zip 38821–0459; tel. 601/256–7111; Robert F. Letson, President and Chief Executive Officer A1 9 10 F7 8 11 12 14 15 16 19 21 22 24 34 35 37 38 39 40 41 44 47 48 49 64 65 71 73 74 P8 | 23 | 10 | 95 | 3368 | 46 | 30420 | 791 | 18673 | 9016 | 328 |

BATESVILLE—Panola County

| SOUTH PANOLA COMMUNITY HOSPITAL, Hospital Drive, Zip 38606, Mailing Address: Box 433, Zip 38606; tel. 601/563–5611; Richard W. Manning, Administrator A9 10 F19 21 22 34 44 65 71 73 P3 7 | 13 | 10 | 70 | 1515 | 18 | 14437 | 0 | 6530 | 3073 | 135 |

BAY SPRINGS—Jasper County

| JASPER GENERAL HOSPITAL, (Includes Jasper County Nursing Home), Sixth Street, Zip 39422, Mailing Address: Box 527, Zip 39422; tel. 601/764–2101; M. Kenneth Posey, FACHE, Administrator (Total facility includes 104 beds in nursing home–type unit) A9 10 F15 32 41 64 65 71 | 13 | 10 | 124 | 303 | 109 | 0 | 0 | — | — | 120 |

BAY ST. LOUIS—Hancock County

| ✠ HANCOCK MEDICAL CENTER, 149 Drinkwater Boulevard, Zip 39520, Mailing Address: P.O. Box 2790, Zip 39521; tel. 601/467–9081; Thomas B. Symonds, Chief Executive Officer A1 9 10 F7 8 11 15 16 17 19 22 34 35 37 40 44 45 46 48 49 65 71 P8 S Quorum Health Group/Quorum Health Resources, Inc., Brentwood, TN | 13 | 10 | 66 | 3547 | 45 | 36643 | 281 | 21225 | 7538 | 303 |

BELZONI—Humphreys County

| ★ HUMPHREYS COUNTY MEMORIAL HOSPITAL, 500 CCC Road, Zip 39038, Mailing Address: P.O. Box 510, Zip 39038; tel. 601/247–3831; Debra L. Griffin, Administrator A9 10 F7 15 21 22 24 26 27 44 52 57 73 | 13 | 10 | 28 | 973 | 15 | 4520 | 2 | 5301 | 2070 | 118 |

BILOXI—Harrison County

□ BILOXI REGIONAL MEDICAL CENTER, 150 Reynoir Street, Zip 39530, Mailing Address: Box 128, Zip 39533; tel. 601/432–1571; Joseph J. Mullany, Executive Director A1 2 9 10 F1 2 7 8 9 10 11 12 14 15 16 17 19 20 21 22 23 24 26 27 31 32 33 34 35 36 37 38 39 40 41 42 43 44 45 46 47 48 49 50 51 52 60 61 63 64 65 66 67 68 69 70 71 72 73 74 P1 5 8 S Health Management Associates, Naples, FL	33	10	153	6421	92	121351	701	34612	13562	473
□ GULF COAST MEDICAL CENTER, 180–A Debuys Road, Zip 39531–4405, Mailing Address: Box 4518, Zip 39531–4518; tel. 601/388–6711; Gary L. Stokes, Chief Executive Officer A1 9 10 F2 3 7 8 11 12 15 16 17 19 21 26 31 32 33 34 35 37 39 40 42 44 46 52 53 54 55 56 57 58 59 63 64 65 67 69 71 73 P1 2 4 5 6 8 S TENET Healthcare Corporation, Santa Barbara, CA	33	10	189	3745	66	181259	133	44882	19665	669
GULF OAKS HOSPITAL, 180–C Debuys Road, Zip 39531; tel. 601/388–0600; Hugh S. Simcoe, III, Administrator (Nonreporting) A9	33	22	45	—	—	—	—	—	—	
✠ VETERANS AFFAIRS MEDICAL CENTER, (Includes Veterans Affairs Medical Center, Gulfport Division, East Beach, Gulfport, Zip 39501; tel. 601/863–1972; George Rodman, Director), 400 Veterans Avenue, Zip 39531–2410; tel. 601/388–5541; George Rodman, Director (Total facility includes 320 beds in nursing home–type unit) (Nonreporting) A1 2 3 5 S Department of Veterans Affairs, Washington, DC	45	10	510	—	—	—	—	—	—	

BOONEVILLE—Prentiss County

| ✠ BAPTIST MEMORIAL HOSPITAL–BOONEVILLE, 100 Hospital Street, Zip 38829; tel. 601/728–5331; Pamela W. Roberts, Administrator A1 9 10 F8 11 15 16 17 19 20 21 22 24 34 37 39 40 44 45 46 51 52 54 57 65 67 71 73 P3 7 S Baptist Memorial Health Care Corporation, Memphis, TN | 21 | 10 | 93 | 2169 | 37 | 21572 | 0 | 10977 | 4198 | 188 |

BRANDON—Rankin County

| ✠ RANKIN MEDICAL CENTER, 350 Crossgates Boulevard, Zip 39042; tel. 601/825–2811; Thomas Wiman, Executive Director A1 2 9 10 F8 11 19 21 22 24 32 34 37 41 42 44 46 47 49 51 52 57 63 65 71 73 P8 S Health Management Associates, Naples, FL | 13 | 10 | 90 | 3092 | 50 | 59594 | 0 | — | — | 577 |

BROOKHAVEN—Lincoln County

| ✠ KING'S DAUGHTERS HOSPITAL, Highway 51 North, Zip 39601, Mailing Address: P.O. Box 948, Zip 39601; tel. 601/833–6011; Wallace Cooper, Chief Executive Officer A1 9 10 F2 7 8 9 10 11 12 15 16 17 19 20 21 22 23 27 31 32 33 34 35 36 37 38 39 40 41 42 43 44 45 47 48 49 51 52 60 61 64 65 66 67 68 69 70 71 72 73 74 S Quorum Health Group/Quorum Health Resources, Inc., Brentwood, TN | 23 | 10 | 102 | 3537 | 48 | 35232 | 593 | 24948 | 10314 | 417 |

Hospital, Address, Telephone, Administrator, Approval, Facility, and Physician Codes, Health Care System, Network	Classi-fication Codes		Utilization Data					Expense (thousands) of dollars		
★ American Hospital Association (AHA) membership □ Joint Commission on Accreditation of Healthcare Organizations (JCAHO) accreditation + American Osteopathic Hospital Association (AOHA) membership ○ American Osteopathic Association (AOA) accreditation △ Commission on Accreditation of Rehabilitation Facilities (CARF) accreditation Control codes 61, 63, 64, 71, 72 and 73 indicate hospitals listed by AOHA, but not registered by AHA. For definition of numerical codes, see page A4	Control	Service	Beds	Admissions	Census	Outpatient Visits	Births	Total	Payroll	Personnel

BRUCE—Calhoun County

BRUCE HOSPITAL, Highway 9 South, Zip 38915, Mailing Address: Box 429, Zip 38915-0429; tel. 601/983-5100; Robert M. Perry, Administrator (Total facility includes 22 beds in nursing home–type unit) (Nonreporting) **A**9 **S** First Health, Inc., Batesville, MS

| | 23 | 10 | 47 | — | — | — | — | — | — | — |

CALHOUN CITY—Calhoun County

HILLCREST HOSPITAL, 140 Burke–Calhoun City Road, Zip 38916-0770, Mailing Address: Route 2, Box 226–A, Burke Road, Zip 38916; tel. 601/628-6611; Charles R. Daugherty, Administrator **A**9 10 **F**15 19 22 34 44 46 65 71

| | 14 | 10 | 30 | 788 | 14 | 6769 | 0 | — | — | 53 |

CANTON—Madison County

MADISON COUNTY MEDICAL CENTER, Highway 16 East, Zip 39046, Mailing Address: P.O. Box 1607, Zip 39046; tel. 601/859-1331; G. Wayne Schuler, Executive Director (Total facility includes 60 beds in nursing home–type unit) **A**9 10 **F**1 2 3 8 16 17 19 20 22 26 31 32 33 34 37 40 44 51 52 54 56 57 58 59 64 65 71 **P**6

| | 13 | 10 | 127 | 1827 | 95 | 18770 | 284 | 11515 | 4265 | 329 |

CARTHAGE—Leake County

LEAKE MEMORIAL HOSPITAL, 300 Ellis Street, Zip 39051-0557, Mailing Address: P.O. Box 557, Zip 39051-0557; tel. 601/267-4511; George Posey, Administrator (Total facility includes 44 beds in nursing home–type unit) **A**9 10 **F**1 14 15 16 19 22 26 34 44 46 64 65 71 73 **P**6

| | 33 | 10 | 76 | 1011 | 64 | 13270 | 0 | — | — | 122 |

CENTREVILLE—Wilkinson County

⊞ FIELD MEMORIAL COMMUNITY HOSPITAL, 270 West Main Street, Zip 39631, Mailing Address: Box 639, Zip 39631-0639; tel. 601/645-5221; Brock A. Slabach, Administrator **A**1 9 10 **F**1 8 12 16 17 19 20 22 31 32 34 39 40 41 44 45 57 61 64 65 69 71 **S** Quorum Health Group/Quorum Health Resources, Inc., Brentwood, TN

| | 13 | 10 | 66 | 1825 | 22 | 8754 | 89 | 7181 | 2915 | 113 |

CHARLESTON—Tallahatchie County

TALLAHATCHIE GENERAL HOSPITAL, 201 South Market, Zip 38921, Mailing Address: P.O. Box 230, Zip 38921-0230; tel. 601/647-5535; F. W. Ergle, Jr., Administrator (Total facility includes 61 beds in nursing home–type unit) **A**9 10 **F**20 22 46 64 65 71 **P**8

| | 13 | 10 | 77 | 487 | 67 | — | 0 | 3335 | 2042 | 126 |

CLARKSDALE—Coahoma County

⊞ NORTHWEST MISSISSIPPI REGIONAL MEDICAL CENTER, 1970 Hospital Drive, Zip 38614, Mailing Address: Box 1218, Zip 38614; tel. 601/624-3401; J. David McCormack, Executive Director (Total facility includes 20 beds in nursing home–type unit) **A**1 5 9 10 **F**11 15 16 17 19 21 22 31 32 37 38 40 44 45 63 64 65 71 73 **S** Health Management Associates, Naples, FL

| | 13 | 10 | 195 | 6747 | 119 | — | 1224 | — | — | 578 |

CLEVELAND—Bolivar County

⊞ BOLIVAR COUNTY HOSPITAL, Highway 8 East, Zip 38732, Mailing Address: P.O. Box 1380, Zip 38732; tel. 601/846-0061; Robert L. Hawley, Jr., Chief Executive Officer (Total facility includes 34 beds in nursing home–type unit) **A**1 9 10 **F**7 8 11 17 19 20 21 22 34 37 40 44 45 46 48 49 64 65 71 73 **P**8 **S** Quorum Health Group/Quorum Health Resources, Inc., Brentwood, TN

| | 13 | 10 | 142 | 4952 | 112 | 31034 | 673 | 20483 | 10321 | 366 |

COLLINS—Covington County

□ COVINGTON COUNTY HOSPITAL, Sixth and Holly Streets, Zip 39428, Mailing Address: P.O. Box 1149, Zip 39428-1149; tel. 601/765-6711; Irving Hitt, Administrator **A**1 9 10 **F**7 8 11 14 15 16 17 19 20 21 22 26 32 33 34 37 40 44 45 46 48 49 52 57 64 65 71 73

| | 13 | 10 | 82 | 1355 | 30 | 17369 | 260 | 7962 | 2738 | 127 |

COLUMBIA—Marion County

METHODIST HOSPITAL OF MARION COUNTY, 1560 Sumrall Road, Zip 39429, Mailing Address: Box 630, Zip 39429; tel. 601/736-6303; Jerry M. Howell, Chief Operating Officer **A**9 10 **F**1 2 7 8 9 10 11 12 15 17 19 20 21 22 23 27 31 32 33 34 35 36 37 38 40 41 43 44 46 47 48 49 51 52 60 61 64 65 66 69 71 72 73

| | 13 | 10 | 79 | 2014 | 35 | 27123 | 3 | — | — | 205 |

COLUMBUS—Lowndes County

⊞ BAPTIST MEMORIAL HOSPITAL–GOLDEN TRIANGLE, 2520 Fifth Street North, Zip 39703-2095, Mailing Address: P.O. Box 1307, Zip 39701-1307; tel. 601/243-1000; J. Stuart Mitchell, III, Administrator **A**1 9 10 **F**1 2 3 7 8 9 10 11 12 15 16 17 19 20 21 22 23 24 26 27 31 32 33 34 35 36 37 38 39 40 41 42 43 44 45 46 47 48 49 51 52 53 54 55 56 57 58 59 61 65 66 67 68 69 71 72 73 74 **P**3 **S** Baptist Memorial Health Care Corporation, Memphis, TN

| | 21 | 10 | 328 | 8348 | 115 | 45448 | 1161 | 54368 | 20449 | 808 |

★ U. S. AIR FORCE HOSPITAL, 201 Independence, Suite 235, Zip 39701-5300; tel. 601/434-2297; Lieutenant Colonel Karen A. Bradway, MSC, USAF, Administrator (Nonreporting) **S** Department of the Air Force, Washington, DC

| | 41 | 10 | 7 | — | — | — | — | — | — | — |

CORINTH—Alcorn County

⊞ MAGNOLIA REGIONAL HEALTH CENTER, 611 Alcorn Drive, Zip 38834; tel. 601/293-1000; Rohn J. Butterfield, Chief Executive Officer **A**1 9 10 **F**7 8 10 11 12 14 15 16 17 19 20 21 22 23 24 32 33 35 37 38 39 40 41 42 46 47 49 52 55 56 58 59 64 65 66 71 73 **P**5 **S** Quorum Health Group/Quorum Health Resources, Inc., Brentwood, TN

| | 15 | 10 | 157 | 6467 | 103 | 124766 | 459 | 46541 | 18512 | 737 |

DE KALB—Kemper County

KEMPER COMMUNITY HOSPITAL, Highway 39 & 16 Intersection, Zip 39328, Mailing Address: Box 246, Zip 39328; tel. 601/743-5851; Tommy Dearing, Administrator (Total facility includes 19 beds in nursing home–type unit) **A**9 10 **F**15 16 33 64 73

| | 33 | 10 | 24 | 29 | 15 | 0 | 0 | — | — | 37 |

DURANT—Holmes County

UNIVERSITY HOSPITAL OF DURANT, 713 North West Avenue, Zip 39063; tel. 601/653-3081; William D. McKinnon, FACHE, Administrator **A**9 10 **F**15 16 20 22 34 46 65 73 **P**6

| | 12 | 10 | 29 | 760 | 16 | 5457 | 0 | — | — | 77 |

Hospital, Address, Telephone, Administrator, Approval, Facility, and Physician Codes, Health Care System, Network	Classi-fication Codes		Utilization Data					Expense (thousands) of dollars		
★ American Hospital Association (AHA) membership □ Joint Commission on Accreditation of Healthcare Organizations (JCAHO) accreditation + American Osteopathic Hospital Association (AOHA) membership ○ American Osteopathic Association (AOA) accreditation △ Commission on Accreditation of Rehabilitation Facilities (CARF) accreditation Control codes 61, 63, 64, 71, 72 and 73 indicate hospitals listed by AOHA, but not registered by AHA. For definition of numerical codes, see page A4	Control	Service	Beds	Admissions	Census	Outpatient Visits	Births	Total	Payroll	Personnel

EUPORA—Webster County

WEBSTER HEALTH SERVICES, 500 Highway 9 South, Zip 39744; tel. 601/258–6221; Harold H. Whitaker, Sr., Administrator (Total facility includes 33 beds in nursing home–type unit) **A**9 10 **F**8 15 16 17 19 21 22 24 32 33 34 44 45 46 48 60 64 65 67 71 **P**4 **S** North Mississippi Health Services, Inc., Tupelo, MS **N** North Mississippi Health Services, Tupelo, MS | 23 | 10 | 76 | 1522 | 54 | 10461 | 0 | 6185 | 2912 | 144

FAYETTE—Jefferson County

JEFFERSON COUNTY HOSPITAL, 809 South Main Street, Zip 39069, Mailing Address: Box 577, Zip 39069; tel. 601/786–3401; Diwana Sanders, Administrator **A**9 10 **F**22 26 35 52 71 | 13 | 10 | 30 | 704 | 8 | 2798 | 0 | — | — | 46

FOREST—Scott County

LACKEY MEMORIAL HOSPITAL, 330 North Broad Street, Zip 39074–0428, Mailing Address: Box 428, Zip 39074–0428; tel. 601/469–4151; Donna Riser, Administrator (Total facility includes 30 beds in nursing home–type unit) **A**9 10 **F**8 14 15 16 17 19 22 26 33 44 45 46 57 64 65 71 73 **P**5 | 23 | 10 | 64 | 1278 | 61 | 6723 | 0 | — | — | 95

GREENVILLE—Washington County

☒ DELTA REGIONAL MEDICAL CENTER, 1400 East Union Street, Zip 38703–3246, Mailing Address: Box 5247, Zip 38704–5247; tel. 601/378–3783; George Repa, Chief Executive Officer **A**1 9 10 **F**2 3 7 8 9 10 11 16 17 19 20 21 22 23 31 32 34 35 37 39 40 42 44 45 49 52 63 65 67 71 73 **P**8 **S** Quorum Health Group/Quorum Health Resources, Inc., Brentwood, TN | 13 | 10 | 159 | 5435 | 97 | 32589 | 556 | 38459 | 16866 | 707

☒ KING'S DAUGHTERS HOSPITAL, 300 Washington Avenue, Zip 38701, Mailing Address: Box 1857, Zip 38702–1857; tel. 601/378–2020; Donald Joe Fisher, Administrator **A**1 9 10 **F**7 9 10 11 14 15 17 19 20 21 22 27 33 34 37 39 40 41 44 45 46 49 65 67 71 73 | 23 | 10 | 103 | 3181 | 46 | 42042 | 685 | 20680 | 8581 | 384

GREENWOOD—Leflore County

☒ GREENWOOD LEFLORE HOSPITAL, 1401 River Road, Zip 38930, Mailing Address: Drawer 1410, Zip 38935–1410; tel. 601/459–7000; Terrell M. Cobb, Executive Director **A**1 9 10 **F**7 8 11 14 16 17 19 20 21 22 23 26 31 34 35 37 39 40 42 44 45 46 52 65 67 71 74 **P**6 8 | 15 | 10 | 210 | 8659 | 128 | 112475 | 754 | — | — | 820

GRENADA—Grenada County

☒ GRENADA LAKE MEDICAL CENTER, 960 Avent Drive, Zip 38901–5094; tel. 601/227–7101; Donald L. Ray, Chief Administrative Officer **A**1 9 10 **F**2 3 7 8 11 15 16 17 19 21 22 24 31 32 33 34 35 36 37 38 40 42 44 46 47 49 54 56 63 65 67 71 73 **P**8 | 13 | 10 | 122 | 4706 | 82 | 27647 | 721 | 23392 | 9445 | 491

GULFPORT—Harrison County

□ BHC SAND HILL BEHAVIORAL HEALTHCARE, (Formerly CPC Sand Hill Behavioral Healthcare), 11150 Highway 49 North, Zip 39503–4110; tel. 601/831–1700; David C. Bell, Chief Operating Officer **A**1 9 10 **F**2 3 9 10 11 12 16 17 20 22 24 27 31 35 37 46 52 53 54 55 56 58 59 65 67 68 71 **S** Behavioral Healthcare Corporation, Nashville, TN | 33 | 22 | 60 | 804 | 34 | 0 | 0 | — | — | 139

☒ COLUMBIA GARDEN PARK HOSPITAL, 1520 Broad Avenue, Zip 39501, Mailing Address: P.O. Box 1240, Zip 39502; tel. 601/864–4210; William E. Peaks, Chief Executive Officer **A**1 9 10 **F**2 7 8 10 11 12 14 15 16 17 19 20 21 22 23 24 26 27 32 33 34 35 37 39 40 41 42 43 44 46 48 49 50 51 52 60 61 63 64 65 66 67 69 71 72 73 74 **P**5 6 7 8 **S** Columbia/HCA Healthcare Corporation, Nashville, TN
CPC SAND HILL BEHAVIORAL HEALTHCARE See BHC Sand Hill Behavioral Healthcare | 33 | 10 | 97 | 2574 | 49 | 20226 | 194 | — | — | 374

☒ △ MEMORIAL HOSPITAL AT GULFPORT, 4500 13th Street, Zip 39501, Mailing Address: Box 1810, Zip 39502–1810; tel. 601/867–4000; W. R. Burton, Administrator **A**1 2 7 9 10 **F**3 7 8 10 11 15 16 17 19 21 22 23 31 33 34 35 37 38 40 41 42 43 44 46 47 48 49 52 54 55 56 58 59 63 65 66 67 71 72 73 74 **P**3 8 | 15 | 10 | 313 | 12705 | 214 | 183831 | 1346 | 112173 | 45331 | 1495

HATTIESBURG—Lamar County

☒ FORREST GENERAL HOSPITAL, 6051 U.S. Highway 49, Zip 39401, Mailing Address: P.O. Box 16389, Zip 39404–6389; tel. 601/288–7000; William C. Oliver, Executive Director **A**1 2 5 9 10 **F**2 3 7 8 10 11 12 14 15 16 17 19 20 21 22 23 32 33 34 35 37 38 39 40 41 42 43 44 45 46 48 49 52 53 54 55 56 58 59 60 63 64 65 66 67 69 71 73 74 **P**8 | 13 | 10 | 537 | 23455 | 372 | 116230 | 2834 | 150194 | 63614 | 2511

☒ METHODIST HOSPITAL OF HATTIESBURG, 5001 Hardy Street, Zip 39402, Mailing Address: Box 16509, Zip 39404–6509; tel. 601/268–8000; William K. Ray, President and Chief Executive Officer **A**1 9 10 **F**7 8 11 12 16 17 19 20 21 22 23 24 27 31 32 34 35 37 38 39 40 41 42 44 45 46 47 48 49 64 65 66 67 71 72 73 74 **P**1 7 | 23 | 10 | 211 | 7991 | 129 | 67744 | 436 | 59514 | 21951 | 907

HAZLEHURST—Copiah County

★ HARDY WILSON MEMORIAL HOSPITAL, 233 Magnolia Street, Zip 39083, Mailing Address: P.O. Box 889, Zip 39083–0889; tel. 601/894–4541; L. Pat Moreland, Administrator **A**9 10 **F**8 20 22 34 40 44 49 57 64 65 71 | 13 | 10 | 49 | 1639 | 31 | 11638 | 221 | — | — | 130

HOLLY SPRINGS—Marshall County

HOLLY SPRINGS MEMORIAL HOSPITAL, 1430 East Salem, Zip 38635, Mailing Address: P.O. Box 6000, Zip 38634–6000; tel. 601/252–1212; Bill Renick, Administrator **A**9 10 **F**15 16 19 22 34 41 44 57 65 71 | 23 | 10 | 40 | 934 | 16 | 21760 | 1 | — | — | 95

HOUSTON—Chickasaw County

□ TRACE REGIONAL HOSPITAL, Highway 8 East, Zip 38851, Mailing Address: P.O. Box 626, Zip 38851; tel. 601/456–3700; Bristol Messer, Chief Executive Officer **A**1 9 10 **F**2 3 8 11 16 19 21 22 24 31 34 37 39 44 52 57 65 71 **P**6 **S** NetCare Health Systems, Inc., Nashville, TN | 33 | 10 | 84 | 1766 | 32 | 13560 | 4 | — | — | 190

Hospital, Address, Telephone, Administrator, Approval, Facility, and Physician Codes, Health Care System, Network	Classi-fication Codes		Utilization Data					Expense (thousands) of dollars		
★ American Hospital Association (AHA) membership □ Joint Commission on Accreditation of Healthcare Organizations (JCAHO) accreditation + American Osteopathic Hospital Association (AOHA) membership ○ American Osteopathic Association (AOA) accreditation △ Commission on Accreditation of Rehabilitation Facilities (CARF) accreditation Control codes 61, 63, 64, 71, 72 and 73 indicate hospitals listed by AOHA, but not registered by AHA. For definition of numerical codes, see page A4	Control	Service	Beds	Admissions	Census	Outpatient Visits	Births	Total	Payroll	Personnel

INDIANOLA—Sunflower County

✠ SOUTH SUNFLOWER COUNTY HOSPITAL, 121 East Baker Street, Zip 38751; tel. 601/887–5235; H. J. Blessitt, Administrator **A**1 9 10 **F**7 11 19 21 22 37 40 44 65 71 **P**1	13	10	69	2134	25	10405	405	—	—	148

IUKA—Tishomingo County

□ IUKA HOSPITAL, 1777 Curtis Drive, Zip 38852, Mailing Address: P.O. Box 860, Zip 38852; tel. 601/423–6051; Robert E. Northern, Administrator **A**1 9 10 **F**2 7 8 10 11 12 14 15 16 17 19 20 21 22 23 24 32 33 34 35 37 38 40 41 42 43 44 45 47 48 49 52 63 64 65 66 67 68 71 72 73 74 **P**3 5 **S** North Mississippi Health Services, Inc., Tupelo, MS **N** North Mississippi Health Services, Tupelo, MS	23	10	48	1988	27	24211	0	—	—	114

JACKSON—Hinds County

□ CHARTER BEHAVIORAL HEALTH SYSTEM, 3531 Lakeland Drive, Zip 39208, Mailing Address: Box 4297, Zip 39296; tel. 601/939–9030; Earl W. Balzen, R.N., Chief Executive Officer **A**1 9 10 **F**2 3 15 22 52 53 54 55 56 57 58 59 65 **P**5 **S** Magellan Health Services, Atlanta, GA	33	22	111	2191	104		0			190
✠ G.V. MONTGOMERY VETERANS AFFAIRS MEDICAL CENTER, (Formerly Veterans Affairs Medical Center), 1500 East Woodrow Wilson Drive, Zip 39216–5199; tel. 601/364–1201; Richard P. Miller, Director (Total facility includes 120 beds in nursing home–type unit) (Nonreporting) **A**1 2 3 5 8 **S** Department of Veterans Affairs, Washington, DC	45	10	443							
✠ METHODIST MEDICAL CENTER, 1850 Chadwick Drive, Zip 39204–3479, Mailing Address: P.O. Box 59001, Zip 39204–9001; tel. 601/376–1000; Thomas L. Harper, President and Chief Executive Officer **A**1 2 5 9 10 **F**7 8 11 14 15 16 17 19 21 22 23 31 32 34 35 37 38 39 40 42 44 45 46 47 48 49 52 54 58 63 64 65 67 71 73 74 **P**8 **S** Methodist Health Systems, Inc., Memphis, TN **N** Methodist Health Systems, Inc., Memphis, TN	23	10	304	12081	195	63656	1552	—	—	1468
✠ MISSISSIPPI BAPTIST MEDICAL CENTER, 1225 North State Street, Zip 39202–2002; tel. 601/968–1000; Kurt W. Metzner, President and Chief Executive Officer **A**1 2 3 5 9 10 **F**2 3 7 8 9 10 11 12 14 15 16 17 20 21 22 23 24 27 31 32 33 35 37 38 39 40 41 42 43 44 45 46 47 48 49 51 54 63 64 65 66 67 68 71 73 74 **P**7 8	23	10	591	19632	336	103543	939	160835	83489	2516
✠ MISSISSIPPI HOSPITAL RESTORATIVE CARE, (Formerly The Restorative Care Hospital at Baptist), (RESTORATIVE CARE), 1225 North State Street, Zip 39202, Mailing Address: P.O. Box 23695, Zip 39225–3695; tel. 601/968–1054; Michael Huseth, Chief Executive Officer **A**1 **F**2 10 11 12 14 15 16 17 19 20 21 22 24 27 31 32 35 37 39 41 42 45 46 47 54 60 63 65 66 67 71 73 74 **P**7 8	23	49	25	162	18	0	0	4331	1487	53
✠ MISSISSIPPI METHODIST HOSPITAL AND REHABILITATION CENTER, 1350 Woodrow Wilson Drive, Zip 39216; tel. 601/364–3462; Mark A. Adams, President and Chief Executive Officer **A**1 10 **F**12 14 15 16 17 19 21 27 32 35 39 41 44 45 46 48 49 65 67 71 73	23	46	121	1646	81	3427	0	31337	16163	642
□ RIVER OAKS EAST–WOMAN'S PAVILION, 1026 North Flowood Drive, Zip 39208–9599, Mailing Address: P.O. Box 4546, Zip 39296–4546; tel. 601/932–1000; Carl Etter, Executive Director **A**1 9 10 **F**7 8 11 12 15 16 17 19 20 21 22 27 31 33 35 37 38 39 40 42 43 44 45 46 47 48 51 52 61 64 65 66 69 70 71 73 74 **P**5 6 7 8	33	44	76	3034	34	4190	1528	21629	8342	292
✠ RIVER OAKS HOSPITAL, 1030 River Oaks Drive, Zip 39208, Mailing Address: P.O. Box 5100, Zip 39296–5100; tel. 601/932–1030; John J. Cleary, President and Chief Executive Officer **A**1 10 **F**7 8 11 12 15 19 20 21 22 27 33 34 37 38 39 40 42 44 45 46 47 52 63 65 71 73 74	33	10	110	7093	79	37913	1183	55665	20966	710
✠ ST. DOMINIC–JACKSON MEMORIAL HOSPITAL, 969 Lakeland Drive, Zip 39216–4699; tel. 601/982–0121; Claude W. Harbarger, President **A**1 2 3 5 9 10 **F**2 3 8 10 11 12 16 17 19 20 21 22 23 24 31 33 34 35 37 39 42 43 44 45 48 49 51 52 55 56 57 58 59 63 65 67 71 73 **P**8 **N** National Cardiovascular Network, Atlanta, GA	23	10	571	13312	302	217305	0	91624	40548	1531
THE RESTORATIVE CARE HOSPITAL AT BAPTIST See Mississippi Hospital Restorative Care										
✠ UNIVERSITY HOSPITALS AND CLINICS, UNIVERSITY OF MISSISSIPPI MEDICAL CENTER, 2500 North State Street, Zip 39216–4505; tel. 601/984–4100; Frederick Woodrell, Associate Vice Chancellor and Director **A**1 2 3 5 8 9 10 **F**7 8 9 10 11 12 15 16 19 20 21 22 23 31 34 35 37 38 39 40 41 42 43 44 45 46 47 48 49 52 55 56 57 58 61 63 64 65 66 67 68 69 70 71 73 **P**6 **S** Quorum Health Group/Quorum Health Resources, Inc., Brentwood, TN	12	10	524	21961	395	178075	3232	—	—	2650
VETERANS AFFAIRS MEDICAL CENTER See G.V. Montgomery Veterans Affairs Medical Center										

KEESLER AFB—Harrison County

✠ U. S. AIR FORCE MEDICAL CENTER KEESLER, 301 Fisher Street, Room 1A132, Zip 39534–2519; tel. 601/377–6510; Colonel William B. Kleefisch, Deputy Commander **A**1 2 3 5 **F**4 7 8 10 11 12 13 14 15 16 17 19 20 21 22 24 25 28 29 30 31 34 35 37 38 39 41 42 43 44 45 46 49 50 51 52 53 54 55 56 57 58 59 60 61 62 63 65 68 69 72 73 74 **S** Department of the Air Force, Washington, DC	41	10	185	9246	98	426029	849	—	—	2306

KILMICHAEL—Montgomery County

KILMICHAEL HOSPITAL, 301 Lamar Avenue, Zip 39747–0188, Mailing Address: P.O. Box 188, Zip 39747–0188; tel. 601/262–4311; Anne S. Ingram, Chief Executive Officer **A**9 10 **F**7 8 11 14 15 16 19 20 21 22 26 27 31 32 33 35 36 37 38 39 40 41 42 44 47 49 51 61 63 65 66 71 73 **P**5 8	13	10	19	625	11	4421	0	1690	765	47

Hospital, Address, Telephone, Administrator, Approval, Facility, and Physician Codes, Health Care System, Network	Classi-fication Codes		Utilization Data					Expense (thousands) of dollars		
★ American Hospital Association (AHA) membership □ Joint Commission on Accreditation of Healthcare Organizations (JCAHO) accreditation + American Osteopathic Hospital Association (AOHA) membership ○ American Osteopathic Association (AOA) accreditation △ Commission on Accreditation of Rehabilitation Facilities (CARF) accreditation Control codes 61, 63, 64, 71, 72 and 73 indicate hospitals listed by AOHA, but not registered by AHA. For definition of numerical codes, see page A4	Control	Service	Beds	Admissions	Census	Outpatient Visits	Births	Total	Payroll	Personnel

KOSCIUSKO—Attala County

MONTFORT JONES MEMORIAL HOSPITAL, Highway 12 West, Zip 39090–3209, Mailing Address: Box 677, Zip 39090–0677; tel. 601/289–4311; Thomas Bland, Administrator **A**9 10 **F**2 8 11 15 19 20 21 22 26 33 34 37 40 44 47 48 49 65 71
13 10 | 72 | 1924 | 38 | 19603 | 215 | 9394 | 3568 | 176

LAUREL—Jones County

✠ SOUTH CENTRAL REGIONAL MEDICAL CENTER, (Includes South Central Extended Care, Ivy Street, Ellisville, Zip 39437; tel. 601/477–9159), 1220 Jefferson, Zip 39440, Mailing Address: P.O. Box 607, Zip 39441; tel. 601/426–4000; G. Douglas Higginbotham, Executive Director (Total facility includes 40 beds in nursing home–type unit) **A**1 9 10 **F**2 7 8 11 14 15 16 17 19 20 21 22 23 24 26 32 33 34 35 37 39 40 41 42 44 45 46 48 49 52 57 63 64 65 66 67 70 71 73 74 **P**8
13 10 | 325 | 9100 | 178 | 67740 | 1045 | 49035 | 23501 | 1369

LEXINGTON—Holmes County

✠ METHODIST HOSPITAL OF MIDDLE MISSISSIPPI, 239 Bowling Green Road, Zip 39095–9332; tel. 601/834–1321; James K. Greer, Administrator **A**1 9 10 **F**7 8 19 21 22 27 34 40 44 46 65 71 73 **S** Methodist Health Systems, Inc., Memphis, TN **N** Methodist Health Systems, Inc., Memphis, TN
23 10 | 80 | 2438 | 39 | 15320 | 123 | — | | 142

LOUISVILLE—Winston County

□ WINSTON MEDICAL CENTER, (Formerly Winston County Community Hospital and Nursing Home), 562 East Main Street, Zip 39339, Mailing Address: Box 967, Zip 39339; tel. 601/773–6211; W. Dale Saulters, Administrator (Total facility includes 120 beds in nursing home–type unit) **A**1 9 10 **F**8 11 19 22 34 37 44 57 64 65 71 73
23 10 | 151 | 1369 | 143 | 18415 | 0 | — | | 144

LUCEDALE—George County

GEORGE COUNTY HOSPITAL, 859 South Winter Street, Zip 39452, Mailing Address: P.O. Box 607, Zip 39452; tel. 601/947–3161; Paul A. Gardner, CPA, Administrator **A**9 10 **F**8 11 15 16 19 21 22 34 37 40 44 49 65 71 73 **P**8
13 10 | 53 | 1956 | 25 | 26516 | 30 | — | | 231

MACON—Noxubee County

★ NOXUBEE GENERAL HOSPITAL, 606 North Jefferson Street, Zip 39341, Mailing Address: Box 480, Zip 39341; tel. 601/726–4231; Arthur Nester, Jr., Administrator (Total facility includes 60 beds in nursing home–type unit) **A**9 10 **F**2 8 9 11 15 19 20 22 27 31 34 37 38 40 44 47 48 52 64 65 70 73
13 10 | 109 | 821 | 71 | 5352 | 0 | 4824 | 2332 | 116

MAGEE—Simpson County

MAGEE GENERAL HOSPITAL, 300 S.E. Third Avenue, Zip 39111; tel. 601/849–5070; Althea H. Crumpton, Administrator **A**9 10 **F**19 21 22 31 34 44 65 71 73
23 10 | 64 | 2380 | 36 | 24118 | 1 | 8616 | 3418 | 169

MAGNOLIA—Pike County

BEACHAM MEMORIAL HOSPITAL, North Cherry Street, Zip 39652–0351; tel. 601/783–2351; Marilyn Speed, Administrator **A**9 10 **F**9 11 16 34 37 47 48 52 64 65 71
15 10 | 37 | 1248 | 24 | 42162 | 0 | — | | 86

MARKS—Quitman County

QUITMAN COUNTY HOSPITAL AND NURSING HOME, 340 Getwell Drive, Zip 38646–9785; tel. 601/326–8031; Richard E. Waller, M.D., Interim Administrator (Total facility includes 60 beds in nursing home–type unit) **A**9 10 **F**2 7 9 10 11 12 15 16 19 20 22 31 33 36 37 38 40 43 44 45 46 47 48 49 52 60 64 65 69 71 73
33 10 | 96 | 959 | 76 | 9612 | 0 | — | | 89

MCCOMB—Pike County

✠ SOUTHWEST MISSISSIPPI REGIONAL MEDICAL CENTER, 215 Marion Avenue, Zip 39648–2798, Mailing Address: P.O. Box 1307, Zip 39648–1307; tel. 601/249–5500; Norman M. Price, FACHE, Administrator **A**1 9 10 **F**1 7 8 10 11 14 15 16 17 19 20 21 22 32 34 35 37 40 44 45 46 48 49 63 64 65 67 70 71 73 74 **P**6
15 10 | 120 | 6825 | 93 | 53524 | 788 | 50191 | 21502 | 897

MEADVILLE—Franklin County

FRANKLIN COUNTY MEMORIAL HOSPITAL, Highway 84, Zip 39653, Mailing Address: Box 636, Zip 39653–0636; tel. 601/384–5801; Semmes Ross, Jr., Administrator **A**9 10 **F**1 2 3 7 8 9 10 11 12 15 16 17 19 20 21 22 23 24 26 27 31 32 33 34 35 36 37 38 39 40 41 42 43 44 45 46 47 48 49 51 52 53 54 55 56 57 58 59 60 61 65 66 67 68 69 71 72 74
13 10 | 40 | 685 | 19 | 15414 | 0 | 5721 | — | 116

MENDENHALL—Simpson County

SIMPSON GENERAL HOSPITAL, 931 Jackson Avenue, Zip 39114; tel. 601/847–2221; Wayne Harris, Administrator **A**9 10 **F**15 16 17 19 20 21 22 31 32 34 44 45 46 48 57 65 67 71 73 **P**5
13 10 | 49 | 1476 | 33 | 12499 | 1 | 8632 | 2917 | 147

MERIDIAN—Lauderdale County

EAST MISSISSIPPI STATE HOSPITAL, 4555 Highland Park Drive, Zip 39307, Mailing Address: Box 4128, West Station, Zip 39304–4128; tel. 601/482–6186; Ramiro J. Martinez, M.D., Director (Total facility includes 248 beds in nursing home–type unit) **F**2 12 14 15 16 20 26 46 52 53 57 64 65 73 **S** Mississippi State Department of Mental Health, Jackson, MS
12 22 | 655 | 1338 | 633 | 0 | 0 | 33640 | 25573 | 805

✠ JEFF ANDERSON REGIONAL MEDICAL CENTER, 2124 14th Street, Zip 39301; tel. 601/483–8811; Mark D. McPhail, Chief Executive Officer **A**1 9 10 **F**7 8 10 11 12 14 15 16 17 19 20 21 22 23 24 31 34 35 37 38 40 41 42 43 44 45 46 47 48 49 52 60 63 65 66 67 71 73 **P**7 8
23 10 | 260 | 8925 | 135 | 48750 | 890 | — | | 788

□ LAUREL WOOD CENTER, 5000 Highway 39 North, Zip 39303; tel. 601/483–6211; Barbara Friday, Administrator **A**1 10 **F**2 3 12 17 35 39 45 46 52 53 54 55 56 57 65 67 71 **P**6
33 22 | 79 | 872 | 31 | 0 | 0 | — | | 110

Hospital, Address, Telephone, Administrator, Approval, Facility, and Physician Codes, Health Care System, Network	Classi-fication Codes		Utilization Data					Expense (thousands) of dollars		
★ American Hospital Association (AHA) membership □ Joint Commission on Accreditation of Healthcare Organizations (JCAHO) accreditation + American Osteopathic Hospital Association (AOHA) membership ○ American Osteopathic Association (AOA) accreditation △ Commission on Accreditation of Rehabilitation Facilities (CARF) accreditation Control codes 61, 63, 64, 71, 72 and 73 indicate hospitals listed by AOHA, but not registered by AHA. For definition of numerical codes, see page A4	Control	Service	Beds	Admissions	Census	Outpatient Visits	Births	Total	Payroll	Personnel
✠ RILEY MEMORIAL HOSPITAL, 1102 21st Avenue, Zip 39301, Mailing Address: Box 1810, Zip 39302–1810; tel. 601/484–3590; Eric E. Weis, FACHE, Chief Executive Officer **A**1 9 10 **F**2 7 8 9 10 11 16 17 19 20 21 22 23 24 31 32 34 35 37 39 40 41 42 44 45 46 47 48 49 51 52 61 63 64 65 67 71 73 74 **P**7 8	23	10	180	6717	101	38101	250	—	—	687
✠ RUSH FOUNDATION HOSPITAL, 1314 19th Avenue, Zip 39301; tel. 601/483–0011; Wallace Strickland, Administrator **A**1 9 10 **F**7 8 10 11 12 15 16 17 19 20 22 23 32 33 35 37 38 40 41 42 44 45 46 49 51 60 64 65 66 67 71 72 73 74 **P**3 5 6 8	23	10	198	9185	139	20657	1218	64042	28242	1305
MONTICELLO—Lawrence County										
LAWRENCE COUNTY HOSPITAL, Highway 84 East, Zip 39654–0788, Mailing Address: Box 788, Zip 39654; tel. 601/587–4051; Deborah Roberts, Administrator **A**9 10 **F**2 9 11 17 20 21 22 32 37 38 45 46 52 65 71	13	10	53	1192	22	—	0	5700	2947	117
NATCHEZ—Adams County										
□ NATCHEZ COMMUNITY HOSPITAL, 129 Jefferson Davis Boulevard, Zip 39120, Mailing Address: Box 1203, Zip 39121; tel. 601/445–6200; Raymond Bane, Executive Director **A**1 9 10 **F**7 8 11 14 16 19 21 22 23 31 34 35 37 40 42 44 49 65 71 73 **P**1 8 **S** Health Management Associates, Naples, FL	33	10	101	3110	40	25115	538	15487	7157	254
✠ NATCHEZ REGIONAL MEDICAL CENTER, Seargent S Prentiss Drive, Zip 39120, Mailing Address: Box 1488, Zip 39121–1488; tel. 601/443–2100; David M. Snyder, Executive Director and Chief Executive Officer **A**1 9 10 **F**1 2 7 8 9 10 11 12 14 15 16 19 20 21 22 23 24 26 27 31 32 33 34 35 36 37 38 39 40 41 42 43 44 47 48 49 51 52 61 64 65 66 67 68 69 71 73 74 **S** Quorum Health Group/Quorum Health Resources, Inc., Brentwood, TN	13	10	121	4037	56	—	596	30312	13724	460
NEW ALBANY—Union County										
✠ BAPTIST MEMORIAL HOSPITAL–UNION COUNTY, 200 Highway 30 West, Zip 38652–3197; tel. 601/538–7631; John Tompkins, Administrator **A**1 9 10 **F**7 8 11 15 17 19 20 21 22 34 35 37 39 40 44 45 46 48 49 63 64 65 67 71 73 74 **S** Baptist Memorial Health Care Corporation, Memphis, TN	21	10	153	6140	64	34476	991	19228	7327	341
OCEAN SPRINGS—Jackson County										
□ OCEAN SPRINGS HOSPITAL, 3109 Bienville Boulevard, Zip 39564; tel. 601/872–1111; Dwight Rimes, Administrator **A**1 **F**2 3 7 8 10 11 12 14 15 16 17 19 20 21 22 23 27 31 32 33 34 35 37 39 40 41 42 43 44 47 48 52 53 54 55 56 57 63 64 65 67 71 **P**3 8 **S** Singing River Hospital System, Pascagoula, MS	13	10	95	4679	69	77838	331	—	—	473
OKOLONA—Chickasaw County										
★ OKOLONA COMMUNITY HOSPITAL, (Includes Shearer–Richardson Memorial Nursing Home), Rockwell Drive, Zip 38860–0420, Mailing Address: P.O. Box 420, Zip 38860–0420; tel. 601/447–3311; Allen J. Lockhart, Administrator (Total facility includes 66 beds in nursing home–type unit) **A**9 10 **F**2 20 23 31 32 33 35 60 64 65 71 73	13	10	76	194	70	0	0	—	—	44
OLIVE BRANCH—De Soto County										
□ CHARTER PARKWOOD BEHAVIORAL HEALTH SYSTEM, (Formerly Parkwood Hospital), 8135 Goodman Road, Zip 38654–2199; tel. 601/895–4900; Kevin E. Blackwell, Chief Executive Officer **A**1 9 10 **F**2 3 11 12 15 16 17 20 22 24 27 33 35 37 39 42 45 47 50 52 53 54 55 56 58 59 63 64 65 67 68 71 72 74	33	22	66	1149	38	0	0	—	—	103
OXFORD—Lafayette County										
✠ BAPTIST MEMORIAL HOSPITAL–NORTH MISSISSIPPI, 2301 South Lamar Boulevard, Zip 38655, Mailing Address: Box 946, Zip 38655; tel. 601/232–8100; James Hahn, Administrator **A**1 9 10 **F**7 8 10 11 12 14 15 16 17 19 20 21 22 24 31 32 33 34 35 37 40 41 42 43 44 45 46 47 48 52 64 65 66 67 71 72 73 74 **P**3 4 5 7 **S** Baptist Memorial Health Care Corporation, Memphis, TN	23	10	158	8942	134	46038	683	50222	15561	737
PASCAGOULA—Jackson County										
✠ SINGING RIVER HOSPITAL, 2809 Denny Avenue, Zip 39581; tel. 601/938–5000; James S. Kaigler, FACHE, Administrator **A**1 2 9 10 **F**2 3 7 8 10 11 12 14 15 16 17 19 20 21 22 23 27 31 32 33 34 35 37 39 40 41 42 43 44 47 48 52 53 54 55 56 57 63 64 65 67 71 **P**3 8 **S** Singing River Hospital System, Pascagoula, MS	13	10	314	11769	197	167399	882	133617	59171	1906
PHILADELPHIA—Neshoba County										
✠ CHOCTAW HEALTH CENTER, Highway 16 West, Zip 39350, Mailing Address: Route 7, Box R–50, Zip 39350; tel. 601/656–2211; Jim Wallace, Executive Director **A**1 10 **F**2 3 4 5 8 9 10 11 12 13 14 15 16 17 18 19 20 21 22 23 27 28 29 30 31 32 33 34 35 37 38 39 40 41 42 43 44 45 46 47 48 49 50 51 52 53 54 55 56 57 58 59 60 61 63 64 65 66 67 68 69 70 71 72 74 **P**6 8 **S** U. S. Public Health Service Indian Health Service, Rockville, MD	47	10	35	613	10	33603	0	—	—	—
NESHOBA COUNTY GENERAL HOSPITAL, 1001 Holland Avenue, Zip 39350, Mailing Address: P.O. Box 648, Zip 39350; tel. 601/663–1200; Lawrence Graeber, Administrator (Total facility includes 118 beds in nursing home–type unit) **A**9 10 **F**8 19 22 27 31 33 34 40 44 64 65 71 **P**8 **S** Quorum Health Group/Quorum Health Resources, Inc., Brentwood, TN	13	10	192	2116	144	27056	6	—	—	156
PICAYUNE—Pearl River County										
CROSBY MEMORIAL HOSPITAL, 801 Goodyear Boulevard, Zip 39466, Mailing Address: Box 909, Zip 39466; tel. 601/798–4711; Calvin Green, Administrator **A**9 10 **F**2 7 8 11 14 15 16 17 19 20 21 24 32 33 34 36 37 39 40 44 45 48 49 52 59 65 66 67 68 71 73 74 **P**8 **S** Quorum Health Group/Quorum Health Resources, Inc., Brentwood, TN	23	10	61	2583	33	34496	324	12373	5914	228

Hospital, Address, Telephone, Administrator, Approval, Facility, and Physician Codes, Health Care System, Network	Classi-fication Codes		Utilization Data					Expense (thousands) of dollars		
★ American Hospital Association (AHA) membership □ Joint Commission on Accreditation of Healthcare Organizations (JCAHO) accreditation + American Osteopathic Hospital Association (AOHA) membership ○ American Osteopathic Association (AOA) accreditation △ Commission on Accreditation of Rehabilitation Facilities (CARF) accreditation Control codes 61, 63, 64, 71, 72 and 73 indicate hospitals listed by AOHA, but not registered by AHA. For definition of numerical codes, see page A4	Control	Service	Beds	Admissions	Census	Outpatient Visits	Births	Total	Payroll	Personnel

PONTOTOC—Pontotoc County

PONTOTOC HOSPITAL AND EXTENDED CARE FACILITY, 176 South Main Street, Zip 38863, Mailing Address: P.O. Box C, Zip 38863; tel. 601/489–5510; Fred B. Hood, Administrator (Total facility includes 44 beds in nursing home–type unit) **A**9 10 **F**8 14 15 16 17 20 22 27 32 33 34 36 39 45 46 48 49 64 65 67 71 73 **P**3 8 **S** North Mississippi Health Services, Inc., Tupelo, MS **N** North Mississippi Health Services, Tupelo, MS

| 23 | 10 | 71 | 737 | 60 | 13573 | 0 | 6810 | 3051 | 99 |

POPLARVILLE—Pearl River County

PEARL RIVER COUNTY HOSPITAL, West Moody Street, Zip 39470, Mailing Address: Box 392, Zip 39470; tel. 601/795–4543; Dorothy C. Bilbo, Acting Administrator (Total facility includes 66 beds in nursing home–type unit) **A**9 10 **F**15 16 34 46 48 49 64 65 73

| 13 | 10 | 90 | 670 | 74 | 0 | 0 | — | — | 85 |

PORT GIBSON—Claiborne County

★ CLAIBORNE COUNTY HOSPITAL, 123 McComb Avenue, Zip 39150, Mailing Address: P.O. Box 1004, Zip 39150; tel. 601/437–5141; Wanda C. Fleming, Administrator **A**9 10 **F**12 16 17 19 22 35 39 40 45 46 52 64 65 71 73

| 13 | 10 | 32 | 776 | 15 | — | 50 | — | — | 53 |

PRENTISS—Jefferson Davis County

JEFFERSON DAVIS COUNTY HOSPITAL, Berry Street, Zip 39474, Mailing Address: P.O. Box 1288, Zip 39474; tel. 601/792–4276; Paul W. Strode, Jr., Administrator (Total facility includes 60 beds in nursing home–type unit) **A**9 10 **F**11 22 34 64 71

| 13 | 10 | 101 | 660 | 68 | 8036 | 0 | 4531 | 2004 | 125 |

QUITMAN—Clarke County

★ H. C. WATKINS MEMORIAL HOSPITAL, 605 South Archusa Avenue, Zip 39355–2398; tel. 601/776–6925; Thomas G. Bartlett, President and Chief Executive Officer (Total facility includes 11 beds in nursing home–type unit) **A**9 10 **F**2 8 11 12 19 20 21 22 31 32 33 34 35 37 44 49 52 64 65 71 **S** Quorum Health Group/Quorum Health Resources, Inc., Brentwood, TN

| 23 | 10 | 43 | 1274 | 38 | 6684 | 0 | | — | 119 |

RICHTON—Perry County

★ PERRY COUNTY GENERAL HOSPITAL, 206 Bay Street, Zip 39476, Mailing Address: Drawer Y, Zip 39476; tel. 601/788–6316; L. K. Peters, Administrator (Total facility includes 66 beds in nursing home–type unit) **A**9 10 **F**22 32 44 49 64 71

| 13 | 10 | 88 | 644 | 67 | — | 0 | — | — | 74 |

RIPLEY—Tippah County

✠ TIPPAH COUNTY HOSPITAL, 1005 City Avenue North, Zip 38663–0499; tel. 601/837–9221; Jerry Green, Administrator (Total facility includes 40 beds in nursing home–type unit) **A**1 9 10 **F**8 11 15 16 19 21 22 27 31 34 37 44 64 65 71 **S** Baptist Memorial Health Care Corporation, Memphis, TN

| 13 | 10 | 110 | 1583 | 59 | 17456 | 0 | 7930 | 4033 | 161 |

RULEVILLE—Sunflower County

NORTH SUNFLOWER COUNTY HOSPITAL, 840 North Oak Avenue, Zip 38771–0369, Mailing Address: P.O. Box 369, Zip 38771–0369; tel. 601/756–2711; Robert Crook, Administrator (Total facility includes 42 beds in nursing home–type unit) **A**9 10 **F**2 15 16 22 26 32 33 34 40 44 54 59 64 65 71 **P**1

| 13 | 10 | 86 | 1391 | 66 | 5670 | 24 | 5698 | 2859 | 160 |

SENATOBIA—Tate County

□ SENATOBIA COMMUNITY HOSPITAL, 401 Getwell Drive, Zip 38668, Mailing Address: P.O. Box 648, Zip 38668; tel. 601/562–3100; James D. Tesar, Administrator **A**1 9 10 **F**7 8 12 19 20 22 31 33 34 40 44 45 46 52 57 65 71 **S** Paracelsus Healthcare Corporation, Houston, TX

| 33 | 10 | 52 | 1194 | 15 | 15141 | 189 | 7567 | 2685 | 120 |

SOUTHAVEN—De Soto County

✠ △ BAPTIST MEMORIAL HOSPITAL–DESOTO, 7601 Southcrest Parkway, Zip 38671; tel. 601/349–4000; Melvin E. Walker, Administrator (Total facility includes 60 beds in nursing home–type unit) **A**1 7 9 10 **F**2 7 8 10 11 12 15 16 17 19 20 21 22 23 24 26 31 32 33 34 35 37 38 39 40 41 42 43 44 45 46 48 49 51 52 60 64 65 66 67 69 71 72 73 74 **P**1 8 **S** Baptist Memorial Health Care Corporation, Memphis, TN

| 23 | 10 | 200 | 5687 | 97 | 37897 | 854 | 33976 | 11974 | 402 |

STARKVILLE—Oktibbeha County

✠ OKTIBBEHA COUNTY HOSPITAL, 400 Hospital Road, Zip 39759, Mailing Address: Drawer 1506, Zip 39760; tel. 601/323–4320; Arthur C. Kelly, Administrator and Chief Executive Officer **A**1 9 10 **F**7 8 11 12 14 15 16 17 19 20 21 22 24 31 33 34 35 37 40 41 44 46 47 49 52 63 65 66 67 69 71 73

| 13 | 10 | 96 | 3634 | 42 | 49874 | 1111 | 20365 | 10340 | 478 |

TUPELO—Lee County

✠ △ NORTH MISSISSIPPI MEDICAL CENTER, 830 South Gloster Street, Zip 38801–4934; tel. 601/841–3000; Jeffrey B. Barber, Dr.PH, President and Chief Executive Officer (Total facility includes 91 beds in nursing home–type unit) **A**1 2 5 7 9 10 **F**2 3 7 8 10 11 12 14 15 16 17 19 21 22 23 24 26 32 33 34 35 37 38 39 40 41 42 43 44 45 46 47 48 49 51 52 53 55 57 58 59 60 63 64 65 66 67 71 73 74 **P**3 6 **S** North Mississippi Health Services, Inc., Tupelo, MS **N** North Mississippi Health Services, Tupelo, MS

| 23 | 10 | 715 | 26638 | 538 | 559053 | 2335 | 208357 | 90971 | 3337 |

TYLERTOWN—Walthall County

WALTHALL COUNTY GENERAL HOSPITAL, 100 Hospital Drive, Zip 39667; tel. 601/876–2122; Jimmy Graves, Administrator **A**9 10 **F**8 12 15 20 22 26 34 44 46 52 57 71 73

| 13 | 10 | 49 | 1701 | 30 | 15551 | 0 | 7518 | 3278 | 124 |

UNION—Newton County

LAIRD HOSPITAL, 25117 Highway 15, Zip 39365; tel. 601/774–8214; James P. Franklin, Executive Director **A**9 10 **F**19 21 22 24 32 33 34 35 37 44 46 65 71 73

| 33 | 10 | 50 | 1851 | 28 | — | 5 | 20176 | 10716 | 433 |

Hospital, Address, Telephone, Administrator, Approval, Facility, and Physician Codes, Health Care System, Network	Classi-fication Codes		Utilization Data					Expense (thousands) of dollars		
★ American Hospital Association (AHA) membership ☐ Joint Commission on Accreditation of Healthcare Organizations (JCAHO) accreditation + American Osteopathic Hospital Association (AOHA) membership ○ American Osteopathic Association (AOA) accreditation △ Commission on Accreditation of Rehabilitation Facilities (CARF) accreditation Control codes 61, 63, 64, 71, 72 and 73 indicate hospitals listed by AOHA, but not registered by AHA. For definition of numerical codes, see page A4	Control	Service	Beds	Admissions	Census	Outpatient Visits	Births	Total	Payroll	Personnel

VICKSBURG—Warren County

☒ COLUMBIA VICKSBURG MEDICAL CENTER, 1111 Frontage Road, Zip 39181–5298; tel. 601/636–2611; William M. Patterson, Administrator **A**1 9 10 **F**7 8 11 12 14 16 17 19 20 21 22 23 31 35 37 39 40 41 44 45 46 47 48 49 51 54 56 57 64 65 67 71 73 **P**6 **S** Columbia/HCA Healthcare Corporation, Nashville, TN	33	10	154	5563	108	32404	353	24387	8786	410
☒ PARKVIEW REGIONAL MEDICAL CENTER, 100 McAuley Drive, Zip 39180–2897, Mailing Address: P.O. Box 590, Zip 39181–0590; tel. 601/631–2131; Charles Mitchener, Jr., Chief Operating Officer and Administrator (Total facility includes 14 beds in nursing home–type unit) **A**1 2 9 10 **F**2 7 8 11 12 19 21 22 23 24 32 34 35 37 39 40 41 44 45 49 52 57 60 64 65 66 67 71 72 73 **P**2 6 **S** Quorum Health Group/Quorum Health Resources, Inc., Brentwood, TN	33	10	197	4755	119	79831	1004	31910	13805	486

WATER VALLEY—Yalobusha County

YALOBUSHA GENERAL HOSPITAL, Highway 7 South, Zip 38965, Mailing Address: Box 728, Zip 38965–0728; tel. 601/473–1411; Edward B. Gilliland, Interim Administrator (Total facility includes 59 beds in nursing home–type unit) **A**9 10 **F**12 14 19 20 39 41 44 64 65 71 **P**4	13	10	91	703	68	—	0	—	—	85

WAYNESBORO—Wayne County

WAYNE GENERAL HOSPITAL, 950 Matthew Drive, Zip 39367, Mailing Address: Box 1249, Zip 39367; tel. 601/735–5151; Donald Hemeter, Administrator **A**9 10 **F**7 8 15 17 19 20 21 22 24 31 32 33 37 40 44 45 47 60 63 65 71 73	13	10	80	3699	51	27889	322	—	—	321

WEST POINT—Clay County

CLAY COUNTY MEDICAL CENTER, 835 Medical Center Drive, Zip 39773; tel. 601/495–2300; David M. Reid, Administrator **A**9 10 **F**7 8 11 15 16 17 19 20 21 22 24 33 34 37 39 40 42 44 45 46 48 49 51 61 65 66 67 71 73 74 **S** North Mississippi Health Services, Inc., Tupelo, MS **N** North Mississippi Health Services, Tupelo, MS	23	10	60	2729	37	21248	371	12292	5327	216

WHITFIELD—Rankin County

★ MISSISSIPPI STATE HOSPITAL, Mailing Address: P.O. Box 157–A, Zip 39193–0157; tel. 601/351–8000; James G. Chastain, Director (Total facility includes 457 beds in nursing home–type unit) **A**9 **F**2 7 8 9 10 11 12 15 19 20 21 22 23 27 31 34 35 37 38 40 42 43 44 45 46 47 48 49 52 53 54 55 56 57 58 59 60 61 64 65 69 73 74 **P**1 **S** Mississippi State Department of Mental Health, Jackson, MS	12	22	1303	1559	1222	6059	0	79988	42214	2075
☐ WHITFIELD MEDICAL SURGICAL HOSPITAL, Zip 39193; tel. 601/351–8023; James I. Morton, FACHE, Administrator and Chief Executive Officer **A**1 9 10 **F**1 2 7 8 9 10 11 12 19 20 21 22 23 24 26 27 31 32 33 34 35 36 37 38 39 40 41 42 43 44 45 47 48 49 50 51 52 60 61 63 64 65 66 67 68 69 70 71 72 73 74	12	10	43	450	13	4347	0	—	—	95

WINONA—Montgomery County

TYLER HOLMES MEMORIAL HOSPITAL, Tyler Holmes Drive, Zip 38967–1599; tel. 601/283–4114; Gary C. Morse, Administrator **A**9 10 **F**1 15 16 17 19 20 21 22 26 27 32 34 36 40 41 44 46 49 52 57 59 61 65 71 **P**8	13	10	49	1530	30	14637	46	7556	2808	149

YAZOO CITY—Yazoo County

KING'S DAUGHTERS HOSPITAL, 823 Grand Avenue, Zip 39194–0329, Mailing Address: Box 329, Zip 39194–0329; tel. 601/746–2261; Noel W. Hart, Administrator **A**9 10 **F**8 11 14 16 19 20 22 24 31 33 34 37 44 46 59 65 71 73	23	10	54	1777	31	38345	0	9349	3335	164

MISSOURI

Resident population 5,324 (in thousands)
Resident population in metro areas 68.1%
Birth rate per 1,000 population 14.4
65 years and over 13.9%
Percent of persons without health insurance 12.2%

Hospital, Address, Telephone, Administrator, Approval, Facility, and Physician Codes, Health Care System, Network	Classi-fication Codes		Utilization Data					Expense (thousands) of dollars		
★ American Hospital Association (AHA) membership □ Joint Commission on Accreditation of Healthcare Organizations (JCAHO) accreditation + American Osteopathic Hospital Association (AOHA) membership ○ American Osteopathic Association (AOA) accreditation △ Commission on Accreditation of Rehabilitation Facilities (CARF) accreditation Control codes 61, 63, 64, 71, 72 and 73 indicate hospitals listed by AOHA, but not registered by AHA. For definition of numerical codes, see page A4	Control	Service	Beds	Admissions	Census	Outpatient Visits	Births	Total	Payroll	Personnel

ALBANY—Gentry County

★ GENTRY COUNTY MEMORIAL HOSPITAL, Clark and College Streets, Zip 64402–1499; tel. 816/726–3941; John W. Richmond, President and Chief Executive Officer (Total facility includes 10 beds in nursing home–type unit) **A**9 10 **F**8 11 12 14 15 16 17 19 22 23 26 27 28 29 30 31 32 33 34 35 37 39 41 42 44 46 48 49 51 63 64 65 66 67 71 73 74 **P**5

| | 23 | 10 | 35 | 864 | 17 | 33159 | 0 | 5858 | 2832 | 104 |

APPLETON CITY—St. Clair County

ELLETT MEMORIAL HOSPITAL, 610 North Ohio Avenue, Zip 64724; tel. 816/476–2111; Sandy Morlan, Administrator **A**9 10 **F**15 16 19 22 29 35 41 44 48 49 65 71

| | 16 | 10 | 25 | 361 | 4 | 1726 | 0 | 1387 | 694 | 40 |

AURORA—Lawrence County

AURORA COMMUNITY HOSPITAL, 500 Porter Street, Zip 65605; tel. 417/678–2122; Don Buchanan, Chief Operating Officer **A**9 10 **F**7 8 11 12 14 17 19 22 24 26 27 28 29 30 32 34 36 37 39 40 41 44 45 46 49 51 64 65 70 71 73 **P**6

| | 14 | 10 | 38 | 1745 | 20 | 20348 | 225 | 9671 | 5101 | 189 |

BELTON—Cass County

★ RESEARCH BELTON HOSPITAL, 17065 South 71 Highway, Zip 64012; tel. 816/348–1200; Daniel F. Sheehan, Administrator (Total facility includes 7 beds in nursing home–type unit) **A**9 **F**1 2 3 4 5 6 7 8 9 10 11 12 13 14 15 16 17 18 19 20 21 22 24 26 28 29 30 31 32 33 34 35 37 38 40 41 42 43 44 46 47 48 49 52 53 54 55 56 57 58 59 60 61 63 64 65 69 70 71 73 74 **P**1 **S** Health Midwest, Kansas City, MO **N** Health Midwest, Kansas City, MO

| | 23 | 10 | 47 | 1459 | 22 | 46027 | 1 | 13104 | 5070 | 124 |

BETHANY—Harrison County

HARRISON COUNTY COMMUNITY HOSPITAL, Highway 69 and 136, Zip 64424, Mailing Address: P.O. Box 428, Zip 64424–0428; tel. 816/425–2211; Dan P. Broyles, Administrator **A**9 10 **F**8 13 14 19 20 21 22 26 27 28 29 30 31 32 33 34 36 37 39 41 42 44 46 49 60 62 64 65 66 67 68 71 73 74 **P**4 5

| | 16 | 10 | 23 | 722 | 8 | 19611 | 0 | 4141 | 1613 | 77 |

BLUE SPRINGS—Jackson County

⊠ △ ST. MARY'S HOSPITAL OF BLUE SPRINGS, 201 West R. D. Mize Road, Zip 64014; tel. 816/228–5900; N. Gary Wages, President and Chief Executive Officer (Total facility includes 10 beds in nursing home–type unit) **A**1 7 9 10 **F**4 7 8 10 12 15 17 19 20 21 22 24 25 26 28 29 30 31 32 33 34 35 37 39 40 41 42 43 44 45 46 48 49 60 63 64 65 66 67 71 72 73 **P**6 7 **S** Carondelet Health System, Saint Louis, MO **N** Carondelet Health, Kansas City, MO

| | 23 | 10 | 102 | 4218 | 60 | 38060 | 824 | 46029 | 20485 | 576 |

BOLIVAR—Polk County

⊠ CITIZENS MEMORIAL HOSPITAL, 1500 North Oakland, Zip 65613–3099; tel. 417/326–6000; Donald J. Babb, Chief Executive Officer **A**1 9 10 **F**7 8 14 15 16 17 19 21 22 26 27 28 29 30 31 32 33 34 35 37 39 40 41 42 44 46 48 49 52 56 57 58 64 65 70 71 73 74 **P**6

| | 16 | 10 | 74 | 2786 | 33 | 27130 | 357 | 29077 | 13272 | 475 |

BONNE TERRE—St. Francois County

BONNE TERRE HOSPITAL See Parkland Health Center, Farmington

PARKLAND HEALTH CENTER–BONNE TERRE See Parkland Health Center, Farmington

BOONVILLE—Cooper County

⊠ COOPER COUNTY MEMORIAL HOSPITAL, 17651 B Highway, Zip 65233, Mailing Address: P.O. Box 88, Zip 65233; tel. 816/882–7461; Wilbert E. Meyer, Administrator (Total facility includes 24 beds in nursing home–type unit) **A**1 9 10 **F**8 12 15 16 17 19 20 22 27 28 29 30 32 34 35 39 41 44 49 54 64 65 67 71 73

| | 13 | 10 | 49 | 717 | 29 | 16183 | 0 | 6723 | 3322 | 152 |

BRANSON—Taney County

⊠ SKAGGS COMMUNITY HEALTH CENTER, (Formerly Skaggs Community Hospital), Business Highway 65 & Skaggs Road, Zip 65616–2035, Mailing Address: P.O. Box 650, Zip 65616–0650; tel. 417/335–7000; Bob Phillips, Administrator (Total facility includes 23 beds in nursing home–type unit) **A**1 9 10 **F**7 8 15 16 17 19 20 22 23 25 26 27 28 29 30 31 32 33 34 35 37 39 40 41 42 44 49 51 64 65 66 67 70 71 72 **P**8

| | 23 | 10 | 99 | 4209 | 55 | 245213 | 425 | 32310 | 14181 | 534 |

BRIDGETON—St. Louis County

ST. VINCENT'S PSYCHIATRIC DIVISION See DePaul Health Center, Saint Louis

BROOKFIELD—Linn County

□ GENERAL JOHN J. PERSHING MEMORIAL HOSPITAL, 130 East Lockling Avenue, Zip 64628–0130, Mailing Address: P.O. Box 408, Zip 64628–0408; tel. 816/258–2222; Phil Hamilton, R.N., Chief Executive Officer **A**1 9 10 **F**7 8 12 14 17 19 22 24 28 29 30 31 32 33 35 39 40 42 44 46 49 51 65 71 73

| | 23 | 10 | 34 | 1162 | 10 | 46141 | 24 | 9407 | 4675 | 181 |

BUTLER—Bates County

BATES COUNTY MEMORIAL HOSPITAL, 615 West Nursery Street, Zip 64730–0370; tel. 816/679–4381; Bob S. Edwards, Jr., Chief Executive Officer (Total facility includes 9 beds in nursing home–type unit) **A**9 10 **F**7 8 19 20 21 22 28 29 30 32 33 34 37 39 40 41 42 44 46 49 54 64 65 67 71 73

| | 13 | 10 | 32 | 1578 | 23 | 16594 | 26 | 8874 | 3746 | 143 |

CAMERON—Clinton County

CAMERON COMMUNITY HOSPITAL, 1015 West Fourth Street, Zip 64429–1498; tel. 816/632–2101; Joseph F. Abrutz, Jr., Administrator **A**9 10 **F**8 11 12 14 15 16 19 20 21 22 24 26 27 28 29 30 31 32 33 34 35 37 39 42 44 45 46 49 54 58 64 65 66 67 71 73 **P**6

| | 23 | 10 | 38 | 1354 | 17 | 23894 | 0 | 12178 | 6442 | 265 |

Hospital, Address, Telephone, Administrator, Approval, Facility, and Physician Codes, Health Care System, Network	Classi-fication Codes		Utilization Data					Expense (thousands) of dollars		
	Control	Service	Beds	Admissions	Census	Outpatient Visits	Births	Total	Payroll	Personnel

★ American Hospital Association (AHA) membership
□ Joint Commission on Accreditation of Healthcare Organizations (JCAHO) accreditation
+ American Osteopathic Hospital Association (AOHA) membership
○ American Osteopathic Association (AOA) accreditation
△ Commission on Accreditation of Rehabilitation Facilities (CARF) accreditation
Control codes 61, 63, 64, 71, 72 and 73 indicate hospitals listed by AOHA, but not registered by AHA. For definition of numerical codes, see page A4

CAPE GIRARDEAU—Cape Girardeau County

✠ △ SAINT FRANCIS MEDICAL CENTER, 211 St. Francis Drive, Zip 63703; tel. 573/335–1251; James J. Sexton, President and Chief Executive Officer (Total facility includes 26 beds in nursing home–type unit) **A**1 2 7 10 **F**3 4 5 8 10 11 12 13 14 15 16 17 19 21 22 23 24 27 28 29 30 31 32 33 35 37 39 41 42 43 44 45 46 47 48 49 63 64 65 66 67 71 73 74 **P**8	23	10	264	7340	134	52735	0	78932	33929	1131
✠ SOUTHEAST MISSOURI HOSPITAL, 1701 Lacey Street, Zip 63701; tel. 573/334–4822; James W. Wente, CPA, CHE, Administrator (Total facility includes 10 beds in nursing home–type unit) **A**1 2 6 10 **F**2 3 4 5 7 8 10 11 12 13 14 15 16 17 18 19 20 21 22 23 24 25 27 28 29 30 31 32 33 34 35 36 37 38 39 40 41 42 43 44 46 47 48 49 52 54 55 56 57 60 63 64 65 66 67 68 70 71 73 74 **P**8	23	10	254	9361	133	108539	1486	82022	32616	1230

CARROLLTON—Carroll County

CARROLL COUNTY MEMORIAL HOSPITAL, 1502 North Jefferson Street, Zip 64633; tel. 816/542–1695; Jack L. Tindle, Chief Executive Officer **A**9 10 **F**8 15 19 22 29 32 34 41 42 44 46 71	23	10	49	444	37	14841	0	2966	1469	69

CARTHAGE—Jasper County

★ MCCUNE–BROOKS HOSPITAL, 627 West Centennial Avenue, Zip 64836–0677; tel. 417/358–8121; James W. McPheeters, III, Administrator (Total facility includes 7 beds in nursing home–type unit) **A**9 10 **F**8 19 21 22 28 29 30 32 33 35 36 37 39 44 49 52 57 64 65 66 67 71 **N** Carondelet Health, Kansas City, MO	14	10	70	1980	38	40996	0	15991	7093	307

CASSVILLE—Barry County

SOUTH BARRY COUNTY MEMORIAL HOSPITAL, 94 Main Street, Zip 65625; tel. 417/847–4115; Deborah Stubbs, Chief Executive Officer **A**9 10 **F**8 12 19 22 24 28 29 30 32 33 34 39 41 44 46 49 51 64 65 71 **P**1 5	16	10	18	633	7	29834	0	6226	2557	127

CHESTERFIELD—St. Louis County

✠ ST. LUKE'S HOSPITAL, 232 South Woods Mill Road, Zip 63017–3480; tel. 314/434–1500; George Tucker, M.D., President (Total facility includes 126 beds in nursing home–type unit) **A**1 2 3 5 9 10 **F**2 3 4 5 6 7 8 9 10 11 12 13 14 15 16 17 18 19 20 21 22 23 24 25 26 27 28 29 30 31 32 33 34 35 36 37 38 39 40 41 42 43 44 45 46 47 48 49 51 52 53 54 55 56 57 58 59 60 61 62 63 64 65 66 67 68 69 70 71 72 73 74 **P**7 8 **S** Sisters of Mercy Health System–St. Louis, Saint Louis, MO **N** Unity Health System, St. Louis, MO	23	10	495	17630	313	125846	2849	176101	87102	1872

CHILLICOTHE—Livingston County

✠ HEDRICK MEDICAL CENTER, 100 Central Avenue, Zip 64601–1599; tel. 816/646–1480; R. Lynn Jackson, Chief Executive Officer **A**1 9 10 **F**7 8 12 14 15 16 17 18 19 22 28 29 30 32 33 34 35 36 37 39 40 41 42 44 45 46 55 58 64 65 67 71 73 **N** BJC Health System, St. Louis, MO; Health Midwest, Kansas City, MO	23	10	80	1885	25	26732	457	14434	6371	191

CLINTON—Henry County

✠ GOLDEN VALLEY MEMORIAL HOSPITAL, 1600 North Second Street, Zip 64735–1197; tel. 816/885–5511; Randy S. Wertz, Administrator (Total facility includes 12 beds in nursing home–type unit) **A**1 9 10 **F**7 8 14 15 17 19 21 22 28 29 30 31 32 33 35 37 39 40 41 42 44 49 52 53 54 55 56 57 58 59 63 64 65 66 67 71 72 73 74	16	10	108	3738	54	11374	367	23167	10517	390

COLUMBIA—Boone County

✠ BOONE HOSPITAL CENTER, 1600 East Broadway, Zip 65201; tel. 573/815–8000; Michael Shirk, President and Senior Executive Officer (Total facility includes 29 beds in nursing home–type unit) **A**1 2 3 5 9 10 **F**4 7 8 10 12 14 15 16 17 19 21 22 24 25 26 28 29 30 31 34 35 37 38 39 40 41 42 43 44 45 46 48 49 52 54 55 56 57 58 59 60 63 64 65 67 69 71 72 73 74 **P**3 5 8 **S** BJC Health System, Saint Louis, MO **N** BJC Health System, St. Louis, MO	23	10	307	12223	191	80405	1206	111899	43722	1197
□ △ COLUMBIA REGIONAL HOSPITAL, 404 Keene Street, Zip 65201–6698; tel. 573/875–9000; Thomas G. Neff, Chief Executive Officer **A**1 2 3 5 7 9 10 **F**4 8 10 12 15 16 18 19 20 22 23 26 28 29 30 31 32 33 34 35 37 39 40 41 42 44 46 48 49 50 52 57 60 63 64 65 66 67 69 71 72 73 74 **P**4 7 8 **S** TENET Healthcare Corporation, Santa Barbara, CA	33	10	265	4922	106	96700	30	62387	22453	806
ELLIS FISCHEL CANCER CENTER, 115 Business Loop 70 West, Zip 65203; tel. 573/882–5460; Keith Weinhold, Director (Nonreporting) **A**2 5	12	49	48	—	—	—	—	—	—	—
✠ HARRY S. TRUMAN MEMORIAL VETERANS HOSPITAL, 800 Hospital Drive, Zip 65201–5297; tel. 573/443–2511; Gary L. Campbell, Director (Total facility includes 44 beds in nursing home–type unit) **A**1 3 5 8 **F**1 2 3 4 5 8 10 11 12 19 20 21 22 26 27 29 30 31 32 33 34 35 37 39 41 42 43 44 45 46 48 49 51 52 54 55 56 57 58 60 63 64 65 67 71 73 74 **P**6 **S** Department of Veterans Affairs, Washington, DC	45	10	230	5946	183	109453	0	—	—	953
□ MID MISSOURI MENTAL HEALTH CENTER, 3 Hospital Drive, Zip 65201; tel. 573/449–2511; Mark Stansberry, Superintendent **A**1 3 5 10 **F**14 15 16 29 52 53 54 55 56 57 58 59 **P**6	12	22	69	1482	55	7873	0	13884	6631	241
□ △ UNIVERSITY HOSPITALS AND CLINICS, (Formerly University & Childrens Hospitals), One Hospital Drive, Zip 65212; tel. 573/882–3737; Patsy J. Hart, Director **A**1 3 5 7 8 9 10 **F**2 4 5 7 8 9 10 11 12 13 15 17 19 20 21 22 23 24 25 26 28 29 30 31 32 34 35 37 38 39 40 41 42 43 44 45 46 47 48 49 51 52 53 54 55 56 57 58 59 60 61 63 65 66 67 68 69 70 71 72 73 74 **P**1	12	10	426	13833	259	407318	1768	213712	94245	3256

CREVE COEUR—St. Louis County

BARNES–JEWISH WEST COUNTY HOSPITAL See Saint Louis

Hospital, Address, Telephone, Administrator, Approval, Facility, and Physician Codes, Health Care System, Network	Classi-fication Codes		Utilization Data					Expense (thousands) of dollars		
	Control	Service	Beds	Admissions	Census	Outpatient Visits	Births	Total	Payroll	Personnel

★ American Hospital Association (AHA) membership
□ Joint Commission on Accreditation of Healthcare Organizations (JCAHO) accreditation
+ American Osteopathic Hospital Association (AOHA) membership
○ American Osteopathic Association (AOA) accreditation
△ Commission on Accreditation of Rehabilitation Facilities (CARF) accreditation
Control codes 61, 63, 64, 71, 72 and 73 indicate hospitals listed by AOHA, but not registered by AHA. For definition of numerical codes, see page A4

CRYSTAL CITY—Jefferson County

□ JEFFERSON MEMORIAL HOSPITAL, Highway 61 South, Zip 63019, Mailing Address: P.O. Box 350, Zip 63019–0350; tel. 314/933–1000; Richard Johansen, Chief Operating Officer and Interim Chief Executive Officer (Total facility includes 28 beds in nursing home–type unit) **A**1 9 10 **F**2 3 7 8 10 11 12 15 16 17 19 21 22 23 25 27 28 29 30 31 32 33 34 35 37 39 40 41 44 46 48 49 52 53 54 55 56 57 58 62 64 65 66 67 71 72 73 **N** BJC Health System, St. Louis, MO | 23 | 10 | 236 | 6889 | 116 | 74289 | 705 | 55331 | 26687 | 887

DEXTER—Stoddard County

□ DEXTER MEMORIAL HOSPITAL, 1200 North One Mile Road, Zip 63841–1099; tel. 573/624–5566; Randal Tennison, Administrator **A**1 9 10 **F**8 11 14 15 19 20 22 25 26 28 29 30 31 32 33 34 37 39 44 45 48 49 51 63 64 65 67 71 73 **P**1 | 23 | 10 | 50 | 935 | 12 | 28642 | 0 | 9053 | 4711 | 178

DONIPHAN—Ripley County

RIPLEY COUNTY MEMORIAL HOSPITAL, 109 Plum Street, Zip 63935; tel. 573/996–2141; Charles Ray Freeman, Administrator **A**9 10 **F**8 15 17 19 22 28 29 30 32 33 34 41 44 45 46 51 53 54 55 57 71 | 13 | 10 | 26 | 605 | 10 | 6121 | 0 | 3093 | 1647 | 81

EL DORADO SPRINGS—Cedar County

CEDAR COUNTY MEMORIAL HOSPITAL, 1401 South Park Street, Zip 64744; tel. 417/876–2511; Jackie Boyles, Administrator **A**9 10 **F**7 8 14 15 16 19 22 28 29 30 31 32 40 41 46 49 64 65 71 73 | 13 | 10 | 34 | 881 | 10 | 6402 | 73 | 5067 | 2701 | 110

ELLINGTON—Reynolds County

REYNOLDS COUNTY GENERAL MEMORIAL HOSPITAL, Highway 21 South, Zip 63638, Mailing Address: P.O. Box 520, Zip 63638; tel. 573/663–2511; Patricia Koppeis, Administrator **A**9 10 **F**8 22 28 29 30 32 34 49 51 **N** BJC Health System, St. Louis, MO | 16 | 10 | 29 | 185 | 2 | 4867 | 0 | 2153 | 862 | 41

EXCELSIOR SPRINGS—Clay County

□ EXCELSIOR SPRINGS MEDICAL CENTER, 1700 Rainbow Boulevard, Zip 64024–1190; tel. 816/630–6081; Sally S. Pannell, Chief Executive Officer (Total facility includes 80 beds in nursing home–type unit) **A**1 9 10 **F**6 8 12 14 15 16 17 19 22 26 28 29 30 32 33 34 35 36 37 39 42 44 46 49 51 64 65 67 71 73 | 14 | 10 | 105 | 818 | 69 | 16554 | 0 | 10299 | 5134 | 145

FAIRFAX—Atchison County

COMMUNITY HOSPITAL ASSOCIATION, Highway 59, Zip 64446–0107; tel. 816/686–2211; Larry S. Goodloe, Administrator **A**9 10 **F**7 8 11 19 20 22 29 30 32 34 35 40 42 44 46 49 58 64 65 71 | 23 | 10 | 44 | 883 | 20 | 10436 | 64 | 6384 | — | 117

FARMINGTON—St. Francois County

+ ○ MINERAL AREA REGIONAL MEDICAL CENTER, 1212 Weber Road, Zip 63640; tel. 573/756–4581; Kenneth C. West, Chief Executive Officer **A**9 10 11 12 13 **F**1 2 3 7 8 16 17 18 19 20 22 28 29 30 31 32 35 37 39 40 42 44 46 49 53 54 56 57 58 59 65 67 70 71 73 **P**6 8 **N** Saint Louis Health Care Network, St. Louis, MO | 23 | 10 | 123 | 4203 | 52 | 94480 | 470 | 28870 | 12520 | 500

⊞ PARKLAND HEALTH CENTER, (Includes Parkland Health Center–Bonne Terre, 7245 Vo–Tech Road, Bonne Terre, Zip 63628; tel. 573/358–1400), 1101 West Liberty Street, Zip 63640–1997; tel. 314/756–6451; Richard L. Conklin, President **A**1 9 10 **F**7 8 14 15 16 19 20 22 28 29 30 32 34 35 36 37 39 40 41 42 44 46 49 51 63 65 69 71 73 **P**5 **S** BJC Health System, Saint Louis, MO **N** BJC Health System, St. Louis, MO | 23 | 10 | 94 | 3120 | 37 | 66052 | 368 | 26508 | 11835 | 385

□ SOUTHEAST MISSOURI MENTAL HEALTH CENTER, 1010 West Columbia, Zip 63640–2997; tel. 314/756–6792; Donald L. Barton, Superintendent **A**1 10 **F**16 17 19 22 24 28 29 34 35 39 41 45 46 52 56 58 65 67 73 | 12 | 22 | 196 | 1280 | 163 | 1648 | 0 | 19803 | 13926 | 605

FLORISSANT—St. Louis County

CHRISTIAN HOSPITAL NORTHWEST See Christian Hospital Northeast–Northwest, Saint Louis

FORT LEONARD WOOD—Pulaski County

⊞ GENERAL LEONARD WOOD ARMY COMMUNITY HOSPITAL, 310 Freedom Drive, Zip 65473–8922; tel. 573/596–0414; Lieutenant Colonel Billy R. Porter, Administrator **A**1 2 **F**3 7 8 12 19 20 21 22 23 29 30 34 35 37 39 40 41 44 45 46 49 51 52 53 54 55 56 57 58 63 65 67 71 73 **S** Department of the Army, Office of the Surgeon General, Falls Church, VA | 42 | 10 | 71 | 4305 | 36 | 233165 | 363 | 56766 | 22617 | 900

FREDERICKTOWN—Madison County

MADISON MEDICAL CENTER, 100 South Wood at West College, Zip 63645, Mailing Address: P.O. Box 431, Zip 63645–0431; tel. 573/783–3341; Floyd D. Bounds, Administrator (Total facility includes 123 beds in nursing home–type unit) **A**9 10 **F**8 14 15 16 17 19 22 28 29 30 32 34 37 39 40 41 44 46 49 51 64 65 71 **N** BJC Health System, St. Louis, MO | 13 | 10 | 147 | 381 | 116 | 15141 | 50 | 8284 | 4253 | 131

FULTON—Callaway County

□ CALLAWAY COMMUNITY HOSPITAL, 10 South Hospital Drive, Zip 65251; tel. 573/642–3376; Gerald M. Torba, Chief Executive Officer **A**1 9 10 **F**7 8 13 14 15 16 17 19 22 24 25 28 29 30 32 34 37 39 40 41 44 46 49 58 65 67 71 | 23 | 10 | 36 | 1161 | 12 | 24112 | 122 | 8443 | 3156 | 148

□ FULTON STATE HOSPITAL, 600 East Fifth Street, Zip 65251; tel. 573/592–4100; Stephen C. Reeves, Superintendent **A**1 10 **F**2 3 12 14 16 20 26 27 28 29 30 33 39 41 45 46 51 52 55 57 64 65 67 73 **P**6 | 12 | 22 | 495 | 729 | 424 | 0 | 0 | 46715 | 28082 | 1177

HANNIBAL—Marion County

□ + HANNIBAL REGIONAL HOSPITAL, Highway 36 West, Zip 63401, Mailing Address: P.O. Box 551, Zip 63401–0551; tel. 573/248–1300; John C. Grossmeier, President and Chief Executive Officer **A**1 2 9 10 **F**3 7 8 10 14 15 16 17 18 19 21 22 23 27 28 29 30 31 32 34 35 37 39 40 41 44 46 49 52 54 55 56 57 58 59 61 63 65 66 67 68 69 71 72 73 74 **P**1 6 | 23 | 10 | 105 | 4226 | 56 | 103507 | 478 | 38618 | 13820 | 702

Hospital, Address, Telephone, Administrator, Approval, Facility, and Physician Codes, Health Care System, Network	Classi-fication Codes		Utilization Data					Expense (thousands) of dollars		
★ American Hospital Association (AHA) membership □ Joint Commission on Accreditation of Healthcare Organizations (JCAHO) accreditation + American Osteopathic Hospital Association (AOHA) membership ○ American Osteopathic Association (AOA) accreditation △ Commission on Accreditation of Rehabilitation Facilities (CARF) accreditation Control codes 61, 63, 64, 71, 72 and 73 indicate hospitals listed by AOHA, but not registered by AHA. For definition of numerical codes, see page A4	Control	Service	Beds	Admissions	Census	Outpatient Visits	Births	Total	Payroll	Personnel

HARRISONVILLE—Cass County

⊠ CASS MEDICAL CENTER, 1800 East Mechanic Street, Zip 64701; tel. 816/884–3291; Alan Freeman, Administrator **A**1 9 10 **F**8 12 14 15 16 19 20 21 22 29 30 33 34 37 39 41 42 44 45 46 49 51 53 54 55 56 57 58 65 66 71 73 **P**6 7 **S** Health Midwest, Kansas City, MO **N** Health Midwest, Kansas City, MO

13 · 10 · 42 · 1237 · 14 · 16266 · 0 · — · — · 168

HAYTI—Pemiscot County

PEMISCOT MEMORIAL HEALTH SYSTEM, Highway 61 and Reed, Zip 63851, Mailing Address: P.O. Box 489, Zip 63851; tel. 314/359–1372; Darrell Jean, Administrator and Chief Executive Officer (Total facility includes 153 beds in nursing home–type unit) **A**10 **F**7 8 11 15 16 19 21 22 25 26 27 28 29 30 31 32 34 35 37 39 40 41 44 49 51 64 65 71 73 74 **P**6

13 · 10 · 216 · 3374 · 158 · 22360 · 177 · 21740 · 11025 · 341

HERMANN—Gasconade County

HERMANN AREA DISTRICT HOSPITAL, Mailing Address: P.O. Box 470, Zip 65041–0470; tel. 573/486–2191; Dan McKinney, Administrator **A**9 10 **F**8 12 15 16 17 19 20 22 28 29 30 32 33 34 35 36 39 40 42 44 46 49 64 65 71 73 **P**6

16 · 10 · 41 · 478 · 27 · 21769 · 26 · 4530 · 2029 · 103

HOUSTON—Texas County

TEXAS COUNTY MEMORIAL HOSPITAL, 1333 Sam Houston Boulevard, Zip 65483–2046; tel. 417/967–3311; Beverly Derrickson, Administrator **A**9 10 **F**8 12 14 16 19 20 22 24 25 27 28 29 30 31 32 33 34 36 37 39 40 41 44 45 46 49 51 64 65 71 73 **P**5 6

13 · 10 · 66 · 2300 · 24 · 10312 · 266 · 9860 · 5023 · 209

INDEPENDENCE—Jackson County

⊠ COLUMBIA INDEPENDENCE REGIONAL HEALTH CENTER, 1509 West Truman Road, Zip 64050; tel. 816/836–8100; Paul F. Herzog, Chief Executive Officer (Total facility includes 82 beds in nursing home–type unit) **A**1 2 5 9 10 **F**1 2 3 4 5 6 7 8 9 10 11 12 13 14 15 16 17 18 19 20 21 22 23 24 26 27 28 29 30 31 32 33 34 35 36 37 38 39 40 41 42 43 44 45 46 47 48 49 51 52 53 54 55 56 57 58 59 60 61 63 64 65 66 67 70 71 73 74 **P**5 6 7 **S** Columbia/HCA Healthcare Corporation, Nashville, TN

33 · 10 · 329 · 9650 · 190 · 160882 · 499 · 80263 · 32925 · 970

⊠ MEDICAL CENTER OF INDEPENDENCE, 17203 East 23rd Street, Zip 64057; tel. 816/478–5000; Michael W. Chappelow, President and Chief Executive Officer (Total facility includes 9 beds in nursing home–type unit) **A**1 9 10 **F**1 2 3 4 5 7 8 9 10 11 12 13 14 15 16 17 18 19 20 21 22 23 24 25 26 27 28 29 30 31 32 33 34 35 36 37 38 39 40 41 42 43 44 45 46 47 48 49 51 52 53 54 55 56 57 58 59 60 61 63 64 65 66 67 68 69 70 71 73 74 **P**1 5 6 **S** Health Midwest, Kansas City, MO **N** Health Midwest, Kansas City, MO

23 · 10 · 123 · 4403 · 56 · 39864 · 831 · 30283 · 13271 · 339

JEFFERSON CITY—Cole County

★ + ○ △ CAPITAL REGION MEDICAL CENTER–MADISON, 1125 Madison Street, Zip 65101–5227, Mailing Address: P.O. Box 1128, Zip 65102–1128; tel. 573/635–7141; Edward F. Farnsworth, President (Total facility includes 16 beds in nursing home–type unit) **A**7 10 11 12 13 **F**1 3 4 7 8 10 12 13 14 15 16 17 18 19 21 22 23 24 25 26 28 29 30 31 32 33 34 35 36 37 39 40 41 42 43 44 45 46 48 49 51 53 54 55 56 57 58 59 60 63 64 65 66 67 71 72 73 **P**5 8

23 · 10 · 41 · 820 · 24 · 38061 · 212 · — · — · 983

⊠ CAPITAL REGION MEDICAL CENTER–SOUTHWEST, 1432 Southwest Boulevard, Zip 65109–4420, Mailing Address: P.O. Box 1128, Zip 65102–1128; tel. 573/635–6811; Edward F. Farnsworth, President **A**1 10 **F**1 3 4 7 8 10 12 13 14 15 16 17 18 19 21 22 23 24 25 26 28 29 30 31 32 33 34 35 36 37 39 40 41 42 43 44 45 46 48 49 52 53 54 55 56 57 58 59 60 63 64 65 66 67 71 72 73 **P**5 8 **N** BJC Health System, St. Louis, MO

23 · 10 · 94 · 4678 · 63 · 41590 · 0 · 66169 · 29749 · 983

⊠ ST. MARYS HEALTH CENTER, 100 St. Marys Medical Plaza, Zip 65101; tel. 573/761–7000; John S. Dubis, President **A**1 2 9 10 **F**4 7 8 10 12 14 15 16 17 18 19 20 21 22 24 28 29 30 31 32 33 34 35 37 39 40 41 42 43 44 45 46 48 49 51 52 54 55 56 57 58 59 60 63 64 65 67 70 71 72 73 74 **P**1 4 **S** SSM Health Care System, Saint Louis, MO

23 · 10 · 151 · 7969 · 95 · 109494 · 1200 · 76013 · 28942 · 946

JOPLIN—Newton County

⊠ + ○ FREEMAN HOSPITALS AND HEALTH SYSTEM, (Includes Freeman Hospital East, 932 East 34th Street, Zip 64804–3999; Freeman Hospital West, 1102 West 32nd Street), 1102 West 32nd Street, Zip 64804–3599; tel. 417/623–2801; Gary D. Duncan, President and Chief Executive Officer (Total facility includes 32 beds in nursing home–type unit) **A**1 9 10 11 12 13 **F**3 4 5 6 7 8 10 12 13 14 15 16 17 18 19 20 21 22 26 27 28 29 30 31 32 33 34 35 37 38 39 40 41 42 43 44 45 46 48 49 51 52 53 54 55 56 57 58 60 61 64 65 66 67 70 71 72 73 74 **P**7 8

23 · 10 · 266 · 13450 · 144 · 131631 · 2194 · 136989 · 59883 · 1426

⊠ △ ST. JOHN'S REGIONAL MEDICAL CENTER, 2727 McClelland Boulevard, Zip 64804; tel. 417/781–2727; Robert G. Brueckner, President and Chief Executive Officer **A**1 2 7 10 **F**4 7 8 10 11 12 15 16 17 18 19 20 21 22 23 25 27 28 29 30 31 32 33 34 35 36 37 39 40 41 42 43 44 45 46 48 49 51 52 54 56 57 58 59 60 61 65 66 67 68 69 70 71 72 73 74 **P**1 **S** Catholic Health Initiatives, Denver, CO **N** Carondelet Health, Kansas City, MO

23 · 10 · 353 · 14428 · 213 · 180799 · 772 · 120196 · 45429 · 1913

KANSAS CITY—Jackson County

⊠ BAPTIST MEDICAL CENTER, 6601 Rockhill Road, Zip 64131–1197; tel. 816/276–7000; Dan H. Anderson, President and Chief Executive Officer (Total facility includes 23 beds in nursing home–type unit) **A**1 2 3 5 9 10 **F**1 2 3 4 5 7 8 9 10 11 12 13 14 15 16 17 18 19 20 21 22 23 24 25 26 27 28 29 30 31 32 33 34 35 36 37 38 39 40 41 42 43 44 45 46 47 48 49 51 52 53 54 55 56 57 58 59 60 61 63 64 65 66 67 68 69 70 71 72 73 74 **P**1 4 5 6 7 **S** Health Midwest, Kansas City, MO **N** Health Midwest, Kansas City, MO

23 · 10 · 315 · 12224 · 209 · 61020 · 1481 · 114105 · 51613 · 1654

Hospital, Address, Telephone, Administrator, Approval, Facility, and Physician Codes, Health Care System, Network	Classi-fication Codes		Utilization Data					Expense (thousands) of dollars		
	Control	Service	Beds	Admissions	Census	Outpatient Visits	Births	Total	Payroll	Personnel

★ American Hospital Association (AHA) membership
□ Joint Commission on Accreditation of Healthcare Organizations (JCAHO) accreditation
+ American Osteopathic Hospital Association (AOHA) membership
○ American Osteopathic Association (AOA) accreditation
△ Commission on Accreditation of Rehabilitation Facilities (CARF) accreditation
Control codes 61, 63, 64, 71, 72 and 73 indicate hospitals listed by AOHA, but not registered by AHA. For definition of numerical codes, see page A4.

Hospital	Control	Service	Beds	Admissions	Census	Outpatient Visits	Births	Total	Payroll	Personnel
⊞ CHILDREN'S MERCY HOSPITAL, 2401 Gillham Road, Zip 64108–9898; tel. 816/234–3000; Randall L. O'Donnell, Ph.D., President and Chief Executive Officer **A**1 2 3 5 8 9 10 **F**4 5 9 10 11 12 13 15 16 17 19 20 21 22 25 28 29 31 32 34 35 37 38 39 41 42 43 44 46 47 49 51 54 58 60 65 67 68 69 70 71 73 **P**4 5 6	23	50	159	6943	115	213255	0	144535	74843	2057
□ CRITTENTON, 10918 Elm Avenue, Zip 64134–4199; tel. 816/765–6600; Robert D. Gray, Ed.D., Chief Executive Officer **A**1 9 10 **F**2 3 12 16 17 18 22 27 29 30 39 41 45 46 52 53 55 56 57 58 59 67 68 70 73 **P**6 7 8 **S** Saint Luke's Shawnee Mission Health System, Kansas City, MO	23	52	28	370	8	16069	0	10126	5882	193
⊞ + ○ PARK LANE MEDICAL CENTER, 5151 Raytown Road, Zip 64133; tel. 816/358–8000; Derell Taloney, President and Chief Executive Officer (Total facility includes 15 beds in nursing home–type unit) **A**1 9 10 11 12 13 **F**1 2 3 4 5 7 8 9 10 11 12 13 14 15 16 17 18 19 20 21 22 23 24 25 26 27 28 29 30 31 32 33 34 35 36 37 38 39 40 41 42 43 44 45 46 47 48 49 51 52 53 54 55 56 57 58 59 60 61 63 64 65 66 67 68 69 70 71 72 73 74 **P**1 4 5 6 7 **S** Health Midwest, Kansas City, MO **N** Health Midwest, Kansas City, MO	23	10	94	2205	39	81878	0	23479	11083	284
★ △ REHABILITATION INSTITUTE, 3011 Baltimore, Zip 64108–3465; tel. 816/751–7900; Ronald L. Herrick, President **A**5 7 9 10 **F**1 2 3 4 5 6 7 8 9 10 11 12 13 14 15 17 18 19 20 21 22 23 24 25 26 27 28 29 30 31 32 33 34 35 36 37 39 40 41 42 43 44 45 46 47 48 49 51 52 53 54 55 56 57 58 59 60 61 64 65 66 67 68 69 70 71 72 73 74 **P**2 5 8 **S** Health Midwest, Kansas City, MO **N** Health Midwest, Kansas City, MO	23	46	22	367	18	11039	0	11525	6354	220
⊞ RESEARCH MEDICAL CENTER, 2316 East Meyer Boulevard, Zip 64132–1199; tel. 816/276–4000; Dan H. Anderson, President and Chief Executive Officer (Total facility includes 35 beds in nursing home–type unit) **A**1 2 3 5 9 10 **F**1 2 3 4 5 7 8 9 10 11 12 13 14 15 16 17 18 19 20 21 22 23 24 25 26 27 28 29 30 31 32 33 34 35 36 37 38 39 40 41 42 43 44 45 46 47 48 49 51 52 53 54 55 56 57 58 59 60 61 63 64 65 66 67 68 69 70 71 72 73 74 **P**1 5 6 **S** Health Midwest, Kansas City, MO **N** Health Midwest, Kansas City, MO	23	10	479	15059	285	70847	1934	191853	81412	1983
⊞ RESEARCH PSYCHIATRIC CENTER, 2323 East 63rd Street, Zip 64130; tel. 816/444–8161; Todd Krass, Administrator and Chief Executive Officer **A**1 9 10 **F**1 2 3 4 5 6 7 8 9 10 11 12 13 15 16 17 18 19 20 22 23 24 26 27 28 29 30 31 32 33 34 35 37 38 39 40 41 42 43 44 45 46 47 48 49 51 52 53 54 55 56 57 58 59 60 61 62 64 65 66 67 68 69 70 71 72 73 74 **P**4 5 8 **S** Columbia/HCA Healthcare Corporation, Nashville, TN **N** Health Midwest, Kansas City, MO	33	22	100	1848	52	3496	0	10445	4744	105
⊞ SAINT JOSEPH HEALTH CENTER, 1000 Carondelet Drive, Zip 64114–4673; tel. 816/942–4400; Richard M. Abell, President and Chief Executive Officer **A**1 2 5 9 10 **F**1 4 5 6 7 8 10 12 13 15 16 17 19 21 22 24 28 29 30 31 32 33 34 35 37 38 39 40 41 42 43 44 45 46 48 49 60 63 64 65 66 67 70 71 72 73 **P**3 4 5 6 7 **S** Carondelet Health System, Saint Louis, MO	23	10	240	11008	166	89760	1870	110449	44130	1150
⊞ SAINT LUKE'S HOSPITAL, 4400 Wornall Road, Zip 64111; tel. 816/932–2000; James M. Brophy, Senior Executive Officer (Total facility includes 30 beds in nursing home–type unit) **A**1 2 3 8 9 10 **F**2 3 4 5 7 8 10 11 12 13 14 15 16 17 18 19 20 21 22 23 24 25 26 27 28 29 30 31 32 33 34 35 37 38 39 40 41 42 43 44 45 46 48 49 51 52 53 54 55 56 57 58 59 60 61 63 64 65 66 67 68 69 70 71 72 73 74 **P**6 8 **S** Saint Luke's Shawnee Mission Health System, Kansas City, MO **N** National Cardiovascular Network, Atlanta, GA	23	10	508	19056	327	177552	2723	223852	93737	2360
SAINT LUKE'S NORTHLAND HOSPITAL, 5830 N.W. Barry Road, Zip 64154–9988; tel. 816/891–6000; James M. Brophy, FACHE, Senior Executive Officer **F**2 3 4 5 7 8 10 11 12 13 14 15 16 17 18 19 20 21 22 24 25 26 27 28 29 30 31 32 33 34 35 37 38 39 40 41 42 43 44 45 46 47 48 49 51 52 53 54 55 56 57 58 59 60 61 63 64 65 66 67 68 69 70 71 72 73 74 **P**6 8 **S** Saint Luke's Shawnee Mission Health System, Kansas City, MO	23	10	55	2961	30	39297	639	28669	10769	275
ST. MARY'S HOSPITAL See Trinity Lutheran Hospital										
⊞ TRINITY LUTHERAN HOSPITAL, (Includes St. Mary's Hospital, 101 Memorial Drive, Zip 64108; tel. 816/751–4600), 3030 Baltimore Avenue, Zip 64108–3404; tel. 816/753–4600; Ronald A. Ommen, President and Chief Executive Officer (Total facility includes 30 beds in nursing home–type unit) **A**1 2 3 5 9 10 **F**1 3 4 5 7 8 9 10 11 12 13 14 15 16 17 18 19 21 22 23 24 25 26 27 28 29 30 31 32 33 34 35 36 37 38 39 40 41 42 43 44 46 47 49 51 52 53 54 55 56 57 58 59 60 64 65 67 68 69 70 71 72 73 74 **P**1 5 6 **S** Health Midwest, Kansas City, MO **N** Health Midwest, Kansas City, MO	23	10	334	8313	159	168869	0	87256	37757	1370
★ △ TRUMAN MEDICAL CENTER–EAST, 7900 Lee's Summit Road, Zip 64139–1241; tel. 816/373–4415; Ross P. Marine, Administrator and Chief Executive Officer (Total facility includes 212 beds in nursing home–type unit) **A**3 5 7 9 10 **F**3 7 8 10 11 12 13 14 15 16 17 18 19 20 21 22 25 26 27 29 30 31 32 34 35 37 38 39 40 41 42 44 45 46 48 49 51 52 53 54 55 56 57 58 59 61 64 65 66 70 71 72 73 74 **S** Truman Medical Center, Kansas City, MO	23	10	302	3607	253	101758	828	41416	20075	678
⊞ TRUMAN MEDICAL CENTER–WEST, 2301 Holmes Street, Zip 64108; tel. 816/556–3000; Rosa L. Miller, R.N., Administrator (Total facility includes 10 beds in nursing home–type unit) **A**1 2 3 5 8 9 10 **F**3 4 7 8 10 14 16 17 19 20 21 22 26 27 28 29 31 34 35 37 38 40 41 42 43 44 45 46 48 49 51 52 53 54 55 56 57 58 59 60 61 63 64 65 66 70 71 73 74 **P**6 7 **S** Truman Medical Center, Kansas City, MO	23	10	229	10770	176	344549	1874	108861	55333	1392
□ TWO RIVERS PSYCHIATRIC HOSPITAL, 5121 Raytown Road, Zip 64133–2141; tel. 816/356–5688; Craig Nuckles, Administrator **A**1 9 10 **F**2 12 14 16 17 18 26 27 29 39 45 46 52 53 54 55 56 57 59 65 67 **S** Universal Health Services, Inc., King of Prussia, PA	33	22	80	1128	41	0	0	8232	3421	—

Hospital, Address, Telephone, Administrator, Approval, Facility, and Physician Codes, Health Care System, Network	Classi-fication Codes		Utilization Data					Expense (thousands) of dollars		
	Control	Service	Beds	Admissions	Census	Outpatient Visits	Births	Total	Payroll	Personnel

Approval/Code Key

★ American Hospital Association (AHA) membership
□ Joint Commission on Accreditation of Healthcare Organizations (JCAHO) accreditation
+ American Osteopathic Hospital Association (AOHA) membership
○ American Osteopathic Association (AOA) accreditation
△ Commission on Accreditation of Rehabilitation Facilities (CARF) accreditation
Control codes 61, 63, 64, 71, 72 and 73 indicate hospitals listed by AOHA, but not registered by AHA. For definition of numerical codes, see page A4

Hospital	Control	Service	Beds	Admissions	Census	Outpatient Visits	Births	Total	Payroll	Personnel
□ VALUEMARK BEHAVIORAL HEALTHCARE SYSTEM OF KANSAS CITY, 4800 N.W. 88th Street, Zip 64154; tel. 816/436–3900; David C. Nissen, Chief Executive Officer (Nonreporting) **A**1 9 10 **S** ValueMark Healthcare Systems, Inc., Atlanta, GA	33	22	72	—	—	—	—	—	—	—
□ △ VENCOR HOSPITAL–KANSAS CITY, (LONG TERM ACUTE CARE), 8701 Troost Avenue, Zip 64131; tel. 816/995–2000; Suzanne R. Wilsey, Administrator (Total facility includes 16 beds in nursing home–type unit) **A**1 7 9 **F**12 14 16 19 21 22 27 29 33 35 37 39 41 42 45 46 50 52 57 60 63 64 65 67 71 73 **P**5 **S** Vencor, Incorporated, Louisville, KY	33	49	100	446	63	231	0	—	—	198
✠ VETERANS AFFAIRS MEDICAL CENTER, 4801 Linwood Boulevard, Zip 64128–2295; tel. 816/861–4700; Hugh F. Doran, Director **A**1 2 3 5 8 9 **F**1 2 3 4 8 9 10 12 16 17 19 20 21 22 23 24 26 27 28 29 30 31 32 33 35 37 39 41 42 43 44 45 46 48 49 51 52 54 55 56 57 58 59 60 63 64 65 67 71 73 74 **S** Department of Veterans Affairs, Washington, DC	45	10	295	7467	201	171078	0	—	—	1145
□ WESTERN MISSOURI MENTAL HEALTH CENTER, 600 East 22nd Street, Zip 64108; tel. 816/512–4000; Gloria Joseph, Superintendent **A**1 3 5 10 **F**3 6 15 18 19 21 22 24 27 29 35 39 41 45 46 52 53 54 55 56 57 58 63 65 67 71 73 **P**6	12	22	110	2916	87	54450	0	26311	14586	672

KENNETT—Dunklin County

Hospital	Control	Service	Beds	Admissions	Census	Outpatient Visits	Births	Total	Payroll	Personnel
□ TWIN RIVERS REGIONAL MEDICAL CENTER, 1301 First Street, Zip 63857; tel. 573/888–4522; Carol Hanes, Chief Executive Officer **A**1 9 10 **F**2 7 8 11 12 13 14 15 16 17 19 21 22 23 24 27 28 29 30 32 33 34 35 37 40 41 42 44 48 49 52 53 56 57 58 59 65 66 71 73 **P**7 **S** TENET Healthcare Corporation, Santa Barbara, CA	33	10	119	2792	39	60287	411	25951	12552	406

KIRKSVILLE—Adair County

Hospital	Control	Service	Beds	Admissions	Census	Outpatient Visits	Births	Total	Payroll	Personnel
□ GRIM–SMITH HOSPITAL AND CLINIC, 112 East Patterson Avenue, Zip 63501; tel. 816/665–7241; Steven E. Clark, Administrator **A**1 9 10 **F**7 8 14 15 16 17 18 19 20 22 24 28 29 30 31 32 34 35 37 39 40 41 42 44 45 46 48 49 54 58 59 65 66 67 70 71 74 **P**5 7 **N** BJC Health System, St. Louis, MO	33	10	75	3586	39	26333	413	26174	11789	379
□ + ○ KIRKSVILLE OSTEOPATHIC MEDICAL CENTER, 800 West Jefferson Street, Zip 63501–1497; tel. 816/626–2121 (Total facility includes 10 beds in nursing home–type unit) (Nonreporting) **A**1 5 9 10 11 12 13	33	10	119	—	—	—	—	—	—	—

LAKE SAINT LOUIS—St. Charles County

Hospital	Control	Service	Beds	Admissions	Census	Outpatient Visits	Births	Total	Payroll	Personnel
★ ST. JOSEPH HOSPITAL WEST, 100 Medical Plaza, Zip 63367–1395; tel. 314/625–5200; Kurt Weinmeister, President (Total facility includes 11 beds in nursing home–type unit) **A**9 10 **F**3 4 5 7 8 10 12 13 14 15 16 17 18 19 20 21 22 23 24 25 26 28 29 30 31 32 33 34 35 37 39 40 41 42 43 44 46 49 51 53 54 55 56 57 58 59 60 61 63 64 65 66 67 68 69 70 71 72 73 74 **P**1 2 4 6 7 **S** SSM Health Care System, Saint Louis, MO **N** Saint Louis Health Care Network, St. Louis, MO	23	10	100	3327	30	19862	484	20443	9472	199

LAMAR—Barton County

Hospital	Control	Service	Beds	Admissions	Census	Outpatient Visits	Births	Total	Payroll	Personnel
★ BARTON COUNTY MEMORIAL HOSPITAL, Second and Gulf Streets, Zip 64759–0626; tel. 417/682–6081; Ronald Morton, Chief Executive Officer (Total facility includes 10 beds in nursing home–type unit) **A**9 10 **F**7 8 11 14 15 16 19 20 21 22 28 29 30 32 34 37 39 40 41 44 48 49 64 65 71	13	10	42	1164	18	23167	90	7398	3007	126

LEBANON—Laclede County

Hospital	Control	Service	Beds	Admissions	Census	Outpatient Visits	Births	Total	Payroll	Personnel
✠ BREECH MEDICAL CENTER, 325 Harwood Avenue, Zip 65536, Mailing Address: P.O. Box N, Zip 65536; tel. 417/532–2136; Gary W. Pulsipher, Chief Executive Officer **A**1 9 10 **F**7 8 17 18 19 20 21 22 27 28 29 30 32 33 34 37 39 40 44 49 61 64 65 71 73	23	10	32	1621	16	19612	285	12486	5768	193

LEES SUMMIT—Jackson County

Hospital	Control	Service	Beds	Admissions	Census	Outpatient Visits	Births	Total	Payroll	Personnel
✠ LEE'S SUMMIT HOSPITAL, 530 North Murray Road, Zip 64081–1497; tel. 816/251–7000; John L. Jacobson, President and Chief Executive Officer **A**1 9 10 **F**3 8 12 14 15 17 18 19 21 22 27 28 29 30 32 34 35 36 37 39 41 42 44 45 46 49 53 54 55 58 63 65 66 67 71 72 73 **P**1 **S** Health Midwest, Kansas City, MO **N** Health Midwest, Kansas City, MO	23	10	77	2922	37	45415	0	23831	9844	270

LEXINGTON—Lafayette County

Hospital	Control	Service	Beds	Admissions	Census	Outpatient Visits	Births	Total	Payroll	Personnel
✠ LAFAYETTE REGIONAL HEALTH CENTER, 1500 State Street, Zip 64067–1199; tel. 816/259–2203; Jeffrey S. Tarrant, Administrator **A**1 9 10 **F**7 8 12 15 16 19 22 25 29 30 32 33 34 37 39 40 41 42 44 45 46 49 51 64 65 71 73 74 **P**4 **S** Health Midwest, Kansas City, MO **N** Health Midwest, Kansas City, MO	23	10	37	1635	18	28146	60	11299	4628	165

LIBERTY—Clay County

Hospital	Control	Service	Beds	Admissions	Census	Outpatient Visits	Births	Total	Payroll	Personnel
✠ LIBERTY HOSPITAL, 2525 Glenn Hendren Drive, Zip 64068–9625; tel. 816/781–7200; Joseph Crossett, Administrator (Total facility includes 20 beds in nursing home–type unit) **A**1 9 10 **F**5 7 8 10 15 16 17 19 21 22 23 26 27 28 29 30 32 33 34 35 36 37 38 39 40 41 42 44 48 49 60 64 65 67 70 71 73 **P**5	16	10	173	7409	107	62490	980	54652	23322	1006

LOUISIANA—Pike County

Hospital	Control	Service	Beds	Admissions	Census	Outpatient Visits	Births	Total	Payroll	Personnel
✠ PIKE COUNTY MEMORIAL HOSPITAL, 2305 West Georgia Street, Zip 63353–0020; tel. 573/754–5531; Thomas E. Lefebvre, President **A**1 9 10 **F**3 7 8 14 15 16 19 22 27 28 29 30 34 35 39 40 44 49 54 55 58 65 67 68 71 73 **P**8 **S** SSM Health Care System, Saint Louis, MO **N** Saint Louis Health Care Network, St. Louis, MO	13	10	25	859	11	14194	105	7620	3567	120

MACON—Macon County

Hospital	Control	Service	Beds	Admissions	Census	Outpatient Visits	Births	Total	Payroll	Personnel
SAMARITAN MEMORIAL HOSPITAL, 1205 North Jackson Street, Zip 63552; tel. 816/385–3151; Bernard A. Orman, Jr., Administrator **A**10 **F**7 8 12 14 15 16 17 19 22 26 28 29 30 31 33 34 39 40 41 42 44 49 51 52 57 59 64 65 69 71 73 74	13	10	35	997	15	19948	19	7865	3273	155

Hospital, Address, Telephone, Administrator, Approval, Facility, and Physician Codes, Health Care System, Network	Classi-fication Codes		Utilization Data					Expense (thousands) of dollars		
★ American Hospital Association (AHA) membership □ Joint Commission on Accreditation of Healthcare Organizations (JCAHO) accreditation + American Osteopathic Hospital Association (AOHA) membership ○ American Osteopathic Association (AOA) accreditation △ Commission on Accreditation of Rehabilitation Facilities (CARF) accreditation Control codes 61, 63, 64, 71, 72 and 73 indicate hospitals listed by AOHA, but not registered by AHA. For definition of numerical codes, see page A4	Control	Service	Beds	Admissions	Census	Outpatient Visits	Births	Total	Payroll	Personnel

MARSHALL—Saline County

★ FITZGIBBON HOSPITAL, 2305 South 65 Highway, Zip 65340–0250, Mailing Address: P.O. Box 250, Zip 65340–0250; tel. 816/886–7431; Ronald A. Ott, Chief Executive Officer (Total facility includes 13 beds in nursing home–type unit) **A**9 10 **F**7 8 14 15 16 17 19 21 22 24 27 28 29 30 32 33 34 35 37 39 40 41 44 46 49 53 54 57 58 59 64 65 66 67 71 74 **P**6 — 23 10 56 1989 25 76900 292 18187 8799 278

MARYVILLE—Nodaway County

✖ ST. FRANCIS HOSPITAL AND HEALTH SERVICES, 2016 South Main Street, Zip 64468–2693; tel. 816/562–2600; Michael Baumgartner, President **A**1 9 10 **F**3 7 8 12 14 15 16 17 18 19 20 21 22 24 27 28 29 30 31 32 33 34 35 39 40 41 42 44 49 51 52 54 55 56 57 58 59 64 65 67 71 73 **P**1 6 7 8 **S** SSM Health Care System, Saint Louis, MO — 23 10 55 1704 18 40357 326 14594 7259 315

MEMPHIS—Scotland County

○ SCOTLAND COUNTY MEMORIAL HOSPITAL, Sigler Avenue, Zip 63555, Mailing Address: Route 1, Box 53, Zip 63555; tel. 816/465–8511; Marcia R. Dial, Administrator **A**9 10 11 **F**5 7 8 12 13 15 16 17 18 19 20 22 26 28 29 30 32 33 34 36 37 39 40 42 44 45 46 48 49 51 64 65 66 67 71 **P**8 — 16 10 32 472 7 10534 34 3081 1305 76

MEXICO—Audrain County

✖ + AUDRAIN MEDICAL CENTER, 620 East Monroe Street, Zip 65265–0858; tel. 573/581–1760; Charles P. Jansen, Administrator (Total facility includes 40 beds in nursing home–type unit) **A**1 9 10 **F**3 7 8 10 12 13 14 15 17 18 19 20 22 23 25 26 28 29 30 32 33 34 35 37 39 40 41 42 44 45 46 49 51 52 53 54 55 56 57 58 59 63 64 65 66 67 68 71 73 74 — 23 10 166 4893 97 143998 252 44314 20002 655

MILAN—Sullivan County

★ SULLIVAN COUNTY MEMORIAL HOSPITAL, 630 West Third Street, Zip 63556; tel. 816/265–4212; Martha Gragg, Chief Executive Officer (Total facility includes 12 beds in nursing home–type unit) **A**10 **F**17 19 20 22 28 29 30 32 33 34 36 44 49 64 65 71 **S** Brim, Inc., Portland, OR — 13 10 47 244 24 10284 0 2847 1335 55

MOBERLY—Randolph County

✖ + MOBERLY REGIONAL MEDICAL CENTER, 1515 Union Avenue, Zip 65270–9449, Mailing Address: P.O. Box 3000, Zip 65270–3000; tel. 816/263–8400; Daniel E. McKay, Executive Director (Total facility includes 21 beds in nursing home–type unit) **A**1 5 9 10 **F**1 7 8 12 14 15 16 17 18 19 20 21 22 24 26 27 28 29 30 32 33 34 37 39 40 41 44 45 46 49 51 52 54 57 59 63 64 65 66 67 68 70 71 73 74 **P**3 6 **S** Community Health Systems, Inc., Brentwood, TN — 33 10 93 2945 38 39348 308 18250 6090 225

MONETT—Barry County

★ COX–MONETT HOSPITAL, 801 Lincoln Avenue, Zip 65708–1698; tel. 417/235–3144; Frank D. Dale, Administrator **A**9 10 **F**8 12 14 15 16 17 19 22 26 27 28 29 30 31 32 33 34 37 39 41 44 45 46 49 51 64 65 67 71 73 **P**1 3 **N** BJC Health System, St. Louis, MO — 23 10 53 933 14 43053 0 8549 3490 169

MOUNT VERNON—Lawrence County

□ △ MISSOURI REHABILITATION CENTER, 600 North Main, Zip 65712–1099; tel. 417/466–3711; Charles A. Drewel, Director **A**1 7 10 **F**3 6 19 21 26 27 29 30 31 33 34 37 39 41 42 46 48 49 51 64 65 67 71 73 **P**6 — 12 10 136 507 72 20638 0 18359 9612 394

MOUNTAIN VIEW—Howell County

✖ ST. FRANCIS HOSPITAL, Highway 60, Zip 65548, Mailing Address: P.O. Box 82, Zip 65548–0082; tel. 417/934–2246; Sister M. Cornelia Blasko, Administrator **A**1 9 10 **F**8 14 15 16 19 22 27 29 32 33 34 39 49 64 65 70 71 **P**5 — 23 10 20 396 5 15408 0 3492 1520 72

NEOSHO—Newton County

FREEMAN NEOSHO HOSPITAL, 113 West Hickory Street, Zip 64850–1799; tel. 417/455–4352; Phil Willcoxon, Administrator **A**9 10 **F**2 3 4 5 7 8 10 11 12 13 17 19 20 21 22 26 27 28 29 30 31 32 33 34 35 37 38 39 40 41 42 43 44 45 46 47 48 49 51 52 53 54 55 56 57 58 59 60 61 63 64 65 66 70 71 72 73 74 **P**4 8 — 23 10 54 1807 30 36341 0 17403 5178 231

NEVADA—Vernon County

□ HEARTLAND BEHAVIORAL HEALTH SERVICES, (Formerly Heartland Hospital), 1500 West Ashland Street, Zip 64772; tel. 417/667–2666; Eugene Hastings, Chief Executive Officer **A**1 10 **F**26 29 52 53 54 55 56 57 59 65 **P**8 **S** Ramsay Health Care, Inc., Coral Gobles, FL — 33 22 60 515 20 4039 0 9209 — 51

✖ NEVADA REGIONAL MEDICAL CENTER, 800 South Ash Street, Zip 64772; tel. 417/667–3355; Michael L. Mullins, President (Total facility includes 10 beds in nursing home–type unit) **A**1 9 10 **F**7 8 15 17 19 22 25 27 28 29 30 31 32 33 34 36 37 39 40 41 42 44 46 49 64 65 71 **P**3 **S** Quorum Health Group/Quorum Health Resources, Inc., Brentwood, TN — 14 10 97 2205 28 24295 281 15542 6141 264

NORTH KANSAS CITY—Clay County

✖ NORTH KANSAS CITY HOSPITAL, 2800 Clay Edwards Drive, Zip 64116–3281; tel. 816/691–2000; Michael E. Payne, President and Chief Executive Officer (Total facility includes 39 beds in nursing home–type unit) **A**1 9 10 **F**2 3 4 7 8 9 10 11 12 14 15 16 17 18 19 20 21 22 23 28 29 30 32 33 34 35 36 37 38 39 40 41 42 43 44 46 47 48 49 52 54 55 56 57 58 59 60 63 64 65 67 70 71 72 73 **P**6 — 14 10 350 12671 226 77747 1323 115104 48722 1277

OSAGE BEACH—Camden County

✖ LAKE OF THE OZARKS GENERAL HOSPITAL, 54 Hospital Drive, Zip 65065; tel. 573/348–8000; Michael E. Henze, Chief Executive Officer (Total facility includes 14 beds in nursing home–type unit) **A**1 9 10 **F**7 8 12 15 16 17 19 20 21 22 23 28 29 30 32 33 34 35 37 39 40 41 42 44 45 46 49 51 53 54 55 56 57 58 59 63 64 65 67 71 73 — 23 10 91 3240 41 66311 601 33974 13470 436

Hospital, Address, Telephone, Administrator, Approval, Facility, and Physician Codes, Health Care System, Network	Classi-fication Codes		Utilization Data					Expense (thousands) of dollars		
★ American Hospital Association (AHA) membership □ Joint Commission on Accreditation of Healthcare Organizations (JCAHO) accreditation + American Osteopathic Hospital Association (AOHA) membership ○ American Osteopathic Association (AOA) accreditation △ Commission on Accreditation of Rehabilitation Facilities (CARF) accreditation Control codes 61, 63, 64, 71, 72 and 73 indicate hospitals listed by AOHA, but not registered by AHA. For definition of numerical codes, see page A4	Control	Service	Beds	Admissions	Census	Outpatient Visits	Births	Total	Payroll	Personnel

OSCEOLA—St. Clair County

✦ SAC–OSAGE HOSPITAL, Junction Highways 13 & Business 13, Zip 64776, Mailing Address: P.O. Box 426, Zip 64776–0426; tel. 417/646–8181; Terry E. Erwine, Administrator **A**1 9 10 **F**7 8 15 16 19 22 28 29 30 31 34 37 39 40 41 42 44 45 46 64 65 67 71 73	16	10	47	1402	22	5866	66	5440	2628	122

PERRYVILLE—Perry County

□ PERRY COUNTY MEMORIAL HOSPITAL, 434 North West Street, Zip 63775–1398; tel. 314/547–2536; Patrick G. Bira, JD, FACHE, Administrator **A**1 9 10 **F**1 7 8 12 14 15 16 17 18 19 22 23 24 26 27 28 29 30 32 33 34 35 39 40 41 42 44 49 53 58 64 65 67 68 71 72 73 **P**8 **N** BJC Health System, St. Louis, MO	13	10	47	1119	14	27361	178	10603	4299	202

PILOT KNOB—Iron County

✦ ARCADIA VALLEY HOSPITAL, Highway 21, Zip 63663, Mailing Address: P.O. Box 548, Zip 63663–0548; tel. 573/546–3924; H. Clark Duncan, Administrator (Total facility includes 24 beds in nursing home–type unit) **A**1 9 10 **F**8 12 15 16 17 19 22 25 26 28 29 30 31 32 33 34 35 37 39 41 44 46 49 64 65 67 71 73 **P**8 **S** SSM Health Care System, Saint Louis, MO **N** Saint Louis Health Care Network, St. Louis, MO	23	10	50	878	35	25056	0	8688	3744	136

POPLAR BLUFF—Butler County

□ △ DOCTORS REGIONAL MEDICAL CENTER, 621 Pine Boulevard, Zip 63901; tel. 573/686–4111; Daniel R. Kelly, Chief Executive Officer (Total facility includes 10 beds in nursing home–type unit) **A**1 2 7 9 10 **F**2 3 7 8 12 14 15 16 17 18 19 20 21 22 23 24 25 28 29 30 31 32 33 34 35 37 39 40 41 42 44 45 48 49 51 52 53 54 55 56 57 58 59 64 65 66 67 70 71 72 73 74 **N** BJC Health System, St. Louis, MO	33	10	187	6459	95	—	470	40221	13161	546
✦ JOHN J. PERSHING VETERANS AFFAIRS MEDICAL CENTER, 1500 North Westwood Boulevard, Zip 63901; tel. 573/686–4151; James W. Roseborough, Director (Total facility includes 49 beds in nursing home–type unit) **A**1 **F**1 2 3 4 5 8 12 15 16 18 19 20 21 22 25 26 27 28 29 30 31 32 34 35 37 39 41 42 43 44 45 46 49 51 52 54 58 59 60 64 65 67 69 71 73 74 **S** Department of Veterans Affairs, Washington, DC	45	10	174	2196	94	50397	0	27281	14671	338
□ △ LUCY LEE HOSPITAL, 2620 North Westwood Boulevard, Zip 63901–2341, Mailing Address: P.O. Box 88, Zip 63901–2341; tel. 573/785–7721; David L. Archer, Chief Executive Officer (Total facility includes 24 beds in nursing home–type unit) **A**1 2 5 7 10 **F**4 5 7 8 11 12 15 17 19 20 21 22 24 25 26 28 29 30 31 32 33 34 35 37 39 40 41 42 44 45 46 48 49 52 53 54 55 56 57 58 59 60 61 64 65 66 67 71 72 73 74 **P**1 7 **S** TENET Healthcare Corporation, Santa Barbara, CA	33	10	185	6610	105	145104	1022	45583	13507	807

POTOSI—Washington County

WASHINGTON COUNTY MEMORIAL HOSPITAL, 300 Health Way, Zip 63664–1499; tel. 314/438–5451; William L. Schwarten, Administrator **A**9 10 **F**8 14 15 16 19 22 25 28 29 30 32 34 37 39 41 44 46 49 65 67 71 74 **N** BJC Health System, St. Louis, MO	13	10	42	461	7	20239	0	6716	2753	145

RICHMOND—Ray County

RAY COUNTY MEMORIAL HOSPITAL, 904 Wollard Boulevard, Zip 64085–2243; tel. 816/776–5432; Tommy L. Hicks, Administrator (Total facility includes 11 beds in nursing home–type unit) **A**9 10 **F**8 15 16 19 22 29 30 32 33 35 37 39 41 42 44 49 64 65 71 73	13	10	50	1189	21	25489	0	9667	4378	189

ROLLA—Phelps County

✦ ○ PHELPS COUNTY REGIONAL MEDICAL CENTER, 1000 West Tenth Street, Zip 65401; tel. 573/364–3100; David Ross, Chief Executive Officer (Total facility includes 32 beds in nursing home–type unit) **A**1 5 9 10 11 12 **F**2 3 7 8 14 15 16 17 18 19 21 22 23 28 29 30 31 33 34 35 37 39 40 41 42 44 46 48 49 52 53 54 55 56 57 58 59 60 64 65 66 67 70 71 72 73 74 **P**1 3 **N** BJC Health System, St. Louis, MO	13	10	227	7122	110	59362	824	49903	19278	599

SAINT CHARLES—St. Charles County

□ BHC SPIRIT OF ST. LOUIS HOSPITAL, (Formerly CPC Spirit of St. Louis Hospital), 5931 Highway 94 South, Zip 63304–5601; tel. 314/441–7300; Larry J. Burge, Chief Executive Officer **A**1 10 **F**2 3 12 18 29 34 52 53 54 55 56 58 59 65 67 **S** Behavioral Healthcare Corporation, Nashville, TN	33	22	75	478	45	270	0	5175	—	75
CPC SPIRIT OF ST. LOUIS HOSPITAL See BHC Spirit of St. Louis Hospital										
✦ ST. JOSEPH HEALTH CENTER, 300 First Capitol Drive, Zip 63301–2835; tel. 314/947–5000; Kurt Weinmeister, President (Total facility includes 24 beds in nursing home–type unit) **A**1 2 9 10 **F**3 4 5 7 8 10 12 13 14 15 16 17 18 19 20 21 22 23 24 25 26 28 29 30 31 32 33 34 35 37 39 40 41 42 43 44 46 48 49 51 52 53 54 55 56 57 58 59 60 61 63 64 65 66 67 68 69 70 71 72 73 74 **P**1 2 4 6 7 **S** SSM Health Care System, Saint Louis, MO **N** Saint Louis Health Care Network, St. Louis, MO; Carondelet Health, Kansas City, MO	23	10	316	11576	145	36553	1010	82996	34778	959

SAINT JOSEPH—Buchanan County

✦ △ HEARTLAND REGIONAL MEDICAL CENTER, (Includes Heartland Hospital East, 5325 Faraon Street, Zip 64506; Heartland Hospital West, 801 Faraon Street, Zip 64501; tel. 816/271–7111; Lowell C. Kruse, President), 5325 Faraon Street, Zip 64506–3398; tel. 816/271–6000; Lowell C. Kruse, President (Total facility includes 210 beds in nursing home–type unit) **A**1 2 5 7 9 10 **F**4 5 7 8 10 11 12 14 15 16 17 18 19 21 22 23 24 25 27 28 30 31 32 33 34 35 37 39 40 41 42 43 44 45 46 48 49 51 52 54 55 56 57 60 65 66 70 71 73 74 **P**6 **N** Northwest Missouri Healthcare Agenda, Albany, MO	12	10	494	15927	373	328687	1513	—	—	2132

Hospital, Address, Telephone, Administrator, Approval, Facility, and Physician Codes, Health Care System, Network	Classi-fication Codes		Utilization Data					Expense (thousands) of dollars		
★ American Hospital Association (AHA) membership □ Joint Commission on Accreditation of Healthcare Organizations (JCAHO) accreditation + American Osteopathic Hospital Association (AOHA) membership ○ American Osteopathic Association (AOA) accreditation △ Commission on Accreditation of Rehabilitation Facilities (CARF) accreditation Control codes 61, 63, 64, 71, 72 and 73 indicate hospitals listed by AOHA, but not registered by AHA. For definition of numerical codes, see page A4	Control	Service	Beds	Admissions	Census	Outpatient Visits	Births	Total	Payroll	Personnel

□ ST. JOSEPH STATE HOSPITAL, 3505 Frederick Avenue, Zip 64506; tel. 816/387–2300; Ron Dittemore, Ed.D., Superintendent (Nonreporting) A1 10	12	22	123	—	—	—	—	—	—	—
SAINT LOUIS—St. Louis County										
□ ALEXIAN BROTHERS HOSPITAL, 3933 South Broadway, Zip 63118–9984; tel. 314/865–3333; Deno E. Fabbre, President and Chief Executive Officer (Total facility includes 40 beds in nursing home–type unit) A1 9 10 F2 3 5 6 8 10 12 14 15 16 17 19 21 22 25 26 27 28 29 30 31 32 33 34 35 36 37 39 41 42 44 45 46 48 49 52 54 55 56 57 58 59 62 63 64 65 67 71 72 73 P5 6 7 8 S Alexian Brothers Health System, Inc., Elk Grove Village, IL	23	10	182	5401	100	36181	0	38954	18336	654
⊞ △ BARNES–JEWISH HOSPITAL, 216 South Kingshighway Boulevard, Zip 63110–1094; tel. 314/362–5000; Alan W. Brass, FACHE, President A1 2 3 5 6 7 8 9 10 F2 3 4 5 7 8 9 10 11 12 13 14 15 16 17 18 19 20 21 22 23 24 25 26 27 28 29 30 31 32 33 34 35 37 38 39 40 41 42 43 44 45 46 47 48 49 50 51 52 53 54 55 56 57 58 59 60 61 63 64 65 66 67 68 69 70 71 72 73 74 P1 4 5 6 7 S BJC Health System, Saint Louis, MO N BJC Health System, St. Louis, MO	23	10	1221	48087	774	309255	3894	629408	264200	7613
⊞ BARNES–JEWISH WEST COUNTY HOSPITAL, 12634 Olive Boulevard, Zip 63141–6354; tel. 314/996–8000; Gregory T. Wozniak, President (Total facility includes 10 beds in nursing home–type unit) A1 9 10 F1 2 3 4 5 6 7 8 9 10 11 12 13 14 15 16 17 18 19 20 21 22 23 24 25 26 27 28 29 30 31 32 33 34 35 36 37 38 39 40 41 42 43 44 45 46 47 48 49 50 51 52 53 54 55 56 57 58 59 60 61 62 63 64 65 66 67 68 69 70 71 72 73 74 P1 5 6 7 8 S BJC Health System, Saint Louis, MO N BJC Health System, St. Louis, MO	23	10	91	2573	43	35475	0	30554	8775	280
⊞ △ BETHESDA GENERAL HOSPITAL, 3655 Vista Avenue, Zip 63110; tel. 314/772–9200; John F. Norwood, President (Total facility includes 28 beds in nursing home–type unit) A1 5 7 9 10 F1 4 6 8 10 12 14 17 19 21 22 23 26 27 28 29 30 32 33 34 35 36 37 39 41 42 44 46 48 49 50 52 54 55 56 57 58 59 60 62 63 64 65 67 71 73	23	10	118	819	38	—	0	15026	6314	151
⊞ CARDINAL GLENNON CHILDREN'S HOSPITAL, 1465 South Grand Boulevard, Zip 63104–1095; tel. 314/577–5600; Douglas A. Ries, President A1 3 5 9 10 F2 3 4 5 6 9 10 12 13 14 15 16 17 18 19 20 21 22 23 25 27 28 29 30 31 32 33 34 35 38 39 41 42 43 44 45 46 47 48 49 50 51 52 53 54 55 56 58 59 60 63 65 66 67 68 69 70 71 72 73 74 P1 6 8 S SSM Health Care System, Saint Louis, MO N Saint Louis Health Care Network, St. Louis, MO	23	50	172	8055	116	170538	0	94144	39520	1095
⊞ △ CHRISTIAN HOSPITAL NORTHEAST–NORTHWEST, (Includes Christian Hospital Northwest, 1225 Graham Road, Florissant, Zip 63031; tel. 314/839–3800), 11133 Dunn Road, Zip 63136–6192; tel. 314/355–2300; W. R. Van Bokkelen, President and Senior Executive Officer (Total facility includes 26 beds in nursing home–type unit) A1 2 5 7 9 10 F1 2 3 4 5 6 7 8 10 11 12 13 14 15 16 17 18 19 20 21 22 23 24 26 28 29 30 31 32 33 34 35 36 37 38 39 40 41 42 43 44 45 46 47 48 49 50 52 53 54 55 56 57 58 59 60 61 62 63 64 65 66 67 68 69 70 71 72 73 74 P4 5 6 7 8 S BJC Health System, Saint Louis, MO N BJC Health System, St. Louis, MO	23	10	542	22157	333	161219	1925	190777	89861	2426
□ △ DEACONESS INCARNATE WORD HEALTH SYSTEM, 6150 Oakland Avenue, Zip 63139–3297; tel. 314/768–3000; Jerry W. Paul, President (Total facility includes 10 beds in nursing home–type unit) A1 2 3 5 7 9 10 12 F1 2 3 4 7 8 10 11 14 16 17 19 21 22 23 26 27 29 30 32 33 34 35 36 37 40 41 42 43 44 48 49 51 52 54 55 56 57 58 59 60 62 64 65 66 67 71 72 73 74 P1 6 7 8	23	10	324	11599	187	95658	1786	127217	59188	1678
+ ○ DEACONESS MEDICAL CENTER–WEST CAMPUS, (Includes Metropolitan Medical Center–West), 2345 Dougherty Ferry Road, Zip 63122; tel. 314/768–3000; Joan D'Ambrose, Executive Vice President and Chief Operating Officer A10 11 12 13 F2 3 4 5 7 8 10 12 13 14 16 17 18 19 21 22 23 25 26 27 29 31 32 33 34 35 36 37 39 40 41 42 43 44 48 49 51 52 54 55 56 57 58 59 60 61 62 63 65 66 67 69 71 72 73 74 P1 6 7 8	23	10	99	2880	44	30687	0	39349	14762	408
⊞ DEPAUL HEALTH CENTER, (Includes St. Anne's Skilled Nursing Division; DePaul Hospital, Bridgeton, St. Vincent's Psychiatric Division, Bridgeton), 12303 DePaul Drive, Zip 63044–2588; tel. 314/344–6000; Robert G. Porter, President (Total facility includes 94 beds in nursing home–type unit) A1 2 5 9 10 F2 3 4 7 8 10 11 12 13 14 15 16 17 18 19 20 21 22 24 25 27 28 29 30 31 32 33 34 35 36 37 38 39 40 41 42 43 44 45 46 47 48 49 51 52 53 54 55 56 57 58 59 60 63 64 65 66 67 68 69 70 71 73 74 P1 3 4 6 S SSM Health Care System, Saint Louis, MO	21	10	371	11981	202	104516	984	108095	48721	1560
⊞ INCARNATE WORD HOSPITAL, 3545 Lafayette Avenue, Zip 63104–9984; tel. 314/865–6500; Linda M. Allin, President and Chief Executive Officer (Total facility includes 56 beds in nursing home–type unit) A1 9 10 F3 4 6 7 8 10 11 12 14 15 16 17 19 20 21 22 23 25 26 27 28 29 30 31 32 33 34 35 36 37 39 40 41 42 43 44 45 46 48 49 52 54 55 56 57 58 59 60 61 62 63 64 65 66 67 71 72 73 P3 5 6 7 8 S Incarnate Word Health Services, San Antonio, TX	21	10	198	5426	131	33920	0	47602	24341	635
□ LUTHERAN MEDICAL CENTER, 2639 Miami Street, Zip 63118–3999; tel. 314/772–1456; Cliff Yeager, Chief Executive Officer (Total facility includes 30 beds in nursing home–type unit) A1 6 10 F2 3 7 8 10 12 14 16 18 19 20 21 22 26 27 28 29 30 31 32 33 34 35 37 39 40 41 42 44 46 48 49 51 52 53 54 55 56 57 58 59 60 61 63 64 65 66 67 71 73 74 P4 5 6 7 8 S TENET Healthcare Corporation, Santa Barbara, CA METROPOLITAN MEDICAL CENTER–WEST See Deaconess Medical Center–West Campus	33	10	232	5051	119	151946	512	47306	22325	499

Hospital, Address, Telephone, Administrator, Approval, Facility, and Physician Codes, Health Care System, Network	Classi-fication Codes		Utilization Data					Expense (thousands) of dollars		
	Control	Service	Beds	Admissions	Census	Outpatient Visits	Births	Total	Payroll	Personnel

★ American Hospital Association (AHA) membership
□ Joint Commission on Accreditation of Healthcare Organizations (JCAHO) accreditation
+ American Osteopathic Hospital Association (AOHA) membership
○ American Osteopathic Association (AOA) accreditation
△ Commission on Accreditation of Rehabilitation Facilities (CARF) accreditation
Control codes 61, 63, 64, 71, 72 and 73 indicate hospitals listed by AOHA, but not registered by AHA. For definition of numerical codes, see page A4

Hospital	Control	Service	Beds	Admissions	Census	Outpatient Visits	Births	Total	Payroll	Personnel
□ METROPOLITAN ST. LOUIS PSYCHIATRIC CENTER, 5351 Delmar, Zip 63116; tel. 314/877–0500; Gregory L. Dale, Chief Executive Officer **A**1 3 5 10 **F**1 2 3 6 12 17 18 20 22 28 29 35 39 41 45 46 52 55 56 57 58 59 62 64 65 67 70 73 **P**6	12	22	125	1578	86	—	0	18473	9091	368
MISSOURI BAPTIST MEDICAL CENTER See Town and Country										
□ SAINT LOUIS UNIVERSITY HOSPITAL, 3635 Vista at Grand Boulevard, Zip 63110–0250, Mailing Address: P.O. Box 15250, Zip 63110–0250; tel. 314/577–8000; James Kimmey, M.D., M.P.H., Chairman and Chief Executive Officer **A**1 3 5 8 9 10 **F**4 5 8 10 11 14 15 19 20 22 23 26 28 29 30 31 32 34 35 37 39 41 42 43 44 45 46 49 50 51 52 53 54 55 56 59 60 61 63 65 67 69 70 71 73 **P**1 4 5 7 **N** National Cardiovascular Network, Atlanta, GA; Saint Louis Health Care Network, St. Louis, MO	23	10	303	11682	212	133880	0	205236	68355	2067
✠ SHRINERS HOSPITALS FOR CHILDREN, ST. LOUIS, 2001 South Lindbergh Boulevard, Zip 63131–3597; tel. 314/432–3600; Carolyn P. Golden, Administrator **A**1 3 5 **F**1 2 3 4 5 6 7 8 9 10 11 12 13 15 17 18 19 20 21 22 23 24 25 26 27 28 29 30 31 32 33 34 35 36 37 38 39 40 41 42 43 44 45 46 47 48 49 50 51 52 53 54 55 56 57 58 59 60 61 62 63 64 65 66 67 68 69 70 71 72 73 74 **S** Shriners Hospitals for Children, Tampa, FL	23	57	76	1757	27	11379	0	—	—	226
✠ △ SSM REHABILITATION INSTITUTE, 6420 Clayton Road, Suite 600, Zip 63117; tel. 314/768–5300; Melinda Clark, President (Total facility includes 20 beds in nursing home–type unit) **A**1 7 9 10 **F**3 4 7 8 10 13 14 15 17 18 19 21 22 24 26 28 29 30 31 32 33 34 35 36 39 41 42 43 44 45 46 48 49 50 51 53 54 55 56 57 58 59 60 62 63 64 65 66 67 68 69 70 71 74 **P**1 2 3 5 6 7 8 **S** SSM Health Care System, Saint Louis, MO **N** Saint Louis Health Care Network, St. Louis, MO	21	46	78	1358	58	85211	0	29156	16081	289
✠ ST. ANTHONY'S MEDICAL CENTER, 10010 Kennerly Road, Zip 63128; tel. 314/525–1000; David P. Seifert, President (Total facility includes 96 beds in nursing home–type unit) **A**1 9 10 **F**1 2 3 4 5 7 8 9 10 11 12 13 14 15 16 17 18 19 20 21 22 23 24 25 26 27 28 29 30 31 32 33 34 35 36 37 38 39 40 41 42 43 44 45 46 47 48 49 51 52 53 54 55 56 57 58 59 60 61 63 64 65 66 67 68 69 70 71 72 73 74 **P**6 8 **S** Sisters of Mercy Health System–St. Louis, Saint Louis, MO **N** Unity Health System, St. Louis, MO	23	10	708	25206	448	136060	1177	174180	77000	2280
✠ △ ST. JOHN'S MERCY MEDICAL CENTER, (Includes St. John's Mercy Hospital, 200 Madison Avenue, Washington, Zip 63090; tel. 314/239–8000), 615 South New Ballas Road, Zip 63141–8277; tel. 314/569–6000; Mark Weber, President (Total facility includes 20 beds in nursing home–type unit) **A**1 2 3 5 7 8 9 10 **F**2 3 4 5 7 8 9 10 11 12 13 14 15 16 17 18 19 20 21 22 23 24 25 26 27 28 29 30 31 32 33 34 35 36 37 38 39 40 41 42 43 44 45 46 47 48 49 50 51 52 53 54 55 56 57 58 59 60 61 63 64 65 66 67 68 69 70 71 72 73 74 **P**1 3 4 5 6 7 8 **S** Sisters of Mercy Health System–St. Louis, Saint Louis, MO **N** Unity Health System, St. Louis, MO	23	10	804	35022	412	347274	7272	308267	138541	4237
✠ ST. JOSEPH HOSPITAL, 525 Couch Avenue, Zip 63122–5594; tel. 314/966–1500; Carla S. Baum, President (Total facility includes 44 beds in nursing home–type unit) **A**1 9 10 **F**2 3 4 5 7 8 9 10 11 12 14 15 16 17 19 21 22 23 28 29 30 31 32 33 34 35 36 37 38 39 40 41 42 43 44 45 47 48 49 52 53 54 55 56 57 58 59 60 63 64 65 66 67 71 73 74 **P**1 4 7 8 **S** SSM Health Care System, Saint Louis, MO	23	10	250	6267	96	107501	865	54492	25505	792
✠ △ ST. LOUIS CHILDREN'S HOSPITAL, One Children's Place, Zip 63110–1077; tel. 314/454–6000; Ted W. Frey, President **A**1 3 5 7 8 10 **F**2 3 4 5 6 7 8 9 10 11 12 13 14 15 16 17 18 19 20 21 22 23 24 25 26 27 28 29 30 31 32 33 34 35 36 37 38 39 40 41 42 43 44 45 46 47 48 49 50 51 52 53 54 55 56 57 58 59 60 61 62 63 64 65 66 67 68 69 70 71 72 73 74 **P**3 4 5 6 7 8 **S** BJC Health System, Saint Louis, MO **N** BJC Health System, St. Louis, MO	23	50	235	11667	139	49986	0	141830	63157	1585
✠ ST. LOUIS REGIONAL MEDICAL CENTER, 5535 Delmar Boulevard, Zip 63112–3095; tel. 314/361–1212; Jean Weeks, Interim President and Chief Executive Officer **A**1 3 5 9 10 **F**4 5 8 10 12 13 14 15 16 17 19 20 22 24 25 26 27 28 29 30 31 32 34 36 37 38 39 40 41 42 44 45 46 49 51 53 54 58 61 63 65 66 67 68 71 72 73 74 **P**6	23	10	153	7189	101	332609	1319	85899	35835	1097
□ ST. LOUIS STATE HOSPITAL, 5400 Arsenal Street, Zip 63139–1494; tel. 314/644–8000; John M. Twiehaus, Ph.D., Superintendent **A**1 10 **F**12 20 24 29 30 39 52 54 55 65 73 **P**6	12	22	215	74	198	0	0	27253	16242	561
✠ ST. MARY'S HEALTH CENTER, 6420 Clayton Road, Zip 63117–1811; tel. 314/768–8000; Michael E. Zilm, President (Total facility includes 50 beds in nursing home–type unit) **A**1 2 3 5 8 9 10 **F**2 3 4 5 7 8 10 11 12 13 14 15 16 17 18 19 20 21 22 23 25 26 27 28 29 30 31 32 33 34 35 36 37 38 39 40 41 42 43 44 45 46 48 49 51 52 53 54 55 56 57 58 59 60 61 63 64 65 66 67 68 69 71 72 73 74 **P**1 6 8 **S** SSM Health Care System, Saint Louis, MO **N** Saint Louis Health Care Network, St. Louis, MO	23	10	440	13714	278	167799	2584	134212	57375	1698
✠ VETERANS AFFAIRS MEDICAL CENTER, Zip 63125; tel. 314/894–6661; Donald L. Ziegenhorn, Director (Total facility includes 129 beds in nursing home–type unit) (Nonreporting) **A**1 2 3 5 8 **S** Department of Veterans Affairs, Washington, DC	45	10	555	—	—	—	—	—	—	—
SAINT PETERS—St. Charles County										
✠ BARNES–JEWISH ST. PETERS HOSPITAL, (Formerly Barnes St. Peters Hospital), 10 Hospital Drive, Zip 63376–1659; tel. 314/916–9000; John Gloss, President **A**1 9 10 **F**2 3 7 8 10 14 15 16 17 19 21 22 26 28 29 30 31 32 33 34 35 37 39 40 41 42 44 49 54 55 58 59 63 65 66 67 71 72 73 74 **P**5 6 8 **S** BJC Health System, Saint Louis, MO **N** BJC Health System, St. Louis, MO	23	10	91	3899	37	68564	903	31219	13646	360

Hospital, Address, Telephone, Administrator, Approval, Facility, and Physician Codes, Health Care System, Network	Classi-fication Codes		Utilization Data					Expense (thousands) of dollars		
★ American Hospital Association (AHA) membership □ Joint Commission on Accreditation of Healthcare Organizations (JCAHO) accreditation + American Osteopathic Hospital Association (AOHA) membership ○ American Osteopathic Association (AOA) accreditation △ Commission on Accreditation of Rehabilitation Facilities (CARF) accreditation Control codes 61, 63, 64, 71, 72 and 73 indicate hospitals listed by AOHA, but not registered by AHA. For definition of numerical codes, see page A4	Control	Service	Beds	Admissions	Census	Outpatient Visits	Births	Total	Payroll	Personnel

SALEM—Dent County

SALEM MEMORIAL DISTRICT HOSPITAL, Highway 72 North, Zip 65560, Mailing Address: P.O. Box 774, Zip 65560; tel. 573/729–6626; Dennis P. Pryor, Administrator (Total facility includes 18 beds in nursing home–type unit) **A**9 10 **F**7 8 12 14 15 16 19 22 27 28 29 30 32 33 34 39 40 41 44 46 49 64 65 66 71	16	10	46	1015	33	16976	56	7291	3115	147

SEDALIA—Pettis County

⊞ BOTHWELL REGIONAL HEALTH CENTER, 601 East 14th Street, Zip 65301–1706, Mailing Address: P.O. Box 1706, Zip 65302–1706; tel. 816/826–8833; James T. Rank, Administrator **A**1 9 10 **F**4 7 8 11 15 16 19 20 21 22 23 29 30 32 33 34 35 37 39 40 41 42 44 49 52 53 56 57 60 65 66 67 71 74	14	10	147	5749	77	39115	590	39360	17205	629

SIKESTON—Scott County

□ MISSOURI DELTA MEDICAL CENTER, 1008 North Main Street, Zip 63801–5099; tel. 573/471–1600; Charles D. Ancell, President (Total facility includes 14 beds in nursing home–type unit) **A**1 9 10 **F**2 3 4 5 6 7 8 10 11 12 15 16 17 18 19 20 21 22 23 24 25 26 27 28 29 30 32 33 34 35 36 37 39 40 41 42 43 44 45 46 48 49 51 53 54 55 56 57 58 59 60 61 62 63 64 65 66 67 69 71 72 73 74 **P**8	23	10	148	4960	86	81644	542	33931	15736	570

SMITHVILLE—Clay County

⊞ SAINT LUKE'S NORTHLAND HOSPITAL–SMITHVILLE CAMPUS, 601 South 169 Highway, Zip 64089; tel. 816/532–3700; Don Sipes, Senior Executive Officer (Total facility includes 16 beds in nursing home–type unit) **A**1 9 10 **F**2 3 4 5 7 8 10 11 12 13 14 15 16 17 18 19 20 21 22 24 25 26 27 28 29 30 31 32 33 34 35 37 38 39 40 41 42 43 44 45 46 48 49 51 52 53 54 55 56 57 58 59 60 61 63 64 65 66 67 68 69 70 71 72 73 74 **P**6 8	23	10	50	780	20	22054	0	6867	3868	113

SPRINGFIELD—Greene County

⊞ ○ COLUMBIA HOSPITAL NORTH AND SOUTH, (Includes Columbia Hospital North, 2828 North National Street, Zip 65801, Mailing Address: Box 783, Jewell Station, Zip 65801–0783; tel. 417/869 5571; Charles M. Boughton, Chief Executive Officer and Administrator; Columbia Hospital South), 3535 South National Avenue, Zip 65807; tel. 417/882–4700; Michelle Fischer, Chief Executive Officer **A**1 10 11 **F**3 7 8 15 16 17 19 21 22 26 27 28 30 32 34 37 39 40 41 44 45 46 48 49 50 51 52 57 58 59 63 64 65 67 71 73 **P**7 **S** Columbia/HCA Healthcare Corporation, Nashville, TN	32	10	195	4277	86	34464	326	39415	18193	—
⊞ △ COX HEALTH SYSTEMS, (Includes Lester E. Cox Medical Center North, Lester E. Cox Medical Center South, 3801 South National Avenue, Zip 65807; tel. 417/885–6000), 1423 North Jefferson Street, Zip 65802–1988; tel. 417/269–3000; Larry D. Wallis, President and Chief Executive Officer (Total facility includes 36 beds in nursing home–type unit) **A**1 2 3 6 7 9 10 **F**1 2 3 4 7 8 10 11 14 15 16 17 19 20 21 22 23 24 25 26 27 28 29 30 31 32 33 34 35 36 37 38 39 40 41 42 43 44 45 46 47 48 49 51 52 53 54 55 56 57 58 59 60 61 63 64 65 66 67 68 70 71 73 74 **P**5 6 8	23	10	676	22703	365	—	3172	247860	117965	3939
DOCTORS HOSPITAL OF SPRINGFIELD See Columbia Hospital North										
□ LAKELAND REGIONAL HOSPITAL, 440 South Market Street, Zip 65806; tel. 417/865–5581; John William Thompson, Ph.D., President and Chief Executive Officer **A**1 10 **F**1 12 19 22 25 29 35 39 45 46 52 53 55 56 58 59 65 67 71 **P**5 6	33	22	112	1935	79	9932	0	9420	4656	161
SPRINGFIELD COMMUNITY HOSPITAL See Columbia Hospital South										
⊞ △ ST. JOHN'S REGIONAL HEALTH CENTER, 1235 East Cherokee Street, Zip 65804–2263; tel. 417/885–2000; Allen L. Shockley, President and Chief Executive Officer (Total facility includes 52 beds in nursing home–type unit) **A**1 2 6 7 10 **F**2 3 4 5 7 8 9 10 11 12 13 14 15 16 17 18 19 20 21 22 23 24 26 27 28 29 30 32 33 34 35 36 37 38 39 40 41 42 43 44 45 46 47 48 49 51 52 53 54 55 56 57 58 59 60 63 64 65 66 67 68 69 70 71 72 73 74 **P**6 **S** Sisters of Mercy Health System–St. Louis, Saint Louis, MO	23	10	813	28789	450	287273	2235	206089	98730	3564
□ U. S. MEDICAL CENTER FOR FEDERAL PRISONERS, 1900 West Sunshine Street, Zip 65808, Mailing Address: P.O. Box 4000, Zip 65808; tel. 417/862–7041; R. H. Rison, Warden (Nonreporting) **A**1	48	10	587	—	—	—	—	—	—	—

STE. GENEVIEVE—Ste. Genevieve County

STE. GENEVIEVE COUNTY MEMORIAL HOSPITAL, Highways 61 and 32, Zip 63670–0468; tel. 314/883–2751; Joseph Moss, Administrator **A**9 10 **F**7 8 14 15 17 18 19 20 22 23 24 26 28 29 30 32 34 35 37 39 40 41 42 44 45 49 65 67 68 71 73	13	10	34	1449	18	37458	95	11090	5081	194

SULLIVAN—Crawford County

★ MISSOURI BAPTIST HOSPITAL OF SULLIVAN, 751 Sappington Bridge Road, Zip 63080, Mailing Address: P.O. Box 190, Zip 63080; tel. 573/468–4186; Davis D. Skinner, Administrator (Total facility includes 6 beds in nursing home–type unit) **A**9 10 **F**7 8 12 14 15 16 17 18 19 20 21 22 26 27 28 29 30 31 32 33 34 35 37 39 40 41 42 44 45 46 49 51 64 65 71 73 **P**5 6 8 **S** BJC Health System, Saint Louis, MO **N** BJC Health System, St. Louis, MO	23	10	60	1659	19	65738	194	13498	5810	186

TOWN AND COUNTRY—St. Louis County

⊞ MISSOURI BAPTIST MEDICAL CENTER, 3015 North Ballas Road, Zip 63131–2374; tel. 314/996–5000; Mark A. Eustis, President **A**1 2 6 9 10 **F**2 3 4 5 7 8 9 10 11 12 13 15 17 18 19 20 21 22 24 25 26 27 28 29 30 31 32 33 34 35 36 37 38 39 40 41 42 43 44 45 46 47 48 49 52 53 54 55 56 57 58 59 60 61 62 63 64 65 66 67 68 69 71 72 73 74 **P**3 4 5 6 7 8 **S** BJC Health System, Saint Louis, MO **N** BJC Health System, St. Louis, MO	23	10	335	13802	189	187205	2438	130367	56320	1692

Hospital, Address, Telephone, Administrator, Approval, Facility, and Physician Codes, Health Care System, Network	Classi-fication Codes		Utilization Data					Expense (thousands) of dollars		
★ American Hospital Association (AHA) membership □ Joint Commission on Accreditation of Healthcare Organizations (JCAHO) accreditation + American Osteopathic Hospital Association (AOHA) membership ○ American Osteopathic Association (AOA) accreditation △ Commission on Accreditation of Rehabilitation Facilities (CARF) accreditation Control codes 61, 63, 64, 71, 72 and 73 indicate hospitals listed by AOHA, but not registered by AHA. For definition of numerical codes, see page A4	Control	Service	Beds	Admissions	Census	Outpatient Visits	Births	Total	Payroll	Personnel
TRENTON—Grundy County										
□ WRIGHT MEMORIAL HOSPITAL, 701 East First Street, Zip 64683–0648, Mailing Address: P.O. Box 628, Zip 64683–0628; tel. 816/359–5621; Johnnye L. Dennis, Chief Executive Officer **A**1 9 10 **F**7 15 19 20 22 26 27 28 29 32 33 34 37 39 40 41 42 43 44 49 51 64 65 67 71 73 **P**5 8 **S** Saint Luke's Shawnee Mission Health System, Kansas City, MO	23	10	48	775	9	21707	12	7893	3990	156
TROY—Lincoln County										
□ LINCOLN COUNTY MEMORIAL HOSPITAL, 1000 East Cherry, Zip 63379; tel. 314/528–8551; Floyd B. Dowell, Jr., Administrator (Total facility includes 8 beds in nursing home–type unit) **A**1 9 10 **F**8 11 12 15 16 17 19 20 21 22 25 28 29 30 32 33 34 35 37 39 41 44 45 46 49 64 65 67 71 **P**1 7 8 **N** Saint Louis Health Care Network, St. Louis, MO	13	10	36	1566	21	31948	0	13680	—	199
WARRENSBURG—Johnson County										
□ WESTERN MISSOURI MEDICAL CENTER, 403 Burkarth Road, Zip 64093–3101; tel. 816/747–2500; Gregory B. Vinardi, President and Chief Executive Officer (Total facility includes 15 beds in nursing home–type unit) **A**1 9 10 **F**7 8 12 13 14 15 16 19 20 21 22 23 24 28 29 30 31 32 33 34 35 36 37 39 40 41 42 44 45 46 61 64 65 66 67 68 71 73 74	13	10	71	2569	34	42081	333	17073	7762	300
WENTZVILLE—St. Charles County										
□ DOCTORS HOSPITAL, 500 Medical Drive, Zip 63385–0711; tel. 314/327–1000; Fred Woody, Chief Executive Officer (Total facility includes 27 beds in nursing home–type unit) **A**1 9 10 **F**7 8 14 15 16 19 21 22 23 28 29 30 32 33 35 37 39 40 41 42 44 46 49 63 64 65 66 67 70 71 72 73 **N** BJC Health System, St. Louis, MO	33	10	94	2029	20	35821	196	16147	5106	150
WEST PLAINS—Howell County										
★ OZARKS MEDICAL CENTER, 1100 Kentucky Avenue, Zip 65775, Mailing Address: P.O. Box 1100, Zip 65775–1100; tel. 417/256–9111; Charles R. Brackney, President and Chief Executive Officer (Total facility includes 16 beds in nursing home–type unit) **A**9 10 **F**7 8 10 12 15 16 19 21 22 28 29 30 31 32 33 34 37 39 40 42 44 45 46 52 53 54 55 56 57 58 60 64 65 67 71 72 73 **P**8 **N** BJC Health System, St. Louis, MO	23	10	120	5382	69	38289	696	44206	20635	846
WHITEMAN AFB—Johnson County										
▣ U. S. AIR FORCE HOSPITAL WHITEMAN, Zip 65305–5001; tel. 816/687–1194; Lieutenant Colonel David Wilmot, USAF, MSC, Administrator **A**1 **F**8 12 15 16 20 24 28 29 30 31 34 39 40 44 45 51 71 74 **P**6 **S** Department of the Air Force, Washington, DC	41	10	20	635	3	71767	217	—	—	296

MONTANA

Resident population 870 (in thousands)
Resident population in metro areas 23.8%
Birth rate per 1,000 population 13.5
65 years and over 13.1%
Percent of persons without health insurance 13.6%

Hospital, Address, Telephone, Administrator, Approval, Facility, and Physician Codes, Health Care System, Network	Classi-fication Codes		Utilization Data					Expense (thousands) of dollars		
	Control	Service	Beds	Admissions	Census	Outpatient Visits	Births	Total	Payroll	Personnel

★ American Hospital Association (AHA) membership
□ Joint Commission on Accreditation of Healthcare Organizations (JCAHO) accreditation
+ American Osteopathic Hospital Association (AOHA) membership
○ American Osteopathic Association (AOA) accreditation
△ Commission on Accreditation of Rehabilitation Facilities (CARF) accreditation
Control codes 61, 63, 64, 71, 72 and 73 indicate hospitals listed by AOHA, but not registered by AHA. For definition of numerical codes, see page A4.

ANACONDA—Deer Lodge County

★ COMMUNITY HOSPITAL OF ANACONDA, 401 West Pennsylvania Street, Zip 59711; tel. 406/563–5261; Sam J. Allen, Administrator (Total facility includes 67 beds in nursing home–type unit) **A**10 **F**19 22 27 33 34 40 44 65 71 **P**6 **S** Quorum Health Group/Quorum Health Resources, Inc., Brentwood, TN

23	10	101	1231	78	137751	51	8832	4244	154

BAKER—Fallon County

FALLON MEDICAL COMPLEX, 202 South 4th Street West, Zip 59313–0820, Mailing Address: P.O. Box 820, Zip 59313–0820; tel. 406/778–3331; David Espeland, Chief Executive Officer (Total facility includes 40 beds in nursing home–type unit) **A**10 **F**7 8 14 15 16 19 20 22 28 30 32 34 35 36 37 40 41 42 49 51 62 64 65 71 73 **P**6 **N** Montana Health Network, Inc., Miles City, MT

23	10	52	298	41	37077	11	4739	2454	118

BIG SANDY—Chouteau County

BIG SANDY MEDICAL CENTER, Mailing Address: P.O. Box 530, Zip 59520–0530; tel. 406/378–2188; Harry Bold, Administrator (Total facility includes 22 beds in nursing home–type unit) **A**10 **F**15 16 22 32 34 49 64

23	10	30	55	21	5476	0	1106	588	32

BIG TIMBER—Rosebud County

PIONEER MEDICAL CENTER, Mailing Address: P.O. Box 1228, Zip 59011; tel. 406/932–4603; Lauri Ann Cooney, Chief Executive Officer (Nonreporting) **A**9

13	49	8	—	—	—	—	—	—	—

BILLINGS—Yellowstone County

⊞ DEACONESS MEDICAL CENTER, 2800 10th Avenue North, Zip 59101–0799, Mailing Address: P.O. Box 37000, Zip 59107–7001; tel. 406/657–4000; Patrick R. Garrett, Administrative Executive Officer **A**1 9 10 **F**2 3 4 6 8 10 11 12 15 16 18 19 20 21 22 23 25 26 27 29 30 31 32 33 34 35 37 39 41 42 43 44 45 48 49 51 52 53 54 55 56 57 58 59 60 62 64 65 66 67 70 71 72 73 74 **P**6 **N** Montana Health Network, Inc., Miles City, MT

23	10	232	9406	149	42754	0	148198	69854	1809

⊞ △ SAINT VINCENT HOSPITAL AND HEALTH CENTER, 1233 North 30th Street, Zip 59101, Mailing Address: P.O. Box 35200, Zip 59107–5200; tel. 406/657–7000; Patrick M. Hermanson, President and Senior Executive **A**1 7 9 10 **F**4 7 8 10 12 15 16 17 18 19 21 22 24 26 28 29 30 31 34 37 38 40 41 42 43 44 45 46 48 49 60 61 64 65 66 67 70 71 73 74 **P**5 / **S** Sisters of Charity of Leavenworth Health Services Corporation, Leavenworth, KS

21	10	257	12171	184	103391	1954	104640	42112	1212

BOZEMAN—Gallatin County

★ BOZEMAN DEACONESS HOSPITAL, 915 Highland Boulevard, Zip 59715; tel. 406/585–5000; John A. Nordwick, President and Chief Executive Officer **A**10 **F**6 7 8 11 12 15 16 17 19 21 23 28 30 32 33 34 35 37 39 40 41 42 44 49 60 62 63 65 66 67 70 71 73

23	10	70	3824	35	53092	699	24302	9689	327

BROWNING—Glacier County

⊞ U. S. PUBLIC HEALTH SERVICE BLACKFEET COMMUNITY HOSPITAL, Mailing Address: P.O. Box 760, Zip 59417–0760; tel. 406/338–6100; Mary Ellen LaFromboise, Service Unit Director (Nonreporting) **A**1 5 10 **S** U. S. Public Health Service Indian Health Service, Rockville, MD

47	10	25	—	—	—	—	—	—	—

BUTTE—Silver Bow County

⊞ ST. JAMES COMMUNITY HOSPITAL, 400 South Clark Street, Zip 59701, Mailing Address: P.O. Box 3300, Zip 59702; tel. 406/723–2500; James T. Paquette, Regional Chief Executive Officer **A**1 9 10 **F**12 15 16 17 19 20 21 22 23 26 28 29 30 33 34 35 37 38 40 42 44 45 46 49 60 63 64 65 66 67 70 71 73 **S** Sisters of Charity of Leavenworth Health Services Corporation, Leavenworth, KS

23	10	103	4278	63	37557	533	34331	13586	405

CHESTER—Liberty County

LIBERTY COUNTY HOSPITAL AND NURSING HOME, Mailing Address: P.O. Box 705, Zip 59522–0705; tel. 406/759–5181; Douglas Faus, Administrator (Total facility includes 55 beds in nursing home–type unit) **A**9 10 **F**6 8 11 22 32 34 37 40 44 49 64 65 71

13	10	66	293	46	6309	23	2753	1418	79

CHOTEAU—Teton County

TETON MEDICAL CENTER, 915 Fourth Street N.W., Zip 59422; tel. 406/466–5763; Jay Pottenger, Administrator (Total facility includes 42 beds in nursing home–type unit) **A**9 10 **F**1 8 16 22 28 30 33 44 49 64

16	10	46	126	36	4703	0	2285	1143	66

CIRCLE—McCone County

MCCONE COUNTY MEDICAL ASSISTANCE FACILITY, Mailing Address: P.O. Box 47, Zip 59215–0047; tel. 406/485–3381; Mike Anderson, Administrator (Total facility includes 38 beds in nursing home–type unit) **A**9 10 **F**1 22 64 65 70 **N** Montana Health Network, Inc., Miles City, MT

23	10	40	47	31	1966	—	1314	635	49

COLUMBUS—Stillwater County

STILLWATER COMMUNITY HOSPITAL, 44 West Fourth Avenue North, Zip 59019, Mailing Address: P.O. Box 959, Zip 59019–0959; tel. 406/322–5316; Tim Russell, Administrator (Total facility includes 9 beds in nursing home–type unit) (Nonreporting) **A**9 10 **N** Montana Health Network, Inc., Miles City, MT

23	10	23	—	—	—	—	—	—	—

CONRAD—Pondera County

★ PONDERA MEDICAL CENTER, 805 Sunset Boulevard, Zip 59425, Mailing Address: P.O. Box 757, Zip 59425–0757; tel. 406/278–3211; L. Carl Hanson, Administrator (Total facility includes 59 beds in nursing home–type unit) **A**9 10 **F**1 7 8 15 16 20 21 22 28 32 33 40 41 44 48 49 64 70 71

13	10	79	673	64	6843	17	5357	2797	129

Hospital, Address, Telephone, Administrator, Approval, Facility, and Physician Codes, Health Care System, Network	Classification Codes		Utilization Data					Expense (thousands) of dollars		
	Control	Service	Beds	Admissions	Census	Outpatient Visits	Births	Total	Payroll	Personnel

★ American Hospital Association (AHA) membership
□ Joint Commission on Accreditation of Healthcare Organizations (JCAHO) accreditation
+ American Osteopathic Hospital Association (AOHA) membership
○ American Osteopathic Association (AOA) accreditation
△ Commission on Accreditation of Rehabilitation Facilities (CARF) accreditation
Control codes 61, 63, 64, 71, 72 and 73 indicate hospitals listed by AOHA, but not registered by AHA. For definition of numerical codes, see page A4

CROW AGENCY—Big Horn County

✠ U. S. PUBLIC HEALTH SERVICE INDIAN HOSPITAL, Mailing Address: Box 9, Zip 59022; tel. 406/638–2626; Tennyson Doney, Service Unit Director **A**1 10 **F**2 3 4 5 6 7 8 10 11 13 14 15 16 17 18 19 20 22 24 25 26 27 28 29 30 31 32 34 35 36 38 39 40 41 42 44 47 48 49 52 53 54 56 57 58 59 60 61 64 65 66 67 68 69 70 71 72 74 **P**6 **S** U. S. Public Health Service Indian Health Service, Rockville, MD	47	10	24	1337	12	82144	224	18383	9194	246

CULBERTSON—Roosevelt County

★ ROOSEVELT MEMORIAL MEDICAL CENTER, (Formerly Roosevelt Medical Center), Mailing Address: P.O. Box 419, Zip 59218; tel. 406/787–6281; Walter Busch, Administrator (Total facility includes 44 beds in nursing home–type unit) **A**9 10 **F**1 8 13 15 22 26 27 28 30 32 34 36 39 41 46 49 51 64 71 73 **P**6 **N** Montana Health Network, Inc., Miles City, MT	23	10	54	182	40	679	0	2678	1647	86

CUT BANK—Glacier County

GLACIER COUNTY MEDICAL CENTER, 802 Second Street S.E., Zip 59427; tel. 406/873–2251; Michael D. Billing, Administrator (Total facility includes 39 beds in nursing home–type unit) **A**9 10 **F**7 8 15 19 20 22 31 32 34 37 40 42 44 56 64 65 71 73 **P**3	13	10	59	519	44	11195	37	3843	1929	—

DEER LODGE—Powell County

★ POWELL COUNTY MEMORIAL HOSPITAL, 1101 Texas Avenue, Zip 59722–1828; tel. 406/846–2212; Tony Pfaff, Chief Executive Officer (Total facility includes 16 beds in nursing home–type unit) **A**9 10 **F**14 15 16 22 32 34 37 40 43 64 **S** Brim, Inc., Portland, OR	23	10	35	260	16	5322	20	3417	1465	69

DILLON—Beaverhead County

★ BARRETT MEMORIAL HOSPITAL, 1260 South Atlantic Street, Zip 59725; tel. 406/683–3000; Jim D. Le Brun, Chief Executive Officer **A**9 10 **F**7 8 14 15 16 17 19 21 22 28 29 30 31 32 33 34 35 39 41 44 45 46 49 61 65 66 71 73 74 **P**5 **S** Brim, Inc., Portland, OR	16	10	31	925	7	21482	87	7675	3325	118

ENNIS—Madison County

MADISON VALLEY HOSPITAL, 217 North Main Street, Zip 59729–0397, Mailing Address: P.O. Box 397, Zip 59729–0397; tel. 406/682–4222; Geri Wilson, Chief Executive Officer **A**9 10 **F**11 15 16 22 25 44	16	10	9	181	1	—	0	1302	—	32

FORSYTH—Rosebud County

★ ROSEBUD HEALTH CARE CENTER, 383 North 17th Avenue, Zip 59327; tel. 406/356–2161; John M. Chioutsis, Chief Executive Officer (Total facility includes 55 beds in nursing home–type unit) (Nonreporting) **A**9 10 **S** Brim, Inc., Portland, OR	23	10	75	—	—	—	—	—	—	—

FORT BENTON—Chouteau County

MISSOURI RIVER MEDICAL CENTER, 1501 St. Charles Street, Zip 59442–0249, Mailing Address: P.O. Box 249, Zip 59442–0249; tel. 406/622–3331; Raymond Bergroos, Administrator (Total facility includes 45 beds in nursing home–type unit) **A**9 10 **F**6 21 22 25 31 32 64 65 **P**6	16	10	50	166	42	6644	0	2557	1375	87

FORT HARRISON—Lewis and Clark County

✠ VETERANS AFFAIRS HOSPITAL, Zip 59636; tel. 406/442–6410; Joseph Underkofler, Director **A**1 **F**2 3 4 8 11 12 19 20 21 22 24 25 26 27 28 29 30 31 34 35 37 39 41 42 44 45 46 49 51 52 54 55 57 58 60 65 67 71 73 74 **P**6 **S** Department of Veterans Affairs, Washington, DC	45	10	88	3003	63	49966	0	29940	14180	341

GLASGOW—Valley County

□ FRANCES MAHON DEACONESS HOSPITAL, 621 Third Street South, Zip 59230; tel. 406/228–4351; Douglas A. McMillan, Chief Executive Officer **A**1 9 10 **F**3 7 8 11 19 21 22 26 28 31 32 34 35 44 45 50 54 63 71 **P**3 **N** Montana Health Network, Inc., Miles City, MT	23	10	36	1058	11	23092	98	11468	4675	185

GLENDIVE—Dawson County

□ GLENDIVE MEDICAL CENTER, 202 Prospect Drive, Zip 59330; tel. 406/365–3306; Paul Hanson, Chief Executive Officer (Total facility includes 75 beds in nursing home–type unit) **A**1 9 10 **F**2 7 8 12 14 15 17 18 19 20 21 22 24 26 27 28 30 31 32 33 34 36 37 39 40 41 42 44 46 48 49 52 58 60 64 65 67 71 73 **P**3 4 **N** Montana Health Network, Inc., Miles City, MT	23	10	104	624	73	14251	73	8808	4123	219

GREAT FALLS—Cascade County

✠ △ BENEFIS HEALTH CARE, (Includes Benefis Health Care–East Campus, 1101 26th Street, Zip 59405; Benefis Health Care–West Campus, 500 15th Avenue South, Zip 59405, Mailing Address: P.O. Box 5013, Zip 59403–5013; tel. 406/727–3333), 500 15th Avenue South, Zip 59403; tel. 406/727–3333; Lloyd V. Smith, President and Chief Executive Officer (Total facility includes 138 beds in nursing home–type unit) (Nonreporting) **A**1 2 7 9 10 **S** Providence Services, Spokane, WA **N** Providence Services, Spokane, WA	23	10	357	—	—	—	—	—	—	—

HAMILTON—Ravalli County

★ MARCUS DALY MEMORIAL HOSPITAL, 1200 Westwood Drive, Zip 59840; tel. 406/363–2211; John M. Bartos, Administrator **A**10 **F**7 8 11 14 15 16 19 21 22 28 30 31 32 33 34 37 39 40 42 44 45 46 49 51 65 66 67 71 73 **P**8	23	10	48	1652	15	62126	218	15284	8161	292

HARDIN—Big Horn County

★ BIG HORN COUNTY MEMORIAL HOSPITAL, 17 North Miles Avenue, Zip 59034, Mailing Address: P.O. Box 430, Zip 59034; tel. 406/665–2310; Raymond T. Hino, Administrator (Total facility includes 37 beds in nursing home–type unit) **A**10 **F**7 8 22 28 30 32 34 40 44 45 49 64 65 71 73 **S** Brim, Inc., Portland, OR	23	10	53	658	38	5672	64	3616	1798	95

HARLEM—Blaine County

✠ U. S. PUBLIC HEALTH SERVICE INDIAN HOSPITAL, Rural Route 1, Box 67, Zip 59526; tel. 406/353–2651; Charles D. Plumage, Director **A**1 10 **F**2 3 4 7 8 9 10 11 12 13 14 15 16 17 18 19 20 21 22 24 27 28 29 30 31 32 34 35 37 38 39 40 42 43 44 45 47 48 49 50 52 53 56 58 60 61 63 65 66 69 70 71 74 **S** U. S. Public Health Service Indian Health Service, Rockville, MD	47	10	12	538	3	40251	0	—	—	80

Hospital, Address, Telephone, Administrator, Approval, Facility, and Physician Codes, Health Care System, Network	Classification Codes		Utilization Data					Expense (thousands) of dollars		
★ American Hospital Association (AHA) membership ☐ Joint Commission on Accreditation of Healthcare Organizations (JCAHO) accreditation + American Osteopathic Hospital Association (AOHA) membership ○ American Osteopathic Association (AOA) accreditation △ Commission on Accreditation of Rehabilitation Facilities (CARF) accreditation Control codes 61, 63, 64, 71, 72 and 73 indicate hospitals listed by AOHA, but not registered by AHA. For definition of numerical codes, see page A4	Control	Service	Beds	Admissions	Census	Outpatient Visits	Births	Total	Payroll	Personnel
HARLOWTON—Wheatland County										
★ WHEATLAND MEMORIAL HOSPITAL, 530 Third Street North, Zip 59036, Mailing Address: Box 287, Zip 59036; tel. 406/632–4351; Craig E. Aasved, Administrator (Total facility includes 33 beds in nursing home–type unit) (Nonreporting) **A**10	13	10	56	—	—	—	—	—	—	—
HAVRE—Hill County										
⊞ NORTHERN MONTANA HOSPITAL, 30 13th Street, Zip 59501, Mailing Address: P.O. Box 1231, Zip 59501; tel. 406/265–2211; David Henry, President and Chief Executive Officer (Total facility includes 33 beds in nursing home–type unit) **A**1 10 **F**2 3 7 8 12 14 15 16 19 21 22 26 28 30 32 34 35 37 39 40 41 44 46 49 51 52 54 56 57 58 59 64 65 66 67 71 73 74 **P**5 **S** Brim, Inc., Portland, OR	23	10	154	3743	68	31322	413	23814	11209	499
HELENA—Lewis and Clark County										
⊞ SHODAIR CHILDREN'S HOSPITAL, 840 Helena Avenue, Zip 59601, Mailing Address: P.O. Box 5539, Zip 59604; tel. 406/444–7500; Jack Casey, Administrator **A**1 10 **F**15 16 52 53 55 58 59 61 65	23	52	66	137	38	8678	0	7720	4675	153
⊞ ST. PETER'S COMMUNITY HOSPITAL, 2475 Broadway, Zip 59601; tel. 406/442–2480; Robert W. Ladenburger, President **A**1 10 **F**7 8 10 12 14 15 16 17 19 21 22 27 28 29 30 31 32 33 34 35 36 37 38 39 40 41 42 44 45 46 49 52 54 55 56 57 58 59 60 63 64 65 67 71 73 **P**8	23	10	80	4887	44	69625	775	42827	19587	499
KALISPELL—Flathead County										
⊞ △ KALISPELL REGIONAL HOSPITAL, 310 Sunnyview Lane, Zip 59901; tel. 406/752–5111; Thomas W. Laux, President and Chief Executive Officer (Total facility includes 92 beds in nursing home–type unit) **A**1 7 10 **F**1 2 3 4 7 8 10 11 12 15 16 17 19 20 21 22 23 24 26 27 28 30 31 32 33 34 35 37 39 40 41 42 44 45 46 48 49 51 52 53 54 55 56 57 58 59 60 63 64 65 66 67 68 71 73 **P**5 6 7 8	23	10	150	6233	69	95535	682	50587	23248	876
LEWISTOWN—Fergus County										
★ CENTRAL MONTANA MEDICAL CENTER, 408 Wendell Avenue, Zip 59457, Mailing Address: P.O. Box 580, Zip 59457; tel. 406/538–7711; David M. Faulkner, Chief Executive Officer and Administrator (Total facility includes 85 beds in nursing home–type unit) **A**10 **F**1 7 8 11 12 19 21 22 28 32 33 34 35 37 39 40 41 44 49 50 63 64 65 66 67 **S** Quorum Health Group/Quorum Health Resources, Inc., Brentwood, TN **N** Montana Health Network, Inc., Miles City, MT	23	10	124	1497	103	29818	137	13184	6110	262
LIBBY—Lincoln County										
★ ST. JOHN'S LUTHERAN HOSPITAL, 350 Louisiana Avenue, Zip 59923; tel. 406/293–7761; Richard L. Palagi, Chief Executive Officer **A**9 10 **F**7 8 11 19 22 30 32 34 37 39 40 41 44 49 66 71 72 **P**7 **S** Brim, Inc., Portland, OR	23	10	27	1034	11	23604	114	7120	3600	133
LIVINGSTON—Park County										
★ LIVINGSTON MEMORIAL HOSPITAL, 504 South 13th Street, Zip 59047; tel. 406/222–3541; Richard V. Brown, Chief Executive Officer **A**10 **F**7 8 11 13 14 15 16 17 19 21 22 24 28 29 30 32 33 34 37 40 42 44 49 63 65 67 68 71 74	23	10	35	1309	13	19155	177	8374	3886	154
MALTA—Phillips County										
PHILLIPS COUNTY HOSPITAL, 417 South Fourth East, Zip 59538, Mailing Address: P.O. Box 640, Zip 59538–0640; tel. 406/654–1100; Larry E. Putnam, Administrator **A**10 **F**16 22 28 30 32 44 49 51 66 71 73 74 **P**3 **N** Montana Health Network, Inc., Miles City, MT	23	10	15	189	1	5585	1	—	—	44
MILES CITY—Custer County										
⊞ HOLY ROSARY HEALTH CENTER, 2600 Wilson, Zip 59301; tel. 406/233–2600; H. Ray Gibbons, President and Chief Executive Officer (Total facility includes 107 beds in nursing home–type unit) **A**1 10 **F**2 3 7 8 11 12 13 14 15 16 17 19 21 22 24 27 28 30 32 35 36 37 39 40 42 44 48 49 52 53 54 55 56 57 58 63 64 65 67 71 73 **P**5 **S** Sisters of Charity of Leavenworth Health Services Corporation, Leavenworth, KS **N** Montana Health Network, Inc., Miles City, MT	21	10	151	1893	97	28305	237	16296	6516	256
⊞ VETERANS AFFAIRS MEDICAL CENTER, 210 South Winchester Avenue, Zip 59301; tel. 406/232–3060; Richard J. Stanley, Director (Total facility includes 30 beds in nursing home–type unit) **A**1 **F**1 2 3 4 8 9 10 11 12 16 17 19 20 21 22 25 26 27 28 30 31 32 34 35 37 39 41 42 43 44 45 46 48 49 50 51 52 54 55 56 57 58 59 60 64 65 69 71 73 74 **S** Department of Veterans Affairs, Washington, DC	45	10	50	643	10	35550	0	—	—	191
MISSOULA—Missoula County										
⊞ △ COMMUNITY MEDICAL CENTER, 2827 Fort Missoula Road, Zip 59801; tel. 406/728–4100; Grant M. Winn, President **A**1 7 10 **F**7 8 11 19 22 30 34 37 38 39 40 41 44 48 49 64 65 71 73 74 **P**6 **S** Brim, Inc., Portland, OR	23	10	115	4853	107	144870	1450	47778	23308	660
⊞ ST. PATRICK HOSPITAL, 500 West Broadway, Zip 59802–4096, Mailing Address: Box 4587, Zip 59806–4587; tel. 406/543–7271; Lawrence L. White, Jr., President (Total facility includes 18 beds in nursing home–type unit) **A**1 9 10 **F**2 3 4 10 11 12 14 15 16 17 19 21 22 23 24 27 29 30 32 33 34 35 36 37 39 41 42 43 44 45 47 49 52 53 54 55 56 57 58 59 60 63 64 65 66 67 68 69 70 71 72 73 **P**6 7 **S** Providence Services, Spokane, WA **N** Northern Rockies Healthcare Network, Missoula, MT; Providence Services, Spokane, WA	21	10	191	8668	113	115052	0	78013	29735	898
PHILIPSBURG—Granite County										
GRANITE COUNTY MEMORIAL HOSPITAL AND NURSING HOME, Mailing Address: P.O. Box 729, Zip 59858–0729; tel. 406/859–3271; Doris White, Administrator (Nonreporting) **A**9 10	13	10	31	—	—	—	—	—	—	—
PLAINS—Sanders County										
★ CLARK FORK VALLEY HOSPITAL, Mailing Address: P.O. Box 768, Zip 59859–0768; tel. 406/826–3601; Tom Mitchell, Chief Executive Officer (Total facility includes 28 beds in nursing home–type unit) **A**9 10 **F**3 4 5 7 8 10 11 14 15 16 22 23 26 28 29 30 31 32 33 34 37 39 41 42 43 44 49 64 67 71 73 **P**6	23	10	44	680	41	—	27	5994	3202	139

Hospital, Address, Telephone, Administrator, Approval, Facility, and Physician Codes, Health Care System, Network	Classification Codes		Utilization Data					Expense (thousands) of dollars		
★ American Hospital Association (AHA) membership □ Joint Commission on Accreditation of Healthcare Organizations (JCAHO) accreditation + American Osteopathic Hospital Association (AOHA) membership ○ American Osteopathic Association (AOA) accreditation △ Commission on Accreditation of Rehabilitation Facilities (CARF) accreditation Control codes 61, 63, 64, 71, 72 and 73 indicate hospitals listed by AOHA, but not registered by AHA. For definition of numerical codes, see page A4	Control	Service	Beds	Admissions	Census	Outpatient Visits	Births	Total	Payroll	Personnel

PLENTYWOOD—Sheridan County

SHERIDAN MEMORIAL HOSPITAL, 440 West Laurel Avenue, Zip 59254; tel. 406/765–1420; Ella Gutzke, Administrator (Total facility includes 78 beds in nursing home–type unit) **A**9 10 **F**7 8 12 15 16 19 22 28 30 31 32 34 37 41 44 46 49 51 64 65 67 71 73 **P**3 **N** Montana Health Network, Inc., Miles City, MT — 23 10 97 651 88 939 41 4683 2505 161

POLSON—Lake County

✠ ST. JOSEPH HOSPITAL, Skyline Drive and 14th Avenue, Zip 59860, Mailing Address: P.O. Box 1010, Zip 59860–1010; tel. 406/883–5377; John W. Glueckert, President **A**1 9 10 **F**7 8 15 22 32 40 44 65 71 73 **S** Providence Services, Spokane, WA **N** Providence Services, Spokane, WA — 21 10 22 654 4 21808 70 4516 2213 71

RED LODGE—Carbon County

★ CARBON COUNTY MEMORIAL HOSPITAL AND NURSING HOME, 600 West 20th Street, Zip 59068, Mailing Address: P.O. Box 590, Zip 59068–0590; tel. 406/446–2345; Kelley Going, Administrator (Total facility includes 30 beds in nursing home–type unit) **A**9 10 **F**7 8 11 12 14 15 16 17 22 24 26 27 28 29 30 32 34 40 41 44 45 46 48 49 51 54 56 57 64 65 66 71 73 **P**5 **N** Montana Health Network, Inc., Miles City, MT — 23 10 52 382 34 — 26 3442 1726 88

RONAN—Lake County

★ ST. LUKE COMMUNITY HOSPITAL, 107 Sixth Avenue S.W., Zip 59864; tel. 406/676–4441; Shane Roberts, Administrator (Total facility includes 75 beds in nursing home–type unit) **A**10 **F**7 8 15 16 22 28 31 34 40 44 64 71 **P**6 — 23 10 99 834 75 25874 114 8694 5010 185

ROUNDUP—Musselshell County

★ ROUNDUP MEMORIAL HOSPITAL, 1202 Third Street West, Zip 59072, Mailing Address: P.O. Box 40, Zip 59072; tel. 406/323–2302; Dave McIvor, Administrator (Total facility includes 37 beds in nursing home–type unit) **A**10 **F**1 8 14 15 16 17 22 28 30 32 34 36 49 64 65 74 **P**6 **S** Brim, Inc., Portland, OR **N** Montana Health Network, Inc., Miles City, MT — 23 10 54 208 39 4335 0 3003 1557 82

SCOBEY—Daniels County

DANIELS MEMORIAL HOSPITAL, 105 Fifth Avenue East, Zip 59263, Mailing Address: P.O. Box 400, Zip 59263–0400; tel. 406/487–2296; Glenn Haugo, Administrator (Total facility includes 48 beds in nursing home–type unit) (Nonreporting) **A**10 **N** Montana Health Network, Inc., Miles City, MT — 23 10 54 — — — — — — —

SHELBY—Toole County

TOOLE COUNTY HOSPITAL AND NURSING HOME, 640 Park Drive, Zip 59474, Mailing Address: P.O. Box 915, Zip 59474; tel. 406/434–5536; Jerry Morasko, Administrator (Total facility includes 68 beds in nursing home–type unit) **A**10 **F**7 8 11 14 19 22 27 32 34 35 37 39 40 42 44 49 64 65 67 71 73 **P**6 — 13 10 88 920 75 9203 73 6764 2826 151

SHERIDAN—Madison County

RUBY VALLEY HOSPITAL, 220 East Crofoot Street, Zip 59749, Mailing Address: Box 336, Zip 59749–0336; tel. 406/842–5453; Steve Lang, Administrator (Nonreporting) **A**10 — 16 10 14 — — — — — — —

SIDNEY—Richland County

SIDNEY HEALTH CENTER, (Formerly Community Memorial Hospital), 216 14th Avenue S.W., Zip 59270, Mailing Address: P.O. Box 1690, Zip 59270–1690; tel. 406/482–2120; Donald J. Rush, Chief Executive Officer **A**9 10 **F**8 11 15 19 21 22 24 30 32 33 35 36 40 42 44 49 65 67 71 73 **N** Montana Health Network, Inc., Miles City, MT — 23 10 42 1410 16 29324 117 13427 5832 227

SUPERIOR—Mineral County

★ MINERAL COMMUNITY HOSPITAL, Roosevelt and Brooklyn, Zip 59872, Mailing Address: P.O. Box 66, Zip 59872–0066; tel. 406/822–4841; Madelyn Faller, Chief Executive Officer (Total facility includes 20 beds in nursing home–type unit) **A**9 10 **F**6 7 8 11 15 21 22 26 28 29 37 44 49 51 64 70 71 **S** Brim, Inc., Portland, OR — 23 10 30 312 25 5657 2 2709 1281 66

TERRY—Prairie County

★ PRAIRIE COMMUNITY MEDICAL ASSISTANCE FACILITY, 312 South Adams Avenue, Zip 59349–0156, Mailing Address: P.O. Box 156, Zip 59349–0156; tel. 406/637–5511; James R. Mantz, Administrator (Total facility includes 19 beds in nursing home–type unit) **A**9 10 **F**8 13 15 22 26 28 36 51 64 — 16 10 21 17 19 981 0 1003 578 31

TOWNSEND—Broadwater County

BROADWATER HEALTH CENTER, 110 North Oak Street, Zip 59644, Mailing Address: P.O. Box 519, Zip 59644; tel. 406/266–3186; Kent Hanawatt, Chief Executive Officer (Total facility includes 32 beds in nursing home–type unit) **A**9 10 **F**1 22 28 32 33 44 48 49 51 64 73 **P**6 — 23 10 44 112 37 7795 5 — — 49

WARM SPRINGS—Deer Lodge County

MONTANA STATE HOSPITAL, Zip 59756; tel. 406/693–7000; Carl Keener, M.D., Medical Director (Nonreporting) — 12 10 32 — — — — — — —

WHITE SULPHUR SPRINGS—Deer Lodge County

MOUNTAINVIEW MEDICAL CENTER, 16 West Main, Zip 59645, Mailing Address: P.O. Box Q, Zip 59645; tel. 406/547–3321; Brian Monsma, Administrator (Total facility includes 31 beds in nursing home–type unit) **A**9 10 **F**13 20 26 28 39 49 64 **P**6 — 23 10 37 99 26 — 0 2038 1124 53

WHITEFISH—Flathead County

★ NORTH VALLEY HOSPITAL, 6575 Highway 93 South, Zip 59937; tel. 406/863–2501; Kenneth E. S. Platou, Chief Executive Officer (Total facility includes 56 beds in nursing home–type unit) **A**9 10 **F**1 7 8 12 13 16 17 19 21 22 26 27 28 29 30 32 34 37 39 40 41 42 44 45 49 54 56 64 65 66 67 71 72 73 74 **P**8 **S** Quorum Health Group/Quorum Health Resources, Inc., Brentwood, TN — 23 10 99 1464 71 31550 185 12629 5991 198

Hospital, Address, Telephone, Administrator, Approval, Facility, and Physician Codes, Health Care System, Network	Classi-fication Codes		Utilization Data					Expense (thousands) of dollars		
	Control	Service	Beds	Admissions	Census	Outpatient Visits	Births	Total	Payroll	Personnel
★ American Hospital Association (AHA) membership □ Joint Commission on Accreditation of Healthcare Organizations (JCAHO) accreditation + American Osteopathic Hospital Association (AOHA) membership ○ American Osteopathic Association (AOA) accreditation △ Commission on Accreditation of Rehabilitation Facilities (CARF) accreditation Control codes 61, 63, 64, 71, 72 and 73 indicate hospitals listed by AOHA, but not registered by AHA. For definition of numerical codes, see page A4										

WOLF POINT—Roosevelt County

    NORTHEAST MONTANA HEALTH SERVICES, (Includes Poplar Community Hospital, H and Court Avenue, Poplar, Zip 59255, Mailing Address: P.O. Box 38, Zip 59255; tel. 406/768–3452; Trinity Hospital, 315 Knapp Street, tel. 406/653–2100), 315 Knapp Street, Zip 59201; tel. 406/653–2110; Earl N. Sheehy, Chief Executive Officer (Total facility includes 82 beds in nursing home–type unit) (Nonreporting) **A**9 10 **N** Montana Health Network, Inc., Miles City, MT

| | 23 | 10 | 128 | — | — | — | — | — | — | — |

NEBRASKA

Resident population 1,637 (in thousands)
Resident population in metro areas 50.7%
Birth rate per 1,000 population 14.4
65 years and over 13.9%
Percent of persons without health insurance 10.7%

Hospital, Address, Telephone, Administrator, Approval, Facility, and Physician Codes, Health Care System, Network	Classi-fication Codes		Utilization Data					Expense (thousands) of dollars		
★ American Hospital Association (AHA) membership ☐ Joint Commission on Accreditation of Healthcare Organizations (JCAHO) accreditation + American Osteopathic Hospital Association (AOHA) membership ○ American Osteopathic Association (AOA) accreditation △ Commission on Accreditation of Rehabilitation Facilities (CARF) accreditation Control codes 61, 63, 64, 71, 72 and 73 indicate hospitals listed by AOHA, but not registered by AHA. For definition of numerical codes, see page A4	Control	Service	Beds	Admissions	Census	Outpatient Visits	Births	Total	Payroll	Personnel

AINSWORTH—Brown County

BROWN COUNTY HOSPITAL, 945 East Zero, Zip 69210; tel. 402/387–2800; Roger Reamer, Administrator **A**9 10 **F**15 19 22 30 31 32 40 44 49 71 73 **N** North Central Hospital Network, Atkinson, NE — 13 10 | 16 | 224 | 2 | 4709 | 26 | 1929 | 851 | 43

ALBION—Boone County

★ BOONE COUNTY HEALTH CENTER, 723 West Fairview Street, Zip 68620, Mailing Address: P.O. Box 151, Zip 68620–0151; tel. 402/395–2191; Gayle E. Primrose, Administrator **A**9 10 **F**1 2 3 6 7 8 11 15 16 17 19 22 24 25 26 28 30 31 32 33 34 35 37 39 40 41 42 44 45 48 49 51 52 53 54 55 57 58 65 66 67 71 73 **P**6 **N** Heartland Health Alliance, Lincoln, NE; Central Nebraska Primary Care Network, Ord, NE — 13 10 | 20 | 776 | 8 | 70632 | 89 | 5975 | 3448 | 126

ALLIANCE—Box Butte County

☐ BOX BUTTE GENERAL HOSPITAL, 2101 Box Butte Avenue, Zip 69301–0810, Mailing Address: P.O. Box 810, Zip 69301–0810; tel. 308/762–6660; Terrance J. Padden, Administrator **A**1 9 10 **F**7 12 15 16 17 18 19 22 28 29 30 33 34 35 37 39 40 41 42 44 46 49 56 65 66 67 71 72 73 **P**3 5 8 **N** Western Nebraska Rural Health Care Network, Chadron, NE — 13 10 | 44 | 752 | 8 | 15128 | 147 | 5767 | 2299 | 97

ALMA—Harlan County

★ HARLAN COUNTY HOSPITAL, 717 North Brown, Zip 68920, Mailing Address: P.O. Box 836, Zip 68920; tel. 308/928–2151; Allen Van Driel, Administrator **A**9 10 **F**8 19 22 31 32 33 34 44 49 71 **P**6 8 **S** Great Plains Health Alliance, Inc., Phillipsburg, KS **N** Heartland Health Alliance, Lincoln, NE; Rural Health Partners, Lexington, NE; Great Plains Health Alliance, Phillipsburg, KS — 13 10 | 25 | 240 | 12 | 6349 | 0 | 2248 | 1161 | 37

ATKINSON—Holt County

WEST HOLT MEMORIAL HOSPITAL, 406 Legion Street, Zip 68713, Mailing Address: Rural Route 1, Box 200, Zip 68713; tel. 402/925–2811; Mel Snow, Administrator **A**9 10 **F**8 11 14 15 16 19 20 22 28 29 32 33 37 40 41 44 49 65 71 **P**3 **N** North Central Hospital Network, Atkinson, NE — 23 10 | 18 | 297 | 3 | 9683 | 20 | 2658 | 1316 | 55

AUBURN—Nemaha County

★ NEMAHA COUNTY HOSPITAL, 2022 13th Street, Zip 68305–1799; tel. 402/274–4366; Glen Krueger, Administrator **A**9 10 **F**8 11 14 15 16 17 19 20 21 22 24 28 30 31 32 35 36 37 40 42 44 49 58 63 65 66 67 71 73 **P**3 **N** Heartland Health Alliance, Lincoln, NE — 13 10 | 34 | 449 | 6 | 16973 | 32 | 3094 | 1504 | 67

AURORA—Hamilton County

MEMORIAL HOSPITAL, 1423 Seventh Street, Zip 68818–1197; tel. 402/694–3171; Eldon A. Wall, Administrator (Total facility includes 53 beds in nursing home–type unit) **A**9 10 **F**7 8 15 22 28 30 32 33 34 36 37 40 41 42 44 49 64 65 66 71 **P**6 **N** Heartland Health Alliance, Lincoln, NE; Blue River Valley Health Network, Brainard, NE — 23 10 | 78 | 617 | 57 | 12970 | 90 | 6662 | 3750 | 144

BASSETT—Rock County

ROCK COUNTY HOSPITAL, Mailing Address: P.O. Box 100, Zip 68714–0100; tel. 402/684–3366; David Stephenson, Administrator (Total facility includes 30 beds in nursing home–type unit) **A**9 10 **F**19 22 44 64 71 **N** North Central Hospital Network, Atkinson, NE — 13 10 | 42 | 207 | 27 | 5231 | 4 | 1972 | 773 | 67

BEATRICE—Gage County

✦ BEATRICE COMMUNITY HOSPITAL AND HEALTH CENTER, 1110 North Tenth Street, Zip 68310, Mailing Address: P.O. Box 278, Zip 68310–0278; tel. 402/228–3344; Kenneth J. Zimmerman, Administrator (Total facility includes 78 beds in nursing home–type unit) **A**1 9 10 **F**7 8 10 11 15 16 17 19 20 21 22 23 26 28 30 31 32 33 34 35 36 37 40 41 42 44 45 46 49 51 54 62 64 65 66 67 71 73 **P**5 **N** Heartland Health Alliance, Lincoln, NE — 23 10 | 138 | 1121 | 84 | 40032 | 166 | 13977 | 7347 | 311

BENKELMAN—Dundy County

DUNDY COUNTY HOSPITAL, North Cheyenne Street, Zip 69021, Mailing Address: P.O. Box 626, Zip 69021–0626; tel. 308/423–2204; Robert L. Sheckler, Administrator **A**9 10 **F**14 28 29 37 44 51 64 71 73 — 13 10 | 15 | 291 | 3 | 6868 | 30 | 2404 | 1200 | —

BLAIR—Washington County

✦ MEMORIAL COMMUNITY HOSPITAL, 810 North 22nd Street, Zip 68008–1199; tel. 402/426–2182; Anton P. Zurbrugg, CHE, President and Chief Executive Officer **A**1 9 10 **F**7 8 14 16 17 18 19 22 28 30 32 33 34 35 36 37 39 40 41 42 44 45 46 49 64 65 67 71 73 — 23 10 | 33 | 1016 | 11 | — | 104 | 8648 | 5026 | 176

BRIDGEPORT—Morrill County

MORRILL COUNTY COMMUNITY HOSPITAL, 1313 South Street, Zip 69336, Mailing Address: P.O. Box 579, Zip 69336; tel. 308/262–1616; Julia Morrow, Administrator (Nonreporting) **A**9 10 **N** Western Nebraska Rural Health Care Network, Chadron, NE — 13 10 | 20 | — | — | — | — | — | — | —

BROKEN BOW—Custer County

JENNIE M. MELHAM MEMORIAL MEDICAL CENTER, 145 Memorial Drive, Zip 68822, Mailing Address: P.O. Box 250, Zip 68822–0250; tel. 308/872–6891; Michael J. Steckler, Chief Executive Officer (Total facility includes 77 beds in nursing home–type unit) **A**9 10 **F**6 7 8 15 16 19 22 32 33 34 35 44 62 64 65 67 71 **N** Heartland Health Alliance, Lincoln, NE — 23 10 | 116 | 1261 | 85 | 10571 | 111 | 6449 | 3141 | 162

Hospital, Address, Telephone, Administrator, Approval, Facility, and Physician Codes, Health Care System, Network	Classi-fication Codes		Utilization Data					Expense (thousands) of dollars		
	Control	Service	Beds	Admissions	Census	Outpatient Visits	Births	Total	Payroll	Personnel

★ American Hospital Association (AHA) membership
□ Joint Commission on Accreditation of Healthcare Organizations (JCAHO) accreditation
+ American Osteopathic Hospital Association (AOHA) membership
○ American Osteopathic Association (AOA) accreditation
△ Commission on Accreditation of Rehabilitation Facilities (CARF) accreditation
Control codes 61, 63, 64, 71, 72 and 73 indicate hospitals listed by AOHA, but not registered by AHA. For definition of numerical codes, see page A4

CALLAWAY—Custer County

★ CALLAWAY DISTRICT HOSPITAL, 211 Kimball, Zip 68825, Mailing Address: P.O. Box 100, Zip 68825; tel. 308/836–2228; Marvin Neth, Administrator **A**9 10 **F**11 15 16 19 22 33 37 40 44 71 **P**3 — 16 10 12 255 3 5695 10 1214 525 27

CAMBRIDGE—Furnas County

★ TRI-VALLEY HEALTH SYSTEM, (Formerly Cambridge Memorial Hospital), West Highway 6 and 34, Zip 69022, Mailing Address: P.O. Box 488, Zip 69022; tel. 308/697–3329; Kristopher H. Marwin, CHE, Chief Executive Officer (Total facility includes 36 beds in nursing home–type unit) **A**9 10 **F**6 7 8 10 11 12 14 15 16 17 22 24 25 27 28 32 33 34 36 37 39 40 42 44 45 49 51 62 65 66 **P**3 **S** Brim, Inc., Portland, OR **N** Heartland Health Alliance, Lincoln, NE; Rural Health Partners, Lexington, NE — 23 10 56 520 40 — 55 7401 3694 130

CENTRAL CITY—Merrick County

LITZENBERG MEMORIAL COUNTY HOSPITAL, 1715 26th Street, Zip 68826, Mailing Address: Route 2, Box 1, Zip 68826; tel. 308/946–3015; Mike Bowman, Administrator (Total facility includes 46 beds in nursing home–type unit) (Nonreporting) **A**9 10 — 13 10 71 — — — — — — —

CHADRON—Dawes County

CHADRON COMMUNITY HOSPITAL, 821 Morehead Street, Zip 69337–2599; tel. 308/432–5586; Harold L. Krueger, Jr., Administrator **A**9 10 **F**6 7 8 12 13 15 16 17 18 19 22 28 30 31 32 33 39 40 42 44 48 61 62 64 65 71 73 **P**5 8 **N** Western Nebraska Rural Health Care Network, Chadron, NE — 23 10 34 800 11 9556 117 6079 2610 133

COLUMBUS—Platte County

✣ COLUMBUS COMMUNITY HOSPITAL, 3020 18th Street, Zip 68602, Mailing Address: P.O. Box 819, Zip 68602–0819; tel. 402/564–7118; Donald H. Zornes, Administrator (Total facility includes 19 beds in nursing home–type unit) **A**1 9 10 **F**7 8 10 11 12 15 16 17 19 20 21 22 28 30 31 32 33 34 35 36 37 38 39 40 41 44 45 46 49 64 65 67 71 73 **P**8 — 23 10 73 2183 36 43408 485 15860 7185 227

COZAD—Dawson County

COZAD COMMUNITY HOSPITAL, 300 East 12th, Zip 69130, Mailing Address: P.O. Box 108, Zip 69130–0108; tel. 308/784–2261; Lyle Davis, Administrator **A**9 10 **F**7 8 15 16 17 19 22 30 32 33 36 37 40 44 45 49 65 71 **P**3 — 16 10 30 641 4 4933 60 3243 1292 64

CRAWFORD—Dawes County

LEGEND BUTTES HEALTH SERVICES, 11 Paddock Street, Zip 69339, Mailing Address: P.O. Box 272, Zip 69339; tel. 308/665–1770; Kim Engel, Chief Executive Officer **A**9 10 **F**8 12 15 19 22 28 30 31 32 51 61 64 **P**5 **N** Rapid City Regional Hospital, Rapid City, SD; Western Nebraska Rural Health Care Network, Chadron, NE — 14 10 10 94 2 1446 1 1036 579 26

CREIGHTON—Knox County

CREIGHTON AREA HEALTH SERVICES, 1503 Main Street, Zip 68729, Mailing Address: P.O. Box 186, Zip 68729; tel. 402/358–3322; Paul Hurd, Chief Executive Officer (Total facility includes 47 beds in nursing home–type unit) **A**9 10 **F**1 7 8 15 16 17 19 22 27 28 30 32 34 35 37 39 40 41 42 44 64 65 71 **N** North Central Hospital Network, Atkinson, NE — 14 10 77 437 54 4033 27 3012 1645 86

CRETE—Saline County

★ CRETE MUNICIPAL HOSPITAL, 1540 Grove Street, Zip 68333–0220, Mailing Address: P.O. Box 220, Zip 68333–0220; tel. 402/826–6800; Joe Lohrman, Administrator (Total facility includes 22 beds in nursing home–type unit) **A**9 10 **F**7 19 21 22 28 32 33 34 42 44 49 64 65 71 **P**3 **N** Heartland Health Alliance, Lincoln, NE; Blue River Valley Health Network, Brainard, NE — 14 10 57 581 45 16335 60 4606 2238 98

DAVID CITY—Butler County

BUTLER COUNTY HEALTH CARE CENTER, 372 South Ninth Street, Zip 68632; tel. 402/367–3115; Roger Reamer, Administrator **A**9 10 **F**1 3 7 8 14 15 16 17 20 22 24 27 28 30 32 34 36 39 40 42 44 45 46 49 51 58 62 64 65 66 67 71 73 **N** Heartland Health Alliance, Lincoln, NE; Blue River Valley Health Network, Brainard, NE — 13 10 31 724 10 17788 111 3717 1894 79

FAIRBURY—Jefferson County

★ JEFFERSON COMMUNITY HEALTH CENTER, Mailing Address: P.O. Box 277, Zip 68352–0277; tel. 402/729–3351; Bill Welch, Administrator (Total facility includes 41 beds in nursing home–type unit) **A**9 10 **F**7 8 15 16 17 19 22 24 28 29 30 32 33 35 41 42 44 49 64 66 67 71 73 **N** Heartland Health Alliance, Lincoln, NE — 23 10 65 613 46 10595 52 4904 2402 114

FALLS CITY—Richardson County

★ COMMUNITY MEDICAL CENTER, 2307 Barada Street, Zip 68355–1599; tel. 402/245–2428; Victor Lee, Chief Executive Officer and Administrator **A**9 10 **F**7 8 15 16 17 19 21 22 26 28 30 32 33 34 35 42 44 45 49 63 64 65 66 71 74 **S** Great Plains Health Alliance, Inc., Phillipsburg, KS **N** Great Plains Health Alliance, Phillipsburg, KS — 23 10 49 944 16 15535 62 5314 2451 119

FRANKLIN—Franklin County

FRANKLIN COUNTY MEMORIAL HOSPITAL, 1406 Q Street, Zip 68939–0315, Mailing Address: P.O. Box 315, Zip 68939–0315; tel. 308/425–6221; Jerrell F. Gerdes, Administrator **A**9 10 **F**15 16 19 22 24 28 33 35 44 71 **P**6 **N** Heartland Health Alliance, Lincoln, NE; Rural Health Partners, Lexington, NE — 13 10 20 274 4 4970 14 2089 993 64

FREMONT—Dodge County

✣ FREMONT AREA MEDICAL CENTER, (Formerly Memorial Hospital of Dodge County), 450 East 23rd Street, Zip 68025–2387; tel. 402/721–1610; Vincent J. O'Connor, Jr., President and Chief Executive Officer (Total facility includes 162 beds in nursing home–type unit) **A**1 2 9 10 **F**1 7 8 11 15 17 19 21 22 26 27 28 29 30 31 32 33 34 35 37 39 40 41 42 44 45 46 48 49 60 63 64 65 66 67 71 73 **P**8 — 13 10 262 3975 194 56734 470 35245 17590 576

Hospital, Address, Telephone, Administrator, Approval, Facility, and Physician Codes, Health Care System, Network	Classi-fication Codes		Utilization Data					Expense (thousands) of dollars		
★ American Hospital Association (AHA) membership ☐ Joint Commission on Accreditation of Healthcare Organizations (JCAHO) accreditation + American Osteopathic Hospital Association (AOHA) membership ○ American Osteopathic Association (AOA) accreditation △ Commission on Accreditation of Rehabilitation Facilities (CARF) accreditation Control codes 61, 63, 64, 71, 72 and 73 indicate hospitals listed by AOHA, but not registered by AHA. For definition of numerical codes, see page A4	Control	Service	Beds	Admissions	Census	Outpatient Visits	Births	Total	Payroll	Personnel

FRIEND—Saline County

| WARREN MEMORIAL HOSPITAL, 905 Second Street, Zip 68359; tel. 402/947–2541; John Ramsay, Administrator (Total facility includes 58 beds in nursing home–type unit) **A**9 10 **F**1 15 16 17 22 26 28 33 36 41 44 49 64 65 67 71 73 **N** Blue River Valley Health Network, Brainard, NE | 14 | 10 | 73 | 80 | 55 | 4081 | 16 | 2060 | 1172 | 81 |

GENEVA—Fillmore County

| FILLMORE COUNTY HOSPITAL, 1325 H Street, Zip 68361–1325, Mailing Address: P.O. Box 193, Zip 68361; tel. 402/759–3167; L. L. Eichelberger, Administrator (Total facility includes 20 beds in nursing home–type unit) **A**9 10 **F**3 7 8 15 19 22 24 26 27 28 29 30 31 32 33 34 35 36 37 39 40 41 42 44 45 46 49 61 64 65 66 67 68 71 73 | 13 | 10 | 53 | 319 | 31 | 10932 | 44 | 3379 | 1543 | 76 |

GENOA—Nance County

| GENOA COMMUNITY HOSPITAL, 706 Ewing Avenue, Zip 68640, Mailing Address: P.O. Box 310, Zip 68640; tel. 402/993–2283; Wade Edwards, Administrator (Total facility includes 59 beds in nursing home–type unit) **A**9 10 **F**7 8 11 14 19 20 21 22 27 28 32 34 36 39 40 44 48 49 64 65 67 71 73 **P**3 6 | 14 | 10 | 99 | 121 | 61 | 3465 | 5 | — | — | 81 |

GORDON—Sheridan County

| ★ GORDON MEMORIAL HOSPITAL DISTRICT, 300 East Eighth Street, Zip 69343–9990; tel. 308/282–0401; Gladys Phemister, Administrator **A**9 10 **F**3 8 11 16 17 19 22 28 30 32 37 40 44 46 61 71 **N** Western Nebraska Rural Health Care Network, Chadron, NE | 16 | 10 | 40 | 824 | 11 | 16069 | 72 | 4020 | 1995 | 91 |

GOTHENBURG—Dawson County

| GOTHENBURG MEMORIAL HOSPITAL, 910 20th Street, Zip 69138, Mailing Address: P.O. Box 469, Zip 69138–0469; tel. 308/537–3661; Roger Heidebrink, Administrator (Total facility includes 34 beds in nursing home–type unit) **A**9 10 **F**32 33 64 **N** Heartland Health Alliance, Lincoln, NE; Rural Health Partners, Lexington, NE | 16 | 10 | 46 | 304 | 36 | 9037 | 45 | 3249 | 1630 | 80 |

GRAND ISLAND—Hall County

| ⊠ SAINT FRANCIS MEDICAL CENTER, (Includes Saint Francis Memorial Health Center, 2116 West Faidley Avenue, Mailing Address: P.O. Box 9804, Zip 68802; tel. 308/384–4600), 2620 West Faidley Avenue, Zip 68803, Mailing Address: P.O. Box 9804, Zip 68802–9804; tel. 308/384–4600; Michael R. Gloor, President and Chief Executive Officer (Total facility includes 36 beds in nursing home–type unit) **A**1 2 3 5 9 10 **F**2 3 7 8 10 11 15 16 17 19 20 21 22 23 27 28 30 32 33 34 35 37 38 39 40 41 42 44 45 49 54 58 60 62 64 65 66 67 71 73 **P**8 **S** Catholic Health Initiatives, Denver, CO | 23 | 10 | 162 | 5832 | 69 | 55352 | 897 | 50821 | 17909 | 757 |
| ⊠ VETERANS AFFAIRS MEDICAL CENTER, 2211 North Broadwell Avenue, Zip 68803–2196; tel. 308/382–3660; Daniel A. Asper, Acting Director (Total facility includes 76 beds in nursing home–type unit) **A**1 **F**1 2 3 8 15 20 21 22 27 28 30 31 32 33 34 37 41 42 44 46 49 51 54 57 58 64 65 67 71 73 74 **S** Department of Veterans Affairs, Washington, DC | 45 | 10 | 142 | 1265 | 82 | 38000 | 0 | 24021 | 11209 | 302 |

GRANT—Perkins County

| PERKINS COUNTY HEALTH SERVICES, (Includes Golden Ours Convalescent Home), 900 Lincoln Avenue, Zip 69140, Mailing Address: Rural Route 1, Box 26, Zip 69140; tel. 308/352–7200; Dan Kelly, Chief Executive Officer (Total facility includes 56 beds in nursing home–type unit) **A**9 10 **F**7 8 11 19 22 26 28 32 34 37 40 42 44 49 64 65 71 **P**3 | 16 | 10 | 76 | 645 | 50 | 5574 | 51 | — | — | — |

HASTINGS—Adams County

| ☐ HASTINGS REGIONAL CENTER, Mailing Address: P.O. Box 579, Zip 68902–0579; tel. 402/463–2471; Michael J. Sheehan, Facility Administrator (Nonreporting) **A**1 10 | 12 | 49 | 232 | — | — | — | — | — | — | — |
| ⊠ MARY LANNING MEMORIAL HOSPITAL, 715 North St. Joseph Avenue, Zip 68901–4497; tel. 402/461–5108; W. Michael Kearney, Pressident (Total facility includes 15 beds in nursing home–type unit) **A**1 2 9 10 **F**3 7 8 10 11 13 15 16 17 19 20 21 22 23 24 28 30 31 32 33 34 35 36 37 38 39 40 41 42 44 45 46 51 52 53 54 55 56 57 58 59 60 62 64 65 66 67 70 71 73 74 **P**6 **N** Heartland Health Alliance, Lincoln, NE; Rural Health Partners, Lexington, NE | 23 | 10 | 125 | 4927 | 63 | 64499 | 607 | 36728 | 18265 | 631 |

HEBRON—Thayer County

| ★ THAYER COUNTY HEALTH SERVICES, (Formerly Thayer County Mem Hospital), 120 Park Avenue, Zip 68370, Mailing Address: P.O. Box 49, Zip 68370; tel. 402/768–6041; Larry E. Leaming, Administrator **A**9 10 **F**7 8 13 15 19 22 28 30 32 35 39 40 41 44 46 49 51 65 66 67 71 73 74 **P**6 | 13 | 10 | 18 | 529 | 4 | 17021 | 45 | 3483 | 1619 | 73 |

HENDERSON—York County

| HENDERSON HEALTH CARE SERVICES, (Formerly Henderson Community Hospital), 1621 Front Street, Zip 68371–0217, Mailing Address: P.O. Box 217, Zip 68371–0217; tel. 402/723–4512; Calvin C. Graber, Chief Executive Officer (Total facility includes 42 beds in nursing home–type unit) **A**9 10 **F**1 7 8 11 14 15 22 25 28 33 36 44 49 64 65 67 71 **P**6 **N** Blue River Valley Health Network, Brainard, NE | 23 | 10 | 51 | 122 | 42 | 3933 | 17 | 2895 | 1750 | 66 |

HOLDREGE—Phelps County

| ⊠ PHELPS MEMORIAL HEALTH CENTER, 1220 Miller Street, Zip 68949, Mailing Address: P.O. Box 828, Zip 68949–0828; tel. 308/995–2211; Jerome Seigfreid, Jr., Chief Executive Officer **A**1 9 10 **F**7 8 10 14 15 16 19 20 22 27 28 30 32 33 35 36 37 44 65 66 67 69 71 73 **P**3 8 **S** Quorum Health Group/Quorum Health Resources, Inc., Brentwood, TN **N** Heartland Health Alliance, Lincoln, NE; Rural Health Partners, Lexington, NE | 23 | 10 | 55 | 1628 | 18 | 15793 | 174 | 8119 | 3604 | 146 |

Hospital, Address, Telephone, Administrator, Approval, Facility, and Physician Codes, Health Care System, Network	Classi-fication Codes		Utilization Data					Expense (thousands) of dollars		
★ American Hospital Association (AHA) membership □ Joint Commission on Accreditation of Healthcare Organizations (JCAHO) accreditation + American Osteopathic Hospital Association (AOHA) membership ○ American Osteopathic Association (AOA) accreditation △ Commission on Accreditation of Rehabilitation Facilities (CARF) accreditation Control codes 61, 63, 64, 71, 72 and 73 indicate hospitals listed by AOHA, but not registered by AHA. For definition of numerical codes, see page A4	Control	Service	Beds	Admissions	Census	Outpatient Visits	Births	Total	Payroll	Personnel

HUMBOLDT—Richardson County

COMMUNITY MEMORIAL HOSPITAL, 1128 Grand Avenue, Zip 68376, Mailing Address: P.O. Box 626, Zip 68376; tel. 402/862–2231; Marlyn Reinitz, Administrator (Nonreporting) **A**9 10

	23	10	20	—	—	—	—	—	—	—

IMPERIAL—Chase County

CHASE COUNTY COMMUNITY HOSPITAL, 600 West 12th Street, Zip 69033; tel. 308/882–7111; James O'Neal, Administrator **A**9 10 **F**7 8 10 19 21 22 28 34 35 37 42 44 49 71 73 **N** Western Nebraska Rural Health Care Network, Chadron, NE

	13	10	26	679	7	10990	61	2891	1341	57

KEARNEY—Buffalo County

★ △ GOOD SAMARITAN HEALTH SYSTEMS, (Includes Richard H. Young Psychiatric Hospital, 4600 17th Avenue, Zip 68847, Mailing Address: P.O. Box 1750, Zip 68848–1705; tel. 308/865–2000), 10 East 31st Street, Zip 68847–2926, Mailing Address: P.O. Box 1990, Zip 68848–1990; tel. 308/865–7100; William Wilson Hendrickson, President and Chief Executive Officer (Total facility includes 22 beds in nursing home–type unit) **A**1 2 3 5 7 9 10 **F**1 2 3 4 5 7 8 9 10 11 12 14 15 16 17 19 21 22 23 24 27 28 29 30 32 33 34 35 36 37 38 39 40 41 42 43 44 45 46 48 49 52 53 54 59 60 64 65 66 67 68 70 71 73 **P**8 **S** Catholic Health Initiatives, Denver, CO

RICHARD H. YOUNG PSYCHIATRIC HOSPITAL See Good Samaritan Health Systems

	21	10	267	7895	138	62160	829	80575	33111	1158

KIMBALL—Kimball County

KIMBALL COUNTY HOSPITAL, 505 South Burg Street, Zip 69145; tel. 308/235–3621; Gerri Linn, Administrator **A**9 10 **F**15 19 22 30 31 32 40 44 49 71 73 **N** Western Nebraska Rural Health Care Network, Chadron, NE

	13	10	16	224	2	4709	26	1929	851	43

LEXINGTON—Dawson County

★ TRI–COUNTY AREA HOSPITAL, 13th and Erie Streets, Zip 68850–0980, Mailing Address: P.O. Box 980, Zip 68850–0980; tel. 308/324–5651; Calvin A. Hiner, Administrator **A**1 9 10 **F**7 8 10 11 16 1/ 19 21 22 28 29 30 32 33 34 35 39 40 42 44 45 49 50 51 62 65 66 67 71 73 **P**1 7 **N** Heartland Health Alliance, Lincoln, NE; Rural Health Partners, Lexington, NE

	16	10	40	1463	16	25157	270	6856	3138	139

LINCOLN—Lancaster County

★ BRYAN MEMORIAL HOSPITAL, 1600 South 48th Street, Zip 68506–1299; tel. 402/489–0200; R. Lynn Wilson, President (Total facility includes 20 beds in nursing home–type unit) **A**1 2 3 5 6 9 10 **F**4 7 8 10 11 12 14 15 16 19 21 22 23 28 29 30 31 32 34 35 37 40 42 43 44 52 54 63 64 65 66 67 69 71 73 **P**8 **N** National Cardiovascular Network, Atlanta, GA; Heartland Health Alliance, Lincoln, NE

	23	10	316	13362	170	184155	1146	133618	49995	1710

★ LINCOLN GENERAL HOSPITAL, 2300 South 16th Street, Zip 68502–3781; tel. 402/475–1011; Arlan L. Stromberg, Administrator **A**1 2 3 5 9 10 **F**1 2 3 7 8 14 15 16 17 18 19 22 23 26 27 29 30 32 33 34 35 37 40 42 44 46 48 49 52 53 54 55 56 57 58 59 60 65 67 68 70 71 72 73 **P**7 8

	14	10	211	6409	98	86304	640	60402	23987	828

□ LINCOLN REGIONAL CENTER, West Prospector Place and Folsom, Zip 68522, Mailing Address: P.O. Box 94949, Zip 68509–4949; tel. 402/471–4444; Barbara Ramsey, Ph.D., Chief Executive Officer **A**1 9 10 **F**14 15 16 20 27 41 52 53 54 55 56 57 58 59 65 67 73 **P**6

	12	22	226	397	211	0	0	20139	13045	508

★ △ MADONNA REHABILITATION HOSPITAL, 5401 South Street, Zip 68506–2134; tel. 402/489–7102; Marsha Lommel Halpern, President and Chief Executive Officer (Total facility includes 182 beds in nursing home–type unit) **A**7 10 **F**1 12 14 15 16 17 19 24 26 27 28 29 30 32 33 34 35 39 41 45 46 48 49 58 64 65 67 71 73 **P**6

	21	46	246	1662	223	—	0	29864	17803	685

★ ST. ELIZABETH COMMUNITY HEALTH CENTER, 555 South 70th Street, Zip 68510–2494; tel. 402/489–7181; Robert J. Lanik, President **A**1 2 3 5 9 10 **F**7 8 9 10 12 14 15 16 19 22 28 30 31 32 33 35 37 38 40 41 42 44 46 49 65 66 67 71 72 73 **P**3 7 **S** Catholic Health Initiatives, Denver, CO

	21	10	162	6623	77	61872	1958	64627	26205	1062

★ VETERANS AFFAIRS MEDICAL CENTER, 600 South 70th Street, Zip 68510–2493; tel. 402/489–3802; David Asper, Director **A**1 3 5 **F**2 3 11 12 15 16 19 20 21 22 23 27 28 29 30 33 34 35 37 41 42 44 45 46 49 51 52 54 58 60 65 71 73 74 **S** Department of Veterans Affairs, Washington, DC

	45	10	73	2215	53	61680	0	—	—	396

LYNCH—Boyd County

NIOBRARA VALLEY HOSPITAL, Mailing Address: P.O. Box 118, Zip 68746; tel. 402/569–2451; E. R. Testerman, Administrator **A**9 10 **F**7 8 19 22 26 27 28 30 32 34 39 40 44 45 49 61 64 71 **P**5 **N** North Central Hospital Network, Atkinson, NE

	23	10	29	748	10	—	2	2308	1138	55

MCCOOK—Red Willow County

★ COMMUNITY HOSPITAL, 1301 East H Street, Zip 69001–1328, Mailing Address: P.O. Box 1328, Zip 69001–1328; tel. 308/345–2650; Gary Bieganski, President **A**1 9 10 **F**7 8 11 14 15 17 19 21 22 28 30 32 37 44 45 65 71 73 74 **N** Heartland Health Alliance, Lincoln, NE; Rural Health Partners, Lexington, NE

	23	10	44	1278	16	39522	126	9762	4174	140

MINDEN—Kearney County

★ KEARNEY COUNTY COMMUNITY HOSPITAL, 727 East First Street, Zip 68959; tel. 308/832–1440; Doug Reiber, Administrator (Total facility includes 42 beds in nursing home–type unit) (Nonreporting) **A**9 10

	13	10	72	—	—	—	—	—	—	—

NEBRASKA CITY—Otoe County

★ ST. MARY'S HOSPITAL, 1314 Third Avenue, Zip 68410; tel. 402/873–3321; Richard W. Waller, Interim Administrator **A**9 10 **F**3 7 8 15 16 19 22 32 35 36 40 44 46 63 65 66 71 73 **S** Catholic Health Initiatives, Denver, CO

	21	10	28	397	9	19446	100	4225	1858	84

Hospital, Address, Telephone, Administrator, Approval, Facility, and Physician Codes, Health Care System, Network	Classi-fication Codes		Utilization Data					Expense (thousands) of dollars		
★ American Hospital Association (AHA) membership □ Joint Commission on Accreditation of Healthcare Organizations (JCAHO) accreditation + American Osteopathic Hospital Association (AOHA) membership ○ American Osteopathic Association (AOA) accreditation △ Commission on Accreditation of Rehabilitation Facilities (CARF) accreditation Control codes 61, 63, 64, 71, 72 and 73 indicate hospitals listed by AOHA, but not registered by AHA. For definition of numerical codes, see page A4	Control	Service	Beds	Admissions	Census	Outpatient Visits	Births	Total	Payroll	Personnel

NELIGH—Antelope County

★ ANTELOPE MEMORIAL HOSPITAL, 102 West Ninth Street, Zip 68756–0229, Mailing Address: P.O. Box 229, Zip 68756–0229; tel. 402/887–4151; Jack W. Green, Administrator **A**9 10 **F**7 8 15 17 19 22 24 30 32 34 39 40 42 44 45 46 49 65 67 71 **N** North Central Hospital Network, Atkinson, NE — 23 10 49 640 13 10402 27 3399 1852 86

NORFOLK—Madison County

✠ FAITH REGIONAL HEALTH SERVICES, (Includes Lutheran Community Hospital, 2700 Norfolk Avenue, Zip 68701, Mailing Address: P.O. Box 869, Zip 68702–0869; tel. 402/371–4880; Our Lady of Lourdes Hospital, 1500 Koenigstein Avenue, Zip 68701–3698; tel. 402/371–3402), 2700 Norfolk Avenue, Zip 68702–0869, Mailing Address: P.O. BOX 869, Zip 68702–0869; tel. 402/371–4880; Robert L. Driewer, Chief Executive Officer **A**1 9 10 **F**3 7 8 12 15 16 17 19 21 22 23 24 28 29 30 32 33 34 35 37 39 40 41 42 44 45 49 52 56 60 65 66 67 71 73 **P**3 7 **S** Missionary Benedictine Sisters American Province, Norfolk, NE — 23 10 155 5421 45 78508 898 36429 15343 1287

LUTHERAN COMMUNITY HOSPITAL See Faith Regional Health Services

□ NORFOLK REGIONAL CENTER, 1700 North Victory Road, Zip 68701, Mailing Address: P.O. Box 1209, Zip 68702–1209; tel. 402/370–3400; Roger W. Steinkruger, Chief Executive Officer **A**1 10 **F**3 12 15 17 18 27 32 34 52 54 55 56 57 58 59 65 67 73 **N** North Central Hospital Network, Atkinson, NE — 12 22 174 450 170 0 0 12859 8314 314

OUR LADY OF LOURDES HOSPITAL See Faith Regional Health Services

NORTH PLATTE—Lincoln County

✠ GREAT PLAINS REGIONAL MEDICAL CENTER, 601 West Leota Street, Zip 69101, Mailing Address: P.O. Box 1167, Zip 69103; tel. 308/534–9310; Lucinda A. Bradley, President **A**1 2 9 10 **F**3 7 8 10 12 15 19 21 23 28 32 33 34 35 37 39 40 42 44 46 48 49 52 53 58 59 60 65 66 71 73 **P**3 8 **S** Quorum Health Group/Quorum Health Resources, Inc., Brentwood, TN **N** Heartland Health Alliance, Lincoln, NE; Rural Health Partners, Lexington, NE — 23 10 99 4079 43 75138 576 37432 15622 484

O'NEILL—Holt County

✠ ST. ANTHONY'S HOSPITAL, Second and Adams Streets, Zip 68763–1597; tel. 402/336–2611; Ronald J. Cork, President and Chief Executive Officer **A**1 9 10 **F**7 8 12 15 16 17 18 19 22 26 28 29 30 31 32 34 35 39 40 42 44 49 54 61 65 66 67 71 73 **P**3 **S** Marycrest Health System, Denver, CO **N** North Central Hospital Network, Atkinson, NE — 21 10 29 853 6 13303 108 6007 2368 97

OAKLAND—Burt County

OAKLAND MEMORIAL HOSPITAL, 601 East Second Street, Zip 68045; tel. 402/685–5601; Karen Vlach, Administrator **A**9 10 **F**7 8 12 15 16 19 22 28 30 32 33 34 36 37 39 40 41 42 44 45 46 49 51 64 71 73 **P**2 — 23 10 23 273 5 — 0 1606 805 38

OFFUTT AFB—Sarpy County

✠ EHRLING BERGQUIST HOSPITAL, 2501 Capehart Road, Zip 68113–2160; tel. 402/294–7312; Colonel John R. Sheehan, Administrator **A**1 3 5 **F**2 3 4 5 7 8 10 11 12 13 14 15 16 18 19 20 21 22 23 24 25 28 29 30 31 32 33 34 35 37 38 39 40 41 42 43 44 45 46 47 48 49 50 51 52 53 54 55 56 57 58 59 60 61 63 64 65 66 69 70 71 72 73 74 **S** Department of the Air Force, Washington, DC — 41 10 45 4490 25 333244 670 — — 759

OGALLALA—Keith County

★ OGALLALA COMMUNITY HOSPITAL, 300 East Tenth Street, Zip 69153; tel. 308/284–4011; Linda Morris, Administrator **A**9 10 **F**1 2 3 4 5 6 7 8 9 10 11 12 13 15 16 17 18 19 20 21 22 23 24 25 26 27 28 29 30 31 32 33 34 35 36 37 38 39 40 41 42 43 44 45 47 48 49 50 51 52 53 54 55 56 57 58 59 60 61 62 63 64 65 67 68 69 70 71 72 74 **P**5 6 8 **S** Lutheran Health Systems, Fargo, ND — 23 10 29 720 7 24002 69 6682 3628 132

OMAHA—Douglas County

✠ ALEGENT HEALTH BERGAN MERCY MEDICAL CENTER, 7500 Mercy Road, Zip 68124; tel. 402/398–6060; Charles J. Marr, Chief Executive Officer (Total facility includes 241 beds in nursing home–type unit) **A**1 2 3 5 9 10 **F**1 2 3 4 5 7 8 10 11 12 15 16 17 18 19 20 21 22 23 24 25 26 27 28 29 30 31 32 33 34 35 36 37 38 39 40 41 42 43 44 45 46 48 49 50 51 52 53 54 55 56 57 58 59 60 61 62 63 64 65 66 67 68 71 72 73 74 **P**8 **S** Catholic Health Initiatives, Denver, CO **N** Alegent Health, Omaha, NE — 21 10 592 16256 483 157681 2573 135126 55433 2498

✠ △ ALEGENT HEALTH IMMANUEL MEDICAL CENTER, (Formerly Immanuel Medical Center), 6901 North 72nd Street, Zip 68122–1799; tel. 402/572–2121; Randall W. Smith, Chief Operating Officer (Total facility includes 200 beds in nursing home–type unit) **A**1 2 5 7 9 10 **F**1 2 3 4 6 7 8 10 11 12 15 16 17 18 19 20 21 22 23 24 25 26 27 28 29 30 31 32 33 34 35 36 37 38 39 40 41 42 43 44 45 46 48 49 50 51 52 53 54 55 56 57 58 59 60 61 62 63 64 65 66 67 68 71 72 73 74 **P**7 8 **N** Alegent Health, Omaha, NE — 23 10 532 5513 371 79408 470 58137 24421 1834

□ BISHOP CLARKSON MEMORIAL HOSPITAL, 4350 Dewey Avenue, Zip 68105–1018, Mailing Address: P.O. Box 3328, Zip 68103–0329; tel. 402/552–2000; Louis Burgher, M.D., Ph.D., President and Chief Executive Officer **A**1 2 3 5 9 10 **F**4 7 8 9 10 12 14 15 17 19 20 21 22 23 24 25 28 29 30 32 34 35 37 39 40 41 42 43 44 45 46 49 51 60 63 64 65 66 67 69 71 72 73 **P**5 6 7 — 23 10 204 7466 109 136977 813 111908 39102 1555

□ BOYS TOWN NATIONAL RESEARCH HOSPITAL, 555 North 30th Street, Zip 68131; tel. 402/498–6511; John K. Arch, Administrator **A**1 3 9 10 **F**16 17 21 25 34 44 46 51 53 73 **P**6 — 23 50 14 1191 4 99563 0 — — 340

Hospital, Address, Telephone, Administrator, Approval, Facility, and Physician Codes, Health Care System, Network	Classi-fication Codes		Utilization Data					Expense (thousands) of dollars		
★ American Hospital Association (AHA) membership □ Joint Commission on Accreditation of Healthcare Organizations (JCAHO) accreditation + American Osteopathic Hospital Association (AOHA) membership ○ American Osteopathic Association (AOA) accreditation △ Commission on Accreditation of Rehabilitation Facilities (CARF) accreditation Control codes 61, 63, 64, 71, 72 and 73 indicate hospitals listed by AOHA, but not registered by AHA. For definition of numerical codes, see page A4	Control	Service	Beds	Admissions	Census	Outpatient Visits	Births	Total	Payroll	Personnel

	Control	Service	Beds	Admissions	Census	Outpatient Visits	Births	Total	Payroll	Personnel
⊠ CHILDREN'S HOSPITAL, 8301 Dodge Street, Zip 68114–4199; tel. 402/354–5400; Gary A. Perkins, President and Chief Executive Officer **A**1 3 5 9 10 **F**10 12 15 17 19 21 22 23 29 32 34 35 38 39 42 43 44 45 47 60 63 65 67 71 72 73 **P**8	23	50	100	4809	67	46797	0	55151	24289	586
○ DOUGLAS COUNTY HOSPITAL, 4102 Woolworth Avenue, Zip 68105–1899; tel. 402/444–7000; James C. Tourville, Administrator (Total facility includes 272 beds in nursing home–type unit) (Nonreporting) **A**9 10 11	13	49	329	—	—	—	—	—	—	—
IMMANUEL MEDICAL CENTER See Alegent Health Immanuel Medical Center										
⊠ METHODIST RICHARD YOUNG, (Includes Richard H. Young Memorial Hospital), 415 South 25th Avenue, Zip 68131; tel. 402/354–6600; Sandra C. Carson, FACHE, President and Chief Executive Officer **A**1 5 9 10 **F**2 3 4 7 8 9 10 11 12 13 15 17 18 19 20 21 22 23 26 27 28 29 30 31 32 33 34 35 37 38 39 40 41 42 44 45 46 47 48 49 51 52 53 54 55 56 57 58 59 60 61 62 64 65 66 67 68 69 70 71 72 73 74 **P**1 3 4 5 6 7	23	22	97	1557	41	—	0	17757	9690	264
⊠ △ NEBRASKA METHODIST HOSPITAL, 8303 Dodge Street, Zip 68114–4199; tel. 402/354–4000; John Martin Fraser, President and Chief Executive Officer (Nonreporting) **A**1 2 3 7 9 10	23	10	250							
RICHARD H. YOUNG MEMORIAL HOSPITAL See Methodist Richard Young										
ST. JOSEPH CENTER FOR MENTAL HEALTH, 819 Dorcas, Zip 68108–1137; tel. 402/449–4000; Robert Caldwell, Chief Operating Officer **A**3 5 9 **F**3 14 16 52 53 54 55 56 57 58 59 65 67 73 **P**1 4 6	33	22	115	2298	70	0	0	18372	8773	222
□ ST. JOSEPH HOSPITAL, 601 North 30th Street, Zip 68131–2197; tel. 402/449–5021; Matthew A. Kurs, President and Chief Executive Officer **A**1 2 3 5 8 10 **F**2 3 4 7 8 10 11 12 15 19 20 21 22 24 25 31 34 35 37 38 40 41 42 43 44 46 47 49 51 52 53 54 55 56 57 58 59 60 63 64 65 69 71 72 73 74 **P**2 5 7 8 **S** TENET Healthcare Corporation, Santa Barbara, CA	33	10	284	10507	159	57620	847	99757	33402	1024
⊠ UNIVERSITY OF NEBRASKA MEDICAL CENTER, 600 South 42nd Street, Zip 68198–4085, Mailing Address: P.O. Box 984085, Zip 68198–4085; tel. 402/559–4000; Joseph Graham, Chief Executive Officer (Total facility includes 30 beds in nursing home–type unit) **A**1 2 3 5 8 9 10 **F**4 5 6 7 8 10 12 13 15 17 18 19 20 21 22 23 24 26 27 28 29 30 31 33 34 35 36 37 38 39 40 41 42 43 44 45 46 47 49 51 52 54 55 56 57 58 59 60 61 63 64 65 66 69 70 71 72 73 **P**1 4 6 7	12	10	302	12684	213	108852	961	171124	62364	1943
⊠ VETERANS AFFAIRS MEDICAL CENTER, 4101 Woolworth Avenue, Zip 68105–1873; tel. 402/449–0600; John J. Phillips, Director **A**1 3 5 8 **F**2 3 4 10 12 17 19 20 21 22 23 26 28 30 31 34 35 37 39 41 42 43 44 45 46 49 50 51 52 54 56 57 58 60 63 65 67 69 71 73 74 **P**1 **S** Department of Veterans Affairs, Washington, DC	45	10	194	5775	139	121699	0	67119	34183	860
ORD—Valley County										
★ VALLEY COUNTY HOSPITAL, 217 Westridge Drive, Zip 68862; tel. 308/728–3211; Nancy Glaubke, Administrator (Total facility includes 70 beds in nursing home–type unit) **A**9 10 **F**7 8 11 19 22 24 27 32 34 35 40 44 64 65 71 **N** Central Nebraska Primary Care Network, Ord, NE	13	10	96	748	69	12168	53	5457	2927	141
OSCEOLA—Polk County										
ANNIE JEFFREY MEMORIAL COUNTY HEALTH CENTER, Mailing Address: P.O. Box 428, Zip 68651; tel. 402/747–2031; Curt Koesterer, Administrator **A**9 10 **F**7 14 15 16 17 19 20 22 24 26 28 29 30 31 32 33 34 35 36 39 40 41 42 44 45 49 64 65 66 71 73 **P**6 **N** Blue River Valley Health Network, Brainard, NE	13	10	21	683	8	9142	23	2788	1211	62
OSHKOSH—Garden County										
GARDEN COUNTY HOSPITAL, Mailing Address: P.O. Box 320, Zip 69154; tel. 308/772–3283; Keith Hillman, Administrator (Total facility includes 36 beds in nursing home–type unit) (Nonreporting) **A**9 10 **N** Western Nebraska Rural Health Care Network, Chadron, NE	13	10	56	—	—	—	—	—	—	—
OSMOND—Pierce County										
★ OSMOND GENERAL HOSPITAL, 5th and Maple Street, Zip 68765–0429, Mailing Address: P.O. Box 429, Zip 68765–0429; tel. 402/748–3393; Celine Mlady, Chief Executive Officer **A**9 10 **F**8 15 19 20 22 28 30 32 33 35 44 49 64 65 71 **P**6 **N** North Central Hospital Network, Atkinson, NE	23	10	30	770	18	4609	0	2555	1454	59
PAPILLION—Sarpy County										
⊠ MIDLANDS COMMUNITY HOSPITAL, 11111 South 84th Street, Zip 68046; tel. 402/593–3000; Diana Smalley, Chief Executive Officer (Total facility includes 10 beds in nursing home–type unit) **A**1 9 10 **F**2 3 7 8 10 16 19 21 22 28 32 34 35 37 40 41 42 44 45 49 52 53 54 55 56 57 58 59 60 63 64 65 66 70 71 72 73 **P**1 5 **S** Quorum Health Group/Quorum Health Resources, Inc., Brentwood, TN	32	10	160	2874	34	29571	364	23758	10013	370
PAWNEE CITY—Pawnee County										
PAWNEE COUNTY MEMORIAL HOSPITAL, 600 I Street, Zip 68420, Mailing Address: P.O. Box 313, Zip 68420; tel. 402/852–2231; James A. Kubik, Administrator (Nonreporting) **A**9 10	13	10	21	—	—	—	—	—	—	—
PENDER—Thurston County										
★ PENDER COMMUNITY HOSPITAL, 603 Earl Street, Zip 68047–0100, Mailing Address: P.O. Box 100, Zip 68047–0100; tel. 402/385–3083; Kevin Kueny, Administrator **A**9 10 **F**7 8 11 15 16 17 19 20 25 26 28 29 30 32 33 34 35 36 40 41 44 46 48 49 51 61 64 65 66 71 72 **P**7 **S** Mercy Health Services, Farmington Hills, MI	16	10	31	811	8	8556	76	3428	1240	—
PLAINVIEW—Pierce County										
PLAINVIEW PUBLIC HOSPITAL, Mailing Address: P.O. Box 489, Zip 68769; tel. 402/582–4245; Donald T. Naiberk, Administrator and Chief Executive Officer (Nonreporting) **A**9 10 **N** North Central Hospital Network, Atkinson, NE	14	10	19	—	—	—	—	—	—	—

Hospital, Address, Telephone, Administrator, Approval, Facility, and Physician Codes, Health Care System, Network	Classi-fication Codes		Utilization Data					Expense (thousands) of dollars		
★ American Hospital Association (AHA) membership □ Joint Commission on Accreditation of Healthcare Organizations (JCAHO) accreditation + American Osteopathic Hospital Association (AOHA) membership ○ American Osteopathic Association (AOA) accreditation △ Commission on Accreditation of Rehabilitation Facilities (CARF) accreditation Control codes 61, 63, 64, 71, 72 and 73 indicate hospitals listed by AOHA, but not registered by AHA. For definition of numerical codes, see page A4	Control	Service	Beds	Admissions	Census	Outpatient Visits	Births	Total	Payroll	Personnel

RED CLOUD—Webster County

WEBSTER COUNTY COMMUNITY HOSPITAL, Sixth Avenue and Franklin Street, Zip 68970–0465; tel. 402/746–2291; Terry L. Hoffart, Administrator **A**9 10 **F**8 19 28 32 37 44 49 66 71 73 **P**3 **N** Heartland Health Alliance, Lincoln, NE; Rural Health Partners, Lexington, NE

	13	10	16	255	5	—	0	1609	705	34

SAINT PAUL—Howard County

★ HOWARD COUNTY COMMUNITY HOSPITAL, 1102 Kendall Street, Zip 68873, Mailing Address: Box 406, Zip 68873; tel. 308/754–4421; Russell W. Swigart, Administrator **A**9 10 **F**7 8 14 19 22 30 33 35 44 45 49 59 64 65 71 73

	13	10	37	478	18	7014	45	2479	1259	64

SARGENT—Custer County

SARGENT DISTRICT HOSPITAL, 1201 West Main, Zip 68874; tel. 308/527–3414; Rajitha Goli, M.D., Medical Director (Nonreporting) **A**9 10

	16	10	18	—	—	—	—	—	—	—

SCHUYLER—Colfax County

ALEGENT HEALTH–MEMORIAL HOSPITAL, 104 West 17th Street, Zip 68661; tel. 402/352–2441; Al Klaasmeyer, Administrator (Total facility includes 31 beds in nursing home–type unit) **A**9 10 **F**7 8 12 15 16 17 22 26 28 30 31 32 33 34 36 39 40 42 44 48 49 56 64 65 66 67 71 **P**8 **N** Alegent Health, Omaha, NE

	23	10	45	214	34	23383	40	2332	1061	117

SCOTTSBLUFF—Scotts Bluff County

⌧ REGIONAL WEST MEDICAL CENTER, 4021 Avenue B, Zip 69361–4695; tel. 308/635–3711; David M. Nitschke, President and Chief Executive Officer (Total facility includes 22 beds in nursing home–type unit) (Nonreporting) **A**1 2 9 10 **N** Western Nebraska Rural Health Care Network, Chadron, NE

	23	10	265	—	—	—	—	—	—	—

SEWARD—Seward County

MEMORIAL HEALTH CARE SYSTEMS, 300 North Columbia Avenue, Zip 68434–9907; tel. 402/643–2971; Ronald D. Waltz, Chief Executive Officer (Total facility includes 120 beds in nursing home–type unit) **A**9 10 **F**1 2 3 4 5 6 7 8 9 10 11 12 13 15 16 17 18 19 20 21 22 23 24 25 26 27 28 29 30 31 32 33 34 35 36 37 38 39 40 41 42 43 44 45 46 47 48 49 50 51 52 53 54 55 56 57 58 59 60 61 62 63 64 65 66 67 68 69 70 71 72 73 74 **P**6 **N** Heartland Health Alliance, Lincoln, NE; Blue River Valley Health Network, Brainard, NE

	23	10	154	522	131	16345	83	10065	5557	141

SIDNEY—Cheyenne County

★ MEMORIAL HEALTH CENTER, 645 Osage Street, Zip 69162; tel. 308/254–5825; Rex D. Walk, Chief Executive Officer (Total facility includes 70 beds in nursing home–type unit) **A**9 10 **F**1 3 7 8 10 11 12 14 15 16 17 18 19 20 22 26 27 28 30 32 34 35 36 37 39 40 41 42 44 49 51 58 64 65 66 67 71 73 **P**8 **N** Western Nebraska Rural Health Care Network, Chadron, NE; High Plains Rural Health Network, Fort Morgan, CO

	23	10	102	1163	81	13735	107	8674	4328	157

SUPERIOR—Nuckolls County

BRODSTONE MEMORIAL HOSPITAL, 520 East Tenth, Zip 68978, Mailing Address: P.O. Box 187, Zip 68978–0187; tel. 402/879–3281; Ronald D. Waggoner, Administrator and Chief Executive Officer **A**9 10 **F**7 8 19 22 27 32 34 35 36 37 40 41 44 49 65 71 **P**8 **N** Heartland Health Alliance, Lincoln, NE; Rural Health Partners, Lexington, NE

	23	10	49	784	12	11605	50	4826	1972	101

SYRACUSE—Otoe County

COMMUNITY MEMORIAL HOSPITAL, 1579 Midland Street, Zip 68446, Mailing Address: P.O. Box N, Zip 68446; tel. 402/269–2011; Ron Anderson, Administrator (Nonreporting) **A**9 10 **N** Heartland Health Alliance, Lincoln, NE

	16	10	18	—	—	—	—	—	—	—

TECUMSEH—Johnson County

★ JOHNSON COUNTY HOSPITAL, 202 High Street, Zip 68450–0599; tel. 402/335–3361; Lavonne M. Rowe, Administrator **A**9 10 **F**1 7 8 14 15 16 17 19 22 28 30 32 33 34 37 40 41 42 44 49 51 71 **N** Heartland Health Alliance, Lincoln, NE

	13	10	30	332	4	4056	28	1903	865	42

TILDEN—Antelope County

TILDEN COMMUNITY HOSPITAL, Mailing Address: P.O. Box 340, Zip 68781; tel. 402/368–5343; LuAnn Barr, Administrator (Nonreporting) **A**9 10

	23	10	20	—	—	—	—	—	—	—

VALENTINE—Cherry County

CHERRY COUNTY HOSPITAL, Highway 12 and Green Street, Zip 69201–0410; tel. 402/376–2525; Brent Peterson, Administrator **A**9 10 **F**8 10 11 14 15 17 19 22 28 29 32 34 35 37 40 44 46 70 71 73 **P**3 6 **N** Heartland Health Alliance, Lincoln, NE

	13	10	27	655	8	7000	217	3471	1551	61

WAHOO—Saunders County

SAUNDERS COUNTY HEALTH SERVICE, 805 West Tenth Street, Zip 68066, Mailing Address: P.O. Box 185, Zip 68066; tel. 402/443–4191; Michael Boyles, Administrator (Total facility includes 73 beds in nursing home–type unit) **A**9 10 **F**8 14 15 16 17 22 28 29 30 32 33 34 36 44 45 49 51 54 61 64 65 66 67 71 **P**6 **N** Blue River Valley Health Network, Brainard, NE

	13	10	103	274	78	8196	0	5350	3079	141

WAYNE—Wayne County

PROVIDENCE MEDICAL CENTER, 1200 Providence Road, Zip 68787; tel. 402/375–3800; Marcile Thomas, Administrator **A**9 10 **F**7 14 15 16 19 22 24 32 33 35 44 49 65 66 71 **S** Missionary Benedictine Sisters American Province, Norfolk, NE

	21	10	34	932	12	7494	99	4583	1967	74

WEST POINT—Cuming County

★ ST. FRANCIS MEMORIAL HOSPITAL, 430 North Monitor Street, Zip 68788–1595; tel. 402/372–2404; Ronald O. Briggs, President **A**9 10 **F**7 8 15 19 22 24 32 34 35 40 44 48 49 66 71 73 **P**6 **S** Franciscan Sisters of Christian Charity HealthCare Ministry, Inc, Manitowoc, WI

	21	10	27	624	7	59643	119	6598	3531	99

Hospital, Address, Telephone, Administrator, Approval, Facility, and Physician Codes, Health Care System, Network	Classi-fication Codes		Utilization Data					Expense (thousands) of dollars		
★ American Hospital Association (AHA) membership □ Joint Commission on Accreditation of Healthcare Organizations (JCAHO) accreditation + American Osteopathic Hospital Association (AOHA) membership ○ American Osteopathic Association (AOA) accreditation △ Commission on Accreditation of Rehabilitation Facilities (CARF) accreditation Control codes 61, 63, 64, 71, 72 and 73 indicate hospitals listed by AOHA, but not registered by AHA. For definition of numerical codes, see page A4	Control	Service	Beds	Admissions	Census	Outpatient Visits	Births	Total	Payroll	Personnel

WINNEBAGO—Thurston County

☒ U. S. PUBLIC HEALTH SERVICE INDIAN HOSPITAL, Zip 68071; tel. 402/878–2231; Shirley A. Poor Thunder, Service Unit Director **A**1 10 **F**2 8 13 14 15 16 18 20 22 24 27 28 30 31 32 34 39 46 49 53 54 56 58 59 65 71 73 **S** U. S. Public Health Service Indian Health Service, Rockville, MD — 47 10 30 557 14 35840 0 6401 2772 89

YORK—York County

★ YORK GENERAL HOSPITAL, 2222 Lincoln Avenue, Zip 68467–1095; tel. 402/362–6671; Charles Schulz, Chief Executive Officer **A**9 10 **F**7 8 11 12 19 21 22 24 28 30 32 33 34 35 36 37 39 40 41 42 44 46 48 49 63 64 65 66 67 71 73 74 **N** Heartland Health Alliance, Lincoln, NE; Blue River Valley Health Network, Brainard, NE — 23 10 48 928 10 29160 159 7595 3460 203

NEVADA

Resident population 1,530 (in thousands)
Resident population in metro areas 85.3%
Birth rate per 1,000 population 16.2
65 years and over 11.4%
Percent of persons without health insurance 15.7%

Hospital, Address, Telephone, Administrator, Approval, Facility, and Physician Codes, Health Care System, Network	Classi-fication Codes		Utilization Data					Expense (thousands) of dollars		
	Control	Service	Beds	Admissions	Census	Outpatient Visits	Births	Total	Payroll	Personnel

★ American Hospital Association (AHA) membership
□ Joint Commission on Accreditation of Healthcare Organizations (JCAHO) accreditation
+ American Osteopathic Hospital Association (AOHA) membership
○ American Osteopathic Association (AOA) accreditation
△ Commission on Accreditation of Rehabilitation Facilities (CARF) accreditation
Control codes 61, 63, 64, 71, 72 and 73 indicate hospitals listed by AOHA, but not registered by AHA. For definition of numerical codes, see page A4

Hospital	Control	Service	Beds	Admissions	Census	Outpatient Visits	Births	Total	Payroll	Personnel
BATTLE MOUNTAIN—Lander County										
BATTLE MOUNTAIN GENERAL HOSPITAL, 535 South Humboldt Street, Zip 89820–1988; tel. 702/635–2550; Kathy Ancho, Administrator **A**10 **F**17 22 34 35 41 45 46 73	13	10	14	150	1	8251	0	3427	1563	69
BOULDER CITY—Clark County										
BOULDER CITY HOSPITAL, 901 Adams Boulevard, Zip 89005; tel. 702/293–4111; Kim O. Crandell, Chief Executive Officer and Administrator (Total facility includes 47 beds in nursing home–type unit) (Nonreporting) **A**10	23	10	67	—	—	—	—	—	—	—
CARSON CITY—Carson City County										
✠ CARSON TAHOE HOSPITAL, 775 Fleischmann Way, Zip 89701, Mailing Address: P.O. Box 2168, Zip 89702–2168; tel. 702/882–1361; Steve Smith, Chief Executive Officer (Total facility includes 125 beds in nursing home–type unit) **A**1 9 10 **F**2 3 7 8 10 12 15 16 17 19 21 22 23 25 26 28 30 32 33 34 35 37 39 40 44 45 46 49 52 54 55 56 57 58 59 60 63 64 65 67 70 71 72 73	15	10	249	6455	190	62223	796	41004	24035	713
ELKO—Elko County										
✠ ELKO GENERAL HOSPITAL, 1297 College Avenue, Zip 89801–3499; tel. 702/753–1999; Anne Rieger, R.N., Administrator **A**1 9 10 **F**7 8 14 17 19 21 22 28 30 35 37 40 41 44 46 49 65 71 73 **P**3 5	13	10	50	2451	19	34425	665	18132	9197	271
ELY—White Pine County										
□ WILLIAM BEE RIRIE HOSPITAL, 1500 Avenue H, Zip 89301–2699; tel. 702/289–3001; Jack T. Wood, Administrator **A**1 9 10 **F**7 8 19 22 25 26 28 32 37 40 44 49 53 55 65 71 73 **P**8	13	10	40	645	6	9950	84	5365	2126	83
FALLON—Churchill County										
★ CHURCHILL COMMUNITY HOSPTIAL, 801 East Williams Avenue, Zip 89406; tel. 702/423–3151; Jeffrey Feike, Administrator (Nonreporting) **A**9 10 **S** Lutheran Health Systems, Fargo, ND	23	10	40	—	—	—	—	—	—	—
HAWTHORNE—Mineral County										
MOUNT GRANT GENERAL HOSPITAL, First and A Street, Zip 89415, Mailing Address: P.O. Box 1510, Zip 89415; tel. 702/945–2461; Richard Munger, Administrator (Total facility includes 20 beds in nursing home–type unit) (Nonreporting) **A**10	16	10	35	—	—	—	—	—	—	—
HENDERSON—Clark County										
✠ ST. ROSE DOMINICAN HOSPITAL, 102 Lake Mead Drive, Zip 89015; tel. 702/564–2622; Rod A. Davis, President and Chief Executive Officer **A**1 9 10 **F**2 3 4 7 8 9 10 11 12 13 14 15 16 17 19 21 22 23 25 26 28 29 30 31 32 33 34 35 37 38 39 40 41 42 43 44 45 46 47 48 49 51 53 55 56 57 58 59 60 64 65 66 67 70 71 72 73 74 **P**3 5 7 **S** Catholic Healthcare West, San Francisco, CA **N** Catholic HealthCare West (CHW), San Francisco, CA	21	10	135	7085	90	101408	1380	51495	20885	622
LAS VEGAS—Clark County										
□ BHC MONTEVISTA HOSPITAL, (Formerly Montevista Hospital), 5900 West Rochelle Avenue, Zip 89103; tel. 702/364–1111; R. Dale Reynolds, Chief Executive Officer and Administrator (Nonreporting) **A**1 10 **S** Behavioral Healthcare Corporation, Nashville, TN	33	22	80	—	—	—	—	—	—	—
□ CHARTER BEHAVIORAL HEALTH SYSTEM OF NEVADA, 7000 West Spring Mountain Road, Zip 89117; tel. 702/876–4357; Lynn M. Rosenbach, Chief Executive Officer (Nonreporting) **A**1 9 10 **S** Magellan Health Services, Atlanta, GA	33	22	84	—	—	—	—	—	—	—
✠ △ COLUMBIA SUNRISE HOSPITAL AND MEDICAL CENTER, 3186 Maryland Parkway, Zip 89109–2306, Mailing Address: P.O. Box 98530, Zip 89193–8530; tel. 702/731–8000; Jerald F. Mitchell, President and Chief Executive Officer **A**1 2 5 7 9 10 **F**4 7 10 11 12 14 15 16 19 21 22 25 29 32 35 37 38 40 41 42 43 44 46 47 48 49 60 64 65 69 71 **S** Columbia/HCA Healthcare Corporation, Nashville, TN	33	10	643	37250	510	—	6329	260987	95405	2160
✠ DESERT SPRINGS HOSPITAL, 2075 East Flamingo Road, Zip 89119, Mailing Address: P.O. Box 19204, Zip 89132; tel. 702/733–8800; Thomas L. Koenig, Chief Executive Officer (Nonreporting) **A**1 10 **S** Quorum Health Group/Quorum Health Resources, Inc., Brentwood, TN	33	10	225	—	—	—	—	—	—	—
✠ MIKE O'CALLAGHAN FEDERAL HOSPITAL, (Formerly Nellis Federal Hospital), 4700 Las Vegas Boulevard North, Suite 2419, Zip 89191–6601; tel. 702/653–2000; Colonel Jack A. Gupton, MSC, USAF, Administrator (Nonreporting) **A**1 **S** Department of the Air Force, Washington, DC	41	10	34	—	—	—	—	—	—	—
MONTEVISTA HOSPITAL See BHC Montevista Hospital										
NELLIS FEDERAL HOSPITAL See Mike O'Callaghan Federal Hospital										
□ THC–LAS VEGAS HOSPITAL, 5100 West Sahara Avenue, Zip 89102; tel. 702/871–1418; Dale A. Kirby, Chief Executive Officer (Nonreporting) **A**1 10 **S** Transitional Hospitals Corporation, Las Vegas, NV	33	49	52	—	—	—	—	—	—	—
□ UNIVERSITY MEDICAL CENTER, 1800 West Charleston Boulevard, Zip 89102; tel. 702/383–2000; William R. Hale, Chief Executive Officer (Nonreporting) **A**1 2 3 5 10	13	10	506	—	—	—	—	—	—	—
□ VALLEY HOSPITAL MEDICAL CENTER, 620 Shadow Lane, Zip 89106; tel. 702/388–4000; Roger Collins, Chief Executive Officer and Managing Director **A**1 9 10 **F**4 7 10 11 12 14 15 16 19 22 25 26 28 32 35 37 38 39 40 41 43 44 52 57 64 65 71 72 73 **P**7 **S** Universal Health Services, Inc., King of Prussia, PA	33	10	365	20358	268	—	2799	133113	46758	1099

Hospital, Address, Telephone, Administrator, Approval, Facility, and Physician Codes, Health Care System, Network	Classi-fication Codes		Utilization Data					Expense (thousands) of dollars		
★ American Hospital Association (AHA) membership □ Joint Commission on Accreditation of Healthcare Organizations (JCAHO) accreditation + American Osteopathic Hospital Association (AOHA) membership ○ American Osteopathic Association (AOA) accreditation △ Commission on Accreditation of Rehabilitation Facilities (CARF) accreditation Control codes 61, 63, 64, 71, 72 and 73 indicate hospitals listed by AOHA, but not registered by AHA. For definition of numerical codes, see page A4	Control	Service	Beds	Admissions	Census	Outpatient Visits	Births	Total	Payroll	Personnel

LOVELOCK—Pershing County

★ PERSHING GENERAL HOSPITAL, 855 Sixth Street, Zip 89419, Mailing Address: P.O. Box 661, Zip 89419; tel. 702/273–2621; Helen Woolley, Administrator (Total facility includes 25 beds in nursing home–type unit) (Nonreporting) **A**9 10 **S** Lutheran Health Systems, Fargo, ND — 16 10 34 — — — — — — —

PERSHING GENERAL HOSPITAL	16	10	34	—	—	—	—	—	—	—

NORTH LAS VEGAS—Clark County

□ LAKE MEAD HOSPITAL MEDICAL CENTER, 1409 East Lake Mead Boulevard, Zip 89030; tel. 702/649–7711; Ernest Libman, Administrator and Chief Executive Officer (Nonreporting) **A**1 10 **S** TENET Healthcare Corporation, Santa Barbara, CA	33	10	140							

OWYHEE—Elko County

⊠ U. S. PUBLIC HEALTH SERVICE OWYHEE COMMUNITY HEALTH FACILITY, Mailing Address: P.O. Box 130, Zip 89832–0130; tel. 702/757–2415; Kay C. Jewett, Administrative Officer **A**1 10 **F**1 2 3 4 5 6 7 8 9 10 11 12 13 14 15 17 18 19 20 21 22 23 24 25 26 27 28 29 30 31 32 33 34 35 36 37 38 39 40 41 42 43 44 45 46 47 48 49 50 51 52 53 54 55 56 57 58 59 60 61 62 63 64 65 66 67 68 69 70 71 72 73 74 **P**5 **S** U. S. Public Health Service Indian Health Service, Rockville, MD	46	10	15	77	1	13047	0	—	—	60

RENO—Washoe County

□ BHC WEST HILLS HOSPITAL, (Formerly West Hills Hospital), 1240 East Ninth Street, Zip 89512, Mailing Address: P.O. Box 30012, Zip 89520; tel. 702/323–0478; Neal Cury, Chief Executive Officer (Nonreporting) **A**1 3 5 9 10 **S** Behavioral Healthcare Corporation, Nashville, TN	33	22	95							
BHC WILLOW SPRINGS RTC, (Formerly Willow Springs Center for Children and Adolescents), 690 Edison Way, Zip 89502; tel. 702/858–3303; Robert Bartlett, Administrator (Nonreporting) **S** Behavioral Healthcare Corporation, Nashville, TN	33	22	74							
⊠ IOANNIS A. LOUGARIS VETERANS AFFAIRS MEDICAL CENTER, 1000 Locust Street, Zip 89520–0111; tel. 702/786–7200; Gary R. Whitfield, Director (Total facility includes 60 beds in nursing home–type unit) **A**1 3 5 **F**1 3 8 10 12 15 17 18 19 20 21 22 24 26 27 28 29 30 31 32 33 34 35 37 39 41 42 44 45 46 49 51 52 54 55 56 57 58 59 60 63 64 65 67 71 72 73 74 **P**6 **S** Department of Veterans Affairs, Washington, DC	45	10	167	3732	118	126133	0	51604	29235	664
△ ST. MARY'S REGIONAL MEDICAL CENTER, 235 West Sixth Street, Zip 89520; tel. 702/323–2041; Jeff K. Bills, Chief Executive Officer (Total facility includes 16 beds in nursing home–type unit) **A**1 7 10 **F**2 3 4 7 8 10 11 12 13 16 17 19 20 21 22 23 25 27 28 29 30 32 33 34 35 37 38 39 40 41 42 43 44 45 46 48 49 61 63 64 65 67 71 72 73 74 **P**3 5 6 8 **N** Saint Mary's Health Network, Reno, NV	21	10	341	13107	185	129299	2220	119250	53512	1881
⊠ WASHOE MEDICAL CENTER, 77 Pringle Way, Zip 89520–0109; tel. 702/328–4777; Robert B. Burn, President and Chief Executive Officer (Total facility includes 19 beds in nursing home–type unit) **A**1 2 3 5 9 10 **F**2 3 4 7 8 10 11 12 13 14 15 16 17 19 22 23 24 25 26 27 28 29 30 31 32 34 35 37 38 39 40 41 42 43 44 45 46 47 49 51 52 54 55 56 57 58 59 60 64 65 67 69 70 71 72 73 74 **P**5 6 7	23	10	436	18714	263	165857	3278	185019	69666	1691

WEST HILLS HOSPITAL See BHC West Hills Hospital

SPARKS—Washoe County

□ NEVADA MENTAL HEALTH INSTITUTE, 480 Galletti Way, Zip 89431–5574; tel. 702/688–2001; David Rosin, M.D., Medical Director **A**1 3 5 10 **F**6 12 34 52 55 56 57 58 59 65 **P**6	12	22	52	1362	44	17079	0	18108	6096	194
□ NORTHERN NEVADA MEDICAL CENTER, 2375 East Prater Way, Zip 89434–9645; tel. 702/331–7000; James R. Pagels, Chief Executive Officer and Managing Director **A**1 10 **F**8 11 12 14 15 16 17 18 20 22 26 28 30 31 34 37 39 44 46 48 49 52 53 54 55 56 59 65 66 69 72 73 **P**5 **S** Universal Health Services, Inc., King of Prussia, PA	32	10	110	2102	39	37027	1	24158	10598	295

TONOPAH—Nye County

NYE REGIONAL MEDICAL CENTER, 825 South Main, Zip 89049, Mailing Address: Box 391, Zip 89049; tel. 702/482–6233; Roger Mayers, Interim Administrator (Total facility includes 24 beds in nursing home–type unit) (Nonreporting) **A**9 10 **S** Quorum Health Group/Quorum Health Resources, Inc., Brentwood, TN	13	10	45	—	—	—	—	—	—	—

WINNEMUCCA—Humboldt County

★ HUMBOLDT GENERAL HOSPITAL, 118 East Haskell Street, Zip 89445; tel. 702/623–5222; Byron Quinton, Administrator (Total facility includes 30 beds in nursing home–type unit) **A**9 10 **F**3 7 8 14 15 19 22 35 37 40 44 64 65 71 73 **P**5	16	10	52	740	23	20418	307	8693	3325	128

YERINGTON—Lyon County

SOUTH LYON MEDICAL CENTER, Surprise at Whitacre Avenue, Zip 89447, Mailing Address: P.O. Box 940, Zip 89447–0940; tel. 702/463–2301; Joan S. Hall, R.N., Administrator (Total facility includes 30 beds in nursing home–type unit) (Nonreporting) **A**9 10	23	10	44	—	—	—	—	—	—	—

NEW HAMPSHIRE

Resident population 1,148 (in thousands)
Resident population in metro areas 59.6%
Birth rate per 1,000 population 13.7
65 years and over 11.9%
Percent of persons without health insurance 11.9%

Hospital, Address, Telephone, Administrator, Approval, Facility, and Physician Codes, Health Care System, Network

★ American Hospital Association (AHA) membership
□ Joint Commission on Accreditation of Healthcare Organizations (JCAHO) accreditation
+ American Osteopathic Hospital Association (AOHA) membership
○ American Osteopathic Association (AOA) accreditation
△ Commission on Accreditation of Rehabilitation Facilities (CARF) accreditation
Control codes 61, 63, 64, 71, 72 and 73 indicate hospitals listed by AOHA, but not registered by AHA. For definition of numerical codes, see page A4

Hospital	Control	Service	Beds	Admissions	Census	Outpatient Visits	Births	Total	Payroll	Personnel
BERLIN—Coos County										
⊞ ANDROSCOGGIN VALLEY HOSPITAL, 59 Page Hill Road, Zip 03570–3531; tel. 603/752–2200; Donald F. Saunders, President **A**1 9 10 **F**7 8 12 14 15 19 21 22 26 28 29 30 31 32 33 34 35 37 40 41 42 44 49 51 52 54 55 56 57 58 64 65 70 71 73 **P**3	23	10	66	2173	39	44244	115	18518	8009	281
CLAREMONT—Sullivan County										
⊞ VALLEY REGIONAL HOSPITAL, 243 Elm Street, Zip 03743–2099; tel. 603/542–7771; Donald R. Holl, President **A**1 9 10 **F**1 3 7 8 12 13 15 16 17 18 19 21 22 23 24 25 26 27 28 29 30 32 33 34 35 37 39 40 41 42 44 45 49 51 52 54 55 56 57 58 59 63 64 65 66 67 68 70 71 72 73 74 **P**7 **N** Partners In Caring, Claremont, NH	23	10	71	1734	24	51810	237	19994	7680	273
COLEBROOK—Coos County										
★ UPPER CONNECTICUT VALLEY HOSPITAL, Corliss Lane, Zip 03576, Mailing Address: RFD 2, Box 13, Zip 03576; tel. 603/237–4971; Deanna S. Howard, Chief Executive Officer **A**9 10 **F**7 8 13 15 16 17 19 22 28 30 32 37 39 40 41 42 44 56 65 71 73	23	10	20	625	8	16566	53	4764	2216	115
CONCORD—Merrimack County										
⊞ CONCORD HOSPITAL, 250 Pleasant Street, Zip 03301–2598; tel. 603/225–2711; Michael B. Green, President **A**1 2 3 5 9 10 **F**3 7 8 10 11 12 13 14 15 16 17 19 20 21 22 23 24 26 29 30 31 32 33 34 35 37 39 40 41 42 44 45 49 51 52 53 54 55 56 57 58 59 63 65 67 68 70 71 72 73 74 **P**6 7 **N** HealthLink, Laconia, NH	23	10	161	8457	111	133268	1335	84754	39769	1057
□ △ HEALTHSOUTH REHABILITATION HOSPITAL, 254 Pleasant Street, Zip 03301; tel. 603/226–9800; Anne M. Fugagli, Administrator (Nonreporting) **A**1 7 9 10 **S** HEALTHSOUTH Corporation, Birmingham, AL	33	46	50	—	—	—	—	—	—	—
□ NEW HAMPSHIRE HOSPITAL, 36 Clinton Street, Zip 03301–3861; tel. 603/271–5200; Chester G. Batchelder, Superintendent (Total facility includes 99 beds in nursing home–type unit) **A**1 3 5 9 10 **F**14 15 16 20 26 28 31 39 41 45 46 52 53 54 55 57 64 65 67 73 **P**4 6	12	22	296	1196	239	0	0	43258	23986	843
DERRY—Rockingham County										
⊞ PARKLAND MEDICAL CENTER, One Parkland Drive, Zip 03038; tel. 603/432–1500; Bruce G. Peters, President and Chief Executive Officer **A**1 9 10 **F**3 4 7 8 10 12 14 15 16 17 19 20 21 22 23 25 26 27 28 29 30 32 33 34 35 37 40 41 42 43 44 45 46 49 50 51 52 53 54 55 57 58 59 60 61 63 65 66 67 68 69 71 72 73 74 **P**1 7 **S** Columbia/HCA Healthcare Corporation, Nashville, TN	33	10	65	3344	41	63355	616	37074	12659	380
DOVER—Strafford County										
SEABORNE HOSPITAL, Seaborne Drive, Zip 03820; tel. 603/742–9300; Michael Torch, Executive Director **A**9 **F**2 3 12 20 22 31 53 54 56 70 **P**6	32	82	44	486	25	0	0	3474	1517	55
⊞ WENTWORTH-DOUGLASS HOSPITAL, 789 Central Avenue, Zip 03820–2589; tel. 603/742–5252; Gregory J. Walker, Chief Executive Officer **A**1 2 9 10 **F**5 7 8 12 13 14 15 16 17 19 21 22 23 24 26 28 29 30 32 33 34 35 37 39 40 41 42 44 45 46 49 51 60 61 63 65 67 70 71 73 **P**5 7 8	23	10	113	3971	50	129041	566	48873	21635	609
DUBLIN—Cheshire County										
BEECH HILL HOSPITAL, New Harrisville Road, Zip 03444, Mailing Address: Box 254, Zip 03444; tel. 603/563–8511; Jeffrey A. Baron, Executive Director (Nonreporting) **A**9	23	82	70	—	—	—	—	—	—	—
EXETER—Rockingham County										
⊞ EXETER HOSPITAL, 10 Buzell Avenue, Zip 03833–2515; tel. 603/778–7311; Kevin J. Callahan, President and Chief Executive Officer (Total facility includes 125 beds in nursing home–type unit) **A**1 2 9 10 **F**4 7 8 10 12 13 14 15 16 17 19 20 21 22 23 24 25 26 27 28 29 30 31 32 33 34 35 37 39 40 41 42 44 45 46 49 51 53 54 55 56 57 58 59 60 61 63 64 65 66 67 70 71 73 74 **P**6 7 8	23	10	218	4205	163	67781	697	52467	22773	636
FRANKLIN—Merrimack County										
⊞ FRANKLIN REGIONAL HOSPITAL, 15 Aiken Avenue, Zip 03235–1299; tel. 603/934–2060; Walter A. Strauch, Executive Director **A**1 9 10 **F**7 8 14 15 16 17 19 22 28 29 30 32 33 34 37 40 41 44 45 46 49 51 54 56 57 64 65 67 68 71 73 74 **P**6 **N** Caring Community Network of the Twin Rivers (CCNTR), Franklin, NH	23	10	49	1640	28	34314	113	16400	8192	240
GREENFIELD—Hillsborough County										
△ CROTCHED MOUNTAIN REHABILITATION CENTER, 1 Verney Drive, Zip 03047; tel. 603/547–3311; Major W. Wheelock, President (Total facility includes 62 beds in nursing home–type unit) **A**7 9 **F**6 12 17 20 24 28 39 48 49 53 64 65 67 73	23	46	146	28	101	0	0	19277	10943	510
HAMPSTEAD—Rockingham County										
□ HAMPSTEAD HOSPITAL, East Road, Zip 03841–2228; tel. 603/329–5311; Phillip Kubiak, President **A**1 9 10 **F**3 6 15 16 18 19 22 25 26 34 35 45 52 53 54 56 57 58 59 65 67 71 **P**1 5 7	33	22	99	1343	39	—	0	8904	5200	117
HANOVER—Grafton County										
★ DARTMOUTH COLLEGE HEALTH SERVICE, 7 Rope Ferry Road, Zip 03755–1421; tel. 603/650–1400; John Turco, M.D., Director **A**9 **F**3 12 15 16 17 18 28 29 30 34 39 41 45 51 54 55 58 59 65 66 67 74	23	11	10	401	2	18850	0	—	—	46

© 1997 AHA Guide

Hospital, Address, Telephone, Administrator, Approval, Facility, and Physician Codes, Health Care System, Network	Classi-fication Codes		Utilization Data					Expense (thousands) of dollars		
	Control	Service	Beds	Admissions	Census	Outpatient Visits	Births	Total	Payroll	Personnel

★ American Hospital Association (AHA) membership
□ Joint Commission on Accreditation of Healthcare Organizations (JCAHO) accreditation
+ American Osteopathic Hospital Association (AOHA) membership
○ American Osteopathic Association (AOA) accreditation
△ Commission on Accreditation of Rehabilitation Facilities (CARF) accreditation
Control codes 61, 63, 64, 71, 72 and 73 indicate hospitals listed by AOHA, but not registered by AHA. For definition of numerical codes, see page A4

KEENE—Cheshire County

✠ △ CHESHIRE MEDICAL CENTER, 580 Court Street, Zip 03431–1718; tel. 603/352–4111; Robert J. Langlais, President and Chief Executive Officer **A**1 2 7 9 10 **F**7 8 11 12 14 15 16 17 18 19 20 21 22 23 24 28 29 30 31 34 35 37 39 40 41 42 44 45 46 48 49 52 53 54 55 56 57 58 60 63 65 66 67 70 71 73
— 23 10 162 4524 78 56181 457 40254 19215 642

LACONIA—Belknap County

★ LAKES REGION GENERAL HOSPITAL, Highland Street, Zip 03246–3298; tel. 603/524–3211; Thomas Clairmont, President **A**2 9 10 **F**3 4 7 8 10 12 13 14 15 16 17 19 20 22 23 26 28 30 31 33 34 35 37 40 41 42 44 45 49 52 53 54 55 56 57 63 65 67 70 71 72 73 74 **P**6 **N** HealthLink, Laconia, NH
— 23 10 117 5200 70 38759 626 48460 23455 710

LANCASTER—Coos County

✠ WEEKS MEMORIAL HOSPITAL, Middle Street, Zip 03584, Mailing Address: Rural Route 1, Box 8, Zip 03584–9702; tel. 603/788–4911; Patsy Pilgrim, Chief Executive Officer **A**1 9 10 **F**7 8 12 14 15 16 17 19 21 22 26 28 29 30 31 34 37 39 40 41 42 44 46 49 56 65 66 67 71 73 **P**6
— 23 10 49 1170 20 60302 92 12853 5673 207

LEBANON—Grafton County

✠ ALICE PECK DAY MEMORIAL HOSPITAL, 125 Mascoma Street, Zip 03766; tel. 603/448–3121; Robert A. Mesropian, President (Total facility includes 50 beds in nursing home–type unit) **A**1 9 10 **F**7 8 12 13 14 15 16 17 19 22 25 26 28 29 30 33 34 39 40 41 42 44 45 46 49 51 64 65 67 70 71 73 74 **P**8
— 23 10 82 631 57 32656 204 12655 6865 204

✠ MARY HITCHCOCK MEMORIAL HOSPITAL, One Medical Center Drive, Zip 03756–0001; tel. 603/650–5000; James W. Varnum, President **A**1 2 3 5 8 9 10 **F**4 8 10 11 12 14 15 16 17 18 19 22 23 26 27 28 29 30 31 32 34 35 37 38 39 40 41 42 43 44 45 46 47 49 51 52 53 54 56 57 58 59 60 61 63 65 66 67 69 70 71 72 73 74 **P**4 5 8 **N** HealthLink, Laconia, NH; Lahey Network, Burlington, MA
— 23 10 352 17666 266 315463 1009 217393 80603 2606

LITTLETON—Grafton County

✠ LITTLETON REGIONAL HOSPITAL, 262 Cottage Street, Zip 03561; tel. 603/444–7731; Robert S. Pearson, Administrator **A**1 2 9 10 **F**7 8 14 15 16 17 19 21 22 23 25 27 28 29 30 31 33 34 35 37 39 40 41 42 44 45 46 61 63 65 67 69 71 73 74 **S** Quorum Health Group/Quorum Health Resources, Inc., Brentwood, TN
— 23 10 49 1346 13 28241 244 14604 5901 183

MANCHESTER—Hillsborough County

✠ △ CATHOLIC MEDICAL CENTER, 100 McGregor Street, Zip 03102–3770; tel. 603/668–3545; Robert Cholette, President and Chief Executive Officer **A**1 2 7 9 10 **F**1 2 3 4 5 6 7 8 10 11 12 14 15 16 17 18 19 20 21 22 23 24 26 27 28 29 30 31 32 33 34 35 36 37 39 40 41 42 43 44 45 46 48 49 52 54 56 57 58 59 60 61 62 65 66 67 71 72 73 74 **P**1 **N** HealthLink, Laconia, NH
— 23 10 262 9345 179 96565 223 122243 42503 1046

✠ ELLIOT HOSPITAL, One Elliot Way, Zip 03103; tel. 603/669–5300; Robert G. Cholette, Chief Executive Officer **A**1 2 9 10 **F**1 3 4 5 6 7 8 10 12 14 15 16 17 18 19 20 21 22 23 24 26 27 28 29 30 31 32 33 34 35 37 38 39 40 41 42 43 44 45 46 49 51 52 54 55 56 57 58 59 60 61 62 63 65 66 67 70 71 72 73 74 **P**1 **N** HealthLink, Laconia, NH
— 23 10 243 9893 138 165300 2360 100078 38004 1213

✠ VETERANS AFFAIRS MEDICAL CENTER, 718 Smyth Road, Zip 03104–4098; tel. 603/624–4366; Paul J. McCool, Director (Total facility includes 120 beds in nursing home–type unit) **A**1 2 5 9 **F**1 2 3 8 11 12 16 19 20 21 22 24 25 26 30 31 32 33 34 37 39 41 42 44 45 46 49 51 54 55 56 58 64 65 67 71 73 74 **P**6 **S** Department of Veterans Affairs, Washington, DC
— 45 10 180 2464 157 99704 0 46352 23242 544

NASHUA—Hillsborough County

□ CHARTER BROOKSIDE BEHAVIORAL HEALTH SYSTEM OF NEW ENGLAND, 29 Northwest Boulevard, Zip 03063; tel. 603/886–5000; Susan A. Cambria, Chief Executive Officer **A**1 9 10 **F**2 3 14 15 16 17 18 19 22 28 29 32 35 52 53 54 55 56 57 58 59 65 67 70 71 **S** Magellan Health Services, Atlanta, GA
— 33 22 100 2291 88 4144 0 15871 5404 160

✠ SOUTHERN NEW HAMPSHIRE REGIONAL MEDICAL CENTER, 8 Prospect Street, Zip 03060, Mailing Address: P.O. Box 2014, Zip 03061–2014; tel. 603/577–2000; Thomas E. Wilhelmsen, Jr., President **A**1 2 9 10 **F**3 7 8 10 12 13 14 15 16 17 18 19 21 22 23 28 29 30 34 35 37 38 39 40 41 42 44 45 46 49 51 52 53 56 57 58 59 60 63 65 67 71 72 73 74 **P**1 3 4 6 7 8 **N** Lahey Network, Burlington, MA
— 23 10 154 6259 73 93315 1381 56309 26443 812

✠ △ ST. JOSEPH HEALTHCARE, 172 Kinsley Street, Zip 03061, Mailing Address: Caller Service 2013, Zip 03061; tel. 603/882–3000; Peter B. Davis, President and Chief Executive Officer **A**1 2 6 7 9 10 **F**1 2 3 7 8 10 11 12 13 14 15 16 17 18 19 20 21 22 23 24 25 26 27 28 29 30 31 32 33 34 35 36 37 39 40 41 42 44 46 48 49 51 52 54 55 56 57 58 59 60 61 63 65 66 67 70 71 72 73 74 **P**6 8 **S** Covenant Health Systems, Inc., Lexington, MA **N** Saint Joseph Health Care, Nashua, NH
— 21 10 208 5773 80 134193 980 59087 27642 751

NEW LONDON—Merrimack County

✠ NEW LONDON HOSPITAL, 270 County Road, Zip 03257; tel. 603/526–2911; Alyson R. Pitman, President and Chief Executive Officer (Total facility includes 56 beds in nursing home–type unit) **A**1 9 10 **F**7 8 13 15 16 17 19 20 22 25 28 30 34 35 37 39 40 41 42 44 45 49 51 64 65 66 67 71 73 74 **P**8
— 23 10 91 1276 72 134539 171 16395 8274 298

NORTH CONWAY—Carroll County

MEMORIAL HOSPITAL, 3073 Main Street, Zip 03860–5001, Mailing Address: P.O. Box 5001, Zip 03860–5001; tel. 603/356–5461; Gary R. Poquette, FACHE, Executive Director (Total facility includes 45 beds in nursing home–type unit) **A**9 10 **F**1 7 8 14 15 16 17 19 20 21 22 29 30 33 34 35 40 41 42 44 45 49 56 59 64 65 66 70 71 73 **P**3
— 23 10 80 1412 61 34239 233 16067 6286 214

Hospital, Address, Telephone, Administrator, Approval, Facility, and Physician Codes, Health Care System, Network	Classi-fication Codes		Utilization Data					Expense (thousands) of dollars		
★ American Hospital Association (AHA) membership □ Joint Commission on Accreditation of Healthcare Organizations (JCAHO) accreditation + American Osteopathic Hospital Association (AOHA) membership ○ American Osteopathic Association (AOA) accreditation △ Commission on Accreditation of Rehabilitation Facilities (CARF) accreditation Control codes 61, 63, 64, 71, 72 and 73 indicate hospitals listed by AOHA, but not registered by AHA. For definition of numerical codes, see page A4	Control	Service	Beds	Admissions	Census	Outpatient Visits	Births	Total	Payroll	Personnel

PETERBOROUGH—Hillsborough County

⊠ MONADNOCK COMMUNITY HOSPITAL, 452 Old Street Road, Zip 03458; tel. 603/924–7191; Frank A. Niro, Chief Executive Officer **A**1 9 10 **F**1 6 7 8 12 13 15 16 17 18 19 20 22 24 28 30 31 32 33 34 36 39 40 41 42 44 45 46 48 49 51 52 54 55 56 57 58 59 63 65 67 69 71 73 74 **P**3 **S** Quorum Health Group/Quorum Health Resources, Inc., Brentwood, TN	23	10	62	1792	24	50379	397	16934	6727	235

PLYMOUTH—Grafton County

SPEARE MEMORIAL HOSPITAL, Hospital Road, Zip 03264–1199; tel. 603/536–1120; David L. Pearse, Executive Director **A**9 10 **F**7 8 12 14 15 17 19 21 22 28 30 33 37 39 40 41 42 44 49 54 56 65 66 67 71 73	23	10	47	1025	11	48728	75	9924	4438	147

PORTSMOUTH—Rockingham County

⊠ PORTSMOUTH REGIONAL HOSPITAL AND PAVILION, (Includes Portsmouth Pavilion), 333 Borthwick Avenue, Zip 03802–7004; tel. 603/436–5110; William J. Schuler, Chief Executive Officer **A**1 9 10 **F**3 4 7 8 10 12 17 18 19 21 22 23 24 26 28 30 32 33 34 35 37 40 41 42 44 49 52 53 56 57 58 59 63 65 71 72 73 **P**1 6 8 **S** Columbia/HCA Healthcare Corporation, Nashville, TN	33	10	179	6930	103	91537	896	—	—	484

ROCHESTER—Strafford County

⊠ FRISBIE MEMORIAL HOSPITAL, 11 Whitehall Road, Zip 03867–3297; tel. 603/332–5211; Alvin D. Felgar, President and Chief Executive Officer **A**1 2 9 10 **F**2 3 7 8 10 11 15 16 17 18 19 21 22 26 30 31 33 34 35 37 39 40 41 42 44 45 49 51 52 54 55 56 57 58 63 65 66 67 71 73 **P**3 5 6 8	23	10	88	3332	50	51613	502	30795	13406	396

SALEM—Rockingham County

□ △ NORTHEAST REHABILITATION HOSPITAL, 70 Butler Street, Zip 03079; tel. 603/893–2900; John F. Prochilo, Chief Executive Officer and Administrator **A**1 7 9 10 **F**1 5 9 12 13 14 15 16 17 24 29 32 34 36 39 41 42 45 48 49 64 65 66 67 71 72 73 74	33	46	80	1163	68	73186	0	21336	11038	387

WOLFEBORO—Carroll County

★ HUGGINS HOSPITAL, 240 South Main Street, Zip 03894, Mailing Address: Box 912, Zip 03894–0912; tel. 603/569–2150; Leslie N. H. MacLeod, President (Total facility includes 27 beds in nursing home–type unit) **A**9 10 **F**1 7 8 15 16 19 21 22 31 35 37 40 41 42 44 45 46 49 64 65 71 74 **P**6	23	10	82	1950	53	49836	113	14909	6716	244

WOODSVILLE—Grafton County

⊠ COTTAGE HOSPITAL, Swiftwater Road, Zip 03785–2001, Mailing Address: P.O. Box 2001, Zip 03785; tel. 603/747–2761; Reginald J. Lavoie, Administrator **A**1 2 9 10 **F**7 8 15 16 19 22 36 37 40 42 54 65 67 71 72 73 74 **P**8	23	10	38	931	13	33160	71	9103	5044	144

NEW JERSEY

Resident population 7,945 (in thousands)
Resident population in metro areas 100%
Birth rate per 1,000 population 15.0
65 years and over 13.7%
Percent of persons without health insurance 13.0%

Hospital, Address, Telephone, Administrator, Approval, Facility, and Physician Codes, Health Care System, Network	Classi-fication Codes		Utilization Data					Expense (thousands) of dollars		
★ American Hospital Association (AHA) membership □ Joint Commission on Accreditation of Healthcare Organizations (JCAHO) accreditation + American Osteopathic Hospital Association (AOHA) membership ○ American Osteopathic Association (AOA) accreditation △ Commission on Accreditation of Rehabilitation Facilities (CARF) accreditation Control codes 61, 63, 64, 71, 72 and 73 indicate hospitals listed by AOHA, but not registered by AHA. For definition of numerical codes, see page A4	Control	Service	Beds	Admissions	Census	Outpatient Visits	Births	Total	Payroll	Personnel

ANCORA—Atlantic County

□ ANCORA PSYCHIATRIC HOSPITAL, 202 Spring Garden Road, Zip 08037–9699; tel. 609/561–1700; Yvonne A. Pressley, Chief Executive Officer **A**1 9 **F**2 3 11 19 20 22 26 35 37 40 44 57 65 71 73 **S** Division of Mental Health Services, Department of Human Services, State of New Jersey, Trenton, NJ
| 12 | 22 | 625 | 983 | 479 | — | — | — | — | 1131 |

ATLANTIC CITY—Atlantic County

✠ ATLANTIC CITY MEDICAL CENTER, 1925 Pacific Avenue, Zip 08401–6713; tel. 609/345–4000; David P. Tilton, President and Chief Executive Officer (Nonreporting) **A**1 2 3 9 10 12 13 **N** AtlantiCare Health System, Egg Harbor Township, NJ
| 23 | 10 | 448 | — | — | — | — | — | — | — |

BAYONNE—Hudson County

✠ BAYONNE HOSPITAL, 29th Street at Avenue E, Zip 07002; tel. 201/858–5000; Michael R. D'Agnes, President and Chief Executive Officer **A**1 2 6 9 10 **F**1 3 7 8 11 12 13 15 16 17 19 20 21 22 26 27 28 29 30 31 33 34 35 37 39 40 42 44 46 48 49 51 52 56 60 63 65 67 71 73 **P**5 7 **N** Qualcare Preferred Providers, Piscataway, NJ
| 23 | 10 | 261 | 9545 | 224 | — | 581 | 75644 | 35230 | 943 |

BELLE MEAD—Somerset County

✠ CARRIER FOUNDATION, County Route 601, P.O. Box 147, Zip 08502; tel. 908/281–1000; C. Richard Sarle, President and Chief Executive Officer **A**1 5 9 10 **F**2 3 14 15 16 46 52 53 54 55 56 57 58 59 65 73 **P**6 **N** Qualcare Preferred Providers, Piscataway, NJ
| 23 | 22 | 100 | 2934 | 87 | 72943 | 0 | — | — | 422 |

BELLEVILLE—Essex County

✠ CLARA MAASS HEALTH SYSTEM, One Clara Maass Drive, Zip 07109; tel. 201/450–2000; Robert S. Curtis, President and Chief Executive Officer (Total facility includes 179 beds in nursing home–type unit) **A**1 2 9 10 **F**1 6 7 8 10 12 13 14 15 16 17 19 21 22 25 26 27 29 30 31 32 33 34 35 37 39 40 41 42 44 45 46 49 51 52 54 55 56 57 60 61 63 64 65 67 71 73 74 **P**3 5 8 **N** First Option Health Plan, Red Bank, NJ; Clara Maass Health System, Belleville, NJ
| 23 | 10 | 644 | 12288 | 372 | 139215 | 984 | 104536 | 54912 | 1386 |

BERKELEY HEIGHTS—Union County

★ RUNNELLS SPECIALIZED HOSPITAL, 40 Watchung Way, Zip 07922–2618; tel. 908/771–5700; Joseph W. Sharp, Administrator (Total facility includes 300 beds in nursing home–type unit) (Nonreporting) **A**9 10
| 13 | 49 | 345 | — | — | — | — | — | — | — |

BERLIN—Camden County

★ WEST JERSEY HOSPITAL–BERLIN, 100 Townsend Avenue, Zip 08009; tel. 609/768–6006; Ellen Guarnieri, Acting Executive Director **A**9 **F**2 3 5 7 8 10 12 13 15 16 17 19 20 21 22 25 26 27 28 29 30 31 32 33 34 35 36 37 38 39 40 41 42 44 45 46 48 49 51 60 61 65 67 71 72 73 74 **P**5 7 **S** West Jersey Health System, Camden, NJ **N** First Option Health Plan, Red Bank, NJ
| 23 | 10 | 79 | 3428 | 58 | 22853 | 0 | 25939 | 13851 | 358 |

BLACKWOOD—Camden County

□ CAMDEN COUNTY HEALTH SERVICES CENTER, Woodbury–Turnersville Road, Zip 08012–2799, Mailing Address: P.O. Box 1639, Zip 08012–2799; tel. 609/374–6500; Anthony Peters, Chief Executive Officer (Total facility includes 275 beds in nursing home–type unit) (Nonreporting) **A**1 3 10
| 13 | 49 | 422 | — | — | — | — | — | — | — |

BOONTON TOWNSHIP—Morris County

ST. CLARES RIVERSIDE HOSPITAL–BOONTON TOWNSHIP CAMPUS See Northwest Covenant Medical Center, Denville

BRIDGETON—Cumberland County

✠ SOUTH JERSEY HOSPITAL, (Includes South Jersey Hospital–Bridgeton, 333 Irving Avenue, tel. 609/451–6600; South Jersey Hospital–Elmer, West Front Street, Elmer, Zip 08318–0516, Mailing Address: P.O. Box 1090, Zip 08318–1090; tel. 609/358–2341; South Jersey Hospital–Millville, 1200 North High, Millville, Zip 08332–2586; tel. 609/825–3500), 333 Irving Avenue, Zip 08302–2100; tel. 609/451–6600; Paul S. Cooper, Chief Executive Officer **A**1 2 9 10 **F**3 7 8 11 12 14 15 16 17 18 19 20 21 22 24 25 28 29 30 32 33 34 36 37 39 40 41 42 44 45 46 49 52 53 54 55 56 57 58 59 60 65 66 67 68 71 73 **N** First Option Health Plan, Red Bank, NJ; Qualcare Preferred Providers, Piscataway, NJ; Fox Chase Network, Rockledge, PA
| 23 | 10 | 375 | 11564 | 190 | 184857 | 834 | 102079 | 46556 | 1332 |

BROWNS MILLS—Burlington County

✠ DEBORAH HEART AND LUNG CENTER, (SPECIALTY HEART & LUNG CENTER), 200 Trenton Road, Zip 08015; tel. 609/893–6611; John R. Ernst, Executive Director **A**1 3 5 9 10 **F**4 10 14 19 21 28 29 30 34 43 45 50 63 65 67 71 73 **P**6
| 23 | 49 | 161 | 5194 | 112 | 29577 | 0 | 121868 | 63357 | 1378 |

CAMDEN—Camden County

○ △ OUR LADY OF LOURDES MEDICAL CENTER, 1600 Haddon Avenue, Zip 08103; tel. 609/757–3500; Alexander J. Hatala, President and Chief Executive Officer **A**1 3 5 7 10 **F**4 7 8 10 11 12 13 14 15 16 17 18 19 20 21 22 26 28 29 30 31 32 34 35 36 37 38 40 41 42 43 44 45 46 47 48 49 51 52 54 55 56 57 58 61 65 67 68 69 70 71 73 74 **P**6 7 **S** Allegany Health System, Tampa, FL **N** First Option Health Plan, Red Bank, NJ
| 23 | 10 | 300 | 13489 | 269 | 183065 | 1282 | 142260 | 62535 | 1832 |

Hospital, Address, Telephone, Administrator, Approval, Facility, and Physician Codes, Health Care System, Network	Classi-fication Codes		Utilization Data					Expense (thousands) of dollars		
★ American Hospital Association (AHA) membership □ Joint Commission on Accreditation of Healthcare Organizations (JCAHO) accreditation + American Osteopathic Hospital Association (AOHA) membership ○ American Osteopathic Association (AOA) accreditation △ Commission on Accreditation of Rehabilitation Facilities (CARF) accreditation Control codes 61, 63, 64, 71, 72 and 73 indicate hospitals listed by AOHA, but not registered by AHA. For definition of numerical codes, see page A4	Control	Service	Beds	Admissions	Census	Outpatient Visits	Births	Total	Payroll	Personnel
☒ THE COOPER HEALTH SYSTEM, One Cooper Plaza, Zip 08103–1489; tel. 609/342–2000; Kevin G. Halpern, President and Chief Executive Officer **A**1 2 3 5 8 9 10 **F**4 7 8 10 11 12 13 14 15 16 17 19 21 22 25 26 28 29 30 31 34 35 37 38 40 41 42 43 44 45 46 47 49 51 52 53 54 55 56 57 58 60 61 63 65 67 69 70 71 73 74 **P**4 6 **N** Qualcare Preferred Providers, Piscataway, NJ	23	10	370	18651	290	363848	1915	288251	164065	3280
☒ WEST JERSEY HOSPITAL–CAMDEN, 1000 Atlantic Avenue, Zip 08104–1595; tel. 609/342–4000; Frederick M. Carey, Executive Director **A**1 2 3 5 9 10 **F**3 5 8 10 12 13 15 16 17 19 20 21 22 25 26 27 28 29 30 31 32 33 34 35 37 39 41 42 44 45 46 49 51 60 61 65 67 68 71 72 73 **P**5 7 **S** West Jersey Health System, Camden, NJ **N** First Option Health Plan, Red Bank, NJ; Qualcare Preferred Providers, Piscataway, NJ	23	10	117	5714	80	49096	0	49565	24736	681
CAPE MAY COURT HOUSE—Cape May County										
☒ BURDETTE TOMLIN MEMORIAL HOSPITAL, Stone Harbor Boulevard, Zip 08210–9990; tel. 609/463–2000; Thomas L. Scott, FACHE, President and Chief Executive Officer **A**1 9 10 **F**3 7 8 13 14 15 16 17 18 19 20 21 22 27 28 30 34 35 37 40 44 45 46 49 56 65 67 71 73 **P**5 7 8 **N** First Option Health Plan, Red Bank, NJ; Cape Advantage Health Alliance, Cape May, NJ	23	10	206	9252	153	83862	660	65601	30693	844
CEDAR GROVE—Essex County										
□ ESSEX COUNTY HOSPITAL CENTER, 125 Fairview Avenue, Zip 07009; tel. 201/228–8200; Robert P. Arnold, Director (Nonreporting) **A**1 10	13	22	400	—						
CHERRY HILL—Camden County										
★ + ○ KENNEDY MEMORIAL HOSPITALS–UNIVERSITY MEDICAL CENTER, (Includes Kennedy Memorial Hospital, 18 East Laurel Road, Stratford, Zip 08084; tel. 609/346–6000; Kennedy Memorial Hospital, 435 Hurffville–Cross Keys Road, Turnersville, Zip 08012; tel. 609/582–2500), 2201 Chapel Avenue West, Zip 08002; tel. 609/488–6500; Joseph W. Devine, Vice President, Hospital Services **A**9 10 11 12 13 **F**2 3 4 6 7 8 10 11 12 13 14 15 16 17 18 19 20 21 22 23 24 25 26 27 28 29 30 31 32 33 34 35 36 37 38 39 40 41 42 43 44 45 46 49 51 52 53 54 55 56 57 58 59 61 63 64 65 66 67 68 69 70 71 73 74 **P**7	23	10	490	21363	332	166282	1797	174486	76979	2477
DENVILLE—Morris County										
☒ NORTHWEST COVENANT MEDICAL CENTER, (Includes Dover General Hospital–Dover Campus, 24 Jardine Street, Dover, Zip 07801–3311; tel. 201/989–3000; St Clares–Riverside Medical Center–Sussex Campus, 20 Walnut Street, Sussex, Zip 07461; tel. 201/702–2200; St. Clares Riverside Hospital–Boonton Township Campus, 130 Powerville Road, Boonton Township, Zip 07005; tel. 201/625–6000; St. Clares Riverside Hospital–Denville Campus, 25 Pocono Road, Zip 07834; tel. 201/625–6000), 25 Pocono Road, Zip 07834–2995; tel. 201/625–6000; Joseph A. Trunfio, President and Chief Executive Officer (Total facility includes 97 beds in nursing home–type unit) **A**1 2 5 9 10 **F**1 2 3 4 5 6 7 8 9 10 12 13 15 16 17 18 19 20 21 22 23 24 25 26 27 28 29 30 31 32 33 34 35 36 37 38 39 40 41 42 43 44 45 46 47 48 49 51 52 53 54 55 56 57 58 59 60 62 63 64 65 66 67 68 70 71 73 74 **P**1 5 6 7 **S** Sisters of the Sorrowful Mother United States Health System, Tulsa, OK **N** Via Caritas Health System, Inc., Wayne, NJ; Qualcare Preferred Providers, Piscataway, NJ	21	10	644	24045	425	294049	2178	217546	102816	2713
DOVER—Morris County										
DOVER GENERAL HOSPITAL–DOVER CAMPUS See Northwest Covenant Medical Center, Denville										
EAST ORANGE—Essex County										
☒ DEPARTMENT OF VETERANS AFFAIRS HEALTH CARE SYSTEM, (Includes Veterans Affairs Medical Center, 385 Tremont Avenue, Veterans Affairs Medical Center, 151 Knollcroft Road, Lyons, Zip 07939–9998; tel. 908/647–0180), 385 Tremont Avenue, Zip 07018–1095; tel. 201/676–1000; Kenneth H. Mizrach, Director (Total facility includes 390 beds in nursing home–type unit) **A**1 2 3 5 8 9 **F**1 2 3 4 5 6 7 8 10 11 12 13 17 18 19 20 21 22 23 24 25 26 27 28 29 30 31 32 33 34 35 36 37 39 41 42 43 44 45 46 48 49 50 51 52 53 54 55 56 57 58 59 60 61 62 63 64 65 66 67 68 69 70 71 72 73 74 **P**6 **S** Department of Veterans Affairs, Washington, DC	45	10	1312	10159	474	359710	0	261673	146933	3261
☒ EAST ORANGE GENERAL HOSPITAL, 300 Central Avenue, Zip 07019–2819; tel. 201/672–8400; Mark Chastang, President and Chief Executive Officer (Nonreporting) **A**1 9 10 **N** First Option Health Plan, Red Bank, NJ VETERANS AFFAIRS MEDICAL CENTER See Department of Veterans Affairs Health Care System	23	10	238	—						
EDISON—Middlesex County										
★ △ JFK JOHNSON REHABILITATION INSTITUTE, 65 James Street, Zip 08818–3059; tel. 908/321–7050; Scott Gebhard, Senior Vice President Operations **A**7 10 **F**1 3 5 7 8 10 11 12 13 15 16 17 18 19 20 22 24 25 26 27 28 29 30 32 33 34 35 36 37 38 39 40 41 42 44 45 46 47 48 49 51 58 60 64 65 66 67 71 72 73 74 **P**7 8 **S** JFK Health Systems, Inc., Edison, NJ	23	46	92	2023	79	—	0	35673	21267	413
☒ JFK MEDICAL CENTER, 65 James Street, Zip 08818; tel. 908/321–7000; John P. McGee, President and Chief Executive Officer (Nonreporting) **A**1 2 3 5 9 **S** JFK Health Systems, Inc., Edison, NJ **N** First Option Health Plan, Red Bank, NJ	23	10	380	—						
ROOSEVELT HOSPITAL, 1 Roosevelt Drive, Zip 08837–2333; tel. 908/321–6800; Thomas Lankey, Acting Superintendent and Chief Executive Officer (Total facility includes 536 beds in nursing home–type unit) (Nonreporting) **A**9 10	13	10	564	—						

Hospital, Address, Telephone, Administrator, Approval, Facility, and Physician Codes, Health Care System, Network	Classi-fication Codes		Utilization Data					Expense (thousands) of dollars		
★ American Hospital Association (AHA) membership □ Joint Commission on Accreditation of Healthcare Organizations (JCAHO) accreditation + American Osteopathic Hospital Association (AOHA) membership ○ American Osteopathic Association (AOA) accreditation △ Commission on Accreditation of Rehabilitation Facilities (CARF) accreditation Control codes 61, 63, 64, 71, 72 and 73 indicate hospitals listed by AOHA, but not registered by AHA. For definition of numerical codes, see page A4	Control	Service	Beds	Admissions	Census	Outpatient Visits	Births	Total	Payroll	Personnel

ELIZABETH—Union County

⊞ ELIZABETH GENERAL MEDICAL CENTER, 925 East Jersey Street, Zip 07201–2728; tel. 908/629–8065; David A. Fletcher, President and Chief Executive Officer (Total facility includes 120 beds in nursing home–type unit) **A**1 2 3 5 6 9 10 **F**1 2 3 7 8 12 15 16 17 18 19 20 21 22 26 28 29 30 31 33 34 37 39 40 41 42 44 45 49 51 52 53 54 55 56 57 58 59 60 64 65 67 71 73 74 **P**5 8 **N** First Option Health Plan, Red Bank, NJ; Qualcare Preferred Providers, Piscataway, NJ | 23 | 10 | 465 | 12975 | 337 | 204357 | 1103 | 120528 | 61209 | 1605

⊞ ST. ELIZABETH HOSPITAL, 225 Williamson Street, Zip 07202–3600; tel. 908/527–5122; Sister Elizabeth Ann Maloney, President and Chief Executive Officer **A**1 2 3 9 10 **F**2 3 7 8 10 12 13 14 15 16 17 19 21 22 24 25 26 27 28 30 31 32 33 34 35 37 39 40 41 42 44 45 49 54 60 63 65 68 71 73 74 **P**5 6 7 **N** The Mount Sinai Health System, New York, NY | 21 | 10 | 266 | 12554 | 201 | 94116 | 1104 | 92739 | 43910 | 1242

ELMER—Salem County

SOUTH JERSEY HOSPITAL–ELMER See South Jersey Hospital, Bridgeton

ENGLEWOOD—Bergen County

⊞ ENGLEWOOD HOSPITAL AND MEDICAL CENTER, 350 Engle Street, Zip 07631; tel. 201/894–3000; Daniel A. Kane, President and Chief Executive Officer **A**1 2 3 5 6 9 10 **F**3 4 5 7 8 10 11 12 13 14 15 16 17 18 19 20 21 22 23 25 26 28 29 30 31 32 33 34 35 36 38 39 40 41 42 44 45 46 49 51 52 53 54 55 56 57 58 59 60 63 65 66 67 68 70 71 73 74 **P**5 6 7 8 **N** The Mount Sinai Health System, New York, NY; First Option Health Plan, Red Bank, NJ | 23 | 10 | 318 | 19264 | 246 | 448680 | 2403 | 146817 | 79198 | 1611

FLEMINGTON—Hunterdon County

⊞ HUNTERDON MEDICAL CENTER, 2100 Wescott Drive, Zip 08822–4604; tel. 908/788–6100; Robert P. Wise, President and Chief Executive Officer **A**1 2 3 5 9 10 **F**1 3 7 8 12 14 15 16 17 18 19 21 22 23 25 26 28 29 30 31 32 33 34 35 36 37 39 40 41 42 44 45 46 49 51 52 53 54 55 56 57 58 59 61 65 66 67 68 69 71 73 74 **P**3 5 6 **N** First Option Health Plan, Red Bank, NJ; Qualcare Preferred Providers, Piscataway, NJ; Fox Chase Network, Rockledge, PA | 23 | 10 | 176 | 7801 | 109 | 221513 | 1292 | 73952 | 36451 | 1062

FLORHAM PARK—Los Angeles County

★ ATLANTIC HEALTH SYSTEM, (Includes Morristown Memorial Hospital, 100 Madison Avenue, Morristown, Zip 07962–1956; tel. 201/971–5000; Jean M. McMahon, R.N., Vice President and General Manager; Mountainside Hospital, Bay and Highland Avenues, Montclair, Zip 07042–4898; tel. 201/429–6000; Robert A. Silver, Senior Vice President and General Manager; Overlook Hospital, 99 Beauvoir Avenue, Summit, Zip 07902–0220; tel. 908/522–2000; David H. Freed, Vice President and General Manager), 325 Columbia Turnpike, Zip 07932, Mailing Address: P.O. Box 959, Zip 07932–0959; tel. 201/660–3100; Richard P. Oths, President and Chief Executive Officer (Total facility includes 410 beds in nursing home–type unit) **A**3 5 6 8 9 10 **F**2 3 4 5 7 8 10 11 12 13 15 16 17 18 19 20 21 22 24 25 26 27 28 29 30 31 32 33 34 35 36 37 38 39 40 41 42 43 44 45 46 47 48 49 51 52 53 54 55 56 57 58 59 60 61 64 65 66 67 68 70 71 72 73 74 **P**3 5 7 8 | 23 | 10 | 1825 | 61577 | 891 | 734559 | 7192 | 576599 | 283120 | 6996

FREEHOLD—Monmouth County

⊞ CENTRASTATE MEDICAL CENTER, 901 West Main Street, Zip 07728–2549; tel. 908/431–2000; Thomas H. Litz, President and Chief Executive Officer **A**1 9 10 **F**3 7 8 11 13 14 15 16 17 19 22 23 25 26 28 29 30 32 33 34 35 37 39 40 41 42 44 45 46 49 51 52 54 55 56 58 61 62 64 65 67 68 71 72 73 74 **P**5 8 **N** First Option Health Plan, Red Bank, NJ; Qualcare Preferred Providers, Piscataway, NJ | 23 | 10 | 240 | 9588 | 178 | 133787 | 1304 | 79678 | 35393 | 1113

GLEN GARDNER—Hunterdon County

□ SENATOR GARRET T. W. HAGEDORN GERO PSYCHIATRIC HOSPITAL, 200 Sanitorium Road, Zip 08826–9752; tel. 908/537–2141; Edna Volpe–Way, Chief Executive Officer (Nonreporting) **A**1 10 **S** Division of Mental Health Services, Department of Human Services, State of New Jersey, Trenton, NJ | 12 | 22 | 181 | — | — | — | — | — | — | —

GREYSTONE PARK—Morris County

⊞ GREYSTONE PARK PSYCHIATRIC HOSPITAL, Central Avenue, Zip 07950, Mailing Address: P.O. Box A, Zip 07950; tel. 201/538–1800; Joseph Jupin, Jr., Chief Executive Officer **A**1 9 10 **F**1 8 9 11 12 15 16 17 19 20 21 22 23 26 27 28 31 34 35 37 38 39 40 42 43 44 46 48 49 50 52 54 55 56 57 58 60 63 65 67 70 71 73 **P**6 **S** Division of Mental Health Services, Department of Human Services, State of New Jersey, Trenton, NJ | 12 | 22 | 605 | 516 | 606 | 0 | 0 | 63505 | 45336 | 1191

HACKENSACK—Bergen County

⊞ HACKENSACK UNIVERSITY MEDICAL CENTER, (Includes Hasbrouck Heights Ambulatory Care Faility, Hasbrouck Heights), 30 Prospect Avenue, Zip 07601–1991; tel. 201/996–2000; John P. Ferguson, President and Chief Executive Officer **A**1 2 3 5 8 9 10 **F**3 4 5 7 8 10 11 12 13 14 15 16 17 18 19 20 21 22 24 25 26 27 28 29 30 31 32 33 34 35 36 37 38 39 40 41 42 43 44 45 46 47 49 51 52 53 54 55 56 57 58 59 60 61 65 66 67 68 69 70 71 72 73 74 **P**7 8 **N** Qualcare Preferred Providers, Piscataway, NJ | 23 | 10 | 614 | 32965 | 478 | 985937 | 3484 | 352440 | 164919 | 3911

HACKETTSTOWN—Warren County

⊞ HACKETTSTOWN COMMUNITY HOSPITAL, 651 Willow Grove Street, Zip 07840–1798; tel. 908/852–5100; Gene C. Milton, President and Chief Executive Officer (Nonreporting) **A**1 2 9 10 **N** First Option Health Plan, Red Bank, NJ | 21 | 10 | 106 | — | — | — | — | — | — | —

HAMILTON—Mercer County

□ ROBERT WOOD JOHNSON UNIVERSITY HOSPITAL AT HAMILTON, One Hamilton Health Place, Zip 08690; tel. 609/586–7900; W. Michael Bryant, President and Chief Executive Officer **A**1 9 10 **F**1 7 8 11 12 14 15 16 17 19 20 21 22 25 26 28 29 30 31 32 33 34 35 36 37 39 40 41 42 44 45 46 49 51 60 61 63 64 65 67 71 73 74 **P**6 7 **N** Qualcare Preferred Providers, Piscataway, NJ | 23 | 10 | 160 | 5659 | 99 | 55678 | 208 | 39004 | 16543 | 693

Hospital, Address, Telephone, Administrator, Approval, Facility, and Physician Codes, Health Care System, Network	Classi-fication Codes		Utilization Data					Expense (thousands) of dollars		
	Control	Service	Beds	Admissions	Census	Outpatient Visits	Births	Total	Payroll	Personnel

★ American Hospital Association (AHA) membership
□ Joint Commission on Accreditation of Healthcare Organizations (JCAHO) accreditation
+ American Osteopathic Hospital Association (AOHA) membership
○ American Osteopathic Association (AOA) accreditation
△ Commission on Accreditation of Rehabilitation Facilities (CARF) accreditation
Control codes 61, 63, 64, 71, 72 and 73 indicate hospitals listed by AOHA, but not registered by AHA. For definition of numerical codes, see page A4

HAMMONTON—Atlantic County

⊠ WILLIAM B. KESSLER MEMORIAL HOSPITAL, 600 South White Horse Pike, Zip 08037–2099; tel. 609/561–6700; Warren E. Gager, Chief Executive Officer (Nonreporting) **A**1 9 10 **N** First Option Health Plan, Red Bank, NJ — 23 10 96 — — — — — — —

HOBOKEN—Hudson County

⊠ ST. MARY HOSPITAL, 308 Willow Avenue, Zip 07030–3889; tel. 201/418–1000; Robert S. Chaloner, President and Chief Executive Officer **A**1 3 9 10 **F**3 8 12 17 18 19 20 21 22 23 26 27 28 30 31 34 37 40 41 42 44 46 47 49 52 53 54 55 56 57 58 59 61 71 72 73 **P**1 4 7 **S** Franciscan Sisters of the Poor Health System, Inc., New York, NY **N** Qualcare Preferred Providers, Piscataway, NJ — 23 10 328 9298 182 84831 1121 84882 37787 1646

HOLMDEL—Monmouth County

⊠ BAYSHORE COMMUNITY HOSPITAL, 727 North Beers Street, Zip 07733; tel. 908/739–5900; Thomas Goldman, President **A**1 9 10 **F**1 3 8 11 12 15 16 17 19 21 22 25 26 28 29 30 32 33 34 35 36 37 39 41 42 44 45 46 49 53 55 57 58 65 67 71 73 **P**5 **N** First Option Health Plan, Red Bank, NJ — 23 10 172 7337 144 — 0 56249 26642 967

IRVINGTON—Essex County

⊠ IRVINGTON GENERAL HOSPITAL, 832 Chancellor Avenue, Zip 07111–0709; tel. 201/399–6000; Thomas A. Biga, Executive Director (Nonreporting) **A**1 9 10 **S** Saint Barnabas Health Care System, Livingston, NJ **N** First Option Health Plan, Red Bank, NJ; Qualcare Preferred Providers, Piscataway, NJ — 23 10 157 — — — — — — —

JERSEY CITY—Hudson County

⊠ CHRIST HOSPITAL, 176 Palisade Avenue, Zip 07306–1196, Mailing Address: P.O. Box J–1, Zip 07306–1196; tel. 201/795–8200; Daniel R. Connell, President **A**1 2 6 9 10 **F**3 7 8 11 12 13 16 17 18 19 20 21 22 23 26 27 28 29 30 31 32 33 34 35 36 37 39 40 41 42 44 45 46 49 50 51 52 53 54 55 56 57 58 59 60 63 65 67 68 71 73 74 **P**5 8 **N** First Option Health Plan, Red Bank, NJ — 23 10 358 18269 310 373697 1179 116364 57307 1057

□ GREENVILLE HOSPITAL, 1825 Kennedy Boulevard, Zip 07305; tel. 201/547–6100; Jonathan M. Metsch, Dr.PH, President and Chief Executive Officer **A**1 9 10 **F**1 2 3 4 7 8 10 11 12 13 15 16 17 18 19 20 21 22 25 26 27 28 30 31 34 37 38 40 42 44 46 47 48 49 52 53 54 55 56 57 58 59 61 63 64 65 66 67 68 70 71 73 74 **P**4 7 **N** The Mount Sinai Health System, New York, NY — 23 10 86 2770 67 16609 0 19020 9511 251

⊠ JERSEY CITY MEDICAL CENTER, 50 Baldwin Avenue, Zip 07304–3199; tel. 201/915–2000; Jonathan M. Metsch, Dr.PH, President and Chief Executive Officer (Nonreporting) **A**1 3 5 9 10 **N** The Mount Sinai Health System, New York, NY — 23 10 487 — — — — — — —

⊠ ST. FRANCIS HOSPITAL, 25 McWilliams Place, Zip 07302–1698; tel. 201/418–1000; Robert S. Chaloner, President and Chief Executive Officer **A**1 6 9 10 **F**2 3 5 8 11 12 17 18 19 20 21 22 23 24 27 28 30 31 32 34 35 37 41 42 44 46 47 48 49 51 52 53 54 56 57 58 59 60 61 65 67 68 70 71 72 73 **P**1 3 4 7 **S** Franciscan Sisters of the Poor Health System, Inc., New York, NY **N** Qualcare Preferred Providers, Piscataway, NJ — 23 10 243 4561 125 28225 0 53795 24918 547

KEARNY—Hudson County

⊠ WEST HUDSON HOSPITAL, 206 Bergen Avenue, Zip 07032; tel. 201/955–7051; Carmen Bruce Alecci, Executive Director (Total facility includes 46 beds in nursing home–type unit) **A**1 9 10 **F**8 12 15 16 17 18 19 21 22 27 28 29 30 31 32 33 34 35 37 39 41 42 44 45 46 49 51 54 56 63 64 65 67 71 73 **P**5 **S** Saint Barnabas Health Care System, Livingston, NJ **N** First Option Health Plan, Red Bank, NJ — 23 10 217 4021 125 35964 0 34778 15992 477

LAKEWOOD—Ocean County

⊠ KIMBALL MEDICAL CENTER, 600 River Avenue, Zip 08701–5281; tel. 908/363–1900; Joanne Carrocino, Executive Director **A**1 9 10 **F**1 2 3 4 7 8 10 11 12 13 14 15 16 17 18 19 20 21 22 24 25 26 27 28 29 30 31 32 33 34 35 36 37 39 40 41 42 43 44 45 46 49 51 52 54 55 56 57 58 59 60 61 64 65 66 67 68 69 71 72 73 74 **P**5 7 **S** Saint Barnabas Health Care System, Livingston, NJ **N** First Option Health Plan, Red Bank, NJ; Qualcare Preferred Providers, Piscataway, NJ — 23 10 292 10897 200 140433 896 97690 45525 1220

LAWRENCEVILLE—Mercer County

⊠ △ ST. LAWRENCE REHABILITATION CENTER, 2381 Lawrenceville Road, Zip 08648; tel. 609/896–9500; Charles L. Brennan, Chief Executive Officer (Total facility includes 30 beds in nursing home–type unit) (Nonreporting) **A**1 7 10 **N** Qualcare Preferred Providers, Piscataway, NJ — 21 46 116 — — — — — — —

LIVINGSTON—Essex County

⊠ ○ SAINT BARNABAS MEDICAL CENTER, 94 Old Short Hills Road, Zip 07039; tel. 201/533–5000; Ronald Del Mauro, Chairman and Chief Executive Officer (Nonreporting) **A**1 2 3 5 8 9 10 11 **S** Saint Barnabas Health Care System, Livingston, NJ **N** First Option Health Plan, Red Bank, NJ; Qualcare Preferred Providers, Piscataway, NJ — 23 10 615 — — — — — — —

LONG BRANCH—Monmouth County

⊠ MONMOUTH MEDICAL CENTER, 300 Second Avenue, Zip 07740–6303; tel. 908/222–5200; Cynthia N. Sparer, Executive Director and Chief Operating Officer (Nonreporting) **A**1 2 3 5 8 9 10 **S** Saint Barnabas Health Care System, Livingston, NJ **N** First Option Health Plan, Red Bank, NJ; Qualcare Preferred Providers, Piscataway, NJ — 23 10 435 — — — — — — —

LYONS—Somerset County

VETERANS AFFAIRS MEDICAL CENTER See Department of Veterans Affairs Health Care System, East Orange

© 1997 AHA Guide

Hospital, Address, Telephone, Administrator, Approval, Facility, and Physician Codes, Health Care System, Network	Classi-fication Codes		Utilization Data					Expense (thousands) of dollars		
★ American Hospital Association (AHA) membership □ Joint Commission on Accreditation of Healthcare Organizations (JCAHO) accreditation + American Osteopathic Hospital Association (AOHA) membership ○ American Osteopathic Association (AOA) accreditation △ Commission on Accreditation of Rehabilitation Facilities (CARF) accreditation Control codes 61, 63, 64, 71, 72 and 73 indicate hospitals listed by AOHA, but not registered by AHA. For definition of numerical codes, see page A4	Control	Service	Beds	Admissions	Census	Outpatient Visits	Births	Total	Payroll	Personnel

MANAHAWKIN—Ocean County

⊞ SOUTHERN OCEAN COUNTY HOSPITAL, 1140 Route 72 West, Zip 08050; tel. 609/978-8910; Steven G. Littleson, President and Chief Executive Officer **A**1 2 9 10 **F**3 8 13 15 17 19 21 22 25 28 29 30 32 33 34 37 42 44 45 46 49 56 63 64 65 66 67 68 71 73 **P**1 5 7 **N** First Option Health Plan, Red Bank, NJ; Qualcare Preferred Providers, Piscataway, NJ	23	10	134	5218	82	69855	0	39870	16130	474

MARLBORO—Monmouth County

□ MARLBORO PSYCHIATRIC HOSPITAL, 546 County Road 520, Zip 07746-1099; tel. 908/946-8100; Gregory Roberts, Chief Executive Officer (Nonreporting) **A**1 9 10 **S** Division of Mental Health Services, Department of Human Services, State of New Jersey, Trenton, NJ	12	22	767	—	—	—	—	—	—	—

MARLTON—Burlington County

★ WEST JERSEY HOSPITAL–MARLTON, Route 73 and Brick Road, Zip 08053; tel. 609/596-3500; Leroy J. Rosenberg, Executive Director **A**9 10 **F**2 3 5 8 10 12 13 15 16 17 19 20 21 22 25 26 27 29 30 31 32 33 34 35 37 41 42 44 45 46 49 51 60 61 65 67 68 71 72 73 **P**5 7 **S** West Jersey Health System, Camden, NJ **N** First Option Health Plan, Red Bank, NJ; Qualcare Preferred Providers, Piscataway, NJ	23	10	167	7775	122	35909	0	59932	29055	792

MILLVILLE—Cumberland County

SOUTH JERSEY HOSPITAL–MILLVILLE See South Jersey Hospital, Bridgeton

MONTCLAIR—Essex County

⊞ MONTCLAIR COMMUNITY HOSPITAL, 120 Harrison Avenue, Zip 07042-2498; tel. 201/744-7300; Emilie M. Murphy, R.N., Director (Nonreporting) **A**1 9 10	23	10	100	—	—	—	—	—	—	—

MOUNTAINSIDE HOSPITAL See Atlantic Health System, Florham Park

MORRISTOWN—Morris County

MORRISTOWN MEMORIAL HOSPITAL See Atlantic Health System, Florham Park

MOUNT HOLLY—Burlington County

⊞ MEMORIAL HOSPITAL OF BURLINGTON COUNTY, 175 Madison Avenue, Zip 08060-2099; tel. 609/267-0700; Chester B. Kaletkowski, President and Chief Executive Officer **A**1 2 3 5 9 10 **F**5 7 8 11 12 13 14 15 16 17 19 21 22 25 26 28 30 31 32 33 34 35 36 37 39 40 41 42 44 45 46 49 51 54 55 57 60 61 65 67 69 71 73 74 **P**2 4 5 7 **N** First Option Health Plan, Red Bank, NJ; Qualcare Preferred Providers, Piscataway, NJ	23	10	413	15309	210	122868	1944	117698	50453	1416

MOUNTAINSIDE—Union County

⊞ △ CHILDREN'S SPECIALIZED HOSPITAL, (Includes Children's Specialized Hospital–Ocean, 94 Stevens Road, Toms River, Zip 08755-1237; tel. 908/914-1100), 150 New Providence Road, Zip 07091-2590; tel. 908/233-3720; Richard B. Ahlfeld, President (Total facility includes 41 beds in nursing home–type unit) **A**1 7 10 **F**12 15 17 20 25 27 28 29 30 34 39 45 46 48 49 51 54 64 65 67 73 **N** Qualcare Preferred Providers, Piscataway, NJ	23	56	117	307	78	86243	0	33026	18814	479

NEPTUNE—Monmouth County

JERSEY SHORE MEDICAL CENTER See Meridian Health System

⊞ △ MERIDIAN HEALTH SYSTEM, (Includes Brick Hospital Division, 425 Jack Martin Boulevard, Brick Township, Zip 08724; tel. 908/840-2200; Jersey Shore Medical Center, 1945 Route 33, Zip 07754-0397; tel. 908/775-5500; Medical Center of Ocean County, 2121 Edgewater Place, Point Pleasant, Zip 08742-2290; tel. 908/892-1100; John T. Gribbin, President and Chief Executive Officer; Point Pleasant Hospital Division, 2121 Edgewater Place, Point Pleasant, Zip 08742; tel. 908/892-1100; Riverview Medical Center, 1 Riverview Plaza, Red Bank, Zip 07701-9982; tel. 908/741-2700; Paul S. Cohen, Executive Director and Chief Operating Officer), 1945 State Highway 33, Zip 07753; tel. 908/776-4215; John K. Lloyd, Chief Executive Officer (Nonreporting) **A**1 2 3 5 6 7 8 9 10 **N** Qualcare Preferred Providers, Piscataway, NJ; National Cardiovascular Network, Atlanta, GA	23	10	1269	—	—	—	—	—	—	—

NEW BRUNSWICK—Middlesex County

HURTADO HEALTH CENTER, 11 Bishop Place, Zip 08903-5069; tel. 908/932-7401; Robert H. Bierman, M.D., Director (Nonreporting)	12	11	27	—	—	—	—	—	—	—
⊞ ROBERT WOOD JOHNSON UNIVERSITY HOSPITAL, 1 Robert Wood Johnson Place, Zip 08903-2601; tel. 908/828-3000; Harvey A. Holzberg, President and Chief Executive Officer (Nonreporting) **A**1 2 3 5 8 9 10 **N** First Option Health Plan, Red Bank, NJ; Qualcare Preferred Providers, Piscataway, NJ	23	10	398	—	—	—	—	—	—	—
⊞ ST. PETER'S MEDICAL CENTER, 254 Easton Avenue, Zip 08901, Mailing Address: P.O. Box 591, Zip 08903-0591; tel. 908/745-8600; John E. Matuska, President and Chief Executive Officer (Nonreporting) **A**1 2 3 5 9 10 **N** First Option Health Plan, Red Bank, NJ; Qualcare Preferred Providers, Piscataway, NJ	23	10	416	—	—	—	—	—	—	—

NEWARK—Essex County

□ COLUMBUS HOSPITAL, 495 North 13th Street, Zip 07107-1397; tel. 201/268-1400; John G. Magliaro, President and Chief Executive Officer **A**1 9 10 **F**3 7 8 11 12 16 19 21 22 25 28 30 31 33 35 37 40 41 42 45 46 49 54 63 65 67 71 73 **P**5 **N** Qualcare Preferred Providers, Piscataway, NJ	23	10	206	8217	137	104623	1042	77535	31569	794
⊞ ○ NEWARK BETH ISRAEL MEDICAL CENTER, 201 Lyons Avenue, Zip 07112-2027; tel. 201/926-7000; Ronald W. Weitz, Executive Director **A**1 2 3 5 8 10 11 12 13 **F**1 4 7 8 9 10 11 12 13 16 17 19 20 21 22 25 26 28 30 31 32 34 35 37 38 39 40 41 42 43 44 46 47 49 51 52 53 54 55 56 58 59 60 61 65 67 69 71 72 73 74 **P**1 5 7 **S** Saint Barnabas Health Care System, Livingston, NJ **N** First Option Health Plan, Red Bank, NJ; Qualcare Preferred Providers, Piscataway, NJ	23	10	451	19559	417	313698	2759	228117	106834	2981

Hospital, Address, Telephone, Administrator, Approval, Facility, and Physician Codes, Health Care System, Network	Classi-fication Codes		Utilization Data					Expense (thousands) of dollars		
★ American Hospital Association (AHA) membership □ Joint Commission on Accreditation of Healthcare Organizations (JCAHO) accreditation + American Osteopathic Hospital Association (AOHA) membership ○ American Osteopathic Association (AOA) accreditation △ Commission on Accreditation of Rehabilitation Facilities (CARF) accreditation Control codes 61, 63, 64, 71, 72 and 73 indicate hospitals listed by AOHA, but not registered by AHA. For definition of numerical codes, see page A4	Control	Service	Beds	Admissions	Census	Outpatient Visits	Births	Total	Payroll	Personnel

□ SAINT JAMES HOSPITAL OF NEWARK, 155 Jefferson Street, Zip 07105; tel. 201/589–1300; Ceu Cirne–Neves, Administrator (Nonreporting) **A**1 3 9 10 **S** Cathedral Healthcare System, Inc., Newark, NJ	21	10	189	—	—	—	—	—	—	—
□ SAINT MICHAEL'S MEDICAL CENTER, 268 Dr. Martin Luther King Jr. Boulevard, Zip 07102–2094; tel. 201/877–5000; Dominick R. Calgi, Senior Vice President and Administrator (Nonreporting) **A**1 3 5 9 10 12 **S** Cathedral Healthcare System, Inc., Newark, NJ	21	10	325	—	—	—	—	—	—	—
✚ UNIVERSITY OF MEDICINE AND DENTISTRY OF NEW JERSEY–UNIVERSITY HOSPITAL, 150 Bergen Street, Zip 07103–2406; tel. 201/982–4300; William L. Vazquez, Vice President and Chief Executive Officer (Nonreporting) **A**1 2 3 5 8 9 10 **N** Qualcare Preferred Providers, Piscataway, NJ	12	10	518	—	—	—	—	—	—	—
NEWTON—Sussex County										
✚ △ NEWTON MEMORIAL HOSPITAL, 175 High Street, Zip 07860–1004; tel. 201/383–2121; Dennis H. Collette, President and Chief Executive Officer **A**1 2 7 9 10 **F**3 7 8 12 15 16 17 18 19 20 21 22 27 28 29 30 31 32 35 37 39 40 41 42 44 45 46 48 49 52 53 54 55 56 57 58 59 61 63 65 67 71 73 **P**5 8 **N** First Option Health Plan, Red Bank, NJ	23	10	162	8634	100	164526	970	51403	23464	576
NORTH BERGEN—Hudson County										
✚ PALISADES GENERAL HOSPITAL, 7600 River Road, Zip 07047–6217; tel. 201/854–5000; Bruce J. Markowitz, President and Chief Executive Officer (Nonreporting) **A**1 9 10 **N** Columbia Presbyterian Regional Network, New York, NY; First Option Health Plan, Red Bank, NJ; Qualcare Preferred Providers, Piscataway, NJ	23	10	202	—	—	—	—	—	—	—
OLD BRIDGE—Middlesex County										
OLD BRIDGE DIVISION See Raritan Bay Medical Center, Perth Amboy										
ORANGE—Essex County										
✚ HOSPITAL CENTER AT ORANGE, (Includes New Jersey Orthopedic Hospital Unit, Orange Memorial Hospital Unit), 188 South Essex Avenue, Zip 07051; tel. 201/266–2200; Paul A. Mertz, President and Chief Executive Officer (Nonreporting) **A**1 2 3 5 9 10 **N** Qualcare Preferred Providers, Piscataway, NJ	23	10	290	—	—	—	—	—	—	—
PARAMUS—Bergen County										
✚ BERGEN PINES COUNTY HOSPITAL, 230 East Ridgewood Avenue, Zip 07652–4131; tel. 201/967–4000; Edward M. Lewis, Chief Executive Officer (Total facility includes 610 beds in nursing home–type unit) (Nonreporting) **A**1 3 5 6 9 10	13	10	1059	—	—	—	—	—	—	—
PASSAIC—Passaic County										
✚ BETH ISRAEL HOSPITAL, 70 Parker Avenue, Zip 07055; tel. 201/365–5000; Jeffrey S. Moll, President and Chief Executive Officer **A**1 2 9 10 **F**3 15 19 21 22 26 31 32 33 34 35 37 41 42 44 45 46 49 60 61 63 65 71 73 74 **N** First Option Health Plan, Red Bank, NJ; Qualcare Preferred Providers, Piscataway, NJ	23	10	223	5625	109	—	0	—	—	711
✚ GENERAL HOSPITAL CENTER AT PASSAIC, 350 Boulevard, Zip 07055–2800; tel. 201/365–4300; Daniel L. Marcantuono, FACHE, President and Chief Executive Officer **A**1 2 9 10 **F**4 8 10 12 13 14 15 16 17 19 21 22 23 24 25 27 28 30 32 34 35 37 39 40 41 42 43 44 46 49 65 67 71 73 74 **P**1 5 **N** General Hospital Center at Passaic, Passaic, NJ	23	10	271	11566	197	99421	1095	105641	50406	1140
✚ ST. MARY'S HOSPITAL, 211 Pennington Avenue, Zip 07055; tel. 201/470–3000; Patricia Peterson, President and Chief Executive Officer **A**1 9 10 **F**4 7 8 11 12 13 15 16 17 18 19 21 22 26 27 28 29 30 31 34 35 37 40 42 44 45 46 49 51 52 53 54 55 56 57 58 59 60 61 65 67 68 69 71 73 74 **P**4 5 8 **N** Via Caritas Health System, Inc., Wayne, NJ	21	10	229	5410	106	104539	792	54338	25615	782
PATERSON—Passaic County										
✚ BARNERT HOSPITAL, 680 Broadway, Zip 07514; tel. 201/977–6600; Fred L. Lang, President and Chief Executive Officer **A**1 9 10 **F**1 3 6 7 8 14 15 16 17 19 21 22 26 27 28 29 30 31 34 36 37 40 41 42 44 45 46 49 52 53 54 55 56 58 59 63 65 67 68 71 73 **P**5 8 **N** First Option Health Plan, Red Bank, NJ	23	10	256	7632	149	182213	910	67806	32491	886
✚ ○ ST. JOSEPH'S HOSPITAL AND MEDICAL CENTER, 703 Main Street, Zip 07503–2691; tel. 201/754–2100; Sister Jane Frances Brady, Chief Executive Officer (Total facility includes 141 beds in nursing home–type unit) **A**1 2 3 5 8 9 10 11 12 **F**1 3 4 5 7 8 9 10 11 12 13 14 15 16 17 18 19 20 21 22 24 25 26 27 28 29 30 31 32 33 34 35 36 37 38 39 40 41 42 43 44 45 46 47 49 50 51 52 53 54 55 56 57 58 59 60 61 64 65 66 67 68 69 70 71 72 73 74 **P**1 5 7 **N** The Mount Sinai Health System, New York, NY; Seton Health Network, Inc., Paterson, NJ; First Option Health Plan, Red Bank, NJ; Via Caritas Health System, Inc., Wayne, NJ; Qualcare Preferred Providers, Piscataway, NJ	21	10	621	27325	434	—	2796	259044	136425	3363
PEAPACK—Somerset County										
✚ MATHENY SCHOOL AND HOSPITAL, (CEREBAL PALSY), Main Street, Zip 07977; tel. 908/234–0011; Robert Schonhorn, President **A**1 10 **F**1 6 12 13 14 15 16 17 20 27 30 32 34 39 45 46 48 49 51 52 54 55 64 65 67 73 **P**6	23	49	99	75	82	150	0	14303	8535	295
PERTH AMBOY—Middlesex County										
✚ RARITAN BAY MEDICAL CENTER, (Includes Old Bridge Division, One Hospital Plaza, Old Bridge, Zip 08857; tel. 908/360–1000; Perth Amboy Division), 530 New Brunswick Avenue, Zip 08861; tel. 908/442–3700; Keith H. McLaughlin, President and Chief Executive Officer **A**1 3 5 6 9 10 **F**2 3 6 7 8 10 12 14 15 16 17 18 19 21 22 23 27 28 29 31 33 34 35 36 39 40 42 44 49 52 54 55 56 58 63 65 67 68 71 73 **P**7 8 **N** Qualcare Preferred Providers, Piscataway, NJ	23	10	415	13929	297	220422	850	135599	72842	1793
PHILLIPSBURG—Warren County										
✚ WARREN HOSPITAL, 185 Roseberry Street, Zip 08865–9955; tel. 908/859–6700; Jeffrey C. Goodwin, President and Chief Executive Officer (Nonreporting) **A**1 2 3 5 9 10 12 13 **N** Qualcare Preferred Providers, Piscataway, NJ	23	10	214	—	—	—	—	—	—	—

Hospital, Address, Telephone, Administrator, Approval, Facility, and Physician Codes, Health Care System, Network	Classi-fication Codes		Utilization Data					Expense (thousands) of dollars		
★ American Hospital Association (AHA) membership □ Joint Commission on Accreditation of Healthcare Organizations (JCAHO) accreditation + American Osteopathic Hospital Association (AOHA) membership ○ American Osteopathic Association (AOA) accreditation △ Commission on Accreditation of Rehabilitation Facilities (CARF) accreditation Control codes 61, 63, 64, 71, 72 and 73 indicate hospitals listed by AOHA, but not registered by AHA. For definition of numerical codes, see page A4	Control	Service	Beds	Admissions	Census	Outpatient Visits	Births	Total	Payroll	Personnel

PISCATAWAY—Middlesex County

UNIVERSITY OF MEDICINE AND DENTISTRY OF NEW JERSEY, UNIVERSITY BEHAVIORAL HEALTHCARE, 671 Hoes Lane, Zip 08854–5633, Mailing Address: P.O. Box 1392, Zip 08855–1392; tel. 908/235–5500; Gary W. Lamson, Vice President and Chief Executive Officer (Nonreporting) **A**3 5 9 10 — 12 22 64 — — — — — — — —

PLAINFIELD—Union County

☒ MUHLENBERG REGIONAL MEDICAL CENTER, Park Avenue and Randolph Road, Zip 07061; tel. 908/668–2000; John R. Kopicki, President and Chief Executive Officer (Nonreporting) **A**1 3 5 6 9 10 **N** First Option Health Plan, Red Bank, NJ — 23 10 261 — — — — — — — —

POINT PLEASANT—Ocean County

MEDICAL CENTER OF OCEAN COUNTY See Meridian Health System, Neptune

POMONA—Atlantic County

☒ △ BACHARACH REHABILITATION HOSPITAL, 61 West Jim Leeds Road, Zip 08240–0723; tel. 609/652–7000; Richard J. Kathrins, Administrator (Nonreporting) **A**1 7 10 — 23 46 80 — — — — — — — —

POMPTON PLAINS—Morris County

☒ CHILTON MEMORIAL HOSPITAL, 97 West Parkway, Zip 07444–1696; tel. 201/831–5000; James J. Doyle, Jr., President and Chief Executive Officer **A**1 2 9 10 **F**7 8 12 13 14 15 16 17 19 20 21 22 25 26 28 29 30 31 32 33 34 35 37 38 39 40 41 42 44 45 47 49 51 52 53 54 55 56 57 60 63 65 66 67 70 71 72 73 74 **P**4 5 7 8 **N** First Option Health Plan, Red Bank, NJ — 23 10 270 9707 149 61276 1441 83062 36437 740

PRINCETON—Mercer County

☒ MEDICAL CENTER AT PRINCETON, (Includes Acute General Hospital, Merwick Unit–Extended Care and Rehabilitation, Princeton House Unit–Community Mental Health and Substance Abuse), 253 Witherspoon Street, Zip 08540–3213; tel. 609/497–4000; Dennis W. Doody, President and Chief Executive Officer (Total facility includes 93 beds in nursing home–type unit) **A**1 2 3 5 9 10 **F**1 2 3 7 8 10 11 12 14 15 16 17 18 19 20 21 22 26 28 29 30 31 32 33 34 35 37 39 40 41 42 44 48 49 52 54 55 56 57 58 59 60 63 64 65 67 71 73 **P**7 8 **N** First Option Health Plan, Red Bank, NJ — 23 10 392 15452 296 193638 1685 111111 53104 1485

PRINCETON UNIVERSITY HEALTH SERVICES, MCCOSH HEALTH CENTER, Washington Road, Zip 08544–1004; tel. 609/258–3129; Pamela Bowen, Director (Nonreporting) — 23 11 21 — — — — — — — —

RAHWAY—Union County

☒ RAHWAY HOSPITAL, 865 Stone Street, Zip 07065; tel. 908/381–4200; Kirk C. Tice, President and Chief Executive Officer (Total facility includes 16 beds in nursing home–type unit) (Nonreporting) **A**1 9 10 **N** Qualcare Preferred Providers, Piscataway, NJ — 23 10 297 — — — — — — — —

RED BANK—Monmouth County

RIVERVIEW MEDICAL CENTER See Meridian Health System, Neptune

RIDGEWOOD—Bergen County

☒ VALLEY HOSPITAL, 223 North Van Dien Avenue, Zip 07450–9982; tel. 201/447–8000; Michael W. Azzara, President **A**1 2 9 10 **F**2 3 4 7 8 10 11 12 13 14 15 16 17 19 20 21 22 25 26 28 29 30 31 32 33 34 35 36 37 38 39 40 41 42 43 44 45 46 49 51 52 53 54 55 56 57 58 59 60 61 65 66 67 68 71 72 73 74 **P**5 6 7 8 **N** Columbia Presbyterian Regional Network, New York, NY; First Option Health Plan, Red Bank, NJ — 23 10 421 36517 383 181132 3221 185455 94142 2205

SALEM—Salem County

☒ MEMORIAL HOSPITAL OF SALEM COUNTY, Salem Woodstown Road, Zip 08079–2080; tel. 609/935–1000; Arnold Kimmel, Interim Chief Executive Officer **A**1 2 9 10 **F**7 8 12 14 16 19 21 22 25 26 28 29 30 31 32 33 35 36 37 39 40 42 44 45 46 49 65 66 71 73 **N** Qualcare Preferred Providers, Piscataway, NJ — 23 10 113 5009 71 91489 448 44105 23503 574

SECAUCUS—Hudson County

□ MEADOWLANDS HOSPITAL MEDICAL CENTER, Meadowland Parkway, Zip 07096–1580; tel. 201/392–3100; Paul V. Cavalli, M.D., President **A**1 9 10 **F**2 3 7 8 10 11 12 13 15 16 17 18 19 20 21 22 24 26 27 28 29 30 31 32 37 38 39 40 41 42 44 46 48 49 52 53 54 55 56 57 58 61 63 65 67 70 71 73 74 **P**7 **N** The Mount Sinai Health System, New York, NY — 23 10 200 6063 93 76295 1181 47515 22488 535

SOMERS POINT—Atlantic County

☒ SHORE MEMORIAL HOSPITAL, 1 East New York Avenue, Zip 08244–2387; tel. 609/653–3500; Richard A. Pitman, President **A**1 2 9 10 **F**3 7 8 12 15 16 19 21 22 26 28 29 30 31 32 33 34 35 37 39 40 41 44 45 46 49 60 63 65 67 71 73 74 **P**2 5 7 **N** First Option Health Plan, Red Bank, NJ; Qualcare Preferred Providers, Piscataway, NJ — 23 10 223 10999 176 81475 1136 97972 44039 1259

SOMERVILLE—Somerset County

☒ SOMERSET MEDICAL CENTER, 110 Rehill Avenue, Zip 08876–2598; tel. 908/685–2200; Michael A. Turner, President and Chief Executive Officer **A**1 2 3 5 9 10 **F**3 4 7 8 11 12 14 15 16 17 19 21 22 26 28 30 31 32 33 34 35 37 39 40 42 44 46 49 51 52 54 55 56 57 58 59 63 65 67 71 73 74 **P**5 7 **N** First Option Health Plan, Red Bank, NJ; Qualcare Preferred Providers, Piscataway, NJ — 23 10 289 12249 188 119931 1041 100170 48847 1277

SOUTH AMBOY—Middlesex County

☒ MEMORIAL MEDICAL CENTER AT SOUTH AMBOY, 540 Bordentown Avenue, Zip 08879; tel. 908/721–1000; Irv J. Diamond, Chief Executive Officer **A**1 9 10 **F**3 8 12 14 15 16 17 18 19 21 22 28 29 30 36 37 39 41 42 44 46 49 52 53 54 55 56 57 58 59 65 67 71 73 — 23 10 161 3368 74 53080 0 30861 16518 518

Hospital, Address, Telephone, Administrator, Approval, Facility, and Physician Codes, Health Care System, Network	Classi-fication Codes		Utilization Data					Expense (thousands) of dollars		
	Control	Service	Beds	Admissions	Census	Outpatient Visits	Births	Total	Payroll	Personnel

★ American Hospital Association (AHA) membership
□ Joint Commission on Accreditation of Healthcare Organizations (JCAHO) accreditation
+ American Osteopathic Hospital Association (AOHA) membership
○ American Osteopathic Association (AOA) accreditation
△ Commission on Accreditation of Rehabilitation Facilities (CARF) accreditation
Control codes 61, 63, 64, 71, 72 and 73 indicate hospitals listed by AOHA, but not registered by AHA. For definition of numerical codes, see page A4

SUMMIT—Union County

□ CHARTER BEHAVIORAL HEALTH SYSTEM OF NEW JERSEY–SUMMIT, 19 Prospect Street, Zip 07902–0100; tel. 908/522–7000; Geoffrey Perselay, Chief Executive Officer (Nonreporting) **A**1 9 10 **S** Magellan Health Services, Atlanta, GA — Control 33 Service 22 Beds 90

OVERLOOK HOSPITAL See Atlantic Health System, Florham Park

SUSSEX—Sussex County

ST CLARES–RIVERSIDE MEDICAL CENTER–SUSSEX CAMPUS See Northwest Covenant Medical Center, Denville

TEANECK—Bergen County

✠ HOLY NAME HOSPITAL, 718 Teaneck Road, Zip 07666; tel. 201/833–3000; Michael Maron, President and Chief Executive Officer (Nonreporting) **A**1 2 3 6 9 10 **N** Columbia Presbyterian Regional Network, New York, NY; First Option Health Plan, Red Bank, NJ; Qualcare Preferred Providers, Piscataway, NJ — 23 10 323

TOMS RIVER—Ocean County

CHILDREN'S SPECIALIZED HOSPITAL–OCEAN See Children's Specialized Hospital, Mountainside

✠ COMMUNITY KIMBALL HEALTH CARE SYSTEM, 99 Highway 37 West, Zip 08755–6423; tel. 908/240–8000; Kevin R. Burchill, Executive Director **A**1 2 9 10 **F**1 2 3 4 7 8 10 11 12 13 14 15 16 17 18 19 20 21 22 24 25 26 27 28 29 30 31 32 33 34 35 36 37 39 40 41 42 43 44 45 46 49 51 52 54 55 56 57 58 59 60 61 63 64 65 66 67 68 69 71 72 73 74 **P**5 7 **S** Saint Barnabas Health Care System, Livingston, NJ **N** First Option Health Plan, Red Bank, NJ; Qualcare Preferred Providers, Piscataway, NJ; Community/Kimball Health Care System, Toms River, NJ — 23 10 510 21005 312 363541 2038 175649 78162 2476

□ △ HEALTHSOUTH REHABILITATION HOSPITAL OF NEW JERSEY, 14 Hospital Drive, Zip 08755; tel. 908/244–3100; Patricia Ostaszewski, Chief Operating Officer and Administrator (Total facility includes 63 beds in nursing home–type unit) **A**1 7 10 **F**6 12 19 21 25 35 41 45 46 48 49 58 59 64 65 66 67 71 73 **P**5 **S** HEALTHSOUTH Corporation, Birmingham, AL — 33 46 155 2408 135 25016 0 23257 13719 402

TRENTON—Mercer County

✠ HELENE FULD MEDICAL CENTER, 750 Brunswick Avenue, Zip 08638; tel. 609/394–6000; Al Maghazehe, President and Chief Executive Officer **A**1 2 3 5 6 9 10 **F**3 7 8 11 12 13 14 15 16 17 18 19 20 21 22 23 27 28 29 30 31 32 33 34 35 36 37 38 39 40 41 42 44 45 46 49 51 52 53 54 55 56 57 58 59 60 61 63 65 66 67 68 69 71 72 73 **P**6 8 **N** Qualcare Preferred Providers, Piscataway, NJ — 23 10 261 10059 191 260384 942 103160 53221 1356

✠ MERCER MEDICAL CENTER, 446 Bellevue Avenue, Zip 08618, Mailing Address: Box 1658, Zip 08607; tel. 609/394–4000; Charles E. Baer, President **A**1 2 6 9 10 **F**1 7 8 11 15 16 17 19 21 22 30 32 34 35 36 37 38 39 40 42 44 46 49 60 61 63 65 66 71 73 **P**5 7 8 **N** First Option Health Plan, Red Bank, NJ — 23 10 318 13256 172 165270 2566 112545 51585 1364

✠ ST. FRANCIS MEDICAL CENTER, 601 Hamilton Avenue, Zip 08629–1986; tel. 609/599–5000; Judith M. Persichilli, President and Chief Executive Officer **A**1 2 3 5 6 9 10 **F**7 8 10 11 12 15 16 17 19 21 22 23 26 27 28 29 30 31 32 33 34 35 36 37 40 42 44 45 46 49 51 52 54 55 56 58 59 60 63 65 67 68 71 72 73 74 **P**5 6 7 8 **S** Catholic Health Initiatives, Denver, CO **N** First Option Health Plan, Red Bank, NJ; Fox Chase Network, Rockledge, PA — 21 10 254 8521 149 134973 364 82158 40162 1012

✠ TRENTON PSYCHIATRIC HOSPITAL, Sullivan Way, Station A, Zip 08625, Mailing Address: P.O. Box 7500, West Trenton, Zip 08628; tel. 609/633–1500; Joseph Jupin, Jr., Chief Executive Officer **A**1 3 9 10 **F**3 6 7 8 9 10 11 12 15 16 17 18 19 20 21 22 23 24 25 26 27 28 29 30 31 32 33 34 35 36 37 39 41 42 43 44 45 46 48 49 50 52 55 56 57 58 59 60 61 63 65 66 67 69 70 71 73 74 **S** Division of Mental Health Services, Department of Human Services, State of New Jersey, Trenton, NJ — 12 22 379 474 294 0 0 35514 — 735

UNION—Union County

✠ + ○ UNION HOSPITAL, 1000 Galloping Hill Road, Zip 07083–1652; tel. 908/687–1900; Kathryn W. Coyne, Executive Director and Chief Operating Officer **A**1 2 9 10 11 12 13 **F**1 2 3 4 5 7 8 9 10 11 12 13 14 15 16 17 18 19 20 21 22 25 26 27 28 29 30 31 32 34 35 37 38 39 40 41 42 43 44 45 46 47 49 51 52 53 54 56 57 58 59 60 61 63 64 65 66 67 68 69 70 71 72 73 74 **P**5 7 8 **S** Saint Barnabas Health Care System, Livingston, NJ **N** First Option Health Plan, Red Bank, NJ; Qualcare Preferred Providers, Piscataway, NJ — 23 10 148 6842 129 127322 0 66720 28034 931

VINELAND—Camden County

✠ NEWCOMB MEDICAL CENTER, 65 South State Street, Zip 08360; tel. 609/691–9000; Joseph A. Ierardi, President and Chief Executive Officer **A**1 2 9 10 **F**7 8 11 12 13 15 17 19 21 22 25 27 28 30 34 35 36 37 38 39 40 41 42 44 45 46 48 49 54 56 65 66 67 69 70 71 73 74 **P**1 3 7 — 23 10 139 5822 84 112095 1193 55106 26559 725

□ VINELAND DEVELOPMENT CENTER HOSPITAL, 1676 East Landis Avenue, Zip 08360; tel. 609/696–6200; Judith L. Sisti, MS, Administrator **A**1 10 **F**8 19 20 21 22 23 27 34 35 42 44 49 51 54 56 57 58 59 65 71 **P**6 — 12 12 100 706 50 7668 0 — — 229

VOORHEES—Camden County

★ WEST JERSEY HOSPITAL–VOORHEES, 101 Carnie Boulevard, Zip 08043–1597; tel. 609/772–5000; Joan T. Meyers, R.N., Executive Director **A**3 5 9 **F**2 3 5 8 10 12 13 15 16 17 19 20 21 22 25 26 27 28 29 30 31 32 33 34 35 37 38 40 41 42 44 45 46 49 51 58 60 61 65 67 71 72 73 74 **P**5 7 **S** West Jersey Health System, Camden, NJ **N** First Option Health Plan, Red Bank, NJ; Qualcare Preferred Providers, Piscataway, NJ — 23 10 253 15547 183 67230 4918 91955 45261 1401

Hospital, Address, Telephone, Administrator, Approval, Facility, and Physician Codes, Health Care System, Network	Classi-fication Codes		Utilization Data					Expense (thousands) of dollars		
★ American Hospital Association (AHA) membership □ Joint Commission on Accreditation of Healthcare Organizations (JCAHO) accreditation + American Osteopathic Hospital Association (AOHA) membership ○ American Osteopathic Association (AOA) accreditation △ Commission on Accreditation of Rehabilitation Facilities (CARF) accreditation Control codes 61, 63, 64, 71, 72 and 73 indicate hospitals listed by AOHA, but not registered by AHA. For definition of numerical codes, see page A4	Control	Service	Beds	Admissions	Census	Outpatient Visits	Births	Total	Payroll	Personnel

WAYNE—Passaic County

☒ WAYNE GENERAL HOSPITAL, 224 Hamburg Turnpike, Zip 07470–2100; tel. 201/942–6900; Kenneth H. Kozloff, Executive Director **A**1 9 10 **F**1 3 7 8 11 12 13 15 16 17 19 21 22 23 25 26 27 28 30 31 32 33 34 35 37 40 41 42 44 45 46 49 51 53 54 55 56 57 58 59 60 63 65 67 71 73 **P**5 8 **S** Saint Barnabas Health Care System, Livingston, NJ **N** Qualcare Preferred Providers, Piscataway, NJ

23 10	146	6943	117	87314	868	65736	32575	783

WEST ORANGE—Essex County

☒ △ KESSLER INSTITUTE FOR REHABILITATION, (Includes East Orange Facility, West Orange Facility, Saddle Brook Facility and Welkind Facility), 1199 Pleasant Valley Way, Zip 07052–1419; tel. 201/731–3600; Kenneth W. Aitchison, President and Chief Executive Officer **A**1 3 5 7 10 **F**1 15 16 32 48 49 67 71 73 **P**6 **N** Qualcare Preferred Providers, Piscataway, NJ

23 46	284	5194	271	141926	0	62350	36359	1420

WESTAMPTON TOWNSHIP—Burlington County

□ HAMPTON HOSPITAL, Rancocas Road, Zip 08073, Mailing Address: P.O. Box 7000, Zip 08073; tel. 609/267–7000; Michael Terwilliger, Acting Chief Executive Officer (Nonreporting) **A**1 9 10 **S** Hospital Group of America, Wayne, PA

33 22	100	—	—	—	—	—	—	—

WESTWOOD—Bergen County

☒ PASCACK VALLEY HOSPITAL, Old Hook Road, Zip 07675–3181; tel. 201/358–3000; Louis R. Ycre, Jr., President and Chief Executive Officer **A**1 2 9 10 **F**7 8 10 11 15 16 17 19 20 21 22 24 26 27 28 29 30 31 32 33 34 35 36 37 39 41 42 44 45 46 49 51 53 54 55 58 60 61 65 67 68 71 72 73 74 **P**1 4 5 7 **N** First Option Health Plan, Red Bank, NJ; Qualcare Preferred Providers, Piscataway, NJ

23 10	237	15067	152	108822	985	91268	42950	947

WILLINGBORO—Burlington County

★ GRADUATE HEALTH SYSTEM–RANCOCAS HOSPITAL, 218–A Sunset Road, Zip 08046–1162; tel. 609/835–2900; Garry L. Scheib, President **A**10 **F**1 3 7 8 11 12 15 16 17 19 20 21 22 23 26 28 30 32 33 35 37 40 41 42 44 46 49 51 52 54 56 57 58 59 60 63 65 66 67 71 73 74 **P**4 5 **S** Allegheny Health, Education and Research Foundation, Pittsburgh, PA

23 10	241	10021	187	92108	1409	75111	35153	1059

WOODBRIDGE—Middlesex County

WOODBRIDGE DEVELOPMENT CENTER, Rahway Avenue, Zip 07095, Mailing Address: P.O. Box 189, Zip 07095; tel. 908/499–5951; Amy R. Bailon, M.D., Medical Director (Nonreporting)

12 12	125	—	—	—	—	—	—	—

WOODBURY—Gloucester County

☒ UNDERWOOD–MEMORIAL HOSPITAL, 509 North Broad Street, Zip 08096–7359, Mailing Address: P.O. Box 359, Zip 08096; tel. 609/845–0100; Steven W. Jackmuff, President and Chief Executive Officer **A**1 3 10 **F**7 8 11 12 15 16 17 18 19 20 21 22 23 26 28 30 31 32 34 35 37 39 40 41 42 44 45 49 51 52 56 58 59 65 67 68 71 73 **N** First Option Health Plan, Red Bank, NJ; Qualcare Preferred Providers, Piscataway, NJ

23 10	232	10740	178	97706	1128	83776	38430	1089

WYCKOFF—Bergen County

☒ RAMAPO RIDGE PSYCHIATRIC HOSPITAL, 301 Sicomac Avenue, Zip 07481–2194; tel. 201/848–5200; Douglas Struyk, President and Chief Executive Officer (Nonreporting) **A**1 10

23 22	80	—	—	—	—	—	—	—

NEW MEXICO

Resident population 1,685 (in thousands)
Resident population in metro areas 56.4%
Birth rate per 1,000 population 17.2
65 years and over 10.9%
Percent of persons without health insurance 23.1%

Hospital, Address, Telephone, Administrator, Approval, Facility, and Physician Codes, Health Care System, Network	Control	Service	Beds	Admissions	Census	Outpatient Visits	Births	Total	Payroll	Personnel
ALAMOGORDO—Otero County										
✠ GERALD CHAMPION MEMORIAL HOSPITAL, 1209 Ninth Street, Zip 88310–0597, Mailing Address: P.O. Box 597, Zip 88311–0597; tel. 505/439–2100; Carl W. Mantey, Administrator **A**1 9 10 **F**7 8 14 15 16 19 21 22 23 24 28 30 33 34 37 40 42 44 65 66 67 71 73 **P**5 **S** Quorum Health Group/Quorum Health Resources, Inc., Brentwood, TN	23	10	74	3385	35	50377	781	21277	7337	247
ALBUQUERQUE—Bernalillo County										
★ CARRIE TINGLEY HOSPITAL, 1127 University Boulevard N.E., Zip 87102–1715; tel. 505/272–5200; Kurt Sams, Interim Administrator (Nonreporting) **A**3 5 9 10 **S** University of New Mexico, Albuquerque, NM	12	57	18	—	—	—	—	—	—	—
☐ CHARTER HEIGHTS BEHAVIORAL HEALTH SYSTEM, (Includes Charter Heights Behavioral Health System Northeast, 103 Hospital Loop N.E., Charter Heights Behavioral Health System Southeast, 5901 Zuni Road S.E., Zip 87108; tel. 505/265–8800), 103 Hospital Loop N.E., Zip 87109; tel. 505/883–8777; Joel A. Hart, FACHE, Chief Executive Officer (Nonreporting) **A**1 9 10 **S** Magellan Health Services, Atlanta, GA	33	22	172	—	—	—	—	—	—	—
DESERT HILLS HOSPITAL, 5310 Sequoia Road N.W., Zip 87120; tel. 505/836–7330; Kay Wade, President and Chief Executive Officer (Nonreporting)	33	22	35	—	—	—	—	—	—	—
☐ △ HEALTHSOUTH REHABILITATION CENTER, 7000 Jefferson N.E., Zip 87109; tel. 505/344–9478; Darby Brockette, Administrator (Nonreporting) **A**1 7 9 10 **S** HEALTHSOUTH Corporation, Birmingham, AL	33	46	60	—	—	—	—	—	—	—
☐ LOVELACE HEALTH SYSTEM, 5400 Gibson Boulevard S.E., Zip 87108; tel. 505/262–7000; Rick Doxtator, Chief Administrative Officer **A**1 2 3 5 9 10 **F**2 3 4 5 7 8 10 11 12 14 15 16 18 19 21 22 25 26 28 29 30 31 32 33 34 35 37 39 40 41 42 43 44 45 46 49 51 53 54 55 56 57 58 59 61 65 66 67 69 70 71 72 73 74 **P**6 **N** Lovelace, Albuquerque, NM	33	10	147	6984	113	955408	1890	278955	119994	2719
☐ MEMORIAL PSYCHIATRIC HOSPITAL, 806 Central Avenue S.E., Zip 87102, Mailing Address: P.O. Box 26568, Zip 87125–6568; tel. 505/247–0220; Richard B. Hiester, Administrator **A**1 10 **F**2 3 14 15 16 22 30 34 52 53 54 55 57 58 59 65 67 70	32	22	58	669	39	—	0	5946	3213	134
✠ PRESBYTERIAN HOSPITAL, 1100 Central Avenue S.E., Zip 87106, Mailing Address: P.O. Box 26666, Zip 87125–6666; tel. 505/841–1234; William Fitzpatrick, M.D., Senior Vice President and Chief Operating Officer **A**1 2 3 5 9 10 **F**3 4 5 7 8 9 10 11 12 13 14 16 17 18 19 21 22 23 24 25 26 28 29 30 32 33 34 35 36 37 38 39 40 41 42 43 44 46 47 48 49 51 53 54 55 56 57 58 59 60 63 64 65 66 67 69 71 72 73 74 **P**1 3 4 5 6 7 **S** Presbyterian Healthcare Services, Albuquerque, NM **N** Presbyterian HealthCare Services, Inc., Albuquerque, NM	23	10	424	27279	299	167748	4030	—	—	4383
★ PRESBYTERIAN KASEMAN HOSPITAL, 8300 Constitution Avenue N.E., Zip 87110, Mailing Address: P.O. Box 26666, Zip 87125–6666; tel. 505/291–2000; Jim Purdy, Administrative Director **A**9 10 **F**2 3 4 5 7 8 9 10 11 12 13 14 16 17 18 19 21 22 23 24 25 26 30 31 32 33 34 35 36 37 38 39 40 41 42 43 44 46 47 49 51 52 53 54 55 56 57 58 59 60 61 63 64 65 66 67 69 70 71 72 73 74 **P**1 4 5 6 7 **S** Presbyterian Healthcare Services, Albuquerque, NM **N** Presbyterian HealthCare Services, Inc., Albuquerque, NM	23	10	120	5240	72	28185	0	—	—	—
✠ PUBLIC HEALTH SERVICE INDIAN HOSPITAL, 801 Vassar Drive N.E., Zip 87106–2799; tel. 505/256–4000; Raymond L. Rodgers, Administrator (Nonreporting) **A**1 10 **S** U. S. Public Health Service Indian Health Service, Rockville, MD	47	10	28	—	—	—	—	—	—	—
✠ ST. JOSEPH MEDICAL CENTER, 601 Martin Luther King Drive N.E., Zip 87102, Mailing Address: P.O. Box 25555, Zip 87125–0555; tel. 505/727–8000; Charles A. Ivy, Vice President (Total facility includes 24 beds in nursing home–type unit) **A**1 2 5 9 10 **F**2 3 4 7 8 10 11 12 19 21 22 23 27 28 30 32 33 34 35 36 37 39 40 41 42 43 44 45 46 48 49 51 52 54 56 57 58 60 61 63 64 65 67 68 70 71 72 73 74 **P**5 6 7 **S** Catholic Health Initiatives, Denver, CO **N** Medical Network of New Mexico, Albuquerque, NM	21	10	204	9007	128	38293	0	74484	26525	1308
✠ ST. JOSEPH NORTHEAST HEIGHTS HOSPITAL, 4701 Montgomery N.E., Zip 87109, Mailing Address: P.O. Box 25555, Zip 87125–0555; tel. 505/727–7800; C. Vincent Townsend, Jr., Vice President, Operations **A**1 9 10 **F**4 7 8 10 11 12 19 21 22 23 27 30 32 33 34 35 36 37 39 40 43 44 46 49 51 54 56 57 58 60 61 63 65 67 68 71 72 73 74 **P**5 6 7 **S** Catholic Health Initiatives, Denver, CO **N** Medical Network of New Mexico, Albuquerque, NM	21	10	71	3509	34	23093	938	17602	6725	328
★ △ ST. JOSEPH REHABILITATION HOSPITAL AND OUTPATIENT CENTER, 505 Elm Street N.E., Zip 87102, Mailing Address: P.O. Box 25555, Zip 87125–2500; tel. 505/727–4700; Mary Lou Coors, Administrator (Total facility includes 17 beds in nursing home–type unit) **A**7 9 10 **F**3 4 7 8 10 11 12 19 21 22 27 28 30 32 33 34 35 36 37 38 39 40 41 42 43 44 45 46 48 49 51 54 56 57 58 60 61 63 64 65 67 68 70 71 72 73 74 **P**5 6 7 **S** Catholic Health Initiatives, Denver, CO **N** Medical Network of New Mexico, Albuquerque, NM	21	46	46	540	33	2980	0	11982	5546	186

Hospital, Address, Telephone, Administrator, Approval, Facility, and Physician Codes, Health Care System, Network	Classi-fication Codes		Utilization Data					Expense (thousands) of dollars		
★ American Hospital Association (AHA) membership □ Joint Commission on Accreditation of Healthcare Organizations (JCAHO) accreditation + American Osteopathic Hospital Association (AOHA) membership ○ American Osteopathic Association (AOA) accreditation △ Commission on Accreditation of Rehabilitation Facilities (CARF) accreditation Control codes 61, 63, 64, 71, 72 and 73 indicate hospitals listed by AOHA, but not registered by AHA. For definition of numerical codes, see page A4	Control	Service	Beds	Admissions	Census	Outpatient Visits	Births	Total	Payroll	Personnel
⊞ ST. JOSEPH WEST MESA HOSPITAL, 10501 Golf Course Road N.W., Zip 87114, Mailing Address: P.O. Box 25555, Zip 87125–0555; tel. 505/893–2003; C. Vincent Townsend, Jr., Vice President, Operations (Total facility includes 22 beds in nursing home–type unit) **A**1 9 10 **F**3 4 7 8 10 12 19 21 22 23 27 30 32 33 34 35 36 37 39 40 42 43 44 46 48 49 51 52 54 56 57 58 61 63 64 65 67 68 71 72 73 74 **P**5 6 7 **S** Catholic Health Initiatives, Denver, CO **N** Medical Network of New Mexico, Albuquerque, NM	21	10	70	2383	30	—	525	15730	5788	281
□ THC–ALBUQUERQUE, 700 High Street N.E., Zip 87102; tel. 505/242–4444; Jean Koester, Chief Executive Officer **A**1 5 10 **F**12 14 15 16 22 28 33 37 39 42 65 67 71 **P**5 **S** Transitional Hospitals Corporation, Las Vegas, NV	33	10	61	417	45	—	0	12390	6243	157
⊞ UNIVERSITY HOSPITAL, 2211 Lomas Boulevard N.E., Zip 87106; tel. 505/272–2121; Stephen McKernan, Chief Executive Officer **A**1 2 3 5 8 9 10 **F**3 4 5 7 8 9 10 12 14 15 16 17 19 21 22 23 24 26 28 29 30 31 32 33 34 35 37 38 40 41 42 43 44 45 46 47 49 54 55 58 60 61 63 65 66 67 68 69 70 71 72 73 74 **S** University of New Mexico, Albuquerque, NM **N** University of New Mexico Health Science Center, Albuquerque, NM	12	10	267	19723	264	355136	3554	185241	78112	2668
★ UNIVERSITY OF NEW MEXICO CHILDREN'S PSYCHIATRIC HOSPITAL, 1001 Yale Boulevard N.E., Zip 87131; tel. 505/272–2945; Christina B. Gunn, Chief Executive Officer (Nonreporting) **A**3 5 9 **S** University of New Mexico, Albuquerque, NM	12	52	53	—	—	—	—	—	—	—
★ UNIVERSITY OF NEW MEXICO MENTAL HEALTH CENTER, 2600 Marble N.E., Zip 87131–2600; tel. 505/272–2870; Christina B. Gunn, Chief Executive Officer (Nonreporting) **A**3 5 9 **S** University of New Mexico, Albuquerque, NM **N** University of New Mexico Health Science Center, Albuquerque, NM	13	22	60	—	—	—	—	—	—	—
⊞ VETERANS AFFAIRS MEDICAL CENTER, 2100 Ridgecrest Drive S.E., Zip 87108; tel. 505/265–1711; Norman E. Browne, Director (Total facility includes 47 beds in nursing home–type unit) **A**1 2 3 5 8 **F**1 2 3 4 5 8 10 12 17 18 19 20 21 22 23 25 26 27 28 29 30 31 32 33 34 35 37 39 41 42 43 44 45 46 48 49 51 52 54 55 56 58 59 60 61 63 64 65 67 71 73 74 **S** Department of Veterans Affairs, Washington, DC	45	10	327	8664	249	322058	0	133837	68553	1722
ARTESIA—Eddy County										
⊞ ARTESIA GENERAL HOSPITAL, 702 North 13th Street, Zip 88210; tel. 505/748–3333; Tony Plantier, Administrator (Nonreporting) **A**1 9 10 **S** Presbyterian Healthcare Services, Albuquerque, NM	16	10	38	—	—	—	—	—	—	—
CANNON AFB—Curry County										
★ U. S. AIR FORCE HOSPITAL, Zip 88103–5300; tel. 505/784–6318; Major Douglas E. Anderson, MSC, USAF, Administrator **F**3 7 8 12 13 14 15 16 1/ 19 20 21 24 28 29 30 31 32 39 40 44 45 46 49 51 53 54 55 56 58 59 61 65 66 67 71 73 74 **P**1 4 5 7 **S** Department of the Air Force, Washington, DC	41	10	5	240	6	100000	360	—	—	—
CARLSBAD—Eddy County										
⊞ COLUMBIA MEDICAL CENTER OF CARLSBAD, 2430 West Pierce Street, Zip 88220–3597; tel. 505/887–4100; Robin E. Lake, Chief Executive Officer (Nonreporting) **A**1 9 10 **S** Columbia/HCA Healthcare Corporation, Nashville, TN	33	10	110	—	—	—	—	—	—	—
CLAYTON—Union County										
★ UNION COUNTY GENERAL HOSPITAL, 301 Harding Street, Zip 88415, Mailing Address: P.O. Box 489, Zip 88415–0489; tel. 505/374–2585; Carrell R. Blakely, Administrator (Nonreporting) **A**9 10 **S** Brim, Inc., Portland, OR	23	10	28	—	—	—	—	—	—	—
CLOVIS—Curry County										
⊞ PLAINS REGIONAL MEDICAL CENTER, (Includes Plains Regional Medical Center–Portales, 1700 South Avenue O, Portales, Zip 88130, Mailing Address: P.O. Drawer 60, Zip 88130; tel. 505/356–4411), 2100 North Thomas Street, Zip 88101, Mailing Address: P.O. Box 1688, Zip 88101–1688; tel. 505/769–2141; Dennis E. Headlee, Administrator (Nonreporting) **A**1 9 10 **S** Presbyterian Healthcare Services, Albuquerque, NM	21	10	84	—	—	—	—	—	—	—
CROWNPOINT—McKinley County										
⊞ U. S. PUBLIC HEALTH SERVICE INDIAN HOSPITAL, Mailing Address: Box 358, Zip 87313–0358; tel. 505/786–5291; Anita Muneta, Chief Executive Officer **A**1 10 **F**2 3 4 6 7 8 9 10 11 12 13 14 15 16 17 18 19 20 21 22 23 24 25 26 27 28 29 30 31 32 33 34 35 36 37 38 39 40 41 42 43 44 45 46 47 48 49 51 52 53 54 55 56 57 58 59 60 61 62 64 65 67 68 69 70 71 72 74 **S** U. S. Public Health Service Indian Health Service, Rockville, MD	44	10	32	942	9	56309	186	16108	8228	247
DEMING—Luna County										
MIMBRES MEMORIAL HOSPITAL, 900 West Ash Street, Zip 88030; tel. 505/546–2761; Harley Smith, Chief Executive Officer (Total facility includes 70 beds in nursing home–type unit) (Nonreporting) **A**9 10 **S** Community Health Systems, Inc., Brentwood, TN	13	10	119	—	—	—	—	—	—	—
ESPANOLA—Rio Arriba County										
⊞ ESPANOLA HOSPITAL, 1010 Spruce Street, Zip 87532; tel. 505/753–7111; Marcella A. Romero, Administrator **A**1 9 10 **F**7 8 12 14 15 16 19 22 28 32 33 34 35 37 40 44 46 49 51 65 71 72 73 **P**3 5 8 **S** Presbyterian Healthcare Services, Albuquerque, NM	23	10	80	2787	20	42201	275	15321	6777	216
FARMINGTON—San Juan County										
⊞ SAN JUAN REGIONAL MEDICAL CENTER, (Includes Interface Rehabilitation Hospital, 525 South Schwartz, tel. 505/327–3422; Jess Hamblen, Administrator), 801 West Maple Street, Zip 87401; tel. 505/325–5011; Donald R. Carlson, President and Chief Executive Officer (Total facility includes 15 beds in nursing home–type unit) **A**1 2 9 10 **F**7 8 12 13 14 15 16 17 19 21 22 23 25 27 28 29 30 32 33 34 35 37 40 41 42 44 46 48 49 54 56 58 59 60 64 65 67 71 72 73 **P**4 5 8	23	10	150	7547	99	81276	1083	62849	26997	845

Hospital, Address, Telephone, Administrator, Approval, Facility, and Physician Codes, Health Care System, Network	Classi-fication Codes		Utilization Data					Expense (thousands) of dollars		
★ American Hospital Association (AHA) membership □ Joint Commission on Accreditation of Healthcare Organizations (JCAHO) accreditation + American Osteopathic Hospital Association (AOHA) membership ○ American Osteopathic Association (AOA) accreditation △ Commission on Accreditation of Rehabilitation Facilities (CARF) accreditation Control codes 61, 63, 64, 71, 72 and 73 indicate hospitals listed by AOHA, but not registered by AHA. For definition of numerical codes, see page A4	Control	Service	Beds	Admissions	Census	Outpatient Visits	Births	Total	Payroll	Personnel

FORT SUMNER—De Baca County

| ★ DEBACA GENERAL HOSPITAL, 500 North Tenth Street, Zip 88119, Mailing Address: P.O. Box 349, Zip 88119; tel. 505/355-2414; Matthew J. Reat, Administrator (Nonreporting) **A**9 10 | 13 | 10 | 21 | — | — | — | — | — | — | — |

GALLUP—McKinley County

| ✠ GALLUP INDIAN MEDICAL CENTER, 516 East Nizhoni Boulevard, Zip 87301-1334, Mailing Address: Box 1337, Zip 87305; tel. 505/722-1000; Timothy G. Fleming, M.D., Chief Executive Officer **A**1 10 **F**3 7 8 12 14 15 16 17 19 20 21 22 25 28 29 30 34 35 37 39 40 44 45 46 49 53 54 56 58 65 68 71 72 74 **S** U. S. Public Health Service Indian Health Service, Rockville, MD | 47 | 10 | 99 | 5395 | 58 | 199585 | 955 | 62342 | 30160 | 727 |
| ✠ REHOBOTH MCKINLEY CHRISTIAN HOSPITAL, 1901 Red Rock Drive, Zip 87301-1901; tel. 505/863-7000; David J. Baltzer, President **A**1 9 10 **F**2 3 7 8 12 13 14 16 17 18 19 21 22 28 30 32 33 34 35 37 40 41 44 45 46 49 51 52 53 54 55 56 58 59 65 67 71 73 74 **P**5 6 | 23 | 10 | 138 | 2800 | 61 | 57641 | 324 | 32144 | 15652 | 543 |

GRANTS—Cibola County

| ✠ CIBOLA GENERAL HOSPITAL, 1212 Bonita Avenue, Zip 87020; tel. 505/287-4446; Polly Pine, Administrator **A**1 9 10 **F**7 8 15 16 19 22 28 32 37 40 44 46 51 65 71 **P**8 **S** Quorum Health Group/Quorum Health Resources, Inc., Brentwood, TN | 23 | 10 | 22 | 1091 | 9 | 10847 | 191 | 6212 | 2838 | 102 |

HOBBS—Lea County

| ✠ COLUMBIA LEA REGIONAL HOSPITAL, 5419 North Lovington Highway, Zip 88240, Mailing Address: P.O. Box 3000, Zip 88240; tel. 505/392-6581; R. Gordon Taylor, Administrator (Nonreporting) **A**1 10 **S** Columbia/HCA Healthcare Corporation, Nashville, TN | 33 | 10 | 250 | — | — | — | — | — | — | — |

HOLLOMAN AFB—Otero County

| ✠ U. S. AIR FORCE HOSPITAL, 280 First Street, Zip 88330-8273; tel. 505/475-5587; Colonel Bruce P. Heseltine, MSC, USAF, Commander **A**1 **F**3 8 12 13 14 15 16 19 20 21 24 28 29 30 34 35 44 65 67 71 73 74 **P**5 **S** Department of the Air Force, Washington, DC | 41 | 10 | 7 | 736 | 3 | 80336 | 0 | — | — | — |

KIRTLAND AFB—Bernalillo County

| ✠ U. S. AIR FORCE HOSPITAL–KIRTLAND, 1951 Second Street S.E., Zip 87117-5559; tel. 505/846-3547; Colonel Paul B. Christianson, USAF, Commander **A**1 3 5 **F**3 4 8 12 19 20 21 22 24 28 29 30 34 39 44 45 46 49 51 54 55 56 58 61 65 71 72 74 **P**1 **S** Department of the Air Force, Washington, DC | 41 | 10 | 10 | 2111 | 9 | 168581 | 0 | 17313 | — | 457 |

LAS CRUCES—Dona Ana County

| □ BHC MESILLA VALLEY HOSPITAL, (Formerly Mesilla Valley Hospital), 3751 Del Rey Boulevard, Zip 88012, Mailing Address: P.O. Box 429, Zip 88004; tel. 505/382-3500; Edward C. Morton, Jr., FACHE, Chief Executive Officer (Nonreporting) **A**1 9 10 **S** Behavioral Healthcare Corporation, Nashville, TN | 32 | 22 | 85 | — | — | — | — | — | — | — |
| ✠ MEMORIAL MEDICAL CENTER, 2450 South Telshor Boulevard, Zip 88011-5076; tel. 505/522-8641; Steven L. Smith, President and Chief Executive Officer (Total facility includes 13 beds in nursing home–type unit) **A**1 5 9 10 **F**4 7 8 10 15 19 21 22 28 35 37 40 42 43 44 49 52 56 60 64 65 70 71 72 73 74 | 15 | 10 | 222 | 11587 | 150 | 104307 | 2671 | 85959 | 34777 | 948 |

LAS VEGAS—San Miguel County

| □ LAS VEGAS MEDICAL CENTER, 3795 Hot Springs Boulevard, Zip 87701, Mailing Address: P.O. Box 1388, Zip 87701; tel. 505/454-2100; Gary Buff, Jr., Administrator (Total facility includes 176 beds in nursing home–type unit) **A**1 **F**12 14 16 17 18 19 20 22 25 27 28 35 39 41 44 45 46 52 53 55 56 57 58 64 65 67 71 73 | 12 | 22 | 410 | 780 | 352 | — | 0 | — | — | 770 |
| ✠ NORTHEASTERN REGIONAL HOSPITAL, 1235 Eighth Street, Zip 87701, Mailing Address: P.O. Box 248, Zip 87701-0238; tel. 505/425-6751; Patricia A. Beelow, Chief Executive Officer **A**1 9 10 **F**7 12 13 15 19 21 22 24 28 30 32 35 37 40 44 52 59 64 65 71 73 **P**3 7 8 **S** Brim, Inc., Portland, OR | 23 | 10 | 56 | 2329 | 25 | — | 449 | 16723 | 6338 | 249 |

LOS ALAMOS—Los Alamos County

| ✠ LOS ALAMOS MEDICAL CENTER, 3917 West Road, Zip 87544; tel. 505/662-4201; Paul J. Wilson, Administrator **A**1 9 10 **F**1 2 3 4 5 6 7 8 9 10 11 12 13 14 15 16 17 18 19 20 21 22 23 24 25 26 27 28 29 30 31 32 33 34 35 36 37 38 39 40 41 42 43 44 45 46 47 48 49 50 51 52 53 54 55 56 57 58 59 60 61 62 63 64 65 66 67 68 69 70 71 72 73 74 **P**3 5 7 8 **S** Lutheran Health Systems, Fargo, ND | 23 | 10 | 47 | 1693 | 15 | 80063 | 258 | 16544 | 6005 | 218 |

LOS LUNAS—Valencia County

| LOS LUNAS HOSPITAL AND TRAINING SCHOOL, Mailing Address: P.O. Box 1269, Zip 87031; tel. 505/865-9611; Matthew McCue, Administrator (Nonreporting) | 12 | 62 | 357 | — | — | — | — | — | — | — |

LOVINGTON—Lea County

| ✠ NOR–LEA GENERAL HOSPITAL, 1600 North Main, Zip 88260; tel. 505/396-6611; David R. Jordan, Ph.D., Administrator and Chief Executive Officer **A**1 9 10 **F**14 17 19 20 22 27 28 32 34 35 41 44 46 64 65 71 | 16 | 10 | 28 | 472 | 5 | 25117 | 0 | 4317 | 1847 | 83 |

MESCALERO—Otero County

| ✠ U. S. PUBLIC HEALTH SERVICE INDIAN HOSPITAL, Mailing Address: Box 210, Zip 88340-0210; tel. 505/671-4441; Joe Wahnee, Jr., Service Unit Director (Nonreporting) **A**1 10 **S** U. S. Public Health Service Indian Health Service, Rockville, MD | 47 | 10 | 13 | — | — | — | — | — | — | — |

PORTALES—Roosevelt County

PLAINS REGIONAL MEDICAL CENTER–PORTALES See Plains Regional Medical Center, Clovis

Hospital, Address, Telephone, Administrator, Approval, Facility, and Physician Codes, Health Care System, Network	Classi-fication Codes		Utilization Data					Expense (thousands) of dollars		
★ American Hospital Association (AHA) membership □ Joint Commission on Accreditation of Healthcare Organizations (JCAHO) accreditation + American Osteopathic Hospital Association (AOHA) membership ○ American Osteopathic Association (AOA) accreditation △ Commission on Accreditation of Rehabilitation Facilities (CARF) accreditation Control codes 61, 63, 64, 71, 72 and 73 indicate hospitals listed by AOHA, but not registered by AHA. For definition of numerical codes, see page A4	Control	Service	Beds	Admissions	Census	Outpatient Visits	Births	Total	Payroll	Personnel

RATON—Colfax County

★ MINERS' COLFAX MEDICAL CENTER, (Includes Miners' Hospital of New Mexico), 200 Hospital Drive, Zip 87740–2099; tel. 505/445–3661; David Antle, Chief Executive Officer (Total facility includes 30 beds in nursing home–type unit) (Nonreporting) **A**9 10

| | 13 | 10 | 68 | — | — | — | — | — | — | — |

ROSWELL—Chaves County

⊞ EASTERN NEW MEXICO MEDICAL CENTER, 405 West Country Club Road, Zip 88201–9981; tel. 505/622–8170; Ronald J. Shafer, President and Chief Executive Officer (Nonreporting) **A**1 9 10

| | 13 | 10 | 158 | — | — | — | — | — | — | — |

□ △ SOUTHERN NEW MEXICO REHABILITATION CENTER, (Formerly New Mexico Rehabilitation Center), (Includes Pecos Valley Lodge), 31 Gail Harris Avenue, Zip 88201; tel. 505/347–5491; Dave Dryden, FACHE, Administrator **A**1 7 9 10 **F**2 3 12 31 48 49 65 **P**6

| | 12 | 46 | 39 | 505 | 28 | 4848 | 0 | 6474 | 3089 | 120 |

RUIDOSO—Lincoln County

⊞ LINCOLN COUNTY MEDICAL CENTER, 211 Sudderth Drive, Zip 88345, Mailing Address: P.O. Drawer 3C/D, Hollywood Station, Zip 88345; tel. 505/257–7381; Valerie Miller, Administrator **A**1 9 10 **F**7 8 12 15 16 17 19 20 22 25 28 30 31 37 40 41 42 44 46 49 71 73 **P**2 8 **S** Presbyterian Healthcare Services, Albuquerque, NM

| | 23 | 10 | 38 | 899 | 7 | 39812 | 222 | 10653 | 4401 | 144 |

SAN FIDEL—Cibola County

⊞ ACOMA–CANONCITO–LAGUNA HOSPITAL, Mailing Address: P.O. Box 130, Zip 87049; tel. 505/552–6634; Richard L. Zephier, Ph.D., Service Unit Director **A**1 10 **F**14 15 16 20 22 34 44 46 49 58 65 71 **P**6 **S** U. S. Public Health Service Indian Health Service, Rockville, MD

| | 47 | 10 | 15 | 465 | 8 | 58146 | 0 | — | — | 188 |

SANTA FE—Santa Fe County

□ BHC PINON HILLS HOSPITAL, (Formerly Pinon Hills Hospital), 313 Camino Alire, Zip 87501; tel. 505/988–8003; Jerry Smith, Chief Executive Officer (Nonreporting) **A**1 9 10 **S** Behavioral Healthcare Corporation, Nashville, TN

| | 33 | 22 | 34 | — | — | — | — | — | — | — |

⊞ PHS SANTA FE INDIAN HOSPITAL, 1700 Cerrillos Road, Zip 87505; tel. 505/988–9821; Lawrence A. Jordan, Director (Nonreporting) **A**1 10 **S** U. S. Public Health Service Indian Health Service, Rockville, MD

| | 47 | 10 | 39 | — | — | — | — | — | — | — |

⊞ △ ST. VINCENT HOSPITAL, 455 St. Michael's Drive, Zip 87505, Mailing Address: P.O. Box 2107, Zip 87504–2107; tel. 505/983–3361; Ronald C. Winger, President and Chief Executive Officer **A**1 2 5 7 9 10 **F**1 3 7 10 11 12 17 18 19 21 22 23 28 30 31 32 33 34 35 37 39 40 41 42 44 45 46 47 48 49 52 53 54 56 57 58 59 60 64 65 67 70 71 72 73 **P**3 8

| | 23 | 10 | 198 | 10883 | 135 | 119749 | 1467 | 83666 | 39985 | 1020 |

SANTA TERESA—Dona Ana County

□ ALLIANCE HOSPITAL OF SANTA TERESA, 100 Laura Court, Zip 88008, Mailing Address: P.O. Box 6, Zip 88008; tel. 505/589–0033; Frank M. Braden, Administrator (Nonreporting) **A**1 10 **S** Bowdon Corporate Offices, Atlanta, GA

| | 33 | 22 | 72 | — | — | — | — | — | — | — |

SHIPROCK—San Juan County

⊞ NORTHERN NAVAJO MEDICAL CENTER, Mailing Address: Box 160, Zip 87420; tel. 505/368–6001; Dee Hutchison, Chief Executive Officer **A**1 10 **F**7 12 13 15 16 17 18 19 20 22 25 28 29 30 31 34 37 39 40 44 46 49 51 53 54 57 58 65 66 68 71 72 74 **S** U. S. Public Health Service Indian Health Service, Rockville, MD

| | 47 | 10 | 59 | 3067 | 31 | 154221 | 788 | 49582 | 22497 | — |

SILVER CITY—Grant County

⊞ GILA REGIONAL MEDICAL CENTER, 1313 East 32nd Street, Zip 88061; tel. 505/538–4000; Alfredo Ontiveros, Administrator **A**1 9 10 **F**3 7 8 16 17 19 21 22 27 30 32 33 35 37 40 41 42 44 49 52 53 58 65 71 73 **P**3 **S** Quorum Health Group/Quorum Health Resources, Inc., Brentwood, TN

| | 13 | 10 | 68 | 3871 | 37 | 54860 | 623 | 25640 | 12707 | 441 |

SOCORRO—Socorro County

⊞ SOCORRO GENERAL HOSPITAL, 1202 Highway 60 West, Zip 87801, Mailing Address: P.O. Box 1009, Zip 87801–1009; tel. 505/835–1140; Jeff Dye, Administrator (Nonreporting) **A**1 9 10 **S** Presbyterian Healthcare Services, Albuquerque, NM

| | 23 | 10 | 30 | — | — | — | — | — | — | — |

TAOS—Taos County

★ HOLY CROSS HOSPITAL, 630 Paseo De Pueblo Sur, Zip 87571, Mailing Address: P.O. Box DD, Zip 87571; tel. 505/758–8883; Rita Campbell, Chief Executive Officer (Nonreporting) **A**9 10 **S** Quorum Health Group/Quorum Health Resources, Inc., Brentwood, TN

| | 23 | 10 | 42 | — | — | — | — | — | — | — |

TRUTH OR CONSEQUENCES—Sierra County

⊞ SIERRA VISTA HOSPITAL, 800 East Ninth Avenue, Zip 87901; tel. 505/894–2111; Domenica Rush, Administrator (Total facility includes 15 beds in nursing home–type unit) **A**1 9 10 **F**7 8 19 22 32 40 44 46 49 64 65 71

| | 15 | 10 | 47 | 351 | 3 | 13403 | 5 | 4732 | 1887 | 91 |

TUCUMCARI—Quay County

★ DR. DAN C. TRIGG MEMORIAL HOSPITAL, 301 East Miel De Luna Avenue, Zip 88401, Mailing Address: P.O. Box 608, Zip 88401; tel. 505/461–0141; Dan Noteware, Administrator **A**9 10 **F**7 8 12 14 15 16 17 19 22 32 34 40 41 44 48 49 51 65 71 73 **S** Presbyterian Healthcare Services, Albuquerque, NM

| | 23 | 10 | 37 | 1241 | 7 | 17647 | 101 | 6064 | 2233 | 90 |

ZUNI—McKinley County

⊞ U. S. PUBLIC HEALTH SERVICE INDIAN HOSPITAL, Mailing Address: P.O. Box 467, Zip 87327; tel. 505/782–4431; Jean Othole, Service Unit Director **A**1 10 **F**1 3 4 5 7 8 10 13 14 15 16 18 19 20 21 22 24 26 27 28 30 35 40 44 46 49 50 51 53 54 55 56 57 58 59 60 63 68 69 72 **S** U. S. Public Health Service Indian Health Service, Rockville, MD

| | 47 | 10 | 29 | 926 | 10 | 60142 | 113 | — | — | 163 |

NEW YORK

Resident population 18,136 (in thousands)
Resident population in metro areas 91.7%
Birth rate per 1,000 population 15.6
65 years and over 13.4%
Percent of persons without health insurance 16.0%

★ American Hospital Association (AHA) membership
□ Joint Commission on Accreditation of Healthcare Organizations (JCAHO) accreditation
+ American Osteopathic Hospital Association (AOHA) membership
○ American Osteopathic Association (AOA) accreditation
△ Commission on Accreditation of Rehabilitation Facilities (CARF) accreditation
Control codes 61, 63, 64, 71, 72 and 73 indicate hospitals listed by AOHA, but not registered by AHA. For definition of numerical codes, see page A4

Hospital, Address, Telephone, Administrator, Approval, Facility, and Physician Codes, Health Care System, Network	Control	Service	Beds	Admissions	Census	Outpatient Visits	Births	Total	Payroll	Personnel
ALBANY—Albany County										
✠ ALBANY MEDICAL CENTER, 43 New Scotland Avenue, Zip 12208; tel. 518/262–3125; Thomas G. Foggo, Executive Vice President Care Delivery and General Director **A**1 2 3 5 8 9 10 12 **F**4 7 8 10 11 12 14 16 17 19 20 21 22 23 25 26 31 32 34 35 37 38 39 40 41 42 43 44 45 46 47 48 49 51 52 53 54 55 56 57 58 59 60 61 63 65 66 67 69 70 71 72 73 74 **N** Greene County Rural Health Network, Catskill, NY; National Cardiovascular Network, Atlanta, GA	23	10	564	24137	479	299783	2461	271642	94950	3073
✠ CAPITAL DISTRICT PSYCHIATRIC CENTER, 75 New Scotland Avenue, Zip 12208; tel. 518/447–9611; Jesse Nixon, Jr., Ph.D., Director (Nonreporting) **A**1 3 5 10 **S** New York State Department of Mental Health, Albany, NY	12	22	200	—	—	—	—	—	—	—
✠ CHILD'S HOSPITAL, 25 Hackett Boulevard, Zip 12208; tel. 518/242–1200; Stephen J. Lauko, Chief Executive Officer (Nonreporting) **A**1 3 5 9 10	23	45	20	—	—	—	—	—	—	—
✠ MEMORIAL HOSPITAL, 600 Northern Boulevard, Zip 12204–1083; tel. 518/471–3221; Bernard Shapiro, Chief Executive Officer (Nonreporting) **A**1 6 9 10 **N** Shared Health Network, Inc., Albany, NY	23	10	212	—	—	—	—	—	—	—
✠ ST. PETER'S HOSPITAL, 315 South Manning Boulevard, Zip 12208–1789; tel. 518/525–1550; Steven P. Boyle, President and Chief Executive Officer **A**1 2 3 5 9 10 **F**2 3 4 6 7 8 10 11 12 13 14 15 16 17 18 20 22 25 26 28 29 30 31 32 33 34 36 37 38 39 40 41 42 43 44 45 46 48 49 51 54 64 **P**5 7 8 **S** Eastern Mercy Health System, Radnor, PA **N** MercyCare Corporation, Albany, NY; Shared Health Network, Inc., Albany, NY	23	10	437	19992	353	458538	2310	161877	75877	2533
✠ △ VETERANS AFFAIRS MEDICAL CENTER, 113 Holland Avenue, Zip 12208–3473; tel. 518/462–3311; Lawrence H. Flesh, M.D., Director (Total facility includes 50 beds in nursing home–type unit) **A**1 2 3 5 7 8 **F**1 3 4 8 10 11 15 16 17 18 19 20 21 22 25 26 28 29 30 31 32 33 34 35 37 39 41 42 44 45 46 48 49 51 52 54 55 56 57 58 59 60 63 64 65 67 71 73 74 **S** Department of Veterans Affairs, Washington, DC	45	10	298	5537	252	218571	0	115060	80557	1320
ALEXANDRIA BAY—Jefferson County										
□ E. J. NOBLE HOSPITAL SAMARITAN, (Formerly E. J. Noble Hospital of Alexandria Bay), 19 Fuller Street, Zip 13607; tel. 315/482–2511; William P. Koughan, President (Total facility includes 27 beds in nursing home–type unit) (Nonreporting) **A**1 9 10 **N** Northern New York Rural Health Care Alliance, Watertown, NY	23	10	52	—	—	—	—	—	—	—
AMITYVILLE—Suffolk County										
□ BRUNSWICK GENERAL HOSPITAL, (Includes Brunswick Hall, 80 Louden Avenue, Zip 11701–2735; tel. 516/789–7100; Brunswick Physical Medicine & Rehabilitation Hospital, 366 Broadway), 366 Broadway, Zip 11701–9820; tel. 516/789–7000; Benjamin M. Stein, M.D., President (Total facility includes 94 beds in nursing home–type unit) **A**1 9 10 **F**3 8 11 15 16 17 19 21 22 26 27 28 30 31 32 33 35 37 39 42 44 46 48 49 52 53 54 55 56 57 58 60 64 65 67 69 71 73 **N** Health First, New York, NY	33	10	474	7078	377	136626	0	85369	44545	1156
□ SOUTH OAKS HOSPITAL, 400 Sunrise Highway, Zip 11701; tel. 516/264–4000; Jean P. Smith, Chief Executive Officer (Nonreporting) **A**1 9 10	33	22	334	—	—	—	—	—	—	—
AMSTERDAM—Montgomery County										
✠ AMSTERDAM MEMORIAL HOSPITAL, 4988 State Highway 30, Zip 12010–1699; tel. 518/842–3100; Cornelio R. Catena, President and Chief Executive Officer (Total facility includes 160 beds in nursing home–type unit) **A**1 9 10 **F**1 11 12 14 15 17 19 20 21 22 25 29 30 34 35 37 39 41 42 44 45 46 49 64 65 66 67 68 71 73 74	23	10	242	2127	197	51386	0	30361	13129	—
✠ ST. MARY'S HOSPITAL, 427 Guy Park Avenue, Zip 12010–1095; tel. 518/842–1900; Peter E. Capobianco, President and Chief Executive Officer **A**1 9 10 **F**2 3 5 7 8 11 14 15 16 17 18 19 22 23 28 29 30 31 32 33 34 35 37 40 41 42 44 45 46 48 49 51 52 53 54 55 56 57 58 59 60 61 65 66 67 71 73 74 **S** Carondelet Health System, Saint Louis, MO **N** Shared Health Network, Inc., Albany, NY	21	10	143	5063	94	158118	707	40948	21725	681
AUBURN—Cayuga County										
✠ AUBURN MEMORIAL HOSPITAL, Lansing Street, Zip 13021; tel. 315/255–7011; Christopher J. Rogers, Administrator (Total facility includes 80 beds in nursing home–type unit) **A**1 5 9 10 **F**7 8 11 16 19 21 22 25 37 40 44 49 52 54 63 64 65 67 71 72 73	23	10	306	7889	228	103837	1379	53895	27829	982
BATAVIA—Genesee County										
✠ GENESEE MEMORIAL HOSPITAL, 127 North Street, Zip 14020–1697; tel. 716/343–6030; Douglas T. Jones, President and Chief Executive Officer **A**1 9 10 **F**7 8 11 15 16 19 22 25 27 28 29 30 33 34 37 39 40 41 42 44 45 51 61 65 67 71 73 74	23	10	70	3190	53	108594	498	24723	11836	415
✠ ST. JEROME HOSPITAL, 16 Bank Street, Zip 14020–2260; tel. 716/343–3131; Charles W. Smith, Jr., Chief Executive Officer **A**1 9 10 **F**2 5 8 11 14 15 16 17 18 19 22 27 28 29 30 32 33 34 35 37 41 44 45 51 60 62 65 66 71 73 **S** Eastern Mercy Health System, Radnor, PA	21	10	96	2986	64	48149	0	—	—	388

Hospital, Address, Telephone, Administrator, Approval, Facility, and Physician Codes, Health Care System, Network	Classi-fication Codes		Utilization Data					Expense (thousands) of dollars		
	Control	Service	Beds	Admissions	Census	Outpatient Visits	Births	Total	Payroll	Personnel

★ American Hospital Association (AHA) membership
☐ Joint Commission on Accreditation of Healthcare Organizations (JCAHO) accreditation
+ American Osteopathic Hospital Association (AOHA) membership
○ American Osteopathic Association (AOA) accreditation
△ Commission on Accreditation of Rehabilitation Facilities (CARF) accreditation
Control codes 61, 63, 64, 71, 72 and 73 indicate hospitals listed by AOHA, but not registered by AHA. For definition of numerical codes, see page A4

Hospital	Control	Service	Beds	Admissions	Census	Outpatient Visits	Births	Total	Payroll	Personnel
✸ VETERANS AFFAIRS WESTERN NEW YORK HEALTHCARE SYSTEM, 222 Richmond Avenue, Zip 14020; tel. 716/343–7500; Richard S. Droske, Director (Total facility includes 70 beds in nursing home–type unit) (Nonreporting) **A**1 5 9 **S** Department of Veterans Affairs, Washington, DC	45	10	158	—	—	—	—	—	—	—
BATH—Steuben County										
✸ IRA DAVENPORT MEMORIAL HOSPITAL, 7571 State Route 54, Zip 14810; tel. 607/776–2141; Timothy F. Reardon, Chief Executive Officer (Total facility includes 120 beds in nursing home–type unit) **A**1 9 10 **F**1 3 7 8 15 16 17 19 20 22 26 30 31 33 34 37 40 42 44 49 51 64 65 67 71 73 **P**3	23	10	186	2176	142	7524	108	16077	8160	310
✸ VETERANS AFFAIRS MEDICAL CENTER, 76 Veterans Avenue, Zip 14810–0842; tel. 607/776–2111; Michael J. Sullivan, Director (Total facility includes 125 beds in nursing home–type unit) **A**1 **F**2 3 4 6 8 10 11 12 14 15 16 17 18 19 20 21 22 23 24 26 27 28 30 31 32 33 34 35 37 39 41 42 43 44 45 46 49 50 51 52 56 57 58 59 60 61 63 64 65 67 71 73 74 **S** Department of Veterans Affairs, Washington, DC	45	10	615	2152	558	57981	0	40881	23775	649
BAY SHORE—Suffolk County										
✸ SOUTHSIDE HOSPITAL, 301 East Main Street, Zip 11706–8458; tel. 516/968–3000; Theodore A. Jospe, President (Nonreporting) **A**1 3 5 9 10 **N** First Choice Network, Inc., Mineola, NY	23	10	463	—	—	—	—	—	—	—
BEACON—Dutchess County										
✸ CRAIG HOUSE CENTER, Howland Avenue, Zip 12508; tel. 914/831–1200; Peter L. Gosline, Administrator (Nonreporting) **A**1 10	33	22	61	—	—	—	—	—	—	—
BELLEROSE—Queens County, See New York City										
BETHPAGE—Nassau County										
☐ MID–ISLAND HOSPITAL, 4295 Hempstead Turnpike, Zip 11714–5769; tel. 516/579–6000; Robert J. Reed, President (Nonreporting) **A**1 9 10	33	10	223	—	—	—	—	—	—	—
BINGHAMTON—Broome County										
BINGHAMTON GENERAL HOSPITAL See United Health Services Hospitals Binghamton										
✸ BINGHAMTON PSYCHIATRIC CENTER, 425 Robinson Street, Zip 13901; tel. 607/724–1391; Margaret R. Dugan, Executive Director **A**1 3 10 **F**15 16 20 25 39 46 52 57 58 65 73 **P**6 **S** New York State Department of Mental Health, Albany, NY	12	22	269	208	273	45141	0	34210	22647	627
✸ OUR LADY OF LOURDES MEMORIAL HOSPITAL, 169 Riverside Drive, Zip 13905–4198; tel. 607/798–5328; Michael G. Guley, President and Chief Executive Officer **A**1 2 9 10 **F**5 6 7 8 12 14 15 16 17 19 22 23 24 25 26 27 28 29 30 31 32 33 34 35 36 37 38 39 40 41 42 44 45 46 49 51 53 60 63 65 66 67 71 72 73 74 **P**5 6 7 **S** Daughters of Charity National Health System, Saint Louis, MO	21	10	170	8997	152	—	1272	90124	42439	1147
✸ ○ UNITED HEALTH SERVICES HOSPITALS–BINGHAMTON, (Includes Binghamton General Hospital, Medicenter, 600 High Avenue, Endicott, Zip 13760; tel. 607/754–7171; Wilson Memorial Regional Medical Center, 33–57 Harrison Street, Johnson City, Zip 13790), 10–42 Mitchell Avenue, Zip 13903; tel. 607/763–6000; Matthew J. Salanger, President and Chief Executive Officer **A**1 2 3 5 8 9 10 11 **F**2 3 4 6 7 8 10 11 12 13 15 16 17 18 19 20 21 22 26 28 29 30 31 32 34 37 38 39 40 41 42 43 44 45 46 48 49 51 52 54 55 56 57 58 61 62 64 65 66 67 70 71 72 73 74 **P**1 6 7	23	10	516	18991	400	200009	1674	181196	77024	2407
BRENTWOOD—Suffolk County										
✸ PILGRIM PSYCHIATRIC CENTER, 998 Crooked Hill Road, Zip 11717–1087; tel. 516/761–2616; Alan M. Weinstock, MS, Chief Executive Officer **A**1 5 10 **F**9 11 12 14 15 16 17 18 19 20 21 22 25 26 34 35 37 39 40 42 43 44 45 46 48 50 52 54 55 56 57 58 60 63 64 65 67 71 73 74 **P**6 **S** New York State Department of Mental Health, Albany, NY	12	22	744	165	695	34703	0	75466	—	1684
BROCKPORT—Monroe County										
✸ LAKESIDE MEMORIAL HOSPITAL, 156 West Avenue, Zip 14420–1286; tel. 716/637–3131; Robert W. Harris, President **A**1 9 10 **F**1 2 3 4 5 6 7 8 9 10 11 12 13 14 15 16 17 18 19 20 21 22 23 24 25 26 27 28 29 30 31 32 33 34 35 36 37 38 39 40 41 42 43 44 45 46 47 48 49 50 51 52 53 54 55 56 57 58 59 60 61 62 63 64 65 66 67 68 69 70 71 72 73 74 **P**3 **N** Lake Ontario Rural Health Network, Medina, NY	23	10	72	2724	47	38232	406	—	—	267
BRONX—Bronx County, See New York City										
BRONXVILLE—Westchester County										
✸ LAWRENCE HOSPITAL, 55 Palmer Avenue, Zip 10708–3491; tel. 914/787–1000; Roger G. Dvorak, President **A**1 2 9 10 **F**7 8 11 12 16 17 19 21 22 26 30 32 33 34 35 36 37 39 40 41 42 44 45 46 48 49 63 65 66 67 71 73 **P**5 8 **N** Healthstar Network, Armonk, NY; The Excelcare System, Inc., Bronxville, NY; Columbia Presbyterian Regional Network, New York, NY	23	10	280	9169	179	29201	1490	68139	35727	868
BROOKLYN—Kings County, See New York City										
BUFFALO—Erie County										
☐ BRYLIN HOSPITALS, 1263 Delaware Avenue, Zip 14209; tel. 716/886–8200; Leonard Pleskow, Chairman **A**1 9 10 **F**2 3 52 53 54 55 56 57 58 59 **P**6	33	22	150	3246	119	24218	0	15256	8937	292
✸ BUFFALO GENERAL HOSPITAL, (Includes Buffalo Columbus Hospital, 300 Niagara Street, Zip 14201; tel. 716/845–4300; Andres Garcia, Chief Executive Officer), 100 High Street, Zip 14203–1154; tel. 716/859–5600; Carrie B. Frank, President and Chief Executive Officer (Total facility includes 242 beds in nursing home–type unit) **A**1 3 5 8 9 10 **F**2 3 4 5 7 8 10 11 12 14 15 16 19 20 21 22 23 26 29 30 31 32 33 34 35 37 38 40 41 42 43 44 46 48 49 50 51 52 53 54 55 56 57 58 60 61 62 64 65 69 71 72 73 74 **P**5 7 **N** Buffalo General Health System, Buffalo, NY	23	10	965	29287	798	265027	1728	269427	135118	3626

		Classi-fication Codes		Utilization Data					Expense (thousands) of dollars		
	Control	Service	Beds	Admissions	Census	Outpatient Visits	Births	Total	Payroll	Personnel

Legend:
★ American Hospital Association (AHA) membership
☐ Joint Commission on Accreditation of Healthcare Organizations (JCAHO) accreditation
+ American Osteopathic Hospital Association (AOHA) membership
○ American Osteopathic Association (AOA) accreditation
△ Commission on Accreditation of Rehabilitation Facilities (CARF) accreditation
Control codes 61, 63, 64, 71, 72 and 73 indicate hospitals listed by AOHA, but not registered by AHA. For definition of numerical codes, see page A4

Hospital	Control	Service	Beds	Admissions	Census	Outpatient Visits	Births	Total	Payroll	Personnel
✠ BUFFALO PSYCHIATRIC CENTER, 400 Forest Avenue, Zip 14213–1298; tel. 716/885–2261; George Molnar, M.D., Executive Director **A**1 10 **F**1 2 3 4 5 6 7 8 9 10 12 15 16 17 19 20 21 22 23 25 26 27 30 31 35 39 40 41 42 43 44 45 46 48 49 50 51 52 54 55 56 57 58 59 60 61 63 64 65 67 69 70 71 73 **P**1 **S** New York State Department of Mental Health, Albany, NY	12	22	323	200	348	68091	0	57594	40687	991
☐ CHILDREN'S HOSPITAL, 219 Bryant Street, Zip 14222–2099; tel. 716/878–7000; Joseph A. Ruffolo, President and Chief Executive Officer (Nonreporting) **A**1 3 5 9 10	23	59	313							
☐ ERIE COUNTY MEDICAL CENTER, 462 Grider Street, Zip 14215; tel. 716/898–3000; Paul J. Candino, Chief Executive Officer (Total facility includes 120 beds in nursing home–type unit) (Nonreporting) **A**1 3 5 9 10	13	10	550							
✠ MERCY HOSPITAL, 565 Abbott Road, Zip 14220; tel. 716/826–7000; James W. Connolly, President and Chief Executive Officer (Total facility includes 74 beds in nursing home–type unit) **A**1 3 5 9 10 **F**7 8 10 11 12 14 15 17 19 20 21 22 25 26 28 29 30 32 33 34 35 37 39 40 41 42 44 46 48 49 51 54 63 64 65 66 67 71 72 73 74 **P**6 8 **S** Eastern Mercy Health System, Radnor, PA	21	10	349	13772	249	274886	2448	110327	52520	1647
✠ MILLARD FILLMORE HEALTH SYSTEM, (Includes Millard Fillmore Suburban Hospital, 1540 Maple Road, Williamsville, Zip 14221; tel. 716/688–3100), 3 Gates Circle, Zip 14209–9986; tel. 716/887–4600; Carol M. Cassell, Executive Vice President and Chief Operating Officer (Total facility includes 75 beds in nursing home–type unit) (Nonreporting) **A**1 3 5 6 8 9 10 **N** Millard Fillmore Health System, Buffalo, NY	23	10	588							
☐ ROSWELL PARK CANCER INSTITUTE, (COMPREHENSIVE CANCER CENTER), Elm and Carlton Streets, Zip 14263–0001; tel. 716/845–2300; David C. Hohn, M.D., President and Chief Executive Officer **A**1 3 5 8 9 10 **F**8 15 16 17 19 20 21 25 28 29 30 31 32 33 34 35 37 39 41 42 44 45 46 49 50 53 54 60 63 65 67 69 71 73 74 **P**6	12	49	136	5240	105	101435	0	—	—	2022
☐ SHEEHAN MEMORIAL HOSPITAL, 425 Michigan Avenue, Zip 14203–2297; tel. 716/848–2000; Olivia Smith-Blackwell, M.D., M.P.H., President and Chief Executive Officer (Nonreporting) **A**1 9 10	23	10	109	—	—	—	—	—	—	—
✠ SISTERS OF CHARITY HOSPITAL OF BUFFALO, 2157 Main Street, Zip 14214–2692; tel. 716/862–1000; John J. Maher, President and Chief Executive Officer (Total facility includes 80 beds in nursing home–type unit) **A**1 3 5 6 9 10 12 13 **F**2 3 7 8 11 12 14 15 16 17 18 19 20 21 22 25 26 28 29 30 32 33 34 35 37 39 40 41 42 44 45 46 48 49 51 60 61 64 65 67 71 72 73 74 **P**3 **S** Daughters of Charity National Health System, Saint Louis, MO	21	10	493	12892	346	515783	2878	103102	50040	1713
✠ VETERANS AFFAIRS WESTERN NEW YORK HEALTHCARE SYSTEM, 3495 Bailey Avenue, Zip 14215–1129; tel. 716/834–9200; Richard S. Droske, Director (Total facility includes 158 beds in nursing home–type unit) **A**1 2 3 5 8 9 **F**1 2 3 4 8 10 11 12 14 17 18 19 20 21 22 24 25 26 27 28 29 30 31 32 33 34 35 37 39 41 42 43 44 45 46 48 49 50 51 52 54 55 56 57 58 59 60 61 63 64 65 67 69 71 72 73 74 **S** Department of Veterans Affairs, Washington, DC	45	10	611	7690	478	319402	0	153965	86452	2022
CAMBRIDGE—Washington County										
☐ MARY MCCLELLAN HOSPITAL, One Myrtle Avenue, Zip 12816; tel. 518/677–2611; Kathleen Lacasse, Chief Executive Officer (Total facility includes 39 beds in nursing home–type unit) (Nonreporting) **A**1 9 10	23	10	113							
CANANDAIGUA—Ontario County										
✠ F. F. THOMPSON HEALTH SYSTEM, 350 Parrish Street, Zip 14424–1793; tel. 716/396–6527; Linda M. Janczak, President and Chief Executive Officer (Total facility includes 188 beds in nursing home–type unit) **A**1 3 9 10 **F**1 7 8 14 15 16 19 21 22 25 28 29 30 34 35 37 39 40 41 42 44 45 49 64 65 66 67 71 72 73 74 **P**3 4 5 8	23	10	301	4394	249	138043	618	44036	23169	557
✠ VETERANS AFFAIRS MEDICAL CENTER, (LONG–TERM MEDICAL & PSYCHIATRY), 400 Fort Hill Avenue, Zip 14424–1197; tel. 716/396–3601; Stuart C. Collyer, Director (Total facility includes 150 beds in nursing home–type unit) **A**1 5 **F**2 3 12 16 17 19 20 22 26 27 28 30 31 33 37 41 46 49 51 52 54 55 56 57 58 59 64 65 67 71 73 74 **P**6 **S** Department of Veterans Affairs, Washington, DC	45	49	626	1990	602	81556	0	63792	41911	1119
CARMEL—Putnam County										
ARMS ACRES, 75 Seminary Hill Road, Zip 10512; tel. 914/225–3400; Edward Spauster, Ph.D., Executive Director (Nonreporting)	33	82	129	—	—	—	—	—	—	—
✠ PUTNAM HOSPITAL CENTER, Stoneleigh Avenue, Zip 10512–9948; tel. 914/279–5711; Rodney N. Hubbers, President and Chief Executive Officer (Nonreporting) **A**1 9 10 **N** Healthstar Network, Armonk, NY; Westchester Health Services Network, Mt Kisco, NY	23	10	164							
CARTHAGE—Jefferson County										
✠ CARTHAGE AREA HOSPITAL, 1001 West Street, Zip 13619–9703; tel. 315/493–1000; Kenn C. Rishel, Administrator and Chief Executive Officer (Total facility includes 30 beds in nursing home–type unit) (Nonreporting) **A**1 9 10 **N** Northern New York Rural Health Care Alliance, Watertown, NY	23	10	78							
CASTLE POINT—Dutchess County										
✠ VETERANS AFFAIRS MEDICAL CENTER, Zip 12511–9999; tel. 914/838–5190; William D. Montague, Acting Medical Center Director (Total facility includes 113 beds in nursing home–type unit) (Nonreporting) **A**1 3 **S** Department of Veterans Affairs, Washington, DC	45	10	233							
CHEEKTOWAGA—Erie County										
✠ ST. JOSEPH HOSPITAL, 2605 Harlem Road, Zip 14225–4097; tel. 716/891–2400; Patrick J. Wiles, Chief Executive Officer **A**1 9 10 **F**4 7 8 10 11 12 15 16 17 19 22 25 28 29 30 31 32 33 35 36 38 41 42 43 44 45 46 49 50 51 60 63 65 69 71 73 74 **P**3 6 8 **S** Eastern Mercy Health System, Radnor, PA	23	10	184	5560	118	194143	0	45866	22265	703

Hospital, Address, Telephone, Administrator, Approval, Facility, and Physician Codes, Health Care System, Network	Classi-fication Codes		Utilization Data					Expense (thousands) of dollars		
★ American Hospital Association (AHA) membership □ Joint Commission on Accreditation of Healthcare Organizations (JCAHO) accreditation + American Osteopathic Hospital Association (AOHA) membership ○ American Osteopathic Association (AOA) accreditation △ Commission on Accreditation of Rehabilitation Facilities (CARF) accreditation Control codes 61, 63, 64, 71, 72 and 73 indicate hospitals listed by AOHA, but not registered by AHA. For definition of numerical codes, see page A4	Control	Service	Beds	Admissions	Census	Outpatient Visits	Births	Total	Payroll	Personnel

CLIFTON SPRINGS—Ontario County
★ CLIFTON SPRINGS HOSPITAL AND CLINIC, 2 Coulter Road, Zip 14432–1189; tel. 315/462–1311; John P. Galati, President and Chief Executive Officer (Total facility includes 108 beds in nursing home–type unit) **A**1 9 10 **F**2 3 4 8 10 14 15 16 17 19 21 22 25 26 27 28 29 30 32 33 34 35 36 37 39 41 42 44 45 46 49 51 52 54 56 57 58 59 60 64 65 66 67 71 73 74 **P**7 | 23 | 10 | 262 | 3432 | 180 | 127924 | 0 | 32720 | 17204 | 641

COBLESKILL—Schoharie County
□ BASSETT HOSPITAL OF SCHOHARIE COUNTY, 41 Grandview Drive, Zip 12043–1331; tel. 518/234–2511; James J. Morrissey, Jr., Administrator (Nonreporting) **A**1 9 10 | 23 | 10 | 40 | — | — | — | — | — | — | —

COOPERSTOWN—Otsego County
★ MARY IMOGENE BASSETT HOSPITAL, (Includes O'Connor Hospital Division, Andes Road, Route 28, Delhi, Zip 13753; tel. 607/746–2371), One Atwell Road, Zip 13326–1394; tel. 607/547–3100; William F. Streck, M.D., President and Chief Executive Officer **A**1 2 3 5 8 9 10 **F**7 8 10 12 14 15 16 19 20 21 22 25 29 30 31 34 35 37 39 40 41 42 44 45 46 49 51 52 53 54 55 56 58 59 60 61 63 65 66 67 70 71 73 **P**6 **N** Bassett Healthcare, Cooperstown, NY | 23 | 10 | 208 | 8283 | 117 | 434253 | 607 | 132800 | 73339 | 1903

CORNING—Steuben County
★ CORNING HOSPITAL, 176 Denison Parkway East, Zip 14830; tel. 607/937–7200; John E. Pignatore, President and Chief Executive Officer (Total facility includes 120 beds in nursing home–type unit) (Nonreporting) **A**1 9 10 | 23 | 10 | 274 | — | — | — | — | — | — | —

CORNWALL—Orange County
★ CORNWALL HOSPITAL, Laurel Avenue, Zip 12518–1499; tel. 914/534–7711; Val S. Gray, Executive Director **A**1 9 10 **F**11 14 15 16 17 19 20 22 28 29 30 35 37 44 49 52 54 56 63 65 67 68 71 73 **N** Columbia Presbyterian Regional Network, New York, NY | 23 | 10 | 125 | 3768 | 80 | 39717 | 0 | 27484 | 14201 | 391

CORTLAND—Cortland County
★ CORTLAND MEMORIAL HOSPITAL, 134 Homer Avenue, Zip 13045–0960; tel. 607/756–3500; Thomas H. Carman, President and Chief Executive Officer (Total facility includes 82 beds in nursing home–type unit) **A**1 9 10 **F**1 7 8 15 17 19 21 22 24 26 28 30 32 35 37 40 41 44 45 46 49 52 54 56 63 64 65 66 67 71 73 74 **P**5 **N** Cortland Area Rural Health Network, Cortland, NY | 23 | 10 | 259 | 5290 | 171 | 117333 | 684 | 38473 | 17983 | 698

CUBA—Allegany County
□ CUBA MEMORIAL HOSPITAL, 140 West Main Street, Zip 14727–1398; tel. 716/968–2000; Darlene D. Bainbridge, Interim Chief Executive Officer (Total facility includes 61 beds in nursing home–type unit) (Nonreporting) **A**1 3 9 | 23 | 10 | 87 | — | — | — | — | — | — | —

DANSVILLE—Livingston County
★ NICHOLAS H. NOYES MEMORIAL HOSPITAL, 111 Clara Barton Street, Zip 14437–9527; tel. 716/335–6001; Diane L. Rogler, President and Chief Executive Officer **A**1 9 10 **F**8 17 19 22 35 36 37 39 40 44 65 71 73 **P**3 | 23 | 10 | 65 | 2583 | 35 | 77790 | 265 | 17833 | 8316 | 322

DELHI—Delaware County
O'CONNOR HOSPITAL DIVISION See Mary Imogene Bassett Hospital, Cooperstown

DIX HILLS—Suffolk County
★ SAGAMORE CHILDREN'S PSYCHIATRIC CENTER, 197 Half Hollow Road, Zip 11746; tel. 516/673–7700; Robert Schweitzer, Ed.D., Executive Director **A**1 **F**12 14 15 16 19 21 22 32 35 39 45 46 52 53 54 55 58 65 71 73 **S** New York State Department of Mental Health, Albany, NY | 12 | 52 | 69 | 201 | 63 | 36068 | 0 | 15767 | 11344 | 238

DOBBS FERRY—Westchester County
□ COMMUNITY HOSPITAL AT DOBBS FERRY, 128 Ashford Avenue, Zip 10522; tel. 914/693–0700; Thomas E. Green, President and Chief Executive Officer (Nonreporting) **A**1 9 10 | 23 | 10 | 50 | — | — | — | — | — | — | —

DUNKIRK—Chautauqua County
★ BROOKS MEMORIAL HOSPITAL, 529 Central Avenue, Zip 14048–2599; tel. 716/366–1111; Richard H. Ketcham, President (Nonreporting) **A**1 9 10 | 23 | 10 | 133 | — | — | — | — | — | — | —

EAST MEADOW—Nassau County
★ NASSAU COUNTY MEDICAL CENTER, 2201 Hempstead Turnpike, Zip 11554–1854; tel. 516/572–0123; Joseph R. Erazo, Chief Executive Officer (Total facility includes 809 beds in nursing home–type unit) (Nonreporting) **A**1 2 3 5 8 9 10 12 **N** Health First, New York, NY | 13 | 10 | 1384 | — | — | — | — | — | — | —

ELIZABETHTOWN—Essex County
★ ELIZABETHTOWN COMMUNITY HOSPITAL, Park Street, Zip 12932–0277; tel. 518/873–6377; Anthony W. Deobil, Administrator **A**1 9 10 **F**1 3 4 7 8 10 12 13 15 17 18 19 21 22 25 26 27 28 30 31 32 33 34 36 37 39 41 42 44 45 46 49 51 60 61 65 66 67 68 71 72 73 74 **P**3 5 7 **N** Eastern Adirondack Health Care Network, Westport, NY | 23 | 10 | 25 | 438 | 15 | 20952 | 0 | 4267 | 2599 | 89

ELLENVILLE—Ulster County
□ ELLENVILLE COMMUNITY HOSPITAL, Route 209, Zip 12428–0668, Mailing Address: P.O. Box 668, Zip 12428–0668; tel. 914/647–6400; Thomas H. Fletcher, Administrator (Nonreporting) **A**1 9 10 | 23 | 10 | 31 | — | — | — | — | — | — | —

ELMHURST—Queens County, See New York City

ELMIRA—Chemung County
★ ARNOT OGDEN MEDICAL CENTER, 600 Roe Avenue, Zip 14905–1629; tel. 607/737–4100; Anthony J. Cooper, President and Chief Executive Officer (Total facility includes 40 beds in nursing home–type unit) **A**1 2 6 9 10 **F**4 7 8 10 11 14 15 16 17 19 21 22 25 26 27 28 29 30 31 34 35 37 38 39 41 42 43 44 45 46 49 51 54 60 63 64 65 67 68 70 71 72 73 74 **P**6 | 23 | 10 | 271 | 7846 | 176 | 179304 | 1296 | 82226 | 40953 | 1129

Hospital, Address, Telephone, Administrator, Approval, Facility, and Physician Codes, Health Care System, Network	Classification Codes		Utilization Data					Expense (thousands) of dollars		
	Control	Service	Beds	Admissions	Census	Outpatient Visits	Births	Total	Payroll	Personnel
★ American Hospital Association (AHA) membership □ Joint Commission on Accreditation of Healthcare Organizations (JCAHO) accreditation + American Osteopathic Hospital Association (AOHA) membership ○ American Osteopathic Association (AOA) accreditation △ Commission on Accreditation of Rehabilitation Facilities (CARF) accreditation Control codes 61, 63, 64, 71, 72 and 73 indicate hospitals listed by AOHA, but not registered by AHA. For definition of numerical codes, see page A4										
◰ ELMIRA PSYCHIATRIC CENTER, 100 Washington Street, Zip 14901–2898; tel. 607/737–4739; Bert W. Pyle, Jr., Director A1 10 F1 12 14 15 16 17 18 20 25 26 34 41 52 53 54 55 56 57 58 59 65 73 P1 S New York State Department of Mental Health, Albany, NY	12	22	161	360	161	4720	0	13882	10723	475
◰ ST. JOSEPH'S HOSPITAL, (Includes Twin Tiers Rehabilitation Center), 555 East Market Street, Zip 14902–1512; tel. 607/733–6541; Sister Marie Castagnaro, President and Chief Executive Officer (Total facility includes 31 beds in nursing home–type unit) A1 2 9 10 F2 3 8 9 11 12 14 15 16 17 18 19 21 22 23 26 28 30 31 33 34 35 37 39 41 42 44 45 46 48 49 51 52 54 55 56 57 58 62 64 65 66 67 69 70 71 73 S Carondelet Health System, Saint Louis, MO	21	10	255	5362	172	92106	0	—	—	794
ENDICOTT—Broome County MEDICENTER See United Health Services Hospitals–Binghamton, Binghamton										
FAR ROCKAWAY—Queens County, See New York City										
FLUSHING—Queens County, See New York City										
FOREST HILLS—Queens County, See New York City										
FULTON—Oswego County ◰ ALBERT LINDLEY LEE MEMORIAL HOSPITAL, 510 South Fourth Street, Zip 13069–2994; tel. 315/592–2224; Dennis A. Casey, Executive Director A1 9 10 F3 4 8 10 16 19 20 21 22 25 28 29 30 31 32 34 37 41 42 44 45 51 53 54 55 56 57 58 59 63 65 66 67 69 71 73 N Oswego County Rural Health Network, Oswego, NY	23	10	67	2326	44	43230	0	17012	8353	288
GENEVA—Ontario County ◰ GENEVA GENERAL HOSPITAL, 196 North Street, Zip 14456–1694; tel. 315/787–4000; James J. Dooley, President (Total facility includes 343 beds in nursing home–type unit) A1 6 9 10 F1 2 4 7 8 10 12 14 15 16 17 19 21 22 25 26 27 28 29 30 31 32 33 34 35 36 37 39 40 41 42 44 46 49 51 54 56 62 64 65 67 68 69 71 72 73 74 N Four Lakes Rural Health Network, Geneva, NY	23	10	479	4783	373	249502	685	51991	23156	858
GLEN COVE—Nassau County ◰ NORTH SHORE UNIVERSITY HOSPITAL AT GLEN COVE, St. Andrews Lane, Zip 11542; tel. 516/674–7300; Mark R. Stenzler, Vice President Administration (Nonreporting) A1 2 3 5 9 10 S North Shore Health System, Manhasset, NY N North Shore Regional Health Systems, Manhasset, NY	23	10	265	—	—	—	—	—	—	—
GLEN OAKS—Queens County, See New York City										
GLENS FALLS—Warren County □ GLENS FALLS HOSPITAL, 100 Park Street, Zip 12801–9898; tel. 518/792–3151; David G. Kruczlnicki, President and Chief Executive Officer (Nonreporting) A1 2 9 10 N Adirondack Rural Health Network, Glens Falls, NY; Shared Health Network, Inc., Albany, NY	23	10	442	—	—	—	—	—	—	—
GLENVILLE—Schenectady County CONIFER PARK, 79 Glenridge Road, Zip 12302; tel. 518/399–6446; Jack Duffy, Executive Director (Nonreporting) A9	33	82	225	—	—	—	—	—	—	—
GLOVERSVILLE—Fulton County □ NATHAN LITTAUER HOSPITAL AND NURSING HOME, 99 East State Street, Zip 12078; tel. 518/725–8621; Thomas J. Dowd, President (Total facility includes 84 beds in nursing home–type unit) A1 5 9 10 F3 4 7 8 10 12 14 15 16 17 18 19 20 21 22 25 26 28 29 30 31 32 33 34 35 37 39 40 41 42 44 45 46 49 51 53 54 55 56 57 58 61 64 65 67 71 73 74 P6 N Shared Health Network, Inc., Albany, NY	23	10	208	4503	152	110044	353	35934	19051	571
GOSHEN—Orange County ◰ ARDEN HILL HOSPITAL, 4 Harriman Drive, Zip 10924–2499; tel. 914/294–5441; A. Gordon McAleer, President A1 9 10 F2 7 8 11 12 15 16 17 19 21 22 28 30 33 34 35 37 40 41 42 44 52 53 54 55 56 57 62 63 65 67 71 73 74 P5 N The Mount Sinai Health System, New York, NY	23	10	176	6591	135	66237	714	42257	20105	580
GOUVERNEUR—St. Lawrence County □ EDWARD JOHN NOBLE HOSPITAL OF GOUVERNEUR, 77 West Barney Street, Zip 13642; tel. 315/287–1000; Charles P. Conole, FACHE, Administrator A1 9 10 F7 8 9 11 12 13 14 15 16 17 18 19 20 21 22 26 28 29 30 32 33 34 35 36 37 38 39 40 41 42 43 44 45 46 47 49 52 53 54 56 57 60 61 65 71 74 P5 N Northern New York Rural Health Care Alliance, Watertown, NY	23	10	47	1508	24	24718	64	9455	4827	189
GOWANDA—Cattaraugus County □ TRI-COUNTY MEMORIAL HOSPITAL, 100 Memorial Drive, Zip 14070–1194; tel. 716/532–3377; Diane J. Osika, Interim Chief Executive Officer A1 9 10 F1 2 3 4 5 6 7 8 9 10 11 12 13 15 16 17 19 20 21 22 23 24 25 26 27 28 30 31 32 33 34 35 37 38 39 40 41 42 43 44 45 46 47 48 49 50 51 52 53 54 55 56 57 58 59 60 61 64 65 67 69 70 71 72 73 74 P5 N Buffalo General Health System, Buffalo, NY	23	10	48	1492	38	44885	0	11414	6250	208
GREENPORT—Suffolk County □ EASTERN LONG ISLAND HOSPITAL, 201 Manor Place, Zip 11944–1298; tel. 516/477–1000; John M. Gwiazda, President and Chief Executive Officer (Nonreporting) A1 9 10 N First Choice Network, Inc., Mineola, NY	23	10	80	—	—	—	—	—	—	—
HAMILTON—Madison County ◰ COMMUNITY MEMORIAL HOSPITAL, Broad Street, Zip 13346–9518; tel. 315/824–1100; David Felton, Administrator (Total facility includes 40 beds in nursing home–type unit) (Nonreporting) A1 9 10 N Hamilton–Bassett–Crouse Rural Health Network, Hamilton, NY	23	10	84	—	—	—	—	—	—	—

Hospital, Address, Telephone, Administrator, Approval, Facility, and Physician Codes, Health Care System, Network	Classi-fication Codes		Utilization Data					Expense (thousands) of dollars		
	Control	Service	Beds	Admissions	Census	Outpatient Visits	Births	Total	Payroll	Personnel

★ American Hospital Association (AHA) membership
□ Joint Commission on Accreditation of Healthcare Organizations (JCAHO) accreditation
+ American Osteopathic Hospital Association (AOHA) membership
○ American Osteopathic Association (AOA) accreditation
△ Commission on Accreditation of Rehabilitation Facilities (CARF) accreditation
Control codes 61, 63, 64, 71, 72 and 73 indicate hospitals listed by AOHA, but not registered by AHA. For definition of numerical codes, see page A4.

HARRIS—Sullivan County

□ COMMUNITY GENERAL HOSPITAL OF SULLIVAN COUNTY, Bushville Road, Zip 12742, Mailing Address: P.O. Box 800, Zip 12742–0800; tel. 914/794–3300; Martin I. Richman, Executive Director (Total facility includes 40 beds in nursing home–type unit) (Nonreporting) **A**1 9 10 **N** Sullivan County Rural Health Network, Harris, NY
23 10 244 — — — — — — —

HEMPSTEAD—Nassau County

□ HEMPSTEAD GENERAL HOSPITAL MEDICAL CENTER, 800 Front Street, Zip 11550–4600; tel. 516/560–1200; Alexander Skutzka, Chief Executive Officer (Nonreporting) **A**1 9 10
32 10 213 — — — — — — —

HOLLISWOOD—Queens County, See New York City

HORNELL—Steuben County

✠ ST. JAMES MERCY HOSPITAL, 411 Canisteo Street, Zip 14843–2197; tel. 607/324–8000; Paul E. Shephard, President and Chief Executive Officer (Total facility includes 55 beds in nursing home–type unit) (Nonreporting) **A**1 6 9 10 **S** Eastern Mercy Health System, Radnor, PA
23 10 200 — — — — — — —

HUDSON—Columbia County

✠ COLUMBIA MEMORIAL HOSPITAL, (Includes Columbia–Greene Long Term Care, 161 Jefferson Heights, Catskill, Zip 12414; tel. 518/943–6363), 71 Prospect Avenue, Zip 12534; tel. 518/828–8244; Jane Ehrlich, President and Chief Executive Officer (Total facility includes 120 beds in nursing home–type unit) (Nonreporting) **A**1 9 10 **N** Greene County Rural Health Network, Catskill, NY
23 10 251 — — — — — — —

HUNTINGTON—Suffolk County

✠ HUNTINGTON HOSPITAL, 270 Park Avenue, Zip 11743–2799; tel. 516/351–2200; J. Ronald Gaudreault, President and Chief Executive Officer **A**1 9 10 **F**4 7 8 11 14 15 16 19 21 22 25 26 28 30 34 36 37 39 40 42 44 46 52 54 60 61 63 65 67 70 71 73 74 **P**5 7 8 **S** North Shore Health System, Manhasset, NY **N** North Shore Regional Health Systems, Manhasset, NY
23 10 269 11908 218 108267 1773 99118 52223 1180

IRVING—Chautauqua County

LAKE SHORE HOSPITAL, 845 Route 5 and 20, Zip 14081–9716; tel. 716/934–2654; James B. Foster, Chief Executive Officer (Total facility includes 120 beds in nursing home–type unit) **A**9 10 **F**1 12 15 16 17 19 22 30 32 33 35 37 44 45 49 52 56 64 65 69 71 **P**3 5 8 **N** Millard Fillmore Health System, Buffalo, NY
23 10 182 2279 169 39993 0 19992 9332 383

ITHACA—Tompkins County

✠ CAYUGA MEDICAL CENTER AT ITHACA, 101 Dates Drive, Zip 14850–1383; tel. 607/274–4011; Bonnie H. Howell, President and Chief Executive Officer **A**1 2 3 5 10 **F**2 7 8 11 14 15 16 17 19 22 24 25 28 29 30 31 32 34 35 36 37 39 40 41 42 44 45 46 47 48 49 51 52 56 57 61 62 65 66 67 71 72 73 74 **P**1 5 7
23 10 142 6246 92 141892 769 42163 18884 616

JACKSON HEIGHTS—Queens County, See New York City

JAMAICA—Queens County, See New York City

JAMESTOWN—Chautauqua County

✠ WOMAN'S CHRISTIAN ASSOCIATION HOSPITAL, 207 Foote Avenue, Zip 14702–9975; tel. 716/487–0141; Mark E. Celmer, President and Chief Executive Officer **A**1 2 9 10 **F**2 3 7 8 12 13 15 16 18 19 20 21 22 25 29 30 31 34 35 37 40 41 42 44 46 48 49 51 52 53 54 55 56 58 59 60 63 65 66 67 69 70 71 73 74 **N** Great Lakes Health Network, Erie, PA
23 10 311 10377 220 184462 819 72729 35642 1354

JOHNSON CITY—Broome County

WILSON MEMORIAL REGIONAL MEDICAL CENTER See United Health Services Hospitals–Binghamton, Binghamton

KATONAH—Westchester County

✠ FOUR WINDS HOSPITAL, 800 Cross River Road, Zip 10536; tel. 914/763–8151; Samuel C. Klagsbrun, M.D., Executive Medical Director **A**1 9 10 **F**3 12 15 16 17 19 21 22 26 27 31 34 35 41 50 52 53 54 55 56 57 58 59 63 65 67 71 73 **P**5 7
33 22 136 1660 129 7935 0 — — —

KENMORE—Erie County

✠ KENMORE MERCY HOSPITAL, 2950 Elmwood Avenue, Zip 14217–1390; tel. 716/447–6100; Sister Mary Joel Schimscheiner, Chief Executive Officer **A**1 9 10 **F**5 8 10 11 12 14 15 16 17 18 19 22 25 26 28 29 30 32 33 34 35 36 39 41 42 44 45 46 49 51 61 65 66 71 73 74 **P**1 5 **S** Eastern Mercy Health System, Radnor, PA
21 10 219 7350 146 172584 0 56233 25787 880

KINGSTON—Ulster County

✠ BENEDICTINE HOSPITAL, 105 Marys Avenue, Zip 12401–5894; tel. 914/338–2500; Sister Louise Garley, President **A**1 3 5 9 10 **F**7 8 11 14 15 16 17 19 21 22 27 30 34 37 40 42 44 46 49 51 52 56 57 63 65 67 71 73 74
21 10 222 7087 144 55618 1036 47381 24320 661

□ KINGSTON HOSPITAL, 396 Broadway, Zip 12401; tel. 914/331–3131; Anthony P. Marmo, Chief Executive Officer (Nonreporting) **A**1 3 5 9 10
23 10 140 — — — — — — —

LACKAWANNA—Erie County

✠ OUR LADY OF VICTORY HOSPITAL, 55 Melroy at Ridge Road, Zip 14218–1687; tel. 716/825–8000; John P. Davanzo, President and Chief Executive Officer (Total facility includes 10 beds in nursing home–type unit) (Nonreporting) **A**1 9 10
21 10 232 — — — — — — —

LEWISTON—Niagara County

✠ MOUNT ST. MARY'S HOSPITAL OF NIAGARA FALLS, 5300 Military Road, Zip 14092–1997; tel. 716/297–4800; Angelo G. Calbone, President and Chief Executive Officer **A**1 10 **F**2 3 7 8 11 14 15 16 19 20 21 22 25 30 31 33 35 37 39 40 44 46 49 51 56 59 61 65 67 71 73 **P**7
21 10 159 5715 118 190521 337 41357 19600 634

Hospital, Address, Telephone, Administrator, Approval, Facility, and Physician Codes, Health Care System, Network	Classification Codes		Utilization Data					Expense (thousands) of dollars		
	Control	Service	Beds	Admissions	Census	Outpatient Visits	Births	Total	Payroll	Personnel

★ American Hospital Association (AHA) membership
□ Joint Commission on Accreditation of Healthcare Organizations (JCAHO) accreditation
+ American Osteopathic Hospital Association (AOHA) membership
○ American Osteopathic Association (AOA) accreditation
△ Commission on Accreditation of Rehabilitation Facilities (CARF) accreditation
Control codes 61, 63, 64, 71, 72 and 73 indicate hospitals listed by AOHA, but not registered by AHA. For definition of numerical codes, see page A4

LITTLE FALLS—Herkimer County

☒ LITTLE FALLS HOSPITAL, 140 Burwell Street, Zip 13365–1725; tel. 315/823–1000; David S. Armstrong, Jr., Administrator (Total facility includes 34 beds in nursing home–type unit) **A**1 9 10 **F**1 3 4 5 6 7 8 10 12 13 14 15 17 18 19 20 21 22 23 24 25 26 27 28 29 30 31 32 33 34 35 36 37 38 39 40 41 42 44 45 46 47 48 49 50 51 52 53 54 55 56 57 58 59 60 61 62 63 64 65 66 67 68 69 70 71 72 73 74 **P**3 4 5 | 23 | 10 | 134 | 3560 | 91 | 63417 | 347 | 18116 | 9687 | 401

LITTLE NECK—Queens County, See New York City
LOCKPORT—Niagara County

☒ LOCKPORT MEMORIAL HOSPITAL, 521 East Avenue, Zip 14094–3299; tel. 716/434–9111; Michael J. Vlosky, President and Chief Executive Officer **A**1 9 10 **F**2 3 8 17 19 22 25 28 29 30 32 33 34 35 37 40 41 42 44 45 46 49 51 65 66 71 73 74 **P**1 5 | 23 | 10 | 134 | 4559 | 74 | 104018 | 433 | 34038 | 14027 | 391

LONG BEACH—Nassau County

☒ LONG BEACH MEDICAL CENTER, 455 East Bay Drive, Zip 11561–2300, Mailing Address: P.O. Box 300, Zip 11561–2300; tel. 516/897–1200; Martin F. Nester, Jr., Chief Executive Officer (Total facility includes 200 beds in nursing home–type unit) **A**1 9 10 12 13 **F**3 4 5 8 11 14 15 16 17 18 19 20 21 22 24 25 26 27 28 29 30 31 32 34 35 37 39 41 44 45 46 48 49 51 52 53 54 55 56 57 58 63 64 65 66 67 68 71 73 74 **P**1 **N** The Mount Sinai Health System, New York, NY | 23 | 10 | 372 | 5848 | 360 | 151514 | 0 | 74759 | 39424 | 931

LONG ISLAND CITY—Queens County, See New York City
LOWVILLE—Lewis County

☒ LEWIS COUNTY GENERAL HOSPITAL, 7785 North State Street, Zip 13367–1297; tel. 315/376–5200; G. William Udovich, Chief Executive Officer and Administrator (Total facility includes 160 beds in nursing home–type unit) (Nonreporting) **A**1 9 10 **S** Brim, Inc., Portland, OR | 13 | 10 | 214 | — | — | — | — | — | — | —

MALONE—Franklin County

☒ ALICE HYDE HOSPITAL ASSOCIATION, 115 Park Street, Zip 12953–0729, Mailing Address: P.O. Box 729, Zip 12953–0729; tel. 518/483–3000; John W. Johnson, President and Chief Executive Officer (Total facility includes 75 beds in nursing home–type unit) **A**1 9 10 **F**1 3 7 8 12 13 15 17 18 19 20 22 23 26 28 30 32 33 34 35 36 37 39 40 41 42 44 46 53 54 56 57 58 60 64 65 67 71 73 | 23 | 10 | 153 | 3791 | 121 | 70299 | 293 | 22914 | 11698 | 379

MANHASSET—Nassau County

MANHASSET AMBULATORY CARE PAVILION See Long Island Jewish Medical Center, New York

☒ NORTH SHORE UNIVERSITY HOSPITAL, 300 Community Drive, Zip 11030; tel. 516/562–0100; John S. T. Gallagher, President (Total facility includes 253 beds in nursing home–type unit) (Nonreporting) **A**1 2 3 5 8 9 10 **S** North Shore Health System, Manhasset, NY **N** North Shore Regional Health Systems, Manhasset, NY | 23 | 10 | 958 | — | — | — | — | — | — | —

MANHATTAN—New York County, See New York City
MARGARETVILLE—Delaware County

□ MARGARETVILLE MEMORIAL HOSPITAL, Route 28, Zip 12455, Mailing Address: P.O. Box 200, Zip 12455; tel. 914/586–2631; Christine Wasyl, Chief Executive Officer (Nonreporting) **A**1 9 10 | 23 | 10 | 22 | — | — | — | — | — | — | —

MASSENA—St. Lawrence County

□ MASSENA MEMORIAL HOSPITAL, One Hospital Drive, Zip 13662; tel. 315/764–1711; Charles F. Fahd, II, Chief Executive Officer (Nonreporting) **A**1 10 | 14 | 10 | 40 | — | — | — | — | — | — | —

MEDINA—Orleans County

☒ MEDINA MEMORIAL HOSPITAL, 200 Ohio Street, Zip 14103; tel. 716/798–2000; Walter S. Becker, Administrator (Total facility includes 30 beds in nursing home–type unit) **A**1 9 10 **F**5 7 8 13 14 15 16 17 19 21 22 25 28 29 30 32 33 34 37 39 40 41 44 45 46 48 49 51 56 64 65 67 68 71 73 **P**3 5 **N** Lake Ontario Rural Health Network, Medina, NY | 23 | 10 | 101 | 2248 | 32 | 91047 | 245 | 18945 | 8626 | 327

MIDDLETOWN—Orange County

☒ △ HORTON MEDICAL CENTER, 60 Prospect Avenue, Zip 10940–4133; tel. 914/343–2424; Paul Dell Uomo, President and Chief Executive Officer **A**1 7 9 10 **F**3 7 8 12 16 17 19 21 22 23 27 28 30 34 35 37 39 40 42 44 46 48 49 51 56 60 61 63 65 67 71 73 74 **P**1 5 **N** Columbia Presbyterian Regional Network, New York, NY | 23 | 10 | 168 | 9698 | 153 | 118393 | 1555 | 72531 | 36518 | 903

☒ MIDDLETOWN PSYCHIATRIC CENTER, 141 Monhagen Avenue, Zip 10940; tel. 914/342–5511; James Bopp, Executive Director **A**1 3 10 **F**2 3 4 8 9 11 12 15 16 18 19 20 21 22 23 25 26 27 30 31 35 37 39 40 41 42 43 44 45 46 48 52 55 56 57 58 59 60 64 65 67 70 71 73 **S** New York State Department of Mental Health, Albany, NY | 12 | 22 | 271 | 199 | 304 | 40767 | 0 | 37169 | 26326 | 630

MINEOLA—Nassau County

☒ WINTHROP–UNIVERSITY HOSPITAL, 259 First Street, Zip 11501; tel. 516/663–2200; Martin J. Delaney, President and Chief Executive Officer **A**1 2 3 5 8 9 10 **F**3 4 7 8 10 12 13 14 15 16 17 18 19 21 22 26 27 28 29 30 31 32 34 35 36 37 38 39 40 41 42 43 44 45 46 49 54 60 61 63 65 67 68 70 71 73 74 **P**5 6 7 **N** First Choice Network, Inc., Mineola, NY | 23 | 10 | 518 | 25435 | 485 | 193012 | 5183 | 279311 | 135965 | 3288

MONTOUR FALLS—Schuyler County

☒ SCHUYLER HOSPITAL, 220 Steuben Street, Zip 14865–9709; tel. 607/535–7121; Robert M. Swinnerton, President and Chief Executive Officer (Total facility includes 120 beds in nursing home–type unit) (Nonreporting) **A**1 9 10 | 23 | 10 | 169 | — | — | — | — | — | — | —

Hospital, Address, Telephone, Administrator, Approval, Facility, and Physician Codes, Health Care System, Network	Classi-fication Codes		Utilization Data					Expense (thousands) of dollars		
★ American Hospital Association (AHA) membership □ Joint Commission on Accreditation of Healthcare Organizations (JCAHO) accreditation + American Osteopathic Hospital Association (AOHA) membership ○ American Osteopathic Association (AOA) accreditation △ Commission on Accreditation of Rehabilitation Facilities (CARF) accreditation Control codes 61, 63, 64, 71, 72 and 73 indicate hospitals listed by AOHA, but not registered by AHA. For definition of numerical codes, see page A4	Control	Service	Beds	Admissions	Census	Outpatient Visits	Births	Total	Payroll	Personnel

MONTROSE—Westchester County

★ FRANKLIN DELANO ROOSEVELT VETERANS AFFAIRS HOSPITAL, Route 9A, Zip 10548; Mailing Address: P.O. Box 100, Zip 10548; tel. 914/737–4400; William D. Montague, Director (Total facility includes 162 beds in nursing home–type unit) **A**1 3 5 **F**1 2 3 4 5 6 8 10 11 12 17 18 19 20 21 22 23 24 26 27 28 29 30 31 32 33 34 35 37 39 41 42 43 44 45 46 48 49 50 51 52 54 55 56 57 58 59 60 63 64 65 67 70 71 73 74 **S** Department of Veterans Affairs, Washington, DC
| | 45 | 22 | 550 | 2903 | 461 | 86185 | 0 | 90919 | 55684 | 1300 |

MOUNT KISCO—Westchester County

★ NORTHERN WESTCHESTER HOSPITAL CENTER, 400 Main Street, Zip 10549; tel. 914/666–1200; Donald W. Davis, President **A**1 2 9 10 **F**7 8 11 12 16 19 21 22 23 26 28 29 30 31 33 35 37 38 39 40 41 42 44 45 46 49 52 53 54 55 56 57 60 61 65 67 71 73 74 **P**7 8 **N** Healthstar Network, Armonk, NY; Westchester Health Services Network, Mt Kisco, NY
| | 23 | 10 | 259 | 9133 | 162 | 61632 | 1731 | 77826 | 38694 | 853 |

MOUNT VERNON—Westchester County

□ MOUNT VERNON HOSPITAL, 12 North Seventh Avenue, Zip 10550; tel. 914/664–8000; Richard L. Petrillo, M.D., Executive Director (Nonreporting) **A**1 3 5 6 9 10
| | 23 | 10 | 182 | — | — | — | — | — | — | — |

NEW HAMPTON—Orange County

□ MID–HUDSON PSYCHIATRIC CENTER, Mailing Address: P.O. Box 158, Zip 10958; tel. 914/374–3171; Richard Bennett, Executive Director **A**1 **F**4 8 9 11 12 19 20 21 22 24 27 29 30 35 37 38 39 40 41 42 43 44 45 46 48 50 52 54 55 60 63 64 65 67 70 71 **P**6
| | 12 | 22 | 279 | 379 | 284 | 0 | 0 | — | — | 529 |

NEW HYDE PARK—Queens County, See New York City

NEW ROCHELLE—Westchester County

★ SOUND SHORE MEDICAL CENTER OF WESTCHESTER, (Formerly New Rochelle Hospital Medical Center), 16 Guion Place, Zip 10802; tel. 914/632–5000; John R. Spicer, President and Chief Executive Officer **A**1 2 3 5 8 9 10 **F**1 3 7 8 12 13 14 15 16 17 18 19 21 22 26 27 28 29 30 31 32 33 34 35 36 37 38 39 40 41 42 44 45 46 48 49 51 53 54 55 56 57 58 60 61 63 64 65 66 67 68 69 70 71 72 73 **P**4 5 6 7 8 **N** Westchester Health Services Network, Mt Kisco, NY
| | 23 | 10 | 257 | 9805 | 186 | 207009 | 1115 | 99682 | 47299 | 1076 |

NEW YORK (Includes all hospitals located within the five boroughs)
    BRONX - Bronx County (Mailing Address - Bronx)
    BROOKLYN - Kings County (Mailing Address - Brooklyn)
    MANHATTAN - New York County (Mailing Address - New York)
    QUEENS - Queens County (Mailing Addresses - Bellerose, Elmhurst, Far Rockaway, Flushing, Forest Hills, Glen Oaks, Holliswood, Jackson Heights, Jamaica, Little Neck, Long Island City, New Hyde Park, and Queens Village)
    RICHMOND VALLEY - Richmond County (Mailing Address - Staten Island)
    ABRAHAM JACOBI GENERAL CARE HOSPITAL AND PSYCHIATIC UNITS See Jacobi Medical Center

★ BAYLEY SETON HOSPITAL, 75 Vanderbilt Avenue, Staten Island, Zip 10304–3850; tel. 718/354–6000; Dominick M. Stanzione, Chief Operating Officer and Executive Vice President **A**1 2 3 5 9 10 **F**2 3 4 5 6 7 8 10 11 12 13 14 15 16 17 18 19 20 21 22 25 26 27 28 29 30 31 32 33 34 35 37 38 39 40 41 42 43 44 45 46 47 49 51 52 53 54 56 57 58 59 60 61 62 64 65 66 67 68 69 70 71 72 73 74 **P**5 7 **S** Sisters of Charity Health Care System Corporation, New York, NY **N** Catholic Health Care Network, Staten Island, NY; Sisters of Charity Health Care System, Staten Island, NY
| | 21 | 10 | 198 | 7835 | 151 | 145693 | 0 | 127325 | 41668 | 838 |

★ BELLEVUE HOSPITAL CENTER, (Includes Bellevue Comprehensive General Care, Bellevue Physical Medicine and Rehabilitation Services, Bellevue Psychiatric Services, Bellevue Tuberculosis Services, Comprehensive Ambulatory Care Services: Level I Trauma Center), First Avenue and 27th Street, Zip 10016; tel. 212/562–4141; Gregory M. Kaladjian, Executive Director **A**1 2 3 5 9 10 **F**1 2 3 4 5 7 8 10 12 13 14 15 16 17 18 19 20 21 22 23 26 28 29 30 31 34 35 38 39 40 41 42 43 44 45 46 48 49 51 52 53 54 55 56 57 58 59 60 61 65 66 67 68 70 71 72 73 74 **P**6 **S** New York City Health and Hospitals Corporation, New York, NY
| | 14 | 10 | 923 | 23866 | 801 | 535005 | 2058 | 406064 | 233632 | 4826 |

★ BETH ISRAEL MEDICAL CENTER, (Includes Beth Israel Medical Center–North Division, 170 East End Avenue, Zip 10128; tel. 212/870–9000), First Avenue and 16th Street, Zip 10003–3803; tel. 212/420–2000; Robert G. Newman, M.D., President **A**1 3 5 6 8 9 10 **F**2 3 4 5 7 8 10 11 12 13 14 15 16 17 18 19 20 21 22 25 26 28 29 30 31 33 34 35 37 38 39 40 41 42 43 44 45 46 48 49 50 51 52 53 54 55 56 57 58 59 60 61 63 64 65 66 67 68 71 73 74 **P**6 **N** Greater Metropolitan Health System, New York, NY; Health First, New York, NY
| | 23 | 10 | 1343 | 54422 | 1058 | 368514 | 5710 | — | — | — |

★ BRONX CHILDREN'S PSYCHIATRIC CENTER, 1000 Waters Place, Bronx, Zip 10461–2799; tel. 718/892–0808; E. Richard Feinberg, M.D., Executive Director (Nonreporting) **A**1 3 **S** New York State Department of Mental Health, Albany, NY
| | 12 | 52 | 75 | — | — | — | — | — | — | — |

★ BRONX PSYCHIATRIC CENTER, 1500 Waters Place, Bronx, Zip 10461; tel. 718/931–0600; LeRoy Carmichael, Executive Director (Nonreporting) **A**1 3 5 10 **S** New York State Department of Mental Health, Albany, NY
| | 12 | 22 | 658 | — | — | — | — | — | — | — |

★ BRONX–LEBANON HOSPITAL CENTER, (Includes Concourse Division, 1650 Grand Concourse, Zip 10457; tel. 212/590–1800; Fulton Division, 1276 Fulton Avenue, tel. 718/590–1800), 1276 Fulton Avenue, Bronx, Zip 10456; tel. 718/590–1800; Miguel A. Fuentes, President and Chief Executive Officer **A**1 2 3 5 8 9 10 **F**1 2 3 4 8 10 11 12 13 15 16 17 18 19 20 21 22 25 26 28 29 30 31 34 35 37 38 39 40 41 42 44 46 47 49 51 52 53 54 55 56 57 58 59 60 61 65 66 67 68 70 71 72 73 74 **P**6 8 **N** Health First, New York, NY
| | 23 | 10 | 576 | 22944 | 505 | 713172 | 2908 | 327084 | 168175 | 3657 |

Hospital, Address, Telephone, Administrator, Approval, Facility, and Physician Codes, Health Care System, Network	Classi-fication Codes		Utilization Data					Expense (thousands) of dollars		
★ American Hospital Association (AHA) membership □ Joint Commission on Accreditation of Healthcare Organizations (JCAHO) accreditation + American Osteopathic Hospital Association (AOHA) membership ○ American Osteopathic Association (AOA) accreditation △ Commission on Accreditation of Rehabilitation Facilities (CARF) accreditation Control codes 61, 63, 64, 71, 72 and 73 indicate hospitals listed by AOHA, but not registered by AHA. For definition of numerical codes, see page A4	Control	Service	Beds	Admissions	Census	Outpatient Visits	Births	Total	Payroll	Personnel
□ BROOKDALE HOSPITAL MEDICAL CENTER, Linden Boulevard at Brookdale Plaza, Brooklyn, Zip 11212–3198; tel. 718/240–5000; Frank J. Maddalena, President and Chief Executive Officer (Total facility includes 448 beds in nursing home–type unit) **A**1 3 5 8 9 10 12 **F**1 4 6 7 8 10 11 12 15 16 17 19 20 21 22 23 25 26 27 28 30 31 32 33 34 35 36 37 38 40 41 42 44 46 47 49 51 52 53 54 55 56 57 58 59 60 61 64 65 66 67 68 70 71 73 **P**5 6 **N** The Mount Sinai Health System, New York, NY	23	10	1048	24726	955	328436	2611	345463	193919	3725
⊞ BROOKLYN HOSPITAL CENTER, (Includes Caledonian Campus, 100 Parkside Avenue, Zip 11226; tel. 718/940–2000; Downtown Campus, 121 DeKalb Avenue, Zip 11201), 121 DeKalb Avenue, Brooklyn, Zip 11201–5493; tel. 718/250–8005; Frederick D. Alley, President and Chief Executive Officer **A**1 2 3 5 8 9 10 **F**1 4 7 8 10 11 12 13 14 15 16 17 19 20 21 22 25 26 27 28 29 30 31 32 33 34 35 37 38 39 40 41 42 43 44 45 46 47 49 51 53 54 55 56 57 58 59 60 61 63 65 67 68 69 70 71 73 74 **P**4 5 8 **N** NYU Medical Center, New York, NY; The Brooklyn Health Network, Brooklyn, NY; Health First, New York, NY	23	10	653	29947	502	189616	4720	268323	150766	3270
⊞ CABRINI MEDICAL CENTER, 227 East 19th Street, Zip 10003–2600; tel. 212/995–6000; Jeffrey Frerichs, President and Chief Executive Officer **A**1 2 3 5 8 9 10 **F**8 11 12 14 15 16 17 19 20 21 22 23 25 26 27 28 29 30 31 32 33 34 35 37 39 42 44 46 48 49 52 56 58 59 60 63 65 70 71 73 74 **P**5 6 8 **N** The Mount Sinai Health System, New York, NY CALEDONIAN CAMPUS See Brooklyn Hospital Center	21	10	493	11980	307	72586	0	171562	87333	1862
⊞ CALVARY HOSPITAL, (SPECIALTY TREATMENT HOSPITAL), 1740 Eastchester Road, Bronx, Zip 10461–2392; tel. 718/863–6900; Frank A. Calamari, President and Chief Executive Officer **A**1 9 10 **F**8 14 16 19 21 22 32 34 39 41 42 45 46 54 60 65 67 70 73 **N** Catholic Health Care Network, Staten Island, NY	21	49	200	2485	177	21923	0	53995	31443	668
⊞ CATHOLIC MEDICAL CENTER OF BROOKLYN AND QUEENS, (Includes Holy Family Home, 1740 84th Street, Brooklyn, Zip 11214; tel. 718/232–3666; Mary Immaculate Hospital, 152–11 89th Avenue, Zip 11432; tel. 718/558–2000; Monsignor James H Fitzpatrick Pavilion for Skilled Nursing Care, 152–11 89th Avenue, Zip 11432; tel. 718/558–2800; St. John's Queens Hospital, tel. 718/558–1000; St. Joseph's Hospital, 158–40 79th Avenue, Flushing, Zip 11366; tel. 212/558–6200; St. Mary's Hospital, 170 Buffalo Avenue, Brooklyn, Zip 11213; tel. 718/221–3000; 88–25 153rd Street, Jamaica, Zip 11432–3731; tel. 718/558–6900; William D. McGuire, President and Chief Executive Officer (Total facility includes 303 beds in nursing home–type unit) (Nonreporting) **A**1 2 3 5 6 8 9 10	21	10	1707	—	—	—	—	—	—	—
⊞ COLER MEMORIAL HOSPITAL, Franklin D. Roosevelt Island, Zip 10044; tel. 212/848–6000; Samuel Lehrfeld, Executive Director (Total facility includes 775 beds in nursing home–type unit) **A**1 10 **F**14 20 26 31 33 41 46 48 54 64 65 73 **P**5 **S** New York City Health and Hospitals Corporation, New York, NY CONCOURSE DIVISION See Bronx–Lebanon Hospital Center	14	48	1025	926	969	0	0	—	—	1571
⊞ CONEY ISLAND HOSPITAL, 2601 Ocean Parkway, Brooklyn, Zip 11235–7795; tel. 718/616–3000; Howard C. Cohen, Executive Director **A**1 3 5 9 10 12 **F**3 4 5 7 8 10 11 12 14 15 16 17 18 19 20 21 22 23 25 26 27 28 30 31 32 34 35 37 39 40 41 42 44 46 48 49 51 53 54 55 56 57 58 59 60 61 65 67 68 69 70 71 73 74 **P**6 **S** New York City Health and Hospitals Corporation, New York, NY	14	10	427	15618	375	391153	1427	222107	128125	2731
CORNERSTONE OF MEDICAL ARTS CENTER HOSPITAL, 57 West 57th Street, Zip 10019; tel. 212/755–0200; Norman J. Sokolow, President (Nonreporting) **A**9	33	82	84	—	—	—	—	—	—	—
⊞ CREEDMOOR PSYCHIATRIC CENTER, Jamaica, Mailing Address: 80–45 Winchester Boulevard, Queens Village, Zip 11427; tel. 718/264–3300; Charlotte Seltzer, Chief Executive Officer **A**1 3 10 **F**16 20 52 58 65 67 73 **S** New York State Department of Mental Health, Albany, NY	12	22	795	877	810	97373	0	18573	—	1611
⊞ DOCTORS' HOSPITAL OF STATEN ISLAND, 1050 Targee Street, Staten Island, Zip 10304; tel. 718/390–1400; Stephen N. F. Anderson, Director (Nonreporting) **A**1 9 10 DOWNTOWN CAMPUS See Brooklyn Hospital Center	33	10	117	—	—	—	—	—	—	—
⊞ △ ELMHURST HOSPITAL CENTER, 79–01 Broadway, Elmhurst, Zip 11373; tel. 718/334–4000; Pete Velez, Executive Director **A**1 2 3 5 7 8 9 10 **F**2 3 4 5 7 8 9 10 11 12 13 14 15 16 17 18 19 20 21 22 23 25 26 27 28 29 30 31 32 34 35 37 38 39 40 41 42 43 44 45 46 47 48 49 50 51 52 53 54 55 56 57 58 59 60 61 63 64 65 66 67 68 69 70 71 73 74 **P**5 6 7 8 **S** New York City Health and Hospitals Corporation, New York, NY **N** Queens Health Network, Elmhurst, NY; The Mount Sinai Health System, New York, NY	14	10	480	19749	429	570552	4401	293354	171045	3634
□ FLUSHING HOSPITAL MEDICAL CENTER, 45th Avenue at Parsons Boulevard, Flushing, Zip 11355; tel. 718/670–5000; Charles J. Pendola, President and Chief Executive Officer **A**1 3 5 9 10 **F**2 3 4 5 7 8 9 10 11 12 13 14 15 16 17 18 19 20 21 22 25 26 27 28 29 30 31 33 34 35 36 37 38 39 40 41 42 43 46 47 48 49 51 52 54 55 56 57 58 60 61 63 64 65 66 67 70 71 72 73 74 **P**5 7 **N** Preferred Health Network, Inc., Flushing, NY; The New York & Presbyterian Hospitals Care Network, Inc., New York, NY FULTON DIVISION See Bronx–Lebanon Hospital Center	23	10	321	18694	320	167213	3120	168824	85430	—
⊞ △ GOLDWATER MEMORIAL HOSPITAL, Franklin D. Roosevelt Island, Zip 10044; tel. 212/318–8000; Samuel Lehrfeld, Executive Director (Total facility includes 544 beds in nursing home–type unit) **A**1 3 5 7 10 **F**14 19 20 31 41 46 48 54 64 65 71 73 **P**6 **S** New York City Health and Hospitals Corporation, New York, NY	14	48	986	1108	937	0	0	99634	43067	1681

Hospital, Address, Telephone, Administrator, Approval, Facility, and Physician Codes, Health Care System, Network	Classi-fication Codes		Utilization Data					Expense (thousands) of dollars		
	Control	Service	Beds	Admissions	Census	Outpatient Visits	Births	Total	Payroll	Personnel

★ American Hospital Association (AHA) membership
□ Joint Commission on Accreditation of Healthcare Organizations (JCAHO) accreditation
+ American Osteopathic Hospital Association (AOHA) membership
○ American Osteopathic Association (AOA) accreditation
△ Commission on Accreditation of Rehabilitation Facilities (CARF) accreditation
Control codes 61, 63, 64, 71, 72 and 73 indicate hospitals listed by AOHA, but not registered by AHA. For definition of numerical codes, see page A4

Hospital	Control	Service	Beds	Admissions	Census	Outpatient Visits	Births	Total	Payroll	Personnel
✦ GRACIE SQUARE HOSPITAL, 420 East 76th Street, Zip 10021–3104; tel. 212/988–4400; Frank Bruno, Chief Executive Officer (Nonreporting) **A**1 9 10 **N** The New York & Presbyterian Hospitals Care Network, Inc., New York, NY	23	22	100	—	—	—	—	—	—	—
✦ △ HARLEM HOSPITAL CENTER, (Includes Harlem General Care Unit and Harlem Psychiatric Unit), 506 Lenox Avenue, Zip 10037–1894; tel. 212/939–1340; Linnette Webb, Senior Vice President and Executive Director **A**1 2 3 5 7 8 9 10 **F**1 2 3 4 5 6 7 8 9 10 11 12 13 15 16 17 18 19 20 21 22 23 25 26 27 28 29 30 31 32 34 35 36 37 38 39 40 41 42 43 44 45 46 47 48 49 50 51 52 53 54 55 56 57 58 59 60 61 63 65 67 69 70 71 72 73 74 **P**1 **S** New York City Health and Hospitals Corporation, New York, NY	14	10	414	15300	373	563820	1220	268861	154667	3472
HILLSIDE HOSPITAL See Long Island Jewish Medical Center										
✦ HOLLISWOOD HOSPITAL, 87–37 Palermo Street, Holliswood, Zip 11423; tel. 718/776–8181; Jeffrey Borenstein, M.D., Chief Executive Officer and Medical Director (Nonreporting) **A**1 9 10	33	22	100	—	—	—	—	—	—	—
✦ △ HOSPITAL FOR JOINT DISEASES ORTHOPEDIC INSTITUTE, (SPECIAL SURG MUSCULOSKELETAL), 301 East 17th Street, Zip 10003–3890; tel. 212/598–6000; John N. Kastanis, FACHE, Chief Executive Officer **A**1 3 5 7 9 10 **F**4 5 7 8 10 11 12 14 15 16 17 19 20 21 22 24 25 26 27 29 30 31 32 34 35 37 38 39 40 41 42 43 44 45 46 47 48 49 51 52 54 55 56 57 60 61 63 65 66 67 69 71 72 73 74 **P**5 7 **N** NYU Medical Center, New York, NY	23	49	163	5805	134	69061	0	—	—	1199
✦ HOSPITAL FOR SPECIAL SURGERY, 535 East 70th Street, Zip 10021–4898; tel. 212/606–1000; John R. Ahearn, President **A**1 3 5 6 8 9 10 **F**1 2 3 4 5 6 7 8 9 10 11 12 13 14 15 17 18 19 20 21 22 23 24 25 26 27 28 29 30 31 32 33 34 35 36 37 38 39 40 41 42 43 44 45 46 47 48 49 50 51 52 53 54 55 56 57 58 59 60 61 63 64 65 66 67 68 69 70 71 72 73 74 **P**5 8 **N** The New York & Presbyterian Hospitals Care Network, Inc., New York, NY	23	47	138	6597	102	151589	0	161573	61817	1187
□ INTERFAITH MEDICAL CENTER, (Includes Brooklyn Jewish Division, 555 Prospect Place, Zip 11238; tel. 718/935–7000; St. John's Episcopal Hospital Division, 1545 Atlantic Avenue, Zip 11213; tel. 718/604–6000), 555 Prospect Place, Brooklyn, Zip 11238–4299; tel. 718/935–7000; Corbett A. Price, Chief Executive Officer **A**1 3 5 6 9 10 **F**1 2 3 4 7 8 10 11 12 13 15 16 17 18 19 20 21 22 25 27 28 30 31 32 34 35 37 38 40 42 43 44 46 49 52 54 55 56 58 59 60 61 65 67 68 69 71 73 74 **P**6 **N** Health First, New York, NY	23	10	455	16149	420	264133	1386	189283	108387	1932
✦ JACOBI MEDICAL CENTER, (Includes Abraham Jacobi General Care Hospital and Psychiatric Units, Van Etten Hospitals), Pelham Parkway South and Eastchester Road, Bronx, Zip 10461; tel. 718/918–8141; Joseph S. Orlando, Executive Director **A**1 3 5 8 10 **F**1 2 3 7 8 9 11 12 13 14 15 16 17 18 19 20 21 22 28 29 30 31 32 34 35 37 38 39 40 41 42 44 45 46 47 48 49 51 52 53 54 55 56 58 60 61 65 67 68 70 71 73 74 **P**6 **S** New York City Health and Hospitals Corporation, New York, NY	14	10	595	21241	486	435335	2608	268228	188885	4251
✦ JAMAICA HOSPITAL MEDICAL CENTER, 8900 Van Wyck Expressway, Jamaica, Zip 11418–2832; tel. 718/206–6000; David P. Rosen, President **A**1 3 5 9 10 12 **F**8 10 12 13 14 15 16 17 19 20 21 22 31 32 34 35 37 40 41 42 44 46 48 49 51 52 53 54 55 56 57 58 59 65 69 70 71 73 74 **P**4 5 **N** NYU Medical Center, New York, NY; Health First, New York, NY	23	10	365	16670	325	164225	2945	160030	95011	2393
✦ KINGS COUNTY HOSPITAL CENTER, 451 Clarkson Avenue, Brooklyn, Zip 11203–2097; tel. 718/245–3131; Jean G. Leon, R.N., Senior Vice President **A**1 2 3 5 9 10 **F**2 3 4 5 7 8 11 12 13 15 17 18 19 20 21 22 24 25 27 28 30 31 34 37 38 39 40 41 42 44 45 46 47 48 49 50 51 52 53 54 55 56 58 60 61 63 65 66 68 70 71 72 73 74 **P**6 **S** New York City Health and Hospitals Corporation, New York, NY	14	10	804	26263	722	715573	2420	—	—	5571
□ KINGS HIGHWAY HOSPITAL CENTER, 3201 Kings Highway, Brooklyn, Zip 11234; tel. 718/252–3000; Samuel Berson, M.D., Executive Director (Nonreporting) **A**1 9 **N** Greater Metropolitan Health System, New York, NY	33	10	212	—	—	—	—	—	—	—
★ KINGSBORO PSYCHIATRIC CENTER, 681 Clarkson Avenue, Brooklyn, Zip 11203; tel. 718/221–7395; Billy E. Jones, M.D., MS, Acting Executive Director **A**3 5 10 **F**1 2 3 4 5 8 9 10 11 12 15 17 18 19 20 21 22 24 25 26 27 28 29 30 31 32 33 35 37 39 40 41 42 43 44 45 46 48 49 50 51 52 54 55 56 57 58 59 60 61 62 63 64 65 68 69 70 71 72 73 74 **S** New York State Department of Mental Health, Albany, NY	12	22	400	624	451	35000	0	57815	41608	1043
✦ △ KINGSBROOK JEWISH MEDICAL CENTER, 585 Schenectady Avenue, Brooklyn, Zip 11203–1891; tel. 718/604–5000; Milton M. Gutman, Chief Executive Officer (Total facility includes 538 beds in nursing home–type unit) **A**1 3 5 7 9 10 **F**1 8 11 12 14 15 16 17 19 20 21 22 25 26 27 28 29 30 32 34 35 37 39 41 44 45 46 48 49 51 52 53 54 55 57 58 64 65 66 71 73 **P**3 5 **N** Health First, New York, NY	23	10	879	8908	829	85203	0	170400	90202	2076
✦ △ LENOX HILL HOSPITAL, 100 East 77th Street, Zip 10021–1883; tel. 212/434–2000; Gladys George, President and Chief Executive Officer **A**1 3 5 7 8 9 10 **F**4 5 7 8 10 11 12 14 15 16 17 19 20 21 22 25 27 28 29 30 31 32 34 35 37 38 39 40 41 42 43 44 45 46 47 49 51 52 53 54 55 56 57 58 60 61 63 65 66 67 68 71 73 74 **P**5 7 8 **N** NYU Medical Center, New York, NY; National Cardiovascular Network, Atlanta, GA	23	10	652	25749	552	268222	3735	311427	144567	3063
✦ △ LINCOLN MEDICAL AND MENTAL HEALTH CENTER, 234 East 149th Street, Bronx, Zip 10451–9998; tel. 718/579–5700; Roberto Rodriguez, Executive Director **A**1 3 9 10 **F**3 7 8 11 14 15 16 17 19 20 21 22 28 29 30 31 32 34 37 38 40 41 42 44 46 47 49 51 52 54 56 58 60 61 65 70 71 73 74 **S** New York City Health and Hospitals Corporation, New York, NY	14	10	470	21354	403	502971	3042	—	—	3708

Hospital, Address, Telephone, Administrator, Approval, Facility, and Physician Codes, Health Care System, Network	Classi-fication Codes		Utilization Data					Expense (thousands) of dollars		
	Control	Service	Beds	Admissions	Census	Outpatient Visits	Births	Total	Payroll	Personnel

★ American Hospital Association (AHA) membership
☐ Joint Commission on Accreditation of Healthcare Organizations (JCAHO) accreditation
+ American Osteopathic Hospital Association (AOHA) membership
○ American Osteopathic Association (AOA) accreditation
△ Commission on Accreditation of Rehabilitation Facilities (CARF) accreditation
Control codes 61, 63, 64, 71, 72 and 73 indicate hospitals listed by AOHA, but not registered by AHA. For definition of numerical codes, see page A4

Hospital	Control	Service	Beds	Admissions	Census	Outpatient Visits	Births	Total	Payroll	Personnel
☐ LONG ISLAND COLLEGE HOSPITAL, 339 Hicks Street, Brooklyn, Zip 11201; tel. 718/780–1000; Donald F. Snell, President and Chief Executive Officer **A**1 2 3 5 8 9 10 **F**2 3 5 7 8 10 11 12 15 16 17 19 20 21 22 23 25 26 27 28 30 31 32 34 35 37 38 39 40 41 42 44 45 46 47 48 49 51 52 53 54 55 56 57 58 60 61 65 66 67 68 71 73 74 **P**5 6 8 **N** The Mount Sinai Health System, New York, NY	23	10	516	19554	372	380333	3163	269813	139548	3069
✦ LONG ISLAND JEWISH MEDICAL CENTER, (Includes Hillside Hospital, 75–59 263rd Street, Glen Oaks, Zip 11004; tel. 718/470–8000; Long Island Jewish Medical Center, tel. 718/470–7000; Manhasset Ambulatory Care Pavilion, 1554 Northern Boulevard, Manhasset, Zip 11030; tel. 516/365–2070; Schneider Children's Hospital, 270–05 76th Avenue, tel. 718/470–3000), 270–05 76th Avenue, New Hyde Park, Zip 11040; tel. 718/470–7000; David R. Dantzker, M.D., President and Chief Executive Officer **A**1 2 3 5 8 9 10 **F**1 3 4 5 6 7 8 10 11 12 13 14 15 16 17 18 19 20 21 22 23 26 27 28 29 30 31 32 34 35 37 38 39 40 41 42 43 44 45 46 47 49 51 52 53 54 55 56 57 58 59 60 61 63 65 66 67 68 69 70 71 72 73 74 **P**5 6 7	23	10	804	33500	699	515000	4623	—	—	4966
LONG ISLAND JEWISH MEDICAL CENTER See Long Island Jewish Medical Center										
✦ LUTHERAN MEDICAL CENTER, 150 55th Street, Brooklyn, Zip 11220–2570; tel. 718/630–7000; Joseph P. Cerni, President and Chief Executive Officer **A**1 3 5 9 10 12 **F**2 3 6 8 11 12 13 14 15 16 17 18 19 20 21 22 23 25 29 30 31 32 34 35 37 39 40 41 42 44 45 46 48 49 51 60 61 62 65 67 71 72 73 74 **P**5 **N** The Mount Sinai Health System, New York, NY	23	10	433	16660	353	433985	2956	—	—	—
✦ MAIMONIDES MEDICAL CENTER, 4802 Tenth Avenue, Brooklyn, Zip 11219–2916; tel. 718/283–6000; Stanley Brezenoff, President (Nonreporting) **A**1 3 5 8 9 10 12 **N** Premier Preferred Care, New York, NY; The Mount Sinai Health System, New York, NY; Health First, New York, NY	23	10	705	—	—	—	—	—	—	—
✦ MANHATTAN EYE, EAR AND THROAT HOSPITAL, 210 East 64th Street, Zip 10021–9885; tel. 212/838–9200; George A. Sarkar, Ph.D., JD, Executive Director (Nonreporting) **A**1 3 5 10	23	45	30	—	—	—	—	—	—	—
✦ MANHATTAN PSYCHIATRIC CENTER–WARD'S ISLAND, 600 East 125th Street, Zip 10035–9998; tel. 212/369–0500; Horace Belton, Executive Director **A**1 3 5 10 **F**3 4 5 7 8 19 21 22 23 24 30 31 32 35 42 43 44 46 50 52 54 55 56 57 58 59 63 65 70 71 73 **S** New York State Department of Mental Health, Albany, NY	12	22	745	193	796	12548	0	—	—	1180
✦ MEMORIAL HOSPITAL FOR CANCER AND ALLIED DISEASES, 1275 York Avenue, Zip 10021; tel. 212/639–2000; John R. Gunn, Executive Vice President (Nonreporting) **A**1 2 3 5 8 9 10	23	49	480	—	—	—	—	—	—	—
✦ METROPOLITAN HOSPITAL CENTER, (Includes Metropolitan General Care Unit, Metropolitan Drug Detoxification and Metropolitan Psychiatric Unit), 1901 First Avenue, Zip 10029; tel. 212/423–6262; Jose R. Sanchez, Executive Director **A**1 3 5 8 9 10 **F**1 2 3 7 8 10 11 12 13 14 15 16 17 18 19 20 21 22 25 26 27 28 29 30 31 32 34 35 37 38 39 40 41 42 44 45 46 47 48 49 51 52 53 54 55 56 57 58 59 60 61 63 65 71 73 74 **S** New York City Health and Hospitals Corporation, New York, NY	14	10	458	13836	435	379788	1701	224587	131218	2920
✦ MONTEFIORE MEDICAL CENTER, (Includes Jack D Weiler Hospital of Albert Einstein College of Medicine, 1825 Eastchester Road, Zip 10461–2373; tel. 718/904–2000; Loeb Center Nursing Rehabilitation, 111 East 210th Street), 111 East 210th Street, Bronx, Zip 10467–2490; tel. 718/920–4321; Spencer Foreman, M.D., President (Total facility includes 80 beds in nursing home–type unit) (Nonreporting) **A**1 2 3 5 8 9 10 **N** Health First, New York, NY	23	10	1141	—	—	—	—	—	—	—
✦ MOUNT SINAI MEDICAL CENTER, One Gustave L. Levy Place, Zip 10029–6574; tel. 212/241–8888; John W. Rowe, M.D., President (Nonreporting) **A**1 3 5 8 9 10 **N** The Mount Sinai Health System, New York, NY; Health First, New York, NY	23	10	1086	—	—	—	—	—	—	—
☐ NEW YORK DOWNTOWN HOSPITAL, 170 William Street, Zip 10038; tel. 212/312–5000; Alan H. Channing, President and Chief Executive Officer (Nonreporting) **A**1 3 5 9 10 **N** NYU Medical Center, New York, NY	23	10	166	—	—	—	—	—	—	—
✦ NEW YORK EYE AND EAR INFIRMARY, 310 East 14th Street, Zip 10003–4201; tel. 212/979–4000; Joseph P. Corcoran, President and Chief Executive Officer **A**1 3 5 9 10 **F**12 17 19 20 25 28 30 34 44 60 65 69 70 71 73 **P**8	23	45	30	3761	20	171693	0	52596	26641	634
✦ NEW YORK HOSPITAL MEDICAL CENTER OF QUEENS, 56–45 Main Street, Flushing, Zip 11355; tel. 718/670–1231; Stephen S. Mills, President and Chief Executive Officer **A**1 2 3 5 9 10 **F**2 3 4 5 7 8 9 10 11 12 13 14 15 16 17 18 19 20 21 22 25 26 27 28 29 30 31 33 34 35 36 37 38 39 40 41 42 43 44 45 46 47 48 49 51 52 54 55 56 57 58 60 61 63 64 65 66 67 70 71 72 73 74 **P**5 7 **N** The New York & Presbyterian Hospitals Care Network, Inc., New York, NY	23	10	421	21346	367	—	2547	225282	104959	2024
✦ NEW YORK METHODIST HOSPITAL, 506 Sixth Street, Brooklyn, Zip 11215; tel. 718/780–3000; Mark J. Mundy, President and Chief Executive Officer (Nonreporting) **A**1 2 3 5 8 9 10 12 **N** The New York & Presbyterian Hospitals Care Network, Inc., New York, NY	23	10	560	—	—	—	—	—	—	—
✦ NEW YORK STATE PSYCHIATRIC INSTITUTE, 722 West 168th Street, Zip 10032; tel. 212/960–2200; John M. Oldham, M.D., Director **A**1 3 5 10 **F**14 15 16 52 53 55 57 58 **S** New York State Department of Mental Health, Albany, NY	12	22	58	345	53	56657	0	—	—	570
✦ △ NEW YORK UNIVERSITY MEDICAL CENTER, (Includes Rusk Institute), 550 First Avenue, Zip 10016–4576; tel. 212/263–7300; Theresa A. Bischoff, Deputy Provost and Executive Vice President **A**1 3 5 7 8 9 10 **F**3 4 5 7 8 10 11 12 13 14 15 16 17 18 19 20 21 22 23 24 25 26 27 28 29 30 31 32 33 34 35 36 37 38 39 40 41 42 43 44 45 46 47 48 49 50 51 52 53 54 55 56 57 58 59 60 61 63 65 66 67 68 69 70 71 72 73 74 **P**5 **N** The Brooklyn Health Network, Brooklyn, NY; Health First, New York, NY	23	10	824	31147	718	87369	2237	524957	245802	4252

Hospital, Address, Telephone, Administrator, Approval, Facility, and Physician Codes, Health Care System, Network	Classi-fication Codes		Utilization Data					Expense (thousands) of dollars		
★ American Hospital Association (AHA) membership □ Joint Commission on Accreditation of Healthcare Organizations (JCAHO) accreditation + American Osteopathic Hospital Association (AOHA) membership ○ American Osteopathic Association (AOA) accreditation △ Commission on Accreditation of Rehabilitation Facilities (CARF) accreditation Control codes 61, 63, 64, 71, 72 and 73 indicate hospitals listed by AOHA, but not registered by AHA. For definition of numerical codes, see page A4	Control	Service	Beds	Admissions	Census	Outpatient Visits	Births	Total	Payroll	Personnel

Hospital	Control	Service	Beds	Admissions	Census	Outpatient Visits	Births	Total	Payroll	Personnel
✚ NORTH CENTRAL BRONX HOSPITAL, 3424 Kossuth Avenue, Bronx, Zip 10467; tel. 718/519–3500; Fay E. Malcolm, R.N., Chief Operating Officer **A**1 3 5 9 10 **F**1 2 3 7 8 9 10 11 12 13 14 15 16 17 18 19 20 21 22 26 28 29 30 31 32 34 35 37 38 39 40 41 42 44 45 46 47 48 49 51 52 53 54 56 58 65 67 68 70 71 73 74 **P**6 **S** New York City Health and Hospitals Corporation, New York, NY	14	10	269	11450	239	251358	3343	133879	92651	2041
✚ NORTH GENERAL HOSPITAL, 1879 Madison Avenue, Zip 10035–2745; tel. 212/423–4000; Eugene McCabe, President (Nonreporting) **A**1 3 5 9 10	23	10	240	—	—	—	—	—	—	—
✚ NORTH SHORE UNIVERSITY HOSPITAL–FOREST HILLS, Flushing, Mailing Address: 102–01 66th Road, Forest Hills, Zip 11375; tel. 718/830–4000; Andrew J. Mitchell, Vice President, Administration (Nonreporting) **A**1 2 3 5 9 10 **N** North Shore Regional Health Systems, Manhasset, NY	23	10	231	—	—	—	—	—	—	—
✚ OUR LADY OF MERCY MEDICAL CENTER, (Includes Florence D'Urso Pavilion, 1870 Pelham Parkway South, Zip 10461; tel. 212/430–6000), 600 East 233rd Street, Bronx, Zip 10466; tel. 718/920–9000; Gary S. Horan, FACHE, President and Chief Executive Officer **A**1 2 3 5 8 9 10 **F**3 7 8 11 12 13 14 15 16 17 19 20 22 25 26 28 30 31 32 34 35 37 38 39 40 42 44 45 46 49 51 52 54 56 57 58 60 61 62 65 66 67 71 73 74 **P**1 **S** Our Lady of Mercy Healthcare System, Inc., New York, NY **N** Catholic Health Care Network, Staten Island, NY	21	10	508	17792	411	251426	2776	190785	99880	2295
✚ PARKWAY HOSPITAL, Flushing, Mailing Address: 70–35 113th Street, Zip 11375; tel. 718/990–4100; Paul E. Svensson, Chief Executive Officer (Nonreporting) **A**1 9 10 **N** The Mount Sinai Health System, New York, NY	33	10	251	—	—	—	—	—	—	—
□ ○ PENINSULA HOSPITAL CENTER, 51–15 Beach Channel Drive, Far Rockaway, Zip 11691–1074; tel. 718/945–7100; Robert V. Levine, President and Chief Executive Officer **A**1 9 10 11 12 13 **F**8 11 15 16 17 18 19 20 21 22 26 28 30 32 33 34 35 37 42 44 45 46 49 51 54 56 60 65 67 70 71 73 **P**5 7 8	23	10	235	5779	188	63677	0	65595	37149	893
✚ △ PRESBYTERIAN HOSPITAL IN THE CITY OF NEW YORK, Columbia–Presbyterian Medical Center, Zip 10032–3784; tel. 212/305–2500; William T. Speck, M.D., President and Chief Executive Officer **A**1 3 5 7 8 9 10 **F**4 7 8 9 10 11 12 13 14 15 16 17 18 19 20 21 22 23 25 26 27 28 29 30 32 34 35 37 38 39 40 41 42 43 44 45 46 47 48 49 50 51 52 53 54 55 56 58 60 63 65 66 67 68 69 71 72 73 74 **P**4 5 7 8 **N** The New York & Presbyterian Hospitals Care Network, Inc., New York, NY	23	10	992	45740	873	599312	5108	—	—	6828
✚ QUEENS CHILDREN'S PSYCHIATRIC CENTER, 74–03 Commonwealth Boulevard, Bellerose, Zip 11426; tel. 718/264–4506; Gloria Faretra, M.D., Executive Director **A**1 **F**12 15 16 17 20 27 52 53 54 55 56 58 59 65 67 73 **P**6 **S** New York State Department of Mental Health, Albany, NY	12	52	106	98	76	30958	0	—	—	362
✚ QUEENS HOSPITAL CENTER, 82–68 164th Street, Jamaica, Zip 11432; tel. 718/883–3000; Gladiola Sampson, Acting Executive Director **A**1 2 3 5 9 10 **F**2 3 4 7 8 10 12 13 14 16 17 19 20 21 22 25 26 31 32 34 35 37 38 40 42 43 44 46 48 49 51 52 53 54 56 57 58 59 60 63 65 67 68 71 73 74 **P**6 **S** New York City Health and Hospitals Corporation, New York, NY **N** Queens Health Network, Elmhurst, NY; The Mount Sinai Health System, New York, NY	14	10	331	12967	291	317533	2020	182489	124231	2462
□ ROCKEFELLER UNIVERSITY HOSPITAL, (CLINICAL RESEARCH), 1230 York Avenue, Zip 10021–6399; tel. 212/327–8000; Emil Gotschlich, M.D., Vice President Medical Sciences **A**1 3 9 10 **F**34 65	23	49	30	274	12	3411	0	—	—	58
✚ SAINT VINCENT'S HOSPITAL AND MEDICAL CENTER OF NEW YORK, (Includes St. Vincent's Hospital, 275 North Street, Zip 10528; tel. 914/925–5300), 153 West 11th Street, Zip 10011–8397; tel. 212/604–7000; Karl P. Adler, M.D., President and Chief Executive Officer (Nonreporting) **A**1 2 3 5 6 8 9 10 **S** Sisters of Charity Center, New York, NY **N** Catholic Health Care Network, Staten Island, NY	21	10	978	—	—	—	—	—	—	—
SCHNEIDER CHILDREN'S HOSPITAL See Long Island Jewish Medical Center										
✚ SOCIETY OF THE NEW YORK HOSPITAL, (Includes New York Hospital, New York Hospital, Westchester Division, Payne Whitney Psychiatric Clinic), 525 East 68th Street, Zip 10021; tel. 212/746–5454; David B. Skinner, M.D., President and Chief Executive Officer (Nonreporting) **A**1 2 3 5 8 10 **N** The New York & Presbyterian Hospitals Care Network, Inc., New York, NY	23	10	1310	—	—	—	—	—	—	—
✚ SOUTH BEACH PSYCHIATRIC CENTER, 777 Seaview Avenue, Staten Island, Zip 10305; tel. 718/667–2300; Lucy Sarkis, M.D., Executive Director **A**1 10 **F**1 3 7 10 15 16 19 21 24 26 31 33 35 41 44 52 53 54 55 56 57 58 59 60 61 71 74 **S** New York State Department of Mental Health, Albany, NY	12	22	325	1279	287	228287	0	70753	50495	1158
□ ○ ST. BARNABAS HOSPITAL, 183rd Street and Third Avenue, Bronx, Zip 10457–9998; tel. 718/960–9000; Ronald Gade, M.D., President (Nonreporting) **A**1 3 5 9 10 11 12 13 **N** The Mount Sinai Health System, New York, NY	23	10	458	—	—	—	—	—	—	—
□ ST. CLARE'S HOSPITAL AND HEALTH CENTER, 415 West 51st Street, Zip 10019; tel. 212/586–1500; Richard N. Yezzo, President **A**1 9 10 12 **F**3 4 7 8 10 11 12 13 16 17 19 20 21 22 26 27 28 31 32 34 35 37 38 40 42 43 44 45 46 47 48 49 51 52 53 54 56 57 58 60 64 65 67 69 70 71 73 74 **P**5 8 **N** Catholic Health Care Network, Staten Island, NY	21	10	236	4720	154	74989	0	76544	43944	908
ST. JOHN'S EPISCOPAL HOSPITAL DIVISION See Interfaith Medical Center										
✚ ○ ST. JOHN'S EPISCOPAL HOSPITAL–SOUTH SHORE, 327 Beach 19th Street, Far Rockaway, Zip 11691–4424; tel. 718/869–7000; Paul J. Connor, III, Administrator (Nonreporting) **A**1 3 5 9 11 **S** Episcopal Health Services Inc., Uniondale, NY **N** Episcopal Health Services, Inc., Uniondale, NY; First Choice Network, Inc., Mineola, NY; The Mount Sinai Health System, New York, NY	21	10	314	—	—	—	—	—	—	—

Hospital, Address, Telephone, Administrator, Approval, Facility, and Physician Codes, Health Care System, Network	Control	Service	Beds	Admissions	Census	Outpatient Visits	Births	Total	Payroll	Personnel

★ American Hospital Association (AHA) membership
□ Joint Commission on Accreditation of Healthcare Organizations (JCAHO) accreditation
+ American Osteopathic Hospital Association (AOHA) membership
○ American Osteopathic Association (AOA) accreditation
△ Commission on Accreditation of Rehabilitation Facilities (CARF) accreditation
Control codes 61, 63, 64, 71, 72 and 73 indicate hospitals listed by AOHA, but not registered by AHA. For definition of numerical codes, see page A4

Hospital	Control	Service	Beds	Admissions	Census	Outpatient Visits	Births	Total	Payroll	Personnel
★ ST. LUKE'S–ROOSEVELT HOSPITAL CENTER, (Includes Roosevelt Hospital, 1000 Tenth Avenue, Zip 10019; tel. 212/523–4000; St. Luke's Hospital Center, 1111 Amsterdam Avenue, tel. 212/523–4000), 1111 Amsterdam Avenue, Zip 10025; tel. 212/523–4295; Ronald C. Ablow, M.D., President and Chief Executive Officer **A**1 3 5 8 9 10 **F**2 3 4 7 8 10 11 12 13 14 15 16 17 18 19 20 21 22 26 28 29 30 31 32 34 35 37 38 39 40 41 42 43 44 45 46 47 48 49 51 52 53 54 55 56 57 58 59 60 61 63 65 67 68 69 70 71 73 74 **P**4 6 7 8 **N** Greater Metropolitan Health System, New York, NY	23	10	715	37307	725	494116	4337	589562	289693	5536
★ ST. VINCENT'S MEDICAL CENTER OF RICHMOND, 355 Bard Avenue, Staten Island, Zip 10310–1699; tel. 718/876–1234; Dominick M. Stanzione, Executive Vice President **A**1 2 3 5 6 9 10 **F**2 3 4 5 6 7 8 10 11 12 13 14 15 16 17 18 19 20 21 22 25 26 27 28 29 30 31 32 33 34 35 37 38 39 40 41 42 43 44 45 46 47 49 51 52 53 54 56 57 58 59 60 61 62 64 65 66 67 68 69 70 71 72 73 74 **S** Sisters of Charity Health Care System Corporation, New York, NY **N** Catholic Health Care Network, Staten Island, NY; Sisters of Charity Health Care System, Staten Island, NY	21	10	440	18298	324	204249	3512	162101	84278	1936
□ △ STATEN ISLAND UNIVERSITY HOSPITAL, 475 Seaview Avenue, Staten Island, Zip 10305–9998; tel. 718/226–9000; Rick J. Varone, President (Nonreporting) **A**1 2 3 5 7 9 10 **N** The Mount Sinai Health System, New York, NY; Health First, New York, NY	23	10	617							
★ THE NEW YORK COMMUNITY HOSPITAL OF BROOKLYN, 2525 Kings Highway, Brooklyn, Zip 11229–1798; tel. 718/692–5300; Lin H. Mo, President and Chief Executive Officer (Nonreporting) **A**1 9 10 **N** The New York & Presbyterian Hospitals Care Network, Inc., New York, NY	23	10	134							
□ UNION HOSPITAL OF THE BRONX, 260 East 188th Street, Bronx, Zip 10458; tel. 718/220–2020; Ronald Gade, M.D., President (Nonreporting) **A**1 9 10	23	10	197							
★ UNIVERSITY HOSPITAL OF BROOKLYN–STATE UNIVERSITY OF NEW YORK HEALTH SCIENCE CENTER AT BROOKLYN, 445 Lenox Road, Brooklyn, Zip 11203–2098; tel. 718/270–2404; Percy Allen, II, FACHE, Vice President Hospital Affairs and Chief Executive Officer **A**1 2 3 5 8 9 10 **F**4 7 8 10 11 12 13 14 15 16 17 19 20 21 25 28 30 31 34 35 37 38 40 41 42 43 44 46 47 48 49 50 51 52 53 54 55 58 59 60 61 63 65 66 69 71 72 73 74 **P**3 6 **N** Health First, New York, NY	12	10	376	11833	264	155144	2354	174814	99193	2057
VAN ETTEN HOSPITALS See Jacobi Medical Center										
★ VETERANS AFFAIRS MEDICAL CENTER, 800 Poly Place, Brooklyn, Zip 11209; tel. 718/630–3500; Michael A. Sabo, Medical Director (Total facility includes 268 beds in nursing home–type unit) **A**1 3 5 8 **F**1 2 3 4 5 8 10 11 14 15 17 19 20 21 22 24 25 26 27 28 30 31 32 33 35 37 39 42 43 44 45 46 49 51 52 56 57 58 59 60 61 64 65 67 69 71 72 73 74 **P**6 **S** Department of Veterans Affairs, Washington, DC	45	10	713	8091	632	374794	0	200509	139195	2172
★ VETERANS AFFAIRS MEDICAL CENTER, 130 West Kingsbridge Road, Bronx, Zip 10468–7511; tel. 718/584–9000; Maryann Musumeci, Director (Total facility includes 120 beds in nursing home–type unit) **A**1 2 3 5 8 **F**2 3 4 8 10 11 12 14 15 16 17 18 19 20 21 22 23 26 27 28 29 30 31 32 33 34 35 37 39 41 42 44 45 46 48 49 51 52 54 55 56 57 58 59 60 63 64 65 66 67 71 72 73 74 **P**6 **S** Department of Veterans Affairs, Washington, DC **N** The Mount Sinai Health System, New York, NY	45	10	482	6071	390	261842	0	—	—	1817
★ VETERANS AFFAIRS MEDICAL CENTER, 423 East 23rd Street, Zip 10010–0070; tel. 212/686–7500; John J. Donnellan, Jr., Director **A**1 2 3 5 8 **F**1 2 3 4 8 10 11 12 16 19 20 21 22 23 26 30 31 32 33 34 35 37 39 42 43 44 45 46 48 49 51 52 54 56 57 58 59 60 63 64 65 67 71 73 74 **S** Department of Veterans Affairs, Washington, DC	45	10	341	7550	316	333195	0	171883	96662	2149
□ VICTORY MEMORIAL HOSPITAL, 9036 Seventh Avenue, Brooklyn, Zip 11228–3625; tel. 718/630–1234; Krishin L. Bhatia, Administrator (Total facility includes 150 beds in nursing home–type unit) (Nonreporting) **A**1 9 10	23	10	410	—	—	—	—	—	—	—
□ WESTCHESTER SQUARE MEDICAL CENTER, 2475 St. Raymond Avenue, Bronx, Zip 10461; tel. 718/430–7300; Alan Kopman, President and Chief Executive Officer **A**1 9 10 **F**11 19 22 34 35 37 42 44 49 65 71 73 **P**5	33	10	205	6814	164	40611	0	53593	26443	621
□ WESTERN QUEENS COMMUNITY HOSPITAL, 25–10 30th Avenue, Astoria Station, Long Island City, Zip 11102–2495; tel. 718/932–1000; Elliot J. Simon, FACHE, Chief Operating Officer (Nonreporting) **A**1 9 10 **N** The Mount Sinai Health System, New York, NY	33	10	208	—	—	—	—	—	—	—
★ WOODHULL MEDICAL AND MENTAL HEALTH CENTER, 760 Broadway, Brooklyn, Zip 11206; tel. 718/963–8101; Cynthia Carrington–Murray, Executive Director **A**1 3 9 10 **F**1 2 3 4 5 7 8 9 10 11 12 14 15 16 17 18 19 20 21 22 24 25 26 27 28 29 30 31 32 33 34 35 37 38 39 40 41 42 43 44 45 46 47 48 49 51 52 53 54 55 56 57 58 59 60 61 63 64 65 67 68 69 70 71 73 74 **P**6 **S** New York City Health and Hospitals Corporation, New York, NY	14	10	413	16933	419	297977	1726	—	—	2858
□ ○ WYCKOFF HEIGHTS MEDICAL CENTER, 374 Stockholm Street, Brooklyn, Zip 11237–4099; tel. 718/963–7102; Charles J. Pendola, President (Nonreporting) **A**1 3 5 9 10 11 12 13 **N** Preferred Health Network, Inc., Flushing, NY; The New York & Presbyterian Hospitals Care Network, Inc., New York, NY	23	10	395	—	—	—	—	—	—	—

NEWARK—Wayne County

Hospital	Control	Service	Beds	Admissions	Census	Outpatient Visits	Births	Total	Payroll	Personnel
★ NEWARK–WAYNE COMMUNITY HOSPITAL, Driving Park Avenue, Zip 14513, Mailing Address: P.O. Box 111, Zip 14513–0111; tel. 315/332–2022; William R. Holman, President (Total facility includes 160 beds in nursing home–type unit) (Nonreporting) **A**1 9 10 **S** Greater Rochester Health System, Inc., Rochester, NY **N** Greater Rochester Health System, Inc., Rochester, NY	23	10	256							

Hospital, Address, Telephone, Administrator, Approval, Facility, and Physician Codes, Health Care System, Network	Control	Service	Beds	Admissions	Census	Outpatient Visits	Births	Total	Payroll	Personnel

NEWBURGH—Orange County
✸ ST. LUKE'S HOSPITAL, 70 Dubois Street, Zip 12550–4898, Mailing Address: P.O. Box 631, Zip 12550; tel. 914/561–4400; Laurence E. Kelly, Senior Vice President **A**1 9 10 **F**3 8 10 11 12 14 16 17 19 21 22 25 27 29 30 31 32 33 34 35 37 39 40 42 43 44 45 46 49 51 60 61 63 65 67 70 71 73 74 **N** Columbia Presbyterian Regional Network, New York, NY | 23 | 10 | 164 | 8427 | 125 | 104000 | 1296 | 51627 | 24722 | 722 |

NEWFANE—Niagara County
INTER–COMMUNITY MEMORIAL HOSPITAL, 2600 William Street, Zip 14108; tel. 716/778–5111; Clare A. Haar, Chief Executive Officer **A**9 10 **F**7 8 11 15 16 17 19 20 25 26 28 29 30 35 37 39 40 41 44 45 49 51 65 71 72 73 74 **P**8 | 23 | 10 | 71 | 2324 | 35 | 50636 | 136 | 14033 | 6193 | 251 |

NIAGARA FALLS—Niagara County
✸ NIAGARA FALLS MEMORIAL MEDICAL CENTER, 621 Tenth Street, Zip 14302–0708, Mailing Address: P.O. Box 708, Zip 14302–0708; tel. 716/278–4000; Timothy J. Finan, FACHE, President **A**1 3 5 9 10 **F**3 11 12 13 14 15 16 18 19 20 21 22 25 27 28 30 31 32 33 35 37 39 40 41 42 44 49 51 52 53 54 55 56 57 58 59 60 63 65 67 71 72 73 **P**3 7 | 23 | 10 | 288 | 8030 | 179 | 291842 | 675 | 63559 | 31262 | 1110 |

NORTH TARRYTOWN—New York County
PHELPS MEMORIAL HOSPITAL CENTER See Sleepy Hollow

NORTH TONAWANDA—Niagara County
▢ DE GRAFF MEMORIAL HOSPITAL, 445 Tremont Street, Zip 14120–0750, Mailing Address: P.O. Box 0750, Zip 14120–0750; tel. 716/694–4500; Thomas F. Schifferli, President and Chief Executive Officer (Total facility includes 80 beds in nursing home–type unit) (Nonreporting) **A**1 9 10 **N** Buffalo General Health System, Buffalo, NY | 23 | 10 | 210 | — | — | — | — | — | — | — |

NORTHPORT—Suffolk County
✸ VETERANS AFFAIRS MEDICAL CENTER, 79 Middleville Road, Zip 11768–2293; tel. 516/261–4400; James A. Clark, Director (Total facility includes 190 beds in nursing home–type unit) **A**1 2 3 5 8 **F**1 2 3 4 6 8 10 11 12 15 16 19 20 21 22 25 26 27 28 29 30 31 32 33 34 35 37 39 41 42 43 44 45 46 48 49 51 52 54 55 56 57 58 59 60 61 63 64 65 67 69 70 71 72 73 74 **P**6 **S** Department of Veterans Affairs, Washington, DC | 45 | 10 | 699 | 5818 | 552 | 385471 | 0 | 139181 | — | 1697 |

NORWICH—Chenango County
▢ CHENANGO MEMORIAL HOSPITAL, 179 North Broad Street, Zip 13815; tel. 607/337–4111; Frank W. Mirabito, President (Total facility includes 80 beds in nursing home–type unit) **A**1 9 10 **F**7 8 12 15 16 17 19 20 21 22 26 28 30 31 32 34 37 39 40 41 42 44 45 46 48 49 51 61 63 64 65 67 71 73 74 **P**6 7 8 **N** Chenango County Rural Health Network, Norwich, NY | 23 | 10 | 138 | 2012 | 102 | 167952 | 274 | 28307 | 13530 | 484 |

NYACK—Rockland County
✸ NYACK HOSPITAL, North Midland Avenue, Zip 10960–1998; tel. 914/348–2000; Greger C. Anderson, President and Chief Executive Officer **A**1 2 9 10 **F**2 9 11 12 14 15 16 17 18 19 21 22 30 31 32 35 37 39 40 41 42 44 45 46 48 49 50 51 52 54 65 70 71 73 74 **P**1 4 5 **N** Columbia Presbyterian Regional Network, New York, NY | 23 | 10 | 317 | 12559 | 207 | 266997 | 1847 | 107727 | 49185 | 1133 |

OCEANSIDE—Nassau County
✸ SOUTH NASSAU COMMUNITIES HOSPITAL, 2445 Oceanside Road, Zip 11572–1500; tel. 516/763–2030; Michael Rodzenko, President and Chief Executive Officer **A**1 2 3 5 9 10 **F**4 5 7 8 9 10 11 14 15 16 17 18 19 21 22 26 27 28 29 30 31 32 34 35 37 38 39 40 41 42 43 44 45 46 47 49 51 52 53 54 55 56 57 58 59 60 63 65 67 68 69 70 71 73 74 **P**3 5 7 | 23 | 10 | 429 | 12377 | 307 | 164446 | 1212 | 102271 | 53091 | 1297 |

OGDENSBURG—St. Lawrence County
▢ HEPBURN MEDICAL CENTER, 214 King Street, Zip 13669–1192; tel. 315/393–3600; Donald C. Lewis, President and Chief Executive Officer (Total facility includes 29 beds in nursing home–type unit) **A**1 9 10 12 **F**4 7 8 14 15 16 17 18 19 21 22 23 24 25 26 28 29 30 33 34 35 39 40 41 42 44 45 46 49 51 52 54 55 56 58 60 63 64 65 67 69 71 73 74 **P**7 | 23 | 10 | 149 | 4692 | 107 | 100429 | 426 | 31319 | 15474 | 459 |

✸ ST. LAWRENCE PSYCHIATRIC CENTER, 1 Chimney Point Drive, Zip 13669–2291; tel. 315/393–3000; John R. Scott, Director (Nonreporting) **A**1 10 **S** New York State Department of Mental Health, Albany, NY | 12 | 22 | 265 | — | — | — | — | — | — | — |

OLEAN—Cattaraugus County
✸ OLEAN GENERAL HOSPITAL, 515 Main Street, Zip 14760–9912; tel. 716/373–2600; Robert A. Catalano, M.D., President and Chief Executive Officer **A**1 3 6 9 10 **F**7 8 9 11 12 15 16 18 19 21 22 23 30 32 33 35 37 38 39 40 41 42 44 45 46 47 49 52 54 56 57 63 64 65 67 71 73 | 23 | 10 | 209 | 7391 | 117 | 131087 | 635 | 43742 | 20699 | 750 |

ONEIDA—Madison County
✸ ONEIDA HEALTHCARE CENTER, 321 Genesee Street, Zip 13421–0321; tel. 315/363–6000; Richard G. Smith, Administrator (Total facility includes 160 beds in nursing home–type unit) (Nonreporting) **A**1 9 10 | 14 | 10 | 263 | — | — | — | — | — | — | — |

ONEONTA—Otsego County
✸ AURELIA OSBORN FOX MEMORIAL HOSPITAL, 1 Norton Avenue, Zip 13820–2697; tel. 607/432–2000; John R. Remillard, President (Total facility includes 131 beds in nursing home–type unit) **A**1 9 10 **F**1 7 8 11 15 17 18 19 21 22 25 26 28 30 32 33 35 36 39 40 41 42 44 45 46 49 51 52 54 56 57 58 63 64 65 71 73 **P**5 **S** Quorum Health Group/Quorum Health Resources, Inc., Brentwood, TN | 23 | 10 | 238 | 4140 | 196 | 118089 | 359 | 42980 | 20181 | 455 |

ORANGEBURG—Rockland County
✸ ROCKLAND CHILDREN'S PSYCHIATRIC CENTER, Convent Road, Zip 10962; tel. 914/359–7400; Marcia Werby, Administrator (Nonreporting) **A**1 3 **S** New York State Department of Mental Health, Albany, NY | 12 | 52 | 54 | — | — | — | — | — | — | — |

Hospital, Address, Telephone, Administrator, Approval, Facility, and Physician Codes, Health Care System, Network	Classi-fication Codes		Utilization Data					Expense (thousands) of dollars		
	Control	Service	Beds	Admissions	Census	Outpatient Visits	Births	Total	Payroll	Personnel

★ American Hospital Association (AHA) membership
□ Joint Commission on Accreditation of Healthcare Organizations (JCAHO) accreditation
+ American Osteopathic Hospital Association (AOHA) membership
○ American Osteopathic Association (AOA) accreditation
△ Commission on Accreditation of Rehabilitation Facilities (CARF) accreditation
Control codes 61, 63, 64, 71, 72 and 73 indicate hospitals listed by AOHA, but not registered by AHA. For definition of numerical codes, see page A4

Hospital	Control	Service	Beds	Admissions	Census	Outpatient Visits	Births	Total	Payroll	Personnel
✠ ROCKLAND PSYCHIATRIC CENTER, 140 Old Orangeburg Road, Zip 10962–0071; tel. 914/359–1000; Stephen N. Lawrence, Ph.D., Chief Executive Officer **A**1 5 10 **F**2 3 4 5 8 9 10 11 12 16 17 18 19 20 21 22 23 25 26 27 28 29 30 31 32 33 34 35 36 37 39 41 42 43 44 45 46 48 49 50 51 52 54 55 56 57 58 59 60 61 63 65 67 70 71 72 73 74 **P**6 **S** New York State Department of Mental Health, Albany, NY	12	22	525	508	581	26171	0	—	—	1079
OSSINING—Westchester County										
OSSINING CORRECTIONAL FACILITIES HOSPITAL, 354 Hunter Street, Zip 10562; tel. 914/941–0108; Benjamin Dyett, M.D., Director (Nonreporting)	12	11	25							
□ STONY LODGE HOSPITAL, 40 Croton Dam Road, Zip 10562, Mailing Address: Box 1250, Briarcliff Manor, Zip 10510; tel. 914/941–7400; Kevin Czipo, Executive Director **A**1 10 **F**14 52 53 **P**1	33	22	55	836	44	0	0	9377	4714	145
OSWEGO—Oswego County										
✠ OSWEGO HOSPITAL, 110 West Sixth Street, Zip 13126–9985; tel. 315/349–5511; Corte J. Spencer, Chief Executive Officer (Total facility includes 38 beds in nursing home–type unit) **A**1 9 10 **F**3 7 8 11 12 13 14 16 17 18 19 20 21 22 25 30 31 32 33 34 36 37 38 39 40 41 42 44 45 49 51 52 53 54 56 58 59 63 64 65 69 71 72 73 74 **N** Oswego County Rural Health Network, Oswego, NY	23	10	202	4876	115	181627	792	33783	17625	562
PATCHOGUE—Suffolk County										
✠ BROOKHAVEN MEMORIAL HOSPITAL MEDICAL CENTER, 101 Hospital Road, Zip 11772–9998; tel. 516/654–7100; Thomas Ockers, President (Nonreporting) **A**1 3 9 10	23	10	321	—	—	—	—	—	—	—
PEEKSKILL—Westchester County										
✠ HUDSON VALLEY HOSPITAL CENTER, 1980 Crompond Road, Zip 10566–4182; tel. 914/737–9000; John C. Federspiel, President and Chief Executive Officer **A**1 9 10 **F**7 8 14 15 16 17 18 19 22 25 26 28 30 34 37 39 40 41 44 46 67 70 71 73 **P**3 4 5 6 7 8 **N** The Excelcare System, Inc., Bronxville, NY; Westchester Health Services Network, Mt Kisco, NY	23	10	120	6136	91	197837	1364	45321	21024	505
PENN YAN—Yates County										
✠ SOLDIERS AND SAILORS MEMORIAL HOSPITAL OF YATES COUNTY, 418 North Main Street, Zip 14527–1085; tel. 315/536–4431; Norman Lindenmuth, M.D., Interim Chief Executive Officer (Total facility includes 152 beds in nursing home–type unit) **A**1 9 10 **F**1 8 14 15 16 17 19 22 25 26 34 37 41 44 51 52 53 54 55 56 57 58 64 65 71 73 **P**6 **N** Four Lakes Rural Health Network, Geneva, NY	23	10	217	1756	182	56146	0	21467	9615	420
PLAINVIEW—Nassau County										
✠ NORTH SHORE UNIVERSITY HOSPITAL AT PLAINVIEW, 888 Old Country Road, Zip 11803–4978; tel. 516/681–8900; Glenn Hirsch, Administrator (Nonreporting) **A**1 2 9 10 **S** North Shore Health System, Manhasset, NY **N** North Shore Regional Health Systems, Manhasset, NY	33	10	279	—	—	—	—	—	—	—
PLATTSBURGH—Clinton County										
✠ CHAMPLAIN VALLEY PHYSICIANS HOSPITAL MEDICAL CENTER, 75 Beekman Street, Zip 12901–1493; tel. 518/561–2000; Kevin J. Carroll, President (Total facility includes 54 beds in nursing home–type unit) **A**1 2 5 9 10 **F**7 8 10 11 12 13 15 16 19 20 21 22 23 24 25 28 30 33 34 35 37 40 41 42 44 46 49 52 56 60 64 65 67 70 71 73 74 **N** Eastern Adirondack Health Care Network, Westport, NY	23	10	410	9351	237	173634	1053	77643	38371	1155
POMONA—Rockland County										
□ DOCTOR ROBERT L. YEAGER HEALTH CENTER, (Includes Summit Park Hospital–Rockland County Infirmary), Sanatorium Road, Zip 10970; tel. 914/364–2700; Peter T. Fella, Commissioner (Total facility includes 300 beds in nursing home–type unit) (Nonreporting) **A**1 10	13	49	408							
PORT CHESTER—Westchester County										
□ UNITED HOSPITAL MEDICAL CENTER, 406 Boston Post Road, Zip 10573; tel. 914/939–7000; Kevin Dahill, President and Chief Executive Officer (Total facility includes 40 beds in nursing home–type unit) (Nonreporting) **A**1 5 9 10 **N** The Excelcare System, Inc., Bronxville, NY; The New York & Presbyterian Hospitals Care Network, Inc., New York, NY	23	10	290	—	—	—	—	—	—	—
PORT JEFFERSON—Suffolk County										
✠ JOHN T. MATHER MEMORIAL HOSPITAL, 75 North Country Road, Zip 11777–2190; tel. 516/473–1320; Kenneth D. Roberts, President **A**1 2 9 10 **F**1 2 3 4 8 11 14 15 16 19 20 21 22 30 31 32 33 34 35 36 37 38 39 40 41 42 44 45 46 47 48 49 52 53 54 55 56 57 58 59 60 61 63 65 67 69 71 73 **P**8	23	10	248	9007	188	90386	0	78749	39381	968
✠ ST. CHARLES HOSPITAL AND REHABILITATION CENTER, 200 Belle Terre Road, Zip 11777; tel. 516/474–6000; Barry T. Zeman, President and Chief Executive Officer (Nonreporting) **A**1 2 3 5 9 10 **N** First Choice Network, Inc., Mineola, NY	21	10	235	—	—	—	—	—	—	—
PORT JERVIS—Orange County										
✠ MERCY COMMUNITY HOSPITAL, 160 East Main Street, Zip 12771–0268, Mailing Address: P.O. Box 1014, Zip 12771; tel. 914/856–5351; R. Andrew Brothers, President and Chief Executive Officer (Total facility includes 46 beds in nursing home–type unit) **A**1 2 9 10 **F**2 7 8 14 .9 20 22 30 35 37 39 40 42 46 49 52 56 64 65 67 71 73 **P**5 8 **S** Franciscan Sisters of the Poor Health System, Inc., New York, NY **N** Tri-State Health System, Suffern, NY	21	10	187	4034	117	63912	241	30749	15391	455
POTSDAM—St. Lawrence County										
✠ CANTON–POTSDAM HOSPITAL, 50 Leroy Street, Zip 13676; tel. 315/265–3300; Bruce C. Potter, President **A**1 9 10 **F**2 7 8 14 16 19 21 22 28 30 35 37 39 40 42 44 46 49 50 65 70 71 73	23	10	94	3664	60	83413	300	24659	12062	457

Hospital, Address, Telephone, Administrator, Approval, Facility, and Physician Codes, Health Care System, Network	Classi- fication Codes		Utilization Data					Expense (thousands) of dollars		
	Control	Service	Beds	Admissions	Census	Outpatient Visits	Births	Total	Payroll	Personnel

★ American Hospital Association (AHA) membership
□ Joint Commission on Accreditation of Healthcare Organizations (JCAHO) accreditation
+ American Osteopathic Hospital Association (AOHA) membership
○ American Osteopathic Association (AOA) accreditation
△ Commission on Accreditation of Rehabilitation Facilities (CARF) accreditation
Control codes 61, 63, 64, 71, 72 and 73 indicate hospitals listed by AOHA, but not registered by AHA. For definition of numerical codes, see page A4.

POUGHKEEPSIE—Dutchess County

Hospital	Control	Service	Beds	Admissions	Census	Outpatient Visits	Births	Total	Payroll	Personnel
✖ HUDSON RIVER PSYCHIATRIC CENTER, Branch B, Zip 12601–1197; tel. 914/452–8000; James Regan, Ph.D., Chief Executive Officer **A**1 5 10 **F**1 3 4 9 11 14 15 16 17 18 19 20 21 22 25 26 28 34 35 37 43 44 45 46 48 49 50 52 55 56 57 58 59 60 63 64 70 71 73 **P**8 **S** New York State Department of Mental Health, Albany, NY	12	22	460	205	530	2000	0	—	—	937
✖ △ SAINT FRANCIS HOSPITAL, (Includes Saint Francis Hospital–Beacon, 60 Delavan Avenue, Beacon, Zip 12508; tel. 914/831–3500), North Road, Zip 12601–1399; tel. 914/471–2000; Sister M. Ann Elizabeth, President **A**1 3 7 9 10 **F**2 3 8 11 13 14 15 16 17 19 20 21 22 23 26 27 28 29 30 31 32 34 35 36 37 39 41 42 44 45 46 48 49 52 53 54 55 56 57 58 63 65 66 70 71 72 73 **N** The Mount Sinai Health System, New York, NY	21	10	317	10720	272	215000	0	98357	49515	1389
✖ VASSAR BROTHERS HOSPITAL, Reade Place, Zip 12601; tel. 914/454–8500; Ronald T. Mullahey, President **A**1 2 3 9 10 **F**2 3 7 8 10 11 12 14 15 16 17 18 19 20 21 23 25 27 28 30 31 32 33 34 35 37 38 39 40 41 42 44 45 46 48 49 52 53 54 55 56 58 59 60 61 65 67 70 71 72 73 74 **N** The Mount Sinai Health System, New York, NY	23	10	257	13064	202	148445	2503	89851	39831	811

QUEENS—Queens County, See New York City
QUEENS VILLAGE—Queens County, See New York City
RHINEBECK—Dutchess County

Hospital	Control	Service	Beds	Admissions	Census	Outpatient Visits	Births	Total	Payroll	Personnel
✖ NORTHERN DUTCHESS HOSPITAL, 10 Springbrook Avenue, Zip 12572–5002, Mailing Address: P.O. Box 5002, Zip 12572–5002; tel. 914/876–3001; Michael C. Mazzarella, Chief Executive Officer (Nonreporting) **A**1 9 10	23	10	71	—	—	—	—	—	—	—

RICHMOND VALLEY—Richmond County, See New York City
RIVERHEAD—Suffolk County

Hospital	Control	Service	Beds	Admissions	Census	Outpatient Visits	Births	Total	Payroll	Personnel
✖ CENTRAL SUFFOLK HOSPITAL, 1300 Roanoke Avenue, Zip 11901–2028; tel. 516/548–6000; Joseph F. Turner, President (Total facility includes 60 beds in nursing home–type unit) **A**1 9 10 **F**4 7 8 14 15 16 19 21 22 28 29 30 32 34 35 37 40 42 44 45 49 64 65 67 71 72 73 **P**7	23	10	196	4723	149	62915	173	48716	22830	530

ROCHESTER—Monroe County

Hospital	Control	Service	Beds	Admissions	Census	Outpatient Visits	Births	Total	Payroll	Personnel
✖ GENESEE HOSPITAL, 224 Alexander Street, Zip 14607–4055; tel. 716/263–6000; Joseph J. DeSilva, FACHE, President and Chief Executive Officer (Total facility includes 40 beds in nursing home–type unit) (Nonreporting) **A**1 2 3 5 8 9 10 **S** Greater Rochester Health System, Inc., Rochester, NY **N** Greater Rochester Health System, Inc., Rochester, NY	23	10	305	—	—	—	—	—	—	—
✖ HIGHLAND HOSPITAL OF ROCHESTER, 1000 South Avenue, Zip 14620; tel. 716/473–2200; Michael J. Weidner, President **A**1 2 3 5 9 10 **F**4 6 7 8 12 14 15 16 19 20 21 22 26 28 29 30 31 32 34 37 39 40 42 44 45 46 49 51 54 60 62 65 67 70 71 73 74	23	10	225	9711	149	175000	2013	86073	43870	1785
□ MONROE COMMUNITY HOSPITAL, 435 East Henrietta Road, Zip 14620–4684; tel. 716/274–7100; Frank Tripodi, Executive Director (Total facility includes 566 beds in nursing home–type unit) (Nonreporting) **A**1 3 5 9 10	13	49	605	—	—	—	—	—	—	—
✖ PARK RIDGE HOSPITAL, 1555 Long Pond Road, Zip 14626–4182; tel. 716/723–7000; Timothy R. McCormick, President **A**1 2 9 10 **F**1 2 3 6 10 12 14 15 16 17 18 19 21 22 26 30 32 33 34 35 37 39 41 42 43 44 45 46 48 49 51 52 53 54 55 56 57 58 59 62 65 66 67 68 69 70 71 72 73 **P**7 **N** Park Ridge Health System, Rochester, NY	23	10	259	8337	195	246986	0	77257	33983	900
✖ ROCHESTER GENERAL HOSPITAL, 1425 Portland Avenue, Zip 14621–3099; tel. 716/338–4000; Richard S. Constantino, M.D., President **A**1 2 3 5 6 8 9 10 **F**1 3 4 5 6 7 8 10 12 13 15 16 17 18 19 20 21 22 24 25 26 28 30 31 32 34 35 37 38 39 40 41 42 43 44 45 46 48 49 51 52 53 54 55 56 57 58 59 60 61 62 63 64 65 66 67 68 70 71 73 74 **P**3 5 7 **S** Greater Rochester Health System, Inc., Rochester, NY **N** Greater Rochester Health System, Inc., Rochester, NY	23	10	476	21539	363	645010	2642	220804	100993	3288
✖ ROCHESTER PSYCHIATRIC CENTER, 1111 Elmwood Avenue, Zip 14620–3005; tel. 716/473–3230; Martin H. Von Holden, Executive Director **A**1 3 5 9 10 **F**1 2 3 4 5 6 7 8 9 10 11 12 13 14 16 17 18 19 20 21 22 23 24 25 26 27 28 29 30 31 32 33 34 35 36 37 38 39 40 41 42 43 44 45 46 47 48 49 50 51 52 53 54 55 56 57 58 59 60 61 62 63 64 65 66 67 68 70 71 72 73 74 **S** New York State Department of Mental Health, Albany, NY	12	22	288	214	313	46030	0	39961	26761	676
✖ △ ST. MARY'S HOSPITAL, 89 Genesee Street, Zip 14611–3285; tel. 716/464–3000; Stewart Putnam, President **A**1 2 3 5 7 9 10 **F**7 8 10 11 12 13 14 15 16 17 19 20 21 22 24 26 28 30 31 34 35 37 39 40 41 42 44 45 46 48 49 51 53 54 55 56 57 58 59 61 65 68 71 72 73 **P**5 6 **S** Daughters of Charity National Health System, Saint Louis, MO	21	10	190	6137	131	295080	676	97507	50660	1371
✖ △ STRONG MEMORIAL HOSPITAL OF THE UNIVERSITY OF ROCHESTER, 601 Elmwood Avenue, Zip 14642; tel. 716/275–2100; Leo P. Brideau, General Director and Chief Executive Officer (Nonreporting) **A**1 3 5 7 8 9 10	23	10	719	—	—	—	—	—	—	—

ROCKVILLE CENTRE—Nassau County

Hospital	Control	Service	Beds	Admissions	Census	Outpatient Visits	Births	Total	Payroll	Personnel
✖ MERCY MEDICAL CENTER, 1000 North Village Avenue, Zip 11570–1098; tel. 516/255–0111; Vincent DiRubbio, Administrator **A**1 2 3 9 10 **F**3 4 7 9 10 11 12 14 15 16 17 19 21 22 23 26 28 30 31 32 33 34 35 37 38 40 41 42 43 44 48 49 52 54 55 56 57 58 59 60 63 64 65 66 67 69 70 71 73 74 **P**6 8	21	10	387	13454	278	184073	2006	124436	61049	1706

ROME—Oneida County

Hospital	Control	Service	Beds	Admissions	Census	Outpatient Visits	Births	Total	Payroll	Personnel
✖ ROME MEMORIAL HOSPITAL, 1500 North James Street, Zip 13440–2898; tel. 315/338–7000; Alvin C. White, President and Chief Executive Officer (Total facility includes 52 beds in nursing home–type unit) **A**1 9 10 **F**3 7 8 14 15 16 19 21 22 28 30 31 32 34 35 37 39 40 41 44 45 49 64 65 66 71 73 74 **P**3 5 7	23	10	164	5427	114	87182	515	33805	16921	633

Hospital, Address, Telephone, Administrator, Approval, Facility, and Physician Codes, Health Care System, Network	Classi-fication Codes		Utilization Data					Expense (thousands) of dollars		
★ American Hospital Association (AHA) membership □ Joint Commission on Accreditation of Healthcare Organizations (JCAHO) accreditation + American Osteopathic Hospital Association (AOHA) membership ○ American Osteopathic Association (AOA) accreditation △ Commission on Accreditation of Rehabilitation Facilities (CARF) accreditation Control codes 61, 63, 64, 71, 72 and 73 indicate hospitals listed by AOHA, but not registered by AHA. For definition of numerical codes, see page A4	Control	Service	Beds	Admissions	Census	Outpatient Visits	Births	Total	Payroll	Personnel

ROSLYN—Nassau County

✠ ST. FRANCIS HOSPITAL, 100 Port Washington Boulevard, Zip 11576–1348; tel. 516/562–6000; Patrick J. Scollard, President and Chief Executive Officer **A**1 5 9 10 **F**3 4 8 10 11 12 14 15 16 17 19 20 21 22 24 28 32 34 35 36 37 39 43 44 45 46 47 49 54 56 65 67 69 71 73 **P**8 **N** Columbia Presbyterian Regional Network, New York, NY

| | 23 | 10 | 247 | 13762 | 305 | 76690 | 0 | 172794 | 78526 | 1612 |

RYE—Westchester County

✠ RYE HOSPITAL CENTER, 754 Boston Post Road, Zip 10580; tel. 914/967–4567; Jack C. Schoenholtz, M.D., Medical Director and Administrator **A**1 10 **F**17 19 20 21 22 35 45 48 50 52 53 55 57 60 63 65 71 73

| | 33 | 22 | 34 | 169 | 28 | 0 | 0 | 4837 | 1876 | 59 |

SARANAC LAKE—Franklin County

✠ ADIRONDACK MEDICAL CENTER, Lake Colby Drive, Zip 12983, Mailing Address: P.O. Box 471, Zip 12983; tel. 518/891–4141; Chandler M. Ralph, President and Chief Executive Officer (Nonreporting) **A**1 9 10 **S** Brim, Inc., Portland, OR

| | 23 | 10 | 100 | — | — | — | — | — | — | — |

SARATOGA SPRINGS—Saratoga County

✠ SARATOGA HOSPITAL, 211 Church Street, Zip 12866–1003; tel. 518/587–3222; David Andersen, President and Chief Executive Officer (Total facility includes 72 beds in nursing home–type unit) **A**1 9 10 **F**7 8 14 16 19 21 22 27 28 30 33 34 35 37 39 40 41 42 44 46 49 52 54 56 63 64 65 67 71 72 73 **N** Shared Health Network, Inc., Albany, NY

| | 23 | 10 | 204 | 6628 | 179 | 106489 | 774 | 47094 | 22401 | 779 |

SCHENECTADY—Schenectady County

✠ BELLEVUE WOMAN'S HOSPITAL, (Formerly Bellevue – The Woman's Hospital), 2210 Troy Road, Zip 12309–4797; tel. 518/346–9400; Michael A. Mangini, Administrator and Chief Executive Officer (Nonreporting) **A**1 9 10

| | 33 | 44 | 40 | — | — | — | — | — | — | — |

✠ ELLIS HOSPITAL, 1101 Nott Street, Zip 12308–2487; tel. 518/382–4124; G. B. Serrill, President and Chief Executive Officer (Total facility includes 82 beds in nursing home–type unit) **A**1 2 3 5 6 9 10 **F**4 5 6 7 8 10 11 12 13 14 15 16 17 18 19 20 21 22 23 25 26 28 29 30 31 32 33 34 35 37 39 40 41 42 43 44 45 46 49 51 52 54 55 56 57 58 59 60 61 63 64 65 67 70 71 73 **S** Quorum Health Group/Quorum Health Resources, Inc., Brentwood, TN **N** Shared Health Network, Inc., Albany, NY

| | 23 | 10 | 434 | 11534 | 301 | 205875 | 419 | 114837 | 53282 | 1588 |

□ ST. CLARE'S HOSPITAL OF SCHENECTADY, 600 McClellan Street, Zip 12304; tel. 518/382–2000; Jerome G. Stewart, President **A**1 3 5 9 10 12 **F**1 2 3 4 5 6 7 8 9 10 11 12 14 15 16 17 19 20 21 22 24 25 26 28 29 30 31 32 34 35 37 38 39 40 42 43 44 45 46 47 48 49 51 52 56 64 65 69 70 71 73 74 **N** Shared Health Network, Inc., Albany, NY

| | 21 | 10 | 200 | 6915 | 118 | 150109 | 675 | 59467 | 29053 | 973 |

✠ △ SUNNYVIEW HOSPITAL AND REHABILITATION CENTER, 1270 Belmont Avenue, Zip 12308–2104; tel. 518/382–4500; Bradford M. Goodwin, President (Nonreporting) **A**1 3 5 7 9 10 **N** Shared Health Network, Inc., Albany, NY

| | 23 | 46 | 92 | — | — | — | — | — | — | — |

SCOTIA—Schenectady County

CONIFER PARK See Glenville

SEAFORD—Nassau County

+ ○ MASSAPEQUA GENERAL HOSPITAL, 750 Hicksville Road, Zip 11783, Mailing Address: Box 20, Zip 11783; tel. 516/520–6000; John P. Breen, Chief Executive Officer (Nonreporting) **A**9 10 11 12 13

| | 33 | 10 | 122 | — | — | — | — | — | — | — |

SIDNEY—Delaware County

✠ THE HOSPITAL, 43 Pearl Street West, Zip 13838; tel. 607/561–2153; Russell A. Test, Chief Executive Officer (Total facility includes 40 beds in nursing home–type unit) **A**1 9 10 **F**7 8 12 19 22 25 30 31 34 37 39 40 41 44 49 51 64 **S** Brim, Inc., Portland, OR

| | 14 | 10 | 87 | 1886 | 63 | 45073 | 169 | 11827 | 5900 | 282 |

SLEEPY HOLLOW—New York County

✠ PHELPS MEMORIAL HOSPITAL CENTER, 701 North Broadway, Zip 10591–1096; tel. 914/366–3000; Keith F. Safian, President and Chief Executive Officer **A**1 9 10 **F**2 3 7 8 9 11 12 14 15 16 17 19 20 21 22 26 27 28 29 30 31 32 33 34 35 36 37 38 39 40 41 42 44 45 46 47 48 49 51 52 54 55 56 57 58 60 61 63 64 65 66 67 68 70 71 72 73 74 **P**1 5 **N** The Excelcare System, Inc., Bronxville, NY; The Mount Sinai Health System, New York, NY

| | 23 | 10 | 235 | 7739 | 139 | 112173 | 680 | 64360 | 32740 | 875 |

SMITHTOWN—Suffolk County

□ COMMUNITY HOSPITAL OF SMITHTOWN, 498 Smithtown By-Pass, Zip 11787–5018; tel. 516/979–9800; Robert M. Jewels, Administrator (Nonreporting) **A**1 9 10

| | 21 | 10 | 112 | — | — | — | — | — | — | — |

✠ ST. JOHN'S EPISCOPAL HOSPITAL–SMITHTOWN, 50 Route 25–A, Zip 11787–1398; tel. 516/862–3000; Laura Righter, Regional Administrator (Nonreporting) **A**1 9 **S** Episcopal Health Services Inc., Uniondale, NY **N** Episcopal Health Services, Inc., Uniondale, NY; First Choice Network, Inc., Mineola, NY; The Mount Sinai Health System, New York, NY

| | 21 | 10 | 366 | — | — | — | — | — | — | — |

SODUS—Wayne County

✠ MYERS COMMUNITY HOSPITAL, 6600 Middle Road, Zip 14551–0310; tel. 315/483–3000; Jane Johnson, President and Chief Executive Officer **A**1 9 10 **F**7 8 11 19 22 30 37 41 44 45 46 49 65 66 71 73 74 **P**5 8

| | 23 | 10 | 54 | 1867 | 24 | 33305 | 214 | 13648 | 5818 | 191 |

SOUTHAMPTON—Suffolk County

□ SOUTHAMPTON HOSPITAL, 240 Meeting House Lane, Zip 11968–5090; tel. 516/726–8555; John J. Ferry, Jr., M.D., President and Chief Executive Officer (Nonreporting) **A**1 9 10 **N** First Choice Network, Inc., Mineola, NY

| | 23 | 10 | 127 | — | — | — | — | — | — | — |

SPRINGVILLE—Erie County

BERTRAND CHAFFEE HOSPITAL, 224 East Main Street, Zip 14141–1497; tel. 716/592–2871; Roger A. Ford, Administrator (Nonreporting) **A**9 10

| | 23 | 10 | 49 | — | — | — | — | — | — | — |

Hospital, Address, Telephone, Administrator, Approval, Facility, and Physician Codes, Health Care System, Network	Classi-fication Codes		Utilization Data					Expense (thousands) of dollars		
★ American Hospital Association (AHA) membership □ Joint Commission on Accreditation of Healthcare Organizations (JCAHO) accreditation + American Osteopathic Hospital Association (AOHA) membership ○ American Osteopathic Association (AOA) accreditation △ Commission on Accreditation of Rehabilitation Facilities (CARF) accreditation Control codes 61, 63, 64, 71, 72 and 73 indicate hospitals listed by AOHA, but not registered by AHA. For definition of numerical codes, see page A4	Control	Service	Beds	Admissions	Census	Outpatient Visits	Births	Total	Payroll	Personnel

STAR LAKE—St. Lawrence County

★ CLIFTON–FINE HOSPITAL, Oswegatchie Trail, Zip 13690, Mailing Address: Box 10, Zip 13690–0010; tel. 315/848–3351; Rodney C. Boula, Administrator (Nonreporting) **A**9 10

	16	10	20	—	—	—	—	—	—	—

STATEN ISLAND—Richmond County, See New York City

STONY BROOK—Suffolk County

✠ UNIVERSITY HOSPITAL, State University of New York, Zip 11794–8410; tel. 516/689–8333; Michael A. Maffetone, Director and Chief Executive Officer **A**1 2 3 5 8 9 10 **F**4 7 8 9 10 11 12 13 14 15 16 17 18 19 20 21 22 23 25 26 28 29 30 31 34 35 37 38 39 40 41 42 43 44 45 46 47 49 51 52 53 54 55 56 58 59 60 61 63 64 65 66 67 68 69 70 71 72 73 74 **P**1 4 6 7 **N** Health First, New York, NY

	12	10	504	23584	395	606936	3555	316018	140616	3815

SUFFERN—Rockland County

□ GOOD SAMARITAN HOSPITAL, 255 Lafayette Avenue, Zip 10901–4869; tel. 914/368–5000; James A. Martin, Chief Executive Officer (Nonreporting) **A**1 9 10 **N** Westchester Health Services Network, Mt Kisco, NY

	21	10	308	—	—	—	—	—	—	—

SYOSSET—Nassau County

✠ NORTH SHORE UNIVERSITY HOSPITAL AT SYOSSET, 221 Jericho Turnpike, Zip 11791–4567; tel. 516/496–6400; Deborah Tascone, R.N., Vice President/Administration (Nonreporting) **A**1 3 9 10

	23	10	186	—	—	—	—	—	—	—

SYRACUSE—Onondaga County

□ BENJAMIN RUSH CENTER, 650 South Salina Street, Zip 13202–3524; tel. 315/476–2161; Robert C. Long, Administrator and Chief Executive Officer **A**1 9 10 **F**2 14 15 16 52 53 55 57 59 **P**6

	31	22	107	1420	61		0			236

✠ COMMUNITY–GENERAL HOSPITAL OF GREATER SYRACUSE, 4900 Broad Road, Zip 13215; tel. 315/492–5011; Kent A. Arnold, President (Total facility includes 50 beds in nursing home–type unit) **A**1 3 5 9 10 **F**4 7 8 12 14 16 19 21 22 25 26 28 29 30 31 34 37 39 40 41 42 44 52 53 54 55 64 65 71 73 **P**6 8

	23	10	356	11585	244	153894	1462	76385	36844	1187

✠ CROUSE HOSPITAL, (Formerly Crouse Irving Memorial Hospital), 736 Irving Avenue, Zip 13210–1690; tel. 315/470–7111; Edward T. Wenzke, President and Chief Executive Officer **A**1 3 5 9 10 **F**2 3 4 7 8 10 11 12 14 15 16 17 19 22 24 25 28 29 30 34 35 37 38 39 40 42 44 45 46 47 49 51 54 65 67 70 71 72 73 74 **P**1 5 7 **N** Hamilton–Bassett–Crouse Rural Health Network, Hamilton, NY

	23	10	490	20177	341	174516	4020	161024	67831	2356

✠ RICHARD H. HUTCHINGS PSYCHIATRIC CENTER, 620 Madison Street, Zip 13210–2319; tel. 315/473–4980; Bryan F. Rudes, Executive Director (Nonreporting) **A**1 3 5 10 **S** New York State Department of Mental Health, Albany, NY

	12	22	184	—	—	—	—	—	—	—

□ ST. JOSEPH'S HOSPITAL HEALTH CENTER, 301 Prospect Avenue, Zip 13203; tel. 315/448–5111; Theodore M. Pasinski, President (Nonreporting) **A**1 3 5 6 9 10 **S** Sisters of the 3rd Franciscan Order, Syracuse, NY

	21	10	431	—	—	—	—	—	—	—

✠ UNIVERSITY HOSPITAL–SUNY HEALTH SCIENCE CENTER AT SYRACUSE, 750 East Adams Street, Zip 13210; tel. 315/464–5540; Ben Moore, III, Executive Director **A**1 2 3 5 8 9 10 **F**4 8 9 10 11 16 17 19 20 21 22 23 26 28 31 35 37 41 42 43 44 46 47 48 49 52 53 54 55 56 57 58 59 60 61 65 68 69 70 71 73 74 **P**5 6 7

	12	10	350	12811	281	264370	0	195705	96736	2682

✠ VETERANS AFFAIRS MEDICAL CENTER, 800 Irving Avenue, Zip 13210; tel. 315/476–7461; Philip P. Thomas, Director (Total facility includes 50 beds in nursing home–type unit) **A**1 3 5 8 **F**1 3 4 8 10 11 12 13 14 15 16 17 18 19 20 22 23 25 26 27 28 30 31 32 33 34 35 37 39 41 42 43 44 45 46 48 49 51 52 54 55 56 57 58 59 61 63 64 65 67 71 72 73 74 **P**6 **S** Department of Veterans Affairs, Washington, DC

	45	10	204	4709	151	167099	0	49547	39881	1049

TICONDEROGA—Essex County

□ MOSES LUDINGTON HOSPITAL, Wicker Street, Zip 12883–1097; tel. 518/585–2831; Diane M. Hart, Chief Executive Officer (Nonreporting) **A**1 9 10 **N** Adirondack Rural Health Network, Glens Falls, NY

	23	10	39	—	—	—	—	—	—	—

TROY—Rensselaer County

□ SAMARITAN HOSPITAL, 2215 Burdett Avenue, Zip 12180; tel. 518/271–3300; Norman E. Dascher, Jr., Chief Operating Officer (Nonreporting) **A**1 6 9 10 **N** Shared Health Network, Inc., Albany, NY; Northern New York Rural Health Care Alliance, Watertown, NY

	23	10	272	—	—	—	—	—	—	—

✠ SETON HEALTH SYSTEM, (Includes Seton Health System–Leonard Hospital, 74 New Turnpike Road, Zip 12182–1498; tel. 518/235–0310; Seton Health System–St. Mary's Hospital, 1300 Massachusetts Avenue), 1300 Massachusetts Avenue, Zip 12180; tel. 518/272–5000; Edward G. Murphy, M.D., President and Chief Executive Officer (Nonreporting) **A**1 9 10 **S** Daughters of Charity National Health System, Saint Louis, MO **N** Seton Health Care System, Troy, NY; Shared Health Network, Inc., Albany, NY

	21	10	344	—	—	—	—	—	—	—

UTICA—Oneida County

✠ FAXTON HOSPITAL, 1676 Sunset Avenue, Zip 13502; tel. 315/738–6200; Keith A. Fenstemacher, President and Chief Executive Officer **A**1 2 9 10 **F**1 7 8 10 11 15 17 19 20 21 22 23 26 28 29 30 32 33 34 35 36 37 38 40 41 42 44 48 49 51 52 56 60 64 65 67 69 70 71 72 73 74 **P**3 **N** MoHawk Valley Network, Inc., Utica, NY

	23	10	166	5691	114	95270	0	43705	20090	662

✠ MOHAWK VALLEY PSYCHIATRIC CENTER, 1400 Noyes at York, Zip 13502–3803; tel. 315/797–6800; Sarah F. Rudes, Executive Director (Nonreporting) **A**1 10 **S** New York State Department of Mental Health, Albany, NY

	12	22	614	—	—	—	—	—	—	—

Hospital, Address, Telephone, Administrator, Approval, Facility, and Physician Codes, Health Care System, Network	Classi-fication Codes		Utilization Data					Expense (thousands) of dollars		
	Control	Service	Beds	Admissions	Census	Outpatient Visits	Births	Total	Payroll	Personnel

★ American Hospital Association (AHA) membership
☐ Joint Commission on Accreditation of Healthcare Organizations (JCAHO) accreditation
+ American Osteopathic Hospital Association (AOHA) membership
○ American Osteopathic Association (AOA) accreditation
△ Commission on Accreditation of Rehabilitation Facilities (CARF) accreditation
Control codes 61, 63, 64, 71, 72 and 73 indicate hospitals listed by AOHA, but not registered by AHA. For definition of numerical codes, see page A4

Hospital	Control	Service	Beds	Admissions	Census	Outpatient Visits	Births	Total	Payroll	Personnel
✉ ST. ELIZABETH MEDICAL CENTER, (Formerly St. Elizabeth Hospital), 2209 Genesee Street, Zip 13501–5999; tel. 315/798–8100; Sister Rose Vincent, President and Chief Executive Officer **A**1 3 6 9 10 12 **F**7 8 10 11 12 13 14 15 16 18 19 21 22 28 30 33 34 35 37 38 39 40 42 44 49 51 52 54 56 57 61 63 65 66 67 69 70 71 72 73 74 **P**6 **S** Sisters of the 3rd Franciscan Order, Syracuse, NY	21	10	201	7462	129	207451	203	58192	28803	1034
✉ ST. LUKE'S MEMORIAL HOSPITAL CENTER, (Includes Allen–Calder Skilled Nursing Facility; Mohawk Valley Division, 295 West Main Street, Ilion, Zip 13357–1599; tel. 315/895–7474; Pearl T. Gentile, Site Administrator), Mailing Address: P.O. Box 479, Zip 13503–0479; tel. 315/798–6000; Andrew E. Peterson, President and Chief Executive Officer (Total facility includes 124 beds in nursing home–type unit) **A**1 9 10 **F**1 4 7 8 10 11 12 14 15 16 19 20 21 22 25 26 28 29 30 31 32 33 34 35 37 40 41 42 44 46 49 51 52 60 63 64 65 70 71 73 74 **P**3 **N** MoHawk Valley Network, Inc., Utica, NY	23	10	379	11557	325	267295	1958	79101	36999	1127
VALHALLA—Westchester County										
✉ BLYTHEDALE CHILDREN'S HOSPITAL, Bradhurst Avenue, Zip 10595–1697; tel. 914/592–7555; Robert Stone, President **A**1 10 **F**14 15 16 20 24 28 29 30 32 34 41 45 46 48 49 53 54 55 58 65 66 67 71 73 **P**6	23	56	92	298	82	—	0	22334	13942	299
☐ WESTCHESTER COUNTY MEDICAL CENTER, Valhalla Campus, Zip 10595; tel. 914/285–7000; Edward A. Stolzenberg, Commissioner **A**1 2 3 5 8 9 10 **F**2 4 5 7 8 9 10 11 17 18 19 20 21 22 23 26 31 33 34 35 37 38 40 41 42 43 44 46 47 48 49 51 52 53 54 56 57 58 60 63 65 66 69 70 71 73 74 **N** Westchester Health Services Network, Mt Kisco, NY	13	10	657	22098	567	94391	11268	—	—	—
VALLEY STREAM—Nassau County										
✉ FRANKLIN HOSPITAL MEDICAL CENTER, 900 Franklin Avenue, Zip 11580–2190; tel. 516/256–6000; Albert Dicker, President and Chief Executive Officer (Total facility includes 120 beds in nursing home–type unit) (Nonreporting) **A**1 2 9 10 **N** North Shore Regional Health Systems, Manhasset, NY	23	10	405	—	—	—	—	—	—	—
WALTON—Delaware County										
☐ DELAWARE VALLEY HOSPITAL, 1 Titus Place, Zip 13856; tel. 607/865–2100; David J. Polge, President and Chief Executive Officer **A**1 9 10 **F**2 7 8 15 17 19 21 22 25 26 27 28 30 33 37 39 40 41 42 44 49 61 63 65 67 71 73 74 **P**6	23	10	42	1379	22	36741	134	10628	5560	185
WARSAW—Wyoming County										
☐ WYOMING COUNTY COMMUNITY HOSPITAL, 400 North Main Street, Zip 14569; tel. 716/786–2233; Lucille K. Sheedy, Administrator and Chief Executive Officer (Total facility includes 160 beds in nursing home–type unit) **A**1 9 10 **F**7 8 14 15 16 19 21 22 25 28 30 33 34 35 37 40 41 42 44 49 52 56 64 65 71 73 74 **P**3 6	13	10	262	3397	214	111049	447	30177	14569	494
WARWICK—Orange County										
✉ ST. ANTHONY COMMUNITY HOSPITAL, 15–19 Maple Avenue, Zip 10990; tel. 914/986–2276; R. Andrew Brothers, President and Chief Executive Officer **A**1 9 10 **F**1 6 7 8 11 16 19 21 22 29 30 33 36 37 40 44 46 64 67 69 71 73 74 **P**5 6 8 **S** Franciscan Sisters of the Poor Health System, Inc., New York, NY **N** Tri–State Health System, Suffern, NY	21	10	73	2453	43	33267	303	18141	—	275
WATERTOWN—Jefferson County										
☐ SAMARITAN MEDICAL CENTER, 830 Washington Street, Zip 13601, Mailing Address: P.O. Box 517, Zip 13601–0517; tel. 315/785–4000; William P. Koughan, President and Chief Executive Officer **A**1 9 10 **F**1 2 3 8 11 14 15 16 17 18 19 21 22 23 24 25 26 27 28 29 30 31 32 33 34 35 37 39 40 42 44 46 47 49 51 52 53 54 55 56 57 58 60 64 65 66 67 71 72 73 74	23	10	239	10660	184	130145	1675	77931	36830	1035
WELLSVILLE—Allegany County										
✉ JONES MEMORIAL HOSPITAL, 191 North Main Street, Zip 14895, Mailing Address: P.O. Box 72, Zip 14895; tel. 716/593–1100; William M. DiBerardino, FACHE, President and Chief Executive Officer **A**1 9 10 **F**7 8 11 12 15 16 17 19 21 22 28 29 30 35 36 37 39 40 41 42 44 45 46 49 51 63 65 66 67 71 73 74 **P**8 **N** Allegany County Health Care Network, Wellsville, NY	23	10	70	2976	35	58354	438	19002	8243	298
WEST BRENTWOOD—Suffolk County										
✉ KINGS PARK PSYCHIATRIC CENTER, 998 Crooked Hill Road, Zip 11717–1089; tel. 516/761–2616; Alan M. Weinstock, MS, Chief Executive Officer **A**1 10 **F**4 7 8 9 10 11 12 14 15 16 18 19 20 21 22 23 25 27 31 34 35 37 39 40 42 43 44 48 50 51 52 55 56 58 60 63 65 69 70 71 73 **P**6 **S** New York State Department of Mental Health, Albany, NY	12	22	777	1266	796	116992	0	96259	65203	1408
WEST HAVERSTRAW—Rockland County										
✉ HELEN HAYES HOSPITAL, Route 9W, Zip 10993–1195; tel. 914/947–3000; Magdalena Ramirez, Director **A**1 3 5 9 10 **F**1 2 3 4 5 6 7 8 9 10 11 12 13 14 16 17 18 19 20 21 22 23 24 25 26 27 28 29 30 31 34 35 36 37 38 39 40 41 42 43 44 45 46 47 48 49 50 51 52 53 54 55 56 57 58 59 60 61 62 63 64 65 66 67 68 69 70 71 72 73 74 **N** Columbia Presbyterian Regional Network, New York, NY	12	46	155	1752	122	32772	0	51391	22868	644
WEST ISLIP—Suffolk County										
✉ GOOD SAMARITAN HOSPITAL MEDICAL CENTER, 1000 Montauk Highway, Zip 11795–4958; tel. 516/376–3000; Daniel P. Walsh, President (Total facility includes 100 beds in nursing home–type unit) (Nonreporting) **A**1 2 9 10 12 13	21	10	525	—	—	—	—	—	—	—
WEST POINT—Orange County										
✉ KELLER ARMY COMMUNITY HOSPITAL, U.S. Military Academy, Zip 10996–1197; tel. 914/938–3305; Colonel Joseph FitzHarris, Commander (Nonreporting) **A**1 3 **S** Department of the Army, Office of the Surgeon General, Falls Church, VA	42	10	49	—	—	—	—	—	—	—

Hospital, Address, Telephone, Administrator, Approval, Facility, and Physician Codes, Health Care System, Network	Classi-fication Codes		Utilization Data					Expense (thousands) of dollars		
★ American Hospital Association (AHA) membership □ Joint Commission on Accreditation of Healthcare Organizations (JCAHO) accreditation + American Osteopathic Hospital Association (AOHA) membership ○ American Osteopathic Association (AOA) accreditation △ Commission on Accreditation of Rehabilitation Facilities (CARF) accreditation Control codes 61, 63, 64, 71, 72 and 73 indicate hospitals listed by AOHA, but not registered by AHA. For definition of numerical codes, see page A4	Control	Service	Beds	Admissions	Census	Outpatient Visits	Births	Total	Payroll	Personnel

WEST SENECA—Erie County

☒ WESTERN NEW YORK CHILDREN'S PSYCHIATRIC CENTER, 1010 East and West Road, Zip 14224; tel. 716/674–9730; Jed M. Cohen, Acting Executive Director **A**1 3 **F**12 13 17 18 20 22 25 27 45 52 53 54 55 56 58 65 67 68 73 **S** New York State Department of Mental Health, Albany, NY

| 12 | 52 | 46 | 103 | 36 | — | 0 | — | — | 163 |

WESTFIELD—Chautauqua County

★ WESTFIELD MEMORIAL HOSPITAL, 189 East Main Street, Zip 14787–1195; tel. 716/326–4921; Barbara A. Malinowski, Administrator and Chief Executive Officer **A**9 10 **F**4 7 8 10 11 14 15 16 17 19 20 21 22 23 25 28 30 33 34 35 37 40 41 42 43 44 49 50 60 61 65 67 71 73 **P**8

| 23 | 10 | 32 | 1325 | 14 | 33794 | 239 | 7409 | 3779 | 135 |

WHITE PLAINS—Westchester County

☒ △ BURKE REHABILITATION HOSPITAL, 785 Mamaroneck Avenue, Zip 10605; tel. 914/948–0050; Mary Beth Walsh, M.D., Chief Executive Officer **A**1 5 7 9 10 **F**5 20 25 26 39 48 49 65 66 67

| 23 | 46 | 150 | 1899 | 126 | 12800 | 0 | 34121 | 19331 | — |

NEW YORK HOSPITAL, WESTCHESTER DIVISION See Society of the New York Hospital, New York

□ ST. AGNES HOSPITAL, (Includes Children's Rehabilitation Center), 305 North Street, Zip 10605; tel. 914/681–4500; Gary S. Horan, FACHE, President and Chief Executive Officer **A**1 3 5 10 **F**2 5 7 8 11 12 13 14 15 16 17 19 20 21 22 27 28 30 32 34 37 39 40 42 44 46 47 49 51 53 54 56 57 58 61 65 66 67 69 71 73 **P**8 **S** Our Lady of Mercy Healthcare System, Inc., New York, NY **N** Catholic Health Care Network, Staten Island, NY

| 21 | 10 | 184 | 7466 | 125 | 79313 | 1056 | 73282 | 31703 | 815 |

☒ WHITE PLAINS HOSPITAL CENTER, Davis Avenue at East Post Road, Zip 10601–4699; tel. 914/681–0600; Jon B. Schandler, President and Chief Executive Officer (Nonreporting) **A**1 2 5 9 10 **N** Healthstar Network, Armonk, NY; Westchester Health Services Network, Mt Kisco, NY; Columbia Presbyterian Regional Network, New York, NY

| 23 | 10 | 301 | — | — | — | — | — | — | — |

WILLIAMSVILLE—Erie County

MILLARD FILLMORE SUBURBAN HOSPITAL See Millard Fillmore Health System, Buffalo

YONKERS—Westchester County

☒ ST. JOHN'S RIVERSIDE HOSPITAL, 967 North Broadway, Zip 10701; tel. 914/964–4444; James Foy, President and Chief Executive Officer (Nonreporting) **A**1 6 9 10 **N** Westchester Health Services Network, Mt Kisco, NY

| 23 | 10 | 273 | — | — | — | — | — | — | — |

☒ ST. JOSEPH'S MEDICAL CENTER, 127 South Broadway, Zip 10701–4080; tel. 914/378–7000; Sister Mary Linehan, President (Total facility includes 200 beds in nursing home–type unit) **A**1 3 5 9 10 **F**1 3 4 7 8 14 15 16 17 19 21 22 25 26 27 29 30 31 32 33 34 35 37 41 42 44 45 46 47 49 51 52 53 54 55 56 57 58 59 60 63 64 65 67 69 71 72 73 74 **P**5 8 **S** Sisters of Charity Center, New York, NY **N** The Excelcare System, Inc., Bronxville, NY; Catholic Health Care Network, Staten Island, NY

| 23 | 10 | 394 | 6759 | 161 | 235790 | 0 | 74218 | 38355 | 933 |

☒ YONKERS GENERAL HOSPITAL, Two Park Avenue, Zip 10703–3497; tel. 914/964–7300; Tibisay A. Guzman, Executive Vice President and Chief Operating Officer **A**1 9 10 **F**2 3 14 15 16 17 18 19 21 22 31 34 37 41 42 44 45 46 54 60 63 65 70 71 73

| 23 | 10 | 190 | 5497 | 115 | 171233 | 0 | 36743 | 22781 | 638 |

NORTH CAROLINA

Resident population 7,195 (in thousands)
Resident population in metro areas 66.6%
Birth rate per 1,000 population 14.6
65 years and over 12.5%
Percent of persons without health insurance 13.3%

Hospital, Address, Telephone, Administrator, Approval, Facility, and Physician Codes, Health Care System, Network	Classification Codes		Utilization Data					Expense (thousands) of dollars		
	Control	Service	Beds	Admissions	Census	Outpatient Visits	Births	Total	Payroll	Personnel

★ American Hospital Association (AHA) membership
□ Joint Commission on Accreditation of Healthcare Organizations (JCAHO) accreditation
+ American Osteopathic Hospital Association (AOHA) membership
○ American Osteopathic Association (AOA) accreditation
△ Commission on Accreditation of Rehabilitation Facilities (CARF) accreditation
Control codes 61, 63, 64, 71, 72 and 73 indicate hospitals listed by AOHA, but not registered by AHA. For definition of numerical codes, see page A4

AHOSKIE—Hertford County

✦ ROANOKE–CHOWAN HOSPITAL, Academy Street, Zip 27910, Mailing Address: Box 1385, Zip 27910; tel. 919/209–3000; Susan S. Lassiter, President **A**1 3 9 10 **F**7 8 12 15 16 19 20 21 22 28 30 32 33 35 37 40 41 42 44 46 49 51 52 54 56 57 58 65 71 73 **P**1 5 6 7 **N** Eastern Carolina Health Network, Greenville, NC	23	10	124	4579	61	183666	516	27832	11960	521

ALBEMARLE—Stanly County

✦ STANLY MEMORIAL HOSPITAL, 301 Yadkin Street, Zip 28001, Mailing Address: Box 1489, Zip 28002; tel. 704/984–4000; Roy M. Hinson, CHE, President and Chief Executive Officer **A**1 9 10 **F**1 7 8 10 11 12 15 19 20 21 22 23 26 28 30 31 32 34 35 36 37 39 40 41 42 44 45 46 48 49 51 52 53 55 56 57 64 65 66 67 71 73 **P**6 **N** Carolinas Hospital Network, Charlotte, NC; Central Carolina Rural Hospital Alliance, Albemarle, NC	23	10	119	4219	57	73693	484	28823	11881	419

ANDREWS—Cherokee County

DISTRICT MEMORIAL HOSPITAL, 71 Whitaker Lane, Zip 28901; tel. 704/321–1291; Daniel C. White, Chief Executive Officer **A**9 10 **F**8 12 14 15 16 17 19 20 21 22 24 28 29 30 32 34 35 37 41 42 44 45 46 49 51 65 67 71 73 **P**5 8	23	10	51	953	36	19736	0	8078	4555	193

ASHEBORO—Randolph County

✦ RANDOLPH HOSPITAL, 364 White Oak Street, Zip 27204, Mailing Address: Box 1048, Zip 27204–1048; tel. 910/625–5151; Robert E. Morrison, President **A**1 9 10 **F**7 8 12 15 16 17 19 20 21 22 28 30 32 34 35 37 39 40 42 44 49 65 71 73 **P**3	23	10	101	4706	54	96063	586	33811	15460	563

ASHEVILLE—Buncombe County

□ CHARTER ASHEVILLE BEHAVIORAL HEALTH SYSTEM, (Formerly Charter Asheville), 60 Caledonia Road, Zip 28803, Mailing Address: P.O. Box 5534, Zip 28813; tel. 704/253–3681; Tammy B. Wood, Chief Executive Officer **A**1 10 **F**2 3 12 14 16 18 19 21 25 34 35 46 50 52 53 54 55 56 57 58 59 63 65 71 **S** Magellan Health Services, Atlanta, GA	33	22	139	1877	54	—	0	—	—	110
✦ MEMORIAL MISSION MEDICAL CENTER, 509 Biltmore Avenue, Zip 28801–4690; tel. 704/255–4000; Robert F. Burgin, President and Chief Executive Officer **A**1 2 3 5 9 10 **F**1 4 6 7 8 10 11 12 13 14 15 16 17 19 20 21 22 23 24 25 26 27 29 30 31 32 33 34 35 37 38 39 40 41 42 44 45 47 49 52 56 57 58 59 60 62 63 64 65 67 70 71 72 73 74 **P**7 **N** Mission & Saint Joseph Health System, Asheville, NC; Western North Carolina Health Network, Asheville, NC	23	10	436	19968	308	164373	3201	199984	83448	2769
✦ ST. JOSEPH'S HOSPITAL, 428 Biltmore Avenue, Zip 28801–4502; tel. 704/255–3100; J. Lewis Daniels, President and Chief Executive Officer (Total facility includes 25 beds in nursing home–type unit) **A**1 2 9 10 **F**1 3 4 6 7 8 10 11 12 13 14 15 16 17 19 20 21 22 23 24 25 26 27 29 30 31 32 33 34 35 37 38 39 40 41 42 43 44 45 47 48 49 52 56 57 58 59 60 61 62 64 65 67 70 71 73 74 **P**7 **N** Mission & Saint Joseph Health System, Asheville, NC; Western North Carolina Health Network, Asheville, NC	21	10	264	10406	172	75706	0	84879	38640	1234
★ △ THOMS REHABILITATION HOSPITAL, 68 Sweeten Creek Road, Zip 28803–1599, Mailing Address: P.O. Box 15025, Zip 28813–0025; tel. 704/274–2400; Charles D. Norvell, President (Nonreporting) **A**7 9 10	23	46	80	—	—	—	—	—	—	—
✦ VETERANS AFFAIRS MEDICAL CENTER, 1100 Tunnel Road, Zip 28805–2087; tel. 704/298–7911; James A. Christian, Director (Total facility includes 120 beds in nursing home–type unit) **A**1 3 5 9 **F**1 2 3 4 8 10 11 12 15 19 20 21 23 26 27 28 30 31 32 33 34 35 37 39 42 43 45 46 49 51 52 54 55 56 57 58 59 60 61 64 65 69 71 73 74 **P**6 **S** Department of Veterans Affairs, Washington, DC	45	10	389	5529	199	95367	0	74234	—	1010

BANNER ELK—Avery County

□ CHARLES A. CANNON JR. MEMORIAL HOSPITAL, 805 Shawneehaw Avenue, Zip 28604, Mailing Address: P.O. Box 8, Zip 28604–0008; tel. 704/898–5111; Edward C. Greene, Jr., Administrator (Total facility includes 10 beds in nursing home–type unit) **A**1 9 10 **F**7 8 16 19 21 22 28 30 33 35 36 37 40 42 44 49 52 56 57 64 65 69 71 73 **P**6 **N** Mountain States Healthcare Network, Johnson City, TN	23	10	50	1737	26	17322	89	11107	6868	196

BELHAVEN—Beaufort County

PUNGO DISTRICT HOSPITAL, 210 East Front Street, Zip 27810–9998; tel. 919/943–2111; Thomas O. Miller, Administrator (Nonreporting) **A**9 10 **N** Eastern Carolina Health Network, Greenville, NC	23	10	44	—	—	—	—	—	—	—

BLACK MOUNTAIN—Buncombe County

ALCOHOL AND DRUG ABUSE TREATMENT CENTER, 301 Tabernacle Road, Zip 28711; tel. 704/669–3402; William A. Rafter, Director (Nonreporting) **A**9	12	82	110	—	—	—	—	—	—	—

BLOWING ROCK—Watauga County

✦ BLOWING ROCK HOSPITAL, (Includes Dr. Charles Davant Rehabilitation and Extended Care Center), Chestnut Street, Zip 28605–0148, Mailing Address: Box 148, Zip 28605–0148; tel. 704/295–3136; Patricia Gray, Administrator and Chief Executive Officer (Total facility includes 72 beds in nursing home–type unit) (Nonreporting) **A**1 9 10	23	10	100	—	—	—	—	—	—	—

Hospital, Address, Telephone, Administrator, Approval, Facility, and Physician Codes, Health Care System, Network	Classi-fication Codes		Utilization Data					Expense (thousands) of dollars		
★ American Hospital Association (AHA) membership □ Joint Commission on Accreditation of Healthcare Organizations (JCAHO) accreditation + American Osteopathic Hospital Association (AOHA) membership ○ American Osteopathic Association (AOA) accreditation △ Commission on Accreditation of Rehabilitation Facilities (CARF) accreditation Control codes 61, 63, 64, 71, 72 and 73 indicate hospitals listed by AOHA, but not registered by AHA. For definition of numerical codes, see page A4	Control	Service	Beds	Admissions	Census	Outpatient Visits	Births	Total	Payroll	Personnel

BOILING SPRINGS—Cleveland County

CRAWLEY MEMORIAL HOSPITAL, 315 West College Avenue, Zip 28017, Mailing Address: Box 996, Zip 28017; tel. 704/434–9466; Daphne Bridges, President (Nonreporting) **A**9 10 **S** Carolinas HealthCare System, Charlotte, NC **N** Carolinas Hospital Network, Charlotte, NC
| | 23 | 10 | 51 | — | — | — | — | — | — | — |

BOONE—Watauga County

☒ WATAUGA MEDICAL CENTER, Deerfield Road, Zip 28607–2600, Mailing Address: P.O. Box 2600, Zip 28607–2600; tel. 704/262–4100; Richard G. Sparks, President (Total facility includes 10 beds in nursing home–type unit) **A**1 9 10 **F**7 8 10 12 14 15 16 17 19 21 22 23 28 29 30 32 35 37 38 40 42 44 45 60 64 65 67 68 71 73 **P**3 8 **N** Carolinas Hospital Network, Charlotte, NC
| | 23 | 10 | 105 | 4870 | 56 | 40041 | 586 | 32054 | 13905 | 461 |

BREVARD—Transylvania County

☒ TRANSYLVANIA COMMUNITY HOSPITAL, Hospital Drive, Zip 28712–1116, Mailing Address: Box 1116, Zip 28712–1116; tel. 704/884–9111; Robert J. Bednarek, Administrator and Chief Executive Officer **A**1 9 10 **F**2 7 8 14 15 16 19 21 22 30 32 33 34 35 36 40 42 44 46 63 65 67 71 73 **P**5 8 **N** Western North Carolina Health Network, Asheville, NC
| | 23 | 10 | 85 | 2314 | 46 | 31345 | 231 | 20161 | 10561 | 419 |

BRYSON CITY—Swain County

□ SWAIN COUNTY HOSPITAL, 45 Plateau Street, Zip 28713; tel. 704/488–2155; Beverly Robinson, Administrator (Nonreporting) **A**1 9 10
| | 23 | 10 | 42 | — | — | — | — | — | — | — |

BURGAW—Pender County

★ PENDER MEMORIAL HOSPITAL, 507 Freemont Street, Zip 28425; tel. 910/259–5451; James L. Jarrett, Chief Executive Officer (Total facility includes 43 beds in nursing home–type unit) **A**9 10 **F**7 8 11 12 15 16 19 22 26 28 30 32 33 35 39 41 44 49 64 65 71 73 **P**5 **S** Quorum Health Group/Quorum Health Resources, Inc., Brentwood, TN
| | 13 | 10 | 86 | 1579 | 46 | 14804 | 4 | 11962 | 5908 | 254 |

BURLINGTON—Alamance County

☒ ALAMANCE REGIONAL MEDICAL CENTER, 1240 Huffman Mill Road, Zip 27216–0202, Mailing Address: P.O. Box 202, Zip 27216–0202; tel. 910/538–7000; Thomas E. Ryan, President (Total facility includes 81 beds in nursing home–type unit) **A**1 2 9 10 **F**2 3 7 8 10 12 14 15 16 17 19 20 21 22 23 26 27 28 29 30 31 32 33 34 35 37 39 40 41 42 44 45 46 48 49 52 53 54 55 56 57 58 59 60 61 63 64 65 67 68 71 73 74 **P**5 7
| | 23 | 10 | 319 | 8775 | 196 | 98397 | 1096 | 80552 | 33585 | 1162 |

BUTNER—Granville County

ALCOHOL AND DRUG ABUSE TREATMENT CENTER, 205 West E Street, Zip 27509; tel. 919/575–7928; Cliff Hood, Director (Nonreporting)
| | 12 | 82 | 80 | — | — | — | — | — | — | — |

□ JOHN UMSTEAD HOSPITAL, 1003 12th Street, Zip 27509–1626; tel. 919/575–7211; Patricia L. Christian, R.N., Ph.D., Director **A**1 3 5 9 10 **F**2 52 53 54 56 57 58 64
| | 12 | 22 | 661 | 4333 | 514 | 4042 | 0 | 61957 | 39310 | 1331 |

CAMP LEJEUNE—Onslow County

☒ NAVAL HOSPITAL, Zip 28547–0100; tel. 910/451–4300; Captain Michael L. Cowan, MC, USN, Commanding Officer (Nonreporting) **A**1 9 **S** Department of Navy, Washington, DC
| | 43 | 10 | 166 | — | — | — | — | — | — | — |

CARY—Jefferson County

WESTERN WAKE MEDICAL CENTER See Wake Medical Center, Raleigh

CHAPEL HILL—Orange County

☒ UNIVERSITY OF NORTH CAROLINA HOSPITALS, (Includes North Carolina Children's Hospital; North Carolina Neurosciences Hospital), 101 Manning Drive, Zip 27514; tel. 919/966–4131; Eric B. Munson, Executive Director **A**1 2 3 5 8 9 10 **F**2 4 5 7 8 9 10 11 12 13 14 15 16 17 19 20 21 22 23 26 30 31 32 33 34 35 37 38 39 40 41 42 43 44 45 46 47 48 49 51 52 53 54 55 56 57 58 60 61 63 64 65 66 67 69 70 71 72 73 74 **P**1 7 **N** UNC Health Network, Chapel Hill, NC
| | 12 | 10 | 659 | 26068 | 469 | 660063 | 2518 | 324735 | 161579 | 4364 |

CHARLOTTE—Mecklenburg County

AMETHYST, 1715 Sharon Road West, Zip 28210, Mailing Address: P.O. Box 32861, Zip 28232–2861; tel. 704/554–8373; Daniel J. Harrison, Assistant Vice President and Administrator (Nonreporting)
| | 16 | 82 | 94 | — | — | — | — | — | — | — |

☒ CAROLINAS MEDICAL CENTER, 1000 Blythe Boulevard, Zip 28203, Mailing Address: P.O. Box 32861, Zip 28232–2861; tel. 704/355–2000; Paul S. Franz, President **A**1 2 3 5 8 9 10 **F**1 2 3 4 5 6 7 8 9 10 11 12 13 14 15 17 18 19 20 21 22 23 24 25 26 27 28 29 30 31 32 33 34 35 36 37 38 39 40 41 42 43 44 45 46 47 48 49 50 51 52 53 54 55 56 57 58 59 60 61 63 64 65 66 67 68 69 70 71 72 73 74 **P**6 7 **S** Carolinas HealthCare System, Charlotte, NC **N** Carolinas Hospital Network, Charlotte, NC
| | 16 | 10 | 843 | 36447 | 606 | 274037 | 5874 | 376379 | 167189 | — |

☒ △ CHARLOTTE INSTITUTE OF REHABILITATION, 1100 Blythe Boulevard, Zip 28203; tel. 704/355–4300; Hollis Hamilton, Administrator (Nonreporting) **A**1 3 7 9 10 **S** Carolinas HealthCare System, Charlotte, NC **N** Carolinas Hospital Network, Charlotte, NC
| | 16 | 46 | 109 | — | — | — | — | — | — | — |

□ CHARTER PINES BEHAVIORAL HEALTH SYSTEM, 3621 Randolph Road, Zip 28211, Mailing Address: P.O. Box 221709, Zip 28222–1709; tel. 704/365–5368; Bruce Chambers, Ph.D., Chief Executive Officer **A**1 9 10 **F**3 16 52 53 54 55 56 57 58 59 **P**5 6 **S** Magellan Health Services, Atlanta, GA
| | 33 | 22 | 60 | 1822 | 36 | 7661 | 0 | — | — | 114 |

☒ △ MERCY HOSPITAL, 2001 Vail Avenue, Zip 28207; tel. 704/379–5000; C. Curtis Copenhaver, Chief Executive Officer **A**1 6 7 9 10 **F**2 3 4 8 10 11 12 14 15 16 19 21 22 28 30 31 32 35 37 39 43 44 48 49 63 65 67 71 73 **P**6 **S** Carolinas HealthCare System, Charlotte, NC **N** Carolinas Hospital Network, Charlotte, NC
| | 16 | 10 | 224 | 7008 | 132 | 255148 | 0 | 70090 | 31207 | 870 |

Hospital, Address, Telephone, Administrator, Approval, Facility, and Physician Codes, Health Care System, Network	Classi-fication Codes		Utilization Data					Expense (thousands) of dollars		
★ American Hospital Association (AHA) membership □ Joint Commission on Accreditation of Healthcare Organizations (JCAHO) accreditation + American Osteopathic Hospital Association (AOHA) membership ○ American Osteopathic Association (AOA) accreditation △ Commission on Accreditation of Rehabilitation Facilities (CARF) accreditation Control codes 61, 63, 64, 71, 72 and 73 indicate hospitals listed by AOHA, but not registered by AHA. For definition of numerical codes, see page A4	Control	Service	Beds	Admissions	Census	Outpatient Visits	Births	Total	Payroll	Personnel
⊞ PRESBYTERIAN HOSPITAL, 200 Hawthorne Lane, Zip 28204, Mailing Address: Box 33549, Zip 28233–3549; tel. 704/384–4000; Paul F. Betzold, President and Chief Executive Officer (Total facility includes 12 beds in nursing home–type unit) **A**1 2 6 9 10 **F**3 4 5 7 8 10 12 13 14 17 18 19 21 22 23 25 26 27 28 29 30 31 32 33 34 35 39 41 42 43 44 45 46 49 51 53 54 55 56 57 58 59 60 61 63 65 67 68 71 72 73 74 **P**1	23	10	481	28252	415	122842	3748	272287	112842	3439
PRESBYTERIAN SPECIALTY HOSPITAL, 1600 East Third Street, Zip 28204, Mailing Address: P.O. Box 34425, Zip 28234–4425; tel. 704/384–6000; Chip Day, Acting Vice President **A**9 10 **F**1 2 3 4 5 6 7 8 9 10 11 12 13 17 18 19 20 21 22 23 24 25 26 27 28 29 30 31 32 33 34 35 36 37 38 39 40 41 42 43 44 45 46 47 48 49 50 51 52 53 54 55 56 57 58 59 60 61 62 63 64 66 67 68 69 70 71 72 73 74 **P**1 6	23	45	15	48	1	4603	0	6926	2519	64
⊞ △ PRESBYTERIAN–ORTHOPAEDIC HOSPITAL, 1901 Randolph Road, Zip 28207; tel. 704/370–1549; Paul M. Jenson, Chief Executive Officer (Nonreporting) **A**1 7 9 10 **S** Columbia/HCA Healthcare Corporation, Nashville, TN	33	47	166	—	—	—	—	—	—	—
□ UNIVERSITY HOSPITAL, 8800 North Tryon Street, Zip 28262, Mailing Address: P.O. Box 560727, Zip 28256; tel. 704/548–6000; W. Spencer Lilly, Administrator **A**1 9 10 **F**2 4 6 7 8 9 10 11 14 16 19 20 21 22 24 28 29 30 31 32 34 35 37 38 39 40 41 42 43 44 47 48 49 50 51 52 53 54 55 56 57 58 59 60 61 63 64 65 66 67 69 70 71 72 73 74 **P**6 7 **S** Carolinas HealthCare System, Charlotte, NC **N** Carolinas Hospital Network, Charlotte, NC	16	10	107	4707	48	69517	1085	33933	14199	425
CHEROKEE—Swain County										
⊞ U. S. PUBLIC HEALTH SERVICE INDIAN HOSPITAL, Hospital Road, Zip 28719; tel. 704/497–9163; Janet Belcourt, Administrator (Nonreporting) **A**1 10 **S** U. S. Public Health Service Indian Health Service, Rockville, MD	47	10	30	—	—	—	—	—	—	—
CLINTON—Sampson County										
⊞ SAMPSON REGIONAL MEDICAL CENTER, (Formerly Sampson County Memorial Hospital), 607 Beaman Street, Zip 28328, Mailing Address: Drawer 258, Zip 28329; tel. 910/592–8511; Lee Pridgen, Jr., Administrator (Total facility includes 30 beds in nursing home–type unit) **A**1 9 10 **F**7 8 14 15 16 19 22 23 32 35 37 40 44 46 49 64 65 71	13	10	146	4208	75	58691	363	28075	14253	544
CLYDE—Haywood County										
⊞ HAYWOOD REGIONAL MEDICAL CENTER, (Formerly Haywood County Hospital), 90 Hospital Drive, Zip 28721–9434; tel. 704/456–7311; David O. Rice, President (Total facility includes 20 beds in nursing home–type unit) **A**1 9 10 **F**7 8 10 12 14 15 16 17 19 21 22 23 24 26 28 29 30 32 33 35 37 40 41 42 44 45 49 54 65 67 71 72 73 74 **P**3 8	13	10	150	5674	86	61092	246	40822	18359	703
COLUMBUS—Polk County										
□ ST. LUKE'S HOSPITAL, 220 Hospital Drive, Zip 28722; tel. 704/894–3311; C. Cameron Highsmith, Jr., President and Chief Executive Officer **A**1 9 10 **F**12 14 16 19 21 22 26 28 30 37 39 44 46 56 57 58 60 64 65 71 73	23	10	73	1926	43	27863	0	12545	6004	354
CONCORD—Cabarrus County										
⊞ CABARRUS MEMORIAL HOSPITAL, 920 Church Street North, Zip 28025–2983; tel. 704/783–3000; Thomas R. Revels, President and Chief Executive Officer **A**1 3 5 6 9 10 **F**4 7 8 10 11 14 15 16 19 21 22 24 30 32 33 35 36 37 38 40 41 42 43 44 58 60 65 72 73 74 **P**3	23	10	322	15585	223	432191	1720	152696	69562	1929
CROSSNORE—Avery County										
⊞ SLOOP MEMORIAL HOSPITAL, One Crossnore Drive, Zip 28616, Mailing Address: Drawer 470, Zip 28616; tel. 704/733–9231; Edward C. Greene, Jr., President **A**1 9 10 **F**7 8 19 21 22 28 30 36 37 40 44 49 52 56 57 64 65 71 73 **P**3 6 **N** Mountain States Healthcare Network, Johnson City, TN	23	10	38	1491	15	26276	88	10997	7163	165
DANBURY—Stokes County										
⊞ STOKES–REYNOLDS MEMORIAL HOSPITAL, Mailing Address: Box 10, Zip 27016–0010; tel. 910/593–2831; Sandra D. Priddy, President (Total facility includes 40 beds in nursing home–type unit) **A**1 9 10 **F**3 8 14 15 16 19 22 25 33 37 44 57 64 65 71 72 73 74 **P**6 7 **N** North Carolina Baptist Hospitals, Inc., Winston–Salem, NC	21	10	93	1050	73	24446	0	10542	5089	239
DUNN—Harnett County										
□ BETSY JOHNSON MEMORIAL HOSPITAL, 800 Tilghman Drive, Zip 28334, Mailing Address: Drawer 1706, Zip 28335; tel. 910/892–7161; Shannon D. Brown, President **A**1 9 10 **F**7 8 14 15 19 22 28 30 34 35 37 40 44 46 63 65 67 71 73	14	10	88	3866	43	48417	486	20263	10155	362
DURHAM—Durham County										
⊞ △ DUKE UNIVERSITY MEDICAL CENTER, (Includes Duke University Hospital), Erwin Road, Zip 27710, Mailing Address: Box 3708, Zip 27710; tel. 919/684–8111; Michael D. Israel, Chief Executive Officer and Vice Chancellor **A**1 2 3 5 7 8 9 10 **F**3 4 7 8 9 10 11 12 13 15 16 17 18 19 20 21 22 23 24 26 27 28 29 30 31 32 34 35 37 38 39 40 41 42 43 44 45 46 47 48 49 50 51 52 53 55 56 57 58 60 61 63 65 66 67 68 69 70 71 72 73 74 **P**1 **N** Duke Health Network, Durham, NC; National Cardiovascular Network, Atlanta, GA	23	10	888	34421	672	706310	2218	573287	222851	5955
⊞ DURHAM REGIONAL HOSPITAL, 3643 North Roxboro Road, Zip 27704–2763; tel. 919/470–4000; Richard L. Myers, President and Chief Executive Officer **A**1 3 5 6 9 10 **F**3 4 7 8 10 11 12 14 15 16 19 21 22 23 24 25 26 27 28 29 30 31 32 34 35 37 39 40 41 42 43 44 45 46 49 51 52 53 54 55 56 57 58 59 60 63 65 67 71 72 73 74 **P**1	13	10	216	13918	182	86296	2632	113105	56512	1830
★ NORTH CAROLINA EYE AND EAR HOSPITAL, 1110 West Main Street, Zip 27701; tel. 919/682–9341; H. Ed Jones, Chief Executive Officer (Nonreporting) **A**9 10	33	45	24	—	—	—	—	—	—	—

Hospital, Address, Telephone, Administrator, Approval, Facility, and Physician Codes, Health Care System, Network	Classi-fication Codes		Utilization Data					Expense (thousands) of dollars		
	Control	Service	Beds	Admissions	Census	Outpatient Visits	Births	Total	Payroll	Personnel

★ American Hospital Association (AHA) membership
□ Joint Commission on Accreditation of Healthcare Organizations (JCAHO) accreditation
+ American Osteopathic Hospital Association (AOHA) membership
○ American Osteopathic Association (AOA) accreditation
△ Commission on Accreditation of Rehabilitation Facilities (CARF) accreditation
   Control codes 61, 63, 64, 71, 72 and 73 indicate hospitals listed by AOHA, but not registered by AHA. For definition of numerical codes, see page A4

Hospital	Control	Service	Beds	Admissions	Census	Outpatient Visits	Births	Total	Payroll	Personnel
✸ VETERANS AFFAIRS MEDICAL CENTER, 508 Fulton Street, Zip 27705; tel. 919/286–0411; Michael B. Phaup, Director (Total facility includes 120 beds in nursing home–type unit) **A**1 3 5 8 9 **F**3 4 8 10 11 15 16 19 20 21 22 26 27 28 29 30 31 32 34 35 37 39 41 42 43 44 45 46 49 51 52 54 55 56 57 58 60 63 64 65 67 69 71 73 74 **S** Department of Veterans Affairs, Washington, DC	45	10	382	8881	278	154679	0	132845	53527	1424
EDEN—Rockingham County										
✸ MOREHEAD MEMORIAL HOSPITAL, 117 East King's Highway, Zip 27288–5299; tel. 910/623–9711; Robert Enders, President (Total facility includes 128 beds in nursing home–type unit) **A**1 9 10 **F**7 8 12 13 15 16 17 19 21 22 23 26 28 30 34 35 36 37 39 40 41 42 44 45 46 49 60 64 65 66 67 68 71 73 74 **S** Quorum Health Group/Quorum Health Resources, Inc., Brentwood, TN	23	10	236	5287	185	96553	772	34925	15492	403
EDENTON—Chowan County										
✸ CHOWAN HOSPITAL, 211 Virginia Road, Zip 27932–0629, Mailing Address: P.O. Box 629, Zip 27932–0629; tel. 919/482–8451; Barbara R. Cale, Administrator (Total facility includes 40 beds in nursing home–type unit) **A**1 9 10 **F**7 8 12 14 15 16 17 19 20 21 22 28 30 31 32 33 34 37 39 40 42 44 45 46 49 52 54 56 58 59 64 65 67 71 73 74 **P**3 **N** Eastern Carolina Health Network, Greenville, NC	13	10	111	2550	64	21551	365	17441	8978	408
ELIZABETH CITY—Pasquotank County										
✸ ALBEMARLE HOSPITAL, 1144 North Road Street, Zip 27909, Mailing Address: Box 1587, Zip 27906–1587; tel. 919/335–0531; Phillip D. Bagby, President and Chief Executive Officer **A**1 9 10 **F**7 8 10 11 12 15 19 20 21 22 23 24 27 28 29 30 34 35 37 39 40 41 42 44 45 46 49 60 65 71 73 **N** Eastern Carolina Health Network, Greenville, NC	13	10	145	6742	110	71648	728	44296	20790	715
ELIZABETHTOWN—Bladen County										
✸ BLADEN COUNTY HOSPITAL, 501 South Poplar Street, Zip 28337–0398, Mailing Address: Box 398, Zip 28337–0398; tel. 910/862–5100; Leo A. Petit, Jr., Chief Executive Officer (Total facility includes 10 beds in nursing home–type unit) **A**1 9 10 **F**7 11 15 16 17 19 21 22 25 28 29 32 33 34 35 37 39 40 44 49 64 65 67 71 72 73 **P**6 7 8 **N** Bladen County Hospital, Elizabethtown, NC	13	10	60	1992	31	39889	243	13124	5942	236
ELKIN—Surry County										
✸ HUGH CHATHAM MEMORIAL HOSPITAL, Parkwood Drive, Zip 28621–0560, Mailing Address: P.O. Box 560, Zip 28621–0560; tel. 910/527–7000; Richard D. Osmus, Chief Executive Officer (Total facility includes 79 beds in nursing home–type unit) **A**1 9 10 **F**6 7 8 10 12 14 15 16 19 21 22 26 28 30 32 33 34 35 37 39 40 41 42 44 45 49 51 61 62 63 64 65 66 67 71 73 74 **P**3 **S** Quorum Health Group/Quorum Health Resources, Inc., Brentwood, TN	23	10	160	4299	136	19913	325	27489	11783	513
ERWIN—Harnett County										
✸ GOOD HOPE HOSPITAL, 410 Denim Drive, Zip 28339–0668, Mailing Address: P.O. Box 668, Zip 28339–0668; tel. 910/897–6151; David T. Boucher, Chief Executive Officer (Nonreporting) **A**1 9 10 **S** Quorum Health Group/Quorum Health Resources, Inc., Brentwood, TN	23	10	72	—	—	—	—	—	—	—
FAYETTEVILLE—Cumberland County										
✸ △ CAPE FEAR VALLEY HEALTH SYSTEM, (Formerly Cape Fear Valley Medical Center), 1638 Owen Drive, Zip 28304, Mailing Address: Box 2000, Zip 28302–2000; tel. 910/609–4000; John T. Carlisle, Chief Executive Officer **A**1 2 3 5 7 9 10 **F**2 3 4 7 8 10 11 12 15 16 17 19 20 21 22 23 25 26 27 28 30 32 33 35 37 38 39 40 41 42 43 44 45 46 48 49 51 53 55 56 57 58 59 60 65 66 67 71 73 74 **P**6	13	10	371	19408	332	265624	4447	170182	66703	2607
✸ COLUMBIA HIGHSMITH–RAINEY MEMORIAL HOSPITAL, 150 Robeson Street, Zip 28301–5570; tel. 910/609–1000; William A. Adams, Chief Executive Officer **A**1 9 10 **F**7 8 11 12 14 15 16 19 21 22 35 37 40 44 46 49 63 71 73 **P**1 2 4 5 6 7 8 **S** Columbia/HCA Healthcare Corporation, Nashville, TN	33	10	133	3613	53	48191	166	27690	12756	450
CUMBERLAND HOSPITAL, 3425 Melrose Road, Zip 28304; tel. 910/609–3000; Edward J. Whitehouse, Administrator (Nonreporting) **A**9 10	13	22	100	—	—	—	—	—	—	—
✸ VETERANS AFFAIRS MEDICAL CENTER, 2300 Ramsey Street, Zip 28301–3899; tel. 910/822–7059; Betty Bolin Brown, Acting Director (Total facility includes 39 beds in nursing home–type unit) **A**1 9 **F**3 8 14 15 16 17 19 20 21 22 24 26 27 28 29 30 31 33 34 35 37 39 41 44 46 48 49 51 52 55 56 57 58 64 65 67 71 73 74 **P**6 **S** Department of Veterans Affairs, Washington, DC	45	10	193	3994	130	113690	0	48900	26719	636
FLETCHER—Henderson County										
✸ PARK RIDGE HOSPITAL, Naples Road, Zip 28732, Mailing Address: P.O. Box 1569, Zip 28732–1569; tel. 704/684–8501; Michael V. Gentry, President **A**1 9 10 **F**7 8 10 11 12 14 15 19 21 22 23 32 33 35 37 39 40 41 44 45 46 52 53 56 57 58 59 65 67 71 73 **P**6 **S** Adventist Health System Sunbelt Health Care Corporation, Winter Park, FL	23	10	89	3197	50	38198	446	31808	14474	493
FORT BRAGG—Cumberland County										
✸ WOMACK ARMY MEDICAL CENTER, Zip 28307–5000; tel. 910/432–4802; Colonel Michael J. Brennan, MSC, M.D., Commander **A**1 3 5 9 **F**2 3 4 5 7 8 9 10 11 12 13 14 15 16 17 18 19 20 21 22 25 26 27 28 29 30 31 34 35 37 38 39 40 41 42 43 44 45 46 47 48 49 51 52 53 54 55 56 58 59 60 61 63 65 66 67 69 71 72 73 74 **P**6 **S** Department of the Army, Office of the Surgeon General, Falls Church, VA	42	10	173	12562	96	880676	2400	102250	25730	1782
FRANKLIN—Macon County										
✸ ANGEL MEDICAL CENTER, Riverview and White Oak Streets, Zip 28734, Mailing Address: P.O. Box 1209, Zip 28734–1209; tel. 704/524–8411; Michael E. Zuliani, Chief Executive Officer (Nonreporting) **A**1 9 10 **S** Quorum Health Group/Quorum Health Resources, Inc., Brentwood, TN	23	10	59	—	—	—	—	—	—	—

Hospital, Address, Telephone, Administrator, Approval, Facility, and Physician Codes, Health Care System, Network	Classi-fication Codes		Utilization Data					Expense (thousands) of dollars		

★ American Hospital Association (AHA) membership
□ Joint Commission on Accreditation of Healthcare Organizations (JCAHO) accreditation
+ American Osteopathic Hospital Association (AOHA) membership
○ American Osteopathic Association (AOA) accreditation
△ Commission on Accreditation of Rehabilitation Facilities (CARF) accreditation
   Control codes 61, 63, 64, 71, 72 and 73 indicate hospitals listed by AOHA, but not registered by AHA. For definition of numerical codes, see page A4

	Control	Service	Beds	Admissions	Census	Outpatient Visits	Births	Total	Payroll	Personnel
FUQUAY–VARINA—Wake County										
SOUTHERN WAKE HOSPITAL See Wake Medical Center, Raleigh										
GASTONIA—Gaston County										
✠ GASTON MEMORIAL HOSPITAL, 2525 Court Drive, Zip 28054, Mailing Address: Box 1747, Zip 28053–1747; tel. 704/834–2000; Wayne F. Shovelin, President and Chief Executive Officer **A**1 2 9 10 **F**3 6 7 8 10 11 15 16 17 18 19 20 21 22 23 24 25 28 29 30 32 33 34 35 37 39 40 41 42 44 45 46 49 52 53 54 55 56 57 58 59 60 63 64 65 67 70 71 72 73 74	23	10	366	16669	252	127136	2210	118310	56357	1721
GOLDSBORO—Wayne County										
□ CHERRY HOSPITAL, Steven Mill Road, Zip 27533–8000, Mailing Address: Caller Box 8000, Zip 27533–8000; tel. 919/731–3200; J. Field Montgomery, Jr., Director (Total facility includes 201 beds in nursing home–type unit) (Nonreporting) **A**1 3 5 9 10	12	22	690	—	—	—	—	—	—	—
✠ WAYNE MEMORIAL HOSPITAL, 2700 Wayne Memorial Drive, Zip 27534–8001, Mailing Address: P.O. Box 8001, Zip 27533–8001; tel. 919/736–1110; James W. Hubbell, President and Chief Executive Officer **A**1 2 9 10 **F**7 8 10 12 14 17 19 21 22 23 26 29 30 31 32 33 34 35 37 39 41 42 44 45 46 49 52 53 54 55 56 57 60 63 65 66 67 71 73 **N** Eastern Carolina Health Network, Greenville, NC	23	10	259	13095	192	77914	1290	75236	31755	1103
GREENSBORO—Guilford County										
□ CHARTER GREENSBORO BEHAVIORAL HEALTH SYSTEM, 700 Walter Reed Drive, Zip 27403–1129, Mailing Address: P.O. Box 10399, Zip 27404–0399; tel. 910/852–4821; Joe Crabtree, Chief Executive Officer (Nonreporting) **A**1 9 10 **S** Magellan Health Services, Atlanta, GA	33	22	68	—	—	—	—	—	—	—
✠ △ MOSES CONE HEALTH SYSTEM, (Includes Women's Hospital of Greensboro, 801 Green Valley Road, Zip 27408; tel. 910/574–6500), 1200 North Elm Street, Zip 27401–1020; tel. 910/574–7000; Dennis R. Barry, President (Total facility includes 150 beds in nursing home–type unit) **A**1 2 3 5 7 8 9 10 **F**4 7 8 10 11 12 14 15 16 17 19 20 21 22 23 25 26 28 29 30 31 32 33 34 35 37 38 39 40 41 42 43 44 45 46 48 49 52 54 55 57 59 60 61 63 64 65 66 67 70 71 73 74 **P**1 7 **N** North Carolina Health Network, Charlotte, NC	23	10	802	28770	617	281426	4315	237132	121733	3385
□ VENCOR HOSPITAL–GREENSBORO, (MEDICALLY COMPLEX LT ACUTE), 2401 Southside Boulevard, Zip 27406; tel. 910/271–2800; James R. Vroom, Chief Executive Officer (Total facility includes 65 beds in nursing home–type unit) **A**1 9 10 **F**12 19 20 21 22 26 27 35 37 39 46 50 54 63 64 65 67 71 73 **S** Vencor, Incorporated, Louisville, KY	33	49	124	596	100	0	0	18194	9453	—
✠ WESLEY LONG COMMUNITY HOSPITAL, 501 North Elam Avenue, Zip 27403, Mailing Address: P.O. Box 2747, Zip 27402; tel. 910/854–6100; Gary L. Park, President **A**1 9 10 **F**4 7 8 10 12 14 15 16 17 19 21 22 28 29 30 31 34 35 37 38 39 40 41 42 44 45 46 48 49 61 63 64 65 67 71 72 73 74 **P**7 8	23	10	157	7712	106	77416	814	65744	27579	785
WOMEN'S HOSPITAL OF GREENSBORO See Moses Cone Health System										
□ YOUTH FOCUS PSYCHIATRIC HOSPITAL, 1601 Huffine Mill Road, Zip 27405–5509; tel. 910/375–8333; David Coleman, Director **A**1 9 **F**14 15 16 52 53 54 55 56 59	23	52	12	172	8	0	0	1399	791	35
GREENVILLE—Pitt County										
✠ △ PITT COUNTY MEMORIAL HOSPITAL–UNIVERSITY MEDICAL CENTER OF EASTERN CAROLINA–PITT COUNTY, 2100 Stantonsburg Road, Zip 27835–6028, Mailing Address: Box 6028, Zip 27835–6028; tel. 919/816–4451; Dave C. McRae, President and Chief Executive Officer **A**1 2 3 5 7 8 9 10 **F**4 7 8 10 11 12 13 14 15 16 17 19 20 21 22 23 24 27 30 31 32 33 34 35 37 38 39 40 41 42 43 44 45 46 47 48 49 51 52 53 54 55 56 57 58 59 60 61 63 65 67 69 70 71 73 74 **P**1 5 7 **N** Eastern Carolina Health Network, Greenville, NC	13	10	680	32692	536	126957	2995	285623	129937	4014
WALTER B. JONES ALCOHOL AND DRUG ABUSE TREATMENT CENTER, 2577 West Fifth Street, Zip 27834; tel. 919/830–3426; Phillip A. Mooring, Director **A**9 **F**2 15 16 **P**6	12	82	76	1083	70	0	0	5819	3232	128
HAMLET—Richmond County										
□ HAMLET HOSPITAL, Rice and Vance Streets, Zip 28345, Mailing Address: Box 1109, Zip 28345; tel. 910/582–3611; Joe D. Howell, Executive Director **A**1 9 10 **F**8 14 16 19 21 22 28 30 31 35 37 39 41 44 46 49 52 56 65 66 71 73 **S** Health Management Associates, Naples, FL	33	10	64	2987	43	16059	0	12728	5179	199
HAVELOCK—Onslow County										
✠ NAVAL HOSPITAL, Zip 28533–0023; tel. 919/466–0266; Captain Paul D. Garst, MC, USN, Commanding Officer **A**1 9 **F**7 8 15 20 22 25 27 28 29 30 40 41 44 45 46 49 51 58 71 72 **S** Department of Navy, Washington, DC	43	10	23	1281	11	148936	549	—	—	391
HENDERSON—Vance County										
✠ MARIA PARHAM HOSPITAL, 566 Ruin Creek Road, Zip 27536–2957; tel. 919/438–4143; Philip S. Lakernick, President and Chief Executive Officer **A**1 9 10 **F**5 7 8 10 11 14 15 16 17 19 20 21 22 23 24 26 28 29 30 31 33 34 35 40 41 42 44 45 46 48 49 56 58 65 66 67 71 72 73 74 **P**1 5 **N** Duke Health Network, Durham, NC	23	10	93	3975	57	76358	665	28216	10773	442
HENDERSONVILLE—Henderson County										
✠ MARGARET R. PARDEE MEMORIAL HOSPITAL, 715 Fleming Street, Zip 28791–2563; tel. 704/696–1000; Frank J. Aaron, Jr., Chief Executive Officer (Total facility includes 40 beds in nursing home–type unit) **A**1 3 9 10 **F**1 7 8 11 12 14 15 16 17 19 22 23 26 28 29 30 32 34 35 37 40 41 42 44 45 49 52 54 55 56 57 58 59 60 61 63 64 65 67 71 72 73 74 **P**1 5 8 **N** Western North Carolina Health Network, Asheville, NC	13	10	228	7251	152	73143	379	53642	24646	892

Hospital, Address, Telephone, Administrator, Approval, Facility, and Physician Codes, Health Care System, Network	Classi-fication Codes		Utilization Data						Expense (thousands) of dollars		
	Control	Service	Beds	Admissions	Census	Outpatient Visits	Births	Total	Payroll	Personnel

★ American Hospital Association (AHA) membership
□ Joint Commission on Accreditation of Healthcare Organizations (JCAHO) accreditation
+ American Osteopathic Hospital Association (AOHA) membership
○ American Osteopathic Association (AOA) accreditation
△ Commission on Accreditation of Rehabilitation Facilities (CARF) accreditation
Control codes 61, 63, 64, 71, 72 and 73 indicate hospitals listed by AOHA, but not registered by AHA. For definition of numerical codes, see page A4

HICKORY—Catawba County

CATAWBA MEMORIAL HOSPITAL, 810 Fairgrove Church Road S.E., Zip 28602; tel. 704/326–3000; J. Anthony Rose, President and Chief Executive Officer A1 5 9 10 F7 8 10 14 15 16 17 19 21 22 23 24 25 26 28 30 31 32 33 34 35 37 40 41 42 44 46 48 49 52 54 55 56 57 58 60 61 65 66 67 71 73 74 P8 N Carolinas Hospital Network, Charlotte, NC — 13 10 190 7177 108 131235 1435 66866 30516 927

△ FRYE REGIONAL MEDICAL CENTER, (Includes Frye Regional Medical Center–South Campus, tel. 704/328–2226), 420 North Center Street, Zip 28601; tel. 704/322–6070; Dennis Phillips, Chief Executive Officer (Nonreporting) A1 7 9 10 S TENET Healthcare Corporation, Santa Barbara, CA — 33 10 355 — — — — — — —

HIGH POINT—Guilford County

HIGH POINT REGIONAL HEALTH SYSTEM, (Formerly High Point Regional Hospital), 601 North Elm Street, Zip 27262, Mailing Address: P.O. Box HP–5, Zip 27261; tel. 910/884–8400; Jeffrey S. Miller, President (Total facility includes 30 beds in nursing home–type unit) A1 2 9 10 F2 3 4 7 8 10 11 12 14 15 16 17 19 20 21 22 23 24 26 28 29 30 31 32 33 35 37 39 40 41 42 43 44 45 46 49 52 54 55 56 57 58 59 60 64 65 66 67 71 72 73 74 P3 5 7 8 — 23 10 321 16213 241 73500 1758 100733 39592 1482

HIGHLANDS—Macon County

HIGHLANDS–CASHIERS HOSPITAL, Hospital Drive, Zip 28741, Mailing Address: P.O. Drawer 190, Zip 28741–0190; tel. 704/526–1200; Phillip E. Fowler, President (Total facility includes 80 beds in nursing home–type unit) A1 9 10 F6 8 15 19 22 28 30 31 32 39 44 45 64 65 71 72 73 — 23 10 104 503 71 12374 0 6611 3015 133

JACKSONVILLE—Onslow County

BRYNN MARR BEHAVIORAL HEALTHCARE SYSTEM, 192 Village Drive, Zip 28546; tel. 910/577–1400; Dale Armstrong, Chief Executive Officer (Nonreporting) A1 9 10 S Ramsay Health Care, Inc., Coral Gobles, FL — 33 22 76 — — — — — — —

ONSLOW MEMORIAL HOSPITAL, 317 Western Boulevard, Zip 28540, Mailing Address: Box 1358, Zip 28540; tel. 910/577–2281; Douglas Kramer, Chief Executive Officer A1 9 10 F7 8 10 12 15 16 19 21 22 23 27 35 40 42 44 45 49 63 71 72 73 P6 7 8 N Eastern Carolina Health Network, Greenville, NC — 16 10 133 7766 91 47446 1933 40277 18647 599

JEFFERSON—Ashe County

ASHE MEMORIAL HOSPITAL, Highway 221 South–Box 8, Zip 28640–0008; tel. 910/246–7101; R. D. Williams, Administrator (Total facility includes 60 beds in nursing home–type unit) A1 9 10 F7 8 14 15 16 19 22 24 28 29 34 35 39 40 41 44 45 49 64 65 71 73 P5 S Quorum Health Group/Quorum Health Resources, Inc., Brentwood, TN — 23 10 115 2154 92 31112 109 12734 5514 244

KENANSVILLE—Duplin County

DUPLIN GENERAL HOSPITAL, 401 North Main Street, Zip 28349–0278, Mailing Address: P.O. Box 278, Zip 28349–0278; tel. 910/296–0941; Richard E. Harrell, President (Total facility includes 20 beds in nursing home–type unit) A1 9 10 F7 8 14 15 16 19 21 22 26 31 37 39 40 42 44 49 51 52 55 56 57 64 65 71 73 74 P6 N Eastern Carolina Health Network, Greenville, NC — 23 10 80 2887 57 32948 551 14413 6826 303

KINGS MOUNTAIN—Cleveland County

KINGS MOUNTAIN HOSPITAL, 706 West King Street, Zip 28086, Mailing Address: P.O. Box 339, Zip 28086; tel. 704/739–3601; Hank Neal, Administrator (Total facility includes 10 beds in nursing home–type unit) A1 9 10 F8 14 19 22 37 44 52 64 65 71 73 S Carolinas HealthCare System, Charlotte, NC N Carolinas Hospital Network, Charlotte, NC — 16 10 70 1804 40 20658 0 10406 4763 174

KINSTON—Lenoir County

CASWELL CENTER, 2415 West Vernon Avenue, Zip 28501; tel. 919/559–5222; Jim S. Woodall, Director A9 F11 14 15 16 20 27 28 31 34 37 39 41 46 65 73 — 12 62 829 47 666 568 0 59187 40800 1675

LENOIR MEMORIAL HOSPITAL, 100 Airport Road, Zip 28501–0678, Mailing Address: P.O. Drawer 1678, Zip 28503–1678; tel. 919/522–7171; Gary E. Black, President and Chief Executive Officer (Total facility includes 26 beds in nursing home–type unit) A1 2 9 10 F7 10 12 14 15 16 17 19 20 21 22 24 28 29 30 34 35 37 39 40 41 42 44 45 46 48 49 56 59 60 64 65 67 70 71 72 73 P5 N Eastern Carolina Health Network, Greenville, NC — 13 10 265 9383 156 63156 789 55484 26336 897

LAURINBURG—Scotland County

SCOTLAND MEMORIAL HOSPITAL, 500 Lauchwood Drive, Zip 28352; tel. 910/291–7000; Gregory C. Wood, Chief Executive Officer (Total facility includes 50 beds in nursing home–type unit) A1 9 10 F1 2 3 7 8 10 18 19 20 21 22 23 27 28 29 30 31 32 33 34 35 36 37 39 40 41 42 44 46 49 60 61 62 63 64 65 67 68 71 72 73 74 P3 8 N Carolinas Hospital Network, Charlotte, NC — 23 10 174 4699 108 60866 601 36436 15822 562

LENOIR—Caldwell County

CALDWELL MEMORIAL HOSPITAL, 321 Mulberry Street S.W., Zip 28645, Mailing Address: P.O. Box 1890, Zip 28645; tel. 704/757–5100; Frederick L. Soule, President and Chief Executive Officer (Total facility includes 10 beds in nursing home–type unit) (Nonreporting) A1 9 10 — 23 10 78 — — — — — — —

LEXINGTON—Davidson County

LEXINGTON MEMORIAL HOSPITAL, 250 Hospital Drive, Zip 27292, Mailing Address: P.O. Box 1817, Zip 27293–1817; tel. 910/248–5161; John A. Cashion, FACHE, President A1 9 10 F3 7 8 15 19 22 25 29 30 32 35 37 39 40 41 42 44 46 49 53 54 55 56 58 59 63 65 67 71 72 73 P2 3 5 8 — 23 10 87 4215 48 67776 708 30967 13103 451

LINCOLNTON—Lincoln County

LINCOLN MEDICAL CENTER, 200 Gamble Drive, Zip 28092–0677, Mailing Address: Box 677, Zip 28093–0677; tel. 704/735–3071; Peter W. Acker, President and Chief Executive Officer A1 9 10 F7 8 14 17 19 21 22 26 27 28 30 34 35 36 39 40 44 49 65 66 67 71 73 P3 7 N Carolinas Hospital Network, Charlotte, NC — 23 10 75 3267 43 42499 430 26788 12727 391

Hospital, Address, Telephone, Administrator, Approval, Facility, and Physician Codes, Health Care System, Network	Classi-fication Codes		Utilization Data					Expense (thousands) of dollars		
★ American Hospital Association (AHA) membership ☐ Joint Commission on Accreditation of Healthcare Organizations (JCAHO) accreditation + American Osteopathic Hospital Association (AOHA) membership ○ American Osteopathic Association (AOA) accreditation △ Commission on Accreditation of Rehabilitation Facilities (CARF) accreditation Control codes 61, 63, 64, 71, 72 and 73 indicate hospitals listed by AOHA, but not registered by AHA. For definition of numerical codes, see page A4	Control	Service	Beds	Admissions	Census	Outpatient Visits	Births	Total	Payroll	Personnel

LOUISBURG—Franklin County

☐ FRANKLIN REGIONAL MEDICAL CENTER, 100 Hospital Drive, Zip 27549, Mailing Address: Box 609, Zip 27549; tel. 919/496–5131; Thomas Hanenburg, Administrator **A**1 9 10 **F**8 10 11 12 15 16 17 19 22 23 25 28 29 30 32 33 35 44 45 46 52 53 54 56 65 66 67 71 73 **P**8 **S** Health Management Associates, Naples, FL

	33	10	85	2582	36	—	0	—	—	200

LUMBERTON—Robeson County

✠ SOUTHEASTERN REGIONAL MEDICAL CENTER, 300 West 27th Street, Zip 28358, Mailing Address: Box 1408, Zip 28359–1408; tel. 910/671–5000; J. L. Welsh, Jr., President **A**1 9 10 **F**1 2 3 7 8 10 14 15 16 17 19 20 21 22 24 28 29 30 31 32 33 34 37 38 39 40 41 42 44 45 46 49 51 52 53 56 57 60 65 66 67 71 73

	23	10	282	11701	194	143133	1481	77029	34853	1255

MARION—McDowell County

✠ MCDOWELL HOSPITAL, 100 Rankin Drive, Zip 28752, Mailing Address: P.O. Box 730, Zip 28752; tel. 704/659–5000; Jeffrey M. Judd, President and Chief Executive Officer **A**1 9 10 **F**7 8 14 17 19 21 22 23 24 30 37 42 44 45 46 49 63 65 67 71 73 74 **P**5 **N** Western North Carolina Health Network, Asheville, NC

	23	10	65	2679	32	34349	317	14218	7406	286

MCCAIN—Hoke County

MCCAIN CORRECTIONAL HOSPITAL, Mailing Address: P.O. Box 5118, Zip 28361–5118; tel. 910/944–2351; F. D. Hubbard, Superintendent (Nonreporting)

	12	11	81	—	—	—	—	—	—	—

MOCKSVILLE—Davie County

✠ DAVIE COUNTY HOSPITAL, 223 Hospital Street, Zip 27028, Mailing Address: P.O. Box 1209, Zip 27028; tel. 704/634–8100; Mike Kimel, Administrator **A**1 9 10 **F**8 11 13 15 16 17 19 22 28 29 30 32 34 35 37 39 41 44 45 46 48 49 65 71 73 **P**6 7 8

	23	10	34	677	14	11081	0	9101	4523	180

MONROE—Union County

✠ UNION REGIONAL MEDICAL CENTER, 600 Hospital Drive, Zip 28112, Mailing Address: P.O. Box 5003, Zip 28111; tel. 704/283–3100; John W. Roberts, President and Chief Executive Officer (Total facility includes 66 beds in nursing home–type unit) **A**1 9 10 **F**2 3 4 5 6 7 8 9 10 11 12 13 14 17 18 19 20 21 22 23 24 25 26 27 28 29 30 31 32 33 34 35 37 38 39 40 41 42 43 44 45 46 47 48 49 50 51 52 53 54 55 56 57 58 59 60 61 62 63 64 65 66 67 68 69 70 71 72 73 74 **P**5 **S** Carolinas HealthCare System, Charlotte, NC **N** Carolinas Hospital Network, Charlotte, NC; Central Carolina Rural Hospital Alliance, Albemarle, NC

	23	10	176	5424	132	84404	852	40108	17838	548

MOORESVILLE—Iredell County

☐ LAKE NORMAN REGIONAL MEDICAL CENTER, 610 East Center Avenue, Zip 28115, Mailing Address: Box 360, Zip 28115; tel. 704/663–1113; P. Paul Smith, Jr., Executive Director **A**1 9 10 **F**7 8 10 12 14 15 16 17 19 22 23 25 26 27 28 30 32 34 35 36 37 39 40 42 44 45 46 49 65 67 71 73 74 **P**8 **S** Health Management Associates, Naples, FL

	33	10	100	3404	41	30692	291	—	—	313

MOREHEAD CITY—Carteret County

✠ CARTERET GENERAL HOSPITAL, 3500 Arendell Street, Zip 28557–1619, Mailing Address: P.O. Box 1619, Zip 28557; tel. 919/247–1616; F. A. Odell, III, FACHE, President (Total facility includes 104 beds in nursing home–type unit) **A**1 9 10 **F**7 8 11 15 16 17 19 21 22 23 25 28 30 32 33 39 40 41 42 44 45 46 49 53 54 56 63 64 65 67 71 72 73 **P**3 4 **N** Eastern Carolina Health Network, Greenville, NC

	13	10	225	5215	173	54477	489	37751	16608	623

MORGANTON—Burke County

☐ BROUGHTON HOSPITAL, 1000 South Sterling Street, Zip 28655–3999; tel. 704/433–2111; Seth P. Hunt, Jr., Director (Total facility includes 44 beds in nursing home–type unit) **A**1 5 9 10 **F**19 20 21 26 28 35 46 52 53 54 55 57 59 60 63 64 65 71 73 **P**6

	12	22	630	3442	487	—	0	89970	35915	1272

✠ GRACE HOSPITAL, 2201 South Sterling Street, Zip 28655–4058; tel. 704/438–2000; V. Otis Wilson, Jr., President (Nonreporting) **A**1 9 10

	23	10	149	—	—	—	—	—	—	—

MOUNT AIRY—Surry County

✠ NORTHERN HOSPITAL OF SURRY COUNTY, 830 Rockford Street, Zip 27030, Mailing Address: Box 1101, Zip 27030–1101; tel. 910/719–7000; William B. James, Chief Executive Officer (Total facility includes 13 beds in nursing home–type unit) **A**1 9 10 **F**7 8 11 12 15 17 19 20 22 25 26 28 29 30 32 33 34 35 37 40 41 42 44 45 49 51 52 56 59 63 64 65 67 71 73 **S** Quorum Health Group/Quorum Health Resources, Inc., Brentwood, TN

	16	10	115	4780	48	68842	568	33287	15542	550

MURPHY—Cherokee County

✠ MURPHY MEDICAL CENTER, 2002 U.S. Highway 64 East, Zip 28906; tel. 704/837–8161; Mike Stevenson, Administrator (Total facility includes 120 beds in nursing home–type unit) **A**1 9 10 **F**7 8 15 16 19 21 22 24 28 29 30 34 35 37 41 42 44 49 60 63 64 65 67 71 73 **P**5 **N** Western North Carolina Health Network, Asheville, NC

	23	10	170	2333	140	27519	261	17532	8568	362

NEW BERN—Craven County

✠ △ CRAVEN REGIONAL MEDICAL AUTHORITY, 2000 Neuse Boulevard, Zip 28560, Mailing Address: Box 12157, Zip 28561; tel. 919/633–8111; Charles H. Ashford, M.D., Interim Chief Executive Officer **A**1 2 7 9 10 **F**4 7 8 10 11 12 14 19 21 22 25 26 27 28 29 30 31 32 34 35 37 39 40 41 42 43 44 48 49 52 55 56 57 59 60 63 64 65 66 71 73 74 **N** Eastern Carolina Health Network, Greenville, NC

	16	10	267	11255	183	97344	1105	93507	37268	1296

Hospital, Address, Telephone, Administrator, Approval, Facility, and Physician Codes, Health Care System, Network	Classi-fication Codes		Utilization Data					Expense (thousands) of dollars		
	Control	Service	Beds	Admissions	Census	Outpatient Visits	Births	Total	Payroll	Personnel

★ American Hospital Association (AHA) membership
□ Joint Commission on Accreditation of Healthcare Organizations (JCAHO) accreditation
+ American Osteopathic Hospital Association (AOHA) membership
○ American Osteopathic Association (AOA) accreditation
△ Commission on Accreditation of Rehabilitation Facilities (CARF) accreditation
Control codes 61, 63, 64, 71, 72 and 73 indicate hospitals listed by AOHA, but not registered by AHA. For definition of numerical codes, see page A4

NORTH WILKESBORO—Wilkes County

✦ WILKES REGIONAL MEDICAL CENTER, 1370 West D Street, Zip 28659, Mailing Address: Box 609, Zip 28659-0609; tel. 910/651-8100; David L. Henson, Chief Executive Officer (Total facility includes 10 beds in nursing home–type unit) **A**1 9 10 **F**7 8 10 12 14 17 19 20 21 22 23 24 26 28 30 32 33 34 35 37 39 40 42 44 49 64 65 71 73 74 — *14 10 130 5139 69 80111 607 35388 16110 —*

OXFORD—Granville County

✦ GRANVILLE MEDICAL CENTER, 1010 College Street, Zip 27565-2507, Mailing Address: Box 947, Zip 27565-0947; tel. 919/690-3000; Andrew Mannich, Administrator (Total facility includes 80 beds in nursing home–type unit) (Nonreporting) **A**1 9 10 **S** Quorum Health Group/Quorum Health Resources, Inc., Brentwood, TN *13 10 146 — — — — — — —*

PINEHURST—Moore County

✦ △ MOORE REGIONAL HOSPITAL, Page Road, Zip 28374, Mailing Address: P.O. Box 3000, Zip 28374-3000; tel. 910/215-1000; Charles T. Frock, President and Chief Executive Officer **A**1 2 7 9 10 **F**2 3 4 7 8 10 11 12 14 15 16 17 19 20 21 22 24 25 27 29 30 31 33 34 35 37 38 39 40 41 42 43 44 45 46 48 49 51 52 54 55 56 57 58 59 60 63 65 67 71 73 74 **P**7 *23 10 330 16013 270 91817 1396 119537 57134 1920*

PINEVILLE—Mecklenburg County

□ BHC CEDAR SPRING HOSPITAL, (Formerly CPC Cedar Spring Hospital), 9600 Pineville–Matthews Road, Zip 28134-7548; tel. 704/541-6676; Steven G. Johnson, Chief Executive Officer **A**1 9 10 **F**1 2 3 12 16 19 27 35 39 52 53 54 55 56 57 58 59 65 **S** Behavioral Healthcare Corporation, Nashville, TN *33 22 70 1052 29 1846 0 4652 2515 85*

PLYMOUTH—Washington County

★ WASHINGTON COUNTY HOSPITAL, 1 Medical Plaza, Zip 27962; tel. 919/793-4135; Lawrence H. McAvoy, Administrator **A**9 10 **F**8 12 15 19 21 22 26 35 37 42 44 49 50 64 71 **S** Quorum Health Group/Quorum Health Resources, Inc., Brentwood, TN **N** Eastern Carolina Health Network, Greenville, NC *13 10 49 832 16 14464 0 6445 2852 166*

RALEIGH—Wake County

CENTRAL PRISON HOSPITAL, 1300 Western Boulevard, Zip 27606-2148; tel. 919/733-0800; Robert Reardon, Hospital Services Administrator **F**19 20 22 27 31 34 35 59 71 **P**6 *12 11 86 1994 66 36037 0 — — 97*

✦ COLUMBIA RALEIGH COMMUNITY HOSPITAL, 3400 Wake Forest Road, Zip 27609-7373, Mailing Address: P.O. Box 28280, Zip 27611; tel. 919/954-3000; James E. Raynor, Chief Executive Officer **A**1 9 10 **F**3 4 7 12 14 15 17 19 21 22 23 24 30 31 32 34 35 37 39 40 41 42 44 45 49 52 53 54 58 59 65 66 71 73 **P**6 **S** Columbia/HCA Healthcare Corporation, Nashville, TN **N** Hospital Alliance for Community Health, Raleigh, NC *33 10 160 5826 77 59024 771 — — 918*

□ DOROTHEA DIX HOSPITAL, 820 South Boylan Avenue, Zip 27603-2176; tel. 919/733-5324; Walter Stelle, Ph.D., Director **A**1 3 5 9 10 **F**8 20 22 26 27 28 29 30 31 37 39 41 42 44 45 46 49 52 53 54 55 57 65 71 73 *12 22 442 4005 402 2763 0 100884 47666 1293*

✦ HOLLY HILL CHARTER BEHAVIORAL HEALTH SYSTEM, 3019 Falstaff Road, Zip 27610; tel. 919/250-7000; James B. Brawley, Chief Executive Officer **A**1 9 10 **F**2 3 12 19 22 26 35 46 52 53 54 55 56 57 58 59 65 67 **S** Columbia/HCA Healthcare Corporation, Nashville, TN *32 22 108 2731 62 0 0 — — —*

✦ REX HEALTHCARE, 4420 Lake Boone Trail, Zip 27607-6599; tel. 919/783-3100; James W. Albright, President and Chief Executive Officer (Total facility includes 140 beds in nursing home–type unit) (Nonreporting) **A**1 2 9 10 **N** Hospital Alliance for Community Health, Raleigh, NC *23 10 534 — — — — — — —*

WAKE COUNTY ALCOHOLISM TREATMENT CENTER, 3000 Falstaff Road, Zip 27610-1897; tel. 919/250-1500; Roy Nickell, Director Substance Abuse Services **A**9 10 **F**2 3 12 16 27 54 56 58 59 65 67 **P**5 *13 82 34 708 27 14201 0 3826 3174 124*

✦ △ WAKE MEDICAL CENTER, (Includes Eastern Wake Day Hospital, 320 Hospital Road, Zebulon, Zip 27597; tel. 919/269-7406; Southern Wake Hospital, 400 West Ranson Street, Fuquay–Varina, Zip 27526; tel. 919/552-2206; Western Wake Medical Center, 1900 Kildaire Farm Road, Cary, Zip 27511; tel. 919/233-2300), 3000 New Bern Avenue, Zip 27610; tel. 919/250-8000; Raymond L. Champ, President (Total facility includes 37 beds in nursing home–type unit) **A**1 3 5 7 9 10 **F**4 5 7 8 10 11 12 13 15 16 17 19 20 21 22 23 24 25 27 28 30 31 32 34 35 37 38 39 40 41 42 43 44 45 46 47 48 49 51 63 64 65 66 67 70 71 72 73 74 **P**3 **N** Hospital Alliance for Community Health, Raleigh, NC *13 10 652 28713 501 308966 3412 250689 107972 3195*

REIDSVILLE—Rockingham County

✦ ANNIE PENN HOSPITAL, 618 South Main Street, Zip 27320-5094; tel. 910/634-1010; Susan H. Fitzgibbon, President and Chief Executive Officer (Total facility includes 42 beds in nursing home–type unit) **A**1 9 10 **F**6 7 8 12 13 14 15 16 17 19 20 21 22 23 26 28 29 30 31 32 33 34 35 37 39 40 41 42 44 45 46 49 54 56 58 64 65 67 68 71 73 74 *23 10 152 3669 87 57303 360 27352 12592 396*

ROANOKE RAPIDS—Halifax County

✦ HALIFAX MEMORIAL HOSPITAL, 250 Smith Church Road, Zip 27870, Mailing Address: P.O. Box 1089, Zip 27870-1089; tel. 919/535-8011; M. E. Gilstrap, President and Chief Executive Officer **A**1 9 10 **F**7 8 12 14 15 17 19 20 21 22 23 28 30 34 35 36 37 40 42 44 45 46 49 51 52 53 55 56 57 58 63 65 67 71 72 73 74 **N** Eastern Carolina Health Network, Greenville, NC *23 10 160 7583 123 60782 794 44841 18297 685*

Hospital, Address, Telephone, Administrator, Approval, Facility, and Physician Codes, Health Care System, Network	Classi-fication Codes		Utilization Data					Expense (thousands) of dollars		
★ American Hospital Association (AHA) membership □ Joint Commission on Accreditation of Healthcare Organizations (JCAHO) accreditation + American Osteopathic Hospital Association (AOHA) membership ○ American Osteopathic Association (AOA) accreditation △ Commission on Accreditation of Rehabilitation Facilities (CARF) accreditation Control codes 61, 63, 64, 71, 72 and 73 indicate hospitals listed by AOHA, but not registered by AHA. For definition of numerical codes, see page A4	Control	Service	Beds	Admissions	Census	Outpatient Visits	Births	Total	Payroll	Personnel

ROCKINGHAM—Richmond County

★ RICHMOND MEMORIAL HOSPITAL, 925 Long Drive, Zip 28379–4815; tel. 910/417–3000; David G. Hohl, Chief Executive Officer (Total facility includes 45 beds in nursing home–type unit) **A**1 9 10 **F**7 8 10 12 14 15 17 19 23 28 30 32 33 34 35 37 39 40 41 42 44 45 49 64 65 67 69 71 73 **P**7 **N** Carolinas Hospital Network, Charlotte, NC; Central Carolina Rural Hospital Alliance, Albemarle, NC | 23 | 10 | 129 | 4420 | 90 | 39728 | 550 | 29562 | 14407 | 483

ROCKY MOUNT—Nash County

□ COMMUNITY HOSPITAL OF ROCKY MOUNT, 1771 Jeffreys Road, Zip 27804; tel. 919/937–5100; Archer R. Ross, Chief Executive Officer (Nonreporting) **A**1 9 10 | 33 | 10 | 50 | — | — | — | — | — | — | —

★ NASH HEALTH CARE SYSTEMS, 2460 Curtis Ellis Drive, Zip 27804–2297; tel. 919/443–8000; Bryant T. Aldridge, President and Chief Executive Officer **A**1 2 9 10 **F**2 3 4 7 8 10 11 12 14 15 16 17 18 19 20 21 22 23 25 28 29 30 32 33 34 35 36 37 39 40 41 42 44 45 46 49 52 53 54 55 56 57 58 59 60 63 65 66 67 70 71 72 73 74 **P**6 7 **N** Eastern Carolina Health Network, Greenville, NC | 13 | 10 | 239 | 9936 | 180 | 84811 | 1011 | 85308 | 38438 | 1213

ROXBORO—Person County

★ PERSON COUNTY MEMORIAL HOSPITAL, 615 Ridge Road, Zip 27573–4630; tel. 910/503–4800; H. James Graham, Administrator (Total facility includes 43 beds in nursing home–type unit) **A**1 9 10 **F**3 6 7 8 11 12 15 16 19 22 26 28 30 35 37 40 41 44 48 49 56 58 59 64 71 73 **S** Quorum Health Group/Quorum Health Resources, Inc., Brentwood, TN | 33 | 10 | 93 | 1647 | 56 | 36029 | — | 13696 | 6093 | 248

RUTHERFORDTON—Rutherford County

★ RUTHERFORD HOSPITAL, 308 South Ridgecrest Avenue, Zip 28139–3097; tel. 704/286–5000; Robert D. Jones, President (Total facility includes 150 beds in nursing home–type unit) **A**1 9 10 **F**1 7 8 11 19 21 22 23 28 30 32 34 35 40 41 42 44 45 46 49 50 52 64 65 71 73 **P**3 **S** Quorum Health Group/Quorum Health Resources, Inc., Brentwood, TN **N** Carolinas Hospital Network, Charlotte, NC; Western North Carolina Health Network, Asheville, NC | 23 | 10 | 293 | 5137 | 208 | 62204 | 665 | 40446 | 19139 | 663

SALISBURY—Rowan County

★ ROWAN REGIONAL MEDICAL CENTER, 612 Mocksville Avenue, Zip 28144–2799; tel. 704/638–1000; James M. Freeman, Chief Executive Officer **A**1 5 9 10 **F**2 3 7 8 10 11 12 14 16 19 22 23 25 26 30 31 32 33 34 35 37 39 40 42 44 45 46 49 52 54 55 56 58 59 63 65 66 67 71 73 74 **P**4 | 23 | 10 | 222 | 9567 | 139 | — | 872 | 60688 | 28858 | 940

★ VETERANS AFFAIRS MEDICAL CENTER, 1601 Brenner Avenue, Zip 28144; tel. 704/638–9000; Bettye W. Story, Ph.D., Director (Total facility includes 120 beds in nursing home–type unit) **A**1 5 9 **F**2 3 4 8 10 12 14 15 17 18 19 20 21 22 23 24 25 26 28 29 30 31 32 33 34 35 37 39 41 42 43 44 45 46 48 49 51 52 54 56 57 58 63 64 65 67 71 73 74 **S** Department of Veterans Affairs, Washington, DC | 45 | 22 | 612 | 3608 | 563 | 117398 | 0 | 102836 | 54188 | 1403

SANFORD—Lee County

□ CENTRAL CAROLINA HOSPITAL, 1135 Carthage Street, Zip 27330; tel. 919/774–2100; L. Glenn Davis, Executive Director **A**1 9 10 **F**7 8 10 11 12 16 19 21 22 23 31 32 33 34 35 36 37 39 40 41 42 44 46 52 65 71 73 **P**1 7 **S** TENET Healthcare Corporation, Santa Barbara, CA | 33 | 10 | 137 | 5848 | 71 | 45461 | 854 | 30574 | 12251 | 506

SCOTLAND NECK—Halifax County

OUR COMMUNITY HOSPITAL, 921 Junior High Road, Zip 27874–0405, Mailing Address: Box 405, Zip 27874–0405; tel. 919/826–4144; T. K. Majure, Administrator (Total facility includes 60 beds in nursing home–type unit) **A**9 10 **F**6 15 20 22 26 27 36 51 64 65 71 73 **P**5 | 23 | 10 | 100 | 181 | 72 | 6314 | 0 | 2986 | 1341 | 81

SEYMOUR JOHNSON AFB—Wayne County

★ U. S. AIR FORCE HOSPITAL SEYMOUR JOHNSON, 1050 Curtiss Avenue, Zip 27531–5300; tel. 919/736–5201; Colonel Michael Lischak, MC, USAF, Commander **A**1 9 **F**8 12 14 15 16 17 20 28 29 34 39 41 44 49 50 51 54 55 56 57 58 65 67 71 74 **P**6 **S** Department of the Air Force, Washington, DC | 41 | 10 | 41 | 1099 | 8 | 127113 | 309 | — | — | 344

SHELBY—Cleveland County

★ CLEVELAND REGIONAL MEDICAL CENTER, 201 Grover Street, Zip 28150; tel. 704/487–3000; John Young, President and Chief Executive Officer (Total facility includes 120 beds in nursing home–type unit) **A**1 2 9 10 **F**7 8 10 11 12 13 15 16 17 19 20 21 22 23 25 26 28 29 30 31 32 33 34 35 37 38 39 40 41 42 44 45 46 47 48 49 51 54 56 60 64 65 67 69 70 71 73 **P**1 7 **S** Carolinas HealthCare System, Charlotte, NC **N** Carolinas Hospital Network, Charlotte, NC | 13 | 10 | 296 | 8022 | 237 | 71868 | 1062 | 62649 | 27854 | 924

SILER CITY—Chatham County

★ CHATHAM HOSPITAL, West Third Street and Ivy Avenue, Zip 27344–2343, Mailing Address: P.O. Box 649, Zip 27344; tel. 919/663–2113; Ted G. Chapin, Chief Executive Officer (Nonreporting) **A**1 5 9 10 **S** Quorum Health Group/Quorum Health Resources, Inc., Brentwood, TN **N** UNC Health Network, Chapel Hill, NC | 23 | 10 | 42 | — | — | — | — | — | — | —

SMITHFIELD—Johnston County

★ JOHNSTON MEMORIAL HOSPITAL, 509 North Bright Leaf Boulevard, Zip 27577–1376, Mailing Address: P.O. Box 1376, Zip 27577–1376; tel. 919/934–8171; Leland E. Farnell, President **A**1 9 10 **F**7 8 10 14 15 16 19 20 21 22 23 25 28 30 32 33 34 35 36 37 40 42 44 49 51 52 54 56 57 65 68 71 73 **P**6 **S** Quorum Health Group/Quorum Health Resources, Inc., Brentwood, TN | 13 | 10 | 127 | 5444 | 63 | 103929 | 677 | 32375 | 14986 | 583

Hospital, Address, Telephone, Administrator, Approval, Facility, and Physician Codes, Health Care System, Network	Classification Codes		Utilization Data					Expense (thousands) of dollars		
	Control	Service	Beds	Admissions	Census	Outpatient Visits	Births	Total	Payroll	Personnel
SOUTHPORT—Brunswick County ✠ J. ARTHUR DOSHER MEMORIAL HOSPITAL, 924 Howe Street, Zip 28461; tel. 910/457–5271; Edgar Haywood, III, Administrator **A**1 9 10 **F**14 15 16 19 22 26 28 32 34 35 41 44 49 65 67 71	16	10	40	1251	14	17384	0	9923	4067	150
SPARTA—Alleghany County ✠ ALLEGHANY COUNTY MEMORIAL HOSPITAL, 233 Doctor's Street, Zip 28675–0009, Mailing Address: P.O. Box 9, Zip 28675–0009; tel. 910/372–5511; James Yarborough, Chief Executive Officer **A**1 9 10 **F**8 12 15 16 19 22 23 29 30 32 35 41 44 46 49 65 71 **S** Quorum Health Group/Quorum Health Resources, Inc., Brentwood, TN	23	10	46	1334	19	9561	36	6858	3925	177
SPRUCE PINE—Mitchell County ☐ SPRUCE PINE COMMUNITY HOSPITAL, 125 Hospital Drive, Zip 28777, Mailing Address: P.O. Drawer 9, Zip 28777; tel. 704/765–4201; Keith S. Holtsclaw, Chief Executive Officer **A**1 9 10 **F**8 11 14 15 16 19 22 24 28 32 33 40 41 42 44 56 65 71 72 73 **P**3 8	23	10	43	1755	17	40435	126	10264	4941	219
STATESVILLE—Iredell County ✠ COLUMBIA DAVIS MEDICAL CENTER, (Formerly Davis Community Hospital), Old Mocksville Road, Zip 28677, Mailing Address: P.O. Box 1823, Zip 28687; tel. 704/873–0281; G. Phillip Lotti, Chief Executive Officer (Total facility includes 13 beds in nursing home–type unit) (Nonreporting) **A**1 9 10 **S** Columbia/HCA Healthcare Corporation, Nashville, TN	33	10	132	—	—	—	—	—	—	—
✠ IREDELL MEMORIAL HOSPITAL, 557 Brookdale Drive, Zip 28677–1828, Mailing Address: P.O. Box 1828, Zip 28687–1828; tel. 704/873–5661; S. Arnold Nunnery, President and Chief Executive Officer (Total facility includes 18 beds in nursing home–type unit) **A**1 2 9 10 **F**7 8 10 11 12 14 15 16 17 19 21 22 23 28 29 30 32 33 35 37 40 41 42 44 45 46 49 51 53 54 55 56 57 58 60 63 64 65 67 71 73 74 **N** Carolinas Hospital Network, Charlotte, NC	23	10	169	7663	107	96005	917	57744	27780	812
SUPPLY—Brunswick County ✠ COLUMBIA BRUNSWICK HOSPITAL, 1 Medical Center Drive, Zip 28462, Mailing Address: P.O. Box 139, Zip 28462; tel. 910/755–8121; C. Mark Gregson, Chief Executive Officer (Nonreporting) **A**1 9 10 **S** Columbia/HCA Healthcare Corporation, Nashville, TN	33	10	56	—	—	—	—	—	—	—
SYLVA—Jackson County ✠ HARRIS REGIONAL HOSPITAL, 68 Hospital Road, Zip 28779–2795; tel. 704/586–7000; Isaac S. Coe, President (Total facility includes 100 beds in nursing home–type unit) **A**1 9 10 **F**7 8 11 12 15 16 17 19 21 22 23 28 29 30 31 32 33 34 35 37 39 40 41 42 44 45 46 49 54 60 63 64 65 71 73 **P**5 7 8 **N** Western North Carolina Health Network, Asheville, NC	23	10	186	4452	133	39583	771	36273	16577	688
TARBORO—Edgecombe County ✠ COLUMBIA HERITAGE HOSPITAL, 111 Hospital Drive, Zip 27886; tel. 919/641–7700; Janet Mullaney, Chief Executive Officer (Total facility includes 10 beds in nursing home–type unit) (Nonreporting) **A**1 9 10 **S** Columbia/HCA Healthcare Corporation, Nashville, TN **N** Eastern Carolina Health Network, Greenville, NC	33	10	127	—	—	—	—	—	—	—
TAYLORSVILLE—Alexander County ✠ ALEXANDER COMMUNITY HOSPITAL, 326 Third Street S.W., Zip 28681–3096; tel. 704/632–4282; Joe W. Pollard, Jr., Administrator (Nonreporting) **A**1 9 10 **S** Quorum Health Group/Quorum Health Resources, Inc., Brentwood, TN	23	10	36	—	—	—	—	—	—	—
THOMASVILLE—Davidson County ✠ COMMUNITY GENERAL HOSPITAL OF THOMASVILLE, 207 Old Lexington Road, Zip 27360, Mailing Address: Box 789, Zip 27361; tel. 910/472–2000; Perry T. Jones, President (Total facility includes 15 beds in nursing home–type unit) **A**1 9 10 **F**7 8 10 11 12 14 15 16 17 19 21 22 28 31 34 36 37 39 40 41 42 44 45 46 52 56 57 63 64 65 67 68 71 73 74 **P**3 5	23	10	123	4636	69	35255	626	24802	12139	459
TROY—Montgomery County ☐ MONTGOMERY MEMORIAL HOSPITAL, 520 Allen Street, Zip 27371, Mailing Address: Box 486, Zip 27371–0486; tel. 910/572–1301; Kerry A. Anderson, R.N., Administrator (Total facility includes 51 beds in nursing home–type unit) **A**1 9 10 **F**8 15 16 19 22 26 30 44 64 65 71 73 74 **P**3	23	10	67	953	53	20352	4	8886	4649	174
VALDESE—Burke County ✠ VALDESE GENERAL HOSPITAL, Mailing Address: Box 700, Zip 28690–0700; tel. 704/874–2251; Lloyd E. Wallace, President and Chief Executive Officer (Total facility includes 120 beds in nursing home–type unit) **A**1 2 9 10 **F**7 8 10 11 12 14 15 16 17 19 21 22 23 26 28 30 32 34 35 37 39 40 41 42 44 46 48 49 60 62 63 64 65 70 71 73 **P**8 **N** Carolinas Hospital Network, Charlotte, NC	16	10	199	3332	157	33177	352	25092	11260	430
WADESBORO—Anson County ✠ ANSON COUNTY HOSPITAL AND SKILLED NURSING FACILITIES, 500 Morven Road, Zip 28170; tel. 704/694–5131; Frederick G. Thompson, Ph.D., Administrator and Chief Executive Officer (Total facility includes 95 beds in nursing home–type unit) **A**1 9 10 **F**8 12 14 15 16 17 19 21 22 29 30 34 41 42 44 45 46 49 64 65 67 71 **N** Carolinas Hospital Network, Charlotte, NC	13	10	125	1526	110	21538	0	13553	6752	306
WASHINGTON—Beaufort County ✠ BEAUFORT COUNTY HOSPITAL, 628 East 12th Street, Zip 27889–3498; tel. 919/975–4100; Kenneth E. Ragland, Administrator **A**1 9 10 **F**3 7 8 11 12 14 15 16 18 19 20 21 22 24 27 28 29 30 32 33 34 35 36 39 41 42 43 44 45 46 49 51 54 55 56 57 62 65 66 67 68 69 70 72 73 74 **P**3 5 **N** Eastern Carolina Health Network, Greenville, NC	23	10	98	3403	42	41126	352	23458	10902	424

Hospital, Address, Telephone, Administrator, Approval, Facility, and Physician Codes, Health Care System, Network	Classi-fication Codes		Utilization Data					Expense (thousands) of dollars		
★ American Hospital Association (AHA) membership □ Joint Commission on Accreditation of Healthcare Organizations (JCAHO) accreditation + American Osteopathic Hospital Association (AOHA) membership ○ American Osteopathic Association (AOA) accreditation △ Commission on Accreditation of Rehabilitation Facilities (CARF) accreditation Control codes 61, 63, 64, 71, 72 and 73 indicate hospitals listed by AOHA, but not registered by AHA. For definition of numerical codes, see page A4	Control	Service	Beds	Admissions	Census	Outpatient Visits	Births	Total	Payroll	Personnel

WHITEVILLE—Columbus County

✠ COLUMBUS COUNTY HOSPITAL, 500 Jefferson Street, Zip 28472–9987; tel. 910/642–8011; William S. Clark, Chief Executive Officer **A**1 9 10 **F**7 10 11 12 14 15 16 17 19 22 23 28 30 34 35 36 37 39 40 44 45 46 49 51 65 66 71 73 **S** Quorum Health Group/Quorum Health Resources, Inc., Brentwood, TN	23	10	117	6030	84	50848	424	33733	15370	547

WILLIAMSTON—Martin County

✠ MARTIN GENERAL HOSPITAL, 310 South McCaskey Road, Zip 27892, Mailing Address: P.O. Box 1128, Zip 27892; tel. 919/809–6121; George H. Brandt, Jr., Administrator **A**1 3 9 10 **F**7 8 15 17 19 20 22 35 37 40 44 49 65 67 71 73 **N** Eastern Carolina Health Network, Greenville, NC	13	10	49	1820	22	29748	248	13100	6549	249

WILMINGTON—New Hanover County

✠ COLUMBIA CAPE FEAR MEMORIAL HOSPITAL, (Formerly Cape Fear Memorial Hospital), 5301 Wrightsville Avenue, Zip 28403, Mailing Address: P.O. Box 4549, Zip 28406–6599; tel. 910/452–8100; C. Mark Gregson, Chief Executive Officer **A**1 9 10 **F**7 8 13 15 16 17 19 21 22 24 25 28 30 34 35 37 39 40 41 44 45 46 49 66 70 71 73 **P**1 2 7 8 **S** Columbia/HCA Healthcare Corporation, Nashville, TN	33	10	109	3859	42	71166	513	—	—	453
✠ NEW HANOVER REGIONAL MEDICAL CENTER, 2131 South 17th Street, Zip 28401, Mailing Address: Box 9000, Zip 28402–9000; tel. 910/343–7000; Jim R. Hobbs, President and Chief Executive Officer **A**1 3 5 9 10 **F**2 4 7 8 10 11 12 15 16 17 18 19 22 23 25 26 27 28 30 31 32 33 34 35 37 38 39 40 42 43 44 45 48 49 51 52 53 54 55 58 59 60 61 63 65 67 68 70 71 73 74	13	10	547	21389	338	231949	2622	203791	86458	2981

WILSON—Wilson County

✠ WILSON MEMORIAL HOSPITAL, 1705 South Tarboro Street, Zip 27893–3428; tel. 919/399–8040; Christopher T. Durrer, President and Chief Executive Officer **A**1 9 10 **F**7 8 10 12 14 15 16 17 19 20 22 23 28 29 30 32 33 34 35 36 37 40 41 42 44 45 46 49 52 53 54 55 56 58 65 67 71 73 **N** Eastern Carolina Health Network, Greenville, NC	23	10	317	7730	123	114630	1139	56989	22931	910

WINDSOR—Bertie County

★ BERTIE COUNTY MEMORIAL HOSPITAL, 401 Sterlingworth Street, Zip 27983–1726, Mailing Address: P.O. Box 40, Zip 27983–1726; tel. 919/794–3141; Anthony F. Mullen, Administrator **A**9 10 **F**8 15 19 22 28 34 44 65 71 **N** Eastern Carolina Health Network, Greenville, NC	23	10	49	495	31	16522	0	4940	2150	97

WINSTON–SALEM—Forsyth County

AMOS COTTAGE REHABILITATION HOSPITAL, 3325 Silas Creek Parkway, Zip 27103; tel. 910/765–9916; Douglas M. Cody, Administrator **A**9 10 **F**12 17 34 39 45 46 49 65 73 **P**6	23	56	31	81	20	—	0	3520	2145	95
□ CHARTER HOSPITAL OF WINSTON–SALEM, 3637 Old Vineyard Road, Zip 27104; tel. 910/768–7710; Marina Cecchini, Chief Executive Officer (Nonreporting) **A**1 9 10 **S** Magellan Health Services, Atlanta, GA	33	22	99	—	—	—	—	—	—	—
✠ △ FORSYTH MEMORIAL HOSPITAL, 3333 Silas Creek Parkway, Zip 27103–3090; tel. 910/718–5000; Paul M. Wiles, President **A**1 2 3 5 7 9 10 **F**3 4 7 8 10 11 12 14 15 16 17 19 20 21 22 23 24 26 28 29 30 31 32 33 34 35 37 38 39 40 41 42 43 44 45 46 48 49 51 52 54 56 57 58 59 60 63 64 65 67 71 73 74 **P**1 6	23	10	747	30725	553	—	5530	252189	126318	3204
✠ MEDICAL PARK HOSPITAL, 1950 South Hawthorne Road, Zip 27103–3993, Mailing Address: P.O. Box 24728, Zip 27114–4728; tel. 910/718–0600; Eduard R. Koehler, Administrator **A**1 2 9 10 **F**2 3 4 7 8 10 11 12 14 15 16 17 19 20 21 22 23 24 25 26 27 28 29 30 31 32 33 34 35 37 38 39 40 41 42 43 44 45 46 48 49 51 52 54 55 56 57 58 59 60 63 64 65 66 67 70 71 72 73 74 **P**6	23	10	59	2340	22	—	0	22920	9746	268
✠ △ NORTH CAROLINA BAPTIST HOSPITAL, Medical Center Boulevard, Zip 27157; tel. 910/716–2011; Len B. Preslar, Jr., President and Chief Executive Officer **A**1 2 3 5 7 8 9 10 **F**2 3 4 5 7 8 9 10 11 12 13 14 15 16 17 19 20 21 22 23 24 26 28 29 30 31 32 34 35 37 38 39 40 41 42 43 44 45 46 47 48 49 50 51 52 53 54 55 56 57 58 59 60 61 63 64 65 66 67 69 70 71 73 74 **P**1 3 4 7 **N** North Carolina Baptist Hospitals, Inc., Winston–Salem, NC	23	10	762	26131	551	95332	0	358500	169615	5139

YADKINVILLE—Yadkin County

✠ HOOTS MEMORIAL HOSPITAL, 624 West Main Street, Zip 27055, Mailing Address: P.O. Box 68, Zip 27055; tel. 910/679–2041; Lance C. Labine, President **A**1 9 10 **F**3 8 15 16 19 22 28 30 31 32 34 35 37 44 49 59 71 73 **P**6 **N** North Carolina Baptist Hospitals, Inc., Winston–Salem, NC	13	10	30	659	7	16660	0	6341	2619	85

ZEBULON—Wake County

EASTERN WAKE DAY HOSPITAL See Wake Medical Center, Raleigh

NORTH DAKOTA

Resident population 641 (in thousands)
Resident population in metro areas 42.1%
Birth rate per 1,000 population 13.6
65 years and over 14.5%
Percent of persons without health insurance 8.4%

Hospital, Address, Telephone, Administrator, Approval, Facility, and Physician Codes, Health Care System, Network	Classi-fication Codes		Utilization Data					Expense (thousands) of dollars		
★ American Hospital Association (AHA) membership □ Joint Commission on Accreditation of Healthcare Organizations (JCAHO) accreditation + American Osteopathic Hospital Association (AOHA) membership ○ American Osteopathic Association (AOA) accreditation △ Commission on Accreditation of Rehabilitation Facilities (CARF) accreditation Control codes 61, 63, 64, 71, 72 and 73 indicate hospitals listed by AOHA, but not registered by AHA. For definition of numerical codes, see page A4	Control	Service	Beds	Admissions	Census	Outpatient Visits	Births	Total	Payroll	Personnel

ASHLEY—McIntosh County

★ ASHLEY MEDICAL CENTER, 612 North Center Avenue, Zip 58413–0556; tel. 701/288–3433; Stephen H. Johnson, Administrator (Total facility includes 44 beds in nursing home–type unit) **A**9 10 **F**7 8 11 14 15 16 19 22 24 27 30 31 32 33 34 37 39 40 44 45 46 49 64 65 66 71 73	23	10	70	259	44	3278	0	3690	1906	112

BELCOURT—Rolette County

✠ U. S. PUBLIC HEALTH SERVICE INDIAN HOSPITAL, Mailing Address: P.O. Box 160, Zip 58316–0130; tel. 701/477–6111; Ray Grandbois, M.P.H., Service Unit Director (Nonreporting) **A**1 5 10 **S** U. S. Public Health Service Indian Health Service, Rockville, MD	47	10	42	—	—	—	—	—	—	—

BISMARCK—Burleigh County

✠ △ MEDCENTER ONE, 300 North Seventh Street, Zip 58501–4439, Mailing Address: P.O. Box 5525, Zip 58506–5525; tel. 701/323–6000; Terrance G. Brosseau, President and Chief Executive Officer (Total facility includes 22 beds in nursing home–type unit) **A**1 2 3 5 7 9 10 **F**2 3 4 5 7 8 10 11 12 13 14 17 18 19 20 21 22 23 24 26 27 28 29 30 31 32 33 34 35 36 37 38 39 40 41 42 43 44 45 46 47 48 49 51 52 53 54 55 56 57 58 59 60 61 62 63 64 65 66 67 68 69 70 71 73 74 **P**1 3 4 **N** Medcenter One, Bismarck, ND	23	10	231	7401	124	432329	533	121341	65681	1510
✠ △ ST. ALEXIUS MEDICAL CENTER, 900 East Broadway, Zip 58501, Mailing Address: P.O. Box 5510, Zip 58506–5510; tel. 701/224–7000; Richard A. Tschider, FACHE, Administrator and Chief Executive Officer **A**1 2 3 5 7 9 10 **F**3 4 5 7 8 10 12 13 14 15 16 17 18 19 20 21 22 23 24 26 27 28 29 30 31 32 33 34 35 37 38 39 40 41 42 43 44 45 47 48 49 51 52 53 54 55 56 57 58 59 61 64 65 66 67 70 71 72 73 74 **P**1 7 **S** Benedictine Sisters of the Annunciation, Bismarck, ND	21	10	269	9681	149	137310	1055	92240	43745	1188

BOTTINEAU—Bottineau County

ST. ANDREW'S HEALTH CENTER, 316 Ohmer Street, Zip 58318–1018; tel. 701/228–2255; Keith Korman, President (Total facility includes 32 beds in nursing home–type unit) **A**5 9 10 **F**6 7 8 15 16 19 26 28 30 32 36 39 40 44 49 53 54 55 57 62 64 65 66 70 71 73 **P**3 **S** Sisters of Mary of the Presentation Health Corporation, Fargo, ND	23	10	67	458	44	5000	10	3434	1585	85

BOWMAN—Bowman County

ST. LUKE'S TRI–STATE HOSPITAL, 202 Sixth Avenue S.W., Zip 58623–0009, Mailing Address: Drawer C, Zip 58623; tel. 701/523–5265; Jim Opdahl, Administrator (Nonreporting) **A**9 10	23	10	17	—	—	—	—	—	—	—

CANDO—Towner County

★ TOWNER COUNTY MEDICAL CENTER, (Formerly Towner County Memorial Hospital), Mailing Address: P.O. Box 688, Zip 58324–0688; tel. 701/968–4411; Timothy J. Tracy, Administrator (Total facility includes 10 beds in nursing home–type unit) (Nonreporting) **A**5 9 10	23	10	32	—	—	—	—	—	—	—

CARRINGTON—Foster County

★ CARRINGTON HEALTH CENTER, 800 North Fourth Street, Zip 58421; tel. 701/652–3141; Paul A. Balerud, Interim Chief Executive Officer (Total facility includes 40 beds in nursing home–type unit) **A**5 9 10 **F**7 8 15 16 19 22 26 28 30 32 34 35 44 49 51 64 65 67 71 73 **P**3 4 **S** Catholic Health Initiatives, Denver, CO	21	10	70	792	52	30297	42	7713	2925	150

CAVALIER—Pembina County

★ PEMBINA COUNTY MEMORIAL HOSPITAL AND WEDGEWOOD MANOR, 301 Mountain Street East, Zip 58220; tel. 701/265–8461; George A. Rohrich, Administrator (Total facility includes 60 beds in nursing home–type unit) **A**5 9 10 **F**7 8 12 15 16 17 19 22 27 28 30 32 33 36 37 39 40 44 46 51 62 64 65 71 **S** Lutheran Health Systems, Fargo, ND	23	10	89	695	67	17785	50	6279	3058	156

COOPERSTOWN—Griggs County

GRIGGS COUNTY HOSPITAL AND NURSING HOME, 1200 Roberts Avenue, Zip 58425, Mailing Address: Box 728, Zip 58425; tel. 701/797–2221; Patrick J. Rafferty, Administrator (Total facility includes 58 beds in nursing home–type unit) (Nonreporting) **A**9 10 **N** MeritCare Health System, Fargo, ND	23	10	69	—	—	—	—	—	—	—

CROSBY—Divide County

ST. LUKE'S HOSPITAL, 702 First Street Southwest, Zip 58730–0010; tel. 701/965–6384; Leslie O. Urvand, Administrator **A**9 10 **F**8 11 14 19 22 28 29 30 32 34 36 41 44 45 46 49 71	23	10	29	323	9	1136	1	2192	885	45

DEVILS LAKE—Ramsey County

✠ MERCY HOSPITAL, 1031 Seventh Street, Zip 58301–2798; tel. 701/662–2131; Marlene Krein, President and Chief Executive Officer **A**1 5 9 10 **F**7 11 14 15 16 17 19 21 22 28 29 30 31 32 33 35 37 39 40 42 44 45 46 49 65 67 68 71 73 **P**5 **S** Catholic Health Initiatives, Denver, CO	21	10	35	1791	20	13602	256	11288	5467	187

DICKINSON—Stark County

✠ ST. JOSEPH'S HOSPITAL AND HEALTH CENTER, 30 Seventh Street West, Zip 58601; tel. 701/225–7200; John S. Studsrud, President **A**1 5 9 10 **F**7 8 14 15 16 17 19 21 22 24 30 32 33 34 35 36 37 40 41 44 46 49 52 53 54 55 56 57 58 59 63 65 66 67 71 73 **S** Catholic Health Initiatives, Denver, CO	21	10	87	2895	35	37095	373	23446	10304	389

Hospital, Address, Telephone, Administrator, Approval, Facility, and Physician Codes, Health Care System, Network	Classi-fication Codes		Utilization Data					Expense (thousands) of dollars		
	Control	Service	Beds	Admissions	Census	Outpatient Visits	Births	Total	Payroll	Personnel

★ American Hospital Association (AHA) membership
□ Joint Commission on Accreditation of Healthcare Organizations (JCAHO) accreditation
+ American Osteopathic Hospital Association (AOHA) membership
○ American Osteopathic Association (AOA) accreditation
△ Commission on Accreditation of Rehabilitation Facilities (CARF) accreditation
Control codes 61, 63, 64, 71, 72 and 73 indicate hospitals listed by AOHA, but not registered by AHA. For definition of numerical codes, see page A4

ELGIN—Grant County

JACOBSON MEMORIAL HOSPITAL CARE CENTER, 601 East Street North, Zip 58533–0376; tel. 701/584–2792; Jacqueline Seibel, Administrator (Total facility includes 25 beds in nursing home–type unit) (Nonreporting) **A**9 10 **N** Medcenter One, Bismarck, ND — 23 10 50 — — — — — — —

FARGO—Cass County

□ △ DAKOTA HEARTLAND HEALTH SYSTEM, (Includes Dakota Heartland Health System–Island Park Campus, 510 Fourth Street South, tel. 701/232–3331; Dakota Heartland Health System–South University Campus, 1720 South University Drive), 1720 South Univeristy Drive, Zip 58103; tel. 701/280–4100; Bruce A. Baldwin, Interim President and Chief Executive Officer (Total facility includes 16 beds in nursing home–type unit) **A**1 2 3 5 7 9 10 **F**3 4 5 6 7 8 10 11 12 13 14 15 16 17 18 19 20 21 22 24 26 27 28 29 30 31 32 33 34 35 36 37 38 40 41 42 43 44 45 46 48 49 51 52 53 54 55 56 58 59 60 61 64 65 66 67 68 69 70 71 72 73 74 **P**5 8 **S** Paracelsus Healthcare Corporation, Houston, TX **N** Heartland Network, Inc., Fargo, ND — 32 10 203 8832 145 160221 1244 74851 31909 1095

⊞ △ MERITCARE HEALTH SYSTEM, 720 Fourth Street North, Zip 58122; tel. 701/234–6000; Roger Gilbertson, M.D., President (Total facility includes 24 beds in nursing home–type unit) **A**1 2 3 5 7 8 9 10 **F**4 7 8 10 11 12 14 15 16 19 21 22 23 24 26 28 29 30 31 32 33 34 35 37 38 39 40 41 42 43 44 45 46 47 48 49 51 52 53 54 55 56 57 58 59 60 61 63 65 66 69 70 71 72 73 74 — 21 10 311 13389 188 53753 1392 120245 41865 1146

⊞ VETERANS AFFAIRS MEDICAL AND REGIONAL OFFICE CENTER, 2101 Elm Street, Zip 58102–2498; tel. 701/232–3241; Douglas M. Kenyon, Director (Total facility includes 50 beds in nursing home–type unit) **A**1 3 5 **F**2 3 8 11 12 17 19 20 21 22 26 27 28 30 31 32 33 35 37 39 41 42 44 46 48 49 51 52 54 55 56 57 58 60 63 64 65 67 71 73 74 **S** Department of Veterans Affairs, Washington, DC — 45 10 153 3180 117 57861 0 43438 21235 511

FORT YATES—Sioux County

⊞ U. S. PUBLIC HEALTH SERVICE INDIAN HOSPITAL, Mailing Address: P.O. Box J, Zip 58538; tel. 701/854–3831; Terry Pourier, Service Unit Director **A**1 5 10 **F**1 2 3 4 5 7 8 10 11 14 15 16 19 20 21 22 26 27 30 31 34 35 37 38 39 40 42 43 44 45 47 48 49 50 51 52 53 54 55 56 57 58 59 60 61 63 65 69 71 **S** U. S. Public Health Service Indian Health Service, Rockville, MD — 47 10 14 397 3 40634 4 8924 3205 94

GARRISON—McLean County

★ GARRISON MEMORIAL HOSPITAL, 407 Third Avenue S.E., Zip 58540–0039; tel. 701/463–2275; Richard Spilovoy, Administrator (Total facility includes 24 beds in nursing home–type unit) **A**5 9 10 **F**8 14 15 16 19 30 32 33 35 49 64 65 70 71 **P**5 8 **S** Benedictine Sisters of the Annunciation, Bismarck, ND — 21 10 54 283 37 1042 0 4416 2063 81

GRAFTON—Walsh County

⊞ UNITY MEDICAL CENTER, 164 West 13th Street, Zip 58237; tel. 701/352–1620; Steve Feltman, Chief Executive Officer **A**1 5 9 10 **F**7 8 15 16 17 19 22 28 29 30 32 34 37 40 41 42 44 49 51 54 65 66 67 71 73 **P**6 — 23 10 27 607 8 30569 42 4769 2711 98

GRAND FORKS—Grand Forks County

⊞ △ UNITED HEALTH SERVICES, (Includes Medical Center Rehabilitation Hospital, 1300 South Columbia Road, Mailing Address: P.O. Box 9017, Zip 58202; tel. 701/780–2311; United Hospital), 1200 South Columbia Road, Zip 58201; tel. 701/780–5000; Rosemary Jacobson, President and Chief Executive Officer **A**1 2 3 5 7 9 10 **F**3 4 6 7 10 12 13 14 15 16 17 18 19 21 22 23 24 26 27 28 30 31 32 33 34 35 36 39 41 42 43 44 45 46 49 50 51 53 54 55 56 57 58 59 60 61 62 63 65 66 67 68 69 70 71 72 73 74 **P**2 **N** United Hospital, Grand Forks, ND — 23 10 291 11227 177 87315 1346 121906 55572 1806

GRAND FORKS AFB—Grand Forks County

★ U. S. AIR FORCE HOSPITAL, Grand Forks SAC, Zip 58205–6332; tel. 701/747–5391; Lieutenant Colonel Stanley E. Hurstell, USAF, MSC, Administrator (Nonreporting) **A**5 **S** Department of the Air Force, Washington, DC — 41 10 15 — — — — — — —

HARVEY—Wells County

★ ST. ALOISIUS MEDICAL CENTER, 325 East Brewster Street, Zip 58341–1605; tel. 701/324–4651; Ronald J. Volk, President (Total facility includes 116 beds in nursing home–type unit) **A**5 9 10 **F**3 6 7 8 19 22 28 32 35 37 40 42 44 49 53 54 58 64 65 67 71 73 **S** Sisters of Mary of the Presentation Health Corporation, Fargo, ND — 21 10 165 704 126 4848 23 6558 3450 125

HAZEN—Mercer County

★ SAKAKAWEA MEDICAL CENTER, 510 Eighth Avenue N.E., Zip 58545–4637; tel. 701/748–2225; Dan Howell, Chief Executive Officer **A**5 9 10 **F**3 7 8 11 15 16 19 22 26 28 30 32 33 35 37 39 40 44 45 62 65 67 71 73 — 23 10 32 756 10 11213 68 4918 2378 112

HETTINGER—Adams County

□ WEST RIVER REGIONAL MEDICAL CENTER, Mailing Address: Rural Route 2, Box 124, Zip 58639–0124; tel. 701/567–4561; Jim K. Long, CPA, Administrator and Chief Executive Officer **A**1 5 9 10 **F**7 8 11 12 13 15 16 17 18 19 20 21 22 27 29 30 32 34 35 37 39 40 41 42 44 46 49 51 58 63 65 66 70 71 73 74 **P**3 — 23 10 45 1500 20 — 125 13114 4525 199

HILLSBORO—Traill County

HILLSBORO COMMUNITY HOSPITAL, 12 Third Street S.E., Zip 58045, Mailing Address: P.O. Box 609, Zip 58045–0609; tel. 701/436–4501; Bruce D. Bowersox, Administrator (Total facility includes 50 beds in nursing home–type unit) (Nonreporting) **A**5 9 10 — 23 10 74 — — — — — — —

JAMESTOWN—Stutsman County

⊞ JAMESTOWN HOSPITAL, 419 Fifth Street N.E., Zip 58401–3360; tel. 701/252–1050; Richard W. Hall, President **A**1 5 9 10 **F**7 8 15 16 19 21 22 30 31 32 33 34 35 37 39 40 41 44 45 46 56 61 63 65 67 71 73 — 23 10 56 1954 22 35103 289 12163 6113 241

Hospital, Address, Telephone, Administrator, Approval, Facility, and Physician Codes, Health Care System, Network	Classi-fication Codes		Utilization Data					Expense (thousands) of dollars		
	Control	Service	Beds	Admissions	Census	Outpatient Visits	Births	Total	Payroll	Personnel

★ American Hospital Association (AHA) membership
☐ Joint Commission on Accreditation of Healthcare Organizations (JCAHO) accreditation
+ American Osteopathic Hospital Association (AOHA) membership
○ American Osteopathic Association (AOA) accreditation
△ Commission on Accreditation of Rehabilitation Facilities (CARF) accreditation
Control codes 61, 63, 64, 71, 72 and 73 indicate hospitals listed by AOHA, but not registered by AHA. For definition of numerical codes, see page A4

Hospital	Control	Service	Beds	Admissions	Census	Outpatient Visits	Births	Total	Payroll	Personnel
⊠ NORTH DAKOTA STATE HOSPITAL, Mailing Address: Box 476, Zip 58402–0476; tel. 701/253–3650; Alex Schweitzer, Administrator **A**1 5 9 10 **F**2 28 29 41 45 46 52 53 54 55 56 57 59 65 67 73 **P**6	12	22	280	1679	223	—	0	24823	15444	573
KENMARE—Ward County										
KENMARE COMMUNITY HOSPITAL, (LONG TERM ACUTE CARE), 317 First Avenue N.W., Zip 58746, Mailing Address: P.O. Box 697, Zip 58746–0697; tel. 701/385–4296; Verlin Buechler, President and Chief Executive Officer (Total facility includes 12 beds in nursing home–type unit) **A**9 10 **F**15 16 17 19 22 26 28 32 33 36 49 53 54 55 57 58 64 65 71 73 **P**5 **S** Marycrest Health System, Denver, CO	21	49	42	142	25	9086	0	1789	948	57
LANGDON—Cavalier County										
★ CAVALIER COUNTY MEMORIAL HOSPITAL, 909 Second Street, Zip 58249; tel. 701/256–6180; Daryl J. Wilkens, Administrator **A**5 9 10 **F**7 8 11 17 19 22 28 29 30 32 34 37 40 44 49 51 65 71 **P**3 6	23	10	28	584	9	17928	23	2747	1510	56
LINTON—Emmons County										
LINTON HOSPITAL, 518 North Broadway, Zip 58552, Mailing Address: P.O. Box 850, Zip 58552; tel. 701/254–4511 (Nonreporting) **A**5 9 10	23	10	25	—	—	—	—	—	—	—
LISBON—Ransom County										
★ LISBON MEDICAL CENTER, (Formerly Community Memorial Hospital), 905 Main Street, Zip 58054–0353, Mailing Address: P.O. Box 353, Zip 58054–0353; tel. 701/683–5241; Jack Jacobs, Administrator (Total facility includes 45 beds in nursing home–type unit) (Nonreporting) **A**5 9 10 **S** Lutheran Health Systems, Fargo, ND	23	10	70	—	—	—	—	—	—	—
MANDAN—Morton County										
★ MEDCENTER ONE MANDAN, 1000 18th Street N.W., Zip 58554–1698; tel. 701/663–6471; James R. Hubbard, Administrator (Total facility includes 120 beds in nursing home–type unit) **A**5 9 10 **F**1 2 4 7 8 10 11 14 15 16 17 19 21 22 23 24 26 27 30 31 32 33 34 35 37 38 39 40 41 42 43 44 47 48 49 51 52 53 54 55 56 57 58 60 61 64 65 66 67 69 71 73 74 **P**1 3 6 **N** Medcenter One, Bismarck, ND	23	10	166	520	137	3609	0	6697	3738	204
MAYVILLE—Traill County										
★ UNION HOSPITAL, 42 Sixth Avenue S.E., Zip 58257–1598; tel. 701/786–3800; James Mackay, Jr., Chief Executive Officer **A**5 9 10 **F**3 7 8 13 14 15 16 19 21 22 24 29 32 33 40 44 65 67 70 71	23	10	28	591	9	12314	28	2751	1378	56
MCVILLE—Nelson County										
COMMUNITY HOSPITAL IN NELSON COUNTY, Main Street, Zip 58254, Mailing Address: P.O. Box H, Zip 58254–0787; tel. 701/322–4328; Jim Opdahl, Administrator (Nonreporting) **A**9 10	23	10	19	—	—	—	—	—	—	—
MINOT—Ward County										
⊠ △ TRINITY MEDICAL CENTER, Burdick Expressway at Main Street, Zip 58701–5020, Mailing Address: P.O. Box 5020, Zip 58702–5020; tel. 701/857–5000; Terry G. Hoff, President (Total facility includes 294 beds in nursing home–type unit) **A**1 2 3 5 7 9 10 **F**1 3 4 6 7 8 10 11 12 13 14 15 16 17 18 19 21 22 23 24 25 26 28 30 31 32 33 34 35 37 38 39 40 41 43 44 45 46 48 49 51 53 54 55 56 57 58 59 61 62 63 64 65 66 67 68 70 71 72 73 74 **P**1 3 4 5 6	23	10	488	5715	397	58127	619	84597	42792	1035
⊠ U. S. AIR FORCE REGIONAL HOSPITAL, 10 Missile Avenue, Zip 58705–5024; tel. 701/723–5103; Colonel Murphy A. Chesney, Commander (Nonreporting) **A**1 5 **S** Department of the Air Force, Washington, DC	41	10	39	—	—	—	—	—	—	—
⊠ UNIMED MEDICAL CENTER, 407 3rd Street S.E., Zip 58702–5001; tel. 701/857–2000; Sister Lona Thorson, Interim Chief Executive Officer **A**1 2 3 5 9 10 **F**2 3 4 7 8 10 11 12 13 17 18 19 20 21 22 24 26 27 28 29 30 31 32 33 34 35 37 38 39 40 41 42 43 44 45 46 49 52 53 54 55 56 57 58 59 60 65 66 67 70 71 73 74 **P**3 7 **S** Marycrest Health System, Denver, CO	21	10	160	5567	86	58165	388	52301	22605	658
NORTHWOOD—Grand Forks County										
★ NORTHWOOD DEACONESS HEALTH CENTER, 4 North Park Street, Zip 58267–0190; tel. 701/587–6459; Larry E. Feickert, Chief Administrative Officer (Total facility includes 112 beds in nursing home–type unit) **A**5 9 10 **F**1 6 7 11 15 17 19 20 22 26 27 28 30 34 35 36 37 39 40 44 45 46 49 51 60 64 71 72 73 74 **P**5	21	10	124	413	106	3407	13	5327	2892	124
OAKES—Dickey County										
⊠ OAKES COMMUNITY HOSPITAL, 314 South Eighth Street, Zip 58474–2099; tel. 701/742–3291; Sister Susan Marie Loeffen, Administrator **A**1 9 10 **F**7 8 15 19 21 22 32 35 37 40 42 44 45 49 66 70 71 **P**5	21	10	30	698	7	27580	57	6561	2438	105
PARK RIVER—Walsh County										
★ ST. ANSGAR'S HEALTH CENTER, 115 Vivian Street, Zip 58270–0708; tel. 701/284–7500; Michael D. Mahrer, President **A**9 10 **F**7 8 15 16 19 22 26 28 31 32 33 34 35 40 41 44 45 61 65 71 **P**5 **S** Catholic Health Initiatives, Denver, CO	21	10	20	326	8	7734	15	3010	1420	61
RICHARDTON—Stark County										
RICHARDTON HEALTH CENTER, Mailing Address: P.O. Box H, Zip 58652; tel. 701/974–3304; Arlene Mack, R.N., Administrator **A**9 10 **F**11 14 15 16 22 24 26 28 29 36 37 49 65 71 73 **N** Medcenter One, Bismarck, ND	23	10	26	82	22	258	0	—	—	33
ROLLA—Rolette County										
PRESENTATION MEDICAL CENTER, 213 Second Avenue N.E., Zip 58367, Mailing Address: P.O. Box 759, Zip 58367–0759; tel. 701/477–3161; Kimber Wraalstad, Chief Executive Officer (Total facility includes 48 beds in nursing home–type unit) **A**5 9 10 **F**7 8 13 19 22 28 30 32 34 36 37 40 41 42 44 45 49 53 54 57 58 64 65 66 71 74 **P**6 **S** Sisters of Mary of the Presentation Health Corporation, Fargo, ND	23	10	102	873	52	8275	112	6697	3661	140

Hospital, Address, Telephone, Administrator, Approval, Facility, and Physician Codes, Health Care System, Network	Classi-fication Codes		Utilization Data					Expense (thousands) of dollars		
	Control	Service	Beds	Admissions	Census	Outpatient Visits	Births	Total	Payroll	Personnel

★   American Hospital Association (AHA) membership
□   Joint Commission on Accreditation of Healthcare Organizations (JCAHO) accreditation
+   American Osteopathic Hospital Association (AOHA) membership
○   American Osteopathic Association (AOA) accreditation
△   Commission on Accreditation of Rehabilitation Facilities (CARF) accreditation
    Control codes 61, 63, 64, 71, 72 and 73 indicate hospitals listed by AOHA, but not
    registered by AHA. For definition of numerical codes, see page A4

Hospital	Control	Service	Beds	Admissions	Census	Outpatient Visits	Births	Total	Payroll	Personnel
RUGBY—Pierce County										
☒ HEART OF AMERICA MEDICAL CENTER, Rugby Heights, Zip 58368, Mailing Address: P.O. Box 197, Zip 58368; tel. 701/776–5261; Jerry E. Jurena, Executive Director (Total facility includes 198 beds in nursing home–type unit) **A**1 5 9 10 **F**3 7 19 21 22 26 28 31 32 33 34 36 37 39 40 41 44 64 65 66 71 73	23	10	236	1023	210	9656	74	10786	5185	242
STANLEY—Mountrail County										
STANLEY COMMUNITY HOSPITAL, 502 Third Street S.E., Zip 58784, Mailing Address: Box 399, Zip 58784–0399; tel. 701/628–2424; David Sandberg, Administrator **A**9 10 **F**7 8 19 22 28 36 **P**8	23	10	25	297	5	3949	3	1669	951	44
TIOGA—Williams County										
★ TIOGA MEDICAL CENTER, 810 North Welo Street, Zip 58852–0159, Mailing Address: P.O. Box 159, Zip 58852–0159; tel. 701/664–3305; Lowell D. Herfindahl, President and Chief Executive Officer (Total facility includes 30 beds in nursing home–type unit) (Nonreporting) **A**5 9 10	23	10	59	—	—	—	—	—	—	—
TURTLE LAKE—McLean County										
COMMUNITY MEMORIAL HOSPITAL, 220 Fifth Avenue, Zip 58575, Mailing Address: P.O. Box 280, Zip 58575; tel. 701/448–2331; Dale Aman, Administrator **A**9 10 **F**8 11 12 14 15 16 19 20 21 22 26 28 30 32 33 35 40 41 44 48 49 50 51 60 63 64 65 71 73 **P**8	21	10	29	319	3	2766	4	1295	746	41
VALLEY CITY—Barnes County										
☒ MERCY HOSPITAL, 570 Chautauqua Boulevard, Zip 58072–3199; tel. 701/845–0440; Greg Hanson, President and Chief Executive Officer **A**1 5 9 10 **F**1 7 8 11 14 15 19 22 26 28 29 30 32 34 35 37 39 40 44 49 65 66 70 71 **S** Catholic Health Initiatives, Denver, CO	21	10	50	1001	38	14255	102	6668	3758	136
WATFORD CITY—McKenzie County										
★ MCKENZIE COUNTY MEMORIAL HOSPITAL, 508 North Main Street, Zip 58854, Mailing Address: P.O. Box 548, Zip 58854–0548; tel. 701/842–3000; Tim Gullingsrud, Administrator **A**9 10 **F**1 7 8 15 16 17 19 21 22 24 26 27 28 30 32 34 40 44 48 64 71 **N** Medcenter One, Bismarck, ND	23	10	24	177	4	6789	9	1545	667	33
WILLISTON—Williams County										
☒ MERCY MEDICAL CENTER, 1301 15th Avenue West, Zip 58801–3896; tel. 701/774–7400; Duane D. Jerde, President and Chief Executive Officer **A**1 9 10 **F**2 3 7 8 12 15 19 21 22 23 24 28 30 32 33 34 35 37 39 40 41 42 44 45 46 49 52 53 58 60 63 65 66 67 68 71 73 74 **S** Catholic Health Initiatives, Denver, CO	21	10	113	2461	52	23738	266	22214	10235	406
WISHEK—McIntosh County										
★ WISHEK COMMUNITY HOSPITAL, 1007 Fourth Avenue South, Zip 58495, Mailing Address: P.O. Box 647, Zip 58495; tel. 701/452–2326; Timothy F. Quinn, Administrator **A**5 9 10 **F**8 11 14 15 16 17 19 21 22 24 25 30 32 34 37 44 45 48 49 53 54 65 71 73 **P**6 8	23	10	22	506	6	12755	0	4169	2288	95

OHIO

Resident population 11,151 (in thousands)
Resident population in metro areas 81.2%
Birth rate per 1,000 population 14.4
65 years and over 13.4%
Percent of persons without health insurance 11.0%

Hospital, Address, Telephone, Administrator, Approval, Facility, and Physician Codes, Health Care System, Network	Classi-fication Codes		Utilization Data					Expense (thousands) of dollars		
	Control	Service	Beds	Admissions	Census	Outpatient Visits	Births	Total	Payroll	Personnel

Codes:
★ American Hospital Association (AHA) membership
□ Joint Commission on Accreditation of Healthcare Organizations (JCAHO) accreditation
+ American Osteopathic Hospital Association (AOHA) membership
○ American Osteopathic Association (AOA) accreditation
△ Commission on Accreditation of Rehabilitation Facilities (CARF) accreditation
Control codes 61, 63, 64, 71, 72 and 73 indicate hospitals listed by AOHA, but not registered by AHA. For definition of numerical codes, see page A4

AKRON—Summit County

AKRON CITY HOSPITAL See Summa Health System

★ AKRON GENERAL MEDICAL CENTER, 400 Wabash Avenue, Zip 44307–2433; tel. 330/384–6000; Michael A. West, President **A**1 2 3 5 9 10 **F**4 7 8 10 11 12 14 16 19 21 22 23 26 28 29 30 31 32 35 37 40 41 42 43 44 45 46 49 51 52 54 56 58 59 60 61 63 65 66 67 69 71 72 73 74 **P**7 8 **N** Northeast Ohio Health Network, Akron, OH; Healthy Connections Network, Akron, OH — 23 10 473 22932 340 251522 2856 221407 101558 2609

★ CHILDREN'S HOSPITAL MEDICAL CENTER OF AKRON, One Perkins Square, Zip 44308–1062; tel. 330/379–8200; William H. Considine, President **A**1 3 5 8 9 10 **F**1 2 3 4 7 8 9 10 11 12 13 14 15 16 17 18 19 20 21 22 24 25 26 27 28 29 30 31 32 33 34 35 37 38 39 40 41 42 43 44 45 46 47 48 49 51 52 53 54 55 56 58 59 60 61 63 64 65 66 67 68 69 70 71 72 73 74 **P**8 **N** Northeast Ohio Health Network, Akron, OH; Cleveland Health Network, Cleveland, OH; Healthy Connections Network, Akron, OH — 23 50 200 6838 111 229397 0 114622 54245 1464

★ △ EDWIN SHAW HOSPITAL, 1621 Flickinger Road, Zip 44312–4495; tel. 330/784–1271; Daniel K. Church, Ph.D., President and Chief Executive Officer (Total facility includes 49 beds in nursing home–type unit) **A**1 5 7 9 10 **F**2 3 12 14 15 16 17 20 26 27 32 34 39 41 46 48 49 53 54 57 58 64 65 67 68 73 — 13 46 188 2553 107 — 0 24833 12943 409

SAINT THOMAS HOSPITAL See Summa Health System

★ SUMMA HEALTH SYSTEM, (Includes Akron City Hospital, 525 East Market Street, Zip 44309–2090, Mailing Address: P.O. Box 2090, Zip 44309–2090; tel. 330/375–3000; Saint Thomas Hospital, 444 North Main Street, Zip 44310; tel. 330/375–3000), Albert F. Gilbert, Ph.D., President and Chief Executive Officer **A**1 2 3 5 6 8 9 10 **F**2 3 4 5 7 8 9 10 11 12 13 15 16 17 18 19 20 21 22 23 25 26 28 29 30 31 33 34 35 36 37 38 39 40 41 42 43 44 45 46 47 48 49 51 52 53 54 56 57 58 59 60 61 65 66 67 69 70 71 73 74 **P**1 3 5 6 7 8 **N** Summa Health System, Akron, OH; Cleveland Health Network, Cleveland, OH; Healthy Connections Network, Akron, OH — 23 10 620 32354 460 454480 3658 — — 4037

ALLIANCE—Stark County

□ △ ALLIANCE COMMUNITY HOSPITAL, 264 East Rice Street, Zip 44601; tel. 216/829–4000; Edward Roth, Chief Executive Officer (Total facility includes 78 beds in nursing home–type unit) **A**1 2 7 9 10 **F**7 8 14 15 17 19 21 22 23 25 28 30 32 33 34 35 36 37 39 40 41 42 44 45 46 48 49 51 64 65 66 67 71 72 73 — 23 10 206 5370 135 101535 681 39679 19412 699

AMHERST—Lorain County

★ ○ EMH AMHERST HOSPITAL, 254 Cleveland Avenue, Zip 44001–1699; tel. 216/988–6000; James L. Keegan, President and Chief Executive Officer **A**1 9 10 11 **F**4 7 8 10 11 14 15 19 21 22 25 26 27 28 30 32 33 34 35 36 37 38 39 40 41 42 43 44 45 46 47 49 51 56 57 59 63 65 66 67 69 71 72 73 74 **P**7 8 **N** Cleveland Health Network, Cleveland, OH; Comprehensive Healthcare of Ohio, Inc., Elyria, OH — 23 10 71 1072 12 27069 223 11447 5427 161

ASHLAND—Ashland County

★ SAMARITAN HOSPITAL, 1025 Center Street, Zip 44805–4098; tel. 419/289–0491; William C. Kelley, Jr., FACHE, President and Chief Executive Officer **A**1 9 10 **F**7 8 15 16 19 21 22 25 28 30 32 34 35 41 42 44 49 59 65 71 72 73 — 23 10 60 2700 28 103678 448 25956 10654 391

ASHTABULA—Ashtabula County

★ ASHTABULA COUNTY MEDICAL CENTER, 2420 Lake Avenue, Zip 44004–4993; tel. 216/997–2262; R. D. Richardson, President and Chief Executive Officer **A**1 9 10 **F**2 3 7 8 14 15 16 19 21 22 27 31 32 33 34 35 37 40 41 42 44 46 49 51 52 53 54 55 56 57 58 59 60 63 64 65 66 71 73 **P**6 **N** Great Lakes Health Network, Erie, PA; Cleveland Health Network, Cleveland, OH — 23 10 163 5653 71 130254 684 46157 20706 704

ATHENS—Athens County

★ + O'BLENESS MEMORIAL HOSPITAL, 55 Hospital Drive, Zip 45701–2302; tel. 614/593–5551; Richard F. Castrop, President **A**1 9 10 12 13 **F**7 8 14 17 19 20 21 22 26 28 30 31 32 34 35 37 39 40 42 44 45 46 48 49 51 56 63 65 67 71 72 73 — 23 10 75 2808 30 57349 507 23438 9866 289

□ SOUTHEAST PSYCHIATRIC HOSPITAL, 100 Hospital Drive, Zip 45701; tel. 614/594–5000; Mark F. McGee, M.D., Chief Clinical Officer (Nonreporting) **A**1 9 10 — 12 22 60 — — — — — — —

BARBERTON—Summit County

★ BARBERTON CITIZENS HOSPITAL, 155 Fifth Street N.E., Zip 44203; tel. 330/745–1611; Mike A. Bernatovicz, Chief Executive Officer (Total facility includes 46 beds in nursing home–type unit) (Nonreporting) **A**1 2 3 5 9 10 **S** Quorum Health Group/Quorum Health Resources, Inc., Brentwood, TN **N** Northeast Ohio Health Network, Akron, OH; Cleveland Health Network, Cleveland, OH — 23 10 272 — — — — — — —

BARNESVILLE—Belmont County

★ BARNESVILLE HOSPITAL ASSOCIATION, 639 West Main Street, Zip 43713–1096, Mailing Address: P.O. Box 309, Zip 43713–0309; tel. 614/425–3941; Richard L. Doan, Chief Executive Officer **A**1 5 9 10 **F**8 13 15 17 19 21 22 27 28 30 31 32 33 34 36 37 39 41 44 45 46 49 54 56 65 67 71 73 **N** Ohio State Health Network, Columbus, OH — 23 10 66 2228 32 35365 0 12536 6286 311

Hospital, Address, Telephone, Administrator, Approval, Facility, and Physician Codes, Health Care System, Network	Classi-fication Codes		Utilization Data					Expense (thousands) of dollars		
	Control	Service	Beds	Admissions	Census	Outpatient Visits	Births	Total	Payroll	Personnel

★ American Hospital Association (AHA) membership
□ Joint Commission on Accreditation of Healthcare Organizations (JCAHO) accreditation
+ American Osteopathic Hospital Association (AOHA) membership
○ American Osteopathic Association (AOA) accreditation
△ Commission on Accreditation of Rehabilitation Facilities (CARF) accreditation
Control codes 61, 63, 64, 71, 72 and 73 indicate hospitals listed by AOHA, but not registered by AHA. For definition of numerical codes, see page A4

BATAVIA—Clermont County

✠ CLERMONT MERCY HOSPITAL, 3000 Hospital Drive, Zip 45103–1998; tel. 513/732–8200; Karen S. Ehrat, Ph.D., President **A**1 9 10 **F**6 7 8 10 12 14 15 17 19 21 22 24 30 32 33 34 35 37 39 41 42 44 46 49 52 53 54 56 57 59 60 63 65 67 71 72 73 74 **P**6 8 **S** Mercy Health System, Cincinnati, OH **N** Mercy Health System, Cincinnati, OH	21	10	133	5061	61	172104	0	44311	20594	529

BEDFORD—Cuyahoga County

✠ UNIVERSITY HOSPITALS HEALTH SYSTEM BEDFORD MEDICAL CENTER, 44 Blaine Avenue, Zip 44146–2799; tel. 216/439–2000; Arlene A. Rak, R.N., President (Nonreporting) **A**1 9 10 **S** University Hospitals Health System, Cleveland, OH **N** University Hospitals Health System, Cleveland, OH	23	10	110	—	—	—	—	—	—	—

BELLAIRE—Belmont County

✠ CITY HOSPITAL, 4697 Harrison Street, Zip 43906–0719, Mailing Address: Box 653, Zip 43906; tel. 614/671–1200; Gary R. Gould, FACHE, Chief Executive Officer **A**1 9 10 **F**4 7 8 10 12 17 19 21 22 23 24 26 27 30 32 33 34 35 37 39 40 41 42 43 44 45 48 49 51 52 53 60 64 65 66 67 70 71 72 73 74 **P**1 2 3 7	23	10	83	2156	31	34692	260	12808	6891	257

BELLEFONTAINE—Logan County

✠ MARY RUTAN HOSPITAL, 205 Palmer Avenue, Zip 43311; tel. 937/592–4015; Ewing H. Crawfis, President (Nonreporting) **A**1 5 9 10 **N** Ohio State Health Network, Columbus, OH	23	10	72	—	—	—	—	—	—	—

BELLEVUE—Huron County

✠ BELLEVUE HOSPITAL, 811 Northwest Street, Zip 44811, Mailing Address: Box 8004, Zip 44811; tel. 419/483–4040; Michael K. Winthrop, President **A**1 2 9 10 **F**7 8 15 16 19 21 22 26 27 30 31 32 33 34 35 37 39 40 41 42 44 49 54 57 63 64 65 66 67 71 73 **P**3 7 8 **N** United Health Partners, Toledo, OH; Lake Erie Health Alliance, Toledo, OH	23	10	59	2381	25	50136	402	18037	7951	266

BOWLING GREEN—Wood County

✠ WOOD COUNTY HOSPITAL, 950 West Wooster Street, Zip 43402–2699; tel. 419/354–8900; Michael A. Miesle, Administrator **A**1 9 10 **F**7 8 10 14 16 19 22 28 31 33 35 36 37 39 40 41 42 43 44 53 54 55 56 57 58 59 63 65 66 69 71 73 **P**8 **N** United Health Partners, Toledo, OH; First Interhealth Network, Toledo, OH; Lake Erie Health Alliance, Toledo, OH	23	10	98	3440	43	95851	516	25397	11884	412

BRYAN—Williams County

□ COMMUNITY HOSPITALS OF WILLIAMS COUNTY, (Includes Bryan Hospital, 433 West High Street, Zip 43506; tel. 419/636–1131; Montpelier Hospital, Snyder and Lincoln Avenue, Montpelier, Zip 43543; tel. 419/485–3154), 433 West High Street, Zip 43506–1680; tel. 419/636–1131; Rusty O. Brunicardi, President (Nonreporting) **A**1 9 10	23	10	121	—	—	—	—	—	—	—

BUCYRUS—Crawford County

✠ BUCYRUS COMMUNITY HOSPITAL, 629 North Sandusky Avenue, Zip 44820–0627, Mailing Address: Box 627, Zip 44820–0627; tel. 419/562–4677; Mark E. Marley, President and Chief Executive Officer **A**1 9 10 **F**7 8 15 16 19 21 22 28 30 32 33 34 35 36 37 39 40 41 42 44 45 49 51 63 65 66 69 71 73 **S** OhioHealth, Columbus, OH	23	10	55	781	17	20548	66	6168	2289	170

CADIZ—Harrison County

□ HARRISON COMMUNITY HOSPITAL, 951 East Market Street, Zip 43907; tel. 614/942–4631; Terry Carson, Chief Executive Officer **A**1 9 10 **F**8 17 19 20 21 22 24 28 30 32 34 35 37 39 41 44 45 48 49 65 67 70 71 73 74 **P**3	23	10	48	772	25	12857	0	6473	3111	163

CAMBRIDGE—Guernsey County

□ APPALACHIAN PSYCHIATRIC HEALTHCARE SYSTEM, (Formerly Cambridge Psychiatric Hospital), 66737 Old 21 Road, Zip 43725–9298; tel. 614/439–1371; Stephen C. Pierson, Ph.D., Chief Executive Officer **A**1 9 10 **F**14 29 30 39 41 45 52 54 55 56 65 67 73	12	22	172	543	108	0	0	26841	15303	401
✠ SOUTHEASTERN OHIO REGIONAL MEDICAL CENTER, 1341 North Clark Street, Zip 43725–0610, Mailing Address: P.O. Box 610, Zip 43725–0610; tel. 614/439–3561; Philip E. Hearing, President and Chief Executive Officer (Total facility includes 20 beds in nursing home–type unit) **A**1 2 9 10 **F**7 8 12 14 15 16 17 19 22 28 29 30 32 34 35 37 39 40 41 44 46 63 64 65 66 67 71 73 74 **P**6 8	23	10	113	4906	66	72875	301	33487	14432	557

CANTON—Stark County

✠ AULTMAN HOSPITAL, 2600 Sixth Street S.W., Zip 44710; tel. 330/452–9911; Richard J. Pryce, President **A**1 2 3 5 6 9 10 **F**4 7 8 10 11 12 14 15 16 17 19 21 22 23 24 25 26 27 28 29 30 31 32 33 34 35 37 38 40 41 42 43 44 45 46 48 49 51 52 54 56 57 58 59 60 61 64 65 66 67 69 71 73 74 **P**7	23	10	736	21184	324	—	2238	—	—	2209
✠ △ COLUMBIA MERCY MEDICAL CENTER, (Formerly Timken Mercy Medical Center), 1320 Mercy Drive N.W., Zip 44708–2641; tel. 330/489–1000; Jack W. Topoleski, President and Chief Executive Officer (Nonreporting) **A**1 2 3 5 7 9 10 **S** Sisters of Charity of St. Augustine Health System, Cleveland, OH TIMKEN MERCY MEDICAL CENTER See Columbia Mercy Medical Center	21	10	416	—	—	—	—	—	—	—

CHAGRIN FALLS—Cuyahoga County

✠ BHC WINDSOR HOSPITAL, (Formerly Windsor Hospital), 115 East Summit Street, Zip 44022; tel. 216/247–5300; Donald K. Sykes, Jr., Chief Executive Officer **A**1 9 10 **F**1 2 3 25 34 46 52 53 54 55 57 58 59 65 67 **P**7 **S** Behavioral Healthcare Corporation, Nashville, TN	33	22	50	973	26	877	0	4975	2407	54

CHARDON—Geauga County

□ △ HEATHER HILL HOSPITAL AND HEALTH CARE CENTER, 12340 Bass Lake Road, Zip 44024; tel. 216/942–6424; Robert Glenn Harr, President (Total facility includes 194 beds in nursing home–type unit) (Nonreporting) **A**1 7 9 10	23	49	250	—	—	—	—	—	—	—

Hospital, Address, Telephone, Administrator, Approval, Facility, and Physician Codes, Health Care System, Network	Classification Codes		Utilization Data					Expense (thousands) of dollars		
	Control	Service	Beds	Admissions	Census	Outpatient Visits	Births	Total	Payroll	Personnel

★ American Hospital Association (AHA) membership
□ Joint Commission on Accreditation of Healthcare Organizations (JCAHO) accreditation
+ American Osteopathic Hospital Association (AOHA) membership
○ American Osteopathic Association (AOA) accreditation
△ Commission on Accreditation of Rehabilitation Facilities (CARF) accreditation
Control codes 61, 63, 64, 71, 72 and 73 indicate hospitals listed by AOHA, but not registered by AHA. For definition of numerical codes, see page A4

✠ UHHS GEAUGA REGIONAL HOSPITAL, 13207 Ravenna Road, Zip 44024; tel. 216/269–6000; Richard J. Frenchie, President and Chief Executive Officer (Total facility includes 21 beds in nursing home–type unit) **A**1 2 9 10 **F**7 8 11 12 14 15 16 19 20 21 22 27 28 30 32 33 34 35 36 37 39 40 41 42 44 45 46 49 63 64 65 66 67 71 73 **P**1 4 5 7 **S** University Hospitals Health System, Cleveland, OH **N** University Hospitals Health System, Cleveland, OH	23	10	121	4820	55	58582	717	34107	15537	396
CHILLICOTHE—Ross County										
✠ ADENA HEALTH SYSTEM, (Formerly Adena Regional Medical Center), 272 Hospital Road, Zip 45601–0708; tel. 614/772–7500; Allen V. Rupiper, President **A**1 5 10 **F**1 7 8 10 12 15 16 17 19 21 22 25 26 28 29 30 31 32 33 34 35 37 39 40 41 42 44 45 46 48 49 51 52 53 54 55 56 57 58 59 60 63 65 67 68 71 72 73 74 **P**2 8 **N** Community Hospitals of Ohio, Newark, OH; Mount Carmel Health System, Columbus, OH	23	10	156	7700	81	101732	880	63667	25788	860
✠ VETERANS AFFAIRS MEDICAL CENTER, 17273 State Route 104, Zip 45601–0999; tel. 614/773–1141; Michael W. Walton, Director (Total facility includes 212 beds in nursing home–type unit) **A**1 5 9 **F**1 2 3 8 12 15 17 19 20 21 22 26 27 28 29 30 31 32 33 34 35 37 41 44 46 49 51 52 54 55 56 57 58 64 65 67 71 73 74 **P**6 **S** Department of Veterans Affairs, Washington, DC	45	22	587	5747	477	90801	0	76226	44745	1235
CINCINNATI—Hamilton County										
✠ BETHESDA NORTH HOSPITAL, 10500 Montgomery Road, Zip 45242; tel. 513/745–1111; Fred Kolb, Site Administrator **A**1 9 10 **F**1 2 3 4 6 7 8 10 11 12 16 17 18 19 21 22 23 24 25 26 27 28 29 30 31 32 33 34 35 37 38 39 40 41 42 43 44 45 46 48 49 51 52 53 54 55 56 57 58 59 60 61 62 63 64 65 66 67 68 69 70 71 72 73 **P**3 7 **S** Bethesda Hospital, Inc., Cincinnati, OH **N** TriHealth, Cincinnati, OH	23	10	353	7266	72	86473	1477	—	—	—
✠ △ BETHESDA OAK HOSPITAL, 619 Oak Street, Zip 45206–1690; tel. 513/569–6111; Linda D. Schaffner, R.N., Vice President and Administrator (Total facility includes 349 beds in nursing home–type unit) **A**1 2 3 5 7 9 10 **F**1 2 3 4 6 7 8 10 11 12 15 16 17 18 19 21 22 23 24 25 26 27 28 29 30 31 32 33 34 35 37 38 39 40 41 42 43 44 45 46 48 49 51 52 53 54 55 56 57 58 59 60 61 62 63 64 65 66 67 68 69 70 71 72 73 **P**3 7 **S** Bethesda Hospital, Inc., Cincinnati, OH **N** First Interhealth Network, Toledo, OH; TriHealth, Cincinnati, OH	23	10	384	5284	100	39831	1577	—	—	—
✠ △ CHILDREN'S HOSPITAL MEDICAL CENTER, (Includes Division of Adolescent Medicine, Cincinnati Center for Developmental Disorders, and Convalescent Hospital for Children; Children's Hospital, tel. 513/636–4200), 3333 Burnet Avenue, Zip 45229–3039; tel. 513/636–4200; James M. Anderson, President and Chief Executive Officer **A**1 2 3 5 7 8 9 10 **F**3 5 10 12 13 15 16 17 18 19 20 21 22 25 28 29 31 32 33 34 35 38 39 42 43 44 45 46 47 48 49 51 52 53 54 55 56 58 60 63 65 66 67 68 69 70 71 72 73 **P**1	23	50	279	14213	200	366618	0	213260	76838	2421
✠ △ CHRIST HOSPITAL, 2139 Auburn Avenue, Zip 45219–2989; tel. 513/369–2000; Claus von Zychlin, Senior Executive Officer (Total facility includes 20 beds in nursing home–type unit) **A**1 2 3 5 6 7 9 10 **F**3 4 8 10 11 14 19 21 22 30 31 32 33 34 35 37 40 41 42 43 44 45 46 48 49 50 52 57 58 59 60 61 64 65 66 69 71 73 74 **P**1 2 6 7 **S** Health Alliance of Greater Cincinnati, Cincinnati, OH **N** National Cardiovascular Network, Atlanta, GA; The Healthcare Alliance of Greater Cincinnati, Cincinnati, OH; CHA Provider Network, Inc., Lexington, KY; Center Care, Bowling Green, KY	23	10	423	21065	279	170837	3725	214834	98986	2966
□ DEACONESS HOSPITAL, 311 Straight Street, Zip 45219–1099; tel. 513/559–2100; E. Anthony Woods, President (Total facility includes 20 beds in nursing home–type unit) (Nonreporting) **A**1 9 10	23	10	219	—	—	—	—	—	—	—
✠ △ DRAKE CENTER, 151 West Galbraith Road, Zip 45216–1096; tel. 513/948–2500; Roberta J. Bradford, President and Chief Executive Officer (Total facility includes 189 beds in nursing home–type unit) **A**1 3 5 7 9 10 **F**12 14 15 16 17 19 20 27 28 29 31 34 35 39 41 48 49 50 64 65 67 71 73 **P**6	23	46	273	983	213	11380	0	42229	20131	606
✠ △ FRANCISCAN HOSPITAL—MOUNT AIRY CAMPUS, (Formerly Providence Hospital), 2446 Kipling Avenue, Zip 45239–6650; tel. 513/853–5000; R. Christopher West, President (Total facility includes 20 beds in nursing home–type unit) **A**1 2 3 5 7 9 10 **F**2 3 6 7 8 10 11 14 15 16 17 19 21 22 24 25 26 27 28 29 30 31 32 33 34 35 36 37 39 40 41 42 44 45 46 48 49 51 52 53 54 55 56 57 58 59 62 64 65 66 67 71 72 73 74 **P**1 4 5 7 **S** Franciscan Sisters of the Poor Health System, Inc., New York, NY	21	10	240	9858	139	92485	134	73302	32737	968
✠ △ FRANCISCAN HOSPITAL—WESTERN HILLS CAMPUS, (Formerly St. Francis–St. George Hospital), 3131 Queen City Avenue, Zip 45238–2396; tel. 513/389–5000; R. Christopher West, President (Total facility includes 20 beds in nursing home–type unit) **A**1 2 7 9 10 **F**1 2 3 6 7 8 10 11 12 14 15 16 17 19 21 22 24 25 26 27 28 29 30 31 32 33 34 35 36 37 39 40 41 42 44 46 48 49 51 52 53 54 55 56 57 58 59 62 64 65 66 67 71 72 73 **P**1 4 5 7 **S** Franciscan Sisters of the Poor Health System, Inc., New York, NY	21	10	226	9088	145	82043	0	60429	26611	734
✠ △ GOOD SAMARITAN HOSPITAL, 375 Dixmyth Avenue, Zip 45220–2489; tel. 513/872–1400; Sister Myra James Bradley, Chairman of the Board of Directors (Total facility includes 15 beds in nursing home–type unit) **A**1 2 3 5 6 7 8 9 10 **F**1 2 3 4 6 7 8 10 11 12 15 16 17 18 19 21 22 23 24 25 26 27 28 29 30 31 32 33 34 35 37 38 39 40 41 42 43 44 45 46 48 49 51 52 53 54 55 56 57 58 59 60 61 62 63 64 65 66 67 70 71 72 73 **P**7 **S** Catholic Health Initiatives, Denver, CO **N** First Interhealth Network, Toledo, OH; TriHealth, Cincinnati, OH; Center Care, Bowling Green, KY	21	10	438	21057	265	143942	5546	194581	86035	2489

Hospital, Address, Telephone, Administrator, Approval, Facility, and Physician Codes, Health Care System, Network	Classi-fication Codes		Utilization Data					Expense (thousands) of dollars		
★ American Hospital Association (AHA) membership □ Joint Commission on Accreditation of Healthcare Organizations (JCAHO) accreditation + American Osteopathic Hospital Association (AOHA) membership ○ American Osteopathic Association (AOA) accreditation △ Commission on Accreditation of Rehabilitation Facilities (CARF) accreditation Control codes 61, 63, 64, 71, 72 and 73 indicate hospitals listed by AOHA, but not registered by AHA. For definition of numerical codes, see page A4	Control	Service	Beds	Admissions	Census	Outpatient Visits	Births	Total	Payroll	Personnel

Hospital	Control	Service	Beds	Admissions	Census	Outpatient Visits	Births	Total	Payroll	Personnel
★ + △ JEWISH HOSPITAL, (Includes Jewish Hospital Kenwood, 4777 East Galbraith Road, Zip 45236; tel. 513/745–2200), 3200 Burnet Avenue, Zip 45229–3099; tel. 513/569–2000; Warren C. Falberg, Senior Executive Officer (Total facility includes 20 beds in nursing home–type unit) A1 2 3 5 7 9 10 F1 2 3 4 5 6 7 8 10 11 12 14 15 16 17 18 19 20 21 22 24 25 26 27 28 29 30 31 32 33 34 35 36 37 38 39 40 41 42 43 44 45 46 48 49 50 51 52 53 54 55 56 57 58 59 60 61 63 64 65 66 67 68 69 70 71 72 73 74 P1 5 6 7 S Health Alliance of Greater Cincinnati, Cincinnati, OH N The Healthcare Alliance of Greater Cincinnati, Cincinnati, OH; CHA Provider Network, Inc., Lexington, KY	23	10	437	12377	185	155231	407	151533	67851	1830
★ MERCY HOSPITAL ANDERSON, 7500 State Road, Zip 45255–2492; tel. 513/624–4500; Karen S. Ehrat, Ph.D., President A1 2 9 10 F6 7 8 10 12 14 15 16 17 19 21 22 28 29 30 32 33 34 35 37 39 40 41 42 44 45 46 49 53 54 56 57 59 60 63 65 66 67 71 72 73 74 P6 8 S Mercy Health System, Cincinnati, OH N Mercy Health System, Cincinnati, OH	21	10	156	8733	87	101137	1674	67341	24796	783
□ PAULINE WARFIELD LEWIS CENTER, 1101 Summit Road, Zip 45237; tel. 513/948–3600; Anthony E. Thompson, Chief Executive Officer (Nonreporting) A1 9 10	12	22	357	—	—	—	—	—	—	—
PROVIDENCE HOSPITAL See Franciscan Hospital–Mount Airy Campus										
★ SHRINERS HOSPITALS FOR CHILDREN, CINCINNATI BURNS INSTITUTE, (PEDIATRIC BURN INJURIES), 3229 Burnet Avenue, Zip 45229–3095; tel. 513/872–6000; Ronald R. Hitzler, Administrator A1 F9 12 19 21 34 35 41 44 45 46 49 50 54 56 63 65 67 69 71 73 S Shriners Hospitals for Children, Tampa, FL	23	59	30	870	19	4723	0	—	—	304
ST. FRANCIS–ST. GEORGE HOSPITAL See Franciscan Hospital–Western Hills Campus										
★ UNIVERISITY HOSPITAL, (Formerly University of Cincinnati Hospital), 234 Goodman Street, Zip 45267–0700; tel. 513/558–1000; Elliot G. Cohen, Senior Executive Officer (Nonreporting) A1 2 3 5 8 9 10 S Health Alliance of Greater Cincinnati, Cincinnati, OH N The Healthcare Alliance of Greater Cincinnati, Cincinnati, OH; CHA Provider Network, Inc., Lexington, KY	12	10	418	—	—	—	—	—	—	—
★ VETERANS AFFAIRS MEDICAL CENTER, 3200 Vine Street, Zip 45220–2288; tel. 513/475–6300; Gary N. Nugent, Medical Director (Total facility includes 64 beds in nursing home–type unit) A1 3 5 8 9 F1 2 3 4 5 8 10 11 12 17 18 19 20 21 22 26 31 32 34 35 37 39 41 42 43 44 45 46 49 51 52 54 56 57 58 60 64 65 71 73 74 S Department of Veterans Affairs, Washington, DC	45	10	240	6581	222	185659	0	90000	—	1244
CIRCLEVILLE—Pickaway County										
★ BERGER HOSPITAL, 600 North Pickaway Street, Zip 43113–1499; tel. 614/474–2126; Brian R. Colfack, CHE, President and Chief Executive Officer (Nonreporting) A1 9 10 N Community Hospitals of Ohio, Newark, OH; Mount Carmel Health System, Columbus, OH	15	10	68	—	—	—	—	—	—	—
CLEVELAND—Cuyahoga County										
CAMPUS HOSPITAL OF CLEVELAND, 18120 Puritas Avenue, Zip 44135; tel. 216/476–0222; Joan Curran, Administrator A9 10 F2 3 12 18 22 52 56 58 59 65 67 P6	33	82	60	958	17	8617	0	7147	3501	64
★ △ CLEVELAND CLINIC HOSPITAL, 9500 Euclid Avenue, Zip 44195–5108; tel. 216/444–2200; Frank L. Lordeman, Chief Operating Officer A1 2 3 5 7 8 9 10 F2 3 4 5 7 8 10 11 12 14 15 16 17 19 20 21 22 24 25 26 27 28 29 30 31 32 33 34 35 37 39 40 41 42 43 44 45 46 47 48 49 50 51 52 53 54 55 56 57 58 59 60 61 63 65 66 67 69 71 73 74 P1 3 5 N Cleveland Health Network, Cleveland, OH	23	10	928	43713	694	1177273	1653	561844	266439	—
□ CLEVELAND PSYCHIATRIC INSTITUTE, 1708 Southpoint Drive, Zip 44109; tel. 216/787–0500; Sandra Rahe, Chief Executive Officer (Nonreporting) A1 3	12	22	175	—	—	—	—	—	—	—
★ COLUMBIA ST. VINCENT CHARITY HOSPITAL, (Formerly St. Vincent Charity Hospital), 2351 East 22nd Street, Zip 44115–3111; tel. 216/861–6200; Samuel H. Turner, Chief Executive Officer (Nonreporting) A1 2 3 5 9 10 S Sisters of Charity of St. Augustine Health System, Cleveland, OH	21	10	266	—	—	—	—	—	—	—
★ DEACONESS HOSPITAL OF CLEVELAND, 4229 Pearl Road, Zip 44109–4218; tel. 216/459–6300; Wayne G. Deschambeau, Chief Executive Officer (Total facility includes 15 beds in nursing home–type unit) (Nonreporting) A1 2 9 10	32	10	212	—	—	—	—	—	—	—
★ △ FAIRVIEW HOSPITAL, (Formerly Fairview General Hospital), 18101 Lorain Avenue, Zip 44111–5656; tel. 216/476–4040; Thomas M. LaMotte, President and Chief Executive Officer (Total facility includes 20 beds in nursing home–type unit) (Nonreporting) A1 3 5 6 7 9 10 S Fairview Hospital System, Cleveland, OH N Cleveland Health Network, Cleveland, OH; Health Cleveland, Cleveland, OH	23	10	428	—	—	—	—	—	—	—
□ GRACE HOSPITAL, 2307 West 14th Street, Zip 44113–3698; tel. 216/687–1500; Robert P. Range, President and Chief Executive Officer A1 9 10 F8 14 15 16 26 27 28 29 30 32 34 37 39 41 44 45 46 49 51 65 71 72 73 P8	23	10	25	130	19	34023	0	9891	4403	165
★ HEALTH HILL HOSPITAL FOR CHILDREN, Mailing Address: 2801 Martin Luther King Jr. Drive, Zip 44104–3865; tel. 216/721–5400; Thomas A. Rathbone, President and Chief Executive Officer A1 9 10 F12 14 16 27 34 39 41 45 46 48 49 53 54 58 65 73	23	56	46	317	31	8240	0	14560	9370	294
□ △ LUTHERAN HOSPITAL, (Formerly Lutheran Medical Center), 2609 Franklin Boulevard, Zip 44113–2992; tel. 216/696–4300; Kenneth T. Misener, Chief Operating Officer (Total facility includes 35 beds in nursing home–type unit) (Nonreporting) A1 3 7 9 10 S Fairview Hospital System, Cleveland, OH N Cleveland Health Network, Cleveland, OH; Health Cleveland, Cleveland, OH	23	10	174	—	—	—	—	—	—	—

Hospital, Address, Telephone, Administrator, Approval, Facility, and Physician Codes, Health Care System, Network	Control	Service	Beds	Admissions	Census	Outpatient Visits	Births	Total	Payroll	Personnel
▣ MERIDIA HILLCREST HOSPITAL, 6780 Mayfield Road, Zip 44124–2202; tel. 216/449–4500; Catherine B. Leary, R.N., Site Administrator, Vice President Clinical Services and Nurse Executive (Nonreporting) A1 2 3 9 10 S Meridia Health System, Mayfield Village, OH N Merida Health System, Mayfield Village, OH	23	10	263	—	—	—	—	—	—	—
▣ MERIDIA HURON HOSPITAL, 13951 Terrace Road, Zip 44112; tel. 216/761–3300; Beverly Lozar, Site Administrator (Total facility includes 20 beds in nursing home–type unit) A1 2 3 5 6 9 10 F3 4 7 8 10 11 12 13 14 15 16 17 19 21 22 23 24 25 26 27 28 29 30 31 32 33 34 35 36 37 38 39 40 41 42 43 44 45 46 48 49 50 51 52 54 55 56 57 58 59 60 61 63 64 65 66 67 68 70 71 72 73 74 P1 3 4 7 8 S Meridia Health System, Mayfield Village, OH N Merida Health System, Mayfield Village, OH	23	10	411	21277	309	195734	3067	215624	65604	1989
▣ △ METROHEALTH MEDICAL CENTER, 2500 Metrohealth Drive, Zip 44109–1998; tel. 216/778–7800; Terry R. White, President and Chief Executive Officer (Total facility includes 291 beds in nursing home–type unit) A1 3 5 6 7 8 9 10 F3 4 5 7 8 9 10 11 12 14 15 16 17 19 20 21 22 23 25 26 27 28 29 30 31 32 33 34 35 37 38 39 40 41 42 43 44 45 46 47 48 49 51 52 53 54 55 56 57 58 59 60 61 63 64 65 70 71 72 73 74 P6 N The MetroHealth System, Cleveland, OH	13	10	811	20488	584	580339	3850	319198	163193	4747
▣ MOUNT SINAI MEDICAL CENTER, One Mt Sinai Drive, Zip 44106–4198; tel. 216/421–4000; Robert A. Schapper, Chief Executive Officer (Nonreporting) A1 2 3 5 8 9 10 N The Mount Sinai Health Care System, Cleveland, OH RAINBOW BABIES AND CHILDREN'S HOSPITAL See University Hospitals of Cleveland	23	10	344	—	—	—	—	—	—	—
□ SAINT LUKE'S MEDICAL CENTER, 11311 Shaker Boulevard, Zip 44104–3805; tel. 216/368–7000; Samuel R. Huston, President and Chief Executive Officer A1 3 5 8 9 10 F1 4 5 7 8 10 12 14 16 17 19 20 21 22 26 31 32 34 35 36 37 38 39 40 42 43 44 46 49 52 53 54 55 56 58 59 60 65 67 69 70 71 73 P1 4 7 S Columbia/HCA Healthcare Corporation, Nashville, TN N Saint Lukes Medical Center, Cleveland, OH	23	10	205	8819	129	131248	1256	92856	42523	1043
▣ SAINT MICHAEL HOSPITAL, (Formerly St. Alexis Hospital Medical Center), 5163 Broadway, Zip 44127–1532; tel. 216/429–8000; Geoffrey D. Moebius, President and Chief Executive Officer (Total facility includes 55 beds in nursing home–type unit) (Nonreporting) A1 2 9 10 ST. ALEXIS HOSPITAL MEDICAL CENTER See Saint Michael Hospital	21	10	188	—	—	—	—	—	—	—
▣ + ○ ST. JOHN WEST SHORE HOSPITAL, 29000 Center Ridge Road, Zip 44145–5219; tel. 216/835–8000; Fred M. DeGrandis, President and Chief Executive Officer (Nonreporting) A1 9 10 11 S Sisters of Charity of St. Augustine Health System, Cleveland, OH ST. VINCENT CHARITY HOSPITAL See Columbia St. Vincent Charity Hospital	21	10	183	—	—	—	—	—	—	—
▣ △ UNIVERSITY HOSPITALS OF CLEVELAND, (Includes Alfred and Norma Lerner Tower, Bolwell Health Center, Hanna Pavilion, Lakeside Hospital, Samuel Mather Pavilion; Rainbow Babies and Children's Hospital, University MacDonald Women's Hospital), 11100 Euclid Avenue, Zip 44106–2602; tel. 216/844–1000; Farah M. Walters, President and Chief Executive Officer A1 2 3 5 7 8 9 10 F3 4 5 7 8 10 11 13 14 16 17 18 19 20 21 22 23 24 25 26 27 28 29 30 31 32 33 34 35 37 38 39 40 41 42 43 44 45 46 47 49 50 51 52 53 54 55 56 57 58 59 60 61 63 64 65 66 67 68 69 70 71 72 73 74 P3 5 6 7 S University Hospitals Health System, Cleveland, OH N University Hospitals Health System, Cleveland, OH UNIVERSITY MACDONALD WOMEN'S HOSPITAL See University Hospitals of Cleveland	23	10	725	36007	550	517835	4827	—	—	5228
▣ VETERANS AFFAIRS MEDICAL CENTER, 10701 East Boulevard, Zip 44106–1702; tel. 216/791–3800; Richard S. Citron, Acting Director (Total facility includes 195 beds in nursing home–type unit) (Nonreporting) A1 3 5 8 9 S Department of Veterans Affairs, Washington, DC	45	10	914	—	—	—	—	—	—	—
COLDWATER—Mercer County										
▣ MERCER COUNTY JOINT TOWNSHIP COMMUNITY HOSPITAL, 800 West Main Street, Zip 45828–1698; tel. 419/678–2341; James W. Isaacs, Chief Executive Officer A1 9 10 F7 8 15 19 21 22 25 28 30 32 33 35 37 40 41 42 44 46 63 65 66 67 71 72 73 N West Central Ohio Regional Healthcare Alliance, Ltd., Lima, OH; LutheranPreferred Network, Fort Wayne, IN	16	10	55	2433	23	45000	443	19145	7958	288
COLUMBUS—Franklin County										
▣ ARTHUR G. JAMES CANCER HOSPITAL AND RESEARCH INSTITUTE, (ACUTE CARE CANCER AND RESEARCH), 300 West Tenth Avenue, Zip 43210; tel. 614/293–5485; David E. Schuller, M.D., Chief Executive Officer A1 2 3 5 8 9 10 F3 4 5 7 8 9 10 11 12 13 14 15 16 17 19 20 21 22 23 24 25 26 28 29 30 31 32 33 34 35 37 38 39 41 42 43 44 45 46 48 49 51 52 53 54 55 56 57 58 59 60 61 63 65 66 67 69 70 71 72 73 74 P5 N Ohio State Health Network, Columbus, OH	12	49	116	5529	97	71645	0	86839	22020	967
□ CENTRAL OHIO PSYCHIATRIC HOSPITAL, 1960 West Broad Street, Zip 43223–1295; tel. 614/752–0333; James Ignelzi, Chief Executive Officer A1 9 10 F14 15 16 45 52 58 65 73 P6	12	22	214	589	169	1300	0	—	—	438
▣ △ CHILDREN'S HOSPITAL, 700 Children's Drive, Zip 43205–2696; tel. 614/722–2000; Thomas N. Hansen, Acting Chief Executive Officer and Medical Director A1 2 3 5 7 9 10 F4 10 12 13 17 19 20 22 24 25 27 28 29 31 32 33 34 35 38 39 42 43 44 45 47 48 49 51 53 54 55 56 58 65 67 68 69 70 71 72 73 P8	23	50	281	10980	166	318717	0	169799	73001	2467

Hospital, Address, Telephone, Administrator, Approval, Facility, and Physician Codes, Health Care System, Network

★ American Hospital Association (AHA) membership
☐ Joint Commission on Accreditation of Healthcare Organizations (JCAHO) accreditation
+ American Osteopathic Hospital Association (AOHA) membership
○ American Osteopathic Association (AOA) accreditation
△ Commission on Accreditation of Rehabilitation Facilities (CARF) accreditation
Control codes 61, 63, 64, 71, 72 and 73 indicate hospitals listed by AOHA, but not registered by AHA. For definition of numerical codes, see page A4

	Classification Codes		Utilization Data					Expense (thousands) of dollars		
	Control	Service	Beds	Admissions	Census	Outpatient Visits	Births	Total	Payroll	Personnel

☐ △ COLUMBUS COMMUNITY HOSPITAL, 1430 South High Street, Zip 43207; tel. 614/445–5000; Bobby Meadows, President and Chief Executive Officer **A**1 7 9 10 **F**2 3 8 14 15 19 22 27 28 32 33 35 37 44 48 64 71 73

| 32 | 10 | 118 | 3445 | 51 | — | 0 | 26063 | 10934 | 333 |

☐ + ○ △ DOCTORS HOSPITAL, (Includes Doctors Hospital West, 5100 West Broad Street, Zip 43228; tel. 614/297–5000), 1087 Dennison Avenue, Zip 43201; tel. 614/297–4000; Richard A. Vincent, President (Nonreporting) **A**1 5 7 9 10 11 12 13 **S** Doctors Hospital, Columbus, OH

| 23 | 10 | 380 | — | — | — | — | — | — | — |

✸ GRANT/RIVERSIDE METHODIST HOSPITALS–GRANT CAMPUS, 111 South Grant Avenue, Zip 43215–1898; tel. 614/461–3232; Jay William Eckersley, Chief Executive Officer **A**1 2 3 5 8 9 10 **F**1 2 3 4 7 8 10 11 12 13 14 15 16 17 19 20 21 22 24 25 26 27 28 29 30 31 32 33 34 35 37 38 39 40 41 42 43 44 45 46 48 49 50 51 53 54 55 56 57 58 59 60 61 63 64 65 66 67 68 70 71 72 73 74 **P**3 4 5 6 7 8 **S** OhioHealth, Columbus, OH

| 21 | 10 | 460 | 19227 | 260 | — | 2852 | — | — | 1958 |

✸ GRANT/RIVERSIDE METHODIST HOSPITALS–RIVERSIDE CAMPUS, 3535 Olentangy River Road, Zip 43214–3998; tel. 614/566–5000; Jay William Eckersley, Chief Executive Officer **A**1 2 3 5 8 9 10 **F**1 2 3 4 7 8 10 11 12 13 15 16 17 18 19 21 22 23 24 25 26 27 28 29 30 32 33 34 35 37 38 39 40 41 42 43 44 45 46 48 49 50 51 52 53 54 55 56 57 58 59 60 61 63 65 66 67 68 69 70 71 72 73 74 **P**3 5 6 7 8 **S** OhioHealth, Columbus, OH

| 21 | 10 | 778 | 37846 | 505 | — | 5986 | — | — | 3942 |

✸ MOUNT CARMEL HEALTH SYSTEM, (Includes Mount Carmel East Hospital, 6001 East Broad Street, Zip 43213; tel. 614/234–6000; Mount Carmel Medical Center, 793 West State Street, Zip 43222; tel. 614/234–5000; St. Ann's Hospital, 500 South Cleveland Avenue, Westerville, Zip 43081–8998; tel. 614/898–4000; Alice M. O'Brien, Senior Vice President of System Operations), 793 West State Street, Zip 43222–1551; tel. 614/225–5000; Dale St. Arnold, President and Chief Executive Officer (Total facility includes 14 beds in nursing home–type unit) **A**1 2 3 5 9 10 **F**7 8 10 11 12 14 15 16 17 19 21 22 23 26 27 28 29 30 31 32 33 34 35 36 37 38 39 40 41 42 43 44 45 46 48 49 50 51 52 54 55 56 57 58 59 60 64 65 66 67 70 71 72 73 74 **P**1 2 3 5 6 7 **S** Holy Cross Health System Corporation, South Bend, IN **N** Mount Carmel Health System, Columbus, OH

| 21 | 10 | 929 | 44165 | 558 | 359518 | 7519 | 389709 | 155445 | 4816 |

✸ △ OHIO STATE UNIVERSITY MEDICAL CENTER, 410 West 10th Avenue, Zip 43210–1240; tel. 614/293–8000; R. Reed Fraley, Associate Vice President for Health Sciences and Chief Executive Officer **A**1 3 5 7 8 9 10 **F**3 4 5 7 8 9 10 11 12 14 15 16 17 19 20 21 22 23 24 25 26 28 29 30 31 32 34 35 37 38 39 40 41 42 43 44 45 46 48 49 51 52 53 54 55 56 57 58 59 60 61 63 65 66 67 69 70 71 72 73 74 **P**5 **N** National Cardiovascular Network, Atlanta, GA; Ohio State Health Network, Columbus, OH

| 12 | 10 | 553 | 23978 | 410 | 305987 | 3138 | 320642 | 125990 | 3576 |

✸ PARK MEDICAL CENTER, 1492 East Broad Street, Zip 43205–1546; tel. 614/251–3000; Cornelius Serle, Chief Executive Officer (Total facility includes 20 beds in nursing home–type unit) (Nonreporting) **A**1 2 3 9 10 **S** Quorum Health Group/Quorum Health Resources, Inc., Brentwood, TN

| 33 | 10 | 145 | — | — | — | — | — | — | — |

CONNEAUT—Ashtabula County

✸ BROWN MEMORIAL HOSPITAL, 158 West Main Road, Zip 44030–2039, Mailing Address: P.O. Box 648, Zip 44030; tel. 216/593–1131; C. Thomas Moore, Chief Executive Officer (Nonreporting) **A**1 9 10 **N** Great Lakes Health Network, Erie, PA

| 23 | 10 | 41 | — | — | — | — | — | — | — |

COSHOCTON—Coshocton County

☐ COSHOCTON COUNTY MEMORIAL HOSPITAL, 1460 Orange Street, Zip 43812–6330, Mailing Address: P.O. Box 1330, Zip 43812–6330; tel. 614/622–6411; Gregory M. Nowak, Administrator (Total facility includes 61 beds in nursing home–type unit) (Nonreporting) **A**1 9 10 **N** Community Hospitals of Ohio, Newark, OH

| 23 | 10 | 151 | — | — | — | — | — | — | — |

CRESTLINE—Crawford County

☐ MEDCENTRAL CRESTLINE HOSPITAL, (Formerly Crestline Memorial Hospital), 700 Columbus Street, Zip 44827, Mailing Address: P.O. Box 350, Zip 44827; tel. 419/683–1212; Robert E. Wirtz, Jr., President and Chief Executive Officer **A**1 9 10 **F**2 3 15 16 19 22 27 28 29 30 32 33 34 39 41 44 46 48 49 64 65 67 73 **P**3 **N** Lake Erie Health Alliance, Toledo, OH

| 23 | 10 | 35 | 809 | 17 | 9639 | 0 | 6695 | 3331 | 133 |

CUYAHOGA FALLS—Summit County

+ ○ CUYAHOGA FALLS GENERAL HOSPITAL, 1900 23rd Street, Zip 44223–1499; tel. 216/971–7000; Fred Anthony, President and Chief Executive Officer **A**9 10 11 12 13 **F**7 8 14 15 16 17 19 20 22 27 28 30 32 35 37 40 41 42 44 49 52 56 58 59 63 65 67 71 73 74 **P**3 8 **N** Northeast Ohio Health Network, Akron, OH

| 23 | 10 | 135 | 4445 | 66 | — | 533 | 45863 | 20935 | 590 |

DAYTON—Montgomery County

✸ CHILDREN'S MEDICAL CENTER, One Children's Plaza, Zip 45404–1815; tel. 937/226–8300; Laurence P. Harkness, President and Chief Executive Officer **A**1 3 5 8 9 10 **F**9 10 13 14 15 16 17 19 20 21 22 25 27 28 30 31 32 34 35 38 39 41 42 44 45 46 47 49 51 53 54 55 58 65 67 68 71 72 73 **P**6

| 23 | 50 | 155 | 6099 | 87 | 205296 | 0 | 72888 | 33561 | 1045 |

DARTMOUTH HOSPITAL See Kettering Medical Center, Kettering

☐ DAYTON MENTAL HEALTH CENTER, 2611 Wayne Avenue, Zip 45420–1800; tel. 513/258–0440; Patricia A. Torvik, Ph.D., Chief Executive Officer **A**1 9 10 **F**19 20 35 39 41 45 46 52 56 57 65 67 71 73 **P**6

| 12 | 22 | 230 | 466 | 216 | 0 | 0 | 26924 | 17026 | 464 |

✸ △ FRANCISCAN MEDICAL CENTER–DAYTON CAMPUS, (Formerly St. Elizabeth Medical Center), One Franciscan Way, Zip 45408–1498; tel. 513/229–6000; James M. Strieby, Chief Executive Officer (Total facility includes 30 beds in nursing home–type unit) **A**1 2 3 5 7 9 10 **F**1 4 6 7 8 10 11 12 14 15 16 17 19 20 21 22 24 26 27 28 29 30 31 34 35 37 39 40 41 42 43 44 45 46 48 49 51 52 53 54 55 56 58 59 60 62 64 65 66 67 70 71 72 73 74 **P**2 4 6 7 8 **S** Franciscan Sisters of the Poor Health System, Inc., New York, NY

| 21 | 10 | 365 | 15640 | 265 | 290231 | 1118 | 143131 | 63891 | 1810 |

Hospital, Address, Telephone, Administrator, Approval, Facility, and Physician Codes, Health Care System, Network	Classi-fication Codes		Utilization Data					Expense (thousands) of dollars		
★ American Hospital Association (AHA) membership ☐ Joint Commission on Accreditation of Healthcare Organizations (JCAHO) accreditation + American Osteopathic Hospital Association (AOHA) membership ○ American Osteopathic Association (AOA) accreditation △ Commission on Accreditation of Rehabilitation Facilities (CARF) accreditation Control codes 61, 63, 64, 71, 72 and 73 indicate hospitals listed by AOHA, but not registered by AHA. For definition of numerical codes, see page A4	Control	Service	Beds	Admissions	Census	Outpatient Visits	Births	Total	Payroll	Personnel

	Control	Service	Beds	Admissions	Census	Outpatient Visits	Births	Total	Payroll	Personnel
⊞ GOOD SAMARITAN HOSPITAL AND HEALTH CENTER, 2222 Philadelphia Drive, Zip 45406–1813; tel. 513/278–2612; K. Douglas Deck, President and Chief Executive Officer **A**1 2 3 5 9 10 **F**2 3 4 7 8 10 11 12 14 15 16 17 18 19 20 21 22 25 26 28 29 30 31 34 35 37 39 40 41 42 43 44 45 46 49 51 52 53 54 55 56 57 58 59 60 65 66 67 71 73 74 **P**6 8 **S** Catholic Health Initiatives, Denver, CO	21	10	428	18091	274	220305	1788	159283	71067	2023
★ ○ GRANDVIEW HOSPITAL AND MEDICAL CENTER, (Includes Southview Hospital and Family Health Center, 1997 Miamisburg–Centerville Road, Zip 45459–3800, Mailing Address: 1997 Miamisburg–Cenerville Road, Zip 45459–3800; tel. 513/439–6000), 405 Grand Avenue, Zip 45405–4796; tel. 513/226–3200; Richard J. Minor, President **A**9 10 11 12 13 **F**2 3 4 7 8 10 11 12 14 15 16 17 18 19 21 22 23 27 28 29 30 31 32 33 34 35 36 37 39 40 41 42 43 44 45 46 48 49 51 52 54 55 56 57 58 65 66 67 68 69 71 72 73 74 **P**4 6 7 8	23	10	320	10157	160	285681	428	132739	64082	1614
KETTERING YOUTH SERVICES See Kettering Medical Center, Kettering										
⊞ △ MIAMI VALLEY HOSPITAL, One Wyoming Street, Zip 45409–2763; tel. 937/208–8000; Thomas G. Breitenbach, President and Chief Executive Officer **A**1 2 3 5 7 8 9 10 **F**1 2 3 4 7 8 9 10 11 12 14 15 16 17 18 19 20 21 22 23 24 25 26 27 28 29 30 31 32 34 35 36 37 38 39 40 41 42 43 44 45 46 48 49 51 54 55 56 57 58 59 60 61 63 65 66 67 68 69 70 71 72 73 74 **P**1 5 7	23	10	714	38443	523	482298	5634	—	—	—
ST. ELIZABETH MEDICAL CENTER See Franciscan Medical Center–Dayton Campus										
⊞ VETERANS AFFAIRS MEDICAL CENTER, 4100 West Third Street, Zip 45428–1002; tel. 937/268–6511; Steven M. Cohen, M.D., Director (Total facility includes 282 beds in nursing home–type unit) **A**1 3 5 8 9 **F**1 2 3 4 8 9 10 12 14 15 16 17 19 20 21 22 23 24 26 27 28 29 30 31 32 33 34 35 37 41 42 43 44 45 46 48 49 51 52 54 58 60 63 64 65 69 71 73 74 **P**6 **S** Department of Veterans Affairs, Washington, DC	45	10	835	6443	661	190688	0	117773	75991	1758
DEFIANCE—Defiance County										
⊞ DEFIANCE HOSPITAL, 1206 East Second Street, Zip 43512–2495; tel. 419/783–6955; Richard C. Sommer, Administrator **A**1 9 10 **F**7 8 11 15 16 19 20 21 22 27 28 29 30 31 32 34 35 36 37 41 42 44 52 55 56 57 58 59 63 65 71 73 **S** Quorum Health Group/Quorum Health Resources, Inc., Brentwood, TN **N** United Health Partners, Toledo, OH; Lake Erie Health Alliance, Toledo, OH; LutheranPreferred Network, Fort Wayne, IN	23	10	96	2969	32	29436	431	21693	8390	271
DELAWARE—Delaware County										
☐ GRADY MEMORIAL HOSPITAL, 561 West Central Avenue, Zip 43015–1485; tel. 614/369–8711; Everett P. Weber, Jr., President and Chief Executive Officer **A**1 2 9 10 **F**7 8 12 14 17 19 21 22 23 26 28 29 30 32 33 34 35 36 37 39 40 41 42 44 45 49 53 54 55 56 58 59 65 66 67 70 71 72 73 **P**7 8 **N** Community Hospitals of Ohio, Newark, OH	23	10	84	2878	29	103000	375	31075	12510	256
DENNISON—Tuscarawas County										
⊞ TWIN CITY HOSPITAL, 819 North First Street, Zip 44621–1098; tel. 614/922–2800; Cheryl Hicks, Chief Executive Officer **A**1 9 10 **F**8 11 12 14 16 17 19 20 21 22 28 29 30 32 33 34 37 39 41 42 44 45 46 48 49 51 63 64 65 66 71 73 74 **P**7	23	10	30	675	8	25710	0	6264	2717	120
DOVER—Tuscarawas County										
⊞ UNION HOSPITAL, 659 Boulevard, Zip 44622–2077; tel. 330/343–3311; William W. Harding, President and Chief Executive Officer **A**1 9 10 **F**7 8 14 15 16 17 19 21 22 28 30 32 33 35 36 37 39 40 42 44 49 53 54 55 56 57 58 63 65 66 67 71 73	23	10	102	3952	43	166476	746	32567	14365	510
EAST LIVERPOOL—Columbiana County										
⊞ EAST LIVERPOOL CITY HOSPITAL, 425 West Fifth Street, Zip 43920–2498; tel. 330/385–7200; Melvin R. Creeley, President (Total facility includes 20 beds in nursing home–type unit) **A**1 9 10 **F**7 8 13 15 16 19 20 21 22 27 28 30 31 32 33 34 35 37 40 42 44 49 52 54 55 56 58 64 65 67 71 72 73 **P**7 8	23	10	186	6339	87	89927	326	35977	15849	531
ELYRIA—Lorain County										
⊞ EMH REGIONAL MEDICAL CENTER, 630 East River Street, Zip 44035–5902; tel. 216/329–7500; James L. Keegan, President and Chief Executive Officer **A**1 2 9 10 **F**4 7 8 10 11 15 16 19 21 22 23 25 26 28 30 32 33 34 35 37 38 39 40 41 42 43 44 49 51 52 56 57 59 63 65 66 67 69 71 72 73 74 **P**7 8 **N** Cleveland Health Network, Cleveland, OH; Comprehensive Healthcare of Ohio, Inc., Elyria, OH	23	10	280	11501	136	180227	1123	96333	38064	1118
EUCLID—Cuyahoga County										
⊞ △ MERIDIA EUCLID HOSPITAL, 18901 Lake Shore Boulevard, Zip 44119–1090; tel. 216/531–9000; Denise Zeman, Site Administrator (Total facility includes 20 beds in nursing home–type unit) **A**1 2 7 9 10 **F**3 4 7 8 10 11 12 13 14 15 16 17 19 21 22 23 24 25 26 27 28 29 30 31 32 33 34 35 36 37 38 39 40 41 42 43 44 45 46 48 49 50 51 52 54 55 56 57 58 59 60 61 63 64 65 66 67 68 70 71 72 73 74 **P**1 3 4 7 8 **S** Meridia Health System, Mayfield Village, OH **N** Merida Health System, Mayfield Village, OH	23	10	214	6332	130	42779	597	64057	20336	685
FAIRFIELD—Butler County										
MERCY HOSPITAL OF FAIRFIELD See Mercy Hospital, Hamilton										
FINDLAY—Hancock County										
⊞ BLANCHARD VALLEY REGIONAL HEALTH CENTER, (Includes Blanchard Valley Regional Health Center–Bluffton Campus, 139 Garau Street, Bluffton, Zip 45817–0048, Mailing Address: P.O. Box 48, Zip 45817–0048; tel. 419/358–9010; Blanchard Valley Regional Health Center–Findlay Campus, 145 West Wallace Street), 145 West Wallace Street, Zip 45840–1299; tel. 419/423–4500; Clifford R. Lehman, Chief Executive Officer **A**1 9 10 **F**1 6 7 8 10 11 12 13 14 15 16 17 19 21 22 25 26 28 29 30 32 33 34 35 37 40 41 42 44 45 49 51 52 59 60 62 65 66 67 71 73 **P**6 **N** Great Lakes Health Network, Erie, PA	23	10	150	6832	82	113326	1093	50397	22593	741

Hospital, Address, Telephone, Administrator, Approval, Facility, and Physician Codes, Health Care System, Network	Classi-fication Codes		Utilization Data					Expense (thousands) of dollars		
	Control	Service	Beds	Admissions	Census	Outpatient Visits	Births	Total	Payroll	Personnel

★ American Hospital Association (AHA) membership
□ Joint Commission on Accreditation of Healthcare Organizations (JCAHO) accreditation
+ American Osteopathic Hospital Association (AOHA) membership
○ American Osteopathic Association (AOA) accreditation
△ Commission on Accreditation of Rehabilitation Facilities (CARF) accreditation
Control codes 61, 63, 64, 71, 72 and 73 indicate hospitals listed by AOHA, but not registered by AHA. For definition of numerical codes, see page A4.

FOSTORIA—Hancock County

| ★ FOSTORIA COMMUNITY HOSPITAL, 501 Van Buren Street, Zip 44830–0907, Mailing Address: P.O. Box 907, Zip 44830–0907; tel. 419/435–7734; Brad A. Higgins, President and Chief Executive Officer **A**1 3 9 10 **F**7 8 11 12 14 15 16 17 19 21 22 24 27 28 29 30 31 32 34 35 36 37 39 40 41 42 44 45 46 49 65 66 67 70 71 73 **N** United Health Partners, Toledo, OH | 23 | 10 | 50 | 1381 | 12 | 33374 | 192 | 13135 | 4999 | 206 |

FREMONT—Sandusky County

| ★ MEMORIAL HOSPITAL, 715 South Taft Avenue, Zip 43420–3200; tel. 419/332–7321; John A. Gorman, Chief Executive Officer **A**1 9 10 **F**1 7 8 15 16 17 19 21 22 27 29 30 32 33 34 35 36 37 39 40 41 42 44 45 49 52 54 55 57 58 59 65 71 73 74 **P**8 **S** Quorum Health Group/Quorum Health Resources, Inc., Brentwood, TN **N** United Health Partners, Toledo, OH; Lake Erie Health Alliance, Toledo, OH | 23 | 10 | 132 | 3587 | 34 | 54000 | 490 | 32507 | 12747 | 394 |

GALION—Crawford County

| ★ GALION COMMUNITY HOSPITAL, Portland Way South, Zip 44833–2314; tel. 419/468–4841; Mark E. Marley, Chief Executive Officer (Total facility includes 29 beds in nursing home–type unit) (Nonreporting) **A**1 9 10 **S** OhioHealth, Columbus, OH | 23 | 10 | 120 | — | — | — | — | — | — | — |

GALLIPOLIS—Gallia County

| ★ △ HOLZER MEDICAL CENTER, 100 Jackson Pike, Zip 45631–1563; tel. 614/446–5000; Charles I. Adkins, Jr., President **A**1 2 5 7 9 10 **F**7 8 11 12 17 19 21 22 23 24 25 26 28 29 30 32 33 35 37 40 41 42 44 46 48 49 58 60 63 64 65 67 69 71 73 74 **P**5 **N** Community Hospitals of Ohio, Newark, OH | 23 | 10 | 269 | 6466 | 91 | 56415 | 830 | 45287 | 18612 | 697 |

GARFIELD HEIGHTS—Cuyahoga County

| ★ MARYMOUNT HOSPITAL, 12300 McCracken Road, Zip 44125–2975; tel. 216/581–0500; Thomas J. Trudell, President and Chief Executive Officer **A**1 2 6 9 10 **F**3 5 6 7 8 10 12 14 15 16 18 19 21 22 23 25 27 28 30 31 32 34 35 36 37 39 40 41 42 44 46 49 52 53 54 55 56 57 58 59 62 63 64 65 66 69 71 72 73 74 **P**1 3 6 7 **N** Cleveland Health Network, Cleveland, OH | 21 | 10 | 213 | 9103 | 152 | 99399 | 963 | 81865 | 36187 | 1105 |

GENEVA—Ashtabula County

| ★ UHHS–MEMORIAL HOSPITAL OF GENEVA, (Formerly Memorial Hospital of Geneva), 870 West Main Street, Zip 44041–1295; tel. 216/466–1141; Gerard D. Klein, Chief Executive Officer **A**1 9 10 **F**8 12 14 15 16 19 22 26 27 28 29 30 34 35 37 41 44 45 46 49 63 65 67 71 73 74 **S** University Hospitals Health System, Cleveland, OH **N** University Hospitals Health System, Cleveland, OH | 23 | 10 | 14 | 809 | 10 | 31297 | 0 | 10058 | 3902 | 157 |

GEORGETOWN—Brown County

| ★ BROWN COUNTY GENERAL HOSPITAL, 425 Home Street, Zip 45121–1407; tel. 513/378–6121; Diana D. Fisher, President and Chief Executive Officer **A**1 9 10 **F**3 7 8 14 19 21 22 28 32 33 35 37 40 41 42 44 45 46 53 54 55 56 57 58 59 65 67 69 71 73 **P**6 | 13 | 10 | 53 | 1570 | 14 | 45282 | 409 | 14608 | 6140 | 226 |

GREEN SPRINGS—Seneca County

| ★ △ ST. FRANCIS HEALTH CARE CENTRE, 401 North Broadway, Zip 44836–9653; tel. 419/639–2626; Gregory T. Storer, Chief Executive Officer (Total facility includes 150 beds in nursing home–type unit) **A**1 7 9 10 **F**12 15 26 31 39 46 48 49 57 58 64 65 67 73 **P**1 **N** Lake Erie Health Alliance, Toledo, OH | 21 | 46 | 186 | 692 | 145 | 10980 | 0 | 15907 | 6581 | 214 |

GREENFIELD—Highland County

| ★ GREENFIELD AREA MEDICAL CENTER, 545 South Street, Zip 45123–1400; tel. 513/981–2116; Mark E. Marchetti, Chief Executive Officer **A**1 9 10 **F**8 15 16 17 19 22 28 29 30 32 33 34 35 41 44 46 48 49 65 71 72 73 **S** Quorum Health Group/Quorum Health Resources, Inc., Brentwood, TN **N** Ohio State Health Network, Columbus, OH | 23 | 10 | 36 | 813 | 16 | 39563 | 0 | 9315 | 3544 | 119 |

GREENVILLE—Darke County

| □ WAYNE HOSPITAL, 835 Sweitzer Street, Zip 45331–1077; tel. 513/548–1141; Raymond E. Laughlin, Jr., President and Chief Executive Officer **A**1 9 10 **F**7 11 15 17 19 21 22 32 33 34 35 40 44 45 49 65 67 71 73 **P**8 | 23 | 10 | 92 | 2790 | 33 | 62552 | 467 | 21385 | 9334 | 289 |

HAMILTON—Butler County

| ★ FORT HAMILTON–HUGHES MEMORIAL HOSPITAL, 630 Eaton Avenue, Zip 45013; tel. 513/867–2000; James A. Kingsbury, President and Chief Executive Officer **A**1 2 9 10 **F**2 3 7 8 10 14 15 16 17 19 21 22 23 25 26 29 30 32 33 34 35 36 37 39 40 41 42 44 45 46 49 52 54 55 56 57 60 62 63 65 67 68 71 72 73 74 **P**7 8 **N** Community Hospitals of Ohio, Newark, OH | 23 | 10 | 193 | 8383 | 100 | 140142 | 1353 | 57331 | 24967 | 871 |
| ★ MERCY HOSPITAL, (Includes Mercy Hospital of Fairfield, 3000 Mack Road, Fairfield, Mercy Hospital of Hamilton, 100 Riverfront Plaza), 100 River Front Plaza, Zip 45011, Mailing Address: P.O. Box 418, Zip 45012–0418; tel. 513/870–7080; Thomas S. Urban, President (Total facility includes 53 beds in nursing home–type unit) **A**1 9 10 **F**4 6 7 8 10 12 14 15 16 17 19 21 22 24 25 26 27 28 29 30 31 32 33 34 35 36 37 39 40 41 42 44 45 46 48 49 53 54 55 56 57 59 60 63 64 65 67 71 72 73 74 **P**6 8 **S** Mercy Health System, Cincinnati, OH **N** Mercy Health System, Cincinnati, OH | 21 | 10 | 248 | 8999 | 143 | 145508 | 312 | 76449 | 30606 | 861 |

HICKSVILLE—Defiance County

| ★ COMMUNITY MEMORIAL HOSPITAL, 208 North Columbus Street, Zip 43526–1299; tel. 419/542–6692; Deryl E. Gulliford, Ph.D., Administrator **A**1 9 10 **F**3 7 12 13 14 15 16 17 18 19 20 22 24 25 28 29 30 31 32 33 34 35 36 39 40 41 44 49 51 63 65 66 71 72 73 74 **P**3 **N** LutheranPreferred Network, Fort Wayne, IN; Sagamore Health Network, Inc., Carmel, IN | 16 | 10 | 28 | 593 | 5 | 22000 | 88 | 5146 | 2133 | 118 |

HILLSBORO—Highland County

| ★ HIGHLAND DISTRICT HOSPITAL, 1275 North High Street, Zip 45133–8571; tel. 513/393–6100; Eloise Moran, Chief Executive Officer **A**1 9 10 **F**7 8 12 14 15 16 17 19 22 32 35 40 42 49 65 66 71 73 | 16 | 10 | 51 | 2138 | 22 | 109815 | 329 | 16321 | 6430 | 241 |

Hospital, Address, Telephone, Administrator, Approval, Facility, and Physician Codes, Health Care System, Network	Classi-fication Codes		Utilization Data					Expense (thousands) of dollars		
★ American Hospital Association (AHA) membership □ Joint Commission on Accreditation of Healthcare Organizations (JCAHO) accreditation + American Osteopathic Hospital Association (AOHA) membership ○ American Osteopathic Association (AOA) accreditation △ Commission on Accreditation of Rehabilitation Facilities (CARF) accreditation Control codes 61, 63, 64, 71, 72 and 73 indicate hospitals listed by AOHA, but not registered by AHA. For definition of numerical codes, see page A4	Control	Service	Beds	Admissions	Census	Outpatient Visits	Births	Total	Payroll	Personnel

IRONTON—Lawrence County

□ RIVER VALLEY HEALTH SYSTEM, (Includes Behavioral Health–Portsmouth Campus, 2201 25th Street, Portsmouth, Zip 45662–3252; tel. 614/354–2804; Rick E. Harlow, Vice President Behavioral Health), 2228 South Ninth Street, Zip 45638–2526; tel. 614/532–3231; Terry L. Vanderhoof, President and Chief Executive Officer (Total facility includes 11 beds in nursing home–type unit) **A**1 5 9 10 **F**2 3 5 7 8 11 12 17 19 20 21 22 25 26 28 29 30 31 32 33 34 35 36 37 39 40 41 42 44 45 46 49 51 52 53 54 55 56 57 58 59 60 64 65 66 68 71 72 73 74 **N** Ohio State Health Network, Columbus, OH ... 13 10 219 3568 61 — 131 — — 405

KENTON—Hardin County

✠ HARDIN MEMORIAL HOSPITAL, 921 East Franklin Street, Zip 43326–2099, Mailing Address: P.O. Box 710, Zip 43326–0710; tel. 419/673–0761; Don J. Sabol, Administrator **A**1 9 10 **F**1 3 4 5 7 8 10 12 13 14 15 16 17 18 19 20 21 22 23 26 27 28 29 30 31 32 33 34 35 36 37 39 40 41 42 43 44 45 46 49 50 51 53 54 55 56 57 58 59 60 61 63 65 66 67 70 71 73 74 **P**3 5 7 8 **S** OhioHealth, Columbus, OH ... 23 10 51 1887 26 45388 149 12988 5187 273

KETTERING—Montgomery County

✠ KETTERING MEDICAL CENTER, (Includes Charles F. Kettering Memorial Hospital, 3535 Southern Boulevard, Zip 45429; tel. 513/298–4331; Kettering Youth Services, 5350 Lamme Road, Dayton, Zip 45439; tel. 513/299–9511; Sycamore Hospital, 2150 Leiter Road, Miamisburg, Zip 45342; tel. 513/866–0551), 3535 Southern Boulevard, Zip 45429–1221; tel. 513/298–4331; Francisco J. Perez, President and Chief Executive Officer **A**1 2 3 5 8 9 10 **F**3 4 5 6 7 8 10 11 12 14 15 16 17 19 21 22 23 24 26 27 28 29 30 32 34 35 37 38 39 40 41 42 43 44 45 46 48 49 50 51 52 53 54 55 56 57 58 59 60 62 63 64 65 66 67 70 71 72 73 74 **P**8 ... 21 10 504 16528 246 123525 1621 200489 88476 2770

LAKEWOOD—Cuyahoga County

✠ LAKEWOOD HOSPITAL, 14519 Detroit Avenue, Zip 44107–4383; tel. 216/521–4200; Jules W. Bouthillet, President and Chief Executive Officer (Total facility includes 45 beds in nursing home–type unit) **A**1 2 9 10 **F**1 4 5 7 8 9 10 11 12 13 14 15 16 17 19 21 22 23 24 25 26 27 28 29 30 31 32 33 34 35 36 37 38 39 40 41 42 43 44 45 46 47 48 49 51 52 53 54 55 56 57 58 59 60 61 63 64 65 66 67 69 70 71 72 73 74 **P**1 3 5 6 7 8 ... 23 10 323 10999 210 138003 550 113763 38282 1127

LANCASTER—Fairfield County

✠ FAIRFIELD MEDICAL CENTER, 401 North Ewing Street, Zip 43130–3371; tel. 614/687–8000; Creighton E. Likes, Jr., President and Chief Executive Officer (Total facility includes 24 beds in nursing home–type unit) **A**1 10 **F**7 8 12 14 16 17 18 19 21 22 24 25 26 28 29 30 32 34 35 37 39 40 41 42 44 45 46 48 49 52 54 55 56 57 58 59 60 63 64 65 66 67 70 71 73 74 **N** Mercy Health System, Cincinnati, OH ... 23 10 225 9164 104 174444 1307 73929 28068 950

LIMA—Allen County

✠ LIMA MEMORIAL HOSPITAL, 1001 Bellefontaine Avenue, Zip 45804–2894; tel. 419/228–3335; John B. White, President and Chief Executive Officer (Total facility includes 17 beds in nursing home–type unit) **A**1 2 9 10 **F**7 8 10 11 12 14 15 19 21 22 23 26 28 29 30 31 32 34 35 36 37 39 40 41 42 44 45 46 48 49 52 54 55 56 57 59 60 63 64 65 66 67 71 73 74 **P**3 7 8 **N** Lake Erie Health Alliance, Toledo, OH; Midwest Health Net, LLC., Fort Wayne, IN ... 23 10 201 6704 96 140891 210 70871 30247 930

OAKWOOD CORRECTIONAL FACILITY, 3200 North West Street, Zip 45801; tel. 419/225–8052; Barbara Brown, Warden **F**12 14 15 16 17 18 30 31 39 45 46 51 52 54 55 56 57 65 67 73 74 ... 12 22 186 372 91 22 0 17895 11222 340

✠ △ ST. RITA'S MEDICAL CENTER, 730 West Market Street, Zip 45801–4670; tel. 419/227–3361; James P. Reber, President **A**1 2 7 9 10 **F**2 3 7 8 10 11 12 13 14 15 16 17 18 19 20 21 22 24 25 26 27 28 29 30 31 32 33 34 35 37 38 39 40 41 42 44 45 46 48 49 52 53 54 55 56 57 58 59 60 63 64 65 66 67 70 71 72 73 **P**8 **S** Mercy Health System, Cincinnati, OH **N** Community Hospitals of Ohio, Newark, OH; West Central Ohio Regional Healthcare Alliance, Ltd., Lima, OH ... 21 10 312 12511 152 233478 2142 114101 51877 1738

LODI—Medina County

✠ LODI COMMUNITY HOSPITAL, 225 Elyria Street, Zip 44254–1096; tel. 330/948–1222; Thomas L. Lockard, President and Chief Executive Officer (Total facility includes 7 beds in nursing home–type unit) **A**1 5 9 10 **F**15 17 19 22 27 28 29 30 32 36 39 41 42 44 49 64 65 71 73 ... 23 10 21 511 8 17565 0 6908 3620 123

LOGAN—Hocking County

✠ HOCKING VALLEY COMMUNITY HOSPITAL, Route 2, State Route 664, Zip 43138–0966, Mailing Address: Box 966, Zip 43138–0966; tel. 614/385–5631; Larry Willard, Administrator (Total facility includes 30 beds in nursing home–type unit) **A**1 9 10 **F**7 8 12 14 15 16 19 22 28 30 34 35 37 40 41 42 44 45 49 51 63 64 65 66 67 71 73 74 **P**1 3 **N** Community Hospitals of Ohio, Newark, OH ... 13 10 92 1689 41 44539 157 15057 6520 257

LONDON—Madison County

✠ MADISON COUNTY HOSPITAL, 210 North Main Street, Zip 43140–1115; tel. 614/852–1372; Gary J. Lehman, President (Total facility includes 11 beds in nursing home–type unit) **A**1 9 10 **F**3 7 8 11 14 15 16 17 19 22 24 26 28 29 30 31 34 35 36 37 39 40 41 42 44 45 49 52 53 54 58 59 64 65 66 67 68 71 73 74 ... 23 10 87 2034 38 20689 238 16944 6873 256

Hospital, Address, Telephone, Administrator, Approval, Facility, and Physician Codes, Health Care System, Network	Classi-fication Codes		Utilization Data					Expense (thousands) of dollars		
★ American Hospital Association (AHA) membership □ Joint Commission on Accreditation of Healthcare Organizations (JCAHO) accreditation + American Osteopathic Hospital Association (AOHA) membership ○ American Osteopathic Association (AOA) accreditation △ Commission on Accreditation of Rehabilitation Facilities (CARF) accreditation Control codes 61, 63, 64, 71, 72 and 73 indicate hospitals listed by AOHA, but not registered by AHA. For definition of numerical codes, see page A4	Control	Service	Beds	Admissions	Census	Outpatient Visits	Births	Total	Payroll	Personnel

LORAIN—Lorain County

✳ △ LORAIN COMMUNITY/ST. JOSEPH REGIONAL HEALTH CENTER, (Includes Lorain Community/St. Joseph Health Center—East Campus, 205 West 20th Street, Zip 44052–3794; tel. 216/233–1000; Lorain Community/St. Joseph Regional Health Center–West Campus, tel. 216/960–3000), 3700 Kolbe Road, Zip 44053–1697; tel. 216/960–3000; Brian C. Lockwood, President and Chief Executive Officer (Total facility includes 16 beds in nursing home–type unit) **A**1 2 7 9 10 **F**1 2 3 4 5 6 7 8 10 12 13 14 15 16 17 18 19 20 21 22 23 24 25 26 27 28 29 30 31 32 33 34 35 36 37 39 40 41 42 43 44 45 46 48 49 50 51 52 53 54 55 56 57 58 59 60 61 62 63 64 65 66 67 68 69 70 71 72 73 74 **P**2 3 7 **S** Mercy Health System, Cincinnati, OH

	23	10	303	13754	206	—	1075	122620	47117	1660

MANSFIELD—Richland County

✳ MEDCENTRAL HEALTH SYSTEM, (Includes Mansfield Hospital, 335 Glessner Avenue, Zip 44903–2265; tel. 419/526–8000; Shelby Hospital, 20 Morris Road, Shelby, Zip 44875–0608; tel. 419/342–5015; Ron Distl, Senior Vice President Health System Management), 335 Glessner Avenue, Zip 44903; tel. 419/526–8000; James E. Meyer, President **A**1 2 6 9 10 **F**7 8 10 11 12 15 16 17 19 20 21 22 25 28 29 30 31 32 33 34 35 36 37 39 40 41 42 44 45 46 48 49 52 53 54 55 56 57 58 60 63 65 66 67 71 73 74 **P**5 7 8

	23	10	280	10802	168	132031	1428	88485	43561	1307

✳ PEOPLES HOSPITAL, 597 Park Avenue East, Zip 44905–2898; tel. 419/526–7300; Philip R. Dever, Chief Executive Officer **A**1 9 10 **F**8 15 16 19 21 30 33 34 35 37 39 44 46 49 65 71 72 73

	23	10	45	1364	20	55659	0	11912	4605	205

✳ RICHLAND HOSPITAL, 1451 Lucas Road, Zip 44901–0637, Mailing Address: Box 637, Zip 44901–0637; tel. 419/589–5511; John Cochran, Administrator (Nonreporting) **A**1 9 10

	23	22	92	—	—	—	—	—	—	—

MARIETTA—Washington County

✳ MARIETTA MEMORIAL HOSPITAL, 401 Matthew Street, Zip 45750–1699; tel. 614/374–1400; Larry J. Unroe, President **A**1 9 10 **F**2 3 4 7 8 12 14 15 16 17 19 21 22 24 26 27 28 29 30 31 32 33 35 37 39 40 41 42 44 45 46 48 49 52 54 55 56 58 59 60 63 64 65 66 67 71 72 73 74 **P**8 **N** Community Hospitals of Ohio, Newark, OH

	23	10	204	5420	67	130171	819	46384	21582	726

★ + ○ SELBY GENERAL HOSPITAL, 1106 Colegate Drive, Zip 45750–1323; tel. 614/373–0582; James J. Cliborne, Jr., Chief Executive Officer **A**9 10 11 12 13 **F**7 8 15 16 19 21 22 30 31 32 34 35 36 37 39 40 41 42 44 49 54 61 65 66 67 71 72 73 74 **P**8 **S** Quorum Health Group/Quorum Health Resources, Inc., Brentwood, TN

	23	10	44	1818	23	23630	49	14315	4900	193

MARION—Marion County

✳ △ MARION GENERAL HOSPITAL, McKinley Park Drive, Zip 43302–6397; tel. 614/383–8400; Frank V. Swinehart, President and Chief Executive Officer **A**1 2 7 9 10 **F**1 7 8 10 14 15 16 17 19 21 22 24 28 30 31 32 33 34 35 37 39 40 41 42 44 45 49 52 53 54 55 58 59 60 65 67 71 73 74 **P**7 8 **S** OhioHealth, Columbus, OH

	23	10	133	6168	69	89978	998	50210	22173	762

□ MEDCENTER HOSPITAL, 1050 Delaware Avenue, Zip 43302–6459; tel. 614/383–7706; Philip W. Smith, Jr., President **A**1 9 10 **F**1 3 10 12 16 19 21 22 30 32 34 35 37 41 42 44 45 48 58 60 63 65 67 73

	23	10	86	3363	46	43369	0	28936	10188	367

MARTINS FERRY—Belmont County

✳ EAST OHIO REGIONAL HOSPITAL, 90 North Fourth Street, Zip 43935–1648; tel. 614/633–1100; Brian K. Felici, Chief Executive Officer (Total facility includes 94 beds in nursing home–type unit) **A**1 9 10 **F**2 3 5 7 8 10 11 12 14 15 16 17 18 19 21 22 23 24 26 27 28 29 30 31 32 33 34 35 37 39 40 41 42 44 45 46 47 48 49 51 52 53 54 55 56 57 58 59 60 61 63 64 65 66 67 70 71 73 74 **P**6 8 **S** Allegheny Health, Education and Research Foundation, Pittsburgh, PA

	23	10	178	4120	133	121381	0	37187	16201	598

MARYSVILLE—Union County

□ MEMORIAL HOSPITAL, 500 London Avenue, Zip 43040–1594; tel. 937/644–6115; Danny L. Boggs, President and Chief Executive Officer (Total facility includes 95 beds in nursing home–type unit) **A**1 9 10 **F**7 8 12 14 15 16 19 21 22 24 27 28 30 31 32 34 35 36 37 39 40 41 42 44 46 49 51 63 64 65 66 67 71 72 73 **P**3 4 7

	13	10	162	2576	103	141623	530	33917	15555	528

MASSILLON—Stark County

★ + ○ DOCTORS HOSPITAL OF STARK COUNTY, 400 Austin Avenue N.W., Zip 44646–3554; tel. 216/837–7200; Thomas E. Cecconi, Chief Executive Officer **A**2 9 10 11 12 13 **F**7 8 10 14 15 16 19 21 22 23 26 27 28 30 32 34 35 37 39 40 41 44 45 49 51 54 60 61 63 65 67 71 73 74 **P**7 **S** Quorum Health Group/Quorum Health Resources, Inc., Brentwood, TN **N** Cleveland Health Network, Cleveland, OH

	23	10	142	3925	58	79816	370	37509	16233	666

✳ △ MASSILLON COMMUNITY HOSPITAL, 875 Eighth Street N.E., Zip 44646–8503, Mailing Address: P.O. Box 805, Zip 44648–8503; tel. 330/832–8761; Mervin F. Strine, President and Chief Executive Officer (Total facility includes 20 beds in nursing home–type unit) **A**1 7 9 10 **F**2 3 4 7 8 10 12 15 16 17 19 20 21 22 23 26 28 29 30 31 32 34 35 37 39 40 41 42 44 45 46 48 49 60 63 64 65 67 71 73 **P**3

	23	10	179	5415	76	102238	277	41430	19494	656

□ MASSILLON PSYCHIATRIC CENTER, 3000 Erie Street, Zip 44646–7993, Mailing Address: Box 540, Zip 44648–0540; tel. 330/833–3135; Cathy L. Cincinat, Acting Chief Executive Officer **A**1 5 10 **F**4 7 8 10 12 14 15 16 17 18 19 20 21 22 35 41 42 44 45 46 51 52 54 55 56 57 65 67 71 73 **P**6

	12	22	184	810	141	0	0	26103	17243	356

MAUMEE—Lucas County

□ CHARTER HOSPITAL OF TOLEDO, 1725 Timber Line Road, Zip 43537–4015; tel. 419/891–9333; Michael Cornelison, Chief Executive Officer (Nonreporting) **A**1 9 10 **S** Magellan Health Services, Atlanta, GA

	33	52	38	—	—	—	—	—	—	—

Hospital, Address, Telephone, Administrator, Approval, Facility, and Physician Codes, Health Care System, Network	Classi-fication Codes		Utilization Data					Expense (thousands) of dollars		
★ American Hospital Association (AHA) membership □ Joint Commission on Accreditation of Healthcare Organizations (JCAHO) accreditation + American Osteopathic Hospital Association (AOHA) membership ○ American Osteopathic Association (AOA) accreditation △ Commission on Accreditation of Rehabilitation Facilities (CARF) accreditation Control codes 61, 63, 64, 71, 72 and 73 indicate hospitals listed by AOHA, but not registered by AHA. For definition of numerical codes, see page A4	Control	Service	Beds	Admissions	Census	Outpatient Visits	Births	Total	Payroll	Personnel

Hospital	Control	Service	Beds	Admissions	Census	Outpatient Visits	Births	Total	Payroll	Personnel
★ ST. LUKE'S HOSPITAL, 5901 Monclova Road, Zip 43537–1899; tel. 419/893–5911; Frank J. Bartell, III, President and Chief Executive Officer (Total facility includes 26 beds in nursing home–type unit) (Nonreporting) **A**1 2 9 10 **N** First Interhealth Network, Toledo, OH	23	10	176	—	—	—	—	—	—	—
MEDINA—Medina County										
★ MEDINA GENERAL HOSPITAL, 1000 East Washington Street, Zip 44256–2170, Mailing Address: P.O. Box 427, Zip 44258–0427; tel. 330/725–1000; Gary D. Hallman, President and Chief Executive Officer **A**1 2 9 10 **F**7 8 12 13 14 15 17 19 20 21 22 28 30 33 34 35 37 39 40 41 42 44 49 51 61 65 66 67 71 73 74 **P**8 **N** Northeast Ohio Health Network, Akron, OH	23	10	118	5261	57	137111	892	47962	21045	774
MIDDLEBURG HEIGHTS—Cuyahoga County										
★ SOUTHWEST GENERAL HEALTH CENTER, 18697 Bagley Road, Zip 44130–3497; tel. 216/816–8000; L. Jon Schurmeier, President and Chief Executive Officer **A**1 2 9 10 **F**2 3 7 8 10 11 12 13 14 15 16 17 18 19 21 22 24 25 26 27 28 29 30 31 32 33 34 35 37 39 40 41 42 44 45 46 49 51 52 53 54 55 56 57 58 59 60 61 63 64 65 66 67 68 70 71 72 73 74 **P**6 8 **N** Cleveland Health Network, Cleveland, OH	23	10	253	12208	150	261812	1641	105389	49406	1782
MIDDLETOWN—Butler County										
★ △ MIDDLETOWN REGIONAL HOSPITAL, 105 McKnight Drive, Zip 45044–4838; tel. 513/424–2111; Douglas W. McNeill, FACHE, President and Chief Executive Officer **A**1 2 7 9 10 **F**3 4 7 8 10 11 12 13 15 16 17 19 21 22 23 24 28 29 30 32 33 34 35 36 37 39 40 41 42 44 46 48 49 52 53 54 55 56 57 58 59 63 64 65 66 71 73 74 **P**8	23	10	174	8442	101	127887	991	71365	30522	886
MILLERSBURG—Holmes County										
□ JOEL POMERENE MEMORIAL HOSPITAL, 981 Wooster Road, Zip 44654–1094; tel. 330/674–1015; Peter Tuerpitz, Administrator and Chief Executive Officer **A**1 9 10 **F**7 8 11 15 19 20 21 22 32 35 37 40 41 44 49 65 71 73 **P**6	13	10	36	1694	14	22531	536	10915	4615	169
MONTPELIER—Williams County										
MONTPELIER HOSPITAL See Community Hospitals of Williams County, Bryan										
MOUNT GILEAD—Morrow County										
★ MORROW COUNTY HOSPITAL, 651 West Marion Road, Zip 43338–1096; tel. 419/946–5015; Alan C. Pauley, Administrator (Total facility includes 38 beds in nursing home–type unit) **A**1 9 10 **F**1 7 8 14 15 17 19 21 22 28 30 34 35 36 37 39 40 42 44 49 51 64 65 71 73 **P**7 8 **S** OhioHealth, Columbus, OH	13	10	75	919	42	—	158	10448	3597	139
MOUNT VERNON—Knox County										
★ KNOX COMMUNITY HOSPITAL, 1330 Coshocton Road, Zip 43050–1495; tel. 614/393–9000; Robert G. Polahar, Chief Executive Officer **A**1 5 9 10 **F**7 14 16 19 22 32 35 37 40 42 44 46 52 59 65 71 73 **P**3 8 **S** Quorum Health Group/Quorum Health Resources, Inc., Brentwood, TN **N** Community Hospitals of Ohio, Newark, OH	23	10	117	4169	48	71547	461	32474	12325	405
NAPOLEON—Henry County										
★ HENRY COUNTY HOSPITAL, 11–600 State Road 424, Zip 43545–9399; tel. 419/592–4015; Robert J. Coholich, Chief Executive Officer **A**1 9 10 **F**3 7 8 11 12 13 14 15 18 19 20 22 24 28 29 30 32 33 34 35 37 39 40 41 42 44 45 46 49 53 58 64 65 67 71 73 74 **N** Lake Erie Health Alliance, Toledo, OH; Midwest Health Net, LLC., Fort Wayne, IN	23	10	39	850	11	33758	146	9049	3490	124
NELSONVILLE—Athens County										
+ ○ DOCTORS HOSPITAL OF NELSONVILLE, 1950 Mount Saint Mary Drive, Zip 45764–1193; tel. 614/753–1931; Mark R. Seckinger, Administrator (Total facility includes 45 beds in nursing home–type unit) (Nonreporting) **A**9 10 11 **S** Doctors Hospital, Columbus, OH	23	10	77	—	—	—	—	—	—	—
NEWARK—Licking County										
★ LICKING MEMORIAL HOSPITAL, 1320 West Main Street, Zip 43055–3699; tel. 614/348–4000; William J. Andrews, President **A**1 9 10 **F**2 3 7 8 10 12 14 15 16 17 19 21 22 28 31 32 35 37 40 41 42 44 45 49 52 54 56 57 58 59 60 63 65 67 71 73 74 **P**6 **N** Community Hospitals of Ohio, Newark, OH	23	10	203	6728	71	172221	1001	53776	25018	727
NORTHFIELD—Summit County										
□ NORTHCOAST BEHAVIORAL HEALTHCARE SYSTEM, 1756 Sagamore Road, Zip 44067, Mailing Address: Box 305, Zip 44067; tel. 216/467–7131; George P. Gintoli, Chief Executive Officer (Nonreporting) **A**1 10	12	22	250	—	—	—	—	—	—	—
NORWALK—Huron County										
★ + ○ FISHER–TITUS MEDICAL CENTER, 272 Benedict Avenue, Zip 44857–2374; tel. 419/668–8101; Richard C. Westhofen, President (Total facility includes 54 beds in nursing home–type unit) **A**1 2 9 10 11 **F**7 8 15 19 20 21 22 23 26 30 32 33 35 36 37 39 40 41 42 44 46 49 53 54 55 56 57 58 59 60 61 63 64 65 66 71 73 74 **P**2 7 8 **N** United Health Partners, Toledo, OH; Lake Erie Health Alliance, Toledo, OH; Midwest Health Net, LLC., Fort Wayne, IN	23	10	166	3382	89	53772	658	32863	14651	459
OAK HILL—Jackson County										
★ OAK HILL COMMUNITY MEDICAL CENTER, 350 Charlotte Avenue, Zip 45656–1326; tel. 614/682–7717; Robert A. Bowers, Chief Executive Officer (Total facility includes 24 beds in nursing home–type unit) **A**1 9 10 **F**1 15 19 22 32 33 37 44 49 64 65 71	23	10	68	620	27	8348	0	5480	—	74
OBERLIN—Lorain County										
★ ALLEN MEMORIAL HOSPITAL, 200 West Lorain Street, Zip 44074–1077; tel. 216/775–1211; James H. Schaum, President and Chief Executive Officer (Total facility includes 16 beds in nursing home–type unit) **A**1 9 10 **F**7 8 14 15 19 20 21 22 30 31 32 33 34 35 36 37 39 40 41 42 44 45 49 61 64 65 66 71 72 73	23	10	91	1957	24	20125	436	14362	6741	209

Hospital, Address, Telephone, Administrator, Approval, Facility, and Physician Codes, Health Care System, Network	Classi-fication Codes		Utilization Data					Expense (thousands) of dollars		
★ American Hospital Association (AHA) membership □ Joint Commission on Accreditation of Healthcare Organizations (JCAHO) accreditation + American Osteopathic Hospital Association (AOHA) membership ○ American Osteopathic Association (AOA) accreditation △ Commission on Accreditation of Rehabilitation Facilities (CARF) accreditation Control codes 61, 63, 64, 71, 72 and 73 indicate hospitals listed by AOHA, but not registered by AHA. For definition of numerical codes, see page A4	Control	Service	Beds	Admissions	Census	Outpatient Visits	Births	Total	Payroll	Personnel

OREGON—Lucas County

✠ △ ST. CHARLES HOSPITAL, 2600 Navarre Avenue, Zip 43616–3297; tel. 419/698–7479; Cathleen K. Nelson, President and Chief Executive Officer **A**1 2 7 9 10 **F**2 3 4 7 8 10 11 12 15 16 17 19 20 21 22 23 24 25 26 27 28 29 30 31 32 33 35 36 37 40 41 42 43 44 49 51 52 53 54 56 57 58 59 60 62 63 64 65 66 67 68 69 70 71 72 73 74 **P**1 3 4 5 6 **S** Mercy Health System, Cincinnati, OH **N** First Interhealth Network, Toledo, OH — 21 10 246 10612 175 181520 833 90059 44822 1534

ORRVILLE—Wayne County

✠ DUNLAP MEMORIAL HOSPITAL, 832 South Main Street, Zip 44667–2208; tel. 330/682–3010; Lynn V. Horner, President and Chief Executive Officer **A**1 9 10 **F**7 8 12 17 19 21 22 27 28 29 30 35 39 40 41 42 44 45 46 49 59 63 65 71 73 — 23 10 38 817 7 22715 272 8342 3350 138

OXFORD—Butler County

✠ MCCULLOUGH–HYDE MEMORIAL HOSPITAL, 110 North Poplar Street, Zip 45056–1292; tel. 513/523–2111; Richard A. Daniels, President and Chief Executive Officer **A**1 9 10 **F**7 8 12 15 16 17 19 21 22 27 28 30 33 34 35 36 37 39 40 42 44 49 63 65 66 67 71 72 73 **P**3 — 23 10 44 2663 22 49449 485 22928 10569 268

PAINESVILLE—Lake County

✠ △ LAKE HOSPITAL SYSTEM, 10 East Washington, Zip 44077–3472; tel. 216/354–2400; Cynthia Ann Moore–Hardy, Interim Chief Executive Officer **A**1 2 7 9 10 **F**4 7 8 10 12 13 14 15 16 17 18 19 20 21 22 25 26 27 29 30 31 32 33 34 35 36 37 39 40 41 42 43 44 45 46 49 60 63 64 65 66 67 71 72 73 74 **P**1 3 **N** Lake Hospital System, Inc., Painesville, OH — 23 10 359 12725 168 347134 1313 121196 50203 1407

PARMA—Cuyahoga County

✠ △ PARMA COMMUNITY GENERAL HOSPITAL, 7007 Powers Boulevard, Zip 44129–5495; tel. 216/888–1800; Thomas A. Selden, President and Chief Executive Officer (Total facility includes 27 beds in nursing home–type unit) **A**1 2 7 9 10 **F**1 7 8 10 11 12 13 14 16 17 19 21 22 24 26 27 28 29 30 31 32 33 34 36 37 39 40 41 42 44 45 46 48 49 52 54 57 59 63 64 65 66 67 71 73 **P**1 7 **N** Cleveland Health Network, Cleveland, OH — 23 10 334 8625 167 133753 531 82839 37991 1140

PAULDING—Paulding County

★ PAULDING COUNTY HOSPITAL, 11558 State Road 111, Zip 45879–9220; tel. 419/399–4080; Joseph M. Dorko, Chief Executive Officer **A**9 10 **F**7 8 19 21 22 28 30 32 34 35 36 39 40 41 44 49 51 71 72 73 **S** Quorum Health Group/Quorum Health Resources, Inc., Brentwood, TN **N** LutheranPreferred Network, Fort Wayne, IN; Midwest Health Net, LLC., Fort Wayne, IN — 13 10 51 810 7 43934 128 9172 4063 138

PIQUA—Miami County

✠ PIQUA MEMORIAL MEDICAL CENTER, 624 Park Avenue, Zip 45356–2098; tel. 513/778–6500; Eva L. Fine, R.N., MS, Assistant Administrator **A**1 2 9 10 **F**3 7 8 10 12 13 15 16 17 18 19 21 22 25 27 28 29 30 31 32 34 35 36 37 39 40 41 42 44 45 46 49 53 54 55 56 57 58 59 60 62 65 66 67 68 71 72 73 74 **P**2 6 **S** Upper Valley Medical Centers, Troy, OH **N** Upper Valley Medical Centers, Inc., Troy, OH — 23 10 85 3454 46 131391 425 45373 17881 635

POMEROY—Meigs County

✠ VETERANS MEMORIAL HOSPITAL OF MEIGS COUNTY, 115 East Memorial Drive, Zip 45769–9572; tel. 614/992–2104; Walter S. Lucas, Administrator (Total facility includes 40 beds in nursing home–type unit) (Nonreporting) **A**1 9 10 — 23 10 69 — — — — — — —

PORT CLINTON—Ottawa County

□ H. B. MAGRUDER MEMORIAL HOSPITAL, 615 Fulton Street, Zip 43452–2034; tel. 419/734–3131; David R. Norwine, President and Chief Executive Officer **A**1 9 10 **F**8 12 14 15 16 17 19 21 22 28 30 34 36 37 39 42 44 45 46 65 66 67 71 **P**6 **N** Lake Erie Health Alliance, Toledo, OH — 23 10 33 1704 17 56583 0 13832 5884 213

PORTSMOUTH—Scioto County

BEHAVIORAL HEALTH–PORTSMOUTH CAMPUS See River Valley Health System, Ironton

MERCY HOSPITAL See Southern Ohio Medical Center

PORTSMOUTH RECEIVING HOSPITAL See River Valley Health System, Ironton

SCIOTO MEMORIAL HOSPITAL See Southern Ohio Medical Center

✠ △ SOUTHERN OHIO MEDICAL CENTER, (Includes Mercy Hospital, 1248 Kinneys Lane, Zip 45662; Scioto Memorial Hospital, 1805 27th Street, Zip 45662), 1805 27th Street, Zip 45662–2400; tel. 614/354–5000; Randal M. Arnett, President and Chief Executive Officer **A**1 7 9 10 **F**7 8 15 17 18 19 20 21 22 24 25 26 28 29 30 31 32 33 34 35 36 37 39 40 41 42 44 45 46 48 49 51 54 55 56 58 60 61 62 63 65 66 67 68 71 72 73 74 **P**3 6 **S** OhioHealth, Columbus, OH — 23 10 281 10621 153 171613 1593 93707 40254 1465

RAVENNA—Portage County

✠ ROBINSON MEMORIAL HOSPITAL, 6847 North Chestnut Street, Zip 44266–1204, Mailing Address: P.O. Box 1204, Zip 44266; tel. 330/297–0811; Stephen Colecchi, President and Chief Executive Officer **A**1 2 5 9 10 **F**7 8 10 11 12 13 15 16 17 19 20 21 22 23 25 26 28 29 30 31 34 35 37 39 40 41 42 44 45 46 49 51 52 54 55 56 59 61 63 65 66 67 71 72 73 74 **P**1 7 **N** Northeast Ohio Health Network, Akron, OH — 13 10 190 8010 100 87102 872 72668 31904 971

RICHMOND HEIGHTS—Cuyahoga County

★ + ○ RICHMOND HEIGHTS GENERAL HOSPITAL, 27100 Chardon Road, Zip 44143–1198; tel. 216/585–6500; Keith J. Petersen, Chief Executive Officer (Nonreporting) **A**9 10 11 12 13 — 23 10 98 — — — — — — —

ROCK CREEK—Ashtabula County

GLENBEIGH HEALTH SOURCES, Route 45, Zip 44084, Mailing Address: P.O. Box 298, Zip 44084; tel. 216/563–3400; Patricia Weston–Hall, Executive Director **A**9 10 **F**2 3 15 16 **P**5 — 23 82 80 896 20 7029 0 — — 54

Hospital, Address, Telephone, Administrator, Approval, Facility, and Physician Codes, Health Care System, Network	Classi-fication Codes		Utilization Data					Expense (thousands) of dollars		
★ American Hospital Association (AHA) membership **□** Joint Commission on Accreditation of Healthcare Organizations (JCAHO) accreditation **+** American Osteopathic Hospital Association (AOHA) membership **○** American Osteopathic Association (AOA) accreditation **△** Commission on Accreditation of Rehabilitation Facilities (CARF) accreditation Control codes 61, 63, 64, 71, 72 and 73 indicate hospitals listed by AOHA, but not registered by AHA. For definition of numerical codes, see page A4	Control	Service	Beds	Admissions	Census	Outpatient Visits	Births	Total	Payroll	Personnel

SAINT CLAIRSVILLE—Belmont County

□ BHC FOX RUN HOSPITAL, (Formerly Fox Run Hospital), 67670 Traco Drive, Zip 43950; tel. 614/695–2131; J. Frank Gallagher, III, Administrator **A**1 10 **F**52 53 57 59 **S** Behavioral Healthcare Corporation, Nashville, TN — 33 22 65 542 34 0 0 3395 1928 90

SAINT MARYS—Auglaize County

⊞ JOINT TOWNSHIP DISTRICT MEMORIAL HOSPITAL, 200 St. Clair Street, Zip 45885–2400; tel. 419/394–3387; James R. Chick, President (Total facility includes 23 beds in nursing home–type unit) **A**1 9 10 **F**7 8 12 15 17 19 21 22 25 27 28 30 32 33 34 35 37 39 40 41 44 46 49 51 64 65 67 71 73 **N** West Central Ohio Regional Healthcare Alliance, Ltd., Lima, OH — 23 10 91 4254 56 61534 355 27077 11974 432

SALEM—Columbiana County

⊞ SALEM COMMUNITY HOSPITAL, 1995 East State Street, Zip 44460–0121; tel. 330/332–1551; Eugene Zentko, Administrator and Chief Executive Officer (Total facility includes 15 beds in nursing home–type unit) **A**1 5 9 10 **F**3 4 7 8 10 12 14 15 19 20 21 22 28 30 34 35 36 37 39 40 41 42 44 45 49 51 60 63 64 65 67 70 71 73 — 23 10 159 5607 73 77741 377 42124 20821 672

SANDUSKY—Erie County

□ + ○ △ FIRELANDS COMMUNITY HOSPITAL, (Includes Firelands Community Hospital–Hayes Avenue, 2020 Hayes Avenue, Zip 44870–8005; tel. 419/626–7400), 1101 Decatur Street, Zip 44870–3335; tel. 419/626–7400; Nelson F. Alward, President and Chief Executive Officer **A**1 2 7 9 10 11 12 13 **F**2 3 7 8 12 14 15 16 17 18 19 20 21 22 27 28 29 30 31 32 33 34 35 36 37 39 40 41 42 44 45 46 48 49 51 52 53 54 55 56 57 58 59 60 65 66 67 71 73 74 **P**8 **N** Cleveland Health Network, Cleveland, OH; Lake Erie Health Alliance, Toledo, OH — 23 10 232 5930 84 199599 856 59457 24470 812

⊞ PROVIDENCE HOSPITAL, 1912 Hayes Avenue, Zip 44870–4736; tel. 419/621–7000; Sister Nancy Linenkugel, FACHE, President and Chief Executive Officer (Total facility includes 46 beds in nursing home–type unit) **A**1 2 6 9 10 **F**2 3 7 8 10 11 12 14 15 16 17 19 20 21 22 23 25 26 27 28 29 30 31 32 33 34 35 37 39 40 41 42 44 45 46 49 52 53 54 55 56 57 58 59 60 63 64 65 66 67 71 73 74 **P**3 8 **S** Franciscan Services Corporation, Sylvania, OH **N** United Health Partners, Toledo, OH — 21 10 170 3674 88 46333 208 38312 15774 457

SIDNEY—Shelby County

⊞ WILSON MEMORIAL HOSPITAL, 915 West Michigan Street, Zip 45365–2491; tel. 937/498–2311; Michael T. Moore, President and Chief Executive Officer **A**1 9 10 **F**7 8 15 16 19 21 22 30 32 33 35 37 39 40 41 44 45 46 49 65 67 71 73 **P**6 **N** West Central Ohio Regional Healthcare Alliance, Ltd., Lima, OH — 23 10 101 3735 41 93696 516 33369 14192 490

SPRINGFIELD—Clark County

⊞ COMMUNITY HOSPITAL, 2615 East High Street, Zip 45501–1422, Mailing Address: Box 1228, Zip 45501–1228; tel. 513/325–0531; Neal E. Kresheck, President (Total facility includes 41 beds in nursing home–type unit) **A**1 6 9 10 **F**7 8 10 11 12 13 14 15 16 17 19 21 22 24 25 26 27 28 29 30 31 32 33 34 35 36 37 39 40 41 42 44 45 46 49 51 60 63 64 65 66 67 71 72 73 74 **P**6 7 — 23 10 201 8478 125 118841 1809 72511 30545 1053

⊞ △ MERCY MEDICAL CENTER, 1343 North Fountain Boulevard, Zip 45501–1380; tel. 513/390–5000; Richard Rogers, Senior Vice President Operations (Total facility includes 20 beds in nursing home–type unit) **A**1 5 7 9 10 **F**1 3 6 8 10 11 12 13 14 15 16 17 18 19 21 22 26 27 28 29 30 31 32 33 34 35 36 37 39 41 42 44 45 46 48 49 51 52 56 60 62 64 65 66 67 71 72 73 74 **P**2 5 6 7 8 **S** Mercy Health System, Cincinnati, OH — 21 10 218 7331 112 139743 0 65920 25661 875

STEUBENVILLE—Jefferson County

⊞ TRINITY HEALTH SYSTEM, (Includes Trinity Medical Center East, 380 Summit Avenue, Zip 43952–2699; tel. 614/283–7000; Trinity Medical Center West, 400 Johnson Road, Zip 43952–2393; tel. 614/264–8000; Angelo G. Calbone, President and Chief Executive Officer), 380 Summit Avenue, Zip 43952; tel. 614/283–7000; Fred B. Brower, President and Chief Executive Officer (Nonreporting) **A**1 2 6 9 10 **S** Franciscan Services Corporation, Sylvania, OH — 21 10 533 — — — — — — —

SYLVANIA—Lucas County

⊞ △ FLOWER HOSPITAL, 5200 Harroun Road, Zip 43560–2196; tel. 419/824–1444; Randall Kelley, Senior Vice President and Chief Operating Officer (Total facility includes 236 beds in nursing home–type unit) **A**1 2 3 5 7 9 10 **F**3 4 5 6 7 8 10 11 12 15 16 17 19 20 21 22 23 25 26 27 28 29 30 32 34 35 37 38 39 40 41 42 43 44 45 46 47 48 49 50 51 52 53 54 56 57 58 59 60 61 62 63 64 65 66 67 68 71 73 74 **P**7 **N** First Interhealth Network, Toledo, OH; Lake Erie Health Alliance, Toledo, OH; Promedica Health System, Toledo, OH — 23 10 375 8542 360 — 994 92460 43319 1233

TIFFIN—Seneca County

⊞ MERCY HOSPITAL, 485 West Market Street, Zip 44883, Mailing Address: Box 727, Zip 44883–0727; tel. 419/447–3130; Mark Shugarman, President **A**1 9 10 **F**4 7 8 11 12 14 15 16 17 19 22 26 27 28 29 30 31 32 34 35 36 39 40 41 42 44 45 46 49 51 56 62 63 65 71 73 **P**8 **S** Mercy Health System, Cincinnati, OH **N** United Health Partners, Toledo, OH; Lake Erie Health Alliance, Toledo, OH — 21 10 60 2591 26 62344 444 23982 10542 363

TOLEDO—Lucas County

⊞ △ MEDICAL COLLEGE HOSPITALS, 3000 Arlington Avenue, Zip 43699–0008, Mailing Address: P.O. Box 10008, Zip 43699–0008; tel. 419/381–4172; Richard C. Sipp, Vice President for Administration **A**1 2 3 5 7 8 10 **F**4 8 10 11 12 19 20 21 22 24 25 26 30 31 35 37 39 41 42 43 44 45 46 47 48 49 52 53 54 55 58 59 60 63 65 66 67 68 69 70 71 73 **P**4 **N** Lake Erie Health Alliance, Toledo, OH; Midwest Health Net, LLC., Fort Wayne, IN — 12 10 240 7993 164 198462 0 136112 55014 1575

Hospital, Address, Telephone, Administrator, Approval, Facility, and Physician Codes, Health Care System, Network	Classi-fication Codes		Utilization Data					Expense (thousands) of dollars		
	Control	Service	Beds	Admissions	Census	Outpatient Visits	Births	Total	Payroll	Personnel

★ American Hospital Association (AHA) membership
□ Joint Commission on Accreditation of Healthcare Organizations (JCAHO) accreditation
+ American Osteopathic Hospital Association (AOHA) membership
○ American Osteopathic Association (AOA) accreditation
△ Commission on Accreditation of Rehabilitation Facilities (CARF) accreditation
Control codes 61, 63, 64, 71, 72 and 73 indicate hospitals listed by AOHA, but not registered by AHA. For definition of numerical codes, see page A4

Hospital	Control	Service	Beds	Admissions	Census	Outpatient Visits	Births	Total	Payroll	Personnel
□ NORTHWEST PSYCHIATRIC HOSPITAL, (Formerly Toledo Mental Health Center), 930 South Detroit Avenue, Zip 43614–2701; tel. 419/381–1881; G. Terrence Smith, Chief Executive Officer **A**1 3 5 9 10 **F**3 4 7 9 10 11 12 14 15 16 17 18 20 27 31 35 37 38 39 40 42 43 45 46 47 48 52 55 56 57 58 65 67 71 73 **P**6	12	22	96	631	94	0	0	16029	—	222
✸ ○ RIVERSIDE HOSPITAL, 1600 North Superior Street, Zip 43604–2199; tel. 419/729–6000; Scott E. Shook, President (Total facility includes 12 beds in nursing home–type unit) **A**1 2 9 10 11 **F**1 7 8 10 11 12 15 16 17 19 21 22 23 24 25 26 27 29 31 32 33 34 35 36 37 38 40 41 42 44 45 46 49 51 52 54 57 58 59 64 65 66 67 71 72 73 **P**1 5	23	10	162	5924	87	81965	791	65557	25786	836
✸ ○ ST. VINCENT MERCY MEDICAL CENTER, (Formerly St. Vincent Medical Center), 2213 Cherry Street, Zip 43608–2691; tel. 419/251–3232; Steven L. Mickus, President and Chief Executive Officer **A**1 2 3 5 6 9 10 11 12 13 **F**2 3 4 7 8 9 10 11 15 16 17 19 21 22 23 24 25 26 28 29 30 31 32 34 35 36 37 38 39 40 41 42 43 44 46 47 48 49 51 52 53 54 55 56 57 58 59 60 63 65 66 67 68 69 70 71 72 73 74 **P**6 8 **S** Mercy Health System, Cincinnati, OH **N** United Health Partners, Toledo, OH; First Interhealth Network, Toledo, OH	21	10	459	19512	296	278606	1990	258973	109847	5180
✸ THE TOLEDO HOSPITAL, 2142 North Cove Boulevard, Zip 43606–3896; tel. 419/471–4000; William W. Glover, President **A**1 2 3 5 8 9 10 **F**3 4 5 6 7 8 10 11 12 15 16 19 20 21 22 23 25 26 27 28 29 30 32 34 35 37 38 39 40 41 42 43 44 45 46 47 48 49 50 51 52 53 54 56 57 58 59 60 61 62 63 64 65 66 67 68 71 73 74 **P**7 8 **N** Promedica Health System, Toledo, OH; Midwest Health Net, LLC., Fort Wayne, IN	23	10	584	24606	358	267070	3786	282343	124376	3538
TROY—Miami County										
✸ DETTMER HOSPITAL, (PSYCHIATRIC & CHEM DEPENDENCE), 3130 North Dixie Highway, Zip 45373–1039; tel. 937/332–7500; Keith Achor, Assistant Administrator **A**1 9 10 **F**2 3 6 7 8 10 11 12 13 14 15 16 17 18 19 20 21 22 23 24 25 26 27 28 29 30 32 34 35 36 37 39 40 41 42 44 45 46 48 49 52 53 54 55 56 57 58 59 62 63 64 65 66 67 68 70 71 72 73 74 **P**5 6 7 8 **S** Upper Valley Medical Centers, Troy, OH **N** Upper Valley Medical Centers, Inc., Troy, OH	23	49	49	1259	22	—	0	10845	5582	210
✸ △ STOUDER MEMORIAL HOSPITAL, 920 Summit Avenue, Zip 45373; tel. 937/332–8500; Patricia Meyer, Assistant Administrator (Total facility includes 18 beds in nursing home–type unit) **A**1 2 7 9 10 **F**1 2 3 7 8 10 13 14 15 16 18 19 20 21 22 24 25 26 27 28 29 30 31 32 33 34 35 36 37 39 40 41 42 44 45 46 48 49 52 53 54 55 56 57 58 59 60 62 63 64 65 66 67 71 72 73 **P**2 6 **S** Upper Valley Medical Centers, Troy, OH **N** Upper Valley Medical Centers, Inc., Troy, OH	23	10	131	3895	50	—	591	50670	18658	515
UPPER SANDUSKY—Wyandot County										
★ WYANDOT MEMORIAL HOSPITAL, 885 North Sandusky Avenue, Zip 43351–1098; tel. 419/294–4991; Joseph A. D'Ettorre, Administrator **A**5 9 10 **F**7 8 11 12 16 19 21 22 33 34 35 40 41 42 44 46 56 71 73 **N** Ohio State Health Network, Columbus, OH	16	10	31	1054	12	30686	133	9549	3557	139
URBANA—Champaign County										
✸ MERCY MEMORIAL HOSPITAL, 904 Scioto Street, Zip 43078–2200; tel. 937/653–5231; Richard Rogers, Senior Vice President **A**1 9 10 **F**3 8 12 13 14 15 16 17 19 22 26 28 29 30 32 33 34 37 39 41 44 46 49 65 67 68 71 73 **P**2 5 6 7 8 **S** Mercy Health System, Cincinnati, OH	21	10	20	997	11	230331	0	21411	7858	324
VAN WERT—Van Wert County										
✸ VAN WERT COUNTY HOSPITAL, 1250 South Washington Street, Zip 45891–2599; tel. 419/238–2390; Mark J. Minick, President and Chief Executive Officer **A**1 9 10 **F**7 8 11 13 14 15 16 17 18 19 22 26 28 29 30 35 37 39 40 41 42 44 46 63 65 66 71 73 **P**1 7 8 **N** West Central Ohio Regional Healthcare Alliance, Ltd., Lima, OH; LutheranPreferred Network, Fort Wayne, IN; Midwest Health Net, LLC., Fort Wayne, IN	23	10	100	1945	17	106405	308	18755	8050	248
WADSWORTH—Medina County										
□ WADSWORTH–RITTMAN HOSPITAL, 195 Wadsworth Road, Zip 44281–9505; tel. 330/334–1504; James W. Brumlow, Jr., President and Chief Executive Officer **A**1 5 9 10 **F**8 17 19 21 22 28 30 32 34 35 37 39 40 41 42 44 48 49 63 65 67 68 71 73 74 **P**7 **N** Cleveland Health Network, Cleveland, OH	23	10	64	1997	21	42505	164	16424	7578	229
WARREN—Trumbull County										
✸ △ HILLSIDE REHABILITATION HOSPITAL, 8747 Squires Lane N.E., Zip 44484–1649; tel. 330/841–3700; Margaret Edwards, Chief Executive Officer **A**1 5 7 9 10 **F**2 3 12 14 16 28 30 39 41 45 48 49 65 73 **P**4	13	46	93	1337	67	20033	0	20307	8793	249
✸ ○ ST. JOSEPH HEALTH CENTER, 667 Eastland Avenue S.E., Zip 44484; tel. 330/841–4000; Robert W. Shroder, Chief Operating Officer (Total facility includes 11 beds in nursing home–type unit) **A**1 9 10 11 12 **F**2 3 4 5 7 8 10 12 14 15 16 17 18 19 21 22 25 26 27 28 29 30 31 32 33 34 35 36 38 39 40 41 42 43 44 45 49 52 54 55 56 57 58 59 60 63 64 65 66 67 69 71 72 73 74 **P**1 5 **S** Mercy Health System, Cincinnati, OH **N** Cleveland Health Network, Cleveland, OH	21	10	170	8073	108	95740	855	71489	30969	750
✸ TRUMBULL MEMORIAL HOSPITAL, 1350 East Market Street, Zip 44482–6628; tel. 330/841–9011; Charles A. Johns, President **A**1 2 5 9 10 **F**7 8 10 11 12 13 14 15 16 19 21 22 24 25 28 29 30 31 32 33 34 35 36 37 39 40 41 42 44 45 49 52 56 57 59 60 63 64 65 66 71 73 **P**8	23	10	322	14159	187	225137	1153	113817	51310	1558
WARRENSVILLE HEIGHTS—Morgan County										
✸ + ○ △ MERIDIA SOUTH POINTE HOSPITAL, 4110 Warrensville Center Road, Zip 44122–7099; tel. 216/491–6000; Kathleen A. Rice, Site Administrator (Nonreporting) **A**1 2 7 9 10 11 12 13 **S** Meridia Health System, Mayfield Village, OH **N** Merida Health System, Mayfield Village, OH	23	10	163	—	—	—	—	—	—	—

Hospital, Address, Telephone, Administrator, Approval, Facility, and Physician Codes, Health Care System, Network	Classi-fication Codes		Utilization Data					Expense (thousands) of dollars		
★ American Hospital Association (AHA) membership □ Joint Commission on Accreditation of Healthcare Organizations (JCAHO) accreditation + American Osteopathic Hospital Association (AOHA) membership ○ American Osteopathic Association (AOA) accreditation △ Commission on Accreditation of Rehabilitation Facilities (CARF) accreditation Control codes 61, 63, 64, 71, 72 and 73 indicate hospitals listed by AOHA, but not registered by AHA. For definition of numerical codes, see page A4	Control	Service	Beds	Admissions	Census	Outpatient Visits	Births	Total	Payroll	Personnel

WASHINGTON COURT HOUSE—Lucas County

✠ FAYETTE COUNTY MEMORIAL HOSPITAL, 1430 Columbus Avenue, Zip 43160–1791; tel. 614/335–1210; Francis G. Albarano, Administrator **A**1 5 9 10 **F**7 8 12 14 15 16 17 19 20 21 22 27 28 29 30 32 33 34 35 36 37 39 40 41 42 44 46 49 56 65 66 67 71 73 **S** Quorum Health Group/Quorum Health Resources, Inc., Brentwood, TN	13	10	48	1338	13	53271	327	15246	6219	228

WAUSEON—Fulton County

✠ FULTON COUNTY HEALTH CENTER, 725 South Shoop Avenue, Zip 43567–1701; tel. 419/335–2015; E. Dean Beck, Administrator **A**1 2 9 10 **F**6 7 8 14 15 19 21 22 23 24 28 30 33 35 36 37 40 41 42 44 49 52 55 56 58 59 65 66 67 71 73 **N** United Health Partners, Toledo, OH; Lake Erie Health Alliance, Toledo, OH	23	10	86	2376	21	89690	321	19229	8647	343

WAVERLY—Pike County

□ PIKE COMMUNITY HOSPITAL, 100 Dawn Lane, Zip 45690–9664; tel. 614/947–2186; Richard E. Sobota, President and Chief Executive Officer **A**1 9 10 **F**8 14 15 16 17 19 21 22 26 27 28 29 30 32 33 34 37 39 44 45 49 63 65 66 71 72 73 **P**5 **N** Ohio State Health Network, Columbus, OH	23	10	40	956	11	—	0	7703	3696	152

WEST UNION—Adams County

□ ADAMS COUNTY HOSPITAL, 210 North Wilson Drive, Zip 45693–1574; tel. 513/544–5571; Philip S. Hanna, Administrator (Total facility includes 18 beds in nursing home–type unit) (Nonreporting) **A**1 9 10	13	10	49	—	—	—	—	—	—	—

WESTERVILLE—Franklin County

ST. ANN'S HOSPITAL See Mount Carmel Health System, Columbus

WILLARD—Huron County

✠ MERCY HOSPITAL–WILLARD, 110 East Howard Street, Zip 44890–1611; tel. 419/933–2931; James O. Detwiler, President **A**1 9 10 **F**7 8 15 16 19 22 23 28 29 30 32 33 34 35 36 37 40 41 42 44 45 49 58 63 65 66 67 71 73 **P**3 8 **S** Mercy Health System, Cincinnati, OH **N** United Health Partners, Toledo, OH	21	10	30	939	8	42756	210	12891	5152	173

WILLOUGHBY—Lake County

□ LAURELWOOD HOSPITAL, 35900 Euclid Avenue, Zip 44094–4648; tel. 216/953–3000; Farshid Afsarifard, Executive Director **A**1 9 10 **F**2 3 12 14 15 16 17 18 25 52 53 54 55 56 57 58 59 65 67 68 73 **P**8 **N** The Mount Sinai Health Care System, Cleveland, OH	23	22	160	2754	65	28768	0	12067	6970	187

WILMINGTON—Clinton County

✠ CLINTON MEMORIAL HOSPITAL, 610 West Main Street, Zip 45177–2194; tel. 513/382–6611; Thomas F. Kurtz, Jr., President and Chief Executive Officer (Total facility includes 12 beds in nursing home–type unit) **A**1 2 9 10 **F**4 7 8 14 15 16 17 19 20 21 22 24 25 26 30 31 32 34 36 37 39 40 41 42 44 45 46 49 54 58 60 64 65 66 67 71 73 74 **P**1 3	13	10	93	3736	42	105533	471	35149	15926	508

WOOSTER—Wayne County

□ WOOSTER COMMUNITY HOSPITAL, 1761 Beall Avenue, Zip 44691–2342; tel. 330/263–8100; William E. Sheron, Chief Executive Officer **A**1 2 9 10 **F**7 8 12 17 19 21 22 28 30 31 32 33 34 35 36 37 39 40 41 42 44 45 46 49 63 65 67 71 73 **P**3 **S** Quorum Health Group/Quorum Health Resources, Inc., Brentwood, TN	14	10	90	4514	48	95252	812	32796	15956	515

WORTHINGTON—Franklin County

□ HARDING HOSPITAL, 445 East Granville Road, Zip 43085–3195; tel. 614/885–5381; S. R. Thorward, M.D., President and Chief Executive Officer **A**1 3 5 9 10 **F**2 3 12 14 15 16 22 32 52 53 54 55 56 57 58 59 **P**6	23	22	56	1286	27	28650	0	13196	8083	248

WRIGHT–PATTERSON AFB—Greene County

✠ U. S. AIR FORCE MEDICAL CENTER WRIGHT–PATTERSON, 4881 Sugar Maple Drive, Zip 45433–5529; tel. 513/257–9913; Brigadier General Earl W. Mabry, II, Commander **A**1 2 3 5 **F**2 3 4 8 10 11 12 13 14 15 16 17 19 20 21 22 24 27 28 29 30 31 34 35 37 38 39 40 41 42 43 44 45 46 51 52 53 54 55 56 57 58 59 60 61 65 66 67 71 73 74 **S** Department of the Air Force, Washington, DC	41	10	135	9433	79	502720	757	—	—	2051

XENIA—Greene County

✠ GREENE MEMORIAL HOSPITAL, 1141 North Monroe Drive, Zip 45385; tel. 513/372–8011; Michael R. Stephens, President (Total facility includes 12 beds in nursing home–type unit) **A**1 2 5 9 10 **F**2 3 6 7 8 10 12 15 16 17 19 21 22 25 26 28 30 32 33 34 35 36 37 39 40 41 42 44 45 46 48 49 51 52 53 54 55 56 57 58 59 60 62 63 64 65 66 67 70 71 72 73 74 **P**6 7 8	23	10	150	4624	71	108855	345	41665	17040	666

YOUNGSTOWN—Mahoning County

BELMONT PINES HOSPITAL See BHC Belmont Pines Hospital

✠ BHC BELMONT PINES HOSPITAL, (Formerly Belmont Pines Hospital), 615 Churchill–Hubbard Road, Zip 44505; tel. 330/759–2700; Al Scott, Ed.D., Administrator **A**1 9 10 **F**14 15 16 17 20 22 34 52 70 **P**5 **S** Behavioral Healthcare Corporation, Nashville, TN	33	22	77	1212	38	1741	0	6183	2269	85

NORTHSIDE MEDICAL CENTER See Western Reserve Care System
SOUTHSIDE MEDICAL CENTER See Western Reserve Care System

✠ ST. ELIZABETH HEALTH CENTER, 1044 Belmont Avenue, Zip 44501, Mailing Address: Box 1790, Zip 44501–1790; tel. 330/759–7484; Kevin E. Nolan, President and Chief Executive Officer **A**1 2 3 5 6 8 9 10 **F**3 4 6 7 8 10 11 12 14 15 16 17 18 19 20 21 22 25 26 27 28 29 30 31 32 34 35 37 38 39 40 41 42 43 44 46 49 51 52 54 55 56 57 58 59 60 61 63 65 67 69 70 71 72 73 74 **S** Mercy Health System, Cincinnati, OH **N** Cleveland Health Network, Cleveland, OH	21	10	318	18532	291	250595	2123	192694	85089	2091

TOD CHILDREN'S HOSPITAL See Western Reserve Care System

Hospital, Address, Telephone, Administrator, Approval, Facility, and Physician Codes, Health Care System, Network	Classi-fication Codes		Utilization Data					Expense (thousands) of dollars		
★ American Hospital Association (AHA) membership □ Joint Commission on Accreditation of Healthcare Organizations (JCAHO) accreditation + American Osteopathic Hospital Association (AOHA) membership ○ American Osteopathic Association (AOA) accreditation △ Commission on Accreditation of Rehabilitation Facilities (CARF) accreditation Control codes 61, 63, 64, 71, 72 and 73 indicate hospitals listed by AOHA, but not registered by AHA. For definition of numerical codes, see page A4	Control	Service	Beds	Admissions	Census	Outpatient Visits	Births	Total	Payroll	Personnel
★ △ WESTERN RESERVE CARE SYSTEM, (Includes Northside Medical Center, 500 Gypsy Lane, Zip 44501–0240; tel. 330/747-1444; Southside Medical Center, 345 Oak Hill Avenue, tel. 330/747-0777; Tod Children's Hospital, 500 Gypsy Lane, Zip 44501–0240; tel. 330/747-6700), 345 Oak Hill Avenue, Zip 44501–0990, Mailing Address: P.O. Box 990, Zip 44501–0990; tel. 330/747-0777; Gary E. Kaatz, President and Chief Executive Officer (Total facility includes 26 beds in nursing home–type unit) **A**1 2 3 7 8 9 10 **F**2 3 4 6 7 8 10 12 13 14 15 16 17 18 19 20 21 22 23 25 26 27 28 30 31 32 33 34 35 36 37 38 39 40 41 42 43 44 46 47 48 49 51 52 53 54 55 56 57 58 59 60 61 63 64 65 66 67 68 71 72 73 74 **P**8	23	10	457	17431	281	190278	1699	190811	93742	2378
+ ○ YOUNGSTOWN OSTEOPATHIC HOSPITAL, 1319 Florencedale Avenue, Zip 44505–2797, Mailing Address: Box 1258, Zip 44501; tel. 330/744-9200; John C. Weir, President and Chief Executive Officer **A**9 10 11 12 13 **F**7 15 19 21 22 30 31 34 37 39 40 44 45 46 49 51 64 66 71 73 **P**8	23	10	88	5089	56	30211	291	25416	10811	246
ZANESVILLE—Muskingum County BETHESDA HOSPITAL See Genesis HealthCare System										
★ △ GENESIS HEALTHCARE SYSTEM, (Includes Bethesda Hospital, 2951 Maple Avenue, Zip 43701–1465; tel. 614/454-4000; Charles D. Hunter, Executive Vice President and Chief Operating Officer; Good Samaritan Medical and Rehabilitation Center, 800 Forest Avenue), 800 Forest Avenue, Zip 43701–2881; tel. 614/454-5000; Thomas L. Sieber, President and Chief Executive Officer (Total facility includes 44 beds in nursing home–type unit) (Nonreporting) **A**1 2 5 7 9 10 **S** Franciscan Sisters of Christian Charity HealthCare Ministry, Inc, Manitowoc, WI **N** Community Hospitals of Ohio, Newark, OH GOOD SAMARITAN MEDICAL AND REHABILITATION CENTER See Genesis HealthCare System	21	10	495	—	—	—	—	—	—	—

OKLAHOMA

Resident population 3,278 (in thousands)
Resident population in metro areas 60.2%
Birth rate per 1,000 population 14.3
65 years and over 13.5%
Percent of persons without health insurance 17.8%

Hospital, Address, Telephone, Administrator, Approval, Facility, and Physician Codes, Health Care System, Network	Classification Codes		Utilization Data					Expense (thousands) of dollars		
	Control	Service	Beds	Admissions	Census	Outpatient Visits	Births	Total	Payroll	Personnel

★ American Hospital Association (AHA) membership
□ Joint Commission on Accreditation of Healthcare Organizations (JCAHO) accreditation
+ American Osteopathic Hospital Association (AOHA) membership
○ American Osteopathic Association (AOA) accreditation
△ Commission on Accreditation of Rehabilitation Facilities (CARF) accreditation
Control codes 61, 63, 64, 71, 72 and 73 indicate hospitals listed by AOHA, but not registered by AHA. For definition of numerical codes, see page A4

ADA—Pontotoc County

✠ CARL ALBERT INDIAN HEALTH FACILITY, 1001 North Country Club Road, Zip 74820–2847; tel. 405/436–3980; Kenneth R. Ross, Administrator (Nonreporting) **A**1 10 **S** U. S. Public Health Service Indian Health Service, Rockville, MD	47	10	53	—	—	—	—	—	—	—
✠ ROLLING HILLS HOSPITAL, 1000 Rolling Hills Lane, Zip 74820; tel. 405/436–3600; Catherine Willner, Executive Director **A**1 9 10 **F**2 3 12 16 19 21 22 34 35 52 53 54 55 57 58 59 **P**6	33	22	40	514	22	4719	0	—	—	—
✠ △ VALLEY VIEW REGIONAL HOSPITAL, 430 North Monta Vista, Zip 74820–4610; tel. 405/332–2323; Philip Fisher, President and Chief Executive Officer **A**1 2 7 9 10 **F**10 12 14 15 17 19 21 22 23 27 28 30 32 33 34 35 36 37 38 39 40 42 44 45 46 48 49 60 63 65 67 70 71 72 73 **P**5 7	23	10	141	5419	81	53674	606	43282	14177	671

ALTUS—Jackson County

✠ JACKSON COUNTY MEMORIAL HOSPITAL, 1200 East Pecan Street, Zip 73521–6192, Mailing Address: Box 8190, Zip 73522–8190; tel. 405/482–4781; William G. Wilson, President and Chief Executive Officer (Total facility includes 25 beds in nursing home–type unit) **A**1 9 10 **F**7 8 11 15 16 17 19 21 22 23 28 30 32 33 34 35 36 37 39 40 41 42 44 45 46 49 51 56 58 59 64 65 66 67 70 71 73 **P**5	16	10	128	4233	74	28645	302	29342	12822	483
★ U. S. AIR FORCE HOSPITAL ALTUS, Altus AFB, Zip 73523–5005; tel. 405/481–5205; Colonel David L. Clark, USAF, Commander **F**3 8 15 18 20 28 29 30 39 40 58 71 **S** Department of the Air Force, Washington, DC	41	10	14	844	5	88323	246	5400	—	261

ALVA—Woods County

★ SHARE MEDICAL CENTER, 800 Share Drive, Zip 73717, Mailing Address: P.O. Box 727, Zip 73717–0727; tel. 405/327–2800; Barbara Oestmann, Chief Executive Officer **A**9 10 **F**1 7 14 15 16 19 20 21 22 28 32 33 34 36 40 42 44 45 51 53 55 56 57 58 65 67 71 73 **S** Quorum Health Group/Quorum Health Resources, Inc., Brentwood, TN	16	10	120	856	78	—	—	5177	2596	—

ANADARKO—Caddo County

ANADARKO MUNICIPAL HOSPITAL, 1002 Central Boulevard East, Zip 73005–4496; tel. 405/247–2551; Leon Torres, Interim Administrator (Nonreporting) **A**9 10	14	10	49	—	—	—	—	—	—	—

ANTLERS—Pushmataha County

PUSHMATAHA COUNTY–TOWN OF ANTLERS HOSPITAL AUTHORITY, 510 East Main Street, Zip 74523, Mailing Address: Box 518, Zip 74523; tel. 405/298–3342; Les Alexander, Administrator **A**9 10 **F**1 2 3 4 6 7 8 9 10 11 12 13 15 17 19 20 21 22 23 24 25 26 27 28 29 30 31 32 33 34 35 36 37 38 39 40 41 42 43 44 45 46 47 48 49 50 51 52 53 54 55 56 57 58 59 60 61 62 63 64 65 66 67 68 69 70 71 72 74 **P**5	15	10	49	1653	22	—	0	7007	3722	—

ARDMORE—Carter County

✠ MERCY MEMORIAL HEALTH CENTER, (Formerly Memorial Hospital of Southern Oklahoma), 1011 14th Street N.W., Zip 73401–1889; tel. 405/223–5400; Bobby G. Thompson, President and Chief Executive Officer **A**1 9 10 **F**3 7 8 10 12 14 15 16 17 19 20 21 22 23 26 28 29 30 31 32 34 35 37 40 41 42 44 45 46 48 49 52 54 55 56 57 59 60 64 65 67 71 73 **P**8 **S** Sisters of Mercy Health System–St. Louis, Saint Louis, MO **N** Mercy Health System, Oklahoma City, OK	23	10	193	7596	104	345214	748	49815	18038	668

ATOKA—Atoka County

★ ATOKA MEMORIAL HOSPITAL, 1501 South Virginia Avenue, Zip 74525; tel. 405/889–3333; Bruce A. Bennett, Administrator and Chief Executive Officer (Nonreporting) **A**9 10 **S** Quorum Health Group/Quorum Health Resources, Inc., Brentwood, TN	16	10	30	—	—	—	—	—	—	—

BARTLESVILLE—Washington County

✠ JANE PHILLIPS MEDICAL CENTER, 3500 East Frank Phillips Boulevard, Zip 74006–2409; tel. 918/333–7200; Larry Minden, Chief Executive Officer (Total facility includes 54 beds in nursing home–type unit) (Nonreporting) **A**1 2 5 9 10	23	10	227	—	—	—	—	—	—	—

BEAVER—Beaver County

BEAVER COUNTY MEMORIAL HOSPITAL, 212 East Eighth Street, Zip 73932, Mailing Address: Box 640, Zip 73932–0640; tel. 405/625–4551; La Vern Melton, Administrator **A**9 10 **F**8 15 16 21 28 44 71	16	10	24	228	2	4140	32	1840	900	29

BETHANY—Oklahoma County

✠ COLUMBIA BETHANY HOSPITAL, 7600 N.W. 23rd Street, Zip 73008; tel. 405/787–3450; David Lundquist, Chief Executive Officer **A**1 9 10 **F**4 10 12 14 15 16 17 19 22 26 28 29 30 32 33 34 36 37 44 46 48 49 52 53 64 65 67 68 71 72 73 **P**3 7 8 **S** Columbia/HCA Healthcare Corporation, Nashville, TN **N** Columbia Oklahoma Division, Inc., Oklahoma City, OK	33	10	75	1996	40	14438	0	16889	7195	283

BLACKWELL—Kay County

★ BLACKWELL REGIONAL HOSPITAL, 710 South 13th Street, Zip 74631; tel. 405/363–2311; Greg Martin, Administrator and Chief Executive Officer **A**9 10 **F**12 16 19 22 28 30 32 34 39 40 44 45 46 65 71 73 **P**3 7 8 **S** INTEGRIS Health, Oklahoma City, OK **N** Integris Health, Oklahoma City, OK	23	10	34	1297	17	—	64	6524	2623	132

Hospital, Address, Telephone, Administrator, Approval, Facility, and Physician Codes, Health Care System, Network	Classi-fication Codes		Utilization Data					Expense (thousands) of dollars		
	Control	Service	Beds	Admissions	Census	Outpatient Visits	Births	Total	Payroll	Personnel

BOISE CITY—Cimarron County

CIMARRON MEMORIAL HOSPITAL, 100 South Ellis, Zip 73933; tel. 405/544–2501; Ronny Lathrop, Chief Executive Officer and Administrator (Total facility includes 44 beds in nursing home–type unit) (Nonreporting) **A**9 10

| | 13 | 10 | 64 | — | — | — | — | — | — | — |

BRISTOW—Creek County

★ BRISTOW MEMORIAL HOSPITAL, Seventh and Spruce Streets, Zip 74010, Mailing Address: Box 780, Zip 74010; tel. 918/367–2215; William L. Legate, Administrator **A**9 10 **F**8 17 19 22 30 32 33 37 44 49 65 71 **P**6 **S** INTEGRIS Health, Oklahoma City, OK **N** Integris Health, Oklahoma City, OK

| | 23 | 10 | 22 | 328 | 3 | 8448 | 0 | 2973 | 1319 | 64 |

BROKEN ARROW—Tulsa County

☐ △ BROKEN ARROW MEDICAL CENTER, 3000 South Elm Place, Zip 74012; tel. 918/455–3535; Bruce Switzer, Administrator **A**1 7 9 10 **F**11 12 15 16 19 21 22 27 32 37 39 41 42 44 48 49 65 71 73

| | 23 | 10 | 70 | 1813 | 31 | 27221 | 2 | 17142 | 8098 | 317 |

BUFFALO—Harper County

HARPER COUNTY COMMUNITY HOSPITAL, Highway 64 North, Zip 73834, Mailing Address: Box 60, Zip 73834; tel. 405/735–2555; Jane McDowell, Chief Executive Officer **A**9 10 **F**8 11 15 17 22 28 29 30 33 36 39 40 44 46 49 64 71

| | 13 | 10 | 25 | 278 | 7 | 1065 | 20 | 1398 | 730 | 47 |

CARNEGIE—Caddo County

★ CARNEGIE TRI–COUNTY MUNICIPAL HOSPITAL, 102 North Broadway, Zip 73015, Mailing Address: Box 97, Zip 73015; tel. 405/654–1050; Phil Hawkins, Administrator (Nonreporting) **A**9 10 **N** First Health West, Lawton, OK

| | 14 | 10 | 28 | | | | | | | |

CHEYENNE—Roger Mills County

★ ROGER MILLS MEMORIAL HOSPITAL, Fifth and L. L Males Avenue, Zip 73628, Mailing Address: Box 219, Zip 73628; tel. 405/497–3336; Marilyn Bryan, Administrator **A**9 10 **F**22 32 33 40 44

| | 13 | 10 | 15 | 155 | 2 | 8049 | 3 | 2149 | 1227 | 46 |

CHICKASHA—Grady County

⊞ GRADY MEMORIAL HOSPITAL, 2220 Iowa, Zip 73018; tel. 405/224–2300; Roger R. Boid, Administrator (Total facility includes 11 beds in nursing home–type unit) **A**1 2 9 10 **F**11 12 19 20 21 22 28 30 32 34 37 39 40 41 44 46 49 56 60 63 64 65 67 71 73

| | 16 | 10 | 147 | 3430 | 48 | 23882 | 399 | 24318 | 11055 | 414 |

CLAREMORE—Rogers County

⊞ COLUMBIA CLAREMORE REGIONAL HOSPITAL, 1202 North Muskogee Place, Zip 74017; tel. 918/341–2556; Ken Seidel, Executive Director (Nonreporting) **A**1 9 10 **S** Columbia/HCA Healthcare Corporation, Nashville, TN **N** Columbia Oklahoma Division, Inc., Oklahoma City, OK

| | 47 | 10 | 50 | — | — | — | — | — | — | — |

⊞ U. S. PUBLIC HEALTH SERVICE COMPREHENSIVE INDIAN HEALTH FACILITY, 101 South Moore Avenue, Zip 74017–5091; tel. 918/342–6434; John Daugherty, Jr., Service Unit Director **A**1 5 10 **F**3 15 16 20 22 34 37 40 44 49 51 61 65 71 **P**6 **S** U. S. Public Health Service Indian Health Service, Rockville, MD

| | 47 | 10 | 50 | 2368 | 26 | 137787 | 687 | 19057 | 12622 | 338 |

CLEVELAND—Pawnee County

CLEVELAND AREA HOSPITAL, 1401 West Pawnee Street, Zip 74020–3019; tel. 918/358–2501; Thomas Henton, Administrator and Chief Executive Officer **A**9 10 **F**28 32 36 44 49 65 71 73

| | 16 | 10 | 25 | 351 | 5 | 10223 | 0 | 3640 | 1848 | 90 |

CLINTON—Custer County

⊞ CLINTON REGIONAL HOSPITAL, 100 North 30th Street, Zip 73601, Mailing Address: Box 1569, Zip 73601; tel. 405/323–2363; George H. Dashner, FACHE, President and Chief Executive Officer **A**1 9 10 **F**7 8 12 15 16 17 19 20 21 22 28 30 32 33 35 37 39 40 41 42 44 49 60 63 65 66 67 71 73

| | 14 | 10 | 49 | 1920 | 22 | 15798 | 245 | 11044 | 5071 | 194 |

⊞ U. S. PUBLIC HEALTH SERVICE INDIAN HOSPITAL, Mailing Address: P.O. Box 279, Zip 73601; tel. 405/323–2884; Thedis V. Mitchell, Director (Nonreporting) **A**1 10 **S** U. S. Public Health Service Indian Health Service, Rockville, MD

| | 47 | 10 | 11 | — | — | — | — | — | — | — |

COALGATE—Coal County

MARY HURLEY HOSPITAL, 6 North Covington Street, Zip 74538–2002; tel. 405/927–2327; Mark Byrd, Chief Executive Officer (Total facility includes 75 beds in nursing home–type unit) **A**9 10 **F**19 22 26 30 32 34 44 49 66 71 73

| | 23 | 10 | 95 | 489 | 68 | 6561 | 2 | 4711 | 2635 | 151 |

CORDELL—Washita County

★ CORDELL MEMORIAL HOSPITAL, 1220 North Glenn English Street, Zip 73632; tel. 405/832–3339; Charles H. Greene, Jr., Administrator **A**9 10 **F**15 22 28 30 44 71 **N** First Health West, Lawton, OK

| | 14 | 10 | 28 | 444 | 5 | 3928 | 0 | 1903 | 914 | 37 |

CUSHING—Payne County

⊞ CUSHING REGIONAL HOSPITAL, 1027 East Cherry, Zip 74023, Mailing Address: Box 1409, Zip 74023–1409; tel. 918/225–2915; Ron Cackler, President and Chief Executive Officer **A**1 9 10 **F**1 3 12 15 17 19 20 21 22 25 26 28 30 32 33 36 37 40 41 42 44 45 46 49 52 54 55 56 57 58 59 64 65 66 67 71 73 **P**8 **S** Quorum Health Group/Quorum Health Resources, Inc., Brentwood, TN **N** Hillcrest Healthcare System, Tulsa, OK

| | 14 | 10 | 75 | 2420 | 36 | 19018 | 428 | 12487 | 4806 | 227 |

DRUMRIGHT—Creek County

★ DRUMRIGHT MEMORIAL HOSPITAL, 501 South Lou Allard Drive, Zip 74030–4899; tel. 918/352–2525; Jerry Jones, Administrator **A**9 10 **F**8 15 16 19 22 25 32 35 37 44 71 73 **P**4 5 8 **S** INTEGRIS Health, Oklahoma City, OK **N** Integris Health, Oklahoma City, OK

| | 23 | 10 | 15 | 560 | 7 | 4657 | 0 | 3721 | 2046 | 95 |

DUNCAN—Stephens County

⊞ DUNCAN REGIONAL HOSPITAL, 1407 Whisenant Drive, Zip 73533, Mailing Address: P.O. Box 2000, Zip 73534–2000; tel. 405/252–5300; David Robertson, Chief Executive Officer (Total facility includes 12 beds in nursing home–type unit) **A**1 9 10 **F**7 8 11 13 14 15 16 17 19 21 22 29 30 32 34 35 37 39 40 41 42 44 45 48 49 64 65 66 71 73 **P**8

| | 23 | 10 | 100 | 4018 | 49 | 44450 | 425 | 24726 | 11081 | 433 |

Hospital, Address, Telephone, Administrator, Approval, Facility, and Physician Codes, Health Care System, Network	Classi-fication Codes		Utilization Data					Expense (thousands) of dollars		
★ American Hospital Association (AHA) membership □ Joint Commission on Accreditation of Healthcare Organizations (JCAHO) accreditation + American Osteopathic Hospital Association (AOHA) membership ○ American Osteopathic Association (AOA) accreditation △ Commission on Accreditation of Rehabilitation Facilities (CARF) accreditation Control codes 61, 63, 64, 71, 72 and 73 indicate hospitals listed by AOHA, but not registered by AHA. For definition of numerical codes, see page A4	Control	Service	Beds	Admissions	Census	Outpatient Visits	Births	Total	Payroll	Personnel

DURANT—Bryan County

□ MEDICAL CENTER OF SOUTHEASTERN OKLAHOMA, 1800 University, Zip 74701, Mailing Address: P.O. Box 1207, Zip 74702; tel. 405/924–3080; Joshua Putter, Executive Director **A**1 9 10 **F**7 8 10 12 14 17 19 20 21 22 23 26 28 30 32 34 35 37 41 44 46 49 61 63 65 67 70 71 73 74 **P**4 **S** Health Management Associates, Naples, FL

| | 33 | 10 | 103 | 4663 | 52 | 25872 | 587 | 20232 | 7435 | 345 |

EDMOND—Oklahoma County

⊞ COLUMBIA EDMOND REGIONAL MEDICAL CENTER, 1 South Bryant Street, Zip 73034–4798; tel. 405/359–5530; Stanley D. Tatum, Chief Executive Officer **A**1 9 10 **F**4 7 8 9 10 11 12 14 15 16 17 18 19 20 21 22 25 26 28 29 30 32 33 34 35 37 38 40 41 42 43 44 45 46 48 49 51 53 54 55 56 58 59 60 61 64 65 66 67 68 71 72 73 74 **P**5 7 8 **S** Columbia/HCA Healthcare Corporation, Nashville, TN **N** Columbia Oklahoma Division, Inc., Oklahoma City, OK

| | 33 | 10 | 75 | 2525 | 33 | 32701 | 315 | 21227 | 7630 | 258 |

HORIZON SPECIALTY HOSPITAL, 1100 East Ninth Street, Zip 73034; tel. 405/341–8150; Joe Smithers, Administrator (Nonreporting) **A**10

| | 33 | 49 | 43 | — | — | — | — | — | — | — |

EL RENO—Canadian County

★ PARK VIEW HOSPITAL, 2115 Parkview Drive, Zip 73036, Mailing Address: P.O. Box 129, Zip 73036–0129; tel. 405/262–2640; Lex Smith, Administrator **A**9 10 **F**7 8 14 15 16 17 20 22 28 29 30 32 33 34 37 39 40 42 44 45 46 48 49 55 57 60 64 65 67 71 73

| | 16 | 10 | 54 | 1874 | 25 | | 168 | 12414 | 6484 | 297 |

ELK CITY—Beckham County

⊞ GREAT PLAINS REGIONAL MEDICAL CENTER, 1705 West Second Street, Zip 73644, Mailing Address: P.O. Box 2339, Zip 73648–2339; tel. 405/225–2511; Tim Francis, Chief Executive Officer **A**1 9 10 **F**8 11 12 14 15 16 17 19 20 21 22 23 26 27 28 29 30 32 33 34 35 37 39 40 41 42 44 45 46 49 51 52 53 54 55 56 57 58 60 63 65 66 71 72 73 74 **P**8

| | 23 | 10 | 78 | 1979 | 31 | 54586 | 176 | 18066 | 7844 | 338 |

ENID—Garfield County

⊞ INTEGRIS BASS BAPTIST HEALTH CENTER, 600 South Monroe, Zip 73701, Mailing Address: Box 3168, Zip 73702; tel. 405/233–2300; W. Eugene Baxter, Dr.PH, Administrator **A**1 3 5 9 10 **F**10 12 15 19 21 22 26 28 29 30 31 32 33 34 35 36 37 38 39 40 41 42 44 46 52 57 60 64 66 67 71 73 74 **P**6 7 **S** INTEGRIS Health, Oklahoma City, OK **N** Integris Health, Oklahoma City, OK

| | 23 | 10 | 119 | 4452 | 72 | 31734 | 729 | 36083 | 14001 | 646 |

□ MEADOWLAKE BEHAVIORAL HEALTH SYSTEM, 2216 South Van Buren, Zip 73703, Mailing Address: P.O. Box 5409, Zip 73702; tel. 405/234–2220; Dave Lamerton, Chief Executive Officer (Nonreporting) **A**1 10 **S** Ramsay Health Care, Inc., Coral Gobles, FL

| | 33 | 22 | 50 | — | — | — | — | — | — | — |

⊞ △ ST. MARY'S MERCY HOSPITAL, 305 South Fifth Street, Zip 73701–5899, Mailing Address: Box 232, Zip 73702–0232; tel. 405/233–6100; Frank Lopez, President and Chief Executive Officer **A**1 2 3 5 7 9 10 **F**7 8 10 12 14 15 16 19 21 22 23 29 30 31 32 34 35 37 38 39 40 41 42 44 45 48 49 64 65 71 72 73 **P**4 5 6 7 **S** Sisters of Mercy Health System–St. Louis, Saint Louis, MO **N** Mercy Health System, Oklahoma City, OK

| | 21 | 10 | 135 | 5197 | 93 | 68993 | 270 | — | — | 578 |

EUFAULA—Mcintosh County

COMMUNITY HOSPITAL–LAKEVIEW, 1 Hospital Drive, Zip 74432, Mailing Address: P.O. Box 629, Zip 74432; tel. 918/689–2535; R. S. Smith, Chief Executive Officer **A**9 10 **F**15 17 19 22 28 30 32 35 44 45 46 63 73

| | 33 | 10 | 33 | 399 | 3 | 8756 | 0 | 3139 | 1206 | 87 |

FAIRFAX—Osage County

★ FAIRFAX MEMORIAL HOSPITAL, Taft Avenue and Highway 18, Zip 74637, Mailing Address: Box 219, Zip 74637; tel. 918/642–3291; Annabeth Murray, Administrator **A**9 10 **F**8 19 22 28 32 34 44 71

| | 14 | 10 | 21 | 376 | 4 | 2654 | 0 | 2620 | 1196 | 57 |

FAIRVIEW—Major County

★ FAIRVIEW HOSPITAL, 523 East State Road, Zip 73737; tel. 405/227–3721; Arthur H. Frable, Administrator **A**9 10 **F**11 14 15 17 19 22 28 30 32 34 36 37 40 44 49 51 65 71 72 73 **P**6

| | 14 | 10 | 31 | 392 | 3 | 1727 | 8 | 2734 | 1626 | 67 |

FORT SILL—Comanche County

⊞ REYNOLDS ARMY COMMUNITY HOSPITAL, 4300 Thomas, Zip 73503–6300; tel. 405/458–3000; Colonel David B. Crandall, Commander (Nonreporting) **A**1 **S** Department of the Army, Office of the Surgeon General, Falls Church, VA

| | 42 | 10 | 116 | — | — | — | — | — | — | — |

FORT SUPPLY—Woodward County

□ WESTERN STATE PSYCHIATRIC CENTER, Mailing Address: P.O. Box 1, Zip 73841–0001; tel. 405/766–2311; Steve Norwood, Director **A**1 10 **F**2 3 12 16 20 41 52 54 55 56 57 58 59 65 73 **P**6 **S** Oklahoma State Department of Mental Health and Substance Abuse Services, Oklahoma City, OK

| | 12 | 22 | 170 | 1084 | 138 | — | 0 | 12203 | 6730 | 283 |

FREDERICK—Tillman County

★ MEMORIAL HOSPITAL, 319 East Josephine, Zip 73542–2299; tel. 405/335–7565; Doug Weaver, Chief Executive Officer **A**9 10 **F**8 12 15 17 19 21 22 28 30 32 34 39 40 44 46 48 49 51 58 64 67 71 73 **P**6

| | 16 | 10 | 32 | 870 | 9 | 16613 | 38 | 5178 | 2648 | 124 |

GROVE—Delaware County

⊞ INTEGRIS GROVE GENERAL HOSPITAL, 1310 South Main Street, Zip 74344–1310; tel. 918/786–2243; Dee Renshaw, Administrator **A**1 9 10 **F**6 7 8 13 15 16 17 19 20 22 26 28 30 32 33 34 42 44 51 62 65 66 67 68 71 73 **P**2 3 5 7 **S** INTEGRIS Health, Oklahoma City, OK **N** Integris Health, Oklahoma City, OK

| | 23 | 10 | 72 | 2919 | 38 | 44737 | 42 | 18995 | 8773 | 410 |

GUTHRIE—Logan County

★ LOGAN HOSPITAL AND MEDICAL CENTER, Highway 33 West at Academy Road, Zip 73044, Mailing Address: P.O. Box 1017, Zip 73044; tel. 405/282–6700; James R. Caton, Chief Executive Officer (Nonreporting) **A**9 10 **S** Quorum Health Group/Quorum Health Resources, Inc., Brentwood, TN

| | 16 | 10 | 32 | — | — | — | — | — | — | — |

Hospital, Address, Telephone, Administrator, Approval, Facility, and Physician Codes, Health Care System, Network	Control	Service	Beds	Admissions	Census	Outpatient Visits	Births	Total	Payroll	Personnel
★ American Hospital Association (AHA) membership ☐ Joint Commission on Accreditation of Healthcare Organizations (JCAHO) accreditation + American Osteopathic Hospital Association (AOHA) membership ○ American Osteopathic Association (AOA) accreditation △ Commission on Accreditation of Rehabilitation Facilities (CARF) accreditation Control codes 61, 63, 64, 71, 72 and 73 indicate hospitals listed by AOHA, but not registered by AHA. For definition of numerical codes, see page A4										
GUYMON—Texas County										
★ MEMORIAL HOSPITAL OF TEXAS COUNTY, 520 Medical Drive, Zip 73942–4438; tel. 405/338–6515; Lu Ann Weldon, Administrator A9 10 F7 8 15 16 19 21 22 28 29 30 32 34 36 40 44 45 46 66 68 71 73	13	10	35	1683	18	10579	186	8987	3424	97
HENRYETTA—Okmulgee County										
⊞ HENRYETTA MEDICAL CENTER, Dewey Bartlett and Main Streets, Zip 74437, Mailing Address: P.O. Box 1269, Zip 74437–1269; tel. 918/652–4463; James P. Bailey, Administrator and Chief Executive Officer (Nonreporting) A1 9 10 S Quorum Health Group/Quorum Health Resources, Inc., Brentwood, TN	16	10	28	—						
HOBART—Kiowa County										
★ ELKVIEW GENERAL HOSPITAL, 429 West Elm Street, Zip 73651–1699; tel. 405/726–3324; J. W. Finch, Jr., Administrator A9 10 F7 8 11 15 19 21 22 30 32 44 45 49 51 56 71 72 73	16	10	40	1250	19	7332	71	—	2710	119
HOLDENVILLE—Hughes County										
★ HOLDENVILLE GENERAL HOSPITAL, 100 Crestview Drive, Zip 74848–9700; tel. 405/379–6631; Joseph J. Mitchell, Chief Executive Officer and Administrator A9 10 F16 19 22 28 32 34 42 44 71 73 S Quorum Health Group/Quorum Health Resources, Inc., Brentwood, TN	14	10	27	791	8	7210	0	5026	2201	89
HOLLIS—Harmon County										
★ HARMON MEMORIAL HOSPITAL, 400 East Chestnut Street, Zip 73550, Mailing Address: P.O. Box 791, Zip 73550; tel. 405/688–3363; Al Allee, Administrator A9 10 F19 22 32 49 65 71 73 N First Health West, Lawton, OK	16	10	18	354	4	3149	0	1319	635	42
HUGO—Choctaw County										
★ CHOCTAW MEMORIAL HOSPITAL, 1405 East Kirk Road, Zip 74743; tel. 405/326–6414; Michael R. Morel, Administrator A9 10 F15 16 19 22 32 34 36 37 39 40 44 46 70 71 73 P5 S INTEGRIS Health, Oklahoma City, OK N Integris Health, Oklahoma City, OK	16	10	41	1239	12	3013	97	5334	2401	102
IDABEL—Mccurtain County										
★ MCCURTAIN MEMORIAL HOSPITAL, 1301 Lincoln, Zip 74745; tel. 405/286–7623; Ronald Campbell, Administrator (Nonreporting) A9 10 S Quorum Health Group/Quorum Health Resources, Inc., Brentwood, TN	23	10	89	—	—	—	—	—	—	—
KINGFISHER—Kingfisher County										
★ KINGFISHER REGIONAL HOSPITAL, 500 South Ninth Street, Zip 73750, Mailing Address: Box 59, Zip 73750–0059; tel. 405/375–3141; Steven G. Daniel, Administrator A9 10 F19 22 32 37 40 51 65 71 P6 S Quorum Health Group/Quorum Health Resources, Inc., Brentwood, TN	23	10	25	1254	12	—	106	6792	3377	137
LAWTON—Comanche County										
⊞ COLUMBIA SOUTHWESTERN MEDICAL CENTER, 5602 S.W. Lee Boulevard, Zip 73505–9635, Mailing Address: P.O. Box 7290, Zip 73506–7290; tel. 405/531–4700; Thomas L. Rine, President and Chief Executive Officer A1 2 9 10 F8 10 11 12 14 15 16 17 19 21 22 28 30 32 34 35 37 38 40 42 44 48 49 51 52 53 58 59 60 65 70 71 72 73 74 P7 S Columbia/HCA Healthcare Corporation, Nashville, TN N Columbia Oklahoma Division, Inc., Oklahoma City, OK	33	10	108	4061	64	63914	475	38355	11097	398
⊞ COMANCHE COUNTY MEMORIAL HOSPITAL, 3401 Gore Boulevard, Zip 73505–0129, Mailing Address: Box 129, Zip 73502–0129; tel. 405/355–8620; Randy Curry, President A1 9 10 F3 4 7 8 10 11 12 14 15 16 19 20 21 22 27 28 29 30 31 32 34 35 37 39 40 41 42 43 44 46 48 49 52 53 56 58 60 63 64 65 66 67 68 71 72 73 74 P3 4 7 N First Health West, OK	16	10	221	7536	147	—	842	97460	43178	1372
MEMORIAL PAVILION, 1602 S.W. 82nd Street, Zip 73505; tel. 405/536–0077; Jim Ivy, Administrator (Nonreporting) A10	33	22	99	—	—	—	—	—	—	—
⊞ U. S. PUBLIC HEALTH SERVICE INDIAN HOSPITAL, 1515 Lawrie Tatum Road, Zip 73507; tel. 405/353–0350; George F. Howell, Service Unit Director (Nonreporting) A1 10 S U. S. Public Health Service Indian Health Service, Rockville, MD	47	10	44	—	—	—	—	—	—	—
LINDSAY—Garvin County										
LINDSAY MUNICIPAL HOSPITAL, Highway 19 West, Zip 73052, Mailing Address: Box 888, Zip 73052; tel. 405/756–4321; Jim Standridge, Administrator (Nonreporting) A9 10	14	10	25	—	—	—	—	—	—	—
MADILL—Marshall County										
MARSHALL MEMORIAL HOSPITAL, 1 Hospital Drive, Zip 73446, Mailing Address: P.O. Box 827, Zip 73446; tel. 405/795–3384; Norma Howard, Administrator A9 10 F15 16 22 28 30 33 34 40 44 65 73 S INTEGRIS Health, Oklahoma City, OK N Integris Health, Oklahoma City, OK	13	10	25	871	10	10802	40	4820	2645	94
MANGUM—Greer County										
MANGUM CITY HOSPITAL, One Wickersham Drive, Zip 73554, Mailing Address: Box 280, Zip 73554; tel. 405/782–3353; Jim Koulovatos, Chief Executive Officer (Nonreporting) A9 10	14	10	40	—	—	—	—	—	—	—
MARIETTA—Love County										
★ LOVE COUNTY HEALTH CENTER, 300 Wanda Street, Zip 73448; tel. 405/276–3347; Richard Barker, Administrator A9 10 F11 12 14 15 16 17 19 26 28 29 30 32 34 71	13	10	30	450	7	9015	0	3670	2438	93
MCALESTER—Pittsburg County										
⊞ △ MCALESTER REGIONAL HEALTH CENTER, One Clark Bass Boulevard, Zip 74501–4267, Mailing Address: P.O. Box 1228, Zip 74502–1228; tel. 918/426–1800; Joel W. Tate, FACHE, Interim Chief Executive Officer A1 7 9 10 F3 4 6 7 8 10 12 15 16 17 18 19 21 22 23 27 28 30 31 32 33 34 35 36 37 39 40 41 42 44 45 46 48 49 63 64 65 66 67 71 73	16	10	198	4725	65	64228	618	31643	13474	624

Hospital, Address, Telephone, Administrator, Approval, Facility, and Physician Codes, Health Care System, Network	Classi-fication Codes		Utilization Data					Expense (thousands) of dollars		
★ American Hospital Association (AHA) membership □ Joint Commission on Accreditation of Healthcare Organizations (JCAHO) accreditation + American Osteopathic Hospital Association (AOHA) membership ○ American Osteopathic Association (AOA) accreditation △ Commission on Accreditation of Rehabilitation Facilities (CARF) accreditation Control codes 61, 63, 64, 71, 72 and 73 indicate hospitals listed by AOHA, but not registered by AHA. For definition of numerical codes, see page A4.	Control	Service	Beds	Admissions	Census	Outpatient Visits	Births	Total	Payroll	Personnel

MIAMI—Ottawa County

Hospital	Control	Service	Beds	Admissions	Census	Outpatient Visits	Births	Total	Payroll	Personnel
⊞ INTEGRIS BAPTIST REGIONAL HEALTH CENTER, 200 Second Street S.W., Zip 74354, Mailing Address: Box 1207, Zip 74355–1207; tel. 918/540–7100; Dee Renshaw, Administrator **A**1 9 10 **F**12 13 14 15 16 17 19 20 21 22 23 26 27 28 29 30 31 32 35 36 37 40 42 44 45 46 49 51 52 56 57 60 63 64 65 66 71 72 73 74 **P**2 4 5 6 7 8 **S** INTEGRIS Health, Oklahoma City, OK **N** Integris Health, Oklahoma City, OK	23	10	124	5564	75	32605	323	28821	13785	520
□ WILLOW CREST HOSPITAL, 130 A Street S.W., Zip 74354; tel. 918/542–1836; Cornelia Willis, Administrator and Chief Executive Officer (Nonreporting) **A**1 9 10 **S** Sterling Healthcare Corporation, Bellevue, WA	33	22	50	—	—	—	—	—	—	—

MIDWEST CITY—Oklahoma County

Hospital	Control	Service	Beds	Admissions	Census	Outpatient Visits	Births	Total	Payroll	Personnel
⊞ MIDWEST CITY REGIONAL MEDICAL CENTER, 2825 Parklawn Drive, Zip 73110–4258; tel. 405/737–4411; Gary D. Newsome, Executive Director and Chief Executive Officer **A**1 2 9 10 **F**4 7 8 10 11 12 15 16 19 21 22 27 28 32 35 37 40 41 42 43 44 45 46 49 52 56 57 63 64 65 67 71 73 74 **P**5 6 **S** Health Management Associates, Naples, FL	33	10	206	6126	122	40759	639	—	—	854

MUSKOGEE—Muskogee County

Hospital	Control	Service	Beds	Admissions	Census	Outpatient Visits	Births	Total	Payroll	Personnel
⊞ △ MUSKOGEE REGIONAL MEDICAL CENTER, 300 Edna M. Rockefeller Drive, Zip 74401; tel. 918/682–5501; Bill R. Kennedy, President and Chief Executive Officer **A**1 2 7 9 10 **F**10 12 14 15 16 19 20 21 22 29 30 32 33 34 35 41 42 44 46 49 58 60 65 67 71 72 73	16	10	225	8897	136	53858	1016	56446	25201	887
⊞ VETERANS AFFAIRS MEDICAL CENTER, Honor Heights Drive, Zip 74401–1399; tel. 918/683–3261; Billy M. Valentine, Director **A**1 3 5 **F**1 3 4 6 8 10 14 15 16 19 20 21 22 25 27 28 31 32 33 34 35 36 39 41 42 44 46 49 51 54 56 58 60 65 67 71 73 74 **P**6 **S** Department of Veterans Affairs, Washington, DC	45	10	99	3728	61	134082	0	—	30783	591

NORMAN—Cleveland County

Hospital	Control	Service	Beds	Admissions	Census	Outpatient Visits	Births	Total	Payroll	Personnel
□ GRIFFIN MEMORIAL HOSPITAL, 900 East Main Street, Zip 73070–0101, Mailing Address: Box 151, Zip 73070; tel. 405/321–4880; William T. Burkett, Superintendent **A**1 3 5 10 **F**19 20 21 22 27 29 34 35 44 46 50 52 56 57 63 65 71 73 **P**6 **S** Oklahoma State Department of Mental Health and Substance Abuse Services, Oklahoma City, OK	12	22	182	2046	181	5641	0	23366	14338	546
J. D. MCCARTY CENTER FOR CHILDREN WITH DEVELOPMENTAL DISABILITIES, 1125 East Alameda, Zip 73071–5264; tel. 405/321–4830; Curtis A. Peters, Chief Executive Officer **A**10 **F**20 34 39 45 46 48 49 54 65 67 73 **P**6	12	56	37	93	26	1076	0	4340	2910	106
⊞ NORMAN REGIONAL HOSPITAL, 901 North Porter Street, Zip 73071, Mailing Address: Box 1308, Zip 73070–1308; tel. 405/321–1700; Craig W. Jones, President and Chief Executive Officer **A**1 2 9 10 **F**4 7 8 10 11 12 15 17 18 19 20 21 22 25 27 28 29 30 31 32 34 35 36 39 40 41 42 43 44 45 46 49 51 52 53 54 55 57 58 59 60 63 64 65 66 67 70 71 72 73 74 **P**3 7 8	16	10	243	11380	163	190547	1182	92683	40779	1422

NOWATA—Nowata County

Hospital	Control	Service	Beds	Admissions	Census	Outpatient Visits	Births	Total	Payroll	Personnel
JANE PHILLIPS NOWATA HEALTH CENTER, 237 South Locust Street, Zip 74048–0426, Mailing Address: P.O. Box 426, Zip 74048–0426; tel. 918/273–3102; Maggie Blevins, Administrator (Nonreporting) **A**9 10	23	10	28	—	—	—	—	—	—	—

OKEENE—Blaine County

Hospital	Control	Service	Beds	Admissions	Census	Outpatient Visits	Births	Total	Payroll	Personnel
OKEENE MUNICIPAL HOSPITAL, 207 East F Street, Zip 73763, Mailing Address: P.O. Box 489, Zip 73763; tel. 405/822–4417; Debbie Howe, Administrator (Total facility includes 44 beds in nursing home–type unit) **A**9 10 **F**6 7 15 19 22 30 32 36 44 49 71	14	10	74	648	36	—	92	3087	1785	103

OKEMAH—Payne County

Hospital	Control	Service	Beds	Admissions	Census	Outpatient Visits	Births	Total	Payroll	Personnel
★ CREEK NATION COMMUNITY HOSPITAL, 309 North 14th Street, Zip 74859; tel. 918/623–1424; Philip Barnoski, Chief Executive Officer **A**10 **F**15 19 27 28 30 31 34 41 44 51 53 54 56 58 65 67 71 **S** U. S. Public Health Service Indian Health Service, Rockville, MD	47	10	34	605	8	1384	0	—	—	111

OKLAHOMA CITY—Oklahoma County

Hospital	Control	Service	Beds	Admissions	Census	Outpatient Visits	Births	Total	Payroll	Personnel
⊞ BONE AND JOINT HOSPITAL, 1111 North Dewey Avenue, Zip 73103–2615; tel. 405/552–9100; James A. Hyde, Administrator (Nonreporting) **A**1 3 5 9 10 **S** SSM Health Care System, Saint Louis, MO	23	47	89	—	—	—	—	—	—	—
CHILDREN'S HOSPITAL OF OKLAHOMA See The University Hospitals										
⊞ COLUMBIA PRESBYTERIAN HOSPITAL, 700 N.E. 13th Street, Zip 73104–5070; tel. 405/271–5100; James O'Loughlin, Chief Executive Officer (Nonreporting) **A**1 2 3 5 9 10 **S** Columbia/HCA Healthcare Corporation, Nashville, TN **N** Columbia Oklahoma Division, Inc., Oklahoma City, OK	33	10	292	—	—	—	—	—	—	—
⊞ DEACONESS HOSPITAL, 5501 North Portland Avenue, Zip 73112–2099; tel. 405/946–5581; Paul Dougherty, Administrator (Total facility includes 22 beds in nursing home–type unit) **A**1 2 9 10 **F**1 3 4 6 7 8 10 12 16 17 18 19 20 21 22 23 25 26 27 28 29 30 31 32 33 34 35 36 37 39 40 41 42 43 44 45 46 49 50 51 52 53 54 55 56 57 58 59 60 61 62 63 64 65 66 67 68 69 70 71 72 73 74	23	10	226	8437	142	—	1128	61189	27781	1040
□ △ HEALTHSOUTH REHABILITATION HOSPITAL, 700 N.W. Seventh Street, Zip 73102–1295; tel. 405/553–1192; Hank Ross, Chief Executive Officer (Nonreporting) **A**1 7 10 **S** HEALTHSOUTH Corporation, Birmingham, AL	33	46	46	—	—	—	—	—	—	—
HIGH POINTE, 6501 N.E. 50th Street, Zip 73141–9613; tel. 405/424–3383; Charlene Arnett, Chief Executive Officer (Nonreporting) **A**10 **S** Century Healthcare Corporation, Tulsa, OK	33	22	68	—	—	—	—	—	—	—
★ + ○ HILLCREST HEALTH CENTER, 2129 S.W. 59th Street, Zip 73119–7001; tel. 405/685–6671; Ray Brazier, President **A**9 10 11 12 13 **F**2 3 4 7 8 10 11 12 16 17 18 19 21 22 26 28 30 32 35 37 39 40 41 42 43 44 45 46 48 49 50 52 53 54 56 58 59 60 64 65 66 70 71 73 74 **P**8 **S** SSM Health Care System, Saint Louis, MO	23	10	181	5965	93	75371	739	45890	19840	518

Hospital, Address, Telephone, Administrator, Approval, Facility, and Physician Codes, Health Care System, Network	Classi-fication Codes		Utilization Data					Expense (thousands) of dollars		
★ American Hospital Association (AHA) membership ☐ Joint Commission on Accreditation of Healthcare Organizations (JCAHO) accreditation + American Osteopathic Hospital Association (AOHA) membership ○ American Osteopathic Association (AOA) accreditation △ Commission on Accreditation of Rehabilitation Facilities (CARF) accreditation Control codes 61, 63, 64, 71, 72 and 73 indicate hospitals listed by AOHA, but not registered by AHA. For definition of numerical codes, see page A4	Control	Service	Beds	Admissions	Census	Outpatient Visits	Births	Total	Payroll	Personnel

Hospital	Control	Service	Beds	Admissions	Census	Outpatient Visits	Births	Total	Payroll	Personnel
⊞ INTEGRIS BAPTIST MEDICAL CENTER, 3300 N.W. Expressway, Zip 73112–4481; tel. 405/949–3011; Thomas R. Rice, President and Chief Operation Officer **A**1 2 3 5 9 10 **F**2 3 4 7 8 9 10 11 12 13 14 15 16 17 18 19 20 21 22 23 25 26 28 29 30 31 32 33 34 35 37 38 39 40 41 42 43 44 45 46 47 48 49 50 51 52 53 54 55 56 57 58 59 60 61 63 64 65 67 68 69 70 71 72 73 74 **P**3 6 7 8 **S** INTEGRIS Health, Oklahoma City, OK **N** Integris Health, Oklahoma City, OK	23	10	424	22230	286	—	2782	224971	80195	—
⊞ △ INTEGRIS SOUTHWEST MEDICAL CENTER, 4401 South Western, Zip 73109–3441; tel. 405/636–7000; Thomas R. Rice, President and Chief Operation Officer **A**1 2 7 9 10 **F**4 7 8 9 10 11 12 14 15 16 17 19 21 22 27 28 29 30 32 33 34 35 36 37 38 39 40 41 42 43 44 45 47 48 49 51 52 53 54 55 56 57 58 59 60 63 64 65 66 67 69 70 71 73 74 **P**5 6 7 **S** INTEGRIS Health, Oklahoma City, OK **N** Integris Health, Oklahoma City, OK	23	10	324	11039	228	140874	974	101622	40518	—
⊞ △ MERCY HEALTH CENTER, 4300 West Memorial Road, Zip 73120–8362; tel. 405/755–1515; Bruce F. Buchanan, FACHE, President and Chief Executive Officer **A**1 2 7 9 10 **F**1 3 4 7 8 10 12 15 16 17 18 19 21 22 26 27 28 29 30 31 32 33 34 35 36 39 41 42 43 44 45 49 53 54 56 58 59 60 65 67 71 73 74 **P**4 6 **S** Sisters of Mercy Health System–St. Louis, Saint Louis, MO **N** Mercy Health System, Oklahoma City, OK	21	10	363	11657	191	230442	1933	108188	46038	1553
☐ NORTHWEST SURGICAL HOSPITAL, 9204 North May, Zip 73120; tel. 405/848–1918; Dan Barnard, Chief Executive Officer **A**1 10 **F**20 22 34 44	33	47	9	361	1	2110	0	—	—	21
⊞ △ ST. ANTHONY HOSPITAL, 1000 North Lee Street, Zip 73102, Mailing Address: Box 205, Zip 73101–0205; tel. 405/272–7000; Steven L. Hunter, President **A**1 2 3 5 7 9 10 **F**1 2 3 4 7 8 10 11 12 15 16 17 19 20 21 22 23 25 26 28 29 30 31 32 33 34 35 37 39 40 41 42 43 44 45 48 49 51 52 53 54 55 56 57 58 59 60 61 63 64 65 66 67 69 71 72 73 74 **P**2 3 5 6 7 8 **S** SSM Health Care System, Saint Louis, MO	21	10	445	11434	205	260540	953	115413	44598	1320
⊞ THE UNIVERSITY HOSPITALS, (Includes Children's Hospital of Oklahoma, 940 N.E. 13th Street, Zip 73104; tel. 405/271–6165; University Hospital, Mailing Address: Box 26307, Zip 73126), 920 N.E. 13th Street, Zip 73104–5068, Mailing Address: P.O. Box 26307, Zip 73126; tel. 405/271–5911; R. Timothy Coussons, M.D., President and Chief Executive Officer **A**1 2 3 5 8 9 10 **F**4 7 8 10 11 12 19 20 21 22 26 34 35 37 38 40 41 42 43 44 46 47 52 53 54 58 59 60 61 63 65 69 70 71 73 74 **P**7 **N** University Hospitals, Oklahoma City, OK UNIVERSITY HOSPITAL See The University Hospitals	12	10	309	15208	232	169946	2069	181236	67375	2716
⊞ VETERANS AFFAIRS MEDICAL CENTER, 921 N.E. 13th Street, Zip 73104–5028; tel. 405/270–0501; Steven J. Gentling, Director (Total facility includes 40 beds in nursing home–type unit) **A**1 3 5 8 9 **F**2 3 4 6 8 10 11 12 15 19 20 21 22 23 25 26 27 28 29 30 31 32 34 35 37 39 41 42 43 44 45 46 48 49 51 52 54 56 58 60 63 64 65 67 69 71 73 74 **P**6 **S** Department of Veterans Affairs, Washington, DC	45	10	277	7570	182	256088	0	123518	54294	1379
OKMULGEE—Okmulgee County										
GEORGE NIGH REHABILITATION INSTITUTE, 900 East Airport Road, Zip 74447, Mailing Address: P.O. Box 1118, Zip 74447; tel. 918/756–9211; Mitchell Townsend, Administrator **A**10 **F**15 16 19 21 28 34 35 41 48 49 65 71 73	12	46	26	249	17	4907	0	3941	1986	86
☐ OMH MEDICAL CENTER, 1401 Morris Drive, Zip 74447, Mailing Address: Box 1038, Zip 74447; tel. 918/756–4233; David D. Rasmussen, Administrator (Nonreporting) **A**1 9 10	23	10	66	—	—	—	—	—	—	—
PAULS VALLEY—Garvin County										
☐ PAULS VALLEY GENERAL HOSPITAL, 100 Valley Drive, Zip 73075–0368, Mailing Address: Box 368, Zip 73075–0368; tel. 405/238–5501; Charles Johnston, Administrator (Total facility includes 8 beds in nursing home–type unit) **A**1 9 10 **F**8 19 22 28 32 34 37 39 40 41 44 49 53 58 59 64 65 71	14	10	42	1792	29	13266	93	7865	3877	166
PAWHUSKA—Osage County										
★ PAWHUSKA HOSPITAL, 1101 East 15th Street, Zip 74056; tel. 918/287–3232; Samuel T. Guild, Administrator (Nonreporting) **A**9 10	14	10	19	—	—	—	—	—	—	—
PAWNEE—Pawnee County										
★ PAWNEE MUNICIPAL HOSPITAL, 1212 Fourth Street, Zip 74058, Mailing Address: Box 467, Zip 74058; tel. 918/762–2577; John Ketring, Administrator **A**9 10 **F**8 19 22 28 30 32 34 39 44 71 73 **S** INTEGRIS Health, Oklahoma City, OK **N** Integris Health, Oklahoma City, OK	23	10	40	808	10	5473	1	—	—	90
PERRY—Noble County										
⊞ PERRY MEMORIAL HOSPITAL, 501 14th Street, Zip 73077–5099; tel. 405/336–3541; Judith K. Feuquay, Chief Executive Officer (Nonreporting) **A**1 9 10 **S** Quorum Health Group/Quorum Health Resources, Inc., Brentwood, TN	16	10	28	—	—	—	—	—	—	—
PONCA CITY—Kay County										
⊞ ST. JOSEPH REGIONAL MEDICAL CENTER OF NORTHERN OKLAHOMA, 14th Street and Hartford Avenue, Zip 74601–2035, Mailing Address: Box 1270, Zip 74602–1270; tel. 405/765–3321; Garry L. England, President and Chief Executive Officer (Total facility includes 10 beds in nursing home–type unit) **A**1 9 10 **F**7 8 13 14 15 16 17 19 21 22 23 27 28 30 31 32 33 35 36 37 40 41 42 44 52 54 56 60 63 64 65 67 70 71 73 **P**5 6 7 **S** Via Christi Health System, Wichita, KS **N** Via Christi Health System, Wichita, KS	21	10	88	3704	52	48453	579	24948	10361	430
POTEAU—Le Flore County										
⊞ EASTERN OKLAHOMA MEDICAL CENTER, 105 Wall Street, Zip 74953, Mailing Address: P.O. Box 1148, Zip 74953; tel. 918/647–8161; Bobby D. Cox, Chief Executive Officer **A**1 9 10 **F**7 8 14 15 16 19 20 21 22 23 28 32 33 37 40 42 44 65 71 73 **P**2 3 4 5 6 7 8 **N** Hillcrest Healthcare System, Tulsa, OK	16	10	84	3111	31	15475	413	16662	6724	305

Hospital, Address, Telephone, Administrator, Approval, Facility, and Physician Codes, Health Care System, Network	Classi-fication Codes		Utilization Data					Expense (thousands) of dollars		
	Control	Service	Beds	Admissions	Census	Outpatient Visits	Births	Total	Payroll	Personnel

PRYOR—Mayes County

✚ MAYES COUNTY MEDICAL CENTER, 129 North Kentucky, Zip 74361, Mailing Address: Box 278, Zip 74362–0278; tel. 918/825–1600; W. Charles Jordan, Administrator **A**1 9 10 **F**10 12 16 17 18 19 22 28 32 33 34 41 42 44 46 65 67 70 71 73 **P**6 7 **S** INTEGRIS Health, Oklahoma City, OK **N** Integris Health, Oklahoma City, OK
| 23 | 10 | 37 | 1190 | 14 | — | 102 | 10107 | 5238 | 221 |

PURCELL—McClain County

★ PURCELL MUNICIPAL HOSPITAL, 1500 North Green Avenue, Zip 73080, Mailing Address: P.O. Box 511, Zip 73080–0511; tel. 405/527–6524; Joe Duerr, Administrator **A**9 10 **F**7 12 14 16 17 19 20 22 25 28 30 32 33 39 40 41 44 45 46 48 49 56 64 65 67 71 73 **P**8 **S** Quorum Health Group/Quorum Health Resources, Inc., Brentwood, TN
| 14 | 10 | 22 | 1351 | 14 | 31328 | 98 | 6743 | 2695 | 132 |

SALLISAW—Sequoyah County

SEQUOYAH MEMORIAL HOSPITAL, 213 East Redwood Street, Zip 74955, Mailing Address: Box 505, Zip 74955–0505; tel. 918/774–1100; Ruth Ann Roark, Administrator (Nonreporting) **A**9 10
| 15 | 10 | 50 | — | — | — | — | — | — | — |

SAPULPA—Creek County

☐ BARTLETT MEMORIAL MEDICAL CENTER, 519 South Division Street, Zip 74066, Mailing Address: Box 1368, Zip 74067–1368; tel. 918/224–4280; W. D. Robinson, Chief Executive Officer **A**1 9 10 **F**7 8 15 16 19 20 21 22 25 28 30 32 33 34 37 40 42 44 45 46 48 49 64 65 69 71 73 **P**5
| 23 | 10 | 113 | 2086 | 27 | 12091 | 70 | 13716 | 7889 | 260 |

SAYRE—Beckham County

★ SAYRE MEMORIAL HOSPITAL, 501 East Washington Street, Zip 73662, Mailing Address: Box 680, Zip 73662; tel. 405/928–5541; Larry Anderson, Administrator **A**9 10 **F**7 19 22 30 32 34 40 44 51 65 71 **P**6 **S** Quorum Health Group/Quorum Health Resources, Inc., Brentwood, TN
| 23 | 10 | 46 | 958 | 10 | — | 106 | 5464 | 3053 | 113 |

SEILING—Dewey County

SEILING HOSPITAL, Highway 60 N.E., Zip 73663, Mailing Address: P.O. Box 720, Zip 73663–0720; tel. 405/922–7361; Chris Mattingly, Administrator **A**9 10 **F**15 19 22 28 32 44 65 71 73
| 14 | 10 | 18 | 350 | 5 | — | 0 | 1659 | 891 | 41 |

SEMINOLE—Seminole County

★ SEMINOLE MUNICIPAL HOSPITAL, 606 West Evans Street, Zip 74868, Mailing Address: P.O. Box 2130, Zip 74818–2130; tel. 405/382–0600; Stephen R. Schoaps, Chief Executive Officer **A**9 10 **F**7 14 15 19 22 32 39 41 44 46 49 51 70 71 73 **S** Quorum Health Group/Quorum Health Resources, Inc., Brentwood, TN
| 14 | 10 | 39 | 658 | 7 | 9561 | 1 | 4344 | 2044 | 110 |

SHATTUCK—Ellis County

✚ NEWMAN MEMORIAL HOSPITAL, 905 South Main Street, Zip 73858–9602, Mailing Address: Box 279, Zip 73858–0279; tel. 405/938–2551; Gary W. Mitchell, Chief Executive Officer **A**1 9 10 **F**7 8 15 17 19 22 27 28 30 32 34 35 36 37 40 42 44 49 65 67 70 71 73 74
| 23 | 10 | 27 | 1069 | 12 | 51680 | 104 | 8255 | 3696 | 155 |

SHAWNEE—Pottawatomie County

✚ MISSION HILL MEMORIAL HOSPITAL, 1900 Gordon Cooper Drive, Zip 74801; tel. 405/273–2240; Thomas G. Honaker, III, Administrator **A**1 9 10 **F**7 8 10 15 19 22 25 30 32 33 35 37 39 40 44 49 65 71 73 **P**4 8 **S** Brim, Inc., Portland, OR
| 32 | 10 | 54 | 1563 | 16 | — | 209 | 9130 | 3789 | 167 |

☐ OAK CREST HOSPITAL AND COUNSELING CENTER, 1601 Gordon Cooper Drive, Zip 74801; tel. 405/275–9610; Eugene Suksi, Administrator (Nonreporting) **A**1 10 **S** Sterling Healthcare Corporation, Bellevue, WA
| 33 | 22 | 50 | — | — | — | — | — | — | — |

✚ SHAWNEE REGIONAL HOSPITAL, 1102 West MacArthur, Zip 74801, Mailing Address: Box 909, Zip 74801; tel. 405/273–2270; Robert F. Maynard, Chief Executive Officer **A**1 2 9 10 **F**7 11 15 16 17 19 21 22 26 28 30 32 33 34 35 40 42 44 45 49 60 63 64 65 67 71 73 74
| 23 | 10 | 116 | 3734 | 45 | 42128 | 662 | 23151 | 10025 | 365 |

SPENCER—Oklahoma County

✚ INTEGRIS MENTAL HEALTH SYSTEM–WILLOW VIEW, (Formerly Willow View Mental Health System), 2601 North Spencer Road, Zip 73084–3699, Mailing Address: P.O. Box 11137, Oklahoma City, Zip 73136–0137; tel. 405/427–2441; Gary L. Watson, President and Chief Operating Officer **A**1 10 **F**3 52 53 54 55 56 57 58 59 67 **P**6 **S** INTEGRIS Health, Oklahoma City, OK
WILLOW VIEW MENTAL HEALTH SYSTEM See Integris Mental Health System–Willow View
| 23 | 22 | 44 | 373 | 43 | 18398 | 0 | 7801 | 5079 | 191 |

STIGLER—Haskell County

★ HASKELL COUNTY HEALTHCARE SYSTEM, (Formerly Haskell County Hospital), 401 N.W. H Street, Zip 74462; tel. 918/967–4682; John C. Neal, Administrator and Chief Executive Officer **A**9 10 **F**17 19 25 27 28 30 32 33 34 39 42 44 49 65 70 71 72 73 **P**5
| 13 | 10 | 31 | 635 | 8 | 6579 | 1 | 4966 | 2737 | 114 |

STILLWATER—Payne County

✚ STILLWATER MEDICAL CENTER, 1323 West Sixth Avenue, Zip 74074, Mailing Address: Box 2408, Zip 74076–2408; tel. 405/372–1480; Jerry G. Moeller, President and Chief Executive Officer (Total facility includes 18 beds in nursing home–type unit) **A**1 9 10 **F**8 10 14 15 16 19 20 21 22 23 31 32 33 34 35 36 37 40 42 44 46 49 56 63 64 65 71 73 **P**8
| 16 | 10 | 92 | 4218 | 58 | 57027 | 719 | 33028 | 14331 | 574 |

STROUD—Lincoln County

★ STROUD MUNICIPAL HOSPITAL, Highway 66 West, Zip 74079, Mailing Address: P.O. Box 530, Zip 74079; tel. 918/968–3571; Jerrell J. Horton, Chief Executive Officer **A**9 10 **F**8 15 22 28 30 32 33 34 37 44 71 73 **P**6 7 8 **S** INTEGRIS Health, Oklahoma City, OK **N** Integris Health, Oklahoma City, OK
| 23 | 10 | 17 | 416 | 6 | 5520 | 16 | 3889 | 1849 | 89 |

Hospital, Address, Telephone, Administrator, Approval, Facility, and Physician Codes, Health Care System, Network	Classi-fication Codes			Utilization Data					Expense (thousands) of dollars		
	Control	Service	Beds	Admissions	Census	Outpatient Visits	Births	Total	Payroll	Personnel

★ American Hospital Association (AHA) membership
□ Joint Commission on Accreditation of Healthcare Organizations (JCAHO) accreditation
+ American Osteopathic Hospital Association (AOHA) membership
○ American Osteopathic Association (AOA) accreditation
△ Commission on Accreditation of Rehabilitation Facilities (CARF) accreditation
  Control codes 61, 63, 64, 71, 72 and 73 indicate hospitals listed by AOHA, but not registered by AHA. For definition of numerical codes, see page A4

SULPHUR—Murray County

	Control	Service	Beds	Admissions	Census	Outpatient Visits	Births	Total	Payroll	Personnel
ARBUCKLE MEMORIAL HOSPITAL, 2011 West Broadway, Zip 73086; tel. 405/622–2161; Mike Pruitt, Administrator (Nonreporting) **A**9 10	13	10	58	—	—	—	—	—	—	—

TAHLEQUAH—Cherokee County

	Control	Service	Beds	Admissions	Census	Outpatient Visits	Births	Total	Payroll	Personnel
✉ TAHLEQUAH CITY HOSPITAL, 1400 East Downing Street, Zip 74464, Mailing Address: Box 1008, Zip 74465–1008; tel. 918/456–0641; L. Gene Matthews, Chief Executive Officer **A**1 9 10 **F**7 8 15 16 19 21 22 26 28 30 32 33 35 37 40 44 52 53 57 65 71 73 **P**5 8 **S** Quorum Health Group/Quorum Health Resources, Inc., Brentwood, TN	16	10	63	2192	28	—	248	16556	7165	300
✉ WILLIAM W. HASTINGS INDIAN HOSPITAL, 100 South Bliss Avenue, Zip 74464–3399; tel. 918/458–3100; Hickory Starr, Jr., Administrator **A**1 10 **F**7 8 12 13 15 17 19 20 22 28 31 32 34 37 39 40 44 52 53 54 55 56 57 58 65 71 73 **P**6 **S** U. S. Public Health Service Indian Health Service, Rockville, MD	47	10	60	3154	29	205440	1211	32682	13921	401

TALIHINA—La Flore County

	Control	Service	Beds	Admissions	Census	Outpatient Visits	Births	Total	Payroll	Personnel
✉ CHOCTAW NATION INDIAN HOSPITAL, Route 2, Box 1725, Zip 74571; tel. 918/567–2211; Rosemary Hooser, Acting Administrator **A**1 10 **F**8 20 22 31 40 44 46 58 65 71 **P**6 **S** U. S. Public Health Service Indian Health Service, Rockville, MD	47	10	44	1176	13	46778	238	17877	7209	316

TINKER AFB—De Kalb County

	Control	Service	Beds	Admissions	Census	Outpatient Visits	Births	Total	Payroll	Personnel
✉ U. S. AIR FORCE HOSPITAL TINKER, 5700 Arnold Street, Zip 73145; tel. 405/736–2237; Colonel David D. Bissell, MC, USAF, Commander **A**1 **F**2 3 4 5 7 8 9 10 11 12 13 14 15 16 17 18 19 20 21 22 23 24 25 26 27 28 29 30 31 32 34 35 36 37 38 39 40 41 42 43 44 45 46 47 48 49 50 51 52 53 54 55 56 57 58 59 60 61 62 63 64 65 66 67 68 69 70 71 72 73 74 **P**1 2 3 4 5 6 7 8 **S** Department of the Air Force, Washington, DC	41	10	25	2362	12	220459	537	21594	3405	635

TISHOMINGO—Johnston County

	Control	Service	Beds	Admissions	Census	Outpatient Visits	Births	Total	Payroll	Personnel
JOHNSTON MEMORIAL HOSPITAL, 1101 South Byrd Street, Zip 73460–3299; tel. 405/371–2327; Garry D. Crain, Administrator and Chief Executive Officer **A**9 10 **F**19 22 34 37 40 44 65 71	13	10	30	681	9	3388	17	4407	2146	108

TULSA—Tulsa County

	Control	Service	Beds	Admissions	Census	Outpatient Visits	Births	Total	Payroll	Personnel
△ BROOKHAVEN HOSPITAL, 201 South Garnett Road, Zip 74128; tel. 918/438–4257; Lance Beard, Chief Executive Officer and Administrator (Nonreporting) **A**7 9 10	31	22	40	—	—	—	—	—	—	—
✉ CHILDREN'S MEDICAL CENTER, 5300 East Skelly Drive, Zip 74135–6599, Mailing Address: Box 35648, Zip 74153–0648; tel. 918/664–6600; Gerard J. Rothlein, Jr., President and Chief Executive Officer (Nonreporting) **A**1 3 5 9 10 **N** Hillcrest Healthcare System, Tulsa, OK	23	59	108							
✉ COLUMBIA DOCTORS HOSPITAL, 2323 South Harvard Avenue, Zip 74114–3370; tel. 918/744–4000; Anthony R. Young, President and Chief Executive Officer **A**1 9 10 **F**7 8 12 16 19 21 22 25 26 27 32 33 34 35 37 40 41 44 48 49 52 57 59 64 65 67 71 73 **P**7 **S** Columbia/HCA Healthcare Corporation, Nashville, TN **N** Eastern Oklahoma Health Network, Tulsa, OK; Columbia Oklahoma Division, Inc., Oklahoma City, OK	33	10	148	3377	59	38361	922	27350	8845	333
✉ + ○ △ COLUMBIA TULSA REGIONAL MEDICAL CENTER, 744 West Ninth Street, Zip 74127–9990; tel. 918/599–5900; James M. MacCallum, President and Chief Executive Officer **A**1 7 9 10 11 12 13 **F**4 7 8 10 11 12 17 18 19 21 22 23 26 30 31 32 35 37 38 40 41 42 43 44 46 48 49 52 53 54 55 56 57 58 59 60 61 64 65 67 70 71 72 73 **P**7 8 **S** Columbia/HCA Healthcare Corporation, Nashville, TN **N** Columbia Oklahoma Division, Inc., Oklahoma City, OK	33	10	264	9889	167	98103	844	81234	33622	1231
✉ △ HILLCREST HEALTHCARE SYSTEM, (Formerly Hillcrest Medical Center), 1120 South Utica, Zip 74104–4090; tel. 918/579–1000; Donald A. Lorack, Jr., President and Chief Executive Officer **A**1 2 3 5 7 9 10 **F**2 3 4 7 8 9 10 11 12 13 14 15 16 17 18 19 21 22 23 25 26 27 28 29 30 31 32 33 34 35 37 38 39 40 41 42 43 44 45 46 48 49 51 52 53 54 55 56 57 58 59 60 61 63 64 65 66 67 68 69 70 71 72 73 74 **P**5 6 7 **N** National Cardiovascular Network, Atlanta, GA; Hillcrest Healthcare System, Tulsa, OK; Eastern Oklahoma Health Network, Tulsa, OK	23	10	385	18925	276	81401	3515	145503	56475	1950
✉ LAUREATE PSYCHIATRIC CLINIC AND HOSPITAL, 6655 South Yale, Zip 74136; tel. 918/481–4000; John L. Fleming, M.D., Interim Chief Executive Officer **A**1 3 5 10 **F**3 4 8 10 11 12 13 14 16 17 18 19 22 25 26 27 29 32 33 34 35 37 38 39 40 41 42 43 44 45 47 48 49 52 53 54 55 56 57 58 59 60 64 65 66 67 68 69 70 71 73	23	22	75	1565	34	17501	0	—	—	234
□ MEMORIAL MEDICAL CENTER AND CANCER TREATMENT CENTER–TULSA, 8181 South Lewis, Zip 74137; tel. 918/496–5000; Sandra Jackson, President **A**1 2 10 **F**8 12 14 15 16 19 21 27 28 30 34 35 37 39 42 44 45 46 60 63 67 73 **P**6 **S** Cancer Treatment Centers of America, Arlington Heights, IL	33	10	65	1100	19	21792	0	33282	9458	325
PARKSIDE HOSPITAL, 1620 East 12th Street, Zip 74120–5499; tel. 918/582–2131; Paul Greever, Interim Chief Executive Officer **A**3 5 9 10 **F**1 2 3 12 17 18 25 31 32 39 52 53 54 55 56 57 58 59 65 67 73 **P**6	23	22	55	1115	15	75346	0	11157	6733	217
✉ SAINT FRANCIS HOSPITAL, 6161 South Yale Avenue, Zip 74136–1992; tel. 918/494–2200; C. T. Thompson, M.D., Interim Chief Executive Officer (Total facility includes 30 beds in nursing home–type unit) **A**1 2 3 5 8 9 10 **F**2 3 4 7 8 10 11 12 13 16 17 18 19 20 21 22 23 26 28 29 30 31 32 33 34 35 36 37 38 39 40 41 42 43 44 45 46 47 48 49 51 52 53 54 55 56 57 58 59 60 63 64 65 66 67 68 69 70 71 73 74 **P**4 5 6	23	10	591	28360	408	374691	2896	209902	85291	3354
□ SHADOW MOUNTAIN HOSPITAL, 6262 South Sheridan Road, Zip 74133–4099; tel. 918/492–8200; Nancy J. Cranton, Chief Executive Officer (Nonreporting) **A**1 9 **S** Healthcare America, Inc., Austin, TX	33	52	100	—	—	—	—	—	—	—

Hospital, Address, Telephone, Administrator, Approval, Facility, and Physician Codes, Health Care System, Network	Classi-fication Codes		Utilization Data					Expense (thousands) of dollars		
★ American Hospital Association (AHA) membership □ Joint Commission on Accreditation of Healthcare Organizations (JCAHO) accreditation + American Osteopathic Hospital Association (AOHA) membership ○ American Osteopathic Association (AOA) accreditation △ Commission on Accreditation of Rehabilitation Facilities (CARF) accreditation Control codes 61, 63, 64, 71, 72 and 73 indicate hospitals listed by AOHA, but not registered by AHA. For definition of numerical codes, see page A4	Control	Service	Beds	Admissions	Census	Outpatient Visits	Births	Total	Payroll	Personnel
✠ △ ST. JOHN MEDICAL CENTER, 1923 South Utica Avenue, Zip 74104–5445; tel. 918/744–2345; Sister M. Therese Gottschalk, President **A**1 2 3 5 7 9 10 **F**1 2 3 4 7 8 10 11 12 14 15 16 17 18 19 20 21 22 23 25 26 27 28 29 30 31 32 33 34 35 37 38 39 40 41 42 43 44 45 47 48 49 52 54 55 56 57 58 59 60 64 65 66 67 69 70 71 73 74 **P**3 5 7 **S** Sisters of the Sorrowful Mother United States Health System, Tulsa, OK	21	10	589	20311	365	98445	1858	185207	60904	3208
VINITA—Craig County										
✠ CRAIG GENERAL HOSPITAL, 735 North Foreman Street, Zip 74301–1418, Mailing Address: Box 326, Zip 74301–0326; tel. 918/256–7551; B. Joe Gunn, FACHE, Administrator and Chief Executive Officer **A**1 9 10 **F**7 8 11 12 15 16 19 21 22 28 32 33 40 44 65 71 73	16	10	28	1000	13	19026	100	7783	3435	141
□ EASTERN STATE HOSPITAL, Mailing Address: P.O. Box 69, Zip 74301; tel. 918/256–7841; Karen Steed, Chief Executive Officer **A**1 10 **F**14 15 16 20 22 27 28 29 30 46 55 65 73 **P**6	12	22	350	2018	317	0	0	24850	15200	607
WAGONER—Wagoner County										
✠ COLUMBIA WAGONER HOSPITAL, (Formerly Columbia Wagoner Community Hospital), 1200 West Cherokee, Zip 74467–4681, Mailing Address: Box 407, Zip 74477–0407; tel. 918/485–5514; John W. Crawford, Chief Executive Officer **A**1 9 10 **F**7 8 12 14 15 16 19 20 21 22 26 28 29 30 31 32 34 37 39 40 42 44 45 46 49 51 52 53 54 55 56 58 65 71 73 74 **P**7 8 **S** Columbia/HCA Healthcare Corporation, Nashville, TN **N** Eastern Oklahoma Health Network, Tulsa, OK; Columbia Oklahoma Division, Inc., Oklahoma City, OK	33	10	100	2536	40	12739	45	20958	8987	252
WATONGA—Blaine County										
★ WATONGA MUNICIPAL HOSPITAL, 500 North Nash Boulevard, Zip 73772–0370, Mailing Address: Box 370, Zip 73772–0370; tel. 405/623–7211; Terry Buckner, Administrator (Nonreporting) **A**9 10 **S** Quorum Health Group/Quorum Health Resources, Inc., Brentwood, TN	16	10	24	—	—	—	—	—	—	—
WAURIKA—Jefferson County										
★ JEFFERSON COUNTY HOSPITAL, Mailing Address: P.O. Box 90, Zip 73573–0090; tel. 405/228–2344; Curtis R. Pryor, Administrator (Nonreporting) **A**9 10 **N** First Health West, Lawton, OK	13	10	28	—	—	—	—	—	—	—
WEATHERFORD—Custer County										
★ SOUTHWESTERN MEMORIAL HOSPITAL, 215 North Kansas Street, Zip 73096–5499; tel. 405/772–5551; Ronnie D. Walker, President **A**9 10 **F**7 8 15 19 28 34 35 44 71 73 **N** First Health West, Lawton, OK	16	10	46	845	7	6906	176	4468	2007	80
WETUMKA—Hughes County										
WETUMKA GENERAL HOSPITAL, 325 South Washita, Zip 74883–5500; tel. 405/452–3276; Carolyn Keesee, Chief Executive Officer **A**9 10 **F**3 15 16 17 22 28 34 64 71	16	10	22	363	8	4512	1	3075	1789	86
WILBURTON—Latimer County										
LATIMER COUNTY GENERAL HOSPITAL, 806 Highway 2 North, Zip 74578; tel. 918/465–2391; Jack Martin, Administrator **A**9 10 **F**14 22 32 44 71 73	13	10	33	543	6	—	0	3209	1735	83
WOODWARD—Woodward County										
✠ WOODWARD HOSPITAL AND HEALTH CENTER, 900 17th Street, Zip 73801; tel. 405/256–5511; Warren K. Spellman, Administrator **A**1 9 10 **F**2 3 7 8 11 12 15 16 17 19 21 22 26 28 30 32 33 35 37 39 40 41 42 44 45 46 48 49 52 57 64 65 66 67 71 72 73 **P**3 4 7 8 **S** Quorum Health Group/Quorum Health Resources, Inc., Brentwood, TN	23	10	68	1698	29	18993	197	15482	6821	275

OREGON

Resident population 3,141 (in thousands)
Resident population in metro areas 70.1%
Birth rate per 1,000 population 13.7
65 years and over 13.6%
Percent of persons without health insurance 13.1%

Hospital, Address, Telephone, Administrator, Approval, Facility, and Physician Codes, Health Care System, Network	Classi-fication Codes		Utilization Data					Expense (thousands) of dollars		
★ American Hospital Association (AHA) membership □ Joint Commission on Accreditation of Healthcare Organizations (JCAHO) accreditation + American Osteopathic Hospital Association (AOHA) membership ○ American Osteopathic Association (AOA) accreditation △ Commission on Accreditation of Rehabilitation Facilities (CARF) accreditation Control codes 61, 63, 64, 71, 72 and 73 indicate hospitals listed by AOHA, but not registered by AHA. For definition of numerical codes, see page A4	Control	Service	Beds	Admissions	Census	Outpatient Visits	Births	Total	Payroll	Personnel

ALBANY—Linn County
☒ ALBANY GENERAL HOSPITAL, 1046 West Sixth Avenue, Zip 97321–1999; tel. 541/812–4000; Richard J. Delano, President **A**1 2 9 10 **F**7 8 15 17 19 21 22 28 29 30 32 33 34 35 37 39 40 41 42 44 46 49 54 59 60 65 67 68 70 71 72 73 **P**5 6 **N** Inter Community Health Network, Corvallis, OR; Health Future, Inc., Medford, OR
| | | 23 | 10 | 71 | 3384 | 30 | 40015 | 668 | 25462 | 11157 | 394 |

ASHLAND—Jackson County
□ ASHLAND COMMUNITY HOSPITAL, 280 Maple Street, Zip 97520, Mailing Address: P.O. Box 98, Zip 97520; tel. 541/482–2441; James R. Watson, Administrator **A**1 9 10 **F**7 8 15 16 19 22 28 30 32 34 36 37 40 41 44 45 46 64 66 70 71 **P**5 **N** Health Future, Inc., Medford, OR
| | | 14 | 10 | 37 | 1429 | 14 | 26675 | 307 | 12973 | 6062 | 193 |

ASTORIA—Clatsop County
☒ COLUMBIA MEMORIAL HOSPITAL, 2111 Exchange Street, Zip 97103; tel. 503/325–4321; Terry O. Finklein, Chief Executive Officer **A**1 9 10 **F**7 8 17 19 21 22 30 32 33 34 37 39 40 41 42 44 49 65 70 71 73 74 **N** Health Future, Inc., Medford, OR
| | | 23 | 10 | 37 | 2375 | 19 | 45196 | 362 | 15817 | 7327 | 236 |

BAKER CITY—Baker County
□ ST. ELIZABETH HEALTH SERVICES, 3325 Pocahontas Road, Zip 97814; tel. 541/523–6461; Robert T. Mannix, Jr., President and Chief Operations Officer (Total facility includes 98 beds in nursing home–type unit) **A**1 9 10 **F**7 8 12 14 19 21 22 26 28 30 32 34 35 37 40 41 44 46 49 64 65 67 70 71 **P**5 **S** Catholic Health Initiatives, Denver, CO
| | | 21 | 10 | 134 | 1462 | 78 | 44471 | 114 | 13257 | 5842 | 208 |

BANDON—Coos County
★ SOUTHERN COOS GENERAL HOSPITAL, 640 West Fourth, Zip 97411; tel. 541/347–2426; James A. Wathen, Chief Executive Officer **A**9 10 **F**8 14 15 20 22 32 34 44 49 65 71
| | | 16 | 10 | 18 | 166 | 2 | 6970 | 0 | 1880 | 915 | 38 |

BEND—Deschutes County
☒ ST. CHARLES MEDICAL CENTER, 2500 N.E. Neff Road, Zip 97701–6015; tel. 541/382–4321; James T. Lussier, President and Chief Executive Officer (Nonreporting) **A**1 2 3 9 10 **N** Central Oregon Hosp Network (CONET), Bend, OR; Health Future, Inc., Medford, OR
| | | 23 | 10 | 181 | — | — | — | — | — | — | — |

BURNS—Harney County
HARNEY DISTRICT HOSPITAL, 557 West Washington Street, Zip 97720–1497; tel. 503/573–7281; David L. Harman, Administrator **A**9 10 **F**7 11 17 19 22 28 29 30 34 37 40 44 70 71 **P**5 8 **N** Central Oregon Hosp Network (CONET), Bend, OR
| | | 16 | 10 | 36 | 453 | 3 | 12824 | 51 | 3937 | 1737 | 58 |

CLACKAMAS—Clackamas County
☒ KAISER SUNNYSIDE MEDICAL CENTER, (Formerly Kaiser Foundation Hospital), 10200 S.E. Sunnyside Road, Zip 97015–9303; tel. 503/652–2880; Alide Chase, Administrator **A**1 2 10 **F**3 4 7 8 10 19 21 22 23 26 29 30 31 32 33 34 35 37 40 41 42 43 44 45 49 53 54 55 56 57 58 59 60 61 65 66 69 71 72 73 **P**6 **S** Kaiser Foundation Hospitals, Oakland, CA **N** Oregon Health System in Collaboration, Lake Oswego, OR
| | | 23 | 10 | 174 | 12462 | 119 | 213015 | 1885 | — | — | 1170 |

COOS BAY—Coos County
☒ BAY AREA HOSPITAL, 1775 Thompson Road, Zip 97420–2198; tel. 541/269–8111; Dale Jessup, President and Chief Executive Officer **A**1 2 9 10 **F**7 11 12 14 16 17 19 21 22 23 28 29 30 31 32 33 35 37 40 41 42 44 45 46 49 52 53 54 56 58 59 60 65 67 70 71 72 73 **P**5 **N** Health Future, Inc., Medford, OR
| | | 16 | 10 | 114 | 7111 | 72 | 49780 | 528 | 47061 | 23561 | 634 |

COQUILLE—Coos County
COQUILLE VALLEY HOSPITAL, 940 East Fifth Street, Zip 97423; tel. 503/396–3101; Edna J. Cotner, Administrator **A**9 10 **F**7 8 22 32 34 40 44 71
| | | 16 | 10 | 30 | 341 | 2 | 9740 | 72 | 3220 | 1315 | 54 |

CORVALLIS—Benton County
☒ GOOD SAMARITAN HOSPITAL CORVALLIS, 3600 N.W. Samaritan Drive, Zip 97330, Mailing Address: P.O. Box 1068, Zip 97339; tel. 541/757–5111; Larry A. Mullins, President and Chief Executive Officer **A**1 2 9 10 **F**4 7 8 10 12 14 15 16 17 19 20 21 22 23 29 30 31 32 34 35 37 39 40 41 42 43 44 45 49 51 52 54 55 56 57 58 60 61 62 63 65 66 67 70 71 73 74 **N** Inter Community Health Network, Corvallis, OR; Health Future, Inc., Medford, OR
| | | 23 | 10 | 124 | 6236 | 67 | 126822 | 1127 | 59159 | 28663 | 685 |

COTTAGE GROVE—Lane County
☒ COTTAGE GROVE HEALTHCARE COMMUNITY, (Formerly Cottage Grove Hospital), 1340 Birch Avenue, Zip 97424; tel. 541/942–0511; William N. Wilber, Chief Executive Officer (Total facility includes 40 beds in nursing home–type unit) **A**1 9 10 **F**8 11 12 19 21 22 26 32 33 34 39 40 41 49 50 65 67 70 71 73 **P**3 6 **S** Brim, Inc., Portland, OR
| | | 23 | 10 | 67 | 1278 | 45 | 51881 | 153 | 11694 | 6281 | 366 |

DALLAS—Polk County
□ VALLEY COMMUNITY HOSPITAL, 550 S.E. Clay Street, Zip 97338, Mailing Address: P.O. Box 378, Zip 97338; tel. 503/623–8301; Stephen A. Bowles, President **A**1 9 10 **F**2 3 7 8 11 12 14 15 16 17 19 21 22 23 28 29 30 34 35 39 40 41 44 45 46 49 65 66 67 70 71 73 **P**5 7
| | | 23 | 10 | 44 | 1229 | 12 | 25170 | 178 | 11170 | 6081 | 188 |

Hospital, Address, Telephone, Administrator, Approval, Facility, and Physician Codes, Health Care System, Network	Classi- fication Codes		Utilization Data					Expense (thousands) of dollars		
★ American Hospital Association (AHA) membership ☐ Joint Commission on Accreditation of Healthcare Organizations (JCAHO) accreditation + American Osteopathic Hospital Association (AOHA) membership ○ American Osteopathic Association (AOA) accreditation △ Commission on Accreditation of Rehabilitation Facilities (CARF) accreditation Control codes 61, 63, 64, 71, 72 and 73 indicate hospitals listed by AOHA, but not registered by AHA. For definition of numerical codes, see page A4	Control	Service	Beds	Admissions	Census	Outpatient Visits	Births	Total	Payroll	Personnel

ENTERPRISE—Wallowa County

★ WALLOWA MEMORIAL HOSPITAL, 401 East First Street, Zip 97828, Mailing Address: P.O. Box 460, Zip 97828; tel. 541/426–3111; Kim Dahlman, Chief Executive Officer (Total facility includes 32 beds in nursing home–type unit) (Nonreporting) **A**9 10 — 16 10 55 — — — — — — —

EUGENE—Lane County

⊞ △ SACRED HEART MEDICAL CENTER, 1255 Hilyard Street, Zip 97401, Mailing Address: P.O. Box 10905, Zip 97440; tel. 541/686–7300; Andrew R. McCulloch, Administrator **A**1 2 7 9 10 **F**4 7 10 11 12 15 16 17 19 22 26 29 30 32 33 34 35 37 38 39 40 41 42 43 44 48 49 52 54 55 56 57 58 64 65 66 67 70 71 73 74 **P**6 **S** PeaceHealth, Bellevue, WA **N** PeaceHealth, Bellevue, WA — 21 10 412 18987 230 265112 2639 182696 72035 2064

SERENITY LANE, 616 East 16th, Zip 97401; tel. 541/687–1110; Neil H. McNaughton, Executive Director and Administrator (Nonreporting) — 23 82 55 — — — — — — —

FLORENCE—Lane County

⊞ PEACE HARBOR HOSPITAL, 400 Ninth Street, Zip 97439, Mailing Address: P.O. Box 580, Zip 97439; tel. 541/997–8412; James Barnhart, Administrator **A**1 9 10 **F**7 8 14 15 16 19 21 22 30 32 33 35 37 40 44 45 49 65 70 71 73 **P**6 **S** PeaceHealth, Bellevue, WA **N** PeaceHealth, Bellevue, WA — 21 10 21 1245 12 22144 94 12199 6227 231

FOREST GROVE—Washington County

⊞ TUALITY FOREST GROVE HOSPITAL, 1809 Maple Street, Zip 97116–1995; tel. 503/357–2173; Dick Stenson, Administrator **A**1 9 10 **F**3 7 8 10 12 13 14 16 17 19 21 22 23 24 25 26 27 28 29 32 33 34 35 37 39 40 41 42 44 45 49 52 57 58 59 64 65 66 67 71 72 73 74 **P**1 7 — 23 10 48 1131 6 41257 330 10520 4224 146

GOLD BEACH—Curry County

CURRY GENERAL HOSPITAL, 94220 Fourth Street, Zip 97444–9990; tel. 541/247–6621; Randall J. Scholten, Chief Executive Officer (Nonreporting) **A**9 10 — 12 10 24 — — — — — — —

GRANTS PASS—Josephine County

⊞ THREE RIVERS COMMUNITY HOSPITAL AND HEALTH CENTER–DIMMICK, 715 N.W. Dimmick Street, Zip 97526–1596; tel. 541/476–6831; John F. Bringhurst, Executive Vice President **A**1 9 10 **F**7 8 11 15 16 17 19 21 22 23 24 28 29 30 32 33 34 35 37 40 41 44 45 46 49 51 54 56 65 67 68 70 71 72 73 **P**3 6 7 **S** Asante Health System, Medford, OR **N** Health Future, Inc., Medford, OR — 23 10 87 3156 26 86649 658 22974 11457 310

☐ THREE RIVERS COMMUNITY HOSPITAL AND HEALTH CENTER–WASHINGTON, 1505 N.W. Washington Boulevard, Zip 97526; tel. 541/479–7531; John F. Bringhurst, Executive Vice President **A**1 9 10 **F**7 8 11 15 16 17 19 21 22 24 29 30 32 33 34 35 37 41 44 45 46 47 49 51 54 56 65 67 68 70 71 72 73 **P**3 6 — 23 10 63 2908 29 59368 0 20311 9731 304

GRESHAM—Multnomah County

⊞ LEGACY MOUNT HOOD MEDICAL CENTER, 24800 S.E. Stark, Zip 97030–0154; tel. 503/667–1122; Jane C. Cummins, President and Chief Executive Officer **A**1 9 10 **F**2 3 7 8 15 17 19 21 22 27 28 30 32 33 35 37 40 41 42 44 45 46 49 60 65 67 71 73 74 **S** Legacy Health System, Portland, OR **N** Oregon Health System in Collaboration, Lake Oswego, OR; Legacy Health System, Portland, OR — 23 10 97 3761 38 40126 598 28619 13035 341

HEPPNER—Linn County

PIONEER MEMORIAL HOSPITAL, 564 East Pioneer Drive, Zip 97836, Mailing Address: P.O. Box 9, Zip 97836; tel. 503/676–9133; Kevin R. Erich, Administrator (Nonreporting) **A**9 10 **S** Adventist Health, Roseville, CA — 16 10 40 — — — — — — —

HERMISTON—Umatilla County

⊞ GOOD SHEPHERD COMMUNITY HOSPITAL, 610 N.W. 11th Street, Zip 97838–9696; tel. 541/567–6483; Dennis E. Burke, Chief Executive Officer **A**1 9 10 **F**7 8 14 15 16 19 22 28 30 32 34 35 37 44 45 46 65 67 70 71 73 **P**5 **N** Health Future, Inc., Medford, OR — 23 10 45 2243 20 36293 440 15864 6815 223

HILLSBORO—Washington County

⊞ TUALITY COMMUNITY HOSPITAL, 335 S.E. Eighth Avenue, Zip 97123, Mailing Address: P.O. Box 309, Zip 97123; tel. 503/681–1111; Richard Stenson, President (Total facility includes 22 beds in nursing home–type unit) **A**1 9 10 **F**7 8 10 12 13 14 16 17 19 21 22 23 24 25 26 27 28 29 30 32 33 34 35 37 39 40 41 42 44 45 49 52 57 58 59 64 65 66 67 71 72 73 74 **P**1 7 — 23 10 129 6281 67 78114 921 50056 15309 492

HOOD RIVER—Hood River County

⊞ HOOD RIVER MEMORIAL HOSPITAL, 13th and May Streets, Zip 97031, Mailing Address: P.O. Box 149, Zip 97031; tel. 541/386–3911; Tim Simmons, Administrator (Nonreporting) **A**1 9 10 — 23 10 21 — — — — — — —

JOHN DAY—Grant County

★ BLUE MOUNTAIN HOSPITAL, 170 Ford Road, Zip 97845; tel. 541/575–1311; David G. Triebes, Administrator (Total facility includes 52 beds in nursing home–type unit) **A**9 10 **F**1 7 8 11 17 19 28 30 34 37 39 40 44 45 48 49 56 64 65 66 67 68 70 71 **P**5 8 **S** Brim, Inc., Portland, OR **N** Central Oregon Hosp Network (CONET), Bend, OR — 16 10 83 529 43 15027 76 6060 2900 67

KLAMATH FALLS—Klamath County

⊞ MERLE WEST MEDICAL CENTER, 2865 Daggett Street, Zip 97601–1180; tel. 541/882–6311; Paul R. Stewart, President and Chief Executive Officer (Total facility includes 108 beds in nursing home–type unit) **A**1 2 3 9 10 **F**4 6 7 8 10 11 12 15 16 17 19 20 21 22 23 27 28 30 31 32 34 35 40 41 42 44 49 51 52 56 58 60 62 63 64 65 66 67 70 71 72 73 **N** Health Future, Inc., Medford, OR — 23 10 239 6878 156 154930 879 64722 32725 993

LA GRANDE—Union County

⊞ GRANDE RONDE HOSPITAL, 900 Sunset Drive, Zip 97850, Mailing Address: P.O. Box 3290, Zip 97850; tel. 541/963–8421; James A. Mattes, President (Total facility includes 14 beds in nursing home–type unit) **A**1 9 10 **F**7 8 11 15 16 17 19 21 22 26 28 30 32 33 34 35 39 40 44 45 46 49 53 54 55 56 57 58 59 63 64 65 67 70 71 73 **P**3 5 8 **N** Health Future, Inc., Medford, OR — 23 10 63 2302 26 36212 361 19228 9274 278

Hospital, Address, Telephone, Administrator, Approval, Facility, and Physician Codes, Health Care System, Network	Classification Codes		Utilization Data					Expense (thousands) of dollars		
	Control	Service	Beds	Admissions	Census	Outpatient Visits	Births	Total	Payroll	Personnel

★ American Hospital Association (AHA) membership
□ Joint Commission on Accreditation of Healthcare Organizations (JCAHO) accreditation
+ American Osteopathic Hospital Association (AOHA) membership
○ American Osteopathic Association (AOA) accreditation
△ Commission on Accreditation of Rehabilitation Facilities (CARF) accreditation
Control codes 61, 63, 64, 71, 72 and 73 indicate hospitals listed by AOHA, but not registered by AHA. For definition of numerical codes, see page A4

LAKEVIEW—Lake County

LAKE DISTRICT HOSPITAL, 700 South J Street, Zip 97630–1679; tel. 503/947–2114; Richard T. Moore, Administrator (Total facility includes 47 beds in nursing home-type unit) (Nonreporting) **A**9 10 **N** Central Oregon Hosp Network (CONET), Bend, OR
16 10 68 — — — — — — —

LEBANON—Linn County

✠ LEBANON COMMUNITY HOSPITAL, 525 North Santiam Highway, Zip 97355, Mailing Address: P.O. Box 739, Zip 97355–0739; tel. 541/258–2101; Alan R. Yordy, Chief Executive Officer **A**1 9 10 **F**7 8 14 15 17 19 22 24 28 29 32 33 34 35 37 40 41 44 49 65 67 70 71 73 **P**3 4 6 **N** Inter Community Health Network, Corvallis, OR; Health Future, Inc., Medford, OR
23 10 49 3323 32 69884 345 20469 10443 395

LINCOLN CITY—Lincoln County

✠ NORTH LINCOLN HOSPITAL, 3043 N.E. 28th Street, Zip 97367–4523, Mailing Address: P.O. Box 767, Zip 97367–0767; tel. 541/994–3661; Eric Buckland, Administrator **A**1 9 10 **F**7 8 19 21 22 23 32 33 35 37 40 41 44 49 70 71 73 **P**5 6
16 10 28 1305 12 70128 174 17547 9057 267

MADRAS—Jefferson County

★ MOUNTAIN VIEW HOSPITAL DISTRICT, 470 N.E. A Street, Zip 97741; tel. 541/475–3882; Ronald W. Barnes, Executive Director (Total facility includes 68 beds in nursing home–type unit) **A**9 10 **F**1 7 14 15 16 19 21 22 28 30 31 32 33 35 37 40 41 44 45 51 64 70 71 **P**5 **S** Brim, Inc., Portland, OR **N** Central Oregon Hosp Network (CONET), Bend, OR
16 10 102 1169 55 16936 192 9512 4937 163

MCMINNVILLE—Yamhill County

✠ COLUMBIA WILLAMETTE VALLEY MEDICAL CENTER, 2700 Three Mile Lane, Zip 97128–6498; tel. 503/472–6131; Rosemari Davis, Chief Executive Officer (Nonreporting) **A**1 9 10 **S** Columbia/HCA Healthcare Corporation, Nashville, TN
33 10 61 — — — — — — —

MEDFORD—Jackson County

✠ PROVIDENCE MEDFORD MEDICAL CENTER, 1111 Crater Lake Avenue, Zip 97504–6241; tel. 541/732–5000; Charles T. Wright, Chief Executive, Southern Oregon Service Area (Nonreporting) **A**1 2 9 10 **S** Sisters of Providence Health System, Seattle, WA **N** Oregon Health System in Collaboration, Lake Oswego, OR; Providence Health System, Portland, OR
21 10 140 — — — — — — —

✠ ROGUE VALLEY MEDICAL CENTER, 2825 East Barnett Road, Zip 97504–8332; tel. 541/608–4900; Gary A. Sherwood, Executive Vice President **A**1 2 9 10 **F**2 3 4 7 10 11 12 14 15 16 17 19 21 22 23 26 27 28 29 30 31 32 33 34 35 37 38 39 40 41 42 43 44 45 46 47 49 51 52 56 57 60 64 65 67 69 70 71 73 74 **P**6 **S** Asante Health System, Medford, OR **N** Health Future, Inc., Medford, OR
23 10 249 11429 144 321939 1650 97595 47517 1390

MILWAUKIE—Clackamas County

✠ PROVIDENCE MILWAUKIE HOSPITAL, 10150 S.E. 32nd Avenue, Zip 97222–6593; tel. 503/652–8300; Janice Burger, Operations Administrator **A**1 2 9 10 **F**1 2 3 4 5 7 8 9 10 11 15 16 17 19 20 22 23 24 26 29 31 32 33 34 35 37 38 39 40 41 42 43 44 47 48 49 51 52 53 56 57 58 60 64 65 66 67 69 70 71 72 73 74 **P**5 **S** Sisters of Providence Health System, Seattle, WA **N** Oregon Health System in Collaboration, Lake Oswego, OR; Providence Health System, Portland, OR
21 10 50 2684 22 159461 419 24452 10110 265

NEWBERG—Yamhill County

✠ PROVIDENCE NEWBERG HOSPITAL, 501 Villa Road, Zip 97132; tel. 503/537–1555; Mark W. Meinert, CHE, Chief Executive, Yamhill Service Area **A**1 9 10 **F**1 7 8 11 12 13 14 15 16 17 19 21 22 26 27 29 32 39 40 41 42 44 65 67 70 71 72 73 **P**4 5 6 **S** Sisters of Providence Health System, Seattle, WA **N** Oregon Health System in Collaboration, Lake Oswego, OR; Providence Health System, Portland, OR
21 10 35 1278 10 64334 257 13886 6486 153

NEWPORT—Lincoln County

✠ PACIFIC COMMUNITIES HOSPITAL, 930 S.W. Abbey Street, Zip 97365–4820, Mailing Address: P.O. Box 945, Zip 97365–4820; tel. 541/265–2244; Michael R. Fraser, Administrator **A**1 9 10 **F**7 8 12 14 19 21 22 23 25 32 33 35 37 39 40 41 44 46 49 63 64 65 67 70 71 **P**6
16 10 41 1876 16 66936 179 18224 8653 248

ONTARIO—Malheur County

✠ HOLY ROSARY MEDICAL CENTER, 351 S.W. Ninth Street, Zip 97914–2693; tel. 541/881–7000; Bruce Jensen, President and Chief Executive Officer **A**1 9 10 **F**7 8 11 15 16 19 21 22 30 31 32 35 40 42 44 45 46 48 49 63 65 66 70 71 73 **P**5 **S** Catholic Health Initiatives, Denver, CO
23 10 74 3815 35 67178 692 25920 10833 382

OREGON CITY—Clackamas County

✠ WILLAMETTE FALLS HOSPITAL, 1500 Division Street, Zip 97045–1597; tel. 503/656–1631; Robert A. Steed, Administrator **A**1 2 9 10 **F**7 8 12 15 19 21 22 25 29 30 32 33 34 35 37 39 40 41 42 44 45 49 51 60 65 66 71 72 73 **P**5 8
23 10 91 5613 40 49798 1067 42020 20011 417

PENDLETON—Umatilla County

EASTERN OREGON PSYCHIATRIC CENTER, 2575 Westgate, Zip 97801; tel. 541/276–4511; Steve Shambaugh, Superintendent (Nonreporting) **A**10
12 22 60 — — — — — — —

✠ ST. ANTHONY HOSPITAL, 1601 S.E. Court Avenue, Zip 97801–3297; tel. 541/276–5121; Jeffrey S. Drop, President and Chief Executive Officer **A**1 2 9 10 **F**7 8 11 12 17 19 20 21 22 28 31 32 33 39 40 41 42 44 46 49 51 65 67 70 71 73 **P**5 **S** Catholic Health Initiatives, Denver, CO
21 10 49 1868 17 28077 441 17274 6672 273

PORTLAND—Multnomah County

✠ ADVENTIST MEDICAL CENTER, 10123 S.E. Market, Zip 97216–2599; tel. 503/257–2500; Larry D. Dodds, President **A**1 2 5 9 10 **F**1 3 4 7 8 10 12 14 15 16 17 19 21 22 23 24 26 28 29 30 32 33 34 35 37 39 40 41 44 45 46 49 52 53 54 55 56 57 58 59 60 61 65 66 67 71 72 73 74 **P**5 6 7 **S** Adventist Health, Roseville, CA
21 10 270 9065 96 118306 1620 98920 44279 1381

DOERNBECHER CHILDREN'S HOSPITAL See University Hospital

Hospital, Address, Telephone, Administrator, Approval, Facility, and Physician Codes, Health Care System, Network	Classi-fication Codes		Utilization Data					Expense (thousands) of dollars		
	Control	Service	Beds	Admissions	Census	Outpatient Visits	Births	Total	Payroll	Personnel

○ EASTMORELAND HOSPITAL, 2900 S.E. Steele Street, Zip 97202; tel. 503/234–0411; Ken Giles, Administrator (Nonreporting) **A**9 10 11 12 13 **S** TENET Healthcare Corporation, Santa Barbara, CA	33	10	77	—	—	—	—	—	—	—
GOOD SAMARITAN HOSPITAL AND MEDICAL CENTER See Legacy Good Samaritan Hospital and Medical Center										
✠ △ LEGACY EMANUEL HOSPITAL AND HEALTH CENTER, 2801 North Gantenbein Avenue, Zip 97227–1674; tel. 503/413–2200; Lowell W. Johnson, Interim President and Chief Executive Officer **A**1 3 5 7 9 10 **F**1 2 3 4 7 8 9 10 11 12 13 14 16 17 19 21 22 23 24 25 26 28 29 30 31 32 33 34 35 37 38 39 40 41 42 43 44 45 46 47 48 49 51 52 53 54 56 57 58 59 60 61 63 64 65 66 67 69 70 71 72 73 74 **S** Legacy Health System, Portland, OR **N** Oregon Health System in Collaboration, Lake Oswego, OR; Legacy Health System, Portland, OR	23	10	411	17108	242	190743	2063	176985	79320	2059
✠ LEGACY GOOD SAMARITAN HOSPITAL AND MEDICAL CENTER, (Includes Good Samaritan Hospital and Medical Center, Rehabilitation Institute of Oregon), 1015 N.W. 22nd Avenue, Zip 97210; tel. 503/413–7711; Lowell W. Johnson, Interim President and Chief Executive Officer **A**1 2 3 5 9 10 **F**1 2 3 4 7 8 9 10 11 12 13 14 16 17 19 21 22 23 24 25 26 28 29 30 31 32 33 34 35 37 38 39 40 41 42 43 44 45 46 47 48 49 51 52 53 54 56 57 58 59 60 61 63 64 65 66 67 69 70 71 72 73 74 **S** Legacy Health System, Portland, OR **N** Oregon Health System in Collaboration, Lake Oswego, OR; Legacy Health System, Portland, OR	23	10	305	11818	153	259949	1684	147127	61442	1558
□ PACIFIC GATEWAY HOSPITAL AND COUNSELING CENTER, 1345 S.E. Harney, Zip 97202; tel. 503/234–5353; W. Michael Johnson, Executive Director (Nonreporting) **A**1 9 10 **S** Sterling Healthcare Corporation, Bellevue, WA	33	22	66	—	—	—	—	—	—	—
✠ △ PROVIDENCE PORTLAND MEDICAL CENTER, 4805 N.E. Glisan Street, Zip 97213–2967; tel. 503/215–1111; David T. Underriner, Operations Administrator (Total facility includes 20 beds in nursing home–type unit) **A**1 2 3 5 7 9 10 **F**1 3 4 5 6 7 8 10 11 12 13 14 15 16 17 18 19 21 22 23 24 26 27 28 29 30 32 33 34 37 38 39 40 41 42 43 44 45 48 49 51 52 53 54 55 56 57 58 59 60 61 62 64 65 66 67 69 71 72 73 74 **P**5 6 **S** Sisters of Providence Health System, Seattle, WA **N** Oregon Health System in Collaboration, Lake Oswego, OR; Providence Health System, Portland, OR	21	10	420	19589	209	770552	2112	186001	75808	2201
✠ PROVIDENCE ST. VINCENT MEDICAL CENTER, 9205 S.W. Barnes Road, Zip 97225–6661; tel. 503/216–1234; Donald Elsom, Operations Administrator **A**1 2 3 5 9 10 **F**1 2 3 4 5 7 8 10 11 12 13 14 15 16 17 18 19 21 22 23 24 25 26 29 30 31 32 33 34 35 37 38 39 40 41 42 43 44 45 46 48 49 51 52 53 54 56 58 59 60 62 63 64 65 66 67 71 72 73 74 **P**4 5 6 **S** Sisters of Providence Health System, Seattle, WA **N** Oregon Health System in Collaboration, Lake Oswego, OR; Providence Health System, Portland, OR	21	10	451	24526	273	488437	4391	229745	92373	2927
REHABILITATION INSTITUTE OF OREGON See Legacy Good Samaritan Hospital and Medical Center										
✠ SHRINERS HOSPITALS FOR CHILDREN, PORTLAND, 3101 S.W. Sam Jackson Park Road, Zip 97201; tel. 503/241–5090; Nancy Jones, Administrator **A**1 3 5 **F**17 34 39 47 49 73 **P**1 6 **S** Shriners Hospitals for Children, Tampa, FL	23	57	25	1205	14	9192	0	—	—	251
✠ UNIVERSITY HOSPITAL, (Includes Doernbecher Children's Hospital, University Hospital), 3181 S.W. Sam Jackson Park Road, Zip 97201–3098; tel. 503/494–8311; Roy G. Vinyard, Chief Administrative Officer **A**1 2 3 5 8 9 10 **F**2 3 4 5 7 8 9 10 11 12 13 15 16 17 18 19 20 21 22 23 25 26 28 29 30 31 32 33 34 35 37 38 39 40 41 42 43 44 45 46 47 48 49 51 52 53 54 55 56 57 58 60 61 63 64 65 66 67 69 70 71 73 74 **P**1 6 7 8 **N** Health Future, Inc., Medford, OR	16	10	380	19075	279	355511	2206	292886	118011	3197
✠ VETERANS AFFAIRS MEDICAL CENTER, 3710 S.W. U.S. Veterans Hospital Road, Zip 97201; tel. 503/220–8262; William Galey, M.D., Chief Executive Officer (Total facility includes 120 beds in nursing home–type unit) (Nonreporting) **A**1 2 3 5 8 **S** Department of Veterans Affairs, Washington, DC	45	10	591	—	—	—	—	—	—	—
□ WOODLAND PARK HOSPITAL, 10300 N.E. Hancock, Zip 97220; tel. 503/257–5500; Jack Dusenbery, Chief Executive Officer (Nonreporting) **A**1 9 10 **S** TENET Healthcare Corporation, Santa Barbara, CA	33	10	123	—	—	—	—	—	—	—
PRINEVILLE—Crook County										
PIONEER MEMORIAL HOSPITAL, 1201 North Elm Street, Zip 97754; tel. 541/447–6254; Donald J. Wee, Executive Director **A**9 10 **F**7 8 15 16 17 28 29 30 32 33 34 37 39 40 44 49 65 67 70 71 74 **P**5 8 **S** Lutheran Health Systems, Fargo, ND **N** Central Oregon Hosp Network (CONET), Bend, OR	23	10	30	918	9	11702	74	8569	3964	119
REDMOND—Deschutes County										
✠ CENTRAL OREGON DISTRICT HOSPITAL, 1253 North Canal Boulevard, Zip 97756–1395; tel. 541/548–8131; James A. Diegel, CHE, Executive Director **A**1 9 10 **F**7 8 11 12 15 16 17 19 21 22 28 29 32 37 39 40 44 45 46 48 49 56 60 65 67 68 71 73 **P**5 **S** Lutheran Health Systems, Fargo, ND **N** Central Oregon Hosp Network (CONET), Bend, OR	16	10	42	1714	12	20407	346	12553	6009	172
REEDSPORT—Douglas County										
LOWER UMPQUA HOSPITAL DISTRICT, 600 Ranch Road, Zip 97467–1795; tel. 541/271–2171; Sandra Reese, Administrator (Total facility includes 22 beds in nursing home–type unit) (Nonreporting) **A**9 10	16	10	43	—	—	—	—	—	—	—
ROSEBURG—Douglas County										
✠ + COLUMBIA DOUGLAS MEDICAL CENTER, 738 West Harvard Boulevard, Zip 97470–2996; tel. 541/673–6641; Christopher L. Boyd, Chief Executive Officer **A**1 2 9 10 **F**4 7 8 10 11 14 15 16 19 22 28 30 32 33 35 39 40 41 42 44 49 70 71 **S** Columbia/HCA Healthcare Corporation, Nashville, TN **N** Health Future, Inc., Medford, OR	33	10	88	3353	36	35348	224	26982	8836	334

Hospital, Address, Telephone, Administrator, Approval, Facility, and Physician Codes, Health Care System, Network	Classi-fication Codes		Utilization Data					Expense (thousands) of dollars		
	Control	Service	Beds	Admissions	Census	Outpatient Visits	Births	Total	Payroll	Personnel

★ American Hospital Association (AHA) membership
☐ Joint Commission on Accreditation of Healthcare Organizations (JCAHO) accreditation
+ American Osteopathic Hospital Association (AOHA) membership
○ American Osteopathic Association (AOA) accreditation
△ Commission on Accreditation of Rehabilitation Facilities (CARF) accreditation
Control codes 61, 63, 64, 71, 72 and 73 indicate hospitals listed by AOHA, but not registered by AHA. For definition of numerical codes, see page A4

Hospital	Control	Service	Beds	Admissions	Census	Outpatient Visits	Births	Total	Payroll	Personnel
⊠ MERCY MEDICAL CENTER, 2700 Stewart Parkway, Zip 97470–1297; tel. 541/673–0611; Victor J. Fresolone, FACHE, President and Chief Executive Officer (Nonreporting) **A**1 2 9 10 **S** Catholic Health Initiatives, Denver, CO **N** Health Future, Inc., Medford, OR	21	10	96	—	—	—	—	—	—	—
⊠ VETERANS AFFAIRS MEDICAL CENTER, 913 N.W. Garden Valley Boulevard, Zip 97470–6513; tel. 541/440–1000; Alan S. Perry, Director (Total facility includes 90 beds in nursing home–type unit) **A**1 **F**2 3 6 8 12 16 17 19 20 21 22 25 26 27 28 30 31 32 35 39 41 44 46 49 51 52 54 55 56 58 59 64 65 67 71 72 73 74 **S** Department of Veterans Affairs, Washington, DC	45	10	229	3914	198	111971	0	51161	26303	682
SALEM—Marion County										
☐ OREGON STATE HOSPITAL, 2600 Center Street N.E., Zip 97310–0530; tel. 503/945–2870; Stanley F. Mazur-Hart, Ph.D., Superintendent **A**1 3 5 10 **F**52 53 57 65 73	12	22	546	600	540	0	0	62867	37780	1030
PSYCHIATRIC MEDICINE CENTER See Salem Hospital										
REGIONAL REHABILITATION CENTER See Salem Hospital										
⊠ SALEM HOSPITAL, (Includes Psychiatric Medicine Center, 1127 Oak Street S.E., Zip 97301; Regional Rehabilitation Center, 2561 Center Street N.E., Zip 97301; tel. 503/370–5986), 665 Winter Street S.E., Zip 97301–3959, Mailing Address: Box 14001, Zip 97309–5014; tel. 503/370–5200; Dennis Noonan, President (Total facility includes 69 beds in nursing home–type unit) (Nonreporting) **A**1 2 9 10	23	10	429	—	—	—	—	—	—	—
SEASIDE—Clatsop County										
⊠ PROVIDENCE SEASIDE HOSPITAL, 725 South Wahanna Road, Zip 97138–7735; tel. 503/717–7000; Ronald Swanson, Chief Executive North Coast Service Area (Nonreporting) **A**1 9 10 **S** Sisters of Providence Health System, Seattle, WA **N** Oregon Health System in Collaboration, Lake Oswego, OR; Providence Health System, Portland, OR	21	10	26	—	—	—	—	—	—	—
SILVERTON—Marion County										
★ SILVERTON HOSPITAL, 342 Fairview Street, Zip 97381; tel. 503/873–1500; William E. Winter, Administrative Director **A**9 10 **F**7 8 11 17 19 22 25 27 28 29 30 34 37 40 41 44 45 46 64 67 70 71 73 **N** Health Future, Inc., Medford, OR	23	10	38	2405	20	34471	752	12858	5717	200
SPRINGFIELD—Lane County										
⊠ MCKENZIE–WILLAMETTE HOSPITAL, 1460 G Street, Zip 97477–4197; tel. 541/726–4400; Roy J. Orr, President and Chief Executive Officer (Nonreporting) **A**1 9 10	23	10	102	—	—	—	—	—	—	—
STAYTON—Marion County										
⊠ SANTIAM MEMORIAL HOSPITAL, 1401 North 10th Avenue, Zip 97383; tel. 503/769–2175; Terry L. Fletchall, Administrator **A**1 9 10 **F**7 8 14 15 16 19 22 27 30 34 39 40 44 49 64 65 71	23	10	40	785	7	18904	112	5899	2766	81
THE DALLES—Wasco County										
⊠ + MID–COLUMBIA MEDICAL CENTER, 1700 East 19th Street, Zip 97058–3316; tel. 541/296–1111; Mark D. Scott, President (Nonreporting) **A**1 9 10 **N** Health Future, Inc., Medford, OR	23	10	49	—	—	—	—	—	—	—
TILLAMOOK—Tillamook County										
⊠ TILLAMOOK COUNTY GENERAL HOSPITAL, 1000 Third Street, Zip 97141–3430; tel. 503/842–4444; Wendell Hesseltine, President (Nonreporting) **A**1 9 10 **S** Adventist Health, Roseville, CA	21	10	20	—	—	—	—	—	—	—
TUALATIN—Washington County										
⊠ LEGACY MERIDIAN PARK HOSPITAL, 19300 S.W. 65th Avenue, Zip 97062–9741; tel. 503/692–1212; Jeff Cushing, Vice President, Administration **A**1 2 9 10 **F**1 2 3 4 7 8 9 10 11 12 17 19 21 22 23 24 26 27 29 30 31 32 33 34 35 37 38 39 40 41 42 43 44 45 46 47 48 49 52 53 54 55 56 57 58 59 60 61 62 63 64 65 67 70 71 73 74 **P**4 5 **S** Legacy Health System, Portland, OR **N** Oregon Health System in Collaboration, Lake Oswego, OR; Legacy Health System, Portland, OR	23	10	116	7149	62	57837	1152	46213	18295	491

PENNSYLVANIA

Resident population 12,072 (in thousands)
Resident population in metro areas 84.7%
Birth rate per 1,000 population 13.4
65 years and over 15.9%
Percent of persons without health insurance 10.6%

Hospital, Address, Telephone, Administrator, Approval, Facility, and Physician Codes, Health Care System, Network	Classi-fication Codes		Utilization Data					Expense (thousands) of dollars		
★ American Hospital Association (AHA) membership □ Joint Commission on Accreditation of Healthcare Organizations (JCAHO) accreditation + American Osteopathic Hospital Association (AOHA) membership ○ American Osteopathic Association (AOA) accreditation △ Commission on Accreditation of Rehabilitation Facilities (CARF) accreditation Control codes 61, 63, 64, 71, 72 and 73 indicate hospitals listed by AOHA, but not registered by AHA. For definition of numerical codes, see page A4	Control	Service	Beds	Admissions	Census	Outpatient Visits	Births	Total	Payroll	Personnel

ABINGTON—Montgomery County

★ ABINGTON MEMORIAL HOSPITAL, 1200 Old York Road, Zip 19001–3788; tel. 215/576–2000; Felix M. Pilla, President and Chief Executive Officer **A**1 2 3 5 6 9 10 **F**1 8 10 11 14 15 16 17 19 20 21 22 24 25 26 27 30 31 32 33 34 35 36 37 38 39 40 41 42 44 46 47 48 49 51 52 53 56 57 58 59 60 61 62 63 64 65 66 67 69 70 71 73 74	23	10	398	20480	300	414678	3292	201978	99269	2618

ALIQUIPPA—Beaver County

★ UNIVERSITY OF PITTSBURGH MEDICAL CENTER, BEAVER VALLEY, (Formerly Aliquippa Hospital), 2500 Hospital Drive, Zip 15001–2191; tel. 412/857–1212; George J. Kobakes, President and Chief Executive Officer (Total facility includes 16 beds in nursing home–type unit) (Nonreporting) **A**1 9 10	23	10	183	—	—	—	—	—	—	—

ALLENTOWN—Lehigh County

+ ○ ALLENTOWN OSTEOPATHIC MEDICAL CENTER, 1736 Hamilton Street, Zip 18104–9990; tel. 610/770–8300; John M. Sherwood, FACHE, President and Chief Executive Officer **A**9 11 12 13 **F**3 4 7 8 10 14 15 16 19 21 22 28 29 30 32 34 35 37 40 42 44 45 46 49 51 58 61 63 65 67 71 73 **P**5 8	23	10	118	4779	63	67257	466	36027	16169	500
□ ALLENTOWN STATE HOSPITAL, 1600 Hanover Avenue, Zip 18103; tel. 610/740–3200; David W. Jay, Superintendent **A**1 9 10 **F**4 8 15 16 19 20 21 27 28 31 35 42 43 44 46 49 50 52 55 57 60 63 65 71 73	12	22	415	183	399	0	0	—	—	569
□ △ GOOD SHEPHERD REHABILITATION HOSPITAL, 543 St. John Street, Zip 18103–3279; tel. 610/776–3120; John V. Cooney, President **A**1 7 9 10 **F**2 5 10 12 14 15 16 17 19 21 22 23 34 35 45 46 48 49 50 52 54 65 67 71 73 **P**6	23	46	75	1679	65	79931	0	26902	—	529
★ LEHIGH VALLEY HOSPITAL, Cedar Crest Boulevard and 1–78, Zip 18103, Mailing Address: P.O. Box 689, Zip 18105–1556; tel. 610/402–8000; Elliot J. Sussman, M.D., President and Chief Executive Officer (Nonreporting) **A**1 2 3 5 8 9 10 12	23	10	647	—	—	—	—	—	—	—
★ SACRED HEART HOSPITAL, Fourth and Chew Streets, Zip 18102–3490; tel. 610/776–4500; Joseph M. Cimerola, FACHE, President and Chief Executive Officer (Total facility includes 22 beds in nursing home–type unit) (Nonreporting) **A**1 2 3 5 9 10 **N** Partnership for Community Health–Lehigh Valley, Allentown, PA; Sacred Heart Health Care System, Allentown, PA	23	10	245	—	—	—	—	—	—	—

ALTOONA—Blair County

ALTOONA CENTER, 1515 Fourth Street, Zip 16601; tel. 814/946–6900; Barry C. Benford, Director (Nonreporting)	12	62	138	—	—	—	—	—	—	—
★ ○ ALTOONA HOSPITAL, 620 Howard Avenue, Zip 16601–4899; tel. 814/946–2011; James W. Barner, President and Chief Executive Officer; Warren Rhyner, Senior Vice President **A**1 2 3 5 6 9 10 11 12 **F**2 3 4 7 8 10 11 14 15 16 18 19 22 23 26 28 30 32 33 34 35 37 40 41 42 43 44 46 49 52 53 54 55 56 57 58 59 60 61 64 65 67 71 73 74 **P**1	23	10	189	12650	185	243944	1330	114296	51208	1397
★ BON SECOURS–HOLY FAMILY REGIONAL HEALTH SYSTEM, (Formerly Mercy Regional Health System), 2500 Seventh Avenue, Zip 16602; tel. 814/944–1681; David J. Davies, Chief Executive Officer **A**1 2 9 10 **F**7 8 14 15 16 17 19 21 22 27 28 30 31 32 33 35 37 40 41 42 44 45 46 48 49 52 54 57 58 59 60 65 66 67 71 73 **P**1 5 **S** Bon Secours Health System, Inc., Marriottsville, MD	23	10	169	5787	108	89278	413	45662	20218	570
□ △ HEALTHSOUTH REHABILITATION HOSPITAL OF ALTOONA, 2005 Valley View Boulevard, Zip 16602; tel. 814/944–3535; Felix Mariani, Administrator (Nonreporting) **A**1 7 9 10 **S** HEALTHSOUTH Corporation, Birmingham, AL	33	46	70	—	—	—	—	—	—	—
★ JAMES E. VAN ZANDT VETERANS AFFAIRS MEDICAL CENTER, 2907 Pleasant Valley Boulevard, Zip 16602–4377; tel. 814/943–8164; Gerald L. Williams, Director (Total facility includes 33 beds in nursing home–type unit) **A**1 **F**3 8 12 14 15 16 17 19 20 21 22 26 27 28 29 30 31 32 33 34 35 37 39 44 45 46 49 51 54 58 64 65 67 71 73 74 **P**6 **S** Department of Veterans Affairs, Washington, DC	45	10	110	2093	86	57795	0	26429	14742	376
MERCY REGIONAL HEALTH SYSTEM See Bon Secours–Holy Family Regional Health System										

AMBLER—Montgomery County

□ HORSHAM CLINIC, 722 East Butler Pike, Zip 19002; tel. 215/643–7800; David A. Baron, D.O., Medical Director; Mark A. Benz, Administrator (Nonreporting) **A**1 5 9 10 **S** Universal Health Services, Inc., King of Prussia, PA	33	22	138	—	—	—	—	—	—	—

ASHLAND—Schuylkill County

□ ASHLAND REGIONAL MEDICAL CENTER, 101 Broad Street, Zip 17921–2198; tel. 717/875–2000; Michael J. Callan, Sr., Chief Executive Officer (Total facility includes 20 beds in nursing home–type unit) **A**1 9 10 **F**8 15 16 19 21 22 26 27 28 29 30 35 37 39 41 44 45 46 49 64 65 66 67 71 73 74	23	10	97	2538	39	—	0	16019	7616	245

BALA CYNWYD—Montgomery County

★ △ MERCY HEALTH SYSTEM OF SOUTHEASTERN PENNSYLVANIA, (Formerly Mercy Health Corporation of Southeastern Pennsylvania), (Includes Mercy Fitzgerald Hospital, 1500 South Lansdowne Avenue, Darby, Zip 19023; tel. 610/237–4020; Mercy Hospital of Philadelphia, 5301 Cedar Avenue, Philadelphia, Zip 19143; tel. 215/748–9000), One Bala Plaza, Suite 402, Zip 19004; tel. 610/660–7440; Plato A. Marinakos, President and Chief Executive Officer (Total facility includes 22 beds in nursing home–type unit) (Nonreporting) **A**1 2 3 5 7 8 9 10 **S** Eastern Mercy Health System, Radnor, PA	21	10	553	—	—	—	—	—	—	—

Hospital, Address, Telephone, Administrator, Approval, Facility, and Physician Codes, Health Care System, Network	Classi-fication Codes		Utilization Data					Expense (thousands) of dollars		
★ American Hospital Association (AHA) membership □ Joint Commission on Accreditation of Healthcare Organizations (JCAHO) accreditation + American Osteopathic Hospital Association (AOHA) membership ○ American Osteopathic Association (AOA) accreditation △ Commission on Accreditation of Rehabilitation Facilities (CARF) accreditation Control codes 61, 63, 64, 71, 72 and 73 indicate hospitals listed by AOHA, but not registered by AHA. For definition of numerical codes, see page A4	Control	Service	Beds	Admissions	Census	Outpatient Visits	Births	Total	Payroll	Personnel

BEAVER—Beaver County

✠ THE MEDICAL CENTER, 1000 Dutch Ridge Road, Zip 15009–9700; tel. 412/728–7000; Larry A. Crowell, President and Chief Executive Officer (Total facility includes 34 beds in nursing home–type unit) **A**1 2 3 5 9 10 **F**4 5 7 8 10 15 16 17 19 20 21 22 23 25 26 28 29 30 31 32 33 34 35 37 39 40 41 42 43 44 45 46 49 51 52 54 56 57 59 60 61 63 64 65 67 71 73 74 **P**6 7
| | 23 | 10 | 470 | 16335 | 264 | 300975 | 1426 | 131800 | 62977 | 1899 |

BENSALEM—Bucks County

LIVENGRIN FOUNDATION, 4833 Hulmeville Road, Zip 19020; tel. 215/638–5200; Richard M. Pine, President and Chief Executive Officer (Nonreporting)
| | 23 | 82 | 76 | — | — | — | — | — | — | — |

BERWICK—Columbia County

✠ BERWICK HOSPITAL CENTER, 701 East 16th Street, Zip 18603–2397; tel. 717/759–5000; Thomas R. Sphatt, President and Chief Executive Officer (Total facility includes 240 beds in nursing home–type unit) **A**1 9 10 **F**2 3 7 8 14 15 16 17 19 21 22 25 26 27 28 30 32 33 34 35 37 39 40 42 44 46 49 58 63 64 65 66 67 71 73 **P**1 **S** Quorum Health Group/Quorum Health Resources, Inc., Brentwood, TN
| | 23 | 10 | 409 | 4019 | 272 | 79305 | 262 | 31384 | 14030 | 599 |

BETHLEHEM—Northampton County

✠ MUHLENBERG HOSPITAL CENTER, 2545 Schoenersville Road, Zip 18017–7384; tel. 610/861–2200; William R. Mason, President and Chief Executive Officer **A**1 9 10 **F**4 8 9 10 12 14 15 16 17 19 20 21 22 28 29 30 32 33 34 35 37 38 40 41 42 43 44 45 46 47 48 49 52 56 57 58 59 60 63 64 65 70 71 73 74 **P**7 8
| | 23 | 10 | 148 | 5823 | 100 | 101011 | 0 | 47289 | 19549 | 602 |

□ ST. LUKE'S HOSPITAL, 801 Ostrum Street, Zip 18015–1014; tel. 610/954–4000; Richard A. Anderson, President (Total facility includes 18 beds in nursing home–type unit) **A**1 2 3 5 6 9 10 12 **F**3 4 7 8 10 11 12 13 14 15 16 17 19 21 22 23 25 26 28 29 30 31 32 33 34 35 37 38 39 40 41 42 43 44 45 49 51 52 54 58 59 60 61 64 65 67 71 72 73 74 **P**8 **N** Fox Chase Network, Rockledge, PA
| | 23 | 10 | 436 | 18346 | 281 | 309509 | 2567 | 153792 | 72538 | 2119 |

BLOOMSBURG—Columbia County

✠ BLOOMSBURG HOSPITAL, 549 East Fair Street, Zip 17815–0340; tel. 717/387–2100; Robert J. Spinelli, Administrator and Chief Executive Officer **A**1 9 10 **F**2 3 7 8 14 15 17 19 21 22 27 28 29 30 32 33 34 35 37 40 41 42 44 46 52 54 55 56 58 59 63 65 67 71 73 **P**3 8
| | 23 | 10 | 125 | 3770 | 47 | 72086 | 580 | 24266 | 9863 | 371 |

BRADDOCK—Allegheny County

□ UNIVERSITY OF PITTSBURGH MEDICAL CENTER, BRADDOCK, (Formerly Braddock Medical Center), 400 Holland Avenue, Zip 15104–1599; tel. 412/636–5000; Richard Wilson Benfer, President **A**1 9 10 **F**2 3 8 11 14 15 16 17 18 19 21 22 23 27 28 29 30 31 33 35 36 37 42 44 49 52 54 55 56 57 63 65 67 71 73 74
| | 23 | 10 | 227 | 7208 | 121 | 92599 | 0 | 38194 | 19008 | 561 |

BRADFORD—McKean County

✠ BRADFORD REGIONAL MEDICAL CENTER, 116–156 Interstate Parkway, Zip 16701–0218; tel. 814/368–4143; George E. Leonhardt, President and Chief Executive Officer (Total facility includes 95 beds in nursing home–type unit) **A**1 9 10 **F**7 8 14 15 16 17 19 21 22 23 24 25 26 28 30 31 32 33 34 35 37 39 40 41 44 45 46 49 51 52 53 54 55 56 57 58 60 63 64 65 66 67 71 73 **N** Great Lakes Health Network, Erie, PA
| | 23 | 10 | 216 | 4699 | 161 | 129563 | 389 | 38694 | 17308 | 615 |

BRIDGEVILLE—Allegheny County

□ MAYVIEW STATE HOSPITAL, 1601 Mayview Road, Zip 15017–1599; tel. 412/257–6500; Shirley J. Dumpman, Superintendent (Total facility includes 92 beds in nursing home–type unit) (Nonreporting) **A**1 5 10
| | 12 | 22 | 826 | — | — | — | — | — | — | — |

BRISTOL—Bucks County

✠ LOWER BUCKS HOSPITAL, 501 Bath Road, Zip 19007–3190; tel. 215/785–9200; Nathan Bosk, FACHE, Chief Executive Officer **A**1 3 9 10 **F**7 8 10 11 12 14 15 16 17 18 19 21 22 24 25 28 29 30 32 34 35 37 38 40 41 42 44 45 46 49 51 52 54 55 56 57 58 63 65 66 67 68 71 73 74 **P**1 5 **N** Temple University Health Network, Philadelphia, PA
| | 23 | 10 | 166 | 8799 | 125 | 135043 | 1430 | 69057 | 31291 | 868 |

BROOKVILLE—Jefferson County

✠ BROOKVILLE HOSPITAL, 100 Hospital Road, Zip 15825–1363; tel. 814/849–2312; Warren J. Bassett, FACHE, President **A**1 9 10 **F**7 8 11 14 15 16 17 19 20 21 22 28 30 32 39 40 41 44 45 49 63 65 66 69 71 **P**5
| | 23 | 10 | 73 | 2158 | 23 | 90366 | 121 | 21173 | 8798 | 325 |

BROWNSVILLE—Fayette County

✠ BROWNSVILLE GENERAL HOSPITAL, 125 Simpson Road, Zip 15417; tel. 412/785–7200; Richard D. Constantine, Chief Executive Officer (Total facility includes 21 beds in nursing home–type unit) (Nonreporting) **A**1 9 10 **S** Quorum Health Group/Quorum Health Resources, Inc., Brentwood, TN
| | 23 | 10 | 116 | — | — | — | — | — | — | — |

BRYN MAWR—Montgomery County

BRYN MAWR COLLEGE INFIRMARY, Bryn Mawr College Campus, Zip 19010; tel. 610/526–7360; Kay Kerr, M.D., Medical Director (Nonreporting)
| | 23 | 11 | 7 | — | — | — | — | — | — | — |

✠ BRYN MAWR HOSPITAL, 130 South Bryn Mawr Avenue, Zip 19010–3160; tel. 610/526–3000; William McCune, Vice President, Administration (Total facility includes 17 beds in nursing home–type unit) **A**1 2 3 5 9 10 **F**3 4 5 7 8 10 11 12 14 15 16 17 19 20 21 22 26 28 29 30 31 32 33 35 36 37 38 39 40 41 42 43 44 45 46 49 51 52 53 54 55 56 57 58 59 60 61 63 64 65 67 68 71 73 74 **P**3 7 8 **S** Jefferson Health System, Radnor, PA **N** Jefferson Health System, Radnor, PA
| | 23 | 10 | 283 | 14208 | 185 | 116237 | 1991 | 131230 | 48191 | 1315 |

BUTLER—Butler County

✠ BUTLER HEALTH SYSTEM, (Formerly Butler Memorial Hospital), 911 East Brady Street, Zip 16001–4697; tel. 412/283–6666; Joseph A. Stewart, President and Chief Executive Officer (Total facility includes 19 beds in nursing home–type unit) **A**1 9 10 **F**2 3 7 8 10 11 13 14 15 16 19 21 22 23 24 27 28 32 33 35 37 40 44 46 49 52 54 56 57 63 64 65 67 71 72 **P**4 5
| | 23 | 10 | 286 | 9639 | 152 | 187790 | 1040 | 70649 | 32398 | 1014 |

Hospital, Address, Telephone, Administrator, Approval, Facility, and Physician Codes, Health Care System, Network	Classi-fication Codes		Utilization Data					Expense (thousands) of dollars		
★ American Hospital Association (AHA) membership □ Joint Commission on Accreditation of Healthcare Organizations (JCAHO) accreditation + American Osteopathic Hospital Association (AOHA) membership ○ American Osteopathic Association (AOA) accreditation △ Commission on Accreditation of Rehabilitation Facilities (CARF) accreditation Control codes 61, 63, 64, 71, 72 and 73 indicate hospitals listed by AOHA, but not registered by AHA. For definition of numerical codes, see page A4	Control	Service	Beds	Admissions	Census	Outpatient Visits	Births	Total	Payroll	Personnel
✠ VETERANS AFFAIRS MEDICAL CENTER, (PRIMARY MEDICAL/LONG TERM CARE), 325 New Castle Road, Zip 16001–2480; tel. 412/287–4781; P. Stajduhar, M.D., Director (Total facility includes 106 beds in nursing home–type unit) **A**1 **F**1 3 4 8 10 11 12 17 18 19 20 21 22 24 26 28 29 30 31 32 34 35 37 39 41 42 43 44 45 46 49 51 52 54 56 58 60 64 65 67 69 71 73 74 **P**6 **S** Department of Veterans Affairs, Washington, DC	45	49	268	1827	227	67285	0	36594	21812	592
CAMP HILL—Cumberland County										
✠ HOLY SPIRIT HOSPITAL, 503 North 21st Street, Zip 17011–2288; tel. 717/763–2100; Sister Romaine Niemeyer, President and Chief Executive Officer **A**1 5 9 10 **F**2 3 4 7 8 10 12 15 17 18 19 21 22 27 28 29 30 31 32 33 34 35 37 39 40 41 42 44 46 51 52 53 54 55 56 57 58 59 60 63 65 67 68 69 71 73 74 **P**8	21	10	317	11622	189	194241	477	84771	42207	1381
STATE CORRECTIONAL INSTITUTION AT CAMP HILL, 2500 Lisbon Road, Zip 17011, Mailing Address: Box 200, Zip 17011, tel. 717/737–4531; Kathy Montag, Administrator Health Care (Nonreporting)	12	49	34	—	—	—	—	—	—	—
CANONSBURG—Washington County										
✠ CANONSBURG GENERAL HOSPITAL, 100 Medical Boulevard, Zip 15317; tel. 412/745–6100; Barbara A. Bensaia, Chief Operating Officer (Total facility includes 28 beds in nursing home–type unit) **A**1 9 10 **F**3 8 10 12 16 17 19 21 22 23 28 30 32 33 34 35 37 39 41 42 44 49 63 64 65 67 71 73 **P**1	23	10	120	3928	66	53852	0	27286	11369	347
CARBONDALE—Lackawanna County										
✠ MARIAN COMMUNITY HOSPITAL, 100 Lincoln Avenue, Zip 18407; tel. 717/281–1000; Sister Jean Coughlin, President and Chief Executive Officer (Nonreporting) **A**1 9 10	21	10	99	—	—	—	—	—	—	—
CARLISLE—Cumberland County										
✠ CARLISLE HOSPITAL, 246 Parker Street, Zip 17013–0310; tel. 717/249–1212; Michael J. Halstead, President and Chief Executive Officer (Nonreporting) **A**1 9 10 **S** Quorum Health Group/Quorum Health Resources, Inc., Brentwood, TN	23	10	183	—	—	—	—	—	—	—
CENTRE HALL—Centre County										
□ MEADOWS PSYCHIATRIC CENTER, Mailing Address: Rural Delivery 1, Box 259, Zip 16828; tel. 814/364–2161; Joseph Barszczewski, Chief Executive Officer **A**1 9 10 **F**1 15 16 52 53 54 55 56 57 58 59 65 **P**7 **S** Universal Health Services, Inc., King of Prussia, PA	33	22	101	1772	91	—	0	—	—	239
CHAMBERSBURG—Franklin County										
✠ △ CHAMBERSBURG HOSPITAL, 112 North Seventh Street, Zip 17201–6005, Mailing Address: P.O. Box 6005, Zip 17201–6005; tel. 717/267–3000; Norman B. Epstein, President **A**1 7 9 10 **F**1 3 7 8 10 11 12 14 15 16 17 18 19 20 21 22 23 24 26 27 28 29 30 31 32 33 34 35 36 37 39 40 41 42 44 45 46 48 49 51 52 54 55 56 57 58 59 60 63 65 67 69 70 71 73 74 **P**6 8	23	10	197	9674	139	157906	1115	70291	33694	948
CHESTER—Delaware County										
✠ ○ COMMUNITY HOSPITAL, DIVISION OF THE CROZER–CHESTER MEDICAL CENTER, Ninth and Wilson Streets, Zip 19013; tel. 610/494–0700 (Nonreporting) **A**1 9 10 11 12 13 **S** Crozer–Keystone Health System, Media, PA	21	10	184	—	—	—	—	—	—	—
KEYSTONE CENTER, 2001 Providence Avenue, Zip 19013–5504; tel. 610/876–9000; Jimmy Patton, Chief Executive Officer and Managing Director (Nonreporting) **S** Universal Health Services, Inc., King of Prussia, PA	33	82	76	—	—	—	—	—	—	—
CLARION—Clarion County										
★ + ○ CLARION HOSPITAL, One Hospital Drive, Zip 16214; tel. 814/226–9500; John J. Shepard, President and Chief Executive Officer **A**9 10 11 12 13 **F**7 8 19 20 21 22 33 34 35 40 41 42 44 49 64 71 **S** Quorum Health Group/Quorum Health Resources, Inc., Brentwood, TN	23	10	88	3318	31	77107	394	20026	9036	349
□ CLARION PSYCHIATRIC CENTER, 2 Hospital Drive, Zip 16214, Mailing Address: Rural Delivery 3, Box 188, Zip 16214; tel. 814/226–9545; Michael R. Keefer, CHE, Chief Executive Officer (Nonreporting) **A**1 9 10 **S** Universal Health Services, Inc., King of Prussia, PA	33	22	52	—	—	—	—	—	—	—
CLARKS SUMMIT—Lackawanna County										
□ CLARKS SUMMIT STATE HOSPITAL, 1451 Hillside Drive, Zip 18411; tel. 717/586–2011; Thomas P. Comerford, Jr., Superintendent (Total facility includes 167 beds in nursing home–type unit) **A**1 10 **F**1 4 8 10 11 12 14 16 17 18 19 20 21 22 26 27 28 30 35 37 39 40 42 44 45 46 48 52 54 55 57 60 61 64 65 67 70 71 73 **P**6	12	22	512	180	417	0	0	35294	19810	579
CLEARFIELD—Clearfield County										
□ CLEARFIELD HOSPITAL, 809 Turnpike Avenue, Zip 16830, Mailing Address: Box 992, Zip 16830; tel. 814/765–5341; Stephen A. Wolfe, President and Chief Executive Officer **A**1 5 9 10 **F**7 8 10 12 14 15 16 17 19 21 22 23 25 28 29 30 32 33 34 35 37 39 40 41 42 44 45 46 49 51 60 63 65 66 67 71 73	23	10	92	4799	57	227288	543	41678	19891	582
COAL TOWNSHIP—Northumberland County										
✠ SHAMOKIN AREA COMMUNITY HOSPITAL, 4200 Hospital Road, Zip 17866–9697; tel. 717/644–4200; Harold C. Warman, Jr., President and Chief Executive Officer (Total facility includes 15 beds in nursing home–type unit) **A**1 9 10 **F**8 14 15 16 17 19 21 22 26 27 28 30 31 34 35 37 41 44 45 46 49 51 57 63 64 65 66 67 71 73 **P**1	23	10	55	1938	25	51977	0	12636	5102	153
COALDALE—Schuylkill County										
✠ MINER'S MEMORIAL MEDICAL CENTER, 360 West Ruddle, Zip 18218–0067, Mailing Address: P.O. Box 67, Zip 18218–0067; tel. 717/645–2131; Michael R. Miller, President and Chief Executive Officer (Total facility includes 48 beds in nursing home–type unit) **A**1 9 10 **F**8 14 15 16 19 21 22 26 30 32 34 35 37 42 44 46 49 56 59 64 65 71 73 **S** Quorum Health Group/Quorum Health Resources, Inc., Brentwood, TN	23	10	110	2583	86	33431	0	25203	12852	349

Hospital, Address, Telephone, Administrator, Approval, Facility, and Physician Codes, Health Care System, Network	Classi-fication Codes		Utilization Data					Expense (thousands) of dollars		
	Control	Service	Beds	Admissions	Census	Outpatient Visits	Births	Total	Payroll	Personnel

★ American Hospital Association (AHA) membership
☐ Joint Commission on Accreditation of Healthcare Organizations (JCAHO) accreditation
+ American Osteopathic Hospital Association (AOHA) membership
○ American Osteopathic Association (AOA) accreditation
△ Commission on Accreditation of Rehabilitation Facilities (CARF) accreditation
Control codes 61, 63, 64, 71, 72 and 73 indicate hospitals listed by AOHA, but not registered by AHA. For definition of numerical codes, see page A4.

COATESVILLE—Chester County

	Control	Service	Beds	Admissions	Census	Outpatient Visits	Births	Total	Payroll	Personnel
⊞ BRANDYWINE HOSPITAL, 201 Reeceville Road, Zip 19320–1536; tel. 610/383–8000; James H. Thorton, President and Chief Executive Officer (Total facility includes 20 beds in nursing home–type unit) **A**1 2 6 9 10 **F**4 5 7 8 10 12 14 15 16 17 18 19 20 21 22 24 25 26 28 29 30 31 32 33 34 35 36 37 39 40 41 42 43 44 45 46 52 56 57 59 64 65 66 67 70 71 73 **P**5 8	23	10	183	7041	103	67132	700	66058	27669	847
⊞ VETERANS AFFAIRS MEDICAL CENTER, Black Horse Hill Road, Zip 19320–9985; tel. 610/384–7711; Gary W. Devansky, Director (Total facility includes 200 beds in nursing home–type unit) **A**1 5 9 **F**1 2 3 6 8 12 15 16 17 18 20 21 24 26 27 30 31 32 34 37 39 41 45 46 49 51 52 54 55 56 57 58 64 65 67 71 73 74 **P**6 **S** Department of Veterans Affairs, Washington, DC	45	22	710	3038	636	95441	0	84986	51173	1352

COLUMBIA—Lancaster County

	Control	Service	Beds	Admissions	Census	Outpatient Visits	Births	Total	Payroll	Personnel
⊞ LANCASTER GENERAL HOSPITAL–SUSQUEHANNA DIVISION, 306 North Seventh Street, Zip 17512, Mailing Address: P.O. Box 926, Zip 17512–0926; tel. 717/684–2841; Scott A. Berlucchi, President and Chief Executive Officer **A**1 9 10 **F**2 3 7 8 14 15 16 17 19 22 30 32 34 39 40 41 44 45 46 49 65 66 67 71 73	23	10	81	1223	29	86179	45	8663	4241	144

CONNELLSVILLE—Fayette County

	Control	Service	Beds	Admissions	Census	Outpatient Visits	Births	Total	Payroll	Personnel
⊞ HIGHLANDS HOSPITAL, 401 East Murphy Avenue, Zip 15425–2797; tel. 412/628–1500; Michael J. Evans, Chief Executive Officer **A**1 9 10 **F**8 11 12 15 16 17 19 21 22 26 28 29 30 31 32 33 35 37 39 41 42 44 46 49 52 53 54 55 56 57 60 63 64 65 67 69 71 73 **P**8	23	10	92	3062	55	44697	0	18645	8524	270

CORRY—Erie County

	Control	Service	Beds	Admissions	Census	Outpatient Visits	Births	Total	Payroll	Personnel
⊞ CORRY MEMORIAL HOSPITAL, 612 West Smith Street, Zip 16407–1196; tel. 814/664–4641; Joseph T. Hodges, President **A**1 9 10 **F**8 14 15 16 19 21 22 27 32 34 37 40 41 44 49 52 57 65 71 73 **P**7 **S** Quorum Health Group/Quorum Health Resources, Inc., Brentwood, TN **N** Great Lakes Health Network, Erie, PA	23	10	55	1945	19	37678	295	11097	4563	187

COUDERSPORT—Potter County

	Control	Service	Beds	Admissions	Census	Outpatient Visits	Births	Total	Payroll	Personnel
⊞ CHARLES COLE MEMORIAL HOSPITAL, U.S. Route 6E, RR 1, Box 205, Zip 16915; tel. 814/274–9300; David B. Acker, Chief Executive Officer (Total facility includes 50 beds in nursing home–type unit) **A**1 9 10 **F**3 11 12 14 15 16 17 19 21 22 24 25 28 32 33 34 35 40 41 44 46 49 51 53 54 55 57 58 63 64 65 66 71 73 74 **P**7	23	10	120	2478	79	76056	331	25197	10189	409

DANVILLE—Montour County

	Control	Service	Beds	Admissions	Census	Outpatient Visits	Births	Total	Payroll	Personnel
☐ DANVILLE STATE HOSPITAL, Zip 17821–0700; tel. 717/275–7011; Paul J. Gritman, Superintendent (Total facility includes 60 beds in nursing home–type unit) **A**1 9 10 **F**1 2 3 4 5 6 7 8 9 10 11 12 13 17 18 20 21 22 23 24 25 26 27 28 29 30 31 32 33 34 35 36 37 38 39 40 41 42 43 44 45 46 47 48 49 50 51 52 53 54 55 56 57 58 59 60 61 62 63 64 65 66 67 68 69 70 71 72 73 74 **P**6	12	22	332	129	258	0	0	31915	19253	518
☐ ○ GEISINGER MEDICAL CENTER, 100 North Academy Avenue, Zip 17822–2201; tel. 717/271–6211; Stuart Heydt, Chief Executive Officer (Nonreporting) **A**1 2 3 5 6 8 9 10 11 12 **S** Geisinger Health System, Danville, PA **N** Geisinger Health System, Danville, PA	23	10	548	—	—	—	—	—	—	—

DEVON—Chester County

	Control	Service	Beds	Admissions	Census	Outpatient Visits	Births	Total	Payroll	Personnel
DEVEREUX FOUNDATION–FRENCH CENTER, 123 Old Lancaster Road, Zip 19333, Mailing Address: Box 400, Zip 19333; tel. 610/964–3215; Richard Warden, Executive Director (Total facility includes 84 beds in nursing home–type unit) (Nonreporting)	23	59	110							

DOWNINGTOWN—Chester County

	Control	Service	Beds	Admissions	Census	Outpatient Visits	Births	Total	Payroll	Personnel
★ ST. JOHN VIANNEY HOSPITAL, 151 Woodbine Road, Zip 19335–3080; tel. 610/269–2600; Louis D. Horvath, Administrator (Nonreporting)	21	22	54	—	—	—	—	—	—	—

DOYLESTOWN—Bucks County

DELAWARE VALLEY MENTAL HEALTH FOUNDATION See Foundations Behavioral Health

	Control	Service	Beds	Admissions	Census	Outpatient Visits	Births	Total	Payroll	Personnel
⊞ △ DOYLESTOWN HOSPITAL, 595 West State Street, Zip 18901; tel. 215/345–2200; Richard A. Reif, President and Chief Executive Officer (Total facility includes 236 beds in nursing home–type unit) **A**1 5 7 9 10 **F**6 7 8 10 12 13 14 15 16 17 18 19 20 21 22 23 25 26 27 28 30 31 32 33 34 35 37 39 40 41 42 44 45 46 48 49 51 52 54 55 56 57 59 61 62 64 65 67 71 73 74 **P**5 6 8	23	10	432	9272	360	188314	1147	90767	43434	1472
☐ FOUNDATIONS BEHAVIORAL HEALTH, (Formerly Delaware Valley Mental Health Foundation), 833 East Butler Avenue, Zip 18901; tel. 215/345–0444; Ronald T. Bernstein, President and Chief Executive Officer **A**1 10 **F**14 15 16 46 52 53 59 65 **P**6	23	22	45	153	36	1271	0	6152	3387	136

DREXEL HILL—Delaware County

	Control	Service	Beds	Admissions	Census	Outpatient Visits	Births	Total	Payroll	Personnel
⊞ ○ DELAWARE COUNTY MEMORIAL HOSPITAL, 501 North Lansdowne Avenue, Zip 19026–1186; tel. 610/284–8100; Joan K. Richards, President **A**1 2 5 9 10 11 **F**1 2 3 4 7 8 10 11 12 13 14 15 16 17 18 19 21 22 23 24 25 26 28 29 30 31 32 33 34 35 36 37 38 39 40 41 42 43 44 45 46 48 49 51 53 54 55 56 57 58 59 60 63 65 66 67 68 70 71 73 74 **P**1 4 5 7 8 **S** Crozer–Keystone Health System, Media, PA **N** Crozer–Keystone Health System, Media, PA; Fox Chase Network, Rockledge, PA	23	10	251	10770	181	—	1082	91778	39347	—

Hospital, Address, Telephone, Administrator, Approval, Facility, and Physician Codes, Health Care System, Network	Control	Service	Beds	Admissions	Census	Outpatient Visits	Births	Total	Payroll	Personnel

★ American Hospital Association (AHA) membership
□ Joint Commission on Accreditation of Healthcare Organizations (JCAHO) accreditation
+ American Osteopathic Hospital Association (AOHA) membership
○ American Osteopathic Association (AOA) accreditation
△ Commission on Accreditation of Rehabilitation Facilities (CARF) accreditation
Control codes 61, 63, 64, 71, 72 and 73 indicate hospitals listed by AOHA, but not registered by AHA. For definition of numerical codes, see page A4

DUBOIS—Philadelphia County

□ DUBOIS REGIONAL MEDICAL CENTER, 100 Hospital Avenue, Zip 15801, Mailing Address: P.O. Box 447, Zip 15801–0447; tel. 814/371–2200; Raymond A. Graeca, President and Chief Executive Officer (Total facility includes 14 beds in nursing home–type unit) **A**1 2 9 10 **F**2 3 7 8 10 13 14 15 16 17 19 21 22 23 25 26 27 28 29 30 32 33 34 35 37 38 39 40 41 42 44 46 48 49 51 52 53 54 55 56 57 58 60 61 64 65 66 67 71 72 73 **P**6 8 **N** Community Benefits Strategy, DuBois, PA	23	10	198	7407	108	225120	708	61711	31055	975

EAGLEVILLE—Montgomery County

★ EAGLEVILLE HOSPITAL, 100 Eagleville Road, Zip 19403–1800, Mailing Address: P.O. Box 45, Zip 19408–0045; tel. 610/539–6000; Kendria Kurtz, Administrator **A**9 10 **F**2 14 15 22 28 29 39 45 54 55 56 65 67 73 74 **P**6	23	82	146	2696	126	143	0	16347	8772	273

EAST STROUDSBURG—Monroe County

⊞ POCONO MEDICAL CENTER, 206 East Brown Street, Zip 18301; tel. 717/421–4000; Marilyn R. Rettaliata, President and Chief Executive Officer **A**1 2 9 10 **F**7 8 11 13 15 19 21 22 25 30 31 35 37 39 40 41 42 44 45 46 49 52 56 60 65 67 71 73 74	23	10	226	9336	147	141504	969	65739	31212	762

EASTON—Northampton County

⊞ EASTON HOSPITAL, 250 South 21st Street, Zip 18042–3892; tel. 610/250–4000; Donna Mulholland, President and Chief Executive Officer **A**1 2 3 5 9 10 **F**1 4 7 8 10 12 15 16 17 19 20 21 22 28 29 30 31 32 33 34 36 37 38 39 40 41 42 43 44 45 46 48 49 54 56 59 60 63 65 67 71 73 74 **P**7 8	23	10	282	13005	233	218187	734	110481	52815	1635

ELKINS PARK—Montgomery County

⊞ ALLEGHENY UNIVERSITY HOSPITAL, ELKINS PARK, 60 East Township Line Road, Zip 19027; tel. 215/663–6000; Margaret M. McGoldrick, Executive Director and Chief Executive Officer **A**1 3 5 9 10 **F**2 3 4 5 7 8 9 10 11 12 13 14 15 16 17 18 19 20 21 22 24 26 27 28 30 31 32 34 35 37 38 39 40 41 42 43 44 45 46 47 48 49 51 52 53 54 55 56 57 58 59 60 61 65 66 67 70 71 73 74 **P**6 7 **S** Allegheny Health, Education and Research Foundation, Pittsburgh, PA	23	10	158	6952	111	55998	1061	53547	22073	659

ELLWOOD CITY—Lawrence County

ELLWOOD CITY HOSPITAL, 724 Pershing Street, Zip 16117–1499; tel. 412/752–0081; Herbert S. Skuba, President and Chief Executive Officer (Total facility includes 23 beds in nursing home–type unit) (Nonreporting) **A**9 10	23	10	118	—	—	—	—	—	—	—

EPHRATA—Lancaster County

□ EPHRATA COMMUNITY HOSPITAL, 169 Martin Avenue, Zip 17522–1724, Mailing Address: P.O. Box 1002, Zip 17522–1002; tel. 717/733–0311; John M. Porter, Jr., President **A**1 9 10 **F**7 8 14 15 16 17 19 21 22 26 29 30 31 32 33 34 35 36 37 39 40 41 42 44 45 46 49 51 52 53 54 55 56 57 58 59 63 64 65 67 71 73 74 **P**6 8	23	10	124	5678	67	141036	593	39436	19480	563

ERIE—Erie County

⊞ HAMOT MEDICAL CENTER, 201 State Street, Zip 16550–0001; tel. 814/877–6000; John T. Malone, President and Chief Executive Officer (Total facility includes 27 beds in nursing home–type unit) **A**1 2 3 5 9 10 **F**2 3 4 5 6 7 8 9 10 12 14 15 16 17 18 19 21 22 23 24 25 26 27 28 29 30 31 32 33 34 35 36 37 38 39 40 41 42 43 44 45 46 49 50 51 52 53 54 55 56 57 58 59 60 61 62 63 64 65 66 67 68 70 71 72 73 74 **P**6 **N** Great Lakes Health Network, Erie, PA; Community Health Net, Erie, PA	23	10	366	14662	232	105298	1437	132919	52479	2199
□ △ HEALTHSOUTH GREAT LAKES REHABILITATION HOSPITAL, 143 East Second Street, Zip 16507; tel. 814/878–1200; William R. Fox, Chief Executive Officer (Nonreporting) **A**1 7 9 10 **S** HEALTHSOUTH Corporation, Birmingham, AL	33	46	108	—	—	—	—	—	—	—
□ △ HEALTHSOUTH LAKE ERIE INSTITUTE OF REHABILITATION, 137 West Second Street, Zip 16507–1403; tel. 814/453–5602; Frank G. DeLisi, III, CHE, Chief Executive Officer and Director Operations (Total facility includes 27 beds in nursing home–type unit) (Nonreporting) **A**1 7 9 10 **S** HEALTHSOUTH Corporation, Birmingham, AL	33	46	99	—	—	—	—	—	—	—
★ ○ METRO HEALTH CENTER, 252 West 11th Street, Zip 16501; tel. 814/870–3400; J. B. Frith, Chief Executive Officer **A**9 10 11 12 13 **F**7 8 14 15 16 19 21 22 28 30 34 35 37 40 41 44 63 65 71 72 73 **P**8 **S** Quorum Health Group/Quorum Health Resources, Inc., Brentwood, TN **N** Community Health Net, Erie, PA	23	10	112	3022	37	41386	240	20093	7197	255
+ ○ MILLCREEK COMMUNITY HOSPITAL, 5515 Peach Street, Zip 16509–2695; tel. 814/864–4031; Mary L. Eckert, President and Chief Executive Officer **A**9 10 11 12 13 **F**2 7 8 14 15 16 19 22 30 35 37 40 42 44 51 65 71 72 73 **N** Vantage Health Care Network, Inc., Meadville, PA	23	10	101	3338	40	44160	242	19327	7342	249
□ SAINT VINCENT HEALTH CENTER, 232 West 25th Street, Zip 16544; tel. 814/452–5000; Sister Catherine Manning, President and Chief Executive Officer **A**1 3 5 6 9 10 **F**3 4 7 8 10 11 15 16 18 19 20 21 22 25 26 28 29 30 32 33 34 35 37 38 40 41 42 43 44 46 48 49 51 52 54 56 57 58 59 63 65 66 67 70 71 72 73 74 **N** Vantage Health Care Network, Inc., Meadville, PA; Saint Vincent Health System, Erie, PA; Community Health Net, Erie, PA	23	10	477	15736	272	165647	1765	139747	61042	1921
⊞ SHRINERS HOSPITALS FOR CHILDREN, ERIE UNIT, 1645 West 8th Street, Zip 16505; tel. 814/875–8700; Richard W. Brzuz, Administrator **A**1 3 **F**5 15 28 34 41 46 48 49 65 71 73 **P**6 **S** Shriners Hospitals for Children, Tampa, FL	23	57	30	733	12	9247	0	—	—	111
⊞ VETERANS AFFAIRS MEDICAL CENTER, 135 East 38th Street, Zip 16504–1596; tel. 814/868–6210; Stephen M. Lucas, Chief Executive Officer (Total facility includes 14 beds in nursing home–type unit) **A**1 **F**1 2 3 8 10 11 14 15 16 17 18 19 20 21 22 26 27 28 29 30 31 32 33 34 35 37 39 41 42 43 44 45 46 48 49 51 52 54 55 56 57 58 59 64 65 67 69 71 73 74 **P**6 **S** Department of Veterans Affairs, Washington, DC	45	10	88	1784	62	79800	0	33193	20197	426

Hospital, Address, Telephone, Administrator, Approval, Facility, and Physician Codes, Health Care System, Network	Classi-fication Codes		Utilization Data					Expense (thousands) of dollars		
★ American Hospital Association (AHA) membership □ Joint Commission on Accreditation of Healthcare Organizations (JCAHO) accreditation + American Osteopathic Hospital Association (AOHA) membership ○ American Osteopathic Association (AOA) accreditation △ Commission on Accreditation of Rehabilitation Facilities (CARF) accreditation Control codes 61, 63, 64, 71, 72 and 73 indicate hospitals listed by AOHA, but not registered by AHA. For definition of numerical codes, see page A4	Control	Service	Beds	Admissions	Census	Outpatient Visits	Births	Total	Payroll	Personnel

EVERETT—Bedford County

☒ MEMORIAL HOSPITAL OF BEDFORD COUNTY, Rural Delivery 1, Box 80, Zip 15537–9513; tel. 814/623–6161; James C. Vreeland, FACHE, President and Chief Executive Officer **A**1 9 10 **F**1 3 4 6 7 8 10 12 13 14 15 16 17 18 19 20 21 22 23 24 26 27 28 29 30 31 32 33 34 35 36 37 39 40 41 42 43 44 49 51 53 54 55 56 57 58 59 60 62 63 65 67 69 70 71 73 **P**8 … 23 10 78 2419 23 69029 274 19422 8500 281

FARRELL—Mercer County

SHENANGO VALLEY CAMPUS See Horizon Hospital System, Greenville

FORT WASHINGTON—Montgomery County

□ NORTHWESTERN INSTITUTE, 450 Bethlehem Pike, Zip 19034–0209; tel. 215/641–5300; Joseph Roynan, Administrator (Nonreporting) **A**1 3 9 10 … 33 22 146 — — — — — — — —

FRANKLIN—Venango County

□ NORTHWEST MEDICAL CENTER, (Includes Northwest Medical Center–Franklin Campus, 1 Spruce Street, tel. 814/437–7000; Northwest Medical Center–Oil City Campus, 174 East Bissell Avenue, Oil City, Zip 16301–0568, Mailing Address: Box 1068, Zip 16301–0568; tel. 814/677–1711), 1 Spruce Street, Zip 16323, Mailing Address: P.O. Box 1068, Oil City, Zip 16301; tel. 814/437–7000; Neil E. Todhunter, Chief Executive Officer (Nonreporting) **A**1 2 9 10 **N** Vantage Health Care Network, Inc., Meadville, PA … 23 10 173 — — — — — — — —

GETTYSBURG—Adams County

☒ GETTYSBURG HOSPITAL, 147 Gettys Street, Zip 17325–9978; tel. 717/334–2121; Steven W. Renner, President and Chief Executive Officer; Richard A. Harley, Vice President Finance **A**1 9 10 **F**3 4 7 8 14 15 16 19 21 22 23 28 30 32 33 34 35 37 39 40 42 44 46 49 56 65 67 71 73 74 **P**8 … 23 10 76 4347 50 97892 582 35431 16401 509

GREENSBURG—Westmoreland County

☒ WESTMORELAND REGIONAL HOSPITAL, 532 West Pittsburgh Street, Zip 15601–2282; tel. 412/832–4000; Joseph J. Peluso, President and Chief Executive Officer (Total facility includes 46 beds in nursing home–type unit) **A**1 2 3 9 10 **F**2 3 4 7 8 10 11 13 14 16 17 19 20 21 22 23 25 26 27 28 29 30 31 32 33 34 35 37 39 40 41 42 43 44 45 46 48 49 52 53 54 55 56 57 58 59 60 61 63 64 65 67 68 71 73 74 **P**7 8 … 23 10 345 13613 248 179986 797 98747 45037 1434

GREENVILLE—Mercer County

□ ○ HORIZON HOSPITAL SYSTEM, (Includes Greenville Campus, 110 North Main Street, Zip 16125–1795; tel. 412/588–2100; Shenango Valley Campus, 2200 Memorial Drive, Farrell, Zip 16121–1398; tel. 412/981–3500), J. Larry Heinike, President and Chief Executive Officer (Total facility includes 28 beds in nursing home–type unit) (Nonreporting) **A**1 2 9 10 11 12 **N** Vantage Health Care Network, Inc., Meadville, PA … 23 10 286 — — — — — — — —

GROVE CITY—Mercer County

☒ + ○ UNITED COMMUNITY HOSPITAL, 631 North Broad Street Extension, Zip 16127–9703; tel. 412/458–5442; Robert J. Turner, Administrator **A**1 9 10 11 **F**3 7 8 11 14 15 16 17 19 21 22 28 30 32 34 35 37 39 40 41 42 44 45 49 56 63 65 67 70 71 73 … 23 10 84 3547 45 72806 331 24099 9643 328

HANOVER—York County

☒ HANOVER GENERAL HOSPITAL, 300 Highland Avenue, Zip 17331–2297; tel. 717/637–3711; William R. Walb, President and Chief Executive Officer **A**1 5 9 10 **F**4 7 8 11 15 16 17 18 19 20 21 22 25 28 30 31 33 34 35 37 39 40 41 42 44 45 49 52 53 63 65 67 71 73 **P**4 8 … 23 10 154 5871 85 125599 612 46747 21159 646

HARRISBURG—Dauphin County

□ + ○ COMMUNITY GENERAL OSTEOPATHIC HOSPITAL, 4300 Londonderry Road, Zip 17109, Mailing Address: P.O. Box 3000, Zip 17105–3000; tel. 717/652–3000; George R. Strohl, Jr., President **A**1 9 10 11 12 13 **F**8 14 15 16 19 21 22 30 33 34 36 37 39 41 42 44 45 49 65 67 71 73 **P**2 … 23 10 115 4308 71 149325 0 44915 19362 547

□ EDGEWATER PSYCHIATRIC CENTER, 1829 North Front Street, Zip 17102–2299; tel. 717/238–8666; Michael J. Dalesio, Ph.D., Acting Executive Director **A**1 9 10 **F**15 16 52 53 55 58 59 **P**6 … 23 22 26 440 17 26103 0 9801 3232 133

□ HARRISBURG STATE HOSPITAL, Cameron and Maclay Streets, Zip 17105–1300, Mailing Address: Pouch A, Zip 17105–1300; tel. 717/772–7455; Bruce Darney, Superintendent **A**1 9 10 **F**14 15 16 20 26 46 52 55 57 65 73 … 12 22 392 115 366 0 0 — — 544

PINNACLEHEALTH AT HARRISBURG HOSPITAL See PinnacleHealth System
PINNACLEHEALTH AT POLYCLINIC HOSPITAL See PinnacleHealth System

☒ PINNACLEHEALTH SYSTEM, (Includes PinnacleHealth at Harrisburg Hospital, 111 South Front Street, Zip 17101–2099; tel. 717/782–3131; Stephen H. Franklin, FACHE, President and Chief Executive Officer; PinnacleHealth at Polyclinic Hospital, 2601 North Third Street, Zip 17110–2098; tel. 717/782–4141; Stephen H. Franklin, FACHE, President and Chief Executive Officer; PinnacleHealth at Seidle Memorial Hospital, 120 South Filbert Street, Mechanicsburg, Zip 17055–6591; tel. 717/795–6760; Stephen H. Franklin, FACHE, President and Chief Executive Officer), 17 South Market Square, Zip 17101, Mailing Address: P.O. Box 8700, Zip 17105–8700; tel. 717/231–8200; John S. Cramer, FACHE, President and Chief Executive Officer (Total facility includes 123 beds in nursing home–type unit) **A**1 2 3 5 9 10 **F**1 3 4 6 7 8 10 11 12 15 16 17 19 20 21 22 23 26 27 28 29 30 31 32 33 34 35 37 38 39 40 41 42 43 44 45 46 48 49 51 52 53 54 57 58 59 60 61 63 64 65 67 69 71 72 73 74 **P**1 3 5 6 7 … 23 10 815 30438 572 422469 4919 271646 124675 3437

HAVERFORD—Delaware County

□ HAVERFORD STATE HOSPITAL, 3500 Darby Road, Zip 19041–1098; tel. 610/526–2600; Frances L. Smith, R.N., MSN, Superintendent **A**1 9 10 **F**14 15 20 41 52 54 55 56 65 73 … 12 22 340 86 290 0 0 31018 18558 493

Hospital, Address, Telephone, Administrator, Approval, Facility, and Physician Codes, Health Care System, Network	Classi-fication Codes		Utilization Data					Expense (thousands) of dollars		
	Control	Service	Beds	Admissions	Census	Outpatient Visits	Births	Total	Payroll	Personnel

HAVERTOWN—Delaware County

✫ MERCY COMMUNITY HOSPITAL, (Formerly Mercy Haverford Hospital), 2000 Old West Chester Pike, Zip 19083; tel. 610/645–3600; Andrew E. Harris, Chief Executive Officer **A**1 9 10 **F**1 2 3 6 7 8 10 15 16 17 19 21 22 23 26 30 32 33 35 37 38 39 40 41 42 46 49 52 56 60 63 64 65 66 71 73 **P**8 **S** Eastern Mercy Health System, Radnor, PA

| | 23 | 10 | 107 | 3933 | 49 | 44000 | 0 | 24332 | 10643 | 317 |

HAZLETON—Luzerne County

✫ HAZLETON GENERAL HOSPITAL, 700 East Broad Street, Zip 18201–6897; tel. 717/450–4357; E. Richard Moore, President **A**1 9 10 **F**8 12 14 15 16 17 19 21 22 28 29 30 31 34 35 37 39 41 42 44 45 46 49 52 54 55 56 57 61 63 65 67 71 73 **P**8

| | 23 | 10 | 152 | 5435 | 111 | 40238 | 0 | 31686 | 13315 | 502 |

✫ HAZLETON–ST. JOSEPH MEDICAL CENTER, 687 North Church Street, Zip 18201–3198; tel. 717/459–4444; Bernard C. Rudegeair, President and Chief Executive Officer (Total facility includes 11 beds in nursing home–type unit) **A**1 9 10 **F**8 14 15 16 17 19 22 24 28 30 32 34 36 37 39 40 41 42 44 45 46 49 51 63 64 65 67 71 72 73 74 **P**5 6

| | 21 | 10 | 122 | 5006 | 86 | 150428 | 487 | 33676 | 15590 | 530 |

HERSHEY—Dauphin County

✫ △ PENN STATE UNIVERSITY HOSPITAL–MILTON S. HERSHEY MEDICAL CENTER, 500 University Drive, Zip 17033, Mailing Address: P.O. Box 850, Zip 17033–0850; tel. 717/531–8521; Bruce H. Hamory, M.D., Executive Director **A**1 2 3 5 7 8 9 10 **F**3 4 5 7 8 10 14 15 16 17 19 21 22 23 24 25 28 29 30 31 34 35 37 38 39 40 41 42 43 44 45 46 47 48 49 51 52 53 54 55 56 57 58 59 60 61 63 65 66 67 69 70 71 72 73 **P**1 6

| | 23 | 10 | 454 | 19656 | 368 | 321245 | 1105 | 254899 | 116951 | 3738 |

HONESDALE—Wayne County

✫ WAYNE MEMORIAL HOSPITAL, 601 Park Street, Zip 18431–1498; tel. 717/253–8100; G. Richard Garman, Executive Director **A**1 9 10 **F**7 8 15 17 19 21 22 24 28 30 31 32 33 34 35 39 40 41 42 44 45 49 53 55 56 57 58 59 60 65 66 67 68 71 73 **P**8

| | 23 | 10 | 95 | 3902 | 68 | 113883 | 508 | 28298 | 13108 | 474 |

HUNTINGDON—Huntingdon County

✫ J. C. BLAIR MEMORIAL HOSPITAL, Warm Springs Avenue, Zip 16652; tel. 814/643–2290; Richard E. D'Alberto, Chief Executive Officer **A**1 9 10 **F**7 8 19 21 22 35 37 40 44 49 58 59 66 71 **P**5 **S** Quorum Health Group/Quorum Health Resources, Inc., Brentwood, TN

| | 23 | 10 | 104 | 3105 | 43 | 81634 | 288 | 25441 | 10589 | 360 |

INDIANA—Indiana County

✫ INDIANA HOSPITAL, Hospital Road, Zip 15701, Mailing Address: P.O. Box 788, Zip 15701; tel. 412/357–7000; Donald D. Sandoval, FACHE, President and Chief Executive Officer (Total facility includes 18 beds in nursing home–type unit) **A**1 9 10 **F**7 8 11 12 13 14 15 16 17 19 20 21 22 23 24 26 28 29 30 32 33 34 35 39 40 41 42 44 45 46 49 51 56 60 63 64 65 67 71 73

| | 23 | 10 | 155 | 6711 | 95 | 159756 | 727 | 54877 | 27447 | 786 |

JEANNETTE—Westmoreland County

☐ JEANNETTE DISTRICT MEMORIAL HOSPITAL, 600 Jefferson Avenue, Zip 15644; tel. 412/527–3551; Robert J. Bulger, President and Chief Executive Officer (Total facility includes 11 beds in nursing home–type unit) **A**1 9 10 **F**4 7 8 15 16 17 19 21 22 29 34 35 37 40 41 42 44 45 48 64 65 71 72 73 **P**1 **N** First Health Alliance, Pittsburgh, PA

| | 23 | 10 | 137 | 5853 | 92 | 83163 | 403 | 35674 | 16408 | 503 |

☐ MONSOUR MEDICAL CENTER, 70 Lincoln Way East, Zip 15644; tel. 412/527–1511; Jerry Joseph, Chief Executive Officer **A**1 9 10 **F**2 7 8 10 12 14 15 16 18 19 22 28 30 31 32 35 37 39 40 42 44 52 53 57 65 71 73

| | 23 | 10 | 146 | 2453 | 57 | 43929 | 51 | 22371 | 10373 | 353 |

JERSEY SHORE—Lycoming County

✫ JERSEY SHORE HOSPITAL, 1020 Thompson Street, Zip 17740–0689; tel. 717/398–0100; Louis A. Ditzel, Jr., President and Chief Executive Officer **A**1 9 10 **F**8 12 14 15 16 17 19 21 22 27 28 29 30 32 34 35 37 39 41 44 45 46 49 50 51 65 66 71 73 **P**6 **S** Quorum Health Group/Quorum Health Resources, Inc., Brentwood, TN

| | 23 | 10 | 64 | 1458 | 16 | 38095 | 0 | 10999 | 4999 | 192 |

JOHNSTOWN—Cambria County

✫ CONEMAUGH MEMORIAL MEDICAL CENTER, 1086 Franklin Street, Zip 15905–4398; tel. 814/534–9000; William F. Casey, President and Chief Executive Officer **A**1 2 3 5 6 9 10 12 **F**4 7 8 10 11 14 15 16 19 20 21 22 23 24 25 26 29 30 31 32 34 35 37 38 39 40 41 42 43 44 45 46 49 51 52 54 55 57 58 60 63 65 67 70 71 72 73 **P**6 8

| | 23 | 10 | 355 | 14695 | 244 | 144107 | 838 | 137430 | 57163 | 1860 |

✫ GOOD SAMARITAN MEDICAL CENTER, 1020 Franklin Street, Zip 15905–4186; tel. 814/533–1000; Steven E. Tucker, Interim President (Total facility includes 73 beds in nursing home–type unit) (Nonreporting) **A**1 9 10

| | 23 | 10 | 240 | — | — | — | — | — | — | — |

☐ LEE HOSPITAL, 320 Main Street, Zip 15901–1694; tel. 814/533–0123; John W. Ungar, President (Total facility includes 18 beds in nursing home–type unit) **A**1 2 9 10 **F**7 8 10 11 12 14 15 16 17 19 21 22 26 27 28 29 30 32 33 34 35 37 39 40 41 42 44 45 48 49 51 56 60 62 64 65 67 71 72 73 74 **P**6 8

| | 23 | 10 | 224 | 7891 | 148 | 97401 | 384 | 72265 | 31951 | 1120 |

KANE—McKean County

☐ KANE COMMUNITY HOSPITAL, North Fraley Street, Zip 16735; tel. 814/837–8585; J. Gary Rhodes, Chief Operating Officer (Nonreporting) **A**1 9 10

| | 23 | 10 | 36 | — | — | — | — | — | — | — |

KINGSTON—Luzerne County

NESBITT MEMORIAL HOSPITAL See Wyoming Valley Health Care System, Wilkes–Barre

KITTANNING—Armstrong County

✫ ARMSTRONG COUNTY MEMORIAL HOSPITAL, One Nolte Drive, Zip 16201–8808; tel. 412/543–8500; Jack D. Hoard, President and Chief Executive Officer (Total facility includes 17 beds in nursing home–type unit) **A**1 9 10 **F**7 8 10 11 12 14 15 17 19 21 22 28 29 32 34 35 37 39 40 41 42 44 46 49 50 51 52 53 54 55 56 57 60 63 64 65 66 67 71 73 **P**4 5

| | 23 | 10 | 215 | 6953 | 119 | 107775 | 498 | 44061 | 19681 | 694 |

Hospital, Address, Telephone, Administrator, Approval, Facility, and Physician Codes, Health Care System, Network	Classi-fication Codes		Utilization Data					Expense (thousands) of dollars		
★ American Hospital Association (AHA) membership □ Joint Commission on Accreditation of Healthcare Organizations (JCAHO) accreditation + American Osteopathic Hospital Association (AOHA) membership ○ American Osteopathic Association (AOA) accreditation △ Commission on Accreditation of Rehabilitation Facilities (CARF) accreditation Control codes 61, 63, 64, 71, 72 and 73 indicate hospitals listed by AOHA, but not registered by AHA. For definition of numerical codes, see page A4	Control	Service	Beds	Admissions	Census	Outpatient Visits	Births	Total	Payroll	Personnel

LAFAYETTE HILL—Montgomery County

□ EUGENIA HOSPITAL, 660 Thomas Road, Zip 19444–1199; tel. 215/836–7700; John P. Ash, FACHE, President and Chief Executive Officer (Nonreporting) **A**1 9 10

| | 33 | 22 | 126 | — | | — | | — | — | — |

LANCASTER—Lancaster County

+ ○ COMMUNITY HOSPITAL OF LANCASTER, 1100 East Orange Street, Zip 17602–3218, Mailing Address: Box 3002, Zip 17604–3002; tel. 717/397–3711; Mark C. Barabas, President **A**9 10 11 12 13 **F**7 8 10 12 14 15 16 17 19 20 21 22 25 28 29 30 31 32 34 35 37 39 40 41 44 48 49 51 52 54 55 56 57 58 63 64 65 67 71 73 74 **P**3 8

| | 23 | 10 | 142 | 5135 | 63 | 42069 | 710 | 36612 | 16248 | 712 |

□ △ LANCASTER GENERAL HOSPITAL, 555 North Duke Street, Zip 17602, Mailing Address: Box 3555, Zip 17604–3555; tel. 717/290–5511; Mark A. Brazitis, President (Total facility includes 30 beds in nursing home–type unit) **A**1 2 3 5 6 7 9 10 **F**3 4 7 8 10 12 14 15 16 19 20 21 22 25 26 27 28 29 30 32 33 34 35 37 38 39 40 41 42 43 44 45 46 48 49 51 52 53 54 56 58 59 60 61 63 64 65 66 67 70 71 73 74 **P**4 7

| | 23 | 10 | 491 | 24009 | 343 | 352108 | 2982 | 204804 | 96930 | 2729 |

⊠ △ ST. JOSEPH HOSPITAL, 250 College Avenue, Zip 17604; tel. 717/291–8211; John Kerr Tolmie, President and Chief Executive Officer (Total facility includes 19 beds in nursing home–type unit) **A**1 2 7 9 10 **F**1 2 3 4 7 8 10 11 12 14 15 16 17 19 21 22 23 24 26 28 29 30 31 32 33 34 35 37 38 39 40 41 42 43 44 45 46 48 49 51 52 53 54 55 56 57 58 59 60 61 63 64 65 67 69 71 73 74 **P**5 6 7 8 **S** Catholic Health Initiatives, Denver, CO

| | 21 | 10 | 256 | 9504 | 115 | 182073 | 1062 | 69098 | 28618 | 804 |

LANGHORNE—Bucks County

+ ○ DELAWARE VALLEY MEDICAL CENTER, 200 Oxford Valley Road, Zip 19047; tel. 215/949–5100; Carl E. Brown, President (Total facility includes 16 beds in nursing home–type unit) **A**10 11 12 13 **F**8 10 11 14 15 16 17 19 21 22 23 26 29 30 31 32 34 35 36 37 39 42 44 45 46 49 52 56 57 59 61 63 64 65 69 71 73

| | 23 | 10 | 160 | 5469 | 87 | — | 0 | 46497 | 21544 | 666 |

⊠ ST. MARY MEDICAL CENTER, Langhorne–Newtown Road, Zip 19047–1295; tel. 215/750–2000; Sister Clare Carty, President and Chief Executive Officer **A**1 2 9 10 **F**7 8 10 11 12 13 14 15 16 17 19 21 22 24 26 28 30 32 35 37 38 39 40 41 42 44 46 48 49 51 56 60 63 65 66 67 70 71 73 74 **P**1 3 6 7 **S** Catholic Health Initiatives, Denver, CO **N** Fox Chase Network, Rockledge, PA

| | 21 | 10 | 263 | 11695 | 164 | 137388 | 1486 | 90686 | 41152 | 1126 |

LANSDALE—Montgomery County

⊠ NORTH PENN HOSPITAL, 100 Medical Campus Drive, Zip 19446–1200; tel. 215/368–2100; Robert H. McKay, President **A**1 2 9 10 **F**7 8 11 14 16 17 19 21 22 28 29 30 34 39 40 41 42 44 46 63 65 66 67 68 71 73 **N** Fox Chase Network, Rockledge, PA

| | 23 | 10 | 150 | 5213 | 63 | 92448 | 838 | 38748 | 17593 | 523 |

LATROBE—Westmoreland County

⊠ LATROBE AREA HOSPITAL, 121 West Second Avenue, Zip 15650–1096; tel. 412/537–1000; Douglas A. Clark, Executive Director **A**1 2 3 5 9 10 **F**5 7 8 10 11 12 15 16 19 21 22 24 25 26 27 28 29 30 31 32 33 34 35 37 39 40 41 42 44 45 49 51 52 53 54 55 56 58 59 60 65 67 68 71 73 74 **P**6

| | 23 | 10 | 226 | 11898 | 158 | 220686 | 857 | 88028 | 47129 | 1230 |

LEBANON—Lebanon County

⊠ GOOD SAMARITAN HOSPITAL, Fourth and Walnut Streets, Zip 17042, Mailing Address: P.O. Box 1281, Zip 17042–1281; tel. 717/270–7500; Robert J. Longo, President and Chief Executive Officer (Total facility includes 19 beds in nursing home–type unit) **A**1 3 5 9 10 **F**4 7 8 10 12 14 15 16 17 18 19 20 21 22 24 27 30 31 32 33 34 35 37 39 40 41 42 44 46 48 49 51 53 54 55 56 57 58 59 60 63 64 65 66 67 71 72 73 74 **P**8

| | 23 | 10 | 195 | 8584 | 127 | 144442 | 1090 | 61433 | 28941 | 933 |

⊠ VETERANS AFFAIRS MEDICAL CENTER, 1700 South Lincoln Avenue, Zip 17042–7597; tel. 717/272–6621; Leonard Washington, Jr., Director (Total facility includes 177 beds in nursing home–type unit) **A**1 3 5 9 **F**2 3 4 8 10 15 17 19 20 21 22 25 26 27 28 30 31 33 34 35 37 39 41 42 43 44 45 46 48 49 50 51 52 54 56 57 58 59 63 64 65 67 71 72 73 74 **P**6 **S** Department of Veterans Affairs, Washington, DC

| | 45 | 10 | 565 | 3191 | 479 | 117302 | 0 | 84137 | 43634 | 1181 |

LEHIGHTON—Carbon County

⊠ GNADEN HUETTEN MEMORIAL HOSPITAL, 211 North 12th Street, Zip 18235; tel. 610/377–1300; Robert J. Clark, FACHE, President and Chief Executive Officer (Total facility includes 91 beds in nursing home–type unit) **A**1 9 10 **F**7 8 14 15 16 17 19 20 21 22 25 26 27 28 30 32 33 35 36 37 39 40 41 42 44 45 46 49 51 52 53 54 55 56 57 58 59 61 64 65 67 71 73 74 **P**5 8

| | 23 | 10 | 200 | 3979 | 146 | 123226 | 323 | 30177 | 14113 | 511 |

LEWISBURG—Union County

EVANGELICAL COMMUNITY HOSPITAL, One Hospital Drive, Zip 17837–9390; tel. 717/522–2000; Michael Daniloff, President **A**9 10 **F**5 7 8 11 12 13 14 15 16 17 18 19 20 21 22 23 24 28 30 32 33 34 35 37 39 40 41 42 44 45 48 49 51 52 53 54 55 56 57 58 61 65 66 67 71 73 74 **P**3 5 8

| | 23 | 10 | 115 | 5661 | 67 | 267050 | 821 | 41560 | 19046 | 681 |

U. S. PENITENTIARY INFIRMARY, (Formerly U. S. Penitentiary Hospital), Route 7, Zip 17837; tel. 717/523–1251; Arnold Reyes, Administrator (Nonreporting)

| | 48 | 11 | 17 | — | | — | | — | — | — |

LEWISTOWN—Mifflin County

⊠ LEWISTOWN HOSPITAL, 400 Highland Avenue, Zip 17044–1198; tel. 717/248–5411; John R. Whitcomb, President and Chief Executive Officer **A**1 2 9 10 12 **F**3 7 8 11 14 19 20 21 22 26 30 33 34 35 37 39 40 41 42 44 49 52 53 54 55 56 57 58 60 63 71 73 **P**3 6

| | 23 | 10 | 163 | 7588 | 103 | 166546 | 710 | 47975 | 22163 | 740 |

LOCK HAVEN—Clinton County

⊠ LOCK HAVEN HOSPITAL, 24 Cree Drive, Zip 17745; tel. 717/893–5000; Gary R. Rhoads, President and Chief Executive Officer (Total facility includes 120 beds in nursing home–type unit) **A**1 9 10 **F**7 8 15 17 19 20 21 22 25 26 27 30 32 33 34 35 37 39 40 41 44 45 46 49 51 53 54 55 56 57 58 59 61 62 63 64 65 71 73 74 **P**8 **S** Quorum Health Group/Quorum Health Resources, Inc., Brentwood, TN

| | 23 | 10 | 195 | 3702 | 149 | 36730 | 341 | 21563 | 9281 | 396 |

Hospital, Address, Telephone, Administrator, Approval, Facility, and Physician Codes, Health Care System, Network	Classi-fication Codes		Utilization Data					Expense (thousands) of dollars		
★ American Hospital Association (AHA) membership □ Joint Commission on Accreditation of Healthcare Organizations (JCAHO) accreditation + American Osteopathic Hospital Association (AOHA) membership ○ American Osteopathic Association (AOA) accreditation △ Commission on Accreditation of Rehabilitation Facilities (CARF) accreditation Control codes 61, 63, 64, 71, 72 and 73 indicate hospitals listed by AOHA, but not registered by AHA. For definition of numerical codes, see page A4	Control	Service	Beds	Admissions	Census	Outpatient Visits	Births	Total	Payroll	Personnel

MALVERN—Chester County

✚ △ BRYN MAWR REHABILITATION HOSPITAL, 414 Paoli Pike, Zip 19355–3300, Mailing Address: P.O. Box 3007, Zip 19355–3300; tel. 610/251–5400; Barry S. Rabner, President (Total facility includes 23 beds in nursing home–type unit) **A**1 7 9 10 **F**4 7 8 10 11 12 15 16 19 22 28 32 34 35 37 38 40 41 42 43 44 46 47 48 49 50 60 64 65 67 71 73 74 **P**5 8 **S** Jefferson Health System, Radnor, PA **N** Jefferson Health System, Radnor, PA — 23 46 141 2480 109 24338 0 30278 15333 451

★ DEVEREUX MAPLETON PSYCHIATRIC INSTITUTE–MAPLETON CENTER, 655 Sugartown Road, Zip 19355–0297, Mailing Address: Box 297, Zip 19355–0297; tel. 610/296–6923; Richard Warden, Administrator (Nonreporting) **S** Devereux Foundation, Devon, PA — 23 22 13 — — — — — — —

MALVERN INSTITUTE, 940 King Road, Zip 19355–2058; tel. 610/647–0330; Valerie Craig, Administrator and Chief Executive Officer **A**9 **F**1 2 3 4 5 6 7 8 9 10 11 12 13 16 17 18 19 20 21 22 23 24 25 26 27 28 29 30 31 32 33 34 35 36 37 38 39 40 41 42 43 44 45 46 47 48 49 50 51 52 53 54 55 56 57 58 59 60 61 62 63 64 65 66 67 68 69 70 71 72 73 74 — 33 82 40 1131 29 1454 0 2175 1259 42

MCCONNELLSBURG—Fulton County

★ FULTON COUNTY MEDICAL CENTER, 216 South First Street, Zip 17233–1399; tel. 717/485–3155; Robert E. Swadley, Chief Executive Officer (Total facility includes 57 beds in nursing home–type unit) **A**9 10 **F**8 11 15 19 22 34 35 40 44 63 64 65 71 — 23 10 96 1069 71 73226 87 9990 4409 223

MCKEES ROCKS—Allegheny County

✚ OHIO VALLEY GENERAL HOSPITAL, 25 Heckel Road, Zip 15136–1694; tel. 412/777–6161; William Provenzano, President **A**1 6 9 10 **F**4 7 8 10 12 13 14 15 16 17 18 19 20 21 22 23 24 25 26 28 29 30 32 33 34 35 36 37 39 40 41 42 44 45 46 49 51 61 65 67 71 72 73 **P**5 **S** Quorum Health Group/Quorum Health Resources, Inc., Brentwood, TN — 23 10 102 5472 81 93210 481 42629 16738 453

MCKEESPORT—Allegheny County

✚ MCKEESPORT HOSPITAL, 1500 Fifth Avenue, Zip 15132–2482; tel. 412/664–2000; Ronald H. Ott, President and Chief Executive Officer (Total facility includes 28 beds in nursing home–type unit) **A**1 3 5 9 10 **F**7 8 10 11 12 13 15 16 17 19 21 22 25 26 27 28 29 30 31 32 33 34 37 39 40 41 42 44 45 46 48 49 51 52 54 55 56 57 60 61 64 65 67 71 73 74 **P**3 — 23 10 320 10156 205 98368 424 80447 38423 1255

MEADOWBROOK—Montgomery County

□ HOLY REDEEMER HOSPITAL AND MEDICAL CENTER, 1648 Huntingdon Pike, Zip 19046–8099; tel. 215/947–3000; Mark T. Jones, President (Total facility includes 15 beds in nursing home–type unit) (Nonreporting) **A**1 5 9 10 — 23 10 217 — — — — — — —

MEADVILLE—Crawford County

✚ MEADVILLE MEDICAL CENTER, (Includes Meadville City Hospital, 751 Liberty Street, tel. 814/333–5000; Spencer Hospital, 1034 Grove Street), 751 Liberty Street, Zip 16335; tel. 814/333–5000; Anthony J. DeFail, President and Chief Executive Officer (Total facility includes 32 beds in nursing home–type unit) **A**1 2 9 10 **F**2 3 7 8 12 14 15 16 17 18 19 20 21 22 30 32 33 35 37 39 40 41 42 44 45 46 48 49 52 53 54 55 56 58 59 61 64 65 67 71 73 74 **P**7 8 **N** Vantage Health Care Network, Inc., Meadville, PA — 23 10 243 8817 152 112107 585 58962 24955 841

MECHANICSBURG—Cumberland County

□ △ HEALTHSOUTH REHABILITATION OF MECHANICSBURG, 175 Lancaster Boulevard, Zip 17055–2016, Mailing Address: P.O. Box 2016, Zip 17055–2016; tel. 717/691–3700; Barbara H. Bowen, Interim Administrator (Nonreporting) **A**1 7 9 10 **S** HEALTHSOUTH Corporation, Birmingham, AL — 33 46 103 — — — — — — —

PINNACLEHEALTH AT SEIDLE MEMORIAL HOSPITAL See PinnacleHealth System, Harrisburg

MEDIA—Delaware County

✚ RIDDLE MEMORIAL HOSPITAL, 1068 West Baltimore Pike, Zip 19063–5177; tel. 610/566–9400; Donald L. Laughlin, President (Total facility includes 22 beds in nursing home–type unit) **A**1 2 9 10 **F**3 7 8 10 12 13 14 17 19 21 22 24 26 28 30 31 32 34 35 37 38 39 40 41 42 44 45 46 49 62 64 65 66 67 71 73 74 **P**5 — 23 10 198 9261 145 74315 867 63078 29536 867

MEYERSDALE—Somerset County

✚ MEYERSDALE MEDICAL CENTER, 200 Hospital Drive, Zip 15552–1247; tel. 814/634–5911; Mary L. Libengood, President **A**1 9 10 **F**8 14 15 19 21 22 28 30 32 37 44 65 67 71 72 73 **P**6 — 23 10 43 617 9 20004 0 4937 2410 104

MONONGAHELA—Washington County

✚ MONONGAHELA VALLEY HOSPITAL, Country Club Road, Route 88, Zip 15063–1095; tel. 412/258–1000; Anthony M. Lombardi, President and Chief Executive Officer **A**1 2 9 10 **F**2 5 7 8 10 11 13 14 15 16 17 19 20 21 22 23 26 28 29 30 31 32 33 34 35 37 39 40 41 42 44 45 46 48 49 52 53 54 56 57 60 61 65 66 67 68 71 73 74 **P**8 — 23 10 282 11577 201 185808 519 70349 33046 1007

MONROEVILLE—Allegheny County

✚ FORBES REGIONAL HOSPITAL, 2570 Haymaker Road, Zip 15146–3592; tel. 412/858–2000; Dana W. Ramish, President and Chief Executive Officer **A**1 2 3 5 9 10 **F**7 8 10 12 14 15 16 17 19 22 24 25 26 28 29 30 33 34 35 36 37 39 40 41 42 44 45 46 49 51 52 54 55 56 57 60 63 65 67 71 72 73 **P**4 5 6 8 **S** Allegheny Health, Education and Research Foundation, Pittsburgh, PA — 23 10 226 14782 226 76497 1410 96452 35889 1053

□ △ HEALTHSOUTH GREATER PITTSBURGH REHABILITATION HOSPITAL, 2380 McGinley Road, Zip 15146; tel. 412/856–2400; Faith A. Deigan, Administrator (Nonreporting) **A**1 7 9 10 **S** HEALTHSOUTH Corporation, Birmingham, AL — 33 46 89 — — — — — — —

Hospital, Address, Telephone, Administrator, Approval, Facility, and Physician Codes, Health Care System, Network	Classi-fication Codes		Utilization Data					Expense (thousands) of dollars		
★ American Hospital Association (AHA) membership □ Joint Commission on Accreditation of Healthcare Organizations (JCAHO) accreditation + American Osteopathic Hospital Association (AOHA) membership ○ American Osteopathic Association (AOA) accreditation △ Commission on Accreditation of Rehabilitation Facilities (CARF) accreditation Control codes 61, 63, 64, 71, 72 and 73 indicate hospitals listed by AOHA, but not registered by AHA. For definition of numerical codes, see page A4	Control	Service	Beds	Admissions	Census	Outpatient Visits	Births	Total	Payroll	Personnel

MONTROSE—Susquehanna County

ENDLESS MOUNTAIN HEALTH SYSTEMS, (Formerly Montrose General Hospital), 1 Grow Avenue, Zip 18801–1199; tel. 717/278–3801; Rex Catlin, Chief Executive Officer (Nonreporting) **A**9 10 — 33 10 34 | — | — | — | — | — | — | —

MOUNT GRETNA—Lebanon County

□ PHILHAVEN, 283 South Butler Road, Zip 17064, Mailing Address: P.O. Box 550, Zip 17064–0550; tel. 717/273–8871; LaVern J. Yutzy, Chief Executive Officer **A**1 9 10 **F**15 16 26 52 53 54 55 56 57 58 59 65 73 74 | 21 | 22 | 106 | 1786 | 62 | 68615 | 0 | 22115 | 14113 | 472

MOUNT PLEASANT—Westmoreland County

✠ FRICK HOSPITAL AND COMMUNITY HEALTH CENTER, 508 South Church Street, Zip 15666–1790; tel. 412/547–1500; Rodney L. Gunderson, Executive Director (Total facility includes 18 beds in nursing home–type unit) **A**1 2 9 10 **F**7 8 10 11 12 14 15 16 17 18 19 20 21 22 26 28 29 30 31 32 33 34 35 37 39 40 41 42 44 45 46 49 53 54 55 56 57 58 59 60 63 64 65 67 69 71 73 | 23 | 10 | 171 | 6081 | 91 | 94816 | 521 | 38689 | 18982 | 565

MUNCY—Lycoming County

MUNCY VALLEY HOSPITAL See Susquehanna Health System, Williamsport

NANTICOKE—Luzerne County

★ MERCY SPECIAL CARE HOSPITAL, (ACUTE LONG TERM CARE), 128 West Washington Street, Zip 18634; tel. 717/735–5000; Robert D. Williams, Administrator **A**9 10 **F**1 3 14 15 16 19 22 26 32 33 34 35 41 42 43 44 45 49 52 53 54 55 56 57 58 59 60 66 71 73 **P**7 8 **S** Mercy Health System, Cincinnati, OH | 23 | 49 | 38 | 416 | 32 | 26406 | 0 | 7845 | 3559 | 91

NATRONA HEIGHTS—Allegheny County

✠ ALLEGHENY VALLEY HOSPITAL, 1301 Carlisle Street, Zip 15065–1192; tel. 412/224–5100; John R. England, President and Chief Executive Officer (Total facility includes 19 beds in nursing home–type unit) **A**1 2 9 10 **F**3 7 8 10 11 15 16 17 19 21 22 28 30 31 32 33 34 35 37 39 40 41 42 44 45 49 52 54 56 60 63 64 65 66 67 71 73 **P**2 7 8 **N** SouthWest Integrated Delivery Network, Pittsburgh, PA | 23 | 10 | 266 | 9568 | 175 | 136935 | 555 | 71436 | 33085 | 963

NEW CASTLE—Lawrence County

✠ △ JAMESON MEMORIAL HOSPITAL, 1211 Wilmington Avenue, Zip 16105–2595; tel. 412/658–9001; Thomas White, President (Total facility includes 20 beds in nursing home–type unit) **A**1 2 6 7 9 10 **F**1 7 8 10 11 12 13 14 15 16 17 19 20 21 22 23 26 28 29 30 32 34 35 37 39 40 41 42 44 45 48 49 54 56 60 61 63 64 65 66 67 71 72 73 74 **P**3 7 8 | 23 | 10 | 183 | 7018 | 113 | 192669 | 525 | 59438 | 26689 | 1017

✠ ST. FRANCIS HOSPITAL OF NEW CASTLE, 1000 South Mercer Street, Zip 16101–4673; tel. 412/658–3511; Sister Donna Zwigart, Chief Executive Officer (Total facility includes 45 beds in nursing home–type unit) **A**1 6 9 10 **F**2 3 5 7 8 11 12 13 14 15 16 17 18 19 20 21 22 23 28 29 30 31 32 33 34 36 39 40 41 42 44 45 46 48 49 52 53 54 55 56 57 58 59 60 61 62 63 64 65 67 71 73 74 **P**5 6 8 **S** St. Francis Health System, Pittsburgh, PA **N** Saint Francis Health System, Pittsburgh, PA | 23 | 10 | 193 | 4340 | 109 | 43864 | 156 | 31156 | 13524 | 517

NEW KENSINGTON—Westmoreland County

□ CITIZENS GENERAL HOSPITAL, 651 Fourth Avenue, Zip 15068–6591; tel. 412/337–3541; Robert E. Marino, Executive Director (Total facility includes 20 beds in nursing home–type unit) **A**1 2 6 9 10 **F**7 8 11 13 14 15 16 18 19 21 22 23 28 29 30 31 32 33 34 35 37 39 40 41 42 44 45 49 60 63 64 65 67 71 73 | 23 | 10 | 120 | 5431 | 86 | 72132 | 311 | 40796 | 17500 | 571

NORRISTOWN—Montgomery County

□ MONTGOMERY COUNTY EMERGENCY SERVICE, 50 Beech Drive, Zip 19404, Mailing Address: Caller Box 3005, Zip 19404–3005; tel. 610/279–6100; Rocio Nell, M.D., Medical and Executive Director (Nonreporting) **A**1 9 10 | 23 | 22 | 53 | — | — | — | — | — | — | —

✠ MONTGOMERY HOSPITAL, 1301 Powell Street, Zip 19404, Mailing Address: P.O. Box 992, Zip 19404–0992; tel. 610/270–2000; Timothy M. Casey, President and Chief Executive Officer (Total facility includes 17 beds in nursing home–type unit) **A**1 2 3 5 9 10 **F**4 7 8 10 11 12 14 15 16 17 19 21 22 27 28 32 33 37 38 39 40 41 42 44 46 49 51 52 54 57 58 59 60 64 65 67 71 73 74 **P**6 **N** Fox Chase Network, Rockledge, PA | 23 | 10 | 256 | 10096 | 158 | 190905 | 659 | 80763 | 39596 | 1051

□ NORRISTOWN STATE HOSPITAL, 1001 Sterigere Street, Zip 19401–5399; tel. 215/270–1000; Albert R. Di Dario, Superintendent **A**1 3 5 9 10 **F**14 20 24 52 57 65 73 | 12 | 22 | 664 | 375 | 587 | 0 | 0 | 69347 | 41575 | 1036

+ ○ SUBURBAN GENERAL HOSPITAL, 2701 DeKalb Pike, Zip 19401; tel. 610/278–2000; Edward R. Solvibile, President (Nonreporting) **A**2 9 10 11 12 13 | 23 | 10 | 118 | — | — | — | — | — | — | —

✠ VALLEY FORGE MEDICAL CENTER AND HOSPITAL, 1033 West Germantown Pike, Zip 19403–3998; tel. 610/539–8500; Marian W. Colcher, President (Nonreporting) **A**1 9 10 | 33 | 10 | 70 | — | — | — | — | — | — | —

NORTH WARREN—Warren County

□ WARREN STATE HOSPITAL, 33 Main Drive, Zip 16365–5099; tel. 814/723–5500; Carmen N. Ferranto, Superintendent **A**1 10 **F**8 10 11 16 19 20 22 31 33 35 37 39 41 42 44 46 48 49 52 55 57 60 65 71 73 | 12 | 22 | 348 | 285 | 300 | 0 | 0 | 36007 | 21365 | 607

OAKDALE—Allegheny County

□ VENCOR HOSPITAL–PITTSBURGH, 7777 Steubenville Pike, Zip 15071; tel. 412/494–5500; Patricia B. Speak, Administrator (Nonreporting) **A**1 10 **S** Vencor, Incorporated, Louisville, KY | 33 | 49 | 63 | — | — | — | — | — | — | —

OIL CITY—Venango County

NORTHWEST MEDICAL CENTER–OIL CITY CAMPUS See Northwest Medical Center, Franklin

Hospital, Address, Telephone, Administrator, Approval, Facility, and Physician Codes, Health Care System, Network	Classi-fication Codes		Utilization Data					Expense (thousands) of dollars		
★ American Hospital Association (AHA) membership □ Joint Commission on Accreditation of Healthcare Organizations (JCAHO) accreditation + American Osteopathic Hospital Association (AOHA) membership ○ American Osteopathic Association (AOA) accreditation △ Commission on Accreditation of Rehabilitation Facilities (CARF) accreditation Control codes 61, 63, 64, 71, 72 and 73 indicate hospitals listed by AOHA, but not registered by AHA. For definition of numerical codes, see page A4	Control	Service	Beds	Admissions	Census	Outpatient Visits	Births	Total	Payroll	Personnel

PALMERTON—Carbon County

□ PALMERTON HOSPITAL, 135 Lafayette Avenue, Zip 18071–9990; tel. 610/826–3141; Peter L. Kern, President and Chief Executive Officer **A**1 9 10 **F**7 8 11 14 15 19 22 30 33 40 44 45 46 65 67 71 — 23 10 70 2611 35 39365 188 16504 7382 263

PAOLI—Chester County

★ PAOLI MEMORIAL HOSPITAL, 255 West Lancaster Avenue, Zip 19301–1792; tel. 610/648–1204; Gail A. Egan, Vice President, Administrator **A**1 2 9 10 **F**3 7 8 10 11 12 14 15 16 17 19 20 21 22 23 26 28 30 32 33 34 35 37 40 41 42 44 46 52 53 54 55 56 57 58 59 60 61 67 71 73 **P**5 7 **S** Jefferson Health System, Radnor, PA **N** Jefferson Health System, Radnor, PA; Fox Chase Network, Rockledge, PA — 23 10 129 7055 78 93850 514 50480 20503 631

PECKVILLE—Lackawanna County

MID–VALLEY HOSPITAL, 1400 Main Street, Zip 18452; tel. 717/383–5500; Gerard H. Warner, Jr., Chief Executive Officer **A**9 10 **F**8 14 15 16 17 19 21 22 30 32 33 34 37 39 42 44 46 49 65 71 73 **P**8 — 23 10 40 1253 21 37505 0 9136 4059 167

PHILADELPHIA—Philadelphia County

□ △ ALBERT EINSTEIN MEDICAL CENTER, (Includes Moss Rehabilitation Hospital, 1200 West Tabor Road, Zip 19141–3099; tel. 215/456–9070), 5501 Old York Road, Zip 19141–3098; tel. 215/456–7890; Martin Goldsmith, President (Total facility includes 102 beds in nursing home–type unit) **A**1 2 3 5 7 8 9 10 13 **F**1 3 4 5 7 8 10 11 12 13 14 15 16 17 18 19 20 21 22 24 25 26 28 29 30 31 33 34 35 37 38 39 40 41 42 43 44 45 46 48 49 51 52 53 54 55 56 57 58 59 60 61 65 67 68 69 70 71 73 **P**6 **S** Albert Einstein Healthcare Network, Philadelphia, PA **N** Albert Einstein Healthcare Network, Philadelphia, PA — 23 10 701 20452 410 130661 1517 — — 3817

★ ALLEGHENY UNIVERSITY HOSPITAL, EAST FALLS, (Formerly Medical College of Pennsylvania Hospital), (Includes Eastern Pennsylvania Psychiatric Institute, 3200 Henry Avenue, tel. 215/842–4000), 3300 Henry Avenue, Zip 19129; tel. 215/842–6000; Margaret M. McGoldrick, Chief Executive Officer **A**1 2 3 5 8 9 10 **F**2 3 4 5 7 8 9 10 11 12 13 14 15 16 17 18 19 20 21 22 24 26 27 28 30 31 32 34 35 37 38 39 40 41 42 43 44 45 46 47 48 49 51 52 53 54 55 56 57 58 59 60 61 65 66 67 69 70 71 73 74 **P**6 7 **S** Allegheny Health, Education and Research Foundation, Pittsburgh, PA — 23 10 369 13289 265 94504 1022 185074 78986 2077

★ ALLEGHENY UNIVERSITY HOSPITALS, HAHNEMANN, (Formerly Hahnemann University Hospital), Broad and Vine Streets, Zip 19102–1192; tel. 215/762–7000; Shelley Gebar, President and Chief Executive Officer **A**1 2 3 5 8 9 10 **F**2 3 4 5 7 8 9 10 11 12 13 14 15 16 17 18 19 20 21 22 24 25 26 27 28 30 31 32 33 34 35 37 38 39 40 41 42 43 44 45 46 47 48 49 51 52 53 54 55 56 57 58 59 60 61 65 66 67 69 70 71 73 74 **P**6 7 **S** Allegheny Health, Education and Research Foundation, Pittsburgh, PA — 23 10 540 20461 392 103467 1549 321303 128001 3238

□ BELMONT CENTER FOR COMPREHENSIVE TREATMENT, 4200 Monument Road, Zip 19131–1689; tel. 215/877–2000; Jack H. Dembow, General Director and Vice President **A**1 3 5 9 10 **F**1 3 12 17 18 19 21 22 34 35 52 53 55 56 57 58 59 60 65 71 73 **P**6 **S** Albert Einstein Healthcare Network, Philadelphia, PA **N** Albert Einstein Healthcare Network, Philadelphia, PA — 23 22 146 3602 115 31668 0 21251 11649 423

□ CHARTER FAIRMOUNT INSTITUTE, 561 Fairthorne Avenue, Zip 19128–2499; tel. 215/487–4000; Paul B. Henry, Administrator (Nonreporting) **A**1 9 10 **S** Magellan Health Services, Atlanta, GA — 33 22 146 — — — — — — —

★ CHESTNUT HILL HOSPITAL, 8835 Germantown Avenue, Zip 19118–2765; tel. 215/248–8200; Cary F. Leptuck, President and Chief Executive Officer **A**1 3 5 9 10 **F**1 4 6 7 8 11 14 15 16 17 19 21 22 25 26 27 28 30 31 33 34 35 36 37 39 40 42 44 45 46 49 51 60 61 62 63 65 67 71 73 74 **P**2 5 7 — 23 10 169 8626 107 93903 1192 58950 27713 802

□ CHILDREN'S HOSPITAL OF PHILADELPHIA, 34th Street and Civic Center Boulevard, Zip 19104–4399; tel. 215/590–1000; Edmond F. Notebaert, President **A**1 2 3 5 8 9 10 **F**10 11 12 13 14 15 16 17 19 20 21 22 25 28 29 30 31 32 34 35 38 39 42 43 44 45 46 47 48 49 51 52 53 54 55 56 58 59 60 65 67 68 69 70 71 73 **P**1 — 23 50 304 16159 232 248855 0 236301 111331 2941

CHILDREN'S REHABILITATION HOSPITAL See Thomas Jefferson University Hospital

□ CHILDREN'S SEASHORE HOUSE, 3405 Civic Center Boulevard, Zip 19104–4388; tel. 215/895–3600; Richard W. Shepherd, President and Chief Executive Officer **A**1 3 5 9 10 **F**5 14 15 19 21 25 27 34 35 48 49 53 54 65 73 **P**5 — 33 56 77 659 60 30699 0 34749 15451 446

EASTERN PENNSYLVANIA PSYCHIATRIC INSTITUTE See Allegheny University Hospital, East Falls

★ EPISCOPAL HOSPITAL, (Includes George L. Harrison Memorial House), 100 East Lehigh Avenue, Zip 19125–1098; tel. 215/427–7000; Mark T. Bateman, President and Chief Executive Officer (Total facility includes 35 beds in nursing home–type unit) **A**1 2 3 5 6 9 10 **F**2 3 5 8 10 12 14 15 16 17 19 20 21 22 25 26 27 28 29 30 31 32 34 35 37 38 39 40 41 42 43 44 45 46 49 51 54 63 64 65 67 68 71 73 74 **P**3 — 23 10 218 8673 159 111820 1366 89927 51876 963

★ FOX CHASE CANCER CENTER–AMERICAN ONCOLOGIC HOSPITAL, (ONCOLOGY), 7701 Burholme Avenue, Zip 19111; tel. 215/728–6900; Robert C. Young, M.D., President **A**1 2 3 5 8 9 10 **F**8 12 14 15 16 17 18 19 20 21 28 29 30 31 32 33 34 35 37 39 41 42 44 45 46 49 54 60 65 67 69 71 73 74 **P**6 **N** Fox Chase Network, Rockledge, PA — 23 49 82 3326 50 37304 0 54855 17990 508

★ FRANKFORD HOSPITAL OF THE CITY OF PHILADELPHIA, (Includes Frankford Campus, Frankford Avenue and Wakeling Street, Zip 19124; tel. 215/831–2000; Torresdale Campus), Knights and Red Lion Roads, Zip 19114–1486; tel. 215/612–4000; Roy A. Powell, President **A**1 3 5 6 8 9 10 **F**2 3 7 8 11 12 13 14 15 16 17 19 21 22 23 24 25 26 27 28 29 30 31 32 34 35 37 38 39 40 41 42 44 45 46 48 49 51 54 59 60 61 65 67 70 71 73 74 **P**7 — 23 10 314 18465 258 169254 1869 163176 72793 1849

Hospital, Address, Telephone, Administrator, Approval, Facility, and Physician Codes, Health Care System, Network	Classi-fication Codes		Utilization Data					Expense (thousands) of dollars		
★ American Hospital Association (AHA) membership □ Joint Commission on Accreditation of Healthcare Organizations (JCAHO) accreditation + American Osteopathic Hospital Association (AOHA) membership ○ American Osteopathic Association (AOA) accreditation △ Commission on Accreditation of Rehabilitation Facilities (CARF) accreditation Control codes 61, 63, 64, 71, 72 and 73 indicate hospitals listed by AOHA, but not registered by AHA. For definition of numerical codes, see page A4	Control	Service	Beds	Admissions	Census	Outpatient Visits	Births	Total	Payroll	Personnel
FRIEDMAN HOSPITAL OF THE HOME FOR THE JEWISH AGED, 5301 Old York Road, Zip 19141–2996; tel. 215/456–2900; Frank Podietz, President (Total facility includes 538 beds in nursing home–type unit) **A**10 **F**1 6 17 20 24 26 27 32 34 48 49 51 54 57 62 64 65 73 **P**6	23	10	566	898	540	52527	0	34988	17665	913
✸ FRIENDS HOSPITAL, 4641 Roosevelt Boulevard, Zip 19124–2399; tel. 215/831–4600; Gary L. Gottlieb, M.D., Chief Executive Officer **A**1 3 9 10 **F**1 3 12 15 16 32 34 52 53 54 55 56 57 58 59 67 73 **P**1 6	23	22	192	3389	160	19719	0	35089	20866	570
✸ GERMANTOWN HOSPITAL AND MEDICAL CENTER, One Penn Boulevard, Zip 19144–1498; tel. 215/951–8000; David A. Ricci, President and Chief Executive Officer (Total facility includes 22 beds in nursing home–type unit) **A**1 3 5 6 9 10 **F**7 8 15 16 17 19 21 22 26 27 28 29 30 32 33 34 35 37 38 39 40 41 42 44 46 47 49 51 60 63 64 65 67 69 71 73 74 **P**8	23	10	158	7471	115	77263	459	58659	28529	649
GIRARD MEDICAL CENTER See North Philadelphia Health System										
★ + ○ GRADUATE HEALTH SYSTEM–CITY AVENUE HOSPITAL, 4150 City Avenue, Zip 19131–1696; tel. 215/871–1000; Melvyn E. Smith, President **A**9 10 11 12 13 **F**4 7 8 10 11 12 17 19 21 22 26 27 28 30 33 35 37 38 40 41 42 43 44 49 51 52 54 56 57 60 61 65 71 73 **P**1 **S** Allegheny Health, Education and Research Foundation, Pittsburgh, PA	23	10	195	6851	106	51960	917	58041	23882	637
GRADUATE HEALTH SYSTEM–PARKVIEW HOSPITAL See Parkview Hospital										
✸ GRADUATE HOSPITAL, One Graduate Plaza, Zip 19146–1497; tel. 215/893–2000; Arnold Berman, M.D., President and Chief Executive Officer **A**1 2 3 5 8 9 10 **F**2 3 4 5 8 10 11 12 15 16 17 19 20 21 22 25 26 27 28 29 30 31 32 33 34 35 37 38 39 40 41 42 43 44 45 46 48 49 51 52 53 54 55 56 57 58 59 60 61 63 64 65 66 67 71 73 74 **P**1 3 5 6 **S** Allegheny Health, Education and Research Foundation, Pittsburgh, PA	23	10	198	10470	165	160242	0	161053	59366	1542
HAHNEMANN UNIVERSITY HOSPITAL See Allegheny University Hospitals, Hahnemann										
✸ △ HOSPITAL OF THE UNIVERSITY OF PENNSYLVANIA, 3400 Spruce Street, Zip 19104–4283; tel. 215/662–4000; William T. Foley, Senior Vice President **A**1 3 5 7 8 9 10 **F**2 3 4 5 7 8 10 11 12 14 15 16 17 19 20 21 22 23 26 28 29 30 31 32 33 34 35 37 38 39 40 41 42 43 44 45 46 48 49 50 51 52 54 55 56 57 58 59 60 61 63 64 65 66 67 69 70 71 73 74 **P**1 3 6 7 **N** University of Pennsylvania Health System, Philadelphia, PA	23	10	644	28277	529	—	2540	495203	179799	5756
✸ JEANES HOSPITAL, 7600 Central Avenue, Zip 19111–2499; tel. 215/728–2000; G. Roger Martin, President and Chief Executive Officer **A**1 9 10 **F**1 7 8 12 14 15 16 17 19 21 22 24 26 28 30 32 33 35 37 38 39 40 41 42 44 46 49 60 61 65 66 67 71 73 74 **N** Temple University Health Network, Philadelphia, PA	23	10	188	8994	143	93125	688	73859	31848	1017
□ JOHN F. KENNEDY MEMORIAL HOSPITAL, Langdon Street and Cheltenham Avenue, Zip 19124–1098; tel. 215/831–7000; James J. Nelson, Chief Executive Officer (Nonreporting) **A**1 9 10	23	10	141	—	—	—	—	—	—	—
□ KENSINGTON HOSPITAL, 136 West Diamond Street, Zip 19122; tel. 215/426–8100; Eileen Hause, Chief Executive Officer **A**1 9 10 **F**3 8 15 16 20 31 44 51 58 65 71	23	10	45	2355	26	8700	0	6313	3552	119
✸ △ MAGEE REHABILITATION HOSPITAL, Six Franklin Plaza, Zip 19102; tel. 215/587–3099; William E. Staas, Jr., President and Medical Director (Nonreporting) **A**1 5 7 9 10	23	46	96	—	—	—	—	—	—	—
MEDICAL COLLEGE OF PENNSYLVANIA HOSPITAL See Allegheny University Hospital, East Falls										
METHODIST HOSPITAL See Thomas Jefferson University Hospital										
✸ MT. SINAI HOSPITAL, 1429 South Fifth Street, Zip 19147–5999; tel. 215/339–3456; Louis Shapiro, Executive Vice President and Chief Operating Officer (Total facility includes 40 beds in nursing home–type unit) **A**1 5 9 10 **F**2 3 4 5 7 8 10 11 12 14 15 16 17 19 20 21 22 25 26 27 28 29 30 31 32 33 34 35 37 38 40 41 42 43 44 45 46 48 49 51 52 53 54 55 56 57 58 59 60 61 64 65 66 67 71 73 74 **P**6 7 8 **S** Allegheny Health, Education and Research Foundation, Pittsburgh, PA	23	10	183	4943	139	20397	0	32512	15241	422
✸ △ NAZARETH HOSPITAL, 2601 Holme Avenue, Zip 19152–2096; tel. 215/335–6000; Daniel J. Sinnott, President and Chief Executive Officer **A**1 7 9 10 **F**7 8 11 12 14 15 16 17 19 21 22 27 28 30 31 34 35 37 38 39 40 41 42 44 45 46 48 49 52 54 56 57 60 63 65 67 71 73 74 **P**5 7 8 **S** Catholic Health Initiatives, Denver, CO	21	10	236	10068	172	144551	574	71623	33680	923
□ NEUMANN MEDICAL CENTER, 1741 Frankford Avenue, Zip 19125–2495; tel. 215/291–2000; Joseph C. Hare, President and Chief Executive Officer **A**1 9 10 **F**8 13 14 15 16 17 19 21 22 25 26 27 28 29 30 34 37 39 42 44 45 46 49 51 52 59 63 65 67 68 71 72 73 74 **N** Temple University Health Network, Philadelphia, PA	23	10	166	2510	87	39562	0	25043	13244	432
□ ○ NORTH PHILADELPHIA HEALTH SYSTEM, (Includes Girard Medical Center, Girard Avenue at Eighth Street, Zip 19122; tel. 215/787–2000; St. Joseph's Hospital, 16th Street and Girard Avenue, tel. 215/787–9000), 16th Street and Girard Avenue, Zip 19130; tel. 215/787–9000; George J. Walmsley, III, President and Chief Executive Officer (Nonreporting) **A**1 5 9 10 11 12 13	23	10	315	—	—	—	—	—	—	—
□ NORTHEASTERN HOSPITAL OF PHILADELPHIA, 2301 East Allegheny Avenue, Zip 19134–4499; tel. 215/291–3000; Jeffrey L. Susi, Executive Director and Chief Executive Officer (Nonreporting) **A**1 2 5 6 9 10 **N** Temple University Health Network, Philadelphia, PA	23	10	166	—	—	—	—	—	—	—
★ PARKVIEW HOSPITAL, (Formerly Graduate Health System–Parkview Hospital), 1331 East Wyoming Avenue, Zip 19124; tel. 215/537–7400; Ernest N. Perilli, Vice President Operations (Total facility includes 19 beds in nursing home–type unit) **A**9 12 13 **F**2 4 7 8 10 11 12 15 16 17 19 21 22 24 27 28 30 32 33 34 35 37 40 41 42 43 44 48 49 52 56 57 58 60 64 65 71 73 74 **S** Allegheny Health, Education and Research Foundation, Pittsburgh, PA	23	10	165	6767	96	45812	845	46704	19049	524

Hospital, Address, Telephone, Administrator, Approval, Facility, and Physician Codes, Health Care System, Network	Classi-fication Codes		Utilization Data					Expense (thousands) of dollars		
★ American Hospital Association (AHA) membership □ Joint Commission on Accreditation of Healthcare Organizations (JCAHO) accreditation + American Osteopathic Hospital Association (AOHA) membership ○ American Osteopathic Association (AOA) accreditation △ Commission on Accreditation of Rehabilitation Facilities (CARF) accreditation Control codes 61, 63, 64, 71, 72 and 73 indicate hospitals listed by AOHA, but not registered by AHA. For definition of numerical codes, see page A4	Control	Service	Beds	Admissions	Census	Outpatient Visits	Births	Total	Payroll	Personnel
⊞ PENNSYLVANIA HOSPITAL, 800 Spruce Street, Zip 19107–6192; tel. 215/829–3000; John R. Ball, M.D., JD, President and Chief Executive Officer (Total facility includes 29 beds in nursing home–type unit) **A**1 2 3 5 8 9 10 **F**1 3 4 7 8 10 11 12 13 14 15 16 17 19 20 21 22 23 24 26 27 28 29 30 31 32 33 34 35 37 38 39 40 41 42 43 44 45 46 49 51 52 53 54 55 56 57 58 59 60 61 64 65 66 67 68 71 73 74 **P**1 6 7	23	10	414	19231	302	161839	3717	226111	95274	2538
⊞ PRESBYTERIAN MEDICAL CENTER OF THE UNIVERSITY OF PENNSYLVANIA HEALTH SYSTEM, (Formerly Presbyterian Medical Center of Philadelphia), 51 North 39th Street, Zip 19104–2699; tel. 215/662–8000; Michele M. Volpe, Chief Operating Officer (Total facility includes 20 beds in nursing home–type unit) (Nonreporting) **A**1 3 5 6 9 10 **N** University of Pennsylvania Health System, Philadelphia, PA	23	10	325	—	—	—	—	—	—	—
□ ROXBOROUGH MEMORIAL HOSPITAL, 5800 Ridge Avenue, Zip 19128–1789; tel. 215/483–9900; John J. Donnelly, Jr., President and Chief Executive Officer (Total facility includes 24 beds in nursing home–type unit) (Nonreporting) **A**1 6 9 10	23	10	129	—	—	—	—	—	—	—
⊞ SHRINERS HOSPITALS FOR CHILDREN, PHILADELPHIA UNIT, 8400 Roosevelt Boulevard, Zip 19152–1299; tel. 215/332–4500; Sharon J. Rajnic, Administrator (Nonreporting) **A**1 3 5 **S** Shriners Hospitals for Children, Tampa, FL	23	57	80	—	—	—	—	—	—	—
⊞ ○ ST. AGNES MEDICAL CENTER, 1900 South Broad Street, Zip 19145; tel. 215/339–4100; Daniel J. Sinnott, President and Chief Executive Officer (Total facility includes 19 beds in nursing home–type unit) **A**1 3 5 9 10 11 **F**1 8 9 11 12 14 15 16 17 19 21 22 24 27 28 30 32 34 37 41 42 44 48 49 63 64 65 71 73 74 **P**4 5 7 8 **S** Catholic Health Initiatives, Denver, CO	21	10	182	5633	120	55211	0	61812	24608	571
⊞ ST. CHRISTOPHER'S HOSPITAL FOR CHILDREN, Erie Avenue at Front Street, Zip 19134–1095; tel. 215/427–5000; Calvin Bland, President and Chief Executive Officer **A**1 3 5 8 9 10 **F**1 2 3 4 5 7 8 9 10 11 12 13 14 15 16 17 18 19 20 21 22 25 26 28 30 31 32 34 35 37 38 39 40 41 42 43 44 45 46 47 48 49 51 52 53 54 55 56 57 58 59 60 61 65 66 67 68 69 70 71 73 74 **P**3 6 **S** Allegheny Health, Education and Research Foundation, Pittsburgh, PA ST. JOSEPH'S HOSPITAL See North Philadelphia Health System	23	50	178	10465	142	108835	0	131677	56852	1243
□ TEMPLE UNIVERSITY HOSPITAL, Broad and Ontario Streets, Zip 19140–5192; tel. 215/707–2000; Paul Boehringer, Executive Director (Total facility includes 16 beds in nursing home–type unit) **A**1 2 3 5 8 9 10 **F**1 4 5 6 7 8 10 11 12 14 15 16 17 18 19 20 21 22 24 25 26 27 28 29 30 31 32 34 35 37 38 39 40 41 42 43 44 45 46 47 48 49 51 52 54 55 56 57 58 59 60 61 62 63 64 65 66 67 69 70 71 72 73 74 **P**1 5 6 **N** Temple University Health Network, Philadelphia, PA	23	10	430	19703	358	164858	1530	274220	125059	2511
⊞ △ THOMAS JEFFERSON UNIVERSITY HOSPITAL, (Includes Methodist Hospital, 2301 South Broad Street, Zip 19148; tel. 215/952–9000; Thomas Jefferson University Hospital–Ford Road Campus, 3905 Ford Road, Zip 19131; tel. 215/578–3630; Diane Peters, Administrator), 111 South 11th Street, Zip 19107–5098; tel. 215/955–7022; Thomas J. Lewis, President and Chief Executive Officer (Total facility includes 120 beds in nursing home–type unit) (Nonreporting) **A**1 2 3 5 6 7 8 9 10 **S** Jefferson Health System, Radnor, PA **N** Health Share, Philadelphia, PA; Jefferson Health System, Radnor, PA THOMAS JEFFERSON UNIVERSITY HOSPITAL–FORD ROAD CAMPUS See Thomas Jefferson University Hospital	23	10	959	—	—	—	—	—	—	—
□ VENCOR HOSPITAL–PHILADELPHIA, 6129 Palmetto Street, Zip 19111; tel. 215/722–8555; Debra Condon, Administrator (Nonreporting) **A**1 10 **S** Vencor, Incorporated, Louisville, KY	33	49	52	—	—	—	—	—	—	—
⊞ VETERANS AFFAIRS MEDICAL CENTER, University and Woodland Avenues, Zip 19104–4594; tel. 215/823–5857; Earl F. Falast, Chief Executive Officer (Total facility includes 180 beds in nursing home–type unit) (Nonreporting) **A**1 3 5 8 9 **S** Department of Veterans Affairs, Washington, DC	45	10	656	—	—	—	—	—	—	—
⊞ WILLS EYE HOSPITAL, (EYE HOSPITAL), 900 Walnut Street, Zip 19107–5598; tel. 215/928–3000; D. McWilliams Kessler, Executive Director **A**1 3 5 9 10 **F**2 3 4 5 6 7 8 10 11 12 13 14 15 16 17 18 19 20 21 22 23 24 25 26 27 28 29 30 31 32 33 34 35 37 38 39 40 41 42 43 44 45 46 47 48 49 50 51 52 53 54 55 56 57 58 59 60 61 62 63 65 66 67 68 69 71 72 73 74	23	49	115	3975	41	62133	0	54883	22734	631
PHOENIXVILLE—Chester County										
⊞ PHOENIXVILLE HOSPITAL, 140 Nutt Road, Zip 19460–0809, Mailing Address: P.O. Box 809, Zip 19460–0809; tel. 610/983–1000; Richard E. Seagrave, President **A**1 9 10 **F**7 8 10 11 13 14 15 16 17 19 20 21 22 26 30 31 32 33 35 37 39 40 42 44 46 49 54 55 56 60 61 63 65 67 71 73	23	10	107	6089	68	112644	1274	43403	19308	584
PITTSBURGH—Allegheny County										
⊞ + ALLEGHENY GENERAL HOSPITAL, 320 East North Avenue, Zip 15212–4772; tel. 412/359–3131; Anthony M. Sanzo, President (Total facility includes 64 beds in nursing home–type unit) **A**1 2 3 5 8 9 10 **F**3 4 7 8 10 11 12 13 14 15 16 17 18 19 20 22 23 24 25 26 27 28 30 31 32 33 34 35 37 38 39 40 41 42 43 44 46 49 50 51 52 53 54 55 56 57 58 59 60 61 63 64 65 66 67 68 69 70 71 73 74 **P**1 2 8 **S** Allegheny Health, Education and Research Foundation, Pittsburgh, PA	23	10	559	28944	515	514783	1556	412868	161235	4493
★ CHILDREN'S HOME OF PITTSBURGH, (TRANSITIONAL INFANT CARE), 5618 Kentucky Avenue, Zip 15232–2696; tel. 412/441–4884; Pamela R. Schanwald, Chief Executive Officer **A**9 10 **F**12 13 15 16 17 19 21 27 31 33 35 38 41 45 50 63 65 71 73	23	59	10	118	6	0	0	2148	1206	43

Hospital, Address, Telephone, Administrator, Approval, Facility, and Physician Codes, Health Care System, Network	Classi-fication Codes		Utilization Data					Expense (thousands) of dollars		
	Control	Service	Beds	Admissions	Census	Outpatient Visits	Births	Total	Payroll	Personnel

★ American Hospital Association (AHA) membership
☐ Joint Commission on Accreditation of Healthcare Organizations (JCAHO) accreditation
+ American Osteopathic Hospital Association (AOHA) membership
○ American Osteopathic Association (AOA) accreditation
△ Commission on Accreditation of Rehabilitation Facilities (CARF) accreditation
Control codes 61, 63, 64, 71, 72 and 73 indicate hospitals listed by AOHA, but not registered by AHA. For definition of numerical codes, see page A4

Hospital	Control	Service	Beds	Admissions	Census	Outpatient Visits	Births	Total	Payroll	Personnel
⊞ CHILDREN'S HOSPITAL OF PITTSBURGH, 3705 Fifth Avenue at De Soto Street, Zip 15213–2583; tel. 412/692–5325; Paul S. Kramer, President and Chief Executive Officer **A**1 2 3 5 8 9 10 **F**4 5 10 15 16 17 19 20 21 22 25 31 32 34 35 38 42 43 44 45 46 47 49 51 64 65 67 68 69 70 71 73 **P**1 **N** Tri–State Network, Pittsburgh, PA; University of Pittsburgh Medical Center, Pittsburgh, PA	23	50	235	12318	162	197622	0	176286	75342	1931
EYE AND EAR HOSPITAL OF PITTSBURGH See University of Pittsburgh Medical Center										
⊞ FORBES METROPOLITAN HOSPITAL, (EXTENDED ACUTE CARE), 225 Penn Avenue, Zip 15221–2173; tel. 412/247–2424; April A. Stevens, R.N., Vice President and Administrator **A**1 9 10 **F**4 7 8 10 11 12 13 15 16 17 19 21 22 24 25 26 27 28 29 30 31 32 33 34 35 36 37 38 39 40 41 42 43 44 45 46 48 49 51 52 54 56 57 59 60 61 64 65 67 71 72 73 74 **P**5 6 8 **S** Allegheny Health, Education and Research Foundation, Pittsburgh, PA	23	49	152	1410	116	36948	1	34684	12654	370
HARMARVILLE REHABILITATION CENTER See Healthsouth Harmarville Rehabilitation Hospital										
☐ △ HEALTHSOUTH HARMARVILLE REHABILITATION HOSPITAL, (Formerly Harmarville Rehabilitation Center), Guys Run Road, Zip 15238–0460, Mailing Address: Box 11460, Guys Run Road, Zip 15238–0460; tel. 412/781–5700; Frank G. DeLisi, III, CHE, Chief Executive Officer and Director Operations (Total facility includes 40 beds in nursing home–type unit) **A**1 3 7 9 10 **F**14 17 19 25 26 34 41 48 49 64 65 66 73 **S** HEALTHSOUTH Corporation, Birmingham, AL	33	46	202	2038	132	49702	0	40919	22565	611
⊞ MAGEE–WOMENS HOSPITAL, 300 Halket Street, Zip 15213–3180; tel. 412/641–1000; Irma E. Goertzen, President and Chief Executive Officer **A**1 2 3 5 8 9 10 **F**2 3 4 7 8 10 11 12 13 14 15 16 17 19 21 22 25 26 27 29 30 31 32 34 35 37 38 39 40 41 42 43 44 45 46 47 48 51 52 54 55 56 57 58 60 61 64 65 66 67 68 69 70 71 73 74 **P**4 7 8 **N** Tri–State Network, Pittsburgh, PA; University of Pittsburgh Medical Center, Pittsburgh, PA	23	44	263	14191	147	60767	8079	118153	52956	2182
☐ △ MERCY HOSPITAL OF PITTSBURGH, 1400 Locust Street, Zip 15219–5166; tel. 412/232–8111; Howard A. Zaren, M.D., FACS, Executive Vice President, Hospital Services (Total facility includes 37 beds in nursing home–type unit) **A**1 2 3 5 6 7 8 9 10 **F**4 6 7 8 9 10 11 12 13 14 15 16 17 18 19 20 21 22 23 24 25 26 27 28 29 30 31 32 33 34 35 37 38 39 40 41 42 43 44 45 46 47 48 49 51 52 53 54 55 56 57 58 60 61 63 64 65 67 68 70 71 72 73 74 **P**5 8 **S** Eastern Mercy Health System, Radnor, PA	23	10	493	19426	353	234662	1271	210570	82179	2264
☐ MERCY PROVIDENCE HOSPITAL, 1004 Arch Street, Zip 15212; tel. 412/323–5600; Thomas Mattei, M.D., Chief Operating Officer **A**1 9 10 **F**8 12 14 15 16 17 18 19 22 27 30 37 39 41 42 44 48 49 52 56 57 58 59 65 71 73 **P**3 5 8 **S** Eastern Mercy Health System, Radnor, PA	21	10	146	4671	100	23506	0	28145	11367	411
MONTEFIORE HOSPITAL See University of Pittsburgh Medical Center										
☐ PASSAVANT HOSPITAL, 9100 Babcock Boulevard, Zip 15237–5842; tel. 412/367–6700; Ralph T. DeStefano, President and Chief Executive Officer **A**1 9 10 **F**4 7 8 10 12 15 16 17 19 22 30 32 34 35 37 39 40 41 42 43 44 45 46 49 51 53 54 55 56 57 58 59 60 63 65 67 69 71 72 73 74 **P**3 5 7 8	23	10	280	9480	137	154651	440	78366	34475	1049
PODIATRY HOSPITAL OF PITTSBURGH, 215 South Negley Avenue, Zip 15206–3594; tel. 412/661–0814; Joseph S. Noviello, Chief Executive Officer (Nonreporting) **A**9 10	23	49	13	—	—	—	—	—	—	—
PRESBYTERIAN UNIVERSITY HOSPITAL See University of Pittsburgh Medical Center										
⊞ △ REHABILITATION INSTITUTE OF PITTSBURGH, 6301 Northumberland Street, Zip 15217–1396; tel. 412/521–9000; John A. Wilson, President and Chief Executive Officer (Total facility includes 25 beds in nursing home–type unit) **A**1 7 9 10 **F**5 12 14 15 16 17 26 32 34 41 46 48 49 53 57 59 64 65 66 73	23	46	115	1410	77	31685	0	23377	12446	383
⊞ SHADYSIDE HOSPITAL, 5230 Centre Avenue, Zip 15232–1304; tel. 412/623–2121; Henry A. Mordoh, President (Total facility includes 145 beds in nursing home–type unit) **A**1 2 3 5 8 9 10 **F**4 7 8 10 11 14 15 16 17 19 21 22 26 27 28 30 31 32 34 35 37 39 40 41 42 43 44 46 49 51 54 60 61 63 64 65 66 67 68 69 71 73 74 **P**1 6 7 **N** Fox Chase Network, Rockledge, PA; National Cardiovascular Network, Atlanta, GA	23	10	508	18987	410	176632	698	197289	77536	2131
SOUTH HILLS HEALTH SYSTEM, Coal Valley Road, Zip 15236–0119, Mailing Address: Box 18119, Zip 15236–0119; tel. 412/469–5000; William R. Jennings, President (Total facility includes 74 beds in nursing home–type unit) (Nonreporting) **A**9 10 **N** Tri–State Network, Pittsburgh, PA	23	10	466							
☐ SOUTHWOOD PSYCHIATRIC HOSPITAL, 2575 Boyce Plaza Road, Zip 15241–3925; tel. 412/257–2290; Alan A. Axelson, M.D., Chief Executive Officer (Nonreporting) **A**1 9 **S** First Hospital Corporation, Norfolk, VA	33	52	50	—	—	—	—	—	—	—
⊞ ST. CLAIR MEMORIAL HOSPITAL, 1000 Bower Hill Road, Zip 15243; tel. 412/561–4900; Benjamin E. Snead, President **A**1 9 10 **F**1 3 4 5 6 7 8 10 11 12 13 14 15 17 18 19 20 21 22 23 24 25 26 27 28 29 30 31 32 33 34 35 37 38 39 40 41 42 43 44 45 46 47 48 49 50 51 52 53 54 55 56 57 58 59 60 61 63 64 65 66 67 68 69 70 71 72 73 74 **P**1 3 7 **N** SouthWest Integrated Delivery Network, Pittsburgh, PA; Alpha Health Network, Pittsburgh, PA	23	10	271	11594	170	112925	1238	81903	40017	1087
⊞ ○ ST. FRANCIS CENTRAL HOSPITAL, 1200 Centre Avenue, Zip 15219–3594; tel. 412/562–3000; Robin Z. Mohr, Chief Executive Officer **A**1 9 10 11 13 **F**2 3 4 5 7 8 10 11 12 13 14 17 18 19 20 21 22 23 25 26 27 28 29 30 31 32 34 35 37 39 40 41 42 43 44 45 46 48 49 51 52 53 54 55 56 57 58 59 60 61 62 63 64 65 66 67 68 71 72 73 74 **P**5 6 **S** St. Francis Health System, Pittsburgh, PA **N** Saint Francis Health System, Pittsburgh, PA	23	10	143	3859	61	51976	0	37465	15010	461

Hospital, Address, Telephone, Administrator, Approval, Facility, and Physician Codes, Health Care System, Network	Classi-fication Codes		Utilization Data					Expense (thousands) of dollars		
★ American Hospital Association (AHA) membership □ Joint Commission on Accreditation of Healthcare Organizations (JCAHO) accreditation + American Osteopathic Hospital Association (AOHA) membership ○ American Osteopathic Association (AOA) accreditation △ Commission on Accreditation of Rehabilitation Facilities (CARF) accreditation Control codes 61, 63, 64, 71, 72 and 73 indicate hospitals listed by AOHA, but not registered by AHA. For definition of numerical codes, see page A4	Control	Service	Beds	Admissions	Census	Outpatient Visits	Births	Total	Payroll	Personnel
✦ △ ST. FRANCIS MEDICAL CENTER, 400 45th Street, Zip 15201–1198; tel. 412/622–4343; Sister Florence Brandt, Chief Executive Officer (Total facility includes 300 beds in nursing home–type unit) **A**1 2 3 5 6 7 8 9 10 **F**2 3 4 5 7 8 10 11 12 14 15 16 19 20 21 22 23 24 25 26 28 30 31 32 34 35 37 39 40 41 42 43 44 45 46 48 49 51 52 53 54 55 56 57 58 59 60 63 64 65 66 67 68 69 71 72 73 74 **S** St. Francis Health System, Pittsburgh, PA	23	10	885	17094	656	290879	714	199553	87079	2280
ST. MARGARET MEMORIAL HOSPITAL See University of Pittsburgh Medical Center, St. Margaret										
STATE CORRECTIONAL INSTITUTION HOSPITAL, Doerr Street, Zip 15233, Mailing Address: Box 99901, Zip 15233; tel. 412/761–1955; Joseph Morrash, Administrator (Nonreporting)	12	11	27	—	—	—	—	—	—	—
□ SUBURBAN GENERAL HOSPITAL, 100 South Jackson Avenue, Zip 15202–3499; tel. 412/734–6000; Thomas H. Prickett, President and Chief Executive Officer (Total facility includes 26 beds in nursing home–type unit) **A**1 9 10 **F**11 14 19 22 32 35 37 41 44 48 49 64 65 71 73	23	10	144	4118	89	53028	0	29716	14243	510
✦ UNIVERSITY OF PITTSBURGH MEDICAL CENTER, (Includes Eye and Ear Hospital of Pittsburgh, 200 Lothrop Street, Zip 15213–2592; tel. 412/647–2345; Montefiore Hospital, 200 Lothrop Street, Zip 15213; tel. 412/647–2345; Presbyterian University Hospital, Western Psychiatric Institute and Clinic, 3811 O'Hara Street, Zip 15213–2593; tel. 412/624–2100), Jeffrey A. Romoff, President **A**1 2 3 5 9 **F**1 2 3 4 5 6 7 8 10 11 12 13 14 15 16 17 18 19 20 21 22 23 24 25 26 27 28 29 30 31 32 33 34 35 36 37 38 39 40 41 42 43 44 45 46 47 48 49 50 51 52 53 54 55 56 57 58 59 60 61 62 63 64 65 66 67 68 69 70 71 72 73 74 **P**1 5 7 **N** Tri–State Network, Pittsburgh, PA; University of Pittsburgh Medical Center, Pittsburgh, PA	23	10	963	32312	751	474449	0	700172	222302	7948
□ UNIVERSITY OF PITTSBURGH MEDICAL CENTER, SOUTH SIDE, 2000 Mary Street, Zip 15203–2095; tel. 412/488–5550; George J. Korbakes, President (Nonreporting) **A**1 9 10	23	10	162	—	—	—	—	—	—	—
✦ UNIVERSITY OF PITTSBURGH MEDICAL CENTER, ST. MARGARET, (Formerly St. Margaret Memorial Hospital), 815 Freeport Road, Zip 15215–3399; tel. 412/784–4000; Stanley J. Kevish, President **A**1 3 5 6 9 10 **F**5 8 10 15 16 17 19 21 22 25 26 28 29 30 31 34 35 37 39 41 42 44 45 46 48 49 56 57 58 60 62 64 65 66 67 71 73 **P**8 **N** Tri–State Network, Pittsburgh, PA; University of Pittsburgh Medical Center, Pittsburgh, PA	23	10	267	8852	145	108274	0	85703	35146	1014
✦ VETERANS AFFAIRS PITTSBURGH HEALTHCARE SYSTEM, (Includes Veterans Affairs Medical Center, 7180 Highland Drive, Zip 15206–1297; tel. 412/365–4900; Veterans Affairs Medical Center, University Drive C, tel. 412/688–6000), Delafield Road, Zip 15240–1001; tel. 412/784–3900; Thomas A. Cappello, Director (Total facility includes 300 beds in nursing home–type unit) **A**1 3 5 8 **F**1 3 4 5 6 8 10 11 12 15 16 17 18 19 20 21 22 23 24 26 27 28 29 30 31 32 34 35 37 39 41 42 43 44 45 46 49 50 51 52 54 55 56 57 58 59 60 63 64 65 67 69 71 73 74 **P**6 **S** Department of Veterans Affairs, Washington, DC	45	22	1172	10912	941	298586	0	205657	134264	2697
✦ WESTERN PENNSYLVANIA HOSPITAL, 4800 Friendship Avenue, Zip 15224; tel. 412/578–5000; Charles M. O'Brien, Jr., President and Chief Executive Officer **A**1 2 3 5 6 8 9 10 **F**4 7 8 9 10 11 12 13 14 15 16 17 18 19 20 21 22 26 27 28 30 31 32 33 34 35 37 38 40 41 42 43 44 45 46 49 50 51 52 54 56 57 60 61 63 65 67 68 69 71 73 74 **P**1 6 7	23	10	462	18463	334	—	1985	204971	87450	2480
WESTERN PSYCHIATRIC INSTITUTE AND CLINIC See University of Pittsburgh Medical Center										
PLEASANT GAP—Centre County										
□ △ HEALTHSOUTH NITTANY VALLEY REHABILITATION HOSPITAL, 550 West College Avenue, Zip 16823–8808; tel. 814/359–3421; Mary Jane Hawkins, Administrator and Chief Executive Officer (Nonreporting) **A**1 7 9 10 **S** HEALTHSOUTH Corporation, Birmingham, AL	33	46	88	—	—	—	—	—	—	—
POTTSTOWN—Montgomery County										
✦ POTTSTOWN MEMORIAL MEDICAL CENTER, 1600 East High Street, Zip 19464–5008; tel. 610/327–7000; John J. Buckley, President and Chief Executive Officer (Total facility includes 21 beds in nursing home–type unit) **A**1 2 9 10 **F**7 8 10 12 13 15 16 17 19 20 22 23 24 28 29 30 32 35 37 39 40 41 42 44 46 49 52 56 59 60 63 64 65 66 67 71 73 74 **P**6	23	10	196	8796	128	—	783	69528	32017	911
POTTSVILLE—Schuylkill County										
✦ GOOD SAMARITAN REGIONAL MEDICAL CENTER, 700 East Norwegian Street, Zip 17901–2798; tel. 717/621–4000; Gino J. Pazzaglini, President and Chief Executive Officer **A**1 2 5 9 10 **F**2 3 4 7 8 11 12 14 15 16 19 21 22 26 28 30 31 32 33 34 35 36 37 39 40 41 42 44 45 46 49 51 60 63 65 67 68 71 73 74 **P**6 **S** Daughters of Charity National Health System, Saint Louis, MO	21	10	197	7922	135	135979	439	48451	23052	690
✦ △ POTTSVILLE HOSPITAL AND WARNE CLINIC, 420 South Jackson Street, Zip 17901–3692; tel. 717/621–5000; Donald R. Gintzig, President and Chief Executive Officer **A**1 2 6 7 9 10 **F**7 8 12 14 15 16 17 19 20 21 22 26 28 30 31 34 35 37 39 40 41 42 44 45 48 49 52 53 55 56 57 58 65 66 71 73 **P**5 **S** Quorum Health Group/Quorum Health Resources, Inc., Brentwood, TN	23	10	196	5836	126	77531	436	44012	19747	737
PUNXSUTAWNEY—Jefferson County										
□ PUNXSUTAWNEY AREA HOSPITAL, 81 Hillcrest Drive, Zip 15767–2616; tel. 814/938–1800; Daniel D. Blough, Jr., Administrator (Total facility includes 14 beds in nursing home–type unit) **A**1 9 10 **F**7 8 15 16 19 21 22 30 31 32 34 37 39 40 44 49 64 65 71	23	10	65	2297	33	68833	215	16811	6753	257

Hospital, Address, Telephone, Administrator, Approval, Facility, and Physician Codes, Health Care System, Network	Classi-fication Codes		Utilization Data					Expense (thousands) of dollars		
★ American Hospital Association (AHA) membership □ Joint Commission on Accreditation of Healthcare Organizations (JCAHO) accreditation + American Osteopathic Hospital Association (AOHA) membership ○ American Osteopathic Association (AOA) accreditation △ Commission on Accreditation of Rehabilitation Facilities (CARF) accreditation Control codes 61, 63, 64, 71, 72 and 73 indicate hospitals listed by AOHA, but not registered by AHA. For definition of numerical codes, see page A4	Control	Service	Beds	Admissions	Census	Outpatient Visits	Births	Total	Payroll	Personnel

QUAKERTOWN—Bucks County

□ ST. LUKE'S QUAKERTOWN HOSPITAL, 1021 Park Avenue, Zip 18951; tel. 215/538–4500; Fred Sprissler, President and Chief Executive Officer (Nonreporting) **A**1 2 9 10

	23	10	71	—	—	—	—	—	—	—

READING—Berks County

□ COMMUNITY GENERAL HOSPITAL, 145 North Sixth Street, Zip 19601, Mailing Address: P.O. Box 1728, Zip 19603–1728; tel. 610/376–2100; S. Michael Francis, President and Chief Executive Officer (Total facility includes 25 beds in nursing home–type unit) (Nonreporting) **A**1 2 9 10 12

	23	10	160	—	—	—	—	—	—	—

✠ READING HOSPITAL AND MEDICAL CENTER, Sixth Avenue and Spruce Street, Zip 19611, Mailing Address: P.O. Box 16052, Zip 19612–6052; tel. 610/378–6000; Charles Sullivan, President and Chief Executive Officer **A**1 2 5 6 9 10 **F**3 4 7 8 10 14 15 16 17 18 19 20 21 22 23 25 26 28 29 30 31 34 35 37 38 39 40 41 42 43 44 45 46 49 51 52 53 54 55 56 57 58 59 60 61 62 65 66 67 68 71 72 73 74 **P**5 8 **N** Fox Chase Network, Rockledge, PA

	23	10	510	23770	368	510748	2603	192346	89677	2651

✠ △ READING REHABILITATION HOSPITAL, 1623 Morgantown Road, Zip 19607–9455; tel. 610/796–6000; Clint Kreitner, President and Chief Executive Officer (Total facility includes 19 beds in nursing home–type unit) **A**1 3 7 9 10 **F**12 14 15 16 26 27 39 41 48 49 64 65 67 73

	21	46	95	1469	59	22631	0	16880	8885	248

✠ ST. JOSEPH MEDICAL CENTER, Twelfth & Walnut Streets, Zip 19603–0316, Mailing Address: P.O. Box 316, Zip 19603–0316; tel. 610/378–2000; Philip G. Dionne, President and Chief Executive Officer **A**1 2 3 5 9 10 **F**1 2 3 4 6 7 8 10 12 13 14 15 16 17 19 20 21 22 24 26 28 30 31 32 33 34 35 37 39 40 41 42 43 44 46 49 51 52 53 54 55 56 60 65 66 67 68 71 72 73 74 **P**1 3 5 7 8 **S** Catholic Health Initiatives, Denver, CO

	21	10	215	9074	123	198205	772	70422	30482	895

RENOVO—Clinton County

BUCKTAIL MEDICAL CENTER, 1001 Pine Street, Zip 17764–1620; tel. 717/923–1000; Lennea F. Brown, Interim Administrator (Total facility includes 41 beds in nursing home–type unit) (Nonreporting) **A**9 10

	23	10	50	—	—	—	—	—	—	—

RIDGWAY—Elk County

□ ELK COUNTY REGIONAL MEDICAL CENTER, 94 Hospital Street, Zip 15853; tel. 814/776–6111; Kenneth G. Turner, CHE, Chief Executive Officer (Nonreporting) **A**1 9 10

	23	10	52	—	—	—	—	—	—	—

RIDLEY PARK—Delaware County

□ TAYLOR HOSPITAL, 175 East Chester Pike, Zip 19078; tel. 610/595–6000; Diane C. Miller, President and Chief Operating Officer (Total facility includes 23 beds in nursing home–type unit) **A**1 2 9 10 **F**8 10 12 15 17 19 20 21 22 30 32 34 35 36 37 39 41 42 44 45 46 48 49 54 64 65 66 67 71 73 **P**2 3 7 8

	23	10	185	6915	107	67488	0	55863	26309	574

ROARING SPRING—Blair County

✠ NASON HOSPITAL, 105 Nason Drive, Zip 16673–1201; tel. 814/224–2141; John P. Kinney, President **A**1 5 9 10 **F**7 8 15 19 21 22 28 29 32 33 34 35 37 40 44 45 49 63 65 67 71 73

	23	10	50	1705	22	41035	212	13265	5538	203

SAINT MARYS—Elk County

✠ ST. MARYS REGIONAL MEDICAL CENTER, 763 Johnsonburg Road, Zip 15857–3417; tel. 814/781–7500; John N. Christenson, President (Total facility includes 138 beds in nursing home–type unit) **A**1 9 10 **F**7 8 12 14 15 17 19 21 22 28 29 30 33 35 37 39 40 41 42 44 45 46 49 62 64 65 66 71 73 74 **N** Great Lakes Health Network, Erie, PA

	23	10	204	3318	163	54144	312	26624	13151	523

SAYRE—Bradford County

✠ ROBERT PACKER HOSPITAL, Guthrie Square, Zip 18840; tel. 717/888–6666; Russell M. Knight, President **A**1 2 3 5 9 10 **F**1 4 6 7 8 10 11 12 13 14 15 16 17 18 19 21 22 23 24 26 27 28 29 30 31 32 33 34 35 36 37 39 40 42 43 44 45 46 49 51 52 53 54 55 56 57 59 61 63 64 65 66 67 68 70 71 72 73 74 **P**5 7 **S** Guthrie Healthcare System, Sayre, PA **N** Guthrie Healthcare System, Sayre, PA

	23	10	265	12106	177	117210	814	102994	38079	1178

SCRANTON—Lackawanna County

✠ △ ALLIED SERVICES REHABILITATION HOSPITAL, 475 Morgan Highway, Zip 18501; tel. 717/348–1300; James L. Brady, President (Nonreporting) **A**1 7 9 10

	23	46	98	—	—	—	—	—	—	—

✠ COMMUNITY MEDICAL CENTER, 1800 Mulberry Street, Zip 18510; tel. 717/969–8000; C. Richard Hartman, M.D., President and Chief Executive Officer **A**1 3 9 10 **F**3 4 6 7 8 10 14 15 16 17 18 19 21 22 25 26 27 30 32 33 34 35 37 38 40 42 43 44 46 49 51 52 53 54 55 56 57 58 59 60 63 64 65 67 68 70 71 72 73 74 **P**8

	23	10	289	11914	194	108737	1782	87793	34793	1082

✠ MERCY HOSPITAL OF SCRANTON, 746 Jefferson Avenue, Zip 18501–0994; tel. 717/348–7100; John L. Nespoli, President and Chief Executive Officer (Total facility includes 20 beds in nursing home–type unit) **A**1 2 3 5 9 10 **F**4 7 8 10 11 12 16 17 19 21 22 23 24 28 29 32 33 34 35 37 38 40 42 43 44 49 51 60 63 64 65 67 71 73 74 **P**8 **S** Mercy Health System, Cincinnati, OH

	21	10	308	12532	229	226129	812	99324	41069	1310

✠ MOSES TAYLOR HOSPITAL, 700 Quincy Avenue, Zip 18510–1724; tel. 717/340–2100; Harold E. Anderson, President and Chief Executive Officer (Total facility includes 32 beds in nursing home–type unit) **A**1 3 5 9 10 **F**8 12 15 19 21 22 23 26 32 33 34 35 37 41 42 44 45 46 49 52 57 64 65 71 73 **P**1 2 6 7

	23	10	222	7545	159	80421	0	61842	22914	746

SELLERSVILLE—Bucks County

✠ △ GRAND VIEW HOSPITAL, 700 Lawn Avenue, Zip 18960–1581; tel. 215/453–4000; Stuart H. Fine, Chief Executive Officer (Total facility includes 20 beds in nursing home–type unit) **A**1 2 5 7 9 10 **F**2 3 7 8 11 12 13 15 16 17 18 19 21 23 24 26 28 29 30 31 32 33 34 36 37 40 41 42 44 45 46 49 52 53 54 56 57 58 59 60 63 64 65 67 71 73 74 **P**1 3 5 7

	23	10	193	8463	116	126892	1144	63073	30075	1041

Hospital, Address, Telephone, Administrator, Approval, Facility, and Physician Codes, Health Care System, Network	Classi-fication Codes		Utilization Data					Expense (thousands) of dollars		
★ American Hospital Association (AHA) membership □ Joint Commission on Accreditation of Healthcare Organizations (JCAHO) accreditation + American Osteopathic Hospital Association (AOHA) membership ○ American Osteopathic Association (AOA) accreditation △ Commission on Accreditation of Rehabilitation Facilities (CARF) accreditation Control codes 61, 63, 64, 71, 72 and 73 indicate hospitals listed by AOHA, but not registered by AHA. For definition of numerical codes, see page A4	Control	Service	Beds	Admissions	Census	Outpatient Visits	Births	Total	Payroll	Personnel

SEWICKLEY—Allegheny County

▣ △ D. T. WATSON REHABILITATION HOSPITAL, Camp Meeting Road, Zip 15143–8773; tel. 412/741–9500; Robert N. Gibson, President and Chief Executive Officer **A**1 7 9 10 **F**12 16 48 49 65 73 **P**6

| | 23 | 46 | 44 | 314 | 14 | 11209 | 0 | 10430 | 4807 | 145 |

▣ SEWICKLEY VALLEY HOSPITAL, (A DIVISION OF VALLEY MEDICAL FACILITIES), 720 Blackburn Road, Zip 15143–1498; tel. 412/741–6600; Donald W. Spalding, President **A**1 6 9 10 **F**4 7 8 10 12 15 17 19 21 22 26 28 29 30 31 32 33 34 36 37 40 41 42 44 48 52 53 54 55 56 57 58 59 60 65 67 71 73 74 **P**6 8 **N** SouthWest Integrated Delivery Network, Pittsburgh, PA

| | 23 | 10 | 184 | 9216 | 119 | 142903 | 863 | 87784 | 37964 | 1098 |

SHARON—Mercer County

▣ △ SHARON REGIONAL HEALTH SYSTEM, 740 East State Street, Zip 16146–7001; tel. 412/983–3911; Wayne W. Johnston, President and Chief Executive Officer (Total facility includes 40 beds in nursing home–type unit) **A**1 6 7 9 10 **F**3 7 8 10 11 13 15 16 17 19 21 22 23 25 26 28 29 30 32 33 34 35 37 39 40 41 42 44 45 48 49 51 52 53 54 55 56 57 58 59 60 63 64 65 66 67 71 72 73 74 **P**8

| | 23 | 10 | 234 | 9091 | 156 | 274516 | 734 | 66568 | 30393 | 1064 |

SHICKSHINNY—Luzerne County

CLEAR BROOK LODGE, Bethel Road, Zip 18655, Mailing Address: Rural Delivery 2, Box 2166, Zip 18655; tel. 717/864–3116; Dave Lombard, President and Chief Executive Officer (Nonreporting)

| | 23 | 82 | 65 | — | — | — | — | — | — | — |

SOMERSET—Somerset County

▣ SOMERSET HOSPITAL CENTER FOR HEALTH, 225 South Center Avenue, Zip 15501–2088; tel. 814/443–5000; Michael J. Farrell, Chief Executive Officer (Total facility includes 15 beds in nursing home–type unit) **A**1 9 10 **F**1 3 7 8 10 13 14 15 16 17 19 20 21 22 23 26 28 29 30 31 32 33 34 35 37 39 40 41 42 44 46 49 52 53 54 55 56 57 58 59 64 65 66 67 71 72 73 74 **P**6

| | 23 | 10 | 130 | 5174 | 83 | 115360 | 506 | 35161 | 15203 | 635 |

SPANGLER—Cambria County

▣ MINERS HOSPITAL NORTHERN CAMBRIA, 2205 Crawford Avenue, Zip 15775; tel. 814/948–7171; Roger P. Winn, Chief Executive Officer **A**1 9 10 **F**8 15 19 21 22 26 28 30 33 34 35 37 39 41 42 44 49 56 65 71 **S** Quorum Health Group/Quorum Health Resources, Inc., Brentwood, TN

| | 23 | 10 | 40 | 1668 | 19 | 35097 | 0 | 10926 | 4702 | 184 |

SPRINGFIELD—Delaware County

▣ SPRINGFIELD HOSPITAL, 190 West Sproul Road, Zip 19064–2097; tel. 610/328–8700 (Nonreporting) **A**1 12 **S** Crozer–Keystone Health System, Media, PA

| | 23 | 10 | 70 | — | — | — | — | — | — | — |

STATE COLLEGE—Centre County

▣ CENTRE COMMUNITY HOSPITAL, 1800 East Park Avenue, Zip 16803–6797; tel. 814/231–7000; Lance H. Rose, FACHE, President and Chief Executive Officer **A**1 2 5 9 10 **F**7 8 14 15 16 19 21 22 23 24 28 32 33 34 35 37 39 40 41 42 44 46 49 52 54 56 57 60 61 63 65 71 73

| | 23 | 10 | 167 | 7879 | 106 | 104196 | 1162 | 55190 | 25868 | 713 |

SUNBURY—Northumberland County

▣ SUNBURY COMMUNITY HOSPITAL, 350 North Eleventh Street, Zip 17801–0737; tel. 717/286–3333; Nicholas A. Prisco, Chief Executive Officer (Total facility includes 29 beds in nursing home–type unit) **A**1 9 10 **F**7 8 10 11 12 13 14 15 16 17 19 20 21 22 23 24 26 28 29 30 31 32 33 34 35 36 39 40 41 42 44 45 49 54 61 64 65 66 67 68 71 73 74 **P**8

| | 23 | 10 | 101 | 3201 | 61 | 76214 | 139 | 19957 | 10201 | 395 |

SUSQUEHANNA—Susquehanna County

BARNES–KASSON COUNTY HOSPITAL, 400 Turnpike Street, Zip 18847–1699; tel. 717/853–3135; Sara C. Iveson, Executive Director (Total facility includes 58 beds in nursing home–type unit) (Nonreporting) **A**9 10

| | 23 | 10 | 105 | — | — | — | — | — | — | — |

TITUSVILLE—Crawford County

★ TITUSVILLE AREA HOSPITAL, 406 West Oak Street, Zip 16354; tel. 814/827–1851; Anthony J. Nasralla, FACHE, President and Chief Executive Officer **A**9 10 **F**7 19 21 22 23 31 32 33 34 35 37 40 42 44 45 46 48 49 61 65 71 73 **N** Vantage Health Care Network, Inc., Meadville, PA

| | 23 | 10 | 90 | 3084 | 32 | 62425 | 331 | 20792 | 8580 | 291 |

TORRANCE—Westmoreland County

□ TORRANCE STATE HOSPITAL, Torrance Road, Zip 15779–0111; tel. 412/459–8000; Richard A. Stillwagon, Superintendent **A**1 10 **F**8 11 14 15 16 19 20 22 35 37 52 57 65 73

| | 12 | 22 | 414 | 291 | 337 | 0 | 0 | 33057 | 18854 | 635 |

TOWANDA—Bradford County

▣ MEMORIAL HOSPITAL, One Hospital Drive, Zip 18848–9767; tel. 717/265–2191; Gary A. Baker, President (Total facility includes 44 beds in nursing home–type unit) **A**1 9 10 **F**1 7 8 9 12 16 17 19 21 22 28 30 31 32 33 34 35 37 38 39 40 41 44 45 46 49 64 65 66 67 70 71 73 **S** Quorum Health Group/Quorum Health Resources, Inc., Brentwood, TN

| | 23 | 10 | 99 | 2114 | 68 | 22718 | 306 | 15006 | 7135 | 282 |

TREVOSE—Bucks County

□ EASTERN STATE SCHOOL AND HOSPITAL, 3740 Lincoln Highway, Zip 19047; tel. 215/953–6000 (Nonreporting) **A**1 5 9 10

| | 12 | 52 | 157 | — | — | — | — | — | — | — |

TROY—Bradford County

★ ○ TROY COMMUNITY HOSPITAL, 100 John Street, Zip 16947; tel. 717/297–2121; Mark A. Webster, President **A**9 10 11 **F**1 4 6 7 8 10 11 12 14 15 19 20 21 22 23 24 26 27 30 32 33 35 37 40 41 42 43 44 45 46 47 49 50 52 54 55 58 60 63 64 65 66 67 70 71 73 74 **P**5 **S** Guthrie Healthcare System, Sayre, PA **N** Guthrie Healthcare System, Sayre, PA

| | 23 | 10 | 35 | 563 | 26 | 27744 | 1 | 8984 | 4779 | 79 |

TUNKHANNOCK—Wyoming County

▣ TYLER MEMORIAL HOSPITAL, Mailing Address: Rural Route 1, Box 273, Zip 18657–9765; tel. 717/836–2161; William M. Milligan, Jr., President and Chief Executive Officer **A**1 2 9 10 **F**7 8 12 14 15 16 17 19 21 22 24 28 30 32 33 35 37 39 41 42 44 45 46 49 65 69 71 73 74 **P**3

| | 23 | 10 | 63 | 2735 | 28 | 38183 | 257 | 13968 | 6415 | 245 |

Hospital, Address, Telephone, Administrator, Approval, Facility, and Physician Codes, Health Care System, Network	Classification Codes		Utilization Data					Expense (thousands) of dollars		
★ American Hospital Association (AHA) membership ☐ Joint Commission on Accreditation of Healthcare Organizations (JCAHO) accreditation + American Osteopathic Hospital Association (AOHA) membership ○ American Osteopathic Association (AOA) accreditation △ Commission on Accreditation of Rehabilitation Facilities (CARF) accreditation Control codes 61, 63, 64, 71, 72 and 73 indicate hospitals listed by AOHA, but not registered by AHA. For definition of numerical codes, see page A4	Control	Service	Beds	Admissions	Census	Outpatient Visits	Births	Total	Payroll	Personnel

TYRONE—Blair County

☒ TYRONE HOSPITAL, One Hospital Drive, Zip 16686–1898; tel. 814/684–1255; Philip J. Stoner, Chief Executive Officer (Nonreporting) **A**1 9 10 **S** Quorum Health Group/Quorum Health Resources, Inc., Brentwood, TN — 23 10 59 — — — — — — —

UNION CITY—Erie County

☒ UNION CITY MEMORIAL HOSPITAL, 130 North Main Street, Zip 16438, Mailing Address: P.O. Box 111, Zip 16438; tel. 814/438–1000; Thomas McLoughlin, President **A**1 9 10 **F**8 12 13 14 15 16 18 19 20 22 25 28 30 32 33 34 37 39 44 45 46 49 65 67 71 73 **P**3 7 **N** Saint Vincent Health System, Erie, PA — 23 10 23 751 12 15333 0 4714 2335 88

UNIONTOWN—Fayette County

☒ UNIONTOWN HOSPITAL, 500 West Berkeley Street, Zip 15401–5596; tel. 412/430–5000; Paul Bacharach, President and Chief Executive Officer **A**1 2 9 10 **F**7 8 14 15 16 19 21 22 30 32 33 34 37 39 40 42 44 46 49 60 62 63 65 71 73 **P**1 6 — 23 10 187 9158 129 118099 904 61300 26042 849

UPLAND—Delaware County

☒ ○ △ CROZER–CHESTER MEDICAL CENTER, One Medical Center Boulevard, Zip 19013–3995; tel. 610/447–2000; Joan K. Richards, President (Nonreporting) **A**1 2 3 5 7 8 9 10 11 **S** Crozer–Keystone Health System, Media, PA **N** Crozer–Keystone Health System, Media, PA — 23 10 527 — — — — — — —

WARMINSTER—Bucks County

☒ ALLEGHENY UNIVERSITY HOSPITAL, BUCKS COUNTY, (Formerly Bucks County Hospital), 225 Newtown Road, Zip 18974; tel. 215/441–6600; Margaret M. McGoldrick, President and Chief Executive Officer **A**1 5 10 **F**2 3 4 5 7 8 9 10 11 12 13 14 15 16 17 18 19 20 21 22 24 27 28 30 31 32 34 35 37 38 39 40 41 42 43 44 45 46 47 48 49 51 52 53 54 55 56 57 58 59 60 61 65 66 67 69 70 71 73 74 **P**6 7 **S** Allegheny Health, Education and Research Foundation, Pittsburgh, PA — 23 10 132 5896 97 69435 379 42561 18166 526

WARREN—Warren County

WARREN GENERAL HOSPITAL, 2 Crescent Park West, Zip 16365; tel. 814/723–3300; Alton M. Schadt, Executive Director **A**9 10 **F**3 6 7 14 15 19 21 22 23 28 29 30 32 33 35 37 40 41 42 44 46 49 51 52 56 60 63 65 66 71 73 **P**3 8 **N** Vantage Health Care Network, Inc., Meadville, PA — 23 10 105 3860 58 75575 448 28618 13035 490

WARREN STATE HOSPITAL See North Warren

WASHINGTON—Washington County

☒ WASHINGTON HOSPITAL, 155 Wilson Avenue, Zip 15301–9986; tel. 412/225–7000; Telford W. Thomas, President and Chief Executive Officer **A**1 2 3 5 6 9 10 **F**3 4 7 8 10 11 12 14 15 16 17 19 20 21 22 23 25 26 28 29 30 32 33 34 35 37 39 40 41 42 43 44 45 49 51 52 54 55 56 57 60 61 63 65 67 68 71 73 74 **P**1 3 7 **N** University of Pittsburgh Medical Center, Pittsburgh, PA — 23 10 334 12441 185 659450 1054 116475 57428 1496

WAYNESBORO—Franklin County

☒ + WAYNESBORO HOSPITAL, 501 East Main Street, Zip 17268–2394; tel. 717/765–4000; William G. George, Senior Vice President **A**1 5 9 10 **F**1 7 8 15 16 17 19 21 22 28 29 30 34 37 39 40 42 44 45 46 65 67 68 71 73 74 **P**8 — 23 10 62 3024 39 51130 434 23085 10562 315

WAYNESBURG—Greene County

☒ GREENE COUNTY MEMORIAL HOSPITAL, Seventh Street and Bonar Avenue, Zip 15370; tel. 412/627–3101; Raoul Walsh, Chief Executive Officer (Total facility includes 20 beds in nursing home–type unit) **A**1 9 10 **F**8 13 14 15 16 19 21 22 23 26 28 30 31 32 34 35 37 41 42 44 45 46 49 52 57 64 65 67 71 73 74 **P**1 — 23 10 92 2732 39 43853 0 22898 8119 292

WELLSBORO—Tioga County

☒ SOLDIERS AND SAILORS MEMORIAL HOSPITAL, 32–36 Central Avenue, Zip 16901–1899; tel. 717/723–7764; Ronald J. Butler, Executive Director **A**1 9 10 **F**1 5 7 8 11 14 15 16 17 19 21 22 25 26 28 30 32 33 34 35 36 37 39 40 41 44 46 49 51 52 53 54 55 56 57 58 59 61 62 64 65 66 71 73 **N** Laurel Health System, Wellsboro, PA — 23 10 103 3627 46 97035 336 22426 10351 333

WERNERSVILLE—Berks County

☐ WERNERSVILLE STATE HOSPITAL, Route 422, Zip 19565–0300, Mailing Address: P.O. Box 300, Zip 19565–0300; tel. 610/670–4111; Thomas V. Sellars, Superintendent **A**1 9 10 **F**4 8 10 19 20 21 31 35 39 42 43 44 45 46 49 52 57 60 65 71 73 — 12 22 371 245 368 0 0 — — 536

WEST CHESTER—Chester County

☒ CHESTER COUNTY HOSPITAL, 701 East Marshall Street, Zip 19380–4412; tel. 610/431–5000; H. L. Perry Pepper, President (Total facility includes 20 beds in nursing home–type unit) **A**1 2 6 9 10 **F**7 8 10 11 12 14 15 16 17 19 21 22 24 26 28 29 30 32 33 34 35 37 38 39 40 41 42 44 45 46 49 60 63 64 65 66 67 71 73 74 **P**8 — 23 10 217 11164 146 147965 2070 76656 33250 991

WEST GROVE—Chester County

☒ SOUTHERN CHESTER COUNTY MEDICAL CENTER, 1011 West Baltimore Pike, Zip 19390–9499; tel. 610/869–1000; Larry K. Spaid, President **A**1 9 10 **F**3 8 12 15 16 17 18 19 21 22 29 30 31 32 33 34 35 37 39 41 42 44 49 51 54 55 56 58 65 67 71 73 **P**1 — 23 10 46 2301 31 60724 0 23388 9502 345

WILKES–BARRE—Luzerne County

CLEAR BROOK MANOR, Road 10 East Northampton Street, Zip 18702; tel. 717/823–1171; Donald Noll, Director (Nonreporting) — 23 82 50 — — — — — — —

Hospital, Address, Telephone, Administrator, Approval, Facility, and Physician Codes, Health Care System, Network	Classi-fication Codes		Utilization Data					Expense (thousands) of dollars		
★ American Hospital Association (AHA) membership □ Joint Commission on Accreditation of Healthcare Organizations (JCAHO) accreditation + American Osteopathic Hospital Association (AOHA) membership ○ American Osteopathic Association (AOA) accreditation △ Commission on Accreditation of Rehabilitation Facilities (CARF) accreditation Control codes 61, 63, 64, 71, 72 and 73 indicate hospitals listed by AOHA, but not registered by AHA. For definition of numerical codes, see page A4	Control	Service	Beds	Admissions	Census	Outpatient Visits	Births	Total	Payroll	Personnel

	Control	Service	Beds	Admissions	Census	Outpatient Visits	Births	Total	Payroll	Personnel
✉ DEPARTMENT OF VETERANS AFFAIRS MEDICAL CENTER, (Formerly Veterans Affairs Medical Center), 1111 East End Boulevard, Zip 18711–0026; tel. 717/824–3521; Reedes Hurt, Chief Executive Officer (Total facility includes 180 beds in nursing home–type unit) **A**1 2 3 5 9 **F**1 2 3 4 5 6 8 10 11 12 14 15 16 17 18 19 20 21 22 23 24 25 26 27 30 31 32 33 34 35 37 39 41 42 44 45 46 49 50 51 52 54 55 56 57 58 59 60 63 64 65 67 69 71 73 74 **S** Department of Veterans Affairs, Washington, DC	45	10	339	4529	330	182292	0	83814	44839	1086
□ FIRST HOSPITAL WYOMING VALLEY, 149 Dana Street, Zip 18702; tel. 717/829–7900; John Kasenchak, Administrator (Nonreporting) **A**1 9 10	33	22	96	—	—	—	—	—	—	—
□ GEISINGER WYOMING VALLEY MEDICAL CENTER, 1000 East Mountain Drive, Zip 18711–0025; tel. 717/826–7300; Conrad W. Schintz, Senior Vice President Operations **A**1 2 9 10 **F**3 7 8 11 14 15 16 19 21 22 28 29 30 33 34 35 37 39 40 41 42 44 45 46 48 49 54 56 60 63 65 67 70 71 73 **P**3 6 8 **S** Geisinger Health System, Danville, PA **N** Geisinger Health System, Danville, PA	23	10	144	6480	97	153438	691	51495	19687	670
✉ △ JOHN HEINZ INSTITUTE OF REHABILITATION MEDICINE, 150 Mundy Street, Zip 18702–6883; tel. 717/826–3800; Thomas E. Pugh, Vice President Rehabilitation Services **A**1 7 9 10 **F**12 14 15 16 17 25 27 28 32 34 39 41 45 46 48 49 65 67 73	23	46	103	2034	99	86054	0	26448	11907	473
✉ MERCY HOSPITAL OF WILKES–BARRE, 25 Church Street, Zip 18765, Mailing Address: Box 658, Zip 18765; tel. 717/826–3100; John L. Nespoli, President and Chief Executive Officer (Nonreporting) **A**1 9 10 **S** Mercy Health System, Cincinnati, OH	21	10	173	—	—	—	—	—	—	—
VETERANS AFFAIRS MEDICAL CENTER See Department of Veterans Affairs Medical Center										
WILKES–BARRE GENERAL HOSPITAL See Wyoming Valley Health Care System										
✉ WYOMING VALLEY HEALTH CARE SYSTEM, (Includes Nesbitt Memorial Hospital, 562 Wyoming Avenue, Kingston, Zip 18704–3784; tel. 717/283–7000; Wilkes–Barre General Hospital, 575 North River Street, tel. 717/829–8111), 575 North River Street, Zip 18764; tel. 717/829–8111; Ron Stern, President and Chief Executive Officer **A**1 5 9 **F**2 3 4 7 8 10 11 14 15 16 17 18 19 21 22 24 25 27 28 30 32 33 34 35 37 39 40 41 42 43 44 46 49 52 53 54 55 56 57 58 59 60 63 64 65 66 67 71 73 74 **P**6 8	23	10	630	21687	373	444319	1882	185650	71575	2491
WYOMING VALLEY HEALTH CARE SYSTEM See										
WILLIAMSBURG—Blair County										
CHARTER BEHAVIORAL HEALTH SYSTEM AT COVE FORGE, New Beginnings Road, Zip 16693; tel. 814/832–2121; Jonathan Wolf, Chief Executive Officer (Nonreporting) **S** Magellan Health Services, Atlanta, GA	33	82	100	—	—	—	—	—	—	—
WILLIAMSPORT—Lycoming County										
✉ △ SUSQUEHANNA HEALTH SYSTEM, (Includes Divine Providence Hospital, 1100 Grampian Boulevard, Zip 17701–1995; tel. 717/320–7006; Kirby O. Smith, President; Muncy Valley Hospital, 215 East Water Street, Muncy, Zip 17756–8700; tel. 717/546–8282; Steven P. Johnson, Senior Vice President/Chief Operating Officer; Williamsport Hospital and Medical Center, 777 Rural Avenue, Zip 17701–3198; tel. 717/321–1000; Steven P. Johnson, Senior Vice President and Chief Operating Officer Hospitals and LTC Operations), 1001 Grampian Boulevard, Zip 17701–1946; tel. 717/320–7000; Donald R. Creamer, President and Chief Executive Officer (Total facility includes 84 beds in nursing home–type unit) **A**1 2 3 5 7 9 10 **F**1 3 4 5 7 8 10 11 12 13 14 15 16 17 19 20 21 22 23 24 25 26 27 28 29 30 31 32 33 34 35 37 39 40 41 42 43 44 45 46 48 52 53 54 55 56 57 58 59 60 61 63 64 65 66 67 68 71 72 73 74 **P**3 7 8	23	10	469	15815	302	435543	1540	138998	63845	2178
WILLIAMSPORT HOSPITAL AND MEDICAL CENTER See Susquehanna Health System										
WILLOW GROVE—Montgomery County										
□ HUNTINGTON HOSPITAL, 240 Fitzwatertown Road, Zip 19090–2399; tel. 215/657–4010; Alan I. Stevens, Administrator (Nonreporting) **A**1 9 10	23	22	31	—	—	—	—	—	—	—
WINDBER—Somerset County										
□ WINDBER HOSPITAL, 600 Somerset Avenue, Zip 15963–1397; tel. 814/467–6611; Nicholas Jacobs, President **A**1 9 10 **F**7 8 14 16 19 21 22 30 32 33 34 35 37 40 41 42 44 48 49 65 67 71 73 74	23	10	67	2081	28	34600	150	15010	6279	287
WYNDMOOR—Philadelphia County										
✉ △ CHESTNUT HILL REHABILITATION HOSPITAL, 8601 Stenton Avenue, Zip 19038; tel. 215/233–6200; James B. McCaslin, Director (Total facility includes 31 beds in nursing home–type unit) **A**1 7 10 **F**1 5 6 7 8 11 12 13 14 15 16 17 19 20 21 22 26 27 28 29 30 32 33 34 35 36 37 39 40 41 42 44 45 46 48 49 50 51 54 56 57 60 61 62 63 64 65 66 67 68 69 71 73 74 **P**4 5 7	23	46	88	1521	61	5971	0	12064	5595	235
WYNNEWOOD—Montgomery County										
✉ LANKENAU HOSPITAL, 100 Lancaster Avenue West, Zip 19096; tel. 610/645–2000; Kenneth Hanover, President and Chief Executive Officer **A**1 3 5 9 10 **F**4 7 8 10 12 14 15 16 17 19 20 21 22 28 29 30 31 32 33 34 35 37 38 39 40 41 42 43 44 45 46 48 49 51 52 54 56 57 59 60 63 65 66 67 68 69 71 73 **P**2 3 5 6 7 8 **S** Jefferson Health System, Radnor, PA **N** Jefferson Health System, Radnor, PA	23	10	263	13700	217	113491	1709	154098	56869	1787
YORK—York County										
□ △ HEALTHSOUTH REHABILITATION HOSPITAL OF YORK, 1850 Normandie Drive, Zip 17404–1534; tel. 717/767–6941; Cheryl Fleming, Chief Operating Officer (Nonreporting) **A**1 7 9 10 **S** HEALTHSOUTH Corporation, Birmingham, AL	33	48	88	—	—	—	—	—	—	—

Hospital, Address, Telephone, Administrator, Approval, Facility, and Physician Codes, Health Care System, Network	Classi-fication Codes		Utilization Data					Expense (thousands) of dollars		
★ American Hospital Association (AHA) membership □ Joint Commission on Accreditation of Healthcare Organizations (JCAHO) accreditation + American Osteopathic Hospital Association (AOHA) membership ○ American Osteopathic Association (AOA) accreditation △ Commission on Accreditation of Rehabilitation Facilities (CARF) accreditation Control codes 61, 63, 64, 71, 72 and 73 indicate hospitals listed by AOHA, but not registered by AHA. For definition of numerical codes, see page A4	Control	Service	Beds	Admissions	Census	Outpatient Visits	Births	Total	Payroll	Personnel

★ + ○	MEMORIAL HOSPITAL, 325 South Belmont Street, Zip 17403–2609, Mailing Address: P.O. Box 15118, Zip 17405–5118; tel. 717/843–8623; Sally J. Dixon, President and Chief Executive Officer **A**9 10 11 12 13 **F**7 8 10 12 14 15 16 17 19 21 22 23 26 28 30 31 32 33 34 35 37 39 40 41 42 44 45 49 51 52 53 56 57 60 63 65 66 67 71 73 **P**2	23	10	131	5827	76	116413	499	45199	21547	664
✶	YORK HOSPITAL, 1001 South George Street, Zip 17405–3676; tel. 717/851–2345; Bruce M. Bartels, President **A**1 2 3 5 8 9 10 **F**3 4 7 8 10 11 12 14 15 16 17 18 19 20 21 22 23 25 26 28 29 30 31 32 34 35 37 38 39 40 41 42 43 44 45 46 49 51 52 53 54 55 56 57 58 59 60 61 63 65 67 68 69 70 71 73 74 **P**6 **S** York Health System, York, PA	23	10	435	23138	334	478778	2892	210264	103280	2771

RHODE ISLAND

Resident population 990 (in thousands)
Resident population in metro areas 93.8%
Birth rate per 1,000 population 14.0
65 years and over 15.7%
Percent of persons without health insurance 11.5%

Hospital, Address, Telephone, Administrator, Approval, Facility, and Physician Codes, Health Care System, Network	Classi- fication Codes		Utilization Data					Expense (thousands) of dollars		
★ American Hospital Association (AHA) membership □ Joint Commission on Accreditation of Healthcare Organizations (JCAHO) accreditation + American Osteopathic Hospital Association (AOHA) membership ○ American Osteopathic Association (AOA) accreditation △ Commission on Accreditation of Rehabilitation Facilities (CARF) accreditation Control codes 61, 63, 64, 71, 72 and 73 indicate hospitals listed by AOHA, but not registered by AHA. For definition of numerical codes, see page A4	Control	Service	Beds	Admissions	Census	Outpatient Visits	Births	Total	Payroll	Personnel

CRANSTON—Providence County

□ ELEANOR SLATER HOSPITAL, (Includes Eleanor Slater Hospital, 2090 Wallum Lake Road, Pascoag, Zip 02859–1813; tel. 401/568–2551; Rhode Island Medical Center, Mailing Address: Box 8269, Zip 02920; tel. 401/464–3085), Mailing Address: P.O. Box 8269, Zip 02920; tel. 401/464–3085; Richard H. Freeman, Chief Executive Officer **A**1 9 10 **F**19 20 21 26 27 31 35 42 48 52 57 64 65 71 73 **P**6 — 12 48 507 180 529 0 0 94828 48569 1206

RHODE ISLAND MEDICAL CENTER See Eleanor Slater Hospital

EAST PROVIDENCE—Providence County

✠ EMMA PENDLETON BRADLEY HOSPITAL, 1011 Veterans Memorial Parkway, Zip 02915–5099; tel. 401/434–3400; Daniel J. Wall, President and Chief Executive Officer **A**1 3 5 9 10 **F**15 16 52 53 54 55 56 58 59 65 **S** Lifespan Corporation, Providence, RI **N** Lifespan, Providence, RI — 23 52 60 745 46 13030 0 22588 13719 —

HOWARD—Providence County

□ INSTITUTE OF MENTAL HEALTH–RHODE ISLAND MEDICAL CENTER, Howard Avenue, Zip 02920, Mailing Address: Box 8281, Cranston, Zip 02920–0281; tel. 401/464–2495; Betty A. Fielder, Clinical Administrative Officer (Nonreporting) **A**1 10 — 12 22 71 — — — — — — — —

NEWPORT—Newport County

✠ △ NEWPORT HOSPITAL, 11 Friendship Street, Zip 02840–2299; tel. 401/846–6400; Arthur J. Sampson, President and Chief Executive Officer **A**1 2 7 9 10 **F**7 8 11 12 15 16 17 19 22 25 26 29 30 34 35 36 37 39 40 41 44 45 46 48 49 52 56 57 59 65 67 71 73 **P**4 **S** Lifespan Corporation, Providence, RI **N** Lifespan, Providence, RI — 23 10 150 5856 81 89086 766 54174 24371 631

NORTH PROVIDENCE—Providence County

✠ ST. JOSEPH HEALTH SERVICES OF RHODE ISLAND, (Includes Our Lady of Fatima Hospital, 200 High Service Avenue, St. Joseph Hospital for Specialty Care, 21 Peace Street, Providence, Zip 02907; tel. 401/456–3000), 200 High Service Avenue, Zip 02904; tel. 401/456–3000; H. John Keimig, President and Chief Executive Officer **A**1 6 9 10 **F**4 6 7 8 10 11 12 13 16 17 19 20 21 22 23 30 34 35 37 39 40 41 42 43 44 46 48 49 51 52 54 55 56 57 58 59 60 65 67 70 71 72 73 **P**8 **N** Lifespan, Providence, RI; Saint Joseph Hospital, Providence, RI — 21 10 307 11585 225 188959 485 109307 58470 1495

PASCOAG—Providence County

ELEANOR SLATER HOSPITAL See Eleanor Slater Hospital, Cranston

PAWTUCKET—Providence County

✠ △ MEMORIAL HOSPITAL OF RHODE ISLAND, 111 Brewster Street, Zip 02860–4499; tel. 401/729–2000; Francis R. Dietz, President **A**1 2 3 5 7 8 9 10 **F**2 4 7 8 9 10 11 12 15 16 17 19 21 22 25 28 29 30 31 32 33 35 36 37 38 39 40 41 42 43 44 45 47 48 49 51 52 53 54 56 57 58 59 60 61 64 65 67 70 71 72 73 74 **P**4 5 6 8 — 23 10 215 7808 122 73411 637 94748 51642 1296

PROVIDENCE—Providence County

✠ BUTLER HOSPITAL, 345 Blackstone Boulevard, Zip 02906–4829; tel. 401/455–6200; Frank A. Delmonico, President and Chief Executive Officer **A**1 3 5 9 10 **F**2 3 4 7 8 10 11 12 15 17 18 19 21 22 23 26 27 29 30 31 32 33 34 35 37 38 39 40 41 42 44 45 46 48 49 51 52 53 54 55 56 57 58 59 61 63 65 67 68 71 73 74 **P**5 6 8 **S** Care New England Health System, Providence, RI **N** Care New England Health System, Providence, RI — 23 22 101 4591 86 41744 0 32756 20771 417

✠ MIRIAM HOSPITAL, 164 Summit Avenue, Zip 02906–2895; tel. 401/331–8500; Steven D. Baron, President and Chief Executive Officer **A**1 2 3 5 8 9 10 **F**2 4 5 8 9 10 11 12 13 14 15 16 17 18 19 20 21 22 23 24 25 26 28 29 30 31 34 35 37 39 41 42 43 44 45 47 49 51 52 53 54 55 56 57 58 60 63 64 65 66 67 70 71 73 74 **P**3 4 5 7 8 **S** Lifespan Corporation, Providence, RI **N** Lifespan, Providence, RI — 23 10 247 11103 163 175198 0 101039 51024 1290

✠ RHODE ISLAND HOSPITAL, 593 Eddy Street, Zip 02903; tel. 401/444–4000; Steven D. Baron, President and Chief Executive Officer **A**1 2 3 5 8 9 10 **F**4 5 8 10 11 12 13 14 15 16 17 18 19 20 21 22 23 24 26 28 29 30 31 32 33 34 35 37 39 41 42 43 44 45 46 47 49 51 52 53 54 55 56 57 58 59 60 63 65 66 67 70 71 73 74 **P**3 4 5 6 7 8 **S** Lifespan Corporation, Providence, RI **N** Lifespan, Providence, RI — 23 10 677 29143 477 447984 0 300578 156974 4322

✠ ROGER WILLIAMS MEDICAL CENTER, 825 Chalkstone Avenue, Zip 02908; tel. 401/456–2000; Robert A. Urciuoli, President and Chief Executive Officer **A**1 2 3 5 8 9 10 **F**2 3 6 8 10 12 15 16 17 19 21 22 25 26 27 28 29 30 32 34 35 37 39 41 42 44 46 49 54 58 60 63 64 65 67 69 71 73 **P**5 8 — 23 10 145 6388 98 138255 0 85115 42927 1086

✠ VETERANS AFFAIRS MEDICAL CENTER, 830 Chalkstone Avenue, Zip 02908–4799; tel. 401/457–3042; Edward H. Seiler, Director **A**1 3 5 9 **F**1 3 4 8 10 16 17 18 19 20 21 22 25 26 27 28 31 32 33 34 35 37 41 42 43 44 46 49 50 51 52 54 55 56 57 58 59 60 61 63 64 65 67 69 71 72 73 74 **S** Department of Veterans Affairs, Washington, DC — 45 10 108 3672 86 189959 0 69491 34570 959

Hospital, Address, Telephone, Administrator, Approval, Facility, and Physician Codes, Health Care System, Network	Classi-fication Codes		Utilization Data					Expense (thousands) of dollars		
	Control	Service	Beds	Admissions	Census	Outpatient Visits	Births	Total	Payroll	Personnel

★ American Hospital Association (AHA) membership
☐ Joint Commission on Accreditation of Healthcare Organizations (JCAHO) accreditation
+ American Osteopathic Hospital Association (AOHA) membership
○ American Osteopathic Association (AOA) accreditation
△ Commission on Accreditation of Rehabilitation Facilities (CARF) accreditation
  Control codes 61, 63, 64, 71, 72 and 73 indicate hospitals listed by AOHA, but not registered by AHA. For definition of numerical codes, see page A4

Hospital	Control	Service	Beds	Admissions	Census	Outpatient Visits	Births	Total	Payroll	Personnel
⊞ WOMEN AND INFANTS HOSPITAL OF RHODE ISLAND, 101 Dudley Street, Zip 02905–2499; tel. 401/274–1100; Thomas G. Parris, Jr., President **A**1 3 5 8 9 10 **F**2 3 4 7 8 10 11 12 15 16 17 18 19 20 21 22 23 24 26 27 29 30 31 32 33 34 35 37 38 39 40 41 42 43 44 45 46 47 48 49 51 52 53 54 55 56 57 58 59 60 61 63 65 66 67 68 70 71 73 74 **P**5 6 8 **S** Care New England Health System, Providence, RI **N** Care New England Health System, Providence, RI	23	44	197	13658	153	54476	8781	127727	65122	1545
WAKEFIELD—Washington County										
⊞ SOUTH COUNTY HOSPITAL, 100 Kenyon Avenue, Zip 02879; tel. 401/782–8000; Patrick L. Muldoon, President and Chief Executive Officer **A**1 9 10 **F**1 3 7 8 11 12 13 14 15 16 17 18 19 20 21 22 24 26 28 29 30 31 32 33 34 35 36 37 39 40 41 42 44 45 46 49 51 53 54 55 56 57 58 59 63 65 66 67 71 72 73 74 **P**2 4 7 8	23	10	100	5045	56	91517	562	42943	19849	557
WARWICK—Kent County										
⊞ KENT COUNTY MEMORIAL HOSPITAL, 455 Tollgate Road, Zip 02886–2770; tel. 401/737–7000; Robert E. Baute, M.D., President and Chief Executive Officer **A**1 2 9 10 **F**2 3 4 7 8 10 12 15 16 17 18 19 21 22 23 26 27 29 30 31 32 33 34 37 39 40 41 42 44 45 46 48 49 50 51 52 53 54 55 56 57 58 59 60 61 62 63 65 66 67 68 71 73 74 **P**5 6 8 **S** Care New England Health System, Providence, RI **N** Care New England Health System, Providence, RI	23	10	291	15654	236	166441	1343	127569	66888	1612
WESTERLY—Washington County										
⊞ WESTERLY HOSPITAL, 25 Wells Street, Zip 02891–2934; tel. 401/596–6000; Michael K. Lally, President and Chief Executive Officer **A**1 9 10 **F**1 3 7 8 9 14 17 19 21 22 26 28 30 32 34 35 36 37 39 40 41 42 44 45 46 48 49 51 61 65 66 67 68 71 72 73 74 **P**7 8	23	10	125	4226	55	220417	559	40759	18936	400
WOONSOCKET—Providence County										
⊞ LANDMARK MEDICAL CENTER, (Includes Landmark Medical Center–Fogarty Unit, Eddie Dowling Highway, North Smithfield, Zip 02896; tel. 401/769–4100; Landmark Medical Center–Woonsocket Unit, 115 Cass Avenue, Zip 02895; tel. 401/769–4100), 115 Cass Avenue, Zip 02895–4731; tel. 401/769–4100; Robert D. Walker, President and Chief Executive Officer **A**1 9 10 **F**7 8 11 15 16 19 21 22 26 28 29 30 32 33 34 35 37 39 40 41 42 44 45 48 49 52 53 54 55 56 57 58 63 65 67 71 72 73 **P**1 6 7	23	10	175	7155	96	160643	471	68236	31305	745

SOUTH CAROLINA

Resident population 3,673 (in thousands)
Resident population in metro areas 69.7%
Birth rate per 1,000 population 14.8
65 years and over 12.0%
Percent of persons without health insurance 14.2%

Hospital, Address, Telephone, Administrator, Approval, Facility, and Physician Codes, Health Care System, Network	Classi-fication Codes		Utilization Data					Expense (thousands) of dollars		
	Control	Service	Beds	Admissions	Census	Outpatient Visits	Births	Total	Payroll	Personnel

★ American Hospital Association (AHA) membership
□ Joint Commission on Accreditation of Healthcare Organizations (JCAHO) accreditation
+ American Osteopathic Hospital Association (AOHA) membership
○ American Osteopathic Association (AOA) accreditation
△ Commission on Accreditation of Rehabilitation Facilities (CARF) accreditation
Control codes 61, 63, 64, 71, 72 and 73 indicate hospitals listed by AOHA, but not registered by AHA. For definition of numerical codes, see page A4

ABBEVILLE—Abbeville County

Hospital	Control	Service	Beds	Admissions	Census	Outpatient Visits	Births	Total	Payroll	Personnel
ABBEVILLE COUNTY MEMORIAL HOSPITAL, Highway 72, Zip 29620–0887, Mailing Address: P.O. Box 887, Zip 29620; tel. 864/459–5011; Bruce P. Bailey, Administrator **A**9 10 **F**7 8 11 15 17 19 22 26 28 29 30 32 34 37 40 41 44 45 46 48 49 56 63 65 69 71 73 74 **P**5 **S** Quorum Health Group/Quorum Health Resources, Inc., Brentwood, TN **N** Premier Health Systems, Inc., Columbia, SC	13	10	48	1184	12	24069	106	8715	4505	179

AIKEN—Aiken County

Hospital	Control	Service	Beds	Admissions	Census	Outpatient Visits	Births	Total	Payroll	Personnel
✚ AIKEN REGIONAL MEDICAL CENTER, (Includes Aurora Pavilion, 655 Medical Park Drive, Zip 29801, Mailing Address: P.O. Box 1073, Zip 29802; tel. 803/641–5900), 202 University Parkway, Zip 29801–2757, Mailing Address: P.O. Box 1117, Zip 29802–1117; tel. 803/641–5000; Richard H. Satcher, Chief Executive Officer **A**1 2 9 10 **F**2 3 4 7 8 10 11 14 15 16 17 19 21 22 23 25 26 28 29 30 31 32 33 34 35 37 39 40 41 42 43 44 45 46 48 49 50 53 54 55 56 57 58 59 60 63 65 67 68 69 70 71 73 74 **P**4 8 **S** Universal Health Services, Inc., King of Prussia, PA	33	10	233	10353	135	86239	1153	—	—	789

ANDERSON—Anderson County

Hospital	Control	Service	Beds	Admissions	Census	Outpatient Visits	Births	Total	Payroll	Personnel
✚ ANDERSON AREA MEDICAL CENTER, 800 North Fant Street, Zip 29621; tel. 864/261–1000; D. K. Oglesby, Jr., President **A**1 2 3 5 9 10 **F**2 3 7 8 9 10 11 14 15 16 17 19 21 22 23 24 25 26 27 28 29 30 31 32 33 34 35 37 38 40 41 42 44 45 46 47 48 49 53 54 55 56 57 58 60 61 63 65 66 67 69 70 71 73 74 **P**4	23	10	371	17170	263	319132	2011	137900	64011	2179

BAMBERG—Bamberg County

Hospital	Control	Service	Beds	Admissions	Census	Outpatient Visits	Births	Total	Payroll	Personnel
★ BAMBERG COUNTY MEMORIAL HOSPITAL AND NURSING CENTER, North and McGee Streets, Zip 29003–0507, Mailing Address: P.O. Box 507, Zip 29003–0507; tel. 803/245–4321; Warren E. Hammett, Administrator (Total facility includes 44 beds in nursing home–type unit) **A**9 10 **F**7 8 15 16 19 22 40 44 46 49 65 71 74 **N** Premier Health Systems, Inc., Columbia, SC	13	10	84	1367	20	10399	106	10211	4372	205

BARNWELL—Barnwell County

Hospital	Control	Service	Beds	Admissions	Census	Outpatient Visits	Births	Total	Payroll	Personnel
★ BARNWELL COUNTY HOSPITAL, Reynolds and Wren Streets, Zip 29812, Mailing Address: Box 588, Zip 29812–0588; tel. 803/259–1000; Tommy R. McDougal, Jr., Administrator and Chief Executive Officer **A**9 10 **F**2 3 4 6 8 10 11 15 16 17 19 21 22 23 24 25 26 27 28 29 30 31 32 33 34 35 37 38 40 41 42 43 44 45 47 48 49 50 51 53 54 55 56 57 58 59 60 63 65 66 69 70 71 73 74 **P**1 2 **N** Premier Health Systems, Inc., Columbia, SC; The Medical Resource Network, L.L.C., Atlanta, GA; University Health, Inc., Augusta, GA	13	10	37	706	13	27629	0	—	—	103

BEAUFORT—Beaufort County

Hospital	Control	Service	Beds	Admissions	Census	Outpatient Visits	Births	Total	Payroll	Personnel
✚ BEAUFORT MEMORIAL HOSPITAL, 955 Ribaut Road, Zip 29902, Mailing Address: P.O. Box 1068, Zip 29901–1068; tel. 803/522–5200; David E. Brown, President and Chief Executive Officer **A**1 9 10 **F**7 8 14 15 16 17 19 21 22 23 24 28 29 30 31 32 33 34 35 37 39 40 41 44 45 46 49 54 55 56 57 63 65 66 69 71 73 74	13	10	162	5914	69	66457	1056	—	—	629
✚ NAVAL HOSPITAL, 1 Pinckney Boulevard, Zip 29902–6148; tel. 803/525–5301; Captain Clint E. Adams, MC, USN, Commanding Officer **A**1 5 9 **F**2 3 4 7 8 9 10 11 12 13 15 16 17 18 19 22 23 25 28 29 30 32 33 34 35 37 38 39 40 42 43 44 45 46 47 48 49 51 52 53 54 55 56 58 59 60 61 63 64 65 66 67 69 70 71 72 73 **P**6 **S** Department of Navy, Washington, DC	43	10	20	1900	11	109023	407	—	—	620

BENNETTSVILLE—Marlboro County

Hospital	Control	Service	Beds	Admissions	Census	Outpatient Visits	Births	Total	Payroll	Personnel
✚ MARLBORO PARK HOSPITAL, 1138 Cheraw Highway, Zip 29512–0738, Mailing Address: Box 738, Zip 29512–0738; tel. 803/479–2881; Stephen Chapman, Executive Director (Total facility includes 7 beds in nursing home–type unit) **A**1 9 10 **F**7 8 11 14 15 17 19 21 22 23 28 29 30 31 33 35 37 39 40 44 45 49 50 63 65 69 71 73 74 **P**5 8 **S** Community Health Systems, Inc., Brentwood, TN **N** Palmetto Community Health Network, Conway, SC; Premier Health Systems, Inc., Columbia, SC	32	10	108	1915	27	13517	122	15394	6400	271

CAMDEN—Kershaw County

Hospital	Control	Service	Beds	Admissions	Census	Outpatient Visits	Births	Total	Payroll	Personnel
✚ KERSHAW COUNTY MEDICAL CENTER, Haile and Roberts Streets, Zip 29020–7003, Mailing Address: P.O. Box 7003, Zip 29020–7003; tel. 803/432–4311; Dennis A. Lofe, FACHE, President (Total facility includes 88 beds in nursing home–type unit) **A**1 9 10 **F**2 3 4 6 7 8 9 10 11 13 14 15 16 17 18 19 20 21 22 26 27 28 29 30 31 32 33 34 35 36 37 38 39 40 41 42 43 44 45 46 47 48 49 51 53 54 55 56 57 58 59 60 61 62 63 65 67 68 69 70 71 73 74 **N** Carolina HealthChoice Network, Columbia, SC; Premier Health Systems, Inc., Columbia, SC	13	10	198	4694	141	60317	329	—	—	550

CHARLESTON—Charleston County

Hospital	Control	Service	Beds	Admissions	Census	Outpatient Visits	Births	Total	Payroll	Personnel
✚ BON SECOURS–ST. FRANCIS XAVIER HOSPITAL, 2095 Henry Tecklenburg Drive, Zip 29414–0001, Mailing Address: P.O. Box 160001, Zip 29414–0001; tel. 803/402–1000; Allen P. Carroll, Chief Executive Officer (Total facility includes 22 beds in nursing home–type unit) **A**1 9 10 **F**2 7 8 10 11 15 16 17 19 21 22 25 26 27 28 30 31 32 33 34 35 36 37 38 40 41 44 45 46 49 54 55 56 57 58 59 60 61 65 69 71 73 74 **S** Bon Secours Health System, Inc., Marriottsville, MD **N** Premier Health Systems, Inc., Columbia, SC	21	10	147	5790	86	52698	966	—	—	678

Hospital, Address, Telephone, Administrator, Approval, Facility, and Physician Codes, Health Care System, Network	Classification Codes		Utilization Data					Expense (thousands) of dollars		
★ American Hospital Association (AHA) membership □ Joint Commission on Accreditation of Healthcare Organizations (JCAHO) accreditation + American Osteopathic Hospital Association (AOHA) membership ○ American Osteopathic Association (AOA) accreditation △ Commission on Accreditation of Rehabilitation Facilities (CARF) accreditation Control codes 61, 63, 64, 71, 72 and 73 indicate hospitals listed by AOHA, but not registered by AHA. For definition of numerical codes, see page A4	Control	Service	Beds	Admissions	Census	Outpatient Visits	Births	Total	Payroll	Personnel

▣ △ CHARLESTON MEMORIAL HOSPITAL, 326 Calhoun Street, Zip 29401–1189; tel. 803/953–8300; Agnes E. Arnold, R.N., CHE, Administrator **A**1 3 5 7 9 10 **F**4 8 10 11 15 16 17 19 22 23 31 32 35 37 44 45 49 54 56 60 65 69 71 73 74	13	10	117	1917	50	45168	0	42442	13092	403
□ CHARTER HOSPITAL OF CHARLESTON, 2777 Speissegger Drive, Zip 29405–8299; tel. 803/747–5830; Todd B. Graybill, Administrator **A**1 10 **F**2 19 21 26 35 52 53 54 55 56 57 58 59 71 **S** Magellan Health Services, Atlanta, GA	33	22	70	1117	25	1743	0	8441	3613	118
▣ COLUMBIA TRIDENT MEDICAL CENTER, 9330 Medical Plaza Drive, Zip 29406–9195; tel. 803/797–7000; Gene B. Wright, President and Chief Executive Officer **A**1 2 9 10 **F**2 4 7 8 9 10 11 15 16 17 19 21 22 23 24 26 28 29 30 31 32 33 34 35 37 38 39 40 41 42 43 44 45 46 47 48 49 53 55 56 57 58 59 60 63 65 66 67 69 70 71 73 74 **P**4 5 **S** Columbia/HCA Healthcare Corporation, Nashville, TN	33	10	286	12775	177	122334	1980	—	—	1115
▣ △ MUSC MEDICAL CENTER OF MEDICAL UNIVERSITY OF SOUTH CAROLINA, 171 Ashley Avenue, Zip 29425–0950; tel. 803/792–2300; Charlene G. Stuart, Vice President Clinical Operations and Chief Executive Officer **A**1 2 3 5 7 8 9 10 **F**2 3 4 5 6 7 8 9 10 11 13 14 15 16 17 18 19 20 21 22 23 24 25 26 27 28 29 30 31 32 33 34 35 36 37 38 39 40 41 42 43 44 45 46 47 48 49 50 51 52 53 54 55 56 57 58 59 60 61 62 63 65 66 67 68 69 70 71 73 74	12	10	575	20389	396	420368	1732	340143	127873	3745
▣ NAVAL HOSPITAL, Zip 29405; tel. 803/743–7000; Captain Kathleen L. Martin, Commanding Officer (Nonreporting) **A**1 3 5 9 **S** Department of Navy, Washington, DC	43	10	40	—	—	—	—	—	—	—
▣ ROPER HOSPITAL, 316 Calhoun Street, Zip 29401–1125; tel. 803/724–2000; James H. Rogers, FACHE, President and Chief Executive Officer (Nonreporting) **A**1 2 5 6 9 10 **N** Premier Health Systems, Inc., Columbia, SC	23	10	398	—	—	—	—	—	—	—
▣ ROPER HOSPITAL NORTH, 2750 Speissegger Drive, Zip 29405–8294; tel. 803/744–2110; John C. Hales, Jr., FACHE, President and Chief Executive Officer **A**1 9 10 **F**2 3 4 8 9 10 11 17 18 19 20 21 22 23 25 26 28 29 30 31 32 34 35 37 38 39 40 41 43 44 45 46 47 48 49 51 54 56 58 60 65 67 69 70 71 74	23	10	104	2218	46	55006	0	—	—	215
▣ VETERANS AFFAIRS MEDICAL CENTER, 109 Bee Street, Zip 29401–5799; tel. 803/577–5011; Dean S. Billik, Director **A**1 2 3 5 8 9 **F**2 3 4 8 10 11 16 17 19 20 21 22 26 28 30 31 32 33 34 35 37 41 42 43 44 45 46 48 49 51 52 54 55 56 57 58 60 63 65 69 71 73 74 **S** Department of Veterans Affairs, Washington, DC	45	10	161	5570	115	174613	0	80959	53394	1009

CHERAW—Chesterfield County

▣ CHESTERFIELD GENERAL HOSPITAL, Highway 9, Zip 29520, Mailing Address: Box 151, Zip 29520–0151; tel. 803/537–7881; Chris Wolf, Chief Executive Officer (Total facility includes 7 beds in nursing home–type unit) **A**1 9 10 **F**6 7 8 11 13 16 17 19 21 22 23 26 27 28 29 30 31 32 33 34 35 37 38 39 40 41 44 45 46 47 48 49 51 63 65 69 71 73 **P**5 **S** Community Health Systems, Inc., Brentwood, TN **N** Palmetto Community Health Network, Conway, SC; Premier Health Systems, Inc., Columbia, SC	32	10	67	2069	27	29212	390	—	—	207

CHESTER—Chester County

□ CHESTER COUNTY HOSPITAL AND NURSING CENTER, 1 Medical Park Drive, Zip 29706–9799; tel. 803/581–3151; William H. Bundy, Acting Administrator (Total facility includes 100 beds in nursing home–type unit) **A**1 9 10 **F**7 8 11 16 17 18 19 21 22 26 27 28 31 32 33 34 36 37 38 39 40 41 44 45 49 62 65 67 68 71 73 74 **N** Carolinas Hospital Network, Charlotte, NC; Premier Health Systems, Inc., Columbia, SC	13	10	170	3021	142	17023	260	23118	10418	338

CLINTON—Laurens County

▣ LAURENS COUNTY HEALTHCARE SYSTEM, (Includes Laurens County Hospital, Mailing Address: P.O. Box 976, Zip 29325; tel. 803/833–9100), Highway 76 West, Zip 29325, Mailing Address: P.O. Box 976, Zip 29325–0976; tel. 864/833–9100; Michael A. Kozar, Chief Executive Officer (Total facility includes 131 beds in nursing home–type unit) **A**1 9 10 **F**7 8 11 13 15 16 17 19 21 22 23 28 29 30 31 32 33 34 35 37 39 40 44 45 46 49 55 56 65 67 69 71 74 **P**3 5 7 **S** Quorum Health Group/Quorum Health Resources, Inc., Brentwood, TN **N** Premier Health Systems, Inc., Columbia, SC	16	10	216	3725	187	44559	395	—	—	486
WHITTEN CENTER INFIRMARY, Whitten Center, Zip 29325, Mailing Address: Drawer 239, Zip 29325; tel. 864/833–2733; George Dellaportas, M.D., Director Professional Services (Nonreporting) **A**9	12	12	24	—	—	—	—	—	—	—

COLUMBIA—Richland County

▣ BAPTIST MEDICAL CENTER/COLUMBIA, Taylor at Marion Street, Zip 29220; tel. 803/771–5010; James M. Bridges, Executive Vice President **A**1 2 9 10 **F**2 3 7 8 10 11 14 15 16 17 19 21 22 23 25 26 28 29 30 31 32 33 34 35 37 38 39 40 41 42 44 45 46 49 53 54 55 56 57 58 59 60 63 65 67 69 71 73 74 **P**4 **S** Baptist Healthcare System of South Carolina, Columbia, SC **N** Premier Health Systems, Inc., Columbia, SC	21	10	387	17894	249	190750	3107	—	—	1999
▣ COLUMBIA PROVIDENCE HOSPITAL, (Formerly Providence Hospital), 2435 Forest Drive, Zip 29204–2098; tel. 803/256–5300; M. John Heydel, President and Chief Executive Officer **A**1 9 10 **F**4 8 10 11 14 15 16 17 19 20 21 22 25 28 29 30 31 34 35 37 41 43 44 45 46 49 54 63 65 67 69 71 73 **S** Sisters of Charity of St. Augustine Health System, Cleveland, OH **N** Premier Health Systems, Inc., Columbia, SC	32	10	214	9765	161	66558	0	—	—	896
CRAFTS–FARROW STATE HOSPITAL, 7901 Farrow Road, Zip 29203–3299; tel. 803/935–7173; Samuel J. Boyd, Administrator **A**9 10 **F**52 57 65 **P**4	12	22	450	236	152	0	0	13287	—	—

Hospital, Address, Telephone, Administrator, Approval, Facility, and Physician Codes, Health Care System, Network	Classi-fication Codes		Utilization Data					Expense (thousands) of dollars		
	Control	Service	Beds	Admissions	Census	Outpatient Visits	Births	Total	Payroll	Personnel

★ American Hospital Association (AHA) membership
□ Joint Commission on Accreditation of Healthcare Organizations (JCAHO) accreditation
+ American Osteopathic Hospital Association (AOHA) membership
○ American Osteopathic Association (AOA) accreditation
△ Commission on Accreditation of Rehabilitation Facilities (CARF) accreditation
Control codes 61, 63, 64, 71, 72 and 73 indicate hospitals listed by AOHA, but not registered by AHA. For definition of numerical codes, see page A4

✠ △ HEALTHSOUTH REHABILITATION HOSPITAL, 2935 Colonial Drive, Zip 29203; tel. 803/254–7777; Mark J. Stepanik, Director Operations **A**1 7 9 10 **F**17 24 26 27 34 39 41 45 46 48 49 65 66 67 73 **S** HEALTHSOUTH Corporation, Birmingham, AL **N** Premier Health Systems, Inc., Columbia, SC	33	46	89	1247	67	9378	—	—	—	234
MIDLANDS CENTER, 8301 Farrow Road, Zip 29203–3294; tel. 803/935–7508; Ronald P. Childs, FACHE, Health Services Administrator **F**2 8 9 10 11 19 21 22 23 25 27 28 30 34 35 37 38 40 41 43 44 45 46 47 48 52 53 54 56 58 60 65 69 70 71 74	12	12	24	282	7	14680	0	—	—	44
✠ RICHLAND MEMORIAL HOSPITAL, Five Richland Medical Park, Zip 29203–6897; tel. 803/434–7000; Kester S. Freeman, Jr., President and Chief Executive Officer **A**1 2 3 5 8 9 10 **F**2 3 4 6 7 8 9 10 11 13 15 16 17 19 20 21 22 24 25 26 27 28 29 30 31 32 33 34 35 37 38 39 40 41 42 43 44 45 46 47 48 49 51 53 54 55 56 57 58 59 60 61 63 65 66 67 68 69 70 71 73 74 **P**4 5 **N** Carolina HealthChoice Network, Columbia, SC; Richland Community Health Partners, Columbia, SC	13	10	609	26103	492	258083	3051	—	—	3371
□ SOUTH CAROLINA STATE HOSPITAL, 2100 Bull Street, Zip 29202, Mailing Address: Box 119, Zip 29202–0119; tel. 803/734–6520; Jaime E. Condom, M.D., Director **A**1 **F**28 29 45 46 49 52 55 56 57 65 73	12	22	350	258	277	0	0	22836	17929	676
✠ WILLIAM JENNINGS BRYAN DORN VETERANS HOSPITAL, 6439 Garners Ferry Road, Zip 29209–1639; tel. 803/776–4000; Brian Heckert, Director **A**1 2 3 5 9 **F**2 3 6 8 10 11 16 17 19 20 21 22 25 26 30 31 32 34 35 37 41 42 44 45 46 48 49 51 54 55 56 57 58 59 63 65 69 71 73 74 **S** Department of Veterans Affairs, Washington, DC	45	10	342	5378	224	887	0	101005	49926	1265
✠ WILLIAM S. HALL PSYCHIATRIC INSTITUTE, 1800 Colonial Drive, Zip 29203, Mailing Address: Box 202, Zip 29202–0202; tel. 803/734–7113; James H. Scully, Jr., M.D., Director **A**1 3 5 9 10 **F**27 34 39 41 45 52 53 54 55 56 57 58 59 65 73	12	22	267	1170	169	0	0	27252	—	513

CONWAY—Horry County

□ COASTAL CAROLINA HOSPITAL, 152 Waccamaw Medical Park Drive, Zip 29526; tel. 803/347–7156; Dale Armstrong, Chief Executive Officer **A**1 10 **F**2 3 14 15 16 17 25 28 30 41 45 46 52 53 54 55 56 57 58 59 65 67 **P**5 **S** Ramsay Health Care, Inc., Coral Gobles, FL	33	22	27	593	16	5134	0	—	—	107
✠ CONWAY HOSPITAL, 300 Singleton Ridge Road, Zip 29528, Mailing Address: Box 829, Zip 29528; tel. 803/347–7111; Philip A. Clayton, President and Chief Executive Officer **A**1 9 10 **F**7 8 10 15 16 17 19 21 22 23 28 30 31 32 35 37 39 40 44 45 48 49 63 65 67 69 70 71 73 74 **N** Palmetto Community Health Network, Conway, SC	23	10	140	8238	90	74753	891	42477	16460	607

DARLINGTON—Darlington County

WILSON MEDICAL CENTER See McLeod Regional Medical Center, Florence

DILLON—Dillon County

✠ SAINT EUGENE COMMUNITY HOSPITAL, 301 East Jackson Street, Zip 29536–2509, Mailing Address: P.O. Box 1327, Zip 29536–1327; tel. 803/774–4111; Ronald W. Webb, President **A**1 9 10 **F**7 8 10 11 13 15 17 19 21 22 24 28 29 30 31 33 34 35 37 40 41 44 45 46 48 49 51 63 65 66 67 68 69 71 73 74 **P**5 **S** SSM Health Care System, Saint Louis, MO **N** Palmetto Community Health Network, Conway, SC	21	10	87	4009	41	27052	271	—	—	277

EASLEY—Pickens County

✠ BAPTIST MEDICAL CENTER EASLEY, 200 Fleetwood Drive, Zip 29640, Mailing Address: P.O. Box 2129, Zip 29641–2129; tel. 864/855–7200; Roddey E. Gettys, III, Executive Vice President **A**1 9 10 **F**7 8 11 13 17 19 20 21 22 23 26 28 29 30 31 34 35 36 37 39 40 41 44 45 46 48 49 65 67 69 71 73 74 **S** Baptist Healthcare System of South Carolina, Columbia, SC **N** Optimum Health Network, Greenville, SC; Premier Health Systems, Inc., Columbia, SC	23	10	93	3726	48	23033	695	31331	13722	463

EDGEFIELD—Edgefield County

□ EDGEFIELD COUNTY HOSPITAL, Bausket Street, Zip 29824, Mailing Address: Box 590, Zip 29824–0590; tel. 803/637–3174; W. Joseph Seel, Administrator **A**1 9 10 **F**8 13 14 16 17 19 22 26 27 28 29 30 31 32 33 39 41 44 45 48 49 51 56 65 67 68 69 71 74 **P**1 **N** Premier Health Systems, Inc., Columbia, SC; Principal Health Care of Georgia, Atlanta, GA; The Medical Resource Network, L.L.C., Atlanta, GA; University Health, Inc., Augusta, GA	13	10	40	871	9	8981	0	—	—	128

FAIRFAX—Allendale County

★ ALLENDALE COUNTY HOSPITAL, Highway 278 West, Zip 29827–0278, Mailing Address: Box 218, Zip 29827–0218; tel. 803/632–3311; M. K. Hiatt, Administrator (Total facility includes 44 beds in nursing home–type unit) **A**9 10 **F**7 8 19 22 28 31 33 40 44 65 69 71 74 **N** Premier Health Systems, Inc., Columbia, SC	13	10	80	796	50	24889	180	6045	2507	139

FLORENCE—Florence County

✠ △ CAROLINAS HOSPITAL SYSTEM, (Includes Bruce Hospital System, 121 East Cedar Street, Florence General Hospital, 512 South Irby Street, Zip 29501–5210; tel. 803/661–3000), 121 East Cedar Street, Zip 29501, Mailing Address: P.O. Box 100550, Zip 29501–0549; tel. 803/661–3000; J. Michael Cowling, Chief Executive Officer **A**1 7 9 10 **F**2 3 4 8 10 11 13 17 19 20 21 22 23 24 25 26 27 28 29 30 31 32 33 34 35 37 38 39 40 41 43 44 45 47 49 51 53 55 57 58 60 62 63 65 66 67 69 71 73 74 **P**2 **S** Quorum Health Group/Quorum Health Resources, Inc., Brentwood, TN	33	10	316	11913	184	108094	—	—	—	1446
□ HEALTHSOUTH REHABILITATION HOSPITAL, 900 East Cheves Street, Zip 29506; tel. 803/679–9000; Oliver J. Booker, Chief Executive Officer (Nonreporting) **A**1 9 10 **S** HEALTHSOUTH Corporation, Birmingham, AL	33	46	88	—	—	—	—	—	—	—

Hospital, Address, Telephone, Administrator, Approval, Facility, and Physician Codes, Health Care System, Network	Classi-fication Codes		Utilization Data					Expense (thousands) of dollars		
	Control	Service	Beds	Admissions	Census	Outpatient Visits	Births	Total	Payroll	Personnel

★ American Hospital Association (AHA) membership
□ Joint Commission on Accreditation of Healthcare Organizations (JCAHO) accreditation
+ American Osteopathic Hospital Association (AOHA) membership
○ American Osteopathic Association (AOA) accreditation
△ Commission on Accreditation of Rehabilitation Facilities (CARF) accreditation
  Control codes 61, 63, 64, 71, 72 and 73 indicate hospitals listed by AOHA, but not registered by AHA. For definition of numerical codes, see page A4.

	C	S	Beds	Adm	Cen	OV	Births	Total	Payroll	Pers
✶ MCLEOD REGIONAL MEDICAL CENTER, (Includes Wilson Medical Center, 701 Cashua Ferry Road, Darlington, Zip 29532, Mailing Address: Box 1859, Zip 29532; tel. 803/395-1100; Debbie Locklair, Administrator), 555 East Cheves Street, Zip 29506-2617, Mailing Address: P.O. Box 100551, Zip 29501-0551; tel. 803/667-2000; J. Bruce Barragan, President and Chief Executive Officer **A**1 2 3 5 9 10 **F**2 3 4 7 8 9 10 11 13 15 17 19 20 21 22 23 25 27 28 29 30 31 32 33 34 35 37 38 39 40 41 42 43 44 45 46 47 48 49 51 52 53 54 55 56 57 58 59 60 63 65 67 69 71 73 74 **P**5 7 8 **N** Palmetto Community Health Network, Conway, SC	23	10	371	20790	302	157017	1920	179135	74223	2842
FORT JACKSON—Richland County										
✶ MONCRIEF ARMY COMMUNITY HOSPITAL, Mailing Address: P.O. Box 500, Zip 29207-5720; tel. 803/751-2284; Colonel Dale Carroll, Commander **A**1 2 5 9 **F**2 3 4 7 8 9 10 11 12 13 14 15 16 17 18 19 20 21 22 25 28 29 30 31 34 35 37 38 39 40 41 42 43 44 45 46 47 48 49 51 52 53 55 56 58 59 60 63 64 65 69 70 71 73 74 **P**6 **S** Department of the Army, Office of the Surgeon General, Falls Church, VA	42	10	91	6775	55	351626	0	39162	12636	470
GAFFNEY—Cherokee County										
□ UPSTATE CAROLINA MEDICAL CENTER, 1530 North Limestone Street, Zip 29340; tel. 803/487-4271; Steve Midkiff, Executive Director (Nonreporting) **A**1 9 10 **S** Health Management Associates, Naples, FL **N** Premier Health Systems, Inc., Columbia, SC	33	10	125							
GEORGETOWN—Georgetown County										
✶ GEORGETOWN MEMORIAL HOSPITAL, 606 Black River Road, Zip 29440, Mailing Address: Drawer 1718, Zip 29442-1718; tel. 803/527-7000; Paul D. Gatens, Sr., Administrator **A**1 9 10 **F**2 5 7 8 9 10 11 14 15 16 17 19 21 22 23 24 25 26 28 29 30 31 34 35 37 39 40 41 42 44 45 46 47 48 49 54 56 59 61 63 65 66 69 70 71 73 74 **S** Quorum Health Group/Quorum Health Resources, Inc., Brentwood, TN **N** Premier Health Systems, Inc., Columbia, SC	23	10	131	6254	81	82014	696	41871	14998	499
GREENVILLE—Greenville County										
✶ GREENVILLE MEMORIAL HOSPITAL, 701 Grove Road, Zip 29605-4295; tel. 864/455-7000; J. Bland Burkhardt, Jr., Senior Vice President and Administrator **A**1 2 5 8 9 10 **F**2 4 8 10 11 13 14 17 19 21 22 25 28 29 30 31 32 33 34 35 37 38 39 40 41 42 43 44 45 46 47 48 52 60 61 63 65 66 67 70 71 73 74 **P**3 6 8 **S** Greenville Hospital System, Greenville, SC **N** Premier Health Systems, Inc., Columbia, SC; Healthfirst of the Greenville Hospital System, Greenville, SC	23	10	620	27063	449	303202	4498	—	—	2840
★ MARSHALL I. PICKENS HOSPITAL, 701 Grove Road, Zip 29605-4295; tel. 864/455-7836; Ryan D. Beaty, Administrator **A**9 **F**2 3 25 30 34 52 53 54 55 56 57 58 59 65 **P**3 6 8 **S** Greenville Hospital System, Greenville, SC **N** Premier Health Systems, Inc., Columbia, SC; Healthfirst of the Greenville Hospital System, Greenville, SC	23	22	106	1932	54	8002	0	—	—	157
★ △ ROGER C. PEACE REHABILITATION HOSPITAL, 701 Grove Road, Zip 29605-4295; tel. 864/455-7000; Ryan D. Beaty, Administrator **A**7 9 **F**2 3 4 5 6 8 10 11 13 14 17 18 19 21 22 23 25 27 28 29 30 31 32 34 35 37 38 40 41 42 43 44 45 46 47 48 51 52 53 54 55 56 57 58 59 60 61 63 65 66 67 70 71 73 74 **P**3 6 8 **S** Greenville Hospital System, Greenville, SC **N** Premier Health Systems, Inc., Columbia, SC; Healthfirst of the Greenville Hospital System, Greenville, SC	23	46	50	651	34	27585	0	—	—	183
✶ SHRINERS HOSPITALS FOR CHILDREN, GREENVILLE, 950 West Faris Road, Zip 29605-4277; tel. 864/271-3444; Gary F. Fraley, Administrator **A**1 3 5 **F**11 15 19 21 22 31 35 38 39 40 47 49 52 53 54 60 65 70 71 73 **S** Shriners Hospitals for Children, Tampa, FL	23	57	60	1059	21	11920	0	—	—	210
✶ △ ST. FRANCIS HEALTH SYSTEM, One St. Francis Drive, Zip 29601-3207; tel. 864/255-1000; Richard C. Neugent, President (Total facility includes 32 beds in nursing home–type unit) **A**1 2 7 9 10 **F**2 3 4 8 10 11 16 17 19 21 22 23 24 25 28 29 30 31 32 33 34 35 37 38 39 40 41 42 43 44 45 46 48 49 52 53 55 57 58 59 60 63 65 66 67 69 71 73 74 **P**1 2 3 **S** Franciscan Sisters of the Poor Health System, Inc., New York, NY **N** Optimum Health Network, Greenville, SC; Saint Francis Health System, Greenville, SC	23	10	269	9133	189	99163	0	—	—	1222
W. J. BARGE MEMORIAL HOSPITAL, Wade Hampton Boulevard, Zip 29614; tel. 803/242-5100; William Brown, Administrator **A**9 **F**22 27 30 34 40 44 45 73 74	23	11	79	1734	9	7001	36	2361	805	58
GREENWOOD—Greenwood County										
✶ SELF MEMORIAL HOSPITAL, 1325 Spring Street, Zip 29646-3860; tel. 864/227-4111; J. L. Dozier, Jr., FACHE, President **A**1 2 3 5 9 10 **F**2 3 7 8 10 11 13 14 15 16 17 18 19 20 21 22 23 24 25 26 28 29 30 31 32 33 34 35 37 38 39 40 41 42 44 45 46 47 49 51 53 54 55 56 57 58 60 63 65 66 67 68 69 70 71 73 74 **P**5 **N** Premier Health Systems, Inc., Columbia, SC	23	10	337	10604	200	143822	2045	84250	40553	1348
GREER—Greenville County										
✶ ALLEN BENNETT HOSPITAL, (Includes Roger Huntington Nursing Center), 313 Memorial Drive, Zip 29650; tel. 864/848-8130; Michael W. Massey, Administrator (Total facility includes 88 beds in nursing home–type unit) **A**1 9 10 **F**2 3 4 7 8 10 11 17 19 21 22 23 24 26 27 30 31 32 33 34 35 36 37 38 39 40 41 42 44 45 46 47 48 49 51 53 54 55 56 57 58 59 60 61 63 65 66 67 68 69 70 71 73 74 **P**2 3 **S** Greenville Hospital System, Greenville, SC **N** Premier Health Systems, Inc., Columbia, SC; Healthfirst of the Greenville Hospital System, Greenville, SC	23	10	146	2706	122	55536	278	25298	9635	298

Hospital, Address, Telephone, Administrator, Approval, Facility, and Physician Codes, Health Care System, Network	Classi-fication Codes		Utilization Data					Expense (thousands) of dollars		
	Control	Service	Beds	Admissions	Census	Outpatient Visits	Births	Total	Payroll	Personnel

Approval codes legend:
- ★ American Hospital Association (AHA) membership
- □ Joint Commission on Accreditation of Healthcare Organizations (JCAHO) accreditation
- + American Osteopathic Hospital Association (AOHA) membership
- ○ American Osteopathic Association (AOA) accreditation
- △ Commission on Accreditation of Rehabilitation Facilities (CARF) accreditation
  Control codes 61, 63, 64, 71, 72 and 73 indicate hospitals listed by AOHA, but not registered by AHA. For definition of numerical codes, see page A4

Hospital	Control	Service	Beds	Admissions	Census	Outpatient Visits	Births	Total	Payroll	Personnel
□ CHARTER GREENVILLE BEHAVIORAL HEALTH SYSTEM, 2700 East Phillips Road, Zip 29650; tel. 864/235–2335; William L. Callison, Chief Executive Officer **A**1 9 10 **F**2 3 14 15 16 17 27 28 29 30 34 45 53 54 55 56 57 58 59 65 67 **S** Magellan Health Services, Atlanta, GA **N** Optimum Health Network, Greenville, SC	33	22	66	2057	50	—	0	7589	—	121
HARTSVILLE—Darlington County										
⊞ BYERLY HOSPITAL, 413 East Carolina Avenue, Zip 29550–4309; tel. 803/339–2100; Page Vaughan, Executive Director **A**1 9 10 **F**7 8 11 13 15 16 17 19 21 22 28 29 30 31 35 36 37 40 44 45 46 49 63 65 67 68 69 71 74 **S** Health Management Associates, Naples, FL	33	10	100	3633	45	35461	461	21957	8205	302
HILTON HEAD ISLAND—Beaufort County										
□ HILTON HEAD MEDICAL CENTER AND CLINICS, (Formerly Hilton Head Hospital), Mailing Address: P.O. Box 21117, Zip 29925–1117; tel. 803/681–6122; Dennis Ray Bruns, President and Chief Executive Officer **A**1 9 10 **F**4 6 7 8 9 10 11 14 15 16 17 19 20 21 22 24 25 26 27 28 29 30 31 32 33 34 36 37 38 39 40 42 44 45 47 48 49 52 53 54 55 56 57 65 66 69 70 71 73 74 **P**4 **S** TENET Healthcare Corporation, Santa Barbara, CA **N** Premier Health Systems, Inc., Columbia, SC; Principal Health Care of Georgia, Atlanta, GA	32	10	68	3191	33	58973	384	—	—	349
KINGSTREE—Williamsburg County										
★ CAROLINAS HOSPITAL SYSTEM–KINGSTREE, (Formerly Williamsburg County Memorial Hospital), 500 Nelson Boulevard, Zip 29556, Mailing Address: P.O. Drawer 568, Zip 29556–0568; tel. 803/354–9661; Richard L. Gamber, Administrator **A**9 10 **F**7 8 11 17 19 22 28 29 30 31 33 34 37 40 41 44 45 46 49 65 71 73 74 **P**7 **S** Quorum Health Group/Quorum Health Resources, Inc., Brentwood, TN	33	10	47	1099	14	23757	74	—	—	152
LAKE CITY—Florence County										
★ CAROLINAS HOSPITAL SYSTEM–LAKE CITY, (Formerly Lake City Community Hospital), U.S. Highway 52 North, Zip 29560–1029, Mailing Address: P.O. Box 1029, Zip 29560–1029; tel. 803/394–2036; Richard L. Gamber, Administrator **A**9 10 **F**8 17 19 22 24 26 28 29 30 31 33 34 35 36 39 41 44 45 46 49 65 66 69 71 73 74 **P**7 **S** Quorum Health Group/Quorum Health Resources, Inc., Brentwood, TN **N** Premier Health Systems, Inc., Columbia, SC	33	10	40	1175	10	30131	0	—	—	172
LANCASTER—Lancaster County										
⊞ SPRINGS MEMORIAL HOSPITAL, 800 West Meeting Street, Zip 29720; tel. 803/286–1214; Robert M. Luther, Executive Director **A**1 9 10 **F**2 3 7 8 10 11 15 16 17 19 21 22 23 28 31 32 33 34 35 37 40 41 44 45 48 49 60 65 69 71 73 74 **P**5 **S** Community Health Systems, Inc., Brentwood, TN	33	10	137	5526	94	96140	596	—	—	514
LOCKHART—Union County										
★ HOPE HOSPITAL, 102 Hope Drive, Zip 29364, Mailing Address: Box 280, Zip 29364–0280; tel. 864/545–6500; Mildred W. Purvis, Administrator **A**9 **F**17 28 45	13	10	10	144	3	0	0	596	294	8
LORIS—Horry County										
⊞ LORIS COMMUNITY HOSPITAL, 3655 Mitchell Street, Zip 29569–2827; tel. 803/756–4011; J. Curtiss Gore, Chief Executive Officer (Total facility includes 88 beds in nursing home–type unit) **A**1 9 10 **F**7 8 11 14 15 16 17 19 21 22 28 30 31 34 37 40 44 45 46 49 63 65 69 70 71 **N** Palmetto Community Health Network, Conway, SC	16	10	193	3244	125	56585	381	—	—	499
MANNING—Clarendon County										
⊞ CLARENDON MEMORIAL HOSPITAL, 10 Hospital Street, Zip 29102, Mailing Address: Box 550, Zip 29102–0550; tel. 803/435–8463; Edward R. Frye, Jr., Administrator **A**1 9 10 **F**7 8 11 14 15 16 17 18 19 20 21 22 25 26 29 30 31 32 33 36 37 39 40 44 45 49 54 65 68 69 71 73 74 **N** Carolina HealthChoice Network, Columbia, SC; Premier Health Systems, Inc., Columbia, SC	16	10	56	1859	31	66350	314	13810	6486	270
MARION—Marion County										
⊞ MARION MEMORIAL HOSPITAL, 1108 North Main Street, Zip 29571, Mailing Address: Box 1150, Zip 29571–1150; tel. 803/423–3210; Thomas E. Fuller, Administrator (Total facility includes 44 beds in nursing home–type unit) **A**1 9 10 **F**7 8 11 14 15 16 17 19 21 22 28 31 34 35 37 40 44 45 49 65 69 71 73 74 **N** Palmetto Community Health Network, Conway, SC	16	10	112	3517	75	15452	541	—	—	396
MOUNT PLEASANT—Charleston County										
□ EAST COOPER REGIONAL MEDICAL CENTER, (Formerly East Cooper Community Hospital), 1200 Johnnie Dodds Boulevard, Zip 29464; tel. 803/881–0100; John Holland, President **A**1 9 10 **F**7 8 10 11 15 16 17 19 22 24 28 29 30 31 34 35 37 39 40 41 44 45 49 56 61 65 66 69 70 71 73 74 **P**4 **S** TENET Healthcare Corporation, Santa Barbara, CA **N** Premier Health Systems, Inc., Columbia, SC	33	10	100	3378	37	37262	1063	—	—	337
MULLINS—Marion County										
⊞ MULLINS HOSPITAL, 518 South Main Street, Zip 29574, Mailing Address: Drawer 849, Zip 29574–0849; tel. 803/464–8211; Donald H. Lloyd, II, Administrator **A**1 9 10 **F**2 3 4 6 10 11 13 14 15 16 17 18 19 20 21 22 23 24 25 26 27 28 29 30 31 32 33 34 35 36 37 38 39 40 41 42 43 44 45 47 48 49 51 52 53 54 55 56 57 58 59 60 63 65 66 67 68 69 70 71 73 74 **P**4 8 **N** Palmetto Community Health Network, Conway, SC	16	10	80	2986	50	19373	0	—	—	244
MYRTLE BEACH—Horry County										
⊞ COLUMBIA GRAND STRAND REGIONAL MEDICAL CENTER, 809 82nd Parkway, Zip 29572–1413; tel. 803/692–1100; Doug White, Chief Executive Officer **A**1 2 9 10 **F**4 7 8 10 11 13 14 15 16 17 19 21 22 23 24 25 26 28 29 30 31 32 33 34 35 37 39 40 41 43 44 45 46 49 60 63 65 66 69 70 71 73 74 **S** Columbia/HCA Healthcare Corporation, Nashville, TN	33	10	168	9072	102	120841	738	40224	—	674

Hospital, Address, Telephone, Administrator, Approval, Facility, and Physician Codes, Health Care System, Network	Classi-fication Codes		Utilization Data					Expense (thousands) of dollars		
	Control	Service	Beds	Admissions	Census	Outpatient Visits	Births	Total	Payroll	Personnel

★ American Hospital Association (AHA) membership
□ Joint Commission on Accreditation of Healthcare Organizations (JCAHO) accreditation
+ American Osteopathic Hospital Association (AOHA) membership
○ American Osteopathic Association (AOA) accreditation
△ Commission on Accreditation of Rehabilitation Facilities (CARF) accreditation
Control codes 61, 63, 64, 71, 72 and 73 indicate hospitals listed by AOHA, but not registered by AHA. For definition of numerical codes, see page A4

NEWBERRY—Newberry County

⊞ NEWBERRY COUNTY MEMORIAL HOSPITAL, 2669 Kinard Street, Zip 29108–0497, Mailing Address: P.O. Box 497, Zip 29108–0497; tel. 803/276–7570; Lynn W. Beasley, President and Chief Executive Officer **A**1 9 10 **F**7 8 11 13 15 16 17 19 21 22 28 29 30 31 37 39 40 44 45 47 49 65 69 71 73 74 **P**4 **S** Quorum Health Group/Quorum Health Resources, Inc., Brentwood, TN **N** Carolina HealthChoice Network, Columbia, SC; Premier Health Systems, Inc., Columbia, SC

	13	10	75	1953	29	34986	204	16382	6450	278

ORANGEBURG—Orangeburg County

⊞ REGIONAL MEDICAL CENTER OF ORANGEBURG AND CALHOUN COUNTIES, 3000 St. Matthews Road, Zip 29118–1470; tel. 803/533–2200; Thomas C. Dandridge, President **A**1 2 9 10 **F**2 3 4 5 6 7 8 9 10 11 13 15 16 17 18 19 20 21 22 23 24 25 26 27 28 29 30 31 32 33 34 35 36 37 38 39 40 41 42 43 44 45 46 47 48 49 50 51 53 54 55 56 57 58 60 61 62 63 65 66 67 68 69 70 71 73 74 **P**5 **S** Quorum Health Group/Quorum Health Resources, Inc., Brentwood, TN **N** Carolina HealthChoice Network, Columbia, SC

	13	10	295	10053	156	42886	1418	67213	27735	1018

PICKENS—Pickens County

⊞ CANNON MEMORIAL HOSPITAL, 123 Medical Park Drive, Zip 29671, Mailing Address: Box 188, Zip 29671–0188; tel. 864/878–4791; Norman G. Rentz, President **A**1 9 10 **F**8 11 13 14 17 19 22 26 28 29 30 31 34 37 44 45 49 65 69 71 **P**5 **N** Premier Health Systems, Inc., Columbia, SC

	23	10	42	1176	16	24606	0	8745	3823	142

RIDGELAND—Jasper County

LOW COUNTRY GENERAL HOSPITAL, Highway 278, Zip 29936, Mailing Address: Drawer 400, Zip 29936–0400; tel. 803/726–8111; Jeffrey L. White, Chief Executive Officer **A**9 10 **F**2 3 4 5 6 7 8 9 10 11 13 15 16 17 19 20 21 22 23 24 25 26 27 28 29 30 31 32 33 34 35 36 37 38 39 40 41 42 43 44 45 46 47 48 49 50 51 52 53 54 55 56 57 58 59 60 61 62 63 65 66 67 68 69 70 71 73 74

	13	10	46	792	9	5274	80	—	—	112

ROCK HILL—York County

□ PIEDMONT HEALTHCARE SYSTEM, 222 Herlong Avenue, Zip 29732; tel. 803/329–1234; Paul A. Walker, President **A**1 9 10 **F**7 11 15 19 21 23 26 31 35 37 38 40 44 48 51 53 54 55 56 57 58 59 60 71 **P**2 **S** TENET Healthcare Corporation, Santa Barbara, CA

	33	10	276	11224	158	91524	1422	74714	28102	1254

SENECA—Oconee County

⊞ OCONEE MEMORIAL HOSPITAL, (Includes Lila Doyle Nursing Care Facility), 298 Memorial Drive, Zip 29672; tel. 864/882–3351; W. H. Hudson, President (Total facility includes 79 beds in nursing home–type unit) **A**1 9 10 **F**7 8 11 15 16 17 19 21 22 23 28 30 31 33 35 37 40 44 45 49 65 67 69 71 73

	23	10	195	6478	149	71914	574	—	—	743

SHAW AFB—Sumter County

⊞ U. S. AIR FORCE HOSPITAL SHAW, 431 Meadowlark Street, Zip 29152–5300; tel. 803/668–2610; Lieutenant Colonel Donald Taylor, Administrator (Nonreporting) **A**1 9 **S** Department of the Air Force, Washington, DC

	41	10	25	—	—	—	—	—	—	—

SIMPSONVILLE—Greenville County

★ HILLCREST HOSPITAL, 729 S.E. Main Street, Zip 29681; tel. 864/967–6100; James Dover, Administrator **A**9 10 **F**2 3 4 8 10 11 15 17 19 21 22 23 24 25 27 28 29 30 31 32 33 34 35 36 37 38 40 41 42 43 44 45 47 48 49 50 53 54 55 56 57 58 59 60 61 63 65 66 69 70 71 73 74 **P**2 3 **S** Greenville Hospital System, Greenville, SC **N** Premier Health Systems, Inc., Columbia, SC; Healthfirst of the Greenville Hospital System, Greenville, SC

	23	10	46	1170	17	41284	0	16439	5191	132

SPARTANBURG—Spartanburg County

⊞ △ MARY BLACK MEMORIAL HOSPITAL, 1700 Skylyn Drive, Zip 29307, Mailing Address: Box 3217, Zip 29304–3217; tel. 864/573–3000; Ronald J. Vigus, Chief Executive Officer **A**1 7 9 10 **F**7 8 10 11 13 14 15 16 17 19 21 22 23 25 28 29 30 31 34 35 37 39 40 41 42 44 45 46 48 49 63 65 67 69 71 73 74 **S** Quorum Health Group/Quorum Health Resources, Inc., Brentwood, TN **N** Optimum Health Network, Greenville, SC; Premier Health Systems, Inc., Columbia, SC

	33	10	197	7995	122	122282	1475	—	—	658

⊞ SPARTANBURG REGIONAL MEDICAL CENTER, 101 East Wood Street, Zip 29303–3016; tel. 864/560–6000; Joseph Michael Oddis, President **A**1 2 3 5 9 10 **F**4 7 8 10 11 14 15 16 17 19 21 22 23 25 26 27 28 29 30 31 32 33 34 35 37 38 39 40 41 43 44 45 46 47 49 51 52 53 54 55 56 57 58 59 60 62 63 65 67 69 70 71 73 74 **P**2 5 6 **S** Spartanburg Regional Healthcare System, Spartanburg, SC

	16	10	471	21555	334	321560	2109	218055	93260	3103

SUMMERVILLE—Dorchester County

★ SUMMERVILLE MEDICAL CENTER, 295 Midland Parkway, Zip 29485; tel. 803/875–3993; James G. Thaw, President and Chief Executive Officer **A**9 **F**2 4 7 8 9 10 15 16 17 19 21 22 24 25 26 28 29 30 31 32 33 34 35 37 38 39 40 41 43 44 45 46 47 48 49 53 55 56 57 58 59 60 63 65 66 69 71 73 74 **P**4 5 **S** Columbia/HCA Healthcare Corporation, Nashville, TN

	33	10	99	2706	39	51786	331	—	—	192

SUMTER—Sumter County

⊞ TUOMEY REGIONAL MEDICAL CENTER, 129 North Washington Street, Zip 29150–4983; tel. 803/778–9000; Jay Cox, President and Chief Executive Officer **A**1 9 10 **F**2 4 7 8 10 11 14 15 16 17 19 21 22 23 25 28 29 30 31 33 34 35 37 38 40 41 42 43 44 45 49 51 53 56 57 60 63 65 67 69 70 71 73 74 **P**5 8 **S** Quorum Health Group/Quorum Health Resources, Inc., Brentwood, TN **N** Carolina HealthChoice Network, Columbia, SC

	23	10	206	8783	147	75823	1263	—	—	1189

Hospital, Address, Telephone, Administrator, Approval, Facility, and Physician Codes, Health Care System, Network	Classi-fication Codes		Utilization Data					Expense (thousands) of dollars		
★ American Hospital Association (AHA) membership □ Joint Commission on Accreditation of Healthcare Organizations (JCAHO) accreditation + American Osteopathic Hospital Association (AOHA) membership ○ American Osteopathic Association (AOA) accreditation △ Commission on Accreditation of Rehabilitation Facilities (CARF) accreditation Control codes 61, 63, 64, 71, 72 and 73 indicate hospitals listed by AOHA, but not registered by AHA. For definition of numerical codes, see page A4	Control	Service	Beds	Admissions	Census	Outpatient Visits	Births	Total	Payroll	Personnel

TRAVELERS REST—Greenville County

□ CHESTNUT HILL PSYCHIATRIC HOSPITAL, One Chestnut Way, Zip 29690; tel. 864/834–8013; Max J. Gorski, Chief Executive Officer **A**1 10 **F**14 16 26 27 45 46 52 54 55 56 57 58 59 65 67

| | 33 | 22 | 44 | 162 | 10 | 0 | 0 | — | — | 65 |

UNION—Union County

⊞ WALLACE THOMSON HOSPITAL, 322 West South Street, Zip 29379–2857, Mailing Address: Box 789, Zip 29379; tel. 864/429–2600; Harrell L. Connelly, Chief Executive Officer **A**1 9 10 **F**8 14 16 17 19 22 27 28 30 32 34 35 36 37 39 40 44 45 46 49 60 63 65 69 71 73 74 **P**5 **S** Quorum Health Group/Quorum Health Resources, Inc., Brentwood, TN

| | 16 | 10 | 107 | 3374 | 47 | 40970 | 104 | 22298 | 9198 | 336 |

VARNVILLE—Hampton County

★ HAMPTON REGIONAL MEDICAL CENTER, 503 Carolina Avenue West, Zip 29944, Mailing Address: P.O. Box 338, Zip 29944–0338; tel. 803/943–2771; Dave H. Hamill, President and Chief Executive Officer **A**9 10 **F**8 14 15 16 17 19 22 28 29 30 34 44 45 65 69 71 73 74

| | 13 | 10 | 36 | 664 | 8 | 7552 | 0 | 5279 | 2747 | 96 |

WALTERBORO—Colleton County

⊞ COLUMBIA COLLETON MEDICAL CENTER, 501 Robertson Boulevard, Zip 29488; tel. 803/549–0600; Rebecca T. Brewer, CHE, Chief Executive Officer (Total facility includes 15 beds in nursing home–type unit) (Nonreporting) **A**1 9 10 **S** Columbia/HCA Healthcare Corporation, Nashville, TN

| | 33 | 10 | 116 | — | — | — | — | — | — | — |

WEST COLUMBIA—Lexington County

□ CHARTER RIVERS BEHAVIORAL HEALTH SYSTEM, 2900 Sunset Boulevard, Zip 29169–3422; tel. 803/796–9911; Brooks Cagle, Chief Executive Officer **A**1 9 10 **F**2 3 14 15 16 17 19 25 26 28 34 35 45 49 52 53 54 55 56 57 58 59 65 73 **S** Magellan Health Services, Atlanta, GA

| | 33 | 22 | 80 | 1424 | 41 | 0 | 0 | 9650 | — | 105 |

⊞ LEXINGTON MEDICAL CENTER, 2720 Sunset Boulevard, Zip 29169–4816; tel. 803/791–2000; Michael J. Biediger, President **A**1 9 10 **F**2 4 6 7 8 10 11 13 15 16 17 18 19 20 21 22 24 25 26 27 28 29 30 31 33 34 35 37 38 39 40 41 42 43 44 45 46 47 48 49 50 51 52 53 54 55 56 57 58 59 60 62 63 65 66 67 69 70 71 73 74 **P**4 **N** Premier Health Systems, Inc., Columbia, SC

| | 16 | 10 | 277 | 12325 | 165 | 170976 | 2171 | 104244 | 41307 | 1323 |

WINNSBORO—Fairfield County

⊞ FAIRFIELD MEMORIAL HOSPITAL, 321 By–Pass, Zip 29180, Mailing Address: Box 620, Zip 29180–0620; tel. 803/635–5548; Brent R. Lammers, Administrator **A**1 5 9 10 **F**2 3 8 16 17 19 22 28 29 32 33 34 39 44 45 49 65 67 69 71 73 **N** Carolina HealthChoice Network, Columbia, SC; Premier Health Systems, Inc., Columbia, SC

| | 13 | 10 | 39 | 1090 | 16 | 25594 | 0 | 9034 | 3825 | 164 |

WOODRUFF—Spartanburg County

★ B.J. WORKMAN MEMORIAL HOSPITAL, 751 East Georgia Street, Zip 29388, Mailing Address: P.O. Box 699, Zip 29388–0699; tel. 864/476–8122; G. Curtis Walker, R.N., Administrator **A**9 10 **F**14 15 16 22 34 44 49 71 74 **P**2 6 **S** Spartanburg Regional Healthcare System, Spartanburg, SC

| | 13 | 10 | 32 | 775 | 9 | 18523 | 0 | — | — | 82 |

SOUTH DAKOTA

Resident population 729 (in thousands)
Resident population in metro areas 33.0%
Birth rate per 1,000 population 15.0
65 years and over 14.4%
Percent of persons without health insurance 10.0%

Hospital, Address, Telephone, Administrator, Approval, Facility, and Physician Codes, Health Care System, Network	Classi-fication Codes		Utilization Data					Expense (thousands) of dollars		
	Control	Service	Beds	Admissions	Census	Outpatient Visits	Births	Total	Payroll	Personnel

★ American Hospital Association (AHA) membership
□ Joint Commission on Accreditation of Healthcare Organizations (JCAHO) accreditation
+ American Osteopathic Hospital Association (AOHA) membership
○ American Osteopathic Association (AOA) accreditation
△ Commission on Accreditation of Rehabilitation Facilities (CARF) accreditation
   Control codes 61, 63, 64, 71, 72 and 73 indicate hospitals listed by AOHA, but not registered by AHA. For definition of numerical codes, see page A4

ABERDEEN—Brown County

✠ △ ST. LUKE'S MIDLAND REGIONAL MEDICAL CENTER, 305 South State Street, Zip 57402–4450; tel. 605/622–5000; Dale J. Stein, President and Chief Executive Officer (Total facility includes 88 beds in nursing home–type unit) **A**1 2 7 9 10 **F**1 2 3 6 7 8 10 12 14 15 16 17 19 21 22 23 26 28 30 31 32 33 34 35 36 37 39 40 41 42 44 45 46 48 49 52 53 54 55 56 57 58 59 60 61 64 65 66 67 71 73 **P**6 7 **S** Presentation Health System, Yankton, SD

| | 21 | 10 | 313 | 7125 | 178 | 154380 | 739 | 62532 | 28278 | 892 |

ARMOUR—Douglas County

DOUGLAS COUNTY MEMORIAL HOSPITAL, 708 Eighth Street, Zip 57313; tel. 605/724–2159; Angelia K. Henry, Administrator **A**9 10 **F**8 16 19 20 22 30 32 34 36 39 44 49 53 57 58 63 71 **N** Missouri Valley Health Network, Yankton, SD

| | 23 | 10 | 9 | 317 | 2 | 4243 | 11 | 1473 | 808 | 46 |

BOWDLE—Edmunds County

★ BOWDLE HOSPITAL, 9051 West Fifth, Zip 57428–0566; tel. 605/285–6146; Bryan Breitling, Administrator and Chief Executive Officer (Total facility includes 41 beds in nursing home–type unit) **A**9 10 **F**8 14 15 19 22 24 27 30 32 33 34 40 44 64 65 71

| | 14 | 10 | 61 | 530 | 48 | 5723 | 12 | 2970 | 1502 | 75 |

BRITTON—Marshall County

MARSHALL COUNTY MEMORIAL HOSPITAL, 413 Ninth Street, Zip 57430–0230, Mailing Address: Box 230, Zip 57430–0230; tel. 605/448–2253; Stephanie Lulewicz, Administrator **A**9 10 **F**8 15 16 19 22 28 30 32 71 **P**5 **S** Presentation Health System, Yankton, SD

| | 23 | 10 | 38 | 485 | 9 | 5476 | 0 | 2038 | 763 | 53 |

BROOKINGS—Brookings County

✠ BROOKINGS HOSPITAL, 300 22nd Avenue, Zip 57006–2496; tel. 605/692–6351; David B. Johnson, Administrator (Total facility includes 79 beds in nursing home–type unit) **A**1 3 9 10 **F**7 12 14 16 17 19 22 26 27 32 33 35 36 37 39 44 45 46 64 65 71 73

| | 14 | 10 | 140 | 1969 | 99 | 35550 | 287 | 12766 | 7006 | 242 |

BURKE—Gregory County

COMMUNITY MEMORIAL HOSPITAL, Mailing Address: P.O. Box 319, Zip 57523; tel. 605/775–2621; Carol A. Varland, Administrator (Nonreporting) **A**9 10 **N** Missouri Valley Health Network, Yankton, SD

| | 23 | 10 | 23 | — | — | — | — | — | — | — |

CANTON—Lincoln County

★ CANTON–INWOOD MEMORIAL HOSPITAL, 440 North Hiawatha Drive, Zip 57013–9404, Mailing Address: Rural Route 3, Box 7, Zip 57013; tel. 605/987–2621; John Devick, Chief Executive Officer **A**9 10 **F**7 8 11 15 16 19 21 22 23 31 33 35 37 40 44 49 50 60 63 65 70 71 **S** Sioux Valley Health System, Sioux Falls, SD **N** Sioux Valley Health System, Sioux Falls, SD

| | 23 | 10 | 25 | 510 | 5 | 9355 | 36 | 2599 | 1127 | 55 |

CHAMBERLAIN—Brule County

★ MID DAKOTA HOSPITAL, 300 South Byron Boulevard, Zip 57325; tel. 605/734–5511; Mick Penticoff, Administrator **A**9 10 **F**7 8 11 17 19 22 28 30 32 33 35 37 40 41 42 44 49 65 71 **P**5 **S** Sioux Valley Health System, Sioux Falls, SD **N** Sioux Valley Health System, Sioux Falls, SD

| | 23 | 10 | 54 | 1531 | 19 | 9331 | 24 | 6128 | 2818 | 119 |

CLEAR LAKE—Deuel County

DEUEL COUNTY MEMORIAL HOSPITAL, 701 Third Avenue South, Zip 57226–1037, Mailing Address: P.O. Box 1037, Zip 57226–1037; tel. 605/874–2141; Robert J. Salmon, Interim Administrator **A**9 10 **F**6 8 13 16 17 19 20 22 24 26 30 32 33 36 42 49 65 71 **P**6 **S** Sioux Valley Health System, Sioux Falls, SD

| | 23 | 10 | 20 | 130 | 4 | 4636 | 0 | 1193 | 513 | 39 |

CUSTER—Custer County

CUSTER COMMUNITY HOSPITAL, 1039 Montgomery Street, Zip 57730; tel. 605/673–2229; Jason Petik, Administrator **A**9 10 **F**7 8 13 15 16 19 22 25 28 32 33 39 40 51 65 71 72

| | 23 | 10 | 12 | 122 | 1 | 7819 | 12 | 2430 | 1136 | 50 |

DE SMET—Kingsbury County

DE SMET MEMORIAL HOSPITAL, 306 Prairie Avenue S.W., Zip 57231–9499; tel. 605/854–3329; John L. Single, Chief Executive Officer and Administrator **A**9 10 **F**8 14 15 16 19 22 30 32 40 44 49 65 71

| | 14 | 10 | 15 | 178 | 2 | 5289 | 0 | 814 | 458 | 15 |

DEADWOOD—Lawrence County

★ NORTHERN HILLS GENERAL HOSPITAL, 61 Charles Street, Zip 57732; tel. 605/578–2313; Richard G. Soukup, Chief Executive Officer **A**9 10 **F**1 2 3 7 8 15 19 22 24 28 29 30 32 33 35 36 37 40 41 44 49 53 54 55 56 57 58 59 64 65 66 71 **N** Regional Hospital Healthcare Network, Deadwood, SD; Rapid City Regional Hospital, Rapid City, SD

| | 23 | 10 | 35 | 861 | 7 | 38754 | 58 | 6247 | 2950 | 117 |

DELL RAPIDS—Minnehaha County

DELL RAPIDS COMMUNITY HOSPITAL, 909 North Iowa Street, Zip 57022; tel. 605/428–5431; Lester Kinstad, Administrator **A**9 10 **F**7 8 11 17 19 20 22 24 30 32 33 34 35 39 40 44 49 71 73

| | 23 | 10 | 19 | 566 | 6 | 6471 | 38 | 2436 | 1312 | 66 |

EAGLE BUTTE—Dewey County

✠ U. S. PUBLIC HEALTH SERVICE INDIAN HOSPITAL, Mailing Address: P.O. Box 1012, Zip 57625–1012; tel. 605/964–3001; Orville Night Pipe, Service Unit Director (Nonreporting) **A**1 10 **S** U. S. Public Health Service Indian Health Service, Rockville, MD

| | 44 | 10 | 27 | — | — | — | — | — | — | — |

Hospital, Address, Telephone, Administrator, Approval, Facility, and Physician Codes, Health Care System, Network	Classi-fication Codes		Utilization Data					Expense (thousands) of dollars		
	Control	Service	Beds	Admissions	Census	Outpatient Visits	Births	Total	Payroll	Personnel

★ American Hospital Association (AHA) membership
□ Joint Commission on Accreditation of Healthcare Organizations (JCAHO) accreditation
+ American Osteopathic Hospital Association (AOHA) membership
○ American Osteopathic Association (AOA) accreditation
△ Commission on Accreditation of Rehabilitation Facilities (CARF) accreditation
Control codes 61, 63, 64, 71, 72 and 73 indicate hospitals listed by AOHA, but not registered by AHA. For definition of numerical codes, see page A4

Hospital	Control	Service	Beds	Admissions	Census	Outpatient Visits	Births	Total	Payroll	Personnel
ELLSWORTH AFB—Meade County										
✠ U. S. AIR FORCE HOSPITAL, Zip 57706; tel. 605/385–3201; Colonel Steven Sem, Commander (Nonreporting) **A**1 **S** Department of the Air Force, Washington, DC	41	10	31	—	—	—	—	—	—	—
EUREKA—McPherson County										
EUREKA COMMUNITY HOSPITAL, 410 Ninth Street, Zip 57437–0517; tel. 605/284–2661; Robert A. Dockter, Administrator **A**9 10 **F**15 19 22 35 44 49 71 **S** Presentation Health System, Yankton, SD	23	10	10	207	2	7073	3	1027	440	28
FAULKTON—Faulk County										
FAULK COUNTY MEMORIAL HOSPITAL, 911 St. John Street, Zip 57438, Mailing Address: P.O. Box 100, Zip 57438; tel. 605/598–6263; Karen Collins, Administrator **A**9 10 **F**6 8 11 12 15 19 22 28 30 32 41 49 51 71	13	10	12	143	2	3307	0	1311	592	26
FLANDREAU—Moody County										
★ FLANDREAU MUNICIPAL HOSPITAL, 214 North Prairie Avenue, Zip 57028–1243; tel. 605/997–2433; Paul Bergman, Administrator (Nonreporting) **A**9 10 **S** Presentation Health System, Yankton, SD	14	10	18	—	—	—	—	—	—	—
FORT MEADE—Meade County										
✠ DEPARTMENT OF VETERANS AFFAIRS BLACK HILLS HEALTH CARE SYSTEM, (Includes Veterans Affairs Medical Center, 113 Comanche Road, Veterans Affairs Medical Center, 500 North Fifth Street, Hot Springs, Zip 57747; tel. 605/745–2052), 113 Comanche Road, Zip 57741–1099; tel. 605/347–2511; Peter P. Henry, Director (Total facility includes 147 beds in nursing home–type unit) (Nonreporting) **A**1 5 9 **S** Department of Veterans Affairs, Washington, DC	45	10	408	—	—	—	—	—	—	—
FREEMAN—Hutchinson County										
★ FREEMAN COMMUNITY HOSPITAL, 510 East Eighth Street, Zip 57029–0370, Mailing Address: P.O. Box 370, Zip 57029–0370; tel. 605/925–4231; James M. Krehbiel, Chief Executive Officer (Total facility includes 59 beds in nursing home–type unit) **A**9 10 **F**1 7 8 14 15 16 17 19 22 26 27 28 29 30 32 33 34 35 36 37 39 40 41 42 44 45 48 49 62 63 64 65 67 71 73 **P**4 **N** Missouri Valley Health Network, Yankton, SD	23	10	85	453	61	7952	38	4107	2174	96
GETTYSBURG—Potter County										
★ GETTYSBURG MEDICAL CENTER, 606 East Garfield, Zip 57442; tel. 605/765–2488; Brian J. McDermott, Administrator (Total facility includes 54 beds in nursing home–type unit) **A**9 10 **F**1 6 8 13 15 17 19 22 24 28 29 30 32 33 34 35 44 45 46 48 49 51 62 64 65 67 71 73 **P**4 5 **S** Catholic Health Initiatives, Denver, CO	23	10	61	218	57	4734	0	2611	1393	30
GREGORY—Gregory County										
★ GREGORY COMMUNITY HOSPITAL, 400 Park Street, Zip 57533–0400, Mailing Address: Box 408, Zip 57533–0408; tel. 605/835–8394; Carol A. Varland, Chief Executive Officer (Total facility includes 58 beds in nursing home–type unit) **A**9 10 **F**1 7 8 11 12 14 15 16 19 20 21 22 24 26 28 29 30 32 35 37 40 42 44 46 58 64 65 66 67 71 **S** Lutheran Health Systems, Fargo, ND **N** Missouri Valley Health Network, Yankton, SD	23	10	86	715	67	18049	30	6061	2854	131
HOT SPRINGS—Fall River County										
★ SOUTHERN HILLS GENERAL HOSPITAL, (Includes Castle Manor), 209 North 16th Street, Zip 57747–1375; tel. 605/745–3159; Linda Iverson, Administrator (Total facility includes 34 beds in nursing home–type unit) (Nonreporting) **A**9 10 **S** Lutheran Health Systems, Fargo, ND **N** Black Hills Healthcare Network, Spearfish, SD	23	10	60	—	—	—	—	—	—	—
HOVEN—Potter County										
★ HOLY INFANT HOSPITAL, Main Street, Zip 57450–0158, Mailing Address: P.O. Box 158, Zip 57450–0158; tel. 605/948–2262; Gavin Hjerleid, Administrator **A**9 10 **F**8 11 19 22 24 32 33 44 65 71	23	10	22	124	13	625	0	1135	415	34
HURON—Beadle County										
✠ HURON REGIONAL MEDICAL CENTER, 172 Fourth Street S.E., Zip 57350–2590; tel. 605/353–6200; John L. Single, Chief Executive Officer **A**1 9 10 **F**6 7 8 14 15 16 19 20 21 22 24 30 32 33 34 35 37 39 40 41 44 45 49 56 65 66 71 73 74 **P**3 **S** Quorum Health Group/Quorum Health Resources, Inc., Brentwood, TN	23	10	55	2646	30	39019	283	17413	7096	243
LEMMON—Perkins County										
FIVE COUNTIES HOSPITAL, 401 Sixth Avenue West, Zip 57638, Mailing Address: Box 479, Zip 57638; tel. 605/374–3871; Helen S. Lindquist, Administrator (Total facility includes 52 beds in nursing home–type unit) **A**9 10 **F**22 64 **N** Rapid City Regional Hospital, Rapid City, SD	23	10	56	62	46	4974	0	1873	903	62
MADISON—Lake County										
✠ MADISON COMMUNITY HOSPITAL, 917 North Washington Avenue, Zip 57042; tel. 605/256–6551; Tamara Miller, Administrator **A**1 9 10 **F**7 8 14 15 17 19 22 28 30 32 33 35 36 37 39 40 41 44 49 65 67 71 73	23	10	49	876	17	11404	74	5208	2725	115
MARTIN—Bennett County										
BENNETT COUNTY COMMUNITY HOSPITAL, Merriman Star Route, Zip 57551, Mailing Address: P.O. Box 70D, Zip 57551; tel. 605/685–6622; James G. Blum, Administrator (Total facility includes 48 beds in nursing home–type unit) **A**9 10 **F**7 8 12 15 22 28 29 32 34 40 49 64	13	10	68	473	50	1525	19	2771	1612	91
MILBANK—Grant County										
□ ST. BERNARD'S PROVIDENCE HOSPITAL, (Includes St. William Home for the Aged), 901 East Virgil Avenue, Zip 57252, Mailing Address: Box 432, Zip 57252; tel. 605/432–4538; Sister Genevieve Karels, Administrator (Total facility includes 82 beds in nursing home–type unit) **A**1 9 10 **F**6 7 8 14 15 16 19 22 30 32 33 34 35 37 39 40 49 64 65 71	23	10	117	483	89	6296	39	5120	2495	83

Hospital, Address, Telephone, Administrator, Approval, Facility, and Physician Codes, Health Care System, Network	Classi-fication Codes		Utilization Data					Expense (thousands) of dollars		
★ American Hospital Association (AHA) membership □ Joint Commission on Accreditation of Healthcare Organizations (JCAHO) accreditation + American Osteopathic Hospital Association (AOHA) membership ○ American Osteopathic Association (AOA) accreditation △ Commission on Accreditation of Rehabilitation Facilities (CARF) accreditation Control codes 61, 63, 64, 71, 72 and 73 indicate hospitals listed by AOHA, but not registered by AHA. For definition of numerical codes, see page A4	Control	Service	Beds	Admissions	Census	Outpatient Visits	Births	Total	Payroll	Personnel

MILLER—Hand County

★ HAND COUNTY MEMORIAL HOSPITAL, 300 West Fifth Street, Zip 57362; tel. 605/853–2421; Clarence A. Lee, Administrator **A**9 10 **F**3 8 11 12 13 14 15 16 17 19 20 21 22 26 27 28 29 30 32 34 36 39 41 42 44 45 46 49 58 63 64 65 66 67 68 70 71 73 74 **P**1 3 4 5 6 8 **S** Presentation Health System, Yankton, SD | 23 | 10 | 23 | 575 | 9 | 3360 | 0 | 2467 | 1179 | 73 |

MITCHELL—Davison County

⊞ QUEEN OF PEACE HOSPITAL, 525 North Foster, Zip 57301–2999; tel. 605/995–2000; Ronald L. Jacobson, President and Chief Executive Officer (Total facility includes 84 beds in nursing home–type unit) **A**1 9 10 **F**1 6 7 8 12 14 15 16 17 19 20 22 23 24 26 27 28 30 32 33 34 35 36 37 39 40 41 42 44 45 49 56 62 64 65 66 67 71 73 74 **P**6 **S** Presentation Health System, Yankton, SD **N** Missouri Valley Health Network, Yankton, SD | 21 | 10 | 183 | 4423 | 138 | 73629 | 484 | 33265 | 15375 | 492 |

MOBRIDGE—Walworth County

★ MOBRIDGE REGIONAL HOSPITAL, Mailing Address: P.O. Box 580, Zip 57601–0580; tel. 605/845–3693; David Anderson, Chief Executive Officer **A**9 10 **F**7 8 14 15 16 19 22 24 26 28 29 30 31 32 34 35 37 40 44 45 49 56 57 65 66 67 71 | 23 | 10 | 48 | 819 | 8 | 7148 | 40 | 4591 | 2361 | 99 |

PARKSTON—Hutchinson County

★ ST. BENEDICT HEALTH CENTER, Glynn Drive, Zip 57366, Mailing Address: P.O. Box B, Zip 57366; tel. 605/928–3311; Gale Walker, Administrator (Total facility includes 75 beds in nursing home–type unit) **A**9 10 **F**1 6 7 8 12 13 15 16 17 19 22 24 25 26 29 32 33 34 36 37 39 40 41 44 45 48 49 51 64 67 71 73 **P**4 **S** Presentation Health System, Yankton, SD **N** Missouri Valley Health Network, Yankton, SD | 21 | 10 | 105 | 732 | 75 | 17611 | 59 | 5044 | 2406 | 114 |

PHILIP—Haakon County

HANS P. PETERSON MEMORIAL HOSPITAL, 603 West Pine, Zip 57567, Mailing Address: P.O. Box 790, Zip 57567; tel. 605/859–2511; David Dick, Administrator (Total facility includes 30 beds in nursing home–type unit) **A**9 10 **F**14 15 16 19 21 22 32 36 39 64 65 **P**6 **N** Rapid City Regional Hospital, Rapid City, SD | 23 | 10 | 50 | 324 | 43 | 1768 | 11 | 1972 | 1071 | 65 |

PIERRE—Hughes County

⊞ ST. MARY'S HOSPITAL, 800 East Dakota Avenue, Zip 57501–3313; tel. 605/224–3100; James D. M. Russell, Chief Executive Officer (Total facility includes 105 beds in nursing home–type unit) **A**1 9 10 **F**8 14 15 16 19 22 30 32 33 34 35 36 37 40 41 42 44 49 62 64 65 71 **P**5 **S** Catholic Health Initiatives, Denver, CO | 23 | 10 | 191 | 2546 | 118 | 16925 | 399 | 19832 | 9855 | 294 |

PINE RIDGE—Shannon County

⊞ U. S. PUBLIC HEALTH SERVICE INDIAN HOSPITAL, Zip 57770–1201; tel. 605/867–5131; Vern F. Donnell, Service Unit Director (Nonreporting) **A**1 10 **S** U. S. Public Health Service Indian Health Service, Rockville, MD | 47 | 10 | 46 | — | — | — | — | — | — | — |

PLATTE—Charles Mix County

★ PLATTE COMMUNITY MEMORIAL HOSPITAL, 609 East Seventh, Zip 57369, Mailing Address: P.O. Box 200, Zip 57369–0200; tel. 605/337–3364; Mark Burket, Chief Executive Officer (Total facility includes 48 beds in nursing home–type unit) **A**9 10 **F**1 7 8 11 14 15 16 17 19 22 24 30 32 33 34 36 41 42 44 45 49 64 65 71 73 **S** Presentation Health System, Yankton, SD **N** Missouri Valley Health Network, Yankton, SD | 23 | 10 | 63 | 334 | 52 | 3391 | 37 | 3469 | 1991 | 95 |

RAPID CITY—Pennington County

⊞ INDIAN HEALTH SERVICE–SIOUX SAN HOSPITAL, 3200 Canyon Lake Drive, Zip 57702; tel. 605/355–2280; James Cournoyer, Director **A**1 10 **F**1 2 3 4 5 6 7 8 9 10 11 12 13 15 16 17 18 19 20 21 22 27 28 29 30 31 33 34 35 37 38 39 40 42 43 44 47 48 49 50 51 52 53 54 55 56 57 58 59 60 63 64 65 67 69 71 72 73 74 **S** U. S. Public Health Service Indian Health Service, Rockville, MD | 47 | 10 | 32 | 545 | 9 | 54673 | 0 | 6809 | 4059 | 151 |

⊞ △ RAPID CITY REGIONAL HOSPITAL, (Includes Black Hills Rehabilitation Hospital, 2908 Fifth Street, Zip 57701; tel. 605/399–1101; Timothy H. Sughrue, Senior Vice President), 353 Fairmont Boulevard, Zip 57701–7393, Mailing Address: P.O. Box 6000, Zip 57709–6000; tel. 605/341–1000; Adil M. Ameer, President and Chief Executive Officer **A**1 2 3 5 7 9 10 **F**1 3 4 7 8 10 12 13 14 15 16 19 20 21 22 23 24 25 26 28 29 30 32 33 34 35 36 37 38 39 40 41 42 43 44 45 46 47 48 49 51 52 53 54 55 56 57 58 59 60 63 65 66 67 71 72 73 **P**6 7 | 23 | 10 | 360 | 14259 | 223 | 152384 | 1699 | 130084 | 58200 | 1643 |

REDFIELD—Spink County

COMMUNITY MEMORIAL HOSPITAL, 110 West Tenth Avenue, Zip 57469–0420, Mailing Address: P.O. Box 420, Zip 57469–0420; tel. 605/472–1111; Daniel Keierleber, Administrator (Nonreporting) **A**9 10 | 14 | 10 | 35 | — | — | — | — | — | — | — |

ROSEBUD—Todd County

⊞ U. S. PUBLIC HEALTH SERVICE INDIAN HOSPITAL, Zip 57570; tel. 605/747–2231; Gayla J. Twiss, Service Unit Director **A**1 10 **F**3 4 7 8 9 10 11 12 13 14 15 16 17 18 19 20 21 22 23 24 27 28 29 30 31 32 33 34 35 37 38 39 40 41 42 43 44 45 46 47 48 49 50 52 53 54 57 58 59 60 61 63 64 65 66 67 69 71 72 74 **P**1 6 **S** U. S. Public Health Service Indian Health Service, Rockville, MD | 47 | 10 | 35 | 865 | 7 | 63856 | 54 | 13241 | 8121 | 207 |

SCOTLAND—Bon Homme County

★ LANDMANN–JUNGMAN MEMORIAL HOSPITAL, 600 Billars Street, Zip 57059; tel. 605/583–2226; William H. Koellner, Administrator **A**9 10 **F**1 8 14 15 16 19 20 22 24 32 33 34 36 39 44 46 49 51 62 65 71 73 **N** Missouri Valley Health Network, Yankton, SD | 23 | 10 | 19 | 346 | 6 | 1720 | 6 | 2265 | 1214 | 63 |

Hospital, Address, Telephone, Administrator, Approval, Facility, and Physician Codes, Health Care System, Network	Classi-fication Codes		Utilization Data					Expense (thousands) of dollars		
★ American Hospital Association (AHA) membership □ Joint Commission on Accreditation of Healthcare Organizations (JCAHO) accreditation + American Osteopathic Hospital Association (AOHA) membership ○ American Osteopathic Association (AOA) accreditation △ Commission on Accreditation of Rehabilitation Facilities (CARF) accreditation Control codes 61, 63, 64, 71, 72 and 73 indicate hospitals listed by AOHA, but not registered by AHA. For definition of numerical codes, see page A4	Control	Service	Beds	Admissions	Census	Outpatient Visits	Births	Total	Payroll	Personnel

SIOUX FALLS—Minnehaha County

□ CHARTER SIOUX FALLS BEHAVIORAL HEALTH SYSTEM, 2812 South Louise Avenue, Zip 57106; tel. 605/361–8111; Patrick G. Kelly, Administrator **A**1 3 5 9 10 **F**2 3 12 16 17 32 52 53 54 55 56 57 58 59 67 **S** Magellan Health Services, Atlanta, GA	33	22	60	789	25	4592	0	5739	2299	91
CHILDRENS CARE HOSPITAL AND SCHOOL, (CHILDREN'S SPECIALTY HOSPITAL), 2501 West 26th Street, Zip 57105–2498; tel. 605/336–1840; Charisse S. Oland, President and Chief Executive Officer **F**12 17 27 34 48 49 64 65 73 **P**8	23	59	96	36	79	0	0	10313	6361	190
☒ △ MCKENNAN HOSPITAL, 800 East 21st Street, Zip 57105, Mailing Address: P.O. Box 5045, Zip 57117–5045; tel. 605/322–8000; Fredrick Slunecka, President and Chief Executive Officer (Total facility includes 196 beds in nursing home–type unit) **A**1 2 3 5 7 9 10 **F**3 4 5 6 7 8 9 10 11 12 13 14 15 16 17 18 19 20 21 22 24 25 26 27 28 29 30 31 32 33 34 35 37 38 39 40 41 42 43 44 45 46 47 48 49 51 52 53 54 55 56 57 58 59 60 62 63 64 65 66 67 68 69 71 73 74 **P**2 6 7 **S** Presentation Health System, Yankton, SD **N** Affiliated Community Health Network, Inc., Willmar, MN	21	10	521	14300	415	183791	1198	142756	61070	1940
☒ ROYAL C. JOHNSON VETERANS MEMORIAL HOSPITAL, 2501 West 22nd Street, Zip 57105, Mailing Address: P.O. Box 5046, Zip 57117–5046; tel. 605/336–3230; R. Vincent Crawford, Director (Total facility includes 78 beds in nursing home–type unit) **A**1 3 5 9 **F**1 2 3 11 12 15 17 19 20 21 22 26 27 28 30 31 32 33 34 37 39 41 42 44 45 46 48 49 51 52 54 55 59 64 65 67 71 73 74 **P**6 **S** Department of Veterans Affairs, Washington, DC	45	10	162	2901	133	74937	0	46997	25004	665
☒ △ SIOUX VALLEY HOSPITAL, 1100 South Euclid Avenue, Zip 57105–0496, Mailing Address: P.O. Box 5039, Zip 57117–5039; tel. 605/333–1000; Kelby K. Krabbenhoft, Chief Executive Officer **A**1 2 3 5 7 9 10 **F**4 7 8 10 11 12 13 14 15 16 17 18 19 20 21 22 24 25 26 27 28 29 30 31 32 33 34 35 37 39 40 41 42 43 44 45 46 47 48 49 51 53 54 55 56 58 61 65 66 67 70 71 72 73 74 **P**6 **S** Sioux Valley Health System, Sioux Falls, SD **N** Southwest Minnesota Health Alliance, Luverne, MN	23	10	504	17956	297	141230	1915	179684	84848	3290

SISSETON—Roberts County

★ COTEAU DES PRAIRIES HOSPITAL, 205 Orchard Drive, Zip 57262; tel. 605/698–7647; Bill Nelson, Administrator (Nonreporting) **A**9 10	23	10	27	—	—	—	—	—	—	—
☒ U. S. PUBLIC HEALTH SERVICE INDIAN HOSPITAL, Chestnut Street, Zip 57262, Mailing Address: P.O. Box 189, Zip 57262; tel. 605/698–7606; Richard Huff, Administrator **A**1 10 **F**3 6 7 8 12 13 14 15 16 17 18 19 20 22 27 28 29 30 31 32 33 34 36 39 40 41 44 45 46 49 51 61 65 67 68 71 73 74 **S** U. S. Public Health Service Indian Health Service, Rockville, MD	47	10	18	333	3	30058	0	—	—	—

SPEARFISH—Lawrence County

★ LOOKOUT MEMORIAL HOSPITAL, 1440 North Main Street, Zip 57783–1504; tel. 605/642–2617; Deb J. Krmpotic, R.N., Administrator **A**9 10 **F**1 7 8 11 12 14 15 16 19 21 22 27 28 30 32 33 34 35 36 37 39 40 41 44 45 46 49 62 63 64 65 66 67 71 73 **P**6 7 **S** Lutheran Health Systems, Fargo, ND **N** Black Hills Healthcare Network, Spearfish, SD	23	10	31	1563	15	38550	330	9128	4064	156

STURGIS—Meade County

★ STURGIS COMMUNITY HEALTH CARE CENTER, 949 Harmon Street, Zip 57785; tel. 605/347–2536; Roger R. Heidt, Administrator (Total facility includes 84 beds in nursing home–type unit) **A**9 10 **F**7 8 12 14 15 16 19 22 28 32 35 37 40 41 44 64 65 67 71 **S** Lutheran Health Systems, Fargo, ND	23	10	114	1021	96	20237	93	8388	3971	112

TYNDALL—Bon Homme County

★ ST. MICHAEL'S HOSPITAL, Douglas Street and Broadway, Zip 57066, Mailing Address: Box 27, Zip 57066; tel. 605/589–3341; Carol Deurmier, Chief Executive Officer (Total facility includes 9 beds in nursing home–type unit) **A**10 **F**7 8 14 15 16 19 22 30 32 33 35 37 40 44 45 54 56 58 64 65 66 71 73 **P**4 **N** Missouri Valley Health Network, Yankton, SD	21	10	34	412	16	13606	20	2453	1342	53

VERMILLION—Clay County

★ DAKOTA MEDICAL CENTER, (Formerly Dakota Hospital), 20 South Plum Street, Zip 57069; tel. 605/624–2611; Larry W. Veitz, Chief Executive Officer (Total facility includes 66 beds in nursing home–type unit) **A**9 10 **F**7 8 10 14 16 17 19 22 28 29 30 32 33 35 37 39 40 41 42 44 45 46 49 64 65 66 67 71 73 **P**3 **S** Sioux Valley Health System, Sioux Falls, SD **N** Sioux Valley Health System, Sioux Falls, SD	23	10	95	939	76	14351	58	6213	3039	78

VIBORG—Turner County

★ PIONEER MEMORIAL HOSPITAL, 315 North Washington Street, Zip 57070, Mailing Address: P.O. Box 368, Zip 57070–0368; tel. 605/326–5161; Georgia Pokorney, Chief Executive Officer (Total facility includes 52 beds in nursing home–type unit) **A**9 10 **F**1 3 4 7 8 10 11 15 19 20 21 22 24 26 28 32 33 34 36 37 38 39 40 42 43 44 45 47 51 62 64 65 67 71 74 **P**5 **S** Sioux Valley Health System, Sioux Falls, SD **N** Sioux Valley Health System, Sioux Falls, SD; Missouri Valley Health Network, Yankton, SD	23	10	77	467	54	8286	5	3429	1748	58

WAGNER—Charles Mix County

★ WAGNER COMMUNITY MEMORIAL HOSPITAL, Third and Walnut, Zip 57380, Mailing Address: P.O. Box 280, Zip 57380–0280; tel. 605/384–3611; Arlene C. Bich, Administrator **A**9 10 **F**7 11 15 16 19 20 22 26 28 29 30 32 33 34 37 40 44 45 49 62 64 65 70 71 **N** Missouri Valley Health Network, Yankton, SD	23	10	20	673	7	7539	8	2753	1215	51

WATERTOWN—Codington County

☒ + PRAIRIE LAKES HOSPITAL AND CARE CENTER, 400 Tenth Avenue N.W., Zip 57201, Mailing Address: P.O. Box 1210, Zip 57201–1210; tel. 605/882–7000; Edmond L. Weiland, President and Chief Executive Officer (Total facility includes 51 beds in nursing home–type unit) **A**1 2 3 9 10 **F**7 8 14 15 16 17 19 22 29 32 33 34 35 37 39 40 41 42 44 45 46 49 56 59 64 65 66 71 73 74 **S** Presentation Health System, Yankton, SD	23	10	122	2938	84	51635	555	24844	9799	352

Hospital, Address, Telephone, Administrator, Approval, Facility, and Physician Codes, Health Care System, Network	Classi-fication Codes		Utilization Data						Expense (thousands) of dollars		
★ American Hospital Association (AHA) membership □ Joint Commission on Accreditation of Healthcare Organizations (JCAHO) accreditation + American Osteopathic Hospital Association (AOHA) membership ○ American Osteopathic Association (AOA) accreditation △ Commission on Accreditation of Rehabilitation Facilities (CARF) accreditation Control codes 61, 63, 64, 71, 72 and 73 indicate hospitals listed by AOHA, but not registered by AHA. For definition of numerical codes, see page A4	Control	Service	Beds	Admissions	Census	Outpatient Visits	Births	Total	Payroll	Personnel

WEBSTER—Day County

★ LAKE AREA HOSPITAL, North First Street, Zip 57274, Mailing Address: P.O. Box 489, Zip 57274–0489; tel. 605/345–3336; Donald J. Finn, Administrator **A**9 10 **F**3 7 8 11 12 15 16 19 21 22 28 30 31 34 40 44 45 49 71 **P**5 **S** Sioux Valley Health System, Sioux Falls, SD

| | | | 23 | 10 | 26 | 592 | 8 | 3849 | 6 | 3019 | 1474 | 66 |

WESSINGTON SPRINGS—Jerauld County

WESKOTA MEMORIAL MEDICAL CENTER, 609 First Street N.E., Zip 57382; tel. 605/539–1201; Thomas V. Richter, Administrator **A**9 10 **F**7 15 19 22 30 32 44 49 71

| | | | 23 | 10 | 28 | 389 | 9 | 3307 | 12 | 1462 | 772 | 34 |

WINNER—Tripp County

★ WINNER REGIONAL HEALTHCARE CENTER, 745 East Eighth Street, Zip 57580–2677, Mailing Address: Box 745, Zip 57580–0745; tel. 605/842–2110; Robert Houser, Chief Executive Officer (Total facility includes 81 beds in nursing home–type unit) **A**9 10 **F**7 8 11 14 15 16 17 19 21 22 26 28 29 30 32 33 34 35 36 39 40 42 44 45 49 50 61 63 64 66 67 69 71 **S** Sioux Valley Health System, Sioux Falls, SD **N** Missouri Valley Health Network, Yankton, SD

| | | | 23 | 10 | 116 | 922 | 87 | 12899 | 167 | 7876 | 4099 | 112 |

YANKTON—Yankton County

✠ △ SACRED HEART HEALTH SERVICES, 501 Summit, Zip 57078–3899; tel. 605/668–8000; Dennis A. Sokol, President and Chief Executive Officer (Total facility includes 113 beds in nursing home–type unit) **A**1 2 5 7 9 10 **F**1 7 8 10 11 12 14 15 16 17 19 21 22 23 24 26 27 29 30 32 33 34 35 36 37 39 40 41 42 44 45 46 48 49 60 63 64 65 66 67 71 73 **P**3 **S** Presentation Health System, Yankton, SD **N** Missouri Valley Health Network, Yankton, SD

| | | | 21 | 10 | 257 | 4897 | 173 | 25102 | 633 | 33206 | 13281 | 421 |

TENNESSEE

Resident population 5,256 (in thousands)
Resident population in metro areas 67.8%
Birth rate per 1,000 population 14.3
65 years and over 12.5%
Percent of persons without health insurance 10.2%

Hospital, Address, Telephone, Administrator, Approval, Facility, and Physician Codes, Health Care System, Network	Classification Codes		Utilization Data					Expense (thousands) of dollars		
	Control	Service	Beds	Admissions	Census	Outpatient Visits	Births	Total	Payroll	Personnel

★ American Hospital Association (AHA) membership
□ Joint Commission on Accreditation of Healthcare Organizations (JCAHO) accreditation
+ American Osteopathic Hospital Association (AOHA) membership
○ American Osteopathic Association (AOA) accreditation
△ Commission on Accreditation of Rehabilitation Facilities (CARF) accreditation
Control codes 61, 63, 64, 71, 72 and 73 indicate hospitals listed by AOHA, but not registered by AHA. For definition of numerical codes, see page A4

Hospital	Control	Service	Beds	Admissions	Census	Outpatient Visits	Births	Total	Payroll	Personnel
ASHLAND CITY—Cheatham County										
★ COLUMBIA CHEATHAM MEDICAL CENTER, 313 North Main Street, Zip 37015; tel. 615/792–3030; Peggy Miller, R.N., Director Nursing and Chief Operating Officer **A**9 **F**8 12 14 15 16 17 19 21 22 28 30 32 33 34 41 44 45 46 49 51 54 65 67 71 73 **P**7 **S** Columbia/HCA Healthcare Corporation, Nashville, TN	33	10	29	1413	16	20427	0	6665	2382	112
ATHENS—McMinn County										
⊞ COLUMBIA ATHENS REGIONAL MEDICAL CENTER, 1114 West Madison Avenue, Zip 37303, Mailing Address: Box 250, Zip 37371–0250; tel. 615/745–1411; Sean S. McMurray, Administrator **A**1 9 10 **F**3 7 8 11 14 15 16 17 19 21 22 23 28 29 30 31 32 33 35 37 39 40 41 42 44 45 46 49 53 54 55 56 57 58 59 61 63 65 67 68 71 72 73 74 **S** Columbia/HCA Healthcare Corporation, Nashville, TN **N** Principal Health Care of Georgia, Atlanta, GA; Chattanooga Healthcare Network, Chattanooga, TN	33	10	97	3051	29	41688	317	14194	6544	232
BOLIVAR—Hardeman County										
⊞ BOLIVAR GENERAL HOSPITAL, 650 Nuckolls Road, Zip 38008; tel. 901/658–3100; George L. Austin, Chief Executive Officer (Nonreporting) **A**1 9 10 **S** West Tennessee Healthcare, Inc., Jackson, TN **N** West Tennessee Healthcare, Inc., Jackson, TN	23	10	47	—	—	—	—	—	—	—
BRISTOL—Sullivan County										
★ WELLMONT HEALTH SYSTEM–BRISTOL, (Formerly Bristol Regional Medical Center), 1 Medical Park Boulevard, Zip 37620; tel. 423/844–4200; Randall M. Olson, Administrator (Total facility includes 30 beds in nursing home–type unit) **A**2 **F**1 4 7 8 10 11 12 14 15 16 17 19 20 21 22 23 24 25 26 28 29 30 31 32 33 34 35 36 37 39 40 41 42 43 44 46 49 51 52 55 56 57 58 59 60 63 65 66 67 70 71 72 73 74 **P**1 4 5 6 7 **S** Quorum Health Group/Quorum Health Resources, Inc., Brentwood, TN **N** Highlands Wellmont Health Network, Inc., Bristol, TN	23	10	339	11800	171	296626	630	109582	45022	1330
BROWNSVILLE—Haywood County										
⊞ METHODIST–HAYWOOD PARK HOSPITAL, 2545 North Washington Avenue, Zip 38012; tel. 901/772–4110; Sandra Bailey, Administrator **A**1 9 10 **F**7 8 14 15 16 17 19 22 27 28 29 30 32 33 39 40 41 44 45 46 49 65 71 73 74 **P**3 6 7 8 **S** Methodist Health Systems, Inc., Memphis, TN	23	10	44	1094	11	12650	226	6046	2649	87
CAMDEN—Benton County										
★ CAMDEN GENERAL HOSPITAL, 175 Hospital Drive, Zip 38320; tel. 901/584–6135; Alfred P. Taylor, Administrator and Chief Executive Officer **A**9 10 **F**8 15 16 19 22 28 30 34 44 71 **S** West Tennessee Healthcare, Inc., Jackson, TN **N** West Tennessee Healthcare, Inc., Jackson, TN	16	10	40	704	9	—	0	4498	2224	93
CARTHAGE—Smith County										
CARTHAGE GENERAL HOSPITAL See Frank T. Rutherford Memorial Hospital										
⊞ COLUMBIA SMITH COUNTY MEMORIAL HOSPITAL, 158 Hospital Drive, Zip 37030–1096; tel. 615/735–1560; Jerry H. Futrell, Chief Executive Officer **A**1 9 10 **F**7 8 12 14 15 16 19 20 22 26 28 32 35 40 44 49 52 57 65 66 71 73 **P**8 **S** Columbia/HCA Healthcare Corporation, Nashville, TN	33	10	53	1744	23	17228	79	9486	3265	134
⊞ FRANK T. RUTHERFORD MEMORIAL HOSPITAL, (Includes Carthage General Hospital, Highway 70 North, Mailing Address: P.O. Box 319, Zip 37030–0319; Wayne Winfree, Administrator; Trousdale Medical Center, 500 Church Street, Hartsville, Zip 37074, Mailing Address: P.O. Box 319, Carthage, Zip 37030; tel. 615/374–2221; 130 Lebanon Highway, Zip 37030, Mailing Address: P.O. Box 319, Zip 37030; tel. 615/735–9815; Wayne Winfree, Chief Executive Officer **A**1 9 10 **F**7 8 12 15 19 22 28 32 44 45 51 65 67 71	23	10	54	2336	25	22333	51	10430	4761	231
CELINA—Clay County										
CUMBERLAND RIVER HOSPITAL NORTH, McArthur Street, Zip 38551, Mailing Address: Box 427, Zip 38551; tel. 615/243–3581; Patrick J. Gray, Chief Executive Officer (Total facility includes 8 beds in nursing home–type unit) (Nonreporting) **A**9 10 **S** Paracelsus Healthcare Corporation, Houston, TX	33	10	36	—	—	—	—	—	—	—
CENTERVILLE—Hickman County										
□ BAPTIST HICKMAN COMMUNITY HOSPITAL, (Formerly Hickman County Health Services), 135 East Swan Street, Zip 37033–1499; tel. 615/729–4271; Jack M. Keller, Administrator (Total facility includes 40 beds in nursing home–type unit) **A**1 9 10 **F**8 14 15 16 19 22 27 28 30 32 33 34 41 49 59 64 65 71	23	10	62	540	45	8317	0	5381	2554	108
CHATTANOOGA—Hamilton County										
⊞ COLUMBIA VALLEY HOSPITAL, (Formerly Valley Psychiatric Hospital), 2200 Morris Hill Road, Zip 37421; tel. 423/894–4220; Solon Boggus, Jr., Chief Executive Officer (Nonreporting) **A**1 10 **S** Columbia/HCA Healthcare Corporation, Nashville, TN **N** Chattanooga Healthcare Network, Chattanooga, TN	33	22	118	—	—	—	—	—	—	—
⊞ ERLANGER MEDICAL CENTER, (Includes Erlanger North Hospital, 632 Morrison Springs Road, Zip 37415; tel. 615/778–3300; T. C. Thompson Children's Hospital, 910 Blackford Street, tel. 615/778–6011; Willie D. Miller Eye Center), 975 East Third Street, Zip 37403; tel. 423/778–7000; Sylvester L. Reeder, III, President and Chief Executive Officer (Nonreporting) **A**1 2 3 5 9 10	16	10	536	—	—	—	—	—	—	—

Hospital, Address, Telephone, Administrator, Approval, Facility, and Physician Codes, Health Care System, Network	Classi-fication Codes		Utilization Data					Expense (thousands) of dollars		
★ American Hospital Association (AHA) membership □ Joint Commission on Accreditation of Healthcare Organizations (JCAHO) accreditation + American Osteopathic Hospital Association (AOHA) membership ○ American Osteopathic Association (AOA) accreditation △ Commission on Accreditation of Rehabilitation Facilities (CARF) accreditation Control codes 61, 63, 64, 71, 72 and 73 indicate hospitals listed by AOHA, but not registered by AHA. For definition of numerical codes, see page A4	Control	Service	Beds	Admissions	Census	Outpatient Visits	Births	Total	Payroll	Personnel
□ HEALTHSOUTH CHATTANOOGA REHABILITATION HOSPITAL, 2412 McCallie Avenue, Zip 37404; tel. 423/698–0221 **A**1 10 **F**5 12 14 16 27 34 41 42 44 48 49 66 **S** HEALTHSOUTH Corporation, Birmingham, AL	33	46	69	922	54	7195	0	9344	5147	147
✠ MEMORIAL HOSPITAL, 2525 De Sales Avenue, Zip 37404–3322; tel. 615/495–2525; L. Clark Taylor, Jr., President and Chief Executive Officer (Nonreporting) **A**1 2 5 9 10 **S** Sisters of Charity of Nazareth Health System, Nazareth, KY **N** Principal Health Care of Georgia, Atlanta, GA	21	10	296	—	—	—	—	—	—	—
□ MOCCASIN BEND MENTAL HEALTH INSTITUTE, 100 Moccasin Bend Road, Zip 37405; tel. 423/785–3400; Russell K. Vatter, Superintendent (Nonreporting) **A**1 10	12	22	200	—	—	—	—	—	—	—
✠ NORTH PARK HOSPITAL, 2051 Hamill Road, Zip 37343–4096; tel. 423/870–6100; Leonard Fant, Administrator (Nonreporting) **A**1 9 10 **S** Healthcorp of Tennessee, Inc., Chattanooga, TN **N** Principal Health Care of Georgia, Atlanta, GA	23	10	83	—	—	—	—	—	—	—
✠ PARKRIDGE MEDICAL CENTER, 2333 McCallie Avenue, Zip 37404–3285; tel. 423/698–6061; Solon Boggus, Jr., Chief Executive Officer (Total facility includes 28 beds in nursing home–type unit) **A**1 9 10 **F**2 3 4 7 8 10 12 14 15 16 19 20 21 22 23 24 26 28 30 31 32 33 34 35 37 38 39 40 41 42 43 44 45 46 49 52 53 54 55 56 57 58 59 60 61 64 65 66 67 71 72 73 74 **P**8 **S** Columbia/HCA Healthcare Corporation, Nashville, TN **N** Principal Health Care of Georgia, Atlanta, GA; Chattanooga Healthcare Network, Chattanooga, TN	33	10	248	7378	129	44728	0	50531	20932	721
✠ △ SISKIN HOSPITAL FOR PHYSICAL REHABILITATION, One Siskin Plaza, Zip 37403; tel. 423/634–1200; Robert P. Main, President and Chief Executive Officer **A**1 7 9 10 **F**12 15 16 17 19 20 21 22 25 26 27 34 35 39 41 48 49 65 67 71 73 **N** Principal Health Care of Georgia, Atlanta, GA	23	46	72	917	66	26801	0	20575	10530	283
□ VENCOR HOSPITAL–CHATTANOOGA, (LONG TERM ACUTE CARE), 709 Walnut Street, Zip 37402; tel. 423/266–7721; Steven E. McGraw, Administrator **A**1 9 10 **F**12 19 21 22 27 35 37 50 63 65 69 71 **S** Vencor, Incorporated, Louisville, KY **N** Principal Health Care of Georgia, Atlanta, GA	33	49	43	228	29	8	0	—	—	217
CLARKSVILLE—Montgomery County										
✠ CLARKSVILLE MEMORIAL HOSPITAL, 1771 Madison Street, Zip 37043, Mailing Address: Box 3160, Zip 37043–3160; tel. 615/552–6622; James Lee Decker, President and Chief Executive Officer **A**1 9 10 **F**8 10 12 16 17 19 21 22 23 26 28 29 30 31 32 33 34 35 37 39 40 41 42 44 45 46 47 49 52 54 56 57 58 59 60 65 67 71 73 74 **P**8 **N** Center Care, Bowling Green, KY; Middle Tennessee Healthcare Network, Nashville, TN	16	10	175	8782	114	77195	1020	59210	24754	939
CLEVELAND—Bradley County										
✠ BRADLEY MEMORIAL HOSPITAL, 2305 Chambliss Avenue N.W., Zip 37311, Mailing Address: Box 3060, Zip 37320–3060; tel. 423/559–6000; Jim Whitlock, Administrator **A**1 9 10 **F**7 8 10 12 14 15 16 17 19 21 22 23 28 30 32 33 34 35 37 39 40 41 42 44 49 52 56 58 59 65 67 68 71 73 74 **N** Principal Health Care of Georgia, Atlanta, GA	13	10	187	8772	92	—	1083	61857	26536	805
□ CLEVELAND COMMUNITY HOSPITAL, 2800 Westside Drive N.W., Zip 37312; tel. 423/339–4100; Phil Rowland, Administrator (Nonreporting) **A**1 9 10 **S** Community Health Systems, Inc., Brentwood, TN **N** Principal Health Care of Georgia, Atlanta, GA	33	10	70	—	—	—	—	—	—	—
COLUMBIA—Maury County										
✠ MAURY REGIONAL HOSPITAL, 1224 Trotwood Avenue, Zip 38401; tel. 615/381–1111; William R. Walter, Administrator **A**1 9 10 **F**3 7 8 10 11 14 19 20 21 22 23 25 27 28 30 31 32 35 37 39 40 41 42 44 45 46 49 51 52 54 56 57 59 60 65 67 71 72 73 74 **N** Middle Tennessee Healthcare Network, Nashville, TN	13	10	275	13355	143	109865	1577	86614	37395	1319
COOKEVILLE—Putnam County										
✠ COOKEVILLE GENERAL HOSPITAL, 142 West Fifth Street, Zip 38501, Mailing Address: P.O. Box 340, Zip 38503–0340; tel. 615/528–2541; Mike Mayes, FACHE, Administrator and Chief Executive Officer **A**1 9 10 **F**4 7 8 10 11 14 15 17 19 22 23 25 28 29 30 32 33 35 37 39 40 41 42 44 45 46 48 49 50 60 65 67 71 73 74 **N** Center Care, Bowling Green, KY; Middle Tennessee Healthcare Network, Nashville, TN	14	10	158	6836	74	96478	1043	48397	20077	784
COPPERHILL—Polk County										
□ COPPER BASIN MEDICAL CENTER, State Highway 68, Zip 37317, Mailing Address: P.O. Box 990, Zip 37317; tel. 423/496–5511; Grady Scott, Administrator **A**1 9 10 **F**8 14 19 22 34 39 65 71	23	10	44	1002	10	12029	0	3560	1973	84
COVINGTON—Tipton County										
✠ BAPTIST MEMORIAL HOSPITAL–TIPTON, 1995 Highway 51 South, Zip 38019; tel. 901/476–2621; William T. Moorer, Administrator **A**1 9 10 **F**3 7 8 14 15 16 19 22 23 24 28 32 33 35 37 39 40 44 46 49 51 63 65 71 **S** Baptist Memorial Health Care Corporation, Memphis, TN	21	10	110	2667	35	34983	361	17145	5368	229
CROSSVILLE—Cumberland County										
✠ CUMBERLAND MEDICAL CENTER, 421 South Main Street, Zip 38555–5031; tel. 615/484–9511; Edwin S. Anderson, President (Nonreporting) **A**1 9 10 **N** Middle Tennessee Healthcare Network, Nashville, TN	23	10	190	—	—	—	—	—	—	—
DAYTON—Rhea County										
★ RHEA MEDICAL CENTER, 7900 Rhea County Highway, Zip 37321; tel. 423/775–1121; Kennedy L. Croom, Jr., Administrator and Chief Executive Officer (Total facility includes 89 beds in nursing home–type unit) **A**9 10 **F**14 15 19 22 35 37 44 64 65 71 73 **S** Quorum Health Group/Quorum Health Resources, Inc., Brentwood, TN	13	10	125	1253	97	29027	0	9759	3804	—

Hospital, Address, Telephone, Administrator, Approval, Facility, and Physician Codes, Health Care System, Network	Classi-fication Codes		Utilization Data					Expense (thousands) of dollars		
★ American Hospital Association (AHA) membership □ Joint Commission on Accreditation of Healthcare Organizations (JCAHO) accreditation + American Osteopathic Hospital Association (AOHA) membership ○ American Osteopathic Association (AOA) accreditation △ Commission on Accreditation of Rehabilitation Facilities (CARF) accreditation Control codes 61, 63, 64, 71, 72 and 73 indicate hospitals listed by AOHA, but not registered by AHA. For definition of numerical codes, see page A4	Control	Service	Beds	Admissions	Census	Outpatient Visits	Births	Total	Payroll	Personnel

DICKSON—Dickson County

★ COLUMBIA HORIZON MEDICAL CENTER, 111 Highway 70 East, Zip 37055–2079; tel. 615/441–2357; Rick Wallace, FACHE, Chief Executive Officer and Administrator (Total facility includes 26 beds in nursing home–type unit) **A**1 9 10 **F**3 4 7 8 10 12 14 15 16 19 21 22 28 30 32 33 34 35 37 40 41 42 44 45 46 49 51 53 54 56 57 58 59 64 65 66 67 71 72 73 74 **P**7 **S** Columbia/HCA Healthcare Corporation, Nashville, TN

| | 33 | 10 | 108 | 4017 | 46 | 63755 | 455 | 38385 | 11633 | 461 |

DYERSBURG—Dyer County

★ METHODIST HOSPITAL OF DYERSBURG, 400 Tickle Street, Zip 38024–3182; tel. 901/285–2410; Richard McCormick, Administrator **A**1 9 10 **F**7 8 12 14 15 19 20 21 22 23 27 28 30 32 33 34 35 37 40 44 45 46 49 60 65 71 73 **P**5 7 8 **S** Methodist Health Systems, Inc., Memphis, TN **N** Methodist Health Systems, Inc., Memphis, TN

| | 23 | 10 | 105 | 3924 | 45 | 43117 | 726 | 28720 | 11175 | 390 |

EAST RIDGE—Hamilton County

★ COLUMBIA EAST RIDGE HOSPITAL, 941 Spring Creek Road, Zip 37412, Mailing Address: P.O. Box 91229, Zip 37412–6229; tel. 423/894–7870; Brenda M. Waltz, CHE, Chief Executive Officer **A**1 9 10 **F**2 3 4 7 8 10 11 14 15 16 18 19 20 21 22 23 24 28 29 30 32 35 37 38 40 42 43 44 45 46 49 51 52 53 54 55 56 57 58 59 60 64 65 66 67 71 72 73 74 **P**4 7 8 **S** Columbia/HCA Healthcare Corporation, Nashville, TN **N** Principal Health Care of Georgia, Atlanta, GA; Chattanooga Healthcare Network, Chattanooga, TN

| | 33 | 10 | 128 | 4577 | 45 | 31699 | 2177 | 26155 | 11187 | 318 |

ELIZABETHTON—Carter County

★ COLUMBIA SYCAMORE SHOALS HOSPITAL, 1501 West Elk Avenue, Zip 37643–1368; tel. 423/542–1300; Larry R. Jeter, Chief Executive Officer (Total facility includes 12 beds in nursing home–type unit) **A**1 9 10 **F**7 8 11 12 14 16 17 19 22 24 26 28 29 30 32 34 35 37 40 42 44 46 47 49 64 65 71 73 74 **P**1 5 7 **S** Columbia/HCA Healthcare Corporation, Nashville, TN

| | 33 | 10 | 112 | 2478 | 30 | 39999 | 455 | 16435 | 6528 | 309 |

ERIN—Houston County

★ COLUMBIA TRINITY HOSPITAL, 353 Main Street, Zip 37061, Mailing Address: P.O. Box 489, Zip 37061–0489; tel. 615/289–4211; Jay Woodall, Chief Executive Officer (Nonreporting) **A**1 9 10 **S** Columbia/HCA Healthcare Corporation, Nashville, TN

| | 33 | 10 | 35 | — | — | — | — | — | — | — |

ERWIN—Unicoi County

★ UNICOI COUNTY MEMORIAL HOSPITAL, Greenway Circle, Zip 37650–2196; tel. 423/743–3141; James L. McMackin, Chief Executive Officer (Total facility includes 46 beds in nursing home–type unit) **A**1 9 10 **F**8 14 17 19 22 28 30 39 44 49 64 65 66 71 **P**5 **N** Mountain States Healthcare Network, Johnson City, TN

| | 16 | 10 | 84 | 1096 | 58 | 23640 | 0 | 8528 | 3860 | 172 |

ETOWAH—McMinn County

★ WOODS MEMORIAL HOSPITAL DISTRICT, Highway 411 North, Zip 37331, Mailing Address: Box 410, Zip 37331; tel. 615/263–3600; Phil Campbell, FACHE, Administrator (Total facility includes 88 beds in nursing home–type unit) (Nonreporting) **A**1 9 10

| | 13 | 10 | 160 | — | — | — | — | — | — | — |

FAYETTEVILLE—Lincoln County

★ LINCOLN REGIONAL HOSPITAL, 700 West Maple Street, Zip 37334; tel. 615/438–1111; Gary G. Kendrick, Chief Executive Officer **A**1 9 10 **F**2 3 7 8 15 17 19 21 22 24 27 28 32 33 34 35 37 40 41 44 49 65 67 71 73 **S** Quorum Health Group/Quorum Health Resources, Inc., Brentwood, TN

| | 13 | 10 | 63 | 2046 | 22 | 29720 | 177 | 11179 | 5661 | 254 |

FRANKLIN—Williamson County

★ WILLIAMSON MEDICAL CENTER, 2021 Carothers Road, Zip 37067, Mailing Address: P.O. Box 681600, Zip 37068–1600; tel. 615/791–0500; Ronald G. Joyner, Chief Executive Officer **A**1 9 10 **F**3 7 8 10 15 19 21 22 23 28 30 33 34 35 37 40 42 44 46 49 54 56 63 65 66 67 71 73 **P**4 **N** Center Care, Bowling Green, KY; Middle Tennessee Healthcare Network, Nashville, TN

| | 13 | 10 | 109 | 5084 | 63 | 80660 | 545 | 43588 | 17729 | 538 |

GAINESBORO—Jackson County

□ CUMBERLAND RIVER HOSPITAL SOUTH, 620 Hospital Drive, Zip 38562, Mailing Address: Box 36, Zip 38562–0036; tel. 615/268–0211; Tim Tapp, Administrator (Nonreporting) **A**1 9 **S** Paracelsus Healthcare Corporation, Houston, TX

| | 33 | 10 | 30 | — | — | — | — | — | — | — |

GALLATIN—Sumner County

★ SUMNER REGIONAL MEDICAL CENTER, 555 Hartsville Pike, Zip 37066, Mailing Address: P.O. Box 1558, Zip 37066–1558; tel. 615/452–4210; William T. Sugg, President and Chief Executive Officer (Nonreporting) **A**1 9 10 **N** Center Care, Bowling Green, KY; Middle Tennessee Healthcare Network, Nashville, TN

| | 23 | 10 | 148 | — | — | — | — | — | — | — |

GERMANTOWN—Shelby County

□ BAPTIST REHABILITATION–GERMANTOWN, 2100 Exeter Road, Zip 38138; tel. 901/757–1350; B. Richard Moseley, Chief Executive Officer **A**1 9 10 **F**5 12 15 16 21 25 27 34 44 45 46 48 49 65 66 67 73 **S** Continental Medical Systems, Inc., Mechanicsburg, PA **N** Arkansas' FirstSource, Little Rock, AR

| | 32 | 46 | 85 | 929 | 49 | 8534 | 0 | 14281 | 6255 | 165 |

GREENEVILLE—Greene County

★ LAUGHLIN MEMORIAL HOSPITAL, 1420 Tusculum Boulevard, Zip 37745; tel. 423/787–5000; Charles H. Whitfield, Jr., Administrator and Chief Operating Officer (Total facility includes 90 beds in nursing home–type unit) **A**1 9 10 **F**7 8 10 12 14 15 16 17 19 21 22 26 28 29 30 32 34 35 37 38 40 41 42 44 45 46 49 60 63 64 65 66 67 71 73 74 **N** Premier Health Network, Johnson City, TN

| | 23 | 10 | 230 | 5070 | 149 | 40498 | 461 | 28022 | 11232 | 421 |

★ TAKOMA ADVENTIST HOSPITAL, 401 Takoma Avenue, Zip 37743; tel. 423/639–3151; Paul Michael Norman, President **A**1 9 10 **F**7 8 11 12 14 15 16 17 18 19 20 21 22 24 26 28 29 30 31 32 33 35 37 38 39 40 41 42 43 44 45 46 47 48 49 51 52 54 55 56 57 58 59 60 63 65 66 67 71 72 73 74 **P**8 **S** Adventist Health System Sunbelt Health Care Corporation, Winter Park, FL **N** Mountain States Healthcare Network, Johnson City, TN

| | 21 | 10 | 80 | 2564 | 34 | 27663 | 266 | 16147 | 5778 | 243 |

Hospital, Address, Telephone, Administrator, Approval, Facility, and Physician Codes, Health Care System, Network	Classi-fication Codes		Utilization Data					Expense (thousands) of dollars		
★ American Hospital Association (AHA) membership □ Joint Commission on Accreditation of Healthcare Organizations (JCAHO) accreditation + American Osteopathic Hospital Association (AOHA) membership ○ American Osteopathic Association (AOA) accreditation △ Commission on Accreditation of Rehabilitation Facilities (CARF) accreditation Control codes 61, 63, 64, 71, 72 and 73 indicate hospitals listed by AOHA, but not registered by AHA. For definition of numerical codes, see page A4	Control	Service	Beds	Admissions	Census	Outpatient Visits	Births	Total	Payroll	Personnel

HARRIMAN—Roane County

□ ROANE MEDICAL CENTER, (Formerly Harriman City Hospital), 412 Devonia Street, Zip 37748–0489, Mailing Address: P.O. Box 489, Zip 37748–0489; tel. 423/882–1323; Jim Gann, Administrator **A**1 9 10 **F**7 8 10 12 15 16 17 19 21 22 24 28 32 35 37 39 40 41 44 46 49 63 65 67 71 73 **P**1	14	10	85	4114	44	35123	105	17195	6712	318

HARTSVILLE—Trousdale County

TROUSDALE MEDICAL CENTER See Frank T. Rutherford Memorial Hospital, Carthage

HENDERSONVILLE—Sumner County

⊞ COLUMBIA HENDERSONVILLE HOSPITAL, 355 New Shackle Island Road, Zip 37075–2393; tel. 615/264–4000; Ron Walker, Chief Executive Officer (Total facility includes 10 beds in nursing home–type unit) **A**1 9 10 **F**7 8 10 12 14 15 17 19 21 22 26 28 29 30 32 33 34 35 37 40 44 46 49 50 51 64 65 66 67 71 72 73 **P**7 **S** Columbia/HCA Healthcare Corporation, Nashville, TN **N** Center Care, Bowling Green, KY	33	10	67	2564	27	56579	472	19303	7543	234

HERMITAGE—Davidson County

⊞ COLUMBIA SUMMIT MEDICAL CENTER, 5655 Frist Boulevard, Zip 37076; tel. 615/316–3000; Bryan K. Dearing, Chief Executive Officer (Total facility includes 16 beds in nursing home–type unit) **A**1 9 10 **F**3 4 6 7 8 9 10 11 12 14 15 16 17 18 19 20 21 22 23 26 27 28 29 30 31 32 33 34 35 37 38 40 41 42 43 44 45 46 47 48 49 50 51 52 53 54 55 56 57 58 59 60 61 62 63 64 65 66 67 69 70 71 72 73 74 **P**5 7 8 **S** Columbia/HCA Healthcare Corporation, Nashville, TN **N** Columbia Healthcare Network, Brentwood, TN	33	10	204	9316	113	79184	1198	51241	22299	795

HUMBOLDT—Gibson County

⊞ HUMBOLDT GENERAL HOSPITAL, 3525 Chere Carol Road, Zip 38343–3699; tel. 901/784–0301; Karen Utley, Administrator (Nonreporting) **A**1 9 10 **S** West Tennessee Healthcare, Inc., Jackson, TN **N** West Tennessee Healthcare, Inc., Jackson, TN	16	10	51							

HUNTINGDON—Carroll County

⊞ BAPTIST MEMORIAL HOSPITAL–HUNTINGDON, 631 R. B. Wilson Drive, Zip 38344; tel. 901/986–4461; Susan M. Breeden, Administrator (Nonreporting) **A**1 9 10 **S** Baptist Memorial Health Care Corporation, Memphis, TN	21	10	70	—	—	—	—	—	—	—

JACKSON—Madison County

⊞ COLUMBIA REGIONAL HOSPITAL OF JACKSON, 367 Hospital Boulevard, Zip 38305–4518, Mailing Address: P.O. Box 3310, Zip 38303–0310; tel. 901/661–2000; Donald H. Wilkerson, Chief Executive Officer **A**1 9 10 **F**4 7 8 10 11 12 17 19 20 21 22 23 26 30 32 33 34 35 37 40 42 44 45 46 49 65 66 71 73 74 **S** Columbia/HCA Healthcare Corporation, Nashville, TN	33	10	103	3865	57	22024	113	32668	12030	389
⊞ △ JACKSON-MADISON COUNTY GENERAL HOSPITAL, 708 West Forest Avenue, Zip 38301–3855; tel. 901/425–5000; James T. Moss, President (Total facility includes 85 beds in nursing home–type unit) **A**1 2 3 5 7 9 10 **F**1 3 4 6 7 8 10 11 12 13 14 15 16 17 18 19 21 22 23 24 25 26 27 28 29 30 31 32 33 34 35 37 38 39 40 41 42 43 44 45 46 49 51 53 54 55 56 57 58 59 60 64 65 66 67 69 71 72 73 74 **P**1 7 **S** West Tennessee Healthcare, Inc., Jackson, TN **N** West Tennessee Healthcare, Inc., Jackson, TN	16	10	567	23368	432	110720	2770	174318	77140	2885
★ PATHWAYS OF TENNESSEE, 238 Summar Drive, Zip 38301; tel. 901/935–8200; James T. Moss, President and Chief Executive Officer **A**10 **F**2 3 4 6 8 10 11 12 13 14 15 16 17 18 19 21 22 25 26 28 29 30 32 33 34 35 37 38 39 40 41 42 43 44 45 46 47 48 49 50 51 52 53 54 55 56 57 58 59 60 61 63 64 65 66 67 71 72 73 74 **P**1 4 7 **S** West Tennessee Healthcare, Inc., Jackson, TN	23	22	57	811	18	94437	0	13589	8490	375

JAMESTOWN—Fentress County

□ FENTRESS COUNTY GENERAL HOSPITAL, Highway 52 West, Zip 38556, Mailing Address: P.O. Box 1500, Zip 38556; tel. 615/879–8171; Curtis B. Courtney, Administrator (Total facility includes 13 beds in nursing home–type unit) (Nonreporting) **A**1 9 10 **S** Paracelsus Healthcare Corporation, Houston, TX	33	10	73	—	—	—	—	—	—	—

JEFFERSON CITY—Jefferson County

⊞ JEFFERSON MEMORIAL HOSPITAL, 1800 Bishop Avenue, Zip 37760, Mailing Address: P.O. Box 560, Zip 37760–0560; tel. 615/475–2091; Michael C. Hicks, Administrator **A**1 9 10 **F**8 15 16 19 21 22 28 30 33 34 37 39 44 45 46 49 51 65 71 73	15	10	51	1990	25	33518	0	10570	4901	221

JELLICO—Campbell County

⊞ JELLICO COMMUNITY HOSPITAL, Mailing Address: Route 1, Box 197, Zip 37762; tel. 423/784–1205; Kenneth R. Mattison, President and Chief Executive Officer **A**1 9 10 **F**7 10 14 15 16 19 21 22 32 35 37 40 41 44 46 49 65 71 **S** Adventist Health System Sunbelt Health Care Corporation, Winter Park, FL	23	10	54	2043	22	33940	264	14474	5193	211

JOHNSON CITY—Washington County

⊞ COLUMBIA JOHNSON CITY SPECIALTY HOSPITAL, 203 East Watauga Avenue, Zip 37601; tel. 615/926–1111; Lori Caudell Fatherree, Chief Executive Officer **A**1 9 10 **F**2 3 4 7 8 10 11 12 14 15 16 17 19 22 23 24 28 30 32 35 37 38 40 41 42 44 48 49 52 53 54 55 56 57 58 59 61 65 66 67 69 70 71 73 74 **P**4 5 7 8 **S** Columbia/HCA Healthcare Corporation, Nashville, TN **N** Premier Health Network, Johnson City, TN	33	10	49	1242	8	12353	729	9897	3903	132
⊞ COLUMBIA NORTH SIDE HOSPITAL, 401 Princeton Road, Zip 37601, Mailing Address: P.O. Box 4900, Zip 37602; tel. 423/854–5900; John B. Crysel, Chief Executive Officer (Total facility includes 13 beds in nursing home–type unit) **A**1 9 10 **F**2 3 4 7 8 10 12 14 15 16 18 21 22 23 24 28 29 30 31 32 33 34 35 37 38 39 40 41 42 43 44 45 47 49 51 54 56 58 59 60 64 65 66 67 68 69 70 71 72 73 74 **P**7 8 **S** Columbia/HCA Healthcare Corporation, Nashville, TN **N** Premier Health Network, Johnson City, TN	33	10	127	4133	52	43060	0	34544	10817	377

Hospital, Address, Telephone, Administrator, Approval, Facility, and Physician Codes, Health Care System, Network	Classi-fication Codes		Utilization Data					Expense (thousands) of dollars		
	Control	Service	Beds	Admissions	Census	Outpatient Visits	Births	Total	Payroll	Personnel

★ American Hospital Association (AHA) membership
□ Joint Commission on Accreditation of Healthcare Organizations (JCAHO) accreditation
+ American Osteopathic Hospital Association (AOHA) membership
○ American Osteopathic Association (AOA) accreditation
△ Commission on Accreditation of Rehabilitation Facilities (CARF) accreditation
Control codes 61, 63, 64, 71, 72 and 73 indicate hospitals listed by AOHA, but not registered by AHA. For definition of numerical codes, see page A4

⊠ △ JOHNSON CITY MEDICAL CENTER HOSPITAL, 400 North State of Franklin Road, Zip 37604–6094; tel. 423/431–6111; Dennis Vonderfecht, President and Chief Executive Officer **A**1 2 3 5 7 8 9 10 **F**2 3 4 7 8 10 12 13 14 15 16 17 19 20 21 22 23 24 25 26 27 28 29 30 32 33 34 35 37 38 39 40 41 42 43 44 45 46 47 48 49 51 52 53 54 55 56 57 58 59 60 63 64 65 66 67 68 69 70 71 72 73 74 **P**3 5 6 7 8 **N** Mountain States Healthcare Network, Johnson City, TN	23	10	407	15696	274	115686	1151	141066	51175	1895
□ △ NORTHEAST TENNESSEE REHABILITATION HOSPITAL, 2511 Wesley Street, Zip 37601; tel. 423/283–0700; Claude Adkins, Chief Executive Officer **A**1 7 9 10 **F**5 12 14 16 17 19 28 29 34 35 39 41 48 49 54 55 60 65 66 67 71 **P**8	32	46	60	480	26	4773	0	9673	—	101
□ WOODRIDGE HOSPITAL, 403 State of Franklin Road, Zip 37604; tel. 423/928–7111; Thomas J. De Martini, Administrator **A**1 3 5 9 10 **F**1 2 3 12 14 15 16 18 19 21 31 35 45 52 53 54 55 56 57 58 59 65 67 71 **P**6 **N** Mountain States Healthcare Network, Johnson City, TN	23	22	65	2869	46	83591	0	14026	8081	142
KINGSPORT—Sullivan County										
□ △ HEALTHSOUTH REHABILITATION HOSPITAL, 113 Cassel Drive, Zip 37660; tel. 423/246–7240; Terry R. Maxhimer, Administrator (Nonreporting) **A**1 7 9 10 **S** HEALTHSOUTH Corporation, Birmingham, AL	33	46	50	—	—	—	—	—	—	—
⊠ INDIAN PATH MEDICAL CENTER, 2000 Brookside Drive, Zip 37660–4604; tel. 615/392–7000; Robert Bauer, Chief Executive Officer (Total facility includes 30 beds in nursing home–type unit) **A**1 9 10 **F**2 3 4 7 8 10 12 14 15 16 19 21 22 23 26 28 30 32 34 35 37 39 40 41 42 44 45 49 54 55 56 57 58 59 61 63 64 65 66 71 73 74 **P**5 6 7 8 **S** Columbia/HCA Healthcare Corporation, Nashville, TN **N** Mountain States Healthcare Network, Johnson City, TN	33	10	130	5595	92	77789	377	45394	16953	812
⊠ INDIAN PATH PAVILION, 2300 Pavilion Drive, Zip 37660–4672; tel. 615/378–7500; Robert Bauer, Chief Executive Officer (Nonreporting) **A**1 10 **S** Columbia/HCA Healthcare Corporation, Nashville, TN **N** Mountain States Healthcare Network, Johnson City, TN	33	22	26	—	—	—	—	—	—	—
★ WELLMONT HEALTH SYSTEM–HOLSTON VALLEY, (Formerly Holston Valley Hospital and Medical Center), West Ravine Street, Zip 37662–0224, Mailing Address: Box 238, Zip 37662–0224; tel. 423/224–5001; Louis H. Bremer, President and Chief Executive Officer (Total facility includes 35 beds in nursing home–type unit) **A**2 5 10 **F**4 7 8 10 11 12 14 15 16 17 19 21 22 23 26 28 30 31 32 33 35 37 38 40 41 42 43 44 46 47 48 49 52 53 54 55 56 57 58 59 60 63 65 66 69 70 71 73 74 **P**4 5 7 8 **S** Quorum Health Group/Quorum Health Resources, Inc., Brentwood, TN **N** CHA Provider Network, Inc., Lexington, KY; Premier Health Network, Johnson City, TN; Highlands Wellmont Health Network, Inc., Bristol, TN	23	10	384	16161	233	130572	1659	148934	59101	1717
KNOXVILLE—Knox County										
⊠ △ BAPTIST HOSPITAL OF EAST TENNESSEE, 137 Blount Avenue S.E., Zip 37920, Mailing Address: Box 1788, Zip 37901–1788; tel. 423/632–5011; Jon Foster, Senior Vice President and Administrator (Nonreporting) **A**1 2 7 9 10 **S** Baptist Health System of Tennessee, Knoxville, TN	21	10	321	—	—	—	—	—	—	—
□ EAST TENNESSEE CHILDREN'S HOSPITAL, 2018 Clinch Avenue, Zip 37916, Mailing Address: P.O. Box 15010, Zip 37901–5010; tel. 615/541–8000; Robert F. Koppel, President and Chief Executive Officer **A**1 9 10 **F**10 13 14 15 16 17 18 19 20 21 22 25 27 28 29 30 31 32 34 35 37 38 39 41 42 44 45 46 47 49 51 53 54 55 56 58 59 65 66 67 68 70 71 72 73 **P**8	23	50	103	4792	63	75958	0	42321	19804	715
⊠ △ FORT SANDERS REGIONAL MEDICAL CENTER, 1901 Clinch Avenue S.W., Zip 37916–2394; tel. 423/541–1111; James R. Burkhart, FACHE, Administrator (Total facility includes 24 beds in nursing home–type unit) **A**1 2 6 7 9 10 **F**2 3 4 7 8 10 11 12 14 15 16 17 18 19 21 22 23 24 25 26 27 28 30 31 32 33 34 35 37 40 41 42 43 44 45 46 48 49 50 52 53 54 55 56 57 58 59 60 61 63 64 65 66 67 68 71 73 74 **P**4 6 7 **N** CHA Provider Network, Inc., Lexington, KY	23	10	419	17055	277	81597	2161	125610	46617	1770
⊠ FORT SANDERS–PARKWEST MEDICAL CENTER, 9352 Park West Boulevard, Zip 37923, Mailing Address: P.O. Box 22993, Zip 37933–0993; tel. 423/694–5700; James R. Burkhart, FACHE, Administrator **A**1 2 9 10 **F**2 3 4 7 8 10 11 12 14 15 16 17 19 21 22 23 24 25 26 27 28 29 30 31 32 33 34 35 37 39 40 41 42 43 44 45 46 48 49 50 51 52 53 54 55 56 57 58 59 60 63 64 65 66 67 71 73 74 **P**1 7 **N** CHA Provider Network, Inc., Lexington, KY	23	10	262	11522	155	84376	674	92173	30064	1050
□ LAKESHORE MENTAL HEALTH INSTITUTE, 5908 Lyons View Drive, Zip 37919; tel. 423/450–5200; Richard Lee Thomas, Superintendent **A**1 10 **F**1 4 5 6 8 10 12 19 20 21 22 25 27 31 35 43 44 46 49 50 52 53 54 55 56 57 58 59 60 63 65 67 69 71 73 **P**6	12	22	277	1572	244	0	0	26703	16027	634
⊠ △ ST. MARY'S HEALTH SYSTEM, 900 East Oak Hill Avenue, Zip 37917–4556; tel. 615/545–8000; Richard C. Williams, President and Chief Executive Officer (Total facility includes 25 beds in nursing home–type unit) **A**1 2 3 7 9 10 **F**1 4 7 10 11 12 16 17 19 21 22 23 24 32 33 35 37 38 40 41 42 44 46 48 49 52 53 54 55 57 58 59 60 64 65 67 71 73 74 **P**1 2 5 6 7 **S** Mercy Health System, Cincinnati, OH	21	10	300	14456	206	182691	1671	124654	50482	1748
⊠ UNIVERSITY OF TENNESSEE MEMORIAL HOSPITAL, 1924 Alcoa Highway, Zip 37920; tel. 615/544–9000; Gene Hall, Administrator **A**1 2 3 9 10 **F**2 3 4 7 8 10 11 13 17 18 19 20 21 22 23 24 28 29 30 31 32 33 34 35 37 38 39 40 41 42 43 44 45 46 47 49 50 51 60 61 63 65 67 69 70 71 73 74 **P**7	23	10	490	21282	337	258287	3066	251216	113960	3723
LA FOLLETTE—Campbell County										
⊠ LA FOLLETTE MEDICAL CENTER, East Avenue, Zip 37766, Mailing Address: Box 1301, Zip 37766–1301; tel. 423/562–2211; J. B. Wright, Administrator (Total facility includes 98 beds in nursing home–type unit) **A**1 9 10 **F**8 14 19 22 32 34 39 44 49 58 59 64 65 71 73	14	10	148	2828	143	108473	0	19267	8822	383

Hospital, Address, Telephone, Administrator, Approval, Facility, and Physician Codes, Health Care System, Network	Classi-fication Codes		Utilization Data					Expense (thousands) of dollars		
★ American Hospital Association (AHA) membership □ Joint Commission on Accreditation of Healthcare Organizations (JCAHO) accreditation + American Osteopathic Hospital Association (AOHA) membership ○ American Osteopathic Association (AOA) accreditation △ Commission on Accreditation of Rehabilitation Facilities (CARF) accreditation Control codes 61, 63, 64, 71, 72 and 73 indicate hospitals listed by AOHA, but not registered by AHA. For definition of numerical codes, see page A4	Control	Service	Beds	Admissions	Census	Outpatient Visits	Births	Total	Payroll	Personnel

LAFAYETTE—Macon County

⊠ MACON COUNTY GENERAL HOSPITAL, 204 Medical Drive, Zip 37083, Mailing Address: P.O. Box 378, Zip 37083; tel. 615/666–2147; Dennis A. Wolford, FACHE, Administrator (Nonreporting) **A**1 9 10 **S** Quorum Health Group/Quorum Health Resources, Inc., Brentwood, TN **N** Center Care, Bowling Green, KY

| 23 | 10 | 43 | — | — | — | — | — | — | — |

LAWRENCEBURG—Lawrence County

⊠ COLUMBIA CROCKETT HOSPITAL, U.S. Highway 43 South, Zip 38464–0847, Mailing Address: Box 847, Zip 38464–0847; tel. 615/762–6571; John A. Marshall, Chief Executive Officer **A**1 9 10 **F**2 7 8 9 10 11 12 15 16 17 19 22 26 28 29 30 34 35 37 38 39 40 41 42 44 45 46 47 48 49 51 52 64 65 66 67 71 **P**7 **S** Columbia/HCA Healthcare Corporation, Nashville, TN

| 33 | 10 | 83 | 2961 | 31 | 37243 | 202 | 15722 | 5887 | 199 |

LEBANON—Wilson County

□ UNIVERSITY MEDICAL CENTER, (Includes McFarland Specialty Hospital, 500 Park Avenue, Zip 37087–3720; tel. 615/449–0500), 1411 Baddour Parkway, Zip 37087; tel. 615/444–8262; Nanette Todd, R.N., Acting Administrator **A**1 9 10 **F**3 7 8 10 12 15 19 21 22 28 29 30 32 34 35 37 39 40 41 42 44 46 48 49 52 57 59 63 64 65 66 71 73 74 **P**5 6 7 **S** TENET Healthcare Corporation, Santa Barbara, CA **N** Center Care, Bowling Green, KY

| 33 | 10 | 225 | 8837 | 128 | 66798 | 831 | 46792 | 16690 | 620 |

LEWISBURG—Marshall County

□ MARSHALL MEDICAL CENTER, 1080 North Ellington Parkway, Zip 37091, Mailing Address: P.O. Box 1609, Zip 37091; tel. 615/359–6241; Steve C. Hoelscher, Administrator **A**1 9 10 **F**7 8 14 15 16 19 21 22 28 29 30 32 34 35 37 39 40 41 44 45 46 65 66 69 71 73

| 13 | 10 | 69 | 1555 | 16 | 29629 | 49 | 9768 | 4370 | 155 |

LEXINGTON—Henderson County

⊠ METHODIST HOSPITAL OF LEXINGTON, 200 West Church Street, Zip 38351, Mailing Address: Box 160, Zip 38351; tel. 901/968–3646; Eugene Ragghianti, Administrator (Nonreporting) **A**1 9 10 **S** Methodist Health Systems, Inc., Memphis, TN **N** Methodist Health Systems, Inc., Memphis, TN

| 21 | 10 | 32 | — | — | — | — | — | — | — |

LINDEN—Perry County

□ BAPTIST PERRY MEMORIAL HOSPITAL, Highway 13 South, Zip 37096, Mailing Address: Route 10, Box 8, Zip 37096; tel. 615/589–2121; John B. Avery, III, Administrator (Nonreporting) **A**1 9 10

| 23 | 10 | 53 | — | — | — | — | — | — | — |

LIVINGSTON—Overton County

⊠ COLUMBIA LIVINGSTON REGIONAL HOSPITAL, 315 Oak Street, Zip 38570, Mailing Address: P.O. Box 550, Zip 38570; tel. 615/823–5611; Timothy W. McGill, Chief Executive Officer (Total facility includes 15 beds in nursing home–type unit) **A**1 9 10 **F**7 8 12 14 15 16 19 20 22 26 28 30 32 33 34 35 37 39 40 42 44 49 64 65 66 67 71 73 74 **P**7 8 **S** Columbia/HCA Healthcare Corporation, Nashville, TN

| 33 | 10 | 85 | 4019 | 47 | 28391 | 275 | 17276 | 6496 | 389 |

LOUDON—Loudon County

⊠ FORT SANDERS LOUDON MEDICAL CENTER, 1125 Grove Street, Zip 37774, Mailing Address: Box 217, Zip 37774–0217; tel. 615/458–8222; Ralph T. Williams, Administrator (Nonreporting) **A**1 9 10 **N** CHA Provider Network, Inc., Lexington, KY

| 23 | 10 | 50 | — | — | — | — | — | — | — |

LOUISVILLE—Blount County

□ PENINSULA HOSPITAL, 2347 Jones Bend Road, Zip 37777, Mailing Address: P.O. Box 2000, Zip 37777; tel. 423/970–9800; David H. McReynolds, Chief Operating Officer and Administrator (Nonreporting) **A**1 9 10 **N** CHA Provider Network, Inc., Lexington, KY

| 33 | 22 | 159 | — | — | — | — | — | — | — |

MADISON—Davidson County

⊠ COLUMBIA NASHVILLE MEMORIAL HOSPITAL, 612 West Due West Avenue, Zip 37115–4474; tel. 615/865–3511; Robert Benson, Chief Executive Officer (Nonreporting) **A**1 2 5 9 10 **S** Columbia/HCA Healthcare Corporation, Nashville, TN **N** Center Care, Bowling Green, KY

| 33 | 10 | 250 | — | — | — | — | — | — | — |

⊠ △ TENNESSEE CHRISTIAN MEDICAL CENTER, (Includes Tennessee Christian Medical Center – Portland, 105 Redbud Drive, Portland, Zip 37148), 500 Hospital Drive, Zip 37115; tel. 615/865–2373; Milton R. Siepman, Ph.D., President and Chief Executive Officer (Total facility includes 50 beds in nursing home–type unit) (Nonreporting) **A**1 7 9 10 **S** Adventist Health System Sunbelt Health Care Corporation, Winter Park, FL **N** Partners for a Healthy Nashville, Nashville, TN; Middle Tennessee Healthcare Network, Nashville, TN

| 21 | 10 | 288 | — | — | — | — | — | — | — |

MANCHESTER—Coffee County

★ COFFEE MEDICAL CENTER, 1001 McArthur Drive, Zip 37355, Mailing Address: P.O. Box 1079, Zip 37355; tel. 615/728–3586; William M. Moore, Administrator (Total facility includes 72 beds in nursing home–type unit) **A**9 10 **F**8 15 17 19 22 26 28 30 33 34 40 41 44 48 49 57 58 59 64 65 67 71 73 **N** Center Care, Bowling Green, KY

| 16 | 10 | 108 | 936 | 79 | 9564 | 38 | 6097 | 2551 | 111 |

○ MEDICAL CENTER OF MANCHESTER, 481 Interstate Drive, Zip 37355, Mailing Address: P.O. Box 1409, Zip 37355; tel. 615/728–6354; Sherry Collier, Chief Nursing Officer and Chief Operating Officer (Nonreporting) **A**9 10 11 **S** TENET Healthcare Corporation, Santa Barbara, CA **N** Center Care, Bowling Green, KY

| 33 | 10 | 49 | — | — | — | — | — | — | — |

MARTIN—Weakley County

⊠ COLUMBIA VOLUNTEER GENERAL HOSPITAL, 161 Mount Pelia Road, Zip 38237, Mailing Address: Box 967, Zip 38237; tel. 901/587–4261; R. Coleman Foss, Chief Executive Officer **A**1 9 10 **F**7 8 12 13 15 16 17 19 21 22 23 24 28 30 32 34 35 37 39 40 42 44 45 46 49 65 66 71 73 **P**6 8 **S** Columbia/HCA Healthcare Corporation, Nashville, TN

| 33 | 10 | 65 | 2678 | 35 | 26307 | 219 | 14807 | 6268 | 232 |

Hospital, Address, Telephone, Administrator, Approval, Facility, and Physician Codes, Health Care System, Network	Classi-fication Codes		Utilization Data					Expense (thousands) of dollars		
	Control	Service	Beds	Admissions	Census	Outpatient Visits	Births	Total	Payroll	Personnel

★ American Hospital Association (AHA) membership
□ Joint Commission on Accreditation of Healthcare Organizations (JCAHO) accreditation
+ American Osteopathic Hospital Association (AOHA) membership
○ American Osteopathic Association (AOA) accreditation
△ Commission on Accreditation of Rehabilitation Facilities (CARF) accreditation
Control codes 61, 63, 64, 71, 72 and 73 indicate hospitals listed by AOHA, but not registered by AHA. For definition of numerical codes, see page A4

MARYVILLE—Blount County

★ BLOUNT MEMORIAL HOSPITAL, 907 East Lamar Alexander Parkway, Zip 37804–5193; tel. 423/983–7211; Joseph M. Dawson, Administrator **A**1 2 6 9 10 **F**2 3 4 7 8 10 11 12 13 14 15 16 17 18 19 21 22 23 24 25 28 30 31 32 33 34 35 37 39 40 41 42 44 46 49 54 55 56 58 59 60 63 65 66 67 70 71 73 **P**8

| | 13 | 10 | 143 | 8125 | 100 | 141579 | 628 | 65230 | 26901 | 979 |

MCKENZIE—Carroll County

★ METHODIST HOSPITAL OF MCKENZIE, 161 Hospital Drive, Zip 38201; tel. 901/352–4170; Randal E. Carson, Administrator **A**1 9 10 **F**7 8 19 22 27 28 30 32 33 39 40 41 44 46 49 66 71 73 **S** Methodist Health Systems, Inc., Memphis, TN **N** Methodist Health Systems, Inc., Memphis, TN

| | 21 | 10 | 27 | 1118 | 9 | 16113 | 375 | 7878 | 3756 | 125 |

MCMINNVILLE—Warren County

★ COLUMBIA RIVER PARK HOSPITAL, 1559 Sparta Road, Zip 37110; tel. 615/815–4000; Jack S. Buck, Chief Executive Officer (Nonreporting) **A**1 9 10 **S** Columbia/HCA Healthcare Corporation, Nashville, TN

| | 33 | 10 | 90 | — | — | — | — | — | — | — |

MEMPHIS—Shelby County

★ △ BAPTIST MEMORIAL HOSPITAL, (Includes Baptist Memorial Hospital East, 6019 Walnut Grove Road, Zip 38119; tel. 901/226–5000; Baptist Memorial Hospital Rehabilitation Center), 899 Madison Avenue, Zip 38146; tel. 901/227–2727; Stephen Curtis Reynolds, President and Chief Executive Officer (Total facility includes 48 beds in nursing home–type unit) **A**1 2 3 5 6 7 9 10 **F**2 3 4 7 8 10 11 12 14 15 16 17 19 21 22 23 24 25 30 32 33 34 35 37 38 39 40 41 42 43 44 45 46 48 49 52 53 54 55 57 58 59 60 63 64 65 66 67 69 70 71 72 73 74 **P**3 7 8 **S** Baptist Memorial Health Care Corporation, Memphis, TN

| | 21 | 10 | 1112 | 42148 | 737 | 198624 | 5163 | 372844 | 123981 | 4039 |

□ CHARTER LAKESIDE BEHAVIORAL HEALTH SYSTEM, 2911 Brunswick Road, Zip 38133, Mailing Address: P.O. Box 341308, Zip 38134; tel. 901/377–4700; Rob S. Waggener, Chief Executive Officer (Nonreporting) **A**1 9 10 **S** Magellan Health Services, Atlanta, GA

| | 33 | 22 | 174 | — | — | — | — | — | — | — |

□ EASTWOOD MEDICAL CENTER, 3000 Getwell Road, Zip 38118; tel. 901/369–8500; Lee A. Simpson, Jr., President and Chief Executive Officer **A**1 9 10 **F**2 3 8 17 19 21 22 26 27 28 29 30 34 35 37 39 42 44 49 51 52 56 57 58 59 63 65 67 71 73 **P**7

| | 33 | 10 | 209 | 3401 | 90 | 22287 | 0 | 26080 | 12090 | 373 |

□ HEALTHSOUTH REHABILITATION HOSPITAL, 1282 Union Avenue, Zip 38104; tel. 901/722–2000; Brenda Antwine, Administrator and Chief Operating Officer (Nonreporting) **A**1 10 **S** HEALTHSOUTH Corporation, Birmingham, AL

| | 32 | 46 | 80 | — | — | — | — | — | — | — |

LE BONHEUR CHILDREN'S MEDICAL CENTER See Methodist Hospitals of Memphis

□ MEMPHIS MENTAL HEALTH INSTITUTE, 865 Poplar Avenue, Zip 38105, Mailing Address: P.O. Box 40966, Zip 38174–0966; tel. 901/524–1201; Elizabeth Banks, Superintendent **A**1 5 9 10 **F**1 2 3 52 56 59 **P**6

| | 12 | 22 | 98 | 1475 | 91 | 0 | 0 | 12672 | 8147 | 311 |

★ METHODIST HOSPITALS OF MEMPHIS, (Includes Le Bonheur Children's Medical Center, One Children's Plaza, Zip 38103–2893; tel. 901/572–3000; James E. Shmerling, President; Methodist Hospital Germantown, 7691 Poplar, Germantown, Zip 38138, Mailing Address: P.O. Box 381588, Zip 38138; tel. 901/754–6418; Cameron J. Welton, Administrator; Methodist Hospitals of Memphis–Central, Methodist Hospitals of Memphis–South Unit, 1300 Wesley Drive, Zip 38116; tel. 901/346–3700; Cecelia Sawyer, Administrator; Methodist North–J. Harris Hospital, 3960 New Covington Pike, Zip 38128; tel. 901/372–5200; Tim Deaton, Administrator), 1265 Union Avenue, Zip 38104–3499; tel. 901/726–7000; Gary S. Shorb, President (Total facility includes 23 beds in nursing home–type unit) **A**1 2 3 5 6 9 10 **F**2 3 4 5 7 8 9 10 11 12 13 15 16 17 18 19 20 21 22 23 24 25 26 27 28 30 31 32 33 34 35 37 38 40 41 42 43 44 45 46 47 48 49 51 52 53 54 57 58 59 60 61 63 64 65 66 67 69 70 71 72 73 74 **P**4 6 7 8 **S** Methodist Health Systems, Inc., Memphis, TN **N** National Cardiovascular Network, Atlanta, GA; Methodist Health Systems, Inc., Memphis, TN

| | 23 | 10 | 1265 | 55875 | 868 | 322208 | 7942 | 395292 | 188141 | 6397 |

□ REGIONAL MEDICAL CENTER AT MEMPHIS, 877 Jefferson Avenue, Zip 38103; tel. 901/545–7100; Burton W. Waller, Jr., President and Chief Executive Officer **A**1 2 3 5 6 8 9 10 **F**7 8 9 12 14 15 16 17 19 20 21 22 28 30 31 34 37 38 39 40 41 42 44 46 49 51 56 60 61 65 68 69 70 71 72 73 74

| | 23 | 10 | 361 | 14150 | 241 | 143530 | 3600 | — | — | 2041 |

□ SAINT FRANCIS HOSPITAL, 5959 Park Avenue, Zip 38119–5198, Mailing Address: P.O. Box 171808, Zip 38187–1808; tel. 901/765–1000; Charles R. Slaton, President and Chief Executive Officer (Total facility includes 197 beds in nursing home–type unit) (Nonreporting) **A**1 2 3 5 9 10 **S** TENET Healthcare Corporation, Santa Barbara, CA

| | 33 | 10 | 559 | — | — | — | — | — | — | — |

★ △ ST. JOSEPH HOSPITAL AND HEALTH CENTERS, 220 Overton Avenue, Zip 38105–2789; tel. 901/577–2700; Joan M. Carlson, President and Chief Executive Officer (Total facility includes 30 beds in nursing home–type unit) **A**1 3 6 7 9 10 **F**2 3 4 8 10 18 19 20 21 22 27 28 30 31 32 34 35 37 39 41 42 43 44 45 46 48 49 52 53 54 55 56 57 58 60 63 64 65 71 73 **P**4 8 **S** Sisters of St. Francis Health Services, Inc., Mishawaka, IN

| | 21 | 10 | 402 | 7604 | 174 | 137548 | 0 | 51982 | 24162 | 910 |

★ ST. JUDE CHILDREN'S RESEARCH HOSPITAL, (PEDIATRIC CATASTROPHIC DISEASE), 332 North Lauderdale Street, Zip 38105–2794, Mailing Address: Box 318, Zip 38101–0318; tel. 901/495–3300; Arthur W. Nienhuis, M.D., Director **A**1 2 3 5 9 10 **F**16 19 20 21 31 34 35 39 42 44 45 46 47 48 49 54 60 63 65 67 69 71 73 **P**6

| | 23 | 59 | 50 | 1872 | 36 | — | 0 | 134390 | 58979 | 1540 |

□ UNIVERSITY BEHAVIORAL HEALTH CENTER, (Formerly University of Tennessee Medical Group Behavioral Health Center), 135 North Pauline Street, Zip 38105; tel. 901/448–2400; Stephen Wilensky, Executive Director **A**1 9 10 **F**3 52 53 54 55 56 57 58 59 **P**1

| | 23 | 22 | 20 | 17 | 11 | 0 | 0 | 2811 | 815 | 20 |

Hospital, Address, Telephone, Administrator, Approval, Facility, and Physician Codes, Health Care System, Network	Classi-fication Codes		Utilization Data					Expense (thousands) of dollars		
★ American Hospital Association (AHA) membership □ Joint Commission on Accreditation of Healthcare Organizations (JCAHO) accreditation + American Osteopathic Hospital Association (AOHA) membership ○ American Osteopathic Association (AOA) accreditation △ Commission on Accreditation of Rehabilitation Facilities (CARF) accreditation Control codes 61, 63, 64, 71, 72 and 73 indicate hospitals listed by AOHA, but not registered by AHA. For definition of numerical codes, see page A4	Control	Service	Beds	Admissions	Census	Outpatient Visits	Births	Total	Payroll	Personnel

□ UNIVERSITY OF TENNESSEE BOWLD HOSPITAL, 951 Court Avenue, Zip 38103–2898; tel. 901/448–4000; Jeffrey R. Woodside, M.D., Executive Director **A**1 2 3 5 9 10 **F**4 10 11 19 20 21 22 26 31 34 35 37 39 42 43 44 45 46 60 61 65 69 71	12	10	111	3675	66	26706	0	42394	15919	475
✠ VETERANS AFFAIRS MEDICAL CENTER, 1030 Jefferson Avenue, Zip 38104–2193; tel. 901/523–8990; K. L. Mulholland, Jr., Director (Total facility includes 120 beds in nursing home–type unit) **A**1 2 3 5 8 **F**2 3 4 10 11 12 14 15 16 17 19 20 21 22 23 24 26 27 30 31 32 33 34 35 37 39 41 42 43 44 45 46 48 49 51 52 54 56 57 58 59 60 63 64 65 67 71 73 74 **P**6 **S** Department of Veterans Affairs, Washington, DC	45	10	631	9912	391	259197	0	—	—	—
MILAN—Gibson County										
✠ CITY OF MILAN HOSPITAL, 4039 South Highland, Zip 38358; tel. 901/686–1591; Mark D. Le Neave, Chief Executive Officer (Total facility includes 13 beds in nursing home–type unit) **A**1 9 10 **F**16 19 21 22 37 44 52 57 64 71 **S** Quorum Health Group/Quorum Health Resources, Inc., Brentwood, TN **N** West Tennessee Healthcare, Inc., Jackson, TN	14	10	62	1053	27	15777	0	6798	2825	114
MILLINGTON—Shelby County										
✠ NAVAL HOSPITAL, 6500 Navy Road, Zip 38054–5201; tel. 901/874–5804; Captain Michael Kilpatrick, MSC, USN, Commanding Officer **A**1 **F**8 15 16 20 21 22 25 27 28 29 30 34 37 39 41 44 45 46 51 52 55 56 58 59 61 65 66 67 71 73 74 **P**6 **S** Department of Navy, Washington, DC	43	10	41	1540	9	163308	0	66924	24892	614
MORRISTOWN—Hamblen County										
□ LAKEWAY REGIONAL HOSPITAL, 726 McFarland Street, Zip 37814–3990; tel. 615/586–2302; Brian E. Dunn, Chief Executive Officer **A**1 9 10 **F**7 8 12 14 19 21 22 26 28 30 35 37 39 40 41 42 44 45 46 48 49 51 52 56 57 63 64 65 71 73 74 **P**8 **S** Community Health Systems, Inc., Brentwood, TN **N** Mountain States Healthcare Network, Johnson City, TN	33	10	135	2935	52	20662	231	18387	5824	236
□ △ MORRISTOWN–HAMBLEN HOSPITAL, 908 West Fourth North Street, Zip 37814–1178; tel. 615/586–4231; Richard L. Clark, Administrator and Chief Executive Officer (Nonreporting) **A**1 7 9 10 **N** Mountain States Healthcare Network, Johnson City, TN	23	10	143	—	—	—	—	—	—	—
MOUNTAIN HOME—Washington County										
✠ JAMES H. QUILLEN VETERANS AFFAIRS MEDICAL CENTER, (Formerly Veterans Affairs Medical Center), Zip 37684; tel. 423/926–1171; Carl J. Gerber, M.D., Ph.D., Director (Total facility includes 120 beds in nursing home–type unit) **A**1 2 3 5 8 **F**1 3 4 5 6 8 10 11 12 14 16 17 18 19 20 21 22 23 24 25 26 27 28 29 30 31 32 33 34 35 37 39 41 42 43 44 45 46 49 51 52 54 55 56 57 58 59 60 63 64 65 67 69 71 73 74 **P**6 **S** Department of Veterans Affairs, Washington, DC	45	10	390	5996	313	193221	0	94311	54946	1406
MURFREESBORO—Rutherford County										
✠ ALVIN C. YORK VETERANS AFFAIRS MEDICAL CENTER, 3400 Lebanon Road, Zip 37129; tel. 615/893–1360; R. Eugene Konik, Director (Total facility includes 166 beds in nursing home–type unit) (Nonreporting) **A**1 3 5 **S** Department of Veterans Affairs, Washington, DC	45	10	631	—	—	—	—	—	—	—
✠ MIDDLE TENNESSEE MEDICAL CENTER, 400 North Highland Avenue, Zip 37130–3854, Mailing Address: P.O. Box 1178, Zip 37133–1178; tel. 615/849–4100; Arthur W. Hastings, President and Chief Executive Officer **A**1 9 10 **F**7 8 10 11 15 16 17 19 21 22 23 24 26 28 29 30 31 32 33 35 37 39 40 42 44 45 46 49 61 65 66 67 71 73 74 **P**5 **N** Middle Tennessee Healthcare Network, Nashville, TN	21	10	191	10018	111	74306	1713	67681	25335	911
NASHVILLE—Davidson County										
✠ BAPTIST HOSPITAL, 2000 Church Street, Zip 37236–0002; tel. 615/329–5555; C. David Stringfield, President (Nonreporting) **A**1 3 5 9 10 **N** Center Care, Bowling Green, KY; Middle Tennessee Healthcare Network, Nashville, TN	23	10	649	—	—	—	—	—	—	—
✠ △ CENTENNIAL MEDICAL CENTER AND PARTHENON PAVILION, 2300 Patterson Street, Zip 37203; tel. 615/342–1000; Ronald J. Elder, President (Total facility includes 24 beds in nursing home–type unit) (Nonreporting) **A**1 2 5 7 9 10 **S** Columbia/HCA Healthcare Corporation, Nashville, TN	33	10	680	—	—	—	—	—	—	—
✠ COLUMBIA SOUTHERN HILLS MEDICAL CENTER, 391 Wallace Road, Zip 37211; tel. 615/781–4000; Lawrence L. Pieretti, Chief Executive Officer (Total facility includes 20 beds in nursing home–type unit) **A**1 9 10 **F**1 2 3 4 5 7 8 10 11 12 13 14 15 16 17 18 19 20 21 22 23 24 25 26 28 29 30 31 32 33 34 35 37 38 39 40 41 42 43 44 45 48 49 50 51 52 53 54 55 56 57 58 59 63 64 65 66 71 73 **P**1 6 7 8 **S** Columbia/HCA Healthcare Corporation, Nashville, TN	33	10	140	7255	78	52487	970	53921	18810	548
✠ METROPOLITAN NASHVILLE GENERAL HOSPITAL, 72 Hermitage Avenue, Zip 37210–2110; tel. 615/862–4490; John M. Stone, Director **A**1 2 3 5 6 9 10 **F**7 8 10 11 13 14 15 17 19 20 21 22 23 30 31 34 35 37 38 39 40 42 43 44 46 49 51 53 54 55 56 57 58 59 60 61 65 69 71 73 **S** Metropolitan Nashville General Hospital, Nashville, TN	15	10	105	4460	69	113261	717	44017	23220	727
□ MIDDLE TENNESSEE MENTAL HEALTH INSTITUTE, 221 Stewarts Ferry Pike, Zip 37214; tel. 615/902–7535; Joseph W. Carobene, Superintendent **A**1 3 10 **F**14 15 16 20 21 39 42 43 52 53 54 55 56 57 65 73	12	22	292	1375	249	0	0	30292	19040	792
★ NASHVILLE METROPOLITAN BORDEAUX HOSPITAL, 1414 County Hospital Road, Zip 37218–3001; tel. 615/862–7000; Wayne Hayes, Administrator (Total facility includes 525 beds in nursing home–type unit) **A**10 **F**15 20 26 27 28 41 46 64 65 67 73 **P**1 **S** Metropolitan Nashville General Hospital, Nashville, TN	15	48	565	590	496	—	0	27486	16930	656

Hospital, Address, Telephone, Administrator, Approval, Facility, and Physician Codes, Health Care System, Network	Classification Codes		Utilization Data					Expense (thousands) of dollars		
	Control	Service	Beds	Admissions	Census	Outpatient Visits	Births	Total	Payroll	Personnel

★ American Hospital Association (AHA) membership
□ Joint Commission on Accreditation of Healthcare Organizations (JCAHO) accreditation
+ American Osteopathic Hospital Association (AOHA) membership
○ American Osteopathic Association (AOA) accreditation
△ Commission on Accreditation of Rehabilitation Facilities (CARF) accreditation
Control codes 61, 63, 64, 71, 72 and 73 indicate hospitals listed by AOHA, but not registered by AHA. For definition of numerical codes, see page A4

Hospital	Control	Service	Beds	Admissions	Census	Outpatient Visits	Births	Total	Payroll	Personnel
★ △ NASHVILLE REHABILITATION HOSPITAL, 610 Gallatin Road, Zip 37206; tel. 615/226–4330; Jane Andrews, Administrator and Chief Executive Officer **A**1 7 9 10 **F**1 12 14 19 22 27 35 41 48 49 65 67 71 73	33	46	28	386	24	2238	0	8082	4221	117
★ PSYCHIATRIC HOSPITAL AT VANDERBILT, 1601 23rd Avenue South, Zip 37212; tel. 615/320–7770; Richard A. Bangert, Chief Executive Officer and Administrator **A**1 3 10 **F**2 3 15 16 17 19 21 22 35 50 52 53 54 55 56 57 58 59 65 70 71 **S** Columbia/HCA Healthcare Corporation, Nashville, TN	32	22	88	2362	44	6628	0	9139	5100	148
★ ST. THOMAS HOSPITAL, 4220 Harding Road, Zip 37205, Mailing Address: Box 380, Zip 37202; tel. 615/222–2111; John F. Tighe, President and Chief Executive Officer **A**1 2 3 5 9 10 **F**4 7 8 10 12 14 15 16 17 19 21 22 24 25 27 28 30 31 32 34 35 37 39 40 41 42 43 44 45 46 49 51 52 54 57 58 59 60 63 65 66 67 69 70 71 73 74 **P**1 3 4 5 6 7 **S** Daughters of Charity National Health System, Saint Louis, MO **N** National Cardiovascular Network, Atlanta, GA; Center Care, Bowling Green, KY; Partners for a Healthy Nashville, Nashville, TN; Middle Tennessee Healthcare Network, Nashville, TN; Saint Thomas Health Services, Nashville, TN	21	10	514	24227	376	119156	683	236562	98034	3569
★ VANDERBILT UNIVERSITY HOSPITAL, 1161 21st Avenue South, Zip 37232–2102; tel. 615/322–5000; Norman B. Urmy, Executive Director (Nonreporting) **A**1 2 3 5 8 9 10 **N** Partners for a Healthy Nashville, Nashville, TN; Middle Tennessee Healthcare Network, Nashville, TN; Saint Thomas Health Services, Nashville, TN	23	10	609	—	—	—	—	—	—	—
★ VETERANS AFFAIRS MEDICAL CENTER, 1310 24th Avenue South, Zip 37212–2637; tel. 615/327–5332; William A. Mountcastle, Director **A**1 2 3 5 8 **F**1 2 3 4 5 6 8 10 11 12 14 15 16 17 18 19 20 21 23 25 26 27 28 29 30 31 32 33 34 35 37 39 41 42 43 44 45 46 49 50 51 52 56 57 58 59 60 63 64 65 67 69 70 71 73 74 **P**6 **S** Department of Veterans Affairs, Washington, DC	45	10	233	7006	175	155851	0	—	—	1674
NEWPORT—Cocke County										
□ BAPTIST HOSPITAL OF COCKE COUNTY, 435 Second Street, Zip 37821; tel. 423/625–2200; Wayne Buckner, Administrator (Total facility includes 56 beds in nursing home–type unit) **A**1 9 10 **F**7 8 15 16 19 20 21 22 26 28 29 30 34 39 40 41 44 45 46 49 61 64 65 71 73 **P**8 **S** Baptist Health System of Tennessee, Knoxville, TN	21	10	109	2772	81	32937	296	17210	7181	260
OAK RIDGE—Anderson County										
□ METHODIST MEDICAL CENTER OF OAK RIDGE, 990 Oak Ridge Turnpike, Zip 37830, Mailing Address: P.O. Box 2529, Zip 37831–2529; tel. 423/481–1000; George A. Mathews, President and Chief Executive Officer **A**1 2 9 10 **F**7 8 10 11 12 14 15 16 19 21 22 28 30 32 33 34 35 37 39 40 41 42 43 44 45 46 49 51 52 54 55 56 57 58 59 61 63 65 66 67 71 73 74	23	10	275	12320	179	84338	1027	90675	46009	1055
□ RIDGEVIEW PSYCHIATRIC HOSPITAL AND CENTER, 240 West Tyrone Road, Zip 37830; tel. 615/482–1076; Robert J. Benning, Chief Executive Officer **A**1 10 **F**3 12 52 53 54 55 56 57 58 59 65 **P**6	23	22	20	556	9	65294	0	6096	4126	163
ONEIDA—Scott County										
□ SCOTT COUNTY HOSPITAL, U.S. Highway 27, Zip 37841–4939, Mailing Address: Box 4939, Zip 37841–4939; tel. 615/569–8521; William N. Grey, Chief Executive Officer **A**1 9 10 **F**2 3 7 8 11 14 15 16 19 22 28 37 39 40 41 42 44 46 49 52 58 59 64 65 66 71 73 **S** Community Health Systems, Inc., Brentwood, TN	33	10	91	3442	38	17292	76	10208	4854	215
PARIS—Henry County										
★ HENRY COUNTY MEDICAL CENTER, Tyson Avenue, Zip 38242–4544, Mailing Address: Box 1030, Zip 38242–1030; tel. 901/644–8537; Thomas H. Gee, Administrator (Total facility includes 172 beds in nursing home–type unit) **A**1 9 10 **F**7 8 19 20 21 22 23 28 30 32 33 35 37 39 40 42 44 46 49 52 53 54 55 56 57 59 60 64 65 67 69 71 73 **N** West Tennessee Healthcare, Inc., Jackson, TN	13	10	267	4500	222	50220	365	27588	12976	533
PARSONS—Decatur County										
DECATUR COUNTY GENERAL HOSPITAL, 1200 Tennessee Avenue South, Zip 38363–0250, Mailing Address: Box 250, Zip 38363–0250; tel. 901/847–3031; Larry N. Lindsey, Administrator (Nonreporting) **A**9 10 **N** West Tennessee Healthcare, Inc., Jackson, TN	13	10	40	—	—	—	—	—	—	—
PIKEVILLE—Bledsoe County										
□ BLEDSOE COUNTY GENERAL HOSPITAL, Mailing Address: P.O. Box 699, Zip 37367–0699; tel. 423/447–2112; Gary Burton, Chief Executive Officer (Nonreporting) **A**1 9 10 **S** Paracelsus Healthcare Corporation, Houston, TX	33	10	26	—	—	—	—	—	—	—
PORTLAND—Sumner County										
TENNESSEE CHRISTIAN MEDICAL CENTER – PORTLAND See Tennessee Christian Medical Center, Madison										
PULASKI—Giles County										
★ COLUMBIA HILLSIDE HOSPITAL, 1265 East College Street, Zip 38478; tel. 615/363–7531; James H. Edmondson, Chief Executive Officer and Administrator (Nonreporting) **A**1 9 10 **S** Columbia/HCA Healthcare Corporation, Nashville, TN	16	10	85	—	—	—	—	—	—	—
RIPLEY—Lauderdale County										
★ BAPTIST MEMORIAL HOSPITAL–LAUDERDALE, 326 Asbury Road, Zip 38063–9701; tel. 901/635–6400; W. Tate Moorer, Administrator **A**1 9 10 **F**2 3 8 15 16 19 22 26 32 34 37 39 41 44 45 46 49 52 54 57 65 71 73 **P**3 7 **S** Baptist Memorial Health Care Corporation, Memphis, TN	21	10	70	1424	22	17245	0	7628	2891	152
ROGERSVILLE—Hawkins County										
★ HAWKINS COUNTY MEMORIAL HOSPITAL, Locust Street, Zip 37857; tel. 423/272–2671; R. Frank Testerman, Administrator **A**1 9 10 **F**8 15 17 19 22 28 30 31 34 35 41 44 45 49 65 69 71 73	13	10	50	1563	22	33640	0	8369	3185	148

Hospital, Address, Telephone, Administrator, Approval, Facility, and Physician Codes, Health Care System, Network	Classi-fication Codes		Utilization Data					Expense (thousands) of dollars		
★ American Hospital Association (AHA) membership □ Joint Commission on Accreditation of Healthcare Organizations (JCAHO) accreditation + American Osteopathic Hospital Association (AOHA) membership ○ American Osteopathic Association (AOA) accreditation △ Commission on Accreditation of Rehabilitation Facilities (CARF) accreditation Control codes 61, 63, 64, 71, 72 and 73 indicate hospitals listed by AOHA, but not registered by AHA. For definition of numerical codes, see page A4	Control	Service	Beds	Admissions	Census	Outpatient Visits	Births	Total	Payroll	Personnel

SAVANNAH—Hardin County

HARDIN COUNTY GENERAL HOSPITAL, 2006 Wayne Road, Zip 38372; tel. 901/925–4954; Charlotte Burns, Administrator and Chief Executive Officer (Total facility includes 73 beds in nursing home–type unit) (Nonreporting) **A**9 10 **N** West Tennessee Healthcare, Inc., Jackson, TN
| | 13 | 10 | 130 | — | — | — | — | — | — | — |

SELMER—McNairy County

✠ MCNAIRY COUNTY GENERAL HOSPITAL, 705 East Poplar Avenue, Zip 38375–1748; tel. 901/645–3221; Rosamond M. Tyler, Administrator **A**1 9 10 **F**7 8 19 21 22 28 29 30 32 33 34 40 44 45 46 49 54 65 69 71 73 **N** West Tennessee Healthcare, Inc., Jackson, TN
| | 13 | 10 | 86 | 1364 | 14 | 21889 | 213 | 6781 | 3077 | 128 |

SEVIERVILLE—Sevier County

✠ FORT SANDERS–SEVIER MEDICAL CENTER, 709 Middle Creek Road, Zip 37862, Mailing Address: P.O. Box 8005, Zip 37864–8005; tel. 423/429–6100; Ralph T. Williams, Administrator (Total facility includes 54 beds in nursing home–type unit) **A**1 9 10 **F**7 8 10 12 15 19 20 21 22 28 30 31 32 33 34 35 37 40 41 44 45 49 63 64 67 71 73 **P**7 **N** CHA Provider Network, Inc., Lexington, KY
| | 23 | 10 | 100 | 2114 | 77 | 60386 | 496 | 16646 | 7074 | 306 |

SEWANEE—Franklin County

COLUMBIA EMERALD–HODGSON HOSPITAL See Columbia Southern Tennessee Medical Center, Winchester

SHELBYVILLE—Bedford County

□ BEDFORD COUNTY GENERAL HOSPITAL, 845 Union Street, Zip 37160–9971; tel. 615/685–5433; Richard L. Graham, Administrator (Total facility includes 107 beds in nursing home–type unit) **A**1 9 10 **F**7 8 12 13 14 15 16 19 20 22 28 29 30 31 32 34 39 40 41 42 44 46 49 64 65 68 69 71 73 **P**8 **N** Center Care, Bowling Green, KY; Middle Tennessee Healthcare Network, Nashville, TN
| | 13 | 10 | 180 | 2401 | 129 | 79367 | 240 | 17061 | 7183 | 311 |

SMITHVILLE—DeKalb County

✠ BAPTIST DEKALB HOSPITAL, 520 West Main Street, Zip 37166, Mailing Address: P.O. Box 640, Zip 37166–0640; tel. 615/597–7171; Alan Markowitz, Ph.D., FACHE, Administrator and Chief Executive Officer **A**1 9 10 **F**7 8 10 12 17 19 21 22 26 28 30 34 35 37 39 40 41 42 44 45 46 48 49 51 52 57 61 65 66 71 **P**5
| | 32 | 10 | 58 | 1742 | 16 | 11944 | 97 | 8334 | 3764 | 136 |

SOMERVILLE—Fayette County

✠ METHODIST HOSPITAL OF FAYETTE, 214 Lakeview Road, Zip 38068–0001, Mailing Address: Box 909, Zip 38068–0001; tel. 901/465–0532; Michael Blome', Administrator **A**1 9 10 **F**2 3 4 5 6 7 8 9 10 11 12 13 14 15 16 17 19 21 22 23 24 25 26 27 28 29 30 31 32 33 34 35 37 38 39 40 41 42 43 44 45 46 47 48 49 51 52 53 54 55 56 57 58 59 60 63 64 65 67 69 71 72 73 **P**1 2 3 4 5 6 7 8 **S** Methodist Health Systems, Inc., Memphis, TN **N** Methodist Health Systems, Inc., Memphis, TN
| | 21 | 10 | 38 | 785 | 10 | 26896 | 55 | 7100 | 2559 | 100 |

SOUTH PITTSBURG—Marion County

✠ COLUMBIA SOUTH PITTSBURG HOSPITAL, 210 West 12th Street, Zip 37380, Mailing Address: P.O. Box 349, Zip 37380–0349; tel. 423/837–6781; Robert Klein, Chief Executive Officer **A**1 9 10 **F**2 3 8 12 15 19 21 22 32 34 35 37 44 45 49 65 71 73 **P**1 **S** Columbia/HCA Healthcare Corporation, Nashville, TN **N** Principal Health Care of Georgia, Atlanta, GA; Chattanooga Healthcare Network, Chattanooga, TN
| | 33 | 10 | 47 | 2498 | 23 | 26687 | 0 | 11159 | 4118 | 165 |

SPARTA—White County

□ WHITE COUNTY COMMUNITY HOSPITAL, 401 Sewell Road, Zip 38583; tel. 615/738–9211; Raymond W. Acker, Administrator (Nonreporting) **A**1 9 10 **S** Community Health Systems, Inc., Brentwood, TN
| | 33 | 10 | 60 | — | — | — | — | — | — | — |

SPRINGFIELD—Robertson County

✠ NORTH CREST MEDICAL CENTER, 100 North Crest Drive, Zip 37172–2984; tel. 615/384–2411; Dennis T. Bynum, Interim Chief Executive Officer **A**1 9 10 **F**7 8 10 11 14 15 16 17 19 21 22 28 30 32 33 35 37 40 42 44 46 48 49 52 53 54 56 57 58 65 67 71 73 74 **P**5
| | 23 | 10 | 100 | 3637 | 44 | 43998 | 501 | 30278 | 11320 | 372 |

SWEETWATER—Monroe County

★ SWEETWATER HOSPITAL, 304 Wright Street, Zip 37874; tel. 423/337–6171; Scott Bowman, Administrator (Nonreporting) **A**9 10
| | 23 | 10 | 59 | — | — | — | — | — | — | — |

TAZEWELL—Claiborne County

✠ CLAIBORNE COUNTY HOSPITAL, 1850 Old Knoxville Road, Zip 37879, Mailing Address: Box 219, Zip 37879; tel. 615/626–4211; Richard Welch, Administrator (Total facility includes 50 beds in nursing home–type unit) **A**1 9 10 **F**12 15 16 17 19 22 27 30 32 33 34 35 37 39 41 44 45 46 49 64 71 **N** CHA Provider Network, Inc., Lexington, KY
| | 13 | 10 | 115 | 3251 | 86 | 33597 | 1 | 13180 | 6350 | 287 |

TRENTON—Gibson County

✠ GIBSON GENERAL HOSPITAL, 200 Hosptial Drive, Zip 38382, Mailing Address: Box 488, Zip 38382; tel. 901/855–2551; Kelly R. Yenawine, Administrator **A**1 9 10 **F**2 14 15 16 19 21 22 28 30 32 33 34 44 49 65 71 73 **P**1 **S** West Tennessee Healthcare, Inc., Jackson, TN **N** West Tennessee Healthcare, Inc., Jackson, TN
| | 15 | 10 | 41 | 909 | 11 | 11744 | 0 | 4169 | 2174 | 82 |

TULLAHOMA—Coffee County

□ HARTON REGIONAL MEDICAL CENTER, 1801 North Jackson Street, Zip 37388, Mailing Address: P.O. Box 460, Zip 37388; tel. 615/393–3000; Brian T. Flynn, Administrator and Chief Executive Officer (Nonreporting) **A**1 9 10 **S** TENET Healthcare Corporation, Santa Barbara, CA **N** Center Care, Bowling Green, KY
| | 33 | 10 | 137 | — | — | — | — | — | — | — |

UNION CITY—Obion County

✠ BAPTIST MEMORIAL HOSPITAL–UNION CITY, 1201 Bishop Street, Zip 38261, Mailing Address: Box 310, Zip 38281–0310; tel. 901/884–8601; Mike Perryman, Administrator **A**1 9 10 **F**2 3 7 8 10 11 12 14 15 16 17 19 21 22 24 28 32 35 37 39 40 41 42 44 46 49 52 53 56 58 60 63 65 67 71 73 **S** Baptist Memorial Health Care Corporation, Memphis, TN
| | 23 | 10 | 133 | 4498 | 56 | 34161 | 329 | 22888 | 8806 | 357 |

Hospital, Address, Telephone, Administrator, Approval, Facility, and Physician Codes, Health Care System, Network	Classi-fication Codes		Utilization Data					Expense (thousands) of dollars		
★ American Hospital Association (AHA) membership □ Joint Commission on Accreditation of Healthcare Organizations (JCAHO) accreditation + American Osteopathic Hospital Association (AOHA) membership ○ American Osteopathic Association (AOA) accreditation △ Commission on Accreditation of Rehabilitation Facilities (CARF) accreditation Control codes 61, 63, 64, 71, 72 and 73 indicate hospitals listed by AOHA, but not registered by AHA. For definition of numerical codes, see page A4	Control	Service	Beds	Admissions	Census	Outpatient Visits	Births	Total	Payroll	Personnel

WAVERLY—Humphreys County

BAPTIST THREE RIVERS HOSPITAL, 451 Highway 13 South, Zip 37185–2149, Mailing Address: P.O. Box 437, Zip 37185–2149; tel. 615/296–4203; Samuel R. Heflin, Jr., Administrator (Total facility includes 10 beds in nursing home–type unit) **A**9 10 **F**19 22 28 32 33 41 44 51 59 64 65 71 73 — 32 10 52 678 9 21792 0 5351 2184 68

WAYNESBORO—Wayne County

□ WAYNE MEDICAL CENTER, (Formerly Wayne County General Hospital), Highway 64 East, Zip 38485, Mailing Address: P.O. Box 580, Zip 38485–0580; tel. 615/722–5411; Shirley Harder, Chief Executive Officer (Total facility includes 61 beds in nursing home–type unit) **A**1 9 10 **F**7 8 19 22 44 64 71 **P**6 — 23 10 110 1022 56 11540 35 5965 2624 155

WESTERN INSTITUTE—Hardeman County

□ WESTERN MENTAL HEALTH INSTITUTE, Highway 64 West, Zip 38074; tel. 901/658–5141; Elizabeth Littlefield, Ed.D., Superintendent **A**1 10 **F**52 53 56 57 — 12 22 247 1009 240 0 0 22041 13750 582

WINCHESTER—Franklin County

⌧ COLUMBIA SOUTHERN TENNESSEE MEDICAL CENTER, (Includes Columbia Emerald–Hodgson Hospital, University Avenue, Sewanee, Zip 37375; tel. 615/598–5691), 185 Hospital Road, Zip 37398; tel. 615/967–8200; Michael W. Garfield, Administrator (Total facility includes 66 beds in nursing home–type unit) **A**1 9 10 **F**7 8 12 14 15 16 19 21 27 30 32 34 35 37 39 40 41 42 44 49 63 64 65 67 71 73 **P**7 8 **S** Columbia/HCA Healthcare Corporation, Nashville, TN **N** Center Care, Bowling Green, KY — 33 10 128 4915 95 47297 494 22691 10211 350

WOODBURY—Cannon County

⌧ COLUMBIA STONES RIVER HOSPITAL, 324 Doolittle Road, Zip 37190, Mailing Address: P.O. Box 458, Zip 37190–0458; tel. 615/563–4001; Terry J. Gunn, Administrator **A**1 9 10 **F**8 12 14 15 17 19 21 22 26 28 29 30 32 35 39 41 44 46 49 51 52 57 63 65 71 73 **P**5 7 8 **S** Columbia/HCA Healthcare Corporation, Nashville, TN — 33 10 55 1411 16 10367 0 5737 2780 118

TEXAS

Resident population 18,724 (in thousands)
Resident population in metro areas 84.1%
Birth rate per 1,000 population 17.9
65 years and over 10.2%
Percent of persons without health insurance 24.2%

Hospital, Address, Telephone, Administrator, Approval, Facility, and Physician Codes, Health Care System, Network	Classi-fication Codes		Utilization Data					Expense (thousands) of dollars		
★ American Hospital Association (AHA) membership □ Joint Commission on Accreditation of Healthcare Organizations (JCAHO) accreditation + American Osteopathic Hospital Association (AOHA) membership ○ American Osteopathic Association (AOA) accreditation △ Commission on Accreditation of Rehabilitation Facilities (CARF) accreditation Control codes 61, 63, 64, 71, 72 and 73 indicate hospitals listed by AOHA, but not registered by AHA. For definition of numerical codes, see page A4	Control	Service	Beds	Admissions	Census	Outpatient Visits	Births	Total	Payroll	Personnel

ABILENE—Taylor County

⊞ ABILENE REGIONAL MEDICAL CENTER, 6250 Highway 83–84 at Antilley Road, Zip 79606; tel. 915/695–9900; Woody Gilliland, Chief Executive Officer (Total facility includes 15 beds in nursing home–type unit) **A**1 9 10 **F**4 7 8 10 11 12 14 15 16 17 19 21 22 24 25 26 28 29 30 32 34 35 37 38 39 40 42 43 44 45 46 49 51 61 64 65 67 71 73 74 **P**6 7 **S** Quorum Health Group/Quorum Health Resources, Inc., Brentwood, TN | 33 | 10 | 160 | 5833 | 89 | 42081 | 523 | 45780 | 17988 | 691 |

⊞ △ HENDRICK HEALTH SYSTEM, (Formerly Hendrick Medical Center), 1242 North 19th Street, Zip 79601–2316; tel. 915/670–2000; Michael C. Waters, President (Total facility includes 49 beds in nursing home–type unit) **A**1 7 9 10 **F**4 5 6 7 8 10 11 12 15 16 17 18 19 20 21 22 23 24 26 27 28 29 30 31 32 33 34 35 37 39 40 41 42 43 44 45 46 47 48 49 56 60 62 63 64 65 66 67 71 73 74 **P**7 8 **N** The Heart Network of Texas, Irving, TX | 21 | 10 | 342 | 13668 | 223 | 125421 | 1708 | 127323 | 56363 | 2272 |

⊞ U. S. AIR FORCE HOSPITAL, 7th Medical Group, Dyess AFB, Zip 79607–1367; tel. 915/696–2345; Lieutenant Colonel Robert W. Blum, MSC, USAF, FACHE, Administrator (Nonreporting) **A**1 **S** Department of the Air Force, Washington, DC | 41 | 10 | 20 | — | — | — | — | — | — | — |

ALBANY—Shackelford County

SHACKELFORD COUNTY HOSPITAL DISTRICT, 840 Greer Street, Zip 76430, Mailing Address: P.O. Box 1507, Zip 76430; tel. 915/762–3313; Melissa Black, Assistant Administrator (Nonreporting) **A**9 10 | 16 | 10 | 24 | — | — | — | — | — | — | — |

ALICE—Jim Wells County

⊞ COLUMBIA ALICE PHYSICIANS AND SURGEONS HOSPITAL, 300 East Third Street, Zip 78332–4794; tel. 512/664–4376; Earl S. Whiteley, CHE, Chief Executive Officer **A**1 9 10 **F**2 3 4 7 8 9 10 11 12 14 15 16 18 19 20 21 22 26 27 28 29 30 31 32 33 34 35 37 38 39 40 42 43 44 45 46 47 49 50 52 53 54 55 56 57 58 59 63 64 65 69 70 71 73 74 **P**3 5 7 8 **S** Columbia/HCA Healthcare Corporation, Nashville, TN **N** Columbia Healthcare – South Texas Division, Corpus Christi, TX | 33 | 10 | 123 | 4167 | 46 | 36489 | 428 | 21634 | 8768 | 326 |

ALPINE—Brewster County

BIG BEND REGIONAL MEDICAL CENTER, 801 East Brown Street, Zip 79830; tel. 915/837–3447; Tom L. Lawson, Administrator **A**9 10 **F**1 3 7 8 12 13 14 17 18 19 22 26 27 28 31 32 33 34 36 39 40 44 45 49 53 54 55 56 57 58 61 62 64 65 67 68 69 70 71 73 **N** Permian Basin Rural Health Network, Fort Stockton, TX | 16 | 10 | 32 | 1213 | 13 | 48228 | 218 | 7486 | 3432 | 144 |

ALVIN—Brazoria County

⊞ COLUMBIA ALVIN MEDICAL CENTER, 301 Medic Lane, Zip 77511; tel. 713/331–6141; Donald A. Shaffett, Chief Executive Officer (Total facility includes 14 beds in nursing home–type unit) **A**1 9 10 **F**8 12 14 15 16 19 22 32 34 35 39 41 44 49 64 65 66 71 73 **P**5 7 8 **S** Columbia/HCA Healthcare Corporation, Nashville, TN | 33 | 10 | 86 | 1233 | 19 | 19023 | 0 | 12024 | 5812 | 125 |

AMARILLO—Potter County

⊞ △ BAPTIST–ST. ANTHONY HEALTH SYSTEM, (Formerly High Plains Baptist Health System), 1600 Wallace Boulevard, Zip 79106; tel. 806/358–5800; John D. Hicks, President and Chief Executive Officer **A**1 2 5 7 9 10 **F**4 5 7 8 10 11 12 14 15 16 19 20 21 22 23 27 28 30 32 34 35 36 37 39 40 41 42 43 44 45 46 49 51 60 65 66 69 71 72 73 74 **P**3 5 7 | 21 | 10 | 361 | 14624 | 206 | 89119 | 1157 | 121884 | 45731 | — |

⊞ BAPTIST–ST. ANTHONY'S HEALTH SYSTEM, (Formerly St. Anthony's Hospital), 200 N.W. Seventh, Zip 79107–9872, Mailing Address: P.O. Box 950, Zip 79176–0950; tel. 806/376–4411; John D. Hicks, President (Total facility includes 38 beds in nursing home–type unit) **A**1 2 3 5 9 10 **F**1 4 7 8 10 11 12 14 15 16 17 19 20 21 22 24 26 28 30 32 33 35 36 37 39 40 41 42 43 44 45 46 48 49 60 64 65 71 72 73 74 **P**3 5 7 **S** Incarnate Word Health Services, San Antonio, TX | 21 | 10 | 349 | 6429 | 102 | 40731 | 105 | 51584 | 20140 | — |

⊞ NORTHWEST TEXAS HEALTHCARE SYSTEM, (Formerly Northwest Texas Hospital), (Includes Psychiatric Pavilion, 7201 Evans, Zip 79106), 1501 South Coulter Avenue, Zip 79106–1790, Mailing Address: P.O. Box 1110, Zip 79175–1110; tel. 806/354–1000; Michael A. Callahan, Chief Executive Officer **A**1 3 5 10 **F**2 3 4 7 8 10 11 12 13 14 15 16 17 18 19 20 21 22 23 24 25 26 29 30 31 32 33 34 35 37 38 39 40 41 42 43 44 45 46 47 48 49 51 52 53 54 55 56 57 58 59 60 61 63 64 65 66 67 71 73 74 **P**3 6 7 **S** Universal Health Services, Inc., King of Prussia, PA
PSYCHIATRIC PAVILION See Northwest Texas Healthcare System | 33 | 10 | 332 | 13794 | 203 | 234713 | 2890 | 135961 | 48075 | 1550 |

⊞ VETERANS AFFAIRS MEDICAL CENTER, 6010 Amarillo Boulevard West, Zip 79106; tel. 806/354–7801; Wallace M. Hopkins, FACHE, Director (Total facility includes 120 beds in nursing home–type unit) **A**1 2 3 5 **F**2 3 8 11 12 16 17 19 20 21 22 24 25 26 28 29 30 31 32 33 34 35 37 39 41 42 44 45 46 48 49 50 51 52 54 55 57 58 59 60 63 64 65 67 71 72 73 74 **P**6 **S** Department of Veterans Affairs, Washington, DC | 45 | 10 | 218 | 3599 | 191 | 177167 | 0 | 55000 | — | 656 |

ANAHUAC—Chambers County

★ BAYSIDE COMMUNITY HOSPITAL, 200 Hospital Drive, Zip 77514, Mailing Address: P.O. Box 398, Zip 77514; tel. 409/267–3143; Stephen M. Goode, Executive Director **A**9 10 **F**22 36 44 **P**6 | 16 | 10 | 17 | 259 | 3 | 5248 | 1 | 2555 | 1103 | 50 |

Hospital, Address, Telephone, Administrator, Approval, Facility, and Physician Codes, Health Care System, Network	Classi-fication Codes		Utilization Data					Expense (thousands) of dollars		

★ American Hospital Association (AHA) membership
□ Joint Commission on Accreditation of Healthcare Organizations (JCAHO) accreditation
+ American Osteopathic Hospital Association (AOHA) membership
○ American Osteopathic Association (AOA) accreditation
△ Commission on Accreditation of Rehabilitation Facilities (CARF) accreditation
Control codes 61, 63, 64, 71, 72 and 73 indicate hospitals listed by AOHA, but not registered by AHA. For definition of numerical codes, see page A4

	Control	Service	Beds	Admissions	Census	Outpatient Visits	Births	Total	Payroll	Personnel
ANDREWS—Andrews County										
✠ PERMIAN GENERAL HOSPITAL, Northeast By–Pass, Zip 79714, Mailing Address: Box 2108, Zip 79714; tel. 915/523–2200; Randy R. Richards, Chief Executive Officer **A**1 9 10 **F**7 8 12 14 15 16 17 18 19 20 21 22 24 28 30 32 34 35 39 40 41 44 45 49 51 64 65 70 71 73 **P**7 **N** Lubbock Methodist Hospital System, Lubbock, TX; Permian Basin Rural Health Network, Fort Stockton, TX	13	10	71	1392	19	48037	271	10876	4910	157
ANGLETON—Brazoria County										
✠ ANGLETON–DANBURY GENERAL HOSPITAL, 132 Hospital Drive, Zip 77515; tel. 409/849–7721; David A. Bleakney, Administrator **A**1 9 10 **F**7 8 10 12 14 15 16 19 21 22 24 28 29 30 31 34 35 37 40 44 45 46 49 65 66 70 71 73 **P**8 **N** Memorial/Sisters of Charity Health Network, Houston, TX	12	10	64	3262	22	—	471	17350	5891	229
ANSON—Jones County										
★ ANSON GENERAL HOSPITAL, 101 Avenue J, Zip 79501; tel. 915/823–3231; Dudley R. White, Administrator **A**9 10 **F**19 20 22 24 32 44 49 71 73 **P**3 8 **N** Lubbock Methodist Hospital System, Lubbock, TX	14	10	30	769	11	38179	1	4801	2405	123
ARANSAS PASS—San Patricio County										
✠ COLUMBIA NORTH BAY HOSPITAL, 1711 West Wheeler Avenue, Zip 78336; tel. 512/758–0502; Steve Sutherlin, Chief Executive Officer **A**1 9 10 **F**2 3 4 7 8 9 10 11 12 13 15 16 17 19 20 21 22 23 24 25 26 27 28 29 30 31 32 33 34 35 37 38 40 41 42 43 44 46 47 48 49 51 52 53 54 55 56 57 58 59 60 61 64 65 66 71 73 74 **P**7 8 **S** Columbia/HCA Healthcare Corporation, Nashville, TN **N** Columbia Healthcare – South Texas Division, Corpus Christi, TX	33	10	69	1736	21	22302	216	16642	6610	229
ARLINGTON—Tarrant County										
✠ ARLINGTON MEMORIAL HOSPITAL, 800 West Randol Mill Road, Zip 76012; tel. 817/548–6100; Rex C. McRae, President **A**1 9 10 **F**4 7 8 10 11 12 14 15 17 19 21 22 23 24 33 34 35 37 38 39 40 41 42 43 44 45 49 60 65 71 73 74 **P**1 **N** Southwest Preferred Network, Dallas, TX	23	10	341	14518	192	104317	2494	97591	40994	1519
□ BHC MILLWOOD HOSPITAL, (Formerly CPC Millwood Hospital), 1011 North Cooper Street, Zip 76011; tel. 817/261–3121; Wayne Hallford, Chief Executive Officer **A**1 9 10 **F**1 3 25 27 34 52 53 54 56 58 59 65 67 **P**8 **S** Behavioral Healthcare Corporation, Nashville, TN	33	22	130	1041	30	6543	0	6030	3199	102
✠ COLUMBIA MEDICAL CENTER OF ARLINGTON, 3301 Matlock Road, Zip 76015; tel. 817/465–3241; John A. Fromhold, Chief Executive Officer **A**1 9 10 **F**3 4 7 8 10 12 14 15 16 17 19 21 22 26 28 29 30 31 32 33 34 35 37 38 39 40 41 42 43 44 45 46 48 49 50 51 52 53 54 55 56 57 58 59 60 63 64 65 66 67 68 71 73 74 **P**5 7 **S** Columbia/HCA Healthcare Corporation, Nashville, TN CPC MILLWOOD HOSPITAL See BHC Millwood Hospital	33	10	165	7467	90	56380	1925	54069	17174	665
□ △ HEALTHSOUTH REHABILITATION HOSPITAL OF ARLINGTON, 3200 Matlock Road, Zip 76015–2911; tel. 817/468–4000; S. Denise Borroni, Administrator and Chief Operating Officer (Total facility includes 18 beds in nursing home–type unit) **A**1 7 9 10 **F**22 34 41 45 48 49 64 65 67 **P**8 **S** HEALTHSOUTH Corporation, Birmingham, AL	33	46	60	670	38	4456	0	10403	3704	127
✠ HUGULEY WILLOW CREEK HOSPITAL, 7000 Highway 287 South, Zip 76017–2805; tel. 817/561–1600; David P. Banks, Chief Executive Officer **A**1 9 10 **F**2 3 14 15 16 17 18 25 52 53 54 55 56 57 58 59 65 67 73 **P**7 **S** Adventist Health System Sunbelt Health Care Corporation, Winter Park, FL	21	22	115	1148	19	—	0	6143	2611	155
□ THC–ARLINGTON, 1000 North Cooper, Zip 76011; tel. 817/543–0200; Darryl S. Dubroca, Administrator (Total facility includes 19 beds in nursing home–type unit) **A**1 10 **F**12 14 16 19 21 22 31 33 34 35 37 39 41 42 49 60 64 65 71 **S** Transitional Hospitals Corporation, Las Vegas, NV	33	10	75	534	48	902	0	13769	7606	173
ASPERMONT—Stonewall County										
★ STONEWALL MEMORIAL HOSPITAL, U.S. Highway 380 & 83 North, Zip 79502, Mailing Address: Drawer C, Zip 79502; tel. 817/989–3551; Scott A. Anderson, Administrator **A**9 10 **F**6 12 15 16 22 28 32 34 41 44 64 71	16	10	16	92	1	3989	0	1663	754	48
ATHENS—Henderson County										
✠ EAST TEXAS MEDICAL CENTER ATHENS, 2000 South Palestine, Zip 75751; tel. 903/675–2216; Patrick L. Wallace, Administrator **A**1 9 10 **F**8 19 21 22 23 27 28 30 32 33 37 40 42 44 49 65 66 67 70 71 **P**7 **S** East Texas Medical Center Regional Healthcare System, Tyler, TX **N** Healthcare Partners of East Texas, Inc., Tyler, TX	23	10	108	5002	54	81184	755	31754	11407	410
ATLANTA—Cass County										
★ ATLANTA MEMORIAL HOSPITAL, Highway 77 at South Williams, Zip 75551, Mailing Address: Box 1049, Zip 75551–1049; tel. 903/796–4151; Tom Crow, Administrator **A**9 10 **F**1 7 8 9 10 11 15 17 19 20 22 26 27 28 30 32 34 37 39 40 42 43 44 45 47 49 57 60 61 65 70 71 72 73 **P**8	16	10	47	1456	17	15632	181	6864	3071	127
BROOKS HOSPITAL, Louise Street, Zip 75551, Mailing Address: P.O. Box 1069, Zip 75551; tel. 903/796–2873; Jesse Brooks, M.D., Administrator **A**9 10 **F**1 3 4 5 6 7 8 10 12 13 17 18 19 20 21 22 23 24 25 26 27 28 29 30 31 32 33 34 35 36 39 41 42 43 44 45 46 49 50 51 53 54 55 56 57 58 59 60 61 62 63 65 66 67 68 69 70 71 72 73 74 **P**1 2 3 4 5 6 7 8	33	10	22	494	7	190	0	—	—	52
AUSTIN—Travis County										
✠ AUSTIN DIAGNOSTIC MEDICAL CENTER, 12221 MoPac Expressway North, Zip 78758; tel. 512/901–1000; Richard E. Salerno, Chief Executive Officer (Total facility includes 18 beds in nursing home–type unit) **A**1 10 **F**1 2 3 4 7 8 10 11 12 14 15 16 17 18 19 21 22 23 24 25 27 28 29 30 31 32 34 35 37 38 39 40 41 42 43 44 45 46 48 49 52 53 54 55 57 58 59 60 61 63 64 65 66 67 68 69 71 72 73 74 **P**1 3 7 8 **S** Columbia/HCA Healthcare Corporation, Nashville, TN	32	10	114	6498	81	148147	718	51195	21843	893

Hospital, Address, Telephone, Administrator, Approval, Facility, and Physician Codes, Health Care System, Network	Classi-fication Codes		Utilization Data					Expense (thousands) of dollars		
★ American Hospital Association (AHA) membership □ Joint Commission on Accreditation of Healthcare Organizations (JCAHO) accreditation + American Osteopathic Hospital Association (AOHA) membership ○ American Osteopathic Association (AOA) accreditation △ Commission on Accreditation of Rehabilitation Facilities (CARF) accreditation Control codes 61, 63, 64, 71, 72 and 73 indicate hospitals listed by AOHA, but not registered by AHA. For definition of numerical codes, see page A4	Control	Service	Beds	Admissions	Census	Outpatient Visits	Births	Total	Payroll	Personnel

Hospital	Control	Service	Beds	Admissions	Census	Outpatient Visits	Births	Total	Payroll	Personnel
□ AUSTIN STATE HOSPITAL, 4110 Guadalupe Street, Zip 78751–4296; tel. 512/452–0381; Diane Faucher, Superintendent **A**1 3 9 10 **F**11 20 37 39 40 52 53 55 56 57 65 73	12	22	352	1666	303	0	0	48889	28103	933
□ BHC SHOAL CREEK HOSPITAL, (Formerly Shoal Creek Hospital), 3501 Mills Avenue, Zip 78731; tel. 512/452–0361; Gail M. Oberta, Administrator and Chief Executive Officer **A**1 9 10 **F**2 3 15 16 19 21 26 27 34 35 52 53 57 58 59 **P**1 **S** Behavioral Healthcare Corporation, Nashville, TN	33	22	118	1576	31	9242	0	6042	3376	80
⊠ BRACKENRIDGE HOSPITAL, (Includes Children's Hospital of Austin), 601 East 15th Street, Zip 78701; tel. 512/476–6461; Charles J. Barnett, President **A**1 2 9 10 **F**4 7 8 10 12 13 15 16 17 19 21 22 23 25 28 29 30 31 32 34 35 37 38 39 40 41 42 43 44 46 47 49 53 56 60 63 64 65 66 67 69 70 71 72 73 74 **P**5 7 8 **S** Daughters of Charity National Health System, Saint Louis, MO	23	10	291	14826	189	143842	2728	142021	50859	1138
□ CHARTER BEHAVIORAL HEALTH SYSTEM OF AUSTIN, 8402 Cross Park Drive, Zip 78754, Mailing Address: P.O. Box 140585, Zip 78714–0585; tel. 512/837–1800; Armin Steege, Chief Executive Officer (Nonreporting) **A**1 9 10 **S** Magellan Health Services, Atlanta, GA	33	22	40	—	—	—	—	—	—	—
CHRISTOPHER HOUSE, (HIV – AIDS), 2820 East Martin Luther King, Zip 78702; tel. 512/370–8500; Carol Cody, Administrator **A**10 **F**14 15 19 21 31 34 35 60 65 71 73 **P**8	23	49	15	253	7	11	0	2442	1130	32
⊠ COLUMBIA ST. DAVID'S HOSPITAL, (Formerly St. David's Hospital), 919 East 32nd Street, Zip 78705, Mailing Address: Box 4039, Zip 78765–4039; tel. 512/476–7111; Cole C. Eslyn, Chief Executive Officer **A**1 2 9 10 **F**1 2 3 4 7 8 10 12 14 15 16 17 18 19 21 22 23 24 25 27 28 29 30 31 32 34 35 36 37 38 39 40 41 42 43 44 45 46 48 49 52 53 54 55 57 58 59 60 61 63 64 65 66 67 68 69 71 72 73 74 **P**1 3 7 8 **S** Columbia/St. David's Medical Center, Austin, TX **N** Columbia Saint David's Health Network, Austin, TX	32	10	296	19416	195	65203	4266	108631	46415	1370
⊠ COLUMBIA ST. DAVID'S SOUTH HOSPITAL, (Formerly Columbia South Austin Medical Center), 901 West Ben White Boulevard, Zip 78704–6903; tel. 512/447–2211; Richard W. Klusmann, Chief Executive Officer **A**1 9 10 **F**4 7 8 10 12 15 19 21 22 23 28 30 33 34 35 37 40 42 43 44 49 60 64 65 67 71 73 74 **P**1 7 **S** Columbia/HCA Healthcare Corporation, Nashville, TN **N** Columbia Saint David's Health Network, Austin, TX	33	10	164	6953	95	206052	890	60364	25084	583
□ △ HEALTHCARE REHABILITATION CENTER, 1106 West Dittmar, Zip 78745–9990, Mailing Address: P.O. Box 150459, Zip 78715–0459; tel. 512/444–4835; James G. Dalzell, Chief Executive Officer **A**1 7 10 **F**12 16 34 39 41 45 46 49 52 65 **S** Healthcare America, Inc., Austin, TX	33	46	30	101	17	3369	0	—	—	35
□ △ HEALTHSOUTH REHABILITATION HOSPITAL OF AUSTIN, 1215 Red River Street, Zip 78701, Mailing Address: P.O. Box 13366, Zip 78711–3366; tel. 512/474–5700; William O. Mitchell, Jr., Chief Executive Officer (Total facility includes 20 beds in nursing home–type unit) **A**1 7 9 10 **F**12 15 16 46 48 49 64 67 73 **S** HEALTHSOUTH Corporation, Birmingham, AL	33	46	70	1129	45	24587	0	12064	6220	231
MERIDELL ACHIEVEMENT CENTER, Mailing Address: P.O. Box 87, Liberty Hill, Zip 78642; tel. 800/366–8656; Scott McAvoy, Managing Director (Nonreporting) **S** Universal Health Services, Inc., King of Prussia, PA	33	52	78							
□ OAKS PSYCHIATRIC HEALTH SYSTEM, (Formerly Oaks Treatment Center), 1407 West Stassney Lane, Zip 78745; tel. 512/464–0400; Mack Wigley, Chief Executive Officer **A**1 **F**1 2 3 6 22 48 49 52 53 54 55 56 57 58 59 64 67 **P**6 7 **S** Healthcare America, Inc., Austin, TX	33	22	118	223	61	0	0	4455	2324	115
⊠ SETON MEDICAL CENTER, 1201 West 38th Street, Zip 78705–1056; tel. 512/323–1000; Charles J. Barnett, President **A**1 2 9 10 **F**4 7 8 10 12 13 15 16 17 19 21 22 23 25 27 28 29 30 31 32 34 35 37 38 39 40 41 42 43 44 46 47 49 53 56 60 61 63 64 65 66 67 69 70 71 72 73 74 **P**6 7 8 **S** Daughters of Charity National Health System, Saint Louis, MO	23	10	472	24436	321	233429	5804	176085	72396	2178
SHOAL CREEK HOSPITAL See BHC Shoal Creek Hospital										
□ SPECIALTY HOSPITAL OF AUSTIN, (LONG TERM ACUTE CARE), 4207 Burnet Road, Zip 78756; tel. 512/706–1900; William R. Cook, Chief Executive Officer **A**1 10 **F**12 14 19 20 22 26 27 35 37 44 60 65 67 69 71 **P**8	33	49	71	382	44	0	0	9754	5025	132
⊠ ST. DAVID'S PAVILION, 1025 East 32nd Street, Zip 78765; tel. 512/867–5800; Cole C. Eslyn, Chief Executive Officer **A**1 9 10 **F**1 3 4 7 8 10 11 12 14 15 16 18 19 21 22 23 24 25 26 27 28 29 30 31 32 34 35 36 37 38 39 40 41 42 43 44 45 46 48 49 52 53 54 55 57 58 59 60 61 63 64 65 66 67 69 71 72 73 74 **P**1 3 7 8 **S** Columbia/St. David's Medical Center, Austin, TX **N** Columbia Saint David's Health Network, Austin, TX	32	22	38	1107	23	4499	0	7458	2573	164
⊠ △ ST. DAVID'S REHABILITATION CENTER, 1005 East 32nd Street, Zip 78705, Mailing Address: P.O. Box 4270, Zip 78765–4270; tel. 512/867–5100; Cole C. Eslyn, Chief Executive Officer (Total facility includes 37 beds in nursing home–type unit) **A**1 7 9 10 **F**1 3 4 7 8 10 11 12 14 15 16 18 19 21 22 23 24 25 26 27 28 29 30 31 32 34 35 36 37 38 39 40 41 42 43 44 45 46 48 49 53 54 55 57 58 59 60 61 63 64 65 66 67 69 71 72 73 74 **P**1 3 7 8 **S** Columbia/St. David's Medical Center, Austin, TX **N** Columbia Saint David's Health Network, Austin, TX	32	46	104	1609	74	31342	0	19854	8631	188

AZLE—Tarrant County

Hospital	Control	Service	Beds	Admissions	Census	Outpatient Visits	Births	Total	Payroll	Personnel
⊠ HARRIS METHODIST NORTHWEST, 108 Denver Trail, Zip 76020; tel. 817/444–8600; Larry Thompson, Vice President and Administrator **A**1 9 10 **F**1 2 3 4 5 7 8 10 11 12 13 14 15 16 17 18 19 21 22 23 24 26 27 28 29 30 32 33 34 35 37 38 39 40 41 42 43 44 45 46 48 49 50 52 53 54 55 56 58 59 60 61 63 64 65 66 67 69 71 72 73 74 **P**2 5 7 **S** Harris Methodist Health System, Fort Worth, TX **N** The Heart Network of Texas, Irving, TX; North Texas Healthcare Network, Dallas, TX	21	10	36	1104	11	20201	1	9167	3740	99

Hospital, Address, Telephone, Administrator, Approval, Facility, and Physician Codes, Health Care System, Network	Classi-fication Codes		Utilization Data					Expense (thousands) of dollars		
★ American Hospital Association (AHA) membership □ Joint Commission on Accreditation of Healthcare Organizations (JCAHO) accreditation + American Osteopathic Hospital Association (AOHA) membership ○ American Osteopathic Association (AOA) accreditation △ Commission on Accreditation of Rehabilitation Facilities (CARF) accreditation Control codes 61, 63, 64, 71, 72 and 73 indicate hospitals listed by AOHA, but not registered by AHA. For definition of numerical codes, see page A4	Control	Service	Beds	Admissions	Census	Outpatient Visits	Births	Total	Payroll	Personnel

BAIRD—Callahan County

□ PINEYWOODS HOSPITAL, 1201 Frank Avenue, Zip 79504, Mailing Address: P.O. Box 1447, Lufkin, Zip 75902–1447; tel. 409/639–7590; Randy Garrett, Administrator **A**1 10 **F**1 2 3 6 12 17 18 22 52 53 55 56 58 65 **P**6 — 12 22 15 414 10 0 0 1476 822 36

BALLINGER—Runnels County

BALLINGER MEMORIAL HOSPITAL, 608 Avenue B, Zip 76821–2499; tel. 915/365–2531; Robert E. Vernor, Administrator **A**9 10 **F**14 15 16 22 24 28 31 65 71 73 — 16 10 16 341 4 7046 1 1970 1001 45

BAY CITY—Matagorda County

✠ MATAGORDA GENERAL HOSPITAL, 1115 Avenue G, Zip 77414–3544; tel. 409/245–6383; Wendell H. Baker, Jr., Chief Executive Officer **A**1 9 10 **F**4 7 8 10 12 16 19 20 21 22 24 26 28 30 31 32 33 34 35 37 39 40 44 54 57 65 67 71 **P**5 8 **S** Matagorda County Hospital District, Bay City, TX — 16 10 61 2292 21 22474 384 22001 10443 239

BAYTOWN—Harris County

□ BAYCOAST MEDICAL CENTER, 1700 James Bowie Drive, Zip 77520, Mailing Address: P.O. Box 1451, Zip 77520; tel. 713/420–6100; Frank T. Beirne, President and Chief Executive Officer **A**1 9 10 **F**7 8 10 11 12 15 16 19 20 21 22 23 28 29 30 32 33 34 35 37 39 40 41 42 44 45 46 48 63 64 65 71 72 73 74 **P**5 7 8 **S** Paracelsus Healthcare Corporation, Houston, TX — 33 10 191 2966 38 39527 537 21362 9178 278

✠ SAN JACINTO METHODIST HOSPITAL, 4401 Garth Road, Zip 77521; tel. 281/420–8600; William Simmons, President and Chief Executive Officer (Total facility includes 45 beds in nursing home–type unit) **A**1 3 5 9 10 **F**1 3 4 6 7 8 10 12 15 19 22 25 27 28 30 32 33 34 35 37 40 41 42 44 45 46 48 49 51 53 54 55 56 58 59 60 64 65 69 71 73 **P**7 8 **S** Methodist Health Care System, Houston, TX **N** Gulf Coast Provider Network, Houston, TX — 21 10 231 8960 139 135154 1213 68790 29151 973

BEAUMONT—Jefferson County

✠ BAPTIST HOSPITAL OF SOUTHEAST TEXAS, College and 11th Streets, Zip 77701, Mailing Address: Drawer 1591, Zip 77704–1491; tel. 409/835–3781; David N. Parmer, President and Chief Executive Officer (Total facility includes 13 beds in nursing home–type unit) **A**1 5 9 10 **F**4 8 10 12 14 15 16 17 19 21 22 23 27 28 30 32 34 35 37 39 41 42 43 44 45 46 47 48 49 60 64 65 67 71 72 73 74 **P**3 5 8 — 23 10 170 6473 123 52055 0 54057 19362 655

✠ COLUMBIA BEAUMONT MEDICAL CENTER, (Formerly Columbia Beaumont Regional Medical Center), (Includes Fannin Pavilion of Beaumont Regional Medical Center, 3250 Fannin Street, tel. 409/833–1411), 3080 College, Zip 77701, Mailing Address: P.O. Box 5817, Zip 77726–5817; tel. 409/833–1411; Luis G. Silva, Chief Executive Officer and Regional Administrator **A**1 9 10 **F**2 3 7 8 12 14 15 16 19 20 22 26 27 28 30 31 32 35 37 38 40 41 42 44 45 52 53 54 55 56 57 58 59 64 65 67 71 73 74 **P**3 7 8 **S** Columbia/HCA Healthcare Corporation, Nashville, TN — 33 10 364 6326 100 46505 1421 41954 19487 540
FANNIN PAVILION OF BEAUMONT REGIONAL MEDICAL CENTER See Columbia Beaumont Medical Center

□ △ SOUTHEAST TEXAS REHABILITATION HOSPITAL, 3340 Plaza 10 Boulevard, Zip 77707; tel. 409/835–0835; David J. Holly, Chief Executive Officer (Total facility includes 18 beds in nursing home–type unit) **A**1 7 9 10 **F**12 19 24 25 27 28 32 34 35 48 49 64 65 67 71 73 **P**5 **S** Continental Medical Systems, Inc., Mechanicsburg, PA — 32 46 60 823 45 17928 0 13275 6112 168

✠ ST. ELIZABETH HOSPITAL, 2830 Calder Avenue, Zip 77702, Mailing Address: P.O. Box 5405, Zip 77726–5405; tel. 409/892–7171; Sister Mary Fatima McCarthy, Administrator (Total facility includes 17 beds in nursing home–type unit) **A**1 2 5 9 10 **F**4 5 7 8 10 11 12 13 14 15 16 17 19 20 21 22 23 24 26 27 28 29 30 31 32 33 34 35 37 38 39 40 41 42 43 44 45 46 47 48 49 51 60 64 65 66 67 71 73 74 **P**2 3 4 5 6 7 8 **S** Sisters of Charity of the Incarnate Word Healthcare System, Houston, TX **N** SouthEast Texas Integrated Community Health Network, Houston, TX — 21 10 480 19629 360 180409 1893 161827 69620 2137

BEDFORD—Tarrant County

✠ HARRIS METHODIST–HEB, (Includes Harris Methodist–Springwood, 1608 Hospital Parkway, Zip 76022; tel. 817/355–7700), 1600 Hospital Parkway, Zip 76022–6913, Mailing Address: P.O. Box 669, Zip 76095; tel. 817/685–4000; Jack McCabe, Senior Vice President and Administrator (Total facility includes 15 beds in nursing home–type unit) **A**1 2 9 10 **F**2 3 4 7 8 10 12 14 15 16 17 18 19 21 22 23 24 28 30 31 32 34 35 37 39 40 41 42 43 44 45 46 48 49 52 53 54 55 56 58 59 60 64 65 67 71 73 74 **P**2 5 7 **S** Harris Methodist Health System, Fort Worth, TX **N** The Heart Network of Texas, Irving, TX; North Texas Healthcare Network, Dallas, TX — 21 10 186 9605 102 60699 1817 82607 31779 1032

BEEVILLE—Bee County

□ SPOHN BEE COUNTY HOSPITAL, (Formerly Bee County Regional Medical Center), 1500 East Houston Street, Zip 78102; tel. 512/354–2125; Andrew E. Anderson, Jr., Administrator **A**1 9 10 **F**8 15 19 22 28 34 35 37 44 45 46 49 65 70 71 73 — 13 10 59 3509 35 34253 391 15204 6738 288

BELLVILLE—Austin County

□ BELLVILLE GENERAL HOSPITAL, 44 North Cummings, Zip 77418–0148, Mailing Address: Box 977, Zip 77418; tel. 409/865–3141; Bob Ellzey, Administrator **A**1 9 10 **F**8 12 19 21 22 26 28 30 32 34 44 49 60 65 71 73 **P**3 — 16 10 30 710 8 22426 110 5429 2337 93

BIG LAKE—Reagan County

REAGAN MEMORIAL HOSPITAL, 805 North Main Street, Zip 76932; tel. 915/884–2561; Ron Galloway, Administrator (Total facility includes 48 beds in nursing home–type unit) **A**9 **F**22 24 26 28 49 64 66 **N** Permian Basin Rural Health Network, Fort Stockton, TX — 16 10 62 122 36 — 1 3007 1612 58

Hospital, Address, Telephone, Administrator, Approval, Facility, and Physician Codes, Health Care System, Network	Classi-fication Codes		Utilization Data					Expense (thousands) of dollars		
★ American Hospital Association (AHA) membership □ Joint Commission on Accreditation of Healthcare Organizations (JCAHO) accreditation + American Osteopathic Hospital Association (AOHA) membership ○ American Osteopathic Association (AOA) accreditation △ Commission on Accreditation of Rehabilitation Facilities (CARF) accreditation Control codes 61, 63, 64, 71, 72 and 73 indicate hospitals listed by AOHA, but not registered by AHA. For definition of numerical codes, see page A4	Control	Service	Beds	Admissions	Census	Outpatient Visits	Births	Total	Payroll	Personnel

BIG SPRING—Howard County

□ BIG SPRING STATE HOSPITAL, Lamesa Highway, Zip 79720, Mailing Address: P.O. Box 231, Zip 79721–0231; tel. 915/267–8216; Edward Moughon, Superintendent **A**1 9 10 **F**14 15 16 17 18 19 20 22 26 35 44 45 49 52 53 55 56 57 65 71 73 **P**5 **N** Permian Basin Rural Health Network, Fort Stockton, TX	12	22	279	888	241	0	0	34902	20296	702
□ SCENIC MOUNTAIN MEDICAL CENTER, 1601 West 11th Place, Zip 79720; tel. 915/263–1211; Kenneth W. Randall, Administrator **A**1 9 10 **F**12 16 19 21 22 23 27 28 31 32 34 35 37 40 41 44 46 48 49 52 57 63 65 71 **P**5 7 8 **S** Community Health Systems, Inc., Brentwood, TN **N** Permian Basin Rural Health Network, Fort Stockton, TX	33	10	113	4093	53	17458	276	19586	7499	272
⊞ VETERANS AFFAIRS MEDICAL CENTER, 300 Veterans Boulevard, Zip 79720–5500; tel. 915/263–7361; Cary D. Brown, Director (Total facility includes 40 beds in nursing home–type unit) (Nonreporting) **A**1 2 3 5 **S** Department of Veterans Affairs, Washington, DC **N** Permian Basin Rural Health Network, Fort Stockton, TX	45	10	189	—	—	—	—	—	—	—

BONHAM—Fannin County

□ NORTHEAST MEDICAL CENTER, 504 Lipscomb Boulevard, Zip 75418–4096, Mailing Address: P.O. Drawer C, Zip 75418; tel. 903/583–8585; Kathleen G. Northcutt, Interim Chief Executive Officer (Total facility includes 10 beds in nursing home–type unit) **A**1 9 10 **F**8 12 19 22 28 32 33 34 35 37 41 42 44 49 60 64 65 67 71 73 **S** Community Health Systems, Inc., Brentwood, TN	32	10	46	1467	22	19799	1	10779	4832	173
⊞ SAM RAYBURN MEMORIAL VETERANS CENTER, 1201 East Ninth Street, Zip 75418; tel. 903/583–2111; Charles C. Freeman, Director (Total facility includes 120 beds in nursing home–type unit) **A**1 **F**3 12 17 20 22 24 26 27 28 34 39 46 49 51 54 57 58 64 65 67 73 74 **P**6 **S** Department of Veterans Affairs, Washington, DC	45	10	374	1389	311	67731	0	24743	14783	385

BORGER—Hutchinson County

⊞ GOLDEN PLAINS COMMUNITY HOSPITAL, 200 South McGee Street, Zip 79007; tel. 806/273–1100; Norman Lambert, Chief Executive Officer **A**1 9 10 **F**7 8 12 15 16 19 22 23 28 32 33 34 35 36 37 40 41 44 46 49 65 67 70 71 73	16	10	49	1239	11	16016	155	9377	3995	148

BOWIE—Montague County

★ BOWIE MEMORIAL HOSPITAL, 705 East Greenwood Avenue, Zip 76230; tel. 817/872–1126; Joyce Crumpler, R.N., Administrator **A**9 10 **F**1 14 15 16 19 28 32 33 37 44 49 65 70 71 **N** Texoma Health Network, Wichita Falls, TX	16	10	44	1345	14	42340	0	8432	4159	152

BRADY—McCulloch County

HEART OF TEXAS MEMORIAL HOSPITAL, Nine Road, Zip 76825–1150, Mailing Address: P.O. Box 1150, Zip 76825–1150; tel. 915/597–2901; Windell M. McCord, Administrator **A**9 10 **F**19 22 24 28 44 49 71 73	16	10	27	718	8	25985	0	4008	1955	83

BRECKENRIDGE—Stephens County

STEPHENS MEMORIAL HOSPITAL, 200 South Geneva Street, Zip 76424; tel. 817/559–2241; James Reese, CHE, Administrator **A**9 10 **F**7 8 15 16 19 22 24 26 28 30 32 34 36 40 44 49 51 65 70 71 73	13	10	33	901	13	22657	55	5402	2679	113

BRENHAM—Washington County

⊞ TRINITY COMMUNITY MEDICAL CENTER OF BRENHAM, 700 Medical Parkway, Zip 77833; tel. 409/836–6173; John L. Simms, President and Chief Executive Officer **A**1 9 10 **F**7 14 15 16 19 20 21 23 26 28 32 44 49 65 70 71 73 **S** Franciscan Services Corporation, Sylvania, OH	21	10	60	2321	27	24531	318	15383	6378	232

BROWNFIELD—Terry County

⊞ BROWNFIELD REGIONAL MEDICAL CENTER, 705 East Felt, Zip 79316–3439; tel. 806/637–3551; Mike Click, Administrator **A**1 9 10 **F**7 8 14 15 16 17 19 21 22 24 28 29 30 31 32 34 40 44 46 49 65 69 70 71 73 **N** Lubbock Methodist Hospital System, Lubbock, TX	16	10	42	726	10	53401	150	7531	3951	166

BROWNSVILLE—Cameron County

□ BROWNSVILLE MEDICAL CENTER, 1040 West Jefferson Street, Zip 78520–5829, Mailing Address: Box 3590, Zip 78523–3590; tel. 210/544–1400; Robert Collete, Chief Executive Officer (Total facility includes 11 beds in nursing home–type unit) **A**1 9 10 **F**4 8 10 14 15 16 19 22 23 27 28 30 32 34 35 37 38 40 41 43 44 46 49 51 64 65 71 72 73 74 **P**1 7 **S** TENET Healthcare Corporation, Santa Barbara, CA	32	10	196	9339	152	57277	1700	60579	21897	733
⊞ COLUMBIA VALLEY REGIONAL MEDICAL CENTER, 1 Ted Hunt Boulevard, Zip 78521, Mailing Address: Box 3710, Zip 78521; tel. 210/831–9611; Pete Delgado, Chief Executive Officer **A**1 9 10 **F**4 7 8 10 11 12 14 15 16 17 21 22 27 28 30 32 34 35 37 38 39 40 41 43 44 48 49 50 54 55 56 64 65 67 71 73 74 **P**5 7 **S** Columbia/HCA Healthcare Corporation, Nashville, TN **N** Columbia Healthcare – South Texas Division, Corpus Christi, TX	33	10	173	7872	100	46681	3076	43262	17719	542

BROWNWOOD—Brown County

⊞ COLUMBIA BROWNWOOD REGIONAL MEDICAL CENTER, 1501 Burnet Drive, Zip 76801, Mailing Address: Box 760, Zip 76804; tel. 915/646–8541; Art Layne, Administrator and Chief Executive Officer (Total facility includes 20 beds in nursing home–type unit) **A**1 9 10 **F**7 8 10 12 14 15 16 17 19 21 22 23 24 25 28 30 32 34 35 36 37 39 40 41 42 44 45 46 48 49 51 52 54 57 58 59 60 63 64 65 67 71 73 74 **P**7 **S** Columbia/HCA Healthcare Corporation, Nashville, TN	33	10	164	6926	96	120050	783	42640	16361	580

BRYAN—Brazos County

⊞ ST. JOSEPH REGIONAL HEALTH CENTER, 2801 Franciscan Drive, Zip 77802; tel. 409/776–3777; Sister Gretchen Kunz, President and Chief Executive Officer (Total facility includes 9 beds in nursing home–type unit) **A**1 3 5 9 10 **F**3 4 7 8 10 11 12 14 15 16 17 19 21 22 23 25 26 28 29 30 31 32 33 34 35 37 39 40 41 42 43 44 45 49 54 55 56 58 60 63 64 65 67 71 72 73 **P**7 8 **S** Franciscan Services Corporation, Sylvania, OH	21	10	195	11248	141	149570	1836	87690	33884	1163

Hospital, Address, Telephone, Administrator, Approval, Facility, and Physician Codes, Health Care System, Network	Classification Codes		Utilization Data					Expense (thousands) of dollars		
	Control	Service	Beds	Admissions	Census	Outpatient Visits	Births	Total	Payroll	Personnel

Key to approval codes:
- ★ American Hospital Association (AHA) membership
- □ Joint Commission on Accreditation of Healthcare Organizations (JCAHO) accreditation
- + American Osteopathic Hospital Association (AOHA) membership
- ○ American Osteopathic Association (AOA) accreditation
- △ Commission on Accreditation of Rehabilitation Facilities (CARF) accreditation

Control codes 61, 63, 64, 71, 72 and 73 indicate hospitals listed by AOHA, but not registered by AHA. For definition of numerical codes, see page A4.

BURLESON—Johnson County

✠ HUGULEY MEMORIAL MEDICAL CENTER, 11801 South Freeway, Zip 76028, Mailing Address: Box 6337, Fort Worth, Zip 76115–0337; tel. 817/293–9110; A. David Jimenez, President and Chief Executive Officer (Total facility includes 33 beds in nursing home–type unit) **A**1 9 10 **F**2 3 7 8 10 11 12 13 14 15 16 17 19 21 22 23 24 25 26 28 29 30 32 33 34 35 37 38 39 40 41 42 44 45 46 47 49 51 52 53 54 55 56 57 58 59 60 62 63 64 65 67 69 71 73 74 **P**1 3 5 6 7 **S** Adventist Health System Sunbelt Health Care Corporation, Winter Park, FL
| | 21 | 10 | 154 | 7016 | 97 | 89427 | 1128 | 66394 | 26173 | 981 |

BURNET—Burnet County

✠ HIGHLAND LAKES MEDICAL CENTER, Highway 281 South, Zip 78611, Mailing Address: P.O. Box 840, Zip 78611; tel. 512/756–6000; James R. Giffin, Interim Administrator **A**1 9 10 **F**19 22 32 33 42 44 71 **S** Quorum Health Group/Quorum Health Resources, Inc., Brentwood, TN
| | 16 | 10 | 42 | 1075 | 12 | 18780 | 1 | 8397 | 3434 | 135 |

CALDWELL—Burleson County

★ BURLESON ST. JOSEPH HEALTH CENTER, 1101 Woodson Drive, Zip 77836, Mailing Address: P.O. Drawer 360, Zip 77836; tel. 409/567–3245; William H. Craig, President and Chief Executive Officer **A**9 10 **F**8 13 14 15 16 17 19 21 22 25 26 28 29 30 32 34 44 46 49 65 71 73 **P**5 7 8 **S** Franciscan Services Corporation, Sylvania, OH
| | 21 | 10 | 30 | 321 | 5 | 14813 | 0 | 5310 | 2105 | 96 |

CAMERON—Milam County

CENTRAL TEXAS HOSPITAL, 806 North Crockett, Zip 76520; tel. 817/697–6591; Louis West, President **A**9 10 **F**14 15 19 22 28 30 37 44 49 71 **N** Central Texas Rural Health Network, Harrietsville, TX; Brazo's Valley Health Network, Waco, TX
| | 23 | 10 | 34 | 491 | 7 | 8141 | 3 | — | — | 60 |

CANADIAN—Hemphill County

HEMPHILL COUNTY HOSPITAL, 1020 South Fourth Street, Zip 79014; tel. 806/323–6422; Robert Ezzell, Administrator **A**9 10 **F**8 12 15 17 26 27 28 32 33 36 39 45 46 49 51 65 70 71
| | 16 | 10 | 19 | 176 | 2 | 13215 | 0 | 3290 | 1549 | 72 |

CANYON—Randall County

✠ PALO DURO HOSPITAL, 2 Hospital Drive, Zip 79015–3199; tel. 806/655–7751; Larry Baggett, Administrator **A**1 9 10 **F**2 3 15 16 19 20 22 26 28 31 32 34 36 39 41 44 45 49 52 54 55 56 58 65 66 67 69 71 73
| | 16 | 10 | 49 | 720 | 5 | — | 0 | 7446 | 3498 | 130 |

CARRIZO SPRINGS—Dimmit County

DIMMIT COUNTY MEMORIAL HOSPITAL, 704 Hospital Drive, Zip 78834; tel. 210/876–2424; Ernest Flores, Jr., Administrator **A**9 10 **F**7 14 15 19 22 28 32 34 37 40 44 61 70 71 **N** Southwest Texas Rural Health Alliance, San Antonio, TX
| | 13 | 10 | 35 | 919 | 11 | 12818 | 107 | 5094 | 2448 | 123 |

CARROLLTON—Denton County

□ TRINITY MEDICAL CENTER, 4343 North Josey Lane, Zip 75010; tel. 214/492–1010; Thomas E. Casaday, President **A**1 9 10 **F**4 7 8 10 12 15 17 19 20 21 22 25 26 28 29 30 32 34 35 37 38 39 40 41 42 43 44 45 46 49 50 58 59 61 63 64 65 66 67 71 72 73 74 **P**3 **S** TENET Healthcare Corporation, Santa Barbara, CA
| | 33 | 10 | 149 | 5134 | 44 | 68105 | 1805 | 40430 | 13118 | 371 |

CARTHAGE—Panola County

□ PANOLA GENERAL HOSPITAL, 409 Cottage Road, Zip 75633, Mailing Address: Box 549, Zip 75633–0549; tel. 903/693–3841; Gary Mikeal Hudson, Administrator **A**1 9 10 **F**8 16 19 22 32 37 44 70 71 73 **N** Healthcare Partners of East Texas, Inc., Tyler, TX; Regional Healthcare Alliance, Tyler, TX
| | 13 | 10 | 30 | 983 | 13 | — | 0 | 8871 | 3979 | 168 |

CENTER—Shelby County

□ MEMORIAL HOSPITAL, 602 Hurst Street, Zip 75935, Mailing Address: Box 1749, Zip 75935–1749; tel. 409/598–2781; Robert V. Deen, Administrator and Chief Executive Officer **A**1 9 10 **F**8 12 15 16 19 21 22 30 32 33 40 44 49 65 70 71 **S** Park Healthcare Company, Nashville, TN **N** Healthcare Partners of East Texas, Inc., Tyler, TX
| | 33 | 10 | 48 | 1264 | 13 | 40022 | 125 | 8361 | 3437 | 131 |

CENTER POINT—Kerr County

□ STARLITE VILLAGE HOSPITAL, Elm Pass Road, Zip 78010, Mailing Address: Box 317, Zip 78010–0317; tel. 210/634–2212; Chas H. Williams, M.D., Administrator **A**1 9 10 **F**2 3 18 22 34 39 52 56 57 58 59 65 67 **P**5
| | 33 | 82 | 42 | 1352 | 20 | 5071 | 0 | 3373 | 1510 | 83 |

CHANNELVIEW—Harris County

SUN BELT REGIONAL MEDICAL CENTER EAST See Columbia East Houston Medical Center, Houston

CHILDRESS—Childress County

□ CHILDRESS REGIONAL MEDICAL CENTER, Highway 83 North, Zip 79201, Mailing Address: Box 1030, Zip 79201; tel. 817/937–6371; Frances T. Smith, Administrator **A**1 9 10 **F**8 12 13 14 15 16 17 19 21 22 26 27 28 29 30 31 32 33 34 39 40 44 45 46 49 51 65 66 67 70 71 73
| | 16 | 10 | 35 | 1019 | 10 | 24789 | 209 | 7287 | 3477 | 167 |

CHILLICOTHE—Hardeman County

CHILLICOTHE HOSPITAL DISTRICT, 303 Avenue I, Zip 79225, Mailing Address: Box 370, Zip 79225; tel. 817/852–5131; Linda Hall, Administrator **A**9 10 **F**12 15 16 19 21 22 28 30 32 35 44 65 69 70 71 73 **N** Texoma Health Network, Wichita Falls, TX
| | 16 | 10 | 12 | 101 | 1 | 491 | 0 | 1222 | 633 | 26 |

CLARKSVILLE—Red River County

✠ EAST TEXAS MEDICAL CENTER–CLARKSVILLE, Highway 82 West, Zip 75426, Mailing Address: Box 1270, Zip 75426; tel. 903/427–3851; Terry Cutler, Executive Director **A**1 9 10 **F**8 14 15 19 22 28 30 32 34 37 39 44 45 46 49 65 71 **S** East Texas Medical Center Regional Healthcare System, Tyler, TX
| | 16 | 10 | 36 | 1292 | 15 | 16036 | 0 | 6609 | 2710 | 120 |

Hospital, Address, Telephone, Administrator, Approval, Facility, and Physician Codes, Health Care System, Network	Classi-fication Codes		Utilization Data					Expense (thousands) of dollars		
★ American Hospital Association (AHA) membership □ Joint Commission on Accreditation of Healthcare Organizations (JCAHO) accreditation + American Osteopathic Hospital Association (AOHA) membership ○ American Osteopathic Association (AOA) accreditation △ Commission on Accreditation of Rehabilitation Facilities (CARF) accreditation Control codes 61, 63, 64, 71, 72 and 73 indicate hospitals listed by AOHA, but not registered by AHA. For definition of numerical codes, see page A4	Control	Service	Beds	Admissions	Census	Outpatient Visits	Births	Total	Payroll	Personnel

CLEBURNE—Johnson County

☒ WALLS REGIONAL HOSPITAL, 201 Walls Drive, Zip 76031; tel. 817/641–2551; Brent D. Magers, FACHE, Chief Executive Officer and Administrator (Total facility includes 12 beds in nursing home–type unit) **A**1 9 10 **F**3 4 7 8 10 12 13 14 15 16 17 19 21 22 23 24 26 27 28 29 30 31 32 33 34 35 37 39 40 41 42 43 44 45 46 49 51 53 54 55 56 58 59 61 63 64 65 66 67 69 70 71 73 74 **P**2 5 7 **S** Harris Methodist Health System, Fort Worth, TX **N** The Heart Network of Texas, Irving, TX; North Texas Healthcare Network, Dallas, TX

| | 21 | 10 | 112 | 3209 | 34 | 81814 | 648 | 21802 | 9166 | 338 |

CLEVELAND—Liberty County

□ CLEVELAND REGIONAL MEDICAL CENTER, 300 East Crockett Street, Zip 77327, Mailing Address: Box 1688, Zip 77328; tel. 713/593–1811; A. C. Buchanon, Administrator (Total facility includes 11 beds in nursing home–type unit) **A**1 9 10 **F**7 8 12 15 16 19 21 22 23 27 28 30 32 33 34 35 37 39 40 41 42 46 49 54 64 65 71 73 **P**7 8 **S** Community Health Systems, Inc., Brentwood, TN

| | 32 | 10 | 115 | 3328 | 36 | 27802 | 428 | 20644 | 8287 | 306 |

CLIFTON—Bosque County

★ GOODALL–WITCHER HOSPITAL, 101 South Avenue T, Zip 76634, Mailing Address: Box 549, Zip 76634; tel. 817/675–8322; Jim B. Smith, President and Chief Executive Officer (Total facility includes 30 beds in nursing home–type unit) **A**9 10 **F**7 8 15 19 21 22 28 30 32 34 37 40 44 49 64 65 70 71 73 **P**3 **N** Central Texas Rural Health Network, Harrietsville, TX; Brazo's Valley Health Network, Waco, TX

| | 23 | 10 | 70 | 1374 | 15 | 28002 | 209 | 10322 | 4283 | 173 |

COLEMAN—Coleman County

COLEMAN COUNTY MEDICAL CENTER, 310 South Pecos Street, Zip 76834; tel. 915/625–2135; Michael Morris, Administrator **A**9 10 **F**14 15 16 19 22 24 34 36 39 44 71 73

| | 16 | 10 | 46 | 724 | 6 | 3653 | 0 | 2929 | 1372 | 58 |

COLLEGE STATION—Brazos County

☒ COLUMBIA MEDICAL CENTER, (Formerly Brazos Valley Medical Center), 1604 Rock Prairie Road, Zip 77845, Mailing Address: P.O. Box 10000, Zip 77842–3500; tel. 409/764–5100; Thomas W. Jackson, Chief Executive Officer (Total facility includes 6 beds in nursing home–type unit) **A**1 5 9 10 **F**7 8 10 12 15 16 19 21 22 23 24 30 31 32 35 37 38 40 41 44 49 64 65 71 **P**8 **S** Columbia/HCA Healthcare Corporation, Nashville, TN

| | 12 | 10 | 106 | 3953 | 40 | 42198 | 1020 | 23918 | 9477 | 298 |

COLORADO CITY—Mitchell County

★ MITCHELL COUNTY HOSPITAL, 1543 Chestnut Street, Zip 79512–3998; tel. 915/728–3431; Joe Wright, Administrator **A**9 10 **F**8 14 15 16 19 24 33 44 49 65 70 71 73 **P**6 **S** Lubbock Methodist Hospital System, Lubbock, TX **N** Lubbock Methodist Hospital System, Lubbock, TX

| | 16 | 10 | 36 | 869 | 10 | 52517 | 73 | 9268 | 5238 | 172 |

COLUMBUS—Colorado County

□ COLUMBUS COMMUNITY HOSPITAL, 110 Shult Drive, Zip 78934, Mailing Address: Box 865, Zip 78934; tel. 409/732–2371; Robert Thomas, Administrator (Nonreporting) **A**1 9 10

| | 23 | 10 | 36 | — | — | — | — | — | — | — |

COMANCHE—Comanche County

COMANCHE COMMUNITY HOSPITAL, 211 South Austin Street, Zip 76442; tel. 915/356–5241; W. Evan Moore, Administrator (Nonreporting) **A**9 10 **N** Lubbock Methodist Hospital System, Lubbock, TX

| | 16 | 10 | 21 | — | — | — | — | — | — | — |

CONROE—Montgomery County

☒ COLUMBIA CONROE REGIONAL MEDICAL CENTER, 504 Medical Boulevard, Zip 77304, Mailing Address: P.O. Box 1538, Zip 77305–1538; tel. 409/539–1111; Larry Kloess, Chief Executive Officer **A**1 3 9 10 **F**4 7 8 10 11 12 14 15 16 19 21 22 23 26 27 28 29 30 32 33 34 35 37 38 39 40 41 42 43 44 45 48 49 50 51 54 60 63 64 65 67 70 71 73 74 **P**2 5 7 8 **S** Columbia/HCA Healthcare Corporation, Nashville, TN

| | 33 | 10 | 242 | 12108 | 134 | 109840 | 1649 | 62269 | 27631 | 771 |

CORPUS CHRISTI—Nueces County

□ CHARTER BEHAVIORAL HEALTH SYSTEM–CORPUS CHRISTI, 3126 Rodd Field Road, Zip 78414; tel. 512/993–8893; Steve Kamber, Chief Executive Officer **A**1 9 10 **F**2 3 15 16 26 52 53 54 55 56 57 58 59 **P**1 7 **S** Magellan Health Services, Atlanta, GA

| | 33 | 22 | 80 | 1303 | 31 | 911 | 0 | 7333 | 3538 | 96 |

☒ COLUMBIA BAY AREA MEDICAL CENTER, 7101 South Padre Island Drive, Zip 78412; tel. 512/985–1200; Kirk G. Wilson, Chief Executive Officer (Total facility includes 16 beds in nursing home–type unit) **A**1 9 10 12 13 **F**3 4 7 8 10 12 15 16 19 21 22 26 28 30 31 32 34 35 39 40 41 42 43 44 49 53 54 55 56 57 59 60 64 65 67 69 71 73 74 **P**1 7 **S** Columbia/HCA Healthcare Corporation, Nashville, TN **N** Columbia Healthcare – South Texas Division, Corpus Christi, TX

| | 32 | 10 | 144 | 7032 | 90 | 36294 | — | 60981 | 21176 | 627 |

☒ COLUMBIA BAYVIEW PSYCHIATRIC CENTER, 6226 Saratoga Boulevard, Zip 78414; tel. 512/993–9700; Janie L. Harwood, Chief Executive Officer **A**1 9 10 **F**2 3 4 5 6 7 8 9 10 11 12 14 15 16 17 18 19 21 22 23 24 25 26 28 29 30 31 32 35 37 38 40 42 43 44 47 48 49 50 51 52 53 54 55 56 57 58 59 60 63 64 70 71 73 74 **P**8 **S** Columbia/HCA Healthcare Corporation, Nashville, TN **N** Columbia Healthcare – South Texas Division, Corpus Christi, TX

| | 33 | 22 | 40 | 1083 | 24 | 3356 | 0 | 5321 | 2635 | 86 |

☒ COLUMBIA DOCTORS REGIONAL MEDICAL CENTER, 3315 South Alameda, Zip 78411, Mailing Address: P.O. Box 3828, Zip 78463–3828; tel. 512/857–1501; Steven Woerner, Chief Executive Officer (Total facility includes 26 beds in nursing home–type unit) **A**1 9 10 **F**2 3 4 7 8 10 11 12 14 15 16 17 18 19 20 21 22 23 25 27 28 29 30 31 32 33 34 35 37 38 39 40 41 42 43 44 45 46 48 49 51 54 55 56 57 58 59 60 65 66 68 69 71 73 74 **P**3 5 7 8 **S** Columbia/HCA Healthcare Corporation, Nashville, TN **N** Columbia Healthcare – South Texas Division, Corpus Christi, TX

| | 32 | 10 | 237 | 10356 | 137 | 32570 | 2765 | 55605 | 21783 | 808 |

Hospital, Address, Telephone, Administrator, Approval, Facility, and Physician Codes, Health Care System, Network	Classification Codes		Utilization Data					Expense (thousands) of dollars		
	Control	Service	Beds	Admissions	Census	Outpatient Visits	Births	Total	Payroll	Personnel

★ American Hospital Association (AHA) membership
□ Joint Commission on Accreditation of Healthcare Organizations (JCAHO) accreditation
+ American Osteopathic Hospital Association (AOHA) membership
○ American Osteopathic Association (AOA) accreditation
△ Commission on Accreditation of Rehabilitation Facilities (CARF) accreditation
Control codes 61, 63, 64, 71, 72 and 73 indicate hospitals listed by AOHA, but not registered by AHA. For definition of numerical codes, see page A4

⊞ COLUMBIA NORTHWEST HOSPITAL, 13725 Farm Road 624, Zip 78410; tel. 512/767–4500; Winston Borland, Chief Executive Officer (Total facility includes 7 beds in nursing home–type unit) A1 9 10 F8 15 19 20 21 22 24 25 28 31 32 34 37 41 44 48 49 63 64 65 66 67 71 S Columbia/HCA Healthcare Corporation, Nashville, TN N Columbia Healthcare – South Texas Division, Corpus Christi, TX	33	10	63	2292	34	190524	0	30963	14739	558
⊞ △ COLUMBIA REHABILITATION HOSPITAL, 6226 Saratoga Boulevard, Zip 78414–3499; tel. 512/991–9690; Jo Ann Baker, Chief Executive Officer A1 7 9 10 F2 3 4 7 8 10 12 15 16 19 20 21 22 25 26 27 28 29 30 31 32 34 35 37 38 39 40 41 42 43 44 45 48 49 52 53 54 55 56 57 58 59 64 65 69 71 73 74 P5 8 S Columbia/HCA Healthcare Corporation, Nashville, TN N Columbia Healthcare – South Texas Division, Corpus Christi, TX	32	46	40	623	28	5516	0	9873	4299	149
⊞ DRISCOLL CHILDREN'S HOSPITAL, 3533 South Alameda Street, Zip 78411, Mailing Address: Box 6530, Zip 78466–6530; tel. 512/850–5000; J. E. Ted Stibbards, Ph.D., President and Chief Executive Officer A1 3 5 9 10 F4 5 10 12 14 15 16 17 19 21 22 25 27 28 29 30 31 34 35 38 39 41 42 43 44 45 47 48 49 51 60 63 65 66 67 68 69 71 72 73 74 N SouthEast Texas Hospital System, Dallas, TX	23	50	180	6908	117	91040	0	65955	27380	1022
⊞ NAVAL HOSPITAL, 10651 E Street, Zip 78419–5131; tel. 512/939–2685; Captain F. G. Barina, Jr., Commanding Officer (Nonreporting) A1 S Department of Navy, Washington, DC	43	10	25	—	—	—	—	—	—	—
⊞ △ SPOHN HEALTH SYSTEM, 600 Elizabeth Street, Zip 78404–2235; tel. 512/881–3000; Jake Henry, Jr., President (Nonreporting) A1 2 7 9 10 S Incarnate Word Health Services, San Antonio, TX	21	10	486	—	—	—	—	—	—	—
⊞ SPOHN MEMORIAL HOSPITAL, (Formerly Memorial Medical Center), 2606 Hospital Boulevard, Zip 78405–1818, Mailing Address: Box 5280, Zip 78465–5280; tel. 512/902–4000; Anthony W. Heep, Vice President and Administrator (Total facility includes 16 beds in nursing home–type unit) A1 3 9 10 F4 5 7 8 9 10 11 12 14 15 16 17 18 19 20 21 22 26 27 28 29 30 31 32 34 35 37 39 40 42 43 44 45 46 49 50 51 52 53 54 55 56 57 58 59 60 63 64 65 69 71 72 73	16	10	253	9027	157	172501	798	104104	41017	1092

CORSICANA—Navarro County
⊞ COLUMBIA NAVARRO REGIONAL HOSPITAL, 3201 West Highway 22, Zip 75110; tel. 903/872–4861; Nancy A. Byrnes, President and Chief Executive Officer A1 9 10 F7 8 10 14 15 16 19 20 22 23 28 30 31 35 37 39 40 41 42 44 48 49 64 65 71 73 P5 S Columbia/HCA Healthcare Corporation, Nashville, TN	33	10	148	4107	66	53429	461	29798	10417	368

CRANE—Crane County
★ CRANE MEMORIAL HOSPITAL, 1310 South Alford, Zip 79731; tel. 915/558–3555; Michele Aguilar, Administrator (Nonreporting) A9 10 N Permian Basin Rural Health Network, Fort Stockton, TX	13	10	28	—	—	—	—	—	—	—

CROCKETT—Houston County
⊞ EAST TEXAS MEDICAL CENTER, 1100 Loop 304 East, Zip 75835–1810; tel. 409/544–2002; Dale E. Clark, Ph.D., Administrator and Chief Executive Officer (Nonreporting) A1 9 10 S East Texas Medical Center Regional Healthcare System, Tyler, TX N Regional Healthcare Alliance, Tyler, TX	16	10	54	—	—	—	—	—	—	—

CROSBYTON—Crosby County
★ CROSBYTON CLINIC HOSPITAL, 710 West Main Street, Zip 79322; tel. 806/675–2382; Michael Johnson, Administrator and Chief Executive Officer A9 10 F2 3 4 7 8 10 11 12 15 16 17 18 19 20 21 22 24 28 29 30 32 34 35 37 38 39 40 41 42 43 44 45 46 47 48 49 51 52 53 54 55 57 58 59 60 64 65 71 73 74 P6 S St. Joseph Health System, Orange, CA	23	10	35	898	11	20369	0	4020	2254	96

CUERO—De Witt County
⊞ CUERO COMMUNITY HOSPITAL, 2550 North Esplanade, Zip 77954; tel. 512/275–6191; James E. Buckner, Jr., Administrator A1 9 10 F7 8 14 15 16 19 21 22 25 28 30 31 32 34 35 37 39 40 44 45 49 51 65 70 71 73 N SouthEast Texas Hospital System, Dallas, TX	16	10	49	2097	27	130089	136	16567	7278	341

DALHART—Dallam County
□ COON MEMORIAL HOSPITAL AND HOME, 1411 Denver Avenue, Zip 79022; tel. 806/249–4571; Leroy Schaffner, Chief Executive Officer A1 9 10 F7 14 15 17 19 22 28 34 36 40 44 45 49 71 73	16	10	28	378	3	10112	7	4188	1733	80

DALLAS—Dallas County
A. WEBB ROBERTS HOSPITAL See Baylor University Medical Center
★ BAYLOR CENTER FOR RESTORATIVE CARE, 3504 Swiss Avenue, Zip 75204; tel. 214/823–1684; Gerry Brueckner, R.N., Executive Director (Nonreporting) A9 10 S Baylor Health Care System, Dallas, TX N Baylor Health Care System Network, Dallas, TX; North Texas Health Network, Irving, TX; North Texas Healthcare Network, Dallas, TX	21	10	74	—	—	—	—	—	—	—
★ △ BAYLOR INSTITUTE FOR REHABILITATION, 3505 Gaston Avenue, Zip 75246–2018; tel. 214/826–7030; Judith C. Waterston, Executive Director A3 7 10 F2 3 4 5 7 8 9 10 11 12 14 15 16 17 19 21 22 23 24 25 26 27 28 29 30 31 32 33 34 35 37 38 39 40 41 42 43 44 45 48 49 51 52 53 56 57 58 60 61 64 65 66 67 69 70 71 73 74 P5 7 S Baylor Health Care System, Dallas, TX N North Texas Health Network, Irving, TX; North Texas Healthcare Network, Dallas, TX	21	46	92	1646	74	8863	0	19904	9958	353

Hospital, Address, Telephone, Administrator, Approval, Facility, and Physician Codes, Health Care System, Network	Classification Codes		Utilization Data					Expense (thousands) of dollars		
	Control	Service	Beds	Admissions	Census	Outpatient Visits	Births	Total	Payroll	Personnel

★ American Hospital Association (AHA) membership
□ Joint Commission on Accreditation of Healthcare Organizations (JCAHO) accreditation
+ American Osteopathic Hospital Association (AOHA) membership
○ American Osteopathic Association (AOA) accreditation
△ Commission on Accreditation of Rehabilitation Facilities (CARF) accreditation
Control codes 61, 63, 64, 71, 72 and 73 indicate hospitals listed by AOHA, but not registered by AHA. For definition of numerical codes, see page A4

Hospital	Control	Service	Beds	Admissions	Census	Outpatient Visits	Births	Total	Payroll	Personnel
⊞ BAYLOR UNIVERSITY MEDICAL CENTER, (Includes A. Webb Roberts Hospital, Erik and Margaret Jonsson Hospital, George W. Truett Memorial Hospital, Karl and Esther Hoblitzelle Memorial Hospital), 3500 Gaston Avenue, Zip 75246–2088; tel. 214/820–0111; Boone Powell, Jr., President **A**1 2 3 5 8 9 10 **F**3 4 5 7 8 10 11 12 15 17 18 19 20 21 22 23 24 26 28 29 30 31 32 33 34 35 36 37 38 39 40 41 42 43 44 45 46 48 49 52 54 55 56 57 58 59 60 61 63 64 65 66 67 69 70 71 73 74 **P**1 5 7 **S** Baylor Health Care System, Dallas, TX **N** National Cardiovascular Network, Atlanta, GA; Baylor Health Care System Network, Dallas, TX; The Heart Network of Texas, Irving, TX; North Texas Health Network, Irving, TX; North Texas Healthcare Network, Dallas, TX	21	10	827	35272	521	358425	3962	389384	159154	4939
⊞ CHARLTON METHODIST HOSPITAL, 3500 West Wheatland Road, Zip 75237–3460, Mailing Address: Box 225357, Zip 75222–5357; tel. 214/947–7500; Kim N. Hollon, FACHE, Executive Director **A**1 3 9 10 **F**4 7 8 10 11 12 14 15 17 19 21 22 24 26 27 28 30 31 32 33 34 35 37 38 39 40 41 42 43 44 48 49 51 54 55 56 60 61 63 64 65 66 67 69 70 71 73 74 **P**1 7 **S** Methodist Hospitals of Dallas, Dallas, TX	23	10	134	7789	97	88639	1409	45313	20531	666
⊞ CHILDREN'S MEDICAL CENTER OF DALLAS, 1935 Motor Street, Zip 75235; tel. 214/640–2000; George D. Farr, President and Chief Executive Officer **A**1 2 3 5 8 9 10 **F**4 10 13 15 16 17 19 20 21 22 25 27 28 30 31 32 34 35 39 41 42 43 44 45 46 47 49 51 52 53 54 55 56 58 59 63 65 66 67 69 71 73	23	50	224	10949	144	182698	0	160133	74790	2028
⊞ △ COLUMBIA HOSPITAL AT MEDICAL CITY DALLAS, (Formerly Medical City Dallas Hospital), 7777 Forest Lane, Zip 75230–2598; tel. 972/566–7000; Stephen Corbeil, President and Chief Executive Officer (Total facility includes 34 beds in nursing home–type unit) **A**1 2 7 9 10 **F**3 4 7 8 10 11 12 14 15 16 17 18 19 20 21 22 23 26 28 29 30 31 32 33 34 35 37 38 39 40 41 42 43 44 45 47 48 49 50 51 53 54 55 56 57 58 59 60 61 63 64 65 67 69 71 73 74 **P**3 5 7 8 **S** Columbia/HCA Healthcare Corporation, Nashville, TN	33	10	543	21586	299	95593	3946	203600	70490	2029
⊞ COLUMBIA MEDICAL ARTS HOSPITAL, (Formerly Medical Arts Hospital), 6161 Harry Hines Boulevard, Zip 75235; tel. 214/688–1111; Al Chapa, Chief Executive Officer **A**1 9 10 **F**12 19 35 44 **P**5 **S** Columbia/HCA Healthcare Corporation, Nashville, TN	33	10	30	264	3	4584	0	5978	1952	73
⊞ ○ COLUMBIA MEDICAL CENTER–DALLAS SOUTHWEST, 2929 South Hampton Road, Zip 75224; tel. 214/330–4611; James B. Warren, Chief Executive Officer **A**1 9 10 11 12 13 **F**2 3 4 7 8 9 10 11 12 14 15 16 19 20 21 22 23 25 26 27 28 29 30 31 32 33 34 35 37 39 40 41 42 43 44 45 46 47 48 49 50 52 53 54 55 56 57 58 59 60 61 63 64 65 66 67 69 70 71 73 74 **P**1 5 7 **S** Columbia/HCA Healthcare Corporation, Nashville, TN **N** Saint Paul Medical Center Affiliate Network, Dallas, TX	33	10	104	2017	25	18518	0	17446	7020	241
⊞ COLUMBIA SPECIALTY HOSPITAL AT MEDICAL ARTS, (LONG TERM ACUTE CARE), 6161 Harry Hines Boulevard, Zip 75235–5306; tel. 214/689–8500; Tim Simmons, Chief Executive Officer **A**1 10 **F**3 4 7 8 10 12 14 15 16 17 19 21 24 25 26 27 28 29 30 31 32 33 34 35 39 41 42 43 44 45 46 49 50 51 53 54 55 56 57 58 59 60 61 62 63 65 66 67 69 71 72 73 74 **P**1 5 7 8 **S** Columbia/HCA Healthcare Corporation, Nashville, TN	33	49	32	205	16	0	0	6695	3301	54
⊞ DALLAS COUNTY HOSPITAL DISTRICT–PARKLAND HEALTH AND HOSPITAL SYSTEM, 5201 Harry Hines Boulevard, Zip 75235–7731; tel. 214/590–8000; Ron J. Anderson, M.D., President and Chief Executive Officer **A**1 2 3 5 8 9 10 **F**4 5 7 8 9 10 11 12 14 15 16 17 18 19 20 21 22 23 25 26 28 29 30 31 34 35 37 38 39 40 41 42 43 44 45 46 48 49 51 52 54 55 56 57 58 60 61 63 65 67 68 69 70 71 73 74	16	10	805	40815	557	825658	13614	518465	193532	6647
□ DOCTORS HOSPITAL OF DALLAS, 9440 Poppy Drive, Zip 75218; tel. 214/324–6100; Robert S. Freymuller, Chief Executive Officer (Total facility includes 18 beds in nursing home–type unit) **A**1 9 10 **F**2 4 7 8 9 10 11 12 14 15 16 19 21 22 23 26 27 30 31 32 33 34 35 37 38 40 41 42 43 44 47 48 49 52 55 56 57 59 60 64 65 66 67 70 71 73 74 **P**5 7 **S** TENET Healthcare Corporation, Santa Barbara, CA ERIK AND MARGARET JONSSON HOSPITAL See Baylor University Medical Center GEORGE W. TRUETT MEMORIAL HOSPITAL See Baylor University Medical Center	33	10	197	8106	130	72852	508	57846	22977	671
□ GREEN OAKS HOSPITAL, 7808 Clodus Fields Drive, Zip 75251; tel. 214/991–9504; Thomas M. Collins, Administrator **A**1 9 10 **F**2 3 15 16 52 53 54 55 56 57 58 59	33	22	106	1952	42	8613	0	10668	4930	167
□ △ HEALTHSOUTH MEDICAL CENTER, 2124 Research Row, Zip 75235; tel. 214/904–6100; Robert M. Smart, Area Manager and Chief Executive Officer **A**1 7 10 **F**5 6 12 14 15 16 19 22 25 26 27 30 32 34 44 45 46 48 49 54 64 65 66 67 71 73 **S** HEALTHSOUTH Corporation, Birmingham, AL KARL AND ESTHER HOBLITZELLE MEMORIAL HOSPITAL See Baylor University Medical Center	33	46	106	1246	56	2782	0	19203	8029	202
★ MARY SHIELS HOSPITAL, 3515 Howell Street, Zip 75204; tel. 214/443–3000; Rob Shiels, Administrator **A**9 10 **F**34 44 45 46 49 MEDICAL ARTS HOSPITAL See Columbia Medical Arts Hospital MEDICAL CITY DALLAS HOSPITAL See Columbia Hospital at Medical City Dallas	33	10	15	393	2	2615	0	5845	2775	66
⊞ METHODIST MEDICAL CENTER, 1441 North Beckley Avenue, Zip 75203, Mailing Address: Box 655999, Zip 75265–5999; tel. 214/947–8181; John W. Carver, FACHE, Executive Director **A**1 2 3 5 8 9 10 **F**4 7 8 10 11 12 14 15 16 19 21 22 23 24 25 26 27 28 30 31 34 35 37 38 39 40 41 42 43 44 46 48 49 54 60 61 63 64 65 66 69 70 71 73 74 **P**1 7 **S** Methodist Hospitals of Dallas, Dallas, TX	23	10	374	13744	252	126950	2052	131691	57532	1698

Hospital, Address, Telephone, Administrator, Approval, Facility, and Physician Codes, Health Care System, Network	Classi-fication Codes		Utilization Data					Expense (thousands) of dollars		
★ American Hospital Association (AHA) membership □ Joint Commission on Accreditation of Healthcare Organizations (JCAHO) accreditation + American Osteopathic Hospital Association (AOHA) membership ○ American Osteopathic Association (AOA) accreditation △ Commission on Accreditation of Rehabilitation Facilities (CARF) accreditation Control codes 61, 63, 64, 71, 72 and 73 indicate hospitals listed by AOHA, but not registered by AHA. For definition of numerical codes, see page A4	Control	Service	Beds	Admissions	Census	Outpatient Visits	Births	Total	Payroll	Personnel
□ △ NORTH DALLAS REHABILITATION HOSPITAL, 8383 Meadow Road, Zip 75231; tel. 214/891–0880; Brian F. Wells, Administrator and Chief Executive Officer **A**1 7 9 10 **F**12 14 15 26 27 32 33 34 39 48 49 54 64 65 67 71 73	33	46	36	113	10	528	0	—	—	42
PEDIATRIC CENTER FOR RESTORATIVE CARE, 3301 Swiss Avenue, Zip 75204; tel. 214/828–4747; Geraldine Brueckner, Administrator (Nonreporting) **A**10 **N** North Texas Health Network, Irving, TX	21	50	26							
✠ △ PRESBYTERIAN HOSPITAL OF DALLAS, 8200 Walnut Hill Lane, Zip 75231–4402; tel. 214/345–6789; Mark H. Merrill, Executive Director (Total facility includes 78 beds in nursing home–type unit) **A**1 2 3 5 7 9 10 **F**4 5 6 7 8 10 11 12 13 14 15 16 17 18 19 21 22 23 24 25 26 27 28 29 30 31 32 33 34 35 36 37 38 39 40 41 42 43 44 45 46 48 49 50 51 52 53 54 55 56 57 58 59 60 61 62 63 64 65 66 67 71 72 73 74 **P**2 7 8 **S** Presbyterian Healthcare System, Dallas, TX **N** Presbyterian Healthcare System, Dallas, TX; North Texas Healthcare Network, Dallas, TX	23	10	637	21395	362	218079	4383	244971	91376	2537
□ RHD MEMORIAL MEDICAL CENTER, Seven Medical Parkway, Zip 75234, Mailing Address: P.O. Box 819094, Zip 75381–9094; tel. 214/247–1000; Thomas E. Casaday, President (Total facility includes 11 beds in nursing home–type unit) **A**1 9 10 **F**4 7 8 10 12 14 15 16 17 19 21 22 26 28 30 31 34 35 37 38 39 40 41 42 43 44 45 46 49 61 64 65 71 73 74 **P**1 3 5 7 8 **S** TENET Healthcare Corporation, Santa Barbara, CA	12	10	117	4205	52	54490	444	50340	13457	426
✠ ST. PAUL MEDICAL CENTER, 5909 Harry Hines Boulevard, Zip 75235; tel. 214/879–1000; Michael A. Austin, CPA, Administrator **A**1 2 3 5 8 9 10 **F**3 4 5 7 8 10 11 12 13 15 16 17 19 21 22 23 24 25 26 27 28 29 30 31 32 33 34 35 37 38 40 41 42 43 44 46 49 52 53 54 55 56 57 58 59 60 61 64 65 67 69 71 73 74 **P**2 3 5 7 **S** Harris Methodist Health System, Fort Worth, TX	21	10	309	13013	213	138180	2394	145225	59973	2012
✠ TEXAS SCOTTISH RITE HOSPITAL FOR CHILDREN, 2222 Welborn Street, Zip 75219–0567, Mailing Address: Box 190567, Zip 75219–0567; tel. 214/521–3168; J. C. Montgomery, Jr., President **A**1 3 5 9 **F**5 19 20 28 34 39 41 44 45 46 60 65 67 71 73 **P**6	23	57	64	2303	24	39269	0	—	—	
□ TIMBERLAWN MENTAL HEALTH SYSTEM, (Formerly Timberlawn Psychiatric Hospital), 4600 Samuell Boulevard, Zip 75228, Mailing Address: Box 151489, Zip 75315–1489; tel. 214/381–7181; Debra S. Lowrance, R.N., Chief Executive Officer and Managing Director **A**1 3 9 10 **F**2 3 15 16 34 52 53 54 55 56 57 58 59 65 **P**1 5 7 8 **S** Universal Health Services, Inc., King of Prussia, PA	33	22	124	2936	82		0	15117	6963	259
□ ○ TRI–CITY HEALTH CENTRE, 7525 Scyene Road, Zip 75227; tel. 214/381–7171; Patti Griffith, R.N., Administrator and Chief Executive Officer **A**1 10 11 12 13 **F**2 3 7 8 10 14 15 16 17 19 21 22 25 26 27 28 30 34 35 37 39 40 42 44 46 49 52 57 58 63 65 71 72 73 **P**1 6 8	23	10	131	3521	51	41504	612	39082	13526	487
□ VENCOR HOSPITAL–DALLAS, (LONG TERM ACUTE CARE), 1600 Abrams Road, Zip 75214–4499; tel. 214/818–2400; Dorothy J. Elford, Administrator **A**1 9 10 **F**22 37 65 **S** Vencor, Incorporated, Louisville, KY	33	49	55	241	33	0	0	9066	4833	254
✠ VETERANS AFFAIRS MEDICAL CENTER, 4500 South Lancaster Road, Zip 75216–7167; tel. 214/376–5451; Alan G. Harper, Director (Total facility includes 120 beds in nursing home–type unit) **A**1 2 3 5 8 **F**1 2 3 4 8 10 11 12 14 15 16 17 18 19 20 21 22 25 26 27 28 29 30 31 32 33 34 35 37 39 41 42 43 44 45 46 48 49 51 52 54 55 56 57 58 59 60 64 65 67 71 72 73 74 **P**1 **S** Department of Veterans Affairs, Washington, DC	45	10	557	11364	419	297801	0	192760	94908	2292
□ △ ZALE LIPSHY UNIVERSITY HOSPITAL, 5151 Harry Hines Boulevard, Zip 75235–7786; tel. 214/590–3000; Robert B. Smith, President and Chief Executive Officer **A**1 3 5 7 8 9 10 **F**4 8 10 12 14 15 19 22 28 32 34 35 37 41 42 43 44 45 46 48 52 54 56 57 59 60 64 65 67 71 73	23	10	146	4585	94	7427	0	72954	27466	490
DE LEON—Comanche County										
✠ DE LEON HOSPITAL, 407 South Texas Avenue, Zip 76444, Mailing Address: Box 319, Zip 76444; tel. 817/893–2011; Michael K. Hare, Administrator **A**1 9 10 **F**8 14 15 16 19 21 22 28 32 33 34 35 44 46 49 65 70 71 73 **N** Lubbock Methodist Hospital System, Lubbock, TX	16	10	14	909	15	20028	6	5026	2149	89
DE SOTO—Dallas County										
□ CEDARS HOSPITAL, 2000 North Old Hickory Trail, Zip 75115; tel. 972/298–7323; Don Johnson, Administrator **A**1 9 10 **F**2 3 14 15 16 26 34 45 52 53 54 55 56 57 58 59 65 **S** Innovative Healthcare Systems, Inc., Birmingham, AL **N** Saint Paul Medical Center Affiliate Network, Dallas, TX; Brazo's Valley Health Network, Waco, TX	33	22	76	736	25	2534	0	6365	2972	103
□ HAVEN HOSPITAL, 800 Kirnwood Drive, Zip 75115–2092; tel. 972/709–3700; Sheila C. Kelly, R.N., MS, Chief Executive Officer **A**1 9 10 **F**2 3 12 14 15 16 26 52 53 57 58 59 67 **S** Ramsay Health Care, Inc., Coral Gobles, FL	33	22	27	620	14	6292	0	5384	2233	145
DECATUR—Wise County										
✠ DECATUR COMMUNITY HOSPITAL, 2000 South FM 51, Zip 76234–9295; tel. 817/627–5921; Steve Summers, Administrator **A**1 9 10 **F**7 12 15 16 19 21 22 24 28 32 34 37 40 44 49 51 65 66 70 71 73	16	10	42	2302	21	66513	362	12534	6154	234
DEL RIO—Val Verde County										
✠ VAL VERDE MEMORIAL HOSPITAL, 801 Bedell Avenue, Zip 78840, Mailing Address: P.O. Box 1527, Zip 78840; tel. 210/775–8566; Scott D. Evans, FACHE, Administrator **A**1 9 10 **F**7 8 15 16 19 21 22 27 28 32 33 34 35 36 37 39 40 44 45 46 49 65 70 71 73 74 **P**5 **N** Memorial/Sisters of Charity Health Network, Houston, TX; Southwest Texas Rural Health Alliance, San Antonio, TX	16	10	78	3228	36	47512	939	18566	8252	361

Hospital, Address, Telephone, Administrator, Approval, Facility, and Physician Codes, Health Care System, Network	Classi-fication Codes		Utilization Data					Expense (thousands) of dollars		
★ American Hospital Association (AHA) membership □ Joint Commission on Accreditation of Healthcare Organizations (JCAHO) accreditation + American Osteopathic Hospital Association (AOHA) membership ○ American Osteopathic Association (AOA) accreditation △ Commission on Accreditation of Rehabilitation Facilities (CARF) accreditation Control codes 61, 63, 64, 71, 72 and 73 indicate hospitals listed by AOHA, but not registered by AHA. For definition of numerical codes, see page A4	Control	Service	Beds	Admissions	Census	Outpatient Visits	Births	Total	Payroll	Personnel

DENISON—Grayson County

☒ TEXOMA HEALTHCARE SYSTEM, (Formerly Texoma Medical Center), 1000 Memorial Drive, Zip 75020, Mailing Address: Box 890, Zip 75021–9988; tel. 903/416–4000; Arthur L. Hohenberger, FACHE, President and Chief Executive Officer **A**1 2 9 10 **F**2 3 4 7 8 10 12 14 15 16 17 19 21 22 23 26 27 28 29 30 32 33 34 35 37 39 40 41 42 43 44 45 46 48 49 51 52 53 54 56 57 58 59 60 65 66 67 71 73 74 **P**1 7 **N** The Heart Network of Texas, Irving, TX

| | 23 | 10 | 205 | 6509 | 94 | 47120 | 446 | 63081 | 24609 | 1029 |

DENTON—Denton County

☒ COLUMBIA MEDICAL CENTER OF DENTON, (Formerly Denton Regional Medical Center), 4405 North Interstate 35, Zip 76207; tel. 817/566–4000; Bob J. Haley, Chief Executive Officer (Total facility includes 25 beds in nursing home–type unit) **A**1 9 10 **F**4 7 8 10 12 16 17 19 20 21 22 23 28 30 32 33 34 35 36 37 40 41 42 43 44 48 49 52 57 59 60 64 65 71 72 73 74 **P**4 5 7 8 **S** Columbia/HCA Healthcare Corporation, Nashville, TN

| | 33 | 10 | 271 | 5900 | 88 | 121820 | 928 | 40202 | 17098 | 679 |

☒ DENTON COMMUNITY HOSPITAL, 207 North Bonnie Brae, Zip 76201; tel. 817/898–7000; Timothy Charles, Chief Executive Officer **A**1 10 **F**4 7 8 10 14 19 21 22 28 30 31 32 35 37 42 44 49 56 63 65 66 67 71 73 74 **P**5 **S** Columbia/HCA Healthcare Corporation, Nashville, TN

| | 33 | 10 | 110 | 3862 | 46 | 32494 | 682 | 26035 | 10321 | 396 |

DENVER CITY—Yoakum County

★ YOAKUM COUNTY HOSPITAL, 412 Mustang Avenue, Zip 79323, Mailing Address: P.O. Drawer 1130, Zip 79323; tel. 806/592–5484; Edward Rodgers, Chief Executive Officer **A**9 10 **F**15 17 22 28 29 30 37 40 44 70 71 73 **P**5 **S** St. Joseph Health System, Orange, CA

| | 13 | 10 | 24 | 508 | 2 | 21500 | 91 | 5287 | 1364 | 62 |

DIMMITT—Castro County

PLAINS MEMORIAL HOSPITAL, 310 West Halsell Street, Zip 79027, Mailing Address: Box 278, Zip 79027; tel. 806/647–2191; Joseph F. Sloan, CHE, Chief Executive Officer **A**9 10 **F**12 15 28 32 33 36 40 44 49 70 71

| | 16 | 10 | 30 | 435 | 4 | 22761 | 71 | 4995 | 1920 | 116 |

DUMAS—Moore County

☒ MEMORIAL HOSPITAL, 224 East Second Street, Zip 79029; tel. 806/935–7171; Scott R. Brown, Administrator and Chief Executive Officer **A**1 9 10 **F**6 7 8 14 15 16 19 20 22 23 26 28 30 32 33 37 40 41 44 49 64 65 71 73 74 **N** Lubbock Methodist Hospital System, Lubbock, TX

| | 16 | 10 | 51 | 1844 | 22 | 22546 | 489 | 10212 | 4196 | 181 |

EAGLE LAKE—Colorado County

□ RICE MEDICAL CENTER, (Formerly Rice District Community Hospital), 600 South Austin Road, Zip 77434–3298, Mailing Address: P.O. Box 277, Zip 77434–0277; tel. 409/234–5571; David N. Keith, Chief Executive Officer **A**1 9 10 **F**7 8 14 15 16 19 22 28 30 32 40 44 49 70 71 73 **P**6

| | 16 | 10 | 38 | 598 | 6 | 19471 | 152 | 5004 | 2205 | 93 |

EAGLE PASS—Maverick County

★ FORT DUNCAN MEDICAL CENTER, 350 South Adams Street, Zip 78852; tel. 210/757–7501; Don Spaulding, Administrator and Chief Executive Officer **A**6 9 10 **F**12 15 19 28 29 30 32 34 37 40 44 45 46 49 64 65 70 71 73 **S** Quorum Health Group/Quorum Health Resources, Inc., Brentwood, TN

| | 16 | 10 | 71 | 4106 | 45 | 18166 | 1040 | 20339 | 8200 | 278 |

EASTLAND—Eastland County

EASTLAND MEMORIAL HOSPITAL, 304 South Daugherty Street, Zip 76448, Mailing Address: Box 897, Zip 76448; tel. 817/629–2601; John Yeary, Administrator **A**9 10 **F**8 15 16 17 19 21 24 26 28 29 30 34 40 44 49 64 67 70 71 73

| | 12 | 10 | 38 | 1304 | 13 | 16669 | 135 | 5371 | 2760 | 137 |

EDEN—Concho County

CONCHO COUNTY HOSPITAL, Eaker and Burleson Streets, Zip 76837, Mailing Address: Box L, Zip 76837; tel. 915/869–5911; Joe Brasig, Administrator **A**9 10 **F**14 15 28 30 32 71 73 **P**5

| | 16 | 10 | 20 | 277 | 2 | 5810 | 0 | 1589 | 826 | 41 |

EDINBURG—Hidalgo County

☒ EDINBURG HOSPITAL, 333 West Freddy Gonzalez Drive, Zip 78539–6199; tel. 210/383–6211; Leon J. Belila, Administrator **A**1 9 10 **F**8 14 15 16 17 19 21 22 28 30 32 34 35 37 40 44 45 48 49 65 70 71 73 **P**1 **S** Universal Health Services, Inc., King of Prussia, PA

| | 33 | 10 | 94 | 4610 | 52 | 31861 | 1329 | 30331 | 12361 | 372 |

EDNA—Jackson County

★ JACKSON COUNTY HOSPITAL, 1013 South Wells Street, Zip 77957–4098; tel. 512/782–5241; Marcella V. Henke, Administrator **A**9 10 **F**8 14 15 16 19 22 32 34 44 57 69 71 73 **N** SouthEast Texas Hospital System, Dallas, TX

| | 16 | 10 | 31 | 361 | 5 | 29965 | 0 | 4951 | 1665 | 63 |

EL CAMPO—Wharton County

☒ EL CAMPO MEMORIAL HOSPITAL, 303 Sandy Corner Road, Zip 77437; tel. 409/543–6251; C. Richard Murphy, Administrator (Nonreporting) **A**1 10 **N** SouthEast Texas Hospital System, Dallas, TX

| | 33 | 10 | 60 | — | — | — | — | — | — | — |

EL PASO—El Paso County

★ COLUMBIA BEHAVIORAL CENTER, 1155 Idaho Street, Zip 79902–1699; tel. 915/544–4000; Joan Courteau, Administrator **A**9 10 **F**1 3 4 7 8 9 10 11 12 14 15 16 18 19 20 21 22 23 24 25 26 27 28 29 30 31 32 33 34 35 37 38 39 40 41 42 43 44 45 46 47 48 49 52 53 54 55 56 57 58 59 60 63 64 65 66 67 71 73 74 **P**1 5 7 **S** Columbia/HCA Healthcare Corporation, Nashville, TN

| | 32 | 22 | 43 | 1194 | 18 | 3277 | 0 | 7059 | 3058 | 112 |

★ △ COLUMBIA MEDICAL CENTER–EAST, (Formerly Columbia Rehabilitation Hospital), 300 Waymore, Zip 77902; tel. 915/577–2600; William G. Collins, Chief Executive Officer (Nonreporting) **A**7 **S** Columbia/HCA Healthcare Corporation, Nashville, TN

| | 33 | 46 | 40 | — | — | — | — | — | — | — |

☒ COLUMBIA MEDICAL CENTER–EAST, 10301 Gateway West, Zip 79925–7798, Mailing Address: P.O. Box 937003, Zip 79937–1690; tel. 915/595–9000; Douglas A. Matney, Senior Vice President Operations (Total facility includes 29 beds in nursing home–type unit) **A**1 9 10 **F**2 3 4 7 8 9 10 11 12 14 15 16 18 19 20 21 22 23 24 25 27 28 29 30 31 32 33 34 35 37 38 39 40 41 42 43 44 45 46 47 48 49 52 53 54 55 56 57 58 59 60 63 64 65 66 67 68 71 73 74 **P**1 5 7 **S** Columbia/HCA Healthcare Corporation, Nashville, TN

| | 32 | 10 | 290 | 12558 | 196 | 98161 | 2123 | 104532 | 37843 | 940 |

Hospital, Address, Telephone, Administrator, Approval, Facility, and Physician Codes, Health Care System, Network	Classi-fication Codes		Utilization Data					Expense (thousands) of dollars		
★ American Hospital Association (AHA) membership ☐ Joint Commission on Accreditation of Healthcare Organizations (JCAHO) accreditation ✛ American Osteopathic Hospital Association (AOHA) membership ○ American Osteopathic Association (AOA) accreditation △ Commission on Accreditation of Rehabilitation Facilities (CARF) accreditation Control codes 61, 63, 64, 71, 72 and 73 indicate hospitals listed by AOHA, but not registered by AHA. For definition of numerical codes, see page A4	Control	Service	Beds	Admissions	Census	Outpatient Visits	Births	Total	Payroll	Personnel

⊞ COLUMBIA MEDICAL CENTER–WEST, 1801 North Oregon Street, Zip 79902; tel. 915/521–1776; Douglas A. Matney, Senior Vice President Operations (Total facility includes 18 beds in nursing home–type unit) **A**1 9 10 **F**2 3 4 7 8 9 10 11 12 14 15 16 18 19 20 21 22 23 24 25 26 27 28 30 31 32 33 34 35 37 38 39 40 41 42 43 44 45 46 47 48 49 52 53 54 55 56 57 58 59 60 63 64 65 66 67 68 71 73 74 **P**1 3 5 7 **S** Columbia/HCA Healthcare Corporation, Nashville, TN	32	10	221	8849	123	85571	1131	91464	30557	924
⊞ PROVIDENCE MEMORIAL HOSPITAL, 2001 North Oregon Street, Zip 79902; tel. 915/577–6011; L. Marcus Fry, Jr., Chief Executive Officer (Total facility includes 34 beds in nursing home–type unit) **A**1 2 5 9 10 **F**4 7 8 10 11 12 15 16 17 19 21 22 25 27 28 29 30 31 32 33 34 35 37 38 40 41 42 43 44 45 46 47 49 51 60 61 63 64 65 66 67 69 71 72 73 74 **P**2 7 8 **S** TENET Healthcare Corporation, Santa Barbara, CA	32	10	348	11416	243	101498	2364	102932	35983	1590
☐ R. E. THOMASON GENERAL HOSPITAL, 4815 Alameda Avenue, Zip 79905, Mailing Address: Box 20009, Zip 79998; tel. 915/544–1200; Pete Duarte, Chief Executive Officer **A**1 2 3 5 9 10 **F**4 8 10 14 15 16 17 19 20 21 22 23 27 28 31 33 35 37 38 39 40 41 42 43 44 45 46 47 49 51 52 54 60 61 63 65 66 68 70 71 73 **P**6	16	10	299	14213	206	354997	5845	101601	39327	1530
⊞ △ RIO VISTA REHABILITATION HOSPITAL, 1740 Curie Drive, Zip 79902; tel. 915/543–6826; Patsy A. Parker, Administrator and Chief Executive Officer (Total facility includes 27 beds in nursing home–type unit) **A**1 7 9 10 **F**4 5 7 8 9 10 11 12 14 15 16 17 19 21 22 25 27 28 30 32 33 34 35 36 37 38 39 40 41 42 43 44 46 47 48 49 60 63 64 65 69 71 73 74 **P**3 5 7 8	33	46	100	1304	60	31185	0	18638	9331	368
☐ SIERRA MEDICAL CENTER, 1625 Medical Center Drive, Zip 79902–5044; tel. 915/747–4000; L. Marcus Fry, Jr., Chief Executive Officer **A**1 2 9 10 **F**4 7 8 10 11 12 16 17 19 20 21 22 28 29 30 31 32 33 34 35 36 37 38 39 40 41 42 43 44 45 46 47 48 49 60 63 64 65 66 67 69 71 73 74 **P**7 8 **S** TENET Healthcare Corporation, Santa Barbara, CA	32	10	365	12055	163	97133	2587	121214	37046	1146
☐ SOUTHWESTERN GENERAL HOSPITAL, 1221 North Cotton, Zip 79902–3096; tel. 915/496–9600; Stephen J. Campbell, Administrator **A**1 9 10 **F**7 11 15 16 17 19 21 22 28 30 34 35 40 44 63 65 71 74	32	10	102	1941	20	15246	118	12366	5616	208
⊞ WILLIAM BEAUMONT ARMY MEDICAL CENTER, 5005 North Piedras Street, Zip 79920–5001; tel. 915/569–2121; Colonel Gordon W. Cho, Chief of Staff (Nonreporting) **A**1 2 3 5 **S** Department of the Army, Office of the Surgeon General, Falls Church, VA	42	10	209	—	—	—	—	—	—	—
ELDORADO—Schleicher County										
SCHLEICHER COUNTY MEDICAL CENTER, 305 Mertzon Highway, Zip 76936, Mailing Address: Box V, Zip 76936; tel. 915/853–2507; Jim B. Roddie, Administrator (Total facility includes 8 beds in nursing home–type unit) **A**9 10 **F**1 22 28 45 49 64 65 73 **P**6	16	10	16	73	5	4568	1	1353	581	41
ELECTRA—Wichita County										
ELECTRA MEMORIAL HOSPITAL, 1207 South Bailey Street, Zip 76360, Mailing Address: Box 1112, Zip 76360–1112; tel. 817/495–3981; Jan A. Reed, CPA, Administrator **A**9 10 **F**8 14 15 16 19 28 32 34 44 70 71 73 **P**7 **N** Texoma Health Network, Wichita Falls, TX	16	10	23	591	7	19553	0	2775	1428	74
FAIRFIELD—Freestone County										
FAIRFIELD MEMORIAL HOSPITAL, 125 Newman Street, Zip 75840; tel. 903/389–2121; Milton W. Meadows, Administrator **A**9 10 **F**15 19 22 25 28 30 34 37 44 71 **N** Healthcare Partners of East Texas, Inc., Tyler, TX; Regional Healthcare Alliance, Tyler, TX	16	10	15	398	6	6908	0	3298	1380	59
FLORESVILLE—Wilson County										
WILSON MEMORIAL HOSPITAL, 1301 Hospital Boulevard, Zip 78114; tel. 210/393–3122; Robert Duffield, Administrator **A**9 10 **F**8 14 19 21 22 28 30 32 33 34 39 44 46 49 65 67 71 73 **N** Southwest Texas Rural Health Alliance, San Antonio, TX	16	10	30	410	5	42051	0	4915	2158	84
FORT HOOD—Bell County										
⊞ DARNALL ARMY COMMUNITY HOSPITAL, Zip 76544–5063; tel. 817/288–8000; Colonel James W. Kirkpatrick, Commander **A**1 2 3 5 **F**1 2 3 4 7 8 10 11 12 13 14 15 16 17 18 19 20 21 22 23 24 25 26 27 28 29 30 31 32 33 34 35 37 38 39 40 41 42 43 44 45 46 47 48 49 51 52 53 54 55 56 57 58 59 60 61 64 65 66 67 71 72 73 74 **P**5 6 8 **S** Department of the Army, Office of the Surgeon General, Falls Church, VA	42	10	169	13020	103	857163	3013	116736	49217	1477
FORT STOCKTON—Pecos County										
⊞ PECOS COUNTY MEMORIAL HOSPITAL, Sanderson Highway, Zip 79735, Mailing Address: Box 1648, Zip 79735; tel. 915/336–2241; David B. Shaw, Administrator and Chief Executive Officer **A**1 9 10 **F**7 12 13 14 15 16 17 19 22 24 28 29 30 32 34 39 40 44 45 46 49 65 67 70 71 72 73 **N** Lubbock Methodist Hospital System, Lubbock, TX; Permian Basin Rural Health Network, Fort Stockton, TX	13	10	31	1101	11	32958	232	9493	4391	196
FORT WORTH—Tarrant County										
☐ ALL SAINTS EPISCOPAL HOSPITAL OF FORT WORTH, 1400 Eighth Avenue, Zip 76104, Mailing Address: P.O. Box 31, Zip 76101; tel. 817/926–2544; James P. Schuessler, President and Chief Executive Officer **A**1 9 10 **F**3 4 8 10 11 12 14 15 16 17 19 21 22 24 25 26 27 28 29 30 32 33 34 35 37 39 40 41 42 43 44 45 46 48 49 52 53 54 55 56 57 58 59 60 61 64 65 66 67 69 71 73 74 **P**1 3 4 5 7	23	10	308	12224	170	—	1478	114797	45348	1199

Hospital, Address, Telephone, Administrator, Approval, Facility, and Physician Codes, Health Care System, Network	Classi-fication Codes		Utilization Data					Expense (thousands) of dollars		
	Control	Service	Beds	Admissions	Census	Outpatient Visits	Births	Total	Payroll	Personnel

★ American Hospital Association (AHA) membership
□ Joint Commission on Accreditation of Healthcare Organizations (JCAHO) accreditation
+ American Osteopathic Hospital Association (AOHA) membership
○ American Osteopathic Association (AOA) accreditation
△ Commission on Accreditation of Rehabilitation Facilities (CARF) accreditation
Control codes 61, 63, 64, 71, 72 and 73 indicate hospitals listed by AOHA, but not registered by AHA. For definition of numerical codes, see page A4

Hospital	Control	Service	Beds	Admissions	Census	Outpatient Visits	Births	Total	Payroll	Personnel
ALL SAINTS HOSPITAL–CITYVIEW, 7100 Oakmont Boulevard, Zip 76132; tel. 817/346–5870; Jean Biacsi, Vice President and Administrator Main Campus **F**2 3 4 7 8 10 11 12 13 14 15 16 17 19 20 21 22 24 26 27 28 29 30 32 33 34 35 37 38 39 40 41 42 43 44 45 46 48 49 51 52 53 54 55 56 57 58 59 60 63 64 65 67 71 73 74 **P**5 6 7	23	10	43	1879	14	—	790	14861	5925	152
⊞ COLUMBIA PLAZA MEDICAL CENTER OF FORT WORTH, 900 Eighth Avenue, Zip 76104–3986; tel. 817/336–2100; Stephen Bernstein, Chief Executive Officer **A**1 9 10 **F**1 2 3 4 5 6 7 8 9 10 11 12 13 17 18 19 20 21 22 23 24 25 26 27 28 29 30 31 32 33 34 35 36 37 38 39 40 41 42 43 44 45 46 47 48 49 50 51 52 53 54 55 56 57 58 59 60 61 62 63 64 65 66 67 68 69 70 71 72 73 74 **P**5 7 8 **S** Columbia/HCA Healthcare Corporation, Nashville, TN	33	10	289	10375	160	28719	887	101170	35975	1163
□ COOK CHILDREN'S MEDICAL CENTER, 801 Seventh Avenue, Zip 76104–2796; tel. 817/885–4000; Russell K. Tolman, President **A**1 3 9 10 **F**10 12 13 15 16 17 18 19 20 21 22 25 27 28 29 30 31 32 34 35 38 39 41 42 43 44 45 46 47 48 49 51 52 53 55 56 58 59 60 63 65 66 67 68 69 70 71 72 73 **P**3 4 6	23	50	181	6929	125	135810	0	113476	48225	1494
□ △ FORT WORTH REHABILITATION HOSPITAL, 6701 Oakmont Boulevard, Zip 76132; tel. 817/370–4700; Robert L. McNew, Chief Executive Officer (Total facility includes 12 beds in nursing home–type unit) **A**1 7 9 10 **F**5 12 14 16 19 21 22 25 27 28 32 34 35 41 45 46 49 50 63 65 71	33	46	62	761	49	7982	0	12773	5204	157
⊞ HARRIS CONTINUED CARE HOSPITAL, (LONG TERM ACUTE CARE), 1301 Pennsylvania Avenue, 4th Floor, Zip 76104, Mailing Address: P.O. Box 3471, Zip 76113; tel. 817/878–5500; Larry Thompson, Administrator **A**1 10 **F**2 3 4 7 8 10 11 12 13 16 17 18 19 21 22 23 24 26 27 28 29 30 31 32 33 34 35 37 38 39 40 41 42 43 44 45 46 48 49 50 52 53 56 58 59 60 61 63 64 65 66 67 69 70 71 72 73 74 **P**2 5 7 **S** Harris Methodist Health System, Fort Worth, TX **N** The Heart Network of Texas, Irving, TX; North Texas Healthcare Network, Dallas, TX	21	49	15	53	6	0	0	5241	1121	21
⊞ HARRIS METHODIST FORT WORTH, 1301 Pennsylvania Avenue, Zip 76104–2895; tel. 817/882–2000; Barclay E. Berdan, Chief Executive Officer (Total facility includes 36 beds in nursing home–type unit) **A**1 2 3 9 10 **F**2 3 4 7 8 10 11 12 13 14 15 16 17 18 19 20 21 22 23 24 25 26 27 28 29 30 31 32 33 34 35 37 38 39 40 41 42 43 44 45 46 47 48 49 51 52 53 54 55 56 57 58 59 60 61 63 64 65 66 67 69 70 71 72 73 74 **P**2 4 5 7 **S** Harris Methodist Health System, Fort Worth, TX **N** The Heart Network of Texas, Irving, TX; North Texas Healthcare Network, Dallas, TX	21	10	499	20745	309	103510	4144	175694	73599	2877
⊞ HARRIS METHODIST SOUTHWEST, 6100 Harris Parkway, Zip 76132; tel. 817/346–5050; David B. Rowe, Vice President and Administrator (Total facility includes 8 beds in nursing home–type unit) **A**1 9 10 **F**2 3 4 7 8 10 11 12 13 14 15 16 17 18 19 20 21 22 23 24 26 27 28 29 30 31 32 33 34 35 37 38 39 40 41 42 43 44 45 46 47 48 49 50 51 52 53 54 55 56 57 58 59 60 61 62 63 64 65 66 67 68 69 70 71 72 73 74 **P**2 5 7 **S** Harris Methodist Health System, Fort Worth, TX **N** The Heart Network of Texas, Irving, TX; North Texas Healthcare Network, Dallas, TX	21	10	70	3714	30	59351	1441	30679	10587	385
□ △ HEALTHSOUTH REHABILITATION HOSPITAL OF FORT WORTH, 1212 West Lancaster, Zip 76102; tel. 817/870–2336; Laura J. Lycan, Administrator and Chief Executive Officer (Total facility includes 15 beds in nursing home–type unit) **A**1 7 9 10 **F**12 16 27 32 34 41 48 49 54 64 65 66 67 **S** HEALTHSOUTH Corporation, Birmingham, AL	33	46	60	608	33	6691	0	6834	3687	121
JOHN PETER SMITH HOSPITAL See Tarrant County Hospital District										
□ + ○ OSTEOPATHIC MEDICAL CENTER OF TEXAS, 1000 Montgomery Street, Zip 76107; tel. 817/731–4311; Ron Stephen, Executive Vice President and Administrator (Total facility includes 19 beds in nursing home–type unit) **A**1 7 9 10 11 12 13 **F**4 7 8 10 11 12 13 14 15 16 17 19 21 22 24 26 27 28 30 31 32 34 35 37 39 40 41 42 43 44 46 48 49 52 53 54 55 56 57 59 61 64 65 66 71 72 73 **P**1 3 5 7	23	10	205	7238	141	64731	642	78611	28274	1011
□ TARRANT COUNTY HOSPITAL DISTRICT, (Includes John Peter Smith Hospital), 1500 South Main Street, Zip 76104–4941; tel. 817/921–3431; Anthony J. Alcini, President and Chief Executive Officer **A**1 3 5 6 9 10 **F**4 7 8 10 12 13 16 17 19 20 21 22 23 25 27 28 30 31 32 33 34 35 37 38 40 41 42 43 44 46 49 51 52 53 54 55 56 58 59 60 61 63 65 67 68 69 71 73 74 **P**5 **S** Tarrant County Hospital District, Fort Worth, TX	16	10	359	19167	233	414467	4820	194516	69398	2322
TARRANT COUNTY PSYCHIATRIC CENTER, 1527 Hemphill Street, Zip 76104; tel. 817/923–6467; Connie Oliverson Perra, Director (Nonreporting) **A**10	16	22	39	—	—	—	—	—	—	—
THC–FORT WORTH, (LONG TERM ACUTE CARE), 7800 Oakmont Boulevard, Zip 76132; tel. 817/346–0094; Barbara Schmidt, Chief Executive Officer (Total facility includes 16 beds in nursing home–type unit) **F**12 14 16 19 21 22 27 31 33 34 35 37 39 41 49 64 65 71 **S** Transitional Hospitals Corporation, Las Vegas, NV	33	49	80	417	33	589	0	10389	5357	113
TRINITY SPRINGS PAVILION–EAST, 1500 South Main Street, Zip 76104–4917; tel. 817/927–3636; Robert N. Bourassa, Executive Director **F**7 8 10 12 13 15 16 19 20 21 22 25 27 28 29 30 31 32 34 41 42 46 49 51 52 53 54 55 56 57 58 59 61 65 67 71 73 74 **P**8 **S** Tarrant County Hospital District, Fort Worth, TX	16	52	34	36	2	1084	0	—	—	44
TWIN OAKS MEDICAL CENTER, 2919 Markum Drive, Zip 76117–4099; tel. 817/831–0311; Lawrence Wedekind, Administrator (Nonreporting) **A**9	33	10	34	—	—	—	—	—	—	—
FREDERICKSBURG—Gillespie County										
⊞ HILL COUNTRY MEMORIAL HOSPITAL, 1020 Kerrville Road, Zip 78624, Mailing Address: Box 835, Zip 78624–0835; tel. 210/997–4353; Jerry L. Durr, Chief Executive Officer **A**1 9 10 **F**7 8 15 17 19 21 22 23 24 30 32 33 34 35 37 39 40 41 42 44 45 46 49 63 64 65 66 67 70 71 73 **P**8 **N** Southwest Texas Rural Health Alliance, San Antonio, TX	23	10	59	2966	33	35343	408	19451	8599	368

Hospital, Address, Telephone, Administrator, Approval, Facility, and Physician Codes, Health Care System, Network	Classification Codes		Utilization Data					Expense (thousands) of dollars		
	Control	Service	Beds	Admissions	Census	Outpatient Visits	Births	Total	Payroll	Personnel

★ American Hospital Association (AHA) membership
□ Joint Commission on Accreditation of Healthcare Organizations (JCAHO) accreditation
+ American Osteopathic Hospital Association (AOHA) membership
○ American Osteopathic Association (AOA) accreditation
△ Commission on Accreditation of Rehabilitation Facilities (CARF) accreditation
Control codes 61, 63, 64, 71, 72 and 73 indicate hospitals listed by AOHA, but not registered by AHA. For definition of numerical codes, see page A4.

FRIONA—Parmer County

PARMER COUNTY COMMUNITY HOSPITAL, 1307 Cleveland Street, Zip 79035; tel. 806/247-2754; Bill J. Neely, Administrator **A**9 10 **F**8 15 19 22 30 32 33 34 36 71 — 23 10 34 489 3 25213 0 3416 1450 61

GAINESVILLE—Cooke County

GAINESVILLE MEMORIAL HOSPITAL, 1016 Ritchey Street, Zip 76240-3539; tel. 817/665-1751; Gerald Culwell, Administrator (Total facility includes 10 beds in nursing home–type unit) **A**9 10 **F**7 8 14 15 16 17 18 19 22 28 30 32 33 34 35 37 39 40 42 44 64 65 71 73 **P**8 — 16 10 50 2051 20 — 318 11898 6484 287

GALVESTON—Galveston County

☒ SHRINERS HOSPITALS FOR CHILDREN, GALVESTON BURNS INSTITUTE, (Formerly Shriners Hospitals for Crippled Children, Galveston Burns Institute), (PEDIATRIC BURN), 815 Market Street, Zip 77550-2725; tel. 409/770-6600; John A. Swartwout, Administrator **A**1 3 5 **F**9 12 19 34 35 44 46 54 65 71 73 **S** Shriners Hospitals for Children, Tampa, FL — 23 59 30 874 19 3090 0 — — 333

☒ UNIVERSITY OF TEXAS MEDICAL BRANCH HOSPITALS, 301 University Boulevard, Zip 77555-0138; tel. 409/772-1011; James F. Arens, M.D., Chief Executive Officer **A**1 2 3 5 8 9 10 **F**1 4 7 8 9 10 11 12 15 16 17 19 20 21 22 23 24 25 26 27 28 30 31 32 33 34 35 37 38 39 40 41 42 43 44 46 47 48 49 51 52 53 54 55 56 57 58 59 60 61 63 65 66 68 69 70 71 72 73 74 **P**5 6 **S** University of Texas System, Austin, TX **N** Gulf Health Network, Galveston, TX — 12 10 858 32369 579 629857 3896 369561 162772 5231

GARLAND—Dallas County

☒ BAYLOR MEDICAL CENTER AT GARLAND, 2300 Marie Curie Boulevard, Zip 75042-5706; tel. 214/487-5000; John B. McWhorter, III, Executive Director (Total facility includes 13 beds in nursing home–type unit) **A**1 3 9 10 **F**4 7 8 10 12 15 16 17 19 20 21 22 24 25 26 27 28 29 30 32 33 35 37 39 40 41 42 43 44 45 46 48 49 50 51 53 54 55 56 60 61 63 64 65 66 67 68 69 70 71 73 74 **P**6 7 8 **S** Baylor Health Care System, Dallas, TX **N** Baylor Health Care System Network, Dallas, TX; North Texas Health Network, Irving, TX; North Texas Healthcare Network, Dallas, TX — 23 10 174 7703 100 90055 1428 60111 27043 973

□ GARLAND COMMUNITY HOSPITAL, 2696 West Walnut Street, Zip 75042; tel. 214/276-7116; K. Dwayne Ray, Administrator and Chief Executive Officer (Total facility includes 10 beds in nursing home–type unit) **A**1 9 10 **F**2 3 15 16 19 21 22 26 27 28 30 32 35 37 39 41 44 49 53 54 55 56 57 58 59 63 65 67 71 73 **S** TENET Healthcare Corporation, Santa Barbara, CA — 32 10 113 2490 38 70070 0 24406 11539 398

GATESVILLE—Coryell County

□ CORYELL MEMORIAL HOSPITAL, 1507 West Main Street, Zip 76528, Mailing Address: P.O. Box 659, Zip 76528; tel. 817/865-8251; David Byrom, Administrator **A**1 9 10 **F**15 16 19 22 32 33 37 44 51 65 71 **P**6 — 16 10 48 893 14 31356 0 9596 4991 242

GEORGETOWN—Williamson County

☒ GEORGETOWN HOSPITAL, 2000 Scenic Drive, Zip 78626; tel. 512/930-5338; Kenneth W. Poteete, President and Chief Executive Officer (Total facility includes 9 beds in nursing home–type unit) **A**1 9 10 **F**7 8 14 15 16 19 21 22 28 30 32 34 37 39 40 41 42 44 49 64 65 67 70 71 73 — 16 10 98 3033 28 30301 719 18060 9096 345

GLEN ROSE—Somervell County

☒ GLEN ROSE MEDICAL CENTER, 1021 Holden Street, Zip 76043, Mailing Address: Box 2099, Zip 76043; tel. 817/897-2215; Gary A. Marks, Administrator (Total facility includes 42 beds in nursing home–type unit) (Nonreporting) **A**1 9 10 — 16 10 104 — — — — — — —

GONZALES—Gonzales County

MEMORIAL HOSPITAL, Highway 90A By-Pass, Zip 78629, Mailing Address: Box 587, Zip 78629; tel. 210/672-7581; Douglas Langley, Administrator **A**9 10 **F**8 14 15 16 17 18 19 22 24 28 29 30 32 34 37 39 40 41 42 44 46 49 51 65 66 67 71 73 **N** Southwest Texas Rural Health Alliance, San Antonio, TX — 16 10 35 1228 14 12653 144 8235 3587 150

☒ △ WARM SPRINGS REHABILITATION HOSPITAL, Mailing Address: P.O. Box 58, Zip 78629-0058; tel. 210/672-6592; John Davis, Administrator **A**1 7 9 10 **F**15 16 32 41 48 49 65 **N** Southwest Texas Rural Health Alliance, San Antonio, TX — 23 46 68 648 38 8138 0 8022 3722 155

GRAHAM—Young County

GRAHAM GENERAL HOSPITAL, 1301 Montgomery Road, Zip 76450, Mailing Address: Box 1390, Zip 76450; tel. 817/549-3400; Blake Kretz, Administrator **A**9 10 **F**7 8 16 19 26 28 30 32 33 34 36 40 41 42 44 57 58 65 70 71 73 **P**5 7 — 14 10 37 1699 16 84795 194 11531 5035 181

GRANBURY—Hood County

☒ HOOD GENERAL HOSPITAL, 1310 Paluxy Road, Zip 76048; tel. 817/573-2683; John V. Villanueva, Chief Executive Officer **A**1 9 10 **F**7 8 12 14 15 16 19 21 22 24 28 32 34 35 37 39 40 42 44 45 49 64 65 69 71 73 **P**3 5 **S** Community Health Systems, Inc., Brentwood, TN — 16 10 49 1387 19 27297 107 16480 6474 254

GRAND PRAIRIE—Dallas County

☒ + ○ DALLAS-FORT WORTH MEDICAL CENTER, 2709 Hospital Boulevard, Zip 75051-1083; tel. 972/641-5000; Robert A. Ficken, Chief Executive Officer and Chief Financial Officer (Total facility includes 11 beds in nursing home–type unit) **A**1 9 10 11 12 13 **F**4 7 8 10 12 13 14 15 16 17 19 21 22 23 24 25 26 28 30 32 34 35 37 38 39 40 41 42 44 48 49 51 52 55 57 64 65 70 71 72 73 74 **P**1 **S** Quorum Health Group/Quorum Health Resources, Inc., Brentwood, TN **N** Saint Paul Medical Center Affiliate Network, Dallas, TX — 23 10 162 4268 58 — 1016 42740 17662 523

GRAND SALINE—Van Zandt County

COZBY-GERMANY HOSPITAL, 707 North Waldrip Street, Zip 75140; tel. 903/962-4242; William Rowton, Chief Executive Officer **A**9 10 **F**14 19 20 22 26 32 34 44 49 59 65 71 **N** Healthcare Partners of East Texas, Inc., Tyler, TX; Regional Healthcare Alliance, Tyler, TX — 23 10 26 404 4 24839 2 2884 1529 64

Hospital, Address, Telephone, Administrator, Approval, Facility, and Physician Codes, Health Care System, Network	Classi-fication Codes		Utilization Data					Expense (thousands) of dollars		
★ American Hospital Association (AHA) membership □ Joint Commission on Accreditation of Healthcare Organizations (JCAHO) accreditation + American Osteopathic Hospital Association (AOHA) membership ○ American Osteopathic Association (AOA) accreditation △ Commission on Accreditation of Rehabilitation Facilities (CARF) accreditation Control codes 61, 63, 64, 71, 72 and 73 indicate hospitals listed by AOHA, but not registered by AHA. For definition of numerical codes, see page A4	Control	Service	Beds	Admissions	Census	Outpatient Visits	Births	Total	Payroll	Personnel

GRAPEVINE—Tarrant County

☒ BAYLOR MEDICAL CENTER AT GRAPEVINE, 1650 West College Street, Zip 76051–1650; tel. 817/329–2500; Mark C. Hood, Executive Director (Total facility includes 9 beds in nursing home–type unit) **A**1 9 10 **F**1 3 4 5 6 7 8 10 11 12 13 15 16 17 18 19 20 21 22 23 24 25 26 27 28 29 30 31 32 33 34 35 36 37 39 40 41 42 43 44 45 46 49 50 51 53 54 55 56 57 58 59 60 61 63 64 65 66 67 69 70 71 73 74 **P**3 5 6 7 8 **S** Baylor Health Care System, Dallas, TX **N** Baylor Health Care System Network, Dallas, TX; North Texas Health Network, Irving, TX; North Texas Healthcare Network, Dallas, TX | 21 | 10 | 68 | 3920 | 39 | 54835 | 850 | — | — | 440

□ CHARTER GRAPEVINE BEHAVIORAL HEALTH SYSTEM, 2300 William D. Tate Avenue, Zip 76051–9964; tel. 817/481–1900; Michael V. Lee, Chief Executive Officer **A**1 9 10 **F**1 2 3 12 19 21 22 27 34 35 46 48 52 53 54 55 56 57 58 59 65 67 70 71 **S** Magellan Health Services, Atlanta, GA | 33 | 22 | 80 | 2209 | 45 | 12384 | 0 | 12824 | 4037 | 99

GREENVILLE—Hunt County

□ GLEN OAKS HOSPITAL, 301 East Division, Zip 75401; tel. 903/454–6000; Thomas E. Rourke, Administrator **A**1 9 10 **F**1 2 3 15 46 52 53 54 55 56 57 58 59 **S** Universal Health Services, Inc., King of Prussia, PA | 33 | 22 | 54 | 931 | 22 | 4878 | 0 | 5496 | 2465 | 71

☒ HUNT MEMORIAL HOSPITAL DISTRICT, (Includes Presbyterian Hospital of Commerce, 2900 Sterling Hart Drive, Commerce, Zip 75428; tel. 903/886–3161; Presbyterian Hospital of Greenville, 4215 Joe Ramsey Boulevard, Zip 75401), Mailing Address: P.O. Drawer 1059, Zip 75403–1059; tel. 903/408–5000; Richard Carter, Chief Executive Officer **A**1 9 **F**7 8 12 14 15 16 19 21 22 28 32 34 35 36 37 39 40 41 44 49 65 67 71 72 73 74 **P**8 **N** Presbyterian Healthcare System, Dallas, TX | 16 | 10 | 118 | 5234 | 56 | 84959 | 793 | 36317 | 16645 | 541

GROESBECK—Limestone County

LIMESTONE MEDICAL CENTER, 900 North Ellis Street, Zip 76642; tel. 817/729–3281; Penny Gray, Administrator and Chief Executive Officer **A**9 10 **F**15 16 19 21 28 32 34 39 46 49 51 65 70 71 73 **N** Central Texas Rural Health Network, Harrietsville, TX; Brazo's Valley Health Network, Waco, TX | 16 | 10 | 38 | 418 | 2 | 2456 | 0 | 3861 | 2255 | 82

GROVES—Jefferson County

★ + ○ DOCTORS HOSPITAL, 5500 39th Street, Zip 77619–9805; tel. 409/962–5733; John Isbell, Chief Executive Officer **A**9 10 11 12 13 **F**3 4 7 8 10 11 12 14 15 19 21 22 26 28 30 32 34 35 37 41 42 43 44 46 49 51 52 53 57 60 63 65 66 70 71 73 **P**1 **S** Quorum Health Group/Quorum Health Resources, Inc., Brentwood, TN | 23 | 10 | 72 | 1974 | 22 | 12705 | 0 | 21017 | 5417 | 175

HALE CENTER—Hale County

☒ HI-PLAINS HOSPITAL, 203 West Fourth Street, Zip 79041, Mailing Address: P.O. Box 1260, Zip 79041; tel. 806/839–2471; Michael J. Keller, Administrator **A**1 9 10 **F**7 14 15 16 17 19 21 24 26 28 29 30 32 40 44 49 61 65 66 70 71 **P**8 | 23 | 10 | 40 | 585 | 5 | 2455 | 79 | 2648 | 1351 | 64

HALLETTSVILLE—Lavaca County

LAVACA MEDICAL CENTER, 1400 North Texana Street, Zip 77964; tel. 512/798–3671; James Vanek, Administrator (Nonreporting) **A**9 10 **N** SouthEast Texas Hospital System, Dallas, TX | 16 | 10 | 31 | — | — | — | — | — | — | —

HAMLIN—Jones County

★ HAMLIN MEMORIAL HOSPITAL, 632 Northwest Second Street, Zip 79520, Mailing Address: P.O. Box 400, Zip 79520; tel. 915/576–3646; Charley C. Latham, Administrator **A**9 10 **F**19 22 34 36 37 44 71 **P**5 | 16 | 10 | 25 | 686 | 10 | — | 0 | 2292 | 1046 | 64

HARLINGEN—Cameron County

□ RIO GRANDE STATE CENTER, 1401 Rangerville Road, Zip 78550; tel. 210/425–8900; Sonia Hernandez–Keeble, Director **A**1 9 **F**15 16 24 28 31 39 45 46 52 55 56 57 65 67 73 | 12 | 22 | 160 | 1484 | 33 | 0 | 0 | 13618 | 9632 | 336

☒ SOUTH TEXAS HOSPITAL, 1301 Rangerville Road, Zip 78552–7609, Mailing Address: P.O. Box 592, Zip 78551–0592; tel. 210/423–3420; James N. Elkins, FACHE, Director **A**1 10 **F**8 12 14 15 16 17 19 20 21 27 28 29 30 31 34 35 39 41 44 45 46 49 51 65 71 73 74 **P**6 **S** Texas Department of Health, Austin, TX | 12 | 10 | 85 | 624 | 34 | 32162 | 0 | 14269 | 6095 | 262

☒ VALLEY BAPTIST MEDICAL CENTER, 2101 Pease Street, Zip 78550, Mailing Address: P.O. Drawer 2588, Zip 78551–2588; tel. 210/421–1100; Ben M. McKibbens, President (Total facility includes 60 beds in nursing home–type unit) **A**1 2 5 9 10 **F**4 7 8 10 11 12 13 15 16 17 18 19 21 22 23 26 28 29 30 32 33 35 37 38 39 40 41 42 43 44 45 46 47 48 49 52 53 54 55 58 59 60 61 63 64 65 67 71 73 74 **P**8 | 21 | 10 | 504 | 19747 | 231 | 97643 | 3776 | 152709 | 60494 | 1906

HASKELL—Haskell County

HASKELL MEMORIAL HOSPITAL, 1 North Avenue N, Zip 79521, Mailing Address: P.O. Box 1117, Zip 79521; tel. 817/864–2621; Bill Nemir, Administrator **A**9 10 **F**14 15 16 19 22 24 27 28 29 32 33 44 46 49 71 73 **P**1 | 16 | 10 | 30 | 396 | 5 | 1977 | 0 | 2484 | 1048 | 59

HEMPHILL—Sabine County

★ SABINE COUNTY HOSPITAL, Highway 83 West, Zip 75948, Mailing Address: P.O. Box 750, Zip 75948; tel. 409/787–3300; Edith McCauley, Administrator **A**9 10 **F**15 19 20 22 28 32 34 40 41 44 49 71 | 16 | 10 | 36 | 528 | 6 | 5368 | 11 | 3637 | 1683 | 69

HENDERSON—Rusk County

☒ HENDERSON MEMORIAL HOSPITAL, 300 Wilson Street, Zip 75652; tel. 903/657–7541; George T. Roberts, Jr., Chief Executive Officer (Total facility includes 16 beds in nursing home–type unit) **A**1 9 10 **F**7 8 12 15 16 19 20 22 28 29 30 31 32 34 35 37 39 40 44 45 46 49 63 64 70 71 **P**8 **S** Quorum Health Group/Quorum Health Resources, Inc., Brentwood, TN **N** Healthcare Partners of East Texas, Inc., Tyler, TX; Regional Healthcare Alliance, Tyler, TX | 23 | 10 | 96 | 3211 | 42 | 56212 | 505 | 17830 | 8336 | 304

Hospital, Address, Telephone, Administrator, Approval, Facility, and Physician Codes, Health Care System, Network	Classification Codes		Utilization Data					Expense (thousands) of dollars		
	Control	Service	Beds	Admissions	Census	Outpatient Visits	Births	Total	Payroll	Personnel

★ American Hospital Association (AHA) membership
□ Joint Commission on Accreditation of Healthcare Organizations (JCAHO) accreditation
+ American Osteopathic Hospital Association (AOHA) membership
○ American Osteopathic Association (AOA) accreditation
△ Commission on Accreditation of Rehabilitation Facilities (CARF) accreditation
Control codes 61, 63, 64, 71, 72 and 73 indicate hospitals listed by AOHA, but not registered by AHA. For definition of numerical codes, see page A4

HENRIETTA—Clay County

CLAY COUNTY MEMORIAL HOSPITAL, 310 West South Street, Zip 76365–3399; tel. 817/538–5621; Edward E. Browning, Administrator **A**9 10 **F**19 22 26 30 32 34 44 57 70 71 **P**8 **N** Texoma Health Network, Wichita Falls, TX	13	10	32	354	5	—	0	2370	1209	50

HEREFORD—Deaf Smith County

✠ HEREFORD REGIONAL MEDICAL CENTER, 801 East Third Street, Zip 79045, Mailing Address: Box 1858, Zip 79045; tel. 806/364–2141; James M. Robinson, Sr., Administrator **A**1 9 10 **F**6 7 8 10 12 13 14 15 16 17 18 19 20 21 24 26 28 29 30 31 32 33 34 36 37 39 40 41 42 43 44 45 46 49 65 67 70 71 73 74 **N** Lubbock Methodist Hospital System, Lubbock, TX	16	10	40	1376	13	25101	351	10025	4711	204

HILLSBORO—Hill County

□ HILL REGIONAL HOSPITAL, 101 Circle Drive, Zip 76645; tel. 817/582–8425; Jan McClure, Chief Executive Officer (Total facility includes 12 beds in nursing home–type unit) **A**1 9 10 **F**7 12 15 16 19 22 26 30 34 35 37 40 41 44 45 46 52 57 64 70 71 73 **S** Community Health Systems, Inc., Brentwood, TN **N** Central Texas Rural Health Network, Harrietsville, TX; Brazo's Valley Health Network, Waco, TX	33	10	73	1600	21	14312	193	8186	3931	102

HONDO—Medina County

MEDINA COMMUNITY HOSPITAL, 3100 Avenue East, Zip 78861; tel. 210/741–4677; Richard D. Arnold, Administrator **A**9 10 **F**7 12 15 16 19 21 22 24 27 28 29 32 33 34 40 41 44 46 49 70 71 73 **P**4 **N** Southwest Texas Rural Health Alliance, San Antonio, TX	15	10	27	921	11	96125	194	13181	6288	271

HOUSTON—Harris County

□ AMERICAN TRANSITIONAL HOSPITAL–HOUSTON MEDICAL CENTER, (LONG TERM ACUTE CARE), 6447 Main Street, Zip 77054, Mailing Address: 6447 Main Street, 6th Floor, Zip 77054; tel. 713/791–9393; Sheila A. Kramer, Chief Executive Officer **A**1 10 **F**12 16 22 39 41 65 67 **P**4 **S** American Transitional Hospitals, Inc., Franklin, TN	33	49	34	373	27	0	0	8267	3600	93
□ △ ATH HEIGHTS HOSPITAL, 1917 Ashland Street, Zip 77008–3994; tel. 713/861–6161; Joe G. Baldwin, Administrator **A**1 7 9 10 **F**12 19 22 37 48 65 71 **S** American Transitional Hospitals, Inc., Franklin, TN	33	10	170	667	63	—	0	19797	7749	189
BEN TAUB GENERAL HOSPITAL See Harris County Hospital District										
★ CASA, A SPECIAL HOSPITAL, (MEDICALLY COMPLEX), 1803 Old Spanish Trail, Zip 77054–2001; tel. 713/796–2272; Gretchen Thorp, R.N., Administrator **A**10 **F**6 12 15 31 42 65 73	32	49	40	644	25	0	0	2886	1233	40
✠ COLUMBIA BELLAIRE MEDICAL CENTER, 5314 Dashwood Street, Zip 77081–4689; tel. 713/512–1200; Walter Leleux, Chief Executive Officer (Total facility includes 15 beds in nursing home–type unit) **A**1 9 10 **F**1 2 3 7 8 12 14 15 16 17 19 21 22 23 26 27 28 30 35 37 40 41 42 44 49 52 53 54 55 56 57 58 59 64 65 67 71 73 74 **P**5 8 **S** Columbia/HCA Healthcare Corporation, Nashville, TN **N** Gulf Coast Provider Network, Houston, TX	33	10	202	5769	93	39332	1424	47830	16451	434
✠ COLUMBIA DOCTORS HOSPITAL AIRLINE, 5815 Airline Drive, Zip 77076; tel. 713/695–6041; Lee Brown, Administrator **A**1 9 **F**8 12 14 15 16 19 20 22 28 30 32 34 37 40 41 44 46 49 65 69 70 71 74 **P**1 5 7 **S** Columbia/HCA Healthcare Corporation, Nashville, TN	32	10	114	3051	51	—	398	13547	6420	248
✠ COLUMBIA DOCTORS HOSPITAL EAST LOOP, 9339 North Loop East, Zip 77029, Mailing Address: Box 24216, Zip 77229; tel. 713/675–3241; John Styles, Jr., Administrator (Nonreporting) **A**1 9 **S** Columbia/HCA Healthcare Corporation, Nashville, TN	32	10	151	—						
✠ COLUMBIA EAST HOUSTON MEDICAL CENTER, (Formerly Columbia Sun Belt Regional Medical Center), (Includes Sun Belt Regional Medical Center East, 15101 East Freeway, Channelview, Zip 77530; tel. 713/452–1511), 13111 East Freeway, Zip 77015; tel. 713/455–6911; Mary Lee Walter, Chief Executive Officer (Total facility includes 9 beds in nursing home–type unit) (Nonreporting) **A**1 9 10 **S** Columbia/HCA Healthcare Corporation, Nashville, TN	33	10	136	—						
✠ COLUMBIA NORTH HOUSTON MEDICAL CENTER, 233 West Parker Road, Zip 77076; tel. 713/697–2831; Mel Bishop, Chief Executive Officer (Total facility includes 21 beds in nursing home–type unit) **A**1 9 **F**3 4 7 8 10 12 14 15 16 19 20 22 23 24 25 26 28 29 30 32 33 34 35 37 39 40 41 42 43 44 45 46 48 49 52 55 57 58 59 64 65 66 67 70 71 73 74 **P**1 5 7 **S** Columbia/HCA Healthcare Corporation, Nashville, TN	33	10	149	7775	110	58573	1333	38973	15788	454
✠ △ COLUMBIA ROSEWOOD MEDICAL CENTER, 9200 Westheimer Road, Zip 77063; tel. 713/780–7900; Pat Currie, Chief Executive Officer (Total facility includes 18 beds in nursing home–type unit) **A**1 7 9 10 **F**2 3 4 5 7 8 10 12 14 16 18 19 20 21 23 24 26 27 28 30 31 32 33 34 35 37 39 40 41 42 43 44 48 49 51 52 53 54 55 56 57 58 59 60 64 65 66 67 71 73 74 **P**5 7 8 **S** Columbia/HCA Healthcare Corporation, Nashville, TN **N** Gulf Coast Provider Network, Houston, TX	33	10	184	5492	78	57406	491	36118	16147	525
✠ △ COLUMBIA SPRING BRANCH MEDICAL CENTER, (Includes Sam Houston Memorial Hospital, 1615 Hillendahl, tel. 713/932–5500), 8850 Long Point Road, Zip 77055; tel. 713/467–6555; Sally E. Jeffcoat, President and Chief Executive Officer (Total facility includes 25 beds in nursing home–type unit) **A**1 2 7 9 10 **F**1 2 3 4 5 7 8 10 11 12 13 14 15 16 17 18 19 20 21 22 23 24 25 26 27 28 29 30 31 32 33 34 35 37 38 39 40 41 42 44 45 46 48 49 51 52 53 54 55 56 57 58 59 60 61 64 65 66 67 68 69 70 71 72 73 74 **P**1 3 5 7 8 **S** Columbia/HCA Healthcare Corporation, Nashville, TN **N** Gulf Coast Provider Network, Houston, TX	33	10	345	10940	164	78035	1411	75974	33277	980
COLUMBIA SUN BELT REGIONAL MEDICAL CENTER See Columbia East Houston Medical Center										

Hospital, Address, Telephone, Administrator, Approval, Facility, and Physician Codes, Health Care System, Network	Classi-fication Codes		Utilization Data					Expense (thousands) of dollars		
★ American Hospital Association (AHA) membership □ Joint Commission on Accreditation of Healthcare Organizations (JCAHO) accreditation + American Osteopathic Hospital Association (AOHA) membership ○ American Osteopathic Association (AOA) accreditation △ Commission on Accreditation of Rehabilitation Facilities (CARF) accreditation Control codes 61, 63, 64, 71, 72 and 73 indicate hospitals listed by AOHA, but not registered by AHA. For definition of numerical codes, see page A4	Control	Service	Beds	Admissions	Census	Outpatient Visits	Births	Total	Payroll	Personnel
▣ COLUMBIA TEXAS ORTHOPEDIC HOSPITAL, (Formerly Texas Orthopedic Hospital), 7401 South Main Street, Zip 77030; tel. 713/799–8600; John J. Jackson, Chief Executive Officer A1 9 10 F2 3 4 5 7 8 10 11 12 13 14 17 18 19 22 23 24 25 26 27 28 30 32 35 37 38 39 40 41 42 43 44 46 47 48 49 50 52 53 54 55 56 57 58 59 60 61 64 65 66 67 68 69 71 72 73 74 P1 5 7 S Columbia/HCA Healthcare Corporation, Nashville, TN	32	47	49	1599	16	25663	0	21213	8123	250
▣ COLUMBIA WEST HOUSTON MEDICAL CENTER, 12141 Richmond Avenue, Zip 77082–2499; tel. 281/558–3444; Janie R. Kauffman, Chief Executive Officer (Total facility includes 18 beds in nursing home–type unit) A1 9 10 F3 4 7 8 10 11 12 16 19 21 22 26 28 29 30 32 33 34 35 37 38 39 40 41 42 43 44 46 48 49 52 57 64 65 66 73 P1 5 7 8 S Columbia/HCA Healthcare Corporation, Nashville, TN N Gulf Coast Provider Network, Houston, TX	33	10	169	6399	92	41451	1236	45064	18243	423
▣ COLUMBIA WOMAN'S HOSPITAL OF TEXAS, 7600 Fannin Street, Zip 77054–1900; tel. 713/790–1234; Linda B. Russell, Chief Executive Officer A1 5 9 10 F2 3 4 7 8 9 12 19 21 22 23 24 25 26 27 30 31 32 34 35 37 38 39 40 41 42 43 44 45 46 47 48 49 51 52 53 54 55 56 57 58 59 60 64 65 66 68 71 73 74 P7 8 S Columbia/HCA Healthcare Corporation, Nashville, TN N Gulf Coast Provider Network, Houston, TX	33	44	148	9552	110	16692	5796	55401	23703	867
□ CYPRESS CREEK HOSPITAL, 17750 Cali Drive, Zip 77090–2700; tel. 713/586–7600; Terry Scovill, Administrator A1 9 10 F2 3 22 52 53 54 55 56 57 58 59 65 67 S Healthcare America, Inc., Austin, TX	33	22	94	1341	35	6983	0	6989	3856	—
▣ CYPRESS FAIRBANKS MEDICAL CENTER, 10655 Steepletop Drive, Zip 77065; tel. 713/890–4285; Bill Klier, Chief Executive Officer (Total facility includes 14 beds in nursing home–type unit) (Nonreporting) A1 9 10 N Gulf Coast Provider Network, Houston, TX	32	10	149	—	—	—	—	—	—	—
▣ DIAGNOSTIC CENTER HOSPITAL, 6447 Main Street, Zip 77030; tel. 713/790–0790; William A. Gregory, Chief Executive Officer (Total facility includes 25 beds in nursing home–type unit) A1 9 10 F2 4 7 8 9 10 11 12 15 16 17 19 20 21 22 23 24 26 27 28 30 31 32 33 34 35 37 38 39 40 41 42 43 44 45 46 47 48 49 50 52 54 55 57 58 60 61 63 64 65 66 67 69 71 73 P3 8 S Methodist Health Care System, Houston, TX	23	10	149	3720	71	13225	0	38984	13742	431
□ FOREST SPRINGS HOSPITAL, 1120 Cypress Station, Zip 77090–3031; tel. 713/893–7200 A1 9 10 F2 3 19 21 35 52 53 54 55 56 58 59 65 S Cambridge International, Inc,, Houston, TX	33	22	48	203	6	237	0	2001	865	73
□ GULF PINES BEHAVIORAL HEALTH SERVICES, 205 Hollow Tree Lane, Zip 77090; tel. 713/537–0700; Lawrence Story, Chief Executive Officer and Administrator A1 9 10 F2 3 12 19 35 46 52 53 54 55 56 57 58 59 71 S Vendell Healthcare, Inc., Nashville, TN	33	22	140	1601	59	7730	0	8583	3613	—
□ HARRIS COUNTY HOSPITAL DISTRICT, (Includes Ben Taub General Hospital, 1504 Taub Loop, Zip 77030; tel. 713/793–2300; Michael R. Bullard, Senior Vice President; Lyndon B Johnson General Hospital, 5656 Kelley, Zip 77026; tel. 713/636–5000; Margo Hilliard, M.D., Senior Vice President; Quentin Mease Hospital, 3601 North MacGregor, Zip 77004; tel. 713/528–1499; Michael R. Bullard, Senior Vice President), 2525 Holly Hall, Zip 77054, Mailing Address: Box 66769, Zip 77266–6769; tel. 713/746–6403; Lois Jean Moore, President and Chief Executive Officer A1 3 5 8 9 10 F3 4 7 8 10 11 12 14 15 17 18 19 20 21 22 23 25 26 27 30 31 32 34 35 37 38 40 42 43 44 47 48 49 52 56 58 59 60 61 63 64 65 67 68 70 71 73 P6	16	10	948	37815	649	807150	10875	387771	151694	5395
▣ HARRIS COUNTY PSYCHIATRIC CENTER, 2800 South MacGregor, Zip 77021, Mailing Address: P.O. Box 20249, Zip 77225–0249; tel. 713/741–5000; Robert W. Guynn, M.D., Executive Director A1 3 5 9 10 F3 12 14 15 16 19 21 27 35 39 46 50 52 53 54 55 56 57 58 63 65 67 71 73 S University of Texas System, Austin, TX	12	22	250	5162	193	0	0	32161	17678	455
▣ △ HERMANN HOSPITAL, 6411 Fannin, Zip 77030–1501; tel. 713/704–4000; David R. Page, President and Chief Executive Officer (Total facility includes 15 beds in nursing home–type unit) A1 3 5 7 8 9 10 F4 7 8 9 10 11 12 14 15 16 17 19 20 21 22 23 24 25 26 27 28 30 31 32 34 35 37 38 39 40 41 42 43 44 45 46 47 48 49 50 51 56 60 61 63 64 65 66 67 68 69 70 71 72 73 74 P7 8 N Gulf Coast Provider Network, Houston, TX	23	10	624	23347	423	212709	2330	338405	127548	3436
▣ HOUSTON NORTHWEST MEDICAL CENTER, 710 FM 1960 West, Zip 77090–3496; tel. 281/440–1000; J. O. Lewis, Chief Executive Officer (Total facility includes 20 beds in nursing home–type unit) A1 2 9 10 F3 4 7 8 9 10 12 15 16 17 19 20 21 22 23 24 28 29 30 33 34 35 37 38 40 41 42 43 44 45 46 49 52 53 54 55 56 57 58 59 60 61 64 65 67 71 72 73 74 P5 7 8 S TENET Healthcare Corporation, Santa Barbara, CA N Gulf Coast Provider Network, Houston, TX	33	10	370	16291	184	151475	3629	130115	49358	1340
▣ △ HOUSTON REHABILITATION INSTITUTE, 17506 Red Oak Drive, Zip 77090, Mailing Address: P.O. Box 73684, Zip 77273–7721; tel. 281/580–1212; Anne R. Leon, Chief Executive Officer (Nonreporting) A1 7 9 10	33	46	68	—	—	—	—	—	—	—
□ INTRACARE MEDICAL CENTER HOSPITAL, 7601 Fannin, Zip 77054; tel. 713/790–0949; Alice Hiniker, Ph.D., Administrator A1 9 10 F2 3 52 53 54 55 56 58 59 65 S Cambridge International, Inc,, Houston, TX	33	22	50	745	27	3951	0	6290	2746	83

LYNDON B JOHNSON GENERAL HOSPITAL See Harris County Hospital District
MEMORIAL HOSPITAL NORTHWEST See Memorial Hospital Southwest

Hospital, Address, Telephone, Administrator, Approval, Facility, and Physician Codes, Health Care System, Network	Classi-fication Codes		Utilization Data					Expense (thousands) of dollars		
★ American Hospital Association (AHA) membership □ Joint Commission on Accreditation of Healthcare Organizations (JCAHO) accreditation + American Osteopathic Hospital Association (AOHA) membership ○ American Osteopathic Association (AOA) accreditation △ Commission on Accreditation of Rehabilitation Facilities (CARF) accreditation Control codes 61, 63, 64, 71, 72 and 73 indicate hospitals listed by AOHA, but not registered by AHA. For definition of numerical codes, see page A4	Control	Service	Beds	Admissions	Census	Outpatient Visits	Births	Total	Payroll	Personnel

MEMORIAL HOSPITAL SOUTHEAST See Memorial Hospital Southwest

★ MEMORIAL HOSPITAL SOUTHWEST, (Includes Memorial Hospital Northwest, 1635 North Loop West, Zip 77008; tel. 713/867–3380; Memorial Hospital Southeast, 11800 Astoria, Zip 77089; tel. 713/929–6100), 7600 Beechnut, Zip 77074–1850; tel. 713/776–5000; James E. Eastham, Administrator, Chief Executive Officer and Vice President (Total facility includes 41 beds in nursing home–type unit) **A**1 2 3 5 9 10 **F**2 3 4 6 7 8 10 11 12 14 15 16 17 19 21 22 23 25 26 27 28 29 30 31 32 33 34 35 37 38 39 40 41 42 43 44 45 46 48 49 51 52 53 54 55 56 57 58 59 60 62 63 64 65 66 67 68 71 72 73 74 **P**3 4 7 **S** Memorial Healthcare System, Houston, TX **N** Memorial/Sisters of Charity Health Network, Houston, TX	23	10	490	21359	296	—	3782	156011	52400	1591
★ MEMORIAL HOSPITAL–MEMORIAL CITY, 920 Frostwood Drive, Zip 77024–9173; tel. 713/932–3000; Jerel T. Humphrey, Vice President, Chief Executive Officer and Administrator (Total facility includes 24 beds in nursing home–type unit) **A**1 2 6 9 10 **F**2 3 4 6 7 8 10 11 12 14 15 16 17 19 21 22 23 25 26 27 28 29 30 31 32 33 34 35 37 38 39 40 41 42 43 44 45 46 48 49 51 52 53 54 55 56 57 58 59 60 62 63 64 65 66 67 68 71 72 73 74 **P**3 4 7 **S** Memorial Healthcare System, Houston, TX **N** Memorial/Sisters of Charity Health Network, Houston, TX	23	10	300	14937	170	—	3129	99161	28417	929
MEMORIAL REHABILITATION HOSPITAL, 3043 Gessner, Zip 77080; tel. 713/462–2515; Roger Truskoloski, Administrator, Chief Executive Officer and Vice President **F**2 3 4 6 7 8 10 11 12 14 15 16 17 19 21 22 23 25 26 27 28 29 30 31 32 33 34 35 37 38 39 40 41 42 43 44 45 46 48 49 51 52 53 54 55 56 57 58 59 60 62 63 64 65 66 67 68 71 72 73 74 **P**3 4 7 **S** Memorial Healthcare System, Houston, TX	23	46	106	668	34	—	0	11467	3412	150
★ MEMORIAL SPRING SHADOWS GLEN, 2801 Gessner, Zip 77080–2599; tel. 713/462–4000; G. Jerry Mueck, Vice President, Chief Executive Officer and Administrator **A**1 9 **F**2 3 4 6 7 8 10 11 12 14 15 16 17 19 21 22 23 25 26 27 28 29 30 31 32 33 34 35 37 38 39 40 41 42 43 44 45 46 48 49 51 52 53 54 55 56 57 58 59 60 62 63 64 65 66 67 68 71 72 73 74 **P**3 4 7 **S** Memorial Healthcare System, Houston, TX **N** Memorial/Sisters of Charity Health Network, Houston, TX	33	22	112	1470	44	673	0	12276	4503	185
NORTHSIDE GENERAL HOSPITAL, 2807 Little York Road, Zip 77093–3495; tel. 713/697–7777; Carole A. Veloso, R.N., President and Chief Executive Officer **A**9 10 **F**11 19 21 22 34 35 44 49 71	33	10	39	1221	13	—	0	6073	1980	100
□ PARK PLAZA HOSPITAL, 1313 Hermann Drive, Zip 77004; tel. 713/527–5000; Judith Novak, President and Chief Executive Officer (Total facility includes 40 beds in nursing home–type unit) **A**1 2 3 5 9 10 **F**4 7 8 10 12 14 15 16 17 19 21 22 26 28 30 31 32 34 35 37 38 40 41 42 43 44 45 46 48 49 52 57 60 61 63 64 65 67 71 73 **P**3 7 **S** TENET Healthcare Corporation, Santa Barbara, CA	32	10	370	9018	189	53151	812	84996	31364	979
QUENTIN MEASE HOSPITAL See Harris County Hospital District										
□ RIVERSIDE GENERAL HOSPITAL, 3204 Ennis, Zip 77004; tel. 713/526–2441; Earnest Gibson, III, Administrator (Nonreporting) **A**1 9 10	23	82	98	—	—	—	—	—	—	—
SAM HOUSTON MEMORIAL HOSPITAL See Columbia Spring Branch Medical Center										
□ SHARPSTOWN GENERAL HOSPITAL, 6700 Bellaire at Tarnef, Zip 77074–4999; Mailing Address: P.O. Box 740389, Zip 77274–0389; tel. 713/774–7611; Glenn Robinson, Chief Executive Officer **A**1 9 10 **F**2 7 8 12 14 15 16 17 19 20 21 22 27 28 30 32 34 35 37 38 40 41 44 49 52 53 57 59 65 71 74 **P**5 7 **S** TENET Healthcare Corporation, Santa Barbara, CA	33	10	121	3985	50	—	1033	28155	13876	378
★ SHRINERS HOSPITALS FOR CHILDREN, HOUSTON, (Formerly Shriners Hospitals for Crippled Children, Houston Unit), 6977 Main Street, Zip 77030; tel. 713/797–1616; Steven B. Reiter, Administrator **A**1 3 5 **F**5 9 12 17 19 20 27 28 34 35 39 44 45 47 48 49 51 54 65 67 71 73 **P**6 **S** Shriners Hospitals for Children, Tampa, FL	23	57	40	670	17	9584	0	—	—	139
★ SPECIALTY HOSPITAL OF HOUSTON, (LONG TERM ACUTE CARE), 5556 Gasmer, Zip 77035; tel. 713/551–5300; Roger W. Wessels, Chief Executive Officer and Administrator **A**1 10 **F**4 8 10 12 14 15 16 17 19 21 22 24 26 30 31 35 37 39 41 42 43 44 45 46 49 50 51 60 63 65 67 71	33	49	44	204	20	0	0	8544	3608	95
★ ST. JOSEPH HOSPITAL, 1919 LaBranch Street, Zip 77002; tel. 713/757–1000; Raymond J. Khoury, Administrator (Total facility includes 29 beds in nursing home–type unit) **A**1 2 3 5 9 10 **F**2 3 4 7 8 10 11 12 13 14 15 16 17 18 19 21 22 23 24 26 28 29 30 31 32 33 34 35 37 38 39 40 41 42 43 44 45 46 48 49 51 52 54 55 56 57 59 60 61 63 64 65 66 67 68 70 71 72 73 74 **P**1 5 6 7 **S** Sisters of Charity of the Incarnate Word Healthcare System, Houston, TX **N** SouthEast Texas Integrated Community Health Network, Houston, TX	23	10	483	17643	268	—	4430	154742	68939	2101
★ ST. LUKE'S EPISCOPAL HOSPITAL, 6720 Bertner Avenue, Zip 77030–2697; Mailing Address: Box 20269, Zip 77225–0269; tel. 713/791–2011; Michael K. Jhin, President and Chief Executive Officer **A**1 2 3 5 8 9 10 **F**4 7 8 10 11 12 14 15 19 21 22 28 29 30 32 34 35 37 39 40 41 42 43 44 45 46 48 49 54 56 61 63 65 67 69 71 73 74 **P**5 7 8	21	10	594	27206	415	182314	2389	332727	126696	3419
★ TEXAS CHILDREN'S HOSPITAL, 6621 Fannin Street, Zip 77030–2399, Mailing Address: Box 300630, Zip 77230–0630; tel. 713/770–1000; Mark A. Wallace, Executive Director and Chief Executive Officer **A**1 3 5 8 9 10 **F**4 5 10 12 13 14 15 16 17 19 20 21 22 24 25 29 30 31 32 34 35 38 39 41 42 43 44 45 46 47 49 50 51 54 55 58 60 63 65 66 67 68 69 70 71 72 73 **P**5 7	23	50	369	18032	315	325307	0	252001	110539	2842

Hospital, Address, Telephone, Administrator, Approval, Facility, and Physician Codes, Health Care System, Network	Classi-fication Codes		Utilization Data					Expense (thousands) of dollars		
★ American Hospital Association (AHA) membership □ Joint Commission on Accreditation of Healthcare Organizations (JCAHO) accreditation + American Osteopathic Hospital Association (AOHA) membership ○ American Osteopathic Association (AOA) accreditation △ Commission on Accreditation of Rehabilitation Facilities (CARF) accreditation Control codes 61, 63, 64, 71, 72 and 73 indicate hospitals listed by AOHA, but not registered by AHA. For definition of numerical codes, see page A4	Control	Service	Beds	Admissions	Census	Outpatient Visits	Births	Total	Payroll	Personnel

☒ △ THE INSTITUTE FOR REHABILITATION AND RESEARCH, 1333 Moursund, Zip 77030–3405; tel. 713/799–5000; Louisa F. Adelung, President and Chief Executive Officer (Nonreporting) **A**1 3 5 7 9 10	23	46	92	—	—	—	—	—	—	—
☒ △ THE METHODIST HOSPITAL, 6565 Fannin, Zip 77030; tel. 713/790–3311; R. G. Girotto, Executive Vice President and Chief Operating Officer (Total facility includes 25 beds in nursing home–type unit) **A**1 2 3 5 7 8 9 10 **F**2 3 4 5 7 8 10 11 12 14 15 16 17 18 19 20 21 22 24 26 28 29 30 31 32 33 34 35 37 39 40 41 42 43 44 45 46 48 49 54 55 56 57 58 59 60 61 63 64 65 66 67 69 71 73 74 **P**2 3 5 7 **S** Methodist Health Care System, Houston, TX	23	10	867	32226	718	285005	2886	442179	156515	5436
□ TWELVE OAKS HOSPITAL, 4200 Portsmouth Street, Zip 77027; tel. 713/623–2500; Steve Altmiller, Chief Executive Officer (Total facility includes 15 beds in nursing home–type unit) **A**1 9 10 **F**3 4 8 10 12 14 16 17 19 21 22 26 27 28 30 31 34 35 37 41 42 43 44 46 48 49 52 54 55 56 58 59 64 65 67 71 73 74 **P**5 **S** TENET Healthcare Corporation, Santa Barbara, CA	32	10	199	5168	115	18604	0	42493	17965	517
□ UNIVERSITY OF TEXAS M. D. ANDERSON CANCER CENTER, (ONCOLOGY COMPREHENSIVE CANCER), 1515 Holcombe Boulevard, Box 506, Zip 77030–4096; tel. 713/461–0529; David J. Bachrach, Professor, Health Services Management **A**1 2 3 5 8 9 10 **F**8 12 14 15 16 17 19 20 21 22 25 27 28 29 30 34 35 37 39 41 42 44 45 46 48 49 50 53 54 55 56 58 60 63 65 67 71 73 **P**6 **S** University of Texas System, Austin, TX	12	49	417	15939	311	422307	0	468243	217911	6584
☒ VENCOR HOSPITAL–HOUSTON, 6441 Main Street, Zip 77030; tel. 713/790–0500; Darrell L. Pile, Administrator **A**1 9 10 **F**12 16 19 21 22 31 35 65 67 71 **S** Vencor, Incorporated, Louisville, KY	32	10	94	484	60	0	0	14768	7492	205
☒ VETERANS AFFAIRS MEDICAL CENTER, 2002 Holcombe Boulevard, Zip 77030–4298; tel. 713/791–1414; Robert F. Stott, Director (Total facility includes 120 beds in nursing home–type unit) **A**1 3 5 8 **F**2 3 4 5 8 10 11 15 16 17 18 19 20 21 22 23 25 26 31 32 35 37 39 41 42 43 44 46 48 49 51 52 54 56 57 58 59 60 64 65 66 67 71 73 74 **P**6 **S** Department of Veterans Affairs, Washington, DC	45	10	859	16356	650	408086	0	—	—	2832
□ WEST OAKS HOSPITAL, 6500 Hornwood, Zip 77074, Mailing Address: Box 741389, Zip 77274; tel. 713/995–0909; Michael Amador, Chief Executive Officer **A**1 9 10 **F**1 2 3 15 16 52 53 55 56 57 58 59 **S** Healthcare America, Inc., Austin, TX	33	22	184	2732	67	—	0	14112	6021	67
☒ YALE CLINIC AND HOSPITAL, 510 West Tidwell Road, Zip 77091; tel. 713/691–1111; Charles Veldekens, Chief Executive Officer **A**1 9 10 **F**4 8 10 12 15 16 17 19 21 22 24 26 27 28 30 31 34 35 37 39 41 44 45 49 51 54 55 57 58 59 61 65 66 67 70 71 **P**5	33	10	43	1082	14	19487	0	5820	2792	98
HUMBLE—Harris County										
□ △ HEALTHSOUTH REHABILITATION HOSPITAL, 19002 McKay Drive, Zip 77338; tel. 281/446–6148; Jessica A. Nantz, Chief Executive Officer (Total facility includes 24 beds in nursing home–type unit) **A**1 7 9 10 **F**1 4 8 12 14 15 16 19 21 22 23 25 26 27 34 35 39 41 44 45 46 48 49 64 65 66 67 71 73 **P**5 **S** HEALTHSOUTH Corporation, Birmingham, AL	33	46	58	547	29	4519	0	5092	2928	107
☒ NORTHEAST MEDICAL CENTER HOSPITAL, 18951 Memorial North, Zip 77338–4297; tel. 713/540–7700; Syble F. Missildine, Administrator (Total facility includes 16 beds in nursing home–type unit) **A**1 2 9 10 **F**1 2 3 4 5 6 7 8 9 10 11 12 13 15 16 17 18 19 20 21 22 23 24 26 27 28 29 30 31 32 33 34 35 36 37 38 39 40 41 42 43 44 45 46 47 48 49 51 52 53 54 55 56 57 58 59 60 61 62 63 64 65 66 67 68 69 70 71 72 73 74 **P**1 5 8	16	10	171	7899	107	112036	1082	67001	25669	686
HUNT—Kerr County										
LA HACIENDA TREATMENT CENTER, FM 1340, Zip 78024, Mailing Address: Box 1, Zip 78024–0001; tel. 210/238–4222; Frank J. Sadlack, Ph.D., Executive Director **A**9 **F**2 3 12 16 17 22 24 30 31 39 41 45 46 54 56 67 **P**1	32	82	90	915	63	1635	0	6596	3060	127
HUNTSVILLE—Walker County										
☒ HUNTSVILLE MEMORIAL HOSPITAL, 3000 I-45, Zip 77340, Mailing Address: P.O. Box 4001, Zip 77342–4001; tel. 409/291–3411; Ralph E. Beaty, Administrator (Total facility includes 11 beds in nursing home–type unit) **A**1 6 9 10 **F**7 8 13 14 17 19 22 28 29 30 32 33 34 35 37 39 40 41 44 45 49 64 65 66 67 71 73 74 **P**8 **S** Quorum Health Group/Quorum Health Resources, Inc., Brentwood, TN **N** Healthcare Partners of East Texas, Inc., Tyler, TX	23	10	130	3637	40	66543	488	24685	11654	404
IRAAN—Pecos County										
□ PECOS COUNTY GENERAL HOSPITAL, 305 West Fifth Street, Zip 79744, Mailing Address: Box 665, Zip 79744; tel. 915/639–2871; David B. Shaw, Administrator and Chief Executive Officer **A**1 9 10 **F**14 15 16 22 28 30 32 34 39 44 49 51 65 **N** Lubbock Methodist Hospital System, Lubbock, TX; Permian Basin Rural Health Network, Fort Stockton, TX	13	10	13	150	1	10433	0	2179	776	27
IRVING—Dallas County										
☒ AMERICAN TRANSITIONAL HOSPITAL–DALLAS/FORT WORTH, (LONG TERM ACUTE CARE), 1745 West Irving Boulevard, Zip 75061; tel. 214/251–2824; LouAnn O. Mathews, Administrator **A**1 10 **F**22 51 65 **S** American Transitional Hospitals, Inc., Franklin, TN	33	49	38	180	14	0	0	5549	1663	75
☒ IRVING HEALTHCARE SYSTEM, 1901 North MacArthur Boulevard, Zip 75061; tel. 972/579–8100; H. J. MacFarland, FACHE, Executive Director (Total facility includes 18 beds in nursing home–type unit) **A**1 2 9 10 **F**1 3 4 7 8 10 11 12 15 16 19 21 22 23 24 25 26 27 28 30 31 32 33 34 35 37 39 40 41 42 43 44 46 48 49 59 60 63 64 65 66 67 71 73 74 **P**1 7 **S** Baylor Health Care System, Dallas, TX **N** Baylor Health Care System Network, Dallas, TX	21	10	231	10836	137	97663	2142	84636	38161	1343

Hospital, Address, Telephone, Administrator, Approval, Facility, and Physician Codes, Health Care System, Network	Control	Service	Beds	Admissions	Census	Outpatient Visits	Births	Total	Payroll	Personnel

★ American Hospital Association (AHA) membership
□ Joint Commission on Accreditation of Healthcare Organizations (JCAHO) accreditation
+ American Osteopathic Hospital Association (AOHA) membership
○ American Osteopathic Association (AOA) accreditation
△ Commission on Accreditation of Rehabilitation Facilities (CARF) accreditation
Control codes 61, 63, 64, 71, 72 and 73 indicate hospitals listed by AOHA, but not registered by AHA. For definition of numerical codes, see page A4

JACKSBORO—Jack County
FAITH COMMUNITY HOSPITAL, 717 Magnolia Street, Zip 76458; tel. 817/567–6633; Don Hopkins, Administrator **A**9 10 **F**19 21 32 33 39 44 49 64 65 71 **P**6 **N** Texoma Health Network, Wichita Falls, TX — 16 10 18 462 4 17433 0 3287 1419 71

JACKSONVILLE—Cherokee County
✠ NAN TRAVIS MEMORIAL HOSPITAL, 501 South Ragsdale Street, Zip 75766; tel. 903/586–3000; Steve Bowen, President (Total facility includes 18 beds in nursing home–type unit) **A**1 9 10 **F**7 8 14 15 16 17 19 22 24 25 28 30 32 34 35 41 42 44 46 49 65 66 67 71 73 74 **P**1 **N** Healthcare Partners of East Texas, Inc., Tyler, TX; Regional Healthcare Alliance, Tyler, TX — 23 10 73 2770 40 36993 317 20058 9500 260

JASPER—Jasper County
✠ JASPER MEMORIAL HOSPITAL, 1275 Marvin Hancock Drive, Zip 75951; tel. 409/384–5461; George N. Miller, Jr., Administrator **A**1 6 9 10 **F**7 8 12 14 18 19 22 25 26 28 29 30 31 32 33 34 37 40 44 45 46 49 51 65 70 71 73 **P**5 7 8 **S** Sisters of Charity of the Incarnate Word Healthcare System, Houston, TX — 16 10 54 2108 18 31497 393 12842 5889 240
LAKES REGIONAL MEDICAL CENTER, (Formerly Mary E. Dickerson Memorial Hospital), 1001 Dickerson Drive, Zip 75951, Mailing Address: P.O. Box 1990, Zip 75951; tel. 409/384–2575; Spencer Guimarin, Administrator **A**9 10 **F**7 8 15 16 19 20 22 32 33 34 40 44 45 46 50 65 71 73 **P**5 — 33 10 35 1199 17 26235 36 6291 3148 139

JOURDANTON—Atascosa County
□ TRI–CITY COMMUNITY HOSPITAL, Highway 97 East, Zip 78026, Mailing Address: Box 189, Zip 78026; tel. 512/769–3515; S. Allen Smith, Administrator **A**1 9 10 **F**8 16 18 19 20 21 22 26 28 30 32 34 35 41 42 44 49 51 57 58 65 66 71 72 **P**5 **N** Southwest Texas Rural Health Alliance, San Antonio, TX — 32 10 30 1731 17 133049 0 16597 6470 319

JUNCTION—Kimble County
KIMBLE HOSPITAL, 2101 Main Street, Zip 76849–2101; tel. 915/446–3321; Ben Snead, Administrator **A**9 10 **F**22 32 34 44 71 **N** Southwest Texas Rural Health Alliance, San Antonio, TX — 16 10 18 276 2 13738 0 2616 1299 51

KATY—Fort Bend County
✠ COLUMBIA KATY MEDICAL CENTER, 5602 Medical Center Drive, Zip 77494; tel. 713/392–1111; Brian S. Barbe, Chief Executive Officer **A**1 9 10 **F**7 8 10 12 16 19 20 21 22 28 29 30 31 32 33 34 35 36 37 40 41 43 44 53 54 55 56 57 58 59 60 65 66 67 69 70 71 73 74 **P**8 **S** Columbia/HCA Healthcare Corporation, Nashville, TN — 33 10 73 4151 33 35673 664 19880 8835 265

KAUFMAN—Kaufman County
✠ PRESBYTERIAN HOSPITAL OF KAUFMAN, 850 Highway 243 West, Zip 75142–9998, Mailing Address: Box 310, Zip 75142; tel. 214/932–7200; Michael J. McBride, CHE, Executive Director (Total facility includes 6 beds in nursing home–type unit) **A**1 9 10 **F**7 8 15 16 17 19 21 22 23 28 34 37 40 42 44 49 61 64 65 71 73 **S** Presbyterian Healthcare System, Dallas, TX **N** Presbyterian Healthcare System, Dallas, TX; North Texas Healthcare Network, Dallas, TX — 23 10 68 2846 35 43640 277 16679 7399 271

KENEDY—Karnes County
OTTO KAISER MEMORIAL HOSPITAL, Highway 181 North, Zip 78119, Mailing Address: Route 1, Box 450, Zip 78119–9718; tel. 210/583–3401; Harold L. Boening, Administrator **A**9 10 **F**19 22 32 37 44 49 71 **N** Southwest Texas Rural Health Alliance, San Antonio, TX — 16 10 30 429 5 27249 0 3786 1670 81

KERMIT—Winkler County
MEMORIAL HOSPITAL, 821 Jeffee Drive, Zip 79745, Mailing Address: Drawer H, Zip 79745; tel. 915/586–5864; Judene Willhelm, Administrator (Nonreporting) **A**9 10 **N** Permian Basin Rural Health Network, Fort Stockton, TX — 13 10 16 — — — — — — —

KERRVILLE—Kerr County
□ KERRVILLE STATE HOSPITAL, 721 Thompson Drive, Zip 78028; tel. 830/896–2211; Gloria P. Olsen, Ph.D., Superintendent **A**1 9 10 **F**14 15 16 20 22 26 30 39 45 52 56 57 65 67 73 — 12 22 213 500 185 0 0 36410 17772 644
✠ SID PETERSON MEMORIAL HOSPITAL, 710 Water Street, Zip 78028–5398; tel. 210/896–4200; F. W. Hall, Jr., Administrator (Total facility includes 28 beds in nursing home–type unit) **A**1 9 10 **F**4 7 8 12 14 15 16 19 21 22 23 28 30 32 34 35 37 40 41 42 44 45 46 49 62 64 65 71 73 74 **P**8 **N** Southwest Texas Rural Health Alliance, San Antonio, TX — 23 10 120 4947 78 84510 456 30537 14278 490
SOUTH TEXAS VETERANS HEALTH CARE SYSTEM, KERRVILLE DIVISION See South Texas Veterans Health Care System, San Antonio

KILGORE—Gregg County
★ ROY H. LAIRD MEMORIAL HOSPITAL, 1612 South Henderson Boulevard, Zip 75662; tel. 903/984–3505; Roderick G. La Grone, President **A**9 10 **F**7 8 19 21 22 26 30 32 34 35 39 40 44 45 71 73 74 **N** Healthcare Partners of East Texas, Inc., Tyler, TX; Regional Healthcare Alliance, Tyler, TX — 14 10 51 1605 13 20982 291 9975 5039 176

KILLEEN—Bell County
✠ METROPLEX HOSPITAL, 2201 South Clear Creek Road, Zip 76542–9305; tel. 817/526–7523 (Total facility includes 13 beds in nursing home–type unit) **A**1 9 10 **F**7 8 10 14 15 16 17 19 21 22 25 28 29 30 32 35 37 39 40 41 42 44 45 46 49 52 53 54 56 57 58 59 63 64 65 67 71 73 **S** Adventist Health System Sunbelt Health Care Corporation, Winter Park, FL **N** Metroplex Health Network, Kileen, TX — 21 10 213 6081 86 — 764 44525 16428 660

KINGSVILLE—Kleberg County
✠ SPOHN KLEBERG MEMORIAL HOSPITAL, 1311 General Cavazos Boulevard, Zip 78363–1197, Mailing Address: P.O. Box 1197, Zip 78363–1197; tel. 512/595–1661; David D. Clark, CHE, Administrator and Vice President (Nonreporting) **A**1 9 10 **S** Incarnate Word Health Services, San Antonio, TX — 21 10 100 — — — — — — —

Hospital, Address, Telephone, Administrator, Approval, Facility, and Physician Codes, Health Care System, Network	Classi-fication Codes		Utilization Data					Expense (thousands) of dollars		
★ American Hospital Association (AHA) membership ☐ Joint Commission on Accreditation of Healthcare Organizations (JCAHO) accreditation + American Osteopathic Hospital Association (AOHA) membership ○ American Osteopathic Association (AOA) accreditation △ Commission on Accreditation of Rehabilitation Facilities (CARF) accreditation Control codes 61, 63, 64, 71, 72 and 73 indicate hospitals listed by AOHA, but not registered by AHA. For definition of numerical codes, see page A4	Control	Service	Beds	Admissions	Census	Outpatient Visits	Births	Total	Payroll	Personnel

KINGWOOD—Harris County

☐ CHARTER BEHAVIORAL HEALTH SYSTEM, 2001 Ladbrook Drive, Zip 77339–3004; tel. 281/358–4501; Mark Micheletti, Chief Executive Officer **A**1 9 10 **F**2 3 18 27 52 53 54 55 56 57 58 59 65 67 **S** Magellan Health Services, Atlanta, GA

| | | 33 | 22 | 80 | 1296 | 29 | 4599 | 0 | 9405 | 2773 | 80 |

✠ COLUMBIA KINGWOOD MEDICAL CENTER, 22999 U.S. Highway 59, Zip 77339; tel. 281/359–7500; Charles D. Schuetz, Chief Executive Officer (Total facility includes 16 beds in nursing home–type unit) (Nonreporting) **A**1 9 10 **S** Columbia/HCA Healthcare Corporation, Nashville, TN

| | | 33 | 10 | 149 | — | — | — | — | — | — | — |

LA GRANGE—Fayette County

✠ FAYETTE MEMORIAL HOSPITAL, 543 North Jackson Street, Zip 78945–2040; tel. 409/968–3166; Marvin E. Cole, President and Chief Executive Officer **A**1 9 10 **F**7 8 12 14 15 16 17 19 22 26 28 29 30 32 34 39 40 41 42 44 49 51 65 71 73 74

| | | 23 | 10 | 45 | 1993 | 24 | 60384 | 310 | 11683 | 4695 | 206 |

LACKLAND AFB—Bexar County

✠ WILFORD HALL MEDICAL CENTER, 2200 Bergquist Drive, Zip 78236–5300; tel. 210/292–7353; Colonel Stephen K. Lecholop, Administrator (Nonreporting) **A**1 2 3 5 **S** Department of the Air Force, Washington, DC

| | | 41 | 10 | 715 | — | — | — | — | — | — | — |

LAKE JACKSON—Brazoria County

✠ △ BRAZOSPORT MEMORIAL HOSPITAL, 100 Medical Drive, Zip 77566–9983; tel. 409/297–4411; Wesley W. Oswald, Chief Executive Officer **A**1 7 9 10 **F**2 3 7 8 10 12 15 19 21 22 23 30 32 35 36 37 40 42 44 48 49 52 53 56 57 59 60 64 65 67 71 73 74 **P**8 **S** Quorum Health Group/Quorum Health Resources, Inc., Brentwood, TN

| | | 23 | 10 | 156 | 5363 | 59 | 59447 | 724 | 34854 | 14792 | 475 |

LAMESA—Dawson County

✠ MEDICAL ARTS HOSPITAL, 1600 North Bryan Avenue, Zip 79331; tel. 806/872–2183; Arla Jeffcoat, Administrator **A**1 9 10 **F**7 8 15 16 17 19 22 23 28 30 32 34 40 44 46 49 65 70 71 73 **N** Lubbock Methodist Hospital System, Lubbock, TX; Permian Basin Rural Health Network, Fort Stockton, TX

| | | 13 | 10 | 44 | 821 | 9 | 16444 | 100 | 7111 | 3715 | 180 |

LANCASTER—Dallas County

✠ COLUMBIA MEDICAL CENTER AT LANCASTER, 2600 West Pleasant Run Road, Zip 75146–1199; tel. 214/223–9600; Ernest C. Lynch, III, Chief Executive Officer (Total facility includes 10 beds in nursing home–type unit) **A**1 9 10 **F**2 3 4 7 8 9 10 11 12 13 16 17 19 20 21 22 23 25 26 28 29 30 31 32 33 34 35 37 38 39 40 41 42 43 44 46 47 48 49 52 57 60 64 65 66 69 70 71 72 73 74 **P**5 7 **S** Columbia/HCA Healthcare Corporation, Nashville, TN

| | | 33 | 10 | 76 | 2564 | 35 | 25737 | 317 | 16655 | 8495 | 281 |

LAREDO—Webb County

✠ COLUMBIA DOCTORS HOSPITAL OF LAREDO, 500 East Mann Road, Zip 78041; tel. 210/723–1131; Benjamin Everett, Chief Executive Officer (Total facility includes 6 beds in nursing home–type unit) **A**1 9 10 **F**8 15 16 19 20 21 22 25 28 30 32 34 35 37 38 39 40 42 44 46 49 60 63 64 65 71 72 73 74 **P**8 **S** Columbia/HCA Healthcare Corporation, Nashville, TN **N** Columbia Healthcare – South Texas Division, Corpus Christi, TX

| | | 32 | 10 | 107 | 5744 | 65 | 57518 | 1875 | 27240 | 11454 | 384 |

✠ MERCY REGIONAL MEDICAL CENTER, 1515 Logan Avenue, Zip 78040, Mailing Address: Drawer 2068, Zip 78044–2068; tel. 210/718–6222; Michael L. Morgan, President and Chief Executive Officer (Total facility includes 30 beds in nursing home–type unit) **A**1 9 10 **F**4 7 8 10 11 12 13 14 15 16 17 19 21 22 25 27 28 30 31 32 34 35 37 38 39 40 43 44 45 47 48 49 63 64 71 72 73 74 **P**8 **S** Sisters of Mercy Health System–St. Louis, Saint Louis, MO

| | | 21 | 10 | 320 | 13521 | 196 | 153943 | 3524 | 85502 | 34031 | 1253 |

LAUGHLIN AFB—Val Verde County

★ U. S. AIR FORCE HOSPITAL, 590 Mitchell Boulevard, Zip 78843–5200; tel. 210/298–6311; Major John G. Wiseman, Administrator (Nonreporting) **S** Department of the Air Force, Washington, DC

| | | 41 | 10 | 8 | — | — | — | — | — | — | — |

LEAGUE CITY—Galveston County

☐ DEVEREUX TEXAS TREATMENT NETWORK, 1150 Devereux Drive, Zip 77573; tel. 713/335–1000; L. Gail Atkinson, Executive Director **A**1 9 10 **F**2 3 12 13 15 16 17 18 22 24 25 30 34 39 45 46 52 53 54 55 56 57 58 59 65 67 68 70 **P**4 **S** Devereux Foundation, Devon, PA

| | | 23 | 22 | 88 | 593 | 48 | 2851 | 0 | 10488 | 5460 | 159 |

LEVELLAND—Hockley County

✠ METHODIST HOSPITAL–LEVELLAND, 1900 South College Avenue, Zip 79336; tel. 806/894–4963; Jerry Osburn, Administrator **A**1 9 10 **F**7 8 14 15 16 17 19 20 21 22 28 29 30 31 32 33 34 36 39 40 43 44 45 46 49 51 53 54 55 56 57 58 59 65 71 73 **P**7 **S** Lubbock Methodist Hospital System, Lubbock, TX

| | | 21 | 10 | 44 | 1585 | 18 | 23406 | 255 | 11159 | 3854 | 171 |

LEWISVILLE—Denton County

✠ COLUMBIA MEDICAL CENTER OF LEWISVILLE, 500 West Main, Zip 75057–3699; tel. 972/420–1000; Raymond M. Dunning, Jr., Chief Executive Officer **A**1 9 10 **F**4 7 8 19 22 32 33 35 37 40 41 42 44 49 64 65 66 67 71 73 74 **S** Columbia/HCA Healthcare Corporation, Nashville, TN

| | | 33 | 10 | 119 | 5985 | 63 | 48409 | 1042 | 47923 | 16040 | 532 |

LIBERTY—Liberty County

☐ LIBERTY–DAYTON HOSPITAL, (Formerly Baptist Hospital Liberty), 1353 North Travis Street, Zip 77575–1353; tel. 409/336–7316; Mynette Dennis, R.N., Administrator **A**1 9 10 **F**12 15 19 21 22 28 30 32 33 34 39 44 46 49 65 71 72 73 **P**3 5 8

| | | 21 | 10 | 29 | 740 | 8 | 14046 | 0 | 5847 | 2539 | 96 |

LINDEN—Cass County

LINDEN MUNICIPAL HOSPITAL, North Kaufman Street, Zip 75563, Mailing Address: Box 32, Zip 75563; tel. 903/756–5561; Fred Wilbanks, Administrator **A**9 10 **F**8 11 16 19 20 22 32 37 44 46 48 49 57 64 71 **N** Healthcare Partners of East Texas, Inc., Tyler, TX

| | | 16 | 10 | 39 | 690 | 8 | 3351 | 0 | 5196 | 2607 | 104 |

Hospital, Address, Telephone, Administrator, Approval, Facility, and Physician Codes, Health Care System, Network	Control	Service	Beds	Admissions	Census	Outpatient Visits	Births	Total	Payroll	Personnel

Classification Codes / **Utilization Data** / **Expense (thousands) of dollars**

★ American Hospital Association (AHA) membership
□ Joint Commission on Accreditation of Healthcare Organizations (JCAHO) accreditation
+ American Osteopathic Hospital Association (AOHA) membership
○ American Osteopathic Association (AOA) accreditation
△ Commission on Accreditation of Rehabilitation Facilities (CARF) accreditation
Control codes 61, 63, 64, 71, 72 and 73 indicate hospitals listed by AOHA, but not registered by AHA. For definition of numerical codes, see page A4

LITTLEFIELD—Lamb County

	Control	Service	Beds	Admissions	Census	Outpatient Visits	Births	Total	Payroll	Personnel
✖ LAMB HEALTHCARE CENTER, 1500 South Sunset, Zip 79339; tel. 806/385–6411; Randall A. Young, Administrator (Nonreporting) **A**1 9 10 **S** Lubbock Methodist Hospital System, Lubbock, TX **N** Lubbock Methodist Hospital System, Lubbock, TX	13	10	41	—	—	—	—	—	—	—

LIVINGSTON—Polk County

MEMORIAL MEDICAL CENTER–LIVINGSTON, 602 East Church Street, Zip 77351–1257, Mailing Address: P.O. Box 1257, Zip 77351–1257; tel. 409/327–4381; James C. Dickson, Administrator **A**9 10 **F**7 8 15 19 22 28 30 34 44 71 73 **N** Healthcare Partners of East Texas, Inc., Tyler, TX	23	10	28	1119	8	—	162	7296	3202	105

LLANO—Llano County

✖ LLANO MEMORIAL HOSPITAL, 200 West Ollie Street, Zip 78643–2628; tel. 915/247–5040; Ernest Parisi, Administrator and Chief Executive Officer **A**1 9 10 **F**7 8 15 16 17 19 21 22 28 30 32 33 41 42 44 49 51 65 71 73 **P**3	13	10	27	1550	13	54519	281	10878	4267	209

LOCKNEY—Floyd County

W. J. MANGOLD MEMORIAL HOSPITAL, 320 North Main Street, Zip 79241–0037, Mailing Address: Box 37, Zip 79241–0037; tel. 806/652–3373; Robin Satterwhite, Administrator **A**9 10 **F**7 22 28 34 40 44 49 51 61 70 71	16	10	27	603	6	21457	136	3060	1493	73

LONGVIEW—Gregg County

✖ COLUMBIA LONGVIEW REGIONAL MEDICAL CENTER, 2901 North Fourth Street, Zip 75605, Mailing Address: P.O. Box 14000, Zip 75607–4000; tel. 903/758–1818; Velinda Stevens, Chief Executive Officer **A**1 9 10 **F**7 8 10 12 15 17 18 19 21 22 23 24 28 30 32 34 35 37 39 40 41 42 44 45 46 48 49 50 60 63 64 65 66 67 71 73 74 **P**5 7 8 **S** Columbia/HCA Healthcare Corporation, Nashville, TN **N** Regional Healthcare Alliance, Tyler, TX	33	10	115	3915	58	44181	420	37417	16944	509
✖ △ GOOD SHEPHERD MEDICAL CENTER, 700 East Marshall Avenue, Zip 75601–5571; tel. 903/236–2000; Jerry D. Adair, President and Chief Executive Officer (Total facility includes 26 beds in nursing home–type unit) **A**1 7 9 10 **F**4 7 8 10 12 14 15 16 17 19 20 21 22 23 25 26 27 28 29 30 31 32 34 35 37 39 40 41 42 43 44 45 46 48 51 56 60 63 64 65 66 69 70 71 73 74 **P**1 **N** Healthcare Partners of East Texas, Inc., Tyler, TX; Good Shepherd Health Network, Longview, TX	23	10	323	14479	218	140956	1726	114126	45700	1709

LUBBOCK—Lubbock County

□ CHARTER PLAINS BEHAVIORAL HEALTH SYSTEM, 801 North Quaker, Zip 79416, Mailing Address: P.O. Box 10560, Zip 79408; tel. 806/744–5505; Karl R. Brady, Chief Executive Officer and Administrator **A**1 5 9 10 **F**2 3 12 34 46 52 53 54 56 57 58 59 65 67 **S** Magellan Health Services, Atlanta, GA	33	22	80	882	20	7480	0	5496	3164	75
□ HIGHLAND MEDICAL CENTER, 2412 50th Street, Zip 79412; tel. 806/788–4060; David Conejo, Chief Executive Officer (Nonreporting) **A**1 2 9 10 **S** Community Health Systems, Inc., Brentwood, TN	33	10	76	—	—	—	—	—	—	—
□ HORIZON SPECIALTY HOSPITAL, 1409 9th Street, Zip 79401; tel. 806/767–9133; Steve Grappe, Administrator **A**1 9 10 **F**12 45 48 65	33	46	30	168	13	0	0	4441	1003	85
★ METHODIST CHILDREN'S HOSPITAL, 3610 21st Street, Zip 79410; tel. 806/784–5040; James P. Houser, President and Chief Executive Officer **A**9 10 **F**4 7 8 10 14 15 16 19 21 22 23 24 26 30 31 32 35 38 41 42 43 44 45 47 49 60 65 69 70 71 **P**7 **S** Lubbock Methodist Hospital System, Lubbock, TX	23	50	65	2306	24	19885	1197	13747	2498	79
✖ △ METHODIST HOSPITAL, 3615 19th Street, Zip 79410–1201, Mailing Address: Box 1201, Zip 79408–1201; tel. 806/792–1011; James P. Houser, President and Chief Executive Officer **A**1 2 6 7 9 10 **F**4 7 8 10 11 14 15 16 17 19 21 22 23 24 26 30 31 32 35 37 38 39 40 41 42 43 44 45 47 49 60 64 65 67 69 70 71 73 74 **P**7 **S** Lubbock Methodist Hospital System, Lubbock, TX	23	10	520	21261	355	—	0	246104	87798	2505
□ SOUTH PARK HOSPITAL, 6610 Quaker Avenue, Zip 79413–5938; tel. 806/791–8000; D. Clinton Matthews, Chief Executive Officer **A**1 9 10 **F**7 8 12 16 17 19 21 22 24 25 30 32 34 35 37 38 39 40 41 42 44 49 61 63 65 66 67 68 71 72 73 74 **P**7 **S** TENET Healthcare Corporation, Santa Barbara, CA	33	10	101	1387	14	19210	372	17640	5578	172
✖ ST. MARY OF THE PLAINS HOSPITAL, 4000 24th Street, Zip 79410; tel. 806/796–6000; Charley O. Trimble, President and Chief Executive Officer **A**1 2 3 5 9 10 **F**2 4 7 8 10 11 12 15 16 17 19 20 21 22 28 29 30 31 32 34 35 37 38 40 41 42 43 44 45 46 47 48 52 56 59 60 64 65 67 71 73 74 **P**3 5 6 7 **S** St. Joseph Health System, Orange, CA	21	10	410	13612	264	—	979	148225	44110	1797
✖ UNIVERSITY MEDICAL CENTER, 602 Indiana Avenue, Zip 79415, Mailing Address: P.O. Box 5980, Zip 79408–5980; tel. 806/743–3111; James P. Courtney, President and Chief Executive Officer **A**1 2 3 5 9 10 **F**4 7 8 9 10 11 12 15 17 19 21 22 23 28 29 30 31 32 35 37 38 40 42 43 44 46 47 48 49 54 56 60 63 64 65 66 67 69 70 71 73 74 **P**7	16	10	312	14457	182	143086	1909	121971	40632	1679

LUFKIN—Angelina County

✖ COLUMBIA WOODLAND HEIGHTS MEDICAL CENTER, 500 Gaslight Boulevard, Zip 75901, Mailing Address: Box 150610, Zip 75915–0610; tel. 409/634–8311; Don H. McBride, Chief Executive Officer (Total facility includes 16 beds in nursing home–type unit) **A**1 9 10 **F**4 7 8 10 11 12 15 16 19 21 22 25 28 30 32 34 35 40 43 44 46 64 65 66 71 73 **P**5 8 **S** Columbia/HCA Healthcare Corporation, Nashville, TN **N** Regional Healthcare Alliance, Tyler, TX	33	10	110	4678	64	44778	476	32800	10998	389
✖ MEMORIAL MEDICAL CENTER OF EAST TEXAS, (Formerly Memorial Health System of Texas), 1201 Frank Street, Zip 75904, Mailing Address: P.O. Box 1447, Zip 75902–1447; tel. 409/634–8111; Gary Lex Whatley, President and Chief Executive Officer (Total facility includes 30 beds in nursing home–type unit) **A**1 2 9 10 **F**7 8 10 11 12 14 15 16 17 18 19 21 22 23 26 27 28 29 30 31 32 33 34 35 37 39 40 41 42 44 45 46 48 49 51 52 54 55 56 57 58 59 60 64 65 67 71 72 73 74 **P**5 7 8 **N** Healthcare Partners of East Texas, Inc., Tyler, TX	23	10	215	8729	132	138101	558	58168	23180	818

Hospital, Address, Telephone, Administrator, Approval, Facility, and Physician Codes, Health Care System, Network	Classi-fication Codes		Utilization Data					Expense (thousands) of dollars		
★ American Hospital Association (AHA) membership □ Joint Commission on Accreditation of Healthcare Organizations (JCAHO) accreditation + American Osteopathic Hospital Association (AOHA) membership ○ American Osteopathic Association (AOA) accreditation △ Commission on Accreditation of Rehabilitation Facilities (CARF) accreditation Control codes 61, 63, 64, 71, 72 and 73 indicate hospitals listed by AOHA, but not registered by AHA. For definition of numerical codes, see page A4	Control	Service	Beds	Admissions	Census	Outpatient Visits	Births	Total	Payroll	Personnel

LULING—Caldwell County

★ EDGAR B. DAVIS MEMORIAL HOSPITAL, 130 Hays Street, Zip 78648, Mailing Address: P.O. Box 510, Zip 78648–0510; tel. 210/875–5643; Neal Kelley, Administrator (Total facility includes 6 beds in nursing home–type unit) **A**9 10 **F**8 12 15 16 19 21 22 27 28 34 35 44 49 53 56 57 58 64 65 71 73 **P**8 **N** Southwest Texas Rural Health Alliance, San Antonio, TX

| | 14 | 10 | 21 | 1005 | 12 | 28755 | 81 | 6002 | 2637 | 96 |

MADISONVILLE—Madison County

✠ ST. FRANCIS HEALTH CENTER, 100 West Cross Street, Zip 77864–0698, Mailing Address: Box 698, Zip 77864–0698; tel. 409/348–2631; James P. Gibson, President and Chief Executive Officer **A**1 9 10 **F**7 8 15 19 21 22 25 28 31 32 34 40 44 49 51 58 65 71 73 **P**6 **S** Franciscan Services Corporation, Sylvania, OH

| | 21 | 10 | 32 | 1103 | 14 | 37971 | 86 | 9185 | 4753 | 263 |

MANSFIELD—Tarrant County

□ VENCOR HOSPITAL–FORT WORTH SOUTH, (LONG TERM ACUTE CARE), (Includes Vencor Hospital – Fort Worth West, 815 Eighth Avenue, Fort Worth, Zip 76104; tel. 817/332–4812), 1802 Highway 157 North, Zip 76063–9555; tel. 817/473–6101 **A**1 9 10 **F**14 16 19 21 22 35 37 39 65 71 73 **S** Vencor, Incorporated, Louisville, KY

| | 33 | 49 | 94 | 471 | 48 | 105 | 0 | 14866 | 7034 | 286 |

MARLIN—Falls County

CENTRAL TEXAS VA HEALTH CARE SYSTEM, MARLIN INTEGRATED CLINICAL FACILITY See Central Texas Veterans Affairs Healthcare System, Temple

FALLS COMMUNITY HOSPITAL AND CLINIC, 322 Coleman Street, Zip 76661–2358, Mailing Address: Box 60, Zip 76661–0060; tel. 817/883–3561; Billy Don York, Administrator **A**9 10 **F**1 3 4 5 6 7 8 10 12 13 17 18 19 20 21 22 23 24 25 26 27 28 29 30 31 32 33 34 35 36 39 41 42 43 44 45 46 49 50 51 53 54 55 56 57 58 59 60 61 62 63 65 66 67 68 69 70 71 72 73 74 **P**5 **N** Central Texas Rural Health Network, Harrietsville, TX; Brazo's Valley Health Network, Waco, TX

| | 23 | 10 | 32 | 986 | 11 | 24331 | 0 | 4409 | 2142 | 104 |

MARSHALL—Harrison County

✠ MARSHALL REGIONAL MEDICAL CENTER, (Formerly Marshall Memorial Hospital), 811 South Washington Avenue, Zip 75670, Mailing Address: P.O. Box 1599, Zip 75671–1599; tel. 903/927–6000; Thomas N. Cammack, Jr., Chief Executive Officer (Total facility includes 10 beds in nursing home–type unit) **A**1 9 10 **F**7 8 12 15 16 17 19 21 22 23 28 31 32 34 35 37 39 40 41 42 44 46 49 64 65 70 71 73 **P**3 7 8

| | 23 | 10 | 103 | 3416 | 48 | 57718 | 609 | 24797 | 10481 | 398 |

MCALLEN—Hidalgo County

□ CHARTER PALMS BEHAVIORAL HEALTH SYSTEM, 1421 East Jackson Avenue, Zip 78501, Mailing Address: P.O. Box 5239, Zip 78502; tel. 210/631–5421; Leslie Bingham, Chief Executive Officer **A**1 9 10 **F**2 3 16 19 34 35 52 53 56 57 58 59 65 71 **S** Magellan Health Services, Atlanta, GA

| | 33 | 22 | 80 | 1052 | 26 | 6591 | 0 | 6231 | 2437 | 78 |

✠ COLUMBIA RIO GRANDE REGIONAL HOSPITAL, 101 East Ridge Road, Zip 78503; tel. 210/632–6000; Randall M. Everts, Chief Executive Officer **A**1 9 10 **F**4 7 8 10 11 12 17 19 20 21 22 23 24 28 29 30 32 34 35 37 39 40 41 42 43 44 46 49 64 65 67 71 73 74 **P**8 **S** Columbia/HCA Healthcare Corporation, Nashville, TN **N** Columbia Healthcare – South Texas Division, Corpus Christi, TX

| | 33 | 10 | 222 | 9661 | 136 | 48566 | 1354 | 55762 | 20850 | 674 |

□ MCALLEN MEDICAL CENTER, 301 West Expressway 83, Zip 78503; tel. 210/632–4000; John L. Mims, Executive Director **A**1 3 9 10 **F**2 4 7 8 10 15 16 17 19 20 21 22 23 24 28 29 30 32 34 35 37 38 39 40 41 42 43 44 45 46 47 48 49 51 52 53 55 56 57 58 59 60 61 64 65 66 67 71 73 **P**8 **S** Universal Health Services, Inc., King of Prussia, PA

| | 33 | 10 | 472 | 22626 | 359 | 82626 | 6378 | 128081 | 52577 | 1487 |

MCCAMEY—Upton County

MCCAMEY HOSPITAL, Highway 305 South, Zip 79752, Mailing Address: Box 1200, Zip 79752–1200; tel. 915/652–8626; Bill Boswell, Chief Executive Officer (Total facility includes 30 beds in nursing home–type unit) **A**9 10 **F**15 22 32 34 44 49 64 **P**5 **N** Permian Basin Rural Health Network, Fort Stockton, TX

| | 16 | 10 | 46 | 114 | 30 | 26353 | 0 | 4196 | 1686 | 49 |

MCKINNEY—Collin County

✠ COLUMBIA MEDICAL CENTER OF MCKINNEY, (Includes North Texas Medical Center–Westpark Campus, 130 South Central Expressway, Zip 75070; tel. 214/548–5300), 1800 North Graves Street, Zip 75069; tel. 214/548–3000; Don S. Ciulla, Chief Executive Officer **A**1 9 10 **F**7 8 12 16 19 22 23 24 26 28 32 34 35 42 44 46 57 65 71 72 73 74 **P**7 8 **S** Columbia/HCA Healthcare Corporation, Nashville, TN

| | 32 | 10 | 150 | 6352 | 85 | 54602 | 1069 | 40111 | 17341 | 611 |

MEMPHIS—Hall County

HALL COUNTY HOSPITAL, 1800 North Boykin Drive, Zip 79245; tel. 806/259–3504; Jody Dixon, Administrator **A**9 10 **F**8 19 22 28 32 33 39 49 64 71 73

| | 16 | 10 | 20 | 313 | 3 | 5819 | 0 | 1661 | 910 | 45 |

MESQUITE—Dallas County

□ MEDICAL CENTER OF MESQUITE, 1011 North Galloway Avenue, Zip 75149; tel. 214/320–7000; Terry J. Fontenot, Administrator **A**1 9 10 **F**4 7 8 10 11 12 14 15 16 17 19 21 22 29 30 32 33 35 37 38 39 40 42 43 44 49 63 64 65 71 73 74 **P**5 8 **S** Paracelsus Healthcare Corporation, Houston, TX **N** Saint Paul Medical Center Affiliate Network, Dallas, TX; Brazo's Valley Health Network, Waco, TX

| | 33 | 10 | 176 | 5609 | 77 | 48807 | 175 | 48286 | 16918 | 488 |

□ MESQUITE COMMUNITY HOSPITAL, 3500 Interstate 30, Zip 75150–2696; tel. 972/698–3300; Raymond P. De Blasi, Chief Executive Officer (Total facility includes 13 beds in nursing home–type unit) **A**1 9 10 **F**7 8 10 15 16 19 20 21 22 26 32 33 34 35 37 39 40 41 42 44 45 49 52 57 64 65 71 73

| | 33 | 10 | 128 | 5766 | 63 | 49322 | 1569 | 30865 | 13710 | 457 |

Hospital, Address, Telephone, Administrator, Approval, Facility, and Physician Codes, Health Care System, Network	Classi-fication Codes		Utilization Data					Expense (thousands) of dollars		
	Control	Service	Beds	Admissions	Census	Outpatient Visits	Births	Total	Payroll	Personnel

American Hospital Association (AHA) membership
□ Joint Commission on Accreditation of Healthcare Organizations (JCAHO) accreditation
+ American Osteopathic Hospital Association (AOHA) membership
○ American Osteopathic Association (AOA) accreditation
△ Commission on Accreditation of Rehabilitation Facilities (CARF) accreditation
Control codes 61, 63, 64, 71, 72 and 73 indicate hospitals listed by AOHA, but not registered by AHA. For definition of numerical codes, see page A4

MEXIA—Limestone County

☒ PARKVIEW REGIONAL HOSPITAL, 312 East Glendale Street, Zip 76667–3608; tel. 817/562–5332; Karl R. Stinson, Administrator **A**1 9 10 **F**8 11 12 13 15 17 19 22 28 30 32 33 34 40 41 44 46 49 65 71 73 **P**1 **S** Principal Hospital Group, Brentwood, TN **N** Central Texas Rural Health Network, Harrietsville, TX; Brazo's Valley Health Network, Waco, TX — 23 10 28 1022 10 22776 132 8649 3372 145

MIDLAND—Midland County

☒ △ MEMORIAL HOSPITAL AND MEDICAL CENTER, (Includes Memorial Rehabilitation Hospital, Zip 79704; tel. 915/697–5200), 2200 West Illinois Avenue, Zip 79701; tel. 915/685–1111; Harold Rubin, President and Chief Executive Officer (Total facility includes 17 beds in nursing home–type unit) **A**1 2 5 7 9 10 **F**4 7 8 10 12 13 14 15 16 17 19 21 22 23 25 28 29 30 31 33 34 35 37 39 40 41 42 43 44 46 48 54 56 60 64 65 67 69 71 72 73 74 **P**3 7 8 **N** Permian Basin Rural Health Network, Fort Stockton, TX — 16 10 270 10188 175 114295 1597 104603 34999 1053

WESTWOOD MEDICAL CENTER, 4214 Andrews Highway, Zip 79703; tel. 915/522–2273; Michael S. Potter, President and Chief Executive Officer **A**9 10 **F**7 8 15 16 19 21 28 31 32 37 39 40 44 46 49 63 71 72 73 74 **P**7 **S** Paracelsus Healthcare Corporation, Houston, TX — 33 10 80 2596 29 35125 231 24949 7303 256

MINERAL WELLS—Palo Pinto County

☒ PALO PINTO GENERAL HOSPITAL, 400 S.W. 25th Avenue, Zip 76067–9685; tel. 817/325–7891; Guy Hazlett, II, FACHE, Chief Executive Officer **A**1 9 10 **F**4 7 8 12 13 14 15 16 19 21 22 29 30 32 33 35 36 37 39 40 44 45 46 49 51 65 66 67 71 73 74 — 16 10 44 2570 29 26409 390 20381 9514 418

MISSION—Hidalgo County

☒ MISSION HOSPITAL, 900 South Bryan Road, Zip 78572; tel. 210/580–9000; Paul H. Ballard, Chief Executive Officer **A**1 9 10 **F**7 8 15 19 28 29 30 34 35 37 40 41 42 44 46 65 67 71 73 **P**7 8 **S** Quorum Health Group/Quorum Health Resources, Inc., Brentwood, TN — 23 10 110 5261 74 32604 1089 30709 12265 547

MISSOURI CITY—Fort Bend County

☒ COLUMBIA FORT BEND HOSPITAL, 3803 FM 1092 at Highway 6, Zip 77459; tel. 713/499–4800; Janie R. Kauffman, Chief Executive Officer (Total facility includes 5 beds in nursing home–type unit) **A**1 9 10 **F**2 3 4 5 6 7 8 9 10 11 12 13 14 15 16 17 18 19 20 21 22 23 24 25 26 28 29 30 31 32 33 34 35 36 37 38 39 40 41 42 43 44 45 46 47 48 49 52 53 54 55 56 57 58 59 60 64 65 66 67 68 69 71 72 73 74 **P**2 5 7 8 **S** Columbia/HCA Healthcare Corporation, Nashville, TN — 33 10 65 3087 33 38857 522 20641 8157 272

MONAHANS—Ward County

☒ WARD MEMORIAL HOSPITAL, 406 South Gary Street, Zip 79756; tel. 915/943–2511; William F. O'Brien, Administrator and Chief Executive Officer **A**1 9 10 **F**2 7 14 15 16 19 22 28 30 32 33 40 44 47 49 52 64 65 67 71 73 **N** Permian Basin Rural Health Network, Fort Stockton, TX — 13 10 39 835 8 14822 38 5410 3024 130

MORTON—Cochran County

★ COCHRAN MEMORIAL HOSPITAL, 201 East Grant Street, Zip 79346; tel. 806/266–5565; Paul McKinney, Administrator **A**9 10 **F**19 25 32 34 44 51 70 71 **P**5 **N** Lubbock Methodist Hospital System, Lubbock, TX — 16 10 30 363 3 7043 0 2539 1040 47

MOUNT PLEASANT—Titus County

☒ TITUS REGIONAL MEDICAL CENTER, 2001 North Jefferson, Zip 75455; tel. 903/577–6000; Steven K. Jacobson, Chief Executive Officer (Total facility includes 20 beds in nursing home–type unit) **A**1 9 10 **F**7 8 10 15 16 17 19 21 22 27 34 35 37 39 40 41 44 48 49 50 63 64 65 66 70 71 73 74 **P**1 **S** Quorum Health Group/Quorum Health Resources, Inc., Brentwood, TN **N** Healthcare Partners of East Texas, Inc., Tyler, TX; Regional Healthcare Alliance, Tyler, TX — 12 10 165 7107 93 22219 1020 38328 16642 640

MOUNT VERNON—Franklin County

☒ EAST TEXAS MEDICAL CENTER—MOUNT VERNON, Highway 37 South, Zip 75457, Mailing Address: Box 477, Zip 75457–0477; tel. 903/537–4552; Charles N. Butts, Administrator (Nonreporting) **A**1 9 10 **S** East Texas Medical Center Regional Healthcare System, Tyler, TX **N** Healthcare Partners of East Texas, Inc., Tyler, TX — 23 10 30 — — — — — — —

MUENSTER—Cooke County

MUENSTER MEMORIAL HOSPITAL, 605 North Maple Street, Zip 76252, Mailing Address: Box 370, Zip 76252; tel. 817/759–2271; Jack R. Endres, Administrator **A**9 10 **F**7 8 15 19 20 21 22 28 30 32 33 34 40 44 49 65 67 71 — 16 10 18 396 4 17436 13 3013 1163 54

MULESHOE—Bailey County

★ MULESHOE AREA MEDICAL CENTER, 708 South First Street, Zip 79347; tel. 806/272–4524; Jim G. Bone, Interim Administrator **A**9 10 **F**14 15 19 32 35 44 49 70 73 **S** Lubbock Methodist Hospital System, Lubbock, TX **N** Lubbock Methodist Hospital System, Lubbock, TX — 16 10 31 506 4 20560 41 4522 2077 108

NACOGDOCHES—Nacogdoches County

□ NACOGDOCHES MEDICAL CENTER, 4920 N.E. Stallings, Zip 75961, Mailing Address: Box 631604, Zip 75963–1604; tel. 409/568–3380; Bryant H. Krenek, Jr., Director **A**1 9 10 **F**4 7 8 10 12 15 16 19 21 22 23 30 32 35 37 40 41 42 43 44 46 49 51 60 64 65 67 71 73 **P**5 **S** TENET Healthcare Corporation, Santa Barbara, CA **N** Regional Healthcare Alliance, Tyler, TX — 32 10 113 5532 68 30987 610 30496 12481 397

☒ △ NACOGDOCHES MEMORIAL HOSPITAL, 1204 North Mound Street, Zip 75961; tel. 409/568–8521; Gary J. Blan, FACHE, President and Chief Executive Officer **A**1 7 9 10 **F**4 7 8 10 14 15 16 19 22 28 30 31 32 33 34 35 37 40 41 42 43 44 45 48 49 65 67 71 73 **P**8 **N** Healthcare Partners of East Texas, Inc., Tyler, TX — 16 10 150 5461 85 37257 810 50394 19172 661

Hospital, Address, Telephone, Administrator, Approval, Facility, and Physician Codes, Health Care System, Network	Classi-fication Codes		Utilization Data					Expense (thousands) of dollars		
★ American Hospital Association (AHA) membership □ Joint Commission on Accreditation of Healthcare Organizations (JCAHO) accreditation + American Osteopathic Hospital Association (AOHA) membership ○ American Osteopathic Association (AOA) accreditation △ Commission on Accreditation of Rehabilitation Facilities (CARF) accreditation Control codes 61, 63, 64, 71, 72 and 73 indicate hospitals listed by AOHA, but not registered by AHA. For definition of numerical codes, see page A4	Control	Service	Beds	Admissions	Census	Outpatient Visits	Births	Total	Payroll	Personnel

□ PINELANDS HOSPITAL, 4632 Northeast Stallings Drive, Zip 75961, Mailing Address: P.O. Box 1004, Zip 79563–1004; tel. 409/560–5900; David Baker, Interim Administrator **A**1 9 10 **F**12 15 17 18 26 52 53 54 55 56 57 58 59 65 67 **P**1 5 7 **N** Healthcare Partners of East Texas, Inc., Tyler, TX; Regional Healthcare Alliance, Tyler, TX	33	22	38	546	17	4098	0	4222	2009	56
NASSAU BAY—Harris County										
✵ ST. JOHN HOSPITAL, 2050 Space Park Drive, Zip 77058; tel. 281/333–5503; Thomas Permetti, Administrator **A**1 9 10 **F**2 3 4 5 7 8 9 10 11 12 14 15 16 17 18 19 20 21 22 24 26 28 29 30 31 32 33 34 35 36 37 38 39 40 41 42 43 44 45 46 47 48 49 50 51 52 53 54 55 56 57 58 59 60 61 63 64 65 66 67 69 71 72 73 74 **P**3 7 8 **S** Sisters of Charity of the Incarnate Word Healthcare System, Houston, TX **N** SouthEast Texas Integrated Community Health Network, Houston, TX	23	10	133	4262	38	102165	639	34238	13265	503
NAVASOTA—Grimes County										
CLC–NAVASOTA REGIONAL HOSPITAL, 210 South Judson Street, Zip 77868, Mailing Address: P.O. Box 1390, Zip 77868–1390; tel. 409/825–6585; Molly Hurst, Administrator (Nonreporting) **A**9	33	10	30	—	—	—	—	—	—	—
NEDERLAND—Jefferson County										
□ MID–JEFFERSON HOSPITAL, Highway 365 and 27th Street, Zip 77627, Mailing Address: P.O. Box 1917, Zip 77627–1917; tel. 409/727–2321; Wilson J. Weber, Chief Executive Officer (Total facility includes 18 beds in nursing home–type unit) **A**1 5 9 10 **F**7 8 12 13 15 16 17 19 21 22 28 29 30 31 32 34 37 40 44 45 46 51 64 71 73 74 **P**3 7 **S** TENET Healthcare Corporation, Santa Barbara, CA	32	10	138	3027	37	58353	439	19953	7203	254
NEW BRAUNFELS—Comal County										
✵ MCKENNA MEMORIAL HOSPITAL, 143 East Garza Street, Zip 78130–4191; tel. 210/606–9111; Marion P. Johnson, FACHE, President and Chief Executive Officer **A**1 9 10 **F**7 8 15 16 17 19 21 22 23 24 30 32 35 37 40 41 42 44 45 46 48 49 65 71 73 74 **P**1 **N** Southwest Texas Rural Health Alliance, San Antonio, TX	23	10	77	4790	46	52999	748	25756	13357	508
NOCONA—Montague County										
★ NOCONA GENERAL HOSPITAL, 100 Park Street, Zip 76255; tel. 817/825–3235; Jamers Brasier, Administrator **A**9 10 **F**8 12 15 16 19 20 22 26 28 32 39 40 41 42 44 49 51 65 70 71 73 **N** Texoma Health Network, Wichita Falls, TX	16	10	36	946	11	9039	82	5835	2775	116
NORTH RICHLAND HILLS—Tarrant County										
✵ COLUMBIA NORTH HILLS HOSPITAL, 4401 Booth Calloway Road, Zip 76180–7399; tel. 817/284–1431; Randy Moresi, Chief Executive Officer (Total facility includes 14 beds in nursing home–type unit) **A**1 9 10 **F**4 7 8 10 11 12 15 16 19 21 22 23 24 28 29 30 32 33 34 35 37 39 40 41 42 43 44 45 46 48 49 64 65 67 71 73 74 **P**5 **S** Columbia/HCA Healthcare Corporation, Nashville, TN	33	10	134	5432	69	49103	789	36818	16626	363
ODESSA—Ector County										
✵ MEDICAL CENTER HOSPITAL, 500 West Fourth Street, Zip 79761–5059, Mailing Address: P.O. Drawer 7239, Zip 79760; tel. 915/640–4000; J. Michael Stephans, Administrator (Total facility includes 25 beds in nursing home–type unit) **A**1 2 3 5 9 10 **F**4 7 8 10 11 16 17 19 21 22 23 25 30 33 34 35 37 38 40 42 43 44 46 49 50 51 60 63 64 65 71 73 **P**8 **N** Permian Basin Rural Health Network, Fort Stockton, TX	16	10	333	11080	218	127645	1380	116962	43130	1539
□ ODESSA REGIONAL HOSPITAL, 520 East Sixth Street, Zip 79761, Mailing Address: Box 4859, Zip 79760; tel. 915/334–8200; Lex A. Guinn, Chief Executive Officer **A**1 9 10 **F**7 8 10 12 14 15 16 19 22 27 28 29 30 32 34 36 37 38 39 40 44 45 46 65 67 70 71 73 74 **P**7 8 **S** TENET Healthcare Corporation, Santa Barbara, CA	32	44	100	4083	41	76867	1392	24787	8800	341
OLNEY—Young County										
★ HAMILTON HOSPITAL, 903 West Hamilton Street, Zip 76374, Mailing Address: Box 158, Zip 76374; tel. 817/564–5521; William R. Smith, Administrator **A**9 10 **F**7 19 22 28 32 33 37 40 44 45 71 73 **P**5 **N** Texoma Health Network, Wichita Falls, TX	16	10	46	916	17	—	36	5402	2595	133
ORANGE—Orange County										
□ BAPTIST HOSPITAL–ORANGE, 608 Strickland, Zip 77630; tel. 409/883–9361; Kevin T. Coleman, Administrator (Total facility includes 16 beds in nursing home–type unit) **A**1 9 10 **F**7 8 12 14 15 16 17 19 21 22 26 27 28 30 31 32 34 35 37 40 41 44 48 49 64 65 67 71 72 73 **P**8	21	10	118	3296	51	50811	299	28376	9235	428
PALACIOS—Matagorda County										
★ WAGNER GENERAL HOSPITAL, 310 Green Street, Zip 77465, Mailing Address: Box 859, Zip 77465; tel. 512/972–2511; Helen Dolezal, Director **A**9 10 **F**8 15 16 19 22 30 32 34 35 44 49 57 65 71 **P**5 **S** Matagorda County Hospital District, Bay City, TX	16	10	6	16	1	4273	0	1405	590	20
PALESTINE—Anderson County										
□ MEMORIAL MOTHER FRANCES HOSPITAL, (Formerly Memorial Hospital), 4000 South Loop 256, Zip 75801, Mailing Address: Box 4070, Zip 75802; tel. 903/731–5000; Stephen M. Erixon, Chief Executive Officer (Nonreporting) **A**1 9 10 **N** Regional Healthcare Alliance, Tyler, TX	23	10	93	—	—	—	—	—	—	—
□ TRINITY VALLEY MEDICAL CENTER, 2900 South Loop 256, Zip 75801; tel. 903/731–1000; Larry C. Bozeman, Chief Executive Officer (Total facility includes 12 beds in nursing home–type unit) **A**1 9 10 **F**7 8 10 12 15 16 19 20 21 22 23 28 29 30 32 34 35 37 40 41 44 45 46 48 49 52 55 56 57 63 64 65 67 71 73 74 **N** Healthcare Partners of East Texas, Inc., Tyler, TX	33	10	150	4657	64	55894	504	32756	12354	475

Hospital, Address, Telephone, Administrator, Approval, Facility, and Physician Codes, Health Care System, Network	Control	Service	Beds	Admissions	Census	Outpatient Visits	Births	Total	Payroll	Personnel

★ American Hospital Association (AHA) membership
□ Joint Commission on Accreditation of Healthcare Organizations (JCAHO) accreditation
+ American Osteopathic Hospital Association (AOHA) membership
○ American Osteopathic Association (AOA) accreditation
△ Commission on Accreditation of Rehabilitation Facilities (CARF) accreditation
Control codes 61, 63, 64, 71, 72 and 73 indicate hospitals listed by AOHA, but not registered by AHA. For definition of numerical codes, see page A4

PAMPA—Gray County

✠ COLUMBIA MEDICAL CENTER OF PAMPA, One Medical Plaza, Zip 79065; tel. 806/663-5500; J. Phillip Young, President and Chief Executive Officer **A**1 9 10 **F**7 8 10 12 15 16 19 21 22 23 26 28 30 32 34 35 39 41 44 46 49 57 61 65 66 67 71 73 **P**7 8 **S** Columbia/HCA Healthcare Corporation, Nashville, TN	33	10	103	3369	47	—	284	22565	10024	469

PARIS—Lamar County

✠ MCCUISTION REGIONAL MEDICAL CENTER, 865 Deshong Drive, Zip 75462, Mailing Address: P.O. Box 160, Zip 75461-0160; tel. 903/737-1111; Anthony A. Daigle, Administrator and Chief Executive Officer **A**1 9 10 **F**7 8 10 11 12 14 15 16 17 19 21 22 23 24 26 28 29 30 31 32 33 34 35 37 41 42 44 45 46 49 52 54 55 56 57 60 65 66 67 71 73 74 **P**1 5 **N** Presbyterian Healthcare System, Dallas, TX	23	10	175	6832	75	45434	832	34020	13523	553
✠ ST. JOSEPH'S HOSPITAL AND HEALTH CENTER, 820 Clarksville Street, Zip 75460-9070, Mailing Address: P.O. Box 9070, Zip 75461-9070; tel. 903/785-4521; Monty E. McLaurin, President **A**1 9 10 **F**3 4 8 10 11 12 14 15 16 19 21 22 23 24 26 28 29 30 31 32 33 34 35 37 39 41 42 43 44 46 48 49 52 54 55 56 57 58 59 60 65 66 70 71 73 **P**7 8 **S** Incarnate Word Health Services, San Antonio, TX **N** Southwest Preferred Network, Dallas, TX	21	10	176	7227	115	39141	0	47362	19639	651

PASADENA—Harris County

✠ COLUMBIA BAYSHORE MEDICAL CENTER, 4000 Spencer Highway, Zip 77504-1294; tel. 713/944-6666; Russell Meyers, Chief Executive Officer (Total facility includes 28 beds in nursing home–type unit) **A**1 2 9 10 **F**2 3 4 7 8 10 11 12 14 15 16 17 19 20 21 22 23 24 26 27 28 29 30 32 33 34 35 37 38 40 41 42 43 44 45 46 48 49 51 52 54 55 56 60 61 64 65 66 67 68 70 71 72 73 74 **P**2 3 4 5 7 8 **S** Columbia/HCA Healthcare Corporation, Nashville, TN **N** Gulf Coast Provider Network, Houston, TX	33	10	353	12888	167	104635	1772	66653	27125	878
□ MEMORIAL HOSPITAL PASADENA, (Formerly Southmore Medical Center), 906 East Southmore Avenue, Zip 77502-1124, Mailing Address: Box 1879, Zip 77502; tel. 713/477-0411; Dennis M. Knox, Vice President and Chief Executive Officer (Total facility includes 22 beds in nursing home–type unit) **A**1 9 10 **F**2 3 4 6 7 8 10 11 12 14 15 16 17 19 21 22 23 25 26 27 28 29 30 31 32 33 34 35 37 38 39 40 41 42 43 44 45 46 48 49 51 52 53 54 55 56 57 58 59 60 62 63 64 65 66 67 68 71 72 73 74 **P**3 4 7 **S** Memorial Healthcare System, Houston, TX	23	10	173	5844	88	—	1220	—	—	465

PEARSALL—Frio County

FRIO HOSPITAL, 320 Berry Ranch Road, Zip 78061; tel. 210/334-3617; Alan D. Holmes, Chief Executive Officer **A**9 10 **F**7 15 16 19 22 32 35 40 44 49 70 71 **N** Southwest Texas Rural Health Alliance, San Antonio, TX	16	10	22	835	9	36654	206	5285	2462	99

PECOS—Reeves County

★ REEVES COUNTY HOSPITAL, 2323 Texas Street, Zip 79772; tel. 915/447-3551; Terry R. Andris, CHE, Interim Chief Executive Officer **A**9 10 **F**7 14 19 22 28 31 40 44 46 65 71 73 **N** Permian Basin Rural Health Network, Fort Stockton, TX	16	10	46	856	9	12442	128	5510	2387	94

PERRYTON—Ochiltree County

OCHILTREE GENERAL HOSPITAL, 3101 Garrett Drive, Zip 79070-5393; tel. 806/435-3606; Wallace N. Boyd, Administrator **A**9 10 **F**7 8 15 19 21 28 29 30 32 33 34 36 37 40 41 44 49 64 65 67 70 71 73 74 **P**1	16	10	45	915	11	12324	192	5633	2897	105

PITTSBURG—Camp County

✠ EAST TEXAS MEDICAL CENTER PITTSBURG, 414 Quitman Street, Zip 75686-1032; tel. 903/856-6663; W. Perry Henderson, Administrator **A**1 9 10 **F**1 8 19 21 22 25 32 44 49 70 71 **P**3 5 **S** East Texas Medical Center Regional Healthcare System, Tyler, TX **N** Healthcare Partners of East Texas, Inc., Tyler, TX	23	10	42	1005	16	101190	0	10352	5117	216

PLAINVIEW—Hale County

✠ METHODIST HOSPITAL PLAINVIEW, 2601 Dimmitt Road, Zip 79072-1833; tel. 806/296-5531; Donald W. Shouse, Administrator **A**1 9 10 **F**2 3 7 8 12 14 15 16 17 18 19 20 21 22 23 25 28 30 31 32 34 35 36 37 39 40 42 44 45 46 49 51 53 54 55 56 57 58 59 65 66 67 70 71 73 **P**3 7 **S** Lubbock Methodist Hospital System, Lubbock, TX	21	10	100	2326	30	60602	423	20308	5975	298

PLANO—Collin County

✠ COLUMBIA MEDICAL CENTER OF PLANO, 3901 West 15th Street, Zip 75075-7799; tel. 214/596-6800; Harvey L. Fishero, President and Chief Executive Officer **A**1 2 9 10 **F**4 7 8 10 11 12 14 15 16 17 18 19 21 22 23 24 28 30 31 32 33 34 35 37 38 40 42 43 44 45 46 49 60 64 65 66 67 71 73 74 **P**3 7 8 **S** Columbia/HCA Healthcare Corporation, Nashville, TN	33	10	259	12819	143	88878	3606	100754	32694	984
✠ △ PLANO REHABILITATION HOSPITAL, 2800 West 15th Street, Zip 75075; tel. 214/612-9000; Laurence J. Frayne, Chief Executive Officer (Total facility includes 8 beds in nursing home–type unit) **A**1 7 9 10 **F**1 5 12 15 16 19 21 22 24 27 32 35 39 41 48 49 50 54 58 63 64 65 66 71 73 74 **P**5	32	46	62	853	54	—	0	14698	6738	290
✠ PRESBYTERIAN HOSPITAL OF PLANO, 6200 West Parker Road, Zip 75093-7914; tel. 972/608-8000; Philip M. Wentworth, FACHE, Executive Director **A**1 9 10 **F**2 7 8 11 12 14 15 16 17 19 21 22 23 27 28 29 30 32 33 34 35 37 38 39 40 44 46 49 52 63 64 65 66 71 73 74 **P**7 8 **S** Presbyterian Healthcare System, Dallas, TX **N** Presbyterian Healthcare System, Dallas, TX; North Texas Health Network, Irving, TX; North Texas Healthcare Network, Dallas, TX	23	10	91	5702	48	35450	1631	50719	14931	499

PORT ARTHUR—Jefferson County

□ PARK PLACE MEDICAL CENTER, 3050 39th Street, Zip 77642, Mailing Address: Box 1648, Zip 77641; tel. 409/983-4951; Bob McCurry, Interim Chief Executive Officer (Total facility includes 21 beds in nursing home–type unit) **A**1 9 10 **F**4 7 8 10 12 15 16 17 19 21 22 23 27 28 29 30 31 34 35 37 38 40 42 43 44 45 46 48 51 59 60 64 65 71 72 73 74 **P**3 7 **S** TENET Healthcare Corporation, Santa Barbara, CA	32	10	219	4798	84	27194	535	35660	12796	359

Hospital, Address, Telephone, Administrator, Approval, Facility, and Physician Codes, Health Care System, Network	Classi-fication Codes		Utilization Data					Expense (thousands) of dollars		
★ American Hospital Association (AHA) membership □ Joint Commission on Accreditation of Healthcare Organizations (JCAHO) accreditation + American Osteopathic Hospital Association (AOHA) membership ○ American Osteopathic Association (AOA) accreditation △ Commission on Accreditation of Rehabilitation Facilities (CARF) accreditation Control codes 61, 63, 64, 71, 72 and 73 indicate hospitals listed by AOHA, but not registered by AHA. For definition of numerical codes, see page A4	Control	Service	Beds	Admissions	Census	Outpatient Visits	Births	Total	Payroll	Personnel

✠ ST. MARY HOSPITAL, 3600 Gates Boulevard, Zip 77642–3601, Mailing Address: P.O. Box 3696, Zip 77643–3696; tel. 409/985–7431; James E. Gardner, Jr., Administrator (Total facility includes 19 beds in nursing home–type unit) **A**1 3 5 9 10 **F**4 7 8 10 12 13 14 15 16 17 19 20 21 22 24 25 27 29 30 32 33 34 35 39 41 42 43 44 46 49 51 54 56 57 58 59 60 65 71 73 74 **P**1 3 4 5 6 7 8 **S** Sisters of Charity of the Incarnate Word Healthcare System, Houston, TX **N** SouthEast Texas Integrated Community Health Network, Houston, TX	21	10	231	9062	127	95634	821	65152	26257	—
PORT LAVACA—Calhoun County										
✠ MEMORIAL MEDICAL CENTER, 815 North Virginia Street, Zip 77979, Mailing Address: P.O. Box 25, Zip 77979; tel. 512/552–6713; Bob L. Bybee, President and Chief Executive Officer **A**1 9 10 **F**7 8 13 14 15 16 19 20 21 22 28 30 31 32 33 37 38 39 40 41 44 45 49 56 65 67 71 73 **N** SouthEast Texas Hospital System, Dallas, TX	13	10	56	1697	20	26552	275	12407	5362	236
QUANAH—Hardeman County										
HARDEMAN COUNTY MEMORIAL HOSPITAL, 402 Mercer Street, Zip 79252, Mailing Address: Box 90, Zip 79252; tel. 817/663–2795; Charles Hurt, Administrator **A**9 10 **F**15 19 22 27 32 34 44 65 70 71 73 **P**3 **N** Texoma Health Network, Wichita Falls, TX	16	10	23	286	5	19548	0	1958	1067	63
QUITMAN—Wood County										
WOOD COUNTY CENTRAL HOSPITAL DISTRICT, 117 Winnsboro Street, Zip 75783, Mailing Address: P.O. Box 1000, Zip 75783–1000; tel. 903/763–4505; Marion W. Stanberry, Administrator **A**9 10 **F**7 8 12 14 15 16 19 21 22 28 30 42 44 46 49 70 71 **P**2 3 7 8 **N** Healthcare Partners of East Texas, Inc., Tyler, TX; Regional Healthcare Alliance, Tyler, TX	16	10	30	1207	14	12047	142	6228	2771	126
RANKIN—Upton County										
RANKIN HOSPITAL DISTRICT, 1105 Elizabeth Street, Zip 79778, Mailing Address: Box 327, Zip 79778; tel. 915/693–2443; John Paul Loyless, Administrator **A**9 10 **F**14 15 16 17 22 32 33 34 39 40 44 46 51 71 73 **N** Permian Basin Rural Health Network, Fort Stockton, TX	16	10	20	87	1	738	17	1666	781	28
REESE AFB—Lubbock County										
★ U. S. AIR FORCE HOSPITAL, 250 13th Street, Zip 79489–5008; tel. 806/885–3542; Major Ward Hinger, MSC, USAF, Administrator (Nonreporting) **A**3 5 **S** Department of the Air Force, Washington, DC	41	10	10	—	—	—	—	—	—	—
REFUGIO—Refugio County										
✠ REFUGIO COUNTY MEMORIAL HOSPITAL, 107 Swift Street, Zip 78377; tel. 512/526–2321; Haskell G. Silkwood, Administrator **A**1 9 10 **F**14 15 16 17 19 22 25 31 34 36 39 44 45 46 49 51 65 66 67 71 73 **P**6 **N** SouthEast Texas Hospital System, Dallas, TX	16	10	20	398	5	14179	0	4822	1834	77
RICHARDSON—Dallas County										
□ BAYLOR RICHARDSON MEDICAL CENTER, 401 West Campbell Road, Zip 75080; tel. 972/498–4000; Ronald L. Boring, President and Chief Executive Officer (Total facility includes 16 beds in nursing home–type unit) **A**1 9 10 **F**2 3 7 8 10 11 12 17 18 19 22 23 26 28 29 30 31 32 33 34 35 37 40 41 42 43 44 45 46 48 49 51 52 53 54 55 56 57 58 59 60 61 64 65 66 67 69 70 71 72 73 74 **P**5 6 7 8 **N** Baylor Health Care System Network, Dallas, TX; North Texas Healthcare Network, Dallas, TX	16	10	113	5236	59	42834	540	40990	15855	570
RICHMOND—Fort Bend County										
✠ POLLY RYON MEMORIAL HOSPITAL, 1705 Jackson Street, Zip 77469–3289; tel. 281/341–3000; Sam L. Steffee, Executive Director and Chief Executive Officer (Total facility includes 34 beds in nursing home–type unit) **A**1 9 10 **F**7 8 14 19 21 22 31 32 33 34 35 37 40 41 44 64 65 66 67 70 71 73 **P**5 8 **N** Memorial/Sisters of Charity Health Network, Houston, TX; Gulf Coast Provider Network, Houston, TX	16	10	138	4592	57	32698	663	26362	11009	339
RIO GRANDE CITY—Starr County										
★ STARR COUNTY MEMORIAL HOSPITAL, Route 1, Zip 78582, Mailing Address: P.O. Box 78, Zip 78582; tel. 210/487–5561; Thalia H. Munoz, Administrator **A**9 10 **F**7 14 15 16 19 22 34 39 40 44 51 65 71	16	10	44	2175	6	52300	957	8723	4088	183
ROCKDALE—Milam County										
RICHARDS MEMORIAL HOSPITAL, 1700 Brazos Street, Zip 76567–2517, Mailing Address: Drawer 1010, Zip 76567–1010; tel. 512/446–2513; Edward F. Lynch, Administrator (Total facility includes 10 beds in nursing home–type unit) **A**9 10 **F**8 15 19 21 25 26 28 32 33 34 41 44 49 64 70 71	16	10	47	602	9	13219	0	4047	1513	81
ROTAN—Fisher County										
FISHER COUNTY HOSPITAL DISTRICT, Roby Highway, Zip 79546, Mailing Address: Drawer F, Zip 79546; tel. 915/735–2256; Ella Raye Helms, Administrator (Total facility includes 7 beds in nursing home–type unit) **A**9 10 **F**8 13 15 16 17 19 22 24 28 30 32 34 39 44 49 51 64 65 70 71 73 **P**6 **S** Lubbock Methodist Hospital System, Lubbock, TX **N** Lubbock Methodist Hospital System, Lubbock, TX	16	10	30	428	11	31665	0	4409	1975	89
ROUND ROCK—Williamson County										
✠ ROUND ROCK HOSPITAL, 2400 Round Rock Avenue, Zip 78681; tel. 512/255–6066; Deborah L. Ryle, Chief Executive Officer (Total facility includes 9 beds in nursing home–type unit) **A**1 9 10 **F**7 12 14 15 16 19 22 23 28 29 30 34 37 40 42 44 49 64 65 71 73 74 **P**7 8 **S** Columbia/HCA Healthcare Corporation, Nashville, TN **N** Columbia Saint David's Health Network, Austin, TX	32	10	75	3671	38	26158	903	25465	9236	286
ROWLETT—Rockwall County										
□ LAKE POINTE MEDICAL CENTER, 6800 Scenic Drive, Zip 75088–1550, Mailing Address: P.O. Box 1550, Zip 75030–1500; tel. 972/412–2273; Kenneth R. Teel, Administrator **A**1 9 10 **F**7 8 11 12 16 19 20 21 22 24 28 29 32 33 34 35 39 40 41 42 44 45 49 64 65 67 71 72 73 **P**8 **S** TENET Healthcare Corporation, Santa Barbara, CA	33	10	92	4250	39	61193	478	27484	11294	310

Hospital, Address, Telephone, Administrator, Approval, Facility, and Physician Codes, Health Care System, Network	Classi-fication Codes		Utilization Data					Expense (thousands) of dollars		
	Control	Service	Beds	Admissions	Census	Outpatient Visits	Births	Total	Payroll	Personnel

★ American Hospital Association (AHA) membership
□ Joint Commission on Accreditation of Healthcare Organizations (JCAHO) accreditation
+ American Osteopathic Hospital Association (AOHA) membership
○ American Osteopathic Association (AOA) accreditation
△ Commission on Accreditation of Rehabilitation Facilities (CARF) accreditation
Control codes 61, 63, 64, 71, 72 and 73 indicate hospitals listed by AOHA, but not registered by AHA. For definition of numerical codes, see page A4

RUSK—Cherokee County

□ EAST TEXAS MEDICAL CENTER RUSK, Copeland and Bonner Streets, Zip 75785, Mailing Address: P.O. Box 317, Zip 75785; tel. 903/683–2273; Don Edd Green, Administrator (Nonreporting) **A**1 9 10 **S** East Texas Medical Center Regional Healthcare System, Tyler, TX **N** Healthcare Partners of East Texas, Inc., Tyler, TX	23	10	25	—	—	—	—	—	—	—
□ RUSK STATE HOSPITAL, Jacksonville Highway North, Zip 75785, Mailing Address: P.O. Box 318, Zip 75785–0318; tel. 903/683–3421; Harold R. Parrish, Superintendent **A**1 10 **F**14 15 16 19 20 21 26 27 28 30 31 35 37 40 44 45 46 48 52 54 55 56 57 65 67 71 73	12	22	386	1594	352	0	0	40279	20871	1004

SAN ANGELO—Tom Green County

★ △ COLUMBIA MEDICAL CENTER OF SAN ANGELO, 3501 Knickerbocker Road, Zip 76904–7698; tel. 915/949–9511; Gregory R. Angle, President and Chief Executive Officer **A**1 2 7 9 10 **F**7 8 10 12 13 17 19 21 22 23 24 25 26 28 29 30 32 37 38 40 42 44 45 46 48 49 51 63 65 66 67 71 72 73 74 **P**3 7 8 **S** Columbia/HCA Healthcare Corporation, Nashville, TN	33	10	138	5217	64	39295	823	35235	13897	—
CONCHO VALLEY REGIONAL HOSPITAL See Shannon Medical Center– St. John's Campus										
□ RIVER CREST HOSPITAL, 1636 Hunters Glen Road, Zip 76901–5016; tel. 915/949–5722; Larry Grimes, Managing Director **A**1 9 10 **F**2 3 12 13 15 16 17 19 21 22 26 27 28 30 35 41 46 49 50 52 53 54 55 56 57 58 59 63 65 67 68 71 **P**5 **S** Universal Health Services, Inc., King of Prussia, PA	33	22	80	1225	29	2948	0	4779	2069	57
★ △ SHANNON MEDICAL CENTER, (Includes Shannon Medical Center– St. John's Campus, 2018 Pulliam Street, Zip 76905–5197; tel. 915/659–7100), 120 East Harris Street, Zip 76903; tel. 915/653–6741; John Geanes, President and Chief Executive Officer (Total facility includes 13 beds in nursing home–type unit) **A**1 2 7 9 10 **F**2 3 4 7 8 10 11 12 14 15 16 17 19 21 22 23 24 25 26 27 28 29 30 32 34 35 37 39 40 41 42 43 44 45 46 48 49 52 53 54 55 56 57 58 59 60 63 64 65 66 67 71 72 73 74 **P**2	23	10	334	12945	181	145637	1160	85123	31919	1314

SAN ANTONIO—Bexar County

★ BAPTIST MEDICAL CENTER, 111 Dallas Street, Zip 78205–1230; tel. 210/222–8431; William W. Webster, Administrator (Total facility includes 31 beds in nursing home–type unit) **A**1 2 3 5 6 9 10 **F**2 3 4 7 8 9 10 11 12 14 15 16 17 19 20 21 22 23 26 28 29 30 31 33 34 35 37 38 39 40 41 42 43 44 45 46 48 49 52 54 55 56 57 59 60 63 64 65 67 69 70 71 73 **P**3 7 8 **S** Baptist Health System, San Antonio, TX	21	10	481	15921	279	68798	2025	118357	65384	2359
★ BROOKE ARMY MEDICAL CENTER, Fort Sam Houston, Zip 78234–6200; tel. 210/916–4141; Colonel Joseph P. Gonzales, MS, USA, Chief of Staff (Nonreporting) **A**1 2 3 5 **S** Department of the Army, Office of the Surgeon General, Falls Church, VA	42	10	464	—	—	—	—	—	—	—
□ CHARTER REAL BEHAVIORAL HEALTH SYSTEM, 8550 Huebner Road, Zip 78240, Mailing Address: P.O. Box 380157, Zip 78280; tel. 210/699–8585; Irving B. Sawyers, Jr., Chief Executive Officer **A**1 9 10 **F**1 2 3 12 14 15 16 25 26 27 31 34 39 41 46 52 53 54 55 56 57 58 59 65 67 **S** Magellan Health Services, Atlanta, GA	33	22	90	1706	49	9672	0	10625	4401	101
□ △ HEALTHSOUTH REHABILITATION INSTITUTE OF SAN ANTONIO, 9119 Cinnamon Hill, Zip 78240; tel. 210/691–0737; Diane B. Lampe, Administrator and Chief Executive Officer **A**1 7 9 10 **F**5 12 14 15 16 19 21 25 26 27 32 35 41 42 44 46 48 49 50 63 65 66 67 71 73 **S** HEALTHSOUTH Corporation, Birmingham, AL	33	46	108	1152	61	14553	0	17200	7019	221
□ HORIZON SPECIALTY HOSPITAL, 7310 Oak Manor Drive, Zip 78229; tel. 210/308–0261; Phylis Muennink, Administrator (Nonreporting) **A**1 9 10	33	49	30	—	—	—	—	—	—	—
★ METHODIST AMBULATORY SURGERY HOSPITAL, (Formerly South Texas Ambulatory Surgery Hospital), 9150 Huebner Road, Zip 78240–1545; tel. 210/561–7250; Elaine F. Morris, Administrator (Total facility includes 16 beds in nursing home–type unit) **A**10 **F**3 4 7 8 10 11 12 17 18 19 21 23 24 25 26 28 29 30 31 32 33 34 35 37 38 39 40 41 42 43 44 45 46 47 48 49 51 54 55 57 60 64 65 66 67 69 71 73 74 **P**8 **S** Columbia/HCA Healthcare Corporation, Nashville, TN	33	10	37	560	8	—	0	12648	4490	—
★ METHODIST WOMEN'S AND CHILDREN'S HOSPITAL, 8109 Fredericksburg Road, Zip 78229–3383; tel. 210/692–5000; Janet Porter, President and Chief Executive Officer **A**1 9 **F**2 3 4 7 8 10 11 12 13 14 15 16 17 18 19 20 21 22 23 24 25 26 27 28 29 30 31 32 33 34 35 36 37 38 39 40 41 42 43 44 45 46 47 48 49 52 54 55 56 57 58 59 60 61 63 64 65 66 67 69 70 71 72 73 74 **P**3 5 6 8 **S** Columbia/HCA Healthcare Corporation, Nashville, TN **N** Methodist Healthcare System of San Antonio, Ltd., San Antonio, TX	32	10	150	7857	69	38147	4518	32831	17951	531
★ METROPOLITAN METHODIST HOSPITAL, 1310 McCullough Avenue, Zip 78212–2617; tel. 210/208–2200; Mark L. Bernard, Chief Executive Officer (Total facility includes 16 beds in nursing home–type unit) **A**1 9 10 **F**2 3 4 7 8 10 11 12 13 14 16 17 19 21 22 23 26 28 30 31 32 33 34 35 37 38 40 41 42 43 44 47 48 49 52 53 54 55 56 57 58 59 60 61 63 64 65 66 67 69 70 71 73 74 **S** Columbia/HCA Healthcare Corporation, Nashville, TN **N** Methodist Healthcare System of San Antonio, Ltd., San Antonio, TX	32	10	232	10783	124	34800	2348	61066	24287	871
□ MISSION VISTA BEHAVIORAL HEALTH SYSTEM, (Formerly Mission Vista Hospital), 14747 Jones Maltsberger, Zip 78247–3713; tel. 210/490–0000; James M. Hunt, Chief Executive Officer **A**1 9 10 **F**2 3 12 14 15 16 18 22 26 34 45 46 52 54 56 57 58 59 65 67 **P**6 **S** Ramsay Health Care, Inc., Coral Gobles, FL	33	22	30	773	14	1888	0	4020	2016	54

Hospital, Address, Telephone, Administrator, Approval, Facility, and Physician Codes, Health Care System, Network	Classi-fication Codes		Utilization Data					Expense (thousands) of dollars		
★ American Hospital Association (AHA) membership □ Joint Commission on Accreditation of Healthcare Organizations (JCAHO) accreditation + American Osteopathic Hospital Association (AOHA) membership ○ American Osteopathic Association (AOA) accreditation △ Commission on Accreditation of Rehabilitation Facilities (CARF) accreditation Control codes 61, 63, 64, 71, 72 and 73 indicate hospitals listed by AOHA, but not registered by AHA. For definition of numerical codes, see page A4	Control	Service	Beds	Admissions	Census	Outpatient Visits	Births	Total	Payroll	Personnel
□ NIX HEALTH CARE SYSTEM, 414 Navarro Street, Zip 78205–2522; tel. 210/271–1800; John F. Strieby, President and Chief Executive Officer (Total facility includes 17 beds in nursing home–type unit) **A**1 3 9 10 **F**4 7 8 10 19 21 28 30 32 34 35 37 39 40 41 42 43 44 45 46 49 52 57 59 60 63 64 65 66 67 69 71 74 **P**1 5 7	33	10	132	3204	56	64960	549	32021	12338	306
NORTHEAST BAPTIST HOSPITAL, 8811 Village Drive, Zip 78217; tel. 210/653–2330; Patricia E. Carey, FACHE, Administrator **F**2 3 4 7 8 9 10 11 12 14 15 16 17 19 20 21 22 23 26 28 29 30 31 33 34 35 37 38 39 40 41 42 43 44 45 46 48 49 52 53 54 55 56 57 59 60 61 63 64 65 67 69 70 71 73 **P**3 7 8 **S** Baptist Health System, San Antonio, TX	21	10	210	9766	129	56540	1759	71241	28677	947
★ NORTHEAST METHODIST HOSPITAL, 12412 Judson Road, Zip 78233, Mailing Address: P.O. Box 659510, Zip 78265–9510; tel. 210/650–4949; Mark L. Bernard, Chief Executive Officer **A**1 9 10 **F**2 3 4 7 8 10 11 12 13 14 15 16 17 19 21 22 23 24 25 26 27 28 29 30 32 33 34 35 37 38 39 40 41 42 43 44 45 46 47 48 49 52 54 55 56 57 58 59 60 61 64 65 66 67 69 71 72 73 74 **P**2 5 7 8 **S** Columbia/HCA Healthcare Corporation, Nashville, TN **N** Methodist Healthcare System of San Antonio, Ltd., San Antonio, TX	32	10	117	3267	48	—	4	30315	11938	388
★ SAN ANTONIO COMMUNITY HOSPITAL, 8026 Floyd Curl Drive, Zip 78229–3915; tel. 210/692–8110; James C. Scoggin, Jr., Chief Executive Officer (Total facility includes 20 beds in nursing home–type unit) **A**1 3 5 9 10 **F**2 3 4 7 8 9 10 12 13 14 15 16 17 18 19 20 21 22 23 24 25 26 27 28 29 30 31 32 33 34 35 37 39 41 42 43 44 45 46 48 49 52 54 55 56 57 58 59 60 61 63 64 65 66 67 69 70 71 72 73 74 **P**3 5 6 7 8 **S** Columbia/HCA Healthcare Corporation, Nashville, TN **N** Methodist Healthcare System of San Antonio, Ltd., San Antonio, TX	32	10	297	7613	119	47198	0	61700	25496	686
□ SAN ANTONIO STATE HOSPITAL, 6711 South New Braunfels, Zip 78223, Mailing Address: Box 23991, Highland Hills Station, Zip 78223–0991; tel. 210/531–7711; Robert C. Arizpe, Superintendent **A**1 9 10 **F**6 8 12 17 18 20 22 27 28 29 30 34 45 46 49 52 53 54 55 56 58 65 67 73 **P**6	12	22	453	2674	390	0	0	64308	33142	1252
★ △ SANTA ROSA HEALTH CARE CORPORATION, 519 West Houston Street, Zip 78207–3108, Mailing Address: Box 7330, Station A, Zip 78207–3108; tel. 210/704–2011; Robert J. Nolan, President and Chief Executive Officer **A**1 2 3 5 7 9 10 **F**2 3 4 5 7 8 10 11 12 13 14 15 16 17 18 19 20 21 22 26 27 28 29 30 31 32 33 34 35 37 38 39 40 41 42 43 44 45 46 47 48 49 51 52 53 54 55 56 57 58 59 60 61 63 64 65 66 67 68 69 71 72 73 74 **P**5 6 7 **S** Incarnate Word Health Services, San Antonio, TX **N** Primary CareNet of Texas, San Antonio, TX	21	10	636	20647	314	124578	2637	183299	63507	2552
SOUTH TEXAS AMBULATORY SURGERY HOSPITAL See Methodist Ambulatory Surgery Hospital										
★ SOUTH TEXAS VETERANS HEALTH CARE SYSTEM, (Includes South Texas Veterans Health Care System, Kerrville Division, 3600 Memorial Boulevard, Kerrville, Zip 78028; tel. 210/896–2020), 7400 Merton Minter Boulevard, Zip 78284–5799; tel. 210/617–5140; Jose R. Coronado, Director (Total facility includes 274 beds in nursing home–type unit) (Nonreporting) **A**1 2 5 8 **S** Department of Veterans Affairs, Washington, DC	45	10	1112	—	—	—	—	—	—	—
SOUTHEAST BAPTIST HOSPITAL, 4214 East Southcross, Zip 78222; tel. 210/337–6900; Harry E. Smith, Administrator **F**2 3 4 7 8 9 10 12 14 15 16 17 19 20 21 22 23 26 28 29 30 31 33 34 35 37 38 39 40 41 42 43 44 45 46 48 49 52 54 55 56 57 59 60 61 63 64 65 67 69 70 71 73 **P**3 7 8 **S** Baptist Health System, San Antonio, TX	21	10	153	5792	81	36567	572	39264	17543	625
□ △ SOUTHWEST GENERAL HOSPITAL, 7400 Barlite Boulevard, Zip 78224–1399; tel. 210/921–2000; Keith Swinney, Chief Executive Officer (Total facility includes 19 beds in nursing home–type unit) **A**1 7 10 **F**7 8 12 15 16 17 19 21 22 26 27 28 32 35 37 40 41 42 44 46 48 49 52 53 54 55 57 60 64 65 71 72 73 74 **P**4 8 **S** TENET Healthcare Corporation, Santa Barbara, CA	33	10	223	5742	109	—	729	44752	22465	822
SOUTHWEST MENTAL HEALTH CENTER, 8535 Tom Slick, Zip 78229–3363; tel. 210/616–0300; Sharon M. Stanush, President **A**3 5 9 **F**12 15 16 20 22 28 29 30 34 45 46 52 53 54 55 56 58 59 65 73 **P**8	23	52	80	74	39	0	0	4702	2361	102
★ SOUTHWEST TEXAS METHODIST HOSPITAL, 7700 Floyd Curl Drive, Zip 78229–3993; tel. 210/692–4000; James C. Scoggin, Jr., Chief Executive Officer **A**1 2 3 5 9 **F**2 3 4 7 8 9 10 11 12 13 14 15 16 17 18 19 20 21 22 23 24 25 26 27 28 29 30 31 32 33 34 35 37 38 39 40 41 42 43 44 45 46 47 48 49 52 53 54 55 56 57 58 59 60 61 63 64 65 66 67 69 70 71 72 73 74 **P**2 3 5 8 **S** Columbia/HCA Healthcare Corporation, Nashville, TN **N** Methodist Healthcare System of San Antonio, Ltd., San Antonio, TX	32	10	585	25663	383	99628	4133	189979	84229	2683
□ ST. LUKE'S BAPTIST HOSPITAL, 7930 Floyd Curl Drive, Zip 78229–0100; tel. 210/692–8703; John Penn Krause, Administrator (Total facility includes 29 beds in nursing home–type unit) **A**1 3 5 9 **F**2 3 4 7 8 9 10 11 12 14 15 16 17 19 20 21 22 23 26 28 29 30 31 33 34 35 37 38 39 40 41 42 43 44 45 46 48 49 52 54 55 57 59 60 63 64 65 67 69 71 73 **P**3 7 8 **S** Baptist Health System, San Antonio, TX	21	10	219	5757	83	—	0	55254	16824	549
★ TEXAS CENTER FOR INFECTIOUS DISEASE, 2303 S.E. Military Drive, Zip 78223–3597; tel. 210/534–8857; James N. Elkins, FACHE, Director **A**1 9 10 **F**8 19 20 21 34 35 46 54 64 65 71 73 **P**6 **S** Texas Department of Health, Austin, TX	12	33	109	214	65	4032	0	13319	6984	327
★ △ UNIVERSITY HEALTH SYSTEM, (Includes University Health Center – Downtown, tel. 210/270–3400; University Hospital, tel. 210/616–4000), 4502 Medical Drive, Zip 78229–4493; tel. 210/616–4000; John A. Guest, President and Chief Executive Officer (Nonreporting) **A**1 3 5 7 8 10	16	10	563	—	—	—	—	—	—	—

Hospital, Address, Telephone, Administrator, Approval, Facility, and Physician Codes, Health Care System, Network	Classi-fication Codes		Utilization Data					Expense (thousands) of dollars		
	Control	Service	Beds	Admissions	Census	Outpatient Visits	Births	Total	Payroll	Personnel

Approval/code legend:

★ American Hospital Association (AHA) membership
☐ Joint Commission on Accreditation of Healthcare Organizations (JCAHO) accreditation
+ American Osteopathic Hospital Association (AOHA) membership
○ American Osteopathic Association (AOA) accreditation
△ Commission on Accreditation of Rehabilitation Facilities (CARF) accreditation
Control codes 61, 63, 64, 71, 72 and 73 indicate hospitals listed by AOHA, but not registered by AHA. For definition of numerical codes, see page A4

Hospital	Control	Service	Beds	Admissions	Census	Outpatient Visits	Births	Total	Payroll	Personnel
★ △ WARM SPRINGS AND BAPTIST REHABILITATION HOSPITAL, 5101 Medical Drive, Zip 78229–6098; tel. 210/616–0100; LeRoy J. Braswell, Administrator **A**1 3 7 9 10 **F**12 15 16 19 21 27 35 41 48 49 50 63 65 67 71 73 **P**7 8	23	46	62	1068	51	10752	0	14857	5471	200
SAN AUGUSTINE—San Augustine County										
MEMORIAL MEDICAL CENTER OF SAN AUGUSTINE, (Formerly San Augustine Memorial Hospital), 511 Hospital Street, Zip 75972, Mailing Address: P.O. Box 658, Zip 75972; tel. 409/275–3446; Richard S. Liszewski, CHE, Administrator **A**9 10 **F**12 15 16 17 22 25 27 28 30 33 34 44 46 49 65 71	16	10	16	535	5	17150	0	3551	1714	78
SAN BENITO—Cameron County										
★ DOLLY VINSANT MEMORIAL HOSPITAL, 400 East Highway 77, Zip 78586, Mailing Address: Box 42, Zip 78586; tel. 210/399–1313; R. William Warren, Chairman and Chief Executive Officer **A**1 9 10 **F**19 21 22 28 34 39 44 45 49 71 73	33	10	49	1187	13	16885	0	7017	3118	140
SAN MARCOS—Hays County										
★ CENTRAL TEXAS MEDICAL CENTER, 1301 Wonder World Drive, Zip 78666; tel. 512/353–8979; Peter M. Weber, President and Chief Executive Officer (Total facility includes 9 beds in nursing home–type unit) **A**1 9 10 **F**7 8 10 12 14 15 16 17 19 20 21 22 24 28 29 30 32 33 35 39 40 41 44 45 46 49 64 65 66 67 71 73 **P**6 8 **S** Adventist Health System Sunbelt Health Care Corporation, Winter Park, FL **N** Southwest Texas Rural Health Alliance, San Antonio, TX	21	10	109	4005	44	52515	870	35787	11791	409
☐ SAN MARCOS TREATMENT CENTER, Bert Brown Road, Zip 78667–0768, Mailing Address: P.O. Box 768, Zip 78667–0768; tel. 512/396–8500; Mack Wigley, Chief Executive Officer **A**1 **F**12 16 20 52 53 **S** Healthcare America, Inc., Austin, TX	33	22	152	161	136	0	0	8830	4749	220
SEGUIN—Guadalupe County										
★ GUADALUPE VALLEY HOSPITAL, 1215 East Court Street, Zip 78155–5189; tel. 210/379–2411; Don L. Richey, Administrator **A**1 9 10 **F**3 7 8 12 14 15 18 19 21 22 28 31 32 33 34 35 37 40 44 45 49 53 55 58 63 65 66 67 70 71 73 **P**3 8 **N** Southwest Texas Rural Health Alliance, San Antonio, TX	15	10	75	3998	48	61513	675	27522	12881	582
SEMINOLE—Gaines County										
★ MEMORIAL HOSPITAL, 209 N.W. Eighth Street, Zip 79360; tel. 915/758–5811; Kirk Cristy, Chief Executive Officer and Administrator **A**9 10 **F**3 4 5 7 8 10 12 13 14 15 16 17 18 19 20 21 22 23 24 26 27 28 29 30 31 32 33 34 35 36 39 40 41 42 43 44 45 46 49 50 51 53 54 55 56 58 59 60 61 63 65 66 67 69 70 71 73 74 **N** Permian Basin Rural Health Network, Fort Stockton, TX	16	10	33	851	8	23170	154	8962	3173	146
SEYMOUR—Baylor County										
★ SEYMOUR HOSPITAL, 200 Stadium Drive, Zip 76380; tel. 817/888–5572; Charles Norris, Administrator **A**9 10 **F**1 8 20 22 25 26 28 30 32 34 37 40 41 44 64 65 70 71 **P**6 **N** Texoma Health Network, Wichita Falls, TX	16	10	34	900	11	6428	79	4656	1884	83
SHAMROCK—Wheeler County										
SHAMROCK GENERAL HOSPITAL, 1000 South Main Street, Zip 79079; tel. 806/256–2114; Allen P. Alberty, Chief Executive Officer (Total facility includes 11 beds in nursing home–type unit) **A**9 10 **F**14 15 16 22 32 33 44 49 64 71 73 74	16	10	43	458	10	11842	2	2936	1486	68
SHEPPARD AFB—Wichita County										
★ U. S. AIR FORCE REGIONAL HOSPITAL–SHEPPARD, 149 Hart Street, Suite 1, Zip 76311–3478; tel. 817/676–2010; Colonel Richard D. Maddox, Administrator **A**1 **F**3 7 12 16 17 20 21 22 25 28 29 30 32 34 35 37 39 41 44 45 46 51 52 53 56 58 65 71 73 74 **P**1 **S** Department of the Air Force, Washington, DC	41	10	65	3638	46	213047	321	—	—	716
SHERMAN—Grayson County										
★ COLUMBIA MEDICAL CENTER OF SHERMAN, 1111 Gallagher Road, Zip 75090; tel. 903/870–7000; John F. Adams, Chief Executive Officer (Total facility includes 22 beds in nursing home–type unit) **A**1 9 10 **F**7 8 12 15 19 21 22 23 26 28 29 30 31 32 33 34 35 37 40 41 42 44 45 46 48 49 52 57 63 64 65 67 71 73 74 **P**1 7 **S** Columbia/HCA Healthcare Corporation, Nashville, TN	33	10	160	2697	46	25125	272	27615	12840	416
★ △ WILSON N. JONES REGIONAL HEALTH SYSTEM, (Formerly Wilson N. Jones Memorial Hospital), 500 North Highland Avenue, Zip 75092, Mailing Address: Box 1258, Zip 75091–1258; tel. 903/870–4611; Harry F. Barnes, FACHE, President and Chief Executive Officer (Total facility includes 29 beds in nursing home–type unit) **A**1 7 9 10 **F**3 7 8 10 11 12 14 15 16 19 21 22 23 24 25 31 32 33 34 35 37 40 41 42 43 44 46 48 49 52 53 56 57 58 63 64 65 66 67 71 73 74 **P**3 5 6 7 8	23	10	197	9051	134	212476	916	83656	29477	924
SILSBEE—Hardin County										
★ COLUMBIA SILSBEE DOCTORS HOSPITAL, Highway 418, Zip 77656, Mailing Address: Box 1208, Zip 77656; tel. 409/385–5531; David Cottey, Chief Executive Officer (Total facility includes 13 beds in nursing home–type unit) **A**9 10 **F**8 12 14 15 16 19 22 25 28 32 34 37 44 45 46 49 51 64 71 73 **S** Columbia/HCA Healthcare Corporation, Nashville, TN	33	10	59	1741	25	80400	0	13126	5972	241
SMITHVILLE—Bastrop County										
SMITHVILLE HOSPITAL, Ninth and Mills Streets, Zip 78957, Mailing Address: Box 359, Zip 78957; tel. 512/237–3214; James W. Langford, Administrator **A**9 10 **F**8 19 22 31 34 44 71 73	16	10	27	1025	10	23000	0	7983	4183	151
SNYDER—Scurry County										
★ D. M. COGDELL MEMORIAL HOSPITAL, 1700 Cogdell Boulevard, Zip 79549–6198; tel. 915/573–6374; Jeff Reecer, Chief Executive Officer (Nonreporting) **A**1 9 10 **S** St. Joseph Health System, Orange, CA	13	10	65	—	—	—	—	—	—	—
SONORA—Sutton County										
LILLIAN M. HUDSPETH MEMORIAL HOSPITAL, 308 Hudspeth Avenue, Zip 76950, Mailing Address: Box 455, Zip 76950–0455; tel. 915/387–2521; Bill Goodrich, Administrator (Total facility includes 39 beds in nursing home–type unit) **A**9 10 **F**14 15 22 28 64	16	10	52	220	28	—	0	2252	1153	37

Hospital, Address, Telephone, Administrator, Approval, Facility, and Physician Codes, Health Care System, Network	Control	Service	Beds	Admissions	Census	Outpatient Visits	Births	Total	Payroll	Personnel

★ American Hospital Association (AHA) membership
☐ Joint Commission on Accreditation of Healthcare Organizations (JCAHO) accreditation
+ American Osteopathic Hospital Association (AOHA) membership
◯ American Osteopathic Association (AOA) accreditation
△ Commission on Accreditation of Rehabilitation Facilities (CARF) accreditation
Control codes 61, 63, 64, 71, 72 and 73 indicate hospitals listed by AOHA, but not registered by AHA. For definition of numerical codes, see page A4

SPEARMAN—Hansford County

★ HANSFORD HOSPITAL, 707 South Roland Street, Zip 79081; tel. 806/659–2535; Anne Snow, Administrator (Total facility includes 84 beds in nursing home–type unit) A9 10 F8 13 14 15 16 17 22 26 27 28 32 33 34 36 41 45 49 64 65 71 73 74 — 16 10 112 196 5 15789 0 2699 1265 52

STAMFORD—Jones County

STAMFORD MEMORIAL HOSPITAL, Highway 6 East, Zip 79553, Mailing Address: Box 911, Zip 79553; tel. 915/773–2725; Craig Haterius, Administrator A9 10 F15 19 20 22 24 32 44 71 P5 — 16 10 35 319 3 2225 0 2859 991 55

STANTON—Martin County

MARTIN COUNTY HOSPITAL DISTRICT, 610 North St. Peter Street, Zip 79782, Mailing Address: Box 640, Zip 79782; tel. 915/756–3345; Rick Jacobus, Administrator A9 10 F15 16 22 40 44 71 P5 N Permian Basin Rural Health Network, Fort Stockton, TX — 16 10 26 344 5 3269 22 2393 1141 45

STEPHENVILLE—Erath County

✠ HARRIS METHODIST–ERATH COUNTY, 411 North Belknap Street, Zip 76401–1399, Mailing Address: Box 1399, Zip 76401; tel. 817/965–1500; Ronald E. Dorris, Administrator A1 9 10 F7 15 16 19 22 23 26 28 29 30 32 33 35 37 39 40 41 42 44 46 49 65 67 70 71 73 74 P2 5 7 S Harris Methodist Health System, Fort Worth, TX N The Heart Network of Texas, Irving, TX; North Texas Healthcare Network, Dallas, TX — 21 10 75 3047 30 15387 465 16491 5761 224

SULPHUR SPRINGS—Hopkins County

✠ HOPKINS COUNTY MEMORIAL HOSPITAL, 115 Airport Road, Zip 75482–0115, Mailing Address: Box 275, Zip 75483–0275; tel. 903/885–7671; Donald R. Magee, Chief Executive Officer A1 9 10 F8 14 15 16 19 22 28 30 31 32 33 34 37 40 42 44 46 49 57 65 71 N Baylor Health Care System Network, Dallas, TX — 16 10 88 3589 38 44335 775 15641 8088 307

SWEENY—Brazoria County

☐ SWEENY COMMUNITY HOSPITAL, 305 North McKinney Street, Zip 77480; tel. 409/548–3311; Herbert A. Turk, FACHE, Administrator A1 9 10 F14 19 22 32 35 37 44 46 49 57 65 67 71 73 — 16 10 22 207 2 3688 1 4753 2128 65

SWEETWATER—Nolan County

✠ ROLLING PLAINS MEMORIAL HOSPITAL, 200 East Arizona Street, Zip 79556, Mailing Address: P.O. Box 690, Zip 79556; tel. 915/235–1701; Thomas F. Kennedy, Administrator A1 9 10 F7 8 14 15 19 20 22 28 31 32 37 40 44 49 65 71 73 — 16 10 54 1747 26 23604 191 10830 4501 180

TAHOKA—Lynn County

LYNN COUNTY HOSPITAL DISTRICT, Brownfield Highway, Zip 79373–1310, Mailing Address: Box 1310, Zip 79373–1310; tel. 806/998–4533; Louise Landers, Administrator (Nonreporting) A9 10 — 16 10 24 — — — — — — —

TAYLOR—Williamson County

☐ JOHNS COMMUNITY HOSPITAL, 305 Mallard Lane, Zip 76574–1208; tel. 512/352–7611; Ernest Balla, Administrator A1 9 10 F8 15 19 21 22 27 28 30 34 37 44 45 49 51 64 65 67 71 P6 — 23 10 46 1225 29 18237 0 7588 4146 143

TEMPLE—Bell County

✠ CENTRAL TEXAS VETERANS AFFAIRS HEALTHCARE SYSTEM, (Includes Central Texas VA Health Care System, 4800 Memorial Drive, Waco, Zip 76711–1397; tel. 817/752–6581; Central Texas VA Health Care System, Marlin Integrated Clinical Facility, 1016 Ward Street, Marlin, Zip 76661–2162; tel. 817/778–4811; Olin E. Teague Veterans' Center), 1901 South First Street, Zip 76504; tel. 817/778–4811; Richard Harwell, Director (Total facility includes 320 beds in nursing home–type unit) (Nonreporting) A1 2 3 5 S Department of Veterans Affairs, Washington, DC — 45 10 1852 — — — — — — —

✠ KING'S DAUGHTERS HOSPITAL, 1901 S.W. H. K. Dodgen Loop, Zip 76502–1896; tel. 817/771–8600; Tucker Bonner, President (Total facility includes 8 beds in nursing home–type unit) A1 9 10 F7 14 15 16 19 20 21 22 23 27 28 30 31 32 33 34 35 37 39 40 41 42 44 45 49 56 63 64 65 67 71 73 P1 N Brazo's Valley Health Network, Waco, TX — 23 10 96 2830 35 34943 405 23831 10019 375

OLIN E. TEAGUE VETERANS' CENTER See Central Texas Veterans Affairs Healthcare System

✠ △ SCOTT AND WHITE MEMORIAL HOSPITAL, 2401 South 31st Street, Zip 76508; tel. 817/724–2111; Dick Sweeden, Administrator (Total facility includes 38 beds in nursing home–type unit) A1 2 3 5 7 8 9 10 F1 2 3 4 7 8 10 11 12 14 15 16 17 19 20 21 22 23 24 25 26 27 28 29 30 31 32 33 35 37 38 40 41 42 43 44 45 46 47 48 49 52 53 54 56 57 58 59 60 61 64 65 66 67 69 71 72 73 74 P6 — 23 10 427 18696 312 98335 2214 193826 139241 3947

TERRELL—Kaufman County

✠ COLUMBIA MEDICAL CENTER AT TERRELL, 1551 Highway 34 South, Zip 75160–4833; tel. 972/563–7611; I. Douglas Streckert, Chief Executive Officer (Total facility includes 18 beds in nursing home–type unit) A1 9 10 F7 8 12 14 15 16 19 21 22 34 35 37 39 40 41 44 45 46 48 64 65 71 73 S Columbia/HCA Healthcare Corporation, Nashville, TN N North Texas Health Network, Irving, TX — 33 10 130 3371 45 29516 327 19339 8430 279

☐ TERRELL STATE HOSPITAL, Brin Street, Zip 75160, Mailing Address: Box 70, Zip 75160–0070; tel. 214/563–6452; Beatrice Butler, Superintendent A1 3 5 9 10 F1 3 4 5 6 7 8 9 10 11 12 13 14 15 16 17 18 19 20 21 22 23 25 26 27 28 29 30 31 34 35 36 37 38 39 40 41 42 43 44 45 46 47 48 49 50 52 53 54 55 56 57 58 59 60 63 64 65 67 68 71 73 P6 — 12 22 425 1693 355 0 0 52176 26021 903

Hospital, Address, Telephone, Administrator, Approval, Facility, and Physician Codes, Health Care System, Network	Classi-fication Codes		Utilization Data					Expense (thousands) of dollars		
★ American Hospital Association (AHA) membership □ Joint Commission on Accreditation of Healthcare Organizations (JCAHO) accreditation + American Osteopathic Hospital Association (AOHA) membership ○ American Osteopathic Association (AOA) accreditation △ Commission on Accreditation of Rehabilitation Facilities (CARF) accreditation Control codes 61, 63, 64, 71, 72 and 73 indicate hospitals listed by AOHA, but not registered by AHA. For definition of numerical codes, see page A4	Control	Service	Beds	Admissions	Census	Outpatient Visits	Births	Total	Payroll	Personnel

TEXARKANA—Bowie County

□ △ HEALTHSOUTH REHABILITATION HOSPITAL OF TEXARKANA, 515 West 12th Street, Zip 75501; tel. 903/793–0088; Jeffrey A. Livingston, Chief Executive Officer **A**1 7 9 10 **F**14 15 16 27 46 48 49 65 66 67 **S** HEALTHSOUTH Corporation, Birmingham, AL — 33 46 | 60 | 856 | 45 | 10211 | 0 | 10512 | 4622 | 174

⊠ MEDICAL ARTS HOSPITAL, 2501 College Drive, Zip 75501–2703, Mailing Address: P.O. Box 6045, Zip 75505–6045; tel. 903/798–5100; Jerry Kincade, Chief Executive Officer **A**1 5 9 10 **F**8 12 14 16 19 20 21 22 25 26 28 30 32 34 35 37 39 42 44 45 46 49 51 64 65 66 71 73 **P**5 7 8 **S** Columbia/HCA Healthcare Corporation, Nashville, TN — 33 10 | 59 | 1122 | 14 | — | 0 | 10276 | 4303 | 262

⊠ ST. MICHAEL HEALTH CARE CENTER, (Includes St. Michael Rehabilitation Hospital, 2400 St. Michael Drive, tel. 903/614–4000; Chris Karam, Administrator), 2600 St. Michael Drive, Zip 75503; tel. 903/614–2009; Don A. Beeler, Chief Executive Officer (Total facility includes 44 beds in nursing home–type unit) **A**1 2 9 10 **F**4 7 8 10 11 12 15 16 17 19 21 22 24 25 27 28 30 32 33 34 35 37 39 40 41 42 43 44 46 48 49 57 58 60 64 65 66 73 **P**3 7 8 **S** Sisters of Charity of the Incarnate Word Healthcare System, Houston, TX **N** Healthcare Partners of East Texas, Inc., Tyler, TX — 21 46 | 80 | 981 | 56 | — | 0 | 16996 | 6987 | 235

⊠ WADLEY REGIONAL MEDICAL CENTER, 1000 Pine Street, Zip 75501–5170, Mailing Address: Box 1878, Zip 75504–1878; tel. 903/798–8000; Hugh R. Hallgren, President and Chief Executive Officer **A**1 2 5 9 10 **F**4 7 8 10 12 13 15 16 17 19 21 22 23 27 28 29 30 31 32 33 34 35 37 39 40 41 42 43 44 45 46 49 50 60 63 64 65 70 71 72 73 74 **P**3 8 **N** The Heart Network of Texas, Irving, TX — 23 10 | 384 | 13010 | 172 | 101739 | 1939 | 91877 | 36468 | 1098

TEXAS CITY—Galveston County

⊠ △ COLUMBIA MAINLAND MEDICAL CENTER, 6801 E F Lowry Expressway, Zip 77591; tel. 409/938–5000; Alice G. Adams, Administrator (Total facility includes 25 beds in nursing home–type unit) (Nonreporting) **A**1 5 7 9 10 **S** Columbia/HCA Healthcare Corporation, Nashville, TN — 33 10 | 171 | — | — | — | — | — | — | —

THE WOODLANDS—Montgomery County

⊠ MEMORIAL HOSPITAL–THE WOODLANDS, 9250 Pinecroft, Zip 77380; tel. 281/364–2300; Steve Sanders, Vice President, Chief Executive Officer and Administrator **A**1 9 **F**3 4 6 7 8 10 12 14 15 16 17 19 21 22 23 25 26 27 28 29 30 31 32 33 34 35 37 39 40 41 42 43 44 45 46 49 51 53 54 55 56 57 58 59 60 62 63 65 66 67 68 71 72 73 74 **P**3 4 7 **S** Memorial Healthcare System, Houston, TX **N** Memorial/Sisters of Charity Health Network, Houston, TX — 23 10 | 68 | 4599 | 35 | 30665 | 1609 | 20972 | 8223 | 275

THROCKMORTON—Throckmorton County

THROCKMORTON COUNTY MEMORIAL HOSPITAL, Seymour Highway, Zip 76483, Mailing Address: P.O. Box 729, Zip 76483; tel. 817/849–2151; Blake Kretz, Administrator (Nonreporting) **A**9 10 **N** Texoma Health Network, Wichita Falls, TX — 13 10 | 20 | — | — | — | — | — | — | —

TOMBALL—Harris County

⊠ △ TOMBALL REGIONAL HOSPITAL, 605 Holderrieth Street, Zip 77375–0889, Mailing Address: Box 889, Zip 77377–0889; tel. 281/351–1623; Robert F. Schaper, President and Chief Executive Officer (Total facility includes 17 beds in nursing home–type unit) **A**1 7 9 10 **F**4 7 8 10 11 12 15 16 19 21 22 23 24 29 30 32 33 34 35 37 39 40 42 43 44 45 46 48 49 52 54 56 57 58 59 64 65 66 67 71 73 **P**8 **N** Memorial/Sisters of Charity Health Network, Houston, TX — 16 10 | 92 | 5975 | 94 | 60212 | 536 | 55065 | 21075 | 687

TRINITY—Trinity County

TRINITY MEMORIAL HOSPITAL, 900 Prospect Drive, Zip 75862–0471, Mailing Address: Box 471, Zip 75862; tel. 409/594–3541; James C. Whitmire, CHE, Administrator **A**9 10 **F**22 32 33 34 44 73 — 16 10 | 22 | 425 | 7 | 6225 | 0 | 3577 | 1771 | 69

TULIA—Swisher County

SWISHER MEMORIAL HOSPITAL DISTRICT, 539 Southeast Second, Zip 79088, Mailing Address: P.O. Box 808, Zip 79088; tel. 806/995–3581; Tony Staynings, Chief Executive Officer **A**9 10 **F**19 22 28 30 32 34 64 71 73 **P**6 **S** St. Joseph Health System, Orange, CA — 16 10 | 25 | 130 | 4 | — | 0 | 2827 | 1335 | 65

TYLER—Smith County

+ DOCTORS MEMORIAL HOSPITAL, 1400 West Southwest Loop 323, Zip 75701; tel. 903/561–3771; Olie E. Clem, Chief Executive Officer **A**9 10 **F**4 10 12 15 19 22 26 28 32 35 40 42 43 44 46 49 60 70 71 **P**7 8 **N** Healthcare Partners of East Texas, Inc., Tyler, TX — 23 10 | 46 | 1493 | 20 | 5867 | 168 | 6302 | 2602 | 143

⊠ △ EAST TEXAS MEDICAL CENTER, (Includes East Texas Medical Center–Psychiatric Unit, 4101 University Boulevard, Zip 75701–6600; tel. 903/566–8668), 1000 South Beckham Street, Zip 75701–1996, Mailing Address: Box 6400, Zip 75711–6400; tel. 903/597–0351 (Total facility includes 34 beds in nursing home–type unit) **A**1 2 7 9 10 **F**4 7 8 10 11 12 14 16 19 21 22 23 26 28 30 32 34 35 37 39 40 41 42 43 44 46 49 52 53 54 55 56 57 58 59 63 64 65 66 69 70 71 73 **P**6 7 8 **S** East Texas Medical Center Regional Healthcare System, Tyler, TX — 23 10 | 338 | 14670 | 206 | 146061 | 503 | 147552 | 51813 | 2480

□ EAST TEXAS MEDICAL CENTER REHABILITATION HOSPITAL, 701 Olympic Plaza Center, Zip 75701–1996; tel. 903/596–3000; Eddie L. Howard, Vice President and Chief Operating Officer **A**1 10 **F**2 3 4 5 7 8 10 11 12 15 16 19 21 24 25 26 27 28 29 30 31 32 34 35 37 39 40 41 42 43 44 45 48 49 52 53 54 55 56 57 58 59 60 61 65 66 67 69 70 71 73 74 **P**7 **S** East Texas Medical Center Regional Healthcare System, Tyler, TX — 23 46 | 49 | 712 | 35 | 121011 | 0 | — | — | 189

⊠ TRINITY MOTHER FRANCES HEALTH SYSTEM, 800 East Dawson, Zip 75701–2093; tel. 903/593–8441; J. Lindsey Bradley, Jr., FACHE, President and Chief Administrative Officer (Total facility includes 17 beds in nursing home–type unit) **A**1 2 3 9 10 **F**4 7 8 10 11 12 13 14 15 16 17 19 21 22 23 24 25 26 28 29 30 32 34 35 37 40 41 42 43 44 45 46 49 51 58 60 64 65 66 67 70 71 72 73 74 **P**5 7 8 **N** The Heart Network of Texas, Irving, TX — 21 10 | 270 | 14460 | 187 | 143701 | 2305 | 146411 | 51480 | 1609

Hospital, Address, Telephone, Administrator, Approval, Facility, and Physician Codes, Health Care System, Network	Classi-fication Codes		Utilization Data					Expense (thousands) of dollars		
★ American Hospital Association (AHA) membership □ Joint Commission on Accreditation of Healthcare Organizations (JCAHO) accreditation + American Osteopathic Hospital Association (AOHA) membership ○ American Osteopathic Association (AOA) accreditation △ Commission on Accreditation of Rehabilitation Facilities (CARF) accreditation Control codes 61, 63, 64, 71, 72 and 73 indicate hospitals listed by AOHA, but not registered by AHA. For definition of numerical codes, see page A4	Control	Service	Beds	Admissions	Census	Outpatient Visits	Births	Total	Payroll	Personnel
□ △ TYLER REHABILITATION HOSPITAL, 3131 Troup Highway, Zip 75701; tel. 903/510–7000; Thomas J. Cook, Chief Executive Officer (Total facility includes 15 beds in nursing home–type unit) **A**1 7 9 10 **F**12 14 15 16 19 21 27 28 30 34 35 39 41 46 48 49 64 65 66 67 71 73 **N** Regional Healthcare Alliance, Tyler, TX	32	46	63	787	56	8034	0	12953	6264	158
✚ UNIVERSITY OF TEXAS HEALTH CENTER AT TYLER, (PULMONARY AND HEART DISEASE), Gladewater Highway, Zip 75708, Mailing Address: Box 2003, Zip 75710–2003; tel. 903/877–3451; George A. Hurst, M.D., Director **A**1 9 10 **F**4 5 7 8 9 10 11 12 13 14 15 16 17 19 21 22 23 24 25 26 28 29 30 31 32 33 34 35 36 37 38 39 40 41 42 43 44 45 47 48 49 51 54 58 60 64 65 66 67 70 71 72 73 74 **P**1 5 6 7 **S** University of Texas System, Austin, TX **N** Regional Healthcare Alliance, Tyler, TX	12	49	117	3272	78	104976	0	58631	32298	1276
UVALDE—Uvalde County										
UVALDE COUNTY HOSPITAL AUTHORITY, 1025 Garner Field Road, Zip 78801–1025; tel. 210/278–6251; Ben M. Durr, Administrator **A**9 10 **F**7 8 15 16 19 21 25 28 32 35 37 40 41 44 45 49 65 70 71 72 73 **N** Southwest Texas Rural Health Alliance, San Antonio, TX	16	10	51	2581	27	37413	610	12832	5889	271
VAN HORN—Culberson County										
CULBERSON HOSPITAL DISTRICT, Eisenhower–Farm Market Road 2185, Zip 79855, Mailing Address: Box 609, Zip 79855–0609; tel. 915/283–2760; Richard Lee, Administrator (Nonreporting) **A**9 10	16	10	25	—	—	—	—	—	—	—
VERNON—Wilbarger County										
□ WILBARGER GENERAL HOSPITAL, 920 Hillcrest Drive, Zip 76384; tel. 817/552–9351; Larry Parsons, Administrator **A**1 9 10 **F**7 12 14 15 16 19 21 22 28 32 34 40 44 45 46 49 54 65 67 70 71 **P**5	16	10	49	1678	24	83353	121	8730	3591	193
VICTORIA—Victoria County										
✚ CITIZENS MEDICAL CENTER, 2701 Hospital Drive, Zip 77901–5749; tel. 512/573–9181; David P. Brown, Administrator (Total facility includes 20 beds in nursing home–type unit) **A**1 2 9 10 **F**4 8 10 12 14 15 16 17 18 19 20 21 22 23 25 26 28 29 30 31 32 33 34 35 37 39 41 42 43 44 45 46 47 49 50 52 54 55 56 57 59 60 63 64 65 67 71 73 **P**8 **N** SouthEast Texas Hospital System, Dallas, TX	12	10	231	7805	137	54386	0	53710	22285	867
✚ COLUMBIA DETAR HOSPITAL, 506 East San Antonio Street, Zip 77901–6060, Mailing Address: Box 2089, Zip 77902–2089; tel. 512/575–7441; William R. Blanchard, Chief Executive Officer (Total facility includes 20 beds in nursing home–type unit) **A**1 9 10 **F**3 4 7 8 10 12 14 15 16 19 22 24 26 27 28 29 30 31 32 33 34 35 36 37 38 39 40 41 42 43 44 45 46 47 48 49 52 53 54 55 56 57 58 64 65 67 71 73 74 **P**2 3 4 5 7 8 **S** Columbia/HCA Healthcare Corporation, Nashville, TN	33	10	251	7187	96	145578	1436	51117	18554	770
★ DEVEREUX–VICTORIA, 120 David Wade Drive, Zip 77902–2666; tel. 512/575–8271; L. Gail Atkinson, Executive Director (Nonreporting) **A**9 **S** Devereux Foundation, Devon, PA	23	52	6	—	—	—	—	—	—	—
□ VICTORIA REGIONAL MEDICAL CENTER, 101 Medical Drive, Zip 77904; tel. 512/573–6100; J. Michael Mastej, Chief Executive Officer and Managing Director **A**1 9 10 **F**3 7 12 14 15 16 19 21 22 28 29 30 31 34 37 40 44 45 46 49 52 53 54 55 56 57 58 59 65 67 71 73 **S** Universal Health Services, Inc., King of Prussia, PA **N** SouthEast Texas Hospital System, Dallas, TX	33	10	108	3555	47	45036	525	29522	10295	424
WACO—McLennan County										
CENTRAL TEXAS VA HEALTH CARE SYSTEM See Central Texas Veterans Affairs Healthcare System, Temple										
✚ △ HILLCREST BAPTIST MEDICAL CENTER, 3000 Herring Avenue, Zip 76708–3299, Mailing Address: Box 5100, Zip 76708–0100; tel. 817/756–8011; Richard E. Scott, President **A**1 2 3 5 7 9 10 **F**1 4 5 7 8 10 11 12 13 15 16 17 19 21 23 24 26 27 28 29 30 31 32 33 34 35 37 38 39 40 41 42 43 44 45 46 48 49 51 56 60 63 65 66 67 68 70 71 72 73 74 **P**6 7 8 **N** The Heart Network of Texas, Irving, TX; Brazo's Valley Health Network, Waco, TX	21	10	282	13281	163	182915	3266	97661	38723	1741
✚ PROVIDENCE HEALTH CENTER, 6901 Medical Parkway, Zip 76712, Mailing Address: P.O. Box 2589, Zip 76702–2589; tel. 817/751–4000; Kent A. Keahey, President **A**1 2 3 5 9 10 **F**3 4 6 8 10 11 14 15 16 17 18 19 21 22 23 26 27 28 30 31 32 33 34 35 39 42 43 44 49 51 52 53 54 55 56 57 58 59 60 63 64 65 67 71 73 **P**8 **S** Daughters of Charity National Health System, Saint Louis, MO	21	10	200	8128	109	37385	0	55667	22462	820
WAXAHACHIE—Ellis County										
✚ BAYLOR MEDICAL CENTER–ELLIS COUNTY, (Includes Baylor Medical Center – Ellis County, 803 West Lampasas Street, Ennis, Zip 75119; tel. 972/875–0900), 1405 West Jefferson Street, Zip 75165; tel. 972/923–7000; James Michael Lee, Executive Director **A**1 9 10 **F**7 8 12 15 19 22 24 27 30 32 35 36 37 39 40 42 44 49 64 65 66 71 73 **P**5 7 8 **S** Baylor Health Care System, Dallas, TX **N** Baylor Health Care System Network, Dallas, TX; North Texas Healthcare Network, Dallas, TX	23	10	91	4707	52	52586	972	39230	15726	515
WEATHERFORD—Parker County										
✚ CAMPBELL HEALTH SYSTEM, (Formerly Campbell Memorial Hospital), 713 East Anderson Street, Zip 76086–9971; tel. 817/596–8751; John B. Millstead, Chief Executive Officer **A**1 9 10 **F**7 8 14 15 16 17 19 21 22 23 24 28 30 31 32 33 34 35 36 37 39 40 41 44 49 65 67 70 71 73 **P**1 **S** Quorum Health Group/Quorum Health Resources, Inc., Brentwood, TN **N** Lubbock Methodist Hospital System, Lubbock, TX	16	10	78	2809	38	77722	542	21651	9303	364

Hospitals, U.S. / TEXAS

Hospital, Address, Telephone, Administrator, Approval, Facility, and Physician Codes, Health Care System, Network	Classification Codes		Utilization Data					Expense (thousands) of dollars		
	Control	Service	Beds	Admissions	Census	Outpatient Visits	Births	Total	Payroll	Personnel

★ American Hospital Association (AHA) membership
□ Joint Commission on Accreditation of Healthcare Organizations (JCAHO) accreditation
+ American Osteopathic Hospital Association (AOHA) membership
○ American Osteopathic Association (AOA) accreditation
△ Commission on Accreditation of Rehabilitation Facilities (CARF) accreditation
Control codes 61, 63, 64, 71, 72 and 73 indicate hospitals listed by AOHA, but not registered by AHA. For definition of numerical codes, see page A4

WEBSTER—Harris County

✸ COLUMBIA CLEAR LAKE REGIONAL MEDICAL CENTER, 500 Medical Center Boulevard, Zip 77598; tel. 713/332–2511; Donald A. Shaffett, Chief Executive Officer (Total facility includes 25 beds in nursing home–type unit) **A**1 9 10 **F**4 7 8 10 11 12 14 15 16 19 21 22 30 32 33 34 35 37 38 40 42 43 44 46 49 57 60 64 71 73 **P**1 7 **S** Columbia/HCA Healthcare Corporation, Nashville, TN **N** Gulf Coast Provider Network, Houston, TX	33	10	434	14326	160	78822	2789	62966	28916	1285

WEIMAR—Colorado County

□ COLORADO–FAYETTE MEDICAL CENTER, 400 Youens Drive, Zip 78962–9561; tel. 409/725–9531; Randy Bacus, Chief Executive Officer (Total facility includes 68 beds in nursing home–type unit) **A**1 9 10 **F**8 19 21 28 32 34 41 44 49 64 65 71 73 **P**3	23	10	106	955	85	29645	1	9393	5052	207

WELLINGTON—Collingsworth County

COLLINGSWORTH GENERAL HOSPITAL, 1014 15th Street, Zip 79095; tel. 806/447–2521; Wiley M. Fires, Administrator **A**9 10 **F**8 12 13 14 15 16 19 22 26 28 30 32 34 46 49 51 71 74 **P**6	16	10	20	317	5	28779	0	2630	1231	69

WESLACO—Hidalgo County

✸ KNAPP MEDICAL CENTER, 1401 East Eighth Street, Zip 78596, Mailing Address: Box 1110, Zip 78599; tel. 210/968–8567; Robert W. Vanderveer, Administrator **A**1 9 10 **F**7 8 14 15 16 19 21 22 26 27 30 32 33 34 35 37 39 40 42 44 45 46 49 63 65 67 71 73 74 **P**3 8	23	10	189	9717	119	52314	1929	50100	21948	757

WEST—McLennan County

WEST COMMUNITY HOSPITAL, 501 Meadow Drive, Zip 76691, Mailing Address: Box 478, Zip 76691; tel. 817/826–7000; Betty York, Executive Director (Nonreporting) **A**9 10 **N** Central Texas Rural Health Network, Harrietsville, TX; Brazo's Valley Health Network, Waco, TX	16	10	21	—	—	—	—	—	—	—

WHARTON—Wharton County

✸ COLUMBIA GULF COAST MEDICAL CENTER, 1400 Highway 59, Zip 77488–3004, Mailing Address: P.O. Box 3004, Zip 77488–3004; tel. 409/532–2500; Michael D. Murphy, Chief Executive Officer (Total facility includes 17 beds in nursing home–type unit) **A**1 2 9 10 **F**7 10 12 14 15 16 19 21 22 23 28 30 32 33 34 37 40 41 42 44 45 46 48 49 60 63 64 65 67 71 73 74 **S** Columbia/HCA Healthcare Corporation, Nashville, TN	33	10	161	3739	58	76090	571	27308	12666	459

WHEELER—Wheeler County

PARKVIEW HOSPITAL, 1000 Sweetwater Street, Zip 79096, Mailing Address: Box 1030, Zip 79096; tel. 806/826–5581; B. W. Robertson, Administrator **A**9 10 **F**8 14 15 16 17 19 22 32 46 65 71	16	10	20	439	7	14878	0	2668	1406	67

WHITNEY—Hill County

LAKE WHITNEY MEDICAL CENTER, 200 North San Jacinto Street, Zip 76692, Mailing Address: P.O. Box 458, Zip 76692; tel. 817/694–3165; Bill A. Johnson, Administrator **A**9 10 **F**2 3 4 6 7 8 9 10 11 12 13 17 18 19 20 21 22 23 24 25 26 27 28 29 30 31 32 33 34 35 36 37 38 40 41 42 43 44 47 48 49 50 52 53 54 55 56 57 58 60 61 63 64 65 66 67 69 70 71 72 73 **N** Central Texas Rural Health Network, Harrietsville, TX; Brazo's Valley Health Network, Waco, TX	16	10	48	562	14	3938	0	2882	1235	71

WICHITA FALLS—Wichita County

✸ BETHANIA REGIONAL HEALTH CARE CENTER, 1600 11th Street, Zip 76301–9988; tel. 817/723–4111; David D. Whitaker, FACHE, President and Chief Executive Officer (Total facility includes 17 beds in nursing home–type unit) **A**1 3 5 9 10 **F**4 7 8 10 11 12 14 15 16 17 19 20 21 22 23 26 28 30 31 32 33 34 35 37 39 40 41 42 43 44 46 49 63 64 65 67 68 71 72 73 74 **P**3 **N** The Heart Network of Texas, Irving, TX; Texoma Health Network, Wichita Falls, TX	21	10	204	7878	111	34698	436	61489	26967	954
□ RED RIVER HOSPITAL, 1505 Eighth Street, Zip 76301–3106; tel. 817/322–3171; Ricky Powell, Administrator **A**1 9 10 **F**2 3 12 19 20 22 52 53 54 55 56 57 58 59 65 **S** Vendell Heralthcare, Inc., Nashville, TN	33	22	50	858	22	5317	0	3680	1874	78
□ WICHITA FALLS STATE HOSPITAL, 6515 Lake Road, Zip 76308–5419, Mailing Address: Box 300, Zip 76307–0300; tel. 817/692–1220; James E. Smith, Superintendent **A**1 9 10 **F**15 16 20 39 41 45 46 52 53 57 65 73 **P**6	12	22	381	1140	349	0	0	47327	25383	1189
✸ WICHITA GENERAL HOSPITAL, 1600 Eighth Street, Zip 76301; tel. 817/723–1461; Jeffrey E. Hausler, President and Chief Executive Officer **A**1 2 3 5 9 10 **F**7 8 10 11 13 14 15 16 17 19 20 21 22 23 28 29 30 31 32 34 35 37 39 40 41 42 44 46 56 60 61 63 64 65 67 68 71 73 74 **P**5 7 8	23	10	225	8089	110	71748	1573	55239	23858	829

WINNIE—Chambers County

□ MEDICAL CENTER OF WINNIE, Broadway at Campbell Road, Zip 77665, Mailing Address: Box 208, Zip 77665; tel. 409/296–2131; J. L. Flotte', Chief Executive Officer (Total facility includes 14 beds in nursing home–type unit) (Nonreporting) **A**1 9 10	23	10	45	—	—	—	—	—	—	—

WINNSBORO—Wood County

✸ PRESBYTERIAN HOSPITAL OF WINNSBORO, 719 West Coke Road, Zip 75494–3098, Mailing Address: P.O. Box 628, Zip 75494–0628; tel. 903/342–5227; Jerry Hopper, FACHE, Executive Director (Total facility includes 8 beds in nursing home–type unit) **A**1 9 10 **F**8 12 15 16 17 19 21 22 27 28 29 30 35 37 41 42 44 46 49 64 65 67 71 73 **P**1 2 3 4 **S** Presbyterian Healthcare System, Dallas, TX **N** Healthcare Partners of East Texas, Inc., Tyler, TX; Presbyterian Healthcare System, Dallas, TX; North Texas Healthcare Network, Dallas, TX	23	10	50	920	12	—	0	8305	4062	128

© 1997 AHA Guide

Hospitals **A431**

Hospital, Address, Telephone, Administrator, Approval, Facility, and Physician Codes, Health Care System, Network	Classi-fication Codes		Utilization Data					Expense (thousands) of dollars		
★ American Hospital Association (AHA) membership □ Joint Commission on Accreditation of Healthcare Organizations (JCAHO) accreditation + American Osteopathic Hospital Association (AOHA) membership ○ American Osteopathic Association (AOA) accreditation △ Commission on Accreditation of Rehabilitation Facilities (CARF) accreditation Control codes 61, 63, 64, 71, 72 and 73 indicate hospitals listed by AOHA, but not registered by AHA. For definition of numerical codes, see page A4	Control	Service	Beds	Admissions	Census	Outpatient Visits	Births	Total	Payroll	Personnel

WINTERS—Runnels County
NORTH RUNNELS HOSPITAL, East Highway 53, Zip 79567, Mailing Address: Box 185, Zip 79567; tel. 915/754–4553; Larry Suit, Administrator **A**9 10 **F**16 19 22 28 30 32 33 44 71

| | 16 | 10 | 21 | 300 | 3 | 17737 | 0 | 2542 | 1539 | 64 |

WOODVILLE—Tyler County
TYLER COUNTY HOSPITAL, 1100 West Bluff Street, Zip 75979, Mailing Address: P.O. Box 549, Zip 75979; tel. 409/283–8141; James W. Gainey, Administrator **A**6 9 10 **F**14 19 22 28 30 32 34 44 70 71 73

| | 16 | 10 | 26 | 984 | 12 | 17085 | 0 | 5139 | 2421 | 111 |

YOAKUM—Lavaca County
⊞ YOAKUM COMMUNITY HOSPITAL, 303 Hubbard Street, Zip 77995, Mailing Address: Box 753, Zip 77995–0753; tel. 512/293–2321; Elwood E. Currier, Jr., CHE, Administrator **A**1 9 10 **F**7 8 12 14 16 17 19 20 22 26 30 32 34 35 39 41 44 45 49 51 57 65 66 67 68 70 71 73 **N** SouthEast Texas Hospital System, Dallas, TX

| | 23 | 10 | 25 | 952 | 12 | 22314 | 151 | 7848 | 3565 | 129 |

UTAH

Resident population 1,951 (in thousands)
Resident population in metro areas 77.3%
Birth rate per 1,000 population 20.0
65 years and over 8.8%
Percent of persons without health insurance 11.5%

Hospital, Address, Telephone, Administrator, Approval, Facility, and Physician Codes, Health Care System, Network	Classi-fication Codes		Utilization Data					Expense (thousands) of dollars		
	Control	Service	Beds	Admissions	Census	Outpatient Visits	Births	Total	Payroll	Personnel

★ American Hospital Association (AHA) membership
□ Joint Commission on Accreditation of Healthcare Organizations (JCAHO) accreditation
+ American Osteopathic Hospital Association (AOHA) membership
○ American Osteopathic Association (AOA) accreditation
△ Commission on Accreditation of Rehabilitation Facilities (CARF) accreditation
 Control codes 61, 63, 64, 71, 72 and 73 indicate hospitals listed by AOHA, but not registered by AHA. For definition of numerical codes, see page A4

AMERICAN FORK—Utah County

Hospital	Control	Service	Beds	Admissions	Census	Outpatient Visits	Births	Total	Payroll	Personnel
✠ AMERICAN FORK HOSPITAL, 1100 East 170 North, Zip 84003–9787; tel. 801/763–3300; Keith N. Alexander, Administrator and Chief Operating Officer **A**1 9 10 **F**7 8 11 12 15 17 19 21 22 28 29 30 35 40 44 45 46 49 64 65 67 70 71 73 74 **P**5 6 **S** Intermountain Health Care, Inc., Salt Lake City, UT **N** Intermountain HealthCare/Amerinet, Salt Lake City, UT	23	10	66	4322	25	73802	2130	20067	9501	400

BEAVER—Beaver County

Hospital	Control	Service	Beds	Admissions	Census	Outpatient Visits	Births	Total	Payroll	Personnel
BEAVER VALLEY HOSPITAL, 85 North 400 East, Zip 84713, Mailing Address: P.O. Box 1670, Zip 84713; tel. 801/438–2531; Craig Val Davidson, CHE, Administrator (Total facility includes 24 beds in nursing home–type unit) **A**9 10 **F**7 14 15 16 20 22 32 44 46 49 62 64 71 73	14	10	36	767	30	6242	110	3654	1569	74

BOUNTIFUL—Davis County

Hospital	Control	Service	Beds	Admissions	Census	Outpatient Visits	Births	Total	Payroll	Personnel
✠ LAKEVIEW HOSPITAL, 630 East Medical Drive, Zip 84010–4996; tel. 801/292–6231; Craig Preston, Chief Executive Officer (Total facility includes 10 beds in nursing home–type unit) **A**1 9 10 **F**1 2 3 4 5 7 8 10 11 12 14 15 16 17 18 19 20 21 22 23 24 25 26 27 28 29 30 31 32 33 34 35 37 38 39 40 41 42 43 44 45 46 47 48 49 51 52 53 54 55 56 57 58 59 60 61 63 64 65 66 67 70 71 72 73 74 **P**4 5 7 8 **S** Columbia/HCA Healthcare Corporation, Nashville, TN	33	10	128	3341	37	51299	788	—	—	482

BRIGHAM CITY—Box Elder County

Hospital	Control	Service	Beds	Admissions	Census	Outpatient Visits	Births	Total	Payroll	Personnel
✠ COLUMBIA BRIGHAM CITY COMMUNITY HOSPITAL, (Formerly Brigham City Community Hospital), 950 South 500 West, Zip 84302; tel. 801/734–9471; Tad A. Morley, Chief Executive Officer (Nonreporting) **A**1 9 10 **S** Columbia/HCA Healthcare Corporation, Nashville, TN	33	10	43	—	—	—	—	—	—	—

CEDAR CITY—Iron County

Hospital	Control	Service	Beds	Admissions	Census	Outpatient Visits	Births	Total	Payroll	Personnel
✠ VALLEY VIEW MEDICAL CENTER, 595 South 75 East, Zip 84720; tel. 801/586–6587; Craig M. Smedley, Administrator **A**1 9 10 **F**7 8 14 15 16 19 21 22 32 37 40 44 49 51 63 64 65 66 71 73 **P**6 **S** Intermountain Health Care, Inc., Salt Lake City, UT **N** Intermountain HealthCare/Amerinet, Salt Lake City, UT	23	10	36	1569	12	63219	490	13150	5979	182

DELTA—Millard County

Hospital	Control	Service	Beds	Admissions	Census	Outpatient Visits	Births	Total	Payroll	Personnel
★ DELTA COMMUNITY MEDICAL CENTER, 126 South White Sage Avenue, Zip 84624; tel. 801/864–5591; James E. Beckstrand, Administrator (Total facility includes 4 beds in nursing home–type unit) **A**9 10 **F**1 3 6 7 8 14 17 18 22 26 28 29 32 33 34 39 40 44 45 46 48 49 53 54 55 56 57 58 64 66 71 73 74 **P**6 7 **S** Intermountain Health Care, Inc., Salt Lake City, UT **N** Intermountain HealthCare/Amerinet, Salt Lake City, UT	23	10	20	416	5	11593	102	3000	1263	45

FILLMORE—Millard County

Hospital	Control	Service	Beds	Admissions	Census	Outpatient Visits	Births	Total	Payroll	Personnel
★ FILLMORE COMMUNITY MEDICAL CENTER, 674 South Highway 99, Zip 84631; tel. 801/743–5591; James E. Beckstrand, Administrator **A**9 10 **F**7 8 11 14 15 18 22 26 28 29 32 33 34 37 39 40 44 45 47 48 49 51 64 65 71 73 **P**6 **S** Intermountain Health Care, Inc., Salt Lake City, UT **N** Intermountain HealthCare/Amerinet, Salt Lake City, UT	23	10	20	297	14	32594	46	2959	1200	53

GUNNISON—Sanpete County

Hospital	Control	Service	Beds	Admissions	Census	Outpatient Visits	Births	Total	Payroll	Personnel
★ GUNNISON VALLEY HOSPITAL, 64 East 100 North, Zip 84634, Mailing Address: P.O. Box 759, Zip 84634; tel. 801/528–7246; Greg Rosenvall, Administrator **A**9 10 **F**3 7 8 13 15 19 21 25 29 30 32 34 40 44 48 49 51 64 67 71 **S** Rural Health Management Corporation, Nephi, UT	16	10	21	713	8	14570	157	5638	2318	99

HEBER CITY—Wasatch County

Hospital	Control	Service	Beds	Admissions	Census	Outpatient Visits	Births	Total	Payroll	Personnel
★ WASATCH COUNTY HOSPITAL, 55 South Fifth East, Zip 84032–1848; tel. 801/654–2500; Randall K. Probst, Administrator **A**9 10 **F**3 7 8 14 15 16 17 20 22 24 26 28 29 30 32 34 36 39 41 44 45 46 49 65 67 71 73 **P**5 **S** Intermountain Health Care, Inc., Salt Lake City, UT **N** Intermountain HealthCare/Amerinet, Salt Lake City, UT	23	10	25	277	5	10816	111	3424	1512	62

HILL AFB—Davis County

Hospital	Control	Service	Beds	Admissions	Census	Outpatient Visits	Births	Total	Payroll	Personnel
✠ U. S. AIR FORCE HOSPITAL, 7321 11th Street, Zip 84056–5012; tel. 801/777–5457; Colonel John A. Reyburn, Jr., Commander **A**1 9 **F**8 12 14 15 16 20 22 29 30 34 39 41 44 45 46 51 54 58 65 71 **S** Department of the Air Force, Washington, DC	41	10	15	1622	8	148886	0	—	—	—

KANAB—Kane County

Hospital	Control	Service	Beds	Admissions	Census	Outpatient Visits	Births	Total	Payroll	Personnel
KANE COUNTY HOSPITAL, 220 West 300 North, Zip 84741; tel. 801/644–5811; Mike Sinclair, Administrator (Nonreporting) **A**9 10	16	10	33	—	—	—	—	—	—	—

LAYTON—Davis County

Hospital	Control	Service	Beds	Admissions	Census	Outpatient Visits	Births	Total	Payroll	Personnel
□ DAVIS HOSPITAL AND MEDICAL CENTER, 1600 West Antelope Drive, Zip 84041–1142; tel. 801/825–9561; Robert Cash, Chief Executive Officer **A**1 9 10 **F**4 7 8 10 11 14 15 16 17 19 21 22 26 28 29 30 32 33 34 35 37 38 39 40 41 42 44 45 46 49 51 52 57 58 60 63 64 65 66 67 71 73 74 **S** Paracelsus Healthcare Corporation, Houston, TX	33	10	126	6035	56	64538	1877	28015	12871	422

LOGAN—Cache County

Hospital	Control	Service	Beds	Admissions	Census	Outpatient Visits	Births	Total	Payroll	Personnel
✠ LOGAN REGIONAL HOSPITAL, 1400 North 500 East, Zip 84341; tel. 801/752–2050; Richard Smith, Administrator (Total facility includes 15 beds in nursing home–type unit) **A**1 9 10 **F**2 3 7 8 10 11 12 15 16 19 21 22 24 28 29 30 32 33 34 35 37 39 40 41 42 44 45 49 51 52 54 56 58 59 64 65 66 67 71 72 73 74 **P**6 7 **S** Intermountain Health Care, Inc., Salt Lake City, UT	23	10	127	6632	54	129726	2177	39640	19017	594

Hospital, Address, Telephone, Administrator, Approval, Facility, and Physician Codes, Health Care System, Network	Classi-fication Codes		Utilization Data					Expense (thousands) of dollars		
★ American Hospital Association (AHA) membership □ Joint Commission on Accreditation of Healthcare Organizations (JCAHO) accreditation + American Osteopathic Hospital Association (AOHA) membership ○ American Osteopathic Association (AOA) accreditation △ Commission on Accreditation of Rehabilitation Facilities (CARF) accreditation Control codes 61, 63, 64, 71, 72 and 73 indicate hospitals listed by AOHA, but not registered by AHA. For definition of numerical codes, see page A4	Control	Service	Beds	Admissions	Census	Outpatient Visits	Births	Total	Payroll	Personnel

MILFORD—Beaver County

★ MILFORD VALLEY MEMORIAL HOSPITAL, 451 North Main Street, Zip 84751–0640, Mailing Address: Box 640, Zip 84751–0640; tel. 801/387–2411; John E. Gledhill, Administrator **A**9 10 **F**1 3 4 5 6 7 8 9 10 11 12 13 14 15 16 17 18 19 20 21 22 23 24 25 26 27 28 29 30 31 32 33 34 35 36 37 38 39 40 41 42 43 44 45 46 47 48 49 50 51 53 54 55 56 57 58 59 60 61 62 63 65 66 67 68 69 70 72 73 74 **P**5 6 **S** Rural Health Management Corporation, Nephi, UT | 16 | 10 | 34 | 467 | 21 | — | 27 | 2828 | 1358 | — |

MOAB—Grand County

★ ALLEN MEMORIAL HOSPITAL, 719 West 400 North Street, Zip 84532, Mailing Address: Box 998, Zip 84532; tel. 801/259–7191; Charles A. Davis, Administrator **A**9 10 **F**7 8 12 14 15 16 17 19 28 30 36 39 40 44 46 48 51 65 67 70 71 73 74 **P**3 **S** Rural Health Management Corporation, Nephi, UT | 16 | 10 | 31 | 638 | 6 | 10642 | 91 | 5465 | 2558 | 112 |

MONTICELLO—San Juan County

★ SAN JUAN HOSPITAL, 364 West First North, Zip 84535, Mailing Address: Box 308, Zip 84535–0308; tel. 801/587–2116; Craig Ambrosiani, Executive Director (Nonreporting) **A**9 10 | 16 | 10 | 25 | — | — | — | — | — | — | — |

MOUNT PLEASANT—Sanpete County

★ SANPETE VALLEY HOSPITAL, 1100 South Medical Drive, Zip 84647; tel. 801/462–2441; George Winn, Administrator **A**9 10 **F**7 8 12 14 17 28 30 32 33 39 42 44 46 49 64 71 **P**6 **S** Intermountain Health Care, Inc., Salt Lake City, UT **N** Intermountain HealthCare/Amerinet, Salt Lake City, UT | 23 | 10 | 20 | 516 | 11 | 61816 | 95 | 6034 | 2965 | 91 |

MURRAY—Salt Lake County

⊞ COTTONWOOD HOSPITAL MEDICAL CENTER, 5770 South 300 East, Zip 84107; tel. 801/262–3461; Douglas R. Fonnesbeck, Administrator **A**1 2 9 10 **F**1 2 3 4 5 6 7 8 9 10 11 12 13 14 15 16 17 18 19 20 21 22 23 24 25 26 27 28 29 30 31 32 33 34 35 36 37 38 39 40 41 42 43 44 45 46 47 48 49 51 52 53 54 55 56 57 58 59 60 61 62 63 64 65 66 67 68 69 70 71 72 73 74 **P**3 4 5 6 **S** Intermountain Health Care, Inc., Salt Lake City, UT **N** Intermountain HealthCare/Amerinet, Salt Lake City, UT | 23 | 10 | 160 | 9779 | 77 | 322559 | 3128 | 75357 | 29902 | 1261 |

NEPHI—Juab County

★ CENTRAL VALLEY MEDICAL CENTER, 549 North 400 East, Zip 84648; tel. 801/623–1242; Mark R. Stoddard, President **A**9 10 **F**8 19 22 28 30 32 34 39 40 44 51 56 64 71 **P**6 **S** Rural Health Management Corporation, Nephi, UT | 23 | 10 | 20 | 556 | 4 | 13920 | 80 | 6031 | 2212 | 68 |

OGDEN—Weber County

⊞ COLUMBIA OGDEN REGIONAL MEDICAL CENTER, (Formerly Ogden Regional Medical Center), 5475 South 500 East, Zip 84405–6978; tel. 801/479–2111; Steven B. Bateman, Chief Executive Officer **A**1 2 9 10 **F**2 3 4 7 8 10 11 12 13 14 15 16 17 18 19 20 21 22 24 26 28 29 30 31 32 34 35 37 38 39 40 41 42 43 44 45 46 49 51 52 53 54 55 56 57 58 59 60 64 65 66 67 68 70 71 72 73 74 **P**4 7 8 **S** Columbia/HCA Healthcare Corporation, Nashville, TN | 33 | 10 | 179 | 6943 | 79 | 51515 | 1891 | — | — | 742 |

⊞ MCKAY–DEE HOSPITAL CENTER, 3939 Harrison Boulevard, Zip 84409–2386, Mailing Address: Box 9370, Zip 84409–0370; tel. 801/627–2800; Thomas Hanrahan, Administrator and Chief Executive Officer **A**1 2 3 5 9 10 **F**2 3 4 7 8 10 11 12 14 15 17 18 19 21 22 24 25 26 28 29 30 31 32 33 34 35 37 38 39 40 41 42 43 44 45 48 49 51 52 53 54 55 56 57 58 59 61 64 65 66 67 70 71 72 73 74 **S** Intermountain Health Care, Inc., Salt Lake City, UT **N** Intermountain HealthCare/Amerinet, Salt Lake City, UT | 23 | 10 | 315 | 12034 | 153 | 126799 | 3635 | 120006 | 50064 | 1682 |

OGDEN REGIONAL MEDICAL CENTER See Columbia Ogden Regional Medical Center

OREM—Utah County

★ OREM COMMUNITY HOSPITAL, 331 North 400 West, Zip 84057; tel. 801/224–4080; Kim Nielsen, Administrator and Chief Executive Officer **A**9 10 **F**2 3 4 7 8 9 10 11 12 14 15 16 17 19 21 22 24 25 28 29 30 31 32 33 35 37 38 40 41 42 43 44 45 47 48 49 52 53 54 55 56 57 58 59 60 63 64 65 66 69 70 71 73 74 **S** Intermountain Health Care, Inc., Salt Lake City, UT **N** Intermountain HealthCare/Amerinet, Salt Lake City, UT | 23 | 10 | 20 | 1015 | 5 | 43646 | 762 | 7335 | 3330 | 125 |

PANGUITCH—Garfield County

★ GARFIELD MEMORIAL HOSPITAL AND CLINICS, 200 North Fourth East, Zip 84759, Mailing Address: P.O. Box 389, Zip 84759–0389; tel. 435/676–8811; Wayne R. Ross, Administrator **A**9 10 **F**7 12 17 20 22 25 32 39 40 44 46 48 64 65 71 73 **P**3 6 **S** Intermountain Health Care, Inc., Salt Lake City, UT **N** Intermountain HealthCare/Amerinet, Salt Lake City, UT | 23 | 10 | 44 | 533 | 27 | 29024 | 38 | 3870 | 2081 | 75 |

PAYSON—Utah County

⊞ MOUNTAIN VIEW HOSPITAL, 1000 East 100 North, Zip 84651–1690; tel. 801/465–7101; Kevin Johnson, Chief Executive Officer **A**1 9 10 **F**2 4 7 8 10 11 12 19 21 22 26 28 30 32 34 35 40 41 44 45 46 48 53 54 55 56 57 58 59 65 70 71 73 74 **P**8 **S** Columbia/HCA Healthcare Corporation, Nashville, TN | 33 | 10 | 127 | 4238 | 40 | 77069 | — | 31514 | 10049 | 384 |

PRICE—Carbon County

⊞ CASTLEVIEW HOSPITAL, 300 North Hospital Drive, Zip 84501; tel. 801/637–4800; L. Allen Penry, Chief Executive Officer (Total facility includes 10 beds in nursing home–type unit) **A**1 9 10 **F**7 8 11 14 15 16 19 21 22 24 27 28 29 30 32 35 37 38 39 40 41 44 46 51 61 63 64 65 66 71 73 74 **P**7 8 **S** Columbia/HCA Healthcare Corporation, Nashville, TN | 33 | 10 | 84 | 2346 | 23 | 76971 | 395 | — | — | 307 |

PROVO—Utah County

□ UTAH STATE HOSPITAL, 1300 East Center Street, Zip 84606, Mailing Address: Box 270, Zip 84603–0270; tel. 801/344–4200; Mark I. Payne, Superintendent **A**1 10 **F**14 15 16 20 22 52 53 54 55 56 57 58 65 | 12 | 22 | 343 | 380 | 310 | 447 | 0 | 28559 | 15830 | 646 |

Hospital, Address, Telephone, Administrator, Approval, Facility, and Physician Codes, Health Care System, Network	Classi-fication Codes		Utilization Data					Expense (thousands) of dollars		
	Control	Service	Beds	Admissions	Census	Outpatient Visits	Births	Total	Payroll	Personnel

Symbol key:
★ American Hospital Association (AHA) membership
□ Joint Commission on Accreditation of Healthcare Organizations (JCAHO) accreditation
+ American Osteopathic Hospital Association (AOHA) membership
○ American Osteopathic Association (AOA) accreditation
△ Commission on Accreditation of Rehabilitation Facilities (CARF) accreditation
Control codes 61, 63, 64, 71, 72 and 73 indicate hospitals listed by AOHA, but not registered by AHA. For definition of numerical codes, see page A4

Hospital	Control	Service	Beds	Admissions	Census	Outpatient Visits	Births	Total	Payroll	Personnel
▣ △ UTAH VALLEY REGIONAL MEDICAL CENTER, 1034 North 500 West, Zip 84605–0390; tel. 801/373–7850; Larry R. Dursteler, Regional Vice President (Total facility includes 14 beds in nursing home–type unit) **A**1 2 7 9 10 **F**4 7 8 10 11 12 14 15 16 17 18 19 20 21 22 24 25 27 28 29 30 31 32 33 34 35 36 37 38 39 40 41 42 43 44 45 46 47 48 49 52 53 54 55 56 57 58 59 60 63 64 65 67 68 70 71 72 73 74 **P**5 6 **S** Intermountain Health Care, Inc., Salt Lake City, UT **N** Intermountain HealthCare/Amerinet, Salt Lake City, UT	23	10	343	16954	182	294468	4156	137575	62000	2468
RICHFIELD—Sevier County										
▣ SEVIER VALLEY HOSPITAL, 1100 North Main Street, Zip 84701; tel. 801/896–8271; Gary E. Beck, Administrator **A**1 9 10 **F**7 8 12 14 15 16 17 19 21 22 28 30 32 33 34 35 39 40 41 44 48 49 51 64 65 71 73 **P**3 5 6 **S** Intermountain Health Care, Inc., Salt Lake City, UT **N** Intermountain HealthCare/Amerinet, Salt Lake City, UT	23	10	25	1502	10	—	217	10699	3792	100
ROOSEVELT—Duchesne County										
★ UINTAH BASIN MEDICAL CENTER, 250 West 300 North, 75–2, Zip 84066–2399; tel. 801/722–6163; Bradley D. LeBaron, Administrator **A**9 10 **F**3 7 8 11 12 14 15 16 17 19 21 24 28 30 32 33 35 37 40 44 49 51 56 61 65 66 67 71 73 **P**5 7 8	13	10	42	1563	14	29628	363	14691	5580	272
SAINT GEORGE—Washington County										
▣ DIXIE REGIONAL MEDICAL CENTER, 544 South 400 East, Zip 84770; tel. 801/634–4000; L. Steven Wilson, Administrator **A**1 2 9 10 **F**4 7 8 10 11 15 16 17 19 21 22 27 28 30 32 33 34 35 39 40 41 42 44 45 46 49 50 51 52 54 60 61 63 65 66 67 68 69 71 72 73 74 **P**5 6 8 **S** Intermountain Health Care, Inc., Salt Lake City, UT **N** Intermountain HealthCare/Amerinet, Salt Lake City, UT	23	10	137	7422	69	215003	1600	50365	19185	623
SALT LAKE CITY—Salt Lake County										
□ BHC OLYMPUS VIEW HOSPITAL, (Formerly CPC Olympus View Hospital), 1430 East 4500 South, Zip 84117–4208; tel. 801/272–8000; Barry W. Woodward, Administrator (Nonreporting) **A**1 10 **S** Behavioral Healthcare Corporation, Nashville, TN	33	22	82	—	—	—	—	—	—	—
▣ COLUMBIA ST. MARK'S HOSPITAL, 1200 East 3900 South, Zip 84124; tel. 801/268–7000; John Hanshaw, Chief Executive Officer (Nonreporting) **A**1 2 3 9 10 **S** Columbia/HCA Healthcare Corporation, Nashville, TN	33	10	203	—	—	—	—	—	—	—
CPC OLYMPUS VIEW HOSPITAL See BHC Olympus View Hospital										
HIGHLAND RIDGE HOSPITAL, 4578 Highland Drive, Zip 84117; tel. 801/272–9851; Richard Bell, Administrator **F**2 3 14 **P**1 **S** Pioneer Healthcare, Peabody, MA	33	82	34	444	25	—	0	3071	1183	43
▣ △ LDS HOSPITAL, Eighth Avenue and C Street, Zip 84143; tel. 801/321–1100; Richard M. Cagen, Chief Executive Officer and Administrator (Total facility includes 32 beds in nursing home–type unit) **A**1 2 3 5 7 9 10 **F**2 3 4 7 8 10 11 12 14 15 16 17 18 19 21 22 24 25 26 28 30 31 32 34 35 37 38 40 41 42 43 44 45 46 47 48 49 51 52 53 54 55 56 57 58 59 60 61 63 64 65 66 67 69 70 71 72 73 74 **P**4 6 **S** Intermountain Health Care, Inc., Salt Lake City, UT	23	10	414	20057	282	597077	3915	235098	94295	2828
▣ PRIMARY CHILDREN'S MEDICAL CENTER, (PEDIATRIC MED/SURG REHAB PSYCH), 100 North Medical Drive, Zip 84113–1100; tel. 801/588–2000; Joseph R. Horton, Chief Executive Officer and Administrator **A**1 3 5 9 10 **F**2 3 4 7 8 10 11 12 13 14 15 17 19 20 21 22 25 26 30 31 32 34 35 37 38 39 40 41 42 43 44 45 46 47 48 49 51 52 53 54 55 56 58 59 60 61 63 64 65 66 67 69 70 71 72 73 74 **S** Intermountain Health Care, Inc., Salt Lake City, UT **N** Intermountain HealthCare/Amerinet, Salt Lake City, UT	23	59	187	9394	143	188918	0	118876	54749	1678
□ SALT LAKE REGIONAL MEDICAL CENTER, 1050 East South Temple, Zip 84102–1599; tel. 801/350–4111; Kay Matsumura, Chief Executive Officer (Nonreporting) **A**1 2 3 5 9 10 **S** Paracelsus Healthcare Corporation, Houston, TX	21	10	200	—	—	—	—	—	—	—
▣ SHRINERS HOSPITALS FOR CHILDREN–INTERMOUNTAIN, (Formerly Shriners Hospitals for Crippled Children, Intermountain Unit), Fairfax Road and Virginia Street, Zip 84103–4399; tel. 801/536–3500; Douglas P. Schweikhart, Administrator **A**1 3 5 **F**12 19 34 35 39 41 47 49 54 65 67 71 73 **S** Shriners Hospitals for Children, Tampa, FL	23	57	40	859	22	5116	0	—	—	161
▣ △ UNIVERSITY OF UTAH HOSPITALS AND CLINICS, 50 North Medical Drive, Zip 84132; tel. 801/581–2377; Christine St. Andre, Executive Director **A**1 2 3 5 7 8 9 10 **F**4 6 7 8 9 10 11 12 14 15 16 17 18 19 20 21 22 23 25 26 28 29 30 31 32 34 35 37 38 40 41 42 43 44 45 46 48 49 51 52 53 54 55 56 57 58 59 60 61 65 66 67 68 69 70 71 72 73 74 **P**5	12	10	380	16165	289	—	2592	223548	89096	3437
□ UNIVERSITY OF UTAH NEUROPSYCHIATRIC INSTITUTE, 501 Chipeta Way, Zip 84108–1225; tel. 801/583–2500; Ross Van Vranken, Chief Executive Officer **A**1 3 5 10 **F**1 2 3 12 14 16 17 19 21 26 35 45 46 52 53 54 55 56 57 58 59 65 67 68 **P**5 8	23	22	90	1840	59	7489	0	12457	5904	187
▣ VETERANS AFFAIRS MEDICAL CENTER, 500 Foothill Drive, Zip 84148; tel. 801/582–1565; Donald F. Moore, Acting Medical Center Director **A**1 2 3 5 8 9 **F**3 4 10 11 12 14 15 16 17 18 19 20 22 24 25 26 27 28 30 31 32 33 34 35 37 39 41 42 43 44 46 48 49 50 51 52 54 55 56 57 58 60 61 63 65 67 69 73 74 **S** Department of Veterans Affairs, Washington, DC	45	10	243	7346	189	164028	0	125365	64523	1477
SANDY—Salt Lake County										
▣ ALTA VIEW HOSPITAL, 9660 South 1300 East, Zip 84094; tel. 801/576–2600; Wes Thompson, Administrator **A**1 9 10 **F**1 2 3 4 5 6 7 8 9 10 11 12 13 14 15 16 17 18 19 20 21 22 24 25 26 27 28 30 31 32 33 35 38 39 40 41 42 43 44 45 46 47 48 49 51 52 53 54 55 56 57 58 59 60 61 62 63 64 65 66 67 68 69 70 71 72 73 74 **P**3 4 5 6 **S** Intermountain Health Care, Inc., Salt Lake City, UT **N** Intermountain HealthCare/Amerinet, Salt Lake City, UT	23	10	68	6207	34	—	1687	32856	14553	—

Hospital, Address, Telephone, Administrator, Approval, Facility, and Physician Codes, Health Care System, Network	Classi-fication Codes		Utilization Data					Expense (thousands) of dollars		
★ American Hospital Association (AHA) membership □ Joint Commission on Accreditation of Healthcare Organizations (JCAHO) accreditation + American Osteopathic Hospital Association (AOHA) membership ○ American Osteopathic Association (AOA) accreditation △ Commission on Accreditation of Rehabilitation Facilities (CARF) accreditation Control codes 61, 63, 64, 71, 72 and 73 indicate hospitals listed by AOHA, but not registered by AHA. For definition of numerical codes, see page A4	Control	Service	Beds	Admissions	Census	Outpatient Visits	Births	Total	Payroll	Personnel
□ △ HEALTHSOUTH REHABILITATION HOSPITAL OF UTAH, 8074 South 1300 East, Zip 84094; tel. 801/561–3400; Richard M. Richards, Administrator (Total facility includes 36 beds in nursing home–type unit) **A**1 7 10 **F**5 12 24 25 27 28 30 32 34 39 41 45 46 48 49 64 65 66 67 73 **P**4 **S** HEALTHSOUTH Corporation, Birmingham, AL	33	46	73	877	42	21465	0	9326	4453	133
TOOELE—Tooele County										
★ TOOELE VALLEY REGIONAL MEDICAL CENTER, 211 South 100 East, Zip 84074–2794; tel. 801/882–1697; Mark F. Dalley, Chief Executive Officer (Total facility includes 84 beds in nursing home–type unit) **A**9 10 **F**3 7 8 11 12 14 15 16 17 18 19 20 22 26 27 28 30 32 37 40 41 44 49 54 56 57 58 64 65 71 73 74 **S** Rural Health Management Corporation, Nephi, UT	13	10	122	498	73	13582	45	9668	4104	174
TREMONTON—Box Elder County										
★ BEAR RIVER VALLEY HOSPITAL, 440 West 600 North, Zip 84337; tel. 801/257–7441; Robert F. Jex, Administrator (Total facility includes 38 beds in nursing home–type unit) **A**9 10 **F**7 12 14 15 17 20 22 32 33 40 44 46 49 64 71 73 **P**3 **S** Intermountain Health Care, Inc., Salt Lake City, UT **N** Intermountain HealthCare/Amerinet, Salt Lake City, UT	23	10	58	619	40	10048	64	3459	1770	51
VERNAL—Uintah County										
★ COLUMBIA ASHLEY VALLEY MEDICAL CENTER, (Formerly Ashley Valley Medical Center), 151 West 200 North, Zip 84078; tel. 801/789–3342; Ronald J. Perry, Chief Executive Officer (Nonreporting) **A**9 10 **S** Columbia/HCA Healthcare Corporation, Nashville, TN	33	10	29	—	—	—	—	—	—	—
WEST JORDAN—Salt Lake County										
□ JORDAN VALLEY HOSPITAL, 3580 West 9000 South, Zip 84088–8811; tel. 801/561–8888; Jeffrey J. Manley, Chief Executive Officer **A**1 9 10 **F**3 5 7 8 10 12 14 18 19 20 21 22 23 26 28 30 31 32 33 35 37 39 40 41 42 43 44 45 48 49 50 51 53 54 55 56 57 58 59 60 61 63 65 66 67 69 71 72 73 74 **P**2 5 7 8 **S** Paracelsus Healthcare Corporation, Houston, TX	33	10	50	2600	18	60564	1200	15876	7493	261
RIVENDELL PSYCHIATRIC CENTER, 5899 West Rivendell Drive, Zip 84088, Mailing Address: P.O. Box 459, Zip 84084; tel. 801/561–3377; Sandy Podley, Chief Executive Officer (Nonreporting) **A**10	33	52	80	—	—	—	—	—	—	—
WEST VALLEY CITY—Salt Lake County										
□ PIONEER VALLEY HOSPITAL, 3460 South Pioneer Parkway, Zip 84120; tel. 801/964–3100; Brian Mottishaw, Chief Executive Officer (Nonreporting) **A**1 2 9 10 **S** Paracelsus Healthcare Corporation, Houston, TX	33	10	127	—	—	—	—	—	—	—
WOODS CROSS—Davis County										
□ BENCHMARK BEHAVIORAL HEALTH SYSTEMS, (Formerly Benchmark Regional Hospital), 592 West 1350 South, Zip 84087–1665; tel. 801/299–5300; Richard O. Hurt, Ph.D., Chief Executive Officer **A**1 9 10 **F**1 2 3 14 15 16 22 52 53 55 56 57 58 59 65 67 **P**6 8 **S** Ramsay Health Care, Inc., Coral Gobles, FL BENCHMARK REGIONAL HOSPITAL See Benchmark Behavioral Health Systems	33	22	68	181	70	1148	0	8721	3547	236

VERMONT

Resident population 585 (in thousands)
Resident population in metro areas 27.2%
Birth rate per 1,000 population 13.0
65 years and over 12.0%
Percent of persons without health insurance 8.6%

Hospital, Address, Telephone, Administrator, Approval, Facility, and Physician Codes, Health Care System, Network	Classi-fication Codes		Utilization Data					Expense (thousands) of dollars		
	Control	Service	Beds	Admissions	Census	Outpatient Visits	Births	Total	Payroll	Personnel

★ American Hospital Association (AHA) membership
□ Joint Commission on Accreditation of Healthcare Organizations (JCAHO) accreditation
+ American Osteopathic Hospital Association (AOHA) membership
○ American Osteopathic Association (AOA) accreditation
△ Commission on Accreditation of Rehabilitation Facilities (CARF) accreditation
Control codes 61, 63, 64, 71, 72 and 73 indicate hospitals listed by AOHA, but not registered by AHA. For definition of numerical codes, see page A4

BARRE—Washington County

☒ CENTRAL VERMONT MEDICAL CENTER, Fisher Road, Zip 05641, Mailing Address: P.O. Box 547, Zip 05641–0547; tel. 802/371–4100; Philo D. Hall, President (Total facility includes 153 beds in nursing home–type unit) **A**1 9 10 **F**7 8 14 15 16 17 19 21 22 23 27 28 30 31 32 33 34 35 37 39 40 41 42 44 45 46 49 51 52 53 54 56 57 58 63 64 65 71 73 **P**6 8 — 23 10 275 4161 209 76419 516 41982 18788 591

BENNINGTON—Bennington County

☒ SOUTHWESTERN VERMONT MEDICAL CENTER, 100 Hospital Drive East, Zip 05201–5013; tel. 802/442–6361; Harvey M. Yorke, President and Chief Executive Officer **A**1 2 9 10 **F**1 3 4 7 8 10 12 14 15 16 17 19 21 22 25 26 27 28 30 32 33 34 35 37 39 40 41 42 44 45 46 49 51 52 54 55 56 57 58 59 60 63 64 65 66 67 69 70 71 72 73 74 **P**5 6 8 — 23 10 93 5033 58 98300 395 38012 18822 475

BRATTLEBORO—Windham County

☒ BRATTLEBORO MEMORIAL HOSPITAL, 9 Belmont Avenue, Zip 05301; tel. 802/257–0341; Brian R. Mitteer, President **A**1 9 10 **F**7 8 11 14 15 16 17 19 21 22 24 28 30 31 37 39 40 41 42 44 46 49 63 65 67 71 73 — 23 10 61 2638 33 51076 373 21608 9514 279

☒ BRATTLEBORO RETREAT, 75 Linden Street, Zip 05301–0803, Mailing Address: P.O. Box 803, Zip 05302; tel. 802/257–7785; Arthur Scott, Interim Director (Total facility includes 117 beds in nursing home–type unit) **A**1 3 5 10 **F**2 3 16 26 27 34 52 53 54 55 56 57 58 59 64 65 67 74 — 23 22 263 2718 90 6000 0 31400 19000 —

BURLINGTON—Chittenden County

☒ FLETCHER ALLEN HEALTH CARE, (Includes Fanny Allen Campus, 101 College Parkway, Colchester, Zip 05446–3035; tel. 802/655–1234; Medical Center Hospital Campus, Colchester Avenue, Zip 05401; tel. 802/656–2345; James H. Taylor, President and Chief Executive Officer), 111 Colchester Avenue, Zip 05401–1429; tel. 802/656–2345; John W. Frymoyer, M.D., Chief Executive Officer **A**1 2 3 5 8 9 10 **F**2 3 4 7 8 9 10 11 12 13 14 15 16 17 18 19 20 21 22 23 25 26 28 29 30 31 32 33 34 35 37 38 39 40 41 42 43 44 45 46 47 48 49 51 52 53 54 55 56 57 58 59 60 63 64 65 66 67 69 70 71 72 73 **P**3 6 8 **N** Fletcher Allen Health Care, Burlington, VT — 23 10 382 20978 364 169527 2311 228242 107323 3100

MIDDLEBURY—Addison County

☒ PORTER HOSPITAL, 75 South Street, Zip 05753–8606; tel. 802/388–4701; James L. Daily, President (Total facility includes 118 beds in nursing home–type unit) **A**1 9 10 **F**8 14 16 17 19 21 22 26 28 30 37 39 40 42 44 45 46 49 63 64 65 67 71 73 — 23 10 163 1515 131 56161 318 18920 8878 432

MORRISVILLE—Lamoille County

☒ COPLEY HOSPITAL, Washington Highway, Zip 05661–9209, Mailing Address: RD 3, Box 760, Zip 05661–9209; tel. 802/888–4231; Carolyn C. Roberts, President **A**1 9 10 **F**7 8 11 14 15 16 17 19 21 22 28 30 33 34 37 39 40 42 44 46 48 49 53 56 58 64 65 66 67 71 73 **P**8 — 23 10 43 1697 20 45463 225 15431 7159 259

NEWPORT—Orleans County

☒ NORTH COUNTRY HOSPITAL AND HEALTH CENTER, Prouty Drive, Zip 05855; tel. 802/334–7331; Sidney A. Toll, President **A**1 9 10 **F**7 8 11 14 15 16 17 19 21 22 28 29 35 37 39 40 41 42 44 46 49 56 65 67 71 73 74 **P**6 — 23 10 37 2013 22 46417 192 19418 10194 285

RANDOLPH—Orange County

☒ GIFFORD MEDICAL CENTER, 44 South Main Street, Zip 05060, Mailing Address: Box 2000, Zip 05060; tel. 802/728–4441; David H. Gregg, Jr., President (Total facility includes 47 beds in nursing home–type unit) **A**1 2 9 10 **F**3 6 7 8 11 12 13 14 15 16 17 18 19 21 22 25 26 27 28 29 30 31 32 33 34 37 39 40 41 42 44 45 46 49 51 53 54 55 56 57 58 61 64 65 67 68 71 72 73 74 **P**6 — 23 10 99 1343 65 74377 260 16782 6973 253

RUTLAND—Rutland County

☒ RUTLAND REGIONAL MEDICAL CENTER, 160 Allen Street, Zip 05701–4595; tel. 802/775–7111; James T. Bowse, President **A**1 2 9 10 **F**4 6 7 8 12 13 14 15 16 19 20 21 22 23 28 30 31 34 35 37 39 40 41 42 44 45 46 48 49 52 54 55 56 58 59 60 63 65 66 67 70 71 72 73 **P**5 8 — 23 10 132 6830 101 98433 688 65517 31076 757

SAINT ALBANS—Franklin County

☒ NORTHWESTERN MEDICAL CENTER, Fairfield Street, Zip 05478–1004, Mailing Address: Box 1370, Zip 05478; tel. 802/524–5911; Peter A. Hofstetter, Chief Executive Officer **A**1 2 9 10 **F**7 8 12 14 15 16 17 19 22 28 29 30 33 34 39 40 41 44 45 46 49 51 65 67 71 73 **P**8 **S** Quorum Health Group/Quorum Health Resources, Inc., Brentwood, TN — 23 10 70 2676 31 22032 440 21992 10010 267

SAINT JOHNSBURY—Caledonia County

☒ NORTHEASTERN VERMONT REGIONAL HOSPITAL, Hospital Drive, Zip 05819–9962, Mailing Address: P.O. Box 905, Zip 05819–9962; tel. 802/748–8141; Paul R. Bengtson, Chief Executive Officer **A**1 9 10 **F**7 8 14 15 16 17 19 21 22 29 30 31 37 39 40 41 42 44 45 46 49 53 54 56 58 63 65 67 71 72 73 74 **P**7 **S** Quorum Health Group/Quorum Health Resources, Inc., Brentwood, TN — 23 10 64 1842 19 64953 258 18870 7415 215

SPRINGFIELD—Windsor County

☒ SPRINGFIELD HOSPITAL, 25 Ridgewood Road, Zip 05156, Mailing Address: P.O. Box 2003, Zip 05156–3057; tel. 802/885–2151; Glenn D. Cordner, Acting Chief Executive Officer **A**1 9 10 **F**3 7 8 12 15 19 21 22 25 26 28 31 33 35 37 40 41 42 44 52 53 56 58 63 65 66 67 71 72 73 **P**4 7 — 23 10 69 2478 29 40958 214 20828 8077 287

Hospital, Address, Telephone, Administrator, Approval, Facility, and Physician Codes, Health Care System, Network	Classi-fication Codes		Utilization Data					Expense (thousands) of dollars		
★ American Hospital Association (AHA) membership □ Joint Commission on Accreditation of Healthcare Organizations (JCAHO) accreditation + American Osteopathic Hospital Association (AOHA) membership ○ American Osteopathic Association (AOA) accreditation △ Commission on Accreditation of Rehabilitation Facilities (CARF) accreditation Control codes 61, 63, 64, 71, 72 and 73 indicate hospitals listed by AOHA, but not registered by AHA. For definition of numerical codes, see page A4	Control	Service	Beds	Admissions	Census	Outpatient Visits	Births	Total	Payroll	Personnel

TOWNSHEND—Windham County

★ GRACE COTTAGE HOSPITAL, (Includes Stratton House Nursing Home), Route 35, Zip 05353, Mailing Address: P.O. Box 216, Zip 05353–0126; tel. 802/365–7357; Albert La Rochelle, Administrator (Total facility includes 30 beds in nursing home–type unit) **A**9 10 **F**1 7 16 22 27 33 36 40 41 44 49 64 65 73

| 23 | 10 | 45 | 367 | 35 | 8036 | 27 | 3921 | 2452 | 69 |

WATERBURY—Washington County

VERMONT STATE HOSPITAL, 103 South Main Street, Zip 05671–2501; tel. 802/241–1000; Bertold Francke, M.D., Interim Executive Director **A**9 10 **F**20 27 52 65 73 **P**6

| 12 | 22 | 70 | 288 | 66 | 0 | 0 | 10059 | 5283 | 175 |

WHITE RIVER JUNCTION—Windsor County

⊞ VETERANS AFFAIRS MEDICAL CENTER, North Hartland Road, Zip 05009–0001; tel. 802/295–9363; Gary M. De Gasta, Director (Total facility includes 22 beds in nursing home–type unit) **A**1 3 5 8 9 **F**1 2 3 4 5 6 8 10 12 14 16 17 18 19 20 21 22 25 26 27 28 29 30 31 32 33 34 35 37 39 41 42 43 44 45 46 48 49 51 52 54 55 56 57 58 59 60 61 64 65 67 71 73 74 **P**6 **S** Department of Veterans Affairs, Washington, DC

| 45 | 10 | 110 | 3229 | 81 | 102447 | 0 | 56380 | 29604 | 669 |

WINDSOR—Windsor County

★ MOUNT ASCUTNEY HOSPITAL AND HEALTH CENTER, Rural Route 1, Box 6, Zip 05089–9702; tel. 802/674–6711; Richard Slusky, Administrator (Total facility includes 66 beds in nursing home–type unit) **A**9 10 **F**8 12 15 16 17 20 22 26 27 29 30 31 32 33 34 36 37 39 41 44 45 46 48 49 54 56 58 64 65 67 71 73 **P**6

| 23 | 10 | 99 | 934 | 87 | 14750 | 0 | 11250 | 5627 | 223 |

VIRGINIA

Resident population 6,618 (in thousands)
Resident population in metro areas 77.7%
Birth rate per 1,000 population 14.7
65 years and over 11.1%
Percent of persons without health insurance 12.0%

Hospital, Address, Telephone, Administrator, Approval, Facility, and Physician Codes, Health Care System, Network	Classi-fication Codes		Utilization Data					Expense (thousands) of dollars		
★ American Hospital Association (AHA) membership □ Joint Commission on Accreditation of Healthcare Organizations (JCAHO) accreditation + American Osteopathic Hospital Association (AOHA) membership ○ American Osteopathic Association (AOA) accreditation △ Commission on Accreditation of Rehabilitation Facilities (CARF) accreditation Control codes 61, 63, 64, 71, 72 and 73 indicate hospitals listed by AOHA, but not registered by AHA. For definition of numerical codes, see page A4	Control	Service	Beds	Admissions	Census	Outpatient Visits	Births	Total	Payroll	Personnel

ABINGDON—Washington County

★ JOHNSTON MEMORIAL HOSPITAL, 351 North Court Street, Zip 24210–2921; tel. 540/676–7000; Clark R. Beil, Chief Executive Officer **A**1 2 9 10 **F**2 3 4 7 8 10 11 12 14 15 16 17 19 20 21 22 23 25 26 27 28 30 31 33 34 37 38 39 40 41 42 43 44 45 46 48 49 51 52 53 54 55 56 57 58 59 63 65 66 67 69 70 71 72 73 74 **P**1 6 8 **N** Mountain States Healthcare Network, Johnson City, TN ... 23 10 135 4716 62 43265 785 32207 13553 493

ALEXANDRIA—Independent City County

★ ALEXANDRIA HOSPITAL, 4320 Seminary Road, Zip 22304–1594; tel. 703/504–3000; H. Patrick Walters, President **A**1 2 3 5 9 10 **F**4 7 8 10 11 12 15 16 19 21 22 26 28 30 31 32 34 35 37 38 39 40 41 42 43 44 45 46 49 52 54 56 59 60 61 63 65 67 71 73 74 **P**5 7 8 ... 23 10 316 14911 208 109965 3432 107116 52291 1352

★ △ INOVA MOUNT VERNON HOSPITAL, (Formerly Mount Vernon Hospital), 2501 Parker's Lane, Zip 22306–3209; tel. 703/664–7000; Susan Herbert, Administrator (Nonreporting) **A**1 2 3 7 9 10 **S** Inova Health System, Springfield, VA **N** Inova Health System, Springfield, VA ... 23 10 229

MOUNT VERNON HOSPITAL See Inova Mount Vernon Hospital

ARLINGTON—Arlington County

★ ARLINGTON HOSPITAL, 1701 North George Mason Drive, Zip 22205–3698; tel. 703/558–5000; James B. Cole, President and Chief Executive Officer **A**1 2 3 5 9 10 **F**3 4 7 8 10 11 17 19 21 22 23 26 28 29 30 31 32 34 35 37 38 40 41 42 43 44 46 49 50 52 53 56 57 58 59 60 63 65 67 71 73 **P**1 7 ... 32 10 256 13723 173 123729 3030 106712 48310 1180

□ HOSPICE OF NORTHERN VIRGINIA, 4715 North 15th Street, Zip 22205; tel. 703/534–7070; David J. English, President and Chief Executive Officer (Nonreporting) **A**1 10 ... 23 49 15 — — — — — — —

□ △ NATIONAL HOSPITAL MEDICAL CENTER, 2455 Army Navy Drive, Zip 22206; tel. 703/920–6700; Ronald E. Yates, Chief Executive Officer **A**1 5 7 9 10 **F**1 3 5 7 8 12 14 15 16 17 18 19 21 22 23 24 25 26 27 28 29 30 31 32 34 35 37 39 41 42 43 44 45 46 48 49 50 51 53 54 55 56 57 58 59 60 62 65 66 67 68 71 72 73 74 **P**4 5 7 8 **S** Columbia/HCA Healthcare Corporation, Nashville, TN ... 23 10 102 1648 26 32135 0 26816 — 190

★ VENCOR HOSPITAL–ARLINGTON, 601 South Carlin Springs Road, Zip 22204–1096; tel. 703/671–1200; Joseph A. Stuber, Administrator (Nonreporting) **A**1 5 9 10 **S** Vencor, Incorporated, Louisville, KY ... 33 10 206 — — — — — — —

BEDFORD—Independent City County

★ CARILION BEDFORD MEMORIAL HOSPITAL, (Formerly Bedford County Memorial Hospital), 1613 Oakwood Street, Zip 24523–0688, Mailing Address: P.O. Box 688, Zip 24523–0688; tel. 540/586–2441; Howard Ainsley, Director (Total facility includes 111 beds in nursing home–type unit) **A**1 9 10 **F**1 6 7 10 11 13 14 15 16 17 19 20 27 28 29 30 32 37 39 40 42 44 49 51 52 53 56 60 64 65 67 71 73 74 **P**6 **S** Carilion Health System, Roanoke, VA **N** Carilion Health System, Roanoke, VA ... 23 10 161 1987 127 11186 303 16422 7375 361

BIG STONE GAP—Wise County

★ LONESOME PINE HOSPITAL, 1990 Holton Avenue East, Zip 24219–0230, Mailing Address: Drawer I, Zip 24219; tel. 540/523–3111; Paul A. Bishop, Administrator **A**1 9 10 **F**7 8 12 14 15 16 17 19 21 22 23 28 30 32 35 37 39 40 44 46 49 63 65 68 71 73 **N** CHA Provider Network, Inc., Lexington, KY; Highlands Wellmont Health Network, Inc., Bristol, TN ... 23 10 60 1992 22 31268 233 13251 5632 222

BLACKSBURG—Montgomery County

★ COLUMBIA MONTGOMERY REGIONAL HOSPITAL, 3700 South Main Street, Zip 24060, Mailing Address: P.O. Box 90004, Zip 24062–9004; tel. 540/953–5101; David R. Williams, Chief Executive Officer (Total facility includes 11 beds in nursing home–type unit) **A**1 9 10 **F**2 3 4 7 8 10 11 12 14 15 16 17 18 19 21 22 23 24 26 28 29 30 31 32 33 34 35 37 38 39 40 41 42 43 44 45 46 48 49 51 52 53 54 55 56 57 58 59 60 61 63 64 65 66 67 70 71 72 73 74 **P**8 **S** Columbia/HCA Healthcare Corporation, Nashville, TN ... 33 10 104 4122 48 51754 583 33001 11654 462

BURKEVILLE—Nottoway County

★ PIEDMONT GERIATRIC HOSPITAL, (GERIATRIC PSYCHIATRY), Highway 460/360, Zip 23922–9999; tel. 804/767–4401; Willard R. Pierce, Jr., Director **A**1 9 10 **F**19 20 22 26 27 35 41 46 52 55 57 60 65 67 71 73 **S** Virginia Department of Mental Health, Richmond, VA ... 12 49 210 116 190 0 0 19377 9298 383

CATAWBA—Roanoke County

□ CATAWBA HOSPITAL, Mailing Address: P.O. Box 200, Zip 24070; tel. 540/375–4200; James S. Reinhard, M.D., Director **A**1 9 10 **F**14 15 16 19 20 26 35 45 46 52 57 65 73 **P**6 ... 12 22 218 421 172 0 0 15227 8671 333

CHARLOTTESVILLE—Independent City County

□ CHARTER BEHAVIORAL HEALTH SYSTEM OF CHARLOTTESVILLE, 2101 Arlington Boulevard, Zip 22903–1593; tel. 804/977–1120; Wayne Adams, Chief Executive Officer **A**1 9 10 **F**3 15 52 53 54 55 56 57 58 59 **S** Magellan Health Services, Atlanta, GA **N** Virginia Health Network, Richmond, VA ... 33 22 62 1066 30 3187 0 — — 103

Hospital, Address, Telephone, Administrator, Approval, Facility, and Physician Codes, Health Care System, Network	Classi-fication Codes		Utilization Data					Expense (thousands) of dollars		
	Control	Service	Beds	Admissions	Census	Outpatient Visits	Births	Total	Payroll	Personnel

★ American Hospital Association (AHA) membership
□ Joint Commission on Accreditation of Healthcare Organizations (JCAHO) accreditation
+ American Osteopathic Hospital Association (AOHA) membership
○ American Osteopathic Association (AOA) accreditation
△ Commission on Accreditation of Rehabilitation Facilities (CARF) accreditation
　Control codes 61, 63, 64, 71, 72 and 73 indicate hospitals listed by AOHA, but not registered by AHA. For definition of numerical codes, see page A4

Hospital	Control	Service	Beds	Admissions	Census	Outpatient Visits	Births	Total	Payroll	Personnel
⊠ MARTHA JEFFERSON HOSPITAL, 459 Locust Avenue, Zip 22902–9940; tel. 804/982–7000; James E. Haden, President and Chief Executive Officer **A**1 2 9 10 **F**7 8 12 14 16 17 19 20 21 22 23 24 25 26 27 28 29 30 31 32 33 34 35 37 39 40 41 42 44 45 46 49 51 60 63 64 65 66 67 71 72 73 74 **P**7 8 **N** Virginia Health Network, Richmond, VA	23	10	156	9194	97	85779	1272	69615	32279	980
⊠ UNIVERSITY OF VIRGINIA MEDICAL CENTER, Jefferson Park Avenue, Zip 22908, Mailing Address: P.O. Box 10050, Zip 22906–0050; tel. 804/924–0211; Michael J. Halseth, Executive Director **A**1 2 3 5 8 9 10 **F**3 4 5 7 8 9 10 11 12 13 14 15 16 17 18 19 20 21 22 23 24 25 26 27 28 29 30 31 32 33 34 35 37 38 39 40 41 42 43 44 45 46 47 48 49 51 52 53 54 55 56 57 58 59 60 61 63 65 66 67 68 69 70 71 72 73 74 **P**3 **N** Central Virginia Health Network, Richmond, VA; National Cardiovascular Network, Atlanta, GA	12	10	604	26936	439	475700	1544	391435	144044	4877
CHESAPEAKE—Independent City County										
⊠ CHESAPEAKE GENERAL HOSPITAL, 736 Battlefield Boulevard North, Zip 23320–4941, Mailing Address: P.O. Box 2028, Zip 23327–2028; tel. 757/547–8121; Donald S. Buckley, FACHE, President **A**1 2 5 9 10 **F**1 4 6 7 8 10 12 14 15 16 17 19 21 22 23 24 26 27 28 29 30 31 32 33 34 35 36 37 39 40 42 44 45 46 52 54 55 57 59 60 61 63 65 66 67 71 73 74 **P**5 8 **N** Virginia Health Network, Richmond, VA	16	10	260	13306	182	130094	2923	94066	41654	1287
CLINTWOOD—Dickenson County										
DICKENSON COUNTY MEDICAL CENTER, Hospital Drive, Zip 24228, Mailing Address: Box 1390, Zip 24228–1390; tel. 540/926–0300; Benjamin A. Peak, Chief Executive Officer **A**9 10 **F**8 14 19 22 26 28 30 32 35 37 44 51 63 65 67 71 73 74 **P**6	33	10	41	1373	16	50711	0	8391	3465	188
CULPEPER—Culpeper County										
⊠ CULPEPER MEMORIAL HOSPITAL, 501 Sunset Lane, Zip 22701–3917, Mailing Address: Box 592, Zip 22701–0592; tel. 540/829–4100; H. Lee Kirk, Jr., President **A**1 9 10 **F**2 7 8 12 14 15 16 17 19 20 22 23 24 28 29 30 32 33 34 35 37 40 41 42 44 46 48 49 52 54 55 57 58 59 63 65 67 71 **P**7 8	23	10	70	3110	33	32287	340	22274	10726	396
DANVILLE—Independent City County										
⊠ DANVILLE REGIONAL MEDICAL CENTER, 142 South Main Street, Zip 24541–2922; tel. 804/799–2100; Larry T. DePriest, President (Total facility includes 60 beds in nursing home–type unit) **A**1 2 3 5 6 9 10 **F**2 3 6 7 8 10 11 12 14 15 16 17 19 21 22 28 29 30 31 32 34 35 37 39 40 41 42 44 45 46 48 49 51 52 54 55 56 58 59 60 61 62 63 64 65 67 71 72 73 74 **P**6 8	23	10	312	12163	261	116487	1166	79687	37172	1076
□ SOUTHERN VIRGINIA MENTAL HEALTH INSTITUTE, 382 Taylor Drive, Zip 24541–4023; tel. 804/799–6220; Constance N. Fletcher, Ph.D., Director **A**1 9 10 **F**15 52 54 55 57 **S** Virginia Department of Mental Health, Richmond, VA	12	22	96	858	84	—	0	7814	5010	171
EMPORIA—Independent City County										
⊠ GREENSVILLE MEMORIAL HOSPITAL, 214 Weaver Avenue, Zip 23847–1482; tel. 804/348–2000; Rosemary C. Check, Chief Executive Officer (Total facility includes 65 beds in nursing home–type unit) **A**1 9 10 **F**7 8 14 19 21 22 28 30 32 33 34 35 36 37 40 42 44 45 46 49 63 64 65 71 73 **S** Quorum Health Group/Quorum Health Resources, Inc., Brentwood, TN **N** Virginia Health Network, Richmond, VA	23	10	130	3309	109	36928	157	18471	8865	302
FAIRFAX—Independent City County										
⊠ INOVA FAIR OAKS HOSPITAL, (Formerly Fair Oaks Hospital), 3600 Joseph Siewick Drive, Zip 22033–1709; tel. 703/391–3600; Steven E. Brown, Administrator **A**1 2 5 9 10 **F**1 2 3 4 6 7 8 10 11 15 16 17 19 20 21 22 29 30 31 32 34 35 37 38 39 40 42 43 44 46 47 48 49 52 53 56 57 58 60 63 64 65 67 69 70 71 72 73 74 **P**3 5 7 8 **S** Inova Health System, Springfield, VA **N** Inova Health System, Springfield, VA	23	10	133	9426	88	61706	2300	66000	26287	671
FALLS CHURCH—Independent City County										
⊠ DOMINION HOSPITAL, 2960 Sleepy Hollow Road, Zip 22044–2001; tel. 703/536–2000; Barbara D. S. Hekimian, Chief Executive Officer **A**1 9 10 **F**15 16 19 35 52 53 54 55 56 57 58 59 65 67 **P**2 4 **S** Columbia/HCA Healthcare Corporation, Nashville, TN	33	22	100	1652	46	6391	0	8782	4473	129
FAIRFAX HOSPITAL See Inova Fairfax Hospital										
⊠ INOVA FAIRFAX HOSPITAL, (Formerly Fairfax Hospital), 3300 Gallows Road, Zip 22046–3300; tel. 703/698–1110; Jolene Tornabeni, Administrator **A**1 2 3 5 8 9 10 **F**1 2 3 4 6 7 8 10 11 12 13 16 17 19 21 22 25 28 29 30 31 34 35 36 37 38 39 40 41 42 43 44 45 46 47 48 49 51 52 53 54 55 56 57 58 59 60 61 63 64 65 66 67 68 69 70 71 72 73 74 **P**1 4 6 7 8 **S** Inova Health System, Springfield, VA **N** Inova Health System, Springfield, VA	23	10	656	43548	555	139128	9555	357458	159751	3321
⊠ NORTHERN VIRGINIA MENTAL HEALTH INSTITUTE, 3302 Gallows Road, Zip 22042–3398; tel. 703/207–7111; Antoni Sulikowski, Facility Director **A**1 9 10 **F**14 15 16 19 20 21 22 35 39 45 50 52 54 55 63 65 67 71 73 **P**1 **S** Virginia Department of Mental Health, Richmond, VA	12	22	62	407	65	0	0	9543	5984	149
FARMVILLE—Prince Edward County										
⊠ SOUTHSIDE COMMUNITY HOSPITAL, 800 Oak Street, Zip 23901–1199; tel. 804/392–8811; John H. Greer, President (Total facility includes 20 beds in nursing home–type unit) **A**1 9 10 **F**7 8 14 15 16 19 20 22 32 37 40 42 44 45 46 49 64 65 66 71 73 **S** Carilion Health System, Roanoke, VA	23	10	108	4498	56	40928	408	24866	11612	397
FISHERSVILLE—Augusta County										
□ AUGUSTA HEALTH CARE, (Formerly Augusta Medical Center), Mailing Address: P.O. Box 1000, Zip 22939; tel. 540/932–4000; Richard H. Graham, President and Chief Executive Officer **A**1 2 10 **F**2 3 7 8 10 12 14 15 16 17 19 20 21 22 23 24 26 27 28 29 30 31 32 33 34 35 36 37 39 40 41 42 44 45 46 48 49 51 52 54 55 56 57 58 59 63 64 65 66 67 71 73 **P**8	23	10	214	11132	137	200710	869	79288	34837	1220

Hospital, Address, Telephone, Administrator, Approval, Facility, and Physician Codes, Health Care System, Network	Classi-fication Codes		Utilization Data						Expense (thousands) of dollars		
	Control	Service	Beds	Admissions	Census	Outpatient Visits	Births	Total	Payroll	Personnel

★ American Hospital Association (AHA) membership
☐ Joint Commission on Accreditation of Healthcare Organizations (JCAHO) accreditation
+ American Osteopathic Hospital Association (AOHA) membership
○ American Osteopathic Association (AOA) accreditation
△ Commission on Accreditation of Rehabilitation Facilities (CARF) accreditation
Control codes 61, 63, 64, 71, 72 and 73 indicate hospitals listed by AOHA, but not registered by AHA. For definition of numerical codes, see page A4

	Control	Service	Beds	Admissions	Census	Outpatient Visits	Births	Total	Payroll	Personnel
☐ △ WOODROW WILSON REHABILITATION CENTER–HOSPITAL, Zip 22939–0100; tel. 703/332–7214; David J. Schwemer, Administrator **A**1 7 10 **F**3 12 19 22 27 34 35 44 48 49 50 65 67 71 73	12	46	30	104	6	3588	0	—	—	118
FORT BELVOIR—Fairfax County										
✚ DEWITT ARMY COMMUNITY HOSPITAL, Zip 22060–5901; tel. 703/805–0510; Colonel Robert C. Harvey, Commander **A**1 3 5 **F**3 4 6 7 8 12 13 14 15 16 17 18 19 20 21 22 23 24 25 26 27 28 29 30 31 34 35 39 40 41 42 43 44 45 46 49 51 53 54 55 56 57 58 59 60 61 65 66 67 69 71 73 74 **S** Department of the Army, Office of the Surgeon General, Falls Church, VA	42	10	62	5863	25	537912	1014	—	—	—
FRANKLIN—Independent City County										
✚ SOUTHAMPTON MEMORIAL HOSPITAL, 100 Fairview Drive, Zip 23851, Mailing Address: P.O. Box 817, Zip 23851–0817; tel. 757/569–6100; Edward J. Patnesky, President and Chief Executive Officer (Total facility includes 131 beds in nursing home–type unit) **A**1 9 10 **F**3 6 7 8 12 14 15 16 19 21 22 23 26 28 30 32 33 34 35 37 39 40 41 42 44 46 49 56 58 62 64 65 66 67 71 73 74 **P**8 **N** Virginia Health Network, Richmond, VA	23	10	207	2955	167	48022	282	25750	11832	466
FREDERICKSBURG—Independent City County										
✚ MARY WASHINGTON HOSPITAL, 1001 Sam Perry Boulevard, Zip 22401; tel. 540/899–1100; Fred M. Rankin, III, President and Chief Executive Officer **A**1 2 9 10 **F**3 4 6 7 8 10 11 12 13 14 15 16 17 18 19 20 21 22 23 25 26 28 29 30 31 32 33 34 35 37 38 39 40 41 42 43 44 45 46 49 52 53 54 55 57 59 60 62 63 65 67 68 71 72 73 **P**5	23	10	290	15105	205	140592	2278	122553	47413	1467
FRONT ROYAL—Warren County										
✚ WARREN MEMORIAL HOSPITAL, 1000 Shenandoah Avenue, Zip 22630–3598; tel. 540/636–0300; Charlie M. Horton, President (Total facility includes 40 beds in nursing home–type unit) **A**1 9 10 **F**7 8 15 16 19 22 26 28 32 33 34 37 39 40 41 44 45 49 63 64 65 66 67 71 73 74 **P**1 5 **N** Valley Health System, Winchester, VA	23	10	86	1693	58	32816	157	15506	6917	215
GALAX—Independent City County										
✚ TWIN COUNTY REGIONAL HOSPITAL, 200 Hospital Drive, Zip 24333; tel. 540/236–8181; Marcus G. Kuhn, President and Chief Executive Officer **A**1 9 10 **F**7 8 10 11 12 19 21 22 24 32 33 34 35 40 41 44 45 46 49 52 54 56 58 59 65 67 71 **P**5	23	10	118	4691	66	55369	420	30392	13680	531
GLOUCESTER—Gloucester County										
☐ RIVERSIDE WALTER REED HOSPITAL, Mailing Address: Route 17, Box 1130, Zip 23061–1130; tel. 804/693–8800; Grady W. Philips, III, Vice President and Administrator (Nonreporting) **A**1 9 10 **S** Riverside Health System, Newport News, VA **N** Virginia Health Network, Richmond, VA	23	10	71	—	—	—	—	—	—	—
GRUNDY—Buchanan County										
✚ BUCHANAN GENERAL HOSPITAL, Mailing Address: Route 5, Box 20, Zip 24614–9611; tel. 540/935–1000; John West, Administrator **A**1 9 10 **F**8 15 19 21 22 23 28 32 35 37 42 44 49 65 71 73 **P**8 **S** Quorum Health Group/Quorum Health Resources, Inc., Brentwood, TN	23	10	99	5095	62	58248	0	24383	9195	341
HAMPTON—Independent City County										
✚ COLUMBIA PENINSULA CENTER FOR BEHAVIORAL HEALTH, 2244 Executive Drive, Zip 23666; tel. 804/827–1001; Rufus S. Hoefer, Administrator (Nonreporting) **A**1 9 10 **S** Columbia/HCA Healthcare Corporation, Nashville, TN	33	22	125	—	—	—	—	—	—	—
✚ SENTARA HAMPTON GENERAL HOSPITAL, 3120 Victoria Boulevard, Zip 23661, Mailing Address: Drawer 640, Zip 23669; tel. 804/727–7000; Les A. Donahue, President and Chief Executive Officer (Total facility includes 26 beds in nursing home–type unit) **A**1 2 9 10 **F**1 4 6 7 8 9 10 11 12 13 14 15 16 17 18 19 20 21 22 23 24 25 26 27 28 29 30 31 32 33 34 35 36 37 38 39 40 41 42 43 44 45 46 48 49 51 52 53 54 55 56 57 58 59 60 61 62 63 64 65 69 70 71 72 73 74 **P**4 5 6 **S** Sentara Health System, Norfolk, VA **N** Sentara Health System, Norfolk, VA	23	10	242	9133	176	146712	1092	67685	25759	898
✚ U. S. AIR FORCE HOSPITAL, 45 Pine Street, Zip 23665–2080; tel. 804/764–6825; Colonel Glenn R. Willauer, Administrator (Nonreporting) **A**1 **S** Department of the Air Force, Washington, DC	41	10	59	—	—	—	—	—	—	—
✚ VETERANS AFFAIRS MEDICAL CENTER, 100 Emancipation Drive, Zip 23667–0001; tel. 804/722–9961; William G. Wright, Director (Total facility includes 120 beds in nursing home–type unit) **A**1 2 3 5 8 **F**3 4 6 8 12 15 16 17 19 20 21 22 23 24 26 27 28 29 30 31 32 33 35 37 39 41 42 43 44 45 46 49 50 51 52 54 55 56 57 58 60 61 63 64 65 69 70 71 72 73 74 **P**6 **S** Department of Veterans Affairs, Washington, DC	45	10	670	4883	314	193994	0	82086	45969	1108
HARRISONBURG—Independent City County										
✚ ROCKINGHAM MEMORIAL HOSPITAL, 235 Cantrell Avenue, Zip 22801–3293; tel. 540/433–4100; Carter Melton, President **A**1 2 9 10 **F**3 7 8 10 11 12 13 14 15 16 17 18 19 20 21 22 23 24 25 28 29 30 31 32 33 34 35 39 40 41 42 44 45 46 49 52 54 55 56 57 58 59 60 63 65 66 67 68 71 73 74 **P**7 8	23	10	265	11304	148	103255	1633	80086	40020	1241
HOPEWELL—Independent City County										
✚ COLUMBIA JOHN RANDOLPH MEDICAL CENTER, 411 West Randolph Road, Zip 23860, Mailing Address: P.O. Box 971, Zip 23860; tel. 804/541–1600; Daniel J. Wetta, Jr., Chief Executive Officer (Total facility includes 124 beds in nursing home–type unit) **A**1 9 10 **F**3 4 7 8 10 11 12 13 14 15 16 17 18 19 21 22 23 24 25 26 28 29 30 31 34 32 33 34 35 36 37 39 40 46 47 48 49 51 52 53 54 55 56 57 58 59 60 63 64 65 66 67 68 69 71 72 73 74 **P**1 5 7 **S** Columbia/HCA Healthcare Corporation, Nashville, TN **N** Preferred Care of Richmond, Richmond, VA	33	10	271	7329	223	88754	526	47561	19081	758

Hospital, Address, Telephone, Administrator, Approval, Facility, and Physician Codes, Health Care System, Network	Classi-fication Codes		Utilization Data					Expense (thousands) of dollars		
★ American Hospital Association (AHA) membership □ Joint Commission on Accreditation of Healthcare Organizations (JCAHO) accreditation + American Osteopathic Hospital Association (AOHA) membership ○ American Osteopathic Association (AOA) accreditation △ Commission on Accreditation of Rehabilitation Facilities (CARF) accreditation Control codes 61, 63, 64, 71, 72 and 73 indicate hospitals listed by AOHA, but not registered by AHA. For definition of numerical codes, see page A4	Control	Service	Beds	Admissions	Census	Outpatient Visits	Births	Total	Payroll	Personnel

HOT SPRINGS—Bath County

★ BATH COUNTY COMMUNITY HOSPITAL, Mailing Address: Drawer Z, Zip 24445; tel. 540/839–7000; Harry M. Lowd, III, Director **A**9 10 **F**8 16 22 28 30 32 37 39 44 45 49 65 71 73 — 23 | 10 | 25 | 606 | 8 | 4092 | 0 | 4873 | 2129 | 81

KILMARNOCK—Lancaster County

✚ RAPPAHANNOCK GENERAL HOSPITAL, 101 Harris Drive, Zip 22482, Mailing Address: P.O. Box 1449, Zip 22482–1449; tel. 804/435–8000; James M. Holmes, President and Chief Executive Officer **A**1 9 10 **F**7 8 14 15 16 19 21 22 31 32 34 35 37 40 42 44 45 46 51 59 63 65 66 71 73 **P**3 4 **N** Central Virginia Health Network, Richmond, VA — 23 | 10 | 76 | 2774 | 36 | 21767 | 276 | 21726 | 10374 | 358

LEBANON—Russell County

□ RUSSELL COUNTY MEDICAL CENTER, Carroll and Tate Streets, Zip 24266; tel. 540/889–1224; Jerry E. Lowery, Executive Director **A**1 9 10 **F**8 11 12 15 16 19 22 23 28 30 32 35 40 41 42 44 46 49 52 55 56 58 59 63 65 71 73 **P**8 **S** Community Health Systems, Inc., Brentwood, TN — 33 | 10 | 78 | 3875 | 54 | 48876 | 77 | 14682 | 6189 | 264

LEESBURG—Loudoun County

□ CHARTER BEHAVIORAL HEALTH SYSTEM AT SPRINGWOOD, 42009 Charter Springwood Lane, Zip 20176; tel. 703/777–0800; Dania O'Connor, Chief Executive Officer (Nonreporting) **A**1 9 **S** Magellan Health Services, Atlanta, GA — 33 | 22 | 77 | — | — | — | — | — | — | —

★ GRAYDON MANOR, 301 Childrens Center Road, Zip 22075–2598; tel. 703/777–3485; Bernard Haberlein, Executive Director **F**16 52 53 55 58 65 — 23 | 52 | 61 | 60 | 52 | 3940 | 0 | 5943 | 4097 | 132

✚ LOUDOUN HOSPITAL CENTER, 224 Cornwall Street N.W., Zip 20176; tel. 703/771–3300; G. T. Dunlop Ecker, President and Chief Executive Officer **A**1 2 9 10 **F**2 3 7 8 12 14 15 16 17 19 20 21 22 25 26 27 28 29 30 31 33 34 35 37 38 39 40 42 44 45 46 48 49 52 53 54 55 56 57 58 59 60 63 64 65 67 71 72 73 **P**6 8 — 23 | 10 | 112 | 4791 | 57 | 37808 | 833 | 43369 | 19830 | 489

LEXINGTON—Independent City County

✚ STONEWALL JACKSON HOSPITAL, 1 Health Circle, Zip 24450–2492; tel. 540/462–1200; William Mahone, V, Administrator (Total facility includes 50 beds in nursing home–type unit) **A**1 9 10 **F**7 8 14 15 16 19 21 22 27 28 30 32 33 34 35 36 37 39 40 41 44 46 49 63 64 65 71 73 **S** Carilion Health System, Roanoke, VA — 23 | 10 | 130 | 2324 | 71 | 38844 | 218 | 15219 | 6852 | 360

LOW MOOR—Alleghany County

✚ COLUMBIA ALLEGHANY REGIONAL HOSPITAL, One ARH Lane, Zip 24457, Mailing Address: P.O. Box 7, Zip 24457–0007; tel. 540/862–6200; Ward W. Stevens, CHE, Chief Executive Officer **A**1 9 10 12 13 **F**7 8 12 17 19 20 21 22 23 28 29 30 32 34 35 36 37 39 40 42 44 45 46 49 56 63 65 66 71 73 74 **S** Columbia/HCA Healthcare Corporation, Nashville, TN — 33 | 10 | 196 | 3950 | 51 | 48094 | 286 | 24683 | 10677 | 409

LURAY—Page County

✚ PAGE MEMORIAL HOSPITAL, 200 Memorial Drive, Zip 22835; tel. 540/743–4561; Donald J. Morgan, Administrator **A**1 9 10 **F**8 14 15 17 19 22 28 30 32 33 35 39 44 45 46 48 49 63 65 67 71 73 74 **P**6 — 23 | 10 | 54 | 1370 | 17 | 42743 | 0 | 8830 | 4240 | 168

LYNCHBURG—Independent City County

✚ LYNCHBURG GENERAL HOSPITAL, 1901 Tate Springs Road, Zip 24501–1167; tel. 804/947–3000; L. Darrell Powers, Senior Vice President (Total facility includes 130 beds in nursing home–type unit) **A**1 2 5 6 9 10 **F**1 2 3 4 8 10 11 14 16 17 18 19 20 21 22 23 24 26 27 28 29 30 33 34 35 37 38 40 41 42 43 44 48 49 52 53 54 55 56 57 58 59 60 63 64 65 67 71 72 73 74 **P**7 8 **S** Centra Health, Inc., Lynchburg, VA — 23 | 10 | 350 | 11468 | 290 | 97894 | 0 | 88624 | 41448 | 1066

✚ △ VIRGINIA BAPTIST HOSPITAL, 3300 Rivermont Avenue, Zip 24503–9989; tel. 804/947–4000; Thomas C. Jividen, Senior Vice President (Total facility includes 36 beds in nursing home–type unit) **A**1 5 7 9 10 **F**1 2 3 4 8 10 11 14 16 17 18 19 20 21 22 23 24 26 27 28 29 30 32 33 34 35 37 38 40 41 42 43 44 48 49 52 53 54 55 56 57 58 59 60 63 64 65 67 71 72 73 74 **P**7 8 **S** Centra Health, Inc., Lynchburg, VA — 23 | 10 | 301 | 9237 | 195 | 39237 | 2285 | 71657 | 39011 | 978

MADISON HEIGHTS—Amherst County

★ CENTRAL VIRGINIA TRAINING CENTER, 210 East Colony Road, Zip 24572, Mailing Address: P.O. Box 1098, Lynchburg, Zip 24505; tel. 804/947–6326; S. J. Butkus, Ph.D., Director (Total facility includes 104 beds in nursing home–type unit) (Nonreporting) **A**10 **S** Virginia Department of Mental Health, Richmond, VA — 12 | 62 | 1112 | — | — | — | — | — | — | —

MANASSAS—Independent City County

✚ PRINCE WILLIAM HOSPITAL, 8700 Sudley Road, Zip 20110–4418, Mailing Address: Box 2610, Zip 20108–0867; tel. 703/369–8000; Kenneth B. Swenson, President **A**1 2 9 10 **F**2 3 7 8 12 14 15 16 17 19 22 23 26 32 34 35 37 38 39 40 41 42 44 45 46 49 53 54 55 56 57 58 59 65 **P**3 — 23 | 10 | 131 | 7280 | 75 | 81114 | 1379 | 51246 | 22967 | 683

MARION—Smyth County

✚ SMYTH COUNTY COMMUNITY HOSPITAL, 700 Park Boulevard, Zip 24354, Mailing Address: P.O. Box 880, Zip 24354–0880; tel. 540/782–1234; Roger W. Cooper, President (Total facility includes 125 beds in nursing home–type unit) **A**1 9 10 **F**3 7 8 19 21 22 23 28 30 32 35 40 42 44 45 49 64 65 66 71 — 23 | 10 | 285 | 3242 | 157 | 40872 | 284 | 25411 | 12448 | 531

✚ SOUTHWESTERN VIRGINIA MENTAL HEALTH INSTITUTE, 502 East Main Street, Zip 24354; tel. 540/783–1200; Gerald E. Deans, Director (Nonreporting) **A**1 9 10 **S** Virginia Department of Mental Health, Richmond, VA — 12 | 22 | 266 | — | — | — | — | — | — | —

MARTINSVILLE—Independent City County

✚ MEMORIAL HOSPITAL OF MARTINSVILLE AND HENRY COUNTY, 320 Hospital Drive, Zip 24112–1981, Mailing Address: Box 4788, Zip 24115–4788; tel. 540/666–7200; Joseph Roach, Executive Director **A**1 2 9 10 **F**7 8 10 11 14 15 16 19 21 22 23 28 29 30 31 32 33 35 37 39 40 41 42 44 45 46 49 52 54 55 56 57 58 59 60 63 65 67 71 73 **P**6 **S** Quorum Health Group/Quorum Health Resources, Inc., Brentwood, TN — 23 | 10 | 152 | 6508 | 93 | 154055 | 486 | 48584 | 22261 | 738

Hospital, Address, Telephone, Administrator, Approval, Facility, and Physician Codes, Health Care System, Network	Classi-fication Codes		Utilization Data					Expense (thousands) of dollars		
★ American Hospital Association (AHA) membership □ Joint Commission on Accreditation of Healthcare Organizations (JCAHO) accreditation + American Osteopathic Hospital Association (AOHA) membership ○ American Osteopathic Association (AOA) accreditation △ Commission on Accreditation of Rehabilitation Facilities (CARF) accreditation Control codes 61, 63, 64, 71, 72 and 73 indicate hospitals listed by AOHA, but not registered by AHA. For definition of numerical codes, see page A4	Control	Service	Beds	Admissions	Census	Outpatient Visits	Births	Total	Payroll	Personnel

NASSAWADOX—Northampton County

☒ NORTHAMPTON–ACCOMACK MEMORIAL HOSPITAL, Mailing Address: P.O. Box 17, Zip 23413–0017; tel. 804/442–8000; Richard A. Brvenik, President and Chief Executive Officer (Total facility includes 13 beds in nursing home–type unit) **A**1 5 9 10 **F**3 7 8 12 13 14 15 16 17 18 19 20 21 22 23 25 26 27 28 30 31 32 33 34 35 36 37 39 40 41 42 44 45 46 49 51 52 53 54 55 56 57 58 59 60 61 63 64 65 66 67 68 69 70 71 72 73 74 **P**4 6 | 23 | 10 | 143 | 5080 | 92 | 48357 | 485 | 23076 | 12773 | 467 |

NEW KENT—New Kent County

□ CUMBERLAND HOSPITAL FOR CHILDREN AND ADOLESCENTS, 9407 Cumberland Road, Zip 23124; tel. 804/966–2242; Elizabeth B. Woodard, Chief Executive Officer **A**1 10 **F**12 15 16 48 53 59 65 **P**5 **S** Healthcare America, Inc., Austin, TX | 33 | 56 | 84 | 155 | 70 | 1152 | 0 | 12890 | 6232 | 212 |

NEWPORT NEWS—Independent City County

□ COLONIAL HOSPITAL, (Formerly Colonial Hospital and Recovery Center), 17579 Warwick Boulevard, Zip 23603; tel. 757/888–0400; Robert J. Lehmann, Chief Executive Officer **A**1 9 10 **F**2 3 14 18 52 53 54 55 56 **P**6 | 33 | 22 | 68 | 766 | 41 | 0 | 0 | 6327 | 3162 | 115 |

☒ MARY IMMACULATE HOSPITAL, (Includes St. Francis Nursing Center), 2 Bernardine Drive, Zip 23602; tel. 757/886–6000; Kirby H. Smith, Jr., Executive Vice President and Chief Executive Officer (Total facility includes 115 beds in nursing home–type unit) **A**1 3 5 9 10 **F**7 8 10 12 14 15 16 17 19 20 21 22 25 27 28 29 30 31 32 33 34 35 37 38 39 40 41 42 44 45 49 63 64 65 67 71 72 73 74 **P**1 7 8 **S** Bon Secours Health System, Inc., Marriottsville, MD **N** Central Virginia Health Network, Richmond, VA | 21 | 10 | 225 | 6095 | 173 | 91050 | 1510 | 43908 | 16302 | 696 |

☒ MCDONALD ARMY COMMUNITY HOSPITAL, Jefferson Avenue, Fort Eustis, Zip 23604–5548; tel. 757/878–7501; Colonel George Weightman, Commander **A**1 **F**8 12 13 15 16 17 18 20 22 27 28 29 30 39 41 44 45 46 49 51 65 71 72 73 74 **P**1 **S** Department of the Army, Office of the Surgeon General, Falls Church, VA | 42 | 10 | 30 | 986 | 5 | 236014 | 0 | — | — | 420 |

□ NEWPORT NEWS GENERAL HOSPITAL, 5100 Marshall Avenue, Zip 23605, Mailing Address: P.O. Box 5769, Zip 23605; tel. 804/247–7200; Lissa B. Hays, Chief Operating Officer (Nonreporting) **A**1 5 9 10 | 23 | 10 | 126 | — | — | — | — | — | — | — |

☒ RIVERSIDE REGIONAL MEDICAL CENTER, (Includes Riverside Psychiatric Institute), 500 J. Clyde Morris Boulevard, Zip 23601–1976; tel. 757/594–2000; Gerald R. Brink, President and Chief Executive Officer (Nonreporting) **A**1 2 3 5 6 9 10 **S** Riverside Health System, Newport News, VA **N** Virginia Health Network, Richmond, VA | 23 | 10 | 576 | — | — | — | — | — | — | — |

NORFOLK—Independent City County

☒ BON SECOURS–DEPAUL MEDICAL CENTER, (Formerly DePaul Medical Center), 150 Kingsley Lane, Zip 23505; tel. 757/889–5000; Sharon M. Tanner, President and Chief Executive Officer (Nonreporting) **A**1 2 3 5 6 9 10 **S** Bon Secours Health System, Inc., Marriottsville, MD **N** Virginia Health Network, Richmond, VA; DePaul Medical Center Group, Norfolk, VA | 21 | 10 | 202 | — | — | — | — | — | — | — |

☒ CHILDREN'S HOSPITAL OF THE KING'S DAUGHTERS, 601 Children's Lane, Zip 23507; tel. 804/668–7700; Robert I. Bonar, Jr., President and Chief Executive Officer **A**1 2 3 5 9 10 **F**10 19 21 22 31 32 34 35 38 39 41 42 43 44 46 47 49 51 65 67 69 71 72 73 **P**1 3 4 6 7 **N** Virginia Health Network, Richmond, VA | 23 | 50 | 146 | 6571 | 128 | 122989 | 0 | 94241 | 40352 | 1284 |

DEPAUL MEDICAL CENTER See Bon Secours–DePaul Medical Center

★ LAKE TAYLOR HOSPITAL, 1309 Kempsville Road, Zip 23502–2286; tel. 757/461–5001; David B. Tate, Jr., President and Chief Executive Officer (Total facility includes 228 beds in nursing home–type unit) **A**9 10 **F**14 20 31 54 57 64 65 73 **S** Riverside Health System, Newport News, VA | 16 | 48 | 304 | 392 | 258 | 0 | 0 | 13413 | 6630 | 285 |

□ NORFOLK COMMUNITY HOSPITAL, 2539 Corprew Avenue, Zip 23504–3994; tel. 757/628–1400; Phillip D. Brooks, President (Nonreporting) **A**1 5 9 10 | 23 | 10 | 103 | — | — | — | — | — | — | — |

□ NORFOLK PSYCHIATRIC CENTER, 860 Kempsville Road, Zip 23502–3980; tel. 757/461–4565; Debra Goldstein, Administrator **A**1 9 10 **F**1 2 3 4 5 6 7 8 9 10 11 12 13 17 18 19 20 21 22 23 24 25 26 27 28 29 30 31 32 33 34 35 36 37 38 39 40 41 42 43 44 45 46 47 48 49 50 51 52 53 55 56 57 58 59 60 61 62 63 64 65 66 67 68 69 70 71 72 73 74 **P**6 **S** Magellan Health Services, Atlanta, GA | 33 | 22 | 77 | 1077 | 55 | 0 | — | — | — | 108 |

★ SENTARA LEIGH HOSPITAL, 830 Kempsville Road, Zip 23502; tel. 757/466–6000; Darleen S. Anderson, R.N., MSN, Site Administrator (Nonreporting) **A**3 5 9 10 **S** Sentara Health System, Norfolk, VA **N** Sentara Health System, Norfolk, VA | 23 | 10 | 220 | — | — | — | — | — | — | — |

☒ SENTARA NORFOLK GENERAL HOSPITAL, 600 Gresham Drive, Zip 23507–1999; tel. 804/668–3000; Roger M. Eitelman, Site Administrator **A**1 2 3 5 6 8 9 10 **F**1 3 4 6 7 8 9 10 11 12 13 14 15 17 18 19 20 21 22 23 24 25 26 28 29 30 31 32 33 34 35 36 37 39 40 41 42 43 44 45 46 48 49 51 52 53 54 55 56 57 58 60 61 63 65 66 67 68 69 70 71 72 73 74 **P**2 5 **S** Sentara Health System, Norfolk, VA **N** Sentara Health System, Norfolk, VA | 23 | 10 | 598 | 22977 | 355 | 307346 | 2494 | 206362 | 77501 | 2690 |

NORTON—Independent City County

□ NORTON COMMUNITY HOSPITAL, 100 15th Street, Zip 24273–1699; tel. 540/679–9700; William Kenley, Administrator and Chief Executive Officer **A**1 9 10 **F**7 8 12 14 15 16 17 19 20 21 22 23 24 25 26 28 30 31 32 33 34 35 37 39 40 41 44 45 46 49 51 63 65 66 67 68 71 72 73 74 **P**5 6 8 **N** Highlands Wellmont Health Network, Inc., Bristol, TN | 23 | 10 | 46 | 3804 | 45 | 50961 | 415 | 21620 | 9023 | 279 |

☒ ST. MARY'S HOSPITAL, Third Street N.E., Zip 24273, Mailing Address: P.O. Box 620, Zip 24273; tel. 540/679–9100; Gary L. DelForge, Administrator (Total facility includes 44 beds in nursing home–type unit) **A**1 9 10 **F**3 7 8 12 13 15 16 19 20 21 22 25 26 28 29 30 32 34 35 37 40 41 42 44 45 46 52 54 55 56 57 58 63 64 65 67 71 73 | 23 | 10 | 133 | 2559 | 68 | 42383 | 93 | 18872 | 7927 | 343 |

Hospital, Address, Telephone, Administrator, Approval, Facility, and Physician Codes, Health Care System, Network	Classi-fication Codes		Utilization Data					Expense (thousands) of dollars		
★ American Hospital Association (AHA) membership □ Joint Commission on Accreditation of Healthcare Organizations (JCAHO) accreditation + American Osteopathic Hospital Association (AOHA) membership ○ American Osteopathic Association (AOA) accreditation △ Commission on Accreditation of Rehabilitation Facilities (CARF) accreditation Control codes 61, 63, 64, 71, 72 and 73 indicate hospitals listed by AOHA, but not registered by AHA. For definition of numerical codes, see page A4	Control	Service	Beds	Admissions	Census	Outpatient Visits	Births	Total	Payroll	Personnel

PEARISBURG—Giles County

★ CARILION GILES MEMORIAL HOSPITAL, (Formerly Giles Memorial Hospital), 1 Taylor Avenue, Zip 24134, Mailing Address: P.O. Box K, Zip 24134; tel. 540/921–6000; Morris D. Reece, Director (Total facility includes 21 beds in nursing home–type unit) **A**1 9 10 **F**3 4 5 6 7 8 10 12 13 14 15 16 17 18 19 20 21 22 23 24 25 26 27 28 29 30 31 32 33 34 35 36 37 39 41 42 43 44 45 46 49 50 51 53 54 55 56 57 58 59 60 61 62 63 64 65 66 67 68 69 70 71 72 73 74 **P**1 2 3 4 5 6 7 8 **S** Carilion Health System, Roanoke, VA **N** Carilion Health System, Roanoke, VA | 23 | 10 | 53 | 1239 | 34 | 24431 | 0 | 12200 | 5795 | 222

PENNINGTON GAP—Lee County

★ LEE COUNTY COMMUNITY HOSPITAL, West Morgan Avenue, Zip 24277, Mailing Address: P.O. Box 70, Zip 24277–0070; tel. 540/546–1440; James L. Davis, Chief Executive Officer (Nonreporting) **A**1 9 10 **N** Mountain States Healthcare Network, Johnson City, TN | 23 | 10 | 80 | — | — | — | — | — | — | —

PETERSBURG—Independent City County

□ CENTRAL STATE HOSPITAL, Mailing Address: Box 4030, Zip 23803–4030; tel. 804/524–7000; James C. Bumpas, Director (Nonreporting) **A**1 5 9 10 | 12 | 22 | 526 | — | — | — | — | — | — | —

★ POPLAR SPRINGS HOSPITAL, 350 Poplar Drive, Zip 23805–4657; tel. 804/733–6874; Anthony J. Vadella, Chief Executive Officer **A**1 9 10 **F**12 16 52 53 54 55 56 57 59 65 **P**5 **N** Preferred Care of Richmond, Richmond, VA | 33 | 22 | 100 | 1569 | 76 | 450 | 0 | 10377 | 4808 | 123

★ SOUTHSIDE REGIONAL MEDICAL CENTER, 801 South Adams Street, Zip 23803–5133; tel. 804/862–5000; David S. Dunham, President (Total facility includes 20 beds in nursing home–type unit) **A**1 6 9 10 **F**7 8 10 12 14 15 16 19 20 21 22 23 25 28 29 30 32 34 35 37 39 40 41 42 44 45 46 49 52 53 54 55 56 57 59 60 63 64 65 67 71 72 73 **P**7 8 **S** Quorum Health Group/Quorum Health Resources, Inc., Brentwood, TN **N** Virginia Health Network, Richmond, VA; Central Virginia Health Network, Richmond, VA | 16 | 10 | 287 | 11418 | 183 | 159712 | 1394 | 77182 | 36362 | 1290

PORTSMOUTH—Independent City County

★ △ BON SECOURS–MARYVIEW MEDICAL CENTER, 3636 High Street, Zip 23707–3236; tel. 804/398–2200; Richard A. Hanson, Acting Administrator (Total facility includes 120 beds in nursing home–type unit) **A**1 2 3 5 7 9 10 **F**3 8 10 11 14 15 16 17 18 19 21 22 23 25 30 32 33 34 35 37 39 40 41 42 44 49 52 53 54 55 56 58 59 60 63 64 65 66 67 71 72 73 **P**8 **S** Bon Secours Health System, Inc., Marriottsville, MD **N** Virginia Health Network, Richmond, VA | 23 | 10 | 441 | 12955 | 294 | 170406 | 744 | 83284 | 36477 | 1338

★ NAVAL MEDICAL CENTER, 620 John Paul Jones Circle, Zip 23708–2197; tel. 757/398–7424; Rear Admiral William R. Rowley, MC, USN, Commander (Nonreporting) **A**1 2 3 5 **S** Department of Navy, Washington, DC | 43 | 10 | 330 | — | — | — | — | — | — | —

★ △ PORTSMOUTH GENERAL HOSPITAL, 850 Crawford Parkway, Zip 23704–2386; tel. 804/398–4000; Nora M. Paffrath, Executive Vice President **A**1 3 5 7 9 10 **F**2 3 4 7 8 10 12 15 16 17 18 19 21 22 23 25 26 27 30 32 34 35 36 37 40 41 42 43 44 45 48 49 50 51 52 53 54 55 56 57 58 59 60 63 64 65 67 69 71 72 73 74 **S** Bon Secours Health System, Inc., Marriottsville, MD **N** Tidewater Health Care, Virginia Beach, VA; Virginia Health Network, Richmond, VA | 23 | 10 | 148 | 2755 | 78 | — | 399 | 20346 | 9121 | 516

PULASKI—Independent City County

★ COLUMBIA PULASKI COMMUNITY HOSPITAL, 2400 Lee Highway, Zip 24301, Mailing Address: P.O. Box 759, Zip 24301–0759; tel. 540/994–8100; Christopher W. Dux, Chief Executive Officer (Total facility includes 12 beds in nursing home–type unit) (Nonreporting) **A**1 9 10 **S** Columbia/HCA Healthcare Corporation, Nashville, TN | 33 | 10 | 74 | — | — | — | — | — | — | —

RADFORD—Independent City County

★ △ CARILION RADFORD COMMUNITY HOSPITAL, (Formerly Radford Community Hospital), 700 Randolph Street, Zip 24141–2430; tel. 540/731–2000; Virginia Ousley, Director (Total facility includes 27 beds in nursing home–type unit) **A**1 7 9 10 **F**7 8 10 13 16 17 19 20 22 23 24 26 27 28 29 30 31 32 34 35 36 37 39 40 41 42 44 45 49 51 53 54 55 56 57 58 59 63 64 65 67 70 71 72 73 74 **P**8 **S** Carilion Health System, Roanoke, VA **N** Carilion Health System, Roanoke, VA | 23 | 10 | 122 | 4535 | 69 | 110462 | 734 | 38032 | 15677 | 580

★ CARILION ST. ALBANS HOSPITAL, (Formerly St. Albans Psychiatric Hospital), Route 11, Lee Highway, Zip 24141, Mailing Address: Box 3608, Zip 24143; tel. 540/639–2481; Janet McKinney Crawford, Administrator **A**1 9 10 **F**3 12 16 52 53 54 57 58 59 65 73 **P**1 3 5 7 8 **S** Carilion Health System, Roanoke, VA **N** Carilion Health System, Roanoke, VA | 23 | 22 | 68 | 1895 | 34 | 8375 | 0 | 10357 | 5648 | 176

RESTON—Fairfax County

★ COLUMBIA RESTON HOSPITAL CENTER, (Formerly Reston Hospital Center), 1850 Town Center Parkway, Zip 20190; tel. 703/689–9023; Thomas D. Miller, President and Chief Executive Officer **A**1 2 5 9 10 **F**2 3 4 7 8 10 12 13 14 15 16 17 18 19 20 21 22 23 24 25 26 28 29 30 32 33 34 35 36 37 38 40 41 42 43 44 45 46 48 49 51 52 53 54 55 56 57 58 59 60 61 63 65 66 67 68 71 72 73 74 **P**4 5 6 8 **S** Columbia/HCA Healthcare Corporation, Nashville, TN | 32 | 10 | 127 | 7561 | 77 | 73204 | 1716 | 44347 | 20830 | 555

RICHLANDS—Tazewell County

★ COLUMBIA CLINCH VALLEY MEDICAL CENTER, 2949 West Front Street, Zip 24641; tel. 540/596–6000; James W. Thweatt, Chief Executive Officer (Total facility includes 22 beds in nursing home–type unit) **A**1 9 10 **F**3 7 8 10 11 12 14 15 17 19 20 21 22 23 28 29 30 31 32 34 35 37 39 40 41 42 44 45 46 48 49 58 60 63 64 65 67 71 73 **S** Columbia/HCA Healthcare Corporation, Nashville, TN **N** Mountain States Healthcare Network, Johnson City, TN | 33 | 10 | 200 | 6862 | 84 | 30822 | 585 | 35013 | 11199 | 506

Hospital, Address, Telephone, Administrator, Approval, Facility, and Physician Codes, Health Care System, Network	Classi-fication Codes		Utilization Data					Expense (thousands) of dollars		
	Control	Service	Beds	Admissions	Census	Outpatient Visits	Births	Total	Payroll	Personnel

★ American Hospital Association (AHA) membership
□ Joint Commission on Accreditation of Healthcare Organizations (JCAHO) accreditation
+ American Osteopathic Hospital Association (AOHA) membership
○ American Osteopathic Association (AOA) accreditation
△ Commission on Accreditation of Rehabilitation Facilities (CARF) accreditation
Control codes 61, 63, 64, 71, 72 and 73 indicate hospitals listed by AOHA, but not registered by AHA. For definition of numerical codes, see page A4

RICHMOND—Independent City County

Hospital	Control	Service	Beds	Admissions	Census	Outpatient Visits	Births	Total	Payroll	Personnel
BON SECOURS–RICHMOND COMMUNITY HOSPITAL, 1500 North 28th Street, Zip 23223–5396, Mailing Address: Box 27184, Zip 23261–7184; tel. 804/225–1700; Samuel F. Lillard, Executive Vice President and Administrator A1 9 10 F8 10 14 15 16 17 19 21 22 30 34 35 37 44 45 46 49 52 54 59 63 65 71 73 S Bon Secours Health System, Inc., Marriottsville, MD N Virginia Health Network, Richmond, VA; Central Virginia Health Network, Richmond, VA	23	10	88	1938	43	9502	0	11417	4387	193
BON SECOURS–STUART CIRCLE, 413 Stuart Circle, Zip 23220; tel. 804/358–7051; Timothy A. Johnson, Executive Vice President and Administrator A1 9 10 F1 2 3 4 6 7 8 10 11 12 15 16 17 19 21 22 23 25 26 27 28 30 32 33 35 37 38 39 40 41 42 43 44 46 47 49 52 56 57 58 59 60 63 64 65 66 67 71 72 73 74 P1 4 5 7 8 S Bon Secours Health System, Inc., Marriottsville, MD N Virginia Health Network, Richmond, VA; Central Virginia Health Network, Richmond, VA	21	10	158	3701	68	24786	0	31952	12194	379
CHARTER WESTBROOK BEHAVIORAL HEALTH SYSTEM, 1500 Westbrook Avenue, Zip 23227; tel. 804/266–9671; Thomas J. Wojick, Chief Executive Officer (Nonreporting) A1 9 10 S Magellan Health Services, Atlanta, GA	33	22	210	—	—	—	—	—	—	—
CHILDREN'S HOSPITAL, 2924 Brook Road, Zip 23220–1298; tel. 804/321–7474; Leslie G. Wyatt, Administrator (Nonreporting) A1 3 5 9	23	57	36	—	—	—	—	—	—	—
△ CHIPPENHAM AND JOHNSTON–WILLIS HOSPITALS, (Includes Chippenham Medical Center, Johnston–Willis Hospital, 1401 Johnston–Willis Drive, Zip 23235; tel. 804/330–2000), 7101 Jahnke Road, Zip 23225; tel. 804/320–3911; Gerard Filicko, Chief Executive Officer A1 2 3 5 7 9 10 F1 2 3 4 6 7 8 10 11 12 13 14 15 16 17 18 19 20 21 22 23 24 25 26 27 28 29 30 31 32 33 34 35 36 37 38 39 40 41 42 43 44 45 46 47 48 49 51 52 53 54 55 56 57 58 59 60 61 63 65 66 67 69 71 72 73 74 P1 3 5 6 7 8 S Columbia/HCA Healthcare Corporation, Nashville, TN N Preferred Care of Richmond, Richmond, VA	33	10	688	27655	489	192584	3544	—	—	2816
△ HEALTHSOUTH MEDICAL CENTER, 7700 East Parham Road, Zip 23294–4301; tel. 804/747–5600; Charles A. Stark, CHE, Administrator, Chief Executive Officer and Director Inpatient Operations A1 5 7 9 10 F5 8 10 11 12 14 15 16 17 19 20 21 22 23 25 26 27 28 29 30 31 33 34 35 37 39 41 42 44 45 46 48 49 51 54 55 56 57 58 63 65 66 67 71 73 74 P7 S HEALTHSOUTH Corporation, Birmingham, AL	33	10	147	3887	68	23312	0	35032	13903	492
□ HEALTHSOUTH REHABILITATION HOSPITAL OF VIRGINIA, 5700 Fitzhugh Avenue, Zip 23226; tel. 804/288–5700; Jeff Ruskan, Administrator (Nonreporting) A1 S HEALTHSOUTH Corporation, Birmingham, AL	33	46	40	—	—	—	—	—	—	—
HENRICO DOCTORS' HOSPITAL, 1602 Skipwith Road, Zip 23229; tel. 804/289–4500; Patrick W. Farrell, Chief Executive Officer A1 2 9 10 F1 2 3 4 7 8 10 11 12 14 15 16 19 21 22 23 24 26 28 29 30 32 33 34 35 37 38 39 40 41 42 43 44 46 47 48 49 52 53 54 55 56 57 58 59 60 61 63 64 65 66 67 69 71 72 73 74 P5 6 7 8 S Columbia/HCA Healthcare Corporation, Nashville, TN N Preferred Care of Richmond, Richmond, VA	33	10	340	14689	215	82321	2967	—	—	1265
HUNTER HOLMES MCGUIRE VETERANS AFFAIRS MEDICAL CENTER, 1201 Broad Rock Boulevard, Zip 23249; tel. 804/675–5000; James W. Dudley, Director (Total facility includes 80 beds in nursing home–type unit) A1 2 3 5 8 F2 3 4 5 6 8 10 11 12 16 17 18 19 20 21 22 23 26 27 28 29 30 31 32 33 34 35 37 39 41 42 43 44 45 46 48 49 51 52 54 56 57 58 60 61 63 64 65 67 69 71 72 73 S Department of Veterans Affairs, Washington, DC	45	10	616	11703	377	231135	0	153640	80829	2500
JOHNSTON–WILLIS HOSPITAL See Chippenham and Johnston–Willis Hospitals										
△ MEDICAL COLLEGE OF VIRGINIA HOSPITALS, VIRGINIA COMMONWEALTH UNIVERSITY, 401 North 12th Street, Zip 23219, Mailing Address: P.O. Box 980510, Zip 23298–0510; tel. 804/828–9000; Carl R. Fischer, Associate Vice President and Chief Executive Officer A1 2 3 5 7 8 9 10 F3 4 7 8 9 10 11 12 14 16 19 20 21 22 23 25 26 27 29 30 31 32 34 35 37 38 40 41 42 43 44 45 46 47 48 49 51 52 53 54 56 57 58 59 60 61 65 66 69 70 71 72 73 74 N Virginia Health Network, Richmond, VA	12	10	715	28755	490	292381	2351	357101	175575	4429
□ METROPOLITAN HOSPITAL, 701 West Grace Street, Zip 23220; tel. 804/775–4100; Priscilla J. Shuler, Chief Executive Officer A1 9 10 F8 16 19 22 32 34 35 37 41 44 52 56 57 65 66 71 73 P7 S Paracelsus Healthcare Corporation, Houston, TX	33	10	131	3020	74	49037	0	17952	8989	207
RETREAT HOSPITAL, 2621 Grove Avenue, Zip 23220–4308; tel. 804/254–5100; Paul L. Baldwin, Chief Operating Officer (Nonreporting) A1 2 9 10 S Columbia/HCA Healthcare Corporation, Nashville, TN N Preferred Care of Richmond, Richmond, VA	33	10	146	—	—	—	—	—	—	—
RICHMOND EYE AND EAR HOSPITAL, 1001 East Marshall Street, Zip 23219; tel. 804/775–4500; William E. Holmes, Chief Executive Officer A1 9 10 F14 15 16 28 30 44 46 65 69 P1 S Quorum Health Group/Quorum Health Resources, Inc., Brentwood, TN	23	45	32	849	4	5747	0	8291	3025	108
RICHMOND MEMORIAL HOSPITAL, 1300 Westwood Avenue, Zip 23227–4699, Mailing Address: Box 26783, Zip 23261–6783; tel. 804/254–6000; Michael–David Robinson, Executive Vice President and Administrator (Total facility includes 20 beds in nursing home–type unit) A1 2 5 6 9 10 F2 4 7 8 10 11 12 14 15 17 19 21 22 25 26 28 29 30 31 32 33 34 35 37 38 39 40 41 42 43 44 46 47 49 52 56 57 60 61 62 63 64 65 71 73 P1 6 S Bon Secours Health System, Inc., Marriottsville, MD N Virginia Health Network, Richmond, VA; Central Virginia Health Network, Richmond, VA	23	10	272	8496	170	310381	0	88377	36054	973

Hospital, Address, Telephone, Administrator, Approval, Facility, and Physician Codes, Health Care System, Network	Classi-fication Codes		Utilization Data						Expense (thousands) of dollars		
	Control	Service	Beds	Admissions	Census	Outpatient Visits	Births	Total	Payroll	Personnel

Legend:
★ American Hospital Association (AHA) membership
□ Joint Commission on Accreditation of Healthcare Organizations (JCAHO) accreditation
+ American Osteopathic Hospital Association (AOHA) membership
○ American Osteopathic Association (AOA) accreditation
△ Commission on Accreditation of Rehabilitation Facilities (CARF) accreditation
Control codes 61, 63, 64, 71, 72 and 73 indicate hospitals listed by AOHA, but not registered by AHA. For definition of numerical codes, see page A4

Hospital	Control	Service	Beds	Admissions	Census	Outpatient Visits	Births	Total	Payroll	Personnel
□ △ SHELTERING ARMS REHABILITATION HOSPITAL, 1311 Palmyra Avenue, Zip 23227–4418; tel. 804/342–4100; Richard C. Craven, President **A**1 7 9 10 **F**4 7 8 10 11 12 17 19 21 22 23 25 26 28 29 30 32 33 34 35 37 38 39 40 41 42 43 44 45 46 47 48 49 51 60 64 65 66 67 70 71 72 73 74 **P**1 **N** Virginia Health Network, Richmond, VA; Central Virginia Health Network, Richmond, VA	23	46	40	822	32	48419	0	19913	12337	303
✚ ST. MARY'S HOSPITAL, 5801 Bremo Road, Zip 23226–1900; tel. 804/285–2011; Ann E. Honeycutt, Executive Vice President and Administrator **A**1 2 3 5 9 10 **F**1 3 4 6 7 8 10 11 12 15 16 17 19 21 22 26 27 29 30 31 32 33 34 35 37 38 39 40 41 42 43 44 45 46 47 49 51 52 56 57 58 59 60 65 66 67 71 72 73 74 **P**1 4 5 7 8 **S** Bon Secours Health System, Inc., Marriottsville, MD **N** Virginia Health Network, Richmond, VA; Central Virginia Health Network, Richmond, VA	21	10	391	20592	265	124520	3060	145549	58360	1804
VALUEMARK WEST END BEHAVIORAL HEALTHCARE SYSTEM, 12800 West Creek Parkway, Zip 23238; tel. 804/784–2200; Jonathan A. Garber, Chief Executive Officer (Nonreporting) **A**9 10 **S** ValueMark Healthcare Systems, Inc., Atlanta, GA	33	22	84							
ROANOKE—Independent City County										
✚ CARILION ROANOKE COMMUNITY HOSPITAL, (Formerly Community Hospital of Roanoke Valley), 101 Elm Avenue S.E., Zip 24013, Mailing Address: P.O. Box 12946, Zip 24029; tel. 540/985–8000; Lucas A. Snipes, Director **A**1 2 3 5 9 10 **F**2 3 4 7 8 10 11 12 13 14 15 16 17 18 19 20 21 22 23 24 25 26 27 29 30 31 32 33 34 35 37 38 40 41 42 43 44 45 46 47 48 49 51 52 54 55 56 57 58 59 60 61 63 64 65 66 67 68 69 71 72 73 74 **P**1 5 **S** Carilion Health System, Roanoke, VA **N** Carilion Health System, Roanoke, VA	23	10	278	10741	139	77226	2475	114660	48905	1499
✚ △ CARILION ROANOKE MEMORIAL HOSPITAL, (Formerly Roanoke Memorial Hospitals), (Includes Roanoke Memorial Rehabilitation Center, South Jefferson and McClanahan Streets, Mailing Address: P.O. Box 13367, Zip 24033), Belleview at Jefferson Street, Zip 24014, Mailing Address: P.O. Box 13367, Zip 24033–3367; tel. 540/981–7000; Lucas A. Snipes, Director **A**1 2 3 5 6 7 9 10 **F**2 4 7 8 10 11 12 13 14 15 16 17 19 20 21 22 23 24 25 26 27 28 29 30 31 32 33 34 35 37 38 40 41 42 43 44 45 47 48 49 51 52 54 55 56 57 58 60 61 63 64 65 66 67 68 69 70 71 72 73 74 **P**8 **S** Carilion Health System, Roanoke, VA **N** Carilion Health System, Roanoke, VA	23	10	388	17843	297	146466	0	185053	66978	2012
ROCKY MOUNT—Franklin County										
✚ CARILION FRANKLIN MEMORIAL HOSPITAL, (Formerly Franklin Memorial Hospital), 180 Floyd Avenue, Zip 24151; tel. 540/483–5277; Matthew J. Perry, Director **A**1 9 10 **F**7 8 11 15 16 17 19 22 30 32 33 39 40 41 42 44 49 65 67 71 73 **P**2 7 8 **S** Carilion Health System, Roanoke, VA **N** Carilion Health System, Roanoke, VA	23	10	37	2586	21	25812	238	14095	5919	210
SALEM—Independent City County										
✚ △ COLUMBIA LEWIS–GALE MEDICAL CENTER, (Formerly Lewis–Gale Medical Center), (Includes Lewis–Gale Psychiatric Center, 1902 Braeburn Drive, Zip 24153–7391; tel. 703/772–2800), 1900 Electric Road, Zip 24153; tel. 540/776–4000; William B. Downey, Administrator (Nonreporting) **A**1 2 7 9 10 **S** Columbia/HCA Healthcare Corporation, Nashville, TN	33	10	521	—	—	—	—	—	—	—
LEWIS–GALE MEDICAL CENTER See Columbia Lewis–Gale Medical Center										
MOUNT REGIS CENTER, 405 Kimball Avenue, Zip 24153; tel. 703/389–4761; Gail S. Basham, Chief Operating Officer **F**2 3 12 17 **P**6 **S** Pioneer Healthcare, Peabody, MA	23	82	25	374	18	—	0	—	—	30
✚ VETERANS AFFAIRS MEDICAL CENTER, 1970 Roanoke Boulevard, Zip 24153; tel. 540/982–2463; John M. Presley, Ph.D., Director (Total facility includes 90 beds in nursing home–type unit) **A**1 2 3 5 8 **F**1 2 3 4 8 10 12 14 15 16 17 19 20 21 22 23 25 26 27 28 29 30 31 32 34 35 37 39 41 42 43 44 45 46 49 51 52 54 55 56 57 58 59 60 63 64 65 67 69 73 74 **S** Department of Veterans Affairs, Washington, DC	45	10	410	6432	316	195531	0	100319	56917	1427
SOUTH BOSTON—Independent City County										
✚ HALIFAX REGIONAL HOSPITAL, 2204 Wilborn Avenue, Zip 24592; tel. 804/575–3100; Chris A. Lumsden, Administrator (Total facility includes 19 beds in nursing home–type unit) **A**1 9 10 **F**7 8 10 11 12 14 15 16 17 19 20 21 22 28 29 30 31 32 34 35 37 40 41 44 45 46 48 49 55 63 64 65 71 73 **P**7 8 **S** Quorum Health Group/Quorum Health Resources, Inc., Brentwood, TN	23	10	157	5607	99	59485	553	34991	13184	517
SOUTH HILL—Mecklenburg County										
✚ COMMUNITY MEMORIAL HEALTHCENTER, 125 Buena Vista Circle, Zip 23970–0090, Mailing Address: P.O. Box 90, Zip 23970–0090; tel. 804/447–3151; Steven G. Kelly, President (Total facility includes 161 beds in nursing home–type unit) **A**1 9 10 **F**2 7 8 11 12 13 14 15 16 17 18 19 21 22 23 26 27 28 30 31 32 33 34 35 36 39 40 41 42 44 45 46 49 52 54 56 57 58 59 63 64 65 66 67 71 72 73 **P**3 8 **N** Virginia Health Network, Richmond, VA; Central Virginia Health Network, Richmond, VA	23	10	284	5234	239	79771	205	34176	15667	723
STAUNTON—Independent City County										
★ DE JARNETTE CENTER, 1355 Richmond Road, Zip 24401–1091, Mailing Address: Box 2309, Zip 24402–2309; tel. 540/332–2100; Andrea C. Newsome, FACHE, Director (Nonreporting) **A**3 9 **S** Virginia Department of Mental Health, Richmond, VA	12	59	60	—	—	—	—	—	—	—
✚ WESTERN STATE HOSPITAL, 1301 Richmond Avenue, Zip 24401, Mailing Address: Box 2500, Zip 24402–2500; tel. 540/332–8000; Lynwood F. Harding, Director **A**1 9 10 **F**2 4 5 8 9 10 11 12 19 20 21 22 23 26 27 30 31 35 37 39 40 41 42 43 44 46 48 49 50 52 57 60 63 65 67 69 71 73 **S** Virginia Department of Mental Health, Richmond, VA	12	22	488	1067	464	0	0	39434	25009	871

Hospital, Address, Telephone, Administrator, Approval, Facility, and Physician Codes, Health Care System, Network	Classi-fication Codes		Utilization Data					Expense (thousands) of dollars		
★ American Hospital Association (AHA) membership □ Joint Commission on Accreditation of Healthcare Organizations (JCAHO) accreditation + American Osteopathic Hospital Association (AOHA) membership ○ American Osteopathic Association (AOA) accreditation △ Commission on Accreditation of Rehabilitation Facilities (CARF) accreditation Control codes 61, 63, 64, 71, 72 and 73 indicate hospitals listed by AOHA, but not registered by AHA. For definition of numerical codes, see page A4	Control	Service	Beds	Admissions	Census	Outpatient Visits	Births	Total	Payroll	Personnel

STUART—Patrick County
★ R. J. REYNOLDS–PATRICK COUNTY MEMORIAL HOSPITAL, Mailing Address: Route 2, Box 71, Zip 24171–9512; tel. 540/694–3151; Alan W. Adkins, Administrator (Total facility includes 25 beds in nursing home–type unit) **A**1 9 10 **F**7 8 14 15 16 17 19 22 28 30 32 33 36 37 39 40 41 44 46 49 64 65 71 73 — 23 | 10 | 59 | 1286 | 33 | 38758 | 142 | 9195 | 4830 | 211

SUFFOLK—Independent City County
★ LOUISE OBICI MEMORIAL HOSPITAL, 1900 North Main Street, Zip 23434, Mailing Address: P.O. Box 1100, Zip 23439; tel. 757/934–4000; William C. Giermak, President and Chief Executive Officer **A**1 2 5 6 9 10 **F**7 8 10 15 16 17 19 22 27 28 30 31 32 34 35 36 37 39 40 41 42 44 45 46 49 52 54 55 59 60 65 67 71 73 74 **P**6 8 **N** Virginia Health Network, Richmond, VA — 23 | 10 | 164 | 6987 | 106 | 83041 | 807 | 49812 | 22662 | 772

TAPPAHANNOCK—Essex County
□ RIVERSIDE TAPPAHANNOCK HOSPITAL, Mailing Address: Route 2, Box 612, Zip 22560; tel. 804/443–3311; Elizabeth J. Martin, Vice President and Administrator (Total facility includes 25 beds in nursing home–type unit) (Nonreporting) **A**1 9 10 **S** Riverside Health System, Newport News, VA **N** Virginia Health Network, Richmond, VA — 23 | 10 | 100 | — | | | | | |

TAZEWELL—Tazewell County
★ TAZEWELL COMMUNITY HOSPITAL, 141 Ben Bolt Avenue, Zip 24651; tel. 540/988–2506; Craig B. James, Administrator **A**1 9 10 **F**8 15 19 22 30 32 34 35 44 46 71 73 **P**1 **S** Carilion Health System, Roanoke, VA — 23 | 10 | 42 | 1258 | 14 | 21595 | 0 | 7793 | 3155 | 136

VIRGINIA BEACH—Independent City County
★ SENTARA BAYSIDE HOSPITAL, 800 Independence Boulevard, Zip 23455–6076; tel. 757/363–6100; Virginia Bogue, Site Administrator **A**1 5 9 10 **F**1 4 6 7 8 9 10 11 12 13 14 15 16 17 18 19 20 22 23 25 26 27 29 30 31 32 33 34 35 37 38 39 40 41 42 43 44 45 46 47 48 49 51 52 56 59 60 61 63 64 65 66 67 69 70 71 72 73 74 **P**4 5 6 **S** Sentara Health System, Norfolk, VA **N** Sentara Health System, Norfolk, VA — 23 | 10 | 141 | 6294 | 69 | 55394 | 1334 | 42302 | 14371 | 524

★ VIRGINIA BEACH GENERAL HOSPITAL, 1060 First Colonial Road, Zip 23454–9000; tel. 804/481–8000; Robert L. Graves, Administrator **A**1 2 3 5 9 10 **F**4 7 8 10 11 12 14 15 16 17 18 19 21 22 23 24 25 28 29 30 31 32 33 34 35 37 38 39 40 41 42 43 44 45 49 56 60 61 63 64 65 66 67 69 70 71 72 73 **P**6 7 8 **N** Tidewater Health Care, Virginia Beach, VA; Virginia Health Network, Richmond, VA — 23 | 10 | 274 | 12339 | 167 | 138880 | 1900 | 88147 | 37141 | 1068

WARRENTON—Fauquier County
★ FAUQUIER HOSPITAL, 500 Hospital Drive, Zip 22186–3099; tel. 540/347–2550; Rodger H. Baker, President and Chief Executive Officer **A**1 9 10 **F**6 7 8 12 14 15 16 17 19 21 22 28 29 30 32 33 34 35 39 41 42 44 45 46 49 63 64 65 67 71 73 **P**6 — 23 | 10 | 83 | 3959 | 44 | 64687 | 406 | 32627 | 15661 | 526

WILLIAMSBURG—Independent City County
★ EASTERN STATE HOSPITAL, Mailing Address: P.O. Box 8791, Zip 23187–8791; tel. 804/253–5161; John M. Favret, Director (Total facility includes 310 beds in nursing home–type unit) (Nonreporting) **A**1 5 9 10 **S** Virginia Department of Mental Health, Richmond, VA — 12 | 22 | 727 | — | | | | | |

★ WILLIAMSBURG COMMUNITY HOSPITAL, 301 Monticello Avenue, Zip 23187–8700, Mailing Address: Box 8700, Zip 23187–8700; tel. 757/259–6000; Les A. Donahue, President and Chief Executive Officer (Nonreporting) **A**1 5 9 10 **S** Sentara Health System, Norfolk, VA **N** Virginia Health Network, Richmond, VA; Sentara Health System, Norfolk, VA — 23 | 10 | 100 | — | | | | | |

WINCHESTER—Independent City County
★ WINCHESTER MEDICAL CENTER, 1840 Amherst Street, Zip 22601–2540, Mailing Address: P.O. Box 3340, Zip 22604–3340; tel. 540/722–8000; George B. Caley, President **A**1 2 9 10 **F**4 7 8 10 11 12 14 15 16 19 21 22 23 28 29 30 32 33 35 36 37 38 39 40 41 42 43 44 46 48 49 52 53 56 58 59 60 63 65 67 69 71 72 73 **P**5 7 8 **N** Valley Health System, Winchester, VA — 23 | 10 | 401 | 18085 | 236 | 189646 | 1671 | 126279 | 56955 | 1647

WISE—Wise County
□ WISE ARH HOSPITAL, Mailing Address: P.O. Box 3267, Zip 24293–3267; tel. 540/328–2511; Louis G. Roe, Jr., Administrator **A**1 9 10 **F**8 11 12 14 15 17 19 21 22 28 29 30 32 37 39 40 41 44 45 46 49 51 65 71 73 **P**4 6 8 **S** Appalachian Regional Healthcare, Lexington, KY **N** CHA Provider Network, Inc., Lexington, KY — 23 | 10 | 41 | 2141 | 24 | 58409 | 41 | 11601 | 5470 | 205

WOODBRIDGE—Prince William County
★ POTOMAC HOSPITAL, 2300 Opitz Boulevard, Zip 22191–3399; tel. 703/670–1313; William Mason Moss, President **A**1 2 9 10 **F**6 7 8 10 11 12 14 15 16 17 19 21 22 28 29 30 31 32 33 34 35 37 38 39 40 41 42 44 46 49 51 52 54 55 56 57 58 59 60 62 63 65 66 67 71 72 73 74 **P**1 — 23 | 10 | 153 | 7227 | 76 | 110641 | 1870 | 57093 | 25352 | 647

WOODSTOCK—Shenandoah County
★ SHENANDOAH MEMORIAL HOSPITAL, 759 South Main Street, Zip 22664, Mailing Address: P.O. Box 508, Zip 22664; tel. 540/459–4021; Floyd Heater, Chief Executive Officer (Total facility includes 34 beds in nursing home–type unit) **A**1 9 10 **F**3 4 7 8 10 12 14 17 19 21 22 23 27 28 30 32 34 35 37 39 40 41 44 45 46 49 50 52 53 54 55 56 57 58 59 60 63 64 65 66 68 69 70 71 73 — 23 | 10 | 129 | 2493 | 61 | 29226 | 227 | 18670 | 8504 | 345

WYTHEVILLE—Wythe County
★ WYTHE COUNTY COMMUNITY HOSPITAL, 600 West Ridge Road, Zip 24382; tel. 540/228–0200; Larry H. Chewning, III, Chief Executive Officer (Total facility includes 8 beds in nursing home–type unit) **A**1 9 10 **F**3 7 8 11 12 14 15 16 17 19 20 21 22 23 26 27 28 29 30 31 32 33 34 35 37 39 40 41 42 44 45 46 48 49 53 54 55 56 57 58 59 61 63 64 65 66 67 71 73 **P**1 6 7 **S** Carilion Health System, Roanoke, VA — 23 | 10 | 75 | 2888 | 36 | 40217 | 254 | 19762 | 8807 | 309

WASHINGTON

Resident population 5,431 (in thousands)
Resident population in metro areas 82.9%
Birth rate per 1,000 population 15.0
65 years and over 11.6%
Percent of persons without health insurance 12.7%

Hospital, Address, Telephone, Administrator, Approval, Facility, and Physician Codes, Health Care System, Network	Classi-fication Codes		Utilization Data					Expense (thousands) of dollars		
★ American Hospital Association (AHA) membership ☐ Joint Commission on Accreditation of Healthcare Organizations (JCAHO) accreditation + American Osteopathic Hospital Association (AOHA) membership ◯ American Osteopathic Association (AOA) accreditation △ Commission on Accreditation of Rehabilitation Facilities (CARF) accreditation Control codes 61, 63, 64, 71, 72 and 73 indicate hospitals listed by AOHA, but not registered by AHA. For definition of numerical codes, see page A4	Control	Service	Beds	Admissions	Census	Outpatient Visits	Births	Total	Payroll	Personnel
ABERDEEN—Grays Harbor County										
✠ GRAYS HARBOR COMMUNITY HOSPITAL, 915 Anderson Drive, Zip 98520; tel. 360/532–8330; Michael J. Madden, Administrator (Total facility includes 60 beds in nursing home–type unit) **A**1 9 10 **F**2 3 7 12 16 19 21 22 25 32 35 37 40 42 44 45 49 54 56 64 65 70 71 73 **P**3 8	23	10	172	4254	102	45801	561	38230	17988	467
ANACORTES—Skagit County										
✠ ISLAND HOSPITAL, 1211 24th Street, Zip 98221–2590; tel. 360/299–1300; C. Philip Sandifer, Administrator **A**1 2 9 10 **F**7 8 12 14 15 16 17 19 21 22 24 28 30 31 32 34 35 37 39 40 42 44 46 49 51 65 67 68 70 71 73 74 **P**7 8	16	10	43	1970	19	—	202	22386	10876	284
ARLINGTON—Snohomish County										
✠ CASCADE VALLEY HOSPITAL, NORTH SNOHOMISH COUNTY HEALTH SYSTEM, 330 South Stillaguamish Avenue, Zip 98223–1642; tel. 360/435–2133; Robert D. Campbell, Jr., Administrator **A**1 9 10 **F**7 8 12 15 19 22 34 35 37 40 42 44 71 **P**5 6 7 8	16	10	48	1908	19	28709	371	18555	8467	292
AUBURN—King County										
☐ AUBURN GENERAL HOSPITAL, 202 North Division, Plaza One, Zip 98001; tel. 206/833–7711; Michael M. Gherardini, Managing Director (Nonreporting) **A**1 2 9 10 **S** Universal Health Services, Inc., King of Prussia, PA	33	10	100	—	—	—	—	—	—	—
BELLEVUE—King County										
✠ OVERLAKE HOSPITAL MEDICAL CENTER, 1035 116th Avenue N.E., Zip 98004; tel. 206/688–5000; Kenneth D. Graham, President and Chief Executive Officer **A**1 2 9 10 **F**4 7 10 11 12 14 15 16 17 19 21 22 26 29 30 31 34 37 39 40 41 42 43 44 45 46 48 49 52 53 54 56 57 59 63 65 67 70 71 73 **P**6	23	10	191	12693	128	81116	2776	100155	46225	907
BELLINGHAM—Whatcom County										
✠ ST. JOSEPH HOSPITAL, 2901 Squalicum Parkway, Zip 98225–1898; tel. 360/734–5400; John Hayward, Administrator **A**1 2 9 10 **F**1 2 3 4 7 10 11 17 19 21 22 28 35 37 40 41 42 43 44 48 49 52 53 54 56 59 60 65 66 70 71 73 **P**1 **S** PeaceHealth, Bellevue, WA **N** PeaceHealth, Bellevue, WA; Dominican Network, Spokane, WA	23	10	206	10548	109	—	1794	89065	40005	985
BREMERTON—Kitsap County										
✠ HARRISON MEMORIAL HOSPITAL, 2520 Cherry Street, Zip 98310–4270; tel. 360/377–3911; David W. Gitch, President and Chief Executive Officer **A**1 2 9 10 **F**4 7 10 12 14 15 16 17 19 21 22 23 25 26 27 28 30 31 32 33 34 35 37 39 40 41 42 44 45 46 49 52 53 54 55 56 57 58 60 61 65 67 70 71 72 73 74 **P**8	23	10	252	12046	129	108635	1917	80869	39548	945
✠ NAVAL HOSPITAL, Boone Road, Zip 98312–1898; tel. 360/479–6600; Captain James A. Johnson, Commanding Officer **A**1 3 5 **F**2 3 7 8 11 12 13 15 16 17 18 19 20 21 22 24 28 29 30 31 34 37 39 40 41 42 44 45 46 49 51 52 54 55 56 58 59 61 65 67 71 72 73 74 **S** Department of Navy, Washington, DC	43	10	76	4855	38	313764	771	79170	39642	883
BREWSTER—Okanogan County										
★ OKANOGAN–DOUGLAS COUNTY HOSPITAL, 703 Northwest Second, Zip 98812, Mailing Address: P.O. Box 577, Zip 98812; tel. 509/689–2517; Howard M. Gamble, Administrator **A**9 10 **F**7 8 11 16 19 25 28 29 30 34 37 40 44 47 49 51 65 66 70 71 **P**8	16	10	43	964	9	15155	194	5821	3134	118
BURIEN—King County										
✠ △ HIGHLINE COMMUNITY HOSPITAL, (Includes Highline Specialty Center, 12844 Military Road Fork, Tukwila, Zip 98168; Mark Benedum, Administrator), 16251 Sylvester Road S.W., Zip 98166; tel. 206/244–9970; Paul Tucker, Administrator (Nonreporting) **A**1 2 7 9 10	23	10	249	—	—	—	—	—	—	—
CENTRALIA—Lewis County										
✠ PROVIDENCE CENTRALIA HOSPITAL, 914 South Scheuber Road, Zip 98531; tel. 360/736–2803; Maureen Comer, Operations Administrator (Total facility includes 41 beds in nursing home–type unit) **A**1 2 9 10 **F**3 6 7 8 12 15 16 17 19 20 21 22 26 28 29 30 32 33 34 35 37 39 40 41 44 45 46 48 49 51 62 64 65 66 67 71 73 74 **P**3 6 8 **S** Sisters of Providence Health System, Seattle, WA	21	10	127	4521	81	112723	557	38092	20405	544
CHELAN—Chelan County										
LAKE CHELAN COMMUNITY HOSPITAL, 503 East Highland Avenue, Zip 98816, Mailing Address: Box 908, Zip 98816; tel. 509/682–2531; Moe Chaudry, Chief Executive Officer **A**9 10 **F**2 3 7 8 14 15 16 17 19 28 30 32 33 36 39 44 46 49 52 65 70 71 73 **P**3	16	10	30	670	11	4523	120	6675	3475	103
CHEWELAH—Stevens County										
★ ST. JOSEPH'S HOSPITAL, 500 East Webster Street, Zip 99109, Mailing Address: P.O. Box 197, Zip 99109; tel. 509/935–8211; Gary V. Peck, Chief Executive Officer (Total facility includes 40 beds in nursing home–type unit) **A**9 10 **F**7 8 14 15 16 17 21 22 28 29 30 34 40 41 44 46 49 51 56 64 65 66 67 71 73 **P**5 8 **S** Providence Services, Spokane, WA **N** Providence Services, Spokane, WA	21	10	65	925	47	13476	71	6798	3167	131
CLARKSTON—Asotin County										
☐ TRI–STATE MEMORIAL HOSPITAL, 1221 Highland Avenue, Zip 99403–0189, Mailing Address: P.O. Box 189, Zip 99403–0189; tel. 509/758–5511; Joseph K. Lillard, Administrator **A**1 9 10 **F**6 8 14 15 16 17 19 22 28 30 32 33 34 37 44 46 62 65 67 69 71 73 **P**5 8	23	10	41	1183	15	26573	0	12886	4874	165

Hospital, Address, Telephone, Administrator, Approval, Facility, and Physician Codes, Health Care System, Network	Classi-fication Codes		Utilization Data					Expense (thousands) of dollars		
★ American Hospital Association (AHA) membership □ Joint Commission on Accreditation of Healthcare Organizations (JCAHO) accreditation + American Osteopathic Hospital Association (AOHA) membership ○ American Osteopathic Association (AOA) accreditation △ Commission on Accreditation of Rehabilitation Facilities (CARF) accreditation Control codes 61, 63, 64, 71, 72 and 73 indicate hospitals listed by AOHA, but not registered by AHA. For definition of numerical codes, see page A4	Control	Service	Beds	Admissions	Census	Outpatient Visits	Births	Total	Payroll	Personnel

COLFAX—Whitman County

★ WHITMAN HOSPITAL AND MEDICAL CENTER, 1200 Almota Road, Zip 99111–5252; tel. 509/397–3435; Gordon C. McLean, Administrator **A**9 10 **F**7 8 12 15 19 22 31 32 33 34 36 40 41 42 44 49 64 65 66 71 **P**3

| 13 | 10 | 32 | 757 | 6 | 10335 | 67 | 4916 | 2153 | 84 |

COLVILLE—Stevens County

✠ MOUNT CARMEL HOSPITAL, 982 East Columbia Street, Zip 99114–0351, Mailing Address: Box 351, Zip 99114–0351; tel. 509/684–2561; Gloria Cooper, Chief Executive Officer **A**1 3 9 10 **F**7 8 12 14 15 16 19 22 34 37 40 41 44 45 46 49 56 65 67 70 71 **P**8 **S** Providence Services, Spokane, WA **N** Dominican Network, Spokane, WA; Providence Services, Spokane, WA

| 21 | 10 | 32 | 1507 | 13 | 26533 | 239 | 10275 | 4783 | 117 |

COUPEVILLE—Island County

✠ WHIDBEY GENERAL HOSPITAL, 101 North Main Street, Zip 98239–0400, Mailing Address: Box 400, Zip 98239–0400; tel. 360/678–5151; Robert Zylstra, Administrator (Nonreporting) **A**1 2 9 10

| 16 | 10 | 51 | — | — | — | — | — | — | — |

DAVENPORT—Lincoln County

★ LINCOLN HOSPITAL, 10 Nichols Street, Zip 99122; tel. 509/725–7101; Thomas J. Martin, Chief Executive Officer (Total facility includes 71 beds in nursing home–type unit) (Nonreporting) **A**9 10 **N** Lincoln County Public Health Coalition, Davenport, WA; Columbian Basin Health Network, Mead, WA

| 16 | 10 | 95 | — | — | — | — | — | — | — |

DAYTON—Columbia County

DAYTON GENERAL HOSPITAL, 1012 South Third Street, Zip 99328; tel. 509/382–2531; Oral R. Compson, Administrator (Nonreporting) **A**9 10

| 16 | 10 | 18 | — | — | — | — | — | — | — |

DEER PARK—Spokane County

★ DEER PARK HEALTH CENTER AND HOSPITAL, East 1015 D Street, Zip 99006; Mailing Address: P.O. Box 742, Zip 99006; tel. 509/276–5061; Cathy Simchuk, Chief Operating Officer (Nonreporting) **A**9 10 **S** Providence Services, Spokane, WA **N** Dominican Network, Spokane, WA

| 33 | 10 | 26 | — | — | — | — | — | — | — |

EDMONDS—Snohomish County

✠ STEVENS HEALTHCARE, (Formerly Stevens Hospital), 21601 76th Avenue West, Zip 98026–7506; tel. 206/640–4000; Steve C. McCary, President and Chief Executive Officer **A**1 2 9 10 **F**4 7 8 10 12 13 16 17 18 19 20 21 22 23 25 26 28 29 30 31 32 33 34 35 39 40 41 42 44 45 46 49 51 52 53 54 55 56 57 58 60 65 66 67 68 71 72 73 74 **P**1 6 7 **N** Health Washington, Seattle, WA

| 16 | 10 | 134 | 7736 | 84 | 223374 | 1380 | 80006 | 38178 | 1001 |

ELLENSBURG—Kittitas County

KITTITAS VALLEY COMMUNITY HOSPITAL, 603 South Chestnut Street, Zip 98926; tel. 509/962–7302; Eric Jensen, Administrator **A**3 9 10 **F**7 8 11 15 16 17 19 22 26 32 33 35 36 37 39 40 41 44 49 65 67 70 71 73

| 16 | 10 | 35 | 1622 | 15 | 37460 | 285 | 12986 | 6412 | 171 |

ENUMCLAW—King County

COMMUNITY MEMORIAL HOSPITAL, 1450 Battersby Avenue, Zip 98022, Mailing Address: P.O. Box 218, Zip 98022–0218; tel. 360/825–2505; Dennis A. Popp, Administrator and Chief Executive Officer **A**9 10 **F**7 19 21 22 24 27 28 33 35 37 40 44 45 63 71 73 74 **P**8

| 23 | 10 | 29 | 1174 | 10 | 20669 | 275 | 11671 | 5362 | 198 |

EPHRATA—Grant County

★ COLUMBIA BASIN HOSPITAL, 200 Southeast Boulevard, Zip 98823–1997; tel. 509/754–4631; Al Beach, Administrator (Total facility includes 29 beds in nursing home–type unit) (Nonreporting) **A**9 10 **N** Columbian Basin Health Network, Mead, WA

| 16 | 10 | 58 | — | — | — | — | — | — | — |

EVERETT—Snohomish County

✠ △ PROVIDENCE GENERAL MEDICAL CENTER, (Includes Providence General Medical Center – Colby Campus, 14th and Colby Avenue, Mailing Address: P.O. Box 1147, Zip 98206; tel. 206/261–2000; Providence General Medical Center – Pacific Campus, tel. 206/258–7123), Pacific and Nassau Streets, Zip 98201, Mailing Address: P.O. Box 1067, Zip 98206–1067; tel. 206/261–2000; Raymond F. Crerand, Interim Chief Executive Northwest Washington Service Area (Total facility includes 12 beds in nursing home–type unit) **A**1 2 7 9 10 **F**2 3 4 7 8 10 12 14 15 16 19 21 22 24 25 26 28 29 30 31 32 33 34 35 39 41 42 43 44 45 46 48 49 50 51 53 56 60 63 64 65 66 67 68 70 71 73 74 **P**6 8 **S** Sisters of Providence Health System, Seattle, WA

| 23 | 10 | 290 | 16321 | 177 | 415231 | 3259 | 149515 | 62879 | 1534 |

FAIRCHILD AFB—Spokane County

★ U. S. AIR FORCE HOSPITAL, 701 Hospital Loop, Zip 99011–8701; tel. 509/247–5217; Colonel Craig G. Hinman, Commander (Nonreporting) **S** Department of the Air Force, Washington, DC

| 41 | 10 | 35 | — | — | — | — | — | — | — |

FEDERAL WAY—King County

✠ ST. FRANCIS HOSPITAL, 34515 Ninth Avenue South, Zip 98003–9710; tel. 206/927–9700; Craig L. Hendrickson, President and Chief Executive Officer **A**1 2 9 10 **F**4 7 8 9 10 12 13 15 16 17 18 19 21 22 23 25 28 29 30 32 33 34 35 37 38 39 40 41 42 43 44 48 49 52 53 55 56 57 63 64 65 67 68 70 71 72 73 74 **P**1 3 5 7 **S** Catholic Health Initiatives, Denver, CO

| 21 | 10 | 67 | 5573 | 43 | 55123 | 1575 | 43270 | 17480 | 397 |

FORKS—Clallam County

FORKS COMMUNITY HOSPITAL, 530 Bogachiel Way, Zip 98331–9699; tel. 360/374–6271; Janet A. Hays, Interim Administrator (Total facility includes 36 beds in nursing home–type unit) **A**9 10 **F**1 3 7 8 13 14 15 16 17 18 21 22 26 28 29 30 31 34 39 44 45 49 51 58 64 65 70 71 73 74

| 16 | 10 | 53 | 384 | 36 | 19728 | 4 | 7841 | 4012 | 156 |

FORT STEILACOOM—Pierce County

□ WESTERN STATE HOSPITAL, Zip 98494; tel. 206/582–8900; Jerry L. Dennis, M.D., Chief Executive Officer **A**1 9 10 **F**16 20 26 27 28 30 39 41 45 52 54 55 56 57 65 71 73 **P**6

| 12 | 22 | 835 | 1704 | 760 | 0 | 0 | 106199 | 62895 | — |

Hospital, Address, Telephone, Administrator, Approval, Facility, and Physician Codes, Health Care System, Network	Classi-fication Codes		Utilization Data					Expense (thousands) of dollars		
	Control	Service	Beds	Admissions	Census	Outpatient Visits	Births	Total	Payroll	Personnel

★ American Hospital Association (AHA) membership
☐ Joint Commission on Accreditation of Healthcare Organizations (JCAHO) accreditation
+ American Osteopathic Hospital Association (AOHA) membership
○ American Osteopathic Association (AOA) accreditation
△ Commission on Accreditation of Rehabilitation Facilities (CARF) accreditation
Control codes 61, 63, 64, 71, 72 and 73 indicate hospitals listed by AOHA, but not registered by AHA. For definition of numerical codes, see page A4

	Control	Service	Beds	Admissions	Census	Outpatient Visits	Births	Total	Payroll	Personnel
GOLDENDALE—Klickitat County										
★ KLICKITAT VALLEY HOSPITAL, 310 South Roosevelt, Zip 98620, Mailing Address: P.O. Box 5, Zip 98620; tel. 509/773–4022; Ron Ingraham, Administrator **A**3 9 10 **F**7 11 15 19 22 28 32 33 35 40 41 42 44 46 51 65 71 74 **P**3 5 8	16	10	31	440	3	16567	55	4057	2114	61
GRAND COULEE—Grant County										
★ COULEE COMMUNITY HOSPITAL, 411 Fortuyn Road, Zip 99133–0840; tel. 509/633–1753; Michael C. Wiltermood, Chief Executive Officer (Total facility includes 29 beds in nursing home–type unit) (Nonreporting) **A**9 10 **S** Brim, Inc., Portland, OR **N** Columbian Basin Health Network, Mead, WA	16	10	48	—	—	—	—	—	—	—
ILWACO—Pacific County										
★ OCEAN BEACH HOSPITAL, Mailing Address: Drawer H, Zip 98624; tel. 360/642–3181; Pamela Ott, R.N., Administrator **A**9 10 **F**11 19 22 34 35 37 44 45 46 65 73	16	10	14	593	6	5925	0	6034	—	110
KENNEWICK—Benton County										
✠ KENNEWICK GENERAL HOSPITAL, 900 South Auburn Street, Zip 99336–0128, Mailing Address: Box 6128, Zip 99336; tel. 509/586–6111; Michael J. Tuohy, Administrator **A**1 2 9 10 **F**7 8 12 15 16 19 21 22 26 30 32 35 37 39 40 41 42 44 46 63 65 66 70 71 72 73 74 **P**8	16	10	70	3784	31	79554	1096	—	—	309
KIRKLAND—King County										
☐ BHC FAIRFAX HOSPITAL, (Formerly CPC Fairfax Hospital), 10200 N.E. 132nd Street, Zip 98034; tel. 206/821–2000; Michelle Egerer, Chief Executive Officer (Nonreporting) **A**1 9 10 **S** Behavioral Healthcare Corporation, Nashville, TN CPC FAIRFAX HOSPITAL See BHC Fairfax Hospital	33	22	133	—	—	—	—	—	—	—
✠ EVERGREEN HOSPITAL MEDICAL CENTER, 12040 N.E. 128th Street, Zip 98034; tel. 206/899–1000; Andrew Fallat, FACHE, Chief Executive Officer (Total facility includes 17 beds in nursing home–type unit) **A**1 2 9 10 **F**1 4 7 8 10 11 12 13 14 15 16 17 18 19 21 22 23 24 26 27 28 29 30 31 32 33 34 35 37 39 40 41 42 44 45 46 49 51 54 56 57 58 60 63 64 65 67 68 70 71 72 73 **P**6 **N** Health Washington, Seattle, WA; PeaceHealth, Bellevue, WA	16	10	149	9468	75	135386	2750	90784	43069	1180
LAKEWOOD—Polk County										
✠ ST. CLARE HOSPITAL, 11315 Bridgeport Way S.W., Zip 98499–0998, Mailing Address: P.O. Box 99998, Zip 98499–0998; tel. 206/588–1711; Craig L. Hendrickson, Regional Hospital Leader **A**1 9 10 **F**2 3 4 6 7 8 9 10 11 12 14 15 16 17 18 19 20 21 22 23 25 26 28 29 30 31 32 33 34 35 37 38 39 41 42 43 44 45 46 47 48 49 52 53 54 55 56 57 58 59 60 61 64 65 66 67 68 69 70 71 72 73 74 **P**5 6 7 8 **S** Catholic Health Initiatives, Denver, CO	23	10	60	3558	31	45891	805	31793	13148	259
LONGVIEW—Cowlitz County										
✠ ST. JOHN MEDICAL CENTER, 1614 East Kessler Boulevard, Zip 98632, Mailing Address: P.O. Box 3002, Zip 98632–0302; tel. 360/423–1530; Mark E. McGourty, Regional Chief Executive Officer **A**1 2 9 10 **F**2 3 6 7 8 10 11 12 14 15 16 17 18 19 20 22 27 34 35 37 38 39 40 41 42 43 44 45 46 49 51 52 60 64 65 67 69 70 71 72 73 **P**6 **S** PeaceHealth, Bellevue, WA **N** PeaceHealth, Bellevue, WA	23	10	178	9758	93	85830	1309	77439	37027	1153
MCCLEARY—Grays Harbor County										
★ MARK REED HOSPITAL, 322 South Birch Street, Zip 98557; tel. 360/495–3244; Jean E. Roberts, Administrator (Nonreporting) **A**9 10 **S** Sisters of Providence Health System, Seattle, WA	16	10	7	—	—	—	—	—	—	—
MEDICAL LAKE—Spokane County										
☐ EASTERN STATE HOSPITAL, Mailing Address: P.O. Box A, Zip 99022–0045; tel. 509/299–4351; C. Jan Gregg, Chief Executive Officer **A**1 9 10 **F**14 15 16 20 27 45 46 52 54 55 56 57 65 73 **P**6	12	22	302	845	269	0	0	40117	23440	562
MONROE—Snohomish County										
✠ VALLEY GENERAL HOSPITAL, 14701 179th S.E., Zip 98272, Mailing Address: P.O. Box 646, Zip 98272–0646; tel. 360/794–7497; Eric Buckland, Chief Executive Officer (Nonreporting) **A**1 9 10	16	10	71	—	—	—	—	—	—	—
MORTON—Lewis County										
★ MORTON GENERAL HOSPITAL, 521 Adams Street, Zip 98356, Mailing Address: Drawer C, Zip 98356; tel. 360/496–5112; Mike Lee, Superintendent (Total facility includes 30 beds in nursing home–type unit) **A**9 10 **F**2 3 7 8 10 11 12 15 17 19 21 22 26 29 32 33 34 35 37 38 39 40 41 42 43 44 45 46 47 48 49 51 52 56 60 62 64 65 67 71 73 74 **P**3 7 8 **S** Sisters of Providence Health System, Seattle, WA	16	10	50	396	34	10410	53	4892	2681	95
MOSES LAKE—Grant County										
✠ SAMARITAN HEALTHCARE, (Formerly Samaritan Hospital), 801 East Wheeler Road, Zip 98837–1899; tel. 509/765–5606; Keith J. Baldwin, Administrator **A**1 9 10 **F**7 11 15 16 17 19 21 22 23 28 29 30 34 35 37 39 40 41 44 45 46 49 51 65 66 67 70 71 73 **P**4 8 **N** Columbian Basin Health Network, Mead, WA	16	10	50	2656	21	30718	921	20389	10098	298
MOUNT VERNON—Skagit County										
✠ AFFILIATED HEALTH SERVICES, (Includes Skagit Valley Hospital, 1415 Kincaid Street, Mailing Address: P.O. Box 1376, Zip 98273–1376; tel. 360/424–4111; Gregg A. Davidson, Associate Administrator and Chief Operating Officer; United General Hospital, 1971 Highway 20, Mailing Address: P.O. Box 1376, Zip 98273–1376; tel. 360/856–6021), 1415 Kincaid Street, Zip 98274, Mailing Address: P.O. Box 1376, Zip 98273–1376; tel. 360/424–4111; Patrick R. Mahoney, Administrator and Chief Executive Officer **A**1 2 9 10 **F**4 5 7 8 10 11 12 14 15 16 17 19 21 22 23 28 29 30 32 33 34 35 36 37 39 40 41 42 44 46 49 52 54 56 58 59 60 63 65 67 70 71 73 74 **P**5 8 UNITED GENERAL HOSPITAL See Affiliated Health Services	16	10	136	7579	74	104430	1230	65103	27084	880

Hospital, Address, Telephone, Administrator, Approval, Facility, and Physician Codes, Health Care System, Network	Classi-fication Codes		Utilization Data					Expense (thousands) of dollars		
★ American Hospital Association (AHA) membership □ Joint Commission on Accreditation of Healthcare Organizations (JCAHO) accreditation + American Osteopathic Hospital Association (AOHA) membership ○ American Osteopathic Association (AOA) accreditation △ Commission on Accreditation of Rehabilitation Facilities (CARF) accreditation Control codes 61, 63, 64, 71, 72 and 73 indicate hospitals listed by AOHA, but not registered by AHA. For definition of numerical codes, see page A4	Control	Service	Beds	Admissions	Census	Outpatient Visits	Births	Total	Payroll	Personnel

NEWPORT—Pend Oreille County

★ NEWPORT COMMUNITY HOSPITAL, 714 West Pine, Zip 99156; tel. 509/447–2441; John R. White, Administrator (Total facility includes 50 beds in nursing home–type unit) (Nonreporting) **A**9 10

| | 16 | 10 | 74 | — | — | — | — | — | — | — |

OAK HARBOR—Island County

⊠ NAVAL HOSPITAL, 3475 North Saratoga Street, Zip 98278–8800; tel. 360/257–9500; Captain Michael W. Benway, Commanding Officer **A**1 **F**7 8 14 15 16 22 28 34 40 41 44 46 49 51 54 58 67 71 73 **P**1 **S** Department of Navy, Washington, DC

| | 43 | 10 | 25 | 1718 | 8 | 154072 | 484 | 14000 | 2879 | 318 |

ODESSA—Lincoln County

★ ODESSA MEMORIAL HOSPITAL, 502 East Amende, Zip 99159, Mailing Address: Box 368, Zip 99159–0368; tel. 509/982–2611; Carol Schott, Administrator (Total facility includes 23 beds in nursing home–type unit) **A**9 10 **F**8 15 16 17 28 32 41 44 64 65 66 67 71 **P**6 **N** Lincoln County Public Health Coalition, Davenport, WA

| | 16 | 10 | 40 | 122 | 30 | 3153 | 0 | 1958 | 1075 | 60 |

OLYMPIA—Thurston County

⊠ COLUMBIA CAPITAL MEDICAL CENTER, 3900 Capital Mall Drive S.W., Zip 98502–8654, Mailing Address: P.O. Box 19002, Zip 98507–0013; tel. 360/754–5858; Garry L. Gause, Chief Executive Officer (Total facility includes 9 beds in nursing home–type unit) **A**1 2 9 10 **F**4 7 8 10 11 12 13 14 15 16 17 19 21 22 23 28 30 31 34 35 37 40 41 42 44 45 46 49 61 64 65 66 71 73 74 **P**5 7 **S** Columbia/HCA Healthcare Corporation, Nashville, TN

| | 33 | 10 | 104 | 3873 | 38 | 49557 | 609 | 26712 | 12162 | 350 |

⊠ △ PROVIDENCE ST. PETER HOSPITAL, 413 Lilly Road N.E., Zip 98506–5166; tel. 360/491–9480; C. Scott Bond, Administrator **A**1 2 3 5 7 9 10 **F**2 3 4 7 8 10 11 12 15 17 18 19 20 21 22 23 24 25 26 27 28 29 30 31 32 33 34 35 37 39 40 41 42 43 44 45 46 48 49 51 52 53 54 55 56 57 58 59 60 63 65 67 70 71 73 **P**6 7 8 **S** Sisters of Providence Health System, Seattle, WA

| | 21 | 10 | 327 | 14373 | 157 | 217014 | 1961 | 134802 | 63010 | 1804 |

OMAK—Okanogan County

★ MID–VALLEY HOSPITAL, 810 Valley Way Road, Zip 98841, Mailing Address: Box 793, Zip 98841; tel. 509/826–1760; Dale F. Payne, Acting Administrator (Nonreporting) **A**3 9 10 **N** Columbian Basin Health Network, Mead, WA

| | 16 | 10 | 32 | — | — | — | — | — | — | — |

OTHELLO—Adams County

★ OTHELLO COMMUNITY HOSPITAL, 315 North 14th Street, Zip 99344; tel. 509/488–2636; Jerry Lane, Administrator **A**9 10 **F**7 8 19 22 27 28 34 36 37 40 41 44 71 **P**1 **N** Columbian Basin Health Network, Mead, WA

| | 16 | 10 | 32 | 861 | 6 | 15973 | 341 | 5023 | 2654 | 74 |

PASCO—Franklin County

⊠ OUR LADY OF LOURDES HEALTH CENTER, 520 North Fourth Avenue, Zip 99301, Mailing Address: P.O. Box 2568, Zip 99302; tel. 509/547–7704; Thomas Corley, Chief Executive Officer (Total facility includes 21 beds in nursing home–type unit) **A**1 2 9 10 **F**2 3 7 8 11 14 15 16 17 19 21 22 32 33 35 37 40 41 42 44 45 47 48 49 52 53 54 55 56 58 59 64 65 66 67 70 71 73 **P**4 5 6 7 8 **S** Carondelet Health System, Saint Louis, MO

| | 21 | 10 | 132 | 3726 | 53 | 35750 | 621 | 31642 | 14247 | 418 |

POMEROY—Garfield County

GARFIELD COUNTY MEMORIAL HOSPITAL, 66th North Sixth Street, Zip 99347–0880, Mailing Address: P.O. Box 880, Zip 99347; tel. 509/843–1591; Harry Aubert, Administrator (Total facility includes 40 beds in nursing home–type unit) **A**9 10 **F**1 13 15 30 51 64 70

| | 16 | 10 | 54 | 59 | 32 | 2000 | 0 | 2013 | 1219 | 77 |

PORT ANGELES—Clallam County

□ OLYMPIC MEMORIAL HOSPITAL, 939 Caroline Street, Zip 98362–3997; tel. 360/417–7000; Tom Stegbauer, Administrator (Nonreporting) **A**1 2 9 10

| | 16 | 10 | 126 | — | — | — | — | — | — | — |

PORT TOWNSEND—Jefferson County

★ JEFFERSON GENERAL HOSPITAL, 834 Sheridan, Zip 98368; tel. 360/385–2200; Victor J. Dirksen, Administrator (Nonreporting) **A**9 10

| | 16 | 10 | 31 | — | — | — | — | — | — | — |

PROSSER—Benton County

★ PROSSER MEMORIAL HOSPITAL, 723 Memorial Street, Zip 99350–1593; tel. 509/786–2222; John E. Rohrer, Administrator (Total facility includes 36 beds in nursing home–type unit) **A**9 10 **F**7 8 16 26 28 32 34 40 44 49 64 65 70 73

| | 16 | 10 | 49 | 738 | 29 | 13041 | 414 | 7492 | 3435 | 120 |

PULLMAN—Whitman County

⊠ PULLMAN MEMORIAL HOSPITAL, N.E. 1125 Washington Avenue, Zip 99163–4742; tel. 509/332–2541; Scott K. Adams, Administrator **A**1 9 10 **F**1 2 3 4 5 6 7 8 9 10 11 12 14 15 16 17 18 19 20 21 22 24 25 26 27 28 29 30 31 32 34 35 37 38 39 40 41 42 43 44 45 46 47 48 49 50 51 53 54 55 56 57 58 59 60 61 62 63 64 65 66 67 68 69 70 71 72 73 74 **P**3 8 **S** Brim, Inc., Portland, OR

| | 16 | 10 | 36 | 1148 | 7 | 38154 | 278 | 11557 | 4973 | 154 |

PUYALLUP—Pierce County

⊠ △ GOOD SAMARITAN COMMUNITY HEALTHCARE, 407 14th Avenue S.E., Zip 98372–0192, Mailing Address: Box 1247, Zip 98371–0192; tel. 206/848–6661; David K. Hamry, President **A**1 2 7 9 10 **F**1 6 7 11 12 14 15 16 17 18 19 21 22 24 25 26 28 29 30 32 33 34 35 37 38 39 40 41 42 44 45 46 48 49 51 53 54 55 56 57 58 59 60 62 63 65 66 67 68 70 71 72 73 **P**1 6 7

| | 21 | 10 | 211 | 9078 | 119 | 377632 | 1390 | 104309 | 60781 | 1639 |

QUINCY—Grant County

QUINCY VALLEY MEDICAL CENTER, (Formerly Quincy Valley Hospital), 908 Tenth Avenue S.W., Zip 98848; tel. 509/787–3531; Jerry Hawley, Administrator (Total facility includes 22 beds in nursing home–type unit) (Nonreporting) **A**9 10 **N** Columbian Basin Health Network, Mead, WA

| | 13 | 10 | 38 | — | — | — | — | — | — | — |

Hospital, Address, Telephone, Administrator, Approval, Facility, and Physician Codes, Health Care System, Network	Classi-fication Codes		Utilization Data					Expense (thousands) of dollars		
★ American Hospital Association (AHA) membership □ Joint Commission on Accreditation of Healthcare Organizations (JCAHO) accreditation + American Osteopathic Hospital Association (AOHA) membership ○ American Osteopathic Association (AOA) accreditation △ Commission on Accreditation of Rehabilitation Facilities (CARF) accreditation Control codes 61, 63, 64, 71, 72 and 73 indicate hospitals listed by AOHA, but not registered by AHA. For definition of numerical codes, see page A4	Control	Service	Beds	Admissions	Census	Outpatient Visits	Births	Total	Payroll	Personnel

REDMOND—King County

★ THE EASTSIDE HOSPITAL, 2700 152nd Avenue N.E., Zip 98052–5560; tel. 206/883–5151; Scott Armstrong, Administrator (Nonreporting) **S** Group Health Cooperative of Puget Sound, Seattle, WA **N** Group Health Cooperative of Puget Sound, Seattle, WA
| | 23 | 10 | 125 | — | — | — | — | — | — | |

RENTON—King County

✠ VALLEY MEDICAL CENTER, 400 South 43rd Street, Zip 98055–9987; tel. 206/228–3450; Richard D. Roodman, Chief Executive Officer (Total facility includes 39 beds in nursing home–type unit) **A**1 2 3 5 9 10 **F**3 4 7 8 10 11 12 13 14 15 16 17 18 19 21 22 23 24 25 27 28 29 30 31 34 35 37 39 40 41 42 44 46 49 51 52 54 56 58 60 64 65 67 68 70 71 73 74 **P**1 6
| | 16 | 10 | 196 | 14830 | 139 | 297591 | 2839 | 120368 | 55350 | 1340 |

REPUBLIC—Ferry County

FERRY COUNTY MEMORIAL HOSPITAL, 36 Klondike Road, Zip 99166; tel. 509/775–3333; Nancy McIntyre, Administrator (Total facility includes 14 beds in nursing home–type unit) **A**9 10 **F**7 8 12 13 15 16 17 18 19 20 26 27 29 30 31 32 33 36 37 39 40 41 44 45 46 49 51 53 54 55 56 57 58 59 61 62 64 65 66 67 68 70 71 73 74
| | 16 | 10 | 25 | 375 | 15 | 5099 | 9 | 2870 | 1299 | 69 |

RICHLAND—Benton County

CARONDELET BEHAVIORAL CARE CENTER See Carondelet Behavioral Health Center

★ CARONDELET BEHAVIORAL HEALTH CENTER, (Formerly Carondelet Behavioral Care Center), 1175 Carondelet Drive, Zip 99352–1175; tel. 509/943–9104; Thomas Corley, Chief Executive Officer **A**9 10 **F**2 3 8 12 19 22 25 26 30 32 34 35 37 40 44 48 49 52 53 54 55 56 57 58 59 64 65 67 71 74 **S** Carondelet Health System, Saint Louis, MO
| | 21 | 22 | 32 | 672 | 23 | 32953 | 0 | 8719 | 4838 | 137 |

✠ KADLEC MEDICAL CENTER, 888 Swift Boulevard, Zip 99352–9974; tel. 509/946–4611; Marcel Loh, President and Chief Executive Officer **A**1 2 9 10 **F**1 7 8 10 12 14 15 19 21 22 23 32 35 37 38 39 40 41 42 44 45 46 48 49 51 60 65 70 71 73 **S** Quorum Health Group/Quorum Health Resources, Inc., Brentwood, TN
| | 23 | 10 | 125 | 6255 | 68 | 66089 | 1271 | 59626 | 24586 | 575 |

RITZVILLE—Adams County

EAST ADAMS RURAL HOSPITAL, 903 South Adams Street, Zip 99169–2298; tel. 509/659–1200; James G. Parrish, Administrator (Nonreporting) **A**9 10 **N** Columbian Basin Health Network, Mead, WA
| | 16 | 10 | 17 | — | — | — | — | — | — | |

SEATTLE—King County

✠ △ CHILDREN'S HOSPITAL AND MEDICAL CENTER, 4800 Sand Point Way N.E., Zip 98105, Mailing Address: Box 5371, Zip 98105–0371; tel. 206/526–2000; Treuman Katz, President and Chief Executive Officer **A**1 2 3 5 7 8 9 10 **F**5 10 12 13 15 16 17 19 20 21 22 28 29 31 32 34 35 38 39 42 43 44 45 47 48 49 51 52 53 54 55 56 58 59 60 61 65 66 67 68 69 70 71 72 73 **P**6 8
| | 23 | 50 | 208 | 10527 | 147 | 133338 | 0 | 135159 | 56096 | 1380 |

✠ GROUP HEALTH COOPERATIVE CENTRAL HOSPITAL, 201 16th Avenue East, Zip 98112–5298; tel. 206/326–3000; Scott Armstrong, Administrator (Nonreporting) **A**1 2 3 5 10 **S** Group Health Cooperative of Puget Sound, Seattle, WA **N** Group Health Cooperative of Puget Sound, Seattle, WA
| | 23 | 10 | 187 | — | — | — | — | — | — | |

✠ △ HARBORVIEW MEDICAL CENTER, 325 Ninth Avenue, Box 359717, Zip 98104–2499; tel. 206/223–3000; David E. Jaffe, Executive Director and Chief Executive Officer **A**1 3 5 7 8 9 10 **F**2 3 4 5 7 8 9 10 11 12 13 15 16 17 18 19 20 21 22 23 25 26 27 28 30 31 32 33 34 35 37 38 39 40 41 42 43 44 45 46 47 48 49 50 51 52 53 54 55 56 57 58 59 60 64 65 66 67 68 69 70 71 72 73 74 **P**3
| | 13 | 10 | 323 | 12484 | 262 | 339394 | 0 | 217630 | 105146 | 2772 |

✠ △ NORTHWEST HOSPITAL, 1550 North 115th Street, Zip 98133–8498; tel. 206/364–0500; James D. Hart, President (Total facility includes 42 beds in nursing home–type unit) (Nonreporting) **A**1 2 3 7 9 10
| | 23 | 10 | 212 | — | — | — | — | — | — | |

✠ △ PROVIDENCE SEATTLE MEDICAL CENTER, 500 17th Avenue, Zip 98122, Mailing Address: P.O. Box 34008, Zip 98124–1008; tel. 206/320–2000; Nancy A. Giunto, Operations Administrator (Total facility includes 51 beds in nursing home–type unit) **A**1 2 3 5 7 9 10 **F**1 4 5 6 7 8 10 11 12 13 15 16 17 18 19 20 21 22 23 24 25 26 27 28 29 30 31 32 33 34 35 37 39 41 42 43 44 45 46 48 49 51 52 54 55 56 57 58 59 60 61 62 64 65 66 67 68 71 72 73 74 **P**6 **S** Sisters of Providence Health System, Seattle, WA
| | 21 | 10 | 334 | 17438 | 208 | 100925 | 1973 | 165625 | 75627 | 2070 |

□ SCHICK SHADEL HOSPITAL, 12101 Ambaum Boulevard S.W., Zip 98146–2699, Mailing Address: Box 48149, Zip 98148–0149; tel. 206/244–8100; Mary Ellen Stewart, Administrator (Nonreporting) **A**1 9 10
| | 33 | 82 | 63 | — | — | — | — | — | — | |

✠ SWEDISH HEALTH SERVICES, (Formerly Swedish Medical Center), (Includes Swedish Medical Center–Ballard, Northwest Market and Barnes, Zip 98107–1507, Mailing Address: Box 70707, Zip 98107; tel. 206/782–2700), 747 Broadway Avenue, Zip 98122–4307; tel. 206/386–6000; Richard H. Peterson, President and Chief Executive Officer (Nonreporting) **A**1 2 3 5 9 10 **N** Health Washington, Seattle, WA
| | 23 | 10 | 558 | — | — | — | — | — | — | |

□ THC–SEATTLE HOSPITAL, 10560 Fifth Avenue N.E., Zip 98125–0977; tel. 206/364–2050; Deborah L. Abrams, Chief Executive Officer (Nonreporting) **A**1 9 10 **S** Transitional Hospitals Corporation, Las Vegas, NV
| | 33 | 10 | 30 | — | — | — | — | — | — | |

✠ △ UNIVERSITY OF WASHINGTON MEDICAL CENTER, 1959 Northeast Pacific Street, Zip 98195–6151, Mailing Address: P.O. Box 356151, Zip 98195–6151; tel. 206/548–3300; Robert H. Muilenburg, Executive Director **A**1 2 3 5 7 8 9 10 **F**4 5 7 8 10 11 14 15 16 19 20 21 22 23 25 28 29 30 31 34 35 37 38 39 40 41 42 43 44 45 46 48 49 50 51 52 54 55 56 57 58 59 60 61 63 65 66 69 71 72 73 74 **P**6
| | 12 | 10 | 266 | 15044 | 252 | 284232 | 1589 | 259035 | 109677 | 2657 |

Hospital, Address, Telephone, Administrator, Approval, Facility, and Physician Codes, Health Care System, Network	Classi-fication Codes		Utilization Data					Expense (thousands) of dollars		
★ American Hospital Association (AHA) membership □ Joint Commission on Accreditation of Healthcare Organizations (JCAHO) accreditation + American Osteopathic Hospital Association (AOHA) membership ○ American Osteopathic Association (AOA) accreditation △ Commission on Accreditation of Rehabilitation Facilities (CARF) accreditation Control codes 61, 63, 64, 71, 72 and 73 indicate hospitals listed by AOHA, but not registered by AHA. For definition of numerical codes, see page A4	Control	Service	Beds	Admissions	Census	Outpatient Visits	Births	Total	Payroll	Personnel

Hospital	Control	Service	Beds	Admissions	Census	Outpatient Visits	Births	Total	Payroll	Personnel
✠ VA PUGET SOUND HEALTH CARE SYSTEM, (Includes VA Puget Sound Health Care System–American Lake Division, Tacoma, Zip 98493; tel. 206/582–8440), 1660 South Columbia Way, Zip 98108–1597; tel. 206/762–1010; Timothy B. Williams, Director (Total facility includes 132 beds in nursing home–type unit) **A**1 3 5 8 **F**2 3 4 8 10 11 12 14 19 20 21 22 24 26 27 30 31 32 33 34 35 37 39 41 42 43 44 45 46 48 49 51 52 54 55 56 57 58 59 60 61 64 65 67 69 71 73 74 **P**6 **S** Department of Veterans Affairs, Washington, DC	45	10	557	11043	333	420223	0	256451	113501	2439
✠ △ VIRGINIA MASON MEDICAL CENTER, 1100 Ninth Avenue, Zip 98111–0900, Mailing Address: P.O. Box 900, Zip 98111–0900; tel. 206/223–6600; J. Michael Rona, Vice President and Executive Administrator (Total facility includes 14 beds in nursing home–type unit) (Nonreporting) **A**1 2 3 5 7 9 10	23	10	210	—	—	—	—	—	—	—
SHELTON—Mason County										
□ MASON GENERAL HOSPITAL, 901 Mountainview Drive, Zip 98584, Mailing Address: P.O. Box 1668, Zip 98584; tel. 360/426–1611; G. Robert Appel, Administrator (Nonreporting) **A**1 9 10	16	10	68	—	—	—	—	—	—	—
SNOQUALMIE—King County										
□ SNOQUALMIE VALLEY HOSPITAL, 9575 Ethan Wade Way S.E., Zip 98065–2021, Mailing Address: P.O. Box 2021, Zip 98065–2021; tel. 206/831–2300; Carol L. Johnson, Administrator **A**1 9 10 **F**7 8 12 14 17 19 22 28 29 30 32 33 34 39 40 41 44 49 65 66 71 73 **P**6	16	10	14	343	3	12786	81	4192	3653	98
SOUTH BEND—Pacific County										
WILLAPA HARBOR HOSPITAL, 800 Alder Street, Zip 98586–0438, Mailing Address: P.O. Box 438, Zip 98586–0438; tel. 360/875–5526; Victor Vander Does, Administrator (Nonreporting) **A**9 10	16	10	18	—	—	—	—	—	—	—
SPOKANE—Spokane County										
□ DEACONESS MEDICAL CENTER–SPOKANE, 800 West Fifth Avenue, Zip 99204, Mailing Address: P.O. Box 248, Zip 99210–0248; tel. 509/458–5800; Thomas J. Zellers, Chief Operating Officer (Nonreporting) **A**1 2 3 5 9 10 **S** Empire Health Services, Spokane, WA	23	10	326	—	—	—	—	—	—	—
✠ HOLY FAMILY HOSPITAL, North 5633 Lidgerwood Avenue, Zip 99220; tel. 509/482–0111; Ronald J. Schurra, Chief Executive Officer **A**1 2 9 10 **F**1 2 7 8 9 10 11 15 16 19 21 22 23 26 28 29 30 32 34 35 37 38 39 40 41 42 43 44 45 46 47 48 49 52 53 54 55 56 57 58 59 60 63 65 66 67 68 69 70 71 72 73 74 **P**7 8 **S** Providence Services, Spokane, WA **N** Dominican Network, Spokane, WA; Providence Services, Spokane, WA	21	10	190	8030	82	70414	1222	53869	26051	783
✠ SACRED HEART MEDICAL CENTER, West 101 Eighth Avenue, Zip 99220, Mailing Address: P.O. Box 2555, Zip 99220–2555; tel. 509/455–3040; Ryland P. Davis, President (Nonreporting) **A**1 2 3 5 9 10 **S** Providence Services, Spokane, WA **N** Providence Services, Spokane, WA	21	10	607	—	—	—	—	—	—	—
✠ SHRINERS HOSPITALS FOR CHILDREN–SPOKANE, 911 West Fifth Avenue, Zip 99204–2901, Mailing Address: P.O. Box 2472, Zip 99210–2472; tel. 509/455–7844; Charles R. Young, Administrator **A**1 3 **F**12 15 17 20 34 39 49 65 73 **S** Shriners Hospitals for Children, Tampa, FL	23	57	30	704	13	6524	0	—	—	119
△ ST. LUKES REHABILITATION INSTITUTE, 711 South Cowley Street, Zip 99202; tel. 509/838–4771; Debra D. Hanks, Administrator (Nonreporting) **A**7 9 10	23	46	72	—	—	—	—	—	—	—
□ VALLEY HOSPITAL AND MEDICAL CENTER, 12606 East Mission Avenue, Zip 99216–9969; tel. 509/924–6650; Michael T. Liepman, Chief Operating Officer (Nonreporting) **A**1 9 10 **S** Empire Health Services, Spokane, WA	23	10	117	—	—	—	—	—	—	—
✠ VETERANS AFFAIRS MEDICAL CENTER, North 4815 Assembly Street, Zip 99205–6197; tel. 509/327–0200; Joseph M. Manley, Director (Total facility includes 60 beds in nursing home–type unit) (Nonreporting) **A**1 **S** Department of Veterans Affairs, Washington, DC	45	10	192	—	—	—	—	—	—	—
SUNNYSIDE—Yakima County										
★ + ○ SUNNYSIDE COMMUNITY HOSPITAL, 10th and Tacoma Avenue, Zip 98944, Mailing Address: P.O. Box 719, Zip 98944–0719; tel. 509/837–1500; Jon D. Smiley, Chief Executive Officer **A**9 10 11 **F**7 8 11 19 20 21 22 23 28 30 32 33 39 40 44 45 46 65 67 70 71 73 **P**4 **S** Brim, Inc., Portland, OR	33	10	30	1856	17	41277	457	14998	6340	164
TACOMA—Pierce County										
□ ALLENMORE HOSPITAL, South 19th and Union Avenue, Zip 98405, Mailing Address: P.O. Box 11414, Zip 98411–0414; tel. 206/572–2323; Charles Hoffman, Administrator **A**1 9 10 **F**1 4 7 8 10 11 12 13 14 17 18 19 20 21 22 23 25 26 28 29 30 31 32 33 34 35 37 38 39 40 41 42 43 44 45 46 47 49 50 51 56 57 60 63 65 67 68 69 70 71 72 73 74 **P**5 6 **S** MultiCare Health System, Tacoma, WA **N** Multicare Health System, Tacoma, WA	23	10	72	2932	33	69394	0	32877	13755	377
✠ MADIGAN ARMY MEDICAL CENTER, Zip 98431–5000; tel. 206/968–1110; Brigadier General George J. Brown, M.D., Commanding General **A**1 2 3 5 **F**3 4 7 8 10 11 12 13 14 15 16 17 19 20 21 22 24 25 27 28 29 30 31 34 35 37 38 39 40 41 42 43 44 45 46 47 49 51 52 54 56 58 60 61 63 65 66 67 71 72 73 74 **S** Department of the Army, Office of the Surgeon General, Falls Church, VA	42	10	216	17483	171	858565	2069	145575	66297	2858
□ MARY BRIDGE CHILDREN'S HOSPITAL AND HEALTH CENTER, 317 Martin Luther King Jr. Way, Zip 98405–0299, Mailing Address: Box 5299, Zip 98405–0299; tel. 206/552–1400; William B. Connoley, President and Chief Executive Officer **A**1 3 5 9 10 **F**1 4 7 8 10 11 12 13 17 18 19 21 22 23 25 26 28 29 30 31 32 33 34 35 37 38 39 40 41 42 43 44 47 49 50 54 60 61 63 65 67 68 70 71 72 73 74 **P**5 6 **S** MultiCare Health System, Tacoma, WA **N** Health Washington, Seattle, WA; Multicare Health System, Tacoma, WA	23	50	72	2655	25	140605	0	27711	12952	313

Hospital, Address, Telephone, Administrator, Approval, Facility, and Physician Codes, Health Care System, Network	Classi-fication Codes		Utilization Data					Expense (thousands) of dollars		
★ American Hospital Association (AHA) membership ☐ Joint Commission on Accreditation of Healthcare Organizations (JCAHO) accreditation + American Osteopathic Hospital Association (AOHA) membership ○ American Osteopathic Association (AOA) accreditation △ Commission on Accreditation of Rehabilitation Facilities (CARF) accreditation Control codes 61, 63, 64, 71, 72 and 73 indicate hospitals listed by AOHA, but not registered by AHA. For definition of numerical codes, see page A4	Control	Service	Beds	Admissions	Census	Outpatient Visits	Births	Total	Payroll	Personnel
☐ PUGET SOUND HOSPITAL, 215 South 36th Street, Zip 98408, Mailing Address: P.O. Box 11412, Zip 98411–0412; tel. 206/474–0561; Bruce Brandler, Administrator (Nonreporting) **A**1 9 10 **S** TENET Healthcare Corporation, Santa Barbara, CA	33	10	146	—	—	—	—	—	—	—
ST. CLARE HOSPITAL See Lakewood										
⊞ △ ST. JOSEPH MEDICAL CENTER, 1717 South J Street, Zip 98405, Mailing Address: P.O. Box 2197, Zip 98401–2197; tel. 206/627–4101; Craig L. Hendrickson, President and Chief Executive Officer **A**1 2 7 9 10 **F**2 4 6 7 8 9 10 11 12 13 14 15 16 17 18 19 20 21 22 23 24 25 26 28 29 30 31 32 33 34 35 36 37 38 39 40 41 42 43 44 45 46 47 48 49 51 52 54 56 57 58 59 60 61 63 64 65 67 69 71 72 73 74 **P**5 7 8 **S** Catholic Health Initiatives, Denver, CO	21	10	271	13191	162	314728	2245	154727	66237	1830
⊞ TACOMA GENERAL HOSPITAL, 315 Martin Luther King Jr. Way, Zip 98405–0299, Mailing Address: P.O. Box 5299, Zip 98405–0299; tel. 206/552–1000; William B. Connoley, President and Chief Executive Officer **A**1 2 3 5 9 10 **F**1 4 7 8 10 11 12 13 14 17 18 19 21 22 24 25 26 28 29 30 31 32 33 34 35 37 38 40 41 42 43 44 45 46 47 49 50 51 60 63 65 67 68 70 71 72 73 74 **P**5 6 **S** MultiCare Health System, Tacoma, WA **N** Health Washington, Seattle, WA; Multicare Health System, Tacoma, WA	23	10	272	12158	161	—	3137	129440	49046	1131
VA PUGET SOUND HEALTH CARE SYSTEM–AMERICAN LAKE DIVISION See VA Puget Sound Health Care System, Seattle										
TONASKET—Okanogan County										
NORTH VALLEY HOSPITAL, Second and Western, Zip 98855, Mailing Address: P.O. Box 488, Zip 98855; tel. 509/486–2151; Donald W. James, Administrator (Total facility includes 70 beds in nursing home–type unit) (Nonreporting) **A**9 10	16	10	92	—	—	—	—	—	—	—
TOPPENISH—Yakima County										
⊞ PROVIDENCE TOPPENISH HOSPITAL, 504 West Fourth Avenue, Zip 98948, Mailing Address: P.O. Box 672, Zip 98948–0672; tel. 509/865–3105; Steve Burdick, Administrator **A**1 9 10 **F**8 14 15 16 19 21 22 32 33 34 37 40 41 44 46 51 65 70 71 73 **S** Sisters of Providence Health System, Seattle, WA	21	10	48	2051	17	52872	680	13356	5896	154
VANCOUVER—Clark County										
⊞ △ SOUTHWEST WASHINGTON MEDICAL CENTER, (Includes Vancouver Memorial Campus, 3400 Main Street, Zip 98663; tel. 206/696–5000), 400 N.E. Mother Joseph Place, Zip 98664, Mailing Address: P.O. Box 1600, Zip 98668; tel. 360/256–2000; Jeffrey D. Selberg, President **A**1 2 3 7 9 10 **F**2 3 4 6 7 8 10 12 14 15 16 17 18 19 21 22 23 24 25 28 29 30 31 32 33 34 35 37 40 41 42 43 44 45 46 48 49 51 52 54 55 56 57 58 59 60 65 67 70 71 72 73 **P**1	23	10	297	15664	163	161292	2856	132878	66183	1799
WALLA WALLA—Walla Walla County										
⊞ JONATHAN M. WAINWRIGHT MEMORIAL VETERANS AFFAIRS MEDICAL CENTER, (Formerly Veterans Affairs Medical Center), 77 Wainwright Drive, Zip 99362–3994; tel. 509/525–5200; George Marnell, Director (Total facility includes 30 beds in nursing home–type unit) **A**1 **F**2 3 12 16 19 20 22 27 28 30 34 44 45 46 52 58 59 64 65 67 71 73 **P**6 **S** Department of Veterans Affairs, Washington, DC	45	10	76	1374	42	45663	0	—	—	310
⊞ △ ST. MARY MEDICAL CENTER, 401 West Poplar Street, Zip 99362, Mailing Address: Box 1477, Zip 99362–0312; tel. 509/525–3320; John A. Isely, President **A**1 2 7 9 10 **F**7 8 14 19 22 28 30 31 32 35 37 38 39 40 41 42 44 48 49 52 56 58 60 70 71 73 74 **P**7 **S** Providence Services, Spokane, WA **N** Providence Services, Spokane, WA	21	10	134	3715	43	52689	483	35581	17045	530
STATE PENITENTIARY HOSPITAL, Mailing Address: Box 520, Zip 99362; tel. 509/525–3610; Barbara Croft, Health Care Manager (Nonreporting)	12	11	36	—	—	—	—	—	—	—
VETERANS AFFAIRS MEDICAL CENTER See Jonathan M. Wainwright Memorial Veterans Affairs Medical Center										
⊞ WALLA WALLA GENERAL HOSPITAL, 1025 South Second Avenue, Zip 99362, Mailing Address: Box 1398, Zip 99362; tel. 509/525–0480; Rodney T. Applegate, President (Nonreporting) **A**1 2 9 10 **S** Adventist Health, Roseville, CA	21	10	72	—	—	—	—	—	—	—
WENATCHEE—Chelan County										
⊞ CENTRAL WASHINGTON HOSPITAL, 1300 Fuller Street, Zip 98801–1948, Mailing Address: Box 1887, Zip 98807–1887; tel. 509/662–1511; Jack T. Evans, Jr., President and Chief Executive Officer (Nonreporting) **A**1 9 10	23	10	152	—	—	—	—	—	—	—
WHITE SALMON—Klickitat County										
SKYLINE HOSPITAL, 211 Skyline Drive, Zip 98672–0099, Mailing Address: Box 99, Zip 98672–0099; tel. 509/493–1101; Lynn Milnes, Administrator and Chief Executive Officer **A**9 10 **F**7 8 12 15 16 22 28 30 32 34 37 40 42 44 46 49 51 56 67 70 71 72 73 **P**1 5	16	10	22	649	5	9626	114	5155	2869	102
YAKIMA—Yakima County										
⊞ PROVIDENCE YAKIMA MEDICAL CENTER, 110 South Ninth Avenue, Zip 98902–3397; tel. 509/575–5000; Barbara A. Hood, Chief Executive Officer Central Washington Service Area (Total facility includes 12 beds in nursing home–type unit) **A**1 2 3 9 10 **F**4 7 8 10 11 15 16 17 19 22 23 28 29 30 32 33 34 35 37 40 41 42 43 44 45 46 48 49 62 64 65 67 70 71 72 73 74 **P**4 5 **S** Sisters of Providence Health System, Seattle, WA	21	10	190	5941	76	234278	460	71113	31086	860
⊞ YAKIMA VALLEY MEMORIAL HOSPITAL, 2811 Tieton Drive, Zip 98902–3799; tel. 509/575–8000; Richard W. Linneweh, Jr., President and Chief Executive Officer **A**1 2 3 9 10 **F**7 8 10 12 13 14 15 16 17 19 21 22 23 28 29 30 32 33 34 35 37 38 39 40 41 42 44 45 46 47 49 52 54 56 58 59 60 63 65 66 67 70 71 73 74	23	10	200	10450	109	166099	2460	78937	32757	913

WEST VIRGINIA

Resident population 1,828 (in thousands)
Resident population in metro areas 41.8%
Birth rate per 1,000 population 12.0
65 years and over 15.3%
Percent of persons without health insurance 16.2%

Hospital, Address, Telephone, Administrator, Approval, Facility, and Physician Codes, Health Care System, Network	Classification Codes		Utilization Data					Expense (thousands) of dollars		
	Control	Service	Beds	Admissions	Census	Outpatient Visits	Births	Total	Payroll	Personnel

★ American Hospital Association (AHA) membership
□ Joint Commission on Accreditation of Healthcare Organizations (JCAHO) accreditation
+ American Osteopathic Hospital Association (AOHA) membership
○ American Osteopathic Association (AOA) accreditation
△ Commission on Accreditation of Rehabilitation Facilities (CARF) accreditation
Control codes 61, 63, 64, 71, 72 and 73 indicate hospitals listed by AOHA, but not registered by AHA. For definition of numerical codes, see page A4

BECKLEY—Raleigh County

Hospital	Control	Service	Beds	Admissions	Census	Outpatient Visits	Births	Total	Payroll	Personnel
□ BECKLEY APPALACHIAN REGIONAL HOSPITAL, 306 Stanaford Road, Zip 25801; tel. 304/255–3000; Norman Wright, Administrator **A**1 9 10 **F**1 3 4 8 11 12 15 16 17 18 19 21 22 26 28 29 30 31 32 33 35 37 39 42 44 45 49 52 53 54 55 56 57 59 63 65 71 73 **P**6 **S** Appalachian Regional Healthcare, Lexington, KY **N** Partners in Health Network, Inc., Charleston, WV; CHA Provider Network, Inc., Lexington, KY	23	10	173	6207	112	19666	0	30547	13283	530
BECKLEY HOSPITAL, 1007 South Oakwood Avenue, Zip 25801; tel. 304/256–1200; Albert M. Tieche, Jr., Administrator **A**9 10 **F**8 12 15 16 19 21 22 31 33 35 37 39 42 44 45 46 50 51 66 71 73 **P**7	33	10	52	2499	45	—	0	18411	7459	—
✖ COLUMBIA RALEIGH GENERAL HOSPITAL, 1710 Harper Road, Zip 25801–3397; tel. 304/256–4100; Brent A. Marsteller, Chief Executive Officer **A**1 9 10 **F**7 8 10 11 12 16 17 19 20 21 22 23 28 30 31 32 34 35 37 38 39 42 44 45 49 52 54 56 65 67 71 72 73 74 **S** Columbia/HCA Healthcare Corporation, Nashville, TN	33	10	251	10320	134	69083	1759	47652	18595	674
✖ VETERANS AFFAIRS MEDICAL CENTER, 200 Veterans Avenue, Zip 25801–6499; tel. 304/255–2121; Gerard P. Husson, Director (Total facility includes 42 beds in nursing home–type unit) **A**1 12 **F**3 15 19 20 22 25 30 31 37 41 42 44 46 49 51 58 60 64 65 71 73 74 **S** Department of Veterans Affairs, Washington, DC	45	10	112	2179	78	56090	0	30204	15400	401

BERKELEY SPRINGS—Morgan County

Hospital	Control	Service	Beds	Admissions	Census	Outpatient Visits	Births	Total	Payroll	Personnel
★ MORGAN COUNTY WAR MEMORIAL HOSPITAL, 1124 Fairfax Street, Zip 25411–1718; tel. 304/258–1234; David A. Sweeney, Administrator (Total facility includes 16 beds in nursing home–type unit) **A**9 10 **F**8 15 16 20 22 27 30 32 33 34 39 44 45 46 49 64 65 71 73	13	10	44	922	30	21776	0	6653	2654	108

BLUEFIELD—Mercer County

Hospital	Control	Service	Beds	Admissions	Census	Outpatient Visits	Births	Total	Payroll	Personnel
✖ BLUEFIELD REGIONAL MEDICAL CENTER, 500 Cherry Street, Zip 24701–3390; tel. 304/327–1100; Eugene P. Pawlowski, President **A**1 9 10 **F**7 8 10 11 12 13 14 15 16 19 21 22 24 30 34 35 37 39 40 41 42 44 45 49 50 60 63 64 65 71 72 73 **P**3 7 8 **N** Southern Virginia Rural Health Network, Bluefield, WV	23	10	265	7442	118	107194	707	57919	25349	856
✖ COLUMBIA ST. LUKE'S HOSPITAL, 1333 Southview Drive, Zip 24701, Mailing Address: P.O. Box 1190, Zip 24701; tel. 304/327–2900; Barry A. Papania, Chief Executive Officer **A**1 9 10 **F**8 12 14 15 16 19 21 22 23 26 32 35 37 44 49 54 56 63 65 71 73 **P**5 7 **S** Columbia/HCA Healthcare Corporation, Nashville, TN	33	10	79	1654	23	25961	0	12872	5100	212

BUCKEYE—Mason County

Hospital	Control	Service	Beds	Admissions	Census	Outpatient Visits	Births	Total	Payroll	Personnel
★ POCAHONTAS MEMORIAL HOSPITAL, Mailing Address: Rural Route 2, Box 52 W, Zip 24924; tel. 304/799–7400; Al Lawson, JD, Chief Executive Officer **A**9 10 **F**14 15 16 21 22 26 28 29 30 32 34 41 44 45 46 49 51 65 71 72 73	13	10	27	689	17	27741	1	3835	1553	84

BUCKHANNON—Upshur County

Hospital	Control	Service	Beds	Admissions	Census	Outpatient Visits	Births	Total	Payroll	Personnel
✖ ST. JOSEPH'S HOSPITAL, Amalia Drive, Zip 26201–2222; tel. 304/473–2000; Wayne B. Griffith, FACHE, Chief Executive Officer (Total facility includes 16 beds in nursing home–type unit) **A**1 9 10 **F**2 7 8 12 14 15 16 17 19 22 28 32 33 34 35 37 40 42 44 46 49 52 56 57 58 59 64 65 67 71 73 **P**7 8 **N** North Central/West Virginia Rural Health Network, Clarksburg, WV	23	10	95	2558	43	38394	183	17380	6768	278

CHARLESTON—Kanawha County

Hospital	Control	Service	Beds	Admissions	Census	Outpatient Visits	Births	Total	Payroll	Personnel
✖ △ CHARLESTON AREA MEDICAL CENTER, (Includes General Division, 501 Morris Street, Mailing Address: Box 1393, Zip 25325; tel. 304/348–5432; Memorial Division, 3200 Maccorkle Avenue S.E., Zip 25304; tel. 304/348–5432; Women and Children's Hospital, 800 Pennsylvania Avenue, Zip 25302; tel. 304/348–5432), 501 Morris Street, Zip 25301, Mailing Address: Box 1547, Zip 25326; tel. 304/348–5432; Phillip H. Goodwin, President and Chief Executive Officer **A**1 2 3 5 7 8 9 10 12 **F**2 3 4 5 7 8 10 11 12 13 14 15 16 17 19 21 22 23 24 25 26 27 28 29 30 31 32 33 34 35 37 38 39 40 41 42 43 44 45 46 47 48 49 51 52 54 55 56 57 58 59 60 61 63 65 66 67 68 69 70 71 72 73 74 **P**3 4 7 8 **S** Camcare, Inc., Charleston, WV **N** Partners in Health Network, Inc., Charleston, WV	23	10	779	34363	553	305846	3796	389123	141401	5421
✖ EYE AND EAR CLINIC OF CHARLESTON, 1306 Kanawha Boulevard East, Zip 25301, Mailing Address: Box 2271, Zip 25328–2271; tel. 304/343–4371; W. Allen Shelton, II, Administrator **A**1 9 10 **F**34 44 65	33	45	26	68	1	6312	0	5917	2182	77
GENERAL DIVISION See Charleston Area Medical Center										
✖ HIGHLAND HOSPITAL, 300 56th Street S.E., Zip 25304, Mailing Address: P.O. Box 4107, Zip 25364–4107; tel. 304/926–1600; David M. McWatters, Administrator **A**1 5 9 10 **F**1 3 12 14 15 16 18 27 30 32 34 39 52 53 54 55 56 57 58 59 65 67	23	22	50	867	32	98	0	6796	3587	144
MEMORIAL DIVISION See Charleston Area Medical Center										
✖ SAINT FRANCIS HOSPITAL, 333 Laidley Street, Zip 25301, Mailing Address: Box 471, Zip 25322; tel. 304/347–6500; David R. Sirk, President and Chief Executive Officer (Total facility includes 30 beds in nursing home–type unit) **A**1 9 10 **F**8 10 12 14 15 19 21 22 25 30 32 34 35 36 37 41 42 44 46 49 51 64 65 71 73 **P**7 **S** Columbia/HCA Healthcare Corporation, Nashville, TN	33	10	155	5180	86	39884	0	49511	15092	510
WOMEN AND CHILDREN'S HOSPITAL See Charleston Area Medical Center										

Hospital, Address, Telephone, Administrator, Approval, Facility, and Physician Codes, Health Care System, Network	Classi-fication Codes		Utilization Data					Expense (thousands) of dollars		
★ American Hospital Association (AHA) membership □ Joint Commission on Accreditation of Healthcare Organizations (JCAHO) accreditation + American Osteopathic Hospital Association (AOHA) membership ○ American Osteopathic Association (AOA) accreditation △ Commission on Accreditation of Rehabilitation Facilities (CARF) accreditation Control codes 61, 63, 64, 71, 72 and 73 indicate hospitals listed by AOHA, but not registered by AHA. For definition of numerical codes, see page A4	Control	Service	Beds	Admissions	Census	Outpatient Visits	Births	Total	Payroll	Personnel

CLARKSBURG—Harrison County

☒ LOUIS A. JOHNSON VETERANS AFFAIRS MEDICAL CENTER, Zip 26301–4199; tel. 304/623–3461; Michael W. Neusch, FACHE, Director (Nonreporting) **A**1 2 3 5 **S** Department of Veterans Affairs, Washington, DC — 45 | 10 | 160 | — | — | — | — | — | — | —

☒ UNITED HOSPITAL CENTER, Route 19 South, Zip 26301, Mailing Address: P.O. Box 1680, Zip 26302–1680; tel. 304/624–2121; Bruce C. Carter, President (Total facility includes 32 beds in nursing home–type unit) **A**1 2 3 5 9 10 12 13 **F**3 7 8 10 11 12 14 15 16 17 19 20 21 22 23 25 29 30 32 33 34 35 37 40 41 42 44 46 49 51 52 53 54 55 56 57 58 60 63 64 65 67 71 72 73 **P**8 **S** West Virginia United Health System, Morgantown, WV **N** Webster Memorial/United Hospital Center EACH/RPCH Network, Webster Springs, WV; North Central/West Virginia Rural Health Network, Clarksburg, WV; Integrated Provider Network, Morgantown, WV | 23 | 10 | 309 | 11475 | 183 | 265112 | 867 | 86255 | 37833 | 1218

ELKINS—Randolph County

☒ DAVIS MEMORIAL HOSPITAL, Gorman Avenue and Reed Street, Zip 26241, Mailing Address: Box 1484, Zip 26241; tel. 304/636–3300; Robert L. Hammer, II, Chief Executive Officer **A**1 9 10 **F**2 3 4 6 7 8 9 10 11 16 19 21 22 23 27 28 29 30 31 32 33 34 35 36 37 38 39 40 41 42 43 44 46 47 48 49 50 52 53 54 55 56 57 58 59 60 63 64 65 69 70 71 73 **P**7 8 | 23 | 10 | 115 | 5793 | 67 | 138825 | 553 | 39677 | 15623 | 587

FAIRMONT—Marion County

☒ FAIRMONT GENERAL HOSPITAL, 1325 Locust Avenue, Zip 26554–1435; tel. 304/367–7100; Richard W. Graham, FACHE, President (Total facility includes 61 beds in nursing home–type unit) **A**1 9 10 **F**2 3 7 8 10 11 12 14 15 16 17 19 21 22 23 28 29 30 32 35 36 39 40 41 42 44 46 49 52 53 54 55 56 57 58 59 63 64 65 66 67 71 73 74 **P**3 7 8 **S** Quorum Health Group/Quorum Health Resources, Inc., Brentwood, TN | 23 | 10 | 249 | 6560 | 144 | 130427 | 526 | 47334 | 21272 | 657

GASSAWAY—Braxton County

★ BRAXTON COUNTY MEMORIAL HOSPITAL, 100 Hoylman Drive, Zip 26624–9308; tel. 304/364–5156; Tony E. Atkins, Administrator **A**9 10 **F**8 13 15 16 19 21 22 24 28 31 32 34 44 65 71 73 74 **S** Camcare, Inc., Charleston, WV **N** Partners in Health Network, Inc., Charleston, WV | 23 | 10 | 30 | 955 | 8 | 21356 | 0 | 7243 | 3691 | 109

GLEN DALE—Marshall County

☒ REYNOLDS MEMORIAL HOSPITAL, 800 Wheeling Avenue, Zip 26038–1697; tel. 304/845–3211; John Sicurella, Chief Executive Officer (Total facility includes 20 beds in nursing home–type unit) **A**1 6 9 10 **F**1 3 7 8 15 16 19 21 22 24 28 29 30 32 33 35 37 39 40 41 42 44 45 46 49 53 54 55 56 57 58 59 60 63 64 65 70 71 73 **P**8 | 23 | 10 | 140 | 3241 | 55 | 51308 | 139 | 26828 | 12374 | 437

GRAFTON—Taylor County

□ GRAFTON CITY HOSPITAL, 500 Market Street, Zip 26354; tel. 304/265–0400; Gary R. Willmon, Administrator (Total facility includes 72 beds in nursing home–type unit) **A**1 9 10 **F**8 11 14 15 16 19 21 22 24 26 28 29 30 34 37 39 44 45 46 49 51 64 65 66 70 71 72 73 74 **P**3 | 14 | 10 | 106 | 1161 | 81 | 24398 | 0 | 8464 | 3550 | 236

GRANTSVILLE—Calhoun County

MINNIE HAMILTON HEALTHCARE CENTER, (Formerly Calhoun General Hospital), High Street, Zip 26147, Mailing Address: Route 1, Box 1A, Zip 26147; tel. 304/354–9244; Barbara Lay, Administrator **A**9 **F**15 16 17 19 21 22 28 30 51 65 71 **P**6 **N** Partners in Health Network, Inc., Charleston, WV | 23 | 10 | 6 | 399 | 2 | 7240 | 0 | 3384 | 1673 | 70

HINTON—Summers County

□ SUMMERS COUNTY APPALACHIAN REGIONAL HOSPITAL, Terrace Street, Zip 25951, Mailing Address: Drawer 940, Zip 25951–0940; tel. 304/466–1000; Clyde E. Bolton, Administrator (Total facility includes 24 beds in nursing home–type unit) **A**1 9 10 **F**8 12 14 15 16 17 19 22 28 30 32 34 35 37 44 46 48 49 51 64 65 70 71 73 **S** Appalachian Regional Healthcare, Lexington, KY **N** Partners in Health Network, Inc., Charleston, WV; CHA Provider Network, Inc., Lexington, KY | 23 | 10 | 50 | 915 | 33 | 50848 | 0 | 9339 | 3350 | 143

HUNTINGTON—Cabell County

☒ + CABELL HUNTINGTON HOSPITAL, 1340 Hal Greer Boulevard, Zip 25701–0195; tel. 304/526–2000; W. Don Smith, II, President and Chief Executive Officer (Total facility includes 15 beds in nursing home–type unit) **A**1 3 5 9 10 **F**4 7 8 9 15 16 19 20 21 22 23 28 29 30 31 32 33 34 35 37 38 39 40 41 42 44 45 46 47 49 51 60 61 63 64 65 67 69 70 71 73 74 **P**5 8 **N** CHA Provider Network, Inc., Lexington, KY | 23 | 10 | 264 | 13857 | 177 | 186815 | 2348 | 99319 | 45543 | 1247

☒ COLUMBIA RIVER PARK HOSPITAL, 1230 Sixth Avenue, Zip 25701, Mailing Address: Box 1875, Zip 25719; tel. 304/526–9111; Scott C. Stamm, Chief Executive Officer **A**1 9 10 **F**1 2 3 14 15 16 52 53 54 55 56 57 58 59 **P**5 **S** Columbia/HCA Healthcare Corporation, Nashville, TN | 33 | 22 | 165 | 2027 | 58 | — | 0 | 10348 | 4373 | 125

☒ △ HEALTHSOUTH REHABILITATION HOSPITAL, 6900 West Country Club Drive, Zip 25705; tel. 304/733–1060; Homer Fowler, Chief Operating Officer (Nonreporting) **A**1 7 10 **S** HEALTHSOUTH Corporation, Birmingham, AL | 33 | 46 | 40 | — | — | — | — | — | — | —

☒ ST. MARY'S HOSPITAL, 2900 First Avenue, Zip 25702; tel. 304/526–1234; J. Thomas Jones, Executive Director (Total facility includes 20 beds in nursing home–type unit) **A**1 2 3 5 6 9 10 **F**2 4 7 8 10 11 12 15 16 17 19 21 22 23 26 28 29 30 31 32 33 34 35 37 39 40 41 42 43 44 45 49 52 53 54 55 56 57 59 60 63 64 65 67 70 71 73 74 **P**2 8 **N** CHA Provider Network, Inc., Lexington, KY | 21 | 10 | 440 | 15649 | 265 | 94169 | 637 | 119900 | 52022 | 1610

☒ VETERANS AFFAIRS MEDICAL CENTER, 1540 Spring Valley Drive, Zip 25704; tel. 304/429–6741; Philip S. Elkins, Director **A**1 3 5 **F**3 4 6 8 10 12 14 15 16 17 18 19 20 21 22 23 24 25 26 27 28 29 30 31 32 33 34 35 37 39 41 42 43 44 45 46 49 50 51 52 54 55 56 57 58 59 60 63 64 65 67 69 71 73 74 **S** Department of Veterans Affairs, Washington, DC | 45 | 10 | 170 | 4486 | 94 | 104373 | 0 | 63691 | 37749 | 777

Hospital, Address, Telephone, Administrator, Approval, Facility, and Physician Codes, Health Care System, Network	Classi-fication Codes		Utilization Data					Expense (thousands) of dollars		
	Control	Service	Beds	Admissions	Census	Outpatient Visits	Births	Total	Payroll	Personnel

★ American Hospital Association (AHA) membership
☐ Joint Commission on Accreditation of Healthcare Organizations (JCAHO) accreditation
✛ American Osteopathic Hospital Association (AOHA) membership
◯ American Osteopathic Association (AOA) accreditation
△ Commission on Accreditation of Rehabilitation Facilities (CARF) accreditation
Control codes 61, 63, 64, 71, 72 and 73 indicate hospitals listed by AOHA, but not registered by AHA. For definition of numerical codes, see page A4

HURRICANE—Putnam County

⊠ PUTNAM GENERAL HOSPITAL, 1400 Hospital Drive, Zip 25526–9210, Mailing Address: P.O. Box 900, Zip 25526–0900; tel. 304/757–1700; Patsy Hardy, Administrator **A**1 9 10 **F**8 11 12 15 16 19 21 22 23 28 32 33 35 39 41 44 49 65 66 71 73 **P**5 7 **S** Columbia/HCA Healthcare Corporation, Nashville, TN	33	10	66	2611	37	36567	0	19544	7028	243

KEYSER—Mineral County

☐ POTOMAC VALLEY HOSPITAL, South Mineral Street, Zip 26726; tel. 304/788–3141; James F. Heitzenrater, Administrator **A**1 9 10 **F**11 14 19 21 22 29 30 31 32 33 37 44 49 63 65 67 71 73	33	10	42	1638	17	40805	3	11138	4092	173

KINGWOOD—Preston County

⊠ PRESTON MEMORIAL HOSPITAL, 300 South Price Street, Zip 26537–1495; tel. 304/329–1400; Raymond E. Wood, President and Chief Executive Officer **A**1 9 10 **F**2 3 7 8 12 17 19 22 24 28 30 32 34 35 40 41 44 49 65 71 73 74 **P**8 **S** Quorum Health Group/Quorum Health Resources, Inc., Brentwood, TN	23	10	60	1344	22	55713	177	9867	4802	184

LOGAN—Logan County

★ GUYAN VALLEY HOSPITAL, 396 Dingess Street, Zip 25601; tel. 304/792–1700; Linda Saunders, Administrator (Nonreporting)	23	10	43	—	—	—	—	—	—	—
☐ LOGAN GENERAL HOSPITAL, 20 Hospital Drive, Zip 25601; tel. 304/792–1101; C. David Morrison, President (Nonreporting) **A**1 10 12 13	23	10	132	—	—	—	—	—	—	—

MADISON—Boone County

⊠ BOONE MEMORIAL HOSPITAL, 701 Madison Avenue, Zip 25130; tel. 304/369–1230; Tommy H. Mullins, Administrator **A**1 9 10 **F**14 15 16 19 21 22 32 33 34 44 45 49 65 71 73 **N** Partners in Health Network, Inc., Charleston, WV; CHA Provider Network, Inc., Lexington, KY	13	10	38	635	15	50576	0	5597	2435	112

MAN—Logan County

☐ MAN ARH HOSPITAL, 700 East McDonald Avenue, Zip 25635–1011; tel. 304/583–8421; Freda Napier, Administrator **A**1 9 10 **F**3 4 7 8 10 11 12 13 14 15 16 17 19 20 21 22 25 28 29 30 32 34 35 37 38 39 42 43 44 45 46 47 49 52 54 56 58 64 65 69 70 71 73 **P**5 **S** Appalachian Regional Healthcare, Lexington, KY **N** Partners in Health Network, Inc., Charleston, WV; CHA Provider Network, Inc., Lexington, KY	23	10	42	867	9	46633	0	12225	5529	216

MARTINSBURG—Berkeley County

⊠ CITY HOSPITAL, Dry Run Road, Zip 25401, Mailing Address: P.O. Box 1418, Zip 25402–1418; tel. 304/264–1000; Peter L. Mulford, Administrator (Total facility includes 19 beds in nursing home–type unit) **A**1 2 9 10 **F**1 3 7 8 12 15 19 22 23 24 26 28 30 32 33 35 37 40 41 42 44 45 46 49 52 53 54 56 57 58 59 64 65 66 67 71 73 74 **P**8 **S** Quorum Health Group/Quorum Health Resources, Inc., Brentwood, TN	23	10	163	7024	113	92800	782	45065	18679	617
⊠ VETERANS AFFAIRS MEDICAL CENTER, Charles Town Road, Zip 25401–0205; tel. 304/263–0811; Richard Pell, Jr., Director (Total facility includes 150 beds in nursing home–type unit) **A**1 3 5 **F**2 3 4 5 8 10 15 16 19 20 21 22 25 26 28 31 33 34 35 37 39 41 42 44 45 46 49 50 51 52 53 54 55 56 57 58 59 60 63 64 65 67 70 71 72 73 74 **S** Department of Veterans Affairs, Washington, DC	45	10	370	4782	289	144768	0	85751	49833	1210

MONTGOMERY—Fayette County

⊠ MONTGOMERY GENERAL HOSPITAL, 401 Sixth Avenue, Zip 25136–0270, Mailing Address: P.O. Box 270, Zip 25136–0270; tel. 304/442–5151; William R. Laird, IV, Interim President (Total facility includes 44 beds in nursing home–type unit) **A**1 9 10 **F**12 14 15 16 19 22 28 32 37 41 44 49 64 65 71 73 **P**6 **N** Partners in Health Network, Inc., Charleston, WV	23	10	90	1609	64	182615	0	21347	9100	247

MORGANTOWN—Monongalia County

☐ CHESTNUT RIDGE HOSPITAL, 930 Chestnut Ridge Road, Zip 26505; tel. 304/293–4000; Lawrence J. Drake, Chief Executive Officer **A**1 5 9 10 **F**2 3 11 19 21 22 35 37 38 40 47 48 52 53 54 56 57 58 59 70 71 **P**6 **S** Ramsay Health Care, Inc., Coral Gobles, FL	33	22	70	1310	37	3276	0	7618	2916	150
☐ △ HEALTHSOUTH MOUNTAIN REGIONAL REHABILITATION HOSPITAL, 1160 Van Voorhis, Zip 26505; tel. 304/598–1100; Sharon Nero, Chief Executive Officer (Nonreporting) **A**1 7 10 **S** HEALTHSOUTH Corporation, Birmingham, AL	33	46	80	—	—	—	—	—	—	—
⊠ MONONGALIA GENERAL HOSPITAL, 1200 J. D. Anderson Drive, Zip 26505; tel. 304/598–1200; Robert P. Ritz, President and Chief Executive Officer (Total facility includes 20 beds in nursing home–type unit) **A**1 3 5 9 10 **F**4 6 7 8 10 11 12 13 14 15 16 17 19 21 22 23 24 25 28 30 31 32 33 34 35 37 39 42 43 44 46 49 51 54 60 61 62 63 64 65 66 67 70 71 72 73 74 **P**5 6 7	23	10	205	8056	115	157708	552	68540	28700	913
⊠ WEST VIRGINIA UNIVERSITY HOSPITALS, Medical Center Drive, Zip 26506–4749; tel. 304/598–4000; Bruce McClymonds, President and Chief Executive Officer **A**1 2 3 5 8 9 10 **F**2 3 4 7 8 10 11 17 18 19 20 21 22 23 25 26 28 29 30 31 32 33 34 35 37 38 40 41 42 43 44 45 46 47 48 49 50 51 52 53 54 55 56 57 58 59 60 61 63 64 65 66 67 69 70 71 73 74 **P**6 **S** West Virginia United Health System, Morgantown, WV **N** Integrated Provider Network, Morgantown, WV	23	10	334	14359	237	368623	1547	172456	65016	2206

NEW MARTINSVILLE—Wetzel County

⊠ WETZEL COUNTY HOSPITAL, 3 East Benjamin Drive, Zip 26155; tel. 304/455–8000; Vincent B. McKee, Chief Executive Officer (Total facility includes 10 beds in nursing home–type unit) **A**1 9 10 **F**7 8 13 14 15 16 17 19 21 22 24 28 30 32 33 34 37 39 40 41 44 45 46 49 64 65 67 70 71 73 **P**4	13	10	66	1747	17	51936	157	14695	6035	186

OAK HILL—Fayette County

☐ PLATEAU MEDICAL CENTER, 430 Main Street, Zip 25901; tel. 304/469–8600 **A**1 9 10 **F**8 12 14 15 16 17 19 20 21 22 27 32 34 37 44 45 46 48 49 63 65 71 73 **P**6 **S** TENET Healthcare Corporation, Santa Barbara, CA **N** Partners in Health Network, Inc., Charleston, WV	33	10	79	2583	39	56127	0	16527	6594	273

Hospital, Address, Telephone, Administrator, Approval, Facility, and Physician Codes, Health Care System, Network	Classi-fication Codes		Utilization Data					Expense (thousands) of dollars		
★ American Hospital Association (AHA) membership □ Joint Commission on Accreditation of Healthcare Organizations (JCAHO) accreditation + American Osteopathic Hospital Association (AOHA) membership ○ American Osteopathic Association (AOA) accreditation △ Commission on Accreditation of Rehabilitation Facilities (CARF) accreditation Control codes 61, 63, 64, 71, 72 and 73 indicate hospitals listed by AOHA, but not registered by AHA. For definition of numerical codes, see page A4	Control	Service	Beds	Admissions	Census	Outpatient Visits	Births	Total	Payroll	Personnel

PARKERSBURG—Wood County

★ CAMDEN–CLARK MEMORIAL HOSPITAL, 800 Garfield Avenue, Zip 26101, Mailing Address: P.O. Box 718, Zip 26102–0718; tel. 304/424–2111; Thomas J. Corder, President and Chief Executive Officer **A**1 2 9 10 **F**7 8 11 12 14 15 16 17 19 21 22 23 24 25 28 30 34 35 37 40 41 42 44 45 46 49 60 63 65 67 71 73 74 **P**7 **N** Mid–Ohio Valley Rural Health Network, Parkersburg, WV
| | 14 | 10 | 212 | 9492 | 126 | 170580 | 824 | 67862 | 28739 | 966 |

□ △ HEALTHSOUTH WESTERN HILLS REGIONAL REHABILITATION HOSPITAL, 3 Western Hills Drive, Zip 26101, Mailing Address: P.O. Box 1428, Zip 26102–1428; tel. 304/420–1300; Thomas Heller, Administrator **A**1 7 9 10 **F**12 14 15 16 27 39 42 48 49 65 66 67 73 **S** HEALTHSOUTH Corporation, Birmingham, AL
| | 33 | 46 | 40 | 638 | 37 | 5646 | 0 | 8866 | 3763 | 105 |

★ ST. JOSEPH'S HOSPITAL, 1824 Murdoch Avenue, Zip 26101, Mailing Address: Box 327, Zip 26102–0327; tel. 304/424–4111; Stephens M. Mundy, Chief Executive Officer (Total facility includes 20 beds in nursing home–type unit) **A**1 9 10 **F**2 3 7 8 10 11 12 14 15 16 17 19 22 23 27 28 29 30 31 32 35 37 40 41 42 44 45 46 48 49 52 53 55 56 57 59 63 64 65 66 67 71 72 73 74 **P**7
| | 32 | 10 | 294 | 8631 | 127 | 132334 | 567 | 57916 | 23716 | 752 |

PETERSBURG—Grant County

★ GRANT MEMORIAL HOSPITAL, Mailing Address: P.O. Box 1019, Zip 26847; tel. 304/257–1026; Robert L. Harman, Administrator (Total facility includes 10 beds in nursing home–type unit) **A**9 10 **F**7 8 12 13 15 17 19 21 22 26 28 29 30 32 33 34 37 40 42 44 49 58 64 65 70 71 74 **N** Eastern Panhandle Integrated Delivery System, Petersburg, WV
| | 13 | 10 | 65 | 2723 | 40 | 62470 | 295 | 15129 | 6945 | 317 |

PHILIPPI—Barbour County

BROADDUS HOSPITAL, College Hill, Zip 26416; tel. 304/457–1760; Susannah Higgins, Chief Executive Officer (Total facility includes 60 beds in nursing home–type unit) **A**9 10 **F**8 12 13 15 17 19 22 26 28 30 32 33 34 35 42 44 51 64 65 71 72 74 **P**3
| | 23 | 10 | 72 | 521 | 62 | 28824 | 0 | 4701 | 2866 | 139 |

POINT PLEASANT—Mason County

★ PLEASANT VALLEY HOSPITAL, 2520 Valley Drive, Zip 25550–2083; tel. 304/675–4340; Michael G. Sellards, Executive Director (Total facility includes 100 beds in nursing home–type unit) **A**1 9 10 **F**7 12 19 22 23 24 28 30 32 33 34 35 37 40 42 44 48 63 64 65 67 71 73 **P**8
| | 23 | 10 | 201 | 3208 | 139 | 54322 | 159 | 37418 | 17706 | 558 |

PRINCETON—Mercer County

★ △ HEALTHSOUTH SOUTHERN HILLS REHABILITATION HOSPITAL, 120 Twelfth Street, Zip 24740; tel. 304/487–8000; Timothy Mitchell, Administrator (Nonreporting) **A**1 7 9 10 **S** HEALTHSOUTH Corporation, Birmingham, AL
| | 33 | 46 | 40 | — | — | — | — | — | — | — |

★ PRINCETON COMMUNITY HOSPITAL, 12th Street, Zip 24740–1369, Mailing Address: P.O. Box 1369, Zip 24740–1369; tel. 304/487–7000; Daniel C. Dunmyer, Chief Executive Officer (Total facility includes 23 beds in nursing home–type unit) **A**1 2 9 10 **F**3 4 7 8 9 11 14 15 16 17 19 20 21 22 23 26 28 30 31 32 33 34 35 37 38 39 40 41 42 44 45 46 47 51 52 53 54 55 56 57 58 60 63 64 65 66 69 71 72 73 **P**2 3 8
| | 14 | 10 | 206 | 7994 | 128 | 94450 | 530 | 57188 | 26405 | 917 |

RANSON—Jefferson County

★ JEFFERSON MEMORIAL HOSPITAL, 300 South Preston Street, Zip 25438–1699; tel. 304/728–1600; Jon D. Applebaum, Administrator **A**1 5 9 10 **F**7 8 14 15 16 17 19 21 22 28 30 32 34 35 37 39 40 41 42 44 45 46 49 54 65 66 67 70 71 73 **P**8
| | 23 | 10 | 56 | 2353 | 24 | 32717 | 248 | 16732 | 7709 | 290 |

RICHWOOD—Nicholas County

RICHWOOD AREA COMMUNITY HOSPITAL, Riverside Addition, Zip 26261; tel. 304/846–2573; D. Parker Haddix, Chief Executive Officer **A**9 **F**19 22 44 71 73 **N** Partners in Health Network, Inc., Charleston, WV
| | 23 | 10 | 6 | 207 | 2 | 10123 | 0 | 3090 | 1335 | 60 |

RIPLEY—Jackson County

★ JACKSON GENERAL HOSPITAL, Pinnell Street, Zip 25271, Mailing Address: P.O. Box 720, Zip 25271; tel. 304/372–2731; Richard L. Rohaley, President and Chief Executive Officer **A**1 9 10 **F**7 8 11 16 19 21 22 28 35 37 40 44 49 65 66 71 **P**3 **N** Partners in Health Network, Inc., Charleston, WV
| | 23 | 10 | 82 | 2273 | 30 | 38183 | 141 | 18214 | 8494 | 319 |

ROMNEY—Hampshire County

HAMPSHIRE MEMORIAL HOSPITAL, 549 Center Avenue, Zip 26757–1199; tel. 304/822–4561; Roberta D. McCauley, Chief Executive Officer (Total facility includes 30 beds in nursing home–type unit) **A**9 10 **F**8 14 15 16 19 22 31 32 44 64 65 71 **P**4
| | 33 | 10 | 47 | 623 | 35 | 25664 | 0 | 5791 | 2167 | 124 |

RONCEVERTE—Greenbrier County

★ GREENBRIER VALLEY MEDICAL CENTER, 202 Maplewood Avenue, Zip 24970–0497, Mailing Address: P.O. Box 497, Zip 24970–0497; tel. 304/647–4411; James B. Wood, Chief Executive Officer **A**1 9 10 12 13 **F**4 7 8 12 16 19 20 21 22 23 26 28 30 32 33 34 35 37 39 40 42 44 46 49 63 65 66 71 73 **S** Columbia/HCA Healthcare Corporation, Nashville, TN
| | 33 | 10 | 122 | 4658 | 59 | 34760 | 495 | 27295 | 9245 | 334 |

SISTERSVILLE—Tyler County

SISTERSVILLE GENERAL HOSPITAL, 314 South Wells Street, Zip 26175; tel. 304/652–2611; Lynn McCormick, Administrator **A**9 **F**8 22 24 28 30 32 33 34 41 44 49 64 65 71 73 **N** Mid–Ohio Valley Rural Health Network, Parkersburg, WV
| | 14 | 10 | 12 | 169 | 2 | 24575 | 0 | 3435 | 1654 | 81 |

SOUTH CHARLESTON—Kanawha County

★ THOMAS MEMORIAL HOSPITAL, 4605 MacCorkle Avenue S.W., Zip 25309–1398; tel. 304/766–3600; Stephen P. Dexter, Chief Executive Officer **A**1 3 5 9 10 **F**2 3 7 8 11 14 15 16 17 19 21 22 24 26 28 29 30 32 33 34 35 36 37 39 40 41 42 44 45 49 52 53 54 55 56 57 58 59 60 63 65 67 71 72 73 74 **P**7
| | 23 | 10 | 216 | 7739 | 119 | 177076 | 386 | 63216 | 26234 | 749 |

Hospital, Address, Telephone, Administrator, Approval, Facility, and Physician Codes, Health Care System, Network	Classi-fication Codes		Utilization Data					Expense (thousands) of dollars		
★ American Hospital Association (AHA) membership □ Joint Commission on Accreditation of Healthcare Organizations (JCAHO) accreditation + American Osteopathic Hospital Association (AOHA) membership ○ American Osteopathic Association (AOA) accreditation △ Commission on Accreditation of Rehabilitation Facilities (CARF) accreditation Control codes 61, 63, 64, 71, 72 and 73 indicate hospitals listed by AOHA, but not registered by AHA. For definition of numerical codes, see page A4	Control	Service	Beds	Admissions	Census	Outpatient Visits	Births	Total	Payroll	Personnel

SPENCER—Roane County

☒ ROANE GENERAL HOSPITAL, 200 Hospital Drive, Zip 25276; tel. 304/927–6200; Andrew Mazon, III, Administrator and Chief Executive Officer (Total facility includes 9 beds in nursing home–type unit) **A**1 9 10 **F**1 7 8 17 19 21 22 28 30 32 34 40 44 45 64 65 71 73 **N** Partners in Health Network, Inc., Charleston, WV

	23	10	55	1270	24	25657	156	10959	5613	222

SUMMERSVILLE—Nicholas County

★ SUMMERSVILLE MEMORIAL HOSPITAL, 400 Fairview Heights Road, Zip 26651–0400; tel. 304/872–2891; Gregory D. Johnson, Administrator (Total facility includes 52 beds in nursing home–type unit) **A**9 10 **F**4 7 8 11 14 17 19 21 22 25 26 30 34 35 37 40 42 44 45 49 64 65 67 70 71 72 73

	14	10	109	2141	79	46977	221	17772	7914	363

WEBSTER SPRINGS—Webster County

★ WEBSTER COUNTY MEMORIAL HOSPITAL, 324 Miller Mountain Drive, Zip 26288; tel. 304/847–5682; Stephen M. Gavalchik, Administrator **A**9 **F**2 4 7 8 9 10 11 14 15 16 17 19 21 22 25 26 28 29 30 32 33 34 35 37 38 40 41 42 44 45 47 49 51 52 54 58 60 64 65 66 67 70 71 72 73 74 **N** Webster Memorial/United Hospital Center EACH/RPCH Network, Webster Springs, WV; North Central/West Virginia Rural Health Network, Clarksburg, WV

	13	10	6	265	2	24707	1	2856	1575	64

WEIRTON—Brooke County

☒ WEIRTON MEDICAL CENTER, 601 Colliers Way, Zip 26062–5091; tel. 304/797–6000; Donald Muhlenthaler, FACHE, President and Chief Executive Officer (Total facility includes 33 beds in nursing home–type unit) **A**1 9 10 **F**7 8 10 11 13 14 15 16 17 19 20 21 22 23 24 25 26 27 28 29 30 31 32 33 34 35 39 40 41 42 44 45 49 52 53 54 55 56 57 58 59 63 64 65 66 67 69 70 71 73 **P**1 **N** Tri–State Community Care Network, Weirton, WV

	23	10	240	6840	110	86235	281	42481	19682	659

WESTON—Lewis County

☒ STONEWALL JACKSON MEMORIAL HOSPITAL, Route 4, Zip 26452, Mailing Address: Route 4, Box 10, Zip 26452; tel. 304/269–8000; David D. Shaffer, Chief Executive Officer (Total facility includes 10 beds in nursing home–type unit) **A**1 9 10 **F**7 8 11 15 19 22 30 32 35 40 42 44 45 49 64 65 71 **P**7 8

	23	10	70	2698	34	61620	224	14680	6342	264

□ WILLIAM R. SHARPE JR. HOSPITAL, Route 33 West, Zip 26452, Mailing Address: P.O. Drawer 1127, Zip 26452; tel. 304/269–1210; Michael A. Todt, Ph.D., Administrator **A**1 5 10 **F**14 15 16 20 26 27 45 46 52 54 55 56 57 65 67 73 **P**6

	12	22	124	1001	93	0	0	19844	8443	404

WHEELING—Ohio County

☒ OHIO VALLEY MEDICAL CENTER, 2000 Eoff Street, Zip 26003; tel. 304/234–0123; Thomas P. Galinski, President and Chief Executive Officer (Total facility includes 172 beds in nursing home–type unit) **A**1 2 3 5 9 10 12 **F**3 5 7 8 10 11 12 14 15 16 17 18 19 21 22 23 24 25 26 27 28 29 30 31 32 34 35 37 39 40 41 42 44 45 47 48 49 51 52 53 54 55 56 57 58 59 60 61 63 64 65 66 67 71 73 74 **P**6 8 **S** Allegheny Health, Education and Research Foundation, Pittsburgh, PA

	23	10	385	7830	259	103983	438	65217	27107	1049

☒ WHEELING HOSPITAL, Medical Park, Zip 26003–0708; tel. 304/243–3000; Donald H. Hofreuter, M.D., Administrator and Chief Executive Officer **A**1 2 3 5 9 10 **F**3 4 7 8 10 11 12 13 15 16 17 19 20 21 22 23 24 26 27 28 29 30 31 32 34 35 37 39 40 41 42 43 44 45 46 49 51 53 54 55 56 57 58 59 60 65 66 67 70 71 72 73 74 **P**3 7 8

	23	10	276	11194	146	209160	1220	96023	42471	1366

WILLIAMSON—Mingo County

□ WILLIAMSON MEMORIAL HOSPITAL, 859 Alderson Street, Zip 25661, Mailing Address: P.O. Box 1980, Zip 25661; tel. 304/235–2500; Roger C. LeDoux, Administrator **A**1 9 10 **F**7 8 12 15 16 19 21 22 23 28 30 31 32 33 34 35 37 39 42 44 46 49 71 **P**6 7 8 **S** Health Management Associates, Naples, FL

	33	10	76	3845	42	28029	241	18823	6619	295

WISCONSIN

Resident population 5,123 (in thousands)
Resident population in metro areas 67.9%
Birth rate per 1,000 population 13.8
65 years and over 13.3%
Percent of persons without health insurance 8.9%

Hospital, Address, Telephone, Administrator, Approval, Facility, and Physician Codes, Health Care System, Network	Classification Codes		Utilization Data					Expense (thousands) of dollars		
★ American Hospital Association (AHA) membership □ Joint Commission on Accreditation of Healthcare Organizations (JCAHO) accreditation + American Osteopathic Hospital Association (AOHA) membership ○ American Osteopathic Association (AOA) accreditation △ Commission on Accreditation of Rehabilitation Facilities (CARF) accreditation Control codes 61, 63, 64, 71, 72 and 73 indicate hospitals listed by AOHA, but not registered by AHA. For definition of numerical codes, see page A4	Control	Service	Beds	Admissions	Census	Outpatient Visits	Births	Total	Payroll	Personnel

AMERY—Polk County

☒ APPLE RIVER HOSPITAL, 230 Deronda Street, Zip 54001–1407; tel. 715/268–7151; Michael Karuschak, Jr., Administrator **A**1 9 10 **F**7 8 11 15 16 19 21 22 27 29 32 34 35 37 39 40 42 44 45 48 49 61 64 65 66 67 71 73 **S** Quorum Health Group/Quorum Health Resources, Inc., Brentwood, TN
| | | 23 | 10 | 10 | 990 | 10 | 12921 | 111 | 7834 | 3103 | 118 |

ANTIGO—Langlade County

□ LANGLADE MEMORIAL HOSPITAL, 112 East Fifth Avenue, Zip 54409–2796; tel. 715/623–2331; David R. Schneider, Executive Director **A**1 9 10 **F**1 2 3 4 7 8 9 10 11 15 16 17 19 21 22 26 29 32 33 34 35 36 37 38 40 42 43 44 45 47 49 52 53 54 55 56 57 58 59 61 63 64 65 67 71 73 **P**7
| | | 21 | 10 | 49 | 1984 | 24 | 27716 | 224 | 16328 | 7392 | 248 |

APPLETON—Outagamie County

☒ APPLETON MEDICAL CENTER, 1818 North Meade Street, Zip 54911; tel. 414/731–4101; Paul E. Macek, Senior Vice President **A**1 2 3 5 9 10 **F**2 3 4 6 7 8 10 11 12 14 15 16 18 19 21 22 23 24 26 29 32 34 35 36 37 38 39 40 41 42 43 44 45 46 48 49 52 53 54 55 56 57 58 59 60 61 62 64 65 66 69 70 71 72 74 **P**6 8 **S** United Health Group, Appleton, WI
| | | 23 | 10 | 146 | 7097 | 86 | 78931 | 1169 | 70905 | 30237 | 941 |

☒ △ ST. ELIZABETH HOSPITAL, 1506 South Oneida Street, Zip 54915–1397; tel. 414/738–2000; Otto L. Cox, President and Chief Executive Officer **A**1 2 3 5 7 10 **F**1 2 3 4 5 6 7 8 9 10 11 12 14 18 19 21 22 23 26 29 32 33 34 35 36 37 38 39 40 41 42 43 44 45 46 47 48 49 52 53 54 55 56 57 58 59 60 61 62 63 64 65 66 70 71 74 **S** Wheaton Franciscan Services, Inc., Wheaton, IL **N** Affinity Health System, Inc., Oshkosh, WI
| | | 21 | 10 | 155 | 7630 | 94 | 163523 | 1164 | 66735 | 29410 | 841 |

ARCADIA—Trempealeau County

☒ FRANCISCAN SKEMP HEALTHCARE–ARCADIA CAMPUS, 464 South St. Joseph Avenue, Zip 54612–1401; tel. 608/323–3341; Robert M. Tracey, Administrator (Total facility includes 75 beds in nursing home–type unit) (Nonreporting) **A**1 9 10 **S** Franciscan Skemp Healthcare, La Crosse, WI **N** Franciscan Skemp Healthcare, LaCrosse, WI
| | | 21 | 10 | 101 | — | — | — | — | — | — | — |

ASHLAND—Ashland County

☒ MEMORIAL MEDICAL CENTER, 1615 Maple Lane, Zip 54806–3689; tel. 715/682–4563; Daniel J. Hymans, President **A**1 9 10 **F**2 3 7 8 11 14 15 17 19 21 22 25 26 28 29 30 33 34 35 37 39 40 41 42 44 45 48 49 52 53 56 57 58 59 61 63 64 65 66 67 71 73 **P**5 6
| | | 23 | 10 | 101 | 3600 | 45 | 29046 | 344 | 24931 | 12631 | 368 |

BALDWIN—St. Croix County

★ BALDWIN HOSPITAL, 730 10th Avenue, Zip 54002–0045; tel. 715/684–3311; Richard L. Range, Administrator **A**9 10 **F**7 8 11 13 15 17 19 20 22 26 27 28 29 30 32 33 34 35 37 40 41 42 44 45 46 48 49 51 61 64 65 66 67 68 71 73
| | | 23 | 10 | 29 | 857 | 8 | 22330 | 55 | 6771 | 2895 | 99 |

BARABOO—Sauk County

☒ ST. CLARE HOSPITAL AND HEALTH SERVICES, 707 14th Street, Zip 53913–1597; tel. 608/356–5561; David B. Jordahl, FACHE, President **A**1 9 10 **F**2 3 7 8 11 12 15 18 19 21 22 24 26 29 31 32 33 34 35 36 37 39 40 41 42 44 45 46 49 61 63 64 65 66 71 **S** SSM Health Care System, Saint Louis, MO **N** Health Care Network of Wisconsin (HCN), Brookfield, WI
| | | 21 | 10 | 76 | 2844 | 30 | 40167 | 261 | 19071 | 8531 | 270 |

BARRON—Barron County

□ BARRON MEMORIAL MEDICAL CENTER AND SKILLED NURSING FACILITY, 1222 Woodland Avenue, Zip 54812; tel. 715/537–3186; Mark D. Wilson, Administrator (Total facility includes 50 beds in nursing home–type unit) **A**1 9 10 **F**7 8 9 11 12 14 15 16 17 19 22 24 29 30 33 34 37 39 40 41 44 45 46 47 49 51 54 55 56 57 58 61 64 65 66 67 71 73 **S** Mayo Foundation, Rochester, MN **N** Luther/Midelfort/Mayo Health System, Eau Claire, WI
| | | 23 | 10 | 92 | 1076 | 60 | 21216 | 78 | 7773 | 3850 | 129 |

BEAVER DAM—Dodge County

☒ BEAVER DAM COMMUNITY HOSPITALS, 707 South University Avenue, Zip 53916–3089; tel. 414/887–7181; John R. Landdeck, President (Total facility includes 123 beds in nursing home–type unit) **A**1 9 10 **F**2 8 11 13 14 15 16 17 19 20 22 26 27 28 29 30 32 33 34 35 37 39 40 41 42 44 45 46 48 49 51 52 61 64 65 66 67 68 71 72 73 74
| | | 23 | 10 | 216 | 3288 | 146 | 60982 | 349 | 27475 | 12962 | — |

BELOIT—Rock County

□ △ BELOIT MEMORIAL HOSPITAL, 1969 West Hart Road, Zip 53511–2299; tel. 608/364–5011; Gregory K. Britton, President and Chief Executive Officer **A**1 7 9 10 **F**5 7 8 9 10 11 12 14 16 17 18 19 20 21 22 23 25 26 27 28 29 30 34 35 37 38 39 40 41 42 44 45 46 47 48 49 51 53 54 55 56 57 58 60 61 63 64 65 66 67 68 69 71 72 73 74
| | | 23 | 10 | 123 | 5263 | 75 | 122573 | 670 | 43842 | 20296 | 680 |

BERLIN—Green Lake County

□ COMMUNITY HEALTH NETWORK, (Includes Berlin Memorial Hospital, Juliette Manor Nursing Home, Community Clinics), 225 Memorial Drive, Zip 54923–1295; tel. 414/361–5580; Craig W. C. Schmidt, President and Chief Executive Officer (Total facility includes 106 beds in nursing home–type unit) **A**1 2 9 10 **F**2 3 4 6 7 8 9 10 11 12 14 15 16 19 21 22 24 25 26 28 29 30 32 33 34 35 36 37 39 40 41 43 45 47 48 49 51 52 53 54 55 56 57 58 59 61 62 63 64 65 66 67 70 71 72 73 74 **P**5 8 **N** Partners Health System, Inc., Berlin, WI
| | | 23 | 10 | 167 | 2362 | 126 | 36926 | 239 | 23556 | 10060 | — |

Hospital, Address, Telephone, Administrator, Approval, Facility, and Physician Codes, Health Care System, Network	Classi-fication Codes		Utilization Data					Expense (thousands) of dollars		
★ American Hospital Association (AHA) membership □ Joint Commission on Accreditation of Healthcare Organizations (JCAHO) accreditation + American Osteopathic Hospital Association (AOHA) membership ○ American Osteopathic Association (AOA) accreditation △ Commission on Accreditation of Rehabilitation Facilities (CARF) accreditation Control codes 61, 63, 64, 71, 72 and 73 indicate hospitals listed by AOHA, but not registered by AHA. For definition of numerical codes, see page A4	Control	Service	Beds	Admissions	Census	Outpatient Visits	Births	Total	Payroll	Personnel

BLACK RIVER FALLS—Jackson County

□ BLACK RIVER MEMORIAL HOSPITAL, 711 West Adams Street, Zip 54615–9113; tel. 715/284–5361; Stanley J. Gaynor, Chief Executive Officer and Administrator **A**1 9 10 **F**2 3 7 12 16 17 19 22 26 28 29 34 35 36 40 41 44 45 49 52 54 61 64 65 66 67 70 71 73 — 23 10 | 38 | 1152 | 11 | 8027 | 164 | 6934 | 3016 | 108

BLOOMER—Chippewa County

✠ BLOOMER COMMUNITY MEMORIAL HOSPITAL AND THE MAPLEWOOD, 1501 Thompson Street, Zip 54724; tel. 715/568–2000; John Perushek, Administrator (Total facility includes 75 beds in nursing home–type unit) (Nonreporting) **A**1 9 10 **S** Mayo Foundation, Rochester, MN **N** Luther/Midelfort/Mayo Health System, Eau Claire, WI — 23 10 | 101 | — | — | — | — | — | — | —

BOSCOBEL—Grant County

BOSCOBEL AREA HEALTH CARE, 205 Parker Street, Zip 53805; tel. 608/375–4112; Steven T. Moburg, Administrator (Total facility includes 85 beds in nursing home–type unit) **A**9 10 **F**1 2 3 7 8 15 17 18 19 22 25 26 29 32 34 35 40 41 42 44 45 49 51 52 53 54 55 56 57 58 59 61 64 65 67 71 72 73 **P**5 8 — 23 10 | 131 | 1292 | 86 | 8462 | 60 | 9333 | 3673 | 129

BROOKFIELD—Waukesha County

✠ △ ELMBROOK MEMORIAL HOSPITAL, 19333 West North Avenue, Zip 53045–4198; tel. 414/785–2000; Kimry A. Johnsrud, President **A**1 7 9 10 **F**2 3 4 5 6 7 8 10 11 12 18 19 21 22 23 25 26 29 31 32 33 34 35 36 37 38 39 40 41 42 43 44 45 46 48 49 52 53 54 55 56 57 58 59 60 61 62 63 65 66 69 70 71 74 **P**2 5 7 8 **S** Wheaton Franciscan Services, Inc., Wheaton, IL **N** Health Care Network of Wisconsin (HCN), Brookfield, WI; Covenant Healthcare System, Inc., Milwaukee, WI — 21 10 | 136 | 5073 | 60 | 51659 | 855 | 44847 | 18687 | 444

BURLINGTON—Racine County

✠ MEMORIAL HOSPITAL CORPORATION OF BURLINGTON, 252 McHenry Street, Zip 53105–1828; tel. 414/763–2411; Paul A. Miller, President and Chief Executive Officer (Nonreporting) **A**1 9 10 **S** Aurora Health Care, Milwaukee, WI **N** Health Care Network of Wisconsin (HCN), Brookfield, WI; Aurora Health Care, Milwaukee, WI — 23 10 | 87 | — | — | — | — | — | — | —

CHILTON—Calumet County

✠ CALUMET MEDICAL CENTER, 614 Memorial Drive, Zip 53014; tel. 414/849–2386; Joseph L. Schumacher, Administrator **A**1 9 10 **F**3 8 10 11 12 15 16 17 18 19 21 22 26 28 29 30 32 33 34 35 36 37 39 41 42 44 45 46 47 49 51 53 54 55 56 57 58 59 61 64 65 66 67 70 71 73 74 **P**1 — 23 10 | 53 | 673 | 8 | 31322 | 0 | 8742 | 4014 | 146

CHIPPEWA FALLS—Chippewa County

✠ ST. JOSEPH'S HOSPITAL, 2661 County Highway I, Zip 54729–1498; tel. 715/723–1811; David B. Fish, Executive Vice President **A**1 9 10 **F**2 3 7 8 11 12 14 15 16 17 19 21 22 26 28 29 30 32 33 34 36 37 39 40 41 42 44 45 46 47 56 61 64 65 67 71 73 **S** Hospital Sisters Health System, Springfield, IL — 21 10 | 127 | 3495 | 56 | 53549 | 365 | 26227 | 13087 | 417

COLUMBUS—Columbia County

✠ COLUMBUS COMMUNITY HOSPITAL, 1515 Park Avenue, Zip 53925; tel. 414/623–2200; Miles Meyer, Administrator **A**1 9 10 **F**7 8 9 11 12 14 15 16 17 19 22 26 28 29 30 34 37 39 40 41 42 44 45 47 49 51 61 63 64 65 71 72 73 74 — 23 10 | 53 | 1641 | 21 | 20734 | 132 | 10561 | 4748 | 153

CUBA CITY—Grant County

CUBA CITY MEDICAL CENTER See Southwest Health Center, Platteville

CUMBERLAND—Barron County

□ CUMBERLAND MEMORIAL HOSPITAL, 1110 Seventh Avenue, Zip 54829, Mailing Address: Box 37, Zip 54829–0037; tel. 715/822–2741; James M. O'Keefe, Administrator (Total facility includes 71 beds in nursing home–type unit) **A**1 9 10 **F**7 12 13 15 16 17 19 20 21 22 26 27 28 29 30 34 35 39 40 42 44 45 46 52 54 56 57 58 61 62 63 64 65 66 67 68 70 71 73 **P**5 **N** Northern Lakes Health Consortium, Duluth, MN — 23 10 | 111 | 1544 | 86 | 7279 | 61 | 7525 | 3911 | 156

DARLINGTON—Lafayette County

MEMORIAL HOSPITAL OF LAFAYETTE COUNTY, 800 Clay Street, Zip 53530, Mailing Address: P.O. Box 70, Zip 53530; tel. 608/776–4466; Don Easley, Administrator **A**9 10 **F**3 7 8 14 15 17 19 22 26 28 29 30 34 35 40 44 45 46 49 56 61 64 65 71 — 13 10 | 28 | 532 | 5 | 17552 | 62 | 4101 | 1603 | 55

DODGEVILLE—Iowa County

✠ MEMORIAL HOSPITAL OF IOWA COUNTY, 825 South Iowa Street, Zip 53533–1999; tel. 608/935–2711; Ray Marmorstone, Administrator (Total facility includes 44 beds in nursing home–type unit) **A**1 9 10 **F**1 7 8 11 12 15 16 19 22 26 29 32 33 34 35 37 39 40 41 42 44 45 46 47 48 49 61 64 65 66 71 72 74 **S** Brim, Inc., Portland, OR — 23 10 | 82 | 1443 | 50 | 30700 | 228 | — | — | 190

DURAND—Pepin County

★ CHIPPEWA VALLEY HOSPITAL AND OAKVIEW CARE CENTER, 1220 Third Avenue West, Zip 54736, Mailing Address: P.O. Box 224, Zip 54736–0224; tel. 715/672–4211; Douglas R. Peterson, President and Chief Executive Officer (Total facility includes 58 beds in nursing home–type unit) **A**9 10 **F**7 8 15 17 19 20 22 24 26 27 28 29 30 32 33 34 36 39 40 41 44 45 46 48 61 64 65 67 71 73 **P**5 — 21 10 | 86 | 711 | 57 | 6205 | 39 | 6024 | 2726 | 103

EAGLE RIVER—Vilas County

★ EAGLE RIVER MEMORIAL HOSPITAL, 201 Hospital Road, Zip 54521; tel. 715/479–7411; Patricia Richardson, President and Chief Operating Officer **A**9 10 **F**2 3 6 8 11 12 13 15 17 19 20 21 22 24 26 28 29 30 32 33 34 35 36 37 39 40 41 42 44 45 46 48 49 51 52 61 62 64 65 66 67 68 71 73 74 **P**4 5 — 23 10 | 8 | 521 | 8 | 15338 | 0 | 5850 | 2714 | 102

Hospital, Address, Telephone, Administrator, Approval, Facility, and Physician Codes, Health Care System, Network	Classi-fication Codes		Utilization Data					Expense (thousands) of dollars		
	Control	Service	Beds	Admissions	Census	Outpatient Visits	Births	Total	Payroll	Personnel

★ American Hospital Association (AHA) membership
□ Joint Commission on Accreditation of Healthcare Organizations (JCAHO) accreditation
+ American Osteopathic Hospital Association (AOHA) membership
○ American Osteopathic Association (AOA) accreditation
△ Commission on Accreditation of Rehabilitation Facilities (CARF) accreditation
Control codes 61, 63, 64, 71, 72 and 73 indicate hospitals listed by AOHA, but not registered by AHA. For definition of numerical codes, see page A4

EAU CLAIRE—Eau Claire County

□ LUTHER HOSPITAL, 1221 Whipple Street, Zip 54702–4105; tel. 715/838–3311; William Rupp, M.D., President and Chief Executive Officer **A**1 2 3 5 9 10 **F**3 4 7 8 9 10 11 12 15 19 21 22 23 29 32 33 34 35 37 38 39 40 41 42 43 44 45 46 47 48 52 53 54 55 56 57 58 59 60 61 63 64 65 66 69 70 71 74 **S** Mayo Foundation, Rochester, MN **N** Luther/Midelfort/Mayo Health System, Eau Claire, WI; Mayo Foundation, Rochester, MN

| | 23 | 10 | 198 | 8009 | 103 | 99160 | 853 | 69237 | 29149 | 1063 |

☒ △ SACRED HEART HOSPITAL, 900 West Clairemont Avenue, Zip 54701–5105; tel. 715/839–4121; Matthew W. Hubler, Executive Vice President **A**1 2 3 5 7 9 10 **F**7 8 10 11 12 13 15 16 17 18 19 20 21 22 23 24 25 26 27 28 29 30 32 33 34 35 36 37 38 39 40 41 42 44 45 46 47 48 49 51 52 53 54 55 56 57 58 59 60 61 62 63 64 65 67 68 70 71 73 74 **P**4 7 8 **S** Hospital Sisters Health System, Springfield, IL

| | 21 | 10 | 261 | 7256 | 96 | 88274 | 773 | 55408 | 25214 | 774 |

EDGERTON—Rock County

MEMORIAL COMMUNITY HOSPITAL, 313 Stoughton Road, Zip 53534–1198; tel. 608/884–3441; Charles E. Bruhn, Chief Executive Officer (Total facility includes 61 beds in nursing home–type unit) **A**9 10 **F**8 11 12 14 15 17 19 22 27 29 30 32 33 34 35 36 37 39 41 42 44 45 46 47 48 49 51 61 62 63 64 65 66 67 68 71 72 73 74 **P**5 7 **S** Brim, Inc., Portland, OR

| | 23 | 10 | 115 | 984 | 76 | 16000 | 0 | — | — | 237 |

ELKHORN—Walworth County

☒ △ LAKELAND MEDICAL CENTER, West 3985 County Road NN, Zip 53121, Mailing Address: P.O. Box 1002, Zip 53121–1002; tel. 414/741–2000; Loren J. Anderson, President and Chief Executive Officer **A**1 7 9 10 **F**2 3 7 8 10 11 12 15 16 17 19 20 21 22 28 29 30 32 33 34 35 37 39 40 41 42 44 45 46 51 52 53 54 56 58 59 61 63 64 65 66 67 71 72 73 74 **P**5 **S** Aurora Health Care, Milwaukee, WI **N** Aurora Health Care, Milwaukee, WI

| | 23 | 10 | 78 | 3524 | 42 | 51687 | 433 | 33207 | 13082 | 385 |

FOND DU LAC—Fond Du Lac County

☒ △ AGNESIAN HEALTHCARE, (Formerly St. Agnes Hospital), 430 East Division Street, Zip 54935–0385; tel. 414/929–2300; Robert A. Fale, President **A**1 2 7 9 10 **F**1 2 3 4 5 7 8 10 11 12 15 16 17 18 19 20 21 22 23 26 28 29 31 32 33 34 35 36 37 39 40 41 42 43 44 45 48 49 52 53 54 55 56 57 58 59 60 61 63 64 65 66 67 70 71 73 74 **P**3 **S** Congregation of St. Agnes, Fond Du Lac, WI **N** Health Care Network of Wisconsin (HCN), Brookfield, WI

ST. AGNES HOSPITAL See Agnesian HealthCare

| | 21 | 10 | 161 | 6716 | 88 | 183408 | 963 | 76101 | 31784 | 786 |

FORT ATKINSON—Jefferson County

☒ FORT ATKINSON MEMORIAL HEALTH SERVICES, 611 East Sherman Avenue, Zip 53538–1998; tel. 414/568–5000; John C. Albaugh, President and Chief Executive Officer **A**1 9 10 **F**3 7 8 9 11 12 15 16 17 19 21 22 23 24 25 26 28 29 30 32 33 34 35 37 39 40 41 42 44 45 46 47 48 49 54 58 61 63 64 65 66 67 68 71 72 73 74 **P**6 7

| | 23 | 10 | 65 | 3880 | 40 | 105438 | 429 | 33912 | 15378 | 458 |

FRIENDSHIP—Adams County

□ ADAMS COUNTY MEMORIAL HOSPITAL AND NURSING CARE UNIT, 402 West Lake Street, Zip 53934, Mailing Address: P.O. Box 40, Zip 53934; tel. 608/339–3331; Allen Teal, Administrator (Total facility includes 18 beds in nursing home–type unit) **A**1 9 10 **F**1 2 3 8 12 13 14 15 16 17 18 19 21 22 25 26 27 28 29 30 32 33 34 35 39 41 42 44 45 48 49 51 55 56 57 61 64 65 66 67 71 **P**5

| | 23 | 10 | 58 | 744 | 25 | 34814 | 0 | 8242 | 4171 | 150 |

GRANTSBURG—Burnett County

BURNETT MEDICAL CENTER, 257 West St. George Avenue, Zip 54840–7827; tel. 715/463–5353; Thomas R. Lemon, Chief Executive Officer (Total facility includes 53 beds in nursing home–type unit) **A**9 10 **F**1 7 8 14 15 16 17 19 21 22 26 28 29 30 34 35 37 39 40 41 42 44 45 46 48 49 61 64 65 66 71 72 73 **S** Brim, Inc., Portland, OR **N** Health Care Network of Wisconsin (HCN), Brookfield, WI

| | 23 | 10 | 64 | 789 | 57 | 8083 | 56 | 4813 | 2373 | 119 |

GREEN BAY—Brown County

☒ BELLIN HOSPITAL, 744 South Webster Avenue, Zip 54301, Mailing Address: P.O. Box 23400, Zip 54305–3400; tel. 414/433–3500; George Kerwin, President **A**1 9 10 **F**4 7 8 10 11 14 15 16 17 19 21 23 24 27 28 29 30 32 33 34 35 37 39 40 41 42 43 44 45 46 51 61 63 64 65 66 67 71 72 73 **P**6

| | 21 | 10 | 167 | 8155 | 91 | 270911 | 1506 | 93745 | 43675 | 1363 |

□ BELLIN PSYCHIATRIC CENTER, 301 East St. Joseph Street, Zip 54301, Mailing Address: P.O. Box 23725, Zip 54305–3725; tel. 414/433–3630; Robert W. Fry, President **A**1 10 **F**2 3 11 14 15 17 19 21 25 26 27 28 29 30 34 35 37 40 45 48 50 51 52 53 54 55 56 57 58 59 61 63 64 65 67 68 71 73

| | 21 | 22 | 60 | 1408 | 30 | 12000 | 0 | 6903 | 3497 | 102 |

BROWN COUNTY MENTAL HEALTH CENTER, 2900 St. Anthony Drive, Zip 54311; tel. 414/468–1136; Mark Quam, Executive Director **A**10 **F**2 3 12 18 25 34 39 52 53 54 55 56 57 58 61 64 65 73

| | 13 | 22 | 74 | 1602 | 38 | 19166 | 0 | 7434 | 4537 | 139 |

☒ ST. MARY'S HOSPITAL MEDICAL CENTER, 1726 Shawano Avenue, Zip 54303–3282; tel. 414/498–4200; James G. Coller, Executive Vice President and Administrator **A**1 9 10 **F**7 8 11 15 16 17 19 21 22 24 29 30 33 34 35 36 37 39 40 42 44 45 46 47 51 56 61 63 64 65 67 70 71 73 **S** Hospital Sisters Health System, Springfield, IL

| | 21 | 10 | 119 | 5021 | 55 | 86618 | 714 | 40878 | 18044 | 509 |

☒ △ ST. VINCENT HOSPITAL, 835 South Van Buren Street, Zip 54307–3508, Mailing Address: P.O. Box 13508, Zip 54307–3508; tel. 414/433–0111; Joseph J. Neidenbach, Administrator and Executive Vice President **A**1 2 7 9 10 **F**4 7 8 10 11 13 17 19 20 21 22 23 26 27 28 29 30 32 33 34 35 36 37 38 39 40 41 42 44 45 46 48 49 51 60 61 63 64 65 66 67 68 70 71 73 **P**1 2 **S** Hospital Sisters Health System, Springfield, IL

| | 21 | 10 | 353 | 12664 | 194 | 101111 | 1737 | 115604 | 55413 | 1618 |

Hospital, Address, Telephone, Administrator, Approval, Facility, and Physician Codes, Health Care System, Network	Classi-fication Codes		Utilization Data					Expense (thousands) of dollars		
★ American Hospital Association (AHA) membership □ Joint Commission on Accreditation of Healthcare Organizations (JCAHO) accreditation + American Osteopathic Hospital Association (AOHA) membership ○ American Osteopathic Association (AOA) accreditation △ Commission on Accreditation of Rehabilitation Facilities (CARF) accreditation Control codes 61, 63, 64, 71, 72 and 73 indicate hospitals listed by AOHA, but not registered by AHA. For definition of numerical codes, see page A4	Control	Service	Beds	Admissions	Census	Outpatient Visits	Births	Total	Payroll	Personnel

GREENFIELD—Milwaukee County

□ THC–MILWAUKEE, 5017 South 110th Street, Zip 53228; tel. 414/427–8282; Lee Jaeger, Chief Executive Officer **A**1 9 10 **F**8 12 16 19 21 22 26 29 35 37 39 42 45 46 57 60 61 64 65 71 **S** Transitional Hospitals Corporation, Las Vegas, NV
| | 33 | 10 | 34 | 169 | 25 | 0 | 0 | 9273 | 2923 | 102 |

HARTFORD—Washington County

✠ HARTFORD MEMORIAL HOSPITAL, 1032 East Sumner Street, Zip 53027; tel. 414/673–2300; Mark Schwartz, President **A**1 9 10 **F**1 7 8 10 11 12 14 15 16 17 19 21 22 24 26 27 28 29 30 32 33 34 35 36 37 39 40 41 42 44 45 49 61 63 64 65 66 67 70 71 73 **S** Aurora Health Care, Milwaukee, WI **N** Health Care Network of Wisconsin (HCN), Brookfield, WI; Aurora Health Care, Milwaukee, WI
| | 23 | 10 | 71 | 1556 | 34 | 49473 | 225 | 17281 | 7629 | 270 |

HAYWARD—Sawyer County

✠ HAYWARD AREA MEMORIAL HOSPITAL AND NURSING HOME, Mailing Address: Route 3, Box 3999, Zip 54843; tel. 715/634–8911; Barbara A. Peickert, R.N., Chief Executive Officer (Total facility includes 76 beds in nursing home–type unit) **A**1 9 10 **F**7 8 15 16 17 19 20 21 22 26 27 28 29 30 33 34 40 41 42 44 45 51 56 61 63 64 65 67 68 71 73 **N** Northern Lakes Health Consortium, Duluth, MN
| | 23 | 10 | 117 | 1112 | 74 | 26165 | 120 | 8427 | 4087 | 145 |

HAZEL GREEN—Grant County

HAZEL GREEN HOSPITAL See Southwest Health Center, Platteville

HILLSBORO—Vernon County

✠ ST. JOSEPH'S MEMORIAL HOSPITAL AND NURSING HOME, 400 Water Avenue, Zip 54634–0527, Mailing Address: P.O. Box 527, Zip 54634–0527; tel. 608/489–2211; Nancy Bauman, Chief Executive Officer (Total facility includes 65 beds in nursing home–type unit) **A**1 9 10 **F**7 8 12 17 19 21 22 26 28 29 30 34 35 36 39 40 41 42 44 45 48 49 54 56 57 61 64 65 66 70 71 73 **S** Brim, Inc., Portland, OR
| | 21 | 10 | 85 | 390 | 67 | 15351 | 53 | 5692 | 2625 | 101 |

HUDSON—St. Croix County

□ HUDSON MEDICAL CENTER, 400 Wisconsin Street, Zip 54016–1600; tel. 715/386–9321; John W. Marnell, Chief Executive Officer **A**1 9 10 **F**1 3 7 8 11 14 15 16 17 19 21 22 24 25 26 27 28 29 30 32 33 34 35 36 37 39 40 41 42 44 45 46 48 49 54 61 64 65 66 67 68 71 73 **P**8 **N** Health Care Network of Wisconsin (HCN), Brookfield, WI
| | 23 | 10 | 39 | 1075 | 19 | 16185 | 168 | 7881 | 3933 | 127 |

JANESVILLE—Rock County

✠ MERCY HEALTH SYSTEM, 1000 Mineral Point Avenue, Zip 53545–5003, Mailing Address: P.O. Box 5003, Zip 53547–5003; tel. 608/756–6000; Javon R. Bea, President and Chief Executive Officer **A**1 3 9 10 **F**1 2 3 4 5 6 7 8 10 11 12 14 16 18 19 21 22 23 24 25 26 29 31 32 33 34 35 36 37 38 39 40 41 42 43 44 45 46 47 48 49 52 53 54 55 56 57 58 59 60 61 62 65 66 70 71 72 74 **P**6 **N** Southern Wisconsin Health Care System, Janesville, WI
| | 23 | 10 | 216 | 9179 | 122 | 395655 | 1387 | 114060 | 59762 | 1353 |

KENOSHA—Kenosha County

✠ KENOSHA HOSPITAL AND MEDICAL CENTER, 6308 Eighth Avenue, Zip 53143; tel. 414/656–2011; Richard O. Schmidt, Jr., President, Chief Executive Officer and General Counsel **A**1 9 10 **F**2 3 4 5 6 7 8 9 10 11 12 14 15 16 19 21 22 23 24 25 26 29 31 32 33 34 35 36 37 38 39 40 41 42 43 44 45 47 48 49 52 53 54 55 56 57 58 61 63 64 65 66 69 70 71 72 73 74 **P**2 4 8 **S** Horizon Healthcare, Inc., Milwaukee, WI **N** Horizon Healthcare, Inc., Milwaukee, WI
| | 23 | 10 | 116 | 5470 | 61 | 125885 | 786 | 62670 | 31627 | 719 |

✠ ST. CATHERINE'S HOSPITAL, 3556 Seventh Avenue, Zip 53140–2595; tel. 414/656–3011; Ryland Davis, Interim Chief Executive Officer **A**1 3 9 10 **F**2 3 7 8 9 10 11 12 14 16 18 19 21 22 25 26 29 32 33 34 35 36 37 38 39 40 41 42 44 45 46 47 48 49 52 54 55 56 57 58 59 60 61 63 64 65 66 69 70 71 74 **P**8 **S** Catholic Health Initiatives, Denver, CO **N** Health Care Network of Wisconsin (HCN), Brookfield, WI
| | 21 | 10 | 148 | 6192 | 83 | 133797 | 737 | 49619 | 22380 | 626 |

KEWAUNEE—Kewaunee County

□ ST. MARY'S KEWAUNEE AREA MEMORIAL HOSPITAL, 810 Lincoln Street, Zip 54216, Mailing Address: P.O. Box 217, Zip 54216–0217; tel. 414/388–2210; Steven H. Spencer, President **A**1 9 10 **F**7 8 15 17 22 25 26 29 30 32 33 34 39 40 44 45 46 51 61 64 65 71 72 73 **N** Aurora Health Care, Milwaukee, WI
| | 23 | 10 | 17 | 256 | 4 | 13708 | 39 | 3076 | 1629 | 57 |

LA CROSSE—La Crosse County

✠ FRANCISCAN SKEMP HEALTHCARE–LA CROSSE CAMPUS, 700 West Avenue South, Zip 54601–4783; tel. 608/785–0940; Ronald R. Paczkowski, Vice President (Nonreporting) **A**1 2 3 9 10 **S** Franciscan Skemp Healthcare, La Crosse, WI **N** Franciscan Skemp Healthcare, LaCrosse, WI
| | 21 | 10 | 226 | — | — | — | — | — | — | — |

✠ △ LUTHERAN HOSPITAL–LA CROSSE, 1910 South Avenue, Zip 54601–9980; tel. 608/785–0530; John N. Katrana, Ph.D., Chief Administrative Officer **A**1 2 5 7 9 10 **F**1 2 3 4 5 6 7 9 10 11 12 13 14 15 16 17 18 19 20 21 22 23 25 26 27 28 29 30 31 32 33 34 35 36 37 38 39 40 41 42 43 44 45 46 47 48 49 51 52 53 54 55 56 57 58 59 60 61 62 63 64 65 66 67 68 69 70 71 72 73 74 **N** Lutheran Health System, LaCrosse, WI
| | 23 | 10 | 293 | 14504 | 174 | 117095 | 1521 | 130167 | 56028 | 1732 |

LADYSMITH—Rusk County

RUSK COUNTY MEMORIAL HOSPITAL AND NURSING HOME, 900 College Avenue West, Zip 54848–2116; tel. 715/532–5561; J. Michael Shaw, Administrator (Total facility includes 99 beds in nursing home–type unit) **A**9 10 **F**2 3 7 8 9 11 19 22 26 28 29 30 34 37 38 39 40 42 44 45 48 51 52 53 54 55 56 57 58 59 61 64 65 67 70 71 73
| | 13 | 10 | 134 | 1370 | 109 | 23265 | 154 | 9549 | 4376 | 162 |

Hospital, Address, Telephone, Administrator, Approval, Facility, and Physician Codes, Health Care System, Network	Classi-fication Codes		Utilization Data					Expense (thousands) of dollars		
★ American Hospital Association (AHA) membership □ Joint Commission on Accreditation of Healthcare Organizations (JCAHO) accreditation + American Osteopathic Hospital Association (AOHA) membership ○ American Osteopathic Association (AOA) accreditation △ Commission on Accreditation of Rehabilitation Facilities (CARF) accreditation Control codes 61, 63, 64, 71, 72 and 73 indicate hospitals listed by AOHA, but not registered by AHA. For definition of numerical codes, see page A4	Control	Service	Beds	Admissions	Census	Outpatient Visits	Births	Total	Payroll	Personnel

LANCASTER—Grant County

✠ LANCASTER MEMORIAL HOSPITAL, 507 South Monroe Street, Zip 53813; tel. 608/723–2143; Larry D. Rentfro, FACHE, Chief Executive Officer **A**1 9 10 **F**7 8 13 14 15 16 17 19 22 24 25 26 28 29 30 32 33 34 35 37 38 39 40 41 42 44 45 48 51 61 64 65 66 67 71 73 74 **P**5 **S** Brim, Inc., Portland, OR	14	10	28	774	6	24042	116	6514	2685	107

MADISON—Dane County

□ MENDOTA MENTAL HEALTH INSTITUTE, 301 Troy Drive, Zip 53704; tel. 608/243–2500; Steve Watters, Chief Executive Officer **A**1 3 5 10 **F**2 12 13 15 17 18 20 22 25 26 27 28 29 30 34 39 45 46 51 52 53 55 56 57 58 61 64 65 67 68 73	12	22	257	689	231	11560	0	35675	21819	655
✠ △ MERITER HOSPITAL, (Includes Meriter–Capitol), 202 South Park Street, Zip 53715–1599; tel. 608/267–6000; Terri L. Potter, President and Chief Executive Officer **A**1 2 3 5 7 9 10 **F**1 2 3 4 5 6 7 8 9 10 11 12 13 15 17 19 20 21 22 23 24 25 26 27 28 29 30 32 33 34 35 36 37 38 39 40 41 42 43 44 45 46 47 48 49 51 52 53 54 55 56 57 58 59 60 61 62 64 65 66 67 68 71 73 74	23	10	426	15505	221	142576	3154	150177	63894	1642
MERITER–CAPITOL See Meriter Hospital										
✠ ST. MARYS HOSPITAL MEDICAL CENTER, 707 South Mills Street, Zip 53715–0450; tel. 608/251–6100; Gerald W. Lefert, President **A**1 3 5 9 10 **F**1 4 7 8 10 11 12 13 15 17 18 19 20 21 22 23 24 25 26 27 28 29 30 32 33 34 35 37 38 39 40 41 43 44 45 46 47 49 51 52 53 54 55 56 57 59 60 61 64 65 66 67 68 70 71 73 **P**5 8 **S** SSM Health Care System, Saint Louis, MO **N** MEDACOM Tri–State, Oakbrook, IL; Health Care Network of Wisconsin (HCN), Brookfield, WI	23	10	319	17190	223	40536	2991	121470	52530	1234
✠ △ UNIVERSITY OF WISCONSIN HOSPITAL AND CLINICS, (Includes University of Wisconsin Children's Hospital), 600 Highland Avenue, Zip 53792; tel. 608/263–6400; Gordon M. Derzon, Chief Executive Officer **A**1 3 5 7 8 9 10 **F**3 4 5 8 9 10 11 12 13 14 16 17 19 20 21 22 23 24 25 26 28 29 30 31 32 34 35 37 39 40 41 42 43 44 45 46 47 48 49 50 51 52 53 54 55 56 57 58 60 61 63 64 65 66 67 69 70 71 72 73 74 **P**1 5 **N** University of Wisconsin Hospitals and Clinics, Madison, WI	12	10	482	19247	350	441912	0	288597	119686	3735
✠ WILLIAM S. MIDDLETON MEMORIAL VETERANS HOSPITAL, 2500 Overlook Terrace, Zip 53705–2286; tel. 608/256–1901; Nathan L. Geraths, Director (Nonreporting) **A**1 3 5 **S** Department of Veterans Affairs, Washington, DC	45	10	200	—	—	—	—	—	—	—

MANITOWOC—Manitowoc County

✠ △ HOLY FAMILY MEMORIAL MEDICAL CENTER, 2300 Western Avenue, Zip 54220, Mailing Address: P.O. Box 1450, Zip 54221–1450; tel. 414/684–2011; Daniel B. McGinty, President and Chief Executive Officer **A**1 7 9 10 **F**2 3 7 8 11 12 14 15 16 17 19 21 22 23 25 26 27 28 29 30 32 33 34 35 36 37 39 40 41 42 44 45 48 49 50 51 52 55 56 58 59 60 61 63 64 65 66 67 71 73 **P**6 **S** Franciscan Sisters of Christian Charity HealthCare Ministry, Inc, Manitowoc, WI	21	10	176	5379	75	135514	464	49815	22656	723

MARINETTE—Marinette County

□ BAY AREA MEDICAL CENTER, 3100 Shore Drive, Zip 54143–4297; tel. 715/735–6621; Rick Ament, President and Chief Executive Officer (Nonreporting) **A**1 9 10	23	10	115	—	—	—	—	—	—	—

MARSHFIELD—Wood County

NORWOOD HEALTH CENTER, 1600 North Chestnut Avenue, Zip 54449–1499; tel. 715/384–2188; Randy Bestul, Administrator **A**10 **F**12 52 53 57 58 61 64 65	13	22	19	530	9	0	0	1490	891	48
✠ △ SAINT JOSEPH'S HOSPITAL, 611 St. Joseph Avenue, Zip 54449–1898; tel. 715/387–1713; Michael A. Schmidt, President and Chief Executive Officer **A**1 2 3 5 7 9 10 **F**2 3 4 5 6 7 9 10 11 13 14 15 16 17 19 21 22 23 25 26 27 28 29 31 32 33 34 35 36 37 38 39 40 41 42 43 44 45 46 47 48 49 51 52 53 56 57 58 59 60 61 63 64 65 66 67 68 69 70 71 73 74 **P**8 **S** Sisters of the Sorrowful Mother United States Health System, Tulsa, OK	21	10	524	16847	270	115114	1060	154819	55564	1514

MAUSTON—Juneau County

□ MILE BLUFF MEDICAL CENTER, 1050 Division Street, Zip 53948; tel. 608/847–6161; Daniel N. Manders, President and Chief Executive Officer (Total facility includes 60 beds in nursing home–type unit) **A**1 9 10 **F**7 8 12 16 17 19 22 26 29 30 32 34 35 39 40 42 44 45 46 49 53 54 55 56 57 58 61 62 64 65 66 67 70 71 72 73 **P**5	23	10	97	2078	77	46208	221	17091	9343	249

MEDFORD—Taylor County

✠ MEMORIAL HOSPITAL OF TAYLOR COUNTY, (Includes Memorial Nursing Home), 135 South Gibson Street, Zip 54451–1696; tel. 715/748–8100; Greg Roraff, President and Chief Executive Officer (Total facility includes 104 beds in nursing home–type unit) **A**1 9 10 **F**1 6 7 8 11 16 17 19 21 22 27 28 29 30 34 35 37 40 41 44 45 46 49 51 54 56 61 63 64 65 67 71 **P**4	23	10	153	1068	114	22871	179	12552	6989	181

MENOMONEE FALLS—Waukesha County

✠ △ COMMUNITY MEMORIAL HOSPITAL, W180 N8085 Town Hall Road, Zip 53051, Mailing Address: P.O. Box 408, Zip 53052–0408; tel. 414/251–1000; Robert Eugene Drisner, President and Chief Executive Officer **A**1 2 7 9 10 **F**2 3 4 5 6 7 8 9 10 11 12 14 15 16 17 18 19 21 22 23 24 25 26 28 29 30 32 33 34 35 36 37 38 39 40 41 42 43 44 45 47 48 49 52 53 54 55 56 57 58 59 60 61 64 65 66 67 68 70 71 73 74 **S** Horizon Healthcare, Inc., Milwaukee, WI **N** Health Care Network of Wisconsin (HCN), Brookfield, WI; Horizon Healthcare, Inc., Milwaukee, WI	23	10	153	6684	83	40309	1002	50680	23352	775

Hospital, Address, Telephone, Administrator, Approval, Facility, and Physician Codes, Health Care System, Network	Control	Service	Beds	Admissions	Census	Outpatient Visits	Births	Total	Payroll	Personnel

Classi-fication Codes | Utilization Data | Expense (thousands) of dollars

★ American Hospital Association (AHA) membership
□ Joint Commission on Accreditation of Healthcare Organizations (JCAHO) accreditation
+ American Osteopathic Hospital Association (AOHA) membership
○ American Osteopathic Association (AOA) accreditation
△ Commission on Accreditation of Rehabilitation Facilities (CARF) accreditation
Control codes 61, 63, 64, 71, 72 and 73 indicate hospitals listed by AOHA, but not registered by AHA. For definition of numerical codes, see page A4

MENOMONIE—Dunn County

□ MYRTLE WERTH HOSPITAL–MAYO HEALTH SYSTEM, 2321 Stout Road, Zip 54751; tel. 715/235–5531; Thomas Miller, III, Chief Executive Officer **A**1 9 10 **F**1 7 8 11 15 19 21 22 34 35 37 39 40 41 44 45 63 65 66 71

| | 23 | 10 | 55 | 1617 | 15 | 28449 | 309 | 8756 | 4088 | 160 |

MEQUON—Ozaukee County

⊞ ST. MARY'S HOSPITAL OZAUKEE, 13111 North Port Washington Road, Zip 53097–2416; tel. 414/243–7300; Therese B. Pandl, Senior Vice President and Chief Operating Officer **A**1 9 10 **F**2 3 4 5 7 8 9 10 11 12 14 15 16 17 18 19 22 25 26 27 28 29 30 32 33 34 35 37 38 39 40 41 42 43 44 45 46 47 48 49 52 53 54 55 56 57 58 59 61 64 65 66 67 70 71 72 73 74 **P**1 2 5 6 7 8 **S** Daughters of Charity National Health System, Saint Louis, MO **N** Columbia – St. Mary's, Inc., Milwaukee, WI; Horizon Healthcare, Inc., Milwaukee, WI

| | 21 | 10 | 82 | 3990 | 49 | 131145 | 635 | 36926 | 17687 | 468 |

MERRILL—Lincoln County

⊞ GOOD SAMARITAN HEALTH CENTER OF MERRILL, 601 Center Avenue South, Zip 54452; tel. 715/536–5511; Michael Hammer, President and Chief Executive Officer **A**1 9 10 **F**1 3 4 5 7 8 9 10 11 12 14 15 17 18 19 21 22 23 26 28 29 30 32 33 34 35 36 37 39 40 41 42 44 45 47 49 53 54 55 56 57 58 59 61 64 65 66 67 68 70 71 73 74 **S** Catholic Health Initiatives, Denver, CO

| | 21 | 10 | 63 | 1578 | 24 | 42868 | 150 | 11108 | 4998 | 158 |

MILWAUKEE—Milwaukee County

CHARTER HOSPITAL OF MILWAUKEE, 11101 West Lincoln Avenue, Zip 53227; tel. 414/327–3000; Gary M. Gilberti, Chief Executive Officer **A**9 10 **F**1 2 3 12 14 15 16 17 18 25 26 28 29 34 39 45 46 52 53 54 55 56 57 58 59 61 64 65 68 **S** Magellan Health Services, Atlanta, GA

| | 33 | 22 | 80 | 1511 | 40 | — | 0 | 8348 | 3730 | 145 |

⊞ CHILDREN'S HOSPITAL OF WISCONSIN, 9000 West Wisconsin Avenue, Zip 53226, Mailing Address: P.O. Box 1997, Zip 53201–1997; tel. 414/266–2000; Jon E. Vice, President and Chief Executive Officer **A**1 3 5 8 9 10 **F**4 5 9 10 11 12 13 14 15 16 17 19 20 21 22 23 25 27 28 29 30 31 32 33 34 35 37 38 39 41 42 43 44 45 46 47 48 49 51 52 53 54 56 58 60 61 63 64 65 67 68 69 70 71 72 73 **P**4 **N** Health Care Network of Wisconsin (HCN), Brookfield, WI

| | 23 | 50 | 222 | 17476 | 171 | 199484 | 0 | 143989 | 49295 | 1403 |

⊞ CLEMENT J. ZABLOCKI VETERANS AFFAIRS MEDICAL CENTER, 5000 West National Avenue, Zip 53295–1000; tel. 414/384–2000; Russell E. Struble, Medical Center Director (Total facility includes 196 beds in nursing home–type unit) (Nonreporting) **A**1 2 3 5 8 **S** Department of Veterans Affairs, Washington, DC

| | 45 | 10 | 566 | — | — | — | — | — | — | — |

⊞ △ COLUMBIA HOSPITAL, 2025 East Newport Avenue, Zip 53211–2990; tel. 414/961–3300; Susan Henckel, Executive Vice President and Chief Executive Officer **A**1 2 3 5 7 9 10 **F**2 3 4 5 7 8 9 10 11 12 13 14 15 16 17 18 19 21 22 23 24 25 26 27 28 29 30 31 32 33 34 35 37 38 40 41 42 43 44 45 46 47 48 49 51 52 53 54 55 56 57 58 59 60 61 63 64 65 66 67 68 70 71 72 73 74 **P**6 **S** Horizon Healthcare, Inc., Milwaukee, WI **N** Health Care Network of Wisconsin (HCN), Brookfield, WI; Columbia – St. Mary's, Inc., Milwaukee, WI; Horizon Healthcare, Inc., Milwaukee, WI

| | 23 | 10 | 337 | 10894 | 170 | 199077 | 923 | 116842 | 48946 | 1378 |

DE PAUL HOSPITAL, 4143 South 13th Street, Zip 53221–1756; tel. 414/281–4400; Kathy M. Olewinski, Administrator **A**9 10 **F**2 3 12 15 17 18 25 29 31 34 39 41 45 51 52 53 58 61 64 65 67 **P**1

| | 23 | 82 | 36 | 768 | 11 | 29000 | 0 | 5731 | 2858 | 153 |

⊞ △ FROEDTERT MEMORIAL LUTHERAN HOSPITAL, 9200 West Wisconsin Avenue, Zip 53226–3596, Mailing Address: P.O. Box 26099, Zip 53226–3596; tel. 414/259–3000; William D. Petasnick, President **A**1 3 5 7 8 9 10 **F**1 2 3 4 5 7 10 11 12 14 16 19 21 22 23 25 26 29 31 32 33 34 35 36 37 39 40 41 42 43 44 45 46 48 49 52 54 55 56 57 58 60 61 62 63 64 65 66 69 70 71 72 74 **S** Horizon Healthcare, Inc., Milwaukee, WI **N** Health Care Network of Wisconsin (HCN), Brookfield, WI; Horizon Healthcare, Inc., Milwaukee, WI

| | 23 | 10 | 459 | 9843 | 172 | 131776 | 0 | 142881 | 39714 | 1206 |

⊞ MILWAUKEE COUNTY MENTAL HEALTH DIVISION, 9455 Watertown Plank Road, Zip 53226–3559; tel. 414/257–6995; M. Kathleen Eilers, Administrator (Total facility includes 340 beds in nursing home–type unit) **A**1 3 5 10 **F**2 3 4 7 9 10 11 12 13 14 17 18 19 20 21 22 23 25 26 27 29 30 31 35 36 38 39 40 42 43 44 45 47 48 51 52 53 56 57 58 59 61 64 65 67 68 69 70 71 72 73

| | 13 | 22 | 578 | 4918 | 457 | 116910 | 0 | 102673 | 55083 | 1313 |

MILWAUKEE PSYCHIATRIC HOSPITAL See Wauwatosa

○ NORTHWEST GENERAL HOSPITAL, 5310 West Capitol Drive, Zip 53216–2299; tel. 414/447–8543; C. Dennis Barr, President and Chief Executive Officer **A**9 10 11 **F**2 3 8 12 13 15 17 19 21 22 28 29 30 34 35 37 39 41 42 44 45 48 49 61 63 64 65 71 72

| | 23 | 10 | 98 | 2224 | 31 | 30599 | 0 | 11457 | 6018 | 213 |

⊞ △ SACRED HEART REHABILITATION INSTITUTE, 2350 North Lake Drive, Zip 53211, Mailing Address: P.O. Box 392, Zip 53201–0392; tel. 414/298–6700; William H. Lange, Administrator and Senior Vice President **A**1 7 9 10 **F**12 13 14 15 16 17 19 21 25 26 27 28 29 30 34 35 39 41 45 46 48 49 51 54 57 61 64 65 66 67 68 71 73 **P**5 6 8 **S** Horizon Healthcare, Inc., Milwaukee, WI **N** Columbia – St. Mary's, Inc., Milwaukee, WI

| | 21 | 46 | 69 | 858 | 45 | 9706 | 0 | 15273 | 8324 | 313 |

⊞ △ SINAI SAMARITAN MEDICAL CENTER, (Includes Sinai Samaritan Medical Center–East Campus, 945 North 12th Street, Sinai Samaritan Medical Center–West Campus, 2000 West Kilbourn Avenue), 945 North 12th Street, Zip 53233, Mailing Address: P.O. Box 342, Zip 53201–0342; tel. 414/219–2000; William I. Jenkins, President and Chief Executive Officer **A**1 2 3 5 7 8 9 10 **F**1 2 3 4 5 7 8 10 11 12 13 14 15 16 17 18 19 20 21 22 23 24 25 26 27 28 29 30 31 32 33 34 35 36 37 38 39 40 41 42 43 44 45 46 47 48 49 51 52 53 54 55 58 59 60 61 63 64 65 66 67 68 70 71 72 73 74 **P**4 7 **S** Aurora Health Care, Milwaukee, WI **N** Health Care Network of Wisconsin (HCN), Brookfield, WI; Aurora Health Care, Milwaukee, WI

| | 23 | 10 | 192 | 15852 | 219 | 275319 | 3860 | 184827 | 67743 | 1932 |

SINAI SAMARITAN MEDICAL CENTER–EAST CAMPUS See Sinai Samaritan Medical Center

SINAI SAMARITAN MEDICAL CENTER–WEST CAMPUS See Sinai Samaritan Medical Center

Hospital, Address, Telephone, Administrator, Approval, Facility, and Physician Codes, Health Care System, Network	Classi-fication Codes		Utilization Data					Expense (thousands) of dollars		
	Control	Service	Beds	Admissions	Census	Outpatient Visits	Births	Total	Payroll	Personnel

★ American Hospital Association (AHA) membership
□ Joint Commission on Accreditation of Healthcare Organizations (JCAHO) accreditation
+ American Osteopathic Hospital Association (AOHA) membership
○ American Osteopathic Association (AOA) accreditation
△ Commission on Accreditation of Rehabilitation Facilities (CARF) accreditation
Control codes 61, 63, 64, 71, 72 and 73 indicate hospitals listed by AOHA, but not registered by AHA. For definition of numerical codes, see page A4

Hospital	Control	Service	Beds	Admissions	Census	Outpatient Visits	Births	Total	Payroll	Personnel
✠ △ ST. FRANCIS HOSPITAL, 3237 South 16th Street, Zip 53215–4592; tel. 414/647–5000; Gregory A. Banaszynski, President **A**1 2 5 7 9 10 **F**2 3 4 5 6 7 8 9 10 11 12 13 14 15 16 17 18 19 20 21 22 23 25 26 27 28 29 30 32 33 34 35 36 37 38 39 40 41 42 43 44 45 46 48 49 51 52 53 54 55 56 57 58 59 60 61 62 63 64 65 66 67 68 70 71 72 73 74 **P**5 6 7 8 **S** Wheaton Franciscan Services, Inc., Wheaton, IL **N** Felician Health Care, Inc., Chicago, IL; Health Care Network of Wisconsin (HCN), Brookfield, WI; Covenant Healthcare System, Inc., Milwaukee, WI	23	10	265	9584	149	97012	1315	86993	35712	1105
✠ ST. JOSEPH'S HOSPITAL, 5000 West Chambers Street, Zip 53210–9988; tel. 414/447–2000; Jon L. Wachs, President **A**1 2 3 5 9 10 **F**1 2 3 4 5 6 7 8 9 10 11 12 13 15 17 18 19 21 22 23 24 25 26 27 28 29 30 31 32 33 34 35 37 38 39 40 41 42 43 44 45 46 48 49 52 53 54 55 56 57 58 59 60 61 63 64 65 66 67 68 70 71 73 74 **P**5 7 **S** Wheaton Franciscan Services, Inc., Wheaton, IL **N** Health Care Network of Wisconsin (HCN), Brookfield, WI; Covenant Healthcare System, Inc., Milwaukee, WI	21	10	484	21217	326	139746	3899	165612	65857	2098
✠ △ ST. LUKE'S MEDICAL CENTER, (Includes St. Luke's South Shore, 5900 South Lake Drive, Cudahy, Zip 53110–8903; tel. 414/769–9000; Terrance E. Wilson, Executive Director), 2900 West Oklahoma Avenue, Zip 53215, Mailing Address: P.O. Box 2901, Zip 53201; tel. 414/649–6000; Mark R. Ambrosius, President (Nonreporting) **A**1 2 3 5 7 8 9 10 **S** Aurora Health Care, Milwaukee, WI **N** National Cardiovascular Network, Atlanta, GA; Health Care Network of Wisconsin (HCN), Brookfield, WI; Aurora Health Care, Milwaukee, WI	23	10	546	—	—	—	—	—	—	—
✠ △ ST. MARY'S HOSPITAL, 2323 North Lake Drive, Zip 53211–9682, Mailing Address: P.O. Box 503, Zip 53201–0503; tel. 414/291–1000; Charles C. Lobeck, Chief Executive Officer **A**1 2 3 5 9 10 **F**3 4 7 8 9 10 11 12 13 14 15 16 17 18 19 21 22 25 26 27 28 29 30 32 34 35 37 38 39 40 41 42 43 44 45 51 53 54 57 58 59 61 63 64 65 66 67 71 72 73 74 **P**5 6 **S** Daughters of Charity National Health System, Saint Louis, MO **N** Health Care Network of Wisconsin (HCN), Brookfield, WI; Columbia – St. Mary's, Inc., Milwaukee, WI; Horizon Healthcare, Inc., Milwaukee, WI	21	10	257	8636	136	271531	2252	121679	56065	1604
✠ △ ST. MICHAEL HOSPITAL, 2400 West Villard Avenue, Zip 53209; tel. 414/527–8000; Jeffrey K. Jenkins, President **A**1 3 5 7 9 10 **F**2 3 4 7 8 10 12 14 16 18 19 21 22 23 24 25 26 29 32 33 34 35 37 38 39 40 41 42 43 44 45 46 48 49 52 53 54 55 56 57 58 59 60 61 63 64 65 66 70 71 74 **P**7 **S** Wheaton Franciscan Services, Inc., Wheaton, IL **N** Health Care Network of Wisconsin (HCN), Brookfield, WI; Covenant Healthcare System, Inc., Milwaukee, WI	21	10	152	9086	132	137254	906	83028	33249	1004
VENCOR HOSPITAL–MILWAUKEE, 5700 West Layton Avenue, Zip 53202; tel. 414/325–5900; E. Kay Gray, Interim Administrator (Nonreporting) **S** Vencor, Incorporated, Louisville, KY	33	49	60	—	—	—	—	—	—	—

MONROE—Green County

Hospital	Control	Service	Beds	Admissions	Census	Outpatient Visits	Births	Total	Payroll	Personnel
□ THE MONROE CLINIC, 515 22nd Avenue, Zip 53566–1598; tel. 608/324–1000; Kenneth Blount, President **A**1 9 10 **F**3 5 7 8 10 11 14 15 16 17 18 19 21 22 23 24 25 26 28 29 30 32 33 34 37 39 40 41 42 44 45 46 47 48 49 51 53 56 57 58 61 63 64 65 66 67 71 72 73 74 **P**6 8 **S** Congregation of St. Agnes, Fond Du Lac, WI	21	10	117	3701	42	219643	365	53797	28295	707

NEENAH—Winnebago County

Hospital	Control	Service	Beds	Admissions	Census	Outpatient Visits	Births	Total	Payroll	Personnel
✠ △ THEDA CLARK MEDICAL CENTER, 130 Second Street, Zip 54956, Mailing Address: P.O. Box 2021, Zip 54957–2021; tel. 414/729–3100; Paul E. Macek, Senior Vice President **A**1 7 9 10 **F**2 3 4 5 6 7 8 10 11 12 14 15 16 17 18 19 21 22 23 24 25 26 28 29 30 32 34 35 36 37 38 39 40 41 42 43 44 45 46 48 49 51 52 53 54 55 56 57 58 59 60 61 62 64 65 66 67 69 70 71 72 73 74 **P**6 8 **S** United Health Group, Appleton, WI	23	10	216	9102	128	62564	1415	67879	32071	997

NEILLSVILLE—Clark County

Hospital	Control	Service	Beds	Admissions	Census	Outpatient Visits	Births	Total	Payroll	Personnel
MEMORIAL MEDICAL CENTER, (Includes Neillsville Memorial Home), 216 Sunset Place, Zip 54456; tel. 715/743–3101; Glen E. Grady, Administrator (Total facility includes 145 beds in nursing home–type unit) **A**9 10 **F**4 6 7 8 10 15 16 17 18 19 21 22 23 24 25 26 28 29 30 32 33 34 35 36 39 40 41 42 43 44 45 46 49 51 53 54 55 56 57 58 59 60 61 62 64 65 70 71 72 73 **P**6	23	10	174	1064	138	39484	29	9222	4970	253

NEW LONDON—Outagamie County

Hospital	Control	Service	Beds	Admissions	Census	Outpatient Visits	Births	Total	Payroll	Personnel
✠ NEW LONDON FAMILY MEDICAL CENTER, 1405 Mill Street, Zip 54961, Mailing Address: P.O. Box 307, Zip 54961; tel. 414/982–5330; Paul E. Gurgel, President and Chief Executive Officer **A**1 9 10 **F**7 8 11 16 17 19 22 26 29 30 34 37 39 40 41 44 45 48 49 61 64 71 72 73	23	10	52	1385	15	55688	136	9427	4196	128

NEW RICHMOND—St. Croix County

Hospital	Control	Service	Beds	Admissions	Census	Outpatient Visits	Births	Total	Payroll	Personnel
★ HOLY FAMILY HOSPITAL, 535 Hospital Road, Zip 54017; tel. 715/246–2101; Jean M. Needham, President **A**9 10 **F**7 8 11 12 15 18 19 21 22 24 26 28 29 30 32 33 34 35 36 39 40 41 42 44 45 46 49 51 61 63 64 65 66 71	21	10	20	1363	12	11471	153	6395	2987	96

OCONOMOWOC—Waukesha County

Hospital	Control	Service	Beds	Admissions	Census	Outpatient Visits	Births	Total	Payroll	Personnel
✠ △ MEMORIAL HOSPITAL OCONOMOWOC, (Formerly Memorial Hospital at Oconomowoc), 791 Summit Avenue, Zip 53066–3896; tel. 414/569–9400; Douglas Guy, President and Chief Executive Officer **A**1 7 9 10 **F**1 2 3 6 7 8 11 13 14 15 16 17 19 20 21 22 24 26 27 28 29 30 31 32 33 34 35 37 39 40 41 42 44 45 46 48 49 51 56 61 63 64 65 67 68 70 71 73 74 **P**5 6 8 **S** Horizon Healthcare, Inc., Milwaukee, WI **N** Health Care Network of Wisconsin (HCN), Brookfield, WI; Horizon Healthcare, Inc., Milwaukee, WI	23	10	73	2845	28	70480	540	30236	14541	391
□ ROGERS MEMORIAL HOSPITAL, 34700 Valley Road, Zip 53066–4599; tel. 414/646–4411; David L. Moulthrop, Ph.D., President and Chief Executive Officer **A**1 9 10 **F**3 12 14 15 16 17 18 19 25 26 27 29 30 34 35 39 45 46 52 53 54 55 56 57 58 59 61 64 65 67	23	22	90	1086	58	4304	0	10440	5394	184

Hospital, Address, Telephone, Administrator, Approval, Facility, and Physician Codes, Health Care System, Network	Classi-fication Codes		Utilization Data					Expense (thousands) of dollars		
★ American Hospital Association (AHA) membership □ Joint Commission on Accreditation of Healthcare Organizations (JCAHO) accreditation + American Osteopathic Hospital Association (AOHA) membership ○ American Osteopathic Association (AOA) accreditation △ Commission on Accreditation of Rehabilitation Facilities (CARF) accreditation Control codes 61, 63, 64, 71, 72 and 73 indicate hospitals listed by AOHA, but not registered by AHA. For definition of numerical codes, see page A4	Control	Service	Beds	Admissions	Census	Outpatient Visits	Births	Total	Payroll	Personnel

OCONTO—Oconto County

★ OCONTO MEMORIAL HOSPITAL, 405 First Street, Zip 54153; tel. 414/834–8800; Steve Dewoody, Chief Executive Officer **A**9 10 **F**1 3 4 5 6 7 8 10 12 15 18 19 21 22 24 26 27 28 29 30 32 33 34 36 39 43 44 45 46 51 53 54 55 56 57 58 59 60 61 62 64 65 66 67 68 71 73 74 **S** Quorum Health Group/Quorum Health Resources, Inc., Brentwood, TN
| 23 | 10 | 17 | 459 | 7 | 12404 | 0 | 3235 | 1575 | 57 |

OCONTO FALLS—Oconto County

COMMUNITY MEMORIAL HOSPITAL, 855 South Main Street, Zip 54154; tel. 414/846–3444; Thomas R. Bayer, Administrator **A**9 10 **F**3 7 8 12 15 17 19 22 25 26 28 29 30 32 34 37 39 40 41 44 45 46 47 48 49 51 61 64 65 67 68 70 71 72 73 74 **P**5 **N** Health Care Network of Wisconsin (HCN), Brookfield, WI
| 23 | 10 | 26 | 881 | 11 | 23798 | 55 | 8254 | 4179 | 139 |

OSCEOLA—Polk County

OSCEOLA MEDICAL CENTER, 301 River Street, Zip 54020, Mailing Address: P.O. Box 218, Zip 54020; tel. 715/294–2111; Jeffrey K. Meyer, Administrator and Chief Executive Officer (Total facility includes 40 beds in nursing home–type unit) **A**9 10 **F**7 8 11 17 19 22 28 29 32 33 34 37 40 41 42 44 45 46 48 49 51 61 64 65 67 71 73 **P**5
| 23 | 10 | 59 | 539 | 44 | 15473 | 70 | 4579 | 2583 | 89 |

OSHKOSH—Winnebago County

⊞ △ MERCY MEDICAL CENTER, 631 Hazel Street, Zip 54902, Mailing Address: P.O. Box 1100, Zip 54902–1100; tel. 414/236–2000; Otto L. Cox, President and Chief Executive Officer **A**1 2 3 7 9 10 **F**3 4 5 7 8 9 10 11 12 18 19 21 22 23 25 26 29 32 33 34 35 36 37 40 41 42 43 44 45 46 47 48 49 52 53 54 55 56 57 58 59 61 63 64 65 66 70 71 72 **P**4 5 **S** Sisters of the Sorrowful Mother United States Health System, Tulsa, OK **N** Affinity Health System, Inc., Oshkosh, WI
| 21 | 10 | 232 | 8068 | 113 | 358439 | 654 | 70093 | 32002 | 940 |

OSSEO—Trempealeau County

OSSEO AREA HOSPITAL AND NURSING HOME, 13025 Eighth Street, Zip 54758, Mailing Address: P.O. Box 70, Zip 54758; tel. 715/597–3121; Bradley D. Groseth, Administrator (Total facility includes 67 beds in nursing home–type unit) **A**10 **F**11 19 22 26 29 32 33 34 37 41 44 45 46 47 49 61 62 64 65 69 71 **P**8 **S** Mayo Foundation, Rochester, MN **N** Luther/Midelfort/Mayo Health System, Eau Claire, WI
| 23 | 10 | 75 | 182 | 62 | 8680 | 0 | — | — | — |

PARK FALLS—Price County

⊞ FLAMBEAU HOSPITAL, 98 Sherry Avenue, Zip 54552, Mailing Address: P.O. Box 310, Zip 54552; tel. 715/762–2484; Curtis A. Johnson, Administrator **A**1 9 10 **F**7 8 9 11 12 15 19 21 22 29 32 33 34 37 38 39 40 42 44 45 46 47 49 61 64 71 **P**8 **S** Sisters of the Sorrowful Mother United States Health System, Tulsa, OK **N** Marshfield Clinic's Regional System, Marshfield, WI; Northern Lakes Health Consortium, Duluth, MN
| 23 | 10 | 42 | 1049 | 14 | 24177 | 116 | 9200 | 4443 | 161 |

PHELPS—Vilas County

NORTHWOODS HOSPITAL, Mailing Address: P.O. Box 126, Zip 54554; tel. 715/545–2313; Judson Schultz, Executive Director (Total facility includes 77 beds in nursing home–type unit) **A**9 10 **F**8 14 16 17 19 20 26 28 29 30 32 34 39 41 44 45 46 48 49 51 61 62 64 65 67 71 72 73 **P**5
| 23 | 10 | 82 | 86 | 70 | 5111 | 0 | — | — | 89 |

PLATTEVILLE—Grant County

⊞ SOUTHWEST HEALTH CENTER, (Includes Cuba City Medical Center, 808 South Washington Street, Cuba City, Zip 53807; tel. 608/744–2161; Hazel Green Hospital, 2110 Church Street, Hazel Green, Zip 53811; tel. 608/854–2231), 1100 Fifth Avenue, Zip 53818; tel. 608/348–2331; Anne K. Klawiter, Chief Executive Officer (Total facility includes 104 beds in nursing home–type unit) **A**1 9 10 **F**6 7 8 15 17 19 20 22 26 28 29 30 32 34 35 36 39 40 44 45 61 64 65 67 71 **S** Brim, Inc., Portland, OR
| 23 | 10 | 118 | 1306 | 105 | 17476 | 165 | 11400 | 4094 | 176 |

PLYMOUTH—Sheboygan County

⊞ VALLEY VIEW MEDICAL CENTER, 901 Reed Street, Zip 53073–2409; tel. 414/893–1771; Patrick J. Trotter, President (Total facility includes 60 beds in nursing home–type unit) **A**1 9 10 **F**7 8 11 12 13 14 15 16 17 19 21 22 26 28 29 30 32 33 34 35 36 37 39 40 41 42 44 45 46 48 49 51 61 62 63 64 65 67 68 70 71 72 74 **P**6 **S** Aurora Health Care, Milwaukee, WI **N** Health Care Network of Wisconsin (HCN), Brookfield, WI; Aurora Health Care, Milwaukee, WI
| 23 | 10 | 92 | 1033 | 70 | 26929 | 160 | 10635 | 4649 | 164 |

PORT WASHINGTON—Ozaukee County

ST. MARY'S HOSPITAL OZAUKEE See Mequon

PORTAGE—Columbia County

⊞ DIVINE SAVIOR HOSPITAL AND NURSING HOME, 1015 West Pleasant Street, Zip 53901–9987, Mailing Address: P.O. Box 387, Zip 53901; tel. 608/742–4131; Michael Decker, President and Chief Executive Officer (Total facility includes 111 beds in nursing home–type unit) **A**1 9 10 **F**2 3 7 8 11 13 15 17 19 20 21 22 25 26 27 28 29 30 34 35 36 37 39 40 41 42 44 45 49 51 56 61 63 64 65 66 67 68 70 71 73 **P**8 **S** Principal Hospital Group, Brentwood, TN
| 21 | 10 | 160 | 2102 | 123 | 36080 | 187 | 18381 | 8313 | 272 |

PRAIRIE DU CHIEN—Crawford County

⊞ PRAIRIE DU CHIEN MEMORIAL HOSPITAL, 705 East Taylor Street, Zip 53821; tel. 608/326–2431; Harold W. Brown, Chief Executive Officer **A**1 9 10 **F**1 2 3 6 7 8 11 12 13 14 15 16 17 19 22 26 27 28 29 30 32 33 34 35 36 37 39 40 41 42 44 45 46 49 53 54 56 58 59 61 62 65 67 68 71 73 **N** Mississippi Valley Health Partnership, Prairie du Chien, WI
| 23 | 10 | 43 | 1419 | 31 | 17645 | 153 | 10206 | 5040 | 184 |

Hospital, Address, Telephone, Administrator, Approval, Facility, and Physician Codes, Health Care System, Network	Classi-fication Codes		Utilization Data					Expense (thousands) of dollars		
	Control	Service	Beds	Admissions	Census	Outpatient Visits	Births	Total	Payroll	Personnel

★ American Hospital Association (AHA) membership
□ Joint Commission on Accreditation of Healthcare Organizations (JCAHO) accreditation
+ American Osteopathic Hospital Association (AOHA) membership
○ American Osteopathic Association (AOA) accreditation
△ Commission on Accreditation of Rehabilitation Facilities (CARF) accreditation
Control codes 61, 63, 64, 71, 72 and 73 indicate hospitals listed by AOHA, but not registered by AHA. For definition of numerical codes, see page A4

PRAIRIE DU SAC—Sauk County

☒ SAUK PRAIRIE MEMORIAL HOSPITAL, 80 First Street, Zip 53578–1550; tel. 608/643–3311; Bobbe Teigen, Administrator **A**1 9 10 **F**2 7 8 11 12 13 14 15 16 17 19 20 21 22 24 25 26 27 28 29 30 31 32 33 34 35 36 37 39 40 41 42 44 45 48 49 51 54 56 57 61 63 64 65 66 67 68 70 71 72 73 **P**8 — 23 10 36 2166 22 36051 193 19772 9356 294

RACINE—Racine County

☒ △ SAINT MARY'S MEDICAL CENTER, 3801 Spring Street, Zip 53405; tel. 414/636–4011; Edward P. Demeulenaere, President and Chief Executive Officer **A**1 7 9 10 **F**2 3 4 7 8 10 11 12 13 14 15 16 17 19 21 22 23 24 25 26 28 29 30 32 33 34 35 37 38 39 40 41 42 43 44 45 46 47 48 49 51 52 53 54 55 56 57 58 59 60 61 64 65 66 67 68 71 72 73 74 **P**6 **S** Wheaton Franciscan Services, Inc., Wheaton, IL **N** All Saints Healthcare System, Racine, WI — 21 10 226 8807 125 213261 0 74536 31897 1846

☒ ST. LUKE'S MEMORIAL HOSPITAL, (Includes St. Luke's Hospital), 1320 Wisconsin Avenue, Zip 53403–1987; tel. 414/636–2011; Edward P. Demeulenaere, President and Chief Executive Officer (Total facility includes 41 beds in nursing home–type unit) **A**1 2 5 9 10 **F**2 3 4 7 10 11 12 14 16 19 21 22 23 24 26 29 32 33 34 35 38 39 40 41 42 43 44 45 46 47 48 49 52 53 54 55 56 57 58 59 60 61 64 65 66 71 72 74 **P**6 **S** Wheaton Franciscan Services, Inc., Wheaton, IL **N** Health Care Network of Wisconsin (HCN), Brookfield, WI; All Saints Healthcare System, Racine, WI — 23 10 183 4565 114 105564 2005 — — —

REEDSBURG—Sauk County

□ REEDSBURG AREA MEDICAL CENTER, 2000 North Dewey Street, Zip 53959; tel. 608/524–6487; George L. Johnson, President (Total facility includes 49 beds in nursing home–type unit) **A**1 9 10 **F**4 7 8 10 11 12 13 15 16 17 18 19 20 21 22 24 27 28 29 30 32 33 34 36 37 39 40 41 42 44 45 47 49 51 61 64 65 66 67 68 70 71 73 **P**5 6 8 — 23 10 71 1969 67 37216 185 15235 6676 212

RHINELANDER—Oneida County

☒ SACRED HEART–ST. MARY'S HOSPITALS, (Includes Sacred Heart Hospital, 216 North Seventh Street, Tomahawk, Zip 54487; tel. 715/453–7700; St. Mary's Hospital, Mailing Address: 1044 Kabel Avenue), 1044 Kabel Avenue, Zip 54501–3998, Mailing Address: P.O. Box 20, Zip 54501; tel. 715/369–6600; Kevin J. O'Donnell, President and Chief Executive Officer **A**1 9 10 **F**2 3 7 8 11 12 15 16 19 22 23 24 26 29 32 33 34 35 36 37 39 40 41 42 44 45 46 49 52 53 54 55 56 57 58 59 60 61 63 64 65 66 71 **P**5 **S** Sisters of the Sorrowful Mother United States Health System, Tulsa, OK — 21 10 51 4651 53 37811 414 34535 16918 559

RICE LAKE—Barron County

☒ LAKEVIEW MEDICAL CENTER, 1100 North Main Street, Zip 54868–1238; tel. 715/234–1515; Edward H. Wolf, Chief Executive Officer **A**1 9 10 **F**7 11 15 16 17 19 22 24 26 29 30 32 33 34 35 36 37 39 40 41 44 45 49 51 61 63 64 65 66 67 68 71 73 **N** Northern Lakes Health Consortium, Duluth, MN — 23 10 68 2801 29 23250 444 17716 8731 255

RICHLAND CENTER—Richland County

□ RICHLAND HOSPITAL, 431 North Park Street, Zip 53581; tel. 608/647–6321; Thomas J. Werner, Administrator (Nonreporting) **A**1 9 10 — 23 10 38 — — — — — — —

RIPON—Fond Du Lac County

☒ RIPON MEDICAL CENTER, 933 Newbury Street, Zip 54971, Mailing Address: P.O. Box 390, Zip 54971–0390; tel. 414/748–3101; Jon W. Baker, Administrator and Chief Executive Officer **A**1 9 10 **F**7 8 11 12 15 16 19 21 22 26 29 34 35 37 39 40 41 42 44 45 46 47 49 54 58 61 63 64 65 66 70 71 72 74 **S** Brim, Inc., Portland, OR — 23 10 29 1104 12 26743 95 9678 3693 128

RIVER FALLS—St. Croix County

☒ RIVER FALLS AREA HOSPITAL, 1629 East Division Street, Zip 54022–1571; tel. 715/425–6155; Sharon Whelan, President **A**1 9 10 **F**7 11 13 14 15 16 17 19 20 21 22 26 27 28 29 30 32 33 34 35 36 37 39 40 44 45 46 47 48 49 51 61 63 65 66 67 68 71 72 73 **P**6 8 **S** Allina Health System, Minneapolis, MN **N** Allina Health System, Minnetonka, MN — 23 10 36 914 8 10250 223 9044 3547 94

SAINT CROIX FALLS—Polk County

□ ST. CROIX VALLEY MEMORIAL HOSPITAL, 204 South Adams Street, Zip 54024; tel. 715/483–3261; Steve L. Urosevich, Chief Executive Officer **A**1 9 10 **F**3 6 7 8 11 15 18 19 21 22 24 26 29 32 33 34 35 37 40 41 42 44 45 46 47 52 53 54 56 57 58 61 63 64 65 66 70 71 74 **N** Health Care Network of Wisconsin (HCN), Brookfield, WI — 23 10 69 1950 16 — 287 11315 5461 168

SHAWANO—Shawano County

☒ SHAWANO MEDICAL CENTER, 309 North Bartlette Street, Zip 54166–2199; tel. 715/526–2111; John J. Kestly, Administrator **A**1 9 10 **F**7 8 10 11 14 15 16 17 19 21 22 26 29 30 32 33 34 35 37 39 40 44 45 46 48 51 56 61 63 64 65 66 67 71 73 74 **P**5 **S** Brim, Inc., Portland, OR — 23 10 46 2525 25 38819 335 14271 6199 214

SHEBOYGAN—Sheboygan County

☒ △ SHEBOYGAN MEMORIAL MEDICAL CENTER, 2629 North Seventh Street, Zip 53083–4998; tel. 414/451–5000; Patrick J. Trotter, President **A**1 2 7 9 10 **F**2 3 5 7 8 10 11 12 15 16 17 19 21 22 23 26 28 29 30 34 35 37 39 40 41 42 44 45 46 47 48 49 52 53 54 55 56 57 58 61 63 64 65 66 67 70 71 73 74 **S** Aurora Health Care, Milwaukee, WI **N** Health Care Network of Wisconsin (HCN), Brookfield, WI; Aurora Health Care, Milwaukee, WI — 23 10 138 5135 60 38021 896 34381 14237 484

☒ △ ST. NICHOLAS HOSPITAL, 1601 North Taylor Drive, Zip 53081–2496; tel. 414/459–8300; Michael J. Stenger, Executive Vice President and Administrator **A**1 2 7 9 10 **F**3 7 8 10 11 12 13 14 16 17 18 19 20 21 22 23 24 26 27 28 29 30 32 33 34 35 36 37 39 40 41 42 44 45 46 48 49 51 54 56 58 60 61 63 64 65 66 67 68 69 70 71 72 73 74 **P**5 **S** Hospital Sisters Health System, Springfield, IL **N** Covenant Healthcare System, Inc., Milwaukee, WI — 21 10 84 3250 44 109328 343 31174 11718 411

Hospital, Address, Telephone, Administrator, Approval, Facility, and Physician Codes, Health Care System, Network	Classi-fication Codes		Utilization Data					Expense (thousands) of dollars		
	Control	Service	Beds	Admissions	Census	Outpatient Visits	Births	Total	Payroll	Personnel

★ American Hospital Association (AHA) membership
☐ Joint Commission on Accreditation of Healthcare Organizations (JCAHO) accreditation
+ American Osteopathic Hospital Association (AOHA) membership
○ American Osteopathic Association (AOA) accreditation
△ Commission on Accreditation of Rehabilitation Facilities (CARF) accreditation
Control codes 61, 63, 64, 71, 72 and 73 indicate hospitals listed by AOHA, but not registered by AHA. For definition of numerical codes, see page A4

SHELL LAKE—Washburn County

☐ INDIANHEAD MEDICAL CENTER, 215 Fourth Avenue West, Zip 54871; tel. 715/468–7833; Larry Abrams, Administrator **A**1 9 10 **F**7 11 15 19 20 22 26 27 28 29 30 34 35 37 40 42 44 45 46 51 61 64 65 67 68 71 73 **P**5	33	10	49	704	7	6231	38	2765	1306	56

SPARTA—Monroe County

✠ FRANCISCAN SKEMP HEALTHCARE–SPARTA CAMPUS, 310 West Main Street, Zip 54656; tel. 608/269–2132; William P. Sexton, Administrator (Total facility includes 30 beds in nursing home–type unit) (Nonreporting) **A**1 9 10 **S** Franciscan Skemp Healthcare, La Crosse, WI **N** Franciscan Skemp Healthcare, LaCrosse, WI	21	10	60	—	—	—	—	—	—	—

SPOONER—Washburn County

✠ COMMUNITY MEMORIAL HOSPITAL AND NURSING HOME, 819 Ash Street, Zip 54801; tel. 715/635–2111; Michael Schafer, Chief Executive Officer (Total facility includes 90 beds in nursing home–type unit) **A**1 9 10 **F**2 7 8 11 12 13 16 17 19 21 22 26 27 28 29 30 32 33 34 36 37 40 41 42 44 45 48 50 51 61 63 64 65 66 67 71 73 **S** Brim, Inc., Portland, OR **N** Northern Lakes Health Consortium, Duluth, MN	23	10	136	1009	98	18604	110	7891	4400	128

STANLEY—Chippewa County

✠ VICTORY MEDICAL CENTER, 230 East Fourth Avenue, Zip 54768; tel. 715/644–5571; Cynthia Eichman, Chief Executive Officer and Administrator (Total facility includes 86 beds in nursing home–type unit) **A**1 9 10 **F**1 7 8 11 15 19 20 21 22 25 28 29 30 32 33 34 37 39 40 41 44 45 46 49 51 56 61 64 65 66 67 69 71 **P**5 8 **S** Sisters of the Sorrowful Mother United States Health System, Tulsa, OK	21	10	127	672	88	18056	55	6403	3317	151

STEVENS POINT—Portage County

✠ SAINT MICHAEL'S HOSPITAL, 900 Illinois Avenue, Zip 54481; tel. 715/346–5000; Jeffrey L. Martin, President and Chief Executive Officer **A**1 9 10 **F**2 7 8 11 14 15 16 17 19 21 22 23 25 26 28 29 30 34 35 36 37 38 39 40 41 42 44 45 46 47 49 51 52 53 54 55 56 57 61 63 64 65 66 67 71 73 **S** Sisters of the Sorrowful Mother United States Health System, Tulsa, OK	21	10	104	4319	45	44967	749	34077	13732	419

STOUGHTON—Dane County

☐ STOUGHTON HOSPITAL ASSOCIATION, 900 Ridge Street, Zip 53589–1896; tel. 608/873–6611; Terrence Brenny, President **A**1 9 10 **F**1 2 3 8 11 14 16 17 19 22 26 28 29 31 32 33 34 37 41 42 44 45 46 48 49 51 54 61 63 64 65 66 67 68 71 72 73	23	10	41	1430	19	39508	0	11935	5155	178

STURGEON BAY—Door County

✠ DOOR COUNTY MEMORIAL HOSPITAL, 330 South 16th Place, Zip 54235–1495; tel. 414/743–5566; Gerald M. Worrick, President and Administrator (Total facility includes 30 beds in nursing home–type unit) **A**1 9 10 **F**1 3 4 7 8 10 11 14 15 16 19 21 22 25 26 29 31 32 33 34 35 37 39 40 41 42 43 44 45 46 48 49 53 54 55 61 64 65 69 70 71 72 73 **P**6	23	10	77	2080	55	28669	185	—	—	343

SUPERIOR—Douglas County

☐ ST. MARY'S HOSPITAL OF SUPERIOR, 3500 Tower Avenue, Zip 54880–5395; tel. 715/392–8281; Terry Jacobson, Administrator (Nonreporting) **A**1 9 10 **S** Benedictine Health System, Duluth, MN **N** Health Care Network of Wisconsin (HCN), Brookfield, WI	23	10	42	—	—	—	—	—	—	—

TOMAH—Monroe County

☐ TOMAH MEMORIAL HOSPITAL, 321 Butts Avenue, Zip 54660, Mailing Address: Box 590, Zip 54660–0590; tel. 608/372–2181; Philip Stuart, Administrator **A**1 9 10 **F**2 3 7 9 11 12 16 17 19 22 26 28 29 30 33 34 35 36 38 39 40 41 44 45 52 61 64 65 67 71 **P**5 **N** Lutheran Health System, LaCrosse, WI	23	10	45	1077	11	21813	197	7734	3526	130
✠ VETERANS AFFAIRS MEDICAL CENTER, 500 East Veterans Street, Zip 54660–9225; tel. 608/372–3971; Stan Johnson, Medical Center Director (Total facility includes 100 beds in nursing home–type unit) (Nonreporting) **A**1 **S** Department of Veterans Affairs, Washington, DC	45	22	569	—	—	—	—	—	—	—

TOMAHAWK—Lincoln County

SACRED HEART HOSPITAL See Sacred Heart–St. Mary's Hospitals, Rhinelander

TWO RIVERS—Manitowoc County

✠ TWO RIVERS COMMUNITY HOSPITAL AND HAMILTON MEMORIAL HOME, 2500 Garfield Street, Zip 54241; tel. 414/793–1178; Steven H. Spencer, President and Chief Executive Officer (Total facility includes 85 beds in nursing home–type unit) **A**1 9 10 **F**7 8 10 11 12 14 15 17 19 22 25 26 28 29 30 33 34 35 36 37 39 40 41 44 45 46 47 48 49 51 61 64 65 67 71 73 **S** Aurora Health Care, Milwaukee, WI **N** Aurora Health Care, Milwaukee, WI	23	10	138	1568	99	20410	283	13814	6299	239

VIROQUA—Vernon County

VERNON MEMORIAL HOSPITAL, 507 South Main Street, Zip 54665; tel. 608/637–2101; Garith W. Steiner, Chief Executive Officer **A**9 10 **F**2 3 7 8 12 13 14 15 16 17 19 22 24 26 28 29 30 32 33 34 39 40 41 42 44 45 46 49 54 55 56 57 58 61 64 65 66 67 70 71 73 **P**5	23	10	21	1557	15	21020	157	11408	5921	175

WATERTOWN—Dodge County

✠ WATERTOWN MEMORIAL HOSPITAL, 125 Hospital Drive, Zip 53098; tel. 414/261–4210; John P. Kosanovich, President **A**1 9 10 **F**1 3 6 8 11 15 17 19 21 22 25 26 27 28 29 30 33 34 35 36 37 39 40 41 42 44 45 46 47 49 51 56 58 61 63 64 65 66 67 68 70 71 72 73 74 **P**8	23	10	45	1695	18	80407	330	20355	9496	285

WAUKESHA—Waukesha County

✠ △ WAUKESHA MEMORIAL HOSPITAL, 725 American Avenue, Zip 53188–5099; tel. 414/544–2011; Rexford W. Titus, III, President and Chief Executive Officer **A**1 2 3 5 7 9 10 **F**2 3 4 6 7 8 10 11 12 13 14 15 17 19 20 21 22 23 25 26 27 28 29 30 32 33 34 35 37 39 40 41 42 43 44 45 46 47 48 49 51 52 53 54 55 56 57 58 59 60 61 62 63 64 65 66 67 68 70 71 72 73 74 **P**1 5 7 **N** Health Care Network of Wisconsin (HCN), Brookfield, WI; Waukesha Hospital System, Inc., Waukesha, WI	23	10	320	11769	162	200975	2046	125107	45750	1081

Hospital, Address, Telephone, Administrator, Approval, Facility, and Physician Codes, Health Care System, Network	Classi-fication Codes		Utilization Data					Expense (thousands) of dollars		
	Control	Service	Beds	Admissions	Census	Outpatient Visits	Births	Total	Payroll	Personnel

★ American Hospital Association (AHA) membership
□ Joint Commission on Accreditation of Healthcare Organizations (JCAHO) accreditation
+ American Osteopathic Hospital Association (AOHA) membership
○ American Osteopathic Association (AOA) accreditation
△ Commission on Accreditation of Rehabilitation Facilities (CARF) accreditation
Control codes 61, 63, 64, 71, 72 and 73 indicate hospitals listed by AOHA, but not registered by AHA. For definition of numerical codes, see page A4

WAUPACA—Waupaca County

✠ RIVERSIDE MEDICAL CENTER, 800 Riverside Drive, Zip 54981–1999; tel. 715/258–1000; Jan V. Carrell, Chief Executive Officer **A**1 9 10 **F**7 8 9 10 11 15 17 19 20 21 22 23 26 27 28 29 30 34 35 37 40 41 42 44 45 46 47 48 51 61 63 64 65 67 71 73 74 **S** Quorum Health Group/Quorum Health Resources, Inc., Brentwood, TN	23	10	40	1629	15	43803	223	14142	6291	202

WAUPUN—Fond Du Lac County

✠ WAUPUN MEMORIAL HOSPITAL, 620 West Brown Street, Zip 53963–1799; tel. 414/324–5581; James E. Baer, FACHE, President and Administrator **A**1 9 10 **F**5 7 8 11 15 16 17 19 21 22 23 25 26 28 29 30 32 33 34 35 36 37 39 40 41 44 45 47 49 51 61 64 65 67 68 71 73 **S** Congregation of St. Agnes, Fond Du Lac, WI **N** Health Care Network of Wisconsin (HCN), Brookfield, WI	21	10	49	1166	13	33583	151	11726	4867	162

WAUSAU—Marathon County

NORTH CENTRAL HEALTH CARE FACILITIES, 1100 Lakeview Drive, Zip 54403–6799; tel. 715/848–4600; Tim A. Steller, Chief Executive Officer (Total facility includes 356 beds in nursing home–type unit) **A**9 10 **F**2 3 12 15 17 19 22 25 26 27 29 34 35 39 45 48 49 52 53 54 55 56 57 58 59 61 64 65 67 73	13	22	406	1542	373	110583	0	38806	20265	589
✠ △ WAUSAU HOSPITAL, 333 Pine Ridge Boulevard, Zip 54401, Mailing Address: P.O. Box 1847, Zip 54402–1847; tel. 715/847–2121; Paul A. Spaude, President and Chief Executive Officer **A**1 2 3 5 7 9 10 **F**2 3 4 7 8 9 10 11 14 15 16 19 21 22 23 25 26 27 28 29 30 32 33 34 35 37 39 40 41 42 43 44 45 46 47 48 49 52 53 54 56 57 58 59 60 61 63 64 65 67 70 71 73 **N** Community Health Care, Inc., Wausau, WI	23	10	221	10895	141	75301	1458	103067	42471	1218

WAUWATOSA—Milwaukee County

+ ○ LAKEVIEW HOSPITAL, 10010 West Blue Mound Road, Zip 53226; tel. 414/259–7200; J. E. Race, Administrator and Chief Executive Officer **A**9 10 11 12 **F**8 11 13 15 17 19 20 21 27 28 29 30 34 35 37 39 41 42 44 45 51 55 61 63 64 65 67 68 71 73 **N** Covenant Healthcare System, Inc., Milwaukee, WI	23	10	72	753	11	10527	0	10118	5568	167
✠ MILWAUKEE PSYCHIATRIC HOSPITAL, 1220 Dewey Avenue, Zip 53213–2598; tel. 414/454–6600; Mark R. Ambrosius, President **A**1 3 5 9 10 **F**1 2 3 4 5 6 7 9 10 11 12 13 15 16 17 18 19 20 21 22 23 24 25 26 27 28 29 30 31 32 33 34 35 36 38 39 40 41 42 43 44 45 46 47 48 49 50 51 52 53 54 55 56 57 58 59 60 61 62 63 64 65 66 67 68 70 71 72 73 74 **P**6 **S** Aurora Health Care, Milwaukee, WI **N** Aurora Health Care, Milwaukee, WI	23	22	80	1652	41	—	0	11874	5543	137

WEST ALLIS—Milwaukee County

CHARTER BEHAVIORAL HEALTH SYSTEM OF MILWAUKEE/WEST ALLIS, 11101 West Lincoln Avenue, Zip 53227; tel. 414/327–3000; Robert Kwech, Chief Executive Officer (Nonreporting)	33	22	80	—	—	—	—	—	—	—
✠ WEST ALLIS MEMORIAL HOSPITAL, 8901 West Lincoln Avenue, Zip 53227–0901, Mailing Address: P.O. Box 27901, Zip 53227–0901; tel. 414/328–6000; Richard A. Kellar, Administrator (Nonreporting) **A**1 2 9 10 **S** Aurora Health Care, Milwaukee, WI **N** Health Care Network of Wisconsin (HCN), Brookfield, WI; Aurora Health Care, Milwaukee, WI	23	10	200	—	—	—	—	—	—	—

WEST BEND—Washington County

✠ ST. JOSEPH'S COMMUNITY HOSPITAL OF WEST BEND, 551 South Silverbrook Drive, Zip 53095–3898; tel. 414/334–5533; Gregory T. Burns, Executive Director **A**1 9 10 **F**7 8 11 12 13 14 15 16 17 18 19 21 22 23 25 26 28 29 30 34 35 36 37 39 40 41 42 44 45 49 52 54 57 61 63 64 65 67 70 71 73 **N** Health Care Network of Wisconsin (HCN), Brookfield, WI	23	10	121	4681	53	45327	692	25309	12374	373

WHITEHALL—Trempealeau County

TRI–COUNTY MEMORIAL HOSPITAL, 18601 Lincoln Street, Zip 54773–0065, Mailing Address: P.O. Box 65, Zip 54773–0065; tel. 715/538–4361; Ronald B. Fields, President (Total facility includes 122 beds in nursing home–type unit) **A**9 10 **F**3 4 5 6 7 8 10 11 14 16 17 19 20 21 22 23 24 26 27 28 29 30 33 34 35 36 37 39 41 42 43 44 45 46 48 49 50 51 53 54 55 56 57 58 59 60 61 63 64 65 66 67 68 69 71 73 74 **N** Lutheran Health System, LaCrosse, WI	23	10	154	586	101	9490	0	6190	3216	161

WILD ROSE—Waushara County

WILD ROSE COMMUNITY MEMORIAL HOSPITAL, Mailing Address: P.O. Box 243, Zip 54984–0243; tel. 414/622–3257; Donald Caves, President **A**9 10 **F**3 6 8 12 16 18 19 22 26 29 32 33 34 37 39 40 41 44 45 49 53 54 56 57 58 61 64 65 66 71 74 **P**5 **N** Partners Health System, Inc., Berlin, WI	23	10	26	423	4	12163	33	4088	1543	74

WINNEBAGO—Winnebago County

□ WINNEBAGO MENTAL HEALTH INSTITUTE, Mailing Address: Box 9, Zip 54985; tel. 414/235–4910; Joann O'Connor, Director **A**1 3 10 **F**2 4 7 8 10 11 19 20 22 24 27 28 29 35 40 41 44 45 46 47 48 50 52 53 55 56 61 63 64 65 70 71 72 73	12	22	330	799	241	262	0	32656	20568	676

WISCONSIN RAPIDS—Wood County

✠ RIVERVIEW HOSPITAL ASSOCIATION, (Includes Riverview Manor), 410 Dewey Street, Zip 54494, Mailing Address: P.O. Box 8080, Zip 54495–8080; tel. 715/423–6060; Celse A. Berard, President (Total facility includes 118 beds in nursing home–type unit) **A**1 9 10 **F**2 7 8 11 14 15 19 21 22 26 29 30 34 35 36 37 39 40 44 45 47 48 49 52 54 61 63 64 65 66 67 71	23	10	197	3586	142	27577	642	—	—	—

WOODRUFF—Oneida County

✠ HOWARD YOUNG MEDICAL CENTER, 240 Maple Street, Zip 54568, Mailing Address: P.O. Box 470, Zip 54568–0470; tel. 715/356–8000; Douglas O. Rosenberg, President and Chief Executive Officer **A**1 9 10 **F**3 6 7 8 9 11 13 15 17 19 21 22 23 24 25 26 27 28 29 30 32 33 34 35 39 40 41 42 44 45 46 47 48 49 51 56 58 61 63 64 65 66 67 71 73	23	10	65	3998	48	43374	267	33818	14534	483

WYOMING

Resident population 480 (in thousands)
Resident population in metro areas 29.8%
Birth rate per 1,000 population 14.0
65 years and over 11.1%
Percent of persons without health insurance 15.4%

Hospital, Address, Telephone, Administrator, Approval, Facility, and Physician Codes, Health Care System, Network	Classi-fication Codes		Utilization Data					Expense (thousands) of dollars		
	Control	Service	Beds	Admissions	Census	Outpatient Visits	Births	Total	Payroll	Personnel

★ American Hospital Association (AHA) membership
□ Joint Commission on Accreditation of Healthcare Organizations (JCAHO) accreditation
+ American Osteopathic Hospital Association (AOHA) membership
○ American Osteopathic Association (AOA) accreditation
△ Commission on Accreditation of Rehabilitation Facilities (CARF) accreditation
Control codes 61, 63, 64, 71, 72 and 73 indicate hospitals listed by AOHA, but not registered by AHA. For definition of numerical codes, see page A4

AFTON—Lincoln County										
★ STAR VALLEY HOSPITAL, 110 Hospital Lane, Zip 83110, Mailing Address: P.O. Box 579, Zip 83110; tel. 307/886–3841; Alberto Vasquez, Chief Executive Officer **A**9 10 **F**7 8 12 15 25 27 28 30 32 34 40 44 46 49 51 65 71 73 **P**6 **S** Intermountain Health Care, Inc., Salt Lake City, UT	16	10	15	547	3	27834	106	3391	1608	48
BUFFALO—Johnson County										
□ JOHNSON COUNTY MEMORIAL HOSPITAL, 497 West Lott Street, Zip 82834; tel. 307/684–5521; Sandy Ward, Administrator (Total facility includes 54 beds in nursing home–type unit) **A**1 9 10 **F**8 19 22 26 28 32 33 35 37 40 44 45 49 64 65 71	16	10	69	568	47	12610	79	6118	3406	126
CASPER—Natrona County										
✉ △ WYOMING MEDICAL CENTER, 1233 East Second Street, Zip 82601; tel. 307/577–7201; Michael E. Schrader, President and Chief Executive Officer **A**1 3 7 9 10 **F**3 4 7 8 10 12 13 14 15 16 17 19 21 22 23 25 27 28 30 31 32 34 35 37 39 40 41 42 43 44 45 46 48 49 51 52 53 54 55 56 58 59 60 61 65 67 71 73 74 **P**3 **N** Wyoming Integrated Network, Casper, WY	23	10	194	7260	89	53098	872	77837	30955	949
CHEYENNE—Laramie County										
★ U. S. AIR FORCE HOSPITAL, 6900 Alden Drive, Zip 82005–3913; tel. 307/775–2045; Major Angela D. Fowler, MSC, USAF, Administrator (Nonreporting) **S** Department of the Air Force, Washington, DC	41	10	15	—	—	—	—	—	—	—
✉ UNITED MEDICAL CENTER, (Includes De Paul Hospital, 2600 East 18th Street, Zip 82001–5511; tel. 307/634–2273), 300 East 23rd Street, Zip 82001–3790; tel. 307/634–2273; Jon M. Gates, Chief Executive Officer **A**1 3 9 10 **F**2 3 4 7 8 10 11 12 15 16 17 19 20 21 22 23 24 28 30 31 32 33 34 37 40 41 42 43 44 45 46 48 49 52 53 54 55 56 57 58 60 63 64 65 66 67 71 73 74 **P**8	13	10	170	7195	88	157827	754	55886	24068	772
✉ VETERANS AFFAIRS MEDICAL CENTER, (Formerly Veterans Affairs Center), 2360 East Pershing Boulevard, Zip 82001–5392; tel. 307/778–7550; David M. Kilpatrick, M.D., Acting Center Director (Total facility includes 50 beds in nursing home–type unit) **A**1 **F**2 3 17 19 20 21 22 25 26 27 28 31 32 33 34 37 44 46 48 49 51 54 56 58 64 65 71 73 74 **S** Department of Veterans Affairs, Washington, DC	45	10	125	1505	68	51623	0	23581	10500	295
CODY—Park County										
✉ WEST PARK HOSPITAL, 707 Sheridan Avenue, Zip 82414; tel. 307/527–7501; Gary Bishop, Administrator (Total facility includes 140 beds in nursing home–type unit) **A**1 9 10 **F**2 3 7 8 15 16 17 19 21 22 26 27 28 32 33 34 35 39 40 41 42 44 45 46 48 49 53 54 55 56 57 58 64 65 66 67 71 73 **S** Quorum Health Group/Quorum Health Resources, Inc., Brentwood, TN	16	10	171	1660	129	—	223	21697	9900	360
DOUGLAS—Converse County										
★ CONVERSE COUNTY MEMORIAL HOSPITAL, 111 South Fifth Street, Zip 82633; tel. 307/358–2122; Fred F. Schroeder, Administrator **A**9 10 **F**7 8 12 14 15 17 19 22 28 32 33 34 35 40 41 44 48 49 54 64 66 68 71 73 **P**5	13	10	34	422	6	24776	83	6417	2798	111
EVANSTON—Uinta County										
✉ EVANSTON REGIONAL HOSPITAL, 190 Arrowhead Drive, Zip 82930; tel. 307/789–3636; Robert W. Allen, Administrator **A**1 9 10 **F**7 8 12 15 16 17 19 20 22 28 29 30 32 33 35 37 39 40 44 46 49 65 67 70 71 73 **S** Intermountain Health Care, Inc., Salt Lake City, UT	23	10	38	1170	10	35989	268	9790	3512	109
WYOMING STATE HOSPITAL, 830 Highway 150 South, Zip 82931, Mailing Address: P.O. Box 177, Zip 82931–0177; tel. 307/789–3464; Pablo Hernandez, M.D., Administrator **A**10 **F**3 6 12 14 15 16 17 18 20 26 27 28 29 45 46 51 52 53 54 55 56 57 58 59 65 67 73	12	22	137	466	115	—	0	15827	8910	443
GILLETTE—Campbell County										
✉ CAMPBELL COUNTY MEMORIAL HOSPITAL, 501 South Burma Avenue, Zip 82716, Mailing Address: Box 3011, Zip 82717; tel. 307/682–8811; David Crow, Chief Executive Officer **A**1 9 10 **F**2 3 7 8 11 12 14 15 16 17 18 19 20 21 22 24 25 28 30 32 33 34 35 36 37 38 39 40 41 42 44 46 49 51 52 53 54 55 56 58 59 63 65 67 71 72 73 74 **P**1 3 **S** Quorum Health Group/Quorum Health Resources, Inc., Brentwood, TN	16	10	119	2030	23	74568	442	29764	12418	516
JACKSON—Teton County										
✉ ST. JOHN'S HOSPITAL AND LIVING CENTER, (Formerly St. John's Hospital and Nursing Home), 625 East Broadway, Zip 83001, Mailing Address: P.O. Box 428, Zip 83001–0428; tel. 307/733–3636; John Valiante, Chief Executive Officer (Total facility includes 60 beds in nursing home–type unit) (Nonreporting) **A**1 9 10 **N** Community Health Care Network, Jackson, WY	16	10	104	—	—	—	—	—	—	—
KEMMERER—Lincoln County										
★ SOUTH LINCOLN MEDICAL CENTER, 711 Onyx Street, Zip 83101, Mailing Address: Box 390, Zip 83101–0390; tel. 307/877–4401; Marla Shelby, Administrator and Chief Executive Officer **A**9 10 **F**7 8 14 22 28 32 40 44 49 71 **P**4	16	10	16	215	2	22183	43	4455	1884	74

Hospital, Address, Telephone, Administrator, Approval, Facility, and Physician Codes, Health Care System, Network	Classi-fication Codes		Utilization Data					Expense (thousands) of dollars		
	Control	Service	Beds	Admissions	Census	Outpatient Visits	Births	Total	Payroll	Personnel

★ American Hospital Association (AHA) membership
☐ Joint Commission on Accreditation of Healthcare Organizations (JCAHO) accreditation
+ American Osteopathic Hospital Association (AOHA) membership
◯ American Osteopathic Association (AOA) accreditation
△ Commission on Accreditation of Rehabilitation Facilities (CARF) accreditation
Control codes 61, 63, 64, 71, 72 and 73 indicate hospitals listed by AOHA, but not registered by AHA. For definition of numerical codes, see page A4

Hospital, Address, Telephone, Administrator, Approval, Facility, and Physician Codes, Health Care System, Network	Control	Service	Beds	Admissions	Census	Outpatient Visits	Births	Total	Payroll	Personnel
LANDER—Fremont County										
☐ LANDER VALLEY MEDICAL CENTER, 1320 Bishop Randall Drive, Zip 82520; tel. 307/332–4420; Andrew Gramlich, Chief Executive Officer (Total facility includes 21 beds in nursing home–type unit) (Nonreporting) **A**1 9 10 **S** TENET Healthcare Corporation, Santa Barbara, CA	33	10	102	—	—	—	—	—	—	—
LARAMIE—Albany County										
✠ IVINSON MEMORIAL HOSPITAL, 255 North 30th Street, Zip 82070–5195; tel. 307/742–2141; Thomas A. Nord, FACHE, President and Chief Executive Officer (Total facility includes 13 beds in nursing home–type unit) **A**1 9 10 **F**7 8 14 15 16 17 18 19 21 22 23 28 30 33 35 37 39 40 41 44 45 46 48 49 52 53 54 55 56 57 58 59 64 65 67 68 71 73 **N** Wyoming Integrated Network, Casper, WY	16	10	65	3160	29	25012	568	26807	12139	327
LOVELL—Big Horn County										
★ NORTH BIG HORN HOSPITAL, 1115 Lane 12, Zip 82431, Mailing Address: P.O. Box 518, Zip 82431; tel. 307/548–2771; Kent Kellersberger, Chief Executive Officer (Total facility includes 95 beds in nursing home–type unit) **A**9 10 **F**1 7 8 11 12 14 15 16 17 22 24 26 28 29 30 31 32 34 37 39 40 44 45 46 49 51 64 65 66 67 71 73	16	10	125	390	91	7921	7	6800	3463	177
LUSK—Niobrara County										
NIOBRARA COUNTY HOSPITAL DISTRICT, 939 Ballencee Avenue, Zip 82225, Mailing Address: P.O. Box 780, Zip 82225; tel. 307/334–2711; Gary W. Robertson, Administrator (Total facility includes 36 beds in nursing home–type unit) **A**9 10 **F**8 14 15 16 19 26 28 29 34 35 44 49 51 64 65 71 **P**6	16	10	46	171	35	—	0	2451	1275	53
NEWCASTLE—Weston County										
WESTON COUNTY MEMORIAL HOSPITAL, 1124 Washington Street, Zip 82701–2996; tel. 307/746–4491; F. Ann Snow, Administrator (Total facility includes 51 beds in nursing home–type unit) **A**9 10 **F**1 7 8 11 14 15 16 19 22 28 30 32 35 37 39 40 44 49 64 67 71 **P**3	13	10	73	318	52	9686	48	4645	2248	106
POWELL—Park County										
✠ POWELL HOSPITAL, 777 Avenue H, Zip 82435; tel. 307/754–2267; Steve Ramsey, Interim Chief Executive Officer (Total facility includes 98 beds in nursing home–type unit) **A**1 9 10 **F**7 8 12 14 15 16 19 21 22 26 27 28 30 32 34 35 39 40 41 44 46 49 51 64 65 66 67 71 73 **S** Brim, Inc., Portland, OR	23	10	138	736	95	15566	190	9576	5126	174
RAWLINS—Carbon County										
☐ MEMORIAL HOSPITAL OF CARBON COUNTY, 2221 West Elm, Zip 82301; tel. 307/324–2221; Richard Johnson, Chief Executive Officer (Total facility includes 10 beds in nursing home–type unit) **A**1 9 10 **F**8 11 12 14 15 17 19 20 22 26 28 32 34 35 37 41 42 44 45 47 48 49 56 64 65 70 71 73 **P**6	13	10	45	1411	21	37033	0	10838	4629	176
RIVERTON—Fremont County										
✠ COLUMBIA RIVERTON MEMORIAL HOSPITAL, 2100 West Sunset Drive, Zip 82501; tel. 307/856–4161; Kenneth H. Armstrong, Chief Executive Officer **A**1 9 10 **F**7 8 11 14 15 19 21 22 23 28 30 31 32 33 34 35 37 39 40 44 45 46 49 65 70 71 73 **P**7 **S** Columbia/HCA Healthcare Corporation, Nashville, TN	33	10	59	1594	16	28049	251	13233	4492	161
ROCK SPRINGS—Sweetwater County										
✠ MEMORIAL HOSPITAL OF SWEETWATER COUNTY, 1200 College Drive, Zip 82901–5868, Mailing Address: Box 1359, Zip 82902–1359; tel. 307/362–3711; John M. Ferry, Executive Director **A**1 9 10 **F**7 8 15 17 19 20 21 22 23 26 28 29 30 31 32 33 34 35 36 37 39 40 42 44 45 46 49 51 58 65 71 73	13	10	99	2415	22	77580	518	21350	8943	314
SHERIDAN—Sheridan County										
☐ MEMORIAL HOSPITAL OF SHERIDAN COUNTY, 1401 West Fifth Street, Zip 82801–2799; tel. 307/672–1000; T. Marvin Goldman, Administrator **A**1 9 10 **F**7 8 11 14 15 19 21 22 23 28 32 33 35 37 40 42 44 46 49 56 60 65 67 71 73 **P**5	13	10	60	2578	33	12471	284	19708	9975	350
✠ VETERANS AFFAIRS MEDICAL CENTER, 1898 Fort Road, Zip 82801; tel. 307/672–3473; J. A. Brinkers, Director (Total facility includes 50 beds in nursing home–type unit) **A**1 **F**2 3 6 8 11 16 18 19 20 21 22 26 27 28 30 32 34 35 39 41 42 44 46 49 51 52 55 56 57 58 60 64 65 67 71 72 73 74 **P**6 **S** Department of Veterans Affairs, Washington, DC	45	22	239	1958	130	32078	0	27562	21316	430
SUNDANCE—Crook County										
CROOK COUNTY MEDICAL SERVICES DISTRICT, 713 Oak Street, Zip 82729, Mailing Address: Box 517, Zip 82729–0517; tel. 307/283–3501; Don A. Nelson, Administrator (Total facility includes 32 beds in nursing home–type unit) **A**9 10 **F**1 14 15 16 22 28 32 33 34 45 46 49 64 65 71 **P**6	16	10	48	216	40	7030	0	3276	2055	79
THERMOPOLIS—Hot Springs County										
✠ HOT SPRINGS COUNTY MEMORIAL HOSPITAL, 150 East Arapahoe, Zip 82443; tel. 307/864–3121; Edward G. Leake, Administrator **A**1 9 10 **F**7 8 11 15 19 22 28 32 34 35 37 39 40 44 45 48 63 65 71 73	13	10	49	1100	11	14203	72	6235	2605	113
TORRINGTON—Goshen County										
✠ COMMUNITY HOSPITAL, 2000 Campbell Drive, Zip 82240; tel. 307/532–4181; Charles Myers, Administrator **A**1 9 10 **F**7 8 11 12 16 17 19 22 26 28 30 32 34 35 36 37 39 40 42 44 49 64 65 66 67 71 **S** Lutheran Health Systems, Fargo, ND	23	10	36	1339	19	28300	142	6736	2828	157
WHEATLAND—Platte County										
✠ PLATTE COUNTY MEMORIAL HOSPITAL, 201 14th Street, Zip 82201, Mailing Address: P.O. Box 848, Zip 82201; tel. 307/322–3636; Dana K. Barnett, Administrator (Total facility includes 43 beds in nursing home–type unit) **A**1 9 10 **F**7 8 11 12 14 15 16 19 22 28 29 32 34 35 37 40 44 64 65 71 73 **S** Lutheran Health Systems, Fargo, ND	23	10	86	1060	68	25722	88	4888	2319	152

Hospital, Address, Telephone, Administrator, Approval, Facility, and Physician Codes, Health Care System, Network	Classi-fication Codes		Utilization Data					Expense (thousands) of dollars		
★ American Hospital Association (AHA) membership ☐ Joint Commission on Accreditation of Healthcare Organizations (JCAHO) accreditation + American Osteopathic Hospital Association (AOHA) membership ○ American Osteopathic Association (AOA) accreditation △ Commission on Accreditation of Rehabilitation Facilities (CARF) accreditation Control codes 61, 63, 64, 71, 72 and 73 indicate hospitals listed by AOHA, but not registered by AHA. For definition of numerical codes, see page A4	Control	Service	Beds	Admissions	Census	Outpatient Visits	Births	Total	Payroll	Personnel

WORLD—Washakie County

☒ WASHAKIE MEMORIAL HOSPITAL, 400 South 15th Street, Zip 82401, Mailing Address: Box 700, Zip 82401; tel. 307/347–3221; John Johnson, Administrator **A**1 9 10 **F**7 8 12 14 15 16 17 19 22 28 29 30 32 35 36 39 40 41 44 45 46 48 49 51 64 65 67 68 71 73 **P**3 **S** Lutheran Health Systems, Fargo, ND

	23	10	30	926	10	36533	85	6714	3008	105

Hospitals in Areas Associated with the United States, by Area

Hospital, Address, Telephone, Administrator, Approval, Facility, and Physician Codes, Health Care System, Network	Classi-fication Codes		Utilization Data					Expense (thousands) of dollars		
★ American Hospital Association (AHA) membership □ Joint Commission on Accreditation of Healthcare Organizations (JCAHO) accreditation + American Osteopathic Hospital Association (AOHA) membership ○ American Osteopathic Association (AOA) accreditation △ Commission on Accreditation of Rehabilitation Facilities (CARF) accreditation Control codes 61, 63, 64, 71, 72 and 73 indicate hospitals listed by AOHA, but not registered by AHA. For definition of numerical codes, see page A4	Control	Service	Beds	Admissions	Census	Outpatient Visits	Births	Total	Payroll	Personnel

AMERICAN SAMOA

PAGO PAGO—American Samoa County

LYNDON B. JOHNSON TROPICAL MEDICAL CENTER, Zip 96799; tel. 684/633–1222; Iotamo T. Saleapaga, M.D., Director Health (Nonreporting) A10	12	10	125	—	—	—	—	—	—	—

GUAM

AGANA—Guam County

✠ U. S. NAVAL HOSPITAL, Mailing Address: Box 7607, FPO, AP, Zip 96538–1600; tel. 671/344–9340; J. M. Ricciardi, Commanding Officer (Nonreporting) A1 S Department of Navy, Washington, DC	43	10	55	—	—	—	—	—	—	—

TAMUNING—Guam County

GUAM MEMORIAL HOSPITAL AUTHORITY, 850 Governor Carlos G. Camacho Road, Zip 96911; tel. 671/646–6711; Helen B. Ripple, Administrator (Total facility includes 29 beds in nursing home–type unit) A10 F7 8 16 19 22 31 34 37 38 39 40 44 45 46 47 48 49 63 64 65 69 71 73	16	10	186	11580	135	—	3621	51955	27871	804

MARSHALL ISLANDS

KWAJALEIN ISLAND—Marshall Islands County

KWAJALEIN HOSPITAL, Mailing Address: Box 1702, APO, AP, Zip 96555–5000; tel. 805/355–2225; Mike Mathews, Administrator F7 8 14 16 17 18 20 22 28 30 34 37 40 41 44 47 49 51 71 P6 S Department of the Army, Office of the Surgeon General, Falls Church, VA	42	10	14	211	2	13689	17	—	—	72

PUERTO RICO

AGUADILLA—Aguadilla County

✠ AGUADILLA GENERAL HOSPITAL, Carr Aguadilla San Juan, Zip 00605, Mailing Address: P.O. Box 4036, Zip 00605; tel. 787/891–3000; William Rodriguez Castro, Executive Director A1 9 10 F7 15 16 20 22 25 39 40 44 65 67 71 73 P1 S Puerto Rico Department of Health, San Juan, PR	12	10	110	6202	73	78970	1800	11828	—	602

AIBONITO—Aibonito County

★ MENNONITE GENERAL HOSPITAL, Mailing Address: Box 1379, Zip 00705; tel. 809/735–8001; Domingo Torres Zayas, Executive Director A9 10 F19 22 33 34 39 42 44 49 56 58 70 71	23	10	131	8658	102	51540	894	20842	8202	531

ARECIBO—Arecibo County

★ ARECIBO REGIONAL HOSPITAL, San Luis Avenue, Zip 00612; tel. 809/878–7272; Jose L. Mirauda, M.D., Executive Director (Nonreporting) A9 10 S Puerto Rico Department of Health, San Juan, PR	12	10	183	—	—	—	—	—	—	—
HOSPITAL DR. SUSONI, 55 Nicomedes Rivera Street, Zip 00612; tel. 809/878–1010; Hector Barreto, M.D., Director (Nonreporting) A9 10	33	10	138	—	—	—	—	—	—	—
★ HOSPITAL EL BUEN PASTOR, 52 De Diego, Zip 00612, Mailing Address: Box 413, Zip 00612; tel. 809/878–2730; Julio Galarce, Administrator (Nonreporting)	33	10	72	—	—	—	—	—	—	—

ARROYO—Arroyo County

★ LAFAYETTE HOSPITAL, Central Lafayette, Zip 00714, Mailing Address: Box 207, Zip 00714; tel. 809/839–3232; Francisco Santiago–Vega, Consultor A9 10 F14 15 16 19 22 34 37 40 64 65 71	33	10	30	1690	19	16173	55	4364	1198	116

Hospital, Address, Telephone, Administrator, Approval, Facility, and Physician Codes, Health Care System, Network	Classi-fication Codes		Utilization Data					Expense (thousands) of dollars		
★ American Hospital Association (AHA) membership □ Joint Commission on Accreditation of Healthcare Organizations (JCAHO) accreditation + American Osteopathic Hospital Association (AOHA) membership ○ American Osteopathic Association (AOA) accreditation △ Commission on Accreditation of Rehabilitation Facilities (CARF) accreditation Control codes 61, 63, 64, 71, 72 and 73 indicate hospitals listed by AOHA, but not registered by AHA. For definition of numerical codes, see page A4	Control	Service	Beds	Admissions	Census	Outpatient Visits	Births	Total	Payroll	Personnel

BAYAMON—Bayamon County

Hospital	Control	Service	Beds	Admissions	Census	Outpatient Visits	Births	Total	Payroll	Personnel
⊞ HOSPITAL HERMANOS MELENDEZ, Route 2, KM 11–7, Zip 00960, Mailing Address: P.O. Box 306, Zip 00960; tel. 809/785–9784; Tomas Martinez, Administrator **A**1 9 10 **F**11 22 37 40 44 51 63 65 67 71 73 **P**8	33	10	205	13541	167	—	1912	32552	11919	613
★ HOSPITAL MATILDE BRENES, Extension Hermanas Davila, Zip 00960, Mailing Address: Box 2957, Zip 00960; tel. 809/786–6315; Manuel J. Vazquez, Administrator (Nonreporting) **A**9 10	33	10	97	—	—	—	—	—	—	—
⊞ HOSPITAL SAN PABLO, Calle San Cruz 70, Zip 00961, Mailing Address: Box 236, Zip 00960; tel. 809/740–4747; Jorge De Jesus, Executive Director (Nonreporting) **A**1 3 5 9 10	33	10	351	—	—	—	—	—	—	—
⊞ HOSPITAL UNIVERSITARIO DR. RAMON RUIZ ARNAU, Avenue Laurel, Santa Juanita, Zip 00956; tel. 809/787–5151; Iris J. Vazquez Rosario, Executive Director **A**1 3 5 9 10 **F**1 3 4 5 6 7 8 10 11 12 13 15 16 17 18 19 20 21 22 23 24 25 26 27 28 29 30 31 32 33 34 35 36 37 38 39 40 41 42 43 44 45 46 47 49 50 51 53 54 55 56 57 58 59 60 61 62 63 65 66 67 68 69 70 71 72 73 74 **P**1 5 **S** Puerto Rico Department of Health, San Juan, PR	16	10	372	14450	245	138361	4825	—	—	1689
⊞ MEPSI CENTER, Carretera Numero 2 K 8–2, Zip 00959–6089, Mailing Address: Call Box 60–89, Zip 00960–6089; tel. 809/793–3030; Manuel G. Mendez, Operating Trustee **A**1 9 10 **F**2 3 14 15 16 19 35 41 46 52 53 55 56 57 59 65 71 **P**1 6	33	22	450	3116	186	—	0	15365	6498	374

CAGUAS—Caguas County

Hospital	Control	Service	Beds	Admissions	Census	Outpatient Visits	Births	Total	Payroll	Personnel
⊞ CAGUAS REGIONAL HOSPITAL, Carretera Caguas A Cidra, Zip 00725, Mailing Address: Box 5729, Zip 00726; tel. 809/744–2500; Noemi Davis Marte, M.D., Medical Director (Nonreporting) **A**1 3 5 9 10	12	10	256	—	—	—	—	—	—	—
□ HOSPITAL INTERAMERICANO DE MEDICINA AVANZADA, Avenida Luis Munoz Marin, Zip 00726, Mailing Address: Apartado 4980, Zip 00726; tel. 787/743–3434; Carlos M. Pineiro, President (Nonreporting) **A**1 9 10	32	10	300	—	—	—	—	—	—	—

CAROLINA—Carolina County

Hospital	Control	Service	Beds	Admissions	Census	Outpatient Visits	Births	Total	Payroll	Personnel
⊞ HOSPITAL DR. FEDERICO TRILLA, 65th Infanteria, KM 8 3, Zip 00984, Mailing Address: P.O. Box 3869, Zip 00984; tel. 787/757–1800; Manuel Soto Tapia, Chief Executive Officer (Nonreporting) **A**1 3 5 9 10	33	10	220	—	—	—	—	—	—	—

CASTANER—Lares County

Hospital	Control	Service	Beds	Admissions	Census	Outpatient Visits	Births	Total	Payroll	Personnel
★ CASTANER GENERAL HOSPITAL, KM 64–2, Route 135, Zip 00631, Mailing Address: Box 1003, Zip 00631; tel. 809/829–5010; Domingo Monroig, Administrator **A**9 10 **F**8 15 16 19 20 22 29 30 31 37 39 40 44 45 51 53 65 70 **P**6	23	10	24	725	8	3710	122	4199	1506	107

CAYEY—Cayey County

Hospital	Control	Service	Beds	Admissions	Census	Outpatient Visits	Births	Total	Payroll	Personnel
★ HOSPITAL MENONITA DE CAYEY, 4 H. Mendoza Street, Zip 00737, Mailing Address: Box 373130, Zip 00737; tel. 787/738–2181; Domingo Torres–Zayas, Executive Director (Nonreporting) **A**9 10	23	10	50	—	—	—	—	—	—	—

CIDRA—Cidra County

Hospital	Control	Service	Beds	Admissions	Census	Outpatient Visits	Births	Total	Payroll	Personnel
⊞ FIRST HOSPITAL PANAMERICANO, State Road 787 KM 1 5, Zip 00739, Mailing Address: P.O. Box 1398, Zip 00739; tel. 809/739–5555; Henry Ruberte', Administrator (Nonreporting) **A**1 5 10 **S** First Hospital Corporation, Norfolk, VA	33	22	165	—	—	—	—	—	—	—

FAJARDO—Fajardo County

Hospital	Control	Service	Beds	Admissions	Census	Outpatient Visits	Births	Total	Payroll	Personnel
★ DOCTORS GUBERN'S HOSPITAL, (Includes Dr. Gubern's Hospital, General Valero Avenue 267 & 261, Mailing Address: Box 846, Zip 00738; tel. 809/792–3495; Antonio R. Barcelo, Director), 110 Antonio R. Barcelo, Zip 00738, Mailing Address: Box 846, Zip 00738; tel. 809/863–0924; Roberto Acevedo, Administrator (Nonreporting) **A**9 10 **S** United Medical Corporation, Windermere, FL	33	10	51	—	—	—	—	—	—	—
⊞ DR. JOSE RAMOS LEBRON HOSPITAL, General Valero Avenue, #194, Zip 00738, Mailing Address: P.O. Box 1283, Zip 00738–1283; tel. 809/863–0505; Victor R. Marrero, Executive Administrator (Nonreporting) **A**1 9 10 **S** Puerto Rico Department of Health, San Juan, PR	33	10	180	—	—	—	—	—	—	—

GUAYAMA—Guayama County

Hospital	Control	Service	Beds	Admissions	Census	Outpatient Visits	Births	Total	Payroll	Personnel
⊞ DR. ALEJANDRO BUITRAGO–GUAYAMA AREA HOSPITAL, Urb La Hacienda, Zip 00785; tel. 809/864–4300; Carlos Rodriguez Mateo, M.D., Medical Director (Nonreporting) **A**1 9 10	12	10	155	—	—	—	—	—	—	—
★ HOSPITAL SANTA ROSA, Veterans Avenue, Zip 00784, Mailing Address: Box 10008, Zip 00785; tel. 787/864–0101; Humberto M. Monserrate, Administrator **A**9 10 **F**7 10 16 19 22 35 37 40 71 **P**8	23	10	89	5076	55	—	601	10399	3137	273

HUMACAO—Humacao County

Hospital	Control	Service	Beds	Admissions	Census	Outpatient Visits	Births	Total	Payroll	Personnel
⊞ FONT MARTELO HOSPITAL, 3 Font Martelo Street, Zip 00792, Mailing Address: Box 639, Zip 00792–0639; tel. 809/852–2424; Julio A. Ortiz, M.D., Chairman (Nonreporting) **A**1 9 10	33	10	64	—	—	—	—	—	—	—
HOSPITAL DR. DOMINGUEZ, 300 Font Martelo Street, Zip 00791, Mailing Address: Box 699, Zip 00792; tel. 787/852–0505; Rogelio Diaz–Reyes, Administrator (Nonreporting) **A**9 10	33	10	54	—	—	—	—	—	—	—
★ HOSPITAL SUB–REGIONAL DR. VICTOR R. NUNEZ, Avenida Tejas, Expreso Cruz Ortiz Stella, Zip 00791; tel. 787/852–2727; Ahmed Alvarez Pabon, Executive Director **F**2 3 4 5 8 9 10 11 12 13 14 15 16 17 18 19 20 21 22 23 28 29 30 31 34 35 37 38 40 41 42 43 44 45 47 48 49 51 52 53 54 55 56 57 58 59 60 61 64 65 69 70 71 73 **P**5	12	10	83	4862	54	50896	1431	16390	6762	406
★ RYDER MEMORIAL HOSPITAL, Mailing Address: P.O. Box 859, Zip 00792; tel. 787/852–0768; Saturnino Pena Flores, Executive Director (Total facility includes 62 beds in nursing home–type unit) **A**9 10 **F**1 6 8 11 12 13 14 15 16 17 19 20 21 22 25 26 27 28 29 30 31 32 33 34 35 37 38 39 40 41 42 44 45 46 49 51 54 56 58 61 62 63 64 65 71 73 **P**8	23	10	209	8995	131	122100	660	32766	13132	1007

Hospital, Address, Telephone, Administrator, Approval, Facility, and Physician Codes, Health Care System, Network	Classi-fication Codes		Utilization Data					Expense (thousands) of dollars		
★ American Hospital Association (AHA) membership □ Joint Commission on Accreditation of Healthcare Organizations (JCAHO) accreditation + American Osteopathic Hospital Association (AOHA) membership ○ American Osteopathic Association (AOA) accreditation △ Commission on Accreditation of Rehabilitation Facilities (CARF) accreditation Control codes 61, 63, 64, 71, 72 and 73 indicate hospitals listed by AOHA, but not registered by AHA. For definition of numerical codes, see page A4	Control	Service	Beds	Admissions	Census	Outpatient Visits	Births	Total	Payroll	Personnel

MANATI—Manati County

★ CLINICA SAN AGUSTIN, Mailing Address: P.O. Box 1118, Zip 00674; tel. 787/854–2091; Astrid Abreu, Administrator (Nonreporting) **A**9 10

	33	10	12	—	—	—	—	—	—	—

★ DOCTORS CENTER, Zip 00674; tel. 787/854–1795; Carla Blanco, Administrator **A**3 9 10 **F**34 37 40 **P**5

	33	10	150	10320	122	62967	1759	21410	8064	496

MAYAGUEZ—Mayaguez County

⊞ BELLA VISTA HOSPITAL, State Road 349, Zip 00680, Mailing Address: P.O. Box 1750, Zip 00681; tel. 787/834–6000; Nemuel O. Artiles, Executive Director (Nonreporting) **A**1 9 10

	21	10	157	—	—	—	—	—	—	—

CLINICA ESPANOLA, Bo La Quinta, Zip 00680; tel. 809/832–0442; Emigdio Inigo–Agostini, M.D., Board President (Nonreporting) **A**9 10

	33	10	69	—	—	—	—	—	—	—

⊞ DR. RAMON E. BETANCES HOSPITAL–MAYAGUEZ MEDICAL CENTER BRANCH, Zip 00680; tel. 809/834–8686; Miguel A. Sepulvida, Administrator (Nonreporting) **A**1 3 5 10

	12	10	253	—	—	—	—	—	—	—

★ HOSPITAL PEREA, 15 Basora Street, Zip 00681, Mailing Address: Box 170, Zip 00681; tel. 809/834–0101; Jaime F. Maestre, Executive Director (Nonreporting) **A**10 **S** United Medical Corporation, Windermere, FL

	33	10	82	—	—	—	—	—	—	—

PONCE—Ponce County

⊞ DR. PILA'S HOSPITAL, Avenida Las Americas, Zip 00731, Mailing Address: Box 1910, Zip 00733–1910; tel. 809/848–5600; Jose Cora, Executive Director and Chief Executive Officer (Nonreporting) **A**1 3 5 9 10

	23	10	172	—	—	—	—	—	—	—

⊞ HOSPITAL DE DAMAS, Ponce by Pass, Zip 00731; tel. 809/840–8686; Roberto A. Rentas, Administrator (Total facility includes 28 beds in nursing home–type unit) (Nonreporting) **A**1 2 3 5 8 9 10

	23	10	334	—	—	—	—	—	—	—

⊞ HOSPITAL EPISCOPAL SAN LUCAS, Guadalupe Street, Zip 00731, Mailing Address: Box 2027, Zip 00733; tel. 809/840–4545; Pedro Brull–Joy, Executive Director (Nonreporting) **A**1 3 5 10

	21	10	160	—	—	—	—	—	—	—

⊞ HOSPITAL ONCOLOGICO ANDRES GRILLASCA, Centro Medico De Ponce, Zip 00733, Mailing Address: Box 1324, Zip 00733; tel. 809/848–0800; Angel M. Franceschi, Administrator (Nonreporting) **A**1 2 3 5 9 10

	23	49	53	—	—	—	—	—	—	—

⊞ PONCE REGIONAL HOSPITAL, Barrio Machuelo, Zip 00731; tel. 809/844–2080; Julio Andino, Executive Director (Nonreporting) **A**1 3 5 9 10 **S** Puerto Rico Department of Health, San Juan, PR

	12	10	407	—	—	—	—	—	—	—

SAN GERMAN—San German County

⊞ HOSPITAL DE LA CONCEPCION, 41 Luna Street, Zip 00683, Mailing Address: Box 285, Zip 00683; tel. 809/892–1860; Herson E. Morales, Administrator (Nonreporting) **A**1 2 3 5 9 10

	21	10	167	—	—	—	—	—	—	—

SAN JUAN—San Juan County

⊞ ASHFORD PRESBYTERIAN COMMUNITY HOSPITAL, 1451 Ashford Avenue Condado, Zip 00907, Mailing Address: P.O. Box 9020032, Zip 00902–0032; tel. 809/721–2160; Jose Cora, Executive Director (Nonreporting) **A**1 9 10

	23	10	180	—	—	—	—	—	—	—

⊞ AUXILIO MUTUO HOSPITAL, Ponce De Leon Avenue, Zip 00919, Mailing Address: Box 191227, Zip 00919–1227; tel. 787/758–2000; Ivan E. Colon, Administrator **A**1 3 9 10 **F**10 11 15 16 19 21 22 33 34 35 37 38 39 40 42 44 46 47 49 56 64 65 69 70 71 73

	23	10	402	20625	352	127640	2064	89613	32024	1852

⊞ BHC HOSPITAL SAN JUAN CAPESTRANO, (Formerly CPC Hosp San Juan Capestrano), Mailing Address: Rural Route 2, Box 11, Zip 00926; tel. 787/760–0222; Laura Vargas, Administrator (Nonreporting) **A**1 10 **S** Behavioral Healthcare Corporation, Nashville, TN

	33	22	88	—	—	—	—	—	—	—

CPC HOSP SAN JUAN CAPESTRANO See BHC Hospital San Juan Capestrano

DOCTORS HOSPITAL, 1395 San Rafael Street, Zip 00910, Mailing Address: Box 11338, Santurce Station, Zip 00910; tel. 809/723–2950; Georgina Mattei de Collazo, Executive Director (Nonreporting) **A**9 10

	33	10	96	—	—	—	—	—	—	—

⊞ FUNDACION HOSPITAL METROPOLITAN, Caparra, Mailing Address: P.O. Box 11981, Zip 00922; tel. 787/793–6200; Ivan Millon, Administrator (Nonreporting) **A**1 9

	23	10	119	—	—	—	—	—	—	—

HATO REY COMMUNITY HOSPITAL, Mailing Address: 435 Ponce De Leon, Hato Rey, Zip 00917; tel. 787/754–0909; Teodoro Muniz, Executive Director **A**9 10 **F**11 19 22 27 40 44 60 65 71

	33	10	105	5389	73	59550	508	13108	4081	312

⊞ HOSPITAL DEL MAESTRO, Domenech Avenue, Zip 00918, Mailing Address: P.O. Box 364708, Zip 00936–4708; tel. 809/758–8383; Maria Mercedes Rivera, Administrator (Nonreporting) **A**1 10

	23	10	214	—	—	—	—	—	—	—

⊞ HOSPITAL PAVIA, 1462 Asia Street, Zip 00909, Mailing Address: Box 11137, Santurce Station, Zip 00910; tel. 809/727–6060; Jose Luis Suarez Fonseca, Executive Director **A**1 9 10 **F**4 7 10 11 15 16 19 21 22 37 38 40 42 43 44 65 71 **S** United Medical Corporation, Windermere, FL

	33	10	183	10336	163	22208	2602	35367	11379	708

★ HOSPITAL SAN FRANCISCO, 371 De Diego Avenue, Zip 00929, Mailing Address: P.O. Box 29025, Zip 00929–0025; tel. 787/767–2528; Domingo Nevarez, Executive Director **A**10 **F**4 8 10 14 15 16 19 22 23 27 28 29 32 33 43 44 45 46 49 64 65 71 73

	33	10	160	7703	121	35311	0	21015	7927	504

⊞ I. GONZALEZ MARTINEZ ONCOLOGIC HOSPITAL, (ONCOLOGY), Puerto Rico Medical Center, Hato Rey, Zip 00935, Mailing Address: Box 191811, Zip 00919–1811; tel. 809/765–2382; Celia Molano, Executive Director **A**1 3 5 9 10 **F**8 12 14 15 16 19 20 21 29 34 35 37 42 44 45 48 49 60 65 71 73

	23	49	80	1723	29	30587	0	9922	4815	182

★ INDUSTRIAL HOSPITAL, Puerto Rico Medical Center, Zip 00936, Mailing Address: Box 5028, Zip 00936; tel. 809/764–3660; Evelyn Vargas–Torres, Administrator **A**3 5 **F**4 9 11 19 21 22 27 34 35 37 39 41 43 44 48 49 65 67 69 70 71 72 **P**8

	12	10	125	3555	88	204409	0	—	—	677

Hospital, Address, Telephone, Administrator, Approval, Facility, and Physician Codes, Health Care System, Network	Classi-fication Codes		Utilization Data					Expense (thousands) of dollars		
★ American Hospital Association (AHA) membership □ Joint Commission on Accreditation of Healthcare Organizations (JCAHO) accreditation + American Osteopathic Hospital Association (AOHA) membership ○ American Osteopathic Association (AOA) accreditation △ Commission on Accreditation of Rehabilitation Facilities (CARF) accreditation Control codes 61, 63, 64, 71, 72 and 73 indicate hospitals listed by AOHA, but not registered by AHA. For definition of numerical codes, see page A4	Control	Service	Beds	Admissions	Census	Outpatient Visits	Births	Total	Payroll	Personnel
★ SAN CARLOS GENERAL HOSPITAL, 1822 Ponce De Leon Avenue, Zip 00919, Mailing Address: Call Box 8410, Zip 00910–8410; tel. 809/727–5858; Pedro Gonzalez, Executive Director (Total facility includes 8 beds in nursing home–type unit) (Nonreporting) **A**9 10	33	10	66	—	—	—	—	—	—	—
★ SAN JORGE CHILDREN'S HOSPITAL, 258 San Jorge Avenue, Zip 00912; tel. 809/727–1000; Domingo Cruz Vivaldi, Administrator (Nonreporting) **A**9 **S** United Medical Corporation, Windermere, FL	33	50	85	—	—	—	—	—	—	—
⊞ SAN JUAN CITY HOSPITAL, Puerto Rico Medical Center, Zip 00928, Mailing Address: Apartado 21405, Rio Piedras, Zip 00928; tel. 787/766–2222; Maritza Espinosa, Chief Executive Officer (Nonreporting) **A**1 3 5 10	14	10	267	—	—	—	—	—	—	—
★ STATE PSYCHIATRIC HOSPITAL, Mailing Address: Call Box 2100, Caparra Heights Station, Zip 00922–2100; tel. 787/766–4646; Guadalupe Alvarez, Administrator (Nonreporting) **A**3 **S** Puerto Rico Department of Health, San Juan, PR	12	22	425	—	—	—	—	—	—	—
⊞ U. S. NAVAL HOSPITAL, Roosevelt Roads, Mailing Address: Box 3007, FPO, AA, Zip 34051–8100; tel. 787/865–6171; Captain W. F. Lorenzen, Commanding Officer **A**1 **F**7 8 14 16 19 20 22 26 30 34 37 40 41 44 46 49 51 54 55 56 58 59 65 71 **P**6 **S** Department of Navy, Washington, DC	43	10	35	1419	8	80289	189	—	—	382
⊞ UNIVERSITY HOSPITAL, Puerto Rico Medical Center, Rio Piedras Station, Zip 00935; tel. 809/754–3654; Roberto Hernandez, Administrator (Nonreporting) **A**1 2 3 5 9 10 **S** Puerto Rico Department of Health, San Juan, PR	12	10	297	—	—	—	—	—	—	—
⊞ UNIVERSITY PEDIATRIC HOSPITAL, Mailing Address: GPO Box 365067, Zip 00910–1079; tel. 809/767–3182; Sylvia Mercado, Chief Executive Officer (Nonreporting) **A**1 3 5 9 10	12	50	135	—	—	—	—	—	—	—
⊞ VETERANS AFFAIRS MEDICAL CENTER, One Veterans Plaza, Zip 00927–5800; tel. 809/766–5665; James A. Palmer, Director (Total facility includes 120 beds in nursing home–type unit) (Nonreporting) **A**1 2 3 5 8 **S** Department of Veterans Affairs, Washington, DC	45	10	693	—	—	—	—	—	—	—
VEGA BAJA—Vega Baja County										
★ WILMA N. VAZQUEZ MEDICAL CENTER, KM 395 Road 2, Call Box 7001, Zip 00694; tel. 787/858–1580; Ramon J. Vilar, Administrator (Total facility includes 68 beds in nursing home–type unit) (Nonreporting) **A**9 10	33	10	150	—	—	—	—	—	—	—
YAUCO—Yauco County										
⊞ HOSPITAL DE AREA DE YAUCO, Carretera 128 KM 1 0, Zip 00698, Mailing Address: Box 68, Zip 00698; tel. 809/856–2105; Miguel A. Solivan, Executive Director **A**1 5 10 **F**8 15 20 22 37 39 40 44 54 65 71	12	10	123	5919	65	67552	1161	13051	5861	460

VIRGIN ISLANDS

CHARLOTTE AMALIE—St. Thomas County
ST. THOMAS HOSPITAL AND COMMUNITY HEALTH SERVICE See Roy Lester Schneider Hospital, Saint Thomas

CHRISTIANSTED—St. Croix County										
⊞ GOVERNOR JUAN F. LOUIS HOSPITAL, (Formerly St. Croix Hospital), 4007 Estate Diamond Ruby, Zip 00820–4421; tel. 809/778–6311; George H. McCoy, Chief Executive Officer (Nonreporting) **A**1 10	12	10	87	—	—	—	—	—	—	—
SAINT THOMAS—St. Thomas County										
ROY LESTER SCHNEIDER HOSPITAL, (Formerly St. Thomas Hospital and Community Health Service), 9048 Sugar Estate, Charlotte Amalie, Zip 00802; tel. 809/774–1300; Evelyn McLaughlin, Acting Chief Executive Officer (Nonreporting) **A**10	12	10	133	—	—	—	—	—	—	—

U.S. Government Hospitals
Outside the United States, by Area

GERMANY

Heidelberg: ★ U. S. Army Hospital, APO, AE 09014
Landstuhl: ★ Landstuhl Army Regional Medical Center, APO, AE 09180
Wurzburg: ★ U. S. Army Hospital, APO, USAMEDDAC Wurzburg, AE 09244

ICELAND

Keflavilk: ★ U. S. Naval Hospital, FPO, Box 8, AE 09728

ITALY

Naples: ★ U. S. Naval Hospital, FPO, AE 09619

JAPAN

Yokosuka: ★ U. S. Naval Hospital, FPO, Box 1487, AP 96350

KOREA

Seoul: ★ U. S. Army Community Hospital Seoul, APO, AP 96205
Yongsan: Medcom 18th Commander, Facilities Division Eamc L EM, APO, AP 96205

PANAMA

Ancon: ★ Gorgas Army Hospital, APO, AA 34004

SPAIN

Rota: ★ U. S. Naval Hospital, Rota, FPO, PSC 819, Box 18, AE 09645–2500

TAIWAN

Taipei: U. S. Naval Hospital Taipei, Taipei, No 300 Shin–Pai Road, Sec 2

★Indicates membership in the American Hospital Association

This section is an index of all hospitals in alphabetical order by hospital name, followed by the city, state and page reference to the hospital's listing in Section A.

A

A. G. HOLLEY STATE HOSPITAL, LANTANA, FL, p. A91
ABBEVILLE COUNTY MEMORIAL HOSPITAL, ABBEVILLE, SC, p. A375
ABBEVILLE GENERAL HOSPITAL, ABBEVILLE, LA, p. A182
ABBOTT NORTHWESTERN HOSPITAL, MINNEAPOLIS, MN, p. A231
ABERDEEN–MONROE COUNTY HOSPITAL, ABERDEEN, MS, p. A237
ABILENE REGIONAL MEDICAL CENTER, ABILENE, TX, p. A398
ABINGTON MEMORIAL HOSPITAL, ABINGTON, PA, p. A353
ABRAHAM LINCOLN MEMORIAL HOSPITAL, LINCOLN, IL, p. A133
ABROM KAPLAN MEMORIAL HOSPITAL, KAPLAN, LA, p. A185
ACADIA HOSPITAL, BANGOR, ME, p. A193
ACADIA–ST. LANDRY HOSPITAL, CHURCH POINT, LA, p. A183
ACOMA–CANONCITO–LAGUNA HOSPITAL, SAN FIDEL, NM, p. A287
ADAIR COUNTY MEMORIAL HOSPITAL, GREENFIELD, IA, p. A154
ADAMS COUNTY HOSPITAL, WEST UNION, OH, p. A337
ADAMS COUNTY MEMORIAL HOSPITAL, DECATUR, IN, p. A141
ADAMS COUNTY MEMORIAL HOSPITAL AND NURSING CARE UNIT, FRIENDSHIP, WI, p. A462
ADCARE HOSPITAL OF WORCESTER, WORCESTER, MA, p. A211
ADDISON COMMUNITY HOSPITAL, ADDISON, MI, p. A212
ADENA HEALTH SYSTEM, CHILLICOTHE, OH, p. A325
ADIRONDACK MEDICAL CENTER, SARANAC LAKE, NY, p. A304
ADVENTIST MEDICAL CENTER, PORTLAND, OR, p. A350
AFFILIATED HEALTH SERVICES, MOUNT VERNON, WA, p. A450
AGNESIAN HEALTHCARE, FOND DU LAC, WI, p. A462
AGUADILLA GENERAL HOSPITAL, AGUADILLA, PR, p. A474
AIKEN REGIONAL MEDICAL CENTER, AIKEN, SC, p. A375
AKRON GENERAL MEDICAL CENTER, AKRON, OH, p. A323
ALAMANCE REGIONAL MEDICAL CENTER, BURLINGTON, NC, p. A309
ALAMEDA COUNTY MEDICAL CENTER, SAN LEANDRO, CA, p. A62
ALAMEDA COUNTY MEDICAL CENTER–HIGHLAND CAMPUS, OAKLAND, CA, p. A55
ALAMEDA HOSPITAL, ALAMEDA, CA, p. A36
ALASKA PSYCHIATRIC HOSPITAL, ANCHORAGE, AK, p. A20
ALBANY AREA HOSPITAL AND MEDICAL CENTER, ALBANY, MN, p. A226
ALBANY GENERAL HOSPITAL, ALBANY, OR, p. A348
ALBANY MEDICAL CENTER, ALBANY, NY, p. A288
ALBEMARLE HOSPITAL, ELIZABETH CITY, NC, p. A311
ALBERT EINSTEIN MEDICAL CENTER, PHILADELPHIA, PA, p. A363
ALBERT LINDLEY LEE MEMORIAL HOSPITAL, FULTON, NY, p. A292
ALCOHOL AND DRUG ABUSE TREATMENT CENTER, BLACK MOUNTAIN, NC, p. A308
ALCOHOL AND DRUG ABUSE TREATMENT CENTER, BUTNER, NC, p. A309
ALCOHOLISM TREATMENT CENTER, WINFIELD, IL, p. A139
ALEGENT HEALTH BERGAN MERCY MEDICAL CENTER, OMAHA, NE, p. A266
ALEGENT HEALTH COMMUNITY MEMORIAL HOSPITAL, MISSOURI VALLEY, IA, p. A157
ALEGENT HEALTH IMMANUEL MEDICAL CENTER, OMAHA, NE, p. A266
ALEGENT HEALTH MERCY HOSPITAL, CORNING, IA, p. A152
ALEGENT HEALTH MERCY HOSPITAL, COUNCIL BLUFFS, IA, p. A153
ALEGENT HEALTH–MEMORIAL HOSPITAL, SCHUYLER, NE, p. A268
ALEXANDER COMMUNITY HOSPITAL, TAYLORSVILLE, NC, p. A317
ALEXANDRIA HOSPITAL, ALEXANDRIA, VA, p. A439
ALEXIAN BROTHERS HOSPITAL, SAN JOSE, CA, p. A62
ALEXIAN BROTHERS HOSPITAL, SAINT LOUIS, MO, p. A253
ALEXIAN BROTHERS MEDICAL CENTER, ELK GROVE VILLAGE, IL, p. A129
ALHAMBRA HOSPITAL, ALHAMBRA, CA, p. A36
ALICE HYDE HOSPITAL ASSOCIATION, MALONE, NY, p. A294
ALICE PECK DAY MEMORIAL HOSPITAL, LEBANON, NH, p. A273
ALL CHILDREN'S HOSPITAL, SAINT PETERSBURG, FL, p. A98
ALL SAINTS EPISCOPAL HOSPITAL OF FORT WORTH, FORT WORTH, TX, p. A409

ALL SAINTS HOSPITAL–CITYVIEW, FORT WORTH, TX, p. A410
ALLEGAN GENERAL HOSPITAL, ALLEGAN, MI, p. A212
ALLEGHANY COUNTY MEMORIAL HOSPITAL, SPARTA, NC, p. A317
ALLEGHENY GENERAL HOSPITAL, PITTSBURGH, PA, p. A365
ALLEGHENY UNIVERSITY HOSPITAL, BUCKS COUNTY, WARMINSTER, PA, p. A370
ALLEGHENY UNIVERSITY HOSPITAL, EAST FALLS, PHILADELPHIA, PA, p. A363
ALLEGHENY UNIVERSITY HOSPITAL, ELKINS PARK, ELKINS PARK, PA, p. A357
ALLEGHENY UNIVERSITY HOSPITALS, HAHNEMANN, PHILADELPHIA, PA, p. A363
ALLEGHENY VALLEY HOSPITAL, NATRONA HEIGHTS, PA, p. A362
ALLEN BENNETT HOSPITAL, GREER, SC, p. A378
ALLEN COUNTY HOSPITAL, IOLA, KS, p. A164
ALLEN MEMORIAL HOSPITAL, WATERLOO, IA, p. A159
ALLEN MEMORIAL HOSPITAL, OBERLIN, OH, p. A333
ALLEN MEMORIAL HOSPITAL, MOAB, UT, p. A434
ALLEN PARISH HOSPITAL, KINDER, LA, p. A186
ALLENDALE COUNTY HOSPITAL, FAIRFAX, SC, p. A377
ALLENMORE HOSPITAL, TACOMA, WA, p. A453
ALLENTOWN OSTEOPATHIC MEDICAL CENTER, ALLENTOWN, PA, p. A353
ALLENTOWN STATE HOSPITAL, ALLENTOWN, PA, p. A353
ALLIANCE COMMUNITY HOSPITAL, ALLIANCE, OH, p. A323
ALLIANCE HOSPITAL OF SANTA TERESA, SANTA TERESA, NM, p. A287
ALLIANT HOSPITALS, LOUISVILLE, KY, p. A177
ALLIED SERVICES REHABILITATION HOSPITAL, SCRANTON, PA, p. A368
ALPENA GENERAL HOSPITAL, ALPENA, MI, p. A212
ALTA BATES MEDICAL CENTER–ASHBY CAMPUS, BERKELEY, CA, p. A38
ALTA DISTRICT HOSPITAL, DINUBA, CA, p. A41
ALTA VIEW HOSPITAL, SANDY, UT, p. A435
ALTON MEMORIAL HOSPITAL, ALTON, IL, p. A123
ALTON MENTAL HEALTH CENTER, ALTON, IL, p. A123
ALTOONA CENTER, ALTOONA, PA, p. A353
ALTOONA HOSPITAL, ALTOONA, PA, p. A353
ALVARADO HOSPITAL MEDICAL CENTER, SAN DIEGO, CA, p. A60
ALVIN C. YORK VETERANS AFFAIRS MEDICAL CENTER, MURFREESBORO, TN, p. A394
AMERICAN FORK HOSPITAL, AMERICAN FORK, UT, p. A433
AMERICAN LEGION HOSPITAL, CROWLEY, LA, p. A184
AMERICAN TRANSITIONAL HOSPITAL–DALLAS/FORT WORTH, IRVING, TX, p. A416
AMERICAN TRANSITIONAL HOSPITAL–HOUSTON MEDICAL CENTER, HOUSTON, TX, p. A413
AMETHYST, CHARLOTTE, NC, p. A309
AMOS COTTAGE REHABILITATION HOSPITAL, WINSTON–SALEM, NC, p. A318
AMSTERDAM MEMORIAL HOSPITAL, AMSTERDAM, NY, p. A288
ANACAPA HOSPITAL, PORT HUENEME, CA, p. A57
ANADARKO MUNICIPAL HOSPITAL, ANADARKO, OK, p. A339
ANAHEIM GENERAL HOSPITAL, ANAHEIM, CA, p. A36
ANAHEIM MEMORIAL HOSPITAL, ANAHEIM, CA, p. A36
ANAMOSA COMMUNITY HOSPITAL, ANAMOSA, IA, p. A151
ANCHOR HOSPITAL, ATLANTA, GA, p. A103
ANCORA PSYCHIATRIC HOSPITAL, ANCORA, NJ, p. A275
ANDERSON AREA MEDICAL CENTER, ANDERSON, SC, p. A375
ANDERSON COUNTY HOSPITAL, GARNETT, KS, p. A163
ANDERSON HOSPITAL, MARYVILLE, IL, p. A133
ANDREW MCFARLAND MENTAL HEALTH CENTER, SPRINGFIELD, IL, p. A138
ANDROSCOGGIN VALLEY HOSPITAL, BERLIN, NH, p. A272
ANGEL MEDICAL CENTER, FRANKLIN, NC, p. A311
ANGLETON–DANBURY GENERAL HOSPITAL, ANGLETON, TX, p. A399
ANNA JAQUES HOSPITAL, NEWBURYPORT, MA, p. A208
ANNE ARUNDEL MEDICAL CENTER, ANNAPOLIS, MD, p. A197
ANNIE JEFFREY MEMORIAL COUNTY HEALTH CENTER, OSCEOLA, NE, p. A267
ANNIE PENN HOSPITAL, REIDSVILLE, NC, p. A315
ANOKA–METROPOLITAN REGIONAL TREATMENT CENTER, ANOKA, MN, p. A226
ANSON COUNTY HOSPITAL AND SKILLED NURSING FACILITIES, WADESBORO, NC, p. A317
ANSON GENERAL HOSPITAL, ANSON, TX, p. A399
ANTELOPE MEMORIAL HOSPITAL, NELIGH, NE, p. A266
ANTELOPE VALLEY HOSPITAL, LANCASTER, CA, p. A48

APPALACHIAN PSYCHIATRIC HEALTHCARE SYSTEM, CAMBRIDGE, OH, p. A324
APPLE RIVER HOSPITAL, AMERY, WI, p. A460
APPLETON MEDICAL CENTER, APPLETON, WI, p. A460
APPLETON MUNICIPAL HOSPITAL AND NURSING HOME, APPLETON, MN, p. A226
APPLING HEALTHCARE SYSTEM, BAXLEY, GA, p. A105
ARBORVIEW HOSPITAL, WARREN, MI, p. A224
ARBOUR HOSPITAL, BOSTON, MA, p. A203
ARBUCKLE MEMORIAL HOSPITAL, SULPHUR, OK, p. A346
ARCADIA VALLEY HOSPITAL, PILOT KNOB, MO, p. A252
ARDEN HILL HOSPITAL, GOSHEN, NY, p. A292
ARECIBO REGIONAL HOSPITAL, ARECIBO, PR, p. A474
ARH REGIONAL MEDICAL CENTER, HAZARD, KY, p. A175
ARIZONA STATE HOSPITAL, PHOENIX, AZ, p. A24
ARKANSAS CHILDREN'S HOSPITAL, LITTLE ROCK, AR, p. A32
ARKANSAS METHODIST HOSPITAL, PARAGOULD, AR, p. A34
ARKANSAS STATE HOSPITAL, LITTLE ROCK, AR, p. A32
ARKANSAS VALLEY REGIONAL MEDICAL CENTER, LA JUNTA, CO, p. A73
ARLINGTON HOSPITAL, ARLINGTON, VA, p. A439
ARLINGTON MEMORIAL HOSPITAL, ARLINGTON, TX, p. A399
ARLINGTON MUNICIPAL HOSPITAL, ARLINGTON, MN, p. A226
ARMS ACRES, CARMEL, NY, p. A290
ARMSTRONG COUNTY MEMORIAL HOSPITAL, KITTANNING, PA, p. A359
ARNOLD MEMORIAL HEALTH CARE CENTER, ADRIAN, MN, p. A226
ARNOT OGDEN MEDICAL CENTER, ELMIRA, NY, p. A291
AROOSTOOK MEDICAL CENTER, PRESQUE ISLE, ME, p. A195
ARROWHEAD COMMUNITY HOSPITAL AND MEDICAL CENTER, GLENDALE, AZ, p. A23
ARROYO GRANDE COMMUNITY HOSPITAL, ARROYO GRANDE, CA, p. A37
ARTESIA GENERAL HOSPITAL, ARTESIA, NM, p. A285
ARTHUR G. JAMES CANCER HOSPITAL AND RESEARCH INSTITUTE, COLUMBUS, OH, p. A327
ASCENSION HOSPITAL, GONZALES, LA, p. A184
ASHE MEMORIAL HOSPITAL, JEFFERSON, NC, p. A313
ASHFORD PRESBYTERIAN COMMUNITY HOSPITAL, SAN JUAN, PR, p. A476
ASHLAND COMMUNITY HOSPITAL, ASHLAND, OR, p. A348
ASHLAND HEALTH CENTER, ASHLAND, KS, p. A161
ASHLAND REGIONAL MEDICAL CENTER, ASHLAND, PA, p. A353
ASHLEY MEDICAL CENTER, ASHLEY, ND, p. A319
ASHLEY MEMORIAL HOSPITAL, CROSSETT, AR, p. A30
ASHTABULA COUNTY MEDICAL CENTER, ASHTABULA, OH, p. A323
ASPEN VALLEY HOSPITAL DISTRICT, ASPEN, CO, p. A70
ATASCADERO STATE HOSPITAL, ATASCADERO, CA, p. A37
ATCHISON HOSPITAL, ATCHISON, KS, p. A161
ATH HEIGHTS HOSPITAL, HOUSTON, TX, p. A413
ATHENS REGIONAL MEDICAL CENTER, ATHENS, GA, p. A103
ATHENS–LIMESTONE HOSPITAL, ATHENS, AL, p. A11
ATHOL MEMORIAL HOSPITAL, ATHOL, MA, p. A203
ATLANTA MEMORIAL HOSPITAL, ATLANTA, TX, p. A399
ATLANTIC CITY MEDICAL CENTER, ATLANTIC CITY, NJ, p. A275
ATLANTIC GENERAL HOSPITAL, BERLIN, MD, p. A198
ATLANTIC HEALTH SYSTEM, FLORHAM PARK, NJ, p. A277
ATLANTICARE MEDICAL CENTER, LYNN, MA, p. A207
ATMORE COMMUNITY HOSPITAL, ATMORE, AL, p. A11
ATOKA MEMORIAL HOSPITAL, ATOKA, OK, p. A339
AUBURN GENERAL HOSPITAL, AUBURN, WA, p. A448
AUBURN MEMORIAL HOSPITAL, AUBURN, NY, p. A288
AUDRAIN MEDICAL CENTER, MEXICO, MO, p. A251
AUDUBON COUNTY MEMORIAL HOSPITAL, AUDUBON, IA, p. A151
AUGUSTA HEALTH CARE, FISHERSVILLE, VA, p. A440
AUGUSTA MEDICAL COMPLEX, AUGUSTA, KS, p. A161
AUGUSTA MENTAL HEALTH INSTITUTE, AUGUSTA, ME, p. A193
AULTMAN HOSPITAL, CANTON, OH, p. A324
AURELIA OSBORN FOX MEMORIAL HOSPITAL, ONEONTA, NY, p. A301
AURORA COMMUNITY HOSPITAL, AURORA, MO, p. A245
AURORA HOSPITAL FOR CHILDREN, DETROIT, MI, p. A214
AUSTEN RIGGS CENTER, STOCKBRIDGE, MA, p. A210
AUSTIN DIAGNOSTIC MEDICAL CENTER, AUSTIN, TX, p. A399
AUSTIN MEDICAL CENTER, AUSTIN, MN, p. A226
AUSTIN STATE HOSPITAL, AUSTIN, TX, p. A400
AUXILIO MUTUO HOSPITAL, SAN JUAN, PR, p. A476
AVALON MUNICIPAL HOSPITAL AND CLINIC, AVALON, CA, p. A37
AVOYELLES HOSPITAL, MARKSVILLE, LA, p. A187

B

B.J. WORKMAN MEMORIAL HOSPITAL, WOODRUFF, SC, p. A381
BACHARACH REHABILITATION HOSPITAL, POMONA, NJ, p. A281
BACON COUNTY HOSPITAL, ALMA, GA, p. A103
BAKERSFIELD MEMORIAL HOSPITAL, BAKERSFIELD, CA, p. A37
BALDPATE HOSPITAL, GEORGETOWN, MA, p. A206
BALDWIN HOSPITAL, BALDWIN, WI, p. A460
BALL MEMORIAL HOSPITAL, MUNCIE, IN, p. A147
BALLINGER MEMORIAL HOSPITAL, BALLINGER, TX, p. A401
BAMBERG COUNTY MEMORIAL HOSPITAL AND NURSING
   CENTER, BAMBERG, SC, p. A375
BANGOR MENTAL HEALTH INSTITUTE, BANGOR, ME, p. A193
BANNOCK REGIONAL MEDICAL CENTER, POCATELLO, ID,
   p. A121
BAPTIST DEKALB HOSPITAL, SMITHVILLE, TN, p. A396
BAPTIST HICKMAN COMMUNITY HOSPITAL, CENTERVILLE, TN,
   p. A387
BAPTIST HOSPITAL, PENSACOLA, FL, p. A96
BAPTIST HOSPITAL, NASHVILLE, TN, p. A394
BAPTIST HOSPITAL EAST, LOUISVILLE, KY, p. A177
BAPTIST HOSPITAL OF COCKE COUNTY, NEWPORT, TN,
   p. A395
BAPTIST HOSPITAL OF EAST TENNESSEE, KNOXVILLE, TN,
   p. A391
BAPTIST HOSPITAL OF MIAMI, MIAMI, FL, p. A92
BAPTIST HOSPITAL OF SOUTHEAST TEXAS, BEAUMONT, TX,
   p. A401
BAPTIST HOSPITAL–ORANGE, ORANGE, TX, p. A422
BAPTIST MEDICAL CENTER, MONTGOMERY, AL, p. A16
BAPTIST MEDICAL CENTER, LITTLE ROCK, AR, p. A32
BAPTIST MEDICAL CENTER, JACKSONVILLE, FL, p. A89
BAPTIST MEDICAL CENTER, KANSAS CITY, MO, p. A248
BAPTIST MEDICAL CENTER, SAN ANTONIO, TX, p. A425
BAPTIST MEDICAL CENTER ARKADELPHIA, ARKADELPHIA, AR,
   p. A29
BAPTIST MEDICAL CENTER EASLEY, EASLEY, SC, p. A377
BAPTIST MEDICAL CENTER HEBER SPRINGS, HEBER SPRINGS,
   AR, p. A31
BAPTIST MEDICAL CENTER–BEACHES, JACKSONVILLE BEACH,
   FL, p. A90
BAPTIST MEDICAL CENTER–NASSAU, FERNANDINA BEACH, FL,
   p. A86
BAPTIST MEDICAL CENTER/COLUMBIA, COLUMBIA, SC,
   p. A376
BAPTIST MEMORIAL HOSPITAL, MEMPHIS, TN, p. A393
BAPTIST MEMORIAL HOSPITAL–BLYTHEVILLE, BLYTHEVILLE,
   AR, p. A29
BAPTIST MEMORIAL HOSPITAL–BOONEVILLE, BOONEVILLE, MS,
   p. A237
BAPTIST MEMORIAL HOSPITAL–DESOTO, SOUTHAVEN, MS,
   p. A243
BAPTIST MEMORIAL HOSPITAL–FORREST CITY, FORREST CITY,
   AR, p. A31
BAPTIST MEMORIAL HOSPITAL–GOLDEN TRIANGLE,
   COLUMBUS, MS, p. A238
BAPTIST MEMORIAL HOSPITAL–HUNTINGDON, HUNTINGDON,
   TN, p. A390
BAPTIST MEMORIAL HOSPITAL–LAUDERDALE, RIPLEY, TN,
   p. A395
BAPTIST MEMORIAL HOSPITAL–NORTH MISSISSIPPI, OXFORD,
   MS, p. A242
BAPTIST MEMORIAL HOSPITAL–OSCEOLA, OSCEOLA, AR,
   p. A34
BAPTIST MEMORIAL HOSPITAL–TIPTON, COVINGTON, TN,
   p. A388
BAPTIST MEMORIAL HOSPITAL–UNION CITY, UNION CITY, TN,
   p. A396
BAPTIST MEMORIAL HOSPITAL–UNION COUNTY, NEW ALBANY,
   MS, p. A242
BAPTIST MEMORIAL MEDICAL CENTER, NORTH LITTLE ROCK,
   AR, p. A34
BAPTIST NORTH HOSPITAL, CUMMING, GA, p. A107
BAPTIST PERRY MEMORIAL HOSPITAL, LINDEN, TN, p. A392
BAPTIST REGIONAL MEDICAL CENTER, CORBIN, KY, p. A173
BAPTIST REHABILITATION INSTITUTE OF ARKANSAS, LITTLE
   ROCK, AR, p. A32
BAPTIST REHABILITATION–GERMANTOWN, GERMANTOWN, TN,
   p. A389
BAPTIST THREE RIVERS HOSPITAL, WAVERLY, TN, p. A397
BAPTIST–ST. ANTHONY HEALTH SYSTEM, AMARILLO, TX,
   p. A398
BAPTIST–ST. ANTHONY'S HEALTH SYSTEM, AMARILLO, TX,
   p. A398
BARAGA COUNTY MEMORIAL HOSPITAL, L'ANSE, MI, p. A219
BARBERTON CITIZENS HOSPITAL, BARBERTON, OH, p. A323
BARLOW RESPIRATORY HOSPITAL, LOS ANGELES, CA, p. A49

BARNERT HOSPITAL, PATERSON, NJ, p. A280
BARNES–JEWISH HOSPITAL, SAINT LOUIS, MO, p. A253
BARNES–JEWISH ST. PETERS HOSPITAL, SAINT PETERS, MO,
   p. A254
BARNES–JEWISH WEST COUNTY HOSPITAL, SAINT LOUIS, MO,
   p. A253
BARNES–KASSON COUNTY HOSPITAL, SUSQUEHANNA, PA,
   p. A369
BARNESVILLE HOSPITAL ASSOCIATION, BARNESVILLE, OH,
   p. A323
BARNSTABLE COUNTY HOSPITAL, POCASSET, MA, p. A209
BARNWELL COUNTY HOSPITAL, BARNWELL, SC, p. A375
BARRETT MEMORIAL HOSPITAL, DILLON, MT, p. A258
BARRON MEMORIAL MEDICAL CENTER AND SKILLED NURSING
   FACILITY, BARRON, WI, p. A460
BARSTOW COMMUNITY HOSPITAL, BARSTOW, CA, p. A37
BARTLETT MEMORIAL MEDICAL CENTER, SAPULPA, OK,
   p. A345
BARTLETT REGIONAL HOSPITAL, JUNEAU, AK, p. A20
BARTON COUNTY MEMORIAL HOSPITAL, LAMAR, MO, p. A250
BARTON MEMORIAL HOSPITAL, SOUTH LAKE TAHOE, CA,
   p. A65
BASCOM PALMER EYE INSTITUTE–ANNE BATES LEACH EYE
   HOSPITAL, MIAMI, FL, p. A92
BASSETT ARMY COMMUNITY HOSPITAL, FORT WAINWRIGHT,
   AK, p. A20
BASSETT HOSPITAL OF SCHOHARIE COUNTY, COBLESKILL, NY,
   p. A291
BATES COUNTY MEMORIAL HOSPITAL, BUTLER, MO, p. A245
BATH COUNTY COMMUNITY HOSPITAL, HOT SPRINGS, VA,
   p. A442
BATON ROUGE GENERAL HEALTH CENTER, BATON ROUGE, LA,
   p. A182
BATON ROUGE GENERAL MEDICAL CENTER, BATON ROUGE,
   LA, p. A182
BATTLE CREEK HEALTH SYSTEM, BATTLE CREEK, MI, p. A212
BATTLE MOUNTAIN GENERAL HOSPITAL, BATTLE MOUNTAIN,
   NV, p. A270
BAUM HARMON MEMORIAL HOSPITAL, PRIMGHAR, IA, p. A158
BAXTER COUNTY REGIONAL HOSPITAL, MOUNTAIN HOME, AR,
   p. A33
BAY AREA HOSPITAL, COOS BAY, OR, p. A348
BAY AREA MEDICAL CENTER, MARINETTE, WI, p. A464
BAY HARBOR HOSPITAL, LOS ANGELES, CA, p. A49
BAY MEDICAL CENTER, PANAMA CITY, FL, p. A96
BAY MEDICAL CENTER, BAY CITY, MI, p. A213
BAY SPECIAL CARE, BAY CITY, MI, p. A213
BAYCOAST MEDICAL CENTER, BAYTOWN, TX, p. A401
BAYFRONT MEDICAL CENTER, SAINT PETERSBURG, FL, p. A98
BAYHEALTH MEDICAL CENTER, MILFORD MEMORIAL CAMPUS,
   MILFORD, DE, p. A80
BAYLEY SETON HOSPITAL, NEW YORK, NY, p. A295
BAYLOR CENTER FOR RESTORATIVE CARE, DALLAS, TX,
   p. A405
BAYLOR INSTITUTE FOR REHABILITATION, DALLAS, TX, p. A405
BAYLOR MEDICAL CENTER AT GARLAND, GARLAND, TX,
   p. A411
BAYLOR MEDICAL CENTER AT GRAPEVINE, GRAPEVINE, TX,
   p. A412
BAYLOR MEDICAL CENTER–ELLIS COUNTY, WAXAHACHIE, TX,
   p. A430
BAYLOR RICHARDSON MEDICAL CENTER, RICHARDSON, TX,
   p. A424
BAYLOR UNIVERSITY MEDICAL CENTER, DALLAS, TX, p. A406
BAYNE–JONES ARMY COMMUNITY HOSPITAL, FORT POLK, LA,
   p. A184
BAYONNE HOSPITAL, BAYONNE, NJ, p. A275
BAYOU OAKS HOSPITAL, HOUMA, LA, p. A185
BAYSHORE COMMUNITY HOSPITAL, HOLMDEL, NJ, p. A278
BAYSIDE COMMUNITY HOSPITAL, ANAHUAC, TX, p. A398
BAYSTATE MEDICAL CENTER, SPRINGFIELD, MA, p. A210
BAYVIEW HOSPITAL AND MENTAL HEALTH SYSTEM, CHULA
   VISTA, CA, p. A40
BEACHAM MEMORIAL HOSPITAL, MAGNOLIA, MS, p. A241
BEAR LAKE MEMORIAL HOSPITAL, MONTPELIER, ID, p. A120
BEAR RIVER VALLEY HOSPITAL, TREMONTON, UT, p. A436
BEAR VALLEY COMMUNITY HOSPITAL, BIG BEAR LAKE, CA,
   p. A38
BEATRICE COMMUNITY HOSPITAL AND HEALTH CENTER,
   BEATRICE, NE, p. A262
BEAUFORT COUNTY HOSPITAL, WASHINGTON, NC, p. A317
BEAUFORT MEMORIAL HOSPITAL, BEAUFORT, SC, p. A375
BEAUREGARD MEMORIAL HOSPITAL, DE RIDDER, LA, p. A184
BEAVER COUNTY MEMORIAL HOSPITAL, BEAVER, OK, p. A339
BEAVER DAM COMMUNITY HOSPITALS, BEAVER DAM, WI,
   p. A460
BEAVER VALLEY HOSPITAL, BEAVER, UT, p. A433
BECKLEY APPALACHIAN REGIONAL HOSPITAL, BECKLEY, WV,
   p. A455
BECKLEY HOSPITAL, BECKLEY, WV, p. A455

BEDFORD COUNTY GENERAL HOSPITAL, SHELBYVILLE, TN,
   p. A396
BEDFORD REGIONAL MEDICAL CENTER, BEDFORD, IN, p. A140
BEEBE MEDICAL CENTER, LEWES, DE, p. A80
BEECH HILL HOSPITAL, DUBLIN, NH, p. A272
BELL MEMORIAL HOSPITAL, ISHPEMING, MI, p. A218
BELLA VISTA HOSPITAL, MAYAGUEZ, PR, p. A476
BELLEVUE HOSPITAL, BELLEVUE, OH, p. A324
BELLEVUE HOSPITAL CENTER, NEW YORK, NY, p. A295
BELLEVUE WOMAN'S HOSPITAL, SCHENECTADY, NY, p. A304
BELLFLOWER MEDICAL CENTER, BELLFLOWER, CA, p. A38
BELLIN HOSPITAL, GREEN BAY, WI, p. A462
BELLIN PSYCHIATRIC CENTER, GREEN BAY, WI, p. A462
BELLVILLE GENERAL HOSPITAL, BELLVILLE, TX, p. A401
BELLWOOD GENERAL HOSPITAL, BELLFLOWER, CA, p. A38
BELMOND COMMUNITY HOSPITAL, BELMOND, IA, p. A151
BELMONT CENTER FOR COMPREHENSIVE TREATMENT,
   PHILADELPHIA, PA, p. A363
BELOIT MEMORIAL HOSPITAL, BELOIT, WI, p. A460
BENCHMARK BEHAVIORAL HEALTH SYSTEMS, WOODS CROSS,
   UT, p. A436
BENEDICTINE HOSPITAL, KINGSTON, NY, p. A293
BENEFIS HEALTH CARE, GREAT FALLS, MT, p. A258
BENEWAH COMMUNITY HOSPITAL, SAINT MARIES, ID, p. A121
BENJAMIN RUSH CENTER, SYRACUSE, NY, p. A305
BENNETT COUNTY COMMUNITY HOSPITAL, MARTIN, SD,
   p. A383
BENSON HOSPITAL, BENSON, AZ, p. A22
BEREA HOSPITAL, BEREA, KY, p. A172
BERGEN PINES COUNTY HOSPITAL, PARAMUS, NJ, p. A280
BERGER HOSPITAL, CIRCLEVILLE, OH, p. A326
BERKSHIRE MEDICAL CENTER, PITTSFIELD, MA, p. A209
BERRIEN COUNTY HOSPITAL, NASHVILLE, GA, p. A112
BERT FISH MEDICAL CENTER, NEW SMYRNA BEACH, FL, p. A94
BERTIE COUNTY MEMORIAL HOSPITAL, WINDSOR, NC, p. A318
BERTRAND CHAFFEE HOSPITAL, SPRINGVILLE, NY, p. A304
BERWICK HOSPITAL CENTER, BERWICK, PA, p. A354
BESSEMER CARRAWAY MEDICAL CENTER, BESSEMER, AL,
   p. A11
BETH ISRAEL DEACONESS MEDICAL CENTER, BOSTON, MA,
   p. A203
BETH ISRAEL HOSPITAL, PASSAIC, NJ, p. A280
BETH ISRAEL MEDICAL CENTER, NEW YORK, NY, p. A295
BETHANIA REGIONAL HEALTH CARE CENTER, WICHITA FALLS,
   TX, p. A431
BETHANY HOSPITAL, CHICAGO, IL, p. A125
BETHANY MEDICAL CENTER, KANSAS CITY, KS, p. A165
BETHESDA GENERAL HOSPITAL, SAINT LOUIS, MO, p. A253
BETHESDA MEMORIAL HOSPITAL, BOYNTON BEACH, FL, p. A84
BETHESDA NORTH HOSPITAL, CINCINNATI, OH, p. A325
BETHESDA OAK HOSPITAL, CINCINNATI, OH, p. A325
BETSY JOHNSON MEMORIAL HOSPITAL, DUNN, NC, p. A310
BEVERLY HOSPITAL, MONTEBELLO, CA, p. A54
BEVERLY HOSPITAL, BEVERLY, MA, p. A203
BHC ALHAMBRA HOSPITAL, ROSEMEAD, CA, p. A59
BHC ASPEN HILL HOSPITAL, FLAGSTAFF, AZ, p. A22
BHC BELMONT HILLS HOSPITAL, BELMONT, CA, p. A38
BHC BELMONT PINES HOSPITAL, YOUNGSTOWN, OH, p. A337
BHC CANYON RIDGE HOSPITAL, CHINO, CA, p. A39
BHC CEDAR SPRING HOSPITAL, PINEVILLE, NC, p. A315
BHC CEDAR VISTA HOSPITAL, FRESNO, CA, p. A43
BHC COLLEGE MEADOWS HOSPITAL, LENEXA, KS, p. A166
BHC EAST LAKE HOSPITAL, NEW ORLEANS, LA, p. A188
BHC FAIRFAX HOSPITAL, KIRKLAND, WA, p. A450
BHC FORT LAUDERDALE HOSPITAL, FORT LAUDERDALE, FL,
   p. A86
BHC FOX RUN HOSPITAL, SAINT CLAIRSVILLE, OH, p. A335
BHC FREMONT HOSPITAL, FREMONT, CA, p. A43
BHC HERITAGE OAKS HOSPITAL, SACRAMENTO, CA, p. A59
BHC HOSPITAL SAN JUAN CAPESTRANO, SAN JUAN, PR,
   p. A476
BHC INTERMOUNTAIN HOSPITAL, BOISE, ID, p. A119
BHC MEADOW WOOD HOSPITAL, BATON ROUGE, LA, p. A182
BHC MESILLA VALLEY HOSPITAL, LAS CRUCES, NM, p. A286
BHC MIDWOOD HOSPITAL, ARLINGTON, TX, p. A399
BHC MONTEVISTA HOSPITAL, LAS VEGAS, NV, p. A270
BHC OLYMPUS VIEW HOSPITAL, SALT LAKE CITY, UT, p. A435
BHC PINNACLE POINTE HOSPITAL, LITTLE ROCK, AR, p. A32
BHC PINON HILLS HOSPITAL, SANTA FE, NM, p. A287
BHC ROSS HOSPITAL, KENTFIELD, CA, p. A46
BHC SAN LUIS REY HOSPITAL, ENCINITAS, CA, p. A42
BHC SAND HILL BEHAVIORAL HEALTHCARE, GULFPORT, MS,
   p. A239
BHC SHOAL CREEK HOSPITAL, AUSTIN, TX, p. A400
BHC SIERRA VISTA HOSPITAL, SACRAMENTO, CA, p. A59
BHC SPIRIT OF ST. LOUIS HOSPITAL, SAINT CHARLES, MO,
   p. A252
BHC ST. JOHNS RIVER HOSPITAL, JACKSONVILLE, FL, p. A89
BHC STREAMWOOD HOSPITAL, STREAMWOOD, IL, p. A138
BHC VALLE VISTA HOSPITAL, GREENWOOD, IN, p. A143

BHC VISTA DEL MAR HOSPITAL, VENTURA, CA, p. A67
BHC WALNUT CREEK HOSPITAL, WALNUT CREEK, CA, p. A68
BHC WEST HILLS HOSPITAL, RENO, NV, p. A271
BHC WILLOW SPRINGS RTC, RENO, NV, p. A271
BHC WINDSOR HOSPITAL, CHAGRIN FALLS, OH, p. A324
BI-COUNTY COMMUNITY HOSPITAL, WARREN, MI, p. A224
BIBB MEDICAL CENTER, CENTREVILLE, AL, p. A13
BIG BEND REGIONAL MEDICAL CENTER, ALPINE, TX, p. A398
BIG HORN COUNTY MEMORIAL HOSPITAL, HARDIN, MT, p. A258
BIG SANDY MEDICAL CENTER, BIG SANDY, MT, p. A257
BIG SPRING STATE HOSPITAL, BIG SPRING, TX, p. A402
BIGGS-GRIDLEY MEMORIAL HOSPITAL, GRIDLEY, CA, p. A45
BILOXI REGIONAL MEDICAL CENTER, BILOXI, MS, p. A237
BINGHAM MEMORIAL HOSPITAL, BLACKFOOT, ID, p. A119
BINGHAMTON PSYCHIATRIC CENTER, BINGHAMTON, NY, p. A289
BIRMINGHAM BAPTIST MEDICAL CENTER–MONTCLAIR CAMPUS, BIRMINGHAM, AL, p. A11
BIRMINGHAM BAPTIST MEDICAL CENTER–PRINCETON, BIRMINGHAM, AL, p. A11
BISHOP CLARKSON MEMORIAL HOSPITAL, OMAHA, NE, p. A266
BIXBY MEDICAL CENTER, ADRIAN, MI, p. A212
BJC MEDICAL CENTER, COMMERCE, GA, p. A107
BLACK RIVER MEMORIAL HOSPITAL, BLACK RIVER FALLS, WI, p. A461
BLACKFORD COUNTY HOSPITAL, HARTFORD CITY, IN, p. A143
BLACKWELL REGIONAL HOSPITAL, BLACKWELL, OK, p. A339
BLADEN COUNTY HOSPITAL, ELIZABETHTOWN, NC, p. A311
BLANCHARD VALLEY REGIONAL HEALTH CENTER, FINDLAY, OH, p. A329
BLECKLEY MEMORIAL HOSPITAL, COCHRAN, GA, p. A106
BLEDSOE COUNTY GENERAL HOSPITAL, PIKEVILLE, TN, p. A395
BLESSING HOSPITAL, QUINCY, IL, p. A136
BLODGETT MEMORIAL MEDICAL CENTER, GRAND RAPIDS, MI, p. A216
BLOOMER COMMUNITY MEMORIAL HOSPITAL AND THE MAPLEWOOD, BLOOMER, WI, p. A461
BLOOMINGTON HOSPITAL, BLOOMINGTON, IN, p. A140
BLOOMSBURG HOSPITAL, BLOOMSBURG, PA, p. A354
BLOSS MEMORIAL HOSPITAL DISTRICT, ATWATER, CA, p. A37
BLOUNT MEMORIAL HOSPITAL, ONEONTA, AL, p. A17
BLOUNT MEMORIAL HOSPITAL, MARYVILLE, TN, p. A393
BLOWING ROCK HOSPITAL, BLOWING ROCK, NC, p. A308
BLUE HILL MEMORIAL HOSPITAL, BLUE HILL, ME, p. A193
BLUE MOUNTAIN HOSPITAL, JOHN DAY, OR, p. A349
BLUEFIELD REGIONAL MEDICAL CENTER, BLUEFIELD, WV, p. A455
BLYTHEDALE CHILDREN'S HOSPITAL, VALHALLA, NY, p. A306
BOAZ–ALBERTVILLE MEDICAL CENTER, BOAZ, AL, p. A12
BOB WILSON MEMORIAL GRANT COUNTY HOSPITAL, ULYSSES, KS, p. A170
BOCA RATON COMMUNITY HOSPITAL, BOCA RATON, FL, p. A83
BOGALUSA COMMUNITY MEDICAL CENTER, BOGALUSA, LA, p. A183
BOLIVAR COUNTY HOSPITAL, CLEVELAND, MS, p. A238
BOLIVAR GENERAL HOSPITAL, BOLIVAR, TN, p. A387
BON SECOURS HOSPITAL, BALTIMORE, MD, p. A197
BON SECOURS HOSPITAL, GROSSE POINTE, MI, p. A217
BON SECOURS–DEPAUL MEDICAL CENTER, NORFOLK, VA, p. A443
BON SECOURS–HOLY FAMILY REGIONAL HEALTH SYSTEM, ALTOONA, PA, p. A353
BON SECOURS–MARYVIEW MEDICAL CENTER, PORTSMOUTH, VA, p. A444
BON SECOURS–RICHMOND COMMUNITY HOSPITAL, RICHMOND, VA, p. A445
BON SECOURS–ST. FRANCIS XAVIER HOSPITAL, CHARLESTON, SC, p. A375
BON SECOURS–ST. JOSEPH HOSPITAL, PORT CHARLOTTE, FL, p. A97
BON SECOURS–STUART CIRCLE, RICHMOND, VA, p. A445
BONE AND JOINT HOSPITAL, OKLAHOMA CITY, OK, p. A343
BONNER GENERAL HOSPITAL, SANDPOINT, ID, p. A121
BOONE COUNTY HEALTH CENTER, ALBION, NE, p. A262
BOONE COUNTY HOSPITAL, BOONE, IA, p. A151
BOONE HOSPITAL CENTER, COLUMBIA, MO, p. A246
BOONE MEMORIAL HOSPITAL, MADISON, WV, p. A457
BOONEVILLE COMMUNITY HOSPITAL, BOONEVILLE, AR, p. A29
BORGESS MEDICAL CENTER, KALAMAZOO, MI, p. A218
BOSCOBEL AREA HEALTH CARE, BOSCOBEL, WI, p. A461
BOSSIER MEDICAL CENTER, BOSSIER CITY, LA, p. A183
BOSTON MEDICAL CENTER, BOSTON, MA, p. A203
BOSTON REGIONAL MEDICAL CENTER, STONEHAM, MA, p. A210
BOTHWELL REGIONAL HEALTH CENTER, SEDALIA, MO, p. A255
BOTSFORD GENERAL HOSPITAL, FARMINGTON HILLS, MI, p. A216

BOULDER CITY HOSPITAL, BOULDER CITY, NV, p. A270
BOULDER COMMUNITY HOSPITAL, BOULDER, CO, p. A70
BOUNDARY COMMUNITY HOSPITAL, BONNERS FERRY, ID, p. A119
BOURNEWOOD HOSPITAL, BROOKLINE, MA, p. A205
BOWDLE HOSPITAL, BOWDLE, SD, p. A382
BOWDON AREA HOSPITAL, BOWDON, GA, p. A105
BOWIE MEMORIAL HOSPITAL, BOWIE, TX, p. A402
BOX BUTTE GENERAL HOSPITAL, ALLIANCE, NE, p. A262
BOYS TOWN NATIONAL RESEARCH HOSPITAL, OMAHA, NE, p. A266
BOZEMAN DEACONESS HOSPITAL, BOZEMAN, MT, p. A257
BRACKENRIDGE HOSPITAL, AUSTIN, TX, p. A400
BRADFORD HEALTH SERVICES AT BIRMINGHAM, BIRMINGHAM, AL, p. A11
BRADFORD HEALTH SERVICES AT HUNTSVILLE, MADISON, AL, p. A15
BRADFORD HEALTH SERVICES AT OAK MOUNTAIN, PELHAM, AL, p. A17
BRADFORD REGIONAL MEDICAL CENTER, BRADFORD, PA, p. A354
BRADLEY COUNTY MEMORIAL HOSPITAL, WARREN, AR, p. A35
BRADLEY MEMORIAL HOSPITAL, CLEVELAND, TN, p. A388
BRADLEY MEMORIAL HOSPITAL AND HEALTH CENTER, SOUTHINGTON, CT, p. A78
BRAINERD REGIONAL HUMAN SERVICES CENTER, BRAINERD, MN, p. A227
BRAINTREE HOSPITAL REHABILITATION NETWORK, BRAINTREE, MA, p. A205
BRANDYWINE HOSPITAL, COATESVILLE, PA, p. A356
BRATTLEBORO MEMORIAL HOSPITAL, BRATTLEBORO, VT, p. A437
BRATTLEBORO RETREAT, BRATTLEBORO, VT, p. A437
BRAXTON COUNTY MEMORIAL HOSPITAL, GASSAWAY, WV, p. A456
BRAZOSPORT MEMORIAL HOSPITAL, LAKE JACKSON, TX, p. A418
BREA COMMUNITY HOSPITAL, BREA, CA, p. A38
BRECKINRIDGE MEMORIAL HOSPITAL, HARDINSBURG, KY, p. A174
BREECH MEDICAL CENTER, LEBANON, MO, p. A250
BRENTWOOD BEHAVIORAL HEALTHCARE, SHREVEPORT, LA, p. A190
BRIDGEPORT HOSPITAL, BRIDGEPORT, CT, p. A76
BRIDGES MEDICAL SERVICES, ADA, MN, p. A226
BRIDGEWATER STATE HOSPITAL, BRIDGEWATER, MA, p. A205
BRIDGEWAY, NORTH LITTLE ROCK, AR, p. A34
BRIGHAM AND WOMEN'S HOSPITAL, BOSTON, MA, p. A204
BRIGHTON CAMPUS OF MAINE MEDICAL CENTER, PORTLAND, ME, p. A195
BRIGHTON HOSPITAL, BRIGHTON, MI, p. A213
BRISTOL HOSPITAL, BRISTOL, CT, p. A76
BRISTOW MEMORIAL HOSPITAL, BRISTOW, OK, p. A340
BROADDUS HOSPITAL, PHILIPPI, WV, p. A458
BROADLAWNS MEDICAL CENTER, DES MOINES, IA, p. A153
BROADWATER HEALTH CENTER, TOWNSEND, MT, p. A260
BROCKTON HOSPITAL, BROCKTON, MA, p. A205
BROCKTON–WEST ROXBURY VETERANS AFFAIRS MEDICAL CENTER, BROCKTON, MA, p. A205
BRODSTONE MEMORIAL HOSPITAL, SUPERIOR, NE, p. A268
BROKEN ARROW MEDICAL CENTER, BROKEN ARROW, OK, p. A340
BROMENN HEALTHCARE, NORMAL, IL, p. A135
BRONSON METHODIST HOSPITAL, KALAMAZOO, MI, p. A218
BRONSON VICKSBURG HOSPITAL, VICKSBURG, MI, p. A224
BRONX CHILDREN'S PSYCHIATRIC CENTER, NEW YORK, NY, p. A295
BRONX PSYCHIATRIC CENTER, NEW YORK, NY, p. A295
BRONX–LEBANON HOSPITAL CENTER, NEW YORK, NY, p. A295
BROOK LANE PSYCHIATRIC CENTER, HAGERSTOWN, MD, p. A200
BROOKDALE HOSPITAL MEDICAL CENTER, NEW YORK, NY, p. A296
BROOKE ARMY MEDICAL CENTER, SAN ANTONIO, TX, p. A425
BROOKHAVEN HOSPITAL, TULSA, OK, p. A346
BROOKHAVEN MEMORIAL HOSPITAL MEDICAL CENTER, PATCHOGUE, NY, p. A302
BROOKINGS HOSPITAL, BROOKINGS, SD, p. A382
BROOKLYN HOSPITAL CENTER, NEW YORK, NY, p. A296
BROOKS COUNTY HOSPITAL, QUITMAN, GA, p. A112
BROOKS HOSPITAL, ATLANTA, TX, p. A399
BROOKS MEMORIAL HOSPITAL, DUNKIRK, NY, p. A291
BROOKSIDE HOSPITAL, SAN PABLO, CA, p. A63
BROOKSVILLE REGIONAL HOSPITAL, BROOKSVILLE, FL, p. A84
BROOKVILLE HOSPITAL, BROOKVILLE, PA, p. A354
BROOKWOOD MEDICAL CENTER, BIRMINGHAM, AL, p. A11
BROTMAN MEDICAL CENTER, CULVER CITY, CA, p. A41
BROUGHTON HOSPITAL, MORGANTON, NC, p. A314
BROWARD GENERAL MEDICAL CENTER, FORT LAUDERDALE, FL, p. A86

BROWN COUNTY GENERAL HOSPITAL, GEORGETOWN, OH, p. A330
BROWN COUNTY HOSPITAL, AINSWORTH, NE, p. A262
BROWN COUNTY MENTAL HEALTH CENTER, GREEN BAY, WI, p. A462
BROWN MEMORIAL HOSPITAL, CONNEAUT, OH, p. A328
BROWNFIELD REGIONAL MEDICAL CENTER, BROWNFIELD, TX, p. A402
BROWNSVILLE GENERAL HOSPITAL, BROWNSVILLE, PA, p. A354
BROWNSVILLE MEDICAL CENTER, BROWNSVILLE, TX, p. A402
BRUCE HOSPITAL, BRUCE, MS, p. A238
BRUNSWICK GENERAL HOSPITAL, AMITYVILLE, NY, p. A288
BRYAN MEMORIAL HOSPITAL, LINCOLN, NE, p. A265
BRYAN W. WHITFIELD MEMORIAL HOSPITAL, DEMOPOLIS, AL, p. A13
BRYCE HOSPITAL, TUSCALOOSA, AL, p. A18
BRYLIN HOSPITALS, BUFFALO, NY, p. A289
BRYN MAWR COLLEGE INFIRMARY, BRYN MAWR, PA, p. A354
BRYN MAWR HOSPITAL, BRYN MAWR, PA, p. A354
BRYN MAWR REHABILITATION HOSPITAL, MALVERN, PA, p. A361
BRYNN MARR BEHAVIORAL HEALTHCARE SYSTEM, JACKSONVILLE, NC, p. A313
BUCHANAN GENERAL HOSPITAL, GRUNDY, VA, p. A441
BUCKTAIL MEDICAL CENTER, RENOVO, PA, p. A368
BUCYRUS COMMUNITY HOSPITAL, BUCYRUS, OH, p. A324
BUENA PARK MEDICAL CENTER, BUENA PARK, CA, p. A38
BUENA VISTA COUNTY HOSPITAL, STORM LAKE, IA, p. A159
BUFFALO GENERAL HOSPITAL, BUFFALO, NY, p. A289
BUFFALO HOSPITAL, BUFFALO, MN, p. A227
BUFFALO PSYCHIATRIC CENTER, BUFFALO, NY, p. A290
BULLHEAD COMMUNITY HOSPITAL, BULLHEAD CITY, AZ, p. A22
BULLOCH MEMORIAL HOSPITAL, STATESBORO, GA, p. A114
BULLOCK COUNTY HOSPITAL, UNION SPRINGS, AL, p. A18
BUNKIE GENERAL HOSPITAL, BUNKIE, LA, p. A183
BURDETTE TOMLIN MEMORIAL HOSPITAL, CAPE MAY COURT HOUSE, NJ, p. A276
BURGESS MEMORIAL HOSPITAL, ONAWA, IA, p. A157
BURKE COUNTY HOSPITAL, WAYNESBORO, GA, p. A116
BURKE REHABILITATION HOSPITAL, WHITE PLAINS, NY, p. A307
BURLESON ST. JOSEPH HEALTH CENTER, CALDWELL, TX, p. A403
BURLINGTON MEDICAL CENTER, BURLINGTON, IA, p. A151
BURNETT MEDICAL CENTER, GRANTSBURG, WI, p. A462
BUTLER COUNTY HEALTH CARE CENTER, DAVID CITY, NE, p. A263
BUTLER HEALTH SYSTEM, BUTLER, PA, p. A354
BUTLER HOSPITAL, PROVIDENCE, RI, p. A373
BUTTERWORTH HOSPITAL, GRAND RAPIDS, MI, p. A216
BYERLY HOSPITAL, HARTSVILLE, SC, p. A379
BYRD REGIONAL HOSPITAL, LEESVILLE, LA, p. A187

C

C. F. MENNINGER MEMORIAL HOSPITAL, TOPEKA, KS, p. A170
CABARRUS MEMORIAL HOSPITAL, CONCORD, NC, p. A310
CABELL HUNTINGTON HOSPITAL, HUNTINGTON, WV, p. A456
CABRINI MEDICAL CENTER, NEW YORK, NY, p. A296
CAGUAS REGIONAL HOSPITAL, CAGUAS, PR, p. A475
CALAIS REGIONAL HOSPITAL, CALAIS, ME, p. A194
CALDWELL COUNTY HOSPITAL, PRINCETON, KY, p. A180
CALDWELL MEMORIAL HOSPITAL, COLUMBIA, LA, p. A183
CALDWELL MEMORIAL HOSPITAL, LENOIR, NC, p. A313
CALEXICO HOSPITAL, CALEXICO, CA, p. A39
CALHOUN MEMORIAL HOSPITAL, ARLINGTON, GA, p. A103
CALHOUN–LIBERTY HOSPITAL, BLOUNTSTOWN, FL, p. A83
CALIFORNIA HOSPITAL MEDICAL CENTER, LOS ANGELES, CA, p. A49
CALIFORNIA MEDICAL FACILITY, VACAVILLE, CA, p. A67
CALIFORNIA MENS COLONY HOSPITAL, SAN LUIS OBISPO, CA, p. A63
CALIFORNIA PACIFIC MEDICAL CENTER, SAN FRANCISCO, CA, p. A61
CALLAWAY COMMUNITY HOSPITAL, FULTON, MO, p. A247
CALLAWAY DISTRICT HOSPITAL, CALLAWAY, NE, p. A263
CALUMET MEDICAL CENTER, CHILTON, WI, p. A461
CALVARY HOSPITAL, NEW YORK, NY, p. A296
CALVERT MEMORIAL HOSPITAL, PRINCE FREDERICK, MD, p. A201
CAMARILLO STATE HOSPITAL AND DEVELOPMENTAL CENTER, CAMARILLO, CA, p. A39
CAMBRIDGE MEDICAL CENTER, CAMBRIDGE, MN, p. A227
CAMBRIDGE PUBLIC HEALTH COMMISSION, CAMBRIDGE, MA, p. A205
CAMDEN COUNTY HEALTH SERVICES CENTER, BLACKWOOD, NJ, p. A275

COCHRAN MEMORIAL HOSPITAL, MORTON, TX, p. A421
COFFEE MEDICAL CENTER, MANCHESTER, TN, p. A392
COFFEE REGIONAL MEDICAL CENTER, DOUGLAS, GA, p. A108
COFFEY COUNTY HOSPITAL, BURLINGTON, KS, p. A161
COFFEYVILLE REGIONAL MEDICAL CENTER, COFFEYVILLE, KS, p. A162
COLEMAN COUNTY MEDICAL CENTER, COLEMAN, TX, p. A404
COLER MEMORIAL HOSPITAL, NEW YORK, NY, p. A296
COLLEGE HOSPITAL, CERRITOS, CA, p. A39
COLLEGE HOSPITAL COSTA MESA, COSTA MESA, CA, p. A41
COLLINGSWORTH GENERAL HOSPITAL, WELLINGTON, TX, p. A431
COLMERY–O'NEIL VETERANS AFFAIRS MEDICAL CENTER, TOPEKA, KS, p. A170
COLONEL FLORENCE A. BLANCHFIELD ARMY COMMUNITY HOSPITAL, FORT CAMPBELL, KY, p. A174
COLONIAL HOSPITAL, NEWPORT NEWS, VA, p. A443
COLORADO MENTAL HEALTH INSTITUTE AT FORT LOGAN, DENVER, CO, p. A71
COLORADO MENTAL HEALTH INSTITUTE AT PUEBLO, PUEBLO, CO, p. A74
COLORADO PLAINS MEDICAL CENTER, FORT MORGAN, CO, p. A72
COLORADO–FAYETTE MEDICAL CENTER, WEIMAR, TX, p. A431
COLQUITT REGIONAL MEDICAL CENTER, MOULTRIE, GA, p. A112
COLUMBIA ALASKA REGIONAL HOSPITAL, ANCHORAGE, AK, p. A20
COLUMBIA ALICE PHYSICIANS AND SURGEONS HOSPITAL, ALICE, TX, p. A398
COLUMBIA ALLEGHANY REGIONAL HOSPITAL, LOW MOOR, VA, p. A442
COLUMBIA ALVIN MEDICAL CENTER, ALVIN, TX, p. A398
COLUMBIA ANDALUSIA HOSPITAL, ANDALUSIA, AL, p. A11
COLUMBIA ASHLEY VALLEY MEDICAL CENTER, VERNAL, UT, p. A436
COLUMBIA ATHENS REGIONAL MEDICAL CENTER, ATHENS, TN, p. A387
COLUMBIA AUDUBON HOSPITAL, LOUISVILLE, KY, p. A177
COLUMBIA AUGUSTA MEDICAL CENTER, AUGUSTA, GA, p. A104
COLUMBIA AVENTURA HOSPITAL AND MEDICAL CENTER, MIAMI, FL, p. A92
COLUMBIA BARROW MEDICAL CENTER, WINDER, GA, p. A116
COLUMBIA BARTOW MEMORIAL HOSPITAL, BARTOW, FL, p. A83
COLUMBIA BASIN HOSPITAL, EPHRATA, WA, p. A449
COLUMBIA BAY AREA MEDICAL CENTER, CORPUS CHRISTI, TX, p. A404
COLUMBIA BAYSHORE MEDICAL CENTER, PASADENA, TX, p. A423
COLUMBIA BAYVIEW PSYCHIATRIC CENTER, CORPUS CHRISTI, TX, p. A404
COLUMBIA BEAUMONT MEDICAL CENTER, BEAUMONT, TX, p. A401
COLUMBIA BEHAVIORAL CENTER, EL PASO, TX, p. A408
COLUMBIA BEHAVIORAL HEALTH CENTER, MIAMI, FL, p. A92
COLUMBIA BELLAIRE MEDICAL CENTER, HOUSTON, TX, p. A413
COLUMBIA BETHANY HOSPITAL, BETHANY, OK, p. A339
COLUMBIA BLAKE MEDICAL CENTER, BRADENTON, FL, p. A84
COLUMBIA BRANDON REGIONAL MEDICAL CENTER, BRANDON, FL, p. A84
COLUMBIA BRIGHAM CITY COMMUNITY HOSPITAL, BRIGHAM CITY, UT, p. A433
COLUMBIA BROWNWOOD REGIONAL MEDICAL CENTER, BROWNWOOD, TX, p. A402
COLUMBIA BRUNSWICK HOSPITAL, SUPPLY, NC, p. A317
COLUMBIA CAPE FEAR MEMORIAL HOSPITAL, WILMINGTON, NC, p. A318
COLUMBIA CAPITAL MEDICAL CENTER, OLYMPIA, WA, p. A451
COLUMBIA CARTERSVILLE MEDICAL CENTER, CARTERSVILLE, GA, p. A106
COLUMBIA CEDARS MEDICAL CENTER, MIAMI, FL, p. A93
COLUMBIA CHEATHAM MEDICAL CENTER, ASHLAND CITY, TN, p. A387
COLUMBIA CHICAGO LAKESHORE HOSPITAL, CHICAGO, IL, p. A125
COLUMBIA CHINO VALLEY MEDICAL CENTER, CHINO, CA, p. A40
COLUMBIA CLAREMORE REGIONAL HOSPITAL, CLAREMORE, OK, p. A340
COLUMBIA CLEAR LAKE REGIONAL MEDICAL CENTER, WEBSTER, TX, p. A431
COLUMBIA CLEARWATER COMMUNITY HOSPITAL, CLEARWATER, FL, p. A84
COLUMBIA CLINCH VALLEY MEDICAL CENTER, RICHLANDS, VA, p. A444
COLUMBIA COLISEUM MEDICAL CENTERS, MACON, GA, p. A111

COLUMBIA COLISEUM PSYCHIATRIC HOSPITAL, MACON, GA, p. A111
COLUMBIA COLLETON MEDICAL CENTER, WALTERBORO, SC, p. A381
COLUMBIA CONROE REGIONAL MEDICAL CENTER, CONROE, TX, p. A404
COLUMBIA CROCKETT HOSPITAL, LAWRENCEBURG, TN, p. A392
COLUMBIA DADE CITY HOSPITAL, DADE CITY, FL, p. A85
COLUMBIA DAUTERIVE HOSPITAL, NEW IBERIA, LA, p. A188
COLUMBIA DAVIS MEDICAL CENTER, STATESVILLE, NC, p. A317
COLUMBIA DE QUEEN REGIONAL MEDICAL CENTER, DE QUEEN, AR, p. A30
COLUMBIA DEERING HOSPITAL, MIAMI, FL, p. A93
COLUMBIA DETAR HOSPITAL, VICTORIA, TX, p. A430
COLUMBIA DOCTORS HOSPITAL, LITTLE ROCK, AR, p. A32
COLUMBIA DOCTORS HOSPITAL, COLUMBUS, GA, p. A107
COLUMBIA DOCTORS HOSPITAL, TULSA, OK, p. A346
COLUMBIA DOCTORS HOSPITAL AIRLINE, HOUSTON, TX, p. A413
COLUMBIA DOCTORS HOSPITAL EAST LOOP, HOUSTON, TX, p. A413
COLUMBIA DOCTORS HOSPITAL OF LAREDO, LAREDO, TX, p. A418
COLUMBIA DOCTORS HOSPITAL OF SARASOTA, SARASOTA, FL, p. A99
COLUMBIA DOCTORS REGIONAL MEDICAL CENTER, CORPUS CHRISTI, TX, p. A404
COLUMBIA DOCTORS' HOSPITAL OF OPELOUSAS, OPELOUSAS, LA, p. A189
COLUMBIA DOUGLAS MEDICAL CENTER, ROSEBURG, OR, p. A351
COLUMBIA DUNWOODY MEDICAL CENTER, ATLANTA, GA, p. A103
COLUMBIA EAST HOUSTON MEDICAL CENTER, HOUSTON, TX, p. A413
COLUMBIA EAST MONTGOMERY MEDICAL CENTER, MONTGOMERY, AL, p. A16
COLUMBIA EAST POINTE HOSPITAL, LEHIGH ACRES, FL, p. A91
COLUMBIA EAST RIDGE HOSPITAL, EAST RIDGE, TN, p. A389
COLUMBIA EASTERN IDAHO REGIONAL MEDICAL CENTER, IDAHO FALLS, ID, p. A120
COLUMBIA EASTSIDE MEDICAL CENTER, SNELLVILLE, GA, p. A114
COLUMBIA EDMOND REGIONAL MEDICAL CENTER, EDMOND, OK, p. A341
COLUMBIA EDWARD WHITE HOSPITAL, SAINT PETERSBURG, FL, p. A98
COLUMBIA EL DORADO HOSPITAL, TUCSON, AZ, p. A27
COLUMBIA ENGLEWOOD COMMUNITY HOSPITAL, ENGLEWOOD, FL, p. A86
COLUMBIA FAIRVIEW PARK HOSPITAL, DUBLIN, GA, p. A108
COLUMBIA FAWCETT MEMORIAL HOSPITAL, PORT CHARLOTTE, FL, p. A97
COLUMBIA FLORENCE HOSPITAL, FLORENCE, AL, p. A14
COLUMBIA FORT BEND HOSPITAL, MISSOURI CITY, TX, p. A421
COLUMBIA FORT WALTON BEACH MEDICAL CENTER, FORT WALTON BEACH, FL, p. A87
COLUMBIA FOUR RIVERS MEDICAL CENTER, SELMA, AL, p. A18
COLUMBIA GARDEN PARK HOSPITAL, GULFPORT, MS, p. A239
COLUMBIA GOOD SAMARITAN HOSPITAL, BAKERSFIELD, CA, p. A37
COLUMBIA GOOD SAMARITAN HOSPITAL, SAN JOSE, CA, p. A62
COLUMBIA GRAND STRAND REGIONAL MEDICAL CENTER, MYRTLE BEACH, SC, p. A379
COLUMBIA GRANT HOSPITAL, CHICAGO, IL, p. A125
COLUMBIA GREENVIEW HOSPITAL, BOWLING GREEN, KY, p. A172
COLUMBIA GULF COAST HOSPITAL, FORT MYERS, FL, p. A87
COLUMBIA GULF COAST MEDICAL CENTER, PANAMA CITY, FL, p. A96
COLUMBIA GULF COAST MEDICAL CENTER, WHARTON, TX, p. A431
COLUMBIA HALSTEAD HOSPITAL, HALSTEAD, KS, p. A163
COLUMBIA HAMILTON MEDICAL CENTER, JASPER, FL, p. A90
COLUMBIA HEALTHONE–BEHAVIORAL HEALTH SERVICES, DENVER, CO, p. A71
COLUMBIA HENDERSONVILLE HOSPITAL, HENDERSONVILLE, TN, p. A390
COLUMBIA HERITAGE HOSPITAL, TARBORO, NC, p. A317
COLUMBIA HIGHLAND HOSPITAL, SHREVEPORT, LA, p. A190
COLUMBIA HIGHSMITH–RAINEY MEMORIAL HOSPITAL, FAYETTEVILLE, NC, p. A311
COLUMBIA HILLSIDE HOSPITAL, PULASKI, TN, p. A395
COLUMBIA HOFFMAN ESTATES MEDICAL CENTER, HOFFMAN ESTATES, IL, p. A132
COLUMBIA HORIZON MEDICAL CENTER, DICKSON, TN, p. A389
COLUMBIA HOSPITAL, WEST PALM BEACH, FL, p. A101

COLUMBIA HOSPITAL, MILWAUKEE, WI, p. A465
COLUMBIA HOSPITAL AT MEDICAL CITY DALLAS, DALLAS, TX, p. A406
COLUMBIA HOSPITAL FOR WOMEN MEDICAL CENTER, WASHINGTON, DC, p. A81
COLUMBIA HOSPITAL FRANKFORT, FRANKFORT, KY, p. A174
COLUMBIA HOSPITAL GEORGETOWN, GEORGETOWN, KY, p. A174
COLUMBIA HOSPITAL LEXINGTON, LEXINGTON, KY, p. A176
COLUMBIA HOSPITAL MAYSVILLE, MAYSVILLE, KY, p. A178
COLUMBIA HOSPITAL NORTH AND SOUTH, SPRINGFIELD, MO, p. A255
COLUMBIA HOSPITAL PARIS, PARIS, KY, p. A179
COLUMBIA HUGHSTON SPORTS MEDICINE HOSPITAL, COLUMBUS, GA, p. A107
COLUMBIA HUNTINGTON BEACH HOSPITAL AND MEDICAL CENTER, HUNTINGTON BEACH, CA, p. A46
COLUMBIA INDEPENDENCE REGIONAL HEALTH CENTER, INDEPENDENCE, MO, p. A248
COLUMBIA J. F. K. MEDICAL CENTER, ATLANTIS, FL, p. A83
COLUMBIA JEFFERSON MEDICAL CENTER, JEFFERSON, LA, p. A185
COLUMBIA JOHN RANDOLPH MEDICAL CENTER, HOPEWELL, VA, p. A441
COLUMBIA JOHNSON CITY SPECIALTY HOSPITAL, JOHNSON CITY, TN, p. A390
COLUMBIA KATY MEDICAL CENTER, KATY, TX, p. A417
COLUMBIA KENDALL MEDICAL CENTER, MIAMI, FL, p. A93
COLUMBIA KINGWOOD MEDICAL CENTER, KINGWOOD, TX, p. A418
COLUMBIA LA GRANGE MEMORIAL HOSPITAL, LA GRANGE, IL, p. A133
COLUMBIA LAKE CITY MEDICAL CENTER, LAKE CITY, FL, p. A90
COLUMBIA LAKE CUMBERLAND REGIONAL HOSPITAL, SOMERSET, KY, p. A180
COLUMBIA LAKELAND MEDICAL CENTER, NEW ORLEANS, LA, p. A188
COLUMBIA LAKESIDE HOSPITAL, METAIRIE, LA, p. A187
COLUMBIA LAKEVIEW REGIONAL MEDICAL CENTER, COVINGTON, LA, p. A183
COLUMBIA LANIER PARK HOSPITAL, GAINESVILLE, GA, p. A109
COLUMBIA LARGO MEDICAL CENTER, LARGO, FL, p. A91
COLUMBIA LAS ENCINAS HOSPITAL, PASADENA, CA, p. A57
COLUMBIA LAWNWOOD REGIONAL MEDICAL CENTER, FORT PIERCE, FL, p. A87
COLUMBIA LEA REGIONAL HOSPITAL, HOBBS, NM, p. A286
COLUMBIA LEWIS–GALE MEDICAL CENTER, SALEM, VA, p. A446
COLUMBIA LIVINGSTON REGIONAL HOSPITAL, LIVINGSTON, TN, p. A392
COLUMBIA LOGAN MEMORIAL HOSPITAL, RUSSELLVILLE, KY, p. A180
COLUMBIA LONGVIEW REGIONAL MEDICAL CENTER, LONGVIEW, TX, p. A419
COLUMBIA LOS ROBLES HOSPITAL AND MEDICAL CENTER, THOUSAND OAKS, CA, p. A66
COLUMBIA MAINLAND MEDICAL CENTER, TEXAS CITY, TX, p. A429
COLUMBIA MEDICAL ARTS HOSPITAL, DALLAS, TX, p. A406
COLUMBIA MEDICAL CENTER, BATON ROUGE, LA, p. A182
COLUMBIA MEDICAL CENTER, COLLEGE STATION, TX, p. A404
COLUMBIA MEDICAL CENTER AT LANCASTER, LANCASTER, TX, p. A418
COLUMBIA MEDICAL CENTER AT TERRELL, TERRELL, TX, p. A428
COLUMBIA MEDICAL CENTER OF ARLINGTON, ARLINGTON, TX, p. A399
COLUMBIA MEDICAL CENTER OF AURORA, AURORA, CO, p. A70
COLUMBIA MEDICAL CENTER OF CARLSBAD, CARLSBAD, NM, p. A285
COLUMBIA MEDICAL CENTER OF DENTON, DENTON, TX, p. A408
COLUMBIA MEDICAL CENTER OF HUNTSVILLE, HUNTSVILLE, AL, p. A15
COLUMBIA MEDICAL CENTER OF LEWISVILLE, LEWISVILLE, TX, p. A418
COLUMBIA MEDICAL CENTER OF MCKINNEY, MCKINNEY, TX, p. A420
COLUMBIA MEDICAL CENTER OF PAMPA, PAMPA, TX, p. A423
COLUMBIA MEDICAL CENTER OF PLANO, PLANO, TX, p. A423
COLUMBIA MEDICAL CENTER OF SAN ANGELO, SAN ANGELO, TX, p. A425
COLUMBIA MEDICAL CENTER OF SHERMAN, SHERMAN, TX, p. A427
COLUMBIA MEDICAL CENTER OF SOUTHWEST LOUISIANA, LAFAYETTE, LA, p. A186
COLUMBIA MEDICAL CENTER PENINSULA, ORMOND BEACH, FL, p. A95
COLUMBIA MEDICAL CENTER PHOENIX, PHOENIX, AZ, p. A24
COLUMBIA MEDICAL CENTER SANFORD, SANFORD, FL, p. A99

COLUMBIA MEDICAL CENTER–DALLAS SOUTHWEST, DALLAS, TX, p. A406

COLUMBIA MEDICAL CENTER–DAYTONA, DAYTONA BEACH, FL, p. A85

COLUMBIA MEDICAL CENTER–EAST, EL PASO, TX, p. A408

COLUMBIA MEDICAL CENTER–EAST, EL PASO, TX, p. A408

COLUMBIA MEDICAL CENTER–OSCEOLA, KISSIMMEE, FL, p. A90

COLUMBIA MEDICAL CENTER–PORT ST. LUCIE, PORT ST. LUCIE, FL, p. A98

COLUMBIA MEDICAL CENTER–WEST, EL PASO, TX, p. A409

COLUMBIA MEMORIAL HOSPITAL, HUDSON, NY, p. A293

COLUMBIA MEMORIAL HOSPITAL, ASTORIA, OR, p. A348

COLUMBIA MEMORIAL HOSPITAL JACKSONVILLE, JACKSONVILLE, FL, p. A89

COLUMBIA MERCY MEDICAL CENTER, CANTON, OH, p. A324

COLUMBIA METROPOLITAN HOSPITAL, ATLANTA, GA, p. A103

COLUMBIA METROWEST MEDICAL CENTER, FRAMINGHAM, MA, p. A206

COLUMBIA MICHAEL REESE HOSPITAL AND MEDICAL CENTER, CHICAGO, IL, p. A125

COLUMBIA MISSION BAY HOSPITAL, SAN DIEGO, CA, p. A60

COLUMBIA MONTGOMERY REGIONAL HOSPITAL, BLACKSBURG, VA, p. A439

COLUMBIA MURRAY MEDICAL CENTER, CHATSWORTH, GA, p. A106

COLUMBIA NASHVILLE MEMORIAL HOSPITAL, MADISON, TN, p. A392

COLUMBIA NAVARRO REGIONAL HOSPITAL, CORSICANA, TX, p. A405

COLUMBIA NEW PORT RICHEY HOSPITAL, NEW PORT RICHEY, FL, p. A94

COLUMBIA NORTH BAY HOSPITAL, ARANSAS PASS, TX, p. A399

COLUMBIA NORTH FLORIDA REGIONAL MEDICAL CENTER, GAINESVILLE, FL, p. A88

COLUMBIA NORTH HILLS HOSPITAL, NORTH RICHLAND HILLS, TX, p. A422

COLUMBIA NORTH HOUSTON MEDICAL CENTER, HOUSTON, TX, p. A413

COLUMBIA NORTH MONROE HOSPITAL, MONROE, LA, p. A187

COLUMBIA NORTH SIDE HOSPITAL, JOHNSON CITY, TN, p. A390

COLUMBIA NORTHLAKE REGIONAL MEDICAL CENTER, ATLANTA, GA, p. A104

COLUMBIA NORTHRIDGE MEDICAL CENTER, PRATTVILLE, AL, p. A17

COLUMBIA NORTHSIDE MEDICAL CENTER, SAINT PETERSBURG, FL, p. A98

COLUMBIA NORTHWEST HOSPITAL, CORPUS CHRISTI, TX, p. A405

COLUMBIA NORTHWEST MEDICAL CENTER, MARGATE, FL, p. A92

COLUMBIA OCALA REGIONAL MEDICAL CENTER, OCALA, FL, p. A95

COLUMBIA OGDEN REGIONAL MEDICAL CENTER, OGDEN, UT, p. A434

COLUMBIA OLYMPIA FIELDS OSTEOPATHIC HOSPITAL AND MEDICAL CENTER, OLYMPIA FIELDS, IL, p. A135

COLUMBIA ORANGE PARK MEDICAL CENTER, ORANGE PARK, FL, p. A95

COLUMBIA OVERLAND PARK REGIONAL MEDICAL CENTER, OVERLAND PARK, KS, p. A168

COLUMBIA PALM DRIVE HOSPITAL, SEBASTOPOL, CA, p. A64

COLUMBIA PALMS WEST HOSPITAL, LOXAHATCHEE, FL, p. A92

COLUMBIA PALMYRA MEDICAL CENTERS, ALBANY, GA, p. A103

COLUMBIA PARADISE VALLEY HOSPITAL, PHOENIX, AZ, p. A24

COLUMBIA PARK MEDICAL CENTER, ORLANDO, FL, p. A95

COLUMBIA PARKWAY MEDICAL CENTER, LITHIA SPRINGS, GA, p. A111

COLUMBIA PEACHTREE REGIONAL HOSPITAL, NEWNAN, GA, p. A112

COLUMBIA PENINSULA CENTER FOR BEHAVIORAL HEALTH, HAMPTON, VA, p. A441

COLUMBIA PINELAKE REGIONAL HOSPITAL, MAYFIELD, KY, p. A178

COLUMBIA PLANTATION GENERAL HOSPITAL, PLANTATION, FL, p. A97

COLUMBIA PLAZA MEDICAL CENTER OF FORT WORTH, FORT WORTH, TX, p. A410

COLUMBIA POLK GENERAL HOSPITAL, CEDARTOWN, GA, p. A106

COLUMBIA POMPANO BEACH MEDICAL CENTER, POMPANO BEACH, FL, p. A97

COLUMBIA PRESBYTERIAN HOSPITAL, OKLAHOMA CITY, OK, p. A343

COLUMBIA PRESBYTERIAN–ST. LUKE'S MEDICAL CENTER, DENVER, CO, p. A71

COLUMBIA PROVIDENCE HOSPITAL, COLUMBIA, SC, p. A376

COLUMBIA PULASKI COMMUNITY HOSPITAL, PULASKI, VA, p. A444

COLUMBIA PUTNAM MEDICAL CENTER, PALATKA, FL, p. A96

COLUMBIA RALEIGH COMMUNITY HOSPITAL, RALEIGH, NC, p. A315

COLUMBIA RALEIGH GENERAL HOSPITAL, BECKLEY, WV, p. A455

COLUMBIA RAULERSON HOSPITAL, OKEECHOBEE, FL, p. A95

COLUMBIA REDMOND REGIONAL MEDICAL CENTER, ROME, GA, p. A113

COLUMBIA REGIONAL HOSPITAL, COLUMBIA, MO, p. A246

COLUMBIA REGIONAL HOSPITAL OF JACKSON, JACKSON, TN, p. A390

COLUMBIA REGIONAL MEDICAL CENTER, MONTGOMERY, AL, p. A16

COLUMBIA REGIONAL MEDICAL CENTER, SPRING HILL, FL, p. A99

COLUMBIA REGIONAL MEDICAL CENTER AT BAYONET POINT, HUDSON, FL, p. A89

COLUMBIA REGIONAL MEDICAL CENTER OF SOUTHWEST FLORIDA, FORT MYERS, FL, p. A87

COLUMBIA REHABILITATION HOSPITAL, CORPUS CHRISTI, TX, p. A405

COLUMBIA RESTON HOSPITAL CENTER, RESTON, VA, p. A444

COLUMBIA RIO GRANDE REGIONAL HOSPITAL, MCALLEN, TX, p. A420

COLUMBIA RIVER PARK HOSPITAL, MCMINNVILLE, TN, p. A393

COLUMBIA RIVER PARK HOSPITAL, HUNTINGTON, WV, p. A456

COLUMBIA RIVEREDGE HOSPITAL, FOREST PARK, IL, p. A130

COLUMBIA RIVERTON MEMORIAL HOSPITAL, RIVERTON, WY, p. A472

COLUMBIA RIVERVIEW MEDICAL CENTER, GONZALES, LA, p. A184

COLUMBIA ROSE MEDICAL CENTER, DENVER, CO, p. A71

COLUMBIA ROSEWOOD MEDICAL CENTER, HOUSTON, TX, p. A413

COLUMBIA SAN CLEMENTE HOSPITAL AND MEDICAL CENTER, SAN CLEMENTE, CA, p. A60

COLUMBIA SAN JOSE MEDICAL CENTER, SAN JOSE, CA, p. A62

COLUMBIA SAN LEANDRO HOSPITAL, SAN LEANDRO, CA, p. A63

COLUMBIA SILSBEE DOCTORS HOSPITAL, SILSBEE, TX, p. A427

COLUMBIA SMITH COUNTY MEMORIAL HOSPITAL, CARTHAGE, TN, p. A387

COLUMBIA SOUTH BAY HOSPITAL, SUN CITY CENTER, FL, p. A100

COLUMBIA SOUTH PITTSBURG HOSPITAL, SOUTH PITTSBURG, TN, p. A396

COLUMBIA SOUTH VALLEY HOSPITAL, GILROY, CA, p. A44

COLUMBIA SOUTHERN HILLS MEDICAL CENTER, NASHVILLE, TN, p. A394

COLUMBIA SOUTHERN TENNESSEE MEDICAL CENTER, WINCHESTER, TN, p. A397

COLUMBIA SOUTHWEST HOSPITAL, LOUISVILLE, KY, p. A177

COLUMBIA SOUTHWESTERN MEDICAL CENTER, LAWTON, OK, p. A342

COLUMBIA SPECIALTY HOSPITAL AT MEDICAL ARTS, DALLAS, TX, p. A406

COLUMBIA SPECIALTY HOSPITAL JACKSONVILLE, JACKSONVILLE, FL, p. A89

COLUMBIA SPRING BRANCH MEDICAL CENTER, HOUSTON, TX, p. A413

COLUMBIA SPRING VIEW HOSPITAL, LEBANON, KY, p. A176

COLUMBIA SPRINGHILL MEDICAL CENTER, SPRINGHILL, LA, p. A191

COLUMBIA ST. DAVID'S HOSPITAL, AUSTIN, TX, p. A400

COLUMBIA ST. DAVID'S SOUTH HOSPITAL, AUSTIN, TX, p. A400

COLUMBIA ST. LUKE'S HOSPITAL, BLUEFIELD, WV, p. A455

COLUMBIA ST. MARK'S HOSPITAL, SALT LAKE CITY, UT, p. A435

COLUMBIA ST. PETERSBURG MEDICAL CENTER, SAINT PETERSBURG, FL, p. A98

COLUMBIA ST. VINCENT CHARITY HOSPITAL, CLEVELAND, OH, p. A326

COLUMBIA STONES RIVER HOSPITAL, WOODBURY, TN, p. A397

COLUMBIA SUBURBAN HOSPITAL, LOUISVILLE, KY, p. A177

COLUMBIA SUMMIT MEDICAL CENTER, HERMITAGE, TN, p. A390

COLUMBIA SUNRISE HOSPITAL AND MEDICAL CENTER, LAS VEGAS, NV, p. A270

COLUMBIA SWEDISH MEDICAL CENTER, ENGLEWOOD, CO, p. A72

COLUMBIA SYCAMORE SHOALS HOSPITAL, ELIZABETHTON, TN, p. A389

COLUMBIA TALLAHASSEE COMMUNITY HOSPITAL, TALLAHASSEE, FL, p. A100

COLUMBIA TERRE HAUTE REGIONAL HOSPITAL, TERRE HAUTE, IN, p. A149

COLUMBIA TEXAS ORTHOPEDIC HOSPITAL, HOUSTON, TX, p. A414

COLUMBIA TRIDENT MEDICAL CENTER, CHARLESTON, SC, p. A376

COLUMBIA TRINITY HOSPITAL, ERIN, TN, p. A389

COLUMBIA TULSA REGIONAL MEDICAL CENTER, TULSA, OK, p. A346

COLUMBIA TWIN CITIES HOSPITAL, NICEVILLE, FL, p. A94

COLUMBIA UNIVERSITY GENERAL HOSPITAL, SEMINOLE, FL, p. A99

COLUMBIA UNIVERSITY HOSPITAL AND MEDICAL CENTER, TAMARAC, FL, p. A100

COLUMBIA VALLEY HOSPITAL, CHATTANOOGA, TN, p. A387

COLUMBIA VALLEY REGIONAL MEDICAL CENTER, BROWNSVILLE, TX, p. A402

COLUMBIA VICKSBURG MEDICAL CENTER, VICKSBURG, MS, p. A244

COLUMBIA VOLUNTEER GENERAL HOSPITAL, MARTIN, TN, p. A392

COLUMBIA WAGONER HOSPITAL, WAGONER, OK, p. A347

COLUMBIA WESLEY MEDICAL CENTER, WICHITA, KS, p. A170

COLUMBIA WEST ANAHEIM MEDICAL CENTER, ANAHEIM, CA, p. A36

COLUMBIA WEST FLORIDA REGIONAL MEDICAL CENTER, PENSACOLA, FL, p. A96

COLUMBIA WEST HILLS MEDICAL CENTER, LOS ANGELES, CA, p. A49

COLUMBIA WEST HOUSTON MEDICAL CENTER, HOUSTON, TX, p. A414

COLUMBIA WEST PACES MEDICAL CENTER, ATLANTA, GA, p. A104

COLUMBIA WEST VALLEY MEDICAL CENTER, CALDWELL, ID, p. A119

COLUMBIA WESTERN PLAINS REGIONAL HOSPITAL, DODGE CITY, KS, p. A162

COLUMBIA WESTSIDE REGIONAL MEDICAL CENTER, PLANTATION, FL, p. A97

COLUMBIA WILLIAMETTE VALLEY MEDICAL CENTER, MCMINNVILLE, OR, p. A350

COLUMBIA WOMAN'S HOSPITAL OF TEXAS, HOUSTON, TX, p. A414

COLUMBIA WOMEN AND CHILDREN'S HOSPITAL–LAKE CHARLES, LAKE CHARLES, LA, p. A186

COLUMBIA WOMEN'S AND CHILDREN'S HOSPITAL, LAFAYETTE, LA, p. A186

COLUMBIA WOMEN'S HOSPITAL–INDIANAPOLIS, INDIANAPOLIS, IN, p. A144

COLUMBIA WOODLAND HEIGHTS MEDICAL CENTER, LUFKIN, TX, p. A419

COLUMBIA WOODLAND HOSPITAL, HOFFMAN ESTATES, IL, p. A132

COLUMBUS COMMUNITY HOSPITAL, COLUMBUS, NE, p. A263

COLUMBUS COMMUNITY HOSPITAL, COLUMBUS, OH, p. A328

COLUMBUS COMMUNITY HOSPITAL, COLUMBUS, TX, p. A404

COLUMBUS COMMUNITY HOSPITAL, COLUMBUS, WI, p. A461

COLUMBUS COUNTY HOSPITAL, WHITEVILLE, NC, p. A318

COLUMBUS HOSPITAL, CHICAGO, IL, p. A125

COLUMBUS HOSPITAL, NEWARK, NJ, p. A279

COLUMBUS REGIONAL HOSPITAL, COLUMBUS, IN, p. A141

COLUSA COMMUNITY HOSPITAL, COLUSA, CA, p. A40

COMANCHE COMMUNITY HOSPITAL, COMANCHE, TX, p. A404

COMANCHE COUNTY HOSPITAL, COLDWATER, KS, p. A162

COMANCHE COUNTY MEMORIAL HOSPITAL, LAWTON, OK, p. A342

COMMMUNITY HOSPITAL OF SAN BERNARDINO, SAN BERNARDINO, CA, p. A60

COMMUNITY GENERAL HOSPITAL, READING, PA, p. A368

COMMUNITY GENERAL HOSPITAL OF SULLIVAN COUNTY, HARRIS, NY, p. A293

COMMUNITY GENERAL HOSPITAL OF THOMASVILLE, THOMASVILLE, NC, p. A317

COMMUNITY GENERAL OSTEOPATHIC HOSPITAL, HARRISBURG, PA, p. A358

COMMUNITY HEALTH CENTER OF BRANCH COUNTY, COLDWATER, MI, p. A214

COMMUNITY HEALTH NETWORK, BERLIN, WI, p. A460

COMMUNITY HOSPITAL, TALLASSEE, AL, p. A18

COMMUNITY HOSPITAL, SANTA ROSA, CA, p. A64

COMMUNITY HOSPITAL, GRAND JUNCTION, CO, p. A73

COMMUNITY HOSPITAL, MUNSTER, IN, p. A147

COMMUNITY HOSPITAL, WATERVLIET, MI, p. A224

COMMUNITY HOSPITAL, CANNON FALLS, MN, p. A227

COMMUNITY HOSPITAL, MCCOOK, NE, p. A265

COMMUNITY HOSPITAL, SPRINGFIELD, OH, p. A335

COMMUNITY HOSPITAL, TORRINGTON, WY, p. A472

COMMUNITY HOSPITAL AND HEALTH CARE CENTER, SAINT PETER, MN, p. A234

COMMUNITY HOSPITAL ASSOCIATION, FAIRFAX, MO, p. A247

COMMUNITY HOSPITAL AT DOBBS FERRY, DOBBS FERRY, NY, p. A291

D

E

F

H

HAXTUN HOSPITAL DISTRICT, HAXTUN, CO, p. A73
HAYES–GREEN–BEACH MEMORIAL HOSPITAL, CHARLOTTE, MI, p. A213
HAYS MEDICAL CENTER, HAYS, KS, p. A164
HAYWARD AREA MEMORIAL HOSPITAL AND NURSING HOME, HAYWARD, WI, p. A463
HAYWOOD REGIONAL MEDICAL CENTER, CLYDE, NC, p. A310
HAZEL HAWKINS MEMORIAL HOSPITAL, HOLLISTER, CA, p. A46
HAZLETON GENERAL HOSPITAL, HAZLETON, PA, p. A359
HAZLETON–ST. JOSEPH MEDICAL CENTER, HAZLETON, PA, p. A359
HEALDSBURG GENERAL HOSPITAL, HEALDSBURG, CA, p. A45
HEALTH ALLIANCE HOSPITALS, LEOMINSTER, MA, p. A207
HEALTH CENTRAL, OCOEE, FL, p. A95
HEALTH FIRST/CAPE CANAVERAL HOSPITAL, COCOA BEACH, FL, p. A85
HEALTH HILL HOSPITAL FOR CHILDREN, CLEVELAND, OH, p. A326
HEALTHCARE REHABILITATION CENTER, AUSTIN, TX, p. A400
HEALTHEAST BETHESDA LUTHERAN HOSPITAL AND REHABILITATION CENTER, SAINT PAUL, MN, p. A234
HEALTHEAST ST. JOHN'S HOSPITAL, MAPLEWOOD, MN, p. A231
HEALTHEAST ST. JOSEPH'S HOSPITAL, SAINT PAUL, MN, p. A234
HEALTHSOURCE SAGINAW, SAGINAW, MI, p. A222
HEALTHSOUTH BAKERSFIELD REHABILITATION HOSPITAL, BAKERSFIELD, CA, p. A37
HEALTHSOUTH CENTRAL GEORGIA REHABILITATION HOSPITAL, MACON, GA, p. A111
HEALTHSOUTH CHATTANOOGA REHABILITATION HOSPITAL, CHATTANOOGA, TN, p. A388
HEALTHSOUTH CHESAPEAKE REHABILITATION HOSPITAL, SALISBURY, MD, p. A201
HEALTHSOUTH DOCTORS' HOSPITAL, CORAL GABLES, FL, p. A85
HEALTHSOUTH GREAT LAKES REHABILITATION HOSPITAL, ERIE, PA, p. A357
HEALTHSOUTH GREATER PITTSBURGH REHABILITATION HOSPITAL, MONROEVILLE, PA, p. A361
HEALTHSOUTH HARMARVILLE REHABILITATION HOSPITAL, PITTSBURGH, PA, p. A366
HEALTHSOUTH LAKE ERIE INSTITUTE OF REHABILITATION, ERIE, PA, p. A357
HEALTHSOUTH LAKESHORE REHABILITATION HOSPITAL, BIRMINGHAM, AL, p. A12
HEALTHSOUTH MEDICAL CENTER, BIRMINGHAM, AL, p. A12
HEALTHSOUTH MEDICAL CENTER, DALLAS, TX, p. A406
HEALTHSOUTH MEDICAL CENTER, RICHMOND, VA, p. A445
HEALTHSOUTH MERIDIAN POINT REHABILITATION HOSPITAL, SCOTTSDALE, AZ, p. A26
HEALTHSOUTH MOUNTAIN REGIONAL REHABILITATION HOSPITAL, MORGANTOWN, WV, p. A457
HEALTHSOUTH NEW ENGLAND REHABILITATION HOSPITAL, WOBURN, MA, p. A211
HEALTHSOUTH NITTANY VALLEY REHABILITATION HOSPITAL, PLEASANT GAP, PA, p. A367
HEALTHSOUTH NORTHERN KENTUCKY REHABILITATION HOSPITAL, EDGEWOOD, KY, p. A173
HEALTHSOUTH REHABILITATION CENTER, ALBUQUERQUE, NM, p. A284
HEALTHSOUTH REHABILITATION HOSPITAL, LARGO, FL, p. A91
HEALTHSOUTH REHABILITATION HOSPITAL, MIAMI, FL, p. A93
HEALTHSOUTH REHABILITATION HOSPITAL, PORTLAND, ME, p. A195
HEALTHSOUTH REHABILITATION HOSPITAL, CONCORD, NH, p. A272
HEALTHSOUTH REHABILITATION HOSPITAL, OKLAHOMA CITY, OK, p. A343
HEALTHSOUTH REHABILITATION HOSPITAL, COLUMBIA, SC, p. A377
HEALTHSOUTH REHABILITATION HOSPITAL, FLORENCE, SC, p. A377
HEALTHSOUTH REHABILITATION HOSPITAL, KINGSPORT, TN, p. A391
HEALTHSOUTH REHABILITATION HOSPITAL, MEMPHIS, TN, p. A393
HEALTHSOUTH REHABILITATION HOSPITAL, HUMBLE, TX, p. A416
HEALTHSOUTH REHABILITATION HOSPITAL, HUNTINGTON, WV, p. A456
HEALTHSOUTH REHABILITATION HOSPITAL OF ALTOONA, ALTOONA, PA, p. A353
HEALTHSOUTH REHABILITATION HOSPITAL OF ARLINGTON, ARLINGTON, TX, p. A399
HEALTHSOUTH REHABILITATION HOSPITAL OF AUSTIN, AUSTIN, TX, p. A400
HEALTHSOUTH REHABILITATION HOSPITAL OF FORT SMITH, FORT SMITH, AR, p. A31

HEALTHSOUTH REHABILITATION HOSPITAL OF FORT WORTH, FORT WORTH, TX, p. A410
HEALTHSOUTH REHABILITATION HOSPITAL OF MONTGOMERY, MONTGOMERY, AL, p. A16
HEALTHSOUTH REHABILITATION HOSPITAL OF NEW JERSEY, TOMS RIVER, NJ, p. A282
HEALTHSOUTH REHABILITATION HOSPITAL OF NORTH ALABAMA, HUNTSVILLE, AL, p. A15
HEALTHSOUTH REHABILITATION HOSPITAL OF SARASOTA, SARASOTA, FL, p. A99
HEALTHSOUTH REHABILITATION HOSPITAL OF SOUTH LOUISIANA, BATON ROUGE, LA, p. A183
HEALTHSOUTH REHABILITATION HOSPITAL OF TALLAHASSEE, TALLAHASSEE, FL, p. A100
HEALTHSOUTH REHABILITATION HOSPITAL OF TEXARKANA, TEXARKANA, TX, p. A429
HEALTHSOUTH REHABILITATION HOSPITAL OF UTAH, SANDY, UT, p. A436
HEALTHSOUTH REHABILITATION HOSPITAL OF VIRGINIA, RICHMOND, VA, p. A445
HEALTHSOUTH REHABILITATION HOSPITAL OF YORK, YORK, PA, p. A371
HEALTHSOUTH REHABILITATION INSTITUTE OF SAN ANTONIO, SAN ANTONIO, TX, p. A425
HEALTHSOUTH REHABILITATION INSTITUTE OF TUCSON, TUCSON, AZ, p. A27
HEALTHSOUTH REHABILITATION OF MECHANICSBURG, MECHANICSBURG, PA, p. A361
HEALTHSOUTH SEA PINES REHABILITATION HOSPITAL, MELBOURNE, FL, p. A92
HEALTHSOUTH SOUTHERN HILLS REHABILITATION HOSPITAL, PRINCETON, WV, p. A458
HEALTHSOUTH SUNRISE REHABILITATION HOSPITAL, FORT LAUDERDALE, FL, p. A87
HEALTHSOUTH TREASURE COAST REHABILITATION HOSPITAL, VERO BEACH, FL, p. A101
HEALTHSOUTH TRI–STATE REHABILITATION HOSPITAL, EVANSVILLE, IN, p. A142
HEALTHSOUTH VALLEY OF THE SUN REHABILITATION HOSPITAL, GLENDALE, AZ, p. A23
HEALTHSOUTH WESTERN HILLS REGIONAL REHABILITATION HOSPITAL, PARKERSBURG, WV, p. A458
HEART OF AMERICA MEDICAL CENTER, RUGBY, ND, p. A322
HEART OF FLORIDA BEHAVIORAL CENTER, LAKELAND, FL, p. A91
HEART OF FLORIDA HOSPITAL, HAINES CITY, FL, p. A88
HEART OF TEXAS MEMORIAL HOSPITAL, BRADY, TX, p. A402
HEART OF THE ROCKIES REGIONAL MEDICAL CENTER, SALIDA, CO, p. A74
HEARTLAND BEHAVIORAL HEALTH SERVICES, NEVADA, MO, p. A251
HEARTLAND REGIONAL MEDICAL CENTER, SAINT JOSEPH, MO, p. A252
HEATHER HILL HOSPITAL AND HEALTH CARE CENTER, CHARDON, OH, p. A324
HEBREW HOME AND HOSPITAL, WEST HARTFORD, CT, p. A79
HEBREW REHABILITATION CENTER FOR AGED, BOSTON, MA, p. A204
HEDRICK MEDICAL CENTER, CHILLICOTHE, MO, p. A246
HEGG MEMORIAL HEALTH CENTER, ROCK VALLEY, IA, p. A158
HELEN ELLIS MEMORIAL HOSPITAL, TARPON SPRINGS, FL, p. A101
HELEN HAYES HOSPITAL, WEST HAVERSTRAW, NY, p. A306
HELEN KELLER HOSPITAL, SHEFFIELD, AL, p. A18
HELEN NEWBERRY JOY HOSPITAL, NEWBERRY, MI, p. A221
HELENA REGIONAL MEDICAL CENTER, HELENA, AR, p. A31
HELENE FULD MEDICAL CENTER, TRENTON, NJ, p. A282
HEMET VALLEY MEDICAL CENTER, HEMET, CA, p. A46
HEMPHILL COUNTY HOSPITAL, CANADIAN, TX, p. A403
HEMPSTEAD GENERAL HOSPITAL MEDICAL CENTER, HEMPSTEAD, NY, p. A293
HENDERSON HEALTH CARE SERVICES, HENDERSON, NE, p. A264
HENDERSON MEMORIAL HOSPITAL, HENDERSON, TX, p. A412
HENDRICK HEALTH SYSTEM, ABILENE, TX, p. A398
HENDRICKS COMMUNITY HOSPITAL, DANVILLE, IN, p. A141
HENDRICKS COMMUNITY HOSPITAL, HENDRICKS, MN, p. A230
HENDRY REGIONAL MEDICAL CENTER, CLEWISTON, FL, p. A85
HENNEPIN COUNTY MEDICAL CENTER, MINNEAPOLIS, MN, p. A232
HENRICO DOCTORS' HOSPITAL, RICHMOND, VA, p. A445
HENRIETTA D. GOODALL HOSPITAL, SANFORD, ME, p. A195
HENRY COUNTY HEALTH CENTER, MOUNT PLEASANT, IA, p. A157
HENRY COUNTY HOSPITAL, NAPOLEON, OH, p. A333
HENRY COUNTY MEDICAL CENTER, PARIS, TN, p. A395
HENRY COUNTY MEMORIAL HOSPITAL, NEW CASTLE, IN, p. A147
HENRY FORD COTTAGE HOSPITAL OF GROSSE POINTE, GROSSE POINTE FARMS, MI, p. A217

HENRY FORD HOSPITAL, DETROIT, MI, p. A214
HENRY FORD WYANDOTTE HOSPITAL, WYANDOTTE, MI, p. A225
HENRY MAYO NEWHALL MEMORIAL HOSPITAL, VALENCIA, CA, p. A67
HENRY MEDICAL CENTER, STOCKBRIDGE, GA, p. A114
HENRYETTA MEDICAL CENTER, HENRYETTA, OK, p. A342
HEPBURN MEDICAL CENTER, OGDENSBURG, NY, p. A301
HEREFORD REGIONAL MEDICAL CENTER, HEREFORD, TX, p. A413
HERINGTON MUNICIPAL HOSPITAL, HERINGTON, KS, p. A164
HERITAGE BEVERLY HILLS HOSPITAL, LECANTO, FL, p. A91
HERMANN AREA DISTRICT HOSPITAL, HERMANN, MO, p. A248
HERMANN HOSPITAL, HOUSTON, TX, p. A414
HERRICK MEMORIAL HOSPITAL, TECUMSEH, MI, p. A224
HERRIN HOSPITAL, HERRIN, IL, p. A131
HEYWOOD HOSPITAL, GARDNER, MA, p. A206
HI–DESERT MEDICAL CENTER, JOSHUA TREE, CA, p. A46
HI–PLAINS HOSPITAL, HALE CENTER, TX, p. A412
HIALEAH HOSPITAL, HIALEAH, FL, p. A88
HIAWATHA COMMUNITY HOSPITAL, HIAWATHA, KS, p. A164
HIGGINS GENERAL HOSPITAL, BREMEN, GA, p. A105
HIGH POINT REGIONAL HEALTH SYSTEM, HIGH POINT, NC, p. A313
HIGH POINTE, OKLAHOMA CITY, OK, p. A343
HIGHLAND COMMUNITY HOSPITAL, BELVIDERE, IL, p. A124
HIGHLAND DISTRICT HOSPITAL, HILLSBORO, OH, p. A330
HIGHLAND HOSPITAL, CHARLESTON, WV, p. A455
HIGHLAND HOSPITAL OF ROCHESTER, ROCHESTER, NY, p. A303
HIGHLAND LAKES MEDICAL CENTER, BURNET, TX, p. A403
HIGHLAND MEDICAL CENTER, LUBBOCK, TX, p. A419
HIGHLAND PARK HOSPITAL, HIGHLAND PARK, IL, p. A131
HIGHLAND RIDGE HOSPITAL, SALT LAKE CITY, UT, p. A435
HIGHLANDS HOSPITAL, CONNELLSVILLE, PA, p. A356
HIGHLANDS REGIONAL MEDICAL CENTER, SEBRING, FL, p. A99
HIGHLANDS REGIONAL MEDICAL CENTER, PRESTONSBURG, KY, p. A180
HIGHLANDS–CASHIERS HOSPITAL, HIGHLANDS, NC, p. A313
HIGHLINE COMMUNITY HOSPITAL, BURIEN, WA, p. A448
HILL COUNTRY MEMORIAL HOSPITAL, FREDERICKSBURG, TX, p. A410
HILL CREST BEHAVIORAL HEALTH SERVICES, BIRMINGHAM, AL, p. A12
HILL REGIONAL HOSPITAL, HILLSBORO, TX, p. A413
HILLCREST BAPTIST MEDICAL CENTER, WACO, TX, p. A430
HILLCREST HEALTH CENTER, OKLAHOMA CITY, OK, p. A343
HILLCREST HEALTHCARE SYSTEM, TULSA, OK, p. A346
HILLCREST HOSPITAL, CALHOUN CITY, MS, p. A238
HILLCREST HOSPITAL, SIMPSONVILLE, SC, p. A380
HILLS AND DALES GENERAL HOSPITAL, CASS CITY, MI, p. A213
HILLSBORO AREA HOSPITAL, HILLSBORO, IL, p. A131
HILLSBORO COMMUNITY HOSPITAL, HILLSBORO, ND, p. A320
HILLSDALE COMMUNITY HEALTH CENTER, HILLSDALE, MI, p. A217
HILLSIDE HOSPITAL, ATLANTA, GA, p. A104
HILLSIDE REHABILITATION HOSPITAL, WARREN, OH, p. A336
HILO MEDICAL CENTER, HILO, HI, p. A117
HILTON HEAD MEDICAL CENTER AND CLINICS, HILTON HEAD ISLAND, SC, p. A379
HINSDALE HOSPITAL, HINSDALE, IL, p. A132
HOAG MEMORIAL HOSPITAL PRESBYTERIAN, NEWPORT BEACH, CA, p. A55
HOCKING VALLEY COMMUNITY HOSPITAL, LOGAN, OH, p. A331
HODGEMAN COUNTY HEALTH CENTER, JETMORE, KS, p. A165
HOLDENVILLE GENERAL HOSPITAL, HOLDENVILLE, OK, p. A342
HOLLAND COMMUNITY HOSPITAL, HOLLAND, MI, p. A218
HOLLISWOOD HOSPITAL, NEW YORK, NY, p. A297
HOLLY HILL CHARTER BEHAVIORAL HEALTH SYSTEM, RALEIGH, NC, p. A315
HOLLY SPRINGS MEMORIAL HOSPITAL, HOLLY SPRINGS, MS, p. A239
HOLLYWOOD COMMUNITY HOSPITAL OF HOLLYWOOD, LOS ANGELES, CA, p. A50
HOLLYWOOD MEDICAL CENTER, LOS ANGELES, FL, p. A88
HOLLYWOOD PAVILION, LOS ANGELES, FL, p. A89
HOLMES REGIONAL MEDICAL CENTER, MELBOURNE, FL, p. A92
HOLTON COMMUNITY HOSPITAL, HOLTON, KS, p. A164
HOLY CROSS HOSPITAL, FORT LAUDERDALE, FL, p. A87
HOLY CROSS HOSPITAL, CHICAGO, IL, p. A125
HOLY CROSS HOSPITAL, DETROIT, MI, p. A215
HOLY CROSS HOSPITAL, TAOS, NM, p. A287
HOLY CROSS HOSPITAL OF SILVER SPRING, SILVER SPRING, MD, p. A202
HOLY FAMILY HEALTH SERVICES, ESTHERVILLE, IA, p. A154
HOLY FAMILY HOSPITAL, SPOKANE, WA, p. A453
HOLY FAMILY HOSPITAL, NEW RICHMOND, WI, p. A466

I

J

K

L

M

MEDFIELD STATE HOSPITAL, MEDFIELD, MA, p. A207
MEDICAL ARTS HOSPITAL, LAMESA, TX, p. A418
MEDICAL ARTS HOSPITAL, TEXARKANA, TX, p. A429
MEDICAL CENTER AT PRINCETON, PRINCETON, NJ, p. A281
MEDICAL CENTER AT SCOTTSVILLE, SCOTTSVILLE, KY,
    p. A180
MEDICAL CENTER EAST, BIRMINGHAM, AL, p. A12
MEDICAL CENTER ENTERPRISE, ENTERPRISE, AL, p. A13
MEDICAL CENTER HOSPITAL, ODESSA, TX, p. A422
MEDICAL CENTER OF CALICO ROCK, CALICO ROCK, AR, p. A29
MEDICAL CENTER OF CENTRAL GEORGIA, MACON, GA, p. A111
MEDICAL CENTER OF DELAWARE, WILMINGTON, DE, p. A80
MEDICAL CENTER OF INDEPENDENCE, INDEPENDENCE, MO,
    p. A248
MEDICAL CENTER OF LOUISIANA AT NEW ORLEANS, NEW
    ORLEANS, LA, p. A188
MEDICAL CENTER OF MANCHESTER, MANCHESTER, TN,
    p. A392
MEDICAL CENTER OF MESQUITE, MESQUITE, TX, p. A420
MEDICAL CENTER OF SOUTH ARKANSAS, EL DORADO, AR,
    p. A30
MEDICAL CENTER OF SOUTHEASTERN OKLAHOMA, DURANT,
    OK, p. A341
MEDICAL CENTER OF SOUTHERN INDIANA, CHARLESTOWN, IN,
    p. A141
MEDICAL CENTER OF WINNIE, WINNIE, TX, p. A431
MEDICAL CENTER SHOALS, MUSCLE SHOALS, AL, p. A17
MEDICAL COLLEGE HOSPITALS, TOLEDO, OH, p. A335
MEDICAL COLLEGE OF GEORGIA HOSPITAL AND CLINICS,
    AUGUSTA, GA, p. A105
MEDICAL COLLEGE OF VIRGINIA HOSPITALS, VIRGINIA
    COMMONWEALTH UNIVERSITY, RICHMOND, VA, p. A445
MEDICAL PARK HOSPITAL, HOPE, AR, p. A31
MEDICAL PARK HOSPITAL, WINSTON-SALEM, NC, p. A318
MEDICINE LODGE MEMORIAL HOSPITAL, MEDICINE LODGE, KS,
    p. A166
MEDINA COMMUNITY HOSPITAL, HONDO, TX, p. A413
MEDINA GENERAL HOSPITAL, MEDINA, OH, p. A333
MEDINA MEMORIAL HOSPITAL, MEDINA, NY, p. A294
MEDIPLEX REHABILITATION HOSPITAL, BOWLING GREEN, KY,
    p. A172
MEDIPLEX REHABILITATION-DENVER, THORNTON, CO, p. A75
MEEKER COUNTY MEMORIAL HOSPITAL, LITCHFIELD, MN,
    p. A230
MELISSA MEMORIAL HOSPITAL, HOLYOKE, CO, p. A73
MELROSE HOSPITAL AND PINE VILLA NURSING HOME,
    MELROSE, MN, p. A231
MEMORIAL CENTER, BAKERSFIELD, CA, p. A37
MEMORIAL COMMUNITY HOSPITAL, BLAIR, NE, p. A262
MEMORIAL COMMUNITY HOSPITAL, EDGERTON, WI, p. A462
MEMORIAL HEALTH CARE, WORCESTER, MA, p. A211
MEMORIAL HEALTH CARE SYSTEMS, SEWARD, NE, p. A268
MEMORIAL HEALTH CENTER, SIDNEY, NE, p. A268
MEMORIAL HEALTHCARE CENTER, OWOSSO, MI, p. A221
MEMORIAL HOSPITAL, COLORADO SPRINGS, CO, p. A70
MEMORIAL HOSPITAL, CRAIG, CO, p. A71
MEMORIAL HOSPITAL, WEISER, ID, p. A122
MEMORIAL HOSPITAL, BELLEVILLE, IL, p. A123
MEMORIAL HOSPITAL, CARTHAGE, IL, p. A124
MEMORIAL HOSPITAL, CHESTER, IL, p. A125
MEMORIAL HOSPITAL, LOGANSPORT, IN, p. A146
MEMORIAL HOSPITAL, SEYMOUR, IN, p. A148
MEMORIAL HOSPITAL, ABILENE, KS, p. A161
MEMORIAL HOSPITAL, MCPHERSON, KS, p. A166
MEMORIAL HOSPITAL, MANCHESTER, KY, p. A178
MEMORIAL HOSPITAL, AURORA, NE, p. A262
MEMORIAL HOSPITAL, NORTH CONWAY, NH, p. A273
MEMORIAL HOSPITAL, ALBANY, NY, p. A288
MEMORIAL HOSPITAL, FREMONT, OH, p. A330
MEMORIAL HOSPITAL, MARYSVILLE, OH, p. A332
MEMORIAL HOSPITAL, FREDERICK, OK, p. A341
MEMORIAL HOSPITAL, TOWANDA, PA, p. A369
MEMORIAL HOSPITAL, YORK, PA, p. A372
MEMORIAL HOSPITAL, CHATTANOOGA, TN, p. A388
MEMORIAL HOSPITAL, CENTER, TX, p. A403
MEMORIAL HOSPITAL, DUMAS, TX, p. A408
MEMORIAL HOSPITAL, GONZALES, TX, p. A411
MEMORIAL HOSPITAL, KERMIT, TX, p. A417
MEMORIAL HOSPITAL, SEMINOLE, TX, p. A427
MEMORIAL HOSPITAL AND HEALTH CARE CENTER, JASPER, IN,
    p. A145
MEMORIAL HOSPITAL AND MANOR, BAINBRIDGE, GA, p. A105
MEMORIAL HOSPITAL AND MEDICAL CENTER, MIDLAND, TX,
    p. A421
MEMORIAL HOSPITAL AND MEDICAL CENTER OF CUMBERLAND,
    CUMBERLAND, MD, p. A199
MEMORIAL HOSPITAL AT EASTON MARYLAND, EASTON, MD,
    p. A200
MEMORIAL HOSPITAL AT EXETER, EXETER, CA, p. A42
MEMORIAL HOSPITAL AT GULFPORT, GULFPORT, MS, p. A239

MEMORIAL HOSPITAL CORPORATION OF BURLINGTON,
    BURLINGTON, WI, p. A461
MEMORIAL HOSPITAL FOR CANCER AND ALLIED DISEASES,
    NEW YORK, NY, p. A298
MEMORIAL HOSPITAL LOS BANOS, LOS BANOS, CA, p. A52
MEMORIAL HOSPITAL OCONOMOWOC, OCONOMOWOC, WI,
    p. A466
MEMORIAL HOSPITAL OF ADEL, ADEL, GA, p. A103
MEMORIAL HOSPITAL OF BEDFORD COUNTY, EVERETT, PA,
    p. A358
MEMORIAL HOSPITAL OF BURLINGTON COUNTY, MOUNT
    HOLLY, NJ, p. A279
MEMORIAL HOSPITAL OF CARBON COUNTY, RAWLINS, WY,
    p. A472
MEMORIAL HOSPITAL OF CARBONDALE, CARBONDALE, IL,
    p. A124
MEMORIAL HOSPITAL OF GARDENA, GARDENA, CA, p. A44
MEMORIAL HOSPITAL OF IOWA COUNTY, DODGEVILLE, WI,
    p. A461
MEMORIAL HOSPITAL OF LAFAYETTE COUNTY, DARLINGTON,
    WI, p. A461
MEMORIAL HOSPITAL OF MARTINSVILLE AND HENRY COUNTY,
    MARTINSVILLE, VA, p. A442
MEMORIAL HOSPITAL OF MICHIGAN CITY, MICHIGAN CITY, IN,
    p. A146
MEMORIAL HOSPITAL OF RHODE ISLAND, PAWTUCKET, RI,
    p. A373
MEMORIAL HOSPITAL OF SALEM COUNTY, SALEM, NJ, p. A281
MEMORIAL HOSPITAL OF SHERIDAN COUNTY, SHERIDAN, WY,
    p. A472
MEMORIAL HOSPITAL OF SOUTH BEND, SOUTH BEND, IN,
    p. A148
MEMORIAL HOSPITAL OF SWEETWATER COUNTY, ROCK
    SPRINGS, WY, p. A472
MEMORIAL HOSPITAL OF TAMPA, TAMPA, FL, p. A100
MEMORIAL HOSPITAL OF TAYLOR COUNTY, MEDFORD, WI,
    p. A464
MEMORIAL HOSPITAL OF TEXAS COUNTY, GUYMON, OK,
    p. A342
MEMORIAL HOSPITAL PASADENA, PASADENA, TX, p. A423
MEMORIAL HOSPITAL PEMBROKE, PEMBROKE PINES, FL,
    p. A96
MEMORIAL HOSPITAL SOUTHWEST, HOUSTON, TX, p. A415
MEMORIAL HOSPITAL WEST, PEMBROKE PINES, FL, p. A96
MEMORIAL HOSPITAL-FLAGLER, BUNNELL, FL, p. A84
MEMORIAL HOSPITAL-MEMORIAL CITY, HOUSTON, TX, p. A415
MEMORIAL HOSPITAL-ORMOND BEACH, ORMOND BEACH, FL,
    p. A96
MEMORIAL HOSPITAL-THE WOODLANDS, THE WOODLANDS,
    TX, p. A429
MEMORIAL HOSPITAL-WEST VOLUSIA, DELAND, FL, p. A86
MEMORIAL HOSPITALS ASSOCIATION, MODESTO, CA, p. A54
MEMORIAL MEDICAL CENTER-LIVINGSTON, LIVINGSTON, TX,
    p. A419
MEMORIAL MEDICAL CENTER, SAVANNAH, GA, p. A114
MEMORIAL MEDICAL CENTER, SPRINGFIELD, IL, p. A138
MEMORIAL MEDICAL CENTER, WOODSTOCK, IL, p. A139
MEMORIAL MEDICAL CENTER, NEW ORLEANS, LA, p. A188
MEMORIAL MEDICAL CENTER, LAS CRUCES, NM, p. A286
MEMORIAL MEDICAL CENTER, PORT LAVACA, TX, p. A424
MEMORIAL MEDICAL CENTER, ASHLAND, WI, p. A460
MEMORIAL MEDICAL CENTER, NEILLSVILLE, WI, p. A466
MEMORIAL MEDICAL CENTER AND CANCER TREATMENT
    CENTER-TULSA, TULSA, OK, p. A346
MEMORIAL MEDICAL CENTER AT SOUTH AMBOY, SOUTH
    AMBOY, NJ, p. A281
MEMORIAL MEDICAL CENTER OF EAST TEXAS, LUFKIN, TX,
    p. A419
MEMORIAL MEDICAL CENTER OF SAN AUGUSTINE, SAN
    AUGUSTINE, TX, p. A427
MEMORIAL MEDICAL CENTER OF WEST MICHIGAN, LUDINGTON,
    MI, p. A219
MEMORIAL MISSION MEDICAL CENTER, ASHEVILLE, NC,
    p. A308
MEMORIAL MOTHER FRANCES HOSPITAL, PALESTINE, TX,
    p. A422
MEMORIAL PAVILION, LAWTON, OK, p. A342
MEMORIAL PSYCHIATRIC HOSPITAL, ALBUQUERQUE, NM,
    p. A284
MEMORIAL REGIONAL HOSPITAL, LOS ANGELES, FL, p. A89
MEMORIAL REHABILITATION HOSPITAL, HOUSTON, TX, p. A415
MEMORIAL SPRING SHADOWS GLEN, HOUSTON, TX, p. A415
MEMPHIS MENTAL HEALTH INSTITUTE, MEMPHIS, TN, p. A393
MENA MEDICAL CENTER, MENA, AR, p. A33
MENDOCINO COAST DISTRICT HOSPITAL, FORT BRAGG, CA,
    p. A43
MENDOTA COMMUNITY HOSPITAL, MENDOTA, IL, p. A134
MENDOTA MENTAL HEALTH INSTITUTE, MADISON, WI, p. A464
MENIFEE VALLEY MEDICAL CENTER, SUN CITY, CA, p. A66
MENNONITE GENERAL HOSPITAL, AIBONITO, PR, p. A474

MENORAH MEDICAL CENTER, OVERLAND PARK, KS, p. A168
MENTAL HEALTH INSTITUTE, CHEROKEE, IA, p. A152
MENTAL HEALTH INSTITUTE, CLARINDA, IA, p. A152
MENTAL HEALTH INSTITUTE, INDEPENDENCE, IA, p. A155
MENTAL HEALTH INSTITUTE, MOUNT PLEASANT, IA, p. A157
MEPSI CENTER, BAYAMON, PR, p. A475
MERCER COUNTY HOSPITAL, ALEDO, IL, p. A123
MERCER COUNTY JOINT TOWNSHIP COMMUNITY HOSPITAL,
    COLDWATER, OH, p. A327
MERCER MEDICAL CENTER, TRENTON, NJ, p. A282
MERCY AMERICAN RIVER/MERCY SAN JUAN HOSPITAL,
    CARMICHAEL, CA, p. A39
MERCY BEHAVIORAL HEALTH, DURANGO, CO, p. A72
MERCY CENTER FOR HEALTH CARE SERVICES, AURORA, IL,
    p. A123
MERCY COMMUNITY HOSPITAL, PORT JERVIS, NY, p. A302
MERCY COMMUNITY HOSPITAL, HAVERTOWN, PA, p. A359
MERCY GENERAL HEALTH PARTNERS-OAK AVENUE CAMPUS,
    MUSKEGON, MI, p. A221
MERCY GENERAL HEALTH PARTNERS-SHERMAN BOULEVARD
    CAMPUS, MUSKEGON, MI, p. A221
MERCY GENERAL HOSPITAL, SACRAMENTO, CA, p. A59
MERCY HEALTH CENTER, DUBUQUE, IA, p. A154
MERCY HEALTH CENTER, OKLAHOMA CITY, OK, p. A344
MERCY HEALTH CENTER OF MANHATTAN, NEW YORK, KS,
    p. A166
MERCY HEALTH SERVICES NORTH-GRAYLING, GRAYLING, MI,
    p. A217
MERCY HEALTH SERVICES-NORTH, CADILLAC, MI, p. A213
MERCY HEALTH SYSTEM, JANESVILLE, WI, p. A463
MERCY HEALTH SYSTEM OF KANSAS, FORT SCOTT, KS,
    p. A163
MERCY HEALTH SYSTEM OF SOUTHEASTERN PENNSYLVANIA,
    BALA CYNWYD, PA, p. A353
MERCY HEALTHCARE-BAKERSFIELD, BAKERSFIELD, CA, p. A37
MERCY HOSPITAL, MIAMI, FL, p. A93
MERCY HOSPITAL, IOWA CITY, IA, p. A155
MERCY HOSPITAL, MOUNDRIDGE, KS, p. A167
MERCY HOSPITAL, SPRINGFIELD, MA, p. A210
MERCY HOSPITAL, DETROIT, MI, p. A215
MERCY HOSPITAL, PORT HURON, MI, p. A222
MERCY HOSPITAL, COON RAPIDS, MN, p. A228
MERCY HOSPITAL, BUFFALO, NY, p. A290
MERCY HOSPITAL, CHARLOTTE, NC, p. A309
MERCY HOSPITAL, DEVILS LAKE, ND, p. A319
MERCY HOSPITAL, VALLEY CITY, ND, p. A322
MERCY HOSPITAL, HAMILTON, OH, p. A330
MERCY HOSPITAL, TIFFIN, OH, p. A335
MERCY HOSPITAL AND HEALTH CARE CENTER, MOOSE LAKE,
    MN, p. A232
MERCY HOSPITAL AND HEALTH SERVICES, MERCED, CA,
    p. A53
MERCY HOSPITAL AND MEDICAL CENTER, CHICAGO, IL,
    p. A126
MERCY HOSPITAL ANDERSON, CINCINNATI, OH, p. A326
MERCY HOSPITAL MEDICAL CENTER, DES MOINES, IA, p. A154
MERCY HOSPITAL OF FOLSOM, FOLSOM, CA, p. A43
MERCY HOSPITAL OF FRANCISCAN SISTERS, OELWEIN, IA,
    p. A157
MERCY HOSPITAL OF PITTSBURGH, PITTSBURGH, PA, p. A366
MERCY HOSPITAL OF SCOTT COUNTY, WALDRON, AR, p. A35
MERCY HOSPITAL OF SCRANTON, SCRANTON, PA, p. A368
MERCY HOSPITAL OF WILKES-BARRE, WILKES-BARRE, PA,
    p. A371
MERCY HOSPITAL PORTLAND, PORTLAND, ME, p. A195
MERCY HOSPITAL-TURNER MEMORIAL, OZARK, AR, p. A34
MERCY HOSPITAL-WILLARD, WILLARD, OH, p. A337
MERCY HOSPITALS OF KANSAS, INDEPENDENCE, KS, p. A164
MERCY MEDICAL, DAPHNE, AL, p. A13
MERCY MEDICAL CENTER, REDDING, CA, p. A58
MERCY MEDICAL CENTER, DURANGO, CO, p. A72
MERCY MEDICAL CENTER, NAMPA, ID, p. A121
MERCY MEDICAL CENTER, CEDAR RAPIDS, IA, p. A152
MERCY MEDICAL CENTER, BALTIMORE, MD, p. A198
MERCY MEDICAL CENTER, ROCKVILLE CENTRE, NY, p. A303
MERCY MEDICAL CENTER, WILLISTON, ND, p. A322
MERCY MEDICAL CENTER, SPRINGFIELD, OH, p. A335
MERCY MEDICAL CENTER, ROSEBURG, OR, p. A352
MERCY MEDICAL CENTER, OSHKOSH, WI, p. A467
MERCY MEDICAL CENTER MOUNT SHASTA, MOUNT SHASTA,
    CA, p. A54
MERCY MEMORIAL HEALTH CENTER, ARDMORE, OK, p. A339
MERCY MEMORIAL HOSPITAL, MONROE, MI, p. A220
MERCY MEMORIAL HOSPITAL, URBANA, OH, p. A336
MERCY PROVIDENCE HOSPITAL, PITTSBURGH, PA, p. A366
MERCY REGIONAL MEDICAL CENTER, LAREDO, TX, p. A418
MERCY SPECIAL CARE HOSPITAL, NANTICOKE, PA, p. A362
MERIDELL ACHIEVEMENT CENTER, AUSTIN, TX, p. A400
MERIDIA EUCLID HOSPITAL, EUCLID, OH, p. A329
MERIDIA HILLCREST HOSPITAL, CLEVELAND, OH, p. A327

MOSES TAYLOR HOSPITAL, SCRANTON, PA, p. A368
MOTION PICTURE AND TELEVISION FUND HOSPITAL AND RESIDENTIAL SERVICES, LOS ANGELES, CA, p. A51
MOUNT ASCUTNEY HOSPITAL AND HEALTH CENTER, WINDSOR, VT, p. A438
MOUNT AUBURN HOSPITAL, CAMBRIDGE, MA, p. A205
MOUNT CARMEL HEALTH SYSTEM, COLUMBUS, OH, p. A328
MOUNT CARMEL HOSPITAL, COLVILLE, WA, p. A449
MOUNT CARMEL MEDICAL CENTER, PITTSBURG, KS, p. A168
MOUNT CLEMENS GENERAL HOSPITAL, MOUNT CLEMENS, MI, p. A220
MOUNT DESERT ISLAND HOSPITAL, BAR HARBOR, ME, p. A193
MOUNT DIABLO MEDICAL CENTER, CONCORD, CA, p. A40
MOUNT GRAHAM COMMUNITY HOSPITAL, SAFFORD, AZ, p. A26
MOUNT GRANT GENERAL HOSPITAL, HAWTHORNE, NV, p. A270
MOUNT REGIS CENTER, SALEM, VA, p. A446
MOUNT SAN RAFAEL HOSPITAL, TRINIDAD, CO, p. A75
MOUNT SINAI HOSPITAL MEDICAL CENTER OF CHICAGO, CHICAGO, IL, p. A126
MOUNT SINAI MEDICAL CENTER, MIAMI BEACH, FL, p. A94
MOUNT SINAI MEDICAL CENTER, NEW YORK, NY, p. A298
MOUNT SINAI MEDICAL CENTER, CLEVELAND, OH, p. A327
MOUNT ST. MARY'S HOSPITAL OF NIAGARA FALLS, LEWISTON, NY, p. A293
MOUNT VERNON HOSPITAL, MOUNT VERNON, NY, p. A295
MOUNTAIN CREST HOSPITAL, FORT COLLINS, CO, p. A72
MOUNTAIN MANOR TREATMENT CENTER, EMMITSBURG, MD, p. A200
MOUNTAIN VIEW HOSPITAL, GADSDEN, AL, p. A14
MOUNTAIN VIEW HOSPITAL, PAYSON, UT, p. A434
MOUNTAIN VIEW HOSPITAL DISTRICT, MADRAS, OR, p. A350
MOUNTAINVIEW MEDICAL CENTER, WHITE SULPHUR SPRINGS, MT, p. A260
MT. SINAI HOSPITAL, PHILADELPHIA, PA, p. A364
MT. WASHINGTON PEDIATRIC HOSPITAL, BALTIMORE, MD, p. A198
MUENSTER MEMORIAL HOSPITAL, MUENSTER, TX, p. A421
MUHLENBERG COMMUNITY HOSPITAL, GREENVILLE, KY, p. A174
MUHLENBERG HOSPITAL CENTER, BETHLEHEM, PA, p. A354
MUHLENBERG REGIONAL MEDICAL CENTER, PLAINFIELD, NJ, p. A281
MULESHOE AREA MEDICAL CENTER, MULESHOE, TX, p. A421
MULLINS HOSPITAL, MULLINS, SC, p. A379
MUNISING MEMORIAL HOSPITAL, MUNISING, MI, p. A220
MUNROE REGIONAL MEDICAL CENTER, OCALA, FL, p. A95
MUNSON ARMY COMMUNITY HOSPITAL, FORT LEAVENWORTH, KS, p. A163
MUNSON MEDICAL CENTER, TRAVERSE CITY, MI, p. A224
MURPHY MEDICAL CENTER, MURPHY, NC, p. A314
MURRAY COUNTY MEMORIAL HOSPITAL, SLAYTON, MN, p. A235
MURRAY–CALLOWAY COUNTY HOSPITAL, MURRAY, KY, p. A179
MUSC MEDICAL CENTER OF MEDICAL UNIVERSITY OF SOUTH CAROLINA, CHARLESTON, SC, p. A376
MUSCATINE GENERAL HOSPITAL, MUSCATINE, IA, p. A157
MUSKOGEE REGIONAL MEDICAL CENTER, MUSKOGEE, OK, p. A343
MYERS COMMUNITY HOSPITAL, SODUS, NY, p. A304
MYRTLE WERTH HOSPITAL–MAYO HEALTH SYSTEM, MENOMONIE, WI, p. A465

N

N. T. ENLOE MEMORIAL HOSPITAL, CHICO, CA, p. A39
NACOGDOCHES MEDICAL CENTER, NACOGDOCHES, TX, p. A421
NACOGDOCHES MEMORIAL HOSPITAL, NACOGDOCHES, TX, p. A421
NAEVE HOSPITAL, ALBERT LEA, MN, p. A226
NAN TRAVIS MEMORIAL HOSPITAL, JACKSONVILLE, TX, p. A417
NANTICOKE MEMORIAL HOSPITAL, SEAFORD, DE, p. A80
NANTUCKET COTTAGE HOSPITAL, NANTUCKET, MA, p. A208
NAPA STATE HOSPITAL, NAPA, CA, p. A55
NAPLES COMMUNITY HOSPITAL, NAPLES, FL, p. A94
NASH HEALTH CARE SYSTEMS, ROCKY MOUNT, NC, p. A316
NASHVILLE METROPOLITAN BORDEAUX HOSPITAL, NASHVILLE, TN, p. A394
NASHVILLE REHABILITATION HOSPITAL, NASHVILLE, TN, p. A395
NASON HOSPITAL, ROARING SPRING, PA, p. A368
NASSAU COUNTY MEDICAL CENTER, EAST MEADOW, NY, p. A291
NATCHAUG HOSPITAL, MANSFIELD CENTER, CT, p. A77
NATCHEZ COMMUNITY HOSPITAL, NATCHEZ, MS, p. A242
NATCHEZ REGIONAL MEDICAL CENTER, NATCHEZ, MS, p. A242

NATCHITOCHES PARISH HOSPITAL, NATCHITOCHES, LA, p. A188
NATHAN LITTAUER HOSPITAL AND NURSING HOME, GLOVERSVILLE, NY, p. A292
NATIONAL HOSPITAL MEDICAL CENTER, ARLINGTON, VA, p. A439
NATIONAL JEWISH MEDICAL AND RESEARCH CENTER, DENVER, CO, p. A71
NATIONAL NAVAL MEDICAL CENTER, BETHESDA, MD, p. A199
NATIONAL PARK MEDICAL CENTER, HOT SPRINGS, AR, p. A31
NATIONAL REHABILITATION HOSPITAL, WASHINGTON, DC, p. A81
NATIVIDAD MEDICAL CENTER, SALINAS, CA, p. A60
NATURE COAST REGIONAL HEALTH NETWORK, WILLISTON, FL, p. A102
NAUKEAG HOSPITAL, ASHBURNHAM, MA, p. A203
NAVAL HOSPITAL, CAMP PENDLETON, CA, p. A39
NAVAL HOSPITAL, LEMOORE, CA, p. A48
NAVAL HOSPITAL, TWENTYNINE PALMS, CA, p. A67
NAVAL HOSPITAL, GROTON, CT, p. A76
NAVAL HOSPITAL, JACKSONVILLE, FL, p. A89
NAVAL HOSPITAL, PENSACOLA, FL, p. A97
NAVAL HOSPITAL, GREAT LAKES, IL, p. A131
NAVAL HOSPITAL, PATUXENT RIVER, MD, p. A201
NAVAL HOSPITAL, CAMP LEJEUNE, NC, p. A309
NAVAL HOSPITAL, HAVELOCK, NC, p. A312
NAVAL HOSPITAL, BEAUFORT, SC, p. A375
NAVAL HOSPITAL, CHARLESTON, SC, p. A376
NAVAL HOSPITAL, MILLINGTON, TN, p. A394
NAVAL HOSPITAL, CORPUS CHRISTI, TX, p. A405
NAVAL HOSPITAL, BREMERTON, WA, p. A448
NAVAL HOSPITAL, OAK HARBOR, WA, p. A451
NAVAL MEDICAL CENTER, SAN DIEGO, CA, p. A60
NAVAL MEDICAL CENTER, PORTSMOUTH, VA, p. A444
NAVAPACHE REGIONAL MEDICAL CENTER, SHOW LOW, AZ, p. A26
NAZARETH HOSPITAL, PHILADELPHIA, PA, p. A364
NEBRASKA METHODIST HOSPITAL, OMAHA, NE, p. A267
NEEDLES–DESERT COMMUNITIES HOSPITAL, NEEDLES, CA, p. A55
NEMAHA COUNTY HOSPITAL, AUBURN, NE, p. A262
NEMAHA VALLEY COMMUNITY HOSPITAL, SENECA, KS, p. A169
NEOSHO MEMORIAL REGIONAL MEDICAL CENTER, CHANUTE, KS, p. A161
NESHOBA COUNTY GENERAL HOSPITAL, PHILADELPHIA, MS, p. A242
NESS COUNTY HOSPITAL NUMBER TWO, NESS CITY, KS, p. A167
NEUMANN MEDICAL CENTER, PHILADELPHIA, PA, p. A364
NEVADA MENTAL HEALTH INSTITUTE, SPARKS, NV, p. A271
NEVADA REGIONAL MEDICAL CENTER, NEVADA, MO, p. A251
NEW BRITAIN GENERAL HOSPITAL, NEW BRITAIN, CT, p. A77
NEW CENTER HOSPITAL, DETROIT, MI, p. A215
NEW ENGLAND BAPTIST HOSPITAL, BOSTON, MA, p. A204
NEW ENGLAND MEDICAL CENTER, BOSTON, MA, p. A204
NEW ENGLAND SINAI HOSPITAL AND REHABILITATION CENTER, STOUGHTON, MA, p. A210
NEW HAMPSHIRE HOSPITAL, CONCORD, NH, p. A272
NEW HANOVER REGIONAL MEDICAL CENTER, WILMINGTON, NC, p. A318
NEW LONDON FAMILY MEDICAL CENTER, NEW LONDON, WI, p. A466
NEW LONDON HOSPITAL, NEW LONDON, NH, p. A273
NEW MILFORD HOSPITAL, NEW MILFORD, CT, p. A78
NEW ORLEANS ADOLESCENT HOSPITAL, NEW ORLEANS, LA, p. A189
NEW ULM MEDICAL CENTER, NEW ULM, MN, p. A232
NEW YORK DOWNTOWN HOSPITAL, NEW YORK, NY, p. A298
NEW YORK EYE AND EAR INFIRMARY, NEW YORK, NY, p. A298
NEW YORK HOSPITAL MEDICAL CENTER OF QUEENS, NEW YORK, NY, p. A298
NEW YORK METHODIST HOSPITAL, NEW YORK, NY, p. A298
NEW YORK STATE PSYCHIATRIC INSTITUTE, NEW YORK, NY, p. A298
NEW YORK UNIVERSITY MEDICAL CENTER, NEW YORK, NY, p. A298
NEWARK BETH ISRAEL MEDICAL CENTER, NEWARK, NJ, p. A279
NEWARK–WAYNE COMMUNITY HOSPITAL, NEWARK, NY, p. A300
NEWBERRY COUNTY MEMORIAL HOSPITAL, NEWBERRY, SC, p. A380
NEWCOMB MEDICAL CENTER, VINELAND, NJ, p. A282
NEWHALL COMMUNITY HOSPITAL, NEWHALL, CA, p. A55
NEWMAN MEMORIAL COUNTY HOSPITAL, EMPORIA, KS, p. A162
NEWMAN MEMORIAL HOSPITAL, SHATTUCK, OK, p. A345
NEWNAN HOSPITAL, NEWNAN, GA, p. A112
NEWPORT COMMUNITY HOSPITAL, NEWPORT, WA, p. A451
NEWPORT HOSPITAL, NEWPORT, RI, p. A373

NEWPORT HOSPITAL AND CLINIC, NEWPORT, AR, p. A33
NEWPORT NEWS GENERAL HOSPITAL, NEWPORT NEWS, VA, p. A443
NEWTON GENERAL HOSPITAL, COVINGTON, GA, p. A107
NEWTON MEDICAL CENTER, NEWTON, KS, p. A167
NEWTON MEMORIAL HOSPITAL, NEWTON, NJ, p. A280
NEWTON–WELLESLEY HOSPITAL, NEWTON, MA, p. A208
NIAGARA FALLS MEMORIAL MEDICAL CENTER, NIAGARA FALLS, NY, p. A301
NICHOLAS COUNTY HOSPITAL, CARLISLE, KY, p. A173
NICHOLAS H. NOYES MEMORIAL HOSPITAL, DANSVILLE, NY, p. A291
NIOBRARA COUNTY HOSPITAL DISTRICT, LUSK, WY, p. A472
NIOBRARA VALLEY HOSPITAL, LYNCH, NE, p. A265
NIX HEALTH CARE SYSTEM, SAN ANTONIO, TX, p. A426
NOBLE HOSPITAL, WESTFIELD, MA, p. A211
NOCONA GENERAL HOSPITAL, NOCONA, TX, p. A422
NOR–LEA GENERAL HOSPITAL, LOVINGTON, NM, p. A286
NORFOLK COMMUNITY HOSPITAL, NORFOLK, VA, p. A443
NORFOLK PSYCHIATRIC CENTER, NORFOLK, VA, p. A443
NORFOLK REGIONAL CENTER, NORFOLK, NE, p. A266
NORMAN REGIONAL HOSPITAL, NORMAN, OK, p. A343
NORRISTOWN STATE HOSPITAL, NORRISTOWN, PA, p. A362
NORTH ADAMS REGIONAL HOSPITAL, NORTH ADAMS, MA, p. A208
NORTH ALABAMA REGIONAL HOSPITAL, DECATUR, AL, p. A13
NORTH ARKANSAS MEDICAL CENTER, HARRISON, AR, p. A31
NORTH ARUNDEL HOSPITAL, GLEN BURNIE, MD, p. A200
NORTH BALDWIN HOSPITAL, BAY MINETTE, AL, p. A11
NORTH BAY MEDICAL CENTER, NEW PORT RICHEY, FL, p. A94
NORTH BIG HORN HOSPITAL, LOVELL, WY, p. A472
NORTH BROWARD MEDICAL CENTER, POMPANO BEACH, FL, p. A97
NORTH CADDO MEDICAL CENTER, VIVIAN, LA, p. A191
NORTH CAROLINA BAPTIST HOSPITAL, WINSTON–SALEM, NC, p. A318
NORTH CAROLINA EYE AND EAR HOSPITAL, DURHAM, NC, p. A310
NORTH CENTRAL BRONX HOSPITAL, NEW YORK, NY, p. A299
NORTH CENTRAL HEALTH CARE FACILITIES, WAUSAU, WI, p. A470
NORTH COAST HEALTH CARE CENTERS–EAST CAMPUS, SANTA ROSA, CA, p. A64
NORTH COLORADO MEDICAL CENTER, GREELEY, CO, p. A73
NORTH COUNTRY HOSPITAL AND HEALTH CENTER, NEWPORT, VT, p. A437
NORTH COUNTRY REGIONAL HOSPITAL, BEMIDJI, MN, p. A226
NORTH CREST MEDICAL CENTER, SPRINGFIELD, TN, p. A396
NORTH DAKOTA STATE HOSPITAL, JAMESTOWN, ND, p. A321
NORTH DALLAS REHABILITATION HOSPITAL, DALLAS, TX, p. A407
NORTH FLORIDA RECEPTION CENTER HOSPITAL, LAKE BUTLER, FL, p. A90
NORTH FULTON REGIONAL HOSPITAL, ROSWELL, GA, p. A113
NORTH GENERAL HOSPITAL, NEW YORK, NY, p. A299
NORTH GEORGIA MEDICAL CENTER AND GILMER NURSING HOME, ELLIJAY, GA, p. A109
NORTH HOLLYWOOD MEDICAL CENTER, LOS ANGELES, CA, p. A51
NORTH IOWA MERCY HEALTH CENTER, MASON CITY, IA, p. A157
NORTH JACKSON HOSPITAL, BRIDGEPORT, AL, p. A12
NORTH KANSAS CITY HOSPITAL, NORTH KANSAS CITY, MO, p. A251
NORTH LINCOLN HOSPITAL, LINCOLN CITY, OR, p. A350
NORTH LOGAN MERCY HOSPITAL, PARIS, AR, p. A34
NORTH LOUISIANA REHABILITATION HOSPITAL, RUSTON, LA, p. A190
NORTH MEMORIAL HEALTH CARE, ROBBINSDALE, MN, p. A233
NORTH MISSISSIPPI MEDICAL CENTER, TUPELO, MS, p. A243
NORTH OAKLAND MEDICAL CENTERS, PONTIAC, MI, p. A221
NORTH OAKS MEDICAL CENTER, HAMMOND, LA, p. A185
NORTH OKALOOSA MEDICAL CENTER, CRESTVIEW, FL, p. A85
NORTH OTTAWA COMMUNITY HOSPITAL, GRAND HAVEN, MI, p. A216
NORTH PARK HOSPITAL, CHATTANOOGA, TN, p. A388
NORTH PENN HOSPITAL, LANSDALE, PA, p. A360
NORTH PHILADELPHIA HEALTH SYSTEM, PHILADELPHIA, PA, p. A364
NORTH RIDGE MEDICAL CENTER, FORT LAUDERDALE, FL, p. A87
NORTH RUNNELS HOSPITAL, WINTERS, TX, p. A432
NORTH SHORE MEDICAL CENTER, MIAMI, FL, p. A93
NORTH SHORE PSYCHIATRIC HOSPITAL, SLIDELL, LA, p. A191
NORTH SHORE UNIVERSITY HOSPITAL, MANHASSET, NY, p. A294
NORTH SHORE UNIVERSITY HOSPITAL AT GLEN COVE, GLEN COVE, NY, p. A292
NORTH SHORE UNIVERSITY HOSPITAL AT PLAINVIEW, PLAINVIEW, NY, p. A302

O

P

PACIFICA HOSPITAL, HUNTINGTON BEACH, CA, p. A46
PACIFICA HOSPITAL OF THE VALLEY, LOS ANGELES, CA, p. A51
PAGE HOSPITAL, PAGE, AZ, p. A24
PAGE MEMORIAL HOSPITAL, LURAY, VA, p. A442
PALISADES GENERAL HOSPITAL, NORTH BERGEN, NJ, p. A280
PALM BEACH GARDENS MEDICAL CENTER, PALM BEACH GARDENS, FL, p. A96
PALM SPRINGS GENERAL HOSPITAL, HIALEAH, FL, p. A88
PALMER LUTHERAN HEALTH CENTER, WEST UNION, IA, p. A160
PALMERTON HOSPITAL, PALMERTON, PA, p. A363
PALMETTO GENERAL HOSPITAL, HIALEAH, FL, p. A88
PALMS OF PASADENA HOSPITAL, SAINT PETERSBURG, FL, p. A98
PALO ALTO COUNTY HOSPITAL, EMMETSBURG, IA, p. A154
PALO DURO HOSPITAL, CANYON, TX, p. A403
PALO PINTO GENERAL HOSPITAL, MINERAL WELLS, TX, p. A421
PALO VERDE HOSPITAL, BLYTHE, CA, p. A38
PALO VERDE MENTAL HEALTH SERVICES, TUCSON, AZ, p. A27
PALOMAR MEDICAL CENTER, ESCONDIDO, CA, p. A42
PALOS COMMUNITY HOSPITAL, PALOS HEIGHTS, IL, p. A135
PAN AMERICAN HOSPITAL, MIAMI, FL, p. A93
PANA COMMUNITY HOSPITAL, PANA, IL, p. A135
PANOLA GENERAL HOSPITAL, CARTHAGE, TX, p. A403
PAOLI MEMORIAL HOSPITAL, PAOLI, PA, p. A363
PARADISE VALLEY HOSPITAL, NATIONAL CITY, CA, p. A55
PARIS COMMUNITY HOSPITAL, PARIS, IL, p. A135
PARK LANE MEDICAL CENTER, KANSAS CITY, MO, p. A249
PARK MEDICAL CENTER, COLUMBUS, OH, p. A328
PARK PLACE MEDICAL CENTER, PORT ARTHUR, TX, p. A423
PARK PLAZA HOSPITAL, HOUSTON, TX, p. A415
PARK RIDGE HOSPITAL, ROCHESTER, NY, p. A303
PARK RIDGE HOSPITAL, FLETCHER, NC, p. A311
PARK VIEW HOSPITAL, EL RENO, OK, p. A341
PARKER COMMUNITY HOSPITAL, PARKER, AZ, p. A24
PARKLAND HEALTH CENTER, FARMINGTON, MO, p. A247
PARKLAND MEDICAL CENTER, DERRY, NH, p. A272
PARKRIDGE MEDICAL CENTER, CHATTANOOGA, TN, p. A388
PARKSIDE HOSPITAL, TULSA, OK, p. A346
PARKVIEW COMMUNITY HOSPITAL MEDICAL CENTER, RIVERSIDE, CA, p. A59
PARKVIEW EPISCOPAL MEDICAL CENTER, PUEBLO, CO, p. A74
PARKVIEW HOSPITAL, BRUNSWICK, ME, p. A194
PARKVIEW HOSPITAL, PHILADELPHIA, PA, p. A364
PARKVIEW HOSPITAL, WHEELER, TX, p. A431
PARKVIEW HOSPITAL OF TOPEKA, TOPEKA, KS, p. A170
PARKVIEW MEMORIAL HOSPITAL, FORT WAYNE, IN, p. A142
PARKVIEW REGIONAL HOSPITAL, MEXIA, TX, p. A421
PARKVIEW REGIONAL MEDICAL CENTER, VICKSBURG, MS, p. A244
PARKWAY HOSPITAL, NEW YORK, NY, p. A299
PARKWAY MEDICAL CENTER HOSPITAL, DECATUR, AL, p. A13
PARKWAY REGIONAL HOSPITAL, FULTON, KY, p. A174
PARKWAY REGIONAL MEDICAL CENTER, NORTH MIAMI BEACH, FL, p. A94
PARKWAY REGIONAL MEDICAL CENTER–WEST, MIAMI, FL, p. A93
PARMA COMMUNITY GENERAL HOSPITAL, PARMA, OH, p. A334
PARMER COUNTY COMMUNITY HOSPITAL, FRIONA, TX, p. A411
PARRISH MEDICAL CENTER, TITUSVILLE, FL, p. A101
PARSONS STATE HOSPITAL AND TRAINING CENTER, PARSONS, KS, p. A168
PASCACK VALLEY HOSPITAL, WESTWOOD, NJ, p. A283
PASSAVANT AREA HOSPITAL, JACKSONVILLE, IL, p. A132
PASSAVANT HOSPITAL, PITTSBURGH, PA, p. A366
PATHWAYS OF TENNESSEE, JACKSON, TN, p. A390
PATTIE A. CLAY HOSPITAL, RICHMOND, KY, p. A180
PATTON STATE HOSPITAL, PATTON, CA, p. A57
PAUL B. HALL REGIONAL MEDICAL CENTER, PAINTSVILLE, KY, p. A179
PAUL OLIVER MEMORIAL HOSPITAL, FRANKFORT, MI, p. A216
PAULDING COUNTY HOSPITAL, PAULDING, OH, p. A334
PAULINE WARFIELD LEWIS CENTER, CINCINNATI, OH, p. A326
PAULS VALLEY GENERAL HOSPITAL, PAULS VALLEY, OK, p. A344
PAWHUSKA HOSPITAL, PAWHUSKA, OK, p. A344
PAWNEE COUNTY MEMORIAL HOSPITAL, PAWNEE CITY, NE, p. A267
PAWNEE MUNICIPAL HOSPITAL, PAWNEE, OK, p. A344
PAYNESVILLE AREA HEALTH CARE SYSTEM, PAYNESVILLE, MN, p. A233
PAYSON REGIONAL MEDICAL CENTER, PAYSON, AZ, p. A24
PEACE HARBOR HOSPITAL, FLORENCE, OR, p. A349
PEACH REGIONAL MEDICAL CENTER, FORT VALLEY, GA, p. A109
PEARL RIVER COUNTY HOSPITAL, POPLARVILLE, MS, p. A243
PECOS COUNTY GENERAL HOSPITAL, IRAAN, TX, p. A416

PECOS COUNTY MEMORIAL HOSPITAL, FORT STOCKTON, TX, p. A409
PEDIATRIC CENTER FOR RESTORATIVE CARE, DALLAS, TX, p. A407
PEKIN HOSPITAL, PEKIN, IL, p. A136
PELLA REGIONAL HEALTH CENTER, PELLA, IA, p. A158
PEMBINA COUNTY MEMORIAL HOSPITAL AND WEDGEWOOD MANOR, CAVALIER, ND, p. A319
PEMBROKE HOSPITAL, PEMBROKE, MA, p. A209
PEMISCOT MEMORIAL HEALTH SYSTEM, HAYTI, MO, p. A248
PENDER COMMUNITY HOSPITAL, PENDER, NE, p. A267
PENDER MEMORIAL HOSPITAL, BURGAW, NC, p. A309
PENDLETON MEMORIAL METHODIST HOSPITAL, NEW ORLEANS, LA, p. A189
PENINSULA HOSPITAL, LOUISVILLE, TN, p. A392
PENINSULA HOSPITAL CENTER, NEW YORK, NY, p. A299
PENINSULA REGIONAL MEDICAL CENTER, SALISBURY, MD, p. A201
PENN STATE UNIVERSITY HOSPITAL–MILTON S. HERSHEY MEDICAL CENTER, HERSHEY, PA, p. A359
PENNOCK HOSPITAL, HASTINGS, MI, p. A217
PENNSYLVANIA HOSPITAL, PHILADELPHIA, PA, p. A365
PENOBSCOT BAY MEDICAL CENTER, ROCKPORT, ME, p. A195
PENOBSCOT VALLEY HOSPITAL, LINCOLN, ME, p. A194
PENROSE–ST. FRANCIS HEALTH SERVICES, COLORADO SPRINGS, CO, p. A70
PEOPLE'S MEMORIAL HOSPITAL OF BUCHANAN COUNTY, INDEPENDENCE, IA, p. A155
PEOPLES HOSPITAL, MANSFIELD, OH, p. A332
PERHAM MEMORIAL HOSPITAL AND HOME, PERHAM, MN, p. A233
PERKINS COUNTY HEALTH SERVICES, GRANT, NE, p. A264
PERMIAN GENERAL HOSPITAL, ANDREWS, TX, p. A399
PERRY COUNTY GENERAL HOSPITAL, RICHTON, MS, p. A243
PERRY COUNTY MEMORIAL HOSPITAL, TELL CITY, IN, p. A149
PERRY COUNTY MEMORIAL HOSPITAL, PERRYVILLE, MO, p. A252
PERRY HOSPITAL, PERRY, GA, p. A112
PERRY MEMORIAL HOSPITAL, PRINCETON, IL, p. A136
PERRY MEMORIAL HOSPITAL, PERRY, OK, p. A344
PERSHING GENERAL HOSPITAL, LOVELOCK, NV, p. A271
PERSON COUNTY MEMORIAL HOSPITAL, ROXBORO, NC, p. A316
PETALUMA VALLEY HOSPITAL, PETALUMA, CA, p. A57
PETERSBURG MEDICAL CENTER, PETERSBURG. AK, p. A21
PHELPS COUNTY REGIONAL MEDICAL CENTER, ROLLA, MO, p. A252
PHELPS MEMORIAL HEALTH CENTER, HOLDREGE, NE, p. A264
PHELPS MEMORIAL HOSPITAL CENTER, SLEEPY HOLLOW, NY, p. A304
PHENIX REGIONAL HOSPITAL, PHENIX CITY, AL, p. A17
PHILHAVEN, MOUNT GRETNA, PA, p. A362
PHILLIPS COUNTY HOSPITAL, PHILLIPSBURG, KS, p. A168
PHILLIPS COUNTY HOSPITAL, MALTA, MT, p. A259
PHILLIPS EYE INSTITUTE, MINNEAPOLIS, MN, p. A232
PHOEBE PUTNEY MEMORIAL HOSPITAL, ALBANY, GA, p. A103
PHOENIX BAPTIST HOSPITAL AND MEDICAL CENTER, PHOENIX, AZ, p. A25
PHOENIX CHILDREN'S HOSPITAL, PHOENIX, AZ, p. A25
PHOENIX GENERAL HOSPITAL AND MEDICAL CENTER, PHOENIX, AZ, p. A25
PHOENIXVILLE HOSPITAL, PHOENIXVILLE, PA, p. A365
PHS SANTA FE INDIAN HOSPITAL, SANTA FE, NM, p. A287
PHYSICIANS MEMORIAL HOSPITAL, LA PLATA, MD, p. A201
PICKENS COUNTY MEDICAL CENTER, CARROLLTON, AL, p. A12
PIEDMONT GERIATRIC HOSPITAL, BURKEVILLE, VA, p. A439
PIEDMONT HEALTHCARE SYSTEM, ROCK HILL, SC, p. A380
PIEDMONT HOSPITAL, ATLANTA, GA, p. A104
PIGGOTT COMMUNITY HOSPITAL, PIGGOTT, AR, p. A34
PIKE COMMUNITY HOSPITAL, WAVERLY, OH, p. A337
PIKE COUNTY MEMORIAL HOSPITAL, MURFREESBORO, AR, p. A33
PIKE COUNTY MEMORIAL HOSPITAL, LOUISIANA, MO, p. A250
PIKEVILLE UNITED METHODIST HOSPITAL OF KENTUCKY, PIKEVILLE, KY, p. A179
PILGRIM PSYCHIATRIC CENTER, BRENTWOOD, NY, p. A289
PINCKNEYVILLE COMMUNITY HOSPITAL, PINCKNEYVILLE, IL, p. A136
PINE MEDICAL CENTER, SANDSTONE, MN, p. A234
PINE REST CHRISTIAN MENTAL HEALTH SERVICES, GRAND RAPIDS, MI, p. A217
PINECREST REHABILITATION HOSPITAL, DELRAY, FL, p. A86
PINELANDS HOSPITAL, NACOGDOCHES, TX, p. A422
PINEVILLE COMMUNITY HOSPITAL ASSOCIATION, PINEVILLE, KY, p. A179
PINEYWOODS HOSPITAL, BAIRD, TX, p. A401
PINNACLEHEALTH SYSTEM, HARRISBURG, PA, p. A358
PIONEER HOSPITAL, ARTESIA, CA, p. A37
PIONEER MEDICAL CENTER, BIG TIMBER, MT, p. A257
PIONEER MEMORIAL HOSPITAL, HEPPNER, OR, p. A349

PIONEER MEMORIAL HOSPITAL, PRINEVILLE, OR, p. A351
PIONEER MEMORIAL HOSPITAL, VIBORG, SD, p. A385
PIONEER VALLEY HOSPITAL, WEST VALLEY CITY, UT, p. A436
PIONEERS HOSPITAL OF RIO BLANCO COUNTY, MEEKER, CO, p. A74
PIONEERS MEMORIAL HEALTHCARE DISTRICT, BRAWLEY, CA, p. A38
PIPESTONE COUNTY MEDICAL CENTER, PIPESTONE, MN, p. A233
PIQUA MEMORIAL MEDICAL CENTER, PIQUA, OH, p. A334
PITT COUNTY MEMORIAL HOSPITAL–UNIVERSITY MEDICAL CENTER OF EASTERN CAROLINA–PITT COUNTY, GREENVILLE, NC, p. A312
PLACENTIA–LINDA HOSPITAL, PLACENTIA, CA, p. A57
PLAINS MEMORIAL HOSPITAL, DIMMITT, TX, p. A408
PLAINS REGIONAL MEDICAL CENTER, CLOVIS, NM, p. A285
PLAINVIEW PUBLIC HOSPITAL, PLAINVIEW, NE, p. A267
PLAINVILLE RURAL HOSPITAL DISTRICT NUMBER ONE, PLAINVILLE, KS, p. A168
PLANO REHABILITATION HOSPITAL, PLANO, TX, p. A423
PLATEAU MEDICAL CENTER, OAK HILL, WV, p. A457
PLATTE COMMUNITY MEMORIAL HOSPITAL, PLATTE, SD, p. A384
PLATTE COUNTY MEMORIAL HOSPITAL, WHEATLAND, WY, p. A472
PLATTE VALLEY MEDICAL CENTER, BRIGHTON, CO, p. A70
PLEASANT VALLEY HOSPITAL, POINT PLEASANT, WV, p. A458
PLUMAS DISTRICT HOSPITAL, QUINCY, CA, p. A58
PMH HEALTH SERVICES NETWORK, PHOENIX, AZ, p. A25
POCAHONTAS COMMUNITY HOSPITAL, POCAHONTAS, IA, p. A158
POCAHONTAS MEMORIAL HOSPITAL, BUCKEYE, WV, p. A455
POCATELLO REGIONAL MEDICAL CENTER, POCATELLO, ID, p. A121
POCONO MEDICAL CENTER, EAST STROUDSBURG, PA, p. A357
PODIATRY HOSPITAL OF PITTSBURGH, PITTSBURGH, PA, p. A366
POINTE COUPEE GENERAL HOSPITAL, NEW ROADS, LA, p. A189
POLLY RYON MEMORIAL HOSPITAL, RICHMOND, TX, p. A424
POMERADO HOSPITAL, POWAY, CA, p. A58
POMONA VALLEY HOSPITAL MEDICAL CENTER, POMONA, CA, p. A57
PONCE REGIONAL HOSPITAL, PONCE, PR, p. A476
PONDERA MEDICAL CENTER, CONRAD, MT, p. A257
PONTIAC OSTEOPATHIC HOSPITAL, PONTIAC, MI, p. A222
PONTOTOC HOSPITAL AND EXTENDED CARE FACILITY, PONTOTOC, MS, p. A243
POPLAR SPRINGS HOSPITAL, PETERSBURG, VA, p. A444
PORT HURON HOSPITAL, PORT HURON, MI, p. A222
PORTAGE HEALTH SYSTEM, HANCOCK, MI, p. A217
PORTER CARE HOSPITAL, DENVER, CO, p. A71
PORTER CARE HOSPITAL–LITTLETON, LITTLETON, CO, p. A73
PORTER HOSPITAL, MIDDLEBURY, VT, p. A437
PORTER MEMORIAL HOSPITAL, VALPARAISO, IN, p. A149
PORTERCARE HOSPITAL–AVISTA, LOUISVILLE, CO, p. A74
PORTERVILLE DEVELOPMENTAL CENTER, PORTERVILLE, CA, p. A57
PORTSMOUTH GENERAL HOSPITAL, PORTSMOUTH, VA, p. A444
PORTSMOUTH REGIONAL HOSPITAL AND PAVILION, PORTSMOUTH, NH, p. A274
POTOMAC HOSPITAL, WOODBRIDGE, VA, p. A447
POTOMAC VALLEY HOSPITAL, KEYSER, WV, p. A457
POTTSTOWN MEMORIAL MEDICAL CENTER, POTTSTOWN, PA, p. A367
POTTSVILLE HOSPITAL AND WARNE CLINIC, POTTSVILLE, PA, p. A367
POUDRE VALLEY HOSPITAL, FORT COLLINS, CO, p. A72
POWELL COUNTY MEMORIAL HOSPITAL, DEER LODGE, MT, p. A258
POWELL HOSPITAL, POWELL, WY, p. A472
PRAIRIE COMMUNITY MEDICAL ASSISTANCE FACILITY, TERRY, MT, p. A260
PRAIRIE DU CHIEN MEMORIAL HOSPITAL, PRAIRIE DU CHIEN, WI, p. A467
PRAIRIE LAKES HOSPITAL AND CARE CENTER, WATERTOWN, SD, p. A385
PRAIRIE VIEW, NEWTON, KS, p. A167
PRATT REGIONAL MEDICAL CENTER, PRATT, KS, p. A168
PRESBYTERIAN HOSPITAL, ALBUQUERQUE, NM, p. A284
PRESBYTERIAN HOSPITAL, CHARLOTTE, NC, p. A310
PRESBYTERIAN HOSPITAL IN THE CITY OF NEW YORK, NEW YORK, NY, p. A299
PRESBYTERIAN HOSPITAL OF DALLAS, DALLAS, TX, p. A407
PRESBYTERIAN HOSPITAL OF KAUFMAN, KAUFMAN, TX, p. A417
PRESBYTERIAN HOSPITAL OF PLANO, PLANO, TX, p. A423
PRESBYTERIAN HOSPITAL OF WINNSBORO, WINNSBORO, TX, p. A431

Q

R

RIVERSIDE GENERAL HOSPITAL, HOUSTON, TX, p. A415
RIVERSIDE GENERAL HOSPITAL–UNIVERSITY MEDICAL CENTER, RIVERSIDE, CA, p. A59
RIVERSIDE HEALTH SYSTEM, WICHITA, KS, p. A171
RIVERSIDE HEALTHCARE, KANKAKEE, IL, p. A132
RIVERSIDE HOSPITAL, TOLEDO, OH, p. A336
RIVERSIDE MEDICAL CENTER, FRANKLINTON, LA, p. A184
RIVERSIDE MEDICAL CENTER, WAUPACA, WI, p. A470
RIVERSIDE OSTEOPATHIC HOSPITAL, TRENTON, MI, p. A224
RIVERSIDE REGIONAL MEDICAL CENTER, NEWPORT NEWS, VA, p. A443
RIVERSIDE TAPPAHANNOCK HOSPITAL, TAPPAHANNOCK, VA, p. A447
RIVERSIDE WALTER REED HOSPITAL, GLOUCESTER, VA, p. A441
RIVERVALLEY BEHAVIORAL HEALTH HOSPITAL, OWENSBORO, KY, p. A179
RIVERVIEW HEALTHCARE ASSOCIATION, CROOKSTON, MN, p. A228
RIVERVIEW HOSPITAL, NOBLESVILLE, IN, p. A147
RIVERVIEW HOSPITAL ASSOCIATION, WISCONSIN RAPIDS, WI, p. A470
RIVERVIEW HOSPITAL FOR CHILDREN, MIDDLETOWN, CT, p. A77
RIVERVIEW REGIONAL MEDICAL CENTER, GADSDEN, AL, p. A14
RIVERWOOD HEALTH CARE CENTER, AITKIN, MN, p. A226
ROANE GENERAL HOSPITAL, SPENCER, WV, p. A459
ROANE MEDICAL CENTER, HARRIMAN, TN, p. A390
ROANOKE–CHOWAN HOSPITAL, AHOSKIE, NC, p. A308
ROBERT F. KENNEDY MEDICAL CENTER, HAWTHORNE, CA, p. A45
ROBERT PACKER HOSPITAL, SAYRE, PA, p. A368
ROBERT WOOD JOHNSON UNIVERSITY HOSPITAL, NEW BRUNSWICK, NJ, p. A279
ROBERT WOOD JOHNSON UNIVERSITY HOSPITAL AT HAMILTON, HAMILTON, NJ, p. A277
ROBINSON MEMORIAL HOSPITAL, RAVENNA, OH, p. A334
ROCHELLE COMMUNITY HOSPITAL, ROCHELLE, IL, p. A137
ROCHESTER GENERAL HOSPITAL, ROCHESTER, NY, p. A303
ROCHESTER METHODIST HOSPITAL, ROCHESTER, MN, p. A233
ROCHESTER PSYCHIATRIC CENTER, ROCHESTER, NY, p. A303
ROCK COUNTY HOSPITAL, BASSETT, NE, p. A262
ROCKCASTLE HOSPITAL, MOUNT VERNON, KY, p. A179
ROCKDALE HOSPITAL, CONYERS, GA, p. A107
ROCKEFELLER UNIVERSITY HOSPITAL, NEW YORK, NY, p. A299
ROCKFORD CENTER, NEWARK, DE, p. A80
ROCKFORD MEMORIAL HOSPITAL, ROCKFORD, IL, p. A137
ROCKINGHAM MEMORIAL HOSPITAL, HARRISONBURG, VA, p. A441
ROCKLAND CHILDREN'S PSYCHIATRIC CENTER, ORANGEBURG, NY, p. A301
ROCKLAND PSYCHIATRIC CENTER, ORANGEBURG, NY, p. A302
ROCKVILLE GENERAL HOSPITAL, VERNON ROCKVILLE, CT, p. A79
ROGER C. PEACE REHABILITATION HOSPITAL, GREENVILLE, SC, p. A378
ROGER MILLS MEMORIAL HOSPITAL, CHEYENNE, OK, p. A340
ROGER WILLIAMS MEDICAL CENTER, PROVIDENCE, RI, p. A373
ROGERS CITY REHABILITATION HOSPITAL, ROGERS CITY, MI, p. A222
ROGERS MEMORIAL HOSPITAL, OCONOMOWOC, WI, p. A466
ROGUE VALLEY MEDICAL CENTER, MEDFORD, OR, p. A350
ROLLING HILLS HOSPITAL, ADA, OK, p. A339
ROLLING PLAINS MEMORIAL HOSPITAL, SWEETWATER, TX, p. A428
ROME MEMORIAL HOSPITAL, ROME, NY, p. A303
ROOSEVELT HOSPITAL, EDISON, NJ, p. A276
ROOSEVELT MEMORIAL MEDICAL CENTER, CULBERTSON, MT, p. A258
ROOSEVELT WARM SPRINGS INSTITUTE FOR REHABILITATION, WARM SPRINGS, GA, p. A115
ROPER HOSPITAL, CHARLESTON, SC, p. A376
ROPER HOSPITAL NORTH, CHARLESTON, SC, p. A376
ROSEAU AREA HOSPITAL AND HOMES, ROSEAU, MN, p. A233
ROSEBUD HEALTH CARE CENTER, FORSYTH, MT, p. A258
ROSELAND COMMUNITY HOSPITAL, CHICAGO, IL, p. A127
ROSWELL PARK CANCER INSTITUTE, BUFFALO, NY, p. A290
ROUND ROCK HOSPITAL, ROUND ROCK, TX, p. A424
ROUNDUP MEMORIAL HOSPITAL, ROUNDUP, MT, p. A260
ROUTT MEMORIAL HOSPITAL, STEAMBOAT SPRINGS, CO, p. A74
ROWAN REGIONAL MEDICAL CENTER, SALISBURY, NC, p. A316
ROXBOROUGH MEMORIAL HOSPITAL, PHILADELPHIA, PA, p. A365
ROY H. LAIRD MEMORIAL HOSPITAL, KILGORE, TX, p. A417
ROY LESTER SCHNEIDER HOSPITAL, SAINT THOMAS, VI, p. A477
ROYAL C. JOHNSON VETERANS MEMORIAL HOSPITAL, SIOUX FALLS, SD, p. A385
RUBY VALLEY HOSPITAL, SHERIDAN, MT, p. A260

RUMFORD COMMUNITY HOSPITAL, RUMFORD, ME, p. A195
RUNNELLS SPECIALIZED HOSPITAL, BERKELEY HEIGHTS, NJ, p. A275
RUSH CITY HOSPITAL, RUSH CITY, MN, p. A234
RUSH COUNTY MEMORIAL HOSPITAL, LA CROSSE, KS, p. A165
RUSH FOUNDATION HOSPITAL, MERIDIAN, MS, p. A242
RUSH MEMORIAL HOSPITAL, RUSHVILLE, IN, p. A148
RUSH NORTH SHORE MEDICAL CENTER, SKOKIE, IL, p. A138
RUSH–PRESBYTERIAN–ST. LUKE'S MEDICAL CENTER, CHICAGO, IL, p. A127
RUSK COUNTY MEMORIAL HOSPITAL AND NURSING HOME, LADYSMITH, WI, p. A463
RUSK STATE HOSPITAL, RUSK, TX, p. A425
RUSSELL COUNTY HOSPITAL, RUSSELL SPRINGS, KY, p. A180
RUSSELL COUNTY MEDICAL CENTER, LEBANON, VA, p. A442
RUSSELL HOSPITAL, ALEXANDER CITY, AL, p. A11
RUSSELL REGIONAL HOSPITAL, RUSSELL, KS, p. A169
RUTHERFORD HOSPITAL, RUTHERFORDTON, NC, p. A316
RUTLAND REGIONAL MEDICAL CENTER, RUTLAND, VT, p. A437
RYDER MEMORIAL HOSPITAL, HUMACAO, PR, p. A475
RYE HOSPITAL CENTER, RYE, NY, p. A304

S

SABETHA COMMUNITY HOSPITAL, SABETHA, KS, p. A169
SABINE COUNTY HOSPITAL, HEMPHILL, TX, p. A412
SABINE MEDICAL CENTER, MANY, LA, p. A187
SAC–OSAGE HOSPITAL, OSCEOLA, MO, p. A252
SACRED HEART HEALTH SERVICES, YANKTON, SD, p. A386
SACRED HEART HOSPITAL, CHICAGO, IL, p. A127
SACRED HEART HOSPITAL, CUMBERLAND, MD, p. A199
SACRED HEART HOSPITAL, ALLENTOWN, PA, p. A353
SACRED HEART HOSPITAL, EAU CLAIRE, WI, p. A462
SACRED HEART HOSPITAL OF PENSACOLA, PENSACOLA, FL, p. A97
SACRED HEART MEDICAL CENTER, EUGENE, OR, p. A349
SACRED HEART MEDICAL CENTER, SPOKANE, WA, p. A453
SACRED HEART REHABILITATION INSTITUTE, MILWAUKEE, WI, p. A465
SACRED HEART–ST. MARY'S HOSPITALS, RHINELANDER, WI, p. A468
SADDLEBACK MEMORIAL MEDICAL CENTER, LAGUNA HILLS, CA, p. A47
SAGAMORE CHILDREN'S PSYCHIATRIC CENTER, DIX HILLS, NY, p. A291
SAGE MEMORIAL HOSPITAL, GANADO, AZ, p. A23
SAGINAW GENERAL HOSPITAL, SAGINAW, MI, p. A222
SAINT AGNES MEDICAL CENTER, FRESNO, CA, p. A44
SAINT ALPHONSUS REGIONAL MEDICAL CENTER, BOISE, ID, p. A119
SAINT ANNE'S HOSPITAL, FALL RIVER, MA, p. A206
SAINT ANTHONY HOSPITAL, CHICAGO, IL, p. A127
SAINT ANTHONY HOSPITAL AND HEALTH CENTERS, MICHIGAN CITY, IN, p. A146
SAINT ANTHONY MEDICAL CENTER, ROCKFORD, IL, p. A137
SAINT ANTHONY'S HEALTH CENTER, ALTON, IL, p. A123
SAINT BARNABAS MEDICAL CENTER, LIVINGSTON, NJ, p. A278
SAINT EUGENE COMMUNITY HOSPITAL, DILLON, SC, p. A377
SAINT FRANCIS HOSPITAL, POUGHKEEPSIE, NY, p. A303
SAINT FRANCIS HOSPITAL, TULSA, OK, p. A346
SAINT FRANCIS HOSPITAL, MEMPHIS, TN, p. A393
SAINT FRANCIS HOSPITAL, CHARLESTON, WV, p. A455
SAINT FRANCIS HOSPITAL AND MEDICAL CENTER, HARTFORD, CT, p. A77
SAINT FRANCIS MEDICAL CENTER, PEORIA, IL, p. A136
SAINT FRANCIS MEDICAL CENTER, CAPE GIRARDEAU, MO, p. A246
SAINT FRANCIS MEDICAL CENTER, GRAND ISLAND, NE, p. A264
SAINT FRANCIS MEMORIAL HOSPITAL, SAN FRANCISCO, CA, p. A61
SAINT JAMES HOSPITAL, PONTIAC, IL, p. A136
SAINT JAMES HOSPITAL OF NEWARK, NEWARK, NJ, p. A280
SAINT JOHN HOSPITAL, LEAVENWORTH, KS, p. A166
SAINT JOHN'S HEALTH SYSTEM, ANDERSON, IN, p. A140
SAINT JOHN'S HOSPITAL AND HEALTH CENTER, SANTA MONICA, CA, p. A64
SAINT JOSEPH COMMUNITY HOSPITAL, NEW HAMPTON, IA, p. A157
SAINT JOSEPH HEALTH CENTER, KANSAS CITY, MO, p. A249
SAINT JOSEPH HOSPITAL, EUREKA, CA, p. A42
SAINT JOSEPH HOSPITAL, DENVER, CO, p. A71
SAINT JOSEPH HOSPITAL, BELVIDERE, IL, p. A124
SAINT JOSEPH HOSPITAL, ELGIN, IL, p. A129
SAINT JOSEPH HOSPITAL & HEALTH CENTER, KOKOMO, IN, p. A145
SAINT JOSEPH MEDICAL CENTER, JOLIET, IL, p. A132

SAINT JOSEPH'S HOSPITAL, MARSHFIELD, WI, p. A464
SAINT JOSEPH'S HOSPITAL OF ATLANTA, ATLANTA, GA, p. A104
SAINT LOUIS UNIVERSITY HOSPITAL, SAINT LOUIS, MO, p. A254
SAINT LOUISE HOSPITAL, MORGAN HILL, CA, p. A54
SAINT LUKE INSTITUTE, SILVER SPRING, MD, p. A202
SAINT LUKE'S HOSPITAL, KANSAS CITY, MO, p. A249
SAINT LUKE'S MEDICAL CENTER, CLEVELAND, OH, p. A327
SAINT LUKE'S NORTHLAND HOSPITAL, KANSAS CITY, MO, p. A249
SAINT LUKE'S NORTHLAND HOSPITAL–SMITHVILLE CAMPUS, SMITHVILLE, MO, p. A255
SAINT MARGARET MERCY HEALTHCARE CENTERS, HAMMOND, IN, p. A143
SAINT MARY MEDICAL CENTER, LONG BEACH, CA, p. A49
SAINT MARY OF NAZARETH HOSPITAL CENTER, CHICAGO, IL, p. A127
SAINT MARY'S HEALTH SERVICES, GRAND RAPIDS, MI, p. A217
SAINT MARY'S MEDICAL CENTER, RACINE, WI, p. A468
SAINT MARY'S REGIONAL MEDICAL CENTER, RUSSELLVILLE, AR, p. A34
SAINT MARYS HOSPITAL, ROCHESTER, MN, p. A233
SAINT MICHAEL HOSPITAL, CLEVELAND, OH, p. A327
SAINT MICHAEL'S HOSPITAL, STEVENS POINT, WI, p. A469
SAINT MICHAEL'S MEDICAL CENTER, NEWARK, NJ, p. A280
SAINT THERESE MEDICAL CENTER, WAUKEGAN, IL, p. A139
SAINT VINCENT HEALTH CENTER, ERIE, PA, p. A357
SAINT VINCENT HOSPITAL, WORCESTER, MA, p. A211
SAINT VINCENT HOSPITAL AND HEALTH CENTER, BILLINGS, MT, p. A257
SAINT VINCENT'S HOSPITAL AND MEDICAL CENTER OF NEW YORK, NEW YORK, NY, p. A299
SAINTS MEMORIAL MEDICAL CENTER, LOWELL, MA, p. A207
SAKAKAWEA MEDICAL CENTER, HAZEN, ND, p. A320
SALEM COMMUNITY HOSPITAL, SALEM, OH, p. A335
SALEM HOSPITAL, HILLSBORO, KS, p. A164
SALEM HOSPITAL, SALEM, MA, p. A209
SALEM HOSPITAL, SALEM, OR, p. A352
SALEM MEMORIAL DISTRICT HOSPITAL, SALEM, MO, p. A255
SALINA REGIONAL HEALTH CENTER, SALINA, KS, p. A169
SALINAS VALLEY MEMORIAL HOSPITAL, SALINAS, CA, p. A60
SALINE COMMUNITY HOSPITAL, SALINE, MI, p. A223
SALINE MEMORIAL HOSPITAL, BENTON, AR, p. A29
SALT LAKE REGIONAL MEDICAL CENTER, SALT LAKE CITY, UT, p. A435
SAM RAYBURN MEMORIAL VETERANS CENTER, BONHAM, TX, p. A402
SAMARITAN BEHAVIORAL HEALTH CENTER–SCOTTSDALE, SCOTTSDALE, AZ, p. A26
SAMARITAN HEALTH SYSTEM, CLINTON, IA, p. A152
SAMARITAN HEALTHCARE, MOSES LAKE, WA, p. A450
SAMARITAN HOSPITAL, TROY, NY, p. A305
SAMARITAN HOSPITAL, ASHLAND, OH, p. A323
SAMARITAN MEDICAL CENTER, WATERTOWN, NY, p. A306
SAMARITAN MEMORIAL HOSPITAL, MACON, MO, p. A250
SAMARITAN–WENDY PAINE O'BRIEN TREATMENT CENTER, PHOENIX, AZ, p. A25
SAMPSON REGIONAL MEDICAL CENTER, CLINTON, NC, p. A310
SAMUEL MAHELONA MEMORIAL HOSPITAL, KAPAA, HI, p. A118
SAMUEL SIMMONDS MEMORIAL HOSPITAL, BARROW, AK, p. A20
SAN ANTONIO COMMUNITY HOSPITAL, UPLAND, CA, p. A67
SAN ANTONIO COMMUNITY HOSPITAL, SAN ANTONIO, TX, p. A426
SAN ANTONIO STATE HOSPITAL, SAN ANTONIO, TX, p. A426
SAN BERNARDINO COUNTY MEDICAL CENTER, SAN BERNARDINO, CA, p. A60
SAN BERNARDINO MOUNTAINS COMMUNITY HOSPITAL DISTRICT, LAKE ARROWHEAD, CA, p. A47
SAN CARLOS GENERAL HOSPITAL, SAN JUAN, PR, p. A477
SAN DIEGO COUNTY PSYCHIATRIC HOSPITAL, SAN DIEGO, CA, p. A61
SAN DIEGO HOSPICE, SAN DIEGO, CA, p. A61
SAN DIMAS COMMUNITY HOSPITAL, SAN DIMAS, CA, p. A61
SAN FRANCISCO GENERAL HOSPITAL MEDICAL CENTER, SAN FRANCISCO, CA, p. A62
SAN GABRIEL VALLEY MEDICAL CENTER, SAN GABRIEL, CA, p. A62
SAN GORGONIO MEMORIAL HOSPITAL, BANNING, CA, p. A37
SAN JACINTO METHODIST HOSPITAL, BAYTOWN, TX, p. A401
SAN JOAQUIN COMMUNITY HOSPITAL, BAKERSFIELD, CA, p. A37
SAN JOAQUIN GENERAL HOSPITAL, FRENCH CAMP, CA, p. A43
SAN JOAQUIN VALLEY REHABILITATION HOSPITAL, FRESNO, CA, p. A44
SAN JORGE CHILDREN'S HOSPITAL, SAN JUAN, PR, p. A477
SAN JUAN CITY HOSPITAL, SAN JUAN, PR, p. A477
SAN JUAN HOSPITAL, MONTICELLO, UT, p. A434

SAN JUAN REGIONAL MEDICAL CENTER, FARMINGTON, NM, p. A285
SAN LUIS OBISPO GENERAL HOSPITAL, SAN LUIS OBISPO, CA, p. A63
SAN LUIS VALLEY REGIONAL MEDICAL CENTER, ALAMOSA, CO, p. A70
SAN MARCOS TREATMENT CENTER, SAN MARCOS, TX, p. A427
SAN MATEO COUNTY GENERAL HOSPITAL, SAN MATEO, CA, p. A63
SAN PEDRO PENINSULA HOSPITAL, LOS ANGELES, CA, p. A51
SAN RAMON REGIONAL MEDICAL CENTER, SAN RAMON, CA, p. A63
SAN VICENTE HOSPITAL, LOS ANGELES, CA, p. A51
SANDWICH COMMUNITY HOSPITAL, SANDWICH, IL, p. A137
SANDYPINES, TEQUESTA, FL, p. A101
SANGER GENERAL HOSPITAL, SANGER, CA, p. A63
SANPETE VALLEY HOSPITAL, MOUNT PLEASANT, UT, p. A434
SANTA ANA HOSPITAL MEDICAL CENTER, SANTA ANA, CA, p. A63
SANTA BARBARA COTTAGE HOSPITAL, SANTA BARBARA, CA, p. A64
SANTA CLARA VALLEY MEDICAL CENTER, SAN JOSE, CA, p. A62
SANTA MARTA HOSPITAL, LOS ANGELES, CA, p. A51
SANTA MONICA–UCLA MEDICAL CENTER, SANTA MONICA, CA, p. A64
SANTA PAULA MEMORIAL HOSPITAL, SANTA PAULA, CA, p. A64
SANTA ROSA HEALTH CARE CORPORATION, SAN ANTONIO, TX, p. A426
SANTA ROSA MEDICAL CENTER, MILTON, FL, p. A94
SANTA ROSA MEMORIAL HOSPITAL, SANTA ROSA, CA, p. A64
SANTA TERESA COMMUNITY HOSPITAL, SAN JOSE, CA, p. A62
SANTA TERESITA HOSPITAL, DUARTE, CA, p. A42
SANTA YNEZ VALLEY COTTAGE HOSPITAL, SOLVANG, CA, p. A65
SANTIAM MEMORIAL HOSPITAL, STAYTON, OR, p. A352
SARAH BUSH LINCOLN HEALTH SYSTEM, MATTOON, IL, p. A133
SARAH D. CULBERTSON MEMORIAL HOSPITAL, RUSHVILLE, IL, p. A137
SARASOTA MEMORIAL HOSPITAL, SARASOTA, FL, p. A99
SARATOGA HOSPITAL, SARATOGA SPRINGS, NY, p. A304
SARGENT DISTRICT HOSPITAL, SARGENT, NE, p. A268
SARTORI MEMORIAL HOSPITAL, CEDAR FALLS, IA, p. A152
SATANTA DISTRICT HOSPITAL, SATANTA, KS, p. A169
SATILLA REGIONAL MEDICAL CENTER, WAYCROSS, GA, p. A116
SAUK PRAIRIE MEMORIAL HOSPITAL, PRAIRIE DU SAC, WI, p. A468
SAUNDERS COUNTY HEALTH SERVICE, WAHOO, NE, p. A268
SAVANNAS HOSPITAL, PORT ST. LUCIE, FL, p. A98
SAVOY MEDICAL CENTER, MAMOU, LA, p. A187
SAYRE MEMORIAL HOSPITAL, SAYRE, OK, p. A345
SCENIC MOUNTAIN MEDICAL CENTER, BIG SPRING, TX, p. A402
SCHEURER HOSPITAL, PIGEON, MI, p. A221
SCHICK SHADEL HOSPITAL, SEATTLE, WA, p. A452
SCHLEICHER COUNTY MEDICAL CENTER, ELDORADO, TX, p. A409
SCHOOLCRAFT MEMORIAL HOSPITAL, MANISTIQUE, MI, p. A220
SCHUMPERT MEDICAL CENTER, SHREVEPORT, LA, p. A190
SCHUYLER HOSPITAL, MONTOUR FALLS, NY, p. A294
SCHWAB REHABILITATION HOSPITAL AND CARE NETWORK, CHICAGO, IL, p. A127
SCOTLAND COUNTY MEMORIAL HOSPITAL, MEMPHIS, MO, p. A251
SCOTLAND MEMORIAL HOSPITAL, LAURINBURG, NC, p. A313
SCOTT AND WHITE MEMORIAL HOSPITAL, TEMPLE, TX, p. A428
SCOTT COUNTY HOSPITAL, SCOTT CITY, KS, p. A169
SCOTT COUNTY HOSPITAL, ONEIDA, TN, p. A395
SCOTT MEDICAL CENTER, SCOTT AFB, IL, p. A137
SCOTT MEMORIAL HOSPITAL, SCOTTSBURG, IN, p. A148
SCOTTISH RITE CHILDREN'S MEDICAL CENTER, ATLANTA, GA, p. A104
SCOTTSDALE MEMORIAL HOSPITAL–NORTH, SCOTTSDALE, AZ, p. A26
SCOTTSDALE MEMORIAL HOSPITAL–OSBORN, SCOTTSDALE, AZ, p. A26
SCREVEN COUNTY HOSPITAL, SYLVANIA, GA, p. A114
SCRIPPS HOSPITAL–EAST COUNTY, EL CAJON, CA, p. A42
SCRIPPS MEMORIAL HOSPITAL–CHULA VISTA, CHULA VISTA, CA, p. A40
SCRIPPS MEMORIAL HOSPITAL–ENCINITAS, ENCINITAS, CA, p. A42
SCRIPPS MEMORIAL HOSPITAL–LA JOLLA, LA JOLLA, CA, p. A47
SCRIPPS MERCY MEDICAL CENTER, SAN DIEGO, CA, p. A61
SEABORNE HOSPITAL, DOVER, NH, p. A272
SEARCY HOSPITAL, MOUNT VERNON, AL, p. A17

SEARHC MT. EDGECUMBE HOSPITAL, SITKA, AK, p. A21
SEBASTIAN RIVER MEDICAL CENTER, SEBASTIAN, FL, p. A99
SEBASTICOOK VALLEY HOSPITAL, PITTSFIELD, ME, p. A195
SEDAN CITY HOSPITAL, SEDAN, KS, p. A169
SEDGWICK COUNTY MEMORIAL HOSPITAL, JULESBURG, CO, p. A73
SEILING HOSPITAL, SEILING, OK, p. A345
SELBY GENERAL HOSPITAL, MARIETTA, OH, p. A332
SELF MEMORIAL HOSPITAL, GREENWOOD, SC, p. A378
SELMA DISTRICT HOSPITAL, SELMA, CA, p. A65
SEMINOLE MUNICIPAL HOSPITAL, SEMINOLE, OK, p. A345
SENATOBIA COMMUNITY HOSPITAL, SENATOBIA, MS, p. A243
SENATOR GARRET T. W. HAGEDORN GERO PSYCHIATRIC HOSPITAL, GLEN GARDNER, NJ, p. A277
SENECA DISTRICT HOSPITAL, CHESTER, CA, p. A39
SENTARA BAYSIDE HOSPITAL, VIRGINIA BEACH, VA, p. A447
SENTARA HAMPTON GENERAL HOSPITAL, HAMPTON, VA, p. A441
SENTARA LEIGH HOSPITAL, NORFOLK, VA, p. A443
SENTARA NORFOLK GENERAL HOSPITAL, NORFOLK, VA, p. A443
SEQUOIA HOSPITAL, REDWOOD CITY, CA, p. A58
SEQUOYAH MEMORIAL HOSPITAL, SALLISAW, OK, p. A345
SERENITY LANE, EUGENE, OR, p. A349
SETON HEALTH SYSTEM, TROY, NY, p. A305
SETON MEDICAL CENTER, DALY CITY, CA, p. A41
SETON MEDICAL CENTER, AUSTIN, TX, p. A400
SETON MEDICAL CENTER COASTSIDE, MOSS BEACH, CA, p. A54
SEVEN RIVERS COMMUNITY HOSPITAL, CRYSTAL RIVER, FL, p. A85
SEVIER VALLEY HOSPITAL, RICHFIELD, UT, p. A435
SEWICKLEY VALLEY HOSPITAL, (A DIVISION OF VALLEY MEDICAL FACILITIES), SEWICKLEY, PA, p. A369
SEYMOUR HOSPITAL, SEYMOUR, TX, p. A427
SHACKELFORD COUNTY HOSPITAL DISTRICT, ALBANY, TX, p. A398
SHADOW MOUNTAIN HOSPITAL, TULSA, OK, p. A346
SHADY GROVE ADVENTIST HOSPITAL, ROCKVILLE, MD, p. A201
SHADYSIDE HOSPITAL, PITTSBURGH, PA, p. A366
SHAMOKIN AREA COMMUNITY HOSPITAL, COAL TOWNSHIP, PA, p. A355
SHAMROCK GENERAL HOSPITAL, SHAMROCK, TX, p. A427
SHANDS AT AGH, GAINESVILLE, FL, p. A88
SHANDS AT LAKE SHORE, LAKE CITY, FL, p. A90
SHANDS AT LIVE OAK, LIVE OAK, FL, p. A91
SHANDS AT STARKE, STARKE, FL, p. A99
SHANDS AT THE UNIVERSITY OF FLORIDA, GAINESVILLE, FL, p. A88
SHANNON MEDICAL CENTER, SAN ANGELO, TX, p. A425
SHARE MEDICAL CENTER, ALVA, OK, p. A339
SHARON HOSPITAL, SHARON, CT, p. A78
SHARON REGIONAL HEALTH SYSTEM, SHARON, PA, p. A369
SHARP CABRILLO HOSPITAL, SAN DIEGO, CA, p. A61
SHARP CHULA VISTA MEDICAL CENTER, CHULA VISTA, CA, p. A40
SHARP CORONADO HOSPITAL, CORONADO, CA, p. A40
SHARP HEALTHCARE MURRIETA, MURRIETA, CA, p. A54
SHARP MEMORIAL HOSPITAL, SAN DIEGO, CA, p. A61
SHARPSTOWN GENERAL HOSPITAL, HOUSTON, TX, p. A415
SHAUGHNESSY–KAPLAN REHABILITATION HOSPITAL, SALEM, MA, p. A209
SHAWANO MEDICAL CENTER, SHAWANO, WI, p. A468
SHAWNEE MISSION MEDICAL CENTER, SHAWNEE MISSION, KS, p. A169
SHAWNEE REGIONAL HOSPITAL, SHAWNEE, OK, p. A345
SHEBOYGAN MEMORIAL MEDICAL CENTER, SHEBOYGAN, WI, p. A468
SHEEHAN MEMORIAL HOSPITAL, BUFFALO, NY, p. A290
SHELBY BAPTIST MEDICAL CENTER, ALABASTER, AL, p. A11
SHELBY COUNTY MYRTUE MEMORIAL HOSPITAL, HARLAN, IA, p. A155
SHELBY MEMORIAL HOSPITAL, SHELBYVILLE, IL, p. A137
SHELTERING ARMS REHABILITATION HOSPITAL, RICHMOND, VA, p. A446
SHENANDOAH MEMORIAL HOSPITAL, SHENANDOAH, IA, p. A158
SHENANDOAH MEMORIAL HOSPITAL, WOODSTOCK, VA, p. A447
SHEPHERD CENTER, ATLANTA, GA, p. A104
SHEPPARD AND ENOCH PRATT HOSPITAL, BALTIMORE, MD, p. A198
SHERIDAN COMMUNITY HOSPITAL, SHERIDAN, MI, p. A223
SHERIDAN COUNTY HOSPITAL, HOXIE, KS, p. A164
SHERIDAN MEMORIAL HOSPITAL, PLENTYWOOD, MT, p. A260
SHERMAN HOSPITAL, ELGIN, IL, p. A129
SHERMAN OAKS HOSPITAL AND HEALTH CENTER, LOS ANGELES, CA, p. A51
SHODAIR CHILDREN'S HOSPITAL, HELENA, MT, p. A259
SHORE MEMORIAL HOSPITAL, SOMERS POINT, NJ, p. A281

SHOSHONE MEDICAL CENTER, KELLOGG, ID, p. A120
SHRINERS HOSPITALS FOR CHILDREN, BURNS INSTITUTE BOSTON UNIT, BOSTON, MA, p. A204
SHRINERS HOSPITALS FOR CHILDREN, CINCINNATI BURNS INSTITUTE, CINCINNATI, OH, p. A326
SHRINERS HOSPITALS FOR CHILDREN, ERIE UNIT, ERIE, PA, p. A357
SHRINERS HOSPITALS FOR CHILDREN, GALVESTON BURNS INSTITUTE, GALVESTON, TX, p. A411
SHRINERS HOSPITALS FOR CHILDREN, GREENVILLE, GREENVILLE, SC, p. A378
SHRINERS HOSPITALS FOR CHILDREN, HONOLULU, HONOLULU, HI, p. A117
SHRINERS HOSPITALS FOR CHILDREN, HOUSTON, HOUSTON, TX, p. A415
SHRINERS HOSPITALS FOR CHILDREN, LOS ANGELES, LOS ANGELES, CA, p. A51
SHRINERS HOSPITALS FOR CHILDREN, PHILADELPHIA UNIT, PHILADELPHIA, PA, p. A365
SHRINERS HOSPITALS FOR CHILDREN, PORTLAND, PORTLAND, OR, p. A351
SHRINERS HOSPITALS FOR CHILDREN, SAN FRANCISCO, SAN FRANCISCO, CA, p. A62
SHRINERS HOSPITALS FOR CHILDREN, SHREVEPORT, SHREVEPORT, LA, p. A191
SHRINERS HOSPITALS FOR CHILDREN, SPRINGFIELD, SPRINGFIELD, MA, p. A210
SHRINERS HOSPITALS FOR CHILDREN, ST. LOUIS, SAINT LOUIS, MO, p. A254
SHRINERS HOSPITALS FOR CHILDREN, TAMPA, TAMPA, FL, p. A100
SHRINERS HOSPITALS FOR CHILDREN, TWIN CITIES UNIT, MINNEAPOLIS, MN, p. A232
SHRINERS HOSPITALS FOR CHILDREN–CHICAGO, CHICAGO, IL, p. A127
SHRINERS HOSPITALS FOR CHILDREN–INTERMOUNTAIN, SALT LAKE CITY, UT, p. A435
SHRINERS HOSPITALS FOR CHILDREN–LEXINGTON UNIT, LEXINGTON, KY, p. A176
SHRINERS HOSPITALS FOR CHILDREN–SPOKANE, SPOKANE, WA, p. A453
SIBLEY MEMORIAL HOSPITAL, WASHINGTON, DC, p. A81
SID PETERSON MEMORIAL HOSPITAL, KERRVILLE, TX, p. A417
SIDNEY HEALTH CENTER, SIDNEY, MT, p. A260
SIERRA MEDICAL CENTER, EL PASO, TX, p. A409
SIERRA NEVADA MEMORIAL HOSPITAL, GRASS VALLEY, CA, p. A45
SIERRA TUCSON, TUCSON, AZ, p. A27
SIERRA VALLEY DISTRICT HOSPITAL, LOYALTON, CA, p. A52
SIERRA VIEW DISTRICT HOSPITAL, PORTERVILLE, CA, p. A58
SIERRA VISTA COMMUNITY HOSPITAL, SIERRA VISTA, AZ, p. A26
SIERRA VISTA HOSPITAL, TRUTH OR CONSEQUENCES, NM, p. A287
SIERRA VISTA REGIONAL MEDICAL CENTER, SAN LUIS OBISPO, CA, p. A63
SIERRA–KINGS DISTRICT HOSPITAL, REEDLEY, CA, p. A58
SILOAM SPRING MEMORIAL HOSPITAL, SILOAM SPRINGS, AR, p. A35
SILVER CROSS HOSPITAL, JOLIET, IL, p. A132
SILVER HILL HOSPITAL, NEW CANAAN, CT, p. A77
SILVERTON HOSPITAL, SILVERTON, OR, p. A352
SIMI VALLEY HOSPITAL AND HEALTH CARE SERVICES, SIMI VALLEY, CA, p. A65
SIMPSON GENERAL HOSPITAL, MENDENHALL, MS, p. A241
SIMPSON INFIRMARY, WELLESLEY COLLEGE, WELLESLEY, MA, p. A211
SINAI HOSPITAL, DETROIT, MI, p. A215
SINAI HOSPITAL OF BALTIMORE, BALTIMORE, MD, p. A198
SINAI SAMARITAN MEDICAL CENTER, MILWAUKEE, WI, p. A465
SINGING RIVER HOSPITAL, PASCAGOULA, MS, p. A242
SIOUX CENTER COMMUNITY HOSPITAL AND HEALTH CENTER, SIOUX CENTER, IA, p. A158
SIOUX VALLEY HOSPITAL, SIOUX FALLS, SD, p. A385
SIOUX VALLEY MEMORIAL HOSPITAL, CHEROKEE, IA, p. A152
SISKIN HOSPITAL FOR PHYSICAL REHABILITATION, CHATTANOOGA, TN, p. A388
SISKIYOU GENERAL HOSPITAL, YREKA, CA, p. A69
SISTERS OF CHARITY HOSPITAL OF BUFFALO, BUFFALO, NY, p. A290
SISTERSVILLE GENERAL HOSPITAL, SISTERSVILLE, WV, p. A458
SITKA COMMUNITY HOSPITAL, SITKA, AK, p. A21
SKAGGS COMMUNITY HEALTH CENTER, BRANSON, MO, p. A245
SKIFF MEDICAL CENTER, NEWTON, IA, p. A157
SKYLINE HOSPITAL, WHITE SALMON, WA, p. A454
SLEEPY EYE MUNICIPAL HOSPITAL, SLEEPY EYE, MN, p. A235
SLIDELL MEMORIAL HOSPITAL AND MEDICAL CENTER, SLIDELL, LA, p. A191

T

U

UNION COUNTY METHODIST HOSPITAL, MORGANFIELD, KY, p. A178
UNION GENERAL HOSPITAL, BLAIRSVILLE, GA, p. A105
UNION GENERAL HOSPITAL, FARMERVILLE, LA, p. A184
UNION HOSPITAL, TERRE HAUTE, IN, p. A149
UNION HOSPITAL, ELKTON, MD, p. A200
UNION HOSPITAL, UNION, NJ, p. A282
UNION HOSPITAL, MAYVILLE, ND, p. A321
UNION HOSPITAL, DOVER, OH, p. A329
UNION HOSPITAL OF THE BRONX, NEW YORK, NY, p. A300
UNION MEMORIAL HOSPITAL, BALTIMORE, MD, p. A198
UNION REGIONAL MEDICAL CENTER, MONROE, NC, p. A314
UNIONTOWN HOSPITAL, UNIONTOWN, PA, p. A370
UNITED COMMUNITY HOSPITAL, GROVE CITY, PA, p. A358
UNITED HEALTH SERVICES, GRAND FORKS, ND, p. A320
UNITED HEALTH SERVICES HOSPITALS–BINGHAMTON, BINGHAMTON, NY, p. A289
UNITED HOSPITAL, SAINT PAUL, MN, p. A234
UNITED HOSPITAL CENTER, CLARKSBURG, WV, p. A456
UNITED HOSPITAL DISTRICT, BLUE EARTH, MN, p. A227
UNITED HOSPITAL MEDICAL CENTER, PORT CHESTER, NY, p. A302
UNITED MEDICAL CENTER, CHEYENNE, WY, p. A471
UNITED MEMORIAL HOSPITAL ASSOCIATION, GREENVILLE, MI, p. A217
UNITED MINE WORKERS OF AMERICA UNION HOSPITAL, WEST FRANKFORT, IL, p. A139
UNITED SAMARITANS MEDICAL CENTER, DANVILLE, IL, p. A128
UNITY HOSPITAL, FRIDLEY, MN, p. A229
UNITY MEDICAL CENTER, GRAFTON, ND, p. A320
UNIVERISITY HOSPITAL, CINCINNATI, OH, p. A326
UNIVERSITY OF COLORADO HOSPITAL, DENVER, CO, p. A72
UNIVERSITY BEHAVIORAL CENTER, ORLANDO, FL, p. A95
UNIVERSITY BEHAVIORAL HEALTH CENTER, MEMPHIS, TN, p. A393
UNIVERSITY COMMUNITY HOSPITAL, TAMPA, FL, p. A101
UNIVERSITY COMMUNITY HOSPITAL–CARROLLWOOD, TAMPA, FL, p. A101
UNIVERSITY HEALTH SERVICES, AMHERST, MA, p. A203
UNIVERSITY HEALTH SYSTEM, SAN ANTONIO, TX, p. A426
UNIVERSITY HOSPITAL, AUGUSTA, GA, p. A105
UNIVERSITY HOSPITAL, CHICAGO, IL, p. A128
UNIVERSITY HOSPITAL, ALBUQUERQUE, NM, p. A285
UNIVERSITY HOSPITAL, STONY BROOK, NY, p. A305
UNIVERSITY HOSPITAL, CHARLOTTE, NC, p. A310
UNIVERSITY HOSPITAL, PORTLAND, OR, p. A351
UNIVERSITY HOSPITAL, SAN JUAN, PR, p. A477
UNIVERSITY HOSPITAL OF ARKANSAS, LITTLE ROCK, AR, p. A33
UNIVERSITY HOSPITAL OF BROOKLYN–STATE UNIVERSITY OF NEW YORK HEALTH SCIENCE CENTER AT BROOKLYN, NEW YORK, NY, p. A300
UNIVERSITY HOSPITAL OF DURANT, DURANT, MS, p. A238
UNIVERSITY HOSPITAL–SUNY HEALTH SCIENCE CENTER AT SYRACUSE, SYRACUSE, NY, p. A305
UNIVERSITY HOSPITALS AND CLINICS, COLUMBIA, MO, p. A246
UNIVERSITY HOSPITALS AND CLINICS, UNIVERSITY OF MISSISSIPPI MEDICAL CENTER, JACKSON, MS, p. A240
UNIVERSITY HOSPITALS HEALTH SYSTEM BEDFORD MEDICAL CENTER, BEDFORD, OH, p. A324
UNIVERSITY HOSPITALS OF CLEVELAND, CLEVELAND, OH, p. A327
UNIVERSITY MEDICAL CENTER, TUCSON, AZ, p. A28
UNIVERSITY MEDICAL CENTER, JACKSONVILLE, FL, p. A90
UNIVERSITY MEDICAL CENTER, LAFAYETTE, LA, p. A186
UNIVERSITY MEDICAL CENTER, LAS VEGAS, NV, p. A270
UNIVERSITY MEDICAL CENTER, LEBANON, TN, p. A392
UNIVERSITY MEDICAL CENTER, LUBBOCK, TX, p. A419
UNIVERSITY MEDICAL CENTER–MESABI, HIBBING, MN, p. A230
UNIVERSITY OF ALABAMA HOSPITAL, BIRMINGHAM, AL, p. A12
UNIVERSITY OF CALIFORNIA LOS ANGELES MEDICAL CENTER, LOS ANGELES, CA, p. A52
UNIVERSITY OF CALIFORNIA LOS ANGELES NEUROPSYCHIATRIC HOSPITAL, LOS ANGELES, CA, p. A52
UNIVERSITY OF CALIFORNIA SAN DIEGO MEDICAL CENTER, SAN DIEGO, CA, p. A61
UNIVERSITY OF CALIFORNIA SAN FRANCISCO MEDICAL CENTER, SAN FRANCISCO, CA, p. A62
UNIVERSITY OF CALIFORNIA, DAVIS MEDICAL CENTER, SACRAMENTO, CA, p. A60
UNIVERSITY OF CALIFORNIA, IRVINE MEDICAL CENTER, ORANGE, CA, p. A56
UNIVERSITY OF CHICAGO HOSPITALS, CHICAGO, IL, p. A128
UNIVERSITY OF CONNECTICUT HEALTH CENTER, JOHN DEMPSEY HOSPITAL, FARMINGTON, CT, p. A76
UNIVERSITY OF ILLINOIS AT CHICAGO MEDICAL CENTER, CHICAGO, IL, p. A128
UNIVERSITY OF IOWA HOSPITALS AND CLINICS, IOWA CITY, IA, p. A155
UNIVERSITY OF KANSAS HOSPITAL, KANSAS CITY, KS, p. A165

UNIVERSITY OF KENTUCKY HOSPITAL, LEXINGTON, KY, p. A176
UNIVERSITY OF LOUISVILLE HOSPITAL, LOUISVILLE, KY, p. A177
UNIVERSITY OF MARYLAND MEDICAL SYSTEM, BALTIMORE, MD, p. A198
UNIVERSITY OF MASSACHUSETTS MEDICAL CENTER, WORCESTER, MA, p. A211
UNIVERSITY OF MEDICINE AND DENTISTRY OF NEW JERSEY, UNIVERSITY BEHAVIORAL HEALTHCARE, PISCATAWAY, NJ, p. A281
UNIVERSITY OF MEDICINE AND DENTISTRY OF NEW JERSEY–UNIVERSITY HOSPITAL, NEWARK, NJ, p. A280
UNIVERSITY OF MIAMI HOSPITAL AND CLINICS, MIAMI, FL, p. A94
UNIVERSITY OF MICHIGAN HOSPITALS, ANN ARBOR, MI, p. A212
UNIVERSITY OF NEBRASKA MEDICAL CENTER, OMAHA, NE, p. A267
UNIVERSITY OF NEW MEXICO CHILDREN'S PSYCHIATRIC HOSPITAL, ALBUQUERQUE, NM, p. A285
UNIVERSITY OF NEW MEXICO MENTAL HEALTH CENTER, ALBUQUERQUE, NM, p. A285
UNIVERSITY OF NORTH CAROLINA HOSPITALS, CHAPEL HILL, NC, p. A309
UNIVERSITY OF PITTSBURGH MEDICAL CENTER, PITTSBURGH, PA, p. A367
UNIVERSITY OF PITTSBURGH MEDICAL CENTER, BEAVER VALLEY, ALIQUIPPA, PA, p. A353
UNIVERSITY OF PITTSBURGH MEDICAL CENTER, BRADDOCK, BRADDOCK, PA, p. A354
UNIVERSITY OF PITTSBURGH MEDICAL CENTER, SOUTH SIDE, PITTSBURGH, PA, p. A367
UNIVERSITY OF PITTSBURGH MEDICAL CENTER, ST. MARGARET, PITTSBURGH, PA, p. A367
UNIVERSITY OF SOUTH ALABAMA KNOLLWOOD PARK HOSPITAL, MOBILE, AL, p. A16
UNIVERSITY OF SOUTH ALABAMA MEDICAL CENTER, MOBILE, AL, p. A16
UNIVERSITY OF SOUTHERN CALIFORNIA–KENNETH NORRIS JR. CANCER HOSPITAL, LOS ANGELES, CA, p. A52
UNIVERSITY OF TENNESSEE BOWLD HOSPITAL, MEMPHIS, TN, p. A394
UNIVERSITY OF TENNESSEE MEMORIAL HOSPITAL, KNOXVILLE, TN, p. A391
UNIVERSITY OF TEXAS HEALTH CENTER AT TYLER, TYLER, TX, p. A430
UNIVERSITY OF TEXAS M. D. ANDERSON CANCER CENTER, HOUSTON, TX, p. A416
UNIVERSITY OF TEXAS MEDICAL BRANCH HOSPITALS, GALVESTON, TX, p. A411
UNIVERSITY OF UTAH HOSPITALS AND CLINICS, SALT LAKE CITY, UT, p. A435
UNIVERSITY OF UTAH NEUROPSYCHIATRIC INSTITUTE, SALT LAKE CITY, UT, p. A435
UNIVERSITY OF VIRGINIA MEDICAL CENTER, CHARLOTTESVILLE, VA, p. A440
UNIVERSITY OF WASHINGTON MEDICAL CENTER, SEATTLE, WA, p. A452
UNIVERSITY OF WISCONSIN HOSPITAL AND CLINICS, MADISON, WI, p. A464
UNIVERSITY PEDIATRIC HOSPITAL, SAN JUAN, PR, p. A477
UNIVERSITY REHABILITATION HOSPITAL, NEW ORLEANS, LA, p. A189
UPPER CONNECTICUT VALLEY HOSPITAL, COLEBROOK, NH, p. A272
UPPER SHORE COMMUNITY MENTAL HEALTH CENTER, CHESTERTOWN, MD, p. A199
UPREACH REHABILITATION HOSPITAL, GAINESVILLE, FL, p. A88
UPSON REGIONAL MEDICAL CENTER, THOMASTON, GA, p. A115
UPSTATE CAROLINA MEDICAL CENTER, GAFFNEY, SC, p. A378
USA DOCTORS HOSPITAL, MOBILE, AL, p. A16
UTAH STATE HOSPITAL, PROVO, UT, p. A434
UTAH VALLEY REGIONAL MEDICAL CENTER, PROVO, UT, p. A435
UVALDE COUNTY HOSPITAL AUTHORITY, UVALDE, TX, p. A430

V

VA CHICAGO HEALTH CARE SYSTEM–LAKESIDE DIVISION, CHICAGO, IL, p. A128
VA CHICAGO HEALTH CARE SYSTEM–WEST SIDE DIVISION, CHICAGO, IL, p. A128
VA MARYLAND HEALTH CARE SYSTEM, PERRY POINT, MD, p. A201
VA PUGET SOUND HEALTH CARE SYSTEM, SEATTLE, WA, p. A453

VACAVALLEY HOSPITAL, VACAVILLE, CA, p. A67
VAIL VALLEY MEDICAL CENTER, VAIL, CO, p. A75
VAL VERDE MEMORIAL HOSPITAL, DEL RIO, TX, p. A407
VALDESE GENERAL HOSPITAL, VALDESE, NC, p. A317
VALDEZ COMMUNITY HOSPITAL, VALDEZ, AK, p. A21
VALLEY BAPTIST MEDICAL CENTER, HARLINGEN, TX, p. A412
VALLEY CHILDREN'S HOSPITAL, FRESNO, CA, p. A44
VALLEY COMMUNITY HOSPITAL, SANTA MARIA, CA, p. A64
VALLEY COMMUNITY HOSPITAL, DALLAS, OR, p. A348
VALLEY COUNTY HOSPITAL, ORD, NE, p. A267
VALLEY FORGE MEDICAL CENTER AND HOSPITAL, NORRISTOWN, PA, p. A362
VALLEY GENERAL HOSPITAL, MONROE, WA, p. A450
VALLEY HOSPITAL, PALMER, AK, p. A21
VALLEY HOSPITAL, RIDGEWOOD, NJ, p. A281
VALLEY HOSPITAL AND MEDICAL CENTER, SPOKANE, WA, p. A453
VALLEY HOSPITAL MEDICAL CENTER, LAS VEGAS, NV, p. A270
VALLEY LUTHERAN HOSPITAL, MESA, AZ, p. A24
VALLEY MEDICAL CENTER, RENTON, WA, p. A452
VALLEY MEDICAL CENTER OF FRESNO, FRESNO, CA, p. A44
VALLEY MEMORIAL HOSPITAL, LIVERMORE, CA, p. A48
VALLEY PRESBYTERIAN HOSPITAL, LOS ANGELES, CA, p. A52
VALLEY REGIONAL HOSPITAL, CLAREMONT, NH, p. A272
VALLEY VIEW HOSPITAL, GLENWOOD SPRINGS, CO, p. A72
VALLEY VIEW MEDICAL CENTER, CEDAR CITY, UT, p. A433
VALLEY VIEW MEDICAL CENTER, PLYMOUTH, WI, p. A467
VALLEY VIEW REGIONAL HOSPITAL, ADA, OK, p. A339
VALLEYCARE MEDICAL CENTER, PLEASANTON, CA, p. A57
VALUEMARK BEHAVIORAL HEALTHCARE OF FLORIDA, ORLANDO, FL, p. A95
VALUEMARK BEHAVIORAL HEALTHCARE SYSTEM OF KANSAS CITY, KANSAS CITY, MO, p. A250
VALUEMARK PINE GROVE BEHAVIORAL HEALTHCARE SYSTEM, LOS ANGELES, CA, p. A52
VALUEMARK WEST END BEHAVIORAL HEALTHCARE SYSTEM, RICHMOND, VA, p. A446
VALUEMARK–BRAWNER BEHAVIORAL HEALTHACARE SYSTEM–NORTH, SMYRNA, GA, p. A114
VAN BUREN COUNTY HOSPITAL, KEOSAUQUA, IA, p. A156
VAN BUREN COUNTY MEMORIAL HOSPITAL, CLINTON, AR, p. A29
VAN NUYS HOSPITAL, LOS ANGELES, CA, p. A52
VAN WERT COUNTY HOSPITAL, VAN WERT, OH, p. A336
VANDERBILT UNIVERSITY HOSPITAL, NASHVILLE, TN, p. A395
VASSAR BROTHERS HOSPITAL, POUGHKEEPSIE, NY, p. A303
VAUGHAN CHILTON MEDICAL CENTER, CLANTON, AL, p. A13
VAUGHAN PERRY HOSPITAL, MARION, AL, p. A16
VAUGHAN REGIONAL MEDICAL CENTER, SELMA, AL, p. A18
VAUGHN JACKSON MEDICAL CENTER, JACKSON, AL, p. A15
VAUGHN THOMASVILLE MEDICAL CENTER, THOMASVILLE, AL, p. A18
VENCOR HOSPITAL–ARLINGTON, ARLINGTON, VA, p. A439
VENCOR HOSPITAL–ATLANTA, ATLANTA, GA, p. A104
VENCOR HOSPITAL–BOSTON, BOSTON, MA, p. A205
VENCOR HOSPITAL–CHATTANOOGA, CHATTANOOGA, TN, p. A388
VENCOR HOSPITAL–CHICAGO NORTH, CHICAGO, IL, p. A128
VENCOR HOSPITAL–CORAL GABLES, CORAL GABLES, FL, p. A85
VENCOR HOSPITAL–DALLAS, DALLAS, TX, p. A407
VENCOR HOSPITAL–DETROIT, LINCOLN PARK, MI, p. A219
VENCOR HOSPITAL–FORT LAUDERDALE, FORT LAUDERDALE, FL, p. A87
VENCOR HOSPITAL–FORT WORTH SOUTH, MANSFIELD, TX, p. A420
VENCOR HOSPITAL–GREENSBORO, GREENSBORO, NC, p. A312
VENCOR HOSPITAL–HOUSTON, HOUSTON, TX, p. A416
VENCOR HOSPITAL–KANSAS CITY, KANSAS CITY, MO, p. A250
VENCOR HOSPITAL–LAGRANGE, LAGRANGE, IN, p. A146
VENCOR HOSPITAL–LOS ANGELES, LOS ANGELES, CA, p. A52
VENCOR HOSPITAL–LOUISVILLE, LOUISVILLE, KY, p. A178
VENCOR HOSPITAL–MILWAUKEE, MILWAUKEE, WI, p. A466
VENCOR HOSPITAL–ONTARIO, ONTARIO, CA, p. A56
VENCOR HOSPITAL–PHILADELPHIA, PHILADELPHIA, PA, p. A365
VENCOR HOSPITAL–PHOENIX, PHOENIX, AZ, p. A25
VENCOR HOSPITAL–PITTSBURGH, OAKDALE, PA, p. A362
VENCOR HOSPITAL–SACRAMENTO, FOLSOM, CA, p. A43
VENCOR HOSPITAL–SAN DIEGO, SAN DIEGO, CA, p. A61
VENCOR HOSPITAL–SAN LEANDRO, SAN LEANDRO, CA, p. A63
VENCOR HOSPITAL–ST PETERSBURG, SAINT PETERSBURG, FL, p. A99
VENCOR HOSPITAL–SYCAMORE, SYCAMORE, IL, p. A138
VENCOR HOSPITAL–TAMPA, TAMPA, FL, p. A101
VENCOR HOSPITAL–TUCSON, TUCSON, AZ, p. A28
VENCOR–NORTH FLORIDA, GREEN COVE SPRINGS, FL, p. A88
VENTURA COUNTY MEDICAL CENTER, VENTURA, CA, p. A68
VERDUGO HILLS HOSPITAL, GLENDALE, CA, p. A45
VERMILION HOSPITAL, LAFAYETTE, LA, p. A186
VERMONT STATE HOSPITAL, WATERBURY, VT, p. A438

VERNON MEMORIAL HOSPITAL, VIROQUA, WI, p. A469
VETERANS AFFAIRS CONNECTICUT HEALTHCARE SYSTEM, WEST HAVEN, CT, p. A79
VETERANS AFFAIRS EDWARD HINES, JR. HOSPITAL, HINES, IL, p. A132
VETERANS AFFAIRS HOSPITAL, FORT HARRISON, MT, p. A258
VETERANS AFFAIRS MEDICAL AND REGIONAL OFFICE CENTER, WICHITA, KS, p. A171
VETERANS AFFAIRS MEDICAL AND REGIONAL OFFICE CENTER, FARGO, ND, p. A320
VETERANS AFFAIRS MEDICAL CENTER, BIRMINGHAM, AL, p. A12
VETERANS AFFAIRS MEDICAL CENTER, MONTGOMERY, AL, p. A16
VETERANS AFFAIRS MEDICAL CENTER, TUSCALOOSA, AL, p. A18
VETERANS AFFAIRS MEDICAL CENTER, TUSKEGEE, AL, p. A18
VETERANS AFFAIRS MEDICAL CENTER, PRESCOTT, AZ, p. A26
VETERANS AFFAIRS MEDICAL CENTER, TUCSON, AZ, p. A28
VETERANS AFFAIRS MEDICAL CENTER, FAYETTEVILLE, AR, p. A30
VETERANS AFFAIRS MEDICAL CENTER, LITTLE ROCK, AR, p. A33
VETERANS AFFAIRS MEDICAL CENTER, FRESNO, CA, p. A44
VETERANS AFFAIRS MEDICAL CENTER, LONG BEACH, CA, p. A49
VETERANS AFFAIRS MEDICAL CENTER, SAN DIEGO, CA, p. A61
VETERANS AFFAIRS MEDICAL CENTER, SAN FRANCISCO, CA, p. A62
VETERANS AFFAIRS MEDICAL CENTER, DENVER, CO, p. A72
VETERANS AFFAIRS MEDICAL CENTER, FORT LYON, CO, p. A72
VETERANS AFFAIRS MEDICAL CENTER, GRAND JUNCTION, CO, p. A73
VETERANS AFFAIRS MEDICAL CENTER, WILMINGTON, DE, p. A80
VETERANS AFFAIRS MEDICAL CENTER, WASHINGTON, DC, p. A81
VETERANS AFFAIRS MEDICAL CENTER, BAY PINES, FL, p. A83
VETERANS AFFAIRS MEDICAL CENTER, GAINESVILLE, FL, p. A88
VETERANS AFFAIRS MEDICAL CENTER, LAKE CITY, FL, p. A91
VETERANS AFFAIRS MEDICAL CENTER, MIAMI, FL, p. A94
VETERANS AFFAIRS MEDICAL CENTER, WEST PALM BEACH, FL, p. A102
VETERANS AFFAIRS MEDICAL CENTER, AUGUSTA, GA, p. A105
VETERANS AFFAIRS MEDICAL CENTER, DECATUR, GA, p. A108
VETERANS AFFAIRS MEDICAL CENTER, DUBLIN, GA, p. A108
VETERANS AFFAIRS MEDICAL CENTER, BOISE, ID, p. A119
VETERANS AFFAIRS MEDICAL CENTER, DANVILLE, IL, p. A128
VETERANS AFFAIRS MEDICAL CENTER, MARION, IL, p. A133
VETERANS AFFAIRS MEDICAL CENTER, NORTH CHICAGO, IL, p. A135
VETERANS AFFAIRS MEDICAL CENTER, DES MOINES, IA, p. A154
VETERANS AFFAIRS MEDICAL CENTER, IOWA CITY, IA, p. A155
VETERANS AFFAIRS MEDICAL CENTER, KNOXVILLE, IA, p. A156
VETERANS AFFAIRS MEDICAL CENTER, NEW ORLEANS, LA, p. A189
VETERANS AFFAIRS MEDICAL CENTER, TOGUS, ME, p. A196
VETERANS AFFAIRS MEDICAL CENTER, BALTIMORE, MD, p. A198
VETERANS AFFAIRS MEDICAL CENTER, FORT HOWARD, MD, p. A200
VETERANS AFFAIRS MEDICAL CENTER, BOSTON, MA, p. A205
VETERANS AFFAIRS MEDICAL CENTER, NORTHAMPTON, MA, p. A208
VETERANS AFFAIRS MEDICAL CENTER, ANN ARBOR, MI, p. A212
VETERANS AFFAIRS MEDICAL CENTER, BATTLE CREEK, MI, p. A213
VETERANS AFFAIRS MEDICAL CENTER, DETROIT, MI, p. A215
VETERANS AFFAIRS MEDICAL CENTER, IRON MOUNTAIN, MI, p. A218
VETERANS AFFAIRS MEDICAL CENTER, SAGINAW, MI, p. A222
VETERANS AFFAIRS MEDICAL CENTER, MINNEAPOLIS, MN, p. A232
VETERANS AFFAIRS MEDICAL CENTER, SAINT CLOUD, MN, p. A234
VETERANS AFFAIRS MEDICAL CENTER, BILOXI, MS, p. A237
VETERANS AFFAIRS MEDICAL CENTER, KANSAS CITY, MO, p. A250
VETERANS AFFAIRS MEDICAL CENTER, SAINT LOUIS, MO, p. A254
VETERANS AFFAIRS MEDICAL CENTER, MILES CITY, MT, p. A259
VETERANS AFFAIRS MEDICAL CENTER, GRAND ISLAND, NE, p. A264
VETERANS AFFAIRS MEDICAL CENTER, LINCOLN, NE, p. A265
VETERANS AFFAIRS MEDICAL CENTER, OMAHA, NE, p. A267

VETERANS AFFAIRS MEDICAL CENTER, MANCHESTER, NH, p. A273
VETERANS AFFAIRS MEDICAL CENTER, ALBUQUERQUE, NM, p. A285
VETERANS AFFAIRS MEDICAL CENTER, ALBANY, NY, p. A288
VETERANS AFFAIRS MEDICAL CENTER, BATH, NY, p. A289
VETERANS AFFAIRS MEDICAL CENTER, CANANDAIGUA, NY, p. A290
VETERANS AFFAIRS MEDICAL CENTER, CASTLE POINT, NY, p. A290
VETERANS AFFAIRS MEDICAL CENTER, NEW YORK, NY, p. A300
VETERANS AFFAIRS MEDICAL CENTER, NEW YORK, NY, p. A300
VETERANS AFFAIRS MEDICAL CENTER, NEW YORK, NY, p. A300
VETERANS AFFAIRS MEDICAL CENTER, NORTHPORT, NY, p. A301
VETERANS AFFAIRS MEDICAL CENTER, SYRACUSE, NY, p. A305
VETERANS AFFAIRS MEDICAL CENTER, ASHEVILLE, NC, p. A308
VETERANS AFFAIRS MEDICAL CENTER, DURHAM, NC, p. A311
VETERANS AFFAIRS MEDICAL CENTER, FAYETTEVILLE, NC, p. A311
VETERANS AFFAIRS MEDICAL CENTER, SALISBURY, NC, p. A316
VETERANS AFFAIRS MEDICAL CENTER, CHILLICOTHE, OH, p. A325
VETERANS AFFAIRS MEDICAL CENTER, CINCINNATI, OH, p. A326
VETERANS AFFAIRS MEDICAL CENTER, CLEVELAND, OH, p. A327
VETERANS AFFAIRS MEDICAL CENTER, DAYTON, OH, p. A329
VETERANS AFFAIRS MEDICAL CENTER, MUSKOGEE, OK, p. A343
VETERANS AFFAIRS MEDICAL CENTER, OKLAHOMA CITY, OK, p. A344
VETERANS AFFAIRS MEDICAL CENTER, PORTLAND, OR, p. A351
VETERANS AFFAIRS MEDICAL CENTER, ROSEBURG, OR, p. A352
VETERANS AFFAIRS MEDICAL CENTER, BUTLER, PA, p. A355
VETERANS AFFAIRS MEDICAL CENTER, COATESVILLE, PA, p. A356
VETERANS AFFAIRS MEDICAL CENTER, ERIE, PA, p. A357
VETERANS AFFAIRS MEDICAL CENTER, LEBANON, PA, p. A360
VETERANS AFFAIRS MEDICAL CENTER, PHILADELPHIA, PA, p. A365
VETERANS AFFAIRS MEDICAL CENTER, SAN JUAN, PR, p. A477
VETERANS AFFAIRS MEDICAL CENTER, PROVIDENCE, RI, p. A373
VETERANS AFFAIRS MEDICAL CENTER, CHARLESTON, SC, p. A376
VETERANS AFFAIRS MEDICAL CENTER, MEMPHIS, TN, p. A394
VETERANS AFFAIRS MEDICAL CENTER, NASHVILLE, TN, p. A395
VETERANS AFFAIRS MEDICAL CENTER, AMARILLO, TX, p. A398
VETERANS AFFAIRS MEDICAL CENTER, BIG SPRING, TX, p. A402
VETERANS AFFAIRS MEDICAL CENTER, DALLAS, TX, p. A407
VETERANS AFFAIRS MEDICAL CENTER, HOUSTON, TX, p. A416
VETERANS AFFAIRS MEDICAL CENTER, SALT LAKE CITY, UT, p. A435
VETERANS AFFAIRS MEDICAL CENTER, WHITE RIVER JUNCTION, VT, p. A438
VETERANS AFFAIRS MEDICAL CENTER, HAMPTON, VA, p. A441
VETERANS AFFAIRS MEDICAL CENTER, SALEM, VA, p. A446
VETERANS AFFAIRS MEDICAL CENTER, SPOKANE, WA, p. A453
VETERANS AFFAIRS MEDICAL CENTER, BECKLEY, WV, p. A455
VETERANS AFFAIRS MEDICAL CENTER, HUNTINGTON, WV, p. A456
VETERANS AFFAIRS MEDICAL CENTER, MARTINSBURG, WV, p. A457
VETERANS AFFAIRS MEDICAL CENTER, TOMAH, WI, p. A469
VETERANS AFFAIRS MEDICAL CENTER, CHEYENNE, WY, p. A471
VETERANS AFFAIRS MEDICAL CENTER, SHERIDAN, WY, p. A472
VETERANS AFFAIRS MEDICAL CENTER–LEXINGTON, LEXINGTON, KY, p. A176
VETERANS AFFAIRS MEDICAL CENTER–LOUISVILLE, LOUISVILLE, KY, p. A178
VETERANS AFFAIRS MEDICAL CENTER–WEST LOS ANGELES, LOS ANGELES, CA, p. A52
VETERANS AFFAIRS NORTHERN INDIANA HEALTH CARE SYSTEM–FORT WAYNE DIVISION, FORT WAYNE, IN, p. A142
VETERANS AFFAIRS NORTHERN INDIANA HEALTH CARE SYSTEM–MARION CAMPUS, MARION, IN, p. A146
VETERANS AFFAIRS PALO ALTO HEALTH CARE SYSTEM, PALO ALTO, CA, p. A56

VETERANS AFFAIRS PITTSBURGH HEALTHCARE SYSTEM, PITTSBURGH, PA, p. A367
VETERANS AFFAIRS WESTERN NEW YORK HEALTHCARE SYSTEM, BATAVIA, NY, p. A289
VETERANS AFFAIRS WESTERN NEW YORK HEALTHCARE SYSTEM, BUFFALO, NY, p. A290
VETERANS HOME AND HOSPITAL, ROCKY HILL, CT, p. A78
VETERANS HOME OF CALIFORNIA, YOUNTVILLE, CA, p. A69
VETERANS MEMORIAL HOSPITAL, WAUKON, IA, p. A159
VETERANS MEMORIAL HOSPITAL OF MEIGS COUNTY, POMEROY, OH, p. A334
VETERANS MEMORIAL MEDICAL CENTER, MERIDEN, CT, p. A77
VIA CHRISTI REGIONAL MEDICAL CENTER, WICHITA, KS, p. A171
VIA CHRISTI REHABILITATION CENTER, WICHITA, KS, p. A171
VICTOR VALLEY COMMUNITY HOSPITAL, VICTORVILLE, CA, p. A68
VICTORIA REGIONAL MEDICAL CENTER, VICTORIA, TX, p. A430
VICTORY MEDICAL CENTER, STANLEY, WI, p. A469
VICTORY MEMORIAL HOSPITAL, WAUKEGAN, IL, p. A139
VICTORY MEMORIAL HOSPITAL, NEW YORK, NY, p. A300
VILLA FELICIANA CHRONIC DISEASE HOSPITAL AND REHABILITATION CENTER, JACKSON, LA, p. A185
VILLA MARIA HOSPITAL, NORTH MIAMI, FL, p. A94
VILLAVIEW COMMUNITY HOSPITAL, SAN DIEGO, CA, p. A61
VILLE PLATTE MEDICAL CENTER, VILLE PLATTE, LA, p. A191
VINELAND DEVELOPMENT CENTER HOSPITAL, VINELAND, NJ, p. A282
VIRGINIA BAPTIST HOSPITAL, LYNCHBURG, VA, p. A442
VIRGINIA BEACH GENERAL HOSPITAL, VIRGINIA BEACH, VA, p. A447
VIRGINIA GAY HOSPITAL, VINTON, IA, p. A159
VIRGINIA MASON MEDICAL CENTER, SEATTLE, WA, p. A453
VIRGINIA REGIONAL MEDICAL CENTER, VIRGINIA, MN, p. A235

W

W. A. FOOTE MEMORIAL HOSPITAL, JACKSON, MI, p. A218
W. J. BARGE MEMORIAL HOSPITAL, GREENVILLE, SC, p. A378
W. J. MANGOLD MEMORIAL HOSPITAL, LOCKNEY, TX, p. A419
WABASH COUNTY HOSPITAL, WABASH, IN, p. A149
WABASH GENERAL HOSPITAL DISTRICT, MOUNT CARMEL, IL, p. A134
WABASH VALLEY HOSPITAL, WEST LAFAYETTE, IN, p. A149
WADLEY REGIONAL MEDICAL CENTER, TEXARKANA, TX, p. A429
WADSWORTH–RITTMAN HOSPITAL, WADSWORTH, OH, p. A336
WAGNER COMMUNITY MEMORIAL HOSPITAL, WAGNER, SD, p. A385
WAGNER GENERAL HOSPITAL, PALACIOS, TX, p. A422
WAHIAWA GENERAL HOSPITAL, WAHIAWA, HI, p. A118
WAKE COUNTY ALCOHOLISM TREATMENT CENTER, RALEIGH, NC, p. A315
WAKE MEDICAL CENTER, RALEIGH, NC, p. A315
WALDO COUNTY GENERAL HOSPITAL, BELFAST, ME, p. A193
WALKER BAPTIST MEDICAL CENTER, JASPER, AL, p. A15
WALLA WALLA GENERAL HOSPITAL, WALLA WALLA, WA, p. A454
WALLACE THOMSON HOSPITAL, UNION, SC, p. A381
WALLOWA MEMORIAL HOSPITAL, ENTERPRISE, OR, p. A349
WALLS REGIONAL HOSPITAL, CLEBURNE, TX, p. A404
WALTER B. JONES ALCOHOL AND DRUG ABUSE TREATMENT CENTER, GREENVILLE, NC, p. A312
WALTER KNOX MEMORIAL HOSPITAL, EMMETT, ID, p. A120
WALTER O. BOSWELL MEMORIAL HOSPITAL, SUN CITY, AZ, p. A26
WALTER OLIN MOSS REGIONAL MEDICAL CENTER, LAKE CHARLES, LA, p. A186
WALTER P. REUTHER PSYCHIATRIC HOSPITAL, WESTLAND, MI, p. A225
WALTER REED HEALTH CARE SYSTEM, WASHINGTON, DC, p. A82
WALTHALL COUNTY GENERAL HOSPITAL, TYLERTOWN, MS, p. A243
WALTON MEDICAL CENTER, MONROE, GA, p. A112
WALTON REGIONAL HOSPITAL, DE FUNIAK SPRINGS, FL, p. A85
WALTON REHABILITATION HOSPITAL, AUGUSTA, GA, p. A105
WAMEGO CITY HOSPITAL, WAMEGO, KS, p. A170
WARD MEMORIAL HOSPITAL, MONAHANS, TX, p. A421
WARM SPRINGS AND BAPTIST REHABILITATION HOSPITAL, SAN ANTONIO, TX, p. A427
WARM SPRINGS REHABILITATION HOSPITAL, GONZALES, TX, p. A411
WARRACK MEDICAL CENTER HOSPITAL, SANTA ROSA, CA, p. A64
WARREN G. MAGNUSON CLINICAL CENTER, NATIONAL INSTITUTES OF HEALTH, BETHESDA, MD, p. A199

Index of Health Care Professionals

This section is an index of the key health care professionals for the hospitals and/or health care systems listed in this publication. The index is in alphabetical order, by individual, followed by the title, institutional affiliation, city, state and page reference to the hospital and/or health care system listing in section A and/or B.

A

AARON Jr., Frank J., Chief Executive Officer, Margaret R. Pardee Memorial Hospital, Hendersonville, NC, p. A312

AASVED, Craig E., Administrator, Wheatland Memorial Hospital, Harlowton, MT, p. A259

ABBOTT, Stephen L., President and Chief Executive Officer, Battle Creek Health System, Battle Creek, MI, p. A212

ABDELHAK, Sherif S., President and Chief Executive Officer, Allegheny Health, Education and Research Foundation, Pittsburgh, PA, p. B64

ABELL, Richard M., President and Chief Executive Officer, Saint Joseph Health Center, Kansas City, MO, p. A249

ABLOW, Ronald C., M.D., President and Chief Executive Officer, St. Luke's–Roosevelt Hospital Center, New York, NY, p. A300

ABRAMS, Deborah L., Chief Executive Officer, THC–Seattle Hospital, Seattle, WA, p. A452

ABRAMS, Larry, Administrator, Indianhead Medical Center, Shell Lake, WI, p. A469

ABREU, Astrid, Administrator, Clinica San Agustin, Manati, PR, p. A476

ABRUTZ Jr., Joseph F., Administrator, Cameron Community Hospital, Cameron, MO, p. A245

ACEVEDO, Roberto, Administrator, Doctors Gubern's Hospital, Fajardo, PR, p. A475

ACHOR, Keith, Assistant Administrator, Dettmer Hospital, Troy, OH, p. A336

ACKER, David B., Chief Executive Officer, Charles Cole Memorial Hospital, Coudersport, PA, p. A356

ACKER, Peter W., President and Chief Executive Officer, Lincoln Medical Center, Lincolnton, NC, p. A313

ACKER, Raymond W., Administrator, White County Community Hospital, Sparta, TN, p. A396

ACKERMAN, Wendy, Administrator, Vaughn Thomasville Medical Center, Thomasville, AL, p. A18

ACKLEY, Michael, Administrator, Fergus Falls Regional Treatment Center, Fergus Falls, MN, p. A229

ACKLEY, Richard Michael, Administrator and Chief Executive Officer, Forest Hospital, Des Plaines, IL, p. A129

ADAIR, Jerry D., President and Chief Executive Officer, Good Shepherd Medical Center, Longview, TX, p. A419

ADAMS, Alice G., Administrator, Columbia Mainland Medical Center, Texas City, TX, p. A429

ADAMS, Daniel F., President and Chief Executive Officer, Presbyterian Intercommunity Hospital, Whittier, CA, p. A68

ADAMS, Jerry W., President, Sumter Regional Hospital, Americus, GA, p. A103

ADAMS, John F., Chief Executive Officer, Columbia Medical Center of Sherman, Sherman, TX, p. A427

ADAMS, Judy, Administrator, Little River Memorial Hospital, Ashdown, AR, p. A29

ADAMS, Mark, Chief Executive Officer, Columbia West Valley Medical Center, Caldwell, ID, p. A119

ADAMS, Mark A., President and Chief Executive Officer, Mississippi Methodist Hospital and Rehabilitation Center, Jackson, MS, p. A240

ADAMS, Scott K., Administrator, Pullman Memorial Hospital, Pullman, WA, p. A451

ADAMS, Wayne, Chief Executive Officer, Charter Behavioral Health System of Charlottesville, Charlottesville, VA, p. A439

ADAMS, William A., Chief Executive Officer, Columbia Highsmith–Rainey Memorial Hospital, Fayetteville, NC, p. A311

ADAMS, Clint E., USN, Commanding Officer, Naval Hospital, Beaufort, SC, p. A375

ADDISON, Wilfred J., Administrator, Inland Hospital, Waterville, ME, p. A196

ADELUNG, Louisa F., President and Chief Executive Officer, The Institute for Rehabilitation and Research, Houston, TX, p. A416

ADKINS, Alan W., Administrator, R. J. Reynolds–Patrick County Memorial Hospital, Stuart, VA, p. A447

ADKINS, Claude, Chief Executive Officer, Northeast Tennessee Rehabilitation Hospital, Johnson City, TN, p. A391

ADKINS Jr., Charles I., President, Holzer Medical Center, Gallipolis, OH, p. A330

ADLER, Karl P., M.D., President and Chief Executive Officer, Saint Vincent's Hospital and Medical Center of New York, New York, NY, p. A299

AFSARIFARD, Farshid, Executive Director, Laurelwood Hospital, Willoughby, OH, p. A337

AGUILAR, Michele, Administrator, Crane Memorial Hospital, Crane, TX, p. A405

AGUILLARD, Daniel, Chief Executive Officer, Methodist Behavioral Resources, New Orleans, LA, p. A188

AHEARN, John R., President, Hospital for Special Surgery, New York, NY, p. A297

AHLFELD, Richard B., President, Children's Specialized Hospital, Mountainside, NJ, p. A279

AINSLEY, Howard, Director, Carilion Bedford Memorial Hospital, Bedford, VA, p. A439

AINSWORTH, Larry K., President and Chief Executive Officer, St. Joseph Hospital, Orange, CA, p. A56

AITCHISON, Kenneth W., President and Chief Executive Officer, Kessler Institute for Rehabilitation, West Orange, NJ, p. A283

AKIN, Dan H., President, Peninsula Regional Medical Center, Salisbury, MD, p. A201

ALBARANO, Francis G., Administrator, Fayette County Memorial Hospital, Washington Court House, OH, p. A337

ALBAUGH, John C., President and Chief Executive Officer, Fort Atkinson Memorial Health Services, Fort Atkinson, WI, p. A462

ALBERT, Anna, Chief Executive Officer, U. S. Public Health Service Phoenix Indian Medical Center, Phoenix, AZ, p. A25

ALBERTY, Allen P., Chief Executive Officer, Shamrock General Hospital, Shamrock, TX, p. A427

ALBRIGHT, James W., President and Chief Executive Officer, Rex Healthcare, Raleigh, NC, p. A315

ALCHESAY–NACHU, Carla, Service Unit Director, U. S. Public Health Service Indian Hospital, Whiteriver, AZ, p. A28

ALCINI, Anthony J.
President and Chief Executive Officer, Tarrant County Hospital District, Fort Worth, TX, p. A410
President and Chief Executive Officer, Tarrant County Hospital District, Fort Worth, TX, p. B139

ALCORN, Velma, Administrator, California Medical Facility, Vacaville, CA, p. A67

ALDRED, Richard, Chief Administrative Officer, St. Dominic's Hospital, Manteca, CA, p. A53

ALDRIDGE, Bryant T., President and Chief Executive Officer, Nash Health Care Systems, Rocky Mount, NC, p. A316

ALECCI, Carmen Bruce, Executive Director, West Hudson Hospital, Kearny, NJ, p. A278

ALEMAN, Ralph A., Chief Executive Officer, Columbia Cedars Medical Center, Miami, FL, p. A93

ALEXANDER, Keith N., Administrator and Chief Operating Officer, American Fork Hospital, American Fork, UT, p. A433

ALEXANDER, Les, Administrator, Pushmataha County–Town of Antlers Hospital Authority, Antlers, OK, p. A339

ALLEE, Al, Administrator, Harmon Memorial Hospital, Hollis, OK, p. A342

ALLEN, Richard L., Chief Executive Officer, Mid–America Rehabilitation Hospital, Overland Park, KS, p. A168

ALLEN, Robert W., Administrator, Evanston Regional Hospital, Evanston, WY, p. A471

ALLEN, Sam J., Administrator, Community Hospital of Anaconda, Anaconda, MT, p. A257

ALLEN, Terry H., Executive Director, 45th Street Mental Health Center, West Palm Beach, FL, p. A101

ALLEN, David M., MSC, Administrator, U. S. Air Force Hospital Dover, Dover AFB, DE, p. A80

ALLEN, Greg, USAF, Commander, U. S. Air Force Hospital, Edwards AFB, CA, p. A42

ALLEN II, Percy, FACHE, Vice President Hospital Affairs and Chief Executive Officer, University Hospital of Brooklyn–State University of New York Health Science Center at Brooklyn, New York, NY, p. A300

ALLEY, Frederick D., President and Chief Executive Officer, Brooklyn Hospital Center, New York, NY, p. A296

ALLEY, Richard S.
Executive Vice President and Chief Executive Officer, Arrowhead Community Hospital and Medical Center, Glendale, AZ, p. A23
Chief Executive Officer, Phoenix Baptist Hospital and Medical Center, Phoenix, AZ, p. A25

ALLIKER, Stanford A., FACHE, President, Levindale Hebrew Geriatric Center and Hospital, Baltimore, MD, p. A198

ALLIN, Linda M., President and Chief Executive Officer, Incarnate Word Hospital, Saint Louis, MO, p. A253

ALLMAN, Roger J., Chief Executive Officer, King's Daughters' Hospital, Madison, IN, p. A146

ALTMILLER, Steve, Chief Executive Officer, Twelve Oaks Hospital, Houston, TX, p. A416

ALTON, Aaron, President, Sisters of Mary of the Presentation Health Corporation, Fargo, ND, p. B134

ALVAREZ, Frank D., Chief Executive Officer, Maricopa Medical Center, Phoenix, AZ, p. A25

ALVAREZ, Guadalupe, Administrator, State Psychiatric Hospital, San Juan, PR, p. A477

ALVIN, William R., President, Henry Ford Wyandotte Hospital, Wyandotte, MI, p. A225

ALVIS, Harry, Chief Executive Officer, Columbia Greenview Hospital, Bowling Green, KY, p. A172

ALVIS, Margaret, R.N., Chief Executive Officer, Earl K. Long Medical Center, Baton Rouge, LA, p. A182

ALWARD, Nelson F., President and Chief Executive Officer, Firelands Community Hospital, Sandusky, OH, p. A335

AMADOR, Michael, Chief Executive Officer, West Oaks Hospital, Houston, TX, p. A416

AMAN, Dale, Administrator, Community Memorial Hospital, Turtle Lake, ND, p. A322

AMBROSIANI, Craig, Executive Director, San Juan Hospital, Monticello, UT, p. A434

AMBROSIUS, Mark R.
President, Milwaukee Psychiatric Hospital, Wauwatosa, WI, p. A470
President, St. Luke's Medical Center, Milwaukee, WI, p. A466

AMEEN, David J., President and Chief Executive Officer, Saint Mary's Health Services, Grand Rapids, MI, p. A217

AMEEN, Lane, M.D., Chief Executive Officer, Elmcrest Psychiatric Institute, Portland, CT, p. A78

AMEER, Adil M., President and Chief Executive Officer, Rapid City Regional Hospital, Rapid City, SD, p. A384

AMENT, Rick, President and Chief Executive Officer, Bay Area Medical Center, Marinette, WI, p. A464

AMOS, James L., President, Margaret Mary Community Hospital, Batesville, IN, p. A140

AMOS, Helen, President and Chief Executive Officer, Mercy Medical Center, Baltimore, MD, p. A198

AMSTUTZ, Terry L., CHE, Chief Executive Officer and Administrator, Medical Center of Calico Rock, Calico Rock, AR, p. A29

ANASTASIO, Lance W., President, Winter Haven Hospital, Winter Haven, FL, p. A102

ANCELL, Charles D., President, Missouri Delta Medical Center, Sikeston, MO, p. A255

ANCHO, Kathy, Administrator, Battle Mountain General Hospital, Battle Mountain, NV, p. A270

ANDERSEN, David, President and Chief Executive Officer, Saratoga Hospital, Saratoga Springs, NY, p. A304

ANDERSEN, Edward, President and Chief Executive Officer, CGH Medical Center, Sterling, IL, p. A138

ANDERSEN, Howard C., Chief Executive Officer, Vail Valley Medical Center, Vail, CO, p. A75

ANDERSON, Dan H.
President and Chief Executive Officer, Baptist Medical Center, Kansas City, MO, p. A248
President and Chief Executive Officer, Research Medical Center, Kansas City, MO, p. A249

ANDERSON, Darleen S., MSN, Site Administrator, Sentara Leigh Hospital, Norfolk, VA, p. A443

ANDERSON, David, Chief Executive Officer, Mobridge Regional Hospital, Mobridge, SD, p. A384

ANDERSON, David S., FACHE, Administrator, Lassen Community Hospital, Susanville, CA, p. A66

ANDERSON, Donald A., President and Chief Executive Officer, Everglades Regional Medical Center, Pahokee, FL, p. A96

ANDERSON, Duane H., President and Chief Executive Officer, Payson Regional Medical Center, Payson, AZ, p. A24

ANDERSON, Edwin S., President, Cumberland Medical Center, Crossville, TN, p. A388

ANDERSON, Greger C., President and Chief Executive Officer, Nyack Hospital, Nyack, NY, p. A301

ANDERSON, H. William, Administrator, Baxter County Regional Hospital, Mountain Home, AR, p. A33

ANDERSON, Harold E., President and Chief Executive Officer, Moses Taylor Hospital, Scranton, PA, p. A368

ANDERSON, J. Kendall, President and Chief Executive Officer, John Muir Medical Center, Walnut Creek, CA, p. A68

ANDERSON, James, Interim Administrator, Madison County Memorial Hospital, Winterset, IA, p. A160

ANDERSON, James M., President and Chief Executive Officer, Children's Hospital Medical Center, Cincinnati, OH, p. A325

ANDERSON, John D., Chief Executive Officer, Columbia Springhill Medical Center, Springhill, LA, p. A191

ANDERSON, Kerry A., R.N., Administrator, Montgomery Memorial Hospital, Troy, NC, p. A317

ANDERSON, Larry, Administrator, Sayre Memorial Hospital, Sayre, OK, p. A345

ANDERSON, Larry W., Administrator, Minnie G. Boswell Memorial Hospital, Greensboro, GA, p. A110

ANDERSON, Loren J., President and Chief Executive Officer, Lakeland Medical Center, Elkhorn, WI, p. A462

ANDERSON, Martin E., Administrator, Lakeshore Community Hospital, Shelby, MI, p. A223

ANDERSON, Melinda, Administrator, Olive View–UCLA Medical Center, Los Angeles, CA, p. A51

ANDERSON, Mike, Administrator, McCone County Medical Assistance Facility, Circle, MT, p. A257

ANDERSON, Paul J., Administrator, Winneshiek County Memorial Hospital, Decorah, IA, p. A153

ANDERSON, Richard A., President, St. Luke's Hospital, Bethlehem, PA, p. A354

ANDERSON, Ron, Administrator, Community Memorial Hospital, Syracuse, NE, p. A268

ANDERSON, Ron J., M.D., President and Chief Executive Officer, Dallas County Hospital District–Parkland Health and Hospital System, Dallas, TX, p. A406

ANDERSON, Scott A., Administrator, Stonewall Memorial Hospital, Aspermont, TX, p. A399

ANDERSON, Scott R., President and Chief Executive Officer, North Memorial Health Care, Robbinsdale, MN, p. A233

ANDERSON, Stephen N. F., Director, Doctors' Hospital of Staten Island, New York, NY, p. A296

ANDERSON, Thomas E., President and Chief Executive Officer, Columbia West Paces Medical Center, Atlanta, GA, p. A104

ANDERSON, William H., Administrator and Chief Executive Officer, South Florida Baptist Hospital, Plant City, FL, p. A97

ANDERSON, William L., Chief Executive Officer, Lutheran Hospital of Indiana, Fort Wayne, IN, p. A142

ANDERSON, Douglas E., USAF, Administrator, U. S. Air Force Hospital, Cannon AFB, NM, p. A285

ANDERSON Jr., Andrew E., Administrator, Spohn Bee County Hospital, Beeville, TX, p. A401

ANDERSON Jr., E. Ratcliffe, M.D., Executive Director, Truman Medical Center, Kansas City, MO, p. B143

ANDINO, Julio, Executive Director, Ponce Regional Hospital, Ponce, PR, p. A476

ANDREWS, Jane, Administrator and Chief Executive Officer, Nashville Rehabilitation Hospital, Nashville, TN, p. A395

ANDREWS, William J., President, Licking Memorial Hospital, Newark, OH, p. A333

ANDREWS, Mary Ann, President and Chief Executive Officer, Sisters of Charity of St. Augustine Health System, Cleveland, OH, p. B134

ANDRIS, Terry R., CHE, Interim Chief Executive Officer, Reeves County Hospital, Pecos, TX, p. A423

ANDRUS, Michael G., Administrator and Chief Executive Officer, Franklin County Medical Center, Preston, ID, p. A121

ANDRUS, Terry W., President, East Alabama Medical Center, Opelika, AL, p. A17

ANDUHA, Manuel, Administrator, Kohala Hospital, Kohala, HI, p. A118

ANEL, Manuel, M.D., Administrator and Chief Executive Officer, Long Beach Doctors Hospital, Long Beach, CA, p. A48

ANGERMEIER, Ingo, FACHE, Administrator and Chief Executive Officer, LSU Medical Center–University Hospital, Shreveport, LA, p. A190

ANGLE, Gregory R., President and Chief Executive Officer, Columbia Medical Center of San Angelo, San Angelo, TX, p. A425

ANNIS, Donald E., Chief Executive Officer, Atlantic General Hospital, Berlin, MD, p. A198

ANTHONY, Fred, President and Chief Executive Officer, Cuyahoga Falls General Hospital, Cuyahoga Falls, OH, p. A328

ANTHONY, Mark, Vice President and Administrator, Oakwood Hospital Annapolis Center, Wayne, MI, p. A224

ANTLE, David, Chief Executive Officer, Miners' Colfax Medical Center, Raton, NM, p. A287

ANTWINE, Brenda, Administrator and Chief Operating Officer, Healthsouth Rehabilitation Hospital, Memphis, TN, p. A393

APPEL, G. Robert, Administrator, Mason General Hospital, Shelton, WA, p. A453

APPEL, Harley B., Chief Executive Officer, Community Memorial Hospital, Marysville, KS, p. A166

APPLEBAUM, Jon D., Administrator, Jefferson Memorial Hospital, Ranson, WV, p. A458

APPLEGATE, Rodney T., President, Walla Walla General Hospital, Walla Walla, WA, p. A454

APRATO, Peter P., Administrator and Chief Operating Officer, Robert F. Kennedy Medical Center, Hawthorne, CA, p. A45

ARBUCKLE, Barry, Ph.D., Chief Operating Officer, Orange Coast Memorial Medical Center, Fountain Valley, CA, p. A43

ARCH, John K., Administrator, Boys Town National Research Hospital, Omaha, NE, p. A266

ARCHBELL, Larry J., Vice President Operations, University Community Hospital–Carrollwood, Tampa, FL, p. A101

ARCHER, David L., Chief Executive Officer, Lucy Lee Hospital, Poplar Bluff, MO, p. A252

ARCHER, Kenneth W., Administrator, Gooding County Memorial Hospital, Gooding, ID, p. A120

ARCIDI, Alfred, M.D., President, Whittier Rehabilitation Hospital, Haverhill, MA, p. A207

ARENS, James F., M.D., Chief Executive Officer, University of Texas Medical Branch Hospitals, Galveston, TX, p. A411

ARISMENDI, Luis, M.D., Administrator, Dameron Hospital, Stockton, CA, p. A65

ARIZPE, Robert C., Superintendent, San Antonio State Hospital, San Antonio, TX, p. A426

ARMADA, Anthony A., Chief Executive Officer, Columbia Chino Valley Medical Center, Chino, CA, p. A40

ARMSTRONG, Anthony W., President, Bay Medical Center, Bay City, MI, p. A213

ARMSTRONG, Dale
Chief Executive Officer, Brynn Marr Behavioral Healthcare System, Jacksonville, NC, p. A313
Chief Executive Officer, Coastal Carolina Hospital, Conway, SC, p. A377

ARMSTRONG, Kenneth H., Chief Executive Officer, Columbia Riverton Memorial Hospital, Riverton, WY, p. A472

ARMSTRONG, Scott
Administrator, Group Health Cooperative Central Hospital, Seattle, WA, p. A452
Administrator, The Eastside Hospital, Redmond, WA, p. A452

ARMSTRONG Jr., David S., Administrator, Little Falls Hospital, Little Falls, NY, p. A294

ARNETT, Charlene, Chief Executive Officer, High Pointe, Oklahoma City, OK, p. A343

ARNETT, Randal M., President and Chief Executive Officer, Southern Ohio Medical Center, Portsmouth, OH, p. A334

ARNOLD, Agnes E., CHE, Administrator, Charleston Memorial Hospital, Charleston, SC, p. A376

ARNOLD, G. Michael, Interim Director, University of California Los Angeles Neuropsychiatric Hospital, Los Angeles, CA, p. A52

ARNOLD, Kent A., President, Community–General Hospital of Greater Syracuse, Syracuse, NY, p. A305

ARNOLD, Margo, Administrator, West Side District Hospital, Taft, CA, p. A66

ARNOLD, Richard D., Administrator, Medina Community Hospital, Hondo, TX, p. A413

ARNOLD, Robert P., Director, Essex County Hospital Center, Cedar Grove, NJ, p. A276

ARNOLD, Thomas B., Chief Operating Officer, Veterans Affairs Medical Center, San Diego, CA, p. A61

ARTILES, Nemuel O., Executive Director, Bella Vista Hospital, Mayaguez, PR, p. A476

ASAY, Grant, Chief Executive Officer, Sitka Community Hospital, Sitka, AK, p. A21

ASH, James L.
President and Chief Executive Officer, Cottage Health System, Santa Barbara, CA, p. B87
President and Chief Executive Officer, Santa Barbara Cottage Hospital, Santa Barbara, CA, p. A64

ASH, John P., FACHE, President and Chief Executive Officer, Eugenia Hospital, Lafayette Hill, PA, p. A360

ASH, Richard M., Administrator, Northern Itasca Health Care Center, Bigfork, MN, p. A227

ASHCRAFT, Steven F., Administrator, Jefferson County Memorial Hospital, Winchester, KS, p. A171

ASHFORD, Charles H., M.D., Interim Chief Executive Officer, Craven Regional Medical Authority, New Bern, NC, p. A314

ASHKIN, David, M.D., Medical Executive Director, A. G. Holley State Hospital, Lantana, FL, p. A91

ASPER, Daniel A., Acting Director, Veterans Affairs Medical Center, Grand Island, NE, p. A264

ASPER, David, Director, Veterans Affairs Medical Center, Lincoln, NE, p. A265

ASSELL, William C., President and Chief Executive Officer, St. Joseph's Mercy Hospital, Centerville, IA, p. A152

ATKINS, Tony E., Administrator, Braxton County Memorial Hospital, Gassaway, WV, p. A456

ATKINSON, Allan, Administrator, Belmond Community Hospital, Belmond, IA, p. A151

ATKINSON, L. Gail
Executive Director, Devereux Texas Treatment Network, League City, TX, p. A418
Executive Director, Devereux–Victoria, Victoria, TX, p. A430

ATKINSON, Robert P., President and Chief Executive Officer, Jefferson Regional Medical Center, Pine Bluff, AR, p. A34

ATKINSON, William K., Ph.D., Chief Executive Officer, Columbia Presbyterian–St. Luke's Medical Center, Denver, CO, p. A71

ATZROTT, Allan Earl, President, Prince George's Hospital Center, Cheverly, MD, p. A199

AUBERT, Harry, Administrator, Garfield County Memorial Hospital, Pomeroy, WA, p. A451

AUMAN, Patrick A., Ph.D., Chief Executive Officer, Transitional Hospital Corporation of Minneapolis, Golden Valley, MN, p. A229

AUSMAN, Dan F., Chief Executive Officer, Monterey Park Hospital, Monterey Park, CA, p. A54

AUSTIN, George L., Chief Executive Officer, Bolivar General Hospital, Bolivar, TN, p. A387

AUSTIN, James D., CHE
  Administrator, Kalkaska Memorial Health Center, Kalkaska, MI, p. A219
  Administrator, Paul Oliver Memorial Hospital, Frankfort, MI, p. A216

AUSTIN, L. Joe, Chief Executive Officer, Huntsville Hospital East, Huntsville, AL, p. A15

AUSTIN, Michael A., CPA, Administrator, St. Paul Medical Center, Dallas, TX, p. A407

AUSTIN, Robert S., President, Gunnison Valley Hospital, Gunnison, CO, p. A73

AVERS, John M., Chief Executive Officer, White County Memorial Hospital, Monticello, IN, p. A147

AVERY, George, Interim Chief Executive Officer, Mayo Regional Hospital, Dover–Foxcroft, ME, p. A194

AVERY III, John B., Administrator, Baptist Perry Memorial Hospital, Linden, TN, p. A392

AXELSON, Alan A., M.D., Chief Executive Officer, Southwood Psychiatric Hospital, Pittsburgh, PA, p. A366

AYRES, Larry J., Administrator and Chief Executive Officer, Pointe Coupee General Hospital, New Roads, LA, p. A189

AZZARA, Michael W., President, Valley Hospital, Ridgewood, NJ, p. A281

B

BABB, Donald J., Chief Executive Officer, Citizens Memorial Hospital, Bolivar, MO, p. A245

BACH, William, M.D., Administrator and Medical Director, RiverValley Behavioral Health Hospital, Owensboro, KY, p. A179

BACHARACH, Paul, President and Chief Executive Officer, Uniontown Hospital, Uniontown, PA, p. A370

BACHRACH, David J., Professor, Health Services Management, University of Texas M. D. Anderson Cancer Center, Houston, TX, p. A416

BACIARELLI, Renato V., Administrator, Mercy Medical Center, Durango, CO, p. A72

BACUS, Randy, Chief Executive Officer, Colorado–Fayette Medical Center, Weimar, TX, p. A431

BADGER Jr., Theodore J., Chief Executive Officer, Beauregard Memorial Hospital, De Ridder, LA, p. A184

BAER, Charles E., President, Mercer Medical Center, Trenton, NJ, p. A282

BAER, James E., FACHE, President and Administrator, Waupun Memorial Hospital, Waupun, WI, p. A470

BAGBY, Phillip D., President and Chief Executive Officer, Albemarle Hospital, Elizabeth City, NC, p. A311

BAGGETT, Larry, Administrator, Palo Duro Hospital, Canyon, TX, p. A403

BAGLEY, Douglas D., Executive Director, LAC–University of Southern California Medical Center, Los Angeles, CA, p. A50

BAHL, Barry I., Associate Director, Veterans Affairs Medical Center, Saint Cloud, MN, p. A234

BAILEY, Bruce P., Administrator, Abbeville County Memorial Hospital, Abbeville, SC, p. A375

BAILEY, Frederick R., Chief Executive Officer, North Fulton Regional Hospital, Roswell, GA, p. A113

BAILEY, James P., Administrator and Chief Executive Officer, Henryetta Medical Center, Henryetta, OK, p. A342

BAILEY, Owen, Administrator, Thomas Hospital, Fairhope, AL, p. A14

BAILEY, Sandra, Administrator, Methodist–Haywood Park Hospital, Brownsville, TN, p. A387

BAILON, Amy R., M.D., Medical Director, Woodbridge Development Center, Woodbridge, NJ, p. A283

BAINBRIDGE, Darlene D., Interim Chief Executive Officer, Cuba Memorial Hospital, Cuba, NY, p. A291

BAIRD, Marvin L., Executive Director, Adams County Memorial Hospital, Decatur, IN, p. A141

BAKER, Bob M., President and Chief Executive Officer, Gratiot Community Hospital, Alma, MI, p. A212

BAKER, David, Interim Administrator, Pinelands Hospital, Nacogdoches, TX, p. A422

BAKER, Gary A., President, Memorial Hospital, Towanda, PA, p. A369

BAKER, Harry M., Chief Executive Officer, Cross County Hospital, Wynne, AR, p. A35

BAKER, Jeannie, Chief Operating Officer, Shands at Starke, Starke, FL, p. A99

BAKER, Jo Ann, Chief Executive Officer, Columbia Rehabilitation Hospital, Corpus Christi, TX, p. A405

BAKER, Jon W., Administrator and Chief Executive Officer, Ripon Medical Center, Ripon, WI, p. A468

BAKER, Rod L., President and Chief Executive Officer, Parrish Medical Center, Titusville, FL, p. A101

BAKER, Rodger H., President and Chief Executive Officer, Fauquier Hospital, Warrenton, VA, p. A447

BAKER, Ronald J., Administrator, Kiowa County Memorial Hospital, Greensburg, KS, p. A163

BAKER Jr., Wendell H.
  Chief Executive Officer, Matagorda County Hospital District, Bay City, TX, p. B112
  Chief Executive Officer, Matagorda General Hospital, Bay City, TX, p. A401

BAKST, Michael D., Ph.D., Executive Director, Community Memorial Hospital of San Buenaventura, Ventura, CA, p. A67

BALCH, Charles M., M.D., President and Chief Executive Officer, City of Hope National Medical Center, Duarte, CA, p. A42

BALDWIN, Bruce A., Interim President and Chief Executive Officer, Dakota Heartland Health System, Fargo, ND, p. A320

BALDWIN, Gilda, Chief Administrative Officer and Chief Operating Officer, Westchester General Hospital, Miami, FL, p. A94

BALDWIN, Joe G., Administrator, ATH Heights Hospital, Houston, TX, p. A413

BALDWIN, Keith J., Administrator, Samaritan Healthcare, Moses Lake, WA, p. A450

BALDWIN, Paul L., Chief Operating Officer, Retreat Hospital, Richmond, VA, p. A445

BALERUD, Paul A., Interim Chief Executive Officer, Carrington Health Center, Carrington, ND, p. A319

BALKCOM, Charles, President, Candler County Hospital, Metter, GA, p. A111

BALL, Donald M., President, Jackson Hospital and Clinic, Montgomery, AL, p. A16

BALL, John R., JD, President and Chief Executive Officer, Pennsylvania Hospital, Philadelphia, PA, p. A365

BALLA, Ernest, Administrator, Johns Community Hospital, Taylor, TX, p. A428

BALLANTYNE III, Reginald M., President, PMH Health Resources, Inc., Phoenix, AZ, p. B121

BALLARD, Bryan M., Executive Director, Delano Regional Medical Center, Delano, CA, p. A41

BALLARD, Paul H., Chief Executive Officer, Mission Hospital, Mission, TX, p. A421

BALLARD, Susan, Administrator, Menifee Valley Medical Center, Sun City, CA, p. A66

BALTZER, David J., President, Rehoboth McKinley Christian Hospital, Gallup, NM, p. A286

BALZEN, Earl W., R.N., Chief Executive Officer, Charter Behavioral Health System, Jackson, MS, p. A240

BAN Jr., Albert, Chief Executive Officer, Fairfield Memorial Hospital, Fairfield, IL, p. A130

BANASZYNSKI, Gregory A., President, St. Francis Hospital, Milwaukee, WI, p. A466

BANE, Raymond, Executive Director, Natchez Community Hospital, Natchez, MS, p. A242

BANGERT, Richard A., Chief Executive Officer and Administrator, Psychiatric Hospital at Vanderbilt, Nashville, TN, p. A395

BANK, Kendall C., President, Northfield Hospital, Northfield, MN, p. A232

BANKS, David P., Chief Executive Officer, Huguley Willow Creek Hospital, Arlington, TX, p. A399

BANKS, Elizabeth, Superintendent, Memphis Mental Health Institute, Memphis, TN, p. A393

BANKSTON, William C., Acting Administrator, Leonard J. Chabert Medical Center, Houma, LA, p. A185

BARABAS, Mark C., President, Community Hospital of Lancaster, Lancaster, PA, p. A360

BARBAKOW, Jeffrey, Chairman and Chief Executive Officer, TENET Healthcare Corporation, Santa Barbara, CA, p. B140

BARBATO, Anthony L., M.D., President and Chief Executive Officer, Loyola University Medical Center, Maywood, IL, p. A133

BARBE, Brian S., Chief Executive Officer, Columbia Katy Medical Center, Katy, TX, p. A417

BARBER, Jeffrey B., Dr.PH
  President and Chief Executive Officer, North Mississippi Health Services, Inc., Tupelo, MS, p. B118
  President and Chief Executive Officer, North Mississippi Medical Center, Tupelo, MS, p. A243

BARBER, Mike, Facility Service Integrator, Clovis Community Hospital, Clovis, CA, p. A40

BARBER, Steve, Administrator, Dorminy Medical Center, Fitzgerald, GA, p. A109

BARBINI, Gerald J., Administrator and Chief Executive Officer, Hubbard Regional Hospital, Webster, MA, p. A210

BARCO, Lawrence F., President, MidMichigan Regional Medical Center–Clare, Clare, MI, p. A213

BARINA Jr., F. G., Commanding Officer, Naval Hospital, Corpus Christi, TX, p. A405

BARKER, Richard, Administrator, Love County Health Center, Marietta, OK, p. A342

BARLOW, Rulon J., Administrator, Central Peninsula General Hospital, Soldotna, AK, p. A21

BARNARD, Dan, Chief Executive Officer, Northwest Surgical Hospital, Oklahoma City, OK, p. A344

BARNER, James W., President and Chief Executive Officer, Altoona Hospital, Altoona, PA, p. A353

BARNES, Harry F., FACHE, President and Chief Executive Officer, Wilson N. Jones Regional Health System, Sherman, TX, p. A427

BARNES, Mary Ann, Administrator, Kaiser Foundation Hospital, Los Angeles, CA, p. A50

BARNES, Ronald W., Executive Director, Mountain View Hospital District, Madras, OR, p. A350

BARNETT, Charles J.
  President, Brackenridge Hospital, Austin, TX, p. A400
  President, Seton Medical Center, Austin, TX, p. A400

BARNETT, Dana K., Administrator, Platte County Memorial Hospital, Wheatland, WY, p. A472

BARNETT, Gary L., President and Chief Executive Officer, Central Kansas Medical Center, Great Bend, KS, p. A163

BARNETT, Timothy, Chief Executive Officer, Yavapai Regional Medical Center, Prescott, AZ, p. A26

BARNETTE, Chris W., President and Chief Executive Officer, Baton Rouge General Medical Center, Baton Rouge, LA, p. A182

BARNHART, James, Administrator, Peace Harbor Hospital, Florence, OR, p. A349

BARNOSKI, Philip, Chief Executive Officer, Creek Nation Community Hospital, Okemah, OK, p. A343

BARON, David A., D.O., Medical Director, Horsham Clinic, Ambler, PA, p. A353

BARON, Jeffrey A., Executive Director, Beech Hill Hospital, Dublin, NH, p. A272

BARON, Steven D.
  President and Chief Executive Officer, Miriam Hospital, Providence, RI, p. A373
  President and Chief Executive Officer, Rhode Island Hospital, Providence, RI, p. A373

BARR, C. Dennis, President and Chief Executive Officer, Northwest General Hospital, Milwaukee, WI, p. A465

BARR, LuAnn, Administrator, Tilden Community Hospital, Tilden, NE, p. A268

BARRAGAN, J. Bruce, President and Chief Executive Officer, McLeod Regional Medical Center, Florence, SC, p. A378

BARRETO, Hector, M.D., Director, Hospital Dr. Susoni, Arecibo, PR, p. A474

BARRETT, Susan
President and Chief Executive Officer, Mercy Health System of Kansas, Fort Scott, KS, p. A163
President and Chief Executive Officer, Mercy Hospitals of Kansas, Independence, KS, p. A164

BARRETTE, Paul Raymond, President and Chief Executive Officer, Maine Coast Memorial Hospital, Ellsworth, ME, p. A194

BARRON, Steven R., Chief Executive Officer, Alexian Brothers Hospital, San Jose, CA, p. A62

BARROW, William F., President and Chief Executive Officer, De Soto Regional Health System, Mansfield, LA, p. A187

BARRY, Dennis R., President, Moses Cone Health System, Greensboro, NC, p. A312

BARRY, R. Michael, Administrator, Plumas District Hospital, Quincy, CA, p. A58

BARSZCZEWSKI, Joseph, Chief Executive Officer, Meadows Psychiatric Center, Centre Hall, PA, p. A355

BARTELL III, Frank J., President and Chief Executive Officer, St. Luke's Hospital, Maumee, OH, p. A333

BARTELS, Bruce M.
President, York Health System, York, PA, p. B149
President, York Hospital, York, PA, p. A372

BARTER, James T., M.D., Director, Metropolitan Children and Adolescent Institute, Chicago, IL, p. A126

BARTLETT, John D., Chief Executive Officer, Palms of Pasadena Hospital, Saint Petersburg, FL, p. A98

BARTLETT, John T., Director, Searcy Hospital, Mount Vernon, AL, p. A17

BARTLETT, Robert, Administrator, BHC Willow Springs RTC, Reno, NV, p. A271

BARTLETT, Thomas G., President and Chief Executive Officer, H. C. Watkins Memorial Hospital, Quitman, MS, p. A243

BARTO Jr., John K., President and Chief Executive Officer, Mercy Center for Health Care Services, Aurora, IL, p. A123

BARTON, Donald L., Superintendent, Southeast Missouri Mental Health Center, Farmington, MO, p. A247

BARTON, Larry O., President, Western Baptist Hospital, Paducah, KY, p. A179

BARTOS, John M., Administrator, Marcus Daly Memorial Hospital, Hamilton, MT, p. A258

BARTZ, Daniel R., Chief Executive Officer, Cloud County Health Center, Concordia, KS, p. A162

BASH, Robert R., Administrator, Booneville Community Hospital, Booneville, AR, p. A29

BASHAM, Gail S., Chief Operating Officer, Mount Regis Center, Salem, VA, p. A446

BASLER, Jack, President, Henry County Memorial Hospital, New Castle, IN, p. A147

BASSETT, Warren J., FACHE, President, Brookville Hospital, Brookville, PA, p. A354

BASTONE, Peter F., President and Chief Executive Officer, Mission Hospital Regional Medical Center, Mission Viejo, CA, p. A53

BATAL, Lucille M., Administrator, Baldpate Hospital, Georgetown, MA, p. A206

BATCHELDER, Chester G., Superintendent, New Hampshire Hospital, Concord, NH, p. A272

BATEMAN, Mark T., President and Chief Executive Officer, Episcopal Hospital, Philadelphia, PA, p. A363

BATEMAN, Steven B., Chief Executive Officer, Columbia Ogden Regional Medical Center, Ogden, UT, p. A434

BATES, Jonathan R., M.D., President and Chief Executive Officer, Arkansas Children's Hospital, Little Rock, AR, p. A32

BATES, Rodney, Administrator, Logan County Hospital, Oakley, KS, p. A167

BATT, Richard A., President and Chief Executive Officer, Franklin Memorial Hospital, Farmington, ME, p. A194

BATULIS, Scott, Administrator, HealthEast Bethesda Lutheran Hospital and Rehabilitation Center, Saint Paul, MN, p. A234

BAUDER, Marianna, President and Chief Executive Officer, Saint Joseph Hospital, Denver, CO, p. A71

BAUER, Clifford J., Chief Executive Officer, Hialeah Hospital, Hialeah, FL, p. A88

BAUER, Robert
Chief Executive Officer, Indian Path Medical Center, Kingsport, TN, p. A391
Chief Executive Officer, Indian Path Pavilion, Kingsport, TN, p. A391

BAUM, Carla S., President, St. Joseph Hospital, Saint Louis, MO, p. A254

BAUMAN, Nancy, Chief Executive Officer, St. Joseph's Memorial Hospital and Nursing Home, Hillsboro, WI, p. A463

BAUMGART, Kris, Administrator, Clarke County Hospital, Osceola, IA, p. A157

BAUMGARTNER, Michael, President, St. Francis Hospital and Health Services, Maryville, MO, p. A251

BAUTE, Robert E., M.D., President and Chief Executive Officer, Kent County Memorial Hospital, Warwick, RI, p. A374

BAXTER, W. Eugene, Dr.PH, Administrator, Integris Bass Baptist Health Center, Enid, OK, p. A341

BAYER, Thomas R., Administrator, Community Memorial Hospital, Oconto Falls, WI, p. A467

BEA, Javon R., President and Chief Executive Officer, Mercy Health System, Janesville, WI, p. A463

BEACH, Al, Administrator, Columbia Basin Hospital, Ephrata, WA, p. A449

BEAMAN Jr., Charles D., President and Chief Executive Officer, Baptist Healthcare System of South Carolina, Columbia, SC, p. B68

BEANE, Donna, Administrator, Needles–Desert Communities Hospital, Needles, CA, p. A55

BEAR, Lawrence P., Administrator, Jersey Community Hospital, Jerseyville, IL, p. A132

BEARD, Joseph W., President and Chief Executive Officer, Covenant Medical Center, Urbana, IL, p. A139

BEARD, Lance, Chief Executive Officer and Administrator, Brookhaven Hospital, Tulsa, OK, p. A346

BEARD, Les, Chief Executive Officer, Columbia Eastside Medical Center, Snellville, GA, p. A114

BEARDSLEY, David L., Administrator, Sandypines, Tequesta, FL, p. A101

BEASLEY, Lynn W., President and Chief Executive Officer, Newberry County Memorial Hospital, Newberry, SC, p. A380

BEATTY, Margaret, President, Sisters of Mercy of the Americas–Regional Community of Baltimore, Baltimore, MD, p. B135

BEATY, Ralph E., Administrator, Huntsville Memorial Hospital, Huntsville, TX, p. A416

BEATY, Ryan D.
Administrator, Marshall I. Pickens Hospital, Greenville, SC, p. A378
Administrator, Roger C. Peace Rehabilitation Hospital, Greenville, SC, p. A378

BEAUCHAMP, Philip K., FACHE
President and Chief Executive Officer, Mease Health Care, Palm Harbor, FL, p. B113
President and Chief Executive Officer, Mease Hospital Dunedin, Dunedin, FL, p. A86

BEBOW, Gary, Administrator and Chief Executive Officer, White River Medical Center, Batesville, AR, p. A29

BECHTOLD, Gregg A., President and Chief Executive Officer, Johnson Memorial Hospital, Franklin, IN, p. A143

BECK, E. Dean, Administrator, Fulton County Health Center, Wauseon, OH, p. A337

BECK, Everett L., Administrator, Mayers Memorial Hospital District, Fall River Mills, CA, p. A42

BECK, Gary E., Administrator, Sevier Valley Hospital, Richfield, UT, p. A435

BECK, Lawrence M., President, Good Samaritan Hospital of Maryland, Baltimore, MD, p. A197

BECK, Walter, Chief Executive Officer, George L. Mee Memorial Hospital, King City, CA, p. A47

BECKER, Gina, Acting Chief Executive Officer, Columbia Northwest Medical Center, Margate, FL, p. A92

BECKER, Lowell L., M.D., President, Cambridge Medical Center, Cambridge, MN, p. A227

BECKER, Walter S., Administrator, Medina Memorial Hospital, Medina, NY, p. A294

BECKSTRAND, James E.
Administrator, Delta Community Medical Center, Delta, UT, p. A433
Administrator, Fillmore Community Medical Center, Fillmore, UT, p. A433

BEDNAREK, Robert J., Administrator and Chief Executive Officer, Transylvania Community Hospital, Brevard, NC, p. A309

BEELER, A. F., Warden, Federal Medical Center, Lexington, KY, p. A176

BEELER, Don A., Chief Executive Officer, St. Michael Health Care Center, Texarkana, TX, p. A429

BEELOW, Patricia A., Chief Executive Officer, Northeastern Regional Hospital, Las Vegas, NM, p. A286

BEEMAN, Barry G.
Chief Executive Officer, Manchester Memorial Hospital, Manchester, CT, p. A77
Chief Executive Officer, Rockville General Hospital, Vernon Rockville, CT, p. A79

BEGLEY, Bruce D., Executive Director, Community Methodist Hospital, Henderson, KY, p. A175

BEHNKE, Bruce, Administrator, Kaiser Foundation Hospital, Honolulu, HI, p. A117

BEHNKE Jr., William C., Chief Executive Officer, Tucson General Hospital, Tucson, AZ, p. A27

BEHRENS, B. Lyn, President, Adventist Health System–Loma Linda, Loma Linda, CA, p. B64

BEHRMANN, John, Administrator and Chief Executive Officer, Kentfield Rehabilitation Hospital, Kentfield, CA, p. A47

BEIL, Clark R., Chief Executive Officer, Johnston Memorial Hospital, Abingdon, VA, p. A439

BEIRNE, Frank T., President and Chief Executive Officer, Baycoast Medical Center, Baytown, TX, p. A401

BELCHER, Edgar L., Administrator, Walton Medical Center, Monroe, GA, p. A112

BELCOURT, Janet, Administrator, U. S. Public Health Service Indian Hospital, Cherokee, NC, p. A310

BELILA, Leon J., Administrator, Edinburg Hospital, Edinburg, TX, p. A408

BELL, Betty, Team Administrator, L. S. Huckabay MD Memorial Hospital, Coushatta, LA, p. A183

BELL, David C., Chief Operating Officer, BHC Sand Hill Behavioral Healthcare, Gulfport, MS, p. A239

BELL, Richard, Administrator, Highland Ridge Hospital, Salt Lake City, UT, p. A435

BELL, Stuart, Administrator, Guthrie County Hospital, Guthrie Center, IA, p. A155

BELTON, Horace, Executive Director, Manhattan Psychiatric Center–Ward's Island, New York, NY, p. A298

BENDER, Ronald, Administrator, Baum Harmon Memorial Hospital, Primghar, IA, p. A158

BENFER, David W., President and Chief Executive Officer, Saint Joseph Medical Center, Joliet, IL, p. A132

BENFER, Richard Wilson, President, University of Pittsburgh Medical Center, Braddock, Braddock, PA, p. A354

BENFORD, Barry C., Director, Altoona Center, Altoona, PA, p. A353

BENGTSON, Paul R., Chief Executive Officer, Northeastern Vermont Regional Hospital, Saint Johnsbury, VT, p. A437

BENJAMIN, Robert C., Chief Executive Officer, Southeast Arizona Medical Center, Douglas, AZ, p. A22

BENN, David P., President and Chief Executive Officer, Memorial Hospitals Association, Modesto, CA, p. A54

BENNETT, Bruce A., Administrator and Chief Executive Officer, Atoka Memorial Hospital, Atoka, OK, p. A339

BENNETT, Jim, Administrator, Columbia Good Samaritan Hospital, Bakersfield, CA, p. A37

BENNETT, Jo Ann, Chief Operating Officer, Healthsouth Bakersfield Rehabilitation Hospital, Bakersfield, CA, p. A37

BENNETT, John, President and Chief Executive Officer, Shelby Memorial Hospital, Shelbyville, IL, p. A137

BENNETT, Richard, Executive Director, Mid–Hudson Psychiatric Center, New Hampton, NY, p. A295

BENNING, Robert J., Chief Executive Officer, Ridgeview Psychiatric Hospital and Center, Oak Ridge, TN, p. A395

BENSAIA, Barbara A., Chief Operating Officer, Canonsburg General Hospital, Canonsburg, PA, p. A355

BENSON, Robert, Chief Executive Officer, Columbia Nashville Memorial Hospital, Madison, TN, p. A392

BENSON, M. J., USN, Commanding Officer, Naval Hospital, Jacksonville, FL, p. A89

BENTLEY, Brian S., Administrator, Sutter Merced Medical Center, Merced, CA, p. A53

BENTON, Earnest E., Chief Executive Officer, Southwest Georgia Regional Medical Center, Cuthbert, GA, p. A107

BENTON, Lowell, Executive Director, Woodland Community Hospital, Cullman, AL, p. A13

BENWAY, Michael W., Commanding Officer, Naval Hospital, Oak Harbor, WA, p. A451

BENZ, Mark A., Administrator, Horsham Clinic, Ambler, PA, p. A353

BERARD, Celse A., President, Riverview Hospital Association, Wisconsin Rapids, WI, p. A470

BERDAN, Barclay E., Chief Executive Officer, Harris Methodist Fort Worth, Fort Worth, TX, p. A410

BERGER, Gerald L., CPA, Chief Operating Officer, Great Lakes Rehabilitation Hospital, Southfield, MI, p. A223

BERGER, Marni, Chief Executive Officer, ValueMark Behavioral Healthcare of Florida, Orlando, FL, p. A95

BERGER, Susan, Prioress, Benedictine Sisters of the Annunciation, Bismarck, ND, p. B70

BERGMAN, Paul, Administrator, Flandreau Municipal Hospital, Flandreau, SD, p. A383

BERGREN, Jeff, Chief Operating Officer and Administrator, BHC Streamwood Hospital, Streamwood, IL, p. A138

BERGROOS, Raymond, Administrator, Missouri River Medical Center, Fort Benton, MT, p. A258

BERHOW, John, President, Continuum, Kendallville, IN, p. B87

BERKLEY, Ralph B., Administrator, Illinois Valley Community Hospital, Peru, IL, p. A136

BERLUCCHI, Scott A., President and Chief Executive Officer, Lancaster General Hospital–Susquehanna Division, Columbia, PA, p. A356

BERMAN, Arnold, M.D., President and Chief Executive Officer, Graduate Hospital, Philadelphia, PA, p. A364

BERMAN, Seth, Executive Director, Hall–Brooke Hospital, A Division of Hall–Brooke Foundation, Westport, CT, p. A79

BERNARD, Mark L.
Chief Executive Officer, Metropolitan Methodist Hospital, San Antonio, TX, p. A425
Chief Executive Officer, Northeast Methodist Hospital, San Antonio, TX, p. A426

BERNARD, Patricia, R.N., Administrator, Osborne County Memorial Hospital, Osborne, KS, p. A167

BERNARD, Peter J.
President and Chief Executive Officer, Caritas Medical Center, Louisville, KY, p. A177
President and Chief Executive Officer, Caritas Peace Center, Louisville, KY, p. A177

BERNATOVICZ, Mike A., Chief Executive Officer, Barberton Citizens Hospital, Barberton, OH, p. A323

BERND, David L., President and Chief Executive Officer, Sentara Health System, Norfolk, VA, p. B131

BERNSTEIN, Martin B., Executive Director, Northern Maine Medical Center, Fort Kent, ME, p. A194

BERNSTEIN, Ronald T., President and Chief Executive Officer, Foundations Behavioral Health, Doylestown, PA, p. A356

BERNSTEIN, Stephen, Chief Executive Officer, Columbia Plaza Medical Center of Fort Worth, Fort Worth, TX, p. A410

BERRETT, Britt, Chief Executive Officer, Sharp Chula Vista Medical Center, Chula Vista, CA, p. A40

BERRY, Stan B., FACHE, President, Hanford Community Medical Center, Hanford, CA, p. A45

BERSON, Samuel, M.D., Executive Director, Kings Highway Hospital Center, New York, NY, p. A297

BERTRAM, Donna L., R.N., Administrator, Penrose–St. Francis Health Services, Colorado Springs, CO, p. A70

BERTSCH, Darrold, Administrator, Central Arizona Medical Center, Florence, AZ, p. A23

BESON, James, Commander, Weed Army Community Hospital, Fort Irwin, CA, p. A43

BESTUL, Randy, Administrator, Norwood Health Center, Marshfield, WI, p. A464

BESWICK, Melinda D., President and Chief Executive Officer, California Hospital Medical Center, Los Angeles, CA, p. A49

BETJEMANN, John H., President, Methodist Hospitals, Gary, IN, p. A143

BETTENDORF, Felix, President, Alexian Brothers Health System, Inc., Elk Grove Village, IL, p. B64

BETTS, Peter J., President and Chief Executive Officer, East Jefferson General Hospital, Metairie, LA, p. A187

BETZOLD, Paul F., President and Chief Executive Officer, Presbyterian Hospital, Charlotte, NC, p. A310

BEVERLY, Ken B., President and Chief Executive Officer, Archbold Medical Center, Thomasville, GA, p. B67

BEVINS, O. David, Chief Executive Officer, Kentucky River Medical Center, Jackson, KY, p. A175

BEYER, Robert L., President and Chief Executive Officer, St. Joseph's Mercy Hospitals and Health Services, Clinton Township, MI, p. A214

BHATIA, Krishin L., Administrator, Victory Memorial Hospital, New York, NY, p. A300

BIACSI, Jean, Vice President and Administrator Main Campus, All Saints Hospital–Cityview, Fort Worth, TX, p. A410

BIANCHI, Charles A., President, Hillsdale Community Health Center, Hillsdale, MI, p. A217

BICH, Arlene C., Administrator, Wagner Community Memorial Hospital, Wagner, SD, p. A385

BICKLING, J. Allan, Chief Executive Officer, Edward W. McCready Memorial Hospital, Crisfield, MD, p. A199

BIEDIGER, Michael J., President, Lexington Medical Center, West Columbia, SC, p. A381

BIEGANSKI, Gary, President, Community Hospital, McCook, NE, p. A265

BIERMAN, Robert H., M.D., Director, Hurtado Health Center, New Brunswick, NJ, p. A279

BIERMAN, Ronald L., Chief Executive Officer, Healthsouth Northern Kentucky Rehabilitation Hospital, Edgewood, KY, p. A173

BIGA, Cathleen D., President and Chief Executive Officer, Columbia La Grange Memorial Hospital, La Grange, IL, p. A133

BIGA, Thomas A., Executive Director, Irvington General Hospital, Irvington, NJ, p. A278

BIGLEY, Robert F.
Chief Executive Officer, Columbia Four Rivers Medical Center, Selma, AL, p. A18
Administrator, Dale Medical Center, Ozark, AL, p. A17

BIGOGNO, James C., FACHE, President and Chief Executive Officer, Howard Community Hospital, Kokomo, IN, p. A145

BIHLDORFF, John P., President and Chief Executive Officer, Newton–Wellesley Hospital, Newton, MA, p. A208

BILBO, Dorothy C., Acting Administrator, Pearl River County Hospital, Poplarville, MS, p. A243

BILL, Charles E., Administrator and Chief Executive Officer, Vencor Hospital–Tucson, Tucson, AZ, p. A28

BILLIK, Dean S., Director, Veterans Affairs Medical Center, Charleston, SC, p. A376

BILLING, Michael D., Administrator, Glacier County Medical Center, Cut Bank, MT, p. A258

BILLS, Jeff K., Chief Executive Officer, St. Mary's Regional Medical Center, Reno, NV, p. A271

BILLS, Robert C., President and Vice Chairman, Valley Presbyterian Hospital, Los Angeles, CA, p. A52

BING, William W., Administrator, Morehouse General Hospital, Bastrop, LA, p. A182

BINGHAM, John, Administrator, Magic Valley Regional Medical Center, Twin Falls, ID, p. A122

BINGHAM, Leslie, Chief Executive Officer, Charter Palms Behavioral Health System, McAllen, TX, p. A420

BIRA, Patrick G., FACHE, Administrator, Perry County Memorial Hospital, Perryville, MO, p. A252

BIRCHELL, Bruce K., Administrator, Bob Wilson Memorial Grant County Hospital, Ulysses, KS, p. A170

BIRD, Kim B., Administrator, Lifecare Hospitals, Shreveport, LA, p. A190

BIRDZELL, JoAnn
President and Chief Executive Officer, St. Catherine Hospital, East Chicago, IN, p. A142
President and Chief Executive Officer, St. Elizabeth's Hospital, Chicago, IL, p. A127

BIRDZELL, John R., FACHE, Chief Executive Officer, Bedford Regional Medical Center, Bedford, IN, p. A140

BISCARO, Ron, Administrator, St. Francis Medical Center of Santa Barbara, Santa Barbara, CA, p. A64

BISCHOFF, Theresa A., Deputy Provost and Executive Vice President, New York University Medical Center, New York, NY, p. A298

BISCONE, Mark A., Executive Director, Waldo County General Hospital, Belfast, ME, p. A193

BISHOP, Gary, Administrator, West Park Hospital, Cody, WY, p. A471

BISHOP, Marvin O., Administrator, Weisbrod Memorial Hospital, Eads, CO, p. A72

BISHOP, Mel, Chief Executive Officer, Columbia North Houston Medical Center, Houston, TX, p. A413

BISHOP, Paul A., Administrator, Lonesome Pine Hospital, Big Stone Gap, VA, p. A439

BISHOP SMITH, Carole, Center Director, Dwight D. Eisenhower Veterans Affairs Medical Center, Leavenworth, KS, p. A165

BISSEGER, Lynda, Chief Executive Officer, Sanger General Hospital, Sanger, CA, p. A63

BISSELL, David D., USAF, Commander, U. S. Air Force Hospital Tinker, Tinker AFB, OK, p. A346

BITTING, Nancy J., President and Chief Executive Officer, Riverside Community Hospital, Riverside, CA, p. A59

BIXLER, David, Administrator, Bascom Palmer Eye Institute–Anne Bates Leach Eye Hospital, Miami, FL, p. A92

BJELICH, Steven C., President and Chief Executive Officer, St. Francis Hospital, Wilmington, DE, p. A80

BLACK, Gary E., President and Chief Executive Officer, Lenoir Memorial Hospital, Kinston, NC, p. A313

BLACK, Melissa, Assistant Administrator, Shackelford County Hospital District, Albany, TX, p. A398

BLACK, Sharon S., R.N., Chief Operating Officer, HEALTHSOUTH Rehabilitation Hospital of South Louisiana, Baton Rouge, LA, p. A183

BLACKMON, James R., Chief Executive Officer, Southeast Alabama Medical Center, Dothan, AL, p. A13

BLACKWELL, Kevin E., Chief Executive Officer, Charter Parkwood Behavioral Health System, Olive Branch, MS, p. A242

BLAIR, John E., President, Ravenswood Hospital Medical Center, Chicago, IL, p. A126

BLAIR, Mardian J., President, Adventist Health System Sunbelt Health Care Corporation, Winter Park, FL, p. B63

BLAKELY, Carrell R., Administrator, Union County General Hospital, Clayton, NM, p. A285

BLAKLEY, Scott F., Administrator, Brentwood Behavioral Healthcare, Shreveport, LA, p. A190

BLAN, Gary J., FACHE, President and Chief Executive Officer, Nacogdoches Memorial Hospital, Nacogdoches, TX, p. A421

BLANCHARD, William R., Chief Executive Officer, Columbia Detar Hospital, Victoria, TX, p. A430

BLANCHETTE, Edward A., M.D., Director, Connecticut Department of Correction's Hospital, Somers, CT, p. A78

BLANCO, Carla, Administrator, Doctors Center, Manati, PR, p. A476

BLAND, Calvin, President and Chief Executive Officer, St. Christopher's Hospital for Children, Philadelphia, PA, p. A365

BLAND, Edward C., Chief Executive Officer, Colusa Community Hospital, Colusa, CA, p. A40

BLAND, Thomas, Administrator, Montfort Jones Memorial Hospital, Kosciusko, MS, p. A241

BLANKENSHIP Jr., Lua R., President and Chief Executive Officer, Children's Hospital, Denver, CO, p. A71

BLASBAND, Charles A., Chief Executive Officer, Citrus Memorial Hospital, Inverness, FL, p. A89

BLASKO, M. Cornelia, Administrator, St. Francis Hospital, Mountain View, MO, p. A251

BLASKO Jr., Joseph, President and Chief Executive Officer, Incarnate Word Health Services, San Antonio, TX, p. B105

BLEAKNEY, David A., Administrator, Angleton–Danbury General Hospital, Angleton, TX, p. A399

BLESSING, William H., President, Mary Free Bed Hospital and Rehabilitation Center, Grand Rapids, MI, p. A217

BLESSITT, H. J., Administrator, South Sunflower County Hospital, Indianola, MS, p. A240

BLEVINS, Maggie, Administrator, Jane Phillips Nowata Health Center, Nowata, OK, p. A343

BLODGETT, Ruth P., Chief Operating Officer, Berkshire Medical Center, Pittsfield, MA, p. A209

BLOME', Michael, Administrator, Methodist Hospital of Fayette, Somerville, TN, p. A396

BLOUGH Jr., Daniel D., Administrator, Punxsutawney Area Hospital, Punxsutawney, PA, p. A367

BLOUNT, Kenneth, President, The Monroe Clinic, Monroe, WI, p. A466

BLUFORD, John W., Administrator, Hennepin County Medical Center, Minneapolis, MN, p. A232

BLUM, James G., Administrator, Bennett County Community Hospital, Martin, SD, p. A383

BLUM, Robert W., FACHE, Administrator, U. S. Air Force Hospital, Abilene, TX, p. A398

BOARDMAN, Debra, Chief Executive Officer, Riverwood Health Care Center, Aitkin, MN, p. A226

BOBB, James R., President, Church Hospital Corporation, Baltimore, MD, p. A197

BOBELDYK, Jerry, Administrator, Murray County Memorial Hospital, Slayton, MN, p. A235

BOEHRINGER, Paul, Executive Director, Temple University Hospital, Philadelphia, PA, p. A365

BOENING, Harold L., Administrator, Otto Kaiser Memorial Hospital, Kenedy, TX, p. A417

BOFF, Michael G., President, Trillium Hospital, Albion, MI, p. A212

BOGAN, James, Chief Executive Officer, Portage Health System, Hancock, MI, p. A217

BOGGS, Danny L., President and Chief Executive Officer, Memorial Hospital, Marysville, OH, p. A332

BOGGS, Michael S., Chief Executive Officer, Columbia Coliseum Medical Centers, Macon, GA, p. A111

BOGGUS Jr., Solon
   Chief Executive Officer, Columbia Valley Hospital, Chattanooga, TN, p. A387
   Chief Executive Officer, Parkridge Medical Center, Chattanooga, TN, p. A388

BOGUE, Virginia, Site Administrator, Sentara Bayside Hospital, Virginia Beach, VA, p. A447

BOHL, Jim, President and Chief Executive Officer, Doctors Hospital, Springfield, IL, p. A138

BOID, Roger R., Administrator, Grady Memorial Hospital, Chickasha, OK, p. A340

BOLD, Harry, Administrator, Big Sandy Medical Center, Big Sandy, MT, p. A257

BOLTON, Clyde E., Administrator, Summers County Appalachian Regional Hospital, Hinton, WV, p. A456

BOMAR–COLE, Shirley, Chief Operating Officer, Provident Hospital of Cook County, Chicago, IL, p. A126

BONAR Jr., Robert I., President and Chief Executive Officer, Children's Hospital of the King's Daughters, Norfolk, VA, p. A443

BOND, C. Scott, Administrator, Providence St. Peter Hospital, Olympia, WA, p. A451

BONDS Jr., Earl, Chief Executive Officer, Healthcare Management Group, Inc., Macon, GA, p. B102

BONE, Jim G., Interim Administrator, Muleshoe Area Medical Center, Muleshoe, TX, p. A421

BONNER, Tucker, President, King's Daughters Hospital, Temple, TX, p. A428

BONNETT, Joseph E., Executive Vice President and Chief Executive Officer, Freeport Memorial Hospital, Freeport, IL, p. A130

BOOKER, Oliver J., Chief Executive Officer, Healthsouth Rehabilitation Hospital, Florence, SC, p. A377

BOONE, Richard, Executive Director, Crawford Memorial Hospital, Van Buren, AR, p. A35

BOOR, Leon J., Chief Executive Officer, Memorial Hospital, Abilene, KS, p. A161

BOOTH, Peter G., President, Henrietta D. Goodall Hospital, Sanford, ME, p. A195

BOPP, James, Executive Director, Middletown Psychiatric Center, Middletown, NY, p. A294

BORDELON, Olive, Chief Executive Officer, St. Frances Cabrini Hospital, Alexandria, LA, p. A182

BORDERS, Douglas, President and Chief Executive Officer, Lourdes Hospital, Paducah, KY, p. A179

BORENSTEIN, Jeffrey, M.D., Chief Executive Officer and Medical Director, Holliswood Hospital, New York, NY, p. A297

BORIES Jr., Robert F., FACHE, Administrator, Shriners Hospitals for Children, Burns Institute Boston Unit, Boston, MA, p. A204

BORING, Ronald L., President and Chief Executive Officer, Baylor Richardson Medical Center, Richardson, TX, p. A424

BORLAND, Winston, Chief Executive Officer, Columbia Northwest Hospital, Corpus Christi, TX, p. A405

BORRONI, S. Denise, Administrator and Chief Operating Officer, Healthsouth Rehabilitation Hospital of Arlington, Arlington, TX, p. A399

BOSK, Nathan, FACHE, Chief Executive Officer, Lower Bucks Hospital, Bristol, PA, p. A354

BOSSARD, Karen L., Administrator, Greene County Medical Center, Jefferson, IA, p. A156

BOSTICK, Roy D., Director, E. A. Conway Medical Center, Monroe, LA, p. A187

BOSTON, Edward D., Chief Executive Officer, Huntsville Hospital System, Huntsville, AL, p. B105

BOSWELL, Bill, Chief Executive Officer, McCamey Hospital, McCamey, TX, p. A420

BOUCHER, David T., Chief Executive Officer, Good Hope Hospital, Erwin, NC, p. A311

BOUFFARD, Rodney, Superintendent, Augusta Mental Health Institute, Augusta, ME, p. A193

BOUIS, Charles, President and Chief Executive Officer, Edward A. Utlaut Memorial Hospital, Greenville, IL, p. A131

BOULA, Rodney C., Administrator, Clifton–Fine Hospital, Star Lake, NY, p. A305

BOULENGER, Bo, Chief Executive Officer, Homestead Hospital, Homestead, FL, p. A89

BOUNDS, Floyd D., Administrator, Madison Medical Center, Fredericktown, MO, p. A247

BOURASSA, Robert N., Executive Director, Trinity Springs Pavilion–East, Fort Worth, TX, p. A410

BOURGEOIS Jr., Milton D., Administrator, St. Anne General Hospital, Raceland, LA, p. A190

BOUTHILLET, Jules W., President and Chief Executive Officer, Lakewood Hospital, Lakewood, OH, p. A331

BOWEN, Barbara H., Interim Administrator, Healthsouth Rehabilitation of Mechanicsburg, Mechanicsburg, PA, p. A361

BOWEN, Claire L., President, Fairview Hospital, Great Barrington, MA, p. A206

BOWEN, Pamela, Director, Princeton University Health Services, McCosh Health Center, Princeton, NJ, p. A281

BOWEN, Steve, President, Nan Travis Memorial Hospital, Jacksonville, TX, p. A417

BOWER, Roger H., USAF, Commander, U. S. Air Force Hospital, MacDill AFB, FL, p. A92

BOWERS, Robert A., Chief Executive Officer, Oak Hill Community Medical Center, Oak Hill, OH, p. A333

BOWERSOX, Bruce D., Administrator, Hillsboro Community Hospital, Hillsboro, ND, p. A320

BOWLES, Stephen A., President, Valley Community Hospital, Dallas, OR, p. A348

BOWLING, John S., President and Chief Executive Officer, South Georgia Medical Center, Valdosta, GA, p. A115

BOWMAN, Leslie C., Regional Administrator, Ancillary Services and Site Administrator, Detroit Receiving Hospital and University Health Center, Detroit, MI, p. A214

BOWMAN, Mike, Administrator, Litzenberg Memorial County Hospital, Central City, NE, p. A263

BOWMAN, Scott, Administrator, Sweetwater Hospital, Sweetwater, TN, p. A396

BOWN, Kathleen, Director, H. C. Solomon Mental Health Center, Lowell, MA, p. A207

BOWSE, James T., President, Rutland Regional Medical Center, Rutland, VT, p. A437

BOYD, Charles E., Administrator, Doctors' Hospital of Shreveport, Shreveport, LA, p. A190

BOYD, Christopher L., Chief Executive Officer, Columbia Douglas Medical Center, Roseburg, OR, p. A351

BOYD, Jerry B., Director, Veterans Affairs Medical Center, Long Beach, CA, p. A49

BOYD, Samuel J., Administrator, Crafts–Farrow State Hospital, Columbia, SC, p. A376

BOYD, Wallace N., Administrator, Ochiltree General Hospital, Perryton, TX, p. A423

BOYER, Gregory E., Chief Executive Officer, Wellington Regional Medical Center, West Palm Beach, FL, p. A102

BOYLE, Jeanne M., R.N., Chief Operating Officer, Middlesex Hospital, Waltham, MA, p. A210

BOYLE, Steven P., President and Chief Executive Officer, St. Peter's Hospital, Albany, NY, p. A288

BOYLES, Jackie, Administrator, Cedar County Memorial Hospital, El Dorado Springs, MO, p. A247

BOYLES, Michael, Administrator, Saunders County Health Service, Wahoo, NE, p. A268

BOYTER, Jerry W., Administrator, Tulare District Hospital, Tulare, CA, p. A67

BOZEMAN, Larry C., Chief Executive Officer, Trinity Valley Medical Center, Palestine, TX, p. A422

BRAAKSMA, Martin P., Executive Director, Wells Community Hospital, Bluffton, IN, p. A140

BRABAND, Jon D., Chief Executive Officer, Glencoe Area Health Center, Glencoe, MN, p. A229

BRACHT, Gerald E., Vice President and Administrator, Scripps Memorial Hospital–Encinitas, Encinitas, CA, p. A42

BRACKIN, D. Wayne, Chief Executive Officer, South Miami Hospital, Miami, FL, p. A93

BRACKNEY, Charles R., President and Chief Executive Officer, Ozarks Medical Center, West Plains, MO, p. A256

BRADEN, Frank M., Administrator, Alliance Hospital of Santa Teresa, Santa Teresa, NM, p. A287

BRADFORD, Roberta J., President and Chief Executive Officer, Drake Center, Cincinnati, OH, p. A325

BRADLEY, David K., Chief Executive Officer, Geary Community Hospital, Junction City, KS, p. A165

BRADLEY, Lucinda A., President, Great Plains Regional Medical Center, North Platte, NE, p. A266

BRADLEY, Richard J., Administrator, G. Pierce Wood Memorial Hospital, Arcadia, FL, p. A83

BRADLEY, Myra James, Chairman of the Board of Directors, Good Samaritan Hospital, Cincinnati, OH, p. A325

BRADLEY Jr., J. Lindsey, FACHE, President and Chief Administrative Officer, Trinity Mother Frances Health System, Tyler, TX, p. A429

BRADSHAW, Dorothy A., Director, Deer's Head Center, Salisbury, MD, p. A201

BRADWAY, Karen A., USAF, Administrator, U. S. Air Force Hospital, Columbus, MS, p. A238

BRADY, James L., President, Allied Services Rehabilitation Hospital, Scranton, PA, p. A368

BRADY, Karl R., Chief Executive Officer and Administrator, Charter Plains Behavioral Health System, Lubbock, TX, p. A419

BRADY, Patrick R., Administrator, Sutter Solano Medical Center, Vallejo, CA, p. A67

BRADY, Jane Frances, Chief Executive Officer, St. Joseph's Hospital and Medical Center, Paterson, NJ, p. A280

BRAILSFORD, Tammie McMann, Administrator, Saint Mary Medical Center, Long Beach, CA, p. A49

BRAMLETT Jr., E. Chandler
   President and Chief Executive Officer, Infirmary Health System, Inc., Mobile, AL, p. B105
   President and Chief Executive Officer, Mobile Infirmary Medical Center, Mobile, AL, p. A16

BRANAMAN, A. Ray, Administrator, Mary Breckinridge Hospital, Hyden, KY, p. A175

BRANDLER, Bruce, Administrator, Puget Sound Hospital, Tacoma, WA, p. A454

BRANDON, David, Chief Executive Officer, Fayette Memorial Hospital, Connersville, IN, p. A141

BRANDT, Stephen, Chief Executive Officer, Columbia West Florida Regional Medical Center, Pensacola, FL, p. A96

BRANDT, Florence, Chief Executive Officer, St. Francis Medical Center, Pittsburgh, PA, p. A367

BRANDT Jr., George H., Administrator, Martin General Hospital, Williamston, NC, p. A318

BRANTLEY, Cheryl Y., Administrator, South Florida Evaluation and Treatment Center, Miami, FL, p. A93

BRASEL, James B., Administrator, Shriners Hospitals for Children, Honolulu, Honolulu, HI, p. A117

BRASIER, Jamers, Administrator, Nocona General Hospital, Nocona, TX, p. A422

BRASIG, Joe, Administrator, Concho County Hospital, Eden, TX, p. A408

BRASS, Alan W., FACHE, President, Barnes–Jewish Hospital, Saint Louis, MO, p. A253

BRASWELL, LeRoy J., Administrator, Warm Springs and Baptist Rehabilitation Hospital, San Antonio, TX, p. A427

BRAUN, Greg, Administrator, Harmony Community Hospital, Harmony, MN, p. A230

BRAWLEY, James B., Chief Executive Officer, Holly Hill Charter Behavioral Health System, Raleigh, NC, p. A315

BRAY, Donald C., President and Chief Executive Officer, University Hospital, Augusta, GA, p. A105

BRAZIER, Ray, President, Hillcrest Health Center, Oklahoma City, OK, p. A343

BRAZITIS, Mark A., President, Lancaster General Hospital, Lancaster, PA, p. A360

BRECKENRIDGE, Bryan L., President, Shady Grove Adventist Hospital, Rockville, MD, p. A201

BREEDEN, James L., Administrator, Kaiser Foundation Hospital, Los Angeles, CA, p. A50

BREEDEN, Susan M., Administrator, Baptist Memorial Hospital–Huntingdon, Huntingdon, TN, p. A390

BREEN, John P., Chief Executive Officer, Massapequa General Hospital, Seaford, NY, p. A304

BREEN, Michael F.
President, Holy Cross Hospital, Detroit, MI, p. A215
President, St. John Health System–Saratoga Campus, Detroit, MI, p. A215

BREGANT Jr., Robert E., Administrator, Ransom Memorial Hospital, Ottawa, KS, p. A168

BREHE, Deborah, Chief Executive Officer, Columbia Mission Bay Hospital, San Diego, CA, p. A60

BREITENBACH, Thomas G., President and Chief Executive Officer, Miami Valley Hospital, Dayton, OH, p. A329

BREITLING, Bryan, Administrator and Chief Executive Officer, Bowdle Hospital, Bowdle, SD, p. A382

BREMER, Louis H., President and Chief Executive Officer, Wellmont Health System–Holston Valley, Kingsport, TN, p. A391

BRENNAN, Charles L., Chief Executive Officer, St. Lawrence Rehabilitation Center, Lawrenceville, NJ, p. A278

BRENNAN, Donald A., President and Chief Executive Officer, Daughters of Charity National Health System, Saint Louis, MO, p. B88

BRENNAN, Michael J., M.D., Commander, Womack Army Medical Center, Fort Bragg, NC, p. A311

BRENNY, Terrence, President, Stoughton Hospital Association, Stoughton, WI, p. A469

BREON, Richard C., President and Chief Executive Officer, St. Mary's Medical Center of Evansville, Evansville, IN, p. A142

BRESSANELLI, Leo A., President and Chief Executive Officer, Genesis Medical Center, Davenport, IA, p. A153

BRETT, C. William, Ph.D., Chief Executive Officer, Psychiatric Hospital of Florida, Clearwater, FL, p. A85

BRETZ, Joy, Administrator, Sheridan County Hospital, Hoxie, KS, p. A164

BREWER, Gary L., Chief Executive Officer, Columbia Tallahassee Community Hospital, Tallahassee, FL, p. A100

BREWER, Jeff, President, Walker Baptist Medical Center, Jasper, AL, p. A15

BREWER, Rebecca T., CHE, Chief Executive Officer, Columbia Colleton Medical Center, Walterboro, SC, p. A381

BREWER, Sally, Chief Executive Officer, Memorial Hospital at Exeter, Exeter, CA, p. A42

BREZENOFF, Stanley, President, Maimonides Medical Center, New York, NY, p. A298

BREZICKA, Donald R., Executive Vice President, Austin Medical Center, Austin, MN, p. A226

BRICKEEN, Jerry W., USN, Commanding Officer, Naval Hospital, Lemoore, CA, p. A48

BRIDEAU, Leo P., General Director and Chief Executive Officer, Strong Memorial Hospital of the University of Rochester, Rochester, NY, p. A303

BRIDGE, Colleen, Administrator, Providence Seward Medical Center, Seward, AK, p. A21

BRIDGES, Daphne, President, Crawley Memorial Hospital, Boiling Springs, NC, p. A309

BRIDGES, James M., Executive Vice President, Baptist Medical Center/Columbia, Columbia, SC, p. A376

BRIGGS, Ronald O., President, St. Francis Memorial Hospital, West Point, NE, p. A268

BRILEY, Ellen, Administrator and Chief Executive Officer, Elba General Hospital, Elba, AL, p. A13

BRIMHALL, Dennis C., President, University of Colorado Hospital, Denver, CO, p. A72

BRINGHURST, John F.
Executive Vice President, Three Rivers Community Hospital and Health Center–Dimmick, Grants Pass, OR, p. A349
Executive Vice President, Three Rivers Community Hospital and Health Center–Washington, Grants Pass, OR, p. A349

BRINK, Gerald R., President and Chief Executive Officer, Riverside Regional Medical Center, Newport News, VA, p. A443

BRINKERS, J. A., Director, Veterans Affairs Medical Center, Sheridan, WY, p. A472

BRINKERT, William K., President, St. John of God Hospital, Brighton, MA, p. A205

BRINKMAN, Carollee, Chief Executive Officer, Graceville Health Center, Graceville, MN, p. A229

BRITT, John H., Executive Director, Massachusetts Hospital School, Canton, MA, p. A206

BRITTON, Gregory K., President and Chief Executive Officer, Beloit Memorial Hospital, Beloit, WI, p. A460

BROADBENT, Ernest J., President and Chief Executive Officer, Braintree Hospital Rehabilitation Network, Braintree, MA, p. A205

BROCCOLINO, Victor A., President and Chief Executive Officer, Howard County General Hospital, Columbia, MD, p. A199

BROCK, John D., Chief Executive Officer, Columbia Spring View Hospital, Lebanon, KY, p. A176

BROCKELMAN, Rodney, Administrator, Jewell County Hospital, Mankato, KS, p. A166

BROCKETTE, Darby, Administrator, Healthsouth Rehabilitation Center, Albuquerque, NM, p. A284

BROCKMANN, William F., President and Chief Executive Officer, Caylor–Nickel Medical Center, Bluffton, IN, p. A140

BRODEUR, Mark S., President, Touchette Regional Hospital, Centreville, IL, p. A125

BRODY, Robert J., President and Chief Executive Officer, St. Francis Hospital and Health Centers, Beech Grove, IN, p. A140

BRODY, Sue G., President, Bayfront Medical Center, Saint Petersburg, FL, p. A98

BROOKER, Ken, Interim Administrator, Brooks County Hospital, Quitman, GA, p. A112

BROOKHART, Duane, Ph.D., President and Chief Executive Officer, Columbia Northridge Medical Center, Prattville, AL, p. A17

BROOKS, Jesse, M.D., Administrator, Brooks Hospital, Atlanta, TX, p. A399

BROOKS, Phillip D., President, Norfolk Community Hospital, Norfolk, VA, p. A443

BROOKS, William P., Superintendent, Winfield State Hospital and Training Center, Winfield, KS, p. A171

BROOKS III, J. Milton, Administrator, Pineville Community Hospital Association, Pineville, KY, p. A179

BROPHY, James M., Senior Executive Officer, Saint Luke's Hospital, Kansas City, MO, p. A249

BROPHY, James M., FACHE, Senior Executive Officer, Saint Luke's Northland Hospital, Kansas City, MO, p. A249

BROSSEAU, Terrance G., President and Chief Executive Officer, MedCenter One, Bismarck, ND, p. A319

BROTHERS, R. Andrew
President and Chief Executive Officer, Mercy Community Hospital, Port Jervis, NY, p. A302
President and Chief Executive Officer, St. Anthony Community Hospital, Warwick, NY, p. A306

BROTMAN, Martin, M.D., President and Chief Executive Officer, California Pacific Medical Center, San Francisco, CA, p. A61

BROUGHTON, Pam McCullough, Chief Executive Officer, Greenbrier Hospital, Covington, LA, p. A184

BROUGHTON, Paul L., FACHE, Senior Vice President, Harper Hospital, Detroit, MI, p. A214

BROWER, Fred B., President and Chief Executive Officer, Trinity Health System, Steubenville, OH, p. A335

BROWN, Barbara, Warden, Oakwood Correctional Facility, Lima, OH, p. A331

BROWN, Betty Bolin, Acting Director, Veterans Affairs Medical Center, Fayetteville, NC, p. A311

BROWN, Carl D., Administrator, Lakeview Community Hospital, Eufaula, AL, p. A13

BROWN, Carl E., President, Delaware Valley Medical Center, Langhorne, PA, p. A360

BROWN, Cary D., Director, Veterans Affairs Medical Center, Big Spring, TX, p. A402

BROWN, David E., President and Chief Executive Officer, Beaufort Memorial Hospital, Beaufort, SC, p. A375

BROWN, David P., Administrator, Citizens Medical Center, Victoria, TX, p. A430

BROWN, Donald G., Chief Executive Officer, Community Memorial Hospital, Monmouth, IL, p. A134

BROWN, Fred L., President and Chief Executive Officer, BJC Health System, Saint Louis, MO, p. B71

BROWN, H. Thomas, Administrator, Cobb Memorial Hospital, Royston, GA, p. A113

BROWN, Harold W., Chief Executive Officer, Prairie Du Chien Memorial Hospital, Prairie Du Chien, WI, p. A467

BROWN, Jerry, Manager, Mercy Behavioral Health, Durango, CO, p. A72

BROWN, Lee, Administrator, Columbia Doctors Hospital Airline, Houston, TX, p. A413

BROWN, Lennea F., Interim Administrator, Bucktail Medical Center, Renovo, PA, p. A368

BROWN, Luella, Service Unit Director, U. S. Public Health Service Indian Hospital, Cass Lake, MN, p. A227

BROWN, Mary W., Executive Vice President and Director, Ochsner Foundation Hospital, New Orleans, LA, p. A189

BROWN, Murray L., Administrator, Neosho Memorial Regional Medical Center, Chanute, KS, p. A161

BROWN, Patricia W., Executive Director, Savannas Hospital, Port St. Lucie, FL, p. A98

BROWN, Rex H., President, Hillsboro Area Hospital, Hillsboro, IL, p. A131

BROWN, Richard V., Chief Executive Officer, Livingston Memorial Hospital, Livingston, MT, p. A259

BROWN, Richard W., President and Chief Executive Officer, Health Midwest, Kansas City, MO, p. B101

BROWN, Robin B., Vice President and Administrator, Scripps Hospital–East County, El Cajon, CA, p. A42

BROWN, Scott R., Administrator and Chief Executive Officer, Memorial Hospital, Dumas, TX, p. A408

BROWN, Shannon D., President, Betsy Johnson Memorial Hospital, Dunn, NC, p. A310

BROWN, Steven E., Administrator, Inova Fair Oaks Hospital, Fairfax, VA, p. A440

BROWN, Terry, Administrator and Chief Executive Officer, Healthsouth Lakeshore Rehabilitation Hospital, Birmingham, AL, p. A12

BROWN, William, Administrator, W. J. Barge Memorial Hospital, Greenville, SC, p. A378

BROWN, George J., M.D., Commanding General, Madigan Army Medical Center, Tacoma, WA, p. A453

BROWN, D. Creager, USAF, Administrator, David Grant Medical Center, Travis AFB, CA, p. A66

BROWN Jr., Michael J., Chief Executive Officer, Charter Behavioral Health System of Northwest Indiana, Hobart, IN, p. A143

BROWNE, J. Timothy, Chief Executive Officer, Columbia Hospital Maysville, Maysville, KY, p. A178

BROWNE, Norman E., Director, Veterans Affairs Medical Center, Albuquerque, NM, p. A285

BROWNING, Edward E., Administrator, Clay County Memorial Hospital, Henrietta, TX, p. A413

BROWNLEE, Walter W., President, Jefferson County Hospital, Fairfield, IA, p. A154

BROYLES, Dan P., Administrator, Harrison County Community Hospital, Bethany, MO, p. A245

BRUCE, Douglas A., Chief Executive Alaska Service Area, Providence Alaska Medical Center, Anchorage, AK, p. A20

BRUCE, Sandra B., President and Chief Executive Officer, Saint Alphonsus Regional Medical Center, Boise, ID, p. A119

BRUECKNER, Geraldine, Administrator, Pediatric Center for Restorative Care, Dallas, TX, p. A407

BRUECKNER, Gerry, R.N., Executive Director, Baylor Center for Restorative Care, Dallas, TX, p. A405

BRUECKNER, Robert G., President and Chief Executive Officer, St. John's Regional Medical Center, Joplin, MO, p. A248

BRUHN, Charles E., Chief Executive Officer, Memorial Community Hospital, Edgerton, WI, p. A462

BRULL–JOY, Pedro, Executive Director, Hospital Episcopal San Lucas, Ponce, PR, p. A476

BRUM, Joseph G., President and Chief Executive Officer, Henry Medical Center, Stockbridge, GA, p. A114

BRUMLOW Jr., James W., President and Chief Executive Officer, Wadsworth–Rittman Hospital, Wadsworth, OH, p. A336

BRUNDIGE, James E., Administrator, Haxtun Hospital District, Haxtun, CO, p. A73

BRUNICARDI, Rusty O., President, Community Hospitals of Williams County, Bryan, OH, p. A324

BRUNO, Frank, Chief Executive Officer, Gracie Square Hospital, New York, NY, p. A297

BRUNS, Dennis Ray, President and Chief Executive Officer, Hilton Head Medical Center and Clinics, Hilton Head Island, SC, p. A379

BRVENIK, Richard A., President and Chief Executive Officer, Northampton–Accomack Memorial Hospital, Nassawadox, VA, p. A443

BRYAN, Marilyn, Administrator, Roger Mills Memorial Hospital, Cheyenne, OK, p. A340

BRYAN–WILLIAMS, Margaret, Administrator, Shriners Hospitals for Children, San Francisco, San Francisco, CA, p. A62

BRYANT, W. Michael, President and Chief Executive Officer, Robert Wood Johnson University Hospital at Hamilton, Hamilton, NJ, p. A277

BRZUZ, Richard W., Administrator, Shriners Hospitals for Children, Erie Unit, Erie, PA, p. A357

BUCHANAN, Bruce F., FACHE, President and Chief Executive Officer, Mercy Health Center, Oklahoma City, OK, p. A344

BUCHANAN, Don, Chief Operating Officer, Aurora Community Hospital, Aurora, MO, p. A245

BUCHANON, A. C., Administrator, Cleveland Regional Medical Center, Cleveland, TX, p. A404

BUCK, Jack S., Chief Executive Officer, Columbia River Park Hospital, McMinnville, TN, p. A393

BUCKLAND, Eric
Administrator, North Lincoln Hospital, Lincoln City, OR, p. A350
Chief Executive Officer, Valley General Hospital, Monroe, WA, p. A450

BUCKLEY, Donald S., FACHE, President, Chesapeake General Hospital, Chesapeake, VA, p. A440

BUCKLEY, Howard R., President, Mercy Hospital Portland, Portland, ME, p. A195

BUCKLEY, Jeffrey L., President and Chief Executive Officer, Gateway Regional Health System, Mount Sterling, KY, p. A179

BUCKLEY, John F., Chief Executive Officer, Columbia Woodland Hospital, Hoffman Estates, IL, p. A132

BUCKLEY, John J., President and Chief Executive Officer, Pottstown Memorial Medical Center, Pottstown, PA, p. A367

BUCKLEY Jr., John J., President, Southern Illinois Hospital Services, Carbondale, IL, p. B137

BUCKNER, Terry, Administrator, Watonga Municipal Hospital, Watonga, OK, p. A347

BUCKNER, Wayne, Administrator, Baptist Hospital of Cocke County, Newport, TN, p. A395

BUCKNER Jr., James E., Administrator, Cuero Community Hospital, Cuero, TX, p. A405

BUDDE, Dale G., President, Marycrest Health System, Denver, CO, p. B112

BUDNICK, Michael J., Administrator and Chief Executive Officer, Gibson General Hospital, Princeton, IN, p. A148

BUDRYS, Ray, President and Chief Executive Officer, Holy Cross Hospital, Fort Lauderdale, FL, p. A87

BUECHLER, Verlin, President and Chief Executive Officer, Kenmare Community Hospital, Kenmare, ND, p. A321

BUFF, Gary, Ed.D., Administrator, Las Vegas Medical Center, Las Vegas, NM, p. A286

BUHRMANN, Henry J., President and Chief Executive Officer, Marin General Hospital, Greenbrae, CA, p. A45

BULGER, Robert J., President and Chief Executive Officer, Jeannette District Memorial Hospital, Jeannette, PA, p. A359

BULL, Jayne R., Administrator, Leelanau Memorial Health Center, Northport, MI, p. A221

BULLARD, Elizabeth A., Administrator, Madison Parish Hospital, Tallulah, LA, p. A191

BULLOCK, Scott B., President, Mid–Maine Medical Center, Waterville, ME, p. A196

BUMPAS, James C., Director, Central State Hospital, Petersburg, VA, p. A444

BUNDY, William H., Acting Administrator, Chester County Hospital and Nursing Center, Chester, SC, p. A376

BUNKER, Stephen P., President and Chief Operating Officer, Holmes Regional Medical Center, Melbourne, FL, p. A92

BURCHILL, Kevin R., Executive Director, Community Kimball Health Care System, Toms River, NJ, p. A282

BURD, Ronald P., President and Chief Exeucutive Officer, Devereux Foundation, Devon, PA, p. B95

BURDICK, Steve, Administrator, Providence Toppenish Hospital, Toppenish, WA, p. A454

BURDIN Jr., John J., President and Chief Executive Officer, Lafayette General Medical Center, Lafayette, LA, p. A186

BURFEIND, Raymond F., President, Covenant Medical Center, Waterloo, IA, p. A159

BURFITT, Gregory H., President and Chief Executive Officer, Brookwood Medical Center, Birmingham, AL, p. A11

BURGE, Larry J., Chief Executive Officer, BHC Spirit of St. Louis Hospital, Saint Charles, MO, p. A252

BURGEOIS, Anne, Interim Chief Executive Officer, Marlborough Hospital, Marlborough, MA, p. A207

BURGER, Janice, Operations Administrator, Providence Milwaukie Hospital, Milwaukie, OR, p. A350

BURGESS, Roger M., Administrator, St. Francis Hospital, Escanaba, MI, p. A215

BURGHER, Louis, Ph.D., President and Chief Executive Officer, Bishop Clarkson Memorial Hospital, Omaha, NE, p. A266

BURGIN, Robert F., President and Chief Executive Officer, Memorial Mission Medical Center, Asheville, NC, p. A308

BURGIO, David E., FACHE, Administrator and Chief Executive Officer, Berea Hospital, Berea, KY, p. A172

BURHARDT, Raye, Acting Administrator, Southern Inyo Healthcare District, Lone Pine, CA, p. A48

BURKE, Dennis E., Chief Executive Officer, Good Shepherd Community Hospital, Hermiston, OR, p. A349

BURKET, Mark, Chief Executive Officer, Platte Community Memorial Hospital, Platte, SD, p. A384

BURKETT, William T., Superintendent, Griffin Memorial Hospital, Norman, OK, p. A343

BURKHARDT Jr., J. Bland, Senior Vice President and Administrator, Greenville Memorial Hospital, Greenville, SC, p. A378

BURKHART, James R., FACHE
Administrator, Fort Sanders Regional Medical Center, Knoxville, TN, p. A391
Administrator, Fort Sanders–Parkwest Medical Center, Knoxville, TN, p. A391

BURN, Robert B., President and Chief Executive Officer, Washoe Medical Center, Reno, NV, p. A271

BURNETTE, W. Scott, Chief Executive Officer, Effingham Hospital, Springfield, GA, p. A114

BURNS, Charlotte, Administrator and Chief Executive Officer, Hardin County General Hospital, Savannah, TN, p. A396

BURNS, Dennis R., Administrator and Chief Executive Officer, Sonoma Valley Hospital, Sonoma, CA, p. A65

BURNS, Gregory T., Executive Director, St. Joseph's Community Hospital of West Bend, West Bend, WI, p. A470

BURNS, Randall, Director, Alaska Psychiatric Hospital, Anchorage, AK, p. A20

BURROUGHS, Michael R., President and Chief Executive Officer, Columbia Northlake Regional Medical Center, Atlanta, GA, p. A104

BURTON, Gary, Chief Executive Officer, Bledsoe County General Hospital, Pikeville, TN, p. A395

BURTON, W. R., Administrator, Memorial Hospital at Gulfport, Gulfport, MS, p. A239

BURZYNSKI, Cheryl A., President, Bay Special Care, Bay City, MI, p. A213

BUSBIN, Patsy, Acting Chief Executive Officer, Bacon County Hospital, Alma, GA, p. A103

BUSCH, Walter, Administrator, Roosevelt Memorial Medical Center, Culbertson, MT, p. A258

BUSER, Kenneth R., President and Chief Executive Officer, Union Memorial Hospital, Baltimore, MD, p. A198

BUSER, Martin B., Executive Vice President Health Services, Scripps Health, San Diego, CA, p. B131

BUSH, Mark E., Executive Vice President, MidMichigan Regional Medical Center–Gladwin, Gladwin, MI, p. A216

BUSHMAIER, Jim E., Administrator and Chief Executive Officer, Stuttgart Regional Medical Center, Stuttgart, AR, p. A35

BUSTELOS Jr., John, President, Griffin Hospital, Derby, CT, p. A76

BUTIKOFER, Lon D., Ph.D., Administrator and Chief Executive Officer, Delaware County Memorial Hospital, Manchester, IA, p. A156

BUTKUS, S. J., Ph.D., Director, Central Virginia Training Center, Madison Heights, VA, p. A442

BUTLER, Beatrice, Superintendent, Terrell State Hospital, Terrell, TX, p. A428

BUTLER, Everett A., Administrator, North Valley Health Center, Warren, MN, p. A236

BUTLER, Frank, Director, University of Kentucky Hospital, Lexington, KY, p. A176

BUTLER, Richard E.
Chief Executive Officer, Fountain Valley Regional Hospital and Medical Center, Fountain Valley, CA, p. A43
Chief Executive Officer, Western Medical Center–Santa Ana, Santa Ana, CA, p. A63

BUTLER, Ronald G., Chief Executive Officer, Columbia Eastern Idaho Regional Medical Center, Idaho Falls, ID, p. A120

BUTLER, Ronald J., Executive Director, Soldiers and Sailors Memorial Hospital, Wellsboro, PA, p. A370

BUTLER Jr., Joe W., Deputy Commander and Administrator, Bayne–Jones Army Community Hospital, Fort Polk, LA, p. A184

BUTTERFIELD, Rohn J., Chief Executive Officer, Magnolia Regional Health Center, Corinth, MS, p. A238

BUTTS, Charles N., Administrator, East Texas Medical Center–Mount Vernon, Mount Vernon, TX, p. A421

BUTTS, Donald E., Chief Executive Officer, Columbia Gulf Coast Medical Center, Panama City, FL, p. A96

BUURMAN, Rita K., Administrator, Sabetha Community Hospital, Sabetha, KS, p. A169

BYBEE, Bob L., President and Chief Executive Officer, Memorial Medical Center, Port Lavaca, TX, p. A424

BYNUM, Dennis T., Interim Chief Executive Officer, North Crest Medical Center, Springfield, TN, p. A396

BYRD, Mark, Chief Executive Officer, Mary Hurley Hospital, Coalgate, OK, p. A340

BYRNE, Frank D., M.D., President, Parkview Memorial Hospital, Fort Wayne, IN, p. A142

BYRNES, Nancy A., President and Chief Executive Officer, Columbia Navarro Regional Hospital, Corsicana, TX, p. A405

BYROM, David, Administrator, Coryell Memorial Hospital, Gatesville, TX, p. A411

C

CACKLER, Ron, President and Chief Executive Officer, Cushing Regional Hospital, Cushing, OK, p. A340

CAGEN, Richard M., Chief Executive Officer and Administrator, LDS Hospital, Salt Lake City, UT, p. A435

CAGLE, Brooks, Chief Executive Officer, Charter Rivers Behavioral Health System, West Columbia, SC, p. A381

CAHILL, Patricia A., Chief Executive Officer, Catholic Health Initiatives, Denver, CO, p. B75

CALAMARI, Frank A., President and Chief Executive Officer, Calvary Hospital, New York, NY, p. A296

CALBONE, Angelo G., President and Chief Executive Officer, Mount St. Mary's Hospital of Niagara Falls, Lewiston, NY, p. A293

CALDERIN, Carolina, Chief Executive Officer, Pan American Hospital, Miami, FL, p. A93

CALDWELL, Darren, Chief Executive Officer, Drew Memorial Hospital, Monticello, AR, p. A33

CALDWELL, Harvey G., Administrator and Chief Executive Officer, Brainerd Regional Human Services Center, Brainerd, MN, p. A227

CALDWELL, Robert, Chief Operating Officer, St. Joseph Center for Mental Health, Omaha, NE, p. A267

CALE, Barbara R., Administrator, Chowan Hospital, Edenton, NC, p. A311

CALEY, George B., President, Winchester Medical Center, Winchester, VA, p. A447

CALGI, Dominick R., Senior Vice President and Administrator, Saint Michael's Medical Center, Newark, NJ, p. A280

CALHOUN, Kevin P., President and Chief Executive Officer, Bell Memorial Hospital, Ishpeming, MI, p. A218

CALICO, Forrest, M.D., President, Appalachian Regional Healthcare, Lexington, KY, p. B66

CALLAHAN, Keith L., Executive Vice President and Administrator, St. Mary's Hospital, Decatur, IL, p. A129

CALLAHAN, Kevin J., President and Chief Executive Officer, Exeter Hospital, Exeter, NH, p. A272

CALLAHAN, Michael A., Chief Executive Officer, Northwest Texas Healthcare System, Amarillo, TX, p. A398

CALLAN Sr., Michael J., Chief Executive Officer, Ashland Regional Medical Center, Ashland, PA, p. A353

CALLAWAY, Warren E., FACHE, Administrator, Carraway Methodist Medical Center, Birmingham, AL, p. A12

CALLISON, William L., Chief Executive Officer, Charter Greenville Behavioral Health System, Greer, SC, p. A379

CALTRIDER, Jerry, Administrator, Bradford Health Services at Oak Mountain, Pelham, AL, p. A17

CAMBRIA, Susan A., Chief Executive Officer, Charter Brookside Behavioral Health System of New England, Nashua, NH, p. A273

CAMERON, Marie, FACHE, President and Chief Executive Officer, Southwest Hospital and Medical Center, Atlanta, GA, p. A104

CAMMACK Jr., Thomas N., Chief Executive Officer, Marshall Regional Medical Center, Marshall, TX, p. A420

CAMPBELL, Bruce C., President, Illinois Masonic Medical Center, Chicago, IL, p. A125

CAMPBELL, C. Scott, Executive Director, Bulloch Memorial Hospital, Statesboro, GA, p. A114

CAMPBELL, David J., President and Chief Executive Officer, Detroit Medical Center, Detroit, MI, p. B94

CAMPBELL, Deborah, Administrator, Thomas H. Boyd Memorial Hospital, Carrollton, IL, p. A124

CAMPBELL, Gary L., Director, Harry S. Truman Memorial Veterans Hospital, Columbia, MO, p. A246

CAMPBELL, H. Neil, Chief Executive Officer, Vendell Healthcare, Inc., Nashville, TN, p. B148

CAMPBELL, Phil, FACHE, Administrator, Woods Memorial Hospital District, Etowah, TN, p. A389

CAMPBELL, Rita, Chief Executive Officer, Holy Cross Hospital, Taos, NM, p. A287

CAMPBELL, Ronald, Administrator, McCurtain Memorial Hospital, Idabel, OK, p. A342

CAMPBELL, Stephen J., Administrator, Southwestern General Hospital, El Paso, TX, p. A409

CAMPBELL, Wayne, Chief Executive Officer, Columbia Fort Walton Beach Medical Center, Fort Walton Beach, FL, p. A87

CAMPBELL, William E., Ph.D., Superintendent, Glenwood State Hospital School, Glenwood, IA, p. A154

CAMPBELL, Paul E., USN, Commanding Officer, Naval Hospital, Patuxent River, MD, p. A201

CAMPBELL Jr., Robert D., Administrator, Cascade Valley Hospital, North Snohomish County Health System, Arlington, WA, p. A448

CAMPION, Brian C., M.D., President and Chief Executive Officer, Franciscan Skemp Healthcare, La Crosse, WI, p. B98

CANDINO, Paul J., Chief Executive Officer, Erie County Medical Center, Buffalo, NY, p. A290

CANISIA, M., Administrator, Saint Francis Medical Center, Peoria, IL, p. A136

CANNINGTON, H. D., Administrator, Jay Hospital, Jay, FL, p. A90

CANTRELL, Dianne, Acting Administrator, Longview General Hospital, Graysville, AL, p. A15

CANTRELL, Gary, President and Chief Executive Officer, Columbia Lawnwood Regional Medical Center, Fort Pierce, FL, p. A87

CAPOBIANCO, Peter E., President and Chief Executive Officer, St. Mary's Hospital, Amsterdam, NY, p. A288

CAPONI, Vincent C., President and Chief Executive Officer, St. Vincent's Hospital, Birmingham, AL, p. A12

CAPPELLO, Thomas A., Director, Veterans Affairs Pittsburgh Healthcare System, Pittsburgh, PA, p. A367

CARBONE, Davide M., Chief Executive Officer, Columbia Aventura Hospital and Medical Center, Miami, FL, p. A92

CARBONE, Nick, Chief Executive Officer, Columbia Regional Medical Center of Southwest Florida, Fort Myers, FL, p. A87

CARDA, Timothy L.
Chief Executive Officer, Anaheim General Hospital, Anaheim, CA, p. A36
Administrator and Chief Executive Officer, Buena Park Medical Center, Buena Park, CA, p. A38

CAREY, Frederick M., Executive Director, West Jersey Hospital–Camden, Camden, NJ, p. A276

CAREY, Patricia E., FACHE, Administrator, Northeast Baptist Hospital, San Antonio, TX, p. A426

CARL, Gerald E.
Administrator, Arnold Memorial Health Care Center, Adrian, MN, p. A226
Administrator, Luverne Community Hospital, Luverne, MN, p. A231

CARLBERG, Duane A., President, Windham Community Memorial Hospital, Willimantic, CT, p. A79

CARLE, Chris, Administrator, St. Elizabeth Medical Center–Grant County, Williamstown, KY, p. A181

CARLISLE, John T., Chief Executive Officer, Cape Fear Valley Health System, Fayetteville, NC, p. A311

CARLSON, Brian J., Administrator, Lake View Memorial Hospital, Two Harbors, MN, p. A235

CARLSON, Donald R., President and Chief Executive Officer, San Juan Regional Medical Center, Farmington, NM, p. A285

CARLSON, Greg L., President and Chief Executive Officer, Owensboro Mercy Health System, Owensboro, KY, p. A179

CARLSON, Joan M., President and Chief Executive Officer, St. Joseph Hospital and Health Centers, Memphis, TN, p. A393

CARLSON, Roland R., Administrator, Sandwich Community Hospital, Sandwich, IL, p. A137

CARLSON, Stephen G., President and Chief Operating Officer, Flagstaff Medical Center, Flagstaff, AZ, p. A23

CARLSTEDT, Nancy S., President, Bloomington Hospital, Bloomington, IN, p. A140

CARMAN, Robert O., President, Wuesthoff Hospital, Rockledge, FL, p. A98

CARMAN, Thomas H., President and Chief Executive Officer, Cortland Memorial Hospital, Cortland, NY, p. A291

CARMICHAEL, LeRoy, Executive Director, Bronx Psychiatric Center, New York, NY, p. A295

CARMONA, Richard, M.D., Chief Executive Officer, Kino Community Hospital, Tucson, AZ, p. A27

CARNETT, William, D.O., Acting Administrator, Hilo Medical Center, Hilo, HI, p. A117

CARNEY, Christopher M., President and Chief Executive Officer, Bon Secours Health System, Inc., Marriottsville, MD, p. B71

CAROBENE, Joseph W., Superintendent, Middle Tennessee Mental Health Institute, Nashville, TN, p. A394

CAROSELLI, Joseph P., Administrator, Idaho Elks Rehabilitation Hospital, Boise, ID, p. A119

CARPENTER, David R., FACHE
Senior Vice President and Administrator, Scottsdale Memorial Hospital–Osborn, Scottsdale, AZ, p. A26
President and Chairman of the Board, UniHealth, Burbank, CA, p. B144

CARR, C. Larry, President, Bakersfield Memorial Hospital, Bakersfield, CA, p. A37

CARR, Wiley N., President and Chief Executive Officer, Porter Memorial Hospital, Valparaiso, IN, p. A149

CARRELL, Jan V., Chief Executive Officer, Riverside Medical Center, Waupaca, WI, p. A470

CARRIER, Patrick Brian, Administrator, Opelousas General Hospital, Opelousas, LA, p. A189

CARRINGTON–MURRAY, Cynthia, Executive Director, Woodhull Medical and Mental Health Center, New York, NY, p. A300

CARROCINO, Joanne, Executive Director, Kimball Medical Center, Lakewood, NJ, p. A278

CARROLL, Allen P., Chief Executive Officer, Bon Secours–St. Francis Xavier Hospital, Charleston, SC, p. A375

CARROLL, James J., Administrator, Community Memorial Hospital and Convalescent and Nursing Care Section, Cloquet, MN, p. A228

CARROLL, Kevin J., President, Champlain Valley Physicians Hospital Medical Center, Plattsburgh, NY, p. A302

CARROLL, Michael W., Administrator, Richland Parish Hospital–Delhi, Delhi, LA, p. A184

CARROLL, Dale, Commander, Moncrief Army Community Hospital, Fort Jackson, SC, p. A378

CARSON, Mitch C., President, Ball Memorial Hospital, Muncie, IN, p. A147

CARSON, Randal E., Administrator, Methodist Hospital of McKenzie, McKenzie, TN, p. A393

CARSON, Sandra C., FACHE, President and Chief Executive Officer, Methodist Richard Young, Omaha, NE, p. A267

CARSON, Terry, Chief Executive Officer, Harrison Community Hospital, Cadiz, OH, p. A324

CARTER, Bruce C., President, United Hospital Center, Clarksburg, WV, p. A456

CARTER, Richard, Chief Executive Officer, Hunt Memorial Hospital District, Greenville, TX, p. A412

CARTY, Clare, President and Chief Executive Officer, St. Mary Medical Center, Langhorne, PA, p. A360

CARVER, John W., FACHE, Executive Director, Methodist Medical Center, Dallas, TX, p. A406

CARY, Roger C., President and Chief Executive Officer, Midwestern Regional Medical Center, Zion, IL, p. A139

CASADAY, Thomas E.
President, RHD Memorial Medical Center, Dallas, TX, p. A407
President, Trinity Medical Center, Carrollton, TX, p. A403

CASCONE, John J., Chief Executive Officer, ValueMark–Brawner Behavioral Healthcare System–North, Smyrna, GA, p. A114

CASEY, Dennis A., Executive Director, Albert Lindley Lee Memorial Hospital, Fulton, NY, p. A292

CASEY, Jack, Administrator, Shodair Children's Hospital, Helena, MT, p. A259

CASEY, Timothy M., President and Chief Executive Officer, Montgomery Hospital, Norristown, PA, p. A362

CASEY, William F., President and Chief Executive Officer, Conemaugh Memorial Medical Center, Johnstown, PA, p. A359

CASEY, Lynn, President and Chief Executive Officer, St. Mary's Hospital and Medical Center, Grand Junction, CO, p. A73

CASH, Robert, Chief Executive Officer, Davis Hospital and Medical Center, Layton, UT, p. A433

CASHION, John A., FACHE, President, Lexington Memorial Hospital, Lexington, NC, p. A313

CASSELL, Carol M., Executive Vice President and Chief Operating Officer, Millard Fillmore Health System, Buffalo, NY, p. A290

CASSIDY, James E., President and Chief Executive Officer, St. Mary's Regional Medical Center, Lewiston, ME, p. A194

CASSIDY, Michael E., Administrator, Stringfellow Memorial Hospital, Anniston, AL, p. A11

CASTAGNARO, Marie, President and Chief Executive Officer, St. Joseph's Hospital, Elmira, NY, p. A292

CASTRO, William Rodriguez, Executive Director, Aguadilla General Hospital, Aguadilla, PR, p. A474

CASTROP, Richard F., President, O'Bleness Memorial Hospital, Athens, OH, p. A323

CATALANO, Robert A., M.D., President and Chief Executive Officer, Olean General Hospital, Olean, NY, p. A301

CATALDO, Vince A., Administrator, Prevost Memorial Hospital, Donaldsonville, LA, p. A184

CATENA, Cornelio R., President and Chief Executive Officer, Amsterdam Memorial Hospital, Amsterdam, NY, p. A288

CATHEY, Shawn, Administrator, Dardanelle Hospital, Dardanelle, AR, p. A30

CATHEY Jr., James E., Chief Executive Officer, North Oaks Medical Center, Hammond, LA, p. A185

CATLIN, Rex, Chief Executive Officer, Endless Mountain Health Systems, Montrose, PA, p. A362

CATON, James R., Chief Executive Officer, Logan Hospital and Medical Center, Guthrie, OK, p. A341

CAVALLI, Paul V., M.D., President, Meadowlands Hospital Medical Center, Secaucus, NJ, p. A281

CAVES, Donald, President, Wild Rose Community Memorial Hospital, Wild Rose, WI, p. A470

CECCHINI, Marina
Chief Executive Officer, Charter Hospital of Winston–Salem, Winston–Salem, NC, p. A318
Chief Executive Officer, Charter Indianapolis Behavioral Health System, Indianapolis, IN, p. A144

CECCONI, Thomas E., Chief Executive Officer, Doctors Hospital of Stark County, Massillon, OH, p. A332

CECERO, David M., President and Chief Executive Officer, West Suburban Hospital Medical Center, Oak Park, IL, p. A135

CELMER, Mark E., President and Chief Executive Officer, Woman's Christian Association Hospital, Jamestown, NY, p. A293

CENTAFANTI, Gary, Vice President and Executive Director, Willough at Naples, Naples, FL, p. A94

CERNI, Joseph P., President and Chief Executive Officer, Lutheran Medical Center, New York, NY, p. A298

CERNY, Ralph J., President and Chief Executive Officer, Munson Medical Center, Traverse City, MI, p. A224

CETTI, Janet E., President and Chief Executive Officer, San Diego Hospice, San Diego, CA, p. A61

CHADDIC, Jim, Chief Executive Officer, Goodland Regional Medical Center, Goodland, KS, p. A163

CHALONER, Robert S.
President and Chief Executive Officer, St. Francis Hospital, Jersey City, NJ, p. A278
President and Chief Executive Officer, St. Mary Hospital, Hoboken, NJ, p. A278

CHAMBERS, Bruce, Ph.D., Chief Executive Officer, Charter Pines Behavioral Health System, Charlotte, NC, p. A309

CHAMP, Raymond L., President, Wake Medical Center, Raleigh, NC, p. A315

CHANDLER, Brue, President and Chief Executive Officer, Saint Joseph's Hospital of Atlanta, Atlanta, GA, p. A104

CHANEY, Dennis R., Administrator, Morgan County Appalachian Regional Hospital, West Liberty, KY, p. A181

CHANNING, Alan H., President and Chief Executive Officer, New York Downtown Hospital, New York, NY, p. A298

CHAPA, Al, Chief Executive Officer, Columbia Medical Arts Hospital, Dallas, TX, p. A406

CHAPIN, Ted G., Chief Executive Officer, Chatham Hospital, Siler City, NC, p. A316

CHAPMAN, Alan G., Administrator and Chief Executive Officer, BHC Aspen Hill Hospital, Flagstaff, AZ, p. A22

CHAPMAN, Richard, Administrator, Trigg County Hospital, Cadiz, KY, p. A172

CHAPMAN, Robert C., FACHE, President and Chief Executive Officer, Eastern Health System, Inc., Birmingham, AL, p. B96

CHAPMAN, Stephen, Executive Director, Marlboro Park Hospital, Bennettsville, SC, p. A375

CHAPPELOW, Michael W., President and Chief Executive Officer, Medical Center of Independence, Independence, MO, p. A248

CHARLES, Timothy, Chief Executive Officer, Denton Community Hospital, Denton, TX, p. A408

CHARYULU, Cindy, Chief Executive Officer, Lost Rivers District Hospital, Arco, ID, p. A119

CHASE, Alide, Administrator, Kaiser Sunnyside Medical Center, Clackamas, OR, p. A348

CHASE, Howard M., FACHE, President and Chief Executive Officer, Methodist Hospitals of Dallas, Dallas, TX, p. B116

CHASTAIN, James G., Director, Mississippi State Hospital, Whitfield, MS, p. A244

CHASTANG, Mark, President and Chief Executive Officer, East Orange General Hospital, East Orange, NJ, p. A276

CHATTERTON, Claude, Chief Executive Officer, Harrisburg Medical Center, Harrisburg, IL, p. A131

CHAUDRY, Moe, Chief Executive Officer, Lake Chelan Community Hospital, Chelan, WA, p. A448

CHECK, Rosemary C., Chief Executive Officer, Greensville Memorial Hospital, Emporia, VA, p. A440

CHERAMIE, Lane M., Chief Executive Officer, Lady of the Sea General Hospital, Cut Off, LA, p. A184

CHESNEY, Murphy A., Commander, U. S. Air Force Regional Hospital, Minot, ND, p. A321

CHESNUT, Arden, Administrator, J. Paul Jones Hospital, Camden, AL, p. A12

CHESTER, Sandra M., Chief Executive Officer, Whittier Hospital Medical Center, Whittier, CA, p. A68

CHEWNING III, Larry H., Chief Executive Officer, Wythe County Community Hospital, Wytheville, VA, p. A447

CHIARAMONTE, Francis P., M.D., Chief Executive Officer, Southern Maryland Hospital, Clinton, MD, p. A199

CHICK, James R., President, Joint Township District Memorial Hospital, Saint Marys, OH, p. A335

CHILDERS Jr., Leo F., FACHE, President, Good Samaritan Regional Health Center, Mount Vernon, IL, p. A134

CHILDS, Ronald P., FACHE, Health Services Administrator, Midlands Center, Columbia, SC, p. A377

CHILL, Martha O'Regan, Administrator and Chief Executive Officer, Pikeville United Methodist Hospital of Kentucky, Pikeville, KY, p. A179

CHILTON, Harold E.
Chief Executive Officer, Sierra Vista Regional Medical Center, San Luis Obispo, CA, p. A63
Chief Executive Officer, Twin Cities Community Hospital, Templeton, CA, p. A66

CHINNERY, H. M., Director, Administration, Naval Hospital, Pensacola, FL, p. A97

CHIOUTSIS, John M., Chief Executive Officer, Rosebud Health Care Center, Forsyth, MT, p. A258

CHIRCOP, Marc, Chief Executive Officer, Daviess County Hospital, Washington, IN, p. A149

CHMURA, Rudy, Superintendent, Soldiers' Home in Holyoke, Holyoke, MA, p. A207

CHO, Gordon W., Chief of Staff, William Beaumont Army Medical Center, El Paso, TX, p. A409

CHODKOWSKI, Paul J.
President and Chief Executive Officer, Redwood Memorial Hospital, Fortuna, CA, p. A43
President and Chief Executive Officer, Saint Joseph Hospital, Eureka, CA, p. A42

CHOLETTE, Robert, President and Chief Executive Officer, Catholic Medical Center, Manchester, NH, p. A273

CHOLETTE, Robert G., Chief Executive Officer, Elliot Hospital, Manchester, NH, p. A273

CHONG, Glenn W.
Senior Vice President and Administrator, Green Hospital of Scripps Clinic, La Jolla, CA, p. A47
Senior Vice President and Administrator, Scripps Memorial Hospital–La Jolla, La Jolla, CA, p. A47

CHRISTENSEN, C. James, Chief Executive Officer, DeWitt Community Hospital, De Witt, IA, p. A153

CHRISTENSEN, Jay, Administrator, Pocahontas Community Hospital, Pocahontas, IA, p. A158

CHRISTENSON, John N., President, St. Marys Regional Medical Center, Saint Marys, PA, p. A368

CHRISTIAN, James A., Director, Veterans Affairs Medical Center, Asheville, NC, p. A308

CHRISTIAN, Patricia L., Ph.D., Director, John Umstead Hospital, Butner, NC, p. A309

CHRISTIANSEN, Gary, President and Chief Executive Officer, Carondelet Health System, Saint Louis, MO, p. B75

CHRISTIANSON, Clark P.
Senior Vice President and Administrator, Memorial Hospital–Flagler, Bunnell, FL, p. A84
Senior Vice President and Administrator, Memorial Hospital–Ormond Beach, Ormond Beach, FL, p. A96

CHRISTIANSON, Del, Administrator, St. Michael's Hospital, Sauk Centre, MN, p. A235

CHRISTIANSON, Paul B., USAF, Commander, U. S. Air Force Hospital–Kirtland, Kirtland AFB, NM, p. A286

CHRISTIE, Arthur P., Administrator, Houston Medical Center, Warner Robins, GA, p. A115

CHRISTISON, Earl L., Administrator, Pocatello Regional Medical Center, Pocatello, ID, p. A121

CHRISTOPHER, William T., President and Chief Executive Officer, Lawrence and Memorial Hospital, New London, CT, p. A78

CHROMIK, James R., Regional Vice President, Administration, North Broward Medical Center, Pompano Beach, FL, p. A97

CHRZAN, Robert A., President and Chief Executive Officer, Children's Hospital and Center for Reconstructive Surgery, Baltimore, MD, p. A197

CHURCH, Daniel K., Ph.D., President and Chief Executive Officer, Edwin Shaw Hospital, Akron, OH, p. A323

CHURCH Jr., John D., Director, Veterans Affairs Medical Center, New Orleans, LA, p. A189

CHURCHILL, Timothy A., President, Stephens Memorial Hospital, Norway, ME, p. A195

CIBRAN, Bert, President and Chief Operating Officer, Ramsay Health Care, Inc., Coral Gobles, FL, p. B129

CIERLIK, Gregory A.
President and Chief Executive Officer, Louis A Weiss Memorial Hospital/University of Chicago Hospitals, Chicago, IL, p. B109
President and Chief Executive Officer, Louis A. Weiss Memorial Hospital, Chicago, IL, p. A126

CIMEROLA, Joseph M., FACHE, President and Chief Executive Officer, Sacred Heart Hospital, Allentown, PA, p. A353

CINCINAT, Cathy L., Acting Chief Executive Officer, Massillon Psychiatric Center, Massillon, OH, p. A332

CIRNE–NEVES, Ceu, Administrator, Saint James Hospital of Newark, Newark, NJ, p. A280

CITRON, Richard S., Acting Director, Veterans Affairs Medical Center, Cleveland, OH, p. A327

CIULLA, Don S., Chief Executive Officer, Columbia Medical Center of McKinney, McKinney, TX, p. A420

CLABOTS, Leland G., President and Chief Executive Officer, Phoenix Children's Hospital, Phoenix, AZ, p. A25

CLAIRMONT, Thomas, President, Lakes Region General Hospital, Laconia, NH, p. A273

CLARK, Barbara J., Vice President and Chief Operating Officer, Michigan Hospital and Medical Center, Detroit, MI, p. A215

CLARK, Dale E., Ph.D., Administrator and Chief Executive Officer, East Texas Medical Center, Crockett, TX, p. A405

CLARK, David D., CHE, Administrator and Vice President, Spohn Kleberg Memorial Hospital, Kingsville, TX, p. A417

CLARK, Douglas A., Executive Director, Latrobe Area Hospital, Latrobe, PA, p. A360

CLARK, Ira C., President, Jackson Memorial Hospital, Miami, FL, p. A93

CLARK, James A., Director, Veterans Affairs Medical Center, Northport, NY, p. A301

CLARK, Kenneth J., Executive Director and Chief Executive Officer, Veterans Affairs Medical Center–West Los Angeles, Los Angeles, CA, p. A52

CLARK, M. Victoria, Administrator, Palo Verde Hospital, Blythe, CA, p. A38

CLARK, Melinda, President, SSM Rehabilitation Institute, Saint Louis, MO, p. A254

CLARK, Michael, Chief Executive Officer, Flint River Community Hospital, Montezuma, GA, p. A112

CLARK, Michael G., Administrator, Yuma District Hospital, Yuma, CO, p. A75

CLARK, Richard L., Administrator and Chief Executive Officer, Morristown–Hamblen Hospital, Morristown, TN, p. A394

CLARK, Robert J., FACHE, President and Chief Executive Officer, Gnaden Huetten Memorial Hospital, Lehighton, PA, p. A360

CLARK, Steven E., Administrator, Grim–Smith Hospital and Clinic, Kirksville, MO, p. A250

CLARK, Thomas, President and Chief Executive Officer, Saints Memorial Medical Center, Lowell, MA, p. A207

CLARK, William S., Chief Executive Officer, Columbus County Hospital, Whiteville, NC, p. A318

CLARK, David L., USAF, Commander, U. S. Air Force Hospital Altus, Altus, OK, p. A339

CLARK Jr., Ralph, President, Helen Keller Hospital, Sheffield, AL, p. A18

CLARKE, Richard W., Chief Executive Officer, Emanuel County Hospital, Swainsboro, GA, p. A114

CLARKE, Robert T.
President and Chief Executive Officer, Memorial Health System, Springfield, IL, p. B113
President and Chief Executive Officer, Memorial Medical Center, Springfield, IL, p. A138

CLASSEN, Howard H., Chief Executive Officer, Natividad Medical Center, Salinas, CA, p. A60

CLAY, Jim, Director, Veterans Affairs Medical Center, Tuskegee, AL, p. A18

CLAYTON, Philip A., President and Chief Executive Officer, Conway Hospital, Conway, SC, p. A377

CLEARY, John J., President and Chief Executive Officer, River Oaks Hospital, Jackson, MS, p. A240

CLEM, Olie E., Chief Executive Officer, Doctors Memorial Hospital, Tyler, TX, p. A429

CLEMENS, Brian L., Chief Executive Officer, North Arkansas Medical Center, Harrison, AR, p. A31

CLEMENT, Mark C., President and Chief Executive Officer, Holy Cross Hospital, Chicago, IL, p. A125

CLEMENT, N. Bruce, Chief Executive Officer, Marquette General Hospital, Marquette, MI, p. A220

CLEMENTS, Larry E., Administrator, Wildwood Lifestyle Center and Hospital, Wildwood, GA, p. A116

CLENDENIN, Harrell E., Vice President and Administrator, Baptist Medical Center Heber Springs, Heber Springs, AR, p. A31

CLIBORNE Jr., James J., Chief Executive Officer, Selby General Hospital, Marietta, OH, p. A332

CLICK, Mike, Administrator, Brownfield Regional Medical Center, Brownfield, TX, p. A402

CLINE, Phillip E., Administrator, Providence Kodiak Island Hospital and Medical Center, Kodiak, AK, p. A21

CLOUGH, Jeanette G., President and Chief Executive Officer, Deaconess Waltham Hospital, Waltham, MA, p. A210

COATES, Cliff, Chief Executive Officer, Community Hospital, Santa Rosa, CA, p. A64

COATES, David M., Ph.D., President and Chief Executive Officer, Reed City Hospital Corporation, Reed City, MI, p. A222

COATS, David B., President, University of California San Diego Medical Center, San Diego, CA, p. A61

COATS, Rodney M., Executive Director, Washington County Memorial Hospital, Salem, IN, p. A148

COBB, Terrell M., Executive Director, Greenwood Leflore Hospital, Greenwood, MS, p. A239

COCHRAN, Barry S.
President, Cherokee Baptist Medical Center, Centre, AL, p. A12
President, DeKalb Baptist Medical Center, Fort Payne, AL, p. A14

COCHRAN, Gloria, Administrator, Burke County Hospital, Waynesboro, GA, p. A116

COCHRAN, John, Administrator, Richland Hospital, Mansfield, OH, p. A332

CODY, Carol, Administrator, Christopher House, Austin, TX, p. A400

CODY, Douglas M., Administrator, Amos Cottage Rehabilitation Hospital, Winston-Salem, NC, p. A318

COE, Isaac S., President, Harris Regional Hospital, Sylva, NC, p. A317

COE, William G., Administrator and Chief Executive Officer, Parker Community Hospital, Parker, AZ, p. A24

COHEN, Elliot G., Senior Executive Officer, Univerisity Hospital, Cincinnati, OH, p. A326

COHEN, Howard C., Executive Director, Coney Island Hospital, New York, NY, p. A296

COHEN, Jed M., Acting Executive Director, Western New York Children's Psychiatric Center, West Seneca, NY, p. A307

COHEN, Philip A., Chief Executive Officer, Garfield Medical Center, Monterey Park, CA, p. A54

COHEN, Steven M., M.D., Director, Veterans Affairs Medical Center, Dayton, OH, p. A329

COHOLICH, Robert J., Chief Executive Officer, Henry County Hospital, Napoleon, OH, p. A333

COKER Jr., Robert J., Administrator, Greene County Hospital, Eutaw, AL, p. A14

COLBERG, Gary R., President and Chief Executive Officer, Hardin Memorial Hospital, Elizabethtown, KY, p. A173

COLBY, Dan, Administrator, Harvard Memorial Hospital, Harvard, IL, p. A131

COLCHER, Marian W., President, Valley Forge Medical Center and Hospital, Norristown, PA, p. A362

COLE, Geoffrey F., President and Chief Executive Officer, Emerson Hospital, Concord, MA, p. A206

COLE, James B., President and Chief Executive Officer, Arlington Hospital, Arlington, VA, p. A439

COLE, James M., President and Chief Executive Officer, Cleo Wallace Center Hospital, Westminster, CO, p. A75

COLE, Marvin E., President and Chief Executive Officer, Fayette Memorial Hospital, La Grange, TX, p. A418

COLECCHI, Stephen, President and Chief Executive Officer, Robinson Memorial Hospital, Ravenna, OH, p. A334

COLEMAN, Dan C., President and Chief Executive Officer, John C. Lincoln Health Network, Phoenix, AZ, p. A25

COLEMAN, David, Director, Youth Focus Psychiatric Hospital, Greensboro, NC, p. A312

COLEMAN, Dennis E., President and Chief Executive Officer, Granada Hills Community Hospital, Los Angeles, CA, p. A50

COLEMAN, James, Director, Kalamazoo Regional Psychiatric Hospital, Kalamazoo, MI, p. A219

COLEMAN, Kevin T., Administrator, Baptist Hospital–Orange, Orange, TX, p. A422

COLFACK, Brian R., CHE, President and Chief Executive Officer, Berger Hospital, Circleville, OH, p. A326

COLLER, James G., Executive Vice President and Administrator, St. Mary's Hospital Medical Center, Green Bay, WI, p. A462

COLLETE, Robert, Chief Executive Officer, Brownsville Medical Center, Brownsville, TX, p. A402

COLLETTE, Dennis H., President and Chief Executive Officer, Newton Memorial Hospital, Newton, NJ, p. A280

COLLIER, C. Thomas, President and Chief Executive Officer, Sierra Nevada Memorial Hospital, Grass Valley, CA, p. A45

COLLIER, Sherry, Chief Nursing Officer and Chief Operating Officer, Medical Center of Manchester, Manchester, TN, p. A392

COLLING, Kenneth F., Administrator, Kaiser Foundation Hospital, San Diego, CA, p. A60

COLLINS, Dale, President and Chief Executive Officer, Baptist Health System of Tennessee, Knoxville, TN, p. B68

COLLINS, Jeffrey A., Chief Executive Officer, Sun Coast Hospital, Largo, FL, p. A91

COLLINS, Karen, Administrator, Faulk County Memorial Hospital, Faulkton, SD, p. A383

COLLINS, Michael F., M.D.
President, Caritas Christi Health Care System, Boston, MA, p. B74
President, St. Elizabeth's Medical Center of Boston, Boston, MA, p. A204

COLLINS, Michael L., Chief Executive Officer, Seven Rivers Community Hospital, Crystal River, FL, p. A85

COLLINS, Roger, Chief Executive Officer and Managing Director, Valley Hospital Medical Center, Las Vegas, NV, p. A270

COLLINS, Thomas J.
President and Chief Executive Officer, Long Beach Memorial Medical Center, Long Beach, CA, p. A48
President and Chief Executive Officer, Memorial Health Services, Long Beach, CA, p. B113

COLLINS, Thomas M., Administrator, Green Oaks Hospital, Dallas, TX, p. A406

COLLINS, William G., Chief Executive Officer, Columbia Medical Center–East, El Paso, TX, p. A408

COLLYER, Stuart C., Director, Veterans Affairs Medical Center, Canandaigua, NY, p. A290

COLON, Ivan E., Administrator, Auxilio Mutuo Hospital, San Juan, PR, p. A476

COLVERT, Charles C., President, Shelby Baptist Medical Center, Alabaster, AL, p. A11

COLVIN, James E., Executive Director, Devereux Hospital and Children's Center of Florida, Melbourne, FL, p. A92

COLVIN, Robert A., President and Chief Executive Officer, Memorial Medical Center, Savannah, GA, p. A114

COLWELL, Loretto Marie, President, St. Francis Hospital and Medical Center, Topeka, KS, p. A170

COMER, Maureen, Operations Administrator, Providence Centralia Hospital, Centralia, WA, p. A448

COMERFORD, Ralph L., Director, Devereux Center–Georgia, Kennesaw, GA, p. A110

COMERFORD Jr., Thomas P., Superintendent, Clarks Summit State Hospital, Clarks Summit, PA, p. A355

COMPSON, Oral R., Administrator, Dayton General Hospital, Dayton, WA, p. A449

COMSTOCK, John M., Chief Executive Officer, Sioux Valley Memorial Hospital, Cherokee, IA, p. A152

CONDOM, Jaime E., M.D., Director, South Carolina State Hospital, Columbia, SC, p. A377

CONDON, Debra, Administrator, Vencor Hospital–Philadelphia, Philadelphia, PA, p. A365

CONEJO, David, Chief Executive Officer, Highland Medical Center, Lubbock, TX, p. A419

CONELL, Marge, R.N., Administrator, Ellinwood District Hospital, Ellinwood, KS, p. A162

CONKLIN, Richard L., President, Parkland Health Center, Farmington, MO, p. A247

CONN, Kevin R., Administrator, Healthsouth Sunrise Rehabilitation Hospital, Fort Lauderdale, FL, p. A87

CONNELL, Daniel R., President, Christ Hospital, Jersey City, NJ, p. A278

CONNELL, Joe M., Chief Executive Officer, Lake Wales Medical Centers, Lake Wales, FL, p. A91

CONNELLY, Harrell L., Chief Executive Officer, Wallace Thomson Hospital, Union, SC, p. A381

CONNELLY, Michael D., President and Chief Executive Officer, Mercy Health System, Cincinnati, OH, p. B115

CONNOLEY, William B.
President and Chief Executive Officer, Mary Bridge Children's Hospital and Health Center, Tacoma, WA, p. A453
President, MultiCare Health System, Tacoma, WA, p. B117
President and Chief Executive Officer, Tacoma General Hospital, Tacoma, WA, p. A454

CONNOLLY, Brian M., President and Chief Executive Officer, Providence Hospital and Medical Centers, Southfield, MI, p. A223

CONNOLLY, James W., President and Chief Executive Officer, Mercy Hospital, Buffalo, NY, p. A290

CONNOR III, Paul J., Administrator, St. John's Episcopal Hospital–South Shore, New York, NY, p. A299

CONOLE, Charles P., FACHE, Administrator, Edward John Noble Hospital of Gouverneur, Gouverneur, NY, p. A292

CONOVER, Jevne, President and Chief Executive Officer, North Ottawa Community Hospital, Grand Haven, MI, p. A216

CONSIDINE, William H., President, Children's Hospital Medical Center of Akron, Akron, OH, p. A323

CONSTANTINE, Richard D., Chief Executive Officer, Brownsville General Hospital, Brownsville, PA, p. A354

CONSTANTINO, Richard S., M.D., President, Rochester General Hospital, Rochester, NY, p. A303

CONTE, Richard L., Chief Executive Officer and Chairman of the Board, Transitional Hospitals Corporation, Las Vegas, NV, p. B142

CONTE, William A., Director, Edith Nourse Rogers Memorial Veterans Hospital, Bedford, MA, p. A203

CONTI, Vincent S., President, Brighton Campus of Maine Medical Center, Portland, ME, p. A195

CONWAY, Jerry, Chief Executive Officer, BHC Vista Del Mar Hospital, Ventura, CA, p. A67

CONWAY, William A., Administrator, McGehee–Desha County Hospital, McGehee, AR, p. A33

CONZEMIUS, James D., President, Flagler Hospital, Saint Augustine, FL, p. A98

COOK, E. Tim, Chief Executive Officer, Columbia Medical Center–Osceola, Kissimmee, FL, p. A90

COOK, Jack M., President and Chief Executive Officer, Health Alliance of Greater Cincinnati, Cincinnati, OH, p. B100

COOK, Richard, Administrator, Columbia Murray Medical Center, Chatsworth, GA, p. A106

COOK, Thomas J., Chief Executive Officer, Tyler Rehabilitation Hospital, Tyler, TX, p. A430

COOK, William R., Chief Executive Officer, Specialty Hospital of Austin, Austin, TX, p. A400

COONEY, John V., President, Good Shepherd Rehabilitation Hospital, Allentown, PA, p. A353

COONEY, Lauri Ann, Chief Executive Officer, Pioneer Medical Center, Big Timber, MT, p. A257

COOPER, Anthony J., President and Chief Executive Officer, Arnot Ogden Medical Center, Elmira, NY, p. A291

COOPER, Chad, Administrator, Sleepy Eye Municipal Hospital, Sleepy Eye, MN, p. A235

COOPER, Gerson I., President, Botsford General Hospital, Farmington Hills, MI, p. A216

COOPER, Gloria, Chief Executive Officer, Mount Carmel Hospital, Colville, WA, p. A449

COOPER, Maxine T.
Chief Executive Officer, Chapman Medical Center, Orange, CA, p. A56
Chief Executive Officer, Placentia–Linda Hospital, Placentia, CA, p. A57

COOPER, Paul S., Chief Executive Officer, South Jersey Hospital, Bridgeton, NJ, p. A275

COOPER, Robert, Chief Executive Officer, Marshalltown Medical and Surgical Center, Marshalltown, IA, p. A156

COOPER, Roger W., President, Smyth County Community Hospital, Marion, VA, p. A442

COOPER, Wallace, Chief Executive Officer, King's Daughters Hospital, Brookhaven, MS, p. A237

COORS, Mary Lou, Administrator, St. Joseph Rehabilitation Hospital and Outpatient Center, Albuquerque, NM, p. A284

COPELAN, H. Neil, President and Chief Executive Officer, South Fulton Medical Center, East Point, GA, p. A108

COPENHAVER, C. Curtis, Chief Executive Officer, Mercy Hospital, Charlotte, NC, p. A309

COPPOL, Michael D., Chief Executive Officer, Charter Behavioral Health System of Indiana at Jefferson, Jeffersonville, IN, p. A145

CORA, Jose
Executive Director, Ashford Presbyterian Community Hospital, San Juan, PR, p. A476
Executive Director and Chief Executive Officer, Dr. Pila's Hospital, Ponce, PR, p. A476

CORBEIL, Stephen, President and Chief Executive Officer, Columbia Hospital at Medical City Dallas, Dallas, TX, p. A406

CORBETT, Clifford L., President and Chief Executive Officer, Morris Hospital, Morris, IL, p. A134

CORCORAN, Joseph P., President and Chief Executive Officer, New York Eye and Ear Infirmary, New York, NY, p. A298

CORDER, Thomas J., President and Chief Executive Officer, Camden–Clark Memorial Hospital, Parkersburg, WV, p. A458

CORDNER, Glenn D., Acting Chief Executive Officer, Springfield Hospital, Springfield, VT, p. A437

CORDOVA, Richard, Executive Director, San Francisco General Hospital Medical Center, San Francisco, CA, p. A62

COREY, Jack M., President, DeKalb Memorial Hospital, Auburn, IN, p. A140

CORK, Ronald J., President and Chief Executive Officer, St. Anthony's Hospital, O'Neill, NE, p. A266

CORLEY, Thomas
Chief Executive Officer, Carondelet Behavioral Health Center, Richland, WA, p. A452
Chief Executive Officer, Our Lady of Lourdes Health Center, Pasco, WA, p. A451

CORLEY, William E., President, Community Hospitals Indianapolis, Indianapolis, IN, p. A144

CORNELISON, Michael, Chief Executive Officer, Charter Hospital of Toledo, Maumee, OH, p. A332

CORNISH, Helen K., Director, Veterans Affairs Medical Center–Lexington, Lexington, KY, p. A176

CORONADO, Jose R., Director, South Texas Veterans Health Care System, San Antonio, TX, p. A426

CORVINO, Frank A., President and Chief Executive Officer, Greenwich Hospital, Greenwich, CT, p. A76

CORY, Clarence, President, Ottumwa Regional Health Center, Ottumwa, IA, p. A158

COSTA, Mark, President, Little Company of Mary Hospital, Torrance, CA, p. A66

COSTELLO Jr., Michael J., Chief Executive Officer, Santa Teresita Hospital, Duarte, CA, p. A42

COTNER, Edna J., Administrator, Coquille Valley Hospital, Coquille, OR, p. A348

COTTEY, David, Chief Executive Officer, Columbia Silsbee Doctors Hospital, Silsbee, TX, p. A427

COUCH, L. C., Board Chairman, Marshall County Health Care Authority, Guntersville, AL, p. B112

COUGHLIN, Jean, President and Chief Executive Officer, Marian Community Hospital, Carbondale, PA, p. A355

COURAGE Jr., Kenneth F., Chief Executive Officer, Psychiatric Institute of Washington, Washington, DC, p. A81

COURNOYER, James, Director, Indian Health Service–Sioux San Hospital, Rapid City, SD, p. A384

COURTEAU, Joan, Administrator, Columbia Behavioral Center, El Paso, TX, p. A408

COURTIER, Steve, Administrator, Monrovia Community Hospital, Monrovia, CA, p. A54

COURTIER, Steven, Chief Executive Officer, Hollywood Community Hospital of Hollywood, Los Angeles, CA, p. A50

COURTNEY, Curtis B., Administrator, Fentress County General Hospital, Jamestown, TN, p. A390

COURTNEY, Hattie, Administrator, Gladys Spellman Specialty Hospital and Nursing Center, Cheverly, MD, p. A199

COURTNEY, James P., President and Chief Executive Officer, University Medical Center, Lubbock, TX, p. A419

COUSER, David G., Administrator, Audubon County Memorial Hospital, Audubon, IA, p. A151

COUSSONS, R. Timothy, M.D., President and Chief Executive Officer, The University Hospitals, Oklahoma City, OK, p. A344

COVA, Charles J., Executive Vice President, Marian Medical Center, Santa Maria, CA, p. A64

COVERT, Michael H., FACHE, President and Chief Executive Officer, Sarasota Memorial Hospital, Sarasota, FL, p. A99

COVERT, Rob, President and Chief Executive Officer, Oaklawn Hospital, Marshall, MI, p. A220

COVINGTON, Steven, Superintendent, Madison State Hospital, Madison, IN, p. A146

COWAN, Michael L., USN, Commanding Officer, Naval Hospital, Camp Lejeune, NC, p. A309

COWLING, J. Michael, Chief Executive Officer, Carolinas Hospital System, Florence, SC, p. A377

COX, Bobby D., Chief Executive Officer, Eastern Oklahoma Medical Center, Poteau, OK, p. A344

COX, Jay, President and Chief Executive Officer, Tuomey Regional Medical Center, Sumter, SC, p. A380

COX, Keith, CHE, Chief Executive Officer, Charter Behavioral Health System, Mobile, AL, p. A16

COX, Leigh, Chief Executive Officer, Navapache Regional Medical Center, Show Low, AZ, p. A26

COX, Otto L.
President and Chief Executive Officer, Mercy Medical Center, Oshkosh, WI, p. A467
President and Chief Executive Officer, St. Elizabeth Hospital, Appleton, WI, p. A460

COX Sr., Arthur J., Director, Florida Center for Addictions and Dual Disorders, Avon Park, FL, p. A83

COXWELL, Loron H., Administrator, Worth County Hospital, Sylvester, GA, p. A114

COYNE, Kathryn W., Executive Director and Chief Operating Officer, Union Hospital, Union, NJ, p. A282

CRABTREE, Joe, Chief Executive Officer, Charter Greensboro Behavioral Health System, Greensboro, NC, p. A312

CRAIG, Larry, Chief Executive Officer, Jane Todd Crawford Memorial Hospital, Greensburg, KY, p. A174

CRAIG, Valerie, Administrator and Chief Executive Officer, Malvern Institute, Malvern, PA, p. A361

CRAIG, William H., President and Chief Executive Officer, Burleson St. Joseph Health Center, Caldwell, TX, p. A403

CRAIGIN, Jane, Chief Executive Officer, St. Vincent Williamsport Hospital, Williamsport, IN, p. A149

CRAIN, Garry D., Administrator and Chief Executive Officer, Johnston Memorial Hospital, Tishomingo, OK, p. A346

CRAIN, Stephen L.
President and Chief Executive Officer, St. Joseph Community Hospital, Mishawaka, IN, p. A147
President, St. Mary Community Hospital, South Bend, IN, p. A148

CRAMER, John S., FACHE, President and Chief Executive Officer, PinnacleHealth System, Harrisburg, PA, p. A358

CRANDALL, David B., Commander, Reynolds Army Community Hospital, Fort Sill, OK, p. A341

CRANDELL, Kim O., Chief Executive Officer and Administrator, Boulder City Hospital, Boulder City, NV, p. A270

CRANE, Margaret W., Chief Executive Officer, Barlow Respiratory Hospital, Los Angeles, CA, p. A49

CRANSTON, Henry J., Chief Operating Officer, Healthsouth Sea Pines Rehabilitation Hospital, Melbourne, FL, p. A92

CRANTON, Nancy J., Chief Executive Officer, Shadow Mountain Hospital, Tulsa, OK, p. A346

CRAVEN, Richard C., President, Sheltering Arms Rehabilitation Hospital, Richmond, VA, p. A446

CRAWFIS, Ewing H., President, Mary Rutan Hospital, Bellefontaine, OH, p. A324

CRAWFORD, Brenita, President and Chief Executive Officer, Mercy Hospital, Detroit, MI, p. A215

CRAWFORD, David E., FACHE, Executive Vice President and Chief Operating Officer, Medical Center East, Birmingham, AL, p. A12

CRAWFORD, E. Mac, President, Chief Executive Officer and Chairman, Magellan Health Services, Atlanta, GA, p. B110

CRAWFORD, Janet McKinney, Administrator, Carilion St. Albans Hospital, Radford, VA, p. A444

CRAWFORD, John W., Chief Executive Officer, Columbia Wagoner Hospital, Wagoner, OK, p. A347

CRAWFORD, R. Vincent, Director, Royal C. Johnson Veterans Memorial Hospital, Sioux Falls, SD, p. A385

CREAMER, Donald R.
President and Chief Executive Officer, Susquehanna Health System, Williamsport, PA, p. A371
President and Chief Executive Officer, Susquehanna Health System, Williamsport, PA, p. B

CREEDEN Jr., Francis V.
President, Providence Medical Center, Kansas City, KS, p. A165
President, Saint John Hospital, Leavenworth, KS, p. A166

CREELEY, Melvin R., President, East Liverpool City Hospital, East Liverpool, OH, p. A329

CRERAND, Raymond F., Interim Chief Executive Northwest Washington Service Area, Providence General Medical Center, Everett, WA, p. A449

CRESS, Michael D., Administrator, Vencor Hospital–San Diego, San Diego, CA, p. A61

CREST, Jerome A., Executive Vice President, Immanuel St. Joseph's–Mayo Health System, Mankato, MN, p. A231

CREWS, James C., President and Chief Executive Officer, Samaritan Health System, Phoenix, AZ, p. B130

CRIPE, Kimberly C., Acting Chief Executive Officer, Children's Hospital of Orange County, Orange, CA, p. A56

CRISTY, Kirk, Chief Executive Officer and Administrator, Memorial Hospital, Seminole, TX, p. A427

CROFT, Barbara, Health Care Manager, State Penitentiary Hospital, Walla Walla, WA, p. A454

CRONBERG, Chris, Chief Executive Officer, Northern Cochise Community Hospital, Willcox, AZ, p. A28

CRONE, William G., President and Chief Executive Officer, Naples Community Hospital, Naples, FL, p. A94

CRONEN, Kathleen, Administrator, Charter North Star Behavioral Health System, Anchorage, AK, p. A20

CRONIN, John C. J., President and Chief Executive Officer, North Adams Regional Hospital, North Adams, MA, p. A208

CROOK, Robert, Administrator, North Sunflower County Hospital, Ruleville, MS, p. A243

CROOM Jr., Kennedy L., Administrator and Chief Executive Officer, Rhea Medical Center, Dayton, TN, p. A388

CROSSETT, Joseph, Administrator, Liberty Hospital, Liberty, MO, p. A250

CROW, David, Chief Executive Officer, Campbell County Memorial Hospital, Gillette, WY, p. A471

CROW, Tom, Administrator, Atlanta Memorial Hospital, Atlanta, TX, p. A399

CROWDER, Jerry W., President and Chief Executive Officer, Bradford Health Services, Birmingham, AL, p. B72

CROWELL, Eric, President and Chief Executive Officer, Trinity Medical Center–West Campus, Rock Island, IL, p. A137

CROWELL, Larry A., President and Chief Executive Officer, The Medical Center, Beaver, PA, p. A354

CROWELL, Lynn, Chief Executive Officer, Howard Memorial Hospital, Nashville, AR, p. A33

CROWLEY, Jane Durney
Chief Executive Officer, Bon Secours Hospital, Baltimore, MD, p. A197
Chief Executive Officer, Liberty Medical Center, Baltimore, MD, p. A198

CROWLEY, Thomas, President, St. Elizabeth Hospital, Wabasha, MN, p. A236

CROWTHER, Bruce K., President and Chief Executive Officer, Northwest Community Hospital, Arlington Heights, IL, p. A123

CRUICKSHANK, James A., Chief Executive Officer, Columbia University Hospital and Medical Center, Tamarac, FL, p. A100

CRUMPLER, Joyce, R.N., Administrator, Bowie Memorial Hospital, Bowie, TX, p. A402

CRUMPTON, Althea H., Administrator, Magee General Hospital, Magee, MS, p. A241

CRYSEL, John B., Chief Executive Officer, Columbia North Side Hospital, Johnson City, TN, p. A390

CUBELLIS, Guido J., Chief Executive Officer, Healthsouth New England Rehabilitation Hospital, Woburn, MA, p. A211

CUCCI, Edward A., President, Swedish Covenant Hospital, Chicago, IL, p. A127

CULBERSON, David, Chief Executive Officer, Columbia West Anaheim Medical Center, Anaheim, CA, p. A36

CULLEN, James J., President, Hospital of Saint Raphael, New Haven, CT, p. A77

CULLEY, James R., Administrator, Valdez Community Hospital, Valdez, AK, p. A21

CULVERN, Rita, Administrator, Jefferson Hospital, Louisville, GA, p. A111

CULWELL, Gerald, Administrator, Gainesville Memorial Hospital, Gainesville, TX, p. A411

CUMMING, Irene M., Chief Executive Officer, University of Kansas Hospital, Kansas City, KS, p. A165

CUMMINGS, Bruce D., Chief Executive Officer, Blue Hill Memorial Hospital, Blue Hill, ME, p. A193

CUMMINS, Jane C., President and Chief Executive Officer, Legacy Mount Hood Medical Center, Gresham, OR, p. A349

CUNNINGHAM, Edward
Executive Director, Crossroads Community Hospital, Mount Vernon, IL, p. A134
Interim Administrator, Marion Memorial Hospital, Marion, IL, p. A133

CURE, DeAnn K., Chief Executive Officer, Kit Carson County Memorial Hospital, Burlington, CO, p. A70

CURLEY, Terrence A., Executive Director, Selma District Hospital, Selma, CA, p. A65

CURRAN, Joan, Administrator, Campus Hospital of Cleveland, Cleveland, OH, p. A326

CURRIE, Pat, Chief Executive Officer, Columbia Rosewood Medical Center, Houston, TX, p. A413

CURRIE, Scott D., Chief Operating Officer, Hayes–Green–Beach Memorial Hospital, Charlotte, MI, p. A213

CURRIER Jr., Elwood E., CHE, Administrator, Yoakum Community Hospital, Yoakum, TX, p. A432

CURRY, Randy, President, Comanche County Memorial Hospital, Lawton, OK, p. A342

CURRY, Robert H.
Senior Vice President and Chief Executive Officer, Maryvale Samaritan Medical Center, Phoenix, AZ, p. A25
Senior Vice President and Chief Executive Officer, Thunderbird Samaritan Medical Center, Glendale, AZ, p. A23

CURTIS, Jeff, President and Chief Executive Officer, H.S.C. Medical Center, Malvern, AR, p. A33

CURTIS, Robert S., President and Chief Executive Officer, Clara Maass Health System, Belleville, NJ, p. A275

CURTISS, Judith A., Administrator, Vencor Hospital–Detroit, Lincoln Park, MI, p. A219

CURY, Neal, Chief Executive Officer, BHC West Hills Hospital, Reno, NV, p. A271

CUSANO, Philip D., President and Chief Executive Officer, Stamford Hospital, Stamford, CT, p. A78

CUSHING, Jeff, Vice President, Administration, Legacy Meridian Park Hospital, Tualatin, OR, p. A352

CUSTER–MITCHELL, Marilyn J., Chief Executive Officer, West Central Community Hospital, Clinton, IN, p. A141

CUTLER, Terry, Executive Director, East Texas Medical Center–Clarksville, Clarksville, TX, p. A403

CWIEK, Mark A., President and Chief Executive Officer, Central Michigan Community Hospital, Mount Pleasant, MI, p. A220

CZIPO, Kevin, Executive Director, Stony Lodge Hospital, Ossining, NY, p. A302

D

D'AGNES, Michael R., President and Chief Executive Officer, Bayonne Hospital, Bayonne, NJ, p. A275

D'AGOSTINO, James P., Chief Executive Officer, Mount San Rafael Hospital, Trinidad, CO, p. A75

D'ALBERTO, Richard E., Chief Executive Officer, J. C. Blair Memorial Hospital, Huntingdon, PA, p. A359

D'AMBROSE, Joan, Executive Vice President and Chief Operating Officer, Deaconess Medical Center–West Campus, Saint Louis, MO, p. A253

D'ERAMO, David, President and Chief Executive Officer, Saint Francis Hospital and Medical Center, Hartford, CT, p. A77

D'ETTORRE, Joseph A., Administrator, Wyandot Memorial Hospital, Upper Sandusky, OH, p. A336

DAGUE, James O., President, Goshen General Hospital, Goshen, IN, p. A143

DAHILL, Kevin, President and Chief Executive Officer, United Hospital Medical Center, Port Chester, NY, p. A302

DAHLBERG, Edwin E., President, St. Luke's Regional Medical Center, Boise, ID, p. A119

DAHLGREN, Ronald E., Chief Executive Officer, Kern Valley Hospital District, Lake Isabella, CA, p. A47

DAHLMAN, Kim, Chief Executive Officer, Wallowa Memorial Hospital, Enterprise, OR, p. A349

DAIGLE, Anthony A., Administrator and Chief Executive Officer, McCuistion Regional Medical Center, Paris, TX, p. A423

DAIKEN, Michael E., Administrator, DeQuincy Memorial Hospital, De Quincy, LA, p. A184

DAILEY, Deborah S., President and Chief Executive Officer, Hospice of Palm Beach County, West Palm Beach, FL, p. A101

DAILY, James L., President, Porter Hospital, Middlebury, VT, p. A437

DAL CIELO, William J., Chief Executive Officer, Alameda Hospital, Alameda, CA, p. A36

DALE, Frank D., Administrator, Cox–Monett Hospital, Monett, MO, p. A251

DALE, Gregory L., Chief Executive Officer, Metropolitan St. Louis Psychiatric Center, Saint Louis, MO, p. A254

DALESIO, Michael J., Ph.D., Acting Executive Director, Edgewater Psychiatric Center, Harrisburg, PA, p. A358

DALLEY, Mark F., Chief Executive Officer, Tooele Valley Regional Medical Center, Tooele, UT, p. A436

DALTON, John, President and Chief Executive Officer, Deaconess–Glover Hospital Corporation, Needham, MA, p. A208

DALTON Jr., James E., President and Chief Executive Officer, Quorum Health Group/Quorum Health Resources, Inc., Brentwood, TN, p. B123

DALY, Michael J., President, Baystate Health Systems, Inc., Springfield, MA, p. B69

DALZELL, James G., Chief Executive Officer, Healthcare Rehabilitation Center, Austin, TX, p. A400

DAMORE, Joseph F., President and Chief Executive Officer, Sparrow Health System, Lansing, MI, p. A219

DAMPIER, Bobby H., Chief Executive Officer, Regional Medical Center of Hopkins County, Madisonville, KY, p. A178

DANDRIDGE, Thomas C., President, Regional Medical Center of Orangeburg and Calhoun Counties, Orangeburg, SC, p. A380

DANIEL, Steven G., Administrator, Kingfisher Regional Hospital, Kingfisher, OK, p. A342

DANIEL, William E., Administrator, Meriwether Regional Hospital, Warm Springs, GA, p. A115

DANIEL, William W., Administrator and Chief Executive Officer, Pioneers Memorial Healthcare District, Brawley, CA, p. A38

DANIELS, Gary J., Ph.D., Superintendent, Parsons State Hospital and Training Center, Parsons, KS, p. A168

DANIELS, Gary R., President, Penobscot Bay Medical Center, Rockport, ME, p. A195

DANIELS, J. Lewis, President and Chief Executive Officer, St. Joseph's Hospital, Asheville, NC, p. A308

DANIELS, John D.
President and Chief Executive Officer, St. Luke's Health System, Inc., Sioux City, IA, p. B138
President and Chief Executive Officer, St. Luke's Regional Medical Center, Sioux City, IA, p. A159

DANIELS, Richard A., President and Chief Executive Officer, McCullough–Hyde Memorial Hospital, Oxford, OH, p. A334

DANILOFF, Michael, President, Evangelical Community Hospital, Lewisburg, PA, p. A360

DANTZKER, David R., M.D., President and Chief Executive Officer, Long Island Jewish Medical Center, New York, NY, p. A298

DARLING, J. Rudy, President and Chief Executive Officer, Carroll Regional Medical Center, Berryville, AR, p. A29

DARNEY, Bruce, Superintendent, Harrisburg State Hospital, Harrisburg, PA, p. A358

DASCHER Jr., Norman E., Chief Operating Officer, Samaritan Hospital, Troy, NY, p. A305

DASHNER, George H., FACHE, President and Chief Executive Officer, Clinton Regional Hospital, Clinton, OK, p. A340

DAUGHERTY, Charles R., Administrator, Hillcrest Hospital, Calhoun City, MS, p. A238

DAUGHERTY, Thomas E., Chief Executive Officer, Mecosta County General Hospital, Big Rapids, MI, p. A213

DAUGHERTY Jr., John, Service Unit Director, U. S. Public Health Service Comprehensive Indian Health Facility, Claremore, OK, p. A340

DAVANZO, John P., President and Chief Executive Officer, Our Lady of Victory Hospital, Lackawanna, NY, p. A293

DAVE, B. J., M.D., Superintendent, Mental Health Institute, Independence, IA, p. A155

DAVENPORT, Neil, Administrator, Decatur County Hospital, Leon, IA, p. A156

DAVIDGE, Robert C., President and Chief Executive Officer, Our Lady of the Lake Regional Medical Center, Baton Rouge, LA, p. A183

DAVIDSON, Craig Val, CHE, Administrator, Beaver Valley Hospital, Beaver, UT, p. A433

DAVIES, David J., Chief Executive Officer, Bon Secours–Holy Family Regional Health System, Altoona, PA, p. A353

DAVIS, Aleen S., Chief Executive Officer, Charter Behavioral Health System of Atlanta at Peachford, Atlanta, GA, p. A103

DAVIS, Charles A., Administrator, Allen Memorial Hospital, Moab, UT, p. A434

DAVIS, Donald W., President, Northern Westchester Hospital Center, Mount Kisco, NY, p. A295

DAVIS, Gary, Service Unit Director, U. S. Public Health Service Indian Hospital, Parker, AZ, p. A24

DAVIS, Glen C., Administrator, Grady General Hospital, Cairo, GA, p. A106

DAVIS, James L., Chief Executive Officer, Lee County Community Hospital, Pennington Gap, VA, p. A444

DAVIS, John, Administrator, Warm Springs Rehabilitation Hospital, Gonzales, TX, p. A411

DAVIS, L. Glenn, Executive Director, Central Carolina Hospital, Sanford, NC, p. A316

DAVIS, Larry R., Chief Executive Officer, United Memorial Hospital Association, Greenville, MI, p. A217

DAVIS, Lary, President, Sonora Community Hospital, Sonora, CA, p. A65

DAVIS, Lyle, Administrator, Cozad Community Hospital, Cozad, NE, p. A263

DAVIS, Michael J., Ph.D., Superintendent, Woodward State Hospital–School, Woodward, IA, p. A160

DAVIS, Pamela Meyer, President and Chief Executive Officer, Edward Hospital, Naperville, IL, p. A134

DAVIS, Paul, Administrator, Gove County Medical Center, Quinter, KS, p. A168

DAVIS, Peter B., President and Chief Executive Officer, St. Joseph Healthcare, Nashua, NH, p. A273

DAVIS, Richard, Foreman Biomedical Equipment Maintenance, U. S. Air Force Hospital, Mather AFB, CA, p. A53

DAVIS, Robert L., President and Chief Executive Officer, North Oakland Medical Centers, Pontiac, MI, p. A221

DAVIS, Rod A., President and Chief Executive Officer, St. Rose Dominican Hospital, Henderson, NV, p. A270

DAVIS, Ronald D., Chief Executive Officer, Washington County Hospital, Washington, IA, p. A159

DAVIS, Rosemari, Chief Executive Officer, Columbia Williamette Valley Medical Center, McMinnville, OR, p. A350

DAVIS, Ryland, Interim Chief Executive Officer, St. Catherine's Hospital, Kenosha, WI, p. A463

DAVIS, Ryland P., President, Sacred Heart Medical Center, Spokane, WA, p. A453

DAVIS, M. Adrian, Ph.D., President and Chief Executive Officer, Memorial Hospital and Health Care Center, Jasper, IN, p. A145

DAVIS Jr., Ray H., Chief Executive Officer, Calais Regional Hospital, Calais, ME, p. A194

DAWES, Dennis W., President, Hendricks Community Hospital, Danville, IN, p. A141

DAWSON, George W., President, Centra Health, Inc., Lynchburg, VA, p. B77

DAWSON, Joseph M., Administrator, Blount Memorial Hospital, Maryville, TN, p. A393

DAY, Chip, Acting Vice President, Presbyterian Specialty Hospital, Charlotte, NC, p. A310

DAY, Robert, Ph.D., Superintendent, Kansas Neurological Institute, Topeka, KS, p. A170

DE BLASI, Raymond P., Chief Executive Officer, Mesquite Community Hospital, Mesquite, TX, p. A420

DE GASTA, Gary M., Director, Veterans Affairs Medical Center, White River Junction, VT, p. A438

DE JEAN, Julie, Administrator, Kansas Rehabilitation Hospital, Topeka, KS, p. A170

DE JESUS, Jorge, Executive Director, Hospital San Pablo, Bayamon, PR, p. A475

DE LA CRUZ, Romel, Administrator, Honokaa Hospital, Honokaa, HI, p. A117

DE MARTINI, Thomas J., Administrator, Woodridge Hospital, Johnson City, TN, p. A391

DE MELECIO, Carmen Feliciano, M.D., Secretary of Health, Puerto Rico Department of Health, San Juan, PR, p. B123

DE NARVAEZ, Denny, Chief Executive Officer, Florida Medical Center Hospital, Fort Lauderdale, FL, p. A87

DE VOSS, Gerald, Acting Administrator, Duane L. Waters Hospital, Jackson, MI, p. A218

DEAN, Harrison M., Senior Vice President and Administrator, Baptist Memorial Medical Center, North Little Rock, AR, p. A34

DEAN, Rhonda, Chief Executive Officer, Columbia El Dorado Hospital, Tucson, AZ, p. A27

DEANS, Gerald E., Director, Southwestern Virginia Mental Health Institute, Marion, VA, p. A442

DEARING, Bryan K., Chief Executive Officer, Columbia Summit Medical Center, Hermitage, TN, p. A390

DEARING, Tommy, Administrator, Kemper Community Hospital, De Kalb, MS, p. A238

DEARTH, Jim, M.D., Chief Executive Officer, Children's Hospital of Alabama, Birmingham, AL, p. A12

DEBOER, Michael D., President and Chief Executive Officer, Baptist Medical Center, Montgomery, AL, p. A16

DEBRUCE, Lucinda, Administrator, Charter Behavioral Health System of Northwest Arkansas, Fayetteville, AR, p. A30

DECK, K. Douglas, President and Chief Executive Officer, Good Samaritan Hospital and Health Center, Dayton, OH, p. A329

DECKER, Dale A., Chief Executive Officer, Sierra Vista Community Hospital, Sierra Vista, AZ, p. A26

DECKER, James Lee, President and Chief Executive Officer, Clarksville Memorial Hospital, Clarksville, TN, p. A388

DECKER, Michael, President and Chief Executive Officer, Divine Savior Hospital and Nursing Home, Portage, WI, p. A467

DEEMS, Andrew W., President and Chief Executive Officer, Eisenhower Memorial Hospital and Betty Ford Center at Eisenhower, Rancho Mirage, CA, p. A58

DEEN, Robert V., Administrator and Chief Executive Officer, Memorial Hospital, Center, TX, p. A403

DEFAIL, Anthony J., President and Chief Executive Officer, Meadville Medical Center, Meadville, PA, p. A361

DEFAUW, Thomas David, President and Chief Executive Officer, Rockford Memorial Hospital, Rockford, IL, p. A137

DEGEORGE–SMITH, Ellen
  Director, Veterans Affairs Medical Center, Des Moines, IA, p. A154
  Acting Director, Veterans Affairs Medical Center, Knoxville, IA, p. A156

DEGINA Jr., Anthony M.
  Chief Executive Officer, Columbia Deering Hospital, Miami, FL, p. A93
  Chief Executive Officer, Columbia Plantation General Hospital, Plantation, FL, p. A97

DEGRAAF, Douglas P., Chief Executive Officer, Winter Park Memorial Hospital, Winter Park, FL, p. A102

DEGRANDIS, Fred M., President and Chief Executive Officer, St. John West Shore Hospital, Cleveland, OH, p. A327

DEIGAN, Faith A., Administrator, Healthsouth Greater Pittsburgh Rehabilitation Hospital, Monroeville, PA, p. A361

DEIKER, Tom, Ph.D., Superintendent, Mental Health Institute, Cherokee, IA, p. A152

DEL MAURO, Ronald
  Chairman and Chief Executive Officer, Saint Barnabas Health Care System, Livingston, NJ, p. B130
  Chairman and Chief Executive Officer, Saint Barnabas Medical Center, Livingston, NJ, p. A278

DELANEY, Martin J., President and Chief Executive Officer, Winthrop–University Hospital, Mineola, NY, p. A294

DELANO, Richard J., President, Albany General Hospital, Albany, OR, p. A348

DELFORGE, Gary L., Administrator, St. Mary's Hospital, Norton, VA, p. A443

DELGADO, Pete, Chief Executive Officer, Columbia Valley Regional Medical Center, Brownsville, TX, p. A402

DELISI III, Frank G., CHE
  Chief Executive Officer and Director Operations, Healthsouth Harmarville Rehabilitation Hospital, Pittsburgh, PA, p. A366
  Chief Executive Officer and Director Operations, Healthsouth Lake Erie Institute of Rehabilitation, Erie, PA, p. A357

DELLAPORTAS, George, M.D., Director Professional Services, Whitten Center Infirmary, Clinton, SC, p. A376

DELLAROCCO, Paul J., President and Chief Executive Officer, Franciscan Children's Hospital and Rehabilitation Center, Boston, MA, p. A204

DELMONICO, Frank A., President and Chief Executive Officer, Butler Hospital, Providence, RI, p. A373

DEMBOW, Jack H., General Director and Vice President, Belmont Center for Comprehensive Treatment, Philadelphia, PA, p. A363

DEMEULENAERE, Edward P.
  President and Chief Executive Officer, Saint Mary's Medical Center, Racine, WI, p. A468
  President and Chief Executive Officer, St. Luke's Memorial Hospital, Racine, WI, p. A468

DEMORALES, Jon, Executive Director, Atascadero State Hospital, Atascadero, CA, p. A37

DENARDO, John J., Director, Veterans Affairs Edward Hines, Jr. Hospital, Hines, IL, p. A132

DENARUAEZ, Denny, Chief Executive Officer, Florida Medical Center South, Plantation, FL, p. A97

DENEY, Robert, Chief Executive Officer, Charter Behavioral Health System–Palm Springs, Cathedral City, CA, p. A39

DENIRO, James C., Director, Veterans Affairs Medical Center, Fresno, CA, p. A44

DENNIS, Daniel, Administrator, Wray Community District Hospital, Wray, CO, p. A75

DENNIS, Jerry L., M.D., Chief Executive Officer, Western State Hospital, Fort Steilacoom, WA, p. A449

DENNIS, Johnnye L., Chief Executive Officer, Wright Memorial Hospital, Trenton, MO, p. A256

DENNIS, Mynette, R.N.
  Administrator, Liberty–Dayton Hospital, Liberty, TX, p. A418
  Administrator, McLean County General Hospital, Calhoun, KY, p. A172

DENNIS Sr., Britton B., Superintendent, Central State Hospital, Milledgeville, GA, p. A112

DENTON, Jack L., President, Eaton Rapids Community Hospital, Eaton Rapids, MI, p. A215

DENTON, Mary M., Administrator, La Salle General Hospital, Jena, LA, p. A185

DEOBIL, Anthony W., Administrator, Elizabethtown Community Hospital, Elizabethtown, NY, p. A291

DEPEW, Joe D., President and Chief Executive Officer, Leesburg Regional Medical Center, Leesburg, FL, p. A91

DEPIERRO, John J., President and Chief Executive Officer, Sisters of Charity Health Care System Corporation, New York, NY, p. B133

DEPRIEST, Larry T., President, Danville Regional Medical Center, Danville, VA, p. A440

DEPUTAT, Robert, President, Oakland General Hospital, Madison Heights, MI, p. A220

DERRICKSON, Beverly, Administrator, Texas County Memorial Hospital, Houston, MO, p. A248

DERZON, Gordon M., Chief Executive Officer, University of Wisconsin Hospital and Clinics, Madison, WI, p. A464

DESANTIS, Daniel, Administrator, Sierra–Kings District Hospital, Reedley, CA, p. A58

DESCHAINE, Terry, Administrator, Fredonia Regional Hospital, Fredonia, KS, p. A163

DESCHAMBEAU, Wayne G., Chief Executive Officer, Deaconess Hospital of Cleveland, Cleveland, OH, p. A326

DESILVA, Joseph J., FACHE, President and Chief Executive Officer, Genesee Hospital, Rochester, NY, p. A303

DESROSIERS, Allan L., President, Anna Jaques Hospital, Newburyport, MA, p. A208

DESTEFANO, Ralph T., President and Chief Executive Officer, Passavant Hospital, Pittsburgh, PA, p. A366

DETWILER, James O., President, Mercy Hospital–Willard, Willard, OH, p. A337

DEURMIER, Carol, Chief Executive Officer, St. Michael's Hospital, Tyndall, SD, p. A385

DEUTSCH, Mel D., Administrator, Larkin Hospital, South Miami, FL, p. A99

DEVANSKY, Gary W., Director, Veterans Affairs Medical Center, Coatesville, PA, p. A356

DEVER, Philip R., Chief Executive Officer, Peoples Hospital, Mansfield, OH, p. A332

DEVICK, John, Chief Executive Officer, Canton–Inwood Memorial Hospital, Canton, SD, p. A382

DEVILLE, Linda, Chief Executive Officer, Ville Platte Medical Center, Ville Platte, LA, p. A191

DEVINE, Joseph W., Vice President, Hospital Services, Kennedy Memorial Hospitals–University Medical Center, Cherry Hill, NJ, p. A276

DEVINS, Thomas, Chief Executive Officer, Clinton Hospital, Clinton, MA, p. A206

DEVITT, ValGene, President and Chief Executive Officer, Ukiah Valley Medical Center, Ukiah, CA, p. A67

DEVOCELLE, Frank H., President and Chief Executive Officer, Olathe Medical Center, Olathe, KS, p. A167

DEWEESE, Tom, Administrator, Metropolitan Nashville General Hospital, Nashville, TN, p. B116

DEWOODY, Steve, Chief Executive Officer, Oconto Memorial Hospital, Oconto, WI, p. A467

DEXTER, Stephen P., Chief Executive Officer, Thomas Memorial Hospital, South Charleston, WV, p. A458

DI DARIO, Albert R., Superintendent, Norristown State Hospital, Norristown, PA, p. A362

DIAL, Marcia R., Administrator, Scotland County Memorial Hospital, Memphis, MO, p. A251

DIAMOND, Eugene C., President and Chief Executive Officer, Saint Margaret Mercy Healthcare Centers, Hammond, IN, p. A143

DIAMOND, Irv J., Chief Executive Officer, Memorial Medical Center at South Amboy, South Amboy, NJ, p. A281

DIAZ, Consuelo C., Chief Executive Officer, LAC–Rancho Los Amigos Medical Center, Downey, CA, p. A41

DIAZ–REYES, Rogelio, Administrator, Hospital Dr. Dominguez, Humacao, PR, p. A475

DIBERARDINO, William M., FACHE, President and Chief Executive Officer, Jones Memorial Hospital, Wellsville, NY, p. A306

DICAPO, Joseph R., Chief Executive Officer, Columbia Medical Center, Baton Rouge, LA, p. A182

DICICCO, Chris, Chief Executive Officer, Doctors Medical Center, Modesto, CA, p. A53

DICK, David, Administrator, Hans P. Peterson Memorial Hospital, Philip, SD, p. A384

DICKER, Albert, President and Chief Executive Officer, Franklin Hospital Medical Center, Valley Stream, NY, p. A306

DICKSON, James C., Administrator, Memorial Medical Center–Livingston, Livingston, TX, p. A419

DICKSON, James J., Administrator and Chief Executive Officer, Coalinga Regional Medical Center, Coalinga, CA, p. A40

DICKSON, Thomas C., Executive Vice President and Chief Operating Officer, Del E. Webb Memorial Hospital, Sun City West, AZ, p. A27

DIEGEL, James A., CHE, Executive Director, Central Oregon District Hospital, Redmond, OR, p. A351

DIEHL, Julie, Administrator, Wichita County Hospital, Leoti, KS, p. A166

DIETZ, Brian E.
President, St. Joseph's Hospital of Marshall County, Plymouth, IN, p. A147
Interim Chief Executive Officer, St. Joseph's Medical Center, South Bend, IN, p. A148

DIETZ, Francis R., President, Memorial Hospital of Rhode Island, Pawtucket, RI, p. A373

DIFEDERICO, William, President, Athol Memorial Hospital, Athol, MA, p. A203

DIFRANCO, Vincent, Chief Executive Officer, Wills Memorial Hospital, Washington, GA, p. A116

DILALLO, Kevin, Executive Director, Highlands Regional Medical Center, Sebring, FL, p. A99

DILLARD, Evan S., President, Marion Baptist Medical Center, Hamilton, AL, p. A15

DILLENSCHNEIDER, Grace Anne, General Superior, Sisters of the 3rd Franciscan Order, Syracuse, NY, p. B136

DILLON, Jerry D., President and Chief Executive Officer, Century Healthcare Corporation, Tulsa, OK, p. B78

DILLON, John M., Chief Executive Officer, Paris Community Hospital, Paris, IL, p. A135

DINAN, Edward M., President and Chief Executive Officer, Sacred Heart Hospital, Cumberland, MD, p. A199

DIONNE, Philip G., President and Chief Executive Officer, St. Joseph Medical Center, Reading, PA, p. A368

DIPISA, Ralph, Chief Executive Officer, Quincy Hospital, Quincy, MA, p. A209

DIRKSEN, Victor J., Administrator, Jefferson General Hospital, Port Townsend, WA, p. A451

DIRUBBIO, Vincent, Administrator, Mercy Medical Center, Rockville Centre, NY, p. A303

DITTEMORE, Ron, Ed.D., Superintendent, St. Joseph State Hospital, Saint Joseph, MO, p. A253

DITZEL Jr., Louis A., President and Chief Executive Officer, Jersey Shore Hospital, Jersey Shore, PA, p. A359

DIX, Dexter D., Director, Veterans Affairs Medical Center, Wilmington, DE, p. A80

DIXON, Jody, Administrator, Hall County Hospital, Memphis, TX, p. A420

DIXON, Robert, President and Chief Executive Officer, Riverside Health System, Wichita, KS, p. A171

DIXON, Sally J., President and Chief Executive Officer, Memorial Hospital, York, PA, p. A372

DIXON, Stephen E.
President and Chief Executive Officer, La Palma Intercommunity Hospital, La Palma, CA, p. A47
President and Chief Executive Officer, Martin Luther Hospital–Anaheim, Anaheim, CA, p. A36

DIXON, Thomas D., Administrator, John and Mary Kirby Hospital, Monticello, IL, p. A134

DIZNEY, Donald R., Chairman, United Medical Corporation, Windermere, FL, p. B145

DOAN, Richard L., Chief Executive Officer, Barnesville Hospital Association, Barnesville, OH, p. A323

DOBBS, Steve, Chief Executive Officer, Columbia Fawcett Memorial Hospital, Port Charlotte, FL, p. A97

DOCKTER, Robert A., Administrator, Eureka Community Hospital, Eureka, SD, p. A383

DODD, Bob A., President, East Pasco Medical Center, Zephyrhills, FL, p. A102

DODDS, Larry D., President, Adventist Medical Center, Portland, OR, p. A350

DOHERTY, Thomas C., Medical Center Director, Veterans Affairs Medical Center, Miami, FL, p. A94

DOISE, Daryl J., Administrator, Columbia Doctors' Hospital of Opelousas, Opelousas, LA, p. A189

DOLEZAL, Helen, Director, Wagner General Hospital, Palacios, TX, p. A422

DOLINS, David, President, Beth Israel Deaconess Medical Center, Boston, MA, p. A203

DONAHUE, Les A.
President and Chief Executive Officer, Sentara Hampton General Hospital, Hampton, VA, p. A441
President and Chief Executive Officer, Williamsburg Community Hospital, Williamsburg, VA, p. A447

DONAHUE, Patrick, Administrator, Union County Methodist Hospital, Morganfield, KY, p. A178

DONALSON III, Walter P., President and Chief Executive Officer, Garrett County Memorial Hospital, Oakland, MD, p. A201

DONEY, Tennyson, Service Unit Director, U. S. Public Health Service Indian Hospital, Crow Agency, MT, p. A258

DONNELL, Vern F., Service Unit Director, U. S. Public Health Service Indian Hospital, Pine Ridge, SD, p. A384

DONNELLAN Jr., John J., Director, Veterans Affairs Medical Center, New York, NY, p. A300

DONNELLY, Leo J., Executive Director, The Friary of Baptist Health Center, Gulf Breeze, FL, p. A88

DONNELLY Jr., John J., President and Chief Executive Officer, Roxborough Memorial Hospital, Philadelphia, PA, p. A365

DONOVAN, Robert A., President and Chief Executive Officer, Lowell General Hospital, Lowell, MA, p. A207

DOODY, Dennis W., President and Chief Executive Officer, Medical Center at Princeton, Princeton, NJ, p. A281

DOODY–CHABRE, Kris, Interim Executive Director, Cary Medical Center, Caribou, ME, p. A194

DOOLEY, James J., President, Geneva General Hospital, Geneva, NY, p. A292

DOOLEY, Jerry, Chief Executive Officer, Columbia Terre Haute Regional Hospital, Terre Haute, IN, p. A149

DOORDAN, Martin L., President, Anne Arundel Medical Center, Annapolis, MD, p. A197

DORAN, Dennis J., President and Chief Executive Officer, United Samaritans Medical Center, Danville, IL, p. A128

DORAN, Hugh F., Director, Veterans Affairs Medical Center, Kansas City, MO, p. A250

DORAN, Jeffrey, Chief Executive Officer, Hale Hospital, Haverhill, MA, p. A207

DORKO, Joseph M., Chief Executive Officer, Paulding County Hospital, Paulding, OH, p. A334

DORRIS, Ronald E., Administrator, Harris Methodist–Erath County, Stephenville, TX, p. A428

DORSEY, Lawrence T., Administrator, University Medical Center, Lafayette, LA, p. A186

DOTSON, Philip E., Administrator and Chief Executive Officer, Athens–Limestone Hospital, Athens, AL, p. A11

DOTY, Elizabeth A., Administrator, Howard County Hospital, Cresco, IA, p. A153

DOUGHERTY, Paul, Administrator, Deaconess Hospital, Oklahoma City, OK, p. A343

DOUGHTERY, Cary, Acting Chief Executive Officer, Louisiana Health Care Authority, Baton Rouge, LA, p. B109

DOUGHTY, Craig, Chief Executive Officer, Mahnomen Health Center, Mahnomen, MN, p. A231

DOVER, Boyd, Executive Director, Desert Hills Center for Youth and Families, Tucson, AZ, p. A27

DOVER, James, Administrator, Hillcrest Hospital, Simpsonville, SC, p. A380

DOVER, James F., Administrator and Executive Vice President, St. Mary's Hospital, Streator, IL, p. A138

DOWD, Thomas J., President, Nathan Littauer Hospital and Nursing Home, Gloversville, NY, p. A292

DOWDELL, Thomas C., Executive Director, Memorial Hospital and Medical Center of Cumberland, Cumberland, MD, p. A199

DOWELL Jr., Floyd B., Administrator, Lincoln County Memorial Hospital, Troy, MO, p. A256

DOWN, Philip, President, Doctors Community Hospital, Lanham, MD, p. A201

DOWNEY, William B., Administrator, Columbia Lewis–Gale Medical Center, Salem, VA, p. A446

DOWNING, Samuel W., Chief Executive Officer, Salinas Valley Memorial Hospital, Salinas, CA, p. A60

DOWNS, Martin, Facility Director, Lincoln Developmental Center, Lincoln, IL, p. A133

DOXTATOR, Rick, Chief Administrative Officer, Lovelace Health System, Albuquerque, NM, p. A284

DOYLE Jr., James J., President and Chief Executive Officer, Chilton Memorial Hospital, Pompton Plains, NJ, p. A281

DOZIER Jr., J. L., FACHE, President, Self Memorial Hospital, Greenwood, SC, p. A378

DOZORETZ, Ronald I., M.D., Chairman, First Hospital Corporation, Norfolk, VA, p. B97

DRAKE, Lawrence J., Chief Executive Officer, Chestnut Ridge Hospital, Morgantown, WV, p. A457

DRANEY, Nolan, Executive Vice President, Saddleback Memorial Medical Center, Laguna Hills, CA, p. A47

DREES, Daniel L., Administrator and Chief Executive Officer, Hegg Memorial Health Center, Rock Valley, IA, p. A158

DREW, John A., President and Chief Executive Officer, Athens Regional Medical Center, Athens, GA, p. A103

DREW, W. David, President and Chief Executive Officer, Atchison Hospital, Atchison, KS, p. A161

DREWA, Marcus E.
President, Methodist Health System, Jacksonville, FL, p. B116
President, Methodist Medical Center, Jacksonville, FL, p. A89
President, Methodist Pathway Center, Jacksonville, FL, p. A89

DREWEL, Charles A., Director, Missouri Rehabilitation Center, Mount Vernon, MO, p. A251

DRIEWER, Robert L., Chief Executive Officer, Faith Regional Health Services, Norfolk, NE, p. A266

DRISNER, Robert Eugene, President and Chief Executive Officer, Community Memorial Hospital, Menomonee Falls, WI, p. A464

DROP, Jeffrey S., President and Chief Executive Officer, St. Anthony Hospital, Pendleton, OR, p. A350

DROSKE, Richard S.
Director, Veterans Affairs Western New York Healthcare System, Batavia, NY, p. A289
Director, Veterans Affairs Western New York Healthcare System, Buffalo, NY, p. A290

DRUCKER, Steven C., President, Loretto Hospital, Chicago, IL, p. A126

DRUE, Margi, Administrator, Kahi Mohala, Ewa Beach, HI, p. A117

DRYDEN, Dave, FACHE, Administrator, Southern New Mexico Rehabilitation Center, Roswell, NM, p. A287

DUARTE, Pete, Chief Executive Officer, R. E. Thomason General Hospital, El Paso, TX, p. A409

DUBIS, John S., President, St. Marys Health Center, Jefferson City, MO, p. A248

DUBROCA, Darryl S., Administrator, THC–Arlington, Arlington, TX, p. A399

DUDLEY, James W., Director, Hunter Holmes McGuire Veterans Affairs Medical Center, Richmond, VA, p. A445

DUERR, Joe, Administrator, Purcell Municipal Hospital, Purcell, OK, p. A345

DUFAULT, Karin, Ph.D., Administrator, Sisters of Providence Health System, Seattle, WA, p. B135

DUFF, James, Administrator, Charter Springs Hospital, Ocala, FL, p. A95

DUFFIELD, Robert, Administrator, Wilson Memorial Hospital, Floresville, TX, p. A409

DUFFY, Charles, President, Decatur County Memorial Hospital, Greensburg, IN, p. A143

DUFFY, Jack, Executive Director, Conifer Park, Glenville, NY, p. A292

DUGAN, Margaret R., Executive Director, Binghamton Psychiatric Center, Binghamton, NY, p. A289

DUKE, Lance B., FACHE
President and Chief Executive Officer, Phenix Regional Hospital, Phenix City, AL, p. A17
President and Chief Executive Officer, The Medical Center, Columbus, GA, p. A107

DUKES, Annie L., JD, Chief Executive Officer, Southeast Colorado Hospital and Long Term Care, Springfield, CO, p. A74

DUMPMAN, Shirley J., Superintendent, Mayview State Hospital, Bridgeville, PA, p. A354

DUNCAN, Darryl L., Chief Executive Officer, Transitional Hospital of Chicago, Chicago, IL, p. A128

DUNCAN, Gary D., President and Chief Executive Officer, Freeman Hospitals and Health System, Joplin, MO, p. A248

DUNCAN, H. Clark, Administrator, Arcadia Valley Hospital, Pilot Knob, MO, p. A252

DUNDON, Mark W., President and Chief Executive Officer, Sisters of Charity of Nazareth Health System, Nazareth, KY, p. B133

DUNHAM, David S., President, Southside Regional Medical Center, Petersburg, VA, p. A444

DUNMYER, Daniel C., Chief Executive Officer, Princeton Community Hospital, Princeton, WV, p. A458

DUNN, Brian E., Chief Executive Officer, Lakeway Regional Hospital, Morristown, TN, p. A394

DUNN, Joseph W., Ph.D.
Chief Executive Officer, Daniel Freeman Marina Hospital, Marina Del Rey, CA, p. A53
Chief Executive Officer, Daniel Freeman Memorial Hospital, Inglewood, CA, p. A46

DUNN, Ronald J., Deputy Commander for Administration, Dwight David Eisenhower Army Medical Center, Fort Gordon, GA, p. A109

DUNNING Jr., Raymond M., Chief Executive Officer, Columbia Medical Center of Lewisville, Lewisville, TX, p. A418

DUPPER, Frank F., President, Adventist Health, Roseville, CA, p. B63

DUPUIS, Burton, Administrator, Gary Memorial Hospital, Breaux Bridge, LA, p. A183

DURHAM, Jeffrey L., Chief Executive Officer, Mediplex Rehabilitation Hospital, Bowling Green, KY, p. A172

DURR, Ben M., Administrator, Uvalde County Hospital Authority, Uvalde, TX, p. A430

DURR, Jerry L., Chief Executive Officer, Hill Country Memorial Hospital, Fredericksburg, TX, p. A410

DURRER, Christopher T., President and Chief Executive Officer, Wilson Memorial Hospital, Wilson, NC, p. A318

DURSTELER, Larry R., Regional Vice President, Utah Valley Regional Medical Center, Provo, UT, p. A435

DUSENBERY, Jack, Chief Executive Officer, Woodland Park Hospital, Portland, OR, p. A351

DUTCHER, Phillip C.
Interim President, Good Samaritan Medical Center, West Palm Beach, FL, p. A101
Interim President and Chief Executive Officer, St. Mary's Hospital, West Palm Beach, FL, p. A101

DUX, Christopher W., Chief Executive Officer, Columbia Pulaski Community Hospital, Pulaski, VA, p. A444

DVORAK, Roger G., President, Lawrence Hospital, Bronxville, NY, p. A289

DWOZAN, C. Richard, President, Habersham County Medical Center, Demorest, GA, p. A108

DYAR, David C., President and Administrator, Westview Hospital, Indianapolis, IN, p. A145

DYE, Jeff, Administrator, Socorro General Hospital, Socorro, NM, p. A287

DYER, Rebecca T., Administrator, Union General Hospital, Blairsville, GA, p. A105

DYETT, Benjamin, M.D., Director, Ossining Correctional Facilities Hospital, Ossining, NY, p. A302

DYKES, Bradford W., Chief Executive Officer, Perry County Memorial Hospital, Tell City, IN, p. A149

DYKES Sr., Kenneth E., Administrator, Emerald Coast Hospital, Apalachicola, FL, p. A83

DYKSTERHOUSE, Trevor J., Administrator, Addison Community Hospital, Addison, MI, p. A212

DYKSTRA, Janet, Chief Executive Officer, Osceola Community Hospital, Sibley, IA, p. A158

E

EAGAR Jr., Dan M., Administrator, Bessemer Carraway Medical Center, Bessemer, AL, p. A11

EASLEY, Don, Administrator, Memorial Hospital of Lafayette County, Darlington, WI, p. A461

EASLEY, Marcia, Chief Operating Officer, Columbia South Bay Hospital, Sun City Center, FL, p. A100

EASTHAM, James E., Administrator, Chief Executive Officer and Vice President, Memorial Hospital Southwest, Houston, TX, p. A415

EATON, Fred R., Administrator, Bannock Regional Medical Center, Pocatello, ID, p. A121

EAZELL, Dale E., Ph.D., President and Chief Executive Officer, Casa Colina Hospital for Rehabilitative Medicine, Pomona, CA, p. A57

EBERLE, Douglas W., President and Chief Executive Officer, St. Elizabeth Medical Center, Lafayette, IN, p. A146

ECHELARD, Paul D., Administrator, Pinecrest Rehabilitation Hospital, Delray, FL, p. A86

ECKENHOFF, Edward A., President and Chief Executive Officer, National Rehabilitation Hospital, Washington, DC, p. A81

ECKER, G. T. Dunlop, President and Chief Executive Officer, Loudoun Hospital Center, Leesburg, VA, p. A442

ECKERSLEY, Jay William
Chief Executive Officer, Grant/Riverside Methodist Hospitals–Grant Campus, Columbus, OH, p. A328
Chief Executive Officer, Grant/Riverside Methodist Hospitals–Riverside Campus, Columbus, OH, p. A328

ECKERT, Mary L., President and Chief Executive Officer, Millcreek Community Hospital, Erie, PA, p. A357

EDGAR, William O., Director, Veterans Affairs Medical Center, Dublin, GA, p. A108

EDMANDS, Clay D., President, Salina Regional Health Center, Salina, KS, p. A169

EDMISSON, Jete, President and Chief Executive Officer, Illini Community Hospital, Pittsfield, IL, p. A136

EDMONDSON, James H., Chief Executive Officer and Administrator, Columbia Hillside Hospital, Pulaski, TN, p. A395

EDWARDS, John R., Chief Executive Officer, Pacific Alliance Medical Center, Los Angeles, CA, p. A51

EDWARDS, Margaret, Chief Executive Officer, Hillside Rehabilitation Hospital, Warren, OH, p. A336

EDWARDS, Mark A., Chief Executive Officer, Blackford County Hospital, Hartford City, IN, p. A143

EDWARDS, Samuel, Administrator, Ventura County Medical Center, Ventura, CA, p. A68

EDWARDS, Thomas I., President and Chief Executive Officer, Chatuge Regional Hospital and Nursing Home, Hiawassee, GA, p. A110

EDWARDS, Wade, Administrator, Genoa Community Hospital, Genoa, NE, p. A264

EDWARDS, Robert P., Administrator, U. S. Air Force Hospital Luke, Glendale, AZ, p. A23

EDWARDS Jr., Bob S., Chief Executive Officer, Bates County Memorial Hospital, Butler, MO, p. A245

EGAN, Gail A., Vice President, Administrator, Paoli Memorial Hospital, Paoli, PA, p. A363

EGERER, Michelle, Chief Executive Officer, BHC Fairfax Hospital, Kirkland, WA, p. A450

EHRAT, Karen S., Ph.D.
President, Clermont Mercy Hospital, Batavia, OH, p. A324
President, Mercy Hospital Anderson, Cincinnati, OH, p. A326

EHRHARDT, Bill E., Executive Director, Bowdon Corporate Offices, Atlanta, GA, p. B72

EHRLICH, Jane, President and Chief Executive Officer, Columbia Memorial Hospital, Hudson, NY, p. A293

EICHELBERGER, L. L., Administrator, Fillmore County Hospital, Geneva, NE, p. A264

EICHER, Kim D., Administrator and Chief Executive Officer, Rehabilitation Hospital of Indiana, Indianapolis, IN, p. A144

EICHMAN, Cynthia, Chief Executive Officer and Administrator, Victory Medical Center, Stanley, WI, p. A469

EILERMAN, Ted, President, St. Elizabeth Medical Center, Granite City, IL, p. A131

EILERS, M. Kathleen, Administrator, Milwaukee County Mental Health Division, Milwaukee, WI, p. A465

EISENMANN, Claudia A., Director Operations, Healthsouth Rehabilitation Hospital of Fort Smith, Fort Smith, AR, p. A31

EISNER, Nina W., Chief Executive Officer, The Pavilion, Champaign, IL, p. A125

EITELMAN, Roger M., Site Administrator, Sentara Norfolk General Hospital, Norfolk, VA, p. A443

ELDER, Ronald J., President, Centennial Medical Center and Parthenon Pavilion, Nashville, TN, p. A394

ELDRIDGE, Ruth A., R.N., Regional Vice President, Administration, Broward General Medical Center, Fort Lauderdale, FL, p. A86

ELFORD, Dorothy J., Administrator, Vencor Hospital–Dallas, Dallas, TX, p. A407

ELHAJ, Ali A., Chief Executive Officer, Charter Ridge Hospital, Lexington, KY, p. A176

ELIZABETH, M. Ann, President, Saint Francis Hospital, Poughkeepsie, NY, p. A303

ELKINS, James N., FACHE
Director, South Texas Hospital, Harlingen, TX, p. A412
Director, Texas Center for Infectious Disease, San Antonio, TX, p. A426

ELKINS, Philip S., Director, Veterans Affairs Medical Center, Huntington, WV, p. A456

ELLERMANN, Michael P., President, Washington County Hospital, Nashville, IL, p. A135

ELLIOTT, Joan, R.N., Chief Operating Officer, Highland Community Hospital, Belvidere, IL, p. A124

ELLIOTT, Maurice W., President, Methodist Health Systems, Inc., Memphis, TN, p. B116

ELLIS, Dan, Administrator, Horn Memorial Hospital, Ida Grove, IA, p. A155

ELLIS, Elmer G., President and Chief Executive Officer, East Texas Medical Center Regional Healthcare System, Tyler, TX, p. B95

ELLZEY, Bob, Administrator, Bellville General Hospital, Bellville, TX, p. A401

ELROD, James K., President, Willis–Knighton Medical Center, Shreveport, LA, p. A191

ELSOM, Donald, Operations Administrator, Providence St. Vincent Medical Center, Portland, OR, p. A351

ELSWICK, P. Shannon, Administrator and Chief Executive Officer, South Lake Hospital, Clermont, FL, p. A85

EMGE, Joann, Chief Executive Officer, Sparta Community Hospital, Sparta, IL, p. A138

EMMONS, Bobby B., Administrator, Fleming County Hospital, Flemingsburg, KY, p. A173

EMRICH, Kathleen, Ed.D., Assistant Vice President and Chief Operating Officer, Kingswood Hospital, Ferndale, MI, p. A216

ENDERS, Robert, President, Morehead Memorial Hospital, Eden, NC, p. A311

ENDRES, Jack R., Administrator, Muenster Memorial Hospital, Muenster, TX, p. A421

ENGEL, Kim, Chief Executive Officer, Legend Buttes Health Services, Crawford, NE, p. A263

ENGELKEN, Joseph T., Chief Executive Officer, Community Hospital Onaga, Onaga, KS, p. A167

ENGER, Mark M.
Senior Vice President and Administrator, Fairview Ridges Hospital, Burnsville, MN, p. A227
Senior Vice President and Administrator, Fairview Southdale Hospital, Minneapolis, MN, p. A231

ENGHOLM, Kari L., Administrator, Humboldt County Memorial Hospital, Humboldt, IA, p. A155

ENGLAND, Garry L., President and Chief Executive Officer, St. Joseph Regional Medical Center of Northern Oklahoma, Ponca City, OK, p. A344

ENGLAND, John R., President and Chief Executive Officer, Allegheny Valley Hospital, Natrona Heights, PA, p. A362

ENGLERTH, Ladonna, Administrator, East Carroll Parish Hospital, Lake Providence, LA, p. A186

ENGLISH, David J., President and Chief Executive Officer, Hospice of Northern Virginia, Arlington, VA, p. A439

EPSTEIN, Norman B., President, Chambersburg Hospital, Chambersburg, PA, p. A355

ERAZO, Joseph R., Chief Executive Officer, Nassau County Medical Center, East Meadow, NY, p. A291

ERB, Myrna, Administrator, Adair County Memorial Hospital, Greenfield, IA, p. A154

ERGLE Jr., F. W., Administrator, Tallahatchie General Hospital, Charleston, MS, p. A238

ERICH, Kevin R., Administrator, Pioneer Memorial Hospital, Heppner, OR, p. A349

ERICKSON, Glenn G., Vice President and Administrator, Fairview Northland Regional Hospital, Princeton, MN, p. A233

ERICKSON, Susan A., Clinical Services Administrator for Women's Services and Site Administrator, Hutzel Hospital, Detroit, MI, p. A215

ERICKSON, Tyler, Administrator, Montrose Memorial Hospital, Montrose, CO, p. A74

ERIXON, Stephen M., Chief Executive Officer, Memorial Mother Frances Hospital, Palestine, TX, p. A422

ERMSHAR, Edwin L., President and Chief Executive Officer, Sierra View District Hospital, Porterville, CA, p. A58

ERNE, Michael H.
Senior Vice President and Administrator, St. Anthony Hospital Central, Denver, CO, p. A71
Senior Vice President and Administrator, St. Anthony Hospital North, Westminster, CO, p. A75

ERNST, John R., Executive Director, Deborah Heart and Lung Center, Browns Mills, NJ, p. A275

ERWINE, Terry E., Administrator, Sac–Osage Hospital, Osceola, MO, p. A252

ESLYN, Cole C.
Chief Executive Officer, Columbia St. David's Hospital, Austin, TX, p. A400
Chief Executive Officer, Columbia/St. David's Medical Center, Austin, TX, p. B85
Chief Executive Officer, St. David's Pavilion, Austin, TX, p. A400
Chief Executive Officer, St. David's Rehabilitation Center, Austin, TX, p. A400

ESPELAND, David, Chief Executive Officer, Fallon Medical Complex, Baker, MT, p. A257

ESPINOSA, Maritza, Chief Executive Officer, San Juan City Hospital, San Juan, PR, p. A477

ESTRADA, Ivette, Administrator, Kaiser Foundation Hospital–West Los Angeles, Los Angeles, CA, p. A50

ETHEREDGE, H. Rex, President and Chief Executive Officer, Columbia Brandon Regional Medical Center, Brandon, FL, p. A84

ETTER, Carl, Executive Director, River Oaks East–Woman's Pavilion, Jackson, MS, p. A240

ETTLINGER, Roy A.
Chief Executive Officer, Arbour Hospital, Boston, MA, p. A203
Chief Executive Officer, H. R. I. Hospital, Brookline, MA, p. A205

EUSTIS, Mark A., President, Missouri Baptist Medical Center, Town and Country, MO, p. A255

EVANS, Don
Chief Executive Officer, Mesa Lutheran Hospital, Mesa, AZ, p. A24
Chief Executive Officer, Valley Lutheran Hospital, Mesa, AZ, p. A24

EVANS, Michael J., Chief Executive Officer, Highlands Hospital, Connellsville, PA, p. A356

EVANS, Scott D., FACHE, Administrator, Val Verde Memorial Hospital, Del Rio, TX, p. A407

EVANS Jr., Jack T., President and Chief Executive Officer, Central Washington Hospital, Wenatchee, WA, p. A454

EVERETT, Benjamin, Chief Executive Officer, Columbia Doctors Hospital of Laredo, Laredo, TX, p. A418

EVERTS, Randall M., Chief Executive Officer, Columbia Rio Grande Regional Hospital, McAllen, TX, p. A420

EZZELL, Robert, Administrator, Hemphill County Hospital, Canadian, TX, p. A403

F

FAAS, Michael D., President and Chief Executive Officer, Metropolitan Hospital, Grand Rapids, MI, p. A217

FABBRE, Deno E., President and Chief Executive Officer, Alexian Brothers Hospital, Saint Louis, MO, p. A253

FAGERSTROM, Charles, Vice President, Norton Sound Regional Hospital, Nome, AK, p. A21

FAHD II, Charles F., Chief Executive Officer, Massena Memorial Hospital, Massena, NY, p. A294

FAHRENBACHER, Fritz, Vice President and Regional Hospital Administrator, Lee Memorial Hospital, Dowagiac, MI, p. A215

FAHS, Melvin H., President, Iroquois Memorial Hospital and Resident Home, Watseka, IL, p. A139

FAILING, Richard J., Chief Executive Officer, Kittson Memorial Hospital, Hallock, MN, p. A230

FAIRFAX, Douglas L., President and Chief Executive Officer, Health Alliance Hospitals, Leominster, MA, p. A207

FAIRMAN, John A., Executive Director, District of Columbia General Hospital, Washington, DC, p. A81

FAJA, Garry C.
President and Chief Executive Officer, Saline Community Hospital, Saline, MI, p. A223
President and Chief Executive Officer, St. Joseph Mercy Health System, Ann Arbor, MI, p. A212

FAJT, John D., Executive Director, Putnam County Hospital, Greencastle, IN, p. A143

FALAST, Earl F., Chief Executive Officer, Veterans Affairs Medical Center, Philadelphia, PA, p. A365

FALATKO, Michael J., President and Chief Executive Officer, Doctors Hospital of Jackson, Jackson, MI, p. A218

FALBERG, Warren C., Senior Executive Officer, Jewish Hospital, Cincinnati, OH, p. A326

FALE, Randall J., President and Chief Executive Officer, St. Joseph's Regional Health Center, Hot Springs, AR, p. A31

FALE, Robert A., President, Agnesian HealthCare, Fond Du Lac, WI, p. A462

FALLAT, Andrew, FACHE, Chief Executive Officer, Evergreen Hospital Medical Center, Kirkland, WA, p. A450

FALLER, Madelyn, Chief Executive Officer, Mineral Community Hospital, Superior, MT, p. A260

FANNING Jr., Robert R., Chief Executive Officer, Beverly Hospital, Beverly, MA, p. A203

FANT, Leonard, Administrator, North Park Hospital, Chattanooga, TN, p. A388

FANTASIA, Sam, Director, Division of Administration and Financial Services, St. Elizabeths Hospital, Washington, DC, p. A81

FARBER, Nancy D., Chief Executive Officer, Washington Township Health Care District, Fremont, CA, p. A43

FARETRA, Gloria, M.D., Executive Director, Queens Children's Psychiatric Center, New York, NY, p. A299

FARNELL, Leland E., President, Johnston Memorial Hospital, Smithfield, NC, p. A316

FARNES, David, Administrator, St. Benedicts Family Medical Center, Jerome, ID, p. A120

FARNSWORTH, Edward F.
President, Capital Region Medical Center–Madison, Jefferson City, MO, p. A248
President, Capital Region Medical Center–Southwest, Jefferson City, MO, p. A248

FARR, George D., President and Chief Executive Officer, Children's Medical Center of Dallas, Dallas, TX, p. A406

FARRELL, Michael J., Chief Executive Officer, Somerset Hospital Center for Health, Somerset, PA, p. A369

FARRELL, Patrick W., Chief Executive Officer, Henrico Doctors' Hospital, Richmond, VA, p. A445

FARRELL Sr., John T., President and Chief Executive Officer, St. Joseph Medical Center of Fort Wayne, Fort Wayne, IN, p. A142

FARRINGTON, Jack N., Ph.D., Executive Vice President, Episcopal Health Services Inc., Uniondale, NY, p. B96

FARRIS, James R., CHE, Chief Executive Officer, Wabash General Hospital District, Mount Carmel, IL, p. A134

FARROW, Gary W., Administrator, North Baldwin Hospital, Bay Minette, AL, p. A11

FASSLER, David, M.D., President, Choate Health Systems, Woburn, MA, p. A211

FATHERREE, Lori Caudell, Chief Executive Officer, Columbia Johnson City Specialty Hospital, Johnson City, TN, p. A390

FAUCHER, Diane, Superintendent, Austin State Hospital, Austin, TX, p. A400

FAULK, A. Donald, FACHE, President, Medical Center of Central Georgia, Macon, GA, p. A111

FAULKNER, David M., Chief Executive Officer and Administrator, Central Montana Medical Center, Lewistown, MT, p. A259

FAULWELL, James A., Administrator, Grundy County Memorial Hospital, Grundy Center, IA, p. A155

FAUS, Douglas, Administrator, Liberty County Hospital and Nursing Home, Chester, MT, p. A257

FAUST, Bill D., Administrator, Floyd County Memorial Hospital, Charles City, IA, p. A152

FAVRET, John M., Director, Eastern State Hospital, Williamsburg, VA, p. A447

FAY, Juliette, President and Chief Executive Officer, Charles River Hospital, Wellesley, MA, p. A211

FEARS, John R., Director, Carl T. Hayden Veterans Affairs Medical Center, Phoenix, AZ, p. A24

FECHTEL Jr., Edward J., President and Chief Executive Officer, St. Mary's Health Care System, Athens, GA, p. A103

FEDERSPIEL, John C., President and Chief Executive Officer, Hudson Valley Hospital Center, Peekskill, NY, p. A302

FEDYK, Mark F., Administrator, Morrison Community Hospital, Morrison, IL, p. A134

FEICKERT, Larry E., Chief Administrative Officer, Northwood Deaconess Health Center, Northwood, ND, p. A321

FEIKE, Jeffrey, Administrator, Churchill Community Hosptial, Fallon, NV, p. A270

FEILER, Kenneth H., Chief Executive Officer, Columbia Rose Medical Center, Denver, CO, p. A71

FEINBERG, E. Richard, M.D., Executive Director, Bronx Children's Psychiatric Center, New York, NY, p. A295

FEINSTEIN, Stephen H., Ph.D., Superintendent, Osawatomie State Hospital, Osawatomie, KS, p. A167

FELDMAN, Janice M., Interim Administrator, Georgetown University Hospital, Washington, DC, p. A81

FELDMAN, Mitchell S., Chief Executive Officer, Delray Community Hospital, Delray Beach, FL, p. A86

FELDT, Roger D., FACHE, President and Chief Executive Officer, Saline Memorial Hospital, Benton, AR, p. A29

FELGAR, Alvin D., President and Chief Executive Officer, Frisbie Memorial Hospital, Rochester, NH, p. A274

FELICI, Brian K., Chief Executive Officer, East Ohio Regional Hospital, Martins Ferry, OH, p. A332

FELLA, Peter T., Commissioner, Doctor Robert L. Yeager Health Center, Pomona, NY, p. A302

FELLMAN, Randall E., USAF, Commanding Officer, U. S. Air Force Hospital Mountain Home, Mountain Home AFB, ID, p. A121

FELTMAN, Steve, Chief Executive Officer, Unity Medical Center, Grafton, ND, p. A320

FELTON, David, Administrator, Community Memorial Hospital, Hamilton, NY, p. A292

FENCEL, Michael M., Chief Executive Officer, Columbia Hospital, West Palm Beach, FL, p. A101

FENSKE, Candace, R.N., Administrator, Madelia Community Hospital, Madelia, MN, p. A231

FENSTEMACHER, Keith A., President and Chief Executive Officer, Faxton Hospital, Utica, NY, p. A305

FENTON, John V.
Chief Executive Officer, Brotman Medical Center, Culver City, CA, p. A41
Chief Executive Officer, Midway Hospital Medical Center, Los Angeles, CA, p. A50

FERGUSON, John P., President and Chief Executive Officer, Hackensack University Medical Center, Hackensack, NJ, p. A277

FERRANTE, Ellen, President and Chief Executive Officer, Fairlawn Rehabilitation Hospital, Worcester, MA, p. A211

FERRANTO, Carmen N., Superintendent, Warren State Hospital, North Warren, PA, p. A362

FERRY, John M., Executive Director, Memorial Hospital of Sweetwater County, Rock Springs, WY, p. A472

FERRY, Thomas P., Administrator and Chief Executive, duPont Hospital for Children, Wilmington, DE, p. A80

FERRY Jr., John J., M.D., President and Chief Executive Officer, Southampton Hospital, Southampton, NY, p. A304

FETH, Joseph S., President, ServantCor, Kankakee, IL, p. B131

FEUQUAY, Judith K., Chief Executive Officer, Perry Memorial Hospital, Perry, OK, p. A344

FEURER, Russell E., Chief Executive, Good Shepherd Hospital, Barrington, IL, p. A123

FEURIG, Thomas L., President and Chief Executive Officer, St. Joseph Mercy Oakland, Pontiac, MI, p. A222

FICKEN, Robert A., Chief Executive Officer and Chief Financial Officer, Dallas–Fort Worth Medical Center, Grand Prairie, TX, p. A411

FICKES, Cathy, R.N., Chief Executive Officer, Mission Community Hospital–San Fernando Campus, San Fernando, CA, p. A61

FICKLIN, Dennis E., Executive Director, Family Health West, Fruita, CO, p. A72

FIELD, Carol, Administrator, Carondolet Holy Cross Hospital, Nogales, AZ, p. A24

FIELDER, Betty A., Clinical Administrative Officer, Institute of Mental Health–Rhode Island Medical Center, Howard, RI, p. A373

FIELDS, Ronald B., President, Tri–County Memorial Hospital, Whitehall, WI, p. A470

FIKE, Ruthita J.
Administrator, Porter Care Hospital, Denver, CO, p. A71
Administrator, Porter Care Hospital–Littleton, Littleton, CO, p. A73

FILICKO, Gerard, Chief Executive Officer, Chippenham and Johnston–Willis Hospitals, Richmond, VA, p. A445

FINAN, Timothy J., FACHE, President, Niagara Falls Memorial Medical Center, Niagara Falls, NY, p. A301

FINAN Jr., John J., President and Chief Executive Officer, Franciscan Missionaries of Our Lady Health System, Inc., Baton Rouge, LA, p. B97

FINCH, Kenneth A., President and Administrator, Castle Medical Center, Kailua, HI, p. A118

FINCH Jr., J. W., Administrator, Elkview General Hospital, Hobart, OK, p. A342

FINCHER, Ron, Chief Executive Officer, Charter Savannah Behavioral Health System, Savannah, GA, p. A113

FINE, Eva L., MS, Assistant Administrator, Piqua Memorial Medical Center, Piqua, OH, p. A334

FINE, Stuart H., Chief Executive Officer, Grand View Hospital, Sellersville, PA, p. A368

FINEGAN, Andrew, Administrator, Charles A. Dean Memorial Hospital, Greenville, ME, p. A194

FINKLEIN, Terry O., Chief Executive Officer, Columbia Memorial Hospital, Astoria, OR, p. A348

FINLAYSON, William C.
President and Chief Executive Officer, O'Connor Hospital, San Jose, CA, p. A62
President and Chief Executive Officer, Saint Louise Hospital, Morgan Hill, CA, p. A54

FINLEY, Alan, Administrator, Van Buren County Memorial Hospital, Clinton, AR, p. A29

FINLEY, Beverly M., Chief Executive Officer, Stanislaus Medical Center, Modesto, CA, p. A54

FINLEY, Ed, Administrator, Stanton County Health Care Facility, Johnson, KS, p. A165

FINN, Donald J., Administrator, Lake Area Hospital, Webster, SD, p. A386

FINNEGAN, John R., Administrator and Chief Operating Officer, Columbia Regional Medical Center, Spring Hill, FL, p. A99

FINUCANE, Mark, Director Health, Los Angeles County–Department of Health Services, Los Angeles, CA, p. B109

FINZEN, Terry S., President, St. Paul–Ramsey Medical Center, Saint Paul, MN, p. A234

FIRES, Wiley M., Administrator, Collingsworth General Hospital, Wellington, TX, p. A431

FISCHER, Carl A., M.D., Director, Western Maryland Center, Hagerstown, MD, p. A200

FISCHER, Carl R., Associate Vice President and Chief Executive Officer, Medical College of Virginia Hospitals, Virginia Commonwealth University, Richmond, VA, p. A445

FISCHER, Joseph, Chief Executive Officer, BHC Pinnacle Pointe Hospital, Little Rock, AR, p. A32

FISCHER, Michelle, Chief Executive Officer, Columbia Hospital North and South, Springfield, MO, p. A255

FISCHER, Robert W., President, Northwest Hospital Center, Randallstown, MD, p. A201

FISH, David B., Executive Vice President, St. Joseph's Hospital, Chippewa Falls, WI, p. A461

FISH, Robert H., President and Chief Executive Officer, Santa Rosa Memorial Hospital, Santa Rosa, CA, p. A64

FISHER, Diana D., President and Chief Executive Officer, Brown County General Hospital, Georgetown, OH, p. A330

FISHER, Donald Joe, Administrator, King's Daughters Hospital, Greenville, MS, p. A239

FISHER, Philip, President and Chief Executive Officer, Valley View Regional Hospital, Ada, OK, p. A339

FISHERO, Harvey L., President and Chief Executive Officer, Columbia Medical Center of Plano, Plano, TX, p. A423

FITZGERALD, Gerald D.
President, Oakwood Healthcare System, Dearborn, MI, p. B119
President and Chief Executive Officer, Oakwood Hospital and Medical Center–Dearborn, Dearborn, MI, p. A214

FITZGIBBON, Susan H., President and Chief Executive Officer, Annie Penn Hospital, Reidsville, NC, p. A315

FITZHARRIS, Joseph, Commander, Keller Army Community Hospital, West Point, NY, p. A306

FITZPATRICK, Daniel, Administrator, Harlan ARH Hospital, Harlan, KY, p. A175

FITZPATRICK, James G., Administrator, Kossuth Regional Health Center, Algona, IA, p. A151

FITZPATRICK, William, M.D., Senior Vice President and Chief Operating Officer, Presbyterian Hospital, Albuquerque, NM, p. A284

FLAHERTY, Tom, Assistant Administrator, Los Angeles County Central Jail Hospital, Los Angeles, CA, p. A50

FLAIG, William G., Administrator, Douglas County Hospital, Alexandria, MN, p. A226

FLAKE, Glenn M., Executive Director, Newnan Hospital, Newnan, GA, p. A112

FLEMING, Cheryl, Chief Operating Officer, Healthsouth Rehabilitation Hospital of York, York, PA, p. A371

FLEMING, John L., M.D., Interim Chief Executive Officer, Laureate Psychiatric Clinic and Hospital, Tulsa, OK, p. A346

FLEMING, Timothy G., M.D., Chief Executive Officer, Gallup Indian Medical Center, Gallup, NM, p. A286

FLEMING, Wanda C., Administrator, Claiborne County Hospital, Port Gibson, MS, p. A243

FLESH, Lawrence H., M.D., Director, Veterans Affairs Medical Center, Albany, NY, p. A288

FLESSNER, Arnold, Administrator, Waverly Municipal Hospital, Waverly, IA, p. A159

FLETCHALL, Terry L., Administrator, Santiam Memorial Hospital, Stayton, OR, p. A352

FLETCHER, Allen P., President, Northeast Alabama Regional Medical Center, Anniston, AL, p. A11

FLETCHER, Constance N., Ph.D., Director, Southern Virginia Mental Health Institute, Danville, VA, p. A440

FLETCHER, David A., President and Chief Executive Officer, Elizabeth General Medical Center, Elizabeth, NJ, p. A277

FLETCHER, Donald C.
President and Chief Executive Officer, Blue Water Health Services Corporation, Port Huron, MI, p. B71
President and Chief Executive Officer, Port Huron Hospital, Port Huron, MI, p. A222

FLETCHER, Thomas H., Administrator, Ellenville Community Hospital, Ellenville, NY, p. A291

FLORES, Saturnino Pena, Executive Director, Ryder Memorial Hospital, Humacao, PR, p. A475

FLORES Jr., Ernest, Administrator, Dimmit County Memorial Hospital, Carrizo Springs, TX, p. A403

FLOTTE', J. L., Chief Executive Officer, Medical Center of Winnie, Winnie, TX, p. A431

FLOWERS, Randel, Ph.D., Administrator, Clinton County Hospital, Albany, KY, p. A172

FLURY, Patricia A., Administrator, Memorial Regional Hospital, Los Angeles, FL, p. A89

FLYNN, Brian T., Administrator and Chief Executive Officer, Harton Regional Medical Center, Tullahoma, TN, p. A396

FLYNN, Patrick D., President and Chief Executive Officer, Washington Regional Medical Center, Fayetteville, AR, p. A30

FLYNN Jr., James H., President and Chief Executive Officer, Franciscan Sisters of the Poor Health System, Inc., New York, NY, p. B98

FOGGO, Thomas G., Executive Vice President Care Delivery and General Director, Albany Medical Center, Albany, NY, p. A288

FOJTASEK, Georgia R., President and Chief Executive Officer, W. A. Foote Memorial Hospital, Jackson, MI, p. A218

FOLEY, William T., Senior Vice President, Hospital of the University of Pennsylvania, Philadelphia, PA, p. A364

FONNESBECK, Douglas R., Administrator, Cottonwood Hospital Medical Center, Murray, UT, p. A434

FONTENOT, Teri G., President and Chief Executive Officer, Woman's Hospital, Baton Rouge, LA, p. A183

FONTENOT, Terry J., Administrator, Medical Center of Mesquite, Mesquite, TX, p. A420

FORD, Ken, Administrator, Tattnall Memorial Hospital, Reidsville, GA, p. A113

FORD, Raymond L., President and Chief Executive Officer, Glenwood Regional Medical Center, West Monroe, LA, p. A191

FORD, Roger A., Administrator, Bertrand Chaffee Hospital, Springville, NY, p. A304

FORD, W. Raymond C., Administrator and Chief Executive Officer, Columbia Specialty Hospital Jacksonville, Jacksonville, FL, p. A89

FOREMAN, Robert, Associate Administrator, Brooksville Regional Hospital, Brooksville, FL, p. A84

FOREMAN, Spencer, M.D., President, Montefiore Medical Center, New York, NY, p. A298

FORMIGONI, Ugo, Metro–West Network Manager, John J. Madden Mental Health Center, Hines, IL, p. A132

FORNOFF, Gerald A., Chief Executive Officer, Columbia Medical Center of Southwest Louisiana, Lafayette, LA, p. A186

FOSDICK, Glenn A., President and Chief Executive Officer, Hurley Medical Center, Flint, MI, p. A216

FOSS, R. Coleman, Chief Executive Officer, Columbia Volunteer General Hospital, Martin, TN, p. A392

FOSSUM, John, Chief Executive Officer, Lac Qui Parle Hospital of Madison, Madison, MN, p. A231

FOSTER, Allen, Administrator, Mizell Memorial Hospital, Opp, AL, p. A17

FOSTER, Barbara J., President and Chief Executive Officer, Pacifica Hospital, Huntington Beach, CA, p. A46

FOSTER, James B., Chief Executive Officer, Lake Shore Hospital, Irving, NY, p. A293

FOSTER, James R., President and Chief Executive Officer, Bert Fish Medical Center, New Smyrna Beach, FL, p. A94

FOSTER, Jon, Senior Vice President and Administrator, Baptist Hospital of East Tennessee, Knoxville, TN, p. A391

FOSTER, Robert T., Deputy Commander for Administrtaion, Ireland Army Community Hospital, Fort Knox, KY, p. A174

FOSTER Jr., Charles L., FACHE, President and Chief Executive Officer, West Georgia Health System, La Grange, GA, p. A110

FOWLER, Homer, Chief Operating Officer, Healthsouth Rehabilitation Hospital, Huntington, WV, p. A456

FOWLER, Phillip E., President, Highlands–Cashiers Hospital, Highlands, NC, p. A313

FOWLER, Angela D., USAF, Administrator, U. S. Air Force Hospital, Cheyenne, WY, p. A471

FOX, David, President, Alcoholism Treatment Center, Winfield, IL, p. A139

FOX, Rosemary
  Acting Administrator, Kaiser Foundation Hospital, San Francisco, CA, p. A61
  Coutinuing Care Leader, Kaiser Foundation Hospital, South San Francisco, CA, p. A65

FOX, Ted, Administrator and Chief Executive Officer, El Centro Regional Medical Center, El Centro, CA, p. A42

FOX, William R., Chief Executive Officer, Healthsouth Great Lakes Rehabilitation Hospital, Erie, PA, p. A357

FOX III, William W., Chief Executive Officer, Middle Georgia Hospital, Macon, GA, p. A111

FOY, James, President and Chief Executive Officer, St. John's Riverside Hospital, Yonkers, NY, p. A307

FRABLE, Arthur H., Administrator, Fairview Hospital, Fairview, OK, p. A341

FRAGALA, M. Richard, M.D., Superintendent, Clifton T. Perkins Hospital Center, Jessup, MD, p. A200

FRAIZER, Frederic L., President and Chief Executive Officer, St. Mary's Medical Center, Saginaw, MI, p. A222

FRALEY, Gary F., Administrator, Shriners Hospitals for Children, Greenville, Greenville, SC, p. A378

FRALEY, R. Reed, Associate Vice President for Health Sciences and Chief Executive Officer, Ohio State University Medical Center, Columbus, OH, p. A328

FRANCES, Richard J., M.D., President and Medical Director, Silver Hill Hospital, New Canaan, CT, p. A77

FRANCESCHI, Angel M., Administrator, Hospital Oncologico Andres Grillasca, Ponce, PR, p. A476

FRANCIS, S. Michael, President and Chief Executive Officer, Community General Hospital, Reading, PA, p. A368

FRANCIS, Talton L., FACHE, President and Chief Executive Officer, Russell Regional Hospital, Russell, KS, p. A169

FRANCIS, Tim, Chief Executive Officer, Great Plains Regional Medical Center, Elk City, OK, p. A341

FRANCKE, Bertold, M.D., Interim Executive Director, Vermont State Hospital, Waterbury, VT, p. A438

FRANDSEN, Jeff, Chief Executive Officer, Columbia Palm Drive Hospital, Sebastopol, CA, p. A64

FRANK, Carrie B., President and Chief Executive Officer, Buffalo General Hospital, Buffalo, NY, p. A289

FRANKLIN, James P., Executive Director, Laird Hospital, Union, MS, p. A243

FRANZ, Charles C., Chief Executive Officer, South Peninsula Hospital, Homer, AK, p. A20

FRANZ, Paul S., President, Carolinas Medical Center, Charlotte, NC, p. A309

FRARACCIO, Robert D., Administrator, Clark Regional Medical Center, Winchester, KY, p. A181

FRASCHETTI, Robert J., President and Chief Executive Officer, St. Jude Medical Center, Fullerton, CA, p. A44

FRASER, John Martin, President and Chief Executive Officer, Nebraska Methodist Hospital, Omaha, NE, p. A267

FRASER, Michael R., Administrator, Pacific Communities Hospital, Newport, OR, p. A350

FRAY, George S., Administrator, Baptist Memorial Hospital–Forrest City, Forrest City, AR, p. A31

FRAYER, Jack F., Administrator, Sylvan Grove Hospital, Jackson, GA, p. A110

FRAYNE, Laurence J., Chief Executive Officer, Plano Rehabilitation Hospital, Plano, TX, p. A423

FREEBORN, Lisa J., Administrator, Wamego City Hospital, Wamego, KS, p. A170

FREEBURG, Eric, Administrator, Memorial Hospital, Chester, IL, p. A125

FREELAND, Franklin, Ed.D., Chief Executive Officer, U. S. Public Health Service Fort Defiance Indian Health Service Hospital, Fort Defiance, AZ, p. A23

FREEMAN, Alan, Administrator, Cass Medical Center, Harrisonville, MO, p. A248

FREEMAN, Carol B., Chief Executive Officer, Columbia Huntington Beach Hospital and Medical Center, Huntington Beach, CA, p. A46

FREEMAN, Charles C., Director, Sam Rayburn Memorial Veterans Center, Bonham, TX, p. A402

FREEMAN, Charles Ray, Administrator, Ripley County Memorial Hospital, Doniphan, MO, p. A247

FREEMAN, James M., Chief Executive Officer, Rowan Regional Medical Center, Salisbury, NC, p. A316

FREEMAN, Richard H., Chief Executive Officer, Eleanor Slater Hospital, Cranston, RI, p. A373

FREEMAN Jr., Kester S., President and Chief Executive Officer, Richland Memorial Hospital, Columbia, SC, p. A377

FREISINGER, Edward, Vice President and Administration, Oakwood Hospital Seaway Center, Trenton, MI, p. A224

FRENCH, Douglas D., President and Chief Executive Officer, St. Vincent Hospitals and Health Services, Indianapolis, IN, p. A144

FRENCH III, George E., Chief Executive Officer, Minden Medical Center, Minden, LA, p. A187

FRENCHIE, Richard J., President and Chief Executive Officer, UHHS Geauga Regional Hospital, Chardon, OH, p. A325

FRERICHS, Jeffrey, President and Chief Executive Officer, Cabrini Medical Center, New York, NY, p. A296

FRESOLONE, Victor J., FACHE, President and Chief Executive Officer, Mercy Medical Center, Roseburg, OR, p. A352

FREY, Ted W., President, St. Louis Children's Hospital, Saint Louis, MO, p. A254

FREYMULLER, Robert S., Chief Executive Officer, Doctors Hospital of Dallas, Dallas, TX, p. A406

FRIDAY, Barbara, Administrator, Laurel Wood Center, Meridian, MS, p. A241

FRIED, Jeffrey M., FACHE, President and Chief Executive Officer, Beebe Medical Center, Lewes, DE, p. A80

FRIEDELL, Peter E., M.D., President, Jackson Park Hospital, Chicago, IL, p. A126

FRIEDMAN, Peter, Administrator, Washington Medical Center, Culver City, CA, p. A41

FRIEDMAN, Steven H., Ph.D., Executive Vice President, Methodist Hospital of Chicago, Chicago, IL, p. A126

FRIEL, John P., President and Chief Executive Officer, Watsonville Community Hospital, Watsonville, CA, p. A68

FRIES, Jack, President, St. Luke's Hospital, San Francisco, CA, p. A62

FRIGO, John S., President, Rush North Shore Medical Center, Skokie, IL, p. A138

FRITH, J. B., Chief Executive Officer, Metro Health Center, Erie, PA, p. A357

FRITTS, Rosemary, Administrator, Pike County Memorial Hospital, Murfreesboro, AR, p. A33

FRITZ, Michael H., President, Carle Foundation Hospital, Urbana, IL, p. A138

FROBENIUS, John, President and Chief Executive Officer, St. Cloud Hospital, Saint Cloud, MN, p. A234

FROCK, Charles T., President and Chief Executive Officer, Moore Regional Hospital, Pinehurst, NC, p. A315

FROEHLICH, Lynette, R.N., Administrator, Arlington Municipal Hospital, Arlington, MN, p. A226

FROMHOLD, John A., Chief Executive Officer, Columbia Medical Center of Arlington, Arlington, TX, p. A399

FRONZA Jr., Leo F., President and Chief Executive Officer, Elmhurst Memorial Hospital, New York, IL, p. A129

FRY, Robert W., President, Bellin Psychiatric Center, Green Bay, WI, p. A462

FRY, Willis F., Executive Director, Broadlawns Medical Center, Des Moines, IA, p. A153

FRY Jr., L. Marcus
  Chief Executive Officer, Providence Memorial Hospital, El Paso, TX, p. A409
  Chief Executive Officer, Sierra Medical Center, El Paso, TX, p. A409

FRYE Jr., Edward R., Administrator, Clarendon Memorial Hospital, Manning, SC, p. A379

FRYMOYER, John W., M.D., Chief Executive Officer, Fletcher Allen Health Care, Burlington, VT, p. A437

FUENTES, Miguel A., President and Chief Executive Officer, Bronx–Lebanon Hospital Center, New York, NY, p. A295

FUGAGLI, Anne M., Administrator, Healthsouth Rehabilitation Hospital, Concord, NH, p. A272

FUHRMAN, Andrew, Chief Executive Officer, BHC Fort Lauderdale Hospital, Fort Lauderdale, FL, p. A86

FULFORD, Richard C., Administrator, Gulf Breeze Hospital, Gulf Breeze, FL, p. A88

FULKS, Jerry, Chief Executive Officer, Columbia Lanier Park Hospital, Gainesville, GA, p. A109

FULL, James M., Chief Executive Officer, Randolph County Hospital, Winchester, IN, p. A150

FULLER, Thomas E., Administrator, Marion Memorial Hospital, Marion, SC, p. A379

FUMAI, Frank L., President and Chief Executive Officer, Cathedral Healthcare System, Inc., Newark, NJ, p. B75

FUQUA, David G., R.N., Chief Executive Officer, Marshall County Hospital, Benton, KY, p. A172

FUREY, Vincent, President, Jackson Brook Institute, South Portland, ME, p. A196

FURSTMAN, Marc A., Chief Executive Officer, Los Angeles Metropolitan Medical Center, Los Angeles, CA, p. A50

FUTRELL, Jerry H., Chief Executive Officer, Columbia Smith County Memorial Hospital, Carthage, TN, p. A387

G

GABOW, Patricia A., M.D., Chief Executive Officer and Medical Director, Denver Health Medical Center, Denver, CO, p. A71

GADE, Ronald, M.D.
President, St. Barnabas Hospital, New York, NY, p. A299
President, Union Hospital of the Bronx, New York, NY, p. A300
GAFFNEY, Betty, Administrator, St. Joseph Memorial Hospital, Murphysboro, IL, p. A134
GAGER, Warren E., Chief Executive Officer, William B. Kessler Memorial Hospital, Hammonton, NJ, p. A278
GAGNE, Michael P., Administrator, Kula Hospital, Kula, HI, p. A118
GAINEY, James W., Administrator, Tyler County Hospital, Woodville, TX, p. A432
GAINTNER, J. Richard, M.D.
Chief Executive Officer, Shands at the University of Florida, Gainesville, FL, p. A88
Chief Executive Officer, Shands Health System, University of Florida Health Science Center, Gainesville, FL, p. B131
GALARCE, Julio, Administrator, Hospital El Buen Pastor, Arecibo, PR, p. A474
GALATI, John P., President and Chief Executive Officer, Clifton Springs Hospital and Clinic, Clifton Springs, NY, p. A291
GALE, Albert J., Chief Executive Officer, Inland Behavioral Health Institute, Coeur D'Alene, ID, p. A119
GALEY, William, M.D., Chief Executive Officer, Veterans Affairs Medical Center, Portland, OR, p. A351
GALINSKI, Thomas P., President and Chief Executive Officer, Ohio Valley Medical Center, Wheeling, WV, p. A459
GALLAGHER, John S. T.
President, North Shore Health System, Manhasset, NY, p. B119
President, North Shore University Hospital, Manhasset, NY, p. A294
GALLAGHER, Catherine C., President, Mercy–Chicago Region Healthcare System, Naperville, IL, p. B115
GALLAGHER III, J. Frank, Administrator, BHC Fox Run Hospital, Saint Clairsville, OH, p. A335
GALLIN, John I., M.D., Director, Warren G. Magnuson Clinical Center, National Institutes of Health, Bethesda, MD, p. A199
GALLOWAY, Ron, Administrator, Reagan Memorial Hospital, Big Lake, TX, p. A401
GAMACHE, Edward L., Director, Veterans Affairs Medical Center, Ann Arbor, MI, p. A212
GAMBER, Richard L.
Administrator, Carolinas Hospital System–Kingstree, Kingstree, SC, p. A379
Administrator, Carolinas Hospital System–Lake City, Lake City, SC, p. A379
GAMBLE, Howard M., Administrator, Okanogan–Douglas County Hospital, Brewster, WA, p. A448
GAMBLE, Joe E., Chief Executive Officer, Carmi Township Hospital, Carmi, IL, p. A124
GAMBRELL Jr., Edward C., Administrator, Stephens County Hospital, Toccoa, GA, p. A115
GAMEL, Richard B., Chief Executive Officer, Citizens Medical Center, Colby, KS, p. A162
GAMMIERE, Thomas A., Vice President and Administrator, Scripps Memorial Hospital–Chula Vista, Chula Vista, CA, p. A40
GANDY Jr., M. P., President, Columbia Lakeside Hospital, Metairie, LA, p. A187
GANN, Jim, Administrator, Roane Medical Center, Harriman, TN, p. A390
GANNON, Frank R., Administrator and Chief Executive Officer, Healthsouth Medical Center, Birmingham, AL, p. A12
GANS, Bruce M., M.D., Senior Vice President, Rehabilitation Institute of Michigan, Detroit, MI, p. A215
GANTNER, Rose K., Chief Executive Officer, Charter Behavioral Health System of Little Rock, Maumelle, AR, p. A33
GANTZ, Daniel L., President, Fayette County Hospital and Long Term Care, Vandalia, IL, p. A139
GARBER, Jeff, Administrator and Chief Executive Officer, Healthsouth Rehabilitation Hospital of Sarasota, Sarasota, FL, p. A99

GARBER, Jonathan A., Chief Executive Officer, ValueMark West End Behavioral Healthcare System, Richmond, VA, p. A446
GARCIA, Louis O., President and Chief Executive Officer, Columbia Medical Center of Aurora, Aurora, CO, p. A70
GARCIA, Martha, Chief Executive Officer, Coral Gables Hospital, Coral Gables, FL, p. A85
GARDESKI, Frances J., Chief Executive Officer, University Medical Center–Mesabi, Hibbing, MN, p. A230
GARDNER, James B., President, Huron Memorial Hospital, Bad Axe, MI, p. A212
GARDNER, Jonathan H., Chief Executive Officer, Veterans Affairs Medical Center, Tucson, AZ, p. A28
GARDNER, Paul A., CPA, Administrator, George County Hospital, Lucedale, MS, p. A241
GARDNER Jr., James E., Administrator, St. Mary Hospital, Port Arthur, TX, p. A424
GARFIELD, Michael W., Administrator, Columbia Southern Tennessee Medical Center, Winchester, TN, p. A397
GARFUNKEL, Sanford M., Medical Center Director, Veterans Affairs Medical Center, Washington, DC, p. A81
GARLEB, Pat, Administrator, Hospital of the California Institution for Men, Chino, CA, p. A40
GARLEY, Louise, President, Benedictine Hospital, Kingston, NY, p. A293
GARMAN, G. Richard, Executive Director, Wayne Memorial Hospital, Honesdale, PA, p. A359
GARNER, Gerald J., Chairman of the Board, Coast Plaza Doctors Hospital, Norwalk, CA, p. A55
GARNER, H. Douglas, Chief Executive Officer, Phoenix General Hospital and Medical Center, Phoenix, AZ, p. A25
GARRETT, Patrick R., Administrative Executive Officer, Deaconess Medical Center, Billings, MT, p. A257
GARRETT, Randy, Administrator, Pineywoods Hospital, Baird, TX, p. A401
GARRETT, Vernon G., Chief Executive Officer, BHC Intermountain Hospital, Boise, ID, p. A119
GARRIGAN, Michael E., President and Chief Executive Officer, St. Francis Hospital, Columbus, GA, p. A107
GARST, Paul D., USN, Commanding Officer, Naval Hospital, Havelock, NC, p. A312
GASCHO, Dwight, President and Chief Executive Officer, Scheurer Hospital, Pigeon, MI, p. A221
GAST, Edwin A., Administrator, Grand River Hospital District, Rifle, CO, p. A74
GASTON, Richard, Administrator, Macon Northside Hospital, Macon, GA, p. A111
GATCH, Donna, Administrator, Gadsden Community Hospital, Quincy, FL, p. A98
GATENS Sr., Paul D., Administrator, Georgetown Memorial Hospital, Georgetown, SC, p. A378
GATES, Jon M., Chief Executive Officer, United Medical Center, Cheyenne, WY, p. A471
GATES, Monica P., Chief Executive Officer, Slidell Memorial Hospital and Medical Center, Slidell, LA, p. A191
GATES, Truman L., Chief Executive Officer, Community Hospital of Los Gatos, Los Gatos, CA, p. A52
GATHRIGHT, Dan, Senior Vice President and Administrator, Baptist Medical Center Arkadelphia, Arkadelphia, AR, p. A29
GATMAITAN, Alfonso W., Chief Executive Officer, Tipton County Memorial Hospital, Tipton, IN, p. A149
GATRELL, Cloyd B., Commander, Munson Army Community Hospital, Fort Leavenworth, KS, p. A163
GAUDREAULT, J. Ronald, President and Chief Executive Officer, Huntington Hospital, Huntington, NY, p. A293
GAUSE, Garry L., Chief Executive Officer, Columbia Capital Medical Center, Olympia, WA, p. A451
GAVALCHIK, Stephen M., Administrator, Webster County Memorial Hospital, Webster Springs, WV, p. A459
GAYER, Alan J., President, Egleston Children's Hospital at Emory University, Atlanta, GA, p. A104
GAYNOR, Stanley J., Chief Executive Officer and Administrator, Black River Memorial Hospital, Black River Falls, WI, p. A461
GEANES, John, President and Chief Executive Officer, Shannon Medical Center, San Angelo, TX, p. A425

GEANEY Jr., Michael J., President, Salem Hospital, Salem, MA, p. A209
GEARY, George A., President, Milton Hospital, Milton, MA, p. A208
GEBAR, Shelley, President and Chief Executive Officer, Allegheny University Hospitals, Hahnemann, Philadelphia, PA, p. A363
GEBHARD, Scott, Senior Vice President Operations, JFK Johnson Rehabilitation Institute, Edison, NJ, p. A276
GEE, Thomas H., Administrator, Henry County Medical Center, Paris, TN, p. A395
GEHANT, David P., President, Boulder Community Hospital, Boulder, CO, p. A70
GEIGER, James F., Administrator, Malcolm Grow Medical Center, Andrews AFB, MD, p. A197
GEISER, Rosann, Corporate Director, Congregation of St. Agnes, Fond Du Lac, WI, p. B87
GEISSLER, Frederick, Chief Executive Officer, Grand View Hospital, Ironwood, MI, p. A218
GELLER, Harold S., Administrator, Jackson County Public Hospital, Maquoketa, IA, p. A156
GENTLING, Steven J., Director, Veterans Affairs Medical Center, Oklahoma City, OK, p. A344
GENTRY, Michael V., President, Park Ridge Hospital, Fletcher, NC, p. A311
GEORGE, Dennis L., Administrator, Coffey County Hospital, Burlington, KS, p. A161
GEORGE, Gladys, President and Chief Executive Officer, Lenox Hill Hospital, New York, NY, p. A297
GEORGE, William G., Senior Vice President, Waynesboro Hospital, Waynesboro, PA, p. A370
GEPFORD, Jon W., President and Chief Executive Officer, Parkview Hospital, Brunswick, ME, p. A194
GERATHS, Nathan L., Director, William S. Middleton Memorial Veterans Hospital, Madison, WI, p. A464
GERBER, Carl J., Ph.D., Director, James H. Quillen Veterans Affairs Medical Center, Mountain Home, TN, p. A394
GERBER, Michael J., Chief Executive Officer, Southern Winds Hospital, Hialeah, FL, p. A88
GERDES, Jerrell F., Administrator, Franklin County Memorial Hospital, Franklin, NE, p. A263
GERLACH, George, President, Granite Falls Municipal Hospital and Manor, Granite Falls, MN, p. A229
GERLACH, John R., Chief Executive Officer/Administrator, DeKalb Medical Center, Decatur, GA, p. A108
GERLACH, Matthew S., Chief Executive Officer and Administrator, Beverly Hospital, Montebello, CA, p. A54
GETTYS III, Roddey E., Executive Vice President, Baptist Medical Center Easley, Easley, SC, p. A377
GHERARDINI, Michael M., Managing Director, Auburn General Hospital, Auburn, WA, p. A448
GIBBONS, H. Ray, President and Chief Executive Officer, Holy Rosary Health Center, Miles City, MT, p. A259
GIBBS, Henry T., Administrator, Bleckley Memorial Hospital, Cochran, GA, p. A106
GIBSON, James P., President and Chief Executive Officer, St. Francis Health Center, Madisonville, TX, p. A420
GIBSON, Robert N., President and Chief Executive Officer, D. T. Watson Rehabilitation Hospital, Sewickley, PA, p. A369
GIBSON, Thomas J., Administrator, USA Doctors Hospital, Mobile, AL, p. A16
GIBSON III, Earnest, Administrator, Riverside General Hospital, Houston, TX, p. A415
GIDDINGS, Lucille C., CHE, President and Chief Executive Officer, Nantucket Cottage Hospital, Nantucket, MA, p. A208
GIEDD, James L., Administrator, Phillips County Hospital, Phillipsburg, KS, p. A168
GIERMAK, William C., President and Chief Executive Officer, Louise Obici Memorial Hospital, Suffolk, VA, p. A447
GIESECKE, Stephan A., MSC, Commander, U. S. Air Force Hospital Moody, Moody AFB, GA, p. A112
GIFFIN, James R., Interim Administrator, Highland Lakes Medical Center, Burnet, TX, p. A403
GILBERT, Albert F., Ph.D., President and Chief Executive Officer, Summa Health System, Akron, OH, p. A323

GILBERT, Brian D., Administrator, Wrangell General Hospital and Long Term Care Facility, Wrangell, AK, p. A21

GILBERT, Thomas D., President and Chief Executive Officer, Columbia Dunwoody Medical Center, Atlanta, GA, p. A103

GILBERT, William L., Chief Executive Officer, French Hospital Medical Center, San Luis Obispo, CA, p. A63

GILBERTI, Gary M., Chief Executive Officer, Charter Hospital of Milwaukee, Milwaukee, WI, p. A465

GILBERTSON, Gerry, President, Fairmont Community Hospital, Fairmont, MN, p. A228

GILBERTSON, Roger, M.D., President, MeritCare Health System, Fargo, ND, p. A320

GILES, Ken, Administrator, Eastmoreland Hospital, Portland, OR, p. A351

GILLIARD, Ronald M., FACHE
Administrator, Mitchell County Hospital, Camilla, GA, p. A106
Administrator, U. S. Air Force Hospital Robins, Robins AFB, GA, p. A113

GILLIHAN, Kerry G., President and Chief Executive Officer, Cardinal Hill Rehabilitation Hospital, Lexington, KY, p. A176

GILLILAND, Edward B., Interim Administrator, Yalobusha General Hospital, Water Valley, MS, p. A244

GILLILAND, Jerry E., President, Park Healthcare Company, Nashville, TN, p. B121

GILLILAND, Woody, Chief Executive Officer, Abilene Regional Medical Center, Abilene, TX, p. A398

GILLMAN, Jerry, President and Chief Executive Officer, Thompson Memorial Medical Center, Burbank, CA, p. A38

GILLS, Karl B., Administrator, North Colorado Medical Center, Greeley, CO, p. A73

GILMORE, Beverly, Chief Executive Officer, Columbia South Valley Hospital, Gilroy, CA, p. A44

GILROY, Gretchen, President and Chief Executive Officer, St. Francis Medical Center–West, Ewa Beach, HI, p. A117

GILSTRAP, M. E., President and Chief Executive Officer, Halifax Memorial Hospital, Roanoke Rapids, NC, p. A315

GINSBERG, Arthur M., Chief Executive Officer, BHC Cedar Vista Hospital, Fresno, CA, p. A43

GINTOLI, George P., Chief Executive Officer, Northcoast Behavioral Healthcare System, Northfield, OH, p. A333

GINTZIG, Donald R., President and Chief Executive Officer, Pottsville Hospital and Warne Clinic, Pottsville, PA, p. A367

GIROTTO, R. G., Executive Vice President and Chief Operating Officer, The Methodist Hospital, Houston, TX, p. A416

GITCH, David W., President and Chief Executive Officer, Harrison Memorial Hospital, Bremerton, WA, p. A448

GITTELMAN, Michael B., Chief Executive Officer, Fair Oaks Hospital, Delray Beach, FL, p. A86

GIUNTO, Nancy A., Operations Administrator, Providence Seattle Medical Center, Seattle, WA, p. A452

GIZZI, James C., President and Chief Executive Officer, St. Francis Hospital of Evanston, Evanston, IL, p. A130

GLASS, Robert, Executive Director, Woodruff Community Hospital, Long Beach, CA, p. A49

GLASS, Sheldon D., M.D., President, Gundry–Glass Hospital, Baltimore, MD, p. A197

GLASSCOCK, Gary M., Administrator, Lloyd Noland Hospital and Health System, Fairfield, AL, p. A14

GLATT, Marie Damian, President, Sisters of Charity of Leavenworth Health Services Corporation, Leavenworth, KS, p. B133

GLAUBKE, Nancy, Administrator, Valley County Hospital, Ord, NE, p. A267

GLAVIS, Edward S., Administrator, Kaiser Foundation Hospital, Fresno, CA, p. A44

GLEDHILL, John E., Administrator, Milford Valley Memorial Hospital, Milford, UT, p. A434

GLOOR, Michael R., President and Chief Executive Officer, Saint Francis Medical Center, Grand Island, NE, p. A264

GLOSS, John, President, Barnes–Jewish St. Peters Hospital, Saint Peters, MO, p. A254

GLOSSY, Bernard, President, Verdugo Hills Hospital, Glendale, CA, p. A45

GLOVER, William W., President, The Toledo Hospital, Toledo, OH, p. A336

GLUECKERT, John W., President, St. Joseph Hospital, Polson, MT, p. A260

GOBLE, Jonathan R., Chief Executive Officer, Muscatine General Hospital, Muscatine, IA, p. A157

GODDARD, Christopher M., Administrator, Marcum and Wallace Memorial Hospital, Irvine, KY, p. A175

GOERING, Melvin, Chief Executive Officer, Prairie View, Newton, KS, p. A167

GOERTZEN, Irma E., President and Chief Executive Officer, Magee–Womens Hospital, Pittsburgh, PA, p. A366

GOESER, Stephen L., Administrator, Shelby County Myrtue Memorial Hospital, Harlan, IA, p. A155

GOETZ, Gary, Director, Children's Psychiatric Hospital of Northern Kentucky, Covington, KY, p. A173

GOFF, James A., FACHE, Director, Veterans Affairs Palo Alto Health Care System, Palo Alto, CA, p. A56

GOING, Kelley, Administrator, Carbon County Memorial Hospital and Nursing Home, Red Lodge, MT, p. A260

GOLD, Larry M., President and Chief Executive Officer, Connecticut Children's Medical Center, Hartford, CT, p. A76

GOLD, Richard, Chief Executive Officer, West Boca Medical Center, Boca Raton, FL, p. A83

GOLDBACH, Peter D., M.D., Chief Executive Officer, Symmes Hospital and Medical Center, Arlington, MA, p. A203

GOLDBERG, Donald H., President, New England Sinai Hospital and Rehabilitation Center, Stoughton, MA, p. A210

GOLDBERG, Edward, President and Chief Executive Officer, Columbia Hoffman Estates Medical Center, Hoffman Estates, IL, p. A132

GOLDBERG, Gerald S., Administrator and Chief Executive Officer, Pacific Hospital of Long Beach, Long Beach, CA, p. A49

GOLDEN, Carolyn P., Administrator, Shriners Hospitals for Children, St. Louis, Saint Louis, MO, p. A254

GOLDFARB, Saul, Chief Executive Officer, Gateways Hospital and Mental Health Center, Los Angeles, CA, p. A50

GOLDMAN, T. Marvin, Administrator, Memorial Hospital of Sheridan County, Sheridan, WY, p. A472

GOLDMAN, Thomas, President, Bayshore Community Hospital, Holmdel, NJ, p. A278

GOLDSMITH, Martin
President, Albert Einstein Healthcare Network, Philadelphia, PA, p. B64
President, Albert Einstein Medical Center, Philadelphia, PA, p. A363

GOLDSTEIN, Debra, Administrator, Norfolk Psychiatric Center, Norfolk, VA, p. A443

GOLDSTEIN, Gary W., M.D., President, Kennedy Krieger Children's Hospital, Baltimore, MD, p. A198

GOLDSTEIN, Steven, Ph.D., Chief Executive Officer, Chestnut Lodge Hospital, Rockville, MD, p. A201

GOLI, Rajitha, M.D., Medical Director, Sargent District Hospital, Sargent, NE, p. A268

GOLSON, Allen, Chief Executive Officer, Columbia Palmyra Medical Centers, Albany, GA, p. A103

GONZALES, Joseph P., USA, Chief of Staff, Brooke Army Medical Center, San Antonio, TX, p. A425

GONZALEZ, Arthur A., Dr.PH, President and Chief Executive Officer, Schumpert Medical Center, Shreveport, LA, p. A190

GONZALEZ, Pedro, Executive Director, San Carlos General Hospital, San Juan, PR, p. A477

GONZALEZ, Sonia I., R.N., Chief Operating Officer, Spring Hill Regional Hospital, Spring Hill, FL, p. A99

GOODE, Galen, Chief Executive Officer, Hamilton Center, Terre Haute, IN, p. A149

GOODE, Stephen M., Executive Director, Bayside Community Hospital, Anahuac, TX, p. A398

GOODLOE, Larry S., Administrator, Community Hospital Association, Fairfax, MO, p. A247

GOODMAN, Carol L., Administrator, Union County Hospital District, Anna, IL, p. A123

GOODMAN, Norman B., President and Chief Executive Officer, Brockton Hospital, Brockton, MA, p. A205

GOODMAN, Terry, Executive Director, Miami Jewish Home and Hospital for Aged, Miami, FL, p. A93

GOODRICH, Bill, Administrator, Lillian M. Hudspeth Memorial Hospital, Sonora, TX, p. A427

GOODSPEED, Ronald B., M.D., President, Southcoast Hospitals Group, Fall River, MA, p. A206

GOODWIN, Bradford M., President, Sunnyview Hospital and Rehabilitation Center, Schenectady, NY, p. A304

GOODWIN, Jeffrey C., President and Chief Executive Officer, Warren Hospital, Phillipsburg, NJ, p. A280

GOODWIN, Phillip H.
President, Camcare, Inc., Charleston, WV, p. B73
President and Chief Executive Officer, Charleston Area Medical Center, Charleston, WV, p. A455

GORDON, Bruce A., Director, Veterans Affairs Medical Center, Northampton, MA, p. A208

GORDON, Michael L., President, Woodlawn Hospital, Rochester, IN, p. A148

GORDON, William G., Chief Executive Officer, Barton Memorial Hospital, South Lake Tahoe, CA, p. A65

GORE, Gary R., Administrator, Guntersville–Arab Medical Center, Guntersville, AL, p. A15

GORE, J. Curtiss, Chief Executive Officer, Loris Community Hospital, Loris, SC, p. A379

GORMAN, John A., Chief Executive Officer, Memorial Hospital, Fremont, OH, p. A330

GORSKI, Max J., Chief Executive Officer, Chestnut Hill Psychiatric Hospital, Travelers Rest, SC, p. A381

GOSLINE, Peter L., Administrator, Craig House Center, Beacon, NY, p. A289

GOSS, Allan S., Director, Department of VA Medical Center–Alexandria, Alexandria, LA, p. A182

GOTSCHLICH, Emil, M.D., Vice President Medical Sciences, Rockefeller University Hospital, New York, NY, p. A299

GOTTLIEB, Gary L., M.D., Chief Executive Officer, Friends Hospital, Philadelphia, PA, p. A364

GOTTSCHALK, M. Therese
President, Sisters of the Sorrowful Mother United States Health System, Tulsa, OK, p. B136
President, St. John Medical Center, Tulsa, OK, p. A347

GOULD, Gary R., FACHE, Chief Executive Officer, City Hospital, Bellaire, OH, p. A324

GOULET, Diana L., Chief Executive Officer, BHC Canyon Ridge Hospital, Chino, CA, p. A39

GOVIER, George A., President and Chief Executive Officer, Mercy Medical Center, Redding, CA, p. A58

GRABER, Calvin C., Chief Executive Officer, Henderson Health Care Services, Henderson, NE, p. A264

GRADY, Glen E., Administrator, Memorial Medical Center, Neillsville, WI, p. A466

GRAEBER, Lawrence, Administrator, Neshoba County General Hospital, Philadelphia, MS, p. A242

GRAECA, Raymond A., President and Chief Executive Officer, DuBois Regional Medical Center, DuBois, PA, p. A357

GRAFF, Sylvester, President and Chief Executive Officer, Queen of Angels–Hollywood Presbyterian Medical Center, Los Angeles, CA, p. A51

GRAGG, Martha, Chief Executive Officer, Sullivan County Memorial Hospital, Milan, MO, p. A251

GRAH, John A., Administrator, Williamson ARH Hospital, South Williamson, KY, p. A180

GRAHAM, George W., President, Torrance Memorial Medical Center, Torrance, CA, p. A66

GRAHAM, H. James, Administrator, Person County Memorial Hospital, Roxboro, NC, p. A316

GRAHAM, John A., President and Chief Executive Officer, Sherman Hospital, Elgin, IL, p. A129

GRAHAM, Joseph, Chief Executive Officer, University of Nebraska Medical Center, Omaha, NE, p. A267

GRAHAM, Kenneth D., President and Chief Executive Officer, Overlake Hospital Medical Center, Bellevue, WA, p. A448

GRAHAM, Larry M., Chief Executive Officer, Chalmette Medical Centers, Chalmette, LA, p. A183

GRAHAM, Richard H., President and Chief Executive Officer, Augusta Health Care, Fishersville, VA, p. A440

GRAHAM, Richard L., Administrator, Bedford County General Hospital, Shelbyville, TN, p. A396

GRAHAM, Richard W., FACHE, President, Fairmont General Hospital, Fairmont, WV, p. A456

GRAHAM, Stewart, Administrator, Charter Behavioral Health Systems, Lafayette, IN, p. A145

GRAJEWSKI, Timothy J., President and Chief Executive Officer, St. John Hospital and Medical Center, Detroit, MI, p. A215

GRAMLEY, Thomas S., Administrator, South Florida State Hospital, Pembroke Pines, FL, p. A96

GRAMLICH, Andrew, Chief Executive Officer, Lander Valley Medical Center, Lander, WY, p. A472

GRAND, Gary S., Chief Executive Officer, Central Louisiana State Hospital, Pineville, LA, p. A190

GRANDBOIS, Ray, M.P.H., Service Unit Director, U. S. Public Health Service Indian Hospital, Belcourt, ND, p. A319

GRANDY, Gary W., Administrator, Petersburg Medical Center, Petersburg, AK, p. A21

GRANGER, Keith, President and Chief Executive Officer, Flowers Hospital, Dothan, AL, p. A13

GRANT, John R., Chief Executive Officer, Columbia Hospital Paris, Paris, KY, p. A179

GRAPPE, Steve, Administrator, Horizon Specialty Hospital, Lubbock, TX, p. A419

GRAVES, Jimmy, Administrator, Walthall County General Hospital, Tylertown, MS, p. A243

GRAVES, Philip G., President, Hutchinson Area Health Care, Hutchinson, MN, p. A230

GRAVES, Robert L., Administrator, Virginia Beach General Hospital, Virginia Beach, VA, p. A447

GRAY, David L., Administrator, Tri County Baptist Hospital, La Grange, KY, p. A175

GRAY, E. Kay, Interim Administrator, Vencor Hospital–Milwaukee, Milwaukee, WI, p. A466

GRAY, Patricia, Administrator and Chief Executive Officer, Blowing Rock Hospital, Blowing Rock, NC, p. A308

GRAY, Patrick J., Chief Executive Officer, Cumberland River Hospital North, Celina, TN, p. A387

GRAY, Penny, Administrator and Chief Executive Officer, Limestone Medical Center, Groesbeck, TX, p. A412

GRAY, Robert D., Ed.D., Chief Executive Officer, Crittenton, Kansas City, MO, p. A249

GRAY, Val S., Executive Director, Cornwall Hospital, Cornwall, NY, p. A291

GRAY Jr., George H., Director, Veterans Affairs Medical Center, Little Rock, AR, p. A33

GRAYBILL, Scott R., Administrator and Chief Executive Officer, Community Hospital of Bremen, Bremen, IN, p. A141

GRAYBILL, Todd B., Administrator, Charter Hospital of Charleston, Charleston, SC, p. A376

GREEN, Calvin, Administrator, Crosby Memorial Hospital, Picayune, MS, p. A242

GREEN, Don Edd, Administrator, East Texas Medical Center Rusk, Rusk, TX, p. A425

GREEN, Jack W., Administrator, Antelope Memorial Hospital, Neligh, NE, p. A266

GREEN, Jerry, Administrator, Tippah County Hospital, Ripley, MS, p. A243

GREEN, John H., Administrator, West Feliciana Parish Hospital, Saint Francisville, LA, p. A190

GREEN, Michael B., President, Concord Hospital, Concord, NH, p. A272

GREEN, Patrick, Administrator, Morgan Memorial Hospital, Madison, GA, p. A111

GREEN, Thomas E., President and Chief Executive Officer, Community Hospital at Dobbs Ferry, Dobbs Ferry, NY, p. A291

GREEN, Warren A., President and Chief Executive Officer, Sinai Hospital of Baltimore, Baltimore, MD, p. A198

GREENBERG, Herman R., Administrator, Maxwell Hospital, Montgomery, AL, p. A16

GREENE, Albert Lawrence, President and Chief Executive Officer, Alta Bates Medical Center–Ashby Campus, Berkeley, CA, p. A38

GREENE, Jerry, Chief Executive Officer, Charter Behavioral Health System of San Diego, San Diego, CA, p. A60

GREENE, Steven J., Chief Executive Officer, Kenner Regional Medical Center, Kenner, LA, p. A185

GREENE, William M., FACHE, President, Santa Paula Memorial Hospital, Santa Paula, CA, p. A64

GREENE Jr., Charles H., Administrator, Cordell Memorial Hospital, Cordell, OK, p. A340

GREENE Jr., Edward C.
Administrator, Charles A. Cannon Jr. Memorial Hospital, Banner Elk, NC, p. A308
President, Sloop Memorial Hospital, Crossnore, NC, p. A310

GREENSPAN, Benn, President and Chief Executive Officer, Mount Sinai Hospital Medical Center of Chicago, Chicago, IL, p. A126

GREENWELL, Maryann J., Executive Director, The Retreat, Sunrise, FL, p. A100

GREENWOOD, Kay, MS, Facility Director, North Alabama Regional Hospital, Decatur, AL, p. A13

GREER, James K., Administrator, Methodist Hospital of Middle Mississippi, Lexington, MS, p. A241

GREER, John H., President, Southside Community Hospital, Farmville, VA, p. A440

GREEVER, Paul, Interim Chief Executive Officer, Parkside Hospital, Tulsa, OK, p. A346

GREGG, C. Jan, Chief Executive Officer, Eastern State Hospital, Medical Lake, WA, p. A450

GREGG Jr., David H., President, Gifford Medical Center, Randolph, VT, p. A437

GREGOIRE, Sharon, Chief Operating Officer, Northwest Hospital, Tucson, AZ, p. A27

GREGORY, Samuel S., Administrator, Upson Regional Medical Center, Thomaston, GA, p. A115

GREGORY, William A., Chief Executive Officer, Diagnostic Center Hospital, Houston, TX, p. A414

GREGSON, C. Mark
Chief Executive Officer, Columbia Brunswick Hospital, Supply, NC, p. A317
Chief Executive Officer, Columbia Cape Fear Memorial Hospital, Wilmington, NC, p. A318

GREY, Joel E.
Chief Executive Officer, Sutter Auburn Faith Hospital, Auburn, CA, p. A37
Chief Executive Officer, Sutter Roseville Medical Center, Roseville, CA, p. A59

GREY, William N., Chief Executive Officer, Scott County Hospital, Oneida, TN, p. A395

GRIFFIN, Debra L., Administrator, Humphreys County Memorial Hospital, Belzoni, MS, p. A237

GRIFFITH, Dennis, Vice President, Decatur General Hospital–West, Decatur, AL, p. A13

GRIFFITH, Patti, R.N., Administrator and Chief Executive Officer, Tri–City Health Centre, Dallas, TX, p. A407

GRIFFITH, Richard L., President and Chief Executive Officer, Queen's Health Systems, Honolulu, HI, p. B123

GRIFFITH, Wayne B., FACHE, Chief Executive Officer, St. Joseph's Hospital, Buckhannon, WV, p. A455

GRIMES, Larry, Managing Director, River Crest Hospital, San Angelo, TX, p. A425

GRIMES, Teresa F., Administrator, Vaughn Jackson Medical Center, Jackson, AL, p. A15

GRIMES III, Thomas F., Executive Vice President and Chief Operating Officer, St. Elizabeth Community Hospital, Red Bluff, CA, p. A58

GRIMM, Steve, Chief Executive Officer, River West Medical Center, Plaquemine, LA, p. A190

GRIPPEN, Glen W., Director, Veterans Affairs Medical Center, Iron Mountain, MI, p. A218

GRISSLER, Brian G., President and Chief Executive Officer, Suburban Hospital, Bethesda, MD, p. A199

GRITMAN, Paul J., Superintendent, Danville State Hospital, Danville, PA, p. A356

GRONEWALD, John E., Chief Operating Officer, Ridgeview Institute, Smyrna, GA, p. A114

GROSETH, Bradley D., Administrator, Osseo Area Hospital and Nursing Home, Osseo, WI, p. A467

GROSS, Dan, Chief Executive Officer, Sharp Memorial Hospital, San Diego, CA, p. A61

GROSS, Diane S., Administrator, Holton Community Hospital, Holton, KS, p. A164

GROSS, Joseph W., President and Chief Executive Officer, St. Elizabeth Medical Center–North, Covington, KY, p. A173

GROSS, Kevin, Interim President and Chief Executive Officer, Columbia Wesley Medical Center, Wichita, KS, p. A170

GROSSMEIER, John C., President and Chief Executive Officer, Hannibal Regional Hospital, Hannibal, MO, p. A247

GROVER Sr., Bradley K.
Chief Executive Officer, Columbia Northside Medical Center, Saint Petersburg, FL, p. A98
President and Chief Executive Officer, Columbia St. Petersburg Medical Center, Saint Petersburg, FL, p. A98

GRUSSING, Mel, Administrator, LAC–High Desert Hospital, Lancaster, CA, p. A48

GUARNIERI, Ellen, Acting Executive Director, West Jersey Hospital–Berlin, Berlin, NJ, p. A275

GUENTHER, Charles, Administrator, Eastern Plumas District Hospital, Portola, CA, p. A58

GUEST, John A., President and Chief Executive Officer, University Health System, San Antonio, TX, p. A426

GUILD, Samuel T., Administrator, Pawhuska Hospital, Pawhuska, OK, p. A344

GUIMARIN, Spencer, Administrator, Lakes Regional Medical Center, Jasper, TX, p. A417

GUINAN, Vincent F., President and Chief Executive Officer, St. Vincent Medical Center, Los Angeles, CA, p. A52

GUINN, Lex A., Chief Executive Officer, Odessa Regional Hospital, Odessa, TX, p. A422

GULEY, Michael G., President and Chief Executive Officer, Our Lady of Lourdes Memorial Hospital, Binghamton, NY, p. A289

GULICK, Margaret S., President and Chief Executive Officer, Memorial Healthcare Center, Owosso, MI, p. A221

GULLIFORD, Deryl E., Ph.D., Administrator, Community Memorial Hospital, Hicksville, OH, p. A330

GULLINGSRUD, Tim, Administrator, McKenzie County Memorial Hospital, Watford City, ND, p. A322

GUNDERSON, Rodney L., Executive Director, Frick Hospital and Community Health Center, Mount Pleasant, PA, p. A362

GUNN, B. Joe, FACHE, Administrator and Chief Executive Officer, Craig General Hospital, Vinita, OK, p. A347

GUNN, Christina B.
Chief Executive Officer, University of New Mexico Children's Psychiatric Hospital, Albuquerque, NM, p. A285
Chief Executive Officer, University of New Mexico Mental Health Center, Albuquerque, NM, p. A285

GUNN, John R., Executive Vice President, Memorial Hospital for Cancer and Allied Diseases, New York, NY, p. A298

GUNN, Terry J., Administrator, Columbia Stones River Hospital, Woodbury, TN, p. A397

GUPTON, Jack A., USAF, Administrator, Mike O'Callaghan Federal Hospital, Las Vegas, NV, p. A270

GURGEL, Paul L., President and Chief Executive Officer, New London Family Medical Center, New London, WI, p. A466

GUSTAFSON, Philip P., Chief Executive Officer, San Ramon Regional Medical Center, San Ramon, CA, p. A63

GUTHMILLER, Martin W., Administrator, Orange City Municipal Hospital, Orange City, IA, p. A157

GUTHRIE, Deborah S., Chief Executive Officer, Columbia Parkway Medical Center, Lithia Springs, GA, p. A111

GUTHRIE, Denise, Chief Executive Officer, Charter Cypress Behavioral Health System, Lafayette, LA, p. A186

GUTMAN, Milton M., Chief Executive Officer, Kingsbrook Jewish Medical Center, New York, NY, p. A297

GUTZKE, Ella, Administrator, Sheridan Memorial Hospital, Plentywood, MT, p. A260

GUY, Douglas, President and Chief Executive Officer, Memorial Hospital Oconomowoc, Oconomowoc, WI, p. A466

GUYNN, Robert W., M.D., Executive Director, Harris County Psychiatric Center, Houston, TX, p. A414

GUZMAN, Tibisay A., Executive Vice President and Chief Operating Officer, Yonkers General Hospital, Yonkers, NY, p. A307

GWIAZDA, John M., President and Chief Executive Officer, Eastern Long Island Hospital, Greenport, NY, p. A292

GYSIN, Joyce, Administrator, Surprise Valley Community Hospital, Cedarville, CA, p. A39

H

HAACK, Frederick W., President, Mille Lacs Health System, Onamia, MN, p. A232

HAAR, Clare A., Chief Executive Officer, Inter–Community Memorial Hospital, Newfane, NY, p. A301

HABERLEIN, Bernard, Executive Director, Graydon Manor, Leesburg, VA, p. A442

HADDIX, D. Parker, Chief Executive Officer, Richwood Area Community Hospital, Richwood, WV, p. A458

HADEN, James E., President and Chief Executive Officer, Martha Jefferson Hospital, Charlottesville, VA, p. A440

HADFIELD, Tomi, Administrator, Riverside General Hospital–University Medical Center, Riverside, CA, p. A59

HAGEN, David F., President and Executive Officer, Roseau Area Hospital and Homes, Roseau, MN, p. A233

HAHN, James, Administrator, Baptist Memorial Hospital–North Mississippi, Oxford, MS, p. A242

HAHN, Richard W., Executive Director, Dunn Memorial Hospital, Bedford, IN, p. A140

HAILS, Robert, Chief Executive Officer, Charter Beacon, Fort Wayne, IN, p. A142

HALE, William R., Chief Executive Officer, University Medical Center, Las Vegas, NV, p. A270

HALES Jr., John C., FACHE, President and Chief Executive Officer, Roper Hospital North, Charleston, SC, p. A376

HALEY, Bob J., Chief Executive Officer, Columbia Medical Center of Denton, Denton, TX, p. A408

HALKO, Mavis B., Administrator, Lakeshore Community Hospital, Dadeville, AL, p. A13

HALL, Amanda M., Administrator, Smith Hospital, Hahira, GA, p. A110

HALL, Dennis A., President, Baptist Health System, Birmingham, AL, p. B68

HALL, Diane S., Administrator, Bullock County Hospital, Union Springs, AL, p. A18

HALL, Gene, Administrator, University of Tennessee Memorial Hospital, Knoxville, TN, p. A391

HALL, Herbert L., Chief Executive Officer, Wellspring Foundation, Bethlehem, CT, p. A76

HALL, Joan S., R.N., Administrator, South Lyon Medical Center, Yerington, NV, p. A271

HALL, Kim, Chief Executive Officer, Charter Behavioral Health System–Glendale, Glendale, AZ, p. A23

HALL, Linda, Administrator, Chillicothe Hospital District, Chillicothe, TX, p. A403

HALL, Marcia K., Chief Executive Officer, Sharp Coronado Hospital, Coronado, CA, p. A40

HALL, Philo D., President, Central Vermont Medical Center, Barre, VT, p. A437

HALL, Richard W., President, Jamestown Hospital, Jamestown, ND, p. A320

HALL, Roger L., Chief Executive Officer, North Okaloosa Medical Center, Crestview, FL, p. A85

HALL, Steve, Chief Executive Officer, Harbor View Medical Center, San Diego, CA, p. A60

HALL II, R. B., Commanding Officer, Naval Hospital, Groton, CT, p. A76

HALL Jr., F. W., Administrator, Sid Peterson Memorial Hospital, Kerrville, TX, p. A417

HALLFORD, Wayne, Chief Executive Officer, BHC Millwood Hospital, Arlington, TX, p. A399

HALLGREN, Hugh R., President and Chief Executive Officer, Wadley Regional Medical Center, Texarkana, TX, p. A429

HALLMAN, Gary D., President and Chief Executive Officer, Medina General Hospital, Medina, OH, p. A333

HALLONQUIST, Frances A., Chief Executive Officer, Kapiolani Medical Center for Women and Children, Honolulu, HI, p. A117

HALPERN, Kevin G., President and Chief Executive Officer, The Cooper Health System, Camden, NJ, p. A276

HALPERN, Marsha Lommel, President and Chief Executive Officer, Madonna Rehabilitation Hospital, Lincoln, NE, p. A265

HALSETH, Michael J., Executive Director, University of Virginia Medical Center, Charlottesville, VA, p. A440

HALSTEAD, Michael J., President and Chief Executive Officer, Carlisle Hospital, Carlisle, PA, p. A355

HAMILL, Dave H., President and Chief Executive Officer, Hampton Regional Medical Center, Varnville, SC, p. A381

HAMILL, James P., President, Holy Cross Hospital of Silver Spring, Silver Spring, MD, p. A202

HAMILTON, Daniel, Chief Executive Officer, Pennock Hospital, Hastings, MI, p. A217

HAMILTON, Hollis, Administrator, Charlotte Institute of Rehabilitation, Charlotte, NC, p. A309

HAMILTON, Michael E., Director, Overton Brooks Veterans Affairs Medical Center, Shreveport, LA, p. A190

HAMILTON, Phil, R.N., Chief Executive Officer, General John J. Pershing Memorial Hospital, Brookfield, MO, p. A245

HAMILTON, Richard C., Chief Executive Officer, Mitchell County Regional Health Center, Osage, IA, p. A157

HAMMACK, Stanley K., Administrator, University of South Alabama Knollwood Park Hospital, Mobile, AL, p. A16

HAMMER, Michael, President and Chief Executive Officer, Good Samaritan Health Center of Merrill, Merrill, WI, p. A465

HAMMER, Pat, Chief Executive Officer, Ten Broeck Hospital, Louisville, KY, p. A177

HAMMER, David L., MC, Commander, U. S. Air Force Academy Hospital, USAF Academy, CO, p. A75

HAMMER II, Robert L., Chief Executive Officer, Davis Memorial Hospital, Elkins, WV, p. A456

HAMMETT, Warren E., Administrator, Bamberg County Memorial Hospital and Nursing Center, Bamberg, SC, p. A375

HAMMOND, Joe, Administrator, Eureka Springs Hospital, Eureka Springs, AR, p. A30

HAMNER, David, Administrator, Hardtner Medical Center, Olla, LA, p. A189

HAMORY, Bruce H., M.D., Executive Director, Penn State University Hospital–Milton S. Hershey Medical Center, Hershey, PA, p. A359

HAMRY, David K., President, Good Samaritan Community Healthcare, Puyallup, WA, p. A451

HANAWATT, Kent, Chief Executive Officer, Broadwater Health Center, Townsend, MT, p. A260

HANCOCK, Edward H., President, Nanticoke Memorial Hospital, Seaford, DE, p. A80

HANDEL, David J., Director, Indiana University Medical Center, Indianapolis, IN, p. A144

HANENBURG, Thomas, Administrator, Franklin Regional Medical Center, Louisburg, NC, p. A314

HANES, Carol, Chief Executive Officer, Twin Rivers Regional Medical Center, Kennett, MO, p. A250

HANEY, T. Mark
Administrator, Promina Paulding Memorial Medical Center, Dallas, GA, p. A107
Administrator, Promina Windy Hill Hospital, Marietta, GA, p. A111

HANKINS, J. William, President and Chief Executive Officer, St. Patrick Hospital of Lake Charles, Lake Charles, LA, p. A186

HANKO, James F., Administrator and Chief Executive Officer, Falls Memorial Hospital, International Falls, MN, p. A230

HANKS, Debra D., Administrator, St. Lukes Rehabilitation Institute, Spokane, WA, p. A453

HANLEY, Richard, Chief Executive Officer, Down East Community Hospital, Machias, ME, p. A195

HANNA, Philip S., Administrator, Adams County Hospital, West Union, OH, p. A337

HANNAN, David T., President and Chief Executive Officer, South Shore Hospital, South Weymouth, MA, p. A209

HANNIG, Virgil, Administrator, Herrin Hospital, Herrin, IL, p. A131

HANOVER, Kenneth, President and Chief Executive Officer, Lankenau Hospital, Wynnewood, PA, p. A371

HANRAHAN, Thomas, Administrator and Chief Executive Officer, McKay–Dee Hospital Center, Ogden, UT, p. A434

HANSEN, Edwin L., Vice President, Yukon–Kuskokwim Delta Regional Hospital, Bethel, AK, p. A20

HANSEN, Irwin C., President and Chief Executive Officer, Summit Medical Center, Oakland, CA, p. A55

HANSEN, Susan M., President and Chief Executive Officer, Columbia Hospital for Women Medical Center, Washington, DC, p. A81

HANSEN, Thomas N., Acting Chief Executive Officer and Medical Director, Children's Hospital, Columbus, OH, p. A327

HANSHAW, John, Chief Executive Officer, Columbia St. Mark's Hospital, Salt Lake City, UT, p. A435

HANSON, Bryant R., President, Floyd Memorial Hospital and Health Services, New Albany, IN, p. A147

HANSON, Craig, Administrator, St. Luke Hospital, Marion, KS, p. A166

HANSON, Greg, President and Chief Executive Officer, Mercy Hospital, Valley City, ND, p. A322

HANSON, Jerry, Administrator, Crawford County Hospital District One, Girard, KS, p. A163

HANSON, L. Carl, Administrator, Pondera Medical Center, Conrad, MT, p. A257

HANSON, Marlin, Administrator, Boaz–Albertville Medical Center, Boaz, AL, p. A12

HANSON, Paul, Chief Executive Officer, Glendive Medical Center, Glendive, MT, p. A258

HANSON, Richard A., Acting Administrator, Bon Secours–Maryview Medical Center, Portsmouth, VA, p. A444

HANSON, Timothy H., President and Chief Executive Officer, HealthEast, Saint Paul, MN, p. B102

HANYAK, Diana C., Chief Executive Officer, Charter Behavioral Health System of Southern California–Corona, Corona, CA, p. A40

HAPPEL, Jerald R., Executive Director, South Bay Medical Center, Redondo Beach, CA, p. A58

HARBARGER, Claude W., President, St. Dominic–Jackson Memorial Hospital, Jackson, MS, p. A240

HARCOURT Jr., John P., President and Chief Executive Officer, Healthcare America, Inc., Austin, TX, p. B101

HARDER, Fred M., President and Chief Executive Officer, Paradise Valley Hospital, National City, CA, p. A55

HARDER, Shirley, Chief Executive Officer, Wayne Medical Center, Waynesboro, TN, p. A397

HARDING, Lynwood F., Director, Western State Hospital, Staunton, VA, p. A446

HARDING, William W., President and Chief Executive Officer, Union Hospital, Dover, OH, p. A329

HARDMAN, R. Kim, Administrator, Decatur County Hospital, Oberlin, KS, p. A167

HARDY, Patsy, Administrator, Putnam General Hospital, Hurricane, WV, p. A457

HARDY, Stephen L., Ph.D., Facility Director, Chester Mental Health Center, Chester, IL, p. A125

HARDY, J. Thomas, Commanding Officer, Irwin Army Community Hospital, Fort Riley, KS, p. A163

HARE, Joseph C., President and Chief Executive Officer, Neumann Medical Center, Philadelphia, PA, p. A364

HARE, Michael K., Administrator, De Leon Hospital, De Leon, TX, p. A407

HARENSKI, Robert J., Chief Executive Officer, Antelope Valley Hospital, Lancaster, CA, p. A48

HARGIS, Paul D., Administrator, Shriners Hospitals for Children, Los Angeles, Los Angeles, CA, p. A51

HARKINS, William D., President and Chief Executive Officer, Ancilla Systems Inc., Hobart, IN, p. B66

HARKNESS, Laurence P., President and Chief Executive Officer, Children's Medical Center, Dayton, OH, p. A328

HARLAN, Thomas M., Chief Executive Officer, Chinese Hospital, San Francisco, CA, p. A61

HARLEY, Richard A., Vice President Finance, Gettysburg Hospital, Gettysburg, PA, p. A358

HARMAN, David L., Administrator, Harney District Hospital, Burns, OR, p. A348

HARMAN, Gerald M., Chief Executive Officer and Executive Vice President, St. Elizabeth's Hospital, Belleville, IL, p. A123

HARMAN, Richmond M., President and Chief Executive Officer, Martin Memorial Health System, Stuart, FL, p. A99

HARMAN, Robert L., Administrator, Grant Memorial Hospital, Petersburg, WV, p. A458

HARMON, Kent, Interim Chief Executive Officer, Rangely District Hospital, Rangely, CO, p. A74

HARMS, Charles F., Administrator, McKee Medical Center, Loveland, CO, p. A74

HARPER, Alan G., Director, Veterans Affairs Medical Center, Dallas, TX, p. A407

HARPER, John D., Administrator, South Shore Hospital, Chicago, IL, p. A127

HARPER, Thomas L., President and Chief Executive Officer, Methodist Medical Center, Jackson, MS, p. A240

HARR, Robert Glenn, President, Heather Hill Hospital and Health Care Center, Chardon, OH, p. A324

HARRELL, David E., President and Chief Executive Officer, Georgia Baptist Health Care System, Atlanta, GA, p. A104

HARRELL, Richard E., President, Duplin General Hospital, Kenansville, NC, p. A313

HARRINGTON, Frank, Administrator, Aberdeen–Monroe County Hospital, Aberdeen, MS, p. A237

HARRINGTON, Joseph P., Chief Executive Officer, Lodi Memorial Hospital, Lodi, CA, p. A48

HARRINGTON, Michael L., Executive Vice President and Administrator, Bon Secours–St. Joseph Hospital, Port Charlotte, FL, p. A97

HARRINGTON, Timothy, President, Victory Memorial Hospital, Waukegan, IL, p. A139

HARRINGTON Jr., John L., FACHE, Administrator, Vencor Hospital–Phoenix, Phoenix, AZ, p. A25

HARRINGTON Jr., Russell D., President, Baptist Health, Little Rock, AR, p. B67

HARRIS, Andrew E., Chief Executive Officer, Mercy Community Hospital, Havertown, PA, p. A359

HARRIS, Frank W., President and Chief Executive Officer, Russell Hospital, Alexander City, AL, p. A11

HARRIS, Jan, Vice President, Maniilaq Health Center, Kotzebue, AK, p. A21

HARRIS, Robert L., President and Chief Executive Officer, Ingalls Memorial Hospital, Harvey, IL, p. A131

HARRIS, Robert W., President, Lakeside Memorial Hospital, Brockport, NY, p. A289

HARRIS, Theresa, Clinical Administrator, Concord Hospital, Baton Rouge, LA, p. A182

HARRIS, Wayne, Administrator, Simpson General Hospital, Mendenhall, MS, p. A241

HARRISON, Daniel J., Assistant Vice President and Administrator, Amethyst, Charlotte, NC, p. A309

HARROD, Pat, Chief Executive Officer, Charter Behavioral Health System of Paducah, Paducah, KY, p. A179

HART, Diane M., Chief Executive Officer, Moses Ludington Hospital, Ticonderoga, NY, p. A305

HART, Gerald L., Chief Executive Officer, State Hospital North, Orofino, ID, p. A121

HART, James D., President, Northwest Hospital, Seattle, WA, p. A452

HART, Joel A., FACHE, Chief Executive Officer, Charter Heights Behavioral Health System, Albuquerque, NM, p. A284

HART, John S., Administrator, Greenleaf Center, Jonesboro, AR, p. A32

HART, Noel W., Administrator, King's Daughters Hospital, Yazoo City, MS, p. A244

HART, Patsy J., Director, University Hospitals and Clinics, Columbia, MO, p. A246

HARTLEY, H. William, Chief Executive Officer, Rush Memorial Hospital, Rushville, IN, p. A148

HARTMAN, C. Richard, M.D., President and Chief Executive Officer, Community Medical Center, Scranton, PA, p. A368

HARTMAN, R. Michael, Chief Executive Officer, Doctors Hospital of Santa Ana, Santa Ana, CA, p. A63

HARVEY, Robert C., Commander, DeWitt Army Community Hospital, Fort Belvoir, VA, p. A441

HARWELL, Richard, Director, Central Texas Veterans Affairs Healthcare System, Temple, TX, p. A428

HARWOOD, Janie L., Chief Executive Officer, Columbia Bayview Psychiatric Center, Corpus Christi, TX, p. A404

HASTINGS, Arthur W., President and Chief Executive Officer, Middle Tennessee Medical Center, Murfreesboro, TN, p. A394

HASTINGS, Eugene, Chief Executive Officer, Heartland Behavioral Health Services, Nevada, MO, p. A251

HASTINGS, G. Richard, President and Chief Executive Officer, Saint Luke's Shawnee Mission Health System, Kansas City, MO, p. B130

HATALA, Alexander J., President and Chief Executive Officer, Our Lady of Lourdes Medical Center, Camden, NJ, p. A275

HATCHER, John M., President, Whitley Memorial Hospital, Columbia City, IN, p. A141

HATERIUS, Craig, Administrator, Stamford Memorial Hospital, Stamford, TX, p. A428

HAUG, William F., FACHE, President and Chief Executive Officer, Motion Picture and Television Fund Hospital and Residential Services, Los Angeles, CA, p. A51

HAUGH, Diana, MS, Superintendent, Larue D. Carter Memorial Hospital, Indianapolis, IN, p. A144

HAUGO, Glenn, Administrator, Daniels Memorial Hospital, Scobey, MT, p. A260

HAUSE, Eileen, Chief Executive Officer, Kensington Hospital, Philadelphia, PA, p. A364

HAUSLER, Jeffrey E., President and Chief Executive Officer, Wichita General Hospital, Wichita Falls, TX, p. A431

HAWKINS, Leslie A., Chief Executive Officer, Mount Desert Island Hospital, Bar Harbor, ME, p. A193

HAWKINS, Mary Jane, Administrator and Chief Executive Officer, Healthsouth Nittany Valley Rehabilitation Hospital, Pleasant Gap, PA, p. A367

HAWKINS, Phil, Administrator, Carnegie Tri–County Municipal Hospital, Carnegie, OK, p. A340

HAWKINS, Robert L., Superintendent, Colorado Mental Health Institute at Pueblo, Pueblo, CO, p. A74

HAWLEY, Jerry, Administrator, Quincy Valley Medical Center, Quincy, WA, p. A451

HAWLEY, Jess, Administrator, Syringa General Hospital, Grangeville, ID, p. A120

HAWLEY Jr., Robert L., Chief Executive Officer, Bolivar County Hospital, Cleveland, MS, p. A238

HAWTHORNE, Connie, Chief Executive Officer, Medical Center Shoals, Muscle Shoals, AL, p. A17

HAWTHORNE, Douglas D., President and Chief Executive Officer, Presbyterian Healthcare System, Dallas, TX, p. B122

HAYES, David R., President, Taylor County Hospital, Campbellsville, KY, p. A173

HAYES, Howard A., President and Chief Executive Officer, St. Joseph Regional Medical Center, Lewiston, ID, p. A120

HAYES, James M., Administrator, Hamilton Memorial Hospital District, McLeansboro, IL, p. A134

HAYES, T. Farrell, President, Healthcorp of Tennessee, Inc., Chattanooga, TN, p. B102

HAYES, Thomas P.
Chief Executive Officer, Fremont Medical Center, Yuba City, CA, p. A69
Chief Executive Officer, Fremont–Rideout Health Group, Yuba City, CA, p. B98
Chief Executive Officer, Rideout Memorial Hospital, Marysville, CA, p. A53

HAYES, Wayne, Administrator, Nashville Metropolitan Bordeaux Hospital, Nashville, TN, p. A394

HAYNES, Jerry, Administrator, McDowell ARH Hospital, McDowell, KY, p. A178

HAYS, Cheryl, Administrator, Lawrence Baptist Medical Center, Moulton, AL, p. A16

HAYS, Janet A., Interim Administrator, Forks Community Hospital, Forks, WA, p. A449

HAYS, Lissa B., Chief Operating Officer, Newport News General Hospital, Newport News, VA, p. A443

HAYWARD, John, Administrator, St. Joseph Hospital, Bellingham, WA, p. A448

HAYWOOD III, Edgar, Administrator, J. Arthur Dosher Memorial Hospital, Southport, NC, p. A317

HAZLETT II, Guy, FACHE, Chief Executive Officer, Palo Pinto General Hospital, Mineral Wells, TX, p. A421

HEAD, William C., USAF, Administrator, U. S. Air Force Regional Hospital, Eglin AFB, FL, p. A86

HEADLEE, Dennis E., Administrator, Plains Regional Medical Center, Clovis, NM, p. A285

HEADLEY, Elwood J., M.D., Director, Veterans Affairs Medical Center, Boston, MA, p. A205

HEARD, William C., Administrator and Chief Executive Officer, Cumberland Hall Hospital, Hopkinsville, KY, p. A175

HEARING, Philip E., President and Chief Executive Officer, Southeastern Ohio Regional Medical Center, Cambridge, OH, p. A324

HEATER, Floyd, Chief Executive Officer, Shenandoah Memorial Hospital, Woodstock, VA, p. A447

HEATH, William J., President and Chief Executive Officer, Saginaw General Hospital, Saginaw, MI, p. A222

HEATHERLY, Neil, Chief Executive Officer, Columbia Metropolitan Hospital, Atlanta, GA, p. A103

HECK III, George L., President and Chief Executive Officer, Coffee Regional Medical Center, Douglas, GA, p. A108

HECKERT, Brian, Director, William Jennings Bryan Dorn Veterans Hospital, Columbia, SC, p. A377

HECKERT Jr., Robert James, MSC, Chief of Staff, Walter Reed Health Care System, Washington, DC, p. A82

HEDDEN, William D., Administrator, Magnolia Hospital, Magnolia, AR, p. A33

HEDRIX, Michael, Chief Executive Officer, Deer River Healthcare Center, Deer River, MN, p. A228

HEEP, Anthony W., Vice President and Administrator, Spohn Memorial Hospital, Corpus Christi, TX, p. A405

HEERAN, Monica F., President and Chief Executive Officer, PeaceHealth, Bellevue, WA, p. B121

HEFLIN Jr., Samuel R., Administrator, Baptist Three Rivers Hospital, Waverly, TN, p. A397

HEIDEBRINK, Roger, Administrator, Gothenburg Memorial Hospital, Gothenburg, NE, p. A264

HEIDT, Roger R., Administrator, Sturgis Community Health Care Center, Sturgis, SD, p. A385

HEIN, Joyce Grove, Chief Executive Officer, Lakewood Medical Center, Morgan City, LA, p. A188

HEINIKE, J. Larry, President and Chief Executive Officer, Horizon Hospital System, Greenville, PA, p. A358

HEISE, Patrick B., Chief Executive Officer, Community Memorial Hospital, Staunton, IL, p. A138

HEITKAMP, Charlotte, Chief Executive Officer, Jackson Medical Center, Jackson, MN, p. A230

HEITZENRATER, James F., Administrator, Potomac Valley Hospital, Keyser, WV, p. A457

HEKIMIAN, Barbara D. S., Chief Executive Officer, Dominion Hospital, Falls Church, VA, p. A440

HELD, Michael J., Administrator, Coral Ridge Psychiatric Hospital, Fort Lauderdale, FL, p. A86

HELIN, Ernie, Interim Administrator, Ashley Memorial Hospital, Crossett, AR, p. A30

HELLER, Thomas, Administrator, Healthsouth Western Hills Regional Rehabilitation Hospital, Parkersburg, WV, p. A458

HELLYER, Nancy R., R.N., Chief Executive Officer, Columbia Grant Hospital, Chicago, IL, p. A125

HELMS, Ella Raye, Administrator, Fisher County Hospital District, Rotan, TX, p. A424

HELMS Jr., Robert N., Divisional Vice President, Operations, Transitional Hospital of Tampa, Tampa, FL, p. A101

HELROID, Michael E., Administrator and Chief Executive Officer, Southern Humboldt Community Healthcare District, Garberville, CA, p. A44

HELZER, James D., Administrator, Veterans Home of California, Yountville, CA, p. A69

HEMETER, Donald, Administrator, Wayne General Hospital, Waynesboro, MS, p. A244

HEMPLING, Randall, Chief Executive Officer, Community Hospital Medical Center, Phoenix, AZ, p. A24

HENCKEL, Susan, Executive Vice President and Chief Executive Officer, Columbia Hospital, Milwaukee, WI, p. A465

HENDERSON, Cynthia T., M.P.H., Interim Hospital Director, Oak Forest Hospital of Cook County, Oak Forest, IL, p. A135

HENDERSON, Donald, Executive Director, Byrd Regional Hospital, Leesville, LA, p. A187

HENDERSON, Jeff, Chief Executive Officer, Rehabilitation Hospital of Baton Rouge, Baton Rouge, LA, p. A183

HENDERSON, W. Perry, Administrator, East Texas Medical Center Pittsburg, Pittsburg, TX, p. A423

HENDRICKSON, Craig L.
Regional Hospital Leader, St. Clare Hospital, Lakewood, WA, p. A450
President and Chief Executive Officer, St. Francis Hospital, Federal Way, WA, p. A449
President and Chief Executive Officer, St. Joseph Medical Center, Tacoma, WA, p. A454
HENDRICKSON, William Wilson, President and Chief Executive Officer, Good Samaritan Health Systems, Kearney, NE, p. A265
HENDRIX, Wayne, President, Kosciusko Community Hospital, Warsaw, IN, p. A149
HENGER, Robert E., Administrator, Carraway Northwest Medical Center, Winfield, AL, p. A19
HENIKOFF, Leo M.
President and Chief Executive Officer, Rush–Presbyterian–St. Luke's Medical Center, Chicago, IL, p. A127
President, Rush–Presbyterian–St. Luke's Medical Center, Chicago, IL, p. B130
HENKE, Marcella V., Administrator, Jackson County Hospital, Edna, TX, p. A408
HENLEY, Darryl E., Administrator, Dos Palos Memorial Hospital, Dos Palos, CA, p. A41
HENLEY, Lavon, Administrator, Atmore Community Hospital, Atmore, AL, p. A11
HENNEY, Jane E., M.D., Vice President Health Sciences, University of New Mexico, Albuquerque, NM, p. B146
HENRY, Angelia K., Administrator, Douglas County Memorial Hospital, Armour, SD, p. A382
HENRY, David, President and Chief Executive Officer, Northern Montana Hospital, Havre, MT, p. A259
HENRY, Paul B., Administrator, Charter Fairmount Institute, Philadelphia, PA, p. A363
HENRY, Peter P., Director, Department of Veterans Affairs Black Hills Health Care System, Fort Meade, SD, p. A383
HENRY, Terry, Interim Administrator, Valley Medical Center of Fresno, Fresno, CA, p. A44
HENRY Jr., Jake, President, Spohn Health System, Corpus Christi, TX, p. A405
HENRY Sr., John Dunklin
Chief Executive Officer, Crawford Long Hospital of Emory University, Atlanta, GA, p. A104
Chief Executive Officer, Emory University Hospital, Atlanta, GA, p. A104
HENSLER, Paul J., Chief Executive Officer, Sutter Lakeside Hospital, Lakeport, CA, p. A47
HENSLEY, Dana S.
President, Birmingham Baptist Medical Center–Montclair Campus, Birmingham, AL, p. A11
President and Chief Executive Officer, Birmingham Baptist Medical Center–Princeton, Birmingham, AL, p. A11
HENSON, Blair W., Administrator, Florala Memorial Hospital, Florala, AL, p. A14
HENSON, David L., Chief Executive Officer, Wilkes Regional Medical Center, North Wilkesboro, NC, p. A315
HENSON, James C., President, United Hospital Corporation, Memphis, TN, p. B144
HENSON, John S., President, Baptist Regional Medical Center, Corbin, KY, p. A173
HENTON, Thomas, Administrator and Chief Executive Officer, Cleveland Area Hospital, Cleveland, OK, p. A340
HENZE, Michael E., Chief Executive Officer, Lake of the Ozarks General Hospital, Osage Beach, MO, p. A251
HERBERT, Susan, Administrator, Inova Mount Vernon Hospital, Alexandria, VA, p. A439
HERDER, David, Administrator, Community Memorial Hospital and Nursing Home, Spring Valley, MN, p. A235
HERFINDAHL, Lowell D., President and Chief Executive Officer, Tioga Medical Center, Tioga, ND, p. A322
HERINGTON, Richard E., President and Chief Executive Officer, Valley Memorial Hospital, Livermore, CA, p. A48
HERLINGER, Daniel R.
President and Chief Executive Officer, St. John's Pleasant Valley Hospital, Camarillo, CA, p. A39
President and Chief Executive Officer, St. John's Regional Medical Center, Oxnard, CA, p. A56

HERMAN, Bernard J., President and Chief Executive Officer, Mercy Healthcare–Bakersfield, Bakersfield, CA, p. A37
HERMAN, Paul, Administrator, San Luis Valley Regional Medical Center, Alamosa, CO, p. A70
HERMANSON, Patrick M., President and Senior Executive, Saint Vincent Hospital and Health Center, Billings, MT, p. A257
HERNANDEZ, Leonard, Administrator, Plainville Rural Hospital District Number One, Plainville, KS, p. A168
HERNANDEZ, Pablo, M.D., Administrator, Wyoming State Hospital, Evanston, WY, p. A471
HERNANDEZ, Roberto, Administrator, University Hospital, San Juan, PR, p. A477
HERNANDEZ–KEEBLE, Sonia, Director, Rio Grande State Center, Harlingen, TX, p. A412
HERRICK, Ronald L., President, Rehabilitation Institute, Kansas City, MO, p. A249
HERRON, John M., Administrator, Baptist North Hospital, Cumming, GA, p. A107
HERRON, Thomas L., FACHE
Chief Executive Officer, Columbia Clearwater Community Hospital, Clearwater, FL, p. A84
President and Chief Executive Officer, Columbia Largo Medical Center, Largo, FL, p. A91
HERSCHBERG, Marvin, Chief Executive Officer, Hawthorne Hospital, Hawthorne, CA, p. A45
HERVEY, Roger D., Administrator, Galena–Stauss Hospital, Galena, IL, p. A130
HERZOG, Paul F., Chief Executive Officer, Columbia Independence Regional Health Center, Independence, MO, p. A248
HESELTINE, Bruce P., USAF, Commander, U. S. Air Force Hospital, Holloman AFB, NM, p. A286
HESS, Carolyn K., Administrator, Grape Community Hospital, Hamburg, IA, p. A155
HESS, Roy, Executive Vice President and Administrator, Bon Secours–Venice Hospital, Venice, FL, p. A101
HESSELMANN, Thomas J., President and Chief Executive Officer, Samaritan Health System, Clinton, IA, p. A152
HESSELTINE, Wendell, President, Tillamook County General Hospital, Tillamook, OR, p. A352
HESTER, Forrest G., President and Chief Executive Officer, Abraham Lincoln Memorial Hospital, Lincoln, IL, p. A133
HEUSER, Keith E., Chief Executive Officer, Memorial Hospital, Carthage, IL, p. A124
HEY, David R., Chief Operating Officer, Westlake Community Hospital, Melrose Park, IL, p. A134
HEYBOER Jr., Lester, President and Chief Executive Officer, HealthSource Saginaw, Saginaw, MI, p. A222
HEYDE, Jorge A., Administrator, Glenoaks Hospital and Medical Center, Glendale Heights, IL, p. A131
HEYDEL, M. John, President and Chief Executive Officer, Columbia Providence Hospital, Columbia, SC, p. A376
HEYDT, Stuart, Chief Executive Officer, Geisinger Medical Center, Danville, PA, p. A356
HIATT, M. K., Administrator, Allendale County Hospital, Fairfax, SC, p. A377
HIBBS, Cathryn A., Chief Executive Officer, Columbia Southwest Hospital, Louisville, KY, p. A177
HICKS, Cheryl, Chief Executive Officer, Twin City Hospital, Dennison, OH, p. A329
HICKS, John D.
President and Chief Executive Officer, Baptist–St. Anthony Health System, Amarillo, TX, p. A398
President, Baptist–St. Anthony's Health System, Amarillo, TX, p. A398
HICKS, John R., Administrator, Platte Valley Medical Center, Brighton, CO, p. A70
HICKS, Kevin J., President and Chief Executive Officer, Columbia Overland Park Regional Medical Center, Overland Park, KS, p. A168
HICKS, Michael C., Administrator, Jefferson Memorial Hospital, Jefferson City, TN, p. A390
HICKS, Tommy L., Administrator, Ray County Memorial Hospital, Richmond, MO, p. A252
HIDDE, A. John, President and Chief Executive Officer, Good Samaritan Hospital, Vincennes, IN, p. A149
HIESTER, Richard B., Administrator, Memorial Psychiatric Hospital, Albuquerque, NM, p. A284

HIETPAS, Bernard G.
Chief Executive Officer, Glenn Medical Center, Willows, CA, p. A69
Administrator, Seneca District Hospital, Chester, CA, p. A39
HIGGINBOTHAM, G. Douglas, Executive Director, South Central Regional Medical Center, Laurel, MS, p. A241
HIGGINS, Brad A., President and Chief Executive Officer, Fostoria Community Hospital, Fostoria, OH, p. A330
HIGGINS, Susannah, Chief Executive Officer, Broaddus Hospital, Philippi, WV, p. A458
HIGH, Cheryl A., Administrator, White Community Hospital, Aurora, MN, p. A226
HIGHSMITH Jr., C. Cameron, President and Chief Executive Officer, St. Luke's Hospital, Columbus, NC, p. A310
HILL, David L., President and Chief Executive Officer, Wahiawa General Hospital, Wahiawa, HI, p. A118
HILL, James C., Chief Executive Officer, Charter Behavioral Health System of Tampa Bay, Tampa, FL, p. A100
HILL, Jim, Chief Executive Officer, Charter Behavioral Health System at Medfield, Largo, FL, p. A91
HILL, Robert B., President, Bethesda Memorial Hospital, Boynton Beach, FL, p. A84
HILL, Thomas E.
Chief Executive Officer, Kennestone Hospital, Marietta, GA, p. A111
Chief Executive Officer, Promina Northwest Health System, Austell, GA, p. B122
HILL, Timothy E., President and Chief Executive Officer, Southwest Hospital, Little Rock, AR, p. A32
HILL, Tom, Chief Executive Officer, Promina Douglas Hospital, Douglasville, GA, p. A108
HILLBOM, Richard, Acting Administrator, Oakwood Hospital Beyer Center–Ypsilanti, Ypsilanti, MI, p. A225
HILLENMEYER, John, President, Orlando Regional Medical Center, Orlando, FL, p. A95
HILLIS, David W., President, Adcare Hospital of Worcester, Worcester, MA, p. A211
HILLMAN, Keith, Administrator, Garden County Hospital, Oshkosh, NE, p. A267
HILTZ, Richard S., President and Chief Executive Officer, Mercy Memorial Hospital, Monroe, MI, p. A220
HINCHEY, Paul P.
President and Chief Executive Officer, Candler Hospital, Savannah, GA, p. A113
President and Chief Executive Officer, St. Joseph's Hospital, Savannah, GA, p. A114
HINDS, Bob, Executive Director, Bradford Health Services at Huntsville, Madison, AL, p. A15
HINER, Calvin A., Administrator, Tri–County Area Hospital, Lexington, NE, p. A265
HINGER, Ward, USAF, Administrator, U. S. Air Force Hospital, Reese AFB, TX, p. A424
HINIKER, Alice, Ph.D., Administrator, Intracare Medical Center Hospital, Houston, TX, p. A414
HINMAN, Craig G., Commander, U. S. Air Force Hospital, Fairchild AFB, WA, p. A449
HINO, Raymond T., Administrator, Big Horn County Memorial Hospital, Hardin, MT, p. A258
HINSDALE, Laurence C., Chief Executive Officer, The Medical Center at Bowling Green, Bowling Green, KY, p. A172
HINSON, Roy M., CHE, President and Chief Executive Officer, Stanly Memorial Hospital, Albemarle, NC, p. A308
HINTON, J. Philip, M.D., Chief Executive Officer, Fresno Community Hospital and Medical Center, Fresno, CA, p. A43
HINTON, James H., President and Chief Executive Officer, Presbyterian Healthcare Services, Albuquerque, NM, p. B121
HINTON, Philip, Chief Executive Officer, Community Hospitals of Central California, Fresno, CA, p. B87
HIRSCH, Glenn, Administrator, North Shore University Hospital at Plainview, Plainview, NY, p. A302
HIRT, Fred D., President and Chief Executive Officer, Mount Sinai Medical Center, Miami Beach, FL, p. A94
HITCHINGS Jr., Roy A., FACHE
President, Cape Cod Hospital, Hyannis, MA, p. A207
President, Falmouth Hospital, Falmouth, MA, p. A206
HITT, Irving, Administrator, Covington County Hospital, Collins, MS, p. A238

HITZLER, Ronald R., Administrator, Shriners Hospitals for Children, Cincinnati Burns Institute, Cincinnati, OH, p. A326

HJERLEID, Gavin, Administrator, Holy Infant Hospital, Hoven, SD, p. A383

HOARD, Jack D., President and Chief Executive Officer, Armstrong County Memorial Hospital, Kittanning, PA, p. A359

HOBBS, Jim R., President and Chief Executive Officer, New Hanover Regional Medical Center, Wilmington, NC, p. A318

HOCKINS, J. Stephen, Administrator, Casa Grande Regional Medical Center, Casa Grande, AZ, p. A22

HODGES, Fredrick W., Chief Executive Officer, Chico Community Hospital, Chico, CA, p. A39

HODGES, Joseph T., President, Corry Memorial Hospital, Corry, PA, p. A356

HOEFER, Rufus S., Administrator, Columbia Peninsula Center for Behavioral Health, Hampton, VA, p. A441

HOELSCHER, Steve C., Administrator, Marshall Medical Center, Lewisburg, TN, p. A392

HOFER, Kathleen
    Chair Person and Chief Executive Officer, Benedictine Health System, Duluth, MN, p. B70
    President, St. Mary's Medical Center, Duluth, MN, p. A228

HOFF, David L., Chief Executive Officer, Iron County Community Hospital, Iron River, MI, p. A218

HOFF, Terry G., President, Trinity Medical Center, Minot, ND, p. A321

HOFFART, Terry L., Administrator, Webster County Community Hospital, Red Cloud, NE, p. A268

HOFFMAN, Charles, Administrator, Allenmore Hospital, Tacoma, WA, p. A453

HOFIUS, Chuck, Administrator, Perham Memorial Hospital and Home, Perham, MN, p. A233

HOFREUTER, Donald H., M.D., Administrator and Chief Executive Officer, Wheeling Hospital, Wheeling, WV, p. A459

HOFSTETTER, Peter A., Chief Executive Officer, Northwestern Medical Center, Saint Albans, VT, p. A437

HOGAN, Karen C., Administrator and Chief Executive Officer, San Diego County Psychiatric Hospital, San Diego, CA, p. A61

HOGAN, Ronald C., Superintendent, Georgia Regional Hospital at Atlanta, Decatur, GA, p. A108

HOGUE, John, Administrator, Covina Valley Community Hospital, West Covina, CA, p. A68

HOHENBERGER, Arthur L., FACHE, President and Chief Executive Officer, Texoma Healthcare System, Denison, TX, p. A408

HOHL, David G., Chief Executive Officer, Richmond Memorial Hospital, Rockingham, NC, p. A316

HOHN, David C., M.D., President and Chief Executive Officer, Roswell Park Cancer Institute, Buffalo, NY, p. A290

HOIDAL, David E.
    Chief Executive Officer, Columbia Jefferson Medical Center, Jefferson, LA, p. A185
    Chief Executive Officer, DePaul/Tulane Behavioral Health Center, New Orleans, LA, p. A188

HOLCOMB, David M., President and Chief Executive Officer, Jennie Edmundson Memorial Hospital, Council Bluffs, IA, p. A153

HOLCOMB, Howard C., Administrator, Washington County Infirmary and Nursing Home, Chatom, AL, p. A13

HOLDEN, R. William, USN, Commanding Officer, Naval Hospital, Great Lakes, IL, p. A131

HOLL, Donald R., President, Valley Regional Hospital, Claremont, NH, p. A272

HOLLAND, John, President, East Cooper Regional Medical Center, Mount Pleasant, SC, p. A379

HOLLON, Kim N., FACHE, Executive Director, Charlton Methodist Hospital, Dallas, TX, p. A406

HOLLOWAY, Roger L., Chief Executive Officer, Kewanee Hospital, Kewanee, IL, p. A132

HOLLY, David J., Chief Executive Officer, Southeast Texas Rehabilitation Hospital, Beaumont, TX, p. A401

HOLM, Richard, Administrator, Cascade Medical Center, Cascade, ID, p. A119

HOLMAN, Donna, Administrator, Jasper Memorial Hospital, Monticello, GA, p. A112

HOLMAN, William R., President, Newark–Wayne Community Hospital, Newark, NY, p. A300

HOLMES, Alan D., Chief Executive Officer, Frio Hospital, Pearsall, TX, p. A423

HOLMES, James M., President and Chief Executive Officer, Rappahannock General Hospital, Kilmarnock, VA, p. A442

HOLMES, James R., President, Redlands Community Hospital, Redlands, CA, p. A58

HOLMES, William E., Chief Executive Officer, Richmond Eye and Ear Hospital, Richmond, VA, p. A445

HOLOM, Randall G., Administrator, Minidoka Memorial Hospital and Extended Care Facility, Rupert, ID, p. A121

HOLT, Rod, Administrator, Kingsburg District Hospital, Kingsburg, CA, p. A47

HOLTER, Lee, Chief Executive Officer, St. James Health Services, Saint James, MN, p. A234

HOLTSCLAW, Keith S., Chief Executive Officer, Spruce Pine Community Hospital, Spruce Pine, NC, p. A317

HOLTZ, Daniel D., FACHE, Administrator and Chief Executive Officer, Hancock Memorial Hospital, Sparta, GA, p. A114

HOLTZ, John, Administrator, Shriners Hospitals for Children, Tampa, Tampa, FL, p. A100

HOLWERDA, Daniel L., President and Chief Executive Officer, Pine Rest Christian Mental Health Services, Grand Rapids, MI, p. A217

HOLZBERG, Harvey A., President and Chief Executive Officer, Robert Wood Johnson University Hospital, New Brunswick, NJ, p. A279

HOLZHAUER, George G., President, Central DuPage Hospital, Winfield, IL, p. A139

HONAKER III, Thomas G., Administrator, Mission Hill Memorial Hospital, Shawnee, OK, p. A345

HONEYCUTT, Ann E., Executive Vice President and Administrator, St. Mary's Hospital, Richmond, VA, p. A446

HONKER, C. Ray, Administrator and Senior Vice President, St. Thomas More Hospital and Progressive Care Center, Canon City, CO, p. A70

HOOD, Barbara A., Chief Executive Officer Central Washington Service Area, Providence Yakima Medical Center, Yakima, WA, p. A454

HOOD, Cliff, Director, Alcohol and Drug Abuse Treatment Center, Butner, NC, p. A309

HOOD, Fred B., Administrator, Pontotoc Hospital and Extended Care Facility, Pontotoc, MS, p. A243

HOOD, Mark C., Executive Director, Baylor Medical Center at Grapevine, Grapevine, TX, p. A412

HOOPER, Ross, Chief Executive Officer, Crittenden Memorial Hospital, West Memphis, AR, p. A35

HOOPES, John L., Administrator and Chief Executive Officer, Cobre Valley Community Hospital, Claypool, AZ, p. A22

HOOSE, Gregory R., Chief Executive Officer, Straith Hospital for Special Surgery, Southfield, MI, p. A223

HOOSER, Rosemary, Acting Administrator, Choctaw Nation Indian Hospital, Talihina, OK, p. A346

HOOVER, Donna, Chief Executive Officer, THC–Orange County, Brea, CA, p. A38

HOOVER, Randall L., Chief Executive Officer, Memorial Medical Center, New Orleans, LA, p. A188

HOPKINS, Don, Administrator, Faith Community Hospital, Jacksboro, TX, p. A417

HOPKINS, Wallace M., FACHE, Director, Veterans Affairs Medical Center, Amarillo, TX, p. A398

HOPPER, Cornelius L., M.D., Vice President Health Affairs, University of California–Systemwide Administration, Oakland, CA, p. B146

HOPPER, Jerry, FACHE, Executive Director, Presbyterian Hospital of Winnsboro, Winnsboro, TX, p. A431

HOPPER, Stephen R., President and Chief Executive Officer, McDonough District Hospital, Macomb, IL, p. A133

HOPSTAD, Kyle, Administrator, Virginia Regional Medical Center, Virginia, MN, p. A235

HORAN, Gary S., FACHE
    President, Our Lady of Mercy Healthcare System, Inc., New York, NY, p. B120
    President and Chief Executive Officer, Our Lady of Mercy Medical Center, New York, NY, p. A299
    President and Chief Executive Officer, St. Agnes Hospital, White Plains, NY, p. A307

HORN, Linda, Administrator, Sutter Delta Medical Center, Antioch, CA, p. A36

HORNER, Lynn V., President and Chief Executive Officer, Dunlap Memorial Hospital, Orrville, OH, p. A334

HORNER, Seward, President, Riverview Hospital, Noblesville, IN, p. A147

HORSTKOTTE, Don A., Chief Executive Officer, Columbia Pinelake Regional Hospital, Mayfield, KY, p. A178

HORTON, Charlie M., President, Warren Memorial Hospital, Front Royal, VA, p. A441

HORTON, Jerrell J., Chief Executive Officer, Stroud Municipal Hospital, Stroud, OK, p. A345

HORTON, Joseph R., Chief Executive Officer and Administrator, Primary Children's Medical Center, Salt Lake City, UT, p. A435

HORVATH, Louis D., Administrator, St. John Vianney Hospital, Downingtown, PA, p. A356

HORWITZ, Fred D., Administrator, Leahi Hospital, Honolulu, HI, p. A117

HORWITZ, Theodore H., FACHE, President, Veterans Memorial Medical Center, Meriden, CT, p. A77

HOSFELD, Anne, Chief Administrative Officer, Novato Community Hospital, Novato, CA, p. A55

HOSS, James R., President and Chief Executive Officer, Mercy Medical Center Mount Shasta, Mount Shasta, CA, p. A54

HOUGHTON, Jack F., Chief Executive Officer, Bossier Medical Center, Bossier City, LA, p. A183

HOUSE, Judy G., Chief Executive Officer, BHC Ross Hospital, Kentfield, CA, p. A46

HOUSER, James P.
    President and Chief Executive Officer, Lubbock Methodist Hospital System, Lubbock, TX, p. B109
    President and Chief Executive Officer, Methodist Children's Hospital, Lubbock, TX, p. A419
    President and Chief Executive Officer, Methodist Hospital, Lubbock, TX, p. A419

HOUSER, Robert, Chief Executive Officer, Winner Regional Healthcare Center, Winner, SD, p. A386

HOUSLEY, Charles E., FACHE, President and Chief Executive Officer, Michigan Health Care Corporation, Southfield, MI, p. B116

HOUSTON, Colleen B., Administrator, Miller County Hospital, Colquitt, GA, p. A106

HOVE, Barton A., Chief Executive Officer, Columbia Hospital Lexington, Lexington, KY, p. A176

HOVE, David R., President and Chief Executive Officer, St Joseph's Area Health Services, Park Rapids, MN, p. A233

HOWARD, Catherine, Chief Executive Officer, Massachusetts Mental Health Center, Boston, MA, p. A204

HOWARD, Deanna S., Chief Executive Officer, Upper Connecticut Valley Hospital, Colebrook, NH, p. A272

HOWARD, Eddie L., Vice President and Chief Operating Officer, East Texas Medical Center Rehabilitation Hospital, Tyler, TX, p. A429

HOWARD, Loy M., Chief Executive Officer, Tanner Medical Center, Carrollton, GA, p. A106

HOWARD, Norma, Administrator, Marshall Memorial Hospital, Madill, OK, p. A342

HOWE, Debbie, Administrator, Okeene Municipal Hospital, Okeene, OK, p. A343

HOWE, G. Edwin, President, Aurora Health Care, Milwaukee, WI, p. B67

HOWELL, Bonnie H., President and Chief Executive Officer, Cayuga Medical Center at Ithaca, Ithaca, NY, p. A293

HOWELL, Dan, Chief Executive Officer, Sakakawea Medical Center, Hazen, ND, p. A320

HOWELL, George F., Service Unit Director, U. S. Public Health Service Indian Hospital, Lawton, OK, p. A342

HOWELL, Jerry M., Chief Operating Officer, Methodist Hospital of Marion County, Columbia, MS, p. A238

HOWELL, Joe D., Executive Director, Hamlet Hospital, Hamlet, NC, p. A312

HOWELL, R. Edward, Director and Chief Executive Officer, University of Iowa Hospitals and Clinics, Iowa City, IA, p. A155

HOYLE, John D., Senior Executive Officer, St. Luke Hospital West, Florence, KY, p. A174

HUBBARD, David, Chief Executive Officer, First Care Medical Services, Fosston, MN, p. A229

HUBBARD, F. D., Superintendent, McCain Correctional Hospital, McCain, NC, p. A314

HUBBARD, James R., Administrator, Medcenter One Mandan, Mandan, ND, p. A321

HUBBARD III, Richard B., President and Chief Executive Officer, Piedmont Hospital, Atlanta, GA, p. A104

HUBBELL, James W., President and Chief Executive Officer, Wayne Memorial Hospital, Goldsboro, NC, p. A312

HUBBERS, Rodney N., President and Chief Executive Officer, Putnam Hospital Center, Carmel, NY, p. A290

HUBER, Michael F., Administrator and Chief Executive Officer, University Hospital, Chicago, IL, p. A128

HUBLER, Matthew W., Executive Vice President, Sacred Heart Hospital, Eau Claire, WI, p. A462

HUDGINS, Thomas J., Administrator, Mary Sherman Hospital, Sullivan, IN, p. A149

HUDSON, Donald C., Vice President and Chief Operating Officer, Mercy Hospital of Folsom, Folsom, CA, p. A43

HUDSON, Gary Mikeal, Administrator, Panola General Hospital, Carthage, TX, p. A403

HUDSON, Jay, President and Chief Executive Officer, Community Hospital of the Monterey Peninsula, Monterey, CA, p. A54

HUDSON, W. H., President, Oconee Memorial Hospital, Seneca, SC, p. A380

HUETER, Diana T., President and Chief Executive Officer, St. Vincent Infirmary Medical Center, Little Rock, AR, p. A32

HUEWE, Helen, President, Mercy Health Center, Dubuque, IA, p. A154

HUEY, Kenneth R., President and Chief Executive Officer, Longmont United Hospital, Longmont, CO, p. A74

HUFF, Richard, Administrator, U. S. Public Health Service Indian Hospital, Sisseton, SD, p. A385

HUFF, William J., Chief Executive Officer, Marshall Browning Hospital, Du Quoin, IL, p. A129

HUFSTEDLER, Jon, Administrator, Walton Regional Hospital, De Funiak Springs, FL, p. A85

HUGHES, Robert C., Healthcare and Hospital Administrator, Pacific Coast Hospital, San Francisco, CA, p. A61

HUGHES Jr., Ned B., President, Gerber Memorial Hospital, Fremont, MI, p. A216

HUMMEL, Joseph Wm, Senior Vice President and Area Manager, Kaiser Foundation Hospital, Los Angeles, CA, p. A50

HUMMER, John Lloyd, Chief Executive Officer and Managing Director, River Parishes Hospital, Laplace, LA, p. A186

HUMPHREY, Jerel T., Vice President, Chief Executive Officer and Administrator, Memorial Hospital–Memorial City, Houston, TX, p. A415

HUMPHREY, Robert J., Administrator, George H. Lanier Memorial Hospital and Health Services, Valley, AL, p. A18

HUNKINS, Theresa, Administrator, Vencor Hospital–Tampa, Tampa, FL, p. A101

HUNSAKER, Susan L., CHE, President and Chief Executive Officer, Physicians Memorial Hospital, La Plata, MD, p. A201

HUNT, James M., Chief Executive Officer, Mission Vista Behavioral Health System, San Antonio, TX, p. A425

HUNT, Roger S., President and Chief Executive Officer, Greater Rochester Health System, Inc., Rochester, NY, p. B99

HUNT Jr., Seth P., Director, Broughton Hospital, Morganton, NC, p. A314

HUNTER, David C., Chief Executive Officer, Wabash County Hospital, Wabash, IN, p. A149

HUNTER, David E. K., Ph.D., Superintendent, Cedarcrest Regional Hospital, Newington, CT, p. A78

HUNTER, Steven L., President, St. Anthony Hospital, Oklahoma City, OK, p. A344

HUPFELD, Stanley F., President and Chief Executive Officer, INTEGRIS Health, Oklahoma City, OK, p. B106

HURD, Paul, Chief Executive Officer, Creighton Area Health Services, Creighton, NE, p. A263

HURON, Bruce C., Interim Chief Executive Officer, Helen Newberry Joy Hospital, Newberry, MI, p. A221

HURST, George A., M.D., Director, University of Texas Health Center at Tyler, Tyler, TX, p. A430

HURST, Molly, Administrator, CLC–Navasota Regional Hospital, Navasota, TX, p. A422

HURSTELL, Stanley E., MSC, Administrator, U. S. Air Force Hospital, Grand Forks AFB, ND, p. A320

HURT, Charles, Administrator, Hardeman County Memorial Hospital, Quanah, TX, p. A424

HURT, Reedes, Chief Executive Officer, Department of Veterans Affairs Medical Center, Wilkes–Barre, PA, p. A371

HURT, Richard O., Ph.D., Chief Executive Officer, Benchmark Behavioral Health Systems, Woods Cross, UT, p. A436

HURTEAU, William J., FACHE, Administrator, Russell County Hospital, Russell Springs, KY, p. A180

HURYSZ, Edwin E., Administrator, Delta County Memorial Hospital, Delta, CO, p. A71

HURZELER, Rosemary Johnson, President and Chief Executive Officer, The Connecticut Hospice, Inc., Branford, CT, p. A76

HUSETH, Michael, Chief Executive Officer, Mississippi Hospital Restorative Care, Jackson, MS, p. A240

HUSSON, Gerard P., Director, Veterans Affairs Medical Center, Beckley, WV, p. A455

HUSTON, Samuel R., President and Chief Executive Officer, Saint Luke's Medical Center, Cleveland, OH, p. A327

HUTCHENRIDER, Ken, President and Chief Executive Officer, Columbia Western Plains Regional Hospital, Dodge City, KS, p. A162

HUTCHINS, Joe T., Chief Executive Officer, Columbia Barrow Medical Center, Winder, GA, p. A116

HUTCHINS, Michael T., Chief Executive Officer, Screven County Hospital, Sylvania, GA, p. A114

HUTCHISON, Dee, Chief Executive Officer, Northern Navajo Medical Center, Shiprock, NM, p. A287

HYDE, James A., Administrator, Bone and Joint Hospital, Oklahoma City, OK, p. A343

HYER, Julie, President and Chief Executive Officer, Dominican Santa Cruz Hospital, Santa Cruz, CA, p. A64

HYMANS, Daniel J., President, Memorial Medical Center, Ashland, WI, p. A460

HYNES, John J., President and Chief Executive Officer, Care New England Health System, Providence, RI, p. B73

I

ICHINOSE, Calvin M., Administrator, Molokai General Hospital, Kaunakakai, HI, p. A118

IDESON, D. Scott, Interim Chief Executive Officer, Woodland Memorial Hospital, Woodland, CA, p. A69

IERARDI, Joseph A., President and Chief Executive Officer, Newcomb Medical Center, Vineland, NJ, p. A282

IGNELZI, James, Chief Executive Officer, Central Ohio Psychiatric Hospital, Columbus, OH, p. A327

ILL, Katherine C., M.D., President, Hospital for Special Care, New Britain, CT, p. A77

INCARNATI, Philip A., President and Chief Executive Officer, McLaren Regional Medical Center, Flint, MI, p. A216

INGRAHAM, Ron, Administrator, Klickitat Valley Hospital, Goldendale, WA, p. A450

INGRAM, Anne S., Chief Executive Officer, Kilmichael Hospital, Kilmichael, MS, p. A240

INIGO–AGOSTINI, Emigdio, M.D., Board President, Clinica Espanola, Mayaguez, PR, p. A476

IRBY, Frank, Chief Executive Officer, Columbia Raulerson Hospital, Okeechobee, FL, p. A95

IRWIN Jr., Richard M., President and Chief Executive Officer, Health Central, Ocoee, FL, p. A95

ISAAC, Richard D., Administrator, Veterans Affairs Medical Center, West Palm Beach, FL, p. A102

ISAACS, James W., Chief Executive Officer, Mercer County Joint Township Community Hospital, Coldwater, OH, p. A327

ISBELL, John, Chief Executive Officer, Doctors Hospital, Groves, TX, p. A412

ISELY, John A., President, St. Mary Medical Center, Walla Walla, WA, p. A454

ISRAEL, Michael D., Chief Executive Officer and Vice Chancellor, Duke University Medical Center, Durham, NC, p. A310

IVERSEN, Dale E., President and Chief Executive Officer, Warrack Medical Center Hospital, Santa Rosa, CA, p. A64

IVERSON, Linda, Administrator, Southern Hills General Hospital, Hot Springs, SD, p. A383

IVES, R. Wayne, Administrator, San Vicente Hospital, Los Angeles, CA, p. A51

IVESON, Sara C., Executive Director, Barnes–Kasson County Hospital, Susquehanna, PA, p. A369

IVY, Charles A., Vice President, St. Joseph Medical Center, Albuquerque, NM, p. A284

IVY, Jim, Administrator, Memorial Pavilion, Lawton, OK, p. A342

J

JACKMAN, Marley D., Administrator, Twin Falls Clinic Hospital, Twin Falls, ID, p. A122

JACKMUFF, Steven W., President and Chief Executive Officer, Underwood–Memorial Hospital, Woodbury, NJ, p. A283

JACKSON, Fred L., Chief Executive Officer, King's Daughters' Medical Center, Ashland, KY, p. A172

JACKSON, Joan, Administrator, Melrose Hospital and Pine Villa Nursing Home, Melrose, MN, p. A231

JACKSON, John J., Chief Executive Officer, Columbia Texas Orthopedic Hospital, Houston, TX, p. A414

JACKSON, R. Lynn, Chief Executive Officer, Hedrick Medical Center, Chillicothe, MO, p. A246

JACKSON, Sandra, President, Memorial Medical Center and Cancer Treatment Center–Tulsa, Tulsa, OK, p. A346

JACKSON, Thomas W., Chief Executive Officer, Columbia Medical Center, College Station, TX, p. A404

JACKSON, Valerie A.
Chief Executive Officer, Columbia East Pointe Hospital, Lehigh Acres, FL, p. A91
Chief Executive Officer, Columbia Gulf Coast Hospital, Fort Myers, FL, p. A87

JACOBS, Jack, Administrator, Lisbon Medical Center, Lisbon, ND, p. A321

JACOBS, Nicholas, President, Windber Hospital, Windber, PA, p. A371

JACOBS, Selby, M.P.H., Director, Connecticut Mental Health Center, New Haven, CT, p. A77

JACOBSEN, David, President, Sterling Healthcare Corporation, Bellevue, WA, p. B138

JACOBSEN, David P., Chief Executive Officer, Tehachapi Hospital, Tehachapi, CA, p. A66

JACOBSON, John L., President and Chief Executive Officer, Lee's Summit Hospital, Lees Summit, MO, p. A250

JACOBSON, Rod, Administrator, Bear Lake Memorial Hospital, Montpelier, ID, p. A120

JACOBSON, Ronald L., President and Chief Executive Officer, Queen of Peace Hospital, Mitchell, SD, p. A384

JACOBSON, Rosemary, President and Chief Executive Officer, United Health Services, Grand Forks, ND, p. A320

JACOBSON, Steven K., Chief Executive Officer, Titus Regional Medical Center, Mount Pleasant, TX, p. A421

JACOBSON, Terry, Administrator, St. Mary's Hospital of Superior, Superior, WI, p. A469

JACOBUS, Rick, Administrator, Martin County Hospital District, Stanton, TX, p. A428

JAEGER, Lee, Chief Executive Officer, THC–Milwaukee, Greenfield, WI, p. A463

JAFFE, David E., Executive Director and Chief Executive Officer, Harborview Medical Center, Seattle, WA, p. A452

JAHN, David B., Administrator and Chief Financial Officer, Schoolcraft Memorial Hospital, Manistique, MI, p. A220

JAMES, Craig B., Administrator, Tazewell Community Hospital, Tazewell, VA, p. A447

JAMES, David, Chief Executive Officer, Sturgis Hospital, Sturgis, MI, p. A223

JAMES, Donald W., Administrator, North Valley Hospital, Tonasket, WA, p. A454

JAMES, William B., Chief Executive Officer, Northern Hospital of Surry County, Mount Airy, NC, p. A314

JAMES Jr., George H., President and Chief Executive Officer, Memorial Hospital, Seymour, IN, p. A148

JANCZAK, Linda M., President and Chief Executive Officer, F. F. Thompson Health System, Canandaigua, NY, p. A290

JANSEN, Charles P., Administrator, Audrain Medical Center, Mexico, MO, p. A251

JARM, Timothy L., President, Jewish Hospital–Shelbyville, Shelbyville, KY, p. A180

JARRETT, James L., Chief Executive Officer, Pender Memorial Hospital, Burgaw, NC, p. A309

JAUDES, Paula, M.D., Interim Director, LaRabida Children's Hospital and Research Center, Chicago, IL, p. A126

JAVOREK, Judeth N., R.N., President and Chief Executive Officer, Holland Community Hospital, Holland, MI, p. A218

JAY, David W., Superintendent, Allentown State Hospital, Allentown, PA, p. A353

JEAN, Darrell, Administrator and Chief Executive Officer, Pemiscot Memorial Health System, Hayti, MO, p. A248

JEANMARD, William C., Chief Executive Officer, Allen Parish Hospital, Kinder, LA, p. A186

JED, Stuart A., Administrator, Villaview Community Hospital, San Diego, CA, p. A61

JEFFCOAT, Arla, Administrator, Medical Arts Hospital, Lamesa, TX, p. A418

JEFFCOAT, Sally E., President and Chief Executive Officer, Columbia Spring Branch Medical Center, Houston, TX, p. A413

JENKINS, Jeffrey K., President, St. Michael Hospital, Milwaukee, WI, p. A466

JENKINS, Mark W., Chief Administrative Officer, Olmsted Medical Center, Rochester, MN, p. A233

JENKINS, William I., President and Chief Executive Officer, Sinai Samaritan Medical Center, Milwaukee, WI, p. A465

JENNINGS, Jan R., President and Chief Executive Officer, Children's Memorial Hospital, Chicago, IL, p. A125

JENNINGS, Peter, Interim Administrator, Rochelle Community Hospital, Rochelle, IL, p. A137

JENNINGS, William R., President, South Hills Health System, Pittsburgh, PA, p. A366

JENSEN, Bruce, President and Chief Executive Officer, Holy Rosary Medical Center, Ontario, OR, p. A350

JENSEN, Eric, Administrator, Kittitas Valley Community Hospital, Ellensburg, WA, p. A449

JENSEN, Jon L., Interim Administrator, Stewart Memorial Community Hospital, Lake City, IA, p. A156

JENSEN, Ronald, Administrator, Weiner Memorial Medical Center, Marshall, MN, p. A231

JENSON, Paul M., Chief Executive Officer, Presbyterian–Orthopaedic Hospital, Charlotte, NC, p. A310

JERDE, Duane D., President and Chief Executive Officer, Mercy Medical Center, Williston, ND, p. A322

JERNIGAN Jr., Robert F., Administrator, South Baldwin Hospital, Foley, AL, p. A14

JERVIS, Charles R., Director, San Bernardino County Medical Center, San Bernardino, CA, p. A60

JESIOLOWSKI, Craig A., Chief Executive Officer, Gibson Community Hospital, Gibson City, IL, p. A130

JESSUP, Dale, President and Chief Executive Officer, Bay Area Hospital, Coos Bay, OR, p. A348

JETER, Larry R., Chief Executive Officer, Columbia Sycamore Shoals Hospital, Elizabethton, TN, p. A389

JEWELS, Robert M., Administrator, Community Hospital of Smithtown, Smithtown, NY, p. A304

JEWETT, Kay C., Administrative Officer, U. S. Public Health Service Owyhee Community Health Facility, Owyhee, NV, p. A271

JEX, Robert F., Administrator, Bear River Valley Hospital, Tremonton, UT, p. A436

JHIN, Michael K., President and Chief Executive Officer, St. Luke's Episcopal Hospital, Houston, TX, p. A415

JIMENEZ, A. David, President and Chief Executive Officer, Huguley Memorial Medical Center, Burleson, TX, p. A403

JIVIDEN, Thomas C., Senior Vice President, Virginia Baptist Hospital, Lynchburg, VA, p. A442

JOHANSEN, Richard, Chief Operating Officer and Interim Chief Executive Officer, Jefferson Memorial Hospital, Crystal City, MO, p. A247

JOHANSON, Blair R., Administrator, Charter Behavioral Health System/Central Georgia, Macon, GA, p. A111

JOHN, Roger S., President and Chief Executive Officer, Great Plains Health Alliance, Inc., Phillipsburg, KS, p. B99

JOHN, Susie, M.D., Chief Executive Officer, Tuba City Indian Medical Center, Tuba City, AZ, p. A27

JOHNS, Charles A., President, Trumbull Memorial Hospital, Warren, OH, p. A336

JOHNSON, Bill A., Administrator, Lake Whitney Medical Center, Whitney, TX, p. A431

JOHNSON, Carol L., Administrator, Snoqualmie Valley Hospital, Snoqualmie, WA, p. A453

JOHNSON, Charles F., President, Lawrence Memorial Hospital of Medford, Medford, MA, p. A207

JOHNSON, Curtis A., Administrator, Flambeau Hospital, Park Falls, WI, p. A467

JOHNSON, Daniel W., Chief Executive Officer, Rivernorth Hospital, Pineville, LA, p. A190

JOHNSON, David B., Administrator, Brookings Hospital, Brookings, SD, p. A382

JOHNSON, Don, Administrator, Cedars Hospital, De Soto, TX, p. A407

JOHNSON, Doyle K., Administrator, Mercy Hospital, Moundridge, KS, p. A167

JOHNSON, Eugene, President and Chief Executive Officer, Satilla Regional Medical Center, Waycross, GA, p. A116

JOHNSON, George L., President, Reedsburg Area Medical Center, Reedsburg, WI, p. A468

JOHNSON, Gregory D., Administrator, Summersville Memorial Hospital, Summersville, WV, p. A459

JOHNSON, James K., Administrator, Anderson County Hospital, Garnett, KS, p. A163

JOHNSON, Jane, President and Chief Executive Officer, Myers Community Hospital, Sodus, NY, p. A304

JOHNSON, Jeanne, Chief Executive Officer, Community Hospital and Health Care Center, Saint Peter, MN, p. A234

JOHNSON, John, Administrator, Washakie Memorial Hospital, Worland, WY, p. A473

JOHNSON, John C., Chief Executive Officer, Palmetto General Hospital, Hialeah, FL, p. A88

JOHNSON, John W., President and Chief Executive Officer, Alice Hyde Hospital Association, Malone, NY, p. A294

JOHNSON, Karen E., Administrator, Hartgrove Hospital, Chicago, IL, p. A125

JOHNSON, Karl E., Chief Executive Officer, Mount Graham Community Hospital, Safford, AZ, p. A26

JOHNSON, Kevin, Chief Executive Officer, Mountain View Hospital, Payson, UT, p. A434

JOHNSON, L. Barney, President and Chief Executive Officer, Harbor Hospital Center, Baltimore, MD, p. A197

JOHNSON, LaQuita, Chief Executive Officer, Oakdale Community Hospital, Oakdale, LA, p. A189

JOHNSON, Laurence E., Administrator, Shriners Hospitals for Children, Twin Cities Unit, Minneapolis, MN, p. A234

JOHNSON, Liz, Chief Executive Officer, Sage Memorial Hospital, Ganado, AZ, p. A23

JOHNSON, Lowell W.
Interim President and Chief Executive Officer, Legacy Emanuel Hospital and Health Center, Portland, OR, p. A351
Interim President and Chief Executive Officer, Legacy Good Samaritan Hospital and Medical Center, Portland, OR, p. A351

JOHNSON, Marion P., FACHE, President and Chief Executive Officer, McKenna Memorial Hospital, New Braunfels, TX, p. A422

JOHNSON, Michael, Administrator and Chief Executive Officer, Crosbyton Clinic Hospital, Crosbyton, TX, p. A405

JOHNSON, Paul H., President and Chief Executive Officer, Gaylord Hospital, Wallingford, CT, p. A79

JOHNSON, Richard, Chief Executive Officer, Memorial Hospital of Carbon County, Rawlins, WY, p. A472

JOHNSON, Robert D., Chief Executive Officer, South Suburban Medical Center, Farmington, MO, p. A229

JOHNSON, Ronald E., Administrator, Meeker County Memorial Hospital, Litchfield, MN, p. A230

JOHNSON, Stan, Medical Center Director, Veterans Affairs Medical Center, Tomah, WI, p. A469

JOHNSON, Stephen H., Administrator, Ashley Medical Center, Ashley, ND, p. A319

JOHNSON, Stephen W., Executive Director, Chattooga County Hospital, Summerville, GA, p. A114

JOHNSON, Steven G., Chief Executive Officer, BHC Cedar Spring Hospital, Pineville, NC, p. A315

JOHNSON, Steven M.
President, Citizens Baptist Medical Center, Talladega, AL, p. A18
President, Coosa Valley Baptist Medical Center, Sylacauga, AL, p. A18

JOHNSON, Terry, Chief Executive Officer, BHC Fremont Hospital, Fremont, CA, p. A43

JOHNSON, Thomas E., Vice President and Administrator, Oakwood Hospital–Heritage Center, Taylor, MI, p. A223

JOHNSON, Thomas M., Chief Executive Officer, Kaweah Delta Healthcare District, Visalia, CA, p. A68

JOHNSON, Timothy A., Executive Vice President and Administrator, Bon Secours–Stuart Circle, Richmond, VA, p. A445

JOHNSON, Van R., President and Chief Executive Officer, Sutter Health, Sacramento, CA, p. B139

JOHNSON, Viola L.
Chief Executive Officer, Huhukam Memorial Hospital, Sacaton, AZ, p. A26
Service Unit Director, U. S. Public Health Service Indian Hospital, San Carlos, AZ, p. A26

JOHNSON, W. Michael, Executive Director, Pacific Gateway Hospital and Counseling Center, Portland, OR, p. A351

JOHNSON, Willard H., President, Chelsea Community Hospital, Chelsea, MI, p. A213

JOHNSON, James A., Commanding Officer, Naval Hospital, Bremerton, WA, p. A448

JOHNSON–PHILLIPPE, Sue E., Chief Executive Officer, LakeView Community Hospital, Paw Paw, MI, p. A221

JOHNSRUD, Kimry A., President, Elmbrook Memorial Hospital, Brookfield, WI, p. A461

JOHNSTON, Charles, Administrator, Pauls Valley General Hospital, Pauls Valley, OK, p. A344

JOHNSTON, R. Joe, President and Chief Executive Officer, Dukes Memorial Hospital, Peru, IN, p. A147

JOHNSTON, Wayne W., President and Chief Executive Officer, Sharon Regional Health System, Sharon, PA, p. A369

JOINER, H. Glenn, Chief Executive Officer, T. J. Samson Community Hospital, Glasgow, KY, p. A174

JOLLY, Jay P., Administrator and Chief Executive Officer, Clay County Hospital, Brazil, IN, p. A141

JONES, Billy E., MS, Acting Executive Director, Kingsboro Psychiatric Center, New York, NY, p. A297

JONES, Craig W., President and Chief Executive Officer, Norman Regional Hospital, Norman, OK, p. A343

JONES, David, President, United Hospital, Saint Paul, MN, p. A234

JONES, Donald J., Administrator, Vaughan Regional Medical Center, Selma, AL, p. A18

JONES, Douglas T., President and Chief Executive Officer, Genesee Memorial Hospital, Batavia, NY, p. A288

JONES, Glen M., Chief Executive Officer, Columbia Florence Hospital, Florence, AL, p. A14

JONES, H. Ed, Chief Executive Officer, North Carolina Eye and Ear Hospital, Durham, NC, p. A310

JONES, J. Thomas, Executive Director, St. Mary's Hospital, Huntington, WV, p. A456

JONES, James S., Director, Veterans Affairs Medical Center, Danville, IL, p. A128

JONES, Jerry, Administrator, Drumright Memorial Hospital, Drumright, OK, p. A340

JONES, Lowell
President, Marymount Medical Center, London, KY, p. A176
Chief Executive Officer, Our Lady of the Way Hospital, Martin, KY, p. A178
JONES, Mark T., President, Holy Redeemer Hospital and Medical Center, Meadowbrook, PA, p. A361
JONES, Nancy, Administrator, Shriners Hospitals for Children, Portland, Portland, OR, p. A351
JONES, Perry T., President, Community General Hospital of Thomasville, Thomasville, NC, p. A317
JONES, Robert D., President, Rutherford Hospital, Rutherfordton, NC, p. A316
JONES, Robert T., M.D., President and Chief Executive Officer, Hutcheson Medical Center, Fort Oglethorpe, GA, p. A109
JORDAHL, David B., FACHE, President, St. Clare Hospital and Health Services, Baraboo, WI, p. A460
JORDAN, Bobby, Chief Executive Officer, Winn Parish Medical Center, Winnfield, LA, p. A192
JORDAN, David R., Ph.D., Administrator and Chief Executive Officer, Nor–Lea General Hospital, Lovington, NM, p. A286
JORDAN, J. Larry, Administrator, Homer Memorial Hospital, Homer, LA, p. A185
JORDAN, Lawrence A., Director, PHS Santa Fe Indian Hospital, Santa Fe, NM, p. A287
JORDAN, Linda U., Administrator, Clay County Hospital, Ashland, AL, p. A11
JORDAN, W. Charles, Administrator, Mayes County Medical Center, Pryor, OK, p. A345
JOSE, Sharon L., R.N., Vice President, Hospital Operations, Pioneer Hospital, Artesia, CA, p. A37
JOSEF, Norma C., M.D., Director, Walter P. Reuther Psychiatric Hospital, Westland, MI, p. A225
JOSEPH, Elliot, Senior Vice President, Oakland Region, Huron Valley Hospital, Commerce Township, MI, p. A214
JOSEPH, Gloria, Superintendent, Western Missouri Mental Health Center, Kansas City, MO, p. A250
JOSEPH, Jerry, Chief Executive Officer, Monsour Medical Center, Jeannette, PA, p. A359
JOSEPH, Michael G., Chief Executive Officer, Columbia Westside Regional Medical Center, Plantation, FL, p. A97
JOSPE, Theodore A., President, Southside Hospital, Bay Shore, NY, p. A289
JOYCE, Michael P., President and Chief Executive Officer, Columbia Medical Center–Port St. Lucie, Port St. Lucie, FL, p. A98
JOYNER, Ronald G., Chief Executive Officer, Williamson Medical Center, Franklin, TN, p. A389
JUBINSKY, Linda, Chief Executive Officer, Columbia Peachtree Regional Hospital, Newnan, GA, p. A112
JUDD, Jeffrey M., President and Chief Executive Officer, McDowell Hospital, Marion, NC, p. A314
JUDD, Russell V., Chief Executive Officer, Barstow Community Hospital, Barstow, CA, p. A37
JUENEMANN, Jean, Chief Executive Officer, Queen of Peace Hospital, New Prague, MN, p. A232
JUENGLING, Craig S., Chief Executive Officer, Charter Behavioral Health System of Potomac Ridge, Rockville, MD, p. A201
JUPIN Jr., Joseph
Chief Executive Officer, Greystone Park Psychiatric Hospital, Greystone Park, NJ, p. A277
Chief Executive Officer, Trenton Psychiatric Hospital, Trenton, NJ, p. A282
JURENA, Jerry E., Executive Director, Heart of America Medical Center, Rugby, ND, p. A322

K

KAATZ, Gary E., President and Chief Executive Officer, Western Reserve Care System, Youngstown, OH, p. A338
KAIGLER, James S., FACHE, Administrator, Singing River Hospital, Pascagoula, MS, p. A242
KAJIWARA, Gary K., President and Chief Executive Officer, Kuakini Medical Center, Honolulu, HI, p. A117
KALADJIAN, Gregory M., Executive Director, Bellevue Hospital Center, New York, NY, p. A295

KALETKOWSKI, Chester B., President and Chief Executive Officer, Memorial Hospital of Burlington County, Mount Holly, NJ, p. A279
KALLEN–ZURY, Karen, Chief Executive Officer, Hollywood Pavilion, Los Angeles, FL, p. A89
KAMBER, Steve, Chief Executive Officer, Charter Behavioral Health System–Corpus Christi, Corpus Christi, TX, p. A404
KANAT, Irvin, DPM, Chief Executive Officer, Kern Hospital for Special Surgery, Warren, MI, p. A224
KANE, Daniel A., President and Chief Executive Officer, Englewood Hospital and Medical Center, Englewood, NJ, p. A277
KANNADY, Donald L., Administrator, Bunkie General Hospital, Bunkie, LA, p. A183
KANTOS, Craig A., Chief Executive Officer, Millinocket Regional Hospital, Millinocket, ME, p. A195
KAPLAN, Lawrence, M.D., President and Chief Executive Officer, Columbia MetroWest Medical Center, Framingham, MA, p. A206
KARELS, Genevieve, Administrator, St. Bernard's Providence Hospital, Milbank, SD, p. A383
KARPF, Michael, M.D., Vice Provost Hospital System and Director Medical Center, University of California Los Angeles Medical Center, Los Angeles, CA, p. A52
KARUSCHAK Jr., Michael, Administrator, Apple River Hospital, Amery, WI, p. A460
KASENCHAK, John, Administrator, First Hospital Wyoming Valley, Wilkes–Barre, PA, p. A371
KASTANIS, John N., FACHE, Chief Executive Officer, Hospital for Joint Diseases Orthopedic Institute, New York, NY, p. A297
KATHRINS, Richard J., Administrator, Bacharach Rehabilitation Hospital, Pomona, NJ, p. A281
KATRANA, John N., Ph.D., Chief Administrative Officer, Lutheran Hospital–La Crosse, La Crosse, WI, p. A463
KATSUDA, Frank, Administrator, Memorial Hospital of Gardena, Gardena, CA, p. A44
KATZ, Stuart A., FACHE, Chief Executive Officer, Hawarden Community Hospital, Hawarden, IA, p. A155
KATZ, Treuman, President and Chief Executive Officer, Children's Hospital and Medical Center, Seattle, WA, p. A452
KAUFFMAN, Janie R.
Chief Executive Officer, Columbia Fort Bend Hospital, Missouri City, TX, p. A421
Chief Executive Officer, Columbia West Houston Medical Center, Houston, TX, p. A414
KAUFMAN, Alan G., Director, Division of Mental Health Services, Department of Human Services, State of New Jersey, Trenton, NJ, p. B95
KAYFES, John A., FACHE, Administrator, Kanabec Hospital, Mora, MN, p. A232
KAYLER, R. S., USN, Commanding Officer, Naval Hospital, Twentynine Palms, CA, p. A67
KEAHEY, Kent A., President, Providence Health Center, Waco, TX, p. A430
KEARNEY, Daniel, Chief Executive Officer, Charter Hospital Orlando South, Kissimmee, FL, p. A90
KEARNEY, W. Michael, Pressident, Mary Lanning Memorial Hospital, Hastings, NE, p. A264
KEARS, David J., Director, Alameda County Health Care Services Agency, San Leandro, CA, p. B64
KECK, Wade E.
Chief Executive Officer, Memorial Health Services, Adel, GA, p. B113
Chief Executive Officer, Memorial Hospital of Adel, Adel, GA, p. A103
KEEFER, Michael R., CHE, Chief Executive Officer, Clarion Psychiatric Center, Clarion, PA, p. A355
KEEGAN, James L.
President and Chief Executive Officer, EMH Amherst Hospital, Amherst, OH, p. A323
President and Chief Executive Officer, EMH Regional Medical Center, Elyria, OH, p. A329
KEEHAN, Carol, President, Providence Hospital, Washington, DC, p. A81
KEEN, Robert C., Ph.D., President and Chief Executive Officer, Hancock Memorial Hospital and Health Services, Greenfield, IN, p. A143
KEENE, Lee D., Administrator, Rockcastle Hospital, Mount Vernon, KY, p. A179

KEENER, Carl, M.D., Medical Director, Montana State Hospital, Warm Springs, MT, p. A260
KEESEE, Carolyn, Chief Executive Officer, Wetumka General Hospital, Wetumka, OK, p. A347
KEIERLEBER, Daniel, Administrator, Community Memorial Hospital, Redfield, SD, p. A384
KEIMIG, H. John, President and Chief Executive Officer, St. Joseph Health Services of Rhode Island, North Providence, RI, p. A373
KEIR, Douglas C., Chief Executive Officer, McDuffie County Hospital, Thomson, GA, p. A115
KEITH, David N., Chief Executive Officer, Rice Medical Center, Eagle Lake, TX, p. A408
KEITH, Judith Marie
President and Chief Executive Officer, Harbor View Mercy Hospital, Fort Smith, AR, p. A31
President and Chief Executive Officer, St. Edward Mercy Medical Center, Fort Smith, AR, p. A31
KEITH, Mary Werner, Administrator, Mercy Hospital–Turner Memorial, Ozark, AR, p. A34
KELLAR, Richard A., Administrator, West Allis Memorial Hospital, West Allis, WI, p. A470
KELLER, Jack M., Administrator, Baptist Hickman Community Hospital, Centerville, TN, p. A387
KELLER, Michael J., Administrator, Hi–Plains Hospital, Hale Center, TX, p. A412
KELLERSBERGER, Kent, Chief Executive Officer, North Big Horn Hospital, Lovell, WY, p. A472
KELLEY, Neal, Administrator, Edgar B. Davis Memorial Hospital, Luling, TX, p. A420
KELLEY, Randall, Senior Vice President and Chief Operating Officer, Flower Hospital, Sylvania, OH, p. A335
KELLEY, Robert C., President and Chief Executive Officer, Madera Community Hospital, Madera, CA, p. A52
KELLEY Jr., William C., FACHE, President and Chief Executive Officer, Samaritan Hospital, Ashland, OH, p. A323
KELLIE, Karen J., President, McCall Memorial Hospital, McCall, ID, p. A120
KELLISON, Jay R., Chief Executive Officer, BHC Walnut Creek Hospital, Walnut Creek, CA, p. A68
KELLY, Arthur C., Administrator and Chief Executive Officer, Oktibbeha County Hospital, Starkville, MS, p. A243
KELLY, Dan, Chief Executive Officer, Perkins County Health Services, Grant, NE, p. A264
KELLY, Daniel R., Chief Executive Officer, Doctors Regional Medical Center, Poplar Bluff, MO, p. A252
KELLY, Frank J., President and Chief Executive Officer, Danbury Hospital, Danbury, CT, p. A76
KELLY, Jeffrey R., President and Chief Executive Officer, Deaconess–Nashoba Hospital, Ayer, MA, p. A203
KELLY, Laurence E., Senior Vice President, St. Luke's Hospital, Newburgh, NY, p. A301
KELLY, Patrick G., Administrator, Charter Sioux Falls Behavioral Health System, Sioux Falls, SD, p. A385
KELLY, Sheila C., MS, Chief Executive Officer, Haven Hospital, De Soto, TX, p. A407
KELLY, Steven G., President, Community Memorial Healthcenter, South Hill, VA, p. A446
KELLY, Timothy A., Ph.D., Commissioner, Virginia Department of Mental Health, Richmond, VA, p. B148
KELLY, Timothy J., M.D., President, Fairbanks Hospital, Indianapolis, IN, p. A144
KELLY Jr., Winfield M., President and Chief Executive Officer, Dimensions Health Corporation, Landover, MD, p. B95
KENDRICK, Gary G., Chief Executive Officer, Lincoln Regional Hospital, Fayetteville, TN, p. A389
KENLEY, William, Administrator and Chief Executive Officer, Norton Community Hospital, Norton, VA, p. A443
KENNEDY, Bill R., President and Chief Executive Officer, Muskogee Regional Medical Center, Muskogee, OK, p. A343
KENNEDY, Christopher S., President and Chief Operating Officer, Health First/Cape Canaveral Hospital, Cocoa Beach, FL, p. A85
KENNEDY, Thomas F., Administrator, Rolling Plains Memorial Hospital, Sweetwater, TX, p. A428

KENNEDY, Philip, President and Chief Executive Officer, Alexian Brothers Medical Center, Elk Grove Village, IL, p. A129

KENNEDY, Michael H., Deputy Commander, Raymond W. Bliss Army Community Hospital, Fort Huachuca, AZ, p. A23

KENNEDY III, Thomas D., President and Chief Executive Officer, Bristol Hospital, Bristol, CT, p. A76

KENT, Robert O., Administrator and Chief Executive Officer, Oneida County Hospital, Malad City, ID, p. A120

KENT, William, Ph.D., Vice President Behavioral Health, Columbia HealthOne–Behavioral Health Services, Denver, CO, p. A71

KENYON, Douglas M., Director, Veterans Affairs Medical and Regional Office Center, Fargo, ND, p. A320

KERCORIAN, Robert A., Chief Executive Officer, Havenwyck Hospital, Auburn Hills, MI, p. A212

KERINS Sr., James J., Administrator, Caverna Memorial Hospital, Horse Cave, KY, p. A175

KERN, Peter L., President and Chief Executive Officer, Palmerton Hospital, Palmerton, PA, p. A363

KERNER, Michael K., President and Chief Executive Officer, Columbia Augusta Medical Center, Augusta, GA, p. A104

KERR, Kay, M.D., Medical Director, Bryn Mawr College Infirmary, Bryn Mawr, PA, p. A354

KERR, Michael D., Chief Executive Officer, Suburban Medical Center, Paramount, CA, p. A56

KERR, Nolan, Administrator, Loma Linda University Behavioral Medicine Center, Redlands, CA, p. A58

KERR, William B., Director, University of California San Francisco Medical Center, San Francisco, CA, p. A62

KERVIN, David D., Administrator, Richardson Medical Center, Rayville, LA, p. A190

KERWIN, George, President, Bellin Hospital, Green Bay, WI, p. A462

KESSEN, Donald J., Administrator, Rawlins County Hospital, Atwood, KS, p. A161

KESSLER, D. McWilliams, Executive Director, Wills Eye Hospital, Philadelphia, PA, p. A365

KESSLER, Warren C., President, Kennebec Valley Medical Center, Augusta, ME, p. A193

KESSLER, William E., President, Saint Anthony's Health Center, Alton, IL, p. A123

KESTLY, John J., Administrator, Shawano Medical Center, Shawano, WI, p. A468

KETCHAM, Mitchel S., Administrator, Manning General Hospital, Manning, IA, p. A156

KETCHAM, Richard H., President, Brooks Memorial Hospital, Dunkirk, NY, p. A291

KETRING, John, Administrator, Pawnee Municipal Hospital, Pawnee, OK, p. A344

KEVISH, Stanley J., President, University of Pittsburgh Medical Center, St. Margaret, Pittsburgh, PA, p. A367

KHAN, Nasir A., M.D., Director, Bournewood Hospital, Brookline, MA, p. A205

KHOURY, Raymond J., Administrator, St. Joseph Hospital, Houston, TX, p. A415

KIECKER, Carol, Chief Executive Officer, Vice President and Area Manager, Kaiser Foundation Hospital, Redwood City, CA, p. A58

KIEF, Brian, President, United Hospital District, Blue Earth, MN, p. A227

KIEFER, Joseph N., Administrator, Helen Ellis Memorial Hospital, Tarpon Springs, FL, p. A101

KIELMAN, Richard C., President and Chief Executive Officer, Dickinson County Memorial Hospital, Spirit Lake, IA, p. A159

KIELY, Robert Gerard, President and Chief Executive Officer, Middlesex Hospital, Middletown, CT, p. A77

KIIL, Julia, Administrator, Chowchilla District Memorial Hospital, Chowchilla, CA, p. A40

KILEY, Dennis, President, Gordon Hospital, Calhoun, GA, p. A106

KILPATRICK, David M., M.D., Acting Center Director, Veterans Affairs Medical Center, Cheyenne, WY, p. A471

KILPATRICK, Michael, USN, Commanding Officer, Naval Hospital, Millington, TN, p. A394

KIMEL, Mike, Administrator, Davie County Hospital, Mocksville, NC, p. A314

KIMMEL, Arnold, Interim Chief Executive Officer, Memorial Hospital of Salem County, Salem, NJ, p. A281

KIMMEY, James, M.P.H., Chairman and Chief Executive Officer, Saint Louis University Hospital, Saint Louis, MO, p. A254

KINCADE, Jerry, Chief Executive Officer, Medical Arts Hospital, Texarkana, TX, p. A429

KINDEL, Dave, President and Chief Executive Officer, Southwest Medical Center, Liberal, KS, p. A166

KINDRED, Bryan, Chief Executive Officer, DCH Healthcare Authority, Tuscaloosa, AL, p. B89

KINDRED, Bryan N., Chief Executive Officer, DCH Regional Medical Center, Tuscaloosa, AL, p. A18

KING, Dennis P., President, Acadia Hospital, Bangor, ME, p. A193

KING, John G., President and Chief Executive Officer, Legacy Health System, Portland, OR, p. B108

KING, Keith R., Chief Executive Officer, Winona Memorial Hospital, Indianapolis, IN, p. A145

KING, Larry R., Administrator, Washington–St. Tammany Regional Medical Center, Bogalusa, LA, p. A183

KING, Michael, Administrator, Winslow Memorial Hospital, Winslow, AZ, p. A28

KING, Randy, Administrator, Baptist Memorial Hospital–Blytheville, Blytheville, AR, p. A29

KINGSBURY, James A., President and Chief Executive Officer, Fort Hamilton–Hughes Memorial Hospital, Hamilton, OH, p. A330

KINGSLEY, Bernard, Chief Operating Officer, Worcester State Hospital, Worcester, MA, p. A211

KINNEY, Charles S., Chief Executive Officer, Martha's Vineyard Hospital, Oak Bluffs, MA, p. A209

KINNEY, John P., President, Nason Hospital, Roaring Spring, PA, p. A368

KINSTAD, Lester, Administrator, Dell Rapids Community Hospital, Dell Rapids, SD, p. A382

KIRBY, Dale A., Chief Executive Officer, THC–Las Vegas Hospital, Las Vegas, NV, p. A270

KIRK, Warren J.
Administrator, Citrus Valley Medical Center Inter–Community Campus, Covina, CA, p. A41
Administrator and Chief Operating Officer, Citrus Valley Medical Center–Queen of the Valley Campus, West Covina, CA, p. A68

KIRK Jr., H. Lee, President, Culpeper Memorial Hospital, Culpeper, VA, p. A440

KIRK Jr., William R., President and Chief Executive Officer, Kent and Queen Anne's Hospital, Chestertown, MD, p. A199

KIRKPATRICK, James W., Commander, Darnall Army Community Hospital, Fort Hood, TX, p. A409

KIRN, Galen, Administrator, California Mens Colony Hospital, San Luis Obispo, CA, p. A63

KIROUSIS, Theodore E.
Area Director, Medfield State Hospital, Medfield, MA, p. A207
Area Director, Westborough State Hospital, Westborough, MA, p. A211

KIRSCHNER, Sidney, President and Chief Executive Officer, Northside Hospital, Atlanta, GA, p. A104

KISER, Greg, Chief Executive Officer, Three Rivers Medical Center, Louisa, KY, p. A176

KITE, Landon, President, Fuller Memorial Hospital, South Attleboro, MA, p. A209

KITTREDGE, Edward F., Chief Executive Officer, Massachusetts Respiratory Hospital, Braintree, MA, p. A205

KIZER, Kenneth W., M.P.H., Under Secretary for Health, Department of Veterans Affairs, Washington, DC, p. B91

KLAASMEYER, Al, Administrator, Alegent Health–Memorial Hospital, Schuyler, NE, p. A268

KLAGSBRUN, Samuel C., M.D., Executive Medical Director, Four Winds Hospital, Katonah, NY, p. A293

KLAWITER, Anne K., Chief Executive Officer, Southwest Health Center, Platteville, WI, p. A467

KLEEFISCH, William B., Deputy Commander, U. S. Air Force Medical Center Keesler, Keesler AFB, MS, p. A240

KLEIN, Ann, Executive Director, Recovery Inn at Menlo Park, Menlo Park, CA, p. A53

KLEIN, Gerard D., Chief Executive Officer, UHHS–Memorial Hospital of Geneva, Geneva, OH, p. A330

KLEIN, Robert, Chief Executive Officer, Columbia South Pittsburg Hospital, South Pittsburg, TN, p. A396

KLEIN, Steven M., President and Chief Executive Officer, North Shore Medical Center, Miami, FL, p. A93

KLIER, Bill, Chief Executive Officer, Cypress Fairbanks Medical Center, Houston, TX, p. A414

KLIMA, Dennis E.
President and Chief Executive Officer, Bayhealth Medical Center, Dover, DE, p. B69
President and Chief Executive Officer, Kent General Hospital, Dover, DE, p. A80

KLINE, Bobbie, R.N., Vice President, Santa Ynez Valley Cottage Hospital, Solvang, CA, p. A65

KLINKENBORG, Verna M., President, Sartori Memorial Hospital, Cedar Falls, IA, p. A152

KLINT, Robert B., M.D., President, SwedishAmerican Hospital, Rockford, IL, p. A137

KLOESS, Larry, Chief Executive Officer, Columbia Conroe Regional Medical Center, Conroe, TX, p. A404

KLUN, James, President, Allegan General Hospital, Allegan, MI, p. A212

KLUSMANN, Richard W., Chief Executive Officer, Columbia St. David's South Hospital, Austin, TX, p. A400

KLUTTZ, James K., President and Chief Executive Officer, Frederick Memorial Hospital, Frederick, MD, p. A200

KNAPP, Dennis L., President, Cameron Memorial Community Hospital, Angola, IN, p. A140

KNAUSS, Albert C., President and Chief Executive Officer, Marion General Hospital, Marion, IN, p. A146

KNEPP, Gerald E.
Chief Executive Officer, Ridgecrest Hospital, Clayton, GA, p. A106
Chief Executive Officer, Woodridge Hospital, Clayton, GA, p. A106

KNIGHT, Alan D., President and Chief Executive Officer, Jordan Hospital, Plymouth, MA, p. A209

KNIGHT, Jimmy M., Administrator and Chief Executive Officer, Corcoran District Hospital, Corcoran, CA, p. A40

KNIGHT, Russell M., President, Robert Packer Hospital, Sayre, PA, p. A368

KNOBLE, James K., President, Methodist Medical Center of Illinois, Peoria, IL, p. A136

KNODE, Scott, Co–Administrator, Community Memorial Hospital, Sumner, IA, p. A159

KNOX, Dennis M., Vice President and Chief Executive Officer, Memorial Hospital Pasadena, Pasadena, TX, p. A423

KNOX, John E., President, River District Hospital, East China, MI, p. A215

KNOX, Jud, President, York Hospital, York, ME, p. A196

KNUEPPEL, Arthur, President and Chief Executive Officer, St. Lawrence Hospital and Healthcare Services, Lansing, MI, p. A219

KNUTSON, Fred, Administrator, Chippewa County Montevideo Hospital, Montevideo, MN, p. A232

KNUTSON, William
Vice President and Administrator, HealthEast St. John's Hospital, Maplewood, MN, p. A231
Vice President and Administrator, HealthEast St. Joseph's Hospital, Saint Paul, MN, p. A234

KOBAKES, George J., President and Chief Executive Officer, University of Pittsburgh Medical Center, Beaver Valley, Aliquippa, PA, p. A353

KOBAN Jr., Michael A., Chief Executive Officer, NetCare Health Systems, Inc., Nashville, TN, p. B117

KOBAYASHI, Bertrand, Deputy Director, State of Hawaii, Department of Health, Honolulu, HI, p. B138

KOCHIS, Thomas, Administrator, Oakwood Hospital Downriver Center–Lincoln Park, Lincoln Park, MI, p. A219

KOEHLER, Eduard R., Administrator, Medical Park Hospital, Winston–Salem, NC, p. A318

KOELLNER, William H., Administrator, Landmann–Jungman Memorial Hospital, Scotland, SD, p. A384

L

LEHMANN, Robert J., Chief Executive Officer, Colonial Hospital, Newport News, VA, p. A443

LEHRFELD, Samuel
Executive Director, Coler Memorial Hospital, New York, NY, p. A296
Executive Director, Goldwater Memorial Hospital, New York, NY, p. A296

LEIS Jr., James L., Administrator and Chief Executive Officer, Charlton Memorial Hospital, Folkston, GA, p. A109

LEISHER, Kenneth W., Deputy Commander, Administration, Evans U. S. Army Community Hospital, Fort Carson, CO, p. A72

LELEUX, Walter, Chief Executive Officer, Columbia Bellaire Medical Center, Houston, TX, p. A413

LEMANSKI, Dennis R., D.O., Vice President and Chief Administrative Officer, Riverside Osteopathic Hospital, Trenton, MI, p. A224

LEMON, Brian J., President, MacNeal Hospital, Berwyn, IL, p. A124

LEMON, Thomas R., Chief Executive Officer, Burnett Medical Center, Grantsburg, WI, p. A462

LENERTZ, Thomas C., President and Chief Executive Officer, Riverview Healthcare Association, Crookston, MN, p. A228

LENNEN, Anthony B., President and Chief Executive Officer, Major Hospital, Shelbyville, IN, p. A148

LENTZ, Stan, Administrator and Chief Executive Officer, Mohave Valley Hospital and Medical Center, Bullhead City, AZ, p. A22

LENZ, Roger W., Administrator, Hamilton County Public Hospital, Webster City, IA, p. A159

LEON, Anne R., Chief Executive Officer, Houston Rehabilitation Institute, Houston, TX, p. A414

LEON, Jean G., R.N., Senior Vice President, Kings County Hospital Center, New York, NY, p. A297

LEONHARD Jr., Robert A., Administrator, University Rehabilitation Hospital, New Orleans, LA, p. A189

LEONHARDT, George E., President and Chief Executive Officer, Bradford Regional Medical Center, Bradford, PA, p. A354

LEONOR, Samuel, President, Florida Hospital–Walker, Avon Park, FL, p. A83

LEOPARD, Jimmy, Chief Executive Officer, Medical Park Hospital, Hope, AR, p. A31

LEPTUCK, Cary F., President and Chief Executive Officer, Chestnut Hill Hospital, Philadelphia, PA, p. A363

LERNER, Holly, Chief Executive Officer, Hollywood Medical Center, Los Angeles, FL, p. A88

LERNER, Wayne M., Dr.PH, President and Chief Executive Officer, Rehabilitation Institute of Chicago, Chicago, IL, p. A126

LERZ, Alfred A., President and Chief Executive Officer, Johnson Memorial Hospital, Stafford Springs, CT, p. A78

LETSON, Robert F., President and Chief Executive Officer, Gilmore Memorial Hospital, Amory, MS, p. A237

LEURCK, Stephen O., President, St. Anthony Medical Center, Crown Point, IN, p. A141

LEVANT, Howard, President and Chief Executive Officer, Queen of the Valley Hospital, Napa, CA, p. A55

LEVENSON, Marvin W., M.D., Administrator and Chief Operating Officer, Pomerado Hospital, Poway, CA, p. A58

LEVINE, Howard H., President and Chief Executive Officer, Columbia West Hills Medical Center, Los Angeles, CA, p. A49

LEVINE, Peter H., M.D., President and Chief Executive Officer, Memorial Health Care, Worcester, MA, p. A211

LEVINE, Robert V., President and Chief Executive Officer, Peninsula Hospital Center, New York, NY, p. A299

LEVINSONN, David, Chief Executive Officer, Sherman Oaks Hospital and Health Center, Los Angeles, CA, p. A51

LEVITSKY, Steven E., Administrator, Vencor Hospital–Boston, Boston, MA, p. A205

LEVY, Shari E., President, Phillips Eye Institute, Minneapolis, MN, p. A232

LEWGOOD, Tony, Administrator, Shriners Hospitals for Children–Lexington Unit, Lexington, KY, p. A176

LEWIS, Donald C., President and Chief Executive Officer, Hepburn Medical Center, Ogdensburg, NY, p. A301

LEWIS, Edward M., Chief Executive Officer, Bergen Pines County Hospital, Paramus, NJ, p. A280

LEWIS, J. O., Chief Executive Officer, Houston Northwest Medical Center, Houston, TX, p. A414

LEWIS, Luther J., Chief Executive Officer, Medical Center of South Arkansas, El Dorado, AR, p. A30

LEWIS, Mary Jo, Chief Executive Officer, Parkway Regional Hospital, Fulton, KY, p. A174

LEWIS, Nick, Administrator, Whitesburg Appalachian Regional Hospital, Whitesburg, KY, p. A181

LEWIS, Rebecca, President, Lexington Hospital, Lexington, KY, p. A176

LEWIS, Theodore M., President and Chief Executive Officer, Fort Washington Hospital, Fort Washington, MD, p. A200

LEWIS, Thomas J., President and Chief Executive Officer, Thomas Jefferson University Hospital, Philadelphia, PA, p. A365

LEWIS, Vickie, Chief Executive Officer, Charter Glade Behavioral Health System, Fort Myers, FL, p. A87

LEWIS, Gordon, Deputy Commander for Administration, Bassett Army Community Hospital, Fort Wainwright, AK, p. A20

LEY, Gary R., President and Chief Executive Officer, Garden City Hospital, Garden City, MI, p. A216

LIBENGOOD, Mary L., President, Meyersdale Medical Center, Meyersdale, PA, p. A361

LIBMAN, Ernest, Administrator and Chief Executive Officer, Lake Mead Hospital Medical Center, North Las Vegas, NV, p. A271

LICHTY, Judy, Administrator, Westbrook Health Center, Westbrook, MN, p. A236

LIEPMAN, Michael T., Chief Operating Officer, Valley Hospital and Medical Center, Spokane, WA, p. A453

LIEVENSE, William C., President and Chief Executive Officer, Columbia Doctors Hospital of Sarasota, Sarasota, FL, p. A99

LIKES Jr., Creighton E., President and Chief Executive Officer, Fairfield Medical Center, Lancaster, OH, p. A331

LILLARD, Joseph K., Administrator, Tri–State Memorial Hospital, Clarkston, WA, p. A448

LILLARD, Samuel F., Executive Vice President and Administrator, Bon Secours–Richmond Community Hospital, Richmond, VA, p. A445

LILLY, W. Spencer, Administrator, University Hospital, Charlotte, NC, p. A310

LINCOLN, David R., President and Chief Executive Officer, Covenant Health Systems, Inc., Lexington, MA, p. B88

LIND, Richard A., President and Chief Executive Officer, Memorial Health Systems, Ormond Beach, FL, p. B113

LINDEN, Todd C., President and Chief Executive Officer, Grinnell Regional Medical Center, Grinnell, IA, p. A155

LINDENMUTH, Norman, M.D., Interim Chief Executive Officer, Soldiers and Sailors Memorial Hospital of Yates County, Penn Yan, NY, p. A302

LINDQUIST, Helen S., Administrator, Five Counties Hospital, Lemmon, SD, p. A383

LINDSEY, Larry N., Administrator, Decatur County General Hospital, Parsons, TN, p. A395

LINEHAN, Mary, President, St. Joseph's Medical Center, Yonkers, NY, p. A307

LINENKUGEL, Nancy, FACHE, President and Chief Executive Officer, Providence Hospital, Sandusky, OH, p. A335

LINGENFELTER, Wayne M., Ed.D., Administrator and Chief Executive Officer, Vencor Hospital–San Leandro, San Leandro, CA, p. A63

LINGLE, Robert L., Executive Director, Singing River Hospital System, Pascagoula, MS, p. B132

LINGOR, John Daniel, President and Chief Executive Officer, Mount Carmel Medical Center, Pittsburg, KS, p. A168

LINN, Gerri, Administrator, Kimball County Hospital, Kimball, NE, p. A265

LINNEWEH Jr., Richard W., President and Chief Executive Officer, Yakima Valley Memorial Hospital, Yakima, WA, p. A454

LINTJER, Gregory W., President, Elkhart General Hospital, Elkhart, IN, p. A142

LIPSON, Manuel J., M.D., President, Spaulding Rehabilitation Hospital, Boston, MA, p. A204

LISCHAK, Michael, USAF, Commander, U. S. Air Force Hospital Seymour Johnson, Seymour Johnson AFB, NC, p. A316

LISTER, Susan, Chief Executive Officer, Charter Winds Hospital, Athens, GA, p. A103

LISZEWSKI, Richard S., CHE, Administrator, Memorial Medical Center of San Augustine, San Augustine, TX, p. A427

LITOS, Dennis M., President and Chief Executive Officer, Michigan Capital Healthcare, Lansing, MI, p. A219

LITTLEFIELD, Elizabeth, Ed.D., Superintendent, Western Mental Health Institute, Western Institute, TN, p. A397

LITTLESON, Steven G., President and Chief Executive Officer, Southern Ocean County Hospital, Manahawkin, NJ, p. A279

LITTRELL, Nancy, Chief Executive Officer, Woodford Hospital, Versailles, KY, p. A181

LITZ, Thomas H., President and Chief Executive Officer, Centrastate Medical Center, Freehold, NJ, p. A277

LIVERMORE, Craig A., President and Chief Executive Officer, Delnor–Community Hospital, Geneva, IL, p. A130

LIVINGSTON, Jeffrey A., Chief Executive Officer, Healthsouth Rehabilitation Hospital of Texarkana, Texarkana, TX, p. A429

LLOYD, John K., Chief Executive Officer, Meridian Health System, Neptune, NJ, p. A279

LLOYD II, Donald H., Administrator, Mullins Hospital, Mullins, SC, p. A379

LOBECK, Charles C., Chief Executive Officer, St. Mary's Hospital, Milwaukee, WI, p. A466

LOCKARD, Thomas L., President and Chief Executive Officer, Lodi Community Hospital, Lodi, OH, p. A331

LOCKHART, Allen J., Administrator, Okolona Community Hospital, Okolona, MS, p. A242

LOCKWOOD, Brian C., President and Chief Executive Officer, Lorain Community/St. Joseph Regional Health Center, Lorain, OH, p. A332

LOEBIG Jr., Wilfred F., President and Chief Executive Officer, Wheaton Franciscan Services, Inc., Wheaton, IL, p. B149

LOEFFEN, Susan Marie, Administrator, Oakes Community Hospital, Oakes, ND, p. A321

LOEWEN, Harold C., President, Oaklawn Psychiatric Center, Inc., Goshen, IN, p. A143

LOFE, Dennis A., FACHE, President, Kershaw County Medical Center, Camden, SC, p. A375

LOFTON, Kevin E., Executive Director and Chief Executive Officer, University of Alabama Hospital, Birmingham, AL, p. A12

LOGAN, Donald B., President and Chief Executive Officer, Southern Regional Medical Center, Riverdale, GA, p. A113

LOGE, Frank J., Director, University of California, Davis Medical Center, Sacramento, CA, p. A60

LOGUE, John W., Executive Vice President and Chief Operating Officer, St. Vincent's Medical Center, Jacksonville, FL, p. A90

LOGUE Jr., Thomas O., Ph.D., Administrator and Chief Executive Officer, Doctor's Memorial Hospital, Perry, FL, p. A97

LOH, Marcel, President and Chief Executive Officer, Kadlec Medical Center, Richland, WA, p. A452

LOHRMAN, Joe, Administrator, Crete Municipal Hospital, Crete, NE, p. A263

LOMBARD, Dave, President and Chief Executive Officer, Clear Brook Lodge, Shickshinny, PA, p. A369

LOMBARDI, Anthony M., President and Chief Executive Officer, Monongahela Valley Hospital, Monongahela, PA, p. A361

LONG, Charles H., Chief Executive Officer, Columbia De Queen Regional Medical Center, De Queen, AR, p. A30

LONG, Jim K., CPA, Administrator and Chief Executive Officer, West River Regional Medical Center, Hettinger, ND, p. A320

LONG, Lawrence C., Chief Executive Officer, Tahoe Forest Hospital District, Truckee, CA, p. A66

LONG, Max, Chief Executive Officer, Walter Knox Memorial Hospital, Emmett, ID, p. A120

LONG, Robert C., Administrator and Chief Executive Officer, Benjamin Rush Center, Syracuse, NY, p. A305

LONGO, Robert J., President and Chief Executive Officer, Good Samaritan Hospital, Lebanon, PA, p. A360

LOPER, Ouida, Administrator, Choctaw County Medical Center, Ackerman, MS, p. A237

LOPEZ, Frank, President and Chief Executive Officer, St. Mary's Mercy Hospital, Enid, OK, p. A341

LORACK Jr., Donald A., President and Chief Executive Officer, Hillcrest Healthcare System, Tulsa, OK, p. A346

LORDEMAN, Frank L., Chief Operating Officer, Cleveland Clinic Hospital, Cleveland, OH, p. A326

LORE, John S., President and Chief Executive Officer, Sisters of St. Joseph Health System, Ann Arbor, MI, p. B136

LORENZEN, W. F., Commanding Officer, U. S. Naval Hospital, Roosevelt Roads, PR, p. A477

LOTHE, Eric L., Chief Executive Officer, Skiff Medical Center, Newton, IA, p. A157

LOTT Jr., Carlos B., Director, Veterans Affairs Medical Center, Detroit, MI, p. A215

LOTTI, G. Phillip, Chief Executive Officer, Columbia Davis Medical Center, Statesville, NC, p. A317

LOUISE, Stella, President and Chief Executive Officer, Saint Mary of Nazareth Hospital Center, Chicago, IL, p. A127

LOVEDAY, William J., President and Chief Executive Officer, Methodist Hospital of Indiana, Indianapolis, IN, p. A144

LOVELL Jr., Charles D., Chief Executive Officer, Muhlenberg Community Hospital, Greenville, KY, p. A174

LOVETT, Juanice, Chief Executive Officer, Sharp Healthcare Murrieta, Murrieta, CA, p. A54

LOVING, David E., Chief Executive Officer, Edge Regional Medical Center, Troy, AL, p. A18

LOWD III, Harry M., Director, Bath County Community Hospital, Hot Springs, VA, p. A442

LOWERY, Jerry E., Executive Director, Russell County Medical Center, Lebanon, VA, p. A442

LOWRANCE, Debra S., R.N., Chief Executive Officer and Managing Director, Timberlawn Mental Health System, Dallas, TX, p. A407

LOWRY, James R., FACHE, Chief Executive Officer, Colquitt Regional Medical Center, Moultrie, GA, p. A112

LOYLESS, John Paul, Administrator, Rankin Hospital District, Rankin, TX, p. A424

LOZAR, Beverly, Site Administrator, Meridia Huron Hospital, Cleveland, OH, p. A327

LUCAS, Stephen M., Chief Executive Officer, Veterans Affairs Medical Center, Erie, PA, p. A357

LUCAS, Walter S., Administrator, Veterans Memorial Hospital of Meigs County, Pomeroy, OH, p. A334

LUCE, Larry D., President, Emory–Adventist Hospital, Smyrna, GA, p. A114

LUCHTEFELD, Daniel J., Director, Eastern State Hospital, Lexington, KY, p. A176

LUCK Jr., James V., M.D., Chief Executive Officer and Medical Director, Orthopaedic Hospital, Los Angeles, CA, p. A51

LUDEKE, Max L., FACHE, Interim Chief Executive Officer, Wood River Township Hospital, Wood River, IL, p. A139

LUKHARD, Kenneth W., President and Chief Executive Officer, Columbia Lake Cumberland Regional Hospital, Somerset, KY, p. A180

LULEWICZ, Stephanie, Administrator, Marshall County Memorial Hospital, Britton, SD, p. A382

LUMSDEN, Chris A., Administrator, Halifax Regional Hospital, South Boston, VA, p. A446

LUND, Mark, Superintendent, Mental Health Institute, Clarinda, IA, p. A152

LUND, Robert S., Administrator, Kaiser Foundation Hospital–Riverside, Riverside, CA, p. A59

LUNDQUIST, David, Chief Executive Officer, Columbia Bethany Hospital, Bethany, OK, p. A339

LUNDSTROM, Greg, Interim Administrator, Lindsborg Community Hospital, Lindsborg, KS, p. A166

LUNSETH, Mark, Administrator, Rush City Hospital, Rush City, MN, p. A234

LUNSFORD, W. Bruce, Board Chairman, President and Chief Executive Officer, Vencor, Incorporated, Louisville, KY, p. B147

LUSE, Robert H., Chief Executive Officer, Mariners Hospital, Tavernier, FL, p. A101

LUSSIER, James T., President and Chief Executive Officer, St. Charles Medical Center, Bend, OR, p. A348

LUTHER, Robert M., Executive Director, Springs Memorial Hospital, Lancaster, SC, p. A379

LUTJEMEIER, Everett, Administrator, Washington County Hospital, Washington, KS, p. A170

LYBARGER, William A., Administrator, Cedar Vale Community Hospital, Cedar Vale, KS, p. A161

LYCAN, Laura J., Administrator and Chief Executive Officer, Healthsouth Rehabilitation Hospital of Fort Worth, Fort Worth, TX, p. A410

LYNCH, Edward F., Administrator, Richards Memorial Hospital, Rockdale, TX, p. A424

LYNCH, Francis P., President and Chief Executive Officer, Mount Auburn Hospital, Cambridge, MA, p. A205

LYNCH III, Ernest C., Chief Executive Officer, Columbia Medical Center at Lancaster, Lancaster, TX, p. A418

LYON, David R., Administrator, ARH Regional Medical Center, Hazard, KY, p. A175

LYONS, Richard D., President and Chief Administrative Officer, Northridge Hospital and Medical Center, Sherman Way Campus, Los Angeles, CA, p. A51

LYSINGER, R. Craig, Administrator, Wabash Valley Hospital, West Lafayette, IN, p. A149

M

MAAS, Lawrence A., Administrator, Sutter Davis Hospital, Davis, CA, p. A41

MABRY, Jerry D., Executive Director, National Park Medical Center, Hot Springs, AR, p. A31

MABRY II, Earl W., Commander, U. S. Air Force Medical Center Wright–Patterson, Wright–Patterson AFB, OH, p. A337

MACCALLUM, James M., President and Chief Executive Officer, Columbia Tulsa Regional Medical Center, Tulsa, OK, p. A346

MACCOOL, W. David, Administrator, Garrard County Memorial Hospital, Lancaster, KY, p. A175

MACDOWELL, Barry S., President, Reid Hospital and Health Care Services, Richmond, IN, p. A148

MACEK, Paul E.
Senior Vice President, Appleton Medical Center, Appleton, WI, p. A460
Senior Vice President, Theda Clark Medical Center, Neenah, WI, p. A466

MACFARLAND, H. J., FACHE, Executive Director, Irving Healthcare System, Irving, TX, p. A416

MACGARD, Elizabeth, Chief Executive Officer, Mendocino Coast District Hospital, Fort Bragg, CA, p. A43

MACK, Arlene, R.N., Administrator, Richardton Health Center, Richardton, ND, p. A321

MACKAY Jr., James, Chief Executive Officer, Union Hospital, Mayville, ND, p. A321

MACKE, Anita, Administrator, Meadowbrook Hospital, Gardner, KS, p. A163

MACKENDER, Daryl, Chief Executive Officer, Knoxville Area Community Hospital, Knoxville, IA, p. A156

MACLAREN, Ron, Chief Executive Officer, Columbia Regional Medical Center, Montgomery, AL, p. A16

MACLEOD, John L., Administrator and Chief Executive Officer, Otsego Memorial Hospital, Gaylord, MI, p. A216

MACLEOD, Leslie N. H., President, Huggins Hospital, Wolfeboro, NH, p. A274

MACRI, William P., Administrator, Franklin–Simpson Memorial Hospital, Franklin, KY, p. A174

MADDALENA, Frank J., President and Chief Executive Officer, Brookdale Hospital Medical Center, New York, NY, p. A296

MADDEN, Michael J.
Administrator, Grays Harbor Community Hospital, Aberdeen, WA, p. A448
Chief Executive Los Angeles Service Area, Providence Holy Cross Medical Center, Los Angeles, CA, p. A51
Chief Executive Los Angeles Service Area, Providence Saint Joseph Medical Center, Burbank, CA, p. A38

MADDEN, Patrick J., President and Chief Executive Officer, Sacred Heart Hospital of Pensacola, Pensacola, FL, p. A97

MADDOCK, Dan S., President, Taylor Regional Hospital, Hawkinsville, GA, p. A110

MADDOX, Jim L., Chief Administrative Officer, North Logan Mercy Hospital, Paris, AR, p. A34

MADDOX, Richard D., Administrator, U. S. Air Force Regional Hospital–Sheppard, Sheppard AFB, TX, p. A427

MADFES, Kenneth, Chief Executive Officer, Healdsburg General Hospital, Healdsburg, CA, p. A45

MADURA, M. Lucille, Provincial Superior, Sisters of the Holy Family of Nazareth–Sacred Heart Province, Des Plaines, IL, p. B136

MAESTRE, Jaime F., Executive Director, Hospital Perea, Mayaguez, PR, p. A476

MAFFETONE, Michael A., Director and Chief Executive Officer, University Hospital, Stony Brook, NY, p. A305

MAGEE, Donald R., Chief Executive Officer, Hopkins County Memorial Hospital, Sulphur Springs, TX, p. A428

MAGERS, Brent D., FACHE, Chief Executive Officer and Administrator, Walls Regional Hospital, Cleburne, TX, p. A404

MAGHAZEHE, Al, President and Chief Executive Officer, Helene Fuld Medical Center, Trenton, NJ, p. A282

MAGLIARO, John G., President and Chief Executive Officer, Columbus Hospital, Newark, NJ, p. A279

MAHADEVAN, Dev, Administrator, Kaiser Foundation Hospital, Los Angeles, CA, p. A50

MAHAFFEY, Robert, Administrator, Heart of Florida Hospital, Haines City, FL, p. A88

MAHAN, Stephen
Chief Executive Officer, Memorial Hospital of Tampa, Tampa, FL, p. A100
Chief Executive Officer, Town and Country Hospital, Tampa, FL, p. A100

MAHER, John J., President and Chief Executive Officer, Sisters of Charity Hospital of Buffalo, Buffalo, NY, p. A290

MAHER, Robert J., President, Our Lady of Bellefonte Hospital, Ashland, KY, p. A172

MAHER Jr., Robert E., President and Chief Executive Officer, Saint Vincent Hospital, Worcester, MA, p. A211

MAHN, Edward F., Chief Executive Officer, Ketchikan General Hospital, Ketchikan, AK, p. A21

MAHONE V, William, Administrator, Stonewall Jackson Hospital, Lexington, VA, p. A442

MAHONEY, Kevin J., President, Wilson Center Psychiatric Facility for Children and Adolescents, Faribault, MN, p. A229

MAHONEY, Michael P., President and Chief Executive Officer, St. Rose Hospital, Hayward, CA, p. A45

MAHONEY, Patrick R., Administrator and Chief Executive Officer, Affiliated Health Services, Mount Vernon, WA, p. A450

MAHRER, Michael D., President, St. Ansgar's Health Center, Park River, ND, p. A321

MAIDLOW, Spencer, President, St. Luke's Hospital, Saginaw, MI, p. A222

MAIER, Harry R., President, Memorial Hospital, Belleville, IL, p. A123

MAIER, Vonnie, President and Chief Executive Officer, Huerfano Medical Center, Walsenburg, CO, p. A75

MAIN, Robert P., President and Chief Executive Officer, Siskin Hospital for Physical Rehabilitation, Chattanooga, TN, p. A388

MAJURE, T. K., Administrator, Our Community Hospital, Scotland Neck, NC, p. A316

MAKI, James W., Chief Executive Officer, Huntington East Valley Hospital, Glendora, CA, p. A45

MAKOWSKI, Peter E., President and Chief Executive Officer, Citrus Valley Health Partners, Covina, CA, p. B78

MALCOLM, Fay E., R.N., Chief Operating Officer, North Central Bronx Hospital, New York, NY, p. A299

MALINOWSKI, Barbara A., Administrator and Chief Executive Officer, Westfield Memorial Hospital, Westfield, NY, p. A307

MALINOWSKI, Mary Norberta, President, St. Joseph Hospital, Bangor, ME, p. A193

MALONE, John T., President and Chief Executive Officer, Hamot Medical Center, Erie, PA, p. A357

MALONEY, Elizabeth Ann, President and Chief Executive Officer, St. Elizabeth Hospital, Elizabeth, NJ, p. A277

MAMOON, Wendy, Chief Operating Officer, The Rock Creek Center, Lemont, IL, p. A133

MANCHUR, Fred, President, San Joaquin Community Hospital, Bakersfield, CA, p. A37

MANCINI, Dorothy J., R.N., Regional Vice President Administration, Imperial Point Medical Center, Fort Lauderdale, FL, p. A87

MANDERNACH, Dianne, Chief Executive Officer, Mercy Hospital and Health Care Center, Moose Lake, MN, p. A232

MANDERS, Daniel N., President and Chief Executive Officer, Mile Bluff Medical Center, Mauston, WI, p. A464

MANDSAGER, Richard, M.D., Director, U. S. Public Health Service Alaska Native Medical Center, Anchorage, AK, p. A20

MANGINI, Michael A., Administrator and Chief Executive Officer, Bellevue Woman's Hospital, Schenectady, NY, p. A304

MANGION, Richard M., President and Chief Executive Officer, Harrington Memorial Hospital, Southbridge, MA, p. A209

MANGOLD, Larry K., Interim President and Chief Executive Officer, Wilcox Memorial Hospital, Lihue, HI, p. A118

MANLEY, Jeffrey J., Chief Executive Officer, Jordan Valley Hospital, West Jordan, UT, p. A436

MANLEY, Joseph M., Director, Veterans Affairs Medical Center, Spokane, WA, p. A453

MANLEY, Warren, Administrator, Camden Medical Center, Saint Marys, GA, p. A113

MANNICH, Andrew, Administrator, Granville Medical Center, Oxford, NC, p. A315

MANNING, Michael, Chief Executive Officer, Jo Ellen Smith Medical Center, New Orleans, LA, p. A188

MANNING, Richard W., Administrator, South Panola Community Hospital, Batesville, MS, p. A237

MANNING, Catherine, President and Chief Executive Officer, Saint Vincent Health Center, Erie, PA, p. A357

MANNIX Jr., Robert T., President and Chief Operations Officer, St. Elizabeth Health Services, Baker City, OR, p. A348

MANSON, Lisa, Administrator, Central Community Hospital, Elkader, IA, p. A154

MANTEY, Carl W., Administrator, Gerald Champion Memorial Hospital, Alamogordo, NM, p. A284

MANTZ, James R., Administrator, Prairie Community Medical Assistance Facility, Terry, MT, p. A260

MAPLES, Ruth, Executive Director, Lanterman Developmental Center, Pomona, CA, p. A57

MARCANTUONO, Daniel L., FACHE, President and Chief Executive Officer, General Hospital Center at Passaic, Passaic, NJ, p. A280

MARCELINE, Alex M., Chief Executive Officer, Columbia Palms West Hospital, Loxahatchee, FL, p. A92

MARCHETTI, Mark E., Chief Executive Officer, Greenfield Area Medical Center, Greenfield, OH, p. A330

MARCOS, Luis R., M.D., President, New York City Health and Hospitals Corporation, New York, NY, p. B117

MARIANI, Felix, Administrator, Healthsouth Rehabilitation Hospital of Altoona, Altoona, PA, p. A353

MARIE, Donna, Chief Executive Officer, Resurrection Medical Center, Chicago, IL, p. A127

MARINAKOS, Plato A., President and Chief Executive Officer, Mercy Health System of Southeastern Pennsylvania, Bala Cynwyd, PA, p. A353

MARINE, Ross P., Administrator and Chief Executive Officer, Truman Medical Center–East, Kansas City, MO, p. A249

MARINO, Robert E., Executive Director, Citizens General Hospital, New Kensington, PA, p. A362

MARION, Ben, Chief Executive Officer, Turning Point Hospital, Moultrie, GA, p. A112

MARK, Richard J., President and Chief Executive Officer, St. Mary's Hospital, East St. Louis, IL, p. A129

MARKELZ, Stephen L., Deputy Commander, Administration, Martin Army Community Hospital, Fort Benning, GA, p. A109

MARKHAM, Patricia, Administrator, Cass County Memorial Hospital, Atlantic, IA, p. A151

MARKIEWICZ, Dennis P., Vice President, Hospital Operations, Crittenton Hospital, Rochester, MI, p. A222

MARKOS, Dennis R., Chief Executive Officer, Ed Fraser Memorial Hospital, MacClenny, FL, p. A92

MARKOWITZ, Alan, FACHE, Administrator and Chief Executive Officer, Baptist DeKalb Hospital, Smithville, TN, p. A396

MARKOWITZ, Bruce J., President and Chief Executive Officer, Palisades General Hospital, North Bergen, NJ, p. A280

MARKS, Craig J., President and Chief Executive Officer, South Haven Community Hospital, South Haven, MI, p. A223

MARKS, Gary A., Administrator, Glen Rose Medical Center, Glen Rose, TX, p. A411

MARLEY, Mark E.
President and Chief Executive Officer, Bucyrus Community Hospital, Bucyrus, OH, p. A324
Chief Executive Officer, Galion Community Hospital, Galion, OH, p. A330

MARMO, Anthony P., Chief Executive Officer, Kingston Hospital, Kingston, NY, p. A293

MARMORSTONE, Ray, Administrator, Memorial Hospital of Iowa County, Dodgeville, WI, p. A461

MARNELL, George, Director, Jonathan M. Wainwright Memorial Veterans Affairs Medical Center, Walla Walla, WA, p. A454

MARNELL, John W., Chief Executive Officer, Hudson Medical Center, Hudson, WI, p. A463

MAROHN, Harold G., Acting Chief Executive Officer, BHC Belmont Hills Hospital, Belmont, CA, p. A38

MARON, Michael, President and Chief Executive Officer, Holy Name Hospital, Teaneck, NJ, p. A282

MARONEY, George, Administrator, Memorial Hospital of Carbondale, Carbondale, IL, p. A124

MAROTTI, Peter A., Chief Executive Officer, McCray Memorial Hospital, Kendallville, IN, p. A145

MARQUARDT, Robert C., FACHE, President, Memorial Medical Center of West Michigan, Ludington, MI, p. A219

MARQUETTE Jr., Gerald Joseph, Administrator, Coffeyville Regional Medical Center, Coffeyville, KS, p. A162

MARQUEZ, Michael, Chief Executive Officer, Manatee Memorial Hospital, Bradenton, FL, p. A84

MARR, Charles J.
Chief Executive Officer, Alegent Health Bergan Mercy Medical Center, Omaha, NE, p. A266
Chief Executive Officer, Alegent Health Mercy Hospital, Council Bluffs, IA, p. A153

MARRERO, Victor R., Executive Administrator, Dr. Jose Ramos Lebron Hospital, Fajardo, PR, p. A475

MARSHALL, Bob, Administrator, North Star Hospital and Counseling Center, Anchorage, AK, p. A20

MARSHALL, James, Chief Executive Officer, Massac Memorial Hospital, Metropolis, IL, p. A134

MARSHALL, John A., Chief Executive Officer, Columbia Crockett Hospital, Lawrenceburg, TN, p. A392

MARSHALL, Mike, Chief Executive Officer, Healthsouth Rehabilitation Hospital of Tallahassee, Tallahassee, FL, p. A100

MARSTELLER, Brent A., Chief Executive Officer, Columbia Raleigh General Hospital, Beckley, WV, p. A455

MARTE, Noemi Davis, M.D., Medical Director, Caguas Regional Hospital, Caguas, PR, p. A475

MARTIN, Andria, MS, Director, University of Connecticut Health Center, John Dempsey Hospital, Farmington, CT, p. A76

MARTIN, D. Wayne, Administrator and Chief Executive Officer, Crisp Regional Hospital, Cordele, GA, p. A107

MARTIN, Elizabeth J., Vice President and Administrator, Riverside Tappahannock Hospital, Tappahannock, VA, p. A447

MARTIN, G. Roger, President and Chief Executive Officer, Jeanes Hospital, Philadelphia, PA, p. A364

MARTIN, Greg, Administrator and Chief Executive Officer, Blackwell Regional Hospital, Blackwell, OK, p. A339

MARTIN, Jack, Administrator, Latimer County General Hospital, Wilburton, OK, p. A347

MARTIN, James A., Chief Executive Officer, Good Samaritan Hospital, Suffern, NY, p. A305

MARTIN, Jeffrey L., President and Chief Executive Officer, Saint Michael's Hospital, Stevens Point, WI, p. A469

MARTIN, Neil, President and Chief Executive Officer, Petaluma Valley Hospital, Petaluma, CA, p. A57

MARTIN, Norm, President and Chief Executive Officer, Parkview Community Hospital Medical Center, Riverside, CA, p. A59

MARTIN, Thomas J., Chief Executive Officer, Lincoln Hospital, Davenport, WA, p. A449

MARTIN, Kathleen L., Commanding Officer, Naval Hospital, Charleston, SC, p. A376

MARTINEZ, Charles, Ph.D., Chief Executive Officer, Community Hospital of Huntington Park, Huntington Park, CA, p. A46

MARTINEZ, Ramiro J., M.D., Director, East Mississippi State Hospital, Meridian, MS, p. A241

MARTINEZ, Tomas, Administrator, Hospital Hermanos Melendez, Bayamon, PR, p. A475

MARTINEZ Jr., Fred, Administrator, St. Charles Parish Hospital, Luling, LA, p. A187

MARTINEZ–LOPEZ, Lester, Director Health Services, Colonel Florence A. Blanchfield Army Community Hospital, Fort Campbell, KY, p. A174

MARWIN, Kristopher H., CHE, Chief Executive Officer, Tri–Valley Health System, Cambridge, NE, p. A263

MASCHING, Frances Marie, President, OSF Healthcare System, Peoria, IL, p. B120

MASON, Bill A., President, Springhill Memorial Hospital, Mobile, AL, p. A16

MASON, James K., Administrator, Jackson County Hospital, Scottsboro, AL, p. A17

MASON, Stephen D., Administrator, Northwest Florida Community Hospital, Chipley, FL, p. A84

MASON, William C., Chief Executive Officer, Baptist Medical Center, Jacksonville, FL, p. A89

MASON, William R., President and Chief Executive Officer, Muhlenberg Hospital Center, Bethlehem, PA, p. A354

MASSA, Lawrence J., Chief Executive Officer, Rice Memorial Hospital, Willmar, MN, p. A236

MASSEY, Charlie L., Administrator, Lane Memorial Hospital, Zachary, LA, p. A192

MASSEY, Michael W., Administrator, Allen Bennett Hospital, Greer, SC, p. A378

MASTEJ, J. Michael, Chief Executive Officer and Managing Director, Victoria Regional Medical Center, Victoria, TX, p. A430

MASTRANGELO, Anthony G., Executive Vice President and Chief Executive Officer, St. Joseph's Hospital, Highland, IL, p. A131

MATARELLI, Steven A., Administrator, Vencor Hospital–Chicago North, Chicago, IL, p. A128

MATEO, Carlos Rodriguez, M.D., Medical Director, Dr. Alejandro Buitrago–Guayama Area Hospital, Guayama, PR, p. A475

MATHER, Kelly, Executive Director, Columbia San Leandro Hospital, San Leandro, CA, p. A63

MATHEWS, George A., President and Chief Executive Officer, Methodist Medical Center of Oak Ridge, Oak Ridge, TN, p. A395

MATHEWS, LouAnn O., Administrator, American Transitional Hospital–Dallas/Fort Worth, Irving, TX, p. A416

MATHEWS, Mike, Administrator, Kwajalein Hospital, Kwajalein Island, MH, p. A474

MATHEWS, Thomas C., Administrator, Columbia Bartow Memorial Hospital, Bartow, FL, p. A83

MATHIS, Larry L., FACHE, President and Chief Executive Officer, Methodist Health Care System, Houston, TX, p. B115

MATNEY, Douglas A.
Senior Vice President Operations, Columbia Medical Center–East, El Paso, TX, p. A408
Senior Vice President Operations, Columbia Medical Center–West, El Paso, TX, p. A409

MATSUMURA, Kay, Chief Executive Officer, Salt Lake Regional Medical Center, Salt Lake City, UT, p. A435

MATT, Jeanine, President, Palmer Lutheran Health Center, West Union, IA, p. A160

MATTEI, Thomas, M.D., Chief Operating Officer, Mercy Providence Hospital, Pittsburgh, PA, p. A366

MATTEI DE COLLAZO, Georgina, Executive Director, Doctors Hospital, San Juan, PR, p. A476

MATTES, James A., President, Grande Ronde Hospital, La Grande, OR, p. A349

MATTHEWS, D. Clinton, Chief Executive Officer, South Park Hospital, Lubbock, TX, p. A419

MATTHEWS, L. Gene, Chief Executive Officer, Tahlequah City Hospital, Tahlequah, OK, p. A346

MATTINGLY, Chris, Administrator, Seiling Hospital, Seiling, OK, p. A345

MATTISON, Kenneth R., President and Chief Executive Officer, Jellico Community Hospital, Jellico, TN, p. A390

MATUSKA, John E., President and Chief Executive Officer, St. Peter's Medical Center, New Brunswick, NJ, p. A279

MAURER, Gregory L., Administrator, Elmore Medical Center, Mountain Home, ID, p. A121

MAXHIMER, Terry R., Administrator, Healthsouth Rehabilitation Hospital, Kingsport, TN, p. A391

MAY, Maurice I., President, Hebrew Rehabilitation Center for Aged, Boston, MA, p. A204

MAYA, Victor, Chief Executive Officer, Columbia Kendall Medical Center, Miami, FL, p. A93

MAYER, Donald A., Chief Executive Officer, Jupiter Medical Center, Jupiter, FL, p. A90

MAYER, Gloria, Executive Director, Friendly Hills Regional Medical Center, La Habra, CA, p. A47

MAYERS, Roger, Interim Administrator, Nye Regional Medical Center, Tonopah, NV, p. A271

MAYES, Mike, FACHE, Administrator and Chief Executive Officer, Cookeville General Hospital, Cookeville, TN, p. A388

MAYNARD, Robert F., Chief Executive Officer, Shawnee Regional Hospital, Shawnee, OK, p. A345

MAYO, Charles M., Administrator, Wheeler County Hospital, Glenwood, GA, p. A109

MAYO, Jim L., Administrator, Baptist Medical Center–Nassau, Fernandina Beach, FL, p. A86

MAYO, Robert, President and Chief Executive Officer, Cancer Treatment Centers of America, Arlington Heights, IL, p. B73

MAZON III, Andrew, Administrator and Chief Executive Officer, Roane General Hospital, Spencer, WV, p. A459

MAZUR–HART, Stanley F., Ph.D., Superintendent, Oregon State Hospital, Salem, OR, p. A352

MAZZARELLA, Michael C., Chief Executive Officer, Northern Dutchess Hospital, Rhinebeck, NY, p. A303

MAZZUCA, Philip J., Executive Director, Parkway Medical Center Hospital, Decatur, AL, p. A13

MCAFEE Jr., James T., Chairman, President and Chief Executive Officer, ValueMark Healthcare Systems, Inc., Atlanta, GA, p. B147

MCALEER, A. Gordon, President, Arden Hill Hospital, Goshen, NY, p. A292

MCALLISTER, C. C., President and Chief Executive Officer, Ouachita Medical Center, Camden, AR, p. A29

MCAVOY, Lawrence H., Administrator, Washington County Hospital, Plymouth, NC, p. A315

MCAVOY, Scott, Managing Director, Meridell Achievement Center, Austin, TX, p. A400

MCBRIDE, Don H., Chief Executive Officer, Columbia Woodland Heights Medical Center, Lufkin, TX, p. A419

MCBRIDE, Michael J., CHE, Executive Director, Presbyterian Hospital of Kaufman, Kaufman, TX, p. A417

MCBRIDE, Norman L., Chief Executive Officer, Valley View Hospital, Glenwood Springs, CO, p. A72

MCCABE, Eugene, President, North General Hospital, New York, NY, p. A299

MCCABE, Jack, Senior Vice President and Administrator, Harris Methodist–HEB, Bedford, TX, p. A401

MCCABE, Steve, Chief Executive Officer, Hill Crest Behavioral Health Services, Birmingham, AL, p. A12

MCCABE Jr., Patrick, Executive Director, Levi Hospital, Hot Springs National Park, AR, p. A31

MCCALL, Gerald A., Administrator, Kaiser Foundation Hospital, Anaheim, CA, p. A36

MCCARTHY, Bridget, President, Mercy American River/Mercy San Juan Hospital, Carmichael, CA, p. A39

MCCARTHY, Mary Fatima, Administrator, St. Elizabeth Hospital, Beaumont, TX, p. A401

MCCARY, Steve C., President and Chief Executive Officer, Stevens Healthcare, Edmonds, WA, p. A449

MCCASLIN, James B., Director, Chestnut Hill Rehabilitation Hospital, Wyndmoor, PA, p. A371

MCCAULEY, Edith, Administrator, Sabine County Hospital, Hemphill, TX, p. A412

MCCAULEY, Roberta D., Chief Executive Officer, Hampshire Memorial Hospital, Romney, WV, p. A458

MCCLELLAN, David A., Executive Director, Riverview Regional Medical Center, Gadsden, AL, p. A14

MCCLINTOCK, Thomas, Chief Executive Officer, Los Angeles Community Hospital, Los Angeles, CA, p. A50

MCCLINTOCK, William T., FACHE, Chief Executive Officer, Boundary Community Hospital, Bonners Ferry, ID, p. A119

MCCLURE, Jan, Chief Executive Officer, Hill Regional Hospital, Hillsboro, TX, p. A413

MCCLYMONDS, Bruce, President and Chief Executive Officer, West Virginia University Hospitals, Morgantown, WV, p. A457

MCCONAHY, Richard L., Chief Executive Officer, Jacksonville Hospital, Jacksonville, AL, p. A15

MCCONKEY, David M., Chief Executive, Good Samaritan Hospital, Downers Grove, IL, p. A129

MCCOOL, Paul J., Director, Veterans Affairs Medical Center, Manchester, NH, p. A273

MCCORD, Windell M., Administrator, Heart of Texas Memorial Hospital, Brady, TX, p. A402

MCCORKLE, Vincent J., President and Chief Executive Officer, Mercy Hospital, Springfield, MA, p. A210

MCCORKLE Jr., Philip H., Chief Executive Officer, Butterworth Hospital, Grand Rapids, MI, p. A216

MCCORMACK, J. David, Executive Director, Northwest Mississippi Regional Medical Center, Clarksdale, MS, p. A238

MCCORMICK, James, Superintendent, Richmond State Hospital, Richmond, IN, p. A148

MCCORMICK, John J., Chief Executive Officer, San Bernardino Mountains Community Hospital District, Lake Arrowhead, CA, p. A47

MCCORMICK, Lynn, Administrator, Sistersville General Hospital, Sistersville, WV, p. A458

MCCORMICK, Richard, Administrator, Methodist Hospital of Dyersburg, Dyersburg, TN, p. A389

MCCORMICK, Timothy R., President, Park Ridge Hospital, Rochester, NY, p. A303

MCCOY, George H., Chief Executive Officer, Governor Juan F. Louis Hospital, Christiansted, VI, p. A477

MCCOY, L. Kent, President, Huntington Memorial Hospital, Huntington, IN, p. A144

MCCOY, Mike, Chief Executive Officer, Saint Mary's Regional Medical Center, Russellville, AR, p. A34

MCCOY, Sherman P., Executive Director and Chief Executive Officer, Howard University Hospital, Washington, DC, p. A81

MCCRACKEN, Clyde T., Administrator, Ness County Hospital Number Two, Ness City, KS, p. A167

MCCRAY, Cindy M., Chief Executive Officer, Hospital District Number Six of Harper County, Anthony, KS, p. A161

MCCUE, Matthew, Administrator, Los Lunas Hospital and Training School, Los Lunas, NM, p. A286

MCCULLOCH, Andrew R., Administrator, Sacred Heart Medical Center, Eugene, OR, p. A349

MCCUNE, William, Vice President, Administration, Bryn Mawr Hospital, Bryn Mawr, PA, p. A354

MCCURRY, Bob, Interim Chief Executive Officer, Park Place Medical Center, Port Arthur, TX, p. A423

MCDANIEL, John P., Chief Executive Officer, Medlantic Healthcare Group, Washington, DC, p. B113

MCDERMOTT, Brian J., Administrator, Gettysburg Medical Center, Gettysburg, SD, p. A383

MCDONALD, William A., President and Chief Executive Officer, Miami Children's Hospital, Miami, FL, p. A93

MCDOUGAL Jr., Tommy R.
Administrator and Chief Executive Officer, Barnwell County Hospital, Barnwell, SC, p. A375
Administrator, Elmore Community Hospital, Wetumpka, AL, p. A18

MCDOWELL, Donald L., President and Chief Executive Officer, Maine Medical Center, Portland, ME, p. A195

MCDOWELL, James W., President and Chief Executive Officer, St. Mary's Hospital, Centralia, IL, p. A124

MCDOWELL, Jane, Chief Executive Officer, Harper County Community Hospital, Buffalo, OK, p. A340

MCELROY, Donald B., Executive Director, Charlotte Regional Medical Center, Punta Gorda, FL, p. A98

MCEWEN, David S., Chief Executive Officer, Marlette Community Hospital, Marlette, MI, p. A220

MCFADDEN, Pamela J., President and Chief Executive Officer, North Coast Health Care Centers–East Campus, Santa Rosa, CA, p. A64

MCGEACHEY, Edward J., President and Chief Executive Officer, Southern Maine Medical Center, Biddeford, ME, p. A193

MCGEE, John P.
President and Chief Executive Officer, JFK Health Systems, Inc., Edison, NJ, p. B107
President and Chief Executive Officer, JFK Medical Center, Edison, NJ, p. A276

MCGEE, Mark F., M.D., Chief Clinical Officer, Southeast Psychiatric Hospital, Athens, OH, p. A323

MCGILL, Richard M., Administrator, Hale County Hospital, Greensboro, AL, p. A15

MCGILL, Timothy W., Chief Executive Officer, Columbia Livingston Regional Hospital, Livingston, TN, p. A392

MCGINTY, Daniel B., President and Chief Executive Officer, Holy Family Memorial Medical Center, Manitowoc, WI, p. A464

MCGINTY Jr., John C., President and Chief Executive Officer, Columbus Regional Hospital, Columbus, IN, p. A141

MCGLASHAN, Thomas H., M.D., Director, Yale Psychiatric Institute, New Haven, CT, p. A77

MCGLEW, Timothy, Chief Executive Officer, Alhambra Hospital, Alhambra, CA, p. A36

MCGOLDRICK, Margaret M.
President and Chief Executive Officer, Allegheny University Hospital, Bucks County, Warminster, PA, p. A370
Chief Executive Officer, Allegheny University Hospital, East Falls, Philadelphia, PA, p. A363
Executive Director and Chief Executive Officer, Allegheny University Hospital, Elkins Park, Elkins Park, PA, p. A357

MCGOURTY, Mark E., Regional Chief Executive Officer, St. John Medical Center, Longview, WA, p. A450

MCGOWAN, Donna, R.N., Administrator, Lane County Hospital, Dighton, KS, p. A162

MCGOWAN, George
Chief Executive Officer, Blount Memorial Hospital, Oneonta, AL, p. A17
Chief Executive Officer, St. Clair Regional Hospital, Pell City, AL, p. A17

MCGRATH, Denise B., Chief Executive Officer, Healthsouth Treasure Coast Rehabilitation Hospital, Vero Beach, FL, p. A101

MCGRAW, Steven E., Administrator, Vencor Hospital–Chattanooga, Chattanooga, TN, p. A388

MCGRIFF III, W. A., President and Chief Executive Officer, University Medical Center, Jacksonville, FL, p. A90

MCGUIRE, William D., President and Chief Executive Officer, Catholic Medical Center of Brooklyn and Queens, New York, NY, p. A296

MCINTYRE, Nancy, Administrator, Ferry County Memorial Hospital, Republic, WA, p. A452

MCINTYRE, Kathleen, President, Little Company of Mary Hospital and Health Care Centers, Evergreen Park, IL, p. A130

MCIVOR, Dave, Administrator, Roundup Memorial Hospital, Roundup, MT, p. A260

MCKAY, Daniel E., Executive Director, Moberly Regional Medical Center, Moberly, MO, p. A251

MCKAY, Robert H., President, North Penn Hospital, Lansdale, PA, p. A360

MCKEE, D. Chet, President, Copley Memorial Hospital, Aurora, IL, p. A123

MCKEE, Vincent B., Chief Executive Officer, Wetzel County Hospital, New Martinsville, WV, p. A457

MCKERNAN, Stephen, Chief Executive Officer, University Hospital, Albuquerque, NM, p. A285

MCKIBBENS, Ben M., President, Valley Baptist Medical Center, Harlingen, TX, p. A412

MCKINNEY, Dan, Administrator, Hermann Area District Hospital, Hermann, MO, p. A248

MCKINNEY, Jim, President, Brim, Inc., Portland, OR, p. B72

MCKINNEY, Paul, Administrator, Cochran Memorial Hospital, Morton, TX, p. A421

MCKINNEY Jr., Buck, Chief Executive Officer, Kiowa District Hospital, Kiowa, KS, p. A165

MCKINNON, Ronald A., Administrator, Benson Hospital, Benson, AZ, p. A22

MCKINNON, William D., FACHE, Administrator, University Hospital of Durant, Durant, MS, p. A238

MCKLEM, Patricia A., Medical Center Director, Veterans Affairs Medical Center, Prescott, AZ, p. A26

MCKNEW, Linda A., R.N., Chief Operating Officer, Shands at Lake Shore, Lake City, FL, p. A90

MCKROW, Dee, Chief Executive Officer, Hills and Dales General Hospital, Cass City, MI, p. A213

MCLAUGHLIN, Evelyn, Acting Chief Executive Officer, Roy Lester Schneider Hospital, Saint Thomas, VI, p. A477

MCLAUGHLIN, Keith H., President and Chief Executive Officer, Raritan Bay Medical Center, Perth Amboy, NJ, p. A280

MCLAURIN, Monty E., President, St. Joseph's Hospital and Health Center, Paris, TX, p. A423

MCLEAN, Gordon C., Administrator, Whitman Hospital and Medical Center, Colfax, WA, p. A449

MCLEAN, Michael A., R.N., Administrator, Fayetteville City Hospital, Fayetteville, AR, p. A30

MCLEOD, Richard D., Administrator, Owen County Memorial Hospital, Owenton, KY, p. A179

MCLOUGHLIN, Thomas, President, Union City Memorial Hospital, Union City, PA, p. A370

MCMACKIN, James L., Chief Executive Officer, Unicoi County Memorial Hospital, Erwin, TN, p. A389

MCMACKIN, Kent W., Chief Executive Officer, Fannin Regional Hospital, Blue Ridge, GA, p. A105

MCMANUS, Joseph S., President and Chief Executive Officer, Lawrence General Hospital, Lawrence, MA, p. A207

MCMANUS, Michael Thomas, President, St. Clement Health Services, Red Bud, IL, p. A136

MCMEEKIN, John C., President and Chief Executive Officer, Crozer–Keystone Health System, Media, PA, p. B88

MCMILLAN, Douglas A., Chief Executive Officer, Frances Mahon Deaconess Hospital, Glasgow, MT, p. A258

MCMILLIN, Alan E., Chief Executive Officer, Columbia Women and Children's Hospital–Lake Charles, Lake Charles, LA, p. A186

MCMULLEN, Ronald B., President, Alton Memorial Hospital, Alton, IL, p. A123

MCMURDO, Timothy B., Chief Executive Officer, San Mateo County General Hospital, San Mateo, CA, p. A63

MCMURRAY, Sean S., Administrator, Columbia Athens Regional Medical Center, Athens, TN, p. A387

MCMURRY, Patricia, Executive Vice President and Chief Executive Officer, HealthSouth Rehabilitation Hospital, Portland, ME, p. A195

MCMURTRY, Roger, Chief Mental Health Bureau, Mississippi State Department of Mental Health, Jackson, MS, p. B117

MCNAIR, Mike H., Chief Executive Officer, Hartselle Medical Center, Hartselle, AL, p. A15

MCNAMARA, Paul E., President, Clinton Memorial Hospital, Saint Johns, MI, p. A222

MCNAUGHTON, Neil H., Executive Director and Administrator, Serenity Lane, Eugene, OR, p. A349

MCNEIL, Greg R., Administrator, Dallas County Hospital, Fordyce, AR, p. A30

MCNEILL, Douglas W., FACHE, President and Chief Executive Officer, Middletown Regional Hospital, Middletown, OH, p. A333

MCNELLY, Mark C., President and Chief Executive Officer, St. Francis Medical Center, Breckenridge, MN, p. A227

MCNEW, Robert L., Chief Executive Officer, Fort Worth Rehabilitation Hospital, Fort Worth, TX, p. A410

MCPHAIL, Mark D., Chief Executive Officer, Jeff Anderson Regional Medical Center, Meridian, MS, p. A241

MCPHEETERS III, James W., Administrator, McCune–Brooks Hospital, Carthage, MO, p. A246

MCPHERSON, Rodney, Administrator, Delta Memorial Hospital, Dumas, AR, p. A30

MCQUEEN, Elbert T., Chief Executive Officer, Healthsouth Central Georgia Rehabilitation Hospital, Macon, GA, p. A111

MCQUOID, Geraldine A., Director, Naukeag Hospital, Ashburnham, MA, p. A203

MCRAE, Arnold F., Administrator and Chief Executive Officer, Healthsouth Rehabilitation Hospital of Montgomery, Montgomery, AL, p. A16

MCRAE, Dave C., President and Chief Executive Officer, Pitt County Memorial Hospital–University Medical Center of Eastern Carolina–Pitt County, Greenville, NC, p. A312

MCRAE, Margaret S., Site Administrator, Cleveland Clinic Hospital, Fort Lauderdale, FL, p. A86

MCRAE, Rex C., President, Arlington Memorial Hospital, Arlington, TX, p. A399

MCREYNOLDS, David H., Chief Operating Officer and Administrator, Peninsula Hospital, Louisville, TN, p. A392

MCVEETY, John A., Chief Executive Officer, Alpena General Hospital, Alpena, MI, p. A212

MCWATTERS, David M., Administrator, Highland Hospital, Charleston, WV, p. A455

MCWHORTER III, John B., Executive Director, Baylor Medical Center at Garland, Garland, TX, p. A411

MEADE, Robert, Chief Executive Officer, Columbia Dade City Hospital, Dade City, FL, p. A85

MEADES, LeVern, Acting Administrator, Lallie Kemp Medical Center, Independence, LA, p. A185

MEADOWS, Bobby, President and Chief Executive Officer, Columbus Community Hospital, Columbus, OH, p. A328

MEADOWS, Deborah T., Administrator, Paul B. Hall Regional Medical Center, Paintsville, KY, p. A179

MEADOWS, Milton W., Administrator, Fairfield Memorial Hospital, Fairfield, TX, p. A409

MECHLER, Kathleen, Chief Executive Officer, Mountain Crest Hospital, Fort Collins, CO, p. A72

MECHTENBERG, David A., Chief Executive Officer, Ridgecrest Community Hospital, Ridgecrest, CA, p. A59

MECKLENBURG, Gary A., President and Chief Executive Officer, Northwestern Memorial Hospital, Chicago, IL, p. A126

MECKSTROTH, David J., President and Chief Executive Officer, Upper Valley Medical Centers, Troy, OH, p. B146

MEDILL, Delmar J., Interim Chief Executive Officer, Jackson Parish Hospital, Jonesboro, LA, p. A185

MEEHAN, John J., President and Chief Executive Officer, Hartford Hospital, Hartford, CT, p. A76

MEEKER, Timothy L., Executive Director, Sonoma Developmental Center, Eldridge, CA, p. A42

MEGARA, John J., Administrator, Anacapa Hospital, Port Hueneme, CA, p. A57

MEHL, Edward J., Chief Executive Officer, Lake Region Hospital Corporation, Fergus Falls, MN, p. A229

MEIBERT, Kenneth A., Chief Executive Officer, BHC Sierra Vista Hospital, Sacramento, CA, p. A59

MEIER, Ernie, President and Chief Executive Officer, Columbia Alaska Regional Hospital, Anchorage, AK, p. A20

MEINERT, Mark W., CHE, Chief Executive, Yamhill Service Area, Providence Newberg Hospital, Newberg, OR, p. A350

MEIS, Fred J., Administrator, Graham County Hospital, Hill City, KS, p. A164

MELBY, Bernette A., Executive Director, University Health Services, Amherst, MA, p. A203

MELCHIORRE Jr., Joseph E., CHE, Executive Administrator, Shriners Hospitals for Children, Tampa, FL, p. B132

MELIN, Craig N., President and Chief Executive Officer, Cooley Dickinson Hospital, Northampton, MA, p. A208

MELTON, Carter, President, Rockingham Memorial Hospital, Harrisonburg, VA, p. A441

MELTON, John W., Chief Executive Officer, Columbia East Montgomery Medical Center, Montgomery, AL, p. A16

MELTON, La Vern, Administrator, Beaver County Memorial Hospital, Beaver, OK, p. A339

MELTON, S. Dean, President and Chief Executive Officer, Morgan County Memorial Hospital, Martinsville, IN, p. A146

MENAUGH, John E., Chief Executive Officer, Sutter Coast Hospital, Crescent City, CA, p. A41

MENDEZ, Lincoln S., Chief Executive Officer, Healthsouth Doctors' Hospital, Coral Gables, FL, p. A85

MENDEZ, Manuel G., Operating Trustee, Mepsi Center, Bayamon, PR, p. A475

MERCADO, Sylvia, Chief Executive Officer, University Pediatric Hospital, San Juan, PR, p. A477

MEREDITH, Stephen L., Chief Executive Officer, Twin Lakes Regional Medical Center, Leitchfield, KY, p. A176

MERRILL, Mark H., Executive Director, Presbyterian Hospital of Dallas, Dallas, TX, p. A407

MERRITT, Tim, Administrator, Elbert Memorial Hospital, Elberton, GA, p. A109

MERTZ, Paul A., President and Chief Executive Officer, Hospital Center at Orange, Orange, NJ, p. A280

MERWIN, Robert W., Chief Executive Officer, Mills–Peninsula Health Services, Burlingame, CA, p. A38

MESMER, Keith, Administrator and Chief Executive Officer, Colorado Plains Medical Center, Fort Morgan, CO, p. A72

MESROPIAN, Robert A., President, Alice Peck Day Memorial Hospital, Lebanon, NH, p. A273

MESSER, Barbara, R.N., Administrator, Capistrano by the Sea Hospital, Dana Point, CA, p. A41

MESSER, Bristol, Chief Executive Officer, Trace Regional Hospital, Houston, MS, p. A239

MESSING, Fred M., Chief Executive Officer, Baptist Hospital of Miami, Miami, FL, p. A92

MESSMER, Joseph, President and Chief Executive Officer, Mercy Medical Center, Nampa, ID, p. A121

METIVIER, Roland, Chief Executive Officer, Columbia Las Encinas Hospital, Pasadena, CA, p. A57

METSCH, Jonathan M., Dr.PH
President and Chief Executive Officer, Greenville Hospital, Jersey City, NJ, p. A278
President and Chief Executive Officer, Jersey City Medical Center, Jersey City, NJ, p. A278

METZ, Roger L., President, Community Memorial Hospital and Convalescent and Rehabilitation Unit, Winona, MN, p. A236

METZNER, Kurt W., President and Chief Executive Officer, Mississippi Baptist Medical Center, Jackson, MS, p. A240

MEYER, Frederick C., President and Chief Executive Officer, Southern California Healthcare System, Pasadena, CA, p. B137

MEYER, James E., President, MedCentral Health System, Mansfield, OH, p. A332

MEYER, Jeffrey K., Administrator and Chief Executive Officer, Osceola Medical Center, Osceola, WI, p. A467

MEYER, Larry L., Vice President and Administrator, Tracy Community Memorial Hospital, Tracy, CA, p. A66

MEYER, Miles, Administrator, Columbus Community Hospital, Columbus, WI, p. A461

MEYER, Patricia, Assistant Administrator, Stouder Memorial Hospital, Troy, OH, p. A336

MEYER, Ralph H., President and Chief Executive Officer, Guthrie Healthcare System, Sayre, PA, p. B100

MEYER, Robert F., M.D., Chief Executive Officer, Samaritan Behavioral Health Center–Scottsdale, Scottsdale, AZ, p. A26

MEYER, Wilbert E., Administrator, Cooper County Memorial Hospital, Boonville, MO, p. A245

MEYERS, Joan T., R.N., Executive Director, West Jersey Hospital–Voorhees, Voorhees, NJ, p. A282

MEYERS, Mark, Chief Executive Officer, Coastal Communities Hospital, Santa Ana, CA, p. A63

MEYERS, Russell, Chief Executive Officer, Columbia Bayshore Medical Center, Pasadena, TX, p. A423

MICHAEL, Barry, Chief Executive Officer, Meadows Regional Medical Center, Vidalia, GA, p. A115

MICHAEL, Max, M.D., Chief Executive Officer and Medical Director, Cooper Green Hospital, Birmingham, AL, p. A12

MICHALSKI, Eugene F., Vice President and Hospital Director, William Beaumont Hospital–Troy, Troy, MI, p. A224

MICHELETTI, Mark, Chief Executive Officer, Charter Behavioral Health System, Kingwood, TX, p. A418

MICHELL, Dyer T., President, Munroe Regional Medical Center, Ocala, FL, p. A95

MICKOSEFF, Tecla A., Administrator, LAC–Harbor–University of California at Los Angeles Medical Center, Torrance, CA, p. A66

MICKUS, Steven L., President and Chief Executive Officer, St. Vincent Mercy Medical Center, Toledo, OH, p. A336

MIDDLEBROOK, Randy, Chief Executive Officer, Aspen Valley Hospital District, Aspen, CO, p. A70

MIDKIFF, Stephen L., Executive Director, Sebastian River Medical Center, Sebastian, FL, p. A99

MIDKIFF, Steve, Executive Director, Upstate Carolina Medical Center, Gaffney, SC, p. A378

MIESLE, Michael A., Administrator, Wood County Hospital, Bowling Green, OH, p. A324

MIGLIARO, John R., Ph.D., Chief Executive Officer, Arizona State Hospital, Phoenix, AZ, p. A24

MIGUEL, Hortense, R.N., Acting Service Unit Director, U. S. Public Health Service Indian Hospital, Winterhaven, CA, p. A69

MIHORA, Michael J., Chief Operating Officer, Herrick Memorial Hospital, Tecumseh, MI, p. A224

MIKLAS, Joanne P., Ph.D., Superintendent, Gracewood State School and Hospital, Gracewood, GA, p. A110

MILANES, Carlos, Executive Vice President and Administrator, Palm Springs General Hospital, Hialeah, FL, p. A88

MILBRANDT, Charles A., Director, Veterans Affairs Medical Center, Minneapolis, MN, p. A232

MILBRATH, Michael, Administrator, Waseca Area Medical Center, Waseca, MN, p. A236

MILES, Paul V., Administrator, Middlesboro Appalachian Regional Hospital, Middlesboro, KY, p. A178

MILEY, Dennis C., Administrator, Tri–County Hospital, Wadena, MN, p. A236

MILLARD, John L., President and Chief Executive Officer, Bethany Medical Center, Kansas City, KS, p. A165

MILLBURG, Charles L., CHE, Chief Executive Officer, Shenandoah Memorial Hospital, Shenandoah, IA, p. A158

MILLER, Alan B., President and Chief Executive Officer, Universal Health Services, Inc., King of Prussia, PA, p. B145

MILLER, Blaine K., Administrator, Minneola District Hospital, Minneola, KS, p. A167

MILLER, Charles F., Chief Executive Officer, Northshore Regional Medical Center, Slidell, LA, p. A191

MILLER, Charles R.
Chief Executive Officer, Northwest Iowa Health Center, Sheldon, IA, p. A158
President and Chief Operating Officer, Paracelsus Healthcare Corporation, Houston, TX, p. B120

MILLER, Diane C., President and Chief Operating Officer, Taylor Hospital, Ridley Park, PA, p. A368

MILLER, Emil P., Chief Executive Officer, North Ridge Medical Center, Fort Lauderdale, FL, p. A87

MILLER, George E., Chief Executive Officer, Columbia North Monroe Hospital, Monroe, LA, p. A187

MILLER, J. Daniel, President and Chief Executive Officer, Columbia Regional Medical Center at Bayonet Point, Hudson, FL, p. A89

MILLER, Jeffrey S., President, High Point Regional Health System, High Point, NC, p. A313

MILLER, Jerry L., Administrator, Baptist Medical Center–Beaches, Jacksonville Beach, FL, p. A90

MILLER, Kevin J., Chief Executive Officer, Medical Center of Southern Indiana, Charlestown, IN, p. A141

MILLER, L. Ned, CHE, Administrator and Chief Executive Officer, Bloss Memorial Hospital District, Atwater, CA, p. A37

MILLER, Michael R., President and Chief Executive Officer, Miner's Memorial Medical Center, Coaldale, PA, p. A355

MILLER, Paul A., President and Chief Executive Officer, Memorial Hospital Corporation of Burlington, Burlington, WI, p. A461

MILLER, Peggy, R.N., Director Nursing and Chief Operating Officer, Columbia Cheatham Medical Center, Ashland City, TN, p. A387

MILLER, Richard, Administrator, Norton County Hospital, Norton, KS, p. A167

MILLER, Richard P.
Director, G.V. Montgomery Veterans Affairs Medical Center, Jackson, MS, p. A240
President and Chief Executive Officer, West Jersey Health System, Camden, NJ, p. B148

MILLER, Robert, Chief Executive Officer, Henry County Health Center, Mount Pleasant, IA, p. A157

MILLER, Rosa L., R.N., Administrator, Truman Medical Center–West, Kansas City, MO, p. A249

MILLER, Tamara, Administrator, Madison Community Hospital, Madison, SD, p. A383

MILLER, Thomas D., President and Chief Executive Officer, Columbia Reston Hospital Center, Reston, VA, p. A444

MILLER, Thomas O., Administrator, Pungo District Hospital, Belhaven, NC, p. A308

MILLER, Valerie, Administrator, Lincoln County Medical Center, Ruidoso, NM, p. A287

MILLER, Wayne T., Administrator, Koala Hospital and Counseling Center, Plymouth, IN, p. A147

MILLER, William P., President and Chief Executive Officer, Caro Community Hospital, Caro, MI, p. A213

MILLER, Mark A., Deputy Commander, Fox Army Community Hospital, Redstone Arsenal, AL, p. A17

MILLER III, Thomas, Chief Executive Officer, Myrtle Werth Hospital–Mayo Health System, Menomonie, WI, p. A465

MILLER Jr., George N., Administrator, Jasper Memorial Hospital, Jasper, TX, p. A417

MILLIGAN Jr., William M., President and Chief Executive Officer, Tyler Memorial Hospital, Tunkhannock, PA, p. A369

MILLIRONS, Dennis C., President and Chief Executive Officer, Riverside Healthcare, Kankakee, IL, p. A132

MILLON, Ivan, Administrator, Fundacion Hospital Metropolitan, Caparra, PR, p. A476

MILLS, Fred R., President and Chief Executive Officer, Baptist Health System, San Antonio, TX, p. B67

MILLS, Stephen S., President and Chief Executive Officer, New York Hospital Medical Center of Queens, New York, NY, p. A298

MILLSTEAD, John B., Chief Executive Officer, Campbell Health System, Weatherford, TX, p. A430

MILNES, Lynn, Administrator and Chief Executive Officer, Skyline Hospital, White Salmon, WA, p. A454

MILTON, Gene C., President and Chief Executive Officer, Hackettstown Community Hospital, Hackettstown, NJ, p. A277

MIMS, John L., Executive Director, McAllen Medical Center, McAllen, TX, p. A420

MINDEN, Larry, Chief Executive Officer, Jane Phillips Medical Center, Bartlesville, OK, p. A339

MINER, Charles B., President and Chief Executive Officer, Meridia Health System, Mayfield Village, OH, p. B115

MINER, Greg, Administrator, Loring Hospital, Sac City, IA, p. A158

MINICK, Mark J., President and Chief Executive Officer, Van Wert County Hospital, Van Wert, OH, p. A336

MINKIN, Robert A., CHE, President and Chief Executive Officer, Desert Hospital, Palm Springs, CA, p. A56

MINNICK, Peggy, Administrator, BHC Alhambra Hospital, Rosemead, CA, p. A59

MINNIS, Vernon, Chief Executive Officer, Hospital District Number Five of Harper County, Harper, KS, p. A164

MINNIX, William L., Chief Executive Officer, Wesley Woods Geriatric Hospital, Atlanta, GA, p. A104

MINOR, Richard J., President, Grandview Hospital and Medical Center, Dayton, OH, p. A329

MIRABITO, Frank W., President, Chenango Memorial Hospital, Norwich, NY, p. A301

MIRAUDA, Jose L., M.D., Executive Director, Arecibo Regional Hospital, Arecibo, PR, p. A474

MIRIN, Steven M., M.D., President and Psychiatrist in Chief, McLean Hospital, Belmont, MA, p. A203

MISENER, Kenneth T.
Vice President and Chief Operating Officer, Fairview Hospital System, Cleveland, OH, p. B97
Chief Operating Officer, Lutheran Hospital, Cleveland, OH, p. A326

MISHLER, Sheila, Chief Executive Officer, BHC Valle Vista Hospital, Greenwood, IN, p. A143

MISSILDINE, Syble F., Administrator, Northeast Medical Center Hospital, Humble, TX, p. A416

MITCHEL, David M., Chief Executive Officer, Avoyelles Hospital, Marksville, LA, p. A187

MITCHELL, Andrew J., Vice President, Administration, North Shore University Hospital–Forest Hills, New York, NY, p. A299

MITCHELL, Gary W., Chief Executive Officer, Newman Memorial Hospital, Shattuck, OK, p. A345

MITCHELL, Jerald F., President and Chief Executive Officer, Columbia Sunrise Hospital and Medical Center, Las Vegas, NV, p. A270

MITCHELL, Jon K., FACHE, President and Chief Executive Officer, Asante Health System, Medford, OR, p. B67

MITCHELL, Joseph J., Chief Executive Officer and Administrator, Holdenville General Hospital, Holdenville, OK, p. A342

MITCHELL, Joseph K., Administrator, Tuolumne General Hospital, Sonora, CA, p. A65

MITCHELL, Kerlene, Administrator, Wedowee Hospital, Wedowee, AL, p. A18

MITCHELL, Sidney E., Executive Director, University of Illinois at Chicago Medical Center, Chicago, IL, p. A128

MITCHELL, Thedis V., Director, U. S. Public Health Service Indian Hospital, Clinton, OK, p. A340

MITCHELL, Timothy, Administrator, Healthsouth Southern Hills Rehabilitation Hospital, Princeton, WV, p. A458

MITCHELL, Tom, Chief Executive Officer, Clark Fork Valley Hospital, Plains, MT, p. A259

MITCHELL, Trish, Chief Executive Officer, Northpointe Behavioral Health System, Tarpon Springs, FL, p. A101

MITCHELL III, J. Stuart, Administrator, Baptist Memorial Hospital–Golden Triangle, Columbus, MS, p. A238

MITCHELL Jr., William O., Chief Executive Officer, Healthsouth Rehabilitation Hospital of Austin, Austin, TX, p. A400

MITCHENER Jr., Charles, Chief Operating Officer and Administrator, Parkview Regional Medical Center, Vicksburg, MS, p. A244

MITTEER, Brian R., President, Brattleboro Memorial Hospital, Brattleboro, VT, p. A437

MIZRACH, Kenneth H., Director, Department of Veterans Affairs Health Care System, East Orange, NJ, p. A276

MLADY, Celine, Chief Executive Officer, Osmond General Hospital, Osmond, NE, p. A267

MO, Lin H., President and Chief Executive Officer, The New York Community Hospital of Brooklyn, New York, NY, p. A300

MOAKLER, Thomas J., Administrator and Chief Executive Officer, Houlton Regional Hospital, Houlton, ME, p. A194

MOBURG, Steven T., Administrator, Boscobel Area Health Care, Boscobel, WI, p. A461

MODDERMAN, Melvin E., Administrator, Lincoln Trail Behavioral Health System, Radcliff, KY, p. A180

MOEBIUS, Geoffrey D., President and Chief Executive Officer, Saint Michael Hospital, Cleveland, OH, p. A327

MOELLER, Jerry G., President and Chief Executive Officer, Stillwater Medical Center, Stillwater, OK, p. A345

MOEN, Daniel P., President and Chief Executive Officer, Heywood Hospital, Gardner, MA, p. A206

MOEN, Robert A., President and Chief Executive Officer, Emanuel Medical Center, Turlock, CA, p. A67

MOHR, Robin Z., Chief Executive Officer, St. Francis Central Hospital, Pittsburgh, PA, p. A366

MOLANO, Celia, Executive Director, I. Gonzalez Martinez Oncologic Hospital, Hato Rey, PR, p. A476

MOLL, Jeffrey S., President and Chief Executive Officer, Beth Israel Hospital, Passaic, NJ, p. A280

MOLNAR, George, M.D., Executive Director, Buffalo Psychiatric Center, Buffalo, NY, p. A290

MONARDO, Greg, President, Davies Medical Center, San Francisco, CA, p. A61

MONFORE Jr., Kenneth E., Administrator, Siskiyou General Hospital, Yreka, CA, p. A69

MONGAN, James J., M.D., President and Chief Operating Officer, Massachusetts General Hospital, Boston, MA, p. A204

MONGE, Peter W., President and Chief Executive Officer, Montgomery General Hospital, Olney, MD, p. A201

MONNAHAN, John E., President and Senior Executive Officer, Clay County Hospital, Flora, IL, p. A130

MONROIG, Domingo, Administrator, Castaner General Hospital, Castaner, PR, p. A475

MONSERRATE, Humberto M., Administrator, Hospital Santa Rosa, Guayama, PR, p. A475

MONSMA, Brian, Administrator, Mountainview Medical Center, White Sulphur Springs, MT, p. A260

MONTAG, Kathy, Administrator Health Care, State Correctional Institution at Camp Hill, Camp Hill, PA, p. A355

MONTAGUE, William D.
Director, Franklin Delano Roosevelt Veterans Affairs Hospital, Montrose, NY, p. A295
Acting Medical Center Director, Veterans Affairs Medical Center, Castle Point, NY, p. A290

MONTGOMERY II, Raymond W., President and Chief Executive Officer, White County Medical Center, Searcy, AR, p. A34

MONTGOMERY Jr., J. C., President, Texas Scottish Rite Hospital for Children, Dallas, TX, p. A407

MONTGOMERY Jr., J. Field, Director, Cherry Hospital, Goldsboro, NC, p. A312

MONTION, Robert M., Administrator, Alta District Hospital, Dinuba, CA, p. A41

MOONEY, Jimmy, Chief Executive Officer, Willingway Hospital, Statesboro, GA, p. A114

MOORE, Alfred, Chief Executive Officer, New Center Hospital, Detroit, MI, p. A215

MOORE, C. Thomas, Chief Executive Officer, Brown Memorial Hospital, Conneaut, OH, p. A328

MOORE, Donald F., Acting Medical Center Director, Veterans Affairs Medical Center, Salt Lake City, UT, p. A435

MOORE, Duncan, President and Chief Executive Officer, Tallahassee Memorial Regional Medical Center, Tallahassee, FL, p. A100

MOORE, E. Richard, President, Hazleton General Hospital, Hazleton, PA, p. A359

MOORE, Gary M., President and Chief Executive Officer, DeSoto Memorial Hospital, Arcadia, FL, p. A83

MOORE, Jason H., President and Chief Executive Officer, John D. Archbold Memorial Hospital, Thomasville, GA, p. A115

MOORE, John, Administrator, Hiawatha Community Hospital, Hiawatha, KS, p. A164

MOORE, Joseph L.
Director, VA Chicago Health Care System–Lakeside Division, Chicago, IL, p. A128
Director, VA Chicago Health Care System–West Side Division, Chicago, IL, p. A128

MOORE, Lois Jean, President and Chief Executive Officer, Harris County Hospital District, Houston, TX, p. A414

MOORE, Michael T., President and Chief Executive Officer, Wilson Memorial Hospital, Sidney, OH, p. A335

MOORE, Richard T., Administrator, Lake District Hospital, Lakeview, OR, p. A350

MOORE, Robert J., CHE, Chief Executive Officer, Pekin Hospital, Pekin, IL, p. A136

MOORE, T. Jerald, President and Chief Executive Officer, American Transitional Hospitals, Inc., Franklin, TN, p. B66

MOORE, Terence F., President, MidMichigan Regional Health System, Midland, MI, p. B116

MOORE, Terry L., Chief Executive Officer, Columbia Englewood Community Hospital, Englewood, FL, p. A86

MOORE, W. Evan, Administrator, Comanche Community Hospital, Comanche, TX, p. A404

MOORE, William M., Administrator, Coffee Medical Center, Manchester, TN, p. A392

MOORE III, Ben, Executive Director, University Hospital–SUNY Health Science Center at Syracuse, Syracuse, NY, p. A305

MOORE–HARDY, Cynthia Ann, Interim Chief Executive Officer, Lake Hospital System, Painesville, OH, p. A334

MOORER, W. Tate, Administrator, Baptist Memorial Hospital–Lauderdale, Ripley, TN, p. A395

MOORER, William T., Administrator, Baptist Memorial Hospital–Tipton, Covington, TN, p. A388

MOORHEAD, J. David, M.D., President, Loma Linda University Medical Center, Loma Linda, CA, p. A48

MOORING, Phillip A., Director, Walter B. Jones Alcohol and Drug Abuse Treatment Center, Greenville, NC, p. A312

MORALES, Herson E., Administrator, Hospital De La Concepcion, San German, PR, p. A476

MORAN, Eloise, Chief Executive Officer, Highland District Hospital, Hillsboro, OH, p. A330

MORASKO, Jerry, Administrator, Toole County Hospital and Nursing Home, Shelby, MT, p. A260

MORASKO, Robert A., Chief Executive Officer, Shoshone Medical Center, Kellogg, ID, p. A120

MORDOH, Henry A., President, Shadyside Hospital, Pittsburgh, PA, p. A366

MOREL, Michael R., Administrator, Choctaw Memorial Hospital, Hugo, OK, p. A342

MORELAND, L. Pat, Administrator, Hardy Wilson Memorial Hospital, Hazlehurst, MS, p. A239

MORESI, Randy, Chief Executive Officer, Columbia North Hills Hospital, North Richland Hills, TX, p. A422

MORGAN, A. Dale, Administrator, Franklin Foundation Hospital, Franklin, LA, p. A184

MORGAN, Charles R., Administrator, Wayne Memorial Hospital, Jesup, GA, p. A110

MORGAN, Craig, Administrator, Knox County General Hospital, Barbourville, KY, p. A172

MORGAN, Donald J., Administrator, Page Memorial Hospital, Luray, VA, p. A442

MORGAN, James E., Director, Huey P. Long Medical Center, Pineville, LA, p. A190

MORGAN, Jean W., Superintendent, Northwest Georgia Regional Hospital, Rome, GA, p. A113

MORGAN, John, President, Gottlieb Memorial Hospital, Melrose Park, IL, p. A134

MORGAN, Kelly C., President and Chief Executive Officer, Mercy Hospital and Health Services, Merced, CA, p. A53

MORGAN, Michael L., President and Chief Executive Officer, Mercy Regional Medical Center, Laredo, TX, p. A418

MORLAN, Sandy, Administrator, Ellett Memorial Hospital, Appleton City, MO, p. A245

MORLEY, Tad A., Chief Executive Officer, Columbia Brigham City Community Hospital, Brigham City, UT, p. A433

MORRASH, Joseph, Administrator, State Correctional Institution Hospital, Pittsburgh, PA, p. A367

MORREL, Robert D., Associate Director, Veterans Affairs Medical and Regional Office Center, Wichita, KS, p. A171

MORRIS, Elaine F., Administrator, Methodist Ambulatory Surgery Hospital, San Antonio, TX, p. A425

MORRIS, Joe, Chief Executive Officer, Kootenai Medical Center, Coeur D'Alene, ID, p. A120

MORRIS, Leigh E., President, La Porte Hospital, La Porte, IN, p. A145

MORRIS, Linda, Administrator, Ogallala Community Hospital, Ogallala, NE, p. A266

MORRIS, Michael, Administrator, Coleman County Medical Center, Coleman, TX, p. A404

MORRIS, Monica, Administrator, Conejos County Hospital, La Jara, CO, p. A73

MORRIS, Randall R., Administrator, West Carroll Memorial Hospital, Oak Grove, LA, p. A189

MORRISON, Ann, R.N., Chief Executive Officer, Sebasticook Valley Hospital, Pittsfield, ME, p. A195

MORRISON, C. David, President, Logan General Hospital, Logan, WV, p. A457

MORRISON, Robert E., President, Randolph Hospital, Asheboro, NC, p. A308

MORRISSEY Jr., James J., Administrator, Bassett Hospital of Schoharie County, Cobleskill, NY, p. A291

MORROW, John, Administrator, Samuel Simmonds Memorial Hospital, Barrow, AK, p. A20

MORROW, Julia, Administrator, Morrill County Community Hospital, Bridgeport, NE, p. A262

MORSE, Brad S., Executive Director, Randolph County Medical Center, Pocahontas, AR, p. A34

MORSE, Gary C., Administrator, Tyler Holmes Memorial Hospital, Winona, MS, p. A244

MORSE, Larry, Administrator, Lawrence Memorial Hospital, Walnut Ridge, AR, p. A35

MORTON, James I., FACHE, Administrator and Chief Executive Officer, Whitfield Medical Surgical Hospital, Whitfield, MS, p. A244

MORTON, Ronald, Chief Executive Officer, Barton County Memorial Hospital, Lamar, MO, p. A250

MORTON Jr., Edward C., FACHE, Chief Executive Officer, BHC Mesilla Valley Hospital, Las Cruces, NM, p. A286

MOSELEY, B. Richard, Chief Executive Officer, Baptist Rehabilitation–Germantown, Germantown, TN, p. A389

MOSS, Dwayne, Administrator, L. V. Stabler Memorial Hospital, Greenville, AL, p. A15

MOSS, James T.
President, Jackson–Madison County General Hospital, Jackson, TN, p. A390
President and Chief Executive Officer, Pathways of Tennessee, Jackson, TN, p. A390
President, West Tennessee Healthcare, Inc., Jackson, TN, p. B148

MOSS, Joseph, Administrator, Ste. Genevieve County Memorial Hospital, Ste. Genevieve, MO, p. A255

MOSS, Paul E., President, Milford Hospital, Milford, CT, p. A77

MOSS, Rod, Chief Executive Officer, Healthsouth Rehabilitation Hospital of North Alabama, Huntsville, AL, p. A15

MOSS, William Mason, President, Potomac Hospital, Woodbridge, VA, p. A447

MOTTISHAW, Brian, Chief Executive Officer, Pioneer Valley Hospital, West Valley City, UT, p. A436

MOTZER, Earl James, FACHE, Chief Executive Officer, The James B. Haggin Memorial Hospital, Harrodsburg, KY, p. A175

MOUGHON, Edward, Superintendent, Big Spring State Hospital, Big Spring, TX, p. A402

MOULTHROP, David L., Ph.D., President and Chief Executive Officer, Rogers Memorial Hospital, Oconomowoc, WI, p. A466

MOUNTCASTLE, William A., Director, Veterans Affairs Medical Center, Nashville, TN, p. A395

MOYLAN, Robert J., CHE, Chief Executive Officer, Hospital for Sick Children, Washington, DC, p. A81

MROSS, Charles D., President and Chief Executive Officer, Franklin Square Hospital Center, Baltimore, MD, p. A197

MUDLER, Gordon A., President and Chief Executive Officer, Hackley Health, Muskegon, MI, p. A220

MUECK, G. Jerry, Vice President, Chief Executive Officer and Administrator, Memorial Spring Shadows Glen, Houston, TX, p. A415

MUELLER, Jens, Chairman, Pacific Health Corporation, Long Beach, CA, p. B120

MUENNINK, Phylis, Administrator, Horizon Specialty Hospital, San Antonio, TX, p. A425

MUHLENTHALER, Donald, FACHE, President and Chief Executive Officer, Weirton Medical Center, Weirton, WV, p. A459

MUILENBURG, Robert H., Executive Director, University of Washington Medical Center, Seattle, WA, p. A452

MULDER, Dale R., President and Chief Executive Officer, St. Joseph's Hospital, Huntingburg, IN, p. A144

MULDOON, Patrick L., President and Chief Executive Officer, South County Hospital, Wakefield, RI, p. A374

MULFORD, Peter L., Administrator, City Hospital, Martinsburg, WV, p. A457

MULHOLLAND, Donna, President and Chief Executive Officer, Easton Hospital, Easton, PA, p. A357

MULHOLLAND Jr., K. L., Director, Veterans Affairs Medical Center, Memphis, TN, p. A394

MULL, Connie, Chief Executive Officer, Cedar Springs Psychiatric Hospital, Colorado Springs, CO, p. A70

MULLAHEY, Ronald T., President, Vassar Brothers Hospital, Poughkeepsie, NY, p. A303

MULLANEY, Garrell S., Superintendent, Connecticut Valley Hospital, Middletown, CT, p. A77

MULLANEY, Janet, Chief Executive Officer, Columbia Heritage Hospital, Tarboro, NC, p. A317

MULLANY, Joseph J., Executive Director, Biloxi Regional Medical Center, Biloxi, MS, p. A237

MULLEN, Anthony F., Administrator, Bertie County Memorial Hospital, Windsor, NC, p. A318

MULLEN, Robert L., Administrator, Rice County Hospital District Number One, Lyons, KS, p. A166

MULLER, A. Gary, FACHE, Regional Vice President Administration, Coral Springs Medical Center, Coral Springs, FL, p. A85

MULLER, Leonard J., President, Oak Park Hospital, Oak Park, IL, p. A135

MULLER, Ralph W., President, University of Chicago Hospitals, Chicago, IL, p. A128

MULLINS, Charles B., Executive Vice Chancellor, University of Texas System, Austin, TX, p. B146

MULLINS, Larry A., President and Chief Executive Officer, Good Samaritan Hospital Corvallis, Corvallis, OR, p. A348

MULLINS, Michael L., President, Nevada Regional Medical Center, Nevada, MO, p. A251

MULLINS, Tommy H., Administrator, Boone Memorial Hospital, Madison, WV, p. A457

MUNDY, Mark J., President and Chief Executive Officer, New York Methodist Hospital, New York, NY, p. A298

MUNDY, Stephens M., Chief Executive Officer, St. Joseph's Hospital, Parkersburg, WV, p. A458

MUNETA, Anita, Chief Executive Officer, U. S. Public Health Service Indian Hospital, Crownpoint, NM, p. A285

MUNGENAST, David, President, Southwestern Michigan Rehabilitation Hospital, Battle Creek, MI, p. A212

MUNGER, Richard, Administrator, Mount Grant General Hospital, Hawthorne, NV, p. A270

MUNIZ, Teodoro, Executive Director, Hato Rey Community Hospital, San Juan, PR, p. A476

MUNOZ, Thalia H., Administrator, Starr County Memorial Hospital, Rio Grande City, TX, p. A424

MUNSON, Eric B., Executive Director, University of North Carolina Hospitals, Chapel Hill, NC, p. A309

MUNTZ, Timothy, President, St. Margaret's Hospital, Spring Valley, IL, p. A138

MURPHY, C. Richard, Administrator, El Campo Memorial Hospital, El Campo, TX, p. A408

MURPHY, Edward G., M.D., President and Chief Executive Officer, Seton Health System, Troy, NY, p. A305

MURPHY, Emilie M., R.N., Director, Montclair Community Hospital, Montclair, NJ, p. A279

MURPHY, Horace W., President, Washington County Hospital Association, Hagerstown, MD, p. A200

MURPHY, Jim, Administrator, Pioneers Hospital of Rio Blanco County, Meeker, CO, p. A74

MURPHY, Joyce A., President and Chief Executive Officer, Carney Hospital, Boston, MA, p. A204

MURPHY, Michael D., Chief Executive Officer, Columbia Gulf Coast Medical Center, Wharton, TX, p. A431

MURPHY, Michael W., Ph.D.
Director, Veterans Affairs Northern Indiana Health Care System–Fort Wayne Division, Fort Wayne, IN, p. A142
Director, Veterans Affairs Northern Indiana Health Care System–Marion Campus, Marion, IN, p. A146

MURPHY, Peter J., President and Chief Executive Officer, St. James Hospital and Health Centers, Chicago Heights, IL, p. A128

MURPHY, Christina, President and Chief Executive Officer, Sisters of Charity of the Incarnate Word Healthcare System, Houston, TX, p. B134

MURPHY III, Frank V., President and Chief Executive Officer, Morton Plant Hospital, Clearwater, FL, p. A84

MURRAY, Annabeth, Administrator, Fairfax Memorial Hospital, Fairfax, OK, p. A341

MURRAY, Joan, R.N., Administrator, St. James Parish Hospital, Lutcher, LA, p. A187

MURRAY, T. Michael, President, South Coast Medical Center, South Laguna, CA, p. A65

MURRAY, Thomas J., President, St. Joseph Hospital, Lexington, KY, p. A176

MURRELL, Joe, Administrator, Vencor Hospital–LaGrange, LaGrange, IN, p. A146

MUSUMECI, Maryann, Director, Veterans Affairs Medical Center, New York, NY, p. A300

MUTCH, Patrick F., President, Laurel Regional Hospital, Laurel, MD, p. A201

MYERS, Charles, Administrator, Community Hospital, Torrington, WY, p. A472

MYERS, Donna L., Administrator and Chief Executive Officer, Rush County Memorial Hospital, La Crosse, KS, p. A165

MYERS, Gary, Administrator, Mammoth Hospital, Mammoth Lakes, CA, p. A53

MYERS, Richard L., President and Chief Executive Officer, Durham Regional Hospital, Durham, NC, p. A310

MYERS, Theodore, M.D., Chief Executive Officer, Naeve Hospital, Albert Lea, MN, p. A226

MYNARK, Richard H., Administrator, Pulaski Memorial Hospital, Winamac, IN, p. A149

N

NABORS, Charles E., Chief Executive Officer and Administrator, Bryan W. Whitfield Memorial Hospital, Demopolis, AL, p. A13

NACHTMAN, Frank, Administrator, Marshall Hospital, Placerville, CA, p. A57

NAGELVOORT, Clarence A., President and Chief Executive Officer, Norwegian–American Hospital, Chicago, IL, p. A126

NAIBERK, Donald T., Administrator and Chief Executive Officer, Plainview Public Hospital, Plainview, NE, p. A267

NAKAYAMA, Makoto
Interim President and Chief Executive Officer, Long Beach Community Medical Center, Long Beach, CA, p. A48
President and Chief Executive Officer, San Gabriel Valley Medical Center, San Gabriel, CA, p. A62

NANTZ, Jessica A., Chief Executive Officer, Healthsouth Rehabilitation Hospital, Humble, TX, p. A416

NAPIER, Freda, Administrator, Man ARH Hospital, Man, WV, p. A457

NAPIER, Randy L., President, Southern Indiana Rehabilitation Hospital, New Albany, IN, p. A147

NAPPER, Rick, Chief Executive Officer, Crittenden County Hospital, Marion, KY, p. A178

NARBUTAS, Virgis, Administrator, Vencor Hospital–Ontario, Ontario, CA, p. A56

NARUM, Larry, President and Chief Executive Officer, Saint Joseph Hospital, Elgin, IL, p. A129

NASRALLA, Anthony J., FACHE, President and Chief Executive Officer, Titusville Area Hospital, Titusville, PA, p. A369

NATHAN, David G., M.D., President, Dana–Farber Cancer Institute, Boston, MA, p. A204

NATHAN, James R., President, Lee Memorial Health System, Fort Myers, FL, p. A87

NATZKE, Kenneth J., Administrator, OSF St. Joseph Medical Center, Bloomington, IL, p. A124

NAY, Clifford D., Executive Director, Scott Memorial Hospital, Scottsburg, IN, p. A148

NEAL, Hank, Administrator, Kings Mountain Hospital, Kings Mountain, NC, p. A313

NEAL, John C., Administrator and Chief Executive Officer, Haskell County Healthcare System, Stigler, OK, p. A345

NEAMAN, Mark R., President and Chief Executive Officer, Evanston Hospital, Evanston, IL, p. A130

NEEDHAM, Jean M., President, Holy Family Hospital, New Richmond, WI, p. A466

NEEDMAN, Herbert G., Administrator and Chief Executive Officer, Temple Community Hospital, Los Angeles, CA, p. A52

NEELY, Bill J., Administrator, Parmer County Community Hospital, Friona, TX, p. A411

NEELY, Cindy, Administrator and Chief Executive Officer, Maude Norton Memorial City Hospital, Columbus, KS, p. A162

NEFF, Mark J., President and Chief Executive Officer, St. Claire Medical Center, Morehead, KY, p. A178

NEFF, Thomas G., Chief Executive Officer, Columbia Regional Hospital, Columbia, MO, p. A246

NEIDENBACH, Joseph J., Administrator and Executive Vice President, St. Vincent Hospital, Green Bay, WI, p. A462

NELL, Rocio, M.D., Medical and Executive Director, Montgomery County Emergency Service, Norristown, PA, p. A362

NELSON, Bill, Administrator, Coteau Des Prairies Hospital, Sisseton, SD, p. A385

NELSON, Brock D.
Chief Executive Officer, Children's Health Care, Minneapolis, Minneapolis, MN, p. A231
Chief Executive Officer, Children's Health Care–St. Paul, Saint Paul, MN, p. A234

NELSON, Cathleen K., President and Chief Executive Officer, St. Charles Hospital, Oregon, OH, p. A334

NELSON, David, Chief Operating Officer, Glendale Adventist Medical Center, Glendale, CA, p. A44

NELSON, David A., President and Chief Executive Officer, Lakewood Health Center, Baudette, MN, p. A226

NELSON, Don A., Administrator, Crook County Medical Services District, Sundance, WY, p. A472

NELSON, Fred, Administrator, Ontonagon Memorial Hospital, Ontonagon, MI, p. A221

NELSON, James J., Chief Executive Officer, John F. Kennedy Memorial Hospital, Philadelphia, PA, p. A364

NELSON, James O., Administrator, Buena Vista County Hospital, Storm Lake, IA, p. A159

NELSON, Kenneth W., Superintendent, Bridgewater State Hospital, Bridgewater, MA, p. A205

NELSON, Rodney M.
President and Chief Executive Officer, Morenci Area Hospital, Morenci, MI, p. A220
President and Chief Executive Officer, Thorn Hospital, Hudson, MI, p. A218

NELSON, R. A., USN, Commander, Naval Medical Center, San Diego, CA, p. A60

NEMIR, Bill, Administrator, Haskell Memorial Hospital, Haskell, TX, p. A412

NERO, Sharon, Chief Executive Officer, Healthsouth Mountain Regional Rehabilitation Hospital, Morgantown, WV, p. A457

NESPOLI, John L.
President and Chief Executive Officer, Mercy Hospital of Scranton, Scranton, PA, p. A368
President and Chief Executive Officer, Mercy Hospital of Wilkes–Barre, Wilkes–Barre, PA, p. A371

NESTER Jr., Arthur, Administrator, Noxubee General Hospital, Macon, MS, p. A241

NESTER Jr., Martin F., Chief Executive Officer, Long Beach Medical Center, Long Beach, NY, p. A294

NETH, Marvin, Administrator, Callaway District Hospital, Callaway, NE, p. A263

NETHERLAND, Ann, Chief Executive Officer, Franklin Medical Center, Winnsboro, LA, p. A192

NEUGENT, Richard C., President, St. Francis Health System, Greenville, SC, p. A378

NEUSCH, Michael W., FACHE, Director, Louis A. Johnson Veterans Affairs Medical Center, Clarksburg, WV, p. A456

NEVAREZ, Domingo, Executive Director, Hospital San Francisco, San Juan, PR, p. A476

NEVILL, David, President and Chief Executive Officer, Columbia Halstead Hospital, Halstead, KS, p. A163

NEWBOLD, Philip A., President and Chief Executive Officer, Memorial Hospital of South Bend, South Bend, IN, p. A148

NEWCOMB, Sherrie, Acting Administrator, Jenkins Community Hospital, Jenkins, KY, p. A175

NEWMAN, Delores, MS, Network Manager, Metro South Network, Tinley Park Mental Health Center, Tinley Park, IL, p. A138

NEWMAN, Douglas, Administrator, Stafford District Hospital, Stafford, KS, p. A169

NEWMAN, Robert G., M.D., President, Beth Israel Medical Center, New York, NY, p. A295

NEWPORT, Errol G., President and Chief Executive Officer, Deaton Specialty Hospital and Home, Baltimore, MD, p. A197

NEWSOME, Andrea C., FACHE, Director, De Jarnette Center, Staunton, VA, p. A446

NEWSOME, Gary D., Executive Director and Chief Executive Officer, Midwest City Regional Medical Center, Midwest City, OK, p. A343

NEWTON, David R., President and Executive Director, Charlotte Hungerford Hospital, Torrington, CT, p. A79

NG, Vincent, Director, Veterans Affairs Connecticut Healthcare System, West Haven, CT, p. A79

NICHOLS, Hugh, Administrator, Vaughan Perry Hospital, Marion, AL, p. A16

NICHOLS, Mark, Chief Executive Officer, Columbia Polk General Hospital, Cedartown, GA, p. A106

NICHOLS, Ralph, Superintendent, Evansville State Hospital, Evansville, IN, p. A142

NICKELL, Roy, Director Substance Abuse Services, Wake County Alcoholism Treatment Center, Raleigh, NC, p. A315

NICKENS III, John R., Chief Executive Officer, Century City Hospital, Los Angeles, CA, p. A49

NICKERSON, Ruth Marie, President and Chief Executive Officer, Saint Agnes Medical Center, Fresno, CA, p. A44

NICO, Vincent O., Regional Vice President, Healthsouth Rehabilitation Hospital, Largo, FL, p. A91

NIEDERPRUEM, Mark L., Administrator, Shriners Hospitals for Children, Springfield, Springfield, MA, p. A210

NIEHM, Sandy, Administrator, Council Community Hospital and Nursing Home, Council, ID, p. A120

NIELSEN, Kim, Administrator and Chief Executive Officer, Orem Community Hospital, Orem, UT, p. A434

NIEMEYER, Romaine, President and Chief Executive Officer, Holy Spirit Hospital, Camp Hill, PA, p. A355

NIENHUIS, Arthur W., M.D., Director, St. Jude Children's Research Hospital, Memphis, TN, p. A393

NIGHT PIPE, Orville, Service Unit Director, U. S. Public Health Service Indian Hospital, Eagle Butte, SD, p. A382

NIRO, Frank A., Chief Executive Officer, Monadnock Community Hospital, Peterborough, NH, p. A274

NISSEN, David C., Chief Executive Officer, ValueMark Behavioral Healthcare System of Kansas City, Kansas City, MO, p. A250

NITSCHKE, David M., President and Chief Executive Officer, Regional West Medical Center, Scottsbluff, NE, p. A268

NIXON Jr., Jesse, Ph.D.
Director, Capital District Psychiatric Center, Albany, NY, p. A288
Director, New York State Department of Mental Health, Albany, NY, p. B118

NOBLE, Stephen H., President, Accord Health Care Corporation, Clearwater, FL, p. B63

NOCE Jr., Walter W., President and Chief Executive Officer, Childrens Hospital of Los Angeles, Los Angeles, CA, p. A49

NOHRE, Allen S., Chief Executive Officer, Desert Vista Behavioral Health Services, Mesa, AZ, p. A24

NOLAN, Kevin E., President and Chief Executive Officer, St. Elizabeth Health Center, Youngstown, OH, p. A337

NOLAN, Michael J., Chief Executive Officer, Ascension Hospital, Gonzales, LA, p. A184

NOLAN, Robert J., President and Chief Executive Officer, Santa Rosa Health Care Corporation, San Antonio, TX, p. A426

NOLAND, Christopher, Chief Executive Officer, Sheridan Community Hospital, Sheridan, MI, p. A223

NOLL, Donald, Director, Clear Brook Manor, Wilkes-Barre, PA, p. A370

NOONAN, Dennis, President, Salem Hospital, Salem, OR, p. A352

NORD, Thomas A., FACHE, President and Chief Executive Officer, Ivinson Memorial Hospital, Laramie, WY, p. A472

NORDWICK, John A., President and Chief Executive Officer, Bozeman Deaconess Hospital, Bozeman, MT, p. A257

NORDWICK, Thomas, President and Chief Executive Officer, Holy Family Health Services, Estherville, IA, p. A154

NOREM, Kathryn J., Executive Director, Starke Memorial Hospital, Knox, IN, p. A145

NOREN, Mary K.
Acting Superintendent, Eastern Shore Hospital Center, Cambridge, MD, p. A199
Acting Administrator and Chief Executive Officer, Upper Shore Community Mental Health Center, Chestertown, MD, p. A199

NORLING, Richard A., President and Chief Executive Officer, Fairview Hospital and Healthcare Services, Minneapolis, MN, p. B97

NORMAN, Alline L., Director, Veterans Affairs Medical Center, Lake City, FL, p. A91

NORMAN, Jeffrey, Chief Executive Officer, PMH Health Services Network, Phoenix, AZ, p. A25

NORMAN, Paul Michael, President, Takoma Adventist Hospital, Greeneville, TN, p. A389

NORRIS, Charles, Administrator, Seymour Hospital, Seymour, TX, p. A427

NORRIS, Doug, Chief Operating Officer, Western Medical Center Hospital Anaheim, Anaheim, CA, p. A36

NORRIS, Gail B., Administrator, Telfair County Hospital, McRae, GA, p. A111

NORRIS, Jim, Executive Director, St. Cloud Hospital, A Division of Orlando Regional Healthcare System, Saint Cloud, FL, p. A98

NORTHCUTT, Kathleen G., Interim Chief Executive Officer, Northeast Medical Center, Bonham, TX, p. A402

NORTHERN, Robert E., Administrator, Iuka Hospital, Iuka, MS, p. A240

NORTHWAY, James D., M.D., President and Chief Executive Officer, Valley Children's Hospital, Fresno, CA, p. A44

NORTON, Charles R., Administrator, Biggs–Gridley Memorial Hospital, Gridley, CA, p. A45

NORVELL, Charles D., President, Thoms Rehabilitation Hospital, Asheville, NC, p. A308

NORWINE, David R., President and Chief Executive Officer, H. B. Magruder Memorial Hospital, Port Clinton, OH, p. A334

NORWOOD, John F., President, Bethesda General Hospital, Saint Louis, MO, p. A253

NORWOOD, Steve, Director, Western State Psychiatric Center, Fort Supply, OK, p. A341

NOSACKA, Mark, Executive Director, Sabine Medical Center, Many, LA, p. A187

NOTEBAERT, Edmond F., President, Children's Hospital of Philadelphia, Philadelphia, PA, p. A363

NOTEWARE, Dan, Administrator, Dr. Dan C. Trigg Memorial Hospital, Tucumcari, NM, p. A287

NOVAK, Edward, President and Chief Executive Officer, Sacred Heart Hospital, Chicago, IL, p. A127

NOVAK, Judith, President and Chief Executive Officer, Park Plaza Hospital, Houston, TX, p. A415

NOVIELLO, Joseph S., Chief Executive Officer, Podiatry Hospital of Pittsburgh, Pittsburgh, PA, p. A366

NOWAK, Gregory M., Administrator, Coshocton County Memorial Hospital, Coshocton, OH, p. A328

NUCKLES, Craig, Administrator, Two Rivers Psychiatric Hospital, Kansas City, MO, p. A249

NUDELMAN, Phil, Ph.D., President and Chief Executive Officer, Group Health Cooperative of Puget Sound, Seattle, WA, p. B100

NUGENT, Gary N., Medical Director, Veterans Affairs Medical Center, Cincinnati, OH, p. A326

NUNAMAKER, E. Michael, President and Chief Executive Officer, Mercy Health Center of Manhattan, New York, KS, p. A166

NUNNERY, S. Arnold, President and Chief Executive Officer, Iredell Memorial Hospital, Statesville, NC, p. A317

NURKIN, Harry A., Ph.D., President and Chief Executive Officer, Carolinas HealthCare System, Charlotte, NC, p. B74

NYE, Richard A., Chief Executive Officer, Labette County Medical Center, Parsons, KS, p. A168

NYP, Randall G., President and Chief Executive Officer, Via Christi Regional Medical Center, Wichita, KS, p. A171

O

O'BRIEN, John, Administrator, Ellsworth Municipal Hospital, Iowa Falls, IA, p. A156

O'BRIEN, John G., Chief Executive Officer, Cambridge Public Health Commission, Cambridge, MA, p. A205

O'BRIEN, Michael C., Administrator, Sarah D. Culbertson Memorial Hospital, Rushville, IL, p. A137

O'BRIEN, William F., Administrator and Chief Executive Officer, Ward Memorial Hospital, Monahans, TX, p. A421

O'BRIEN Jr., Charles M., President and Chief Executive Officer, Western Pennsylvania Hospital, Pittsburgh, PA, p. A367

O'CONNELL, John W., President, Franciscan Services Corporation, Sylvania, OH, p. B97

O'CONNELL, Rick, Chief Executive Officer, Columbia Park Medical Center, Orlando, FL, p. A95

O'CONNOR, Dania, Chief Executive Officer, Charter Behavioral Health System at Springwood, Leesburg, VA, p. A442

O'CONNOR, Joann, Director, Winnebago Mental Health Institute, Winnebago, WI, p. A470

O'CONNOR, Maureen, Interim Administrator and Chief Operating Officer, St. Bernardine Medical Center, San Bernardino, CA, p. A60

O'CONNOR, William D., President and Chief Executive Officer, Rehabilitation Hospital of the Pacific, Honolulu, HI, p. A117

O'CONNOR Jr., Vincent J., President and Chief Executive Officer, Fremont Area Medical Center, Fremont, NE, p. A263

O'DONNELL, Kevin J., President and Chief Executive Officer, Sacred Heart–St. Mary's Hospitals, Rhinelander, WI, p. A468

O'DONNELL, Randall L., Ph.D., President and Chief Executive Officer, Children's Mercy Hospital, Kansas City, MO, p. A249

O'DONNELL Jr., Thomas F., FACS, President and Chief Executive Officer, New England Medical Center, Boston, MA, p. A204

O'GRADY Jr., Michael J., President and Chief Executive Officer, Indian River Memorial Hospital, Vero Beach, FL, p. A101

O'KEEFE, James M., Administrator, Cumberland Memorial Hospital, Cumberland, WI, p. A461

O'LOUGHLIN, James, Chief Executive Officer, Columbia Presbyterian Hospital, Oklahoma City, OK, p. A343

O'MALLEY, Dennis, President, Craig Hospital, Englewood, CO, p. A72

O'NEAL, James, Administrator, Chase County Community Hospital, Imperial, NE, p. A265

O'NEIL, John D., Executive Vice President and Administrator, St. Mary's Hospital Warrick, Boonville, IN, p. A140

O'ROURKE, Terrence Michael, President, Blodgett Memorial Medical Center, Grand Rapids, MI, p. A216

O'SHEA, James E., Administrator, Greenbrier Hospital, Brooksville, FL, p. A84

OAKEY, James A., President and Chief Executive Officer, Helix Health, Lutherville, MD, p. B104

OBERTA, Gail M., Administrator and Chief Executive Officer, BHC Shoal Creek Hospital, Austin, TX, p. A400

OCHS, David, Administrator, Saint James Hospital, Pontiac, IL, p. A136

OCHS, Kristine, R.N., Administrator, Grisell Memorial Hospital District One, Ransom, KS, p. A168

OCKERS, Thomas, President, Brookhaven Memorial Hospital Medical Center, Patchogue, NY, p. A302

ODDIS, Joseph Michael
President, Spartanburg Regional Healthcare System, Spartanburg, SC, p. B137
President, Spartanburg Regional Medical Center, Spartanburg, SC, p. A380

ODELL III, F. A., FACHE, President, Carteret General Hospital, Morehead City, NC, p. A314

OESTMANN, Barbara, Chief Executive Officer, Share Medical Center, Alva, OK, p. A339

OGLESBY, Darrell M., Administrator, Putnam General Hospital, Eatonton, GA, p. A109

OGLESBY Jr., D. K., President, Anderson Area Medical Center, Anderson, SC, p. A375

OHLEN, Robert B., President and Chief Executive Officer, Lawrence Memorial Hospital, Lawrence, KS, p. A165

OKINAKA, Cynthia, Administrator, St. Francis Medical Center, Honolulu, HI, p. A117

OLAND, Charisse S., President and Chief Executive Officer, Childrens Care Hospital and School, Sioux Falls, SD, p. A385

OLANDER, Laura, Chief Executive Officer, Franklin General Hospital, Hampton, IA, p. A155

OLDHAM, John M., M.D., Director, New York State Psychiatric Institute, New York, NY, p. A298

OLEWINSKI, Kathy M., Administrator, De Paul Hospital, Milwaukee, WI, p. A465

OLIVER, William C., Executive Director, Forrest General Hospital, Hattiesburg, MS, p. A239

OLIVERIUS, Maynard F.
President and Chief Executive Officer, Stormont–Vail HealthCare, Topeka, KS, p. A170
President and Chief Executive Officer, Stormont–Vail HealthCare, Topeka, KS, p. B139

OLSEN, Gloria P., Ph.D., Superintendent, Kerrville State Hospital, Kerrville, TX, p. A417

OLSEN, Robert T., Chief Executive Officer, Yuma Regional Medical Center, Yuma, AZ, p. A28

OLSON, JoAline, R.N., President and Chief Executive Officer, St. Helena Hospital, Deer Park, CA, p. A41

OLSON, Lynn W., Administrator and Chief Executive Officer, Regina Medical Center, Hastings, MN, p. A230

OLSON, Nathan C., President and Chief Executive Officer, Hammond–Henry Hospital, Geneseo, IL, p. A130

OLSON, Neva M., Administrator, Samuel Mahelona Memorial Hospital, Kapaa, HI, p. A118

OLSON, Randall M., Administrator, Wellmont Health System–Bristol, Bristol, TN, p. A387

OMMEN, Ronald A., President and Chief Executive Officer, Trinity Lutheran Hospital, Kansas City, MO, p. A249

ONO, Sidney, Administrator, Desert Valley Hospital, Victorville, CA, p. A68

ONTIVEROS, Alfredo, Administrator, Gila Regional Medical Center, Silver City, NM, p. A287

OPDAHL, Jim
Administrator, Community Hospital in Nelson County, McVille, ND, p. A321
Administrator, St. Luke's Tri–State Hospital, Bowman, ND, p. A319

OPPEGARD, Stanley C., Vice President and Chief Operating Officer, Methodist Hospital, Sacramento, CA, p. A59

ORAVEC Jr., Andrew, Administrator, Columbia New Port Richey Hospital, New Port Richey, FL, p. A94

ORDWAY, Lynn, Administrator, Edgemont Hospital, Los Angeles, CA, p. A49

ORFGEN, Lynn C., Chief Executive Officer, St. Charles General Hospital, New Orleans, LA, p. A189

ORLANDO, Joseph S., Executive Director, Jacobi Medical Center, New York, NY, p. A297

ORMAN Jr., Bernard A., Administrator, Samaritan Memorial Hospital, Macon, MO, p. A250

ORME, Cliff, Executive Director, Valley Hospital, Palmer, AK, p. A21

ORMOND, Evalyn
Administrator, Sterlington Hospital, Sterlington, LA, p. A191
Administrator, Union General Hospital, Farmerville, LA, p. A184

ORR, Jon, Administrator, Mountain View Hospital, Gadsden, AL, p. A14

ORR, Lindell W., Chief Executive Officer, Columbia Blake Medical Center, Bradenton, FL, p. A84

ORR, Roy J., President and Chief Executive Officer, McKenzie–Willamette Hospital, Springfield, OR, p. A352

ORR, Steven R., Chairman and Chief Executive Officer, Lutheran Health Systems, Fargo, ND, p. B110

ORRICK, Charles H., Administrator, Donalsonville Hospital, Donalsonville, GA, p. A108

ORTEGO, Craig A., Administrator, Moosa Memorial Hospital, Eunice, LA, p. A184

ORTENZIO, Robert, President and Chief Executive Officer, Continental Medical Systems, Inc., Mechanicsburg, PA, p. B87

ORTIZ, Julio A., M.D., Chairman, Font Martelo Hospital, Humacao, PR, p. A475

OSBORNE, David W., President and Chief Executive Officer, Norwalk Hospital, Norwalk, CT, p. A78

OSBORNE, Doug, Interim Superintendent, Georgia Regional Hospital at Savannah, Savannah, GA, p. A113

OSBURN, Jerry, Administrator, Methodist Hospital–Levelland, Levelland, TX, p. A418

OSIKA, Diane J., Interim Chief Executive Officer, Tri–County Memorial Hospital, Gowanda, NY, p. A292

OSMUS, Richard D., Chief Executive Officer, Hugh Chatham Memorial Hospital, Elkin, NC, p. A311

OSSE, John M., Administrator, Mitchell County Hospital, Beloit, KS, p. A161

OSTASZEWSKI, Patricia, Chief Operating Officer and Administrator, Healthsouth Rehabilitation Hospital of New Jersey, Toms River, NJ, p. A282

OSWALD, Wesley W., Chief Executive Officer, Brazosport Memorial Hospital, Lake Jackson, TX, p. A418

OTAKE, Stanley, Chief Executive Officer, Bellflower Medical Center, Bellflower, CA, p. A38

OTHOLE, Jean, Service Unit Director, U. S. Public Health Service Indian Hospital, Zuni, NM, p. A287

OTHS, Richard P., President and Chief Executive Officer, Atlantic Health System, Florham Park, NJ, p. A277

OTT, Pamela, R.N., Administrator, Ocean Beach Hospital, Ilwaco, WA, p. A450

OTT, Ronald A., Chief Executive Officer, Fitzgibbon Hospital, Marshall, MO, p. A251

OTT, Ronald H., President and Chief Executive Officer, McKeesport Hospital, McKeesport, PA, p. A361

OTTEN, Jeffrey, President, Brigham and Women's Hospital, Boston, MA, p. A204

OUSLEY, Virginia, Director, Carilion Radford Community Hospital, Radford, VA, p. A444

OVIEDA, James G., President and Chief Executive Officer, Santa Marta Hospital, Los Angeles, CA, p. A51

OWEN, Ronald S., Chief Executive Officer, Huntsville Hospital, Huntsville, AL, p. A15

OWEN, Steve N., Chief Executive Officer, Union Hospital, Elkton, MD, p. A200

OWENS, Ben E., President, St. Bernards Regional Medical Center, Jonesboro, AR, p. A32

OXLEY, Donald, Vice President, Area Manager and Chief Executive Officer, Kaiser Foundation Hospital, Oakland, CA, p. A55

P

PAAP, Antonie H., President and Chief Executive Officer, Children's Hospital Oakland, Oakland, CA, p. A55

PABON, Ahmed Alvarez, Executive Director, Hospital Sub–Regional Dr. Victor R. Nunez, Humacao, PR, p. A475

PACINI, Carol, Provincialate Superior, Little Company of Mary Sisters Healthcare System, Evergreen Park, IL, p. B109

PACKER, Richard, Administrator, Cassia Regional Medical Center, Burley, ID, p. A119

PACKNETT, Michael J., President and Chief Executive Officer, St. Mary–Rogers Memorial Hospital, Rogers, AR, p. A34

PACZKOWSKI, Ronald R., Vice President, Franciscan Skemp Healthcare–La Crosse Campus, La Crosse, WI, p. A463

PADDEN, Terrance J., Administrator, Box Butte General Hospital, Alliance, NE, p. A262

PAFFRATH, Nora M., Executive Vice President, Portsmouth General Hospital, Portsmouth, VA, p. A444

PAGE, Dan B., President, Greenleaf Health Systems, Inc., Chattanooga, TN, p. B99

PAGE, David R., President and Chief Executive Officer, Hermann Hospital, Houston, TX, p. A414

PAGE, Susan M., President and Chief Executive Officer, Pratt Regional Medical Center, Pratt, KS, p. A168

PAGELS, James R., Chief Executive Officer and Managing Director, Northern Nevada Medical Center, Sparks, NV, p. A271

PALAGI, Richard L., Chief Executive Officer, St. John's Lutheran Hospital, Libby, MT, p. A259

PALMER, James A., Director, Veterans Affairs Medical Center, San Juan, PR, p. A477

PALMER, Mary, President and Chief Executive Officer, Columbia Riveredge Hospital, Forest Park, IL, p. A130

PALMER, William H., President, Miller Dwan Medical Center, Duluth, MN, p. A228

PANDL, Therese B., Senior Vice President and Chief Operating Officer, St. Mary's Hospital Ozaukee, Mequon, WI, p. A465

PANICEK, John M., Administrator, Saint Marys Hospital, Rochester, MN, p. A233

PANNELL, Sally S., Chief Executive Officer, Excelsior Springs Medical Center, Excelsior Springs, MO, p. A247

PAPANIA, Barry A., Chief Executive Officer, Columbia St. Luke's Hospital, Bluefield, WV, p. A455

PAPIN, Tom, Administrator, Itasca Medical Center, Grand Rapids, MN, p. A229

PAQUETTE, James T., Regional Chief Executive Officer, St. James Community Hospital, Butte, MT, p. A257

PARENTE, William D., Director and Chief Executive Officer, Santa Monica–UCLA Medical Center, Santa Monica, CA, p. A64

PARIS, David, Administrator, Georgiana Doctors Hospital, Georgiana, AL, p. A14

PARIS, Gregory A., Administrator, Monroe County Hospital, Albia, IA, p. A151

PARIS, Herbert, President, Mid Coast Hospital, Bath, ME, p. A193

PARISI, Ernest, Administrator and Chief Executive Officer, Llano Memorial Hospital, Llano, TX, p. A419

PARK, Darlene, Executive Director, Rogers City Rehabilitation Hospital, Rogers City, MI, p. A222

PARK, Gary L., President, Wesley Long Community Hospital, Greensboro, NC, p. A312

PARKER, Douglas M., Chief Executive Officer, R. T. Jones Hospital, Canton, GA, p. A106

PARKER, Douglas W., Chief Executive Officer, St. Vincent–North Rehabilitation Hospital, Sherwood, AR, p. A35

PARKER, Patsy A., Administrator and Chief Executive Officer, Rio Vista Rehabilitation Hospital, El Paso, TX, p. A409

PARKER, Phillip L.
Administrator, D. W. McMillan Memorial Hospital, Brewton, AL, p. A12
Administrator, Escambia County Health Care Authority, Brewton, AL, p. B96

PARKER, Scott S., President, Intermountain Health Care, Inc., Salt Lake City, UT, p. B106

PARKER, Tim, Chief Executive Officer, Miami Heart Institute, Miami, FL, p. A93

PARKS, Ralph L., Administrator and Chief Executive Officer, Victor Valley Community Hospital, Victorville, CA, p. A68

PARKS III, Burton O., Administrator, West Shore Hospital, Manistee, MI, p. A220

PARMER, David N., President and Chief Executive Officer, Baptist Hospital of Southeast Texas, Beaumont, TX, p. A401

PARRIS, Y. C., Director, Veterans Affairs Medical Center, Birmingham, AL, p. A12

PARRIS Jr., Thomas G., President, Women and Infants Hospital of Rhode Island, Providence, RI, p. A374

PARRISH, Harold R., Superintendent, Rusk State Hospital, Rusk, TX, p. A425

PARRISH, James G., Administrator, East Adams Rural Hospital, Ritzville, WA, p. A452

PARSONS, Ann C., Interim Administrator, St. Vincent Mercy Hospital, Elwood, IN, p. A142

PARSONS, Karla, R.N., Administrator, Avalon Municipal Hospital and Clinic, Avalon, CA, p. A37

PARSONS, Larry, Administrator, Wilbarger General Hospital, Vernon, TX, p. A430

PARTON, Gerald L., Chief Executive Officer, Doctors Hospital of Jefferson, Metairie, LA, p. A187
PASCUALY, Rodrigo A.
    Administrator, Palo Verde Mental Health Services, Tucson, AZ, p. A27
    Administrator, Tucson Medical Center, Tucson, AZ, p. A27
PASINSKI, Theodore M., President, St. Joseph's Hospital Health Center, Syracuse, NY, p. A305
PASSAMA, Gary J., President and Chief Executive Officer, NorthBay Healthcare System, Fairfield, CA, p. B119
PATE, Alfred S., Director, Veterans Affairs Medical Center, North Chicago, IL, p. A135
PATNESKY, Edward J., President and Chief Executive Officer, Southampton Memorial Hospital, Franklin, VA, p. A441
PATOUT, John P., Administrator, Vermilion Hospital, Lafayette, LA, p. A186
PATSEY, Lois K., Administrator and Chief Executive Officer, East Bay Hospital, Richmond, CA, p. A59
PATTEN, Bill, Administrator, Sedgwick County Memorial Hospital, Julesburg, CO, p. A73
PATTERSON, Donald E., Administrator, Siloam Spring Memorial Hospital, Siloam Springs, AR, p. A35
PATTERSON, Patti J., Commissioner, Texas Department of Health, Austin, TX, p. B142
PATTERSON, William M., Administrator, Columbia Vicksburg Medical Center, Vicksburg, MS, p. A244
PATTON, David W., Chief Executive Officer, Kona Community Hospital, Kealakekua, HI, p. A118
PATTON, Jimmy, Chief Executive Officer and Managing Director, Keystone Center, Chester, PA, p. A355
PATTULLO, Douglas E., Chief Executive Officer, Tolfree Memorial Hospital, West Branch, MI, p. A225
PATZ, Stephen M.
    Chief Executive Officer, Parkway Regional Medical Center, North Miami Beach, FL, p. A94
    Chief Executive Officer, Parkway Regional Medical Center–West, Miami, FL, p. A93
PAUGH, J. William, President and Chief Executive Officer, St. Joseph Hospital, Augusta, GA, p. A105
PAUL, Jerry W., President, Deaconess Incarnate Word Health System, Saint Louis, MO, p. A253
PAUL, Kevin, Administrator, Dooly Medical Center, Vienna, GA, p. A115
PAULDING, Ralph, Administrator, Wirth Regional Hospital, Oakland City, IN, p. A147
PAULEY, Alan C., Administrator, Morrow County Hospital, Mount Gilead, OH, p. A333
PAULSON, Mark E., Administrator, Appleton Municipal Hospital and Nursing Home, Appleton, MN, p. A226
PAUTLER, J. Stephen, CHE, Administrator, Windom Area Hospital, Windom, MN, p. A236
PAWLAK, Paul, President, Silver Cross Hospital, Joliet, IL, p. A132
PAWLOWSKI, Eugene P., President, Bluefield Regional Medical Center, Bluefield, WV, p. A455
PAYNE, Dale F., Acting Administrator, Mid–Valley Hospital, Omak, WA, p. A451
PAYNE, Mark I., Superintendent, Utah State Hospital, Provo, UT, p. A434
PAYNE, Michael E., President and Chief Executive Officer, North Kansas City Hospital, North Kansas City, MO, p. A251
PAZZAGLINI, Gino J., President and Chief Executive Officer, Good Samaritan Regional Medical Center, Pottsville, PA, p. A367
PEACE, Thomas, Ph.D., Commissioner, Oklahoma State Department of Mental Health and Substance Abuse Services, Oklahoma City, OK, p. B119
PEACH, Paul E., Medical Director, Roosevelt Warm Springs Institute for Rehabilitation, Warm Springs, GA, p. A115
PEAK, Benjamin A., Chief Executive Officer, Dickenson County Medical Center, Clintwood, VA, p. A440
PEAK, James G., Director, Memorial Hospital and Manor, Bainbridge, GA, p. A105
PEAKS, William E., Chief Executive Officer, Columbia Garden Park Hospital, Gulfport, MS, p. A239
PEARSE, David L., Executive Director, Speare Memorial Hospital, Plymouth, NH, p. A274

PEARSON, Bruce E., Vice President and Chief Executive Officer, Desert Samaritan Medical Center, Mesa, AZ, p. A23
PEARSON, Diane, Administrator, Cook County North Shore Hospital, Grand Marais, MN, p. A229
PEARSON, Gerald P., President, Franciscan Sisters Health Care Corporation, Frankfort, IL, p. B98
PEARSON, Robert S., Administrator, Littleton Regional Hospital, Littleton, NH, p. A273
PEARSON, Roger W., Administrator, Ellsworth County Hospital, Ellsworth, KS, p. A162
PECK, Gary V., Chief Executive Officer, St. Joseph's Hospital, Chewelah, WA, p. A448
PECK, Richard H., Administrator, Eliza Coffee Memorial Hospital, Florence, AL, p. A14
PECK, Theresa
    President and Chief Executive Officer, Catholic Health Partners, Chicago, IL, p. B76
    President and Chief Executive Officer, Columbus Hospital, Chicago, IL, p. A125
    President and Chief Executive Officer, Saint Anthony Hospital, Chicago, IL, p. A127
    President and Chief Executive Officer, St. Joseph Hospital, Chicago, IL, p. A127
PECOT, L. J., Administrator, St. Helena Parish Hospital, Greensburg, LA, p. A184
PEDERSEN, William L., Chief Executive Officer, St. Peter Regional Treatment Center, Saint Peter, MN, p. A234
PEED, Nancy, Administrator, Peach Regional Medical Center, Fort Valley, GA, p. A109
PEEK, Scott, Administrator, Chambers Memorial Hospital, Danville, AR, p. A30
PEEPLES, Lewis T., Chief Executive Officer, Jennie Stuart Medical Center, Hopkinsville, KY, p. A175
PEICKERT, Barbara A., R.N., Chief Executive Officer, Hayward Area Memorial Hospital and Nursing Home, Hayward, WI, p. A463
PEIFFER, Paul V., Chief Executive Officer, Kokomo Rehabilitation Hospital, Kokomo, IN, p. A145
PELHAM, Judith, President and Chief Executive Officer, Mercy Health Services, Farmington Hills, MI, p. B114
PELL Jr., Richard, Director, Veterans Affairs Medical Center, Martinsburg, WV, p. A457
PELLEY, Catherine M., President and Chief Executive Officer, St. Mary Regional Medical Center, Apple Valley, CA, p. A36
PELUSO, Joseph J., President and Chief Executive Officer, Westmoreland Regional Hospital, Greensburg, PA, p. A358
PENDOLA, Charles J.
    President and Chief Executive Officer, Flushing Hospital Medical Center, New York, NY, p. A296
    President, Wyckoff Heights Medical Center, New York, NY, p. A300
PENLAND, Victoria M.
    Administrator and Chief Operating Officer, Palomar Medical Center, Escondido, CA, p. A42
    Interim President and Chief Executive Officer, Palomar Pomerado Health System, San Diego, CA, p. B120
PENRY, L. Allen, Chief Executive Officer, Castleview Hospital, Price, UT, p. A434
PENTICOFF, Mick, Administrator, Mid Dakota Hospital, Chamberlain, SD, p. A382
PENTZ, Thomas R.
    Chief Executive Officer, Columbia Medical Center Peninsula, Ormond Beach, FL, p. A95
    Chief Executive Officer, Columbia Medical Center–Daytona, Daytona Beach, FL, p. A85
PEPPER, H. L. Perry, President, Chester County Hospital, West Chester, PA, p. A370
PEREZ, Francisco J., President and Chief Executive Officer, Kettering Medical Center, Kettering, OH, p. A331
PEREZ, George, Executive Vice President and Chief Operating Officer, Walter O. Boswell Memorial Hospital, Sun City, AZ, p. A26
PERILLI, Ernest N., Vice President Operations, Parkview Hospital, Philadelphia, PA, p. A364
PERKINS, Gary A., President and Chief Executive Officer, Children's Hospital, Omaha, NE, p. A267
PERMETTI, Thomas, Administrator, St. John Hospital, Nassau Bay, TX, p. A422

PERNAU, James O., Administrator, Sterling Regional Medcenter, Sterling, CO, p. A75
PERRA, Connie Oliverson, Director, Tarrant County Psychiatric Center, Fort Worth, TX, p. A410
PERREAULT, Robert A., Director, Veterans Affairs Medical Center, Decatur, GA, p. A108
PERRY, Alan S., Director, Veterans Affairs Medical Center, Roseburg, OR, p. A352
PERRY, George H., Ph.D., Chief Executive Officer, Bayou Oaks Hospital, Houma, LA, p. A185
PERRY, Matthew J., Director, Carilion Franklin Memorial Hospital, Rocky Mount, VA, p. A446
PERRY, Mike, Chief Executive Officer, Westbridge Treatment Center, Phoenix, AZ, p. A25
PERRY, Robert M., Administrator, Bruce Hospital, Bruce, MS, p. A238
PERRY, Ronald J., Chief Executive Officer, Columbia Ashley Valley Medical Center, Vernal, UT, p. A436
PERRYMAN, Margaret, Chief Executive Officer, Gillette Children's Specialty Healthcare, Saint Paul, MN, p. A234
PERRYMAN, Mike, Administrator, Baptist Memorial Hospital–Union City, Union City, TN, p. A396
PERSELAY, Geoffrey, Chief Executive Officer, Charter Behavioral Health System of New Jersey–Summit, Summit, NJ, p. A282
PERSICHILLI, Judith M., President and Chief Executive Officer, St. Francis Medical Center, Trenton, NJ, p. A282
PERUSHEK, John, Administrator, Bloomer Community Memorial Hospital and the MapleWood, Bloomer, WI, p. A461
PETASNICK, William D., President, Froedtert Memorial Lutheran Hospital, Milwaukee, WI, p. A465
PETERS, Anthony, Chief Executive Officer, Camden County Health Services Center, Blackwood, NJ, p. A275
PETERS, Bruce G., President and Chief Executive Officer, Parkland Medical Center, Derry, NH, p. A272
PETERS, Curtis A., Chief Executive Officer, J. D. McCarty Center for Children With Developmental Disabilities, Norman, OK, p. A343
PETERS, Douglas S., President and Chief Executive Officer, Jefferson Health System, Radnor, PA, p. B107
PETERS, J. Robert, Executive Director, Memorial Hospital, Colorado Springs, CO, p. A70
PETERS, L. K., Administrator, Perry County General Hospital, Richton, MS, p. A243
PETERSEN, Gary L., Administrator, Crawford County Memorial Hospital, Denison, IA, p. A153
PETERSEN, Keith J., Chief Executive Officer, Richmond Heights General Hospital, Richmond Heights, OH, p. A334
PETERSEN, Thomas A., Vice President and Chief Operating Officer, Mercy General Hospital, Sacramento, CA, p. A59
PETERSON, Andrew E., President and Chief Executive Officer, St. Luke's Memorial Hospital Center, Utica, NY, p. A306
PETERSON, Brent, Administrator, Cherry County Hospital, Valentine, NE, p. A268
PETERSON, Bruce D., Administrator, Mercer County Hospital, Aledo, IL, p. A123
PETERSON, Clayton R., President, Long Prairie Memorial Hospital and Home, Long Prairie, MN, p. A230
PETERSON, David A., President and Chief Executive Officer, Aroostook Medical Center, Presque Isle, ME, p. A195
PETERSON, Douglas R., President and Chief Executive Officer, Chippewa Valley Hospital and Oakview Care Center, Durand, WI, p. A461
PETERSON, Frederick, Administrator, Ortonville Area Health Services, Ortonville, MN, p. A233
PETERSON, Larry, Chief Executive Officer, San Dimas Community Hospital, San Dimas, CA, p. A61
PETERSON, Leland W., President and Chief Executive Officer, Sun Health Corporation, Sun City, AZ, p. B139
PETERSON, Patricia, President and Chief Executive Officer, St. Mary's Hospital, Passaic, NJ, p. A280

POSEY, George, Administrator, Leake Memorial Hospital, Carthage, MS, p. A238

POSEY, M. Kenneth, FACHE, Administrator, Jasper General Hospital, Bay Springs, MS, p. A237

POSTON, Stuart, President, Murray–Calloway County Hospital, Murray, KY, p. A179

POTEETE, Kenneth W., President and Chief Executive Officer, Georgetown Hospital, Georgetown, TX, p. A411

POTTENGER, Jay, Administrator, Teton Medical Center, Choteau, MT, p. A257

POTTER, Bruce C., President, Canton–Potsdam Hospital, Potsdam, NY, p. A302

POTTER, Michael S., President and Chief Executive Officer, Westwood Medical Center, Midland, TX, p. A421

POTTER, Terri L., President and Chief Executive Officer, Meriter Hospital, Madison, WI, p. A464

POTTER, B. B., Commanding Officer, Naval Hospital, Camp Pendleton, CA, p. A39

POTTS, Jeffrey, Administrator, Vaughan Chilton Medical Center, Clanton, AL, p. A13

POURIER, Terry, Service Unit Director, U. S. Public Health Service Indian Hospital, Fort Yates, ND, p. A320

POWELL, Denny W., Chief Executive Officer, Columbia Medical Center Phoenix, Phoenix, AZ, p. A24

POWELL, Ricky, Administrator, Red River Hospital, Wichita Falls, TX, p. A431

POWELL, Roy A., President, Frankford Hospital of the City of Philadelphia, Philadelphia, PA, p. A363

POWELL Jr., Boone
President, Baylor Health Care System, Dallas, TX, p. B69
President, Baylor University Medical Center, Dallas, TX, p. A406

POWERS, L. Darrell, Senior Vice President, Lynchburg General Hospital, Lynchburg, VA, p. A442

POWERS, Michael K., Administrator, Fairbanks Memorial Hospital, Fairbanks, AK, p. A20

POWERS, Shirley B., Senior Executive Officer, Alliant Hospitals, Louisville, KY, p. A177

POWERS, Terry C., Administrator, Fort Logan Hospital, Stanford, KY, p. A180

PRESLAR Jr., Len B., President and Chief Executive Officer, North Carolina Baptist Hospital, Winston–Salem, NC, p. A318

PRESLEY, John M., Ph.D., Director, Veterans Affairs Medical Center, Salem, VA, p. A446

PRESSLEY, Yvonne A., Chief Executive Officer, Ancora Psychiatric Hospital, Ancora, NJ, p. A275

PRESTON, Craig, Chief Executive Officer, Lakeview Hospital, Bountiful, UT, p. A433

PRIBYL, Stephen J., USAF, Administrator, Scott Medical Center, Scott AFB, IL, p. A137

PRICE, Corbett A., Chief Executive Officer, Interfaith Medical Center, New York, NY, p. A297

PRICE, Floyd N., Administrator, Grove Hill Memorial Hospital, Grove Hill, AL, p. A15

PRICE, Norman M., FACHE, Administrator, Southwest Mississippi Regional Medical Center, McComb, MS, p. A241

PRICE, William E., Interim Chief Executive Officer, Ojai Valley Community Hospital, Ojai, CA, p. A56

PRICE Jr., Eston, Administrator, Evans Memorial Hospital, Claxton, GA, p. A106

PRICE Jr., Warren T.
Chief Executive Officer, East Louisiana State Hospital, Jackson, LA, p. A185
Chief Executive Officer, Greenwell Springs Hospital, Greenwell Springs, LA, p. A184

PRICKETT, Thomas H., President and Chief Executive Officer, Suburban General Hospital, Pittsburgh, PA, p. A367

PRIDDY, Sandra D., President, Stokes–Reynolds Memorial Hospital, Danbury, NC, p. A310

PRIDGEN Jr., Lee, Administrator, Sampson Regional Medical Center, Clinton, NC, p. A310

PRIMEAUX, Elizabeth A., Chief Executive Officer, Greater El Monte Community Hospital, South El Monte, CA, p. A65

PRIMROSE, Gayle E., Administrator, Boone County Health Center, Albion, NE, p. A262

PRISCO, Nicholas A., Chief Executive Officer, Sunbury Community Hospital, Sunbury, PA, p. A369

PRISELAC, Thomas M., President and Chief Executive Officer, Cedars–Sinai Medical Center, Los Angeles, CA, p. A49

PRISTER, James Richard, Chief Operating Officer, Suburban Hospital, Hinsdale, IL, p. A132

PRITCHARD, Eugene, President, Condell Medical Center, Libertyville, IL, p. A133

PRITCHETT, Beverly, Executive Officer, Department of the Army, Office of the Surgeon General, Falls Church, VA, p. B90

PROBST, Randall K., Administrator, Wasatch County Hospital, Heber City, UT, p. A433

PROCHILO, John F., Chief Executive Officer and Administrator, Northeast Rehabilitation Hospital, Salem, NH, p. A274

PROPHIT, Alice M., Chief Executive Officer, North Louisiana Rehabilitation Hospital, Ruston, LA, p. A190

PROUT, John S., President and Chief Executive Officer, St. Joseph Medical Center, Towson, MD, p. A202

PROVENZANO, William, President, Ohio Valley General Hospital, McKees Rocks, PA, p. A361

PRUITT, Mike, Administrator, Arbuckle Memorial Hospital, Sulphur, OK, p. A346

PRUSAK, Thomas K., President, St. Joseph's Medical Center, Brainerd, MN, p. A227

PRYCE, Richard J., President, Aultman Hospital, Canton, OH, p. A324

PRYOR, Curtis R., Administrator, Jefferson County Hospital, Waurika, OK, p. A347

PRYOR, Dennis P., Administrator, Salem Memorial District Hospital, Salem, MO, p. A255

PUGH, Larry W., President and Chief Executive Officer, Allen Memorial Hospital, Waterloo, IA, p. A159

PUGH, Richard E., President and Chief Executive Officer, New Milford Hospital, New Milford, CT, p. A78

PUGH, Thomas E., Vice President Rehabilitation Services, John Heinz Institute of Rehabilitation Medicine, Wilkes–Barre, PA, p. A371

PUGLISI Jr., Frank J., Executive Director, Merrithew Memorial Hospital, Martinez, CA, p. A53

PULSIPHER, Gary W., Chief Executive Officer, Breech Medical Center, Lebanon, MO, p. A250

PUNG, Dawn S., Administrator, Kau Hospital, Pahala, HI, p. A118

PURCELL Jr., Howard J., President, Community Memorial Hospital, Cheboygan, MI, p. A213

PURDY, Jim, Administrative Director, Presbyterian Kaseman Hospital, Albuquerque, NM, p. A284

PURVIS, Mildred W., Administrator, Hope Hospital, Lockhart, SC, p. A379

PUTNAM, Larry E., Administrator, Phillips County Hospital, Malta, MT, p. A259

PUTNAM, Stewart, President, St. Mary's Hospital, Rochester, NY, p. A303

PUTTER, Joshua, Executive Director, Medical Center of Southeastern Oklahoma, Durant, OK, p. A341

PYLE, Joseph, Administrator, Meadow Wood Behavioral Health System, New Castle, DE, p. A80

PYLE Jr., Bert W., Director, Elmira Psychiatric Center, Elmira, NY, p. A292

Q

QUAM, Mark, Executive Director, Brown County Mental Health Center, Green Bay, WI, p. A462

QUIGLEY, T. Richard, President and Chief Executive Officer, Youville Lifecare, Cambridge, MA, p. A205

QUINLAN, Richard S., President and Chief Executive Officer, UniCare Health System, Melrose, MA, p. A208

QUINLIVAN, Thomas J., Administrator, Tracy Municipal Hospital, Tracy, MN, p. A235

QUINN, Timothy F., Administrator, Wishek Community Hospital, Wishek, ND, p. A322

QUINN, Robert G., FACHE, Administrator, U. S. Air Force Hospital, Beale AFB, CA, p. A37

QUINTON, Byron, Administrator, Humboldt General Hospital, Winnemucca, NV, p. A271

R

RAAB, Daniel J., President and Chief Executive Officer, St. Vincent Memorial Hospital, Taylorville, IL, p. A138

RABJOHNS, Eric, Chief Executive Officer, College Hospital Costa Mesa, Costa Mesa, CA, p. A41

RABKIN, Mitchell T., Chief Executive Officer, CareGroup, Boston, MA, p. B74

RABNER, Barry S., President, Bryn Mawr Rehabilitation Hospital, Malvern, PA, p. A361

RABUKA, Mickey M., Administrator, North Georgia Medical Center and Gilmer Nursing Home, Ellijay, GA, p. A109

RACE, J. E., Administrator and Chief Executive Officer, Lakeview Hospital, Wauwatosa, WI, p. A470

RADKE, Sam, Interim Chief Executive Officer, St. Vincent General Hospital, Leadville, CO, p. A73

RAFFERTY, Patrick J., Administrator, Griggs County Hospital and Nursing Home, Cooperstown, ND, p. A319

RAFTER, William A., Director, Alcohol and Drug Abuse Treatment Center, Black Mountain, NC, p. A308

RAGGHIANTI, Eugene, Administrator, Methodist Hospital of Lexington, Lexington, TN, p. A392

RAGLAND, James H., Administrator, Marengo Memorial Hospital, Marengo, IA, p. A156

RAGLAND, Kenneth E., Administrator, Beaufort County Hospital, Washington, NC, p. A317

RAHE, Sandra, Chief Executive Officer, Cleveland Psychiatric Institute, Cleveland, OH, p. A326

RAHN, Douglas L., Chief Executive Officer, Community Health Center of Branch County, Coldwater, MI, p. A214

RAJNIC, Sharon J., Administrator, Shriners Hospitals for Children, Philadelphia Unit, Philadelphia, PA, p. A365

RAK, Arlene A., R.N., President, University Hospitals Health System Bedford Medical Center, Bedford, OH, p. A324

RALEY, Ana, Administrator, Hadley Memorial Hospital, Washington, DC, p. A81

RALPH, Chandler M., President and Chief Executive Officer, Adirondack Medical Center, Saranac Lake, NY, p. A304

RALPH, Stephen A., President and Chief Executive Officer, Huntington Memorial Hospital, Pasadena, CA, p. A57

RAMIREZ, Magdalena, Director, Helen Hayes Hospital, West Haverstraw, NY, p. A306

RAMISH, Dana W., President and Chief Executive Officer, Forbes Regional Hospital, Monroeville, PA, p. A361

RAMPAGE, Bruce E., President and Chief Executive Officer, Saint Anthony Hospital and Health Centers, Michigan City, IN, p. A146

RAMSAY, John, Administrator, Warren Memorial Hospital, Friend, NE, p. A264

RAMSEY, Barbara, Ph.D., Chief Executive Officer, Lincoln Regional Center, Lincoln, NE, p. A265

RAMSEY, Steve, Interim Chief Executive Officer, Powell Hospital, Powell, WY, p. A472

RANDALL, Foster, Administrator and Chief Executive Officer, LAC–King–Drew Medical Center, Los Angeles, CA, p. A50

RANDALL, Kenneth W., Administrator, Scenic Mountain Medical Center, Big Spring, TX, p. A402

RANDALL, Malcom, Director, Veterans Affairs Medical Center, Gainesville, FL, p. A88

RANERI, Joni K., Administrator, Healthsouth Rehabilitation Institute of Tucson, Tucson, AZ, p. A27

RANEY, James Edward, President and Chief Executive Officer, United Health Group, Appleton, WI, p. B144

RANGE, Richard L., Administrator, Baldwin Hospital, Baldwin, WI, p. A460

RANGE, Robert P., President and Chief Executive Officer, Grace Hospital, Cleveland, OH, p. A326

RANK, James T., Administrator, Bothwell Regional Health Center, Sedalia, MO, p. A255

RANKIN III, Fred M., President and Chief Executive Officer, Mary Washington Hospital, Fredericksburg, VA, p. A441

RANSDELL, Lewis A., Administrator, Vencor Hospital–Fort Lauderdale, Fort Lauderdale, FL, p. A87

RAPAPORT, Gary D., Administrator and Chief Executive Officer, Oak Valley District Hospital, Oakdale, CA, p. A55

RAPAPORT, Morton I., M.D., President and Chief Executive Officer, University of Maryland Medical System, Baltimore, MD, p. A198

RAPP, Larry, Chief Medical and Executive Officer, Grant County Health Center, Elbow Lake, MN, p. A228

RAPP, Peter, Senior Vice President and Administrator, Fairview–University Medical Center, Minneapolis, MN, p. A231

RAPP, Phillip J., President and Chief Executive Officer, St. Francis at Salina, Salina, KS, p. A169

RASH, Marty, President and Chief Executive Officer, Principal Hospital Group, Brentwood, TN, p. B122

RASMUSSEN, David J., Administrator, OMH Medical Center, Okmulgee, OK, p. A344

RASMUSSEN, Kyle, Administrator, Bridges Medical Services, Ada, MN, p. A226

RASMUSSEN, William C., Chief Executive Officer, Valley Community Hospital, Santa Maria, CA, p. A64

RATHBONE, Thomas A., President and Chief Executive Officer, Health Hill Hospital for Children, Cleveland, OH, p. A326

RAU, John, President, Stevens Community Medical Center, Morris, MN, p. A232

RAVENBERG, Larry, Administrator, Ely–Bloomenson Community Hospital, Ely, MN, p. A228

RAY, Donald L., Chief Administrative Officer, Grenada Lake Medical Center, Grenada, MS, p. A239

RAY, K. Dwayne, Administrator and Chief Executive Officer, Garland Community Hospital, Garland, TX, p. A411

RAY, William K., President and Chief Executive Officer, Methodist Hospital of Hattiesburg, Hattiesburg, MS, p. A239

RAYNOR, James E., Chief Executive Officer, Columbia Raleigh Community Hospital, Raleigh, NC, p. A315

READ, J. Larry, President, St. Luke's Hospital, Jacksonville, FL, p. A89

REAGAN, Jim, M.D., Administrator, Morris County Hospital, Council Grove, KS, p. A162

REAMER, Roger
Administrator, Brown County Hospital, Ainsworth, NE, p. A262
Administrator, Butler County Health Care Center, David City, NE, p. A263

REAMS, Betty J., Executive Director, Piggott Community Hospital, Piggott, AR, p. A34

REARDON, Robert, Hospital Services Administrator, Central Prison Hospital, Raleigh, NC, p. A315

REARDON, Timothy F., Chief Executive Officer, Ira Davenport Memorial Hospital, Bath, NY, p. A289

REASBECK, Suzanne, President and Chief Executive Officer, Flaget Memorial Hospital, Bardstown, KY, p. A172

REAT, Matthew J., Administrator, DeBaca General Hospital, Fort Sumner, NM, p. A286

REBER, James P., President, St. Rita's Medical Center, Lima, OH, p. A331

REDDING, Jim D.
Chief Executive Officer, Memorial Medical Center, Woodstock, IL, p. A139
Chief Executive Officer, Northern Illinois Medical Center, McHenry, IL, p. A134

REDDISH, Robert R., Administrator and Chief Executive Officer, Chicot County Memorial Hospital, Lake Village, AR, p. A32

REDDOCH Jr., James F., Director, Bryce Hospital, Tuscaloosa, AL, p. A18

REDMOND, Lisa, Chief Executive Officer, BHC College Meadows Hospital, Lenexa, KS, p. A166

REECE, David A., President, MidMichigan Regional Medical Center, Midland, MI, p. A220

REECE, Morris D., Director, Carilion Giles Memorial Hospital, Pearisburg, VA, p. A444

REECER, Jeff, Chief Executive Officer, D. M. Cogdell Memorial Hospital, Snyder, TX, p. A427

REED, Greg, Administrator, Eldora Regional Medical Center, Eldora, IA, p. A154

REED, Harold, Administrator, Fayette Medical Center, Fayette, AL, p. A14

REED, Jan A., CPA, Administrator, Electra Memorial Hospital, Electra, TX, p. A409

REED, Joy, R.N., Administrator, Ottawa County Hospital, Minneapolis, KS, p. A167

REED, Robert J., President, Mid–Island Hospital, Bethpage, NY, p. A289

REED, Ronald R., President and Chief Executive Officer, Mercy Hospital, Iowa City, IA, p. A155

REED, Steven B., President and Chief Executive Officer, Columbia Women's Hospital–Indianapolis, Indianapolis, IN, p. A144

REED, Timothy A., Administrator, Kaiser Foundation Hospital, Bellflower, CA, p. A38

REEDER, Steve, Chief Executive Officer, Helena Regional Medical Center, Helena, AR, p. A31

REEDER III, Sylvester L., President and Chief Executive Officer, Erlanger Medical Center, Chattanooga, TN, p. A387

REEK, Thomas F., Chief Executive Officer, Cuyuna Regional Medical Center, Crosby, MN, p. A228

REES, Ron R., Administrator, Halifax Community Health System, Daytona Beach, FL, p. A85

REESE, James, CHE, Administrator, Stephens Memorial Hospital, Breckenridge, TX, p. A402

REESE, Sandra, Administrator, Lower Umpqua Hospital District, Reedsport, OR, p. A351

REEVES, Becky, Administrator, North Shore Psychiatric Hospital, Slidell, LA, p. A191

REEVES, Luther E., Chief Executive Officer, Appling Healthcare System, Baxley, GA, p. A105

REEVES, Stephen C., Superintendent, Fulton State Hospital, Fulton, MO, p. A247

REGAN, James, Ph.D., Chief Executive Officer, Hudson River Psychiatric Center, Poughkeepsie, NY, p. A303

REGEHR, Stan, President and Chief Executive Officer, Memorial Hospital, McPherson, KS, p. A166

REGLING, Anne M., Regional Executive, Grace Hospital, Detroit, MI, p. A214

REIBER, Doug, Administrator, Kearney County Community Hospital, Minden, NE, p. A265

REID, David M., Administrator, Clay County Medical Center, West Point, MS, p. A244

REIF, Richard A., President and Chief Executive Officer, Doylestown Hospital, Doylestown, PA, p. A356

REINER, Steven S., Administrator, Kearny County Hospital, Lakin, KS, p. A165

REINERTSEN, James, M.D., Chief Executive Officer, Methodist Hospital HealthSystem Minnesota, Saint Louis Park, MN, p. A234

REINHARD, James S., M.D., Director, Catawba Hospital, Catawba, VA, p. A439

REINHARDT, J. Rudy, Administrator, Hendry Regional Medical Center, Clewiston, FL, p. A85

REINITZ, Marlyn, Administrator, Community Memorial Hospital, Humboldt, NE, p. A265

REITER, Steven B., Administrator, Shriners Hospitals for Children, Houston, Houston, TX, p. A415

REITINGER, Thomas A., President and Chief Executive Officer, Mercy Hospital Medical Center, Des Moines, IA, p. A154

REKER, Douglas J., Administrator and Chief Executive Officer, Glacial Ridge Hospital, Glenwood, MN, p. A229

REMBIS, Michael A., Chief Executive Officer, John F. Kennedy Memorial Hospital, Indio, CA, p. A46

REMILLARD, John R., President, Aurelia Osborn Fox Memorial Hospital, Oneonta, NY, p. A301

RENANDER, Dennis J.
President and Chief Executive Officer, Mercy Health Services North–Grayling, Grayling, MI, p. A217
President and Chief Executive Officer, Mercy Health Services–North, Cadillac, MI, p. A213

RENFORD, Edward J., President and Chief Executive Officer, Grady Memorial Hospital, Atlanta, GA, p. A104

RENICK, Bill, Administrator, Holly Springs Memorial Hospital, Holly Springs, MS, p. A239

RENNER, Steven W., President and Chief Executive Officer, Gettysburg Hospital, Gettysburg, PA, p. A358

RENSHAW, Dee
Administrator, Integris Baptist Regional Health Center, Miami, OK, p. A343
Administrator, Integris Grove General Hospital, Grove, OK, p. A341

RENTAS, Roberto A., Administrator, Hospital De Damas, Ponce, PR, p. A476

RENTFRO, Larry D., FACHE, Chief Executive Officer, Lancaster Memorial Hospital, Lancaster, WI, p. A464

RENTZ, Norman G., President, Cannon Memorial Hospital, Pickens, SC, p. A380

REPA, George, Chief Executive Officer, Delta Regional Medical Center, Greenville, MS, p. A239

RESNICK, Peter V., Executive Director, Dearborn County Hospital, Lawrenceburg, IN, p. A146

RESSLER, Rickie L., R.N., Interim President, New Ulm Medical Center, New Ulm, MN, p. A232

RETTALIATA, Marilyn R., President and Chief Executive Officer, Pocono Medical Center, East Stroudsburg, PA, p. A357

REVELS, Thomas R., President and Chief Executive Officer, Cabarrus Memorial Hospital, Concord, NC, p. A310

REYBURN Jr., John A.
Commander, U. S. Air Force Hospital, Hill AFB, UT, p. A433
Commander, U. S. Air Force Hospital, Vandenberg AFB, CA, p. A67

REYES, Arnold, Administrator, U. S. Penitentiary Infirmary, Lewisburg, PA, p. A360

REYNOLDS, Britt T., Chief Executive Officer, Columbia Hospital Georgetown, Georgetown, KY, p. A174

REYNOLDS, R. Dale, Chief Executive Officer and Administrator, BHC Montevista Hospital, Las Vegas, NV, p. A270

REYNOLDS, Stephen Curtis
President and Chief Executive Officer, Baptist Memorial Health Care Corporation, Memphis, TN, p. B68
President and Chief Executive Officer, Baptist Memorial Hospital, Memphis, TN, p. A393

RHEAULT, LeRoy E., President and Chief Executive Officer, Via Christi Health System, Wichita, KS, p. B148

RHINE, Scott, Administrator and Chief Executive Officer, Lompoc District Hospital, Lompoc, CA, p. A48

RHINEHART, Jennie, Administrator, Community Hospital, Tallassee, AL, p. A18

RHOADS, Gary R., President and Chief Executive Officer, Lock Haven Hospital, Lock Haven, PA, p. A360

RHODES, J. Gary, Chief Operating Officer, Kane Community Hospital, Kane, PA, p. A359

RHYNE, Robert R., D.D.S., Director, Veterans Affairs Medical Center, Grand Junction, CO, p. A73

RHYNER, Warren, Senior Vice President, Altoona Hospital, Altoona, PA, p. A353

RICCI, David A., President and Chief Executive Officer, Germantown Hospital and Medical Center, Philadelphia, PA, p. A364

RICCIARDI, J. M., Commanding Officer, U. S. Naval Hospital, Agana, GU, p. A474

RICE, Alan J., President, Simi Valley Hospital and Health Care Services, Simi Valley, CA, p. A65

RICE, David O., President, Haywood Regional Medical Center, Clyde, NC, p. A310

RICE, Kathleen A., Site Administrator, Meridia South Pointe Hospital, Warrensville Heights, OH, p. A336

RICE, Thomas R.
President and Chief Operation Officer, Integris Baptist Medical Center, Oklahoma City, OK, p. A344
President and Chief Operation Officer, Integris Southwest Medical Center, Oklahoma City, OK, p. A344

RICE, Tim, Administrator, Greater Staples Hospital and Care Center, Staples, MN, p. A235

RICHARD, Robert J., Administrator, People's Memorial Hospital of Buchanan County, Independence, IA, p. A155

RICHARDS, Joan K.
President, Crozer–Chester Medical Center, Upland, PA, p. A370
President, Delaware County Memorial Hospital, Drexel Hill, PA, p. A356

RICHARDS, Randy R., Chief Executive Officer, Permian General Hospital, Andrews, TX, p. A399

RICHARDS, Richard M., Administrator, Healthsouth Rehabilitation Hospital of Utah, Sandy, UT, p. A436

RICHARDS, Tom, Facility Director, Choate Mental Health and Developmental Center, Anna, IL, p. A123

RICHARDSON, A. D., Administrator, Hood Memorial Hospital, Amite, LA, p. A182

RICHARDSON, Darrel C., Chief Operating Officer, Kanakanak Hospital, Dillingham, AK, p. A20

RICHARDSON, J. E., Chief Executive Officer, Savoy Medical Center, Mamou, LA, p. A187

RICHARDSON, Mark D., President and Chief Executive Officer, Burlington Medical Center, Burlington, IA, p. A151

RICHARDSON, Patricia, President and Chief Operating Officer, Eagle River Memorial Hospital, Eagle River, WI, p. A461

RICHARDSON, R. D., President and Chief Executive Officer, Ashtabula County Medical Center, Ashtabula, OH, p. A323

RICHARDSON, William T., President and Chief Executive Officer, Tift General Hospital, Tifton, GA, p. A115

RICHEY, Don L., Administrator, Guadalupe Valley Hospital, Seguin, TX, p. A427

RICHMAN, Martin I., Executive Director, Community General Hospital of Sullivan County, Harris, NY, p. A293

RICHMOND, John W., President and Chief Executive Officer, Gentry County Memorial Hospital, Albany, MO, p. A245

RICHMOND, Kenneth A., President and Chief Executive Officer, Dorchester General Hospital, Cambridge, MD, p. A199

RICHTER, Thomas V., Administrator, Weskota Memorial Medical Center, Wessington Springs, SD, p. A386

RICKS, Charles S., D.D.S., President and Chief Executive Officer, Boston Regional Medical Center, Stoneham, MA, p. A210

RIDDELL, Andrew J., President and Chief Executive Officer, Atlanticare Medical Center, Lynn, MA, p. A207

RIDDLE, Brian L., Chief Executive Officer, Oconee Regional Medical Center, Milledgeville, GA, p. A112

RIDDLE, Marilyn M., Chief Executive Officer, Olympus Specialty Hospital–Springfield, Springfield, MA, p. A210

RIDENOUR, Richard T., USN, Commander, National Naval Medical Center, Bethesda, MD, p. A199

RIDLEY, Keith R., Chief Executive Officer, Kahuku Hospital, Kahuku, HI, p. A118

RIEDMANN, Gary P., President and Chief Executive Officer, St. Anthony Regional Hospital, Carroll, IA, p. A151

RIEGE, Michael J., Administrator, Virginia Gay Hospital, Vinton, IA, p. A159

RIEGER, Anne, R.N., Administrator, Elko General Hospital, Elko, NV, p. A270

RIES, Douglas A., President, Cardinal Glennon Children's Hospital, Saint Louis, MO, p. A253

RIES, William G., President, Lake Forest Hospital, Lake Forest, IL, p. A133

RIGDON, Henry, Executive Vice President, Northeast Georgia Medical Center, Gainesville, GA, p. A109

RIGHTER, Laura, Regional Administrator, St. John's Episcopal Hospital–Smithtown, Smithtown, NY, p. A304

RILEY, Carolyn E., Chief Executive Officer, Monroe County Medical Center, Tompkinsville, KY, p. A180

RILEY, Vernette, Administrator and Chief Executive Officer, Dallas County Hospital, Perry, IA, p. A158

RIMES, Dwight, Administrator, Ocean Springs Hospital, Ocean Springs, MS, p. A242

RINE, Thomas L., President and Chief Executive Officer, Columbia Southwestern Medical Center, Lawton, OK, p. A342

RINEHARDT, Mark, Chief Executive Officer, Lake City Hospital, Lake City, MN, p. A230

RINKER, Franklin M., President and Chief Executive Officer, Promina Gwinnett Hospital System, Lawrenceville, GA, p. A111

RIORDAN, William J.
President and Chief Executive Officer, St. Joseph Medical Center, Stamford, CT, p. A78
President and Chief Executive Officer, St. Vincent's Medical Center, Bridgeport, CT, p. A76

RIPPLE, Helen B., Administrator, Guam Memorial Hospital Authority, Tamuning, GU, p. A474

RISER, Donna, Administrator, Lackey Memorial Hospital, Forest, MS, p. A239

RISHEL, Kenn C., Administrator and Chief Executive Officer, Carthage Area Hospital, Carthage, NY, p. A290

RISK, Richard R., President and Chief Executive Officer, Advocate Health Care, Oakbrook, IL, p. B64

RISON, R. H., Warden, U. S. Medical Center for Federal Prisoners, Springfield, MO, p. A255

RITER, Pamela M., R.N., Administrator, Vencor Hospital–St Petersburg, Saint Petersburg, FL, p. A99

RITTENHOUSE, Vivian M., Vice President and Market Leader, Kaiser Foundation Hospital and Rehabilitation Center, Vallejo, CA, p. A67

RITZ, Robert P., President and Chief Executive Officer, Monongalia General Hospital, Morgantown, WV, p. A457

RIVERA, Maria Mercedes, Administrator, Hospital Del Maestro, San Juan, PR, p. A476

ROACH, Joseph, Executive Director, Memorial Hospital of Martinsville and Henry County, Martinsville, VA, p. A442

ROADMAN II, Charles H., Deputy Surgeon General, Department of the Air Force, Washington, DC, p. B89

ROARK, Ruth Ann, Administrator, Sequoyah Memorial Hospital, Sallisaw, OK, p. A345

ROBBINS, Alan H., M.D., President, New England Baptist Hospital, Boston, MA, p. A204

ROBBINS, B. C., Superintendent, Georgia Mental Health Institute, Atlanta, GA, p. A104

ROBBINS, Wes, Chief Executive Officer, Charter by–the–Sea Behavioral Health System, Saint Simons Island, GA, p. A113

ROBERSON, Madeleine L., Chief Executive Officer, Columbia Women's and Children's Hospital, Lafayette, LA, p. A186

ROBERTS, Carolyn C., President, Copley Hospital, Morrisville, VT, p. A437

ROBERTS, Deborah, Administrator, Lawrence County Hospital, Monticello, MS, p. A242

ROBERTS, Gregory, Chief Executive Officer, Marlboro Psychiatric Hospital, Marlboro, NJ, p. A279

ROBERTS, Jean E., Administrator, Mark Reed Hospital, McCleary, WA, p. A450

ROBERTS, John W., President and Chief Executive Officer, Union Regional Medical Center, Monroe, NC, p. A314

ROBERTS, Jonathan, Dr.PH, President and Chief Executive Officer, Medical Center of Louisiana at New Orleans, New Orleans, LA, p. A188

ROBERTS, Kenneth D., President, John T. Mather Memorial Hospital, Port Jefferson, NY, p. A302

ROBERTS, Pamela W., Administrator, Baptist Memorial Hospital–Booneville, Booneville, MS, p. A237

ROBERTS, Shane, Administrator, St. Luke Community Hospital, Ronan, MT, p. A260

ROBERTS, Shirley R., Administrator, Washington County Regional Hospital, Sandersville, GA, p. A113

ROBERTS, David W., Commanding Officer, Kimbrough Army Community Hospital, Fort George G Meade, MD, p. A200

ROBERTS Jr., George T., Chief Executive Officer, Henderson Memorial Hospital, Henderson, TX, p. A412

ROBERTSON, B. W., Administrator, Parkview Hospital, Wheeler, TX, p. A431

ROBERTSON, Bob, Administrator, Trinity Hospital, Weaverville, CA, p. A68

ROBERTSON, David, Chief Executive Officer, Duncan Regional Hospital, Duncan, OK, p. A340

ROBERTSON, Gary W., Administrator, Niobrara County Hospital District, Lusk, WY, p. A472

ROBERTSON, Jeffrey J., Administrator, Lakeview Hospital, Stillwater, MN, p. A235

ROBERTSON, John L., Chief Executive Officer, Medical Center Enterprise, Enterprise, AL, p. A13

ROBERTSON, Thomas L., President and Chief Executive Officer, Carilion Health System, Roanoke, VA, p. B74

ROBERTSON, William G., Senior Executive Officer, Shawnee Mission Medical Center, Shawnee Mission, KS, p. A169

ROBERTSON Jr., James E., Chief Executive Officer, Clearwater Valley Hospital, Orofino, ID, p. A121

ROBERTSTAD, John R., President and Chief Executive Officer, Bixby Medical Center, Adrian, MI, p. A212

ROBINSON, Anna, Administrator, Kaiser Foundation Hospital, Walnut Creek, CA, p. A68

ROBINSON, Beverly, Administrator, Swain County Hospital, Bryson City, NC, p. A309

ROBINSON, Brian C., Chief Executive Officer, Columbia North Florida Regional Medical Center, Gainesville, FL, p. A88

ROBINSON, Edward P., Administrator, Community Hospital, Munster, IN, p. A147

ROBINSON, Glenn, Chief Executive Officer, Sharpstown General Hospital, Houston, TX, p. A415

ROBINSON, Margaret, Administrator, Anamosa Community Hospital, Anamosa, IA, p. A151

ROBINSON, Michael–David, Executive Vice President and Administrator, Richmond Memorial Hospital, Richmond, VA, p. A445

ROBINSON, Phillip D., Chief Executive Officer, Columbia J. F. K. Medical Center, Atlantis, FL, p. A83

ROBINSON, Richard F., Director, Veterans Affairs Medical Center, Fayetteville, AR, p. A30

ROBINSON, Richard H., Chief Executive Officer, Irvine Medical Center, Irvine, CA, p. A46

ROBINSON, W. D., Chief Executive Officer, Bartlett Memorial Medical Center, Sapulpa, OK, p. A345

ROBINSON Sr., James M., Administrator, Hereford Regional Medical Center, Hereford, TX, p. A413

ROBY, William J., Executive Vice President, Mountain Manor Treatment Center, Emmitsburg, MD, p. A200

ROCKER, Watson W., President and Chief Executive Officer, Jenkins County Hospital, Millen, GA, p. A112

ROCKLAGE, Mary Roch, President and Chief Executive Officer, Sisters of Mercy Health System–St. Louis, Saint Louis, MO, p. B134

ROCKWOOD Jr., John M., President, Munson Healthcare, Traverse City, MI, p. B117

RODDIE, Jim B., Administrator, Schleicher County Medical Center, Eldorado, TX, p. A409

RODGERS, Edward, Chief Executive Officer, Yoakum County Hospital, Denver City, TX, p. A408

RODGERS, Raymond L., Administrator, Public Health Service Indian Hospital, Albuquerque, NM, p. A284

RODMAN, George, Director, Veterans Affairs Medical Center, Biloxi, MS, p. A237

RODNEY, Nelson, Administrator, Harbor View, Miami, FL, p. A93

RODRIGUEZ, Roberto, Executive Director, Lincoln Medical and Mental Health Center, New York, NY, p. A297

RODRIGUEZ, Roy, Chief Executive Officer, Bayview Hospital and Mental Health System, Chula Vista, CA, p. A40

RODZENKO, Michael, President and Chief Executive Officer, South Nassau Communities Hospital, Oceanside, NY, p. A301

ROE Jr., Louis G., Administrator, Wise ARH Hospital, Wise, VA, p. A447

ROEBACK, Jason, President, Frazier Rehabilitation Center, Louisville, KY, p. A177

ROEDER, John R., President, Providence Hospital, Mobile, AL, p. A16

ROGAN, Peter G., Chief Executive Officer, Edgewater Medical Center, Chicago, IL, p. A125

ROGERS, Bryan R., President and Chief Executive Officer, Foothill Presbyterian Hospital–Morris L. Johnston Memorial, Glendora, CA, p. A45

ROGERS, Charles L., President, Cushing Memorial Hospital, Leavenworth, KS, p. A165

ROGERS, Christopher J., Administrator, Auburn Memorial Hospital, Auburn, NY, p. A288

ROGERS, James E., President and Chief Executive Officer, Columbia Audubon Hospital, Louisville, KY, p. A177

ROGERS, James H., FACHE, President and Chief Executive Officer, Roper Hospital, Charleston, SC, p. A376

ROGERS, Joel P., Chief Executive Officer, Westbrook Community Hospital, Westbrook, ME, p. A196

ROGERS, Richard
Senior Vice President Operations, Mercy Medical Center, Springfield, OH, p. A335
Senior Vice President, Mercy Memorial Hospital, Urbana, OH, p. A336

ROGERS, Tracy A., President and Chief Executive Officer, Columbia Suburban Hospital, Louisville, KY, p. A177

ROGERSON, R. E., Warden, Iowa Medical and Classification Center, Oakdale, IA, p. A157

ROGLER, Diane L., President and Chief Executive Officer, Nicholas H. Noyes Memorial Hospital, Dansville, NY, p. A291

ROGOLS, Kevin L., President and Chief Executive Officer, Finley Hospital, Dubuque, IA, p. A154

ROHALEY, Richard L., President and Chief Executive Officer, Jackson General Hospital, Ripley, WV, p. A458

ROHAN, Heather J., Chief Executive Officer, Columbia Pompano Beach Medical Center, Pompano Beach, FL, p. A97

ROHRER, John E., Administrator, Prosser Memorial Hospital, Prosser, WA, p. A451

ROHRICH, George A., Administrator, Pembina County Memorial Hospital and Wedgewood Manor, Cavalier, ND, p. A319

ROJEK, Kenneth J., Chief Executive, Lutheran General Hospital, Park Ridge, IL, p. A136

ROME, Philip H., Administrator, Walter Olin Moss Regional Medical Center, Lake Charles, LA, p. A186

ROMERO, Dudley, President and Chief Executive Officer, Our Lady of Lourdes Regional Medical Center, Lafayette, LA, p. A186

ROMERO, Marcella A., Administrator, Espanola Hospital, Espanola, NM, p. A285

ROMOFF, Jeffrey A., President, University of Pittsburgh Medical Center, Pittsburgh, PA, p. A367

RONA, J. Michael, Vice President and Executive Administrator, Virginia Mason Medical Center, Seattle, WA, p. A453

RONSTROM, Stephen F., President and Chief Executive Officer, Hays Medical Center, Hays, KS, p. A164

ROODMAN, Richard D., Chief Executive Officer, Valley Medical Center, Renton, WA, p. A452

ROONEY, Ronald K., President, Arkansas Methodist Hospital, Paragould, AR, p. A34

ROOT, Darwin E., Administrator, Harrison Memorial Hospital, Cynthiana, KY, p. A173

RORAFF, Greg, President and Chief Executive Officer, Memorial Hospital of Taylor County, Medford, WI, p. A464

ROSASCO Jr., Edward J., President, Mercy Hospital, Miami, FL, p. A93

ROSE, J. Anthony, President and Chief Executive Officer, Catawba Memorial Hospital, Hickory, NC, p. A313

ROSE, Lance H., FACHE, President and Chief Executive Officer, Centre Community Hospital, State College, PA, p. A369

ROSE, Renee, President and Chief Executive Officer, Horizon Healthcare, Inc., Milwaukee, WI, p. B104

ROSEBOROUGH, James W., Director, John J. Pershing Veterans Affairs Medical Center, Poplar Bluff, MO, p. A252

ROSEN, David P., President, Jamaica Hospital Medical Center, New York, NY, p. A297

ROSENBACH, Lynn M., Chief Executive Officer, Charter Behavioral Health System of Nevada, Las Vegas, NV, p. A270

ROSENBERG, Douglas O., President and Chief Executive Officer, Howard Young Medical Center, Woodruff, WI, p. A470

ROSENBERG, Leroy J., Executive Director, West Jersey Hospital–Marlton, Marlton, NJ, p. A279

ROSENTHAL, David S., M.D., Director, Stillman Infirmary, Harvard University Health Services, Cambridge, MA, p. A205

ROSENVALL, Greg, Administrator, Gunnison Valley Hospital, Gunnison, UT, p. A433

ROSIN, David, M.D., Medical Director, Nevada Mental Health Institute, Sparks, NV, p. A271

ROSS, Archer R., Chief Executive Officer, Community Hospital of Rocky Mount, Rocky Mount, NC, p. A316

ROSS, David, Chief Executive Officer, Phelps County Regional Medical Center, Rolla, MO, p. A252

ROSS, David J., Administrator, White Mountain Communities Hospital, Springerville, AZ, p. A26

ROSS, Hank, Chief Executive Officer, Healthsouth Rehabilitation Hospital, Oklahoma City, OK, p. A343

ROSS, Harvey, Executive Director and Chief Executive Officer, Mediplex Rehabilitation–Denver, Thornton, CO, p. A75

ROSS, James E., FACHE, Chief Executive Officer, James Lawrence Kernan Hospital, Baltimore, MD, p. A197

ROSS, Joseph P., President and Chief Executive Officer, Memorial Hospital at Easton Maryland, Easton, MD, p. A200

ROSS, Kenneth R., Administrator, Carl Albert Indian Health Facility, Ada, OK, p. A339

ROSS, Miriam, Acting Administrator, Madison County Memorial Hospital, Madison, FL, p. A92

ROSS, Wayne R., Administrator, Garfield Memorial Hospital and Clinics, Panguitch, UT, p. A434

ROSS, Zeff, Administrator, Memorial Hospital West, Pembroke Pines, FL, p. A96

ROSS Jr., Semmes, Administrator, Franklin County Memorial Hospital, Meadville, MS, p. A241

ROSSETTI, Stephen J., Ph.D., President and Chief Executive Officer, Saint Luke Institute, Silver Spring, MD, p. A202

ROSSFELD, John, Administrator, University of Miami Hospital and Clinics, Miami, FL, p. A94

ROSSI, L. J., M.D., Chief Executive Officer, Hopedale Medical Complex, Hopedale, IL, p. A132

ROSSOW, James C., Administrator, Divine Providence Health Center, Ivanhoe, MN, p. A230

ROTERT, James, Administrator, Tyler Healthcare Center, Tyler, MN, p. A235

ROTH, Edward, Chief Executive Officer, Alliance Community Hospital, Alliance, OH, p. A323

ROTH, Gregory P., Executive Director, University Behavioral Center, Orlando, FL, p. A95

ROTH, Linda, Administrator, Keefe Memorial Hospital, Cheyenne Wells, CO, p. A70

ROTHLEIN Jr., Gerard J., President and Chief Executive Officer, Children's Medical Center, Tulsa, OK, p. A346

ROTHMAN, William, Chief Executive Officer, Healthsouth Chesapeake Rehabilitation Hospital, Salisbury, MD, p. A201

ROTHSTEIN, Ruth M.
Chief, Cook County Bureau of Health Services, Chicago, IL, p. B87
Hospital Director, Cook County Hospital, Chicago, IL, p. A125

ROURKE, Thomas E., Administrator, Glen Oaks Hospital, Greenville, TX, p. A412

ROWAN, John R., Director, Veterans Affairs Medical Center, Montgomery, AL, p. A16

ROWE, David B., Vice President and Administrator, Harris Methodist Southwest, Fort Worth, TX, p. A410

ROWE, Gary L., President and Chief Executive Officer, St. Catherine Hospital, Garden City, KS, p. A163

ROWE, John W., M.D., President, Mount Sinai Medical Center, New York, NY, p. A298

ROWE, Lavonne M., Administrator, Johnson County Hospital, Tecumseh, NE, p. A268

ROWLAND, Phil, Administrator, Cleveland Community Hospital, Cleveland, TN, p. A388

ROWLEY, William R., USN, Commander, Naval Medical Center, Portsmouth, VA, p. A444

ROWTON, William, Chief Executive Officer, Cozby–Germany Hospital, Grand Saline, TX, p. A411

ROYNAN, Joseph, Administrator, Northwestern Institute, Fort Washington, PA, p. A358

ROZEK, Thomas M., Senior Vice President, Children's Hospital of Michigan, Detroit, MI, p. A214

RUBERTE', Henry, Administrator, First Hospital Panamericano, Cidra, PR, p. A475

RUBIN, Harold, President and Chief Executive Officer, Memorial Hospital and Medical Center, Midland, TX, p. A421

RUCKDESCHEL, John C., M.D., Director and Chief Executive Officer, H. Lee Moffitt Cancer Center and Research Institute, Tampa, FL, p. A100

RUDEGEAIR, Bernard C., President and Chief Executive Officer, Hazleton–St. Joseph Medical Center, Hazleton, PA, p. A359

RUDES, Bryan F., Executive Director, Richard H. Hutchings Psychiatric Center, Syracuse, NY, p. A305

RUDES, Sarah F., Executive Director, Mohawk Valley Psychiatric Center, Utica, NY, p. A305

RUDNICK, Barry, M.D., Acting Clinical Director, Crownsville Hospital Center, Crownsville, MD, p. A199

RUELAS, Raul D., M.D., Administrator, Gulf Coast Treatment Center, Fort Walton Beach, FL, p. A87

RUFFERTY, Patrick W., Chief Executive Officer, Doctors Hospital of Manteca, Manteca, CA, p. A53

RUFFIN, Edward W., Administrator, Columbia Coliseum Psychiatric Hospital, Macon, GA, p. A111

RUFFNER, John, Administrator, Hemet Valley Medical Center, Hemet, CA, p. A46

RUFFOLO, Joseph A., President and Chief Executive Officer, Children's Hospital, Buffalo, NY, p. A290

RUMLEY, Darrell, Service Unit Director, U. S. Public Health Service Indian Hospital, Sells, AZ, p. A26

RUPIPER, Allen V., President, Adena Health System, Chillicothe, OH, p. A325

RUPP, William, M.D., President and Chief Executive Officer, Luther Hospital, Eau Claire, WI, p. A462

RUPPERT, James C., Regional Administrator, Alegent Health Mercy Hospital, Corning, IA, p. A152

RUSH, Domenica, Administrator, Sierra Vista Hospital, Truth or Consequences, NM, p. A287

RUSH, Donald J., Chief Executive Officer, Sidney Health Center, Sidney, MT, p. A260

RUSHING, R. Lynn, Chief Executive Officer, Brook Lane Psychiatric Center, Hagerstown, MD, p. A200

RUSHING, Winston, President, Columbia Memorial Hospital Jacksonville, Jacksonville, FL, p. A89

RUSKAN, Jeff, Administrator, Healthsouth Rehabilitation Hospital of Virginia, Richmond, VA, p. A445

RUSSEL, Kimberly A., President and Chief Executive Officer, Mary Greeley Medical Center, Ames, IA, p. A151

RUSSELL, Daniel F., President and Chief Executive Officer, Eastern Mercy Health System, Radnor, PA, p. B96

RUSSELL, James D. M., Chief Executive Officer, St. Mary's Hospital, Pierre, SD, p. A384

RUSSELL, Linda B., Chief Executive Officer, Columbia Woman's Hospital of Texas, Houston, TX, p. A414

RUSSELL, Mark R., President and Chief Executive Officer, Hospital Group of America, Wayne, PA, p. B104

RUSSELL, Tim, Administrator, Stillwater Community Hospital, Columbus, MT, p. A257

RUSSELL, Webster T., Chief Executive Officer, South Central Kansas Regional Medical Center, Arkansas City, KS, p. A161

RUTENBERG, Jack, Administrator, Villa Maria Hospital, North Miami, FL, p. A94

RUTKOWSKI, Robert, Chief Executive, South Suburban Hospital, Hazel Crest, IL, p. A131

RUTTER, David E., Administrator, Mahaska County Hospital, Oskaloosa, IA, p. A158

RUYLE, W. Kenneth, Director, Veterans Affairs Medical Center, Tuscaloosa, AL, p. A18

RUZYCKI, Frank C., Executive Director, Roosevelt Warm Springs Institute for Rehabilitation, Warm Springs, GA, p. A115

RYAN, Michael J., President and Chief Executive Officer, Nemaha Valley Community Hospital, Seneca, KS, p. A169

RYAN, Thomas E., President, Alamance Regional Medical Center, Burlington, NC, p. A309

RYAN, Timothy J., JD
President and Chief Executive Officer, Detroit–Macomb Hospital Corporation, Warren, MI, p. B95
President and Chief Executive Officer, Macomb Hospital Center, Warren, MI, p. A224

RYAN, Mary Jean, President and Chief Executive Officer, SSM Health Care System, Saint Louis, MO, p. B137

RYLE, Deborah L., Chief Executive Officer, Round Rock Hospital, Round Rock, TX, p. A424

S

SABA, Francis M., President and Chief Executive Officer, Milford–Whitinsville Regional Hospital, Milford, MA, p. A208

SABIN, Margaret D., Chief Executive Officer, Routt Memorial Hospital, Steamboat Springs, CO, p. A74

SABIN, Robert H., Medical Center Director, Veterans Affairs Medical Center, Saginaw, MI, p. A222

SABO, Michael A., Medical Director, Veterans Affairs Medical Center, New York, NY, p. A300

SABOL, Don J., Administrator, Hardin Memorial Hospital, Kenton, OH, p. A331

SACCO, Frank V., FACHE, Chief Executive Officer, Memorial Healthcare System, Los Angeles, FL, p. B114

SACKETT, John, Administrator, PorterCare Hospital–Avista, Louisville, CO, p. A74

SACKETT, Ronald, President, Hinsdale Hospital, Hinsdale, IL, p. A132

SACKETT, Walter, Senior Vice President and Administrator, St. Mary–Corwin Regional Medical Center, Pueblo, CO, p. A74

SADLACK, Frank J., Ph.D., Executive Director, La Hacienda Treatment Center, Hunt, TX, p. A416

SADLER, Blair L., President, Children's Hospital and Health Center, San Diego, CA, p. A60

SADVARY, Thomas J., FACHE, Senior Vice President and Administrator, Scottsdale Memorial Hospital–North, Scottsdale, AZ, p. A26

SAFIAN, Keith F., President and Chief Executive Officer, Phelps Memorial Hospital Center, Sleepy Hollow, NY, p. A304

SAGO, Glenn R., Administrator, Arkansas State Hospital, Little Rock, AR, p. A32

SAINER, Elliot A., President and Chief Executive Officer, College Health Enterprises, Huntington Beach, CA, p. B78

SALA Jr., Anthony S., Chief Executive Officer, Columbia Highland Hospital, Shreveport, LA, p. A190

SALANGER, Matthew J., President and Chief Executive Officer, United Health Services Hospitals–Binghamton, Binghamton, NY, p. A289

SALBER, M. Agnes, Prioress, Missionary Benedictine Sisters American Province, Norfolk, NE, p. B116

SALEAPAGA, Iotamo T., M.D., Director Health, Lyndon B. Johnson Tropical Medical Center, Pago Pago, AS, p. A474

SALERNO, Richard E., Chief Executive Officer, Austin Diagnostic Medical Center, Austin, TX, p. A399

SALERNO, Thomas A., Chief Executive Officer, Tempe St. Luke's Hospital, Tempe, AZ, p. A27

SALISBURY, Roger, Administrator, Hodgeman County Health Center, Jetmore, KS, p. A165

SALMON, Robert J.
Chief Executive Officer, Canby Community Health Services, Canby, MN, p. A227
Interim Administrator, Deuel County Memorial Hospital, Clear Lake, SD, p. A382

SALVANT, Darlene, Chief Executive Officer, BHC East Lake Hospital, New Orleans, LA, p. A188

SAMET, Kenneth A., President, Washington Hospital Center, Washington, DC, p. A82

SAMPLE, James L., Chief Executive Officer, Columbia Andalusia Hospital, Andalusia, AL, p. A11

SAMPSON, Arthur J., President and Chief Executive Officer, Newport Hospital, Newport, RI, p. A373

SAMPSON, Gladiola, Acting Executive Director, Queens Hospital Center, New York, NY, p. A299

SAMS, Kurt, Interim Administrator, Carrie Tingley Hospital, Albuquerque, NM, p. A284

SANCHEZ, Jose R., Executive Director, Metropolitan Hospital Center, New York, NY, p. A298

SANDBERG, David, Administrator, Stanley Community Hospital, Stanley, ND, p. A322

SANDER, Larry J., FACHE, Director, Veterans Affairs Medical Center–Louisville, Louisville, KY, p. A178

SANDERS, Diwana, Administrator, Jefferson County Hospital, Fayette, MS, p. A239

SANDERS, Steve, Vice President, Chief Executive Officer and Administrator, Memorial Hospital–The Woodlands, The Woodlands, TX, p. A429

SANDERS, Jimmy, Administrator, Winn Army Community Hospital, Fort Stewart, GA, p. A109

SANDIFER, C. Philip, Administrator, Island Hospital, Anacortes, WA, p. A448

SANDLIN, Keith, Chief Executive Officer, Columbia Cartersville Medical Center, Cartersville, GA, p. A106

SANDOVAL, Donald D., FACHE, President and Chief Executive Officer, Indiana Hospital, Indiana, PA, p. A359

SANNER, Charlotte K., M.D., Director Health Service, Simpson Infirmary, Wellesley College, Wellesley, MA, p. A211

SANTIAGO–VEGA, Francisco, Consultor, Lafayette Hospital, Arroyo, PR, p. A474

SANZO, Anthony M., President, Allegheny General Hospital, Pittsburgh, PA, p. A365

SANZONE, Raymond D., Executive Director, Tewksbury Hospital, Tewksbury, MA, p. A210

SARDONE, Frank J.
President and Chief Executive Officer, Bronson Healthcare Group, Inc., Kalamazoo, MI, p. B73
President and Chief Executive Officer, Bronson Methodist Hospital, Kalamazoo, MI, p. A218
President, Bronson Vicksburg Hospital, Vicksburg, MI, p. A224

SARKAR, George A., JD, Executive Director, Manhattan Eye, Ear and Throat Hospital, New York, NY, p. A298

SARKIS, Lucy, M.D., Executive Director, South Beach Psychiatric Center, New York, NY, p. A299

SARLE, C. Richard, President and Chief Executive Officer, Carrier Foundation, Belle Mead, NJ, p. A275

SASSER, Wayne, Administrator, Crenshaw Baptist Hospital, Luverne, AL, p. A15

SATALA, Taylor, Service Unit Director, U. S. Public Health Services Indian Hospital, Keams Canyon, AZ, p. A23

SATCHER, Richard H., Chief Executive Officer, Aiken Regional Medical Center, Aiken, SC, p. A375

SATO, Jim, Chief Executive Officer, Bear Valley Community Hospital, Big Bear Lake, CA, p. A38

SATTERWHITE, Robin, Administrator, W. J. Mangold Memorial Hospital, Lockney, TX, p. A419

SATZGER, Bruce G., Administrator and Chief Executive Officer, Commmunity Hospital of San Bernardino, San Bernardino, CA, p. A60

SAULS, Randy
Interim Administrator, Clinch Memorial Hospital, Homerville, GA, p. A110
Administrator, Louis Smith Memorial Hospital, Lakeland, GA, p. A110

SAULTERS, W. Dale, Administrator, Winston Medical Center, Louisville, MS, p. A241

SAUNDERS, Donald F., President, Androscoggin Valley Hospital, Berlin, NH, p. A272

SAUNDERS, Linda, Administrator, Guyan Valley Hospital, Logan, WV, p. A457

SAWYER, Thomas H., President and Chief Executive Officer, General Health System, Baton Rouge, LA, p. B98

SAWYERS Jr., Irving B., Chief Executive Officer, Charter Real Behavioral Health System, San Antonio, TX, p. A425

SCHADT, Alton M., Executive Director, Warren General Hospital, Warren, PA, p. A370

SCHAENGOLD, Phillip S., JD, Chief Executive Officer, George Washington University Hospital, Washington, DC, p. A81

SCHAFER, Michael, Chief Executive Officer, Community Memorial Hospital and Nursing Home, Spooner, WI, p. A469

SCHAFFER, Arnold R., Chief Executive Officer, Encino–Tarzana Regional Medical Center, Los Angeles, CA, p. A49

SCHAFFNER, Leroy, Chief Executive Officer, Coon Memorial Hospital and Home, Dalhart, TX, p. A405

SCHAFFNER, Linda D., R.N., Vice President and Administrator, Bethesda Oak Hospital, Cincinnati, OH, p. A325

SCHANDLER, Jon B., President and Chief Executive Officer, White Plains Hospital Center, White Plains, NY, p. A307

SCHANWALD, Pamela R., Chief Executive Officer, Children's Home of Pittsburgh, Pittsburgh, PA, p. A365

SCHAPER, Robert F., President and Chief Executive Officer, Tomball Regional Hospital, Tomball, TX, p. A429

SCHAPPER, Robert A., Chief Executive Officer, Mount Sinai Medical Center, Cleveland, OH, p. A327

SCHAUM, James H., President and Chief Executive Officer, Allen Memorial Hospital, Oberlin, OH, p. A333

SCHEFFER, Richard H., President, Wing Memorial Hospital and Medical Centers, Palmer, MA, p. A209

SCHEIB, Garry L., President, Graduate Health System–Rancocas Hospital, Willingboro, NJ, p. A283

SCHERLIN, Marlys, Administrator, Greater Community Hospital, Creston, IA, p. A153

SCHERR, Morris L., Executive Vice President, Taylor Manor Hospital, Ellicott City, MD, p. A200

SCHERTZ, David A.
Administrator, Saint Anthony Medical Center, Rockford, IL, p. A137
Administrator, Saint Joseph Hospital, Belvidere, IL, p. A124

SCHIFFERLI, Thomas F., President and Chief Executive Officer, De Graff Memorial Hospital, North Tonawanda, NY, p. A301

SCHIMSCHEINER, Mary Joel, Chief Executive Officer, Kenmore Mercy Hospital, Kenmore, NY, p. A293

SCHINTZ, Conrad W., Senior Vice President Operations, Geisinger Wyoming Valley Medical Center, Wilkes–Barre, PA, p. A371

SCHIRMER, William E., FACHE, Interim Chief Executive Officer, Crawford Memorial Hospital, Robinson, IL, p. A137

SCHLAUTMAN, Jacolyn M., Executive Vice President and Administrator, St. Joseph's Hospital, Breese, IL, p. A124

SCHMELTER, Robert, President, Community Hospital of Ottawa, Ottawa, IL, p. A135

SCHMIDT, Barbara, Chief Executive Officer, THC–Fort Worth, Fort Worth, TX, p. A410

SCHMIDT, Craig W. C., President and Chief Executive Officer, Community Health Network, Berlin, WI, p. A460

SCHMIDT, Gene E., President, Hutchinson Hospital Corporation, Hutchinson, KS, p. A164

SCHMIDT, Michael A., President and Chief Executive Officer, Saint Joseph's Hospital, Marshfield, WI, p. A464

SCHMIDT, Paul R., President and Chief Executive Officer, Tawas St. Joseph Hospital, Tawas City, MI, p. A223

SCHMIDT, Richard T., Executive Director, Decatur Hospital, Decatur, GA, p. A108

SCHMIDT, Robert, Chief Executive Officer, Tweeten Lutheran Health Care Center, Spring Grove, MN, p. A235

SCHMIDT, Steve, Administrator and Chief Executive Officer, Lancaster Community Hospital, Lancaster, CA, p. A48

SCHMIDT, Timothy E., Interim Chief Executive Officer, Harris Hospital, Newport, AR, p. A33

SCHMIDT Jr., Richard O., President, Chief Executive Officer and General Counsel, Kenosha Hospital and Medical Center, Kenosha, WI, p. A463

SCHMOYER, Carol, Administrator, Wickenburg Regional Hospital, Wickenburg, AZ, p. A28

SCHNEDLER, Lisa Wagner, Administrator, Van Buren County Hospital, Keosauqua, IA, p. A156

SCHNEIDER, Barry S., President and Chief Executive Officer, Columbia Olympia Fields Osteopathic Hospital and Medical Center, Olympia Fields, IL, p. A135

SCHNEIDER, Carol, Chief Executive, Christ Hospital and Medical Center, Oak Lawn, IL, p. A135

SCHNEIDER, Charles F., President, Day Kimball Hospital, Putnam, CT, p. A78

SCHNEIDER, Cynthia K., Administrator, Greeley County Hospital, Tribune, KS, p. A170

SCHNEIDER, David R., Executive Director, Langlade Memorial Hospital, Antigo, WI, p. A460

SCHNEIDER, Mark E., Chief Executive Officer, Rivendell Psychiatric Center, Benton, AR, p. A29

SCHNEIDER, Thomas R., Administrator, Shriners Hospitals for Children, Shreveport, Shreveport, LA, p. A191

SCHOAPS, Stephen R., Chief Executive Officer, Seminole Municipal Hospital, Seminole, OK, p. A345

SCHOEN, William J., President, Health Management Associates, Naples, FL, p. B100

SCHOENHOLTZ, Jack C., M.D., Medical Director and Administrator, Rye Hospital Center, Rye, NY, p. A304

SCHOLTEN, Randall J., Chief Executive Officer, Curry General Hospital, Gold Beach, OR, p. A349

SCHON, John, Administrator and Chief Executive Officer, Dickinson County Healthcare System, Iron Mountain, MI, p. A218

SCHONHORN, Robert, President, Matheny School and Hospital, Peapack, NJ, p. A280

SCHOPPMAN, Billie Anne, R.N., Administrator, Vencor Hospital–Los Angeles, Los Angeles, CA, p. A52

SCHOTT, Carol, Administrator, Odessa Memorial Hospital, Odessa, WA, p. A451

SCHRADER, Michael E., President and Chief Executive Officer, Wyoming Medical Center, Casper, WY, p. A471

SCHRECK, Edward, President and Chief Executive Officer, Eden Hospital Medical Center, Castro Valley, CA, p. A39

SCHREEG, Timothy M., President and Chief Executive Officer, Jasper County Hospital, Rensselaer, IN, p. A148

SCHROEDER, Edward G., President and Chief Executive Officer, St. Joseph's Medical Center, Stockton, CA, p. A66

SCHROEDER, Fred F., Administrator, Converse County Memorial Hospital, Douglas, WY, p. A471

SCHRUPP, Richard, President and Chief Executive Officer, Mercy Hospital of Franciscan Sisters, Oelwein, IA, p. A157

SCHUBERT, John D., Administrator and Chief Executive Officer, Pinckneyville Community Hospital, Pinckneyville, IL, p. A136

SCHUESSLER, James P., President and Chief Executive Officer, All Saints Episcopal Hospital of Fort Worth, Fort Worth, TX, p. A409

SCHUETZ, Charles D., Chief Executive Officer, Columbia Kingwood Medical Center, Kingwood, TX, p. A418

SCHULER, G. Wayne, Executive Director, Madison County Medical Center, Canton, MS, p. A238

SCHULER, William J., Chief Executive Officer, Portsmouth Regional Hospital and Pavilion, Portsmouth, NH, p. A274

SCHULLER, David E., M.D., Chief Executive Officer, Arthur G. James Cancer Hospital and Research Institute, Columbus, OH, p. A327

SCHULTE, James E., Administrator, Redwood Falls Municipal Hospital, Redwood Falls, MN, p. A233

SCHULTZ, Judson, Executive Director, Northwoods Hospital, Phelps, WI, p. A467

SCHULTZ, Michael, Chief Executive Officer, Redbud Community Hospital, Clearlake, CA, p. A40

SCHULZ, Charles, Chief Executive Officer, York General Hospital, York, NE, p. A269

SCHULZ, Larry A., President and Chief Executive Officer, St. Gabriel's Hospital, Little Falls, MN, p. A230

SCHUMACHER, Joseph L., Administrator, Calumet Medical Center, Chilton, WI, p. A461

SCHURMAN, Bruce A., President, Marianjoy Rehabilitation Hospital and Clinics, Wheaton, IL, p. A139

SCHURMEIER, L. Jon, President and Chief Executive Officer, Southwest General Health Center, Middleburg Heights, OH, p. A333

SCHURRA, Ronald J., Chief Executive Officer, Holy Family Hospital, Spokane, WA, p. A453

SCHUSTER, Emmett, Administrator and Chief Executive Officer, Greenwood County Hospital, Eureka, KS, p. A163

SCHWARTEN, William L., Administrator, Washington County Memorial Hospital, Potosi, MO, p. A252

SCHWARTZ, John N., Chief Executive Officer, Trinity Hospital, Chicago, IL, p. A128

SCHWARTZ, Mark, President, Hartford Memorial Hospital, Hartford, WI, p. A463

SCHWARZ, Donald E., President and Chief Executive Officer, Jewish Memorial Hospital and Rehabilitation Center, Boston, MA, p. A204

SCHWEIKHART, Douglas P., Administrator, Shriners Hospitals for Children–Intermountain, Salt Lake City, UT, p. A435

SCHWEITZER, Alex, Administrator, North Dakota State Hospital, Jamestown, ND, p. A321

SCHWEITZER, Robert, Ed.D., Executive Director, Sagamore Children's Psychiatric Center, Dix Hills, NY, p. A291

SCHWEMER, David J., Administrator, Woodrow Wilson Rehabilitation Center–Hospital, Fishersville, VA, p. A441

SCHWIENTEK, Barbara, Executive Director, Monticello Big Lake Hospital, Monticello, MN, p. A232

SCHWIND, Mary, MS, Chief Executive Officer, Columbia San Jose Medical Center, San Jose, CA, p. A62

SCIOLA, Anthony, President and Chief Executive Officer, Shaughnessy–Kaplan Rehabilitation Hospital, Salem, MA, p. A209

SCOGGIN Jr., James C.
 Chief Executive Officer, San Antonio Community Hospital, San Antonio, TX, p. A426
 Chief Executive Officer, Southwest Texas Methodist Hospital, San Antonio, TX, p. A426

SCOGGINS, T. Henry, FACHE, President, Memorial Hospital, Manchester, KY, p. A178

SCOLLARD, Patrick J., President and Chief Executive Officer, St. Francis Hospital, Roslyn, NY, p. A304

SCOTT, Al, Ed.D., Administrator, BHC Belmont Pines Hospital, Youngstown, OH, p. A337

SCOTT, Arthur, Interim Director, Brattleboro Retreat, Brattleboro, VT, p. A437

SCOTT, Camille, Administrator, Benewah Community Hospital, Saint Maries, ID, p. A121

SCOTT, Charles Francis, President, St. Joseph's Hospital, Tampa, FL, p. A100

SCOTT, Grady, Administrator, Copper Basin Medical Center, Copperhill, TN, p. A388

SCOTT, John R., Director, St. Lawrence Psychiatric Center, Ogdensburg, NY, p. A301

SCOTT, Mark D., President, Mid–Columbia Medical Center, The Dalles, OR, p. A352

SCOTT, Richard E., President, Hillcrest Baptist Medical Center, Waco, TX, p. A430

SCOTT, Richard L., Chairman and Chief Executive Officer, Columbia/HCA Healthcare Corporation, Nashville, TN, p. B78

SCOTT, Thomas L., FACHE, President and Chief Executive Officer, Burdette Tomlin Memorial Hospital, Cape May Court House, NJ, p. A276

SCOVILL, Terry, Administrator, Cypress Creek Hospital, Houston, TX, p. A414

SCROGGY, Ron, Interim Group Administrator, Inner Harbour Hospitals, Douglasville, GA, p. A108

SCULLY Jr., James H., M.D., Director, William S. Hall Psychiatric Institute, Columbia, SC, p. A377

SCURR, David J., Superintendent, Mental Health Institute, Mount Pleasant, IA, p. A157

SEABERG, Lynn, Administrator and Chief Executive Officer, Indian Valley Hospital District, Greenville, CA, p. A45

SEAGRAVE, Richard E., President, Phoenixville Hospital, Phoenixville, PA, p. A365

SEALE, Corey A., Chief Executive Officer, Fallbrook Hospital District, Fallbrook, CA, p. A43

SEAVER, Roger E.
 President and Chief Executive Officer, Glendale Memorial Hospital and Health Center, Glendale, CA, p. A44
 President and Chief Executive Officer, Northridge Hospital Medical Center–Roscoe Boulevard Campus, Los Angeles, CA, p. A51

SECKINGER, Mark R., Administrator, Doctors Hospital of Nelsonville, Nelsonville, OH, p. A333

SEEL, W. Joseph, Administrator, Edgefield County Hospital, Edgefield, SC, p. A377

SEELY, E. T., Acting Administrator and Chief Financial Officer, Ferrell Hospital, Eldorado, IL, p. A129

SEIBEL, Jacqueline, Administrator, Jacobson Memorial Hospital Care Center, Elgin, ND, p. A320

SEIDEL, Ken, Executive Director, Columbia Claremore Regional Hospital, Claremore, OK, p. A340

SEIDLER, Richard A., Chief Executive Officer, Davenport Medical Center, Davenport, IA, p. A153

SEIFERT, David P., President, St. Anthony's Medical Center, Saint Louis, MO, p. A254

SEIGFREID Jr., Jerome, Chief Executive Officer, Phelps Memorial Health Center, Holdrege, NE, p. A264

SEILER, Edward H., Director, Veterans Affairs Medical Center, Providence, RI, p. A373

SEILER, Steven L., Senior Vice President and Chief Executive Officer, Good Samaritan Regional Medical Center, Phoenix, AZ, p. A24

SELBERG, Jeffrey D., President, Southwest Washington Medical Center, Vancouver, WA, p. A454

SELDEN, Thomas A., President and Chief Executive Officer, Parma Community General Hospital, Parma, OH, p. A334

SELLARDS, Michael G., Executive Director, Pleasant Valley Hospital, Point Pleasant, WV, p. A458

SELLARS, Thomas V., Superintendent, Wernersville State Hospital, Wernersville, PA, p. A370

SELTZER, Charlotte, Chief Executive Officer, Creedmoor Psychiatric Center, New York, NY, p. A296

SELZ, Timothy P., President, Saint Therese Medical Center, Waukegan, IL, p. A139

SELZER, Stephen R., Administrator, Southwest Memorial Hospital, Cortez, CO, p. A71

SEM, Steven, Commander, U. S. Air Force Hospital, Ellsworth AFB, SD, p. A383

SENNEFF, Robert G., Chief Executive Officer, Salem Hospital, Hillsboro, KS, p. A164

SENSOR, Wayne E., Chief Executive Officer, Northeast Arkansas Rehabilitation Hospital, Jonesboro, AR, p. A32

SEPULVIDA, Miguel A., Administrator, Dr. Ramon E. Betances Hospital–Mayaguez Medical Center Branch, Mayaguez, PR, p. A476

SERILLA, Michael, Acting Executive Vice President and Administrator, Bon Secours Hospital, Grosse Pointe, MI, p. A217

SERLE, Cornelius, Chief Executive Officer, Park Medical Center, Columbus, OH, p. A328

SERNULKA, John M., President and Chief Executive Officer, Carroll County General Hospital, Westminster, MD, p. A202

SERRILL, G. B., President and Chief Executive Officer, Ellis Hospital, Schenectady, NY, p. A304

SESSIONS, David, President, St. John Hospital–Macomb Center, Harrison Township, MI, p. A217

SEWARD Jr., James P., Executive Director, Berrien County Hospital, Nashville, GA, p. A112

SEXTON, J. Dennis, President, All Children's Hospital, Saint Petersburg, FL, p. A98

SEXTON, James J., President and Chief Executive Officer, Saint Francis Medical Center, Cape Girardeau, MO, p. A246

SEXTON, William P., Administrator, Franciscan Skemp Healthcare–Sparta Campus, Sparta, WI, p. A469

SEYMOUR, James A., Regional Administrator, Alegent Health Community Memorial Hospital, Missouri Valley, IA, p. A157

SHAFER, Ronald J., President and Chief Executive Officer, Eastern New Mexico Medical Center, Roswell, NM, p. A287

SHAFFER, David D., Chief Executive Officer, Stonewall Jackson Memorial Hospital, Weston, WV, p. A459

SHAFFETT, Donald A.
 Chief Executive Officer, Columbia Alvin Medical Center, Alvin, TX, p. A398
 Chief Executive Officer, Columbia Clear Lake Regional Medical Center, Webster, TX, p. A441

SHAMBAUGH, Steve, Superintendent, Eastern Oregon Psychiatric Center, Pendleton, OR, p. A350

SHAPIRO, Bernard, Chief Executive Officer, Memorial Hospital, Albany, NY, p. A288

SHAPIRO, Edward R., M.D., Medical Director and Chief Executive Officer, Austen Riggs Center, Stockbridge, MA, p. A210

SHAPIRO, Louis, Executive Vice President and Chief Operating Officer, Mt. Sinai Hospital, Philadelphia, PA, p. A364

SHAPIRO, Marcia S., Administrator and Chief Executive Officer, Columbia Chicago Lakeshore Hospital, Chicago, IL, p. A125

SHARFSTEIN, Steven S., M.D., President, Medical Director and Chief Executive Officer, Sheppard and Enoch Pratt Hospital, Baltimore, MD, p. A198

SHARMA, Timothy, M.D., President, Cambridge International, Inc,, Houston, TX, p. B73

SHARP, Joseph
 Administrator, Bellwood General Hospital, Bellflower, CA, p. A38
 Acting Administrator, Orange County Community Hospital of Buena Park, Buena Park, CA, p. A38

SHARP, Joseph W., Administrator, Runnells Specialized Hospital, Berkeley Heights, NJ, p. A275

SHARPE, Diane, Chief Executive Officer, ValueMark Pine Grove Behavioral Healthcare System, Los Angeles, CA, p. A52

SHAW, David B.
Administrator and Chief Executive Officer, Pecos County General Hospital, Iraan, TX, p. A416
Administrator and Chief Executive Officer, Pecos County Memorial Hospital, Fort Stockton, TX, p. A409

SHAW, Douglas E., President, Jewish Hospital, Louisville, KY, p. A177

SHAW, J. Michael, Administrator, Rusk County Memorial Hospital and Nursing Home, Ladysmith, WI, p. A463

SHAW, Phil, Executive Director, Spalding Regional Hospital, Griffin, GA, p. A110

SHEAR, Bruce A., President and Chief Executive Officer, Pioneer Healthcare, Peabody, MA, p. B121

SHECKLER, Robert L., Administrator, Dundy County Hospital, Benkelman, NE, p. A262

SHEEDY, Lucille K., Administrator and Chief Executive Officer, Wyoming County Community Hospital, Warsaw, NY, p. A306

SHEEHAN, Daniel F., Administrator, Research Belton Hospital, Belton, MO, p. A245

SHEEHAN, Michael J., Facility Administrator, Hastings Regional Center, Hastings, NE, p. A264

SHEEHAN, John R., Administrator, Ehrling Bergquist Hospital, Offutt AFB, NE, p. A266

SHEEHY, Earl N., Chief Executive Officer, Northeast Montana Health Services, Wolf Point, MT, p. A261

SHEETZ, Douglas A., Chief Executive Officer, Keokuk County Health Center, Sigourney, IA, p. A158

SHELBY, Dennis R., Chief Executive Officer, Northwest Arkansas Rehabilitation Hospital, Fayetteville, AR, p. A30

SHELBY, Marla, Administrator and Chief Executive Officer, South Lincoln Medical Center, Kemmerer, WY, p. A471

SHELDEN, Roy R., Administrator and Chief Executive Officer, Chemical Dependency Institute of Northern California, Campbell, CA, p. A39

SHELDON, Lyle Ernest
Executive Vice President and Chief Operating Officer, Fallston General Hospital, Fallston, MD, p. A200
President and Chief Executive Officer, Harford Memorial Hospital, Havre De Grace, MD, p. A200
President and Chief Executive Officer, Upper Chesapeake Health System, Fallston, MD, p. B146

SHELTON, Frank, President, Union Hospital, Terre Haute, IN, p. A149

SHELTON II, W. Allen, Administrator, Eye and Ear Clinic of Charleston, Charleston, WV, p. A455

SHEMBERGER, Kaylor E., President and Chief Executive Officer, Chandler Regional Hospital, Chandler, AZ, p. A22

SHEPARD, John J., President and Chief Executive Officer, Clarion Hospital, Clarion, PA, p. A355

SHEPARD, R. Coert, President, Anderson Hospital, Maryville, IL, p. A133

SHEPHARD, Paul E., President and Chief Executive Officer, St. James Mercy Hospital, Hornell, NY, p. A293

SHEPHERD, Richard W., President and Chief Executive Officer, Children's Seashore House, Philadelphia, PA, p. A363

SHERON, William E., Chief Executive Officer, Wooster Community Hospital, Wooster, OH, p. A337

SHERROD, Rhonda, Administrator, Shands at Live Oak, Live Oak, FL, p. A91

SHERWOOD, Gary A., Executive Vice President, Rogue Valley Medical Center, Medford, OR, p. A350

SHERWOOD, John M., FACHE, President and Chief Executive Officer, Allentown Osteopathic Medical Center, Allentown, PA, p. A353

SHIELDS, Lena L., Chief Executive, Bethany Hospital, Chicago, IL, p. A125

SHIELS, Rob, Administrator, Mary Shiels Hospital, Dallas, TX, p. A406

SHIMONO, Jiro R., Director, Delaware Psychiatric Center, New Castle, DE, p. A80

SHIPPY, Janice, R.N., Administrator, Sedan City Hospital, Sedan, KS, p. A169

SHIRK, Michael, President and Senior Executive Officer, Boone Hospital Center, Columbia, MO, p. A246

SHIRTCLIFF, Christine, Executive Vice President, Mary Lane Hospital, Ware, MA, p. A210

SHOCKLEY, Allen L., President and Chief Executive Officer, St. John's Regional Health Center, Springfield, MO, p. A255

SHONKA, Marie Madeleine, President, Saint John's Hospital and Health Center, Santa Monica, CA, p. A64

SHOOK, Scott E., President, Riverside Hospital, Toledo, OH, p. A336

SHORB, Gary S., President, Methodist Hospitals of Memphis, Memphis, TN, p. A393

SHOSTAK, G. Peter, Administrator, University of Southern California–Kenneth Norris Jr. Cancer Hospital, Los Angeles, CA, p. A52

SHOUSE, Donald W., Administrator, Methodist Hospital Plainview, Plainview, TX, p. A423

SHOVELIN, Wayne F., President and Chief Executive Officer, Gaston Memorial Hospital, Gastonia, NC, p. A312

SHRODER, Robert W., Chief Operating Officer, St. Joseph Health Center, Warren, OH, p. A336

SHUFFIELD, Charles R., President, Sparks Regional Medical Center, Fort Smith, AR, p. A31

SHUGARMAN, Mark, President, Mercy Hospital, Tiffin, OH, p. A335

SHULER, Priscilla J., Chief Executive Officer, Metropolitan Hospital, Richmond, VA, p. A445

SHUMAKER, Revonda L., R.N., President, St. Anthony's Hospital, Saint Petersburg, FL, p. A99

SHYAVITZ, Linda, President and Chief Executive Officer, Sturdy Memorial Hospital, Attleboro, MA, p. A203

SICURELLA, John, Chief Executive Officer, Reynolds Memorial Hospital, Glen Dale, WV, p. A456

SIEBER, Thomas L., President and Chief Executive Officer, Genesis HealthCare System, Zanesville, OH, p. A338

SIEGEL, Bruce, M.P.H., President and Chief Executive Officer, Tampa General Healthcare, Tampa, FL, p. A100

SIEGEL, Patricia, Senior Vice President, Health Plan, Hospitals and Inland Empire Area Manager, Kaiser Foundation Hospital, Fontana, CA, p. A43

SIEGWALD–MAYS, Cheryl, Administrator, Columbia Behavioral Health Center, Miami, FL, p. A92

SIEMEN–MESSING, Pauline, R.N., President and Chief Executive Officer, Harbor Beach Community Hospital, Harbor Beach, MI, p. A217

SIEMERS, Thomas R., Chief Executive Officer, Rebsamen Regional Medical Center, Jacksonville, AR, p. A31

SIEPMAN, Milton R., Ph.D., President and Chief Executive Officer, Tennessee Christian Medical Center, Madison, TN, p. A392

SILBERNAGEL, Gil, Administrator, Memorial Hospital Los Banos, Los Banos, CA, p. A52

SILKWOOD, Haskell G., Administrator, Refugio County Memorial Hospital, Refugio, TX, p. A424

SILLEN, Robert, Executive Director, Santa Clara Valley Medical Center, San Jose, CA, p. A62

SILLS, Doug, President and Chief Executive Officer, Columbia Medical Center Sanford, Sanford, FL, p. A99

SILVA, Luis G., Chief Executive Officer and Regional Administrator, Columbia Beaumont Medical Center, Beaumont, TX, p. A401

SILVA, William G., Administrator, Metropolitan State Hospital, Norwalk, CA, p. A55

SILVER, Richard A., Director, James A. Haley Veterans Hospital, Tampa, FL, p. A100

SILVERNALE, Vern, Administrator, Johnson Memorial Health Services, Dawson, MN, p. A228

SILVIA, Clarence J., President, Bradley Memorial Hospital and Health Center, Southington, CT, p. A78

SIMCHUK, Cathy, Chief Operating Officer, Deer Park Health Center and Hospital, Deer Park, WA, p. A449

SIMCOE III, Hugh S., Administrator, Gulf Oaks Hospital, Biloxi, MS, p. A237

SIMMONS, Preston M., Administrator, Page Hospital, Page, AZ, p. A24

SIMMONS, Randy, Administrator, Davis County Hospital, Bloomfield, IA, p. A151

SIMMONS, Stephen H.
Senior Administrator, University of South Alabama Hospitals, Mobile, AL, p. B146
Administrator, University of South Alabama Medical Center, Mobile, AL, p. A16

SIMMONS, Tim
Chief Executive Officer, Columbia Specialty Hospital at Medical Arts, Dallas, TX, p. A406
Administrator, Hood River Memorial Hospital, Hood River, OR, p. A349

SIMMONS, W. Clay, Executive Director, Bradford Health Services at Birmingham, Birmingham, AL, p. A11

SIMMONS, William, President and Chief Executive Officer, San Jacinto Methodist Hospital, Baytown, TX, p. A401

SIMMS, John L., President and Chief Executive Officer, Trinity Community Medical Center of Brenham, Brenham, TX, p. A402

SIMON, Elliot J., FACHE, Chief Operating Officer, Western Queens Community Hospital, New York, NY, p. A300

SIMON, James K., President and Chief Executive Officer, Lower Florida Keys Health System, Key West, FL, p. A90

SIMON, Mary Alvera, Administrator, Mercy Hospital of Scott County, Waldron, AR, p. A35

SIMONIN, Steve J., Chief Executive Officer, Community Memorial Hospital, Clarion, IA, p. A152

SIMPATICO, Thomas, M.D., Facility Director and Network System Manager, Chicago–Read Mental Health Center, Chicago, IL, p. A125

SIMPSON, Tim, Administrator, Vencor–North Florida, Green Cove Springs, FL, p. A88

SIMPSON Jr., Lee A., President and Chief Executive Officer, Eastwood Medical Center, Memphis, TN, p. A393

SIMS, Norman L., USAF, Commander, U. S. Air Force Hospital Little Rock, Jacksonville, AR, p. A32

SIMS Jr., John H., Director, Veterans Affairs Medical Center, Togus, ME, p. A196

SINCLAIR, Mike, Administrator, Kane County Hospital, Kanab, UT, p. A433

SINGLE, John L.
Chief Executive Officer and Administrator, De Smet Memorial Hospital, De Smet, SD, p. A382
Chief Executive Officer, Huron Regional Medical Center, Huron, SD, p. A383

SINGLETON, J. Knox, President, Inova Health System, Springfield, VA, p. B105

SINNOTT, Daniel J.
President and Chief Executive Officer, Nazareth Hospital, Philadelphia, PA, p. A364
President and Chief Executive Officer, St. Agnes Medical Center, Philadelphia, PA, p. A365

SIPES, Don, Senior Executive Officer, Saint Luke's Northland Hospital–Smithville Campus, Smithville, MO, p. A255

SIPKOSKI, Michael, Executive Vice President and Chief Executive Officer, St. Francis Hospital, Litchfield, IL, p. A133

SIPP, Richard C., Vice President for Administration, Medical College Hospitals, Toledo, OH, p. A335

SIRK, David R., President and Chief Executive Officer, Saint Francis Hospital, Charleston, WV, p. A455

SISSON, William G., President, Central Baptist Hospital, Lexington, KY, p. A176

SISTI, Judith L., MS, Administrator, Vineland Development Center Hospital, Vineland, NJ, p. A282

SKELLEY, Dennis B., President and Chief Executive Officer, Walton Rehabilitation Hospital, Augusta, GA, p. A105

SKINNER, David B., M.D., President and Chief Executive Officer, Society of the New York Hospital, New York, NY, p. A299

SKINNER, Davis D., Administrator, Missouri Baptist Hospital of Sullivan, Sullivan, MO, p. A255

SKINNER, Sandra, Chief Executive Officer, First Health, Inc., Batesville, MS, p. B97

SKJERVEN, John, Interim Chief Executive Officer, North Country Regional Hospital, Bemidji, MN, p. A226

SKOGSBERGH, James H.
President, Iowa Lutheran Hospital, Des Moines, IA, p. A153
President, Iowa Methodist Medical Center, Des Moines, IA, p. A153

SKOMOROCH, Orianna A., Administrator, Kauai Veterans Memorial Hospital, Waimea, HI, p. A118

SKUBA, Herbert S., President and Chief Executive Officer, Ellwood City Hospital, Ellwood City, PA, p. A357

SKUTZKA, Alexander, Chief Executive Officer, Hempstead General Hospital Medical Center, Hempstead, NY, p. A293

SLABACH, Brock A., Administrator, Field Memorial Community Hospital, Centreville, MS, p. A238

SLAGTER, Dean G., Administrator, Renville County Hospital, Olivia, MN, p. A232

SLATON, Charles R., President and Chief Executive Officer, Saint Francis Hospital, Memphis, TN, p. A393

SLAUBAUGH, D. Ray, President, Graham Hospital, Canton, IL, p. A124

SLAVIERO, Ron, Administrator, Franklin Hospital and Skilled Nursing Care Unit, Benton, IL, p. A124

SLAVIERO, Ronald, Administrator, United Mine Workers of America Union Hospital, West Frankfort, IL, p. A139

SLIETER, Richard G., President, Owatonna Hospital, Owatonna, MN, p. A233

SLOAN, Gary, Chief Executive Officer, Doctors Hospital of Pinole, Pinole, CA, p. A57

SLOAN, Joseph F., CHE, Chief Executive Officer, Plains Memorial Hospital, Dimmitt, TX, p. A408

SLOAN, Robert L., Chief Executive Officer, Sibley Memorial Hospital, Washington, DC, p. A81

SLUNECKA, Fredrick, President and Chief Executive Officer, McKennan Hospital, Sioux Falls, SD, p. A385

SLUSKY, Richard, Administrator, Mount Ascutney Hospital and Health Center, Windsor, VT, p. A438

SMALLEY, Diana, Chief Executive Officer, Midlands Community Hospital, Papillion, NE, p. A267

SMART, Michael, Chief Executive Officer, Alameda County Medical Center–Highland Campus, Oakland, CA, p. A55

SMART, Michael G., Chief Executive Officer, Alameda County Medical Center, San Leandro, CA, p. A62

SMART, Robert M., Area Manager and Chief Executive Officer, Healthsouth Medical Center, Dallas, TX, p. A406

SMEDLEY, Craig M., Administrator, Valley View Medical Center, Cedar City, UT, p. A433

SMIGELSKI, Daniel R., Chief Executive Officer, Gritman Medical Center, Moscow, ID, p. A121

SMILEY, Jon D., Chief Executive Officer, Sunnyside Community Hospital, Sunnyside, WA, p. A453

SMILEY, W. David, Chief Executive Officer, San Joaquin Valley Rehabilitation Hospital, Fresno, CA, p. A44

SMITH, Alex B., Ph.D., Executive Director, Terrebonne General Medical Center, Houma, LA, p. A185

SMITH, Arthur R., Chief Executive Officer and Administrator, Hamilton County Hospital, Syracuse, KS, p. A169

SMITH, Bernadette, Chief Operating Officer, Seton Medical Center, Daly City, CA, p. A41

SMITH, C. W., President, Parkview Episcopal Medical Center, Pueblo, CO, p. A74

SMITH, Charles M., M.D., President and Chief Executive Officer, Medical Center of Delaware, Wilmington, DE, p. A80

SMITH, Connie, Senior Vice President, Medical Center at Scottsville, Scottsville, KY, p. A180

SMITH, David M., FACHE, President and Chief Executive Officer, West Jefferson Medical Center, Marrero, LA, p. A187

SMITH, Dennis H.
Director, VA Maryland Health Care System, Perry Point, MD, p. A201
Director, Veterans Affairs Medical Center, Baltimore, MD, p. A198
Director, Veterans Affairs Medical Center, Fort Howard, MD, p. A200

SMITH, F. Curtis, President, Massachusetts Eye and Ear Infirmary, Boston, MA, p. A204

SMITH, Frances L., MSN, Superintendent, Haverford State Hospital, Haverford, PA, p. A358

SMITH, Frances T., Administrator, Childress Regional Medical Center, Childress, TX, p. A403

SMITH, G. Terrence, Chief Executive Officer, Northwest Psychiatric Hospital, Toledo, OH, p. A336

SMITH, Gordon, Administrator, Merrill Pioneer Community Hospital, Rock Rapids, IA, p. A158

SMITH, Gordon L., Administrator, Eye Foundation Hospital, Birmingham, AL, p. A12

SMITH, H. Gerald, President and Chief Executive Officer, St. Francis Medical Center, Monroe, LA, p. A187

SMITH, H. Randolph, Administrator, Wiregrass Hospital, Geneva, AL, p. A14

SMITH, Harlan J., President, Franklin Medical Center, Greenfield, MA, p. A206

SMITH, Harley, Chief Executive Officer, Mimbres Memorial Hospital, Deming, NM, p. A285

SMITH, Harry E., Administrator, Southeast Baptist Hospital, San Antonio, TX, p. A426

SMITH, James E., Superintendent, Wichita Falls State Hospital, Wichita Falls, TX, p. A431

SMITH, Jean P., Chief Executive Officer, South Oaks Hospital, Amityville, NY, p. A288

SMITH, Jeffrey H., Ph.D., Superintendent, Logansport State Hospital, Logansport, IN, p. A146

SMITH, Jerry, Chief Executive Officer, BHC Pinon Hills Hospital, Santa Fe, NM, p. A287

SMITH, Jim B., President and Chief Executive Officer, Goodall–Witcher Hospital, Clifton, TX, p. A404

SMITH, Joe E., Administrator and Chief Executive Officer, DeWitt City Hospital, De Witt, AR, p. A30

SMITH, Johnson L., Chief Executive Officer and Administrator, Conway County Hospital, Morrilton, AR, p. A33

SMITH, Joseph S., Chief Executive Officer, Boone County Hospital, Boone, IA, p. A151

SMITH, Lex, Administrator, Park View Hospital, El Reno, OK, p. A341

SMITH, Lloyd V., President and Chief Executive Officer, Benefis Health Care, Great Falls, MT, p. A258

SMITH, Melvyn E., President, Graduate Health System–City Avenue Hospital, Philadelphia, PA, p. A364

SMITH, Meredith H., Administrator, Dodge County Hospital, Eastman, GA, p. A108

SMITH, Michael N., Director Healthcare Services, San Joaquin General Hospital, French Camp, CA, p. A43

SMITH, R. S., Chief Executive Officer, Community Hospital–Lakeview, Eufaula, OK, p. A341

SMITH, Randall W., Chief Operating Officer, Alegent Health Immanuel Medical Center, Omaha, NE, p. A266

SMITH, Randolph R., Administrator, Calexico Hospital, Calexico, CA, p. A39

SMITH, Raymond N., Chief Executive Officer, Community Hospital of Gardena, Gardena, CA, p. A44

SMITH, Richard, Administrator, Logan Regional Hospital, Logan, UT, p. A433

SMITH, Richard G., Administrator, Oneida Healthcare Center, Oneida, NY, p. A301

SMITH, Robbie, Administrator, Higgins General Hospital, Bremen, GA, p. A105

SMITH, Robert B., President and Chief Executive Officer, Zale Lipshy University Hospital, Dallas, TX, p. A407

SMITH, Robert L., President and Chief Executive Officer, Decatur General Hospital, Decatur, AL, p. A13

SMITH, Ronald L., President, Harris Methodist Health System, Fort Worth, TX, p. B100

SMITH, S. Allen, Administrator, Tri–City Community Hospital, Jourdanton, TX, p. A417

SMITH, Steve, Chief Executive Officer, Carson Tahoe Hospital, Carson City, NV, p. A270

SMITH, Steven L., President and Chief Executive Officer, Memorial Medical Center, Las Cruces, NM, p. A286

SMITH, Terry J., Administrator, Bibb Medical Center, Centreville, AL, p. A13

SMITH, Thomas G., Administrator, Parkview Hospital of Topeka, Topeka, KS, p. A170

SMITH, Thomas W., President and Chief Executive Officer, Ephraim McDowell Regional Medical Center, Danville, KY, p. A173

SMITH, Timothy, President and Chief Executive Officer, Garden Grove Hospital and Medical Center, Garden Grove, CA, p. A44

SMITH, Todd A., Chief Executive Officer, Charter Behavioral Health System of Southern California–Charter Oak, Covina, CA, p. A41

SMITH, Tommy J., President and Chief Executive Officer, Baptist Healthcare System, Louisville, KY, p. B68

SMITH, W. David, Director, Veterans Affairs Medical Center, Fort Lyon, CO, p. A72

SMITH, Wayne T., President, Community Health Systems, Inc., Brentwood, TN, p. B86

SMITH, William C., Chief Executive Officer, Livingston Hospital and Healthcare Services, Salem, KY, p. A180

SMITH, William R., Administrator, Hamilton Hospital, Olney, TX, p. A422

SMITH II, W. Don, President and Chief Executive Officer, Cabell Huntington Hospital, Huntington, WV, p. A456

SMITH Jr., Charles W., Chief Executive Officer, St. Jerome Hospital, Batavia, NY, p. A288

SMITH Jr., Kirby H., Executive Vice President and Chief Executive Officer, Mary Immaculate Hospital, Newport News, VA, p. A443

SMITH Jr., P. Paul, Executive Director, Lake Norman Regional Medical Center, Mooresville, NC, p. A314

SMITH Jr., Philip W., President, MedCenter Hospital, Marion, OH, p. A332

SMITH–BLACKWELL, Olivia, M.P.H., President and Chief Executive Officer, Sheehan Memorial Hospital, Buffalo, NY, p. A290

SMITHERS, Joe, Administrator, Horizon Specialty Hospital, Edmond, OK, p. A341

SMITHHISLER, John, CHE, Chief Executive Officer, Centinela Hospital Medical Center, Inglewood, CA, p. A46

SMITHMIER, Kenneth L., President and Chief Executive Officer, Decatur Memorial Hospital, Decatur, IL, p. A128

SNEAD, Ben, Administrator, Kimble Hospital, Junction, TX, p. A417

SNEAD, Benjamin E., President, St. Clair Memorial Hospital, Pittsburgh, PA, p. A366

SNEDIGAR, Rudy, Administrator, Clarinda Regional Health Center, Clarinda, IA, p. A152

SNELL, Donald F., President and Chief Executive Officer, Long Island College Hospital, New York, NY, p. A298

SNIPES, Lucas A.
Director, Carilion Roanoke Community Hospital, Roanoke, VA, p. A446
Director, Carilion Roanoke Memorial Hospital, Roanoke, VA, p. A446

SNOW, Anne, Administrator, Hansford Hospital, Spearman, TX, p. A428

SNOW, F. Ann, Administrator, Weston County Memorial Hospital, Newcastle, WY, p. A472

SNOW, Mel, Administrator, West Holt Memorial Hospital, Atkinson, NE, p. A262

SNYDER, David M., Executive Director and Chief Executive Officer, Natchez Regional Medical Center, Natchez, MS, p. A242

SOBOTA, Richard E., President and Chief Executive Officer, Pike Community Hospital, Waverly, OH, p. A337

SODOMKA, Patricia, Executive Director, Medical College of Georgia Hospital and Clinics, Augusta, GA, p. A105

SOILEAU, Joseph L., Chief Executive Officer, South Cameron Memorial Hospital, Cameron, LA, p. A183

SOK, James E., President, Sharon Hospital, Sharon, CT, p. A78

SOKOL, Dennis A., President and Chief Executive Officer, Sacred Heart Health Services, Yankton, SD, p. A386

SOKOLOW, Norman J., President, Cornerstone of Medical Arts Center Hospital, New York, NY, p. A296

SOLARE, Frank A., President and Chief Executive Officer, Thorek Hospital and Medical Center, Chicago, IL, p. A127

SOLBERG, Bradley, President and Chief Executive Officer, Three Rivers Area Hospital, Three Rivers, MI, p. A224

SOLHEIM, John H., Chief Executive Officer, St. Mary's Regional Health Center, Detroit Lakes, MN, p. A228

SOLIVAN, Miguel A., Executive Director, Hospital De Area De Yauco, Yauco, PR, p. A477

SOLNIT, Albert J., M.D., Commissioner, Connecticut State Department of Mental Health, Hartford, CT, p. B87

SOLVIBILE, Edward R., President, Suburban General Hospital, Norristown, PA, p. A362

SOMMER, Richard C., Administrator, Defiance Hospital, Defiance, OH, p. A329

SONDECKER, James, Administrator, St. Joseph's Behavioral Health Center, Stockton, CA, p. A65

SONDUCK, Allan C., President and Chief Executive Officer, St. Mary's Hospital, Kankakee, IL, p. A132

SOPO, Deborah A., President, Brighton Hospital, Brighton, MI, p. A213

SOUKUP, Richard G., Chief Executive Officer, Northern Hills General Hospital, Deadwood, SD, p. A382

SOULE, Frederick L., President and Chief Executive Officer, Caldwell Memorial Hospital, Lenoir, NC, p. A313

SOYUGENC, Marjorie Z., President and Chief Executive Officer, Welborn Memorial Baptist Hospital, Evansville, IN, p. A142

SPAETH, Ronald G., President and Chief Executive Officer, Highland Park Hospital, Highland Park, IL, p. A131

SPAID, Larry K., President, Southern Chester County Medical Center, West Grove, PA, p. A370

SPALDING, Donald W., President, Sewickley Valley Hospital, (A Division of Valley Medical Facilities), Sewickley, PA, p. A369

SPANG, A. James, Administrator, Shriners Hospitals for Children–Chicago, Chicago, IL, p. A127

SPARER, Cynthia N., Executive Director and Chief Operating Officer, Monmouth Medical Center, Long Branch, NJ, p. A278

SPARKMAN, Ronald L., Administrator, Carraway Burdick West Medical Center, Haleyville, AL, p. A15

SPARKS, Richard G., President, Watauga Medical Center, Boone, NC, p. A309

SPARROW, William T., Chief Executive Officer, BHC San Luis Rey Hospital, Encinitas, CA, p. A42

SPARTZ, Gregory G., Chief Executive Officer, Willmar Regional Treatment Center, Willmar, MN, p. A236

SPAUDE, Paul A., President and Chief Executive Officer, Wausau Hospital, Wausau, WI, p. A470

SPAULDING, Don, Administrator and Chief Executive Officer, Fort Duncan Medical Center, Eagle Pass, TX, p. A408

SPAUSTER, Edward, Ph.D., Executive Director, Arms Acres, Carmel, NY, p. A290

SPEAK, Patricia B., Administrator, Vencor Hospital–Pittsburgh, Oakdale, PA, p. A362

SPEARS, Leonard J., Administrator, American Legion Hospital, Crowley, LA, p. A184

SPECK, William T., M.D., President and Chief Executive Officer, Presbyterian Hospital in the City of New York, New York, NY, p. A299

SPEED, Marilyn, Administrator, Beacham Memorial Hospital, Magnolia, MS, p. A241

SPELLMAN, Warren K., Administrator, Woodward Hospital and Health Center, Woodward, OK, p. A347

SPENCER, Corte J., Chief Executive Officer, Oswego Hospital, Oswego, NY, p. A302

SPENCER, Herman J., Administrator, Northern Inyo Hospital, Bishop, CA, p. A38

SPENCER, Steven H.
President, St. Mary's Kewaunee Area Memorial Hospital, Kewaunee, WI, p. A463
President and Chief Executive Officer, Two Rivers Community Hospital and Hamilton Memorial Home, Two Rivers, WI, p. A469

SPHATT, Thomas R., President and Chief Executive Officer, Berwick Hospital Center, Berwick, PA, p. A354

SPICER, John R., President and Chief Executive Officer, Sound Shore Medical Center of Westchester, New Rochelle, NY, p. A295

SPIEGEL, Robert W., President and Chief Executive Officer, Charles River Hospital–West, Chicopee, MA, p. A206

SPILLMAN, Eugene, Executive Director, Natchitoches Parish Hospital, Natchitoches, LA, p. A188

SPILOVOY, Richard, Administrator, Garrison Memorial Hospital, Garrison, ND, p. A320

SPINELLI, Robert J., Administrator and Chief Executive Officer, Bloomsburg Hospital, Bloomsburg, PA, p. A354

SPINNER, Robert K., President, Abbott Northwestern Hospital, Minneapolis, MN, p. A231

SPITLER III, William H., President, Perry Memorial Hospital, Princeton, IL, p. A136

SPIVEY, Sue, Administrator, Irwin County Hospital, Ocilla, GA, p. A112

SPOELMAN, Roger
Chief Executive Officer, Mercy General Health Partners–Oak Avenue Campus, Muskegon, MI, p. A221
Chief Executive Officer, Mercy General Health Partners–Sherman Boulevard Campus, Muskegon, MI, p. A221

SPRAY, William Russell, Chief Executive Officer, Gadsden Regional Medical Center, Gadsden, AL, p. A14

SPRENGER, Gordon M., Executive Officer, Allina Health System, Minneapolis, MN, p. B65

SPRENGER, Jay, Commander, U. S. Air Force Hospital, Panama City, FL, p. A96

SPRINGER, Kay H., Administrator, Steele Memorial Hospital, Salmon, ID, p. A121

SPRISSLER, Fred, President and Chief Executive Officer, St. Luke's Quakertown Hospital, Quakertown, PA, p. A368

SPYHALSKI, Richard A., Chief Executive Officer, Northwest Medical Center, Thief River Falls, MN, p. A235

ST. ANDRE, Christine, Executive Director, University of Utah Hospitals and Clinics, Salt Lake City, UT, p. A435

ST. ARNOLD, Dale, President and Chief Executive Officer, Mount Carmel Health System, Columbus, OH, p. A328

ST. CLAIR, Marvin O., Administrator, Hawaii State Hospital, Kaneohe, HI, p. A118

ST. CLAIR, Nelson L., President, Riverside Health System, Newport News, VA, p. B129

STAAS Jr., William E., President and Medical Director, Magee Rehabilitation Hospital, Philadelphia, PA, p. A364

STACEY, Bryan, Administrator, Ashland Health Center, Ashland, KS, p. A161

STACEY, Rulon F., President, Poudre Valley Hospital, Fort Collins, CO, p. A72

STACK, Edward A., President, Behavioral Healthcare Corporation, Nashville, TN, p. B69

STACK, R. Timothy, FACHE, President and Chief Executive Officer, Borgess Medical Center, Kalamazoo, MI, p. A218

STAJDUHAR, P., M.D., Director, Veterans Affairs Medical Center, Butler, PA, p. A355

STAMM, Scott C., Chief Executive Officer, Columbia River Park Hospital, Huntington, WV, p. A456

STANBERRY, Marion W., Administrator, Wood County Central Hospital District, Quitman, TX, p. A424

STANDRIDGE, Jim, Administrator, Lindsay Municipal Hospital, Lindsay, OK, p. A342

STANLEY, Richard J., Director, Veterans Affairs Medical Center, Miles City, MT, p. A259

STANLEY, Robert R., Chief Executive Officer, Iberia General Hospital and Medical Center, New Iberia, LA, p. A188

STANSBERRY, Mark, Superintendent, Mid Missouri Mental Health Center, Columbia, MO, p. A246

STANUSH, Sharon M., President, Southwest Mental Health Center, San Antonio, TX, p. A426

STANZIONE, Dominick M.
Chief Operating Officer and Executive Vice President, Bayley Seton Hospital, New York, NY, p. A295
Executive Vice President, St. Vincent's Medical Center of Richmond, New York, NY, p. A300

STAPLES, Nancy, MS, Administrator, Elgin Mental Health Center, Elgin, IL, p. A129

STARK, Charles A., CHE, Administrator, Chief Executive Officer and Director Inpatient Operations, Healthsouth Medical Center, Richmond, VA, p. A445

STARMANN–HARRISON, Mary, FACHE, Chief Executive Officer, St. Luke's Medical Center, Phoenix, AZ, p. A25

STARNES, Gregory D., Chief Executive Officer, Culver Union Hospital, Crawfordsville, IN, p. A141

STARR, Gerald A., Chief Executive Officer, Kern Medical Center, Bakersfield, CA, p. A37

STARR Jr., Hickory, Administrator, William W. Hastings Indian Hospital, Tahlequah, OK, p. A346

STATUTO, Richard, Chief Executive Officer, St. Joseph Health System, Orange, CA, p. B138

STAYNINGS, Tony, Chief Executive Officer, Swisher Memorial Hospital District, Tulia, TX, p. A429

STEBBINS, Deborah E., FACHE, President and Chief Executive Officer, Seton Medical Center Coastside, Moss Beach, CA, p. A54

STECKLER, Michael J., Chief Executive Officer, Jennie M. Melham Memorial Medical Center, Broken Bow, NE, p. A262

STEED, Karen, Chief Executive Officer, Eastern State Hospital, Vinita, OK, p. A347

STEED, Larry N., Administrator, Tanner Medical Center–Villa Rica, Villa Rica, GA, p. A115

STEED, Robert A., Administrator, Willamette Falls Hospital, Oregon City, OR, p. A350

STEEGE, Armin, Chief Executive Officer, Charter Behavioral Health System of Austin, Austin, TX, p. A400

STEFFEE, Sam L., Executive Director and Chief Executive Officer, Polly Ryon Memorial Hospital, Richmond, TX, p. A424

STEGBAUER, Tom, Administrator, Olympic Memorial Hospital, Port Angeles, WA, p. A451

STEIDER, Norman D., President, Memorial Hospital of Michigan City, Michigan City, IN, p. A146

STEIN, Benjamin M., M.D., President, Brunswick General Hospital, Amityville, NY, p. A288

STEIN, Dale J., President and Chief Executive Officer, St. Luke's Midland Regional Medical Center, Aberdeen, SD, p. A382

STEIN, Gary M., President and Chief Executive Officer, Touro Infirmary, New Orleans, LA, p. A189

STEIN, Norman V., President, University Community Hospital, Tampa, FL, p. A101

STEINER, Garith W., Chief Executive Officer, Vernon Memorial Hospital, Viroqua, WI, p. A469

STEINER, Keith M., Chief Executive Officer, Madison Memorial Hospital, Rexburg, ID, p. A121

STEINHAUER, Bruce W., M.D., Chief Executive Officer, Lahey Hitchcock Clinic, Burlington, MA, p. A205

STEINHOFF, Earl J., Chief Executive Officer, Prowers Medical Center, Lamar, CO, p. A73

STEINIG, Norman, Administrator, Eastern Ozarks Regional Health System, Cherokee Village, AR, p. A29

STEINKRUGER, Roger W., Chief Executive Officer, Norfolk Regional Center, Norfolk, NE, p. A266

STEITZ, David P.
Chief Executive Officer, Columbia Hospital Frankfort, Frankfort, KY, p. A174
Chief Executive Officer, Columbia Lake City Medical Center, Lake City, FL, p. A90

STELLE, Walter, Ph.D., Director, Dorothea Dix Hospital, Raleigh, NC, p. A315

STELLER, Tim A., Chief Executive Officer, North Central Health Care Facilities, Wausau, WI, p. A470

STENBERG, Scott, Chief Executive Officer, Sutter Amador Hospital, Jackson, CA, p. A46

STENGER, Michael J., Executive Vice President and Administrator, St. Nicholas Hospital, Sheboygan, WI, p. A468

STENSON, Dick, Administrator, Tuality Forest Grove Hospital, Forest Grove, OR, p. A349

STENSON, Richard, President, Tuality Community Hospital, Hillsboro, OR, p. A349

STENSRUD, Kirk, Administrator, Hendricks Community Hospital, Hendricks, MN, p. A230

STENZLER, Mark R., Vice President Administration, North Shore University Hospital at Glen Cove, Glen Cove, NY, p. A292

STEPANIK, Mark J., Director Operations, Healthsouth Rehabilitation Hospital, Columbia, SC, p. A377

STEPHANS, J. Michael, Administrator, Medical Center Hospital, Odessa, TX, p. A422

STEPHEN, Ron, Executive Vice President and Administrator, Osteopathic Medical Center of Texas, Fort Worth, TX, p. A410

STEPHENS, James H., President and Chief Executive Officer, Saint John's Health System, Anderson, IN, p. A140

STEPHENS, Michael D., President and Chief Executive Officer, Hoag Memorial Hospital Presbyterian, Newport Beach, CA, p. A55

STEPHENS, Michael R., President, Greene Memorial Hospital, Xenia, OH, p. A337

STEPHENS, Terry A., Executive Director, Sierra Tucson, Tucson, AZ, p. A27

STEPHENS Jr., Jack T., President and Chief Executive Officer, Lakeland Regional Medical Center, Lakeland, FL, p. A91

STEPHENSON, David, Administrator, Rock County Hospital, Bassett, NE, p. A262

STEPP, Merle E., President and Chief Executive Officer, Clark Memorial Hospital, Jeffersonville, IN, p. A145

STERN, Ron, President and Chief Executive Officer, Wyoming Valley Health Care System, Wilkes–Barre, PA, p. A371

STEVENS, Alan I., Administrator, Huntington Hospital, Willow Grove, PA, p. A371

STEVENS, April A., R.N., Vice President and Administrator, Forbes Metropolitan Hospital, Pittsburgh, PA, p. A366

STEVENS, Essimae, Service Unit Director, U.S. Public Health Service Indian Hospital, Redlake, MN, p. A233

STEVENS, Harry H., Administrator, Bradley County Memorial Hospital, Warren, AR, p. A35

STEVENS, Robert, President and Chief Executive Officer, Ridgeview Medical Center, Waconia, MN, p. A236

STEVENS, Velinda, Chief Executive Officer, Columbia Longview Regional Medical Center, Longview, TX, p. A419

STEVENS, Ward W., CHE, Chief Executive Officer, Columbia Alleghany Regional Hospital, Low Moor, VA, p. A442

STEVENS Jr., Vernon R., Administrator, Riverland Medical Center, Ferriday, LA, p. A184

STEVENSON, Alan, Administrator, Wood River Medical Center, Los Angeles, ID, p. A122

STEVENSON, Mike, Administrator, Murphy Medical Center, Murphy, NC, p. A314

STEWART, Charles L., Administrator, Northport Hospital–DCH, Northport, AL, p. A17

STEWART, Christine R., President and Chief Executive Officer, Northwest Medical Center, Russellville, AL, p. A17

STEWART, Diane Gail, Administrator, Sutter Center for Psychiatry, Sacramento, CA, p. A59

STEWART, Jerome G., President, St. Clare's Hospital of Schenectady, Schenectady, NY, p. A304

STEWART, Joseph A., President and Chief Executive Officer, Butler Health System, Butler, PA, p. A354

STEWART, Lawrence C., Director, Veterans Affairs Medical Center, San Francisco, CA, p. A62

STEWART, Mary Ellen, Administrator, Schick Shadel Hospital, Seattle, WA, p. A452

STEWART, Paul R., President and Chief Executive Officer, Merle West Medical Center, Klamath Falls, OR, p. A349

STIBBARDS, J. E. Ted, Ph.D., President and Chief Executive Officer, Driscoll Children's Hospital, Corpus Christi, TX, p. A405

STILLWAGON, Richard A., Superintendent, Torrance State Hospital, Torrance, PA, p. A369

STILLWELL, James M., Director, Impact Drug and Alcohol Treatment Center, Pasadena, CA, p. A57

STINDT, John, Chief Executive Officer, Swift County–Benson Hospital, Benson, MN, p. A227

STINSON, Karl R., Administrator, Parkview Regional Hospital, Mexia, TX, p. A421

STOCK, Greg K., Chief Executive Officer, Thibodaux Regional Medical Center, Thibodaux, LA, p. A191

STOCKTON, Eddy R., Administrator, Wayne County Hospital, Monticello, KY, p. A178

STODDARD, Mark R.
President, Central Valley Medical Center, Nephi, UT, p. A434

President, Rural Health Management Corporation, Nephi, UT, p. B130

STOECKEL, Craig, Interim Administrator, St. John's Regional Health Center, Red Wing, MN, p. A233

STOKER, Teresa, Executive Director, Hillside Hospital, Atlanta, GA, p. A104

STOKES, Barry S.
Chief Executive Officer, Columbia Edward White Hospital, Saint Petersburg, FL, p. A98

Chief Operating Officer, Columbia University General Hospital, Seminole, FL, p. A99

STOKES, Gary L., Chief Executive Officer, Gulf Coast Medical Center, Biloxi, MS, p. A237

STOLL, Dale D., Chief Executive Officer, Arkansas Valley Regional Medical Center, La Junta, CO, p. A73

STOLZENBERG, Edward A., Commissioner, Westchester County Medical Center, Valhalla, NY, p. A306

STONE, John M., Director, Metropolitan Nashville General Hospital, Nashville, TN, p. A394

STONE, Robert, President, Blythedale Children's Hospital, Valhalla, NY, p. A306

STONE, Thomas J., Administrator, St. Tammany Parish Hospital, Covington, LA, p. A184

STONER, Philip J., Chief Executive Officer, Tyrone Hospital, Tyrone, PA, p. A370

STORDAHL, Dean R., Director, Jerry L. Pettis Memorial Veterans Medical Center, Loma Linda, CA, p. A48

STORER, Gregory T., Chief Executive Officer, St. Francis Health Care Centre, Green Springs, OH, p. A330

STORY, Bettye W., Ph.D., Director, Veterans Affairs Medical Center, Salisbury, NC, p. A316

STORY, Lawrence, Chief Executive Officer and Administrator, Gulf Pines Behavioral Health Services, Houston, TX, p. A414

STOTT, Robert F., Director, Veterans Affairs Medical Center, Houston, TX, p. A416

STOTTS, Cathy, Chief Executive Officer, Lucas County Health Center, Chariton, IA, p. A152

STOVALL, Ed, Administrative Officer, Northville Psychiatric Hospital, Northville, MI, p. A221

STRACK, J. Gary, Chairman and Chief Executive Officer, Orlando Regional Healthcare System, Orlando, FL, p. B119

STRANGE, John, President and Chief Executive Officer, St. Luke's Hospital, Duluth, MN, p. A228

STRASSHEIM, Dale S., President, BroMenn Healthcare, Normal, IL, p. A135

STRAUCH, Walter A., Executive Director, Franklin Regional Hospital, Franklin, NH, p. A272

STRECK, William F., M.D., President and Chief Executive Officer, Mary Imogene Bassett Hospital, Cooperstown, NY, p. A291

STRECKERT, I. Douglas, Chief Executive Officer, Columbia Medical Center at Terrell, Terrell, TX, p. A428

STREET, Jackie, President, Idaho Falls Recovery Center, Idaho Falls, ID, p. A120

STRICKLAND, Samuel A., Administrator, Hart County Hospital, Hartwell, GA, p. A110

STRICKLAND, Wallace, Administrator, Rush Foundation Hospital, Meridian, MS, p. A242

STRIEBY, James M., Chief Executive Officer, Franciscan Medical Center–Dayton Campus, Dayton, OH, p. A328

STRIEBY, John F., President and Chief Executive Officer, Nix Health Care System, San Antonio, TX, p. A426

STRIEPE, James L., Administrator, Spencer Municipal Hospital, Spencer, IA, p. A159

STRINE, Mervin F., President and Chief Executive Officer, Massillon Community Hospital, Massillon, OH, p. A332

STRINGFIELD, C. David, President, Baptist Hospital, Nashville, TN, p. A394

STRODE Jr., Paul W., Administrator, Jefferson Davis County Hospital, Prentiss, MS, p. A243

STROHL Jr., George R., President, Community General Osteopathic Hospital, Harrisburg, PA, p. A358

STROMBERG, Arlan L., Administrator, Lincoln General Hospital, Lincoln, NE, p. A265

STRONG, Patricia, Administrator, Aurora Hospital for Children, Detroit, MI, p. A214

STROTE, Ted, Administrator, Stevens County Hospital, Hugoton, KS, p. A164

STROUD, Bridget K., Chief Executive Officer, Faribault Regional Center, Faribault, MN, p. A229

STRUBLE, Russell E., Medical Center Director, Clement J. Zablocki Veterans Affairs Medical Center, Milwaukee, WI, p. A465

STRUTHERS, Tony, Chief Executive Officer, Columbia San Clemente Hospital and Medical Center, San Clemente, CA, p. A60

STRUYK, Douglas, President and Chief Executive Officer, Ramapo Ridge Psychiatric Hospital, Wyckoff, NJ, p. A283

STUART, Charlene G., Vice President Clinical Operations and Chief Executive Officer, MUSC Medical Center of Medical University of South Carolina, Charleston, SC, p. A376

STUART, Philip, Administrator, Tomah Memorial Hospital, Tomah, WI, p. A469

STUBBS, Deborah, Chief Executive Officer, South Barry County Memorial Hospital, Cassville, MO, p. A246

STUBER, Joseph A., Administrator, Vencor Hospital–Arlington, Arlington, VA, p. A439

STUDER, Quinton, President, Baptist Hospital, Pensacola, FL, p. A96

STUDSRUD, John S., President, St. Joseph's Hospital and Health Center, Dickinson, ND, p. A319

STUENKEL, Kurt, FACHE, President and Chief Executive Officer, Floyd Medical Center, Rome, GA, p. A113

STYLES Jr., John, Administrator, Columbia Doctors Hospital East Loop, Houston, TX, p. A413

SUAREZ FONSECA, Jose Luis, Executive Director, Hospital Pavia, San Juan, PR, p. A476

SUDDERS, Marylou, Commissioner, Massachusetts Department of Mental Health, Boston, MA, p. B112

SUGG, William T., President and Chief Executive Officer, Sumner Regional Medical Center, Gallatin, TN, p. A389

SUGIYAMA, Deborah
President, NorthBay Medical Center, Fairfield, CA, p. A42

President, Vacavalley Hospital, Vacaville, CA, p. A67

SUH, Young S., President and Chief Executive Officer, Genesys Regional Medical Center, Grand Blanc, MI, p. A216

SUIT, Larry, Administrator, North Runnels Hospital, Winters, TX, p. A432

SUKSI, Eugene, Administrator, Oak Crest Hospital and Counseling Center, Shawnee, OK, p. A345

SULIKOWSKI, Antoni, Facility Director, Northern Virginia Mental Health Institute, Falls Church, VA, p. A440

SULLIVAN, Charles, President and Chief Executive Officer, Reading Hospital and Medical Center, Reading, PA, p. A368

SULLIVAN, John, Chief Executive Officer, Our Lady of the Resurrection Medical Center, Chicago, IL, p. A126

SULLIVAN, Michael J., Director, Veterans Affairs Medical Center, Bath, NY, p. A289

SULLIVAN, Marie Celeste, President and Chief Executive Officer, Allegany Health System, Tampa, FL, p. B64

SUMMERS, Steve, Administrator, Decatur Community Hospital, Decatur, TX, p. A407

SUMMERS, William L., Executive Director, Patton State Hospital, Patton, CA, p. A57

SUMMERSETT III, James A., FACHE, President and Chief Executive Officer, Conway Regional Medical Center, Conway, AR, p. A30

SUROWITZ, Dale, President and Chief Executive Officer, North Hollywood Medical Center, Los Angeles, CA, p. A51

SUSI, Jeffrey L., Executive Director and Chief Executive Officer, Northeastern Hospital of Philadelphia, Philadelphia, PA, p. A364

SUSSMAN, Elliot J., M.D., President and Chief Executive Officer, Lehigh Valley Hospital, Allentown, PA, p. A353

SUSSMAN, Michael H., Acting Chief Executive Officer, Santa Ana Hospital Medical Center, Santa Ana, CA, p. A63

SUTHERLIN, Steve, Chief Executive Officer, Columbia North Bay Hospital, Aransas Pass, TX, p. A399

SUTTERER, Larry J., USAF, Administrator, U. S. Air Force Regional Hospital, Elmendorf AFB, AK, p. A20

SVENSSON, Paul E., Chief Executive Officer, Parkway Hospital, New York, NY, p. A299

SVOBODA, John, Chief Executive Officer, Caldwell County Hospital, Princeton, KY, p. A180

SWADLEY, Robert E., Chief Executive Officer, Fulton County Medical Center, McConnellsburg, PA, p. A361

SWANSON, Ronald, Chief Executive North Coast Service Area, Providence Seaside Hospital, Seaside, OR, p. A352

SWANSON, Vivian, Interim Administrator, Pine Medical Center, Sandstone, MN, p. A234

SWARTWOUT, John A., Administrator, Shriners Hospitals for Children, Galveston Burns Institute, Galveston, TX, p. A411

SWEARINGEN, Lawrence L., President, Blessing Hospital, Quincy, IL, p. A136

SWEEDEN, Dick, Administrator, Scott and White Memorial Hospital, Temple, TX, p. A428

SWEENEY, David A., Administrator, Morgan County War Memorial Hospital, Berkeley Springs, WV, p. A455

SWENSON, Kenneth B., President, Prince William Hospital, Manassas, VA, p. A442

SWIGART, Russell W., Administrator, Howard County Community Hospital, Saint Paul, NE, p. A268

SWINEHART, Frank V., President and Chief Executive Officer, Marion General Hospital, Marion, OH, p. A332

SWINIARSKI, Wayne A., FACHE, Chief Executive Officer, West Calcasieu Cameron Hospital, Sulphur, LA, p. A191

SWINNERTON, Robert M., President and Chief Executive Officer, Schuyler Hospital, Montour Falls, NY, p. A294

SWINNEY, Keith, Chief Executive Officer, Southwest General Hospital, San Antonio, TX, p. A426

SWISHER, Charles D., Executive Director, Kendrick Memorial Hospital, Mooresville, IN, p. A147

SWITZER, Bruce, Administrator, Broken Arrow Medical Center, Broken Arrow, OK, p. A340

SWORD, Russ D., President and Chief Executive Officer, Northwest Medical Center, Springdale, AR, p. A35

SYKES Jr., Donald K., Chief Executive Officer, BHC Windsor Hospital, Chagrin Falls, OH, p. A324

SYMONDS, Thomas B., Chief Executive Officer, Hancock Medical Center, Bay St. Louis, MS, p. A237

SYPNIEWSKI, Al, Administrator, Baptist Memorial Hospital–Osceola, Osceola, AR, p. A34

T

TALLEY, James J., Administrator, Wheaton Community Hospital, Wheaton, MN, p. A236

TALLY, James E., Ph.D., President and Chief Executive Officer, Scottish Rite Children's Medical Center, Atlanta, GA, p. A104

TALMO, Michael, Chief Executive Officer, Rivendell of Michigan, Saint Johns, MI, p. A223

TALONEY, Derell, President and Chief Executive Officer, Park Lane Medical Center, Kansas City, MO, p. A249

TAMAR, Earl, Executive Director and System Vice President, Cape Coral Hospital, Cape Coral, FL, p. A84

TAMLYN, Mary E., Administrator, Mackinac Straits Hospital and Health Center, Saint Ignace, MI, p. A222

TAMME, Paula, Chief Executive Officer, Central State Hospital, Louisville, KY, p. A177

TAMME, Susan Stout, President, Baptist Hospital East, Louisville, KY, p. A177

TAN, Bienvenido, M.D., Chief Executive Officer, Newhall Community Hospital, Newhall, CA, p. A55

TAN–LACHICA, Nieves, M.D., Superintendent, Andrew McFarland Mental Health Center, Springfield, IL, p. A138

TANNER, Anthony J., Executive Vice President, HEALTHSOUTH Corporation, Birmingham, AL, p. B102

TANNER, Gale V., Administrator, Monroe County Hospital, Forsyth, GA, p. A109

TANNER, Laurence A., President and Chief Executive Officer, New Britain General Hospital, New Britain, CT, p. A77

TANNER, Sharon M., President and Chief Executive Officer, Bon Secours–DePaul Medical Center, Norfolk, VA, p. A443

TAPIA, Manuel Soto, Chief Executive Officer, Hospital Dr. Federico Trilla, Carolina, PR, p. A475

TAPP, Tim, Administrator, Cumberland River Hospital South, Gainesboro, TN, p. A389

TARBET, Michele T., R.N., Chief Executive Officer, Grossmont Hospital, La Mesa, CA, p. A47

TARR, Judith, Chief Executive Officer, Miles Memorial Hospital, Damariscotta, ME, p. A194

TARRANT, Jeffrey S., Administrator, Lafayette Regional Health Center, Lexington, MO, p. A250

TASCONE, Deborah, R.N., Vice President/Administration, North Shore University Hospital at Syosset, Syosset, NY, p. A305

TATE, Joel W., FACHE, Interim Chief Executive Officer, McAlester Regional Health Center, McAlester, OK, p. A342

TATE Jr., David B., President and Chief Executive Officer, Lake Taylor Hospital, Norfolk, VA, p. A443

TATUM, Stanley D., Chief Executive Officer, Columbia Edmond Regional Medical Center, Edmond, OK, p. A341

TAUSSIG, Lynn M., M.D., President and Chief Executive Officer, National Jewish Medical and Research Center, Denver, CO, p. A71

TAVARY, Jim, Chief Executive Officer and Administrator, Copper Queen Community Hospital, Bisbee, AZ, p. A22

TAVERNIER, Patrice L., Administrator, Fishermen's Hospital, Marathon, FL, p. A92

TAYLOR, Alfred P., Administrator and Chief Executive Officer, Camden General Hospital, Camden, TN, p. A387

TAYLOR, Dennis A., Administrator, North Bay Medical Center, New Port Richey, FL, p. A94

TAYLOR, James H., President and Chief Executive Officer, University of Louisville Hospital, Louisville, KY, p. A177

TAYLOR, Meredith, Administrator, Vencor Hospital–Sacramento, Folsom, CA, p. A43

TAYLOR, R. Gordon, Administrator, Columbia Lea Regional Hospital, Hobbs, NM, p. A286

TAYLOR, Steven L., Chief Executive Officer, Harrison County Hospital, Corydon, IN, p. A141

TAYLOR, Wayne, Director, Western State Hospital, Hopkinsville, KY, p. A175

TAYLOR, Donald, Administrator, U. S. Air Force Hospital Shaw, Shaw AFB, SC, p. A380

TAYLOR Jr., L. Clark, President and Chief Executive Officer, Memorial Hospital, Chattanooga, TN, p. A388

TEAGUE, M. E., Chief Executive Officer, Louisiana State Hospitals, New Orleans, LA, p. B109

TEAGUE, Michael E., Chief Executive Officer, New Orleans Adolescent Hospital, New Orleans, LA, p. A189

TEAL, Allen, Administrator, Adams County Memorial Hospital and Nursing Care Unit, Friendship, WI, p. A462

TEEL, Kenneth R., Administrator, Lake Pointe Medical Center, Rowlett, TX, p. A424

TEEL, Kerry, President and Chief Executive Officer, Innovative Healthcare Systems, Inc., Birmingham, AL, p. B105

TEIGEN, Bobbe, Administrator, Sauk Prairie Memorial Hospital, Prairie Du Sac, WI, p. A468

TEMBREULL, John P., Administrator, Baraga County Memorial Hospital, L'Anse, MI, p. A219

TENBARGE, Ronald W., Executive Vice President and Chief Executive Officer, Bullhead Community Hospital, Bullhead City, AZ, p. A22

TENNISON, Randal, Administrator, Dexter Memorial Hospital, Dexter, MO, p. A247

TERLESKI, Deirdre, Chief Executive Officer, Memorial Center, Bakersfield, CA, p. A37

TERREBONNE, Terry J., Administrator, Jennings American Legion Hospital, Jennings, LA, p. A185

TERRILL, John, Administrator, Smith County Memorial Hospital, Smith Center, KS, p. A169

TERWILLIGER, Michael, Acting Chief Executive Officer, Hampton Hospital, Westampton Township, NJ, p. A283

TESAR, James D., Administrator, Senatobia Community Hospital, Senatobia, MS, p. A243

TEST, Russell A., Chief Executive Officer, The Hospital, Sidney, NY, p. A304

TESTERMAN, E. R., Administrator, Niobrara Valley Hospital, Lynch, NE, p. A265

TESTERMAN, R. Frank, Administrator, Hawkins County Memorial Hospital, Rogersville, TN, p. A395

THACHER, Frederick J., Chairman, Community Care Systems, Inc., Wellesley Hills, MA, p. B86

THAMES, Barbara H., Chief Executive Officer, Santa Rosa Medical Center, Milton, FL, p. A94

THAW, James G., President and Chief Executive Officer, Summerville Medical Center, Summerville, SC, p. A380

THEBEAU, Robert S., President, Kishwaukee Community Hospital, De Kalb, IL, p. A128

THEROULT, Thomas N., Administrator, Koala Behavioral Health–Columbus Campus, Columbus, IN, p. A141

THIER, Samuel O., M.D., Chief Executive Officer, Partners HealthCare System, Boston, MA, p. B121

THOMAS, E. Daniel, Administrator and Chief Executive Officer, Del Amo Hospital, Torrance, CA, p. A66

THOMAS, James R., Chief Executive Officer, Columbia Redmond Regional Medical Center, Rome, GA, p. A113

THOMAS, Marcile, Administrator, Providence Medical Center, Wayne, NE, p. A268

THOMAS, Michael P., Administrator, Meade District Hospital, Meade, KS, p. A166

THOMAS, Philip P., Director, Veterans Affairs Medical Center, Syracuse, NY, p. A305

THOMAS, Richard Lee, Superintendent, Lakeshore Mental Health Institute, Knoxville, TN, p. A391

THOMAS, Richard M., President, Pattie A. Clay Hospital, Richmond, KY, p. A180

THOMAS, Robert, Administrator, Columbus Community Hospital, Columbus, TX, p. A404

THOMAS, Telford W., President and Chief Executive Officer, Washington Hospital, Washington, PA, p. A370

THOMPSON, Anthony E., Chief Executive Officer, Pauline Warfield Lewis Center, Cincinnati, OH, p. A326

THOMPSON, Bobby G., President and Chief Executive Officer, Mercy Memorial Health Center, Ardmore, OK, p. A339

THOMPSON, C. T., M.D., Interim Chief Executive Officer, Saint Francis Hospital, Tulsa, OK, p. A346

THOMPSON, Charlotte, Administrator, Tri–Ward General Hospital, Bernice, LA, p. A183

THOMPSON, Frederick G., Ph.D., Administrator and Chief Executive Officer, Anson County Hospital and Skilled Nursing Facilities, Wadesboro, NC, p. A317

THOMPSON, Harriet, Administrator, Hancock County Memorial Hospital, Britt, IA, p. A151

THOMPSON, John William, Ph.D., President and Chief Executive Officer, Lakeland Regional Hospital, Springfield, MO, p. A255

THOMPSON, Larry
  Administrator, Harris Continued Care Hospital, Fort Worth, TX, p. A410
  Vice President and Administrator, Harris Methodist Northwest, Azle, TX, p. A400

THOMPSON, Mark, Chief Executive Officer, Cumberland County Hospital, Burkesville, KY, p. A172

THOMPSON, Mary L., Administrator, Lincoln Community Hospital and Nursing Home, Hugo, CO, p. A73

THOMPSON, Royce C., President, Florida Hospital Waterman, Eustis, FL, p. A86

THOMPSON, Thomas, President, Saint Joseph Community Hospital, New Hampton, IA, p. A157

THOMPSON, Wes, Administrator, Alta View Hospital, Sandy, UT, p. A435

THOMPSON, William D., Commandant, Lawrence F. Quigley Memorial Hospital, Chelsea, MA, p. A206

THORESON, Scott, Administrator, Springfield Community Hospital, Springfield, MN, p. A235

THORP, Gretchen, R.N., Administrator, Casa, A Special Hospital, Houston, TX, p. A413

THORSLAND Jr., Ed, Director, Veterans Affairs Medical Center, Denver, CO, p. A72

THORSON, Lona, Interim Chief Executive Officer, UniMed Medical Center, Minot, ND, p. A321

THORTON, James H., President and Chief Executive Officer, Brandywine Hospital, Coatesville, PA, p. A356

THORWARD, S. R., M.D., President and Chief Executive Officer, Harding Hospital, Worthington, OH, p. A337

THWEATT, James W., Chief Executive Officer, Columbia Clinch Valley Medical Center, Richlands, VA, p. A444

TIBBITTS, Tom, President, Trinity Regional Hospital, Fort Dodge, IA, p. A154

TICE, Kirk C., President and Chief Executive Officer, Rahway Hospital, Rahway, NJ, p. A281

TIECHE Jr., Albert M., Administrator, Beckley Hospital, Beckley, WV, p. A455

TIGHE, John F., President and Chief Executive Officer, St. Thomas Hospital, Nashville, TN, p. A395

TILLER, Gary L., Administrator, Kingman Community Hospital, Kingman, KS, p. A165

TILTON, David P., President and Chief Executive Officer, Atlantic City Medical Center, Atlantic City, NJ, p. A275

TINDLE, Jack L., Chief Executive Officer, Carroll County Memorial Hospital, Carrollton, MO, p. A246

TINKER, A. James, President and Chief Executive Officer, Mercy Medical Center, Cedar Rapids, IA, p. A152

TIPPETS, Wayne C., Director, Veterans Affairs Medical Center, Boise, ID, p. A119

TITUS III, Rexford W., President and Chief Executive Officer, Waukesha Memorial Hospital, Waukesha, WI, p. A469

TOBIN, John H., President, Waterbury Hospital, Waterbury, CT, p. A79

TODD, Mike, Chief Executive Officer, Samaritan–Wendy Paine O'Brien Treatment Center, Phoenix, AZ, p. A25

TODD, Nanette, R.N., Acting Administrator, University Medical Center, Lebanon, TN, p. A392

TODD Jr., Warren A., MSC, Commander, Tripler Army Medical Center, Honolulu, HI, p. A117

TODHUNTER, Neil E., Chief Executive Officer, Northwest Medical Center, Franklin, PA, p. A358

TODT, Michael A., Ph.D., Administrator, William R. Sharpe Jr. Hospital, Weston, WV, p. A459

TOEBBE, Nelson, Chief Executive Officer, Rockdale Hospital, Conyers, GA, p. A107

TOERING, Marla, Administrator, Sioux Center Community Hospital and Health Center, Sioux Center, IA, p. A158

TOLL, Sidney A., President, North Country Hospital and Health Center, Newport, VT, p. A437

TOLMAN, Russell K., President, Cook Children's Medical Center, Fort Worth, TX, p. A410

TOLMIE, John Kerr, President and Chief Executive Officer, St. Joseph Hospital, Lancaster, PA, p. A360

TOLOSKY, Mark R., Chief Executive Officer, Baystate Medical Center, Springfield, MA, p. A210

TOMPKINS, John, Administrator, Baptist Memorial Hospital–Union County, New Albany, MS, p. A242

TOMT, Gene, FACHE, Chief Executive Officer, Bonner General Hospital, Sandpoint, ID, p. A121

TONG, Dalton A., FACHE, President and Chief Executive Officer, Greater Southeast Healthcare System, Washington, DC, p. B99

TOPOLESKI, Jack W., President and Chief Executive Officer, Columbia Mercy Medical Center, Canton, OH, p. A324

TORBA, Gerald M., Chief Executive Officer, Callaway Community Hospital, Fulton, MO, p. A247

TORCH, Michael, Executive Director, Seaborne Hospital, Dover, NH, p. A272

TORCHIA, Jude, Chief Executive Officer, HEALTHSOUTH Rehabilitation Hospital, Miami, FL, p. A93

TORNABENI, Jolene, Administrator, Inova Fairfax Hospital, Falls Church, VA, p. A440

TORRES, Leon, Interim Administrator, Anadarko Municipal Hospital, Anadarko, OK, p. A339

TORRES–ZAYAS, Domingo, Executive Director, Hospital Menonita De Cayey, Cayey, PR, p. A475

TORRESCANO, Bob, Administrator, North Florida Reception Center Hospital, Lake Butler, FL, p. A90

TORVIK, Patricia A., Ph.D., Chief Executive Officer, Dayton Mental Health Center, Dayton, OH, p. A328

TOTH, Cynthia M., Administrator, Upreach Rehabilitation Hospital, Gainesville, FL, p. A88

TOURVILLE, James C., Administrator, Douglas County Hospital, Omaha, NE, p. A267

TOWNSEND, Mitchell, Administrator, George Nigh Rehabilitation Institute, Okmulgee, OK, p. A344

TOWNSEND, Stanley, Administrator, Stone County Medical Center, Mountain View, AR, p. A33

TOWNSEND Jr., C. Vincent
Vice President, Operations, St. Joseph Northeast Heights Hospital, Albuquerque, NM, p. A284
Vice President, Operations, St. Joseph West Mesa Hospital, Albuquerque, NM, p. A285

TRACEY, Robert M., Administrator, Franciscan Skemp Healthcare–Arcadia Campus, Arcadia, WI, p. A460

TRACY, Timothy J., Administrator, Towner County Medical Center, Cando, ND, p. A319

TRAHAN, Alcus, Administrator, Acadia–St. Landry Hospital, Church Point, LA, p. A183

TRAHAN, Lyman, Administrator, Abrom Kaplan Memorial Hospital, Kaplan, LA, p. A185

TRAMP, Francis, President, Burgess Memorial Hospital, Onawa, IA, p. A157

TRAUM, Clarence, President and Chief Executive Officer, Highlands Regional Medical Center, Prestonsburg, KY, p. A180

TRAVERSE, Bruce L., President, Carson City Hospital, Carson City, MI, p. A213

TREFRY, Robert J., President and Chief Executive Officer, Bridgeport Hospital, Bridgeport, CT, p. A76

TREMBULAK, Frank J., Executive Vice President and Chief Operating Officer, Geisinger Health System, Danville, PA, p. B98

TRENT, William, USAF, Commanding Officer, U. S. Air Force Hospital, Patrick AFB, FL, p. A96

TRIANA, Milton, President and Chief Executive Officer, St. Mary Medical Center, Hobart, IN, p. A144

TRIEBES, David G., Administrator, Blue Mountain Hospital, John Day, OR, p. A349

TRIMBLE, Charley O., President and Chief Executive Officer, St. Mary of the Plains Hospital, Lubbock, TX, p. A419

TRIMMER, Mary R., President and Chief Executive Officer, Mercy Hospital, Port Huron, MI, p. A222

TRIPODI, Frank, Executive Director, Monroe Community Hospital, Rochester, NY, p. A303

TROTTER, Patrick J.
President, Sheboygan Memorial Medical Center, Sheboygan, WI, p. A468
President, Valley View Medical Center, Plymouth, WI, p. A467

TROWER, G. Wil, President and Chief Executive Officer, North Broward Hospital District, Fort Lauderdale, FL, p. B118

TRSTENSKY, Jomary, President, Hospital Sisters Health System, Springfield, IL, p. B105

TRUDELL, Thomas J., President and Chief Executive Officer, Marymount Hospital, Garfield Heights, OH, p. A330

TRUELOVE, Lynn, President, Rapides Regional Medical Center, Alexandria, LA, p. A182

TRUJILLO, Michael, M.P.H., Director, U. S. Public Health Service Indian Health Service, Rockville, MD, p. B143

TRULL, David J., President and Chief Executive Officer, Faulkner Hospital, Boston, MA, p. A204

TRUNFIO, Joseph A., President and Chief Executive Officer, Northwest Covenant Medical Center, Denville, NJ, p. A276

TRUSKOLOSKI, Roger, Administrator, Chief Executive Officer and Vice President, Memorial Rehabilitation Hospital, Houston, TX, p. A415

TSCHIDER, Richard A., FACHE, Administrator and Chief Executive Officer, St. Alexius Medical Center, Bismarck, ND, p. A319

TSCHOPP, Edward C., Administrator, Lakeview Regional Hospital, West Monroe, LA, p. A191

TSO, Ronald, Chief Executive Officer, Chinle Comprehensive Health Care Facility, Chinle, AZ, p. A22

TUCKER, Edgar, Director, Colmery–O'Neil Veterans Affairs Medical Center, Topeka, KS, p. A170

TUCKER, George, M.D., President, St. Luke's Hospital, Chesterfield, MO, p. A246

TUCKER, Joseph R., President, St. Claude Medical Center, New Orleans, LA, p. A189

TUCKER, Paul, Administrator, Highline Community Hospital, Burien, WA, p. A448

TUCKER, Steven E., Interim President, Good Samaritan Medical Center, Johnstown, PA, p. A359

TUERPITZ, Peter, Administrator and Chief Executive Officer, Joel Pomerene Memorial Hospital, Millersburg, OH, p. A333

TUNGATE, Rex A., Administrator, Westlake Regional Hospital, Columbia, KY, p. A173

TUOHY, Michael J., Administrator, Kennewick General Hospital, Kennewick, WA, p. A450

TURCO, John, M.D., Director, Dartmouth College Health Service, Hanover, NH, p. A272

TURK, Herbert A., FACHE, Administrator, Sweeny Community Hospital, Sweeny, TX, p. A428

TURLEY, Frank, Ph.D., Executive Director, Napa State Hospital, Napa, CA, p. A55

TURNBULL, James, Administrator and Chief Executive Officer, Clara Barton Hosptial, Hoisington, KS, p. A164

TURNER, Howard D., Administrator and Chief Executive Officer, Heart of the Rockies Regional Medical Center, Salida, CO, p. A74

TURNER, Joseph F., President, Central Suffolk Hospital, Riverhead, NY, p. A303

TURNER, Kenneth G., CHE, Chief Executive Officer, Elk County Regional Medical Center, Ridgway, PA, p. A368

TURNER, Michael A., President and Chief Executive Officer, Somerset Medical Center, Somerville, NJ, p. A281

TURNER, Robert J., Administrator, United Community Hospital, Grove City, PA, p. A358

TURNER, Samuel H., Chief Executive Officer, Columbia St. Vincent Charity Hospital, Cleveland, OH, p. A326

TURNEY, Brian, Chief Executive Officer, Kingman Regional Medical Center, Kingman, AZ, p. A23

TURNEY, Dennis, Chief Executive Officer, Community Hospital, Watervliet, MI, p. A224

TUTEN, Amelia, R.N., Administrator, Columbia Hamilton Medical Center, Jasper, FL, p. A90

TUTEN, E. Allen, Administrator, Lincoln General Hospital, Ruston, LA, p. A190

TWIEHAUS, John M., Ph.D., Superintendent, St. Louis State Hospital, Saint Louis, MO, p. A254

TWISS, Gayla J., Service Unit Director, U. S. Public Health Service Indian Hospital, Rosebud, SD, p. A384

TYLER, Rosamond M., Administrator, McNairy County General Hospital, Selmer, TN, p. A396

U

UCHMAN, Stanley F., Commander, U. S. Air Force Hospital, Davis–Monthan AFB, AZ, p. A22

UDOVICH, G. William, Chief Executive Officer and Administrator, Lewis County General Hospital, Lowville, NY, p. A294

UFFER, Mark, Chief Executive Officer, St. Luke Medical Center, Pasadena, CA, p. A57

UHLING, Casey, Administrator, St. Mary's Hospital, Cottonwood, ID, p. A120

ULAND, Jonas S., Executive Director, Greene County General Hospital, Linton, IN, p. A146

ULICNY, Gary R., Ph.D., President and Chief Executive Officer, Shepherd Center, Atlanta, GA, p. A104

ULLIAN, Elaine S., President and Chief Executive Officer, Boston Medical Center, Boston, MA, p. A203

ULMER, Evonne G., Chief Executive Officer, Ionia County Memorial Hospital, Ionia, MI, p. A218

ULSETH, Randy, Interim Administrator, Community Hospital, Cannon Falls, MN, p. A227

UMBDENSTOCK, Richard J., President and Chief Executive Officer, Providence Services, Spokane, WA, p. B123

UNDERKOFLER, Joseph, Director, Veterans Affairs Hospital, Fort Harrison, MT, p. A258

UNDERRINER, David T., Operations Administrator, Providence Portland Medical Center, Portland, OR, p. A351

UNDERWOOD, Benjamin H., FAAMA, President and Chief Executive Officer, Anchor Hospital, Atlanta, GA, p. A103

UNDERWOOD, Della, Chief Executive Officer, THC–Boston, Peabody, MA, p. A209

UNGAR, John W., President, Lee Hospital, Johnstown, PA, p. A359

UNROE, Larry J., President, Marietta Memorial Hospital, Marietta, OH, p. A332

UNRUH, Greg, Chief Executive Officer, Scott County Hospital, Scott City, KS, p. A169

UOMO, Paul Dell, President and Chief Executive Officer, Horton Medical Center, Middletown, NY, p. A294

UPTON, Brian, Administrator and Chief Executive Officer, Gulf Pines Hospital, Port St. Joe, FL, p. A97
UPTON, Terry, Chief Executive Officer, Columbia Ocala Regional Medical Center, Ocala, FL, p. A95
URBAN, Thomas S., President, Mercy Hospital, Hamilton, OH, p. A330
URCIUOLI, Robert A., President and Chief Executive Officer, Roger Williams Medical Center, Providence, RI, p. A373
URMY, Norman B., Executive Director, Vanderbilt University Hospital, Nashville, TN, p. A395
UROSEVICH, Steve L., Chief Executive Officer, St. Croix Valley Memorial Hospital, Saint Croix Falls, WI, p. A468
URSO, Susan, Administrator, Mendota Community Hospital, Mendota, IL, p. A134
URVAND, Leslie O., Administrator, St. Luke's Hospital, Crosby, ND, p. A319
USHIJIMA, Arthur A., President and Chief Executive Officer, Queen's Medical Center, Honolulu, HI, p. A117
UTLEY, Karen, Administrator, Humboldt General Hospital, Humboldt, TN, p. A390

V

VAAGENES, Carl P., Administrator, Pipestone County Medical Center, Pipestone, MN, p. A233
VADELLA, Anthony J., Chief Executive Officer, Poplar Springs Hospital, Petersburg, VA, p. A444
VALDESPINO, Gustavo A.
   Chief Executive Officer, Lakewood Regional Medical Center, Lakewood, CA, p. A47
   Chief Executive Officer, Los Alamitos Medical Center, Los Alamitos, CA, p. A49
VALENTINE, Billy M., Director, Veterans Affairs Medical Center, Muskogee, OK, p. A343
VALERIUS, Thomas J., Chief Executive Officer, Jay County Hospital, Portland, IN, p. A148
VALIANTE, John, Chief Executive Officer, St. John's Hospital and Living Center, Jackson, WY, p. A471
VALLIANT, Robert F., Administrator, Bartlett Regional Hospital, Juneau, AK, p. A20
VAN BOKKELEN, W. R., President and Senior Executive Officer, Christian Hospital Northeast–Northwest, Saint Louis, MO, p. A253
VAN DRIEL, Allen, Administrator, Harlan County Hospital, Alma, NE, p. A262
VAN ETTEN, Peter
   President, Lucile Salter Packard Children's Hospital at Stanford, Palo Alto, CA, p. A56
   President and Chief Executive Officer, Stanford University Hospital, Stanford, CA, p. A65
VAN GORDER, Chris D., President and Chief Executive Officer, Anaheim Memorial Hospital, Anaheim, CA, p. A36
VAN HOY, Page, Chief Executive Officer, Tustin Rehabilitation Hospital, Tustin, CA, p. A67
VAN STRATEN, Elizabeth, President and Chief Executive Officer, St. Bernard Hospital and Health Care Center, Chicago, IL, p. A127
VAN VOORHIS, Donald, Administrator, Vencor Hospital–Sycamore, Sycamore, IL, p. A138
VAN VRANKEN, Ross, Chief Executive Officer, University of Utah Neuropsychiatric Institute, Salt Lake City, UT, p. A435
VANDENBERG, Patricia, President and Chief Executive Officer, Holy Cross Health System Corporation, South Bend, IN, p. B104
VANDER DOES, Victor, Administrator, Willapa Harbor Hospital, South Bend, WA, p. A453
VANDERGRIFT, Patricia, Administrator, BHC St. Johns River Hospital, Jacksonville, FL, p. A89
VANDERHOOF, Terry L., President and Chief Executive Officer, River Valley Health System, Ironton, OH, p. A331
VANDERVEER, Robert W., Administrator, Knapp Medical Center, Weslaco, TX, p. A431
VANDERVORT, Darryl L., President and Chief Executive Officer, Katherine Shaw Bethea Hospital, Dixon, IL, p. A129

VANEK, James, Administrator, Lavaca Medical Center, Hallettsville, TX, p. A412
VANNESS II, William C., M.D., Chief Executive Officer, Community Hospital of Anderson and Madison County, Anderson, IN, p. A140
VANOURNY, Stephen E., M.D., President, St. Luke's Hospital, Cedar Rapids, IA, p. A152
VARGAS, Laura, Administrator, BHC Hospital San Juan Capestrano, San Juan, PR, p. A476
VARGAS–TORRES, Evelyn, Administrator, Industrial Hospital, San Juan, PR, p. A476
VARLAND, Carol A.
   Administrator, Community Memorial Hospital, Burke, SD, p. A382
   Chief Executive Officer, Gregory Community Hospital, Gregory, SD, p. A383
VARNUM, James W., President, Mary Hitchcock Memorial Hospital, Lebanon, NH, p. A273
VARONE, Rick J., President, Staten Island University Hospital, New York, NY, p. A300
VASKELIS, Glenna L., Administrator, Sequoia Hospital, Redwood City, CA, p. A58
VASQUEZ, Alberto, Chief Executive Officer, Star Valley Hospital, Afton, WY, p. A471
VASSE, Gregory J., President and Chief Executive Officer, Henry Ford Cottage Hospital of Grosse Pointe, Grosse Pointe Farms, MI, p. A217
VATTER, Russell K., Superintendent, Moccasin Bend Mental Health Institute, Chattanooga, TN, p. A388
VAUGHAN, Page, Executive Director, Byerly Hospital, Hartsville, SC, p. A379
VAUGHT, Richard H., Administrator, William Newton Memorial Hospital, Winfield, KS, p. A171
VAZQUEZ, Manuel J., Administrator, Hospital Matilde Brenes, Bayamon, PR, p. A475
VAZQUEZ, William L., Vice President and Chief Executive Officer, University of Medicine and Dentistry of New Jersey–University Hospital, Newark, NJ, p. A280
VAZQUEZ ROSARIO, Iris J., Executive Director, Hospital Universitario Dr. Ramon Ruiz Arnau, Bayamon, PR, p. A475
VEENSTRA, Henry A., President, Zeeland Community Hospital, Zeeland, MI, p. A225
VEITZ, Larry W., Chief Executive Officer, Dakota Medical Center, Vermillion, SD, p. A385
VELDEKENS, Charles, Chief Executive Officer, Yale Clinic and Hospital, Houston, TX, p. A416
VELEZ, Pete, Executive Director, Elmhurst Hospital Center, New York, NY, p. A296
VELICK, Stephen H., Chief Executive Officer, Henry Ford Hospital, Detroit, MI, p. A214
VELLINGA, David H., President and Chief Executive Officer, North Iowa Mercy Health Center, Mason City, IA, p. A157
VELOSO, Carole A., R.N., President and Chief Executive Officer, Northside General Hospital, Houston, TX, p. A415
VELTE, Carl J., Chief Executive Officer, Munising Memorial Hospital, Munising, MI, p. A220
VENTURA, N. Lawrence, Superintendent, Bangor Mental Health Institute, Bangor, ME, p. A193
VERMAELEN, Elizabeth A., President, Sisters of Charity Center, New York, NY, p. B133
VERNOR, Robert E., Administrator, Ballinger Memorial Hospital, Ballinger, TX, p. A401
VIATOR, Kyle J., Chief Executive Officer, Columbia Dauterive Hospital, New Iberia, LA, p. A188
VICE, Jon E., President and Chief Executive Officer, Children's Hospital of Wisconsin, Milwaukee, WI, p. A465
VICKERY, James F., President, Baptist Health Care Corporation, Pensacola, FL, p. B67
VICTORY, Ronald D., Administrator, Penobscot Valley Hospital, Lincoln, ME, p. A194
VIGUS, Ronald J., Chief Executive Officer, Mary Black Memorial Hospital, Spartanburg, SC, p. A380
VILAR, Ramon J., Administrator, Wilma N. Vazquez Medical Center, Vega Baja, PR, p. A477
VILLANUEVA, John V., Chief Executive Officer, Hood General Hospital, Granbury, TX, p. A411
VINARDI, Gregory B., President and Chief Executive Officer, Western Missouri Medical Center, Warrensburg, MO, p. A256

VINCENT, Richard A.
   President, Doctors Hospital, Columbus, OH, p. A328
   President, Doctors Hospital, Columbus, OH, p. B95
VINCENT, Rose, President and Chief Executive Officer, St. Elizabeth Medical Center, Utica, NY, p. A306
VINSON, Daniel M., CPA, Senior Executive Officer, St. Luke Hospital East, Fort Thomas, KY, p. A174
VINTURELLA, Joseph C., Chief Executive Officer, Southeast Louisiana Hospital, Abita Springs, LA, p. A182
VINYARD, Roy G., Chief Administrative Officer, University Hospital, Portland, OR, p. A351
VISALLI, Charles, Administrator, Heritage Beverly Hills Hospital, Lecanto, FL, p. A91
VIVALDI, Domingo Cruz, Administrator, San Jorge Children's Hospital, San Juan, PR, p. A477
VLACH, Karen, Administrator, Oakland Memorial Hospital, Oakland, NE, p. A266
VLOSKY, Michael J., President and Chief Executive Officer, Lockport Memorial Hospital, Lockport, NY, p. A294
VODENICKER, Johnette L., Senior Vice President and Administrator, Memorial Hospital–West Volusia, DeLand, FL, p. A86
VOGT, Allen J., Administrator, Cook Hospital and Convalescent Nursing Care Unit, Cook, MN, p. A228
VOLK, Ronald J., President, St. Aloisius Medical Center, Harvey, ND, p. A320
VOLPE, Michele M., Chief Operating Officer, Presbyterian Medical Center of the University of Pennsylvania Health System, Philadelphia, PA, p. A365
VOLPE–WAY, Edna, Chief Executive Officer, Senator Garret T. W. Hagedorn Gero Psychiatric Hospital, Glen Gardner, NJ, p. A277
VON HOLDEN, Martin H., Executive Director, Rochester Psychiatric Center, Rochester, NY, p. A303
VON ZYCHLIN, Claus, Senior Executive Officer, Christ Hospital, Cincinnati, OH, p. A325
VONDERFECHT, Dennis, President and Chief Executive Officer, Johnson City Medical Center Hospital, Johnson City, TN, p. A391
VONDRAK, Darrell E., Administrator, Palo Alto County Hospital, Emmetsburg, IA, p. A154
VOZEL, Gerald F., Administrator and Chief Executive Officer, Healthsouth Tri–State Rehabilitation Hospital, Evansville, IN, p. A142
VREELAND, James C., FACHE, President and Chief Executive Officer, Memorial Hospital of Bedford County, Everett, PA, p. A358
VROOM, James R., Chief Executive Officer, Vencor Hospital–Greensboro, Greensboro, NC, p. A312
VYVERBERG, Robert W., Ed.D., Director, George A. Zeller Mental Health Center, Peoria, IL, p. A136
VYVERBERGER, Robert, Acting Facility Director and Network Manager, H. Douglas Singer Mental Health and Developmental Center, Rockford, IL, p. A137

W

WAACK, Ronald L., President, Masonic Geriatric Healthcare Center, Wallingford, CT, p. A79
WACHS, Jon L., President, St. Joseph's Hospital, Milwaukee, WI, p. A466
WADE, Kay, President and Chief Executive Officer, Desert Hills Hospital, Albuquerque, NM, p. A284
WAGES, N. Gary, President and Chief Executive Officer, St. Mary's Hospital of Blue Springs, Blue Springs, MO, p. A245
WAGGENER, Rob S., Chief Executive Officer, Charter Lakeside Behavioral Health System, Memphis, TN, p. A393
WAGGONER, Ronald D., Administrator and Chief Executive Officer, Brodstone Memorial Hospital, Superior, NE, p. A268
WAGNER, Anthony G., Executive Administrator, Laguna Honda Hospital and Rehabilitation Center, San Francisco, CA, p. A61
WAGNER, Henry C., President, Jewish Hospital Healthcare Services, Louisville, KY, p. B107
WAGNON, Ronnie, Administrator, Caldwell Memorial Hospital, Columbia, LA, p. A183

WAHLER, Darryl, Administrator, Hoopeston Community Memorial Hospital, Hoopeston, IL, p. A132

WAHLMEIER, James, Administrator, Trego County–Lemke Memorial Hospital, Wakeeney, KS, p. A170

WAHNEE Jr., Joe, Service Unit Director, U. S. Public Health Service Indian Hospital, Mescalero, NM, p. A286

WAITE, Sally, Acting Administrator, Dr. John Warner Hospital, Clinton, IL, p. A128

WAITE, Marguerite, President and Chief Executive Officer, St. Mary's Hospital, Waterbury, CT, p. A79

WAITE III, Ralph J., Chief Executive Officer, BHC Meadow Wood Hospital, Baton Rouge, LA, p. A182

WAKEFIELD Jr., Robert D., Executive Director, Lemuel Shattuck Hospital, Boston, MA, p. A204

WAKEMAN, Daniel, Chief Executive Officer, Chippewa County War Memorial Hospital, Sault Ste. Marie, MI, p. A223

WALB, William R., President and Chief Executive Officer, Hanover General Hospital, Hanover, PA, p. A358

WALDHOFF, Stephen C., Administrator, Rochester Methodist Hospital, Rochester, MN, p. A233

WALDROUP, Gerald E., Administrator, Lawrence County Memorial Hospital, Lawrenceville, IL, p. A133

WALK, Rex D., Chief Executive Officer, Memorial Health Center, Sidney, NE, p. A268

WALKER, Benjamin H., Acting Superintendent, Georgia Regional Hospital at Augusta, Augusta, GA, p. A105

WALKER, G. Curtis, R.N., Administrator, B.J. Workman Memorial Hospital, Woodruff, SC, p. A381

WALKER, Gale, Administrator, St. Benedict Health Center, Parkston, SD, p. A384

WALKER, Gregory J., Chief Executive Officer, Wentworth–Douglass Hospital, Dover, NH, p. A272

WALKER, James R., FACHE, President and Chief Executive Officer, North Arundel Hospital, Glen Burnie, MD, p. A200

WALKER, John E., Chief Executive Officer, Riverside Medical Center, Franklinton, LA, p. A184

WALKER, Melvin E., Administrator, Baptist Memorial Hospital–Desoto, Southaven, MS, p. A243

WALKER, Paul A., President, Piedmont Healthcare System, Rock Hill, SC, p. A380

WALKER, Robert D., President and Chief Executive Officer, Landmark Medical Center, Woonsocket, RI, p. A374

WALKER, Robert J., President, Frank R. Howard Memorial Hospital, Willits, CA, p. A69

WALKER, Ron, Chief Executive Officer, Columbia Hendersonville Hospital, Hendersonville, TN, p. A390

WALKER, Ronnie D., President, Southwestern Memorial Hospital, Weatherford, OK, p. A347

WALKLEY Jr., Philip H., Chief Executive Officer, Methodist Hospital of Jonesboro, Jonesboro, AR, p. A32

WALL, Daniel J., President and Chief Executive Officer, Emma Pendleton Bradley Hospital, East Providence, RI, p. A373

WALL, Eldon A., Administrator, Memorial Hospital, Aurora, NE, p. A262

WALL, Michael L., President and Chief Executive Officer, Mount Diablo Medical Center, Concord, CA, p. A40

WALLACE, Archie T., Chief Executive Officer, Thomas B. Finan Center, Cumberland, MD, p. A199

WALLACE, Jim, Executive Director, Choctaw Health Center, Philadelphia, MS, p. A242

WALLACE, Lloyd E., President and Chief Executive Officer, Valdese General Hospital, Valdese, NC, p. A317

WALLACE, Mark A., Executive Director and Chief Executive Officer, Texas Children's Hospital, Houston, TX, p. A415

WALLACE, Michael S., Administrator and Chief Executive Officer, Healthsouth Valley of the Sun Rehabilitation Hospital, Glendale, AZ, p. A23

WALLACE, Patrick L., Administrator, East Texas Medical Center Athens, Athens, TX, p. A399

WALLACE, Richard B., Chief Executive Officer, Rabun County Memorial Hospital, Clayton, GA, p. A106

WALLACE, Rick, FACHE, Chief Executive Officer and Administrator, Columbia Horizon Medical Center, Dickson, TN, p. A389

WALLACE, Samuel T., President, Iowa Health System, Des Moines, IA, p. B106

WALLER, Richard E., M.D., Interim Administrator, Quitman County Hospital and Nursing Home, Marks, MS, p. A241

WALLER, Richard W., Interim Administrator, St. Mary's Hospital, Nebraska City, NE, p. A265

WALLER, Robert R., M.D., President and Chief Executive Officer, Mayo Foundation, Rochester, MN, p. B112

WALLER Jr., Burton W., President and Chief Executive Officer, Regional Medical Center at Memphis, Memphis, TN, p. A393

WALLING, John R., President and Chief Executive Officer, Lafayette Home Hospital, Lafayette, IN, p. A145

WALLIS, Larry D., President and Chief Executive Officer, Cox Health Systems, Springfield, MO, p. A255

WALLMAN, Gerald H., Administrator, Doctors Hospital of West Covina, West Covina, CA, p. A68

WALMSLEY III, George J., President and Chief Executive Officer, North Philadelphia Health System, Philadelphia, PA, p. A364

WALSH, Daniel C., President, Good Samaritan Hospital Medical Center, West Islip, NY, p. A306

WALSH, Mary Beth, M.D., Chief Executive Officer, Burke Rehabilitation Hospital, White Plains, NY, p. A307

WALSH, Maura, President and Chief Executive Officer, Columbia Doctors Hospital, Little Rock, AR, p. A32

WALSH, Raoul, Chief Executive Officer, Greene County Memorial Hospital, Waynesburg, PA, p. A370

WALTER, Mary Lee, Chief Executive Officer, Columbia East Houston Medical Center, Houston, TX, p. A413

WALTER, William R., Administrator, Maury Regional Hospital, Columbia, TN, p. A388

WALTERS, Farah M.
President and Chief Executive Officer, University Hospitals Health System, Cleveland, OH, p. B146
President and Chief Executive Officer, University Hospitals of Cleveland, Cleveland, OH, p. A327

WALTERS, H. Patrick, President, Alexandria Hospital, Alexandria, VA, p. A439

WALTON, Michael W., Director, Veterans Affairs Medical Center, Chillicothe, OH, p. A325

WALTZ, Brenda M., CHE, Chief Executive Officer, Columbia East Ridge Hospital, East Ridge, TN, p. A389

WALTZ, Ronald D., Chief Executive Officer, Memorial Health Care Systems, Seward, NE, p. A268

WALZ, George, CHE, Chief Executive Officer, Breckinridge Memorial Hospital, Hardinsburg, KY, p. A174

WANGER, David S.
Chief Executive Officer, General Hospital, Eureka, CA, p. A42
Chief Executive Officer, Lindsay District Hospital, Lindsay, CA, p. A48

WARD, Sandy, Administrator, Johnson County Memorial Hospital, Buffalo, WY, p. A471

WARDEN, Gail L., President and Chief Executive Officer, Henry Ford Health System, Detroit, MI, p. B104

WARDEN, Richard
Executive Director, Devereux Foundation–French Center, Devon, PA, p. A356
Administrator, Devereux Mapleton Psychiatric Institute–Mapleton Center, Malvern, PA, p. A361

WARMAN Jr., Harold C., President and Chief Executive Officer, Shamokin Area Community Hospital, Coal Township, PA, p. A355

WARNER, Donald L., Chief Operating Officer, Arborview Hospital, Warren, MI, p. A224

WARNER Jr., Gerard H., Chief Executive Officer, Mid–Valley Hospital, Peckville, PA, p. A363

WARREN, James B., Chief Executive Officer, Columbia Medical Center–Dallas Southwest, Dallas, TX, p. A406

WARREN, Larry, Interim Executive Director, University of Michigan Hospitals, Ann Arbor, MI, p. A212

WARREN, R. William, Chairman and Chief Executive Officer, Dolly Vinsant Memorial Hospital, San Benito, TX, p. A427

WARREN, Roger D., M.D., Administrator, Hanover Hospital, Hanover, KS, p. A163

WASHINGTON, W. Pearl, MSN, Administrator, C. F. Menninger Memorial Hospital, Topeka, KS, p. A170

WASHINGTON Jr., Leonard, Director, Veterans Affairs Medical Center, Lebanon, PA, p. A360

WASSERMAN, Joseph A.
President and Chief Executive Officer, Lakeland Medical Center–Niles, Niles, MI, p. A221
President and Chief Executive Officer, Lakeland Medical Center–St. Joseph, Saint Joseph, MI, p. A223
President and Chief Executive Officer, Lakeland Regional Health System, Inc., Saint Joseph, MI, p. B108

WASSERMAN, Neil
Director, Clinton Valley Center, Pontiac, MI, p. A221
Director, Hawthorn Center, Northville, MI, p. A221

WASSON, Ted D., President and Chief Executive Officer, William Beaumont Hospital Corporation, Royal Oak, MI, p. B149

WASYL, Christine, Chief Executive Officer, Margaretville Memorial Hospital, Margaretville, NY, p. A294

WATERHOUSE, Blake E., M.D., President and Chief Executive Officer, Straub Clinic and Hospital, Honolulu, HI, p. A117

WATERS, Michael C., President, Hendrick Health System, Abilene, TX, p. A398

WATERS, W. Charles, President, Newton Medical Center, Newton, KS, p. A167

WATERSTON, Judith C., Executive Director, Baylor Institute for Rehabilitation, Dallas, TX, p. A405

WATFORD, Rodney C., Administrator, North Jackson Hospital, Bridgeport, AL, p. A12

WATHEN, James A., Chief Executive Officer, Southern Coos General Hospital, Bandon, OR, p. A348

WATKINS, John R., Chief Executive Officer, THC–New Orleans, New Orleans, LA, p. A189

WATSON, Duffy, President and Chief Executive Officer, Henry Mayo Newhall Memorial Hospital, Valencia, CA, p. A67

WATSON, Gary L., President and Chief Operating Officer, Integris Mental Health System–Willow View, Spencer, OK, p. A345

WATSON, James R., Administrator, Ashland Community Hospital, Ashland, OR, p. A348

WATSON, Randy J., Administrator, Charter Forest Behavioral Health System, Shreveport, LA, p. A190

WATSON, Virgil, Administrator, Sumner County Hospital District One, Caldwell, KS, p. A161

WATTERS, Steve, Chief Executive Officer, Mendota Mental Health Institute, Madison, WI, p. A464

WAUGH, Patrick D., Chief Executive Officer, St. Luke's Behavioral Health Center, Phoenix, AZ, p. A25

WAXLER, Richard A., Administrator, Greenleaf Center, Fort Oglethorpe, GA, p. A109

WEADICK, James F., Administrator and Chief Executive Officer, Newton General Hospital, Covington, GA, p. A107

WEARMOUTH, Chris, Administrator, Nature Coast Regional Health Network, Williston, FL, p. A102

WEATHERLY, Jesse O., Administrator, Cullman Regional Medical Center, Cullman, AL, p. A13

WEATHERSON, Billie, Administrator, Sierra Valley District Hospital, Loyalton, CA, p. A52

WEAVER, Doug, Chief Executive Officer, Memorial Hospital, Frederick, OK, p. A341

WEAVER, Thomas H., FACHE, Director, Veterans Affairs Medical Center, Bay Pines, FL, p. A83

WEBB, Linnette, Senior Vice President and Executive Director, Harlem Hospital Center, New York, NY, p. A297

WEBB, Ronald W., President, Saint Eugene Community Hospital, Dillon, SC, p. A377

WEBB Jr., Charles L., Administrator, Charter louisville Behavioral Health System, Louisville, KY, p. A177

WEBER, Mark, President, St. John's Mercy Medical Center, Saint Louis, MO, p. A254

WEBER, Peter M., President and Chief Executive Officer, Central Texas Medical Center, San Marcos, TX, p. A427

WEBER, Wilson J., Chief Executive Officer, Mid–Jefferson Hospital, Nederland, TX, p. A422

WEBER Jr., Everett P., President and Chief Executive Officer, Grady Memorial Hospital, Delaware, OH, p. A329

WEBSTER, Mark A., President, Troy Community Hospital, Troy, PA, p. A369

WEBSTER, William W., Administrator, Baptist Medical Center, San Antonio, TX, p. A425

WEDEKIND, Lawrence, Administrator, Twin Oaks Medical Center, Fort Worth, TX, p. A410

WEE, Donald J., Executive Director, Pioneer Memorial Hospital, Prineville, OR, p. A351

WEEKS, Jean, Interim President and Chief Executive Officer, St. Louis Regional Medical Center, Saint Louis, MO, p. A254

WEEKS, Lin C., R.N., Director, University of Massachusetts Medical Center, Worcester, MA, p. A211

WEEKS, Steven Douglas, Vice President and Administrator, Baptist Rehabilitation Institute of Arkansas, Little Rock, AR, p. A32

WEEMS, Nadine L., Administrator, Perry Hospital, Perry, GA, p. A112

WEIBLEN, Jack W., FACHE, Chief Executive Officer, Bay Harbor Hospital, Los Angeles, CA, p. A49

WEIDNER, Michael J., President, Highland Hospital of Rochester, Rochester, NY, p. A303

WEIGHTMAN, George, Commander, McDonald Army Community Hospital, Newport News, VA, p. A443

WEILAND, Edmond L., President and Chief Executive Officer, Prairie Lakes Hospital and Care Center, Watertown, SD, p. A385

WEILER, Joseph W., President, McKenzie Memorial Hospital, Sandusky, MI, p. A223

WEINBAUM, Barry G., Chief Executive Officer, Alvarado Hospital Medical Center, San Diego, CA, p. A60

WEINBERG, Arnold N., M.D., Director, M. I. T. Medical Department, Cambridge, MA, p. A205

WEINER, David Stephen, President, Children's Hospital, Boston, MA, p. A204

WEINHOLD, Keith, Director, Ellis Fischel Cancer Center, Columbia, MO, p. A246

WEINMEISTER, Kurt
President, St. Joseph Health Center, Saint Charles, MO, p. A252
President, St. Joseph Hospital West, Lake Saint Louis, MO, p. A250

WEINSTEIN, Jay S., Chief Executive Officer, North Suburban Medical Center, Thornton, CO, p. A75

WEINSTEIN, Stephen M., President and Chief Executive Officer, Doctors Hospital of Hyde Park, Chicago, IL, p. A125

WEINSTOCK, Alan M., MS
Chief Executive Officer, Kings Park Psychiatric Center, West Brentwood, NY, p. A306
Chief Executive Officer, Pilgrim Psychiatric Center, Brentwood, NY, p. A289

WEIR, John C., President and Chief Executive Officer, Youngstown Osteopathic Hospital, Youngstown, OH, p. A338

WEIR, Silas M., Chief Executive Officer, Centura Special Care Hospital, Denver, CO, p. A71

WEIS, Eric E., FACHE, Chief Executive Officer, Riley Memorial Hospital, Meridian, MS, p. A242

WEISS, Thomas M., Chief Executive Officer, Columbia Medical Center of Huntsville, Huntsville, AL, p. A15

WEITZ, Ronald W., Executive Director, Newark Beth Israel Medical Center, Newark, NJ, p. A279

WELCH, Bill, Administrator, Jefferson Community Health Center, Fairbury, NE, p. A263

WELCH, Richard, Administrator, Claiborne County Hospital, Tazewell, TN, p. A396

WELDING, Theodore, Chief Executive Officer, Vencor Hospital–Coral Gables, Coral Gables, FL, p. A85

WELDON, Lu Ann, Administrator, Memorial Hospital of Texas County, Guymon, OK, p. A342

WELLINGER, M. Rosita, President and Chief Executive Officer, St. Francis Health System, Pittsburgh, PA, p. B138

WELLMAN, Roxann A., Chief Executive Officer, Minnewaska District Hospital, Starbuck, MN, p. A235

WELLS, Brian F., Administrator and Chief Executive Officer, North Dallas Rehabilitation Hospital, Dallas, TX, p. A407

WELLS, Mary Ellen, President, Buffalo Hospital, Buffalo, MN, p. A227

WELSH, John H., Chief Executive Officer, Rumford Community Hospital, Rumford, ME, p. A195

WELSH Jr., J. L., President, Southeastern Regional Medical Center, Lumberton, NC, p. A314

WELTZIN, Richard, USAF, Administrator, U. S. Air Force Hospital, Shreveport, LA, p. A191

WENDLING, Jeffrey T., President, Northern Michigan Hospital, Petoskey, MI, p. A221

WENTE, James J., Administrator, Nicholas County Hospital, Carlisle, KY, p. A173

WENTE, James W., CHE, Administrator, Southeast Missouri Hospital, Cape Girardeau, MO, p. A246

WENTWORTH, Philip M., FACHE, Executive Director, Presbyterian Hospital of Plano, Plano, TX, p. A423

WENTZ, Robert J., President and Chief Executive Officer, Oroville Hospital, Oroville, CA, p. A56

WENZKE, Edward T., President and Chief Executive Officer, Crouse Hospital, Syracuse, NY, p. A305

WERBY, Marcia, Administrator, Rockland Children's Psychiatric Center, Orangeburg, NY, p. A301

WERNER, Thomas J., Administrator, Richland Hospital, Richland Center, WI, p. A468

WERNER, Thomas L., President, Florida Hospital, Orlando, FL, p. A95

WERNICK, Joel, President and Chief Executive Officer, Phoebe Putney Memorial Hospital, Albany, GA, p. A103

WERNKE, Dale P., Chief Executive Officer, Jennings Community Hospital, North Vernon, IN, p. A147

WERTZ, Randy S., Administrator, Golden Valley Memorial Hospital, Clinton, MO, p. A246

WESOLOWSKI, Jaime A., Chief Executive Officer, Meadowcrest Hospital, Gretna, LA, p. A185

WESP, James H.
Administrator, Lakeview Rehabilitation Hospital, Elizabethtown, KY, p. A173
Administrator, Vencor Hospital–Louisville, Louisville, KY, p. A178

WESSELS, Roger W., Chief Executive Officer and Administrator, Specialty Hospital of Houston, Houston, TX, p. A415

WEST, John, Administrator, Buchanan General Hospital, Grundy, VA, p. A441

WEST, Kenneth C., Chief Executive Officer, Mineral Area Regional Medical Center, Farmington, MO, p. A247

WEST, Louis, President, Central Texas Hospital, Cameron, TX, p. A403

WEST, Michael A., President, Akron General Medical Center, Akron, OH, p. A323

WEST, R. Christopher
President, Franciscan Hospital–Mount Airy Campus, Cincinnati, OH, p. A325
President, Franciscan Hospital–Western Hills Campus, Cincinnati, OH, p. A325

WEST, Steven J., President and Chief Executive Officer, Galesburg Cottage Hospital, Galesburg, IL, p. A130

WEST, Warren Kyle, Administrator and Chief Executive Officer, Healthsouth Meridian Point Rehabilitation Hospital, Scottsdale, AZ, p. A26

WESTFALL, Bernard G., President, West Virginia United Health System, Morgantown, WV, p. B149

WESTHOFEN, Richard C., President, Fisher–Titus Medical Center, Norwalk, OH, p. A333

WESTHOFF, Thomas G., Chief Executive Officer, Standish Community Hospital, Standish, MI, p. A223

WESTIN, Charles A., FACHE, Administrator, Republic County Hospital, Belleville, KS, p. A161

WESTON–HALL, Patricia, Executive Director, Glenbeigh Health Sources, Rock Creek, OH, p. A334

WETTA Jr., Daniel J., Chief Executive Officer, Columbia John Randolph Medical Center, Hopewell, VA, p. A441

WHALEN, David
President and Chief Executive Officer, Columbia Putnam Medical Center, Palatka, FL, p. A96
Chief Executive Officer, Columbia Twin Cities Hospital, Niceville, FL, p. A94

WHATLEY, David, Director, Veterans Affairs Medical Center, Augusta, GA, p. A105

WHATLEY, Gary Lex, President and Chief Executive Officer, Memorial Medical Center of East Texas, Lufkin, TX, p. A419

WHEELER, Michael K., Director, Veterans Affairs Medical Center, Battle Creek, MI, p. A213

WHEELOCK, Major W., President, Crotched Mountain Rehabilitation Center, Greenfield, NH, p. A272

WHELAN, Sharon, President, River Falls Area Hospital, River Falls, WI, p. A468

WHELAN–WILLIAMS, Sue, Site Administrator, South Seminole Hospital, Longwood, FL, p. A91

WHIPKEY, Neil, Administrator, Campbellton Graceville Hospital, Graceville, FL, p. A88

WHIPPLE, Ingrid L., Chief Executive Officer, BHC Heritage Oaks Hospital, Sacramento, CA, p. A59

WHISENANT, Betty, Site Manager, Promina Cobb Hospital, Austell, GA, p. A105

WHITAKER, David D., FACHE, President and Chief Executive Officer, Bethania Regional Health Care Center, Wichita Falls, TX, p. A431

WHITAKER, E. Berton, President and Chief Executive Officer, Southeast Georgia Regional Medical Center, Brunswick, GA, p. A106

WHITAKER, James B., President, Circles of Care, Melbourne, FL, p. A92

WHITAKER Sr., Harold H., Administrator, Webster Health Services, Eupora, MS, p. A239

WHITCOMB, John R., President and Chief Executive Officer, Lewistown Hospital, Lewistown, PA, p. A360

WHITE, Alvin C., President and Chief Executive Officer, Rome Memorial Hospital, Rome, NY, p. A303

WHITE, Daniel C., Chief Executive Officer, District Memorial Hospital, Andrews, NC, p. A308

WHITE, Daryl Sue, R.N., Managing Director, River Oaks Hospital, New Orleans, LA, p. A189

WHITE, Doris, Administrator, Granite County Memorial Hospital and Nursing Home, Philipsburg, MT, p. A259

WHITE, Doug, Chief Executive Officer, Columbia Grand Strand Regional Medical Center, Myrtle Beach, SC, p. A379

WHITE, Dudley R., Administrator, Anson General Hospital, Anson, TX, p. A399

WHITE, James W., Chief Executive Officer, Columbia Riverview Medical Center, Gonzales, LA, p. A184

WHITE, Jeffrey L., Chief Executive Officer, Low Country General Hospital, Ridgeland, SC, p. A380

WHITE, Joan C., Chief Executive Officer, Columbia Good Samaritan Hospital, San Jose, CA, p. A62

WHITE, John B., President and Chief Executive Officer, Lima Memorial Hospital, Lima, OH, p. A331

WHITE, John R., Administrator, Newport Community Hospital, Newport, WA, p. A451

WHITE, Kevin A., Administrator, Medicine Lodge Memorial Hospital, Medicine Lodge, KS, p. A166

WHITE, Mary M., President and Chief Executive Officer, Columbia Swedish Medical Center, Englewood, CO, p. A72

WHITE, Stephen J., FACHE, President and Chief Executive Officer, Witham Memorial Hospital, Lebanon, IN, p. A146

WHITE, Terry R., President and Chief Executive Officer, Metrohealth Medical Center, Cleveland, OH, p. A327

WHITE, Thomas, President, Jameson Memorial Hospital, New Castle, PA, p. A362

WHITE, Thomas M., President, Empire Health Services, Spokane, WA, p. B96

WHITE Jr., Lawrence L., President, St. Patrick Hospital, Missoula, MT, p. A259

WHITEBORN, Jeffrey T., Chief Executive Officer, Columbia Fairview Park Hospital, Dublin, GA, p. A108

WHITEHOUSE, Edward J., Administrator, Cumberland Hospital, Fayetteville, NC, p. A311

WHITELEY, Earl S., CHE, Chief Executive Officer, Columbia Alice Physicians and Surgeons Hospital, Alice, TX, p. A398

WHITFIELD, Gary R., Director, Ioannis A. Lougaris Veterans Affairs Medical Center, Reno, NV, p. A271

WHITFIELD Jr., Charles H., Administrator and Chief Operating Officer, Laughlin Memorial Hospital, Greeneville, TN, p. A389

WHITING, Joseph K., Executive Vice President and Chief Operating Officer, Bayhealth Medical Center, Milford Memorial Campus, Milford, DE, p. A80

WHITLOCK, Jim, Administrator, Bradley Memorial Hospital, Cleveland, TN, p. A388

WHITMIRE, James C., CHE, Administrator, Trinity Memorial Hospital, Trinity, TX, p. A429

WHITSON, Charles P., Chief Executive Officer, Charter Behavioral Health System of Lake Charles, Lake Charles, LA, p. A186

WHITTINGTON, Terry G., Chief Executive Officer and Administrator, Bogalusa Community Medical Center, Bogalusa, LA, p. A183

WICK, Timothy J., Chief Executive Officer, Guttenberg Municipal Hospital, Guttenberg, IA, p. A155

WIDENER, Stephen G., President and Chief Executive Officer, Chestatee Regional Hospital, Dahlonega, GA, p. A107

WIEBE, John F., Chief Executive Officer, Clay County Hospital, Clay Center, KS, p. A162

WIESENDANGER, John, President, Northern Cumberland Memorial Hospital, Bridgton, ME, p. A194

WIESNER, Gerald, Vice President and Chief Operating Officer, Miami County Medical Center, Paola, KS, p. A168

WIGGINS, Gary K., Chief Executive Officer, Central Valley General Hospital, Hanford, CA, p. A45

WIGGINS, Louise, Administrator, Summit Hospital of Northwest Louisiana, Bossier City, LA, p. A183

WIGLEY, Mack
Chief Executive Officer, Oaks Psychiatric Health System, Austin, TX, p. A400
Chief Executive Officer, San Marcos Treatment Center, San Marcos, TX, p. A427

WILBANKS, Fred, Administrator, Linden Municipal Hospital, Linden, TX, p. A418

WILBER, William N., Chief Executive Officer, Cottage Grove Healthcare Community, Cottage Grove, OR, p. A348

WILBURN Jr., L. Thomas, Chairman, Bethesda Hospital, Inc., Cincinnati, OH, p. B71

WILCZEK, Joseph W., President, Saint Anne's Hospital, Fall River, MA, p. A206

WILDER, Steve, President and Chief Executive Officer, Central Community Hospital, Clifton, IL, p. A128

WILENSKY, Stephen, Executive Director, University Behavioral Health Center, Memphis, TN, p. A393

WILES, Patrick J., Chief Executive Officer, St. Joseph Hospital, Cheektowaga, NY, p. A290

WILES, Paul M., President, Forsyth Memorial Hospital, Winston–Salem, NC, p. A318

WILEY, John E., Chief Executive Officer and Administrator, First Hospital Vallejo, Vallejo, CA, p. A67

WILFORD, Dan S., President, Memorial Healthcare System, Houston, TX, p. B114

WILFORD, Ned B., President and Chief Executive Officer, Hamilton Medical Center, Dalton, GA, p. A107

WILHELM, Mary Eileen, President and Chief Executive Officer, Mercy Medical, Daphne, AL, p. A13

WILHELMSEN Jr., Thomas E., President, Southern New Hampshire Regional Medical Center, Nashua, NH, p. A273

WILKENS, Daryl J., Administrator, Cavalier County Memorial Hospital, Langdon, ND, p. A321

WILKERSON, Donald H., Chief Executive Officer, Columbia Regional Hospital of Jackson, Jackson, TN, p. A390

WILKERSON, Larry D., Chief Executive Officer, Augusta Medical Complex, Augusta, KS, p. A161

WILKINS, Patricia S., Administrator, North Caddo Medical Center, Vivian, LA, p. A191

WILKINS, William W., President and Chief Executive Officer, OhioHealth, Columbus, OH, p. B119

WILKINSON, Gary L., Director, Veterans Affairs Medical Center, Iowa City, IA, p. A155

WILKINSON, Steven D., Chief Executive Officer, Menorah Medical Center, Overland Park, KS, p. A168

WILL, Daniel, Administrator, Zumbrota Health Care, Zumbrota, MN, p. A236

WILLARD, Larry, Administrator, Hocking Valley Community Hospital, Logan, OH, p. A331

WILLAUER, Glenn R., Administrator, U. S. Air Force Hospital, Hampton, VA, p. A441

WILLCOXON, Phil, Administrator, Freeman Neosho Hospital, Neosho, MO, p. A251

WILLERT, Todd, Administrator, Story County Hospital and Long Term Care Facility, Nevada, IA, p. A157

WILLERT, St. Joan
President and Chief Executive Officer, Carondelet St. Joseph's Hospital, Tucson, AZ, p. A27
President and Chief Executive Officer, Carondelet St. Mary's Hospital, Tucson, AZ, p. A27

WILLETT, Allan Brock, M.D., Director, Colorado Mental Health Institute at Fort Logan, Denver, CO, p. A71

WILLETT, Richard, Chief Executive Officer, Redington–Fairview General Hospital, Skowhegan, ME, p. A195

WILLHELM, Judene, Administrator, Memorial Hospital, Kermit, TX, p. A417

WILLIAMS, Charlotte, Interim Administrator, Deckerville Community Hospital, Deckerville, MI, p. A214

WILLIAMS, Chas H., M.D., Administrator, Starlite Village Hospital, Center Point, TX, p. A403

WILLIAMS, David R., Chief Executive Officer, Columbia Montgomery Regional Hospital, Blacksburg, VA, p. A439

WILLIAMS, Denise R., President, Roseland Community Hospital, Chicago, IL, p. A127

WILLIAMS, Gerald L., Director, James E. Van Zandt Veterans Affairs Medical Center, Altoona, PA, p. A353

WILLIAMS, John G.
President and Chief Executive Officer, Saint Francis Memorial Hospital, San Francisco, CA, p. A61
President, St. Mary's Medical Center, San Francisco, CA, p. A62

WILLIAMS, Miriam K., Administrator, Charter Hospital of Pasco, Lutz, FL, p. A92

WILLIAMS, Oreta, Administrator, Jeff Davis Hospital, Hazlehurst, GA, p. A110

WILLIAMS, R. D., Administrator, Ashe Memorial Hospital, Jefferson, NC, p. A313

WILLIAMS, Ralph T.
Administrator, Fort Sanders Loudon Medical Center, Loudon, TN, p. A392
Administrator, Fort Sanders–Sevier Medical Center, Sevierville, TN, p. A396

WILLIAMS, Richard C., President and Chief Executive Officer, St. Mary's Health System, Knoxville, TN, p. A391

WILLIAMS, Robert B.
Administrator, Florida State Hospital, Chattahoochee, FL, p. A84
Administrator, Shands at AGH, Gainesville, FL, p. A88

WILLIAMS, Robert D., Administrator, Mercy Special Care Hospital, Nanticoke, PA, p. A362

WILLIAMS, Roby D., Administrator, Hardin County General Hospital, Rosiclare, IL, p. A137

WILLIAMS, Roger, Chief Executive Officer, Carroll County Memorial Hospital, Carrollton, KY, p. A173

WILLIAMS, Stephen A., President, Alliant Health System, Louisville, KY, p. B65

WILLIAMS, Timothy B., Director, VA Puget Sound Health Care System, Seattle, WA, p. A453

WILLIAMS, Trude, R.N., Administrator, Pacifica Hospital of the Valley, Los Angeles, CA, p. A51

WILLIAMS III, Raymond, President and Chief Executive Officer, Sumner Regional Medical Center, Wellington, KS, p. A170

WILLIAMS Jr., Elton L., CPA, President, Lake Charles Memorial Hospital, Lake Charles, LA, p. A186

WILLIAMS Jr., John F., M.D., Director, Wishard Health Services, Indianapolis, IN, p. A145

WILLIS, Cornelia, Administrator and Chief Executive Officer, Willow Crest Hospital, Miami, OK, p. A343

WILLIS, Yvonne, Administrator, Bowdon Area Hospital, Bowdon, GA, p. A105

WILLMAN, Arthur C., Vice President Operations, Searhc MT. Edgecumbe Hospital, Sitka, AK, p. A21

WILLMON, Gary R., Administrator, Grafton City Hospital, Grafton, WV, p. A456

WILLNER, Catherine, Executive Director, Rolling Hills Hospital, Ada, OK, p. A339

WILLS, Andrew, Chief Executive Officer, Estes Park Medical Center, Estes Park, CO, p. A72

WILMOT, David, MSC, Administrator, U. S. Air Force Hospital Whiteman, Whiteman AFB, MO, p. A256

WILSEY, Suzanne R., Administrator, Vencor Hospital–Kansas City, Kansas City, MO, p. A250

WILSON, Bill D., Administrator, Wayne County Hospital, Corydon, IA, p. A152

WILSON, Bob L., Administrator, Villa Feliciana Chronic Disease Hospital and Rehabilitation Center, Jackson, LA, p. A185

WILSON, Franklin K., Administrator, Allen County Hospital, Iola, KS, p. A164

WILSON, Geri, Chief Executive Officer, Madison Valley Hospital, Ennis, MT, p. A258

WILSON, Hugh D.
Chief Executive Officer, Columbia Doctors Hospital, Columbus, GA, p. A107
Chief Executive Officer, Columbia Hughston Sports Medicine Hospital, Columbus, GA, p. A107

WILSON, Jim, President and Chief Executive Officer, Susan B. Allen Memorial Hospital, El Dorado, KS, p. A162

WILSON, John A., President and Chief Executive Officer, Rehabilitation Institute of Pittsburgh, Pittsburgh, PA, p. A366

WILSON, John M., President, San Pedro Peninsula Hospital, Los Angeles, CA, p. A51

WILSON, Kirk G., Chief Executive Officer, Columbia Bay Area Medical Center, Corpus Christi, TX, p. A404

WILSON, L. Steven, Administrator, Dixie Regional Medical Center, Saint George, UT, p. A435

WILSON, Mark D., Administrator, Barron Memorial Medical Center and Skilled Nursing Facility, Barron, WI, p. A460

WILSON, Nancy, Senior Vice President and Regional Administrator, Scripps Mercy Medical Center, San Diego, CA, p. A61

WILSON, Paul J., Administrator, Los Alamos Medical Center, Los Alamos, NM, p. A286

WILSON, R. Lynn, President, Bryan Memorial Hospital, Lincoln, NE, p. A265

WILSON, Ralph J., Administrator, Red Bay Hospital, Red Bay, AL, p. A17

WILSON, Stephen K., President, Genesis Rehabilitation Hospital, Jacksonville, FL, p. A89

WILSON, William G., President and Chief Executive Officer, Jackson County Memorial Hospital, Altus, OK, p. A339

WILSON Jr., V. Otis, President, Grace Hospital, Morganton, NC, p. A314

WILTERMOOD, Michael C., Chief Executive Officer, Coulee Community Hospital, Grand Coulee, WA, p. A450

WIMAN, Thomas, Executive Director, Rankin Medical Center, Brandon, MS, p. A237

WINFREE, Wayne, Chief Executive Officer, Frank T. Rutherford Memorial Hospital, Carthage, TN, p. A387

WINFREY, Robert C., President and Chief Operating Officer, Greater Southeast Community Hospital, Washington, DC, p. A81

WINGER, Ronald C., President and Chief Executive Officer, St. Vincent Hospital, Santa Fe, NM, p. A287

WINKLER, Gordon W., Administrator, Ringgold County Hospital, Mount Ayr, IA, p. A157

WINN, George, Administrator, Sanpete Valley Hospital, Mount Pleasant, UT, p. A434

WINN, Grant M., President, Community Medical Center, Missoula, MT, p. A259

WINN, Roger P., Chief Executive Officer, Miners Hospital Northern Cambria, Spangler, PA, p. A369

WINSLOW, F. Scott, President and Chief Executive Officer, Columbia Michael Reese Hospital and Medical Center, Chicago, IL, p. A125

WINTER, William E., Administrative Director, Silverton Hospital, Silverton, OR, p. A352

WINTHROP, Michael K., President, Bellevue Hospital, Bellevue, OH, p. A324

WIRTZ Jr., Robert E., President and Chief Executive Officer, MedCentral Crestline Hospital, Crestline, OH, p. A328

WISBY, Diane, Vice President, Goleta Valley Cottage Hospital, Santa Barbara, CA, p. A63

WISE, Franklin E., Administrator, Fulton County Hospital, Salem, AR, p. A34

WISE, Jerry R., Administrator, Stewart–Webster Hospital, Richland, GA, p. A113

WISE, Robert P., President and Chief Executive Officer, Hunterdon Medical Center, Flemington, NJ, p. A277

WISEMAN, Richard J., Ph.D., Superintendent, Riverview Hospital for Children, Middletown, CT, p. A77

WISEMAN, John G., Administrator, U. S. Air Force Hospital, Laughlin AFB, TX, p. A418

WISSINK, Gerald L., President and Chief Executive Officer, Baptist Hospitals and Health Systems, Inc., Phoenix, AZ, p. B68

WITT, Stephen, Chief Executive Officer, College Hospital, Cerritos, CA, p. A39

WOERNER, Steven, Chief Executive Officer, Columbia Doctors Regional Medical Center, Corpus Christi, TX, p. A404

WOJICK, Thomas J., Chief Executive Officer, Charter Westbrook Behavioral Health System, Richmond, VA, p. A445

WOLF, Chris, Chief Executive Officer, Chesterfield General Hospital, Cheraw, SC, p. A376

WOLF, Edward H., Chief Executive Officer, Lakeview Medical Center, Rice Lake, WI, p. A468

WOLF, James N., Chief Executive Officer, District One Hospital, Faribault, MN, p. A229

WOLF, Jonathan, Chief Executive Officer, Charter Behavioral Health System at Cove Forge, Williamsburg, PA, p. A371

WOLF, Laura J., President, Franciscan Sisters of Christian Charity HealthCare Ministry, Inc, Manitowoc, WI, p. B98

WOLFE, Philip R., Executive Director, N. T. Enloe Memorial Hospital, Chico, CA, p. A39

WOLFE, Stephen A., President and Chief Executive Officer, Clearfield Hospital, Clearfield, PA, p. A355

WOLFF, Ronald V., President and Chief Executive Officer, Bay Medical Center, Panama City, FL, p. A96

WOLFORD, Dennis A., FACHE, Administrator, Macon County General Hospital, Lafayette, TN, p. A392

WOLIN, Harry, Administrator and Chief Executive Officer, Mason District Hospital, Havana, IL, p. A131

WOOD, Alice, Director, Richard L. Roudebush Veterans Affairs Medical Center, Indianapolis, IN, p. A144

WOOD, Glen A., Chief Executive Officer, Morton County Health System, Elkhart, KS, p. A162

WOOD, Gregory C., Chief Executive Officer, Scotland Memorial Hospital, Laurinburg, NC, p. A313

WOOD, Jack T., Administrator, William Bee Ririe Hospital, Ely, NV, p. A270

WOOD, James B., Chief Executive Officer, Greenbrier Valley Medical Center, Ronceverte, WV, p. A458

WOOD, James R., Chairman and Chief Executive Officer, Maryland General Hospital, Baltimore, MD, p. A198

WOOD, Kenneth R., Administrator, Johnson Regional Medical Center, Clarksville, AR, p. A29

WOOD, Raymond E., President and Chief Executive Officer, Preston Memorial Hospital, Kingwood, WV, p. A457

WOOD, Sharon R., Administrator, Veterans Home and Hospital, Rocky Hill, CT, p. A78

WOOD, Tammy B., Chief Executive Officer, Charter Asheville Behavioral Health System, Asheville, NC, p. A308

WOODALL, Jay, Chief Executive Officer, Columbia Trinity Hospital, Erin, TN, p. A389

WOODALL, Jim S., Director, Caswell Center, Kinston, NC, p. A313

WOODARD, Elizabeth B., Chief Executive Officer, Cumberland Hospital for Children and Adolescents, New Kent, VA, p. A443

WOODRELL, Frederick, Associate Vice Chancellor and Director, University Hospitals and Clinics, University of Mississippi Medical Center, Jackson, MS, p. A240

WOODS, Daniel J., Administrator, Veterans Memorial Hospital, Waukon, IA, p. A159

WOODS, E. Anthony, President, Deaconess Hospital, Cincinnati, OH, p. A325

WOODSIDE, Jeffrey R., M.D., Executive Director, University of Tennessee Bowld Hospital, Memphis, TN, p. A394

WOODWARD, Barry W., Administrator, BHC Olympus View Hospital, Salt Lake City, UT, p. A435

WOODWORTH, Marlene, Chief Executive Officer, Corona Regional Medical Center, Corona, CA, p. A40

WOODY, Fred, Chief Executive Officer, Doctors Hospital, Wentzville, MO, p. A256

WOOLLEY, Helen, Administrator, Pershing General Hospital, Lovelock, NV, p. A271

WOOLSLAYER, Richard N., Chief Executive Officer, Arroyo Grande Community Hospital, Arroyo Grande, CA, p. A37

WOOTEN, Richard L., Administrator, Jackson Hospital, Marianna, FL, p. A92

WORDELMAN, Scott, President and Chief Executive Officer, Chisago Health Services, Chisago City, MN, p. A227

WORKMAN, Dennis, M.D., Medical Director, Charter Behavioral Health System of Atlanta, Atlanta, GA, p. A103

WORLEY, Steve, President and Chief Executive Officer, Children's Hospital, New Orleans, LA, p. A188

WORRELL, Robert, Chief Executive Officer, Redgate Memorial Hospital, Long Beach, CA, p. A49

WORRICK, Gerald M., President and Administrator, Door County Memorial Hospital, Sturgeon Bay, WI, p. A469

WORSHAM, Sharon, Administrator, Charter Centennial Peaks Health System, Louisville, CO, p. A74

WOZNIAK, Gregory T., President, Barnes–Jewish West County Hospital, Saint Louis, MO, p. A253

WRAALSTAD, Kimber, Chief Executive Officer, Presentation Medical Center, Rolla, ND, p. A321

WRAY, Christine R., Chief Executive Officer, St. Mary's Hospital, Leonardtown, MD, p. A201

WRIGHT, Charles T., Chief Executive, Southern Oregon Service Area, Providence Medford Medical Center, Medford, OR, p. A350

WRIGHT, Gene B., President and Chief Executive Officer, Columbia Trident Medical Center, Charleston, SC, p. A376

WRIGHT, J. B., Administrator, La Follette Medical Center, La Follette, TN, p. A391

WRIGHT, Joe, Administrator, Mitchell County Hospital, Colorado City, TX, p. A404

WRIGHT, Norman, Administrator, Beckley Appalachian Regional Hospital, Beckley, WV, p. A455

WRIGHT, Rick, CPA, President and Chief Executive Officer, Keweenaw Memorial Medical Center, Laurium, MI, p. A219

WRIGHT, Roy W., Chief Executive Officer, Des Moines General Hospital, Des Moines, IA, p. A153

WRIGHT, Skip, Administrator, Vencor Hospital–Atlanta, Atlanta, GA, p. A104

WRIGHT, William G., Director, Veterans Affairs Medical Center, Hampton, VA, p. A441

WRIGHT, Margaret, President, Palos Community Hospital, Palos Heights, IL, p. A135

WYATT, Leslie G., Administrator, Children's Hospital, Richmond, VA, p. A445

WYNN, Chester A., President and Chief Executive Officer, Passavant Area Hospital, Jacksonville, IL, p. A132

X

XINIS, James J., President and Chief Executive Officer, Calvert Memorial Hospital, Prince Frederick, MD, p. A201

Y

YAGER, Jolene, R.N., Administrator, Lincoln County Hospital, Lincoln, KS, p. A166

YANOS, Craig J., Administrator, Madison Community Hospital, Madison Heights, MI, p. A220

YARBOROUGH, James, Chief Executive Officer, Alleghany County Memorial Hospital, Sparta, NC, p. A317

YARBROUGH, Kathy, Administrator, Mark Twain St. Joseph's Hospital, San Andreas, CA, p. A60

YARBROUGH, Mary G., President and Chief Executive Officer, St. Joseph's Hospital and Medical Center, Phoenix, AZ, p. A25

YATES, Ronald E., Chief Executive Officer, National Hospital Medical Center, Arlington, VA, p. A439

YCRE Jr., Louis R., President and Chief Executive Officer, Pascack Valley Hospital, Westwood, NJ, p. A283

YEAGER, Cliff, Chief Executive Officer, Lutheran Medical Center, Saint Louis, MO, p. A253

YEAGER, Dave, Chief Executive Officer, Brea Community Hospital, Brea, CA, p. A38

YEARY, John, Administrator, Eastland Memorial Hospital, Eastland, TX, p. A408

YENAWINE, Kelly R., Administrator, Gibson General Hospital, Trenton, TN, p. A396

YEZZO, Richard N., President, St. Clare's Hospital and Health Center, New York, NY, p. A299

YIM, Herbert K., Administrator, Lanai Community Hospital, Lanai City, HI, p. A118

YOCHUM, Richard E., President, Pomona Valley Hospital Medical Center, Pomona, CA, p. A57

YOKOBOSKY Jr., Walter J., Chief Executive Officer, Rockford Center, Newark, DE, p. A80

YORDY, Alan R., Chief Executive Officer, Lebanon Community Hospital, Lebanon, OR, p. A350

YORK, Betty, Executive Director, West Community Hospital, West, TX, p. A431

YORK, Billy Don, Administrator, Falls Community Hospital and Clinic, Marlin, TX, p. A420

YORK, Russell W., President and Chief Executive Officer, Spalding Rehabilitation Hospital, Aurora, CO, p. A70

YORKE, Harvey M., President and Chief Executive Officer, Southwestern Vermont Medical Center, Bennington, VT, p. A437

YOSKO, Kathleen C., President and Chief Executive Officer, Schwab Rehabilitation Hospital and Care Network, Chicago, IL, p. A127

YOUNG, Anthony R., President and Chief Executive Officer, Columbia Doctors Hospital, Tulsa, OK, p. A346

YOUNG, Charles R., Administrator, Shriners Hospitals for Children–Spokane, Spokane, WA, p. A453

YOUNG, J. Phillip, President and Chief Executive Officer, Columbia Medical Center of Pampa, Pampa, TX, p. A423

YOUNG, John, President and Chief Executive Officer, Cleveland Regional Medical Center, Shelby, NC, p. A316

YOUNG, Michael, Administrator, Mad River Community Hospital, Arcata, CA, p. A36

YOUNG, Randall A., Administrator, Lamb Healthcare Center, Littlefield, TX, p. A419

YOUNG, Richard T., Administrator, Detroit Riverview Hospital, Detroit, MI, p. A214

YOUNG, Robert C., M.D., President, Fox Chase Cancer Center–American Oncologic Hospital, Philadelphia, PA, p. A363

YOUNG Jr., Frederick C., President, Pendleton Memorial Methodist Hospital, New Orleans, LA, p. A189

YOUNG Jr., William W., President, Central Maine Medical Center, Lewiston, ME, p. A194

YUTZY, LaVern J., Chief Executive Officer, Philhaven, Mount Gretna, PA, p. A362

Z

ZACCAGNINO, Joseph A., President and Chief Executive Officer, Yale–New Haven Hospital, New Haven, CT, p. A77

ZACHARY, Beth D., Chief Operating Officer, White Memorial Medical Center, Los Angeles, CA, p. A52

ZAGER, Joe, Chief Executive Officer, Monroe County Hospital, Monroeville, AL, p. A16

ZAREN, Howard A., FACS, Executive Vice President, Hospital Services, Mercy Hospital of Pittsburgh, Pittsburgh, PA, p. A366

ZASTROW, Allan, FACHE, Chief Executive Officer, Keokuk Area Hospital, Keokuk, IA, p. A156

ZAYAS, Domingo Torres, Executive Director, Mennonite General Hospital, Aibonito, PR, p. A474

ZECHMAN Jr., Edwin K., President and Chief Executive Officer, Children's National Medical Center, Washington, DC, p. A81

ZEH, Brian R., Executive Director, Clinton County Hospital, Frankfort, IN, p. A143

ZELLERS, Thomas J., Chief Operating Officer, Deaconess Medical Center–Spokane, Spokane, WA, p. A453

ZEMAN, Barry T., President and Chief Executive Officer, St. Charles Hospital and Rehabilitation Center, Port Jefferson, NY, p. A302

ZEMAN, Denise, Site Administrator, Meridia Euclid Hospital, Euclid, OH, p. A329

ZENTKO, Eugene, Administrator and Chief Executive Officer, Salem Community Hospital, Salem, OH, p. A335

ZEPEDA, Susan G., Ph.D., Administrator, San Luis Obispo General Hospital, San Luis Obispo, CA, p. A63

ZEPHIER, Richard L., Ph.D., Service Unit Director, Acoma–Canoncito–Laguna Hospital, San Fidel, NM, p. A287

ZIEGENHORN, Donald L., Director, Veterans Affairs Medical Center, Saint Louis, MO, p. A254

ZILM, Michael E., President, St. Mary's Health Center, Saint Louis, MO, p. A254

ZIMMERMAN, Joann, Vice President Patient Services and Chief Operating Officer, Camino Healthcare, Mountain View, CA, p. A54

ZIMMERMAN, Kenneth J., Administrator, Beatrice Community Hospital and Health Center, Beatrice, NE, p. A262

ZIMMERMAN, Nancy, Administrator, Comanche County Hospital, Coldwater, KS, p. A162

ZIOMEK, Janice, Administrator, Moreno Valley Community Hospital, Moreno Valley, CA, p. A54

ZORNES, Donald H., Administrator, Columbus Community Hospital, Columbus, NE, p. A263

ZUBER, Eugene, Administrator, Newport Hospital and Clinic, Newport, AR, p. A33

ZUBKOFF, William, Ph.D., Chief Executive Officer, South Shore Hospital and Medical Center, Miami Beach, FL, p. A94

ZULIANI, Michael E., Chief Executive Officer, Angel Medical Center, Franklin, NC, p. A311

ZUMWALT, Roger C., Executive Director, Community Hospital, Grand Junction, CO, p. A73

ZURBRUGG, Anton P., CHE, President and Chief Executive Officer, Memorial Community Hospital, Blair, NE, p. A262

ZWIGART, Donna, Chief Executive Officer, St. Francis Hospital of New Castle, New Castle, PA, p. A362

ZYLSTRA, Robert, Administrator, Whidbey General Hospital, Coupeville, WA, p. A449

AHA Membership Categories

The American Hospital Association is primarily an organization of hospitals and related institutions. Its object, according to its bylaws, is "to promote high–quality health care and health services for all the people through leadership in the development of public policy, leadership in the representation and advocacy of hospital and health care organization interests, and leadership in the provision of services to assist hospitals and health care organizations in meeting the health care needs of their communities."

The major source of income for the AHA is its membership dues, which are established by the membership through the House of Delegates. The types of membership and the basis for dues for each type are described in the following paragraphs.

Institutional Members

Type I–A and I–B, Hospitals

General and special hospitals that care for patients with conditions requiring a comparatively short stay. Type I–A includes short–term hospitals that are freestanding or which are operating units of health care systems not holding type III membership. Type I–B are short–term hospitals that are operating units of health care systems holding type III membership.

Type II–A and II–B, Hospitals

All other hospitals that provide inpatient care. Type II–A includes long–term hospitals that are freestanding or which are operating units of helath care systems not holding type III membership. Type II–B includes longer–term hospitals that are operating units of health care systems holding type III membership.

Type III, Health Care Systems

Only those organizations (corporate headquarters, or similar entity) operating two or more hospitals or a single hospital owning, leasing, or sponsoring at least three operating entities of nonhospital preacute and postacute health care organizations can be classified as type III institutions. Headquarters of health care systems are eligible for type III membership when 90 percent of their owned, leased, managed, or sponsored hospitals are AHA members.

Membership dues are computed individually for each hospital and are based on total reported operating expenses for the most recent 12–month period. Type III members pay no dues other than those dues paid by their type B member units.

Type IV, Nonhospital Preacute and Postacute Health Care Organizations

Type IV–A, and IV–B organizations are defined as nonhospital preacute and postacute organizations that are responsible for delivery or delivery and financing of health care services. Health care delivery, for purposes of this definition, is the availability of professional health care staff during all hours of the organization's operations. Type IV–C members shall be limited to educational organizations.

Provisional Members

Hospitals that are in the planning or construction stage and that, on completion, will be eligible for institutional membership type I or type II. Provisional membership may also be granted to applicant institutions that cannot, at present, meet the requirements of type I or type II membership.

Government Institution Group Members

Groups of government hospitals operated by the same unit of government may obtain institutional membership under a group plan. Membership dues are based on a special schedule set forth in the bylaws of the AHA.

Contracting Hospitals

The AHA also provides membership services to certain hospitals that are prevented from holding membership because of legal or other restrictions. Contracting hospitals pay dues on the same basis as if they were classified as type I or II members.

Associate Members

Associate members are organizations interested in the objectives of the AHA but not eligible for institution membership. Membership dues are a fixed annual sum, depending on the location (inside or outside the United States and Canada) of the organization.

Types I and II

Hospitals

U.S. hospitals and hospitals in areas associated with the U.S. that are type I (short–term) or type II (long–term) members of the American Hospital Association are included in the list of hospitals in section A. Canadian types I and II members of the American Hospital Association are listed below.

Canada

ALBERTA

Edmonton: MISERICORDIA COMMUNITY HEALTH CENTRE, 16940 87th Avenue, Zip T5R 4H5; tel. 403/930–5611; Douglas C. Perry, M.D., Chief Corporate Officer
ROYAL ALEXANDRA HOSPITAL, 10240 Kingsway, Zip T5H 3V9; tel. 403/477–4111; Leslee Thompson, Senior Operating Officer
UNIVERSITY OF ALBERTA HOSPITAL, 8440 112 Street, Zip T6G 2B7; tel. 403/492–8822; Lynn Cook, Site Administrator
Lamont: LAMONT HEALTH CARE CENTRE, 5216–53rd Street, Zip T0B 2R0; tel. 403/895–2211; Harold James, Chief Executive Officer
St. Albert: STURGEON COMMUNITY HEALTH CENTRE, 201 Boudreau Road, Zip T8N 6C4; tel. 403/460–6200; Wendy Hill, Network Administrator
Stony Plain: STONY PLAIN MUNICIPAL HOSPITAL, 4800 55th Avenue, Zip T7Z 1P9; tel. 403/963–2241; Myrene Couves, Administrator

BRITISH COLUMBIA

Langley: LANGLEY MEMORIAL HOSPITAL, 22051 Fraser Highway, Zip V3A 4H4; tel. 604/534–4121; Pat E. Zanon, President and Chief Executive Officer
North Vancouver: LIONS GATE HOSPITAL, 231 East 15th Street, Zip V7L 2L7; tel. 604/988–3131; L. Best, Chief Operating Officer
Vancouver: BRITISH COLUMBIA'S CHILDREN'S HOSPITAL, 4480 Oak Street, Zip V6H 3V4; tel. 604/875–2345; John H. Tegenfeldt, President

MANITOBA

Portage La Prarie: PORTAGE DISTRICT GENERAL HOSPITAL, 524 Fifth Street S.E., Zip R1N 3A8; tel. 204/239–2211; Garry C. Mattin, Executive Director
Winnipeg: RIVERVIEW HEALTH CENTRE, 1 Morley Avenue East, Zip R3L 2P4; tel. 204/452–3411; Norman R. Kasian, President
ST. BONIFACE GENERAL HOSPITAL, 409 Tache Avenue, Zip R2H 2A6; tel. 204/233–8563; J. T. Litvak, President and Chief Executive Officer

VICTORIA GENERAL HOSPITAL, 2340 Pembina Highway, Zip R3T 2E8; tel. 204/269–3570; Marion Suski, President and Chief Executive Officer

NOVA SCOTIA

North Sydney: NORTHSIDE HARBOR VIEW HOSPITAL, P.O. Box 399, Zip B2A 3M4; tel. 902/794–8521; Mary S. MacIsaac, Chief Executive Officer
Sydney: CAPE BRETON REGIONAL HOSPITAL, 1482 George Street, Zip B1P 1P3; tel. 902/567–8000; John Malcom, Chief Executive Officer

ONTARIO

Brantford: ST. JOSEPH'S HOSPITAL, 99 Wayne Gretzky Parkway, Zip N3S 6T6; tel. 519/753–8641; Romeo Cercone, President and Chief Executive Officer
Brockville: ST. VINCENT DE PAUL HOSPITAL, 42 Garden Street, Zip K6V 2C3; tel. 613/342–4461; Thomas P. Harrington, Chief Executive Officer
Chatham: PUBLIC GENERAL HOSPITAL, 106 Emma Street, Zip N7L 1A8; tel. 519/352–6400; H. David Vigar, Executive Director
Etobicoke: QUEENSWAY GENERAL HOSPITAL, 150 Sherway Drive, Zip M9C 1A5; tel. 416/259–6671; John J. Penaligon, President and Chief Executive Officer
Guelph: HOMEWOOD HEALTH CENTER, 150 Delhi Street, Zip N1E 6K9; tel. 519/824–1010; Ronald A. Pond, M.D., President and Chief Executive Officer
London: ST. MARYS' HOSPITAL CAMPUS, P.O. Box 5777, Zip N6A 1Y6; tel. 613/646–6000; Philip C. Hassen, President
North York: BAYCREST CENTRE–GERIATRIC CARE, 3560 Bathurst Street, Zip M6A 2E1; tel. 416/789–5131; Stephen W. Herbert, President and Chief Executive Officer
NORTH YORK BRANSON HOSPITAL, 555 Finch Avenue West, Zip M2R 1N5; tel. 416/633–9420; Jack A. Gallup, President and Chief Executive Officer
Ottawa: ROYAL OTTAWA HOSPITAL, 1145 Carling Avenue, Zip K1Z 7K4; tel. 613/722–6521; George F. Langill, Executive Director
Parry Sound: WEST PARRY SOUND HEALTH CENTRE, 10 James Street, Zip P2A 1T3; tel. 705/746–9321; Norman Maciver, Chief Executive Officer

Renfrew: RENFREW VICTORIA HOSPITAL, 499 Raglan Street North, Zip K7V 1P6; tel. 613/432–4851; Randy V. Penney, Executive Director
Strathroy: STRATHROY MIDDLESEX GENERAL HOSPITAL, 395 Carrie Street, Zip N7G 3C9; tel. 519/245–1550; Thomas M. Enright, Executive Director
Sudbury: SUDBURY MEMORIAL HOSPITAL, 865 Regent Street South, Zip P3E 3Y9; tel. 705/671–1000; Esko J. Vainio, Executive Director
Thornhill: SHOULDICE HOSPITAL, P.O. Box 370, Zip L3T 4A3; tel. 905/889–1125; Alan O'Dell, Administrator
Toronto: CENTRAL HOSPITAL, 333 Sherbourne Street, Zip M5A 2F5; tel. 416/969–4111; Sandra Jelenich, Acting President and Chief Executive Officer
DOCTORS HOSPITAL, 45 Brunswick Avenue, Zip M5S 2M1; tel. 416/923–5411; Brian McFarlane, President and Chief Executive Officer
MOUNT SINAI HOSPITAL, 600 University Avenue, Zip M5G 1X5; tel. 416/596–4200; Theodore J. Freedman, President and Chief Executive Officer
QUEEN ELIZABETH HOSPITAL, 550 University Avenue, Zip M5G 2A2; tel. 416/597–5111; Clifford A. Nordal, President and Chief Executive Officer
ST. JOSEPH'S HEALTH CENTRE, 30 the Queensway, Zip M6R 1B5; tel. 416/534–9531; Leo N. Steven, President and Chief Executive Officer
WOMEN'S COLLEGE HOSPITAL, 76 Grenville Street, Zip M5S 1B2; tel. 416/323–6400; W. B. MacLeod, President and Chief Executive Officer

QUEBEC

Montreal: HOPITAL NOTRE DAME, 1560 Rue Sherbrooke Est, Zip H2L 4M1; tel. 514/876–6421; David Levine, Director General
MONTREAL CHILDREN'S HOSPITAL, 2300 Tupper Street, Zip H3H 1P3; tel. 514/934–4400; Elizabeth Riley, Executive Director
MOUNT SINAI HOSPITAL CENTER, 5690 Cavendish Cote St–Luc', Zip H4W 1S7; tel. 514/369–2222; Joseph Rothbart, Executive Director
REDDY MEMORIAL HOSPITAL, 4039 Tupper Street, Zip H3Z 1T5; tel. 514/933–7511; Rejean Plante, Executive Director
Sherbrooke: SHERBROOKE HOSPITAL, 375 Argyle Street, Zip J1J 3H5; tel. 819/569–3661; Daniel Bergeron, Director General

Type III

Health Care Systems

Health Care Systems that are type III members of the American Hospital Association are included in the lists of health care systems in section B of this guide. Membership is indicated by a star (★) preceding the name of the system.

Type IV

Type IV members of the American Hospital Association include Nonhospital Precute and Postacute Health Care Organizations. These organizations are responsible for delivery or delivery and financing of health care services.
Type IV members also include Associated University Programs in Health Administration and Hospital Schools of Nursing.

Associated University Programs in Health Administration

ALABAMA

Birmingham: UNIVERSITY OF ALABAMA AT BIRMINGHAM, Zip 35294; tel. 205/934–5661; Charles L. Joiner, Ph.D., Dean

ARIZONA

Tempe: SCHOOL OF HEALTH ADMINISTRATION AND POLICY, ARIZONA STATE UNIVERSITY, P.O. Box 874506, Zip 85287–4506; tel. 602/965–7778; Frank G. Williams, Ph.D., Professor

CALIFORNIA

Los Angeles: UCLA SCHOOL OF PUBLIC HEALTH, University of California, Zip 90024; Ronald Andersen, Chairman

San Francisco: GOLDEN GATE UNIVERSITY, 536 Mission Street, General Library, Zip 94105; tel. 415/442–0777; Steven Dunlap, Assistant Librarian

DISTRICT OF COLUMBIA

Washington: SCHOOL OF PUBLIC HEALTH AND HEALTH SERVICES, THE GEORGE WASHINGTON UNIVERSITY, 600 21st Street N.W., Zip 20052; tel. 202/676–6220; Richard F. Southby, Ph.D., Associate Dean Health Services

GEORGIA

Atlanta: GEORGIA STATE UNIVERSITY, INSTITUTE OF HEALTH ADMINISTRATION, University Plaza, Zip 30303; tel. 404/651–2000; Everett A. Johnson, Director

ILLINOIS

Carbondale: SOUTHERN ILLINOIS UNIVERSITY, COLLEGE OF APPLIED SCIENCES AND ARTS, Zip 62901; tel. 618/536–6682; Frederic L. Morgan, Ph.D., Chair Health Care Professions

Chicago: UNIVERSITY OF CHICAGO, GRADUATE PROGRAM IN HEALTH ADMINISTRATION AND POLICY, 969 East 60th Street, Zip 60637; tel. 312/753–4191; Edward Lawlor, Ph.D., Director

Evanston: HEALTH SERVICE MANAGEMENT PROGRAM, KELLOGG GRADUATE SCHOOL OF MANAGEMENT, NORTHWESTERN UNIVERSITY, 2001 Sheridan Road, Zip 60208; tel. 847/492–5540; Joel Shalowitz, M.D., Professor and Director

University Park: PROGRAM IN HEALTH SERVICE ADMINISTRATION, SCHOOL OF HEALTH PROFESSIONS, GOVERNORS STATE UNIVERSITY, Zip 60466; tel. 847/534–4030; Sang–O Rhee, Chairman

IOWA

Calmar: NORTHEAST IOWA COMMUNITY COLLEGE, Box 400, Zip 52132; tel. 319/562–3263; Melinda Hanson, R.N., Chairperson Health and Human Services

Iowa City: GRADUATE PROGRAM IN HOSPITAL AND HEALTH ADMINISTRATION, UNIVERSITY OF IOWA, 2700 Steindler Building, Zip 52242; tel. 319/356–2593; Douglas Wakefield, Interim Head

MARYLAND

Bethesda: NAVAL SCHOOL OF HEALTH SCIENCES, Naval Medical Command, National Region, Zip 20889–5611; tel. 301/295–1251; Captain Harry Coffey, Commanding Officer

MISSOURI

Saint Louis: PROGRAM IN HOSPITAL AND HEALTH CARE ADMINISTRATION, ST. LOUIS UNIVERSITY, 3525 Caroline Street, Zip 63104; tel. 314/577–8000; Michael Counte, Ph.D., Chairman

WASHINGTON UNIVERSITY, SCHOOL OF MEDICINE, 4547 Clayton Avenue, Zip 63110; tel. 314/362–2477; James O. Hepner, Ph.D., Director Health Administration Program

NEW YORK

Valhalla: NEW YORK MEDICAL COLLEGE, Administration Building, Zip 10595; tel. 914/347–5044; Reverend Harry C. Barrett, M.P.H., President and Chief Executive Officer

OHIO

Columbus: GRADUATE PROGRAM IN HEALTH SERVICES MANAGEMENT AND POLICY, OHIO STATE UNIVERSITY, 1583 Perry Street, Room 246 Samp, Zip 43210; tel. 614/292–9708; Stephen F. Loebs, Ph.D., Chairman and Associate Professor

PENNSYLVANIA

Philadelphia: TEMPLE UNIVERSITY, DEPARTMENT OF HEALTH ADMINISTRATION, SCHOOL OF BUSINESS ADMINISTRATION, Zip 19122–6083; tel. 215/787–8082; William Aaronson, Professor and Chairman

University Park: PENNSYLVANIA STATE UNIVERSITY, 116 Henderson Building, Zip 16802; tel. 814/863–2859; Diane Brannon, Ph.D., Interim Department Head, Health Policy and Administration

TEXAS

Fort Sam Houston: ARMY–BAYLOR UNIVERSITY PROGRAM IN HEALTH CARE ADMINISTRATION, Academy of Health Sciences–USA, Zip 78234; tel. 512/221–5009

San Antonio: OUR LADY OF THE LAKE UNIVERSITY – GRADUATE PROGRAM IN HEALTH CARE MANAGEMENT, 411 S.W. 24th Street, Zip 78207–4666; tel. 210/434–6711; Paul Brooke, M.D., Health Care Coordinator

TRINITY UNIVERSITY, 715 Stadium Drive, Suite 58, Zip 78212–7200; tel. 210/736–8107; Niccie McKay, Ph.D., Chairman

Sheppard AFB: U. S. AIR FORCE SCHOOL OF HEALTH CARE SCIENCES, Building 1900, MSTL/114, Academic Library, Zip 76311; tel. 817/851–2511

PUERTO RICO

San Juan: SCHOOL OF PUBLIC HEALTH, P.O. Box 5067, Zip 00936; tel. 809/767–9626; Orlando Nieves, Dean

Hospital Schools of Nursing

ARKANSAS

Little Rock: BAPTIST MEDICAL SYSTEM School of Nursing
Pine Bluff: JEFFERSON REGIONAL MEDICAL CENTER School of Nursing

CALIFORNIA

Los Angeles: LOS ANGELES COUNTY–UNIVERSITY OF SOUTHERN CALIFORNIA MEDICAL CENTER School of Nursing

CONNECTICUT

Bridgeport: ST. VINCENT'S COLLEGE
Hartford: SAINT FRANCIS HOSPITAL AND MEDICAL CENTER School of Nursing
Middletown: MIDDLESEX MEMORIAL HOSPITAL ONA M. WILCOX School of Nursing
Waterbury: ST. MARY'S HOSPITAL School of Nursing

DELAWARE

Lewes: BEEBE MEDICAL CENTER School of Nursing

FLORIDA

Miami: JAMES M. JACKSON MEMORIAL HOSPITAL School of Nursing

GEORGIA

Atlanta: GEORGIA BAPTIST MEDICAL CENTER School of Nursing

ILLINOIS

Canton: GRAHAM HOSPITAL School of Nursing
Chicago: RAVENSWOOD HOSPITAL MEDICAL CENTER School of Nursing
Danville: LAKEVIEW MEDICAL CENTER School of Nursing
Evanston: ST. FRANCIS HOSPITAL School of Nursing
Peoria: METHODIST HOSPITAL OF CENTRAL ILLINOIS School of Nursing

INDIANA

Lafayette: ST. ELIZABETH HOSPITAL MEDICAL CENTER School of Nursing

IOWA

Council Bluffs: JENNIE EDMUNDSON MEMORIAL HOSPITAL School of Nursing
Des Moines: IOWA METHODIST HOSPITAL School of Nursing
MERCY HOSPITAL MEDICAL CENTER School of Nursing
Sioux City: ST. LUKE'S REGIONAL MEDICAL CENTER School of Nursing

LOUISIANA

Baton Rouge: BATON ROUGE GENERAL MEDICAL CENTER School of Nursing
OUR LADY OF LAKE REGIONAL MEDICAL CENTER School of Nursing

MARYLAND

Baltimore: UNION MEMORIAL HOSPITAL School of Nursing
Easton: MEMORIAL HOSPITAL AT EASTON MARYLAND School of Nursing

MASSACHUSETTS

Boston: NEW ENGLAND BAPTIST HOSPITAL School of Nursing
Brockton: BROCKTON HOSPITAL School of Nursing
Medford: LAWRENCE MEMORIAL HOSPITAL OF MEDFORD School of Nursing

Springfield: BAYSTATE MEDICAL CENTER School of Nursing

MICHIGAN

Detroit: HENRY FORD HOSPITAL School of Nursing
Kalamazoo: BRONSON METHODIST HOSPITAL School of Nursing

MISSOURI

Saint Louis: BARNES HOSPITAL School of Nursing
LUTHERAN MEDICAL CENTER School of Nursing
Springfield: LESTER E. COX MEDICAL CENTERS School of Nursing
ST JOHN'S School of Nursing
Town & Country: MISSOURI BAPTIST MEDICAL CENTER School of Nursing

NEBRASKA

Lincoln: BRYAN MEMORIAL HOSPITAL School of Nursing

NEW JERSEY

Camden: OUR LADY OF LOURDES MEDICAL CENTER School of Nursing
Elizabeth: ELIZABETH GENERAL MEDICAL CENTER School of Nursing
Englewood: ENGLEWOOD HOSPITAL AND MEDICAL CENTER School of Nursing
Jersey City: CHRIST HOSPITAL School of Nursing
Montclair: MOUNTAINSIDE HOSPITAL School of Nursing
Neptune: ANN MAY School of Nursing
Plainfield: MUHLENBERG REGIONAL MEDICAL CENTER School of Nursing
Teaneck: HOLY NAME HOSPITAL School of Nursing
Trenton: HELENE FULD MEDICAL CENTER School of Nursing
MERCER MEDICAL CENTER School of Nursing
ST. FRANCIS MEDICAL CENTER School of Nursing

NEW YORK

Buffalo: SISTERS OF CHARITY HOSPITAL School of Nursing
Elmira: ARNOT–OGDEN MEMORIAL HOSPITAL School of Nursing
New York: ST. VINCENT'S HOSPITAL AND MEDICAL CENTER OF NEW YORK School of Nursing
Staten Island: ST. VINCENT'S MEDICAL CENTER School of Nursing
Utica: ST. ELIZABETH HOSPITAL School of Nursing
Yonkers: ST. JOHN'S RIVERSIDE HOSPITAL COCHRAN School of Nursing

NORTH CAROLINA

Charlotte: MERCY HOSPITAL School of Nursing
PRESBYTERIAN HOSPITAL School of Nursing
Concord: CABARRUS MEMORIAL HOSPITAL School of Nursing
Durham: WATTS School of Nursing WATTS School of Nursing

NORTH DAKOTA

Bismarck: MEDCENTER ONE School of Nursing
Minot: TRINITY MEDICAL CENTER School of Nursing

OHIO

Akron: AKRON CITY HOSPITAL IDABELLE FIRESTONE School of Nursing
SUMMA ST. THOMAS School of Nursing
Canton: AULTMAN HOSPITAL School of Nursing
Cincinnati: CHRIST HOSPITAL School of Nursing
GOOD SAMARITAN HOSPITAL School of Nursing
Cleveland: FAIRVIEW GENERAL HOSPITAL School of Nursing

METROHEALTH MEDICAL CENTER School of Nursing
Sandusky: PROVIDENCE HOSPITAL School of Nursing
Springfield: COMMUNITY HOSPITAL OF SPRINGFIELD AND CLARK COUNTY School of Nursing
Toledo: MERCY HOSPITAL School of Nursing
ST. VINCENT MEDICAL CENTER School of Nursing

PENNSYLVANIA

Altoona: ALTOONA HOSPITAL School of Nursing
Johnstown: CONEMAUGH VALLEY MEMORIAL HOSPITAL School of Nursing
New Castle: JAMESON MEMORIAL HOSPITAL School of Nursing
ST. FRANCIS HOSPITAL OF NEW CASTLE School of Nursing
Philadelphia: EPISCOPAL HOSPITAL School of Nursing
GERMANTOWN HOSPITAL AND MEDICAL CENTER School of Nursing
METHODIST HOSPITAL School of Nursing
Pittsburgh: SHADYSIDE HOSPITAL School of Nursing
ST. FRANCIS MEDICAL CENTER School of Nursing
ST. MARGARET MEMORIAL HOSPITAL LOUISE SUYDAM MCCLINTIC School of Nursing
WESTERN PENNSYLVANIA HOSPITAL School of Nursing
Pottsville: POTTSVILLE HOSPITAL AND WARNE CLINIC School of Nursing
Sewickley: SEWICKLEY VALLEY HOSPITAL School of Nursing
Sharon: SHARON REGIONAL HEALTH SYSTEM School of Nursing
Washington: WASHINGTON HOSPITAL School of Nursing
West Chester: CHESTER COUNTY HOSPITAL School of Nursing

RHODE ISLAND

North Providence: ST. JOSEPH HOSPITAL School of Nursing

TENNESSEE

Knoxville: FORT SANDERS REGIONAL MEDICAL CENTER School of Nursing
Memphis: BAPTIST MEMORIAL HOSPITAL School of Nursing
METHODIST HOSPITALS OF MEMPHIS–CENTRAL School of Nursing
ST. JOSEPH HOSPITAL School of Nursing

TEXAS

Lubbock: METHODIST HOSPITAL School of Nursing
San Antonio: BAPTIST MEDICAL CENTER School of Nursing

VIRGINIA

Danville: MEMORIAL HOSPITAL OF DANVILLE School of Nursing
Lynchburg: LYNCHBURG GENERAL–MARSHALL LODGE HOSPITAL School of Nursing
Newport News: RIVERSIDE REGIONAL MEDICAL CENTER School of Nursing
Norfolk: DEPAUL MEDICAL CENTER School of Nursing
SENTARA NORFOLK GENERAL HOSPITAL School of Nursing
Petersburg: SOUTHSIDE REGIONAL MEDICAL CENTER School of Nursing
Richmond: RICHMOND MEMORIAL HOSPITAL School of Nursing
Suffolk: OBICI HOSPITAL School of Nursing

WEST VIRGINIA

Huntington: ST. MARY'S HOSPITAL School of Nursing

Nonhospital Preacute and Postacute Care Facilities

ALABAMA

Birmingham: HEALTH PARTNERS OF ALABAMA, INC., 600 Beacon Parkway West, Zip 35209; tel. 205/942–5787; Jim Ludwig, President and Chief Executive Officer

ALASKA

Anchorage: DEPARTMENT OF VETERANS AFFAIRS ALASKA MEDICAL AND REGIONAL OFFICE CENTER, 2925 Debarr Road, Zip 99508–2989; tel. 907/257–6930; Alonzo M. Poteet, III, Director

ARIZONA

Phoenix: CAMELBACK FAMILY MEDICINE, 5040 North 15th Avenue, Zip 85015; tel. 602/238–3314; Reginald M. Ballantyne, III, President
JESSE OWENS MEMORIAL MEDICAL CENTER, 325 East Baseline Road, Zip 85040; tel. 602/238–3314; Reginald M. Ballantyne, III, President
WEST MCDOWELL FAMILY MEDICAL CENTER, 5030 West McDowell Road, Zip 85035; tel. 602/2383314; Peter J. Martin, Chief Executive Officer

ARKANSAS

Little Rock: CENTRAL ARKANSAS RADIATION THERAPY INSTITUTE, P.O. Box 55050, Zip 72215; tel. 501/664–8573; Janice E. Burford, President and Chief Executive Officer

CALIFORNIA

Long Beach: NAVAL MEDICAL CLINIC, Reeves Avenue, Building 831, Zip 90822–5073; tel. 310/521–4201; Captain J. M. Lamdin, Commanding Officer
Los Angeles: DEPARTMENT OF VETERANS AFFAIRS, OUTPATIENT CLINIC, 351 East Temple Street, Room A–102, Zip 90012; tel. 213/253–5000
Port Hueneme: NAVAL MEDICAL CLINIC, Zip 93043; tel. 805/982–4501
San Francisco: VETERANS AFFAIRS OUTPATIENT CLINIC, 4150 Clement Street, Zip 94121; tel. 415/221–4810; Lawrence C. Stewart, Director
Sepulveda: VETERANS AFFAIRS MEDICAL CENTER, 16111 Plummer Street, Zip 91343; tel. 818/891–7711; Perry C. Norman, Director

CONNECTICUT

Stamford: THE REHABILITATION CENTER, 26 Palmer's Hill Road, Zip 06902; tel. 203/325–1544; Kathleen Murphy, President

FLORIDA

Key West: NAVAL REGIONAL MEDICAL CLINIC, Roosevelt Boulevard, Zip 33040; tel. 305/296–2461; W. A. Nacrelli, Commanding Officer
Miami: VITAS HEALTHCARE CORPORATION, 100 South Biscayne Boulevard, Zip 33131; tel. 305/374–4143; J. R. Williams, M.D., Executive Director
Riverview: TAMPA BAY ACADEMY, 12012 Boyette Road, Zip 33569; tel. 813/677–6700; Edward C. Hoefle, Administrator

HAWAII

Honolulu: VETERANS AFFAIRS MEDICAL REGIONAL OFFICE, P.O. Box 50188, Zip 96850; tel. 808/541–1582
Pearl Harbor: NAVAL REGIONAL MEDICAL CLINIC, Box 121, Building 1750, Zip 96860–5080; tel. 808/471–3025; Captain Robert Murphy, M.D., MSC, USN, Commanding Officer

ILLINOIS

Des Plaines: GOLF SURGICAL CENTER, 8901 Golf Road, Zip 60616; tel. 847/299–2273; Mary Lou Emmons, M.D., Administrator
Westchester: CRS REHABILITATION SPECIALISTS, 2245 Enterprise Drive, Suite 4514, Zip 60154; tel. 708/531–0099; Lori K. Danis, President and Chief Executive Officer

INDIANA

Kendallville: COMPRECARE HOME HEALTH AND HOSPICE, P.O. Box 517, Zip 46755; tel. 219/347–6340; Marilyn Alligood, R.N., Chief Executive Officer
NOBLE COUNTY EMERGENCY MEDICAL SERVICES, P.O. Box 249, Zip 46755; tel. 219/347–6307
OCCUPATIONAL HEALTH MANAGEMENT, P.O. Box 249, Zip 46755; tel. 219/347–6309; Marylyn Asher, Chief Executive Officer

KANSAS

Wichita: U. S. AIR FORCE HOSPITAL, 59570 Leavenworth Street, Suite 6E4, Zip 67221–5300; tel. 316/652–5000; Lieutenant Colonel Bruce A. Harma, Administrator

LOUISIANA

New Orleans: NAVAL MEDICAL CLINIC, Zip 70142; tel. 504/678–2400; Lieutenant Colonel Deborah Auth, Director, Administration

MARYLAND

Annapolis: NAVAL MEDICAL CLINIC, Zip 21402; tel. 410/293–1330
Baltimore: TOTAL HEALTH CARE, INC., 1501 Division Street, Zip 21217; tel. 410/383–8300; Claude D. Hill, M.D., Chief Executive Officer

MASSACHUSETTS

Falmouth: GOSNOLD ON CAPE COD, 200 Ter Heun Drive, Box CC, Zip 02540; tel. 508/540–6550; Raymond Tamasi, Chief Executive Officer

MICHIGAN

Port Huron: TRI–HOSPITAL E.M.S., 309 Grand River Street, Zip 48060; tel. 313/985–7115; Ken Cummings, Chief Executive Officer
WILLOW ENTERPRISES, INC., 1221 Pine Grove Avenue, Zip 48060; tel. 313/989–3737
Sault Sainte Marie: SAULT SAINTE MARIE TRIBAL HEALTH AND HUMAN SERVICES CENTER, 2864 Ashmun Street, Zip 49783; tel. 906/495–5651; Russell Vizina, Division Director Health

MISSOURI

Independence: SURGI–CARE CENTER OF INDEPENDENCE, 2311 Redwood Avenue, Zip 64057; tel. 816/373–7995; Michael W. Chappelow, President and Chief Executive Officer
Saint Louis: IRENE WALTER JOHNSON INSTITUTE OF REHABILITATION, P.O. Box 8062, Zip 63110; tel. 314/362–6979; Denise McCartney, Administrative Director

MONTANA

Malmstrom AFB: U. S. AIR FORCE CLINIC, Zip 59402–5300; tel. 406/731–3863; Lieutenant Colonel Gary D. McMannon, FACHE, USAF, Administrator

NEVADA

Las Vegas: VETERANS AFFAIRS–OUTPATIENT CLINIC, 1703 West Charleston Boulevard, Zip 89102; tel. 702/389–3700; Ramon J. Reevey, Director

NEW HAMPSHIRE

Portsmouth: NAVAL MEDICAL CLINIC, Building H–1, Zip 03801; tel. 207/439–1000; Captain F. M. Richardson, Commanding Officer

NEW MEXICO

Fort Bayard: FORT BAYARD MEDICAL CENTER, P.O. Box 36219, Zip 88036; tel. 505/537–3302; Marquita George, Administrator

NEW YORK

Lake Placid: CAMELOT, 50 Riverside Drive, Zip 12946; tel. 518/523–3605; Reverend Carlos J. Caguiat, FACHE, Vice President
New York: STATE UNIVERSITY OF NEW YORK, UNIVERSITY OPTOMETRIC CENTER, 100 East 24th Street, Zip 10010; tel. 212/780–4930; Richard C. Weber, Executive Director
Rochester: ROCHESTER REHABILITATION CENTER, 1000 Elmwood Avenue, Zip 14620; tel. 716/271–2520; George H. Gieselman, President

NORTH CAROLINA

Winston Salem: QUALCHOICE OF NORTH CAROLINA, INC., 2000 West First Street, Suite 210, Zip 27104; tel. 910/716–0900; Douglas G. Cueny, President

OHIO

Cleveland: KAISER PERMANENTE, 1001 Lakeside, Zip 44114; tel. 216/362–2000; Greg Palmer, Chief Executive Officer
Columbus: VETERANS AFFAIRS OUTPATIENT CLINIC, 2090 Kenny Road, Zip 43221; tel. 614/469–5663; Troy E. Page, Director

OKLAHOMA

Enid: U. S. AIR FORCE CLINIC, Vance AFB, Building 810, Zip 73705–5000; tel. 405/249–7494; Lieutenant Colonel Andrew F. Love, MSC, USAF, Commander Medical Group

OREGON

Portland: BESS KAISER FOUNDATION HOSPITAL, 5055 North Greeley Avenue, Zip 97217–3591; tel. 503/285–9321; Alide Chase, Administrator

PENNSYLVANIA

Pittsburgh: HEALTH ASSISTANCE PROGRAM FOR PERSONNEL IN INDUSTRY, 4221 Penn Avenue, Zip 15224; tel. 412/622–4994; Eugene Ginchereau, M.D., Director
HEALTHAMERICA PENNSYLVANIA, INC., Five Gateway Center, Zip 15222; tel. 412/553–7305; Daniel J. Felush, Executive Vice President, Medical Delivery System
York: YORK HEALTH CARE SERVICES, 1001 South George Street, Zip 17405; tel. 717/851–2121; Brian A. Gragnolati, President
YORK HEALTH PLAN, 1803 Mount Rose Avenue, Zip 17403; tel. 717/741–9511; Charles H. Chodroff, M.D., Executive Director
YORK HEALTH SYSTEM MEDICAL GROUP, Zip 17403; tel. 717/741–8125; William R. Richards, Executive Director

RHODE ISLAND

Newport: NAVAL HOSPITAL, Zip 02841–1002; tel. 401/841–3915; Captain C. Henderson, III, MSC, USN, Commanding Officer

TEXAS

El Paso: VETERANS AFFAIRS HEALTHCARE CENTER, 5001 North Piedras Street, Zip 79930–4211; tel. 915/564–6100; Edward Valenzuela, Director

Houston: CHAMPION'S RESIDENTIAL TREATMENT CENTER, 14320 Walters Road, Zip 77014; tel. 713/537–5050; Brad Thompson, Chief Executive Officer

San Antonio: U. S. AIR FORCE CLINIC BROOKS, Building 615, Zip 78235–5300; tel. 210/536–2087; Major Edward M. Jenkins, Administrator

VIRGINIA

Fort Lee: KENNER ARMY HEALTH CLINIC, Zip 23801–1716; tel. 804/734–9256; Colonel John J. Moore, M.D., MC, USA, Commanding Officer

Quantico: NAVAL REGIONAL MEDICAL CLINIC, Zip 22134; tel. 703/640–2236; Captain William L. Roach, Jr., MSC, USN, Commanding Officer

WASHINGTON

Seattle: NAVAL REGIONAL MEDICAL CLINIC, 7500 Sand Point Way, Zip 98105; tel. 206/526–3515

WEST VIRGINIA

Clarksburg: SUMMIT CENTER FOR HUMAN DEVELOPMENT, INC., 6 Hospital Plaza, Zip 26301; tel. 304/623–5666; Les Delpizzo, Executive Director

WISCONSIN

Green Bay: UNITY HOSPICE, P.O. Box 22395, Zip 54305–2395; tel. 414/433–7470; Donald Seibel, Executive Director

Milwaukee: EYE INSTITUTE–MEDICAL COLLEGE OF WISCONSIN, 925 North 87th Street, Zip 53226–3595; tel. 414/257–5541; James N. Browne, Chief Executive Officer

Associate Members

Ambulatory Centers and Home Care Agencies

United States

FLORIDA

NEMOURS CHILDREN'S CLINIC, 807 Nira Street, Jacksonville, Zip 32207; tel. 904/390–3600; Barry P. Sales, Administrator

NEW YORK

INTERNATIONAL CENTER FOR THE DISABLED, 340 East 24th Street, New York, Zip 10010; tel. 212/679–0100; Robert J. Allen, Executive Director

WESTFALL SURGERY CENTER, 919 Westfall Road, Rochester, Zip 14618; tel. 716/256–1330; Gary J. Scott, Administrative Director

PENNSYLVANIA

CRAIG HOUSE–TECHNOMA, 751 North Negley Avenue, Pittsburgh, Zip 15206; tel. 412/361–2801; Richard L. Kerchnner, Administrator

TEXAS

CANCER THERAPY AND RESEARCH FOUNDATION OF SOUTH TEXAS, 7979 Wurzbach Drive, San Antonio, Zip 78229; tel. 512/690–1111; Diane Roberts, Chief Operating Officer Clinical Services

WISCONSIN

CURATIVE REHABILITATION CENTER, 1000 North 92nd Street, Wauwatosa, Zip 53226; tel. 414/259–1414; Robert H. Coons, Jr., President

Philippines

DEPARTMENT OF VETERANS AFFAIRS, OUTPATIENT CLINIC, Manila, Zip 96440; tel. 632/521–7116

Blue Cross Plans

United States

ARIZONA

BLUE CROSS AND BLUE SHIELD OF ARIZONA, Box 13466, Phoenix, Zip 85002–3466; tel. 602/864–4400; Robert B. Bulla, President and Chief Executive Officer

DISTRICT OF COLUMBIA

BLUE CROSS AND BLUE SHIELD OF THE NATIONAL CAPITAL AREA, 550 12th Street S.W., Washington, Zip 20065; tel. 202/479–8000; Larry C. Glasscock, President and Chief Executive Officer

FLORIDA

BLUE CROSS AND BLUE SHIELD OF FLORIDA, INC., P.O. Box 1798, Jacksonville, Zip 32231–0014; tel. 904/791–8081; William E. Flaherty, Chairman and Chief Executive Officer

ILLINOIS

BLUE CROSS–BLUE SHIELD OF ILLINOIS, P.O. Box 1364, Chicago, Zip 60690; tel. 312/819–1220; Raymond F. McCaskey, President and Chief Executive Officer

NEW YORK

BLUE CROSS AND BLUE SHIELD OF CENTRAL NEW YORK, Box 4809, Syracuse, Zip 13221–4809; tel. 315/448–3902; Albert F. Antonini, President and Chief Executive Officer

BLUE CROSS AND BLUE SHIELD OF THE ROCHESTER AREA, 150 East Main Street, Rochester, Zip 14647; tel. 716/454–1700; Howard J. Berman, President and Chief Executive Officer

OHIO

ANTHEM BLUE CROSS & BLUE SHIELD, 1351 William Howard Taft Road, Cincinnati, Zip 45206; tel. 513/977–8811; Dwayne Hauser, Chief Executive Officer

OKLAHOMA

BLUE CROSS AND BLUE SHIELD OF OKLAHOMA, Box 3283, Tulsa, Zip 74102; tel. 918/583–0861; Ronald F. King, President and Chief Executive Officer

PENNSYLVANIA

BLUE CROSS OF NORTHEASTERN PENNSYLVANIA, 70 North Main Street, Wilkes–Barre, Zip 18711; tel. 717/831–3676; Art Menichillo, Senior Director

BLUE CROSS OF WESTERN PENNSYLVANIA, 120 Fifth Avenue Place, Suite 3111, Pittsburgh, Zip 15222; tel. 412/255–7000; William M. Lowry, Chief Executive Officer

CAPITAL BLUE CROSS, 2500 Elmerton Avenue, Harrisburg, Zip 17110; tel. 717/541–7000; James M. Mead, President

TENNESSEE

BLUE CROSS AND BLUE SHIELD OF MEMPHIS, P.O. Box 98, Memphis, Zip 38101; tel. 901/544–2111; Gene Holcomb, President and Chief Executive Officer

TEXAS

BLUE CROSS AND BLUE SHIELD OF TEXAS, INC., Box 655730, Dallas, Zip 75265–5730; tel. 214/766–6900; Rogers Coleman, M.D., President

Canada

ONTARIO

ONTARIO BLUE CROSS, P.O. Box 2000, Don Mills, Zip M9C 5P1; tel. 416/626–1688; Andrew Yorke, Chief Operating Officer

Healthcare Management

HAWAII

KAISER FOUNDATION HEALTH PLAN, INC., 711
Kapiolani Boulevard, Honolulu, Zip 96813;
tel. 808/529–5296; Cora M. Tellez, Vice President

Health System Agencies

MICHIGAN

ALLIANCE FOR HEALTH, 72 Monroe Center N.W., Suite
200, Grand Rapids, Zip 49503–2816;
tel. 616/459–1323; Lody Zwarensteyn, President

GREATER DETROIT HEALTH HOSPITAL COUNCIL, INC.,
645 Griswold Street, Suite 4100, Detroit,
Zip 48226–4209; tel. 313/963–4990; James B.
Kenney, Ph.D., President and Chief Executive Officer

Other Inpatient Care Institutions

ONTARIO

HILLCREST HOSPITAL, 47 Austin Terrace, Toronto,
Zip M5R 1Y8; tel. 416/537–3421; Frank Martin
Markel, President and Chief Executive Officer

Shared Services Organizations

INDIANA

HOLY CROSS SERVICES CORPORATION, Saint Mary's,
Lourdes Hall, Notre Dame, Zip 46556–5014;
tel. 219/284–4615; David L. Burk, Chief Executive
Officer

KENTUCKY

WESTERN KENTUCKY HOSPITAL SERVICES, P.O. Box
1127, Madisonville, Zip 42431; Richard V. Harris,
Executive Vice President

MARYLAND

DAUGHTERS OF CHARITY HEALTH SYSTEM EAST, 1302
Concourse Drive, Suite 300, Linthicum Heights,
Zip 21090–1025; tel. 301/850–9000; James E.
Small, President and Chief Executive Officer

PENNSYLVANIA

HOSPITAL CENTRAL SERVICES, INC., 2171 28th Street
S.W., Allentown, Zip 18103; tel. 215/791–2222; J.
Michael Lee, President

RHODE ISLAND

VECTOR HEALTHSYSTEMS, INC., Box 9427, Providence,
Zip 02940; tel. 401/453–8300; Stephen Saucier,
President

TEXAS

TEXAS HOSPITAL ASSOCIATION, Box 15587, Austin,
Zip 78761–5587; tel. 512/453–7204; Terry
Townsend, President and Chief Executive Officer

Other Associate Members

U.S. government hospitals in areas outside the United States that are members of the American Hospital Association are not shown here, but are included in the list of such hospitals in section A of this guide, where membership is indicated by a star (★) preceeding the name of the individual hospital.

UNITED STATES

ARCHITECTURE:

BURT HILL KOSAR RITTELMANN ASSOCIATES, 400 Morgan Center, Butler, Pennsylvania Zip 16001–5977; tel. 412/285–4761; John E. Brock, Principal

CRSS CONSTRUCTORS, INC., 2500 Michelson Drive, Suite 100, Irvine, California Zip 92715; tel. 714/476–2900; Gordon D. Davis, Vice President

EARL SWENSSON ASSOCIATES, INC., 2100 West End Avenue, Suite 1200, Nashville, Tennessee Zip 37203; tel. 615/329–9445; Richard L. Miller, President

EASON, EARL AND ASSOCIATES, INC., 75 Beattie Place, Suite 600, Greenville, South Carolina Zip 29601; tel. 864/233–0003; Richard R. Earl, Principal

ENGBERG ANDERSON DESIGN PARTNERSHIP, INC., 611 North Broadway, Suite 517, Milwaukee, Wisconsin Zip 53202; tel. 414/276–6600; Scott M. Smith, Architect

GREENWELL GOETZ ARCHITECTS, PC., 1310 G Street N.W., Suite 600, Washington, District of Columbia Zip 20005; tel. 202/682–0700; James W. Greenwell, Principal

HENNINGSON, DURHAM AND RICHARDSON, 8404 Indian Hills Drive, Omaha, Nebraska Zip 68114; tel. 402/391–0123; Lynn E. Bonge, Executive Vice President

JCM GROUP, 10866 Wilshire Boulevard, Suite 600, Los Angeles, California Zip 90024; tel. 310/474–6868; Wayne C. Twedell, President

LEGAT MEDICAL ARCHITECTS, 24 North Chapel, Waukegan, Illinois Zip 60085; tel. 847/605–0234; Casimir Frankiewicz, President

MARSHALL CRAFT ASSOCIATES, INC., 6112 York Road, Baltimore, Maryland Zip 21212; tel. 301/532–3131; Richard S. Abbott, Secretary

MATTHEI AND COLIN ASSOCIATES, 332 South Michigan Avenue, Suite 614, Chicago, Illinois Zip 60604; tel. 312/939–4002; Ronald G. Kobold, Managing Partner

PERKINS & WILL, One Park Avenue, New York, New York Zip 10016; tel. 212/251–7000; Donald Blair, Principal

SKIDMORE, OWINGS & MERRILL, 220 East 42nd Street, New York, New York Zip 10017; tel. 212/309–9500; Edward A. Carroll, Associate Partner

SVERDRUP FACILITIES CORPORATION, 801 North 11th Street, Saint Louis, Missouri Zip 63101–1015; tel. 314/997–0300; Nicholas J. Varrone, Vice President

THE RITCHIE ORGANIZATION, 80 Bridge Street, Newton, Massachusetts Zip 02158; tel. 617/969–9400; Wendell R. Morgan, Jr., President

WILLIAM A. BERRY & SON, INC., 100 Conifer Hill Drive, Danvers, Massachusetts Zip 01923; tel. 508/774–1057; Ronda Paradis, Vice President

CERTIFIED PUBLIC ACCOUNTANT:

DELOITTE & TOUCHE, 2200 Ross Avenue, Suite 1600, Dallas, Texas Zip 75201; tel. 214/777–7655; Karen Earwood, Senior Manager

HERBERTH AND NETTLETON, 4447 Stoneridge Drive, Pleasanton, California Zip 94588–8325; tel. 510/417–0900; Leonard Herberth, Principal

COMMUNICATION SYSTEMS ORGANIZATION:

A. T. & T. CONSUMER COMMUNICATIONS SERVICES, 20 Independence Boulevard, Room 3A38, Warren, New Jersey Zip 07059; tel. 908/580–8883; Ron Bozek, Manager

IMED LINK, INC., 19491 Old Georgetown Road, 408, Bethesda, Maryland Zip 20814; tel. 301/897–0011; Jerold J. Principato, President and Chief Executive Officer

SOUTHWESTERN BELL, One Bell Center, Room 11–E–2, Saint Louis, Missouri Zip 63101–3099; tel. 314/235–2446; William C. Winter, Manager Market Healthcare

SPRINT HEALTHCARE SYSTEMS, 9393 West 110th Street, Overland Park, Kansas Zip 66210; tel. 913/624–1027; Rod Corn, Director

UNGERMANN–BASS, 3990 Freedom Circle, Santa Clara, California Zip 95052; tel. 408/562–5525; Bruce W. Brown, Executive Vice President

CONSTRUCTION FIRM:

ELLERBE BECKET, 800 La Salle Avenue, Minneapolis, Minnesota Zip 55402–2014; tel. 612/853–2537; Jon Buggy, Marketing Director

HBE CORPORATION, P.O. Box 27339, Saint Louis, Missouri Zip 63141; tel. 314/567–9000; John Wodoslawsky, Executive Vice President Sales

LEO A. DALY COMPANY, 8600 Indian Hills Drive, Omaha, Nebraska Zip 68114; tel. 402/391–8111; James M. Ingram, Senior Vice President

CONSULTING FIRM:

A.P.M., INCORPORATED, 1675 Broadway, 18th Floor, New York, New York Zip 10019; tel. 212/903–9300; Karen Flaherty, Coordinator Marketing

AIG HELATHCARE MANAGEMENT SERVICES, 70 Pine Street, 60th Floor, New York, New York Zip 10270; tel. 212/770–3745; Charles G. Benda, Ph.D., Senior Vice President

ARAMARK HEALTHCARE SUPPORT SERVICES, 1101 Market Street, Philadelphia, Pennsylvania Zip 19107; tel. 215/238–3000; Constance B. Girard–diCarlo, President

ARTHUR ANDERSEN & COMPANY, 33 West Monroe Street, Chicago, Illinois Zip 60603; tel. 312/580–0033; James Kackley, Managing Partner

AXIS RECEIVABLES SOLUTIONS, INC., 999 East Touhy Avenue, Suite 225, Des Plaines, Illinois Zip 60018; tel. 847/635–3300; Brad Gustin, Executive Vice President

BOSTON CONSULTING GROUP, 135 East 57th Street, New York, New York Zip 10022; tel. 212/446–2800; Lurie Regan, Healthcare Researcher

CAMPBELL WILSON, 9400 Central Expressway, Suite 613, Dallas, Texas Zip 75231; tel. 214/373–7077; Danna J. Wilson, Principal

CHANCELLOR GROUP, INCORPORATED, 800 Marquette Avenue, Suite 1300, Minneapolis, Minnesota Zip 55402–2877; tel. 612/835–5123; David Allen, Partner

CHI LABORATORY SYSTEMS, INC., 3135 South State Street, Suite 300, Ann Arbor, Michigan Zip 48108; tel. 313/662–6363; John W. Craft, Principal

CHI SYSTEMS, INC., 130 South First Street, Ann Arbor, Michigan Zip 48104; tel. 313/761–3912; Karl G. Bartscht, Chief Executive Officer

COFFEY COMMUNICATIONS, INC., 1505 Business One Circle, Walla Walla, Washington Zip 99362; tel. 509/525–0101; Alan H. Coffey, Chief Executive Officer

COOPERS & LYBRAND, L.L.P., 203 North LaSalle Street, Chicago, Illinois Zip 60601; tel. 312/701–5893; Robert McDonald, Chairman, National Healthcare Industry

CROSS COUNTRY STAFFING, 7771 West Oakland Park Boulevard, Suite 100, Fort Lauderdale, Florida Zip 33351; tel. 561/394–0088

D.J. SULLIVAN & ASSOCIATES, INC., 2155 Jackson Avenue, Ann Arbor, Michigan Zip 48103–3917; tel. 313/662–7500; Claudia Eminger, Director Operations

DELOITTE & TOUCHE, 180 North Stetson Avenue, Chicago, Illinois Zip 60601; tel. 312/946–3215; Michael A. Engelhart, National Director Health Care Services

EJJ OLSON & ASSOCIATES, 2266 North Prospect Avenue, Milwaukee, Wisconsin Zip 53202; tel. 414/271–3553; Edward Olson, President

ENVIRONMENTAL COMPLIANCE TESTING, INC., 565 Rounseville Road, Box 7, Rochester, Massachusetts Zip 02770; tel. 508/763–5919; Ann Fournier, President

ERNST & YOUNG, 925 Euclid Avenue, Cleveland, Ohio Zip 44115–1405; tel. 216/861–5000; Richard L. Marrapese, Partner

ERNST AND YOUNG, 2001 Market Street, Suite 4000, Philadelphia, Pennsylvania Zip 19103–7096; tel. 215/448–5000; Thomas K. Shaffert, Partner

FIRST CONSULTING GROUP, 100 East Wadlow Road, Long Beach, California Zip 90807; tel. 310/595–5291; Patricia Robinson, Director Training and Education

GOBBELL HAYS PARTNERS, INC., 217 Fifth Avenue North, Nashville, Tennessee Zip 37219; tel. 615/254–8500; Nicholas R. Ganick, Vice President

HAMILTON–KSA, 1355 Peachtree Street N.E., Suite 900, Atlanta, Georgia Zip 30309–0900; tel. 404/892–0321; W. Barry Moore, National Director

HBO & COMPANY, 301 Perimeter Center North, Atlanta, Georgia Zip 30346; tel. 404/393–6000; Arthur J. Keegan, Vice President Corporate Accounts

HEALTH DIMENSIONS, 7100 Northland Circle, Suite 205, Minneapolis, Minnesota Zip 55428; Betty Ice, Director Client Relations

HEALTHCARE FINANCIAL ENTERPRISES, INC., 1475 West Cypress Creek Road, 204, Fort Lauderdale, Florida Zip 33309; tel. 954/772–7878; Peter A. Carvalho, President

HEIDRICK AND STRUGGLES, 233 South Wacker, Suite 7000, Chicago, Illinois Zip 60606; tel. 312/372–8811; Richard P. Gustafson, Partner

HRADVANTAGE, 3550 North McAree Road, Waukegan, Illinois Zip 60087; tel. 847/599–9800; Scott Hamilton, Managing Director

INFOCARE CONSULTING SERVICES, 6300 Glenwood, Suite 12, Overland Park, Kansas Zip 66202; tel. 913/432–3600; Richard Khoury, President and Chief Executive Officer

INPHYNET MEDICAL MANAGEMENT, 1200 South Pine Island Road, Suite 600, Fort Lauderdale, Florida Zip 33324; tel. 305/475–1300; Marta Prado, Vice President

JAMES RUSSELL, INC., P.O. Box 427, Bloomington, Illinois Zip 61702–0427; tel. 309/663–9467; Billy D. Adkisson, President

JANNOTTA, BRAY AND ASSOCIATES, 30 Oak Hollow, Suite 100, Southfield, Michigan Zip 48034–7467; tel. 313/827–4510; Joan Hanpeter, Managing Director

JAROS, BAUM AND BOLLES, 345 Park Avenue, New York, New York Zip 10154; Donald E. Ross, Partner

JOHN NUVEEN AND CO. INCORPORATED, 333 West Wacker Drive, Chicago, Illinois Zip 60606; tel. 312/917–7700; Terence M. Mieling, Vice President and National Director Health Care

JURAN INSTITUTE, 11 River Road, Wilton, Connecticut Zip 06897; tel. 203/834–1700; Sally Georgen Archer, Account Executive

KASET INTERNATIONAL, 8875 Hidden River Parkway, Suite 400, Tampa, Florida Zip 33637; tel. 813/977–8875; Beth Z. Potter, Marketing Manager

KPMG PEAT MARWICK, 650 Town Center Drive, Costa Mesa, California Zip 92692; tel. 714/850–4450; Ronald Merriman, Partner

LAMMERS & GERSHON ASSOCIATES, INC., 1801 Alexander Bell Drive, Suite 600, Reston, Virginia Zip 22091; tel. 703/476–8400; Howard J. Gershon, Executive Vice President

LAW & ECONOMICS CONSULTING GROUP, 1603 Orrington Avenue, Evanston, Illinois Zip 60202; tel. 847/475–1566; Eva Temkin, Research Analyst

MARITZ PERFORMANCE IMPROVEMENT COMPANY, 1400 South Highway Drive, Fenton, Missouri Zip 63099; tel. 314/827–2473; Barbara Sutton, Process Manager

MARSHALL ERDMAN & ASSOCIATES, INC., 5117 University Avenue, Madison, Wisconsin Zip 53705; tel. 608/238–0211; Ron R. Halverson, Senior Vice President Sales and Marketing

MCFAUL & LYONS, INC., 306 Horizon Center, Trenton, New Jersey Zip 08691; tel. 609/588–4900; William McFaul, Chairman of the Board

METRICOR, INC., 620 West Main Street, Suite 200, Louisville, Kentucky Zip 40202–2922; tel. 502/561–8400; Craig M. Johnson, Vice President Finance

MMI COMPANIES, INC., 540 Lake Cook Road, Deerfield, Illinois Zip 60015–5290; tel. 847/940–7550; Anna Marie Hajek, Executive Vice President

MORGAN SERVICES, INC., 323 North Michigan Avenue, Chicago, Illinois Zip 60601; tel. 312/346–3181; Timothy A. Simmons, Vice President

PEDIATRIX MEDICAL GROUP, 1455 North Park Drive, Fort Lauderdale, Florida Zip 33326; tel. 305/384–0175; Julia Stones, Director Marketing

PHASE II CONSULTING, 10 West Broadway, Salt Lake City, Utah 84101; tel. 801/596–2127; N. M. Balay, Business Manager

PRESS, GANEY ASSOCIATES, INC., 1657 Commerce Drive, South Bend, Indiana Zip 46628; tel. 219/232–3387; Mary Patricia Malone, MS, JD, Vice President Corporate Development

RURAL HEALTH CONSULTANTS, 2500 West Sixth, Suite H, Lawrence, Kansas Zip 66049; tel. 913/832–8778; Tina Shoemaker, Senior Consultant

SECURITY FIRST GROUP, 11365 West Olympic Boulevard, Los Angeles, California Zip 90064; tel. 310/312–5010; June Koss, Director Marketing Support

SHERLOCK, SMITH AND ADAMS, INC., 3047 Carter Hill Road, Montgomery, Alabama Zip 36111; tel. 205/263–6481; Roland H. Vaughan, President

SIMIONE CENTRAL, INC., P.O. Box 5248, Hamden, Connecticut Zip 06518; tel. 203/281–0540; William J. Simione, Jr., President

THE CIT GROUP, INDUSTRIAL FINANCING, 650 Cit Drive, Livingston, New Jersey Zip 07039; tel. 201/740–5594; Anthony Pacchiano, Vice President

TIBER GROUP, INC., 200 South Wacker Drive, Suite 2620, Chicago, Illinois Zip 60601; tel. 312/609–9900; Joe Burik, Librarian

TOFT WOLFF FARROW, INC., 282 Second Street, San Francisco, California Zip 94105; tel. 415/247–8700; Lawrence S. Wolff, President

TOWERS PERRIN, 100 Summit Lake Drive, Valhalla, New York Zip 10595; tel. 212/309–3400; Leslie Tobias, Information Specialist

TRANSCRIPTIONS, LTD./MEDQUIST, INC., State Highway 73 North, Suite 311, Marlton, New Jersey Zip 08053–3422; tel. 609/596–8877; David Cohen, President

VICTOR KRAMER COMPANY, INC., 405 Murray Hill Parkway, Suite 1040, East Rutherford, New Jersey Zip 07073; tel. 201/935–0414; Thomas Mara, President

WEST HUDSON AND COMPANY, INC., 5230 Pacific Concourse Drive, Suite 400, Los Angeles, California Zip 90045; tel. 310/297–4200; Adrianne Court, Operations Manager

WHITMAN GARVEY, INC., 1191 Second Avenue, Suite 1800, Seattle, Washington Zip 98101–2939; tel. 206/628–3763; James T. Whitman, President

YAFFE AND COMPANY, INC., 2119 Caves Road, Owings Mills, Maryland Zip 21117; tel. 301/332–1166; Rian M. Yaffe, President

EDUCATIONAL SERVICES:

AMERICAN ASSOCIATION FOR MEDICAL TRANSCRIPTION, P.O. Box 576187, Modesto, California Zip 95357–6187; tel. 209/551–0883; Claudia J. Tessier, Executive Director

AMERICAN OVERSEAS BOOK COMPANY, INCORPORATED, 550 Walnut Street, Norwood, New Jersey Zip 07648; tel. 201/767–7600; Hale R. Gaffney, President

CALIFORNIA COLLEGE FOR HEALTH SCIENCES, 222 West 24th Street, National City, California Zip 91950; tel. 619/477–4800; Dale K. Bean, Program Director

FACILITIES MANAGEMENT:

AMERICAN UTILITIES, P.O. Box 1214, Orem, Utah Zip 84059–1214; Ellen Burkett, President

DYNAMIC HEALTH, INC., 777 South Harbor Island Boulevard, Suite 890, Tampa, Florida Zip 33609–1037; tel. 813/287–5001; John J. Silver, Jr., President and Chief Executive Officer

JOHNSON CONTROLS, INC., 3354 Perimeter Hill Drive, Suite 105, Nashville, Tennessee Zip 37211; tel. 615/333–9304; C. Patrick Hardwick, Business Development Manager

MEDICAL PLANNING ASSOCIATES, 22762 Pacific Coast Highway, Malibu, California Zip 90265; tel. 310/456–2084; Daniel Logan, President

PRISON HEALTH SERVICES, INC., 3565 Piedmont Road, Building 2–410, Brentwood, Tennessee Zip 37027; Denise King, Manager Marketing Services

SCRIBCOR, INC., 400 North Michigan Avenue, Suite 415, Chicago, Illinois Zip 60611; tel. 312/923–8000; Stephen T. Kardel, President

SERVICEMASTER COMPANY, One Servicemaster Way, Downers Grove, Illinois Zip 60515; tel. 708/964–1300; C. William Pollard, Chairman

SPECTRUM HEALTHCARE SERVICES, 12647 Olive Boulevard, Saint Louis, Missouri Zip 63141; tel. 314/878–2280; Tony Bevilacqua, Vice President Marketing

HEALTH CARE ALLIANCE:

PREMIER, INC., 3 Westbrook Corporate Center, 9th Floor, Westchester, Illinois Zip 60154–5735; tel. 708/409–4100; Alan Weinstein, President

UNIVERSITY HEALTH SYSTEM OF NEW JERSEY, 317 George Street, New Brunswick, New Jersey Zip 08901; tel. 908/235–7000; Thomas E. Terrill, Ph.D., President

UNIVERSITY HEALTHSYSTEM CONSORTIUM, INC., 2001 Spring Road, Suite 700, Oak Brook, Illinois Zip 60521; tel. 708/954–1700; Robert J. Baker, President and Chief Executive Officer

VHA, INC., P.O. Box 140909, Irving, Texas Zip 75014–0909; tel. 214/830–0000; C. Thomas Smith, President and Chief Executive Officer

INFORMATION SYSTEMS:

ALLTELL INFORMATION SERVICES, INC., 200 Ashford Center North, Atlanta, Georgia Zip 30338; tel. 404/847–5000; Katie G. Mazzuckelli, Director Market Planning, Research and Communications

CCSI, 8612 Watershed Court, Gaithersburg, Maryland Zip 20877–3751; tel. 301/948–3579; Carlos B. Arostegui, President

CERNER CORPORATION, 2800 Rockcreek Parkway, Kansas City, Missouri Zip 64117; tel. 816/221–1024; C. S. Runnion, III, Executive Vice President

EPI–SYSTEMATICS, INC., 2711 Park Windsor Drive, Suite 304, Fort Myers, Florida Zip 33901; tel. 813/936–4774; Michael Reardon, Vice President Client Services

FIRST COAST SYSTEMS, 6430 Southpoint Parkway, Suite 250, Jacksonville, Florida Zip 32216–0978; tel. 904/296–4200; Charles R. Gibbs, President

H.C.I.A., INC., 300 East Lombard Street, Baltimore, Maryland Zip 21202; tel. 410/576–9600; Jean Chenoweth, Senior Vice President Industry Relations

I.B.M. CORPORATION, 122 Morningside Circle, Parkersburg, West Virginia Zip 26101; tel. 304/428–3268; Jeff Lantz, Health Industry Specialist

I.B.M. CORPORATION, 2345 Grand Avenue, Kansas City, Missouri Zip 64108; tel. 816/556–6696; Donna K. Long, Manager

I.B.M. CORPORATION, P.O. Box 2150, Atlanta, Georgia Zip 30301–2150; tel. 404/238–4671; Wendy Rubel, Communications Senior Program Administrator

IMS AMERICA, LTD., 660 West Germantown Pike, Plymouth Meeting, Pennsylvania Zip 19462; tel. 215/834–5000; Ann Murphy, Senior Information Manager

MEDICUS SYSTEMS CORPORATION, One Rotary Center, Suite 400, Evanston, Illinois Zip 60201; tel. 847/570–7500; Patrick C. Sommers, President and Chief Executive Officer

MICROMEDEX, INC., 6200 South Syracuse Way, Suite 300, Englewood, Colorado Zip 80111–4740; tel. 303/486–6400; A. C. Howerton, Vice President Sales and Marketing

MOTOROLA EMTEK HEALTHCARE DIVISION, 1501 West Fountainhead Parkway, Suite 190, Tempe, Arizona Zip 85282; tel. 602/902–2600; Al DeStefano, President and General Manager

PHAMIS, INC., 401 Second Avenue South, Suite 200, Seattle, Washington Zip 98154–1144; tel. 206/622–9558; Frank Sample, President and Chief Executive Officer

PROFESSIONAL ON–LINE COMPUTERS, INCORPORATED, 4835 Towne Centre Road, Suite 201, Saginaw, Michigan Zip 48604; tel. 517/790–0970; Trisha Hegler, Marketing Representative

RESOURCE INFORMATION MANAGEMENT SYSTEMS, P.O. Box 3094, Naperville, Illinois Zip 60566–2599; tel. 708/369–5300; Jeff Heimsoth, Market Analyst

REUTERS HEALTH INFORMATION SERVICES, 825 Eighth Avenue, Suite 3100, New York, New York Zip 10019; tel. 212/474–6000; Kathy Bogomolov, Manager Sales Information

SCIENCE APPLICATIONS INTERNATIONAL CORPORATION, 10260 Campus Point Drive, San Diego, California Zip 92121–1578; tel. 619/535–7738; David Cox, Sector Vice President, Health Care Technology Sector

SOCIETE WATKINS LIMITED, P.O. Box 908, Roswell, Georgia Zip 30077; tel. 404/998–0900; Thomas H. Watkins, Managing Principal

SUPERIOR CONSULTANT COMPANY, INC., 4000 Town Center, Suite 1100, Southfield, Michigan Zip 48075; tel. 810/386–8300; Richard D. Helppie, President

TANDEM COMPUTERS, INC., 1302 Concourse Drive, Suite 200, Linthicum Heights, Maryland Zip 21090–2916; tel. 410/859–8800; Gloria Parker, Manager Healthcare Solutions

THE COMPUCARE COMPANY, 12110 Sunset Hills Road, Reston, Virginia Zip 22090; tel. 703/709–2300; Ron Bernier, President

VECTOR RESEARCH, INC., P.O. Box 1506, Ann Arbor, Michigan Zip 48106; tel. 313/973–9210; Kevin J. Dombkowski, Program Scientist

XEROX CORPORATION, 7900 Westpark Drive, Suite 400, McLean, Virginia Zip 22101; tel. 703/442–6704; Jack Bowie, Healthcare Marketing Manager

INSURANCE BROKER:

ACORDIA HEALTH INDUSTRY BENEFITS, INC., 6802 Hillsdale Court, Indianapolis, Indiana Zip 46250–2001; tel. 317/488–6000; Russell Sherlock, Chief Operating Officer

AETNA RETIREMENT SERVICES, 151 Farmington Avenue–TNA1, Hartford, Connecticut Zip 06156; tel. 203/273–3291; Robert H. Barley, Vice President

AFLAC, 1932 Wynnton Road, Columbus, Georgia Zip 31999; tel. 706/660–7034; J. Thomas Moore, II, Manager

AMERICAN HOME ASSURANCE COMPANY, 70 Pine Street, 7th Floor, New York, New York Zip 10270; tel. 212/770–5480; Mary Anne Eddy, President, Healthcare Division

CLAIMS ADMINISTRATION CORPORATION, FEDERAL MARKETS, GROUP OPERATIONS DIVISION, 7361 Calhoun Place, Rockville, Maryland Zip 20855; tel. 301/738–1216; Andrea Andrus, Senior Vice President Operations

GREAT–WEST LIFE AND ANNUITY INSURANCE COMPANY, 8505 East Orchard Road, Englewood, Colorado Zip 80111; tel. 303/689–3940; Sandra Shively, Secretary Benefit Payment Field Operations

HEALTHCARE UNDERWRITERS MUTUAL INSURANCE COMPANY, 8 British American Boulevard, Latham, New York Zip 12110; tel. 518/786–2700; Gerald J. Cassidy, President and Chief Executive Officer

JOHN ALDEN LIFE INSURANCE COMPANY, 5200 Blue Lagoon Drive, Suite 470, Miami, Florida Zip 33126; tel. 305/263–8166; James S. Wells, Director Product Development

KEMPER NATIONAL INSURANCE COMPANIES, One Kemper Drive, D–7, Long Grove, Illinois Zip 60049–0001; tel. 847/540–2059; Richard C. Lunt, Manager Property Valuation and Appraisal

LOCKTON COMPANIES, 7400 State Line Road, Prairie Village, Kansas Zip 66208; tel. 913/676–9546; Becky Sullivan, Vice President Unit Manager

PHICO INSURANCE COMPANY, P.O. Box 85, Mechanicsburg, Pennsylvania Zip 17055–0085; tel. 717/766–1122; Barry Persofsky, President and Chief Executive Officer

PRINCIPAL FINANCIAL GROUP, 711 High Street, Des Moines, Iowa Zip 50392–4620; tel. 515/247–5222; Joan Burns, Technical Senior Consultant

ROLLINS HUDIG HALL HEALTHCARE RISK, INC., 201 Alhambra Circle, Suite 800, Coral Gables, Florida Zip 33134; tel. 305/441–8770; Larry Corcoran, Executive Vice President

VALIC, 2919 Allen Parkway (L13–05), Houston, Texas Zip 77019; tel. 713/831–5311; Carol Melville, Associate Director Healthcare Marketing

WASHINGTON CASUALTY COMPANY–NORTHWEST HEALTHCARE INSURANCE SERVICES, 14100 S.E. 36th Street, Bellevue, Washington Zip 98006–1568; tel. 206/455–2282; Mark D. Judy, President and Chief Executive Officer

INVESTMENT BROKER:

KIRKPATRICK PETTIS, 745 Craig Road, Suite 220, Saint Louis, Missouri Zip 63141; tel. 314/872–8871; Arlan Dohrmann, Manager Healthcare

STEPHENS, INC., 111 Center Street, Little Rock, Arkansas Zip 72201; tel. 501/377–8125; Nancy Weaver, Research Analyst

LABORATORY FACILITY:

PATHOLOGISTS REFERENCE LABORATORY, 402 South Boulevard, Tampa, Florida Zip 33606; tel. 813/253–0101; Terry Farrell, Administrator

MANUFACTURER / SUPPLIER:

ABBOTT LABORATORIES, One Abbott Park Road, Abbott Park, Illinois Zip 60064; tel. 847/937–2692; William M. Dwyer, Senior Director Strategic Marketing

ALM SURGICAL EQUIPMENT, INC., 1820 North Lemon Street, Anaheim, California Zip 92801–1009; tel. 714/578–1234; George E. Crispin, President

AMERICAN SEATING COMPANY, 401 American Seating Center, Grand Rapids, Michigan Zip 49504; tel. 616/732–6597; David De Marse, Director Channel Development

AMGEN, 1840 Dehavilland Drive, Department 631, Thousand Oaks, California Zip 91320–1789; tel. 805/499–5725; Teresa Romney, Revenue Analyst

AMGEN, 1885 33rd Street, Boulder, Colorado Zip 80301; tel. 303/541–1440

BAXTER HEALTHCARE CORPORATION, 26 Wiggins Avenue, Bedford, Massachusetts Zip 01730; tel. 617/275–1100; Stewart Randle, New England Regional President

BAXTER INTERNATIONAL, INC., One Baxter Parkway, 32W, Deerfield, Illinois Zip 60015; tel. 847/940–6511; Mari-Anne Hechmann, Manager Customer Relations

BAXTER PERFUSION SERVICES, 16818 Via Del Campo Court, San Diego, California Zip 92127; tel. 619/485–5599; Jeffrey C. Crowley, Vice President Clinical Operations

BECKMAN INSTRUMENTS, INC., 200 South Kraemer Boulevard, Brea, California Zip 92821; tel. 714/993–5821; David E. Todd, Manager Market Research

BERLEX LABORATORIES, 300 Fairfield Road, Wayne, New Jersey Zip 07470–7358; tel. 201/695–4100; Larry W. Tobias, Senior Market Research Analyst

BFI MEDICAL WASTE SYSTEMS, 757 North Eldridge, Houston, Texas Zip 77077; tel. 713/870–7013; Steven Fields, Vice President

BIC CORPORATION, 500 Bic Drive, Milford, Connecticut Zip 06460; tel. 203/783–2105; Gregory D. Young, Assistant Product Manager

BOEHRINGER INGELHEIM PHARMACEUTICALS, INC., P.O. Box 368, Ridgefield, Connecticut Zip 06877; tel. 203/798–9988; Nancy A. Cunniff

BOSTON SCIENTIFIC CORPORATION, One Boston Scientific Place, Natick, Massachusetts Zip 01760; tel. 617/972–4406; John Abele, Chairman

CARL ZEISS, INC., One Zeiss Drive, Thornwood, New York Zip 10594; tel. 914/747–1800; Catherine A. Lewis, Manager

CORNING NICHOLS INSTITUTE, 33608 Ortega Highway, San Juan Capistrano, California Zip 92690; tel. 714/728–4000; Judy Kildow, Associate Director Market Development

DEPUY, INC., P.O. Box 988, Warsaw, Indiana Zip 46581–0988; tel. 219/267–8143; Jan Deaton, Manager Marketing Research

DEVON INDUSTRIES, INC., 9530 DeSoto Avenue, Chatsworth, California Zip 91311; tel. 818/709–6880; Kathleen Baffone, Market Research Analyst

DIAGNOSTIC HEALTH SERVICES, 2777 Stemmons Freeway, Suite 1525, Dallas, Texas Zip 75207; tel. 214/634–0403; James Kirker, Vice President

DUPONT MERCK PHARMACEUTICAL COMPANY, P.O. Box 80723, Wilmington, Delaware Zip 19880–0723; tel. 302/992–5040; Margaret M. Summers, Process Support Team Leader

FIELDCREST CANNON, INC., P.O. Box 107, Kannapolis, North Carolina Zip 28081; tel. 704/939–2000; J. G. Coles, Vice President

GENERAL ELECTRIC MEDICAL SYSTEMS, P.O. Box 414, W-428, Milwaukee, Wisconsin Zip 53201–0414; tel. 414/548–2369; Tim Butler, Manager Marketing

HILL-ROM, 1069 State Route 46 East, Batesville, Indiana Zip 47006; tel. 812/934–8285; Fay Bohlke, Marketing

HOLLISTER INCORPORATED, 2000 Hollister Drive, Libertyville, Illinois Zip 60048; tel. 847/680–1000; Elizabeth Cunningham, Librarian

HONEYWELL, INC., P.O. Box 524, MN 27–3246, Minneapolis, Minnesota Zip 55440; tel. 612/951–3718; Martin Greimel, Director Healthcare Business Unit

HORIZON MEDICAL PRODUCTS, INC., P.O. Box 627, Manchester, Georgia Zip 31816; tel. 404/264–2600; Lauren L. Long, Product Manager

I-STAT CORPORATION, 303 College Road East, Princeton, New Jersey Zip 08540; tel. 800/827–7828; Peter Devlin, Product Manager

IMMUNEX CORPORATION, 51 University Street, Seattle, Washington Zip 98101; tel. 206/587–0430; Michael L. Kleinberg, Director Professional Services

INTERMEDICS, INC., 4000 Technology Drive, Angleton, Texas Zip 77515; tel. 409/848–4000; Richard R. Ames, Vice President Sales

JOHNSON AND JOHNSON, P.O. Box 6800, Piscataway, New Jersey Zip 08855–6800; tel. 908/562–3510; Susan Barrett, Director Segment Marketing

MANAGEMENT SCIENCE ASSOCIATES, INC., 4801 Cliff Avenue, Independence, Missouri Zip 64055; tel. 816/795–1947; Kenneth J. McDonald, President

MEDTRONIC, INC., 7000 Central Avenue N.E., Minneapolis, Minnesota Zip 55432; tel. 612/574–3486; Steve Rasmussen, Manager Information Resources

MERCK U. S. HUMAN HEALTH, WP35–150, West Point, Pennsylvania Zip 19486; tel. 215/652–5000; Phyllis Rausch, President

METROPOLITAN GAS SERVICES, INC., 3334 South S.W. Loop 323, Suite 119, Tyler, Texas Zip 75701; tel. 903/581–1360; C. Greg Downum, Operations Manager

MICROTEK MEDICAL, INC., 512 Lehmberg Road, Columbus, Mississippi Zip 39702; tel. 601/327–1863; Kathy W. Zachry, Vice President Marketing and Sales

MILCARE, INC., A. HERMAN MILLER COMPANY, 8500 Byron Road, Zeeland, Michigan Zip 49464; tel. 616/654–8000; David Reid, Senior Vice President and General Manager

MILLIKEN AND COMPANY, 201 Lubben Industrial Drive West, La Grange, Georgia Zip 30240; tel. 706/880–5500; Charles R. Ball, Vice President

NEMSCHOFF CHAIRS, INC., P.O. Box 129, Sheboygan, Wisconsin Zip 53082–0129; tel. 414/457–7726; David Stinson, Vice President

NOVARTIS PHARMACEUTICALS CORPORATION, 556 Morris Avenue, D3114, Summit, New Jersey Zip 07901; tel. 908/277–7363; William J. Hix, Head Headquarters Sales

OHMEDA, P.O. Box 7550, Madison, Wisconsin Zip 53707–7550; tel. 608/221–1551; Paul J. Gibler, Marketing Communications Manager

OTSUKA AMERICA PHARMACEUTICAL, INC., 2440 Research Boulevard, Suite 500, Rockville, Maryland Zip 20850; tel. 301/990–0030; Rio Iwanaga, Vice President Sales

PACESETTER, INC., P.O. Box 9221, Sylmar, California Zip 91392–9221; tel. 818/362–6822; Lori Hallmark, Manager Accounting

PFIZER U.S. PHARMACEUTICALS GROUP, 235 East 42nd Street, New York, New York Zip 10017; tel. 212/573–7877; Daniel J. Coakley, Director Trade Development and Industry Affairs

PROCTER & GAMBLE, Two Procter & Gamble Plaza, Cincinnati, Ohio Zip 45202; tel. 513/983–6248; James L. Knepler, Manager Patient Care Professional Relations Health Care Products

ROCHE LABORATORIES, 340 Kingsland Street, Nutley, New Jersey Zip 07110; tel. 201/235–4353; S. Rebecca Miller, Director, External Affairs

SHERWOOD – DAVIS & GECK, 1915 Olive Street, Saint Louis, Missouri Zip 63103–1642; tel. 314/241–5700; Robert C. Egan, Executive Vice President

SIEMENS MEDICAL SYSTEMS, INC., 186 Wood Avenue South, Iselin, New Jersey Zip 08830; tel. 908/321–3427; James Mazalewski, Manager Market and Sales Analysis

SIGMA–TAU PHARMACEUTICALS, INC., 800 South Frederick Avenue, Suite 300, Gaithersburg, Maryland Zip 20877; tel. 301/948–1041; C. Kenneth Mehrling, Executive Vice President and General Manager

THE MEDSTAT GROUP/INFORUM, 424 Church Street, Suite 2600, Nashville, Tennessee Zip 37219; tel. 800/829–0600; Roland Keistler, Director Marketing

TREMCO, INC., 10701 Shaker Boulevard, Cleveland, Ohio Zip 44104; tel. 216/292–5000; Dick McOwen, National Sales Manager

UARCO NATIONAL HEALTH CARE, 10 South Riverside Plaza, Suite 747, Barrington, Illinois Zip 60010; tel. 847/381–7000; Gene Tierney, Area Vice President

W. W. GRAINGER, INC., 333 Knightsbridge Parkway, Lincolnshire, Illinois Zip 60069; tel. 847/913–8333; Kolleen K. Schulze, Associate Marketing Manager

ZENECA PHARMACEUTICALS GROUP, P.O. Box 15437, Wilmington, Delaware Zip 19850–5437; tel. 302/886–3167; Zahirr Ladhani, Strategy Manager

METRO HEALTH CARE ASSOCIATION:

HEALTHCARE ASSOCIATION OF SOUTHERN CALIFORNIA, 201 North Figueroa Street, 4th Floor, Los Angeles, California Zip 90071–3322; tel. 213/538–0700; James Barber, President

OTHER:

ABTOX, INC., 104 Terrace Drive, Mundelein, Illinois Zip 60060; tel. 847/949–0552; Ross A. Caputo, Ph.D., Presdient

ACCUCHECK, INC., 13921A West Greenfield Avenue, New Berlin, Wisconsin Zip 53151; tel. 414/827–9099; Donald B. Turtenwald, Chief Executive Officer

ADVISORY BOARD COMPANY, 600 New Hampshire Avenue N.W., Washington, District of Columbia Zip 20037–2403; tel. 202/672–5600; David Bradley, President

AFFILIATED HEALTHCARE, INC., 11200 Westheimer, Suite 700, Houston, Texas Zip 77042; tel. 713/782–4555; Tony Quintanilla, Vice President

AGOURON PHARMACEUTICALS, 10350 North Torrey Pines Road, La Jolla, California Zip 92037; tel. 619/622–8093; Ramon D. Seva, Jr., Marketing Manager

AMERICA'S BLOOD CENTERS, 725 15th Street N.W., Suite 700, Washington, District of Columbia Zip 20005; tel. 202/393–5725; Jim MacPherson, Executive Director

AMERICAN ASSOCIATION OF NURSE ANESTHETISTS, 222 South Prospect Avenue, Park Ridge, Illinois Zip 60068–4001; tel. 847/692–7050; John F. Garde, Executive Director

AMERICAN BOARD OF MEDICAL SPECIALTIES, 1007 Church Street, Suite 404, Evanston, Illinois Zip 60201–5913; tel. 847/491–9091; J. Lee Dockery, M.D., Executive Vice President

AMERICAN ELECTRIC POWER, P.O. Box 2021, Roanoke, Virginia Zip 24022; tel. 540/985–2750; Jon F. Williams, Healthcare Segment Manager

AMERICAN HEALTH PROPERTIES, INC., 6400 South Fiddlers Green Circle, Suite 1800, Englewood, Colorado Zip 80111–4961; tel. 303/796–9793; Greg Schonert, Vice President

AMERICAN SCHOOLS OF PROFESSIONAL PSYCHOLOGY, 20 South Clark Street, Chicago, Illinois Zip 60603; tel. 312/899–9900; Daniel Lorence, Director, Graduate Program in Health Services Administration

AMERICAN SOCIETY OF HOSPITAL PHARMACISTS, 7272 Wisconsin Avenue, Bethesda, Maryland Zip 20814; tel. 301/657–3000; Joseph A. Oddis, Executive Vice President

ANTHEM HEALTH COMPANIES, 4040 Vincennes Circle, Indianapolis, Indiana Zip 46268–3027; tel. 317/298–6600; Teresa Milenbaugh, Research Specialist

AON HEALTHCARE ALLIANCE, 101 Westpark Drive, Suite 160, Brentwood, Tennessee Zip 37027; tel. 615/371–5449; Corbette S. Doyle, President and Chief Executive Officer

APPLIED MEDICAL RESOURCES, 26051 Merit Circle, Building 103, Laguna Hills, California Zip 92653; tel. 714/582–6120; Anne Rose, Marketing and Sales Coordinator

APPLIED MEDICAL TECHNOLOGIES, 1036 East Skyline Drive, Suite F., Phoenix, Arizona Zip 85012; tel. 602/248–2810; Jeff Zander, Vice President

ARMED FORCES INSTITUTE OF PATHOLOGY, 6825 16th Street N.W., Building 54, Washington, District of Columbia Zip 20306–6000; tel. 202/782–2100; Colonel Michael Dickerson, Director

ARMED FORCES MEDICAL LIBRARY, 5109 Leesburg Pike, Room 670, Falls Church, Virginia Zip 22041–3258; tel. 703/756–8028; D. Zehnpfennig, Administrative Librarian

ARMSTRONG MEDICAL INDUSTRIES, INC., 575 Knightsbridge Parkway, Lincolnshire, Illinois Zip 60069; tel. 847/913–0101; Warren Armstrong, Chief Executive Officer

ASSOCIATION OF OPERATING ROOM NURSES, 2170 South Parker Road, Suite 300, Denver, Colorado Zip 80231–5711; tel. 303/755–6304; Sara Katsh, Librarian

ASSOCIATION OF UNIVERSITY PROGRAMS IN HEALTH ADMINISTRATION, 1911 North Fort Myer Drive, Suite 503, Arlington, Virginia Zip 22209; tel. 703/524–0511; Henry Fernandez, President

BEATTY, HARVEY AND ASSOCIATES, 12 West 32nd Street, New York, New York Zip 10001; tel. 212/563–0565; Arthur Peckerar, Associate

BEECH STREET, 173 Technology, Irvine, California Zip 92618; tel. 714/727–1359; Doreen Corwin, Vice President Network Development

BELL ENVIRONMENTAL SERVICES, INC., 229 New Road, Parsippany, New Jersey Zip 07054; tel. 201/575–7800; Philip M. Waldorf, President

BERGEN BRUNSWIG CORPORATION, 4000 Metropolitan Drive, Orange, California Zip 92868; tel. 714/385–6903; Shannon J. Jager, Librarian

BERGMANN ASSOCIATES, One South Washington Street, Rochester, New York Zip 14614; tel. 716/232–5135; Manfred W. Wolters, Director, Health Care Services

BLANK ROME COMISKY AND MCCAULEY, 1200 Four Penn Center Plaza, Philadelphia, Pennsylvania Zip 19103; tel. 215/569–5520; Harry D. Madonna, Attorney

BLUE CROSS AND BLUE SHIELD ASSOCIATION, 676 North St. Clair, Chicago, Illinois Zip 60611; tel. 312/440–6000; Patrick G. Hays, President

BLUE SHIELD OF CALIFORNIA, 6701 Center Drive West, Suite 800, Los Angeles, California Zip 90045; tel. 310/568–5460; Alan Puzarne, Senior Vice President and Chief Executive Southern Region

BREITNER, CLARK AND HALL, INC., 63 South Main Street, Randolph, Massachusetts Zip 02368; tel. 617/986–0011; Owen Breitner, Partner

BROADCAST MUSIC, INC., 10 Music Square East, Nashville, Tennessee Zip 37203–4399; tel. 615/401–2000; Paul E. Bell, Director Industry Relations

BROCKTON MULTI SERVICE CENTER, 165 Quincy Street, Brockton, Massachusetts Zip 02402; tel. 508/580–0800; John P. Sullivan, Ph.D., Area Director

CABOT MARSH CORPORATION, 40 Bethlehem Plaza, Bethlehem, Pennsylvania Zip 18017; tel. 610/882–3080; Edward Pfeiffer, Director Marketing

CAREPLEX GROUP, 197 First Avenue, Needham Heights, Massachusetts Zip 02194; tel. 617/433–1000; Michael M. Gosman, Executive Vice President

CARTER HEALTHCARE FACILITIES, 1275 Peachtree Street N.E., Atlanta, Georgia Zip 30367–1801; tel. 404/888–3148; Earnest M. Curtis, III, Vice President

CES/WAY INTERNATIONAL, INC., 5308 Ashbrook, Houston, Texas Zip 77081; tel. 713/666–3541; Michael D. Leach, President and Chief Executive Officer

COMMUNITY BLOOD CENTER, 349 South Main Street, Dayton, Ohio Zip 45402; tel. 513/461–3450; Jodi L. Minneman, Chief Operating Officer

CONNECTICUT HOSPITAL ASSOCIATION, Box 90, Wallingford, Connecticut Zip 06492–0090; tel. 203/265–7611; Dennis P. May, President

COPELCO CAPITAL, INC., 700 East Gate Drive, Mount Laurel, New Jersey Zip 08054; tel. 800/257–8451; Kevin Ward, Division Manager

COUNTRY VILLA HEALTH SERVICES, 4551 Glencoe Avenue, 3rd Floor, Marina Del Rey, California Zip 90292; tel. 310/574–3733; John H. Libby, Executive Vice President

CREDITEK CORPORATION, 7 Entin Road, Parsippany, New Jersey Zip 07054–0454; tel. 201/515–4900; Joseph W. Delaney, Sales Consultant healthcare Services Division

CURBELL, INC., ELECTRONICS DIVISION, 7 Cobham Drive, Orchard Park, New York Zip 14127–4180; tel. 716/667–3377; Michael P. Donovan, Marketing Manager

CUTLER–HAMMER, P.O. Drawer 2258, Sumter, South Carolina Zip 29151; tel. 803/481–6695; Bernard S. Gaudi, Institutional Sales Manager

DATASTREAM SYSTEMS, 1200 Woodruff Road, Suite C–40, Greenville, South Carolina Zip 29605; tel. 800/955–6775; Andrew Jeffries, Direct Marketing Manager

DELMARVA FOUNDATION FOR MEDICAL CARE, INC., 9240 Centreville Road, Easton, Maryland Zip 21601; tel. 410/822–0697; Timothy G. Jones, Chief Financial Officer

DEPARTMENT OF AIR FORCE MEDICAL SERVICE, HQ USAF/SG, Bolling AFB, District of Columbia Zip 20332–6188; tel. 202/545–6700

DEPARTMENT OF THE ARMY, OFFICE OF THE SURGEON GENERAL, Washington, District of Columbia Zip 20310; tel. 202/690–6467; Commander James Bemberg, Administrative Officer

DEPARTMENT OF THE NAVY, BUREAU OF MEDICINE AND SURGERY, Navy Department, Washington, District of Columbia Zip 20372; tel. 202/545–6700

DEPARTMENT OF VETERANS AFFAIRS, 301 Howard Street, Suite 700, San Francisco, California Zip 94105; Linda Pierce, Director, Sierra Pacific Network

DEPARTMENT OF VETERANS AFFAIRS, 810 Vermont Avenue N.W., Washington, District of Columbia Zip 20420; tel. 202/273–5400; Jesse Brown, Secretary

DHHS, PUBLIC HEALTH SERVICE, DIVISION OF INDIAN HEALTH, HEALTH CARE ADMINISTRATION BRANCH, 5600 Fisher Lane, Room 6A–25, Rockville, Maryland Zip 20857; tel. 301/443–1085; Susanne Caviness, M.D., Chief Patient Registration and Quality Management

DIABETES TREATMENT CENTERS OF AMERICA, One Burton Hills Boulevard, Suite 300, Nashville, Tennessee Zip 37215; tel. 615/665–1133; Kathryn J. Kirk, Senior Vice President

DIAMOND CRYSTAL SPECIALTY FOODS, INC., 10 Burlington Avenue, Wilmington, Massachusetts Zip 01887–3997; tel. 617/944–3977; Denise C. Kelly, Marketing Manager

DIVERSIFIED INVESTMENT ADVISORS, 4 Manhattanville Road, Purchase, New York Zip 10577; tel. 914/697–8552; Cherith Harrison, Vice President

DU PONT CORIAN, P.O. Box 80702, Room 1243, Wilmington, Delaware Zip 19880–0702; tel. 302/999–5447; Todd Sutton, Manager

DUKE ENDOWMENT, 100 North Tryon Street, Suite 3500, Charlotte, North Carolina Zip 28202–4000; tel. 704/376–0291; Jere W. Witherspoon, Executive Director

DUN & BRADSTREET, 899 Eaton Avenue, Bethlehem, Pennsylvania Zip 18025; tel. 610/882–6502; Kathleen Attinello, Divisional Manager

EDAP TECHNOMED, INC., 179 Sidney Street, Cambridge, Massachusetts Zip 02139; tel. 617/441–9212; Christine Meehan, Vice President Marketing

EMCARE, INC., 4333 Edmondson, Dallas, Texas Zip 75205; tel. 214/712–2037; Gary L. Gaddy, Vice President Marketing and Sales

EMERGENCY PRACTICE ASSOCIATES, P.O. Box 1260, Waterloo, Iowa Zip 50706; tel. 319/236–3858; Margo Grimm, Senior vice President

ENRON CAPITAL & TRADE RESOURCES, 1400 Smith Street, EB2535B, Houston, Texas Zip 77002–7361; tel. 713/853–5696; Jamie Ginsberg, Manager

ENVIRO GUARD, LTD., P.O. Box 983, Holly Springs, North Carolina Zip 27540; tel. 919/363–0550; Dan Farmer, Technical Director

ERGODYNE, 1410 Energy Park Drive, Suite 1, Saint Paul, Minnesota Zip 55108; tel. 612/642–9889; Michelle Lee, Marketing Manager

EXECUTIVE RISK MANAGEMENT ASSOCIATES, 82 Hopmeadow Street, Simsbury, Connecticut Zip 06070; tel. 203/244–8900; Paul Romano, Manager

FINOVA, P.O. Box 5075, Costa Mesa, California Zip 92628–5075; tel. 714/751–0991; Janet Smith, Manager Business Development Center

FORUM GROUP, INC., 11320 Random Hills Road, Suite 400, Fairfax, Virginia Zip 22030; tel. 703/277–7000; Brian C. Swinton, Senior Vice President

GALLEON TRADERS, INC., 55 Dawson Drive, Needham, Massachusetts Zip 02192; tel. 617/449–2055; Greg J. Catenza, President

GENERAL MEDICAL CORPORATION, 8741 Landmark Road, Richmond, Virginia Zip 23228; tel. 804/264–3184; Marie Miller, Director Acute Care Marketing

GENEVA COMPANIES, 5 Park Plaza, Suite 1900, Irvine, California Zip 92174; tel. 714/756–2200; Danielle C. Bialek, Senior Research Associate

GERIATRIC HEALTH VENTURES, INC., 3626 North Hall Street, Suite 826, Dallas, Texas Zip 75219–5133; tel. 214/522–2544; Wilkes L. Kothmann, President

GLAXO, INC., 5 Moore Drive, Research Triangle Park, North Carolina Zip 27709; tel. 919/248–7797; Candy Hodge, Senior Manager

GLOBAL MED–NET, INC., 1751 West Diehl Road, Suite 400, Naperville, Illinois Zip 60563; tel. 630/717–6700; Patricia A. Schneider, Vice President Medical Provider Relations

GOJO INDUSTRIES, INC., 3783 State Road, Cuyahoga Falls, Ohio Zip 44223; tel. 330/920–8100; Donna Santoro, Vice President Market Development

GROUP HEALTH INC., 441 Ninth Avenue, 8th Floor, New York, New York Zip 10001–1601; tel. 212/615–0780; Louis Massari, Manager

GUIDANT CORPORATION/CPI, 4100 Hamline Avenue North, Saint Paul, Minnesota Zip 55112; tel. 612/582–4017; Eva R. Shipley, Supervisor, Library Information Center

HARVARD PILGRIM HEALTH CARE, 10 Brookline Place West, Brookline, Massachusetts Zip 02146; tel. 617/730–4747; Beauregard Stubblefield–Tave, Director Health Care Policy

HAWAII MEDICAL SERVICE ASSOCIATION, P.O. Box 860, Honolulu, Hawaii Zip 96808–0860; tel. 808/948–5482; Waynette Wong–Chu, Manager Facility Reimbursement

HAWAII STATE DEPARTMENT OF HEALTH, Box 3378, Honolulu, Hawaii Zip 96801; tel. 808/961–4255; Bertrand Kobayashi, Deputy Director

HCIA/LBA HEALTH MANAGEMENT, INC., 6300 South Syracuse Way, Suite 630, Englewood, Colorado Zip 80111; tel. 303/740–7779; Ray A. Padilla, Vice President

HEALTH CARE PROPERTY INVESTORS, INC., 10990 Wilshire Boulevard, Suite 1200, Los Angeles, California Zip 90024; tel. 213/473–1990; Kenneth B. Roath, President and Chief Executive Officer

HEALTH FOUNDATION OF SOUTH FLORIDA, 1400 N.W. 12th Avenue, Miami, Florida Zip 33136; tel. 305/325–5405; Anthony C. Defurio, Managing Director

HEALTH PARTNERS OF PHILADELPHIA, 4700 Wissahickon Avenue, Suite 118, Philadelphia, Pennsylvania Zip 19144–4283; tel. 215/849–9606; Barbara Plager, President and Chief Executive Officer

HEALTHCARE COMPARE CORPORATION, 3200 Highland Avenue, Downers Grove, Illinois Zip 60515; tel. 708/719–9000; James C. Smith, President and Chief Executive Officer

HEALTHCARE REALTY MANAGEMENT, 1400 Urban Center Drive, Suite 400, Birmingham, Alabama Zip 35242; tel. 205/970–7770; Cindy Rasco, Librarian

HEALTHCARE REALTY TRUST, INC., 3310 West End Avenue, Nashville, Tennessee Zip 37203; tel. 615/269–8175; David R. Emery, Chairman

HEALTHCARE RESEARCH SYSTEM, 1650 Lakeshore Drive, Suite 300, Columbus, Ohio Zip 43204; tel. 614/487–6300; A. Kevin Honne, Senior Account Executive, Provider Development

HEALTHTASK, 3535 Piedmont Road N.E., Suite 408, Atlanta, Georgia Zip 30305; tel. 404/240–3832; Michael C. Thuerk, Vice President Marketing

HELPMATE ROBOTICS, INC., Shelton Rock Lane, Danbury, Connecticut Zip 06810; tel. 203/798–8988; Thomas K. Sweeny, President and Chief Executive Officer

HMH SERVIDES, INC., 1340 Old Chain Bridge Road, Suite 202, Vienna, Virginia Zip 22182; Jack DeVaney, Executive Director

HOECHST MARION ROUSSEL, P.O. Box 9627, Kansas City, Missouri Zip 64134–0627; tel. 816/966–4000; Matt Kerr, Market Manager

IMPAC HEALTH CARE, DIVISION OF INTERGRATED CONTROL SYSTEMS, INC., 231 Beach Street, Litchfield, Connecticut Zip 06759; tel. 203/567–0135; Christopher J. Hyland, Vice President Health Care

IMV LTD., 6411 Ivy Lane, Suite 714, Greenbelt, Maryland Zip 20770; tel. 301/345–2866; Ashok Shah, Vice President

INSTITUTE OF PHYSICAL MEDICINE AND REHABILITATION, 6501 North Sheridan Road, Peoria, Illinois Zip 61614; tel. 309/692–8110; Richard Erickson, President

INTEGRAL, INC., 1 Brattle Square, 4th Floor, Cambridge, Massachusetts Zip 02138; tel. 617/349–0640; Dalayna Williams, Project Assistant

INTERFACE FLOORING SYSTEMS, INC., 1503 Orchard Hill Road, La Grange, Georgia Zip 30241; tel. 706/882–1891; Scott Mahan, Market Research Manager

INTERNATIONAL ASSOCIATION FOR HEALTHCARE SECURITY AND SAFETY, P.O. Box 637, Lombard, Illinois Zip 60148; tel. 630/953–0990; Nancy Felesena, Executive Assistant

J. STEPHENS MAYHUGH AND ASSOCIATES, INC., P.O. Box 900, New Roads, Louisiana Zip 70760; tel. 800/426–2349; Janet Stephens Mayhugh, Chief Executive Officer

JANZEN, JOHNSTON AND ROCKWELL, EMERGENCY MEDICINE MANAGEMENT SERVICES, INC., 4551 Glencoe Avenue, Suite 260, Marina Del Rey, California Zip 90292; tel. 310/301–2030; Richard W. Sanders, Vice President Marketing

JULIEN J. STUDLEY, INC., 300 Paric Avenue, New York, New York Zip 10022; tel. 212/326–1000; Nicholas E. Borg, Executive Vice President and Chief Operating Officer

K–MEDIC, INC., 190 Veterans Drive, Northvale, New Jersey Zip 07647; tel. 201/767–4002; Blair Engelken, Marketing Manager

KANSAS HEALTH FOUNDATION, 309 East Douglas, Wichita, Kansas Zip 67202; tel. 316/262–7676; Don Stewart, Vice President and Senior Advisor

LANDIS AND STAEFA, INC., 1000 Deerfield Parkway, Buffalo Grove, Illinois Zip 60089; tel. 847/215–1050; Dana F. Coliano, Healthcare Market Manager

LIBERTY HEALTHCARE CORPORATION, 401 City Avenue, Suite 820, Bala Cynwyd, Pennsylvania Zip 19004; tel. 610/668–8800; Herbert T. Caskey, M.D., President

LIVING HOPE INSTITUTE, 600 South McKinley, Suite 400, Little Rock, Arkansas Zip 72205; tel. 501/663-7878; D. Kimbro Stephens, Vice President

LOGICAL SOLUTIONS COMPANY, INC., 1 Pope Road, Windham, Maine Zip 04062; tel. 207/892-7536; Marc J. Roy, Vice President

LOGIN BROTHERS BOOK COMPANY, INC., 1436 West Randolph Street, Chicago, Illinois Zip 60607; tel. 312/733-6424; Geoff Gustafson, Manager Operations

M D ANDERSON CANCER CENTER OUTREACH CORPORATION, 7505 South Main Street, Suite 250, Houston, Texas Zip 77030; tel. 713/794-5000; Robert N. Shaw, President

MANAGED CARE INFORMATION SYSTEMS, INC., 4505 Las Virgenes, Suite 102, Calabasas, California Zip 91302; tel. 818/880-1379; Paul Garziano, Senior Vice President

MCDONALD'S CORPORATION, 711 Jorie Boulevard, Dept 093, Oak Brook, Illinois Zip 60521; tel. 708/575-3000; Laura Ramirez, Senior Manager Specials

MEDFORCE, A DIVISION OF MJP, INC., 3501 North Causeway, 6th Floor, Metairie, Louisiana Zip 70002; tel. 504/833-4796; Patrick E. Haggerty, President

MEDICAL INFORMATION MANAGEMENT SYSTEM, INC., 511 Union Street, Suite 1800, Nashville, Tennessee Zip 37219; tel. 615/259-3400; James R. Stratman, Vice President

MEDICAL MANAGEMENT DEVELOPMENT ASSOCIATES, INC., California tel. 619/674-1460; Mary Ann Martin, R.N., President

MEDICAL PROTECTIVE COMPANY, 5814 Reed Road, Fort Wayne, Indiana Zip 46835; tel. 219/486-0424; Kathleen M. Roman, Director Risk Management

MODERN HEALTHCARE, 740 North Rush Street, Chicago, Illinois Zip 60611; tel. 312/368-6644; Charles S. Lauer, Corporate Vice President

MONTGOMERY SECURITIES, 600 Montgomery Street, San Francisco, California Zip 94111; tel. 415/627-2324; Amy de Rham, Principal

MORRISON HEALTH CARE, INC., 1955 Lake Park Drive, Suite 400, Smyrna, Georgia Zip 30080-8855; tel. 770/437-3300; Glenn Davenport, President and Chief Executive Officer

NALC HEALTH BENEFIT PLAN, 20547 Waverly Court, Ashburn, Virginia Zip 22093-0001; tel. 703/729-4677; Harry D. Boteler, Administrator

NATIONAL ASSOCIATION OF HEALTH UNIT COORDINATORS, INC., 1821 University Avenue, Suite 162 South, Renton, Washington Zip 98059-6022; tel. 206/235-1129; Florence Frye, President and Chief Executive Officer

NATIONAL HEALTHCARE LINEN SERVICES, 1420 Peachtree Street N.E., Atlanta, Georgia Zip 30309; tel. 404/853-6142; William Gallagher, Business Manager

NATIONAL HEALTHCARE, L.P., P.O. Box 1398, Murfreesboro, Tennessee Zip 37133; tel. 615/890-2020; Laura E. McCoy, Census Development Corporate Director

NAVAL REGIONAL MEDICAL CENTER, PSC 1005, Box 36, FPO, APO/FPO Europe Zip 09593-0136

NETCO COMMUNICATIONS CORPORATION, 333 North Washington Avenue, Minneapolis, Minnesota Zip 55401; tel. 612/204-3100; Kelly J. Brown, Director Medical Products

NEW AMERICAN HEALTHCARE CORPORTION, P.O. Box 3689, Brentwood, Tennessee Zip 37024; tel. 615/221-5070; Dana C. McLendon, Jr., Senior Vice President

NIPSCO INDUSTRIES HEALTH CARE MARKETING AND SALES, 5265 Hohman Avenue, Hammond, Indiana Zip 46320; tel. 219/647-6413; John McKee, Manager Health Care Segment

NURSING MANAGEMENT SERVICES, INC., 3423 Piedmont Road, Suite 500, Atlanta, Georgia Zip 30305; tel. 404/816-8678; Lynne Ashford, Vice President Operations

OFFICE OF CIVILIAN HEALTH & MEDICAL PROGRAMS OF THE UNIFORMED SERVICES, Ochampus Library, Aurora, Colorado Zip 80045; tel. 303/361-3901

OLYMPUS AMERICA, INC., 2 Corporte Center Drive, Melville, New York Zip 11747; tel. 516/844-5435; Steven K. Wendt, Senior Manager National Accounts

OMNIFLIGHT HELICOPTERS, INC., 4650 Airport Parkway, Dallas, Texas Zip 75248; tel. 214/233-6464; JoAnn Parker, Assistant

ORCA MEDICAL SYSTEMS, 22125 17th Avenue S.E., Suite 105, Bothell, Washington Zip 98021; tel. 206/489-2611; Mark R. Willig, Vice President Sales and Marketing

ORGANON, INC., 375 Mount Pleasant Avenue, West Orange, New Jersey Zip 07052; tel. 201/325-4610; Jeanne Lampasona, Senior Market Research Analyst

OSMONICS, INC., 5951 Clearwater Drive, Minnetonka, Minnesota Zip 55343-8995; tel. 612/933-2277; Roger Miller, Vice President

OWEN HEALTHCARE, INC., 9800 Centre Parkway, Suite 1100, Houston, Texas Zip 77036; tel. 713/777-8173; Wendy Gold, Communications Coordinator

PDI COMMUNICATION SYSTEMS DIVISION, 40 Greenwood Lane, Springboro, Ohio Zip 45066; tel. 513/743-6010; Donald R. Rettich, President and Chief Executive Officer

PERFORMANCE PROMOTIONS GROUP, 740 North Lakeview Parkway, Vernon Hills, Illinois Zip 60061; tel. 847/634-8950; Donna L. McMillin, Operations Manager

PRECISION THERAPY, 2901 N.E. 185th Street, North Miami Beach, Florida Zip 33180; tel. 305/682-8118; Steve Nathasingh, Vice President Corporate Development

PRICE WATERHOUSE, 200 East Randolph, Chicago, Illinois Zip 60601; tel. 312/540-2606; Ronald J. Bukovac, Manager

PRIORITY MANAGEMENT SYSTEMS, INC., 500-108th Avenue N.E., Suite 1740, Bellevue, Washington Zip 98004; tel. 206/454-7686; Larry Senechal, Vice President Global and National Accounts

PRUDENTIAL HEALTHCARE, 240 Gibraltar Road, Horsham, Pennsylvania Zip 19044; tel. 215/443-4475; Maureen MacCoy, Director Clinical Administration

QUANTUM SOLUTIONS, 1250 Capital of Texas Highway South, Austin, Texas Zip 78746; tel. 512/329-8880; Kevin Rioux, Associate

RABOBANK NEDERLAND, 300 South Wacker Drive, Suite 3500, Chicago, Illinois Zip 60606; tel. 312/408-8213; Lydia Crowson, Vice President

RCS USA, INC., 2201 Cantu Court, Suite 200, Sarasota, Florida Zip 34232; tel. 941/378-0557; Roy Ferris, President

READING'S FUN, LTD., 123 North Main Street, Fairfield, Iowa Zip 52556; tel. 515/469-6257; Sheila Atchley, Trade Show Manager

REHABWORKS, 521 South Greenwood Avenue, Clearwater, Florida Zip 34616; tel. 813/442-6450; Jack Egan, President

RENFREW CENTER, 475 Spring Lane, Philadelphia, Pennsylvania Zip 19128; tel. 215/482-5353; Samuel Menaged, President

RURAL/METRO CORPORATION, 8401 East Indian School Road, Scottsdale, Arizona Zip 85251; tel. 602/994-3886; Michel A. Sucher, M.D., Vice President, Medical Affairs

SAINT JOSEPH'S CARE GROUP, INC., P.O. Box 1935, South Bend, Indiana Zip 46634; tel. 219/237-7111; Dennis W. Heck, Chief Executive Officer

SGS INTERNATIONAL CERTIFICATION SERVICES, INC., 301 Route 17 North, Rutherford, New Jersey Zip 07070; tel. 201/935-1500; Laura DeVincentis, Healthmark Manager

SHAMROCK SCIENTIFIC SPECIALTY SYSTEM, INC., 34 Davis Drive, Bellwood, Illinois Zip 60104; tel. 800/323-0249; Maryann Mueller, Office Manager

SHARED MEDICAL SYSTEMS, 51 Valley Stream Parkway, Malvern, Pennsylvania Zip 19355; tel. 215/296-6300; Susan B. West, Manager Communications

SHERIDAN HEALTHCORPORATION, 4651 Sheridan Street, Suite 400, Hollywood, Florida Zip 33021; tel. 305/987-3077; Charles Fotsch, Executive Vice President

SNELLING SEARCH MEDICAL GROUP, 1500 Louisville Avenue, Suite 102, Monroe, Louisiana Zip 71201; tel. 318/387-0099; Gil Johnson, General Manager

SPECTRUM COMPREHENSIVE CARE, INC., 12300 Ford Road, Suite 300, Dallas, Texas Zip 75234; tel. 214/243-6279; Joseph Rosenfield, President and Chief Executive Officer

STAFF RELIEF, INC., 409 King Street, 3rd Floor, Charleston, South Carolina Zip 29403; tel. 803/853-4100; Gerard D. Burns, Director Business Development

STEPHENS, LYNN, KLEIN AND MCNICHOLAS, P.A., 9130 South Dadeland Boulevard, Miami, Florida Zip 33156; tel. 305/670-3700; Oscar J. Cabanas, Partner

STRATEGIC PERSUASIONS, 535 Barnett Avenue, Suite 300, San Francisco, California Zip 94131; tel. 415/285-4560; Michael Crawford, Principal

SYNDICATED OFFICE SYSTEMS, 3 Imperial Promenade, Suite 1100, Santa Ana, California Zip 92707; tel. 714/438-6500; Arnold M. Robin, President

SYNTELLECT, INC., 20401 North 29th Avenue, Phoenix, Arizona Zip 85027; tel. 602/789-2834; Robyn Cochran, Product Marketing Manager-Healthcare

TERRY S. WARD AND ASSOCIATES, 5300 Hollister, Suite 200, Houston, Texas Zip 77040; tel. 713/690-1000; Terry S. Ward, President

TEXAS MEDICAL CENTER, 406 Jesse Jones Library Building, Houston, Texas Zip 77030; tel. 713/791-8805; Richard E. Wainerdi, President

THE CANNON CORPORATION, 2170 Whitehaven Road, Grand Island, New York Zip 14072; tel. 716/773-6800; Christopher B. Miovski, Principal

THE HILLIER GROUP, 500 Alexander Park CN23, Princeton, New Jersey Zip 08543-0023; tel. 609/452-8888; Jan L. Bishop, Director Health Care Studio

THE LINC GROUP, 303 East Wacker Drive, 1000, Chicago, Illinois Zip 60601; tel. 312/946-7300; Martin E. Zimmerman, President

THE MEADOWS, 1655 North Tegner Street, Wickenburg, Arizona Zip 85390; tel. 602/684-3926; Patrick Mellody, Executive Director

THE REHAB GROUP, 109 West Park Drive, Suite 340, Brentwood, Tennessee Zip 37027; tel. 615/3715203; Tony Reed, Chief Executive Officer

THE RENFREW CENTER, 7700 Renfrew Lane, Coconut Creek, Florida Zip 33073; tel. 305/698-9222; Barbara Peterson, Executive Director

THE VINCENT ASSOCIATION, 10015 Technology Boulevard West, Suite 151, Dallas, Texas Zip 75220-4339; tel. 214/351-5400; F. Andrew Gerdes, Project Manager

THE WOOD COMPANY, 6081 Hamilton Boulevard, Allentown, Pennsylvania Zip 18106; tel. 610/395-3800; Bill Gazgano, Vice President

TRANSCEND SERVICES, INC., 3335 Peachtree Road N.E., Suite 1000, Atlanta, Georgia Zip 30326; tel. 404/364-8000; G. Scott Dillon, Chief Development Officer

TRANSLOGIC CORPORATION, 10825 East 47th Avenue, Denver, Colorado Zip 80239; tel. 800/525-1841; Jim Patrician, President

TRI-DIM FILTER CORPORATION, 999 Raymond Street, Elgin, Illinois Zip 60120; tel. 847/695-2600; Bob McDonald, Midwest Regional Manager

U. S. AIR FORCE SCHOOL OF AEROSPACE MEDICINE, USAFSAM-CCE, Brooks AFB, Texas Zip 78235-5301; tel. 512/536-3342

U. S. ARMY MEDICAL COMMAND, Fort Sam Houston, Texas Zip 78234; tel. 210/221-1211

U. S. NURSING CORPORATION, 3888 East Mexico Avenue, Suite 129, Denver, Colorado Zip 80210; tel. 303/692-8550; Thomas D. Frey, R.N., Director Nursing

U.S. ARMY AND AIR FORCE JOINT MEDICAL LIBRARY, 5109 Leesburg Pike, Suite 670, Falls Church, Virginia Zip 22041; tel. 703/756-8032; Timothy Gasper, Library Technician

UNITED HOSPITAL FUND OF NEW YORK, 350 Fifth Avenue, 23rd Floor, New York, New York Zip 10118; tel. 212/494-0700; James R. Tallon, Jr., President

UNIVA HEALTH NETWORK, 10503 Timberwood Circle, 200, Louisville, Kentucky Zip 40223; tel. 502/394-4000; Bill T. Zavaglia, President and Chief Executive Officer

VETERANS AFFAIRS CENTRAL REGION OFFICE, P.O. Box 134002, Ann Arbor, Michigan Zip 48113-4002; Linda Belton, Network Director

VETERANS AFFAIRS EASTERN REGION OFFICE, 9600 North Point Road, Fort Howard, Maryland Zip 21052

VETERANS AFFAIRS SOUTHERN REGION, 1461 Lakeover Road, Jackson, Mississippi Zip 39213; tel. 601/364-7920; John R. Higgins, M.D., Network Director

VISITING NURSES ASSOCIATION, 1710 Union Boulevard, Allentown, Pennsylvania Zip 18103; tel. 610/434-6134; Patricia Frenbuto, President

WESCOM, INC., 9446 Phillips Highway, Jacksonville, Florida Zip 32256; tel. 904/260-6334; Pamela Wilson, Sales Administrator

YAMANOUCHI USA, INC., 10 Bank Street, Suite 790, White Plains, New York Zip 10606; tel. 914/686-0556; Koki Ohashi, Marketing Manager

OTHER COMMERCIAL INSURER:

BLUE CROSS AND BLUE SHIELD OF OHIO, P.O. Box 94624, Cleveland, Ohio Zip 44101; tel. 216/687-7000; John Burry, Jr., Chairman and Chief Executive Officer

PREFERRED PROVIDER ORGANIZATION:

USA HEALTHNET, INC, 7301 North 16th Street, Suite 201, Phoenix, Arizona Zip 85020; tel. 602/371-3880; Beatrice E. Hughes, Executive Vice President

RECRUITMENT SERVICES:

DIVERSIFIED SEARCH COMPANIES, 2005 Market Street, 33rd Floor, Philadelphia, Pennsylvania Zip 19103; tel. 215/732-6666; Judith M. von Seldeneck, Chief Executive Officer

SCHOOL OF NURSING:

NORTHEASTERN HOSPITAL OF PHILADELPHIA SCHOOL OF NURSING, 2301 East Allegheny Avenue, Philadelphia, Pennsylvania Zip 19134; tel. 215/291-3000; Shirley L. Hickman, Ph.D., Director School of Nursing

STATE AGENCY FOR HEALTH:

OFFICE OF HOSPITAL AND PATIENT DATA SYSTEMS–WASHINGTON STATE DEPARTMENT OF HEALTH, P.O. Box 47811, Olympia, Washington Zip 98504-7811; tel. 206/705-6000; Hank Brown, Acting Office Director

WASTE MANAGEMENT:

WASTE MANAGEMENT OF NORTH AMERICA, 3003 Butterfield Road, Oakbrook, Illinois Zip 60521; tel. 708/572-8800; Bill Plunkett, Vice President

INFORMATION SYSTEMS:

INFOMEDIKA, INC., 40 Mayaguez Street, Hato Rey, Puerto Rico Zip 00918; tel. 809/751-2080; Luis M. Ramirez Ronda, President

CANADA

ARCHITECTURE:

ARCHITECTURA– WAISMAN DEWAR GROUT CARTER, INC., 500-1500 West Georgia Street, Vancouver, British Columbia Zip V6G 2Z6; tel. 604/662-8000; Ian Carter, Principal

CULHAM, PEDERSEN & VALENTINE, ARCHITECTS & ENGINEERS, 500 404 Sixth Avenue S.W., Calgery, Alberta Zip T2P 059; tel. 403/262-5511; Peter Traverso, Partner

G + G PARTNERHIP ARCHITECTS, 205 Richmond Street, Suite 705, Toronto, Ontario Zip M5V 1V3; tel. 416/596-0654; Girish Ghatalia, Architect

MANUFACTURER / SUPPLIER:

B.H.M. MEDICAL INC., C. P. 697, Magog, Quebec Zip J1X 5A8; tel. 819/868-0441; Robert Lajoie, Sales and Marketing Director

IBEX TECHNOLOGIES, 5485 Pare, Montreal, Quebec Zip H4P 1P7; tel. 514/344-4004; Celine Houser, Product Director

OTHER:

ALBERTA HEALTH–LIBRARY SERVICES BRANCH, P.O. Box 2222, Edmonton, Alberta Zip T5J 2P4; tel. 403/427-8720; Peggy Yeh, Librarian

CANADIAN COORDINATING OFFICE FOR HEALTH TECHNOLOGY ASSESSMENT, 110–Green Valley Crescent, Ottawa, Ontario Zip K2C 3V4; tel. 613/226-2553; Annie Hall, Information Specialist

CANADIAN INSTITUTE FOR HEALTH INFORMATION, 377 Dalhousie Street, Suite 200, Ottawa, Ontario Zip K1N 9N8; tel. 613/241-7860; Rheal LeBlanc, President and Chief Executive Officer

COMCARE CANADA, LTD., 744 East Broadway, Vancouver, British Columbia Zip V5L 2X9; tel. 604/873-6451; Patricia Turner, Administrator

COMCARE SOCIETE DU QUEBEC, INC., 4619 Rue St–Denis, Montreal, Quebec Zip H2J 2L4; tel. 514/932-1481; Kristine Audette, Corporate Supervisor

COMCARE, LTD, 18 Spadina Road, Toronto, Ontario Zip M5R 2S7; tel. 416/929-3364; Lewis Nickerson, Executive Vice President

DARCOR CASTERS, 7 Staffordshire Place, Toronto, Ontario Zip M8W 1T1; tel. 416/255-8563; Cyril J. Muhic, Regional Sales Manager

DESJARDINS LIFE INSURANCE, 200 Avenue Des Commandeurs, Levis, Quebec Zip G6V 6R2; tel. 800/465-6390; Louise Des Ormeaux, Director

ELECTROLINE EQUIPMENT, 8265 St. Michel, Montreal, Quebec Zip H1Z 3E4; tel. 514/374-6335; Beth Leve, Manager

FIRST GROUP. INC, 110 Cremazie West, 14th Floor, Montreal, Quebec Zip H2P 1B9; tel. 514/383-1611; Lise Boivin, Administrative Assistant

INSTANTEL, INC., 362 Terry Fox Drive, Kanata, Ontario Zip K2K 2P5; tel. 613/592-4642; Steve Mildenberger, Business Manager

M.D.S. NORDION, 447 March Road, Kanata, Ontario Zip K2K 1X8; tel. 613/592-2790; Dan Aitkenhead, Marketing Associate

MEDIREX SYSTEMS, 499 Queen Street East, Toronto, Ontario Zip M5A 1V1; tel. 416/363-9313; Mark D. Caskenette, Consultant

MITEL CORPORATION, P.O. Box 13089, Kanata, Ontario Zip K2K 1X3; tel. 613/592-2122; Michael F. Branchaud, Health Care Manager

PROVINCIAL HEALTH AUTHORITIES OF ALBERTA, 44 Capital Boulevard, 200, 10044-108 Street N.W., Edmonton, Alberta Zip T5J 3S7; tel. 403/426-8500; Michael Higgins, Executive Director

SASKATCHEWAN ASSOCIATION OF HEALTH ORGANIZATIONS, 1445 Park Street, Regina, Saskatchewan Zip S4N 4C5; tel. 306/525-2741; John Carter, Education Services Director

SASKATCHEWAN HEALTH RESOURCE CENTRE, 3475 Albert Street, Regina, Saskatchewan Zip S4S 6X6; tel. 306/565-2345

ST. JOSEPH'S HEALTH CARE SYSTEM, P.O. Box 155, LCD 1, Hamilton, Ontario Zip L8L 7V7; tel. 905/528-0138; Brian Guest, Executive Director

TOTAL CARE TECHNOLOGIES, INC., 1708 Dolphin Avenue, 5th Floor, Kewwna, British Columbia Zip V1Y 9S4; tel. 604/763-0034; Al Hildebrandt, President

STATE HEALTH PLANNING/DEVELOPMENT AGENCY:

GREATER VANCOUVER REGIONAL HOSPITAL DISTRICT, 4330 Kingsway Street, Burnaby, British Columbia Zip V5H 4G8; tel. 604/731-1155; Greg Stump, Administrator

FOREIGN

AUSTRALIA

OTHER:

AUSTRALIAN HOSPITAL ASSOCIATION, P.O. Box 54, Deakin West, Peter Baulderstone, National Director

AUSTRALIAN INSTITUTE OF HEALTH AND WELFARE, GPO Box 570, Canberra, Judith Abercromby, Librarian

AUSTRALIAN PRIVATE HOSPITALS ASSOCIATION LTD., 25 Napier Close, Suite 1, Deakin, Ian Chalmers, Executive Director

CEDAR COURT REHABILITATION HOSPITAL, 888 Toorak Road, Camberwell, Victoria, Zip 3124; tel. 613/809-2444; Rodney G. Nissen, General Manager

THE VICTORIAN HEALTHCARE ASSOCIATION LIMITED, P.O. Box 365, South Melbourne, Zip 3205; tel. 613/266-3691; John Popper, Managing Director

PROVINCIAL HOSPITAL ASSOCIATION:

HEALTH SERVICES ASSOCIATION OF NEW SOUTH WALES, Unit 1, 3 Wharf Road, Leichhardt, Sydney, Zip 2040; tel. 029/818-3344; Rod Young, Executive Director

BAHAMAS

OTHER:

PRINCESS MARGARET HOSPITAL, P.O. Box N 3730, Nassau, tel. 809/322-2861; Andil LaRoda, Aministrator

BAHRAIN

OTHER:

INTERNATIONAL HOSPITAL OF BAHRAIN, P.O. Box 1084, Manama, F. S. Zeerah, M.D., President

BERMUDA

OTHER:

KING EDWARD VII MEMORIAL HOSPITAL, P.O. Box HM1023, Hamilton, L. Keitha Bassett, Health Sciences Librarian

BRAZIL

CONSULTING FIRM:

HOSPITALIUM–PLANNING AND HOSPITAL ADMINISTRATION, Rua Dos Pinheiros, 498–CJ, 61, San Paulo, Zip 05422–000; Edson G. Santos, Director and Partner

OTHER:

CLINICA SAO VICENTE, Rua Joao Borges 204 – Gavea, Dogue, Luiz Roberto Londres, President

SOC BEN SAO CAMILO–GHSUL, R. Prof Ivocorsevil, 273, Porto Algre–RS, Zip 90 460–051; Nairio A. Augusto P. Santos, Director

SOCIEDADE HOSPITAL SAMARITANO, Rua Conselheiro Brotero, 1486, Sao Paulo, tel. 000/825–1122; Edson M. Dos Santos, General Superintendent

CHILE

OTHER:

CLINICA SANTA MARIA, Avenida Santa Maria 0410, Santiago, Pedro Navarrete, Chief Executive Officer

SCHOOL OF MEDICINE:

PONTIFICIA UNIVERSIDAD CATOLICA DE CHILE FACULTAD DE MEDICINA, Lira 44, Santiago, Jamie Bellolio Rodriguez, Economic Vice Dean–Faculty of Medicine

COLUMBIA

OTHER:

FUNDACION SANTA FE DE BOGOTA, Calle 116 9–02, Santa Fe De Bogota, Ana Catalina Vesquez Quintero, Manager

FUNDACION SANTA FE DE BOGOTA, Apartado Aereo, Bogota, Roberto Esguerra, M.D., Director

GERMANY

OTHER:

CARENET HOSPITAL MANAGEMENT SERVICE, AM Kronberger Hang 5, Schwalbach An Taunus, Zip 65824; Claude Salmona Ricci, Summit Consultant

GREAT BRITAIN

OTHER:

ST. PAUL INTERNATIONAL INSURANCE COMPANY, 4 Austin Avenue, Hartburn, Stockton on Tees, Zip TS18 3QN; Ian Warren, Manager

TOTUTTI LIMITED, 43 Portland Place, London, Zip W1N 4LN; R. Kadiwar, M.D., Director

GREECE

OTHER:

DIAGNOSTIC AND THERAPEUTIC CENTRE OF ATHENS HYGEIA, S A, 4 Erythrou Stavrou & Kifissiap, Athens, C. Kitsionas, Executive Director

IASO S.A. DIAGNOSTIC THERAPEUTIC AND RESEARCH CENTER, OBSTETRICS AND GYNECOLOGY HOSPITAL, 37–39 Kifissias Avenue, Maroussi Athens, Zip 15123; Constantin Mavros, Ph.D., Managing Director and Chief Executive Officer

ONASSIS CARDIAC SURGERY CENTER, 356 Sygrou Avenue, Athens, Zip 17674; Alexandra Briassouli, Public Relations Manager

INDIA

OTHER:

JOSCO HOSPITAL PRIVETE LIMITED, Iranikudy Post, Pandalam, Alleppey, Kerala Sta, Mercy Jose, Managing Director

MANGALAM HOSPITALS PVT. LTD., Baker Junction, Kottayam 68606, Saji Varghese, M.D., President

ISRAEL

OTHER:

HADASSAH MEDICAL ORGANIZATION, Box 12000, Jerusalem, Zip 91120; Shmuel Penchas, M.D., Director General

S.A.R.E.L. SUPPLIES AND SERVICES FOR MEDICINE LTD., 15 Yehuda & Noah Mozes Street, Tel Aviv, Moshe Modai, Ph.D., Chief Executive Officer

JAPAN

CONSULTING FIRM:

SYSTEM ENVIRONMENTAL RESEARCH INSTITUTE, CO., Kishiya Boulevard, 1–13–35 Hirao, Chuo–ku, Fukuoka, Zip 810; Yukitoshi Yamamoto, President

OTHER:

NAVAL REGIONAL MEDICAL CENTER, FPO, Zip 96362

ST. LUKE'S INTERNATIONAL HOSPITAL, 10–1 Akashi–Cho, Chuo–Ku, Tokyo 104, Shigeaki Hinohara, M.D., Honorary President

KOREA

CONSULTING FIRM:

INSTITUTE OF MODERN HOSPITAL MANAGEMENT, Sinsawong 636–14–4FE Building, Seoul, Key Sung Jung, Director General

LEBANON

OTHER:

AMERICAN UNIVERSITY OF BEIRUT MEDICAL CENTER, 850 Third Avenue, 18th Floor, New York, Zip 10022; Dieter Kuntz, Executive Director

MAKASSED GENERAL HOSPITAL, P.O. Box 6301, Beirut, Moh'd Firikh, Director

MALAYSIA

OTHER:

GLENEAGLES MEDICAL CENTRE, 1 Jalan Pangkor, Penang 10050, Albert Phua Siaw Seng, Senior Administrator

JOHOR SPECIALIST HOSPITAL, 39–B, Jalan Abdul Samad, 80100 Johor Bahru, tel. 07/227–8118; Puan Siti Sa'diah Sa–Diah Bakir, Director and Administrator

MEXICO

OTHER:

HOSPITAL MEXICO–AMERICANO, Calle Colomos 2110, Guadalajara, Omar Nicolas Aguilar, M.D., General Manager

SHRINERS HOSPITAL FOR CHILDREN, Suchil 152, Colonel El Rosario, Mexico City, Carmen G. Solorzano, Administrator

OTHER INPATIENT CARE:

OASIS HOSPITAL, 2247 San Diego Avenue, Suite 235, San Ysidro, Zip 92143; tel. 800/700–1850; Francisco Contreras, Director

PAKISTAN

FACILITIES MANAGEMENT:

SHAUKAT KHANUM MEMORIAL CANCER HOSPITAL AND RESEARCH CENTER, 29 Shah Jamal, Lahore 54600, David Wood, Director

PERU

OTHER:

ASOCIACION BENEFICA ANGLO AMERICANA, Avenue Alfredo Salazar 3 Era, Lima 27, Gonzalo Garrido–Lecca, Director

SOUTHERN PERU COPPER CORPORATION, 1612 N.W. 84th Avenue, Miami, Zip 33126–1032; Rod G. Guzman, Medical Division Superintendent

PHILIPPINES

FACILITIES MANAGEMENT:

WATEROUS MEDICAL CORPORATION, 166 Pilar Street, San Juan, Manila, Eleanor M. Santiago, M.D., M.P.H., Vice Chairperson

OTHER:

ST. LUKE'S MEDICAL CENTER, 279 East Rodriguez Sr Boulevard, Quezon City, Jose F. G. Ledesma, Chief Executive Officer

PORTUGAL

OTHER:

HOSPITAL DE EGAS MONIZ, Rua Da Junqueira, Lisbon 300

SAUDI ARABIA

FACILITIES MANAGEMENT:

SAUDI CATERING AND CONTRACTING, P.O. Box 308, Riyadh 11411, Samir S. Layous, Regional Regional Manager

OTHER:

AL–SALAMA HOSPITAL, P.O. Box 40030, Jeddah, Atef S. Salloum, M.D., Director Development and Planning

GREEN CRESCENT HEALTH SERVICES, P.O. Box 3096, Riyadh, Zip 11471; Wail Buraik, M.D., President

MUHAMMAD S BASHARAHIL HOSPITAL, P.O. Box 10505, Makkah, Sameer M. Basharahil, Vice President

PRINCE FAHD BIN SULTAN HOSPITAL, P.O. Box 254, Tabuk, Rajai M. Dajani, Director

SAUDI ARAMCO MEDICAL SERVICES, 9009 West Loop South, MS–549, Houston, Zip 77096; Harris Worchel, Supervisor Information and Image Services

SINGAPORE

CONSULTING FIRM:

JOHNSON & JOHNSON MEDICAL SINGAPORE, 3 International Road, Jurong 619619, Donna Loo, Clinical Education Consultant

SPAIN

OTHER:

ESCUELA INTERNACIONAL DE ALTA DIRECCION HOSPITALARIO, Alcala 114, 1, Madrid 28009, Enrique Marochi Rodriguez, Chairman

TAIWAN

OTHER:

CHANG GUNG MEMORIAL HOSPITAL, 199 Tun Hwa North Road, Taipei, Yi–Chou Chuang, Director Administration Center

MACKAY MEMORIAL HOSPITAL, 92–Sec–2 North Chung San Road, Taipei, Rick C. C. Huang, Vice Superintendent

NATIONAL TAIWAN UNIVERSITY HOSPITAL, 1 Chang–Te Street, Taipei, Tung–Yuan Tai, M.D., Director

TURKEY

OTHER:

BAYRAKTAR GAYRIMENKUL GELLSTIRME A. S., Buyukdere Caddesi, 106, Esentepe–Istanbul, A. Oktay Cini, M.D., Vice President

UNITED ARAB EMIRATES

OTHER:

AMERICAN HOSPITAL–DUBAI, P.O. Box 59, Dubai, Saeed M. Almulla, Chairman

MINISTRY OF HEALTH, Box 848, Abu Dhabi, tel. 971/234–1478; Abdul Rahim Jaffar, M.D., Assistant Undersecretary

B

Networks, Health Care Systems and Alliances

Section B

Introduction

This section includes listings for networks, health care systems and alliances.

Networks

The *AHA Guide* shows listings of networks. A network is defined as a group of hospitals, physicians, other providers, insurers and/or community agencies that work together to coordinate and deliver a broad spectrum of services to their community. Organizations listed represent the lead or hub of the network activity. Networks are listed by state, then alphabetically by name including participating partners.

The network identification process has purposely been designed to capture networks of varying organization type. Sources include but are not limited to the following: *AHA Annual Survey,* national, state and metropolitan associations, national news and periodical searches, and the networks and their health care providers themselves. Therefore, networks are included regardless of whether a hospital or healthcare system is the network lead. When an individual hospital does appear in the listing, it is indicative of the role the hospital plays as the network lead. In addition, the network listing is **not** mutually exclusive of the hospital, health care system or alliance listings within this publication.

Networks are very fluid in their composition as goals evolve and partners change. Therefore, some of the networks included in this listing may have dissolved, reformed, or simply been renamed as this section was being produced for publication. It is our hope that you will use the integrated health delivery network update/correction form provided to keep us informed of any changes that have occurred. Simply tear out the perforated form, complete and return to the address listed at the bottom.

The network identification process is an ongoing and responsive initiative. As more information is collected and validated, it will be made available in other venues, in addition to the *AHA Guide.* For more information concerning the network identification process, please contact Healthcare InfoSource, Inc. a subsidiary of the American Hospital Association at 312/422–2100.

Health Care Systems

To reflect the diversity that exists among health care organizations, this publication uses the term health care system to identify both multihospital and diversified single hospital systems.

Multihospital Systems

A multihospital health care system is two or more hospitals owned, leased, sponsored, or contract managed by a central organization.

Single Hospital Systems

Single, freestanding member hospitals may be categorized as health care systems by bringing into Type IV–A membership three or more, and at least 25 percent, of their owned or leased non–hospital preacute and postacute health care organizations. (For purposes of definition, health care delivery is the availability of professional healthcare staff during all hours of the organization's operations). Type IV–A organizations provide, or provide and finance, diagnostic, therapeutic, and/or consultative patient or client services that normally precede or follow acute, inpatient, hospitalization; or that serve to prevent or substitute for such hospitalization. These services are provided in either a freestanding facility not eligible for licensure as a hospital understate statue or through one that is a subsidiary of a hospital.

The first part of this section is an alphabetical list of multihospital health care systems. Each system listed contains two or more hospitals, which are listed under the system by state. Data for this section were compiled from the 1996 *Annual Survey* and the membership information base as published in section A of the *AHA Guide.*

One of the following codes appears after the name of each system listed to indicate the type of organizational control reported by that system:

CC	Catholic (Roman) church–related system, not–for–profit
CO	Other church–related system, not–for–profit
NP	Other not–for–profit system, including nonfederal, governmental systems
IO	Investor–owned, for profit system
FG	Federal Government

One of the following codes appears after the name of each hospital to indicate how that hospital is related to the system:

O	Owned
L	Leased
S	Sponsored
CM	Contract–managed

The second part of this section lists health care systems indexed geographically by state and city. Every effort has been made to be as inclusive and accurate as possible. However, as in all efforts of this type, there may be omissions. For further information, write to the section for Health Care Systems, American Hospital Association, One North Franklin, Chicago, IL 60606–3401.

Alliances

An alliance is a formal organization, usually owned by shareholders/members, that works on behalf of its individual members in the provision of services and products and in the promotion of activities and ventures. The organization functions under a set of bylaws or other written rules to which each member agrees to abide.

Alliances are listed alphabetically by name. Its members are listed alphabetically by state, city, and then by member name.

Networks and their Hospitals

ALABAMA

ALABAMA HEALTH SERVICES
48 Medical Park East Drive, Suite 450, Birmingham, AL 35235–2407; tel. 205/838–3999; Robert C. Chapman, President & Chief Executive Officer

BLOUNT MEMORIAL HOSPITAL, 1000 Lincoln Avenue, Oneonta, AL, Zip 35121, Mailing Address: P.O. Box 220, Zip 35121; tel. 205/625–3511; George McGowan, Chief Executive Officer

BROOKWOOD MEDICAL CENTER, 2010 Brookwood Medical Center Drive, Birmingham, AL, Zip 35209; tel. 205/877–1000; Gregory H. Burfitt, President and Chief Executive Officer

LLOYD NOLAND HOSPITAL AND HEALTH SYSTEM, 701 Lloyd Noland Parkway, Fairfield, AL, Zip 35064–2699; tel. 205/783–5106; Gary M. Glasscock, Administrator

MEDICAL CENTER EAST, 50 Medical Park East Drive, Birmingham, AL, Zip 35235–9987; tel. 205/838–3000; David E. Crawford, FACHE, Executive Vice President and Chief Operating Officer

ST. CLAIR REGIONAL HOSPITAL, 2805 Hospital Drive, Pell City, AL, Zip 35125; tel. 205/338–3301; George McGowan, Chief Executive Officer

BAPTIST HEALTH SYSTEM
P.O. Box 830605, Birmingham, AL 35283–0605; tel. 205/715–5000; Carl Sather, Senior Vice President

BIRMINGHAM BAPTIST MEDICAL CENTER–MONTCLAIR CAMPUS, 800 Montclair Road, Birmingham, AL, Zip 35213; tel. 205/592–1000; Dana S. Hensley, President

BIRMINGHAM BAPTIST MEDICAL CENTER–PRINCETON, 701 Princeton Avenue S.W., Birmingham, AL, Zip 35211–1305; tel. 205/783–3000; Dana S. Hensley, President and Chief Executive Officer

CHEROKEE BAPTIST MEDICAL CENTER, 400 Northwood Drive, Centre, AL, Zip 35960–1023; tel. 205/927–5531; Barry S. Cochran, President

CITIZENS BAPTIST MEDICAL CENTER, 604 Stone Avenue, Talladega, AL, Zip 35160, Mailing Address: P.O. Box 978, Zip 35161; tel. 205/362–8111; Steven M. Johnson, President

COOSA VALLEY BAPTIST MEDICAL CENTER, 315 West Hickory Street, Sylacauga, AL, Zip 35150–2996; tel. 205/249–5000; Steven M. Johnson, President

CULLMAN REGIONAL MEDICAL CENTER, 1912 Alabama Highway 157, Cullman, AL, Zip 35055, Mailing Address: P.O. Box 1108, Zip 35056–1108; tel. 205/737–2000; Jesse O. Weatherly, Administrator

DEKALB BAPTIST MEDICAL CENTER, 200 Medical Center Drive, Fort Payne, AL, Zip 35967, Mailing Address: P.O. Box 778, Zip 35967–0778; tel. 205/845–3150; Barry S. Cochran, President

LAWRENCE BAPTIST MEDICAL CENTER, 202 Hospital Street, Moulton, AL, Zip 35650–0039, Mailing Address: P.O. Box 39, Zip 35650–0039; tel. 205/974–2200; Cheryl Hays, Administrator

MARION BAPTIST MEDICAL CENTER, 1315 Military Street South, Hamilton, AL, Zip 35570; tel. 205/921–7861; Evan S. Dillard, President

SHELBY BAPTIST MEDICAL CENTER, 1000 First Street North, Alabaster, AL, Zip 35007–0488, Mailing Address: Box 488, Zip 35007–0488; tel. 205/620–8100; Charles C. Colvert, President

WALKER BAPTIST MEDICAL CENTER, 3400 Highway 78 East, Jasper, AL, Zip 35501, Mailing Address: Box 3547, Zip 35502–3547; tel. 205/387–4000; Jeff Brewer, President

HEALTHGROUP OF ALABAMA, L.L.C.
P.O. Box 1246, Madison, AL 35758; tel. 205/772–4155; Edward D. Boston, Chief Executive Officer

ATHENS–LIMESTONE HOSPITAL, 700 West Market Street, Athens, AL, Zip 35611, Mailing Address: Box 999, Zip 35611; tel. 205/233–9292; Philip E. Dotson, Administrator and Chief Executive Officer

DECATUR GENERAL HOSPITAL, 1201 Seventh Street S.E., Decatur, AL, Zip 35601, Mailing Address: Box 2239, Zip 35609–2239; tel. 205/341–2000; Robert L. Smith, President and Chief Executive Officer

DECATUR GENERAL HOSPITAL–WEST, 2205 Beltline Road S.W., Decatur, AL, Zip 35602, Mailing Address: P.O. Box 2240, Zip 35609–2240; tel. 205/350–1450; Dennis Griffith, Vice President

ELIZA COFFEE MEMORIAL HOSPITAL, 205 Marengo Street, Florence, AL, Zip 35630, Mailing Address: Box 818, Zip 35631; tel. 205/767–9191; Richard H. Peck, Administrator

HUNTSVILLE HOSPITAL, 101 Sivley Road, Huntsville, AL, Zip 35801–9990; tel. 205/517–8123; Ronald S. Owen, Chief Executive Officer

HUNTSVILLE HOSPITAL EAST, 911 Big Cove Road S.E., Huntsville, AL, Zip 35801–3784; tel. 205/517–8020; L. Joe Austin, Chief Executive Officer

PROVIDER OF RURAL HEALTH NETWORK
P.O. Box 11126, Montgomery, AL 36111; tel. 334/260–8600; Tommy McDougal, President

BRYAN W. WHITFIELD MEMORIAL HOSPITAL, Highway 80 West, Demopolis, AL, Zip 36732, Mailing Address: Box 890, Zip 36732; tel. 334/289–4000; Charles E. Nabors, Chief Executive Officer and Administrator

UNIVERSITY OF ALABAMA HOSPITAL/UAB HEALTH SYSTEM
701 South 20th Street, Suite 720, Birmingham, AL 35233; tel. 205/934–5199; Dr. Michael Geheb, Chief Executive Officer

UNIVERSITY OF ALABAMA HOSPITAL, 619 South 19th Street, Birmingham, AL, Zip 35233–6505; tel. 205/934–4011; Kevin E. Lofton, Executive Director and Chief Executive Officer

ALASKA

KETCHIKAN GENERAL HOSPITAL
3100 Tongass Avenue, Ketchikan, AK 99901; tel. 907/225–5171; Ed Mahn, President

KETCHIKAN GENERAL HOSPITAL, 3100 Tongass Avenue, Ketchikan, AK, Zip 99901–5746; tel. 907/225–5171; Edward F. Mahn, Chief Executive Officer

NORTH STAR HOSPITAL AND COUNSELING CENTER, 1650 South Bragaw, Anchorage, AK, Zip 99508–3467; tel. 907/277–1522; Bob Marshall, Administrator

NORTON SOUND REGIONAL HOSPITAL
P.O. Box 966, Nome, AK 99762; tel. 907/443–3311; H. Mack, Network Contact

NORTON SOUND REGIONAL HOSPITAL, Bering Street, Nome, AK, Zip 99762, Mailing Address: Box 966, Zip 99762; tel. 907/443–3311; Charles Fagerstrom, Vice President

ARIZONA

ARIZONA VOLUNTARY HOSPITAL FEDERATION
1430 West Broadway, Suite A110, Tempe, AZ 85282; tel. 602/968–5622; Lew Harper, Network Contact

CASA GRANDE REGIONAL MEDICAL CENTER, 1800 East Florence Boulevard, Casa Grande, AZ, Zip 85222; tel. 520/426–6300; J. Stephen Hockins, Administrator

CHANDLER REGIONAL HOSPITAL, 475 South Dobson Road, Chandler, AZ, Zip 85224–4230; tel. 602/963–4561; Kaylor E. Shemberger, President and Chief Executive Officer

FLAGSTAFF MEDICAL CENTER, 1200 North Beaver Street, Flagstaff, AZ, Zip 86001; tel. 602/779–3366; Stephen G. Carlson, President and Chief Operating Officer

KINGMAN REGIONAL MEDICAL CENTER, 3269 Stockton Hill Road, Kingman, AZ, Zip 86401; tel. 520/757–0602; Brian Turney, Chief Executive Officer

PAYSON REGIONAL MEDICAL CENTER, 807 South Ponderosa Street, Payson, AZ, Zip 85541; tel. 520/474–3222; Duane H. Anderson, President and Chief Executive Officer

PMH HEALTH SERVICES NETWORK, 1201 South Seventh Avenue, Phoenix, AZ, Zip 85007–3995; tel. 602/258–5111; Jeffrey Norman, Chief Executive Officer

UNIVERSITY MEDICAL CENTER, 1501 North Campbell Avenue, Tucson, AZ, Zip 85724; tel. 602/694–0111; Gregory A. Pivirotto, President and Chief Executive Officer

YAVAPAI REGIONAL MEDICAL CENTER, 1003 Willow Creek Road, Prescott, AZ, Zip 86301; tel. 520/445–2700; Timothy Barnett, Chief Executive Officer

YUMA REGIONAL MEDICAL CENTER, 2400 Avenue A, Yuma, AZ, Zip 85364–7170; tel. 520/344–2000; Robert T. Olsen, Chief Executive Officer

BAPTIST HOSPITALS AND HEALTH SYSTEMS
2224 West Northern Avenue, D–300, Phoenix, AZ 85021; tel. 602/864–5260; Michael L. Purvis, Executive Vice President

ARROWHEAD COMMUNITY HOSPITAL AND MEDICAL CENTER, 18701 North 67th Avenue, Glendale, AZ, Zip 85308–5722; tel. 602/561–1000; Richard S. Alley, Executive Vice President and Chief Executive Officer

BULLHEAD COMMUNITY HOSPITAL, 2735 Silver Creek Road, Bullhead City, AZ, Zip 86442; tel. 520/763–2273; Ronald W. Tenbarge, Executive Vice President and Chief Executive Officer

PHOENIX BAPTIST HOSPITAL AND MEDICAL CENTER, 6025 North 20th Avenue, Phoenix, AZ, Zip 85015; tel. 602/249–0212; Richard S. Alley, Chief Executive Officer

CARONDELET HEALTH NETWORK, INC.
1601 West Saint Mary's Road, Tucson, AZ 85745; tel. 602/622–5833; Sister Saint Joan Willert, President & Chief Executive Officer

CARONDELET ST. JOSEPH'S HOSPITAL, 350 North Wilmot Road, Tucson, AZ, Zip 85711; tel. 520/296–3211; Sister St. Joan Willert, President and Chief Executive Officer

CARONDELET ST. MARY'S HOSPITAL, 1601 West St. Mary's Road, Tucson, AZ, Zip 85745–2682; tel. 602/622–5833; Sister St. Joan Willert, President and Chief Executive Officer

CARONDOLET HOLY CROSS HOSPITAL, 1171 Target Range Road, Nogales, AZ, Zip 85621; tel. 520/287–2771; Carol Field, Administrator

HEALTH PARTNERS OF SOUTHERN ARIZONA
5301 East Grant, Tucson, AZ 85712; tel. 412/243–2940; Hank Walker, President & Chief Executive Officer

PALO VERDE MENTAL HEALTH SERVICES, 2695 North Craycroft, Tucson, AZ, Zip 85712, Mailing Address: P.O. Box 40030, Zip 85717–0030; tel. 520/324–5438; Rodrigo A. Pascualy, Administrator

TUCSON MEDICAL CENTER, 5301 East Grant Road, Tucson, AZ, Zip 85712–2874, Mailing Address: Box 42195, Zip 85733–2195; tel. 520/324–5438; Rodrigo A. Pascualy, Administrator

LUTHERAN HEALTHCARE NETWORK
500 West Tenth Place, Mesa, AZ 85201; tel. 602/461–2157; Don Evans, Chief Executive Officer

Section B

MESA LUTHERAN HOSPITAL, 525 West Brown Road, Mesa, AZ, Zip 85201–3299; tel. 602/834–1211; Don Evans, Chief Executive Officer

VALLEY LUTHERAN HOSPITAL, 6644 Baywood Avenue, Mesa, AZ, Zip 85206; tel. 602/981–4100; Don Evans, Chief Executive Officer

MARICOPA INTEGRATED HEALTH SYSTEM
2601 East Roosevelt Street, Phoenix, AZ
85008; tel. 602/267–5011; Frank D. Alvarez,
Chief Executive Officer

MARICOPA MEDICAL CENTER, 2601 East Roosevelt Street, Phoenix, AZ, Zip 85008, Mailing Address: P.O. Box 5099, Zip 85010; tel. 602/267–5011; Frank D. Alvarez, Chief Executive Officer

NORTHERN ARIZONA HEALTHCARE
1200 North Beaver Street, Flagstaff, AZ
86001; tel. 520/779–3366; Joseph M.
Kortum, President and Chief Executive Officer

FLAGSTAFF MEDICAL CENTER, 1200 North Beaver Street, Flagstaff, AZ, Zip 86001; tel. 602/779–3366; Stephen G. Carlson, President and Chief Operating Officer

MARCUS J. LAWRENCE MEDICAL CENTER, 202 South Willard Street, Cottonwood, AZ, Zip 86326; tel. 520/634–2251; Rita M. Poindexter, President and Chief Operating Officer

SAINT LUKES HEALTH SYSTEM
1800 East Van Buren Street, Phoenix, AZ
85006; tel. 602/784–5509; Tom Salerno,
Chief Executive Officer

ST. LUKE'S BEHAVIORAL HEALTH CENTER, 1800 East Van Buren, Phoenix, AZ, Zip 85006–3742; tel. 602/251–8484; Patrick D. Waugh, Chief Executive Officer

ST. LUKE'S MEDICAL CENTER, 1800 East Van Buren Street, Phoenix, AZ, Zip 85006–3742; tel. 602/251–8100; Mary Starmann–Harrison, FACHE, Chief Executive Officer

TEMPE ST. LUKE'S HOSPITAL, 1500 South Mill Avenue, Tempe, AZ, Zip 85281–6699; tel. 602/784–5501; Thomas A. Salerno, Chief Executive Officer

SAMARITAN HEALTH SERVICES
1441 North 12th Street, Phoenix, AZ 85006;
tel. 602/230–1555; Phyllis Biedess, President

COLUMBIA SAN CLEMENTE HOSPITAL AND MEDICAL CENTER, 654 Camino De Los Mares, San Clemente, CA, Zip 92673; tel. 714/496–1122; Tony Struthers, Chief Executive Officer

DESERT SAMARITAN MEDICAL CENTER, 1400 South Dobson Road, Mesa, AZ, Zip 85202–9879; tel. 602/835–3000; Bruce E. Pearson, Vice President and Chief Executive Officer

GOOD SAMARITAN REGIONAL MEDICAL CENTER, 1111 East McDowell Road, Phoenix, AZ, Zip 85006, Mailing Address: Box 2989, Zip 85062; tel. 602/239–2000; Steven L. Seiler, Senior Vice President and Chief Executive Officer

HAVASU SAMARITAN REGIONAL HOSPITAL, 101 Civic Center Lane, Lake Havasu City, AZ, Zip 86403; tel. 520/855–8185; Kevin P. Poorten, Vice President and Chief Executive Officer

MARYVALE SAMARITAN MEDICAL CENTER, 5102 West Campbell Avenue, Phoenix, AZ, Zip 85031; tel. 602/848–5101; Robert H. Curry, Senior Vice President and Chief Executive Officer

NEEDLES–DESERT COMMUNITIES HOSPITAL, 1401 Bailey Avenue, Needles, CA, Zip 92363; tel. 619/326–4531; Donna Beane, Administrator

SAMARITAN BEHAVIORAL HEALTH CENTER–DESERT SAMARITAN MEDICAL CENTER, 2225 West Southern Avenue, Mesa, AZ, Zip 85202; tel. 602/464–4000

SAMARITAN BEHAVIORAL HEALTH CENTER–SCOTTSDALE, 7575 East Earll Drive, Scottsdale, AZ, Zip 85251–6998; tel. 602/941–7500; Robert F. Meyer, M.D., Chief Executive Officer

SAMARITAN–WENDY PAINE O'BRIEN TREATMENT CENTER, 5055 North 34th Street, Phoenix, AZ, Zip 85018; tel. 602/955–6200; Mike Todd, Chief Executive Officer

THUNDERBIRD SAMARITAN MEDICAL CENTER, 5555 West Thunderbird Road, Glendale, AZ, Zip 85306; tel. 602/588–5555; Robert H. Curry, Senior Vice President and Chief Executive Officer

WHITE MOUNTAIN COMMUNITIES HOSPITAL, 118 South Mountain Avenue, Springerville, AZ, Zip 85938, Mailing Address: Box 880, Zip 85938–0471; tel. 520/333–4368; David J. Ross, Administrator

SUN HEALTH CORPORATION
13180 North 103rd Drive, Sun City, AZ
85351; tel. 602/876–5352; Leland W.
Peterson, President & Chief Executive Officer

DEL E. WEBB MEMORIAL HOSPITAL, 14502 West Meeker Boulevard, Sun City West, AZ, Zip 85375, Mailing Address: P.O. Box 5169, Zip 85375; tel. 602/214–4000; Thomas C. Dickson, Executive Vice President and Chief Operating Officer

WALTER O. BOSWELL MEMORIAL HOSPITAL, 10401 West Thunderbird Boulevard, Sun City, AZ, Zip 85351, Mailing Address: Box 1690, Zip 85372; tel. 602/977–7211; George Perez, Executive Vice President and Chief Operating Officer

ARKANSAS

ARKANSAS NETWORK
5106 McClanahan, Suite E, North Little Rock,
AR 72116; tel. 501/666–1200; Mike Gross,
Network Director

BATES MEDICAL CENTER, 602 North Walton Boulevard, Bentonville, AR, Zip 72712; tel. 501/273–2481; Thomas P. O'Neal, Executive Vice President and Chief Operating Officer

CHICOT COUNTY MEMORIAL HOSPITAL, 2729 Highway 65 and 82 South, Lake Village, AR, Zip 71653–0000, Mailing Address: Box 512, Zip 71653–0441; tel. 501/265–5351; Robert R. Reddish, Administrator and Chief Executive Officer

DELTA MEMORIAL HOSPITAL, 300 East Pickens Street, Dumas, AR, Zip 71639, Mailing Address: Box 887, Zip 71639–0887; tel. 501/382–4303; Rodney McPherson, Administrator

HOWARD MEMORIAL HOSPITAL, 800 West Leslie Street, Nashville, AR, Zip 71852–0381, Mailing Address: Box 381, Zip 71852–0381; tel. 501/845–4400; Lynn Crowell, Chief Executive Officer

MENA MEDICAL CENTER, 311 North Morrow Street, Mena, AR, Zip 71953; tel. 501/394–6100; Albert Pilkington, III, Administrator and Chief Executive Officer

NORTHWEST MEDICAL CENTER, 609 West Maple Avenue, Springdale, AR, Zip 72764, Mailing Address: P.O. Box 47, Zip 72765; tel. 501/751–5711; Russ D. Sword, President and Chief Executive Officer

OUACHITA MEDICAL CENTER, 638 California Street, Camden, AR, Zip 71701, Mailing Address: Box 797, Zip 71701; tel. 501/836–1000; C. C. McAllister, President and Chief Executive Officer

REBSAMEN REGIONAL MEDICAL CENTER, 1400 West Braden Street, Jacksonville, AR, Zip 72076; tel. 501/985–7000; Thomas R. Siemers, Chief Executive Officer

SALINE MEMORIAL HOSPITAL, 1 Medical Park Drive, Benton, AR, Zip 72015; tel. 501/776–6000; Roger D. Feldt, FACHE, President and Chief Executive Officer

SILOAM SPRING MEMORIAL HOSPITAL, 205 East Jefferson Street, Siloam Springs, AR, Zip 72761; tel. 501/524–4141; Donald E. Patterson, Administrator

ST. VINCENT INFIRMARY MEDICAL CENTER, Two St. Vincent Circle, Little Rock, AR, Zip 72205–5499; tel. 501/660–3000; Diana T. Hueter, President and Chief Executive Officer

ARKANSAS' FIRSTSOURCE
P.O. Box 2181, Little Rock, AR 72203–2181;
tel. 501/378–2000; Mike Brown, Executive
Director

ARKANSAS CHILDREN'S HOSPITAL, 800 Marshall Street, Little Rock, AR, Zip 72202–3591; tel. 501/320–8000; Jonathan R. Bates, M.D., President and Chief Executive Officer

ARKANSAS METHODIST HOSPITAL, 900 West Kingshighway, Paragould, AR, Zip 72450, Mailing Address: Box 339, Zip 72450; tel. 501/239–7000; Ronald K. Rooney, President

BAPTIST MEDICAL CENTER, 9601 Interstate 630, Exit 7, Little Rock, AR, Zip 72205–7299; tel. 501/202–2000; Steven B. Lampkin, Senior Vice President and Administrator

BAPTIST MEDICAL CENTER ARKADELPHIA, 3050 Twin Rivers Drive, Arkadelphia, AR, Zip 71923; tel. 501/245–1100; Dan Gathright, Senior Vice President and Administrator

BAPTIST MEDICAL CENTER HEBER SPRINGS, Highway 110 West, Heber Springs, AR, Zip 72543–1087, Mailing Address: P.O. Box 1087, Zip 72543–1087; tel. 501/362–3121; Harrell E. Clendenin, Vice President and Administrator

BAPTIST MEMORIAL HOSPITAL–BLYTHEVILLE, 1520 North Division Street, Blytheville, AR, Zip 72315, Mailing Address: P.O. Box 108, Zip 72316–0108; tel. 501/762–3300; Randy King, Administrator

BAPTIST MEMORIAL HOSPITAL–FORREST CITY, 1601 Newcastle Road, Forrest City, AR, Zip 72335, Mailing Address: P.O. Box 667, Zip 72336–0667; tel. 501/633–2020; George S. Fray, Administrator

BAPTIST MEMORIAL HOSPITAL–OSCEOLA, 611 West Lee Avenue, Osceola, AR, Zip 72370, Mailing Address: Box 607, Zip 72370–0607; tel. 501/563–7000; Al Sypniewski, Administrator

BAPTIST MEMORIAL MEDICAL CENTER, One Pershing Circle, North Little Rock, AR, Zip 72114–1899; tel. 501/202–3000; Harrison M. Dean, Senior Vice President and Administrator

BAPTIST REHABILITATION INSTITUTE OF ARKANSAS, 9601 Interstate 630, Exit 7, Little Rock, AR, Zip 72205–7249; tel. 501/202–7000; Steven Douglas Weeks, Vice President and Administrator

BAPTIST REHABILITATION–GERMANTOWN, 2100 Exeter Road, Germantown, TN, Zip 38138; tel. 901/757–1350; B. Richard Moseley, Chief Executive Officer

BAXTER COUNTY REGIONAL HOSPITAL, 624 Hospital Drive, Mountain Home, AR, Zip 72653; tel. 501/424–1000; H. William Anderson, Administrator

BOONEVILLE COMMUNITY HOSPITAL, 880 West Main, Booneville, AR, Zip 72927, Mailing Address: P.O. Box 290, Zip 72927; tel. 501/675–2800; Robert R. Bash, Administrator

BRADLEY COUNTY MEMORIAL HOSPITAL, 404 South Bradley Street, Warren, AR, Zip 71671; tel. 501/226–3731; Harry H. Stevens, Administrator

CARROLL REGIONAL MEDICAL CENTER, 214 Carter Street, Berryville, AR, Zip 72616, Mailing Address: P.O. Box 387, Zip 72616; tel. 501/423–5230; J. Rudy Darling, President and Chief Executive Officer

CHAMBERS MEMORIAL HOSPITAL, Highway 10 at Detroit, Danville, AR, Zip 72833, Mailing Address: P.O. Box 639, Zip 72833–0639; tel. 501/495–2241; Scott Peek, Administrator

CHICOT COUNTY MEMORIAL HOSPITAL, 2729 Highway 65 and 82 South, Lake Village, AR, Zip 71653–0000, Mailing Address: Box 512, Zip 71653–0441; tel. 501/265–5351; Robert R. Reddish, Administrator and Chief Executive Officer

COLUMBIA DE QUEEN REGIONAL MEDICAL CENTER, 1306 Collin Raye Drive, De Queen, AR, Zip 71832–2198; tel. 501/584–4111; Charles H. Long, Chief Executive Officer

CONWAY COUNTY HOSPITAL, 4 Hospital Drive, Morrilton, AR, Zip 72110–4510; tel. 501/354–3512; Johnson L. Smith, Chief Executive Officer and Administrator

CONWAY REGIONAL MEDICAL CENTER, 2302 College Avenue, Conway, AR, Zip 72032–6297; tel. 501/329–3831; James A. Summersett, III, FACHE, President and Chief Executive Officer

CRAWFORD MEMORIAL HOSPITAL, East Main & South 20th Streets, Van Buren, AR, Zip 72956, Mailing Address: Box 409, Zip 72956; tel. 501/474–3401; Richard Boone, Executive Director

CRITTENDEN MEMORIAL HOSPITAL, 200 Tyler Street, West Memphis, AR, Zip 72301, Mailing Address: Box 2248, Zip 72303–2248; tel. 501/735–1500; Ross Hooper, Chief Executive Officer

CROSS COUNTY HOSPITAL, 310 South Falls Boulevard, Wynne, AR, Zip 72396, Mailing Address: P.O. Box 590, Zip 72396; tel. 501/238–3300; Harry M. Baker, Chief Executive Officer

DELTA MEMORIAL HOSPITAL, 300 East Pickens Street, Dumas, AR, Zip 71639, Mailing Address: Box 887, Zip 71639–0887; tel. 501/382–4303; Rodney McPherson, Administrator

DEWITT CITY HOSPITAL, Highway 1 and Madison Street, De Witt, AR, Zip 72042, Mailing Address: Box 32, Zip 72042; tel. 501/946–3571; Joe E. Smith, Administrator and Chief Executive Officer

DREW MEMORIAL HOSPITAL, 778 Scogin Drive, Monticello, AR, Zip 71655–5728; tel. 501/367–2411; Darren Caldwell, Chief Executive Officer

EASTERN OZARKS REGIONAL HEALTH SYSTEM, 122 South Allegheny Drive, Cherokee Village, AR, Zip 72529; tel. 501/257–4101; Norman Steinig, Administrator

EUREKA SPRINGS HOSPITAL, 24 Norris Street, Eureka Springs, AR, Zip 72632; tel. 501/253–7400; Joe Hammond, Administrator

FULTON COUNTY HOSPITAL, Highway 9, Salem, AR, Zip 72576, Mailing Address: P.O. Box 517, Zip 72576; tel. 501/895–2691; Franklin E. Wise, Administrator

GRAVETTE MEDICAL CENTER HOSPITAL, 1101 Jackson Street S.W., Gravette, AR, Zip 72736–0470, Mailing Address: P.O. Box 470, Zip 72736–0470; tel. 501/787–5291; John F. Phillips, Administrator

GREENLEAF CENTER, 2712 East Johnson, Jonesboro, AR, Zip 72401; tel. 501/932–2800; John S. Hart, Administrator

H.S.C. MEDICAL CENTER, 1001 Schneider Drive, Malvern, AR, Zip 72104; tel. 501/337–4911; Jeff Curtis, President and Chief Executive Officer

HARBOR VIEW MERCY HOSPITAL, 10301 Mayo Road, Fort Smith, AR, Zip 72903, Mailing Address: P.O. Box 17000, Zip 72917–7000; tel. 501/484–5550; Sister Judith Marie Keith, President and Chief Executive Officer

HARRIS HOSPITAL, 1205 McLain Street, Newport, AR, Zip 72112; tel. 501/523–8911; Timothy E. Schmidt, Interim Chief Executive Officer

HELENA REGIONAL MEDICAL CENTER, 155 Newman Drive, Helena, AR, Zip 72342, Mailing Address: Box 788, Zip 72342–0788; tel. 501/338–5800; Steve Reeder, Chief Executive Officer

HOWARD MEMORIAL HOSPITAL, 800 West Leslie Street, Nashville, AR, Zip 71852–0381, Mailing Address: Box 381, Zip 71852–0381; tel. 501/845–4400; Lynn Crowell, Chief Executive Officer

JEFFERSON REGIONAL MEDICAL CENTER, 1515 West 42nd Avenue, Pine Bluff, AR, Zip 71603–7089; tel. 501/541–7100; Robert P. Atkinson, President and Chief Executive Officer

JOHNSON REGIONAL MEDICAL CENTER, 1100 East Poplar Street, Clarksville, AR, Zip 72830, Mailing Address: P.O. Box 738, Zip 72830–0738; tel. 501/754–5454; Kenneth R. Wood, Administrator

LAWRENCE MEMORIAL HOSPITAL, 1309 West Main, Walnut Ridge, AR, Zip 72476–0839, Mailing Address: Box 839, Zip 72476; tel. 501/886–1200; Larry Morse, Administrator

LITTLE RIVER MEMORIAL HOSPITAL, Fifth and Locke Streets, Ashdown, AR, Zip 71822–0577, Mailing Address: Box 577, Zip 71822; tel. 501/898–5011; Judy Adams, Administrator

MAGNOLIA HOSPITAL, 101 Hospital Drive, Magnolia, AR, Zip 71753–2416, Mailing Address: Box 629, Zip 71753–0629; tel. 501/235–3000; William D. Hedden, Administrator

MCGEHEE–DESHA COUNTY HOSPITAL, 900 South Third, McGehee, AR, Zip 71654–0351, Mailing Address: Box 351, Zip 71654–0351; tel. 501/222–5600; William A. Conway, Administrator

MEDICAL CENTER OF CALICO ROCK, 103 Grasse Street, Calico Rock, AR, Zip 72519; tel. 501/297–3726; Terry L. Amstutz, CHE, Chief Executive Officer and Administrator

MEDICAL CENTER OF SOUTH ARKANSAS, 700 West Grove, El Dorado, AR, Zip 71730, Mailing Address: P.O. Box 1998, Zip 71731–1998; tel. 501/864–3200; Luther J. Lewis, Chief Executive Officer

MEDICAL PARK HOSPITAL, 2001 South Main Street, Hope, AR, Zip 71801; tel. 501/777–2323; Jimmy Leopard, Chief Executive Officer

MENA MEDICAL CENTER, 311 North Morrow Street, Mena, AR, Zip 71953; tel. 501/394–6100; Albert Pilkington, III, Administrator and Chief Executive Officer

MERCY HOSPITAL OF SCOTT COUNTY, Highways 71 and 80, Waldron, AR, Zip 72958–9984, Mailing Address: Box 2230, Zip 72958–2230; tel. 501/637–4135; Sister Mary Alvera Simon, Administrator

MERCY HOSPITAL–TURNER MEMORIAL, 801 West River, Ozark, AR, Zip 72949; tel. 501/667–4138; Sister Mary Werner Keith, Administrator

NEWPORT HOSPITAL AND CLINIC, 2000 McLain, Newport, AR, Zip 72112; tel. 501/523–6721; Eugene Zuber, Administrator

NORTH ARKANSAS MEDICAL CENTER, 620 North Willow Street, Harrison, AR, Zip 72601; tel. 501/365–2000; Brian L. Clemens, Chief Executive Officer

NORTH LOGAN MERCY HOSPITAL, 500 East Academy, Paris, AR, Zip 72855–4099; tel. 501/963–6101; Jim L. Maddox, Chief Administrative Officer

NORTHEAST ARKANSAS REHABILITATION HOSPITAL, 1201 Fleming Avenue, Jonesboro, AR, Zip 72401, Mailing Address: P.O. Box 1680, Zip 72403–1680; tel. 501/932–0440; Wayne E. Sensor, Chief Executive Officer

OUACHITA MEDICAL CENTER, 638 California Street, Camden, AR, Zip 71701, Mailing Address: Box 797, Zip 71701; tel. 501/836–1000; C. C. McAllister, President and Chief Executive Officer

PIGGOTT COMMUNITY HOSPITAL, 1206 Gordon Duckworth Drive, Piggott, AR, Zip 72454; tel. 501/598–3881; Betty J. Reams, Executive Director

PIKE COUNTY MEMORIAL HOSPITAL, 315 East 13th Street, Murfreesboro, AR, Zip 71958; tel. 501/285–3182; Rosemary Fritts, Administrator

RANDOLPH COUNTY MEDICAL CENTER, 2801 Medical Center Drive, Pocahontas, AR, Zip 72455; tel. 501/892–4511; Brad S. Morse, Executive Director

REBSAMEN REGIONAL MEDICAL CENTER, 1400 West Braden Street, Jacksonville, AR, Zip 72076; tel. 501/985–7000; Thomas R. Siemers, Chief Executive Officer

SAINT MARY'S REGIONAL MEDICAL CENTER, 1808 West Main Street, Russellville, AR, Zip 72801; tel. 501/968–2841; Mike McCoy, Chief Executive Officer

SALINE MEMORIAL HOSPITAL, 1 Medical Park Drive, Benton, AR, Zip 72015; tel. 501/776–6000; Roger D. Feldt, FACHE, President and Chief Executive Officer

SILOAM SPRING MEMORIAL HOSPITAL, 205 East Jefferson Street, Siloam Springs, AR, Zip 72761; tel. 501/524–4141; Donald E. Patterson, Administrator

ST. BERNARDS REGIONAL MEDICAL CENTER, 224 East Matthews Street, Jonesboro, AR, Zip 72401, Mailing Address: P.O. Box 9320, Zip 72403–9320; tel. 501/972–4100; Ben E. Owens, President

ST. EDWARD MERCY MEDICAL CENTER, 7301 Rogers Avenue, Fort Smith, AR, Zip 72903, Mailing Address: P.O. Box 17000, Zip 72917–7000; tel. 501/484–6000; Sister Judith Marie Keith, President and Chief Executive Officer

ST. JOSEPH'S REGIONAL HEALTH CENTER, 300 Werner Street, Hot Springs, AR, Zip 71913; tel. 501/622–1000; Randall J. Fale, President and Chief Executive Officer

ST. MARY–ROGERS MEMORIAL HOSPITAL, 1200 West Walnut Street, Rogers, AR, Zip 72756–3599; tel. 501/636–0200; Michael J. Packnett, President and Chief Executive Officer

STONE COUNTY MEDICAL CENTER, Highway 14 East, Mountain View, AR, Zip 72560–0510, Mailing Address: P.O. Box 510, Zip 72560; tel. 501/269–4361; Stanley Townsend, Administrator

STUTTGART REGIONAL MEDICAL CENTER, North Buerkle Road, Stuttgart, AR, Zip 72160, Mailing Address: Box 1905, Zip 72160; tel. 501/673–3511; Jim E. Bushmaier, Administrator and Chief Executive Officer

VAN BUREN COUNTY MEMORIAL HOSPITAL, Highway 65 South, Clinton, AR, Zip 72031, Mailing Address: Box 206, Zip 72031; tel. 501/745–2401; Alan Finley, Administrator

WASHINGTON REGIONAL MEDICAL CENTER, 1125 North College Avenue, Fayetteville, AR, Zip 72703; tel. 501/442–1000; Patrick D. Flynn, President and Chief Executive Officer

WHITE COUNTY MEDICAL CENTER, 3214 East Race, Searcy, AR, Zip 72143–4847; tel. 501/268–6121; Raymond W. Montgomery, II, President and Chief Executive Officer

WHITE RIVER MEDICAL CENTER, 1710 Harrison Street, Batesville, AR, Zip 72501, Mailing Address: P.O. Box 2197, Zip 72503–2197; tel. 501/793–1200; Gary Bebow, Administrator and Chief Executive Officer

BAPTIST HEALTH
9601 Interstate 630, Exit 7, Little Rock, AR 72205; tel. 501/227–2015; Dewey Freeman, Vice President

BAPTIST MEDICAL CENTER, 9601 Interstate 630, Exit 7, Little Rock, AR, Zip 72205–7299; tel. 501/202–2000; Steven B. Lampkin, Senior Vice President and Administrator

BAPTIST MEDICAL CENTER ARKADELPHIA, 3050 Twin Rivers Drive, Arkadelphia, AR, Zip 71923; tel. 501/245–1100; Dan Gathright, Senior Vice President and Administrator

BAPTIST MEMORIAL MEDICAL CENTER, One Pershing Circle, North Little Rock, AR, Zip 72114–1899; tel. 501/202–3000; Harrison M. Dean, Senior Vice President and Administrator

BAPTIST REHABILITATION INSTITUTE OF ARKANSAS, 9601 Interstate 630, Exit 7, Little Rock, AR, Zip 72205–7249; tel. 501/202–7000; Steven Douglas Weeks, Vice President and Administrator

SAINT EDWARD MERCY MEDICAL CENTER
7301 Rogers Avenue, Fort Smith, AR 72917–7000; tel. 501/484–6000; Larry Goss, Vice President

HARBOR VIEW MERCY HOSPITAL, 10301 Mayo Road, Fort Smith, AR, Zip 72903, Mailing Address: P.O. Box 17000, Zip 72917–7000; tel. 501/484–5550; Sister Judith Marie Keith, President and Chief Executive Officer

MERCY HOSPITAL OF SCOTT COUNTY, Highways 71 and 80, Waldron, AR, Zip 72958–9984, Mailing Address: Box 2230, Zip 72958–2230; tel. 501/637–4135; Sister Mary Alvera Simon, Administrator

MERCY HOSPITAL–TURNER MEMORIAL, 801 West River, Ozark, AR, Zip 72949; tel. 501/667–4138; Sister Mary Werner Keith, Administrator

NORTH LOGAN MERCY HOSPITAL, 500 East Academy, Paris, AR, Zip 72855–4099; tel. 501/963–6101; Jim L. Maddox, Chief Administrative Officer

ST. EDWARD MERCY MEDICAL CENTER, 7301 Rogers Avenue, Fort Smith, AR, Zip 72903, Mailing Address: P.O. Box 17000, Zip 72917–7000; tel. 501/484–6000; Sister Judith Marie Keith, President and Chief Executive Officer

CALIFORNIA

ADVENTIST HEALTH SYSTEM–LOMA LINDA
11161 Anderson Street, Loma Linda, CA 92350; tel. 909/824–4540; B. Lyn Behrens, MB, BS, President

LOMA LINDA UNIVERSITY BEHAVIORAL MEDICINE CENTER, 1710 Barton Road, Redlands, CA, Zip 92373; tel. 909/793-9333; Nolan Kerr, Administrator

LOMA LINDA UNIVERSITY MEDICAL CENTER, 11234 Anderson Street, Loma Linda, CA, Zip 92354-2870, Mailing Address: P.O. Box 2000, Zip 92354-0200; tel. 909/824-0800; J. David Moorhead, M.D., President

ADVENTIST HEALTH–NORTHERN CALIFORNIA
363 Highland Avenue, Deer Park, CA 94576;
tel. 707/963-6240; Everett Gooch,
President & Chief Executive Officer

FEATHER RIVER HOSPITAL, 5974 Pentz Road, Paradise, CA, Zip 95969-5593; tel. 916/877-9361; George Pifer, President

FRANK R. HOWARD MEMORIAL HOSPITAL, 1 Madrone Street, Willits, CA, Zip 95490; tel. 707/459-6801; Robert J. Walker, President

ST. HELENA HOSPITAL, 650 Sanitarium Road, Deer Park, CA, Zip 94576, Mailing Address: P.O. Box 250, Zip 94576; tel. 707/963-3611; JoAline Olson, R.N., President and Chief Executive Officer

UKIAH VALLEY MEDICAL CENTER, 275 Hospital Drive, Ukiah, CA, Zip 95482; tel. 707/462-3111; ValGene Devitt, President and Chief Executive Officer

ADVENTIST HEALTH–SOUTHERN CALIFORNIA
1509 Wilson Terrace, Glendale, CA 91206;
tel. 818/409-8300; Bob Carmen, President &
Chief Executive Officer

GLENDALE ADVENTIST MEDICAL CENTER, 1509 Wilson Terrace, Glendale, CA, Zip 91206-4007; tel. 818/409-8000; David Nelson, Chief Operating Officer

SIMI VALLEY HOSPITAL AND HEALTH CARE SERVICES, 2975 North Sycamore Drive, Simi Valley, CA, Zip 93065-1277; tel. 805/527-2462; Alan J. Rice, President

WHITE MEMORIAL MEDICAL CENTER, 1720 Cesar E Chavez Avenue, Los Angeles, CA, Zip 90033-2481; tel. 213/268-5000; Beth D. Zachary, Chief Operating Officer

CATHOLIC HEALTHCARE WEST (CHW)
1700 Montgomery Street, Suite 300, San
Francisco, CA 94111; tel. 415/438-5500;
Debbie Cantu, Director of Corporate
Communications

BAKERSFIELD MEMORIAL HOSPITAL, 420 34th Street, Bakersfield, CA, Zip 93301, Mailing Address: Box 1888, Zip 93303-1888; tel. 805/327-1792; C. Larry Carr, President

DOMINICAN SANTA CRUZ HOSPITAL, 1555 Soquel Drive, Santa Cruz, CA, Zip 95065-1794; tel. 408/462-7700; Sister Julie Hyer, President and Chief Executive Officer

MARK TWAIN ST. JOSEPH'S HOSPITAL, 768 Mountain Ranch Road, San Andreas, CA, Zip 95249-9710; tel. 209/754-3521; Kathy Yarbrough, Administrator

MERCY AMERICAN RIVER/MERCY SAN JUAN HOSPITAL, 6501 Coyle Avenue, Carmichael, CA, Zip 95608, Mailing Address: P.O. Box 479, Zip 95608; tel. 916/537-5000; Sister Bridget McCarthy, President

MERCY GENERAL HOSPITAL, 4001 J Street, Sacramento, CA, Zip 95819; tel. 916/453-4950; Thomas A. Petersen, Vice President and Chief Operating Officer

MERCY HEALTHCARE–BAKERSFIELD, 2215 Truxtun Avenue, Bakersfield, CA, Zip 93301, Mailing Address: Box 119, Zip 93302; tel. 805/632-5000; Bernard J. Herman, President and Chief Executive Officer

MERCY HOSPITAL AND HEALTH SERVICES, 2740 M Street, Merced, CA, Zip 95340-2880; tel. 209/384-6444; Kelly C. Morgan, President and Chief Executive Officer

MERCY HOSPITAL OF FOLSOM, 1650 Creekside Drive, Folsom, CA, Zip 95630-3405; tel. 916/983-7400; Donald C. Hudson, Vice President and Chief Operating Officer

MERCY MEDICAL CENTER, 2175 Rosaline Avenue, Redding, CA, Zip 96001, Mailing Address: Box 496009, Zip 96049-6009; tel. 916/225-6000; George A. Govier, President and Chief Executive Officer

MERCY MEDICAL CENTER MOUNT SHASTA, 914 Pine Street, Mount Shasta, CA, Zip 96067, Mailing Address: P.O. Box 239, Zip 96067-0239; tel. 916/926-6111; James R. Hoss, President and Chief Executive Officer

METHODIST HOSPITAL, 7500 Hospital Drive, Sacramento, CA, Zip 95823-5477; tel. 916/423-3000; Stanley C. Oppegard, Vice President and Chief Operating Officer

O'CONNOR HOSPITAL, 2105 Forest Avenue, San Jose, CA, Zip 95128-1471; tel. 408/947-2500; William C. Finlayson, President and Chief Executive Officer

ROBERT F. KENNEDY MEDICAL CENTER, 4500 West 116th Street, Hawthorne, CA, Zip 90250; tel. 310/973-1711; Peter P. Aprato, Administrator and Chief Operating Officer

SAINT FRANCIS MEMORIAL HOSPITAL, 900 Hyde Street, San Francisco, CA, Zip 94109, Mailing Address: Box 7726, Zip 94120-7726; tel. 415/353-6000; John G. Williams, President and Chief Executive Officer

SAINT LOUISE HOSPITAL, 18500 Saint Louise Drive, Morgan Hill, CA, Zip 95037; tel. 408/779-1500; William C. Finlayson, President and Chief Executive Officer

SAINT MARY MEDICAL CENTER, 1050 Linden Avenue, Long Beach, CA, Zip 90801, Mailing Address: P.O. Box 887, Zip 90801; tel. 310/491-9000; Tammie McMann Brailsford, Administrator

SEQUOIA HOSPITAL, 170 Alameda De Las Pulgas, Redwood City, CA, Zip 94062-2799; tel. 415/367-5561; Glenna L. Vaskelis, Administrator

SETON MEDICAL CENTER, 1900 Sullivan Avenue, Daly City, CA, Zip 94015-2229; tel. 415/992-4000; Bernadette Smith, Chief Operating Officer

SETON MEDICAL CENTER COASTSIDE, 600 Marine Boulevard, Moss Beach, CA, Zip 94038; tel. 415/728-5521; Deborah E. Stebbins, FACHE, President and Chief Executive Officer

SIERRA NEVADA MEMORIAL HOSPITAL, 155 Glasson Way, Grass Valley, CA, Zip 95945-5792, Mailing Address: Box 1029, Zip 95945-5792; tel. 916/274-6000; C. Thomas Collier, President and Chief Executive Officer

ST. BERNARDINE MEDICAL CENTER, 2101 North Waterman Avenue, San Bernardino, CA, Zip 92404; tel. 909/883-8711; Maureen O'Connor, Interim Administrator and Chief Operating Officer

ST. DOMINIC'S HOSPITAL, 1777 West Yosemite Avenue, Manteca, CA, Zip 95337; tel. 209/825-3500; Richard Aldred, Chief Administrative Officer

ST. ELIZABETH COMMUNITY HOSPITAL, 2550 Sister Mary Columba Drive, Red Bluff, CA, Zip 96080-4397; tel. 916/529-8005; Thomas F. Grimes, III, Executive Vice President and Chief Operating Officer

ST. FRANCIS MEDICAL CENTER, 3630 East Imperial Highway, Lynwood, CA, Zip 90262; tel. 310/603-6000; Gerald T. Kozai, Administrator and Chief Operating Officer

ST. JOHN'S PLEASANT VALLEY HOSPITAL, 2309 Antonio Avenue, Camarillo, CA, Zip 93010-1459; tel. 805/389-5800; Daniel R. Herlinger, President and Chief Executive Officer

ST. JOHN'S REGIONAL MEDICAL CENTER, 1600 North Rose Avenue, Oxnard, CA, Zip 93030; tel. 805/988-2500; Daniel R. Herlinger, President and Chief Executive Officer

ST. JOSEPH'S BEHAVIORAL HEALTH CENTER, 2510 North California Street, Stockton, CA, Zip 95204-5568; tel. 209/948-2100; James Sondecker, Administrator

ST. JOSEPH'S HOSPITAL AND MEDICAL CENTER, 350 West Thomas Road, Phoenix, AZ, Zip 85013, Mailing Address: Box 2071, Zip 85001-2071; tel. 602/406-3100; Mary G. Yarbrough, President and Chief Executive Officer

ST. JOSEPH'S MEDICAL CENTER, 1800 North California Street, Stockton, CA, Zip 95204-6088, Mailing Address: P.O. Box 213008, Zip 95213-9008; tel. 209/943-2000; Edward G. Schroeder, President and Chief Executive Officer

ST. MARY'S MEDICAL CENTER, 450 Stanyan Street, San Francisco, CA, Zip 94117-1079; tel. 415/668-1000; John G. Williams, President

ST. ROSE DOMINICAN HOSPITAL, 102 Lake Mead Drive, Henderson, NV, Zip 89015; tel. 702/564-2622; Rod A. Davis, President and Chief Executive Officer

ST. VINCENT MEDICAL CENTER, 2131 West Third Street, Los Angeles, CA, Zip 90057-0992, Mailing Address: P.O. Box 57992, Zip 90057; tel. 213/484-7111; Vincent F. Guinan, President and Chief Executive Officer

WOODLAND MEMORIAL HOSPITAL, 1325 Cottonwood Street, Woodland, CA, Zip 95695-5199; tel. 916/662-3961; D. Scott Ideson, Interim Chief Executive Officer

CEDARS–SINAI HEALTH SYSTEM
8700 Beverly Boulevard, Los Angeles, CA
90048; tel. 310/855-5000; Thomas M.
Priselac, President & Chief Executive Officer

CEDARS–SINAI MEDICAL CENTER, 8700 Beverly Boulevard, Los Angeles, CA, Zip 90048-0750, Mailing Address: Box 48750, Zip 90048-0750; tel. 310/855-5000; Thomas M. Priselac, President and Chief Executive Officer

EAST BAY MEDICAL NETWORK
2000 Powell Street, 9th Floor, Emeryville, CA
94608; tel. 510/450-9850; Blake Kirk,
Provider Relations

ALAMEDA HOSPITAL, 2070 Clinton Avenue, Alameda, CA, Zip 94501; tel. 510/522-3700; William J. Dal Cielo, Chief Executive Officer

ALTA BATES MEDICAL CENTER–ASHBY CAMPUS, 2450 Ashby Avenue, Berkeley, CA, Zip 94705; tel. 510/204-4444; Albert Lawrence Greene, President and Chief Executive Officer

COLUMBIA SAN LEANDRO HOSPITAL, 13855 East 14th Street, San Leandro, CA, Zip 94578-0398; tel. 510/667-4510; Kelly Mather, Executive Director

MOUNT DIABLO MEDICAL CENTER, 2540 East Street, Concord, CA, Zip 94520, Mailing Address: P.O. Box 4110, Zip 94524-4110; tel. 510/682-8200; Michael L. Wall, President and Chief Executive Officer

PATTON STATE HOSPITAL, 3102 East Highland Avenue, Patton, CA, Zip 92369; tel. 909/425-7000; William L. Summers, Executive Director

SUTTER DELTA MEDICAL CENTER, 3901 Lone Tree Way, Antioch, CA, Zip 94509; tel. 510/779-7200; Linda Horn, Administrator

WASHINGTON TOWNSHIP HEALTH CARE DISTRICT, 2000 Mowry Avenue, Fremont, CA, Zip 94538-1716; tel. 510/797-1111; Nancy D. Farber, Chief Executive Officer

ESSENTIAL HEALTHCARE NETWORK
525 North Garfield Park, Monterey Park, CA
91754; tel. 818/573-2222; A. Schaffer,
Acting Executive Director

COMMUNITY HOSPITAL OF HUNTINGTON PARK, 2623 East Slauson Avenue, Huntington Park, CA, Zip 90255; tel. 213/583-1931; Charles Martinez, Ph.D., Chief Executive Officer

GARFIELD MEDICAL CENTER, 525 North Garfield Avenue, Monterey Park, CA, Zip 91754; tel. 818/573-2222; Philip A. Cohen, Chief Executive Officer

GREATER EL MONTE COMMUNITY HOSPITAL, 1701 South Santa Anita Avenue, South El Monte, CA, Zip 91733-9918; tel. 818/579-7777; Elizabeth A. Primeaux, Chief Executive Officer

PACIFIC ALLIANCE MEDICAL CENTER, 531 West College Street, Los Angeles, CA, Zip 90012; tel. 213/624-8411; John R. Edwards, Chief Executive Officer

QUEEN OF ANGELS–HOLLYWOOD PRESBYTERIAN MEDICAL CENTER, 1300 North Vermont Avenue, Los Angeles, CA, Zip 90027–0069; tel. 213/413–3000; Sylvester Graff, President and Chief Executive Officer

ROBERT F. KENNEDY MEDICAL CENTER, 4500 West 116th Street, Hawthorne, CA, Zip 90250; tel. 310/973–1711; Peter P. Aprato, Administrator and Chief Operating Officer

SANTA MARTA HOSPITAL, 319 North Humphreys Avenue, Los Angeles, CA, Zip 90022; tel. 213/266–6500; James G. Ovieda, President and Chief Executive Officer

ST. FRANCIS MEDICAL CENTER, 3630 East Imperial Highway, Lynwood, CA, Zip 90262; tel. 310/603–6000; Gerald T. Kozai, Administrator and Chief Operating Officer

SUBURBAN MEDICAL CENTER, 16453 South Colorado Avenue, Paramount, CA, Zip 90723; tel. 310/531–3110; Michael D. Kerr, Chief Executive Officer

FREMONT–RIDEOUT HEALTH GROUP
989 Plumas Street, Yuba City, CA 95991; tel. 916/751–4226; Thomas P. Hayes, Chief Executive Officer

FREMONT MEDICAL CENTER, 970 Plumas Street, Yuba City, CA, Zip 95991; tel. 916/751–4000; Thomas P. Hayes, Chief Executive Officer

RIDEOUT MEMORIAL HOSPITAL, 726 Fourth Street, Marysville, CA, Zip 95901–2128, Mailing Address: Box 2128, Zip 95901–2128; tel. 916/749–4300; Thomas P. Hayes, Chief Executive Officer

FRIENDLY HILLS HEALTHCARE NETWORK
931 South Beach, LaHabra, CA 90631; tel. 310/694–4711; Albert Barnett, M.D., Chairman & Chief Executive Officer

FRIENDLY HILLS REGIONAL MEDICAL CENTER, 1251 West Lambert Road, La Habra, CA, Zip 90631; tel. 310/694–3838; Gloria Mayer, Executive Director

ST. JUDE MEDICAL CENTER, 101 East Valencia Mesa Drive, Fullerton, CA, Zip 92635; tel. 714/992–3000; Robert J. Fraschetti, President and Chief Executive Officer

HEALTH FIRST NETWORK
4020 5th Avenue, 3rd Floor, San Diego, CA 92103; tel. 619/293–0986; Roger Burke, President

PALOMAR MEDICAL CENTER, 555 East Valley Parkway, Escondido, CA, Zip 92025–3084; tel. 619/739–3000; Victoria M. Penland, Administrator and Chief Operating Officer

POMERADO HOSPITAL, 15615 Pomerado Road, Poway, CA, Zip 92064; tel. 619/485–4600; Marvin W. Levenson, M.D., Administrator and Chief Operating Officer

INTERMOUNTAIN HEALTHCARE NETWORK
228 McDowell Street, Alturas, CA 96101; tel. 916/233–5131; Donna Donald, Network Contact

INDIAN VALLEY HOSPITAL DISTRICT, 174 Hot Springs Road, Greenville, CA, Zip 95947; tel. 916/284–7191; Lynn Seaberg, Administrator and Chief Executive Officer

MAYERS MEMORIAL HOSPITAL DISTRICT, Highway 299 East, Fall River Mills, CA, Zip 96028, Mailing Address: Box 459, Zip 96028; tel. 916/336–5511; Everett L. Beck, Administrator

MODOC MEDICAL CENTER, 228 McDowell Street, Alturas, CA, Zip 96101; tel. 916/233–5131; Woody J. Laughnan, Chief Executive Officer

SURPRISE VALLEY COMMUNITY HOSPITAL, Main and Washington Streets, Cedarville, CA, Zip 96104, Mailing Address: P.O. Box 246, Zip 96104–0246; tel. 916/279–6111; Joyce Gysin, Administrator

KAISER FOUNDATION HEALTH PLAN OF NORTHERN CALIFORNIA
1950 Franklin Street, Oakland, CA 94612; tel. 510/987–1000; David Pockell, Executive Regional Vice President

KAISER FOUNDATION HOSPITAL, 2425 Geary Boulevard, San Francisco, CA, Zip 94115; tel. 415/202–2000; Rosemary Fox, Acting Administrator

KAISER FOUNDATION HOSPITAL, 280 West MacArthur Boulevard, Oakland, CA, Zip 94611; tel. 510/596–1000; Donald Oxley, Vice President, Area Manager and Chief Executive Officer

KAISER FOUNDATION HOSPITAL, 1425 South Main Street, Walnut Creek, CA, Zip 94596; tel. 510/295–4000; Anna Robinson, Administrator

KAISER FOUNDATION HOSPITAL, 27400 Hesperian Boulevard, Hayward, CA, Zip 94545–4297; tel. 510/784–4313; Lisa Koltun, Administrator

KAISER FOUNDATION HOSPITAL, 1150 Veterans Boulevard, Redwood City, CA, Zip 94063–2087; tel. 415/299–2000; Carol Kiecker, Chief Executive Officer, Vice President and Area Manager

KAISER FOUNDATION HOSPITAL, 6600 Bruceville Road, Sacramento, CA, Zip 95823; tel. 916/688–2430; Sarah Krevans, Area Manager

KAISER FOUNDATION HOSPITAL, 99 Montecillo Road, San Rafael, CA, Zip 94903–3397; tel. 415/444–2000; Richard R. Pettingill, Chief Executive Officer

KAISER FOUNDATION HOSPITAL, 900 Kiely Boulevard, Santa Clara, CA, Zip 95051–5386; tel. 408/236–6400

KAISER FOUNDATION HOSPITAL, 1200 El Camino Real, South San Francisco, CA, Zip 94080–3299; tel. 415/742–2547; Rosemary Fox, Coutinuing Care Leader

KAISER FOUNDATION HOSPITAL AND REHABILITATION CENTER, 975 Sereno Drive, Vallejo, CA, Zip 94589; tel. 707/648–6230; Vivian M. Rittenhouse, Vice President and Market Leader

REDDING MEDICAL CENTER, 1100 Butte Street, Redding, CA, Zip 96001–0853, Mailing Address: Box 496072, Zip 96049–6072; tel. 916/244–5454; Jeff Koury, Chief Executive Officer

LITTLE COMPANY OF MARY HEALTH SERVICES
4101 Torrance Boulevard, Torrance, CA 90503; tel. 310/540–7676; James Lester, President

LITTLE COMPANY OF MARY HOSPITAL, 4101 Torrance Boulevard, Torrance, CA, Zip 90503–4698; tel. 310/540–7676; Mark Costa, President

SAN PEDRO PENINSULA HOSPITAL, 1300 West Seventh Street, San Pedro, CA, Zip 90732; tel. 310/832–3311; John M. Wilson, President

NORTHBAY HEALTHCARE SYSTEM
1200 B Gale Wilson Boulevard, Fairfield, CA 94533; tel. 707/429–7817; Gary J. Passama, President & Chief Executive Officer

NORTHBAY MEDICAL CENTER, 1200 B. Gale Wilson Boulevard, Fairfield, CA, Zip 94533–3587; tel. 707/429–3600; Deborah Sugiyama, President

VACAVALLEY HOSPITAL, 1000 Nut Tree Road, Vacaville, CA, Zip 95687; tel. 707/446–5716; Deborah Sugiyama, President

PROVIDENCE HEALTH SYSTEM IN CALIFORNIA
501 South Buena Vista Street, Burbank, CA 91505; tel. 818/843–5111; Michael Madden, Chairman

PROVIDENCE HOLY CROSS MEDICAL CENTER, 15031 Rinaldi Street, Mission Hills, CA, Zip 91345–1285; tel. 818/365–8051; Michael J. Madden, Chief Executive Los Angeles Service Area

PROVIDENCE SAINT JOSEPH MEDICAL CENTER, 501 South Buena Vista Street, Burbank, CA, Zip 91505–4866; tel. 818/843–5111; Michael J. Madden, Chief Executive Los Angeles Service Area

SAINT JOSEPH HEALTH SYSTEM
440 South Batavia Street, Orange, CA 92668–3995; tel. 714/997–7690; Jim Dake, Manager of Technical Services

QUEEN OF THE VALLEY HOSPITAL, 1000 Trancas Street, Napa, CA, Zip 94558, Mailing Address: Box 2340, Zip 94558; tel. 707/252–4411; Howard Levant, President and Chief Executive Officer

REDWOOD MEMORIAL HOSPITAL, 3300 Renner Drive, Fortuna, CA, Zip 95540; tel. 707/725–3361; Paul J. Chodkowski, President and Chief Executive Officer

SAINT JOSEPH HOSPITAL, 2700 Dolbeer Street, Eureka, CA, Zip 95501; tel. 707/445–8121; Paul J. Chodkowski, President and Chief Executive Officer

SANTA ROSA MEMORIAL HOSPITAL, 1165 Montgomery Drive, Santa Rosa, CA, Zip 95405, Mailing Address: Box 522, Zip 95402; tel. 707/546–3210; Robert H. Fish, President and Chief Executive Officer

ST. MARY REGIONAL MEDICAL CENTER, 18300 Highway 18, Apple Valley, CA, Zip 92307–0725, Mailing Address: Box 7025, Zip 92307–0725; tel. 619/242–2311; Catherine M. Pelley, President and Chief Executive Officer

ST. JOSEPH HOSPITAL, 1100 West Stewart Drive, Orange, CA, Zip 92668, Mailing Address: P.O. Box 5600, Zip 92613–5600; tel. 714/633–9111; Larry K. Ainsworth, President and Chief Executive Officer

ST. JUDE MEDICAL CENTER, 101 East Valencia Mesa Drive, Fullerton, CA, Zip 92635; tel. 714/992–3000; Robert J. Fraschetti, President and Chief Executive Officer

SCRIPPSHEALTH
4275 Campus Point Court, San Diego, CA 92121; tel. 619/678–6111; Kay Alexander, Executive Assistant

GREEN HOSPITAL OF SCRIPPS CLINIC, 10666 North Torrey Pines Road, La Jolla, CA, Zip 92037–1093; tel. 619/455–9100; Glenn W. Chong, Senior Vice President and Administrator

SCRIPPS HOSPITAL–EAST COUNTY, 1688 East Main Street, El Cajon, CA, Zip 92021; tel. 619/593–5600; Robin B. Brown, Vice President and Administrator

SCRIPPS MEMORIAL HOSPITAL–CHULA VISTA, 435 H Street, Chula Vista, CA, Zip 91912–1537, Mailing Address: Box 1537, Zip 91910–1537; tel. 619/691–7000; Thomas A. Gammiere, Vice President and Administrator

SCRIPPS MEMORIAL HOSPITAL–ENCINITAS, 354 Santa Fe Drive, Encinitas, CA, Zip 92024, Mailing Address: P.O. Box 817, Zip 92023; tel. 619/753–6501; Gerald E. Bracht, Vice President and Administrator

SCRIPPS MEMORIAL HOSPITAL–LA JOLLA, 9888 Genesee Avenue, La Jolla, CA, Zip 92037–1276, Mailing Address: Box 28, Zip 92038–0028; tel. 619/626–4123; Glenn W. Chong, Senior Vice President and Administrator

SCRIPPS MERCY MEDICAL CENTER, 4077 Fifth Avenue, San Diego, CA, Zip 92103–2180; tel. 619/260–7101; Nancy Wilson, Senior Vice President and Regional Administrator

SHARP HEALTHCARE
3131 Berger Avenue, Suite 100, San Diego, CA 92123; tel. 619/541–4000; Mike Murphy, President & Chief Executive Officer

GROSSMONT HOSPITAL, 5555 Grossmont Center Drive, La Mesa, CA, Zip 91942, Mailing Address: Box 158, Zip 91944–0158; tel. 619/465–0711; Michele T. Tarbet, R.N., Chief Executive Officer

SHARP CABRILLO HOSPITAL, 3475 Kenyon Street, San Diego, CA, Zip 92110–5067; tel. 619/221–3400; Randi Larsson, Senior Vice President and Administrator

SHARP CHULA VISTA MEDICAL CENTER, 751 Medical Center Court, Chula Vista, CA, Zip 91911, Mailing Address: Box 1297, Zip 91912; tel. 619/482–5800; Britt Berrett, Chief Executive Officer

SHARP HEALTHCARE MURRIETA, 25500 Medical Center Drive, Murrieta, CA, Zip 92562–5966; tel. 909/696–6000; Juanice Lovett, Chief Executive Officer

Section B

SHARP MEMORIAL HOSPITAL, 7901 Frost Street, San Diego, CA, Zip 92123–2788; tel. 619/541–3400; Dan Gross, Chief Executive Officer

SOUTHERN CALIFORNIA HEALTHCARE SYSTEMS
1300 East Green Street, Pasadena, CA 91106; tel. 818/397–2900; Frederick C. Meyer, President & Chief Executive Officer

BEVERLY HOSPITAL, 309 West Beverly Boulevard, Montebello, CA, Zip 90640; tel. 213/726–1222; Matthew S. Gerlach, Chief Executive Officer and Administrator

HUNTINGTON EAST VALLEY HOSPITAL, 150 West Alosta Avenue, Glendora, CA, Zip 91740–4398; tel. 818/335–0231; James W. Maki, Chief Executive Officer

HUNTINGTON MEMORIAL HOSPITAL, 100 West California Boulevard, Pasadena, CA, Zip 91105, Mailing Address: P.O. Box 7013, Zip 91109–7013; tel. 818/397–5000; Stephen A. Ralph, President and Chief Executive Officer

METHODIST HOSPITAL OF SOUTHERN CALIFORNIA, 300 West Huntington Drive, Arcadia, CA, Zip 91007, Mailing Address: P.O. Box 60016, Zip 91066–6016; tel. 818/445–4441; Dennis M. Lee, President

VERDUGO HILLS HOSPITAL, 1812 Verdugo Boulevard, Glendale, CA, Zip 91208, Mailing Address: P.O. Box 1431, Zip 91209–1431; tel. 818/790–7100; Bernard Glossy, President

SUTTER\CHS
P.O. Box 160727, Sacramento, CA 95816; tel. 916/733–8800; Van Johnson, President & Chief Executive Officer

ALTA BATES MEDICAL CENTER–ASHBY CAMPUS, 2450 Ashby Avenue, Berkeley, CA, Zip 94705; tel. 510/204–4444; Albert Lawrence Greene, President and Chief Executive Officer

CALIFORNIA PACIFIC MEDICAL CENTER, Clay at Buchanan Street, San Francisco, CA, Zip 94115, Mailing Address: P.O. Box 7999, Zip 94120; tel. 415/563–4321; Martin Brotman, M.D., President and Chief Executive Officer

COMMUNITY HOSPITAL, 3325 Chanate Road, Santa Rosa, CA, Zip 95404; tel. 707/576–4000; Cliff Coates, Chief Executive Officer

DAMERON HOSPITAL, 525 West Acacia Street, Stockton, CA, Zip 95203; tel. 209/944–5550; Luis Arismendi, M.D., Administrator

EDEN HOSPITAL MEDICAL CENTER, 20103 Lake Chabot Road, Castro Valley, CA, Zip 94546; tel. 510/537–1234; Edward Schreck, President and Chief Executive Officer

MARIN GENERAL HOSPITAL, 250 Bon Air Road, Greenbrae, CA, Zip 94904, Mailing Address: Box 8010, San Rafael, Zip 94912–8010; tel. 415/925–7000; Henry J. Buhrmann, President and Chief Executive Officer

MEMORIAL HOSPITAL LOS BANOS, 520 West I Street, Los Banos, CA, Zip 93635; tel. 209/826–0591; Gil Silbernagel, Administrator

MEMORIAL HOSPITALS ASSOCIATION, Modesto, CA, Mailing Address: P.O. Box 942, Zip 95353; tel. 209/526–4500; David P. Benn, President and Chief Executive Officer

MILLS–PENINSULA HEALTH SERVICES, 1783 El Camino Real, Burlingame, CA, Zip 94010–3205; tel. 415/696–5400; Robert W. Merwin, Chief Executive Officer

NOVATO COMMUNITY HOSPITAL, 1625 Hill Road, Novato, CA, Zip 94947, Mailing Address: P.O. Box 1108, Zip 94948; tel. 415/897–3111; Anne Hosfeld, Chief Administrative Officer

OAK VALLEY DISTRICT HOSPITAL, 350 South Oak Street, Oakdale, CA, Zip 95361; tel. 209/847–3011; Gary D. Rapaport, Administrator and Chief Executive Officer

SUTTER AMADOR HOSPITAL, 810 Court Street, Jackson, CA, Zip 95642–2379; tel. 209/223–7500; Scott Stenberg, Chief Executive Officer

SUTTER AUBURN FAITH HOSPITAL, 11815 Education Street, Auburn, CA, Zip 95604, Mailing Address: Box 8992, Zip 95604–8992; tel. 916/888–4518; Joel E. Grey, Chief Executive Officer

SUTTER CENTER FOR PSYCHIATRY, 7700 Folsom Boulevard, Sacramento, CA, Zip 95826–2608; tel. 916/386–3000; Diane Gail Stewart, Administrator

SUTTER COAST HOSPITAL, 800 East Washington Boulevard, Crescent City, CA, Zip 95531; tel. 707/464–8511; John E. Menaugh, Chief Executive Officer

SUTTER COMMUNITY HOSPITALS, 5151 F Street, Sacramento, CA, Zip 95819–3295; tel. 916/454–3333; Lou Lazatin, Chief Executive Officer

SUTTER DAVIS HOSPITAL, 2000 Sutter Place, Davis, CA, Zip 95616, Mailing Address: P.O. Box 1617, Zip 95617; tel. 916/756–6440; Lawrence A. Maas, Administrator

SUTTER DELTA MEDICAL CENTER, 3901 Lone Tree Way, Antioch, CA, Zip 94509; tel. 510/779–7200; Linda Horn, Administrator

SUTTER LAKESIDE HOSPITAL, 5176 Hill Road East, Lakeport, CA, Zip 95453–6111; tel. 707/262–5001; Paul J. Hensler, Chief Executive Officer

SUTTER MERCED MEDICAL CENTER, 301 East 13th Street, Merced, CA, Zip 95340–6211, Mailing Address: Box 231, Zip 95341–0231; tel. 209/385–7000; Brian S. Bentley, Administrator

SUTTER ROSEVILLE MEDICAL CENTER, One Medical Plaza, Roseville, CA, Zip 95661–3477; tel. 916/781–1000; Joel E. Grey, Chief Executive Officer

SUTTER SOLANO MEDICAL CENTER, 300 Hospital Drive, Vallejo, CA, Zip 94589–2517, Mailing Address: P.O. Box 3189, Zip 94589; tel. 707/554–4444; Patrick R. Brady, Administrator

TRACY COMMUNITY MEMORIAL HOSPITAL, 1420 North Tracy Boulevard, Tracy, CA, Zip 95376–3497; tel. 209/835–1500; Larry L. Meyer, Vice President and Administrator

TENET HEALTHCARE CORPORATION
3820 State Street, Santa Barbara, CA 93105; tel. 805/563–7000; Jeffrey C. Barbakow, Chairman & Chief Executive Officer

ALVARADO HOSPITAL MEDICAL CENTER, 6655 Alvarado Road, San Diego, CA, Zip 92120–5298; tel. 619/229–3100; Barry G. Weinbaum, Chief Executive Officer

CENTURY CITY HOSPITAL, 2070 Century Park East, Los Angeles, CA, Zip 90067; tel. 310/553–6211; John R. Nickens, III, Chief Executive Officer

COMMUNITY HOSPITAL OF LOS GATOS, 815 Pollard Road, Los Gatos, CA, Zip 95030; tel. 408/378–6131; Truman L. Gates, Chief Executive Officer

DOCTORS HOSPITAL OF MANTECA, 1205 East North Street, Manteca, CA, Zip 95336, Mailing Address: Box 191, Zip 95336; tel. 209/823–3111; Patrick W. Rufferty, Chief Executive Officer

DOCTORS HOSPITAL OF PINOLE, 2151 Appian Way, Pinole, CA, Zip 94564; tel. 510/724–5000; Gary Sloan, Chief Executive Officer

DOCTORS MEDICAL CENTER, 1441 Florida Avenue, Modesto, CA, Zip 95350–4418, Mailing Address: P.O. Box 4138, Zip 95352–4138; tel. 209/578–1211; Chris DiCicco, Chief Executive Officer

ENCINO–TARZANA REGIONAL MEDICAL CENTER, 18321 Clark Street, Tarzana, CA, Zip 91356; tel. 818/881–0800; Arnold R. Schaffer, Chief Executive Officer

GARDEN GROVE HOSPITAL AND MEDICAL CENTER, 12601 Garden Grove Boulevard, Garden Grove, CA, Zip 92843–1959; tel. 714/741–2700; Timothy Smith, President and Chief Executive Officer

GARFIELD MEDICAL CENTER, 525 North Garfield Avenue, Monterey Park, CA, Zip 91754; tel. 818/573–2222; Philip A. Cohen, Chief Executive Officer

IRVINE MEDICAL CENTER, 16200 Sand Canyon Avenue, Irvine, CA, Zip 92618–3714; tel. 714/753–2000; Richard H. Robinson, Chief Executive Officer

JOHN F. KENNEDY MEMORIAL HOSPITAL, 47–111 Monroe Street, Indio, CA, Zip 92201, Mailing Address: P.O. Drawer LLLL, Zip 92202–2558; tel. 619/347–6191; Michael A. Rembis, Chief Executive Officer

LAKEWOOD REGIONAL MEDICAL CENTER, 3700 East South Street, Lakewood, CA, Zip 90712; tel. 310/531–2550; Gustavo A. Valdespino, Chief Executive Officer

LOS ALAMITOS MEDICAL CENTER, 3751 Katella Avenue, Los Alamitos, CA, Zip 90720; tel. 310/598–1311; Gustavo A. Valdespino, Chief Executive Officer

NORTH HOLLYWOOD MEDICAL CENTER, 12629 Riverside Drive, North Hollywood, CA, Zip 91607–3495; tel. 818/980–9200; Dale Surowitz, President and Chief Executive Officer

PLACENTIA–LINDA HOSPITAL, 1301 Rose Drive, Placentia, CA, Zip 92870; tel. 714/993–2000; Maxine T. Cooper, Chief Executive Officer

REDDING MEDICAL CENTER, 1100 Butte Street, Redding, CA, Zip 96001–0853, Mailing Address: Box 496072, Zip 96049–6072; tel. 916/244–5454; Jeff Koury, Chief Executive Officer

SAN DIMAS COMMUNITY HOSPITAL, 1350 West Covina Boulevard, San Dimas, CA, Zip 91773–0308; tel. 909/599–6811; Larry Peterson, Chief Executive Officer

SAN RAMON REGIONAL MEDICAL CENTER, 6001 Norris Canyon Road, San Ramon, CA, Zip 94583; tel. 510/275–9200; Philip P. Gustafson, Chief Executive Officer

SIERRA VISTA REGIONAL MEDICAL CENTER, 1010 Murray Street, San Luis Obispo, CA, Zip 93405, Mailing Address: Box 1367, Zip 93406–1367; tel. 805/546–7600; Harold E. Chilton, Chief Executive Officer

SOUTH BAY MEDICAL CENTER, 514 North Prospect Avenue, Redondo Beach, CA, Zip 90277; tel. 310/376–9474; Jerald R. Happel, Executive Director

TWIN CITIES COMMUNITY HOSPITAL, 1100 Las Tablas Road, Templeton, CA, Zip 93465; tel. 805/434–3500; Harold E. Chilton, Chief Executive Officer

UNIHEALTH
4100 West Alameda, Burbank, CA 91505; tel. 818/238–6000; Terry Hartshorn, President

CALIFORNIA HOSPITAL MEDICAL CENTER, 1401 South Grand Avenue, Los Angeles, CA, Zip 90015; tel. 213/748–2411; Melinda D. Beswick, President and Chief Executive Officer

GLENDALE MEMORIAL HOSPITAL AND HEALTH CENTER, 1420 South Central Avenue, Glendale, CA, Zip 91204–2594; tel. 818/502–1900; Roger E. Seaver, President and Chief Executive Officer

LA PALMA INTERCOMMUNITY HOSPITAL, 7901 Walker Street, La Palma, CA, Zip 90623–5850, Mailing Address: P.O. Box 5850, Buena Park, Zip 90622; tel. 714/670–7400; Stephen E. Dixon, President and Chief Executive Officer

LINDSAY DISTRICT HOSPITAL, 740 North Sequoia Avenue, Lindsay, CA, Zip 93247, Mailing Address: Box 40, Zip 93247; tel. 209/562–4955; David S. Wanger, Chief Executive Officer

LONG BEACH COMMUNITY MEDICAL CENTER, 1720 Termino Avenue, Long Beach, CA, Zip 90804; tel. 310/498–1000; Makoto Nakayama, Interim President and Chief Executive Officer

MARTIN LUTHER HOSPITAL–ANAHEIM, 1830 West Romneya Drive, Anaheim, CA, Zip 92801–1854; tel. 714/491–5200; Stephen E. Dixon, President and Chief Executive Officer

NORTHRIDGE HOSPITAL AND MEDICAL CENTER, SHERMAN WAY CAMPUS, 14500 Sherman Circle, Van Nuys, CA, Zip 91405; tel. 818/997–0101; Richard D. Lyons, President and Chief Administrative Officer

NORTHRIDGE HOSPITAL MEDICAL CENTER–ROSCOE BOULEVARD CAMPUS, 18300 Roscoe Boulevard, Northridge, CA, Zip 91328; tel. 818/885–8500; Roger E. Seaver, President and Chief Executive Officer

SAN GABRIEL VALLEY MEDICAL CENTER, 218 South Santa Anita Street, San Gabriel, CA, Zip 91776, Mailing Address: P.O. Box 1507, Zip 91778–1507; tel. 818/289–5454; Makoto Nakayama, President and Chief Executive Officer

SANTA MONICA–UCLA MEDICAL CENTER, 1250 16th Street, Santa Monica, CA, Zip 90404–1200; tel. 310/319–4000; William D. Parente, Director and Chief Executive Officer

COLORADO

CENTURA PENROSE–ST FRANCIS HEALTH SERVICES 2215 N. Cascade Avenue, P.O. Box 7021, Colorado Springs, CO 80933; tel. 719/776–5000; Donna L. Bertram, Administrator

PENROSE–ST. FRANCIS HEALTH SERVICES, 2215 North Cascade Avenue, Colorado Springs, CO, Zip 80907; tel. 719/776–5000; Donna L. Bertram, R.N., Administrator

COLUMBIA – HEALTH ONE 8200 East Belleview Avenue, Room 202, Englewood, CO 80111; tel. 303/267–8509; Chris Ives, Systems Director

COLUMBIA MEDICAL CENTER OF AURORA, 1501 South Potomac Street, Aurora, CO, Zip 80012; tel. 303/695–2600; Louis O. Garcia, President and Chief Executive Officer

COLUMBIA PRESBYTERIAN–ST. LUKE'S MEDICAL CENTER, 1719 East 19th Avenue, Denver, CO, Zip 80218; tel. 303/839–6000; William K. Atkinson, Ph.D., Chief Executive Officer

COLUMBIA ROSE MEDICAL CENTER, 4567 East Ninth Avenue, Denver, CO, Zip 80220; tel. 303/320–2101; Kenneth H. Feiler, Chief Executive Officer

COLUMBIA SWEDISH MEDICAL CENTER, 501 East Hampden Avenue, Englewood, CO, Zip 80110–0101, Mailing Address: P.O. Box 2901, Zip 80150–0101; tel. 303/788–5000; Mary M. White, President and Chief Executive Officer

NORTH SUBURBAN MEDICAL CENTER, 9191 Grant Street, Thornton, CO, Zip 80229; tel. 303/451–7800; Jay S. Weinstein, Chief Executive Officer

COMMUNITY HEALTH PROVIDERS ORGANIZATION 2021 North 12th Street, Grand Junction, CO 81501; tel. 970/256–6200; Roger C. Zumwalt, Chief Executive Officer

COMMUNITY HOSPITAL, 2021 North 12th Street, Grand Junction, CO, Zip 81501; tel. 970/242–0920; Roger C. Zumwalt, Executive Director

HEALTH & MEDICAL NETWORK OF COLORADO 555 East Pikes Peak, Suite 108, Colorado Springs, CO 80903; tel. 719/475–5025; Ron Burnside, President & Chief Executive Officer

MEMORIAL HOSPITAL, 1400 East Boulder Street, Colorado Springs, CO, Zip 80909–5599, Mailing Address: Box 1326, Zip 80901; tel. 719/475–5000; J. Robert Peters, Executive Director

HIGH PLAINS RURAL HEALTH NETWORK 218 East Kiowa Avenue, Fort Morgan, CO 80701; tel. 303/867–6195; Peter Caplan, Executive Director

CHEYENNE COUNTY HOSPITAL, 210 West First Street, Saint Francis, KS, Zip 67756, Mailing Address: P.O. Box 547, Zip 67756–0547; tel. 913/332–2104; Leslie Lacy, Administrator

COLORADO PLAINS MEDICAL CENTER, 1000 Lincoln Street, Fort Morgan, CO, Zip 80701; tel. 970/867–3391; Keith Mesmer, Administrator and Chief Executive Officer

EAST MORGAN COUNTY HOSPITAL, 2400 West Edison, Brush, CO, Zip 80723; tel. 970/842–5151; Anne Platt, Administrator

ESTES PARK MEDICAL CENTER, 555 Prospect, Estes Park, CO, Zip 80517, Mailing Address: P.O. Box 2740, Zip 80517–2740; tel. 970/586–2317; Andrew Wills, Chief Executive Officer

HAXTUN HOSPITAL DISTRICT, 235 West Fletcher Street, Haxtun, CO, Zip 80731–0308, Mailing Address: Box 308, Zip 80731–0308; tel. 970/774–6123; James E. Brundige, Administrator

HAYS MEDICAL CENTER, 2220 Canterbury Road, Hays, KS, Zip 67601–2323, Mailing Address: P.O. Box 8100, Zip 67601; tel. 913/623–5407; Stephen F. Ronstrom, President and Chief Executive Officer

KEEFE MEMORIAL HOSPITAL, 602 North Sixth Street West, Cheyenne Wells, CO, Zip 80810, Mailing Address: P.O. Box 578, Zip 80810; tel. 719/767–5661; Linda Roth, Administrator

KIT CARSON COUNTY MEMORIAL HOSPITAL, 286 16th Street, Burlington, CO, Zip 80807–1697; tel. 719/346–5311; DeAnn K. Cure, Chief Executive Officer

LINCOLN COMMUNITY HOSPITAL AND NURSING HOME, 111 Sixth Street, Hugo, CO, Zip 80821, Mailing Address: Box 248, Zip 80821; tel. 719/743–2421; Mary L. Thompson, Administrator

MELISSA MEMORIAL HOSPITAL, 505 South Baxter Avenue, Holyoke, CO, Zip 80734–1496; tel. 970/854–2241; Geo V. Larson, II, Administrator

MEMORIAL HEALTH CENTER, 645 Osage Street, Sidney, NE, Zip 69162; tel. 308/254–5825; Rex D. Walk, Chief Executive Officer

NORTH COLORADO MEDICAL CENTER, 1801 16th Street, Greeley, CO, Zip 80631–5199; tel. 970/350–6000; Karl B. Gills, Administrator

PROWERS MEDICAL CENTER, 401 Kendall Drive, Lamar, CO, Zip 81052–3993; tel. 719/336–4343; Earl J. Steinhoff, Chief Executive Officer

RAWLINS COUNTY HOSPITAL, 707 Grant Street, Atwood, KS, Zip 67730–4700, Mailing Address: Box 47, Zip 67730–4700; tel. 913/626–3211; Donald J. Kessen, Administrator

STERLING REGIONAL MEDCENTER, 615 Fairhurst, Sterling, CO, Zip 80751–0500, Mailing Address: Box 3500, Zip 80751; tel. 970/522–0122; James O. Pernau, Administrator

WRAY COMMUNITY DISTRICT HOSPITAL, 1017 West 7th Street, Wray, CO, Zip 80758–1420; tel. 970/332–4811; Daniel Dennis, Administrator

YUMA DISTRICT HOSPITAL, 910 South Main Street, Yuma, CO, Zip 80759–3098, Mailing Address: P.O. Box 306, Zip 80759–0306; tel. 970/848–5405; Michael G. Clark, Administrator

PRIMERA HEALTH CARE 600 Grant Street, Suite 700, Denver, CO 80203–3525; tel. 303/813–5000; David Cooke, Chief Operating Officer

LUTHERAN MEDICAL CENTER, 8300 West 38th Avenue, Wheat Ridge, CO, Zip 80033–6005; tel. 303/425–4500; Kay R. Phillips, President and Chief Executive Officer

SAINT JOSEPH HOSPITAL, 1835 Franklin Street, Denver, CO, Zip 80218; tel. 303/837–7111; Sister Marianna Bauder, President and Chief Executive Officer

QUORUM HEALTH NETWORK OF COLORADO 4450 Arapahoe Avenue, Suite 200, Boulder, CO 80303; tel. 303/440–5511; John Leavitt, Executive Director

GRAND RIVER HOSPITAL DISTRICT, 701 East Fifth Street, Rifle, CO, Zip 81650–2970, Mailing Address: P.O. Box 912, Zip 81650–0912; tel. 970/625–1510; Edwin A. Gast, Administrator

PIONEERS HOSPITAL OF RIO BLANCO COUNTY, 345 Cleveland Street, Meeker, CO, Zip 81641–0000; tel. 970/878–5047; Jim Murphy, Administrator

THE CHILDREN'S HOSPITAL 1056 East 19th Avenue, Denver, CO 80218; tel. 303/861–8888; Lua R. Blankenship, President

CHILDREN'S HOSPITAL, 1056 East 19th Avenue, Denver, CO, Zip 80218–1088; tel. 303/861–8888; Lua R. Blankenship, Jr., President and Chief Executive Officer

CONNECTICUT

CONNECTICUT HEALTH SYSTEM, INC. 80 Seymour Street, Hartford, CT 06102–5037; tel. 860/545–5000; John Meehan, President & Chief Executive Officer

GAYLORD HOSPITAL, Gaylord Farm Road, Wallingford, CT, Zip 06492–7049, Mailing Address: P.O. Box 400, Zip 06492–0400; tel. 203/284–2801; Paul H. Johnson, President and Chief Executive Officer

HOSPITAL OF SAINT RAPHAEL, 1450 Chapel Street, New Haven, CT, Zip 06511–1450; tel. 203/789–3000; James J. Cullen, President

EASTERN CONNECTICUT HEALTH NETWORK 71 Haynes Street, Manchester, CT 06040; tel. 203/872–0501; Michael Gallacher, President

MANCHESTER MEMORIAL HOSPITAL, 71 Haynes Street, Manchester, CT, Zip 06040–4188; tel. 860/646–1222; Barry G. Beeman, Chief Executive Officer

ROCKVILLE GENERAL HOSPITAL, 31 Union Street, Vernon Rockville, CT, Zip 06066–3160; tel. 860/872–0501; Barry G. Beeman, Chief Executive Officer

SAINT FRANCIS PHYSICIAN HOSPITAL ORGANIZATION 1000 Asylum Avenue – Suite 3214, Hartford, CT 06105–1299; tel. 860/714–5606; Jess Kupec, PHO President

SAINT FRANCIS HOSPITAL AND MEDICAL CENTER, 114 Woodland Street, Hartford, CT, Zip 06105–1299; tel. 860/714–4000; David D'Eramo, President and Chief Executive Officer

SAINT MARY'S HOSPITAL 56 Franklin Street, Waterbury, CT 06706; tel. 203/574–6000; Jack Dobbins, Executive Vice President

ST. MARY'S HOSPITAL, 56 Franklin Street, Waterbury, CT, Zip 06706–1200; tel. 203/574–6000; Sister Marguerite Waite, President and Chief Executive Officer

DELAWARE

MEDICAL CENTER OF DELAWARE FOUNDATION P.O. Box 1668, Wilmington, DE 19899; tel. 302/733–1321; James F. Caldas, Executive Vice President

MEDICAL CENTER OF DELAWARE, 501 West 14th Street, Wilmington, DE, Zip 19801, Mailing Address: P.O. Box 1668, Zip 19899–1668; tel. 302/733–1000; Charles M. Smith, M.D., President and Chief Executive Officer

NANTICOKE HEALTH SERVICES 801 Middleford Road, Seaford, DE 19973; tel. 302/629–6611; Edward H. Hancock, President

NANTICOKE MEMORIAL HOSPITAL, 801 Middleford Road, Seaford, DE, Zip 19973–3698; tel. 302/629–6611; Edward H. Hancock, President

DISTRICT OF COLUMBIA

MEDLANTIC HEALTHCARE GROUP 100 Irving Street, NorthWest, Washington, DC 20010; tel. 202/877–7800; Ken Samet, President

NATIONAL REHABILITATION HOSPITAL, 102 Irving Street N.W., Washington, DC, Zip 20010–2949; tel. 202/877–1000; Edward A. Eckenhoff, President and Chief Executive Officer

WASHINGTON HOSPITAL CENTER, 110 Irving Street N.W., Washington, DC, Zip 20010–2975; tel. 202/877–7000; Kenneth A. Samet, President

FLORIDA

ADVENTIST HEALTH SYSTEM 111 North Orlando Avenue, Winter Park, FL 32789–3675; tel. 407/647–4400; Mardian J. Blair, President

EAST PASCO MEDICAL CENTER, 7050 Gall
Boulevard, Zephyrhills, FL, Zip 33541–1399;
tel. 813/788–0411; Bob A. Dodd, President

FLORIDA HOSPITAL, 601 East Rollins Street, Orlando,
FL, Zip 32803–1489; tel. 407/896–6611;
Thomas L. Werner, President

FLORIDA HOSPITAL WATERMAN, 201 North Eustis
Street, Eustis, FL, Zip 32726, Mailing Address:
P.O. Box B, Zip 32727–0377;
tel. 352/589–3333; Royce C. Thompson,
President

FLORIDA HOSPITAL–WALKER, 2501 U.S. Highway 27
North, Avon Park, FL, Zip 33825–1200, Mailing
Address: P.O. Box 1200, Zip 33826–1200;
tel. 941/453–7511; Samuel Leonor, President

ALLEGANY HEALTH SYSTEM
**6200 Courtney Campbell Causeway, Tampa,
FL 33607–1458; tel. 813/281–9098; Debbie
Coakley, Network Contact**

ST. ANTHONY'S HOSPITAL, 1200 Seventh Avenue
North, Saint Petersburg, FL, Zip 33705, Mailing
Address: P.O. Box 12588, Zip 33733;
tel. 813/825–1100; Revonda L. Shumaker,
R.N., President

ST. JOSEPH'S HOSPITAL, 3001 West Martin Luther
King Boulevard, Tampa, FL, Zip 33607–6387,
Mailing Address: P.O. Box 4227,
Zip 33677–4227; tel. 813/870–4000; Charles
Francis Scott, President

ST. MARY'S HOSPITAL, 901 45th Street, West Palm
Beach, FL, Zip 33407–2495, Mailing Address:
P.O. Box 24620, Zip 33416–4620;
tel. 561/844–6300; Phillip C. Dutcher, Interim
President and Chief Executive Officer

BAPTIST HEALTH CARE, INC.
**1000 West Moreno, Pensacola, FL 32501;
tel. 904/434–4011; Alfred G. Stubblefield,
Executive Vice President**

BAPTIST HOSPITAL, 1000 West Moreno, Pensacola,
FL, Zip 32501–2393, Mailing Address: P.O. Box
17500, Zip 32522–7500; tel. 904/469–2313;
Quinton Studer, President

GULF BREEZE HOSPITAL, 1110 Gulf Breeze Parkway,
Gulf Breeze, FL, Zip 32561–1110, Mailing
Address: P.O. Box 159, Zip 32562–0159;
tel. 904/934–2000; Richard C. Fulford,
Administrator

JAY HOSPITAL, 221 South Alabama Street, Jay, FL,
Zip 32565, Mailing Address: P.O. Box 397,
Zip 32565; tel. 904/675–8000; H. D.
Cannington, Administrator

MIZELL MEMORIAL HOSPITAL, 702 Main Street, Opp,
AL, Zip 36467–1626, Mailing Address: P.O. Box
1010, Zip 36467–1010; tel. 334/493–3541;
Allen Foster, Administrator

BAPTIST/ST. VINCENT'S HEALTH SYSTEM
**1301 Riverplace Boulevard, Jacksonville, FL
32207; tel. 904/202–4000; William C. Mason,
Chief Executive Officer**

BAPTIST MEDICAL CENTER, 800 Prudential Drive,
Jacksonville, FL, Zip 32207–8203;
tel. 904/202–2000; William C. Mason, Chief
Executive Officer

BAPTIST MEDICAL CENTER–BEACHES, 1350 13th
Avenue South, Jacksonville Beach, FL,
Zip 32250–3205; tel. 904/247–2900; Jerry L.
Miller, Administrator

BAPTIST MEDICAL CENTER–NASSAU, 1250 South
18th Street, Fernandina Beach, FL, Zip 32034;
tel. 904/321–3501; Jim L. Mayo, Administrator

ST. VINCENT'S MEDICAL CENTER, 1800 Barrs Street,
Jacksonville, FL, Zip 32204, Mailing Address:
P.O. Box 2982, Zip 32203–2982;
tel. 904/308–7300; John W. Logue, Executive
Vice President and Chief Operating Officer

BAYCARE HEALTH NETWORK, INC.
**17757 U.S. Highway 19 North, Suite 100,
Clearwater, FL 34624; tel. 813/535–3335;
John K. Vretas, President & Chief Executive
Officer**

ALL CHILDREN'S HOSPITAL, 801 Sixth Street South,
Saint Petersburg, FL, Zip 33701–4899;
tel. 813/898–7451; J. Dennis Sexton, President

BAYFRONT MEDICAL CENTER, 701 Sixth Street
South, Saint Petersburg, FL, Zip 33701–4891;
tel. 813/823–1234; Sue G. Brody, President

BROOKSVILLE REGIONAL HOSPITAL, 55 Ponce De
Leon Boulevard, Brooksville, FL,
Zip 34601–0037, Mailing Address: Box 37,
Zip 34605–0037; tel. 352/796–5111; Robert
Foreman, Associate Administrator

EAST PASCO MEDICAL CENTER, 7050 Gall
Boulevard, Zephyrhills, FL, Zip 33541–1399;
tel. 813/788–0411; Bob A. Dodd, President

MANATEE MEMORIAL HOSPITAL, 206 Second Street
East, Bradenton, FL, Zip 34208;
tel. 941/745–7373; Michael Marquez, Chief
Executive Officer

MEASE COUNTRYSIDE HOSPITAL, 3231
McMullen–Booth Road, Safety Harbor, FL,
Zip 34695–1098, Mailing Address: P.O. 1098,
Zip 34695–1098; tel. 813/725–6111; James A.
Pfeiffer, Chief Administrative Officer

MEASE HOSPITAL DUNEDIN, 601 Main Street,
Dunedin, FL, Zip 34698, Mailing Address: P.O.
Box 760, Zip 34697–0760; tel. 813/733–1111;
Philip K. Beauchamp, FACHE, President and
Chief Executive Officer

MORTON PLANT HOSPITAL, 323 Jeffords Street,
Clearwater, FL, Zip 34616–3892, Mailing
Address: Box 210, Zip 34617–0210;
tel. 813/462–7000; Frank V. Murphy, III,
President and Chief Executive Officer

NORTH BAY MEDICAL CENTER, 6600 Madison Street,
New Port Richey, FL, Zip 34652;
tel. 813/842–8468; Dennis A. Taylor,
Administrator

SOUTH FLORIDA BAPTIST HOSPITAL, 301 North
Alexander Street, Plant City, FL,
Zip 33566–9058, Mailing Address: Drawer H,
Zip 33564–9058; tel. 813/757–1200; William
H. Anderson, Administrator and Chief Executive
Officer

SPRING HILL REGIONAL HOSPITAL, 10461 Quality
Drive, Spring Hill, FL, Zip 34609;
tel. 904/688–3053; Sonia I. Gonzalez, R.N.,
Chief Operating Officer

ST. ANTHONY'S HOSPITAL, 1200 Seventh Avenue
North, Saint Petersburg, FL, Zip 33705, Mailing
Address: P.O. Box 12588, Zip 33733;
tel. 813/825–1100; Revonda L. Shumaker,
R.N., President

ST. JOSEPH'S HOSPITAL, 3001 West Martin Luther
King Boulevard, Tampa, FL, Zip 33607–6387,
Mailing Address: P.O. Box 4227,
Zip 33677–4227; tel. 813/870–4000; Charles
Francis Scott, President

UNIVERSITY COMMUNITY HOSPITAL, 3100 East
Fletcher Avenue, Tampa, FL, Zip 33613–4688;
tel. 813/971–6000; Norman V. Stein, President

UNIVERSITY COMMUNITY HOSPITAL–CARROLLWOOD,
7171 North Dale Mabry Highway, Tampa, FL,
Zip 33614–2699; tel. 813/558–8001; Larry J.
Archbell, Vice President Operations

COLUMBIA/HCA CENTRAL FLORIDA DIVISION
**2111 Glenwood Drive, Suite 100, Winter Park,
FL 32792–3309; tel. 407/646–7505; Joseph
R. Swedish, President**

COLUMBIA LAWNWOOD REGIONAL MEDICAL CENTER,
1700 South 23rd Street, Fort Pierce, FL,
Zip 34950–0188; tel. 561/461–4000; Gary
Cantrell, President and Chief Executive Officer

COLUMBIA MEDICAL CENTER SANFORD, 1401 West
Seminole Boulevard, Sanford, FL,
Zip 32771–6764; tel. 407/321–4500; Doug
Sills, President and Chief Executive Officer

COLUMBIA MEDICAL CENTER–DAYTONA, 400 North
Clyde Morris Boulevard, Daytona Beach, FL,
Zip 32114, Mailing Address: Box 9000,
Zip 32120; tel. 904/239–5000; Thomas R.
Pentz, Chief Executive Officer

COLUMBIA MEDICAL CENTER–OSCEOLA, 700 West
Oak Street, Kissimmee, FL, Zip 34741, Mailing
Address: P.O. Box 422589, Zip 34742–2589;
tel. 407/846–2266; E. Tim Cook, Chief
Executive Officer

COLUMBIA MEDICAL CENTER–PORT ST. LUCIE, 1800
S.E. Tiffany Avenue, Port St. Lucie, FL,
Zip 34952–7580; tel. 407/335–4000; Michael
P. Joyce, President and Chief Executive Officer

COLUMBIA PARK MEDICAL CENTER, 818 South Main
Lane, Orlando, FL, Zip 32801;
tel. 407/649–6111; Rick O'Connell, Chief
Executive Officer

COLUMBIA RAULERSON HOSPITAL, 1796 Highway
441 North, Okeechobee, FL, Zip 34972, Mailing
Address: Box 1307, Zip 34973–1307;
tel. 941/763–2151; Frank Irby, Chief Executive
Officer

SOUTH SEMINOLE HOSPITAL, 555 West State Road
434, Longwood, FL, Zip 32750;
tel. 407/767–1200; Sue Whelan–Williams, Site
Administrator

WINTER PARK MEMORIAL HOSPITAL, 200 North
Lakemont Avenue, Winter Park, FL,
Zip 32792–3273; tel. 407/646–7000; Douglas
P. DeGraaf, Chief Executive Officer

**COLUMBIA/HCA NORTH & NORTHEAST FLORIDA
DIVISION**
**3627 University Boulevard South, Suite 800,
Jacksonville, FL 32216; tel. 904/399–6695;
Charles Evans, President**

COLUMBIA FORT WALTON BEACH MEDICAL CENTER,
1000 Mar–Walt Drive, Fort Walton Beach, FL,
Zip 32547–6708; tel. 904/862–1111; Wayne
Campbell, Chief Executive Officer

COLUMBIA GULF COAST MEDICAL CENTER, 449
West 23rd Street, Panama City, FL, Zip 32405,
Mailing Address: P.O. Box 15309,
Zip 32406–5309; tel. 904/769–8341; Donald
E. Butts, Chief Executive Officer

COLUMBIA HAMILTON MEDICAL CENTER, 506 N.W.
Fourth Street, Jasper, FL, Zip 32052;
tel. 904/792–7200; Amelia Tuten, R.N.,
Administrator

COLUMBIA LAKE CITY MEDICAL CENTER, 1701 West
U.S. Highway 90, Lake City, FL, Zip 32055;
tel. 904/752–2922; David P. Steitz, Chief
Executive Officer

COLUMBIA MEMORIAL HOSPITAL JACKSONVILLE,
3625 University Boulevard South, Jacksonville,
FL, Zip 32216, Mailing Address: Box 16325,
Zip 32216; tel. 904/399–6111; Winston
Rushing, President

COLUMBIA NORTH FLORIDA REGIONAL MEDICAL
CENTER, 6500 Newberry Road, Gainesville, FL,
Zip 32605–4392, Mailing Address: P.O. Box
147006, Zip 32614–7006; tel. 352/333–4000;
Brian C. Robinson, Chief Executive Officer

COLUMBIA OCALA REGIONAL MEDICAL CENTER,
1431 S.W. First Avenue, Ocala, FL, Zip 34474,
Mailing Address: Box 2200, Zip 34478–2200;
tel. 352/401–1000; Terry Upton, Chief
Executive Officer

COLUMBIA ORANGE PARK MEDICAL CENTER, 2001
Kingsley Avenue, Orange Park, FL,
Zip 32073–5156; tel. 904/276–8500; Robert
M. Krieger, Chief Executive Officer

COLUMBIA PUTNAM MEDICAL CENTER, Highway 20
West, Palatka, FL, Zip 32177, Mailing Address:
P.O. Box 778, Zip 32178–0778;
tel. 904/328–5711; David Whalen, President
and Chief Executive Officer

COLUMBIA SPECIALTY HOSPITAL JACKSONVILLE,
4901 Richard Street, Jacksonville, FL,
Zip 32207; tel. 904/737–3120; W. Raymond C.
Ford, Administrator and Chief Executive Officer

COLUMBIA TALLAHASSEE COMMUNITY HOSPITAL,
2626 Capital Medical Boulevard, Tallahassee,
FL, Zip 32308; tel. 904/656–5000; Gary L.
Brewer, Chief Executive Officer

COLUMBIA TWIN CITIES HOSPITAL, 2190 Highway 85
North, Niceville, FL, Zip 32578;
tel. 904/678–4131; David Whalen, Chief
Executive Officer

COLUMBIA WEST FLORIDA REGIONAL MEDICAL
CENTER, 8383 North Davis Highway, Pensacola,
FL, Zip 32514, Mailing Address: P.O. Box
18900, Zip 32523–8900; tel. 904/494–4000;
Stephen Brandt, Chief Executive Officer

NORTH OKALOOSA MEDICAL CENTER, 151 Redstone
Avenue S.E., Crestview, FL, Zip 32539–6026;
tel. 904/689–8100; Roger L. Hall, Chief
Executive Officer

SANTA ROSA MEDICAL CENTER, 1450 Berryhill Road,
Milton, FL, Zip 32570, Mailing Address: P.O. Box
648, Zip 32572; tel. 904/626–7762; Barbara
H. Thames, Chief Executive Officer

COLUMBIA/HCA SOUTH FLORIDA DIVISION
7975 NorthWest 154th Street, Suite 400A, Miami Lakes, FL 33016; tel. 305/364–1202; Chuck Hall, President

COLUMBIA AVENTURA HOSPITAL AND MEDICAL CENTER, 20900 Biscayne Boulevard, Miami, FL, Zip 33180–1407; tel. 305/682–7100; Davide M. Carbone, Chief Executive Officer

COLUMBIA CEDARS MEDICAL CENTER, 1400 N.W. 12th Avenue, Miami, FL, Zip 33136–1003; tel. 305/325–5511; Ralph A. Aleman, Chief Executive Officer

COLUMBIA DEERING HOSPITAL, 9333 S.W. 152nd Street, Miami, FL, Zip 33157; tel. 305/256–5100; Anthony M. Degina, Jr., Chief Executive Officer

COLUMBIA KENDALL MEDICAL CENTER, 11750 Bird Road, Miami, FL, Zip 33175–3530; tel. 305/223–3000; Victor Maya, Chief Executive Officer

COLUMBIA NORTHWEST MEDICAL CENTER, 2801 North State Road 7, Margate, FL, Zip 33063, Mailing Address: P.O. Box 639002, Zip 33063–9002; tel. 305/978–4000; Gina Becker, Acting Chief Executive Officer

COLUMBIA PALMS WEST HOSPITAL, 13001 Southern Boulevard, Loxahatchee, FL, Zip 33470–1150; tel. 407/798–3300; Alex M. Marceline, Chief Executive Officer

COLUMBIA PLANTATION GENERAL HOSPITAL, 401 N.W. 42nd Avenue, Plantation, FL, Zip 33317–2882; tel. 954/587–5010; Anthony M. Degina, Jr., Chief Executive Officer

COLUMBIA POMPANO BEACH MEDICAL CENTER, 600 S.W. Third Street, Pompano Beach, FL, Zip 33060–6979; tel. 954/782–2000; Heather J. Rohan, Chief Executive Officer

COLUMBIA UNIVERSITY HOSPITAL AND MEDICAL CENTER, 7201 North University Drive, Tamarac, FL, Zip 33321; tel. 305/721–2200; James A. Cruickshank, Chief Executive Officer

COLUMBIA WESTSIDE REGIONAL MEDICAL CENTER, 8201 West Broward Boulevard, Plantation, FL, Zip 33324–9937; tel. 954/473–6600; Michael G. Joseph, Chief Executive Officer

MEMORIAL HOSPITAL PEMBROKE, 2301 University Drive, Pembroke Pines, FL, Zip 33024; tel. 954/962–9650; J. E. Piriz, Administrator

MIAMI HEART INSTITUTE, 4701 Meridian Avenue, Miami, FL, Zip 33140–2910; tel. 305/674–3114; Tim Parker, Chief Executive Officer

COLUMBIA/HCA SOUTHWEST FLORIDA DIVISION
2000 Main Street, Suite 600, Fort Myers, FL 33901; tel. 305/364–1202; Charles Hall, President

COLUMBIA DOCTORS HOSPITAL OF SARASOTA, 5731 Bee Ridge Road, Sarasota, FL, Zip 34233; tel. 941/342–1100; William C. Lievense, President and Chief Executive Officer

COLUMBIA EAST POINTE HOSPITAL, 1500 Lee Boulevard, Lehigh Acres, FL, Zip 33936; tel. 941/369–2101; Valerie A. Jackson, Chief Executive Officer

COLUMBIA ENGLEWOOD COMMUNITY HOSPITAL, 700 Medical Boulevard, Englewood, FL, Zip 34223; tel. 941/475–6571; Terry L. Moore, Chief Executive Officer

COLUMBIA FAWCETT MEMORIAL HOSPITAL, 21298 Olean Boulevard, Port Charlotte, FL, Zip 33952–6765, Mailing Address: P.O. Box 4028, Punta Gorda, Zip 33949–4028; tel. 941/629–1181; Steve Dobbs, Chief Executive Officer

COLUMBIA GULF COAST HOSPITAL, 13681 Doctors Way, Fort Myers, FL, Zip 33912; tel. 941/768–5000; Valerie A. Jackson, Chief Executive Officer

COLUMBIA REGIONAL MEDICAL CENTER OF SOUTHWEST FLORIDA, 2727 Winkler Avenue, Fort Myers, FL, Zip 33901–9396; tel. 941/939–1147; Nick Carbone, Chief Executive Officer

COLUMBIA/HCA TAMPA BAY DIVISION
6200 Courtney Campbell Causeway, Tampa, FL 33607; tel. 813/286–6000; William Hussey, President

COLUMBIA BLAKE MEDICAL CENTER, 2020 59th Street West, Bradenton, FL, Zip 34209, Mailing Address: P.O. Box 25004, Zip 34206–5004; tel. 941/792–6611; Lindell W. Orr, Chief Executive Officer

COLUMBIA BRANDON REGIONAL MEDICAL CENTER, 119 Oakfield Drive, Brandon, FL, Zip 33511–5799; tel. 813/681–5551; H. Rex Etheredge, President and Chief Executive Officer

COLUMBIA CLEARWATER COMMUNITY HOSPITAL, 1521 Druid Road East, Clearwater, FL, Zip 34616–6193, Mailing Address: P.O. Box 9068, Zip 34618–9068; tel. 813/447–4571; Thomas L. Herron, FACHE, Chief Executive Officer

COLUMBIA DADE CITY HOSPITAL, 13100 Fort King Road, Dade City, FL, Zip 33525–5294; tel. 904/521–1100; Robert Meade, Chief Executive Officer

COLUMBIA EDWARD WHITE HOSPITAL, 2323 Ninth Avenue North, Saint Petersburg, FL, Zip 33713, Mailing Address: P.O. Box 12018, Zip 33733–2018; tel. 813/323–1111; Barry S. Stokes, Chief Executive Officer

COLUMBIA LARGO MEDICAL CENTER, 201 14th Street S.W., Largo, FL, Zip 33770, Mailing Address: P.O. Box 2905, Zip 33779; tel. 813/586–1411; Thomas L. Herron, FACHE, President and Chief Executive Officer

COLUMBIA NEW PORT RICHEY HOSPITAL, 5637 Marine Parkway, New Port Richey, FL, Zip 34652, Mailing Address: Box 996, Zip 34656–0996; tel. 813/848–1733; Andrew Oravec, Jr., Administrator

COLUMBIA NORTHSIDE MEDICAL CENTER, 6000 49th Street North, Saint Petersburg, FL, Zip 33709; tel. 813/521–4411; Bradley K. Grover, Sr., Chief Executive Officer

COLUMBIA REGIONAL MEDICAL CENTER, 11375 Cortez Boulevard, Spring Hill, FL, Zip 34613, Mailing Address: P.O. Box 5300, Zip 34606; tel. 904/596–6632; John R. Finnegan, Administrator and Chief Operating Officer

COLUMBIA REGIONAL MEDICAL CENTER AT BAYONET POINT, 14000 Fivay Road, Hudson, FL, Zip 34667–7199; tel. 813/863–2411; J. Daniel Miller, President and Chief Executive Officer

COLUMBIA SOUTH BAY HOSPITAL, 4016 State Road 674, Sun City Center, FL, Zip 33573–5298; tel. 813/634–3301; Marcia Easley, Chief Operating Officer

COLUMBIA ST. PETERSBURG MEDICAL CENTER, 6500 38th Avenue North, Saint Petersburg, FL, Zip 33710; tel. 813/384–1414; Bradley K. Grover, Sr., President and Chief Executive Officer

COMMUNITY HEALTH NETWORK OF INDIAN RIVER COUNTY
1000 36th Street, Vero Beach, FL 32960; tel. 561/567–4311; Gerard J. Koziel, Sr Vice President–Planning & Development

INDIAN RIVER MEMORIAL HOSPITAL, 1000 36th Street, Vero Beach, FL, Zip 32960–6592; tel. 407/567–4311; Michael J. O'Grady, Jr., President and Chief Executive Officer

COMMUNITY HEALTH NETWORK OF SOUTH FLORIDA
4725 North Federal Highway, Ft Lauderdale, FL 33308; tel. 305/771–8000; Raymond Budrys, President

BROWARD GENERAL MEDICAL CENTER, 1600 South Andrews Avenue, Fort Lauderdale, FL, Zip 33316–2510; tel. 954/355–4400; Ruth A. Eldridge, R.N., Regional Vice President, Administration

CORAL SPRINGS MEDICAL CENTER, 3000 Coral Hills Drive, Coral Springs, FL, Zip 33065; tel. 954/344–3000; A. Gary Muller, FACHE, Regional Vice President Administration

HOLY CROSS HOSPITAL, 4725 North Federal Highway, Fort Lauderdale, FL, Zip 33308, Mailing Address: Box 23460, Zip 33307; tel. 305/771–8000; Ray Budrys, President and Chief Executive Officer

IMPERIAL POINT MEDICAL CENTER, 6401 North Federal Highway, Fort Lauderdale, FL, Zip 33308–1495; tel. 954/776–8500; Dorothy J. Mancini, R.N., Regional Vice President Administration

MEMORIAL HOSPITAL WEST, 703 North Flamingo Road, Pembroke Pines, FL, Zip 33028; tel. 954/436–5000; Zeff Ross, Administrator

NORTH BROWARD MEDICAL CENTER, 201 Sample Road, Pompano Beach, FL, Zip 33064–3502; tel. 954/941–8300; James R. Chromik, Regional Vice President, Administration

DIMENSIONS HEALTH/BAPTIST HEALTH SYSTEMS
8900 North Kendall Drive, Miami, FL 33176; tel. 305/596–1960; Brian Keeley, President

BAPTIST HOSPITAL OF MIAMI, 8900 North Kendall Drive, Miami, FL, Zip 33176–2197; tel. 305/596–6503; Fred M. Messing, Chief Executive Officer

HOMESTEAD HOSPITAL, 160 N.W. 13th Street, Homestead, FL, Zip 33030–4299; tel. 305/248–3232; Bo Boulenger, Chief Executive Officer

MARINERS HOSPITAL, 50 High Point Road, Tavernier, FL, Zip 33070; tel. 305/852–4418; Robert H. Luse, Chief Executive Officer

SOUTH MIAMI HOSPITAL, 6200 S.W. 73rd Street, Miami, FL, Zip 33143–9990; tel. 305/661–4611; D. Wayne Brackin, Chief Executive Officer

FLORIDA HEALTH CHOICE
5300 West Atlantic Avenue, Suite 302, Del Ray Beach, FL 33486; tel. 407/496–0505; D. Nat West, President

BOCA RATON COMMUNITY HOSPITAL, 800 Meadows Road, Boca Raton, FL, Zip 33486–2368; tel. 561/395–7100; Randolph J. Pierce, President and Chief Executive Officer

FLORIDA HOSPITAL HEALTH NETWORK
601 East Rollins Street, Orlando, FL 32803; tel. 407/896–6611; Thomas L. Werner, President

FLORIDA HOSPITAL, 601 East Rollins Street, Orlando, FL, Zip 32803–1489; tel. 407/896–6611; Thomas L. Werner, President

FLORIDA HOSPITAL WATERMAN, 201 North Eustis Street, Eustis, FL, Zip 32726, Mailing Address: P.O. Box B, Zip 32727–0377; tel. 352/589–3333; Royce C. Thompson, President

GENESIS HEALTH, INC.
3627 University Boulevard South, Jacksonville, FL 32216; tel. 904/391–1201; Douglas Baer, Vice President

GENESIS REHABILITATION HOSPITAL, 3599 University Boulevard South, Jacksonville, FL, Zip 32216–4211, Mailing Address: P.O. Box 16406, Zip 32245–6406; tel. 904/858–7600; Stephen K. Wilson, President

LAKE OKEECHOBEE RURAL HEALTH NETWORK
1500 NorthWest Avenue L, Belle Glade, FL 33430; tel. 407/996–0216; Andrew Behrman, Chief Executive Officer

COLUMBIA J. F. K. MEDICAL CENTER, 5301 South Congress Avenue, Atlantis, FL, Zip 33462; tel. 561/965–7300; Phillip D. Robinson, Chief Executive Officer

GLADES GENERAL HOSPITAL, 1201 South Main Street, Belle Glade, FL, Zip 33430; tel. 561/996–6571; Michael G. Layfield, Chief Executive Officer

HENDRY REGIONAL MEDICAL CENTER, 500 West Sugarland Highway, Clewiston, FL, Zip 33440; tel. 941/983–9121; J. Rudy Reinhardt, Administrator

MARTIN MEMORIAL HEALTH SYSTEM, 300 S.E. Hospital Drive, Stuart, FL, Zip 34994, Mailing Address: P.O. Box 9010, Zip 34995–9010; tel. 561/223–5945; Richmond M. Harman, President and Chief Executive Officer

MED CONNECT
4901 NorthWest 17th Way, Suite 304, Ft Lauderdale, FL 33309; tel. 305/938–9755; Bill Gil, Chief Executive Officer

COLUMBIA PALMS WEST HOSPITAL, 13001 Southern Boulevard, Loxahatchee, FL, Zip 33470–1150; tel. 407/798–3300; Alex M. Marceline, Chief Executive Officer

COLUMBIA PLANTATION GENERAL HOSPITAL, 401 N.W. 42nd Avenue, Plantation, FL, Zip 33317–2882; tel. 954/587–5010; Anthony M. Degina, Jr., Chief Executive Officer

FLORIDA MEDICAL CENTER HOSPITAL, 5000 West Oakland Park Boulevard, Fort Lauderdale, FL, Zip 33313–1585; tel. 305/735–6000; Denny De Narvaez, Chief Executive Officer

GOOD SAMARITAN MEDICAL CENTER, Flagler Drive at Palm Beach Lakes Boulevard, West Palm Beach, FL, Zip 33401; tel. 561/655–5511; Phillip C. Dutcher, Interim President

NORTH RIDGE MEDICAL CENTER, 5757 North Dixie Highway, Fort Lauderdale, FL, Zip 33334; tel. 305/776–6000; Emil P. Miller, Chief Executive Officer

PALM BEACH GARDENS MEDICAL CENTER, 3360 Burns Road, Palm Beach Gardens, FL, Zip 33410–4304; tel. 407/622–1411

ST. MARY'S HOSPITAL, 901 45th Street, West Palm Beach, FL, Zip 33407–2495, Mailing Address: P.O. Box 24620, Zip 33416–4620; tel. 561/844–6300; Phillip C. Dutcher, Interim President and Chief Executive Officer

MEMORIAL HEALTHCARE SYSTEM
3501 Johnson Street, Hollywood, FL 33021; tel. 954/967–2918; Paul Betz, Administrative Resident

MEMORIAL HOSPITAL PEMBROKE, 2301 University Drive, Pembroke Pines, FL, Zip 33024; tel. 954/962–9650; J. E. Piriz, Administrator

MEMORIAL HOSPITAL WEST, 703 North Flamingo Road, Pembroke Pines, FL, Zip 33028; tel. 954/436–5000; Zeff Ross, Administrator

MEMORIAL REGIONAL HOSPITAL, 3501 Johnson Street, Hollywood, FL, Zip 33021–5421; tel. 954/987–2000; Patricia A. Flury, Administrator

METHODIST HEALTH SYSTEMS
580 West Eighth Street, Jacksonville, FL 32209; tel. 904/798–8000; Marcus Drewa, President

METHODIST MEDICAL CENTER, 580 West Eighth Street, Jacksonville, FL, Zip 32209–6553; tel. 904/798–8000; Marcus E. Drewa, President

METHODIST PATHWAY CENTER, 580 West Eighth Street, Jacksonville, FL, Zip 32209–6553; tel. 904/798–8250; Marcus E. Drewa, President

MID–FLORIDA MEDICAL SERVICES, INC.
200 Avenue 'F', Northeast, Winter Haven, FL 33881; tel. 941/293–1121; Lance Anastasio, President

LAKE WALES MEDICAL CENTERS, 410 South 11th Street, Lake Wales, FL, Zip 33853, Mailing Address: P.O. Box 3460, Zip 33859–3460; tel. 941/676–1433; Joe M. Connell, Chief Executive Officer

WINTER HAVEN HOSPITAL, 200 Avenue F N.E., Winter Haven, FL, Zip 33881; tel. 941/297–1899; Lance W. Anastasio, President

MORTON PLANT MEASE HEALTH CARE
833 Milwaukee Avenue, Dunedin, FL 34698; tel. 813/734–6498; Ginger Lay, Director, Managed Care

MEASE COUNTRYSIDE HOSPITAL, 3231 McMullen–Booth Road, Safety Harbor, FL, Zip 34695–1098, Mailing Address: P.O. 1098, Zip 34695–1098; tel. 813/725–6111; James A. Pfeiffer, Chief Administrative Officer

MEASE HOSPITAL DUNEDIN, 601 Main Street, Dunedin, FL, Zip 34698, Mailing Address: P.O. Box 760, Zip 34697–0760; tel. 813/733–1111; Philip K. Beauchamp, FACHE, President and Chief Executive Officer

MORTON PLANT HOSPITAL, 323 Jeffords Street, Clearwater, FL, Zip 34616–3892, Mailing Address: Box 210, Zip 34617–0210; tel. 813/462–7000; Frank V. Murphy, III, President and Chief Executive Officer

ORLANDO REGIONAL HEALTHCARE SYSTEM
1414 Kuhl Avenue, Orlando, FL 32806; tel. 407/841–5111; Gary Strack, Chairman & Chief Executive Officer

ORLANDO REGIONAL MEDICAL CENTER, 1414 Kuhl Avenue, Orlando, FL, Zip 32806–2093; tel. 407/841–5111; John Hillenmeyer, President

SOUTH LAKE HOSPITAL, 847 Eighth Street, Clermont, FL, Zip 34711; tel. 352/394–4071; P. Shannon Elswick, Administrator and Chief Executive Officer

SOUTH SEMINOLE HOSPITAL, 555 West State Road 434, Longwood, FL, Zip 32750; tel. 407/767–1200; Sue Whelan–Williams, Site Administrator

ST. CLOUD HOSPITAL, A DIVISION OF ORLANDO REGIONAL HEALTHCARE SYSTEM, 2906 17th Street, Saint Cloud, FL, Zip 34769–6099; tel. 407/892–2135; Jim Norris, Executive Director

PANHANDLE AREA HEALTH NETWORK
Box 1608, Marianna, FL 32447; tel. 904/482–9254; Lucia Maxwell, Executive Director

CALHOUN–LIBERTY HOSPITAL, 424 Burns Avenue, Blountstown, FL, Zip 32424–1097; tel. 904/674–5411; Josh Plummer, Administrator

CAMPBELLTON GRACEVILLE HOSPITAL, 5429 College Drive, Graceville, FL, Zip 32440; tel. 904/263–4431; Neil Whipkey, Administrator

DOCTORS MEMORIAL HOSPITAL, 401 East Byrd Avenue, Bonifay, FL, Zip 32425, Mailing Address: Box 188, Zip 32425; tel. 904/547–1120; Dale Larson, Executive Director

JACKSON HOSPITAL, 4250 Hospital Drive, Marianna, FL, Zip 32446, Mailing Address: P.O. Box 1608, Zip 32447–1608; tel. 904/526–2200; Richard L. Wooten, Administrator

NORTHWEST FLORIDA COMMUNITY HOSPITAL, 1360 Brickyard Road, Chipley, FL, Zip 32428–5010, Mailing Address: P.O. Box 889, Zip 32428; tel. 904/638–1610; Stephen D. Mason, Administrator

TENET SOUTH FLORIDA HEALTH SYSTEM NETWORK
500 West Cypress Creek Road, Suite 370, Fort Lauderdale, FL 33309; tel. 954/351–7757; Don Steigman, Senior Vice President

DELRAY COMMUNITY HOSPITAL, 5352 Linton Boulevard, Delray Beach, FL, Zip 33484; tel. 407/498–4440; Mitchell S. Feldman, Chief Executive Officer

HIALEAH HOSPITAL, 651 East 25th Street, Hialeah, FL, Zip 33013–3878; tel. 305/693–6100; Clifford J. Bauer, Chief Executive Officer

HOLLYWOOD MEDICAL CENTER, 3600 Washington Street, Hollywood, FL, Zip 33021; tel. 954/966–4500; Holly Lerner, Chief Executive Officer

MEMORIAL HOSPITAL OF TAMPA, 2901 Swann Avenue, Tampa, FL, Zip 33609–4057; tel. 813/873–6400; Stephen Mahan, Chief Executive Officer

PALM BEACH GARDENS MEDICAL CENTER, 3360 Burns Road, Palm Beach Gardens, FL, Zip 33410–4304; tel. 407/622–1411

PALMETTO GENERAL HOSPITAL, 2001 West 68th Street, Hialeah, FL, Zip 33016; tel. 305/823–5000; John C. Johnson, Chief Executive Officer

PALMS OF PASADENA HOSPITAL, 1501 Pasadena Avenue South, Saint Petersburg, FL, Zip 33707; tel. 813/381–1000; John D. Bartlett, Chief Executive Officer

SHRINERS HOSPITALS FOR CHILDREN, TAMPA, 12502 North Pine Drive, Tampa, FL, Zip 33612–9499; tel. 813/972–2250; John Holtz, Administrator

TOWN AND COUNTRY HOSPITAL, 6001 Webb Road, Tampa, FL, Zip 33615–3291; tel. 813/885–6666; Stephen Mahan, Chief Executive Officer

WEST BOCA MEDICAL CENTER, 21644 State Road 7, Boca Raton, FL, Zip 33428–1899; tel. 407/488–8000; Richard Gold, Chief Executive Officer

THE HEALTH ADVANTAGE NETWORK
2111 Glenwood Drive, Suite 202, Winter Park, FL 32792; tel. 407/646–7800; Elizabeth Abely, Network Contact

COLUMBIA AVENTURA HOSPITAL AND MEDICAL CENTER, 20900 Biscayne Boulevard, Miami, FL, Zip 33180–1407; tel. 305/682–7100; Davide M. Carbone, Chief Executive Officer

COLUMBIA BLAKE MEDICAL CENTER, 2020 59th Street West, Bradenton, FL, Zip 34209, Mailing Address: P.O. Box 25004, Zip 34206–5004; tel. 941/792–6611; Lindell W. Orr, Chief Executive Officer

COLUMBIA BRANDON REGIONAL MEDICAL CENTER, 119 Oakfield Drive, Brandon, FL, Zip 33511–5799; tel. 813/681–5551; H. Rex Etheredge, President and Chief Executive Officer

COLUMBIA CEDARS MEDICAL CENTER, 1400 N.W. 12th Avenue, Miami, FL, Zip 33136–1003; tel. 305/325–5511; Ralph A. Aleman, Chief Executive Officer

COLUMBIA CLEARWATER COMMUNITY HOSPITAL, 1521 Druid Road East, Clearwater, FL, Zip 34616–6193, Mailing Address: P.O. Box 9068, Zip 34618–9068; tel. 813/447–4571; Thomas L. Herron, FACHE, Chief Executive Officer

COLUMBIA DADE CITY HOSPITAL, 13100 Fort King Road, Dade City, FL, Zip 33525–5294; tel. 904/521–1100; Robert Meade, Chief Executive Officer

COLUMBIA DEERING HOSPITAL, 9333 S.W. 152nd Street, Miami, FL, Zip 33157; tel. 305/256–5100; Anthony M. Degina, Jr., Chief Executive Officer

COLUMBIA DOCTORS HOSPITAL OF SARASOTA, 5731 Bee Ridge Road, Sarasota, FL, Zip 34233; tel. 941/342–1100; William C. Lievense, President and Chief Executive Officer

COLUMBIA EAST POINTE HOSPITAL, 1500 Lee Boulevard, Lehigh Acres, FL, Zip 33936; tel. 941/369–2101; Valerie A. Jackson, Chief Executive Officer

COLUMBIA EDWARD WHITE HOSPITAL, 2323 Ninth Avenue North, Saint Petersburg, FL, Zip 33713, Mailing Address: P.O. Box 12018, Zip 33733–2018; tel. 813/323–1111; Barry S. Stokes, Chief Executive Officer

COLUMBIA ENGLEWOOD COMMUNITY HOSPITAL, 700 Medical Boulevard, Englewood, FL, Zip 34223; tel. 941/475–6571; Terry L. Moore, Chief Executive Officer

COLUMBIA FAWCETT MEMORIAL HOSPITAL, 21298 Olean Boulevard, Port Charlotte, FL, Zip 33952–6765, Mailing Address: P.O. Box 4028, Punta Gorda, Zip 33949–4028; tel. 941/629–1181; Steve Dobbs, Chief Executive Officer

COLUMBIA FORT WALTON BEACH MEDICAL CENTER, 1000 Mar–Walt Drive, Fort Walton Beach, FL, Zip 32547–6708; tel. 904/862–1111; Wayne Campbell, Chief Executive Officer

COLUMBIA GULF COAST HOSPITAL, 13681 Doctors Way, Fort Myers, FL, Zip 33912; tel. 941/768–5000; Valerie A. Jackson, Chief Executive Officer

COLUMBIA GULF COAST MEDICAL CENTER, 449 West 23rd Street, Panama City, FL, Zip 32405, Mailing Address: P.O. Box 15309, Zip 32406–5309; tel. 904/769–8341; Donald E. Butts, Chief Executive Officer

COLUMBIA HAMILTON MEDICAL CENTER, 506 N.W. Fourth Street, Jasper, FL, Zip 32052; tel. 904/792–7200; Amelia Tuten, R.N., Administrator

COLUMBIA KENDALL MEDICAL CENTER, 11750 Bird Road, Miami, FL, Zip 33175–3530; tel. 305/223–3000; Victor Maya, Chief Executive Officer

COLUMBIA LAKE CITY MEDICAL CENTER, 1701 West U.S. Highway 90, Lake City, FL, Zip 32055; tel. 904/752–2922; David P. Steitz, Chief Executive Officer

COLUMBIA LARGO MEDICAL CENTER, 201 14th Street S.W., Largo, FL, Zip 33770, Mailing Address: P.O. Box 2905, Zip 33779; tel. 813/586–1411; Thomas L. Herron, FACHE, President and Chief Executive Officer

COLUMBIA LAWNWOOD REGIONAL MEDICAL CENTER, 1700 South 23rd Street, Fort Pierce, FL, Zip 34950–0188; tel. 561/461–4000; Gary Cantrell, President and Chief Executive Officer

COLUMBIA MEDICAL CENTER SANFORD, 1401 West Seminole Boulevard, Sanford, FL, Zip 32771–6764; tel. 407/321–4500; Doug Sills, President and Chief Executive Officer

COLUMBIA MEDICAL CENTER–DAYTONA, 400 North Clyde Morris Boulevard, Daytona Beach, FL, Zip 32114, Mailing Address: Box 9000, Zip 32120; tel. 904/239–5000; Thomas R. Pentz, Chief Executive Officer

COLUMBIA MEDICAL CENTER–OSCEOLA, 700 West Oak Street, Kissimmee, FL, Zip 34741, Mailing Address: P.O. Box 422589, Zip 34742–2589; tel. 407/846–2266; E. Tim Cook, Chief Executive Officer

COLUMBIA MEDICAL CENTER–PORT ST. LUCIE, 1800 S.E. Tiffany Avenue, Port St. Lucie, FL, Zip 34952–7580; tel. 407/335–4000; Michael P. Joyce, President and Chief Executive Officer

COLUMBIA MEMORIAL HOSPITAL JACKSONVILLE, 3625 University Boulevard South, Jacksonville, FL, Zip 32216, Mailing Address: Box 16325, Zip 32216; tel. 904/399–6111; Winston Rushing, President

COLUMBIA NEW PORT RICHEY HOSPITAL, 5637 Marine Parkway, New Port Richey, FL, Zip 34652, Mailing Address: Box 996, Zip 34656–0996; tel. 813/848–1733; Andrew Oravec, Jr., Administrator

COLUMBIA NORTH FLORIDA REGIONAL MEDICAL CENTER, 6500 Newberry Road, Gainesville, FL, Zip 32605–4392, Mailing Address: P.O. Box 147006, Zip 32614–7006; tel. 352/333–4000; Brian C. Robinson, Chief Executive Officer

COLUMBIA NORTHSIDE MEDICAL CENTER, 6000 49th Street North, Saint Petersburg, FL, Zip 33709; tel. 813/521–4411; Bradley K. Grover, Sr., Chief Executive Officer

COLUMBIA NORTHWEST MEDICAL CENTER, 2801 North State Road 7, Margate, FL, Zip 33063, Mailing Address: P.O. Box 639002, Zip 33063–9002; tel. 305/978–4000; Gina Becker, Acting Chief Executive Officer

COLUMBIA OCALA REGIONAL MEDICAL CENTER, 1431 S.W. First Avenue, Ocala, FL, Zip 34474, Mailing Address: Box 2200, Zip 34478–2200; tel. 352/401–1000; Terry Upton, Chief Executive Officer

COLUMBIA ORANGE PARK MEDICAL CENTER, 2001 Kingsley Avenue, Orange Park, FL, Zip 32073–5156; tel. 904/276–8500; Robert M. Krieger, Chief Executive Officer

COLUMBIA PALMS WEST HOSPITAL, 13001 Southern Boulevard, Loxahatchee, FL, Zip 33470–1150; tel. 407/798–3300; Alex M. Marceline, Chief Executive Officer

COLUMBIA PARK MEDICAL CENTER, 818 South Main Lane, Orlando, FL, Zip 32801; tel. 407/649–6111; Rick O'Connell, Chief Executive Officer

COLUMBIA PLANTATION GENERAL HOSPITAL, 401 N.W. 42nd Avenue, Plantation, FL, Zip 33317–2882; tel. 954/587–5010; Anthony M. Degina, Jr., Chief Executive Officer

COLUMBIA POMPANO BEACH MEDICAL CENTER, 600 S.W. Third Street, Pompano Beach, FL, Zip 33060–6979; tel. 954/782–2000; Heather J. Rohan, Chief Executive Officer

COLUMBIA PUTNAM MEDICAL CENTER, Highway 20 West, Palatka, FL, Zip 32177, Mailing Address: P.O. Box 778, Zip 32178–0778; tel. 904/328–5711; David Whalen, President and Chief Executive Officer

COLUMBIA RAULERSON HOSPITAL, 1796 Highway 441 North, Okeechobee, FL, Zip 34972, Mailing Address: Box 1307, Zip 34973–1307; tel. 941/763–2151; Frank Irby, Chief Executive Officer

COLUMBIA REGIONAL MEDICAL CENTER, 11375 Cortez Boulevard, Spring Hill, FL, Zip 34613, Mailing Address: P.O. Box 5300, Zip 34606; tel. 904/596–6632; John R. Finnegan, Administrator and Chief Operating Officer

COLUMBIA REGIONAL MEDICAL CENTER AT BAYONET POINT, 14000 Fivay Road, Hudson, FL, Zip 34667–7199; tel. 813/863–2411; J. Daniel Miller, President and Chief Executive Officer

COLUMBIA REGIONAL MEDICAL CENTER OF SOUTHWEST FLORIDA, 2727 Winkler Avenue, Fort Myers, FL, Zip 33901–9396; tel. 941/939–1147; Nick Carbone, Chief Executive Officer

COLUMBIA SOUTH BAY HOSPITAL, 4016 State Road 674, Sun City Center, FL, Zip 33573–5298; tel. 813/634–3301; Marcia Easley, Chief Operating Officer

COLUMBIA SPECIALTY HOSPITAL JACKSONVILLE, 4901 Richard Street, Jacksonville, FL, Zip 32207; tel. 904/737–3120; W. Raymond C. Ford, Administrator and Chief Executive Officer

COLUMBIA ST. PETERSBURG MEDICAL CENTER, 6500 38th Avenue North, Saint Petersburg, FL, Zip 33710; tel. 813/384–1414; Bradley K. Grover, Sr., President and Chief Executive Officer

COLUMBIA TALLAHASSEE COMMUNITY HOSPITAL, 2626 Capital Medical Boulevard, Tallahassee, FL, Zip 32308; tel. 904/656–5000; Gary L. Brewer, Chief Executive Officer

COLUMBIA TWIN CITIES HOSPITAL, 2190 Highway 85 North, Niceville, FL, Zip 32578; tel. 904/678–4131; David Whalen, Chief Executive Officer

COLUMBIA UNIVERSITY HOSPITAL AND MEDICAL CENTER, 7201 North University Drive, Tamarac, FL, Zip 33321; tel. 305/721–2200; James A. Cruickshank, Chief Executive Officer

COLUMBIA WEST FLORIDA REGIONAL MEDICAL CENTER, 8383 North Davis Highway, Pensacola, FL, Zip 32514, Mailing Address: P.O. Box 18900, Zip 32523–8900; tel. 904/494–4000; Stephen Brandt, Chief Executive Officer

COLUMBIA WESTSIDE REGIONAL MEDICAL CENTER, 8201 West Broward Boulevard, Plantation, FL, Zip 33324–9937; tel. 954/473–6600; Michael G. Joseph, Chief Executive Officer

MEMORIAL HOSPITAL PEMBROKE, 2301 University Drive, Pembroke Pines, FL, Zip 33024; tel. 954/962–9650; J. E. Piriz, Administrator

MIAMI HEART INSTITUTE, 4701 Meridian Avenue, Miami, FL, Zip 33140–2910; tel. 305/674–3114; Tim Parker, Chief Executive Officer

NORTH OKALOOSA MEDICAL CENTER, 151 Redstone Avenue S.E., Crestview, FL, Zip 32539–6026; tel. 904/689–8100; Roger L. Hall, Chief Executive Officer

SANTA ROSA MEDICAL CENTER, 1450 Berryhill Road, Milton, FL, Zip 32570, Mailing Address: P.O. Box 648, Zip 32572; tel. 904/626–7762; Barbara H. Thames, Chief Executive Officer

SOUTH SEMINOLE HOSPITAL, 555 West State Road 434, Longwood, FL, Zip 32750; tel. 407/767–1200; Sue Whelan–Williams, Site Administrator

WINTER PARK MEMORIAL HOSPITAL, 200 North Lakemont Avenue, Winter Park, FL, Zip 32792–3273; tel. 407/646–7000; Douglas P. DeGraaf, Chief Executive Officer

GEORGIA

CANDLER HEALTH SYSTEM
5353 Reynolds Street, Savannah, GA 31412; tel. 912/692–2018; Thomas E. Hassett, Chief Executive Officer

APPLING HEALTHCARE SYSTEM, 301 East Tollison Street, Baxley, GA, Zip 31513; tel. 912/367–9841; Luther E. Reeves, Chief Executive Officer

CANDLER COUNTY HOSPITAL, Cedar Road, Metter, GA, Zip 30439, Mailing Address: Box 597, Zip 30439–0597; tel. 912/685–5741; Charles Balkcom, President

CANDLER HOSPITAL, 5353 Reynolds Street, Savannah, GA, Zip 31405, Mailing Address: Box 9787, Zip 31412–9787; tel. 912/692–6000; Paul P. Hinchey, President and Chief Executive Officer

EFFINGHAM HOSPITAL, 459 Highway 119 South, Springfield, GA, Zip 31329, Mailing Address: Box 386, Zip 31329–0386; tel. 912/754–6451; W. Scott Burnette, Chief Executive Officer

EMORY UNIVERSITY HOSPITAL, 1364 Clifton Road N.E., Atlanta, GA, Zip 30322–1102; tel. 404/727–7021; John Dunklin Henry, Sr., Chief Executive Officer

LIBERTY REGIONAL MEDICAL CENTER, 112 East Oglethorpe Boulevard, Hinesville, GA, Zip 31313, Mailing Address: Box 919, Zip 31313; tel. 912/369–9400; H. Scott Kroell, Jr., Chief Executive Officer

MEADOWS REGIONAL MEDICAL CENTER, 1703 Meadows Lane, Vidalia, GA, Zip 30475, Mailing Address: P.O. Box 1048, Zip 30474; tel. 912/537–8921; Barry Michael, Chief Executive Officer

WILLINGWAY HOSPITAL, 311 Jones Mill Road, Statesboro, GA, Zip 30458; tel. 912/764–6236; Jimmy Mooney, Chief Executive Officer

CHATTAHOOCHEE HEALTH NETWORK
P.O. Box 3274, Gainesville, GA 30503–3274; tel. 770/503–3552; R. Fleming Weaver, Executive Director

COLUMBIA LANIER PARK HOSPITAL, 675 White Sulphur Road, Gainesville, GA, Zip 30505, Mailing Address: P.O. Box 1354, Zip 30503; tel. 770/503–3000; Jerry Fulks, Chief Executive Officer

COLUMBUS REGIONAL HEALTHCARE SYSTEM, INC.
P.O. Box 790, Columbus, GA 31902–0790; tel. 706/660–6103; Larry Sanders, Chairman & Chief Executive Officer

PHENIX REGIONAL HOSPITAL, 1707 21st Avenue, Phenix City, AL, Zip 36867, Mailing Address: Box 190, Zip 36868–0190; tel. 334/291–8502; Lance B. Duke, FACHE, President and Chief Executive Officer

THE MEDICAL CENTER, 710 Center Street, Columbus, GA, Zip 31902, Mailing Address: Box 951, Zip 31902; tel. 706/571–1000; Lance B. Duke, FACHE, President and Chief Executive Officer

COMMUNITY HEALTHCARE NETWORK
707 Center Street, Suite 400, Columbus, GA 31902–0790; tel. 706/660–6110; Kevin Sass, Executive Director & Vice President

MERIWETHER REGIONAL HOSPITAL, Warm Springs, GA, Mailing Address: P.O. Box 8, Zip 31830; tel. 706/655–3331; William E. Daniel, Administrator

SOUTHWEST GEORGIA REGIONAL MEDICAL CENTER, 109 Randolph Street, Cuthbert, GA, Zip 31740–1338; tel. 912/732–2181; Earnest E. Benton, Chief Executive Officer

THE MEDICAL CENTER, 710 Center Street, Columbus, GA, Zip 31902, Mailing Address: Box 951, Zip 31902; tel. 706/571–1000; Lance B. Duke, FACHE, President and Chief Executive Officer

WEST GEORGIA HEALTH SYSTEM, 1514 Vernon Road, La Grange, GA, Zip 30240–4199; tel. 706/882–1411; Charles L. Foster, Jr., FACHE, President and Chief Executive Officer

EMORY UNIVERSITY SYSTEM OF HEALTHCARE AFFILIATE NETWORK
1365 Clifton Road Northeast, Atlanta, GA 30322; tel. 404/778–3623; Don Wells, Director of Business Development

COLUMBIA FAIRVIEW PARK HOSPITAL, 200 Industrial Boulevard, Dublin, GA, Zip 31021, Mailing Address: Box 1408, Zip 31040; tel. 912/275–2000; Jeffrey T. Whiteborn, Chief Executive Officer

HANCOCK MEMORIAL HOSPITAL, 453 Boland Street, Sparta, GA, Zip 31087, Mailing Address: P.O. Box 490, Zip 31087; tel. 706/444–7006; Daniel D. Holtz, FACHE, Administrator and Chief Executive Officer

TIFT GENERAL HOSPITAL, 901 East 18th Street, Tifton, GA, Zip 31794, Mailing Address: Drawer 747, Zip 31793; tel. 912/382–7120; William T. Richardson, President and Chief Executive Officer

Section B

WESLEY WOODS GERIATRIC HOSPITAL, 1821 Clifton Road N.E., Atlanta, GA, Zip 30329–5102; tel. 404/728–6200; William L. Minnix, Chief Executive Officer

GEORGIA 1ST, INC.
150 E. Ponce de Leon Avenue Suite 490, Decatur, GA 30030; tel. 404/778–4939; Russ Toal, President & Chief Executive Officer

APPLING HEALTHCARE SYSTEM, 301 East Tollison Street, Baxley, GA, Zip 31513; tel. 912/367–9841; Luther E. Reeves, Chief Executive Officer

ATHENS REGIONAL MEDICAL CENTER, 1199 Prince Avenue, Athens, GA, Zip 30606–2793; tel. 706/549–9977; John A. Drew, President and Chief Executive Officer

BROOKS COUNTY HOSPITAL, 903 North Court Street, Quitman, GA, Zip 31643, Mailing Address: P.O. Box 5000, Zip 31643; tel. 912/263–4171; Ken Brooker, Interim Administrator

CAMDEN MEDICAL CENTER, 2000 Dan Proctor Drive, Saint Marys, GA, Zip 31558–0805, Mailing Address: Box 805, Zip 31558–0805; tel. 912/576–4200; Warren Manley, Administrator

CANDLER COUNTY HOSPITAL, Cedar Road, Metter, GA, Zip 30439, Mailing Address: Box 597, Zip 30439–0597; tel. 912/685–5741; Charles Balkcom, President

CANDLER HOSPITAL, 5353 Reynolds Street, Savannah, GA, Zip 31405, Mailing Address: Box 9787, Zip 31412–9787; tel. 912/692–6000; Paul P. Hinchey, President and Chief Executive Officer

COLUMBIA EASTSIDE MEDICAL CENTER, 1700 Medical Way, Snellville, GA, Zip 30278, Mailing Address: P.O. Box 587, Zip 30278; tel. 770/979–0200; Les Beard, Chief Executive Officer

COLUMBIA FAIRVIEW PARK HOSPITAL, 200 Industrial Boulevard, Dublin, GA, Zip 31021, Mailing Address: Box 1408, Zip 31040; tel. 912/275–2000; Jeffrey T. Whiteborn, Chief Executive Officer

COLUMBIA PALMYRA MEDICAL CENTERS, 2000 Palmyra Road, Albany, GA, Zip 31701, Mailing Address: Box 1908, Zip 31702–1908; tel. 912/434–2000; Allen Golson, Chief Executive Officer

CRAWFORD LONG HOSPITAL OF EMORY UNIVERSITY, 550 Peachtree Street N.E., Atlanta, GA, Zip 30365–2225; tel. 404/686–4411; John Dunklin Henry, Sr., Chief Executive Officer

CRISP REGIONAL HOSPITAL, 902 North Seventh Street, Cordele, GA, Zip 31015–5007; tel. 912/276–3100; D. Wayne Martin, Administrator and Chief Executive Officer

EARLY MEMORIAL HOSPITAL, 630 Columbia Street, Blakely, GA, Zip 31723; tel. 912/723–4241

EFFINGHAM HOSPITAL, 459 Highway 119 South, Springfield, GA, Zip 31329, Mailing Address: Box 386, Zip 31329–0386; tel. 912/754–6451; W. Scott Burnette, Chief Executive Officer

EGLESTON CHILDREN'S HOSPITAL AT EMORY UNIVERSITY, 1405 Clifton Road N.E., Atlanta, GA, Zip 30322–1101; tel. 404/325–6000; Alan J. Gayer, President

ELBERT MEMORIAL HOSPITAL, 4 Medical Drive, Elberton, GA, Zip 30635–1897; tel. 706/283–3151; Tim Merritt, Administrator

EMORY UNIVERSITY HOSPITAL, 1364 Clifton Road N.E., Atlanta, GA, Zip 30322–1102; tel. 404/727–7021; John Dunklin Henry, Sr., Chief Executive Officer

EMORY–ADVENTIST HOSPITAL, 3949 South Cobb Drive, Smyrna, GA, Zip 30080; tel. 770/434–0710; Larry D. Luce, President

FLOYD MEDICAL CENTER, 304 Turner McCall Boulevard, Rome, GA, Zip 30165, Mailing Address: Box 233, Zip 30162–0233; tel. 706/802–2000; Kurt Stuenkel, FACHE, President and Chief Executive Officer

GRADY GENERAL HOSPITAL, 1155 Fifth Street S.E., Cairo, GA, Zip 31728, Mailing Address: P.O. Box 360, Zip 31728; tel. 912/377–1150; Glen C. Davis, Administrator

HABERSHAM COUNTY MEDICAL CENTER, Highway 441, Demorest, GA, Zip 30535, Mailing Address: Box 37, Zip 30535; tel. 706/754–2161; C. Richard Dwozan, President

HIGGINS GENERAL HOSPITAL, 200 Allen Memorial Drive, Bremen, GA, Zip 30110, Mailing Address: Box 655, Zip 30110; tel. 770/537–5851; Robbie Smith, Administrator

HOUSTON MEDICAL CENTER, 1601 Watson Boulevard, Warner Robins, GA, Zip 31093–3431, Mailing Address: Box 2886, Zip 31099–2886; tel. 912/922–4281; Arthur P. Christie, Administrator

JOHN D. ARCHBOLD MEMORIAL HOSPITAL, 910 South Broad Street, Thomasville, GA, Zip 31792, Mailing Address: P.O. Box 1018, Zip 31799; tel. 912/228–2000; Jason H. Moore, President and Chief Executive Officer

LIBERTY REGIONAL MEDICAL CENTER, 112 East Oglethorpe Boulevard, Hinesville, GA, Zip 31313, Mailing Address: Box 919, Zip 31313; tel. 912/369–9400; H. Scott Kroell, Jr., Chief Executive Officer

LOUIS SMITH MEMORIAL HOSPITAL, 852 West Thigpen Avenue, Lakeland, GA, Zip 31635–1099; tel. 912/482–3110; Randy Sauls, Administrator

MEDICAL CENTER OF CENTRAL GEORGIA, 777 Hemlock Street, Macon, GA, Zip 31201, Mailing Address: Box 6000, Zip 31208; tel. 912/633–1000; A. Donald Faulk, FACHE, President

MEDICAL COLLEGE OF GEORGIA HOSPITAL AND CLINICS, 1120 15th Street, Augusta, GA, Zip 30912–5000; tel. 706/721–0211; Patricia Sodomka, Executive Director

MITCHELL COUNTY HOSPITAL, 90 Stephens Street, Camilla, GA, Zip 31730, Mailing Address: P.O. Box 639, Zip 31730; tel. 912/336–5284; Ronald M. Gilliard, FACHE, Administrator

NEWTON GENERAL HOSPITAL, 5126 Hospital Drive, Covington, GA, Zip 30209; tel. 770/786–7053; James F. Weadick, Administrator and Chief Executive Officer

NORTH FULTON REGIONAL HOSPITAL, 3000 Hospital Boulevard, Roswell, GA, Zip 30076–9930; tel. 404/751–2500; Frederick R. Bailey, Chief Executive Officer

NORTHEAST GEORGIA MEDICAL CENTER, 743 Spring Street N.E., Gainesville, GA, Zip 30501–3899; tel. 770/535–3553; Henry Rigdon, Executive Vice President

NORTHSIDE HOSPITAL, 1000 Johnson Ferry Road N.E., Atlanta, GA, Zip 30342–1611; tel. 404/851–8000; Sidney Kirschner, President and Chief Executive Officer

OCONEE REGIONAL MEDICAL CENTER, 821 North Cobb Street, Milledgeville, GA, Zip 31061, Mailing Address: Box 690, Zip 31061; tel. 912/454–3500; Brian L. Riddle, Chief Executive Officer

SOUTH GEORGIA MEDICAL CENTER, 2501 North Patterson Street, Valdosta, GA, Zip 31602, Mailing Address: Box 1727, Zip 31603–1727; tel. 912/333–1000; John S. Bowling, President and Chief Executive Officer

SOUTHEAST GEORGIA REGIONAL MEDICAL CENTER, 3100 Kemble Avenue, Brunswick, GA, Zip 31520, Mailing Address: Box 1518, Zip 31521; tel. 912/264–7000; E. Berton Whitaker, President and Chief Executive Officer

SOUTHERN REGIONAL MEDICAL CENTER, 11 Upper Riverdale Road S.W., Riverdale, GA, Zip 30274–2600; tel. 770/991–8000; Donald B. Logan, President and Chief Executive Officer

SPALDING REGIONAL HOSPITAL, 601 South Eighth Street, Griffin, GA, Zip 30224, Mailing Address: P.O. Drawer V, Zip 30224–1168; tel. 770/228–2721; Phil Shaw, Executive Director

SUMTER REGIONAL HOSPITAL, 100 Wheatley Drive, Americus, GA, Zip 31709; tel. 912/924–6011; Jerry W. Adams, President

TANNER MEDICAL CENTER, 705 Dixie Street, Carrollton, GA, Zip 30117–3818; tel. 770/836–9666; Loy M. Howard, Chief Executive Officer

TANNER MEDICAL CENTER–VILLA RICA, 601 Dallas Road, Villa Rica, GA, Zip 30180, Mailing Address: Box 638, Zip 30180; tel. 770/459–7100; Larry N. Steed, Administrator

THE MEDICAL CENTER, 710 Center Street, Columbus, GA, Zip 31902, Mailing Address: Box 951, Zip 31902; tel. 706/571–1000; Lance B. Duke, FACHE, President and Chief Executive Officer

TIFT GENERAL HOSPITAL, 901 East 18th Street, Tifton, GA, Zip 31794, Mailing Address: Drawer 747, Zip 31793; tel. 912/382–7120; William T. Richardson, President and Chief Executive Officer

UPSON REGIONAL MEDICAL CENTER, 801 West Gordon Street, Thomaston, GA, Zip 30286–2831, Mailing Address: Box 1059, Zip 30286; tel. 706/647–8111; Samuel S. Gregory, Administrator

WALTON MEDICAL CENTER, 330 Alcovy Street, Monroe, GA, Zip 30655, Mailing Address: Box 1346, Zip 30655; tel. 770/267–8461; Edgar L. Belcher, Administrator

WEST GEORGIA HEALTH SYSTEM, 1514 Vernon Road, La Grange, GA, Zip 30240–4199; tel. 706/882–1411; Charles L. Foster, Jr., FACHE, President and Chief Executive Officer

GRADY HEALTH SYSTEM
80 Butler Street, Atlanta, GA 30335; tel. 404/616–4307; Edward Renford, President

GRADY MEMORIAL HOSPITAL, 80 Butler Street S.E., Atlanta, GA, Zip 30335–3801, Mailing Address: P.O. Box 26189, Zip 30335–3801; tel. 404/616–4252; Edward J. Renford, President and Chief Executive Officer

NATIONAL CARDIOVASCULAR NETWORK
3390 Peachtree Road, Suite 300, Atlanta, GA 30326–1108; tel. 404/848–1911; Michael Lanzilotta, President

ABBOTT NORTHWESTERN HOSPITAL, 800 East 28th Street, Minneapolis, MN, Zip 55407–3799; tel. 612/863–4203; Robert K. Spinner, President

ALBANY MEDICAL CENTER, 43 New Scotland Avenue, Albany, NY, Zip 12208; tel. 518/262–3125; Thomas G. Foggo, Executive Vice President Care Delivery and General Director

BAYLOR UNIVERSITY MEDICAL CENTER, 3500 Gaston Avenue, Dallas, TX, Zip 75246–2088; tel. 214/820–0111; Boone Powell, Jr., President

BIRMINGHAM BAPTIST MEDICAL CENTER–MONTCLAIR CAMPUS, 800 Montclair Road, Birmingham, AL, Zip 35213; tel. 205/592–1000; Dana S. Hensley, President

BRYAN MEMORIAL HOSPITAL, 1600 South 48th Street, Lincoln, NE, Zip 68506–1299; tel. 402/489–0200; R. Lynn Wilson, President

CEDARS–SINAI MEDICAL CENTER, 8700 Beverly Boulevard, Los Angeles, CA, Zip 90048–0750, Mailing Address: Box 48750, Zip 90048–0750; tel. 310/855–5000; Thomas M. Priselac, President and Chief Executive Officer

CHRIST HOSPITAL, 2139 Auburn Avenue, Cincinnati, OH, Zip 45219–2989; tel. 513/369–2000; Claus von Zychlin, Senior Executive Officer

COLUMBIA MEDICAL CENTER PHOENIX, 1947 East Thomas Road, Phoenix, AZ, Zip 85016; tel. 602/650–7600; Denny W. Powell, Chief Executive Officer

DUKE UNIVERSITY MEDICAL CENTER, Erwin Road, Durham, NC, Zip 27710, Mailing Address: Box 3708, Zip 27710; tel. 919/684–8111; Michael D. Israel, Chief Executive Officer and Vice Chancellor

EMORY UNIVERSITY HOSPITAL, 1364 Clifton Road N.E., Atlanta, GA, Zip 30322–1102; tel. 404/727–7021; John Dunklin Henry, Sr., Chief Executive Officer

FLORIDA HOSPITAL, 601 East Rollins Street, Orlando, FL, Zip 32803–1489; tel. 407/896–6611; Thomas L. Werner, President

GOOD SAMARITAN HOSPITAL, 3815 Highland Avenue, Downers Grove, IL, Zip 60515; tel. 630/275–5900; David M. McConkey, Chief Executive

HILLCREST HEALTHCARE SYSTEM, 1120 South Utica, Tulsa, OK, Zip 74104–4090; tel. 918/579–1000; Donald A. Lorack, Jr., President and Chief Executive Officer

JEWISH HOSPITAL, 217 East Chestnut Street, Louisville, KY, Zip 40202–1886; tel. 502/587–4011; Douglas E. Shaw, President

LENOX HILL HOSPITAL, 100 East 77th Street, New York, NY, Zip 10021–1883; tel. 212/434–2000; Gladys George, President and Chief Executive Officer

MAINE MEDICAL CENTER, 22 Bramhall Street, Portland, ME, Zip 04102; tel. 207/871–0111; Donald L. McDowell, President and Chief Executive Officer

MERCY GENERAL HOSPITAL, 4001 J Street, Sacramento, CA, Zip 95819; tel. 916/453–4950; Thomas A. Petersen, Vice President and Chief Operating Officer

MERIDIAN HEALTH SYSTEM, 1945 State Highway 33, Neptune, NJ, Zip 07753; tel. 908/776–4215; John K. Lloyd, Chief Executive Officer

METHODIST HOSPITALS OF MEMPHIS, 1265 Union Avenue, Memphis, TN, Zip 38104–3499; tel. 901/726–7000; Gary S. Shorb, President

MORRISTOWN MEMORIAL HOSPITAL, 100 Madison Avenue, Morristown, NJ, Zip 07962–1956; tel. 201/971–5000; Jean M. McMahon, R.N., Vice President and General Manager

NEW ENGLAND MEDICAL CENTER, 750 Washington Street, Boston, MA, Zip 02111–1845; tel. 617/636–5000; Thomas F. O'Donnell, Jr., M.D., FACS, President and Chief Executive Officer

NORTH RIDGE MEDICAL CENTER, 5757 North Dixie Highway, Fort Lauderdale, FL, Zip 33334; tel. 305/776–6000; Emil P. Miller, Chief Executive Officer

OHIO STATE UNIVERSITY MEDICAL CENTER, 410 West 10th Avenue, Columbus, OH, Zip 43210–1240; tel. 614/293–8000; R. Reed Fraley, Associate Vice President for Health Sciences and Chief Executive Officer

SAINT LOUIS UNIVERSITY HOSPITAL, 3635 Vista at Grand Boulevard, Saint Louis, MO, Zip 63110–0250, Mailing Address: P.O. Box 15250, Zip 63110–0250; tel. 314/577–8000; James Kimmey, M.D., M.P.H., Chairman and Chief Executive Officer

SAINT LUKE'S HOSPITAL, 4400 Wornall Road, Kansas City, MO, Zip 64111; tel. 816/932–2000; James M. Brophy, Senior Executive Officer

SHADYSIDE HOSPITAL, 5230 Centre Avenue, Pittsburgh, PA, Zip 15232–1304; tel. 412/623–2121; Henry A. Mordoh, President

SINAI HOSPITAL OF BALTIMORE, 2401 West Belvedere Avenue, Baltimore, MD, Zip 21215–5271; tel. 410/601–9000; Warren A. Green, President and Chief Executive Officer

ST. DOMINIC–JACKSON MEMORIAL HOSPITAL, 969 Lakeland Drive, Jackson, MS, Zip 39216–4699; tel. 601/982–0121; Claude W. Harbarger, President

ST. FRANCIS HOSPITAL OF EVANSTON, 355 Ridge Avenue, Evanston, IL, Zip 60202–3399; tel. 847/316–4000; James C. Gizzi, President and Chief Executive Officer

ST. JOHN'S HOSPITAL, 800 East Carpenter Street, Springfield, IL, Zip 62769; tel. 217/544–6464; Allison C. Laabs, Executive Vice President and Administrator

ST. LUKE'S MEDICAL CENTER, 2900 West Oklahoma Avenue, Milwaukee, WI, Zip 53215, Mailing Address: P.O. Box 2901, Zip 53201; tel. 414/649–6000; Mark R. Ambrosius, President

ST. THOMAS HOSPITAL, 4220 Harding Road, Nashville, TN, Zip 37205, Mailing Address: Box 380, Zip 37202; tel. 615/222–2111; John F. Tighe, President and Chief Executive Officer

ST. VINCENT HOSPITALS AND HEALTH SERVICES, 2001 West 86th Street, Indianapolis, IN, Zip 46260, Mailing Address: Box 40970, Zip 46240–0970; tel. 317/338–2345; Douglas D. French, President and Chief Executive Officer

ST. VINCENT INFIRMARY MEDICAL CENTER, Two St. Vincent Circle, Little Rock, AR, Zip 72205–5499; tel. 501/660–3000; Diana T. Hueter, President and Chief Executive Officer

UNIVERSITY OF VIRGINIA MEDICAL CENTER, Jefferson Park Avenue, Charlottesville, VA, Zip 22908, Mailing Address: P.O. Box 10050, Zip 22906–0050; tel. 804/924–0211; Michael J. Halseth, Executive Director

WASHINGTON HOSPITAL CENTER, 110 Irving Street N.W., Washington, DC, Zip 20010–2975; tel. 202/877–7000; Kenneth A. Samet, President

WILLIAM BEAUMONT HOSPITAL–ROYAL OAK, 3601 West Thirteen Mile Road, Royal Oak, MI, Zip 48073–6769; tel. 810/551–5000; John D. Labriola, Vice President and Director

NORTHWEST GEORGIA HEALTHCARE PARTNERSHIP
P.O. Box 308, Dalton, GA 30722;
tel. 706/272–6013; Nancy Kennedy,
Executive Director

COLUMBIA MURRAY MEDICAL CENTER, 707 Old Ellijay Road, Chatsworth, GA, Zip 30705, Mailing Address: P.O. Box 1406, Zip 30705; tel. 706/695–4564; Richard Cook, Administrator

HAMILTON MEDICAL CENTER, 1200 Memorial Drive, Dalton, GA, Zip 30720, Mailing Address: P.O. Box 1168, Zip 30722–1168; tel. 706/272–6000; Ned B. Wilford, President and Chief Executive Officer

PRINCIPAL HEALTH CARE OF GEORGIA
3715 Northside Parkway – Suite 4300,
Atlanta, GA 30327; tel. 404/231–9911; Ken Bryant, Executive Director

APPLING HEALTHCARE SYSTEM, 301 East Tollison Street, Baxley, GA, Zip 31513; tel. 912/367–9841; Luther E. Reeves, Chief Executive Officer

BERRIEN COUNTY HOSPITAL, 1221 East McPherson Street, Nashville, GA, Zip 31639, Mailing Address: P.O. Box 665, Zip 31639; tel. 912/686–7471; James P. Seward, Jr., Executive Director

BRADLEY MEMORIAL HOSPITAL, 2305 Chambliss Avenue N.W., Cleveland, TN, Zip 37311, Mailing Address: Box 3060, Zip 37320–3060; tel. 423/559–6000; Jim Whitlock, Administrator

BULLOCH MEMORIAL HOSPITAL, 500 East Grady Street, Statesboro, GA, Zip 30458, Mailing Address: P.O. Box 1048, Zip 30459–1048; tel. 912/764–6671; C. Scott Campbell, Executive Director

BURKE COUNTY HOSPITAL, 351 Liberty Street, Waynesboro, GA, Zip 30830; tel. 706/554–4435; Gloria Cochran, Administrator

CANDLER COUNTY HOSPITAL, Cedar Road, Metter, GA, Zip 30439, Mailing Address: Box 597, Zip 30439–0597; tel. 912/685–5741; Charles Balkcom, President

CANDLER HOSPITAL, 5353 Reynolds Street, Savannah, GA, Zip 31405, Mailing Address: Box 9787, Zip 31412–9787; tel. 912/692–6000; Paul P. Hinchey, President and Chief Executive Officer

CLEVELAND COMMUNITY HOSPITAL, 2800 Westside Drive N.W., Cleveland, TN, Zip 37312; tel. 423/339–4100; Phil Rowland, Administrator

COBB MEMORIAL HOSPITAL, 577 Franklin Springs Street, Royston, GA, Zip 30662, Mailing Address: Box 589, Zip 30662–0589; tel. 706/245–5034; H. Thomas Brown, Administrator

COLUMBIA ATHENS REGIONAL MEDICAL CENTER, 1114 West Madison Avenue, Athens, TN, Zip 37303, Mailing Address: Box 250, Zip 37371–0250; tel. 615/745–1411; Sean S. McMurray, Administrator

COLUMBIA CARTERSVILLE MEDICAL CENTER, 960 Joe Frank Harris Parkway, Cartersville, GA, Zip 30120, Mailing Address: P.O. Box 200008, Zip 30120–9001; tel. 770/382–1530; Keith Sandlin, Chief Executive Officer

COLUMBIA COLISEUM MEDICAL CENTERS, 350 Hospital Drive, Macon, GA, Zip 31213; tel. 912/765–7000; Michael S. Boggs, Chief Executive Officer

COLUMBIA DOCTORS HOSPITAL, 616 19th Street, Columbus, GA, Zip 31901–1528, Mailing Address: P.O. Box 2188, Zip 31902–2188; tel. 706/571–4262; Hugh D. Wilson, Chief Executive Officer

COLUMBIA EAST RIDGE HOSPITAL, 941 Spring Creek Road, East Ridge, TN, Zip 37412, Mailing Address: P.O. Box 91229, Zip 37412–6229; tel. 423/894–7870; Brenda M. Waltz, CHE, Chief Executive Officer

COLUMBIA FAIRVIEW PARK HOSPITAL, 200 Industrial Boulevard, Dublin, GA, Zip 31021, Mailing Address: Box 1408, Zip 31040; tel. 912/275–2000; Jeffrey T. Whiteborn, Chief Executive Officer

COLUMBIA PALMYRA MEDICAL CENTERS, 2000 Palmyra Road, Albany, GA, Zip 31701, Mailing Address: Box 1908, Zip 31702–1908; tel. 912/434–2000; Allen Golson, Chief Executive Officer

COLUMBIA PEACHTREE REGIONAL HOSPITAL, 60 Hospital Road, Newnan, GA, Zip 30264, Mailing Address: Box 2228, Zip 30264; tel. 770/253–1912; Linda Jubinsky, Chief Executive Officer

COLUMBIA SOUTH PITTSBURG HOSPITAL, 210 West 12th Street, South Pittsburg, TN, Zip 37380, Mailing Address: P.O. Box 349, Zip 37380–0349; tel. 423/837–6781; Robert Klein, Chief Executive Officer

DECATUR HOSPITAL, 450 North Candler Street, Decatur, GA, Zip 30030, Mailing Address: Box 40, Zip 30031; tel. 404/377–0221; Richard T. Schmidt, Executive Director

DEKALB MEDICAL CENTER, 2701 North Decatur Road, Decatur, GA, Zip 30033; tel. 404/501–1000; John R. Gerlach, Chief Executive Officer/Administrator

DODGE COUNTY HOSPITAL, 715 Griffin Street, Eastman, GA, Zip 31023, Mailing Address: Box 4309, Zip 31023; tel. 912/374–4000; Meredith H. Smith, Administrator

DOOLY MEDICAL CENTER, 1300 Union Street, Vienna, GA, Zip 31092, Mailing Address: Box 278, Zip 31092; tel. 912/268–4141; Kevin Paul, Administrator

EDGEFIELD COUNTY HOSPITAL, Bausket Street, Edgefield, SC, Zip 29824, Mailing Address: Box 590, Zip 29824–0590; tel. 803/637–3174; W. Joseph Seel, Administrator

EFFINGHAM HOSPITAL, 459 Highway 119 South, Springfield, GA, Zip 31329, Mailing Address: Box 386, Zip 31329–0386; tel. 912/754–6451; W. Scott Burnette, Chief Executive Officer

EGLESTON CHILDREN'S HOSPITAL AT EMORY UNIVERSITY, 1405 Clifton Road N.E., Atlanta, GA, Zip 30322–1101; tel. 404/325–6000; Alan J. Gayer, President

EMANUEL COUNTY HOSPITAL, 117 Kite Road, Swainsboro, GA, Zip 30401, Mailing Address: P.O. Box 879, Zip 30401; tel. 912/237–9911; Richard W. Clarke, Chief Executive Officer

FLOYD MEDICAL CENTER, 304 Turner McCall Boulevard, Rome, GA, Zip 30165, Mailing Address: Box 233, Zip 30162–0233; tel. 706/802–2000; Kurt Stuenkel, FACHE, President and Chief Executive Officer

GORDON HOSPITAL, 1035 Red Bud Road, Calhoun, GA, Zip 30701, Mailing Address: P.O. Box 12938, Zip 30703–7013; tel. 706/629–2895; Dennis Kiley, President

HART COUNTY HOSPITAL, Gibson and Cade Streets, Hartwell, GA, Zip 30643–0280, Mailing Address: P.O. Box 280, Zip 30643–0280; tel. 706/856–6100; Samuel A. Strickland, Administrator

HIGGINS GENERAL HOSPITAL, 200 Allen Memorial Drive, Bremen, GA, Zip 30110, Mailing Address: Box 655, Zip 30110; tel. 770/537–5851; Robbie Smith, Administrator

HILTON HEAD MEDICAL CENTER AND CLINICS, Hilton Head Island, SC, Mailing Address: P.O. Box 21117, Zip 29925–1117; tel. 803/681–6122; Dennis Ray Bruns, President and Chief Executive Officer

HUTCHESON MEDICAL CENTER, 100 Gross Crescent Circle, Fort Oglethorpe, GA, Zip 30742; tel. 706/858–2000; Robert T. Jones, M.D., President and Chief Executive Officer

JEFFERSON HOSPITAL, 1067 Peachtree Street, Louisville, GA, Zip 30434; tel. 912/625–7000; Rita Culvern, Administrator

LIBERTY REGIONAL MEDICAL CENTER, 112 East Oglethorpe Boulevard, Hinesville, GA, Zip 31313, Mailing Address: Box 919, Zip 31313; tel. 912/369–9400; H. Scott Kroell, Jr., Chief Executive Officer

LOUIS SMITH MEMORIAL HOSPITAL, 852 West Thigpen Avenue, Lakeland, GA, Zip 31635–1099; tel. 912/482–3110; Randy Sauls, Administrator

MCDUFFIE COUNTY HOSPITAL, 521 Hill Street S.W., Thomson, GA, Zip 30824; tel. 706/595–1411; Douglas C. Keir, Chief Executive Officer

MEADOWS REGIONAL MEDICAL CENTER, 1703 Meadows Lane, Vidalia, GA, Zip 30475, Mailing Address: P.O. Box 1048, Zip 30474; tel. 912/537–8921; Barry Michael, Chief Executive Officer

MEMORIAL HOSPITAL, 2525 De Sales Avenue, Chattanooga, TN, Zip 37404–3322; tel. 615/495–2525; L. Clark Taylor, Jr., President and Chief Executive Officer

MEMORIAL HOSPITAL AND MANOR, 1500 East Shotwell Street, Bainbridge, GA, Zip 31717; tel. 912/246–3500; James G. Peak, Director

MEMORIAL MEDICAL CENTER, 4700 Waters Avenue, Savannah, GA, Zip 31404, Mailing Address: Box 23089, Zip 31403–3089; tel. 912/350–8000; Robert A. Colvin, President and Chief Executive Officer

NEWTON GENERAL HOSPITAL, 5126 Hospital Drive, Covington, GA, Zip 30209; tel. 770/786–7053; James F. Weadick, Administrator and Chief Executive Officer

NORTH GEORGIA MEDICAL CENTER AND GILMER NURSING HOME, Jasper Road, Ellijay, GA, Zip 30540–0346, Mailing Address: Box 346, Zip 30540–0346; tel. 706/276–4741; Mickey M. Rabuka, Administrator

NORTH PARK HOSPITAL, 2051 Hamill Road, Chattanooga, TN, Zip 37343–4096; tel. 423/870–6100; Leonard Fant, Administrator

NORTHEAST GEORGIA MEDICAL CENTER, 743 Spring Street N.E., Gainesville, GA, Zip 30501–3899; tel. 770/535–3553; Henry Rigdon, Executive Vice President

NORTHSIDE HOSPITAL, 1000 Johnson Ferry Road N.E., Atlanta, GA, Zip 30342–1611; tel. 404/851–8000; Sidney Kirschner, President and Chief Executive Officer

OCONEE REGIONAL MEDICAL CENTER, 821 North Cobb Street, Milledgeville, GA, Zip 31061, Mailing Address: Box 690, Zip 31061; tel. 912/454–3500; Brian L. Riddle, Chief Executive Officer

PARKRIDGE MEDICAL CENTER, 2333 McCallie Avenue, Chattanooga, TN, Zip 37404–3285; tel. 423/698–6061; Solon Boggus, Jr., Chief Executive Officer

PHENIX REGIONAL HOSPITAL, 1707 21st Avenue, Phenix City, AL, Zip 36867, Mailing Address: Box 190, Zip 36868–0190; tel. 334/291–8502; Lance B. Duke, FACHE, President and Chief Executive Officer

PIEDMONT HOSPITAL, 1968 Peachtree Road N.W., Atlanta, GA, Zip 30309–1231; tel. 404/605–5000; Richard B. Hubbard, III, President and Chief Executive Officer

PROMINA COBB HOSPITAL, 3950 Austell Road, Austell, GA, Zip 30001–1121; tel. 770/732–4000; Betty Whisenant, Site Manager

PROMINA DOUGLAS HOSPITAL, 8954 Hospital Drive, Douglasville, GA, Zip 30134–2282; tel. 770/949–1500; Tom Hill, Chief Executive Officer

PROMINA GWINNETT HOSPITAL SYSTEM, Lawrenceville, GA, Mailing Address: Box 348, Zip 30246–0348; tel. 770/995–4321; Franklin M. Rinker, President and Chief Executive Officer

PROMINA PAULDING MEMORIAL MEDICAL CENTER, 600 West Memorial Drive, Dallas, GA, Zip 30132–1335; tel. 770/445–4411; T. Mark Haney, Administrator

PROMINA WINDY HILL HOSPITAL, 2540 Windy Hill Road, Marietta, GA, Zip 30067; tel. 770/644–1000; T. Mark Haney, Administrator

PUTNAM GENERAL HOSPITAL, Lake Oconee Parkway, Eatonton, GA, Zip 31024–4330, Mailing Address: Box 4330, Zip 31024–4330; tel. 706/485–2711; Darrell M. Oglesby, Administrator

R. T. JONES HOSPITAL, 201 Hospital Road, Canton, GA, Zip 30114, Mailing Address: P.O. Box 906, Zip 30114; tel. 770/720–5100; Douglas M. Parker, Chief Executive Officer

RIDGECREST HOSPITAL, 393 Ridgecrest Circle, Clayton, GA, Zip 30525; tel. 706/782–4297; Gerald E. Knepp, Chief Executive Officer

ROCKDALE HOSPITAL, 1412 Milstead Avenue N.E., Conyers, GA, Zip 30207–9990; tel. 770/918–3000; Nelson Toebbe, Chief Executive Officer

SATILLA REGIONAL MEDICAL CENTER, 410 Darling Avenue, Waycross, GA, Zip 31501, Mailing Address: P.O. Box 139, Zip 31502–0139; tel. 912/283–3030; Eugene Johnson, President and Chief Executive Officer

SCOTTISH RITE CHILDREN'S MEDICAL CENTER, 1001 Johnson Ferry Road N.E., Atlanta, GA, Zip 30342; tel. 404/256–5252; James E. Tally, Ph.D., President and Chief Executive Officer

SHEPHERD CENTER, 2020 Peachtree Road N.W., Atlanta, GA, Zip 30309–1465; tel. 404/352–2020; Gary R. Ulicny, Ph.D., President and Chief Executive Officer

SISKIN HOSPITAL FOR PHYSICAL REHABILITATION, One Siskin Plaza, Chattanooga, TN, Zip 37403; tel. 423/634–1200; Robert P. Main, President and Chief Executive Officer

SOUTH FULTON MEDICAL CENTER, 1170 Cleveland Avenue, East Point, GA, Zip 30344; tel. 404/305–3500; H. Neil Copelan, President and Chief Executive Officer

SOUTH GEORGIA MEDICAL CENTER, 2501 North Patterson Street, Valdosta, GA, Zip 31602, Mailing Address: Box 1727, Zip 31603–1727; tel. 912/333–1000; John S. Bowling, President and Chief Executive Officer

SOUTHEAST ALABAMA MEDICAL CENTER, 1108 Ross Clark Circle, Dothan, AL, Zip 36301, Mailing Address: P.O. Box 6987, Zip 36302; tel. 334/793–8111; James R. Blackmon, Chief Executive Officer

SOUTHEAST GEORGIA REGIONAL MEDICAL CENTER, 3100 Kemble Avenue, Brunswick, GA, Zip 31520, Mailing Address: Box 1518, Zip 31521; tel. 912/264–7000; E. Berton Whitaker, President and Chief Executive Officer

SOUTHERN REGIONAL MEDICAL CENTER, 11 Upper Riverdale Road S.W., Riverdale, GA, Zip 30274–2600; tel. 770/991–8000; Donald B. Logan, President and Chief Executive Officer

SPALDING REGIONAL HOSPITAL, 601 South Eighth Street, Griffin, GA, Zip 30224, Mailing Address: P.O. Drawer V, Zip 30224–1168; tel. 770/228–2721; Phil Shaw, Executive Director

ST. MARY'S HEALTH CARE SYSTEM, 1230 Baxter Street, Athens, GA, Zip 30606–3791; tel. 706/548–7581; Edward J. Fechtel, Jr., President and Chief Executive Officer

STEPHENS COUNTY HOSPITAL, 2003 Falls Road, Toccoa, GA, Zip 30577; tel. 706/886–6841; Edward C. Gambrell, Jr., Administrator

SUMTER REGIONAL HOSPITAL, 100 Wheatley Drive, Americus, GA, Zip 31709; tel. 912/924–6011; Jerry W. Adams, President

TANNER MEDICAL CENTER, 705 Dixie Street, Carrollton, GA, Zip 30117–3818; tel. 770/836–9666; Loy M. Howard, Chief Executive Officer

TANNER MEDICAL CENTER–VILLA RICA, 601 Dallas Road, Villa Rica, GA, Zip 30180, Mailing Address: Box 638, Zip 30180; tel. 770/459–7100; Larry N. Steed, Administrator

TAYLOR REGIONAL HOSPITAL, Macon Highway, Hawkinsville, GA, Zip 31036; tel. 912/783–0200; Dan S. Maddock, President

THE MEDICAL CENTER, 710 Center Street, Columbus, GA, Zip 31902, Mailing Address: Box 951, Zip 31902; tel. 706/571–1000; Lance B. Duke, FACHE, President and Chief Executive Officer

UNIVERSITY HOSPITAL, 1350 Walton Way, Augusta, GA, Zip 30901–2629; tel. 706/722–9011; Donald C. Bray, President and Chief Executive Officer

UPSON REGIONAL MEDICAL CENTER, 801 West Gordon Street, Thomaston, GA, Zip 30286–2831, Mailing Address: Box 1059, Zip 30286; tel. 706/647–8111; Samuel S. Gregory, Administrator

VENCOR HOSPITAL–CHATTANOOGA, 709 Walnut Street, Chattanooga, TN, Zip 37402; tel. 423/266–7721; Steven E. McGraw, Administrator

WALTON REHABILITATION HOSPITAL, 1355 Independence Drive, Augusta, GA, Zip 30901–1037; tel. 706/823–8505; Dennis B. Skelley, President and Chief Executive Officer

WASHINGTON COUNTY REGIONAL HOSPITAL, 610 Sparta Highway, Sandersville, GA, Zip 31082, Mailing Address: Box 636, Zip 31082; tel. 912/552–3901; Shirley R. Roberts, Administrator

WAYNE MEMORIAL HOSPITAL, 865 South First Street, Jesup, GA, Zip 31598, Mailing Address: Box 408, Zip 31598; tel. 912/427–6811; Charles R. Morgan, Administrator

PROMINA HEALTH SYSTEM, INC.
2000 South Park Place, Atlanta, GA 30339; tel. 770/956–6010; Eric P. Norwood, Vice President System

DECATUR HOSPITAL, 450 North Candler Street, Decatur, GA, Zip 30030, Mailing Address: Box 40, Zip 30031; tel. 404/377–0221; Richard T. Schmidt, Executive Director

DEKALB MEDICAL CENTER, 2701 North Decatur Road, Decatur, GA, Zip 30033; tel. 404/501–1000; John R. Gerlach, Chief Executive Officer/Administrator

KENNESTONE HOSPITAL, 677 Church Street, Marietta, GA, Zip 30060; tel. 770/793–5000; Thomas E. Hill, Chief Executive Officer

PIEDMONT HOSPITAL, 1968 Peachtree Road N.W., Atlanta, GA, Zip 30309–1231; tel. 404/605–5000; Richard B. Hubbard, III, President and Chief Executive Officer

PROMINA COBB HOSPITAL, 3950 Austell Road, Austell, GA, Zip 30001–1121; tel. 770/732–4000; Betty Whisenant, Site Manager

PROMINA GWINNETT HOSPITAL SYSTEM, Lawrenceville, GA, Mailing Address: Box 348, Zip 30246–0348; tel. 770/995–4321; Franklin M. Rinker, President and Chief Executive Officer

SOUTHERN REGIONAL MEDICAL CENTER, 11 Upper Riverdale Road S.W., Riverdale, GA, Zip 30274–2600; tel. 770/991–8000; Donald B. Logan, President and Chief Executive Officer

SAINT JOSEPH'S HOSPITAL OF ATLANTA
5665 Peachtree, Dunwoody Road, Northeast, Atlanta, GA 30342; tel. 404/851–7543; Brian Tisher, Planning Specialist

SAINT JOSEPH'S HOSPITAL OF ATLANTA, 5665 Peachtree Dunwoody Road N.E., Atlanta, GA, Zip 30342–1764; tel. 404/851–7001; Brue Chandler, President and Chief Executive Officer

THE MEDICAL RESOURCE NETWORK, L.L.C.
900 Circle 75 Parkway, Suite 1400, Atlanta, GA 30339; tel. 770/980–2340; David Record, Executive Vice President & COO

APPLING HEALTHCARE SYSTEM, 301 East Tollison Street, Baxley, GA, Zip 31513; tel. 912/367–9841; Luther E. Reeves, Chief Executive Officer

ATHENS REGIONAL MEDICAL CENTER, 1199 Prince Avenue, Athens, GA, Zip 30606–2793; tel. 706/549–9977; John A. Drew, President and Chief Executive Officer

BARNWELL COUNTY HOSPITAL, Reynolds and Wren Streets, Barnwell, SC, Zip 29812, Mailing Address: Box 588, Zip 29812–0588; tel. 803/259–1000; Tommy R. McDougal, Jr., Administrator and Chief Executive Officer

BERRIEN COUNTY HOSPITAL, 1221 East McPherson Street, Nashville, GA, Zip 31639, Mailing Address: P.O. Box 665, Zip 31639; tel. 912/686–7471; James P. Seward, Jr., Executive Director

BROOKS COUNTY HOSPITAL, 903 North Court Street, Quitman, GA, Zip 31643, Mailing Address: P.O. Box 5000, Zip 31643; tel. 912/263–4171; Ken Brooker, Interim Administrator

BURKE COUNTY HOSPITAL, 351 Liberty Street, Waynesboro, GA, Zip 30830; tel. 706/554–4435; Gloria Cochran, Administrator

CALHOUN MEMORIAL HOSPITAL, 209 Academy & Carswell Streets, Arlington, GA, Zip 31713, Mailing Address: Drawer R, Zip 31713; tel. 912/725–4272; Peggy Pierce, Administrator

CANDLER COUNTY HOSPITAL, Cedar Road, Metter, GA, Zip 30439, Mailing Address: Box 597, Zip 30439–0597; tel. 912/685–5741; Charles Balkcom, President

CANDLER HOSPITAL, 5353 Reynolds Street, Savannah, GA, Zip 31405, Mailing Address: Box 9787, Zip 31412–9787; tel. 912/692–6000; Paul P. Hinchey, President and Chief Executive Officer

CHATTOOGA COUNTY HOSPITAL, 1010 Highland Avenue, Summerville, GA, Zip 30747, Mailing Address: Box 449, Zip 30747–0449; tel. 706/857–4761; Stephen W. Johnson, Executive Director

CHEROKEE BAPTIST MEDICAL CENTER, 400 Northwood Drive, Centre, AL, Zip 35960–1023; tel. 205/927–5531; Barry S. Cochran, President

CRISP REGIONAL HOSPITAL, 902 North Seventh Street, Cordele, GA, Zip 31015–5007; tel. 912/276–3100; D. Wayne Martin, Administrator and Chief Executive Officer

DECATUR HOSPITAL, 450 North Candler Street, Decatur, GA, Zip 30030, Mailing Address: Box 40, Zip 30031; tel. 404/377–0221; Richard T. Schmidt, Executive Director

DEKALB MEDICAL CENTER, 2701 North Decatur Road, Decatur, GA, Zip 30033; tel. 404/501–1000; John R. Gerlach, Chief Executive Officer/Administrator

DODGE COUNTY HOSPITAL, 715 Griffin Street, Eastman, GA, Zip 31023, Mailing Address: Box 4309, Zip 31023; tel. 912/374–4000; Meredith H. Smith, Administrator

DONALSONVILLE HOSPITAL, Hospital Circle, Donalsonville, GA, Zip 31745, Mailing Address: Box 677, Zip 31745; tel. 912/524–5217; Charles H. Orrick, Administrator

DOOLY MEDICAL CENTER, 1300 Union Street, Vienna, GA, Zip 31092, Mailing Address: Box 278, Zip 31092; tel. 912/268–4141; Kevin Paul, Administrator

EARLY MEMORIAL HOSPITAL, 630 Columbia Street, Blakely, GA, Zip 31723; tel. 912/723–4241

EDGEFIELD COUNTY HOSPITAL, Bausket Street, Edgefield, SC, Zip 29824, Mailing Address: Box 590, Zip 29824–0590; tel. 803/637–3174; W. Joseph Seel, Administrator

EFFINGHAM HOSPITAL, 459 Highway 119 South, Springfield, GA, Zip 31329, Mailing Address: Box 386, Zip 31329–0386; tel. 912/754–6451; W. Scott Burnette, Chief Executive Officer

EGLESTON CHILDREN'S HOSPITAL AT EMORY UNIVERSITY, 1405 Clifton Road N.E., Atlanta, GA, Zip 30322–1101; tel. 404/325–6000; Alan J. Gayer, President

EMANUEL COUNTY HOSPITAL, 117 Kite Road, Swainsboro, GA, Zip 30401, Mailing Address: P.O. Box 879, Zip 30401; tel. 912/237–9911; Richard W. Clarke, Chief Executive Officer

FLOYD MEDICAL CENTER, 304 Turner McCall Boulevard, Rome, GA, Zip 30162, Mailing Address: Box 233, Zip 30162–0233; tel. 706/802–2000; Kurt Stuenkel, FACHE, President and Chief Executive Officer

GORDON HOSPITAL, 1035 Red Bud Road, Calhoun, GA, Zip 30701, Mailing Address: P.O. Box 12938, Zip 30703–7013; tel. 706/629–2895; Dennis Kiley, President

GRADY GENERAL HOSPITAL, 1155 Fifth Street S.E., Cairo, GA, Zip 31728, Mailing Address: P.O. Box 360, Zip 31728; tel. 912/377–1150; Glen C. Davis, Administrator

HAMILTON MEDICAL CENTER, 1200 Memorial Drive, Dalton, GA, Zip 30720, Mailing Address: P.O. Box 1168, Zip 30722–1168; tel. 706/272–6000; Ned B. Wilford, President and Chief Executive Officer

HEALTHSOUTH CENTRAL GEORGIA REHABILITATION HOSPITAL, 3351 Northside Drive, Macon, GA, Zip 31210; tel. 912/471–3536; Elbert T. McQueen, Chief Executive Officer

HIGGINS GENERAL HOSPITAL, 200 Allen Memorial Drive, Bremen, GA, Zip 30110, Mailing Address: Box 655, Zip 30110; tel. 770/537–5851; Robbie Smith, Administrator

HOUSTON MEDICAL CENTER, 1601 Watson Boulevard, Warner Robins, GA, Zip 31093–3431, Mailing Address: Box 2886, Zip 31099–2886; tel. 912/922–4281; Arthur P. Christie, Administrator

JEFFERSON HOSPITAL, 1067 Peachtree Street, Louisville, GA, Zip 30434; tel. 912/625–7000; Rita Culvern, Administrator

JOHN D. ARCHBOLD MEMORIAL HOSPITAL, 910 South Broad Street, Thomasville, GA, Zip 31792, Mailing Address: P.O. Box 1018, Zip 31799; tel. 912/228–2000; Jason H. Moore, President and Chief Executive Officer

KENNESTONE HOSPITAL, 677 Church Street, Marietta, GA, Zip 30060; tel. 770/793–5000; Thomas E. Hill, Chief Executive Officer

LIBERTY REGIONAL MEDICAL CENTER, 112 East Oglethorpe Boulevard, Hinesville, GA, Zip 31313, Mailing Address: Box 919, Zip 31313; tel. 912/369–9400; H. Scott Kroell, Jr., Chief Executive Officer

MCDUFFIE COUNTY HOSPITAL, 521 Hill Street S.W., Thomson, GA, Zip 30824; tel. 706/595–1411; Douglas C. Keir, Chief Executive Officer

MEDICAL CENTER OF CENTRAL GEORGIA, 777 Hemlock Street, Macon, GA, Zip 31201, Mailing Address: Box 6000, Zip 31208; tel. 912/633–1000; A. Donald Faulk, FACHE, President

MINNIE G. BOSWELL MEMORIAL HOSPITAL, 1201 Siloam Highway, Greensboro, GA, Zip 30642, Mailing Address: P.O. Box 329, Zip 30642; tel. 706/453–7331; Larry W. Anderson, Administrator

MITCHELL COUNTY HOSPITAL, 90 Stephens Street, Camilla, GA, Zip 31730, Mailing Address: P.O. Box 639, Zip 31730; tel. 912/336–5284; Ronald M. Gilliard, FACHE, Administrator

MONROE COUNTY HOSPITAL, 88 Martin Luther King Jr. Drive, Forsyth, GA, Zip 31029, Mailing Address: Box 1068, Zip 31029–1068; tel. 912/994–2521; Gale V. Tanner, Administrator

NORTHEAST GEORGIA MEDICAL CENTER, 743 Spring Street N.E., Gainesville, GA, Zip 30501–3899; tel. 770/535–3553; Henry Rigdon, Executive Vice President

NORTHSIDE HOSPITAL, 1000 Johnson Ferry Road N.E., Atlanta, GA, Zip 30342–1611; tel. 404/851–8000; Sidney Kirschner, President and Chief Executive Officer

OCONEE REGIONAL MEDICAL CENTER, 821 North Cobb Street, Milledgeville, GA, Zip 31061, Mailing Address: Box 690, Zip 31061; tel. 912/454–3500; Brian L. Riddle, Chief Executive Officer

PEACH REGIONAL MEDICAL CENTER, 601 North Camellia Boulevard, Fort Valley, GA, Zip 31030–4599; tel. 912/825–8691; Nancy Peed, Administrator

PERRY HOSPITAL, 1120 Morningside Drive, Perry, GA, Zip 31069, Mailing Address: Drawer 1004, Zip 31069–1004; tel. 912/987–3600; Nadine L. Weems, Administrator

PHENIX REGIONAL HOSPITAL, 1707 21st Avenue, Phenix City, AL, Zip 36867, Mailing Address: Box 190, Zip 36868–0190; tel. 334/291–8502; Lance B. Duke, FACHE, President and Chief Executive Officer

PHOEBE PUTNEY MEMORIAL HOSPITAL, 417 Third Avenue, Albany, GA, Zip 31701–1828, Mailing Address: P.O. Box 1828, Zip 31703–1828; tel. 912/883–1800; Joel Wernick, President and Chief Executive Officer

PIEDMONT HOSPITAL, 1968 Peachtree Road N.W., Atlanta, GA, Zip 30309–1231; tel. 404/605–5000; Richard B. Hubbard, III, President and Chief Executive Officer

PROMINA COBB HOSPITAL, 3950 Austell Road, Austell, GA, Zip 30001–1121; tel. 770/732–4000; Betty Whisenant, Site Manager

PROMINA DOUGLAS HOSPITAL, 8954 Hospital Drive, Douglasville, GA, Zip 30134–2282; tel. 770/949–1500; Tom Hill, Chief Executive Officer

PROMINA PAULDING MEMORIAL MEDICAL CENTER, 600 West Memorial Drive, Dallas, GA, Zip 30132–1335; tel. 770/445–4411; T. Mark Haney, Administrator

PROMINA WINDY HILL HOSPITAL, 2540 Windy Hill Road, Marietta, GA, Zip 30067; tel. 770/644–1000; T. Mark Haney, Administrator

PUTNAM GENERAL HOSPITAL, Lake Oconee Parkway, Eatonton, GA, Zip 31024–4330, Mailing Address: Box 4330, Zip 31024–4330; tel. 706/485–2711; Darrell M. Oglesby, Administrator

SHEPHERD CENTER, 2020 Peachtree Road N.W., Atlanta, GA, Zip 30309–1465; tel. 404/352–2020; Gary R. Ulicny, Ph.D., President and Chief Executive Officer

SOUTH FULTON MEDICAL CENTER, 1170 Cleveland Avenue, East Point, GA, Zip 30344; tel. 404/305–3500; H. Neil Copelan, President and Chief Executive Officer

SOUTH GEORGIA MEDICAL CENTER, 2501 North Patterson Street, Valdosta, GA, Zip 31602, Mailing Address: Box 1727, Zip 31603–1727; tel. 912/333–1000; John S. Bowling, President and Chief Executive Officer

SOUTHWEST GEORGIA REGIONAL MEDICAL CENTER, 109 Randolph Street, Cuthbert, GA, Zip 31740–1338; tel. 912/732–2181; Earnest E. Benton, Chief Executive Officer

TAYLOR REGIONAL HOSPITAL, Macon Highway, Hawkinsville, GA, Zip 31036; tel. 912/783–0200; Dan S. Maddock, President

THE MEDICAL CENTER, 710 Center Street, Columbus, GA, Zip 31902, Mailing Address: Box 951, Zip 31902; tel. 706/571–1000; Lance B. Duke, FACHE, President and Chief Executive Officer

UNIVERSITY HOSPITAL, 1350 Walton Way, Augusta, GA, Zip 30901–2629; tel. 706/722–9011; Donald C. Bray, President and Chief Executive Officer

UPSON REGIONAL MEDICAL CENTER, 801 West Gordon Street, Thomaston, GA, Zip 30286–2831, Mailing Address: Box 1059, Zip 30286; tel. 706/647–8111; Samuel S. Gregory, Administrator

WILLINGWAY HOSPITAL, 311 Jones Mill Road, Statesboro, GA, Zip 30458; tel. 912/764–6236; Jimmy Mooney, Chief Executive Officer

UNIVERSITY HEALTH, INC.
1350 Walton Way, Augusta, GA 30901;
tel. 706/722–9011; Donald C. Bray, President

BARNWELL COUNTY HOSPITAL, Reynolds and Wren Streets, Barnwell, SC, Zip 29812, Mailing Address: Box 588, Zip 29812–0588; tel. 803/259–1000; Tommy R. McDougal, Jr., Administrator and Chief Executive Officer

BURKE COUNTY HOSPITAL, 351 Liberty Street, Waynesboro, GA, Zip 30830; tel. 706/554–4435; Gloria Cochran, Administrator

EDGEFIELD COUNTY HOSPITAL, Bausket Street, Edgefield, SC, Zip 29824, Mailing Address: Box 590, Zip 29824–0590; tel. 803/637–3174; W. Joseph Seel, Administrator

EMANUEL COUNTY HOSPITAL, 117 Kite Road, Swainsboro, GA, Zip 30401, Mailing Address: P.O. Box 879, Zip 30401; tel. 912/237–9911; Richard W. Clarke, Chief Executive Officer

JEFFERSON HOSPITAL, 1067 Peachtree Street, Louisville, GA, Zip 30434; tel. 912/625–7000; Rita Culvern, Administrator

MCDUFFIE COUNTY HOSPITAL, 521 Hill Street S.W., Thomson, GA, Zip 30824; tel. 706/595–1411; Douglas C. Keir, Chief Executive Officer

MINNIE G. BOSWELL MEMORIAL HOSPITAL, 1201 Siloam Highway, Greensboro, GA, Zip 30642, Mailing Address: P.O. Box 329, Zip 30642; tel. 706/453–7331; Larry W. Anderson, Administrator

UNIVERSITY HOSPITAL, 1350 Walton Way, Augusta, GA, Zip 30901–2629; tel. 706/722–9011; Donald C. Bray, President and Chief Executive Officer

WILLS MEMORIAL HOSPITAL, 120 Gordon Street, Washington, GA, Zip 30673, Mailing Address: Box 370, Zip 30673–0370; tel. 706/678–2151; Vincent DiFranco, Chief Executive Officer

HAWAII

PACIFIC HEALTH CARE
1946 Young Street, Honolulu, HI 96826; tel. 808/547–9712; Gary Kajiwara, President & Chief Executive Officer

KUAKINI MEDICAL CENTER, 347 North Kuakini Street, Honolulu, HI, Zip 96817–2381; tel. 808/536–2236; Gary K. Kajiwara, President and Chief Executive Officer

ST. FRANCIS MEDICAL CENTER, 2230 Liliha Street, Honolulu, HI, Zip 96817–9979, Mailing Address: P.O. Box 30100, Zip 96820–0100; tel. 808/547–6011; Cynthia Okinaka, Administrator

QUEENS HEALTH SYSTEMS
1301 Punchbowl Street, Honolulu, HI 96813; tel. 808/532–6100; Richard Griffith, President & Chief Executive Officer

MOLOKAI GENERAL HOSPITAL, Kaunakakai, HI, Mailing Address: P.O. Box 408, Zip 96748–0408; tel. 808/553–5331; Calvin M. Ichinose, Administrator

QUEEN'S MEDICAL CENTER, 1301 Punchbowl Street, Honolulu, HI, Zip 96813; tel. 808/538–9011; Arthur A. Ushijima, President and Chief Executive Officer

IDAHO

NORTH IDAHO RURAL HEALTH CONSORTIUM
700 Ironwood Drive, Suite 220, Coeur d'Alene, ID 83814; tel. 208/666–3863; Carol Wilson, Program Coordinator

BENEWAH COMMUNITY HOSPITAL, 229 South Seventh Street, Saint Maries, ID, Zip 83861; tel. 208/245–5551; Camille Scott, Administrator

BONNER GENERAL HOSPITAL, 520 North Third Avenue, Sandpoint, ID, Zip 83864–0877, Mailing Address: Box 1448, Zip 83864–0877; tel. 208/263–1441; Gene Tomt, FACHE, Chief Executive Officer

BOUNDARY COMMUNITY HOSPITAL, 6640 Kaniksu Street, Bonners Ferry, ID, Zip 83805, Mailing Address: HCR 61, Box 61A, Zip 83805; tel. 208/267–3141; William T. McClintock, FACHE, Chief Executive Officer

KOOTENAI MEDICAL CENTER, 2003 Lincoln Way, Coeur D'Alene, ID, Zip 83814; tel. 208/666–2000; Joe Morris, Chief Executive Officer

SHOSHONE MEDICAL CENTER, 3 Jacobs Gulch, Kellogg, ID, Zip 83837–2096; tel. 208/784–1221; Robert A. Morasko, Chief Executive Officer

SOUTH CENTRAL HEALTH NETWORK
P.O. Box 547, Twin Falls, ID 83303; tel. 208/734–5900; Connie Perry, Project Coordinator

GOODING COUNTY MEMORIAL HOSPITAL, 1120 Montana Street, Gooding, ID, Zip 83330; tel. 208/934–4433; Kenneth W. Archer, Administrator

MAGIC VALLEY REGIONAL MEDICAL CENTER, 650 Addison Avenue West, Twin Falls, ID, Zip 83301, Mailing Address: Box 409, Zip 83303–0409; tel. 208/737–2000; John Bingham, Administrator

MINIDOKA MEMORIAL HOSPITAL AND EXTENDED CARE FACILITY, 1224 Eighth Street, Rupert, ID, Zip 83350; tel. 208/436–0481; Randall G. Holom, Administrator

ST. BENEDICTS FAMILY MEDICAL CENTER, 709 North Lincoln Avenue, Jerome, ID, Zip 83338, Mailing Address: Box 586, Zip 83338–0586; tel. 208/324–4301; David Farnes, Administrator

TWIN FALLS CLINIC HOSPITAL, 666 Shoshone Street East, Twin Falls, ID, Zip 83301, Mailing Address: Box 1233, Zip 83301; tel. 208/733–3700; Marley D. Jackman, Administrator

WOOD RIVER MEDICAL CENTER, Sun Valley Road, Sun Valley, ID, Zip 83353, Mailing Address: P.O. Box 86, Zip 83353; tel. 208/622–3333; Alan Stevenson, Administrator

ILLINOIS

ADVOCATE HEALTH CARE
2025 Windsor Drive, Oak Brook, IL 60521–0222; tel. 708/572–9393; Richard R. Risk, President & Chief Executive Officer

BETHANY HOSPITAL, 3435 West Van Buren, Chicago, IL, Zip 60624; tel. 773/265–7700; Lena L. Shields, Chief Executive

CHRIST HOSPITAL AND MEDICAL CENTER, 4440 West 95th Street, Oak Lawn, IL, Zip 60453–2699; tel. 708/425–8000; Carol Schneider, Chief Executive

GOOD SAMARITAN HOSPITAL, 3815 Highland Avenue, Downers Grove, IL, Zip 60515; tel. 630/275–5900; David M. McConkey, Chief Executive

GOOD SHEPHERD HOSPITAL, 450 West Highway 22, Barrington, IL, Zip 60010–1999; tel. 847/381–9600; Russell E. Feurer, Chief Executive

LUTHERAN GENERAL HOSPITAL, 1775 Dempster Street, Park Ridge, IL, Zip 60068–1174; tel. 847/723–2210; Kenneth J. Rojek, Chief Executive

RAVENSWOOD HOSPITAL MEDICAL CENTER, 4550 North Winchester Avenue, Chicago, IL, Zip 60640–5205; tel. 773/878–4300; John E. Blair, President

SOUTH SUBURBAN HOSPITAL, 17800 South Kedzie Avenue, Hazel Crest, IL, Zip 60429; tel. 708/799–8000; Robert Rutkowski, Chief Executive

TRINITY MEDICAL CENTER–WEST CAMPUS, 2701 17th Street, Rock Island, IL, Zip 61201; tel. 309/757–3822; Eric Crowell, President and Chief Executive Officer

ALEXIAN BROTHERS HEALTH SYSTEM, INC.
600 Alexian Way, Elk Grove Village, IL 60007; tel. 847/640–7550; Brother Felix Bettendorf, President

ALEXIAN BROTHERS MEDICAL CENTER, 800 Biesterfield Road, Elk Grove Village, IL, Zip 60007–3397; tel. 847/437–5500; Brother Philip Kennedy, President and Chief Executive Officer

CATHOLIC HEALTH PARTNERS
2520 North Lakeview Avenue, Chicago, IL 60614; tel. 312/883–7300; Lee Domanico, Chief Exectve Officer

COLUMBUS HOSPITAL, 2520 North Lakeview Avenue, Chicago, IL, Zip 60614; tel. 773/883–7300; Sister Theresa Peck, President and Chief Executive Officer

SAINT ANTHONY HOSPITAL, 2875 West 19th Street, Chicago, IL, Zip 60623; tel. 773/521–1710; Sister Theresa Peck, President and Chief Executive Officer

ST. JOSEPH HOSPITAL, 2900 North Lake Shore Drive, Chicago, IL, Zip 60657–6274; tel. 773/665–3000; Sister Theresa Peck, President and Chief Executive Officer

CENTEGRA HEALTH SYSTEM
4309 Medical Center Drive, Suite B202, McHenry, IL 60090; tel. 815/759–8100; Gail Bumgarner, Vice President

MEMORIAL MEDICAL CENTER, Highway 14 and Doty Road, Woodstock, IL, Zip 60098–3797, Mailing Address: P.O. Box 1990, Zip 60098; tel. 815/338–2500; Jim D. Redding, Chief Executive Officer

NORTHERN ILLINOIS MEDICAL CENTER, 4201 Medical Center Drive, McHenry, IL, Zip 60050–9506; tel. 815/344–5000; Jim D. Redding, Chief Executive Officer

FAMILY HEALTH NETWORK, INC.
910 W. Van Buren – 6th Floor, Chicago, IL 60607; tel. 312/491–1956; Mary Ader, Vice President of Provider Services

COLUMBUS HOSPITAL, 2520 North Lakeview Avenue, Chicago, IL, Zip 60614; tel. 773/883–7300; Sister Theresa Peck, President and Chief Executive Officer

MOUNT SINAI HOSPITAL MEDICAL CENTER OF CHICAGO, California Avenue and 15th Street, Chicago, IL, Zip 60608–1610; tel. 312/542–2000; Benn Greenspan, President and Chief Executive Officer

NORWEGIAN–AMERICAN HOSPITAL, 1044 North Francisco Avenue, Chicago, IL, Zip 60622; tel. 773/292–8200; Clarence A. Nagelvoort, President and Chief Executive Officer

SAINT ANTHONY HOSPITAL, 2875 West 19th Street, Chicago, IL, Zip 60623; tel. 773/521–1710; Sister Theresa Peck, President and Chief Executive Officer

SCHWAB REHABILITATION HOSPITAL AND CARE NETWORK, 1401 South California Boulevard, Chicago, IL, Zip 60608–1612; tel. 773/522–2010; Kathleen C. Yosko, President and Chief Executive Officer

ST. BERNARD HOSPITAL AND HEALTH CARE CENTER, 64th & Dan Ryan Expressway, Chicago, IL, Zip 60621; tel. 773/962–3900; Sister Elizabeth Van Straten, President and Chief Executive Officer

ST. ELIZABETH'S HOSPITAL, 1431 North Claremont Avenue, Chicago, IL, Zip 60622; tel. 773/278–2000; JoAnn Birdzell, President and Chief Executive Officer

ST. JOSEPH HOSPITAL, 2900 North Lake Shore Drive, Chicago, IL, Zip 60657–6274; tel. 773/665–3000; Sister Theresa Peck, President and Chief Executive Officer

FELICIAN HEALTH CARE, INC.
3800 Peterson Avenue, Chicago, IL 60659; tel. 414/647–5622; Sister Mary Clarette, CSSF

ST. FRANCIS HOSPITAL, 3237 South 16th Street, Milwaukee, WI, Zip 53215–4592; tel. 414/647–5000; Gregory A. Banaszynski, President

ST. MARY'S HOSPITAL, 400 North Pleasant Avenue, Centralia, IL, Zip 62801–3091; tel. 618/532–6731; James W. McDowell, President and Chief Executive Officer

FREEPORT REGIONAL HEALTH PLAN
1045 West Stephenson Street, Freeport, IL 61032; tel. 815/235–0272; Shelly Dunham, Provider and Member Service Coordinator

FREEPORT MEMORIAL HOSPITAL, 1045 West Stephenson Street, Freeport, IL, Zip 61032; tel. 815/235–4131; Joseph E. Bonnett, Executive Vice President and Chief Executive Officer

MEDACOM TRI–STATE
1315 West 22nd Street, Suite 300, Oakbrook, IL 60521; tel. 630/954–1880; Elizabeth Kerr, Network Coordinator

BETHANY HOSPITAL, 3435 West Van Buren, Chicago, IL, Zip 60624; tel. 773/265–7700; Lena L. Shields, Chief Executive

CHRIST HOSPITAL AND MEDICAL CENTER, 4440 West 95th Street, Oak Lawn, IL, Zip 60453–2699; tel. 708/425–8000; Carol Schneider, Chief Executive

COLUMBIA LA GRANGE MEMORIAL HOSPITAL, 5101 South Willow Springs Road, La Grange, IL, Zip 60525–2680; tel. 708/352–1200; Cathleen D. Biga, President and Chief Executive Officer

DELNOR–COMMUNITY HOSPITAL, 300 Randall Road, Geneva, IL, Zip 60134–4200; tel. 630/208–3000; Craig A. Livermore, President and Chief Executive Officer

GENESIS MEDICAL CENTER, 1227 East Rusholme Street, Davenport, IA, Zip 52803; tel. 319/421–6000; Leo A. Bressanelli, President and Chief Executive Officer

GOOD SAMARITAN HOSPITAL, 3815 Highland Avenue, Downers Grove, IL, Zip 60515; tel. 630/275–5900; David M. McConkey, Chief Executive

GOOD SAMARITAN REGIONAL HEALTH CENTER, 605 North 12th Street, Mount Vernon, IL, Zip 62864; tel. 618/242–4600; Leo F. Childers, Jr., FACHE, President

GOOD SHEPHERD HOSPITAL, 450 West Highway 22, Barrington, IL, Zip 60010–1999; tel. 847/381–9600; Russell E. Feurer, Chief Executive

LOYOLA UNIVERSITY MEDICAL CENTER, 2160 South First Avenue, Maywood, IL, Zip 60153–5585; tel. 708/216–9000; Anthony L. Barbato, M.D., President and Chief Executive Officer

SAINT JOSEPH HOSPITAL, 77 North Airlite Street, Elgin, IL, Zip 60123–4912; tel. 847/695–3200; Larry Narum, President and Chief Executive Officer

SAINT JOSEPH MEDICAL CENTER, 333 North Madison Street, Joliet, IL, Zip 60435–6595; tel. 815/741–7236; David W. Benfer, President and Chief Executive Officer

SAINT THERESE MEDICAL CENTER, 2615 Washington Street, Waukegan, IL, Zip 60085–4988; tel. 847/249–3900; Timothy P. Selz, President

SOUTH SUBURBAN HOSPITAL, 17800 South Kedzie Avenue, Hazel Crest, IL, Zip 60429; tel. 708/799–8000; Robert Rutkowski, Chief Executive

ST. FRANCIS HOSPITAL AND HEALTH CENTER, 12935 South Gregory Street, Blue Island, IL, Zip 60406–2470; tel. 708/597–2000; Jay E. Kreuzer, President

ST. JAMES HOSPITAL AND HEALTH CENTERS, 1423 Chicago Road, Chicago Heights, IL, Zip 60411–9934; tel. 708/756–1000; Peter J. Murphy, President and Chief Executive Officer

ST. MARYS HOSPITAL MEDICAL CENTER, 707 South Mills Street, Madison, WI, Zip 53715–0450; tel. 608/251–6100; Gerald W. Lefert, President

SWEDISHAMERICAN HOSPITAL, 1400 Charles Street, Rockford, IL, Zip 61104–2298; tel. 815/968–4400; Robert B. Klint, M.D., President

TRINITY HOSPITAL, 2320 East 93rd Street, Chicago, IL, Zip 60617; tel. 773/978–2000; John N. Schwartz, Chief Executive Officer

UNITED SAMARITANS MEDICAL CENTER, 812 North Logan, Danville, IL, Zip 61832–3788; tel. 217/442–6300; Dennis J. Doran, President and Chief Executive Officer

MERCER COUNTY COMMUNITY CARE NETWORK
409 NorthWest Ninth Avenue, Aledo, IL 61231; tel. 309/582–5301; Bruce D. Peterson, Administrator

MERCER COUNTY HOSPITAL, 409 N.W. Ninth Avenue, Aledo, IL, Zip 61231; tel. 309/582–5301; Bruce D. Peterson, Administrator

NORTHWESTERN HEALTH CARE NETWORK
980 North Michigan Avenue, Suite 1500, Chicago, IL 60611; tel. 312/335–6000; Amy Kosifas, Assistant Vice President–Planning

CHILDREN'S MEMORIAL HOSPITAL, 2300 Children's Plaza, Chicago, IL, Zip 60614; tel. 773/880–4000; Jan R. Jennings, President and Chief Executive Officer

EVANSTON HOSPITAL, 2650 Ridge Avenue, Evanston, IL, Zip 60201; tel. 847/570–2000; Mark R. Neaman, President and Chief Executive Officer

HIGHLAND PARK HOSPITAL, 718 Glenview Avenue, Highland Park, IL, Zip 60035–2497; tel. 847/432–8000; Ronald G. Spaeth, President and Chief Executive Officer

INGALLS MEMORIAL HOSPITAL, One Ingalls Drive, Harvey, IL, Zip 60426–3591; tel. 708/333–2300; Robert L. Harris, President and Chief Executive Officer

NORTHWEST COMMUNITY HOSPITAL, 800 West Central Road, Arlington Heights, IL, Zip 60005–2392; tel. 847/618–1000; Bruce K. Crowther, President and Chief Executive Officer

NORTHWESTERN MEMORIAL HOSPITAL, Superior Street and Fairbanks Court, Chicago, IL, Zip 60611–2950; tel. 312/908–2000; Gary A. Mecklenburg, President and Chief Executive Officer

SILVER CROSS HOSPITAL, 1200 Maple Road, Joliet, IL, Zip 60432; tel. 815/740–1100; Paul Pawlak, President

SWEDISH COVENANT HOSPITAL, 5145 North California Avenue, Chicago, IL, Zip 60625–3688; tel. 773/878–8200; Edward A. Cucci, President

RUSH SYSTEM FOR HEALTH
1725 West Congress Parkway, Chicago, IL 60612; tel. 312/942–7091; Avery S. Miller, Vice President

COPLEY MEMORIAL HOSPITAL, 2000 Ogden Avenue, Aurora, IL, Zip 60504–4206; tel. 630/978–6200; D. Chet McKee, President

HOLY FAMILY MEDICAL CENTER, 100 North River Road, Des Plaines, IL, Zip 60016; tel. 847/297–1800; Sister Patricia Ann Koschalke, President and Chief Executive Officer

ILLINOIS MASONIC MEDICAL CENTER, 836 West Wellington Avenue, Chicago, IL, Zip 60657–5193; tel. 773/975–1600; Bruce C. Campbell, President

LAKE FOREST HOSPITAL, 660 North Westmoreland Road, Lake Forest, IL, Zip 60045–1696; tel. 847/234–5600; William G. Ries, President

OAK PARK HOSPITAL, 520 South Maple Avenue, Oak Park, IL, Zip 60304–1097; tel. 708/383–9300; Leonard J. Muller, President

RIVERSIDE HEALTHCARE, 350 North Wall Street, Kankakee, IL, Zip 60901–0749; tel. 815/933–1671; Dennis C. Millirons, President and Chief Executive Officer

RUSH NORTH SHORE MEDICAL CENTER, 9600 Gross Point Road, Skokie, IL, Zip 60076–1257; tel. 847/677–9600; John S. Frigo, President

RUSH–PRESBYTERIAN–ST. LUKE'S MEDICAL CENTER, 1653 West Congress Parkway, Chicago, IL, Zip 60612–3833; tel. 312/942–5000; Leo M. Henikoff, President and Chief Executive Officer

WESTLAKE COMMUNITY HOSPITAL, 1225 Lake Street, Melrose Park, IL, Zip 60160; tel. 708/681–3000; David R. Hey, Chief Operating Officer

SERVANTCOR
335 East Fifth Avenue, Clifton, IL 60927; tel. 815/937–2034; Joseph F. Feth, President

CENTRAL COMMUNITY HOSPITAL, 335 East Fifth Avenue, Clifton, IL, Zip 60927, Mailing Address: Box 68, Zip 60927; tel. 815/694–2392; Steve Wilder, President and Chief Executive Officer

COVENANT MEDICAL CENTER, 1400 West Park Street, Urbana, IL, Zip 61801; tel. 217/337–2000; Joseph W. Beard, President and Chief Executive Officer

ST. MARY'S HOSPITAL, 500 West Court Street, Kankakee, IL, Zip 60901; tel. 815/937–2400; Allan C. Sonduck, President and Chief Executive Officer

SWEDISHAMERICAN HEALTH SYSTEM
1313 East State Street, Rockford, IL 61104; tel. 815/968–4400; Thomas Myers, Vice President–Marketing

SWEDISHAMERICAN HOSPITAL, 1400 Charles Street, Rockford, IL, Zip 61104–2298; tel. 815/968–4400; Robert B. Klint, M.D., President

SYNERGON HEALTH SYSTEM
520 South Maple Avenue, Oak Park, IL 60304; tel. 708/660–2060; Julie Stasiak, Director of Planning

OAK PARK HOSPITAL, 520 South Maple Avenue, Oak Park, IL, Zip 60304–1097; tel. 708/383–9300; Leonard J. Muller, President

WESTLAKE COMMUNITY HOSPITAL, 1225 Lake Street, Melrose Park, IL, Zip 60160; tel. 708/681–3000; David R. Hey, Chief Operating Officer

THE CARLE FOUNDATION
611 West Park Street, Urbana, IL 61801; tel. 217/383–3311; Karen Shelby, Network Contact

CARLE FOUNDATION HOSPITAL, 611 West Park Street, Urbana, IL, Zip 61801–2595; tel. 217/383–3311; Michael H. Fritz, President

THE PAVILION, 809 West Church Street, Champaign, IL, Zip 61820; tel. 217/373–1700; Nina W. Eisner, Chief Executive Officer

UNIFIED HEALTH CARE NETWORK
2160 South 1st Avenue, Building 105, Room 3922, Maywood, IL 60153; tel. 708/216–9190; Burton VanderLaan, M.D., President

LOYOLA UNIVERSITY MEDICAL CENTER, 2160 South First Avenue, Maywood, IL, Zip 60153–5585; tel. 708/216–9000; Anthony L. Barbato, M.D., President and Chief Executive Officer

OUR LADY OF THE RESURRECTION MEDICAL CENTER, 5645 West Addison Street, Chicago, IL, Zip 60634–4455; tel. 312/282–7000; John Sullivan, Chief Executive Officer

RESURRECTION MEDICAL CENTER, 7435 West Talcott Avenue, Chicago, IL, Zip 60631–3746; tel. 773/774–8000; Sister Donna Marie, Chief Executive Officer

SAINT FRANCIS MEDICAL CENTER, 530 N.E. Glen Oak Avenue, Peoria, IL, Zip 61637; tel. 309/655–2000; Sister M. Canisia, Administrator

SAINT JAMES HOSPITAL, 610 East Water Street, Pontiac, IL, Zip 61764; tel. 815/842–2828; David Ochs, Administrator

SAINT MARY OF NAZARETH HOSPITAL CENTER, 2233 West Division Street, Chicago, IL, Zip 60622–3086; tel. 312/770–2000; Sister Stella Louise, President and Chief Executive Officer

ST. BERNARD HOSPITAL AND HEALTH CARE CENTER, 64th & Dan Ryan Expressway, Chicago, IL, Zip 60621; tel. 773/962–3900; Sister Elizabeth Van Straten, President and Chief Executive Officer

UNIVERSITY OF CHICAGO HOSPITALS & HEALTH SYSTEM
5841 South Maryland Avenue, Chicago, IL 60637; tel. 773/702–1000; Ralph Muller, President

LOUIS A. WEISS MEMORIAL HOSPITAL, 4646 North Marine Drive, Chicago, IL, Zip 60640–1501; tel. 773/878–8700; Gregory A. Cierlik, President and Chief Executive Officer

UNIVERSITY OF CHICAGO HOSPITALS, 5841 South Maryland, Chicago, IL, Zip 60637–1470; tel. 773/702–1000; Ralph W. Muller, President

INDIANA

ANCILLA SYSTEMS, INC.
1000 South Lake Park Avenue, Hobart, IN 46342; tel. 219/947–8500; William D. Harkins, President

COMMUNITY HOSPITAL OF BREMEN, 411 South Whitlock Street, Bremen, IN, Zip 46506–1699; tel. 219/546–2211; Scott R. Graybill, Administrator and Chief Executive Officer

ST. CATHERINE HOSPITAL, 4321 Fir Street, East Chicago, IN, Zip 46312; tel. 219/392–7000; JoAnn Birdzell, President and Chief Executive Officer

ST. JOSEPH COMMUNITY HOSPITAL, 215 West Fourth Street, Mishawaka, IN, Zip 46544; tel. 219/259–2431; Stephen L. Crain, President and Chief Executive Officer

ST. JOSEPH MEDICAL CENTER OF FORT WAYNE, 700 Broadway, Fort Wayne, IN, Zip 46802; tel. 219/425–3000; John T. Farrell, Sr., President and Chief Executive Officer

ST. MARY COMMUNITY HOSPITAL, 2515 East Jefferson Boulevard, South Bend, IN, Zip 46615–2691; tel. 219/288–8311; Stephen L. Crain, President

ST. MARY'S MEDICAL CENTER OF EVANSVILLE, 3700 Washington Avenue, Evansville, IN, Zip 47750; tel. 812/485–4000; Richard C. Breon, President and Chief Executive Officer

HEALTH QUEST
One Caylor–Nickel Square, Bluffton, IN 46714; tel. 219/824–3500; William F. Brockman, Chief Executive Officer

CAYLOR–NICKEL MEDICAL CENTER, One Caylor–Nickel Square, Bluffton, IN, Zip 46714; tel. 219/824–3500; William F. Brockmann, President and Chief Executive Officer

JAY COUNTY HOSPITAL, 500 West Votaw Street, Portland, IN, Zip 47371–1322; tel. 219/726–7131; Thomas J. Valerius, Chief Executive Officer

RANDOLPH COUNTY HOSPITAL, 325 South Oak Street, Winchester, IN, Zip 47394, Mailing Address: P.O. Box 407, Zip 47394; tel. 765/584–9001; James M. Full, Chief Executive Officer

HOLY CROSS HEALTH SYSTEM
3606 East Jefferson Boulevard, South Bend, IN 46615–3097; tel. 219/233–8558; Sister Pat Vandenburg, President & Chief Executive Officer

SAINT JOHN'S HEALTH SYSTEM, 2015 Jackson Street, Anderson, IN, Zip 46016–4339; tel. 765/649–2511; James H. Stephens, President and Chief Executive Officer

ST. JOSEPH'S HOSPITAL OF MARSHALL COUNTY, 1915 Lake Avenue, Plymouth, IN, Zip 46563–9905, Mailing Address: P.O. Box 670, Zip 46563–9905; tel. 219/936–3181; Brian E. Dietz, President

ST. JOSEPH'S MEDICAL CENTER, 801 East LaSalle, South Bend, IN, Zip 46617, Mailing Address: Box 1935, Zip 46634; tel. 219/237–7111; Brian E. Dietz, Interim Chief Executive Officer

LUTHERANPREFERRED NETWORK
7950 West Jefferson Boulevard, Fort Wayne, IN 46804; tel. 219/435–7001; Michael Schatzlein, Vice President

ADAMS COUNTY MEMORIAL HOSPITAL, 805 High Street, Decatur, IN, Zip 46733, Mailing Address: P.O. Box 151, Zip 46733; tel. 219/724–2145; Marvin L. Baird, Executive Director

BLACKFORD COUNTY HOSPITAL, 503 East Van Cleve Street, Hartford City, IN, Zip 47348; tel. 765/348–0300; Mark A. Edwards, Chief Executive Officer

CAMERON MEMORIAL COMMUNITY HOSPITAL, 416 East Maumee Street, Angola, IN, Zip 46703; tel. 219/665–2141; Dennis L. Knapp, President

CAYLOR–NICKEL MEDICAL CENTER, One Caylor–Nickel Square, Bluffton, IN, Zip 46714; tel. 219/824–3500; William F. Brockmann, President and Chief Executive Officer

COMMUNITY MEMORIAL HOSPITAL, 208 North Columbus Street, Hicksville, OH, Zip 43526–1299; tel. 419/542–6692; Deryl E. Gulliford, Ph.D., Administrator

DEFIANCE HOSPITAL, 1206 East Second Street, Defiance, OH, Zip 43512–2495; tel. 419/783–6955; Richard C. Sommer, Administrator

DEKALB MEMORIAL HOSPITAL, 1316 East Seventh Street, Auburn, IN, Zip 46706–0542, Mailing Address: P.O. Box 542, Zip 46706; tel. 219/925–4600; Jack M. Corey, President

DUKES MEMORIAL HOSPITAL, Grant and Boulevard, Peru, IN, Zip 46970–1698; tel. 765/473–6621; R. Joe Johnston, President and Chief Executive Officer

HUNTINGTON MEMORIAL HOSPITAL, 1215 Etna Avenue, Huntington, IN, Zip 46750–3696; tel. 219/356–3000; L. Kent McCoy, President

INDIANA UNIVERSITY MEDICAL CENTER, 550 North University Boulevard, Indianapolis, IN, Zip 46202–5262; tel. 317/274–5000; David J. Handel, Director

JAY COUNTY HOSPITAL, 500 West Votaw Street, Portland, IN, Zip 47371–1322; tel. 219/726–7131; Thomas J. Valerius, Chief Executive Officer

KOSCIUSKO COMMUNITY HOSPITAL, 2101 East Dubois Drive, Warsaw, IN, Zip 46580; tel. 219/267–3200; Wayne Hendrix, President

LUTHERAN HOSPITAL OF INDIANA, 7950 West Jefferson Boulevard, Fort Wayne, IN, Zip 46804–1677; tel. 219/435–7001; William L. Anderson, Chief Executive Officer

MCCRAY MEMORIAL HOSPITAL, 951 East Hospital Drive, Kendallville, IN, Zip 46755, Mailing Address: P.O. Box 249, Zip 46755; tel. 219/347–1100; Peter A. Marotti, Chief Executive Officer

MERCER COUNTY JOINT TOWNSHIP COMMUNITY HOSPITAL, 800 West Main Street, Coldwater, OH, Zip 45828–1698; tel. 419/678–2341; James W. Isaacs, Chief Executive Officer

PAULDING COUNTY HOSPITAL, 11558 State Road 111, Paulding, OH, Zip 45879–9220; tel. 419/399–4080; Joseph M. Dorko, Chief Executive Officer

VAN WERT COUNTY HOSPITAL, 1250 South Washington Street, Van Wert, OH, Zip 45891–2599; tel. 419/238–2390; Mark J. Minick, President and Chief Executive Officer

WABASH COUNTY HOSPITAL, 710 North East Street, Wabash, IN, Zip 46992, Mailing Address: Box 548, Zip 46992–0548; tel. 219/563–3131; David C. Hunter, Chief Executive Officer

WELLS COMMUNITY HOSPITAL, 1100 South Main Street, Bluffton, IN, Zip 46714; tel. 219/824–3210; Martin P. Braaksma, Executive Director

MEMORIAL HEALTH SYSTEM, INC.
707 North Michigan Street, Suite 100, South Bend, IN 46601; tel. 219/284–3699; David Sage, Chief Operating Officer

ELKHART GENERAL HOSPITAL, 600 East Boulevard, Elkhart, IN, Zip 46514, Mailing Address: Box 1329, Zip 46515; tel. 219/294–2621; Gregory W. Lintjer, President

LA PORTE HOSPITAL, State and Madison Streets, La Porte, IN, Zip 46350–0250, Mailing Address: P.O. Box 250, Zip 46352–0250; tel. 219/326–1234; Leigh E. Morris, President

LUTHERAN HOSPITAL OF INDIANA, 7950 West Jefferson Boulevard, Fort Wayne, IN, Zip 46804–1677; tel. 219/435–7001; William L. Anderson, Chief Executive Officer

ST. JOSEPH COMMUNITY HOSPITAL, 215 West Fourth Street, Mishawaka, IN, Zip 46544; tel. 219/259–2431; Stephen L. Crain, President and Chief Executive Officer

METHODIST HOSPITAL OF INDIANA
P.O. Box 1367, Indianapolis, IN 46202; tel. 317/929–2000; William J. Loveday, President & Chief Executive Officer

METHODIST HOSPITAL OF INDIANA, 1701 North Senate Boulevard, Indianapolis, IN, Zip 46202, Mailing Address: I. 65 at 21st Street, P.O. Box 1367, Zip 46206–1367; tel. 317/929–2000; William J. Loveday, President and Chief Executive Officer

REHABILITATION HOSPITAL OF INDIANA, 4141 Shore Drive, Indianapolis, IN, Zip 46254–2607; tel. 317/329–2000; Kim D. Eicher, Administrator and Chief Executive Officer

MIDWEST HEALTH NET, LLC.
6202 Constitution Drive, Fort Wayne, IN 46804; tel. 219/436–7879; Thomas C. Henry, President

BEDFORD REGIONAL MEDICAL CENTER, 2900 West 16th Street, Bedford, IN, Zip 47421; tel. 812/275–1200; John R. Birdzell, FACHE, Chief Executive Officer

CAMERON MEMORIAL COMMUNITY HOSPITAL, 416 East Maumee Street, Angola, IN, Zip 46703; tel. 219/665–2141; Dennis L. Knapp, President

CAYLOR–NICKEL MEDICAL CENTER, One Caylor–Nickel Square, Bluffton, IN, Zip 46714; tel. 219/824–3500; William F. Brockmann, President and Chief Executive Officer

CLINTON COUNTY HOSPITAL, 1300 South Jackson Street, Frankfort, IN, Zip 46041–3394, Mailing Address: P.O. Box 669, Zip 46041–0669; tel. 765/659–4731; Brian R. Zeh, Executive Director

COMMUNITY HOSPITAL OF ANDERSON AND MADISON COUNTY, 1515 North Madison Avenue, Anderson, IN, Zip 46011–3453; tel. 765/642–8011; William C. Vanness, II, M.D., Chief Executive Officer

DECATUR COUNTY MEMORIAL HOSPITAL, 720 North Lincoln Street, Greensburg, IN, Zip 47240–1398; tel. 812/663–4331; Charles Duffy, President

DEKALB MEMORIAL HOSPITAL, 1316 East Seventh Street, Auburn, IN, Zip 46706–0542, Mailing Address: P.O. Box 542, Zip 46706; tel. 219/925–4600; Jack M. Corey, President

DOCTORS HOSPITAL OF JACKSON, 110 North Elm Avenue, Jackson, MI, Zip 49202–3595; tel. 517/787–1440; Michael J. Falatko, President and Chief Executive Officer

DUKES MEMORIAL HOSPITAL, Grant and Boulevard, Peru, IN, Zip 46970–1698; tel. 765/473–6621; R. Joe Johnston, President and Chief Executive Officer

FISHER–TITUS MEDICAL CENTER, 272 Benedict Avenue, Norwalk, OH, Zip 44857–2374; tel. 419/668–8101; Richard C. Westhofen, President

GREENE COUNTY GENERAL HOSPITAL, Rural Route 1, Box 1000, Linton, IN, Zip 47441–9457; tel. 812/847–2281; Jonas S. Uland, Executive Director

HANCOCK MEMORIAL HOSPITAL AND HEALTH SERVICES, 801 North State Street, Greenfield, IN, Zip 46140–2537, Mailing Address: Box 827, Zip 46140; tel. 317/462–5544; Robert C. Keen, Ph.D., President and Chief Executive Officer

HENRY COUNTY HOSPITAL, 11–600 State Road 424, Napoleon, OH, Zip 43545–9399; tel. 419/592–4015; Robert J. Coholich, Chief Executive Officer

HENRY COUNTY MEMORIAL HOSPITAL, 1000 North 16th Street, New Castle, IN, Zip 47362–4319, Mailing Address: Box 490, Zip 47362–0490; tel. 765/521–0890; Jack Basler, President

HOWARD COMMUNITY HOSPITAL, 3500 South La Fountain Street, Kokomo, IN, Zip 46904–9011; tel. 765/453–0702; James C. Bigogno, FACHE, President and Chief Executive Officer

HUNTINGTON MEMORIAL HOSPITAL, 1215 Etna Avenue, Huntington, IN, Zip 46750–3696; tel. 219/356–3000; L. Kent McCoy, President

JOHNSON MEMORIAL HOSPITAL, 1125 West Jefferson Street, Franklin, IN, Zip 46131–2140, Mailing Address: P.O. Box 549, Zip 46131–0549; tel. 317/736–3300; Gregg A. Bechtold, President and Chief Executive Officer

KOSCIUSKO COMMUNITY HOSPITAL, 2101 East Dubois Drive, Warsaw, IN, Zip 46580; tel. 219/267–3200; Wayne Hendrix, President

LIMA MEMORIAL HOSPITAL, 1001 Bellefontaine Avenue, Lima, OH, Zip 45804–2894; tel. 419/228–3335; John B. White, President and Chief Executive Officer

MCCRAY MEMORIAL HOSPITAL, 951 East Hospital Drive, Kendallville, IN, Zip 46755, Mailing Address: P.O. Box 249, Zip 46755; tel. 219/347–1100; Peter A. Marotti, Chief Executive Officer

MEDICAL COLLEGE HOSPITALS, 3000 Arlington Avenue, Toledo, OH, Zip 43699–0008, Mailing Address: P.O. Box 10008, Zip 43699–0008; tel. 419/381–4172; Richard C. Sipp, Vice President for Administration

MERCY MEMORIAL HOSPITAL, 740 North Macomb Street, Monroe, MI, Zip 48161–9974, Mailing Address: P.O. Box 67, Zip 48161–0067; tel. 313/241–1700; Richard S. Hiltz, President and Chief Executive Officer

METHODIST HOSPITAL OF INDIANA, 1701 North Senate Boulevard, Indianapolis, IN, Zip 46202, Mailing Address: I. 65 at 21st Street, P.O. Box 1367, Zip 46206–1367; tel. 317/929–2000; William J. Loveday, President and Chief Executive Officer

MORGAN COUNTY MEMORIAL HOSPITAL, 2209 John R. Wooden Drive, Martinsville, IN, Zip 46151, Mailing Address: P.O. Box 1717, Zip 46151; tel. 765/349–6501; S. Dean Melton, President and Chief Executive Officer

PARKVIEW MEMORIAL HOSPITAL, 2200 Randallia Drive, Fort Wayne, IN, Zip 46805; tel. 219/484–6636; Frank D. Byrne, M.D., President

PAULDING COUNTY HOSPITAL, 11558 State Road 111, Paulding, OH, Zip 45879–9220; tel. 419/399–4080; Joseph M. Dorko, Chief Executive Officer

RANDOLPH COUNTY HOSPITAL, 325 South Oak Street, Winchester, IN, Zip 47394, Mailing Address: P.O. Box 407, Zip 47394; tel. 765/584–9001; James M. Full, Chief Executive Officer

RIVERVIEW HOSPITAL, 395 Westfield Road, Noblesville, IN, Zip 46060–1425, Mailing Address: P.O. Box 220, Zip 46061–0220; tel. 317/773–0760; Seward Horner, President

ST. CATHERINE HOSPITAL, 4321 Fir Street, East Chicago, IN, Zip 46312; tel. 219/392–7000; JoAnn Birdzell, President and Chief Executive Officer

ST. ELIZABETH'S HOSPITAL, 1431 North Claremont Avenue, Chicago, IL, Zip 60622; tel. 773/278–2000; JoAnn Birdzell, President and Chief Executive Officer

ST. JOSEPH COMMUNITY HOSPITAL, 215 West Fourth Street, Mishawaka, IN, Zip 46544; tel. 219/259–2431; Stephen L. Crain, President and Chief Executive Officer

ST. JOSEPH MEDICAL CENTER OF FORT WAYNE, 700 Broadway, Fort Wayne, IN, Zip 46802; tel. 219/425–3000; John T. Farrell, Sr., President and Chief Executive Officer

ST. MARY COMMUNITY HOSPITAL, 2515 East Jefferson Boulevard, South Bend, IN, Zip 46615–2691; tel. 219/288–8311; Stephen L. Crain, President

ST. MARY MEDICAL CENTER, 1500 South Lake Park Avenue, Hobart, IN, Zip 46342; tel. 219/942–0551; Milton Triana, President and Chief Executive Officer

ST. MARY'S HOSPITAL, 129 North Eighth Street, East St. Louis, IL, Zip 62201–2999; tel. 618/274–1900; Richard J. Mark, President and Chief Executive Officer

THE TOLEDO HOSPITAL, 2142 North Cove Boulevard, Toledo, OH, Zip 43606–3896; tel. 419/471–4000; William W. Glover, President

TIPTON COUNTY MEMORIAL HOSPITAL, 1000 South Main Street, Tipton, IN, Zip 46072–9799; tel. 317/675–8500; Alfonso W. Gatmaitan, Chief Executive Officer

VAN WERT COUNTY HOSPITAL, 1250 South Washington Street, Van Wert, OH, Zip 45891–2599; tel. 419/238–2390; Mark J. Minick, President and Chief Executive Officer

WABASH COUNTY HOSPITAL, 710 North East Street, Wabash, IN, Zip 46992, Mailing Address: Box 548, Zip 46992–0548; tel. 219/563–3131; David C. Hunter, Chief Executive Officer

WELLS COMMUNITY HOSPITAL, 1100 South Main Street, Bluffton, IN, Zip 46714; tel. 219/824–3210; Martin P. Braaksma, Executive Director

WESTVIEW HOSPITAL, 3630 Guion Road, Indianapolis, IN, Zip 46222–1699; tel. 317/924–6661; David C. Dyar, President and Administrator

WHITE COUNTY MEMORIAL HOSPITAL, 1101 O'Connor Boulevard, Monticello, IN, Zip 47960; tel. 219/583–7111; John M. Avers, Chief Executive Officer

WHITLEY MEMORIAL HOSPITAL, 353 North Oak Street, Columbia City, IN, Zip 46725; tel. 219/244–6191; John M. Hatcher, President

WITHAM MEMORIAL HOSPITAL, 1124 North Lebanon Street, Lebanon, IN, Zip 46052–1776, Mailing Address: P.O. Box 1200, Zip 46052–3005; tel. 317/482–2700; Stephen J. White, FACHE, President and Chief Executive Officer

PARKVIEW HEALTH SYSTEM
146 Chestnut Street, Fort Wayne, IN 46805; tel. 219/484–6636; David Ridderheim, President & Chief Executive Officer

HUNTINGTON MEMORIAL HOSPITAL, 1215 Etna Avenue, Huntington, IN, Zip 46750–3696; tel. 219/356–3000; L. Kent McCoy, President

PARKVIEW MEMORIAL HOSPITAL, 2200 Randallia Drive, Fort Wayne, IN, Zip 46805; tel. 219/484–6636; Frank D. Byrne, M.D., President

WHITLEY MEMORIAL HOSPITAL, 353 North Oak Street, Columbia City, IN, Zip 46725; tel. 219/244–6191; John M. Hatcher, President

SAGAMORE HEALTH NETWORK, INC.
11555 North Meridian, Suite 400, Carmel, IN 46032; tel. 317/573–2903; William R. Ealy, President

ADAMS COUNTY MEMORIAL HOSPITAL, 805 High Street, Decatur, IN, Zip 46733, Mailing Address: P.O. Box 151, Zip 46733; tel. 219/724–2145; Marvin L. Baird, Executive Director

CAMERON MEMORIAL COMMUNITY HOSPITAL, 416 East Maumee Street, Angola, IN, Zip 46703; tel. 219/665–2141; Dennis L. Knapp, President

CLAY COUNTY HOSPITAL, 1206 East National Avenue, Brazil, IN, Zip 47834–2797; tel. 812/448–2675; Jay P. Jolly, Administrator and Chief Executive Officer

CLINTON COUNTY HOSPITAL, 1300 South Jackson Street, Frankfort, IN, Zip 46041–3394, Mailing Address: P.O. Box 669, Zip 46041–0669; tel. 765/659–4731; Brian R. Zeh, Executive Director

COMMUNITY HOSPITAL OF BREMEN, 411 South Whitlock Street, Bremen, IN, Zip 46506–1699; tel. 219/546–2211; Scott R. Graybill, Administrator and Chief Executive Officer

COMMUNITY MEMORIAL HOSPITAL, 208 North Columbus Street, Hicksville, OH, Zip 43526–1299; tel. 419/542–6692; Deryl E. Gulliford, Ph.D., Administrator

DUKES MEMORIAL HOSPITAL, Grant and Boulevard, Peru, IN, Zip 46970–1698; tel. 765/473–6621; R. Joe Johnston, President and Chief Executive Officer

DUNN MEMORIAL HOSPITAL, 1600 23rd Street, Bedford, IN, Zip 47421–4704; tel. 812/275–3331; Richard W. Hahn, Executive Director

FAIRBANKS HOSPITAL, 8102 Clearvista Parkway, Indianapolis, IN, Zip 46256–4698; tel. 317/849–8222; Timothy J. Kelly, M.D., President

FLOYD MEMORIAL HOSPITAL AND HEALTH SERVICES, 1850 State Street, New Albany, IN, Zip 47150; tel. 812/949–5500; Bryant R. Hanson, President

GIBSON GENERAL HOSPITAL, 1808 Sherman Drive, Princeton, IN, Zip 47670–1043; tel. 812/385–3401; Michael J. Budnick, Administrator and Chief Executive Officer

GREENE COUNTY GENERAL HOSPITAL, Rural Route 1, Box 1000, Linton, IN, Zip 47441–9457; tel. 812/847–2281; Jonas S. Uland, Executive Director

HANCOCK MEMORIAL HOSPITAL AND HEALTH SERVICES, 801 North State Street, Greenfield, IN, Zip 46140–2537, Mailing Address: Box 827, Zip 46140; tel. 317/462–5544; Robert C. Keen, Ph.D., President and Chief Executive Officer

HENDRICKS COMMUNITY HOSPITAL, 1000 East Main Street, Danville, IN, Zip 46122–0409, Mailing Address: P.O. Box 409, Zip 46122–0409; tel. 317/745–4451; Dennis W. Dawes, President

HENRY COUNTY MEMORIAL HOSPITAL, 1000 North 16th Street, New Castle, IN, Zip 47362–4319, Mailing Address: Box 490, Zip 47362–0490; tel. 765/521–0890; Jack Basler, President

HUNTINGTON MEMORIAL HOSPITAL, 1215 Etna Avenue, Huntington, IN, Zip 46750–3696; tel. 219/356–3000; L. Kent McCoy, President

INDIANA UNIVERSITY MEDICAL CENTER, 550 North University Boulevard, Indianapolis, IN, Zip 46202–5262; tel. 317/274–5000; David J. Handel, Director

JOHNSON MEMORIAL HOSPITAL, 1125 West Jefferson Street, Franklin, IN, Zip 46131–2140, Mailing Address: P.O. Box 549, Zip 46131–0549; tel. 317/736–3300; Gregg A. Bechtold, President and Chief Executive Officer

KENDRICK MEMORIAL HOSPITAL, 1201 Hadley Road N.W., Mooresville, IN, Zip 46158–1789; tel. 317/831–1160; Charles D. Swisher, Executive Director

KOSCIUSKO COMMUNITY HOSPITAL, 2101 East Dubois Drive, Warsaw, IN, Zip 46580; tel. 219/267–3200; Wayne Hendrix, President

LA PORTE HOSPITAL, State and Madison Streets, La Porte, IN, Zip 46350–0250, Mailing Address: P.O. Box 250, Zip 46352–0250; tel. 219/326–1234; Leigh E. Morris, President

MARY SHERMAN HOSPITAL, 320 North Section Street, Sullivan, IN, Zip 47882, Mailing Address: P.O. Box 10, Zip 47882–0010; tel. 812/268–4311; Thomas J. Hudgins, Administrator

MCCRAY MEMORIAL HOSPITAL, 951 East Hospital Drive, Kendallville, IN, Zip 46755, Mailing Address: P.O. Box 249, Zip 46755; tel. 219/347–1100; Peter A. Marotti, Chief Executive Officer

MEDICAL CENTER OF SOUTHERN INDIANA, 2200 Market Street, Charlestown, IN, Zip 47111–0069, Mailing Address: P.O. Box 69, Zip 47111–0069; tel. 812/256–3301; Kevin J. Miller, Chief Executive Officer

MEMORIAL HOSPITAL, 1101 Michigan Avenue, Logansport, IN, Zip 46947–1596, Mailing Address: P.O. Box 7013, Zip 46947–7013; tel. 219/753–7541; George W. Poor, President and Chief Executive Officer

METHODIST HOSPITAL OF INDIANA, 1701 North Senate Boulevard, Indianapolis, IN, Zip 46202, Mailing Address: I. 65 at 21st Street, P.O. Box 1367, Zip 46206–1367; tel. 317/929–2000; William J. Loveday, President and Chief Executive Officer

MORGAN COUNTY MEMORIAL HOSPITAL, 2209 John R. Wooden Drive, Martinsville, IN, Zip 46151, Mailing Address: P.O. Box 1717, Zip 46151; tel. 765/349–6501; S. Dean Melton, President and Chief Executive Officer

OAKLAWN PSYCHIATRIC CENTER, INC., 330 Lakeview Drive, Goshen, IN, Zip 46526–9365, Mailing Address: P.O. Box 809, Zip 46527–0809; tel. 219/533–1234; Harold C. Loewen, President

ORANGE COUNTY HOSPITAL, 642 West Hospital Road, Paoli, IN, Zip 47454–0499, Mailing Address: P.O. Box 499, Zip 47454–0499; tel. 812/723–2811; James W. Pope, Chief Executive Officer

PARKVIEW MEMORIAL HOSPITAL, 2200 Randallia Drive, Fort Wayne, IN, Zip 46805; tel. 219/484–6636; Frank D. Byrne, M.D., President

PULASKI MEMORIAL HOSPITAL, 616 East 13th Street, Winamac, IN, Zip 46996–1117; tel. 219/946–6131; Richard H. Mynark, Administrator

PUTNAM COUNTY HOSPITAL, 1542 Bloomington Street, Greencastle, IN, Zip 46135; tel. 765/653–5121; John D. Fajt, Executive Director

RANDOLPH COUNTY HOSPITAL, 325 South Oak Street, Winchester, IN, Zip 47394, Mailing Address: P.O. Box 407, Zip 47394; tel. 765/584–9001; James M. Full, Chief Executive Officer

REHABILITATION HOSPITAL OF INDIANA, 4141 Shore Drive, Indianapolis, IN, Zip 46254–2607; tel. 317/329–2000; Kim D. Eicher, Administrator and Chief Executive Officer

RIVERVIEW HOSPITAL, 395 Westfield Road, Noblesville, IN, Zip 46060–1425, Mailing Address: P.O. Box 220, Zip 46061–0220; tel. 317/773–0760; Seward Horner, President

Section B

Networks / Sagamore Health Network, Inc.

RUSH MEMORIAL HOSPITAL, 1300 North Main Street, Rushville, IN, Zip 46173–1198; tel. 765/932–4111; H. William Hartley, Chief Executive Officer

SAINT ANTHONY HOSPITAL AND HEALTH CENTERS, 301 West Homer Street, Michigan City, IN, Zip 46360–4358; tel. 219/879–8511; Bruce E. Rampage, President and Chief Executive Officer

SAINT JOHN'S HEALTH SYSTEM, 2015 Jackson Street, Anderson, IN, Zip 46016–4339; tel. 765/649–2511; James H. Stephens, President and Chief Executive Officer

SAINT MARGARET MERCY HEALTHCARE CENTERS, 5454 Hohman Avenue, Hammond, IN, Zip 46320; tel. 219/933–2074; Eugene C. Diamond, President and Chief Executive Officer

ST. ANTHONY MEDICAL CENTER, 1201 South Main Street, Crown Point, IN, Zip 46307–8483; tel. 219/738–2100; Stephen O. Leurck, President

ST. CATHERINE HOSPITAL, 4321 Fir Street, East Chicago, IN, Zip 46312; tel. 219/392–7000; JoAnn Birdzell, President and Chief Executive Officer

ST. FRANCIS HOSPITAL AND HEALTH CENTERS, 1600 Albany Street, Beech Grove, IN, Zip 46107–1593; tel. 317/787–3311; Robert J. Brody, President and Chief Executive Officer

ST. JOSEPH COMMUNITY HOSPITAL, 215 West Fourth Street, Mishawaka, IN, Zip 46544; tel. 219/259–2431; Stephen L. Crain, President and Chief Executive Officer

ST. JOSEPH MEDICAL CENTER OF FORT WAYNE, 700 Broadway, Fort Wayne, IN, Zip 46802; tel. 219/425–3000; John T. Farrell, Sr., President and Chief Executive Officer

ST. JOSEPH'S HOSPITAL OF MARSHALL COUNTY, 1915 Lake Avenue, Plymouth, IN, Zip 46563–9905, Mailing Address: P.O. Box 670, Zip 46563–9905; tel. 219/936–3181; Brian E. Dietz, President

ST. JOSEPH'S MEDICAL CENTER, 801 East LaSalle, South Bend, IN, Zip 46617, Mailing Address: Box 1935, Zip 46634; tel. 219/237–7111; Brian E. Dietz, Interim Chief Executive Officer

ST. MARY COMMUNITY HOSPITAL, 2515 East Jefferson Boulevard, South Bend, IN, Zip 46615–2691; tel. 219/288–8311; Stephen L. Crain, President

ST. MARY MEDICAL CENTER, 1500 South Lake Park Avenue, Hobart, IN, Zip 46342; tel. 219/942–0551; Milton Triana, President and Chief Executive Officer

ST. MARY'S HOSPITAL WARRICK, 1116 Millis Avenue, Boonville, IN, Zip 47601–0629, Mailing Address: Box 629, Zip 47601–0629; tel. 812/897–4800; John D. O'Neil, Executive Vice President and Administrator

ST. MARY'S MEDICAL CENTER OF EVANSVILLE, 3700 Washington Avenue, Evansville, IN, Zip 47750; tel. 812/485–4000; Richard C. Breon, President and Chief Executive Officer

ST. VINCENT HOSPITALS AND HEALTH SERVICES, 2001 West 86th Street, Indianapolis, IN, Zip 46260, Mailing Address: Box 40970, Zip 46240–0970; tel. 317/338–2345; Douglas D. French, President and Chief Executive Officer

ST. VINCENT MERCY HOSPITAL, 1331 South A Street, Elwood, IN, Zip 46036–1942; tel. 765/552–4600; Ann C. Parsons, Interim Administrator

STARKE MEMORIAL HOSPITAL, 102 East Culver Road, Knox, IN, Zip 46534–2299; tel. 219/772–6231; Kathryn J. Norem, Executive Director

TIPTON COUNTY MEMORIAL HOSPITAL, 1000 South Main Street, Tipton, IN, Zip 46072–9799; tel. 317/675–8500; Alfonso W. Gatmaitan, Chief Executive Officer

UNION HOSPITAL, 1606 North Seventh Street, Terre Haute, IN, Zip 47804–2780; tel. 812/238–7000; Frank Shelton, President

WABASH COUNTY HOSPITAL, 710 North East Street, Wabash, IN, Zip 46992, Mailing Address: Box 548, Zip 46992–0548; tel. 219/563–3131; David C. Hunter, Chief Executive Officer

WELLS COMMUNITY HOSPITAL, 1100 South Main Street, Bluffton, IN, Zip 46714; tel. 219/824–3210; Martin P. Braaksma, Executive Director

WESTVIEW HOSPITAL, 3630 Guion Road, Indianapolis, IN, Zip 46222–1699; tel. 317/924–6661; David C. Dyar, President and Administrator

WHITE COUNTY MEMORIAL HOSPITAL, 1101 O'Connor Boulevard, Monticello, IN, Zip 47960; tel. 219/583–7111; John M. Avers, Chief Executive Officer

WHITLEY MEMORIAL HOSPITAL, 353 North Oak Street, Columbia City, IN, Zip 46725; tel. 219/244–6191; John M. Hatcher, President

WITHAM MEMORIAL HOSPITAL, 1124 North Lebanon Street, Lebanon, IN, Zip 46052–1776, Mailing Address: P.O. Box 1200, Zip 46052–3005; tel. 317/482–2700; Stephen J. White, FACHE, President and Chief Executive Officer

SAINT VINCENT HOSPITALS AND HEALTH SERVICES, INC.
2001 West 86th Street, Indianapolis, IN 40970; tel. 317/338–7000; Douglas D. French, President & Chief Executive Officer

JENNINGS COMMUNITY HOSPITAL, 301 Henry Street, North Vernon, IN, Zip 47265; tel. 812/346–6200; Dale P. Wernke, Chief Executive Officer

SAINT JOSEPH HOSPITAL & HEALTH CENTER, 1907 West Sycamore Street, Kokomo, IN, Zip 46904–9010; tel. 765/456–5300; Kathleen Korbelak, President and Chief Executive Officer

ST. VINCENT MERCY HOSPITAL, 1331 South A Street, Elwood, IN, Zip 46036–1942; tel. 765/552–4600; Ann C. Parsons, Interim Administrator

ST. VINCENT WILLIAMSPORT HOSPITAL, 412 North Monroe Street, Williamsport, IN, Zip 47993–0215; tel. 765/762–2496; Jane Craigin, Chief Executive Officer

SELECT HEALTH NETWORK
P.O. Box 1197, South Bend, IN 46624; tel. 219/237–7822; Len Strezelecki, Chief Executive Officer

ST. JOSEPH'S MEDICAL CENTER, 801 East LaSalle, South Bend, IN, Zip 46617, Mailing Address: Box 1935, Zip 46634; tel. 219/237–7111; Brian E. Dietz, Interim Chief Executive Officer

SUBURBAN HEALTH ORGANIZATION
1 American Square – Suite 2245, Indianapolis, IN 46282; tel. 317/692–5222; Julie M. Carmichael, President

CLINTON COUNTY HOSPITAL, 1300 South Jackson Street, Frankfort, IN, Zip 46041–3394, Mailing Address: P.O. Box 669, Zip 46041–0669; tel. 765/659–4731; Brian R. Zeh, Executive Director

HANCOCK MEMORIAL HOSPITAL AND HEALTH SERVICES, 801 North State Street, Greenfield, IN, Zip 46140–2537, Mailing Address: Box 827, Zip 46140; tel. 317/462–5544; Robert C. Keen, Ph.D., President and Chief Executive Officer

HENDRICKS COMMUNITY HOSPITAL, 1000 East Main Street, Danville, IN, Zip 46122–0409, Mailing Address: P.O. Box 409, Zip 46122–0409; tel. 317/745–4451; Dennis W. Dawes, President

HENRY COUNTY MEMORIAL HOSPITAL, 1000 North 16th Street, New Castle, IN, Zip 47362–4319, Mailing Address: Box 490, Zip 47362–0490; tel. 765/521–0890; Jack Basler, President

JOHNSON MEMORIAL HOSPITAL, 1125 West Jefferson Street, Franklin, IN, Zip 46131–2140, Mailing Address: P.O. Box 549, Zip 46131–0549; tel. 317/736–3300; Gregg A. Bechtold, President and Chief Executive Officer

MORGAN COUNTY MEMORIAL HOSPITAL, 2209 John R. Wooden Drive, Martinsville, IN, Zip 46151, Mailing Address: P.O. Box 1717, Zip 46151; tel. 765/349–6501; S. Dean Melton, President and Chief Executive Officer

PUTNAM COUNTY HOSPITAL, 1542 Bloomington Street, Greencastle, IN, Zip 46135; tel. 765/653–5121; John D. Fajt, Executive Director

RIVERVIEW HOSPITAL, 395 Westfield Road, Noblesville, IN, Zip 46060–1425, Mailing Address: P.O. Box 220, Zip 46061–0220; tel. 317/773–0760; Seward Horner, President

TIPTON COUNTY MEMORIAL HOSPITAL, 1000 South Main Street, Tipton, IN, Zip 46072–9799; tel. 317/675–8500; Alfonso W. Gatmaitan, Chief Executive Officer

WESTVIEW HOSPITAL, 3630 Guion Road, Indianapolis, IN, Zip 46222–1699; tel. 317/924–6661; David C. Dyar, President and Administrator

WITHAM MEMORIAL HOSPITAL, 1124 North Lebanon Street, Lebanon, IN, Zip 46052–1776, Mailing Address: P.O. Box 1200, Zip 46052–3005; tel. 317/482–2700; Stephen J. White, FACHE, President and Chief Executive Officer

IOWA

GENESIS HEALTH SYSTEM
1227 East Rushmore Street, Davenport, IA 52803; tel. 319/326–6512; Leo Bressanelli, Chief Executive Officer

DEWITT COMMUNITY HOSPITAL, 1118 11th Street, De Witt, IA, Zip 52742; tel. 319/659–3241; C. James Christensen, Chief Executive Officer

GENESIS MEDICAL CENTER, 1227 East Rusholme Street, Davenport, IA, Zip 52803; tel. 319/421–6000; Leo A. Bressanelli, President and Chief Executive Officer

ILLINI HOSPITAL, 801 Hospital Road, Silvis, IL, Zip 61282; tel. 309/792–9363; Gary E. Larson, Chief Executive Officer

MERCY NETWORK OF HEALTH SERVICES
400 University Drive, Des Moines, IA 50309; tel. 515/247–8372; Sara Drobnick, Vice President

ADAIR COUNTY MEMORIAL HOSPITAL, 609 S.E. Kent Street, Greenfield, IA, Zip 50849; tel. 515/743–2123; Myrna Erb, Administrator

AUDUBON COUNTY MEMORIAL HOSPITAL, 515 Pacific Street, Audubon, IA, Zip 50025–1099; tel. 712/563–2611; David G. Couser, Administrator

DAVIS COUNTY HOSPITAL, 507 North Madison Street, Bloomfield, IA, Zip 52537–1299; tel. 515/664–2145; Randy Simmons, Administrator

HAMILTON COUNTY PUBLIC HOSPITAL, 800 Ohio Street, Webster City, IA, Zip 50595; tel. 515/832–9400; Roger W. Lenz, Administrator

MANNING GENERAL HOSPITAL, 410 Main Street, Manning, IA, Zip 51455; tel. 712/653–2072; Mitchel S. Ketcham, Administrator

MERCY HOSPITAL MEDICAL CENTER, 400 University Avenue, Des Moines, IA, Zip 50314; tel. 515/247–4278; Thomas A. Reitinger, President and Chief Executive Officer

MONROE COUNTY HOSPITAL, RR 3, Box 311–11, Albia, IA, Zip 52531; tel. 515/932–2134; Gregory A. Paris, Administrator

RINGGOLD COUNTY HOSPITAL, 211 Shellway Drive, Mount Ayr, IA, Zip 50854; tel. 515/464–3226; Gordon W. Winkler, Administrator

ST. ANTHONY REGIONAL HOSPITAL, South Clark Street, Carroll, IA, Zip 51401; tel. 712/792–8231; Gary P. Riedmann, President and Chief Executive Officer

ST. JOSEPH'S MERCY HOSPITAL, 1 St. Joseph's Drive, Centerville, IA, Zip 52544; tel. 515/437–3411; William C. Assell, President and Chief Executive Officer

STORY COUNTY HOSPITAL AND LONG TERM CARE FACILITY, 630 Sixth Street, Nevada, IA, Zip 50201; tel. 515/382–2111; Todd Willert, Administrator

WAYNE COUNTY HOSPITAL, 417 South East Street, Corydon, IA, Zip 50060, Mailing Address: Box 305, Zip 50060; tel. 515/872–2260; Bill D. Wilson, Administrator

NORTH IOWA MERCY HEALTH NETWORK
84 Beaumont Drive, Mason City, IA 50401; tel. 515/424–7481; David Ross, President

Section B

B22 Networks, Health Care Systems and Alliances

© 1997 AHA Guide

BELMOND COMMUNITY HOSPITAL, 403 First Street S.E., Belmond, IA, Zip 50421–0326, Mailing Address: P.O. Box 326, Zip 50421; tel. 515/444–3223; Allan Atkinson, Administrator

ELDORA REGIONAL MEDICAL CENTER, 2413 Edgington Avenue, Eldora, IA, Zip 50627–1541; tel. 515/858–5416; Greg Reed, Administrator

FRANKLIN GENERAL HOSPITAL, 1720 Central Avenue East, Hampton, IA, Zip 50441–1859; tel. 515/456–4721; Laura Olander, Chief Executive Officer

HANCOCK COUNTY MEMORIAL HOSPITAL, 531 Second Street N.W., Britt, IA, Zip 50423, Mailing Address: Box 68, Zip 50423–0068; tel. 515/843–3801; Harriet Thompson, Administrator

HOWARD COUNTY HOSPITAL, 235 Eighth Avenue West, Cresco, IA, Zip 52136–1098; tel. 319/547–2101; Elizabeth A. Doty, Administrator

KOSSUTH REGIONAL HEALTH CENTER, 1515 South Phillips Street, Algona, IA, Zip 50511; tel. 515/295–2451; James G. Fitzpatrick, Administrator

MITCHELL COUNTY REGIONAL HEALTH CENTER, 616 North Eighth Street, Osage, IA, Zip 50461–1498; tel. 515/732–3781; Richard C. Hamilton, Chief Executive Officer

NORTH IOWA MERCY HEALTH CENTER, 1000 Fourth Street S.W., Mason City, IA, Zip 50401; tel. 515/422–7000; David H. Vellinga, President and Chief Executive Officer

ST LUKES/IOWA HEALTH SYSTEM
700 East University Avenue, Des Moines, IA 50316; tel. 515/263–5399; Barry C. Spear, Vice President of System Development

IOWA METHODIST MEDICAL CENTER, 1200 Pleasant Street, Des Moines, IA, Zip 50309–9976; tel. 515/241–6212; James H. Skogsbergh, President

MARENGO MEMORIAL HOSPITAL, 300 West May Street, Marengo, IA, Zip 52301, Mailing Address: Box 228, Zip 52301; tel. 319/642–5543; James H. Ragland, Administrator

VIRGINIA GAY HOSPITAL, 502 North Ninth Avenue, Vinton, IA, Zip 52349; tel. 319/472–2348; Michael J. Riege, Administrator

KANSAS

COMMUNITY HEALTH ALLIANCE
Route 1, Box 1, Winchester, KS 66097; tel. 816/276–7580; Steven Ashcroft, Administrator

COMMUNITY HOSPITAL ONAGA, 120 West Eighth Street, Onaga, KS, Zip 66521–0120; tel. 913/889–4272; Joseph T. Engelken, Chief Executive Officer

COMMUNITY MEMORIAL HOSPITAL, 708 North 18th Street, Marysville, KS, Zip 66508–1399; tel. 913/562–2311; Harley B. Appel, Chief Executive Officer

GEARY COMMUNITY HOSPITAL, Ash and St. Mary's Road, Junction City, KS, Zip 66441, Mailing Address: Box 490, Zip 66441–0490; tel. 913/238–4131; David K. Bradley, Chief Executive Officer

HOLTON COMMUNITY HOSPITAL, 510 Kansas Avenue, Holton, KS, Zip 66436; tel. 913/364–2116; Diane S. Gross, Administrator

HORTON HEALTH FOUNDATION, 240 West 18th Street, Horton, KS, Zip 66439; tel. 913/486–2642

JEFFERSON COUNTY MEMORIAL HOSPITAL, 408 Delaware Street, Winchester, KS, Zip 66097, Mailing Address: Rural Route 1, Box 1, Zip 66097; tel. 913/774–4340; Steven F. Ashcraft, Administrator

MERCY HEALTH CENTER OF MANHATTAN, Manhattan, KS, Mailing Address: 1823 College Avenue, Zip 66502; E. Michael Nunamaker, President and Chief Executive Officer

MORRIS COUNTY HOSPITAL, 600 North Washington Street, Council Grove, KS, Zip 66846, Mailing Address: P.O. Box 275, Zip 66846; tel. 316/767–6811; Jim Reagan, M.D., Administrator

NEMAHA VALLEY COMMUNITY HOSPITAL, 1600 Community Drive, Seneca, KS, Zip 66538; tel. 913/336–6181; Michael J. Ryan, President and Chief Executive Officer

ST. FRANCIS HOSPITAL AND MEDICAL CENTER, 1700 West Seventh Street, Topeka, KS, Zip 66606–1690; tel. 913/295–8000; Sister Loretto Marie Colwell, President

GREAT PLAINS HEALTH ALLIANCE
P.O. Box 366, Phillipsburg, KS 67661; tel. 913/543–2111; Roger John, President

ASHLAND HEALTH CENTER, 709 Oak Street, Ashland, KS, Zip 67831, Mailing Address: P.O. Box 188, Zip 67831; tel. 316/635–2241; Bryan Stacey, Administrator

CHEYENNE COUNTY HOSPITAL, 210 West First Street, Saint Francis, KS, Zip 67756, Mailing Address: P.O. Box 547, Zip 67756–0547; tel. 913/332–2104; Leslie Lacy, Administrator

COMMUNITY MEDICAL CENTER, 2307 Barada Street, Falls City, NE, Zip 68355–1599; tel. 402/245–2428; Victor Lee, Chief Executive Officer and Administrator

ELLINWOOD DISTRICT HOSPITAL, 605 North Main Street, Ellinwood, KS, Zip 67526; tel. 316/564–2548; Marge Conell, R.N., Administrator

FREDONIA REGIONAL HOSPITAL, 1527 Madison Street, Fredonia, KS, Zip 66736, Mailing Address: Box 579, Zip 66736; tel. 316/378–2121; Terry Deschaine, Administrator

GREELEY COUNTY HOSPITAL, 506 Third Street, Tribune, KS, Zip 67879, Mailing Address: Box 338, Zip 67879; tel. 316/376–4221; Cynthia K. Schneider, Administrator

GRISELL MEMORIAL HOSPITAL DISTRICT ONE, 210 South Vermont, Ransom, KS, Zip 67572–0268, Mailing Address: P.O. Box 268, Zip 67572–0268; tel. 913/731–2231; Kristine Ochs, R.N., Administrator

HARLAN COUNTY HOSPITAL, 717 North Brown, Alma, NE, Zip 68920, Mailing Address: P.O. Box 836, Zip 68920; tel. 308/928–2151; Allen Van Driel, Administrator

KIOWA COUNTY MEMORIAL HOSPITAL, 501 South Walnut Street, Greensburg, KS, Zip 67054; tel. 316/723–3341; Ronald J. Baker, Administrator

LANE COUNTY HOSPITAL, 243 South Second, Dighton, KS, Zip 67839, Mailing Address: Box 969, Zip 67839; tel. 316/397–5321; Donna McGowan, R.N., Administrator

LINCOLN COUNTY HOSPITAL, 624 North Second Street, Lincoln, KS, Zip 67455, Mailing Address: P.O. Box 406, Zip 67455; tel. 913/524–4403; Jolene Yager, R.N., Administrator

MEDICINE LODGE MEMORIAL HOSPITAL, 710 North Walnut Street, Medicine Lodge, KS, Zip 67104, Mailing Address: P.O. Drawer C, Zip 67104; tel. 316/886–3771; Kevin A. White, Administrator

MINNEOLA DISTRICT HOSPITAL, 212 Main Street, Minneola, KS, Zip 67865; tel. 316/885–4264; Blaine K. Miller, Administrator

MITCHELL COUNTY HOSPITAL, 400 West Eighth, Beloit, KS, Zip 67420, Mailing Address: P.O. Box 399, Zip 67420; tel. 913/738–2266; John M. Osse, Administrator

OSBORNE COUNTY MEMORIAL HOSPITAL, 424 West New Hampshire Street, Osborne, KS, Zip 67473–0070, Mailing Address: P.O. Box 70, Zip 67473–0070; tel. 913/346–2121; Patricia Bernard, R.N., Administrator

OTTAWA COUNTY HOSPITAL, 215 East Eighth, Minneapolis, KS, Zip 67467, Mailing Address: Box 209, Zip 67467; tel. 913/392–2122; Joy Reed, R.N., Administrator

PHILLIPS COUNTY HOSPITAL, 1150 State Street, Phillipsburg, KS, Zip 67661, Mailing Address: Box 607, Zip 67661; tel. 913/543–5226; James L. Giedd, Administrator

RAWLINS COUNTY HOSPITAL, 707 Grant Street, Atwood, KS, Zip 67730–4700; tel. 913/626–3211; Donald J. Kessen, Administrator

REPUBLIC COUNTY HOSPITAL, 2420 G Street, Belleville, KS, Zip 66935; tel. 913/527–2255; Charles A. Westin, FACHE, Administrator

SABETHA COMMUNITY HOSPITAL, 14th and Oregon Streets, Sabetha, KS, Zip 66534, Mailing Address: P.O. Box 229, Zip 66534; tel. 913/284–2121; Rita K. Buurman, Administrator

SALEM HOSPITAL, 701 South Main Street, Hillsboro, KS, Zip 67063–9981; tel. 316/947–3114; Robert G. Senneff, Chief Executive Officer

SATANTA DISTRICT HOSPITAL, 401 South Cheyenne Street, Satanta, KS, Zip 67870, Mailing Address: P.O. Box 159, Zip 67870–0159; tel. 316/649–2761; T. G. Lee, Administrator

SMITH COUNTY MEMORIAL HOSPITAL, 614 South Main Street, Smith Center, KS, Zip 66967–0349, Mailing Address: P.O. Box 349, Zip 66967–0349; tel. 913/282–6845; John Terrill, Administrator

TREGO COUNTY–LEMKE MEMORIAL HOSPITAL, 320 13th Street, Wakeeney, KS, Zip 67672–2099; tel. 913/743–2182; James Wahlmeier, Administrator

HAYS MEDICAL CENTER
201 East 7th Street, Hays, KS 67601; tel. 913/623–5116; Jodi Schmidt, Vice President–Regional Partnerships

CHEYENNE COUNTY HOSPITAL, 210 West First Street, Saint Francis, KS, Zip 67756, Mailing Address: P.O. Box 547, Zip 67756–0547; tel. 913/332–2104; Leslie Lacy, Administrator

DWIGHT D. EISENHOWER VETERANS AFFAIRS MEDICAL CENTER, 4101 South Fourth Street Trafficway, Leavenworth, KS, Zip 66048–5055; tel. 913/682–2000; Carole Bishop Smith, Center Director

GRISELL MEMORIAL HOSPITAL DISTRICT ONE, 210 South Vermont, Ransom, KS, Zip 67572–0268, Mailing Address: P.O. Box 268, Zip 67572–0268; tel. 913/731–2231; Kristine Ochs, R.N., Administrator

PHILLIPS COUNTY HOSPITAL, 1150 State Street, Phillipsburg, KS, Zip 67661, Mailing Address: Box 607, Zip 67661; tel. 913/543–5226; James L. Giedd, Administrator

RAWLINS COUNTY HOSPITAL, 707 Grant Street, Atwood, KS, Zip 67730–4700, Mailing Address: Box 47, Zip 67730–4700; tel. 913/626–3211; Donald J. Kessen, Administrator

SATANTA DISTRICT HOSPITAL, 401 South Cheyenne Street, Satanta, KS, Zip 67870, Mailing Address: P.O. Box 159, Zip 67870–0159; tel. 316/649–2761; T. G. Lee, Administrator

TREGO COUNTY–LEMKE MEMORIAL HOSPITAL, 320 13th Street, Wakeeney, KS, Zip 67672–2099; tel. 913/743–2182; James Wahlmeier, Administrator

HEART OF AMERICA NETWORK
929 North Saint Francis, Wichita, KS 67214; tel. 316/268–5000; Bruce Carmichael, Vice President Regional Development

ST. FRANCIS HOSPITAL AND MEDICAL CENTER, 1700 West Seventh Street, Topeka, KS, Zip 66606–1690; tel. 913/295–8000; Sister Loretto Marie Colwell, President

VIA CHRISTI REGIONAL MEDICAL CENTER, 929 North St. Francis Street, Wichita, KS, Zip 67214–3882; tel. 316/268–5000; Randall G. Nyp, President and Chief Executive Officer

JAYHAWK HEALTH ALLIANCE
20333 West 151st Street, Olathe, KS 66061; tel. 913/791–4200; Frank H. Devocelle, Network Contact

ANDERSON COUNTY HOSPITAL, 421 South Maple, Garnett, KS, Zip 66032, Mailing Address: Box 309, Zip 66032; tel. 913/448–3131; James K. Johnson, Administrator

LAWRENCE MEMORIAL HOSPITAL, 325 Maine, Lawrence, KS, Zip 66044–1393; tel. 913/749–6100; Robert B. Ohlen, President and Chief Executive Officer

Section B

MIAMI COUNTY MEDICAL CENTER, 2100 Baptiste, Paola, KS, Zip 66071–0365, Mailing Address: P.O. Box 365, Zip 66071–0365; tel. 913/294–2327; Gerald Wiesner, Vice President and Chief Operating Officer

OLATHE MEDICAL CENTER, 20333 West 151st Street, Olathe, KS, Zip 66061–5352; tel. 913/791–4200; Frank H. Devocelle, President and Chief Executive Officer

PROVIDENCE MEDICAL CENTER, 8929 Parallel Parkway, Kansas City, KS, Zip 66112–0430; tel. 913/596–4000; Francis V. Creeden, Jr., President

SAINT JOHN HOSPITAL, 3500 South Fourth Street, Leavenworth, KS, Zip 66048–5092; tel. 913/680–6000; Francis V. Creeden, Jr., President

UNIVERSITY OF KANSAS HOSPITAL, 3901 Rainbow Boulevard, Kansas City, KS, Zip 66160–7200; tel. 913/588–5000; Irene M. Cumming, Chief Executive Officer

MED-OP
202 Center Avenue, Oakley, KS 67748–1714; tel. 913/672–3540; Andrew Draper, Executive Director

CITIZENS MEDICAL CENTER, 100 East College Drive, Colby, KS, Zip 67701–3799; tel. 913/462–7511; Richard B. Gamel, Chief Executive Officer

DECATUR COUNTY HOSPITAL, 810 West Columbia, Oberlin, KS, Zip 67749, Mailing Address: P.O. Box 268, Zip 67749; tel. 913/475–2208; R. Kim Hardman, Administrator

GOODLAND REGIONAL MEDICAL CENTER, 220 West Second Street, Goodland, KS, Zip 67735–1602; tel. 913/899–3625; Jim Chaddic, Chief Executive Officer

GOVE COUNTY MEDICAL CENTER, Fifth and Garfield Streets, Quinter, KS, Zip 67752; tel. 913/754–3341; Paul Davis, Administrator

GRAHAM COUNTY HOSPITAL, 304 West Prout Street, Hill City, KS, Zip 67642, Mailing Address: P.O. Box 339, Zip 67642; tel. 913/421–2121; Fred J. Meis, Administrator

HAYS MEDICAL CENTER, 2220 Canterbury Road, Hays, KS, Zip 67601–2323, Mailing Address: P.O. Box 8100, Zip 67601; tel. 913/623–5407; Stephen F. Ronstrom, President and Chief Executive Officer

LOGAN COUNTY HOSPITAL, 211 Cherry Street, Oakley, KS, Zip 67748; tel. 913/672–3211; Rodney Bates, Administrator

NESS COUNTY HOSPITAL NUMBER TWO, 312 East Custer Street, Ness City, KS, Zip 67560; tel. 913/798–2291; Clyde T. McCracken, Administrator

NORTON COUNTY HOSPITAL, 102 East Holme, Norton, KS, Zip 67654–0250, Mailing Address: P.O. Box 250, Zip 67654–0250; tel. 913/877–3351; Richard Miller, Administrator

PLAINVILLE RURAL HOSPITAL DISTRICT NUMBER ONE, 304 South Colorado Avenue, Plainville, KS, Zip 67663; tel. 913/434–4553; Leonard Hernandez, Administrator

RUSH COUNTY MEMORIAL HOSPITAL, Eighth and Locust Streets, La Crosse, KS, Zip 67548, Mailing Address: P.O. Box 520, Zip 67548–0520; tel. 913/222–2545; Donna L. Myers, Administrator and Chief Executive Officer

SCOTT COUNTY HOSPITAL, 310 East Third Street, Scott City, KS, Zip 67871; tel. 316/872–5811; Greg Unruh, Chief Executive Officer

SHERIDAN COUNTY HOSPITAL, 826 18th Street, Hoxie, KS, Zip 67740–0167, Mailing Address: P.O. Box 167, Zip 67740–0167; tel. 913/675–3281; Joy Bretz, Administrator

PIONEER NETWORK
P.O. Box 159, Santana, KS 67870; tel. 316/649–2761; Tom Lee, Administrator

SATANTA DISTRICT HOSPITAL, 401 South Cheyenne Street, Satanta, KS, Zip 67870, Mailing Address: P.O. Box 159, Zip 67870–0159; tel. 316/649–2761; T. G. Lee, Administrator

SOUTHEAST KANSAS NETWORK
1400 West 4th Street, Coffeyville, KS 67337; tel. 316/251–1200; Jerry Marquette, President

ALLEN COUNTY HOSPITAL, 101 South First Street, Iola, KS, Zip 66749, Mailing Address: P.O. Box 540, Zip 66749–0540; tel. 316/365–3131; Franklin K. Wilson, Administrator

COFFEYVILLE REGIONAL MEDICAL CENTER, 1400 West Fourth, Coffeyville, KS, Zip 67337–3306; tel. 316/251–1200; Gerald Joseph Marquette, Jr., Administrator

FREDONIA REGIONAL HOSPITAL, 1527 Madison Street, Fredonia, KS, Zip 66736, Mailing Address: Box 579, Zip 66736; tel. 316/378–2121; Terry Deschaine, Administrator

LABETTE COUNTY MEDICAL CENTER, 1902 South U.S. Highway 59, Parsons, KS, Zip 67357, Mailing Address: P.O. Box 956, Zip 67357; tel. 316/421–4880; Richard A. Nye, Chief Executive Officer

MAUDE NORTON MEMORIAL CITY HOSPITAL, 220 North Pennsylvania Street, Columbus, KS, Zip 66725–1197; tel. 316/429–2545; Cindy Neely, Administrator and Chief Executive Officer

MERCY HEALTH SYSTEM OF KANSAS, 821 Burke Street, Fort Scott, KS, Zip 66701; tel. 316/223–2200; Susan Barrett, President and Chief Executive Officer

MOUNT CARMEL MEDICAL CENTER, Centennial and Rouse Streets, Pittsburg, KS, Zip 66762–6686; tel. 316/231–6100; John Daniel Lingor, President and Chief Executive Officer

NEOSHO MEMORIAL REGIONAL MEDICAL CENTER, 629 South Plummer, Chanute, KS, Zip 66720; tel. 316/431–4000; Murray L. Brown, Administrator

RICE COUNTY HOSPITAL DISTRICT NUMBER ONE, 619 South Clark Street, Lyons, KS, Zip 67554, Mailing Address: P.O. Box 828, Zip 67554; tel. 316/257–5173; Robert L. Mullen, Administrator

WILSON COUNTY HOSPITAL, 205 Mill Street, Neodesha, KS, Zip 66757, Mailing Address: Box 360, Zip 66757; tel. 316/325–2611; Deanna Pittman, Administrator

SUNFLOWER HEALTH NETWORK, INC.
P.O. Box 2568, Salina, KS 67402–2568; tel. 913/452–7028; Sheryl Dority, Operations Coordinator

CLAY COUNTY HOSPITAL, 617 Liberty Street, Clay Center, KS, Zip 67432; tel. 913/632–2144; John F. Wiebe, Chief Executive Officer

CLOUD COUNTY HEALTH CENTER, 1100 Highland Drive, Concordia, KS, Zip 66901–3997; tel. 913/243–1234; Daniel R. Bartz, Chief Executive Officer

ELLSWORTH COUNTY HOSPITAL, 300 Kingsley Street, Ellsworth, KS, Zip 67439, Mailing Address: Drawer 87, Zip 67439; tel. 913/472–3111; Roger W. Pearson, Administrator

HERINGTON MUNICIPAL HOSPITAL, 100 East Helen Street, Herington, KS, Zip 67449; tel. 913/258–2207; William D. Peterson, Administrator

JEWELL COUNTY HOSPITAL, 100 Crestvue, Mankato, KS, Zip 66956, Mailing Address: Box 327, Zip 66956–0327; tel. 913/378–3137; Rodney Brockelman, Administrator

LINCOLN COUNTY HOSPITAL, 624 North Second Street, Lincoln, KS, Zip 67455, Mailing Address: P.O. Box 406, Zip 67455; tel. 913/524–4403; Jolene Yager, R.N., Administrator

LINDSBORG COMMUNITY HOSPITAL, 605 West Lincoln Street, Lindsborg, KS, Zip 67456–2399; tel. 913/227–3308; Greg Lundstrom, Interim Administrator

MEMORIAL HOSPITAL, 511 N.E. Tenth Street, Abilene, KS, Zip 67410, Mailing Address: P.O. Box 219, Zip 67410–0219; tel. 913/263–2100; Leon J. Boor, Chief Executive Officer

MEMORIAL HOSPITAL, 1000 Hospital Drive, McPherson, KS, Zip 67460–2321; tel. 316/241–2250; Stan Regehr, President and Chief Executive Officer

MITCHELL COUNTY HOSPITAL, 400 West Eighth, Beloit, KS, Zip 67420, Mailing Address: P.O. Box 399, Zip 67420; tel. 913/738–2266; John M. Osse, Administrator

OSBORNE COUNTY MEMORIAL HOSPITAL, 424 West New Hampshire Street, Osborne, KS, Zip 67473–0070, Mailing Address: P.O. Box 70, Zip 67473–0070; tel. 913/346–2121; Patricia Bernard, R.N., Administrator

OTTAWA COUNTY HOSPITAL, 215 East Eighth, Minneapolis, KS, Zip 67467, Mailing Address: Box 209, Zip 67467; tel. 913/392–2122; Joy Reed, R.N., Administrator

REPUBLIC COUNTY HOSPITAL, 2420 G Street, Belleville, KS, Zip 66935; tel. 913/527–2255; Charles A. Westin, FACHE, Administrator

RUSSELL REGIONAL HOSPITAL, 200 South Main Street, Russell, KS, Zip 67665; tel. 913/483–3131; Talton L. Francis, FACHE, President and Chief Executive Officer

SALINA REGIONAL HEALTH CENTER, 400 South Santa Fe Avenue, Salina, KS, Zip 67401, Mailing Address: P.O. Box 5080, Zip 67401; tel. 913/452–7000; Clay D. Edmands, President

SMITH COUNTY MEMORIAL HOSPITAL, 614 South Main Street, Smith Center, KS, Zip 66967–0349, Mailing Address: P.O. Box 349, Zip 66967–0349; tel. 913/282–6845; John Terrill, Administrator

VIA CHRISTI HEALTH SYSTEM
929 North Saint Francis, Wichita, KS 67214; tel. 316/268–5101; LeRoy Rheau, President and Chief Executive Officer

CLOUD COUNTY HEALTH CENTER, 1100 Highland Drive, Concordia, KS, Zip 66901–3997; tel. 913/243–1234; Daniel R. Bartz, Chief Executive Officer

MERCY HEALTH CENTER OF MANHATTAN, Manhattan, KS, Mailing Address: 1823 College Avenue, Zip 66502; E. Michael Nunamaker, President and Chief Executive Officer

MOUNT CARMEL MEDICAL CENTER, Centennial and Rouse Streets, Pittsburg, KS, Zip 66762–6686; tel. 316/231–6100; John Daniel Lingor, President and Chief Executive Officer

SALINA REGIONAL HEALTH CENTER, 400 South Santa Fe Avenue, Salina, KS, Zip 67401, Mailing Address: P.O. Box 5080, Zip 67401; tel. 913/452–7000; Clay D. Edmands, President

ST. JOSEPH REGIONAL MEDICAL CENTER OF NORTHERN OKLAHOMA, 14th Street and Hartford Avenue, Ponca City, OK, Zip 74601–2035, Mailing Address: Box 1270, Zip 74602–1270; tel. 405/765–3321; Garry L. England, President and Chief Executive Officer

VIA CHRISTI REGIONAL MEDICAL CENTER, 929 North St. Francis Street, Wichita, KS, Zip 67214–3882; tel. 316/268–5000; Randall G. Nyp, President and Chief Executive Officer

KENTUCKY

ALLIANT HEALTH SYSTEM
P.O. Box 35070, Louisville, KY 40232–5070; tel. 502/629–8025; Steven A. Williams, President

ALLIANT HOSPITALS, 200 East Chestnut Street, Louisville, KY, Zip 40202, Mailing Address: Box 35070, Zip 40232–5070; tel. 502/629–8000; Shirley B. Powers, Senior Executive Officer

BAPTIST HEALTHCARE SYSTEM
4007 Kresge Way, Louisville, KY 40207; tel. 502/896–5000; Tom Smith, President & Chief Executive Officer

BAPTIST HOSPITAL EAST, 4000 Kresge Way, Louisville, KY, Zip 40207–4676; tel. 502/897–8100; Susan Stout Tamme, President

BAPTIST REGIONAL MEDICAL CENTER, 1 Trillium Way, Corbin, KY, Zip 40701–8420; tel. 606/528–1212; John S. Henson, President

CARITAS MEDICAL CENTER, 1850 Bluegrass Avenue, Louisville, KY, Zip 40215–1199; tel. 502/361–6000; Peter J. Bernard, President and Chief Executive Officer

CARITAS PEACE CENTER, 2020 Newburg Road, Louisville, KY, Zip 40205; tel. 502/451–3330; Peter J. Bernard, President and Chief Executive Officer

CENTRAL BAPTIST HOSPITAL, 1740 Nicholasville Road, Lexington, KY, Zip 40503; tel. 606/275–6100; William G. Sisson, President

TRI COUNTY BAPTIST HOSPITAL, 1025 New Moody Lane, La Grange, KY, Zip 40031–0559; tel. 502/222–5388; David L. Gray, Administrator

WESTERN BAPTIST HOSPITAL, 2501 Kentucky Avenue, Paducah, KY, Zip 42003; tel. 502/575–2100; Larry O. Barton, President

BLUE GRASS FAMILY HEALTH PLAN
651 Perimeter Park, Suite 2B, Lexington, KY 40517; tel. 606/269–4475; Katherine Schaefer, Network Coordinator

BAPTIST REGIONAL MEDICAL CENTER, 1 Trillium Way, Corbin, KY, Zip 40701–8420; tel. 606/528–1212; John S. Henson, President

BEREA HOSPITAL, 305 Estill Street, Berea, KY, Zip 40403; tel. 606/986–3151; David E. Burgio, FACHE, Administrator and Chief Executive Officer

CENTRAL BAPTIST HOSPITAL, 1740 Nicholasville Road, Lexington, KY, Zip 40503; tel. 606/275–6100; William G. Sisson, President

CLARK REGIONAL MEDICAL CENTER, West Lexington Avenue, Winchester, KY, Zip 40391, Mailing Address: P.O. Box 630, Zip 40392–0630; tel. 606/745–3500; Robert D. Fraraccio, Administrator

COLUMBIA HOSPITAL FRANKFORT, 299 King's Daughters Drive, Frankfort, KY, Zip 40601–4186; tel. 502/875–5240; David P. Steitz, Chief Executive Officer

COLUMBIA HOSPITAL GEORGETOWN, 1140 Lexington Road, Georgetown, KY, Zip 40324; tel. 502/868–1100; Britt T. Reynolds, Chief Executive Officer

COLUMBIA HOSPITAL MAYSVILLE, 989 Medical Park Drive, Maysville, KY, Zip 41056; tel. 606/759–5311; J. Timothy Browne, Chief Executive Officer

COLUMBIA HOSPITAL PARIS, 9 Linville Drive, Paris, KY, Zip 40361; tel. 606/987–1000; John R. Grant, Chief Executive Officer

FORT LOGAN HOSPITAL, 124 Portman Avenue, Stanford, KY, Zip 40484–1200; tel. 606/365–2187; Terry C. Powers, Administrator

GARRARD COUNTY MEMORIAL HOSPITAL, 308 West Maple Avenue, Lancaster, KY, Zip 40444–1098; tel. 606/792–6844; W. David MacCool, Administrator

HARRISON MEMORIAL HOSPITAL, Cynthiana, KY, Mailing Address: P.O. Box 250, Zip 41031–0250; tel. 606/234–2300; Darwin E. Root, Administrator

KNOX COUNTY GENERAL HOSPITAL, 321 High Street, Barbourville, KY, Zip 40906, Mailing Address: P.O. Box 160, Zip 40906; tel. 606/546–4175; Craig Morgan, Administrator

MARCUM AND WALLACE MEMORIAL HOSPITAL, 60 Mercy Court, Irvine, KY, Zip 40336, Mailing Address: P.O. Box 928, Zip 40336; tel. 606/723–2115; Christopher M. Goddard, Administrator

MARYMOUNT MEDICAL CENTER, 310 East Ninth Street, London, KY, Zip 40741–1299; tel. 606/878–6520; Lowell Jones, President

OWEN COUNTY MEMORIAL HOSPITAL, 330 Roland Avenue, Owenton, KY, Zip 40359; tel. 502/484–3441; Richard D. McLeod, Administrator

PATTIE A. CLAY HOSPITAL, EKU By–Pass, Richmond, KY, Zip 40475, Mailing Address: P.O. Box 1600, Zip 40476–2603; tel. 606/625–3131; Richard M. Thomas, President

ST. JOSEPH HOSPITAL, One St. Joseph Drive, Lexington, KY, Zip 40504; tel. 606/278–3436; Thomas J. Murray, President

THE JAMES B. HAGGIN MEMORIAL HOSPITAL, 464 Linden Avenue, Harrodsburg, KY, Zip 40330–1862; tel. 606/734–5441; Earl James Motzer, Ph.D., FACHE, Chief Executive Officer

WOODFORD HOSPITAL, 360 Amsden Avenue, Versailles, KY, Zip 40383–1286; tel. 606/873–3111; Nancy Littrell, Chief Executive Officer

CARITAS HEALTH SERVICES
1850 Bluegrass Avenue, Louisville, KY 40215–1199; tel. 502/361–6140; Conrad H. Thorne, Chief of Network Operations

CARITAS MEDICAL CENTER, 1850 Bluegrass Avenue, Louisville, KY, Zip 40215–1199; tel. 502/361–6000; Peter J. Bernard, President and Chief Executive Officer

CARITAS PEACE CENTER, 2020 Newburg Road, Louisville, KY, Zip 40205; tel. 502/451–3330; Peter J. Bernard, President and Chief Executive Officer

CENTER CARE
800 Park Street, Bowling Green, KY 42101; tel. 502/745–1517; John M. Fones, Senior Vice President

BAPTIST HOSPITAL, 2000 Church Street, Nashville, TN, Zip 37236–0002; tel. 615/329–5555; C. David Stringfield, President

BAPTIST HOSPITAL EAST, 4000 Kresge Way, Louisville, KY, Zip 40207–4676; tel. 502/897–8100; Susan Stout Tamme, President

BAPTIST REGIONAL MEDICAL CENTER, 1 Trillium Way, Corbin, KY, Zip 40701–8420; tel. 606/528–1212; John S. Henson, President

BEDFORD COUNTY GENERAL HOSPITAL, 845 Union Street, Shelbyville, TN, Zip 37160–9971; tel. 615/685–5433; Richard L. Graham, Administrator

CAVERNA MEMORIAL HOSPITAL, 1501 South Dixie Street, Horse Cave, KY, Zip 42749; tel. 502/786–2191; James J. Kerins, Sr., Administrator

CENTRAL BAPTIST HOSPITAL, 1740 Nicholasville Road, Lexington, KY, Zip 40503; tel. 606/275–6100; William G. Sisson, President

CHRIST HOSPITAL, 2139 Auburn Avenue, Cincinnati, OH, Zip 45219–2989; tel. 513/369–2000; Claus von Zychlin, Senior Executive Officer

CLARKSVILLE MEMORIAL HOSPITAL, 1771 Madison Street, Clarksville, TN, Zip 37043, Mailing Address: Box 3160, Zip 37043–3160; tel. 615/552–6622; James Lee Decker, President and Chief Executive Officer

CLINTON COUNTY HOSPITAL, 723 Burkesville Road, Albany, KY, Zip 42602; tel. 606/387–6421; Randel Flowers, Ph.D., Administrator

COFFEE MEDICAL CENTER, 1001 McArthur Drive, Manchester, TN, Zip 37355, Mailing Address: P.O. Box 1079, Zip 37355; tel. 615/728–3586; William M. Moore, Administrator

COLUMBIA DAUTERIVE HOSPITAL, 600 North Lewis Street, New Iberia, LA, Zip 70560, Mailing Address: P.O. Box 11210, Zip 70562–1210; tel. 318/365–7311; Kyle J. Viator, Chief Executive Officer

COLUMBIA DOCTORS' HOSPITAL OF OPELOUSAS, 5101 Highway 167 South, Opelousas, LA, Zip 70570; tel. 318/948–2100; Daryl J. Doise, Administrator

COLUMBIA HENDERSONVILLE HOSPITAL, 355 New Shackle Island Road, Hendersonville, TN, Zip 37075–2393; tel. 615/264–4000; Ron Walker, Chief Executive Officer

COLUMBIA HOSPITAL MAYSVILLE, 989 Medical Park Drive, Maysville, KY, Zip 41056; tel. 606/759–5311; J. Timothy Browne, Chief Executive Officer

COLUMBIA LOGAN MEMORIAL HOSPITAL, 1625 South Nashville Road, Russellville, KY, Zip 42276–0010, Mailing Address: P.O. Box 10, Zip 42276; tel. 502/726–4011

COLUMBIA MEDICAL CENTER OF SOUTHWEST LOUISIANA, 2810 Ambassador Caffery Parkway, Lafayette, LA, Zip 70506; tel. 318/981–2949; Gerald A. Fornoff, Chief Executive Officer

COLUMBIA NASHVILLE MEMORIAL HOSPITAL, 612 West Due West Avenue, Madison, TN, Zip 37115–4474; tel. 615/865–3511; Robert Benson, Chief Executive Officer

COLUMBIA PINELAKE REGIONAL HOSPITAL, 1099 Medical Center Circle, Mayfield, KY, Zip 42066, Mailing Address: P.O. Box 1099, Zip 42066; tel. 502/251–4100; Don A. Horstkotte, Chief Executive Officer

COLUMBIA SOUTHERN TENNESSEE MEDICAL CENTER, 185 Hospital Road, Winchester, TN, Zip 37398; tel. 615/967–8200; Michael W. Garfield, Administrator

COLUMBIA WOMEN'S AND CHILDREN'S HOSPITAL, 4600 Ambassador Caffery Parkway, Lafayette, LA, Zip 70508, Mailing Address: P.O. Box 88030, Zip 70598–8030; tel. 318/981–9100; Madeleine L. Roberson, Chief Executive Officer

COOKEVILLE GENERAL HOSPITAL, 142 West Fifth Street, Cookeville, TN, Zip 38501, Mailing Address: P.O. Box 340, Zip 38503–0340; tel. 615/528–2541; Mike Mayes, FACHE, Administrator and Chief Executive Officer

CUMBERLAND COUNTY HOSPITAL, Highway 90 West, Burkesville, KY, Zip 42717–0280, Mailing Address: P.O. Box 280, Zip 42717–0280; tel. 502/864–2511; Mark Thompson, Chief Executive Officer

FRANKLIN–SIMPSON MEMORIAL HOSPITAL, Brookhaven Road, Franklin, KY, Zip 42135–2929, Mailing Address: P.O. Box 2929, Zip 42135–2929; tel. 502/586–3253; William P. Macri, Administrator

GOOD SAMARITAN HOSPITAL, 375 Dixmyth Avenue, Cincinnati, OH, Zip 45220–2489; tel. 513/872–1400; Sister Myra James Bradley, Chairman of the Board of Directors

HARTON REGIONAL MEDICAL CENTER, 1801 North Jackson Street, Tullahoma, TN, Zip 37388, Mailing Address: P.O. Box 460, Zip 37388; tel. 615/393–3000; Brian T. Flynn, Administrator and Chief Executive Officer

JEWISH HOSPITAL, 217 East Chestnut Street, Louisville, KY, Zip 40202–1886; tel. 502/587–4011; Douglas E. Shaw, President

LAKEVIEW REHABILITATION HOSPITAL, 134 Heartland Drive, Elizabethtown, KY, Zip 42701; tel. 502/769–3100; James H. Wesp, Administrator

MACON COUNTY GENERAL HOSPITAL, 204 Medical Drive, Lafayette, TN, Zip 37083, Mailing Address: P.O. Box 378, Zip 37083; tel. 615/666–2147; Dennis A. Wolford, FACHE, Administrator

MEDICAL CENTER AT SCOTTSVILLE, 456 Burnley Road, Scottsville, KY, Zip 42164; tel. 502/622–2800; Connie Smith, Senior Vice President

MEDICAL CENTER OF MANCHESTER, 481 Interstate Drive, Manchester, TN, Zip 37355, Mailing Address: P.O. Box 1409, Zip 37355; tel. 615/728–6354; Sherry Collier, Chief Nursing Officer and Chief Operating Officer

MONROE COUNTY MEDICAL CENTER, 529 Capp Harlan Road, Tompkinsville, KY, Zip 42167; tel. 502/487–9231; Carolyn E. Riley, Chief Executive Officer

MUHLENBERG COMMUNITY HOSPITAL, 440 Hopkinsville Street, Greenville, KY, Zip 42345, Mailing Address: P.O. Box 387, Zip 42345; tel. 502/338–8000; Charles D. Lovell, Jr., Chief Executive Officer

NORTH OAKS MEDICAL CENTER, 15790 Medical Center Drive, Hammond, LA, Zip 70403, Mailing Address: Box 2668, Zip 70404; tel. 504/345–2700; James E. Cathey, Jr., Chief Executive Officer

OHIO COUNTY HOSPITAL, 1211 Main Street, Hartford, KY, Zip 42347; tel. 502/298–7411; Blaine Pieper, Administrator

OWENSBORO MERCY HEALTH SYSTEM, 811 East Parrish Avenue, Owensboro, KY, Zip 42303, Mailing Address: P.O. Box 20007, Zip 42303; tel. 502/688–2000; Greg L. Carlson, President and Chief Executive Officer

PIKEVILLE UNITED METHODIST HOSPITAL OF KENTUCKY, 911 South Bypass, Pikeville, KY, Zip 41501–1595; tel. 606/437–3500; Martha O'Regan Chill, Administrator and Chief Executive Officer

ST. ELIZABETH MEDICAL CENTER–GRANT COUNTY, 238 Barnes Road, Williamstown, KY, Zip 41097; tel. 606/824–2400; Chris Carle, Administrator

ST. ELIZABETH MEDICAL CENTER–NORTH, 401 East 20th Street, Covington, KY, Zip 41014; tel. 606/292–4000; Joseph W. Gross, President and Chief Executive Officer

ST. JOSEPH HOSPITAL, One St. Joseph Drive, Lexington, KY, Zip 40504; tel. 606/278–3436; Thomas J. Murray, President

ST. THOMAS HOSPITAL, 4220 Harding Road, Nashville, TN, Zip 37205, Mailing Address: Box 380, Zip 37202; tel. 615/222–2111; John F. Tighe, President and Chief Executive Officer

SUMNER REGIONAL MEDICAL CENTER, 555 Hartsville Pike, Gallatin, TN, Zip 37066, Mailing Address: P.O. Box 1558, Zip 37066–1558; tel. 615/452–4210; William T. Sugg, President and Chief Executive Officer

T. J. SAMSON COMMUNITY HOSPITAL, 1301 North Race Street, Glasgow, KY, Zip 42141–3483; tel. 502/651–4444; H. Glenn Joiner, Chief Executive Officer

THE JAMES B. HAGGIN MEMORIAL HOSPITAL, 464 Linden Avenue, Harrodsburg, KY, Zip 40330–1862; tel. 606/734–5441; Earl James Motzer, Ph.D., FACHE, Chief Executive Officer

THE MEDICAL CENTER AT BOWLING GREEN, 250 Park Street, Bowling Green, KY, Zip 42101, Mailing Address: Box 90010, Zip 42102–9010; tel. 502/745–1000; Laurence C. Hinsdale, Chief Executive Officer

TWIN LAKES REGIONAL MEDICAL CENTER, 910 Wallace Avenue, Leitchfield, KY, Zip 42754; tel. 502/259–9400; Stephen L. Meredith, Chief Executive Officer

UNIVERSITY MEDICAL CENTER, 1411 Baddour Parkway, Lebanon, TN, Zip 37087; tel. 615/444–8262; Nanette Todd, R.N., Acting Administrator

WESTLAKE REGIONAL HOSPITAL, Westlake Drive, Columbia, KY, Zip 42728, Mailing Address: P.O. Box 468, Zip 42728–0468; tel. 502/384–4753; Rex A. Tungate, Administrator

WILLIAMSON MEDICAL CENTER, 2021 Carothers Road, Franklin, TN, Zip 37067, Mailing Address: P.O. Box 681600, Zip 37068–1600; tel. 615/791–0500; Ronald G. Joyner, Chief Executive Officer

CHA PROVIDER NETWORK, INC.
P.O. Box 22171, Lexington, KY 40522–2171; tel. 606/272–5820; Michael G. Strother, Director of Network

ARH REGIONAL MEDICAL CENTER, 100 Medical Center Drive, Hazard, KY, Zip 41701–1000; tel. 606/439–6610; David R. Lyon, Administrator

BECKLEY APPALACHIAN REGIONAL HOSPITAL, 306 Stanaford Road, Beckley, WV, Zip 25801; tel. 304/255–3000; Norman Wright, Administrator

BEREA HOSPITAL, 305 Estill Street, Berea, KY, Zip 40403; tel. 606/986–3151; David E. Burgio, FACHE, Administrator and Chief Executive Officer

BOONE MEMORIAL HOSPITAL, 701 Madison Avenue, Madison, WV, Zip 25130; tel. 304/369–1230; Tommy H. Mullins, Administrator

CABELL HUNTINGTON HOSPITAL, 1340 Hal Greer Boulevard, Huntington, WV, Zip 25701–0195; tel. 304/526–2000; W. Don Smith, II, President and Chief Executive Officer

CARDINAL HILL REHABILITATION HOSPITAL, 2050 Versailles Road, Lexington, KY, Zip 40504–1499; tel. 606/254–5701; Kerry G. Gillihan, President and Chief Executive Officer

CHARTER RIDGE HOSPITAL, 3050 Rio Dosa Drive, Lexington, KY, Zip 40509–9990; tel. 606/269–2325; Ali A. Elhaj, Chief Executive Officer

CHRIST HOSPITAL, 2139 Auburn Avenue, Cincinnati, OH, Zip 45219–2989; tel. 513/369–2000; Claus von Zychlin, Senior Executive Officer

CLAIBORNE COUNTY HOSPITAL, 1850 Old Knoxville Road, Tazewell, TN, Zip 37879, Mailing Address: Box 219, Zip 37879; tel. 615/626–4211; Richard Welch, Administrator

CLARK REGIONAL MEDICAL CENTER, West Lexington Avenue, Winchester, KY, Zip 40391, Mailing Address: P.O. Box 630, Zip 40392–0630; tel. 606/745–3500; Robert D. Fraraccio, Administrator

FORT LOGAN HOSPITAL, 124 Portman Avenue, Stanford, KY, Zip 40484–1200; tel. 606/365–2187; Terry C. Powers, Administrator

FORT SANDERS LOUDON MEDICAL CENTER, 1125 Grove Street, Loudon, TN, Zip 37774, Mailing Address: Box 217, Zip 37774–0217; tel. 615/458–8222; Ralph T. Williams, Administrator

FORT SANDERS REGIONAL MEDICAL CENTER, 1901 Clinch Avenue S.W., Knoxville, TN, Zip 37916–2394; tel. 423/541–1111; James R. Burkhart, FACHE, Administrator

FORT SANDERS–PARKWEST MEDICAL CENTER, 9352 Park West Boulevard, Knoxville, TN, Zip 37923, Mailing Address: P.O. Box 22993, Zip 37933–0993; tel. 423/694–5700; James R. Burkhart, FACHE, Administrator

FORT SANDERS–SEVIER MEDICAL CENTER, 709 Middle Creek Road, Sevierville, TN, Zip 37862, Mailing Address: P.O. Box 8005, Zip 37864–8005; tel. 423/429–6100; Ralph T. Williams, Administrator

GARRARD COUNTY MEMORIAL HOSPITAL, 308 West Maple Avenue, Lancaster, KY, Zip 40444–1098; tel. 606/792–6844; W. David MacCool, Administrator

HARLAN ARH HOSPITAL, 81 Ball Park Road, Harlan, KY, Zip 40831–1792; tel. 606/573–8100; Daniel Fitzpatrick, Administrator

HARRISON MEMORIAL HOSPITAL, Cynthiana, KY, Mailing Address: P.O. Box 250, Zip 41031–0250; tel. 606/234–2300; Darwin E. Root, Administrator

HIGHLANDS REGIONAL MEDICAL CENTER, 5000 Kentucky Route 321, Prestonsburg, KY, Zip 41653, Mailing Address: Box 668, Zip 41653–0668; tel. 606/886–8511; Clarence Traum, President and Chief Executive Officer

JENKINS COMMUNITY HOSPITAL, Main Street, Jenkins, KY, Zip 41537, Mailing Address: P.O. Box 472, Zip 41537; tel. 606/832–2171; Sherrie Newcomb, Acting Administrator

JEWISH HOSPITAL, 3200 Burnet Avenue, Cincinnati, OH, Zip 45229–3099; tel. 513/569–2000; Warren C. Falberg, Senior Executive Officer

KNOX COUNTY GENERAL HOSPITAL, 321 High Street, Barbourville, KY, Zip 40906, Mailing Address: P.O. Box 160, Zip 40906; tel. 606/546–4175; Craig Morgan, Administrator

LONESOME PINE HOSPITAL, 1990 Holton Avenue East, Big Stone Gap, VA, Zip 24219–0230, Mailing Address: Drawer I, Zip 24219; tel. 540/523–3111; Paul A. Bishop, Administrator

MAN ARH HOSPITAL, 700 East McDonald Avenue, Man, WV, Zip 25635–1011; tel. 304/583–8421; Freda Napier, Administrator

MARCUM AND WALLACE MEMORIAL HOSPITAL, 60 Mercy Court, Irvine, KY, Zip 40336, Mailing Address: P.O. Box 928, Zip 40336; tel. 606/723–2115; Christopher M. Goddard, Administrator

MARY BRECKINRIDGE HOSPITAL, Hospital Drive, Hyden, KY, Zip 41749–0000; tel. 606/672–2901; A. Ray Branaman, Administrator

MCDOWELL ARH HOSPITAL, Route 122, McDowell, KY, Zip 41647, Mailing Address: Box 247, Zip 41647; tel. 606/377–3400; Jerry Haynes, Administrator

MEMORIAL HOSPITAL, 401 Memorial Drive, Manchester, KY, Zip 40962–9156; tel. 606/598–5104; T. Henry Scoggins, FACHE, President

MIDDLESBORO APPALACHIAN REGIONAL HOSPITAL, 3600 West Cumberland Avenue, Middlesboro, KY, Zip 40965, Mailing Address: Box 340, Zip 40965–0340; tel. 606/242–1101; Paul V. Miles, Administrator

MORGAN COUNTY APPALACHIAN REGIONAL HOSPITAL, 476 Liberty Road, West Liberty, KY, Zip 41472, Mailing Address: Box 579, Zip 41472–0579; tel. 606/743–3186; Dennis R. Chaney, Administrator

NICHOLAS COUNTY HOSPITAL, 2323 Concrete Road, Carlisle, KY, Zip 40311, Mailing Address: Box 232, Zip 40311; tel. 606/289–7181; James J. Wente, Administrator

OUR LADY OF BELLEFONTE HOSPITAL, St. Christopher Drive, Ashland, KY, Zip 41105–0789, Mailing Address: P.O. Box 789, Zip 41105–0789; tel. 606/833–3333; Robert J. Maher, President

OUR LADY OF THE WAY HOSPITAL, 11022 Main Street, Martin, KY, Zip 41649–0910; tel. 606/285–5181; Lowell Jones, Chief Executive Officer

OWEN COUNTY MEMORIAL HOSPITAL, 330 Roland Avenue, Owenton, KY, Zip 40359; tel. 502/484–3441; Richard D. McLeod, Administrator

PATTIE A. CLAY HOSPITAL, EKU By–Pass, Richmond, KY, Zip 40475, Mailing Address: P.O. Box 1600, Zip 40476–2603; tel. 606/625–3131; Richard M. Thomas, President

PENINSULA HOSPITAL, 2347 Jones Bend Road, Louisville, TN, Zip 37777, Mailing Address: P.O. Box 2000, Zip 37777; tel. 423/970–9800; David H. McReynolds, Chief Operating Officer and Administrator

PINEVILLE COMMUNITY HOSPITAL ASSOCIATION, Riverview Avenue, Pineville, KY, Zip 40977–0850; tel. 606/337–3051; J. Milton Brooks, III, Administrator

ROCKCASTLE HOSPITAL, 145 Newcomb Avenue, Mount Vernon, KY, Zip 40456, Mailing Address: P.O. Box 1310, Zip 40456; tel. 606/256–2195; Lee D. Keene, Administrator

ST. CLAIRE MEDICAL CENTER, 222 Medical Circle, Morehead, KY, Zip 40351–1180; tel. 606/783–6500; Mark J. Neff, President and Chief Executive Officer

ST. LUKE HOSPITAL EAST, 85 North Grand Avenue, Fort Thomas, KY, Zip 41075–1796; tel. 606/572–3100; Daniel M. Vinson, CPA, Senior Executive Officer

ST. LUKE HOSPITAL WEST, 7380 Turfway Road, Florence, KY, Zip 41042; tel. 606/525–5200; John D. Hoyle, Senior Executive Officer

ST. MARY'S HOSPITAL, 2900 First Avenue, Huntington, WV, Zip 25702; tel. 304/526–1234; J. Thomas Jones, Executive Director

SUMMERS COUNTY APPALACHIAN REGIONAL HOSPITAL, Terrace Street, Hinton, WV, Zip 25951, Mailing Address: Drawer 940, Zip 25951–0940; tel. 304/466–1000; Clyde E. Bolton, Administrator

THE JAMES B. HAGGIN MEMORIAL HOSPITAL, 464 Linden Avenue, Harrodsburg, KY, Zip 40330–1862; tel. 606/734–5441; Earl James Motzer, Ph.D., FACHE, Chief Executive Officer

THREE RIVERS MEDICAL CENTER, Highway 644, Louisa, KY, Zip 41230, Mailing Address: Box 769, Zip 41230; tel. 606/638–9451; Greg Kiser, Chief Executive Officer

UNIVERISITY HOSPITAL, 234 Goodman Street, Cincinnati, OH, Zip 45267–0700; tel. 513/558–1000; Elliot G. Cohen, Senior Executive Officer

UNIVERSITY OF KENTUCKY HOSPITAL, 800 Rose Street, Lexington, KY, Zip 40536–0084; tel. 606/323–5000; Frank Butler, Director

WELLMONT HEALTH SYSTEM–HOLSTON VALLEY, West Ravine Street, Kingsport, TN, Zip 37662–0224, Mailing Address: Box 238, Zip 37662–0224; tel. 423/224–5001; Louis H. Bremer, President and Chief Executive Officer

WHITESBURG APPALACHIAN REGIONAL HOSPITAL, 550 Jenkins Road, Whitesburg, KY, Zip 41858; tel. 606/633–3600; Nick Lewis, Administrator

WILLIAMSON ARH HOSPITAL, 260 Hospital Drive, South Williamson, KY, Zip 41503; tel. 606/237–1700; John A. Grah, Administrator

WISE ARH HOSPITAL, Wise, VA, Mailing Address: P.O. Box 3267, Zip 24293–3267; tel. 540/328–2511; Louis G. Roe, Jr., Administrator

WOODFORD HOSPITAL, 360 Amsden Avenue, Versailles, KY, Zip 40383–1286; tel. 606/873–3111; Nancy Littrell, Chief Executive Officer

COMMUNITY CARE NETWORK
1305 North Elm Street, Henderson, KY 42420; tel. 502/827–7380; LeaAnn H. Martin, Director of Marketing

CALDWELL COUNTY HOSPITAL, 101 Hospital Drive, Princeton, KY, Zip 42445–0410, Mailing Address: Box 410, Zip 42445–0410; tel. 502/365–0300; John Svoboda, Chief Executive Officer

COMMUNITY METHODIST HOSPITAL, 1305 North Elm Street, Henderson, KY, Zip 42420, Mailing Address: Box 48, Zip 42420–0048; tel. 502/827–7700; Bruce D. Begley, Executive Director

CRITTENDEN COUNTY HOSPITAL, Highway 60 South, Marion, KY, Zip 42064–0386, Mailing Address: Box 386, Zip 42064; tel. 502/965–5281; Rick Napper, Chief Executive Officer

FRANKLIN–SIMPSON MEMORIAL HOSPITAL, Brookhaven Road, Franklin, KY, Zip 42135–2929, Mailing Address: P.O. Box 2929, Zip 42135–2929; tel. 502/586–3253; William P. Macri, Administrator

JENNIE STUART MEDICAL CENTER, 320 West 18th Street, Hopkinsville, KY, Zip 42240–6315; tel. 502/887–0100; Lewis T. Peeples, Chief Executive Officer

LIVINGSTON HOSPITAL AND HEALTHCARE SERVICES, 131 Hospital Drive, Salem, KY, Zip 42078, Mailing Address: Box 138, Zip 42078; tel. 502/988–2299; William C. Smith, Chief Executive Officer

MUHLENBERG COMMUNITY HOSPITAL, 440 Hopkinsville Street, Greenville, KY, Zip 42345, Mailing Address: P.O. Box 387, Zip 42345; tel. 502/338–8000; Charles D. Lovell, Jr., Chief Executive Officer

MURRAY–CALLOWAY COUNTY HOSPITAL, 803 Poplar Street, Murray, KY, Zip 42071–2432; tel. 502/762–1100; Stuart Poston, President

OWENSBORO MERCY HEALTH SYSTEM, 811 East Parrish Avenue, Owensboro, KY, Zip 42303, Mailing Address: P.O. Box 20007, Zip 42303; tel. 502/688–2000; Greg L. Carlson, President and Chief Executive Officer

REGIONAL MEDICAL CENTER OF HOPKINS COUNTY, 900 Hospital Drive, Madisonville, KY, Zip 42431–1694; tel. 502/825–5100; Bobby H. Dampier, Chief Executive Officer

UNION COUNTY METHODIST HOSPITAL, 4604 Highway 60 West, Morganfield, KY, Zip 42437–9570; tel. 502/389–3030; Patrick Donahue, Administrator

COMMUNITY HEALTH DELIVERY SYSTEM, INC.
2020 Newburg Road, Louisville, KY 40205; tel. 502/451–3330; Fran Dotson, Network Contact

ALLIANT HOSPITALS, 200 East Chestnut Street, Louisville, KY, Zip 40202, Mailing Address: Box 35070, Zip 40232–5070; tel. 502/629–8000; Shirley B. Powers, Senior Executive Officer

BAPTIST HOSPITAL EAST, 4000 Kresge Way, Louisville, KY, Zip 40207–4676; tel. 502/897–8100; Susan Stout Tamme, President

BAPTIST REGIONAL MEDICAL CENTER, 1 Trillium Way, Corbin, KY, Zip 40701–8420; tel. 606/528–1212; John S. Henson, President

BRECKINRIDGE MEMORIAL HOSPITAL, 1011 Old Highway 60, Hardinsburg, KY, Zip 40143–2597; tel. 502/756–7000; George Walz, CHE, Chief Executive Officer

CALDWELL COUNTY HOSPITAL, 101 Hospital Drive, Princeton, KY, Zip 42445–0410, Mailing Address: Box 410, Zip 42445–0410; tel. 502/365–0300; John Svoboda, Chief Executive Officer

CARITAS MEDICAL CENTER, 1850 Bluegrass Avenue, Louisville, KY, Zip 40215–1199; tel. 502/361–6000; Peter J. Bernard, President and Chief Executive Officer

CARITAS PEACE CENTER, 2020 Newburg Road, Louisville, KY, Zip 40205; tel. 502/451–3330; Peter J. Bernard, President and Chief Executive Officer

CARROLL COUNTY MEMORIAL HOSPITAL, 309 11th Street, Carrollton, KY, Zip 41008; tel. 502/732–4321; Roger Williams, Chief Executive Officer

CAVERNA MEMORIAL HOSPITAL, 1501 South Dixie Street, Horse Cave, KY, Zip 42749; tel. 502/786–2191; James J. Kerins, Sr., Administrator

CENTRAL BAPTIST HOSPITAL, 1740 Nicholasville Road, Lexington, KY, Zip 40503; tel. 606/275–6100; William G. Sisson, President

FLAGET MEMORIAL HOSPITAL, 201 Cathedral Manor, Bardstown, KY, Zip 40004–1299; tel. 502/348–3923; Suzanne Reasbeck, President and Chief Executive Officer

JANE TODD CRAWFORD MEMORIAL HOSPITAL, 202–206 Milby Street, Greensburg, KY, Zip 42743, Mailing Address: P.O. Box 220, Zip 42743; tel. 502/932–4211; Larry Craig, Chief Executive Officer

MARYMOUNT MEDICAL CENTER, 310 East Ninth Street, London, KY, Zip 40741–1299; tel. 606/878–6520; Lowell Jones, President

ST. ELIZABETH MEDICAL CENTER–GRANT COUNTY, 238 Barnes Road, Williamstown, KY, Zip 41097; tel. 606/824–2400; Chris Carle, Administrator

ST. ELIZABETH MEDICAL CENTER–NORTH, 401 East 20th Street, Covington, KY, Zip 41014; tel. 606/292–4000; Joseph W. Gross, President and Chief Executive Officer

ST. JOSEPH HOSPITAL, One St. Joseph Drive, Lexington, KY, Zip 40504; tel. 606/278–3436; Thomas J. Murray, President

TRI COUNTY BAPTIST HOSPITAL, 1025 New Moody Lane, La Grange, KY, Zip 40031–0559; tel. 502/222–5388; David L. Gray, Administrator

TRIGG COUNTY HOSPITAL, Highway 68 East, Cadiz, KY, Zip 42211, Mailing Address: Box 312, Zip 42211; tel. 502/522–3215; Richard Chapman, Administrator

TWIN LAKES REGIONAL MEDICAL CENTER, 910 Wallace Avenue, Leitchfield, KY, Zip 42754; tel. 502/259–9400; Stephen L. Meredith, Chief Executive Officer

WESTERN BAPTIST HOSPITAL, 2501 Kentucky Avenue, Paducah, KY, Zip 42003; tel. 502/575–2100; Larry O. Barton, President

JEWISH HOSPITAL HEALTHCARE SERVICES
217 East Chestnut Street, Louisville, KY 40202; tel. 502/587–4011; Greg Pugh, Data Analyst

CLARK MEMORIAL HOSPITAL, 1220 Missouri Avenue, Jeffersonville, IN, Zip 47130–3743, Mailing Address: Box 69, Zip 47131–0069; tel. 812/282–6631; Merle E. Stepp, President and Chief Executive Officer

FRAZIER REHABILITATION CENTER, 220 Abraham Flexner Way, Louisville, KY, Zip 40202–1887; tel. 502/582–7400; Jason Roeback, President

HARDIN MEMORIAL HOSPITAL, 913 North Dixie Highway, Elizabethtown, KY, Zip 42701–2599; tel. 502/737–1212; Gary R. Colberg, President and Chief Executive Officer

JEWISH HOSPITAL, 217 East Chestnut Street, Louisville, KY, Zip 40202–1886; tel. 502/587–4011; Douglas E. Shaw, President

JEWISH HOSPITAL–SHELBYVILLE, 727 Hospital Drive, Shelbyville, KY, Zip 40065; tel. 502/647–4301; Timothy L. Jarm, President

LEXINGTON HOSPITAL, 150 North Eagle Creek Drive, Lexington, KY, Zip 40509–1807; tel. 606/268–4800; Rebecca Lewis, President

PATTIE A. CLAY HOSPITAL, EKU By–Pass, Richmond, KY, Zip 40475, Mailing Address: P.O. Box 1600, Zip 40476–2603; tel. 606/625–3131; Richard M. Thomas, President

SCOTT MEMORIAL HOSPITAL, 1415 North Gardner Street, Scottsburg, IN, Zip 47170–0456, Mailing Address: Box 430, Zip 47170–0430; tel. 812/752–8500; Clifford D. Nay, Executive Director

TAYLOR COUNTY HOSPITAL, 1700 Old Lebanon Road, Campbellsville, KY, Zip 42718; tel. 502/465–3561; David R. Hayes, President

WASHINGTON COUNTY MEMORIAL HOSPITAL, 911 North Shelby Street, Salem, IN, Zip 47167; tel. 812/883–5881; Rodney M. Coats, Executive Director

SAINT ELIZABETH MEDICAL CENTER
1 Medical Village Drive, Covington, KY 41017; tel. 606/344–2000; Joseph W. Gross, President & Chief Executive Officer

ST. ELIZABETH MEDICAL CENTER–GRANT COUNTY, 238 Barnes Road, Williamstown, KY, Zip 41097; tel. 606/824–2400; Chris Carle, Administrator

ST. ELIZABETH MEDICAL CENTER–NORTH, 401 East 20th Street, Covington, KY, Zip 41014; tel. 606/292–4000; Joseph W. Gross, President and Chief Executive Officer

LOUISIANA

COLUMBIA LAKEVIEW REGIONAL MEDICAL CENTER
95 East Fairway Drive, Covington, LA 70433; tel. 504/867–3800; Scott Koenig, Chief Executive Officer

COLUMBIA LAKEVIEW REGIONAL MEDICAL CENTER, 95 East Fairway Drive, Covington, LA, Zip 70433; tel. 504/876–3800; Scott Koenig, Chief Executive Officer

FRANCISCAN MISSIONARIES OF OUR LADY HEALTH NETWORK
4200 Essen Lane, Baton Rouge, LA 70809; tel. 504/923–2701; Charles Thoele, Interim Vice President

OUR LADY OF LOURDES REGIONAL MEDICAL CENTER, 611 St. Landry Street, Lafayette, LA, Zip 70506–4697, Mailing Address: Box 4027, Zip 70502–4027; tel. 318/289–2000; Dudley Romero, President and Chief Executive Officer

OUR LADY OF THE LAKE REGIONAL MEDICAL CENTER, 5000 Henessy Boulevard, Baton Rouge, LA, Zip 70808–4350; tel. 504/765–6565; Robert C. Davidge, President and Chief Executive Officer

ST. FRANCIS MEDICAL CENTER, 309 Jackson Street, Monroe, LA, Zip 71201, Mailing Address: Box 1901, Zip 71210–1901; tel. 318/327–4000; H. Gerald Smith, President and Chief Executive Officer

HEALTHCARE ADVANTAGE, INC.
829 Saint Charles Avenue, New Orleans, LA 70103; tel. 504/568–9009; Jane Cooper, President

DOCTORS HOSPITAL OF JEFFERSON, 4320 Houma Boulevard, Metairie, LA, Zip 70006–2973; tel. 504/456–5800; Gerald L. Parton, Chief Executive Officer

EAST JEFFERSON GENERAL HOSPITAL, 4200 Houma Boulevard, Metairie, LA, Zip 70011–9987; tel. 504/454–4000; Peter J. Betts, President and Chief Executive Officer

PENDLETON MEMORIAL METHODIST HOSPITAL, 5620 Read Boulevard, New Orleans, LA, Zip 70127–3154; tel. 504/244–5100; Frederick C. Young, Jr., President

WEST JEFFERSON MEDICAL CENTER, 1101 Medical Center Boulevard, Marrero, LA, Zip 70072–3191; tel. 504/347–5511; David M. Smith, FACHE, President and Chief Executive Officer

LOUISIANA HEALTH CARE AUTHORITY
8550 United Plaza Boulevard, Baton Rouge, LA 70809; tel. 504/342–2964; Carolyn Mattis, Director of Networks

E. A. CONWAY MEDICAL CENTER, 4864 Jackson Street, Monroe, LA, Zip 71202, Mailing Address: P.O. Box 1881, Zip 71210–8005; tel. 318/330–7000; Roy D. Bostick, Director

Section B

EARL K. LONG MEDICAL CENTER, 5825 Airline Highway, Baton Rouge, LA, Zip 70805; tel. 504/358–1000; Margaret Alvis, MSN, R.N., Chief Executive Officer

HUEY P. LONG MEDICAL CENTER, 352 Hospital Boulevard, Pineville, LA, Zip 71360, Mailing Address: Box 5352, Zip 71361–5352; tel. 318/448–0811; James E. Morgan, Director

LALLIE KEMP MEDICAL CENTER, 52579 Highway 51 South, Independence, LA, Zip 70443; tel. 504/878–9421; LeVern Meades, Acting Administrator

LEONARD J. CHABERT MEDICAL CENTER, 1978 Industrial Boulevard, Houma, LA, Zip 70363; tel. 504/873–2200; William C. Bankston, Acting Administrator

MEDICAL CENTER OF LOUISIANA AT NEW ORLEANS, 2021 Perdido Street, New Orleans, LA, Zip 70112–1396; tel. 504/588–3000; Jonathan Roberts, Dr.PH, President and Chief Executive Officer

UNIVERSITY MEDICAL CENTER, 2390 West Congress Street, Lafayette, LA, Zip 70506, Mailing Address: P.O. Box 4016–C, Zip 70502–4016; tel. 318/261–6004; Lawrence T. Dorsey, Administrator

WALTER OLIN MOSS REGIONAL MEDICAL CENTER, 1000 Walters Street, Lake Charles, LA, Zip 70605; tel. 318/475–8100; Philip H. Rome, Administrator

WASHINGTON–ST. TAMMANY REGIONAL MEDICAL CENTER, 400 Memphis Street, Bogalusa, LA, Zip 70427–0040, Mailing Address: Box 40, Zip 70429–0040; tel. 504/735–1322; Larry R. King, Administrator

OCHSNER/SISTERS OF CHARITY HEALTH NETWORK
One Galleria Boulevard, Suite 1224, New Orleans, LA 70001; tel. 504/836–8064; Jim Pittman, Director of Networks

BEAUREGARD MEMORIAL HOSPITAL, 600 South Pine Street, De Ridder, LA, Zip 70634, Mailing Address: P.O. Box 730, Zip 70634–0730; tel. 318/462–7100; Theodore J. Badger, Jr., Chief Executive Officer

BUNKIE GENERAL HOSPITAL, Evergreen Highway, Bunkie, LA, Zip 71322, Mailing Address: Box 380, Zip 71322–0380; tel. 318/346–6681; Donald L. Kannady, Administrator

BYRD REGIONAL HOSPITAL, 1020 Fertitta Boulevard, Leesville, LA, Zip 71446; tel. 318/239–9041; Donald Henderson, Executive Director

COLUMBIA MEDICAL CENTER, 17000 Medical Center Drive, Baton Rouge, LA, Zip 70816–3224; tel. 504/755–4800; Joseph R. Dicapo, Chief Executive Officer

DE SOTO REGIONAL HEALTH SYSTEM, 207 Jefferson Street, Mansfield, LA, Zip 71052, Mailing Address: P.O. Box 672, Zip 71052; tel. 318/872–4610; William F. Barrow, President and Chief Executive Officer

HOMER MEMORIAL HOSPITAL, 620 East College Street, Homer, LA, Zip 71040; tel. 318/927–2024; J. Larry Jordan, Administrator

JENNINGS AMERICAN LEGION HOSPITAL, 1634 Elton Road, Jennings, LA, Zip 70546; tel. 318/821–4151; Terry J. Terrebonne, Administrator

LADY OF THE SEA GENERAL HOSPITAL, 200 West 134th Place, Cut Off, LA, Zip 70345; tel. 504/632–6401; Lane M. Cheramie, Chief Executive Officer

LANE MEMORIAL HOSPITAL, 6300 Main Street, Zachary, LA, Zip 70791–9990; tel. 504/658–4000; Charlie L. Massey, Administrator

MINDEN MEDICAL CENTER, 1 Medical Plaza, Minden, LA, Zip 71055; tel. 318/377–2321; George E. French, III, Chief Executive Officer

NATCHITOCHES PARISH HOSPITAL, 501 Keyser Avenue, Natchitoches, LA, Zip 71457, Mailing Address: Box 2009, Zip 71457–2009; tel. 318/352–1200; Eugene Spillman, Executive Director

NORTHSHORE REGIONAL MEDICAL CENTER, 100 Medical Center Drive, Slidell, LA, Zip 70461–8572; tel. 504/649–7070; Charles F. Miller, Chief Executive Officer

OCHSNER FOUNDATION HOSPITAL, 1516 Jefferson Highway, New Orleans, LA, Zip 70121; tel. 504/842–3000; Mary W. Brown, Executive Vice President and Director

PENDLETON MEMORIAL METHODIST HOSPITAL, 5620 Read Boulevard, New Orleans, LA, Zip 70127–3154; tel. 504/244–5100; Frederick C. Young, Jr., President

RIVER WEST MEDICAL CENTER, 59355 River West Drive, Plaquemine, LA, Zip 70764–9543; tel. 504/687–9222; Steve Grimm, Chief Executive Officer

RIVERLAND MEDICAL CENTER, 1700 North E 'E' Wallace Boulevard, Ferriday, LA, Zip 71334, Mailing Address: Box 111, Zip 71334; tel. 318/757–6551; Vernon R. Stevens, Jr., Administrator

RIVERNORTH HOSPITAL, 5505 Shreveport Highway, Pineville, LA, Zip 71360; tel. 318/640–0222; Daniel W. Johnson, Chief Executive Officer

SABINE MEDICAL CENTER, 240 Highland Drive, Many, LA, Zip 71449–3718; tel. 318/256–5691; Mark Nosacka, Executive Director

SCHUMPERT MEDICAL CENTER, One St. Mary Place, Shreveport, LA, Zip 71101, Mailing Address: P.O. Box 21976, Zip 71120–1076; tel. 318/681–4500; Arthur A. Gonzalez, Dr.PH, President and Chief Executive Officer

ST. ANNE GENERAL HOSPITAL, Highway 1 and Twin Oaks Drive, Raceland, LA, Zip 70394, Mailing Address: Box 440, Zip 70394; tel. 504/537–6841; Milton D. Bourgeois, Jr., Administrator

ST. FRANCES CABRINI HOSPITAL, 3330 Masonic Drive, Alexandria, LA, Zip 71301; tel. 318/487–1122; Sister Olive Bordelon, Chief Executive Officer

ST. PATRICK HOSPITAL OF LAKE CHARLES, 524 South Ryan Street, Lake Charles, LA, Zip 70601, Mailing Address: P.O. Box 3401, Zip 70602–3401; tel. 318/436–2511; J. William Hankins, President and Chief Executive Officer

WEST CALCASIEU CAMERON HOSPITAL, Cypress Street, Sulphur, LA, Zip 70663, Mailing Address: P.O. Box 2509, Zip 70664–2509; tel. 318/527–4240; Wayne A. Swiniarski, FACHE, Chief Executive Officer

WEST JEFFERSON MEDICAL CENTER, 1101 Medical Center Boulevard, Marrero, LA, Zip 70072–3191; tel. 504/347–5511; David M. Smith, FACHE, President and Chief Executive Officer

TENET LOUISIANA HEALTH SYSTEM NETWORK
111 Veterans Boulevard, Suite 1424, Metairie, LA 70005; tel. 504/833–1495; Richard S. Freeman, Senior Vice President of Operations

DOCTORS HOSPITAL OF JEFFERSON, 4320 Houma Boulevard, Metairie, LA, Zip 70006–2973; tel. 504/456–5800; Gerald L. Parton, Chief Executive Officer

JO ELLEN SMITH MEDICAL CENTER, 4444 General Meyer Avenue, New Orleans, LA, Zip 70131; tel. 504/363–7011; Michael Manning, Chief Executive Officer

KENNER REGIONAL MEDICAL CENTER, 180 West Esplanade Avenue, Kenner, LA, Zip 70065; tel. 504/468–8600; Steven J. Greene, Chief Executive Officer

MEADOWCREST HOSPITAL, 2500 Belle Chase Highway, Gretna, LA, Zip 70056; tel. 504/392–3131; Jaime A. Wesolowski, Chief Executive Officer

MEDICAL CENTER OF LOUISIANA AT NEW ORLEANS, 2021 Perdido Street, New Orleans, LA, Zip 70112–1396; tel. 504/588–3000; Jonathan Roberts, Dr.PH, President and Chief Executive Officer

NORTHSHORE REGIONAL MEDICAL CENTER, 100 Medical Center Drive, Slidell, LA, Zip 70461–8572; tel. 504/649–7070; Charles F. Miller, Chief Executive Officer

ST. CHARLES GENERAL HOSPITAL, 3700 St. Charles Avenue, New Orleans, LA, Zip 70115; tel. 504/899–7441; Lynn C. Orfgen, Chief Executive Officer

MAINE

BLUE HILL MEMORIAL HOSPITAL FOUNDATION
Water Street, Blue Hill, ME 04614; tel. 207/374–2836; Bruce D. Cummings, Chief Executive Officer

BLUE HILL MEMORIAL HOSPITAL, Water Street, Blue Hill, ME, Zip 04614–0823, Mailing Address: P.O. Box 823, Zip 04614–0823; tel. 207/374–2836; Bruce D. Cummings, Chief Executive Officer

CENTRAL MAINE HEALTHCARE CORP
304 Cambridge Road, Lewiston, ME 94240; tel. 207/795–2303; William W. Young, Jr., President & Chief Executive Officer

NORTHERN CUMBERLAND MEMORIAL HOSPITAL, South High Street, Bridgton, ME, Zip 04009, Mailing Address: P.O. Box 230, Zip 04009–0230; tel. 207/647–8841; John Wiesendanger, President

RUMFORD COMMUNITY HOSPITAL, 420 Franklin Street, Rumford, ME, Zip 04276, Mailing Address: P.O. Box 619, Zip 04276; tel. 207/364–4581; John H. Welsh, Chief Executive Officer

STEPHENS MEMORIAL HOSPITAL, 80 Main Street, Norway, ME, Zip 04268–1297; tel. 207/743–5933; Timothy A. Churchill, President

HEALTH NET, INC.
One Merchants Plaza, 5th Floor, Bangor, ME 04401; tel. 207/942–2844; Paul Brough, Executive Director

ACADIA HOSPITAL, 268 Stillwater Avenue, Bangor, ME, Zip 04401, Mailing Address: P.O. Box 422, Zip 04402–0422; tel. 207/973–6100; Dennis P. King, President

EASTERN MAINE MEDICAL CENTER, 489 State Street, Bangor, ME, Zip 04401, Mailing Address: P.O. Box 404, Zip 04402–0404; tel. 207/973–7000; Norman A. Ledwin, President and Chief Executive Officer

SYNERNET
222 Saint John Street, Suite 329, Portland, ME 04102; tel. 207/775–6081; Maxine Adams, Vice President of Network

BLUE HILL MEMORIAL HOSPITAL, Water Street, Blue Hill, ME, Zip 04614–0823, Mailing Address: P.O. Box 823, Zip 04614–0823; tel. 207/374–2836; Bruce D. Cummings, Chief Executive Officer

BRIGHTON CAMPUS OF MAINE MEDICAL CENTER, 335 Brighton Avenue, Portland, ME, Zip 04102–9735, Mailing Address: P.O. Box 9735, Zip 04102–9735; tel. 207/879–8000; Vincent S. Conti, President

FRANKLIN MEMORIAL HOSPITAL, One Hospital Drive, Farmington, ME, Zip 04938–9990; tel. 207/778–6031; Richard A. Batt, President and Chief Executive Officer

HENRIETTA D. GOODALL HOSPITAL, 25 June Street, Sanford, ME, Zip 04073–2645; tel. 207/324–4310; Peter G. Booth, President

INLAND HOSPITAL, Kennedy Memorial Drive, Waterville, ME, Zip 04901; tel. 207/861–3000; Wilfred J. Addison, Administrator

MERCY HOSPITAL PORTLAND, 144 State Street, Portland, ME, Zip 04101–3795; tel. 207/879–3000; Howard R. Buckley, President

MID COAST HOSPITAL, 1356 Washington Street, Bath, ME, Zip 04530–2897; tel. 207/443–5524; Herbert Paris, President

MILES MEMORIAL HOSPITAL, Bristol Road, Damariscotta, ME, Zip 04543, Mailing Address: Rural Route 2, Box 4500, Zip 04543; tel. 207/563–1234; Judith Tarr, Chief Executive Officer

MOUNT DESERT ISLAND HOSPITAL, Wayman Lane, Bar Harbor, ME, Zip 04609–0008, Mailing Address: P.O. Box 8, Zip 04609–0008; tel. 207/288–5081; Leslie A. Hawkins, Chief Executive Officer

NORTHERN CUMBERLAND MEMORIAL HOSPITAL, South High Street, Bridgton, ME, Zip 04009, Mailing Address: P.O. Box 230, Zip 04009–0230; tel. 207/647–8841; John Wiesendanger, President

NORTHERN MAINE MEDICAL CENTER, 143 East Main Street, Fort Kent, ME, Zip 04743; tel. 207/834–3155; Martin B. Bernstein, Executive Director

PENOBSCOT BAY MEDICAL CENTER, 6 Glen Cove Drive, Rockport, ME, Zip 04856–4241; tel. 207/596–8000; Gary R. Daniels, President

REDINGTON–FAIRVIEW GENERAL HOSPITAL, Fairview Avenue, Skowhegan, ME, Zip 04976, Mailing Address: P.O. Box 468, Zip 04976; tel. 207/474–5121; Richard Willett, Chief Executive Officer

RUMFORD COMMUNITY HOSPITAL, 420 Franklin Street, Rumford, ME, Zip 04276, Mailing Address: P.O. Box 619, Zip 04276; tel. 207/364–4581; John H. Welsh, Chief Executive Officer

SEBASTICOOK VALLEY HOSPITAL, 99 Grove Street, Pittsfield, ME, Zip 04967–1199; tel. 207/487–5141; Ann Morrison, R.N., Chief Executive Officer

SOUTHERN MAINE MEDICAL CENTER, One Medical Center Drive, Biddeford, ME, Zip 04005, Mailing Address: P.O. Box 626, Zip 04005–0626; tel. 207/283–7000; Edward J. McGeachey, President and Chief Executive Officer

ST. JOSEPH HOSPITAL, 360 Broadway, Bangor, ME, Zip 04401–3897, Mailing Address: P.O. Box 403, Zip 04402–0403; tel. 207/262–1100; Sister Mary Norberta Malinowski, President

ST. MARY'S REGIONAL MEDICAL CENTER, 45 Golder Street, Lewiston, ME, Zip 04240, Mailing Address: P.O. Box 291, Zip 04243–0291; tel. 207/777–8100; James E. Cassidy, President and Chief Executive Officer

STEPHENS MEMORIAL HOSPITAL, 80 Main Street, Norway, ME, Zip 04268–1297; tel. 207/743–5933; Timothy A. Churchill, President

WALDO COUNTY GENERAL HOSPITAL, Northport Avenue, Belfast, ME, Zip 04915, Mailing Address: P.O. Box 287, Zip 04915–0287; tel. 207/338–2500; Mark A. Biscone, Executive Director

WESTBROOK COMMUNITY HOSPITAL, 40 Park Road, Westbrook, ME, Zip 04092; tel. 207/854–8464; Joel P. Rogers, Chief Executive Officer

YORK HOSPITAL, 15 Hospital Drive, York, ME, Zip 03909–1099; tel. 207/363–4321; Jud Knox, President

MARYLAND

DIMENSIONS HEALTHCARE SYSTEM
9200 Basil Court, Landover, MD 20785; tel. 301/925–7000; Winfield M. Kelly, Jr., President & Chief Executive Officer

PRINCE GEORGE'S HOSPITAL CENTER, 3001 Hospital Drive, Cheverly, MD, Zip 20785–1189; tel. 301/618–2000; Allan Earl Atzrott, President

HELIX HEALTH SYSTEM
2330 West Joppa Road, Suite 301, Lutherville, MD 21093; tel. 410/296–6050; Michael R. Merson, President & Chief Executive Officer

CHURCH HOSPITAL CORPORATION, 100 North Broadway, Baltimore, MD, Zip 21231–1593; tel. 410/522–8000; James R. Bobb, President

FRANKLIN SQUARE HOSPITAL CENTER, 9000 Franklin Square Drive, Baltimore, MD, Zip 21237–3998; tel. 410/682–7000; Charles D. Mross, President and Chief Executive Officer

GOOD SAMARITAN HOSPITAL OF MARYLAND, 5601 Loch Raven Boulevard, Baltimore, MD, Zip 21239–2995; tel. 410/532–8000; Lawrence M. Beck, President

UNION MEMORIAL HOSPITAL, 201 East University Parkway, Baltimore, MD, Zip 21218–2391; tel. 410/554–2000; Kenneth R. Buser, President and Chief Executive Officer

JOHNS HOPKINS HEALTH SYSTEM
600 North Wolfe Street, Baltimore, MD 21287; tel. 410/955–9540; Ronald R. Peterson, President

JOHNS HOPKINS BAYVIEW MEDICAL CENTER, 4940 Eastern Avenue, Baltimore, MD, Zip 21224–2780; tel. 410/550–0100; Ronald R. Peterson, President

JOHNS HOPKINS HOSPITAL, 600 North Wolfe Street, Baltimore, MD, Zip 21287; tel. 410/955–5000; Ronald R. Peterson, President

MARYLAND HEALTH NETWORK
10440 Little Patuxent, Columbia, MD 21044; tel. 410/715–6601; Peter Clay, President

GREATER BALTIMORE MEDICAL CENTER, 6701 North Charles Street, Baltimore, MD, Zip 21204–6892; tel. 410/828–2000; Robert P. Kowal, President

HOLY CROSS HOSPITAL OF SILVER SPRING, 1500 Forest Glen Road, Silver Spring, MD, Zip 20910; tel. 301/754–7000; James P. Hamill, President

MONTGOMERY GENERAL HOSPITAL, 18101 Prince Philip Drive, Olney, MD, Zip 20832–1512; tel. 301/774–8882; Peter W. Monge, President and Chief Executive Officer

NORTHWEST HOSPITAL CENTER, 5401 Old Court Road, Randallstown, MD, Zip 21133–5185; tel. 410/521–2200; Robert W. Fischer, President

ST. AGNES HEALTHCARE, 900 Caton Avenue, Baltimore, MD, Zip 21229–5299; tel. 410/368–6000; Robert E. Pezzoli, President and Chief Executive Officer

UNIVERSITY OF MARYLAND MEDICAL SYSTEM
22 South Greene Street, Baltimore, MD 21201; tel. 410/328–8667; Morton I. Rapoport, M.D., President & Chief Executive Officer

DEATON SPECIALTY HOSPITAL AND HOME, 611 South Charles Street, Baltimore, MD, Zip 21230–3898; tel. 410/547–8500; Errol G. Newport, President and Chief Executive Officer

JAMES LAWRENCE KERNAN HOSPITAL, 2200 Kernan Drive, Baltimore, MD, Zip 21207–6697; tel. 410/448–2500; James E. Ross, FACHE, Chief Executive Officer

UNIVERSITY OF MARYLAND MEDICAL SYSTEM, 22 South Greene Street, Baltimore, MD, Zip 21201–1595; tel. 410/328–8667; Morton I. Rapoport, M.D., President and Chief Executive Officer

MASSACHUSETTS

BAYSTATE HEALTH SYSTEM
759 Chestnut Street, Springfield, MA 01199; tel. 413/784–0000; Michael J. Daly, President & Chief Executive Officer

BAYSTATE MEDICAL CENTER, 759 Chestnut Street, Springfield, MA, Zip 01199–0001; tel. 413/784–0000; Mark R. Tolosky, Chief Executive Officer

FRANKLIN MEDICAL CENTER, 164 High Street, Greenfield, MA, Zip 01301; tel. 413/773–0211; Harlan J. Smith, President

MARY LANE HOSPITAL, 85 South Street, Ware, MA, Zip 01082; tel. 413/967–6211; Christine Shirtcliff, Executive Vice President

BERKSHIRE HEALTH SYSTEM
725 North Street, Pittsfield, MA 01201; tel. 413/447–2000; David Phelps, President

BERKSHIRE MEDICAL CENTER, 725 North Street, Pittsfield, MA, Zip 01201; tel. 413/447–2000; Ruth P. Blodgett, Chief Operating Officer

FAIRVIEW HOSPITAL, 29 Lewis Avenue, Great Barrington, MA, Zip 01230–1713; tel. 413/528–0790; Claire L. Bowen, President

CAPE COD HEALTHCARE, INC.
27 Park Street, Hyannisport, MA 02601; tel. 508/771–1800; Jim Lyons, Chief Executive Officer

CAPE COD HOSPITAL, 27 Park Street, Hyannis, MA, Zip 02601; tel. 508/771–1800; Roy A. Hitchings, Jr., FACHE, President

FALMOUTH HOSPITAL, 100 Ter Heun Drive, Falmouth, MA, Zip 02540–2599; tel. 508/457–3500; Roy A. Hitchings, Jr., FACHE, President

CAREGROUP
375 Longwood Avenue, Boston, MA 02215; tel. 617/975–5400; Mitchell T. Rabkin, M.D., Chief Executive Officer

BETH ISRAEL DEACONESS MEDICAL CENTER, 330 Brookline Avenue, Boston, MA, Zip 02215; tel. 617/667–2000; David Dolins, President

DEACONESS WALTHAM HOSPITAL, Hope Avenue, Waltham, MA, Zip 02254–9116; tel. 617/647–6000; Jeanette G. Clough, President and Chief Executive Officer

DEACONESS–GLOVER HOSPITAL CORPORATION, 148 Chestnut Street, Needham, MA, Zip 02192–2483; tel. 617/444–5600; John Dalton, President and Chief Executive Officer

DEACONESS–NASHOBA HOSPITAL, 200 Groton Road, Ayer, MA, Zip 01432; tel. 508/772–0200; Jeffrey R. Kelly, President and Chief Executive Officer

MOUNT AUBURN HOSPITAL, 330 Mount Auburn Street, Cambridge, MA, Zip 02238; tel. 617/492–3500; Francis P. Lynch, President and Chief Executive Officer

NEW ENGLAND BAPTIST HOSPITAL, 125 Parker Hill Avenue, Boston, MA, Zip 02120–3297; tel. 617/738–5800; Alan H. Robbins, M.D., President

CARITAS CHRISTI HEALTH NETWORK
736 Cambridge Street, Boston, MA 02135; tel. 617/789–2500; Michael F. Collins, M.D., President & Chief Executive Officer

GOOD SAMARITAN MEDICAL CENTER, 235 North Pearl Street, Brockton, MA, Zip 02401; tel. 508/427–3000; Frank J. Larkin, President and Chief Executive Officer

HOLY FAMILY HOSPITAL AND MEDICAL CENTER, 70 East Street, Methuen, MA, Zip 01844–4597; tel. 508/687–0151; William L. Lane, President

SAINT ANNE'S HOSPITAL, 795 Middle Street, Fall River, MA, Zip 02721–1798; tel. 508/674–5741; Joseph W. Wilczek, President

ST. ELIZABETH'S MEDICAL CENTER OF BOSTON, 736 Cambridge Street, Boston, MA, Zip 02135; tel. 617/789–3000; Michael F. Collins, M.D., President

ST. JOHN OF GOD HOSPITAL, 296 Allston Street, Brighton, MA, Zip 02146–1659; tel. 617/277–5750; William K. Brinkert, President

CHILDREN'S HOSPITAL
300 Longwood Avenue, Boston, MA 02115; tel. 617/355–7156; Deborah C. Jackson, Vice President of Network Development

CHILDREN'S HOSPITAL, 300 Longwood Avenue, Boston, MA, Zip 02115; tel. 617/355–6000; David Stephen Weiner, President

CONTINUUM OF CARE NETWORK
57 Union Street, Marlborough, MA 01752; tel. 508/481–5000; Cheryl Herberg, Network Coordinator

MARLBOROUGH HOSPITAL, 57 Union Street, Marlborough, MA, Zip 01752; tel. 508/481–5000; Anne Burgeois, Interim Chief Executive Officer

FALLON HEALTHCARE SYSTEM
10 Chestnut Street, Worcester, MA 01608; tel. 508/799–2100; Margaret McKenna, Director of Provider Relations

ATHOL MEMORIAL HOSPITAL, 2033 Main Street, Athol, MA, Zip 01331–3598; tel. 508/249–3511; William DiFederico, President

BETH ISRAEL DEACONESS MEDICAL CENTER, 330 Brookline Avenue, Boston, MA, Zip 02215; tel. 617/667–2000; David Dolins, President

BOSTON REGIONAL MEDICAL CENTER, 5 Woodland Road, Stoneham, MA, Zip 02180, Mailing Address: P.O. Box 9102, Zip 02180–9102; tel. 617/979–7000; Charles S. Ricks, D.D.S., President and Chief Executive Officer

BRIGHAM AND WOMEN'S HOSPITAL, 75 Francis Street, Boston, MA, Zip 02115–6195; tel. 617/732–5500; Jeffrey Otten, President

CHILDREN'S HOSPITAL, 300 Longwood Avenue, Boston, MA, Zip 02115; tel. 617/355–6000; David Stephen Weiner, President

CLINTON HOSPITAL, 201 Highland Street, Clinton, MA, Zip 01510; tel. 508/368–3000; Thomas Devins, Chief Executive Officer

DANA–FARBER CANCER INSTITUTE, 44 Binney Street, Boston, MA, Zip 02115–6084; tel. 617/632–3000; David G. Nathan, M.D., President

DEACONESS WALTHAM HOSPITAL, Hope Avenue, Waltham, MA, Zip 02254–9116; tel. 617/647–6000; Jeanette G. Clough, President and Chief Executive Officer

DEACONESS–GLOVER HOSPITAL CORPORATION, 148 Chestnut Street, Needham, MA, Zip 02192–2483; tel. 617/444–5600; John Dalton, President and Chief Executive Officer

DEACONESS–NASHOBA HOSPITAL, 200 Groton Road, Ayer, MA, Zip 01432; tel. 508/772–0200; Jeffrey R. Kelly, President and Chief Executive Officer

HARRINGTON MEMORIAL HOSPITAL, 100 South Street, Southbridge, MA, Zip 01550–4045; tel. 508/765–9771; Richard M. Mangion, President and Chief Executive Officer

HEALTH ALLIANCE HOSPITALS, 60 Hospital Road, Leominster, MA, Zip 01453–8004; tel. 508/537–4811; Douglas L. Fairfax, President and Chief Executive Officer

HOLY FAMILY HOSPITAL AND MEDICAL CENTER, 70 East Street, Methuen, MA, Zip 01844–4597; tel. 508/687–0151; William L. Lane, President

HUBBARD REGIONAL HOSPITAL, 340 Thompson Road, Webster, MA, Zip 01570–0608; tel. 508/943–2600; Gerald J. Barbini, Administrator and Chief Executive Officer

LAWRENCE GENERAL HOSPITAL, 1 General Street, Lawrence, MA, Zip 01842–0389, Mailing Address: P.O. Box 189, Zip 01842–0389; tel. 508/683–4000; Joseph S. McManus, President and Chief Executive Officer

MARLBOROUGH HOSPITAL, 57 Union Street, Marlborough, MA, Zip 01752; tel. 508/481–5000; Anne Burgeois, Interim Chief Executive Officer

MASSACHUSETTS GENERAL HOSPITAL, 55 Fruit Street, Boston, MA, Zip 02114; tel. 617/726–2000; James J. Mongan, M.D., President and Chief Operating Officer

MILFORD–WHITINSVILLE REGIONAL HOSPITAL, 14 Prospect Street, Milford, MA, Zip 01757; tel. 508/473–1190; Francis M. Saba, President and Chief Executive Officer

NEW ENGLAND BAPTIST HOSPITAL, 125 Parker Hill Avenue, Boston, MA, Zip 02120–3297; tel. 617/738–5800; Alan H. Robbins, M.D., President

SAINT VINCENT HOSPITAL, 25 Winthrop Street, Worcester, MA, Zip 01604–4593; tel. 508/798–1234; Robert E. Maher, Jr., President and Chief Executive Officer

SAINTS MEMORIAL MEDICAL CENTER, One Hospital Drive, Lowell, MA, Zip 01852; tel. 508/458–1411; Thomas Clark, President and Chief Executive Officer

UNIVERSITY OF MASSACHUSETTS MEDICAL CENTER, 55 Lake Avenue North, Worcester, MA, Zip 01655; tel. 508/856–0011; Lin C. Weeks, Dr.PH, R.N., Director

LAHEY NETWORK
41 Mall Road, Burlington, MA 01805; tel. 617/273–8223; Bruce Steinhauer, M.D., President

ATLANTICARE MEDICAL CENTER, 500 Lynnfield Street, Lynn, MA, Zip 01904–1487; tel. 617/581–9200; Andrew J. Riddell, President and Chief Executive Officer

LAHEY HITCHCOCK CLINIC, 41 Mall Road, Burlington, MA, Zip 01805–0001; tel. 617/744–5100; Bruce W. Steinhauer, M.D., Chief Executive Officer

MARY HITCHCOCK MEMORIAL HOSPITAL, One Medical Center Drive, Lebanon, NH, Zip 03756–0001; tel. 603/650–5000; James W. Varnum, President

SOUTHERN NEW HAMPSHIRE REGIONAL MEDICAL CENTER, 8 Prospect Street, Nashua, NH, Zip 03060, Mailing Address: P.O. Box 2014, Zip 03061–2014; tel. 603/577–2000; Thomas E. Wilhelmsen, Jr., President

WING MEMORIAL HOSPITAL AND MEDICAL CENTERS, 40 Wright Street, Palmer, MA, Zip 01069–1138; tel. 413/283–7651; Richard H. Scheffer, President

NEW ENGLAND HEALTH PARTNERSHIP
34 Washington Street, Suite 320, Waltham, MA 02181–1903; tel. 617/431–0300; Dick Lefebvre, President

BOSTON MEDICAL CENTER, One Boston Medical Ctr Place, Boston, MA, Zip 02118–2393; tel. 617/638–8000; Elaine S. Ullian, President and Chief Executive Officer

HALE HOSPITAL, 140 Lincoln Avenue, Haverhill, MA, Zip 01830; tel. 508/374–2000; Jeffrey Doran, Chief Executive Officer

HUBBARD REGIONAL HOSPITAL, 340 Thompson Road, Webster, MA, Zip 01570–0608; tel. 508/943–2600; Gerald J. Barbini, Administrator and Chief Executive Officer

LAHEY HITCHCOCK CLINIC, 41 Mall Road, Burlington, MA, Zip 01805–0001; tel. 617/744–5100; Bruce W. Steinhauer, M.D., Chief Executive Officer

MALDEN HOSPITAL, 100 Hospital Road, Malden, MA, Zip 02148–3591; tel. 617/322–7560; Stanley W. Krygowski, President

QUINCY HOSPITAL, 114 Whitwell Street, Quincy, MA, Zip 02169–1899; tel. 617/773–6100; Ralph DiPisa, Chief Executive Officer

NORTHEAST HEALTH SYSTEMS
85 Herrick Street, Beverly, MA 01915; tel. 508/922–3000; Bradford H. Silsby, Vice President of Strategic Planning

ADDISON GILBERT HOSPITAL, 298 Washington Street, Gloucester, MA, Zip 01930–4887; tel. 508/283–4000; Robert L. Shafner, President

BEVERLY HOSPITAL, 85 Herrrick Street, Beverly, MA, Zip 01915–1777; tel. 508/922–3000; Robert R. Fanning, Jr., Chief Executive Officer

PARTNERS HEALTHCARE SYSTEM
32 Fruit Street, Boston, MA 02114; tel. 617/732–5500; John McGonagle, Director of Community Health Services

BRIGHAM AND WOMEN'S HOSPITAL, 75 Francis Street, Boston, MA, Zip 02115–6195; tel. 617/732–5500; Jeffrey Otten, President

MASSACHUSETTS GENERAL HOSPITAL, 55 Fruit Street, Boston, MA, Zip 02114; tel. 617/726–2000; James J. Mongan, M.D., President and Chief Operating Officer

SALEM HOSPITAL, 81 Highland Avenue, Salem, MA, Zip 01970; tel. 508/741–1200; Michael J. Geaney, Jr., President

SHAUGHNESSY–KAPLAN REHABILITATION HOSPITAL, Dove Avenue, Salem, MA, Zip 01970; tel. 508/745–9000; Anthony Sciola, President and Chief Executive Officer

SISTERS OF PROVIDENCE HEALTH SYSTEM
146 Chestnut Street, Springfield, MA 01103; tel. 413/731–5548; Bob Suchecki, Director of Managed Care

MERCY HOSPITAL, 271 Carew Street, Springfield, MA, Zip 01104, Mailing Address: P.O. Box 9012, Zip 01102–9012; tel. 413/748–9000; Vincent J. McCorkle, President and Chief Executive Officer

SOUTHCOAST HEALTH SYSTEM
101 Page Street, New Bedford, MA 02740; tel. 508/679–7003; C. Tod Allen, Vice President Planning

CHARLTON MEMORIAL HOSPITAL, 363 Highland Avenue, Fall River, MA, Zip 02720–3794; tel. 508/679–7013

ST. LUKE'S HOSPITAL OF NEW BEDFORD, 101 Page Street, New Bedford, MA, Zip 02740, Mailing Address: P.O. Box H–3000, Zip 02741–3000; tel. 508/997–1515

TOBEY HOSPITAL, 43 High Street, Wareham, MA, Zip 02571; tel. 508/295–0880

MICHIGAN
BATTLE CREEK HEALTH SYSTEM
300 North Avenue, Battle Creek, MI 49016; tel. 616/966–8000; Stephen L. Abbott, President & Chief Executive Officer

BATTLE CREEK HEALTH SYSTEM, 300 North Avenue, Battle Creek, MI, Zip 49016–3396; tel. 616/966–8000; Stephen L. Abbott, President and Chief Executive Officer

BUTTERWORTH HEALTH SYSTEM
100 Michigan Street, SouthEast, Grand Rapids, MI 49503; tel. 616/776–2008; Carol Sarosik, Regional Vice President

BUTTERWORTH HOSPITAL, 100 Michigan Street N.E., Grand Rapids, MI, Zip 49503–2551; tel. 616/391–1774; Philip H. McCorkle, Jr., Chief Executive Officer

CARSON CITY HOSPITAL, 406 East Elm Street, Carson City, MI, Zip 48811–0879, Mailing Address: P.O. Box 879, Zip 48811–0879; tel. 517/584–3131; Bruce L. Traverse, President

GERBER MEMORIAL HOSPITAL, 212 South Sullivan Street, Fremont, MI, Zip 49412; tel. 616/924–3300; Ned B. Hughes, Jr., President

METROPOLITAN HOSPITAL, 1919 Boston Street S.E., Grand Rapids, MI, Zip 49506, Mailing Address: P.O. Box 158, Zip 49501–0158; tel. 616/247–7200; Michael D. Faas, President and Chief Executive Officer

PINE REST CHRISTIAN MENTAL HEALTH SERVICES, 300 68th Street S.E., Grand Rapids, MI, Zip 49501–0165, Mailing Address: P.O. Box 165, Zip 49501–0165; tel. 616/455–5000; Daniel L. Holwerda, President and Chief Executive Officer

UNITED MEMORIAL HOSPITAL ASSOCIATION, 615 South Bower Street, Greenville, MI, Zip 48838–2614, Mailing Address: P.O. Box 430, Zip 48838–0430; tel. 616/754–4691; Larry R. Davis, Chief Executive Officer

ZEELAND COMMUNITY HOSPITAL, 100 South Pine Street, Zeeland, MI, Zip 49464; tel. 616/772–4644; Henry A. Veenstra, President

DETROIT MEDICAL CENTER
4201 Saint Antoine Boulevard, Detroit, MI 48201; tel. 313/745–3605; Douglas Keegan, Vice President Planning

CHILDREN'S HOSPITAL OF MICHIGAN, 3901 Beaubien, Detroit, MI, Zip 48201–9985; tel. 313/745–0073; Thomas M. Rozek, Senior Vice President

DETROIT RECEIVING HOSPITAL AND UNIVERSITY HEALTH CENTER, 4201 St. Antoine Boulevard, Detroit, MI, Zip 48201–2194; tel. 313/745–3605; Leslie C. Bowman, Regional Administrator, Ancillary Services and Site Administrator

GRACE HOSPITAL, 6071 West Outer Drive, Detroit, MI, Zip 48235; tel. 313/966–3300; Anne M. Regling, Regional Executive

HARPER HOSPITAL, 3990 John R, Detroit, MI, Zip 48201–9027; tel. 313/745–8040; Paul L. Broughton, FACHE, Senior Vice President

HURON VALLEY HOSPITAL, 1601 East Commerce Road, Commerce Township, MI, Zip 48382; tel. 810/360–3300; Elliot Joseph, Senior Vice President, Oakland Region

HUTZEL HOSPITAL, 4707 St. Antoine Boulevard, Detroit, MI, Zip 48201–0154; tel. 313/745–7555; Susan A. Erickson, Clinical Services Administrator for Women's Services and Site Administrator

REHABILITATION INSTITUTE OF MICHIGAN, 261 Mack Boulevard, Detroit, MI, Zip 48201; tel. 313/745–1203; Bruce M. Gans, M.D., Senior Vice President

DETROIT–MACOMB HOSPITAL CORP
12000 E. 12 Mile Road, Warren, MI 48093–3570; tel. 313/573–5914; Timothy J. Ryan, President & Chief Executive Officer

DETROIT RIVERVIEW HOSPITAL, 7733 East Jefferson Avenue, Detroit, MI, Zip 48214; tel. 313/499–3000; Richard T. Young, Administrator

MACOMB HOSPITAL CENTER, 11800 East Twelve Mile Road, Warren, MI, Zip 48093; tel. 810/573–5000; Timothy J. Ryan, JD, President and Chief Executive Officer

FIRST CHOICE NETWORK
Medical Park Drive, Watervliet, MI 49098; tel. 616/463–8427; John P. Isaia, Director of Business Development

BORGESS MEDICAL CENTER, 1521 Gull Road, Kalamazoo, MI, Zip 49001–1640; tel. 616/226–7000; R. Timothy Stack, FACHE, President and Chief Executive Officer

COMMUNITY HOSPITAL, Medical Park Drive, Watervliet, MI, Zip 49098–0158, Mailing Address: Box 158, Zip 49098; tel. 616/463–3111; Dennis Turney, Chief Executive Officer

LEE MEMORIAL HOSPITAL, 420 West High Street, Dowagiac, MI, Zip 49047–1907; tel. 616/782–8681; Fritz Fahrenbacher, Vice President and Regional Hospital Administrator

GREAT LAKES HEALTH NETWORK
P.O. Box 5153, Southfield, MI 48086; tel. 810/356–3460; Barbara Potter, Network Coordinator

BI-COUNTY COMMUNITY HOSPITAL, 13355 East Ten Mile Road, Warren, MI, Zip 48089–2065; tel. 810/759–7300; Gary W. Popiel, Vice President and Chief Administrative Officer

BOTSFORD GENERAL HOSPITAL, 28050 Grand River Avenue, Farmington Hills, MI, Zip 48336–5933; tel. 248/471–8000; Gerson I. Cooper, President

GARDEN CITY HOSPITAL, 6245 North Inkster Road, Garden City, MI, Zip 48135; tel. 313/421–3300; Gary R. Ley, President and Chief Executive Officer

MOUNT CLEMENS GENERAL HOSPITAL, 1000 Harrington Boulevard, Mount Clemens, MI, Zip 48043–2992; tel. 810/493–8000; Ralph J. La Gro, President and Chief Executive Officer

OAKLAND GENERAL HOSPITAL, 27351 Dequindre, Madison Heights, MI, Zip 48071; tel. 810/967–7000; Robert Deputat, President

PONTIAC OSTEOPATHIC HOSPITAL, 50 North Perry Street, Pontiac, MI, Zip 48342; tel. 810/338–5000; Patrick Lamberti, Chief Executive Officer

RIVERSIDE OSTEOPATHIC HOSPITAL, 150 Truax Street, Trenton, MI, Zip 48183–2151; tel. 313/676–4200; Dennis R. Lemanski, D.O., Vice President and Chief Administrative Officer

HENRY FORD HEALTH SYSTEM
1 Ford Place, Detroit, MI 48202; tel. 313/876–8708; Peter Butler, Chief Administrative Officer

HENRY FORD COTTAGE HOSPITAL OF GROSSE POINTE, 159 Kercheval Avenue, Grosse Pointe Farms, MI, Zip 48236–3692; tel. 313/640–1000; Gregory J. Vasse, President and Chief Executive Officer

HENRY FORD HOSPITAL, 2799 West Grand Boulevard, Detroit, MI, Zip 48202–2689; tel. 313/876–2600; Stephen H. Velick, Chief Executive Officer

HENRY FORD WYANDOTTE HOSPITAL, 2333 Biddle Avenue, Wyandotte, MI, Zip 48192; tel. 313/284–2400; William R. Alvin, President

KINGSWOOD HOSPITAL, 10300 West Eight Mile Road, Ferndale, MI, Zip 48220; tel. 810/398–3200; Kathleen Emrich, R.N., Ed.D., Assistant Vice President and Chief Operating Officer

HOSPITAL NETWORK INC.
One Healthcare Plaza, Kalamazoo, MI 49007; tel. 616/341–8888; Richard M. Fluke, President & Chief Executive Officer

ALLEGAN GENERAL HOSPITAL, 555 Linn Street, Allegan, MI, Zip 49010–1594; tel. 616/673–8424; James Klun, President

BRONSON METHODIST HOSPITAL, 252 East Lovell Street, Kalamazoo, MI, Zip 49007–5345; tel. 616/341–6000; Frank J. Sardone, President and Chief Executive Officer

BRONSON VICKSBURG HOSPITAL, 13326 North Boulevard, Vicksburg, MI, Zip 49097–1099; tel. 616/649–2321; Frank J. Sardone, President

OAKLAWN HOSPITAL, 200 North Madison Street, Marshall, MI, Zip 49068; tel. 616/781–4271; Rob Covert, President and Chief Executive Officer

STURGIS HOSPITAL, 916 Myrtle, Sturgis, MI, Zip 49091–2001; tel. 616/659–4400; David James, Chief Executive Officer

LAKELAND REGIONAL HEALTH SYSTEM
1234 Napier Avenue, St. Joseph, MI 49085; tel. 616/927–5363; Sam Ocampo, Manager Strategic Planning

BRONSON METHODIST HOSPITAL, 252 East Lovell Street, Kalamazoo, MI, Zip 49007–5345; tel. 616/341–6000; Frank J. Sardone, President and Chief Executive Officer

LAKELAND MEDICAL CENTER, BERRIEN CENTER, 6418 Dean's Hill Road, Berrien Center, MI, Zip 49102–9704; tel. 616/471–7761

LAKELAND MEDICAL CENTER–NILES, 31 North St. Joseph Avenue, Niles, MI, Zip 49120–2287; tel. 616/683–5510; Joseph A. Wasserman, President and Chief Executive Officer

LAKELAND MEDICAL CENTER–ST. JOSEPH, 1234 Napier Avenue, Saint Joseph, MI, Zip 49085; tel. 616/983–8300; Joseph A. Wasserman, President and Chief Executive Officer

SOUTH HAVEN COMMUNITY HOSPITAL, 955 South Bailey Avenue, South Haven, MI, Zip 49090; tel. 616/637–5271; Craig J. Marks, President and Chief Executive Officer

MERCY GENERAL HEALTH PARTNERS
1500 E. Sherman Boulevard, P.O. Box 358, Muskegon, MI 49443; tel. 616/739–3901; Roger Spoelman, President & Chief Executive Officer

MERCY GENERAL HEALTH PARTNERS–OAK AVENUE CAMPUS, 1700 Oak Avenue, Muskegon, MI, Zip 49442; tel. 616/773–3311; Roger Spoelman, Chief Executive Officer

MERCY GENERAL HEALTH PARTNERS–SHERMAN BOULEVARD CAMPUS, 1500 East Sherman Boulevard, Muskegon, MI, Zip 49443, Mailing Address: P.O. Box 358, Zip 49443–0358; tel. 616/739–9341; Roger Spoelman, Chief Executive Officer

MERCY HEALTH SERVICES
34605 Twelve Mile Road, Farmington Hills, MI 48331–3221; tel. 810/489–6783; Robert Laverty, Executive VP System Integration

BATTLE CREEK HEALTH SYSTEM, 300 North Avenue, Battle Creek, MI, Zip 49016–3396; tel. 616/966–8000; Stephen L. Abbott, President and Chief Executive Officer

DECKERVILLE COMMUNITY HOSPITAL, 3559 Pine Street, Deckerville, MI, Zip 48427–0126, Mailing Address: P.O. Box 126, Zip 48427–0126; tel. 810/376–2835; Charlotte Williams, Interim Administrator

MCPHERSON HOSPITAL, 620 Byron Road, Howell, MI, Zip 48843–1093; tel. 517/545–6000; C. W. Lauderbach, Jr., Chief Operating Officer

MERCY GENERAL HEALTH PARTNERS–OAK AVENUE CAMPUS, 1700 Oak Avenue, Muskegon, MI, Zip 49442; tel. 616/773–3311; Roger Spoelman, Chief Executive Officer

MERCY HEALTH SERVICES NORTH–GRAYLING, 1100 Michigan Avenue, Grayling, MI, Zip 49738–1398; tel. 517/348–5461; Dennis J. Renander, President and Chief Executive Officer

MERCY HEALTH SERVICES–NORTH, 400 Hobart Street, Cadillac, MI, Zip 49601–9596; tel. 616/876–7200; Dennis J. Renander, President and Chief Executive Officer

MERCY HOSPITAL, 5555 Conner Avenue, Detroit, MI, Zip 48213–3499; tel. 313/579–4000; Brenita Crawford, President and Chief Executive Officer

MERCY HOSPITAL, 2601 Electric Avenue, Port Huron, MI, Zip 48061–6518; tel. 810/985–1510; Mary R. Trimmer, President and Chief Executive Officer

SAINT MARY'S HEALTH SERVICES, 200 Jefferson Avenue S.E., Grand Rapids, MI, Zip 49503; tel. 616/752–6090; David J. Ameen, President and Chief Executive Officer

SALINE COMMUNITY HOSPITAL, 400 West Russell Street, Saline, MI, Zip 48176–1101; tel. 313/429–1500; Garry C. Faja, President and Chief Executive Officer

ST. JOSEPH MERCY HEALTH SYSTEM, 5301 East Huron River Drive, Ann Arbor, MI, Zip 48106, Mailing Address: Box 995, Zip 48106–0992; tel. 313/712–3456; Garry C. Faja, President and Chief Executive Officer

ST. JOSEPH MERCY OAKLAND, 900 Woodward Avenue, Pontiac, MI, Zip 48341–2985; tel. 810/858–3000; Thomas L. Feurig, President and Chief Executive Officer

ST. JOSEPH'S MERCY HOSPITALS AND HEALTH SERVICES, Clinton Township, MI, Robert L. Beyer, President and Chief Executive Officer

ST. LAWRENCE HOSPITAL AND HEALTHCARE SERVICES, 1210 West Saginaw Street, Lansing, MI, Zip 48915–1999; tel. 517/372–3610; Arthur Knueppel, President and Chief Executive Officer

MICHIGAN CAPITAL HEALTHCARE
401 West Greenlawn, Lansing, MI 48910; tel. 517/334–2969; Lee Hladki, Vice President Network

MICHIGAN CAPITAL HEALTHCARE, 401 West Greenlawn Avenue, Lansing, MI, Zip 48910–2819; tel. 517/334–2121; Dennis M. Litos, President and Chief Executive Officer

MUNSON HEALTHCARE
1105 Sixth Street, Traverse City, MI 49684; tel. 616/935–6000; John M. Rockwood, President & Chief Executive Officer

KALKASKA MEMORIAL HEALTH CENTER, 419 Coral Street, Kalkaska, MI, Zip 49646, Mailing Address: P.O. Box 249, Zip 49646–0249; tel. 616/258–9142; James D. Austin, CHE, Administrator

LEELANAU MEMORIAL HEALTH CENTER, 215 South High Street, Northport, MI, Zip 49670, Mailing Address: P.O. Box 217, Zip 49670; tel. 616/386–5101; Jayne R. Bull, Administrator

PAUL OLIVER MEMORIAL HOSPITAL, 224 Park Avenue, Frankfort, MI, Zip 49635; tel. 616/352–9621; James D. Austin, CHE, Administrator

PORT HURON HOSPITAL/BLUE WATER HEALTH SERVICES
1221 Pine Grove Avenue, Port Huron, MI 48060–5011; tel. 810/989–3708; Gary LeRoy, Consultant

PORT HURON HOSPITAL, 1221 Pine Grove Avenue, Port Huron, MI, Zip 48061–5011; tel. 810/987–5000; Donald C. Fletcher, President and Chief Executive Officer

RIVER DISTRICT HOSPITAL, 4100 South River Road, East China, MI, Zip 48054; tel. 810/329–7111; John E. Knox, President

ST. JOHN HOSPITAL AND MEDICAL CENTER, 22101 Moross Road, Detroit, MI, Zip 48236–2172; tel. 313/343–4000; Timothy J. Grajewski, President and Chief Executive Officer

YALE COMMUNITY HOSPITAL, 420 North Street, Yale, MI, Zip 48097, Mailing Address: P.O. Box 129, Zip 48097–0129; tel. 810/387–3211; Joyce Laupichler, Administrator

SAINT JOHN HEALTH SYSTEM
22101 Moross Road, Detroit, MI 48236; tel. 313/343–7529; Mark J. Brady, Senior Planning Analyst

HOLY CROSS HOSPITAL, 4777 East Outer Drive, Detroit, MI, Zip 48234–0401; tel. 313/369–9100; Michael F. Breen, President

OAKLAND GENERAL HOSPITAL, 27351 Dequindre, Madison Heights, MI, Zip 48071; tel. 810/967–7000; Robert Deputat, President

PORT HURON HOSPITAL, 1221 Pine Grove Avenue, Port Huron, MI, Zip 48061–5011; tel. 810/987–5000; Donald C. Fletcher, President and Chief Executive Officer

RIVER DISTRICT HOSPITAL, 4100 South River Road, East China, MI, Zip 48054; tel. 810/329–7111; John E. Knox, President

ST. JOHN HEALTH SYSTEM–SARATOGA CAMPUS, 15000 Gratiot Avenue, Detroit, MI, Zip 48205–1999; tel. 313/245–1200; Michael F. Breen, President

ST. JOHN HOSPITAL AND MEDICAL CENTER, 22101 Moross Road, Detroit, MI, Zip 48236–2172; tel. 313/343–4000; Timothy J. Grajewski, President and Chief Executive Officer

ST. JOHN HOSPITAL–MACOMB CENTER, 26755 Ballard Road, Harrison Township, MI, Zip 48045–2458; tel. 810/465–5501; David Sessions, President

WILLIAM BEAUMONT HOSPITAL CORP
3601 West Thirteen Mile Road, Royal Oak, MI 48073; tel. 248/551–0673; David Ladd, Director of Planning

MOUNT CLEMENS GENERAL HOSPITAL, 1000 Harrington Boulevard, Mount Clemens, MI, Zip 48043–2992; tel. 810/493–8000; Ralph J. La Gro, President and Chief Executive Officer

NORTH OAKLAND MEDICAL CENTERS, 461 West Huron Street, Pontiac, MI, Zip 48341–1651; tel. 810/857–7200; Robert L. Davis, President and Chief Executive Officer

ST. MARY HOSPITAL, 36475 West Five Mile Road, Livonia, MI, Zip 48154–1988; tel. 313/655–4800; Sister Mary Modesta Piwowar, President and Chief Executive Officer

WILLIAM BEAUMONT HOSPITAL–ROYAL OAK, 3601 West Thirteen Mile Road, Royal Oak, MI, Zip 48073–6769; tel. 810/551–5000; John D. Labriola, Vice President and Director

WILLIAM BEAUMONT HOSPITAL–TROY, 44201 Dequindre Road, Troy, MI, Zip 48098–1198; tel. 810/828–5100; Eugene F. Michalski, Vice President and Hospital Director

MINNESOTA

AFFILIATED COMMUNITY HEALTH NETWORK, INC.
101 Wilmar Avenue, SouthWest, Willmar, MN 56201; tel. 612/231–6719; Burnell J. Mellema, M.D., President

MCKENNAN HOSPITAL, 800 East 21st Street, Sioux Falls, SD, Zip 57105, Mailing Address: P.O. Box 5045, Zip 57117–5045; tel. 605/322–8000; Fredrick Slunecka, President and Chief Executive Officer

REDWOOD FALLS MUNICIPAL HOSPITAL, 100 Fallwood Road, Redwood Falls, MN, Zip 56283–1828; tel. 507/637–2907; James E. Schulte, Administrator

RICE MEMORIAL HOSPITAL, 301 Becker Avenue S.W., Willmar, MN, Zip 56201–3395; tel. 320/231–4227; Lawrence J. Massa, Chief Executive Officer

WEINER MEMORIAL MEDICAL CENTER, 300 South Bruce Street, Marshall, MN, Zip 56258–1934; tel. 507/532–9661; Ronald Jensen, Administrator

WILLMAR REGIONAL TREATMENT CENTER, North Highway 71, Willmar, MN, Zip 56201–1128, Mailing Address: Box 1128, Zip 56201–1128; tel. 612/231–5100; Gregory G. Spartz, Chief Executive Officer

ALLINA HEALTH SYSTEM
5601 Smetana Drive, Minnetonka, MN 55343; tel. 612/992–3357; Mary Onstad, Network Contact

ABBOTT NORTHWESTERN HOSPITAL, 800 East 28th Street, Minneapolis, MN, Zip 55407–3799; tel. 612/863–4203; Robert K. Spinner, President

BUFFALO HOSPITAL, 303 Catlin Street, Buffalo, MN, Zip 55313–1947, Mailing Address: P.O. Box 609, Zip 55313–0609; tel. 612/682–7180; Mary Ellen Wells, President

CAMBRIDGE MEDICAL CENTER, 701 South Dellwood Street, Cambridge, MN, Zip 55008–1920; tel. 612/689–7700; Lowell L. Becker, M.D., President

FAIRMONT COMMUNITY HOSPITAL, 835 Johnson Street, Fairmont, MN, Zip 56031–4523, Mailing Address: P.O. Box 835, Zip 56031–0835; tel. 507/238–4254; Gerry Gilbertson, President

GRANITE FALLS MUNICIPAL HOSPITAL AND MANOR, 345 Tenth Avenue, Granite Falls, MN, Zip 56241–1499; tel. 320/564–3111; George Gerlach, President

HUTCHINSON AREA HEALTH CARE, 1095 Highway 15 South, Hutchinson, MN, Zip 55350–3182; tel. 320/234–5000; Philip G. Graves, President

LONG PRAIRIE MEMORIAL HOSPITAL AND HOME, 20 Ninth Street S.E., Long Prairie, MN, Zip 56347–1404; tel. 320/732–2141; Clayton R. Peterson, President

MILLE LACS HEALTH SYSTEM, 200 North Elm Street, Onamia, MN, Zip 56359–7978; tel. 320/532–3154; Frederick W. Haack, President

NEW ULM MEDICAL CENTER, 1324 Fifth Street North, New Ulm, MN, Zip 56073–1553, Mailing Address: P.O. Box 577, Zip 56073; tel. 507/354–2111; Rickie L. Ressler, R.N., Interim President

NORTHFIELD HOSPITAL, 801 West First Street, Northfield, MN, Zip 55057–1697; tel. 507/645–6661; Kendall C. Bank, President

OWATONNA HOSPITAL, 903 Oak Street South, Owatonna, MN, Zip 55060–3234; tel. 507/451–3850; Richard G. Slieter, President

PHILLIPS EYE INSTITUTE, 2215 Park Avenue, Minneapolis, MN, Zip 55404–3756; tel. 612/336–6000; Shari E. Levy, President

RIVER FALLS AREA HOSPITAL, 1629 East Division Street, River Falls, WI, Zip 54022–1571; tel. 715/425–6155; Sharon Whelan, President

ST. FRANCIS REGIONAL MEDICAL CENTER, 1455 St. Francis Avenue, Shakopee, MN, Zip 55379–1228; tel. 612/403–3000; Venetia Kudrle, President

STEVENS COUNTY HOSPITAL, 1006 South Jackson Street, Hugoton, KS, Zip 67951, Mailing Address: Box 10, Zip 67951; tel. 316/544–8511; Ted Strote, Administrator

UNITED HOSPITAL, 333 North Smith Street, Saint Paul, MN, Zip 55102–2389; tel. 612/220–8000; David Jones, President

UNITED HOSPITAL DISTRICT, 515 South Moore Street, Blue Earth, MN, Zip 56013–2158, Mailing Address: P.O. Box 160, Zip 56013–0160; tel. 507/526–3273; Brian Kief, President

BENEDICTINE HEALTH SYSTEM
503 East Third Street, Duluth, MN 55805; tel. 218/720–2370; Barry J. Halm, President

ITASCA MEDICAL CENTER, 126 First Avenue S.E., Grand Rapids, MN, Zip 55744–3698; tel. 218/326–3401; Tom Papin, Administrator

ST. FRANCIS REGIONAL MEDICAL CENTER, 1455 St. Francis Avenue, Shakopee, MN, Zip 55379–1228; tel. 612/403–3000; Venetia Kudrle, President

FAIRVIEW HEALTH SYSTEM
2450 Riverside Avenue, Minneapolis, MN 53454; tel. 612/672–6876; Barbara G. Nye, Vice President

CHISAGO HEALTH SERVICES, 11685 Lake Boulevard North, Chisago City, MN, Zip 55013–9540; tel. 612/257–8400; Scott Wordelman, President and Chief Executive Officer

FAIRVIEW NORTHLAND REGIONAL HOSPITAL, 911 Northland Drive, Princeton, MN, Zip 55371; tel. 612/389–1313; Glenn G. Erickson, Vice President and Administrator

FAIRVIEW RIDGES HOSPITAL, 201 East Nicollet Boulevard, Burnsville, MN, Zip 55337–5799; tel. 612/892–2000; Mark M. Enger, Senior Vice President and Administrator

FAIRVIEW SOUTHDALE HOSPITAL, 6401 France Avenue South, Minneapolis, MN, Zip 55435–2199; tel. 612/924–5000; Mark M. Enger, Senior Vice President and Administrator

FAIRVIEW–UNIVERSITY MEDICAL CENTER, 2450 Riverside Avenue, Minneapolis, MN, Zip 55454–1400; tel. 612/672–6300; Peter Rapp, Senior Vice President and Administrator

HEALTHEAST
1700 University Avenue, St. Paul, MN 55104; tel. 612/232–5615; Tim Hanson, President

HEALTHEAST BETHESDA LUTHERAN HOSPITAL AND REHABILITATION CENTER, 559 Capitol Boulevard, Saint Paul, MN, Zip 55103; tel. 612/232–2133; Scott Batulis, Administrator

HEALTHEAST ST. JOHN'S HOSPITAL, 1575 Beam Avenue, Maplewood, MN, Zip 55109; tel. 612/232–7000; William Knutson, Vice President and Administrator

HEALTHEAST ST. JOSEPH'S HOSPITAL, 69 West Exchange Street, Saint Paul, MN, Zip 55102; tel. 612/232–3000; William Knutson, Vice President and Administrator

HEALTHPARTNERS
8100 34th Avenue South, Minneapolis, MN 55440; tel. 612/883–5585; George Halvorson, President

ST. PAUL–RAMSEY MEDICAL CENTER, 640 Jackson Street, Saint Paul, MN, Zip 55101–2595; tel. 612/221–3456; Terry S. Finzen, President

I-35 CORRIDOR HEALTH NETWORK
600 East Superior Street, Suite 404, Duluth, MN 55802; tel. 218/727–9393; Lynn S. Clayton, Administrator

CHISAGO HEALTH SERVICES, 11685 Lake Boulevard North, Chisago City, MN, Zip 55013–9540; tel. 612/257–8400; Scott Wordelman, President and Chief Executive Officer

FAIRVIEW–UNIVERSITY MEDICAL CENTER, 2450 Riverside Avenue, Minneapolis, MN, Zip 55454–1400; tel. 612/672–6300; Peter Rapp, Senior Vice President and Administrator

KANABEC HOSPITAL, 300 Clark Street, Mora, MN, Zip 55051; tel. 320/679–1212; John A. Kayfes, FACHE, Administrator

MERCY HOSPITAL AND HEALTH CARE CENTER, 710 South Kenwood Avenue, Moose Lake, MN, Zip 55767; tel. 218/485–4481; Dianne Mandernach, Chief Executive Officer

PINE MEDICAL CENTER, 109 Court Avenue South, Sandstone, MN, Zip 55072; tel. 612/245–2212; Vivian Swanson, Interim Administrator

RUSH CITY HOSPITAL, 760 West Fourt Street, Rush City, MN, Zip 55069; tel. 612/358–4708; Mark Lunseth, Administrator

ITASCA PARTNERSHIP FOR QUALITY HEALTHCARE
126 1st Avenue Southeast, Grand Rapids, MN 55744; tel. 218/326–7513; Lee Jess, D.D.S., President

DEER RIVER HEALTHCARE CENTER, 1002 Comstock Drive, Deer River, MN, Zip 56636; tel. 218/246–2900; Michael Hedrix, Chief Executive Officer

ITASCA MEDICAL CENTER, 126 First Avenue S.E., Grand Rapids, MN, Zip 55744–3698; tel. 218/326–3401; Tom Papin, Administrator

NORTHERN ITASCA HEALTH CARE CENTER, 258 Pine Tree Drive, Bigfork, MN, Zip 56628, Mailing Address: P.O. Box 258, Zip 56628–0258; tel. 218/743–3177; Richard M. Ash, Administrator

MAYO FOUNDATION
200 SouthWest First Street, Rochester, MN 55905; tel. 507/284–8860; Dave Sperling, President

AUSTIN MEDICAL CENTER, 1000 First Drive N.W., Austin, MN, Zip 55912; tel. 507/437–4551; Donald R. Brezicka, Executive Vice President

LUTHER HOSPITAL, 1221 Whipple Street, Eau Claire, WI, Zip 54702–4105; tel. 715/838–3311; William Rupp, M.D., President and Chief Executive Officer

ROCHESTER METHODIST HOSPITAL, 201 West Center Street, Rochester, MN, Zip 55902–3084; tel. 507/266–7180; Stephen C. Waldhoff, Administrator

SAINT MARYS HOSPITAL, 1216 Second Street S.W., Rochester, MN, Zip 55902–1970; tel. 507/255–5123; John M. Panicek, Administrator

MINNESOTA RURAL HEALTH COOPERATIVE
P.O. Box 104, Willmar, MN 56201;
tel. 320/231–3849; Lyle Munneke, M.D.,
President & Chairperson

APPLETON MUNICIPAL HOSPITAL AND NURSING HOME, 30 South Behl Street, Appleton, MN, Zip 56208–1699; tel. 612/289–2422; Mark E. Paulson, Administrator

CANBY COMMUNITY HEALTH SERVICES, 112 St. Olaf Avenue South, Canby, MN, Zip 56220–1433; tel. 507/223–7277; Robert J. Salmon, Chief Executive Officer

CHIPPEWA COUNTY MONTEVIDEO HOSPITAL, 824 North 11th Street, Montevideo, MN, Zip 56265; tel. 320/269–8877; Fred Knutson, Administrator

DIVINE PROVIDENCE HEALTH CENTER, 312 East George Street, Ivanhoe, MN, Zip 56142–0136, Mailing Address: P.O. Box G, Zip 56142–0136; tel. 507/694–1414; James C. Rossow, Administrator

GRACEVILLE HEALTH CENTER, 115 West Second Street, Graceville, MN, Zip 56240–0157, Mailing Address: P.O. Box 157, Zip 56240–0157; tel. 320/748–7223; Carollee Brinkman, Chief Executive Officer

GRANITE FALLS MUNICIPAL HOSPITAL AND MANOR, 345 Tenth Avenue, Granite Falls, MN, Zip 56241–1499; tel. 320/564–3111; George Gerlach, President

HENDRICKS COMMUNITY HOSPITAL, 503 East Lincoln Street, Hendricks, MN, Zip 56136; tel. 507/275–3134; Kirk Stensrud, Administrator

JOHNSON MEMORIAL HEALTH SERVICES, 1282 Walnut Street, Dawson, MN, Zip 56232; tel. 612/769–4323; Vern Silvernale, Administrator

LAC QUI PARLE HOSPITAL OF MADISON, 820 Third Avenue, Madison, MN, Zip 56256, Mailing Address: P.O. Box 184, Zip 56256; tel. 320/598–7556; John Fossum, Chief Executive Officer

ORTONVILLE AREA HEALTH SERVICES, 750 Eastvold Avenue, Ortonville, MN, Zip 56278; tel. 320/839–2502; Frederick Peterson, Administrator

REDWOOD FALLS MUNICIPAL HOSPITAL, 100 Fallwood Road, Redwood Falls, MN, Zip 56283–1828; tel. 507/637–2907; James E. Schulte, Administrator

RENVILLE COUNTY HOSPITAL, 611 East Fairview Avenue, Olivia, MN, Zip 56277–1397; tel. 612/523–1261; Dean G. Slagter, Administrator

RICE MEMORIAL HOSPITAL, 301 Becker Avenue S.W., Willmar, MN, Zip 56201–3395; tel. 320/231–4227; Lawrence J. Massa, Chief Executive Officer

SWIFT COUNTY–BENSON HOSPITAL, 1815 Wisconsin Avenue, Benson, MN, Zip 56215–1653; tel. 320/843–4232; John Stindt, Chief Executive Officer

TYLER HEALTHCARE CENTER, 240 Willow Street, Tyler, MN, Zip 56178–0280; tel. 507/247–5521; James Rotert, Administrator

WEINER MEMORIAL MEDICAL CENTER, 300 South Bruce Street, Marshall, MN, Zip 56258–1934; tel. 507/532–9661; Ronald Jensen, Administrator

NORTHERN LAKES HEALTH CONSORTIUM
600 East Superior Street, Suite 404, Duluth,
MN 55802; tel. 218/727–9393; Terry J. Hill,
Executive Director

COMMUNITY MEMORIAL HOSPITAL AND CONVALESCENT AND NURSING CARE SECTION, 512 Skyline Boulevard, Cloquet, MN, Zip 55720–1199; tel. 218/879–4641; James J. Carroll, Administrator

COMMUNITY MEMORIAL HOSPITAL AND NURSING HOME, 819 Ash Street, Spooner, WI, Zip 54801; tel. 715/635–2111; Michael Schafer, Chief Executive Officer

COOK COUNTY NORTH SHORE HOSPITAL, Grand Marais, MN, Mailing Address: P.O. Box 10, Zip 55604–0010; tel. 218/387–1500; Diane Pearson, Administrator

COOK HOSPITAL AND CONVALESCENT NURSING CARE UNIT, 10 South Fifth Street East, Cook, MN, Zip 55723; tel. 218/666–5945; Allen J. Vogt, Administrator

CUMBERLAND MEMORIAL HOSPITAL, 1110 Seventh Avenue, Cumberland, WI, Zip 54829, Mailing Address: Box 37, Zip 54829–0037; tel. 715/822–2741; James M. O'Keefe, Administrator

CUYUNA REGIONAL MEDICAL CENTER, 320 East Main Street, Crosby, MN, Zip 56441; tel. 218/546–7000; Thomas F. Reek, Chief Executive Officer

DEER RIVER HEALTHCARE CENTER, 1002 Comstock Drive, Deer River, MN, Zip 56636; tel. 218/246–2900; Michael Hedrix, Chief Executive Officer

ELY–BLOOMENSON COMMUNITY HOSPITAL, 328 West Conan Street, Ely, MN, Zip 55731–1198; tel. 218/365–3271; Larry Ravenberg, Administrator

FALLS MEMORIAL HOSPITAL, 1400 Highway 71, International Falls, MN, Zip 56649–2189; tel. 218/283–4481; James F. Hanko, Administrator and Chief Executive Officer

FLAMBEAU HOSPITAL, 98 Sherry Avenue, Park Falls, WI, Zip 54552, Mailing Address: P.O. Box 310, Zip 54552; tel. 715/762–2484; Curtis A. Johnson, Administrator

GRAND VIEW HOSPITAL, N10561 Grand View Lane, Ironwood, MI, Zip 49938–9622; tel. 906/932–2525; Frederick Geissler, Chief Executive Officer

HAYWARD AREA MEMORIAL HOSPITAL AND NURSING HOME, Hayward, WI, Mailing Address: Route 3, Box 3999, Zip 54843; tel. 715/634–8911; Barbara A. Peickert, R.N., Chief Executive Officer

ITASCA MEDICAL CENTER, 126 First Avenue S.E., Grand Rapids, MN, Zip 55744–3698; tel. 218/326–3401; Tom Papin, Administrator

LAKE VIEW MEMORIAL HOSPITAL, 325 11th Avenue, Two Harbors, MN, Zip 55616–1298; tel. 218/834–7300; Brian J. Carlson, Administrator

LAKEVIEW MEDICAL CENTER, 1100 North Main Street, Rice Lake, WI, Zip 54868–1238; tel. 715/234–1515; Edward H. Wolf, Chief Executive Officer

MERCY HOSPITAL AND HEALTH CARE CENTER, 710 South Kenwood Avenue, Moose Lake, MN, Zip 55767; tel. 218/485–4481; Dianne Mandernach, Chief Executive Officer

MILLE LACS HEALTH SYSTEM, 200 North Elm Street, Onamia, MN, Zip 56359–7978; tel. 320/532–3154; Frederick W. Haack, President

MILLER DWAN MEDICAL CENTER, 502 East Second Street, Duluth, MN, Zip 55805–1982; tel. 218/727–8762; William H. Palmer, President

NORTHERN ITASCA HEALTH CARE CENTER, 258 Pine Tree Drive, Bigfork, MN, Zip 56628, Mailing Address: P.O. Box 258, Zip 56628–0258; tel. 218/743–3177; Richard M. Ash, Administrator

ONTONAGON MEMORIAL HOSPITAL, 601 Seventh Street, Ontonagon, MI, Zip 49953; tel. 906/884–4134; Fred Nelson, Administrator

PINE MEDICAL CENTER, 109 Court Avenue South, Sandstone, MN, Zip 55072; tel. 612/245–2212; Vivian Swanson, Interim Administrator

RIVERWOOD HEALTH CARE CENTER, 301 Minnesota Avenue South, Aitkin, MN, Zip 56431–1626; tel. 218/927–2121; Debra Boardman, Chief Executive Officer

RUSH CITY HOSPITAL, 760 West Fourt Street, Rush City, MN, Zip 55069; tel. 612/358–4708; Mark Lunseth, Administrator

ST. LUKE'S HOSPITAL, 915 East First Street, Duluth, MN, Zip 55805–2193; tel. 218/726–5555; John Strange, President and Chief Executive Officer

UNIVERSITY MEDICAL CENTER–MESABI, 750 East 34th Street, Hibbing, MN, Zip 55746; tel. 218/262–4881; Frances J. Gardeski, Chief Executive Officer

VIRGINIA REGIONAL MEDICAL CENTER, 901 Ninth Street North, Virginia, MN, Zip 55792–2398; tel. 218/741–3340; Kyle Hopstad, Administrator

WHITE COMMUNITY HOSPITAL, 5211 Highway 110, Aurora, MN, Zip 55705; tel. 218/229–2211; Cheryl A. High, Administrator

NORTHSTAR HEALTH CONSORTIUM
715 Delmore Drive, Roseau, MN 56751;
tel. 218/463–2500; Dave Hagen, Chairman

KITTSON MEMORIAL HOSPITAL, 1010 South Birch Street, Hallock, MN, Zip 56728, Mailing Address: P.O. Box 700, Zip 56728; tel. 218/843–3612; Richard J. Failing, Chief Executive Officer

LAKEWOOD HEALTH CENTER, 600 South Main Avenue, Baudette, MN, Zip 56623, Mailing Address: Route 1, Box 2120, Zip 56623; tel. 218/634–2120; David A. Nelson, President and Chief Executive Officer

NORTH VALLEY HEALTH CENTER, 109 South Minnesota Street, Warren, MN, Zip 56762–1499; tel. 218/745–4211; Everett A. Butler, Administrator

ROSEAU AREA HOSPITAL AND HOMES, 715 Delmore Avenue, Roseau, MN, Zip 56751; tel. 218/463–2500; David F. Hagen, President and Executive Officer

QUALITY HEALTH ALLIANCE
501 Holly Lane – Sr. 11A, Mankato, MN
56001; tel. 507/389–4715; Todd Erik Henry,
Executive Director

NEW ULM MEDICAL CENTER, 1324 Fifth Street North, New Ulm, MN, Zip 56073–1553, Mailing Address: P.O. Box 577, Zip 56073; tel. 507/354–2111; Rickie L. Ressler, R.N., Interim President

SLEEPY EYE MUNICIPAL HOSPITAL, 400 Fourth Avenue N.W., Sleepy Eye, MN, Zip 56085; tel. 507/794–3571; Chad Cooper, Administrator

SPRINGFIELD COMMUNITY HOSPITAL, 625 North Jackson, Springfield, MN, Zip 56087, Mailing Address: Box 146, Zip 56087; tel. 507/723–6201; Scott Thoreson, Administrator

ST. JAMES HEALTH SERVICES, 1207 Sixth Avenue South, Saint James, MN, Zip 56081; tel. 507/375–3261; Lee Holter, Chief Executive Officer

ST. PETER REGIONAL TREATMENT CENTER, 100 Freeman Drive, Saint Peter, MN, Zip 56082–1599; tel. 507/931–7100; William L. Pedersen, Chief Executive Officer

UNITED HOSPITAL DISTRICT, 515 South Moore Street, Blue Earth, MN, Zip 56013–2158, Mailing Address: P.O. Box 160, Zip 56013–0160; tel. 507/526–3273; Brian Kief, President

WASECA AREA MEDICAL CENTER, 100 Fifth Avenue N.W., Waseca, MN, Zip 56093–2422; tel. 507/835–1210; Michael Milbrath, Administrator

QUALITY HEALTH NETWORK, INC.
910 Main Street, Suite 202, Redwing, MN
55066; tel. 612/388–0750; Ronald
Schiemann, Administrator

FAIRVIEW–UNIVERSITY MEDICAL CENTER, 2450 Riverside Avenue, Minneapolis, MN, Zip 55454–1400; tel. 612/672–6300; Peter Rapp, Senior Vice President and Administrator

ST. JOHN'S REGIONAL HEALTH CENTER, 1407 West Fourth Street, Red Wing, MN, Zip 55066–2198; tel. 612/388–6721; Craig Stoeckel, Interim Administrator

SOUTHWEST MINNESOTA HEALTH ALLIANCE
305 East Luverne Street, Luverne, MN 56156;
tel. 507/283–2775; Jeff Stevenson, President

Section B

CANBY COMMUNITY HEALTH SERVICES, 112 St. Olaf Avenue South, Canby, MN, Zip 56220–1433; tel. 507/223–7277; Robert J. Salmon, Chief Executive Officer

LUVERNE COMMUNITY HOSPITAL, 305 East Luverne Street, Luverne, MN, Zip 56156–2519, Mailing Address: P.O. Box 1019, Zip 56156; tel. 507/283–2321; Gerald E. Carl, Administrator

MURRAY COUNTY MEMORIAL HOSPITAL, 2042 Juniper Avenue, Slayton, MN, Zip 56172; tel. 507/836–6111; Jerry Bobeldyk, Administrator

SIOUX VALLEY HOSPITAL, 1100 South Euclid Avenue, Sioux Falls, SD, Zip 57105–0496, Mailing Address: P.O. Box 5039, Zip 57117–5039; tel. 605/333–1000; Kelby K. Krabbenhoft, Chief Executive Officer

TRACY MUNICIPAL HOSPITAL, 251 Fifth Street East, Tracy, MN, Zip 56175–1536; tel. 507/629–3200; Thomas J. Quinlivan, Administrator

WINDOM AREA HOSPITAL, Highways 60 and 71 North, Windom, MN, Zip 56101, Mailing Address: P.O. Box 339, Zip 56101; tel. 507/831–2400; J. Stephen Pautler, CHE, Administrator

WORTHINGTON REGIONAL HOSPITAL, 1018 Sixth Avenue, Worthington, MN, Zip 56187, Mailing Address: P.O. Box 997, Zip 56187; tel. 507/372–2941; Melvin J. Platt, Administrator

MISSISSIPPI

NORTH MISSISSIPPI HEALTH SERVICES
830 South Gloster Street, Tupelo, MS 38801; tel. 601/841–3000; Jeffrey B. Barber, President & Chief Executive Officer

CLAY COUNTY MEDICAL CENTER, 835 Medical Center Drive, West Point, MS, Zip 39773; tel. 601/495–2300; David M. Reid, Administrator

IUKA HOSPITAL, 1777 Curtis Drive, Iuka, MS, Zip 38852, Mailing Address: P.O. Box 860, Zip 38852; tel. 601/423–6051; Robert E. Northern, Administrator

NORTH MISSISSIPPI MEDICAL CENTER, 830 South Gloster Street, Tupelo, MS, Zip 38801–4934; tel. 601/841–3000; Jeffrey B. Barber, Dr.PH, President and Chief Executive Officer

PONTOTOC HOSPITAL AND EXTENDED CARE FACILITY, 176 South Main Street, Pontotoc, MS, Zip 38863, Mailing Address: P.O. Box C, Zip 38863; tel. 601/489–5510; Fred B. Hood, Administrator

WEBSTER HEALTH SERVICES, 500 Highway 9 South, Eupora, MS, Zip 39744; tel. 601/258–6221; Harold H. Whitaker, Sr., Administrator

MISSOURI

BJC HEALTH SYSTEM
4444 Forest Park Avenue, Suite 500, St. Louis, MO 63108–2259; tel. 314/286–2085; Patrick N. Lee, Management Associate

ALTON MEMORIAL HOSPITAL, One Memorial Drive, Alton, IL, Zip 62002–6722; tel. 618/463–7311; Ronald B. McMullen, President

BARNES–JEWISH HOSPITAL, 216 South Kingshighway Boulevard, Saint Louis, MO, Zip 63110–1094; tel. 314/362–5000; Alan W. Brass, FACHE, President

BARNES–JEWISH ST. PETERS HOSPITAL, 10 Hospital Drive, Saint Peters, MO, Zip 6337–1659; tel. 314/916–9000; John Gloss, President

BARNES–JEWISH WEST COUNTY HOSPITAL, 12634 Olive Boulevard, Saint Louis, MO, Zip 63141–6354; tel. 314/996–8000; Gregory T. Wozniak, President

BOONE HOSPITAL CENTER, 1600 East Broadway, Columbia, MO, Zip 65201; tel. 573/815–8000; Michael Shirk, President and Senior Executive Officer

CAPITAL REGION MEDICAL CENTER–SOUTHWEST, 1432 Southwest Boulevard, Jefferson City, MO, Zip 65109–4420, Mailing Address: P.O. Box 1128, Zip 65102–1128; tel. 573/635–6811; Edward F. Farnsworth, President

CHRISTIAN HOSPITAL NORTHEAST–NORTHWEST, 11133 Dunn Road, Saint Louis, MO, Zip 63136–6192; tel. 314/355–2300; W. R. Van Bokkelen, President and Senior Executive Officer

CLAY COUNTY HOSPITAL, 700 North Mill Street, Flora, IL, Zip 62839, Mailing Address: P.O. Box 280, Zip 62839; tel. 618/662–2131; John E. Monnahan, President and Senior Executive Officer

COX–MONETT HOSPITAL, 801 Lincoln Avenue, Monett, MO, Zip 65708–1698; tel. 417/235–3144; Frank D. Dale, Administrator

DOCTORS HOSPITAL, 500 Medical Drive, Wentzville, MO, Zip 63385–0711; tel. 314/327–1000; Fred Woody, Chief Executive Officer

DOCTORS REGIONAL MEDICAL CENTER, 621 Pine Boulevard, Poplar Bluff, MO, Zip 63901; tel. 573/686–4111; Daniel R. Kelly, Chief Executive Officer

FAYETTE COUNTY HOSPITAL AND LONG TERM CARE, Seventh and Taylor Streets, Vandalia, IL, Zip 62471–1296; tel. 618/283–1231; Daniel L. Gantz, President

GRIM–SMITH HOSPITAL AND CLINIC, 112 East Patterson Avenue, Kirksville, MO, Zip 63501; tel. 816/665–7241; Steven E. Clark, Administrator

HEDRICK MEDICAL CENTER, 100 Central Avenue, Chillicothe, MO, Zip 64601–1599; tel. 816/646–1480; R. Lynn Jackson, Chief Executive Officer

JEFFERSON MEMORIAL HOSPITAL, Highway 61 South, Crystal City, MO, Zip 63019, Mailing Address: P.O. Box 350, Zip 63019–0350; tel. 314/933–1000; Richard Johansen, Chief Operating Officer and Interim Chief Executive Officer

KEOKUK AREA HOSPITAL, 1600 Morgan Street, Keokuk, IA, Zip 52632; tel. 319/524–7150; Allan Zastrow, FACHE, Chief Executive Officer

MADISON MEDICAL CENTER, 100 South Wood at West College, Fredericktown, MO, Zip 63645, Mailing Address: P.O. Box 431, Zip 63645–0431; tel. 573/783–3341; Floyd D. Bounds, Administrator

MEMORIAL HOSPITAL, 1900 State Street, Chester, IL, Zip 62233–0609, Mailing Address: Box 609, Zip 62233; tel. 618/826–4581; Eric Freeburg, Administrator

MISSOURI BAPTIST HOSPITAL OF SULLIVAN, 751 Sappington Bridge Road, Sullivan, MO, Zip 63080, Mailing Address: P.O. Box 190, Zip 63080; tel. 573/468–4186; Davis D. Skinner, Administrator

MISSOURI BAPTIST MEDICAL CENTER, 3015 North Ballas Road, Town and Country, MO, Zip 63131–2374; tel. 314/996–5000; Mark A. Eustis, President

OZARKS MEDICAL CENTER, 1100 Kentucky Avenue, West Plains, MO, Zip 65775, Mailing Address: P.O. Box 1100, Zip 65775–1100; tel. 417/256–9111; Charles R. Brackney, President and Chief Executive Officer

PARKLAND HEALTH CENTER, 1101 West Liberty Street, Farmington, MO, Zip 63640–1997; tel. 314/756–6451; Richard L. Conklin, President

PERRY COUNTY MEMORIAL HOSPITAL, 434 North West Street, Perryville, MO, Zip 63775–1398; tel. 314/547–2536; Patrick G. Bira, JD, FACHE, Administrator

PHELPS COUNTY REGIONAL MEDICAL CENTER, 1000 West Tenth Street, Rolla, MO, Zip 65401; tel. 573/364–3100; David Ross, Chief Executive Officer

PINCKNEYVILLE COMMUNITY HOSPITAL, 101 North Walnut Street, Pinckneyville, IL, Zip 62274; tel. 618/357–2187; John D. Schubert, Administrator and Chief Executive Officer

PUBLIC HOSPITAL OF THE TOWN OF SALEM, 1201 Ricker Drive, Salem, IL, Zip 62881–6250, Mailing Address: P.O. Box 1250, Zip 62881–1250; tel. 618/548–3194; Clarence E. Lay, Chief Executive Officer

REYNOLDS COUNTY GENERAL MEMORIAL HOSPITAL, Highway 21 South, Ellington, MO, Zip 63638, Mailing Address: P.O. Box 520, Zip 63638; tel. 573/663–2511; Patricia Koppeis, Administrator

ST. CLEMENT HEALTH SERVICES, One St. Clement Boulevard, Red Bud, IL, Zip 62278–1194; tel. 618/282–3831; Michael Thomas McManus, President

ST. LOUIS CHILDREN'S HOSPITAL, One Children's Place, Saint Louis, MO, Zip 63110–1077; tel. 314/454–6000; Ted W. Frey, President

WASHINGTON COUNTY MEMORIAL HOSPITAL, 300 Health Way, Potosi, MO, Zip 63664–1499; tel. 314/438–5451; William L. Schwarten, Administrator

CARONDELET HEALTH
P.O. Box 8510, Kansas City, MO 64114; tel. 816/943–2673; Richard M. Abell, Chief Executive Officer

MCCUNE–BROOKS HOSPITAL, 627 West Centennial Avenue, Carthage, MO, Zip 64836–0677; tel. 417/358–8121; James W. McPheeters, III, Administrator

ST. JOHN'S REGIONAL MEDICAL CENTER, 2727 McClelland Boulevard, Joplin, MO, Zip 64804; tel. 417/781–2727; Robert G. Brueckner, President and Chief Executive Officer

ST. JOSEPH HEALTH CENTER, 300 First Capitol Drive, Saint Charles, MO, Zip 63301–2835; tel. 314/947–5000; Kurt Weinmeister, President

ST. MARY'S HOSPITAL OF BLUE SPRINGS, 201 West R. D. Mize Road, Blue Springs, MO, Zip 64014; tel. 816/228–5900; N. Gary Wages, President and Chief Executive Officer

HEALTH MIDWEST
2304 East Meyer Boulevard, A–20, Kansas City, MO 64132; tel. 816/276–9181; Richard W. Brown, President

ALLEN COUNTY HOSPITAL, 101 South First Street, Iola, KS, Zip 66749, Mailing Address: P.O. Box 540, Zip 66749–0540; tel. 316/365–3131; Franklin K. Wilson, Administrator

BAPTIST MEDICAL CENTER, 6601 Rockhill Road, Kansas City, MO, Zip 64131–1197; tel. 816/276–7000; Dan H. Anderson, President and Chief Executive Officer

CASS MEDICAL CENTER, 1800 East Mechanic Street, Harrisonville, MO, Zip 64701; tel. 816/884–3291; Alan Freeman, Administrator

HEDRICK MEDICAL CENTER, 100 Central Avenue, Chillicothe, MO, Zip 64601–1599; tel. 816/646–1480; R. Lynn Jackson, Chief Executive Officer

LAFAYETTE REGIONAL HEALTH CENTER, 1500 State Street, Lexington, MO, Zip 64067–1199; tel. 816/259–2203; Jeffrey S. Tarrant, Administrator

LEE'S SUMMIT HOSPITAL, 530 North Murray Road, Lees Summit, MO, Zip 64081–1497; tel. 816/251–7000; John L. Jacobson, President and Chief Executive Officer

MEDICAL CENTER OF INDEPENDENCE, 17203 East 23rd Street, Independence, MO, Zip 64057; tel. 816/478–5000; Michael W. Chappelow, President and Chief Executive Officer

PARK LANE MEDICAL CENTER, 5151 Raytown Road, Kansas City, MO, Zip 64133; tel. 816/358–8000; Derell Taloney, President and Chief Executive Officer

REHABILITATION INSTITUTE, 3011 Baltimore, Kansas City, MO, Zip 64108–3465; tel. 816/751–7900; Ronald L. Herrick, President

RESEARCH BELTON HOSPITAL, 17065 South 71 Highway, Belton, MO, Zip 64012; tel. 816/348–1200; Daniel F. Sheehan, Administrator

RESEARCH MEDICAL CENTER, 2316 East Meyer Boulevard, Kansas City, MO, Zip 64132–1199; tel. 816/276–4000; Dan H. Anderson, President and Chief Executive Officer

RESEARCH PSYCHIATRIC CENTER, 2323 East 63rd Street, Kansas City, MO, Zip 64130; tel. 816/444–8161; Todd Krass, Administrator and Chief Executive Officer

TRINITY LUTHERAN HOSPITAL, 3030 Baltimore Avenue, Kansas City, MO, Zip 64108–3404; tel. 816/753–4600; Ronald A. Ommen, President and Chief Executive Officer

NORTHWEST MISSOURI HEALTHCARE AGENDA
705 North College Avenue, Albany, MO 64402; tel. 816/726–3941; John Richmond, Chairman

HEARTLAND REGIONAL MEDICAL CENTER, 5325 Faraon Street, Saint Joseph, MO, Zip 64506–3398; tel. 816/271–6000; Lowell C. Kruse, President

SAINT LOUIS HEALTH CARE NETWORK
477 North Lindbergh Boulevard, St. Louis, MO 63141; tel. 314/994–7800; Stephanie McCutcheon, President & Chief Executive Officer

ARCADIA VALLEY HOSPITAL, Highway 21, Pilot Knob, MO, Zip 63663, Mailing Address: P.O. Box 548, Zip 63663–0548; tel. 573/546–3924; H. Clark Duncan, Administrator

CARDINAL GLENNON CHILDREN'S HOSPITAL, 1465 South Grand Boulevard, Saint Louis, MO, Zip 63104–1095; tel. 314/577–5600; Douglas A. Ries, President

LINCOLN COUNTY MEMORIAL HOSPITAL, 1000 East Cherry, Troy, MO, Zip 63379; tel. 314/528–8551; Floyd B. Dowell, Jr., Administrator

MINERAL AREA REGIONAL MEDICAL CENTER, 1212 Weber Road, Farmington, MO, Zip 63640; tel. 573/756–4581; Kenneth C. West, Chief Executive Officer

PIKE COUNTY MEMORIAL HOSPITAL, 2305 West Georgia Street, Louisiana, MO, Zip 63353–0020; tel. 573/754–5531; Thomas E. Lefebvre, President

SAINT LOUIS UNIVERSITY HOSPITAL, 3635 Vista at Grand Boulevard, Saint Louis, MO, Zip 63110–0250, Mailing Address: P.O. Box 15250, Zip 63110–0250; tel. 314/577–8000; James Kimmey, M.D., M.P.H., Chairman and Chief Executive Officer

SSM REHABILITATION INSTITUTE, 6420 Clayton Road, Suite 600, Saint Louis, MO, Zip 63117; tel. 314/768–5300; Melinda Clark, President

ST. JOSEPH HEALTH CENTER, 300 First Capitol Drive, Saint Charles, MO, Zip 63301–2835; tel. 314/947–5000; Kurt Weinmeister, President

ST. JOSEPH HOSPITAL WEST, 100 Medical Plaza, Lake Saint Louis, MO, Zip 63367–1395; tel. 314/625–5200; Kurt Weinmeister, President

ST. MARY'S HEALTH CENTER, 6420 Clayton Road, Saint Louis, MO, Zip 63117–1811; tel. 314/768–8000; Michael E. Zilm, President

ST. MARY'S HOSPITAL, 129 North Eighth Street, East St. Louis, IL, Zip 62201–2999; tel. 618/274–1900; Richard J. Mark, President and Chief Executive Officer

WASHINGTON COUNTY HOSPITAL, 705 South Grand Street, Nashville, IL, Zip 62263–1532; tel. 618/327–8236; Michael P. Ellermann, President

UNITY HEALTH SYSTEM
1655 Des Peres Road, Suite 301, St. Louis, MO 63131; tel. 314/909–3300; James R. (Jay) Hardman, Chief Executive Officer

COMMUNITY MEMORIAL HOSPITAL, 400 Caldwell Street, Staunton, IL, Zip 62088–1499; tel. 618/635–2200; Patrick B. Heise, Chief Executive Officer

SAINT ANTHONY'S HEALTH CENTER, Saint Anthony's Way, Alton, IL, Zip 62002, Mailing Address: P.O. Box 340, Zip 62002–0340; tel. 618/465–2571; William E. Kessler, President

ST. ANTHONY'S MEDICAL CENTER, 10010 Kennerly Road, Saint Louis, MO, Zip 63128; tel. 314/525–1000; David P. Seifert, President

ST. CLEMENT HEALTH SERVICES, One St. Clement Boulevard, Red Bud, IL, Zip 62278–1194; tel. 618/282–3831; Michael Thomas McManus, President

ST. ELIZABETH MEDICAL CENTER, 2100 Madison Avenue, Granite City, IL, Zip 62040; tel. 618/798–3000; Ted Eilerman, President

ST. ELIZABETH'S HOSPITAL, 211 South Third Street, Belleville, IL, Zip 62222–0694; tel. 618/234–2120; Gerald M. Harman, Chief Executive Officer and Executive Vice President

ST. JOHN'S MERCY MEDICAL CENTER, 615 South New Ballas Road, Saint Louis, MO, Zip 63141–8277; tel. 314/569–6000; Mark Weber, President

ST. JOSEPH'S HOSPITAL, 1515 Main Street, Highland, IL, Zip 62249–1656; tel. 618/654–7421; Anthony G. Mastrangelo, Executive Vice President and Chief Executive Officer

ST. LUKE'S HOSPITAL, 232 South Woods Mill Road, Chesterfield, MO, Zip 63017–3480; tel. 314/434–1500; George Tucker, M.D., President

MONTANA

MONTANA HEALTH NETWORK, INC.
11 South 7th Street, Suite 160, Miles City, MT 59301; tel. 406/232–1420; Janet Bastian, Chief Executive Officer

CARBON COUNTY MEMORIAL HOSPITAL AND NURSING HOME, 600 West 20th Street, Red Lodge, MT, Zip 59068, Mailing Address: P.O. Box 590, Zip 59068–0590; tel. 406/446–2345; Kelley Going, Administrator

CENTRAL MONTANA MEDICAL CENTER, 408 Wendell Avenue, Lewistown, MT, Zip 59457, Mailing Address: P.O. Box 580, Zip 59457; tel. 406/538–7711; David M. Faulkner, Chief Executive Officer and Administrator

DANIELS MEMORIAL HOSPITAL, 105 Fifth Avenue East, Scobey, MT, Zip 59263, Mailing Address: P.O. Box 400, Zip 59263–0400; tel. 406/487–2296; Glenn Haugo, Administrator

DEACONESS MEDICAL CENTER, 2800 10th Avenue North, Billings, MT, Zip 59101–0799, Mailing Address: P.O. Box 37000, Zip 59107–7001; tel. 406/657–4000; Patrick R. Garrett, Administrative Executive Officer

FALLON MEDICAL COMPLEX, 202 South 4th Street West, Baker, MT, Zip 59313–0820, Mailing Address: P.O. Box 820, Zip 59313–0820; tel. 406/778–3331; David Espeland, Chief Executive Officer

FRANCES MAHON DEACONESS HOSPITAL, 621 Third Street South, Glasgow, MT, Zip 59230; tel. 406/228–4351; Douglas A. McMillan, Chief Executive Officer

GLENDIVE MEDICAL CENTER, 202 Prospect Drive, Glendive, MT, Zip 59330; tel. 406/365–3306; Paul Hanson, Chief Executive Officer

HOLY ROSARY HEALTH CENTER, 2600 Wilson, Miles City, MT, Zip 59301; tel. 406/233–2600; H. Ray Gibbons, President and Chief Executive Officer

MCCONE COUNTY MEDICAL ASSISTANCE FACILITY, Circle, MT, Mailing Address: P.O. Box 47, Zip 59215–0047; tel. 406/485–3381; Mike Anderson, Administrator

NORTHEAST MONTANA HEALTH SERVICES, 315 Knapp Street, Wolf Point, MT, Zip 59201; tel. 406/653–2110; Earl N. Sheehy, Chief Executive Officer

PHILLIPS COUNTY HOSPITAL, 417 South Fourth East, Malta, MT, Zip 59538, Mailing Address: P.O. Box 640, Zip 59538–0640; tel. 406/654–1100; Larry E. Putnam, Administrator

ROOSEVELT MEMORIAL MEDICAL CENTER, Culbertson, MT, Mailing Address: P.O. Box 419, Zip 59218; tel. 406/787–6281; Walter Busch, Administrator

ROUNDUP MEMORIAL HOSPITAL, 1202 Third Street West, Roundup, MT, Zip 59072, Mailing Address: P.O. Box 40, Zip 59072; tel. 406/323–2302; Dave McIvor, Administrator

SHERIDAN MEMORIAL HOSPITAL, 440 West Laurel Avenue, Plentywood, MT, Zip 59254; tel. 406/765–1420; Ella Gutzke, Administrator

SIDNEY HEALTH CENTER, 216 14th Avenue S.W., Sidney, MT, Zip 59270, Mailing Address: P.O. Box 1690, Zip 59270–1690; tel. 406/482–2120; Donald J. Rush, Chief Executive Officer

STILLWATER COMMUNITY HOSPITAL, 44 West Fourth Avenue North, Columbus, MT, Zip 59019, Mailing Address: P.O. Box 959, Zip 59019–0959; tel. 406/322–5316; Tim Russell, Administrator

NORTHERN ROCKIES HEALTHCARE NETWORK
P.O. Box 4587, Missoula, MT 59806; tel. 406/542–0001; Lorrie Boehnke, Network Coordinator

ST. PATRICK HOSPITAL, 500 West Broadway, Missoula, MT, Zip 59802–4096, Mailing Address: Box 4587, Zip 59806–4587; tel. 406/543–7271; Lawrence L. White, Jr., President

NEBRASKA

ALEGENT HEALTH
1010 North 96th Street, Omaha, NE 68114; tel. 402/255–1661; Robert Azar, President of Public Health Information

ALEGENT HEALTH BERGAN MERCY MEDICAL CENTER, 7500 Mercy Road, Omaha, NE, Zip 68124; tel. 402/398–6060; Charles J. Marr, Chief Executive Officer

ALEGENT HEALTH COMMUNITY MEMORIAL HOSPITAL, 631 North Eighth Street, Missouri Valley, IA, Zip 51555–1199; tel. 712/642–2784; James A. Seymour, Regional Administrator

ALEGENT HEALTH IMMANUEL MEDICAL CENTER, 6901 North 72nd Street, Omaha, NE, Zip 68122–1799; tel. 402/572–2121; Randall W. Smith, Chief Operating Officer

ALEGENT HEALTH MERCY HOSPITAL, Rosary Drive, Corning, IA, Zip 50841, Mailing Address: Box 368, Zip 50841; tel. 515/322–3121; James C. Ruppert, Regional Administrator

ALEGENT HEALTH MERCY HOSPITAL, 800 Mercy Drive, Council Bluffs, IA, Zip 51503, Mailing Address: Box 1C, Zip 51502; tel. 712/328–5000; Charles J. Marr, Chief Executive Officer

ALEGENT HEALTH–MEMORIAL HOSPITAL, 104 West 17th Street, Schuyler, NE, Zip 68661; tel. 402/352–2441; Al Klaasmeyer, Administrator

BLUE RIVER VALLEY HEALTH NETWORK
P.O. Box 156, Brainard, NE 68626; tel. 402/545–2728; JoEllen Urba, Network Coordinator

ANNIE JEFFREY MEMORIAL COUNTY HEALTH CENTER, Osceola, NE, Mailing Address: P.O. Box 428, Zip 68651; tel. 402/747–2031; Curt Koesterer, Administrator

BUTLER COUNTY HEALTH CARE CENTER, 372 South Ninth Street, David City, NE, Zip 68632; tel. 402/367–3115; Roger Reamer, Administrator

CRETE MUNICIPAL HOSPITAL, 1540 Grove Street, Crete, NE, Zip 68333–0220, Mailing Address: P.O. Box 220, Zip 68333–0220; tel. 402/826–6800; Joe Lohrman, Administrator

HENDERSON HEALTH CARE SERVICES, 1621 Front Street, Henderson, NE, Zip 68371–0217, Mailing Address: P.O. Box 217, Zip 68371–0217; tel. 402/723–4512; Calvin C. Graber, Chief Executive Officer

MEMORIAL HEALTH CARE SYSTEMS, 300 North Columbia Avenue, Seward, NE, Zip 68434–9907; tel. 402/643–2971; Ronald D. Waltz, Chief Executive Officer

MEMORIAL HOSPITAL, 1423 Seventh Street, Aurora, NE, Zip 68818–1197; tel. 402/694–3171; Eldon A. Wall, Administrator

SAUNDERS COUNTY HEALTH SERVICE, 805 West Tenth Street, Wahoo, NE, Zip 68066, Mailing Address: P.O. Box 185, Zip 68066; tel. 402/443–4191; Michael Boyles, Administrator

WARREN MEMORIAL HOSPITAL, 905 Second Street, Friend, NE, Zip 68359; tel. 402/947–2541; John Ramsay, Administrator

YORK GENERAL HOSPITAL, 2222 Lincoln Avenue, York, NE, Zip 68467–1095; tel. 402/362–6671; Charles Schulz, Chief Executive Officer

**CENTRAL NEBRASKA PRIMARY CARE NETWORK
1518 J Street, Ord, NE 68862;
tel. 308/728–3011; Barbara Weems,
Foundation President**

BOONE COUNTY HEALTH CENTER, 723 West Fairview Street, Albion, NE, Zip 68620, Mailing Address: P.O. Box 151, Zip 68620–0151; tel. 402/395–2191; Gayle E. Primrose, Administrator

VALLEY COUNTY HOSPITAL, 217 Westridge Drive, Ord, NE, Zip 68862; tel. 308/728–3211; Nancy Glaubke, Administrator

**HEARTLAND HEALTH ALLIANCE
1600 South 48th Street, Lincoln, NE 68506;
tel. 402/483–3111; R. Lynn Wilson, President**

BEATRICE COMMUNITY HOSPITAL AND HEALTH CENTER, 1110 North Tenth Street, Beatrice, NE, Zip 68310, Mailing Address: P.O. Box 278, Zip 68310–0278; tel. 402/228–3344; Kenneth J. Zimmerman, Administrator

BOONE COUNTY HEALTH CENTER, 723 West Fairview Street, Albion, NE, Zip 68620, Mailing Address: P.O. Box 151, Zip 68620–0151; tel. 402/395–2191; Gayle E. Primrose, Administrator

BRODSTONE MEMORIAL HOSPITAL, 520 East Tenth, Superior, NE, Zip 68978, Mailing Address: P.O. Box 187, Zip 68978–0187; tel. 402/879–3281; Ronald D. Waggoner, Administrator and Chief Executive Officer

BRYAN MEMORIAL HOSPITAL, 1600 South 48th Street, Lincoln, NE, Zip 68506–1299; tel. 402/489–0200; R. Lynn Wilson, President

BUTLER COUNTY HEALTH CARE CENTER, 372 South Ninth Street, David City, NE, Zip 68632; tel. 402/367–3115; Roger Reamer, Administrator

CHERRY COUNTY HOSPITAL, Highway 12 and Green Street, Valentine, NE, Zip 69201–0410; tel. 402/376–2525; Brent Peterson, Administrator

COMMUNITY HOSPITAL, 1301 East H Street, McCook, NE, Zip 69001–1328, Mailing Address: P.O. Box 1328, Zip 69001–1328; tel. 308/345–2650; Gary Biegansk, President

COMMUNITY MEMORIAL HOSPITAL, 1579 Midland Street, Syracuse, NE, Zip 68446, Mailing Address: P.O. Box N, Zip 68446; tel. 402/269–2011; Ron Anderson, Administrator

CRETE MUNICIPAL HOSPITAL, 1540 Grove Street, Crete, NE, Zip 68333–0220, Mailing Address: P.O. Box 220, Zip 68333–0220; tel. 402/826–6800; Joe Lohrman, Administrator

FRANKLIN COUNTY MEMORIAL HOSPITAL, 1406 Q Street, Franklin, NE, Zip 68939–0315, Mailing Address: P.O. Box 315, Zip 68939–0315; tel. 308/425–6221; Jerrell F. Gerdes, Administrator

GOTHENBURG MEMORIAL HOSPITAL, 910 20th Street, Gothenburg, NE, Zip 69138, Mailing Address: P.O. Box 469, Zip 69138–0469; tel. 308/537–3661; Roger Heidebrink, Administrator

GREAT PLAINS REGIONAL MEDICAL CENTER, 601 West Leota Street, North Platte, NE, Zip 69101, Mailing Address: P.O. Box 1167, Zip 69103; tel. 308/534–9310; Lucinda A. Bradley, President

HARLAN COUNTY HOSPITAL, 717 North Brown, Alma, NE, Zip 68920, Mailing Address: P.O. Box 836, Zip 68920; tel. 308/928–2151; Allen Van Driel, Administrator

JEFFERSON COMMUNITY HEALTH CENTER, Fairbury, NE, Mailing Address: P.O. Box 277, Zip 68352–0277; tel. 402/729–3351; Bill Welch, Administrator

JENNIE M. MELHAM MEMORIAL MEDICAL CENTER, 145 Memorial Drive, Broken Bow, NE, Zip 68822, Mailing Address: P.O. Box 250, Zip 68822–0250; tel. 308/872–6891; Michael J. Steckler, Chief Executive Officer

JOHNSON COUNTY HOSPITAL, 202 High Street, Tecumseh, NE, Zip 68450–0599; tel. 402/335–3361; Lavonne M. Rowe, Administrator

MARY LANNING MEMORIAL HOSPITAL, 715 North St. Joseph Avenue, Hastings, NE, Zip 68901–4497; tel. 402/461–5108; W. Michael Kearney, Pressident

MEMORIAL HEALTH CARE SYSTEMS, 300 North Columbia Avenue, Seward, NE, Zip 68434–9907; tel. 402/643–2971; Ronald D. Waltz, Chief Executive Officer

MEMORIAL HOSPITAL, 1423 Seventh Street, Aurora, NE, Zip 68818–1197; tel. 402/694–3171; Eldon A. Wall, Administrator

NEMAHA COUNTY HOSPITAL, 2022 13th Street, Auburn, NE, Zip 68305–1799; tel. 402/274–4366; Glen Krueger, Administrator

PHELPS MEMORIAL HEALTH CENTER, 1220 Miller Street, Holdrege, NE, Zip 68949, Mailing Address: P.O. Box 828, Zip 68949–0828; tel. 308/995–2211; Jerome Seigfried, Jr., Chief Executive Officer

TRI–COUNTY AREA HOSPITAL, 13th and Erie Streets, Lexington, NE, Zip 68850–0980, Mailing Address: P.O. Box 980, Zip 68850–0980; tel. 308/324–5651; Calvin A. Hiner, Administrator

TRI–VALLEY HEALTH SYSTEM, West Highway 6 and 34, Cambridge, NE, Zip 69022, Mailing Address: P.O. Box 488, Zip 69022; tel. 308/697–3329; Kristopher H. Marwin, CHE, Chief Executive Officer

WEBSTER COUNTY COMMUNITY HOSPITAL, Sixth Avenue and Franklin Street, Red Cloud, NE, Zip 68970–0465; tel. 402/746–2291; Terry L. Hoffart, Administrator

YORK GENERAL HOSPITAL, 2222 Lincoln Avenue, York, NE, Zip 68467–1095; tel. 402/362–6671; Charles Schulz, Chief Executive Officer

**NORTH CENTRAL HOSPITAL NETWORK
R.R.I. Box 200, Atkinson, NE 68713–0200;
tel. 402/925–2811; Mel Snow, President**

ANTELOPE MEMORIAL HOSPITAL, 102 West Ninth Street, Neligh, NE, Zip 68756–0229, Mailing Address: P.O. Box 229, Zip 68756–0229; tel. 402/887–4151; Jack W. Green, Administrator

BROWN COUNTY HOSPITAL, 945 East Zero, Ainsworth, NE, Zip 69210; tel. 402/387–2800; Roger Reamer, Administrator

CREIGHTON AREA HEALTH SERVICES, 1503 Main Street, Creighton, NE, Zip 68729, Mailing Address: P.O. Box 186, Zip 68729; tel. 402/358–3322; Paul Hurd, Chief Executive Officer

LUTHERAN COMMUNITY HOSPITAL, 2700 Norfolk Avenue, Norfolk, NE, Zip 68701, Mailing Address: P.O. Box 869, Zip 68702–0869; tel. 402/371–4880

NIOBRARA VALLEY HOSPITAL, Lynch, NE, Mailing Address: P.O. Box 118, Zip 68746; tel. 402/569–2451; E. R. Testerman, Administrator

NORFOLK REGIONAL CENTER, 1700 North Victory Road, Norfolk, NE, Zip 68701, Mailing Address: P.O. Box 1209, Zip 68702–1209; tel. 402/370–3400; Roger W. Steinkruger, Chief Executive Officer

OSMOND GENERAL HOSPITAL, 5th and Maple Street, Osmond, NE, Zip 68765–0429, Mailing Address: P.O. Box 429, Zip 68765–0429; tel. 402/748–3393; Celine Mlady, Chief Executive Officer

PLAINVIEW PUBLIC HOSPITAL, Plainview, NE, Mailing Address: P.O. Box 489, Zip 68769; tel. 402/582–4245; Donald T. Naiberk, Administrator and Chief Executive Officer

ROCK COUNTY HOSPITAL, Bassett, NE, Mailing Address: P.O. Box 100, Zip 68714–0100; tel. 402/684–3366; David Stephenson, Administrator

ST. ANTHONY'S HOSPITAL, Second and Adams Streets, O'Neill, NE, Zip 68763–1597; tel. 402/336–2611; Ronald J. Cork, President and Chief Executive Officer

WEST HOLT MEMORIAL HOSPITAL, 406 Legion Street, Atkinson, NE, Zip 68713, Mailing Address: Rural Route 1, Box 200, Zip 68713; tel. 402/925–2811; Mel Snow, Administrator

**RURAL HEALTH PARTNERS
513 North Grant Street, Suite 5, Lexington, NE
68850; tel. 308/324–3050; Sheila Rowe,
Executive Director**

BRODSTONE MEMORIAL HOSPITAL, 520 East Tenth, Superior, NE, Zip 68978, Mailing Address: P.O. Box 187, Zip 68978–0187; tel. 402/879–3281; Ronald D. Waggoner, Administrator and Chief Executive Officer

COMMUNITY HOSPITAL, 1301 East H Street, McCook, NE, Zip 69001–1328, Mailing Address: P.O. Box 1328, Zip 69001–1328; tel. 308/345–2650; Gary Bieganski, President

FRANKLIN COUNTY MEMORIAL HOSPITAL, 1406 Q Street, Franklin, NE, Zip 68939–0315, Mailing Address: P.O. Box 315, Zip 68939–0315; tel. 308/425–6221; Jerrell F. Gerdes, Administrator

GOTHENBURG MEMORIAL HOSPITAL, 910 20th Street, Gothenburg, NE, Zip 69138, Mailing Address: P.O. Box 469, Zip 69138–0469; tel. 308/537–3661; Roger Heidebrink, Administrator

GREAT PLAINS REGIONAL MEDICAL CENTER, 601 West Leota Street, North Platte, NE, Zip 69101, Mailing Address: P.O. Box 1167, Zip 69103; tel. 308/534–9310; Lucinda A. Bradley, President

HARLAN COUNTY HOSPITAL, 717 North Brown, Alma, NE, Zip 68920, Mailing Address: P.O. Box 836, Zip 68920; tel. 308/928–2151; Allen Van Driel, Administrator

MARY LANNING MEMORIAL HOSPITAL, 715 North St. Joseph Avenue, Hastings, NE, Zip 68901–4497; tel. 402/461–5108; W. Michael Kearney, Pressident

PHELPS MEMORIAL HEALTH CENTER, 1220 Miller Street, Holdrege, NE, Zip 68949, Mailing Address: P.O. Box 828, Zip 68949–0828; tel. 308/995–2211; Jerome Seigfried, Jr., Chief Executive Officer

TRI–COUNTY AREA HOSPITAL, 13th and Erie Streets, Lexington, NE, Zip 68850–0980, Mailing Address: P.O. Box 980, Zip 68850–0980; tel. 308/324–5651; Calvin A. Hiner, Administrator

TRI–VALLEY HEALTH SYSTEM, West Highway 6 and 34, Cambridge, NE, Zip 69022, Mailing Address: P.O. Box 488, Zip 69022; tel. 308/697–3329; Kristopher H. Marwin, CHE, Chief Executive Officer

WEBSTER COUNTY COMMUNITY HOSPITAL, Sixth Avenue and Franklin Street, Red Cloud, NE, Zip 68970–0465; tel. 402/746–2291; Terry L. Hoffart, Administrator

**WESTERN NEBRASKA RURAL HEALTH CARE NETWORK
821 Morehead Street, Chadron, NE 69337;
tel. 308/432–5586; Harold Krueger, Chief
Executive Officer**

BOX BUTTE GENERAL HOSPITAL, 2101 Box Butte Avenue, Alliance, NE, Zip 69301–0810, Mailing Address: P.O. Box 810, Zip 69301–0810; tel. 308/762–6660; Terrance J. Padden, Administrator

CHADRON COMMUNITY HOSPITAL, 821 Morehead Street, Chadron, NE, Zip 69337–2599; tel. 308/432–5586; Harold L. Krueger, Jr., Administrator

CHASE COUNTY COMMUNITY HOSPITAL, 600 West 12th Street, Imperial, NE, Zip 69033; tel. 308/882–7111; James O'Neal, Administrator

GARDEN COUNTY HOSPITAL, Oshkosh, NE, Mailing Address: P.O. Box 320, Zip 69154; tel. 308/772–3283; Keith Hillman, Administrator

GORDON MEMORIAL HOSPITAL DISTRICT, 300 East Eighth Street, Gordon, NE, Zip 69343–9990; tel. 308/282–0401; Gladys Phemister, Administrator

KIMBALL COUNTY HOSPITAL, 505 South Burg Street, Kimball, NE, Zip 69145; tel. 308/235–3621; Gerri Linn, Administrator

LEGEND BUTTES HEALTH SERVICES, 11 Paddock Street, Crawford, NE, Zip 69339, Mailing Address: P.O. Box 272, Zip 69339; tel. 308/665–1770; Kim Engel, Chief Executive Officer

MEMORIAL HEALTH CENTER, 645 Osage Street, Sidney, NE, Zip 69162; tel. 308/254–5825; Rex D. Walk, Chief Executive Officer

MORRILL COUNTY COMMUNITY HOSPITAL, 1313 South Street, Bridgeport, NE, Zip 69336, Mailing Address: P.O. Box 579, Zip 69336; tel. 308/262–1616; Julia Morrow, Administrator

REGIONAL WEST MEDICAL CENTER, 4021 Avenue B, Scottsbluff, NE, Zip 69361–4695; tel. 308/635–3711; David M. Nitschke, President and Chief Executive Officer

NEVADA

SAINT MARY'S HEALTH NETWORK
1155 West Fourth Street – Suite 216, Reno, NV 89520; tel. 702/789–3004; Jeff K. Bills, President & Chief Executive Officer

ST. MARY'S REGIONAL MEDICAL CENTER, 235 West Sixth Street, Reno, NV, Zip 89520; tel. 702/323–2041; Jeff K. Bills, Chief Executive Officer

NEW HAMPSHIRE

CARING COMMUNITY NETWORK OF THE TWIN RIVERS (CCNTR)
15 Aiken Avenue, Franklin, NH 03235; tel. 603/934–2060; Walter A. Strauch, Chairperson

FRANKLIN REGIONAL HOSPITAL, 15 Aiken Avenue, Franklin, NH, Zip 03235–1299; tel. 603/934–2060; Walter A. Strauch, Executive Director

HEALTHLINK
80 Highland Street, Laconia, NH 03246; tel. 603/527–2910; Sharon Swanson, Network Contact

CATHOLIC MEDICAL CENTER, 100 McGregor Street, Manchester, NH, Zip 03102–3770; tel. 603/668–3545; Robert Cholette, President and Chief Executive Officer

CONCORD HOSPITAL, 250 Pleasant Street, Concord, NH, Zip 03301–2598; tel. 603/225–2711; Michael B. Green, President

ELLIOT HOSPITAL, One Elliot Way, Manchester, NH, Zip 03103; tel. 603/669–5300; Robert G. Cholette, Chief Executive Officer

LAKES REGION GENERAL HOSPITAL, Highland Street, Laconia, NH, Zip 03246–3298; tel. 603/524–3211; Thomas Clairmont, President

MARY HITCHCOCK MEMORIAL HOSPITAL, One Medical Center Drive, Lebanon, NH, Zip 03756–0001; tel. 603/650–5000; James W. Varnum, President

PARTNERS IN CARING
243 Elm Street, Claremont, NH 03743; tel. 603/542–7771; Joan Churchill, Chairperson

VALLEY REGIONAL HOSPITAL, 243 Elm Street, Claremont, NH, Zip 03743–2099; tel. 603/542–7771; Donald R. Holl, President

SAINT JOSEPH HEALTH CARE
172 Kinsley Street, Nashua, NH 03061; tel. 603/882–3000; Peter B. Davis, President

ST. JOSEPH HEALTHCARE, 172 Kinsley Street, Nashua, NH, Zip 03061, Mailing Address: Caller Service 2013, Zip 03061; tel. 603/882–3000; Peter B. Davis, President and Chief Executive Officer

NEW JERSEY

ATLANTICARE HEALTH SYSTEM
6725 Delilah Road, Egg Harbor Township, NJ 08234; tel. 609/272–6311; Dominic S. Moffa, Vice President–Administration

ATLANTIC CITY MEDICAL CENTER, 1925 Pacific Avenue, Atlantic City, NJ, Zip 08401–6713; tel. 609/345–4000; David P. Tilton, President and Chief Executive Officer

CAPE ADVANTAGE HEALTH ALLIANCE
Two Stone Harbor Boulevard, Cape May, NJ 08210; tel. 609/463–2480; Tom Scott, President & Chief Executive Officer

BURDETTE TOMLIN MEMORIAL HOSPITAL, Stone Harbor Boulevard, Cape May Court House, NJ, Zip 08210–9990; tel. 609/463–2000; Thomas L. Scott, FACHE, President and Chief Executive Officer

CLARA MAASS HEALTH SYSTEM
One Franklin Avenue, Belleville, NJ 07109; tel. 201/450–2000; Robert S. Curtis, President

CLARA MAASS HEALTH SYSTEM, One Clara Maass Drive, Belleville, NJ, Zip 07109; tel. 201/450–2000; Robert S. Curtis, President and Chief Executive Officer

COMMUNITY/KIMBALL HEALTH CARE SYSTEM
99 Highway 37 West, Toms River, NJ 08755; tel. 908/240–8000; Mark Pilla, President

COMMUNITY KIMBALL HEALTH CARE SYSTEM, 99 Highway 37 West, Toms River, NJ, Zip 08755–6423; tel. 908/240–8000; Kevin R. Burchill, Executive Director

FIRST OPTION HEALTH PLAN
2 Bridge Street, Red Bank, NJ 07701; tel. 908/842–5000; Michele Severin, Director Network Development

BARNERT HOSPITAL, 680 Broadway, Paterson, NJ, Zip 07514; tel. 201/977–6600; Fred L. Lang, President and Chief Executive Officer

BAYSHORE COMMUNITY HOSPITAL, 727 North Beers Street, Holmdel, NJ, Zip 07733; tel. 908/739–5900; Thomas Goldman, President

BETH ISRAEL HOSPITAL, 70 Parker Avenue, Passaic, NJ, Zip 07055; tel. 201/365–5000; Jeffrey S. Moll, President and Chief Executive Officer

BURDETTE TOMLIN MEMORIAL HOSPITAL, Stone Harbor Boulevard, Cape May Court House, NJ, Zip 08210–9990; tel. 609/463–2000; Thomas L. Scott, FACHE, President and Chief Executive Officer

CENTRASTATE MEDICAL CENTER, 901 West Main Street, Freehold, NJ, Zip 07728–2549; tel. 908/431–2000; Thomas H. Litz, President and Chief Executive Officer

CHILTON MEMORIAL HOSPITAL, 97 West Parkway, Pompton Plains, NJ, Zip 07444–1696; tel. 201/831–5000; James J. Doyle, Jr., President and Chief Executive Officer

CHRIST HOSPITAL, 176 Palisade Avenue, Jersey City, NJ, Zip 07306–1196, Mailing Address: P.O. Box J–1, Zip 07306–1196; tel. 201/795–8200; Daniel R. Connell, President

CLARA MAASS HEALTH SYSTEM, One Clara Maass Drive, Belleville, NJ, Zip 07109; tel. 201/450–2000; Robert S. Curtis, President and Chief Executive Officer

COMMUNITY KIMBALL HEALTH CARE SYSTEM, 99 Highway 37 West, Toms River, NJ, Zip 08755–6423; tel. 908/240–8000; Kevin R. Burchill, Executive Director

EAST ORANGE GENERAL HOSPITAL, 300 Central Avenue, East Orange, NJ, Zip 07019–2819; tel. 201/672–8400; Mark Chastang, President and Chief Executive Officer

ELIZABETH GENERAL MEDICAL CENTER, 925 East Jersey Street, Elizabeth, NJ, Zip 07201–2728; tel. 908/629–8065; David A. Fletcher, President and Chief Executive Officer

ENGLEWOOD HOSPITAL AND MEDICAL CENTER, 350 Engle Street, Englewood, NJ, Zip 07631; tel. 201/894–3000; Daniel A. Kane, President and Chief Executive Officer

HACKETTSTOWN COMMUNITY HOSPITAL, 651 Willow Grove Street, Hackettstown, NJ, Zip 07840–1798; tel. 908/852–5100; Gene C. Milton, President and Chief Executive Officer

HOLY NAME HOSPITAL, 718 Teaneck Road, Teaneck, NJ, Zip 07666; tel. 201/833–3000; Michael Maron, President and Chief Executive Officer

HUNTERDON MEDICAL CENTER, 2100 Wescott Drive, Flemington, NJ, Zip 08822–4604; tel. 908/788–6100; Robert P. Wise, President and Chief Executive Officer

IRVINGTON GENERAL HOSPITAL, 832 Chancellor Avenue, Irvington, NJ, Zip 07111–0709; tel. 201/399–6000; Thomas A. Biga, Executive Director

JFK MEDICAL CENTER, 65 James Street, Edison, NJ, Zip 08818; tel. 908/321–7000; John P. McGee, President and Chief Executive Officer

KIMBALL MEDICAL CENTER, 600 River Avenue, Lakewood, NJ, Zip 08701–5281; tel. 908/363–1900; Joanne Carrocino, Executive Director

MEDICAL CENTER AT PRINCETON, 253 Witherspoon Street, Princeton, NJ, Zip 08540–3213; tel. 609/497–4000; Dennis W. Doody, President and Chief Executive Officer

MEMORIAL HOSPITAL OF BURLINGTON COUNTY, 175 Madison Avenue, Mount Holly, NJ, Zip 08060–2099; tel. 609/267–0700; Chester B. Kaletkowski, President and Chief Executive Officer

MERCER MEDICAL CENTER, 446 Bellevue Avenue, Trenton, NJ, Zip 08618, Mailing Address: Box 1658, Zip 08607; tel. 609/394–4000; Charles E. Baer, President

MONMOUTH MEDICAL CENTER, 300 Second Avenue, Long Branch, NJ, Zip 07740–6303; tel. 908/222–5200; Cynthia N. Sparer, Executive Director and Chief Operating Officer

MORRISTOWN MEMORIAL HOSPITAL, 100 Madison Avenue, Morristown, NJ, Zip 07962–1956; tel. 201/971–5000; Jean M. McMahon, R.N., Vice President and General Manager

MUHLENBERG REGIONAL MEDICAL CENTER, Park Avenue and Randolph Road, Plainfield, NJ, Zip 07061; tel. 908/668–2000; John R. Kopicki, President and Chief Executive Officer

NEWARK BETH ISRAEL MEDICAL CENTER, 201 Lyons Avenue, Newark, NJ, Zip 07112–2027; tel. 201/926–7000; Ronald W. Weitz, Executive Director

NEWTON MEMORIAL HOSPITAL, 175 High Street, Newton, NJ, Zip 07860–1004; tel. 201/383–2121; Dennis H. Collette, President and Chief Executive Officer

OUR LADY OF LOURDES MEDICAL CENTER, 1600 Haddon Avenue, Camden, NJ, Zip 08103; tel. 609/757–3500; Alexander J. Hatala, President and Chief Executive Officer

PALISADES GENERAL HOSPITAL, 7600 River Road, North Bergen, NJ, Zip 07047–6217; tel. 201/854–5000; Bruce J. Markowitz, President and Chief Executive Officer

PASCACK VALLEY HOSPITAL, Old Hook Road, Westwood, NJ, Zip 07675–3181; tel. 201/358–3000; Louis R. Ycre, Jr., President and Chief Executive Officer

RIVERVIEW MEDICAL CENTER, 1 Riverview Plaza, Red Bank, NJ, Zip 07701–9982; tel. 908/741–2700; Paul S. Cohen, Executive Director and Chief Operating Officer

ROBERT WOOD JOHNSON UNIVERSITY HOSPITAL, 1 Robert Wood Johnson Place, New Brunswick, NJ, Zip 08903–2601; tel. 908/828–3000; Harvey A. Holzberg, President and Chief Executive Officer

SAINT BARNABAS MEDICAL CENTER, 94 Old Short Hills Road, Livingston, NJ, Zip 07039; tel. 201/533–5000; Ronald Del Mauro, Chairman and Chief Executive Officer

SHORE MEMORIAL HOSPITAL, 1 East New York Avenue, Somers Point, NJ, Zip 08244–2387; tel. 609/653–3500; Richard A. Pitman, President

SOMERSET MEDICAL CENTER, 110 Rehill Avenue, Somerville, NJ, Zip 08876–2598; tel. 908/685–2200; Michael A. Turner, President and Chief Executive Officer

SOUTH JERSEY HOSPITAL, 333 Irving Avenue, Bridgeton, NJ, Zip 08302–2100; tel. 609/451–6600; Paul S. Cooper, Chief Executive Officer

SOUTHERN OCEAN COUNTY HOSPITAL, 1140 Route 72 West, Manahawkin, NJ, Zip 08050; tel. 609/978–8910; Steven G. Littleson, President and Chief Executive Officer

ST. FRANCIS MEDICAL CENTER, 601 Hamilton Avenue, Trenton, NJ, Zip 08629–1986; tel. 609/599–5000; Judith M. Persichilli, President and Chief Executive Officer

Section B

ST. JOSEPH'S HOSPITAL AND MEDICAL CENTER, 703 Main Street, Paterson, NJ, Zip 07503–2691; tel. 201/754–2100; Sister Jane Frances Brady, Chief Executive Officer

ST. PETER'S MEDICAL CENTER, 254 Easton Avenue, New Brunswick, NJ, Zip 08901, Mailing Address: P.O. Box 591, Zip 08903–0591; tel. 908/745–8600; John E. Matuska, President and Chief Executive Officer

UNDERWOOD–MEMORIAL HOSPITAL, 509 North Broad Street, Woodbury, NJ, Zip 08096–7359, Mailing Address: P.O. Box 359, Zip 08096; tel. 609/845–0100; Steven W. Jackmuff, President and Chief Executive Officer

UNION HOSPITAL, 1000 Galloping Hill Road, Union, NJ, Zip 07083–1652; tel. 908/687–1900; Kathryn W. Coyne, Executive Director and Chief Operating Officer

VALLEY HOSPITAL, 223 North Van Dien Avenue, Ridgewood, NJ, Zip 07450–9982; tel. 201/447–8000; Michael W. Azzara, President

WEST HUDSON HOSPITAL, 206 Bergen Avenue, Kearny, NJ, Zip 07032; tel. 201/955–7051; Carmen Bruce Alecci, Executive Director

WEST JERSEY HOSPITAL–BERLIN, 100 Townsend Avenue, Berlin, NJ, Zip 08009; tel. 609/768–6006; Ellen Guarnieri, Acting Executive Director

WEST JERSEY HOSPITAL–CAMDEN, 1000 Atlantic Avenue, Camden, NJ, Zip 08104–1595; tel. 609/342–4000; Frederick M. Carey, Executive Director

WEST JERSEY HOSPITAL–MARLTON, Route 73 and Brick Road, Marlton, NJ, Zip 08053; tel. 609/596–3500; Leroy J. Rosenberg, Executive Director

WEST JERSEY HOSPITAL–VOORHEES, 101 Carnie Boulevard, Voorhees, NJ, Zip 08043–1597; tel. 609/772–5000; Joan T. Meyers, R.N., Executive Director

WILLIAM B. KESSLER MEMORIAL HOSPITAL, 600 South White Horse Pike, Hammonton, NJ, Zip 08037–2099; tel. 609/561–6700; Warren E. Gager, Chief Executive Officer

GENERAL HOSPITAL CENTER AT PASSAIC, 350 Boulevard, Passaic, NJ 07055; tel. 201/365–4300; Daniel L. Marcantuono, President & Chief Executive Officer

GENERAL HOSPITAL CENTER AT PASSAIC, 350 Boulevard, Passaic, NJ, Zip 07055–2800; tel. 201/365–4300; Daniel L. Marcantuono, FACHE, President and Chief Executive Officer

QUALCARE PREFERRED PROVIDERS 242 Old Brunswick Road, Piscataway, NJ 08854; tel. 908/562–2800; Concetta Klucsik, Director of Marketing

BAYONNE HOSPITAL, 29th Street at Avenue E, Bayonne, NJ, Zip 07002; tel. 201/858–5000; Michael R. D'Agnes, President and Chief Executive Officer

BETH ISRAEL HOSPITAL, 70 Parker Avenue, Passaic, NJ, Zip 07055; tel. 201/365–5000; Jeffrey S. Moll, President and Chief Executive Officer

CARRIER FOUNDATION, County Route 601, P.O. Box 147, Belle Mead, NJ, Zip 08502; tel. 908/281–1000; C. Richard Sarle, President and Chief Executive Officer

CENTRASTATE MEDICAL CENTER, 901 West Main Street, Freehold, NJ, Zip 07728–2549; tel. 908/431–2000; Thomas H. Litz, President and Chief Executive Officer

CHILDREN'S SPECIALIZED HOSPITAL, 150 New Providence Road, Mountainside, NJ, Zip 07091–2590; tel. 908/233–3720; Richard B. Ahlfeld, President

COLUMBUS HOSPITAL, 495 North 13th Street, Newark, NJ, Zip 07107–1397; tel. 201/268–1400; John G. Magliaro, President and Chief Executive Officer

COMMUNITY KIMBALL HEALTH CARE SYSTEM, 99 Highway 37 West, Toms River, NJ, Zip 08755–6423; tel. 908/240–8000; Kevin R. Burchill, Executive Director

ELIZABETH GENERAL MEDICAL CENTER, 925 East Jersey Street, Elizabeth, NJ, Zip 07201–2728; tel. 908/629–8065; David A. Fletcher, President and Chief Executive Officer

HACKENSACK UNIVERSITY MEDICAL CENTER, 30 Prospect Avenue, Hackensack, NJ, Zip 07601–1991; tel. 201/996–2000; John P. Ferguson, President and Chief Executive Officer

HELENE FULD MEDICAL CENTER, 750 Brunswick Avenue, Trenton, NJ, Zip 08638; tel. 609/394–6000; Al Maghazehe, President and Chief Executive Officer

HOLY NAME HOSPITAL, 718 Teaneck Road, Teaneck, NJ, Zip 07666; tel. 201/833–3000; Michael Maron, President and Chief Executive Officer

HOSPITAL CENTER AT ORANGE, 188 South Essex Avenue, Orange, NJ, Zip 07051; tel. 201/266–2200; Paul A. Mertz, President and Chief Executive Officer

HUNTERDON MEDICAL CENTER, 2100 Wescott Drive, Flemington, NJ, Zip 08822–4604; tel. 908/788–6100; Robert P. Wise, President and Chief Executive Officer

IRVINGTON GENERAL HOSPITAL, 832 Chancellor Avenue, Irvington, NJ, Zip 07111–0709; tel. 201/399–6000; Thomas A. Biga, Executive Director

KESSLER INSTITUTE FOR REHABILITATION, 1199 Pleasant Valley Way, West Orange, NJ, Zip 07052–1419; tel. 201/731–3600; Kenneth W. Aitchison, President and Chief Executive Officer

KIMBALL MEDICAL CENTER, 600 River Avenue, Lakewood, NJ, Zip 08701–5281; tel. 908/363–1900; Joanne Carrocino, Executive Director

MEDICAL CENTER OF OCEAN COUNTY, 2121 Edgewater Place, Point Pleasant, NJ, Zip 08742–2290; tel. 908/892–1100; John T. Gribbin, President and Chief Executive Officer

MEMORIAL HOSPITAL OF BURLINGTON COUNTY, 175 Madison Avenue, Mount Holly, NJ, Zip 08060–2099; tel. 609/267–0700; Chester B. Kaletkowski, President and Chief Executive Officer

MEMORIAL HOSPITAL OF SALEM COUNTY, Salem Woodstown Road, Salem, NJ, Zip 08079–2080; tel. 609/935–1000; Arnold Kimmel, Interim Chief Executive Officer

MERIDIAN HEALTH SYSTEM, 1945 State Highway 33, Neptune, NJ, Zip 07753; tel. 908/776–4215; John K. Lloyd, Chief Executive Officer

MONMOUTH MEDICAL CENTER, 300 Second Avenue, Long Branch, NJ, Zip 07740–6303; tel. 908/222–5200; Cynthia N. Sparer, Executive Director and Chief Operating Officer

MORRISTOWN MEMORIAL HOSPITAL, 100 Madison Avenue, Morristown, NJ, Zip 07962–1956; tel. 201/971–5000; Jean M. McMahon, R.N., Vice President and General Manager

MOUNTAINSIDE HOSPITAL, Bay and Highland Avenues, Montclair, NJ, Zip 07042–4898; tel. 201/429–6000; Robert A. Silver, Senior Vice President and General Manager

NEWARK BETH ISRAEL MEDICAL CENTER, 201 Lyons Avenue, Newark, NJ, Zip 07112–2027; tel. 201/926–7000; Ronald W. Weitz, Executive Director

NORTHWEST COVENANT MEDICAL CENTER, 25 Pocono Road, Denville, NJ, Zip 07834–2995; tel. 201/625–6000; Joseph A. Trunfio, President and Chief Executive Officer

OVERLOOK HOSPITAL, 99 Beauvoir Avenue, Summit, NJ, Zip 07902–0220; tel. 908/522–2000; David H. Freed, Vice President and General Manager

PALISADES GENERAL HOSPITAL, 7600 River Road, North Bergen, NJ, Zip 07047–6217; tel. 201/854–5000; Bruce J. Markowitz, President and Chief Executive Officer

PASCACK VALLEY HOSPITAL, Old Hook Road, Westwood, NJ, Zip 07675–3181; tel. 201/358–3000; Louis R. Ycre, Jr., President and Chief Executive Officer

RAHWAY HOSPITAL, 865 Stone Street, Rahway, NJ, Zip 07065; tel. 908/381–4200; Kirk C. Tice, President and Chief Executive Officer

RARITAN BAY MEDICAL CENTER, 530 New Brunswick Avenue, Perth Amboy, NJ, Zip 08861; tel. 908/442–3700; Keith H. McLaughlin, President and Chief Executive Officer

RIVERVIEW MEDICAL CENTER, 1 Riverview Plaza, Red Bank, NJ, Zip 07701–9982; tel. 908/741–2700; Paul S. Cohen, Executive Director and Chief Operating Officer

ROBERT WOOD JOHNSON UNIVERSITY HOSPITAL, 1 Robert Wood Johnson Place, New Brunswick, NJ, Zip 08903–2601; tel. 908/828–3000; Harvey A. Holzberg, President and Chief Executive Officer

ROBERT WOOD JOHNSON UNIVERSITY HOSPITAL AT HAMILTON, One Hamilton Health Place, Hamilton, NJ, Zip 08690; tel. 609/586–7900; W. Michael Bryant, President and Chief Executive Officer

SAINT BARNABAS MEDICAL CENTER, 94 Old Short Hills Road, Livingston, NJ, Zip 07039; tel. 201/533–5000; Ronald Del Mauro, Chairman and Chief Executive Officer

SHORE MEMORIAL HOSPITAL, 1 East New York Avenue, Somers Point, NJ, Zip 08244–2387; tel. 609/653–3500; Richard A. Pitman, President

SOMERSET MEDICAL CENTER, 110 Rehill Avenue, Somerville, NJ, Zip 08876–2598; tel. 908/685–2200; Michael A. Turner, President and Chief Executive Officer

SOUTH JERSEY HOSPITAL, 333 Irving Avenue, Bridgeton, NJ, Zip 08302–2100; tel. 609/451–6600; Paul S. Cooper, Chief Executive Officer

SOUTHERN OCEAN COUNTY HOSPITAL, 1140 Route 72 West, Manahawkin, NJ, Zip 08050; tel. 609/978–8910; Steven G. Littleson, President and Chief Executive Officer

ST. FRANCIS HOSPITAL, 25 McWilliams Place, Jersey City, NJ, Zip 07302–1698; tel. 201/418–1000; Robert S. Chaloner, President and Chief Executive Officer

ST. JOSEPH'S HOSPITAL AND MEDICAL CENTER, 703 Main Street, Paterson, NJ, Zip 07503–2691; tel. 201/754–2100; Sister Jane Frances Brady, Chief Executive Officer

ST. LAWRENCE REHABILITATION CENTER, 2381 Lawrenceville Road, Lawrenceville, NJ, Zip 08648; tel. 609/896–9500; Charles L. Brennan, Chief Executive Officer

ST. MARY HOSPITAL, 308 Willow Avenue, Hoboken, NJ, Zip 07030–3889; tel. 201/418–1000; Robert S. Chaloner, President and Chief Executive Officer

ST. PETER'S MEDICAL CENTER, 254 Easton Avenue, New Brunswick, NJ, Zip 08901, Mailing Address: P.O. Box 591, Zip 08903–0591; tel. 908/745–8600; John E. Matuska, President and Chief Executive Officer

THE COOPER HEALTH SYSTEM, One Cooper Plaza, Camden, NJ, Zip 08103–1489; tel. 609/342–2000; Kevin G. Halpern, President and Chief Executive Officer

UNDERWOOD–MEMORIAL HOSPITAL, 509 North Broad Street, Woodbury, NJ, Zip 08096–7359, Mailing Address: P.O. Box 359, Zip 08096; tel. 609/845–0100; Steven W. Jackmuff, President and Chief Executive Officer

UNION HOSPITAL, 1000 Galloping Hill Road, Union, NJ, Zip 07083–1652; tel. 908/687–1900; Kathryn W. Coyne, Executive Director and Chief Operating Officer

UNIVERSITY OF MEDICINE AND DENTISTRY OF NEW JERSEY–UNIVERSITY HOSPITAL, 150 Bergen Street, Newark, NJ, Zip 07103–2406; tel. 201/982–4300; William L. Vazquez, Vice President and Chief Executive Officer

WARREN HOSPITAL, 185 Roseberry Street, Phillipsburg, NJ, Zip 08865–9955; tel. 908/859–6700; Jeffrey C. Goodwin, President and Chief Executive Officer

WAYNE GENERAL HOSPITAL, 224 Hamburg Turnpike, Wayne, NJ, Zip 07470–2100; tel. 201/942–6900; Kenneth H. Kozloff, Executive Director

WEST JERSEY HOSPITAL–CAMDEN, 1000 Atlantic Avenue, Camden, NJ, Zip 08104–1595; tel. 609/342–4000; Frederick M. Carey, Executive Director

WEST JERSEY HOSPITAL–MARLTON, Route 73 and
Brick Road, Marlton, NJ, Zip 08053;
tel. 609/596–3500; Leroy J. Rosenberg,
Executive Director

WEST JERSEY HOSPITAL–VOORHEES, 101 Carnie
Boulevard, Voorhees, NJ, Zip 08043–1597;
tel. 609/772–5000; Joan T. Meyers, R.N.,
Executive Director

SETON HEALTH NETWORK, INC.
703 Main Street, Paterson, NJ 07503;
tel. 201/754–2790; Anthony Losardo, M.D.,
President

ST. JOSEPH'S HOSPITAL AND MEDICAL CENTER, 703
Main Street, Paterson, NJ, Zip 07503–2691;
tel. 201/754–2100; Sister Jane Frances Brady,
Chief Executive Officer

VIA CARITAS HEALTH SYSTEM, INC.
57 Willowbrook Boulevard, Suite 205, Wayne,
NJ 07470; tel. 201/625–6505; Joseph A.
Trunfio, Ph.D, President

NORTHWEST COVENANT MEDICAL CENTER, 25
Pocono Road, Denville, NJ, Zip 07834–2995;
tel. 201/625–6000; Joseph A. Trunfio, President
and Chief Executive Officer

ST. JOSEPH'S HOSPITAL AND MEDICAL CENTER, 703
Main Street, Paterson, NJ, Zip 07503–2691;
tel. 201/754–2100; Sister Jane Frances Brady,
Chief Executive Officer

ST. MARY'S HOSPITAL, 211 Pennington Avenue,
Passaic, NJ, Zip 07055; tel. 201/470–3000;
Patricia Peterson, President and Chief Executive
Officer

NEW MEXICO

LOVELACE
5400 Gibson Boulevard, SouthEast,
Albuquerque, NM 87108; tel. 505/262–7000;
John Lucas, M.D., Chief Executive Officer

LOVELACE HEALTH SYSTEM, 5400 Gibson Boulevard
S.E., Albuquerque, NM, Zip 87108;
tel. 505/262–7000; Rick Doxtator, Chief
Administrative Officer

MEDICAL NETWORK OF NEW MEXICO
7850 Jefferson, Northeast, Albuquerque, NM
87109; tel. 505/727–8076; Marian Lowe,
Executive Director

ST. JOSEPH MEDICAL CENTER, 601 Martin Luther
King Drive N.E., Albuquerque, NM, Zip 87102,
Mailing Address: P.O. Box 25555,
Zip 87125–0555; tel. 505/727–8000; Charles
A. Ivy, Vice President

ST. JOSEPH NORTHEAST HEIGHTS HOSPITAL, 4701
Montgomery N.E., Albuquerque, NM, Zip 87109,
Mailing Address: P.O. Box 25555,
Zip 87125–0555; tel. 505/727–7800; C.
Vincent Townsend, Jr., Vice President,
Operations

ST. JOSEPH REHABILITATION HOSPITAL AND
OUTPATIENT CENTER, 505 Elm Street N.E.,
Albuquerque, NM, Zip 87102, Mailing Address:
P.O. Box 25555, Zip 87125–2500;
tel. 505/727–4700; Mary Lou Coors,
Administrator

ST. JOSEPH WEST MESA HOSPITAL, 10501 Golf
Course Road N.W., Albuquerque, NM,
Zip 87114, Mailing Address: P.O. Box 25555,
Zip 87125–0555; tel. 505/893–2003; C.
Vincent Townsend, Jr., Vice President,
Operations

PRESBYTERIAN HEALTHCARE SERVICES, INC.
P.O. Box 27489, Albuquerque, NM
87125–7489; tel. 505/923–5280; Kim
Hedrick, Director–Network Provider Services

PRESBYTERIAN HOSPITAL, 1100 Central Avenue S.E.,
Albuquerque, NM, Zip 87106, Mailing Address:
P.O. Box 26666, Zip 87125–6666;
tel. 505/841–1234; William Fitzpatrick, M.D.,
Senior Vice President and Chief Operating Officer

PRESBYTERIAN KASEMAN HOSPITAL, 8300
Constitution Avenue N.E., Albuquerque, NM,
Zip 87110, Mailing Address: P.O. Box 26666,
Zip 87125–6666; tel. 505/291–2000; Jim
Purdy, Administrative Director

UNIVERSITY OF NEW MEXICO HEALTH SCIENCE
CENTER
2211 Lomas Boulevard, NorthEast,
Albuquerque, NM 87106; tel. 505/843–2121;
William H. Johnson, Chief Executive

UNIVERSITY HOSPITAL, 2211 Lomas Boulevard N.E.,
Albuquerque, NM, Zip 87106;
tel. 505/272–2121; Stephen McKernan, Chief
Executive Officer

UNIVERSITY OF NEW MEXICO MENTAL HEALTH
CENTER, 2600 Marble N.E., Albuquerque, NM,
Zip 87131–2600; tel. 505/272–2870; Christina
B. Gunn, Chief Executive Officer

NEW YORK

ADIRONDACK RURAL HEALTH NETWORK
100 Park Street, Glens Falls, NY 12801;
tel. 518/792–3151; David Kruczlnicki,
President

GLENS FALLS HOSPITAL, 100 Park Street, Glens
Falls, NY, Zip 12801–9898; tel. 518/792–3151;
David G. Kruczlnicki, President and Chief
Executive Officer

MOSES LUDINGTON HOSPITAL, Wicker Street,
Ticonderoga, NY, Zip 12883–1097;
tel. 518/585–2831; Diane M. Hart, Chief
Executive Officer

ALLEGANY COUNTY HEALTH CARE NETWORK
191 North Main Street, Wellsville, NY 14895;
tel. 716/593–1100; William M. DiBerardino,
President & Chief Executive Officer

JONES MEMORIAL HOSPITAL, 191 North Main Street,
Wellsville, NY, Zip 14895, Mailing Address: P.O.
Box 72, Zip 14895; tel. 716/593–1100; William
M. DiBerardino, FACHE, President and Chief
Executive Officer

BASSETT HEALTHCARE
1 Atwell Road, Cooperstown, NY 13326;
tel. 607/547–3100; William F. Streck, M.D.,
President

MARY IMOGENE BASSETT HOSPITAL, One Atwell
Road, Cooperstown, NY, Zip 13326–1394;
tel. 607/547–3100; William F. Streck, M.D.,
President and Chief Executive Officer

BUFFALO GENERAL HEALTH SYSTEM
100 High Street, Buffalo, NY 14203;
tel. 716/845–2732; John L. Friedlander,
President & Chief Executive Officer

BUFFALO GENERAL HOSPITAL, 100 High Street,
Buffalo, NY, Zip 14203–1154;
tel. 716/859–5600; Carrie B. Frank, President
and Chief Executive Officer

DE GRAFF MEMORIAL HOSPITAL, 445 Tremont
Street, North Tonawanda, NY, Zip 14120–0750,
Mailing Address: P.O. Box 25555,
Zip 14120–0750; tel. 716/694–4500; Thomas
F. Schifferli, President and Chief Executive
Officer

TRI–COUNTY MEMORIAL HOSPITAL, 100 Memorial
Drive, Gowanda, NY, Zip 14070–1194;
tel. 716/532–3377; Diane J. Osika, Interim Chief
Executive Officer

CATHOLIC HEALTH CARE NETWORK
75 Vanderbilt Avenue, Staten Island, NY
10304; tel. 718/390–5080; John DePierro,
President & Chief Executive Officer

BAYLEY SETON HOSPITAL, 75 Vanderbilt Avenue,
Staten Island, NY, Zip 10304–3850;
tel. 718/354–6000; Dominick M. Stanzione,
Chief Operating Officer and Executive Vice
President

CALVARY HOSPITAL, 1740 Eastchester Road, Bronx,
NY, Zip 10461–2392; tel. 718/863–6900;
Frank A. Calamari, President and Chief Executive
Officer

OUR LADY OF MERCY MEDICAL CENTER, 600 East
233rd Street, Bronx, NY, Zip 10466;
tel. 718/920–9000; Gary S. Horan, FACHE,
President and Chief Executive Officer

SAINT VINCENT'S HOSPITAL AND MEDICAL CENTER
OF NEW YORK, 153 West 11th Street, New
York, NY, Zip 10011–8397; tel. 212/604–7000;
Karl P. Adler, M.D., President and Chief
Executive Officer

ST. AGNES HOSPITAL, 305 North Street, White
Plains, NY, Zip 10605; tel. 914/681–4500; Gary
S. Horan, FACHE, President and Chief Executive
Officer

ST. CLARE'S HOSPITAL AND HEALTH CENTER, 415
West 51st Street, New York, NY, Zip 10019;
tel. 212/586–1500; Richard N. Yezzo, President

ST. JOSEPH'S MEDICAL CENTER, 127 South
Broadway, Yonkers, NY, Zip 10701–4080;
tel. 914/378–7000; Sister Mary Linehan,
President

ST. VINCENT'S MEDICAL CENTER OF RICHMOND,
355 Bard Avenue, Staten Island, NY,
Zip 10310–1699; tel. 718/876–1234; Dominick
M. Stanzione, Executive Vice President

CHENANGO COUNTY RURAL HEALTH NETWORK
179 North Broad Street, Norwich, NY 13815;
tel. 607/335–4111; Frank W. Mirabito,
President

CHENANGO MEMORIAL HOSPITAL, 179 North Broad
Street, Norwich, NY, Zip 13815;
tel. 607/337–4111; Frank W. Mirabito, President

COLUMBIA PRESBYTERIAN REGIONAL NETWORK
161 Fort Washington Avenue, 14th FL, New
York, NY 10032–3784; tel. 212/305–2500;
Marc H. Lory, Executive Vice President & COO

CORNWALL HOSPITAL, Laurel Avenue, Cornwall, NY,
Zip 12518–1499; tel. 914/534–7711; Val S.
Gray, Executive Director

HELEN HAYES HOSPITAL, Route 9W, West
Haverstraw, NY, Zip 10993–1195;
tel. 914/947–3000; Magdalena Ramirez,
Director

HOLY NAME HOSPITAL, 718 Teaneck Road, Teaneck,
NJ, Zip 07666; tel. 201/833–3000; Michael
Maron, President and Chief Executive Officer

HORTON MEDICAL CENTER, 60 Prospect Avenue,
Middletown, NY, Zip 10940–4133;
tel. 914/343–2424; Paul Dell Uomo, President
and Chief Executive Officer

LAWRENCE HOSPITAL, 55 Palmer Avenue, Bronxville,
NY, Zip 10708–3491; tel. 914/787–1000;
Roger G. Dvorak, President

NEW MILFORD HOSPITAL, 21 Elm Street, New
Milford, CT, Zip 06776–2993;
tel. 860/355–2611; Richard E. Pugh, President
and Chief Executive Officer

NYACK HOSPITAL, North Midland Avenue, Nyack, NY,
Zip 10960–1998; tel. 914/348–2000; Greger
C. Anderson, President and Chief Executive
Officer

PALISADES GENERAL HOSPITAL, 7600 River Road,
North Bergen, NJ, Zip 07047–6217;
tel. 201/854–5000; Bruce J. Markowitz,
President and Chief Executive Officer

ST. FRANCIS HOSPITAL, 100 Port Washington
Boulevard, Roslyn, NY, Zip 11576–1348;
tel. 516/562–6000; Patrick J. Scollard,
President and Chief Executive Officer

ST. LUKE'S HOSPITAL, 70 Dubois Street, Newburgh,
NY, Zip 12550–4898, Mailing Address: P.O. Box
631, Zip 12550; tel. 914/561–4400; Laurence
E. Kelly, Senior Vice President

VALLEY HOSPITAL, 223 North Van Dien Avenue,
Ridgewood, NJ, Zip 07450–9982;
tel. 201/447–8000; Michael W. Azzara,
President

WHITE PLAINS HOSPITAL CENTER, Davis Avenue at
East Post Road, White Plains, NY,
Zip 10601–4699; tel. 914/681–0600; Jon B.
Schandler, President and Chief Executive Officer

CORTLAND AREA RURAL HEALTH NETWORK
134 Homer Avenue, Cortland, NY 13045;
tel. 607/756–3500; Thomas H. Carman,
President & Chief Executive Officer

CORTLAND MEMORIAL HOSPITAL, 134 Homer
Avenue, Cortland, NY, Zip 13045–0960;
tel. 607/756–3500; Thomas H. Carman,
President and Chief Executive Officer

EASTERN ADIRONDACK HEALTH CARE NETWORK
P.O. Box 466, Westport, NY 12993;
tel. 518/962–2313; Lynn Edmonds, Network
Coordinator

Section B

CHAMPLAIN VALLEY PHYSICIANS HOSPITAL MEDICAL CENTER, 75 Beekman Street, Plattsburgh, NY, Zip 12901–1493; tel. 518/561–2000; Kevin J. Carroll, President

ELIZABETHTOWN COMMUNITY HOSPITAL, Park Street, Elizabethtown, NY, Zip 12932–0277; tel. 518/873–6377; Anthony W. Deobil, Administrator

EPISCOPAL HEALTH SERVICES, INC.
333 Earle Ovington Boulevard, Uniondale, NY 11787; tel. 516/228–6100; Jack Farrington, Ph.d, Executive Director

ST. JOHN'S EPISCOPAL HOSPITAL–SMITHTOWN, 50 Route 25–A, Smithtown, NY, Zip 11787–1398; tel. 516/862–3000; Laura Righter, Regional Administrator

ST. JOHN'S EPISCOPAL HOSPITAL–SOUTH SHORE, 327 Beach 19th Street, Far Rockaway, NY, Zip 11691–4424; tel. 718/869–7000; Paul J. Connor, III, Administrator

FIRST CHOICE NETWORK, INC.
288 Old Country Road, Mineola, NY 11501; tel. 516/663–8536; Thomas McCabe, Marketing Director

EASTERN LONG ISLAND HOSPITAL, 201 Manor Place, Greenport, NY, Zip 11944–1298; tel. 516/477–1000; John M. Gwiazda, President and Chief Executive Officer

SOUTHAMPTON HOSPITAL, 240 Meeting House Lane, Southampton, NY, Zip 11968–5090; tel. 516/726–8555; John J. Ferry, Jr., M.D., President and Chief Executive Officer

SOUTHSIDE HOSPITAL, 301 East Main Street, Bay Shore, NY, Zip 11706–8458; tel. 516/968–3000; Theodore A. Jospe, President

ST. CHARLES HOSPITAL AND REHABILITATION CENTER, 200 Belle Terre Road, Port Jefferson, NY, Zip 11777; tel. 516/474–6000; Barry T. Zeman, President and Chief Executive Officer

ST. JOHN'S EPISCOPAL HOSPITAL–SMITHTOWN, 50 Route 25–A, Smithtown, NY, Zip 11787–1398; tel. 516/862–3000; Laura Righter, Regional Administrator

ST. JOHN'S EPISCOPAL HOSPITAL–SOUTH SHORE, 327 Beach 19th Street, Far Rockaway, NY, Zip 11691–4424; tel. 718/869–7000; Paul J. Connor, III, Administrator

WINTHROP–UNIVERSITY HOSPITAL, 259 First Street, Mineola, NY 11501; tel. 516/663–2200; Martin J. Delaney, President and Chief Executive Officer

FOUR LAKES RURAL HEALTH NETWORK
196 North Street, Geneva, NY 14456; tel. 315/787–4000; James J. Dooley, President & Chief Executive Officer

GENEVA GENERAL HOSPITAL, 196 North Street, Geneva, NY, Zip 14456–1694; tel. 315/787–4000; James J. Dooley, President

SOLDIERS AND SAILORS MEMORIAL HOSPITAL OF YATES COUNTY, 418 North Main Street, Penn Yan, NY, Zip 14527–1085; tel. 315/536–4431; Norman Lindenmuth, M.D., Interim Chief Executive Officer

GREATER METROPOLITAN HEALTH SYSTEM
First Avenue at East 16th Street, New York, NY 10003; tel. 212/420–2873; Robert G. Newman, M.D., President & Chief Executive Officer

BETH ISRAEL MEDICAL CENTER, First Avenue and 16th Street, New York, NY, Zip 10003–3803; tel. 212/420–2000; Robert G. Newman, M.D., President

KINGS HIGHWAY HOSPITAL CENTER, 3201 Kings Highway, Brooklyn, NY, Zip 11234; tel. 718/252–3000; Samuel Berson, M.D., Executive Director

ST. LUKE'S–ROOSEVELT HOSPITAL CENTER, 1111 Amsterdam Avenue, New York, NY, Zip 10025; tel. 212/523–4295; Ronald C. Ablow, M.D., President and Chief Executive Officer

GREATER ROCHESTER HEALTH SYSTEM, INC.
1040 University Avenue, Rochester, NY 14607; tel. 716/756–4280; Roger S. Hunt, President & CEO

GENESEE HOSPITAL, 224 Alexander Street, Rochester, NY, Zip 14607–4055; tel. 716/263–6000; Joseph J. DeSilva, FACHE, President and Chief Executive Officer

NEWARK–WAYNE COMMUNITY HOSPITAL, Driving Park Avenue, Newark, NY, Zip 14513, Mailing Address: P.O. Box 111, Zip 14513–0111; tel. 315/332–2022; William R. Holman, President

ROCHESTER GENERAL HOSPITAL, 1425 Portland Avenue, Rochester, NY, Zip 14621–3099; tel. 716/338–4000; Richard S. Constantino, M.D., President

GREENE COUNTY RURAL HEALTH NETWORK
71 Prospect Avenue, Catskill, NY 12534; tel. 518/828–7601; Andrew E. Toga, Acting Chief Executive Officer

ALBANY MEDICAL CENTER, 43 New Scotland Avenue, Albany, NY, Zip 12208; tel. 518/262–3125; Thomas G. Foggo, Executive Vice President Care Delivery and General Director

COLUMBIA MEMORIAL HOSPITAL, 71 Prospect Avenue, Hudson, NY, Zip 12534; tel. 518/828–8244; Jane Ehrlich, President and Chief Executive Officer

HAMILTON–BASSETT–CROUSE RURAL HEALTH NETWORK
150 Broad Street, Hamilton, NY 13346; tel. 315/824–6080; David W. Felton, Chief Executive Officer

COMMUNITY MEMORIAL HOSPITAL, Broad Street, Hamilton, NY, Zip 13346–9518; tel. 315/824–1100; David Felton, Administrator

CROUSE HOSPITAL, 736 Irving Avenue, Syracuse, NY, Zip 13210–1690; tel. 315/470–7111; Edward T. Wenzke, President and Chief Executive Officer

HEALTH FIRST
555 West 57th Street, Suite 1520, New York, NY 10019; tel. 212/801–1500; Paul Dickstein, Network Contact

BETH ISRAEL MEDICAL CENTER, First Avenue and 16th Street, New York, NY, Zip 10003–3803; tel. 212/420–2000; Robert G. Newman, M.D., President

BRONX–LEBANON HOSPITAL CENTER, 1276 Fulton Avenue, Bronx, NY, Zip 10456; tel. 718/590–1800; Miguel A. Fuentes, President and Chief Executive Officer

BROOKLYN HOSPITAL CENTER, 121 DeKalb Avenue, Brooklyn, NY, Zip 11201–5493; tel. 718/250–8005; Frederick D. Alley, President and Chief Executive Officer

BRUNSWICK GENERAL HOSPITAL, 366 Broadway, Amityville, NY, Zip 11701–9820; tel. 516/789–7000; Benjamin M. Stein, M.D., President

INTERFAITH MEDICAL CENTER, 555 Prospect Place, Brooklyn, NY, Zip 11238–4299; tel. 718/935–7000; Corbett A. Price, Chief Executive Officer

JAMAICA HOSPITAL MEDICAL CENTER, 8900 Van Wyck Expressway, Jamaica, NY, Zip 11418–2832; tel. 718/206–6000; David P. Rosen, President

KINGSBROOK JEWISH MEDICAL CENTER, 585 Schenectady Avenue, Brooklyn, NY, Zip 11203–1891; tel. 718/604–5000; Milton M. Gutman, Chief Executive Officer

MAIMONIDES MEDICAL CENTER, 4802 Tenth Avenue, Brooklyn, NY, Zip 11219–2916; tel. 718/283–6000; Stanley Brezenoff, President

MONTEFIORE MEDICAL CENTER, 111 East 210th Street, Bronx, NY, Zip 10467–2490; tel. 718/920–4321; Spencer Foreman, M.D., President

MOUNT SINAI MEDICAL CENTER, One Gustave L. Levy Place, New York, NY, Zip 10029–6574; tel. 212/241–8888; John W. Rowe, M.D., President

NASSAU COUNTY MEDICAL CENTER, 2201 Hempstead Turnpike, East Meadow, NY, Zip 11554–1854; tel. 516/572–0123; Joseph R. Erazo, Chief Executive Officer

NEW YORK UNIVERSITY MEDICAL CENTER, 550 First Avenue, New York, NY, Zip 10016–4576; tel. 212/263–7300; Theresa A. Bischoff, Deputy Provost and Executive Vice President

STATEN ISLAND UNIVERSITY HOSPITAL, 475 Seaview Avenue, Staten Island, NY, Zip 10305–9998; tel. 718/226–9000; Rick J. Varone, President

UNIVERSITY HOSPITAL, State University of New York, Stony Brook, NY, Zip 11794–8410; tel. 516/689–8333; Michael A. Maffetone, Director and Chief Executive Officer

UNIVERSITY HOSPITAL OF BROOKLYN–STATE UNIVERSITY OF NEW YORK HEALTH SCIENCE CENTER AT BROOKLYN, 445 Lenox Road, Brooklyn, NY, Zip 11203–2098; tel. 718/270–2404; Percy Allen, II, FACHE, Vice President Hospital Affairs and Chief Executive Officer

HEALTHSTAR NETWORK
1 North Greenwich Road, Armonk, NY 10504; tel. 914/273–5454; Kevin G. Murphy, Vice President & Chief Financial Officer

LAWRENCE HOSPITAL, 55 Palmer Avenue, Bronxville, NY, Zip 10708–3491; tel. 914/787–1000; Roger G. Dvorak, President

NORTHERN WESTCHESTER HOSPITAL CENTER, 400 Main Street, Mount Kisco, NY, Zip 10549; tel. 914/666–1200; Donald W. Davis, President

PUTNAM HOSPITAL CENTER, Stoneleigh Avenue, Carmel, NY, Zip 10512–9948; tel. 914/279–5711; Rodney N. Hubbers, President and Chief Executive Officer

WHITE PLAINS HOSPITAL CENTER, Davis Avenue at East Post Road, White Plains, NY, Zip 10601–4699; tel. 914/681–0600; Jon B. Schandler, President and Chief Executive Officer

LAKE ONTARIO RURAL HEALTH NETWORK
200 Ohio Street, Medina, NY 14103; tel. 716/798–2000; Walter S. Becker, Administrator

LAKESIDE MEMORIAL HOSPITAL, 156 West Avenue, Brockport, NY, Zip 14420–1286; tel. 716/637–3131; Robert W. Harris, President

MEDINA MEMORIAL HOSPITAL, 200 Ohio Street, Medina, NY, Zip 14103; tel. 716/798–2000; Walter S. Becker, Administrator

MERCYCARE CORPORATION
315 South Manning Boulevard, Albany, NY 12208; tel. 518/454–1550; Steven P. Boyle, President

ST. PETER'S HOSPITAL, 315 South Manning Boulevard, Albany, NY, Zip 12208–1789; tel. 518/525–1550; Steven P. Boyle, President and Chief Executive Officer

MILLARD FILLMORE HEALTH SYSTEM
901 Washington Street, Buffalo, NY 14203; tel. 716/843–7308; Jan Fuller, Director of Planning

LAKE SHORE HOSPITAL, 845 Route 5 and 20, Irving, NY, Zip 14081–9716; tel. 716/934–2654; James B. Foster, Chief Executive Officer

MILLARD FILLMORE HEALTH SYSTEM, 3 Gates Circle, Buffalo, NY, Zip 14209–9986; tel. 716/887–4600; Carol M. Cassell, Executive Vice President and Chief Operating Officer

MOHAWK VALLEY NETWORK, INC.
P.O. Box 5068, Utica, NY 13502–5068; tel. 315/798–6386; Fred Asforth, Network Vice President

FAXTON HOSPITAL, 1676 Sunset Avenue, Utica, NY, Zip 13502; tel. 315/738–6200; Keith A. Fenstemacher, President and Chief Executive Officer

ST. LUKE'S MEMORIAL HOSPITAL CENTER, Utica, NY, Mailing Address: P.O. Box 479, Zip 13503–0479; tel. 315/798–6000; Andrew E. Peterson, President and Chief Executive Officer

NORTH SHORE REGIONAL HEALTH SYSTEMS
300 Community Drive, Manhasset, NY 11030; tel. 516/562–0100; John Gallagher, President

FRANKLIN HOSPITAL MEDICAL CENTER, 900 Franklin Avenue, Valley Stream, NY, Zip 11580–2190; tel. 516/256–6000; Albert Dicker, President and Chief Executive Officer

HUNTINGTON HOSPITAL, 270 Park Avenue, Huntington, NY, Zip 11743–2799; tel. 516/351–2200; J. Ronald Gaudreault, President and Chief Executive Officer

NORTH SHORE UNIVERSITY HOSPITAL, 300 Community Drive, Manhasset, NY, Zip 11030; tel. 516/562–0100; John S. T. Gallagher, President

NORTH SHORE UNIVERSITY HOSPITAL AT GLEN COVE, St. Andrews Lane, Glen Cove, NY, Zip 11542; tel. 516/674–7300; Mark R. Stenzler, Vice President Administration

NORTH SHORE UNIVERSITY HOSPITAL AT PLAINVIEW, 888 Old Country Road, Plainview, NY, Zip 11803–4978; tel. 516/681–8900; Glenn Hirsch, Administrator

NORTH SHORE UNIVERSITY HOSPITAL–FOREST HILLS, Flushing, NY, Mailing Address: 102–01 66th Road, Forest Hills, Zip 11375; tel. 718/830–4000; Andrew J. Mitchell, Vice President, Administration

NORTHERN NEW YORK RURAL HEALTH CARE ALLIANCE
200 Woolworth Building, Watertown, NY 13601; tel. 315/786–0565; Janice Charles, Chairman

CARTHAGE AREA HOSPITAL, 1001 West Street, Carthage, NY, Zip 13619–9703; tel. 315/493–1000; Kenn C. Rishel, Administrator and Chief Executive Officer

E. J. NOBLE HOSPITAL SAMARITAN, 19 Fuller Street, Alexandria Bay, NY, Zip 13607; tel. 315/482–2511; William P. Koughan, President

EDWARD JOHN NOBLE HOSPITAL OF GOUVERNEUR, 77 West Barney Street, Gouverneur, NY, Zip 13642; tel. 315/287–1000; Charles P. Conole, FACHE, Administrator

SAMARITAN HOSPITAL, 2215 Burdett Avenue, Troy, NY, Zip 12180; tel. 518/271–3300; Norman E. Dascher, Jr., Chief Operating Officer

NYU MEDICAL CENTER
550 First Avenue, New York, NY 10016; tel. 212/263–5500; John P. Harney, Senior Administrator, Hospital Operation

BROOKLYN HOSPITAL CENTER, 121 DeKalb Avenue, Brooklyn, NY, Zip 11201–5493; tel. 718/250–8005; Frederick D. Alley, President and Chief Executive Officer

HOSPITAL FOR JOINT DISEASES ORTHOPEDIC INSTITUTE, 301 East 17th Street, New York, NY, Zip 10003–3890; tel. 212/598–6000; John N. Kastanis, FACHE, Chief Executive Officer

JAMAICA HOSPITAL MEDICAL CENTER, 8900 Van Wyck Expressway, Jamaica, NY, Zip 11418–2832; tel. 718/206–6000; David P. Rosen, President

LENOX HILL HOSPITAL, 100 East 77th Street, New York, NY, Zip 10021–1883; tel. 212/434–2000; Gladys George, President and Chief Executive Officer

NEW YORK DOWNTOWN HOSPITAL, 170 William Street, New York, NY, Zip 10038; tel. 212/312–5000; Alan H. Channing, President and Chief Executive Officer

OSWEGO COUNTY RURAL HEALTH NETWORK
110 West Sixth Avenue, Oswego, NY 13126; tel. 315/349–5511; Corte Spencer, Co–Chairman

ALBERT LINDLEY LEE MEMORIAL HOSPITAL, 510 South Fourth Street, Fulton, NY, Zip 13069–2994; tel. 315/592–2224; Dennis A. Casey, Executive Director

OSWEGO HOSPITAL, 110 West Sixth Street, Oswego, NY, Zip 13126–9985; tel. 315/349–5511; Corte J. Spencer, Chief Executive Officer

PARK RIDGE HEALTH SYSTEM
1555 Long Pond Road, Rochester, NY 14626; tel. 716/723–7000; Timothy R. McCormick, President

PARK RIDGE HOSPITAL, 1555 Long Pond Road, Rochester, NY, Zip 14626–4182; tel. 716/723–7000; Timothy R. McCormick, President

PREFERRED HEALTH NETWORK, INC.
45 Avenue & Parsons Boulevard, Flushing, NY 11355; tel. 718/963–7102; Charles J. Pandola, President

FLUSHING HOSPITAL MEDICAL CENTER, 45th Avenue at Parsons Boulevard, Flushing, NY, Zip 11355; tel. 718/670–5000; Charles J. Pendola, President and Chief Executive Officer

WYCKOFF HEIGHTS MEDICAL CENTER, 374 Stockholm Street, Brooklyn, NY, Zip 11237–4099; tel. 718/963–7102; Charles J. Pendola, President

PREMIER PREFERRED CARE
441 Lexington Avenue, New York, NY 10017; tel. 908/205–0100; Jeff Nelson, President

MAIMONIDES MEDICAL CENTER, 4802 Tenth Avenue, Brooklyn, NY, Zip 11219–2916; tel. 718/283–6000; Stanley Brezenoff, President

QUEENS HEALTH NETWORK
79–01 Broadway, Elmhurst, NY 11373; tel. 718/334–4000; Pete Velez, Network Senior Vice President

ELMHURST HOSPITAL CENTER, 79–01 Broadway, Elmhurst, NY, Zip 11373; tel. 718/334–4000; Pete Velez, Executive Director

QUEENS HOSPITAL CENTER, 82–68 164th Street, Jamaica, NY, Zip 11432; tel. 718/883–3000; Gladiola Sampson, Acting Executive Director

SETON HEALTH CARE SYSTEM
1300 Massachusetts Avenue, Troy, NY 12180; tel. 518/270–2520; Edward Murphy, President

SETON HEALTH SYSTEM, 1300 Massachusetts Avenue, Troy, NY, Zip 12180; tel. 518/272–5000; Edward G. Murphy, M.D., President and Chief Executive Officer

SHARED HEALTH NETWORK, INC.
125 Wolf Road, Suite 404, Albany, NY 12205; tel. 518/458–8607; Eugene Stearns, Executive Director

ELLIS HOSPITAL, 1101 Nott Street, Schenectady, NY, Zip 12308–2487; tel. 518/382–4124; G. B. Serrill, President and Chief Executive Officer

GLENS FALLS HOSPITAL, 100 Park Street, Glens Falls, NY, Zip 12801–9898; tel. 518/792–3151; David G. Kruczlnicki, President and Chief Executive Officer

MEMORIAL HOSPITAL, 600 Northern Boulevard, Albany, NY, Zip 12204–1083; tel. 518/471–3221; Bernard Shapiro, Chief Executive Officer

NATHAN LITTAUER HOSPITAL AND NURSING HOME, 99 East State Street, Gloversville, NY, Zip 12078; tel. 518/725–8621; Thomas J. Dowd, President

SAMARITAN HOSPITAL, 2215 Burdett Avenue, Troy, NY, Zip 12180; tel. 518/271–3300; Norman E. Dascher, Jr., Chief Operating Officer

SARATOGA HOSPITAL, 211 Church Street, Saratoga Springs, NY, Zip 12866–1003; tel. 518/587–3222; David Andersen, President and Chief Executive Officer

SETON HEALTH SYSTEM, 1300 Massachusetts Avenue, Troy, NY, Zip 12180; tel. 518/272–5000; Edward G. Murphy, M.D., President and Chief Executive Officer

ST. CLARE'S HOSPITAL OF SCHENECTADY, 600 McClellan Street, Schenectady, NY, Zip 12304; tel. 518/382–2000; Jerome G. Stewart, President

ST. MARY'S HOSPITAL, 427 Guy Park Avenue, Amsterdam, NY, Zip 12010–1095; tel. 518/842–1900; Peter E. Capobianco, President and Chief Executive Officer

ST. PETER'S HOSPITAL, 315 South Manning Boulevard, Albany, NY, Zip 12208–1789; tel. 518/525–1550; Steven P. Boyle, President and Chief Executive Officer

SUNNYVIEW HOSPITAL AND REHABILITATION CENTER, 1270 Belmont Avenue, Schenectady, NY, Zip 12308–2104; tel. 518/382–4500; Bradford M. Goodwin, President

SISTERS OF CHARITY HEALTH CARE SYSTEM
75 Vanderbilt Avenue, Staten Island, NY 10304; tel. 718/390–5080; John J. DePierro, President & Chief Executive Officer

BAYLEY SETON HOSPITAL, 75 Vanderbilt Avenue, Staten Island, NY, Zip 10304–3850; tel. 718/354–6000; Dominick M. Stanzione, Chief Operating Officer and Executive Vice President

ST. VINCENT'S MEDICAL CENTER OF RICHMOND, 355 Bard Avenue, Staten Island, NY, Zip 10310–1699; tel. 718/876–1234; Dominick M. Stanzione, Executive Vice President

SULLIVAN COUNTY RURAL HEALTH NETWORK
Bushville Road, Harris, NY 12742; tel. 914/794–3300; Martin I. Richman, Executive Director

COMMUNITY GENERAL HOSPITAL OF SULLIVAN COUNTY, Bushville Road, Harris, NY, Zip 12742, Mailing Address: P.O. Box 800, Zip 12742–0800; tel. 914/794–3300; Martin I. Richman, Executive Director

THE BROOKLYN HEALTH NETWORK
121 DeKalb Avenue, Brooklyn, NY 11201; tel. 718/250–8000; Fred Alley, President & Chief Executive Officer

BROOKLYN HOSPITAL CENTER, 121 DeKalb Avenue, Brooklyn, NY, Zip 11201–5493; tel. 718/250–8005; Frederick D. Alley, President and Chief Executive Officer

NEW YORK UNIVERSITY MEDICAL CENTER, 550 First Avenue, New York, NY, Zip 10016–4576; tel. 212/263–7300; Theresa A. Bischoff, Deputy Provost and Executive Vice President

THE EXCELCARE SYSTEM, INC.
33 Palmer Avenue, Bronxville, NY 10708; tel. 914/787–3000; Donald S. Broas, President & Chief Executive Officer

HUDSON VALLEY HOSPITAL CENTER, 1980 Crompond Road, Peekskill, NY, Zip 10566–4182; tel. 914/737–9000; John C. Federspiel, President and Chief Executive Officer

LAWRENCE HOSPITAL, 55 Palmer Avenue, Bronxville, NY, Zip 10708–3491; tel. 914/787–1000; Roger G. Dvorak, President

PHELPS MEMORIAL HOSPITAL CENTER, 701 North Broadway, Sleepy Hollow, NY, Zip 10591–1096; tel. 914/366–3000; Keith F. Safian, President and Chief Executive Officer

ST. JOSEPH'S MEDICAL CENTER, 127 South Broadway, Yonkers, NY, Zip 10701–4080; tel. 914/378–7000; Sister Mary Linehan, President

UNITED HOSPITAL MEDICAL CENTER, 406 Boston Post Road, Port Chester, NY, Zip 10573; tel. 914/939–7000; Kevin Dahill, President and Chief Executive Officer

THE MOUNT SINAI HEALTH SYSTEM
One Gustave L. Levy Place, New York, NY 10029; tel. 212/241–2700; Gary Rosenburg, Ph.D., Senior Vice President

ARDEN HILL HOSPITAL, 4 Harriman Drive, Goshen, NY, Zip 10924–2499; tel. 914/294–5441; A. Gordon McAleer, President

BROOKDALE HOSPITAL MEDICAL CENTER, Linden Boulevard at Brookdale Plaza, Brooklyn, NY, Zip 11212–3198; tel. 718/240–5000; Frank J. Maddalena, President and Chief Executive Officer

CABRINI MEDICAL CENTER, 227 East 19th Street, New York, NY, Zip 10003–2600; tel. 212/995–6000; Jeffrey Frerichs, President and Chief Executive Officer

ELMHURST HOSPITAL CENTER, 79–01 Broadway, Elmhurst, NY, Zip 11373; tel. 718/334–4000; Pete Velez, Executive Director

ENGLEWOOD HOSPITAL AND MEDICAL CENTER, 350 Engle Street, Englewood, NJ, Zip 07631; tel. 201/894–3000; Daniel A. Kane, President and Chief Executive Officer

Section B

GREENVILLE HOSPITAL, 1825 Kennedy Boulevard, Jersey City, NJ, Zip 07305; tel. 201/547–6100; Jonathan M. Metsch, Dr.PH, President and Chief Executive Officer

JERSEY CITY MEDICAL CENTER, 50 Baldwin Avenue, Jersey City, NJ, Zip 07304–3199; tel. 201/915–2000; Jonathan M. Metsch, Dr.PH, President and Chief Executive Officer

LONG BEACH MEDICAL CENTER, 455 East Bay Drive, Long Beach, NY, Zip 11561–2300, Mailing Address: P.O. Box 300, Zip 11561–2300; tel. 516/897–1200; Martin F. Nester, Jr., Chief Executive Officer

LONG ISLAND COLLEGE HOSPITAL, 339 Hicks Street, Brooklyn, NY, Zip 11201; tel. 718/780–1000; Donald F. Snell, President and Chief Executive Officer

LUTHERAN MEDICAL CENTER, 150 55th Street, Brooklyn, NY, Zip 11220–2570; tel. 718/630–7000; Joseph P. Cerni, President and Chief Executive Officer

MAIMONIDES MEDICAL CENTER, 4802 Tenth Avenue, Brooklyn, NY, Zip 11219–2916; tel. 718/283–6000; Stanley Brezenoff, President

MEADOWLANDS HOSPITAL MEDICAL CENTER, Meadowland Parkway, Secaucus, NJ, Zip 07096–1580; tel. 201/392–3100; Paul V. Cavalli, M.D., President

MOUNT SINAI MEDICAL CENTER, One Gustave L. Levy Place, New York, NY, Zip 10029–6574; tel. 212/241–8888; John W. Rowe, M.D., President

PARKWAY HOSPITAL, Flushing, NY, Mailing Address: 70–35 113th Street, Zip 11375; tel. 718/990–4100; Paul E. Svensson, Chief Executive Officer

PHELPS MEMORIAL HOSPITAL CENTER, 701 North Broadway, Sleepy Hollow, NY, Zip 10591–1096; tel. 914/366–3000; Keith F. Safian, President and Chief Executive Officer

QUEENS HOSPITAL CENTER, 82–68 164th Street, Jamaica, NY, Zip 11432; tel. 718/883–3000; Gladiola Sampson, Acting Executive Director

SAINT FRANCIS HOSPITAL, North Road, Poughkeepsie, NY, Zip 12601–1399; tel. 914/471–2000; Sister M. Ann Elizabeth, President

ST. BARNABAS HOSPITAL, 183rd Street and Third Avenue, Bronx, NY, Zip 10457–9998; tel. 718/960–9000; Ronald Gade, M.D., President

ST. ELIZABETH HOSPITAL, 225 Williamson Street, Elizabeth, NJ, Zip 07202–3600; tel. 908/527–5122; Sister Elizabeth Ann Maloney, President and Chief Executive Officer

ST. JOHN'S EPISCOPAL HOSPITAL–SMITHTOWN, 50 Route 25–A, Smithtown, NY, Zip 11787–1398; tel. 516/862–3000; Laura Righter, Regional Administrator

ST. JOHN'S EPISCOPAL HOSPITAL–SOUTH SHORE, 327 Beach 19th Street, Far Rockaway, NY, Zip 11691–4424; tel. 718/869–7000; Paul J. Connor, III, Administrator

ST. JOSEPH'S HOSPITAL AND MEDICAL CENTER, 703 Main Street, Paterson, NJ, Zip 07503–2691; tel. 201/754–2100; Sister Jane Frances Brady, Chief Executive Officer

ST. MARY'S HOSPITAL, 901 45th Street, West Palm Beach, FL, Zip 33407–2495, Mailing Address: P.O. Box 24620, Zip 33416–4620; tel. 561/844–6300; Phillip C. Dutcher, Interim President and Chief Executive Officer

STATEN ISLAND UNIVERSITY HOSPITAL, 475 Seaview Avenue, Staten Island, NY, Zip 10305–9998; tel. 718/226–9000; Rick J. Varone, President

VASSAR BROTHERS HOSPITAL, Reade Place, Poughkeepsie, NY, Zip 12601; tel. 914/454–8500; Ronald T. Mullahey, President

VETERANS AFFAIRS MEDICAL CENTER, 130 West Kingsbridge Road, Bronx, NY, Zip 10468–7511; tel. 718/584–9000; Maryann Musumeci, Director

WESTERN QUEENS COMMUNITY HOSPITAL, 25–10 30th Avenue, Astoria Station, Long Island City, NY, Zip 11102–2495; tel. 718/932–1000; Elliot J. Simon, FACHE, Chief Operating Officer

THE NEW YORK & PRESBYTERIAN HOSPITALS CARE NETWORK, INC.
525 East 68th Street, New York, NY 10021; tel. 212/746–4030; George A. Vecchione, President

FLUSHING HOSPITAL MEDICAL CENTER, 45th Avenue at Parsons Boulevard, Flushing, NY, Zip 11355; tel. 718/670–5000; Charles J. Pendola, President and Chief Executive Officer

GRACIE SQUARE HOSPITAL, 420 East 76th Street, New York, NY, Zip 10021–3104; tel. 212/988–4400; Frank Bruno, Chief Executive Officer

HOSPITAL FOR SPECIAL SURGERY, 535 East 70th Street, New York, NY, Zip 10021–4898; tel. 212/606–1000; John R. Ahearn, President

NEW YORK HOSPITAL MEDICAL CENTER OF QUEENS, 56–45 Main Street, Flushing, NY, Zip 11355; tel. 718/670–1231; Stephen S. Mills, President and Chief Executive Officer

NEW YORK METHODIST HOSPITAL, 506 Sixth Street, Brooklyn, NY, Zip 11215; tel. 718/780–3000; Mark J. Mundy, President and Chief Executive Officer

PRESBYTERIAN HOSPITAL IN THE CITY OF NEW YORK, Columbia–Presbyterian Medical Center, New York, NY, Zip 10032–3784; tel. 212/305–2500; William T. Speck, M.D., President and Chief Executive Officer

SOCIETY OF THE NEW YORK HOSPITAL, 525 East 68th Street, New York, NY, Zip 10021; tel. 212/746–5454; David B. Skinner, M.D., President and Chief Executive Officer

THE NEW YORK COMMUNITY HOSPITAL OF BROOKLYN, 2525 Kings Highway, Brooklyn, NY, Zip 11229–1798; tel. 718/692–5300; Lin H. Mo, President and Chief Executive Officer

UNITED HOSPITAL MEDICAL CENTER, 406 Boston Post Road, Port Chester, NY, Zip 10573; tel. 914/939–7000; Kevin Dahill, President and Chief Executive Officer

WYCKOFF HEIGHTS MEDICAL CENTER, 374 Stockholm Street, Brooklyn, NY, Zip 11237–4099; tel. 718/963–7102; Charles J. Pendola, President

TRI–STATE HEALTH SYSTEM
255 Lafayette Aven, Suffern, NY 10901; tel. 914/368–5000; James A. Martin, President

MERCY COMMUNITY HOSPITAL, 160 East Main Street, Port Jervis, NY, Zip 12771–0268, Mailing Address: P.O. Box 1014, Zip 12771; tel. 914/856–5351; R. Andrew Brothers, President and Chief Executive Officer

ST. ANTHONY COMMUNITY HOSPITAL, 15–19 Maple Avenue, Warwick, NY, Zip 10990; tel. 914/986–2276; R. Andrew Brothers, President and Chief Executive Officer

WESTCHESTER HEALTH SERVICES NETWORK
116 Radio Circle Drive, Mt Kisco, NY 10549; tel. 914/244–1085; Frank Hemeon, President & Chief Executive Officer

GOOD SAMARITAN HOSPITAL, 255 Lafayette Avenue, Suffern, NY, Zip 10901–4869; tel. 914/368–5000; James A. Martin, Chief Executive Officer

HUDSON VALLEY HOSPITAL CENTER, 1980 Crompond Road, Peekskill, NY, Zip 10566–4182; tel. 914/737–9000; John C. Federspiel, President and Chief Executive Officer

NORTHERN WESTCHESTER HOSPITAL CENTER, 400 Main Street, Mount Kisco, NY, Zip 10549; tel. 914/666–1200; Donald W. Davis, President

PUTNAM HOSPITAL CENTER, Stoneleigh Avenue, Carmel, NY, Zip 10512–9948; tel. 914/279–5711; Rodney N. Hubbers, President and Chief Executive Officer

SOUND SHORE MEDICAL CENTER OF WESTCHESTER, 16 Guion Place, New Rochelle, NY, Zip 10802; tel. 914/632–5000; John R. Spicer, President and Chief Executive Officer

ST. JOHN'S RIVERSIDE HOSPITAL, 967 North Broadway, Yonkers, NY, Zip 10701; tel. 914/964–4444; James Foy, President and Chief Executive Officer

STAMFORD HOSPITAL, Shelburne Road and West Broad Street, Stamford, CT, Zip 06902, Mailing Address: P.O. Box 9317, Zip 06904–9317; tel. 203/325–7000; Philip D. Cusano, President and Chief Executive Officer

WESTCHESTER COUNTY MEDICAL CENTER, Valhalla Campus, Valhalla, NY, Zip 10595; tel. 914/285–7000; Edward A. Stolzenberg, Commissioner

WHITE PLAINS HOSPITAL CENTER, Davis Avenue at East Post Road, White Plains, NY, Zip 10601–4699; tel. 914/681–0600; Jon B. Schandler, President and Chief Executive Officer

NORTH CAROLINA

BLADEN COUNTY HOSPITAL
Clarkton Road, Elizabethtown, NC 28337; tel. 919/862–5100; Leo A. Petit, Jr., Chief Executive Officer

BLADEN COUNTY HOSPITAL, 501 South Poplar Street, Elizabethtown, NC, Zip 28337–0398, Mailing Address: Box 398, Zip 28337–0398; tel. 910/862–5100; Leo A. Petit, Jr., Chief Executive Officer

CAROLINAS HOSPITAL NETWORK
P.O. Box 32861, Charlotte, NC 28232–2861; tel. 704/355–8625; Austin Letson, President

ANSON COUNTY HOSPITAL AND SKILLED NURSING FACILITIES, 500 Morven Road, Wadesboro, NC, Zip 28170; tel. 704/694–5131; Frederick G. Thompson, Ph.D., Administrator and Chief Executive Officer

CAROLINAS MEDICAL CENTER, 1000 Blythe Boulevard, Charlotte, NC, Zip 28203, Mailing Address: P.O. Box 32861, Zip 28232–2861; tel. 704/355–2000; Paul S. Franz, President

CATAWBA MEMORIAL HOSPITAL, 810 Fairgrove Church Road S.E., Hickory, NC, Zip 28602; tel. 704/326–3000; J. Anthony Rose, President and Chief Executive Officer

CHARLOTTE INSTITUTE OF REHABILITATION, 1100 Blythe Boulevard, Charlotte, NC, Zip 28203; tel. 704/355–4300; Hollis Hamilton, Administrator

CHESTER COUNTY HOSPITAL AND NURSING CENTER, 1 Medical Park Drive, Chester, SC, Zip 29706–9799; tel. 803/581–3151; William H. Bundy, Acting Administrator

CLEVELAND REGIONAL MEDICAL CENTER, 201 Grover Street, Shelby, NC, Zip 28150; tel. 704/487–3000; John Young, President and Chief Executive Officer

CRAWLEY MEMORIAL HOSPITAL, 315 West College Avenue, Boiling Springs, NC, Zip 28017, Mailing Address: Box 996, Zip 28017; tel. 704/434–9466; Daphne Bridges, President

IREDELL MEMORIAL HOSPITAL, 557 Brookdale Drive, Statesville, NC, Zip 28677–1828, Mailing Address: P.O. Box 1828, Zip 28687–1828; tel. 704/873–5661; S. Arnold Nunnery, President and Chief Executive Officer

KINGS MOUNTAIN HOSPITAL, 706 West King Street, Kings Mountain, NC, Zip 28086, Mailing Address: P.O. Box 339, Zip 28086; tel. 704/739–3601; Hank Neal, Administrator

LINCOLN MEDICAL CENTER, 200 Gamble Drive, Lincolnton, NC, Zip 28092–0677, Mailing Address: Box 677, Zip 28093–0677; tel. 704/735–3071; Peter W. Acker, President and Chief Executive Officer

MERCY HOSPITAL, 2001 Vail Avenue, Charlotte, NC, Zip 28207; tel. 704/379–5000; C. Curtis Copenhaver, Chief Executive Officer

RICHMOND MEMORIAL HOSPITAL, 925 Long Drive, Rockingham, NC, Zip 28379–4815; tel. 910/417–3000; David G. Hohl, Chief Executive Officer

RUTHERFORD HOSPITAL, 308 South Ridgecrest Avenue, Rutherfordton, NC, Zip 28139–3097; tel. 704/286–5000; Robert D. Jones, President

SCOTLAND MEMORIAL HOSPITAL, 500 Lauchwood Drive, Laurinburg, NC, Zip 28352; tel. 910/291–7000; Gregory C. Wood, Chief Executive Officer

Section B

STANLY MEMORIAL HOSPITAL, 301 Yadkin Street, Albemarle, NC, Zip 28001, Mailing Address: Box 1489, Zip 28002; tel. 704/984-4000; Roy M. Hinson, CHE, President and Chief Executive Officer

UNION REGIONAL MEDICAL CENTER, 600 Hospital Drive, Monroe, NC, Zip 28112, Mailing Address: P.O. Box 5003, Zip 28111; tel. 704/283-3100; John W. Roberts, President and Chief Executive Officer

UNIVERSITY HOSPITAL, 8800 North Tryon Street, Charlotte, NC, Zip 28262, Mailing Address: P.O. Box 560727, Zip 28256; tel. 704/548-6000; W. Spencer Lilly, Administrator

VALDESE GENERAL HOSPITAL, Valdese, NC, Mailing Address: Box 700, Zip 28690-0700; tel. 704/874-2251; Lloyd E. Wallace, President and Chief Executive Officer

WATAUGA MEDICAL CENTER, Deerfield Road, Boone, NC, Zip 28607-2600, Mailing Address: P.O. Box 2600, Zip 28607-2600; tel. 704/262-4100; Richard G. Sparks, President

CENTRAL CAROLINA RURAL HOSPITAL ALLIANCE
P.O. Box 938, Albemarle, NC 28002; tel. 704/983-8955; Robert Smith, Executive Director

RICHMOND MEMORIAL HOSPITAL, 925 Long Drive, Rockingham, NC, Zip 28379-4815; tel. 910/417-3000; David G. Hohl, Chief Executive Officer

STANLY MEMORIAL HOSPITAL, 301 Yadkin Street, Albemarle, NC, Zip 28001, Mailing Address: Box 1489, Zip 28002; tel. 704/984-4000; Roy M. Hinson, CHE, President and Chief Executive Officer

UNION REGIONAL MEDICAL CENTER, 600 Hospital Drive, Monroe, NC, Zip 28112, Mailing Address: P.O. Box 5003, Zip 28111; tel. 704/283-3100; John W. Roberts, President and Chief Executive Officer

DUKE HEALTH NETWORK
3100 Tower Building, Suite 600, Durham, NC 27707; tel. 919/419-5001; Paul Rosenberg, Chief Operating Officer

DUKE UNIVERSITY MEDICAL CENTER, Erwin Road, Durham, NC, Zip 27710, Mailing Address: Box 3708, Zip 27710; tel. 919/684-8111; Michael D. Israel, Chief Executive Officer and Vice Chancellor

MARIA PARHAM HOSPITAL, 566 Ruin Creek Road, Henderson, NC, Zip 27536-2957; tel. 919/438-4143; Philip S. Lakernick, President and Chief Executive Officer

EASTERN CAROLINA HEALTH NETWORK
P.O. Box 8468, Greenville, NC 27835-8468; tel. 919/816-6750; Randall H.H. Madry, Chief Executive Officer

ALBEMARLE HOSPITAL, 1144 North Road Street, Elizabeth City, NC, Zip 27909, Mailing Address: Box 1587, Zip 27906-1587; tel. 919/335-0531; Phillip D. Bagby, President and Chief Executive Officer

BEAUFORT COUNTY HOSPITAL, 628 East 12th Street, Washington, NC, Zip 27889-3498; tel. 919/975-4100; Kenneth E. Ragland, Administrator

BERTIE COUNTY MEMORIAL HOSPITAL, 401 Sterlingworth Street, Windsor, NC, Zip 27983-1726, Mailing Address: P.O. Box 40, Zip 27983-1726; tel. 919/794-3141; Anthony F. Mullen, Administrator

CARTERET GENERAL HOSPITAL, 3500 Arendell Street, Morehead City, NC, Zip 28557-1619, Mailing Address: P.O. Box 1619, Zip 28557; tel. 919/247-1616; F. A. Odell, III, FACHE, President

CHOWAN HOSPITAL, 211 Virginia Road, Edenton, NC, Zip 27932-0629, Mailing Address: P.O. Box 629, Zip 27932-0629; tel. 919/482-8451; Barbara R. Cale, Administrator

COLUMBIA HERITAGE HOSPITAL, 111 Hospital Drive, Tarboro, NC, Zip 27886; tel. 919/641-7700; Janet Mullaney, Chief Executive Officer

CRAVEN REGIONAL MEDICAL AUTHORITY, 2000 Neuse Boulevard, New Bern, NC, Zip 28560, Mailing Address: Box 12157, Zip 28561; tel. 919/633-8111; Charles H. Ashford, M.D., Interim Chief Executive Officer

DUPLIN GENERAL HOSPITAL, 401 North Main Street, Kenansville, NC, Zip 28349-0278, Mailing Address: P.O. Box 278, Zip 28349-0278; tel. 910/296-0941; Richard E. Harrell, President

HALIFAX MEMORIAL HOSPITAL, 250 Smith Church Road, Roanoke Rapids, NC, Zip 27870, Mailing Address: P.O. Box 1089, Zip 27870-1089; tel. 919/535-8011; M. E. Gilstrap, President and Chief Executive Officer

LENOIR MEMORIAL HOSPITAL, 100 Airport Road, Kinston, NC, Zip 28501-0678, Mailing Address: P.O. Drawer 1678, Zip 28503-1678; tel. 919/522-7171; Gary E. Black, President and Chief Executive Officer

MARTIN GENERAL HOSPITAL, 310 South McCaskey Road, Williamston, NC, Zip 27892, Mailing Address: P.O. Box 1128, Zip 27892; tel. 919/809-6121; George H. Brandt, Jr., Administrator

NASH HEALTH CARE SYSTEMS, 2460 Curtis Ellis Drive, Rocky Mount, NC, Zip 27804-2297; tel. 919/443-8000; Bryant T. Aldridge, President and Chief Executive Officer

ONSLOW MEMORIAL HOSPITAL, 317 Western Boulevard, Jacksonville, NC, Zip 28540, Mailing Address: Box 1358, Zip 28540; tel. 910/577-2281; Douglas Kramer, Chief Executive Officer

PITT COUNTY MEMORIAL HOSPITAL-UNIVERSITY MEDICAL CENTER OF EASTERN CAROLINA-PITT COUNTY, 2100 Stantonsburg Road, Greenville, NC, Zip 27835-6028, Mailing Address: Box 6028, Zip 27835-6028; tel. 919/816-4451; Dave C. McRae, President and Chief Executive Officer

PUNGO DISTRICT HOSPITAL, 210 East Front Street, Belhaven, NC, Zip 27810-9998; tel. 919/943-2111; Thomas O. Miller, Administrator

ROANOKE-CHOWAN HOSPITAL, Academy Street, Ahoskie, NC, Zip 27910, Mailing Address: Box 1385, Zip 27910; tel. 919/209-3000; Susan S. Lassiter, President

WASHINGTON COUNTY HOSPITAL, 1 Medical Plaza, Plymouth, NC, Zip 27962; tel. 919/793-4135; Lawrence H. McAvoy, Administrator

WAYNE MEMORIAL HOSPITAL, 2700 Wayne Memorial Drive, Goldsboro, NC, Zip 27534-8001, Mailing Address: P.O. Box 8001, Zip 27533-8001; tel. 919/736-1110; James W. Hubbell, President and Chief Executive Officer

WILSON MEMORIAL HOSPITAL, 1705 South Tarboro Street, Wilson, NC, Zip 27893-3428; tel. 919/399-8040; Christopher T. Durrer, President and Chief Executive Officer

HOSPITAL ALLIANCE FOR COMMUNITY HEALTH
P.O. Box 14049, 10 Sunnybrook Road, Raleigh, NC 27620-4049; tel. 919/250-3813; Peter J. Morris, M.D., Secretary

COLUMBIA RALEIGH COMMUNITY HOSPITAL, 3400 Wake Forest Road, Raleigh, NC, Zip 27609-7373, Mailing Address: P.O. Box 28280, Zip 27611; tel. 919/954-3000; James E. Raynor, Chief Executive Officer

REX HEALTHCARE, 4420 Lake Boone Trail, Raleigh, NC, Zip 27607-6599; tel. 919/783-3100; James W. Albright, President and Chief Executive Officer

WAKE MEDICAL CENTER, 3000 New Bern Avenue, Raleigh, NC, Zip 27610; tel. 919/250-8000; Raymond L. Champ, President

MISSION & SAINT JOSEPH HEALTH SYSTEM
509 Biltmore Avenue, Asheville, NC 28801; tel. 704/255-3100; Robert F. Burgin, President and Chief Executive Officer

MEMORIAL MISSION MEDICAL CENTER, 509 Biltmore Avenue, Asheville, NC, Zip 28801-4690; tel. 704/255-4000; Robert F. Burgin, President and Chief Executive Officer

ST. JOSEPH'S HOSPITAL, 428 Biltmore Avenue, Asheville, NC, Zip 28801-4502; tel. 704/255-3100; J. Lewis Daniels, President and Chief Executive Officer

NORTH CAROLINA BAPTIST HOSPITALS, INC.
Medical Center Boulevard, Winston-Salem, NC 27157; tel. 910/716-7840; Douglas Atkinson, Vice President of Networking

HOOTS MEMORIAL HOSPITAL, 624 West Main Street, Yadkinville, NC, Zip 27055, Mailing Address: P.O. Box 68, Zip 27055; tel. 910/679-2041; Lance C. Labine, President

NORTH CAROLINA BAPTIST HOSPITAL, Medical Center Boulevard, Winston-Salem, NC, Zip 27157; tel. 910/716-2011; Len B. Preslar, Jr., President and Chief Executive Officer

STOKES-REYNOLDS MEMORIAL HOSPITAL, Danbury, NC, Mailing Address: Box 10, Zip 27016-0010; tel. 910/593-2831; Sandra D. Priddy, President

NORTH CAROLINA HEALTH NETWORK
P.O. Box 668800, Charlotte, NC 28266-8800; tel. 704/529-3300; Rose Duncan, Interim Director

MOSES CONE HEALTH SYSTEM, 1200 North Elm Street, Greensboro, NC, Zip 27401-1020; tel. 910/574-7000; Dennis R. Barry, President

UNC HEALTH NETWORK
101 Manning Drive, Chapel Hill, NC 27514; tel. 919/966-4131; Mary Beck, Director of Planning

CHATHAM HOSPITAL, West Third Street and Ivy Avenue, Siler City, NC, Zip 27344-2343, Mailing Address: P.O. Box 649, Zip 27344; tel. 919/663-2113; Ted G. Chapin, Chief Executive Officer

UNIVERSITY OF NORTH CAROLINA HOSPITALS, 101 Manning Drive, Chapel Hill, NC, Zip 27514; tel. 919/966-4131; Eric B. Munson, Executive Director

WESTERN NORTH CAROLINA HEALTH NETWORK
509 Biltmore Avenue, Asheville, NC 28801; tel. 704/255-4495; MaryAnn Digman, Adminstrator of Regional Services

HARRIS REGIONAL HOSPITAL, 68 Hospital Road, Sylva, NC, Zip 28779-2795; tel. 704/586-7000; Isaac S. Coe, President

MARGARET R. PARDEE MEMORIAL HOSPITAL, 715 Fleming Street, Hendersonville, NC, Zip 28791-2563; tel. 704/696-1000; Frank J. Aaron, Jr., Chief Executive Officer

MCDOWELL HOSPITAL, 100 Rankin Drive, Marion, NC, Zip 28752, Mailing Address: P.O. Box 730, Zip 28752; tel. 704/659-5000; Jeffrey M. Judd, President and Chief Executive Officer

MEMORIAL MISSION MEDICAL CENTER, 509 Biltmore Avenue, Asheville, NC, Zip 28801-4690; tel. 704/255-4000; Robert F. Burgin, President and Chief Executive Officer

MURPHY MEDICAL CENTER, 2002 U.S. Highway 64 East, Murphy, NC, Zip 28906; tel. 704/837-8161; Mike Stevenson, Administrator

RUTHERFORD HOSPITAL, 308 South Ridgecrest Avenue, Rutherfordton, NC, Zip 28139-3097; tel. 704/286-5000; Robert D. Jones, President

ST. JOSEPH'S HOSPITAL, 428 Biltmore Avenue, Asheville, NC, Zip 28801-4502; tel. 704/255-3100; J. Lewis Daniels, President and Chief Executive Officer

TRANSYLVANIA COMMUNITY HOSPITAL, Hospital Drive, Brevard, NC, Zip 28712-1116, Mailing Address: Box 1116, Zip 28712-1116; tel. 704/884-9111; Robert J. Bednarek, Administrator and Chief Executive Officer

NORTH DAKOTA

HEARTLAND NETWORK, INC.
510 South 4th Street, Fargo, ND 58103; tel. 701/241-7077; Walter Rogers, President & Chief Executive Officer

DAKOTA HEARTLAND HEALTH SYSTEM, 1720 South Univeristy Drive, Fargo, ND, Zip 58103; tel. 701/280-4100; Bruce A. Baldwin, Interim President and Chief Executive Officer

MEDCENTER ONE
300 North Seventh Street, Bismarck, ND
58506–5525; tel. 701/224–6000; Terrance G.
Brosseau, President and Chief Executive
Officer

JACOBSON MEMORIAL HOSPITAL CARE CENTER, 601 East Street North, Elgin, ND, Zip 58533–0376; tel. 701/584–2792; Jacqueline Seibel, Administrator

MCKENZIE COUNTY MEMORIAL HOSPITAL, 508 North Main Street, Watford City, ND, Zip 58854, Mailing Address: P.O. Box 548, Zip 58854–0548; tel. 701/842–3000; Tim Gullingsrud, Administrator

MEDCENTER ONE, 300 North Seventh Street, Bismarck, ND, Zip 58501–4439, Mailing Address: P.O. Box 5525, Zip 58506–5525; tel. 701/323–6000; Terrance G. Brosseau, President and Chief Executive Officer

MEDCENTER ONE MANDAN, 1000 18th Street N.W., Mandan, ND, Zip 58554–1698; tel. 701/663–6471; James R. Hubbard, Administrator

RICHARDTON HEALTH CENTER, Richardton, ND, Mailing Address: P.O. Box H, Zip 58652; tel. 701/974–3304; Arlene Mack, R.N., Administrator

MERITCARE HEALTH SYSTEM
720 Fourth Street, North, Fargo, ND 58122;
tel. 701/234–6000; Roger Gilbertson, M.D.,
President

GRIGGS COUNTY HOSPITAL AND NURSING HOME, 1200 Roberts Avenue, Cooperstown, ND, Zip 58425, Mailing Address: Box 728, Zip 58425; tel. 701/797–2221; Patrick J. Rafferty, Administrator

UNITED HOSPITAL
1200 South Columbia Road, Grand Forks, ND
58201; tel. 701/780–5000; Rosemary
Jacobson, President & Chief Executive Officer

UNITED HEALTH SERVICES, 1200 South Columbia Road, Grand Forks, ND, Zip 58201; tel. 701/780–5000; Rosemary Jacobson, President and Chief Executive Officer

OHIO

CLEVELAND HEALTH NETWORK
9500 Euclid Avenue, H18, Cleveland, OH
44195; tel. 216/444–2300; Floyd D. Loop,
M.D., Chairman

ASHTABULA COUNTY MEDICAL CENTER, 2420 Lake Avenue, Ashtabula, OH, Zip 44004–4993; tel. 216/997–2262; R. D. Richardson, President and Chief Executive Officer

BARBERTON CITIZENS HOSPITAL, 155 Fifth Street N.E., Barberton, OH, Zip 44203; tel. 330/745–1611; Mike A. Bernatovicz, Chief Executive Officer

CHILDREN'S HOSPITAL MEDICAL CENTER OF AKRON, One Perkins Square, Akron, OH, Zip 44308–1062; tel. 330/379–8200; William H. Considine, President

CLEVELAND CLINIC HOSPITAL, 9500 Euclid Avenue, Cleveland, OH, Zip 44195–5108; tel. 216/444–2200; Frank L. Lordeman, Chief Operating Officer

DOCTORS HOSPITAL OF STARK COUNTY, 400 Austin Avenue N.W., Massillon, OH, Zip 44646–3554; tel. 216/837–7200; Thomas E. Cecconi, Chief Executive Officer

EMH AMHERST HOSPITAL, 254 Cleveland Avenue, Amherst, OH, Zip 44001–1699; tel. 216/988–6000; James L. Keegan, President and Chief Executive Officer

EMH REGIONAL MEDICAL CENTER, 630 East River Street, Elyria, OH, Zip 44035–5902; tel. 216/329–7500; James L. Keegan, President and Chief Executive Officer

FAIRVIEW HOSPITAL, 18101 Lorain Avenue, Cleveland, OH, Zip 44111–5656; tel. 216/476–4040; Thomas M. LaMotte, President and Chief Executive Officer

FIRELANDS COMMUNITY HOSPITAL, 1101 Decatur Street, Sandusky, OH, Zip 44870–3335; tel. 419/626–7400; Nelson F. Alward, President and Chief Executive Officer

LUTHERAN HOSPITAL, 2609 Franklin Boulevard, Cleveland, OH, Zip 44113–2992; tel. 216/696–4300; Kenneth T. Misener, Chief Operating Officer

MARYMOUNT HOSPITAL, 12300 McCracken Road, Garfield Heights, OH, Zip 44125–2975; tel. 216/581–0500; Thomas J. Trudell, President and Chief Executive Officer

PARMA COMMUNITY GENERAL HOSPITAL, 7007 Powers Boulevard, Parma, OH, Zip 44129–5495; tel. 216/888–1800; Thomas A. Selden, President and Chief Executive Officer

SOUTHWEST GENERAL HEALTH CENTER, 18697 Bagley Road, Middleburg Heights, OH, Zip 44130–3497; tel. 216/816–8000; L. Jon Schurmeier, President and Chief Executive Officer

ST. ELIZABETH HEALTH CENTER, 1044 Belmont Avenue, Youngstown, OH, Zip 44501, Mailing Address: Box 1790, Zip 44501–1790; tel. 330/759–7484; Kevin E. Nolan, President and Chief Executive Officer

ST. JOSEPH HEALTH CENTER, 667 Eastland Avenue S.E., Warren, OH, Zip 44484; tel. 330/841–4000; Robert W. Shroder, Chief Operating Officer

SUMMA HEALTH SYSTEM, Akron, OH, Albert F. Gilbert, Ph.D., President and Chief Executive Officer

WADSWORTH–RITTMAN HOSPITAL, 195 Wadsworth Road, Wadsworth, OH, Zip 44281–9505; tel. 330/334–1504; James W. Brumlow, Jr., President and Chief Executive Officer

COMMUNITY HOSPITALS OF OHIO
1320 West Main Street, Newark, OH
43055–3699; tel. 614/348–4000; William J.
Andrews, President

ADENA HEALTH SYSTEM, 272 Hospital Road, Chillicothe, OH, Zip 45601–0708; tel. 614/772–7500; Allen V. Rupiper, President

BERGER HOSPITAL, 600 North Pickaway Street, Circleville, OH, Zip 43113–1499; tel. 614/474–2126; Brian R. Colfack, CHE, President and Chief Executive Officer

COSHOCTON COUNTY MEMORIAL HOSPITAL, 1460 Orange Street, Coshocton, OH, Zip 43812–6330, Mailing Address: P.O. Box 1330, Zip 43812–6330; tel. 614/622–6411; Gregory M. Nowak, Administrator

FORT HAMILTON–HUGHES MEMORIAL HOSPITAL, 630 Eaton Avenue, Hamilton, OH, Zip 45013; tel. 513/867–2000; James A. Kingsbury, President and Chief Executive Officer

GENESIS HEALTHCARE SYSTEM, 800 Forest Avenue, Zanesville, OH, Zip 43701–2881; tel. 614/454–5000; Thomas L. Sieber, President and Chief Executive Officer

GRADY MEMORIAL HOSPITAL, 561 West Central Avenue, Delaware, OH, Zip 43015–1485; tel. 614/369–8711; Everett P. Weber, Jr., President and Chief Executive Officer

HOCKING VALLEY COMMUNITY HOSPITAL, Route 2, State Route 664, Logan, OH, Zip 43138–0966, Mailing Address: Box 966, Zip 43138–0966; tel. 614/385–5631; Larry Willard, Administrator

HOLZER MEDICAL CENTER, 100 Jackson Pike, Gallipolis, OH, Zip 45631–1563; tel. 614/446–5000; Charles I. Adkins, Jr., President

KNOX COMMUNITY HOSPITAL, 1330 Coshocton Road, Mount Vernon, OH, Zip 43050–1495; tel. 614/393–9000; Robert G. Polahar, Chief Executive Officer

LICKING MEMORIAL HOSPITAL, 1320 West Main Street, Newark, OH, Zip 43055–3699; tel. 614/348–4000; William J. Andrews, President

MARIETTA MEMORIAL HOSPITAL, 401 Matthew Street, Marietta, OH, Zip 45750–1699; tel. 614/374–1400; Larry J. Unroe, President

ST. RITA'S MEDICAL CENTER, 730 West Market Street, Lima, OH, Zip 45801–4670; tel. 419/227–3361; James P. Reber, President

COMPREHENSIVE HEALTHCARE OF OHIO, INC.
630 East River Street, Elyria, OH 44035;
tel. 216/329–7500; James Keegan,
President & Chief Executive Officer

EMH AMHERST HOSPITAL, 254 Cleveland Avenue, Amherst, OH, Zip 44001–1699; tel. 216/988–6000; James L. Keegan, President and Chief Executive Officer

EMH REGIONAL MEDICAL CENTER, 630 East River Street, Elyria, OH, Zip 44035–5902; tel. 216/329–7500; James L. Keegan, President and Chief Executive Officer

FIRST INTERHEALTH NETWORK
3454 Oak Alley Court, Suite 510, Toledo, OH
43606; tel. 419/534–2000; Christine Pilliod,
Director of Marketing

BETHESDA OAK HOSPITAL, 619 Oak Street, Cincinnati, OH, Zip 45206–1690; tel. 513/569–6111; Linda D. Schaffner, R.N., Vice President and Administrator

FLOWER HOSPITAL, 5200 Harroun Road, Sylvania, OH, Zip 43560–2196; tel. 419/824–1444; Randall Kelley, Senior Vice President and Chief Operating Officer

GOOD SAMARITAN HOSPITAL, 375 Dixmyth Avenue, Cincinnati, OH, Zip 45220–2489; tel. 513/872–1400; Sister Myra James Bradley, Chairman of the Board of Directors

ST. CHARLES HOSPITAL, 2600 Navarre Avenue, Oregon, OH, Zip 43616–3297; tel. 419/698–7479; Cathleen K. Nelson, President and Chief Executive Officer

ST. LUKE'S HOSPITAL, 5901 Monclova Road, Maumee, OH, Zip 43537–1899; tel. 419/893–5911; Frank J. Bartell, III, President and Chief Executive Officer

ST. VINCENT MERCY MEDICAL CENTER, 2213 Cherry Street, Toledo, OH, Zip 43608–2691; tel. 419/251–3232; Steven L. Mickus, President and Chief Executive Officer

WOOD COUNTY HOSPITAL, 950 West Wooster Street, Bowling Green, OH, Zip 43402–2699; tel. 419/354–8900; Michael A. Miesle, Administrator

HEALTH CLEVELAND
18101 Lorain Avenue, Cleveland, OH 44111;
tel. 216/476–7020; Kenneth Misener,
Executive Vice President

FAIRVIEW HOSPITAL, 18101 Lorain Avenue, Cleveland, OH, Zip 44111–5656; tel. 216/476–4040; Thomas M. LaMotte, President and Chief Executive Officer

LUTHERAN HOSPITAL, 2609 Franklin Boulevard, Cleveland, OH, Zip 44113–2992; tel. 216/696–4300; Kenneth T. Misener, Chief Operating Officer

HEALTHY CONNECTIONS NETWORK
P.O. Box 2090, Akron, OH 44309–2090;
tel. 216/375–3000; Patricia Thomas, Director
Community Services

AKRON GENERAL MEDICAL CENTER, 400 Wabash Avenue, Akron, OH, Zip 44307–2433; tel. 330/384–6000; Michael A. West, President

CHILDREN'S HOSPITAL MEDICAL CENTER OF AKRON, One Perkins Square, Akron, OH, Zip 44308–1062; tel. 330/379–8200; William H. Considine, President

SUMMA HEALTH SYSTEM, Akron, OH, Albert F. Gilbert, Ph.D., President and Chief Executive Officer

LAKE ERIE HEALTH ALLIANCE
2142 North Cove Boulevard, Toledo, OH
43606; tel. 419/471–3450; John E. Horns,
President

BELLEVUE HOSPITAL, 811 Northwest Street, Bellevue, OH, Zip 44811, Mailing Address: Box 8004, Zip 44811; tel. 419/483–4040; Michael K. Winthrop, President

DEFIANCE HOSPITAL, 1206 East Second Street, Defiance, OH, Zip 43512–2495; tel. 419/783–6955; Richard C. Sommer, Administrator

FIRELANDS COMMUNITY HOSPITAL, 1101 Decatur Street, Sandusky, OH, Zip 44870–3335; tel. 419/626–7400; Nelson F. Alward, President and Chief Executive Officer

FISHER–TITUS MEDICAL CENTER, 272 Benedict Avenue, Norwalk, OH, Zip 44857–2374; tel. 419/668–8101; Richard C. Westhofen, President

FLOWER HOSPITAL, 5200 Harroun Road, Sylvania, OH, Zip 43560–2196; tel. 419/824–1444; Randall Kelley, Senior Vice President and Chief Operating Officer

FULTON COUNTY HEALTH CENTER, 725 South Shoop Avenue, Wauseon, OH, Zip 43567–1701; tel. 419/335–2015; E. Dean Beck, Administrator

H. B. MAGRUDER MEMORIAL HOSPITAL, 615 Fulton Street, Port Clinton, OH, Zip 43452–2034; tel. 419/734–3131; David R. Norwine, President and Chief Executive Officer

HENRY COUNTY HOSPITAL, 11–600 State Road 424, Napoleon, OH, Zip 43545–9399; tel. 419/592–4015; Robert J. Coholich, Chief Executive Officer

LIMA MEMORIAL HOSPITAL, 1001 Bellefontaine Avenue, Lima, OH, Zip 45804–2894; tel. 419/228–3335; John B. White, President and Chief Executive Officer

MEDCENTRAL CRESTLINE HOSPITAL, 700 Columbus Street, Crestline, OH, Zip 44827, Mailing Address: P.O. Box 350, Zip 44827; tel. 419/683–1212; Robert E. Wirtz, Jr., President and Chief Executive Officer

MEDICAL COLLEGE HOSPITALS, 3000 Arlington Avenue, Toledo, OH, Zip 43699–0008, Mailing Address: P.O. Box 10008, Zip 43699–0008; tel. 419/381–4172; Richard C. Sipp, Vice President for Administration

MEMORIAL HOSPITAL, 715 South Taft Avenue, Fremont, OH, Zip 43420–3200; tel. 419/332–7321; John A. Gorman, Chief Executive Officer

MERCY HOSPITAL, 485 West Market Street, Tiffin, OH, Zip 44883, Mailing Address: Box 727, Zip 44883–0727; tel. 419/447–3130; Mark Shugarman, President

MERCY MEMORIAL HOSPITAL, 740 North Macomb Street, Monroe, MI, Zip 48161–9974, Mailing Address: P.O. Box 67, Zip 48161–0067; tel. 313/241–1700; Richard S. Hiltz, President and Chief Executive Officer

ST. FRANCIS HEALTH CARE CENTRE, 401 North Broadway, Green Springs, OH, Zip 44836–9653; tel. 419/639–2626; Gregory T. Storer, Chief Executive Officer

WOOD COUNTY HOSPITAL, 950 West Wooster Street, Bowling Green, OH, Zip 43402–2699; tel. 419/354–8900; Michael A. Miesle, Administrator

LAKE HOSPITAL SYSTEM, INC.
10 East Washington, Painesville, OH 44077; tel. 216/354–1698; Ralph W. Sorrell, Sr., President & Chief Executive Officer

LAKE HOSPITAL SYSTEM, 10 East Washington, Painesville, OH, Zip 44077–3472; tel. 216/354–2400; Cynthia Ann Moore–Hardy, Interim Chief Executive Officer

MERCY HEALTH SYSTEM
4340 Glendale–Millford Road, Suite 100, Cincinnati, OH 45242; tel. 513/483–5200; Julie Hanser, President and Chief Executive Officer

CLERMONT MERCY HOSPITAL, 3000 Hospital Drive, Batavia, OH, Zip 45103–1998; tel. 513/732–8200; Karen S. Ehrat, Ph.D., President

FAIRFIELD MEDICAL CENTER, 401 North Ewing Street, Lancaster, OH, Zip 43130–3371; tel. 614/687–8000; Creighton E. Likes, Jr., President and Chief Executive Officer

MERCY HOSPITAL, 100 River Front Plaza, Hamilton, OH, Zip 45011, Mailing Address: P.O. Box 418, Zip 45012–0418; tel. 513/870–7080; Thomas S. Urban, President

MERCY HOSPITAL ANDERSON, 7500 State Road, Cincinnati, OH, Zip 45255–2492; tel. 513/624–4500; Karen S. Ehrat, Ph.D., President

MERIDA HEALTH SYSTEM
6700 Beta Drive, Suite 200, Mayfield Village, OH 44143; tel. 216/446–8000; Charles B. Miner, President & Chief Executive Officer

MERIDIA EUCLID HOSPITAL, 18901 Lake Shore Boulevard, Euclid, OH, Zip 44119–1090; tel. 216/531–9000; Denise Zeman, Site Administrator

MERIDIA HILLCREST HOSPITAL, 6780 Mayfield Road, Cleveland, OH, Zip 44124–2202; tel. 216/449–4500; Catherine B. Leary, R.N., Site Administrator, Vice President Clinical Services and Nurse Executive

MERIDIA HURON HOSPITAL, 13951 Terrace Road, Cleveland, OH, Zip 44112; tel. 216/761–3300; Beverly Lozar, Site Administrator

MERIDIA SOUTH POINTE HOSPITAL, 4110 Warrensville Center Road, Warrensville Heights, OH, Zip 44122–7099; tel. 216/491–6000; Kathleen A. Rice, Site Administrator

MOUNT CARMEL HEALTH SYSTEM
793 West State Street, Columbus, OH 43222; tel. 614/234–5000; Dale St. Arnold, President & Chief Executive Officer

ADENA HEALTH SYSTEM, 272 Hospital Road, Chillicothe, OH, Zip 45601–0708; tel. 614/772–7500; Allen V. Rupiper, President

BERGER HOSPITAL, 600 North Pickaway Street, Circleville, OH, Zip 43113–1499; tel. 614/474–2126; Brian R. Colfack, CHE, President and Chief Executive Officer

MOUNT CARMEL HEALTH SYSTEM, 793 West State Street, Columbus, OH, Zip 43222–1551; tel. 614/225–5000; Dale St. Arnold, President and Chief Executive Officer

ST. ANN'S HOSPITAL, 500 South Cleveland Avenue, Westerville, OH, Zip 43081–8998; tel. 614/898–4000; Alice M. O'Brien, Senior Vice President of System Operations

NORTHEAST OHIO HEALTH NETWORK
400 Wabash Avenue, Akron, OH 44307; tel. 330/384–6781; David Kantor, Executive Director

AKRON GENERAL MEDICAL CENTER, 400 Wabash Avenue, Akron, OH, Zip 44307–2433; tel. 330/384–6000; Michael A. West, President

BARBERTON CITIZENS HOSPITAL, 155 Fifth Street N.E., Barberton, OH, Zip 44203; tel. 330/745–1611; Mike A. Bernatovicz, Chief Executive Officer

CHILDREN'S HOSPITAL MEDICAL CENTER OF AKRON, One Perkins Square, Akron, OH, Zip 44308–1062; tel. 330/379–8200; William H. Considine, President

CUYAHOGA FALLS GENERAL HOSPITAL, 1900 23rd Street, Cuyahoga Falls, OH, Zip 44223–1499; tel. 216/971–7000; Fred Anthony, President and Chief Executive Officer

MEDINA GENERAL HOSPITAL, 1000 East Washington Street, Medina, OH, Zip 44256–2170, Mailing Address: P.O. Box 427, Zip 44258–0427; tel. 330/725–1000; Gary D. Hallman, President and Chief Executive Officer

ROBINSON MEMORIAL HOSPITAL, 6847 North Chestnut Street, Ravenna, OH, Zip 44266–1204, Mailing Address: P.O. Box 1204, Zip 44266; tel. 330/297–0811; Stephen Colecchi, President and Chief Executive Officer

OHIO STATE HEALTH NETWORK
941 Chatham Lane, Suite 3200, Columbus, OH 43221; tel. 614/293–3685; Ewing Crawfis, Board Chairman

ARTHUR G. JAMES CANCER HOSPITAL AND RESEARCH INSTITUTE, 300 West Tenth Avenue, Columbus, OH, Zip 43210; tel. 614/293–5485; David E. Schuller, M.D., Chief Executive Officer

BARNESVILLE HOSPITAL ASSOCIATION, 639 West Main Street, Barnesville, OH, Zip 43713–1096, Mailing Address: P.O. Box 309, Zip 43713–0309; tel. 614/425–3941; Richard L. Doan, Chief Executive Officer

GREENFIELD AREA MEDICAL CENTER, 545 South Street, Greenfield, OH, Zip 45123–1400; tel. 513/981–2116; Mark E. Marchetti, Chief Executive Officer

MARY RUTAN HOSPITAL, 205 Palmer Avenue, Bellefontaine, OH, Zip 43311; tel. 937/592–4015; Ewing H. Crawfis, President

OHIO STATE UNIVERSITY MEDICAL CENTER, 410 West 10th Avenue, Columbus, OH, Zip 43210–1240; tel. 614/293–8000; R. Reed Fraley, Associate Vice President for Health Sciences and Chief Executive Officer

PIKE COMMUNITY HOSPITAL, 100 Dawn Lane, Waverly, OH, Zip 45690–9664; tel. 614/947–2186; Richard E. Sobota, President and Chief Executive Officer

RIVER VALLEY HEALTH SYSTEM, 2228 South Ninth Street, Ironton, OH, Zip 45638–2526; tel. 614/532–3231; Terry L. Vanderhoof, President and Chief Executive Officer

WYANDOT MEMORIAL HOSPITAL, 885 North Sandusky Avenue, Upper Sandusky, OH, Zip 43351–1098; tel. 419/294–4991; Joseph A. D'Ettorre, Administrator

PROMEDICA HEALTH SYSTEM
2121 Hughes Drive, Toledo, OH 43606; tel. 419/291–3686; William Glover, Acting President & CEO

FLOWER HOSPITAL, 5200 Harroun Road, Sylvania, OH, Zip 43560–2196; tel. 419/824–1444; Randall Kelley, Senior Vice President and Chief Operating Officer

THE TOLEDO HOSPITAL, 2142 North Cove Boulevard, Toledo, OH, Zip 43606–3896; tel. 419/471–4000; William W. Glover, President

SAINT LUKES MEDICAL CENTER
11311 Shaker Boulevard, Cleveland, OH 44104; tel. 216/368–7354; James L. Heffernan, Senior Vice President

SAINT LUKE'S MEDICAL CENTER, 11311 Shaker Boulevard, Cleveland, OH, Zip 44104–3805; tel. 216/368–7000; Samuel R. Huston, President and Chief Executive Officer

SUMMA HEALTH SYSTEM
525 East Market Street, Akron, OH 44309; tel. 330/375–3000; Albert Gilbert, Ph.d., President

SUMMA HEALTH SYSTEM, Akron, OH, Albert F. Gilbert, Ph.D., President and Chief Executive Officer

THE HEALTHCARE ALLIANCE OF GREATER CINCINNATI
2060 Reading Road, Cincinnati, OH 45219; tel. 513/632–3700; Jack Cook, Chief Executive Officer

CHRIST HOSPITAL, 2139 Auburn Avenue, Cincinnati, OH, Zip 45219–2989; tel. 513/369–2000; Claus von Zychlin, Senior Executive Officer

JEWISH HOSPITAL, 3200 Burnet Avenue, Cincinnati, OH, Zip 45229–3099; tel. 513/569–2000; Warren C. Falberg, Senior Executive Officer

ST. LUKE HOSPITAL EAST, 85 North Grand Avenue, Fort Thomas, KY, Zip 41075–1796; tel. 606/572–3100; Daniel M. Vinson, CPA, Senior Executive Officer

ST. LUKE HOSPITAL WEST, 7380 Turfway Road, Florence, KY, Zip 41042; tel. 606/525–5200; John D. Hoyle, Senior Executive Officer

UNIVERISITY HOSPITAL, 234 Goodman Street, Cincinnati, OH, Zip 45267–0700; tel. 513/558–1000; Elliot G. Cohen, Senior Executive Officer

THE METROHEALTH SYSTEM
2500 MetroHealth Drive, Cleveland, OH 44109–1998; tel. 216/398–6000; Terry White, President & Chief Executive Officer

METROHEALTH MEDICAL CENTER, 2500 Metrohealth Drive, Cleveland, OH, Zip 44109–1998; tel. 216/778–7800; Terry R. White, President and Chief Executive Officer

THE MOUNT SINAI HEALTH CARE SYSTEM
One Mount Sinai Drive, Cleveland, OH 44106; tel. 216/421–4000; Robert Shakno, President & Chief Executive Officer

LAURELWOOD HOSPITAL, 35900 Euclid Avenue, Willoughby, OH, Zip 44094–4648; tel. 216/953–3000; Farshid Afsarifard, Executive Director

MOUNT SINAI MEDICAL CENTER, One Mt Sinai Drive, Cleveland, OH, Zip 44106–4198; tel. 216/421–4000; Robert A. Schapper, Chief Executive Officer

Section B

TRIHEALTH
619 Oak Street, Cincinnati, OH 45206; tel. 513/569-6141; L. Thomas Wilburn Jr., President & Chief Executive Officer

BETHESDA NORTH HOSPITAL, 10500 Montgomery Road, Cincinnati, OH, Zip 45242; tel. 513/745-1111; Fred Kolb, Site Administrator

BETHESDA OAK HOSPITAL, 619 Oak Street, Cincinnati, OH, Zip 45206-1690; tel. 513/569-6111; Linda D. Schaffner, R.N., Vice President and Administrator

GOOD SAMARITAN HOSPITAL, 375 Dixmyth Avenue, Cincinnati, OH, Zip 45220-2489; tel. 513/872-1400; Sister Myra James Bradley, Chairman of the Board of Directors

UNITED HEALTH PARTNERS
2213 Cherry Street, Toledo, OH 43608; tel. 419/321-3232; David Crane, Vice President of Marketing

BELLEVUE HOSPITAL, 811 Northwest Street, Bellevue, OH, Zip 44811, Mailing Address: Box 8004, Zip 44811; tel. 419/483-4040; Michael K. Winthrop, President

DEFIANCE HOSPITAL, 1206 East Second Street, Defiance, OH, Zip 43512-2495; tel. 419/783-6955; Richard C. Sommer, Administrator

FISHER-TITUS MEDICAL CENTER, 272 Benedict Avenue, Norwalk, OH, Zip 44857-2374; tel. 419/668-8101; Richard C. Westhofen, President

FOSTORIA COMMUNITY HOSPITAL, 501 Van Buren Street, Fostoria, OH, Zip 44830-0907, Mailing Address: P.O. Box 907, Zip 44830-0907; tel. 419/435-7734; Brad A. Higgins, President and Chief Executive Officer

FULTON COUNTY HEALTH CENTER, 725 South Shoop Avenue, Wauseon, OH, Zip 43567-1701; tel. 419/335-2015; E. Dean Beck, Administrator

MEMORIAL HOSPITAL, 715 South Taft Avenue, Fremont, OH, Zip 43420-3200; tel. 419/332-7321; John A. Gorman, Chief Executive Officer

MERCY HOSPITAL, 485 West Market Street, Tiffin, OH, Zip 44883, Mailing Address: Box 727, Zip 44883-0727; tel. 419/447-3130; Mark Shugarman, President

MERCY HOSPITAL-WILLARD, 110 East Howard Street, Willard, OH, Zip 44890-1611; tel. 419/933-2931; James O. Detwiler, President

PROVIDENCE HOSPITAL, 1912 Hayes Avenue, Sandusky, OH, Zip 44870-4736; tel. 419/621-7000; Sister Nancy Linenkugel, FACHE, President and Chief Executive Officer

ST. VINCENT MERCY MEDICAL CENTER, 2213 Cherry Street, Toledo, OH, Zip 43608-2691; tel. 419/251-3232; Steven L. Mickus, President and Chief Executive Officer

WOOD COUNTY HOSPITAL, 950 West Wooster Street, Bowling Green, OH, Zip 43402-2699; tel. 419/354-8900; Michael A. Miesle, Administrator

UNIVERSITY HOSPITALS HEALTH SYSTEM
11100 Euclid Avenue, Cleveland, OH 44106; tel. 216/844-1000; James G. Lubetkin, Vice President Corporate Communications

UHHS GEAUGA REGIONAL HOSPITAL, 13207 Ravenna Road, Chardon, OH, Zip 44024; tel. 216/269-6000; Richard J. Frenchie, President and Chief Executive Officer

UHHS-MEMORIAL HOSPITAL OF GENEVA, 870 West Main Street, Geneva, OH, Zip 44041-1295; tel. 216/466-1141; Gerard D. Klein, Chief Executive Officer

UNIVERSITY HOSPITALS HEALTH SYSTEM BEDFORD MEDICAL CENTER, 44 Blaine Avenue, Bedford, OH, Zip 44146-2799; tel. 216/439-2000; Arlene A. Rak, R.N., President

UNIVERSITY HOSPITALS OF CLEVELAND, 11100 Euclid Avenue, Cleveland, OH, Zip 44106-2602; tel. 216/844-1000; Farah M. Walters, President and Chief Executive Officer

UPPER VALLEY MEDICAL CENTERS, INC.
3130 North Dixie Highway, Troy, OH 45373; tel. 937/332-7858; Michele Elam, Financial Coordinator

DETTMER HOSPITAL, 3130 North Dixie Highway, Troy, OH, Zip 45373-1039; tel. 937/332-7500; Keith Achor, Assistant Administrator

PIQUA MEMORIAL MEDICAL CENTER, 624 Park Avenue, Piqua, OH, Zip 45356-2098; tel. 513/778-6500; Eva L. Fine, R.N., MS, Assistant Administrator

STOUDER MEMORIAL HOSPITAL, 920 Summit Avenue, Troy, OH, Zip 45373; tel. 937/332-8500; Patricia Meyer, Assistant Administrator

WEST CENTRAL OHIO REGIONAL HEALTHCARE ALLIANCE, LTD.
730 West Market Street, Lima, OH 45801; tel. 419/226-9085; P. Anthony Long, Executive Director

JOINT TOWNSHIP DISTRICT MEMORIAL HOSPITAL, 200 St. Clair Street, Saint Marys, OH, Zip 45885-2400; tel. 419/394-3387; James R. Chick, President

MERCER COUNTY JOINT TOWNSHIP COMMUNITY HOSPITAL, 800 West Main Street, Coldwater, OH, Zip 45828-1698; tel. 419/678-2341; James W. Isaacs, Chief Executive Officer

ST. RITA'S MEDICAL CENTER, 730 West Market Street, Lima, OH, Zip 45801-4670; tel. 419/227-3361; James P. Reber, President

VAN WERT COUNTY HOSPITAL, 1250 South Washington Street, Van Wert, OH, Zip 45891-2599; tel. 419/238-2390; Mark J. Minick, President and Chief Executive Officer

WILSON MEMORIAL HOSPITAL, 915 West Michigan Street, Sidney, OH, Zip 45365-2491; tel. 937/498-2311; Michael T. Moore, President and Chief Executive Officer

OKLAHOMA

COLUMBIA OKLAHOMA DIVISION, INC.
6501 North Broadway, Suite 200, Oklahoma City, OK 73116; tel. 405/879-0960; David Dunlap, President

COLUMBIA BETHANY HOSPITAL, 7600 N.W. 23rd Street, Bethany, OK, Zip 73008; tel. 405/787-3450; David Lundquist, Chief Executive Officer

COLUMBIA CLAREMORE REGIONAL HOSPITAL, 1202 North Muskogee Place, Claremore, OK, Zip 74017; tel. 918/341-2556; Ken Seidel, Executive Director

COLUMBIA DOCTORS HOSPITAL, 2323 South Harvard Avenue, Tulsa, OK, Zip 74114-3370; tel. 918/744-4000; Anthony R. Young, President and Chief Executive Officer

COLUMBIA EDMOND REGIONAL MEDICAL CENTER, 1 South Bryant Street, Edmond, OK, Zip 73034-4798; tel. 405/359-5530; Stanley D. Tatum, Chief Executive Officer

COLUMBIA PRESBYTERIAN HOSPITAL, 700 N.E. 13th Street, Oklahoma City, OK, Zip 73104-5070; tel. 405/271-5100; James O'Loughlin, Chief Executive Officer

COLUMBIA SOUTHWESTERN MEDICAL CENTER, 5602 S.W. Lee Boulevard, Lawton, OK, Zip 73505-9635, Mailing Address: P.O. Box 7290, Zip 73506-7290; tel. 405/531-4700; Thomas L. Rine, President and Chief Executive Officer

COLUMBIA TULSA REGIONAL MEDICAL CENTER, 744 West Ninth Street, Tulsa, OK, Zip 74127-9990; tel. 918/599-5900; James M. MacCallum, President and Chief Executive Officer

COLUMBIA WAGONER HOSPITAL, 1200 West Cherokee, Wagoner, OK, Zip 74467-4681, Mailing Address: Box 407, Zip 74477-0407; tel. 918/485-5514; John W. Crawford, Chief Executive Officer

EASTERN OKLAHOMA HEALTH NETWORK
P.O. Box 14147, Tulsa, OK 74114; tel. 918/579-1000; Thomas P. Hadley, Executive Vice President

COLUMBIA DOCTORS HOSPITAL, 2323 South Harvard Avenue, Tulsa, OK, Zip 74114-3370; tel. 918/744-4000; Anthony R. Young, President and Chief Executive Officer

COLUMBIA WAGONER HOSPITAL, 1200 West Cherokee, Wagoner, OK, Zip 74467-4681, Mailing Address: Box 407, Zip 74477-0407; tel. 918/485-5514; John W. Crawford, Chief Executive Officer

HILLCREST HEALTHCARE SYSTEM, 1120 South Utica, Tulsa, OK, Zip 74104-4090; tel. 918/579-1000; Donald A. Lorack, Jr., President and Chief Executive Officer

FIRST HEALTH WEST
4411 West Gore Boulevard, Lawton, OK 73505; tel. 405/355-8620; Tanya Case, Director of Networks

CARNEGIE TRI-COUNTY MUNICIPAL HOSPITAL, 102 North Broadway, Carnegie, OK, Zip 73015, Mailing Address: Box 97, Zip 73015; tel. 405/654-1050; Phil Hawkins, Administrator

COMANCHE COUNTY MEMORIAL HOSPITAL, 3401 Gore Boulevard, Lawton, OK, Zip 73505-0129, Mailing Address: Box 129, Zip 73502-0129; tel. 405/355-8620; Randy Curry, President

CORDELL MEMORIAL HOSPITAL, 1220 North Glenn English Street, Cordell, OK, Zip 73632; tel. 405/832-3339; Charles H. Greene, Jr., Administrator

ELKVIEW GENERAL HOSPITAL, 429 West Elm Street, Hobart, OK, Zip 73651-1699; tel. 405/726-3324; J. W. Finch, Jr., Administrator

HARMON MEMORIAL HOSPITAL, 400 East Chestnut Street, Hollis, OK, Zip 73550, Mailing Address: P.O. Box 791, Zip 73550; tel. 405/688-3363; Al Allee, Administrator

JEFFERSON COUNTY HOSPITAL, Waurika, OK, Mailing Address: P.O. Box 90, Zip 73573-0090; tel. 405/228-2344; Curtis R. Pryor, Administrator

SOUTHWESTERN MEMORIAL HOSPITAL, 215 North Kansas Street, Weatherford, OK, Zip 73096-5499; tel. 405/772-5551; Ronnie D. Walker, Administrator

HILLCREST HEALTHCARE SYSTEM
1120 South Utica Avenue, Tulsa, OK 74104-4090; tel. 918/579-1000; Donald A. Lorack, Jr, President & Chief Executive Officer

CHILDREN'S MEDICAL CENTER, 5300 East Skelly Drive, Tulsa, OK, Zip 74135-6599, Mailing Address: Box 35648, Zip 74153-0648; tel. 918/664-6600; Gerard J. Rothlein, Jr., President and Chief Executive Officer

CUSHING REGIONAL HOSPITAL, 1027 East Cherry, Cushing, OK, Zip 74023, Mailing Address: Box 1409, Zip 74023-1409; tel. 918/225-2915; Ron Cackler, President and Chief Executive Officer

EASTERN OKLAHOMA MEDICAL CENTER, 105 Wall Street, Poteau, OK, Zip 74953, Mailing Address: P.O. Box 1148, Zip 74953; tel. 918/647-8161; Bobby D. Cox, Chief Executive Officer

HILLCREST HEALTHCARE SYSTEM, 1120 South Utica, Tulsa, OK, Zip 74104-4090; tel. 918/579-1000; Donald A. Lorack, Jr., President and Chief Executive Officer

INTEGRIS HEALTH
3366 Northwest Expressway, Oklahoma City, OK 73112; tel. 405/949-6066; Stanley Hupfeld, President & Chief Executive Officer

BLACKWELL REGIONAL HOSPITAL, 710 South 13th Street, Blackwell, OK, Zip 74631; tel. 405/363-2311; Greg Martin, Administrator and Chief Executive Officer

BRISTOW MEMORIAL HOSPITAL, Seventh and Spruce Streets, Bristow, OK, Zip 74010, Mailing Address: Box 780, Zip 74010; tel. 918/367-2215; William L. Legate, Administrator

CHOCTAW MEMORIAL HOSPITAL, 1405 East Kirk Road, Hugo, OK, Zip 74743; tel. 405/326-6414; Michael R. Morel, Administrator

DRUMRIGHT MEMORIAL HOSPITAL, 501 South Lou Allard Drive, Drumright, OK, Zip 74030–4899; tel. 918/352–2525; Jerry Jones, Administrator

INTEGRIS BAPTIST MEDICAL CENTER, 3300 N.W. Expressway, Oklahoma City, OK, Zip 73112–4481; tel. 405/949–3011; Thomas R. Rice, President and Chief Operation Officer

INTEGRIS BAPTIST REGIONAL HEALTH CENTER, 200 Second Street S.W., Miami, OK, Zip 74354, Mailing Address: Box 1207, Zip 74355–1207; tel. 918/540–7100; Dee Renshaw, Administrator

INTEGRIS BASS BAPTIST HEALTH CENTER, 600 South Monroe, Enid, OK, Zip 73701, Mailing Address: Box 3168, Zip 73702; tel. 405/233–2300; W. Eugene Baxter, Dr.PH, Administrator

INTEGRIS GROVE GENERAL HOSPITAL, 1310 South Main Street, Grove, OK, Zip 74344–1310; tel. 918/786–2243; Dee Renshaw, Administrator

INTEGRIS SOUTHWEST MEDICAL CENTER, 4401 South Western, Oklahoma City, OK, Zip 73109–3441; tel. 405/636–7000; Thomas R. Rice, President and Chief Operation Officer

MARSHALL MEMORIAL HOSPITAL, 1 Hospital Drive, Madill, OK, Zip 73446, Mailing Address: P.O. Box 827, Zip 73446; tel. 405/795–3384; Norma Howard, Administrator

MAYES COUNTY MEDICAL CENTER, 129 North Kentucky, Pryor, OK, Zip 74361, Mailing Address: Box 278, Zip 74362–0278; tel. 918/825–1600; W. Charles Jordan, Administrator

PAWNEE MUNICIPAL HOSPITAL, 1212 Fourth Street, Pawnee, OK, Zip 74058, Mailing Address: Box 467, Zip 74058; tel. 918/762–2577; John Ketring, Administrator

STROUD MUNICIPAL HOSPITAL, Highway 66 West, Stroud, OK, Zip 74079, Mailing Address: P.O. Box 530, Zip 74079; tel. 918/968–3571; Jerrell J. Horton, Chief Executive Officer

MERCY HEALTH SYSTEM
4300 West Memorial Road, Oklahoma City, OK 73120; tel. 405/752–3754; Bruce F. Buchanan, President & Chief Executive Officer

MERCY HEALTH CENTER, 4300 West Memorial Road, Oklahoma City, OK, Zip 73120–8362; tel. 405/755–1515; Bruce F. Buchanan, FACHE, President and Chief Executive Officer

MERCY MEMORIAL HEALTH CENTER, 1011 14th Street N.W., Ardmore, OK, Zip 73401–1889; tel. 405/223–5400; Bobby G. Thompson, President and Chief Executive Officer

ST. MARY'S MERCY HOSPITAL, 305 South Fifth Street, Enid, OK, Zip 73701–5899, Mailing Address: Box 232, Zip 73702–0232; tel. 405/233–6100; Frank Lopez, President and Chief Executive Officer

UNIVERSITY HOSPITALS
P.O. Box 26307, Oklahoma City, OK 73126; tel. 405/271–5911; R. Tim Cousson, MD, Chief Executive Officer

THE UNIVERSITY HOSPITALS, 920 N.E. 13th Street, Oklahoma City, OK, Zip 73104–5068, Mailing Address: P.O. Box 26307, Zip 73126; tel. 405/271–5911; R. Timothy Coussons, M.D., President and Chief Executive Officer

OREGON

CENTRAL OREGON HOSP NETWORK (CONET)
2500 NorthEast Neff Road, Bend, OR 97701; tel. 541/388–7702; James T. Lussier, Chief Executive Officer

BLUE MOUNTAIN HOSPITAL, 170 Ford Road, John Day, OR, Zip 97845; tel. 541/575–1311; David G. Triebes, Administrator

CENTRAL OREGON DISTRICT HOSPITAL, 1253 North Canal Boulevard, Redmond, OR, Zip 97756–1395; tel. 541/548–8131; James A. Diegel, CHE, Executive Director

HARNEY DISTRICT HOSPITAL, 557 West Washington Street, Burns, OR, Zip 97720–1497; tel. 503/573–7281; David L. Harman, Administrator

LAKE DISTRICT HOSPITAL, 700 South J Street, Lakeview, OR, Zip 97630–1679; tel. 503/947–2114; Richard T. Moore, Administrator

MOUNTAIN VIEW HOSPITAL DISTRICT, 470 N.E. A Street, Madras, OR, Zip 97741; tel. 541/475–3882; Ronald W. Barnes, Executive Director

PIONEER MEMORIAL HOSPITAL, 1201 North Elm Street, Prineville, OR, Zip 97754; tel. 541/447–6254; Donald J. Wee, Executive Director

ST. CHARLES MEDICAL CENTER, 2500 N.E. Neff Road, Bend, OR, Zip 97701–6015; tel. 541/382–4321; James T. Lussier, President and Chief Executive Officer

HEALTH FUTURE, INC.
825 East Main Street, Suite D, Medford, OR 97504; tel. 503/772–3062; John Meenaghan, Executive Director

ALBANY GENERAL HOSPITAL, 1046 West Sixth Avenue, Albany, OR, Zip 97321–1999; tel. 541/812–4000; Richard J. Delano, President

ASHLAND COMMUNITY HOSPITAL, 280 Maple Street, Ashland, OR, Zip 97520, Mailing Address: P.O. Box 98, Zip 97520; tel. 541/482–2441; James R. Watson, Administrator

BAY AREA HOSPITAL, 1775 Thompson Road, Coos Bay, OR, Zip 97420–2198; tel. 541/269–8111; Dale Jessup, President and Chief Executive Officer

COLUMBIA DOUGLAS MEDICAL CENTER, 738 West Harvard Boulevard, Roseburg, OR, Zip 97470–2996; tel. 541/673–6641; Christopher L. Boyd, Chief Executive Officer

COLUMBIA MEMORIAL HOSPITAL, 2111 Exchange Street, Astoria, OR, Zip 97103; tel. 503/325–4321; Terry O. Finklein, Chief Executive Officer

GOOD SAMARITAN HOSPITAL CORVALLIS, 3600 N.W. Samaritan Drive, Corvallis, OR, Zip 97330, Mailing Address: P.O. Box 1068, Zip 97339; tel. 541/757–5111; Larry A. Mullins, President and Chief Executive Officer

GOOD SHEPHERD COMMUNITY HOSPITAL, 610 N.W. 11th Street, Hermiston, OR, Zip 97838–9696; tel. 541/567–6483; Dennis E. Burke, Chief Executive Officer

GRANDE RONDE HOSPITAL, 900 Sunset Drive, La Grande, OR, Zip 97850, Mailing Address: P.O. Box 3290, Zip 97850; tel. 541/963–8421; James A. Mattes, President

LEBANON COMMUNITY HOSPITAL, 525 North Santiam Highway, Lebanon, OR, Zip 97355, Mailing Address: P.O. Box 739, Zip 97355–0739; tel. 541/258–2101; Alan R. Yordy, Chief Executive Officer

MERCY MEDICAL CENTER, 2700 Stewart Parkway, Roseburg, OR, Zip 97470–1297; tel. 541/673–0611; Victor J. Fresolone, FACHE, President and Chief Executive Officer

MERLE WEST MEDICAL CENTER, 2865 Daggett Street, Klamath Falls, OR, Zip 97601–1180; tel. 541/882–6311; Paul R. Stewart, President and Chief Executive Officer

MID–COLUMBIA MEDICAL CENTER, 1700 East 19th Street, The Dalles, OR, Zip 97058–3316; tel. 541/296–1111; Mark D. Scott, President

ROGUE VALLEY MEDICAL CENTER, 2825 East Barnett Road, Medford, OR, Zip 97504–8332; tel. 541/608–4900; Gary A. Sherwood, Executive Vice President

SILVERTON HOSPITAL, 342 Fairview Street, Silverton, OR, Zip 97381; tel. 503/873–1500; William E. Winter, Administrative Director

ST. CHARLES MEDICAL CENTER, 2500 N.E. Neff Road, Bend, OR, Zip 97701–6015; tel. 541/382–4321; James T. Lussier, President and Chief Executive Officer

THREE RIVERS COMMUNITY HOSPITAL AND HEALTH CENTER–DIMMICK, 715 N.W. Dimmick Street, Grants Pass, OR, Zip 97526–1596; tel. 541/476–6831; John F. Bringhurst, Executive Vice President

UNIVERSITY HOSPITAL, 3181 S.W. Sam Jackson Park Road, Portland, OR, Zip 97201–3098; tel. 503/494–8311; Roy G. Vinyard, Chief Administrative Officer

INTER COMMUNITY HEALTH NETWORK
3600 North Samaritan Drive, Corvallis, OR 97339; tel. 503/757–5111; Larry Mullins, Chairman

ALBANY GENERAL HOSPITAL, 1046 West Sixth Avenue, Albany, OR, Zip 97321–1999; tel. 541/812–4000; Richard J. Delano, President

GOOD SAMARITAN HOSPITAL CORVALLIS, 3600 N.W. Samaritan Drive, Corvallis, OR, Zip 97330, Mailing Address: P.O. Box 1068, Zip 97339; tel. 541/757–5111; Larry A. Mullins, President and Chief Executive Officer

LEBANON COMMUNITY HOSPITAL, 525 North Santiam Highway, Lebanon, OR, Zip 97355, Mailing Address: P.O. Box 739, Zip 97355–0739; tel. 541/258–2101; Alan R. Yordy, Chief Executive Officer

LEGACY HEALTH SYSTEM
1919 NorthWest Lovejoy Street, Portland, OR 97209; tel. 503/415–8600; John G. King, President & Chief Executive Officer

LEGACY EMANUEL HOSPITAL AND HEALTH CENTER, 2801 North Gantenbein Avenue, Portland, OR, Zip 97227–1674; tel. 503/413–2200; Lowell W. Johnson, Interim President and Chief Executive Officer

LEGACY GOOD SAMARITAN HOSPITAL AND MEDICAL CENTER, 1015 N.W. 22nd Avenue, Portland, OR, Zip 97210; tel. 503/413–7711; Lowell W. Johnson, Interim President and Chief Executive Officer

LEGACY MERIDIAN PARK HOSPITAL, 19300 S.W. 65th Avenue, Tualatin, OR, Zip 97062–9741; tel. 503/692–1212; Jeff Cushing, Vice President, Administration

LEGACY MOUNT HOOD MEDICAL CENTER, 24800 S.E. Stark, Gresham, OR, Zip 97030–0154; tel. 503/667–1122; Jane C. Cummins, President and Chief Executive Officer

OREGON HEALTH SYSTEM IN COLLABORATION
4000 Kruse Way Place B2–100, Lake Oswego, OR 97035; tel. 503/636–2204; Kent Ballantyne, Project Coordinator

KAISER SUNNYSIDE MEDICAL CENTER, 10200 S.E. Sunnyside Road, Clackamas, OR, Zip 97015–9303; tel. 503/652–2880; Alide Chase, Administrator

LEGACY EMANUEL HOSPITAL AND HEALTH CENTER, 2801 North Gantenbein Avenue, Portland, OR, Zip 97227–1674; tel. 503/413–2200; Lowell W. Johnson, Interim President and Chief Executive Officer

LEGACY GOOD SAMARITAN HOSPITAL AND MEDICAL CENTER, 1015 N.W. 22nd Avenue, Portland, OR, Zip 97210; tel. 503/413–7711; Lowell W. Johnson, Interim President and Chief Executive Officer

LEGACY MERIDIAN PARK HOSPITAL, 19300 S.W. 65th Avenue, Tualatin, OR, Zip 97062–9741; tel. 503/692–1212; Jeff Cushing, Vice President, Administration

LEGACY MOUNT HOOD MEDICAL CENTER, 24800 S.E. Stark, Gresham, OR, Zip 97030–0154; tel. 503/667–1122; Jane C. Cummins, President and Chief Executive Officer

PROVIDENCE MEDFORD MEDICAL CENTER, 1111 Crater Lake Avenue, Medford, OR, Zip 97504–6241; tel. 541/732–5000; Charles T. Wright, Chief Executive, Southern Oregon Service Area

PROVIDENCE MILWAUKIE HOSPITAL, 10150 S.E. 32nd Avenue, Milwaukie, OR, Zip 97222–6593; tel. 503/652–8300; Janice Burger, Operations Administrator

PROVIDENCE NEWBERG HOSPITAL, 501 Villa Road, Newberg, OR, Zip 97132; tel. 503/537–1555; Mark W. Meinert, CHE, Chief Executive, Yamhill Service Area

PROVIDENCE PORTLAND MEDICAL CENTER, 4805 N.E. Glisan Street, Portland, OR, Zip 97213–2967; tel. 503/215–1111; David T. Underriner, Operations Administrator

PROVIDENCE SEASIDE HOSPITAL, 725 South Wahanna Road, Seaside, OR, Zip 97138–7735; tel. 503/717–7000; Ronald Swanson, Chief Executive North Coast Service Area

PROVIDENCE ST. VINCENT MEDICAL CENTER, 9205 S.W. Barnes Road, Portland, OR, Zip 97225–6661; tel. 503/216–1234; Donald Elsom, Operations Administrator

PROVIDENCE HEALTH SYSTEM
1235 NorthEast 47th Avenue, Portland, OR 97213; tel. 503/215–4700; John Lee, Regional Vice President

PROVIDENCE MEDFORD MEDICAL CENTER, 1111 Crater Lake Avenue, Medford, OR, Zip 97504–6241; tel. 541/732–5000; Charles T. Wright, Chief Executive, Southern Oregon Service Area

PROVIDENCE MILWAUKIE HOSPITAL, 10150 S.E. 32nd Avenue, Milwaukie, OR, Zip 97222–6593; tel. 503/652–8300; Janice Burger, Operations Administrator

PROVIDENCE NEWBERG HOSPITAL, 501 Villa Road, Newberg, OR, Zip 97132; tel. 503/537–1555; Mark W. Meinert, CHE, Chief Executive, Yamhill Service Area

PROVIDENCE PORTLAND MEDICAL CENTER, 4805 N.E. Glisan Street, Portland, OR, Zip 97213–2967; tel. 503/215–1111; David T. Underriner, Operations Administrator

PROVIDENCE SEASIDE HOSPITAL, 725 South Wahanna Road, Seaside, OR, Zip 97138–7735; tel. 503/717–7000; Ronald Swanson, Chief Executive North Coast Service Area

PROVIDENCE ST. VINCENT MEDICAL CENTER, 9205 S.W. Barnes Road, Portland, OR, Zip 97225–6661; tel. 503/216–1234; Donald Elsom, Operations Administrator

PENNSYLVANIA

ALBERT EINSTEIN HEALTHCARE NETWORK
5501 Old York Road, Philadelphia, PA 19141–3098; tel. 215/456–7890; Martin Goldsmith, President & Chief Executive Officer

ALBERT EINSTEIN MEDICAL CENTER, 5501 Old York Road, Philadelphia, PA, Zip 19141–3098; tel. 215/456–7890; Martin Goldsmith, President

BELMONT CENTER FOR COMPREHENSIVE TREATMENT, 4200 Monument Road, Philadelphia, PA, Zip 19131–1689; tel. 215/877–2000; Jack H. Dembow, General Director and Vice President

ALPHA HEALTH NETWORK
Foster Plaza, Pittsburgh, PA 15220; tel. 412/937–1396; Rich Chiocchi, Network Contact

ST. CLAIR MEMORIAL HOSPITAL, 1000 Bower Hill Road, Pittsburgh, PA, Zip 15243; tel. 412/561–4900; Benjamin E. Snead, President

COMMUNITY BENEFITS STRATEGY
P.O. Box 447, DuBois, PA 15801; tel. 814/375–3495; Diane Skroba, Public Relations Manager

DUBOIS REGIONAL MEDICAL CENTER, 100 Hospital Avenue, DuBois, PA, Zip 15801, Mailing Address: P.O. Box 447, Zip 15801–0447; tel. 814/371–2200; Raymond A. Graeca, President and Chief Executive Officer

COMMUNITY HEALTH NET
1202 State Street, Erie, PA 16501; tel. 814/454–4530; Darleen Collen, Chief Executive Officer

HAMOT MEDICAL CENTER, 201 State Street, Erie, PA, Zip 16550–0001; tel. 814/877–6000; John T. Malone, President and Chief Executive Officer

METRO HEALTH CENTER, 252 West 11th Street, Erie, PA, Zip 16501; tel. 814/870–3400; J. B. Frith, Chief Executive Officer

SAINT VINCENT HEALTH CENTER, 232 West 25th Street, Erie, PA, Zip 16544; tel. 814/452–5000; Sister Catherine Manning, President and Chief Executive Officer

CROZER–KEYSTONE HEALTH SYSTEM
1400 North Providence Road, Media, PA 19063; tel. 610/892–8000; John C. McMeekin, President & Chief Executive Officer

CROZER–CHESTER MEDICAL CENTER, One Medical Center Boulevard, Upland, PA, Zip 19013–3995; tel. 610/447–2000; Joan K. Richards, President

DELAWARE COUNTY MEMORIAL HOSPITAL, 501 North Lansdowne Avenue, Drexel Hill, PA, Zip 19026–1186; tel. 610/284–8100; Joan K. Richards, President

FIRST HEALTH ALLIANCE
10 Duff Road, Suite 211, Pittsburgh, PA 15235; tel. 412/243–2940; Don Hutchinson, President

JEANNETTE DISTRICT MEMORIAL HOSPITAL, 600 Jefferson Avenue, Jeannette, PA, Zip 15644; tel. 412/527–3551; Robert J. Bulger, President and Chief Executive Officer

FOX CHASE NETWORK
8 Huntingdon Pike, 3rd Floor, Rockledge, PA 19046; tel. 215/728–4773; Susan A. Higman, Vice President

DELAWARE COUNTY MEMORIAL HOSPITAL, 501 North Lansdowne Avenue, Drexel Hill, PA, Zip 19026–1186; tel. 610/284–8100; Joan K. Richards, President

FOX CHASE CANCER CENTER–AMERICAN ONCOLOGIC HOSPITAL, 7701 Burholme Avenue, Philadelphia, PA, Zip 19111; tel. 215/728–6900; Robert C. Young, M.D., President

HUNTERDON MEDICAL CENTER, 2100 Wescott Drive, Flemington, NJ, Zip 08822–4604; tel. 908/788–6100; Robert P. Wise, President and Chief Executive Officer

MONTGOMERY HOSPITAL, 1301 Powell Street, Norristown, PA, Zip 19404, Mailing Address: P.O. Box 992, Zip 19404–0992; tel. 610/270–2000; Timothy M. Casey, President and Chief Executive Officer

NORTH PENN HOSPITAL, 100 Medical Campus Drive, Lansdale, PA, Zip 19446–1200; tel. 215/368–2100; Robert H. McKay, President

PAOLI MEMORIAL HOSPITAL, 255 West Lancaster Avenue, Paoli, PA, Zip 19301–1792; tel. 610/648–1204; Gail A. Egan, Vice President, Administrator

PINNACLEHEALTH AT POLYCLINIC HOSPITAL, 2601 North Third Street, Harrisburg, PA, Zip 17110–2098; tel. 717/782–4141; Stephen H. Franklin, FACHE, President and Chief Executive Officer

READING HOSPITAL AND MEDICAL CENTER, Sixth Avenue and Spruce Street, Reading, PA, Zip 19611, Mailing Address: P.O. Box 16052, Zip 19612–6052; tel. 610/378–6000; Charles Sullivan, President and Chief Executive Officer

RIVERVIEW MEDICAL CENTER, 1 Riverview Plaza, Red Bank, NJ, Zip 07701–9982; tel. 908/741–2700; Paul S. Cohen, Executive Director and Chief Operating Officer

SHADYSIDE HOSPITAL, 5230 Centre Avenue, Pittsburgh, PA, Zip 15232–1304; tel. 412/623–2121; Henry A. Mordoh, President

SOUTH JERSEY HOSPITAL, 333 Irving Avenue, Bridgeton, NJ, Zip 08302–2100; tel. 609/451–6600; Paul S. Cooper, Chief Executive Officer

ST. FRANCIS MEDICAL CENTER, 601 Hamilton Avenue, Trenton, NJ, Zip 08629–1986; tel. 609/599–5000; Judith M. Persichilli, President and Chief Executive Officer

ST. LUKE'S HOSPITAL, 801 Ostrum Street, Bethlehem, PA, Zip 18015–1014; tel. 610/954–4000; Richard A. Anderson, President

ST. MARY MEDICAL CENTER, Langhorne–Newtown Road, Langhorne, PA, Zip 19047–1295; tel. 215/750–2000; Sister Clare Carty, President and Chief Executive Officer

GEISINGER HEALTH SYSTEM
100 North Academy Avenue, Danville, PA 17822; tel. 717/271–6211; Frank J. Trembulak, Executive Vice President & COO

GEISINGER MEDICAL CENTER, 100 North Academy Avenue, Danville, PA, Zip 17822–2201; tel. 717/271–6211; Stuart Heydt, Chief Executive Officer

GEISINGER WYOMING VALLEY MEDICAL CENTER, 1000 East Mountain Drive, Wilkes–Barre, PA, Zip 18711–0025; tel. 717/826–7300; Conrad W. Schintz, Senior Vice President Operations

GREAT LAKES HEALTH NETWORK
201 State Street, Erie, PA 16550; tel. 814/877–7053; Andrew J. Glass, President

ASHTABULA COUNTY MEDICAL CENTER, 2420 Lake Avenue, Ashtabula, OH, Zip 44004–4993; tel. 216/997–2262; R. D. Richardson, President and Chief Executive Officer

BLANCHARD VALLEY REGIONAL HEALTH CENTER, 145 West Wallace Street, Findlay, OH, Zip 45840–1299; tel. 419/423–4500; Clifford R. Lehman, Chief Executive Officer

BRADFORD REGIONAL MEDICAL CENTER, 116–156 Interstate Parkway, Bradford, PA, Zip 16701–0218; tel. 814/368–4143; George E. Leonhardt, President and Chief Executive Officer

BROWN MEMORIAL HOSPITAL, 158 West Main Road, Conneaut, OH, Zip 44030–2039, Mailing Address: P.O. Box 648, Zip 44030; tel. 216/593–1131; C. Thomas Moore, Chief Executive Officer

CORRY MEMORIAL HOSPITAL, 612 West Smith Street, Corry, PA, Zip 16407–1196; tel. 814/664–4641; Joseph T. Hodges, President

HAMOT MEDICAL CENTER, 201 State Street, Erie, PA, Zip 16550–0001; tel. 814/877–6000; John T. Malone, President and Chief Executive Officer

ST. MARYS REGIONAL MEDICAL CENTER, 763 Johnsonburg Road, Saint Marys, PA, Zip 15857–3417; tel. 814/781–7500; John N. Christenson, President

WOMAN'S CHRISTIAN ASSOCIATION HOSPITAL, 207 Foote Avenue, Jamestown, NY, Zip 14702–9975; tel. 716/487–0141; Mark E. Celmer, President and Chief Executive Officer

GUTHRIE HEALTHCARE SYSTEM
One Guthrie Square, Sayre, PA 18840; tel. 717/882–6666; Antionette Arnold, Adminstrative Resident

ROBERT PACKER HOSPITAL, Guthrie Square, Sayre, PA, Zip 18840; tel. 717/888–6666; Russell M. Knight, President

TROY COMMUNITY HOSPITAL, 100 John Street, Troy, PA, Zip 16947; tel. 717/297–2121; Mark A. Webster, President

HEALTH SHARE
111 South 11th Street, Philadelphia, PA 19107; tel. 215/955–6000; Carmhill Brown, Associate Vice President of Marketing

THOMAS JEFFERSON UNIVERSITY HOSPITAL, 111 South 11th Street, Philadelphia, PA, Zip 19107–5098; tel. 215/955–7022; Thomas J. Lewis, President and Chief Executive Officer

JEFFERSON HEALTH SYSTEM
259 Radnor–Chestnut Road, Radnor, PA 19087; tel. 610/225–6200; Douglas S. Peters, President & Chief Executive Officer

BRYN MAWR HOSPITAL, 130 South Bryn Mawr Avenue, Bryn Mawr, PA, Zip 19010–3160; tel. 610/526–3000; William McCune, Vice President, Administration

BRYN MAWR REHABILITATION HOSPITAL, 414 Paoli Pike, Malvern, PA, Zip 19355–3300, Mailing Address: P.O. Box 3007, Zip 19355–3300; tel. 610/251–5400; Barry S. Rabner, President

LANKENAU HOSPITAL, 100 Lancaster Avenue West, Wynnewood, PA, Zip 19096; tel. 610/645–2000; Kenneth Hanover, President and Chief Executive Officer

METHODIST HOSPITAL, 2301 South Broad Street, Philadelphia, PA, Zip 19148; tel. 215/952–9000

PAOLI MEMORIAL HOSPITAL, 255 West Lancaster Avenue, Paoli, PA, Zip 19301–1792; tel. 610/648–1204; Gail A. Egan, Vice President, Administrator

THOMAS JEFFERSON UNIVERSITY HOSPITAL, 111 South 11th Street, Philadelphia, PA, Zip 19107–5098; tel. 215/955–7022; Thomas J. Lewis, President and Chief Executive Officer

LAUREL HEALTH SYSTEM
15 Meade Street, Wellsboro, PA 16901–1813; tel. 717/723–0501; Robert Morris, President & Chief Executive Officer

SOLDIERS AND SAILORS MEMORIAL HOSPITAL, 32–36 Central Avenue, Wellsboro, PA, Zip 16901–1899; tel. 717/723–7764; Ronald J. Butler, Executive Director

PARTNERSHIP FOR COMMUNITY HEALTH–LEHIGH VALLEY
P.O. Box 689, Allentown, PA 18105; tel. 610/954–7550; Leo Conners, Chairman

SACRED HEART HOSPITAL, Fourth and Chew Streets, Allentown, PA, Zip 18102–3490; tel. 610/776–4500; Joseph M. Cimerola, FACHE, President and Chief Executive Officer

PRIME CARE
2601 North 3rd Street, Harrisburg, PA 17110; tel. 717/782–4141; Alan Davidson, President

PINNACLEHEALTH AT POLYCLINIC HOSPITAL, 2601 North Third Street, Harrisburg, PA, Zip 17110–2098; tel. 717/782–4141; Stephen H. Franklin, FACHE, President and Chief Executive Officer

PROVIDENCE HEALTH SYSTEM
1100 Grampian Boulevard, Williamsport, PA 17701; tel. 717/326–8181; Anthony W. Deobil, President

MUNCY VALLEY HOSPITAL, 215 East Water Street, Muncy, PA, Zip 17756–8700; tel. 717/546–8282; Steven P. Johnson, Senior Vice President/Chief Operating Officer

WILLIAMSPORT HOSPITAL AND MEDICAL CENTER, 777 Rural Avenue, Williamsport, PA, Zip 17701–3198; tel. 717/321–1000; Steven P. Johnson, Senior Vice President and Chief Operating Officer Hospitals and LTC Operations

SACRED HEART HEALTH CARE SYSTEM
421 Chew Street, Allentown, PA 18102; tel. 610/776–4500; Joseph M. Cimerola, FACHE

SACRED HEART HOSPITAL, Fourth and Chew Streets, Allentown, PA, Zip 18102–3490; tel. 610/776–4500; Joseph M. Cimerola, FACHE, President and Chief Executive Officer

SAINT FRANCIS HEALTH SYSTEM
4410 Penn Avenue, Pittsburgh, PA 15224; tel. 412/622–4214; Sister M. Rosita Wellinger, President and Chief Executive Officer

ST. FRANCIS CENTRAL HOSPITAL, 1200 Centre Avenue, Pittsburgh, PA, Zip 15219–3594; tel. 412/562–3000; Robin Z. Mohr, Chief Executive Officer

ST. FRANCIS HOSPITAL OF NEW CASTLE, 1000 South Mercer Street, New Castle, PA, Zip 16101–4673; tel. 412/658–3511; Sister Donna Zwigart, Chief Executive Officer

SAINT VINCENT HEALTH SYSTEM
232 West 25th Street, Erie, PA 16544; tel. 814/452–5000; Dorothy Law, Program Leader Mrktng & Communications

SAINT VINCENT HEALTH CENTER, 232 West 25th Street, Erie, PA, Zip 16544; tel. 814/452–5000; Sister Catherine Manning, President and Chief Executive Officer

UNION CITY MEMORIAL HOSPITAL, 130 North Main Street, Union City, PA, Zip 16438, Mailing Address: P.O. Box 111, Zip 16438; tel. 814/438–1000; Thomas McLoughlin, President

SOUTHWEST INTEGRATED DELIVERY NETWORK
501 Holiday Drive, Pittsburgh, PA 15220; tel. 412/937–1396; Annette Fetchko, Vice President, Network Development

ALLEGHENY VALLEY HOSPITAL, 1301 Carlisle Street, Natrona Heights, PA, Zip 15065–1192; tel. 412/224–5100; John R. England, President and Chief Executive Officer

SEWICKLEY VALLEY HOSPITAL, (A DIVISION OF VALLEY MEDICAL FACILITIES), 720 Blackburn Road, Sewickley, PA, Zip 15143–1498; tel. 412/741–6600; Donald W. Spalding, President

ST. CLAIR MEMORIAL HOSPITAL, 1000 Bower Hill Road, Pittsburgh, PA, Zip 15243; tel. 412/561–4900; Benjamin E. Snead, President

TEMPLE UNIVERSITY HEALTH NETWORK
3401 North Broad St., 1st FL Parkinson, Philadelphia, PA 19140; tel. 215/707–8000; Leon S. Malmud, M.D., President

JEANES HOSPITAL, 7600 Central Avenue, Philadelphia, PA, Zip 19111–2499; tel. 215/728–2000; G. Roger Martin, President and Chief Executive Officer

LOWER BUCKS HOSPITAL, 501 Bath Road, Bristol, PA, Zip 19007–3190; tel. 215/785–9200; Nathan Bosk, FACHE, Chief Executive Officer

NEUMANN MEDICAL CENTER, 1741 Frankford Avenue, Philadelphia, PA, Zip 19125–2495; tel. 215/291–2000; Joseph C. Hare, President and Chief Executive Officer

NORTHEASTERN HOSPITAL OF PHILADELPHIA, 2301 East Allegheny Avenue, Philadelphia, PA, Zip 19134–4499; tel. 215/291–3000; Jeffrey L. Susi, Executive Director and Chief Executive Officer

TEMPLE UNIVERSITY HOSPITAL, Broad and Ontario Streets, Philadelphia, PA, Zip 19140–5192; tel. 215/707–2000; Paul Boehringer, Executive Director

TRI-STATE NETWORK
81 Highland Avenue, Pittsburgh, PA 15213; tel. 412/692–7107; Nanci Case, Director of Planning/Marketing

CHILDREN'S HOSPITAL OF PITTSBURGH, 3705 Fifth Avenue at De Soto Street, Pittsburgh, PA, Zip 15213–2583; tel. 412/692–5325; Paul S. Kramer, President and Chief Executive Officer

MAGEE–WOMENS HOSPITAL, 300 Halket Street, Pittsburgh, PA, Zip 15213–3180; tel. 412/641–1000; Irma E. Goertzen, President and Chief Executive Officer

SOUTH HILLS HEALTH SYSTEM, Coal Valley Road, Pittsburgh, PA, Zip 15236–0119, Mailing Address: Box 18119, Zip 15236–0119; tel. 412/469–5000; William R. Jennings, President

UNIVERSITY OF PITTSBURGH MEDICAL CENTER, Pittsburgh, PA, Jeffrey A. Romoff, President

UNIVERSITY OF PITTSBURGH MEDICAL CENTER, ST. MARGARET, 815 Freeport Road, Pittsburgh, PA, Zip 15215–3399; tel. 412/784–4000; Stanley J. Kevish, President

UNIVERSITY OF PENNSYLVANIA HEALTH SYSTEM
21 Penn Tower, 399 South 34th Street, Philadelphia, PA 19104; tel. 215/898–5181; William N. Kelley, M.D., Chief Executive Officer

HOSPITAL OF THE UNIVERSITY OF PENNSYLVANIA, 3400 Spruce Street, Philadelphia, PA, Zip 19104–4283; tel. 215/662–4000; William T. Foley, Senior Vice President

PRESBYTERIAN MEDICAL CENTER OF THE UNIVERSITY OF PENNSYLVANIA HEALTH SYSTEM, 51 North 39th Street, Philadelphia, PA, Zip 19104–2699; tel. 215/662–8000; Michele M. Volpe, Chief Operating Officer

UNIVERSITY OF PITTSBURGH MEDICAL CENTER
3811 O'Hara Street, Pittsburgh, PA 15213; tel. 412/647–3000; Jeffrey Romoff, President

CHILDREN'S HOSPITAL OF PITTSBURGH, 3705 Fifth Avenue at De Soto Street, Pittsburgh, PA, Zip 15213–2583; tel. 412/692–5325; Paul S. Kramer, President and Chief Executive Officer

MAGEE–WOMENS HOSPITAL, 300 Halket Street, Pittsburgh, PA, Zip 15213–3180; tel. 412/641–1000; Irma E. Goertzen, President and Chief Executive Officer

UNIVERSITY OF PITTSBURGH MEDICAL CENTER, Pittsburgh, PA, Jeffrey A. Romoff, President

UNIVERSITY OF PITTSBURGH MEDICAL CENTER, ST. MARGARET, 815 Freeport Road, Pittsburgh, PA, Zip 15215–3399; tel. 412/784–4000; Stanley J. Kevish, President

WASHINGTON HOSPITAL, 155 Wilson Avenue, Washington, PA, Zip 15301–9986; tel. 412/225–7000; Telford W. Thomas, President and Chief Executive Officer

VANTAGE HEALTH CARE NETWORK, INC.
265 Conneaut Lake Road, Meadville, PA 16335; tel. 814/337–0000; Gerald P. Alonge, Executive Director

HORIZON HOSPITAL SYSTEM, Greenville, PA, J. Larry Heinike, President and Chief Executive Officer

MEADVILLE MEDICAL CENTER, 751 Liberty Street, Meadville, PA, Zip 16335; tel. 814/333–5000; Anthony J. DeFail, President and Chief Executive Officer

MILLCREEK COMMUNITY HOSPITAL, 5515 Peach Street, Erie, PA, Zip 16509–2695; tel. 814/864–4031; Mary L. Eckert, President and Chief Executive Officer

NORTHWEST MEDICAL CENTER, 1 Spruce Street, Franklin, PA, Zip 16323, Mailing Address: P.O. Box 1068, Oil City, Zip 16301; tel. 814/437–7000; Neil E. Todhunter, Chief Executive Officer

SAINT VINCENT HEALTH CENTER, 232 West 25th Street, Erie, PA, Zip 16544; tel. 814/452–5000; Sister Catherine Manning, President and Chief Executive Officer

TITUSVILLE AREA HOSPITAL, 406 West Oak Street, Titusville, PA, Zip 16354; tel. 814/827–1851; Anthony J. Nasralla, FACHE, President and Chief Executive Officer

WARREN GENERAL HOSPITAL, 2 Crescent Park West, Warren, PA, Zip 16365; tel. 814/723–3300; Alton M. Schadt, Executive Director

RHODE ISLAND

CARE NEW ENGLAND HEALTH SYSTEM
45 Willard Avenue, Providence, RI 02905; tel. 401/453–7900; John J. Hynes, Esq., President and Chief Executive Officer

BUTLER HOSPITAL, 345 Blackstone Boulevard, Providence, RI, Zip 02906–4829; tel. 401/455–6200; Frank A. Delmonico, President and Chief Executive Officer

KENT COUNTY MEMORIAL HOSPITAL, 455 Tollgate Road, Warwick, RI, Zip 02886–2770; tel. 401/737–7000; Robert E. Baute, M.D., President and Chief Executive Officer

WOMEN AND INFANTS HOSPITAL OF RHODE ISLAND, 101 Dudley Street, Providence, RI, Zip 02905–2499; tel. 401/274–1100; Thomas G. Parris, Jr., President

LIFESPAN
167 Point Street, Coro Building, Providence, RI 02903; tel. 401/444–2023; Joseph S. Lubiner, Network Contact

EMMA PENDLETON BRADLEY HOSPITAL, 1011 Veterans Memorial Parkway, East Providence, RI, Zip 02915–5099; tel. 401/434–3400; Daniel J. Wall, President and Chief Executive Officer

MIRIAM HOSPITAL, 164 Summit Avenue, Providence, RI, Zip 02906–2895; tel. 401/331–8500; Steven D. Baron, President and Chief Executive Officer

NEWPORT HOSPITAL, 11 Friendship Street, Newport, RI, Zip 02840–2299; tel. 401/846–6400; Arthur J. Sampson, President and Chief Executive Officer

RHODE ISLAND HOSPITAL, 593 Eddy Street, Providence, RI, Zip 02903; tel. 401/444–4000; Steven D. Baron, President and Chief Executive Officer

ST. JOSEPH HEALTH SERVICES OF RHODE ISLAND, 200 High Service Avenue, North Providence, RI, Zip 02904; tel. 401/456–3000; H. John Keimig, President and Chief Executive Officer

SAINT JOSEPH HOSPITAL
200 High Service Avenue, Providence, RI 02904; tel. 401/456–4419; Kathy Monteith, Network Coordinator

ST. JOSEPH HEALTH SERVICES OF RHODE ISLAND, 200 High Service Avenue, North Providence, RI, Zip 02904; tel. 401/456–3000; H. John Keimig, President and Chief Executive Officer

SOUTH CAROLINA

CAROLINA HEALTHCHOICE NETWORK
1718 Saint Julian Place, Columbia, SC 29204; tel. 803/254–0984; Suzanne H. Catalano, Executive Director

CLARENDON MEMORIAL HOSPITAL, 10 Hospital Street, Manning, SC, Zip 29102, Mailing Address: Box 550, Zip 29102–0550; tel. 803/435–8463; Edward R. Frye, Jr., Administrator

FAIRFIELD MEMORIAL HOSPITAL, 321 By-Pass, Winnsboro, SC, Zip 29180, Mailing Address: Box 620, Zip 29180–0620; tel. 803/635–5548; Brent R. Lammers, Administrator

KERSHAW COUNTY MEDICAL CENTER, Haile and Roberts Streets, Camden, SC, Zip 29020–7003, Mailing Address: P.O. Box 7003, Zip 29020–7003; tel. 803/432–4311; Dennis A. Lofe, FACHE, President

NEWBERRY COUNTY MEMORIAL HOSPITAL, 2669 Kinard Street, Newberry, SC, Zip 29108–0497, Mailing Address: P.O. Box 497, Zip 29108–0497; tel. 803/276–7570; Lynn W. Beasley, President and Chief Executive Officer

REGIONAL MEDICAL CENTER OF ORANGEBURG AND CALHOUN COUNTIES, 3000 St. Matthews Road, Orangeburg, SC, Zip 29118–1470; tel. 803/533–2200; Thomas C. Dandridge, President

RICHLAND MEMORIAL HOSPITAL, Five Richland Medical Park, Columbia, SC, Zip 29203–6897; tel. 803/434–7000; Kester S. Freeman, Jr., President and Chief Executive Officer

TUOMEY REGIONAL MEDICAL CENTER, 129 North Washington Street, Sumter, SC, Zip 29150–4983; tel. 803/778–9000; Jay Cox, President and Chief Executive Officer

HEALTHFIRST OF THE GREENVILLE HOSPITAL SYSTEM
701 Grove Road, Greenville, SC 29605; tel. 803/455–5716; Paul Briggs, Senior Vice President

ALLEN BENNETT HOSPITAL, 313 Memorial Drive, Greer, SC, Zip 29650; tel. 864/848–8130; Michael W. Massey, Administrator

GREENVILLE MEMORIAL HOSPITAL, 701 Grove Road, Greenville, SC, Zip 29605–4295; tel. 864/455–7000; J. Bland Burkhardt, Jr., Senior Vice President and Administrator

HILLCREST HOSPITAL, 729 S.E. Main Street, Simpsonville, SC, Zip 29681; tel. 864/967–6100; James Dover, Administrator

MARSHALL I. PICKENS HOSPITAL, 701 Grove Road, Greenville, SC, Zip 29605–4295; tel. 864/455–7836; Ryan D. Beaty, Administrator

ROGER C. PEACE REHABILITATION HOSPITAL, 701 Grove Road, Greenville, SC, Zip 29605–4295; tel. 864/455–7000; Ryan D. Beaty, Administrator

OPTIMUM HEALTH NETWORK
1 Saint Francis Drive, Greenville, SC 29601; tel. 803/220–4986; Paul D. Hovey, Vice President

BAPTIST MEDICAL CENTER EASLEY, 200 Fleetwood Drive, Easley, SC, Zip 29640, Mailing Address: P.O. Box 2129, Zip 29641–2129; tel. 864/855–7200; Roddey E. Gettys, III, Executive Vice President

CHARTER GREENVILLE BEHAVIORAL HEALTH SYSTEM, 2700 East Phillips Road, Greer, SC, Zip 29650; tel. 864/235–2335; William L. Callison, Chief Executive Officer

MARY BLACK MEMORIAL HOSPITAL, 1700 Skylyn Drive, Spartanburg, SC, Zip 29307, Mailing Address: Box 3217, Zip 29304–3217; tel. 864/573–3000; Ronald J. Vigus, Chief Executive Officer

ST. FRANCIS HEALTH SYSTEM, One St. Francis Drive, Greenville, SC, Zip 29601–3207; tel. 864/255–1000; Richard C. Neugent, President

PALMETTO COMMUNITY HEALTH NETWORK
900 C Main Street, Conway, SC 29526; tel. 803/248–5296; Edward V. Schlaefer, Executive Director

CHESTERFIELD GENERAL HOSPITAL, Highway 9, Cheraw, SC, Zip 29520, Mailing Address: Box 151, Zip 29520–0151; tel. 803/537–7881; Chris Wolf, Chief Executive Officer

CONWAY HOSPITAL, 300 Singleton Ridge Road, Conway, SC, Zip 29528, Mailing Address: Box 829, Zip 29528; tel. 803/347–7111; Philip A. Clayton, President and Chief Executive Officer

LORIS COMMUNITY HOSPITAL, 3655 Mitchell Street, Loris, SC, Zip 29569–2827; tel. 803/756–4011; J. Curtiss Gore, Chief Executive Officer

MARION MEMORIAL HOSPITAL, 1108 North Main Street, Marion, SC, Zip 29571, Mailing Address: Box 1150, Zip 29571–1150; tel. 803/423–3210; Thomas E. Fuller, Administrator

MARLBORO PARK HOSPITAL, 1138 Cheraw Highway, Bennettsville, SC, Zip 29512–0738, Mailing Address: Box 738, Zip 29512–0738; tel. 803/479–2881; Stephen Chapman, Executive Director

MCLEOD REGIONAL MEDICAL CENTER, 555 East Cheves Street, Florence, SC, Zip 29506–2617, Mailing Address: P.O. Box 100551, Zip 29501–0551; tel. 803/667–2000; J. Bruce Barragan, President and Chief Executive Officer

MULLINS HOSPITAL, 518 South Main Street, Mullins, SC, Zip 29574, Mailing Address: Drawer 849, Zip 29574–0849; tel. 803/464–8211; Donald H. Lloyd, II, Administrator

SAINT EUGENE COMMUNITY HOSPITAL, 301 East Jackson Street, Dillon, SC, Zip 29536–2509, Mailing Address: P.O. Box 1327, Zip 29536–1327; tel. 803/774–4111; Ronald W. Webb, President

PREMIER HEALTH SYSTEMS, INC.
1400 Pickens Street, Suite 300, Columbia, SC 29201; tel. 803/988–8999; Frank Riley, President & Chief Executive Officer

ABBEVILLE COUNTY MEMORIAL HOSPITAL, Highway 72, Abbeville, SC, Zip 29620–0887, Mailing Address: P.O. Box 887, Zip 29620; tel. 864/459–5011; Bruce P. Bailey, Administrator

ALLEN BENNETT HOSPITAL, 313 Memorial Drive, Greer, SC, Zip 29650; tel. 864/848–8130; Michael W. Massey, Administrator

ALLENDALE COUNTY HOSPITAL, Highway 278 West, Fairfax, SC, Zip 29827–0278, Mailing Address: Box 218, Zip 29827–0218; tel. 803/632–3311; M. K. Hiatt, Administrator

BAMBERG COUNTY MEMORIAL HOSPITAL AND NURSING CENTER, North and McGee Streets, Bamberg, SC, Zip 29003–0507, Mailing Address: P.O. Box 507, Zip 29003–0507; tel. 803/245–4321; Warren E. Hammett, Administrator

BAPTIST MEDICAL CENTER EASLEY, 200 Fleetwood Drive, Easley, SC, Zip 29640, Mailing Address: P.O. Box 2129, Zip 29641–2129; tel. 864/855–7200; Roddey E. Gettys, III, Executive Vice President

BAPTIST MEDICAL CENTER/COLUMBIA, Taylor at Marion Street, Columbia, SC, Zip 29220; tel. 803/771–5010; James M. Bridges, Executive Vice President

BARNWELL COUNTY HOSPITAL, Reynolds and Wren Streets, Barnwell, SC, Zip 29812, Mailing Address: Box 588, Zip 29812–0588; tel. 803/259–1000; Tommy R. McDougal, Jr., Administrator and Chief Executive Officer

BON SECOURS–ST. FRANCIS XAVIER HOSPITAL, 2095 Henry Tecklenburg Drive, Charleston, SC, Zip 29414–0001, Mailing Address: P.O. Box 160001, Zip 29414–0001; tel. 803/402–1000; Allen P. Carroll, Chief Executive Officer

CANNON MEMORIAL HOSPITAL, 123 Medical Park Drive, Pickens, SC, Zip 29671, Mailing Address: Box 188, Zip 29671–0188; tel. 864/878–4791; Norman G. Rentz, President

CAROLINAS HOSPITAL SYSTEM–LAKE CITY, U.S. Highway 52 North, Lake City, SC, Zip 29560–1029, Mailing Address: P.O. Box 1029, Zip 29560–1029; tel. 803/394–2036; Richard L. Gamber, Administrator

CHESTER COUNTY HOSPITAL AND NURSING CENTER, 1 Medical Park Drive, Chester, SC, Zip 29706–9799; tel. 803/581–3151; William H. Bundy, Acting Administrator

CHESTERFIELD GENERAL HOSPITAL, Highway 9, Cheraw, SC, Zip 29520, Mailing Address: Box 151, Zip 29520–0151; tel. 803/537–7881; Chris Wolf, Chief Executive Officer

CLARENDON MEMORIAL HOSPITAL, 10 Hospital Street, Manning, SC, Zip 29102, Mailing Address: Box 550, Zip 29102–0550; tel. 803/435–8463; Edward R. Frye, Jr., Administrator

COLUMBIA PROVIDENCE HOSPITAL, 2435 Forest Drive, Columbia, SC, Zip 29204–2098; tel. 803/256–5300; M. John Heydel, President and Chief Executive Officer

EAST COOPER REGIONAL MEDICAL CENTER, 1200 Johnnie Dodds Boulevard, Mount Pleasant, SC, Zip 29464; tel. 803/881–0100; John Holland, President

EDGEFIELD COUNTY HOSPITAL, Bausket Street, Edgefield, SC, Zip 29824, Mailing Address: Box 590, Zip 29824–0590; tel. 803/637–3174; W. Joseph Seel, Administrator

FAIRFIELD MEMORIAL HOSPITAL, 321 By-Pass, Winnsboro, SC, Zip 29180, Mailing Address: Box 620, Zip 29180–0620; tel. 803/635–5548; Brent R. Lammers, Administrator

GEORGETOWN MEMORIAL HOSPITAL, 606 Black River Road, Georgetown, SC, Zip 29440, Mailing Address: Drawer 1718, Zip 29442–1718; tel. 803/527–7000; Paul D. Gatens, Sr., Administrator

GREENVILLE MEMORIAL HOSPITAL, 701 Grove Road, Greenville, SC, Zip 29605–4295; tel. 864/455–7000; J. Bland Burkhardt, Jr., Senior Vice President and Administrator

HEALTHSOUTH REHABILITATION HOSPITAL, 2935 Colonial Drive, Columbia, SC, Zip 29203; tel. 803/254–7777; Mark J. Stepanik, Director Operations

HILLCREST HOSPITAL, 729 S.E. Main Street, Simpsonville, SC, Zip 29681; tel. 864/967–6100; James Dover, Administrator

HILTON HEAD MEDICAL CENTER AND CLINICS, Hilton Head Island, SC, Mailing Address: P.O. Box 21117, Zip 29925–1117; tel. 803/681–6122; Dennis Ray Bruns, President and Chief Executive Officer

KERSHAW COUNTY MEDICAL CENTER, Haile and Roberts Streets, Camden, SC, Zip 29020–7003, Mailing Address: P.O. Box 7003, Zip 29020–7003; tel. 803/432–4311; Dennis A. Lofe, FACHE, President

LAURENS COUNTY HEALTHCARE SYSTEM, Highway 76 West, Clinton, SC, Zip 29325, Mailing Address: P.O. Box 976, Zip 29325–0976; tel. 864/833–9100; Michael A. Kozar, Chief Executive Officer

LEXINGTON MEDICAL CENTER, 2720 Sunset Boulevard, West Columbia, SC, Zip 29169–4816; tel. 803/791–2000; Michael J. Biediger, President

MARLBORO PARK HOSPITAL, 1138 Cheraw Highway, Bennettsville, SC, Zip 29512–0738, Mailing Address: Box 738, Zip 29512–0738; tel. 803/479–2881; Stephen Chapman, Executive Director

MARSHALL I. PICKENS HOSPITAL, 701 Grove Road, Greenville, SC, Zip 29605–4295; tel. 864/455–7836; Ryan D. Beaty, Administrator

MARY BLACK MEMORIAL HOSPITAL, 1700 Skylyn Drive, Spartanburg, SC, Zip 29307, Mailing Address: Box 3217, Zip 29304–3217; tel. 864/573–3000; Ronald J. Vigus, Chief Executive Officer

NEWBERRY COUNTY MEMORIAL HOSPITAL, 2669 Kinard Street, Newberry, SC, Zip 29108–0497, Mailing Address: P.O. Box 497, Zip 29108–0497; tel. 803/276–7570; Lynn W. Beasley, President and Chief Executive Officer

ROGER C. PEACE REHABILITATION HOSPITAL, 701 Grove Road, Greenville, SC, Zip 29605–4295; tel. 864/455–7000; Ryan D. Beaty, Administrator

ROPER HOSPITAL, 316 Calhoun Street, Charleston, SC, Zip 29401–1125; tel. 803/724–2000; James H. Rogers, FACHE, President and Chief Executive Officer

SELF MEMORIAL HOSPITAL, 1325 Spring Street, Greenwood, SC, Zip 29646–3860; tel. 864/227–4111; J. L. Dozier, Jr., FACHE, President

ST. JOSEPH'S HOSPITAL, 11705 Mercy Boulevard, Savannah, GA, Zip 31419–1791; tel. 912/927–5404; Paul P. Hinchey, President and Chief Executive Officer

UPSTATE CAROLINA MEDICAL CENTER, 1530 North Limestone Street, Gaffney, SC, Zip 29340; tel. 803/487–4271; Steve Midkiff, Executive Director

WILLINGWAY HOSPITAL, 311 Jones Mill Road, Statesboro, GA, Zip 30458; tel. 912/764–6236; Jimmy Mooney, Chief Executive Officer

RICHLAND COMMUNITY HEALTH PARTNERS
3 Richland Medical Park, Suite 100, Columbia, SC 29203; tel. 803/434–3100; Tom Brown, Director

RICHLAND MEMORIAL HOSPITAL, Five Richland Medical Park, Columbia, SC, Zip 29203–6897; tel. 803/434–7000; Kester S. Freeman, Jr., President and Chief Executive Officer

SAINT FRANCIS HEALTH SYSTEM
One Saint Francis Drive, Greenville, SC 29601; tel. 803/255–1000; Richard C. Neugent, Chief Executive Officer

ST. FRANCIS HEALTH SYSTEM, One St. Francis Drive, Greenville, SC, Zip 29601–3207; tel. 864/255–1000; Richard C. Neugent, President

SOUTH DAKOTA

BLACK HILLS HEALTHCARE NETWORK
930 10th Street, Spearfish, SD 57783; tel. 605/642–4641; Ellen D. Holley, Director of Marketing/Communications

LOOKOUT MEMORIAL HOSPITAL, 1440 North Main Street, Spearfish, SD, Zip 57783–1504; tel. 605/642–2617; Deb J. Krmpotic, R.N., Administrator

SOUTHERN HILLS GENERAL HOSPITAL, 209 North 16th Street, Hot Springs, SD, Zip 57747–1375; tel. 605/745–3159; Linda Iverson, Administrator

STURGIS COMMUNITY HEALTH CARE CENTER, 949 Harmon Street, Sturgis, SD, Zip 57785; tel. 605/347–2536; Roger R. Heidt, Administrator

MISSOURI VALLEY HEALTH NETWORK
1017 West 5th Street, Yankton, SD 57078; tel. 605/665–9005; Lanette Hinchly, Office Manager

COMMUNITY MEMORIAL HOSPITAL, Burke, SD, Mailing Address: P.O. Box 319, Zip 57523; tel. 605/775–2621; Carol A. Varland, Administrator

DOUGLAS COUNTY MEMORIAL HOSPITAL, 708 Eighth Street, Armour, SD, Zip 57313; tel. 605/724–2159; Angelia K. Henry, Administrator

FREEMAN COMMUNITY HOSPITAL, 510 East Eighth Street, Freeman, SD, Zip 57029–0370, Mailing Address: P.O. Box 370, Zip 57029–0370; tel. 605/925–4231; James M. Krehbiel, Chief Executive Officer

GREGORY COMMUNITY HOSPITAL, 400 Park Street, Gregory, SD, Zip 57533–0400, Mailing Address: Box 408, Zip 57533–0408; tel. 605/835–8394; Carol A. Varland, Chief Executive Officer

LANDMANN–JUNGMAN MEMORIAL HOSPITAL, 600 Billars Street, Scotland, SD, Zip 57059; tel. 605/583–2226; William H. Koellner, Administrator

PIONEER MEMORIAL HOSPITAL, 315 North Washington Street, Viborg, SD, Zip 57070, Mailing Address: P.O. Box 368, Zip 57070–0368; tel. 605/326–5161; Georgia Pokorney, Chief Executive Officer

PLATTE COMMUNITY MEMORIAL HOSPITAL, 609 East Seventh, Platte, SD, Zip 57369, Mailing Address: P.O. Box 200, Zip 57369–0200; tel. 605/337–3364; Mark Burket, Chief Executive Officer

QUEEN OF PEACE HOSPITAL, 525 North Foster, Mitchell, SD, Zip 57301–2999; tel. 605/995–2000; Ronald L. Jacobson, President and Chief Executive Officer

SACRED HEART HEALTH SERVICES, 501 Summit, Yankton, SD, Zip 57078–3899; tel. 605/668–8000; Dennis A. Sokol, President and Chief Executive Officer

ST. BENEDICT HEALTH CENTER, Glynn Drive, Parkston, SD, Zip 57366, Mailing Address: P.O. Box B, Zip 57366; tel. 605/928–3311; Gale Walker, Administrator

ST. MICHAEL'S HOSPITAL, Douglas Street and Broadway, Tyndall, SD, Zip 57066, Mailing Address: Box 27, Zip 57066; tel. 605/589–3341; Carol Deurmier, Chief Executive Officer

WAGNER COMMUNITY MEMORIAL HOSPITAL, Third and Walnut, Wagner, SD, Zip 57380, Mailing Address: P.O. Box 280, Zip 57380–0280; tel. 605/384–3611; Arlene C. Bich, Administrator

WINNER REGIONAL HEALTHCARE CENTER, 745 East Eighth Street, Winner, SD, Zip 57580–2677, Mailing Address: Box 745, Zip 57580–0745; tel. 605/842–2110; Robert Houser, Chief Executive Officer

RAPID CITY REGIONAL HOSPITAL
353 Fairmont Boulevard, Rapid City, SD 57709; tel. 605/341–1000; Carolyn Helfenstein, Director of Marketing

FIVE COUNTIES HOSPITAL, 401 Sixth Avenue West, Lemmon, SD, Zip 57638, Mailing Address: Box 479, Zip 57638; tel. 605/374–3871; Helen S. Lindquist, Administrator

HANS P. PETERSON MEMORIAL HOSPITAL, 603 West Pine, Philip, SD, Zip 57567, Mailing Address: P.O. Box 790, Zip 57567; tel. 605/859–2511; David Dick, Administrator

LEGEND BUTTES HEALTH SERVICES, 11 Paddock Street, Crawford, NE, Zip 69339, Mailing Address: P.O. Box 272, Zip 69339; tel. 308/665–1770; Kim Engel, Chief Executive Officer

NORTHERN HILLS GENERAL HOSPITAL, 61 Charles Street, Deadwood, SD, Zip 57732; tel. 605/578–2313; Richard G. Soukup, Chief Executive Officer

REGIONAL HOSPITAL HEALTHCARE NETWORK
61 Charles Street, Deadwood, SD 57732; tel. 605/578–2313; Wendall Rawling, Interim Chief Executive Officer

NORTHERN HILLS GENERAL HOSPITAL, 61 Charles Street, Deadwood, SD, Zip 57732; tel. 605/578–2313; Richard G. Soukup, Chief Executive Officer

SIOUX VALLEY HEALTH SYSTEM
300 Main Street, Sioux Falls, SD 57117; tel. 605/333–1531; Tom Evans, Vice President of Rural Health

CANBY COMMUNITY HEALTH SERVICES, 112 St. Olaf Avenue South, Canby, MN, Zip 56220–1433; tel. 507/223–7277; Robert J. Salmon, Chief Executive Officer

CANTON–INWOOD MEMORIAL HOSPITAL, 440 North Hiawatha Drive, Canton, SD, Zip 57013–9404, Mailing Address: Rural Route 3, Box 7, Zip 57013; tel. 605/987–2621; John Devick, Chief Executive Officer

DAKOTA MEDICAL CENTER, 20 South Plum Street, Vermillion, SD, Zip 57069; tel. 605/624–2611; Larry W. Veitz, Chief Executive Officer

MERRILL PIONEER COMMUNITY HOSPITAL, 801 South Greene Street, Rock Rapids, IA, Zip 51246–1998; tel. 712/472–2591; Gordon Smith, Administrator

MID DAKOTA HOSPITAL, 300 South Byron Boulevard, Chamberlain, SD, Zip 57325; tel. 605/734–5511; Mick Penticoff, Administrator

MURRAY COUNTY MEMORIAL HOSPITAL, 2042 Juniper Avenue, Slayton, MN, Zip 56172; tel. 507/836–6111; Jerry Bobeldyk, Administrator

NORTHWEST IOWA HEALTH CENTER, 118 North Seventh Avenue, Sheldon, IA, Zip 51201; tel. 712/324–5041; Charles R. Miller, Chief Executive Officer

PIONEER MEMORIAL HOSPITAL, 315 North Washington Street, Viborg, SD, Zip 57070, Mailing Address: P.O. Box 368, Zip 57070–0368; tel. 605/326–5161; Georgia Pokorney, Chief Executive Officer

TRACY MUNICIPAL HOSPITAL, 251 Fifth Street East, Tracy, MN, Zip 56175–1536; tel. 507/629–3200; Thomas J. Quinlivan, Administrator

WESTBROOK HEALTH CENTER, 920 Bell Avenue, Westbrook, MN, Zip 56183, Mailing Address: P.O. Box 188, Zip 56183–0188; tel. 507/274–6121; Judy Lichty, Administrator

WINDOM AREA HOSPITAL, Highways 60 and 71 North, Windom, MN, Zip 56101, Mailing Address: P.O. Box 339, Zip 56101; tel. 507/831–2400; J. Stephen Pautler, CHE, Administrator

TENNESSEE

CHATTANOOGA HEALTHCARE NETWORK
401 Chestnut Street, Suite 222, Chattanooga, TN 37402; tel. 423/266–5174; Judy Clay, Network Contact

COLUMBIA ATHENS REGIONAL MEDICAL CENTER, 1114 West Madison Avenue, Athens, TN, Zip 37303, Mailing Address: Box 250, Zip 37371–0250; tel. 615/745–1411; Sean S. McMurray, Administrator

COLUMBIA EAST RIDGE HOSPITAL, 941 Spring Creek Road, East Ridge, TN, Zip 37412, Mailing Address: P.O. Box 91229, Zip 37412–6229; tel. 423/894–7870; Brenda M. Waltz, CHE, Chief Executive Officer

COLUMBIA SOUTH PITTSBURG HOSPITAL, 210 West 12th Street, South Pittsburg, TN, Zip 37380, Mailing Address: P.O. Box 349, Zip 37380–0349; tel. 423/837–6781; Robert Klein, Chief Executive Officer

COLUMBIA VALLEY HOSPITAL, 2200 Morris Hill Road, Chattanooga, TN, Zip 37421; tel. 423/894–4220; Solon Boggus, Jr., Chief Executive Officer

PARKRIDGE MEDICAL CENTER, 2333 McCallie Avenue, Chattanooga, TN, Zip 37404–3285; tel. 423/698–6061; Solon Boggus, Jr., Chief Executive Officer

COLUMBIA HEALTHCARE NETWORK
Two Maryland Farms, Suite 300, Brentwood, TN 37027; tel. 615/661–7200; Luis A. Rosa, Chief Executive Officer

COLUMBIA SUMMIT MEDICAL CENTER, 5655 Frist Boulevard, Hermitage, TN, Zip 37076; tel. 615/316–3000; Bryan K. Dearing, Chief Executive Officer

HIGHLANDS WELLMONT HEALTH NETWORK, INC.
1 Medical Park Boulevard, P.O. Box 989, Bristol, TN 37621–0989; tel. 423/844–4186; Dave Nowiski, Executive VP System Development

LONESOME PINE HOSPITAL, 1990 Holton Avenue East, Big Stone Gap, VA, Zip 24219–0230, Mailing Address: Drawer I, Zip 24219; tel. 540/523–3111; Paul A. Bishop, Administrator

NORTON COMMUNITY HOSPITAL, 100 15th Street, Norton, VA, Zip 24273–1699; tel. 540/679–9700; William Kenley, Administrator and Chief Executive Officer

WELLMONT HEALTH SYSTEM–BRISTOL, 1 Medical Park Boulevard, Bristol, TN, Zip 37620; tel. 423/844–4200; Randall M. Olson, Administrator

WELLMONT HEALTH SYSTEM–HOLSTON VALLEY, West Ravine Street, Kingsport, TN, Zip 37662–0224, Mailing Address: Box 238, Zip 37662–0224; tel. 423/224–5001; Louis H. Bremer, President and Chief Executive Officer

METHODIST HEALTH SYSTEMS, INC.
1211 Union Avenue, Memphis, TN 38104;
tel. 901/726–8273; Maurice Elliott, President

METHODIST HOSPITAL OF DYERSBURG, 400 Tickle Street, Dyersburg, TN, Zip 38024–3182; tel. 901/285–2410; Richard McCormick, Administrator

METHODIST HOSPITAL OF FAYETTE, 214 Lakeview Road, Somerville, TN, Zip 38068–0001, Mailing Address: Box 909, Zip 38068–0001; tel. 901/465–0532; Michael Blome', Administrator

METHODIST HOSPITAL OF LEXINGTON, 200 West Church Street, Lexington, TN, Zip 38351, Mailing Address: Box 160, Zip 38351; tel. 901/968–3646; Eugene Ragghianti, Administrator

METHODIST HOSPITAL OF MCKENZIE, 161 Hospital Drive, McKenzie, TN, Zip 38201; tel. 901/352–4170; Randal E. Carson, Administrator

METHODIST HOSPITAL OF MIDDLE MISSISSIPPI, 239 Bowling Green Road, Lexington, MS, Zip 39095–9332; tel. 601/834–1321; James K. Greer, Administrator

METHODIST HOSPITALS OF MEMPHIS, 1265 Union Avenue, Memphis, TN, Zip 38104–3499; tel. 901/726–7000; Gary S. Shorb, President

METHODIST MEDICAL CENTER, 1850 Chadwick Drive, Jackson, MS, Zip 39204–3479, Mailing Address: P.O. Box 59001, Zip 39204–9001; tel. 601/376–1000; Thomas L. Harper, President and Chief Executive Officer

MIDDLE TENNESSEE HEALTHCARE NETWORK
3401 West End Avenue, Suite 120, Nashville,
TN 37203; tel. 615/386–2680; Roy Wright,
President & Chief Executive Officer

BAPTIST HOSPITAL, 2000 Church Street, Nashville, TN, Zip 37236–0002; tel. 615/329–5555; C. David Stringfield, President

BEDFORD COUNTY GENERAL HOSPITAL, 845 Union Street, Shelbyville, TN, Zip 37160–9971; tel. 615/685–5433; Richard L. Graham, Administrator

CARTHAGE GENERAL HOSPITAL, Highway 70 North, Carthage, TN, Zip 37030, Mailing Address: P.O. Box 319, Zip 37030–0319; Wayne Winfree, Administrator

CLARKSVILLE MEMORIAL HOSPITAL, 1771 Madison Street, Clarksville, TN, Zip 37043, Mailing Address: Box 3160, Zip 37043–3160; tel. 615/552–6622; James Lee Decker, President and Chief Executive Officer

COOKEVILLE GENERAL HOSPITAL, 142 West Fifth Street, Cookeville, TN, Zip 38501, Mailing Address: P.O. Box 340, Zip 38503–0340; tel. 615/528–2541; Mike Mayes, FACHE, Administrator and Chief Executive Officer

CUMBERLAND MEDICAL CENTER, 421 South Main Street, Crossville, TN, Zip 38555–5031; tel. 615/484–9511; Edwin S. Anderson, President

MAURY REGIONAL HOSPITAL, 1224 Trotwood Avenue, Columbia, TN, Zip 38401; tel. 615/381–1111; William R. Walter, Administrator

MIDDLE TENNESSEE MEDICAL CENTER, 400 North Highland Avenue, Murfreesboro, TN, Zip 37130–3854, Mailing Address: P.O. Box 1178, Zip 37133–1178; tel. 615/849–4100; Arthur W. Hastings, President and Chief Executive Officer

ST. THOMAS HOSPITAL, 4220 Harding Road, Nashville, TN, Zip 37205, Mailing Address: Box 380, Zip 37202; tel. 615/222–2111; John F. Tighe, President and Chief Executive Officer

SUMNER REGIONAL MEDICAL CENTER, 555 Hartsville Pike, Gallatin, TN, Zip 37066, Mailing Address: P.O. Box 1558, Zip 37066–1558; tel. 615/452–4210; William T. Sugg, President and Chief Executive Officer

TENNESSEE CHRISTIAN MEDICAL CENTER, 500 Hospital Drive, Madison, TN, Zip 37115; tel. 615/865–2373; Milton R. Siepman, Ph.D., President and Chief Executive Officer

VANDERBILT UNIVERSITY HOSPITAL, 1161 21st Avenue South, Nashville, TN, Zip 37232–2102; tel. 615/322–5000; Norman B. Urmy, Executive Director

WILLIAMSON MEDICAL CENTER, 2021 Carothers Road, Franklin, TN, Zip 37067, Mailing Address: P.O. Box 681600, Zip 37068–1600; tel. 615/791–0500; Ronald G. Joyner, Chief Executive Officer

MOUNTAIN STATES HEALTHCARE NETWORK
400 North State of Franklin Road, Johnson
City, TN 37604; tel. 423/431–6810; Patricia
Holtsclaw, Executive Director

CHARLES A. CANNON JR. MEMORIAL HOSPITAL, 805 Shawneehaw Avenue, Banner Elk, NC, Zip 28604, Mailing Address: P.O. Box 8, Zip 28604–0008; tel. 704/898–5111; Edward C. Greene, Jr., Administrator

COLUMBIA CLINCH VALLEY MEDICAL CENTER, 2949 West Front Street, Richlands, VA, Zip 24641; tel. 540/596–6000; James W. Thweatt, Chief Executive Officer

INDIAN PATH MEDICAL CENTER, 2000 Brookside Drive, Kingsport, TN, Zip 37660–4604; tel. 615/392–7000; Robert Bauer, Chief Executive Officer

INDIAN PATH PAVILION, 2300 Pavilion Drive, Kingsport, TN, Zip 37660–4672; tel. 615/378–7500; Robert Bauer, Chief Executive Officer

JOHNSON CITY MEDICAL CENTER HOSPITAL, 400 North State of Franklin Road, Johnson City, TN, Zip 37604–6094; tel. 423/431–6111; Dennis Vonderfecht, President and Chief Executive Officer

JOHNSTON MEMORIAL HOSPITAL, 351 North Court Street, Abingdon, VA, Zip 24210–2921; tel. 540/676–7000; Clark R. Beil, Chief Executive Officer

LAKEWAY REGIONAL HOSPITAL, 726 McFarland Street, Morristown, TN, Zip 37814–3990; tel. 615/586–2302; Brian E. Dunn, Chief Executive Officer

LEE COUNTY COMMUNITY HOSPITAL, West Morgan Avenue, Pennington Gap, VA, Zip 24277, Mailing Address: P.O. Box 70, Zip 24277–0070; tel. 540/546–1440; James L. Davis, Chief Executive Officer

MORRISTOWN–HAMBLEN HOSPITAL, 908 West Fourth North Street, Morristown, TN, Zip 37814–1178; tel. 615/586–4231; Richard L. Clark, Administrator and Chief Executive Officer

SLOOP MEMORIAL HOSPITAL, One Crossnore Drive, Crossnore, NC, Zip 28616, Mailing Address: Drawer 470, Zip 28616; tel. 704/733–9231; Edward C. Greene, Jr., President

TAKOMA ADVENTIST HOSPITAL, 401 Takoma Avenue, Greeneville, TN, Zip 37743; tel. 423/639–3151; Paul Michael Norman, President

UNICOI COUNTY MEMORIAL HOSPITAL, Greenway Circle, Erwin, TN, Zip 37650–2196; tel. 423/743–3141; James L. McMackin, Chief Executive Officer

WOODRIDGE HOSPITAL, 403 State of Franklin Road, Johnson City, TN, Zip 37604; tel. 423/928–7111; Thomas J. De Martini, Administrator

PARTNERS FOR A HEALTHY NASHVILLE
161 Fourth Avenue North, Nashville, TN
37219; tel. 615/259–4728; Joanne F. Pulles,
Executive Director

ST. THOMAS HOSPITAL, 4220 Harding Road, Nashville, TN, Zip 37205, Mailing Address: Box 380, Zip 37202; tel. 615/222–2111; John F. Tighe, President and Chief Executive Officer

TENNESSEE CHRISTIAN MEDICAL CENTER, 500 Hospital Drive, Madison, TN, Zip 37115; tel. 615/865–2373; Milton R. Siepman, Ph.D., President and Chief Executive Officer

VANDERBILT UNIVERSITY HOSPITAL, 1161 21st Avenue South, Nashville, TN, Zip 37232–2102; tel. 615/322–5000; Norman B. Urmy, Executive Director

PREMIER HEALTH NETWORK
313 Princeton Road, Suite 7, Johnson City, TN
37601; tel. 615/844–4205; Eddie George,
Chief Executive Officer

COLUMBIA JOHNSON CITY SPECIALTY HOSPITAL, 203 East Watauga Avenue, Johnson City, TN, Zip 37601; tel. 615/926–1111; Lori Caudell Fatherree, Chief Executive Officer

COLUMBIA NORTH SIDE HOSPITAL, 401 Princeton Road, Johnson City, TN, Zip 37601, Mailing Address: P.O. Box 4900, Zip 37602; tel. 423/854–5900; John B. Crysel, Chief Executive Officer

LAUGHLIN MEMORIAL HOSPITAL, 1420 Tusculum Boulevard, Greeneville, TN, Zip 37745; tel. 423/787–5000; Charles H. Whitfield, Jr., Administrator and Chief Operating Officer

WELLMONT HEALTH SYSTEM–HOLSTON VALLEY, West Ravine Street, Kingsport, TN, Zip 37662–0224, Mailing Address: Box 238, Zip 37662–0224; tel. 423/224–5001; Louis H. Bremer, President and Chief Executive Officer

SAINT THOMAS HEALTH SERVICES
P.O. Box 380 – 4220 Harding Road, Nashville,
TN 37202; tel. 615/222–6800; Susan R.
Russell, Vice President of Community Relations

ST. THOMAS HOSPITAL, 4220 Harding Road, Nashville, TN, Zip 37205, Mailing Address: Box 380, Zip 37202; tel. 615/222–2111; John F. Tighe, President and Chief Executive Officer

VANDERBILT UNIVERSITY HOSPITAL, 1161 21st Avenue South, Nashville, TN, Zip 37232–2102; tel. 615/322–5000; Norman B. Urmy, Executive Director

WEST TENNESSEE HEALTHCARE, INC.
708 West Forest, Jackson, TN 38301;
tel. 901/425–6730; Jim Moss, Chief Executive
Officer

BOLIVAR GENERAL HOSPITAL, 650 Nuckolls Road, Bolivar, TN, Zip 38008; tel. 901/658–3100; George L. Austin, Chief Executive Officer

CAMDEN GENERAL HOSPITAL, 175 Hospital Drive, Camden, TN, Zip 38320; tel. 901/584–6135; Alfred P. Taylor, Administrator and Chief Executive Officer

CITY OF MILAN HOSPITAL, 4039 South Highland, Milan, TN, Zip 38358; tel. 901/686–1591; Mark D. Le Neave, Chief Executive Officer

DECATUR COUNTY GENERAL HOSPITAL, 1200 Tennessee Avenue South, Parsons, TN, Zip 38363–0250, Mailing Address: Box 250, Zip 38363–0250; tel. 901/847–3031; Larry N. Lindsey, Administrator

GIBSON GENERAL HOSPITAL, 200 Hosptial Drive, Trenton, TN, Zip 38382, Mailing Address: Box 488, Zip 38382; tel. 901/855–2551; Kelly R. Yenawine, Administrator

HARDIN COUNTY GENERAL HOSPITAL, 2006 Wayne Road, Savannah, TN, Zip 38372; tel. 901/925–4954; Charlotte Burns, Administrator and Chief Executive Officer

HENRY COUNTY MEDICAL CENTER, Tyson Avenue, Paris, TN, Zip 38242–4544, Mailing Address: Box 1030, Zip 38242–1030; tel. 901/644–8537; Thomas H. Gee, Administrator

HUMBOLDT GENERAL HOSPITAL, 3525 Chere Carol Road, Humboldt, TN, Zip 38343–3699; tel. 901/784–0301; Karen Utley, Administrator

JACKSON–MADISON COUNTY GENERAL HOSPITAL, 708 West Forest Avenue, Jackson, TN, Zip 38301–3855; tel. 901/425–5000; James T. Moss, President

MCNAIRY COUNTY GENERAL HOSPITAL, 705 East Poplar Avenue, Selmer, TN, Zip 38375–1748; tel. 901/645–3221; Rosamond M. Tyler, Administrator

TEXAS

BAYLOR HEALTH CARE SYSTEM NETWORK
3600 Gaston Avenue, Suite 150, Dallas, TX
75246; tel. 214/820–2731; Boone Powell, Jr.,
President & Chief Executive Officer

BAYLOR CENTER FOR RESTORATIVE CARE, 3504 Swiss Avenue, Dallas, TX, Zip 75204; tel. 214/823–1684; Gerry Brueckner, R.N., Executive Director

Section B

BAYLOR MEDICAL CENTER AT GARLAND, 2300 Marie Curie Boulevard, Garland, TX, Zip 75042–5706; tel. 214/487–5000; John B. McWhorter, III, Executive Director

BAYLOR MEDICAL CENTER AT GRAPEVINE, 1650 West College Street, Grapevine, TX, Zip 76051–1650; tel. 817/329–2500; Mark C. Hood, Executive Director

BAYLOR MEDICAL CENTER–ELLIS COUNTY, 1405 West Jefferson Street, Waxahachie, TX, Zip 75165; tel. 972/923–7000; James Michael Lee, Executive Director

BAYLOR RICHARDSON MEDICAL CENTER, 401 West Campbell Road, Richardson, TX, Zip 75080; tel. 972/498–4000; Ronald L. Boring, President and Chief Executive Officer

BAYLOR UNIVERSITY MEDICAL CENTER, 3500 Gaston Avenue, Dallas, TX, Zip 75246–2088; tel. 214/820–0111; Boone Powell, Jr., President

HOPKINS COUNTY MEMORIAL HOSPITAL, 115 Airport Road, Sulphur Springs, TX, Zip 75482–0115, Mailing Address: Box 275, Zip 75483–0275; tel. 903/885–7671; Donald R. Magee, Chief Executive Officer

IRVING HEALTHCARE SYSTEM, 1901 North MacArthur Boulevard, Irving, TX, Zip 75061; tel. 972/579–8100; H. J. MacFarland, FACHE, Executive Director

BRAZO'S VALLEY HEALTH NETWORK
3115 Pine Avenue, Waco, TX 76708; tel. 817/757–3882; Don Reeves, Executive Director

CEDARS HOSPITAL, 2000 North Old Hickory Trail, De Soto, TX, Zip 75115; tel. 972/298–7323; Don Johnson, Administrator

CENTRAL TEXAS HOSPITAL, 806 North Crockett, Cameron, TX, Zip 76520; tel. 817/697–6591; Louis West, President

FALLS COMMUNITY HOSPITAL AND CLINIC, 322 Coleman Street, Marlin, TX, Zip 76661–2358, Mailing Address: Box 60, Zip 76661–0060; tel. 817/883–3561; Billy Don York, Administrator

GOODALL–WITCHER HOSPITAL, 101 South Avenue T, Clifton, TX, Zip 76634, Mailing Address: Box 549, Zip 76634; tel. 817/675–8322; Jim B. Smith, President and Chief Executive Officer

HILL REGIONAL HOSPITAL, 101 Circle Drive, Hillsboro, TX, Zip 76645; tel. 817/582–8425; Jan McClure, Chief Executive Officer

HILLCREST BAPTIST MEDICAL CENTER, 3000 Herring Avenue, Waco, TX, Zip 76708–3299, Mailing Address: Box 5100, Zip 76708–0100; tel. 817/756–8011; Richard E. Scott, President

KING'S DAUGHTERS HOSPITAL, 1901 S.W. H. K. Dodgen Loop, Temple, TX, Zip 76502–1896; tel. 817/771–8600; Tucker Bonner, President

LAKE WHITNEY MEDICAL CENTER, 200 North San Jacinto Street, Whitney, TX, Zip 76692, Mailing Address: P.O. Box 458, Zip 76692; tel. 817/694–3165; Bill A. Johnson, Administrator

LIMESTONE MEDICAL CENTER, 900 North Ellis Street, Groesbeck, TX, Zip 76642; tel. 817/729–3281; Penny Gray, Administrator and Chief Executive Officer

MEDICAL CENTER OF MESQUITE, 1011 North Galloway Avenue, Mesquite, TX, Zip 75149; tel. 214/320–7000; Terry J. Fontenot, Administrator

PARKVIEW REGIONAL HOSPITAL, 312 East Glendale Street, Mexia, TX, Zip 76667–3608; tel. 817/562–5332; Karl R. Stinson, Administrator

WEST COMMUNITY HOSPITAL, 501 Meadow Drive, West, TX, Zip 76691, Mailing Address: Box 478, Zip 76691; tel. 817/826–7000; Betty York, Executive Director

CENTRAL TEXAS RURAL HEALTH NETWORK
503 East 4th Street, Harrietsville, TX 77964–2824; tel. 512/798–2302; Marcella V. Henke, Executive Director

CENTRAL TEXAS HOSPITAL, 806 North Crockett, Cameron, TX, Zip 76520; tel. 817/697–6591; Louis West, President

FALLS COMMUNITY HOSPITAL AND CLINIC, 322 Coleman Street, Marlin, TX, Zip 76661–2358, Mailing Address: Box 60, Zip 76661–0060; tel. 817/883–3561; Billy Don York, Administrator

GOODALL–WITCHER HOSPITAL, 101 South Avenue T, Clifton, TX, Zip 76634, Mailing Address: Box 549, Zip 76634; tel. 817/675–8322; Jim B. Smith, President and Chief Executive Officer

HILL REGIONAL HOSPITAL, 101 Circle Drive, Hillsboro, TX, Zip 76645; tel. 817/582–8425; Jan McClure, Chief Executive Officer

LAKE WHITNEY MEDICAL CENTER, 200 North San Jacinto Street, Whitney, TX, Zip 76692, Mailing Address: P.O. Box 458, Zip 76692; tel. 817/694–3165; Bill A. Johnson, Administrator

LIMESTONE MEDICAL CENTER, 900 North Ellis Street, Groesbeck, TX, Zip 76642; tel. 817/729–3281; Penny Gray, Administrator and Chief Executive Officer

PARKVIEW REGIONAL HOSPITAL, 312 East Glendale Street, Mexia, TX, Zip 76667–3608; tel. 817/562–5332; Karl R. Stinson, Administrator

WEST COMMUNITY HOSPITAL, 501 Meadow Drive, West, TX, Zip 76691, Mailing Address: Box 478, Zip 76691; tel. 817/826–7000; Betty York, Executive Director

COLUMBIA HEALTHCARE – SOUTH TEXAS DIVISION
6629 Wooldridge Road, Corpus Christi, TX 78414; tel. 512/985–5200; Donald Stewart, President

COLUMBIA ALICE PHYSICIANS AND SURGEONS HOSPITAL, 300 East Third Street, Alice, TX, Zip 78332–4794; tel. 512/664–4376; Earl S. Whiteley, CHE, Chief Executive Officer

COLUMBIA BAY AREA MEDICAL CENTER, 7101 South Padre Island Drive, Corpus Christi, TX, Zip 78412; tel. 512/985–1200; Kirk G. Wilson, Chief Executive Officer

COLUMBIA BAYVIEW PSYCHIATRIC CENTER, 6226 Saratoga Boulevard, Corpus Christi, TX, Zip 78414; tel. 512/993–9700; Janie L. Harwood, Chief Executive Officer

COLUMBIA DOCTORS HOSPITAL OF LAREDO, 500 East Mann Road, Laredo, TX, Zip 78041; tel. 210/723–1131; Benjamin Everett, Chief Executive Officer

COLUMBIA DOCTORS REGIONAL MEDICAL CENTER, 3315 South Alameda, Corpus Christi, TX, Zip 78411, Mailing Address: P.O. Box 3828, Zip 78463–3828; tel. 512/857–1501; Steven Woerner, Chief Executive Officer

COLUMBIA NORTH BAY HOSPITAL, 1711 West Wheeler Avenue, Aransas Pass, TX, Zip 78336; tel. 512/758–0502; Steve Sutherlin, Chief Executive Officer

COLUMBIA NORTHWEST HOSPITAL, 13725 Farm Road 624, Corpus Christi, TX, Zip 78410; tel. 512/767–4500; Winston Borland, Chief Executive Officer

COLUMBIA REHABILITATION HOSPITAL, 6226 Saratoga Boulevard, Corpus Christi, TX, Zip 78414–3499; tel. 512/991–9690; Jo Ann Baker, Chief Executive Officer

COLUMBIA RIO GRANDE REGIONAL HOSPITAL, 101 East Ridge Road, McAllen, TX, Zip 78503; tel. 210/632–6000; Randall M. Everts, Chief Executive Officer

COLUMBIA VALLEY REGIONAL MEDICAL CENTER, 1 Ted Hunt Boulevard, Brownsville, TX, Zip 78521, Mailing Address: Box 3710, Zip 78521; tel. 210/831–9611; Pete Delgado, Chief Executive Officer

COLUMBIA SAINT DAVID'S HEALTH NETWORK
98 San Jacinto Boulevard, Austin, TX 78731; tel. 512/482–4135; Sharon J. Alvis, Executive Director

COLUMBIA ST. DAVID'S HOSPITAL, 919 East 32nd Street, Austin, TX, Zip 78705, Mailing Address: Box 4039, Zip 78765–4039; tel. 512/476–7111; Cole C. Eslyn, Chief Executive Officer

COLUMBIA ST. DAVID'S SOUTH HOSPITAL, 901 West Ben White Boulevard, Austin, TX, Zip 78704–6903; tel. 512/447–2211; Richard W. Klusmann, Chief Executive Officer

ROUND ROCK HOSPITAL, 2400 Round Rock Avenue, Round Rock, TX, Zip 78681; tel. 512/255–6066; Deborah L. Ryle, Chief Executive Officer

ST. DAVID'S PAVILION, 1025 East 32nd Street, Austin, TX, Zip 78765; tel. 512/867–5800; Cole C. Eslyn, Chief Executive Officer

ST. DAVID'S REHABILITATION CENTER, 1005 East 32nd Street, Austin, TX, Zip 78705, Mailing Address: P.O. Box 4270, Zip 78765–4270; tel. 512/867–5100; Cole C. Eslyn, Chief Executive Officer

GOOD SHEPERD HEALTH NETWORK
700 East Marshall, Longview, TX 75601–5571; tel. 903/236–2000; Dr. Rebecca Burrow, Executive Director

GOOD SHEPHERD MEDICAL CENTER, 700 East Marshall Avenue, Longview, TX, Zip 75601–5571; tel. 903/236–2000; Jerry D. Adair, President and Chief Executive Officer

GULF COAST PROVIDER NETWORK
2900 North Loop West, Suite 1230, Houston, TX 77092; tel. 713/956–4992; Susan D. Cowan, President

COLUMBIA BAYSHORE MEDICAL CENTER, 4000 Spencer Highway, Pasadena, TX, Zip 77504–1294; tel. 713/944–6666; Russell Meyers, Chief Executive Officer

COLUMBIA BELLAIRE MEDICAL CENTER, 5314 Dashwood Street, Houston, TX, Zip 77081–4689; tel. 713/512–1200; Walter Leleux, Chief Executive Officer

COLUMBIA CLEAR LAKE REGIONAL MEDICAL CENTER, 500 Medical Center Boulevard, Webster, TX, Zip 77598; tel. 713/332–2511; Donald A. Shaffett, Chief Executive Officer

COLUMBIA ROSEWOOD MEDICAL CENTER, 9200 Westheimer Road, Houston, TX, Zip 77063; tel. 713/780–7900; Pat Currie, Chief Executive Officer

COLUMBIA SPRING BRANCH MEDICAL CENTER, 8850 Long Point Road, Houston, TX, Zip 77055; tel. 713/467–6555; Sally E. Jeffcoat, President and Chief Executive Officer

COLUMBIA WEST HOUSTON MEDICAL CENTER, 12141 Richmond Avenue, Houston, TX, Zip 77082–2499; tel. 281/558–3444; Janie R. Kauffman, Chief Executive Officer

COLUMBIA WOMAN'S HOSPITAL OF TEXAS, 7600 Fannin Street, Houston, TX, Zip 77054–1900; tel. 713/790–1234; Linda B. Russell, Chief Executive Officer

CYPRESS FAIRBANKS MEDICAL CENTER, 10655 Steepletop Drive, Houston, TX, Zip 77065; tel. 713/890–4285; Bill Klier, Chief Executive Officer

HERMANN HOSPITAL, 6411 Fannin, Houston, TX, Zip 77030–1501; tel. 713/704–4000; David R. Page, President and Chief Executive Officer

HOUSTON NORTHWEST MEDICAL CENTER, 710 FM 1960 West, Houston, TX, Zip 77090–3496; tel. 281/440–1000; J. O. Lewis, Chief Executive Officer

POLLY RYON MEMORIAL HOSPITAL, 1705 Jackson Street, Richmond, TX, Zip 77469–3289; tel. 281/341–3000; Sam L. Steffee, Executive Director and Chief Executive Officer

SAN JACINTO METHODIST HOSPITAL, 4401 Garth Road, Baytown, TX, Zip 77521; tel. 281/420–8600; William Simmons, President and Chief Executive Officer

GULF HEALTH NETWORK
701 University Boulevard, Suite 229, Galveston, TX 77550; tel. 401/766–4235; Jim Shallock, President

UNIVERSITY OF TEXAS MEDICAL BRANCH HOSPITALS, 301 University Boulevard, Galveston, TX, Zip 77555–0138; tel. 409/772–1011; James F. Arens, M.D., Chief Executive Officer

HEALTHCARE PARTNERS OF EAST TEXAS, INC.
P.O. Box 6340, Tyler, TX 75711;
tel. 903/533–0684; Cindy Martinez, Executive
Director & President

COZBY–GERMANY HOSPITAL, 707 North Waldrip
Street, Grand Saline, TX, Zip 75140;
tel. 903/962–4242; William Rowton, Chief
Executive Officer

DOCTORS MEMORIAL HOSPITAL, 1400 West
Southwest Loop 323, Tyler, TX, Zip 75701;
tel. 903/561–3771; Olie E. Clem, Chief
Executive Officer

EAST TEXAS MEDICAL CENTER ATHENS, 2000 South
Palestine, Athens, TX, Zip 75751;
tel. 903/675–2216; Patrick L. Wallace,
Administrator

EAST TEXAS MEDICAL CENTER PITTSBURG, 414
Quitman Street, Pittsburg, TX, Zip 75686–1032;
tel. 903/856–6663; W. Perry Henderson,
Administrator

EAST TEXAS MEDICAL CENTER RUSK, Copeland and
Bonner Streets, Rusk, TX, Zip 75785, Mailing
Address: P.O. Box 317, Zip 75785;
tel. 903/683–2273; Don Edd Green,
Administrator

EAST TEXAS MEDICAL CENTER–MOUNT VERNON,
Highway 37 South, Mount Vernon, TX,
Zip 75457, Mailing Address: Box 477,
Zip 75457–0477; tel. 903/537–4552; Charles
N. Butts, Administrator

FAIRFIELD MEMORIAL HOSPITAL, 125 Newman
Street, Fairfield, TX, Zip 75840;
tel. 903/389–2121; Milton W. Meadows,
Administrator

GOOD SHEPHERD MEDICAL CENTER, 700 East
Marshall Avenue, Longview, TX,
Zip 75601–5571; tel. 903/236–2000; Jerry D.
Adair, President and Chief Executive Officer

HENDERSON MEMORIAL HOSPITAL, 300 Wilson
Street, Henderson, TX, Zip 75652;
tel. 903/657–7541; George T. Roberts, Jr.,
Chief Executive Officer

HUNTSVILLE MEMORIAL HOSPITAL, 3000 I–45,
Huntsville, TX, Zip 77340, Mailing Address: P.O.
Box 4001, Zip 77342–4001;
tel. 409/291–3411; Ralph E. Beaty,
Administrator

LINDEN MUNICIPAL HOSPITAL, North Kaufman Street,
Linden, TX, Zip 75563, Mailing Address: Box 32,
Zip 75563; tel. 903/756–5561; Fred Wilbanks,
Administrator

MEMORIAL HOSPITAL, 602 Hurst Street, Center, TX,
Zip 75935, Mailing Address: Box 1749,
Zip 75935–1749; tel. 409/598–2781; Robert V.
Deen, Administrator and Chief Executive Officer

MEMORIAL MEDICAL CENTER–LIVINGSTON, 602 East
Church Street, Livingston, TX, Zip 77351–1257,
Mailing Address: P.O. Box 1257,
Zip 77351–1257; tel. 409/327–4381; James C.
Dickson, Administrator

MEMORIAL MEDICAL CENTER OF EAST TEXAS, 1201
Frank Street, Lufkin, TX, Zip 75904, Mailing
Address: P.O. Box 1447, Zip 75902–1447;
tel. 409/634–8111; Gary Lex Whatley, President
and Chief Executive Officer

NACOGDOCHES MEMORIAL HOSPITAL, 1204 North
Mound Street, Nacogdoches, TX, Zip 75961;
tel. 409/568–8521; Gary J. Blan, FACHE,
President and Chief Executive Officer

NAN TRAVIS MEMORIAL HOSPITAL, 501 South
Ragsdale Street, Jacksonville, TX, Zip 75766;
tel. 903/586–3000; Steve Bowen, President

PANOLA GENERAL HOSPITAL, 409 Cottage Road,
Carthage, TX, Zip 75633, Mailing Address: Box
549, Zip 75633–0549; tel. 903/693–3841;
Gary Mikeal Hudson, Administrator

PINELANDS HOSPITAL, 4632 Northeast Stallings
Drive, Nacogdoches, TX, Zip 75961, Mailing
Address: P.O. Box 1004, Zip 75963–1004;
tel. 409/560–5900; David Baker, Interim
Administrator

PRESBYTERIAN HOSPITAL OF WINNSBORO, 719 West
Coke Road, Winnsboro, TX, Zip 75494–3098,
Mailing Address: P.O. Box 628,
Zip 75494–0628; tel. 903/342–5227; Jerry
Hopper, FACHE, Executive Director

ROY H. LAIRD MEMORIAL HOSPITAL, 1612 South
Henderson Boulevard, Kilgore, TX, Zip 75662;
tel. 903/984–3505; Roderick G. La Grone,
President

ST. MICHAEL HEALTH CARE CENTER, 2600 St.
Michael Drive, Texarkana, TX, Zip 75503;
tel. 903/614–2009; Don A. Beeler, Chief
Executive Officer

TITUS REGIONAL MEDICAL CENTER, 2001 North
Jefferson, Mount Pleasant, TX, Zip 75455;
tel. 903/577–6000; Steven K. Jacobson, Chief
Executive Officer

TRINITY VALLEY MEDICAL CENTER, 2900 South Loop
256, Palestine, TX, Zip 75801;
tel. 903/731–1000; Larry C. Bozeman, Chief
Executive Officer

WOOD COUNTY CENTRAL HOSPITAL DISTRICT, 117
Winnsboro Street, Quitman, TX, Zip 75783,
Mailing Address: P.O. Box 1000,
Zip 75783–1000; tel. 903/763–4505; Marion
W. Stanberry, Administrator

LUBBOCK METHODIST HOSPITAL SYSTEM
3615 19th Street, Lubbock, TX 79410;
tel. 806/793–4217; William D. Pateet, III,
President & Chief Executive Officer

ANSON GENERAL HOSPITAL, 101 Avenue J, Anson,
TX, Zip 79501; tel. 915/823–3231; Dudley R.
White, Administrator

BROWNFIELD REGIONAL MEDICAL CENTER, 705 East
Felt, Brownfield, TX, Zip 79316–3439;
tel. 806/637–3551; Mike Click, Administrator

CAMPBELL HEALTH SYSTEM, 713 East Anderson
Street, Weatherford, TX, Zip 76086–9971;
tel. 817/596–8751; John B. Millstead, Chief
Executive Officer

COCHRAN MEMORIAL HOSPITAL, 201 East Grant
Street, Morton, TX, Zip 79346;
tel. 806/266–5565; Paul McKinney,
Administrator

COMANCHE COMMUNITY HOSPITAL, 211 South
Austin Street, Comanche, TX, Zip 76442;
tel. 915/356–5241; W. Evan Moore,
Administrator

DE LEON HOSPITAL, 407 South Texas Avenue, De
Leon, TX, Zip 76444, Mailing Address: Box 319,
Zip 76444; tel. 817/893–2011; Michael K.
Hare, Administrator

FISHER COUNTY HOSPITAL DISTRICT, Roby Highway,
Rotan, TX, Zip 79546, Mailing Address: Drawer
F, Zip 79546; tel. 915/735–2256; Ella Raye
Helms, Administrator

HEREFORD REGIONAL MEDICAL CENTER, 801 East
Third Street, Hereford, TX, Zip 79045, Mailing
Address: Box 1858, Zip 79045;
tel. 806/364–2141; James M. Robinson, Sr.,
Administrator

LAMB HEALTHCARE CENTER, 1500 South Sunset,
Littlefield, TX, Zip 79339; tel. 806/385–6411;
Randall A. Young, Administrator

MEDICAL ARTS HOSPITAL, 1600 North Bryan Avenue,
Lamesa, TX, Zip 79331; tel. 806/872–2183;
Arla Jeffcoat, Administrator

MEMORIAL HOSPITAL, 224 East Second Street,
Dumas, TX, Zip 79029; tel. 806/935–7171;
Scott R. Brown, Administrator and Chief
Executive Officer

MITCHELL COUNTY HOSPITAL, 1543 Chestnut Street,
Colorado City, TX, Zip 79512–3998;
tel. 915/728–3431; Joe Wright, Administrator

MULESHOE AREA MEDICAL CENTER, 708 South First
Street, Muleshoe, TX, Zip 79347;
tel. 806/272–4524; Jim G. Bone, Interim
Administrator

PECOS COUNTY GENERAL HOSPITAL, 305 West Fifth
Street, Iraan, TX, Zip 79744, Mailing Address:
Box 665, Zip 79744; tel. 915/639–2871; David
B. Shaw, Administrator and Chief Executive
Officer

PECOS COUNTY MEMORIAL HOSPITAL, Sanderson
Highway, Fort Stockton, TX, Zip 79735, Mailing
Address: Box 1648, Zip 79735;
tel. 915/336–2241; David B. Shaw,
Administrator and Chief Executive Officer

PERMIAN GENERAL HOSPITAL, Northeast By–Pass,
Andrews, TX, Zip 79714, Mailing Address: Box
2108, Zip 79714; tel. 915/523–2200; Randy R.
Richards, Chief Executive Officer

MEMORIAL/SISTERS OF CHARITY HEALTH NETWORK
7737 SouthWest Freeway, Suite 200, Houston,
TX 77074; tel. 713/776–6992; Dan Wilford,
President

ANGLETON–DANBURY GENERAL HOSPITAL, 132
Hospital Drive, Angleton, TX, Zip 77515;
tel. 409/849–7721; David A. Bleakney,
Administrator

MEMORIAL HOSPITAL SOUTHWEST, 7600 Beechnut,
Houston, TX, Zip 77074–1850;
tel. 713/776–5000; James E. Eastham,
Administrator, Chief Executive Officer and Vice
President

MEMORIAL HOSPITAL–MEMORIAL CITY, 920
Frostwood Drive, Houston, TX, Zip 77024–9173;
tel. 713/932–3000; Jerel T. Humphrey, Vice
President, Chief Executive Officer and
Administrator

MEMORIAL HOSPITAL–THE WOODLANDS, 9250
Pinecroft, The Woodlands, TX, Zip 77380;
tel. 281/364–2300; Steve Sanders, Vice
President, Chief Executive Officer and
Administrator

MEMORIAL SPRING SHADOWS GLEN, 2801 Gessner,
Houston, TX, Zip 77080–2599;
tel. 713/462–4000; G. Jerry Mueck, Vice
President, Chief Executive Officer and
Administrator

POLLY RYON MEMORIAL HOSPITAL, 1705 Jackson
Street, Richmond, TX, Zip 77469–3289;
tel. 281/341–3000; Sam L. Steffee, Executive
Director and Chief Executive Officer

TOMBALL REGIONAL HOSPITAL, 605 Holderrieth
Street, Tomball, TX, Zip 77375–0889, Mailing
Address: Box 889, Zip 77377–0889;
tel. 281/351–1623; Robert F. Schaper,
President and Chief Executive Officer

VAL VERDE MEMORIAL HOSPITAL, 801 Bedell
Avenue, Del Rio, TX, Zip 78840, Mailing
Address: P.O. Box 1527, Zip 78840;
tel. 210/775–8566; Scott D. Evans, FACHE,
Administrator

METHODIST HEALTHCARE SYSTEM OF SAN ANTONIO, LTD.
7550 IH 10 West, Suite 1000, San Antonio, TX
78229; tel. 210/377–1647; John E. Hornbeak,
President

METHODIST WOMEN'S AND CHILDREN'S HOSPITAL,
8109 Fredericksburg Road, San Antonio, TX,
Zip 78229–3383; tel. 210/692–5000; Janet
Porter, President and Chief Executive Officer

METROPOLITAN METHODIST HOSPITAL, 1310
McCullough Avenue, San Antonio, TX,
Zip 78212–2617; tel. 210/208–2200; Mark L.
Bernard, Chief Executive Officer

NORTHEAST METHODIST HOSPITAL, 12412 Judson
Road, San Antonio, TX, Zip 78233, Mailing
Address: P.O. Box 659510, Zip 78265–9510;
tel. 210/650–4949; Mark L. Bernard, Chief
Executive Officer

SAN ANTONIO COMMUNITY HOSPITAL, 8026 Floyd
Curl Drive, San Antonio, TX, Zip 78229–3915;
tel. 210/692–8110; James C. Scoggin, Jr.,
Chief Executive Officer

SOUTHWEST TEXAS METHODIST HOSPITAL, 7700
Floyd Curl Drive, San Antonio, TX,
Zip 78229–3993; tel. 210/692–4000; James C.
Scoggin, Jr., Chief Executive Officer

METROPLEX HEALTH NETWORK
2201 South Cleer Creek Road, Kileen, TX
75642; tel. 817/519–8218; Vicki Carlson,
Director of Managed Care

METROPLEX HOSPITAL, 2201 South Clear Creek
Road, Killeen, TX, Zip 76542–9305;
tel. 817/526–7523

NORTH TEXAS HEALTH NETWORK
5601 MacArthur, Suite 300, Irving, TX 75038;
tel. 214/751–0047; Charlie Coil, President

BAYLOR CENTER FOR RESTORATIVE CARE, 3504
Swiss Avenue, Dallas, TX, Zip 75204;
tel. 214/823–1684; Gerry Brueckner, R.N.,
Executive Director

BAYLOR INSTITUTE FOR REHABILITATION, 3505
Gaston Avenue, Dallas, TX, Zip 75246–2018;
tel. 214/826–7030; Judith C. Waterston,
Executive Director

BAYLOR MEDICAL CENTER AT GARLAND, 2300 Marie Curie Boulevard, Garland, TX, Zip 75042–5706; tel. 214/487–5000; John B. McWhorter, III, Executive Director

BAYLOR MEDICAL CENTER AT GRAPEVINE, 1650 West College Street, Grapevine, TX, Zip 76051–1650; tel. 817/329–2500; Mark C. Hood, Executive Director

BAYLOR UNIVERSITY MEDICAL CENTER, 3500 Gaston Avenue, Dallas, TX, Zip 75246–2088; tel. 214/820–0111; Boone Powell, Jr., President

COLUMBIA MEDICAL CENTER AT TERRELL, 1551 Highway 34 South, Terrell, TX, Zip 75160–4833; tel. 972/563–7611; I. Douglas Streckert, Chief Executive Officer

PEDIATRIC CENTER FOR RESTORATIVE CARE, 3301 Swiss Avenue, Dallas, TX, Zip 75204; tel. 214/828–4747; Geraldine Brueckner, Administrator

PRESBYTERIAN HOSPITAL OF PLANO, 6200 West Parker Road, Plano, TX, Zip 75093–7914; tel. 972/608–8000; Philip M. Wentworth, FACHE, Executive Director

NORTH TEXAS HEALTHCARE NETWORK
3333 Lee Parkway, Suite 900, Dallas, TX 75919; tel. 214/820–3425; Bill Cook, President

BAYLOR CENTER FOR RESTORATIVE CARE, 3504 Swiss Avenue, Dallas, TX, Zip 75204; tel. 214/823–1684; Gerry Brueckner, R.N., Executive Director

BAYLOR INSTITUTE FOR REHABILITATION, 3505 Gaston Avenue, Dallas, TX, Zip 75246–2018; tel. 214/826–7030; Judith C. Waterston, Executive Director

BAYLOR MEDICAL CENTER AT GARLAND, 2300 Marie Curie Boulevard, Garland, TX, Zip 75042–5706; tel. 214/487–5000; John B. McWhorter, III, Executive Director

BAYLOR MEDICAL CENTER AT GRAPEVINE, 1650 West College Street, Grapevine, TX, Zip 76051–1650; tel. 817/329–2500; Mark C. Hood, Executive Director

BAYLOR MEDICAL CENTER–ELLIS COUNTY, 1405 West Jefferson Street, Waxahachie, TX, Zip 75165; tel. 972/923–7000; James Michael Lee, Executive Director

BAYLOR RICHARDSON MEDICAL CENTER, 401 West Campbell Road, Richardson, TX, Zip 75080; tel. 972/498–4000; Ronald L. Boring, President and Chief Executive Officer

BAYLOR UNIVERSITY MEDICAL CENTER, 3500 Gaston Avenue, Dallas, TX, Zip 75246–2088; tel. 214/820–0111; Boone Powell, Jr., President

HARRIS CONTINUED CARE HOSPITAL, 1301 Pennsylvania Avenue, 4th Floor, Fort Worth, TX, Zip 76104, Mailing Address: P.O. Box 3471, Zip 76113; tel. 817/878–5500; Larry Thompson, Administrator

HARRIS METHODIST FORT WORTH, 1301 Pennsylvania Avenue, Fort Worth, TX, Zip 76104–2895; tel. 817/882–2000; Barclay E. Berdan, Chief Executive Officer

HARRIS METHODIST NORTHWEST, 108 Denver Trail, Azle, TX, Zip 76020; tel. 817/444–8600; Larry Thompson, Vice President and Administrator

HARRIS METHODIST SOUTHWEST, 6100 Harris Parkway, Fort Worth, TX, Zip 76132; tel. 817/346–5050; David B. Rowe, Vice President and Administrator

HARRIS METHODIST–ERATH COUNTY, 411 North Belknap Street, Stephenville, TX, Zip 76401–1399, Mailing Address: Box 1399, Zip 76401; tel. 817/965–1500; Ronald E. Dorris, Administrator

HARRIS METHODIST–HEB, 1600 Hospital Parkway, Bedford, TX, Zip 76022–6913, Mailing Address: P.O. Box 669, Zip 76095; tel. 817/685–4000; Jack McCabe, Senior Vice President and Administrator

PRESBYTERIAN HOSPITAL OF DALLAS, 8200 Walnut Hill Lane, Dallas, TX, Zip 75231–4402; tel. 214/345–6789; Mark H. Merrill, Executive Director

PRESBYTERIAN HOSPITAL OF KAUFMAN, 850 Highway 243 West, Kaufman, TX, Zip 75142–9998, Mailing Address: Box 310, Zip 75142; tel. 214/932–7200; Michael J. McBride, CHE, Executive Director

PRESBYTERIAN HOSPITAL OF PLANO, 6200 West Parker Road, Plano, TX, Zip 75093–7914; tel. 972/608–8000; Philip M. Wentworth, FACHE, Executive Director

PRESBYTERIAN HOSPITAL OF WINNSBORO, 719 West Coke Road, Winnsboro, TX, Zip 75494–3098, Mailing Address: P.O. Box 628, Zip 75494–0628; tel. 903/342–5227; Jerry Hopper, FACHE, Executive Director

WALLS REGIONAL HOSPITAL, 201 Walls Drive, Cleburne, TX, Zip 76031; tel. 817/641–2551; Brent D. Magers, FACHE, Chief Executive Officer and Administrator

PERMIAN BASIN RURAL HEALTH NETWORK
P.O. Box 1648, Fort Stockton, TX 79735; tel. 915/336–2241; George Miller, Jr., President

BIG BEND REGIONAL MEDICAL CENTER, 801 East Brown Street, Alpine, TX, Zip 79830; tel. 915/837–3447; Tom L. Lawson, Administrator

BIG SPRING STATE HOSPITAL, Lamesa Highway, Big Spring, TX, Zip 79720, Mailing Address: P.O. Box 231, Zip 79721–0231; tel. 915/267–8216; Edward Moughon, Superintendent

CRANE MEMORIAL HOSPITAL, 1310 South Alford, Crane, TX, Zip 79731; tel. 915/558–3555; Michele Aguilar, Administrator

MARTIN COUNTY HOSPITAL DISTRICT, 610 North St. Peter Street, Stanton, TX, Zip 79782, Mailing Address: Box 640, Zip 79782; tel. 915/756–3345; Rick Jacobus, Administrator

MCCAMEY HOSPITAL, Highway 305 South, McCamey, TX, Zip 79752, Mailing Address: Box 1200, Zip 79752–1200; tel. 915/652–8626; Bill Boswell, Chief Executive Officer

MEDICAL ARTS HOSPITAL, 1600 North Bryan Avenue, Lamesa, TX, Zip 79331; tel. 806/872–2183; Arla Jeffcoat, Administrator

MEDICAL CENTER HOSPITAL, 500 West Fourth Street, Odessa, TX, Zip 79761–5059, Mailing Address: P.O. Drawer 7239, Zip 79760; tel. 915/640–4000; J. Michael Stephans, Administrator

MEMORIAL HOSPITAL, 821 Jeffee Drive, Kermit, TX, Zip 79745, Mailing Address: Drawer H, Zip 79745; tel. 915/586–5864; Judene Willhelm, Administrator

MEMORIAL HOSPITAL, 209 N.W. Eighth Street, Seminole, TX, Zip 79360; tel. 915/758–5811; Kirk Cristy, Chief Executive Officer and Administrator

MEMORIAL HOSPITAL AND MEDICAL CENTER, 2200 West Illinois Avenue, Midland, TX, Zip 79701; tel. 915/685–1111; Harold Rubin, President and Chief Executive Officer

PECOS COUNTY GENERAL HOSPITAL, 305 West Fifth Street, Iraan, TX, Zip 79744, Mailing Address: Box 665, Zip 79744; tel. 915/639–2871; David B. Shaw, Administrator and Chief Executive Officer

PECOS COUNTY MEMORIAL HOSPITAL, Sanderson Highway, Fort Stockton, TX, Zip 79735, Mailing Address: Box 1648, Zip 79735; tel. 915/336–2241; David B. Shaw, Administrator and Chief Executive Officer

PERMIAN GENERAL HOSPITAL, Northeast By-Pass, Andrews, TX, Zip 79714, Mailing Address: Box 2108, Zip 79714; tel. 915/523–2200; Randy R. Richards, Chief Executive Officer

RANKIN HOSPITAL DISTRICT, 1105 Elizabeth Street, Rankin, TX, Zip 79778, Mailing Address: Box 327, Zip 79778; tel. 915/693–2443; John Paul Loyless, Administrator

REAGAN MEMORIAL HOSPITAL, 805 North Main Street, Big Lake, TX, Zip 76932; tel. 915/884–2561; Ron Galloway, Administrator

REEVES COUNTY HOSPITAL, 2323 Texas Street, Pecos, TX, Zip 79772; tel. 915/447–3551; Terry R. Andris, CHE, Interim Chief Executive Officer

SCENIC MOUNTAIN MEDICAL CENTER, 1601 West 11th Place, Big Spring, TX, Zip 79720; tel. 915/263–1211; Kenneth W. Randall, Administrator

VETERANS AFFAIRS MEDICAL CENTER, 300 Veterans Boulevard, Big Spring, TX, Zip 79720–5500; tel. 915/263–7361; Cary D. Brown, Director

WARD MEMORIAL HOSPITAL, 406 South Gary Street, Monahans, TX, Zip 79756; tel. 915/943–2511; William F. O'Brien, Administrator and Chief Executive Officer

PRESBYTERIAN HEALTHCARE SYSTEM
8200 Walnut Hill Lane, Dallas, TX 75231; tel. 214/345–8486; Douglas Hawthorne, President

HUNT MEMORIAL HOSPITAL DISTRICT, Greenville, TX, Mailing Address: P.O. Drawer 1059, Zip 75403–1059; tel. 903/408–5000; Richard Carter, Chief Executive Officer

MCCUISTION REGIONAL MEDICAL CENTER, 865 Deshong Drive, Paris, TX, Zip 75462, Mailing Address: P.O. Box 160, Zip 75461–0160; tel. 903/737–1111; Anthony A. Daigle, Administrator and Chief Executive Officer

PRESBYTERIAN HOSPITAL OF DALLAS, 8200 Walnut Hill Lane, Dallas, TX, Zip 75231–4402; tel. 214/345–6789; Mark H. Merrill, Executive Director

PRESBYTERIAN HOSPITAL OF KAUFMAN, 850 Highway 243 West, Kaufman, TX, Zip 75142–9998, Mailing Address: Box 310, Zip 75142; tel. 214/932–7200; Michael J. McBride, CHE, Executive Director

PRESBYTERIAN HOSPITAL OF PLANO, 6200 West Parker Road, Plano, TX, Zip 75093–7914; tel. 972/608–8000; Philip M. Wentworth, FACHE, Executive Director

PRESBYTERIAN HOSPITAL OF WINNSBORO, 719 West Coke Road, Winnsboro, TX, Zip 75494–3098, Mailing Address: P.O. Box 628, Zip 75494–0628; tel. 903/342–5227; Jerry Hopper, FACHE, Executive Director

PRIMARY CARENET OF TEXAS
6243 IH 10 West, Suite 1001, San Antonio, TX 78201; tel. 210/704–4800; Susan Ginnity, Vice President Marketing & Sales

SANTA ROSA HEALTH CARE CORPORATION, 519 West Houston Street, San Antonio, TX, Zip 78207–3108, Mailing Address: Box 7330, Station A, Zip 78207–3108; tel. 210/704–2011; Robert J. Nolan, President and Chief Executive Officer

REGIONAL HEALTHCARE ALLIANCE
800 East Dawson, Tyler, TX 75701; tel. 903/531–4449; John Webb, President

COLUMBIA LONGVIEW REGIONAL MEDICAL CENTER, 2901 North Fourth Street, Longview, TX, Zip 75605, Mailing Address: P.O. Box 14000, Zip 75607–4000; tel. 903/758–1818; Velinda Stevens, Chief Executive Officer

COLUMBIA WOODLAND HEIGHTS MEDICAL CENTER, 500 Gaslight Boulevard, Lufkin, TX, Zip 75901, Mailing Address: Box 150610, Zip 75915–0610; tel. 409/634–8311; Don H. McBride, Chief Executive Officer

COZBY–GERMANY HOSPITAL, 707 North Waldrip Street, Grand Saline, TX, Zip 75140; tel. 903/962–4242; William Rowton, Chief Executive Officer

EAST TEXAS MEDICAL CENTER, 1100 Loop 304 East, Crockett, TX, Zip 75835–1810; tel. 409/544–2002; Dale E. Clark, Ph.D., Administrator and Chief Executive Officer

FAIRFIELD MEMORIAL HOSPITAL, 125 Newman Street, Fairfield, TX, Zip 75840; tel. 903/389–2121; Milton W. Meadows, Administrator

HENDERSON MEMORIAL HOSPITAL, 300 Wilson Street, Henderson, TX, Zip 75652; tel. 903/657–7541; George T. Roberts, Jr., Chief Executive Officer

MEMORIAL MOTHER FRANCES HOSPITAL, 4000 South Loop 256, Palestine, TX, Zip 75801, Mailing Address: Box 4070, Zip 75802; tel. 903/731–5000; Stephen M. Erixon, Chief Executive Officer

NACOGDOCHES MEDICAL CENTER, 4920 N.E. Stallings, Nacogdoches, TX, Zip 75961, Mailing Address: Box 631604, Zip 75963–1604; tel. 409/568–3380; Bryant H. Krenek, Jr., Director

NAN TRAVIS MEMORIAL HOSPITAL, 501 South Ragsdale Street, Jacksonville, TX, Zip 75766; tel. 903/586–3000; Steve Bowen, President

PANOLA GENERAL HOSPITAL, 409 Cottage Road, Carthage, TX, Zip 75633, Mailing Address: Box 549, Zip 75633–0549; tel. 903/693–3841; Gary Mikeal Hudson, Administrator

PINELANDS HOSPITAL, 4632 Northeast Stallings Drive, Nacogdoches, TX, Zip 75961, Mailing Address: P.O. Box 1004, Zip 79563–1004; tel. 409/560–5900; David Baker, Interim Administrator

ROY H. LAIRD MEMORIAL HOSPITAL, 1612 South Henderson Boulevard, Kilgore, TX, Zip 75662; tel. 903/984–3505; Roderick G. La Grone, President

TITUS REGIONAL MEDICAL CENTER, 2001 North Jefferson, Mount Pleasant, TX, Zip 75455; tel. 903/577–6000; Steven K. Jacobson, Chief Executive Officer

TYLER REHABILITATION HOSPITAL, 3131 Troup Highway, Tyler, TX, Zip 75701; tel. 903/510–7000; Thomas J. Cook, Chief Executive Officer

UNIVERSITY OF TEXAS HEALTH CENTER AT TYLER, Gladewater Highway, Tyler, TX, Zip 75708, Mailing Address: Box 2003, Zip 75710–2003; tel. 903/877–3451; George A. Hurst, M.D., Director

WOOD COUNTY CENTRAL HOSPITAL DISTRICT, 117 Winnsboro Street, Quitman, TX, Zip 75783, Mailing Address: P.O. Box 1000, Zip 75783–1000; tel. 903/763–4505; Marion W. Stanberry, Administrator

SAINT PAUL MEDICAL CENTER AFFILIATE NETWORK
5909 Harry Hines Boulevard, Dallas, TX 75235; tel. 214/879–3100; R. Chris Christy, Network Coordinator

CEDARS HOSPITAL, 2000 North Old Hickory Trail, De Soto, TX, Zip 75115; tel. 972/298–7323; Don Johnson, Administrator

COLUMBIA MEDICAL CENTER–DALLAS SOUTHWEST, 2929 South Hampton Road, Dallas, TX, Zip 75224; tel. 214/330–4611; James B. Warren, Chief Executive Officer

DALLAS–FORT WORTH MEDICAL CENTER, 2709 Hospital Boulevard, Grand Prairie, TX, Zip 75051–1083; tel. 972/641–5000; Robert A. Ficken, Chief Executive Officer and Chief Financial Officer

MEDICAL CENTER OF MESQUITE, 1011 North Galloway Avenue, Mesquite, TX, Zip 75149; tel. 214/320–7000; Terry J. Fontenot, Administrator

SOUTHEAST TEXAS HOSPITAL SYSTEM
233 West 10th Street, Dallas, TX 75208; tel. 800/776–6959; Bob McElearney, Interim President

CITIZENS MEDICAL CENTER, 2701 Hospital Drive, Victoria, TX, Zip 77901–5749; tel. 512/573–9181; David P. Brown, Administrator

CUERO COMMUNITY HOSPITAL, 2550 North Esplanade, Cuero, TX, Zip 77954; tel. 512/275–6191; James E. Buckner, Jr., Administrator

DRISCOLL CHILDREN'S HOSPITAL, 3533 South Alameda Street, Corpus Christi, TX, Zip 78411, Mailing Address: Box 6530, Zip 78466–6530; tel. 512/850–5000; J. E. Ted Stibbards, Ph.D., President and Chief Executive Officer

EL CAMPO MEMORIAL HOSPITAL, 303 Sandy Corner Road, El Campo, TX, Zip 77437; tel. 409/543–6251; C. Richard Murphy, Administrator

JACKSON COUNTY HOSPITAL, 1013 South Wells Street, Edna, TX, Zip 77957–4098; tel. 512/782–5241; Marcella V. Henke, Administrator

LAVACA MEDICAL CENTER, 1400 North Texana Street, Hallettsville, TX, Zip 77964; tel. 512/798–3671; James Vanek, Administrator

MEMORIAL MEDICAL CENTER, 815 North Virginia Street, Port Lavaca, TX, Zip 77979, Mailing Address: P.O. Box 25, Zip 77979; tel. 512/552–6713; Bob L. Bybee, President and Chief Executive Officer

REFUGIO COUNTY MEMORIAL HOSPITAL, 107 Swift Street, Refugio, TX, Zip 78377; tel. 512/526–2321; Haskell G. Silkwood, Administrator

VICTORIA REGIONAL MEDICAL CENTER, 101 Medical Drive, Victoria, TX, Zip 77904; tel. 512/573–6100; J. Michael Mastej, Chief Executive Officer and Managing Director

YOAKUM COMMUNITY HOSPITAL, 303 Hubbard Street, Yoakum, TX, Zip 77995, Mailing Address: Box 753, Zip 77995–0753; tel. 512/293–2321; Elwood E. Currier, Jr., CHE, Administrator

SOUTHEAST TEXAS INTEGRATED COMMUNITY HEALTH NETWORK
2600 North Loop, Houston, TX 77092; tel. 713/681–8877; Stanley T. Urban, President & Chief Executive Officer

ST. ELIZABETH HOSPITAL, 2830 Calder Avenue, Beaumont, TX, Zip 77702, Mailing Address: P.O. Box 5405, Zip 77726–5405; tel. 409/892–7171; Sister Mary Fatima McCarthy, Administrator

ST. JOHN HOSPITAL, 2050 Space Park Drive, Nassau Bay, TX, Zip 77058; tel. 281/333–5503; Thomas Permetti, Administrator

ST. JOSEPH HOSPITAL, 1919 LaBranch Street, Houston, TX, Zip 77002; tel. 713/757–1000; Raymond J. Khoury, Administrator

ST. MARY HOSPITAL, 3600 Gates Boulevard, Port Arthur, TX, Zip 77642–3601, Mailing Address: P.O. Box 3696, Zip 77643–3696; tel. 409/985–7431; James E. Gardner, Jr., Administrator

SOUTHWEST PREFERRED NETWORK
14901 Quorum Drive, Suite 200, Dallas, TX 75240; tel. 214/866–7400; Ron Lutz, President & Chief Executive Officer

ARLINGTON MEMORIAL HOSPITAL, 800 West Randol Mill Road, Arlington, TX, Zip 76012; tel. 817/548–6100; Rex C. McRae, President

ST. JOSEPH'S HOSPITAL AND HEALTH CENTER, 820 Clarksville Street, Paris, TX, Zip 75460–9070, Mailing Address: P.O. Box 9070, Zip 75461–9070; tel. 903/785–4521; Monty E. McLaurin, President

SOUTHWEST TEXAS RURAL HEALTH ALLIANCE
900 Northeast Loop 410, Suite 500, San Antonio, TX 78209; tel. 210/829–0009; Kay Peck, President

CENTRAL TEXAS MEDICAL CENTER, 1301 Wonder World Drive, San Marcos, TX, Zip 78666; tel. 512/353–8979; Peter M. Weber, President and Chief Executive Officer

DIMMIT COUNTY MEMORIAL HOSPITAL, 704 Hospital Drive, Carrizo Springs, TX, Zip 78834; tel. 210/876–2424; Ernest Flores, Jr., Administrator

EDGAR B. DAVIS MEMORIAL HOSPITAL, 130 Hays Street, Luling, TX, Zip 78648, Mailing Address: P.O. Box 510, Zip 78648–0510; tel. 210/875–5643; Neal Kelley, Administrator

FRIO HOSPITAL, 320 Berry Ranch Road, Pearsall, TX, Zip 78061; tel. 210/334–3617; Alan D. Holmes, Chief Executive Officer

GUADALUPE VALLEY HOSPITAL, 1215 East Court Street, Seguin, TX, Zip 78155–5189; tel. 210/379–2411; Don L. Richey, Administrator

HILL COUNTRY MEMORIAL HOSPITAL, 1020 Kerrville Road, Fredericksburg, TX, Zip 78624, Mailing Address: Box 835, Zip 78624–0835; tel. 210/997–4353; Jerry L. Durr, Chief Executive Officer

KIMBLE HOSPITAL, 2101 Main Street, Junction, TX, Zip 76849–2101; tel. 915/446–3321; Ben Snead, Administrator

MCKENNA MEMORIAL HOSPITAL, 143 East Garza Street, New Braunfels, TX, Zip 78130–4191; tel. 210/606–9111; Marion P. Johnson, FACHE, President and Chief Executive Officer

MEDINA COMMUNITY HOSPITAL, 3100 Avenue East, Hondo, TX, Zip 78861; tel. 210/741–4677; Richard D. Arnold, Administrator

MEMORIAL HOSPITAL, Highway 90A By-Pass, Gonzales, TX, Zip 78629, Mailing Address: Box 587, Zip 78629; tel. 210/672–7581; Douglas Langley, Administrator

OTTO KAISER MEMORIAL HOSPITAL, Highway 181 North, Kenedy, TX, Zip 78119, Mailing Address: Route 1, Box 450, Zip 78119–9718; tel. 210/583–3401; Harold L. Boening, Administrator

SID PETERSON MEMORIAL HOSPITAL, 710 Water Street, Kerrville, TX, Zip 78028–5398; tel. 210/896–4200; F. W. Hall, Jr., Administrator

TRI-CITY COMMUNITY HOSPITAL, Highway 97 East, Jourdanton, TX, Zip 78026, Mailing Address: Box 189, Zip 78026; tel. 512/769–3515; S. Allen Smith, Administrator

UVALDE COUNTY HOSPITAL AUTHORITY, 1025 Garner Field Road, Uvalde, TX, Zip 78801–1025; tel. 210/278–6251; Ben M. Durr, Administrator

VAL VERDE MEMORIAL HOSPITAL, 801 Bedell Avenue, Del Rio, TX, Zip 78840, Mailing Address: P.O. Box 1527, Zip 78840; tel. 210/775–8566; Scott D. Evans, FACHE, Administrator

WARM SPRINGS REHABILITATION HOSPITAL, Gonzales, TX, Mailing Address: P.O. Box 58, Zip 78629–0058; tel. 210/672–6592; John Davis, Administrator

WILSON MEMORIAL HOSPITAL, 1301 Hospital Boulevard, Floresville, TX, Zip 78114; tel. 210/393–3122; Robert Duffield, Administrator

TEXOMA HEALTH NETWORK
1600 11th Street, Wichita Falls, TX 76301; tel. 817/872–1126; David Whitaker, Executive Director

BETHANIA REGIONAL HEALTH CARE CENTER, 1600 11th Street, Wichita Falls, TX, Zip 76301–9988; tel. 817/723–4111; David D. Whitaker, FACHE, President and Chief Executive Officer

BOWIE MEMORIAL HOSPITAL, 705 East Greenwood Avenue, Bowie, TX, Zip 76230; tel. 817/872–1126; Joyce Crumpler, R.N., Administrator

CHILLICOTHE HOSPITAL DISTRICT, 303 Avenue I, Chillicothe, TX, Zip 79225, Mailing Address: Box 370, Zip 79225; tel. 817/852–5131; Linda Hall, Administrator

CLAY COUNTY MEMORIAL HOSPITAL, 310 West South Street, Henrietta, TX, Zip 76365–3399; tel. 817/538–5621; Edward E. Browning, Administrator

ELECTRA MEMORIAL HOSPITAL, 1207 South Bailey Street, Electra, TX, Zip 76360, Mailing Address: Box 1112, Zip 76360–1112; tel. 817/495–3981; Jan A. Reed, CPA, Administrator

FAITH COMMUNITY HOSPITAL, 717 Magnolia Street, Jacksboro, TX, Zip 76458; tel. 817/567–6633; Don Hopkins, Administrator

HAMILTON HOSPITAL, 903 West Hamilton Street, Olney, TX, Zip 76374, Mailing Address: Box 158, Zip 76374; tel. 817/564–5521; William R. Smith, Administrator

HARDEMAN COUNTY MEMORIAL HOSPITAL, 402 Mercer Street, Quanah, TX, Zip 79252, Mailing Address: Box 90, Zip 79252; tel. 817/663–2795; Charles Hurt, Administrator

NOCONA GENERAL HOSPITAL, 100 Park Street, Nocona, TX, Zip 76255; tel. 817/825–3235; Jamers Brasier, Administrator

SEYMOUR HOSPITAL, 200 Stadium Drive, Seymour, TX, Zip 76380; tel. 817/888–5572; Charles Norris, Administrator

THROCKMORTON COUNTY MEMORIAL HOSPITAL, Seymour Highway, Throckmorton, TX, Zip 76483, Mailing Address: P.O. Box 729, Zip 76483; tel. 817/849–2151; Blake Kretz, Administrator

THE HEART NETWORK OF TEXAS
511 East John Carpenter Freeway, Suite 440, Irving, TX '75062; tel. 972/409–9100; Daniel Hanzlik, Executive Director

Section B

BAYLOR UNIVERSITY MEDICAL CENTER, 3500 Gaston Avenue, Dallas, TX, Zip 75246–2088; tel. 214/820–0111; Boone Powell, Jr., President

BETHANIA REGIONAL HEALTH CARE CENTER, 1600 11th Street, Wichita Falls, TX, Zip 76301–9988; tel. 817/723–4111; David D. Whitaker, FACHE, President and Chief Executive Officer

HARRIS CONTINUED CARE HOSPITAL, 1301 Pennsylvania Avenue, 4th Floor, Fort Worth, TX, Zip 76104, Mailing Address: P.O. Box 3471, Zip 76113; tel. 817/878–5500; Larry Thompson, Administrator

HARRIS METHODIST FORT WORTH, 1301 Pennsylvania Avenue, Fort Worth, TX, Zip 76104–2895; tel. 817/882–2000; Barclay E. Berdan, Chief Executive Officer

HARRIS METHODIST NORTHWEST, 108 Denver Trail, Azle, TX, Zip 76020; tel. 817/444–8600; Larry Thompson, Vice President and Administrator

HARRIS METHODIST SOUTHWEST, 6100 Harris Parkway, Fort Worth, TX, Zip 76132; tel. 817/346–5050; David B. Rowe, Vice President and Administrator

HARRIS METHODIST–ERATH COUNTY, 411 North Belknap Street, Stephenville, TX, Zip 76401–1399, Mailing Address: Box 1399, Zip 76401; tel. 817/965–1500; Ronald E. Dorris, Administrator

HARRIS METHODIST–HEB, 1600 Hospital Parkway, Bedford, TX, Zip 76022–6913, Mailing Address: P.O. Box 669, Zip 76095; tel. 817/685–4000; Jack McCabe, Senior Vice President and Administrator

HENDRICK HEALTH SYSTEM, 1242 North 19th Street, Abilene, TX, Zip 79601–2316; tel. 915/670–2000; Michael C. Waters, President

HILLCREST BAPTIST MEDICAL CENTER, 3000 Herring Avenue, Waco, TX, Zip 76708–3299, Mailing Address: Box 5100, Zip 76708–0100; tel. 817/756–8011; Richard E. Scott, President

TEXOMA HEALTHCARE SYSTEM, 1000 Memorial Drive, Denison, TX, Zip 75020, Mailing Address: Box 890, Zip 75021–9988; tel. 903/416–4000; Arthur L. Hohenberger, FACHE, President and Chief Executive Officer

TRINITY MOTHER FRANCES HEALTH SYSTEM, 800 East Dawson, Tyler, TX, Zip 75701–2093; tel. 903/593–8441; J. Lindsey Bradley, Jr., FACHE, President and Chief Administrative Officer

WADLEY REGIONAL MEDICAL CENTER, 1000 Pine Street, Texarkana, TX, Zip 75501–5170, Mailing Address: Box 1878, Zip 75504–1878; tel. 903/798–8000; Hugh R. Hallgren, President and Chief Executive Officer

WALLS REGIONAL HOSPITAL, 201 Walls Drive, Cleburne, TX, Zip 76031; tel. 817/641–2551; Brent D. Magers, FACHE, Chief Executive Officer and Administrator

UTAH

INTERMOUNTAIN HEALTHCARE/AMERINET 36 South State Street, 22nd Floor, Salt Lake City, UT 84111; tel. 801/442–2000; Scott Parker, President

ALTA VIEW HOSPITAL, 9660 South 1300 East, Sandy, UT, Zip 84094; tel. 801/576–2600; Wes Thompson, Administrator

AMERICAN FORK HOSPITAL, 1100 East 170 North, American Fork, UT, Zip 84003–9787; tel. 801/763–3300; Keith N. Alexander, Administrator and Chief Operating Officer

BEAR RIVER VALLEY HOSPITAL, 440 West 600 North, Tremonton, UT, Zip 84337; tel. 801/257–7441; Robert F. Jex, Administrator

CASSIA REGIONAL MEDICAL CENTER, 1501 Hiland Avenue, Burley, ID, Zip 83318; tel. 208/678–4444; Richard Packer, Administrator

COTTONWOOD HOSPITAL MEDICAL CENTER, 5770 South 300 East, Murray, UT, Zip 84107; tel. 801/262–3461; Douglas R. Fonnesbeck, Administrator

DELTA COMMUNITY MEDICAL CENTER, 126 South White Sage Avenue, Delta, UT, Zip 84624; tel. 801/864–5591; James E. Beckstrand, Administrator

DIXIE REGIONAL MEDICAL CENTER, 544 South 400 East, Saint George, UT, Zip 84770; tel. 801/634–4000; L. Steven Wilson, Administrator

FILLMORE COMMUNITY MEDICAL CENTER, 674 South Highway 99, Fillmore, UT, Zip 84631; tel. 801/743–5591; James E. Beckstrand, Administrator

GARFIELD MEMORIAL HOSPITAL AND CLINICS, 200 North Fourth East, Panguitch, UT, Zip 84759, Mailing Address: P.O. Box 389, Zip 84759–0389; tel. 435/676–8811; Wayne R. Ross, Administrator

MCKAY–DEE HOSPITAL CENTER, 3939 Harrison Boulevard, Ogden, UT, Zip 84409–2386, Mailing Address: Box 9370, Zip 84409–0370; tel. 801/627–2800; Thomas Hanrahan, Administrator and Chief Executive Officer

OREM COMMUNITY HOSPITAL, 331 North 400 West, Orem, UT, Zip 84057; tel. 801/224–4080; Kim Nielsen, Administrator and Chief Executive Officer

POCATELLO REGIONAL MEDICAL CENTER, 777 Hospital Way, Pocatello, ID, Zip 83201; tel. 208/234–0777; Earl L. Christison, Administrator

PRIMARY CHILDREN'S MEDICAL CENTER, 100 North Medical Drive, Salt Lake City, UT, Zip 84113–1100; tel. 801/588–2000; Joseph R. Horton, Chief Executive Officer and Administrator

SANPETE VALLEY HOSPITAL, 1100 South Medical Drive, Mount Pleasant, UT, Zip 84647; tel. 801/462–2441; George Winn, Administrator

SEVIER VALLEY HOSPITAL, 1100 North Main Street, Richfield, UT, Zip 84701; tel. 801/896–8271; Gary E. Beck, Administrator

UTAH VALLEY REGIONAL MEDICAL CENTER, 1034 North 500 West, Provo, UT, Zip 84605–0390; tel. 801/373–7850; Larry R. Dursteler, Regional Vice President

VALLEY VIEW MEDICAL CENTER, 595 South 75 East, Cedar City, UT, Zip 84720; tel. 801/586–6587; Craig M. Smedley, Administrator

WASATCH COUNTY HOSPITAL, 55 South Fifth East, Heber City, UT, Zip 84032–1848; tel. 801/654–2500; Randall K. Probst, Administrator

VERMONT

FLETCHER ALLEN HEALTH CARE 111 Colchester Avenue, Burlington, VT 05401; tel. 802/865–5191; Jim Taylor, President

FLETCHER ALLEN HEALTH CARE, 111 Colchester Avenue, Burlington, VT, Zip 05401–1429; tel. 802/656–2345; John W. Frymoyer, M.D., Chief Executive Officer

VIRGINIA

CARILION HEALTH SYSTEM 101 Elm Avenue, Roanoke, VA 24013; tel. 540/981–7900; Shirley Hollard, Vice President

CARILION BEDFORD MEMORIAL HOSPITAL, 1613 Oakwood Street, Bedford, VA, Zip 24523–0688, Mailing Address: P.O. Box 688, Zip 24523–0688; tel. 540/586–2441; Howard Ainsley, Director

CARILION FRANKLIN MEMORIAL HOSPITAL, 180 Floyd Avenue, Rocky Mount, VA, Zip 24151; tel. 540/483–5277; Matthew J. Perry, Director

CARILION GILES MEMORIAL HOSPITAL, 1 Taylor Avenue, Pearisburg, VA, Zip 24134, Mailing Address: P.O. Box K, Zip 24134; tel. 540/921–6000; Morris D. Reece, Director

CARILION RADFORD COMMUNITY HOSPITAL, 700 Randolph Street, Radford, VA, Zip 24141–2430; tel. 540/731–2000; Virginia Ousley, Director

CARILION ROANOKE COMMUNITY HOSPITAL, 101 Elm Avenue S.E., Roanoke, VA, Zip 24013, Mailing Address: P.O. Box 12946, Zip 24029; tel. 540/985–8000; Lucas A. Snipes, Director

CARILION ROANOKE MEMORIAL HOSPITAL, Belleview at Jefferson Street, Roanoke, VA, Zip 24014, Mailing Address: P.O. Box 13367, Zip 24033–3367; tel. 540/981–7000; Lucas A. Snipes, Director

CARILION ST. ALBANS HOSPITAL, Route 11, Lee Highway, Radford, VA, Zip 24141, Mailing Address: Box 3608, Zip 24143; tel. 540/639–2481; Janet McKinney Crawford, Administrator

CENTRAL VIRGINIA HEALTH NETWORK 8100 Three Chopt Road, Suite 209, Richmond, VA 23229; tel. 804/673–2846; Michael B. Matthews, Chief Executive Officer

BON SECOURS–RICHMOND COMMUNITY HOSPITAL, 1500 North 28th Street, Richmond, VA, Zip 23223–5396, Mailing Address: Box 27184, Zip 23261–7184; tel. 804/225–1700; Samuel F. Lillard, Executive Vice President and Administrator

BON SECOURS–STUART CIRCLE, 413 Stuart Circle, Richmond, VA, Zip 23220; tel. 804/358–7051; Timothy A. Johnson, Executive Vice President and Administrator

COMMUNITY MEMORIAL HEALTHCENTER, 125 Buena Vista Circle, South Hill, VA, Zip 23970–0090, Mailing Address: P.O. Box 90, Zip 23970–0090; tel. 804/447–3151; Steven G. Kelly, President

MARY IMMACULATE HOSPITAL, 2 Bernardine Drive, Newport News, VA, Zip 23602; tel. 757/886–6000; Kirby H. Smith, Jr., Executive Vice President and Chief Executive Officer

RAPPAHANNOCK GENERAL HOSPITAL, 101 Harris Drive, Kilmarnock, VA, Zip 22482, Mailing Address: P.O. Box 1449, Zip 22482–1449; tel. 804/435–8000; James M. Holmes, President and Chief Executive Officer

RICHMOND MEMORIAL HOSPITAL, 1300 Westwood Avenue, Richmond, VA, Zip 23227–4699, Mailing Address: Box 26783, Zip 23261–6783; tel. 804/254–6000; Michael–David Robinson, Executive Vice President and Administrator

SHELTERING ARMS REHABILITATION HOSPITAL, 1311 Palmyra Avenue, Richmond, VA, Zip 23227–4418; tel. 804/342–4100; Richard C. Craven, President

SOUTHSIDE REGIONAL MEDICAL CENTER, 801 South Adams Street, Petersburg, VA, Zip 23803–5133; tel. 804/862–5000; David S. Dunham, President

ST. MARY'S HOSPITAL, 5801 Bremo Road, Richmond, VA, Zip 23226–1900; tel. 804/285–2011; Ann E. Honeycutt, Executive Vice President and Administrator

UNIVERSITY OF VIRGINIA MEDICAL CENTER, Jefferson Park Avenue, Charlottesville, VA, Zip 22908, Mailing Address: P.O. Box 10050, Zip 22906–0050; tel. 804/924–0211; Michael J. Halseth, Executive Director

DEPAUL MEDICAL CENTER GROUP 150 Kingsley Lane, Norfolk, VA 23505; tel. 804/889–5000; Kevin P. Conlin, President & Chief Executive Officer

BON SECOURS–DEPAUL MEDICAL CENTER, 150 Kingsley Lane, Norfolk, VA, Zip 23505; tel. 757/889–5000; Sharon M. Tanner, President and Chief Executive Officer

INOVA HEALTH SYSTEM 8001 Braddock Road, Springfield, VA 22151; tel. 703/321–4213; J. Knox Singleton, President & Chief Executive Officer

INOVA FAIR OAKS HOSPITAL, 3600 Joseph Siewick Drive, Fairfax, VA, Zip 22033–1709; tel. 703/391–3600; Steven E. Brown, Administrator

INOVA FAIRFAX HOSPITAL, 3300 Gallows Road, Falls Church, VA, Zip 22046–3300; tel. 703/698–1110; Jolene Tornabeni, Administrator

INOVA MOUNT VERNON HOSPITAL, 2501 Parker's Lane, Alexandria, VA, Zip 22306–3209; tel. 703/664–7000; Susan Herbert, Administrator

PREFERRED CARE OF RICHMOND 9100 Arboretum Parkway, Richmond, VA 23236; tel. 804/560–4160; Sheri Duff, Network Coordinator

Section B

CHIPPENHAM AND JOHNSTON–WILLIS HOSPITALS, 7101 Jahnke Road, Richmond, VA, Zip 23225; tel. 804/320–3911; Gerard Filicko, Chief Executive Officer

COLUMBIA JOHN RANDOLPH MEDICAL CENTER, 411 West Randolph Road, Hopewell, VA, Zip 23860, Mailing Address: P.O. Box 971, Zip 23860; tel. 804/541–1600; Daniel J. Wetta, Jr., Chief Executive Officer

HENRICO DOCTORS' HOSPITAL, 1602 Skipwith Road, Richmond, VA, Zip 23229; tel. 804/289–4500; Patrick W. Farrell, Chief Executive Officer

POPLAR SPRINGS HOSPITAL, 350 Poplar Drive, Petersburg, VA, Zip 23805–4657; tel. 804/733–6874; Anthony J. Vadella, Chief Executive Officer

RETREAT HOSPITAL, 2621 Grove Avenue, Richmond, VA, Zip 23220–4308; tel. 804/254–5100; Paul L. Baldwin, Chief Operating Officer

SENTARA HEALTH SYSTEM
  6015 Poplar Hall Drive, Suite 306, Norfolk, VA 23502; tel. 804/455–7000; Glenn R. Mitchell, President

SENTARA BAYSIDE HOSPITAL, 800 Independence Boulevard, Virginia Beach, VA, Zip 23455–6076; tel. 757/363–6100; Virginia Bogue, Site Administrator

SENTARA HAMPTON GENERAL HOSPITAL, 3120 Victoria Boulevard, Hampton, VA, Zip 23661, Mailing Address: Drawer 640, Zip 23669; tel. 804/727–7000; Les A. Donahue, President and Chief Executive Officer

SENTARA LEIGH HOSPITAL, 830 Kempsville Road, Norfolk, VA, Zip 23502; tel. 757/466–6000; Darleen S. Anderson, R.N., MSN, Site Administrator

SENTARA NORFOLK GENERAL HOSPITAL, 600 Gresham Drive, Norfolk, VA, Zip 23507–1999; tel. 804/668–3000; Roger M. Eitelman, Site Administrator

WILLIAMSBURG COMMUNITY HOSPITAL, 301 Monticello Avenue, Williamsburg, VA, Zip 23187–8700, Mailing Address: Box 8700, Zip 23187–8700; tel. 757/259–6000; Les A. Donahue, President and Chief Executive Officer

TIDEWATER HEALTH CARE
  1080 First Colonial Road, Virginia Beach, VA 23454; tel. 804/496–6200; Douglas L. Johnson, Ph.D., President and Chief Executive Officer

PORTSMOUTH GENERAL HOSPITAL, 850 Crawford Parkway, Portsmouth, VA, Zip 23704–2386; tel. 804/398–4000; Nora M. Paffrath, Executive Vice President

VIRGINIA BEACH GENERAL HOSPITAL, 1060 First Colonial Road, Virginia Beach, VA, Zip 23454–9000; tel. 804/481–8000; Robert L. Graves, Administrator

VALLEY HEALTH SYSTEM
  P.O. Box 3340, Winchester, VA 22604; tel. 540/722–8000; David W. Goff, Chief Executive Officer

WARREN MEMORIAL HOSPITAL, 1000 Shenandoah Avenue, Front Royal, VA, Zip 22630–3598; tel. 540/636–0300; Charlie M. Horton, President

WINCHESTER MEDICAL CENTER, 1840 Amherst Street, Winchester, VA, Zip 22601–2540, Mailing Address: P.O. Box 3340, Zip 22604–3340; tel. 540/722–8000; George B. Caley, President

VIRGINIA HEALTH NETWORK
  7400 Beaufont Springs Drive, Suite 505, Richmond, VA 23225; tel. 804/320–3837; David Keplinger, Marketing Vice President

BON SECOURS–DEPAUL MEDICAL CENTER, 150 Kingsley Lane, Norfolk, VA, Zip 23505; tel. 757/889–5000; Sharon M. Tanner, President and Chief Executive Officer

BON SECOURS–MARYVIEW MEDICAL CENTER, 3636 High Street, Portsmouth, VA, Zip 23707–3236; tel. 804/398–2200; Richard A. Hanson, Acting Administrator

BON SECOURS–RICHMOND COMMUNITY HOSPITAL, 1500 North 28th Street, Richmond, VA, Zip 23223–5396, Mailing Address: Box 27184, Zip 23261–7184; tel. 804/225–1700; Samuel F. Lillard, Executive Vice President and Administrator

BON SECOURS–STUART CIRCLE, 413 Stuart Circle, Richmond, VA, Zip 23220; tel. 804/358–7051; Timothy A. Johnson, Executive Vice President and Administrator

CHARTER BEHAVIORAL HEALTH SYSTEM OF CHARLOTTESVILLE, 2101 Arlington Boulevard, Charlottesville, VA, Zip 22903–1593; tel. 804/977–1120; Wayne Adams, Chief Executive Officer

CHESAPEAKE GENERAL HOSPITAL, 736 Battlefield Boulevard North, Chesapeake, VA, Zip 23320–4941, Mailing Address: P.O. Box 2028, Zip 23327–2028; tel. 757/547–8121; Donald S. Buckley, FACHE, President

CHILDREN'S HOSPITAL OF THE KING'S DAUGHTERS, 601 Children's Lane, Norfolk, VA, Zip 23507; tel. 804/668–7700; Robert I. Bonar, Jr., President and Chief Executive Officer

COMMUNITY MEMORIAL HEALTHCENTER, 125 Buena Vista Circle, South Hill, VA, Zip 23970–0090, Mailing Address: P.O. Box 90, Zip 23970–0090; tel. 804/447–3151; Steven G. Kelly, President

GREENSVILLE MEMORIAL HOSPITAL, 214 Weaver Avenue, Emporia, VA, Zip 23847–1482; tel. 804/348–2000; Rosemary C. Check, Chief Executive Officer

LOUISE OBICI MEMORIAL HOSPITAL, 1900 North Main Street, Suffolk, VA, Zip 23434, Mailing Address: P.O. Box 1100, Zip 23439; tel. 757/934–4000; William C. Giermak, President and Chief Executive Officer

MARTHA JEFFERSON HOSPITAL, 459 Locust Avenue, Charlottesville, VA, Zip 22902–9940; tel. 804/982–7000; James E. Haden, President and Chief Executive Officer

MEDICAL COLLEGE OF VIRGINIA HOSPITALS, VIRGINIA COMMONWEALTH UNIVERSITY, 401 North 12th Street, Richmond, VA, Zip 23219, Mailing Address: P.O. Box 980510, Zip 23298–0510; tel. 804/828–9000; Carl R. Fischer, Associate Vice President and Chief Executive Officer

PORTSMOUTH GENERAL HOSPITAL, 850 Crawford Parkway, Portsmouth, VA, Zip 23704–2386; tel. 804/398–4000; Nora M. Paffrath, Executive Vice President

RICHMOND MEMORIAL HOSPITAL, 1300 Westwood Avenue, Richmond, VA, Zip 23227–4699, Mailing Address: Box 26783, Zip 23261–6783; tel. 804/254–6000; Michael–David Robinson, Executive Vice President and Administrator

RIVERSIDE REGIONAL MEDICAL CENTER, 500 J. Clyde Morris Boulevard, Newport News, VA, Zip 23601–1976; tel. 757/594–2000; Gerald R. Brink, President and Chief Executive Officer

RIVERSIDE TAPPAHANNOCK HOSPITAL, Tappahannock, VA, Mailing Address: Route 2, Box 612, Zip 22560; tel. 804/443–3311; Elizabeth J. Martin, Vice President and Administrator

RIVERSIDE WALTER REED HOSPITAL, Gloucester, VA, Mailing Address: Route 17, Box 1130, Zip 23061–1130; tel. 804/693–8800; Grady W. Philips, III, Vice President and Administrator

SHELTERING ARMS REHABILITATION HOSPITAL, 1311 Palmyra Avenue, Richmond, VA, Zip 23227–4418; tel. 804/342–4100; Richard C. Craven, President

SOUTHAMPTON MEMORIAL HOSPITAL, 100 Fairview Drive, Franklin, VA, Zip 23851, Mailing Address: P.O. Box 817, Zip 23851–0817; tel. 757/569–6100; Edward J. Patnesky, President and Chief Executive Officer

SOUTHSIDE REGIONAL MEDICAL CENTER, 801 South Adams Street, Petersburg, VA, Zip 23803–5133; tel. 804/862–5000; David S. Dunham, President

ST. MARY'S HOSPITAL, 5801 Bremo Road, Richmond, VA, Zip 23226–1900; tel. 804/285–2011; Ann E. Honeycutt, Executive Vice President and Administrator

VIRGINIA BEACH GENERAL HOSPITAL, 1060 First Colonial Road, Virginia Beach, VA, Zip 23454–9000; tel. 804/481–8000; Robert L. Graves, Administrator

WILLIAMSBURG COMMUNITY HOSPITAL, 301 Monticello Avenue, Williamsburg, VA, Zip 23187–8700, Mailing Address: Box 8700, Zip 23187–8700; tel. 757/259–6000; Les A. Donahue, President and Chief Executive Officer

WASHINGTON

COLUMBIAN BASIN HEALTH NETWORK
  P.O. Box 185, Mead, WA 99021; tel. 509/238–2167; Jamie Norr, Network Contact

COLUMBIA BASIN HOSPITAL, 200 Southeast Boulevard, Ephrata, WA, Zip 98823–1997; tel. 509/754–4631; Al Beach, Administrator

COULEE COMMUNITY HOSPITAL, 411 Fortuyn Road, Grand Coulee, WA, Zip 99133–0840; tel. 509/633–1753; Michael C. Wiltermood, Chief Executive Officer

EAST ADAMS RURAL HOSPITAL, 903 South Adams Street, Ritzville, WA, Zip 99169–2298; tel. 509/659–1200; James G. Parrish, Administrator

LINCOLN HOSPITAL, 10 Nichols Street, Davenport, WA, Zip 99122; tel. 509/725–7101; Thomas J. Martin, Chief Executive Officer

MID–VALLEY HOSPITAL, 810 Valley Way Road, Omak, WA, Zip 98841, Mailing Address: Box 793, Zip 98841; tel. 509/826–1760; Dale F. Payne, Acting Administrator

OTHELLO COMMUNITY HOSPITAL, 315 North 14th Street, Othello, WA, Zip 99344; tel. 509/488–2636; Jerry Lane, Administrator

QUINCY VALLEY MEDICAL CENTER, 908 Tenth Avenue S.W., Quincy, WA, Zip 98848; tel. 509/787–3531; Jerry Hawley, Administrator

SAMARITAN HEALTHCARE, 801 East Wheeler Road, Moses Lake, WA, Zip 98837–1899; tel. 509/765–5606; Keith J. Baldwin, Administrator

DOMINICAN NETWORK
  5633 North Lidgerwood, Spokane, WA 99207; tel. 509/482–2458; Ron Schurra, President

DEER PARK HEALTH CENTER AND HOSPITAL, East 1015 D Street, Deer Park, WA, Zip 99006, Mailing Address: P.O. Box 742, Zip 99006; tel. 509/276–5061; Cathy Simchuk, Chief Operating Officer

HOLY FAMILY HOSPITAL, North 5633 Lidgerwood Avenue, Spokane, WA, Zip 99220; tel. 509/482–0111; Ronald J. Schurra, Chief Executive Officer

MOUNT CARMEL HOSPITAL, 982 East Columbia Street, Colville, WA, Zip 99114–0351, Mailing Address: Box 351, Zip 99114–0351; tel. 509/684–2561; Gloria Cooper, Chief Executive Officer

ST. JOSEPH HOSPITAL, 2901 Squalicum Parkway, Bellingham, WA, Zip 98225–1898; tel. 360/734–5400; John Hayward, Administrator

GROUP HEALTH COOPERATIVE OF PUGET SOUND
  521 Wall Street, Seattle, WA 98121; tel. 206/448–3000; Phil Nudelman, Ph.D, President & Chief Executive Officer

GROUP HEALTH COOPERATIVE CENTRAL HOSPITAL, 201 16th Avenue East, Seattle, WA, Zip 98112–5298; tel. 206/326–3000; Scott Armstrong, Administrator

THE EASTSIDE HOSPITAL, 2700 152nd Avenue N.E., Redmond, WA, Zip 98052–5560; tel. 206/883–5151; Scott Armstrong, Administrator

HEALTH WASHINGTON
  P.O. Box 14999, Seattle, WA 98104–5044; tel. 206/386–3462; Joe Leinonen, President & Chief Executive Officer

EVERGREEN HOSPITAL MEDICAL CENTER, 12040 N.E. 128th Street, Kirkland, WA, Zip 98034; tel. 206/899–1000; Andrew Fallat, FACHE, Chief Executive Officer

MARY BRIDGE CHILDREN'S HOSPITAL AND HEALTH CENTER, 317 Martin Luther King Jr. Way, Tacoma, WA, Zip 98405–0299, Mailing Address: Box 5299, Zip 98405–0299; tel. 206/552–1400; William B. Connoley, President and Chief Executive Officer

STEVENS HEALTHCARE, 21601 76th Avenue West, Edmonds, WA, Zip 98026–7506; tel. 206/640–4000; Steve C. McCary, President and Chief Executive Officer

SWEDISH HEALTH SERVICES, 747 Broadway Avenue, Seattle, WA, Zip 98122–4307; tel. 206/386–6000; Richard H. Peterson, President and Chief Executive Officer

TACOMA GENERAL HOSPITAL, 315 Martin Luther King Jr. Way, Tacoma, WA, Zip 98405–0299, Mailing Address: P.O. Box 5299, Zip 98405–0299; tel. 206/552–1000; William B. Connoley, President and Chief Executive Officer

LINCOLN COUNTY PUBLIC HEALTH COALITION
22 Bramhall Street, Davenport, WA 99122; tel. 509/725–1001; Diane Martin, Administrator

LINCOLN HOSPITAL, 10 Nichols Street, Davenport, WA, Zip 99122; tel. 509/725–7101; Thomas J. Martin, Chief Executive Officer

ODESSA MEMORIAL HOSPITAL, 502 East Amende, Odessa, WA, Zip 99159, Mailing Address: Box 368, Zip 99159–0368; tel. 509/982–2611; Carol Schott, Administrator

MULTICARE HEALTH SYSTEM
P.O. Box 5299, Tacoma, WA 98405; tel. 206/552–1000; William B. Connoley, President & Chief Executive Officer

ALLENMORE HOSPITAL, South 19th and Union Avenue, Tacoma, WA, Zip 98405, Mailing Address: P.O. Box 11414, Zip 98411–0414; tel. 206/572–2323; Charles Hoffman, Administrator

MARY BRIDGE CHILDREN'S HOSPITAL AND HEALTH CENTER, 317 Martin Luther King Jr. Way, Tacoma, WA, Zip 98405–0299, Mailing Address: Box 5299, Zip 98405–0299; tel. 206/552–1400; William B. Connoley, President and Chief Executive Officer

TACOMA GENERAL HOSPITAL, 315 Martin Luther King Jr. Way, Tacoma, WA, Zip 98405–0299, Mailing Address: P.O. Box 5299, Zip 98405–0299; tel. 206/552–1000; William B. Connoley, President and Chief Executive Officer

PEACEHEALTH
15325 Southeast 30th Place, Suite 300, Bellevue, WA 98007; tel. 206/747–1711; Sister Monica Heeran, Chief Executive Officer

EVERGREEN HOSPITAL MEDICAL CENTER, 12040 N.E. 128th Street, Kirkland, WA, Zip 98034; tel. 206/899–1000; Andrew Fallat, FACHE, Chief Executive Officer

KETCHIKAN GENERAL HOSPITAL, 3100 Tongass Avenue, Ketchikan, AK, Zip 99901–5746; tel. 907/225–5171; Edward F. Mahn, Chief Executive Officer

PEACE HARBOR HOSPITAL, 400 Ninth Street, Florence, OR, Zip 97439, Mailing Address: P.O. Box 580, Zip 97439; tel. 541/997–8412; James Barnhart, Administrator

SACRED HEART MEDICAL CENTER, 1255 Hilyard Street, Eugene, OR, Zip 97401, Mailing Address: P.O. Box 10905, Zip 97440; tel. 541/686–7300; Andrew R. McCulloch, Administrator

ST. JOHN MEDICAL CENTER, 1614 East Kessler Boulevard, Longview, WA, Zip 98632, Mailing Address: P.O. Box 3002, Zip 98632–0302; tel. 360/423–1530; Mark E. McGourty, Regional Chief Executive Officer

ST. JOSEPH HOSPITAL, 2901 Squalicum Parkway, Bellingham, WA, Zip 98225–1898; tel. 360/734–5400; John Hayward, Administrator

PROVIDENCE SERVICES
9 East 9th Avenue, Spokane, WA 99202; tel. 509/742–7337; Richard J. Umdenstock, President & Chief Executive Officer

BENEFIS HEALTH CARE, 500 15th Avenue South, Great Falls, MT, Zip 59403; tel. 406/727–3333; Lloyd V. Smith, President and Chief Executive Officer

HOLY FAMILY HOSPITAL, North 5633 Lidgerwood Avenue, Spokane, WA, Zip 99220; tel. 509/482–0111; Ronald J. Schurra, Chief Executive Officer

MOUNT CARMEL HOSPITAL, 982 East Columbia Street, Colville, WA, Zip 99114–0351, Mailing Address: Box 351, Zip 99114–0351; tel. 509/684–2561; Gloria Cooper, Chief Executive Officer

SACRED HEART MEDICAL CENTER, West 101 Eighth Avenue, Spokane, WA, Zip 99220, Mailing Address: P.O. Box 2555, Zip 99220–2555; tel. 509/455–3040; Ryland P. Davis, President

ST. JOSEPH HOSPITAL, Skyline Drive and 14th Avenue, Polson, MT, Zip 59860, Mailing Address: P.O. Box 1010, Zip 59860–1010; tel. 406/883–5377; John W. Glueckert, President

ST. JOSEPH'S HOSPITAL, 500 East Webster Street, Chewelah, WA, Zip 99109, Mailing Address: P.O. Box 197, Zip 99109; tel. 509/935–8211; Gary V. Peck, Chief Executive Officer

ST. MARY MEDICAL CENTER, 401 West Poplar Street, Walla Walla, WA, Zip 99362, Mailing Address: Box 1477, Zip 99362–0312; tel. 509/525–3320; John A. Isely, President

ST. PATRICK HOSPITAL, 500 West Broadway, Missoula, MT, Zip 59802–4096, Mailing Address: Box 4587, Zip 59806–4587; tel. 406/543–7271; Lawrence L. White, Jr., President

WEST VIRGINIA

EASTERN PANHANDLE INTEGRATED DELIVERY SYSTEM
P.O. Box 1019, Petersburg, WV 26847; tel. 304/257–1026; Robert L. Harman, Chairman

GRANT MEMORIAL HOSPITAL, Petersburg, WV, Mailing Address: P.O. Box 1019, Zip 26847; tel. 304/257–1026; Robert L. Harman, Administrator

INTEGRATED PROVIDER NETWORK
7000 Hampton Center, Suite F, Morgantown, WV 26505; tel. 304/598–3911; Brad Minton, Network Contact

UNITED HOSPITAL CENTER, Route 19 South, Clarksburg, WV, Zip 26301, Mailing Address: P.O. Box 1680, Zip 26302–1680; tel. 304/624–2121; Bruce C. Carter, President

WEST VIRGINIA UNIVERSITY HOSPITALS, Medical Center Drive, Morgantown, WV, Zip 26506–4749; tel. 304/598–4000; Bruce McClymonds, President and Chief Executive Officer

MID–OHIO VALLEY RURAL HEALTH NETWORK
P.O. Box 718, Parkersburg, WV 26102; tel. 304/424–2111; Iris McCrady, Network Contact

CAMDEN–CLARK MEMORIAL HOSPITAL, 800 Garfield Avenue, Parkersburg, WV, Zip 26101, Mailing Address: P.O. Box 718, Zip 26102–0718; tel. 304/424–2111; Thomas J. Corder, President and Chief Executive Officer

SISTERSVILLE GENERAL HOSPITAL, 314 South Wells Street, Sistersville, WV, Zip 26175; tel. 304/652–2611; Lynn McCormick, Administrator

NORTH CENTRAL/WEST VIRGINIA RURAL HEALTH NETWORK
P.O. Box 1680, Clarksburg, WV 26302; tel. 304/473–2000; Louise Reese, Network Contact

ST. JOSEPH'S HOSPITAL, Amalia Drive, Buckhannon, WV, Zip 26201–2222; tel. 304/473–2000; Wayne B. Griffith, FACHE, Chief Executive Officer

UNITED HOSPITAL CENTER, Route 19 South, Clarksburg, WV, Zip 26301, Mailing Address: P.O. Box 1680, Zip 26302–1680; tel. 304/624–2121; Bruce C. Carter, President

WEBSTER COUNTY MEMORIAL HOSPITAL, 324 Miller Mountain Drive, Webster Springs, WV, Zip 26288; tel. 304/847–5682; Stephen M. Gavalchik, Administrator

PARTNERS IN HEALTH NETWORK, INC.
P.O. Box 1547, Charleston, WV 25326; tel. 304/348–3072; Scot Mitchell, Executive Director

BECKLEY APPALACHIAN REGIONAL HOSPITAL, 306 Stanaford Road, Beckley, WV, Zip 25801; tel. 304/255–3000; Norman Wright, Administrator

BOONE MEMORIAL HOSPITAL, 701 Madison Avenue, Madison, WV, Zip 25130; tel. 304/369–1230; Tommy H. Mullins, Administrator

BRAXTON COUNTY MEMORIAL HOSPITAL, 100 Hoylman Drive, Gassaway, WV, Zip 26624–9308; tel. 304/364–5156; Tony E. Atkins, Administrator

CHARLESTON AREA MEDICAL CENTER, 501 Morris Street, Charleston, WV, Zip 25301, Mailing Address: Box 1547, Zip 25326; tel. 304/348–5432; Phillip H. Goodwin, President and Chief Executive Officer

JACKSON GENERAL HOSPITAL, Pinnell Street, Ripley, WV, Zip 25271, Mailing Address: P.O. Box 720, Zip 25271; tel. 304/372–2731; Richard L. Rohaley, President and Chief Executive Officer

MAN ARH HOSPITAL, 700 East McDonald Avenue, Man, WV, Zip 25635–1011; tel. 304/583–8421; Freda Napier, Administrator

MINNIE HAMILTON HEALTHCARE CENTER, High Street, Grantsville, WV, Zip 26147, Mailing Address: Route 1, Box 1A, Zip 26147; tel. 304/354–9244; Barbara Lay, Administrator

MONTGOMERY GENERAL HOSPITAL, 401 Sixth Avenue, Montgomery, WV, Zip 25136–0270, Mailing Address: P.O. Box 270, Zip 25136–0270; tel. 304/442–5151; William R. Laird, IV, Interim President

PLATEAU MEDICAL CENTER, 430 Main Street, Oak Hill, WV, Zip 25901; tel. 304/469–8600

RICHWOOD AREA COMMUNITY HOSPITAL, Riverside Addition, Richwood, WV, Zip 26261; tel. 304/846–2573; D. Parker Haddix, Chief Executive Officer

ROANE GENERAL HOSPITAL, 200 Hospital Drive, Spencer, WV, Zip 25276; tel. 304/927–6200; Andrew Mazon, Ill, Administrator and Chief Executive Officer

SUMMERS COUNTY APPALACHIAN REGIONAL HOSPITAL, Terrace Street, Hinton, WV, Zip 25951, Mailing Address: Drawer 940, Zip 25951–0940; tel. 304/466–1000; Clyde E. Bolton, Administrator

WILLIAMSON ARH HOSPITAL, 260 Hospital Drive, South Williamson, KY, Zip 41503; tel. 606/237–1700; John A. Grah, Administrator

SOUTHERN VIRGINIA RURAL HEALTH NETWORK
500 Cherry Street, Bluefield, WV 24701; tel. 304/327–1714; Mark A. Vestich, Network Contact

BLUEFIELD REGIONAL MEDICAL CENTER, 500 Cherry Street, Bluefield, WV, Zip 24701–3390; tel. 304/327–1100; Eugene P. Pawlowski, President

TRI–STATE COMMUNITY CARE NETWORK
601 Colliers Way, Weirton, WV 26062; tel. 304/797–6413; Cynthia R. Nixon, Chief Financial Officer

WEIRTON MEDICAL CENTER, 601 Colliers Way, Weirton, WV, Zip 26062–5091; tel. 304/797–6000; Donald Muhlenthaler, FACHE, President and Chief Executive Officer

WEBSTER MEMORIAL/UNITED HOSPITAL CENTER EACH/RPCH NETWORK
324 Miller Mountain Drive, Webster Springs, WV 26288; tel. 304/847–5682; Steve Gavalchik, President

UNITED HOSPITAL CENTER, Route 19 South, Clarksburg, WV, Zip 26301, Mailing Address: P.O. Box 1680, Zip 26302–1680; tel. 304/624–2121; Bruce C. Carter, President

WEBSTER COUNTY MEMORIAL HOSPITAL, 324 Miller Mountain Drive, Webster Springs, WV, Zip 26288; tel. 304/847–5682; Stephen M. Gavalchik, Administrator

WISCONSIN

AFFINITY HEALTH SYSTEM, INC.
631 Hazel Street, Oshkosh, WI 54902–5677; tel. 414/236–2010; Otto L. Cox, Chief Executive Officer

MERCY MEDICAL CENTER, 631 Hazel Street, Oshkosh, WI, Zip 54902, Mailing Address: P.O. Box 1100, Zip 54902–1100; tel. 414/236–2000; Otto L. Cox, President and Chief Executive Officer

ST. ELIZABETH HOSPITAL, 1506 South Oneida Street, Appleton, WI, Zip 54915–1397; tel. 414/738–2000; Otto L. Cox, President and Chief Executive Officer

ALL SAINTS HEALTHCARE SYSTEM
3801 Spring Street, Racine, WI 53405; tel. 414/636–4860; Ed DeMeulenaere, President Chief Executive Officer

SAINT MARY'S MEDICAL CENTER, 3801 Spring Street, Racine, WI, Zip 53405; tel. 414/636–4011; Edward P. Demeulenaere, President and Chief Executive Officer

ST. LUKE'S MEMORIAL HOSPITAL, 1320 Wisconsin Avenue, Racine, WI, Zip 53403–1987; tel. 414/636–2011; Edward P. Demeulenaere, President and Chief Executive Officer

AURORA HEALTH CARE
P.O. Box 343910, Milwaukee, WI 53234–3910; tel. 414/647–3000; G. Edwin Howe, President

HARTFORD MEMORIAL HOSPITAL, 1032 East Sumner Street, Hartford, WI, Zip 53027; tel. 414/673–2300; Mark Schwartz, President

LAKELAND MEDICAL CENTER, West 3985 County Road NN, Elkhorn, WI, Zip 53121, Mailing Address: P.O. Box 1002, Zip 53121–1002; tel. 414/741–2000; Loren J. Anderson, President and Chief Executive Officer

MEMORIAL HOSPITAL CORPORATION OF BURLINGTON, 252 McHenry Street, Burlington, WI, Zip 53105–1828; tel. 414/763–2411; Paul A. Miller, President and Chief Executive Officer

MILWAUKEE PSYCHIATRIC HOSPITAL, 1220 Dewey Avenue, Wauwatosa, WI, Zip 53213–2598; tel. 414/454–6600; Mark R. Ambrosius, President

SHEBOYGAN MEMORIAL MEDICAL CENTER, 2629 North Seventh Street, Sheboygan, WI, Zip 53083–4998; tel. 414/451–5000; Patrick J. Trotter, President

SINAI SAMARITAN MEDICAL CENTER, 945 North 12th Street, Milwaukee, WI, Zip 53233, Mailing Address: P.O. Box 342, Zip 53201–0342; tel. 414/219–2000; William I. Jenkins, President and Chief Executive Officer

ST. LUKE'S MEDICAL CENTER, 2900 West Oklahoma Avenue, Milwaukee, WI, Zip 53215, Mailing Address: P.O. Box 2901, Zip 53201; tel. 414/649–6000; Mark R. Ambrosius, President

ST. MARY'S KEWAUNEE AREA MEMORIAL HOSPITAL, 810 Lincoln Street, Kewaunee, WI, Zip 54216, Mailing Address: P.O. Box 217, Zip 54216–0217; tel. 414/388–2210; Steven H. Spencer, President

TWO RIVERS COMMUNITY HOSPITAL AND HAMILTON MEMORIAL HOME, 2500 Garfield Street, Two Rivers, WI, Zip 54241; tel. 414/793–1178; Steven H. Spencer, President and Chief Executive Officer

VALLEY VIEW MEDICAL CENTER, 901 Reed Street, Plymouth, WI, Zip 53073–2409; tel. 414/893–1771; Patrick J. Trotter, President

WEST ALLIS MEMORIAL HOSPITAL, 8901 West Lincoln Avenue, West Allis, WI, Zip 53227–0901, Mailing Address: P.O. Box 27901, Zip 53227–0901; tel. 414/328–6000; Richard A. Kellar, Administrator

COLUMBIA – ST. MARY'S, INC.
2025 East Newport Avenue, Milwaukee, WI 53211; tel. 414/961–3638; John Schuler, President & Chief Executive Officer

COLUMBIA HOSPITAL, 2025 East Newport Avenue, Milwaukee, WI, Zip 53211–2990; tel. 414/961–3300; Susan Henckel, Executive Vice President and Chief Executive Officer

SACRED HEART REHABILITATION INSTITUTE, 2350 North Lake Drive, Milwaukee, WI, Zip 53211, Mailing Address: P.O. Box 392, Zip 53201–0392; tel. 414/298–6700; William H. Lange, Administrator and Senior Vice President

ST. MARY'S HOSPITAL, 2323 North Lake Drive, Milwaukee, WI, Zip 53211–9682, Mailing Address: P.O. Box 503, Zip 53201–0503; tel. 414/291–1000; Charles C. Lobeck, Chief Executive Officer

ST. MARY'S HOSPITAL OZAUKEE, 13111 North Port Washington Road, Mequon, WI, Zip 53097–2416; tel. 414/243–7300; Therese B. Pandl, Senior Vice President and Chief Operating Officer

COMMUNITY HEALTH CARE, INC.
425 Pine Ridge Boulevard, Wausau, WI 54401; tel. 715/847–2117; Donald C. Sibery, President

WAUSAU HOSPITAL, 333 Pine Ridge Boulevard, Wausau, WI, Zip 54401, Mailing Address: P.O. Box 1847, Zip 54402–1847; tel. 715/847–2121; Paul A. Spaude, President and Chief Executive Officer

COVENANT HEALTHCARE SYSTEM, INC.
1126 South 70th Street, Suite 306, Milwaukee, WI 53214–0970; tel. 414/456–2300; E. Thomas Sheahan, President & Chief Executive Officer

ELMBROOK MEMORIAL HOSPITAL, 19333 West North Avenue, Brookfield, WI, Zip 53045–4198; tel. 414/785–2000; Kimry A. Johnsrud, President

LAKEVIEW HOSPITAL, 10010 West Blue Mound Road, Wauwatosa, WI, Zip 53226; tel. 414/259–7200; J. E. Race, Administrator and Chief Executive Officer

ST. FRANCIS HOSPITAL, 3237 South 16th Street, Milwaukee, WI, Zip 53215–4592; tel. 414/647–5000; Gregory A. Banaszynski, President

ST. JOSEPH'S HOSPITAL, 5000 West Chambers Street, Milwaukee, WI, Zip 53210–9988; tel. 414/447–2000; Jon L. Wachs, President

ST. MICHAEL HOSPITAL, 2400 West Villard Avenue, Milwaukee, WI, Zip 53209; tel. 414/527–8000; Jeffrey K. Jenkins, President

ST. NICHOLAS HOSPITAL, 1601 North Taylor Drive, Sheboygan, WI, Zip 53081–2496; tel. 414/459–8300; Michael J. Stenger, Executive Vice President and Administrator

FRANCISCAN SKEMP HEALTHCARE
700 West Avenue South, LaCrosse, WI 54601; tel. 608/791–9703; Brian C. Campion, M.D., President & Chief Executive Officer

FRANCISCAN SKEMP HEALTHCARE–ARCADIA CAMPUS, 464 South St. Joseph Avenue, Arcadia, WI, Zip 54612–1401; tel. 608/323–3341; Robert M. Tracey, Administrator

FRANCISCAN SKEMP HEALTHCARE–LA CROSSE CAMPUS, 700 West Avenue South, La Crosse, WI, Zip 54601–4783; tel. 608/785–0940; Ronald R. Paczkowski, Vice President

FRANCISCAN SKEMP HEALTHCARE–SPARTA CAMPUS, 310 West Main Street, Sparta, WI, Zip 54656; tel. 608/269–2132; William P. Sexton, Administrator

HEALTH CARE NETWORK OF WISCONSIN (HCN)
250 Bishops Way, Suite 300, Brookfield, WI 53005–6222; tel. 414/784–0223; Jim Wrocklage, Chief Executive Officer

AGNESIAN HEALTHCARE, 430 East Division Street, Fond Du Lac, WI, Zip 54935–0385; tel. 414/929–2300; Robert A. Fale, President

BURNETT MEDICAL CENTER, 257 West St. George Avenue, Grantsburg, WI, Zip 54840–7827; tel. 715/463–5353; Thomas R. Lemon, Chief Executive Officer

CHILDREN'S HOSPITAL OF WISCONSIN, 9000 West Wisconsin Avenue, Milwaukee, WI, Zip 53226, Mailing Address: P.O. Box 1997, Zip 53201–1997; tel. 414/266–2000; Jon E. Vice, President and Chief Executive Officer

COLUMBIA HOSPITAL, 2025 East Newport Avenue, Milwaukee, WI, Zip 53211–2990; tel. 414/961–3300; Susan Henckel, Executive Vice President and Chief Executive Officer

COMMUNITY MEMORIAL HOSPITAL, W180 N8085 Town Hall Road, Menomonee Falls, WI, Zip 53051, Mailing Address: P.O. Box 408, Zip 53052–0408; tel. 414/251–1000; Robert Eugene Drisner, President and Chief Executive Officer

COMMUNITY MEMORIAL HOSPITAL, 855 South Main Street, Oconto Falls, WI, Zip 54154; tel. 414/846–3444; Thomas R. Bayer, Administrator

ELMBROOK MEMORIAL HOSPITAL, 19333 West North Avenue, Brookfield, WI, Zip 53045–4198; tel. 414/785–2000; Kimry A. Johnsrud, President

FROEDTERT MEMORIAL LUTHERAN HOSPITAL, 9200 West Wisconsin Avenue, Milwaukee, WI, Zip 53226–3596, Mailing Address: P.O. Box 26099, Zip 53226–3596; tel. 414/259–3000; William D. Petasnick, President

HARTFORD MEMORIAL HOSPITAL, 1032 East Sumner Street, Hartford, WI, Zip 53027; tel. 414/673–2300; Mark Schwartz, President

HUDSON MEDICAL CENTER, 400 Wisconsin Street, Hudson, WI, Zip 54016–1600; tel. 715/386–9321; John W. Marnell, Chief Executive Officer

MEMORIAL HOSPITAL CORPORATION OF BURLINGTON, 252 McHenry Street, Burlington, WI, Zip 53105–1828; tel. 414/763–2411; Paul A. Miller, President and Chief Executive Officer

MEMORIAL HOSPITAL OCONOMOWOC, 791 Summit Avenue, Oconomowoc, WI, Zip 53066–3896; tel. 414/569–9400; Douglas Guy, President and Chief Executive Officer

SHEBOYGAN MEMORIAL MEDICAL CENTER, 2629 North Seventh Street, Sheboygan, WI, Zip 53083–4998; tel. 414/451–5000; Patrick J. Trotter, President

SINAI SAMARITAN MEDICAL CENTER, 945 North 12th Street, Milwaukee, WI, Zip 53233, Mailing Address: P.O. Box 342, Zip 53201–0342; tel. 414/219–2000; William I. Jenkins, President and Chief Executive Officer

ST. CATHERINE'S HOSPITAL, 3556 Seventh Avenue, Kenosha, WI, Zip 53140–2595; tel. 414/656–3011; Ryland Davis, Interim Chief Executive Officer

ST. CLARE HOSPITAL AND HEALTH SERVICES, 707 14th Street, Baraboo, WI, Zip 53913–1597; tel. 608/356–5561; David B. Jordahl, FACHE, President

ST. CROIX VALLEY MEMORIAL HOSPITAL, 204 South Adams Street, Saint Croix Falls, WI, Zip 54024; tel. 715/483–3261; Steve L. Urosevich, Chief Executive Officer

ST. FRANCIS HOSPITAL, 3237 South 16th Street, Milwaukee, WI, Zip 53215–4592; tel. 414/647–5000; Gregory A. Banaszynski, President

ST. JOSEPH'S COMMUNITY HOSPITAL OF WEST BEND, 551 South Silverbrook Drive, West Bend, WI, Zip 53095–3898; tel. 414/334–5533; Gregory T. Burns, Executive Director

ST. JOSEPH'S HOSPITAL, 5000 West Chambers Street, Milwaukee, WI, Zip 53210–9988; tel. 414/447–2000; Jon L. Wachs, President

ST. LUKE'S MEDICAL CENTER, 2900 West Oklahoma Avenue, Milwaukee, WI, Zip 53215, Mailing Address: P.O. Box 2901, Zip 53201; tel. 414/649–6000; Mark R. Ambrosius, President

ST. LUKE'S MEMORIAL HOSPITAL, 1320 Wisconsin Avenue, Racine, WI, Zip 53403–1987; tel. 414/636–2011; Edward P. Demeulenaere, President and Chief Executive Officer

ST. MARY'S HOSPITAL, 2323 North Lake Drive, Milwaukee, WI, Zip 53211–9682, Mailing Address: P.O. Box 503, Zip 53201–0503; tel. 414/291–1000; Charles C. Lobeck, Chief Executive Officer

ST. MARY'S HOSPITAL OF SUPERIOR, 3500 Tower Avenue, Superior, WI, Zip 54880–5395; tel. 715/392–8281; Terry Jacobson, Administrator

ST. MARYS HOSPITAL MEDICAL CENTER, 707 South Mills Street, Madison, WI, Zip 53715–0450; tel. 608/251–6100; Gerald W. Lefert, President

ST. MICHAEL HOSPITAL, 2400 West Villard Avenue, Milwaukee, WI, Zip 53209; tel. 414/527–8000; Jeffrey K. Jenkins, President

VALLEY VIEW MEDICAL CENTER, 901 Reed Street, Plymouth, WI, Zip 53073–2409; tel. 414/893–1771; Patrick J. Trotter, President

WAUKESHA MEMORIAL HOSPITAL, 725 American Avenue, Waukesha, WI, Zip 53188–5099; tel. 414/544–2011; Rexford W. Titus, III, President and Chief Executive Officer

WAUPUN MEMORIAL HOSPITAL, 620 West Brown Street, Waupun, WI, Zip 53963–1799; tel. 414/324–5581; James E. Baer, FACHE, President and Administrator

WEST ALLIS MEMORIAL HOSPITAL, 8901 West Lincoln Avenue, West Allis, WI, Zip 53227–0901, Mailing Address: P.O. Box 27901, Zip 53227–0901; tel. 414/328–6000; Richard A. Kellar, Administrator

HORIZON HEALTHCARE, INC.
2300 North Mayfair Road, Suite 550, Milwaukee, WI 53226; tel. 414/257–3888; Kurt W. Metzner, President & Chief Executive Officer

COLUMBIA HOSPITAL, 2025 East Newport Avenue, Milwaukee, WI, Zip 53211–2990; tel. 414/961–3300; Susan Henckel, Executive Vice President and Chief Executive Officer

COMMUNITY MEMORIAL HOSPITAL, W180 N8085 Town Hall Road, Menomonee Falls, WI, Zip 53051, Mailing Address: P.O. Box 408, Zip 53052–0408; tel. 414/251–1000; Robert Eugene Drisner, President and Chief Executive Officer

FROEDTERT MEMORIAL LUTHERAN HOSPITAL, 9200 West Wisconsin Avenue, Milwaukee, WI, Zip 53226–3596, Mailing Address: P.O. Box 26099, Zip 53226–3596; tel. 414/259–3000; William D. Petasnick, President

KENOSHA HOSPITAL AND MEDICAL CENTER, 6308 Eighth Avenue, Kenosha, WI, Zip 53143; tel. 414/656–2011; Richard O. Schmidt, Jr., President, Chief Executive Officer and General Counsel

MEMORIAL HOSPITAL OCONOMOWOC, 791 Summit Avenue, Oconomowoc, WI, Zip 53066–3896; tel. 414/569–9400; Douglas Guy, President and Chief Executive Officer

ST. MARY'S HOSPITAL, 2323 North Lake Drive, Milwaukee, WI, Zip 53211–9682, Mailing Address: P.O. Box 503, Zip 53201–0503; tel. 414/291–1000; Charles C. Lobeck, Chief Executive Officer

ST. MARY'S HOSPITAL OZAUKEE, 13111 North Port Washington Road, Mequon, WI, Zip 53097–2416; tel. 414/243–7300; Therese B. Pandl, Senior Vice President and Chief Operating Officer

LUTHER/MIDELFORT/MAYO HEALTH SYSTEM
733 West Clairmont, Eau Claire, WI 54701; tel. 715/838–6732; William C. Rupp, President & Chief Executive Officer

BARRON MEMORIAL MEDICAL CENTER AND SKILLED NURSING FACILITY, 1222 Woodland Avenue, Barron, WI, Zip 54812; tel. 715/537–3186; Mark D. Wilson, Administrator

BLOOMER COMMUNITY MEMORIAL HOSPITAL AND THE MAPLEWOOD, 1501 Thompson Street, Bloomer, WI, Zip 54724; tel. 715/568–2000; John Perushek, Administrator

LUTHER HOSPITAL, 1221 Whipple Street, Eau Claire, WI, Zip 54702–4105; tel. 715/838–3311; William Rupp, M.D., President and Chief Executive Officer

OSSEO AREA HOSPITAL AND NURSING HOME, 13025 Eighth Street, Osseo, WI, Zip 54758, Mailing Address: P.O. Box 70, Zip 54758; tel. 715/597–3121; Bradley D. Groseth, Administrator

LUTHERAN HEALTH SYSTEM
1910 South Avenue, LaCrosse, WI 54601; tel. 608/785–0530; John Katrana, Chief Executive Officer

LUTHERAN HOSPITAL–LA CROSSE, 1910 South Avenue, La Crosse, WI, Zip 54601–9980; tel. 608/785–0530; John N. Katrana, Ph.D., Chief Administrative Officer

TOMAH MEMORIAL HOSPITAL, 321 Butts Avenue, Tomah, WI, Zip 54660, Mailing Address: Box 590, Zip 54660–0590; tel. 608/372–2181; Philip Stuart, Administrator

TRI–COUNTY MEMORIAL HOSPITAL, 18601 Lincoln Street, Whitehall, WI, Zip 54773–0065, Mailing Address: P.O. Box 65, Zip 54773–0065; tel. 715/538–4361; Ronald B. Fields, President

MARSHFIELD CLINIC'S REGIONAL SYSTEM
1000 North Oak Avenue, Marshfield, WI 54449; tel. 715/389–4884; John Smylie, Director of Regional Operations

FLAMBEAU HOSPITAL, 98 Sherry Avenue, Park Falls, WI, Zip 54552, Mailing Address: P.O. Box 310, Zip 54552; tel. 715/762–2484; Curtis A. Johnson, Administrator

MISSISSIPPI VALLEY HEALTH PARTNERSHIP
705 East Taylor Street, Prairie du Chien, WI 53821; tel. 608/326–2431; Harold W. Brown, Chief Executive Officer

PRAIRIE DU CHIEN MEMORIAL HOSPITAL, 705 East Taylor Street, Prairie Du Chien, WI, Zip 53821; tel. 608/326–2431; Harold W. Brown, Chief Executive Officer

PARTNERS HEALTH SYSTEM, INC.
225 Memorial Drive, Berlin, WI 54923; tel. 414/361–5580; Craig W. C. Schmidt, Chairman & Chief Executive Officer

COMMUNITY HEALTH NETWORK, 225 Memorial Drive, Berlin, WI, Zip 54923–1295; tel. 414/361–5580; Craig W. C. Schmidt, President and Chief Executive Officer

WILD ROSE COMMUNITY MEMORIAL HOSPITAL, Wild Rose, WI, Mailing Address: P.O. Box 243, Zip 54984–0243; tel. 414/622–3257; Donald Caves, President

SOUTHERN WISCONSIN HEALTH CARE SYSTEM
1000 Mineral Point Avenue, Janesville, WI 53545–5003; tel. 608/756–6625; Javon R. Bea, President & Chief Executive Officer

MERCY HEALTH SYSTEM, 1000 Mineral Point Avenue, Janesville, WI, Zip 53545–5003, Mailing Address: P.O. Box 5003, Zip 53547–5003; tel. 608/756–6000; Javon R. Bea, President and Chief Executive Officer

UNIVERSITY OF WISCONSIN HOSPITALS AND CLINICS
600 Highland Avenue, Madison, WI 53792; tel. 608/263–6400; Gordon Derzon, Chief Executive Officer

UNIVERSITY OF WISCONSIN HOSPITAL AND CLINICS, 600 Highland Avenue, Madison, WI, Zip 53792; tel. 608/263–6400; Gordon M. Derzon, Chief Executive Officer

WAUKESHA HOSPITAL SYSTEM, INC.
725 American Avenue, Waukesha, WI 53188; tel. 414/544–2011; Donald Fundingsland, President

WAUKESHA MEMORIAL HOSPITAL, 725 American Avenue, Waukesha, WI, Zip 53188–5099; tel. 414/544–2011; Rexford W. Titus, III, President and Chief Executive Officer

WYOMING

COMMUNITY HEALTH CARE NETWORK
P.O. Box 428, Jackson, WY 83001; tel. 307/733–3636; Nancy Johnsen, Wellness Coordinator

ST. JOHN'S HOSPITAL AND LIVING CENTER, 625 East Broadway, Jackson, WY, Zip 83001, Mailing Address: P.O. Box 428, Zip 83001–0428; tel. 307/733–3636; John Valiante, Chief Executive Officer

WYOMING INTEGRATED NETWORK
1233 East 2nd Street, Casper, WY 82601; tel. 307/577–2153; Fred Schroeder, Network Contact

IVINSON MEMORIAL HOSPITAL, 255 North 30th Street, Laramie, WY, Zip 82070–5195; tel. 307/742–2141; Thomas A. Nord, FACHE, President and Chief Executive Officer

WYOMING MEDICAL CENTER, 1233 East Second Street, Casper, WY, Zip 82601; tel. 307/577–7201; Michael E. Schrader, President and Chief Executive Officer

Section B

Statistics for Multihospital Health Care Systems and their Hospitals

The following tables describing multihospital health care systems refer to information in section B of the 1997 *AHA Guide*.

Table 1 shows the number of multihospital health care systems by type of control. Table 2 provides a breakdown of the number of systems that own, lease, sponsor or contract manage hospitals within each control category. Table 3 gives the number of hospitals and beds in each control category as well as total hospitals and beds. Finally, Table 4 shows the percentage of hospitals and beds in each control category.

For more information on multihospital health care systems, please write to the Section for Health Care Systems, One North Franklin, Chicago, Illinois 60606–3401 or call 312/422–3000.

Table 1. Multihospital Health Care Systems, by Type of Organizaton Control

Type of Control	Code	Number of Systems
Catholic (Roman) church–related	CC	55
Other church–related	CO	13
Subtotal, church–related		68
Other not–for–profit	NP	163
Subtotal, not–for–profit		231
Investor Owned	IO	44
Federal Government	FG	5
Total		280

Table 2. Multihospital Health Care Systems, by Type of Ownership and Control

Type of Ownership	Catholic Church–Related (CC)	Other Church–Related (CO)	Total Church–Related (CC + CO)	Other Not–for–Profit (NP)	Total Not–for–Profit (CC, CO, + NP)	Investor–Owned (IO)	Federal Govern–ment	All Systems
Systems that only own, lease or sponsor	42	11	53	131	184	36	5	225
Systems that only contract–manage	0	0	0	2	2	1	0	3
Systems that contract–manage, own, lease, or sponsor	13	2	15	30	45	7	0	52
Total	55	13	68	163	231	44	5	280

Table 3. Hospitals and Beds in Multihospital Health Care Systems, by Type of Ownership and Control

Type of Ownership	Catholic Church–Related (CC) H	B	Other Church–Related (CO) H	B	Total Church–Related (CC + CO) H	B	Other Not–for–Profit (NP) H	B	Total Not–for–Profit (CC, CO, + NP) H	B	Investor–Owned (IO) H	B	Federal Govern–ment H	B	All Systems H	B
Owned, leased or sponsored	465	110,104	90	19,392	555	129,496	788	179,720	1,343	309,216	887	119,466	295	73,042	2,525	501,724
Contract–managed	51	3,223	3	122	54	3,345	117	9,556	171	12,901	301	28,963	0	0	472	41,864
Total	516	113,327	93	19,514	609	132,841	905	189,276	1,514	322,117	1,188	148,429	295	73,042	2,997	543,588

H = hospitals; B = beds.

Table 4. Hospitals and Beds in Multihospital Health Care Systems, by Type of Ownership and Control, as a Percentage of All Systems

Type of Ownership	Catholic Church–Related (CC) H	B	Other Church–Related (CO) H	B	Total Church–Related (CC + CO) H	B	Other Not–for–Profit (NP) H	B	Total Not–for–Profit (CC, CO, + NP) H	B	Investor–Owned (IO) H	B	Federal Govern–ment H	B	All Systems H	B
Owned, leased or sponsored	18.4	21.9	3.6	3.9	22.0	25.8	31.2	35.8	53.2	61.6	35.1	23.8	11.7	14.6	100.0	100.0
Contract–managed	10.8	7.7	0.6	0.3	11.4	8.0	24.8	22.8	36.2	30.8	63.8	69.2	0.0	0.0	100.0	100.0
Total	17.2	20.8	3.1	3.6	20.3	24.4	30.2	34.8	50.5	59.3	39.6	27.3	9.8	13.4	100.0	100.0

H = hospitals; B = beds.
*Please note that figures may not always equal the provided subtotal or total percentages due to rounding.

0071: ACCORD HEALTH CARE CORPORATION (IO)
3696 Ulmerton Road, Clearwater, FL Zip 34622;
tel. 813/573–1755; Stephen H. Noble, President

GEORGIA: STEWART–WEBSTER HOSPITAL (O, 25 beds) 300 Alston Street,
Richland, GA Zip 31825, Mailing Address: Box 190, Zip 31825;
tel. 912/887–3366; Jerry R. Wise, Administrator

WHEELER COUNTY HOSPITAL (O, 30 beds) Third Street, Glenwood, GA
Zip 30428, Mailing Address: P.O. Box 398, Zip 30428; tel. 912/523–5113;
Charles M. Mayo, Administrator

Owned, leased, sponsored:	2 hospitals	55 beds
Contract–managed:	0 hospitals	0 beds
Totals:	2 hospitals	55 beds

★0235: ADVENTIST HEALTH (CO)
2100 Douglas Boulevard, Roseville, CA Zip 95661–3898, Mailing
Address: P.O. Box 619002, Zip 95661–9002; tel. 916/781–2000;
Frank F. Dupper, President

CALIFORNIA: FEATHER RIVER HOSPITAL (O, 122 beds) 5974 Pentz Road,
Paradise, CA Zip 95969–5593; tel. 916/877–9361; George Pifer,
President

FRANK R. HOWARD MEMORIAL HOSPITAL (L, 28 beds) 1 Madrone Street,
Willits, CA Zip 95490; tel. 707/459–6801; Robert J. Walker, President

GLENDALE ADVENTIST MEDICAL CENTER (O, 396 beds) 1509 Wilson
Terrace, Glendale, CA Zip 91206–4007; tel. 818/409–8000; David Nelson,
Chief Operating Officer

HANFORD COMMUNITY MEDICAL CENTER (O, 59 beds) 450 Greenfield
Avenue, Hanford, CA Zip 93230–0240, Mailing Address: Box 240, Zip
93232–0240; tel. 209/582–9000; Stan B. Berry, FACHE, President

PARADISE VALLEY HOSPITAL (O, 130 beds) 2400 East Fourth Street,
National City, CA Zip 91950; tel. 619/470–4321; Fred M. Harder, President
and Chief Executive Officer

REDBUD COMMUNITY HOSPITAL (O, 34 beds) 18th Avenue and Highway 53,
Clearlake, CA Zip 95422, Mailing Address: Box 6720, Zip 95422;
tel. 707/994–6486; Michael Schultz, Chief Executive Officer

SAN JOAQUIN COMMUNITY HOSPITAL (O, 178 beds) 2615 Eye Street,
Bakersfield, CA Zip 93301, Mailing Address: Box 2615, Zip 93303–2615;
tel. 805/395–3000; Fred Manchur, President

SIMI VALLEY HOSPITAL AND HEALTH CARE SERVICES (O, 225 beds) 2975
North Sycamore Drive, Simi Valley, CA Zip 93065–1277; tel. 805/527–2462;
Alan J. Rice, President

SONORA COMMUNITY HOSPITAL (O, 113 beds) 1 South Forest Road, Sonora,
CA Zip 95370; tel. 209/532–3161; Lary Davis, President

ST. HELENA HOSPITAL (O, 168 beds) 650 Sanitarium Road, Deer Park, CA
Zip 94576, Mailing Address: P.O. Box 250, Zip 94576; tel. 707/963–3611;
JoAline Olson, R.N., President and Chief Executive Officer

UKIAH VALLEY MEDICAL CENTER (O, 101 beds) 275 Hospital Drive, Ukiah,
CA Zip 95482; tel. 707/462–3111; ValGene Devitt, President and Chief
Executive Officer

WHITE MEMORIAL MEDICAL CENTER (O, 354 beds) 1720 Cesar E Chavez
Avenue, Los Angeles, CA Zip 90033–2481; tel. 213/268–5000; Beth D.
Zachary, Chief Operating Officer

HAWAII: CASTLE MEDICAL CENTER (O, 150 beds) 640 Ulukahiki Street,
Kailua, HI Zip 96734–4498; tel. 808/263–5500; Kenneth A. Finch,
President and Administrator

OREGON: ADVENTIST MEDICAL CENTER (O, 270 beds) 10123 S.E. Market,
Portland, OR Zip 97216–2599; tel. 503/257–2500; Larry D. Dodds,
President

PIONEER MEMORIAL HOSPITAL (C, 40 beds) 564 East Pioneer Drive,
Heppner, OR Zip 97836, Mailing Address: P.O. Box 9, Zip 97836;
tel. 503/676–9133; Kevin R. Erich, Administrator

TILLAMOOK COUNTY GENERAL HOSPITAL (L, 20 beds) 1000 Third Street,
Tillamook, OR Zip 97141–3430; tel. 503/842–4444; Wendell Hesseltine,
President

WASHINGTON: WALLA WALLA GENERAL HOSPITAL (O, 72 beds) 1025 South
Second Avenue, Walla Walla, WA Zip 99362, Mailing Address: Box 1398,
Zip 99362; tel. 509/525–0480; Rodney T. Applegate, President

Owned, leased, sponsored:	16 hospitals	2420 beds
Contract–managed:	1 hospital	40 beds
Totals:	17 hospitals	2460 beds

★4165: ADVENTIST HEALTH SYSTEM SUNBELT HEALTH CARE CORPORATION (CO)
111 North Orlando Avenue, Winter Park, FL Zip 32789–3675;
tel. 407/975–1417; Mardian J. Blair, President

FLORIDA: EAST PASCO MEDICAL CENTER (O, 120 beds) 7050 Gall
Boulevard, Zephyrhills, FL Zip 33541–1399; tel. 813/788–0411; Bob A.
Dodd, President

FLORIDA HOSPITAL (O, 1406 beds) 601 East Rollins Street, Orlando, FL
Zip 32803–1489; tel. 407/896–6611; Thomas L. Werner, President

FLORIDA HOSPITAL WATERMAN (O, 182 beds) 201 North Eustis Street,
Eustis, FL Zip 32726, Mailing Address: P.O. Box B, Zip 32727–0377;
tel. 352/589–3333; Royce C. Thompson, President

FLORIDA HOSPITAL–WALKER (O, 151 beds) 2501 U.S. Highway 27 North,
Avon Park, FL Zip 33825–1200, Mailing Address: P.O. Box 1200, Zip
33826–1200; tel. 941/453–7511; Samuel Leonor, President

GEORGIA: EMORY–ADVENTIST HOSPITAL (O, 54 beds) 3949 South Cobb
Drive, Smyrna, GA Zip 30080; tel. 770/434–0710; Larry D. Luce,
President

GORDON HOSPITAL (O, 50 beds) 1035 Red Bud Road, Calhoun, GA
Zip 30701, Mailing Address: P.O. Box 12938, Zip 30703–7013;
tel. 706/629–2895; Dennis Kiley, President

KENTUCKY: MEMORIAL HOSPITAL (O, 55 beds) 401 Memorial Drive,
Manchester, KY Zip 40962–9156; tel. 606/598–5104; T. Henry
Scoggins, FACHE, President

NORTH CAROLINA: PARK RIDGE HOSPITAL (O, 89 beds) Naples Road,
Fletcher, NC Zip 28732, Mailing Address: P.O. Box 1569, Zip
28732–1569; tel. 704/684–8501; Michael V. Gentry, President

TENNESSEE: JELLICO COMMUNITY HOSPITAL (L, 54 beds) Jellico, TN Mailing
Address: Route 1, Box 197, Zip 37762; tel. 423/784–1205; Kenneth R.
Mattison, President and Chief Executive Officer

TAKOMA ADVENTIST HOSPITAL (O, 80 beds) 401 Takoma Avenue,
Greeneville, TN Zip 37743; tel. 423/639–3151; Paul Michael Norman,
President

TENNESSEE CHRISTIAN MEDICAL CENTER (O, 288 beds) 500 Hospital Drive,
Madison, TN Zip 37115; tel. 615/865–2373; Milton R. Siepman, Ph.D.,
President and Chief Executive Officer

TEXAS: CENTRAL TEXAS MEDICAL CENTER (O, 109 beds) 1301 Wonder
World Drive, San Marcos, TX Zip 78666; tel. 512/353–8979; Peter M.
Weber, President and Chief Executive Officer

HUGULEY MEMORIAL MEDICAL CENTER (O, 154 beds) 11801 South
Freeway, Burleson, TX Zip 76028, Mailing Address: Box 6337, Fort Worth,
Zip 76115–0337; tel. 817/293–9110; A. David Jimenez, President and Chief
Executive Officer

HUGULEY WILLOW CREEK HOSPITAL (O, 115 beds) 7000 Highway 287
South, Arlington, TX Zip 76017–2805; tel. 817/561–1600; David P. Banks,
Chief Executive Officer

For explanation of codes following names, see page B2.
★ Indicates Type III membership in the American Hospital Association.

Section B

METROPLEX HOSPITAL (O, 213 beds) 2201 South Clear Creek Road, Killeen, TX Zip 76542–9305; tel. 817/526–7523

Owned, leased, sponsored:	15 hospitals	3120 beds
Contract–managed:	0 hospitals	0 beds
Totals:	15 hospitals	3120 beds

2175: ADVENTIST HEALTH SYSTEM–LOMA LINDA (NP)
11161 Anderson Street, Loma Linda, CA Zip 92350; tel. 909/824–4540; B. Lyn Behrens, President

CALIFORNIA: LOMA LINDA UNIVERSITY BEHAVIORAL MEDICINE CENTER (O, 89 beds) 1710 Barton Road, Redlands, CA Zip 92373; tel. 909/793–9333; Nolan Kerr, Administrator

LOMA LINDA UNIVERSITY MEDICAL CENTER (O, 729 beds) 11234 Anderson Street, Loma Linda, CA Zip 92354–2870, Mailing Address: P.O. Box 2000, Zip 92354–0200; tel. 909/824–0800; J. David Moorhead, M.D., President

Owned, leased, sponsored:	2 hospitals	818 beds
Contract–managed:	0 hospitals	0 beds
Totals:	2 hospitals	818 beds

★0064: ADVOCATE HEALTH CARE (NP)
2025 Windsor Drive, Oakbrook, IL Zip 60521–0222; tel. 708/990–5003; Richard R. Risk, President and Chief Executive Officer

ILLINOIS: BETHANY HOSPITAL (O, 120 beds) 3435 West Van Buren, Chicago, IL Zip 60624; tel. 773/265–7700; Lena L. Shields, Chief Executive

CHRIST HOSPITAL AND MEDICAL CENTER (O, 800 beds) 4440 West 95th Street, Oak Lawn, IL Zip 60453–2699; tel. 708/425–8000; Carol Schneider, Chief Executive

GOOD SAMARITAN HOSPITAL (O, 259 beds) 3815 Highland Avenue, Downers Grove, IL Zip 60515; tel. 630/275–5900; David M. McConkey, Chief Executive

GOOD SHEPHERD HOSPITAL (O, 154 beds) 450 West Highway 22, Barrington, IL Zip 60010–1999; tel. 847/381–9600; Russell E. Feurer, Chief Executive

LUTHERAN GENERAL HOSPITAL (O, 559 beds) 1775 Dempster Street, Park Ridge, IL Zip 60068–1174; tel. 847/723–2210; Kenneth J. Rojek, Chief Executive

RAVENSWOOD HOSPITAL MEDICAL CENTER (O, 301 beds) 4550 North Winchester Avenue, Chicago, IL Zip 60640–5205; tel. 773/878–4300; John E. Blair, President

SOUTH SUBURBAN HOSPITAL (O, 216 beds) 17800 South Kedzie Avenue, Hazel Crest, IL Zip 60429; tel. 708/799–8000; Robert Rutkowski, Chief Executive

TRINITY HOSPITAL (O, 218 beds) 2320 East 93rd Street, Chicago, IL Zip 60617; tel. 773/978–2000; John N. Schwartz, Chief Executive Officer

Owned, leased, sponsored:	8 hospitals	2627 beds
Contract–managed:	0 hospitals	0 beds
Totals:	8 hospitals	2627 beds

0225: ALAMEDA COUNTY HEALTH CARE SERVICES AGENCY (NP)
1850 Fairway Drive, San Leandro, CA Zip 94577; tel. 510/618–3452; David J. Kears, Director

CALIFORNIA: ALAMEDA COUNTY MEDICAL CENTER (O, 193 beds) 15400 Foothill Boulevard, San Leandro, CA Zip 94578–1091; tel. 510/667–7920; Michael G. Smart, Chief Executive Officer

ALAMEDA COUNTY MEDICAL CENTER–HIGHLAND CAMPUS (O, 247 beds) 1411 East 31st Street, Oakland, CA Zip 94602; tel. 510/437–5081; Michael Smart, Chief Executive Officer

Owned, leased, sponsored:	2 hospitals	440 beds
Contract–managed:	0 hospitals	0 beds
Totals:	2 hospitals	440 beds

1685: ALBERT EINSTEIN HEALTHCARE NETWORK (NP)
5501 Old York Road, Philadelphia, PA Zip 19141–3098; tel. 215/456–7890; Martin Goldsmith, President

PENNSYLVANIA: ALBERT EINSTEIN MEDICAL CENTER (O, 701 beds) 5501 Old York Road, Philadelphia, PA Zip 19141–3098; tel. 215/456–7890; Martin Goldsmith, President

BELMONT CENTER FOR COMPREHENSIVE TREATMENT (O, 146 beds) 4200 Monument Road, Philadelphia, PA Zip 19131–1689; tel. 215/877–2000; Jack H. Dembow, General Director and Vice President

Owned, leased, sponsored:	2 hospitals	847 beds
Contract–managed:	0 hospitals	0 beds
Totals:	2 hospitals	847 beds

0065: ALEXIAN BROTHERS HEALTH SYSTEM, INC. (CC)
600 Alexian Way, Elk Grove Village, IL Zip 60007–3395; tel. 847/640–7550; Brother Felix Bettendorf, President

CALIFORNIA: ALEXIAN BROTHERS HOSPITAL (O, 192 beds) 225 North Jackson Avenue, San Jose, CA Zip 95116–1691; tel. 408/259–5000; Steven R. Barron, Chief Executive Officer

ILLINOIS: ALEXIAN BROTHERS MEDICAL CENTER (O, 391 beds) 800 Biesterfield Road, Elk Grove Village, IL Zip 60007–3397; tel. 847/437–5500; Brother Philip Kennedy, President and Chief Executive Officer

MISSOURI: ALEXIAN BROTHERS HOSPITAL (O, 182 beds) 3933 South Broadway, Saint Louis, MO Zip 63118–9984; tel. 314/865–3333; Deno E. Fabbre, President and Chief Executive Officer

Owned, leased, sponsored:	3 hospitals	765 beds
Contract–managed:	0 hospitals	0 beds
Totals:	3 hospitals	765 beds

★1385: ALLEGANY HEALTH SYSTEM (CC)
6200 Courtney Campbell Causeway, Tampa, FL Zip 33607–1458; tel. 813/281–9098; Sister Marie Celeste Sullivan, President and Chief Executive Officer

FLORIDA: GOOD SAMARITAN MEDICAL CENTER (O, 341 beds) Flagler Drive at Palm Beach Lakes Boulevard, West Palm Beach, FL Zip 33401; tel. 561/655–5511; Phillip C. Dutcher, Interim President

ST. ANTHONY'S HOSPITAL (O, 329 beds) 1200 Seventh Avenue North, Saint Petersburg, FL Zip 33705, Mailing Address: P.O. Box 12588, Zip 33733; tel. 813/825–1100; Revonda L. Shumaker, R.N., President

ST. JOSEPH'S HOSPITAL (O, 883 beds) 3001 West Martin Luther King Boulevard, Tampa, FL Zip 33607–6387, Mailing Address: P.O. Box 4227, Zip 33677–4227; tel. 813/870–4000; Charles Francis Scott, President

ST. MARY'S HOSPITAL (O, 433 beds) 901 45th Street, West Palm Beach, FL Zip 33407–2495, Mailing Address: P.O. Box 24620, Zip 33416–4620; tel. 561/844–6300; Phillip C. Dutcher, Interim President and Chief Executive Officer

NEW JERSEY: OUR LADY OF LOURDES MEDICAL CENTER (O, 300 beds) 1600 Haddon Avenue, Camden, NJ Zip 08103; tel. 609/757–3500; Alexander J. Hatala, President and Chief Executive Officer

Owned, leased, sponsored:	5 hospitals	2286 beds
Contract–managed:	0 hospitals	0 beds
Totals:	5 hospitals	2286 beds

★2305: ALLEGHENY HEALTH, EDUCATION AND RESEARCH FOUNDATION (NP)
120 Fifth Avenue, Pittsburgh, PA Zip 15222; tel. 412/359–8800; Sherif S. Abdelhak, President and Chief Executive Officer

GRADUATE HEALTH SYSTEM–RANCOCAS HOSPITAL (O, 241 beds) 218–A Sunset Road, Willingboro, NJ Zip 08046–1162; tel. 609/835–2900; Garry L. Scheib, President

OHIO: EAST OHIO REGIONAL HOSPITAL (C, 178 beds) 90 North Fourth Street, Martins Ferry, OH Zip 43935–1648; tel. 614/633–1100; Brian K. Felici, Chief Executive Officer

For explanation of codes following names, see page B2.
★ Indicates Type III membership in the American Hospital Association.

PENNSYLVANIA: ALLEGHENY GENERAL HOSPITAL (O, 559 beds) 320 East North Avenue, Pittsburgh, PA Zip 15212–4772; tel. 412/359–3131; Anthony M. Sanzo, President

ALLEGHENY UNIVERSITY HOSPITAL, BUCKS COUNTY (O, 132 beds) 225 Newtown Road, Warminster, PA Zip 18974; tel. 215/441–6600; Margaret M. McGoldrick, President and Chief Executive Officer

ALLEGHENY UNIVERSITY HOSPITAL, EAST FALLS (O, 369 beds) 3300 Henry Avenue, Philadelphia, PA Zip 19129; tel. 215/842–6000; Margaret M. McGoldrick, Chief Executive Officer

ALLEGHENY UNIVERSITY HOSPITAL, ELKINS PARK (O, 158 beds) 60 East Township Line Road, Elkins Park, PA Zip 19027; tel. 215/663–6000; Margaret M. McGoldrick, Executive Director and Chief Executive Officer

ALLEGHENY UNIVERSITY HOSPITALS, HAHNEMANN (O, 540 beds) Broad and Vine Streets, Philadelphia, PA Zip 19102–1192; tel. 215/762–7000; Shelley Gebar, President and Chief Executive Officer

FORBES METROPOLITAN HOSPITAL (O, 152 beds) 225 Penn Avenue, Pittsburgh, PA Zip 15221–2173; tel. 412/247–2424; April A. Stevens, R.N., Vice President and Administrator

FORBES REGIONAL HOSPITAL (O, 226 beds) 2570 Haymaker Road, Monroeville, PA Zip 15146–3592; tel. 412/858–2000; Dana W. Ramish, President and Chief Executive Officer

GRADUATE HEALTH SYSTEM–CITY AVENUE HOSPITAL (O, 195 beds) 4150 City Avenue, Philadelphia, PA Zip 19131–1696; tel. 215/871–1000; Melvyn E. Smith, President

GRADUATE HOSPITAL (O, 198 beds) One Graduate Plaza, Philadelphia, PA Zip 19146–1497; tel. 215/893–2000; Arnold Berman, M.D., President and Chief Executive Officer

MT. SINAI HOSPITAL (O, 183 beds) 1429 South Fifth Street, Philadelphia, PA Zip 19147–5999; tel. 215/339–3456; Louis Shapiro, Executive Vice President and Chief Operating Officer

PARKVIEW HOSPITAL (O, 165 beds) 1331 East Wyoming Avenue, Philadelphia, PA Zip 19124; tel. 215/537–7400; Ernest N. Perilli, Vice President Operations

ST. CHRISTOPHER'S HOSPITAL FOR CHILDREN (O, 178 beds) Erie Avenue at Front Street, Philadelphia, PA Zip 19134–1095; tel. 215/427–5000; Calvin Bland, President and Chief Executive Officer

WEST VIRGINIA: OHIO VALLEY MEDICAL CENTER (C, 385 beds) 2000 Eoff Street, Wheeling, WV Zip 26003; tel. 304/234–0123; Thomas P. Galinski, President and Chief Executive Officer

Owned, leased, sponsored:	13 hospitals	3296 beds
Contract–managed:	2 hospitals	563 beds
Totals:	15 hospitals	3859 beds

★2285: ALLIANT HEALTH SYSTEM (NP)
234 East Gray Street, Suite 225, Louisville, KY Zip 40202, Mailing Address: P.O. Box 35070, Zip 40232–5070; tel. 502/629–8025; Stephen A. Williams, President

ILLINOIS: FAIRFIELD MEMORIAL HOSPITAL (C, 185 beds) 303 N.W. 11th Street, Fairfield, IL Zip 62837; tel. 618/842–2611; Albert Ban Jr., Chief Executive Officer

MASSAC MEMORIAL HOSPITAL (C, 31 beds) 28 Chick Street, Metropolis, IL Zip 62960–2481, Mailing Address: P.O. Box 850, Zip 62960–0850; tel. 618/524–2176; James Marshall, Chief Executive Officer

PARIS COMMUNITY HOSPITAL (C, 49 beds) 721 East Court Street, Paris, IL Zip 61944–2420; tel. 217/465–4141; John M. Dillon, Chief Executive Officer

WABASH GENERAL HOSPITAL DISTRICT (C, 56 beds) 1418 College Drive, Mount Carmel, IL Zip 62863; tel. 618/262–8621; James R. Farris, CHE, Chief Executive Officer

INDIANA: BLACKFORD COUNTY HOSPITAL (C, 36 beds) 503 East Van Cleve Street, Hartford City, IN Zip 47348; tel. 765/348–0300; Mark A. Edwards, Chief Executive Officer

DECATUR COUNTY MEMORIAL HOSPITAL (C, 75 beds) 720 North Lincoln Street, Greensburg, IN Zip 47240–1398; tel. 812/663–4331; Charles Duffy, President

GIBSON GENERAL HOSPITAL (C, 109 beds) 1808 Sherman Drive, Princeton, IN Zip 47670–1043; tel. 812/385–3401; Michael J. Budnick, Administrator and Chief Executive Officer

HARRISON COUNTY HOSPITAL (C, 46 beds) 245 Atwood Street, Corydon, IN Zip 47112–1774; tel. 812/738–4251; Steven L. Taylor, Chief Executive Officer

JAY COUNTY HOSPITAL (C, 55 beds) 500 West Votaw Street, Portland, IN Zip 47371–1322; tel. 219/726–7131; Thomas J. Valerius, Chief Executive Officer

PERRY COUNTY MEMORIAL HOSPITAL (C, 38 beds) 1 Hospital Road, Tell City, IN Zip 47586–0362; tel. 812/547–7011; Bradford W. Dykes, Chief Executive Officer

RANDOLPH COUNTY HOSPITAL (C, 27 beds) 325 South Oak Street, Winchester, IN Zip 47394, Mailing Address: P.O. Box 407, Zip 47394; tel. 765/584–9001; James M. Full, Chief Executive Officer

RUSH MEMORIAL HOSPITAL (C, 52 beds) 1300 North Main Street, Rushville, IN Zip 46173–1198; tel. 765/932–4111; H. William Hartley, Chief Executive Officer

WABASH COUNTY HOSPITAL (C, 75 beds) 710 North East Street, Wabash, IN Zip 46992, Mailing Address: Box 548, Zip 46992–0548; tel. 219/563–3131; David C. Hunter, Chief Executive Officer

KENTUCKY: ALLIANT HOSPITALS (O, 709 beds) 200 East Chestnut Street, Louisville, KY Zip 40202, Mailing Address: Box 35070, Zip 40232–5070; tel. 502/629–8000; Shirley B. Powers, Senior Executive Officer

BRECKINRIDGE MEMORIAL HOSPITAL (C, 45 beds) 1011 Old Highway 60, Hardinsburg, KY Zip 40143–2597; tel. 502/756–7000; George Walz, CHE, Chief Executive Officer

CALDWELL COUNTY HOSPITAL (C, 15 beds) 101 Hospital Drive, Princeton, KY Zip 42445–0410, Mailing Address: Box 410, Zip 42445–0410; tel. 502/365–0300; John Svoboda, Chief Executive Officer

CARROLL COUNTY MEMORIAL HOSPITAL (L, 39 beds) 309 11th Street, Carrollton, KY Zip 41008; tel. 502/732–4321; Roger Williams, Chief Executive Officer

CAVERNA MEMORIAL HOSPITAL (C, 28 beds) 1501 South Dixie Street, Horse Cave, KY Zip 42749; tel. 502/786–2191; James J. Kerins Sr., Administrator

RUSSELL COUNTY HOSPITAL (C, 45 beds) Dowell Road, Russell Springs, KY Zip 42642, Mailing Address: P.O. Box 1610, Zip 42642; tel. 502/866–4141; William J. Hurteau, FACHE, Administrator

THE JAMES B. HAGGIN MEMORIAL HOSPITAL (C, 59 beds) 464 Linden Avenue, Harrodsburg, KY Zip 40330–1862; tel. 606/734–5441; Earl James Motzer, Ph.D., FACHE, Chief Executive Officer

TWIN LAKES REGIONAL MEDICAL CENTER (C, 75 beds) 910 Wallace Avenue, Leitchfield, KY Zip 42754; tel. 502/259–9400; Stephen L. Meredith, Chief Executive Officer

Owned, leased, sponsored:	2 hospitals	748 beds
Contract–managed:	19 hospitals	1101 beds
Totals:	21 hospitals	1849 beds

★0041: ALLINA HEALTH SYSTEM (NP)
5601 Smetana Drive, Minneapolis, MN Zip 55440, Mailing Address: P.O. Box 9310, Zip 55440–9310; tel. 612/992–2000; Gordon M. Sprenger, Executive Officer

MINNESOTA: ABBOTT NORTHWESTERN HOSPITAL (O, 612 beds) 800 East 28th Street, Minneapolis, MN Zip 55407–3799; tel. 612/863–4203; Robert K. Spinner, President

BUFFALO HOSPITAL (O, 30 beds) 303 Catlin Street, Buffalo, MN Zip 55313–1947, Mailing Address: P.O. Box 609, Zip 55313–0609; tel. 612/682–7180; Mary Ellen Wells, President

CAMBRIDGE MEDICAL CENTER (O, 81 beds) 701 South Dellwood Street, Cambridge, MN Zip 55008–1920; tel. 612/689–7700; Lowell L. Becker, M.D., President

FAIRMONT COMMUNITY HOSPITAL (C, 108 beds) 835 Johnson Street, Fairmont, MN Zip 56031–4523, Mailing Address: P.O. Box 835, Zip 56031–0835; tel. 507/238–4254; Gerry Gilbertson, President

For explanation of codes following names, see page B2.
★ Indicates Type III membership in the American Hospital Association.

Section B

GRANITE FALLS MUNICIPAL HOSPITAL AND MANOR (C, 87 beds) 345 Tenth Avenue, Granite Falls, MN Zip 56241–1499; tel. 320/564–3111; George Gerlach, President

HUTCHINSON AREA HEALTH CARE (C, 187 beds) 1095 Highway 15 South, Hutchinson, MN Zip 55350–3182; tel. 320/234–5000; Philip G. Graves, President

LONG PRAIRIE MEMORIAL HOSPITAL AND HOME (O, 141 beds) 20 Ninth Street S.E., Long Prairie, MN Zip 56347–1404; tel. 320/732–2141; Clayton R. Peterson, President

MERCY HOSPITAL (O, 194 beds) 4050 Coon Rapids Boulevard, Coon Rapids, MN Zip 55433–2586; tel. 612/422–4500

MILLE LACS HEALTH SYSTEM (C, 98 beds) 200 North Elm Street, Onamia, MN Zip 56359–7978; tel. 320/532–3154; Frederick W. Haack, President

NEW ULM MEDICAL CENTER (O, 47 beds) 1324 Fifth Street North, New Ulm, MN Zip 56073–1553, Mailing Address: P.O. Box 577, Zip 56073; tel. 507/354–2111; Rickie L. Ressler, R.N., Interim President

NORTHFIELD HOSPITAL (C, 69 beds) 801 West First Street, Northfield, MN Zip 55057–1697; tel. 507/645–6661; Kendall C. Bank, President

OWATONNA HOSPITAL (O, 66 beds) 903 Oak Street South, Owatonna, MN Zip 55060–3234; tel. 507/451–3850; Richard G. Slieter, President

PHILLIPS EYE INSTITUTE (O, 10 beds) 2215 Park Avenue, Minneapolis, MN Zip 55404–3756; tel. 612/336–6000; Shari E. Levy, President

ST. FRANCIS REGIONAL MEDICAL CENTER (O, 63 beds) 1455 St. Francis Avenue, Shakopee, MN Zip 55379–1228; tel. 612/403–3000; Venetia Kudrle, President

STEVENS COMMUNITY MEDICAL CENTER (C, 37 beds) 400 East First Street, Morris, MN Zip 56267–1407, Mailing Address: P.O. Box 660, Zip 56267; tel. 612/589–1313; John Rau, President

UNITED HOSPITAL (O, 386 beds) 333 North Smith Street, Saint Paul, MN Zip 55102–2389; tel. 612/220–8000; David Jones, President

UNITED HOSPITAL DISTRICT (C, 43 beds) 515 South Moore Street, Blue Earth, MN Zip 56013–2158, Mailing Address: P.O. Box 160, Zip 56013–0160; tel. 507/526–3273; Brian Kief, President

UNITY HOSPITAL (O, 190 beds) 550 Osborne Road N.E., Fridley, MN Zip 55432–2799; tel. 612/422–4500

WISCONSIN: RIVER FALLS AREA HOSPITAL (O, 36 beds) 1629 East Division Street, River Falls, WI Zip 54022–1571; tel. 715/425–6155; Sharon Whelan, President

Owned, leased, sponsored:	12 hospitals	1856 beds
Contract–managed:	7 hospitals	629 beds
Totals:	19 hospitals	2485 beds

0074: AMERICAN TRANSITIONAL HOSPITALS, INC. (IO)
112 Second Avenue North, Franklin, TN Zip 37064; tel. 615/791–7099; T. Jerald Moore, President and Chief Executive Officer

TEXAS: ATH HEIGHTS HOSPITAL (O, 170 beds) 1917 Ashland Street, Houston, TX Zip 77008–3994; tel. 713/861–6161; Joe G. Baldwin, Administrator

AMERICAN TRANSITIONAL HOSPITAL–DALLAS/FORT WORTH (O, 38 beds) 1745 West Irving Boulevard, Irving, TX Zip 75061; tel. 214/251–2824; LouAnn O. Mathews, Administrator

AMERICAN TRANSITIONAL HOSPITAL–HOUSTON MEDICAL CENTER (O, 34 beds) 6447 Main Street, Houston, TX Zip 77054, Mailing Address: 6447 Main Street, 6th Floor, Zip 77054; tel. 713/791–9393; Sheila A. Kramer, Chief Executive Officer

Owned, leased, sponsored:	3 hospitals	242 beds
Contract–managed:	0 hospitals	0 beds
Totals:	3 hospitals	242 beds

★**0135: ANCILLA SYSTEMS INC.** (CC)
1000 South Lake Park Avenue, Hobart, IN Zip 46342; tel. 219/947–8500; William D. Harkins, President and Chief Executive Officer

ILLINOIS: ST. ELIZABETH'S HOSPITAL (O, 240 beds) 1431 North Claremont Avenue, Chicago, IL Zip 60622; tel. 773/278–2000; JoAnn Birdzell, President and Chief Executive Officer

ST. MARY'S HOSPITAL (O, 119 beds) 129 North Eighth Street, East St. Louis, IL Zip 62201–2999; tel. 618/274–1900; Richard J. Mark, President and Chief Executive Officer

INDIANA: COMMUNITY HOSPITAL OF BREMEN (C, 28 beds) 411 South Whitlock Street, Bremen, IN Zip 46506–1699; tel. 219/546–2211; Scott R. Graybill, Administrator and Chief Executive Officer

ST. CATHERINE HOSPITAL (O, 204 beds) 4321 Fir Street, East Chicago, IN Zip 46312; tel. 219/392–7000; JoAnn Birdzell, President and Chief Executive Officer

ST. JOSEPH COMMUNITY HOSPITAL (O, 187 beds) 215 West Fourth Street, Mishawaka, IN Zip 46544; tel. 219/259–2431; Stephen L. Crain, President and Chief Executive Officer

ST. JOSEPH MEDICAL CENTER OF FORT WAYNE (O, 194 beds) 700 Broadway, Fort Wayne, IN Zip 46802; tel. 219/425–3000; John T. Farrell Sr., President and Chief Executive Officer

ST. MARY COMMUNITY HOSPITAL (O, 70 beds) 2515 East Jefferson Boulevard, South Bend, IN Zip 46615–2691; tel. 219/288–8311; Stephen L. Crain, President

ST. MARY MEDICAL CENTER (O, 102 beds) 1500 South Lake Park Avenue, Hobart, IN Zip 46342; tel. 219/942–0551; Milton Triana, President and Chief Executive Officer

Owned, leased, sponsored:	7 hospitals	1116 beds
Contract–managed:	1 hospital	28 beds
Totals:	8 hospitals	1144 beds

0145: APPALACHIAN REGIONAL HEALTHCARE (NP)
1220 Harrodsburg Road, Lexington, KY Zip 40504, Mailing Address: Box 8086, Zip 40533–8086; tel. 606/226–2440; Forrest Calico, M.D., President

KENTUCKY: ARH REGIONAL MEDICAL CENTER (O, 288 beds) 100 Medical Center Drive, Hazard, KY Zip 41701–1000; tel. 606/439–6610; David R. Lyon, Administrator

HARLAN ARH HOSPITAL (O, 125 beds) 81 Ball Park Road, Harlan, KY Zip 40831–1792; tel. 606/573–8100; Daniel Fitzpatrick, Administrator

MCDOWELL ARH HOSPITAL (O, 74 beds) Route 122, McDowell, KY Zip 41647, Mailing Address: Box 247, Zip 41647; tel. 606/377–3400; Jerry Haynes, Administrator

MIDDLESBORO APPALACHIAN REGIONAL HOSPITAL (O, 96 beds) 3600 West Cumberland Avenue, Middlesboro, KY Zip 40965, Mailing Address: Box 340, Zip 40965–0340; tel. 606/242–1101; Paul V. Miles, Administrator

MORGAN COUNTY APPALACHIAN REGIONAL HOSPITAL (L, 55 beds) 476 Liberty Road, West Liberty, KY Zip 41472, Mailing Address: Box 579, Zip 41472–0579; tel. 606/743–3186; Dennis R. Chaney, Administrator

WHITESBURG APPALACHIAN REGIONAL HOSPITAL (O, 71 beds) 550 Jenkins Road, Whitesburg, KY Zip 41858; tel. 606/633–3600; Nick Lewis, Administrator

WILLIAMSON ARH HOSPITAL (O, 148 beds) 260 Hospital Drive, South Williamson, KY Zip 41503; tel. 606/237–1700; John A. Grah, Administrator

VIRGINIA: WISE ARH HOSPITAL (O, 41 beds) Wise, VA Mailing Address: P.O. Box 3267, Zip 24293–3267; tel. 540/328–2511; Louis G. Roe Jr., Administrator

WEST VIRGINIA: BECKLEY APPALACHIAN REGIONAL HOSPITAL (O, 173 beds) 306 Stanaford Road, Beckley, WV Zip 25801; tel. 304/255–3000; Norman Wright, Administrator

MAN ARH HOSPITAL (O, 42 beds) 700 East McDonald Avenue, Man, WV Zip 25635–1011; tel. 304/583–8421; Freda Napier, Administrator

SUMMERS COUNTY APPALACHIAN REGIONAL HOSPITAL (L, 50 beds) Terrace Street, Hinton, WV Zip 25951, Mailing Address: Drawer 940, Zip 25951–0940; tel. 304/466–1000; Clyde E. Bolton, Administrator

For explanation of codes following names, see page B2.
★ Indicates Type III membership in the American Hospital Association.

Section B

Owned, leased, sponsored:	11 hospitals	1163 beds
Contract–managed:	0 hospitals	0 beds
Totals:	11 hospitals	1163 beds

0104: ARCHBOLD MEDICAL CENTER (NP)

910 South Broad Street, Thomasville, GA Zip 31792;
tel. 912/228–2739; Ken B. Beverly, President and Chief Executive
Officer

GEORGIA: BROOKS COUNTY HOSPITAL (L, 35 beds) 903 North Court Street,
Quitman, GA Zip 31643, Mailing Address: P.O. Box 5000, Zip 31643;
tel. 912/263–4171; Ken Brooker, Interim Administrator

EARLY MEMORIAL HOSPITAL (L, 176 beds) 630 Columbia Street, Blakely, GA
Zip 31723; tel. 912/723–4241

GRADY GENERAL HOSPITAL (L, 45 beds) 1155 Fifth Street S.E., Cairo, GA
Zip 31728, Mailing Address: P.O. Box 360, Zip 31728; tel. 912/377–1150;
Glen C. Davis, Administrator

JOHN D. ARCHBOLD MEMORIAL HOSPITAL (O, 328 beds) 910 South Broad
Street, Thomasville, GA Zip 31792, Mailing Address: P.O. Box 1018, Zip
31799; tel. 912/228–2000; Jason H. Moore, President and Chief Executive
Officer

MITCHELL COUNTY HOSPITAL (L, 182 beds) 90 Stephens Street, Camilla, GA
Zip 31730, Mailing Address: P.O. Box 639, Zip 31730; tel. 912/336–5284;
Ronald M. Gilliard, FACHE, Administrator

Owned, leased, sponsored:	5 hospitals	766 beds
Contract–managed:	0 hospitals	0 beds
Totals:	5 hospitals	766 beds

★0094: ASANTE HEALTH SYSTEM (NP)

2650 Siskiyou Boulevard, Suite 200, Medford, OR Zip 97504–8389;
tel. 541/608–4100; Jon K. Mitchell, FACHE, President and Chief
Executive Officer

OREGON: ROGUE VALLEY MEDICAL CENTER (O, 249 beds) 2825 East
Barnett Road, Medford, OR Zip 97504–8332; tel. 541/608–4900; Gary
A. Sherwood, Executive Vice President

THREE RIVERS COMMUNITY HOSPITAL AND HEALTH CENTER–DIMMICK (O,
87 beds) 715 N.W. Dimmick Street, Grants Pass, OR Zip 97526–1596;
tel. 541/476–6831; John F. Bringhurst, Executive Vice President

Owned, leased, sponsored:	2 hospitals	336 beds
Contract–managed:	0 hospitals	0 beds
Totals:	2 hospitals	336 beds

★2215: AURORA HEALTH CARE (NP)

3000 West Montana, Milwaukee, WI Zip 53215–3268, Mailing
Address: P.O. Box 343910, Zip 53234–3910; tel. 414/647–3000;
G. Edwin Howe, President

WISCONSIN: HARTFORD MEMORIAL HOSPITAL (O, 71 beds) 1032 East
Sumner Street, Hartford, WI Zip 53027; tel. 414/673–2300; Mark
Schwartz, President

LAKELAND MEDICAL CENTER (O, 78 beds) West 3985 County Road NN,
Elkhorn, WI Zip 53121, Mailing Address: P.O. Box 1002, Zip 53121–1002;
tel. 414/741–2000; Loren J. Anderson, President and Chief Executive Officer

MEMORIAL HOSPITAL CORPORATION OF BURLINGTON (O, 87 beds) 252
McHenry Street, Burlington, WI Zip 53105–1828; tel. 414/763–2411; Paul A.
Miller, President and Chief Executive Officer

MILWAUKEE PSYCHIATRIC HOSPITAL (O, 80 beds) 1220 Dewey Avenue,
Wauwatosa, WI Zip 53213–2598; tel. 414/454–6600; Mark R. Ambrosius,
President

SHEBOYGAN MEMORIAL MEDICAL CENTER (O, 138 beds) 2629 North
Seventh Street, Sheboygan, WI Zip 53083–4998; tel. 414/451–5000;
Patrick J. Trotter, President

SINAI SAMARITAN MEDICAL CENTER (O, 192 beds) 945 North 12th Street,
Milwaukee, WI Zip 53233, Mailing Address: P.O. Box 342, Zip 53201–0342;
tel. 414/219–2000; William I. Jenkins, President and Chief Executive Officer

ST. LUKE'S MEDICAL CENTER (O, 546 beds) 2900 West Oklahoma Avenue,
Milwaukee, WI Zip 53215, Mailing Address: P.O. Box 2901, Zip 53201;
tel. 414/649–6000; Mark R. Ambrosius, President

TWO RIVERS COMMUNITY HOSPITAL AND HAMILTON MEMORIAL HOME (O,
138 beds) 2500 Garfield Street, Two Rivers, WI Zip 54241;
tel. 414/793–1178; Steven H. Spencer, President and Chief Executive
Officer

VALLEY VIEW MEDICAL CENTER (O, 92 beds) 901 Reed Street, Plymouth, WI
Zip 53073–2409; tel. 414/893–1771; Patrick J. Trotter, President

WEST ALLIS MEMORIAL HOSPITAL (O, 200 beds) 8901 West Lincoln Avenue,
West Allis, WI Zip 53227–0901, Mailing Address: P.O. Box 27901, Zip
53227–0901; tel. 414/328–6000; Richard A. Kellar, Administrator

Owned, leased, sponsored:	10 hospitals	1622 beds
Contract–managed:	0 hospitals	0 beds
Totals:	10 hospitals	1622 beds

★0355: BAPTIST HEALTH (NP)

9601 Interstate 630, Exit 7, Little Rock, AR Zip 72205–7299;
tel. 501/202–2000; Russell D. Harrington Jr., President

ARKANSAS: BAPTIST MEDICAL CENTER (O, 635 beds) 9601 Interstate 630,
Exit 7, Little Rock, AR Zip 72205–7299; tel. 501/202–2000; Steven B.
Lampkin, Senior Vice President and Administrator

BAPTIST MEDICAL CENTER ARKADELPHIA (L, 57 beds) 3050 Twin Rivers
Drive, Arkadelphia, AR Zip 71923; tel. 501/245–1100; Dan Gathright, Senior
Vice President and Administrator

BAPTIST MEDICAL CENTER HEBER SPRINGS (L, 22 beds) Highway 110 West,
Heber Springs, AR Zip 72543–1087, Mailing Address: P.O. Box 1087, Zip
72543–1087; tel. 501/362–3121; Harrell E. Clendenin, Vice President and
Administrator

BAPTIST MEMORIAL MEDICAL CENTER (L, 200 beds) One Pershing Circle,
North Little Rock, AR Zip 72114–1899; tel. 501/202–3000; Harrison M.
Dean, Senior Vice President and Administrator

BAPTIST REHABILITATION INSTITUTE OF ARKANSAS (O, 100 beds) 9601
Interstate 630, Exit 7, Little Rock, AR Zip 72205–7249; tel. 501/202–7000;
Steven Douglas Weeks, Vice President and Administrator

Owned, leased, sponsored:	5 hospitals	1014 beds
Contract–managed:	0 hospitals	0 beds
Totals:	5 hospitals	1014 beds

0185: BAPTIST HEALTH CARE CORPORATION (NP)

1717 North E Street, Suite 320, Pensacola, FL Zip 32501–6335;
tel. 904/469–2337; James F. Vickery, President

ALABAMA: MIZELL MEMORIAL HOSPITAL (O, 57 beds) 702 Main Street, Opp,
AL Zip 36467–1626, Mailing Address: P.O. Box 1010, Zip 36467–1010;
tel. 334/493–3541; Allen Foster, Administrator

FLORIDA: BAPTIST HOSPITAL (O, 521 beds) 1000 West Moreno, Pensacola,
FL Zip 32501–2393, Mailing Address: P.O. Box 17500, Zip 32522–7500;
tel. 904/469–2313; Quinton Studer, President

GULF BREEZE HOSPITAL (O, 45 beds) 1110 Gulf Breeze Parkway, Gulf
Breeze, FL Zip 32561–1110, Mailing Address: P.O. Box 159, Zip
32562–0159; tel. 904/934–2000; Richard C. Fulford, Administrator

JAY HOSPITAL (L, 47 beds) 221 South Alabama Street, Jay, FL Zip 32565,
Mailing Address: P.O. Box 397, Zip 32565; tel. 904/675–8000; H. D.
Cannington, Administrator

Owned, leased, sponsored:	4 hospitals	670 beds
Contract–managed:	0 hospitals	0 beds
Totals:	4 hospitals	670 beds

0265: BAPTIST HEALTH SYSTEM (CO)

660 North Main Street, Suite 300, San Antonio, TX Zip 78205–1222;
tel. 210/302–3000; Fred R. Mills, President and Chief Executive
Officer

TEXAS: BAPTIST MEDICAL CENTER (O, 481 beds) 111 Dallas Street, San
Antonio, TX Zip 78205–1230; tel. 210/222–8431; William W. Webster,
Administrator

For explanation of codes following names, see page B2.
★ Indicates Type III membership in the American Hospital Association.

Section B

NORTHEAST BAPTIST HOSPITAL (O, 210 beds) 8811 Village Drive, San Antonio, TX Zip 78217; tel. 210/653–2330; Patricia E. Carey, FACHE, Administrator

SOUTHEAST BAPTIST HOSPITAL (O, 153 beds) 4214 East Southcross, San Antonio, TX Zip 78222; tel. 210/337–6900; Harry E. Smith, Administrator

ST. LUKE'S BAPTIST HOSPITAL (O, 219 beds) 7930 Floyd Curl Drive, San Antonio, TX Zip 78229–0100; tel. 210/692–8703; John Penn Krause, Administrator

Owned, leased, sponsored:	4 hospitals	1063 beds
Contract–managed:	0 hospitals	0 beds
Totals:	4 hospitals	1063 beds

★0345: BAPTIST HEALTH SYSTEM (CO)

3500 Blue Lake Drive, Suite 100, Birmingham, AL Zip 35243, Mailing Address: P.O. Box 830605, Zip 35283–0605; tel. 205/715–5319; Dennis A. Hall, President

ALABAMA: BIRMINGHAM BAPTIST MEDICAL CENTER–MONTCLAIR CAMPUS (O, 1023 beds) 800 Montclair Road, Birmingham, AL Zip 35213; tel. 205/592–1000; Dana S. Hensley, President

BIRMINGHAM BAPTIST MEDICAL CENTER–PRINCETON (O, 1033 beds) 701 Princeton Avenue S.W., Birmingham, AL Zip 35211–1305; tel. 205/783–3000; Dana S. Hensley, President and Chief Executive Officer

CHEROKEE BAPTIST MEDICAL CENTER (O, 45 beds) 400 Northwood Drive, Centre, AL Zip 35960–1023; tel. 205/927–5531; Barry S. Cochran, President

CITIZENS BAPTIST MEDICAL CENTER (O, 97 beds) 604 Stone Avenue, Talladega, AL Zip 35160, Mailing Address: P.O. Box 978, Zip 35161; tel. 205/362–8111; Steven M. Johnson, President

COOSA VALLEY BAPTIST MEDICAL CENTER (O, 176 beds) 315 West Hickory Street, Sylacauga, AL Zip 35150–2996; tel. 205/249–5000; Steven M. Johnson, President

CULLMAN REGIONAL MEDICAL CENTER (O, 115 beds) 1912 Alabama Highway 157, Cullman, AL Zip 35055, Mailing Address: P.O. Box 1108, Zip 35056–1108; tel. 205/737–2000; Jesse O. Weatherly, Administrator

DEKALB BAPTIST MEDICAL CENTER (O, 91 beds) 200 Medical Center Drive, Fort Payne, AL Zip 35967, Mailing Address: P.O. Box 778, Zip 35967–0778; tel. 205/845–3150; Barry S. Cochran, President

LAWRENCE BAPTIST MEDICAL CENTER (L, 30 beds) 202 Hospital Street, Moulton, AL Zip 35650–0039, Mailing Address: P.O. Box 39, Zip 35650–0039; tel. 205/974–2200; Cheryl Hays, Administrator

MARION BAPTIST MEDICAL CENTER (L, 112 beds) 1315 Military Street South, Hamilton, AL Zip 35570; tel. 205/921–7861; Evan S. Dillard, President

SHELBY BAPTIST MEDICAL CENTER (O, 228 beds) 1000 First Street North, Alabaster, AL Zip 35007–0488, Mailing Address: Box 488, Zip 35007–0488; tel. 205/620–8100; Charles C. Colvert, President

WALKER BAPTIST MEDICAL CENTER (O, 267 beds) 3400 Highway 78 East, Jasper, AL Zip 35501, Mailing Address: Box 3547, Zip 35502–3547; tel. 205/387–4000; Jeff Brewer, President

Owned, leased, sponsored:	11 hospitals	3217 beds
Contract–managed:	0 hospitals	0 beds
Totals:	11 hospitals	3217 beds

2155: BAPTIST HEALTH SYSTEM OF TENNESSEE (NP)

137 Blount Avenue S.E., Knoxville, TN Zip 37920, Mailing Address: Box 1788, Zip 37901; tel. 615/632–5099; Dale Collins, President and Chief Executive Officer

TENNESSEE: BAPTIST HOSPITAL OF COCKE COUNTY (O, 109 beds) 435 Second Street, Newport, TN Zip 37821; tel. 423/625–2200; Wayne Buckner, Administrator

BAPTIST HOSPITAL OF EAST TENNESSEE (O, 321 beds) 137 Blount Avenue S.E., Knoxville, TN Zip 37920, Mailing Address: Box 1788, Zip 37901–1788; tel. 423/632–5011; Jon Foster, Senior Vice President and Administrator

Owned, leased, sponsored:	2 hospitals	430 beds
Contract–managed:	0 hospitals	0 beds
Totals:	2 hospitals	430 beds

★0315: BAPTIST HEALTHCARE SYSTEM (CO)

4007 Kresge Way, Louisville, KY Zip 40207–4677; tel. 502/896–5000; Tommy J. Smith, President and Chief Executive Officer

KENTUCKY: BAPTIST HOSPITAL EAST (O, 407 beds) 4000 Kresge Way, Louisville, KY Zip 40207–4676; tel. 502/897–8100; Susan Stout Tamme, President

BAPTIST REGIONAL MEDICAL CENTER (O, 255 beds) 1 Trillium Way, Corbin, KY Zip 40701–8420; tel. 606/528–1212; John S. Henson, President

CENTRAL BAPTIST HOSPITAL (O, 321 beds) 1740 Nicholasville Road, Lexington, KY Zip 40503; tel. 606/275–6100; William G. Sisson, President

TRI COUNTY BAPTIST HOSPITAL (O, 120 beds) 1025 New Moody Lane, La Grange, KY Zip 40031–0559; tel. 502/222–5388; David L. Gray, Administrator

WESTERN BAPTIST HOSPITAL (O, 310 beds) 2501 Kentucky Avenue, Paducah, KY Zip 42003; tel. 502/575–2100; Larry O. Barton, President

Owned, leased, sponsored:	5 hospitals	1413 beds
Contract–managed:	0 hospitals	0 beds
Totals:	5 hospitals	1413 beds

★4155: BAPTIST HEALTHCARE SYSTEM OF SOUTH CAROLINA (CO)

Taylor at Marion Street, Columbia, SC Zip 29220; tel. 803/771–5010; Charles D. Beaman Jr., President and Chief Executive Officer

SOUTH CAROLINA: BAPTIST MEDICAL CENTER EASLEY (O, 93 beds) 200 Fleetwood Drive, Easley, SC Zip 29640, Mailing Address: P.O. Box 2129, Zip 29641–2129; tel. 864/855–7200; Roddey E. Gettys III, Executive Vice President

BAPTIST MEDICAL CENTER/COLUMBIA (O, 387 beds) Taylor at Marion Street, Columbia, SC Zip 29220; tel. 803/771–5010; James M. Bridges, Executive Vice President

Owned, leased, sponsored:	2 hospitals	480 beds
Contract–managed:	0 hospitals	0 beds
Totals:	2 hospitals	480 beds

★8810: BAPTIST HOSPITALS AND HEALTH SYSTEMS, INC. (NP)

2224 West Northern Avenue, Suite D–300, Phoenix, AZ Zip 85021; tel. 602/864–1184; Gerald L. Wissink, President and Chief Executive Officer

ARIZONA: ARROWHEAD COMMUNITY HOSPITAL AND MEDICAL CENTER (O, 80 beds) 18701 North 67th Avenue, Glendale, AZ Zip 85308–5722; tel. 602/561–1000; Richard S. Alley, Executive Vice President and Chief Executive Officer

BULLHEAD COMMUNITY HOSPITAL (O, 182 beds) 2735 Silver Creek Road, Bullhead City, AZ Zip 86442; tel. 520/763–2273; Ronald W. Tenbarge, Executive Vice President and Chief Executive Officer

PHOENIX BAPTIST HOSPITAL AND MEDICAL CENTER (O, 222 beds) 6025 North 20th Avenue, Phoenix, AZ Zip 85015; tel. 602/249–0212; Richard S. Alley, Chief Executive Officer

Owned, leased, sponsored:	3 hospitals	484 beds
Contract–managed:	0 hospitals	0 beds
Totals:	3 hospitals	484 beds

★1625: BAPTIST MEMORIAL HEALTH CARE CORPORATION (NP)

899 Madison Avenue, Memphis, TN Zip 38146; tel. 901/227–2727; Stephen Curtis Reynolds, President and Chief Executive Officer

For explanation of codes following names, see page B2.
★ Indicates Type III membership in the American Hospital Association.

Section B

ARKANSAS: BAPTIST MEMORIAL HOSPITAL–BLYTHEVILLE (L, 210 beds) 1520 North Division Street, Blytheville, AR Zip 72315, Mailing Address: P.O. Box 108, Zip 72316–0108; tel. 501/762–3300; Randy King, Administrator

BAPTIST MEMORIAL HOSPITAL–FORREST CITY (L, 86 beds) 1601 Newcastle Road, Forrest City, AR Zip 72335, Mailing Address: P.O. Box 667, Zip 72336–0667; tel. 501/633–2020; George S. Fray, Administrator

BAPTIST MEMORIAL HOSPITAL–OSCEOLA (L, 59 beds) 611 West Lee Avenue, Osceola, AR Zip 72370, Mailing Address: Box 607, Zip 72370–0607; tel. 501/563–7000; Al Sypniewski, Administrator

MISSISSIPPI: BAPTIST MEMORIAL HOSPITAL–BOONEVILLE (L, 93 beds) 100 Hospital Street, Booneville, MS Zip 38829; tel. 601/728–5331; Pamela W. Roberts, Administrator

BAPTIST MEMORIAL HOSPITAL–DESOTO (O, 200 beds) 7601 Southcrest Parkway, Southaven, MS Zip 38671; tel. 601/349–4000; Melvin E. Walker, Administrator

BAPTIST MEMORIAL HOSPITAL–GOLDEN TRIANGLE (L, 328 beds) 2520 Fifth Street North, Columbus, MS Zip 39703–2095, Mailing Address: P.O. Box 1307, Zip 39701–1307; tel. 601/243–1000; J. Stuart Mitchell III, Administrator

BAPTIST MEMORIAL HOSPITAL–NORTH MISSISSIPPI (L, 158 beds) 2301 South Lamar Boulevard, Oxford, MS Zip 38655, Mailing Address: Box 946, Zip 38655; tel. 601/232–8100; James Hahn, Administrator

BAPTIST MEMORIAL HOSPITAL–UNION COUNTY (L, 153 beds) 200 Highway 30 West, New Albany, MS Zip 38652–3197; tel. 601/538–7631; John Tompkins, Administrator

TIPPAH COUNTY HOSPITAL (C, 110 beds) 1005 City Avenue North, Ripley, MS Zip 38663–0499; tel. 601/837–9221; Jerry Green, Administrator

TENNESSEE: BAPTIST MEMORIAL HOSPITAL (O, 1112 beds) 899 Madison Avenue, Memphis, TN Zip 38146; tel. 901/227–2727; Stephen Curtis Reynolds, President and Chief Executive Officer

BAPTIST MEMORIAL HOSPITAL–HUNTINGDON (O, 70 beds) 631 R. B. Wilson Drive, Huntingdon, TN Zip 38344; tel. 901/986–4461; Susan M. Breeden, Administrator

BAPTIST MEMORIAL HOSPITAL–LAUDERDALE (O, 70 beds) 326 Asbury Road, Ripley, TN Zip 38063–9701; tel. 901/635–6400; W. Tate Moorer, Administrator

BAPTIST MEMORIAL HOSPITAL–TIPTON (O, 110 beds) 1995 Highway 51 South, Covington, TN Zip 38019; tel. 901/476–2621; William T. Moorer, Administrator

BAPTIST MEMORIAL HOSPITAL–UNION CITY (O, 133 beds) 1201 Bishop Street, Union City, TN Zip 38261, Mailing Address: Box 310, Zip 38281–0310; tel. 901/884–8601; Mike Perryman, Administrator

Owned, leased, sponsored:	13 hospitals	2782 beds
Contract–managed:	1 hospital	110 beds
Totals:	14 hospitals	2892 beds

★0107: BAYHEALTH MEDICAL CENTER (NP)
640 South State Street, Dover, DE Zip 19901; Dennis E. Klima, President and Chief Executive Officer

DELAWARE: BAYHEALTH MEDICAL CENTER, MILFORD MEMORIAL CAMPUS (O, 130 beds) 21 West Clarke Avenue, Milford, DE Zip 19963, Mailing Address: P.O. Box 199, Zip 19963–0199; tel. 302/424–5613; Joseph K. Whiting, Executive Vice President and Chief Operating Officer

KENT GENERAL HOSPITAL (O, 193 beds) 640 South State Street, Dover, DE Zip 19901–3597; tel. 302/674–4700; Dennis E. Klima, President and Chief Executive Officer

Owned, leased, sponsored:	2 hospitals	323 beds
Contract–managed:	0 hospitals	0 beds
Totals:	2 hospitals	323 beds

★0095: BAYLOR HEALTH CARE SYSTEM (CO)
3500 Gaston Avenue, Dallas, TX Zip 75226; tel. 214/820–0111; Boone Powell Jr., President

TEXAS: BAYLOR CENTER FOR RESTORATIVE CARE (O, 74 beds) 3504 Swiss Avenue, Dallas, TX Zip 75204; tel. 214/823–1684; Gerry Brueckner, R.N., Executive Director

BAYLOR INSTITUTE FOR REHABILITATION (O, 92 beds) 3505 Gaston Avenue, Dallas, TX Zip 75246–2018; tel. 214/826–7030; Judith C. Waterston, Executive Director

BAYLOR MEDICAL CENTER AT GARLAND (O, 174 beds) 2300 Marie Curie Boulevard, Garland, TX Zip 75042–5706; tel. 214/487–5000; John B. McWhorter III, Executive Director

BAYLOR MEDICAL CENTER AT GRAPEVINE (O, 68 beds) 1650 West College Street, Grapevine, TX Zip 76051–1650; tel. 817/329–2500; Mark C. Hood, Executive Director

BAYLOR MEDICAL CENTER–ELLIS COUNTY (O, 91 beds) 1405 West Jefferson Street, Waxahachie, TX Zip 75165; tel. 972/923–7000; James Michael Lee, Executive Director

BAYLOR UNIVERSITY MEDICAL CENTER (O, 827 beds) 3500 Gaston Avenue, Dallas, TX Zip 75246–2088; tel. 214/820–0111; Boone Powell Jr., President

IRVING HEALTHCARE SYSTEM (L, 231 beds) 1901 North MacArthur Boulevard, Irving, TX Zip 75061; tel. 972/579–8100; H. J. MacFarland, FACHE, Executive Director

Owned, leased, sponsored:	7 hospitals	1557 beds
Contract–managed:	0 hospitals	0 beds
Totals:	7 hospitals	1557 beds

★1095: BAYSTATE HEALTH SYSTEMS, INC. (NP)
759 Chestnut Street, Springfield, MA Zip 01199–0001; tel. 413/784–0000; Michael J. Daly, President

MASSACHUSETTS: BAYSTATE MEDICAL CENTER (O, 660 beds) 759 Chestnut Street, Springfield, MA Zip 01199–0001; tel. 413/784–0000; Mark R. Tolosky, Chief Executive Officer

FRANKLIN MEDICAL CENTER (O, 105 beds) 164 High Street, Greenfield, MA Zip 01301; tel. 413/773–0211; Harlan J. Smith, President

MARY LANE HOSPITAL (O, 35 beds) 85 South Street, Ware, MA Zip 01082; tel. 413/967–6211; Christine Shirtcliff, Executive Vice President

Owned, leased, sponsored:	3 hospitals	800 beds
Contract–managed:	0 hospitals	0 beds
Totals:	3 hospitals	800 beds

0069: BEHAVIORAL HEALTHCARE CORPORATION (IO)
102 Woodmont Boulevard, Suite 500, Nashville, TN Zip 37205; tel. 615/269–3492; Edward A. Stack, President

ARIZONA: BHC ASPEN HILL HOSPITAL (O, 26 beds) 305 West Forest Avenue, Flagstaff, AZ Zip 86001–1464; tel. 520/773–1060; Alan G. Chapman, Administrator and Chief Executive Officer

ARKANSAS: BHC PINNACLE POINTE HOSPITAL (O, 98 beds) 11501 Financial Center Parkway, Little Rock, AR Zip 72211–3715; tel. 501/223–3322; Joseph Fischer, Chief Executive Officer

CALIFORNIA: BHC ALHAMBRA HOSPITAL (O, 98 beds) 4619 North Rosemead Boulevard, Rosemead, CA Zip 91770–1498, Mailing Address: P.O. Box 369, Zip 91770; tel. 818/286–1191; Peggy Minnick, Administrator

BHC BELMONT HILLS HOSPITAL (O, 53 beds) 1301 Ralston Avenue, Belmont, CA Zip 94002; tel. 415/593–2143; Harold G. Marohn, Acting Chief Executive Officer

BHC CANYON RIDGE HOSPITAL (O, 59 beds) 5353 G Street, Chino, CA Zip 91710; tel. 909/590–3700; Diana L. Goulet, Chief Executive Officer

BHC CEDAR VISTA HOSPITAL (O, 61 beds) 7171 North Cedar Avenue, Fresno, CA Zip 93720; tel. 209/449–8000; Arthur M. Ginsberg, Chief Executive Officer

BHC FREMONT HOSPITAL (O, 78 beds) 39001 Sundale Drive, Fremont, CA Zip 94538; tel. 510/796–1100; Terry Johnson, Chief Executive Officer

BHC HERITAGE OAKS HOSPITAL (O, 76 beds) 4250 Auburn Boulevard, Sacramento, CA Zip 95841; tel. 916/489–3336; Ingrid L. Whipple, Chief Executive Officer

For explanation of codes following names, see page B2.
★ Indicates Type III membership in the American Hospital Association.

BHC ROSS HOSPITAL (O, 56 beds) 1111 Sir Francis Drake Boulevard, Kentfield, CA Zip 94904; tel. 415/258–6900; Judy G. House, Chief Executive Officer

BHC SAN LUIS REY HOSPITAL (O, 117 beds) 335 Saxony Road, Encinitas, CA Zip 92024–2723; tel. 619/753–1245; William T. Sparrow, Chief Executive Officer

BHC SIERRA VISTA HOSPITAL (O, 72 beds) 8001 Bruceville Road, Sacramento, CA Zip 95823; tel. 916/423–2000; Kenneth A. Meibert, Chief Executive Officer

BHC VISTA DEL MAR HOSPITAL (O, 87 beds) 801 Seneca Street, Ventura, CA Zip 93001; tel. 805/653–6434; Jerry Conway, Chief Executive Officer

BHC WALNUT CREEK HOSPITAL (O, 108 beds) 175 La Casa Via, Walnut Creek, CA Zip 94598; tel. 510/933–7990; Jay R. Kellison, Chief Executive Officer

FLORIDA: BHC FORT LAUDERDALE HOSPITAL (O, 100 beds) 1601 East Las Olas Boulevard, Fort Lauderdale, FL Zip 33301–2393; tel. 954/463–4321; Andrew Fuhrman, Chief Executive Officer

BHC ST. JOHNS RIVER HOSPITAL (O, 60 beds) 6300 Beach Boulevard, Jacksonville, FL Zip 32216; tel. 904/724–9202; Patricia Vandergrift, Administrator

IDAHO: BHC INTERMOUNTAIN HOSPITAL (O, 75 beds) 303 North Allumbaugh Street, Boise, ID Zip 83704–9266; tel. 208/377–8400; Vernon G. Garrett, Chief Executive Officer

ILLINOIS: BHC STREAMWOOD HOSPITAL (O, 100 beds) 1400 East Irving Park Road, Streamwood, IL Zip 60107; tel. 630/837–9000; Jeff Bergren, Chief Operating Officer and Administrator

INDIANA: BHC VALLE VISTA HOSPITAL (O, 96 beds) 898 East Main Street, Greenwood, IN Zip 46143; tel. 317/887–1348; Sheila Mishler, Chief Executive Officer

KANSAS: BHC COLLEGE MEADOWS HOSPITAL (O, 120 beds) 14425 College Boulevard, Lenexa, KS Zip 66215; tel. 913/469–1100; Lisa Redmond, Chief Executive Officer

LOUISIANA: BHC EAST LAKE HOSPITAL (O, 72 beds) 5650 Read Boulevard, New Orleans, LA Zip 70127–3145; tel. 504/241–0888; Darlene Salvant, Chief Executive Officer

BHC MEADOW WOOD HOSPITAL (O, 55 beds) 9032 Perkins Road, Baton Rouge, LA Zip 70810; tel. 504/766–8553; Ralph J. Waite III, Chief Executive Officer

DEPAUL/TULANE BEHAVIORAL HEALTH CENTER (O, 102 beds) 1040 Calhoun Street, New Orleans, LA Zip 70118; tel. 504/899–8282; David E. Hoidal, Chief Executive Officer

MISSISSIPPI: BHC SAND HILL BEHAVIORAL HEALTHCARE (O, 60 beds) 11150 Highway 49 North, Gulfport, MS Zip 39503–4110; tel. 601/831–1700; David C. Bell, Chief Operating Officer

MISSOURI: BHC SPIRIT OF ST. LOUIS HOSPITAL (O, 75 beds) 5931 Highway 94 South, Saint Charles, MO Zip 63304–5601; tel. 314/441–7300; Larry J. Burge, Chief Executive Officer

NEVADA: BHC MONTEVISTA HOSPITAL (O, 80 beds) 5900 West Rochelle Avenue, Las Vegas, NV Zip 89103; tel. 702/364–1111; R. Dale Reynolds, Chief Executive Officer and Administrator

BHC WEST HILLS HOSPITAL (O, 95 beds) 1240 East Ninth Street, Reno, NV Zip 89512, Mailing Address: P.O. Box 30012, Zip 89520; tel. 702/323–0478; Neal Cury, Chief Executive Officer

BHC WILLOW SPRINGS RTC (O, 74 beds) 690 Edison Way, Reno, NV Zip 89502; tel. 702/858–3303; Robert Bartlett, Administrator

NEW MEXICO: BHC MESILLA VALLEY HOSPITAL (O, 85 beds) 3751 Del Rey Boulevard, Las Cruces, NM Zip 88012, Mailing Address: P.O. Box 429, Zip 88004; tel. 505/382–3500; Edward C. Morton Jr., FACHE, Chief Executive Officer

BHC PINON HILLS HOSPITAL (O, 34 beds) 313 Camino Alire, Santa Fe, NM Zip 87501; tel. 505/988–8003; Jerry Smith, Chief Executive Officer

NORTH CAROLINA: BHC CEDAR SPRING HOSPITAL (O, 70 beds) 9600 Pineville–Matthews Road, Pineville, NC Zip 28134–7548; tel. 704/541–6676; Steven G. Johnson, Chief Executive Officer

OHIO: BHC BELMONT PINES HOSPITAL (O, 77 beds) 615 Churchill–Hubbard Road, Youngstown, OH Zip 44505; tel. 330/759–2700; Al Scott, Ed.D., Administrator

BHC FOX RUN HOSPITAL (O, 65 beds) 67670 Traco Drive, Saint Clairsville, OH Zip 43950; tel. 614/695–2131; J. Frank Gallagher III, Administrator

BHC WINDSOR HOSPITAL (O, 50 beds) 115 East Summit Street, Chagrin Falls, OH Zip 44022; tel. 216/247–5300; Donald K. Sykes Jr., Chief Executive Officer

PUERTO RICO: BHC HOSPITAL SAN JUAN CAPESTRANO (O, 88 beds) San Juan, PR Mailing Address: Rural Route 2, Box 11, Zip 00926; tel. 787/760–0222; Laura Vargas, Administrator

TEXAS: BHC MILLWOOD HOSPITAL (O, 130 beds) 1011 North Cooper Street, Arlington, TX Zip 76011; tel. 817/261–3121; Wayne Hallford, Chief Executive Officer

BHC SHOAL CREEK HOSPITAL (O, 118 beds) 3501 Mills Avenue, Austin, TX Zip 78731; tel. 512/452–0361; Gail M. Oberta, Administrator and Chief Executive Officer

UTAH: BHC OLYMPUS VIEW HOSPITAL (O, 82 beds) 1430 East 4500 South, Salt Lake City, UT Zip 84117–4208; tel. 801/272–8000; Barry W. Woodward, Administrator

WASHINGTON: BHC FAIRFAX HOSPITAL (O, 133 beds) 10200 N.E. 132nd Street, Kirkland, WA Zip 98034; tel. 206/821–2000; Michelle Egerer, Chief Executive Officer

Owned, leased, sponsored:	38 hospitals	3085 beds
Contract–managed:	0 hospitals	0 beds
Totals:	38 hospitals	3085 beds

0515: BENEDICTINE HEALTH SYSTEM (CC)
503 East Third Street, Duluth, MN Zip 55805–1964; tel. 218/720–2370; Sister Kathleen Hofer, Chair Person and Chief Executive Officer

IDAHO: ST. MARY'S HOSPITAL (O, 28 beds) Lewiston and North Streets, Cottonwood, ID Zip 83522, Mailing Address: P.O. Box 137, Zip 83522–0137; tel. 208/962–3251; Casey Uhling, Administrator

MINNESOTA: ST. JOSEPH'S MEDICAL CENTER (O, 153 beds) 523 North Third Street, Brainerd, MN Zip 56401–3098; tel. 218/829–2861; Thomas K. Prusak, President

ST. MARY'S MEDICAL CENTER (O, 286 beds) 407 East Third Street, Duluth, MN Zip 55805–1984; tel. 218/726–4000; Sister Kathleen Hofer, President

ST. MARY'S REGIONAL HEALTH CENTER (O, 167 beds) 1027 Washington Avenue, Detroit Lakes, MN Zip 56501–3598; tel. 218/847–5611; John H. Solheim, Chief Executive Officer

WISCONSIN: ST. MARY'S HOSPITAL OF SUPERIOR (O, 42 beds) 3500 Tower Avenue, Superior, WI Zip 54880–5395; tel. 715/392–8281; Terry Jacobson, Administrator

Owned, leased, sponsored:	5 hospitals	676 beds
Contract–managed:	0 hospitals	0 beds
Totals:	5 hospitals	676 beds

0545: BENEDICTINE SISTERS OF THE ANNUNCIATION (CC)
7520 University Drive, Bismarck, ND Zip 58504–9653; tel. 701/255–1520; Sister Susan Berger, Prioress

NORTH DAKOTA: GARRISON MEMORIAL HOSPITAL (S, 54 beds) 407 Third Avenue S.E., Garrison, ND Zip 58540–0039; tel. 701/463–2275; Richard Spilovoy, Administrator

ST. ALEXIUS MEDICAL CENTER (S, 269 beds) 900 East Broadway, Bismarck, ND Zip 58501, Mailing Address: P.O. Box 5510, Zip 58506–5510; tel. 701/224–7000; Richard A. Tschider, FACHE, Administrator and Chief Executive Officer

Owned, leased, sponsored:	2 hospitals	323 beds
Contract–managed:	0 hospitals	0 beds
Totals:	2 hospitals	323 beds

★2435: BERKSHIRE HEALTH SYSTEMS, INC. (NP)
725 North Street, Pittsfield, MA Zip 01201; tel. 413/447–2743; David E. Phelps, President and Chief Executive Officer

For explanation of codes following names, see page B2.
★ Indicates Type III membership in the American Hospital Association.

Section B

MASSACHUSETTS: BERKSHIRE MEDICAL CENTER (O, 330 beds) 725 North Street, Pittsfield, MA Zip 01201; tel. 413/447–2000; Ruth P. Blodgett, Chief Operating Officer

FAIRVIEW HOSPITAL (O, 34 beds) 29 Lewis Avenue, Great Barrington, MA Zip 01230–1713; tel. 413/528–0790; Claire L. Bowen, President

Owned, leased, sponsored:	2 hospitals	364 beds
Contract–managed:	0 hospitals	0 beds
Totals:	2 hospitals	364 beds

★0415:   BETHESDA HOSPITAL, INC. (NP)
619 Oak Street, Cincinnati, OH Zip 45206–1690; tel. 513/569–6141; L. Thomas Wilburn Jr., Chairman

OHIO: BETHESDA NORTH HOSPITAL (O, 353 beds) 10500 Montgomery Road, Cincinnati, OH Zip 45242; tel. 513/745–1111; Fred Kolb, Site Administrator

BETHESDA OAK HOSPITAL (O, 384 beds) 619 Oak Street, Cincinnati, OH Zip 45206–1690; tel. 513/569–6111; Linda D. Schaffner, R.N., Vice President and Administrator

Owned, leased, sponsored:	2 hospitals	737 beds
Contract–managed:	0 hospitals	0 beds
Totals:	2 hospitals	737 beds

★0051:   BJC HEALTH SYSTEM (NP)
4444 Forest Park Avenue, Saint Louis, MO Zip 63108–2259; tel. 314/286–2030; Fred L. Brown, President and Chief Executive Officer

ILLINOIS: ALTON MEMORIAL HOSPITAL (O, 224 beds) One Memorial Drive, Alton, IL Zip 62002–6722; tel. 618/463–7311; Ronald B. McMullen, President

CLAY COUNTY HOSPITAL (C, 31 beds) 700 North Mill Street, Flora, IL Zip 62839, Mailing Address: P.O. Box 280, Zip 62839; tel. 618/662–2131; John E. Monnahan, President and Senior Executive Officer

FAYETTE COUNTY HOSPITAL AND LONG TERM CARE (L, 133 beds) Seventh and Taylor Streets, Vandalia, IL Zip 62471–1296; tel. 618/283–1231; Daniel L. Gantz, President

MISSOURI: BARNES–JEWISH HOSPITAL (O, 1221 beds) 216 South Kingshighway Boulevard, Saint Louis, MO Zip 63110–1094; tel. 314/362–5000; Alan W. Brass, FACHE, President

BARNES–JEWISH ST. PETERS HOSPITAL (O, 91 beds) 10 Hospital Drive, Saint Peters, MO Zip 63376–1659; tel. 314/916–9000; John Gloss, President

BARNES–JEWISH WEST COUNTY HOSPITAL (O, 91 beds) 12634 Olive Boulevard, Saint Louis, MO Zip 63141–6354; tel. 314/996–8000; Gregory T. Wozniak, President

BOONE HOSPITAL CENTER (L, 307 beds) 1600 East Broadway, Columbia, MO Zip 65201; tel. 573/815–8000; Michael Shirk, President and Senior Executive Officer

CHRISTIAN HOSPITAL NORTHEAST–NORTHWEST (O, 542 beds) 11133 Dunn Road, Saint Louis, MO Zip 63136–6192; tel. 314/355–2300; W. R. Van Bokkelen, President and Senior Executive Officer

MISSOURI BAPTIST HOSPITAL OF SULLIVAN (O, 60 beds) 751 Sappington Bridge Road, Sullivan, MO Zip 63080, Mailing Address: P.O. Box 190, Zip 63080; tel. 573/468–4186; Davis D. Skinner, Administrator

MISSOURI BAPTIST MEDICAL CENTER (O, 335 beds) 3015 North Ballas Road, Town and Country, MO Zip 63131–2374; tel. 314/996–5000; Mark A. Eustis, President

PARKLAND HEALTH CENTER (O, 94 beds) 1101 West Liberty Street, Farmington, MO Zip 63640–1997; tel. 314/756–6451; Richard L. Conklin, President

ST. LOUIS CHILDREN'S HOSPITAL (O, 235 beds) One Children's Place, Saint Louis, MO Zip 63110–1077; tel. 314/454–6000; Ted W. Frey, President

Owned, leased, sponsored:	11 hospitals	3333 beds
Contract–managed:	1 hospital	31 beds
Totals:	12 hospitals	3364 beds

●★0053:   BLUE WATER HEALTH SERVICES CORPORATION (NP)
1221 Pine Grove Avenue, Port Huron, MI Zip 48060; tel. 810/989–3717; Donald C. Fletcher, President and Chief Executive Officer

MICHIGAN: PORT HURON HOSPITAL (O, 184 beds) 1221 Pine Grove Avenue, Port Huron, MI Zip 48061–5011; tel. 810/987–5000; Donald C. Fletcher, President and Chief Executive Officer

Owned, leased, sponsored:	1 hospital	184 beds
Contract–managed:	0 hospitals	0 beds
Totals:	1 hospital	184 beds

★5085:   BON SECOURS HEALTH SYSTEM, INC. (CC)
1505 Marriottsville Road, Marriottsville, MD Zip 21104–1399; tel. 410/442–5511; Christopher M. Carney, President and Chief Executive Officer

FLORIDA: BON SECOURS–ST. JOSEPH HOSPITAL (O, 313 beds) 2500 Harbor Boulevard, Port Charlotte, FL Zip 33952–5396; tel. 941/625–4122; Michael L. Harrington, Executive Vice President and Administrator

BON SECOURS–VENICE HOSPITAL (O, 390 beds) 540 The Rialto, Venice, FL Zip 34285; tel. 941/485–7711; Roy Hess, Executive Vice President and Administrator

MARYLAND: BON SECOURS HOSPITAL (O, 148 beds) 2000 West Baltimore Street, Baltimore, MD Zip 21223–1597; tel. 410/362–3000; Jane Durney Crowley, Chief Executive Officer

LIBERTY MEDICAL CENTER (O, 160 beds) 2600 Liberty Heights Avenue, Baltimore, MD Zip 21215; tel. 410/383–4000; Jane Durney Crowley, Chief Executive Officer

MICHIGAN: BON SECOURS HOSPITAL (O, 242 beds) 468 Cadieux Road, Grosse Pointe, MI Zip 48230; tel. 313/343–1000; Michael Serilla, Acting Executive Vice President and Administrator

PENNSYLVANIA: BON SECOURS–HOLY FAMILY REGIONAL HEALTH SYSTEM (O, 169 beds) 2500 Seventh Avenue, Altoona, PA Zip 16602; tel. 814/944–1681; David J. Davies, Chief Executive Officer

SOUTH CAROLINA: BON SECOURS–ST. FRANCIS XAVIER HOSPITAL (O, 147 beds) 2095 Henry Tecklenburg Drive, Charleston, SC Zip 29414–0001, Mailing Address: P.O. Box 160001, Zip 29414–0001; tel. 803/402–1000; Allen P. Carroll, Chief Executive Officer

VIRGINIA: BON SECOURS–DEPAUL MEDICAL CENTER (O, 202 beds) 150 Kingsley Lane, Norfolk, VA Zip 23505; tel. 757/889–5000; Sharon M. Tanner, President and Chief Executive Officer

BON SECOURS–MARYVIEW MEDICAL CENTER (O, 441 beds) 3636 High Street, Portsmouth, VA Zip 23707–3236; tel. 804/398–2200; Richard A. Hanson, Acting Administrator

BON SECOURS–RICHMOND COMMUNITY HOSPITAL (O, 88 beds) 1500 North 28th Street, Richmond, VA Zip 23223–5396, Mailing Address: Box 27184, Zip 23261–7184; tel. 804/225–1700; Samuel F. Lillard, Executive Vice President and Administrator

BON SECOURS–STUART CIRCLE (O, 158 beds) 413 Stuart Circle, Richmond, VA Zip 23220; tel. 804/358–7051; Timothy A. Johnson, Executive Vice President and Administrator

MARY IMMACULATE HOSPITAL (O, 225 beds) 2 Bernardine Drive, Newport News, VA Zip 23602; tel. 757/886–6000; Kirby H. Smith Jr., Executive Vice President and Chief Executive Officer

PORTSMOUTH GENERAL HOSPITAL (O, 148 beds) 850 Crawford Parkway, Portsmouth, VA Zip 23704–2386; tel. 804/398–4000; Nora M. Paffrath, Executive Vice President

RICHMOND MEMORIAL HOSPITAL (O, 272 beds) 1300 Westwood Avenue, Richmond, VA Zip 23227–4699, Mailing Address: Box 26783, Zip 23261–6783; tel. 804/254–6000; Michael–David Robinson, Executive Vice President and Administrator

For explanation of codes following names, see page B2.
★ Indicates Type III membership in the American Hospital Association.
● Single hospital health care system

© 1997 AHA Guide

Networks, Health Care Systems and Alliances   **B71**

ST. MARY'S HOSPITAL (O, 391 beds) 5801 Bremo Road, Richmond, VA Zip 23226–1900; tel. 804/285–2011; Ann E. Honeycutt, Executive Vice President and Administrator

Owned, leased, sponsored:	15 hospitals	3494 beds
Contract–managed:	0 hospitals	0 beds
Totals:	15 hospitals	3494 beds

0073: BOWDON CORPORATE OFFICES (IO)

4250 Perimeter Park South, Suite 102, Atlanta, GA Zip 30341; tel. 770/452–1221; Bill E. Ehrhardt, Executive Director

GEORGIA: BOWDON AREA HOSPITAL (O, 41 beds) 501 Mitchell Avenue, Bowdon, GA Zip 30108; tel. 770/258–7207; Yvonne Willis, Administrator

NEW MEXICO: ALLIANCE HOSPITAL OF SANTA TERESA (L, 72 beds) 100 Laura Court, Santa Teresa, NM Zip 88008, Mailing Address: P.O. Box 6, Zip 88008; tel. 505/589–0033; Frank M. Braden, Administrator

Owned, leased, sponsored:	2 hospitals	113 beds
Contract–managed:	0 hospitals	0 beds
Totals:	2 hospitals	113 beds

2455: BRADFORD HEALTH SERVICES (IO)

2101 Magnolia Avenue South, Suite 518, Birmingham, AL Zip 35205; tel. 205/251–7753; Jerry W. Crowder, President and Chief Executive Officer

ALABAMA: BRADFORD HEALTH SERVICES AT HUNTSVILLE (O, 84 beds) 1600 Browns Ferry Road, Madison, AL Zip 35758, Mailing Address: P.O. Box 176, Zip 35758–0176; tel. 205/461–7272; Bob Hinds, Executive Director

BRADFORD HEALTH SERVICES AT OAK MOUNTAIN (O, 84 beds) 2280 Highway 35, Pelham, AL Zip 35124; tel. 205/664–3460; Jerry Caltrider, Administrator

Owned, leased, sponsored:	2 hospitals	168 beds
Contract–managed:	0 hospitals	0 beds
Totals:	2 hospitals	168 beds

★0585: BRIM, INC. (IO)

305 N.E. 102nd Avenue, Portland, OR Zip 97220–4199; tel. 503/256–2070; Jim McKinney, President

ARIZONA: COBRE VALLEY COMMUNITY HOSPITAL (C, 38 beds) One Hospital Drive, Claypool, AZ Zip 85532, Mailing Address: P.O. Box 3261, Zip 85532–3261; tel. 520/425–3261; John L. Hoopes, Administrator and Chief Executive Officer

NAVAPACHE REGIONAL MEDICAL CENTER (C, 54 beds) 2200 Show Low Lake Road, Show Low, AZ Zip 85901; tel. 520/537–4375; Leigh Cox, Chief Executive Officer

NORTHERN COCHISE COMMUNITY HOSPITAL (C, 48 beds) 901 West Rex Allen Drive, Willcox, AZ Zip 85643; tel. 520/384–3541; Chris Cronberg, Chief Executive Officer

CALIFORNIA: BEAR VALLEY COMMUNITY HOSPITAL (C, 30 beds) 41870 Garstin Road, Big Bear Lake, CA Zip 92315, Mailing Address: P.O. Box 1649, Zip 92315–1649; tel. 909/866–6501; Jim Sato, Chief Executive Officer

HAZEL HAWKINS MEMORIAL HOSPITAL (C, 86 beds) 911 Sunset Drive, Hollister, CA Zip 95023–5695; tel. 408/637–5711; Louis D. Kraml, Administrator

NEEDLES–DESERT COMMUNITIES HOSPITAL (C, 39 beds) 1401 Bailey Avenue, Needles, CA Zip 92363; tel. 619/326–4531; Donna Beane, Administrator

PIONEERS MEMORIAL HEALTHCARE DISTRICT (C, 80 beds) 207 West Legion Road, Brawley, CA Zip 92227–9699; tel. 619/351–3333; William W. Daniel, Administrator and Chief Executive Officer

SAN GORGONIO MEMORIAL HOSPITAL (C, 68 beds) 600 North Highland Springs Avenue, Banning, CA Zip 92220; tel. 909/845–1121; Kay Lang, Chief Executive Officer

IDAHO: CLEARWATER VALLEY HOSPITAL (C, 23 beds) 301 Cedar, Orofino, ID Zip 83544–9029; tel. 208/476–4555; James E. Robertson Jr., Chief Executive Officer

ILLINOIS: HAMMOND–HENRY HOSPITAL (C, 105 beds) 210 West Elk Street, Geneseo, IL Zip 61254–1099; tel. 309/944–6431; Nathan C. Olson, President and Chief Executive Officer

HILLSBORO AREA HOSPITAL (C, 95 beds) 1200 East Tremont Street, Hillsboro, IL Zip 62049; tel. 217/532–6111; Rex H. Brown, President

SPARTA COMMUNITY HOSPITAL (C, 39 beds) 818 East Broadway Street, Sparta, IL Zip 62286–0297, Mailing Address: P.O. Box 297, Zip 62286–0297; tel. 618/443–2177; Joann Emge, Chief Executive Officer

WOOD RIVER TOWNSHIP HOSPITAL (C, 128 beds) 101 East Edwardsville Road, Wood River, IL Zip 62095–1332; tel. 618/254–3821; Max L. Ludeke, FACHE, Interim Chief Executive Officer

INDIANA: WIRTH REGIONAL HOSPITAL (C, 11 beds) Highway 64 West, Oakland City, IN Zip 47660–9379, Mailing Address: Rural Route 3, Box 14A, Zip 47660–9379; tel. 812/749–6111; Ralph Paulding, Administrator

IOWA: GUTTENBERG MUNICIPAL HOSPITAL (C, 29 beds) Second and Main Street, Guttenberg, IA Zip 52052–0550, Mailing Address: Box 550, Zip 52052–0550; tel. 319/252–1121; Timothy J. Wick, Chief Executive Officer

LOUISIANA: JACKSON PARISH HOSPITAL (C, 59 beds) 165 Beech Springs Road, Jonesboro, LA Zip 71251; tel. 318/259–4435; Delmar J. Medill, Interim Chief Executive Officer

LADY OF THE SEA GENERAL HOSPITAL (C, 55 beds) 200 West 134th Place, Cut Off, LA Zip 70345; tel. 504/632–6401; Lane M. Cheramie, Chief Executive Officer

MICHIGAN: CHIPPEWA COUNTY WAR MEMORIAL HOSPITAL (C, 130 beds) 500 Osborn Boulevard, Sault Ste. Marie, MI Zip 49783–4467; tel. 906/635–4460; Daniel Wakeman, Chief Executive Officer

MINNESOTA: SWIFT COUNTY–BENSON HOSPITAL (C, 31 beds) 1815 Wisconsin Avenue, Benson, MN Zip 56215–1653; tel. 320/843–4232; John Stindt, Chief Executive Officer

MISSOURI: SULLIVAN COUNTY MEMORIAL HOSPITAL (C, 47 beds) 630 West Third Street, Milan, MO Zip 63556; tel. 816/265–4212; Martha Gragg, Chief Executive Officer

MONTANA: BARRETT MEMORIAL HOSPITAL (C, 31 beds) 1260 South Atlantic Street, Dillon, MT Zip 59725; tel. 406/683–3000; Jim D. Le Brun, Chief Executive Officer

BIG HORN COUNTY MEMORIAL HOSPITAL (C, 53 beds) 17 North Miles Avenue, Hardin, MT Zip 59034, Mailing Address: P.O. Box 430, Zip 59034; tel. 406/665–2310; Raymond T. Hino, Administrator

COMMUNITY MEDICAL CENTER (C, 115 beds) 2827 Fort Missoula Road, Missoula, MT Zip 59801; tel. 406/728–4100; Grant M. Winn, President

MINERAL COMMUNITY HOSPITAL (C, 30 beds) Roosevelt and Brooklyn, Superior, MT Zip 59872, Mailing Address: P.O. Box 66, Zip 59872–0066; tel. 406/822–4841; Madelyn Faller, Chief Executive Officer

NORTHERN MONTANA HOSPITAL (C, 154 beds) 30 13th Street, Havre, MT Zip 59501, Mailing Address: P.O. Box 1231, Zip 59501; tel. 406/265–2211; David Henry, President and Chief Executive Officer

POWELL COUNTY MEMORIAL HOSPITAL (C, 35 beds) 1101 Texas Avenue, Deer Lodge, MT Zip 59722–1828; tel. 406/846–2212; Tony Pfaff, Chief Executive Officer

ROSEBUD HEALTH CARE CENTER (C, 75 beds) 383 North 17th Avenue, Forsyth, MT Zip 59327; tel. 406/356–2161; John M. Chioutsis, Chief Executive Officer

ROUNDUP MEMORIAL HOSPITAL (C, 54 beds) 1202 Third Street West, Roundup, MT Zip 59072, Mailing Address: P.O. Box 40, Zip 59072; tel. 406/323–2302; Dave McIvor, Administrator

ST. JOHN'S LUTHERAN HOSPITAL (C, 27 beds) 350 Louisiana Avenue, Libby, MT Zip 59923; tel. 406/293–7761; Richard L. Palagi, Chief Executive Officer

NEBRASKA: TRI–VALLEY HEALTH SYSTEM (C, 56 beds) West Highway 6 and 34, Cambridge, NE Zip 69022, Mailing Address: P.O. Box 488, Zip 69022; tel. 308/697–3329; Kristopher H. Marwin, CHE, Chief Executive Officer

For explanation of codes following names, see page B2.
★ Indicates Type III membership in the American Hospital Association.

NEW MEXICO: NORTHEASTERN REGIONAL HOSPITAL (C, 56 beds) 1235 Eighth Street, Las Vegas, NM Zip 87701, Mailing Address: P.O. Box 248, Zip 87701–0238; tel. 505/425–6751; Patricia A. Beelow, Chief Executive Officer

UNION COUNTY GENERAL HOSPITAL (O, 28 beds) 301 Harding Street, Clayton, NM Zip 88415, Mailing Address: P.O. Box 489, Zip 88415–0489; tel. 505/374–2585; Carrell R. Blakely, Administrator

NEW YORK: ADIRONDACK MEDICAL CENTER (C, 100 beds) Lake Colby Drive, Saranac Lake, NY Zip 12983, Mailing Address: P.O. Box 471, Zip 12983; tel. 518/891–4141; Chandler M. Ralph, President and Chief Executive Officer

LEWIS COUNTY GENERAL HOSPITAL (C, 214 beds) 7785 North State Street, Lowville, NY Zip 13367–1297; tel. 315/376–5200; G. William Udovich, Chief Executive Officer and Administrator

THE HOSPITAL (C, 87 beds) 43 Pearl Street West, Sidney, NY Zip 13838; tel. 607/561–2153; Russell A. Test, Chief Executive Officer

OKLAHOMA: MISSION HILL MEMORIAL HOSPITAL (C, 54 beds) 1900 Gordon Cooper Drive, Shawnee, OK Zip 74801; tel. 405/273–2240; Thomas G. Honaker III, Administrator

OREGON: BLUE MOUNTAIN HOSPITAL (C, 83 beds) 170 Ford Road, John Day, OR Zip 97845; tel. 541/575–1311; David G. Triebes, Administrator

COTTAGE GROVE HEALTHCARE COMMUNITY (C, 67 beds) 1340 Birch Avenue, Cottage Grove, OR Zip 97424; tel. 541/942–0511; William N. Wilber, Chief Executive Officer

MOUNTAIN VIEW HOSPITAL DISTRICT (C, 102 beds) 470 N.E. A Street, Madras, OR Zip 97741; tel. 541/475–3882; Ronald W. Barnes, Executive Director

WASHINGTON: COULEE COMMUNITY HOSPITAL (C, 48 beds) 411 Fortuyn Road, Grand Coulee, WA Zip 99133–0840; tel. 509/633–1753; Michael C. Wiltermood, Chief Executive Officer

PULLMAN MEMORIAL HOSPITAL (C, 36 beds) N.E. 1125 Washington Avenue, Pullman, WA Zip 99163–4742; tel. 509/332–2541; Scott K. Adams, Administrator

SUNNYSIDE COMMUNITY HOSPITAL (C, 30 beds) 10th and Tacoma Avenue, Sunnyside, WA Zip 98944, Mailing Address: P.O. Box 719, Zip 98944–0719; tel. 509/837–1500; Jon D. Smiley, Chief Executive Officer

WISCONSIN: BURNETT MEDICAL CENTER (C, 64 beds) 257 West St. George Avenue, Grantsburg, WI Zip 54840–7827; tel. 715/463–5353; Thomas R. Lemon, Chief Executive Officer

COMMUNITY MEMORIAL HOSPITAL AND NURSING HOME (C, 136 beds) 819 Ash Street, Spooner, WI Zip 54801; tel. 715/635–2111; Michael Schafer, Chief Executive Officer

LANCASTER MEMORIAL HOSPITAL (C, 28 beds) 507 South Monroe Street, Lancaster, WI Zip 53813; tel. 608/723–2143; Larry D. Rentfro, FACHE, Chief Executive Officer

MEMORIAL COMMUNITY HOSPITAL (C, 115 beds) 313 Stoughton Road, Edgerton, WI Zip 53534–1198; tel. 608/884–3441; Charles E. Bruhn, Chief Executive Officer

MEMORIAL HOSPITAL OF IOWA COUNTY (C, 82 beds) 825 South Iowa Street, Dodgeville, WI Zip 53533–1999; tel. 608/935–2711; Ray Marmorstone, Administrator

RIPON MEDICAL CENTER (C, 29 beds) 933 Newbury Street, Ripon, WI Zip 54971, Mailing Address: P.O. Box 390, Zip 54971–0390; tel. 414/748–3101; Jon W. Baker, Administrator and Chief Executive Officer

SHAWANO MEDICAL CENTER (C, 46 beds) 309 North Bartlette Street, Shawano, WI Zip 54166–2199; tel. 715/526–2111; John J. Kestly, Administrator

SOUTHWEST HEALTH CENTER (C, 118 beds) 1100 Fifth Avenue, Platteville, WI Zip 53818; tel. 608/348–2331; Anne K. Klawiter, Chief Executive Officer

ST. JOSEPH'S MEMORIAL HOSPITAL AND NURSING HOME (C, 85 beds) 400 Water Avenue, Hillsboro, WI Zip 54634–0527, Mailing Address: P.O. Box 527, Zip 54634–0527; tel. 608/489–2211; Nancy Bauman, Chief Executive Officer

WYOMING: POWELL HOSPITAL (C, 138 beds) 777 Avenue H, Powell, WY Zip 82435; tel. 307/754–2267; Steve Ramsey, Interim Chief Executive Officer

Owned, leased, sponsored:	1 hospital	28 beds
Contract–managed:	51 hospitals	3543 beds
Totals:	52 hospitals	3571 beds

★0595: BRONSON HEALTHCARE GROUP, INC. (NP)
One Healthcare Plaza, Kalamazoo, MI Zip 49007–5345; tel. 616/341–6000; Frank J. Sardone, President and Chief Executive Officer

MICHIGAN: BRONSON METHODIST HOSPITAL (O, 314 beds) 252 East Lovell Street, Kalamazoo, MI Zip 49007–5345; tel. 616/341–6000; Frank J. Sardone, President and Chief Executive Officer

BRONSON VICKSBURG HOSPITAL (O, 41 beds) 13326 North Boulevard, Vicksburg, MI Zip 49097–1099; tel. 616/649–2321; Frank J. Sardone, President

Owned, leased, sponsored:	2 hospitals	355 beds
Contract–managed:	0 hospitals	0 beds
Totals:	2 hospitals	355 beds

0077: CAMBRIDGE INTERNATIONAL, INC, (IO)
7505 Fannin, Suite 680, Houston, TX Zip 77225; tel. 713/790–1153; Timothy Sharma, M.D., President

TEXAS: FOREST SPRINGS HOSPITAL (O, 48 beds) 1120 Cypress Station, Houston, TX Zip 77090–3031; tel. 713/893–7200

INTRACARE MEDICAL CENTER HOSPITAL (O, 50 beds) 7601 Fannin, Houston, TX Zip 77054; tel. 713/790–0949; Alice Hiniker, Ph.D., Administrator

Owned, leased, sponsored:	2 hospitals	98 beds
Contract–managed:	0 hospitals	0 beds
Totals:	2 hospitals	98 beds

★0955: CAMCARE, INC. (NP)
501 Morris Street, Charleston, WV Zip 25301, Mailing Address: P.O. Box 1547, Zip 25326; tel. 304/348–5432; Phillip H. Goodwin, President

WEST VIRGINIA: BRAXTON COUNTY MEMORIAL HOSPITAL (C, 30 beds) 100 Hoylman Drive, Gassaway, WV Zip 26624–9308; tel. 304/364–5156; Tony E. Atkins, Administrator

CHARLESTON AREA MEDICAL CENTER (O, 779 beds) 501 Morris Street, Charleston, WV Zip 25301, Mailing Address: Box 1547, Zip 25326; tel. 304/348–5432; Phillip H. Goodwin, President and Chief Executive Officer

Owned, leased, sponsored:	1 hospital	779 beds
Contract–managed:	1 hospital	30 beds
Totals:	2 hospitals	809 beds

0113: CANCER TREATMENT CENTERS OF AMERICA (IO)
3455 West Salt Creek Lane, Arlington Heights, IL Zip 60005–1080; tel. 847/342–7400; Robert Mayo, President and Chief Executive Officer

ILLINOIS: MIDWESTERN REGIONAL MEDICAL CENTER (O, 70 beds) 2501 Emmaus Avenue, Zion, IL Zip 60099–2587; tel. 847/872–4561; Roger C. Cary, President and Chief Executive Officer

OKLAHOMA: MEMORIAL MEDICAL CENTER AND CANCER TREATMENT CENTER–TULSA (O, 65 beds) 8181 South Lewis, Tulsa, OK Zip 74137; tel. 918/496–5000; Sandra Jackson, President

Owned, leased, sponsored:	2 hospitals	135 beds
Contract–managed:	0 hospitals	0 beds
Totals:	2 hospitals	135 beds

★0099: CARE NEW ENGLAND HEALTH SYSTEM (NP)
45 Willard Avenue, Providence, RI Zip 02905; tel. 401/453–7900; John J. Hynes, President and Chief Executive Officer

For explanation of codes following names, see page B2.
★ Indicates Type III membership in the American Hospital Association.

RHODE ISLAND: BUTLER HOSPITAL (O, 101 beds) 345 Blackstone Boulevard, Providence, RI Zip 02906–4829; tel. 401/455–6200; Frank A. Delmonico, President and Chief Executive Officer

KENT COUNTY MEMORIAL HOSPITAL (O, 291 beds) 455 Tollgate Road, Warwick, RI Zip 02886–2770; tel. 401/737–7000; Robert E. Baute, M.D., President and Chief Executive Officer

WOMEN AND INFANTS HOSPITAL OF RHODE ISLAND (O, 197 beds) 101 Dudley Street, Providence, RI Zip 02905–2499; tel. 401/274–1100; Thomas G. Parris Jr., President

Owned, leased, sponsored:	3 hospitals	589 beds
Contract–managed:	0 hospitals	0 beds
Totals:	3 hospitals	589 beds

★0096: CAREGROUP (NP)
375 Longwood Avenue, Boston, MA Zip 02215; tel. 617/667–2222; Mitchell T. Rabkin, Chief Executive Officer

MASSACHUSETTS: BETH ISRAEL DEACONESS MEDICAL CENTER (O, 671 beds) 330 Brookline Avenue, Boston, MA Zip 02215; tel. 617/667–2000; David Dolins, President

DEACONESS WALTHAM HOSPITAL (O, 198 beds) Hope Avenue, Waltham, MA Zip 02254–9116; tel. 617/647–6000; Jeanette G. Clough, President and Chief Executive Officer

DEACONESS–GLOVER HOSPITAL CORPORATION (O, 54 beds) 148 Chestnut Street, Needham, MA Zip 02192–2483; tel. 617/444–5600; John Dalton, President and Chief Executive Officer

DEACONESS–NASHOBA HOSPITAL (O, 49 beds) 200 Groton Road, Ayer, MA Zip 01432; tel. 508/772–0200; Jeffrey R. Kelly, President and Chief Executive Officer

MOUNT AUBURN HOSPITAL (O, 172 beds) 330 Mount Auburn Street, Cambridge, MA Zip 02238; tel. 617/492–3500; Francis P. Lynch, President and Chief Executive Officer

NEW ENGLAND BAPTIST HOSPITAL (O, 141 beds) 125 Parker Hill Avenue, Boston, MA Zip 02120–3297; tel. 617/738–5800; Alan H. Robbins, M.D., President

Owned, leased, sponsored:	6 hospitals	1285 beds
Contract–managed:	0 hospitals	0 beds
Totals:	6 hospitals	1285 beds

★0070: CARILION HEALTH SYSTEM (NP)
1212 Third Street S.W., Roanoke, VA Zip 24016, Mailing Address: P.O. Box 13727, Zip 24036–3727; tel. 540/981–7000; Thomas L. Robertson, President and Chief Executive Officer

VIRGINIA: CARILION BEDFORD MEMORIAL HOSPITAL (O, 161 beds) 1613 Oakwood Street, Bedford, VA Zip 24523–0688, Mailing Address: P.O. Box 688, Zip 24523–0688; tel. 540/586–2441; Howard Ainsley, Director

CARILION FRANKLIN MEMORIAL HOSPITAL (O, 37 beds) 180 Floyd Avenue, Rocky Mount, VA Zip 24151; tel. 540/483–5277; Matthew J. Perry, Director

CARILION GILES MEMORIAL HOSPITAL (O, 53 beds) 1 Taylor Avenue, Pearisburg, VA Zip 24134, Mailing Address: P.O. Box K, Zip 24134; tel. 540/921–6000; Morris D. Reece, Director

CARILION RADFORD COMMUNITY HOSPITAL (O, 122 beds) 700 Randolph Street, Radford, VA Zip 24141–2430; tel. 540/731–2000; Virginia Ousley, Director

CARILION ROANOKE COMMUNITY HOSPITAL (O, 278 beds) 101 Elm Avenue S.E., Roanoke, VA Zip 24013, Mailing Address: P.O. Box 12946, Zip 24029; tel. 540/985–8000; Lucas A. Snipes, Director

CARILION ROANOKE MEMORIAL HOSPITAL (O, 388 beds) Belleview at Jefferson Street, Roanoke, VA Zip 24014, Mailing Address: P.O. Box 13367, Zip 24033–3367; tel. 540/981–7000; Lucas A. Snipes, Director

CARILION ST. ALBANS HOSPITAL (O, 68 beds) Route 11, Lee Highway, Radford, VA Zip 24141, Mailing Address: Box 3608, Zip 24143; tel. 540/639–2481; Janet McKinney Crawford, Administrator

SOUTHSIDE COMMUNITY HOSPITAL (C, 108 beds) 800 Oak Street, Farmville, VA Zip 23901–1199; tel. 804/392–8811; John H. Greer, President

STONEWALL JACKSON HOSPITAL (C, 130 beds) 1 Health Circle, Lexington, VA Zip 24450–2492; tel. 540/462–1200; William Mahone V, Administrator

TAZEWELL COMMUNITY HOSPITAL (C, 42 beds) 141 Ben Bolt Avenue, Tazewell, VA Zip 24651; tel. 540/988–2506; Craig B. James, Administrator

WYTHE COUNTY COMMUNITY HOSPITAL (C, 75 beds) 600 West Ridge Road, Wytheville, VA Zip 24382; tel. 540/228–0200; Larry H. Chewning III, Chief Executive Officer

Owned, leased, sponsored:	7 hospitals	1107 beds
Contract–managed:	4 hospitals	355 beds
Totals:	11 hospitals	1462 beds

★1125: CARITAS CHRISTI HEALTH CARE SYSTEM (NP)
736 Cambridge Street, Boston, MA Zip 02135; tel. 617/789–2500; Michael F. Collins, M.D., President

MASSACHUSETTS: CARNEY HOSPITAL (S, 194 beds) 2100 Dorchester Avenue, Boston, MA Zip 02124–5666; tel. 617/296–4000; Joyce A. Murphy, President and Chief Executive Officer

GOOD SAMARITAN MEDICAL CENTER (S, 218 beds) 235 North Pearl Street, Brockton, MA Zip 02401; tel. 508/427–3000; Frank J. Larkin, President and Chief Executive Officer

HOLY FAMILY HOSPITAL AND MEDICAL CENTER (S, 247 beds) 70 East Street, Methuen, MA Zip 01844–4597; tel. 508/687–0151; William L. Lane, President

SAINT ANNE'S HOSPITAL (S, 165 beds) 795 Middle Street, Fall River, MA Zip 02721–1798; tel. 508/674–5741; Joseph W. Wilczek, President

ST. ELIZABETH'S MEDICAL CENTER OF BOSTON (S, 256 beds) 736 Cambridge Street, Boston, MA Zip 02135; tel. 617/789–3000; Michael F. Collins, M.D., President

ST. JOHN OF GOD HOSPITAL (S, 31 beds) 296 Allston Street, Brighton, MA Zip 02146–1659; tel. 617/277–5750; William K. Brinkert, President

Owned, leased, sponsored:	6 hospitals	1111 beds
Contract–managed:	0 hospitals	0 beds
Totals:	6 hospitals	1111 beds

0705: CAROLINAS HEALTHCARE SYSTEM (NP)
1000 Blythe Boulevard, Charlotte, NC Zip 28203, Mailing Address: Box 32861, Zip 28232–2861; tel. 704/355–2000; Harry A. Nurkin, Ph.D., President and Chief Executive Officer

NORTH CAROLINA: CAROLINAS MEDICAL CENTER (O, 843 beds) 1000 Blythe Boulevard, Charlotte, NC Zip 28203, Mailing Address: P.O. Box 32861, Zip 28232–2861; tel. 704/355–2000; Paul S. Franz, President

CHARLOTTE INSTITUTE OF REHABILITATION (O, 109 beds) 1100 Blythe Boulevard, Charlotte, NC Zip 28203; tel. 704/355–4300; Hollis Hamilton, Administrator

CLEVELAND REGIONAL MEDICAL CENTER (C, 296 beds) 201 Grover Street, Shelby, NC Zip 28150; tel. 704/487–3000; John Young, President and Chief Executive Officer

CRAWLEY MEMORIAL HOSPITAL (C, 51 beds) 315 West College Avenue, Boiling Springs, NC Zip 28017, Mailing Address: Box 996, Zip 28017; tel. 704/434–9466; Daphne Bridges, President

KINGS MOUNTAIN HOSPITAL (O, 70 beds) 706 West King Street, Kings Mountain, NC Zip 28086, Mailing Address: P.O. Box 339, Zip 28086; tel. 704/739–3601; Hank Neal, Administrator

MERCY HOSPITAL (O, 224 beds) 2001 Vail Avenue, Charlotte, NC Zip 28207; tel. 704/379–5000; C. Curtis Copenhaver, Chief Executive Officer

UNION REGIONAL MEDICAL CENTER (L, 176 beds) 600 Hospital Drive, Monroe, NC Zip 28112, Mailing Address: P.O. Box 5003, Zip 28111; tel. 704/283–3100; John W. Roberts, President and Chief Executive Officer

UNIVERSITY HOSPITAL (O, 107 beds) 8800 North Tryon Street, Charlotte, NC Zip 28262, Mailing Address: P.O. Box 560727, Zip 28256; tel. 704/548–6000; W. Spencer Lilly, Administrator

For explanation of codes following names, see page B2.
★ Indicates Type III membership in the American Hospital Association.

Owned, leased, sponsored:	6 hospitals	1529 beds
Contract–managed:	2 hospitals	347 beds
Totals:	8 hospitals	1876 beds

★**5945: CARONDELET HEALTH SYSTEM** (CC)
13801 Riverport Drive, Suite 300, Saint Louis, MO Zip 63043–4810; tel. 314/770–0333; Gary Christiansen, President and Chief Executive Officer

ARIZONA: CARONDELET ST. JOSEPH'S HOSPITAL (O, 287 beds) 350 North Wilmot Road, Tucson, AZ Zip 85711; tel. 520/296–3211; Sister St. Joan Willert, President and Chief Executive Officer

CARONDELET ST. MARY'S HOSPITAL (O, 345 beds) 1601 West St. Mary's Road, Tucson, AZ Zip 85745–2682; tel. 602/622–5833; Sister St. Joan Willert, President and Chief Executive Officer

CARONDOLET HOLY CROSS HOSPITAL (O, 80 beds) 1171 Target Range Road, Nogales, AZ Zip 85621; tel. 520/287–2771; Carol Field, Administrator

CALIFORNIA: DANIEL FREEMAN MARINA HOSPITAL (O, 180 beds) 4650 Lincoln Boulevard, Marina Del Rey, CA Zip 90292–6360; tel. 310/823–8911; Joseph W. Dunn, Ph.D., Chief Executive Officer

DANIEL FREEMAN MEMORIAL HOSPITAL (O, 365 beds) 333 North Prairie Avenue, Inglewood, CA Zip 90301–4514; tel. 310/674–7050; Joseph W. Dunn, Ph.D., Chief Executive Officer

SANTA MARTA HOSPITAL (O, 110 beds) 319 North Humphreys Avenue, Los Angeles, CA Zip 90022; tel. 213/266–6500; James G. Ovieda, President and Chief Executive Officer

GEORGIA: ST. JOSEPH HOSPITAL (O, 145 beds) 2260 Wrightsboro Road, Augusta, GA Zip 30904–4726; tel. 706/481–7000; J. William Paugh, President and Chief Executive Officer

WALTON REHABILITATION HOSPITAL (C, 58 beds) 1355 Independence Drive, Augusta, GA Zip 30901–1037; tel. 706/823–8505; Dennis B. Skelley, President and Chief Executive Officer

IDAHO: ST. JOSEPH REGIONAL MEDICAL CENTER (O, 156 beds) 415 Sixth Street, Lewiston, ID Zip 83501–0816; tel. 208/743–2511; Howard A. Hayes, President and Chief Executive Officer

MISSOURI: SAINT JOSEPH HEALTH CENTER (O, 240 beds) 1000 Carondelet Drive, Kansas City, MO Zip 64114–4673; tel. 816/942–4400; Richard M. Abell, President and Chief Executive Officer

ST. MARY'S HOSPITAL OF BLUE SPRINGS (O, 102 beds) 201 West R. D. Mize Road, Blue Springs, MO Zip 64014; tel. 816/228–5900; N. Gary Wages, President and Chief Executive Officer

NEW YORK: ST. JOSEPH'S HOSPITAL (O, 255 beds) 555 East Market Street, Elmira, NY Zip 14902–1512; tel. 607/733–6541; Sister Marie Castagnaro, President and Chief Executive Officer

ST. MARY'S HOSPITAL (O, 143 beds) 427 Guy Park Avenue, Amsterdam, NY Zip 12010–1095; tel. 518/842–1900; Peter E. Capobianco, President and Chief Executive Officer

WASHINGTON: CARONDELET BEHAVIORAL HEALTH CENTER (O, 32 beds) 1175 Carondelet Drive, Richland, WA Zip 99352–1175; tel. 509/943–9104; Thomas Corley, Chief Executive Officer

OUR LADY OF LOURDES HEALTH CENTER (O, 132 beds) 520 North Fourth Avenue, Pasco, WA Zip 99301, Mailing Address: P.O. Box 2568, Zip 99302; tel. 509/547–7704; Thomas Corley, Chief Executive Officer

Owned, leased, sponsored:	14 hospitals	2572 beds
Contract–managed:	1 hospital	58 beds
Totals:	15 hospitals	2630 beds

6545: CATHEDRAL HEALTHCARE SYSTEM, INC. (CC)
219 Chestnut Street, Newark, NJ Zip 07105–1558; tel. 201/690–3600; Frank L. Fumai, President and Chief Executive Officer

NEW JERSEY: SAINT JAMES HOSPITAL OF NEWARK (O, 189 beds) 155 Jefferson Street, Newark, NJ Zip 07105; tel. 201/589–1300; Ceu Cirne–Neves, Administrator

SAINT MICHAEL'S MEDICAL CENTER (O, 325 beds) 268 Dr. Martin Luther King Jr. Boulevard, Newark, NJ Zip 07102–2094; tel. 201/877–5000; Dominick R. Calgi, Senior Vice President and Administrator

Owned, leased, sponsored:	2 hospitals	514 beds
Contract–managed:	0 hospitals	0 beds
Totals:	2 hospitals	514 beds

★**0092: CATHOLIC HEALTH INITIATIVES** (CC)
1999 Broadway, Suite 2605, Denver, CO Zip 80202; tel. 303/298–9100; Patricia A. Cahill, Chief Executive Officer

COLORADO: MERCY MEDICAL CENTER (S, 92 beds) 375 East Park Avenue, Durango, CO Zip 81301; tel. 970/247–4311; Renato V. Baciarelli, Administrator

PENROSE–ST. FRANCIS HEALTH SERVICES (S, 522 beds) 2215 North Cascade Avenue, Colorado Springs, CO Zip 80907; tel. 719/776–5000; Donna L. Bertram, R.N., Administrator

ST. ANTHONY HOSPITAL CENTRAL (S, 238 beds) 4231 West 16th Avenue, Denver, CO Zip 80204–4098; tel. 303/629–3511; Michael H. Erne, Senior Vice President and Administrator

ST. ANTHONY HOSPITAL NORTH (S, 110 beds) 2551 West 84th Avenue, Westminster, CO Zip 80030; tel. 303/426–2151; Michael H. Erne, Senior Vice President and Administrator

ST. MARY–CORWIN REGIONAL MEDICAL CENTER (S, 261 beds) 1008 Minnequa Avenue, Pueblo, CO Zip 81004–3798; tel. 719/560–4000; Walter Sackett, Senior Vice President and Administrator

ST. THOMAS MORE HOSPITAL AND PROGRESSIVE CARE CENTER (S, 218 beds) 1338 Phay Avenue, Canon City, CO Zip 81212–2221; tel. 719/269–2000; C. Ray Honker, Administrator and Senior Vice President

DELAWARE: ST. FRANCIS HOSPITAL (S, 277 beds) Seventh and Clayton Streets, Wilmington, DE Zip 19805–0500, Mailing Address: P.O. Box 2500, Zip 19805–0500; tel. 302/421–4100; Steven C. Bjelich, President and Chief Executive Officer

IDAHO: MERCY MEDICAL CENTER (S, 144 beds) 1512 12th Avenue Road, Nampa, ID Zip 83686–6008; tel. 208/467–1171; Joseph Messmer, President and Chief Executive Officer

IOWA: ALEGENT HEALTH MERCY HOSPITAL (S, 24 beds) Rosary Drive, Corning, IA Zip 50841, Mailing Address: Box 368, Zip 50841; tel. 515/322–3121; James C. Ruppert, Regional Administrator

ALEGENT HEALTH MERCY HOSPITAL (S, 194 beds) 800 Mercy Drive, Council Bluffs, IA Zip 51503, Mailing Address: Box 1C, Zip 51502; tel. 712/328–5000; Charles J. Marr, Chief Executive Officer

MERCY HOSPITAL MEDICAL CENTER (S, 584 beds) 400 University Avenue, Des Moines, IA Zip 50314; tel. 515/247–4278; Thomas A. Reitinger, President and Chief Executive Officer

ST. JOSEPH'S MERCY HOSPITAL (S, 58 beds) 1 St. Joseph's Drive, Centerville, IA Zip 52544; tel. 515/437–3411; William C. Assell, President and Chief Executive Officer

KANSAS: CENTRAL KANSAS MEDICAL CENTER (S, 175 beds) 3515 Broadway Street, Great Bend, KS Zip 67530; tel. 316/792–2511; Gary L. Barnett, President and Chief Executive Officer

ST. CATHERINE HOSPITAL (S, 99 beds) 410 East Walnut, Garden City, KS Zip 67846–5672; tel. 316/272–2222; Gary L. Rowe, President and Chief Executive Officer

KENTUCKY: OUR LADY OF THE WAY HOSPITAL (S, 39 beds) 11022 Main Street, Martin, KY Zip 41649–0910; tel. 606/285–5181; Lowell Jones, Chief Executive Officer

MARYLAND: ST. JOSEPH MEDICAL CENTER (S, 460 beds) 7620 York Road, Towson, MD Zip 21204–7582; tel. 410/337–1000; John S. Prout, President and Chief Executive Officer

MINNESOTA: ALBANY AREA HOSPITAL AND MEDICAL CENTER (S, 13 beds) 300 Third Avenue, Albany, MN Zip 56307; tel. 320/845–2121; Ben Koppelman, Administrator

LAKEWOOD HEALTH CENTER (S, 73 beds) 600 South Main Avenue, Baudette, MN Zip 56623, Mailing Address: Route 1, Box 2120, Zip 56623; tel. 218/634–2120; David A. Nelson, President and Chief Executive Officer

For explanation of codes following names, see page B2.
★ Indicates Type III membership in the American Hospital Association.

ST JOSEPH'S AREA HEALTH SERVICES (S, 42 beds) 600 Pleasant Avenue, Park Rapids, MN Zip 56470; tel. 218/732-3311; David R. Hove, President and Chief Executive Officer

ST. FRANCIS MEDICAL CENTER (S, 171 beds) 415 Oak Street, Breckenridge, MN Zip 56520; tel. 218/643-3000; Mark C. McNelly, President and Chief Executive Officer

ST. GABRIEL'S HOSPITAL (S, 205 beds) 815 Second Street S.E., Little Falls, MN Zip 56345-3596; tel. 320/632-5441; Larry A. Schulz, President and Chief Executive Officer

MISSOURI: ST. JOHN'S REGIONAL MEDICAL CENTER (S, 353 beds) 2727 McClelland Boulevard, Joplin, MO Zip 64804; tel. 417/781-2727; Robert G. Brueckner, President and Chief Executive Officer

NEBRASKA: ALEGENT HEALTH BERGAN MERCY MEDICAL CENTER (S, 592 beds) 7500 Mercy Road, Omaha, NE Zip 68124; tel. 402/398-6060; Charles J. Marr, Chief Executive Officer

GOOD SAMARITAN HEALTH SYSTEMS (S, 267 beds) 10 East 31st Street, Kearney, NE Zip 68847-2926, Mailing Address: P.O. Box 1990, Zip 68848-1990; tel. 308/865-7100; William Wilson Hendrickson, President and Chief Executive Officer

SAINT FRANCIS MEDICAL CENTER (S, 162 beds) 2620 West Faidley Avenue, Grand Island, NE Zip 68803, Mailing Address: P.O. Box 9804, Zip 68802-9804; tel. 308/384-4600; Michael R. Gloor, President and Chief Executive Officer

ST. ELIZABETH COMMUNITY HEALTH CENTER (S, 162 beds) 555 South 70th Street, Lincoln, NE Zip 68510-2494; tel. 402/489-7181; Robert J. Lanik, President

ST. MARY'S HOSPITAL (S, 28 beds) 1314 Third Avenue, Nebraska City, NE Zip 68410; tel. 402/873-3321; Richard W. Waller, Interim Administrator

NEW JERSEY: ST. FRANCIS MEDICAL CENTER (S, 254 beds) 601 Hamilton Avenue, Trenton, NJ Zip 08629-1986; tel. 609/599-5000; Judith M. Persichilli, President and Chief Executive Officer

NEW MEXICO: ST. JOSEPH MEDICAL CENTER (S, 204 beds) 601 Martin Luther King Drive N.E., Albuquerque, NM Zip 87102, Mailing Address: P.O. Box 25555, Zip 87125-0555; tel. 505/727-8000; Charles A. Ivy, Vice President

ST. JOSEPH NORTHEAST HEIGHTS HOSPITAL (S, 71 beds) 4701 Montgomery N.E., Albuquerque, NM Zip 87109, Mailing Address: P.O. Box 25555, Zip 87125-0555; tel. 505/727-7800; C. Vincent Townsend Jr., Vice President, Operations

ST. JOSEPH REHABILITATION HOSPITAL AND OUTPATIENT CENTER (S, 46 beds) 505 Elm Street N.E., Albuquerque, NM Zip 87102, Mailing Address: P.O. Box 25555, Zip 87125-2500; tel. 505/727-4700; Mary Lou Coors, Administrator

ST. JOSEPH WEST MESA HOSPITAL (S, 70 beds) 10501 Golf Course Road N.W., Albuquerque, NM Zip 87114, Mailing Address: P.O. Box 25555, Zip 87125-0555; tel. 505/893-2003; C. Vincent Townsend Jr., Vice President, Operations

NORTH DAKOTA: CARRINGTON HEALTH CENTER (S, 70 beds) 800 North Fourth Street, Carrington, ND Zip 58421; tel. 701/652-3141; Paul A. Balerud, Interim Chief Executive Officer

MERCY HOSPITAL (S, 35 beds) 1031 Seventh Street, Devils Lake, ND Zip 58301-2798; tel. 701/662-2131; Marlene Krein, President and Chief Executive Officer

MERCY HOSPITAL (S, 50 beds) 570 Chautauqua Boulevard, Valley City, ND Zip 58072-3199; tel. 701/845-0440; Greg Hanson, President and Chief Executive Officer

MERCY MEDICAL CENTER (S, 113 beds) 1301 15th Avenue West, Williston, ND Zip 58801-3896; tel. 701/774-7400; Duane D. Jerde, President and Chief Executive Officer

ST. ANSGAR'S HEALTH CENTER (S, 20 beds) 115 Vivian Street, Park River, ND Zip 58270-0708; tel. 701/284-7500; Michael D. Mahrer, President

ST. JOSEPH'S HOSPITAL AND HEALTH CENTER (S, 87 beds) 30 Seventh Street West, Dickinson, ND Zip 58601; tel. 701/225-7200; John S. Studsrud, President

OHIO: GOOD SAMARITAN HOSPITAL (S, 438 beds) 375 Dixmyth Avenue, Cincinnati, OH Zip 45220-2489; tel. 513/872-1400; Sister Myra James Bradley, Chairman of the Board of Directors

GOOD SAMARITAN HOSPITAL AND HEALTH CENTER (S, 428 beds) 2222 Philadelphia Drive, Dayton, OH Zip 45406-1813; tel. 513/278-2612; K. Douglas Deck, President and Chief Executive Officer

OREGON: HOLY ROSARY MEDICAL CENTER (S, 74 beds) 351 S.W. Ninth Street, Ontario, OR Zip 97914-2693; tel. 541/881-7000; Bruce Jensen, President and Chief Executive Officer

MERCY MEDICAL CENTER (S, 96 beds) 2700 Stewart Parkway, Roseburg, OR Zip 97470-1297; tel. 541/673-0611; Victor J. Fresolone, FACHE, President and Chief Executive Officer

ST. ANTHONY HOSPITAL (S, 49 beds) 1601 S.E. Court Avenue, Pendleton, OR Zip 97801-3297; tel. 541/276-5121; Jeffrey S. Drop, President and Chief Executive Officer

ST. ELIZABETH HEALTH SERVICES (S, 134 beds) 3325 Pocahontas Road, Baker City, OR Zip 97814; tel. 541/523-6461; Robert T. Mannix Jr., President and Chief Operations Officer

PENNSYLVANIA: NAZARETH HOSPITAL (S, 236 beds) 2601 Holme Avenue, Philadelphia, PA Zip 19152-2096; tel. 215/335-6000; Daniel J. Sinnott, President and Chief Executive Officer

ST. AGNES MEDICAL CENTER (S, 182 beds) 1900 South Broad Street, Philadelphia, PA Zip 19145; tel. 215/339-4100; Daniel J. Sinnott, President and Chief Executive Officer

ST. JOSEPH HOSPITAL (S, 256 beds) 250 College Avenue, Lancaster, PA Zip 17604; tel. 717/291-8211; John Kerr Tolmie, President and Chief Executive Officer

ST. JOSEPH MEDICAL CENTER (S, 215 beds) Twelfth & Walnut Streets, Reading, PA Zip 19603-0316, Mailing Address: P.O. Box 316, Zip 19603-0316; tel. 610/378-2000; Philip G. Dionne, President and Chief Executive Officer

ST. MARY MEDICAL CENTER (S, 263 beds) Langhorne-Newtown Road, Langhorne, PA Zip 19047-1295; tel. 215/750-2000; Sister Clare Carty, President and Chief Executive Officer

SOUTH DAKOTA: GETTYSBURG MEDICAL CENTER (S, 61 beds) 606 East Garfield, Gettysburg, SD Zip 57442; tel. 605/765-2488; Brian J. McDermott, Administrator

ST. MARY'S HOSPITAL (S, 191 beds) 800 East Dakota Avenue, Pierre, SD Zip 57501-3313; tel. 605/224-3100; James D. M. Russell, Chief Executive Officer

WASHINGTON: ST. CLARE HOSPITAL (S, 60 beds) 11315 Bridgeport Way S.W., Lakewood, WA Zip 98499-0998, Mailing Address: P.O. Box 99998, Zip 98499-0998; tel. 206/588-1711; Craig L. Hendrickson, Regional Hospital Leader

ST. FRANCIS HOSPITAL (S, 67 beds) 34515 Ninth Avenue South, Federal Way, WA Zip 98003-9710; tel. 206/927-9700; Craig L. Hendrickson, President and Chief Executive Officer

ST. JOSEPH MEDICAL CENTER (S, 271 beds) 1717 South J Street, Tacoma, WA Zip 98405, Mailing Address: P.O. Box 2197, Zip 98401-2197; tel. 206/627-4101; Craig L. Hendrickson, President and Chief Executive Officer

WISCONSIN: GOOD SAMARITAN HEALTH CENTER OF MERRILL (S, 63 beds) 601 Center Avenue South, Merrill, WI Zip 54452; tel. 715/536-5511; Michael Hammer, President and Chief Executive Officer

ST. CATHERINE'S HOSPITAL (S, 148 beds) 3556 Seventh Avenue, Kenosha, WI Zip 53140-2595; tel. 414/656-3011; Ryland Davis, Interim Chief Executive Officer

Owned, leased, sponsored:	56 hospitals	9815 beds
Contract-managed:	0 hospitals	0 beds
Totals:	56 hospitals	9815 beds

★0079: CATHOLIC HEALTH PARTNERS (CC)
2913 North Commonwealth, Chicago, IL Zip 60657; tel. 773/665-3170; Sister Theresa Peck, President and Chief Executive Officer

ILLINOIS: COLUMBUS HOSPITAL (O, 291 beds) 2520 North Lakeview Avenue, Chicago, IL Zip 60614; tel. 773/883-7300; Sister Theresa Peck, President and Chief Executive Officer

For explanation of codes following names, see page B2.
★ Indicates Type III membership in the American Hospital Association.

SAINT ANTHONY HOSPITAL (O, 186 beds) 2875 West 19th Street, Chicago, IL Zip 60623; tel. 773/521–1710; Sister Theresa Peck, President and Chief Executive Officer

ST. JOSEPH HOSPITAL (S, 347 beds) 2900 North Lake Shore Drive, Chicago, IL Zip 60657–6274; tel. 773/665–3000; Sister Theresa Peck, President and Chief Executive Officer

Owned, leased, sponsored:	3 hospitals	824 beds
Contract–managed:	0 hospitals	0 beds
Totals:	3 hospitals	824 beds

★5205: CATHOLIC HEALTHCARE WEST (CC)
1700 Montgomery Street, Suite 300, San Francisco, CA Zip 94111–9603; tel. 415/438–5500; Richard J. Kramer, President and Chief Executive Officer

ARIZONA: ST. JOSEPH'S HOSPITAL AND MEDICAL CENTER (S, 514 beds) 350 West Thomas Road, Phoenix, AZ Zip 85013, Mailing Address: Box 2071, Zip 85001–2071; tel. 602/406–3100; Mary G. Yarbrough, President and Chief Executive Officer

CALIFORNIA: BAKERSFIELD MEMORIAL HOSPITAL (S, 379 beds) 420 34th Street, Bakersfield, CA Zip 93301, Mailing Address: Box 1888, Zip 93303–1888; tel. 805/327–1792; C. Larry Carr, President

DOMINICAN SANTA CRUZ HOSPITAL (S, 284 beds) 1555 Soquel Drive, Santa Cruz, CA Zip 95065–1794; tel. 408/462–7700; Sister Julie Hyer, President and Chief Executive Officer

MARK TWAIN ST. JOSEPH'S HOSPITAL (S, 33 beds) 768 Mountain Ranch Road, San Andreas, CA Zip 95249–9710; tel. 209/754–3521; Kathy Yarbrough, Administrator

MERCY AMERICAN RIVER/MERCY SAN JUAN HOSPITAL (S, 352 beds) 6501 Coyle Avenue, Carmichael, CA Zip 95608, Mailing Address: P.O. Box 479, Zip 95608; tel. 916/537–5000; Sister Bridget McCarthy, President

MERCY GENERAL HOSPITAL (S, 405 beds) 4001 J Street, Sacramento, CA Zip 95819; tel. 916/453–4950; Thomas A. Petersen, Vice President and Chief Operating Officer

MERCY HEALTHCARE–BAKERSFIELD (S, 261 beds) 2215 Truxtun Avenue, Bakersfield, CA Zip 93301, Mailing Address: Box 119, Zip 93302; tel. 805/632–5000; Bernard J. Herman, President and Chief Executive Officer

MERCY HOSPITAL AND HEALTH SERVICES (S, 101 beds) 2740 M Street, Merced, CA Zip 95340–2880; tel. 209/384–6444; Kelly C. Morgan, President and Chief Executive Officer

MERCY HOSPITAL OF FOLSOM (S, 95 beds) 1650 Creekside Drive, Folsom, CA Zip 95630–3405; tel. 916/983–7400; Donald C. Hudson, Vice President and Chief Operating Officer

MERCY MEDICAL CENTER (S, 220 beds) 2175 Rosaline Avenue, Redding, CA Zip 96001, Mailing Address: Box 496009, Zip 96049–6009; tel. 916/225–6000; George A. Govier, President and Chief Executive Officer

MERCY MEDICAL CENTER MOUNT SHASTA (S, 80 beds) 914 Pine Street, Mount Shasta, CA Zip 96067, Mailing Address: P.O. Box 239, Zip 96067–0239; tel. 916/926–6111; James R. Hoss, President and Chief Executive Officer

METHODIST HOSPITAL (S, 303 beds) 7500 Hospital Drive, Sacramento, CA Zip 95823–5477; tel. 916/423–3000; Stanley C. Oppegard, Vice President and Chief Operating Officer

O'CONNOR HOSPITAL (S, 141 beds) 2105 Forest Avenue, San Jose, CA Zip 95128–1471; tel. 408/947–2500; William C. Finlayson, President and Chief Executive Officer

ROBERT F. KENNEDY MEDICAL CENTER (S, 195 beds) 4500 West 116th Street, Hawthorne, CA Zip 90250; tel. 310/973–1711; Peter P. Aprato, Administrator and Chief Operating Officer

SAINT FRANCIS MEMORIAL HOSPITAL (S, 190 beds) 900 Hyde Street, San Francisco, CA Zip 94109, Mailing Address: Box 7726, Zip 94120–7726; tel. 415/353–6000; John G. Williams, President and Chief Executive Officer

SAINT LOUISE HOSPITAL (S, 40 beds) 18500 Saint Louise Drive, Morgan Hill, CA Zip 95037; tel. 408/779–1500; William C. Finlayson, President and Chief Executive Officer

SAINT MARY MEDICAL CENTER (S, 479 beds) 1050 Linden Avenue, Long Beach, CA Zip 90801, Mailing Address: P.O. Box 887, Zip 90801; tel. 310/491–9000; Tammie McMann Brailsford, Administrator

SEQUOIA HOSPITAL (S, 249 beds) 170 Alameda De Las Pulgas, Redwood City, CA Zip 94062–2799; tel. 415/367–5561; Glenna L. Vaskelis, Administrator

SETON MEDICAL CENTER (S, 279 beds) 1900 Sullivan Avenue, Daly City, CA Zip 94015–2229; tel. 415/992–4000; Bernadette Smith, Chief Operating Officer

SETON MEDICAL CENTER COASTSIDE (S, 121 beds) 600 Marine Boulevard, Moss Beach, CA Zip 94038; tel. 415/728–5521; Deborah E. Stebbins, FACHE, President and Chief Executive Officer

SIERRA NEVADA MEMORIAL HOSPITAL (S, 111 beds) 155 Glasson Way, Grass Valley, CA Zip 95945–5792, Mailing Address: Box 1029, Zip 95945–5792; tel. 916/274–6000; C. Thomas Collier, President and Chief Executive Officer

ST. BERNARDINE MEDICAL CENTER (S, 447 beds) 2101 North Waterman Avenue, San Bernardino, CA Zip 92404; tel. 909/883–8711; Maureen O'Connor, Interim Administrator and Chief Operating Officer

ST. DOMINIC'S HOSPITAL (S, 40 beds) 1777 West Yosemite Avenue, Manteca, CA Zip 95337; tel. 209/825–3500; Richard Aldred, Chief Administrative Officer

ST. ELIZABETH COMMUNITY HOSPITAL (S, 53 beds) 2550 Sister Mary Columba Drive, Red Bluff, CA Zip 96080–4397; tel. 916/529–8005; Thomas F. Grimes III, Executive Vice President and Chief Operating Officer

ST. FRANCIS MEDICAL CENTER (S, 414 beds) 3630 East Imperial Highway, Lynwood, CA Zip 90262; tel. 310/603–6000; Gerald T. Kozai, Administrator and Chief Operating Officer

ST. JOHN'S PLEASANT VALLEY HOSPITAL (S, 153 beds) 2309 Antonio Avenue, Camarillo, CA Zip 93010–1459; tel. 805/389–5800; Daniel R. Herlinger, President and Chief Executive Officer

ST. JOHN'S REGIONAL MEDICAL CENTER (S, 230 beds) 1600 North Rose Avenue, Oxnard, CA Zip 93030; tel. 805/988–2500; Daniel R. Herlinger, President and Chief Executive Officer

ST. JOSEPH'S BEHAVIORAL HEALTH CENTER (S, 35 beds) 2510 North California Street, Stockton, CA Zip 95204–5568; tel. 209/948–2100; James Sondecker, Administrator

ST. JOSEPH'S MEDICAL CENTER (S, 312 beds) 1800 North California Street, Stockton, CA Zip 95204–6088, Mailing Address: P.O. Box 213008, Zip 95213–9008; tel. 209/943–2000; Edward G. Schroeder, President and Chief Executive Officer

ST. MARY'S MEDICAL CENTER (S, 256 beds) 450 Stanyan Street, San Francisco, CA Zip 94117–1079; tel. 415/668–1000; John G. Williams, President

ST. VINCENT MEDICAL CENTER (S, 350 beds) 2131 West Third Street, Los Angeles, CA Zip 90057–0992, Mailing Address: P.O. Box 57992, Zip 90057; tel. 213/484–7111; Vincent F. Guinan, President and Chief Executive Officer

WOODLAND MEMORIAL HOSPITAL (S, 103 beds) 1325 Cottonwood Street, Woodland, CA Zip 95695–5199; tel. 916/662–3961; D. Scott Ideson, Interim Chief Executive Officer

NEVADA: ST. ROSE DOMINICAN HOSPITAL (S, 135 beds) 102 Lake Mead Drive, Henderson, NV Zip 89015; tel. 702/564–2622; Rod A. Davis, President and Chief Executive Officer

Owned, leased, sponsored:	33 hospitals	7360 beds
Contract–managed:	0 hospitals	0 beds
Totals:	33 hospitals	7360 beds

★2265: CENTRA HEALTH, INC. (NP)
1920 Atherholt Road, Lynchburg, VA Zip 24501–1104; tel. 804/947–4700; George W. Dawson, President

VIRGINIA: LYNCHBURG GENERAL HOSPITAL (O, 350 beds) 1901 Tate Springs Road, Lynchburg, VA Zip 24501–1167; tel. 804/947–3000; L. Darrell Powers, Senior Vice President

For explanation of codes following names, see page B2.
★ Indicates Type III membership in the American Hospital Association.

Section B

VIRGINIA BAPTIST HOSPITAL (O, 301 beds) 3300 Rivermont Avenue, Lynchburg, VA Zip 24503–9989; tel. 804/947–4000; Thomas C. Jividen, Senior Vice President

Owned, leased, sponsored:	2 hospitals	651 beds
Contract–managed:	0 hospitals	0 beds
Totals:	2 hospitals	651 beds

0665: CENTURY HEALTHCARE CORPORATION (IO)
5555 East 71st Street, Suite 9220, Tulsa, OK Zip 74136–6540; tel. 918/491–0775; Jerry D. Dillon, President and Chief Executive Officer

ARIZONA: WESTBRIDGE TREATMENT CENTER (O, 78 beds) 1830 East Roosevelt, Phoenix, AZ Zip 85006; tel. 602/254–0884; Mike Perry, Chief Executive Officer

OKLAHOMA: HIGH POINTE (O, 68 beds) 6501 N.E. 50th Street, Oklahoma City, OK Zip 73141–9613; tel. 405/424–3383; Charlene Arnett, Chief Executive Officer

Owned, leased, sponsored:	2 hospitals	146 beds
Contract–managed:	0 hospitals	0 beds
Totals:	2 hospitals	146 beds

0101: CITRUS VALLEY HEALTH PARTNERS (NP)
210 West San Bernardino Road, Covina, CA Zip 91723; tel. 818/938–7577; Peter E. Makowski, President and Chief Executive Officer

CALIFORNIA: CITRUS VALLEY MEDICAL CENTER INTER–COMMUNITY CAMPUS (O, 252 beds) 210 West San Bernardino Road, Covina, CA Zip 91723–1901; tel. 818/331–7331; Warren J. Kirk, Administrator

CITRUS VALLEY MEDICAL CENTER–QUEEN OF THE VALLEY CAMPUS (O, 263 beds) 1115 South Sunset Avenue, West Covina, CA Zip 91790, Mailing Address: Box 1980, Zip 91793; tel. 818/962–4011; Warren J. Kirk, Administrator and Chief Operating Officer

FOOTHILL PRESBYTERIAN HOSPITAL–MORRIS L. JOHNSTON MEMORIAL (O, 106 beds) 250 South Grand Avenue, Glendora, CA Zip 91741; tel. 818/857–3235; Bryan R. Rogers, President and Chief Executive Officer

Owned, leased, sponsored:	3 hospitals	621 beds
Contract–managed:	0 hospitals	0 beds
Totals:	3 hospitals	621 beds

0076: COLLEGE HEALTH ENTERPRISES (IO)
7711 Center Avenue, Suite 300, Huntington Beach, CA Zip 92647; tel. 714/891–5000; Elliot A. Sainer, President and Chief Executive Officer

COLLEGE HOSPITAL (O, 125 beds) 10802 College Place, Cerritos, CA Zip 90703–1579; tel. 562/924–9581; Stephen Witt, Chief Executive Officer

COLLEGE HOSPITAL COSTA MESA (O, 119 beds) 301 Victoria Street, Costa Mesa, CA Zip 92627; tel. 714/642–2607; Eric Rabjohns, Chief Executive Officer

Owned, leased, sponsored:	2 hospitals	244 beds
Contract–managed:	0 hospitals	0 beds
Totals:	2 hospitals	244 beds

★0048: COLUMBIA/HCA HEALTHCARE CORPORATION (IO)
One Park Plaza, Nashville, TN Zip 37203; tel. 615/320–2000; Richard L. Scott, Chairman and Chief Executive Officer

ALABAMA: COLUMBIA ANDALUSIA HOSPITAL (O, 101 beds) 849 South Three Notch Street, Andalusia, AL Zip 36420–0760, Mailing Address: Box 760, Zip 36420; tel. 334/222–8466; James L. Sample, Chief Executive Officer

COLUMBIA EAST MONTGOMERY MEDICAL CENTER (O, 150 beds) 400 Taylor Road, Montgomery, AL Zip 36117, Mailing Address: P.O. Box 241267, Zip 36124–1267; tel. 334/277–8330; John W. Melton, Chief Executive Officer

COLUMBIA FLORENCE HOSPITAL (O, 155 beds) 2111 Cloyd Boulevard, Florence, AL Zip 35630, Mailing Address: Box 2010, Zip 35631; tel. 205/767–8700; Glen M. Jones, Chief Executive Officer

COLUMBIA FOUR RIVERS MEDICAL CENTER (O, 150 beds) 1015 Medical Center Parkway, Selma, AL Zip 36701; tel. 334/872–8461; Robert F. Bigley, Chief Executive Officer

COLUMBIA MEDICAL CENTER OF HUNTSVILLE (O, 120 beds) One Hospital Drive, Huntsville, AL Zip 35801–3403; tel. 205/882–3100; Thomas M. Weiss, Chief Executive Officer

COLUMBIA NORTHRIDGE MEDICAL CENTER (O, 50 beds) 124 South Memorial Drive, Prattville, AL Zip 36067; tel. 334/365–0651; Duane Brookhart, Ph.D., President and Chief Executive Officer

COLUMBIA REGIONAL MEDICAL CENTER (O, 250 beds) 301 South Ripley Street, Montgomery, AL Zip 36104–4495; tel. 334/269–8000; Ron MacLaren, Chief Executive Officer

MEDICAL CENTER SHOALS (O, 128 beds) 201 Avalon Avenue, Muscle Shoals, AL Zip 35661, Mailing Address: P.O. Box 3359, Zip 35662; tel. 205/386–1600; Connie Hawthorne, Chief Executive Officer

NORTHWEST MEDICAL CENTER (O, 100 beds) Highway 43 By–Pass, Russellville, AL Zip 35653, Mailing Address: P.O. Box 1089, Zip 35653; tel. 205/332–1611; Christine R. Stewart, President and Chief Executive Officer

ALASKA: COLUMBIA ALASKA REGIONAL HOSPITAL (O, 238 beds) 2801 Debarr Road, Anchorage, AK Zip 99508, Mailing Address: P.O. Box 143889, Zip 99514–3889; tel. 907/276–1131; Ernie Meier, President and Chief Executive Officer

ARIZONA: COLUMBIA EL DORADO HOSPITAL (O, 166 beds) 1400 North Wilmot, Tucson, AZ Zip 85712, Mailing Address: Box 13070, Zip 85732; tel. 520/886–6361; Rhonda Dean, Chief Executive Officer

COLUMBIA MEDICAL CENTER PHOENIX (O, 295 beds) 1947 East Thomas Road, Phoenix, AZ Zip 85016; tel. 602/650–7600; Denny W. Powell, Chief Executive Officer

COLUMBIA PARADISE VALLEY HOSPITAL (O, 140 beds) 3929 East Bell Road, Phoenix, AZ Zip 85032; tel. 602/867–1881; Rebecca C. Kuhn, R.N., President and Chief Executive Officer

NORTHWEST HOSPITAL (O, 152 beds) 6200 North La Cholla Boulevard, Tucson, AZ Zip 85741; tel. 520/742–9000; Sharon Gregoire, Chief Operating Officer

ARKANSAS: COLUMBIA DE QUEEN REGIONAL MEDICAL CENTER (O, 75 beds) 1306 Collin Raye Drive, De Queen, AR Zip 71832–2198; tel. 501/584–4111; Charles H. Long, Chief Executive Officer

COLUMBIA DOCTORS HOSPITAL (O, 308 beds) 6101 West Capitol, Little Rock, AR Zip 72205–5331; tel. 501/661–4000; Maura Walsh, President and Chief Executive Officer

MEDICAL CENTER OF SOUTH ARKANSAS (O, 195 beds) 700 West Grove, El Dorado, AR Zip 71730, Mailing Address: P.O. Box 1998, Zip 71731–1998; tel. 501/864–3200; Luther J. Lewis, Chief Executive Officer

MEDICAL PARK HOSPITAL (O, 75 beds) 2001 South Main Street, Hope, AR Zip 71801; tel. 501/777–2323; Jimmy Leopard, Chief Executive Officer

CALIFORNIA: COLUMBIA CHINO VALLEY MEDICAL CENTER (O, 104 beds) 5451 Walnut Avenue, Chino, CA Zip 91710; tel. 909/464–8600; Anthony A. Armada, Chief Executive Officer

COLUMBIA GOOD SAMARITAN HOSPITAL (O, 64 beds) 901 Olive Drive, Bakersfield, CA Zip 93308–4137; tel. 805/399–4461; Jim Bennett, Administrator

COLUMBIA GOOD SAMARITAN HOSPITAL (O, 348 beds) 2425 Samaritan Drive, San Jose, CA Zip 95124, Mailing Address: P.O. Box 240002, Zip 95154–2402; tel. 408/559–2011; Joan C. White, Chief Executive Officer

COLUMBIA HUNTINGTON BEACH HOSPITAL AND MEDICAL CENTER (O, 135 beds) 17772 Beach Boulevard, Huntington Beach, CA Zip 92647–9932; tel. 714/842–1473; Carol B. Freeman, Chief Executive Officer

COLUMBIA LAS ENCINAS HOSPITAL (O, 138 beds) 2900 East Del Mar Boulevard, Pasadena, CA Zip 91107–4375; tel. 818/795–9901; Roland Metivier, Chief Executive Officer

COLUMBIA LOS ROBLES HOSPITAL AND MEDICAL CENTER (O, 185 beds) 215 West Janss Road, Thousand Oaks, CA Zip 91360–1899; tel. 805/497–2727; Ronald C. Phelps, Chief Executive Officer

For explanation of codes following names, see page B2.
★ Indicates Type III membership in the American Hospital Association.

B78 Networks, Health Care Systems and Alliances

© 1997 AHA Guide

COLUMBIA MISSION BAY HOSPITAL (O, 117 beds) 3030 Bunker Hill Street, San Diego, CA Zip 92109–5780; tel. 619/274–7721; Deborah Brehe, Chief Executive Officer

COLUMBIA PALM DRIVE HOSPITAL (O, 48 beds) 501 Petaluma Avenue, Sebastopol, CA Zip 95472; tel. 707/823–8511; Jeff Frandsen, Chief Executive Officer

COLUMBIA SAN JOSE MEDICAL CENTER (O, 327 beds) 675 East Santa Clara Street, San Jose, CA Zip 95112, Mailing Address: P.O. Box 240003, Zip 95154–2403; tel. 408/998–3212; Mary Schwind, R.N., MS, Chief Executive Officer

COLUMBIA SAN LEANDRO HOSPITAL (O, 136 beds) 13855 East 14th Street, San Leandro, CA Zip 94578–0398; tel. 510/667–4510; Kelly Mather, Executive Director

COLUMBIA SOUTH VALLEY HOSPITAL (O, 93 beds) 9400 No Name Uno, Gilroy, CA Zip 95020–2368; tel. 408/848–2000; Beverly Gilmore, Chief Executive Officer

COLUMBIA WEST ANAHEIM MEDICAL CENTER (O, 219 beds) 3033 West Orange Avenue, Anaheim, CA Zip 92804–3184; tel. 714/827–3000; David Culberson, Chief Executive Officer

COLUMBIA WEST HILLS MEDICAL CENTER (O, 236 beds) 7300 Medical Center Drive, West Hills, CA Zip 91307, Mailing Address: P.O. Box 7937, Zip 91309–7937; tel. 818/712–4110; Howard H. Levine, President and Chief Executive Officer

HEALDSBURG GENERAL HOSPITAL (O, 49 beds) 1375 University Avenue, Healdsburg, CA Zip 95448; tel. 707/431–6500; Kenneth Madfes, Chief Executive Officer

WESTLAKE MEDICAL CENTER (O, 60 beds) 4415 South Lakeview Canyon Road, Westlake Village, CA Zip 91361; tel. 818/706–8000; Ronald C. Phelps, Chief Executive Officer

COLORADO: COLUMBIA HEALTHONE–BEHAVIORAL HEALTH SERVICES (O, 86 beds) 4400 East Iliff Avenue, Denver, CO Zip 80222; tel. 303/758–1514; William Kent, Ph.D., Vice President Behavioral Health

COLUMBIA MEDICAL CENTER OF AURORA (O, 334 beds) 1501 South Potomac Street, Aurora, CO Zip 80012; tel. 303/695–2600; Louis O. Garcia, President and Chief Executive Officer

COLUMBIA PRESBYTERIAN–ST. LUKE'S MEDICAL CENTER (O, 479 beds) 1719 East 19th Avenue, Denver, CO Zip 80218; tel. 303/839–6000; William K. Atkinson, Ph.D., Chief Executive Officer

COLUMBIA ROSE MEDICAL CENTER (O, 250 beds) 4567 East Ninth Avenue, Denver, CO Zip 80220; tel. 303/320–2101; Kenneth H. Feiler, Chief Executive Officer

COLUMBIA SWEDISH MEDICAL CENTER (O, 328 beds) 501 East Hampden Avenue, Englewood, CO Zip 80110–0101, Mailing Address: P.O. Box 2901, Zip 80150–0101; tel. 303/788–5000; Mary M. White, President and Chief Executive Officer

NORTH SUBURBAN MEDICAL CENTER (O, 125 beds) 9191 Grant Street, Thornton, CO Zip 80229; tel. 303/451–7800; Jay S. Weinstein, Chief Executive Officer

SPALDING REHABILITATION HOSPITAL (O, 176 beds) 900 Potomac Street, Aurora, CO Zip 80011; tel. 303/367–1166; Russell W. York, President and Chief Executive Officer

DELAWARE: ROCKFORD CENTER (O, 70 beds) 100 Rockford Drive, Newark, DE Zip 19713; tel. 302/996–5480; Walter J. Yokobosky Jr., Chief Executive Officer

FLORIDA: COLUMBIA AVENTURA HOSPITAL AND MEDICAL CENTER (O, 407 beds) 20900 Biscayne Boulevard, Miami, FL Zip 33180–1407; tel. 305/682–7100; Davide M. Carbone, Chief Executive Officer

COLUMBIA BARTOW MEMORIAL HOSPITAL (O, 88 beds) 1239 East Main Street, Bartow, FL Zip 33830–5005, Mailing Address: Box 1050, Zip 33830–1050; tel. 941/533–8111; Thomas C. Mathews, Administrator

COLUMBIA BEHAVIORAL HEALTH CENTER (O, 88 beds) 11100 N.W. 27th Street, Miami, FL Zip 33172; tel. 305/591–3230; Cheryl Siegwald–Mays, Administrator

COLUMBIA BLAKE MEDICAL CENTER (O, 284 beds) 2020 59th Street West, Bradenton, FL Zip 34209, Mailing Address: P.O. Box 25004, Zip 34206–5004; tel. 941/792–6611; Lindell W. Orr, Chief Executive Officer

COLUMBIA BRANDON REGIONAL MEDICAL CENTER (O, 225 beds) 119 Oakfield Drive, Brandon, FL Zip 33511–5799; tel. 813/681–5551; H. Rex Etheredge, President and Chief Executive Officer

COLUMBIA CEDARS MEDICAL CENTER (O, 500 beds) 1400 N.W. 12th Avenue, Miami, FL Zip 33136–1003; tel. 305/325–5511; Ralph A. Aleman, Chief Executive Officer

COLUMBIA CLEARWATER COMMUNITY HOSPITAL (O, 133 beds) 1521 Druid Road East, Clearwater, FL Zip 34616–6193, Mailing Address: P.O. Box 9068, Zip 34618–9068; tel. 813/447–4571; Thomas L. Herron, FACHE, Chief Executive Officer

COLUMBIA DADE CITY HOSPITAL (O, 120 beds) 13100 Fort King Road, Dade City, FL Zip 33525–5294; tel. 904/521–1100; Robert Meade, Chief Executive Officer

COLUMBIA DEERING HOSPITAL (O, 233 beds) 9333 S.W. 152nd Street, Miami, FL Zip 33157; tel. 305/256–5100; Anthony M. Degina Jr., Chief Executive Officer

COLUMBIA DOCTORS HOSPITAL OF SARASOTA (O, 147 beds) 5731 Bee Ridge Road, Sarasota, FL Zip 34233; tel. 941/342–1100; William C. Lievense, President and Chief Executive Officer

COLUMBIA EAST POINTE HOSPITAL (O, 88 beds) 1500 Lee Boulevard, Lehigh Acres, FL Zip 33936; tel. 941/369–2101; Valerie A. Jackson, Chief Executive Officer

COLUMBIA EDWARD WHITE HOSPITAL (O, 134 beds) 2323 Ninth Avenue North, Saint Petersburg, FL Zip 33713, Mailing Address: P.O. Box 12018, Zip 33733–2018; tel. 813/323–1111; Barry S. Stokes, Chief Executive Officer

COLUMBIA ENGLEWOOD COMMUNITY HOSPITAL (O, 100 beds) 700 Medical Boulevard, Englewood, FL Zip 34223; tel. 941/475–6571; Terry L. Moore, Chief Executive Officer

COLUMBIA FAWCETT MEMORIAL HOSPITAL (O, 249 beds) 21298 Olean Boulevard, Port Charlotte, FL Zip 33952–6765, Mailing Address: P.O. Box 4028, Punta Gorda, Zip 33949–4028; tel. 941/629–1181; Steve Dobbs, Chief Executive Officer

COLUMBIA FORT WALTON BEACH MEDICAL CENTER (O, 247 beds) 1000 Mar–Walt Drive, Fort Walton Beach, FL Zip 32547–6708; tel. 904/862–1111; Wayne Campbell, Chief Executive Officer

COLUMBIA GULF COAST HOSPITAL (O, 120 beds) 13681 Doctors Way, Fort Myers, FL Zip 33912; tel. 941/768–5000; Valerie A. Jackson, Chief Executive Officer

COLUMBIA GULF COAST MEDICAL CENTER (O, 176 beds) 449 West 23rd Street, Panama City, FL Zip 32405, Mailing Address: P.O. Box 15309, Zip 32406–5309; tel. 904/769–8341; Donald E. Butts, Chief Executive Officer

COLUMBIA HAMILTON MEDICAL CENTER (O, 42 beds) 506 N.W. Fourth Street, Jasper, FL Zip 32052; tel. 904/792–7200; Amelia Tuten, R.N., Administrator

COLUMBIA HOSPITAL (O, 250 beds) 2201 45th Street, West Palm Beach, FL Zip 33407–2069; tel. 561/842–6141; Michael M. Fencel, Chief Executive Officer

COLUMBIA J. F. K. MEDICAL CENTER (O, 363 beds) 5301 South Congress Avenue, Atlantis, FL Zip 33462; tel. 561/965–7300; Phillip D. Robinson, Chief Executive Officer

COLUMBIA KENDALL MEDICAL CENTER (O, 235 beds) 11750 Bird Road, Miami, FL Zip 33175–3530; tel. 305/223–3000; Victor Maya, Chief Executive Officer

COLUMBIA LAKE CITY MEDICAL CENTER (O, 75 beds) 1701 West U.S. Highway 90, Lake City, FL Zip 32055; tel. 904/752–2922; David P. Steitz, Chief Executive Officer

COLUMBIA LARGO MEDICAL CENTER (O, 243 beds) 201 14th Street S.W., Largo, FL Zip 33770, Mailing Address: P.O. Box 2905, Zip 33779; tel. 813/586–1411; Thomas L. Herron, FACHE, President and Chief Executive Officer

COLUMBIA LAWNWOOD REGIONAL MEDICAL CENTER (O, 363 beds) 1700 South 23rd Street, Fort Pierce, FL Zip 34950–0188; tel. 561/461–4000; Gary Cantrell, President and Chief Executive Officer

COLUMBIA MEDICAL CENTER PENINSULA (O, 119 beds) 264 South Atlantic Avenue, Ormond Beach, FL Zip 32176–8192; tel. 904/672–4161; Thomas R. Pentz, Chief Executive Officer

For explanation of codes following names, see page B2.
★ Indicates Type III membership in the American Hospital Association.

COLUMBIA MEDICAL CENTER SANFORD (O, 226 beds) 1401 West Seminole Boulevard, Sanford, FL Zip 32771–6764; tel. 407/321–4500; Doug Sills, President and Chief Executive Officer

COLUMBIA MEDICAL CENTER–DAYTONA (O, 214 beds) 400 North Clyde Morris Boulevard, Daytona Beach, FL Zip 32114, Mailing Address: Box 9000, Zip 32120; tel. 904/239–5000; Thomas R. Pentz, Chief Executive Officer

COLUMBIA MEDICAL CENTER–OSCEOLA (O, 156 beds) 700 West Oak Street, Kissimmee, FL Zip 34741, Mailing Address: P.O. Box 422589, Zip 34742–2589; tel. 407/846–2266; E. Tim Cook, Chief Executive Officer

COLUMBIA MEDICAL CENTER–PORT ST. LUCIE (O, 150 beds) 1800 S.E. Tiffany Avenue, Port St. Lucie, FL Zip 34952–7580; tel. 407/335–4000; Michael P. Joyce, President and Chief Executive Officer

COLUMBIA MEMORIAL HOSPITAL JACKSONVILLE (O, 310 beds) 3625 University Boulevard South, Jacksonville, FL Zip 32216, Mailing Address: Box 16325, Zip 32216; tel. 904/399–6111; Winston Rushing, President

COLUMBIA NEW PORT RICHEY HOSPITAL (O, 414 beds) 5637 Marine Parkway, New Port Richey, FL Zip 34652, Mailing Address: Box 996, Zip 34656–0996; tel. 813/848–1733; Andrew Oravec Jr., Administrator

COLUMBIA NORTH FLORIDA REGIONAL MEDICAL CENTER (O, 278 beds) 6500 Newberry Road, Gainesville, FL Zip 32605–4392, Mailing Address: P.O. Box 147006, Zip 32614–7006; tel. 352/333–4000; Brian C. Robinson, Chief Executive Officer

COLUMBIA NORTHSIDE MEDICAL CENTER (O, 301 beds) 6000 49th Street North, Saint Petersburg, FL Zip 33709; tel. 813/521–4411; Bradley K. Grover Sr., Chief Executive Officer

COLUMBIA NORTHWEST MEDICAL CENTER (O, 150 beds) 2801 North State Road 7, Margate, FL Zip 33063, Mailing Address: P.O. Box 639002, Zip 33063–9002; tel. 305/978–4000; Gina Becker, Acting Chief Executive Officer

COLUMBIA OCALA REGIONAL MEDICAL CENTER (O, 216 beds) 1431 S.W. First Avenue, Ocala, FL Zip 34474, Mailing Address: Box 2200, Zip 34478–2200; tel. 352/401–1000; Terry Upton, Chief Executive Officer

COLUMBIA ORANGE PARK MEDICAL CENTER (O, 196 beds) 2001 Kingsley Avenue, Orange Park, FL Zip 32073–5156; tel. 904/276–8500; Robert M. Krieger, Chief Executive Officer

COLUMBIA PALMS WEST HOSPITAL (O, 117 beds) 13001 Southern Boulevard, Loxahatchee, FL Zip 33470–1150; tel. 407/798–3300; Alex M. Marceline, Chief Executive Officer

COLUMBIA PARK MEDICAL CENTER (O, 267 beds) 818 South Main Lane, Orlando, FL Zip 32801; tel. 407/649–6111; Rick O'Connell, Chief Executive Officer

COLUMBIA PLANTATION GENERAL HOSPITAL (O, 264 beds) 401 N.W. 42nd Avenue, Plantation, FL Zip 33317–2882; tel. 954/587–5010; Anthony M. Degina Jr., Chief Executive Officer

COLUMBIA POMPANO BEACH MEDICAL CENTER (O, 80 beds) 600 S.W. Third Street, Pompano Beach, FL Zip 33060–6979; tel. 954/782–2000; Heather J. Rohan, Chief Executive Officer

COLUMBIA PUTNAM MEDICAL CENTER (O, 161 beds) Highway 20 West, Palatka, FL Zip 32177, Mailing Address: P.O. Box 778, Zip 32178–0778; tel. 904/328–5711; David Whalen, President and Chief Executive Officer

COLUMBIA RAULERSON HOSPITAL (O, 101 beds) 1796 Highway 441 North, Okeechobee, FL Zip 34972, Mailing Address: Box 1307, Zip 34973–1307; tel. 941/763–2151; Frank Irby, Chief Executive Officer

COLUMBIA REGIONAL MEDICAL CENTER (O, 204 beds) 11375 Cortez Boulevard, Spring Hill, FL Zip 34613, Mailing Address: P.O. Box 5300, Zip 34606; tel. 904/596–6632; John R. Finnegan, Administrator and Chief Operating Officer

COLUMBIA REGIONAL MEDICAL CENTER AT BAYONET POINT (O, 256 beds) 14000 Fivay Road, Hudson, FL Zip 34667–7199; tel. 813/863–2411; J. Daniel Miller, President and Chief Executive Officer

COLUMBIA REGIONAL MEDICAL CENTER OF SOUTHWEST FLORIDA (O, 400 beds) 2727 Winkler Avenue, Fort Myers, FL Zip 33901–9396; tel. 941/939–1147; Nick Carbone, Chief Executive Officer

COLUMBIA SOUTH BAY HOSPITAL (O, 112 beds) 4016 State Road 674, Sun City Center, FL Zip 33573–5298; tel. 813/634–3301; Marcia Easley, Chief Operating Officer

COLUMBIA SPECIALTY HOSPITAL JACKSONVILLE (O, 61 beds) 4901 Richard Street, Jacksonville, FL Zip 32207; tel. 904/737–3120; W. Raymond C. Ford, Administrator and Chief Executive Officer

COLUMBIA ST. PETERSBURG MEDICAL CENTER (O, 199 beds) 6500 38th Avenue North, Saint Petersburg, FL Zip 33710; tel. 813/384–1414; Bradley K. Grover Sr., President and Chief Executive Officer

COLUMBIA TALLAHASSEE COMMUNITY HOSPITAL (O, 180 beds) 2626 Capital Medical Boulevard, Tallahassee, FL Zip 32308; tel. 904/656–5000; Gary L. Brewer, Chief Executive Officer

COLUMBIA TWIN CITIES HOSPITAL (O, 60 beds) 2190 Highway 85 North, Niceville, FL Zip 32578; tel. 904/678–4131; David Whalen, Chief Executive Officer

COLUMBIA UNIVERSITY GENERAL HOSPITAL (O, 152 beds) 10200 Seminole Boulevard, Seminole, FL Zip 34642–0005, Mailing Address: P.O. Box 4005, Zip 34642–0005; tel. 813/397–5511; Barry S. Stokes, Chief Operating Officer

COLUMBIA UNIVERSITY HOSPITAL AND MEDICAL CENTER (O, 211 beds) 7201 North University Drive, Tamarac, FL Zip 33321; tel. 305/721–2200; James A. Cruickshank, Chief Executive Officer

COLUMBIA WEST FLORIDA REGIONAL MEDICAL CENTER (O, 531 beds) 8383 North Davis Highway, Pensacola, FL Zip 32514, Mailing Address: P.O. Box 18900, Zip 32523–8900; tel. 904/494–4000; Stephen Brandt, Chief Executive Officer

COLUMBIA WESTSIDE REGIONAL MEDICAL CENTER (O, 204 beds) 8201 West Broward Boulevard, Plantation, FL Zip 33324–9937; tel. 954/473–6600; Michael G. Joseph, Chief Executive Officer

MIAMI HEART INSTITUTE (O, 278 beds) 4701 Meridian Avenue, Miami, FL Zip 33140–2910; tel. 305/674–3114; Tim Parker, Chief Executive Officer

WINTER PARK MEMORIAL HOSPITAL (O, 339 beds) 200 North Lakemont Avenue, Winter Park, FL Zip 32792–3273; tel. 407/646–7000; Douglas P. DeGraaf, Chief Executive Officer

GEORGIA: COLUMBIA AUGUSTA MEDICAL CENTER (O, 284 beds) 3651 Wheeler Road, Augusta, GA Zip 30909–6426; tel. 706/651–3232; Michael K. Kerner, President and Chief Executive Officer

COLUMBIA BARROW MEDICAL CENTER (O, 60 beds) 316 North Broad Street, Winder, GA Zip 30680, Mailing Address: Box 768, Zip 30680; tel. 770/867–3400; Joe T. Hutchins, Chief Executive Officer

COLUMBIA CARTERSVILLE MEDICAL CENTER (O, 80 beds) 960 Joe Frank Harris Parkway, Cartersville, GA Zip 30120, Mailing Address: P.O. Box 200008, Zip 30120–9001; tel. 770/382–1530; Keith Sandlin, Chief Executive Officer

COLUMBIA COLISEUM MEDICAL CENTERS (O, 188 beds) 350 Hospital Drive, Macon, GA Zip 31213; tel. 912/765–7000; Michael S. Boggs, Chief Executive Officer

COLUMBIA COLISEUM PSYCHIATRIC HOSPITAL (O, 92 beds) 340 Hospital Drive, Macon, GA Zip 31201–8002; tel. 912/741–1355; Edward W. Ruffin, Administrator

COLUMBIA DOCTORS HOSPITAL (O, 219 beds) 616 19th Street, Columbus, GA Zip 31901–1528, Mailing Address: P.O. Box 2188, Zip 31902–2188; tel. 706/571–4262; Hugh D. Wilson, Chief Executive Officer

COLUMBIA DUNWOODY MEDICAL CENTER (O, 122 beds) 4575 North Shallowford Road, Atlanta, GA Zip 30338; tel. 770/454–2000; Thomas D. Gilbert, President and Chief Executive Officer

COLUMBIA EASTSIDE MEDICAL CENTER (O, 114 beds) 1700 Medical Way, Snellville, GA Zip 30278, Mailing Address: P.O. Box 587, Zip 30278; tel. 770/979–0200; Les Beard, Chief Executive Officer

COLUMBIA FAIRVIEW PARK HOSPITAL (O, 190 beds) 200 Industrial Boulevard, Dublin, GA Zip 31021, Mailing Address: Box 1408, Zip 31040; tel. 912/275–2000; Jeffrey T. Whiteborn, Chief Executive Officer

COLUMBIA HUGHSTON SPORTS MEDICINE HOSPITAL (O, 100 beds) 100 Frist Court, Columbus, GA Zip 31908–7188, Mailing Address: P.O. Box 7188, Zip 31908–7188; tel. 706/576–2100; Hugh D. Wilson, Chief Executive Officer

COLUMBIA LANIER PARK HOSPITAL (O, 124 beds) 675 White Sulphur Road, Gainesville, GA Zip 30505, Mailing Address: P.O. Box 1354, Zip 30503; tel. 770/503–3000; Jerry Fulks, Chief Executive Officer

COLUMBIA METROPOLITAN HOSPITAL (O, 64 beds) 3223 Howell Mill Road N.W., Atlanta, GA Zip 30327; tel. 404/351–0500; Neil Heatherly, Chief Executive Officer

For explanation of codes following names, see page B2.
★ Indicates Type III membership in the American Hospital Association.

COLUMBIA MURRAY MEDICAL CENTER (O, 42 beds) 707 Old Ellijay Road, Chatsworth, GA Zip 30705, Mailing Address: P.O. Box 1406, Zip 30705; tel. 706/695-4564; Richard Cook, Administrator

COLUMBIA NORTHLAKE REGIONAL MEDICAL CENTER (O, 120 beds) 1455 Montreal Road, Atlanta, GA Zip 30084, Mailing Address: P.O. Box 450000, Zip 31145; tel. 770/270-3000; Michael R. Burroughs, President and Chief Executive Officer

COLUMBIA PALMYRA MEDICAL CENTERS (O, 156 beds) 2000 Palmyra Road, Albany, GA Zip 31701, Mailing Address: Box 1908, Zip 31702-1908; tel. 912/434-2000; Allen Golson, Chief Executive Officer

COLUMBIA PARKWAY MEDICAL CENTER (O, 233 beds) 1000 Thornton Road, Lithia Springs, GA Zip 30057, Mailing Address: P.O. Box 570, Zip 30057; tel. 770/732-7777; Deborah S. Guthrie, Chief Executive Officer

COLUMBIA PEACHTREE REGIONAL HOSPITAL (O, 144 beds) 60 Hospital Road, Newnan, GA Zip 30264, Mailing Address: Box 2228, Zip 30264; tel. 770/253-1912; Linda Jubinsky, Chief Executive Officer

COLUMBIA REDMOND REGIONAL MEDICAL CENTER (O, 188 beds) 501 Redmond Road, Rome, GA Zip 30165-7001, Mailing Address: Box 107001, Zip 30164-7001; tel. 706/291-0291; James R. Thomas, Chief Executive Officer

COLUMBIA WEST PACES MEDICAL CENTER (O, 294 beds) 3200 Howell Mill Road N.W., Atlanta, GA Zip 30327-4101; tel. 404/351-0351; Thomas E. Anderson, President and Chief Executive Officer

IDAHO: COLUMBIA EASTERN IDAHO REGIONAL MEDICAL CENTER (O, 286 beds) 3100 Channing Way, Idaho Falls, ID Zip 83404, Mailing Address: P.O. Box 2077, Zip 83403-2077; tel. 208/529-6111; Ronald G. Butler, Chief Executive Officer

COLUMBIA WEST VALLEY MEDICAL CENTER (O, 122 beds) 1717 Arlington, Caldwell, ID Zip 83605-4864; tel. 208/459-4641; Mark Adams, Chief Executive Officer

ILLINOIS: COLUMBIA CHICAGO LAKESHORE HOSPITAL (O, 102 beds) 4840 North Marine Drive, Chicago, IL Zip 60640; tel. 773/907-4601; Marcia S. Shapiro, Administrator and Chief Executive Officer

COLUMBIA GRANT HOSPITAL (O, 213 beds) 550 West Webster Avenue, Chicago, IL Zip 60614-9980; tel. 773/883-2000; Nancy R. Hellyer, R.N., Chief Executive Officer

COLUMBIA HOFFMAN ESTATES MEDICAL CENTER (O, 195 beds) 1555 North Barrington Road, Hoffman Estates, IL Zip 60194; tel. 847/843-2000; Edward Goldberg, President and Chief Executive Officer

COLUMBIA LA GRANGE MEMORIAL HOSPITAL (O, 231 beds) 5101 South Willow Springs Road, La Grange, IL Zip 60525-2680; tel. 708/352-1200; Cathleen D. Biga, President and Chief Executive Officer

COLUMBIA MICHAEL REESE HOSPITAL AND MEDICAL CENTER (O, 523 beds) 2929 South Ellis Avenue, Chicago, IL Zip 60616; tel. 312/791-2000; F. Scott Winslow, President and Chief Executive Officer

COLUMBIA OLYMPIA FIELDS OSTEOPATHIC HOSPITAL AND MEDICAL CENTER (O, 174 beds) 20201 Crawford Avenue, Olympia Fields, IL Zip 60461-1080; tel. 708/747-4000; Barry S. Schneider, President and Chief Executive Officer

COLUMBIA RIVEREDGE HOSPITAL (O, 120 beds) 8311 West Roosevelt Road, Forest Park, IL Zip 60130-2500; tel. 708/771-7000; Mary Palmer, President and Chief Executive Officer

COLUMBIA WOODLAND HOSPITAL (O, 94 beds) 1650 Moon Lake Boulevard, Hoffman Estates, IL Zip 60194-5000; tel. 847/882-1600; John F. Buckley, Chief Executive Officer

INDIANA: COLUMBIA TERRE HAUTE REGIONAL HOSPITAL (O, 236 beds) 3901 South Seventh Street, Terre Haute, IN Zip 47802-4299; tel. 812/232-0021; Jerry Dooley, Chief Executive Officer

COLUMBIA WOMEN'S HOSPITAL–INDIANAPOLIS (O, 132 beds) 8111 Township Line Road, Indianapolis, IN Zip 46260-8043; tel. 317/875-5994; Steven B. Reed, President and Chief Executive Officer

KANSAS: COLUMBIA HALSTEAD HOSPITAL (O, 137 beds) 328 Poplar Street, Halstead, KS Zip 67056-2099; tel. 316/835-2651; David Nevill, President and Chief Executive Officer

COLUMBIA OVERLAND PARK REGIONAL MEDICAL CENTER (O, 287 beds) 10500 Quivira Road, Overland Park, KS Zip 66215-2373, Mailing Address: P.O. Box 15959, Zip 66215; tel. 913/541-5000; Kevin J. Hicks, President and Chief Executive Officer

COLUMBIA WESLEY MEDICAL CENTER (O, 553 beds) 550 North Hillside Avenue, Wichita, KS Zip 67214-4976; tel. 316/688-2468; Kevin Gross, Interim President and Chief Executive Officer

COLUMBIA WESTERN PLAINS REGIONAL HOSPITAL (O, 85 beds) 3001 Avenue A, Dodge City, KS Zip 67801, Mailing Address: Box 1478, Zip 67801; tel. 316/225-8401; Ken Hutchenrider, President and Chief Executive Officer

KENTUCKY: COLUMBIA AUDUBON HOSPITAL (O, 480 beds) One Audubon Plaza Drive, Louisville, KY Zip 40217-1397, Mailing Address: Box 17550, Zip 40217-0550; tel. 502/636-7111; James E. Rogers, President and Chief Executive Officer

COLUMBIA GREENVIEW HOSPITAL (O, 211 beds) 1801 Ashley Circle, Bowling Green, KY Zip 42104, Mailing Address: Box 90024, Zip 42102-9024; tel. 502/793-1000; Harry Alvis, Chief Executive Officer

COLUMBIA HOSPITAL FRANKFORT (O, 147 beds) 299 King's Daughters Drive, Frankfort, KY Zip 40601-4186; tel. 502/875-5240; David P. Steitz, Chief Executive Officer

COLUMBIA HOSPITAL GEORGETOWN (O, 61 beds) 1140 Lexington Road, Georgetown, KY Zip 40324; tel. 502/868-1100; Britt T. Reynolds, Chief Executive Officer

COLUMBIA HOSPITAL LEXINGTON (O, 219 beds) 310 South Limestone Street, Lexington, KY Zip 40508-3008; tel. 606/252-6612; Barton A. Hove, Chief Executive Officer

COLUMBIA HOSPITAL MAYSVILLE (O, 90 beds) 989 Medical Park Drive, Maysville, KY Zip 41056; tel. 606/759-5311; J. Timothy Browne, Chief Executive Officer

COLUMBIA HOSPITAL PARIS (O, 58 beds) 9 Linville Drive, Paris, KY Zip 40361; tel. 606/987-1000; John R. Grant, Chief Executive Officer

COLUMBIA LAKE CUMBERLAND REGIONAL HOSPITAL (O, 227 beds) 305 Langdon Street, Somerset, KY Zip 42501, Mailing Address: Box 620, Zip 42502-2750; tel. 606/679-7441; Kenneth W. Lukhard, President and Chief Executive Officer

COLUMBIA LOGAN MEMORIAL HOSPITAL (O, 64 beds) 1625 South Nashville Road, Russellville, KY Zip 42276-0010, Mailing Address: P.O. Box 10, Zip 42276; tel. 502/726-4011

COLUMBIA PINELAKE REGIONAL HOSPITAL (O, 106 beds) 1099 Medical Center Circle, Mayfield, KY Zip 42066, Mailing Address: P.O. Box 1099, Zip 42066; tel. 502/251-4100; Don A. Horstkotte, Chief Executive Officer

COLUMBIA SOUTHWEST HOSPITAL (O, 150 beds) 9820 Third Street Road, Louisville, KY Zip 40272-9984; tel. 502/933-8100; Cathryn A. Hibbs, Chief Executive Officer

COLUMBIA SPRING VIEW HOSPITAL (O, 113 beds) 320 Loretto Road, Lebanon, KY Zip 40033-0320; tel. 502/692-3161; John D. Brock, Chief Executive Officer

COLUMBIA SUBURBAN HOSPITAL (O, 380 beds) 4001 Dutchmans Lane, Louisville, KY Zip 40207; tel. 502/893-1000; Tracy A. Rogers, President and Chief Executive Officer

LOUISIANA: AVOYELLES HOSPITAL (O, 55 beds) 4231 Highway 1192, Marksville, LA Zip 71351, Mailing Address: Box 255, Zip 71351; tel. 318/253-8611; David M. Mitchel, Chief Executive Officer

COLUMBIA DAUTERIVE HOSPITAL (O, 92 beds) 600 North Lewis Street, New Iberia, LA Zip 70560, Mailing Address: P.O. Box 11210, Zip 70562-1210; tel. 318/365-7311; Kyle J. Viator, Chief Executive Officer

COLUMBIA DOCTORS' HOSPITAL OF OPELOUSAS (O, 105 beds) 5101 Highway 167 South, Opelousas, LA Zip 70570; tel. 318/948-2100; Daryl J. Doise, Administrator

COLUMBIA HIGHLAND HOSPITAL (O, 121 beds) 1453 East Bert Kouns Industrial Loop, Shreveport, LA Zip 71105-6050; tel. 318/798-4300; Anthony S. Sala Jr., Chief Executive Officer

COLUMBIA JEFFERSON MEDICAL CENTER (O, 108 beds) 1221 South Clearview Parkway, Jefferson, LA Zip 70121; tel. 504/734-1900; David E. Hoidal, Chief Executive Officer

COLUMBIA LAKELAND MEDICAL CENTER (O, 130 beds) 6000 Bullard Avenue, New Orleans, LA Zip 70128; tel. 504/241-6335; Trudy Land, Chief Executive Officer

COLUMBIA LAKESIDE HOSPITAL (O, 99 beds) 4700 I-10 Service Road, Metairie, LA Zip 70001-1269; tel. 504/885-3333; M. P. Gandy Jr., President

Section B

For explanation of codes following names, see page B2.
★ Indicates Type III membership in the American Hospital Association.

© 1997 AHA Guide   Networks, Health Care Systems and Alliances   **B81**

COLUMBIA LAKEVIEW REGIONAL MEDICAL CENTER (O, 163 beds) 95 East Fairway Drive, Covington, LA Zip 70433; tel. 504/876–3800; Scott Koenig, Chief Executive Officer

COLUMBIA MEDICAL CENTER (O, 183 beds) 17000 Medical Center Drive, Baton Rouge, LA Zip 70816–3224; tel. 504/755–4800; Joseph R. Dicapo, Chief Executive Officer

COLUMBIA MEDICAL CENTER OF SOUTHWEST LOUISIANA (O, 107 beds) 2810 Ambassador Caffery Parkway, Lafayette, LA Zip 70506; tel. 318/981–2949; Gerald A. Fornoff, Chief Executive Officer

COLUMBIA NORTH MONROE HOSPITAL (O, 210 beds) 3421 Medical Park Drive, Monroe, LA Zip 71203; tel. 318/388–1946; George E. Miller, Chief Executive Officer

COLUMBIA RIVERVIEW MEDICAL CENTER (O, 104 beds) 1125 West Louisiana Highway 30, Gonzales, LA Zip 70737; tel. 504/647–5000; James W. White, Chief Executive Officer

COLUMBIA SPRINGHILL MEDICAL CENTER (O, 86 beds) 2001 Doctors Drive, Springhill, LA Zip 71075, Mailing Address: Box 920, Zip 71075–0920; tel. 318/539–1000; John D. Anderson, Chief Executive Officer

COLUMBIA WOMEN AND CHILDREN'S HOSPITAL–LAKE CHARLES (O, 72 beds) 4200 Nelson Road, Lake Charles, LA Zip 70605; tel. 318/474–6370; Alan E. McMillin, Chief Executive Officer

COLUMBIA WOMEN'S AND CHILDREN'S HOSPITAL (O, 96 beds) 4600 Ambassador Caffery Parkway, Lafayette, LA Zip 70508, Mailing Address: P.O. Box 88030, Zip 70598–8030; tel. 318/981–9100; Madeleine L. Roberson, Chief Executive Officer

OAKDALE COMMUNITY HOSPITAL (O, 60 beds) 130 North Hospital Drive, Oakdale, LA Zip 71463, Mailing Address: Box 629, Zip 71463; tel. 318/335–3700; LaQuita Johnson, Chief Executive Officer

RAPIDES REGIONAL MEDICAL CENTER (O, 359 beds) 211 Fourth Street, Alexandria, LA Zip 71301–8421, Mailing Address: Box 30101, Zip 71301–8421; tel. 318/473–3000; Lynn Truelove, President

SAVOY MEDICAL CENTER (O, 503 beds) 801 Poinciana Avenue, Mamou, LA Zip 70554; tel. 318/468–5261; J. E. Richardson, Chief Executive Officer

TULANE UNIVERSITY HOSPITAL AND CLINIC (O, 259 beds) 1415 Tulane Avenue, New Orleans, LA Zip 70112–2632; tel. 504/588–5263; Stephen A. Pickett, President and Chief Executive Officer

WINN PARISH MEDICAL CENTER (O, 103 beds) 301 West Boundary Street, Winnfield, LA Zip 71483, Mailing Address: Box 152, Zip 71483; tel. 318/628–2721; Bobby Jordan, Chief Executive Officer

MASSACHUSETTS: COLUMBIA METROWEST MEDICAL CENTER (O, 423 beds) 115 Lincoln Street, Framingham, MA Zip 01701; tel. 508/383–1000; Lawrence Kaplan, M.D., President and Chief Executive Officer

MISSISSIPPI: COLUMBIA GARDEN PARK HOSPITAL (O, 97 beds) 1520 Broad Avenue, Gulfport, MS Zip 39501, Mailing Address: P.O. Box 1240, Zip 39502; tel. 601/864–4210; William E. Peaks, Chief Executive Officer

COLUMBIA VICKSBURG MEDICAL CENTER (O, 154 beds) 1111 Frontage Road, Vicksburg, MS Zip 39181–5298; tel. 601/636–2611; William M. Patterson, Administrator

MISSOURI: COLUMBIA HOSPITAL NORTH AND SOUTH (O, 195 beds) 3535 South National Avenue, Springfield, MO Zip 65807; tel. 417/882–4700; Michelle Fischer, Chief Executive Officer

COLUMBIA INDEPENDENCE REGIONAL HEALTH CENTER (O, 329 beds) 1509 West Truman Road, Independence, MO Zip 64050; tel. 816/836–8100; Paul F. Herzog, Chief Executive Officer

RESEARCH PSYCHIATRIC CENTER (O, 100 beds) 2323 East 63rd Street, Kansas City, MO Zip 64130; tel. 816/444–8161; Todd Krass, Administrator and Chief Executive Officer

NEVADA: COLUMBIA SUNRISE HOSPITAL AND MEDICAL CENTER (O, 643 beds) 3186 Maryland Parkway, Las Vegas, NV Zip 89109–2306, Mailing Address: P.O. Box 98530, Zip 89193–8530; tel. 702/731–8000; Jerald F. Mitchell, President and Chief Executive Officer

NEW HAMPSHIRE: PARKLAND MEDICAL CENTER (O, 65 beds) One Parkland Drive, Derry, NH Zip 03038; tel. 603/432–1500; Bruce G. Peters, President and Chief Executive Officer

PORTSMOUTH REGIONAL HOSPITAL AND PAVILION (O, 179 beds) 333 Borthwick Avenue, Portsmouth, NH Zip 03802–7004; tel. 603/436–5110; William J. Schuler, Chief Executive Officer

NEW MEXICO: COLUMBIA LEA REGIONAL HOSPITAL (O, 250 beds) 5419 North Lovington Highway, Hobbs, NM Zip 88240, Mailing Address: P.O. Box 3000, Zip 88240; tel. 505/392–6581; R. Gordon Taylor, Administrator

COLUMBIA MEDICAL CENTER OF CARLSBAD (O, 110 beds) 2430 West Pierce Street, Carlsbad, NM Zip 88220–3597; tel. 505/887–4100; Robin E. Lake, Chief Executive Officer

NORTH CAROLINA: COLUMBIA BRUNSWICK HOSPITAL (O, 56 beds) 1 Medical Center Drive, Supply, NC Zip 28462, Mailing Address: P.O. Box 139, Zip 28462; tel. 910/755–8121; C. Mark Gregson, Chief Executive Officer

COLUMBIA CAPE FEAR MEMORIAL HOSPITAL (O, 109 beds) 5301 Wrightsville Avenue, Wilmington, NC Zip 28403, Mailing Address: P.O. Box 4549, Zip 28406–6599; tel. 910/452–8100; C. Mark Gregson, Chief Executive Officer

COLUMBIA DAVIS MEDICAL CENTER (O, 132 beds) Old Mocksville Road, Statesville, NC Zip 28677, Mailing Address: P.O. Box 1823, Zip 28687; tel. 704/873–0281; G. Phillip Lotti, Chief Executive Officer

COLUMBIA HERITAGE HOSPITAL (O, 127 beds) 111 Hospital Drive, Tarboro, NC Zip 27886; tel. 919/641–7700; Janet Mullaney, Chief Executive Officer

COLUMBIA HIGHSMITH–RAINEY MEMORIAL HOSPITAL (O, 133 beds) 150 Robeson Street, Fayetteville, NC Zip 28301–5570; tel. 910/609–1000; William A. Adams, Chief Executive Officer

COLUMBIA RALEIGH COMMUNITY HOSPITAL (O, 160 beds) 3400 Wake Forest Road, Raleigh, NC Zip 27609–7373, Mailing Address: P.O. Box 28280, Zip 27611; tel. 919/954–3000; James E. Raynor, Chief Executive Officer

HOLLY HILL CHARTER BEHAVIORAL HEALTH SYSTEM (O, 108 beds) 3019 Falstaff Road, Raleigh, NC Zip 27610; tel. 919/250–7000; James B. Brawley, Chief Executive Officer

PRESBYTERIAN–ORTHOPAEDIC HOSPITAL (O, 166 beds) 1901 Randolph Road, Charlotte, NC Zip 28207; tel. 704/370–1549; Paul M. Jenson, Chief Executive Officer

OHIO: SAINT LUKE'S MEDICAL CENTER (O, 205 beds) 11311 Shaker Boulevard, Cleveland, OH Zip 44104–3805; tel. 216/368–7000; Samuel R. Huston, President and Chief Executive Officer

OKLAHOMA: COLUMBIA BETHANY HOSPITAL (L, 75 beds) 7600 N.W. 23rd Street, Bethany, OK Zip 73008; tel. 405/787–3450; David Lundquist, Chief Executive Officer

COLUMBIA CLAREMORE REGIONAL HOSPITAL (O, 50 beds) 1202 North Muskogee Place, Claremore, OK Zip 74017; tel. 918/341–2556; Ken Seidel, Executive Director

COLUMBIA DOCTORS HOSPITAL (O, 148 beds) 2323 South Harvard Avenue, Tulsa, OK Zip 74114–3370; tel. 918/744–4000; Anthony R. Young, President and Chief Executive Officer

COLUMBIA EDMOND REGIONAL MEDICAL CENTER (O, 75 beds) 1 South Bryant Street, Edmond, OK Zip 73034–4798; tel. 405/359–5530; Stanley D. Tatum, Chief Executive Officer

COLUMBIA PRESBYTERIAN HOSPITAL (O, 292 beds) 700 N.E. 13th Street, Oklahoma City, OK Zip 73104–5070; tel. 405/271–5100; James O'Loughlin, Chief Executive Officer

COLUMBIA SOUTHWESTERN MEDICAL CENTER (O, 108 beds) 5602 S.W. Lee Boulevard, Lawton, OK Zip 73505–9635, Mailing Address: P.O. Box 7290, Zip 73506–7290; tel. 405/531–4700; Thomas L. Rine, President and Chief Executive Officer

COLUMBIA TULSA REGIONAL MEDICAL CENTER (O, 264 beds) 744 West Ninth Street, Tulsa, OK Zip 74127–9990; tel. 918/599–5900; James M. MacCallum, President and Chief Executive Officer

COLUMBIA WAGONER HOSPITAL (O, 100 beds) 1200 West Cherokee, Wagoner, OK Zip 74467–4681, Mailing Address: Box 407, Zip 74477–0407; tel. 918/485–5514; John W. Crawford, Chief Executive Officer

OREGON: COLUMBIA DOUGLAS MEDICAL CENTER (O, 88 beds) 738 West Harvard Boulevard, Roseburg, OR Zip 97470–2996; tel. 541/673–6641; Christopher L. Boyd, Chief Executive Officer

COLUMBIA WILLIAMETTE VALLEY MEDICAL CENTER (O, 61 beds) 2700 Three Mile Lane, McMinnville, OR Zip 97128–6498; tel. 503/472–6131; Rosemari Davis, Chief Executive Officer

SOUTH CAROLINA: COLUMBIA COLLETON MEDICAL CENTER (O, 116 beds) 501 Robertson Boulevard, Walterboro, SC Zip 29488; tel. 803/549–0600; Rebecca T. Brewer, CHE, Chief Executive Officer

---

For explanation of codes following names, see page B2.
★ Indicates Type III membership in the American Hospital Association.

COLUMBIA GRAND STRAND REGIONAL MEDICAL CENTER (O, 168 beds) 809 82nd Parkway, Myrtle Beach, SC Zip 29572–1413; tel. 803/692–1100; Doug White, Chief Executive Officer

COLUMBIA TRIDENT MEDICAL CENTER (O, 286 beds) 9330 Medical Plaza Drive, Charleston, SC Zip 29406–9195; tel. 803/797–7000; Gene B. Wright, President and Chief Executive Officer

SUMMERVILLE MEDICAL CENTER (O, 99 beds) 295 Midland Parkway, Summerville, SC Zip 29485; tel. 803/875–3993; James G. Thaw, President and Chief Executive Officer

TENNESSEE: CENTENNIAL MEDICAL CENTER AND PARTHENON PAVILION (O, 680 beds) 2300 Patterson Street, Nashville, TN Zip 37203; tel. 615/342–1000; Ronald J. Elder, President

COLUMBIA ATHENS REGIONAL MEDICAL CENTER (O, 97 beds) 1114 West Madison Avenue, Athens, TN Zip 37303, Mailing Address: Box 250, Zip 37371–0250; tel. 615/745–1411; Sean S. McMurray, Administrator

COLUMBIA CHEATHAM MEDICAL CENTER (O, 29 beds) 313 North Main Street, Ashland City, TN Zip 37015; tel. 615/792–3030; Peggy Miller, R.N., Director Nursing and Chief Operating Officer

COLUMBIA CROCKETT HOSPITAL (O, 83 beds) U.S. Highway 43 South, Lawrenceburg, TN Zip 38464–0847, Mailing Address: Box 847, Zip 38464–0847; tel. 615/762–6571; John A. Marshall, Chief Executive Officer

COLUMBIA EAST RIDGE HOSPITAL (O, 128 beds) 941 Spring Creek Road, East Ridge, TN Zip 37412, Mailing Address: P.O. Box 91229, Zip 37412–6229; tel. 423/894–7870; Brenda M. Waltz, CHE, Chief Executive Officer

COLUMBIA HENDERSONVILLE HOSPITAL (O, 67 beds) 355 New Shackle Island Road, Hendersonville, TN Zip 37075–2393; tel. 615/264–4000; Ron Walker, Chief Executive Officer

COLUMBIA HILLSIDE HOSPITAL (O, 85 beds) 1265 East College Street, Pulaski, TN Zip 38478; tel. 615/363–7531; James H. Edmondson, Chief Executive Officer and Administrator

COLUMBIA HORIZON MEDICAL CENTER (O, 108 beds) 111 Highway 70 East, Dickson, TN Zip 37055–2079; tel. 615/441–2357; Rick Wallace, FACHE, Chief Executive Officer and Administrator

COLUMBIA JOHNSON CITY SPECIALTY HOSPITAL (O, 49 beds) 203 East Watauga Avenue, Johnson City, TN Zip 37601; tel. 615/926–1111; Lori Caudell Fatherree, Chief Executive Officer

COLUMBIA LIVINGSTON REGIONAL HOSPITAL (O, 85 beds) 315 Oak Street, Livingston, TN Zip 38570, Mailing Address: P.O. Box 550, Zip 38570; tel. 615/823–5611; Timothy W. McGill, Chief Executive Officer

COLUMBIA NASHVILLE MEMORIAL HOSPITAL (O, 250 beds) 612 West Due West Avenue, Madison, TN Zip 37115–4474; tel. 615/865–3511; Robert Benson, Chief Executive Officer

COLUMBIA NORTH SIDE HOSPITAL (O, 127 beds) 401 Princeton Road, Johnson City, TN Zip 37601, Mailing Address: P.O. Box 4900, Zip 37602; tel. 423/854–5900; John B. Crysel, Chief Executive Officer

COLUMBIA REGIONAL HOSPITAL OF JACKSON (O, 103 beds) 367 Hospital Boulevard, Jackson, TN Zip 38305–4518, Mailing Address: P.O. Box 3310, Zip 38303–0310; tel. 901/661–2000; Donald H. Wilkerson, Chief Executive Officer

COLUMBIA RIVER PARK HOSPITAL (O, 90 beds) 1559 Sparta Road, McMinnville, TN Zip 37110; tel. 615/815–4000; Jack S. Buck, Chief Executive Officer

COLUMBIA SMITH COUNTY MEMORIAL HOSPITAL (O, 53 beds) 158 Hospital Drive, Carthage, TN Zip 37030–1096; tel. 615/735–1560; Jerry H. Futrell, Chief Executive Officer

COLUMBIA SOUTH PITTSBURG HOSPITAL (O, 47 beds) 210 West 12th Street, South Pittsburg, TN Zip 37380, Mailing Address: P.O. Box 349, Zip 37380–0349; tel. 423/837–6781; Robert Klein, Chief Executive Officer

COLUMBIA SOUTHERN HILLS MEDICAL CENTER (O, 140 beds) 391 Wallace Road, Nashville, TN Zip 37211; tel. 615/781–4000; Lawrence L. Pieretti, Chief Executive Officer

COLUMBIA SOUTHERN TENNESSEE MEDICAL CENTER (O, 128 beds) 185 Hospital Road, Winchester, TN Zip 37398; tel. 615/967–8200; Michael W. Garfield, Administrator

COLUMBIA STONES RIVER HOSPITAL (O, 55 beds) 324 Doolittle Road, Woodbury, TN Zip 37190, Mailing Address: P.O. Box 458, Zip 37190–0458; tel. 615/563–4001; Terry J. Gunn, Administrator

COLUMBIA SUMMIT MEDICAL CENTER (O, 204 beds) 5655 Frist Boulevard, Hermitage, TN Zip 37076; tel. 615/316–3000; Bryan K. Dearing, Chief Executive Officer

COLUMBIA SYCAMORE SHOALS HOSPITAL (O, 112 beds) 1501 West Elk Avenue, Elizabethton, TN Zip 37643–1368; tel. 423/542–1300; Larry R. Jeter, Chief Executive Officer

COLUMBIA TRINITY HOSPITAL (O, 35 beds) 353 Main Street, Erin, TN Zip 37061, Mailing Address: P.O. Box 489, Zip 37061–0489; tel. 615/289–4211; Jay Woodall, Chief Executive Officer

COLUMBIA VALLEY HOSPITAL (O, 118 beds) 2200 Morris Hill Road, Chattanooga, TN Zip 37421; tel. 423/894–4220; Solon Boggus Jr., Chief Executive Officer

COLUMBIA VOLUNTEER GENERAL HOSPITAL (O, 65 beds) 161 Mount Pelia Road, Martin, TN Zip 38237, Mailing Address: Box 967, Zip 38237; tel. 901/587–4261; R. Coleman Foss, Chief Executive Officer

INDIAN PATH MEDICAL CENTER (O, 130 beds) 2000 Brookside Drive, Kingsport, TN Zip 37660–4604; tel. 615/392–7000; Robert Bauer, Chief Executive Officer

INDIAN PATH PAVILION (O, 26 beds) 2300 Pavilion Drive, Kingsport, TN Zip 37660–4672; tel. 615/378–7500; Robert Bauer, Chief Executive Officer

PARKRIDGE MEDICAL CENTER (O, 248 beds) 2333 McCallie Avenue, Chattanooga, TN Zip 37404–3285; tel. 423/698–6061; Solon Boggus Jr., Chief Executive Officer

PSYCHIATRIC HOSPITAL AT VANDERBILT (O, 88 beds) 1601 23rd Avenue South, Nashville, TN Zip 37212; tel. 615/320–7770; Richard A. Bangert, Chief Executive Officer and Administrator

TEXAS: AUSTIN DIAGNOSTIC MEDICAL CENTER (O, 114 beds) 12221 MoPac Expressway North, Austin, TX Zip 78758; tel. 512/901–1000; Richard E. Salerno, Chief Executive Officer

COLUMBIA ALICE PHYSICIANS AND SURGEONS HOSPITAL (O, 123 beds) 300 East Third Street, Alice, TX Zip 78332–4794; tel. 512/664–4376; Earl S. Whiteley, CHE, Chief Executive Officer

COLUMBIA ALVIN MEDICAL CENTER (O, 86 beds) 301 Medic Lane, Alvin, TX Zip 77511; tel. 713/331–6141; Donald A. Shaffett, Chief Executive Officer

COLUMBIA BAY AREA MEDICAL CENTER (O, 144 beds) 7101 South Padre Island Drive, Corpus Christi, TX Zip 78412; tel. 512/985–1200; Kirk G. Wilson, Chief Executive Officer

COLUMBIA BAYSHORE MEDICAL CENTER (O, 353 beds) 4000 Spencer Highway, Pasadena, TX Zip 77504–1294; tel. 713/944–6666; Russell Meyers, Chief Executive Officer

COLUMBIA BAYVIEW PSYCHIATRIC CENTER (O, 40 beds) 6226 Saratoga Boulevard, Corpus Christi, TX Zip 78414; tel. 512/993–9700; Janie L. Harwood, Chief Executive Officer

COLUMBIA BEAUMONT MEDICAL CENTER (O, 364 beds) 3080 College, Beaumont, TX Zip 77701, Mailing Address: P.O. Box 5817, Zip 77726–5817; tel. 409/833–1411; Luis G. Silva, Chief Executive Officer and Regional Administrator

COLUMBIA BEHAVIORAL CENTER (O, 43 beds) 1155 Idaho Street, El Paso, TX Zip 79902–1699; tel. 915/544–4000; Joan Courteau, Administrator

COLUMBIA BELLAIRE MEDICAL CENTER (O, 202 beds) 5314 Dashwood Street, Houston, TX Zip 77081–4689; tel. 713/512–1200; Walter Leleux, Chief Executive Officer

COLUMBIA BROWNWOOD REGIONAL MEDICAL CENTER (O, 164 beds) 1501 Burnet Drive, Brownwood, TX Zip 76801, Mailing Address: Box 760, Zip 76804; tel. 915/646–8541; Art Layne, Administrator and Chief Executive Officer

COLUMBIA CLEAR LAKE REGIONAL MEDICAL CENTER (O, 434 beds) 500 Medical Center Boulevard, Webster, TX Zip 77598; tel. 713/332–2511; Donald A. Shaffett, Chief Executive Officer

COLUMBIA CONROE REGIONAL MEDICAL CENTER (O, 242 beds) 504 Medical Boulevard, Conroe, TX Zip 77304, Mailing Address: P.O. Box 1538, Zip 77305–1538; tel. 409/539–1111; Larry Kloess, Chief Executive Officer

COLUMBIA DETAR HOSPITAL (O, 251 beds) 506 East San Antonio Street, Victoria, TX Zip 77901–6060, Mailing Address: Box 2089, Zip 77902–2089; tel. 512/575–7441; William R. Blanchard, Chief Executive Officer

COLUMBIA DOCTORS HOSPITAL AIRLINE (O, 114 beds) 5815 Airline Drive, Houston, TX Zip 77076; tel. 713/695–6041; Lee Brown, Administrator

For explanation of codes following names, see page B2.
★ Indicates Type III membership in the American Hospital Association.

Section B

COLUMBIA DOCTORS HOSPITAL EAST LOOP (O, 151 beds) 9339 North Loop East, Houston, TX Zip 77029, Mailing Address: Box 24216, Zip 77229; tel. 713/675–3241; John Styles Jr., Administrator

COLUMBIA DOCTORS HOSPITAL OF LAREDO (O, 107 beds) 500 East Mann Road, Laredo, TX Zip 78041; tel. 210/723–1131; Benjamin Everett, Chief Executive Officer

COLUMBIA DOCTORS REGIONAL MEDICAL CENTER (O, 237 beds) 3315 South Alameda, Corpus Christi, TX Zip 78411, Mailing Address: P.O. Box 3828, Zip 78463–3828; tel. 512/857–1501; Steven Woerner, Chief Executive Officer

COLUMBIA EAST HOUSTON MEDICAL CENTER (O, 136 beds) 13111 East Freeway, Houston, TX Zip 77015; tel. 713/455–6911; Mary Lee Walter, Chief Executive Officer

COLUMBIA FORT BEND HOSPITAL (O, 65 beds) 3803 FM 1092 at Highway 6, Missouri City, TX Zip 77459; tel. 713/499–4800; Janie R. Kauffman, Chief Executive Officer

COLUMBIA GULF COAST MEDICAL CENTER (O, 161 beds) 1400 Highway 59, Wharton, TX Zip 77488–3004, Mailing Address: P.O. Box 3004, Zip 77488–3004; tel. 409/532–2500; Michael D. Murphy, Chief Executive Officer

COLUMBIA HOSPITAL AT MEDICAL CITY DALLAS (O, 543 beds) 7777 Forest Lane, Dallas, TX Zip 75230–2598; tel. 972/566–7000; Stephen Corbeil, President and Chief Executive Officer

COLUMBIA KATY MEDICAL CENTER (O, 73 beds) 5602 Medical Center Drive, Katy, TX Zip 77494; tel. 713/392–1111; Brian S. Barbe, Chief Executive Officer

COLUMBIA KINGWOOD MEDICAL CENTER (O, 149 beds) 22999 U.S. Highway 59, Kingwood, TX Zip 77339; tel. 281/359–7500; Charles D. Schuetz, Chief Executive Officer

COLUMBIA LONGVIEW REGIONAL MEDICAL CENTER (O, 115 beds) 2901 North Fourth Street, Longview, TX Zip 75605, Mailing Address: P.O. Box 14000, Zip 75607–4000; tel. 903/758–1818; Velinda Stevens, Chief Executive Officer

COLUMBIA MAINLAND MEDICAL CENTER (O, 171 beds) 6801 E F Lowry Expressway, Texas City, TX Zip 77591; tel. 409/938–5000; Alice G. Adams, Administrator

COLUMBIA MEDICAL ARTS HOSPITAL (O, 30 beds) 6161 Harry Hines Boulevard, Dallas, TX Zip 75235; tel. 214/688–1111; Al Chapa, Chief Executive Officer

COLUMBIA MEDICAL CENTER (O, 106 beds) 1604 Rock Prairie Road, College Station, TX Zip 77845, Mailing Address: P.O. Box 10000, Zip 77842–3500; tel. 409/764–5100; Thomas W. Jackson, Chief Executive Officer

COLUMBIA MEDICAL CENTER AT LANCASTER (O, 76 beds) 2600 West Pleasant Run Road, Lancaster, TX Zip 75146–1199; tel. 214/223–9600; Ernest C. Lynch III, Chief Executive Officer

COLUMBIA MEDICAL CENTER AT TERRELL (O, 130 beds) 1551 Highway 34 South, Terrell, TX Zip 75160–4833; tel. 972/563–7611; I. Douglas Streckert, Chief Executive Officer

COLUMBIA MEDICAL CENTER OF ARLINGTON (O, 165 beds) 3301 Matlock Road, Arlington, TX Zip 76015; tel. 817/465–3241; John A. Fromhold, Chief Executive Officer

COLUMBIA MEDICAL CENTER OF DENTON (O, 271 beds) 4405 North Interstate 35, Denton, TX Zip 76207; tel. 817/566–4000; Bob J. Haley, Chief Executive Officer

COLUMBIA MEDICAL CENTER OF LEWISVILLE (O, 119 beds) 500 West Main, Lewisville, TX Zip 75057–3699; tel. 972/420–1000; Raymond M. Dunning Jr., Chief Executive Officer

COLUMBIA MEDICAL CENTER OF MCKINNEY (O, 150 beds) 1800 North Graves Street, McKinney, TX Zip 75069; tel. 214/548–3000; Don S. Ciulla, Chief Executive Officer

COLUMBIA MEDICAL CENTER OF PAMPA (O, 103 beds) One Medical Plaza, Pampa, TX Zip 79065; tel. 806/663–5500; J. Phillip Young, President and Chief Executive Officer

COLUMBIA MEDICAL CENTER OF PLANO (O, 259 beds) 3901 West 15th Street, Plano, TX Zip 75075–7799; tel. 214/596–6800; Harvey L. Fishero, President and Chief Executive Officer

COLUMBIA MEDICAL CENTER OF SAN ANGELO (O, 138 beds) 3501 Knickerbocker Road, San Angelo, TX Zip 76904–7698; tel. 915/949–9511; Gregory R. Angle, President and Chief Executive Officer

COLUMBIA MEDICAL CENTER OF SHERMAN (O, 160 beds) 1111 Gallagher Road, Sherman, TX Zip 75090; tel. 903/870–7000; John F. Adams, Chief Executive Officer

COLUMBIA MEDICAL CENTER–DALLAS SOUTHWEST (O, 104 beds) 2929 South Hampton Road, Dallas, TX Zip 75224; tel. 214/330–4611; James B. Warren, Chief Executive Officer

COLUMBIA MEDICAL CENTER–EAST (O, 40 beds) 300 Waymore, El Paso, TX Zip 77902; tel. 915/577–2600; William G. Collins, Chief Executive Officer

COLUMBIA MEDICAL CENTER–EAST (O, 290 beds) 10301 Gateway West, El Paso, TX Zip 79925–7798, Mailing Address: P.O. Box 937003, Zip 79937–1690; tel. 915/595–9000; Douglas A. Matney, Senior Vice President Operations

COLUMBIA MEDICAL CENTER–WEST (O, 221 beds) 1801 North Oregon Street, El Paso, TX Zip 79902; tel. 915/521–1776; Douglas A. Matney, Senior Vice President Operations

COLUMBIA NAVARRO REGIONAL HOSPITAL (O, 148 beds) 3201 West Highway 22, Corsicana, TX Zip 75110; tel. 903/872–4861; Nancy A. Byrnes, President and Chief Executive Officer

COLUMBIA NORTH BAY HOSPITAL (O, 69 beds) 1711 West Wheeler Avenue, Aransas Pass, TX Zip 78336; tel. 512/758–0502; Steve Sutherlin, Chief Executive Officer

COLUMBIA NORTH HILLS HOSPITAL (O, 134 beds) 4401 Booth Calloway Road, North Richland Hills, TX Zip 76180–7399; tel. 817/284–1431; Randy Moresi, Chief Executive Officer

COLUMBIA NORTH HOUSTON MEDICAL CENTER (O, 149 beds) 233 West Parker Road, Houston, TX Zip 77076; tel. 713/697–2831; Mel Bishop, Chief Executive Officer

COLUMBIA NORTHWEST HOSPITAL (O, 63 beds) 13725 Farm Road 624, Corpus Christi, TX Zip 78410; tel. 512/767–4500; Winston Borland, Chief Executive Officer

COLUMBIA PLAZA MEDICAL CENTER OF FORT WORTH (O, 289 beds) 900 Eighth Avenue, Fort Worth, TX Zip 76104–3986; tel. 817/336–2100; Stephen Bernstein, Chief Executive Officer

COLUMBIA REHABILITATION HOSPITAL (O, 40 beds) 6226 Saratoga Boulevard, Corpus Christi, TX Zip 78414–3499; tel. 512/991–9690; Jo Ann Baker, Chief Executive Officer

COLUMBIA RIO GRANDE REGIONAL HOSPITAL (O, 222 beds) 101 East Ridge Road, McAllen, TX Zip 78503; tel. 210/632–6000; Randall M. Everts, Chief Executive Officer

COLUMBIA ROSEWOOD MEDICAL CENTER (O, 184 beds) 9200 Westheimer Road, Houston, TX Zip 77063; tel. 713/780–7900; Pat Currie, Chief Executive Officer

COLUMBIA SILSBEE DOCTORS HOSPITAL (O, 59 beds) Highway 418, Silsbee, TX Zip 77656, Mailing Address: Box 1208, Zip 77656; tel. 409/385–5531; David Cottey, Chief Executive Officer

COLUMBIA SPECIALTY HOSPITAL AT MEDICAL ARTS (O, 32 beds) 6161 Harry Hines Boulevard, Dallas, TX Zip 75235–5306; tel. 214/689–8500; Tim Simmons, Chief Executive Officer

COLUMBIA SPRING BRANCH MEDICAL CENTER (O, 345 beds) 8850 Long Point Road, Houston, TX Zip 77055; tel. 713/467–6555; Sally E. Jeffcoat, President and Chief Executive Officer

COLUMBIA ST. DAVID'S SOUTH HOSPITAL (O, 164 beds) 901 West Ben White Boulevard, Austin, TX Zip 78704–6903; tel. 512/447–2211; Richard W. Klusmann, Chief Executive Officer

COLUMBIA TEXAS ORTHOPEDIC HOSPITAL (O, 49 beds) 7401 South Main Street, Houston, TX Zip 77030; tel. 713/799–8600; John J. Jackson, Chief Executive Officer

COLUMBIA VALLEY REGIONAL MEDICAL CENTER (O, 173 beds) 1 Ted Hunt Boulevard, Brownsville, TX Zip 78521, Mailing Address: Box 3710, Zip 78521; tel. 210/831–9611; Pete Delgado, Chief Executive Officer

COLUMBIA WEST HOUSTON MEDICAL CENTER (O, 169 beds) 12141 Richmond Avenue, Houston, TX Zip 77082–2499; tel. 281/558–3444; Janie R. Kauffman, Chief Executive Officer

For explanation of codes following names, see page B2.
★ Indicates Type III membership in the American Hospital Association.

COLUMBIA WOMAN'S HOSPITAL OF TEXAS (O, 148 beds) 7600 Fannin Street, Houston, TX Zip 77054–1900; tel. 713/790–1234; Linda B. Russell, Chief Executive Officer

COLUMBIA WOODLAND HEIGHTS MEDICAL CENTER (O, 110 beds) 500 Gaslight Boulevard, Lufkin, TX Zip 75901, Mailing Address: Box 150610, Zip 75915–0610; tel. 409/634–8311; Don H. McBride, Chief Executive Officer

DENTON COMMUNITY HOSPITAL (O, 110 beds) 207 North Bonnie Brae, Denton, TX Zip 76201; tel. 817/898–7000; Timothy Charles, Chief Executive Officer

MEDICAL ARTS HOSPITAL (O, 59 beds) 2501 College Drive, Texarkana, TX Zip 75501–2703, Mailing Address: P.O. Box 6045, Zip 75505–6045; tel. 903/798–5100; Jerry Kincade, Chief Executive Officer

METHODIST AMBULATORY SURGERY HOSPITAL (O, 37 beds) 9150 Huebner Road, San Antonio, TX Zip 78240–1545; tel. 210/561–7250; Elaine F. Morris, Administrator

METHODIST WOMEN'S AND CHILDREN'S HOSPITAL (O, 150 beds) 8109 Fredericksburg Road, San Antonio, TX Zip 78229–3383; tel. 210/692–5000; Janet Porter, President and Chief Executive Officer

METROPOLITAN METHODIST HOSPITAL (O, 232 beds) 1310 McCullough Avenue, San Antonio, TX Zip 78212–2617; tel. 210/208–2200; Mark L. Bernard, Chief Executive Officer

NORTHEAST METHODIST HOSPITAL (O, 117 beds) 12412 Judson Road, San Antonio, TX Zip 78233, Mailing Address: P.O. Box 659510, Zip 78265–9510; tel. 210/650–4949; Mark L. Bernard, Chief Executive Officer

ROUND ROCK HOSPITAL (O, 75 beds) 2400 Round Rock Avenue, Round Rock, TX Zip 78681; tel. 512/255–6066; Deborah L. Ryle, Chief Executive Officer

SAN ANTONIO COMMUNITY HOSPITAL (O, 297 beds) 8026 Floyd Curl Drive, San Antonio, TX Zip 78229–3915; tel. 210/692–8110; James C. Scoggin Jr., Chief Executive Officer

SOUTHWEST TEXAS METHODIST HOSPITAL (O, 585 beds) 7700 Floyd Curl Drive, San Antonio, TX Zip 78229–3993; tel. 210/692–4000; James C. Scoggin Jr., Chief Executive Officer

UTAH: CASTLEVIEW HOSPITAL (O, 84 beds) 300 North Hospital Drive, Price, UT Zip 84501; tel. 801/637–4800; L. Allen Penry, Chief Executive Officer

COLUMBIA ASHLEY VALLEY MEDICAL CENTER (O, 29 beds) 151 West 200 North, Vernal, UT Zip 84078; tel. 801/789–3342; Ronald J. Perry, Chief Executive Officer

COLUMBIA BRIGHAM CITY COMMUNITY HOSPITAL (O, 43 beds) 950 South 500 West, Brigham City, UT Zip 84302; tel. 801/734–9471; Tad A. Morley, Chief Executive Officer

COLUMBIA OGDEN REGIONAL MEDICAL CENTER (O, 179 beds) 5475 South 500 East, Ogden, UT Zip 84405–6978; tel. 801/479–2111; Steven B. Bateman, Chief Executive Officer

COLUMBIA ST. MARK'S HOSPITAL (O, 203 beds) 1200 East 3900 South, Salt Lake City, UT Zip 84124; tel. 801/268–7000; John Hanshaw, Chief Executive Officer

LAKEVIEW HOSPITAL (O, 128 beds) 630 East Medical Drive, Bountiful, UT Zip 84010–4996; tel. 801/292–6231; Craig Preston, Chief Executive Officer

MOUNTAIN VIEW HOSPITAL (O, 127 beds) 1000 East 100 North, Payson, UT Zip 84651–1690; tel. 801/465–7101; Kevin Johnson, Chief Executive Officer

VIRGINIA: CHIPPENHAM AND JOHNSTON–WILLIS HOSPITALS (O, 688 beds) 7101 Jahnke Road, Richmond, VA Zip 23225; tel. 804/320–3911; Gerard Filicko, Chief Executive Officer

COLUMBIA ALLEGHANY REGIONAL HOSPITAL (O, 196 beds) One ARH Lane, Low Moor, VA Zip 24457, Mailing Address: P.O. Box 7, Zip 24457–0007; tel. 540/862–6200; Ward W. Stevens, CHE, Chief Executive Officer

COLUMBIA CLINCH VALLEY MEDICAL CENTER (O, 200 beds) 2949 West Front Street, Richlands, VA Zip 24641; tel. 540/596–6000; James W. Thweatt, Chief Executive Officer

COLUMBIA JOHN RANDOLPH MEDICAL CENTER (O, 271 beds) 411 West Randolph Road, Hopewell, VA Zip 23860, Mailing Address: P.O. Box 971, Zip 23860; tel. 804/541–1600; Daniel J. Wetta Jr., Chief Executive Officer

COLUMBIA LEWIS–GALE MEDICAL CENTER (O, 521 beds) 1900 Electric Road, Salem, VA Zip 24153; tel. 540/776–4000; William B. Downey, Administrator

COLUMBIA MONTGOMERY REGIONAL HOSPITAL (O, 104 beds) 3700 South Main Street, Blacksburg, VA Zip 24060, Mailing Address: P.O. Box 90004, Zip 24062–9004; tel. 540/953–5101; David R. Williams, Chief Executive Officer

COLUMBIA PENINSULA CENTER FOR BEHAVIORAL HEALTH (O, 125 beds) 2244 Executive Drive, Hampton, VA Zip 23666; tel. 804/827–1001; Rufus S. Hoefer, Administrator

COLUMBIA PULASKI COMMUNITY HOSPITAL (O, 74 beds) 2400 Lee Highway, Pulaski, VA Zip 24301, Mailing Address: P.O. Box 759, Zip 24301–0759; tel. 540/994–8100; Christopher W. Dux, Chief Executive Officer

COLUMBIA RESTON HOSPITAL CENTER (O, 127 beds) 1850 Town Center Parkway, Reston, VA Zip 20190; tel. 703/689–9023; Thomas D. Miller, President and Chief Executive Officer

DOMINION HOSPITAL (O, 100 beds) 2960 Sleepy Hollow Road, Falls Church, VA Zip 22044–2001; tel. 703/536–2000; Barbara D. S. Hekimian, Chief Executive Officer

HENRICO DOCTORS' HOSPITAL (O, 340 beds) 1602 Skipwith Road, Richmond, VA Zip 23229; tel. 804/289–4500; Patrick W. Farrell, Chief Executive Officer

NATIONAL HOSPITAL MEDICAL CENTER (C, 102 beds) 2455 Army Navy Drive, Arlington, VA Zip 22206; tel. 703/920–6700; Ronald E. Yates, Chief Executive Officer

RETREAT HOSPITAL (O, 146 beds) 2621 Grove Avenue, Richmond, VA Zip 23220–4308; tel. 804/254–5100; Paul L. Baldwin, Chief Operating Officer

WASHINGTON: COLUMBIA CAPITAL MEDICAL CENTER (O, 104 beds) 3900 Capital Mall Drive S.W., Olympia, WA Zip 98502–8654, Mailing Address: P.O. Box 19002, Zip 98507–0013; tel. 360/754–5858; Garry L. Gause, Chief Executive Officer

WEST VIRGINIA: COLUMBIA RALEIGH GENERAL HOSPITAL (O, 251 beds) 1710 Harper Road, Beckley, WV Zip 25801–3397; tel. 304/256–4100; Brent A. Marsteller, Chief Executive Officer

COLUMBIA RIVER PARK HOSPITAL (O, 165 beds) 1230 Sixth Avenue, Huntington, WV Zip 25701, Mailing Address: Box 1875, Zip 25719; tel. 304/526–9111; Scott C. Stamm, Chief Executive Officer

COLUMBIA ST. LUKE'S HOSPITAL (O, 79 beds) 1333 Southview Drive, Bluefield, WV Zip 24701, Mailing Address: P.O. Box 1190, Zip 24701; tel. 304/327–2900; Barry A. Papania, Chief Executive Officer

GREENBRIER VALLEY MEDICAL CENTER (O, 122 beds) 202 Maplewood Avenue, Ronceverte, WV Zip 24970–0497, Mailing Address: P.O. Box 497, Zip 24970–0497; tel. 304/647–4411; James B. Wood, Chief Executive Officer

PUTNAM GENERAL HOSPITAL (O, 66 beds) 1400 Hospital Drive, Hurricane, WV Zip 25526–9210, Mailing Address: P.O. Box 900, Zip 25526–0900; tel. 304/757–1700; Patsy Hardy, Administrator

SAINT FRANCIS HOSPITAL (O, 155 beds) 333 Laidley Street, Charleston, WV Zip 25301, Mailing Address: Box 471, Zip 25322; tel. 304/347–6500; David R. Sirk, President and Chief Executive Officer

WYOMING: COLUMBIA RIVERTON MEMORIAL HOSPITAL (O, 59 beds) 2100 West Sunset Drive, Riverton, WY Zip 82501; tel. 307/856–4161; Kenneth H. Armstrong, Chief Executive Officer

Owned, leased, sponsored:	322 hospitals	55337 beds
Contract–managed:	1 hospital	102 beds
Totals:	323 hospitals	55439 beds

★**0003: COLUMBIA/ST. DAVID'S MEDICAL CENTER** (IO)
919 East 32nd Street, Austin, TX Zip 78705, Mailing Address: P.O. Box 4039, Zip 78765; tel. 512/397–4265; Cole C. Eslyn, Chief Executive Officer

TEXAS: COLUMBIA ST. DAVID'S HOSPITAL (O, 296 beds) 919 East 32nd Street, Austin, TX Zip 78705, Mailing Address: Box 4039, Zip 78765–4039; tel. 512/476–7111; Cole C. Eslyn, Chief Executive Officer

ST. DAVID'S PAVILION (O, 38 beds) 1025 East 32nd Street, Austin, TX Zip 78765; tel. 512/867–5800; Cole C. Eslyn, Chief Executive Officer

For explanation of codes following names, see page B2.
★ Indicates Type III membership in the American Hospital Association.

Section B

ST. DAVID'S REHABILITATION CENTER (O, 104 beds) 1005 East 32nd Street, Austin, TX Zip 78705, Mailing Address: P.O. Box 4270, Zip 78765–4270; tel. 512/867–5100; Cole C. Eslyn, Chief Executive Officer

Owned, leased, sponsored:	3 hospitals	438 beds
Contract–managed:	0 hospitals	0 beds
Totals:	3 hospitals	438 beds

0215: COMMUNITY CARE SYSTEMS, INC. (IO)

15 Walnut Street, Wellesley Hills, MA Zip 02181–0001; tel. 617/431–3000; Frederick J. Thacher, Chairman

MAINE: JACKSON BROOK INSTITUTE (O, 106 beds) 175 Running Hill Road, South Portland, ME Zip 04106; tel. 207/761–2200; Vincent Furey, President

MASSACHUSETTS: CHARLES RIVER HOSPITAL (O, 62 beds) 203 Grove Street, Wellesley, MA Zip 02181; tel. 617/235–8400; Juliette Fay, President and Chief Executive Officer

CHARLES RIVER HOSPITAL–WEST (O, 90 beds) 350 Memorial Drive, Chicopee, MA Zip 01020–5025; tel. 413/594–2211; Robert W. Spiegel, President and Chief Executive Officer

Owned, leased, sponsored:	3 hospitals	258 beds
Contract–managed:	0 hospitals	0 beds
Totals:	3 hospitals	258 beds

0080: COMMUNITY HEALTH SYSTEMS, INC. (IO)

155 Franklin Road, Suite 400, Brentwood, TN Zip 37027–4600, Mailing Address: P.O. Box 217, Zip 37024–0217; tel. 615/373–9600; Wayne T. Smith, President

ALABAMA: EDGE REGIONAL MEDICAL CENTER (O, 87 beds) 1330 Highway 231 South, Troy, AL Zip 36081–1224; tel. 334/670–5000; David E. Loving, Chief Executive Officer

HARTSELLE MEDICAL CENTER (O, 150 beds) 201 Pine Street N.W., Hartselle, AL Zip 35640, Mailing Address: P.O. Box 969, Zip 35640; tel. 205/773–6511; Mike H. McNair, Chief Executive Officer

L. V. STABLER MEMORIAL HOSPITAL (O, 74 beds) Highway 10 West, Greenville, AL Zip 36037–0915, Mailing Address: Box 1000, Zip 36037–0915; tel. 334/382–2676; Dwayne Moss, Administrator

PARKWAY MEDICAL CENTER HOSPITAL (O, 94 beds) 1874 Beltline Road S.W., Decatur, AL Zip 35601, Mailing Address: P.O. Box 2211, Zip 35609; tel. 205/350–2211; Philip J. Mazzuca, Executive Director

WOODLAND COMMUNITY HOSPITAL (O, 67 beds) 1910 Cherokee Avenue S.E., Cullman, AL Zip 35055; tel. 205/739–3500; Lowell Benton, Executive Director

ARKANSAS: HARRIS HOSPITAL (O, 88 beds) 1205 McLain Street, Newport, AR Zip 72112; tel. 501/523–8911; Timothy E. Schmidt, Interim Chief Executive Officer

RANDOLPH COUNTY MEDICAL CENTER (L, 50 beds) 2801 Medical Center Drive, Pocahontas, AR Zip 72455; tel. 501/892–4511; Brad S. Morse, Executive Director

CALIFORNIA: BARSTOW COMMUNITY HOSPITAL (L, 56 beds) 555 South Seventh Avenue, Barstow, CA Zip 92311; tel. 619/256–1761; Russell V. Judd, Chief Executive Officer

FLORIDA: DOCTORS MEMORIAL HOSPITAL (L, 34 beds) 401 East Byrd Avenue, Bonifay, FL Zip 32425, Mailing Address: Box 188, Zip 32425; tel. 904/547–1120; Dale Larson, Executive Director

NORTH OKALOOSA MEDICAL CENTER (O, 91 beds) 151 Redstone Avenue S.E., Crestview, FL Zip 32539–6026; tel. 904/689–8100; Roger L. Hall, Chief Executive Officer

GEORGIA: BERRIEN COUNTY HOSPITAL (O, 155 beds) 1221 East McPherson Street, Nashville, GA Zip 31639, Mailing Address: P.O. Box 665, Zip 31639; tel. 912/686–7471; James P. Seward Jr., Executive Director

FANNIN REGIONAL HOSPITAL (O, 46 beds) Highway 5 North, Blue Ridge, GA Zip 30513, Mailing Address: Box 1549, Zip 30513; tel. 706/632–3711; Kent W. McMackin, Chief Executive Officer

ILLINOIS: CROSSROADS COMMUNITY HOSPITAL (O, 49 beds) 8 Doctors Park Road, Mount Vernon, IL Zip 62864; tel. 618/244–5500; Edward Cunningham, Executive Director

MARION MEMORIAL HOSPITAL (L, 84 beds) 917 West Main Street, Marion, IL Zip 62959; tel. 618/997–5341; Edward Cunningham, Interim Administrator

KENTUCKY: KENTUCKY RIVER MEDICAL CENTER (L, 55 beds) 540 Jett Drive, Jackson, KY Zip 41339–9620; tel. 606/666–4971; O. David Bevins, Chief Executive Officer

PARKWAY REGIONAL HOSPITAL (O, 70 beds) 2000 Holiday Lane, Fulton, KY Zip 42041; tel. 502/472–2522; Mary Jo Lewis, Chief Executive Officer

THREE RIVERS MEDICAL CENTER (O, 90 beds) Highway 644, Louisa, KY Zip 41230, Mailing Address: Box 769, Zip 41230; tel. 606/638–9451; Greg Kiser, Chief Executive Officer

LOUISIANA: BYRD REGIONAL HOSPITAL (O, 59 beds) 1020 Fertitta Boulevard, Leesville, LA Zip 71446; tel. 318/239–9041; Donald Henderson, Executive Director

RIVER WEST MEDICAL CENTER (O, 119 beds) 59355 River West Drive, Plaquemine, LA Zip 70764–9543; tel. 504/687–9222; Steve Grimm, Chief Executive Officer

RIVERNORTH HOSPITAL (O, 53 beds) 5505 Shreveport Highway, Pineville, LA Zip 71360; tel. 318/640–0222; Daniel W. Johnson, Chief Executive Officer

SABINE MEDICAL CENTER (O, 68 beds) 240 Highland Drive, Many, LA Zip 71449–3718; tel. 318/256–5691; Mark Nosacka, Executive Director

MISSOURI: MOBERLY REGIONAL MEDICAL CENTER (O, 93 beds) 1515 Union Avenue, Moberly, MO Zip 65270–9449, Mailing Address: P.O. Box 3000, Zip 65270–3000; tel. 816/263–8400; Daniel E. McKay, Executive Director

NEW MEXICO: MIMBRES MEMORIAL HOSPITAL (L, 119 beds) 900 West Ash Street, Deming, NM Zip 88030; tel. 505/546–2761; Harley Smith, Chief Executive Officer

SOUTH CAROLINA: CHESTERFIELD GENERAL HOSPITAL (O, 67 beds) Highway 9, Cheraw, SC Zip 29520, Mailing Address: Box 151, Zip 29520–0151; tel. 803/537–7881; Chris Wolf, Chief Executive Officer

MARLBORO PARK HOSPITAL (O, 108 beds) 1138 Cheraw Highway, Bennettsville, SC Zip 29512–0738, Mailing Address: Box 738, Zip 29512–0738; tel. 803/479–2881; Stephen Chapman, Executive Director

SPRINGS MEMORIAL HOSPITAL (O, 137 beds) 800 West Meeting Street, Lancaster, SC Zip 29720; tel. 803/286–1214; Robert M. Luther, Executive Director

TENNESSEE: CLEVELAND COMMUNITY HOSPITAL (O, 70 beds) 2800 Westside Drive N.W., Cleveland, TN Zip 37312; tel. 423/339–4100; Phil Rowland, Administrator

LAKEWAY REGIONAL HOSPITAL (O, 135 beds) 726 McFarland Street, Morristown, TN Zip 37814–3990; tel. 615/586–2302; Brian E. Dunn, Chief Executive Officer

SCOTT COUNTY HOSPITAL (L, 91 beds) U.S. Highway 27, Oneida, TN Zip 37841–4939, Mailing Address: Box 4939, Zip 37841–4939; tel. 615/569–8521; William N. Grey, Chief Executive Officer

WHITE COUNTY COMMUNITY HOSPITAL (O, 60 beds) 401 Sewell Road, Sparta, TN Zip 38583; tel. 615/738–9211; Raymond W. Acker, Administrator

TEXAS: CLEVELAND REGIONAL MEDICAL CENTER (O, 115 beds) 300 East Crockett Street, Cleveland, TX Zip 77327, Mailing Address: Box 1688, Zip 77328; tel. 713/593–1811; A. C. Buchanon, Administrator

HIGHLAND MEDICAL CENTER (O, 76 beds) 2412 50th Street, Lubbock, TX Zip 79412; tel. 806/788–4060; David Conejo, Chief Executive Officer

HILL REGIONAL HOSPITAL (O, 73 beds) 101 Circle Drive, Hillsboro, TX Zip 76645; tel. 817/582–8425; Jan McClure, Chief Executive Officer

HOOD GENERAL HOSPITAL (L, 49 beds) 1310 Paluxy Road, Granbury, TX Zip 76048; tel. 817/573–2683; John V. Villanueva, Chief Executive Officer

NORTHEAST MEDICAL CENTER (O, 46 beds) 504 Lipscomb Boulevard, Bonham, TX Zip 75418–4096, Mailing Address: P.O. Drawer C, Zip 75418; tel. 903/583–8585; Kathleen G. Northcutt, Interim Chief Executive Officer

SCENIC MOUNTAIN MEDICAL CENTER (O, 113 beds) 1601 West 11th Place, Big Spring, TX Zip 79720; tel. 915/263–1211; Kenneth W. Randall, Administrator

For explanation of codes following names, see page B2.
★ Indicates Type III membership in the American Hospital Association.

VIRGINIA: RUSSELL COUNTY MEDICAL CENTER (O, 78 beds) Carroll and Tate Streets, Lebanon, VA Zip 24266; tel. 540/889–1224; Jerry E. Lowery, Executive Director

Owned, leased, sponsored:	37 hospitals	3069 beds
Contract–managed:	0 hospitals	0 beds
Totals:	37 hospitals	3069 beds

1085: COMMUNITY HOSPITALS OF CENTRAL CALIFORNIA (NP)
Fresno and R Streets, Fresno, CA Zip 93721, Mailing Address: P.O. Box 1232, Zip 93721; tel. 209/442–6000; Philip Hinton, Chief Executive Officer

CALIFORNIA: CLOVIS COMMUNITY HOSPITAL (O, 143 beds) 2755 Herndon Avenue, Clovis, CA Zip 93611; tel. 209/323–4060; Mike Barber, Facility Service Integrator

FRESNO COMMUNITY HOSPITAL AND MEDICAL CENTER (O, 375 beds) Fresno and R Streets, Fresno, CA Zip 93721, Mailing Address: Box 1232, Zip 93715; tel. 209/442–6000; J. Philip Hinton, M.D., Chief Executive Officer

Owned, leased, sponsored:	2 hospitals	518 beds
Contract–managed:	0 hospitals	0 beds
Totals:	2 hospitals	518 beds

5695: CONGREGATION OF ST. AGNES (CC)
475 Gillett Street, Fond Du Lac, WI Zip 54935–4598; tel. 414/923–0804; Rosann Geiser, Corporate Director

WISCONSIN: AGNESIAN HEALTHCARE (S, 161 beds) 430 East Division Street, Fond Du Lac, WI Zip 54935–0385; tel. 414/929–2300; Robert A. Fale, President

THE MONROE CLINIC (S, 117 beds) 515 22nd Avenue, Monroe, WI Zip 53566–1598; tel. 608/324–1000; Kenneth Blount, President

WAUPUN MEMORIAL HOSPITAL (S, 49 beds) 620 West Brown Street, Waupun, WI Zip 53963–1799; tel. 414/324–5581; James E. Baer, FACHE, President and Administrator

Owned, leased, sponsored:	3 hospitals	327 beds
Contract–managed:	0 hospitals	0 beds
Totals:	3 hospitals	327 beds

0014: CONNECTICUT STATE DEPARTMENT OF MENTAL HEALTH (NP)
90 Washington Street, Hartford, CT Zip 06106; tel. 203/566–3650; Albert J. Solnit, M.D., Commissioner

CONNECTICUT: CEDARCREST REGIONAL HOSPITAL (O, 146 beds) 525 Russell Road, Newington, CT Zip 06111–1595; tel. 203/666–4613; David E. K. Hunter, Ph.D., Superintendent

CONNECTICUT MENTAL HEALTH CENTER (O, 49 beds) 34 Park Street, New Haven, CT Zip 06519, Mailing Address: Box 1842, Zip 06508–1842; tel. 203/789–7290; Selby Jacobs, M.D., M.P.H., Director

CONNECTICUT VALLEY HOSPITAL (O, 418 beds) Eastern Drive, Middletown, CT Zip 06457–7023, Mailing Address: P.O. Box 351, Zip 06457–7023; Garrell S. Mullaney, Superintendent

GREATER BRIDGEPORT COMMUNITY MENTAL HEALTH CENTER (O, 62 beds) 1635 Central Avenue, Bridgeport, CT Zip 06610–0902, Mailing Address: Box 5117, Zip 06610; tel. 203/579–6646; James M. Lehane III, Director

Owned, leased, sponsored:	4 hospitals	675 beds
Contract–managed:	0 hospitals	0 beds
Totals:	4 hospitals	675 beds

1715: CONTINENTAL MEDICAL SYSTEMS, INC. (IO)
600 Wilson Lane, Mechanicsburg, PA Zip 17055–0715, Mailing Address: P.O. Box 715, Zip 17055–0715; tel. 717/790–8300; Robert Ortenzio, President and Chief Executive Officer

ARKANSAS: NORTHWEST ARKANSAS REHABILITATION HOSPITAL (O, 60 beds) 153 Monte Painter Drive, Fayetteville, AR Zip 72703; tel. 501/444–2200; Dennis R. Shelby, Chief Executive Officer

ST. VINCENT–NORTH REHABILITATION HOSPITAL (O, 60 beds) 2201 Wildwood Avenue, Sherwood, AR Zip 72120–5074, Mailing Address: P.O. Box 6930, Zip 72124–6930; tel. 501/834–1800; Douglas W. Parker, Chief Executive Officer

CALIFORNIA: KENTFIELD REHABILITATION HOSPITAL (O, 60 beds) 1125 Sir Francis Drake Boulevard, Kentfield, CA Zip 94904, Mailing Address: P.O. Box 338, Zip 94914–0338; tel. 415/456–9680; John Behrmann, Administrator and Chief Executive Officer

KANSAS: WESLEY REHABILITATION HOSPITAL (O, 65 beds) 8338 West 13th Street North, Wichita, KS Zip 67212–2984; tel. 316/729–9999; Joseph F. Pitingolo Jr., Chief Executive Officer

MASSACHUSETTS: BRAINTREE HOSPITAL REHABILITATION NETWORK (O, 187 beds) 250 Pond Street, Braintree, MA Zip 02185; tel. 617/848–5353; Ernest J. Broadbent, President and Chief Executive Officer

TENNESSEE: BAPTIST REHABILITATION–GERMANTOWN (C, 85 beds) 2100 Exeter Road, Germantown, TN Zip 38138; tel. 901/757–1350; B. Richard Moseley, Chief Executive Officer

TEXAS: SOUTHEAST TEXAS REHABILITATION HOSPITAL (O, 60 beds) 3340 Plaza 10 Boulevard, Beaumont, TX Zip 77707; tel. 409/835–0835; David J. Holly, Chief Executive Officer

Owned, leased, sponsored:	6 hospitals	492 beds
Contract–managed:	1 hospital	85 beds
Totals:	7 hospitals	577 beds

•★0098: CONTINUUM (NP)
111 Cedar Street, Kendallville, IN Zip 46755, Mailing Address: P.O. Box 249, Zip 46755; tel. 219/347–6344; John Berhow, President

INDIANA: MCCRAY MEMORIAL HOSPITAL (O, 51 beds) 951 East Hospital Drive, Kendallville, IN Zip 46755, Mailing Address: P.O. Box 249, Zip 46755; tel. 219/347–1100; Peter A. Marotti, Chief Executive Officer

Owned, leased, sponsored:	1 hospital	51 beds
Contract–managed:	0 hospitals	0 beds
Totals:	1 hospital	51 beds

0016: COOK COUNTY BUREAU OF HEALTH SERVICES (NP)
1835 West Harrison Street, Chicago, IL Zip 60612; tel. 312/633–8533; Ruth M. Rothstein, Chief

ILLINOIS: COOK COUNTY HOSPITAL (O, 770 beds) 1835 West Harrison Street, Chicago, IL Zip 60612; tel. 312/633–6000; Ruth M. Rothstein, Hospital Director

OAK FOREST HOSPITAL OF COOK COUNTY (O, 627 beds) 15900 South Cicero Avenue, Oak Forest, IL Zip 60452; tel. 708/687–7200; Cynthia T. Henderson, M.D., M.P.H., Interim Hospital Director

PROVIDENT HOSPITAL OF COOK COUNTY (O, 100 beds) 500 East 51st Street, Chicago, IL Zip 60615; tel. 773/572–1200; Shirley Bomar–Cole, Chief Operating Officer

Owned, leased, sponsored:	3 hospitals	1497 beds
Contract–managed:	0 hospitals	0 beds
Totals:	3 hospitals	1497 beds

0103: COTTAGE HEALTH SYSTEM (NP)
Pueblo at Bath Streets, Santa Barbara, CA Zip 93102, Mailing Address: P.O. Box 689, Zip 93102; tel. 805/682–7111; James L. Ash, President and Chief Executive Officer

CALIFORNIA: GOLETA VALLEY COTTAGE HOSPITAL (O, 79 beds) 351 South Patterson Avenue, Santa Barbara, CA Zip 93111, Mailing Address: Box 6306, Zip 93160; tel. 805/967–3411; Diane Wisby, Vice President

SANTA BARBARA COTTAGE HOSPITAL (O, 307 beds) Pueblo at Bath Streets, Santa Barbara, CA Zip 93105, Mailing Address: Box 689, Zip 93102; tel. 805/682–7111; James L. Ash, President and Chief Executive Officer

For explanation of codes following names, see page B2.
★ Indicates Type III membership in the American Hospital Association.
• Single hospital health care system

SANTA YNEZ VALLEY COTTAGE HOSPITAL (O, 20 beds) 700 Alamo Pintado Road, Solvang, CA Zip 93463; tel. 805/688–6431; Bobbie Kline, R.N., Vice President

Owned, leased, sponsored:	3 hospitals	406 beds
Contract–managed:	0 hospitals	0 beds
Totals:	3 hospitals	406 beds

★5885: **COVENANT HEALTH SYSTEMS, INC.** (CC)
420 Bedford Street, Lexington, MA Zip 02173–1502; tel. 617/862–1634; David R. Lincoln, President and Chief Executive Officer

MAINE: ST. MARY'S REGIONAL MEDICAL CENTER (O, 173 beds) 45 Golder Street, Lewiston, ME Zip 04240, Mailing Address: P.O. Box 291, Zip 04243–0291; tel. 207/777–8100; James E. Cassidy, President and Chief Executive Officer

MASSACHUSETTS: YOUVILLE LIFECARE (O, 286 beds) 1575 Cambridge Street, Cambridge, MA Zip 02138–4398; tel. 617/876–4344; T. Richard Quigley, President and Chief Executive Officer

NEW HAMPSHIRE: ST. JOSEPH HEALTHCARE (O, 208 beds) 172 Kinsley Street, Nashua, NH Zip 03061, Mailing Address: Caller Service 2013, Zip 03061; tel. 603/882–3000; Peter B. Davis, President and Chief Executive Officer

Owned, leased, sponsored:	3 hospitals	667 beds
Contract–managed:	0 hospitals	0 beds
Totals:	3 hospitals	667 beds

★0008: **CROZER–KEYSTONE HEALTH SYSTEM** (NP)
1400 North Providence Road, Suite 4010, Media, PA Zip 19063–2049; tel. 610/892–8000; John C. McMeekin, President and Chief Executive Officer

PENNSYLVANIA: COMMUNITY HOSPITAL, DIVISION OF THE CROZER–CHESTER MEDICAL CENTER (O, 184 beds) Ninth and Wilson Streets, Chester, PA Zip 19013; tel. 610/494–0700

CROZER–CHESTER MEDICAL CENTER (O, 527 beds) One Medical Center Boulevard, Upland, PA Zip 19013–3995; tel. 610/447–2000; Joan K. Richards, President

DELAWARE COUNTY MEMORIAL HOSPITAL (O, 251 beds) 501 North Lansdowne Avenue, Drexel Hill, PA Zip 19026–1186; tel. 610/284–8100; Joan K. Richards, President

SPRINGFIELD HOSPITAL (O, 70 beds) 190 West Sproul Road, Springfield, PA Zip 19064–2097; tel. 610/328–8700

Owned, leased, sponsored:	4 hospitals	1032 beds
Contract–managed:	0 hospitals	0 beds
Totals:	4 hospitals	1032 beds

★1855: **DAUGHTERS OF CHARITY NATIONAL HEALTH SYSTEM** (CC)
4600 Edmundson Road, Saint Louis, MO Zip 63134, Mailing Address: P.O. Box 45998, Zip 63145–5998; tel. 314/253–6700; Donald A. Brennan, President and Chief Executive Officer

ALABAMA: PROVIDENCE HOSPITAL (S, 349 beds) 6801 Airport Boulevard, Mobile, AL Zip 36608, Mailing Address: P.O. Box 850429, Zip 36685; tel. 334/633–1000; John R. Roeder, President

ST. VINCENT'S HOSPITAL (S, 338 beds) 810 St. Vincent's Drive, Birmingham, AL Zip 35205, Mailing Address: P.O. Box 12407, Zip 35202–2407; tel. 205/939–7000; Vincent C. Caponi, President and Chief Executive Officer

CONNECTICUT: ST. VINCENT'S MEDICAL CENTER (S, 289 beds) 2800 Main Street, Bridgeport, CT Zip 06606–4292; tel. 203/576–6000; William J. Riordan, President and Chief Executive Officer

DISTRICT OF COLUMBIA: PROVIDENCE HOSPITAL (S, 556 beds) 1150 Varnum Street N.E., Washington, DC Zip 20017–2180; tel. 202/269–7000; Sister Carol Keehan, President

FLORIDA: SACRED HEART HOSPITAL OF PENSACOLA (S, 520 beds) 5151 North Ninth Avenue, Pensacola, FL Zip 32504, Mailing Address: P.O. Box 2700, Zip 32513–2700; tel. 904/416–7000; Patrick J. Madden, President and Chief Executive Officer

ST. VINCENT'S MEDICAL CENTER (S, 756 beds) 1800 Barrs Street, Jacksonville, FL Zip 32204, Mailing Address: P.O. Box 2982, Zip 32203–2982; tel. 904/308–7300; John W. Logue, Executive Vice President and Chief Operating Officer

INDIANA: SAINT JOSEPH HOSPITAL & HEALTH CENTER (S, 157 beds) 1907 West Sycamore Street, Kokomo, IN Zip 46904–9010; tel. 765/456–5300; Kathleen Korbelak, President and Chief Executive Officer

ST. MARY'S HOSPITAL WARRICK (S, 36 beds) 1116 Millis Avenue, Boonville, IN Zip 47601–0629, Mailing Address: Box 629, Zip 47601–0629; tel. 812/897–4800; John D. O'Neil, Executive Vice President and Administrator

ST. MARY'S MEDICAL CENTER OF EVANSVILLE (S, 549 beds) 3700 Washington Avenue, Evansville, IN Zip 47750; tel. 812/485–4000; Richard C. Breon, President and Chief Executive Officer

ST. VINCENT HOSPITALS AND HEALTH SERVICES (S, 427 beds) 2001 West 86th Street, Indianapolis, IN Zip 46260, Mailing Address: Box 40970, Zip 46240–0970; tel. 317/338–2345; Douglas D. French, President and Chief Executive Officer

MARYLAND: SACRED HEART HOSPITAL (S, 272 beds) 900 Seton Drive, Cumberland, MD Zip 21502–1874; tel. 301/759–4200; Edward M. Dinan, President and Chief Executive Officer

ST. AGNES HEALTHCARE (S, 422 beds) 900 Caton Avenue, Baltimore, MD Zip 21229–5299; tel. 410/368–6000; Robert E. Pezzoli, President and Chief Executive Officer

MICHIGAN: PROVIDENCE HOSPITAL AND MEDICAL CENTERS (S, 351 beds) 16001 West Nine Mile Road, Southfield, MI Zip 48075–4854, Mailing Address: Box 2043, Zip 48037–2043; tel. 810/424–3000; Brian M. Connolly, President and Chief Executive Officer

ST. MARY'S MEDICAL CENTER (S, 268 beds) 830 South Jefferson Avenue, Saginaw, MI Zip 48601–2594; tel. 517/776–8000; Frederic L. Fraizer, President and Chief Executive Officer

NEW YORK: OUR LADY OF LOURDES MEMORIAL HOSPITAL (S, 170 beds) 169 Riverside Drive, Binghamton, NY Zip 13905–4198; tel. 607/798–5328; Michael G. Guley, President and Chief Executive Officer

SETON HEALTH SYSTEM (S, 344 beds) 1300 Massachusetts Avenue, Troy, NY Zip 12180; tel. 518/272–5000; Edward G. Murphy, M.D., President and Chief Executive Officer

SISTERS OF CHARITY HOSPITAL OF BUFFALO (S, 493 beds) 2157 Main Street, Buffalo, NY Zip 14214–2692; tel. 716/862–1000; John J. Maher, President and Chief Executive Officer

ST. MARY'S HOSPITAL (S, 190 beds) 89 Genesee Street, Rochester, NY Zip 14611–3285; tel. 716/464–3000; Stewart Putnam, President

PENNSYLVANIA: GOOD SAMARITAN REGIONAL MEDICAL CENTER (S, 197 beds) 700 East Norwegian Street, Pottsville, PA Zip 17901–2798; tel. 717/621–4000; Gino J. Pazzaglini, President and Chief Executive Officer

TENNESSEE: ST. THOMAS HOSPITAL (S, 514 beds) 4220 Harding Road, Nashville, TN Zip 37205, Mailing Address: Box 380, Zip 37202; tel. 615/222–2111; John F. Tighe, President and Chief Executive Officer

TEXAS: BRACKENRIDGE HOSPITAL (L, 291 beds) 601 East 15th Street, Austin, TX Zip 78701; tel. 512/476–6461; Charles J. Barnett, President

PROVIDENCE HEALTH CENTER (S, 200 beds) 6901 Medical Parkway, Waco, TX Zip 76712, Mailing Address: P.O. Box 2589, Zip 76702–2589; tel. 817/751–4000; Kent A. Keahey, President

SETON MEDICAL CENTER (S, 472 beds) 1201 West 38th Street, Austin, TX Zip 78705–1056; tel. 512/323–1000; Charles J. Barnett, President

WISCONSIN: ST. MARY'S HOSPITAL (S, 257 beds) 2323 North Lake Drive, Milwaukee, WI Zip 53211–9682, Mailing Address: P.O. Box 503, Zip 53201–0503; tel. 414/291–1000; Charles C. Lobeck, Chief Executive Officer

For explanation of codes following names, see page B2.
★ Indicates Type III membership in the American Hospital Association.

ST. MARY'S HOSPITAL OZAUKEE (S, 82 beds) 13111 North Port Washington Road, Mequon, WI Zip 53097–2416; tel. 414/243–7300; Therese B. Pandl, Senior Vice President and Chief Operating Officer

Owned, leased, sponsored:	25 hospitals	8500 beds
Contract–managed:	0 hospitals	0 beds
Totals:	25 hospitals	8500 beds

★1825: DCH HEALTHCARE AUTHORITY (NP)

809 University Boulevard East, Tuscaloosa, AL Zip 35401; tel. 205/759–7111; Bryan Kindred, Chief Executive Officer

ALABAMA: DCH REGIONAL MEDICAL CENTER (O, 476 beds) 809 University Boulevard East, Tuscaloosa, AL Zip 35401–9961; tel. 205/759–7111; Bryan N. Kindred, Chief Executive Officer

FAYETTE MEDICAL CENTER (L, 162 beds) 1653 Temple Avenue North, Fayette, AL Zip 35555, Mailing Address: P.O. Drawer 878, Zip 35555; tel. 205/932–5966; Harold Reed, Administrator

NORTHPORT HOSPITAL–DCH (O, 132 beds) 2700 Hospital Drive, Northport, AL Zip 35476; tel. 205/333–4500; Charles L. Stewart, Administrator

Owned, leased, sponsored:	3 hospitals	770 beds
Contract–managed:	0 hospitals	0 beds
Totals:	3 hospitals	770 beds

9655: DEPARTMENT OF NAVY (FG)

Washington, DC Zip 20066

CALIFORNIA: NAVAL HOSPITAL (O, 25 beds) 930 Franklin Avenue, Lemoore, CA Zip 93246–5000; tel. 209/998–4201; Captain Jerry W. Brickeen, MSC, USN, Commanding Officer

NAVAL HOSPITAL (O, 209 beds) Camp Pendleton, CA Mailing Address: Box 555191, Zip 92055–5191; tel. 619/725–1288; Captain B. B. Potter, Commanding Officer

NAVAL HOSPITAL (O, 29 beds) Twentynine Palms, CA Mailing Address: Box 788250, MCAGCC, Zip 92278–8250; tel. 619/830–2492; Captain R. S. Kayler, MSC, USN, Commanding Officer

NAVAL MEDICAL CENTER (O, 386 beds) 34800 Bob Wilson Drive, San Diego, CA Zip 92134–5000; tel. 619/532–6400; Rear Admiral R. A. Nelson, MC, USN, Commander

CONNECTICUT: NAVAL HOSPITAL (O, 25 beds) 1 Wahoo Drive, Box 600, Groton, CT Zip 06349–5600; tel. 860/449–3261; Captain R. B. Hall II, Commanding Officer

FLORIDA: NAVAL HOSPITAL (O, 96 beds) 2080 Child Street, Jacksonville, FL Zip 32214–5000; tel. 904/777–7300; Captain M. J. Benson, MSC, USN, Commanding Officer

NAVAL HOSPITAL (O, 104 beds) 6000 West Highway 98, Pensacola, FL Zip 32512–0003; tel. 904/452–6413; Commander H. M. Chinnery, Director, Administration

GUAM: U. S. NAVAL HOSPITAL (O, 55 beds) Agana, GU Mailing Address: Box 7607, FPO, APZip 96538–1600; tel. 671/344–9340; J. M. Ricciardi, Commanding Officer

ILLINOIS: NAVAL HOSPITAL (O, 136 beds) Great Lakes, IL Zip 60088–5230; tel. 847/688–4560; Captain R. William Holden, MC, USN, Commanding Officer

MARYLAND: NATIONAL NAVAL MEDICAL CENTER (O, 217 beds) Bethesda, MD Zip 20889–5600; tel. 301/295–5800; Rear Admiral Richard T. Ridenour, MC, USN, Commander

NAVAL HOSPITAL (O, 5 beds) Patuxent River, MD Zip 20670–5370; tel. 301/342–1418; Captain Paul E. Campbell, MSC, USN, Commanding Officer

NORTH CAROLINA: NAVAL HOSPITAL (O, 166 beds) Camp Lejeune, NC Zip 28547–0100; tel. 910/451–4300; Captain Michael L. Cowan, MC, USN, Commanding Officer

NAVAL HOSPITAL (O, 23 beds) Havelock, NC Zip 28533–0023; tel. 919/466–0266; Captain Paul D. Garst, MC, USN, Commanding Officer

PUERTO RICO: U. S. NAVAL HOSPITAL (O, 35 beds) Roosevelt Roads, PR Mailing Address: Box 3007, FPO, AAZip 34051–8100; tel. 787/865–6171; Captain W. F. Lorenzen, Commanding Officer

SOUTH CAROLINA: NAVAL HOSPITAL (O, 20 beds) 1 Pinckney Boulevard, Beaufort, SC Zip 29902–6148; tel. 803/525–5301; Captain Clint E. Adams, MC, USN, Commanding Officer

NAVAL HOSPITAL (O, 40 beds) Charleston, SC Zip 29405; tel. 803/743–7000; Captain Kathleen L. Martin, Commanding Officer

TENNESSEE: NAVAL HOSPITAL (O, 41 beds) 6500 Navy Road, Millington, TN Zip 38054–5201; tel. 901/874–5804; Captain Michael Kilpatrick, MSC, USN, Commanding Officer

TEXAS: NAVAL HOSPITAL (O, 25 beds) 10651 E Street, Corpus Christi, TX Zip 78419–5131; tel. 512/939–2685; Captain F. G. Barina Jr., Commanding Officer

VIRGINIA: NAVAL MEDICAL CENTER (O, 330 beds) 620 John Paul Jones Circle, Portsmouth, VA Zip 23708–2197; tel. 757/398–7424; Rear Admiral William R. Rowley, MC, USN, Commander

WASHINGTON: NAVAL HOSPITAL (O, 76 beds) Boone Road, Bremerton, WA Zip 98312–1898; tel. 360/479–6600; Captain James A. Johnson, Commanding Officer

NAVAL HOSPITAL (O, 25 beds) 3475 North Saratoga Street, Oak Harbor, WA Zip 98278–8800; tel. 360/257–9500; Captain Michael W. Benway, Commanding Officer

Owned, leased, sponsored:	21 hospitals	2068 beds
Contract–managed:	0 hospitals	0 beds
Totals:	21 hospitals	2068 beds

9495: DEPARTMENT OF THE AIR FORCE (FG)

Washington, DC Zip 20333; tel. 202/767–5066; Major General Charles H. Roadman II, Deputy Surgeon General

ALABAMA: MAXWELL HOSPITAL (O, 30 beds) 330 Kirkpatrick Avenue East, Montgomery, AL Zip 36112–6219; tel. 334/953–7801; Colonel Herman R. Greenberg, Administrator

ALASKA: U. S. AIR FORCE REGIONAL HOSPITAL (O, 64 beds) 24800 Hospital Drive, Elmendorf AFB, AK Zip 99506–3700; tel. 907/552–4033; Colonel Larry J. Sutterer, MSC, USAF, Administrator

ARIZONA: U. S. AIR FORCE HOSPITAL (O, 20 beds) 4175 South Alamo Avenue, Davis–Monthan AFB, AZ Zip 85707–4405; tel. 520/228–2930; Colonel Stanley F. Uchman, Commander

U. S. AIR FORCE HOSPITAL LUKE (O, 23 beds) Luke AFB, Glendale, AZ Zip 85309–1525; tel. 602/856–7501; Colonel Robert P. Edwards, Administrator

ARKANSAS: U. S. AIR FORCE HOSPITAL LITTLE ROCK (O, 12 beds) Little Rock AFB, Jacksonville, AR Zip 72099–5057; tel. 501/988–7411; Colonel Norman L. Sims, MSC, USAF, Commander

CALIFORNIA: DAVID GRANT MEDICAL CENTER (O, 185 beds) 101 Bodin Circle, Travis AFB, CA Zip 94535–1800; tel. 707/423–7300; Colonel D. Creager Brown, MSC, USAF, Administrator

U. S. AIR FORCE HOSPITAL (O, 8 beds) 338 South Dakota, Vandenberg AFB, CA Zip 93437–6307; tel. 805/734–8232; Colonel John A. Reyburn Jr., Commander

U. S. AIR FORCE HOSPITAL (O, 6 beds) 15301 Warren Shingle Road, Beale AFB, CA Zip 95903–1907; tel. 916/634–4838; Lieutenant Colonel Robert G. Quinn, MSC, USAF, FACHE, Administrator

U. S. AIR FORCE HOSPITAL (O, 10 beds) 30 Hospital Road, Building 5500, Edwards AFB, CA Zip 93524–1730; tel. 805/277–2010; Major Greg Allen, MSC, USAF, Commander

COLORADO: U. S. AIR FORCE ACADEMY HOSPITAL (O, 46 beds) 4102 Pinion Drive, USAF Academy, CO Zip 80840–4000; tel. 719/333–5111; Colonel David L. Hammer, USAF, MC, Commander

DELAWARE: U. S. AIR FORCE HOSPITAL DOVER (O, 16 beds) 307 Tuskegee Boulevard, Dover AFB, DE Zip 19902–7307; tel. 302/677–2525; Major David M. Allen, MSC, Administrator

FLORIDA: U. S. AIR FORCE HOSPITAL (O, 15 beds) 1381 South Patrick Drive, Patrick AFB, FL Zip 32925–3606; tel. 407/494–8102; Colonel William Trent, MSC, USAF, Commanding Officer

U. S. AIR FORCE HOSPITAL (O, 25 beds) Tyndall AFB, Panama City, FL Zip 32403–5300; tel. 904/283–7515; Colonel Jay Sprenger, Commander

For explanation of codes following names, see page B2.
★ Indicates Type III membership in the American Hospital Association.

U. S. AIR FORCE HOSPITAL (O, 50 beds) 8415 Bayshore Boulevard, MacDill AFB, FL Zip 33621-1607; tel. 813/828-3258; Colonel Roger H. Bower, MC, USAF, Commander

U. S. AIR FORCE REGIONAL HOSPITAL (O, 85 beds) 307 Boatner Road, Suite 114, Eglin AFB, FL Zip 32542-1282; tel. 904/883-8221; Colonel William C. Head, MSC, USAF, Administrator

GEORGIA: U. S. AIR FORCE HOSPITAL MOODY (O, 16 beds) 3278 Mitchell Boulevard, Moody AFB, GA Zip 31699-1500; tel. 912/257-3772; Colonel Stephan A. Giesecke, USAF, MSC, Commander

U. S. AIR FORCE HOSPITAL ROBINS (O, 32 beds) Robins AFB, GA Zip 31098-2227; tel. 912/926-9381; Lieutenant Colonel Ronald M. Gilliard, MSC, USAF, FACHE, Administrator

IDAHO: U. S. AIR FORCE HOSPITAL MOUNTAIN HOME (O, 29 beds) Mountain Home AFB, ID Zip 83648-5300; tel. 208/828-7600; Lieutenant Colonel Randall E. Fellman, MC, USAF, Commanding Officer

ILLINOIS: SCOTT MEDICAL CENTER (O, 59 beds) Scott AFB, IL Zip 62225-5252; tel. 618/256-7012; Colonel Stephen J. Pribyl, MSC, USAF, Administrator

LOUISIANA: U. S. AIR FORCE HOSPITAL (O, 25 beds) Barksdale AFB, Shreveport, LA Zip 71110-5300; tel. 318/456-6004; Colonel Richard Weltzin, MSC, USAF, Administrator

MARYLAND: MALCOLM GROW MEDICAL CENTER (O, 185 beds) 1050 West Perimeter, Suite A1-19, Andrews AFB, MD Zip 20748, Mailing Address: Andrews AFB, Washington, DC Zip 20331-6600; tel. 301/981-3002; Colonel James F. Geiger, Administrator

MISSISSIPPI: U. S. AIR FORCE HOSPITAL (O, 7 beds) 201 Independence, Suite 235, Columbus, MS Zip 39701-5300; tel. 601/434-2297; Lieutenant Colonel Karen A. Bradway, MSC, USAF, Administrator

U. S. AIR FORCE MEDICAL CENTER KEESLER (O, 185 beds) 301 Fisher Street, Room 1A132, Keesler AFB, MS Zip 39534-2519; tel. 601/377-6510; Colonel William B. Kleefisch, Deputy Commander

MISSOURI: U. S. AIR FORCE HOSPITAL WHITEMAN (O, 20 beds) Whiteman AFB, MO Zip 65305-5001; tel. 816/687-1194; Lieutenant Colonel David Wilmot, USAF, MSC, Administrator

NEBRASKA: EHRLING BERGQUIST HOSPITAL (O, 45 beds) 2501 Capehart Road, Offutt AFB, NE Zip 68113-2160; tel. 402/294-7312; Colonel John R. Sheehan, Administrator

NEVADA: MIKE O'CALLAGHAN FEDERAL HOSPITAL (O, 34 beds) 4700 Las Vegas Boulevard North, Suite 2419, Las Vegas, NV Zip 89191-6601; tel. 702/653-2000; Colonel Jack A. Gupton, MSC, USAF, Administrator

NEW MEXICO: U. S. AIR FORCE HOSPITAL (O, 7 beds) 280 First Street, Holloman AFB, NM Zip 88330-8273; tel. 505/475-5587; Colonel Bruce P. Heseltine, MSC, USAF, Commander

U. S. AIR FORCE HOSPITAL (O, 5 beds) Cannon AFB, NM Zip 88103-5300; tel. 505/784-6318; Major Douglas E. Anderson, MSC, USAF, Administrator

U. S. AIR FORCE HOSPITAL-KIRTLAND (O, 10 beds) 1951 Second Street S.E., Kirtland AFB, NM Zip 87117-5559; tel. 505/846-3547; Colonel Paul B. Christianson, USAF, Commander

NORTH CAROLINA: U. S. AIR FORCE HOSPITAL SEYMOUR JOHNSON (O, 41 beds) 1050 Curtiss Avenue, Seymour Johnson AFB, NC Zip 27531-5300; tel. 919/736-5201; Colonel Michael Lischak, MC, USAF, Commander

NORTH DAKOTA: U. S. AIR FORCE HOSPITAL (O, 15 beds) Grand Forks SAC, Grand Forks AFB, ND Zip 58205-6332; tel. 701/747-5391; Lieutenant Colonel Stanley E. Hurstell, USAF, MSC, Administrator

U. S. AIR FORCE REGIONAL HOSPITAL (O, 39 beds) 10 Missile Avenue, Minot, ND Zip 58705-5024; tel. 701/723-5103; Colonel Murphy A. Chesney, Commander

OHIO: U. S. AIR FORCE MEDICAL CENTER WRIGHT-PATTERSON (O, 135 beds) 4881 Sugar Maple Drive, Wright-Patterson AFB, OH Zip 45433-5529; tel. 513/257-9913; Brigadier General Earl W. Mabry II, Commander

OKLAHOMA: U. S. AIR FORCE HOSPITAL ALTUS (O, 14 beds) Altus AFB, Altus, OK Zip 73523-5005; tel. 405/481-5205; Colonel David L. Clark, USAF, Commander

U. S. AIR FORCE HOSPITAL TINKER (O, 25 beds) 5700 Arnold Street, Tinker AFB, OK Zip 73145; tel. 405/736-2237; Colonel David D. Bissell, MC, USAF, Commander

SOUTH CAROLINA: U. S. AIR FORCE HOSPITAL SHAW (O, 25 beds) 431 Meadowlark Street, Shaw AFB, SC Zip 29152-5300; tel. 803/668-2610; Lieutenant Colonel Donald Taylor, Administrator

SOUTH DAKOTA: U. S. AIR FORCE HOSPITAL (O, 31 beds) Ellsworth AFB, SD Zip 57706; tel. 605/385-3201; Colonel Steven Sem, Commander

TEXAS: U. S. AIR FORCE HOSPITAL (O, 20 beds) 7th Medical Group, Dyess AFB, Abilene, TX Zip 79607-1367; tel. 915/696-2345; Lieutenant Colonel Robert W. Blum, MSC, USAF, FACHE, Administrator

U. S. AIR FORCE HOSPITAL (O, 8 beds) 590 Mitchell Boulevard, Laughlin AFB, TX Zip 78843-5200; tel. 210/298-6311; Major John G. Wiseman, Administrator

U. S. AIR FORCE HOSPITAL (O, 10 beds) 250 13th Street, Reese AFB, TX Zip 79489-5008; tel. 806/885-3542; Major Ward Hinger, MSC, USAF, Administrator

U. S. AIR FORCE REGIONAL HOSPITAL-SHEPPARD (O, 65 beds) 149 Hart Street, Suite 1, Sheppard AFB, TX Zip 76311-3478; tel. 817/676-2010; Colonel Richard D. Maddox, Administrator

WILFORD HALL MEDICAL CENTER (O, 715 beds) 2200 Bergquist Drive, Lackland AFB, TX Zip 78236-5300; tel. 210/292-7353; Colonel Stephen K. Lecholop, Administrator

UTAH: U. S. AIR FORCE HOSPITAL (O, 15 beds) 7321 11th Street, Hill AFB, UT Zip 84056-5012; tel. 801/777-5457; Colonel John A. Reyburn Jr., Commander

VIRGINIA: U. S. AIR FORCE HOSPITAL (O, 59 beds) 45 Pine Street, Hampton, VA Zip 23665-2080; tel. 804/764-6825; Colonel Glenn R. Willauer, Administrator

WASHINGTON: U. S. AIR FORCE HOSPITAL (O, 35 beds) 701 Hospital Loop, Fairchild AFB, WA Zip 99011-8701; tel. 509/247-5217; Colonel Craig G. Hinman, Commander

WYOMING: U. S. AIR FORCE HOSPITAL (O, 15 beds) 6900 Alden Drive, Cheyenne, WY Zip 82005-3913; tel. 307/775-2045; Major Angela D. Fowler, MSC, USAF, Administrator

Owned, leased, sponsored:	46 hospitals	2521 beds
Contract-managed:	0 hospitals	0 beds
Totals:	46 hospitals	2521 beds

9395: DEPARTMENT OF THE ARMY, OFFICE OF THE SURGEON GENERAL (FG)
5109 Leesburg Pike, Falls Church, VA Zip 22041; tel. 703/681-3114; Major Beverly Pritchett, Executive Officer

ALABAMA: FOX ARMY COMMUNITY HOSPITAL (O, 29 beds) Redstone Arsenal, AL Zip 35809-7000; tel. 205/876-4147; Major Mark A. Miller, Deputy Commander

LYSTER U. S. ARMY COMMUNITY HOSPITAL (O, 42 beds) U.S. Army Aeromedical Center, Fort Rucker, AL Zip 36362-5333; tel. 334/255-7360; Lieutenant Colonel Melvin Leggett Jr., Deputy Commander, Administration

ALASKA: BASSETT ARMY COMMUNITY HOSPITAL (O, 43 beds) Fort Wainwright, Fort Wainwright, AK Zip 99703-7400; tel. 907/353-5108; Lieutenant Colonel Gordon Lewis, Deputy Commander for Administration

ARIZONA: RAYMOND W. BLISS ARMY COMMUNITY HOSPITAL (O, 30 beds) Fort Huachuca, AZ Zip 85613-7040; tel. 520/533-2350; Lieutenant Colonel Michael H. Kennedy, Deputy Commander

CALIFORNIA: WEED ARMY COMMUNITY HOSPITAL (O, 27 beds) Fort Irwin, CA Zip 92310-5065; tel. 619/380-3108; Colonel James Beson, Commander

COLORADO: EVANS U. S. ARMY COMMUNITY HOSPITAL (O, 103 beds) Fort Carson, CO Zip 80913-5101; tel. 719/526-7200; Colonel Kenneth W. Leisher, Deputy Commander, Administration

DISTRICT OF COLUMBIA: WALTER REED HEALTH CARE SYSTEM (O, 474 beds) Washington, DC Zip 20307-5001; tel. 202/782-6393; Colonel Robert James Heckert Jr., MSC, Chief of Staff

GEORGIA: DWIGHT DAVID EISENHOWER ARMY MEDICAL CENTER (O, 313 beds) Fort Gordon, GA Zip 30905-5650; tel. 706/787-8192; Colonel Ronald J. Dunn, Deputy Commander for Administration

For explanation of codes following names, see page B2.
★ Indicates Type III membership in the American Hospital Association.

MARTIN ARMY COMMUNITY HOSPITAL (O, 126 beds) Fort Benning, GA Zip 31905–6100; tel. 706/544–2041; Colonel Stephen L. Markelz, Deputy Commander, Administration

WINN ARMY COMMUNITY HOSPITAL (O, 100 beds) Fort Stewart, GA Zip 31314–5300; tel. 912/370–6001; Lieutenant Colonel Jimmy Sanders, Administrator

HAWAII: TRIPLER ARMY MEDICAL CENTER (O, 354 beds) Honolulu, HI Zip 96859–5000; tel. 808/433–6661; Brigadier General Warren A. Todd Jr., MSC, Commander

KANSAS: IRWIN ARMY COMMUNITY HOSPITAL (O, 56 beds) Building 600, Fort Riley, KS Zip 66442; tel. 913/239–7100; Colonel J. Thomas Hardy, Commanding Officer

MUNSON ARMY COMMUNITY HOSPITAL (O, 20 beds) 550 Pope Avenue, Fort Leavenworth, KS Zip 66027–2332; tel. 913/684–6420; Colonel Cloyd B. Gatrell, Commander

KENTUCKY: COLONEL FLORENCE A. BLANCHFIELD ARMY COMMUNITY HOSPITAL (O, 107 beds) 650 Joel Drive, Fort Campbell, KY Zip 42223–5349; tel. 502/798–8040; Colonel Lester Martinez–Lopez, Director Health Services

IRELAND ARMY COMMUNITY HOSPITAL (O, 76 beds) 851 Ireland Loop, Fort Knox, KY Zip 40121–5520; tel. 502/624–9020; Lieutenant Colonel Robert T. Foster, Deputy Commander for Administrtaion

LOUISIANA: BAYNE–JONES ARMY COMMUNITY HOSPITAL (O, 52 beds) Fort Polk, LA Zip 71459–6000; tel. 318/531–3928; Colonel Joe W. Butler Jr., Deputy Commander and Administrator

MARSHALL ISLANDS: KWAJALEIN HOSPITAL (O, 14 beds) Kwajalein Island, MH Mailing Address: Box 1702, APO, APZip 96555–5000; tel. 805/355–2225; Mike Mathews, Administrator

MARYLAND: KIMBROUGH ARMY COMMUNITY HOSPITAL (O, 22 beds) Fort George G Meade, MD Zip 20755; tel. 301/677–4171; Colonel David W. Roberts, Commanding Officer

MISSOURI: GENERAL LEONARD WOOD ARMY COMMUNITY HOSPITAL (O, 71 beds) 310 Freedom Drive, Fort Leonard Wood, MO Zip 65473–8922; tel. 573/596–0414; Lieutenant Colonel Billy R. Porter, Administrator

NEW YORK: KELLER ARMY COMMUNITY HOSPITAL (O, 49 beds) U.S. Military Academy, West Point, NY Zip 10996–1197; tel. 914/938–3305; Colonel Joseph FitzHarris, Commander

NORTH CAROLINA: WOMACK ARMY MEDICAL CENTER (O, 173 beds) Fort Bragg, NC Zip 28307–5000; tel. 910/432–4802; Colonel Michael J. Brennan, MSC, M.D., Commander

OKLAHOMA: REYNOLDS ARMY COMMUNITY HOSPITAL (O, 116 beds) 4300 Thomas, Fort Sill, OK Zip 73503–6300; tel. 405/458–3000; Colonel David B. Crandall, Commander

SOUTH CAROLINA: MONCRIEF ARMY COMMUNITY HOSPITAL (O, 91 beds) Fort Jackson, SC Mailing Address: P.O. Box 500, Zip 29207–5720; tel. 803/751–2284; Colonel Dale Carroll, Commander

TEXAS: BROOKE ARMY MEDICAL CENTER (O, 464 beds) Fort Sam Houston, San Antonio, TX Zip 78234–6200; tel. 210/916–4141; Colonel Joseph P. Gonzales, MS, USA, Chief of Staff

DARNALL ARMY COMMUNITY HOSPITAL (O, 169 beds) Fort Hood, TX Zip 76544–5063; tel. 817/288–8000; Colonel James W. Kirkpatrick, Commander

WILLIAM BEAUMONT ARMY MEDICAL CENTER (O, 209 beds) 5005 North Piedras Street, El Paso, TX Zip 79920–5001; tel. 915/569–2121; Colonel Gordon W. Cho, Chief of Staff

VIRGINIA: DEWITT ARMY COMMUNITY HOSPITAL (O, 62 beds) Fort Belvoir, VA Zip 22060–5901; tel. 703/805–0510; Colonel Robert C. Harvey, Commander

MCDONALD ARMY COMMUNITY HOSPITAL (O, 30 beds) Jefferson Avenue, Fort Eustis, Newport News, VA Zip 23604–5548; tel. 757/878–7501; Colonel George Weightman, Commander

WASHINGTON: MADIGAN ARMY MEDICAL CENTER (O, 216 beds) Tacoma, WA Zip 98431–5000; tel. 206/968–1110; Brigadier General George J. Brown, M.D., Commanding General

Owned, leased, sponsored:	29 hospitals	3638 beds
Contract–managed:	0 hospitals	0 beds
Totals:	29 hospitals	3638 beds

9295: DEPARTMENT OF VETERANS AFFAIRS (FG)
810 Vermont Avenue N.W., Washington, DC Zip 20420; tel. 202/273–5781; Kenneth W. Kizer, M.D., M.P.H., Under Secretary for Health

ALABAMA: VETERANS AFFAIRS MEDICAL CENTER (O, 317 beds) 700 South 19th Street, Birmingham, AL Zip 35233–1996; tel. 205/933–8101; Y. C. Parris, Director

VETERANS AFFAIRS MEDICAL CENTER (O, 124 beds) 215 Perry Hill Road, Montgomery, AL Zip 36109–3798; tel. 334/272–4670; John R. Rowan, Director

VETERANS AFFAIRS MEDICAL CENTER (O, 307 beds) 3701 Loop Road, Tuscaloosa, AL Zip 35404–9983; tel. 205/554–2000; W. Kenneth Ruyle, Director

VETERANS AFFAIRS MEDICAL CENTER (O, 679 beds) 2400 Hospital Road, Tuskegee, AL Zip 36083–5001; tel. 334/727–0550; Jim Clay, Director

ARIZONA: CARL T. HAYDEN VETERANS AFFAIRS MEDICAL CENTER (O, 422 beds) 650 East Indian School Road, Phoenix, AZ Zip 85012–1894; tel. 602/277–5551; John R. Fears, Director

VETERANS AFFAIRS MEDICAL CENTER (O, 288 beds) 3601 South 6th Avenue, Tucson, AZ Zip 85723; tel. 520/792–1450; Jonathan H. Gardner, Chief Executive Officer

VETERANS AFFAIRS MEDICAL CENTER (O, 287 beds) 500 Highway 89 North, Prescott, AZ Zip 86313; tel. 520/445–4860; Patricia A. McKlem, Medical Center Director

ARKANSAS: VETERANS AFFAIRS MEDICAL CENTER (O, 94 beds) 1100 North College Avenue, Fayetteville, AR Zip 72703–6995; tel. 501/443–4301; Richard F. Robinson, Director

VETERANS AFFAIRS MEDICAL CENTER (O, 830 beds) 4300 West Seventh Street, Little Rock, AR Zip 72205–5484; tel. 501/661–1202; George H. Gray Jr., Director

CALIFORNIA: JERRY L. PETTIS MEMORIAL VETERANS MEDICAL CENTER (O, 315 beds) 11201 Benton Street, Loma Linda, CA Zip 92357; tel. 909/825–7084; Dean R. Stordahl, Director

VETERANS AFFAIRS MEDICAL CENTER (O, 220 beds) 2615 East Clinton Avenue, Fresno, CA Zip 93703; tel. 209/225–6100; James C. DeNiro, Director

VETERANS AFFAIRS MEDICAL CENTER (O, 1131 beds) 5901 East Seventh Street, Long Beach, CA Zip 90822–5201; tel. 562/494–5400; Jerry B. Boyd, Director

VETERANS AFFAIRS MEDICAL CENTER (O, 269 beds) 3350 LaJolla Village Drive, San Diego, CA Zip 92161; tel. 619/552–8585; Thomas B. Arnold, Chief Operating Officer

VETERANS AFFAIRS MEDICAL CENTER (O, 372 beds) 4150 Clement Street, San Francisco, CA Zip 94121–1598; tel. 415/750–2041; Lawrence C. Stewart, Director

VETERANS AFFAIRS MEDICAL CENTER–WEST LOS ANGELES (O, 1327 beds) 11301 Wilshire Boulevard, Los Angeles, CA Zip 90073–0275; tel. 310/268–3132; Kenneth J. Clark, Executive Director and Chief Executive Officer

VETERANS AFFAIRS PALO ALTO HEALTH CARE SYSTEM (O, 1028 beds) 3801 Miranda Avenue, Palo Alto, CA Zip 94304–1207; tel. 415/493–5000; James A. Goff, FACHE, Director

COLORADO: VETERANS AFFAIRS MEDICAL CENTER (O, 336 beds) 1055 Clermont Street, Denver, CO Zip 80220–3877; tel. 303/399–8020; Ed Thorsland Jr., Director

VETERANS AFFAIRS MEDICAL CENTER (O, 299 beds) Fort Lyon, CO Zip 81038; tel. 719/456–1260; W. David Smith, Director

VETERANS AFFAIRS MEDICAL CENTER (O, 116 beds) 2121 North Avenue, Grand Junction, CO Zip 81501–6499; tel. 970/242–0731; Robert R. Rhyne, D.D.S., Director

CONNECTICUT: VETERANS AFFAIRS CONNECTICUT HEALTHCARE SYSTEM (O, 343 beds) 950 Campbell Avenue, West Haven, CT Zip 06516; tel. 203/932–5711; Vincent Ng, Director

DELAWARE: VETERANS AFFAIRS MEDICAL CENTER (O, 210 beds) 1601 Kirkwood Highway, Wilmington, DE Zip 19805–4989; tel. 302/633–5201; Dexter D. Dix, Director

DISTRICT OF COLUMBIA: VETERANS AFFAIRS MEDICAL CENTER (O, 451 beds) 50 Irving Street N.W., Washington, DC Zip 20422; tel. 202/745–8100; Sanford M. Garfunkel, Medical Center Director

FLORIDA: JAMES A. HALEY VETERANS HOSPITAL (O, 640 beds) 13000 Bruce B. Downs Boulevard, Tampa, FL Zip 33612–4798; tel. 813/972–2000; Richard A. Silver, Director

VETERANS AFFAIRS MEDICAL CENTER (O, 773 beds) 10000 Bay Pines Boulevard, Bay Pines, FL Zip 33744, Mailing Address: P.O. Box 5005, Zip 33744; tel. 813/398–6661; Thomas H. Weaver, FACHE, Director

VETERANS AFFAIRS MEDICAL CENTER (O, 242 beds) 7305 North Military Trail, West Palm Beach, FL Zip 33410–6400; tel. 561/882–8262; Richard D. Isaac, Administrator

VETERANS AFFAIRS MEDICAL CENTER (O, 669 beds) 1201 N.W. 16th Street, Miami, FL Zip 33125–1624; tel. 305/324–4455; Thomas C. Doherty, Medical Center Director

VETERANS AFFAIRS MEDICAL CENTER (O, 384 beds) 1601 S.W. Archer Road, Gainesville, FL Zip 32608–1197; tel. 352/376–1611; Malcom Randall, Director

VETERANS AFFAIRS MEDICAL CENTER (O, 360 beds) 801 South Marion Street, Lake City, FL Zip 32025–5898; tel. 904/755–3016; Alline L. Norman, Director

GEORGIA: VETERANS AFFAIRS MEDICAL CENTER (O, 378 beds) 1670 Clairmont Road, Decatur, GA Zip 30033–4098; tel. 404/728–7600; Robert A. Perreault, Director

VETERANS AFFAIRS MEDICAL CENTER (O, 587 beds) 1 Freedom Way, Augusta, GA Zip 30904–6285; tel. 706/733–0188; David Whatley, Director

VETERANS AFFAIRS MEDICAL CENTER (O, 253 beds) 1826 Veterans Boulevard, Dublin, GA Zip 31021; tel. 912/277–2701; William O. Edgar, Director

IDAHO: VETERANS AFFAIRS MEDICAL CENTER (O, 176 beds) 500 West Fort Street, Boise, ID Zip 83702–4598; tel. 208/422–1000; Wayne C. Tippets, Director

ILLINOIS: VA CHICAGO HEALTH CARE SYSTEM–LAKESIDE DIVISION (O, 252 beds) 333 East Huron Street, Chicago, IL Zip 60611–3004; tel. 312/640–2100; Joseph L. Moore, Director

VA CHICAGO HEALTH CARE SYSTEM–WEST SIDE DIVISION (O, 323 beds) 820 South Damen Avenue, Chicago, IL Zip 60612, Mailing Address: Box 8195, Zip 60680; tel. 312/666–6500; Joseph L. Moore, Director

VETERANS AFFAIRS EDWARD HINES, JR. HOSPITAL (O, 896 beds) Fifth Avenue & Roosevelt Road, Hines, IL Zip 60141–5000, Mailing Address: P.O. Box 5000, Zip 60141–5000; tel. 708/343–7200; John J. DeNardo, Director

VETERANS AFFAIRS MEDICAL CENTER (O, 531 beds) 1900 East Main Street, Danville, IL Zip 61832; tel. 217/442–8000; James S. Jones, Director

VETERANS AFFAIRS MEDICAL CENTER (O, 836 beds) 3001 Green Bay Road, North Chicago, IL Zip 60064; tel. 847/688–1900; Alfred S. Pate, Director

VETERANS AFFAIRS MEDICAL CENTER (O, 162 beds) 2401 West Main Street, Marion, IL Zip 62959–1194; tel. 618/997–5311; Linda Kurz, Director

INDIANA: RICHARD L. ROUDEBUSH VETERANS AFFAIRS MEDICAL CENTER (O, 197 beds) 1481 West Tenth Street, Indianapolis, IN Zip 46202; tel. 317/635–7401; Alice Wood, Director

VETERANS AFFAIRS NORTHERN INDIANA HEALTH CARE SYSTEM–FORT WAYNE DIVISION (O, 568 beds) 2121 Lake Avenue, Fort Wayne, IN Zip 46805–5347; tel. 219/426–5431; Michael W. Murphy, Ph.D., Director

VETERANS AFFAIRS NORTHERN INDIANA HEALTH CARE SYSTEM–MARION CAMPUS (O, 580 beds) 1700 East 38th Street, Marion, IN Zip 46953–4589; tel. 765/674–3351; Michael W. Murphy, Ph.D., Director

IOWA: VETERANS AFFAIRS MEDICAL CENTER (O, 99 beds) 3600 30th Street, Des Moines, IA Zip 50310–5774; tel. 515/255–2173; Ellen DeGeorge–Smith, Director

VETERANS AFFAIRS MEDICAL CENTER (O, 159 beds) Highway 6 West, Iowa City, IA Zip 52246–2208; tel. 319/338–0581; Gary L. Wilkinson, Director

VETERANS AFFAIRS MEDICAL CENTER (O, 565 beds) 1515 West Pleasant, Knoxville, IA Zip 50138–3399; tel. 515/842–3101; Ellen DeGeorge–Smith, Acting Director

KANSAS: COLMERY–O'NEIL VETERANS AFFAIRS MEDICAL CENTER (O, 437 beds) 2200 Gage Boulevard, Topeka, KS Zip 66622; tel. 913/350–3111; Edgar Tucker, Director

DWIGHT D. EISENHOWER VETERANS AFFAIRS MEDICAL CENTER (O, 122 beds) 4101 South Fourth Street Trafficway, Leavenworth, KS Zip 66048–5055; tel. 913/682–2000; Carole Bishop Smith, Center Director

VETERANS AFFAIRS MEDICAL AND REGIONAL OFFICE CENTER (O, 83 beds) 5500 East Kellogg, Wichita, KS Zip 67218; tel. 316/685–2221; Robert D. Morrel, Associate Director

KENTUCKY: VETERANS AFFAIRS MEDICAL CENTER–LEXINGTON (O, 613 beds) 2250 Leestown Pike, Lexington, KY Zip 40511–1093; tel. 606/233–4511; Helen K. Cornish, Director

VETERANS AFFAIRS MEDICAL CENTER–LOUISVILLE (O, 229 beds) 800 Zorn Avenue, Louisville, KY Zip 40206–1499; tel. 502/895–3401; Larry J. Sander, FACHE, Director

LOUISIANA: DEPARTMENT OF VA MEDICAL CENTER–ALEXANDRIA (O, 401 beds) Shreveport Highway, Alexandria, LA Zip 71306–6002; tel. 318/473–0010; Allan S. Goss, Director

OVERTON BROOKS VETERANS AFFAIRS MEDICAL CENTER (O, 197 beds) 510 East Stoner Avenue, Shreveport, LA Zip 71101–4295; tel. 318/221–8411; Michael E. Hamilton, Director

VETERANS AFFAIRS MEDICAL CENTER (O, 285 beds) 1601 Perdido Street, New Orleans, LA Zip 70146; tel. 504/568–0811; John D. Church Jr., Director

MAINE: VETERANS AFFAIRS MEDICAL CENTER (O, 241 beds) Togus, ME Zip 04330; tel. 207/623–8411; John H. Sims Jr., Director

MARYLAND: VA MARYLAND HEALTH CARE SYSTEM (O, 526 beds) Circle Drive, Perry Point, MD Zip 21902; tel. 410/642–2411; Dennis H. Smith, Director

VETERANS AFFAIRS MEDICAL CENTER (O, 897 beds) 10 North Greene Street, Baltimore, MD Zip 21201–1524; tel. 410/605–7001; Dennis H. Smith, Director

VETERANS AFFAIRS MEDICAL CENTER (O, 245 beds) 9600 North Point Road, Fort Howard, MD Zip 21052–9989; tel. 410/477–1800; Dennis H. Smith, Director

MASSACHUSETTS: BROCKTON–WEST ROXBURY VETERANS AFFAIRS MEDICAL CENTER (O, 765 beds) 940 Belmont Street, Brockton, MA Zip 02401; tel. 508/583–4500; Michael E. Lawson, Director

EDITH NOURSE ROGERS MEMORIAL VETERANS HOSPITAL (O, 680 beds) 200 Springs Road, Bedford, MA Zip 01730; tel. 617/687–2000; William A. Conte, Director

VETERANS AFFAIRS MEDICAL CENTER (O, 418 beds) Boston, MA Mailing Address: 150 South Huntington Avenue, Jamaica Plain Station, Zip 02130–4820; tel. 617/232–9500; Elwood J. Headley, M.D., Director

VETERANS AFFAIRS MEDICAL CENTER (O, 361 beds) Route 9, Northampton, MA Zip 01060–1288; tel. 413/584–4040; Bruce A. Gordon, Director

MICHIGAN: VETERANS AFFAIRS MEDICAL CENTER (O, 238 beds) 2215 Fuller Road, Ann Arbor, MI Zip 48105; tel. 313/769–7100; Edward L. Gamache, Director

VETERANS AFFAIRS MEDICAL CENTER (O, 640 beds) 5500 Armstrong Road, Battle Creek, MI Zip 49016; tel. 616/966–5600; Michael K. Wheeler, Director

VETERANS AFFAIRS MEDICAL CENTER (O, 432 beds) 4646 John R Street, Detroit, MI Zip 48201; tel. 313/576–1000; Carlos B. Lott Jr., Director

VETERANS AFFAIRS MEDICAL CENTER (O, 133 beds) 325 East H Street, Iron Mountain, MI Zip 49801–4792; tel. 906/774–3300; Glen W. Grippen, Director

VETERANS AFFAIRS MEDICAL CENTER (O, 215 beds) 1500 Weiss Street, Saginaw, MI Zip 48602; tel. 517/793–2340; Robert H. Sabin, Medical Center Director

For explanation of codes following names, see page B2.
★ Indicates Type III membership in the American Hospital Association.

MINNESOTA: VETERANS AFFAIRS MEDICAL CENTER (O, 519 beds) One Veterans Drive, Minneapolis, MN Zip 55417–2399; tel. 612/725–2000; Charles A. Milbrandt, Director

VETERANS AFFAIRS MEDICAL CENTER (O, 570 beds) 4801 Eighth Street North, Saint Cloud, MN Zip 56303–2099; tel. 320/252–1670; Barry I. Bahl, Associate Director

MISSISSIPPI: G.V. MONTGOMERY VETERANS AFFAIRS MEDICAL CENTER (O, 443 beds) 1500 East Woodrow Wilson Drive, Jackson, MS Zip 39216–5199; tel. 601/364–1201; Richard P. Miller, Director

VETERANS AFFAIRS MEDICAL CENTER (O, 510 beds) 400 Veterans Avenue, Biloxi, MS Zip 39531–2410; tel. 601/388–5541; George Rodman, Director

MISSOURI: HARRY S. TRUMAN MEMORIAL VETERANS HOSPITAL (O, 230 beds) 800 Hospital Drive, Columbia, MO Zip 65201–5297; tel. 573/443–2511; Gary L. Campbell, Director

JOHN J. PERSHING VETERANS AFFAIRS MEDICAL CENTER (O, 174 beds) 1500 North Westwood Boulevard, Poplar Bluff, MO Zip 63901; tel. 573/686–4151; James W. Roseborough, Director

VETERANS AFFAIRS MEDICAL CENTER (O, 555 beds) Saint Louis, MO Zip 63125; tel. 314/894–6661; Donald L. Ziegenhorn, Director

VETERANS AFFAIRS MEDICAL CENTER (O, 295 beds) 4801 Linwood Boulevard, Kansas City, MO Zip 64128–2295; tel. 816/861–4700; Hugh F. Doran, Director

MONTANA: VETERANS AFFAIRS HOSPITAL (O, 88 beds) Fort Harrison, MT Zip 59636; tel. 406/442–6410; Joseph Underkofler, Director

VETERANS AFFAIRS MEDICAL CENTER (O, 50 beds) 210 South Winchester Avenue, Miles City, MT Zip 59301; tel. 406/232–3060; Richard J. Stanley, Director

NEBRASKA: VETERANS AFFAIRS MEDICAL CENTER (O, 142 beds) 2211 North Broadwell Avenue, Grand Island, NE Zip 68803–2196; tel. 308/382–3660; Daniel A. Asper, Acting Director

VETERANS AFFAIRS MEDICAL CENTER (O, 73 beds) 600 South 70th Street, Lincoln, NE Zip 68510–2493; tel. 402/489–3802; David Asper, Director

VETERANS AFFAIRS MEDICAL CENTER (O, 194 beds) 4101 Woolworth Avenue, Omaha, NE Zip 68105–1873; tel. 402/449–0600; John J. Phillips, Director

NEVADA: IOANNIS A. LOUGARIS VETERANS AFFAIRS MEDICAL CENTER (O, 167 beds) 1000 Locust Street, Reno, NV Zip 89520–0111; tel. 702/786–7200; Gary R. Whitfield, Director

NEW HAMPSHIRE: VETERANS AFFAIRS MEDICAL CENTER (O, 180 beds) 718 Smyth Road, Manchester, NH Zip 03104–4098; tel. 603/624–4366; Paul J. McCool, Director

NEW JERSEY: DEPARTMENT OF VETERANS AFFAIRS HEALTH CARE SYSTEM (O, 1312 beds) 385 Tremont Avenue, East Orange, NJ Zip 07018–1095; tel. 201/676–1000; Kenneth H. Mizrach, Director

NEW MEXICO: VETERANS AFFAIRS MEDICAL CENTER (O, 327 beds) 2100 Ridgecrest Drive S.E., Albuquerque, NM Zip 87108; tel. 505/265–1711; Norman E. Browne, Director

NEW YORK: FRANKLIN DELANO ROOSEVELT VETERANS AFFAIRS HOSPITAL (O, 550 beds) Route 9A, Montrose, NY Zip 10548, Mailing Address: P.O. Box 100, Zip 10548; tel. 914/737–4400; William D. Montague, Director

VETERANS AFFAIRS MEDICAL CENTER (O, 298 beds) 113 Holland Avenue, Albany, NY Zip 12208–3473; tel. 518/462–3311; Lawrence H. Flesh, M.D., Director

VETERANS AFFAIRS MEDICAL CENTER (O, 615 beds) 76 Veterans Avenue, Bath, NY Zip 14810–0842; tel. 607/776–2111; Michael J. Sullivan, Director

VETERANS AFFAIRS MEDICAL CENTER (O, 713 beds) 800 Poly Place, Brooklyn, NY Zip 11209; tel. 718/630–3500; Michael A. Sabo, Medical Director

VETERANS AFFAIRS MEDICAL CENTER (O, 626 beds) 400 Fort Hill Avenue, Canandaigua, NY Zip 14424–1197; tel. 716/396–3601; Stuart C. Collyer, Director

VETERANS AFFAIRS MEDICAL CENTER (O, 233 beds) Castle Point, NY Zip 12511–9999; tel. 914/838–5190; William D. Montague, Acting Medical Center Director

VETERANS AFFAIRS MEDICAL CENTER (O, 482 beds) 130 West Kingsbridge Road, Bronx, NY Zip 10468–7511; tel. 718/584–9000; Maryann Musumeci, Director

VETERANS AFFAIRS MEDICAL CENTER (O, 341 beds) 423 East 23rd Street, New York, NY Zip 10010–0070; tel. 212/686–7500; John J. Donnellan Jr., Director

VETERANS AFFAIRS MEDICAL CENTER (O, 699 beds) 79 Middleville Road, Northport, NY Zip 11768–2293; tel. 516/261–4400; James A. Clark, Director

VETERANS AFFAIRS MEDICAL CENTER (O, 204 beds) 800 Irving Avenue, Syracuse, NY Zip 13210; tel. 315/476–7461; Philip P. Thomas, Director

VETERANS AFFAIRS WESTERN NEW YORK HEALTHCARE SYSTEM (O, 158 beds) 222 Richmond Avenue, Batavia, NY Zip 14020; tel. 716/343–7500; Richard S. Droske, Director

VETERANS AFFAIRS WESTERN NEW YORK HEALTHCARE SYSTEM (O, 611 beds) 3495 Bailey Avenue, Buffalo, NY Zip 14215–1129; tel. 716/834–9200; Richard S. Droske, Director

NORTH CAROLINA: VETERANS AFFAIRS MEDICAL CENTER (O, 382 beds) 508 Fulton Street, Durham, NC Zip 27705; tel. 919/286–0411; Michael B. Phaup, Director

VETERANS AFFAIRS MEDICAL CENTER (O, 193 beds) 2300 Ramsey Street, Fayetteville, NC Zip 28301–3899; tel. 910/822–7059; Betty Bolin Brown, Acting Director

VETERANS AFFAIRS MEDICAL CENTER (O, 389 beds) 1100 Tunnel Road, Asheville, NC Zip 28805–2087; tel. 704/298–7911; James A. Christian, Director

VETERANS AFFAIRS MEDICAL CENTER (O, 612 beds) 1601 Brenner Avenue, Salisbury, NC Zip 28144; tel. 704/638–9000; Bettye W. Story, Ph.D., Director

NORTH DAKOTA: VETERANS AFFAIRS MEDICAL AND REGIONAL OFFICE CENTER (O, 153 beds) 2101 Elm Street, Fargo, ND Zip 58102–2498; tel. 701/232–3241; Douglas M. Kenyon, Director

OHIO: VETERANS AFFAIRS MEDICAL CENTER (O, 914 beds) 10701 East Boulevard, Cleveland, OH Zip 44106–1702; tel. 216/791–3800; Richard S. Citron, Acting Director

VETERANS AFFAIRS MEDICAL CENTER (O, 587 beds) 17273 State Route 104, Chillicothe, OH Zip 45601–0999; tel. 614/773–1141; Michael W. Walton, Director

VETERANS AFFAIRS MEDICAL CENTER (O, 240 beds) 3200 Vine Street, Cincinnati, OH Zip 45220–2288; tel. 513/475–6300; Gary N. Nugent, Medical Director

VETERANS AFFAIRS MEDICAL CENTER (O, 835 beds) 4100 West Third Street, Dayton, OH Zip 45428–1002; tel. 937/268–6511; Steven M. Cohen, M.D., Director

OKLAHOMA: VETERANS AFFAIRS MEDICAL CENTER (O, 99 beds) Honor Heights Drive, Muskogee, OK Zip 74401–1399; tel. 918/683–3261; Billy M. Valentine, Director

VETERANS AFFAIRS MEDICAL CENTER (O, 277 beds) 921 N.E. 13th Street, Oklahoma City, OK Zip 73104–5028; tel. 405/270–0501; Steven J. Gentling, Director

OREGON: VETERANS AFFAIRS MEDICAL CENTER (O, 591 beds) 3710 S.W. U.S. Veterans Hospital Road, Portland, OR Zip 97201; tel. 503/220–8262; William Galey, M.D., Chief Executive Officer

VETERANS AFFAIRS MEDICAL CENTER (O, 229 beds) 913 N.W. Garden Valley Boulevard, Roseburg, OR Zip 97470–6513; tel. 541/440–1000; Alan S. Perry, Director

PENNSYLVANIA: DEPARTMENT OF VETERANS AFFAIRS MEDICAL CENTER (O, 339 beds) 1111 East End Boulevard, Wilkes–Barre, PA Zip 18711–0026; tel. 717/824–3521; Reedes Hurt, Chief Executive Officer

JAMES E. VAN ZANDT VETERANS AFFAIRS MEDICAL CENTER (O, 110 beds) 2907 Pleasant Valley Boulevard, Altoona, PA Zip 16602–4377; tel. 814/943–8164; Gerald L. Williams, Director

VETERANS AFFAIRS MEDICAL CENTER (O, 268 beds) 325 New Castle Road, Butler, PA Zip 16001–2480; tel. 412/287–4781; P. Stajduhar, M.D., Director

VETERANS AFFAIRS MEDICAL CENTER (O, 710 beds) Black Horse Hill Road, Coatesville, PA Zip 19320–9985; tel. 610/384–7711; Gary W. Devansky, Director

For explanation of codes following names, see page B2.
★ Indicates Type III membership in the American Hospital Association.

VETERANS AFFAIRS MEDICAL CENTER (O, 88 beds) 135 East 38th Street, Erie, PA Zip 16504–1596; tel. 814/868–6210; Stephen M. Lucas, Chief Executive Officer

VETERANS AFFAIRS MEDICAL CENTER (O, 565 beds) 1700 South Lincoln Avenue, Lebanon, PA Zip 17042–7597; tel. 717/272–6621; Leonard Washington Jr., Director

VETERANS AFFAIRS MEDICAL CENTER (O, 656 beds) University and Woodland Avenues, Philadelphia, PA Zip 19104–4594; tel. 215/823–5857; Earl F. Falast, Chief Executive Officer

VETERANS AFFAIRS PITTSBURGH HEALTHCARE SYSTEM (O, 1172 beds) Delafield Road, Pittsburgh, PA Zip 15240–1001; tel. 412/784–3900; Thomas A. Cappello, Director

PUERTO RICO: VETERANS AFFAIRS MEDICAL CENTER (O, 693 beds) One Veterans Plaza, San Juan, PR Zip 00927–5800; tel. 809/766–5665; James A. Palmer, Director

RHODE ISLAND: VETERANS AFFAIRS MEDICAL CENTER (O, 108 beds) 830 Chalkstone Avenue, Providence, RI Zip 02908–4799; tel. 401/457–3042; Edward H. Seiler, Director

SOUTH CAROLINA: VETERANS AFFAIRS MEDICAL CENTER (O, 161 beds) 109 Bee Street, Charleston, SC Zip 29401–5799; tel. 803/577–5011; Dean S. Billik, Director

WILLIAM JENNINGS BRYAN DORN VETERANS HOSPITAL (O, 342 beds) 6439 Garners Ferry Road, Columbia, SC Zip 29209–1639; tel. 803/776–4000; Brian Heckert, Director

SOUTH DAKOTA: DEPARTMENT OF VETERANS AFFAIRS BLACK HILLS HEALTH CARE SYSTEM (O, 408 beds) 113 Comanche Road, Fort Meade, SD Zip 57741–1099; tel. 605/347–2511; Peter P. Henry, Director

ROYAL C. JOHNSON VETERANS MEMORIAL HOSPITAL (O, 162 beds) 2501 West 22nd Street, Sioux Falls, SD Zip 57105, Mailing Address: P.O. Box 5046, Zip 57117–5046; tel. 605/336–3230; R. Vincent Crawford, Director

TENNESSEE: ALVIN C. YORK VETERANS AFFAIRS MEDICAL CENTER (O, 631 beds) 3400 Lebanon Road, Murfreesboro, TN Zip 37129; tel. 615/893–1360; R. Eugene Konik, Director

JAMES H. QUILLEN VETERANS AFFAIRS MEDICAL CENTER (O, 390 beds) Mountain Home, TN Zip 37684; tel. 423/926–1171; Carl J. Gerber, M.D., Ph.D., Director

VETERANS AFFAIRS MEDICAL CENTER (O, 631 beds) 1030 Jefferson Avenue, Memphis, TN Zip 38104–2193; tel. 901/523–8990; K. L. Mulholland Jr., Director

VETERANS AFFAIRS MEDICAL CENTER (O, 233 beds) 1310 24th Avenue South, Nashville, TN Zip 37212–2637; tel. 615/327–5332; William A. Mountcastle, Director

TEXAS: CENTRAL TEXAS VETERANS AFFAIRS HEALTHCARE SYSTEM (O, 1852 beds) 1901 South First Street, Temple, TX Zip 76504; tel. 817/778–4811; Richard Harwell, Director

SAM RAYBURN MEMORIAL VETERANS CENTER (O, 374 beds) 1201 East Ninth Street, Bonham, TX Zip 75418; tel. 903/583–2111; Charles C. Freeman, Director

SOUTH TEXAS VETERANS HEALTH CARE SYSTEM (O, 1112 beds) 7400 Merton Minter Boulevard, San Antonio, TX Zip 78284–5799; tel. 210/617–5140; Jose R. Coronado, Director

VETERANS AFFAIRS MEDICAL CENTER (O, 218 beds) 6010 Amarillo Boulevard West, Amarillo, TX Zip 79106; tel. 806/354–7801; Wallace M. Hopkins, FACHE, Director

VETERANS AFFAIRS MEDICAL CENTER (O, 189 beds) 300 Veterans Boulevard, Big Spring, TX Zip 79720–5500; tel. 915/263–7361; Cary D. Brown, Director

VETERANS AFFAIRS MEDICAL CENTER (O, 557 beds) 4500 South Lancaster Road, Dallas, TX Zip 75216–7167; tel. 214/376–5451; Alan G. Harper, Director

VETERANS AFFAIRS MEDICAL CENTER (O, 859 beds) 2002 Holcombe Boulevard, Houston, TX Zip 77030–4298; tel. 713/791–1414; Robert F. Stott, Director

UTAH: VETERANS AFFAIRS MEDICAL CENTER (O, 243 beds) 500 Foothill Drive, Salt Lake City, UT Zip 84148; tel. 801/582–1565; Donald F. Moore, Acting Medical Center Director

VERMONT: VETERANS AFFAIRS MEDICAL CENTER (O, 110 beds) North Hartland Road, White River Junction, VT Zip 05009–0001; tel. 802/295–9363; Gary M. De Gasta, Director

VIRGINIA: HUNTER HOLMES MCGUIRE VETERANS AFFAIRS MEDICAL CENTER (O, 616 beds) 1201 Broad Rock Boulevard, Richmond, VA Zip 23249; tel. 804/675–5000; James W. Dudley, Director

VETERANS AFFAIRS MEDICAL CENTER (O, 670 beds) 100 Emancipation Drive, Hampton, VA Zip 23667–0001; tel. 804/722–9961; William G. Wright, Director

VETERANS AFFAIRS MEDICAL CENTER (O, 410 beds) 1970 Roanoke Boulevard, Salem, VA Zip 24153; tel. 540/982–2463; John M. Presley, Ph.D., Director

WASHINGTON: JONATHAN M. WAINWRIGHT MEMORIAL VETERANS AFFAIRS MEDICAL CENTER (O, 76 beds) 77 Wainwright Drive, Walla Walla, WA Zip 99362–3994; tel. 509/525–5200; George Marnell, Director

VA PUGET SOUND HEALTH CARE SYSTEM (O, 557 beds) 1660 South Columbia Way, Seattle, WA Zip 98108–1597; tel. 206/762–1010; Timothy B. Williams, Director

VETERANS AFFAIRS MEDICAL CENTER (O, 192 beds) North 4815 Assembly Street, Spokane, WA Zip 99205–6197; tel. 509/327–0200; Joseph M. Manley, Director

WEST VIRGINIA: LOUIS A. JOHNSON VETERANS AFFAIRS MEDICAL CENTER (O, 160 beds) Clarksburg, WV Zip 26301–4199; tel. 304/623–3461; Michael W. Neusch, FACHE, Director

VETERANS AFFAIRS MEDICAL CENTER (O, 112 beds) 200 Veterans Avenue, Beckley, WV Zip 25801–6499; tel. 304/255–2121; Gerard P. Husson, Director

VETERANS AFFAIRS MEDICAL CENTER (O, 170 beds) 1540 Spring Valley Drive, Huntington, WV Zip 25704; tel. 304/429–6741; Philip S. Elkins, Director

VETERANS AFFAIRS MEDICAL CENTER (O, 370 beds) Charles Town Road, Martinsburg, WV Zip 25401–0205; tel. 304/263–0811; Richard Pell Jr., Director

WISCONSIN: CLEMENT J. ZABLOCKI VETERANS AFFAIRS MEDICAL CENTER (O, 566 beds) 5000 West National Avenue, Milwaukee, WI Zip 53295–1000; tel. 414/384–2000; Russell E. Struble, Medical Center Director

VETERANS AFFAIRS MEDICAL CENTER (O, 569 beds) 500 East Veterans Street, Tomah, WI Zip 54660–9225; tel. 608/372–3971; Stan Johnson, Medical Center Director

WILLIAM S. MIDDLETON MEMORIAL VETERANS HOSPITAL (O, 200 beds) 2500 Overlook Terrace, Madison, WI Zip 53705–2286; tel. 608/256–1901; Nathan L. Geraths, Director

WYOMING: VETERANS AFFAIRS MEDICAL CENTER (O, 125 beds) 2360 East Pershing Boulevard, Cheyenne, WY Zip 82001–5392; tel. 307/778–7550; David M. Kilpatrick, M.D., Acting Center Director

VETERANS AFFAIRS MEDICAL CENTER (O, 239 beds) 1898 Fort Road, Sheridan, WY Zip 82801; tel. 307/672–3473; J. A. Brinkers, Director

Owned, leased, sponsored:	149 hospitals	62626 beds
Contract–managed:	0 hospitals	0 beds
Totals:	149 hospitals	62626 beds

★**2145: DETROIT MEDICAL CENTER** (NP)
4201 St. Antoine Boulevard, Detroit, MI Zip 48201–2194; tel. 313/745–5192; David J. Campbell, President and Chief Executive Officer

MICHIGAN: CHILDREN'S HOSPITAL OF MICHIGAN (O, 245 beds) 3901 Beaubien, Detroit, MI Zip 48201–9985; tel. 313/745–0073; Thomas M. Rozek, Senior Vice President

DETROIT RECEIVING HOSPITAL AND UNIVERSITY HEALTH CENTER (O, 290 beds) 4201 St. Antoine Boulevard, Detroit, MI Zip 48201–2194; tel. 313/745–3605; Leslie C. Bowman, Regional Administrator, Ancillary Services and Site Administrator

GRACE HOSPITAL (O, 352 beds) 6071 West Outer Drive, Detroit, MI Zip 48235; tel. 313/966–3300; Anne M. Regling, Regional Executive

For explanation of codes following names, see page B2.
★ Indicates Type III membership in the American Hospital Association.

Section B

HARPER HOSPITAL (O, 427 beds) 3990 John R, Detroit, MI Zip 48201–9027; tel. 313/745–8040; Paul L. Broughton, FACHE, Senior Vice President

HURON VALLEY HOSPITAL (O, 139 beds) 1601 East Commerce Road, Commerce Township, MI Zip 48382; tel. 810/360–3300; Elliot Joseph, Senior Vice President, Oakland Region

HUTZEL HOSPITAL (O, 243 beds) 4707 St. Antoine Boulevard, Detroit, MI Zip 48201–0154; tel. 313/745–7555; Susan A. Erickson, Clinical Services Administrator for Women's Services and Site Administrator

REHABILITATION INSTITUTE OF MICHIGAN (O, 96 beds) 261 Mack Boulevard, Detroit, MI Zip 48201; tel. 313/745–1203; Bruce M. Gans, M.D., Senior Vice President

SINAI HOSPITAL (O, 469 beds) 6767 West Outer Drive, Detroit, MI Zip 48235–2899; tel. 313/493–6800

Owned, leased, sponsored:	8 hospitals	2261 beds
Contract–managed:	0 hospitals	0 beds
Totals:	8 hospitals	2261 beds

★0042:   DETROIT–MACOMB HOSPITAL CORPORATION (NP)
12000 East Twelve Mile Road, Warren, MI Zip 48093; tel. 810/573–5914; Timothy J. Ryan, JD, President and Chief Executive Officer

DETROIT RIVERVIEW HOSPITAL (O, 230 beds) 7733 East Jefferson Avenue, Detroit, MI Zip 48214; tel. 313/499–3000; Richard T. Young, Administrator

MACOMB HOSPITAL CENTER (O, 297 beds) 11800 East Twelve Mile Road, Warren, MI Zip 48093; tel. 810/573–5000; Timothy J. Ryan, JD, President and Chief Executive Officer

Owned, leased, sponsored:	2 hospitals	527 beds
Contract–managed:	0 hospitals	0 beds
Totals:	2 hospitals	527 beds

0845:   DEVEREUX FOUNDATION (NP)
19 South Waterloo Road, Devon, PA Zip 19333, Mailing Address: Box 400, Zip 19333; tel. 610/964–3000; Ronald P. Burd, President and Chief Exeuctive Officer

FLORIDA: DEVEREUX HOSPITAL AND CHILDREN'S CENTER OF FLORIDA (O, 100 beds) 8000 Devereux Drive, Melbourne, FL Zip 32940–7907; tel. 407/242–9100; James E. Colvin, Executive Director

GEORGIA: DEVEREUX CENTER–GEORGIA (O, 115 beds) 1291 Stanley Road, Kennesaw, GA Zip 30152; tel. 770/427–0147; Ralph L. Comerford, Director

PENNSYLVANIA: DEVEREUX MAPLETON PSYCHIATRIC INSTITUTE–MAPLETON CENTER (O, 13 beds) 655 Sugartown Road, Malvern, PA Zip 19355–0297, Mailing Address: Box 297, Zip 19355–0297; tel. 610/296–6923; Richard Warden, Administrator

TEXAS: DEVEREUX TEXAS TREATMENT NETWORK (O, 88 beds) 1150 Devereux Drive, League City, TX Zip 77573; tel. 713/335–1000; L. Gail Atkinson, Executive Director

DEVEREUX–VICTORIA (O, 6 beds) 120 David Wade Drive, Victoria, TX Zip 77902–2666; tel. 512/575–8271; L. Gail Atkinson, Executive Director

Owned, leased, sponsored:	5 hospitals	322 beds
Contract–managed:	0 hospitals	0 beds
Totals:	5 hospitals	322 beds

★0029:   DIMENSIONS HEALTH CORPORATION (NP)
9200 Basil Court, Landover, MD Zip 20785; tel. 301/925–7000; Winfield M. Kelly Jr., President and Chief Executive Officer

MARYLAND: LAUREL REGIONAL HOSPITAL (O, 185 beds) 7300 Van Dusen Road, Laurel, MD Zip 20707–9266; tel. 301/725–4300; Patrick F. Mutch, President

PRINCE GEORGE'S HOSPITAL CENTER (O, 370 beds) 3001 Hospital Drive, Cheverly, MD Zip 20785–1189; tel. 301/618–2000; Allan Earl Atzrott, President

Owned, leased, sponsored:	2 hospitals	555 beds
Contract–managed:	0 hospitals	0 beds
Totals:	2 hospitals	555 beds

0010:   DIVISION OF MENTAL HEALTH SERVICES, DEPARTMENT OF HUMAN SERVICES, STATE OF NEW JERSEY (NP)
Capital Center, CN 727, Trenton, NJ Zip 08625–0727; tel. 609/777–0702; Alan G. Kaufman, Director

NEW JERSEY: ANCORA PSYCHIATRIC HOSPITAL (O, 625 beds) 202 Spring Garden Road, Ancora, NJ Zip 08037–9699; tel. 609/561–1700; Yvonne A. Pressley, Chief Executive Officer

GREYSTONE PARK PSYCHIATRIC HOSPITAL (O, 605 beds) Central Avenue, Greystone Park, NJ Zip 07950, Mailing Address: P.O. Box A, Zip 07950; tel. 201/538–1800; Joseph Jupin Jr., Chief Executive Officer

MARLBORO PSYCHIATRIC HOSPITAL (O, 767 beds) 546 County Road 520, Marlboro, NJ Zip 07746–1099; tel. 908/946–8100; Gregory Roberts, Chief Executive Officer

SENATOR GARRET T. W. HAGEDORN GERO PSYCHIATRIC HOSPITAL (O, 181 beds) 200 Sanitorium Road, Glen Gardner, NJ Zip 08826–9752; tel. 908/537–2141; Edna Volpe–Way, Chief Executive Officer

TRENTON PSYCHIATRIC HOSPITAL (O, 379 beds) Sullivan Way, Station A, Trenton, NJ Zip 08625, Mailing Address: P.O. Box 7500, West Trenton, Zip 08628; tel. 609/633–1500; Joseph Jupin Jr., Chief Executive Officer

Owned, leased, sponsored:	5 hospitals	2557 beds
Contract–managed:	0 hospitals	0 beds
Totals:	5 hospitals	2557 beds

1045:   DOCTORS HOSPITAL (NP)
1087 Dennison Avenue, Columbus, OH Zip 43201; tel. 614/297–4000; Richard A. Vincent, President

OHIO: DOCTORS HOSPITAL (O, 380 beds) 1087 Dennison Avenue, Columbus, OH Zip 43201; tel. 614/297–4000; Richard A. Vincent, President

DOCTORS HOSPITAL OF NELSONVILLE (O, 77 beds) 1950 Mount Saint Mary Drive, Nelsonville, OH Zip 45764–1193; tel. 614/753–1931; Mark R. Seckinger, Administrator

Owned, leased, sponsored:	2 hospitals	457 beds
Contract–managed:	0 hospitals	0 beds
Totals:	2 hospitals	457 beds

1895:   EAST TEXAS MEDICAL CENTER REGIONAL HEALTHCARE SYSTEM (NP)
1000 South Beckham Street, Tyler, TX Zip 75701–1996, Mailing Address: P.O. Drawer 6400, Zip 75711–6400; tel. 903/535–6211; Elmer G. Ellis, President and Chief Executive Officer

TEXAS: EAST TEXAS MEDICAL CENTER (O, 338 beds) 1000 South Beckham Street, Tyler, TX Zip 75701–1996, Mailing Address: Box 6400, Zip 75711–6400; tel. 903/597–0351

EAST TEXAS MEDICAL CENTER (L, 54 beds) 1100 Loop 304 East, Crockett, TX Zip 75835–1810; tel. 409/544–2002; Dale E. Clark, Ph.D., Administrator and Chief Executive Officer

EAST TEXAS MEDICAL CENTER ATHENS (L, 108 beds) 2000 South Palestine, Athens, TX Zip 75751; tel. 903/675–2216; Patrick L. Wallace, Administrator

EAST TEXAS MEDICAL CENTER PITTSBURG (L, 42 beds) 414 Quitman Street, Pittsburg, TX Zip 75686–1032; tel. 903/856–6663; W. Perry Henderson, Administrator

EAST TEXAS MEDICAL CENTER REHABILITATION HOSPITAL (O, 49 beds) 701 Olympic Plaza Center, Tyler, TX Zip 75701–1996; tel. 903/596–3000; Eddie L. Howard, Vice President and Chief Operating Officer

EAST TEXAS MEDICAL CENTER RUSK (L, 25 beds) Copeland and Bonner Streets, Rusk, TX Zip 75785, Mailing Address: P.O. Box 317, Zip 75785; tel. 903/683–2273; Don Edd Green, Administrator

EAST TEXAS MEDICAL CENTER–CLARKSVILLE (L, 36 beds) Highway 82 West, Clarksville, TX Zip 75426, Mailing Address: Box 1270, Zip 75426; tel. 903/427–3851; Terry Cutler, Executive Director

For explanation of codes following names, see page B2.
★ Indicates Type III membership in the American Hospital Association.

Networks, Health Care Systems and Alliances

EAST TEXAS MEDICAL CENTER–MOUNT VERNON (L, 30 beds) Highway 37 South, Mount Vernon, TX Zip 75457, Mailing Address: Box 477, Zip 75457–0477; tel. 903/537–4552; Charles N. Butts, Administrator

Owned, leased, sponsored:	8 hospitals	682 beds
Contract–managed:	0 hospitals	0 beds
Totals:	8 hospitals	682 beds

★**0100: EASTERN HEALTH SYSTEM, INC.** (NP)
48 Medical Park East Drive, 450, Birmingham, AL Zip 35235; tel. 205/838–3999; Robert C. Chapman, FACHE, President and Chief Executive Officer

ALABAMA: BLOUNT MEMORIAL HOSPITAL (L, 57 beds) 1000 Lincoln Avenue, Oneonta, AL Zip 35121, Mailing Address: P.O. Box 220, Zip 35121; tel. 205/625–3511; George McGowan, Chief Executive Officer

MEDICAL CENTER EAST (O, 282 beds) 50 Medical Park East Drive, Birmingham, AL Zip 35235–9987; tel. 205/838–3000; David E. Crawford, FACHE, Executive Vice President and Chief Operating Officer

ST. CLAIR REGIONAL HOSPITAL (C, 51 beds) 2805 Hospital Drive, Pell City, AL Zip 35125; tel. 205/338–3301; George McGowan, Chief Executive Officer

Owned, leased, sponsored:	2 hospitals	339 beds
Contract–managed:	1 hospital	51 beds
Totals:	3 hospitals	390 beds

★**0555: EASTERN MAINE HEALTHCARE** (NP)
489 State Street, Bangor, ME Zip 04401, Mailing Address: P.O. Box 404, Zip 04402–0404; tel. 207/973–7051; Norman A. Ledwin, President

MAINE: ACADIA HOSPITAL (O, 72 beds) 268 Stillwater Avenue, Bangor, ME Zip 04401, Mailing Address: P.O. Box 422, Zip 04402–0422; tel. 207/973–6100; Dennis P. King, President

EASTERN MAINE MEDICAL CENTER (O, 344 beds) 489 State Street, Bangor, ME Zip 04401, Mailing Address: P.O. Box 404, Zip 04402–0404; tel. 207/973–7000; Norman A. Ledwin, President and Chief Executive Officer

Owned, leased, sponsored:	2 hospitals	416 beds
Contract–managed:	0 hospitals	0 beds
Totals:	2 hospitals	416 beds

★**3595: EASTERN MERCY HEALTH SYSTEM** (CC)
3 Radnor Corporate Center, Suite 220, Radnor, PA Zip 19087; tel. 610/971–9770; Daniel F. Russell, President and Chief Executive Officer

ALABAMA: MERCY MEDICAL (S, 157 beds) 101 Villa Drive, Daphne, AL Zip 36526, Mailing Address: P.O. Box 1090, Zip 36526; tel. 334/626–2694; Sister Mary Eileen Wilhelm, President and Chief Executive Officer

FLORIDA: HOLY CROSS HOSPITAL (S, 437 beds) 4725 North Federal Highway, Fort Lauderdale, FL Zip 33308, Mailing Address: Box 23460, Zip 33307; tel. 305/771–8000; Ray Budrys, President and Chief Executive Officer

GEORGIA: SAINT JOSEPH'S HOSPITAL OF ATLANTA (S, 346 beds) 5665 Peachtree Dunwoody Road N.E., Atlanta, GA Zip 30342–1764; tel. 404/851–7001; Brue Chandler, President and Chief Executive Officer

MAINE: MERCY HOSPITAL PORTLAND (S, 159 beds) 144 State Street, Portland, ME Zip 04101–3795; tel. 207/879–3000; Howard R. Buckley, President

NEW YORK: KENMORE MERCY HOSPITAL (S, 219 beds) 2950 Elmwood Avenue, Kenmore, NY Zip 14217–1390; tel. 716/447–6100; Sister Mary Joel Schimscheiner, Chief Executive Officer

MERCY HOSPITAL (S, 349 beds) 565 Abbott Road, Buffalo, NY Zip 14220; tel. 716/826–7000; James W. Connolly, President and Chief Executive Officer

ST. JAMES MERCY HOSPITAL (S, 200 beds) 411 Canisteo Street, Hornell, NY Zip 14843–2197; tel. 607/324–8000; Paul E. Shephard, President and Chief Executive Officer

ST. JEROME HOSPITAL (S, 96 beds) 16 Bank Street, Batavia, NY Zip 14020–2260; tel. 716/343–3131; Charles W. Smith Jr., Chief Executive Officer

ST. JOSEPH HOSPITAL (S, 184 beds) 2605 Harlem Road, Cheektowaga, NY Zip 14225–4097; tel. 716/891–2400; Patrick J. Wiles, Chief Executive Officer

ST. PETER'S HOSPITAL (S, 437 beds) 315 South Manning Boulevard, Albany, NY Zip 12208–1789; tel. 518/525–1550; Steven P. Boyle, President and Chief Executive Officer

PENNSYLVANIA: MERCY COMMUNITY HOSPITAL (S, 107 beds) 2000 Old West Chester Pike, Havertown, PA Zip 19083; tel. 610/645–3600; Andrew E. Harris, Chief Executive Officer

MERCY HEALTH SYSTEM OF SOUTHEASTERN PENNSYLVANIA (S, 553 beds) One Bala Plaza, Suite 402, Bala Cynwyd, PA Zip 19004; tel. 610/660–7440; Plato A. Marinakos, President and Chief Executive Officer

MERCY HOSPITAL OF PITTSBURGH (S, 493 beds) 1400 Locust Street, Pittsburgh, PA Zip 15219–5166; tel. 412/232–8111; Howard A. Zaren, M.D., FACS, Executive Vice President, Hospital Services

MERCY PROVIDENCE HOSPITAL (S, 146 beds) 1004 Arch Street, Pittsburgh, PA Zip 15212; tel. 412/323–5600; Thomas Mattei, M.D., Chief Operating Officer

Owned, leased, sponsored:	14 hospitals	3883 beds
Contract–managed:	0 hospitals	0 beds
Totals:	14 hospitals	3883 beds

0945: EMPIRE HEALTH SERVICES (NP)
West 800 Fifth Avenue, Spokane, WA Zip 99204, Mailing Address: P.O. Box 248, Zip 99210–0248; tel. 509/458–7960; Thomas M. White, President

WASHINGTON: DEACONESS MEDICAL CENTER–SPOKANE (O, 326 beds) 800 West Fifth Avenue, Spokane, WA Zip 99204, Mailing Address: P.O. Box 248, Zip 99210–0248; tel. 509/458–5800; Thomas J. Zellers, Chief Operating Officer

VALLEY HOSPITAL AND MEDICAL CENTER (O, 117 beds) 12606 East Mission Avenue, Spokane, WA Zip 99216–9969; tel. 509/924–6650; Michael T. Liepman, Chief Operating Officer

Owned, leased, sponsored:	2 hospitals	443 beds
Contract–managed:	0 hospitals	0 beds
Totals:	2 hospitals	443 beds

★**0735: EPISCOPAL HEALTH SERVICES INC.** (CO)
333 Earle Ovington Boulevard, Uniondale, NY Zip 11553–3645; tel. 516/228–6100; Jack N. Farrington, Ph.D., Executive Vice President

NEW YORK: ST. JOHN'S EPISCOPAL HOSPITAL–SMITHTOWN (O, 366 beds) 50 Route 25–A, Smithtown, NY Zip 11787–1398; tel. 516/862–3000; Laura Righter, Regional Administrator

ST. JOHN'S EPISCOPAL HOSPITAL–SOUTH SHORE (O, 314 beds) 327 Beach 19th Street, Far Rockaway, NY Zip 11691–4424; tel. 718/869–7000; Paul J. Connor III, Administrator

Owned, leased, sponsored:	2 hospitals	680 beds
Contract–managed:	0 hospitals	0 beds
Totals:	2 hospitals	680 beds

1255: ESCAMBIA COUNTY HEALTH CARE AUTHORITY (NP)
1301 Belleville Avenue, Brewton, AL Zip 36426; tel. 334/368–2500; Phillip L. Parker, Administrator

ALABAMA: ATMORE COMMUNITY HOSPITAL (O, 51 beds) 401 Medical Park Drive, Atmore, AL Zip 36502; tel. 334/368–2500; Lavon Henley, Administrator

D. W. MCMILLAN MEMORIAL HOSPITAL (O, 83 beds) 1301 Belleville Avenue, Brewton, AL Zip 36426, Mailing Address: Box 908, Zip 36427; tel. 334/867–8061; Phillip L. Parker, Administrator

---

For explanation of codes following names, see page B2.
★ Indicates Type III membership in the American Hospital Association.

Owned, leased, sponsored:	2 hospitals	134 beds
Contract–managed:	0 hospitals	0 beds
Totals:	2 hospitals	134 beds

★1325: FAIRVIEW HOSPITAL AND HEALTHCARE SERVICES (NP)

2450 Riverside Avenue, Minneapolis, MN Zip 55454–1400; tel. 612/672–6300; Richard A. Norling, President and Chief Executive Officer

MINNESOTA: CHISAGO HEALTH SERVICES (O, 89 beds) 11685 Lake Boulevard North, Chisago City, MN Zip 55013–9540; tel. 612/257–8400; Scott Wordelman, President and Chief Executive Officer

DISTRICT MEMORIAL HOSPITAL (O, 44 beds) 246 11th Avenue S.E., Forest Lake, MN Zip 55025–1898; tel. 612/464–3341; John F. Lannon, Administrator

FAIRVIEW NORTHLAND REGIONAL HOSPITAL (O, 41 beds) 911 Northland Drive, Princeton, MN Zip 55371; tel. 612/389–1313; Glenn G. Erickson, Vice President and Administrator

FAIRVIEW RIDGES HOSPITAL (O, 124 beds) 201 East Nicollet Boulevard, Burnsville, MN Zip 55337–5799; tel. 612/892–2000; Mark M. Enger, Senior Vice President and Administrator

FAIRVIEW SOUTHDALE HOSPITAL (O, 390 beds) 6401 France Avenue South, Minneapolis, MN Zip 55435–2199; tel. 612/924–5000; Mark M. Enger, Senior Vice President and Administrator

FAIRVIEW–UNIVERSITY MEDICAL CENTER (O, 1362 beds) 2450 Riverside Avenue, Minneapolis, MN Zip 55454–1400; tel. 612/672–6300; Peter Rapp, Senior Vice President and Administrator

UNIVERSITY MEDICAL CENTER–MESABI (O, 132 beds) 750 East 34th Street, Hibbing, MN Zip 55746; tel. 218/262–4881; Frances J. Gardeski, Chief Executive Officer

Owned, leased, sponsored:	7 hospitals	2182 beds
Contract–managed:	0 hospitals	0 beds
Totals:	7 hospitals	2182 beds

2515: FAIRVIEW HOSPITAL SYSTEM (NP)

18101 Lorain Avenue, Cleveland, OH Zip 44111–5656; tel. 216/476–7000; Kenneth T. Misener, Vice President and Chief Operating Officer

OHIO: FAIRVIEW HOSPITAL (O, 428 beds) 18101 Lorain Avenue, Cleveland, OH Zip 44111–5656; tel. 216/476–4040; Thomas M. LaMotte, President and Chief Executive Officer

LUTHERAN HOSPITAL (O, 174 beds) 2609 Franklin Boulevard, Cleveland, OH Zip 44113–2992; tel. 216/696–4300; Kenneth T. Misener, Chief Operating Officer

Owned, leased, sponsored:	2 hospitals	602 beds
Contract–managed:	0 hospitals	0 beds
Totals:	2 hospitals	602 beds

1275: FIRST HEALTH, INC. (IO)

107 Public Square, Batesville, MS Zip 38606; tel. 601/563–7676; Sandra Skinner, Chief Executive Officer

KENTUCKY: JENKINS COMMUNITY HOSPITAL (O, 60 beds) Main Street, Jenkins, KY Zip 41537, Mailing Address: P.O. Box 472, Zip 41537; tel. 606/832–2171; Sherrie Newcomb, Acting Administrator

MISSISSIPPI: BRUCE HOSPITAL (O, 47 beds) Highway 9 South, Bruce, MS Zip 38915, Mailing Address: Box 429, Zip 38915–0429; tel. 601/983–5100; Robert M. Perry, Administrator

Owned, leased, sponsored:	2 hospitals	107 beds
Contract–managed:	0 hospitals	0 beds
Totals:	2 hospitals	107 beds

2635: FIRST HOSPITAL CORPORATION (IO)

240 Corporate Boulevard, Norfolk, VA Zip 23502; tel. 757/459–5100; Ronald I. Dozoretz, M.D., Chairman

CALIFORNIA: FIRST HOSPITAL VALLEJO (O, 61 beds) 525 Oregon Street, Vallejo, CA Zip 94590; tel. 707/648–2200; John E. Wiley, Chief Executive Officer and Administrator

PENNSYLVANIA: SOUTHWOOD PSYCHIATRIC HOSPITAL (O, 50 beds) 2575 Boyce Plaza Road, Pittsburgh, PA Zip 15241–3925; tel. 412/257–2290; Alan A. Axelson, M.D., Chief Executive Officer

PUERTO RICO: FIRST HOSPITAL PANAMERICANO (O, 165 beds) State Road 787 KM 1 5, Cidra, PR Zip 00739, Mailing Address: P.O. Box 1398, Zip 00739; tel. 809/739–5555; Henry Ruberte', Administrator

Owned, leased, sponsored:	3 hospitals	276 beds
Contract–managed:	0 hospitals	0 beds
Totals:	3 hospitals	276 beds

★1475: FRANCISCAN MISSIONARIES OF OUR LADY HEALTH SYSTEM, INC. (CC)

4200 Essen Lane, Baton Rouge, LA Zip 70809; tel. 504/923–2701; John J. Finan Jr., President and Chief Executive Officer

LOUISIANA: OUR LADY OF LOURDES REGIONAL MEDICAL CENTER (O, 293 beds) 611 St. Landry Street, Lafayette, LA Zip 70506–4697, Mailing Address: Box 4027, Zip 70502–4027; tel. 318/289–2000; Dudley Romero, President and Chief Executive Officer

OUR LADY OF THE LAKE REGIONAL MEDICAL CENTER (O, 660 beds) 5000 Henessy Boulevard, Baton Rouge, LA Zip 70808–4350; tel. 504/765–6565; Robert C. Davidge, President and Chief Executive Officer

ST. FRANCIS MEDICAL CENTER (O, 385 beds) 309 Jackson Street, Monroe, LA Zip 71201, Mailing Address: Box 1901, Zip 71210–1901; tel. 318/327–4000; H. Gerald Smith, President and Chief Executive Officer

Owned, leased, sponsored:	3 hospitals	1338 beds
Contract–managed:	0 hospitals	0 beds
Totals:	3 hospitals	1338 beds

★5375: FRANCISCAN SERVICES CORPORATION (CC)

6832 Convent Boulevard, Sylvania, OH Zip 43560–2897; tel. 419/882–8373; John W. O'Connell, President

OHIO: PROVIDENCE HOSPITAL (S, 170 beds) 1912 Hayes Avenue, Sandusky, OH Zip 44870–4736; tel. 419/621–7000; Sister Nancy Linenkugel, FACHE, President and Chief Executive Officer

TRINITY HEALTH SYSTEM (S, 533 beds) 380 Summit Avenue, Steubenville, OH Zip 43952; tel. 614/283–7000; Fred B. Brower, President and Chief Executive Officer

TEXAS: BURLESON ST. JOSEPH HEALTH CENTER (S, 30 beds) 1101 Woodson Drive, Caldwell, TX Zip 77836, Mailing Address: P.O. Drawer 360, Zip 77836; tel. 409/567–3245; William H. Craig, President and Chief Executive Officer

ST. FRANCIS HEALTH CENTER (S, 32 beds) 100 West Cross Street, Madisonville, TX Zip 77864–0698, Mailing Address: Box 698, Zip 77864–0698; tel. 409/348–2631; James P. Gibson, President and Chief Executive Officer

ST. JOSEPH REGIONAL HEALTH CENTER (S, 195 beds) 2801 Franciscan Drive, Bryan, TX Zip 77802; tel. 409/776–3777; Sister Gretchen Kunz, President and Chief Executive Officer

TRINITY COMMUNITY MEDICAL CENTER OF BRENHAM (S, 60 beds) 700 Medical Parkway, Brenham, TX Zip 77833; tel. 409/836–6173; John L. Simms, President and Chief Executive Officer

Owned, leased, sponsored:	6 hospitals	1020 beds
Contract–managed:	0 hospitals	0 beds
Totals:	6 hospitals	1020 beds

For explanation of codes following names, see page B2.
★ Indicates Type III membership in the American Hospital Association.

Section B

★1415: FRANCISCAN SISTERS HEALTH CARE CORPORATION (CC)
9223 West St. Francis Road, Frankfort, IL Zip 60423–8334; tel. 815/469–4888; Gerald P. Pearson, President

ILLINOIS: SAINT JOSEPH HOSPITAL (O, 202 beds) 77 North Airlite Street, Elgin, IL Zip 60123–4912; tel. 847/695–3200; Larry Narum, President and Chief Executive Officer

SAINT JOSEPH MEDICAL CENTER (O, 505 beds) 333 North Madison Street, Joliet, IL Zip 60435–6595; tel. 815/741–7236; David W. Benfer, President and Chief Executive Officer

SAINT THERESE MEDICAL CENTER (O, 254 beds) 2615 Washington Street, Waukegan, IL Zip 60085–4988; tel. 847/249–3900; Timothy P. Selz, President

UNITED SAMARITANS MEDICAL CENTER (O, 308 beds) 812 North Logan, Danville, IL Zip 61832–3788; tel. 217/442–6300; Dennis J. Doran, President and Chief Executive Officer

Owned, leased, sponsored:	4 hospitals	1269 beds
Contract–managed:	0 hospitals	0 beds
Totals:	4 hospitals	1269 beds

★1455: FRANCISCAN SISTERS OF CHRISTIAN CHARITY HEALTHCARE MINISTRY, INC (CC)
2409 South Alverno Road, Manitowoc, WI Zip 54220–9320; tel. 920/684–7071; Sister Laura J. Wolf, President

NEBRASKA: ST. FRANCIS MEMORIAL HOSPITAL (O, 27 beds) 430 North Monitor Street, West Point, NE Zip 68788–1595; tel. 402/372–2404; Ronald O. Briggs, President

OHIO: GENESIS HEALTHCARE SYSTEM (O, 495 beds) 800 Forest Avenue, Zanesville, OH Zip 43701–2881; tel. 614/454–5000; Thomas L. Sieber, President and Chief Executive Officer

WISCONSIN: HOLY FAMILY MEMORIAL MEDICAL CENTER (O, 176 beds) 2300 Western Avenue, Manitowoc, WI Zip 54220, Mailing Address: P.O. Box 1450, Zip 54221–1450; tel. 414/684–2011; Daniel B. McGinty, President and Chief Executive Officer

Owned, leased, sponsored:	3 hospitals	698 beds
Contract–managed:	0 hospitals	0 beds
Totals:	3 hospitals	698 beds

★1485: FRANCISCAN SISTERS OF THE POOR HEALTH SYSTEM, INC. (CC)
708 Third Avenue, Suite 200, New York, NY Zip 10017; tel. 212/818–1987; James H. Flynn Jr., President and Chief Executive Officer

KENTUCKY: OUR LADY OF BELLEFONTE HOSPITAL (S, 194 beds) St. Christopher Drive, Ashland, KY Zip 41105–0789, Mailing Address: P.O. Box 789, Zip 41105–0789; tel. 606/833–3333; Robert J. Maher, President

NEW JERSEY: ST. FRANCIS HOSPITAL (S, 243 beds) 25 McWilliams Place, Jersey City, NJ Zip 07302–1698; tel. 201/418–1000; Robert S. Chaloner, President and Chief Executive Officer

ST. MARY HOSPITAL (S, 328 beds) 308 Willow Avenue, Hoboken, NJ Zip 07030–3889; tel. 201/418–1000; Robert S. Chaloner, President and Chief Executive Officer

NEW YORK: MERCY COMMUNITY HOSPITAL (O, 187 beds) 160 East Main Street, Port Jervis, NY Zip 12771–0268, Mailing Address: P.O. Box 1014, Zip 12771; tel. 914/856–5351; R. Andrew Brothers, President and Chief Executive Officer

ST. ANTHONY COMMUNITY HOSPITAL (S, 73 beds) 15–19 Maple Avenue, Warwick, NY Zip 10990; tel. 914/986–2276; R. Andrew Brothers, President and Chief Executive Officer

OHIO: FRANCISCAN HOSPITAL–MOUNT AIRY CAMPUS (S, 240 beds) 2446 Kipling Avenue, Cincinnati, OH Zip 45239–6650; tel. 513/853–5000; R. Christopher West, President

FRANCISCAN HOSPITAL–WESTERN HILLS CAMPUS (S, 226 beds) 3131 Queen City Avenue, Cincinnati, OH Zip 45238–2396; tel. 513/389–5000; R. Christopher West, President

FRANCISCAN MEDICAL CENTER–DAYTON CAMPUS (S, 365 beds) One Franciscan Way, Dayton, OH Zip 45408–1498; tel. 513/229–6000; James M. Strieby, Chief Executive Officer

SOUTH CAROLINA: ST. FRANCIS HEALTH SYSTEM (S, 269 beds) One St. Francis Drive, Greenville, SC Zip 29601–3207; tel. 864/255–1000; Richard C. Neugent, President

Owned, leased, sponsored:	9 hospitals	2125 beds
Contract–managed:	0 hospitals	0 beds
Totals:	9 hospitals	2125 beds

★9650: FRANCISCAN SKEMP HEALTHCARE (CC)
700 West Avenue South, La Crosse, WI Zip 54601; tel. 608/791–9710; Brian C. Campion, M.D., President and Chief Executive Officer

WISCONSIN: FRANCISCAN SKEMP HEALTHCARE–ARCADIA CAMPUS (O, 101 beds) 464 South St. Joseph Avenue, Arcadia, WI Zip 54612–1401; tel. 608/323–3341; Robert M. Tracey, Administrator

FRANCISCAN SKEMP HEALTHCARE–LA CROSSE CAMPUS (O, 226 beds) 700 West Avenue South, La Crosse, WI Zip 54601–4783; tel. 608/785–0940; Ronald R. Paczkowski, Vice President

FRANCISCAN SKEMP HEALTHCARE–SPARTA CAMPUS (O, 60 beds) 310 West Main Street, Sparta, WI Zip 54656; tel. 608/269–2132; William P. Sexton, Administrator

Owned, leased, sponsored:	3 hospitals	387 beds
Contract–managed:	0 hospitals	0 beds
Totals:	3 hospitals	387 beds

2115: FREMONT–RIDEOUT HEALTH GROUP (NP)
989 Plumas Street, Yuba City, CA Zip 95991; tel. 916/751–4010; Thomas P. Hayes, Chief Executive Officer

CALIFORNIA: FREMONT MEDICAL CENTER (O, 92 beds) 970 Plumas Street, Yuba City, CA Zip 95991; tel. 916/751–4000; Thomas P. Hayes, Chief Executive Officer

RIDEOUT MEMORIAL HOSPITAL (O, 97 beds) 726 Fourth Street, Marysville, CA Zip 95901–2128, Mailing Address: Box 2128, Zip 95901–2128; tel. 916/749–4300; Thomas P. Hayes, Chief Executive Officer

Owned, leased, sponsored:	2 hospitals	189 beds
Contract–managed:	0 hospitals	0 beds
Totals:	2 hospitals	189 beds

5570: GEISINGER HEALTH SYSTEM (NP)
100 North Academy Avenue, Danville, PA Zip 17822; tel. 717/271–6211; Frank J. Trembulak, Executive Vice President and Chief Operating Officer

PENNSYLVANIA: GEISINGER MEDICAL CENTER (O, 548 beds) 100 North Academy Avenue, Danville, PA Zip 17822–2201; tel. 717/271–6211; Stuart Heydt, Chief Executive Officer

GEISINGER WYOMING VALLEY MEDICAL CENTER (O, 144 beds) 1000 East Mountain Drive, Wilkes–Barre, PA Zip 18711–0025; tel. 717/826–7300; Conrad W. Schintz, Senior Vice President Operations

Owned, leased, sponsored:	2 hospitals	692 beds
Contract–managed:	0 hospitals	0 beds
Totals:	2 hospitals	692 beds

★0775: GENERAL HEALTH SYSTEM (NP)
3849 North Boulevard, Suite 200, Baton Rouge, LA Zip 70806; tel. 504/387–7810; Thomas H. Sawyer, President and Chief Executive Officer

LOUISIANA: BATON ROUGE GENERAL HEALTH CENTER (O, 72 beds) 8585 Picardy Avenue, Baton Rouge, LA Zip 70809, Mailing Address: P.O. Box 84330, Zip 70884–4330; tel. 504/763–4000; Linda Lee, Administrator

For explanation of codes following names, see page B2.
★ Indicates Type III membership in the American Hospital Association.

BATON ROUGE GENERAL MEDICAL CENTER (O, 355 beds) 3600 Florida Street, Baton Rouge, LA Zip 70806, Mailing Address: P.O. Box 2511, Zip 70821–2511; tel. 504/387–7770; Chris W. Barnette, President and Chief Executive Officer

VERMILION HOSPITAL (O, 54 beds) 2520 North University, Lafayette, LA Zip 70507, Mailing Address: P.O. Box 91526, Zip 70509–1526; tel. 318/234–5614; John P. Patout, Administrator

Owned, leased, sponsored:	3 hospitals	481 beds
Contract–managed:	0 hospitals	0 beds
Totals:	3 hospitals	481 beds

★1535: GREAT PLAINS HEALTH ALLIANCE, INC. (NP)
625 Third, Phillipsburg, KS Zip 67661, Mailing Address: P.O. Box 366, Zip 67661–0366; tel. 913/543–2111; Roger S. John, President and Chief Executive Officer

KANSAS: ASHLAND HEALTH CENTER (C, 48 beds) 709 Oak Street, Ashland, KS Zip 67831, Mailing Address: P.O. Box 188, Zip 67831; tel. 316/635–2241; Bryan Stacey, Administrator

CHEYENNE COUNTY HOSPITAL (L, 23 beds) 210 West First Street, Saint Francis, KS Zip 67756, Mailing Address: P.O. Box 547, Zip 67756–0547; tel. 913/332–2104; Leslie Lacy, Administrator

ELLINWOOD DISTRICT HOSPITAL (L, 12 beds) 605 North Main Street, Ellinwood, KS Zip 67526; tel. 316/564–2548; Marge Conell, R.N., Administrator

FREDONIA REGIONAL HOSPITAL (C, 42 beds) 1527 Madison Street, Fredonia, KS Zip 66736, Mailing Address: Box 579, Zip 66736; tel. 316/378–2121; Terry Deschaine, Administrator

GREELEY COUNTY HOSPITAL (L, 49 beds) 506 Third Street, Tribune, KS Zip 67879, Mailing Address: Box 338, Zip 67879; tel. 316/376–4221; Cynthia K. Schneider, Administrator

GRISELL MEMORIAL HOSPITAL DISTRICT ONE (C, 46 beds) 210 South Vermont, Ransom, KS Zip 67572–0268, Mailing Address: P.O. Box 268, Zip 67572–0268; tel. 913/731–2231; Kristine Ochs, R.N., Administrator

KIOWA COUNTY MEMORIAL HOSPITAL (O, 38 beds) 501 South Walnut Street, Greensburg, KS Zip 67054; tel. 316/723–3341; Ronald J. Baker, Administrator

LANE COUNTY HOSPITAL (C, 31 beds) 243 South Second, Dighton, KS Zip 67839, Mailing Address: Box 969, Zip 67839; tel. 316/397–5321; Donna McGowan, R.N., Administrator

LINCOLN COUNTY HOSPITAL (C, 34 beds) 624 North Second Street, Lincoln, KS Zip 67455, Mailing Address: P.O. Box 406, Zip 67455; tel. 913/524–4403; Jolene Yager, R.N., Administrator

MEDICINE LODGE MEMORIAL HOSPITAL (C, 42 beds) 710 North Walnut Street, Medicine Lodge, KS Zip 67104, Mailing Address: P.O. Drawer C, Zip 67104; tel. 316/886–3771; Kevin A. White, Administrator

MINNEOLA DISTRICT HOSPITAL (C, 15 beds) 212 Main Street, Minneola, KS Zip 67865; tel. 316/885–4264; Blaine K. Miller, Administrator

MITCHELL COUNTY HOSPITAL (L, 89 beds) 400 West Eighth, Beloit, KS Zip 67420, Mailing Address: P.O. Box 399, Zip 67420; tel. 913/738–2266; John M. Osse, Administrator

OSBORNE COUNTY MEMORIAL HOSPITAL (C, 29 beds) 424 West New Hampshire Street, Osborne, KS Zip 67473–0070, Mailing Address: P.O. Box 70, Zip 67473–0070; tel. 913/346–2121; Patricia Bernard, R.N., Administrator

OTTAWA COUNTY HOSPITAL (L, 53 beds) 215 East Eighth, Minneapolis, KS Zip 67467, Mailing Address: Box 209, Zip 67467; tel. 913/392–2122; Joy Reed, R.N., Administrator

PHILLIPS COUNTY HOSPITAL (L, 62 beds) 1150 State Street, Phillipsburg, KS Zip 67661, Mailing Address: Box 607, Zip 67661; tel. 913/543–5226; James L. Giedd, Administrator

RAWLINS COUNTY HOSPITAL (C, 24 beds) 707 Grant Street, Atwood, KS Zip 67730–4700, Mailing Address: Box 47, Zip 67730–4700; tel. 913/626–3211; Donald J. Kessen, Administrator

REPUBLIC COUNTY HOSPITAL (L, 86 beds) 2420 G Street, Belleville, KS Zip 66935; tel. 913/527–2255; Charles A. Westin, FACHE, Administrator

SABETHA COMMUNITY HOSPITAL (L, 27 beds) 14th and Oregon Streets, Sabetha, KS Zip 66534, Mailing Address: P.O. Box 229, Zip 66534; tel. 913/284–2121; Rita K. Buurman, Administrator

SALEM HOSPITAL (C, 86 beds) 701 South Main Street, Hillsboro, KS Zip 67063–9981; tel. 316/947–3114; Robert G. Senneff, Chief Executive Officer

SATANTA DISTRICT HOSPITAL (C, 42 beds) 401 South Cheyenne Street, Satanta, KS Zip 67870, Mailing Address: P.O. Box 159, Zip 67870–0159; tel. 316/649–2761; T. G. Lee, Administrator

SMITH COUNTY MEMORIAL HOSPITAL (L, 54 beds) 614 South Main Street, Smith Center, KS Zip 66967–0349, Mailing Address: P.O. Box 349, Zip 66967–0349; tel. 913/282–6845; John Terrill, Administrator

TREGO COUNTY–LEMKE MEMORIAL HOSPITAL (C, 73 beds) 320 13th Street, Wakeeney, KS Zip 67672–2099; tel. 913/743–2182; James Wahlmeier, Administrator

NEBRASKA: COMMUNITY MEDICAL CENTER (C, 49 beds) 2307 Barada Street, Falls City, NE Zip 68355–1599; tel. 402/245–2428; Victor Lee, Chief Executive Officer and Administrator

HARLAN COUNTY HOSPITAL (C, 25 beds) 717 North Brown, Alma, NE Zip 68920, Mailing Address: P.O. Box 836, Zip 68920; tel. 308/928–2151; Allen Van Driel, Administrator

Owned, leased, sponsored:	10 hospitals	493 beds
Contract–managed:	14 hospitals	586 beds
Totals:	24 hospitals	1079 beds

★0046: GREATER ROCHESTER HEALTH SYSTEM, INC. (NP)
1040 University Avenue, Rochester, NY Zip 14607; tel. 716/756–4280; Roger S. Hunt, President and Chief Executive Officer

NEW YORK: GENESEE HOSPITAL (O, 305 beds) 224 Alexander Street, Rochester, NY Zip 14607–4055; tel. 716/263–6000; Joseph J. DeSilva, FACHE, President and Chief Executive Officer

NEWARK–WAYNE COMMUNITY HOSPITAL (O, 256 beds) Driving Park Avenue, Newark, NY Zip 14513, Mailing Address: P.O. Box 111, Zip 14513–0111; tel. 315/332–2022; William R. Holman, President

ROCHESTER GENERAL HOSPITAL (O, 476 beds) 1425 Portland Avenue, Rochester, NY Zip 14621–3099; tel. 716/338–4000; Richard S. Constantino, M.D., President

Owned, leased, sponsored:	3 hospitals	1037 beds
Contract–managed:	0 hospitals	0 beds
Totals:	3 hospitals	1037 beds

★2015: GREATER SOUTHEAST HEALTHCARE SYSTEM (NP)
1310 Southern Avenue S.E., Washington, DC Zip 20032; tel. 202/574–6926; Dalton A. Tong, CPA, FACHE, President and Chief Executive Officer

DISTRICT OF COLUMBIA: GREATER SOUTHEAST COMMUNITY HOSPITAL (O, 305 beds) 1310 Southern Avenue S.E., Washington, DC Zip 20032–4699; tel. 202/574–6000; Robert C. Winfrey, President and Chief Operating Officer

MARYLAND: FORT WASHINGTON HOSPITAL (O, 33 beds) 11711 Livingston Road, Fort Washington, MD Zip 20744–5164; tel. 301/292–7000; Theodore M. Lewis, President and Chief Executive Officer

Owned, leased, sponsored:	2 hospitals	338 beds
Contract–managed:	0 hospitals	0 beds
Totals:	2 hospitals	338 beds

1155: GREENLEAF HEALTH SYSTEMS, INC. (IO)
One Northgate Park, Chattanooga, TN Zip 37415; tel. 423/870–5110; Dan B. Page, President

ARKANSAS: GREENLEAF CENTER (O, 40 beds) 2712 East Johnson, Jonesboro, AR Zip 72401; tel. 501/932–2800; John S. Hart, Administrator

---

For explanation of codes following names, see page B2.
★ Indicates Type III membership in the American Hospital Association.

GEORGIA: GREENLEAF CENTER (C, 90 beds) 500 Greenleaf Circle, Fort Oglethorpe, GA Zip 30742; tel. 706/861–4357; Richard A. Waxler, Administrator

GREENLEAF CENTER (O, 70 beds) 2209 Pineview Drive, Valdosta, GA Zip 31602; tel. 912/247–4357; Michael Lane, Administrator and Chief Executive Officer

Owned, leased, sponsored:	2 hospitals	110 beds
Contract–managed:	1 hospital	90 beds
Totals:	3 hospitals	200 beds

★1555: GREENVILLE HOSPITAL SYSTEM (NP)
701 Grove Road, Greenville, SC Zip 29605–4211; tel. 864/455–7000; Frank D. Pinckney, President

SOUTH CAROLINA: ALLEN BENNETT HOSPITAL (O, 146 beds) 313 Memorial Drive, Greer, SC Zip 29650; tel. 864/848–8130; Michael W. Massey, Administrator

GREENVILLE MEMORIAL HOSPITAL (O, 620 beds) 701 Grove Road, Greenville, SC Zip 29605–4295; tel. 864/455–7000; J. Bland Burkhardt Jr., Senior Vice President and Administrator

HILLCREST HOSPITAL (O, 46 beds) 729 S.E. Main Street, Simpsonville, SC Zip 29681; tel. 864/967–6100; James Dover, Administrator

MARSHALL I. PICKENS HOSPITAL (O, 106 beds) 701 Grove Road, Greenville, SC Zip 29605–4295; tel. 864/455–7836; Ryan D. Beaty, Administrator

ROGER C. PEACE REHABILITATION HOSPITAL (O, 50 beds) 701 Grove Road, Greenville, SC Zip 29605–4295; tel. 864/455–7000; Ryan D. Beaty, Administrator

Owned, leased, sponsored:	5 hospitals	968 beds
Contract–managed:	0 hospitals	0 beds
Totals:	5 hospitals	968 beds

★9995: GROUP HEALTH COOPERATIVE OF PUGET SOUND (NP)
521 Wall Street, Seattle, WA Zip 98121–1536; tel. 206/326–3000; Phil Nudelman, Ph.D., President and Chief Executive Officer

WASHINGTON: GROUP HEALTH COOPERATIVE CENTRAL HOSPITAL (O, 187 beds) 201 16th Avenue East, Seattle, WA Zip 98112–5298; tel. 206/326–3000; Scott Armstrong, Administrator

THE EASTSIDE HOSPITAL (O, 125 beds) 2700 152nd Avenue N.E., Redmond, WA Zip 98052–5560; tel. 206/883–5151; Scott Armstrong, Administrator

Owned, leased, sponsored:	2 hospitals	312 beds
Contract–managed:	0 hospitals	0 beds
Totals:	2 hospitals	312 beds

★0675: GUTHRIE HEALTHCARE SYSTEM (NP)
Guthrie Square, Sayre, PA Zip 18840; tel. 717/882–4312; Ralph H. Meyer, President and Chief Executive Officer

PENNSYLVANIA: ROBERT PACKER HOSPITAL (O, 265 beds) Guthrie Square, Sayre, PA Zip 18840; tel. 717/888–6666; Russell M. Knight, President

TROY COMMUNITY HOSPITAL (O, 35 beds) 100 John Street, Troy, PA Zip 16947; tel. 717/297–2121; Mark A. Webster, President

Owned, leased, sponsored:	2 hospitals	300 beds
Contract–managed:	0 hospitals	0 beds
Totals:	2 hospitals	300 beds

★2345: HARRIS METHODIST HEALTH SYSTEM (CO)
6000 Western Place, Suite 200, Fort Worth, TX Zip 76107; tel. 817/570–8900; Ronald L. Smith, President

TEXAS: HARRIS CONTINUED CARE HOSPITAL (O, 15 beds) 1301 Pennsylvania Avenue, 4th Floor, Fort Worth, TX Zip 76104, Mailing Address: P.O. Box 3471, Zip 76113; tel. 817/878–5500; Larry Thompson, Administrator

HARRIS METHODIST FORT WORTH (O, 499 beds) 1301 Pennsylvania Avenue, Fort Worth, TX Zip 76104–2895; tel. 817/882–2000; Barclay E. Berdan, Chief Executive Officer

HARRIS METHODIST NORTHWEST (O, 36 beds) 108 Denver Trail, Azle, TX Zip 76020; tel. 817/444–8600; Larry Thompson, Vice President and Administrator

HARRIS METHODIST SOUTHWEST (O, 70 beds) 6100 Harris Parkway, Fort Worth, TX Zip 76132; tel. 817/346–5050; David B. Rowe, Vice President and Administrator

HARRIS METHODIST–ERATH COUNTY (O, 75 beds) 411 North Belknap Street, Stephenville, TX Zip 76401–1399, Mailing Address: Box 1399, Zip 76401; tel. 817/965–1500; Ronald E. Dorris, Administrator

HARRIS METHODIST–HEB (O, 186 beds) 1600 Hospital Parkway, Bedford, TX Zip 76022–6913, Mailing Address: P.O. Box 669, Zip 76095; tel. 817/685–4000; Jack McCabe, Senior Vice President and Administrator

ST. PAUL MEDICAL CENTER (O, 309 beds) 5909 Harry Hines Boulevard, Dallas, TX Zip 75235; tel. 214/879–1000; Michael A. Austin, CPA, Administrator

WALLS REGIONAL HOSPITAL (O, 112 beds) 201 Walls Drive, Cleburne, TX Zip 76031; tel. 817/641–2551; Brent D. Magers, FACHE, Chief Executive Officer and Administrator

Owned, leased, sponsored:	8 hospitals	1302 beds
Contract–managed:	0 hospitals	0 beds
Totals:	8 hospitals	1302 beds

★0082: HEALTH ALLIANCE OF GREATER CINCINNATI (NP)
2060 Reading Road, Suite 400, Cincinnati, OH Zip 45202–1456; tel. 513/632–3700; Jack M. Cook, President and Chief Executive Officer

KENTUCKY: ST. LUKE HOSPITAL EAST (O, 221 beds) 85 North Grand Avenue, Fort Thomas, KY Zip 41075–1796; tel. 606/572–3100; Daniel M. Vinson, CPA, Senior Executive Officer

ST. LUKE HOSPITAL WEST (O, 152 beds) 7380 Turfway Road, Florence, KY Zip 41042; tel. 606/525–5200; John D. Hoyle, Senior Executive Officer

OHIO: CHRIST HOSPITAL (O, 423 beds) 2139 Auburn Avenue, Cincinnati, OH Zip 45219–2989; tel. 513/369–2000; Claus von Zychlin, Senior Executive Officer

JEWISH HOSPITAL (O, 437 beds) 3200 Burnet Avenue, Cincinnati, OH Zip 45229–3099; tel. 513/569–2000; Warren C. Falberg, Senior Executive Officer

UNIVERISITY HOSPITAL (O, 418 beds) 234 Goodman Street, Cincinnati, OH Zip 45267–0700; tel. 513/558–1000; Elliot G. Cohen, Senior Executive Officer

Owned, leased, sponsored:	5 hospitals	1651 beds
Contract–managed:	0 hospitals	0 beds
Totals:	5 hospitals	1651 beds

1775: HEALTH MANAGEMENT ASSOCIATES (IO)
5811 Pelican Bay Boulevard, Suite 500, Naples, FL Zip 33963–2710; tel. 941/598–3175; William J. Schoen, President

ALABAMA: RIVERVIEW REGIONAL MEDICAL CENTER (O, 281 beds) 600 South Third Street, Gadsden, AL Zip 35901, Mailing Address: P.O. Box 268, Zip 35999–0268; tel. 205/543–5200; David A. McClellan, Executive Director

STRINGFELLOW MEMORIAL HOSPITAL (L, 66 beds) 301 East 18th Street, Anniston, AL Zip 36207; tel. 205/235–8900; Michael E. Cassidy, Administrator

ARKANSAS: CRAWFORD MEMORIAL HOSPITAL (L, 103 beds) East Main & South 20th Streets, Van Buren, AR Zip 72956, Mailing Address: Box 409, Zip 72956; tel. 501/474–3401; Richard Boone, Executive Director

FLORIDA: CHARLOTTE REGIONAL MEDICAL CENTER (O, 148 beds) 809 East Marion Avenue, Punta Gorda, FL Zip 33950–3898; tel. 941/637–3128; Donald B. McElroy, Executive Director

FISHERMEN'S HOSPITAL (L, 58 beds) 3301 Overseas Highway, Marathon, FL Zip 33050–0068; tel. 305/743–5533; Patrice L. Tavernier, Administrator

HEART OF FLORIDA BEHAVIORAL CENTER (O, 66 beds) 2510 North Florida Avenue, Lakeland, FL Zip 33805; tel. 941/682–6105; David M. Polunas, Administrator and Chief Executive Officer

For explanation of codes following names, see page B2.
★ Indicates Type III membership in the American Hospital Association.

HEART OF FLORIDA HOSPITAL (L, 51 beds) Tenth Street and Wood Avenue, Haines City, FL Zip 33844, Mailing Address: Box 67, Zip 33844; tel. 813/422–4971; Robert Mahaffey, Administrator

HIGHLANDS REGIONAL MEDICAL CENTER (L, 126 beds) 3600 South Highlands Avenue, Sebring, FL Zip 33870–5495, Mailing Address: Drawer 2066, Zip 33871–2066; tel. 941/385–6101; Kevin Dilallo, Executive Director

SANDYPINES (O, 60 beds) 11301 S.E. Tequesta Terrace, Tequesta, FL Zip 33469; tel. 407/744–0211; David L. Beardsley, Administrator

SEBASTIAN RIVER MEDICAL CENTER (O, 133 beds) 13695 North U.S. Highway 1, Sebastian, FL Zip 32958, Mailing Address: Box 780838, Zip 32978; tel. 561/589–3186; Stephen L. Midkiff, Executive Director

UNIVERSITY BEHAVIORAL CENTER (O, 100 beds) 2500 Discovery Drive, Orlando, FL Zip 32826; tel. 407/281–7000; Gregory P. Roth, Executive Director

GEORGIA: BULLOCH MEMORIAL HOSPITAL (O, 158 beds) 500 East Grady Street, Statesboro, GA Zip 30458, Mailing Address: P.O. Box 1048, Zip 30459–1048; tel. 912/764–6671; C. Scott Campbell, Executive Director

KANSAS: PARKVIEW HOSPITAL OF TOPEKA (O, 60 beds) 3707 S.W. Sixth Street, Topeka, KS Zip 66606; tel. 913/295–3000; Thomas G. Smith, Administrator

KENTUCKY: PAUL B. HALL REGIONAL MEDICAL CENTER (O, 72 beds) 625 James S Trimble Boulevard, Paintsville, KY Zip 41240, Mailing Address: P.O. Box 1487, Zip 41240; tel. 606/789–3511; Deborah T. Meadows, Administrator

MISSISSIPPI: BILOXI REGIONAL MEDICAL CENTER (L, 153 beds) 150 Reynoir Street, Biloxi, MS Zip 39530, Mailing Address: Box 128, Zip 39533; tel. 601/432–1571; Joseph J. Mullany, Executive Director

NATCHEZ COMMUNITY HOSPITAL (O, 101 beds) 129 Jefferson Davis Boulevard, Natchez, MS Zip 39120, Mailing Address: Box 1203, Zip 39121; tel. 601/445–6200; Raymond Bane, Executive Director

NORTHWEST MISSISSIPPI REGIONAL MEDICAL CENTER (L, 195 beds) 1970 Hospital Drive, Clarksdale, MS Zip 38614, Mailing Address: Box 1218, Zip 38614; tel. 601/624–3401; J. David McCormack, Executive Director

RANKIN MEDICAL CENTER (L, 90 beds) 350 Crossgates Boulevard, Brandon, MS Zip 39042; tel. 601/825–2811; Thomas Wiman, Executive Director

NORTH CAROLINA: FRANKLIN REGIONAL MEDICAL CENTER (O, 85 beds) 100 Hospital Drive, Louisburg, NC Zip 27549, Mailing Address: Box 609, Zip 27549; tel. 919/496–5131; Thomas Hanenburg, Administrator

HAMLET HOSPITAL (O, 64 beds) Rice and Vance Streets, Hamlet, NC Zip 28345, Mailing Address: Box 1109, Zip 28345; tel. 910/582–3611; Joe D. Howell, Executive Director

LAKE NORMAN REGIONAL MEDICAL CENTER (O, 100 beds) 610 East Center Avenue, Mooresville, NC Zip 28115, Mailing Address: Box 360, Zip 28115; tel. 704/663–1113; P. Paul Smith Jr., Executive Director

OKLAHOMA: MEDICAL CENTER OF SOUTHEASTERN OKLAHOMA (O, 103 beds) 1800 University, Durant, OK Zip 74701, Mailing Address: P.O. Box 1207, Zip 74702; tel. 405/924–3080; Joshua Putter, Executive Director

MIDWEST CITY REGIONAL MEDICAL CENTER (L, 206 beds) 2825 Parklawn Drive, Midwest City, OK Zip 73110–4258; tel. 405/737–4411; Gary D. Newsome, Executive Director and Chief Executive Officer

SOUTH CAROLINA: BYERLY HOSPITAL (L, 100 beds) 413 East Carolina Avenue, Hartsville, SC Zip 29550–4309; tel. 803/339–2100; Page Vaughan, Executive Director

UPSTATE CAROLINA MEDICAL CENTER (O, 125 beds) 1530 North Limestone Street, Gaffney, SC Zip 29340; tel. 803/487–4271; Steve Midkiff, Executive Director

WEST VIRGINIA: WILLIAMSON MEMORIAL HOSPITAL (O, 76 beds) 859 Alderson Street, Williamson, WV Zip 25661, Mailing Address: P.O. Box 1980, Zip 25661; tel. 304/235–2500; Roger C. LeDoux, Administrator

Owned, leased, sponsored:	26 hospitals	2880 beds
Contract–managed:	0 hospitals	0 beds
Totals:	26 hospitals	2880 beds

★8815:   HEALTH MIDWEST (NP)
2304 East Meyer Boulevard, Suite A–20, Kansas City, MO Zip 64132–4104; tel. 816/276–9181; Richard W. Brown, President and Chief Executive Officer

KANSAS: ALLEN COUNTY HOSPITAL (L, 41 beds) 101 South First Street, Iola, KS Zip 66749, Mailing Address: P.O. Box 540, Zip 66749–0540; tel. 316/365–3131; Franklin K. Wilson, Administrator

MENORAH MEDICAL CENTER (O, 70 beds) 5721 West 119th Street, Overland Park, KS Zip 66209; tel. 913/498–6000; Steven D. Wilkinson, Chief Executive Officer

MISSOURI: BAPTIST MEDICAL CENTER (O, 315 beds) 6601 Rockhill Road, Kansas City, MO Zip 64131–1197; tel. 816/276–7000; Dan H. Anderson, President and Chief Executive Officer

CASS MEDICAL CENTER (C, 42 beds) 1800 East Mechanic Street, Harrisonville, MO Zip 64701; tel. 816/884–3291; Alan Freeman, Administrator

LAFAYETTE REGIONAL HEALTH CENTER (L, 37 beds) 1500 State Street, Lexington, MO Zip 64067–1199; tel. 816/259–2203; Jeffrey S. Tarrant, Administrator

LEE'S SUMMIT HOSPITAL (O, 77 beds) 530 North Murray Road, Lees Summit, MO Zip 64081–1497; tel. 816/251–7000; John L. Jacobson, President and Chief Executive Officer

MEDICAL CENTER OF INDEPENDENCE (O, 123 beds) 17203 East 23rd Street, Independence, MO Zip 64057; tel. 816/478–5000; Michael W. Chappelow, President and Chief Executive Officer

PARK LANE MEDICAL CENTER (O, 94 beds) 5151 Raytown Road, Kansas City, MO Zip 64133; tel. 816/358–8000; Derell Taloney, President and Chief Executive Officer

REHABILITATION INSTITUTE (O, 22 beds) 3011 Baltimore, Kansas City, MO Zip 64108–3465; tel. 816/751–7900; Ronald L. Herrick, President

RESEARCH BELTON HOSPITAL (O, 47 beds) 17065 South 71 Highway, Belton, MO Zip 64012; tel. 816/348–1200; Daniel F. Sheehan, Administrator

RESEARCH MEDICAL CENTER (O, 479 beds) 2316 East Meyer Boulevard, Kansas City, MO Zip 64132–1199; tel. 816/276–4000; Dan H. Anderson, President and Chief Executive Officer

TRINITY LUTHERAN HOSPITAL (O, 334 beds) 3030 Baltimore Avenue, Kansas City, MO Zip 64108–3404; tel. 816/753–4600; Ronald A. Ommen, President and Chief Executive Officer

Owned, leased, sponsored:	11 hospitals	1639 beds
Contract–managed:	1 hospital	42 beds
Totals:	12 hospitals	1681 beds

0395:   HEALTHCARE AMERICA, INC. (IO)
1407 West Stassney Lane, Austin, TX Zip 78745, Mailing Address: P.O. Box 4008, Zip 78765–4008; tel. 512/464–0200; John P. Harcourt Jr., President and Chief Executive Officer

COLORADO: CEDAR SPRINGS PSYCHIATRIC HOSPITAL (O, 101 beds) 2135 Southgate Road, Colorado Springs, CO Zip 80906–2693; tel. 719/633–4114; Connie Mull, Chief Executive Officer

OKLAHOMA: SHADOW MOUNTAIN HOSPITAL (O, 100 beds) 6262 South Sheridan Road, Tulsa, OK Zip 74133–4099; tel. 918/492–8200; Nancy J. Cranton, Chief Executive Officer

TEXAS: CYPRESS CREEK HOSPITAL (O, 94 beds) 17750 Cali Drive, Houston, TX Zip 77090–2700; tel. 713/586–7600; Terry Scovill, Administrator

HEALTHCARE REHABILITATION CENTER (O, 30 beds) 1106 West Dittmar, Austin, TX Zip 78745–9990, Mailing Address: P.O. Box 150459, Zip 78715–0459; tel. 512/444–4835; James G. Dalzell, Chief Executive Officer

OAKS PSYCHIATRIC HEALTH SYSTEM (O, 118 beds) 1407 West Stassney Lane, Austin, TX Zip 78745; tel. 512/464–0400; Mack Wigley, Chief Executive Officer

SAN MARCOS TREATMENT CENTER (O, 152 beds) Bert Brown Road, San Marcos, TX Zip 78667–0768, Mailing Address: P.O. Box 768, Zip 78667–0768; tel. 512/396–8500; Mack Wigley, Chief Executive Officer

WEST OAKS HOSPITAL (O, 184 beds) 6500 Hornwood, Houston, TX Zip 77074, Mailing Address: Box 741389, Zip 77274; tel. 713/995–0909; Michael Amador, Chief Executive Officer

Section B

For explanation of codes following names, see page B2.
★ Indicates Type III membership in the American Hospital Association.

VIRGINIA: CUMBERLAND HOSPITAL FOR CHILDREN AND ADOLESCENTS (O, 84 beds) 9407 Cumberland Road, New Kent, VA Zip 23124; tel. 804/966–2242; Elizabeth B. Woodard, Chief Executive Officer

Owned, leased, sponsored:	8 hospitals	863 beds
Contract–managed:	0 hospitals	0 beds
Totals:	8 hospitals	863 beds

1585: HEALTHCARE MANAGEMENT GROUP, INC. (IO)
776 Baconsfield Drive, Suite 209, Macon, GA Zip 31211–0101; tel. 912/743–5606; Earl Bonds Jr., Chief Executive Officer

GEORGIA: MORGAN MEMORIAL HOSPITAL (L, 26 beds) Canterbury Park, Madison, GA Zip 30650, Mailing Address: Box 860, Zip 30650; tel. 706/342–1667; Patrick Green, Administrator

SYLVAN GROVE HOSPITAL (L, 28 beds) 1050 McDonough Road, Jackson, GA Zip 30233; tel. 404/775–7861; Jack F. Frayer, Administrator

Owned, leased, sponsored:	2 hospitals	54 beds
Contract–managed:	0 hospitals	0 beds
Totals:	2 hospitals	54 beds

2795: HEALTHCORP OF TENNESSEE, INC. (IO)
735 Broad Street, Chattanooga, TN Zip 37402; tel. 615/267–8406; T. Farrell Hayes, President

ALABAMA: LAKESHORE COMMUNITY HOSPITAL (C, 27 beds) 201 Mariarden Road, Dadeville, AL Zip 36853, Mailing Address: P.O. Box 248, Zip 36853; tel. 205/825–7821; Mavis B. Halko, Administrator

LAKEVIEW COMMUNITY HOSPITAL (C, 74 beds) 820 West Washington Street, Eufaula, AL Zip 36027; tel. 205/687–5761; Carl D. Brown, Administrator

VAUGHAN CHILTON MEDICAL CENTER (L, 45 beds) 1010 Lay Dam Road, Clanton, AL Zip 35045; tel. 205/755–2500; Jeffrey Potts, Administrator

ARKANSAS: DALLAS COUNTY HOSPITAL (O, 32 beds) 201 Clifton Street, Fordyce, AR Zip 71742; tel. 501/352–3155; Greg R. McNeil, Administrator

TENNESSEE: NORTH PARK HOSPITAL (C, 83 beds) 2051 Hamill Road, Chattanooga, TN Zip 37343–4096; tel. 423/870–6100; Leonard Fant, Administrator

Owned, leased, sponsored:	2 hospitals	77 beds
Contract–managed:	3 hospitals	184 beds
Totals:	5 hospitals	261 beds

★2185: HEALTHEAST (NP)
559 Capitol Boulevard, 6–South, Saint Paul, MN Zip 55103–0000; tel. 612/232–2300; Timothy H. Hanson, President and Chief Executive Officer

MINNESOTA: HEALTHEAST BETHESDA LUTHERAN HOSPITAL AND REHABILITATION CENTER (O, 127 beds) 559 Capitol Boulevard, Saint Paul, MN Zip 55103; tel. 612/232–2133; Scott Batulis, Administrator

HEALTHEAST ST. JOHN'S HOSPITAL (O, 150 beds) 1575 Beam Avenue, Maplewood, MN Zip 55109; tel. 612/232–7000; William Knutson, Vice President and Administrator

HEALTHEAST ST. JOSEPH'S HOSPITAL (O, 292 beds) 69 West Exchange Street, Saint Paul, MN Zip 55102; tel. 612/232–3000; William Knutson, Vice President and Administrator

Owned, leased, sponsored:	3 hospitals	569 beds
Contract–managed:	0 hospitals	0 beds
Totals:	3 hospitals	569 beds

0023: HEALTHSOUTH CORPORATION (IO)
One Healthsouth Parkway, Birmingham, AL Zip 35243; tel. 205/967–7116; Anthony J. Tanner, Executive Vice President

ALABAMA: HEALTHSOUTH LAKESHORE REHABILITATION HOSPITAL (O, 100 beds) 3800 Ridgeway Drive, Birmingham, AL Zip 35209; tel. 205/868–2000; Terry Brown, Administrator and Chief Executive Officer

HEALTHSOUTH MEDICAL CENTER (O, 201 beds) 1201 11th Avenue South, Birmingham, AL Zip 35205; tel. 205/930–7000; Frank R. Gannon, Administrator and Chief Executive Officer

HEALTHSOUTH REHABILITATION HOSPITAL OF MONTGOMERY (O, 80 beds) 4465 Narrow Lane Road, Montgomery, AL Zip 36116; tel. 334/284–7700; Arnold F. McRae, Administrator and Chief Executive Officer

HEALTHSOUTH REHABILITATION HOSPITAL OF NORTH ALABAMA (O, 50 beds) 107 Governors Drive, Huntsville, AL Zip 35801; tel. 205/535–2300; Rod Moss, Chief Executive Officer

ARIZONA: HEALTHSOUTH MERIDIAN POINT REHABILITATION HOSPITAL (O, 43 beds) 11250 North 92nd Street, Scottsdale, AZ Zip 85260–6148; tel. 602/860–0671; Warren Kyle West, Administrator and Chief Executive Officer

HEALTHSOUTH REHABILITATION INSTITUTE OF TUCSON (O, 80 beds) 2650 North Wyatt Drive, Tucson, AZ Zip 85712; tel. 520/325–1300; Joni K. Raneri, Administrator

HEALTHSOUTH VALLEY OF THE SUN REHABILITATION HOSPITAL (O, 42 beds) 13460 North 67th Avenue, Glendale, AZ Zip 85304; tel. 602/878–8800; Michael S. Wallace, Administrator and Chief Executive Officer

ARKANSAS: HEALTHSOUTH REHABILITATION HOSPITAL OF FORT SMITH (O, 80 beds) 1401 South J Street, Fort Smith, AR Zip 72901; tel. 501/785–3300; Claudia A. Eisenmann, Director Operations

CALIFORNIA: HEALTHSOUTH BAKERSFIELD REHABILITATION HOSPITAL (O, 60 beds) 5001 Commerce Drive, Bakersfield, CA Zip 93309; tel. 805/323–5500; Jo Ann Bennett, Chief Operating Officer

FLORIDA: HEALTHSOUTH REHABILITATION HOSPITAL (O, 45 beds) 20601 Old Cutler Road, Miami, FL Zip 33189; tel. 305/251–3800; Jude Torchia, Chief Executive Officer

HEALTHSOUTH DOCTORS' HOSPITAL (O, 157 beds) 5000 University Drive, Coral Gables, FL Zip 33146–2094; tel. 305/666–2111; Lincoln S. Mendez, Chief Executive Officer

HEALTHSOUTH REHABILITATION HOSPITAL (O, 60 beds) 901 North Clearwater–Largo Road, Largo, FL Zip 34640–1955; tel. 813/586–2999; Vincent O. Nico, Regional Vice President

HEALTHSOUTH REHABILITATION HOSPITAL OF SARASOTA (O, 60 beds) 3251 Proctor Road, Sarasota, FL Zip 34231–8538; tel. 941/921–8600; Jeff Garber, Administrator and Chief Executive Officer

HEALTHSOUTH REHABILITATION HOSPITAL OF TALLAHASSEE (O, 70 beds) 1675 Riggins Road, Tallahassee, FL Zip 32308–5315; tel. 904/656–4800; Mike Marshall, Chief Executive Officer

HEALTHSOUTH SEA PINES REHABILITATION HOSPITAL (O, 80 beds) 101 East Florida Avenue, Melbourne, FL Zip 32901–9966; tel. 407/984–4600; Henry J. Cranston, Chief Operating Officer

HEALTHSOUTH SUNRISE REHABILITATION HOSPITAL (O, 108 beds) 4399 Nob Hill Road, Fort Lauderdale, FL Zip 33351–5899; tel. 305/749–0300; Kevin R. Conn, Administrator

HEALTHSOUTH TREASURE COAST REHABILITATION HOSPITAL (O, 70 beds) 1600 37th Street, Vero Beach, FL Zip 32960–6549; tel. 407/778–2100; Denise B. McGrath, Chief Executive Officer

GEORGIA: HEALTHSOUTH CENTRAL GEORGIA REHABILITATION HOSPITAL (O, 50 beds) 3351 Northside Drive, Macon, GA Zip 31210; tel. 912/471–3536; Elbert T. McQueen, Chief Executive Officer

INDIANA: HEALTHSOUTH TRI–STATE REHABILITATION HOSPITAL (O, 80 beds) 4100 Covert Avenue, Evansville, IN Zip 47714, Mailing Address: P.O. Box 5349, Zip 47716–5349; tel. 812/476–9983; Gerald F. Vozel, Administrator and Chief Executive Officer

KENTUCKY: HEALTHSOUTH NORTHERN KENTUCKY REHABILITATION HOSPITAL (O, 40 beds) 201 Medical Village Drive, Edgewood, KY Zip 41017; tel. 606/341–2044; Ronald L. Bierman, Chief Executive Officer

LOUISIANA: HEALTHSOUTH REHABILITATION HOSPITAL OF SOUTH LOUISIANA (O, 40 beds) 4040 North Boulevard, Baton Rouge, LA Zip 70806–3829; tel. 504/383–5055; Sharon S. Black, R.N., Chief Operating Officer

MAINE: HEALTHSOUTH REHABILITATION HOSPITAL (O, 76 beds) 13 Charles Street, Portland, ME Zip 04102–9924; tel. 207/775–4000; Patricia McMurry, Executive Vice President and Chief Executive Officer

For explanation of codes following names, see page B2.
★ Indicates Type III membership in the American Hospital Association.

MARYLAND: HEALTHSOUTH CHESAPEAKE REHABILITATION HOSPITAL (O, 42 beds) 220 Tilghman Road, Salisbury, MD Zip 21804; tel. 410/546–4600; William Rothman, Chief Executive Officer

MASSACHUSETTS: FAIRLAWN REHABILITATION HOSPITAL (O, 110 beds) 189 May Street, Worcester, MA Zip 01602–4399; tel. 508/791–6351; Ellen Ferrante, President and Chief Executive Officer

HEALTHSOUTH NEW ENGLAND REHABILITATION HOSPITAL (O, 198 beds) Two Rehabilitation Way, Woburn, MA Zip 01801–6098; tel. 617/935–5050; Guido J. Cubellis, Chief Executive Officer

REHABILITATION HOSPITAL OF WESTERN MASSACHUSETTS (O, 40 beds) 14 Chestnut Place, Ludlow, MA Zip 01056; tel. 413/589–7581; Mark D. Kramer, Administrator

NEW HAMPSHIRE: HEALTHSOUTH REHABILITATION HOSPITAL (O, 50 beds) 254 Pleasant Street, Concord, NH Zip 03301; tel. 603/226–9800; Anne M. Fugagli, Administrator

NEW JERSEY: HEALTHSOUTH REHABILITATION HOSPITAL OF NEW JERSEY (O, 155 beds) 14 Hospital Drive, Toms River, NJ Zip 08755; tel. 908/244–3100; Patricia Ostaszewski, Chief Operating Officer and Administrator

NEW MEXICO: HEALTHSOUTH REHABILITATION CENTER (O, 60 beds) 7000 Jefferson N.E., Albuquerque, NM Zip 87109; tel. 505/344–9478; Darby Brockette, Administrator

OKLAHOMA: HEALTHSOUTH REHABILITATION HOSPITAL (O, 46 beds) 700 N.W. Seventh Street, Oklahoma City, OK Zip 73102–1295; tel. 405/553–1192; Hank Ross, Chief Executive Officer

PENNSYLVANIA: HEALTHSOUTH GREAT LAKES REHABILITATION HOSPITAL (O, 108 beds) 143 East Second Street, Erie, PA Zip 16507; tel. 814/878–1200; William R. Fox, Chief Executive Officer

HEALTHSOUTH GREATER PITTSBURGH REHABILITATION HOSPITAL (O, 89 beds) 2380 McGinley Road, Monroeville, PA Zip 15146; tel. 412/856–2400; Faith A. Deigan, Administrator

HEALTHSOUTH HARMARVILLE REHABILITATION HOSPITAL (O, 202 beds) Guys Run Road, Pittsburgh, PA Zip 15238–0460, Mailing Address: Box 11460, Guys Run Road, Zip 15238–0460; tel. 412/781–5700; Frank G. DeLisi III, CHE, Chief Executive Officer and Director Operations

HEALTHSOUTH LAKE ERIE INSTITUTE OF REHABILITATION (O, 99 beds) 137 West Second Street, Erie, PA Zip 16507–1403; tel. 814/453–5602; Frank G. DeLisi III, CHE, Chief Executive Officer and Director Operations

HEALTHSOUTH NITTANY VALLEY REHABILITATION HOSPITAL (O, 88 beds) 550 West College Avenue, Pleasant Gap, PA Zip 16823–8808; tel. 814/359–3421; Mary Jane Hawkins, Administrator and Chief Executive Officer

HEALTHSOUTH REHABILITATION HOSPITAL OF ALTOONA (O, 70 beds) 2005 Valley View Boulevard, Altoona, PA Zip 16602; tel. 814/944–3535; Felix Mariani, Administrator

HEALTHSOUTH REHABILITATION HOSPITAL OF YORK (O, 88 beds) 1850 Normandie Drive, York, PA Zip 17404–1534; tel. 717/767–6941; Cheryl Fleming, Chief Operating Officer

HEALTHSOUTH REHABILITATION OF MECHANICSBURG (O, 103 beds) 175 Lancaster Boulevard, Mechanicsburg, PA Zip 17055–2016, Mailing Address: P.O. Box 2016, Zip 17055–2016; tel. 717/691–3700; Barbara H. Bowen, Interim Administrator

SOUTH CAROLINA: HEALTHSOUTH REHABILITATION HOSPITAL (O, 89 beds) 2935 Colonial Drive, Columbia, SC Zip 29203; tel. 803/254–7777; Mark J. Stepanik, Director Operations

HEALTHSOUTH REHABILITATION HOSPITAL (O, 88 beds) 900 East Cheves Street, Florence, SC Zip 29506; tel. 803/679–9000; Oliver J. Booker, Chief Executive Officer

TENNESSEE: HEALTHSOUTH CHATTANOOGA REHABILITATION HOSPITAL (O, 69 beds) 2412 McCallie Avenue, Chattanooga, TN Zip 37404; tel. 423/698–0221

HEALTHSOUTH REHABILITATION HOSPITAL (O, 50 beds) 113 Cassel Drive, Kingsport, TN Zip 37660; tel. 423/246–7240; Terry R. Maxhimer, Administrator

HEALTHSOUTH REHABILITATION HOSPITAL (O, 80 beds) 1282 Union Avenue, Memphis, TN Zip 38104; tel. 901/722–2000; Brenda Antwine, Administrator and Chief Operating Officer

TEXAS: HEALTHSOUTH MEDICAL CENTER (O, 106 beds) 2124 Research Row, Dallas, TX Zip 75235; tel. 214/904–6100; Robert M. Smart, Area Manager and Chief Executive Officer

HEALTHSOUTH REHABILITATION HOSPITAL (O, 58 beds) 19002 McKay Drive, Humble, TX Zip 77338; tel. 281/446–6148; Jessica A. Nantz, Chief Executive Officer

HEALTHSOUTH REHABILITATION HOSPITAL OF ARLINGTON (O, 60 beds) 3200 Matlock Road, Arlington, TX Zip 76015–2911; tel. 817/468–4000; S. Denise Borroni, Administrator and Chief Operating Officer

HEALTHSOUTH REHABILITATION HOSPITAL OF AUSTIN (O, 70 beds) 1215 Red River Street, Austin, TX Zip 78701, Mailing Address: P.O. Box 13366, Zip 78711–3366; tel. 512/474–5700; William O. Mitchell Jr., Chief Executive Officer

HEALTHSOUTH REHABILITATION HOSPITAL OF FORT WORTH (O, 60 beds) 1212 West Lancaster, Fort Worth, TX Zip 76102; tel. 817/870–2336; Laura J. Lycan, Administrator and Chief Executive Officer

HEALTHSOUTH REHABILITATION HOSPITAL OF TEXARKANA (O, 60 beds) 515 West 12th Street, Texarkana, TX Zip 75501; tel. 903/793–0088; Jeffrey A. Livingston, Chief Executive Officer

HEALTHSOUTH REHABILITATION INSTITUTE OF SAN ANTONIO (O, 108 beds) 9119 Cinnamon Hill, San Antonio, TX Zip 78240; tel. 210/691–0737; Diane B. Lampe, Administrator and Chief Executive Officer

UTAH: HEALTHSOUTH REHABILITATION HOSPITAL OF UTAH (O, 73 beds) 8074 South 1300 East, Sandy, UT Zip 84094; tel. 801/561–3400; Richard M. Richards, Administrator

VIRGINIA: HEALTHSOUTH MEDICAL CENTER (O, 147 beds) 7700 East Parham Road, Richmond, VA Zip 23294–4301; tel. 804/747–5600; Charles A. Stark, CHE, Administrator, Chief Executive Officer and Director Inpatient Operations

HEALTHSOUTH REHABILITATION HOSPITAL OF VIRGINIA (O, 40 beds) 5700 Fitzhugh Avenue, Richmond, VA Zip 23226; tel. 804/288–5700; Jeff Ruskan, Administrator

WEST VIRGINIA: HEALTHSOUTH MOUNTAIN REGIONAL REHABILITATION HOSPITAL (O, 80 beds) 1160 Van Voorhis, Morgantown, WV Zip 26505; tel. 304/598–1100; Sharon Nero, Chief Executive Officer

HEALTHSOUTH REHABILITATION HOSPITAL (O, 40 beds) 6900 West Country Club Drive, Huntington, WV Zip 25705; tel. 304/733–1060; Homer Fowler, Chief Operating Officer

HEALTHSOUTH SOUTHERN HILLS REHABILITATION HOSPITAL (O, 40 beds) 120 Twelfth Street, Princeton, WV Zip 24740; tel. 304/487–8000; Timothy Mitchell, Administrator

HEALTHSOUTH WESTERN HILLS REGIONAL REHABILITATION HOSPITAL (O, 40 beds) 3 Western Hills Drive, Parkersburg, WV Zip 26101, Mailing Address: P.O. Box 1428, Zip 26102–1428; tel. 304/420–1300; Thomas Heller, Administrator

Owned, leased, sponsored:	57 hospitals	4578 beds
Contract–managed:	0 hospitals	0 beds
Totals:	57 hospitals	4578 beds

1985: HEALTHSYSTEM MINNESOTA (NP) 6500 Excelsior Boulevard, Saint Louis Park, MN Zip 55426–4702; tel. 612/932–6300

MINNESOTA: GLENCOE AREA HEALTH CENTER (C, 149 beds) 705 East 18th Street, Glencoe, MN Zip 55336–1499; tel. 320/864–3121; Jon D. Braband, Chief Executive Officer

METHODIST HOSPITAL HEALTHSYSTEM MINNESOTA (O, 376 beds) 6500 Excelsior Boulevard, Saint Louis Park, MN Zip 55426–4702, Mailing Address: Box 650, Minneapolis, Zip 55440–0650; tel. 612/993–5000; James Reinertsen, M.D., Chief Executive Officer

Owned, leased, sponsored:	1 hospital	376 beds
Contract–managed:	1 hospital	149 beds
Totals:	2 hospitals	525 beds

For explanation of codes following names, see page B2.
★ Indicates Type III membership in the American Hospital Association.

★2355: HELIX HEALTH (NP)
2330 West Joppa Road, Suite 301, Lutherville, MD Zip 21093; tel. 410/847–6700; James A. Oakey, President and Chief Executive Officer

MARYLAND: CHURCH HOSPITAL CORPORATION (O, 165 beds) 100 North Broadway, Baltimore, MD Zip 21231–1593; tel. 410/522–8000; James R. Bobb, President

FRANKLIN SQUARE HOSPITAL CENTER (O, 405 beds) 9000 Franklin Square Drive, Baltimore, MD Zip 21237–3998; tel. 410/682–7000; Charles D. Mross, President and Chief Executive Officer

GOOD SAMARITAN HOSPITAL OF MARYLAND (O, 274 beds) 5601 Loch Raven Boulevard, Baltimore, MD Zip 21239–2995; tel. 410/532–8000; Lawrence M. Beck, President

HARBOR HOSPITAL CENTER (O, 176 beds) 3001 South Hanover Street, Baltimore, MD Zip 21225–1290; tel. 410/347–3200; L. Barney Johnson, President and Chief Executive Officer

UNION MEMORIAL HOSPITAL (O, 378 beds) 201 East University Parkway, Baltimore, MD Zip 21218–2391; tel. 410/554–2000; Kenneth R. Buser, President and Chief Executive Officer

Owned, leased, sponsored:	5 hospitals	1398 beds
Contract–managed:	0 hospitals	0 beds
Totals:	5 hospitals	1398 beds

★9505: HENRY FORD HEALTH SYSTEM (NP)
One Ford Place, Detroit, MI Zip 48202; tel. 313/876–8715; Gail L. Warden, President and Chief Executive Officer

MICHIGAN: BI–COUNTY COMMUNITY HOSPITAL (O, 152 beds) 13355 East Ten Mile Road, Warren, MI Zip 48089–2065; tel. 810/759–7300; Gary W. Popiel, Vice President and Chief Administrative Officer

HENRY FORD COTTAGE HOSPITAL OF GROSSE POINTE (O, 144 beds) 159 Kercheval Avenue, Grosse Pointe Farms, MI Zip 48236–3692; tel. 313/640–1000; Gregory J. Vasse, President and Chief Executive Officer

HENRY FORD HOSPITAL (O, 605 beds) 2799 West Grand Boulevard, Detroit, MI Zip 48202–2689; tel. 313/876–2600; Stephen H. Velick, Chief Executive Officer

HENRY FORD WYANDOTTE HOSPITAL (O, 355 beds) 2333 Biddle Avenue, Wyandotte, MI Zip 48192; tel. 313/284–2400; William R. Alvin, President

KINGSWOOD HOSPITAL (O, 64 beds) 10300 West Eight Mile Road, Ferndale, MI Zip 48220; tel. 810/398–3200; Kathleen Emrich, R.N., Ed.D., Assistant Vice President and Chief Operating Officer

RIVERSIDE OSTEOPATHIC HOSPITAL (O, 148 beds) 150 Truax Street, Trenton, MI Zip 48183–2151; tel. 313/676–4200; Dennis R. Lemanski, D.O., Vice President and Chief Administrative Officer

Owned, leased, sponsored:	6 hospitals	1468 beds
Contract–managed:	0 hospitals	0 beds
Totals:	6 hospitals	1468 beds

★5585: HOLY CROSS HEALTH SYSTEM CORPORATION (CC)
3606 East Jefferson Boulevard, South Bend, IN Zip 46615–3097; tel. 219/233–8558; Sister Patricia Vandenberg, President and Chief Executive Officer

CALIFORNIA: SAINT AGNES MEDICAL CENTER (O, 326 beds) 1303 East Herndon Avenue, Fresno, CA Zip 93720–3397; tel. 209/449–3000; Sister Ruth Marie Nickerson, President and Chief Executive Officer

IDAHO: CASCADE MEDICAL CENTER (C, 10 beds) 402 Old State Highway, Cascade, ID Zip 83611, Mailing Address: P.O. Box 151, Zip 83611; tel. 208/382–4242; Richard Holm, Administrator

ELMORE MEDICAL CENTER (C, 78 beds) 895 North Sixth East Street, Mountain Home, ID Zip 83647, Mailing Address: P.O. Box 1270, Zip 83647–0348; tel. 208/587–8401; Gregory L. Maurer, Administrator

MCCALL MEMORIAL HOSPITAL (C, 12 beds) 1000 State Street, McCall, ID Zip 83638, Mailing Address: P.O. Box 906, Zip 83638; tel. 208/634–2221; Karen J. Kellie, President

SAINT ALPHONSUS REGIONAL MEDICAL CENTER (O, 287 beds) 1055 North Curtis Road, Boise, ID Zip 83706–1370; tel. 208/378–2121; Sandra B. Bruce, President and Chief Executive Officer

ST. BENEDICTS FAMILY MEDICAL CENTER (C, 65 beds) 709 North Lincoln Avenue, Jerome, ID Zip 83338, Mailing Address: Box 586, Zip 83338–0586; tel. 208/324–4301; David Farnes, Administrator

INDIANA: SAINT JOHN'S HEALTH SYSTEM (O, 371 beds) 2015 Jackson Street, Anderson, IN Zip 46016–4339; tel. 765/649–2511; James H. Stephens, President and Chief Executive Officer

ST. JOSEPH'S HOSPITAL OF MARSHALL COUNTY (O, 58 beds) 1915 Lake Avenue, Plymouth, IN Zip 46563–9905, Mailing Address: P.O. Box 670, Zip 46563–9905; tel. 219/936–3181; Brian E. Dietz, President

ST. JOSEPH'S MEDICAL CENTER (O, 289 beds) 801 East LaSalle, South Bend, IN Zip 46617, Mailing Address: Box 1935, Zip 46634; tel. 219/237–7111; Brian E. Dietz, Interim Chief Executive Officer

MARYLAND: HOLY CROSS HOSPITAL OF SILVER SPRING (O, 434 beds) 1500 Forest Glen Road, Silver Spring, MD Zip 20910; tel. 301/754–7000; James P. Hamill, President

OHIO: MOUNT CARMEL HEALTH SYSTEM (O, 929 beds) 793 West State Street, Columbus, OH Zip 43222–1551; tel. 614/225–5000; Dale St. Arnold, President and Chief Executive Officer

Owned, leased, sponsored:	7 hospitals	2694 beds
Contract–managed:	4 hospitals	165 beds
Totals:	11 hospitals	2859 beds

★0027: HORIZON HEALTHCARE, INC. (NP)
2300 North Mayfair Road, Suite 550, Milwaukee, WI Zip 53226–1508; tel. 414/257–3888; Sister Renee Rose, President and Chief Executive Officer

WISCONSIN: COLUMBIA HOSPITAL (O, 337 beds) 2025 East Newport Avenue, Milwaukee, WI Zip 53211–2990; tel. 414/961–3300; Susan Henckel, Executive Vice President and Chief Executive Officer

COMMUNITY MEMORIAL HOSPITAL (O, 153 beds) W180 N8085 Town Hall Road, Menomonee Falls, WI Zip 53051, Mailing Address: P.O. Box 408, Zip 53052–0408; tel. 414/251–1000; Robert Eugene Drisner, President and Chief Executive Officer

FROEDTERT MEMORIAL LUTHERAN HOSPITAL (O, 459 beds) 9200 West Wisconsin Avenue, Milwaukee, WI Zip 53226–3596, Mailing Address: P.O. Box 26099, Zip 53226–3596; tel. 414/259–3000; William D. Petasnick, President

KENOSHA HOSPITAL AND MEDICAL CENTER (O, 116 beds) 6308 Eighth Avenue, Kenosha, WI Zip 53143; tel. 414/656–2011; Richard O. Schmidt Jr., President, Chief Executive Officer and General Counsel

MEMORIAL HOSPITAL OCONOMOWOC (O, 73 beds) 791 Summit Avenue, Oconomowoc, WI Zip 53066–3896; tel. 414/569–9400; Douglas Guy, President and Chief Executive Officer

SACRED HEART REHABILITATION INSTITUTE (O, 69 beds) 2350 North Lake Drive, Milwaukee, WI Zip 53211, Mailing Address: P.O. Box 392, Zip 53201–0392; tel. 414/298–6700; William H. Lange, Administrator and Senior Vice President

Owned, leased, sponsored:	6 hospitals	1207 beds
Contract–managed:	0 hospitals	0 beds
Totals:	6 hospitals	1207 beds

0455: HOSPITAL GROUP OF AMERICA (IO)
1265 Drummers Lane, Suite 107, Wayne, PA Zip 19087; tel. 610/687–5151; Mark R. Russell, President and Chief Executive Officer

DELAWARE: MEADOW WOOD BEHAVIORAL HEALTH SYSTEM (O, 50 beds) 575 South Dupont Highway, New Castle, DE Zip 19720; tel. 302/328–3330; Joseph Pyle, Administrator

ILLINOIS: HARTGROVE HOSPITAL (O, 119 beds) 520 North Ridgeway Avenue, Chicago, IL Zip 60624; tel. 773/722–3113; Karen E. Johnson, Administrator

For explanation of codes following names, see page B2.
★ Indicates Type III membership in the American Hospital Association.

© 1997 AHA Guide

NEW JERSEY: HAMPTON HOSPITAL (O, 100 beds) Rancocas Road, Westampton Township, NJ Zip 08073, Mailing Address: P.O. Box 7000, Zip 08073; tel. 609/267–7000; Michael Terwilliger, Acting Chief Executive Officer

Owned, leased, sponsored:	3 hospitals	269 beds
Contract–managed:	0 hospitals	0 beds
Totals:	3 hospitals	269 beds

★5355: HOSPITAL SISTERS HEALTH SYSTEM (CC)
Springfield, IL Mailing Address: P.O. Box 19431, Zip 62794–9431; tel. 217/523–4747; Sister Jomary Trstensky, President

ILLINOIS: ST. ANTHONY'S MEMORIAL HOSPITAL (O, 131 beds) 503 North Maple Street, Effingham, IL Zip 62401–2099; tel. 217/347–1495; Anthony D. Pfitzer, Administrator

ST. ELIZABETH'S HOSPITAL (O, 379 beds) 211 South Third Street, Belleville, IL Zip 62222–0694; tel. 618/234–2120; Gerald M. Harman, Chief Executive Officer and Executive Vice President

ST. FRANCIS HOSPITAL (O, 97 beds) 1215 East Union Avenue, Litchfield, IL Zip 62056–1215, Mailing Address: P.O. Box 1215, Zip 62056–1215; tel. 217/324–2191; Michael Sipkoski, Executive Vice President and Chief Executive Officer

ST. JOHN'S HOSPITAL (O, 580 beds) 800 East Carpenter Street, Springfield, IL Zip 62769; tel. 217/544–6464; Allison C. Laabs, Executive Vice President and Administrator

ST. JOSEPH'S HOSPITAL (O, 57 beds) 9515 Holy Cross Lane, Breese, IL Zip 62230–0099, Mailing Address: P.O. Box 99, Zip 62230–0099; tel. 618/526–4511; Jacolyn M. Schlautman, Executive Vice President and Administrator

ST. JOSEPH'S HOSPITAL (O, 76 beds) 1515 Main Street, Highland, IL Zip 62249–1656; tel. 618/654–7421; Anthony G. Mastrangelo, Executive Vice President and Chief Executive Officer

ST. MARY'S HOSPITAL (O, 205 beds) 1800 East Lake Shore Drive, Decatur, IL Zip 62521–3883; tel. 217/464–2966; Keith L. Callahan, Executive Vice President and Administrator

ST. MARY'S HOSPITAL (O, 170 beds) 111 East Spring Street, Streator, IL Zip 61364; tel. 815/673–2311; James F. Dover, Administrator and Executive Vice President

WISCONSIN: SACRED HEART HOSPITAL (O, 261 beds) 900 West Clairemont Avenue, Eau Claire, WI Zip 54701–5105; tel. 715/839–4121; Matthew W. Hubler, Executive Vice President

ST. JOSEPH'S HOSPITAL (O, 127 beds) 2661 County Highway I, Chippewa Falls, WI Zip 54729–1498; tel. 715/723–1811; David B. Fish, Executive Vice President

ST. MARY'S HOSPITAL MEDICAL CENTER (O, 119 beds) 1726 Shawano Avenue, Green Bay, WI Zip 54303–3282; tel. 414/498–4200; James G. Coller, Executive Vice President and Administrator

ST. NICHOLAS HOSPITAL (O, 84 beds) 1601 North Taylor Drive, Sheboygan, WI Zip 53081–2496; tel. 414/459–8300; Michael J. Stenger, Executive Vice President and Administrator

ST. VINCENT HOSPITAL (O, 353 beds) 835 South Van Buren Street, Green Bay, WI Zip 54307–3508, Mailing Address: P.O. Box 13508, Zip 54307–3508; tel. 414/433–0111; Joseph J. Neidenbach, Administrator and Executive Vice President

Owned, leased, sponsored:	13 hospitals	2639 beds
Contract–managed:	0 hospitals	0 beds
Totals:	13 hospitals	2639 beds

0117: HUNTSVILLE HOSPITAL SYSTEM (NP)
101 Silvey Road, Huntsville, AL Zip 35801; tel. 205/517–8020; Edward D. Boston, Chief Executive Officer

ALABAMA: HUNTSVILLE HOSPITAL (O, 558 beds) 101 Sivley Road, Huntsville, AL Zip 35801–9990; tel. 205/517–8123; Ronald S. Owen, Chief Executive Officer

HUNTSVILLE HOSPITAL EAST (O, 223 beds) 911 Big Cove Road S.E., Huntsville, AL Zip 35801–3784; tel. 205/517–8020; L. Joe Austin, Chief Executive Officer

Owned, leased, sponsored:	2 hospitals	781 beds
Contract–managed:	0 hospitals	0 beds
Totals:	2 hospitals	781 beds

★5565: INCARNATE WORD HEALTH SERVICES (CC)
9311 San Pedro, Suite 1250, San Antonio, TX Zip 78216–4469; tel. 210/524–4100; Joseph Blasko Jr., President and Chief Executive Officer

MISSOURI: INCARNATE WORD HOSPITAL (O, 198 beds) 3545 Lafayette Avenue, Saint Louis, MO Zip 63104–9984; tel. 314/865–6500; Linda M. Allin, President and Chief Executive Officer

TEXAS: BAPTIST–ST. ANTHONY'S HEALTH SYSTEM (O, 349 beds) 200 N.W. Seventh, Amarillo, TX Zip 79107–9872, Mailing Address: P.O. Box 950, Zip 79176–0950; tel. 806/376–4411; John D. Hicks, President

SANTA ROSA HEALTH CARE CORPORATION (O, 636 beds) 519 West Houston Street, San Antonio, TX Zip 78207–3108, Mailing Address: Box 7330, Station A, Zip 78207–3108; tel. 210/704–2011; Robert J. Nolan, President and Chief Executive Officer

SPOHN HEALTH SYSTEM (O, 486 beds) 600 Elizabeth Street, Corpus Christi, TX Zip 78404–2235; tel. 512/881–3000; Jake Henry Jr., President

SPOHN KLEBERG MEMORIAL HOSPITAL (O, 100 beds) 1311 General Cavazos Boulevard, Kingsville, TX Zip 78363–1197, Mailing Address: P.O. Box 1197, Zip 78363–1197; tel. 512/595–1661; David D. Clark, CHE, Administrator and Vice President

ST. JOSEPH'S HOSPITAL AND HEALTH CENTER (O, 176 beds) 820 Clarksville Street, Paris, TX Zip 75460–9070, Mailing Address: P.O. Box 9070, Zip 75461–9070; tel. 903/785–4521; Monty E. McLaurin, President

Owned, leased, sponsored:	6 hospitals	1945 beds
Contract–managed:	0 hospitals	0 beds
Totals:	6 hospitals	1945 beds

2025: INFIRMARY HEALTH SYSTEM, INC. (NP)
3 Mobile Infirmary Circle, Mobile, AL Zip 36607; tel. 334/431–5500; E. Chandler Bramlett Jr., President and Chief Executive Officer

ALABAMA: GROVE HILL MEMORIAL HOSPITAL (C, 46 beds) 295 South Jackson Street, Grove Hill, AL Zip 36451, Mailing Address: P.O. Box 935, Zip 36451; tel. 334/275–3191; Floyd N. Price, Administrator

MOBILE INFIRMARY MEDICAL CENTER (O, 550 beds) 5 Mobile Infirmary Drive North, Mobile, AL Zip 36604, Mailing Address: P.O. Box 2144, Zip 36652–2144; tel. 334/431–4700; E. Chandler Bramlett Jr., President and Chief Executive Officer

WASHINGTON COUNTY INFIRMARY AND NURSING HOME (C, 88 beds) St. Stephens Avenue, Chatom, AL Zip 36518, Mailing Address: Box 597, Zip 36518–0597; tel. 334/847–2223; Howard C. Holcomb, Administrator

Owned, leased, sponsored:	1 hospital	550 beds
Contract–managed:	2 hospitals	134 beds
Totals:	3 hospitals	684 beds

0089: INNOVATIVE HEALTHCARE SYSTEMS, INC. (IO)
1900 International Park Drive, Suite 220, Birmingham, AL Zip 35243; tel. 205/967–3455; Kerry Teel, President and Chief Executive Officer

LOUISIANA: LAKEVIEW REGIONAL HOSPITAL (O, 60 beds) 6200 Cypress Street, West Monroe, LA Zip 71291–9012; tel. 318/396–5900; Edward C. Tschopp, Administrator

TEXAS: CEDARS HOSPITAL (O, 76 beds) 2000 North Old Hickory Trail, De Soto, TX Zip 75115; tel. 972/298–7323; Don Johnson, Administrator

Owned, leased, sponsored:	2 hospitals	136 beds
Contract–managed:	0 hospitals	0 beds
Totals:	2 hospitals	136 beds

★1305: INOVA HEALTH SYSTEM (NP)
8001 Braddock Road, Springfield, VA Zip 22151–2150; tel. 703/321–4213; J. Knox Singleton, President

For explanation of codes following names, see page B2.
★ Indicates Type III membership in the American Hospital Association.

Section B

VIRGINIA: INOVA FAIR OAKS HOSPITAL (O, 133 beds) 3600 Joseph Siewick Drive, Fairfax, VA Zip 22033–1709; tel. 703/391–3600; Steven E. Brown, Administrator

INOVA FAIRFAX HOSPITAL (O, 656 beds) 3300 Gallows Road, Falls Church, VA Zip 22046–3300; tel. 703/698–1110; Jolene Tornabeni, Administrator

INOVA MOUNT VERNON HOSPITAL (O, 229 beds) 2501 Parker's Lane, Alexandria, VA Zip 22306–3209; tel. 703/664–7000; Susan Herbert, Administrator

Owned, leased, sponsored:	3 hospitals	1018 beds
Contract–managed:	0 hospitals	0 beds
Totals:	3 hospitals	1018 beds

★**0305: INTEGRIS HEALTH** (NP)
3366 Northwest Expressway, Oklahoma City, OK Zip 73112; tel. 405/949–6068; Stanley F. Hupfeld, President and Chief Executive Officer

OKLAHOMA: BLACKWELL REGIONAL HOSPITAL (L, 34 beds) 710 South 13th Street, Blackwell, OK Zip 74631; tel. 405/363–2311; Greg Martin, Administrator and Chief Executive Officer

BRISTOW MEMORIAL HOSPITAL (L, 22 beds) Seventh and Spruce Streets, Bristow, OK Zip 74010, Mailing Address: Box 780, Zip 74010; tel. 918/367–2215; William L. Legate, Administrator

CHOCTAW MEMORIAL HOSPITAL (C, 41 beds) 1405 East Kirk Road, Hugo, OK Zip 74743; tel. 405/326–6414; Michael R. Morel, Administrator

DRUMRIGHT MEMORIAL HOSPITAL (L, 15 beds) 501 South Lou Allard Drive, Drumright, OK Zip 74030–4899; tel. 918/352–2525; Jerry Jones, Administrator

INTEGRIS BAPTIST MEDICAL CENTER (O, 424 beds) 3300 N.W. Expressway, Oklahoma City, OK Zip 73112–4481; tel. 405/949–3011; Thomas R. Rice, President and Chief Operation Officer

INTEGRIS BAPTIST REGIONAL HEALTH CENTER (O, 124 beds) 200 Second Street S.W., Miami, OK Zip 74354, Mailing Address: Box 1207, Zip 74355–1207; tel. 918/540–7100; Dee Renshaw, Administrator

INTEGRIS BASS BAPTIST HEALTH CENTER (O, 119 beds) 600 South Monroe, Enid, OK Zip 73701, Mailing Address: Box 3168, Zip 73702; tel. 405/233–2300; W. Eugene Baxter, Dr.PH, Administrator

INTEGRIS GROVE GENERAL HOSPITAL (O, 72 beds) 1310 South Main Street, Grove, OK Zip 74344–1310; tel. 918/786–2243; Dee Renshaw, Administrator

INTEGRIS MENTAL HEALTH SYSTEM–WILLOW VIEW (O, 44 beds) 2601 North Spencer Road, Spencer, OK Zip 73084–3699, Mailing Address: P.O. Box 11137, Oklahoma City, Zip 73136–0137; tel. 405/427–2441; Gary L. Watson, President and Chief Operating Officer

INTEGRIS SOUTHWEST MEDICAL CENTER (O, 324 beds) 4401 South Western, Oklahoma City, OK Zip 73109–3441; tel. 405/636–7000; Thomas R. Rice, President and Chief Operation Officer

MARSHALL MEMORIAL HOSPITAL (C, 25 beds) 1 Hospital Drive, Madill, OK Zip 73446, Mailing Address: P.O. Box 827, Zip 73446; tel. 405/795–3384; Norma Howard, Administrator

MAYES COUNTY MEDICAL CENTER (L, 37 beds) 129 North Kentucky, Pryor, OK Zip 74361, Mailing Address: Box 278, Zip 74362–0278; tel. 918/825–1600; W. Charles Jordan, Administrator

PAWNEE MUNICIPAL HOSPITAL (L, 40 beds) 1212 Fourth Street, Pawnee, OK Zip 74058, Mailing Address: Box 467, Zip 74058; tel. 918/762–2577; John Ketring, Administrator

STROUD MUNICIPAL HOSPITAL (L, 17 beds) Highway 66 West, Stroud, OK Zip 74079, Mailing Address: P.O. Box 530, Zip 74079; tel. 918/968–3571; Jerrell J. Horton, Chief Executive Officer

Owned, leased, sponsored:	12 hospitals	1272 beds
Contract–managed:	2 hospitals	66 beds
Totals:	14 hospitals	1338 beds

★**1815: INTERMOUNTAIN HEALTH CARE, INC.** (NP)
36 South State Street, 22nd Floor, Salt Lake City, UT Zip 84111; tel. 801/442–2000; Scott S. Parker, President

IDAHO: CASSIA REGIONAL MEDICAL CENTER (O, 87 beds) 1501 Hiland Avenue, Burley, ID Zip 83318; tel. 208/678–4444; Richard Packer, Administrator

POCATELLO REGIONAL MEDICAL CENTER (O, 87 beds) 777 Hospital Way, Pocatello, ID Zip 83201; tel. 208/234–0777; Earl L. Christison, Administrator

UTAH: ALTA VIEW HOSPITAL (O, 68 beds) 9660 South 1300 East, Sandy, UT Zip 84094; tel. 801/576–2600; Wes Thompson, Administrator

AMERICAN FORK HOSPITAL (O, 66 beds) 1100 East 170 North, American Fork, UT Zip 84003–9787; tel. 801/763–3300; Keith N. Alexander, Administrator and Chief Operating Officer

BEAR RIVER VALLEY HOSPITAL (O, 58 beds) 440 West 600 North, Tremonton, UT Zip 84337; tel. 801/257–7441; Robert F. Jex, Administrator

COTTONWOOD HOSPITAL MEDICAL CENTER (O, 160 beds) 5770 South 300 East, Murray, UT Zip 84107; tel. 801/262–3461; Douglas R. Fonnesbeck, Administrator

DELTA COMMUNITY MEDICAL CENTER (O, 20 beds) 126 South White Sage Avenue, Delta, UT Zip 84624; tel. 801/864–5591; James E. Beckstrand, Administrator

DIXIE REGIONAL MEDICAL CENTER (O, 137 beds) 544 South 400 East, Saint George, UT Zip 84770; tel. 801/634–4000; L. Steven Wilson, Administrator

FILLMORE COMMUNITY MEDICAL CENTER (O, 20 beds) 674 South Highway 99, Fillmore, UT Zip 84631; tel. 801/743–5591; James E. Beckstrand, Administrator

GARFIELD MEMORIAL HOSPITAL AND CLINICS (O, 44 beds) 200 North Fourth East, Panguitch, UT Zip 84759, Mailing Address: P.O. Box 389, Zip 84759–0389; tel. 435/676–8811; Wayne R. Ross, Administrator

LDS HOSPITAL (O, 414 beds) Eighth Avenue and C Street, Salt Lake City, UT Zip 84143; tel. 801/321–1100; Richard M. Cagen, Chief Executive Officer and Administrator

LOGAN REGIONAL HOSPITAL (O, 127 beds) 1400 North 500 East, Logan, UT Zip 84341; tel. 801/752–2050; Richard Smith, Administrator

MCKAY–DEE HOSPITAL CENTER (O, 315 beds) 3939 Harrison Boulevard, Ogden, UT Zip 84409–2386, Mailing Address: Box 9370, Zip 84409–0370; tel. 801/627–2800; Thomas Hanrahan, Administrator and Chief Executive Officer

OREM COMMUNITY HOSPITAL (O, 20 beds) 331 North 400 West, Orem, UT Zip 84057; tel. 801/224–4080; Kim Nielsen, Administrator and Chief Executive Officer

PRIMARY CHILDREN'S MEDICAL CENTER (O, 187 beds) 100 North Medical Drive, Salt Lake City, UT Zip 84113–1100; tel. 801/588–2000; Joseph R. Horton, Chief Executive Officer and Administrator

SANPETE VALLEY HOSPITAL (O, 20 beds) 1100 South Medical Drive, Mount Pleasant, UT Zip 84647; tel. 801/462–2441; George Winn, Administrator

SEVIER VALLEY HOSPITAL (O, 25 beds) 1100 North Main Street, Richfield, UT Zip 84701; tel. 801/896–8271; Gary E. Beck, Administrator

UTAH VALLEY REGIONAL MEDICAL CENTER (O, 343 beds) 1034 North 500 West, Provo, UT Zip 84605–0390; tel. 801/373–7850; Larry R. Dursteler, Regional Vice President

VALLEY VIEW MEDICAL CENTER (O, 36 beds) 595 South 75 East, Cedar City, UT Zip 84720; tel. 801/586–6587; Craig M. Smedley, Administrator

WASATCH COUNTY HOSPITAL (L, 25 beds) 55 South Fifth East, Heber City, UT Zip 84032–1848; tel. 801/654–2500; Randall K. Probst, Administrator

WYOMING: EVANSTON REGIONAL HOSPITAL (O, 38 beds) 190 Arrowhead Drive, Evanston, WY Zip 82930; tel. 307/789–3636; Robert W. Allen, Administrator

STAR VALLEY HOSPITAL (C, 15 beds) 110 Hospital Lane, Afton, WY Zip 83110, Mailing Address: P.O. Box 579, Zip 83110; tel. 307/886–3841; Alberto Vasquez, Chief Executive Officer

Owned, leased, sponsored:	21 hospitals	2297 beds
Contract–managed:	1 hospital	15 beds
Totals:	22 hospitals	2312 beds

★**0061: IOWA HEALTH SYSTEM** (NP)
1200 Pleasant Street, Des Moines, IA Zip 50309–1453; tel. 515/241–6212; Samuel T. Wallace, President

For explanation of codes following names, see page B2.
★ Indicates Type III membership in the American Hospital Association.

IOWA: ALLEN MEMORIAL HOSPITAL (O, 176 beds) 1825 Logan Avenue, Waterloo, IA Zip 50703; tel. 319/235–3941; Larry W. Pugh, President and Chief Executive Officer

ANAMOSA COMMUNITY HOSPITAL (L, 18 beds) 104 Broadway Place, Anamosa, IA Zip 52205; tel. 319/462–6131; Margaret Robinson, Administrator

CLARKE COUNTY HOSPITAL (C, 48 beds) 800 South Fillmore Street, Osceola, IA Zip 50213–0427, Mailing Address: P.O. Box 427, Zip 50213–0427; tel. 515/342–2184; Kris Baumgart, Administrator

COMMUNITY MEMORIAL HOSPITAL (C, 33 beds) 1316 South Main Street, Clarion, IA Zip 50525–0429; tel. 515/532–2811; Steve J. Simonin, Chief Executive Officer

IOWA LUTHERAN HOSPITAL (O, 243 beds) 700 East University Avenue, Des Moines, IA Zip 50316–2392; tel. 515/263–5612; James H. Skogsbergh, President

IOWA METHODIST MEDICAL CENTER (O, 557 beds) 1200 Pleasant Street, Des Moines, IA Zip 50309–9976; tel. 515/241–6212; James H. Skogsbergh, President

LORING HOSPITAL (C, 54 beds) Highland Avenue, Sac City, IA Zip 50583–0217; tel. 712/662–7105; Greg Miner, Administrator

MAHASKA COUNTY HOSPITAL (C, 53 beds) 1229 C Avenue East, Oskaloosa, IA Zip 52577; tel. 515/672–3100; David E. Rutter, Administrator

ST. LUKE'S HOSPITAL (O, 406 beds) 1026 A Avenue N.E., Cedar Rapids, IA Zip 52402–3026, Mailing Address: P.O. Box 3026, Zip 52406–3026; tel. 319/369–7211; Stephen E. Vanourny, M.D., President

ST. LUKE'S REGIONAL MEDICAL CENTER (O, 192 beds) 2720 Stone Park Boulevard, Sioux City, IA Zip 51104–2000· tel. 712/279–3500; John D. Daniels, President and Chief Executive Officer

VIRGINIA GAY HOSPITAL (C, 97 beds) 502 North Ninth Avenue, Vinton, IA Zip 52349; tel. 319/472–2348; Michael J. Riege, Administrator

Owned, leased, sponsored:	6 hospitals	1592 beds
Contract–managed:	5 hospitals	285 beds
Totals:	11 hospitals	1877 beds

★7775: JEFFERSON HEALTH SYSTEM (NP)
259 Radnor–Chester Road, Suite 290, Radnor, PA Zip 19087–5260; tel. 610/293–8200; Douglas S. Peters, President and Chief Executive Officer

PENNSYLVANIA: BRYN MAWR HOSPITAL (O, 283 beds) 130 South Bryn Mawr Avenue, Bryn Mawr, PA Zip 19010–3160; tel. 610/526–3000; William McCune, Vice President, Administration

BRYN MAWR REHABILITATION HOSPITAL (O, 141 beds) 414 Paoli Pike, Malvern, PA Zip 19355–3300, Mailing Address: P.O. Box 3007, Zip 19355–3300; tel. 610/251–5400; Barry S. Rabner, President

LANKENAU HOSPITAL (O, 263 beds) 100 Lancaster Avenue West, Wynnewood, PA Zip 19096; tel. 610/645–2000; Kenneth Hanover, President and Chief Executive Officer

PAOLI MEMORIAL HOSPITAL (O, 129 beds) 255 West Lancaster Avenue, Paoli, PA Zip 19301–1792; tel. 610/648–1204; Gail A. Egan, Vice President, Administrator

THOMAS JEFFERSON UNIVERSITY HOSPITAL (O, 959 beds) 111 South 11th Street, Philadelphia, PA Zip 19107–5098; tel. 215/955–7022; Thomas J. Lewis, President and Chief Executive Officer

Owned, leased, sponsored:	5 hospitals	1775 beds
Contract–managed:	0 hospitals	0 beds
Totals:	5 hospitals	1775 beds

★0052: JEWISH HOSPITAL HEALTHCARE SERVICES (NP)
217 East Chestnut Street, Louisville, KY Zip 40202; tel. 502/587–4011; Henry C. Wagner, President

INDIANA: CLARK MEMORIAL HOSPITAL (C, 265 beds) 1220 Missouri Avenue, Jeffersonville, IN Zip 47130–3743, Mailing Address: Box 69, Zip 47131–0069; tel. 812/282–6631; Merle E. Stepp, President and Chief Executive Officer

SCOTT MEMORIAL HOSPITAL (C, 40 beds) 1415 North Gardner Street, Scottsburg, IN Zip 47170–0456, Mailing Address: Box 430, Zip 47170–0430; tel. 812/752–8500; Clifford D. Nay, Executive Director

SOUTHERN INDIANA REHABILITATION HOSPITAL (O, 60 beds) 3104 Blackiston Boulevard, New Albany, IN Zip 47150; tel. 812/941–8300; Randy L. Napier, President

WASHINGTON COUNTY MEMORIAL HOSPITAL (C, 50 beds) 911 North Shelby Street, Salem, IN Zip 47167; tel. 812/883–5881; Rodney M. Coats, Executive Director

KENTUCKY: FRAZIER REHABILITATION CENTER (O, 93 beds) 220 Abraham Flexner Way, Louisville, KY Zip 40202–1887; tel. 502/582–7400; Jason Roeback, President

HARDIN MEMORIAL HOSPITAL (C, 276 beds) 913 North Dixie Highway, Elizabethtown, KY Zip 42701–2599; tel. 502/737–1212; Gary R. Colberg, President and Chief Executive Officer

JEWISH HOSPITAL (O, 404 beds) 217 East Chestnut Street, Louisville, KY Zip 40202–1886; tel. 502/587–4011; Douglas E. Shaw, President

JEWISH HOSPITAL–SHELBYVILLE (O, 66 beds) 727 Hospital Drive, Shelbyville, KY Zip 40065; tel. 502/647–4301; Timothy L. Jarm, President

LEXINGTON HOSPITAL (C, 174 beds) 150 North Eagle Creek Drive, Lexington, KY Zip 40509–1807; tel. 606/268–4800; Rebecca Lewis, President

PATTIE A. CLAY HOSPITAL (C, 96 beds) EKU By–Pass, Richmond, KY Zip 40475, Mailing Address: P.O. Box 1600, Zip 40476–2603; tel. 606/625–3131; Richard M. Thomas, President

TAYLOR COUNTY HOSPITAL (C, 80 beds) 1700 Old Lebanon Road, Campbellsville, KY Zip 42718; tel. 502/465–3561; David R. Hayes, President

UNIVERSITY OF LOUISVILLE HOSPITAL (C, 269 beds) 530 South Jackson Street, Louisville, KY Zip 40202–3611; tel. 502/562–3000; James H. Taylor, President and Chief Executive Officer

Owned, leased, sponsored:	4 hospitals	623 beds
Contract–managed:	8 hospitals	1250 beds
Totals:	12 hospitals	1873 beds

★8855: JFK HEALTH SYSTEMS, INC. (NP)
80 James Street, 2nd Floor, Edison, NJ Zip 08820–3998; tel. 908/632–1500; John P. McGee, President and Chief Executive Officer

NEW JERSEY: JFK JOHNSON REHABILITATION INSTITUTE (O, 92 beds) 65 James Street, Edison, NJ Zip 08818–3059; tel. 908/321–7050; Scott Gebhard, Senior Vice President Operations

JFK MEDICAL CENTER (O, 380 beds) 65 James Street, Edison, NJ Zip 08818; tel. 908/321–7000; John P. McGee, President and Chief Executive Officer

Owned, leased, sponsored:	2 hospitals	472 beds
Contract–managed:	0 hospitals	0 beds
Totals:	2 hospitals	472 beds

★1015: JOHNS HOPKINS HEALTH SYSTEM (NP)
600 North Wolfe Street, Baltimore, MD Zip 21287–1193; tel. 410/955–9540; Ronald R. Peterson, President

MARYLAND: JOHNS HOPKINS BAYVIEW MEDICAL CENTER (O, 667 beds) 4940 Eastern Avenue, Baltimore, MD Zip 21224–2780; tel. 410/550–0100; Ronald R. Peterson, President

JOHNS HOPKINS HOSPITAL (O, 886 beds) 600 North Wolfe Street, Baltimore, MD Zip 21287; tel. 410/955–5000; Ronald R. Peterson, President

Owned, leased, sponsored:	2 hospitals	1553 beds
Contract–managed:	0 hospitals	0 beds
Totals:	2 hospitals	1553 beds

★2105: KAISER FOUNDATION HOSPITALS (NP)
One Kaiser Plaza, Oakland, CA Zip 94612–3600; tel. 510/271–5910; David M. Lawrence, M.D., Chairman and Chief Executive Officer

For explanation of codes following names, see page B2.
★ Indicates Type III membership in the American Hospital Association.

CALIFORNIA: KAISER FOUNDATION HOSPITAL (O, 210 beds) 2425 Geary Boulevard, San Francisco, CA Zip 94115; tel. 415/202–2000; Rosemary Fox, Acting Administrator

KAISER FOUNDATION HOSPITAL (O, 117 beds) 401 Bicentennial Way, Santa Rosa, CA Zip 95403; tel. 707/571–4000; Richard R. Pettingill, President and Chief Executive Officer

KAISER FOUNDATION HOSPITAL (O, 311 beds) 4747 Sunset Boulevard, Los Angeles, CA Zip 90027; tel. 213/783–4011; Joseph Wm Hummel, Senior Vice President and Area Manager

KAISER FOUNDATION HOSPITAL (O, 89 beds) 7300 North Fresno Street, Fresno, CA Zip 93720; tel. 209/448–4500; Edward S. Glavis, Administrator

KAISER FOUNDATION HOSPITAL (O, 263 beds) 280 West MacArthur Boulevard, Oakland, CA Zip 94611; tel. 510/596–1000; Donald Oxley, Vice President, Area Manager and Chief Executive Officer

KAISER FOUNDATION HOSPITAL (O, 268 beds) 1425 South Main Street, Walnut Creek, CA Zip 94596; tel. 510/295–4000; Anna Robinson, Administrator

KAISER FOUNDATION HOSPITAL (O, 131 beds) 441 North Lakeview Avenue, Anaheim, CA Zip 92807; tel. 714/279–4100; Gerald A. McCall, Administrator

KAISER FOUNDATION HOSPITAL (O, 248 beds) 9400 East Rosecrans Avenue, Bellflower, CA Zip 90706–2246; tel. 310/461–3000; Timothy A. Reed, Administrator

KAISER FOUNDATION HOSPITAL (O, 287 beds) 9961 Sierra Avenue, Fontana, CA Zip 92335–6794; tel. 909/427–5000; Patricia Siegel, Senior Vice President, Health Plan, Hospitals and Inland Empire Area Manager

KAISER FOUNDATION HOSPITAL (O, 179 beds) 25825 South Vermont Avenue, Harbor City, CA Zip 90710; tel. 310/325–5111; Mary Ann Barnes, Administrator

KAISER FOUNDATION HOSPITAL (O, 190 beds) 27400 Hesperian Boulevard, Hayward, CA Zip 94545–4297; tel. 510/784–4313; Lisa Koltun, Administrator

KAISER FOUNDATION HOSPITAL (O, 277 beds) 4647 Zion Avenue, San Diego, CA Zip 92120; tel. 619/528–5000; Kenneth F. Colling, Administrator

KAISER FOUNDATION HOSPITAL (O, 144 beds) 1150 Veterans Boulevard, Redwood City, CA Zip 94063–2087; tel. 415/299–2000; Carol Kiecker, Chief Executive Officer, Vice President and Area Manager

KAISER FOUNDATION HOSPITAL (O, 304 beds) 2025 Morse Avenue, Sacramento, CA Zip 95825–2115; tel. 916/978–1710; Sarah Krevans, Administrator

KAISER FOUNDATION HOSPITAL (O, 221 beds) 6600 Bruceville Road, Sacramento, CA Zip 95823; tel. 916/688–2430; Sarah Krevans, Area Manager

KAISER FOUNDATION HOSPITAL (O, 119 beds) 99 Montecillo Road, San Rafael, CA Zip 94903–3397; tel. 415/444–2000; Richard R. Pettingill, Chief Executive Officer

KAISER FOUNDATION HOSPITAL (O, 249 beds) 900 Kiely Boulevard, Santa Clara, CA Zip 95051–5386; tel. 408/236–6400

KAISER FOUNDATION HOSPITAL (O, 79 beds) 1200 El Camino Real, South San Francisco, CA Zip 94080–3299; tel. 415/742–2547; Rosemary Fox, Coutinuing Care Leader

KAISER FOUNDATION HOSPITAL (O, 269 beds) 13652 Cantara Street, Panorama City, CA Zip 91402; tel. 818/375–2000; Dev Mahadevan, Administrator

KAISER FOUNDATION HOSPITAL (O, 139 beds) 5601 DeSoto Avenue, Woodland Hills, CA Zip 91365–4084; tel. 818/719–2000; James L. Breeden, Administrator

KAISER FOUNDATION HOSPITAL AND REHABILITATION CENTER (O, 219 beds) 975 Sereno Drive, Vallejo, CA Zip 94589; tel. 707/648–6230; Vivian M. Rittenhouse, Vice President and Market Leader

KAISER FOUNDATION HOSPITAL–RIVERSIDE (O, 121 beds) 10800 Magnolia Avenue, Riverside, CA Zip 92505–3000; tel. 909/353–4600; Robert S. Lund, Administrator

KAISER FOUNDATION HOSPITAL–WEST LOS ANGELES (O, 161 beds) 6041 Cadillac Avenue, Los Angeles, CA Zip 90034; tel. 213/857–2201; Ivette Estrada, Administrator

SANTA TERESA COMMUNITY HOSPITAL (O, 178 beds) 250 Hospital Parkway, San Jose, CA Zip 95119; tel. 408/972–7000

HAWAII: KAISER FOUNDATION HOSPITAL (O, 198 beds) 3288 Moanalua Road, Honolulu, HI Zip 96819; tel. 808/834–5333; Bruce Behnke, Administrator

OREGON: KAISER SUNNYSIDE MEDICAL CENTER (O, 174 beds) 10200 S.E. Sunnyside Road, Clackamas, OR Zip 97015–9303; tel. 503/652–2880; Alide Chase, Administrator

Owned, leased, sponsored:	26 hospitals	5145 beds
Contract–managed:	0 hospitals	0 beds
Totals:	26 hospitals	5145 beds

★0056: LAKELAND REGIONAL HEALTH SYSTEM, INC. (NP) 1234 Napier Avenue, Saint Joseph, MI Zip 49085–2158; tel. 616/983–8300; Joseph A. Wasserman, President and Chief Executive Officer

MICHIGAN: LAKELAND MEDICAL CENTER–NILES (O, 106 beds) 31 North St. Joseph Avenue, Niles, MI Zip 49120–2287; tel. 616/683–5510; Joseph A. Wasserman, President and Chief Executive Officer

LAKELAND MEDICAL CENTER–ST. JOSEPH (O, 254 beds) 1234 Napier Avenue, Saint Joseph, MI Zip 49085; tel. 616/983–8300; Joseph A. Wasserman, President and Chief Executive Officer

Owned, leased, sponsored:	2 hospitals	360 beds
Contract–managed:	0 hospitals	0 beds
Totals:	2 hospitals	360 beds

★2755: LEGACY HEALTH SYSTEM (NP) 1919 N.W. Lovejoy Street, Portland, OR Zip 97209–1503; tel. 503/415–5600; John G. King, President and Chief Executive Officer

OREGON: LEGACY EMANUEL HOSPITAL AND HEALTH CENTER (O, 411 beds) 2801 North Gantenbein Avenue, Portland, OR Zip 97227–1674; tel. 503/413–2200; Lowell W. Johnson, Interim President and Chief Executive Officer

LEGACY GOOD SAMARITAN HOSPITAL AND MEDICAL CENTER (O, 305 beds) 1015 N.W. 22nd Avenue, Portland, OR Zip 97210; tel. 503/413–7711; Lowell W. Johnson, Interim President and Chief Executive Officer

LEGACY MERIDIAN PARK HOSPITAL (O, 116 beds) 19300 S.W. 65th Avenue, Tualatin, OR Zip 97062–9741; tel. 503/692–1212; Jeff Cushing, Vice President, Administration

LEGACY MOUNT HOOD MEDICAL CENTER (O, 97 beds) 24800 S.E. Stark, Gresham, OR Zip 97030–0154; tel. 503/667–1122; Jane C. Cummins, President and Chief Executive Officer

Owned, leased, sponsored:	4 hospitals	929 beds
Contract–managed:	0 hospitals	0 beds
Totals:	4 hospitals	929 beds

★0060: LIFESPAN CORPORATION (NP) 167 Point Street, Providence, RI Zip 02903; tel. 401/444–6699; William Kreykes, President and Chief Executive Officer

RHODE ISLAND: EMMA PENDLETON BRADLEY HOSPITAL (O, 60 beds) 1011 Veterans Memorial Parkway, East Providence, RI Zip 02915–5099; tel. 401/434–3400; Daniel J. Wall, President and Chief Executive Officer

MIRIAM HOSPITAL (O, 247 beds) 164 Summit Avenue, Providence, RI Zip 02906–2895; tel. 401/331–8500; Steven D. Baron, President and Chief Executive Officer

NEWPORT HOSPITAL (O, 150 beds) 11 Friendship Street, Newport, RI Zip 02840–2299; tel. 401/846–6400; Arthur J. Sampson, President and Chief Executive Officer

RHODE ISLAND HOSPITAL (O, 677 beds) 593 Eddy Street, Providence, RI Zip 02903; tel. 401/444–4000; Steven D. Baron, President and Chief Executive Officer

For explanation of codes following names, see page B2.
★ Indicates Type III membership in the American Hospital Association.

Owned, leased, sponsored:	4 hospitals	1134 beds
Contract–managed:	0 hospitals	0 beds
Totals:	4 hospitals	1134 beds

2295: LITTLE COMPANY OF MARY SISTERS HEALTHCARE SYSTEM (CC)

9350 South California Avenue, Evergreen Park, IL Zip 60805; tel. 708/229–5491; Sister Carol Pacini, Provincialate Superior

CALIFORNIA: LITTLE COMPANY OF MARY HOSPITAL (O, 335 beds) 4101 Torrance Boulevard, Torrance, CA Zip 90503–4698; tel. 310/540–7676; Mark Costa, President

ILLINOIS: LITTLE COMPANY OF MARY HOSPITAL AND HEALTH CARE CENTERS (O, 372 beds) 2800 West 95th Street, Evergreen Park, IL Zip 60805–2795; tel. 708/422–6200; Sister Kathleen McIntyre, President

INDIANA: MEMORIAL HOSPITAL AND HEALTH CARE CENTER (O, 125 beds) 800 West Ninth Street, Jasper, IN Zip 47546–2516; tel. 812/482–2345; Sister M. Adrian Davis, Ph.D., President and Chief Officer

Owned, leased, sponsored:	3 hospitals	832 beds
Contract–managed:	0 hospitals	0 beds
Totals:	3 hospitals	832 beds

5755: LOS ANGELES COUNTY–DEPARTMENT OF HEALTH SERVICES (NP)

313 North Figueroa Street, Room 912, Los Angeles, CA Zip 90012; tel. 213/240–8101; Mark Finucane, Director Health

CALIFORNIA: LAC–HARBOR–UNIVERSITY OF CALIFORNIA AT LOS ANGELES MEDICAL CENTER (O, 455 beds) 1000 West Carson Street, Torrance, CA Zip 90509; tel. 310/222–2101; Tecla A. Mickoseff, Administrator

LAC–HIGH DESERT HOSPITAL (O, 76 beds) 44900 North 60th Street West, Lancaster, CA Zip 93536; tel. 805/945–8461; Mel Grussing, Administrator

LAC–KING–DREW MEDICAL CENTER (O, 264 beds) 12021 South Wilmington Avenue, Los Angeles, CA Zip 90059; tel. 310/668–4321; Foster Randall, Administrator and Chief Executive Officer

LAC–RANCHO LOS AMIGOS MEDICAL CENTER (O, 300 beds) 7601 East Imperial Highway, Downey, CA Zip 90242; tel. 562/401–7022; Consuelo C. Diaz, Chief Executive Officer

LAC–UNIVERSITY OF SOUTHERN CALIFORNIA MEDICAL CENTER (O, 1157 beds) 1200 North State Street, Los Angeles, CA Zip 90033–1084; tel. 213/226–2622; Douglas D. Bagley, Executive Director

OLIVE VIEW–UCLA MEDICAL CENTER (O, 241 beds) 14445 Olive View Drive, Sylmar, CA Zip 91342–1495; tel. 818/364–1555; Melinda Anderson, Administrator

Owned, leased, sponsored:	6 hospitals	2493 beds
Contract–managed:	0 hospitals	0 beds
Totals:	6 hospitals	2493 beds

★0058: LOUIS A WEISS MEMORIAL HOSPITAL/UNIVERSITY OF CHICAGO HOSPITALS (NP)

4646 North Marine Drive, Chicago, IL Zip 60640; tel. 773/878–8700; Gregory A. Cierlik, President and Chief Executive Officer

ILLINOIS: LOUIS A. WEISS MEMORIAL HOSPITAL (O, 200 beds) 4646 North Marine Drive, Chicago, IL Zip 60640–1501; tel. 773/878–8700; Gregory A. Cierlik, President and Chief Executive Officer

UNIVERSITY OF CHICAGO HOSPITALS (O, 526 beds) 5841 South Maryland, Chicago, IL Zip 60637–1470; tel. 773/702–1000; Ralph W. Muller, President

Owned, leased, sponsored:	2 hospitals	726 beds
Contract–managed:	0 hospitals	0 beds
Totals:	2 hospitals	726 beds

0715: LOUISIANA HEALTH CARE AUTHORITY (NP)

8550 United Plaza Boulevard, 4th Floor, Baton Rouge, LA Zip 70809; tel. 504/922–0488; Cary Doughtery, Acting Chief Executive Officer

LOUISIANA: E. A. CONWAY MEDICAL CENTER (O, 223 beds) 4864 Jackson Street, Monroe, LA Zip 71202, Mailing Address: P.O. Box 1881, Zip 71210–8005; tel. 318/330–7000; Roy D. Bostick, Director

EARL K. LONG MEDICAL CENTER (O, 204 beds) 5825 Airline Highway, Baton Rouge, LA Zip 70805; tel. 504/358–1000; Margaret Alvis, MSN, R.N., Chief Executive Officer

HUEY P. LONG MEDICAL CENTER (O, 143 beds) 352 Hospital Boulevard, Pineville, LA Zip 71360, Mailing Address: Box 5352, Zip 71361–5352; tel. 318/448–0811; James E. Morgan, Director

LALLIE KEMP MEDICAL CENTER (O, 68 beds) 52579 Highway 51 South, Independence, LA Zip 70443; tel. 504/878–9421; LeVern Meades, Acting Administrator

LEONARD J. CHABERT MEDICAL CENTER (O, 151 beds) 1978 Industrial Boulevard, Houma, LA Zip 70363; tel. 504/873–2200; William C. Bankston, Acting Administrator

UNIVERSITY MEDICAL CENTER (O, 161 beds) 2390 West Congress Street, Lafayette, LA Zip 70506, Mailing Address: P.O. Box 4016–C, Zip 70502–4016; tel. 318/261–6004; Lawrence T. Dorsey, Administrator

WALTER OLIN MOSS REGIONAL MEDICAL CENTER (O, 66 beds) 1000 Walters Street, Lake Charles, LA Zip 70605; tel. 318/475–8100; Philip H. Rome, Administrator

WASHINGTON–ST. TAMMANY REGIONAL MEDICAL CENTER (O, 55 beds) 400 Memphis Street, Bogalusa, LA Zip 70427–0040, Mailing Address: Box 40, Zip 70429–0040; tel. 504/735–1322; Larry R. King, Administrator

Owned, leased, sponsored:	8 hospitals	1071 beds
Contract–managed:	0 hospitals	0 beds
Totals:	8 hospitals	1071 beds

0047: LOUISIANA STATE HOSPITALS (NP)

210 State Street, New Orleans, LA Zip 70118; tel. 504/897–3400; M. E. Teague, Chief Executive Officer

CENTRAL LOUISIANA STATE HOSPITAL (O, 280 beds) 242 West Shamrock Avenue, Pineville, LA Zip 71360, Mailing Address: P.O. Box 5031, Zip 71361–5031; tel. 318/484–6200; Gary S. Grand, Chief Executive Officer

EAST LOUISIANA STATE HOSPITAL (O, 452 beds) Jackson, LA Mailing Address: P.O. Box 498, Zip 70748; tel. 504/634–0100; Warren T. Price Jr., Chief Executive Officer

GREENWELL SPRINGS HOSPITAL (O, 104 beds) 23260 Greenwell Springs Road, Greenwell Springs, LA Zip 70739, Mailing Address: P.O. Box 549, Zip 70739–0549; tel. 504/261–2730; Warren T. Price Jr., Chief Executive Officer

NEW ORLEANS ADOLESCENT HOSPITAL (O, 99 beds) 210 State Street, New Orleans, LA Zip 70118; tel. 504/897–3400; Michael E. Teague, Chief Executive Officer

SOUTHEAST LOUISIANA HOSPITAL (O, 251 beds) Abita Springs, LA Mailing Address: P.O. Box 3850, Mandeville, Zip 70470–3850; tel. 504/626–6300; Joseph C. Vinturella, Chief Executive Officer

Owned, leased, sponsored:	5 hospitals	1186 beds
Contract–managed:	0 hospitals	0 beds
Totals:	5 hospitals	1186 beds

★0036: LUBBOCK METHODIST HOSPITAL SYSTEM (NP)

3615 19th Street, Lubbock, TX Zip 79410–1201; tel. 806/792–1011; James P. Houser, President and Chief Executive Officer

TEXAS: FISHER COUNTY HOSPITAL DISTRICT (C, 30 beds) Roby Highway, Rotan, TX Zip 79546, Mailing Address: Drawer F, Zip 79546; tel. 915/735–2256; Ella Raye Helms, Administrator

LAMB HEALTHCARE CENTER (C, 41 beds) 1500 South Sunset, Littlefield, TX Zip 79339; tel. 806/385–6411; Randall A. Young, Administrator

METHODIST CHILDREN'S HOSPITAL (O, 65 beds) 3610 21st Street, Lubbock, TX Zip 79410; tel. 806/784–5040; James P. Houser, President and Chief Executive Officer

For explanation of codes following names, see page B2.
★ Indicates Type III membership in the American Hospital Association.

Networks, Health Care Systems and Alliances

Section B

METHODIST HOSPITAL (O, 520 beds) 3615 19th Street, Lubbock, TX Zip 79410–1201, Mailing Address: Box 1201, Zip 79408–1201; tel. 806/792–1011; James P. Houser, President and Chief Executive Officer

METHODIST HOSPITAL PLAINVIEW (L, 100 beds) 2601 Dimmitt Road, Plainview, TX Zip 79072–1833; tel. 806/296–5531; Donald W. Shouse, Administrator

METHODIST HOSPITAL–LEVELLAND (L, 44 beds) 1900 South College Avenue, Levelland, TX Zip 79336; tel. 806/894–4963; Jerry Osburn, Administrator

MITCHELL COUNTY HOSPITAL (C, 36 beds) 1543 Chestnut Street, Colorado City, TX Zip 79512–3998; tel. 915/728–3431; Joe Wright, Administrator

MULESHOE AREA MEDICAL CENTER (C, 31 beds) 708 South First Street, Muleshoe, TX Zip 79347; tel. 806/272–4524; Jim G. Bone, Interim Administrator

Owned, leased, sponsored:	4 hospitals	729 beds
Contract–managed:	4 hospitals	138 beds
Totals:	8 hospitals	867 beds

★2235: LUTHERAN HEALTH SYSTEMS (NP)
4310 17th Avenue S.W., Fargo, ND Zip 58103, Mailing Address: P.O. Box 6200, Zip 58106–6200; tel. 701/277–7500; Steven R. Orr, Chairman and Chief Executive Officer

ALASKA: CENTRAL PENINSULA GENERAL HOSPITAL (C, 58 beds) 250 Hospital Place, Soldotna, AK Zip 99669; tel. 907/262–4404; Rulon J. Barlow, Administrator

FAIRBANKS MEMORIAL HOSPITAL (L, 200 beds) 1650 Cowles Street, Fairbanks, AK Zip 99701; tel. 907/452–8181; Michael K. Powers, Administrator

PROVIDENCE KODIAK ISLAND HOSPITAL AND MEDICAL CENTER (C, 44 beds) 1915 East Rezanof Drive, Kodiak, AK Zip 99615; tel. 907/486–3281; Phillip E. Cline, Administrator

ARIZONA: MESA LUTHERAN HOSPITAL (O, 278 beds) 525 West Brown Road, Mesa, AZ Zip 85201–3299; tel. 602/834–1211; Don Evans, Chief Executive Officer

VALLEY LUTHERAN HOSPITAL (O, 172 beds) 6644 Baywood Avenue, Mesa, AZ Zip 85206; tel. 602/981–4100; Don Evans, Chief Executive Officer

CALIFORNIA: LASSEN COMMUNITY HOSPITAL (C, 59 beds) 560 Hospital Lane, Susanville, CA Zip 96130–4809; tel. 916/257–5325; David S. Anderson, FACHE, Administrator

COLORADO: EAST MORGAN COUNTY HOSPITAL (L, 29 beds) 2400 West Edison, Brush, CO Zip 80723; tel. 970/842–5151; Anne Platt, Administrator

MCKEE MEDICAL CENTER (O, 109 beds) 2000 Boise Avenue, Loveland, CO Zip 80538–4281; tel. 970/669–4640; Charles F. Harms, Administrator

NORTH COLORADO MEDICAL CENTER (L, 262 beds) 1801 16th Street, Greeley, CO Zip 80631–5199; tel. 970/350–6000; Karl B. Gills, Administrator

STERLING REGIONAL MEDCENTER (O, 36 beds) 615 Fairhurst, Sterling, CO Zip 80751–0500, Mailing Address: Box 3500, Zip 80751; tel. 970/522–0122; James O. Pernau, Administrator

IOWA: CENTRAL COMMUNITY HOSPITAL (C, 29 beds) 901 Davidson Street, Elkader, IA Zip 52043–9799; tel. 319/245–2250; Lisa Manson, Administrator

KANSAS: DECATUR COUNTY HOSPITAL (L, 74 beds) 810 West Columbia, Oberlin, KS Zip 67749, Mailing Address: P.O. Box 268, Zip 67749; tel. 913/475–2208; R. Kim Hardman, Administrator

ST. LUKE HOSPITAL (L, 54 beds) 1014 East Melvin, Marion, KS Zip 66861; tel. 316/382–2179; Craig Hanson, Administrator

MINNESOTA: ORTONVILLE AREA HEALTH SERVICES (C, 105 beds) 750 Eastvold Avenue, Ortonville, MN Zip 56278; tel. 320/839–2502; Frederick Peterson, Administrator

NEBRASKA: OGALLALA COMMUNITY HOSPITAL (L, 29 beds) 300 East Tenth Street, Ogallala, NE Zip 69153; tel. 308/284–4011; Linda Morris, Administrator

NEVADA: CHURCHILL COMMUNITY HOSPTIAL (O, 40 beds) 801 East Williams Avenue, Fallon, NV Zip 89406; tel. 702/423–3151; Jeffrey Feike, Administrator

PERSHING GENERAL HOSPITAL (C, 34 beds) 855 Sixth Street, Lovelock, NV Zip 89419, Mailing Address: P.O. Box 661, Zip 89419; tel. 702/273–2621; Helen Woolley, Administrator

NEW MEXICO: LOS ALAMOS MEDICAL CENTER (O, 47 beds) 3917 West Road, Los Alamos, NM Zip 87544; tel. 505/662–4201; Paul J. Wilson, Administrator

NORTH DAKOTA: LISBON MEDICAL CENTER (O, 70 beds) 905 Main Street, Lisbon, ND Zip 58054–0353, Mailing Address: P.O. Box 353, Zip 58054–0353; tel. 701/683–5241; Jack Jacobs, Administrator

PEMBINA COUNTY MEMORIAL HOSPITAL AND WEDGEWOOD MANOR (L, 89 beds) 301 Mountain Street East, Cavalier, ND Zip 58220; tel. 701/265–8461; George A. Rohrich, Administrator

OREGON: CENTRAL OREGON DISTRICT HOSPITAL (C, 42 beds) 1253 North Canal Boulevard, Redmond, OR Zip 97756–1395; tel. 541/548–8131; James A. Diegel, CHE, Executive Director

PIONEER MEMORIAL HOSPITAL (C, 30 beds) 1201 North Elm Street, Prineville, OR Zip 97754; tel. 541/447–6254; Donald J. Wee, Executive Director

SOUTH DAKOTA: GREGORY COMMUNITY HOSPITAL (O, 86 beds) 400 Park Street, Gregory, SD Zip 57533–0400, Mailing Address: Box 408, Zip 57533–0408; tel. 605/835–8394; Carol A. Varland, Chief Executive Officer

LOOKOUT MEMORIAL HOSPITAL (O, 31 beds) 1440 North Main Street, Spearfish, SD Zip 57783–1504; tel. 605/642–2617; Deb J. Krmpotic, R.N., Administrator

SOUTHERN HILLS GENERAL HOSPITAL (O, 60 beds) 209 North 16th Street, Hot Springs, SD Zip 57747–1375; tel. 605/745–3159; Linda Iverson, Administrator

STURGIS COMMUNITY HEALTH CARE CENTER (O, 114 beds) 949 Harmon Street, Sturgis, SD Zip 57785; tel. 605/347–2536; Roger R. Heidt, Administrator

WYOMING: COMMUNITY HOSPITAL (O, 36 beds) 2000 Campbell Drive, Torrington, WY Zip 82240; tel. 307/532–4181; Charles Myers, Administrator

PLATTE COUNTY MEMORIAL HOSPITAL (L, 86 beds) 201 14th Street, Wheatland, WY Zip 82201, Mailing Address: P.O. Box 848, Zip 82201; tel. 307/322–3636; Dana K. Barnett, Administrator

WASHAKIE MEMORIAL HOSPITAL (L, 30 beds) 400 South 15th Street, Worland, WY Zip 82401, Mailing Address: Box 700, Zip 82401; tel. 307/347–3221; John Johnson, Administrator

Owned, leased, sponsored:	21 hospitals	1932 beds
Contract–managed:	8 hospitals	401 beds
Totals:	29 hospitals	2333 beds

0695: MAGELLAN HEALTH SERVICES (IO)
3414 Peachtree Road N.E., Suite 1400, Atlanta, GA Zip 30326; tel. 404/841–9200; E. Mac Crawford, President, Chief Executive Officer and Chairman

ALABAMA: CHARTER BEHAVIORAL HEALTH SYSTEM (O, 94 beds) 5800 Southland Drive, Mobile, AL Zip 36693, Mailing Address: P.O. Box 991800, Zip 36691; tel. 334/661–3001; Keith Cox, CHE, Chief Executive Officer

ALASKA: CHARTER NORTH STAR BEHAVIORAL HEALTH SYSTEM (O, 80 beds) 2530 Debarr Road, Anchorage, AK Zip 99508; tel. 907/258–7575; Kathleen Cronen, Administrator

ARIZONA: CHARTER BEHAVIORAL HEALTH SYSTEM–EAST VALLEY (O, 80 beds) 2190 North Grace Boulevard, Chandler, AZ Zip 85224; tel. 602/899–8989; James Plummer, Chief Executive Officer

CHARTER BEHAVIORAL HEALTH SYSTEM–GLENDALE (O, 90 beds) 6015 West Peoria Avenue, Glendale, AZ Zip 85302; tel. 602/878–7878; Kim Hall, Chief Executive Officer

ARKANSAS: CHARTER BEHAVIORAL HEALTH SYSTEM OF LITTLE ROCK (O, 60 beds) 1601 Murphy Drive, Maumelle, AR Zip 72113; tel. 501/851–8700; Rose K. Gantner, Chief Executive Officer

CHARTER BEHAVIORAL HEALTH SYSTEM OF NORTHWEST ARKANSAS (O, 49 beds) 4253 Crossover Road, Fayetteville, AR Zip 72702; tel. 501/521–5731; Lucinda DeBruce, Administrator

For explanation of codes following names, see page B2.
★ Indicates Type III membership in the American Hospital Association.

© 1997 AHA Guide

CALIFORNIA: CHARTER BEHAVIORAL HEALTH SYSTEM OF SAN DIEGO (O, 80 beds) 11878 Avenue of Industry, San Diego, CA Zip 92128; tel. 619/487–3200; Jerry Greene, Chief Executive Officer

CHARTER BEHAVIORAL HEALTH SYSTEM OF SOUTHERN CALIFORNIA–CHARTER OAK (O, 95 beds) 1161 East Covina Boulevard, Covina, CA Zip 91724–1161; tel. 818/966–1632; Todd A. Smith, Chief Executive Officer

CHARTER BEHAVIORAL HEALTH SYSTEM OF SOUTHERN CALIFORNIA–CORONA (O, 92 beds) 2055 Kellogg Avenue, Corona, CA Zip 91719; tel. 909/735–2910; Diana C. Hanyak, Chief Executive Officer

CHARTER BEHAVIORAL HEALTH SYSTEM OF SOUTHERN CALIFORNIA/MISSION VIEJO (O, 80 beds) 23228 Madero, Mission Viejo, CA Zip 92691; tel. 714/830–4800; James S. Plummer, Chief Executive Officer

CHARTER BEHAVIORAL HEALTH SYSTEM–PALM SPRINGS (O, 80 beds) 69–696 Ramon Road, Cathedral City, CA Zip 92234; tel. 619/321–2000; Robert Deney, Chief Executive Officer

COLORADO: CHARTER CENTENNIAL PEAKS HEALTH SYSTEM (O, 72 beds) 2255 South 88th Street, Louisville, CO Zip 80027; tel. 303/673–9990; Sharon Worsham, Administrator

CONNECTICUT: ELMCREST PSYCHIATRIC INSTITUTE (O, 92 beds) 25 Marlborough Street, Portland, CT Zip 06480–1829; tel. 860/342–0480; Lane Ameen, M.D., Chief Executive Officer

FLORIDA: CHARTER BEHAVIORAL HEALTH SYSTEM AT MEDFIELD (O, 64 beds) 12891 Seminole Boulevard, Largo, FL Zip 34648–2300; tel. 813/587–6000; Jim Hill, Chief Executive Officer

CHARTER BEHAVIORAL HEALTH SYSTEM OF TAMPA BAY (O, 146 beds) 4004 North Riverside Drive, Tampa, FL Zip 33603; tel. 813/238–8671; James C. Hill, Chief Executive Officer

CHARTER GLADE BEHAVIORAL HEALTH SYSTEM (O, 104 beds) 3550 Colonial Boulevard, Fort Myers, FL Zip 33912, Mailing Address: P.O. Box 60120, Zip 33906; tel. 813/939–0403; Vickie Lewis, Chief Executive Officer

CHARTER HOSPITAL ORLANDO SOUTH (O, 60 beds) 206 Park Place Drive, Kissimmee, FL Zip 34741; tel. 407/846–0444; Daniel Kearney, Chief Executive Officer

CHARTER HOSPITAL OF PASCO (O, 72 beds) 21808 State Road 54, Lutz, FL Zip 33549; tel. 813/948–2441; Miriam K. Williams, Administrator

CHARTER SPRINGS HOSPITAL (O, 92 beds) 3130 S.W. 27th Avenue, Ocala, FL Zip 34474, Mailing Address: P.O. Box 3338, Zip 34478; tel. 352/237–7293; James Duff, Administrator

GEORGIA: CHARTER BEHAVIORAL HEALTH SYSTEM OF ATLANTA (O, 40 beds) 811 Juniper Street N.E., Atlanta, GA Zip 30308; tel. 404/881–5800; Dennis Workman, M.D., Medical Director

CHARTER BEHAVIORAL HEALTH SYSTEM OF ATLANTA AT PEACHFORD (O, 224 beds) 2151 Peachford Road, Atlanta, GA Zip 30338; tel. 770/455–3200; Aleen S. Davis, Chief Executive Officer

CHARTER BEHAVIORAL HEALTH SYSTEM/CENTRAL GEORGIA (O, 118 beds) 3500 Riverside Drive, Macon, GA Zip 31210; tel. 912/474–6200; Blair R. Johanson, Administrator

CHARTER SAVANNAH BEHAVIORAL HEALTH SYSTEM (O, 112 beds) 1150 Cornell Avenue, Savannah, GA Zip 31406; tel. 912/354–3911; Ron Fincher, Chief Executive Officer

CHARTER WINDS HOSPITAL (O, 80 beds) 240 Mitchell Bridge Road, Athens, GA Zip 30606; tel. 706/546–7277; Susan Lister, Chief Executive Officer

CHARTER BY–THE–SEA BEHAVIORAL HEALTH SYSTEM (O, 101 beds) 2927 Demere Road, Saint Simons Island, GA Zip 31522–1620; tel. 912/638–1999; Wes Robbins, Chief Executive Officer

INDIANA: CHARTER BEACON (O, 97 beds) 1720 Beacon Street, Fort Wayne, IN Zip 46805; tel. 219/423–3651; Robert Hails, Chief Executive Officer

CHARTER BEHAVIORAL HEALTH SYSTEM OF INDIANA AT JEFFERSON (O, 100 beds) 2700 River City Park Road, Jeffersonville, IN Zip 47130; tel. 812/284–3400; Michael D. Coppol, Chief Executive Officer

CHARTER BEHAVIORAL HEALTH SYSTEM OF NORTHWEST INDIANA (O, 60 beds) 101 West 61st Avenue and State Road 51, Hobart, IN Zip 46342; tel. 219/947–4464; Michael J. Brown Jr., Chief Executive Officer

CHARTER BEHAVIORAL HEALTH SYSTEMS (O, 64 beds) 3700 Rome Drive, Lafayette, IN Zip 47905, Mailing Address: P.O. Box 5969, Zip 47903; tel. 765/448–6999; Stewart Graham, Administrator

CHARTER INDIANAPOLIS BEHAVIORAL HEALTH SYSTEM (O, 80 beds) 5602 Caito Drive, Indianapolis, IN Zip 46226; tel. 317/545–2111; Marina Cecchini, Chief Executive Officer

KENTUCKY: CHARTER BEHAVIORAL HEALTH SYSTEM OF PADUCAH (O, 56 beds) 435 Berger Road, Paducah, KY Zip 42001, Mailing Address: P.O. Box 7609, Zip 42002–7609; tel. 502/444–0444; Pat Harrod, Chief Executive Officer

CHARTER RIDGE HOSPITAL (O, 110 beds) 3050 Rio Dosa Drive, Lexington, KY Zip 40509–9990; tel. 606/269–2325; Ali A. Elhaj, Chief Executive Officer

CHARTER LOUISVILLE BEHAVIORAL HEALTH SYSTEM (O, 66 beds) 1405 Browns Lane, Louisville, KY Zip 40207; tel. 502/896–0495; Charles L. Webb Jr., Administrator

LOUISIANA: CHARTER BEHAVIORAL HEALTH SYSTEM OF LAKE CHARLES (O, 60 beds) 4250 Fifth Avenue South, Lake Charles, LA Zip 70605–3812; tel. 318/474–6133; Charles P. Whitson, Chief Executive Officer

CHARTER CYPRESS BEHAVIORAL HEALTH SYSTEM (O, 70 beds) 302 Dulles Drive, Lafayette, LA Zip 70506; tel. 318/233–9024; Denise Guthrie, Chief Executive Officer

CHARTER FOREST BEHAVIORAL HEALTH SYSTEM (O, 60 beds) 9320 Linwood Avenue, Shreveport, LA Zip 71106, Mailing Address: P.O. Box 18130, Zip 71138–1130; tel. 318/688–3930; Randy J. Watson, Administrator

MARYLAND: CHARTER BEHAVIORAL HEALTH SYSTEM OF POTOMAC RIDGE (O, 140 beds) 14901 Broschart Road, Rockville, MD Zip 20850–3321; tel. 301/251–4500; Craig S. Juengling, Chief Executive Officer

MISSISSIPPI: CHARTER BEHAVIORAL HEALTH SYSTEM (O, 111 beds) 3531 Lakeland Drive, Jackson, MS Zip 39208, Mailing Address: Box 4297, Zip 39296; tel. 601/939–9030; Earl W. Balzen, R.N., Chief Executive Officer

NEVADA: CHARTER BEHAVIORAL HEALTH SYSTEM OF NEVADA (O, 84 beds) 7000 West Spring Mountain Road, Las Vegas, NV Zip 89117; tel. 702/876–4357; Lynn M. Rosenbach, Chief Executive Officer

NEW HAMPSHIRE: CHARTER BROOKSIDE BEHAVIORAL HEALTH SYSTEM OF NEW ENGLAND (O, 100 beds) 29 Northwest Boulevard, Nashua, NH Zip 03063; tel. 603/886–5000; Susan A. Cambria, Chief Executive Officer

NEW JERSEY: CHARTER BEHAVIORAL HEALTH SYSTEM OF NEW JERSEY–SUMMIT (O, 90 beds) 19 Prospect Street, Summit, NJ Zip 07902–0100; tel. 908/522–7000; Geoffrey Perselay, Chief Executive Officer

NEW MEXICO: CHARTER HEIGHTS BEHAVIORAL HEALTH SYSTEM (O, 172 beds) 103 Hospital Loop N.E., Albuquerque, NM Zip 87109; tel. 505/883–8777; Joel A. Hart, FACHE, Chief Executive Officer

NORTH CAROLINA: CHARTER ASHEVILLE BEHAVIORAL HEALTH SYSTEM (O, 139 beds) 60 Caledonia Road, Asheville, NC Zip 28803, Mailing Address: P.O. Box 5534, Zip 28813; tel. 704/253–3681; Tammy B. Wood, Chief Executive Officer

CHARTER GREENSBORO BEHAVIORAL HEALTH SYSTEM (O, 68 beds) 700 Walter Reed Drive, Greensboro, NC Zip 27403–1129, Mailing Address: P.O. Box 10399, Zip 27404–0399; tel. 910/852–4821; Joe Crabtree, Chief Executive Officer

CHARTER HOSPITAL OF WINSTON–SALEM (O, 99 beds) 3637 Old Vineyard Road, Winston–Salem, NC Zip 27104; tel. 910/768–7710; Marina Cecchini, Chief Executive Officer

CHARTER PINES BEHAVIORAL HEALTH SYSTEM (O, 60 beds) 3621 Randolph Road, Charlotte, NC Zip 28211, Mailing Address: P.O. Box 221709, Zip 28222–1709; tel. 704/365–5368; Bruce Chambers, Ph.D., Chief Executive Officer

OHIO: CHARTER HOSPITAL OF TOLEDO (O, 38 beds) 1725 Timber Line Road, Maumee, OH Zip 43537–4015; tel. 419/891–9333; Michael Cornelison, Chief Executive Officer

PENNSYLVANIA: CHARTER BEHAVIORAL HEALTH SYSTEM AT COVE FORGE (O, 100 beds) New Beginnings Road, Williamsburg, PA Zip 16693; tel. 814/832–2121; Jonathan Wolf, Chief Executive Officer

CHARTER FAIRMOUNT INSTITUTE (O, 146 beds) 561 Fairthorne Avenue, Philadelphia, PA Zip 19128–2499; tel. 215/487–4000; Paul B. Henry, Administrator

SOUTH CAROLINA: CHARTER GREENVILLE BEHAVIORAL HEALTH SYSTEM (O, 66 beds) 2700 East Phillips Road, Greer, SC Zip 29650; tel. 864/235–2335; William L. Callison, Chief Executive Officer

For explanation of codes following names, see page B2.
★ Indicates Type III membership in the American Hospital Association.

CHARTER HOSPITAL OF CHARLESTON (O, 70 beds) 2777 Speissegger Drive, Charleston, SC Zip 29405-8299; tel. 803/747-5830; Todd B. Graybill, Administrator

CHARTER RIVERS BEHAVIORAL HEALTH SYSTEM (O, 80 beds) 2900 Sunset Boulevard, West Columbia, SC Zip 29169-3422; tel. 803/796-9911; Brooks Cagle, Chief Executive Officer

SOUTH DAKOTA: CHARTER SIOUX FALLS BEHAVIORAL HEALTH SYSTEM (O, 60 beds) 2812 South Louise Avenue, Sioux Falls, SD Zip 57106; tel. 605/361-8111; Patrick G. Kelly, Administrator

TENNESSEE: CHARTER LAKESIDE BEHAVIORAL HEALTH SYSTEM (O, 174 beds) 2911 Brunswick Road, Memphis, TN Zip 38133, Mailing Address: P.O. Box 341308, Zip 38134; tel. 901/377-4700; Rob S. Waggener, Chief Executive Officer

TEXAS: CHARTER BEHAVIORAL HEALTH SYSTEM (O, 80 beds) 2001 Ladbrook Drive, Kingwood, TX Zip 77339-3004; tel. 281/358-4501; Mark Micheletti, Chief Executive Officer

CHARTER BEHAVIORAL HEALTH SYSTEM OF AUSTIN (O, 40 beds) 8402 Cross Park Drive, Austin, TX Zip 78754, Mailing Address: P.O. Box 140585, Zip 78714-0585; tel. 512/837-1800; Armin Steege, Chief Executive Officer

CHARTER BEHAVIORAL HEALTH SYSTEM–CORPUS CHRISTI (O, 80 beds) 3126 Rodd Field Road, Corpus Christi, TX Zip 78414; tel. 512/993-8893; Steve Kamber, Chief Executive Officer

CHARTER GRAPEVINE BEHAVIORAL HEALTH SYSTEM (O, 80 beds) 2300 William D. Tate Avenue, Grapevine, TX Zip 76051-9964; tel. 817/481-1900; Michael V. Lee, Chief Executive Officer

CHARTER PALMS BEHAVIORAL HEALTH SYSTEM (O, 80 beds) 1421 East Jackson Avenue, McAllen, TX Zip 78501, Mailing Address: P.O. Box 5239, Zip 78502; tel. 210/631-5421; Leslie Bingham, Chief Executive Officer

CHARTER PLAINS BEHAVIORAL HEALTH SYSTEM (O, 80 beds) 801 North Quaker, Lubbock, TX Zip 79416, Mailing Address: P.O. Box 10560, Zip 79408; tel. 806/744-5505; Karl R. Brady, Chief Executive Officer and Administrator

CHARTER REAL BEHAVIORAL HEALTH SYSTEM (O, 90 beds) 8550 Huebner Road, San Antonio, TX Zip 78240, Mailing Address: P.O. Box 380157, Zip 78280; tel. 210/699-8585; Irving B. Sawyers Jr., Chief Executive Officer

VIRGINIA: CHARTER BEHAVIORAL HEALTH SYSTEM AT SPRINGWOOD (O, 77 beds) 42009 Charter Springwood Lane, Leesburg, VA Zip 20176; tel. 703/777-0800; Dania O'Connor, Chief Executive Officer

CHARTER BEHAVIORAL HEALTH SYSTEM OF CHARLOTTESVILLE (O, 62 beds) 2101 Arlington Boulevard, Charlottesville, VA Zip 22903-1593; tel. 804/977-1120; Wayne Adams, Chief Executive Officer

CHARTER WESTBROOK BEHAVIORAL HEALTH SYSTEM (O, 210 beds) 1500 Westbrook Avenue, Richmond, VA Zip 23227; tel. 804/266-9671; Thomas J. Wojick, Chief Executive Officer

NORFOLK PSYCHIATRIC CENTER (O, 77 beds) 860 Kempsville Road, Norfolk, VA Zip 23502-3980; tel. 757/461-4565; Debra Goldstein, Administrator

WISCONSIN: CHARTER HOSPITAL OF MILWAUKEE (O, 80 beds) 11101 West Lincoln Avenue, Milwaukee, WI Zip 53227; tel. 414/327-3000; Gary M. Gilberti, Chief Executive Officer

Owned, leased, sponsored:	66 hospitals	5913 beds
Contract-managed:	0 hospitals	0 beds
Totals:	66 hospitals	5913 beds

1975: MARSHALL COUNTY HEALTH CARE AUTHORITY (NP)
8000 Alabama Highway 69, Guntersville, AL Zip 35976; tel. 205/753-8000; L. C. Couch, Board Chairman

ALABAMA: BOAZ-ALBERTVILLE MEDICAL CENTER (O, 102 beds) U.S. Highway 431 North, Boaz, AL Zip 35957-0999, Mailing Address: Drawer Z, Zip 35957-0999; tel. 205/593-8310; Marlin Hanson, Administrator

GUNTERSVILLE-ARAB MEDICAL CENTER (O, 90 beds) 8000 Alabama Highway 69, Guntersville, AL Zip 35976; tel. 205/753-8000; Gary R. Gore, Administrator

Owned, leased, sponsored:	2 hospitals	192 beds
Contract-managed:	0 hospitals	0 beds
Totals:	2 hospitals	192 beds

5395: MARYCREST HEALTH SYSTEM (CC)
2861 West 52nd Avenue, Denver, CO Zip 80221-1259; tel. 303/458-8611; Dale G. Budde, President

NEBRASKA: ST. ANTHONY'S HOSPITAL (O, 29 beds) Second and Adams Streets, O'Neill, NE Zip 68763-1597; tel. 402/336-2611; Ronald J. Cork, President and Chief Executive Officer

NORTH DAKOTA: KENMARE COMMUNITY HOSPITAL (O, 42 beds) 317 First Avenue N.W., Kenmare, ND Zip 58746, Mailing Address: P.O. Box 697, Zip 58746-0697; tel. 701/385-4296; Verlin Buechler, President and Chief Executive Officer

UNIMED MEDICAL CENTER (O, 160 beds) 407 3rd Street S.E., Minot, ND Zip 58702-5001; tel. 701/857-2000; Sister Lona Thorson, Interim Chief Executive Officer

Owned, leased, sponsored:	3 hospitals	231 beds
Contract-managed:	0 hospitals	0 beds
Totals:	3 hospitals	231 beds

0013: MASSACHUSETTS DEPARTMENT OF MENTAL HEALTH (NP)
25 Staniford Street, Boston, MA Zip 02114; tel. 617/727-5600; Marylou Sudders, Commissioner

MASSACHUSETTS: LEMUEL SHATTUCK HOSPITAL (O, 230 beds) 170 Morton Street, Jamaica Plain, Boston, MA Zip 02130-3787; tel. 617/522-8110; Robert D. Wakefield Jr., Executive Director

MASSACHUSETTS MENTAL HEALTH CENTER (O, 27 beds) 74 Fenwood Road, Boston, MA Zip 02115; tel. 617/734-1300; Catherine Howard, Chief Executive Officer

MEDFIELD STATE HOSPITAL (O, 212 beds) 45 Hospital Road, Medfield, MA Zip 02052; tel. 508/359-7312; Theodore E. Kirousis, Area Director

TAUNTON STATE HOSPITAL (O, 185 beds) 60 Hodges Avenue Extension, Taunton, MA Zip 02780, Mailing Address: P.O. Box 4007, Zip 02780; tel. 508/824-7551; Gary Phillips, Administrator and Chief Operating Officer

TEWKSBURY HOSPITAL (O, 527 beds) East Street, Tewksbury, MA Zip 01876-1998; tel. 508/851-7321; Raymond D. Sanzone, Executive Director

WESTBOROUGH STATE HOSPITAL (O, 220 beds) Westborough, MA Mailing Address: P.O. Box 288, Zip 01581; tel. 617/727-9830; Theodore E. Kirousis, Area Director

WORCESTER STATE HOSPITAL (O, 176 beds) 305 Belmont Street, Worcester, MA Zip 01604; tel. 508/752-4681; Bernard Kingsley, Chief Operating Officer

Owned, leased, sponsored:	7 hospitals	1577 beds
Contract-managed:	0 hospitals	0 beds
Totals:	7 hospitals	1577 beds

2505: MATAGORDA COUNTY HOSPITAL DISTRICT (NP)
1115 Avenue G, Bay City, TX Zip 77414; tel. 409/245-6383; Wendell H. Baker Jr., Chief Executive Officer

TEXAS: MATAGORDA GENERAL HOSPITAL (O, 61 beds) 1115 Avenue G, Bay City, TX Zip 77414-3544; tel. 409/245-6383; Wendell H. Baker Jr., Chief Executive Officer

WAGNER GENERAL HOSPITAL (O, 6 beds) 310 Green Street, Palacios, TX Zip 77465, Mailing Address: Box 859, Zip 77465; tel. 512/972-2511; Helen Dolezal, Director

Owned, leased, sponsored:	2 hospitals	67 beds
Contract-managed:	0 hospitals	0 beds
Totals:	2 hospitals	67 beds

★1875: MAYO FOUNDATION (NP)
200 S.W. First Street, Rochester, MN Zip 55905; tel. 507/284-2511; Robert R. Waller, M.D., President and Chief Executive Officer

FLORIDA: ST. LUKE'S HOSPITAL (O, 220 beds) 4201 Belfort Road, Jacksonville, FL Zip 32216; tel. 904/296-3700; J. Larry Read, President

For explanation of codes following names, see page B2.
★ Indicates Type III membership in the American Hospital Association.

Section B

IOWA: FLOYD COUNTY MEMORIAL HOSPITAL (C, 29 beds) 800 Eleventh Street, Charles City, IA Zip 50616–3499; tel. 515/228–6830; Bill D. Faust, Administrator

MINNESOTA: AUSTIN MEDICAL CENTER (O, 108 beds) 1000 First Drive N.W., Austin, MN Zip 55912; tel. 507/437–4551; Donald R. Brezicka, Executive Vice President

IMMANUEL ST. JOSEPH'S–MAYO HEALTH SYSTEM (O, 147 beds) 1025 Marsh Street, Mankato, MN Zip 56001, Mailing Address: P.O. Box 8673, Zip 56002–8673; tel. 507/625–4031; Jerome A. Crest, Executive Vice President

NAEVE HOSPITAL (O, 72 beds) 404 West Fountain Street, Albert Lea, MN Zip 56007–2473; tel. 507/373–2384; Theodore Myers, M.D., Chief Executive Officer

ROCHESTER METHODIST HOSPITAL (O, 335 beds) 201 West Center Street, Rochester, MN Zip 55902–3084; tel. 507/266–7180; Stephen C. Waldhoff, Administrator

SAINT MARYS HOSPITAL (O, 797 beds) 1216 Second Street S.W., Rochester, MN Zip 55902–1970; tel. 507/255–5123; John M. Panicek, Administrator

WISCONSIN: BARRON MEMORIAL MEDICAL CENTER AND SKILLED NURSING FACILITY (C, 92 beds) 1222 Woodland Avenue, Barron, WI Zip 54812; tel. 715/537–3186; Mark D. Wilson, Administrator

BLOOMER COMMUNITY MEMORIAL HOSPITAL AND THE MAPLEWOOD (C, 101 beds) 1501 Thompson Street, Bloomer, WI Zip 54724; tel. 715/568–2000; John Perushek, Administrator

LUTHER HOSPITAL (O, 198 beds) 1221 Whipple Street, Eau Claire, WI Zip 54702–4105; tel. 715/838–3311; William Rupp, M.D., President and Chief Executive Officer

OSSEO AREA HOSPITAL AND NURSING HOME (C, 75 beds) 13025 Eighth Street, Osseo, WI Zip 54758, Mailing Address: P.O. Box 70, Zip 54758; tel. 715/597–3121; Bradley D. Groseth, Administrator

Owned, leased, sponsored:	7 hospitals	1877 beds
Contract–managed:	4 hospitals	297 beds
Totals:	11 hospitals	2174 beds

1335:   MEASE HEALTH CARE (NP)
135 Annwood Road, Palm Harbor, FL Zip 34648; tel. 813/733–1111; Philip K. Beauchamp, FACHE, President and Chief Executive Officer

FLORIDA: MEASE COUNTRYSIDE HOSPITAL (O, 100 beds) 3231 McMullen–Booth Road, Safety Harbor, FL Zip 34695–1098, Mailing Address: P.O. 1098, Zip 34695–1098; tel. 813/725–6111; James A. Pfeiffer, Chief Administrative Officer

MEASE HOSPITAL DUNEDIN (O, 258 beds) 601 Main Street, Dunedin, FL Zip 34698, Mailing Address: P.O. Box 760, Zip 34697–0760; tel. 813/733–1111; Philip K. Beauchamp, FACHE, President and Chief Executive Officer

Owned, leased, sponsored:	2 hospitals	358 beds
Contract–managed:	0 hospitals	0 beds
Totals:	2 hospitals	358 beds

★6615:   MEDLANTIC HEALTHCARE GROUP (NP)
100 Irving Street N.W., Washington, DC Zip 20010–2975; tel. 202/877–6006; John P. McDaniel, Chief Executive Officer

DISTRICT OF COLUMBIA: NATIONAL REHABILITATION HOSPITAL (O, 160 beds) 102 Irving Street N.W., Washington, DC Zip 20010–2949; tel. 202/877–1000; Edward A. Eckenhoff, President and Chief Executive Officer

WASHINGTON HOSPITAL CENTER (O, 772 beds) 110 Irving Street N.W., Washington, DC Zip 20010–2975; tel. 202/877–7000; Kenneth A. Samet, President

Owned, leased, sponsored:	2 hospitals	932 beds
Contract–managed:	0 hospitals	0 beds
Totals:	2 hospitals	932 beds

0084:   MEMORIAL HEALTH SERVICES (NP)
2801 Atlantic Avenue, Long Beach, CA Zip 90801, Mailing Address: P.O. Box 1428, Zip 90801–1428; tel. 562/933–2000; Thomas J. Collins, President and Chief Executive Officer

CALIFORNIA: ANAHEIM MEMORIAL HOSPITAL (O, 192 beds) 1111 West La Palma Avenue, Anaheim, CA Zip 92801, Mailing Address: Box 3005, Zip 92803; tel. 714/774–1450; Chris D. Van Gorder, President and Chief Executive Officer

LONG BEACH MEMORIAL MEDICAL CENTER (O, 726 beds) 2801 Atlantic Avenue, Long Beach, CA Zip 90806, Mailing Address: Box 1428, Zip 90801–1428; tel. 562/933–2000; Thomas J. Collins, President and Chief Executive Officer

ORANGE COAST MEMORIAL MEDICAL CENTER (O, 230 beds) 9920 Talbert Avenue, Fountain Valley, CA Zip 92708; tel. 714/378–7000; Barry Arbuckle, Ph.D., Chief Operating Officer

SADDLEBACK MEMORIAL MEDICAL CENTER (O, 220 beds) 24451 Health Center Drive, Laguna Hills, CA Zip 92653; tel. 714/837–4500; Nolan Draney, Executive Vice President

Owned, leased, sponsored:	4 hospitals	1368 beds
Contract–managed:	0 hospitals	0 beds
Totals:	4 hospitals	1368 beds

2335:   MEMORIAL HEALTH SERVICES (IO)
706 North Parrish Avenue, Adel, GA Zip 31620, Mailing Address: Box 677, Zip 31620; tel. 912/896–2251; Wade E. Keck, Chief Executive Officer

GEORGIA: BLECKLEY MEMORIAL HOSPITAL (C, 45 beds) 408 Peacock Street, Cochran, GA Zip 31014–1559, Mailing Address: Box 536, Zip 31014–0536; tel. 912/934–6211; Henry T. Gibbs, Administrator

MEMORIAL HOSPITAL OF ADEL (C, 155 beds) 706 North Parrish Avenue, Adel, GA Zip 31620–0677, Mailing Address: Box 677, Zip 31620–0677; tel. 912/896–2251; Wade E. Keck, Chief Executive Officer

SMITH HOSPITAL (C, 71 beds) 117 East Main Street, Hahira, GA Zip 31632, Mailing Address: P.O. Box 337, Zip 31632; tel. 912/794–2502; Amanda M. Hall, Administrator

TELFAIR COUNTY HOSPITAL (C, 52 beds) U.S. 341 South, McRae, GA Zip 31055, Mailing Address: P.O. Box 150, Zip 31055; tel. 912/868–5621; Gail B. Norris, Administrator

Owned, leased, sponsored:	0 hospitals	0 beds
Contract–managed:	4 hospitals	323 beds
Totals:	4 hospitals	323 beds

★0086:   MEMORIAL HEALTH SYSTEM (NP)
800 North Rutledge Street, Springfield, IL Zip 62781–0001; tel. 217/788–3000; Robert T. Clarke, President and Chief Executive Officer

ILLINOIS: ABRAHAM LINCOLN MEMORIAL HOSPITAL (O, 47 beds) 315 8th Street, Lincoln, IL Zip 62656–2698; tel. 217/732–2161; Forrest G. Hester, President and Chief Executive Officer

MEMORIAL MEDICAL CENTER (O, 455 beds) 800 North Rutledge Street, Springfield, IL Zip 62781–0001; tel. 217/788–3000; Robert T. Clarke, President and Chief Executive Officer

ST. VINCENT MEMORIAL HOSPITAL (S, 149 beds) 201 East Pleasant Street, Taylorville, IL Zip 62568–1597; tel. 217/824–3331; Daniel J. Raab, President and Chief Executive Officer

Owned, leased, sponsored:	3 hospitals	651 beds
Contract–managed:	0 hospitals	0 beds
Totals:	3 hospitals	651 beds

★2615:   MEMORIAL HEALTH SYSTEMS (NP)
875 Sterthaus Avenue, Ormond Beach, FL Zip 32174–5197; tel. 904/676–6114; Richard A. Lind, President and Chief Executive Officer

Section B

FLORIDA: MEMORIAL HOSPITAL–FLAGLER (O, 81 beds) Moody Boulevard, Bunnell, FL Zip 32110, Mailing Address: HCR1, Box 2, Zip 32110; tel. 904/437–2211; Clark P. Christianson, Senior Vice President and Administrator

MEMORIAL HOSPITAL–ORMOND BEACH (O, 205 beds) 875 Sterthaus Avenue, Ormond Beach, FL Zip 32174–5197; tel. 904/676–6000; Clark P. Christianson, Senior Vice President and Administrator

MEMORIAL HOSPITAL–WEST VOLUSIA (L, 156 beds) 701 West Plymouth Avenue, DeLand, FL Zip 32720, Mailing Address: Box 509, Zip 32721–0509; tel. 904/734–3320; Johnette L. Vodenicker, Senior Vice President and Administrator

Owned, leased, sponsored:	3 hospitals	442 beds
Contract–managed:	0 hospitals	0 beds
Totals:	3 hospitals	442 beds

★**0083: MEMORIAL HEALTHCARE SYSTEM** (NP)
3501 Johnson Street, Hollywood, FL Zip 33021; tel. 954/985–5805; Frank V. Sacco, FACHE, Chief Executive Officer

MEMORIAL HOSPITAL PEMBROKE (L, 301 beds) 2301 University Drive, Pembroke Pines, FL Zip 33024; tel. 954/962–9650; J. E. Piriz, Administrator

MEMORIAL HOSPITAL WEST (O, 110 beds) 703 North Flamingo Road, Pembroke Pines, FL Zip 33028; tel. 954/436–5000; Zeff Ross, Administrator

MEMORIAL REGIONAL HOSPITAL (O, 792 beds) 3501 Johnson Street, Hollywood, FL Zip 33021–5421; tel. 954/987–2000; Patricia A. Flury, Administrator

Owned, leased, sponsored:	3 hospitals	1203 beds
Contract–managed:	0 hospitals	0 beds
Totals:	3 hospitals	1203 beds

★**2645: MEMORIAL HEALTHCARE SYSTEM** (NP)
7737 S.W. Freeway, Suite 200, Houston, TX Zip 77074–1800; tel. 713/776–6992; Dan S. Wilford, President

TEXAS: MEMORIAL HOSPITAL PASADENA (O, 173 beds) 906 East Southmore Avenue, Pasadena, TX Zip 77502–1124, Mailing Address: Box 1879, Zip 77502; tel. 713/477–0411; Dennis M. Knox, Vice President and Chief Executive Officer

MEMORIAL HOSPITAL SOUTHWEST (O, 490 beds) 7600 Beechnut, Houston, TX Zip 77074–1850; tel. 713/776–5000; James E. Eastham, Administrator, Chief Executive Officer and Vice President

MEMORIAL HOSPITAL–MEMORIAL CITY (L, 300 beds) 920 Frostwood Drive, Houston, TX Zip 77024–9173; tel. 713/932–3000; Jerel T. Humphrey, Vice President, Chief Executive Officer and Administrator

MEMORIAL HOSPITAL–THE WOODLANDS (O, 68 beds) 9250 Pinecroft, The Woodlands, TX Zip 77380; tel. 281/364–2300; Steve Sanders, Vice President, Chief Executive Officer and Administrator

MEMORIAL REHABILITATION HOSPITAL (L, 106 beds) 3043 Gessner, Houston, TX Zip 77080; tel. 713/462–2515; Roger Truskoloski, Administrator, Chief Executive Officer and Vice President

MEMORIAL SPRING SHADOWS GLEN (L, 112 beds) 2801 Gessner, Houston, TX Zip 77080–2599; tel. 713/462–4000; G. Jerry Mueck, Vice President, Chief Executive Officer and Administrator

Owned, leased, sponsored:	6 hospitals	1249 beds
Contract–managed:	0 hospitals	0 beds
Totals:	6 hospitals	1249 beds

★**5165: MERCY HEALTH SERVICES** (CC)
34605 Twelve Mile Road, Farmington Hills, MI Zip 48331–3221; tel. 810/489–6000; Judith Pelham, President and Chief Executive Officer

ILLINOIS: MORRISON COMMUNITY HOSPITAL (C, 114 beds) 303 North Jackson Street, Morrison, IL Zip 61270–3042; tel. 815/772–4003; Mark F. Fedyk, Administrator

IOWA: BAUM HARMON MEMORIAL HOSPITAL (C, 19 beds) 255 North Welch Avenue, Primghar, IA Zip 51245, Mailing Address: P.O. Box 528, Zip 51245; tel. 712/757–3905; Ronald Bender, Administrator

BELMOND COMMUNITY HOSPITAL (C, 22 beds) 403 First Street S.E., Belmond, IA Zip 50421–0326, Mailing Address: P.O. Box 326, Zip 50421; tel. 515/444–3223; Allan Atkinson, Administrator

ELDORA REGIONAL MEDICAL CENTER (C, 18 beds) 2413 Edgington Avenue, Eldora, IA Zip 50627–1541; tel. 515/858–5416; Greg Reed, Administrator

ELLSWORTH MUNICIPAL HOSPITAL (C, 40 beds) 110 Rocksylvania Avenue, Iowa Falls, IA Zip 50126–2431; tel. 515/648–4631; John O'Brien, Administrator

FRANKLIN GENERAL HOSPITAL (C, 82 beds) 1720 Central Avenue East, Hampton, IA Zip 50441–1859; tel. 515/456–4721; Laura Olander, Chief Executive Officer

HANCOCK COUNTY MEMORIAL HOSPITAL (C, 26 beds) 531 Second Street N.W., Britt, IA Zip 50423, Mailing Address: Box 68, Zip 50423–0068; tel. 515/843–3801; Harriet Thompson, Administrator

HAWARDEN COMMUNITY HOSPITAL (C, 19 beds) 1111 11th Street, Hawarden, IA Zip 51023; tel. 712/552–3100; Stuart A. Katz, FACHE, Chief Executive Officer

HOWARD COUNTY HOSPITAL (C, 32 beds) 235 Eighth Avenue West, Cresco, IA Zip 52136–1098; tel. 319/547–2101; Elizabeth A. Doty, Administrator

KOSSUTH REGIONAL HEALTH CENTER (C, 29 beds) 1515 South Phillips Street, Algona, IA Zip 50511; tel. 515/295–2451; James G. Fitzpatrick, Administrator

MARIAN HEALTH CENTER (O, 267 beds) 801 Fifth Street, Sioux City, IA Zip 51102, Mailing Address: Box 3168, Zip 51102; tel. 712/279–2010

MERCY HEALTH CENTER (O, 385 beds) 250 Mercy Drive, Dubuque, IA Zip 52001–7360; tel. 319/589–8000; Sister Helen Huewe, President

MITCHELL COUNTY REGIONAL HEALTH CENTER (C, 40 beds) 616 North Eighth Street, Osage, IA Zip 50461–1498; tel. 515/732–3781; Richard C. Hamilton, Chief Executive Officer

NORTH IOWA MERCY HEALTH CENTER (O, 285 beds) 1000 Fourth Street S.W., Mason City, IA Zip 50401; tel. 515/422–7000; David H. Vellinga, President and Chief Executive Officer

PALO ALTO COUNTY HOSPITAL (C, 54 beds) 3201 First Street, Emmetsburg, IA Zip 50536; tel. 712/852–2434; Darrell E. Vondrak, Administrator

SAINT JOSEPH COMMUNITY HOSPITAL (O, 55 beds) 308 North Maple Avenue, New Hampton, IA Zip 50659; tel. 515/394–4121; Thomas Thompson, President

SAMARITAN HEALTH SYSTEM (O, 360 beds) 1410 North Fourth Street, Clinton, IA Zip 52732, Mailing Address: P.O. Box 2960, Zip 52733–2960; tel. 319/244–5555; Thomas J. Hesselmann, President and Chief Executive Officer

MICHIGAN: BATTLE CREEK HEALTH SYSTEM (O, 402 beds) 300 North Avenue, Battle Creek, MI Zip 49016–3396; tel. 616/966–8000; Stephen L. Abbott, President and Chief Executive Officer

DECKERVILLE COMMUNITY HOSPITAL (C, 17 beds) 3559 Pine Street, Deckerville, MI Zip 48427–0126, Mailing Address: P.O. Box 126, Zip 48427–0126; tel. 810/376–2835; Charlotte Williams, Interim Administrator

MCPHERSON HOSPITAL (O, 63 beds) 620 Byron Road, Howell, MI Zip 48843–1093; tel. 517/545–6000; C. W. Lauderbach Jr., Chief Operating Officer

MERCY GENERAL HEALTH PARTNERS–OAK AVENUE CAMPUS (C, 127 beds) 1700 Oak Avenue, Muskegon, MI Zip 49442; tel. 616/773–3311; Roger Spoelman, Chief Executive Officer

MERCY GENERAL HEALTH PARTNERS–SHERMAN BOULEVARD CAMPUS (O, 123 beds) 1500 East Sherman Boulevard, Muskegon, MI Zip 49443, Mailing Address: P.O. Box 358, Zip 49443–0358; tel. 616/739–9341; Roger Spoelman, Chief Executive Officer

MERCY HEALTH SERVICES NORTH–GRAYLING (O, 98 beds) 1100 Michigan Avenue, Grayling, MI Zip 49738–1398; tel. 517/348–5461; Dennis J. Renander, President and Chief Executive Officer

MERCY HEALTH SERVICES–NORTH (O, 89 beds) 400 Hobart Street, Cadillac, MI Zip 49601–9596; tel. 616/876–7200; Dennis J. Renander, President and Chief Executive Officer

MERCY HOSPITAL (O, 248 beds) 5555 Conner Avenue, Detroit, MI Zip 48213–3499; tel. 313/579–4000; Brenita Crawford, President and Chief Executive Officer

For explanation of codes following names, see page B2.
★ Indicates Type III membership in the American Hospital Association.

MERCY HOSPITAL (O, 119 beds) 2601 Electric Avenue, Port Huron, MI Zip 48061–6518; tel. 810/985–1510; Mary R. Trimmer, President and Chief Executive Officer

SAINT MARY'S HEALTH SERVICES (O, 287 beds) 200 Jefferson Avenue S.E., Grand Rapids, MI Zip 49503; tel. 616/752–6090; David J. Ameen, President and Chief Executive Officer

SALINE COMMUNITY HOSPITAL (O, 48 beds) 400 West Russell Street, Saline, MI Zip 48176–1101; tel. 313/429–1500; Garry C. Faja, President and Chief Executive Officer

ST. JOSEPH MERCY HEALTH SYSTEM (O, 481 beds) 5301 East Huron River Drive, Ann Arbor, MI Zip 48106, Mailing Address: Box 995, Zip 48106–0992; tel. 313/712–3456; Garry C. Faja, President and Chief Executive Officer

ST. JOSEPH MERCY OAKLAND (O, 417 beds) 900 Woodward Avenue, Pontiac, MI Zip 48341–2985; tel. 810/858–3000; Thomas L. Feurig, President and Chief Executive Officer

ST. JOSEPH'S MERCY HOSPITALS AND HEALTH SERVICES (O, 380 beds) Clinton Township, MI Robert L. Beyer, President and Chief Executive Officer

ST. LAWRENCE HOSPITAL AND HEALTHCARE SERVICES (O, 375 beds) 1210 West Saginaw Street, Lansing, MI Zip 48915–1999; tel. 517/372–3610; Arthur Knueppel, President and Chief Executive Officer

NEBRASKA: PENDER COMMUNITY HOSPITAL (C, 31 beds) 603 Earl Street, Pender, NE Zip 68047–0100, Mailing Address: P.O. Box 100, Zip 68047–0100; tel. 402/385–3083; Kevin Kueny, Administrator

Owned, leased, sponsored:	18 hospitals	4482 beds
Contract–managed:	15 hospitals	670 beds
Totals:	33 hospitals	5152 beds

★5155: MERCY HEALTH SYSTEM (CC)

2335 Grandview Avenue, 4th Floor, Cincinnati, OH Zip 45206–2280; tel. 513/221–2736; Michael D. Connelly, President and Chief Executive Officer

KENTUCKY: LOURDES HOSPITAL (S, 290 beds) 1530 Lone Oak Road, Paducah, KY Zip 42002, Mailing Address: P.O. Box 7100, Zip 42002–7100; tel. 502/444–2444; Douglas Borders, President and Chief Executive Officer

MARCUM AND WALLACE MEMORIAL HOSPITAL (S, 16 beds) 60 Mercy Court, Irvine, KY Zip 40336, Mailing Address: P.O. Box 928, Zip 40336; tel. 606/723–2115; Christopher M. Goddard, Administrator

OHIO: CLERMONT MERCY HOSPITAL (S, 133 beds) 3000 Hospital Drive, Batavia, OH Zip 45103–1998; tel. 513/732–8200; Karen S. Ehrat, Ph.D., President

LORAIN COMMUNITY/ST. JOSEPH REGIONAL HEALTH CENTER (S, 303 beds) 3700 Kolbe Road, Lorain, OH Zip 44053–1697; tel. 216/960–3000; Brian C. Lockwood, President and Chief Executive Officer

MERCY HOSPITAL (S, 248 beds) 100 River Front Plaza, Hamilton, OH Zip 45011, Mailing Address: P.O. Box 418, Zip 45012–0418; tel. 513/870–7080; Thomas S. Urban, President

MERCY HOSPITAL (S, 60 beds) 485 West Market Street, Tiffin, OH Zip 44883, Mailing Address: Box 727, Zip 44883–0727; tel. 419/447–3130; Mark Shugarman, President

MERCY HOSPITAL ANDERSON (S, 156 beds) 7500 State Road, Cincinnati, OH Zip 45255–2492; tel. 513/624–4500; Karen S. Ehrat, Ph.D., President

MERCY HOSPITAL–WILLARD (S, 30 beds) 110 East Howard Street, Willard, OH Zip 44890–1611; tel. 419/933–2931; James O. Detwiler, President

MERCY MEDICAL CENTER (S, 218 beds) 1343 North Fountain Boulevard, Springfield, OH Zip 45501–1380; tel. 513/390–5000; Richard Rogers, Senior Vice President Operations

MERCY MEMORIAL HOSPITAL (S, 20 beds) 904 Scioto Street, Urbana, OH Zip 43078–2200; tel. 937/653–5231; Richard Rogers, Senior Vice President

ST. CHARLES HOSPITAL (S, 246 beds) 2600 Navarre Avenue, Oregon, OH Zip 43616–3297; tel. 419/698–7479; Cathleen K. Nelson, President and Chief Executive Officer

ST. ELIZABETH HEALTH CENTER (S, 318 beds) 1044 Belmont Avenue, Youngstown, OH Zip 44501, Mailing Address: Box 1790, Zip 44501–1790; tel. 330/759–7484; Kevin E. Nolan, President and Chief Executive Officer

ST. JOSEPH HEALTH CENTER (S, 170 beds) 667 Eastland Avenue S.E., Warren, OH Zip 44484; tel. 330/841–4000; Robert W. Shroder, Chief Operating Officer

ST. RITA'S MEDICAL CENTER (S, 312 beds) 730 West Market Street, Lima, OH Zip 45801–4670; tel. 419/227–3361; James P. Reber, President

ST. VINCENT MERCY MEDICAL CENTER (S, 459 beds) 2213 Cherry Street, Toledo, OH Zip 43608–2691; tel. 419/251–3232; Steven L. Mickus, President and Chief Executive Officer

PENNSYLVANIA: MERCY HOSPITAL OF SCRANTON (S, 308 beds) 746 Jefferson Avenue, Scranton, PA Zip 18501–0994; tel. 717/348–7100; John L. Nespoli, President and Chief Executive Officer

MERCY HOSPITAL OF WILKES–BARRE (S, 173 beds) 25 Church Street, Wilkes–Barre, PA Zip 18765, Mailing Address: Box 658, Zip 18765; tel. 717/826–3100; John L. Nespoli, President and Chief Executive Officer

MERCY SPECIAL CARE HOSPITAL (S, 38 beds) 128 West Washington Street, Nanticoke, PA Zip 18634; tel. 717/735–5000; Robert D. Williams, Administrator

TENNESSEE: ST. MARY'S HEALTH SYSTEM (S, 300 beds) 900 East Oak Hill Avenue, Knoxville, TN Zip 37917–4556; tel. 615/545–8000; Richard C. Williams, President and Chief Executive Officer

Owned, leased, sponsored:	19 hospitals	3798 beds
Contract–managed:	0 hospitals	0 beds
Totals:	19 hospitals	3798 beds

5215: MERCY–CHICAGO REGION HEALTHCARE SYSTEM (CC)

55 Shuman Boulevard, Suite 150, Naperville, IL Zip 60563–8469; tel. 708/778–2164; Sister Catherine C. Gallagher, President

ILLINOIS: MERCY CENTER FOR HEALTH CARE SERVICES (S, 193 beds) 1325 North Highland Avenue, Aurora, IL Zip 60506; tel. 630/859–2222; John K. Barto Jr., President and Chief Executive Officer

MERCY HOSPITAL AND MEDICAL CENTER (S, 392 beds) Stevenson Expressway at King Drive, Chicago, IL Zip 60616–2477; tel. 312/567–2006; Winkle Lee, Chief Executive Officer

IOWA: MERCY HOSPITAL (S, 240 beds) 500 East Market Street, Iowa City, IA Zip 52245; tel. 319/339–0300; Ronald R. Reed, President and Chief Executive Officer

Owned, leased, sponsored:	3 hospitals	825 beds
Contract–managed:	0 hospitals	0 beds
Totals:	3 hospitals	825 beds

★8835: MERIDIA HEALTH SYSTEM (NP)

6700 Beta Drive, Suite 200, Mayfield Village, OH Zip 44143; tel. 216/446–8000; Charles B. Miner, President and Chief Executive Officer

OHIO: MERIDIA EUCLID HOSPITAL (O, 214 beds) 18901 Lake Shore Boulevard, Euclid, OH Zip 44119–1090; tel. 216/531–9000; Denise Zeman, Site Administrator

MERIDIA HILLCREST HOSPITAL (O, 263 beds) 6780 Mayfield Road, Cleveland, OH Zip 44124–2202; tel. 216/449–4500; Catherine B. Leary, R.N., Site Administrator, Vice President Clinical Services and Nurse Executive

MERIDIA HURON HOSPITAL (O, 411 beds) 13951 Terrace Road, Cleveland, OH Zip 44112; tel. 216/761–3300; Beverly Lozar, Site Administrator

MERIDIA SOUTH POINTE HOSPITAL (O, 163 beds) 4110 Warrensville Center Road, Warrensville Heights, OH Zip 44122–7099; tel. 216/491–6000; Kathleen A. Rice, Site Administrator

Owned, leased, sponsored:	4 hospitals	1051 beds
Contract–managed:	0 hospitals	0 beds
Totals:	4 hospitals	1051 beds

★7235: METHODIST HEALTH CARE SYSTEM (CO)

6565 Fannin Street, D–200, Houston, TX Zip 77030; tel. 713/790–2221; Larry L. Mathis, FACHE, President and Chief Executive Officer

For explanation of codes following names, see page B2.
★ Indicates Type III membership in the American Hospital Association.

TEXAS: DIAGNOSTIC CENTER HOSPITAL (O, 149 beds) 6447 Main Street, Houston, TX Zip 77030; tel. 713/790-0790; William A. Gregory, Chief Executive Officer

SAN JACINTO METHODIST HOSPITAL (O, 231 beds) 4401 Garth Road, Baytown, TX Zip 77521; tel. 281/420-8600; William Simmons, President and Chief Executive Officer

THE METHODIST HOSPITAL (O, 867 beds) 6565 Fannin, Houston, TX Zip 77030; tel. 713/790-3311; R. G. Girotto, Executive Vice President and Chief Operating Officer

Owned, leased, sponsored:	3 hospitals	1247 beds
Contract-managed:	0 hospitals	0 beds
Totals:	3 hospitals	1247 beds

2715: METHODIST HEALTH SYSTEM (CO)
580 West Eighth Street, Jacksonville, FL Zip 32209-6553; tel. 904/798-8000; Marcus E. Drewa, President

FLORIDA: METHODIST MEDICAL CENTER (O, 160 beds) 580 West Eighth Street, Jacksonville, FL Zip 32209-6553; tel. 904/798-8000; Marcus E. Drewa, President

METHODIST PATHWAY CENTER (O, 25 beds) 580 West Eighth Street, Jacksonville, FL Zip 32209-6553; tel. 904/798-8250; Marcus E. Drewa, President

Owned, leased, sponsored:	2 hospitals	185 beds
Contract-managed:	0 hospitals	0 beds
Totals:	2 hospitals	185 beds

★9345: METHODIST HEALTH SYSTEMS, INC. (CO)
1211 Union Avenue, Suite 700, Memphis, TN Zip 38104; tel. 901/726-2300; Maurice W. Elliott, President

MISSISSIPPI: METHODIST HOSPITAL OF MIDDLE MISSISSIPPI (O, 80 beds) 239 Bowling Green Road, Lexington, MS Zip 39095-9332; tel. 601/834-1321; James K. Greer, Administrator

METHODIST MEDICAL CENTER (L, 304 beds) 1850 Chadwick Drive, Jackson, MS Zip 39204-3479, Mailing Address: P.O. Box 59001, Zip 39204-9001; tel. 601/376-1000; Thomas L. Harper, President and Chief Executive Officer

TENNESSEE: METHODIST HOSPITAL OF DYERSBURG (O, 105 beds) 400 Tickle Street, Dyersburg, TN Zip 38024-3182; tel. 901/285-2410; Richard McCormick, Administrator

METHODIST HOSPITAL OF FAYETTE (O, 38 beds) 214 Lakeview Road, Somerville, TN Zip 38068-0001, Mailing Address: Box 909, Zip 38068-0001; tel. 901/465-0532; Michael Blome', Administrator

METHODIST HOSPITAL OF LEXINGTON (O, 32 beds) 200 West Church Street, Lexington, TN Zip 38351, Mailing Address: Box 160, Zip 38351; tel. 901/968-3646; Eugene Ragghianti, Administrator

METHODIST HOSPITAL OF MCKENZIE (O, 27 beds) 161 Hospital Drive, McKenzie, TN Zip 38201; tel. 901/352-4170; Randal E. Carson, Administrator

METHODIST HOSPITALS OF MEMPHIS (O, 1265 beds) 1265 Union Avenue, Memphis, TN Zip 38104-3499; tel. 901/726-7000; Gary S. Shorb, President

METHODIST-HAYWOOD PARK HOSPITAL (O, 44 beds) 2545 North Washington Avenue, Brownsville, TN Zip 38012; tel. 901/772-4110; Sandra Bailey, Administrator

Owned, leased, sponsored:	8 hospitals	1895 beds
Contract-managed:	0 hospitals	0 beds
Totals:	8 hospitals	1895 beds

★2735: METHODIST HOSPITALS OF DALLAS (NP)
1441 North Beckley, Dallas, TX Zip 75203, Mailing Address: P.O. Box 655999, Zip 75265-5999; tel. 214/947-8181; Howard M. Chase, FACHE, President and Chief Executive Officer

TEXAS: CHARLTON METHODIST HOSPITAL (O, 134 beds) 3500 West Wheatland Road, Dallas, TX Zip 75237-3460, Mailing Address: Box 225357, Zip 75222-5357; tel. 214/947-7500; Kim N. Hollon, FACHE, Executive Director

METHODIST MEDICAL CENTER (O, 374 beds) 1441 North Beckley Avenue, Dallas, TX Zip 75203, Mailing Address: Box 655999, Zip 75265-5999; tel. 214/947-8181; John W. Carver, FACHE, Executive Director

Owned, leased, sponsored:	2 hospitals	508 beds
Contract-managed:	0 hospitals	0 beds
Totals:	2 hospitals	508 beds

0022: METROPOLITAN NASHVILLE GENERAL HOSPITAL (NP)
215 Second Avenue North, Nashville, TN Zip 37201; tel. 615/862-4000; Tom Deweese, Administrator

TENNESSEE: METROPOLITAN NASHVILLE GENERAL HOSPITAL (O, 105 beds) 72 Hermitage Avenue, Nashville, TN Zip 37210-2110; tel. 615/862-4490; John M. Stone, Director

NASHVILLE METROPOLITAN BORDEAUX HOSPITAL (O, 565 beds) 1414 County Hospital Road, Nashville, TN Zip 37218-3001; tel. 615/862-7000; Wayne Hayes, Administrator

Owned, leased, sponsored:	2 hospitals	670 beds
Contract-managed:	0 hospitals	0 beds
Totals:	2 hospitals	670 beds

2055: MICHIGAN HEALTH CARE CORPORATION (NP)
23100 Providence Drive, Suite 300, Southfield, MI Zip 48075; tel. 810/304-3400; Charles E. Housley, FACHE, President and Chief Executive Officer

MICHIGAN: AURORA HOSPITAL FOR CHILDREN (O, 80 beds) 3737 Lawton, Detroit, MI Zip 48208; tel. 313/361-7600; Patricia Strong, Administrator

MICHIGAN HOSPITAL AND MEDICAL CENTER (O, 416 beds) 2700 Martin Luther King Jr. Boulevard, Detroit, MI Zip 48208; tel. 313/361-8112; Barbara J. Clark, Vice President and Chief Operating Officer

Owned, leased, sponsored:	2 hospitals	496 beds
Contract-managed:	0 hospitals	0 beds
Totals:	2 hospitals	496 beds

★0001: MIDMICHIGAN REGIONAL HEALTH SYSTEM (NP)
4005 Orchard Drive, Midland, MI Zip 48670; tel. 517/839-3000; Terence F. Moore, President

MIDMICHIGAN REGIONAL MEDICAL CENTER (O, 221 beds) 4005 Orchard Drive, Midland, MI Zip 48670; tel. 517/839-3000; David A. Reece, President

MIDMICHIGAN REGIONAL MEDICAL CENTER-CLARE (O, 64 beds) 104 West Sixth Street, Clare, MI Zip 48617-1409; tel. 517/386-9951; Lawrence F. Barco, President

MIDMICHIGAN REGIONAL MEDICAL CENTER-GLADWIN (O, 32 beds) 455 South Quarter Street, Gladwin, MI Zip 48624; tel. 517/426-9286; Mark E. Bush, Executive Vice President

Owned, leased, sponsored:	3 hospitals	317 beds
Contract-managed:	0 hospitals	0 beds
Totals:	3 hospitals	317 beds

2855: MISSIONARY BENEDICTINE SISTERS AMERICAN PROVINCE (CC)
300 North 18th Street, Norfolk, NE Zip 68701; tel. 402/371-3438; Sister M. Agnes Salber, Prioress

NEBRASKA: FAITH REGIONAL HEALTH SERVICES (O, 155 beds) 2700 Norfolk Avenue, Norfolk, NE Zip 68702-0869, Mailing Address: P.O. BOX 869, Zip 68702-0869; tel. 402/371-4880; Robert L. Driewer, Chief Executive Officer

PROVIDENCE MEDICAL CENTER (O, 34 beds) 1200 Providence Road, Wayne, NE Zip 68787; tel. 402/375-3800; Marcile Thomas, Administrator

---

For explanation of codes following names, see page B2.
★ Indicates Type III membership in the American Hospital Association.

Section B

Owned, leased, sponsored:	2 hospitals	189 beds
Contract–managed:	0 hospitals	0 beds
Totals:	2 hospitals	189 beds

0017: MISSISSIPPI STATE DEPARTMENT OF MENTAL HEALTH (NP)
1101 Robert E Lee Building, Jackson, MS Zip 39201–1101; tel. 601/359–1288; Roger McMurtry, Chief Mental Health Bureau

MISSISSIPPI: EAST MISSISSIPPI STATE HOSPITAL (O, 655 beds) 4555 Highland Park Drive, Meridian, MS Zip 39307, Mailing Address: Box 4128, West Station, Zip 39304–4128; tel. 601/482–6186; Ramiro J. Martinez, M.D., Director

MISSISSIPPI STATE HOSPITAL (O, 1303 beds) Whitfield, MS Mailing Address: P.O. Box 157–A, Zip 39193–0157; tel. 601/351–8000; James G. Chastain, Director

Owned, leased, sponsored:	2 hospitals	1958 beds
Contract–managed:	0 hospitals	0 beds
Totals:	2 hospitals	1958 beds

6555: MULTICARE HEALTH SYSTEM (NP)
315 Martin Luther King Jr. Way, Tacoma, WA Zip 98405, Mailing Address: P.O. Box 5299, Zip 98405–0299; tel. 206/552–1000; William B. Connoley, President

WASHINGTON: ALLENMORE HOSPITAL (O, 72 beds) South 19th and Union Avenue, Tacoma, WA Zip 98405, Mailing Address: P.O. Box 11414, Zip 98411–0414; tel. 206/572–2323; Charles Hoffman, Administrator

MARY BRIDGE CHILDREN'S HOSPITAL AND HEALTH CENTER (O, 72 beds) 317 Martin Luther King Jr. Way, Tacoma, WA Zip 98405–0299, Mailing Address: Box 5299, Zip 98405–0299; tel. 206/552–1400; William B. Connoley, President and Chief Executive Officer

TACOMA GENERAL HOSPITAL (O, 272 beds) 315 Martin Luther King Jr. Way, Tacoma, WA Zip 98405–0299, Mailing Address: P.O. Box 5299, Zip 98405–0299; tel. 206/552–1000; William B. Connoley, President and Chief Executive Officer

Owned, leased, sponsored:	3 hospitals	416 beds
Contract–managed:	0 hospitals	0 beds
Totals:	3 hospitals	416 beds

★1465: MUNSON HEALTHCARE (NP)
1105 Sixth Street, Traverse City, MI Zip 49684–2386; tel. 616/935–6502; John M. Rockwood Jr., President

MICHIGAN: KALKASKA MEMORIAL HEALTH CENTER (C, 76 beds) 419 Coral Street, Kalkaska, MI Zip 49646, Mailing Address: P.O. Box 249, Zip 49646–0249; tel. 616/258–9142; James D. Austin, CHE, Administrator

LEELANAU MEMORIAL HEALTH CENTER (C, 91 beds) 215 South High Street, Northport, MI Zip 49670, Mailing Address: P.O. Box 217, Zip 49670; tel. 616/386–5101; Jayne R. Bull, Administrator

MUNSON MEDICAL CENTER (O, 368 beds) 1105 Sixth Street, Traverse City, MI Zip 49684–2386; tel. 616/935–5000; Ralph J. Cerny, President and Chief Executive Officer

PAUL OLIVER MEMORIAL HOSPITAL (O, 48 beds) 224 Park Avenue, Frankfort, MI Zip 49635; tel. 616/352–9621; James D. Austin, CHE, Administrator

Owned, leased, sponsored:	2 hospitals	416 beds
Contract–managed:	2 hospitals	167 beds
Totals:	4 hospitals	583 beds

3175: NEPONSET VALLEY HEALTH SYSTEM (NP)
800 Washington Street, Norwood, MA Zip 02062–3487; tel. 617/769–4000; Yolanda Landrau, R.N., Ed.D., President and Chief Executive Officer

MASSACHUSETTS: NORWOOD HOSPITAL (O, 150 beds) 800 Washington Street, Norwood, MA Zip 02062; tel. 617/769–4000; Yolanda Landrau, R.N., Ed.D., President and Chief Executive Officer

SOUTHWOOD COMMUNITY HOSPITAL (O, 182 beds) 111 Dedham Street, Norfolk, MA Zip 02056; tel. 508/668–0385; Yolanda Landrau, R.N., Ed.D., President and Chief Executive Officer

Owned, leased, sponsored:	2 hospitals	332 beds
Contract–managed:	0 hospitals	0 beds
Totals:	2 hospitals	332 beds

0116: NETCARE HEALTH SYSTEMS, INC. (IO)
424 Church Street, Suite 2100, Nashville, TN Zip 37219; tel. 615/742–8500; Michael A. Koban Jr., Chief Executive Officer

GEORGIA: CHATUGE REGIONAL HOSPITAL AND NURSING HOME (O, 116 beds) 110 Main Street, Hiawassee, GA Zip 30546, Mailing Address: Box 509, Zip 30546–0509; tel. 706/896–2222; Thomas I. Edwards, President and Chief Executive Officer

CHESTATEE REGIONAL HOSPITAL (O, 52 beds) 1111 Mountain Drive, Dahlonega, GA Zip 30533; tel. 706/864–6136; Stephen G. Widener, President and Chief Executive Officer

NORTH GEORGIA MEDICAL CENTER AND GILMER NURSING HOME (O, 150 beds) Jasper Road, Ellijay, GA Zip 30540–0346, Mailing Address: Box 346, Zip 30540–0346; tel. 706/276–4741; Mickey M. Rabuka, Administrator

MISSISSIPPI: TRACE REGIONAL HOSPITAL (O, 84 beds) Highway 8 East, Houston, MS Zip 38851, Mailing Address: P.O. Box 626, Zip 38851; tel. 601/456–3700; Bristol Messer, Chief Executive Officer

Owned, leased, sponsored:	4 hospitals	402 beds
Contract–managed:	0 hospitals	0 beds
Totals:	4 hospitals	402 beds

3075: NEW YORK CITY HEALTH AND HOSPITALS CORPORATION (NP)
125 Worth Street, Room 514, New York, NY Zip 10013; tel. 212/788–3321; Luis R. Marcos, M.D., President

NEW YORK: BELLEVUE HOSPITAL CENTER (O, 923 beds) First Avenue and 27th Street, New York, NY Zip 10016; tel. 212/562–4141; Gregory M. Kaladjian, Executive Director

COLER MEMORIAL HOSPITAL (O, 1025 beds) Franklin D. Roosevelt Island, New York, NY Zip 10044; tel. 212/848–6000; Samuel Lehrfeld, Executive Director

CONEY ISLAND HOSPITAL (O, 427 beds) 2601 Ocean Parkway, Brooklyn, NY Zip 11235–7795; tel. 718/616–3000; Howard C. Cohen, Executive Director

ELMHURST HOSPITAL CENTER (O, 480 beds) 79–01 Broadway, Elmhurst, NY Zip 11373; tel. 718/334–4000; Pete Velez, Executive Director

GOLDWATER MEMORIAL HOSPITAL (O, 986 beds) Franklin D. Roosevelt Island, New York, NY Zip 10044; tel. 212/318–8000; Samuel Lehrfeld, Executive Director

HARLEM HOSPITAL CENTER (O, 414 beds) 506 Lenox Avenue, New York, NY Zip 10037–1894; tel. 212/939–1340; Linnette Webb, Senior Vice President and Executive Director

JACOBI MEDICAL CENTER (O, 595 beds) Pelham Parkway South and Eastchester Road, Bronx, NY Zip 10461; tel. 718/918–8141; Joseph S. Orlando, Executive Director

KINGS COUNTY HOSPITAL CENTER (O, 804 beds) 451 Clarkson Avenue, Brooklyn, NY Zip 11203–2097; tel. 718/245–3131; Jean G. Leon, R.N., Senior Vice President

LINCOLN MEDICAL AND MENTAL HEALTH CENTER (O, 470 beds) 234 East 149th Street, Bronx, NY Zip 10451–9998; tel. 718/579–5700; Roberto Rodriguez, Executive Director

METROPOLITAN HOSPITAL CENTER (O, 458 beds) 1901 First Avenue, New York, NY Zip 10029; tel. 212/423–6262; Jose R. Sanchez, Executive Director

NORTH CENTRAL BRONX HOSPITAL (O, 269 beds) 3424 Kossuth Avenue, Bronx, NY Zip 10467; tel. 718/519–3500; Fay E. Malcolm, R.N., Chief Operating Officer

QUEENS HOSPITAL CENTER (O, 331 beds) 82–68 164th Street, Jamaica, NY Zip 11432; tel. 718/883–3000; Gladiola Sampson, Acting Executive Director

For explanation of codes following names, see page B2.
★ Indicates Type III membership in the American Hospital Association.

WOODHULL MEDICAL AND MENTAL HEALTH CENTER (O, 413 beds) 760 Broadway, Brooklyn, NY Zip 11206; tel. 718/963-8101; Cynthia Carrington-Murray, Executive Director

Owned, leased, sponsored:	13 hospitals	7595 beds
Contract-managed:	0 hospitals	0 beds
Totals:	13 hospitals	7595 beds

0009: NEW YORK STATE DEPARTMENT OF MENTAL HEALTH (NP)

44 Holland Avenue, Albany, NY Zip 12229; tel. 518/447-9611; Jesse Nixon Jr., Ph.D., Director

BINGHAMTON PSYCHIATRIC CENTER (O, 269 beds) 425 Robinson Street, Binghamton, NY Zip 13901; tel. 607/724-1391; Margaret R. Dugan, Executive Director

BRONX CHILDREN'S PSYCHIATRIC CENTER (O, 75 beds) 1000 Waters Place, Bronx, NY Zip 10461-2799; tel. 718/892-0808; E. Richard Feinberg, M.D., Executive Director

BRONX PSYCHIATRIC CENTER (O, 658 beds) 1500 Waters Place, Bronx, NY Zip 10461; tel. 718/931-0600; LeRoy Carmichael, Executive Director

BUFFALO PSYCHIATRIC CENTER (O, 323 beds) 400 Forest Avenue, Buffalo, NY Zip 14213-1298; tel. 716/885-2261; George Molnar, M.D., Executive Director

CAPITAL DISTRICT PSYCHIATRIC CENTER (O, 200 beds) 75 New Scotland Avenue, Albany, NY Zip 12208; tel. 518/447-9611; Jesse Nixon Jr., Ph.D., Director

CREEDMOOR PSYCHIATRIC CENTER (O, 795 beds) Jamaica, NY Mailing Address: 80-45 Winchester Boulevard, Queens Village, Zip 11427; tel. 718/264-3300; Charlotte Seltzer, Chief Executive Officer

ELMIRA PSYCHIATRIC CENTER (O, 161 beds) 100 Washington Street, Elmira, NY Zip 14901-2898; tel. 607/737-4739; Bert W. Pyle Jr., Director

HUDSON RIVER PSYCHIATRIC CENTER (O, 460 beds) Branch B, Poughkeepsie, NY Zip 12601-1197; tel. 914/452-8000; James Regan, Ph.D., Chief Executive Officer

KINGS PARK PSYCHIATRIC CENTER (O, 777 beds) 998 Crooked Hill Road, West Brentwood, NY Zip 11717-1089; tel. 516/761-2616; Alan M. Weinstock, MS, Chief Executive Officer

KINGSBORO PSYCHIATRIC CENTER (O, 400 beds) 681 Clarkson Avenue, Brooklyn, NY Zip 11203; tel. 718/221-7395; Billy E. Jones, M.D., MS, Acting Executive Director

MANHATTAN PSYCHIATRIC CENTER-WARD'S ISLAND (O, 745 beds) 600 East 125th Street, New York, NY Zip 10035-9998; tel. 212/369-0500; Horace Belton, Executive Director

MIDDLETOWN PSYCHIATRIC CENTER (O, 271 beds) 141 Monhagen Avenue, Middletown, NY Zip 10940; tel. 914/342-5511; James Bopp, Executive Director

MOHAWK VALLEY PSYCHIATRIC CENTER (O, 614 beds) 1400 Noyes at York, Utica, NY Zip 13502-3803; tel. 315/797-6800; Sarah F. Rudes, Executive Director

NEW YORK STATE PSYCHIATRIC INSTITUTE (O, 58 beds) 722 West 168th Street, New York, NY Zip 10032; tel. 212/960-2200; John M. Oldham, M.D., Director

PILGRIM PSYCHIATRIC CENTER (O, 744 beds) 998 Crooked Hill Road, Brentwood, NY Zip 11717-1087; tel. 516/761-2616; Alan M. Weinstock, MS, Chief Executive Officer

QUEENS CHILDREN'S PSYCHIATRIC CENTER (O, 106 beds) 74-03 Commonwealth Boulevard, Bellerose, NY Zip 11426; tel. 718/264-4506; Gloria Faretra, M.D., Executive Director

RICHARD H. HUTCHINGS PSYCHIATRIC CENTER (O, 184 beds) 620 Madison Street, Syracuse, NY Zip 13210-2319; tel. 315/473-4980; Bryan F. Rudes, Executive Director

ROCHESTER PSYCHIATRIC CENTER (O, 288 beds) 1111 Elmwood Avenue, Rochester, NY Zip 14620-3005; tel. 716/473-3230; Martin H. Von Holden, Executive Director

ROCKLAND CHILDREN'S PSYCHIATRIC CENTER (O, 54 beds) Convent Road, Orangeburg, NY Zip 10962; tel. 914/359-7400; Marcia Werby, Administrator

ROCKLAND PSYCHIATRIC CENTER (O, 525 beds) 140 Old Orangeburg Road, Orangeburg, NY Zip 10962-0071; tel. 914/359-1000; Stephen N. Lawrence, Ph.D., Chief Executive Officer

SAGAMORE CHILDREN'S PSYCHIATRIC CENTER (O, 69 beds) 197 Half Hollow Road, Dix Hills, NY Zip 11746; tel. 516/673-7700; Robert Schweitzer, Ed.D., Executive Director

SOUTH BEACH PSYCHIATRIC CENTER (O, 325 beds) 777 Seaview Avenue, Staten Island, NY Zip 10305; tel. 718/667-2300; Lucy Sarkis, M.D., Executive Director

ST. LAWRENCE PSYCHIATRIC CENTER (O, 265 beds) 1 Chimney Point Drive, Ogdensburg, NY Zip 13669-2291; tel. 315/393-3000; John R. Scott, Director

WESTERN NEW YORK CHILDREN'S PSYCHIATRIC CENTER (O, 46 beds) 1010 East and West Road, West Seneca, NY Zip 14224; tel. 716/674-9730; Jed M. Cohen, Acting Executive Director

Owned, leased, sponsored:	24 hospitals	8412 beds
Contract-managed:	0 hospitals	0 beds
Totals:	24 hospitals	8412 beds

★3115: NORTH BROWARD HOSPITAL DISTRICT (NP)

303 S.E. 17th Street, Fort Lauderdale, FL Zip 33316-2510; tel. 305/355-5100; G. Wil Trower, President and Chief Executive Officer

FLORIDA: BROWARD GENERAL MEDICAL CENTER (O, 548 beds) 1600 South Andrews Avenue, Fort Lauderdale, FL Zip 33316-2510; tel. 954/355-4400; Ruth A. Eldridge, R.N., Regional Vice President, Administration

CORAL SPRINGS MEDICAL CENTER (O, 167 beds) 3000 Coral Hills Drive, Coral Springs, FL Zip 33065; tel. 954/344-3000; A. Gary Muller, FACHE, Regional Vice President Administration

IMPERIAL POINT MEDICAL CENTER (O, 154 beds) 6401 North Federal Highway, Fort Lauderdale, FL Zip 33308-1495; tel. 954/776-8500; Dorothy J. Mancini, R.N., Regional Vice President Administration

NORTH BROWARD MEDICAL CENTER (O, 334 beds) 201 Sample Road, Pompano Beach, FL Zip 33064-3502; tel. 954/941-8300; James R. Chromik, Regional Vice President, Administration

Owned, leased, sponsored:	4 hospitals	1203 beds
Contract-managed:	0 hospitals	0 beds
Totals:	4 hospitals	1203 beds

0032: NORTH MISSISSIPPI HEALTH SERVICES, INC. (NP)

830 South Gloster Street, Tupelo, MS Zip 38801; tel. 601/841-3136; Jeffrey B. Barber, Dr.PH, President and Chief Executive Officer

MISSISSIPPI: CLAY COUNTY MEDICAL CENTER (O, 60 beds) 835 Medical Center Drive, West Point, MS Zip 39773; tel. 601/495-2300; David M. Reid, Administrator

IUKA HOSPITAL (O, 48 beds) 1777 Curtis Drive, Iuka, MS Zip 38852, Mailing Address: P.O. Box 860, Zip 38852; tel. 601/423-6051; Robert E. Northern, Administrator

NORTH MISSISSIPPI MEDICAL CENTER (O, 715 beds) 830 South Gloster Street, Tupelo, MS Zip 38801-4934; tel. 601/841-3000; Jeffrey B. Barber, Dr.PH, President and Chief Executive Officer

PONTOTOC HOSPITAL AND EXTENDED CARE FACILITY (L, 71 beds) 176 South Main Street, Pontotoc, MS Zip 38863, Mailing Address: P.O. Box C, Zip 38863; tel. 601/489-5510; Fred B. Hood, Administrator

WEBSTER HEALTH SERVICES (L, 76 beds) 500 Highway 9 South, Eupora, MS Zip 39744; tel. 601/258-6221; Harold H. Whitaker Sr., Administrator

Owned, leased, sponsored:	5 hospitals	970 beds
Contract-managed:	0 hospitals	0 beds
Totals:	5 hospitals	970 beds

For explanation of codes following names, see page B2.
★ Indicates Type III membership in the American Hospital Association.

★0062: NORTH SHORE HEALTH SYSTEM (NP)
300 Community Drive, Manhasset, NY Zip 11030;
tel. 516/562–4060; John S. T. Gallagher, President

NEW YORK: HUNTINGTON HOSPITAL (C, 269 beds) 270 Park Avenue,
Huntington, NY Zip 11743–2799; tel. 516/351–2200; J. Ronald
Gaudreault, President and Chief Executive Officer

NORTH SHORE UNIVERSITY HOSPITAL (O, 958 beds) 300 Community Drive,
Manhasset, NY Zip 11030; tel. 516/562–0100; John S. T. Gallagher,
President

NORTH SHORE UNIVERSITY HOSPITAL AT GLEN COVE (O, 265 beds) St.
Andrews Lane, Glen Cove, NY Zip 11542; tel. 516/674–7300; Mark R.
Stenzler, Vice President Administration

NORTH SHORE UNIVERSITY HOSPITAL AT PLAINVIEW (O, 279 beds) 888 Old
Country Road, Plainview, NY Zip 11803–4978; tel. 516/681–8900; Glenn
Hirsch, Administrator

Owned, leased, sponsored:	3 hospitals	1502 beds
Contract–managed:	1 hospital	269 beds
Totals:	4 hospitals	1771 beds

★2075: NORTHBAY HEALTHCARE SYSTEM (NP)
1200 B Gale Wilson Boulevard, Fairfield, CA Zip 94533–3587;
tel. 707/429–3600; Gary J. Passama, President and Chief Executive
Officer

CALIFORNIA: NORTHBAY MEDICAL CENTER (O, 92 beds) 1200 B. Gale
Wilson Boulevard, Fairfield, CA Zip 94533–3587; tel. 707/429–3600;
Deborah Sugiyama, President

VACAVALLEY HOSPITAL (O, 35 beds) 1000 Nut Tree Road, Vacaville, CA
Zip 95687; tel. 707/446–5716; Deborah Sugiyama, President

Owned, leased, sponsored:	2 hospitals	127 beds
Contract–managed:	0 hospitals	0 beds
Totals:	2 hospitals	127 beds

★1165: OAKWOOD HEALTHCARE SYSTEM (NP)
18101 Oakwood Boulevard, Dearborn, MI Zip 48124, Mailing
Address: P.O. Box 2500, Zip 48123–2500; tel. 313/593–7000;
Gerald D. Fitzgerald, President

MICHIGAN: OAKWOOD HOSPITAL ANNAPOLIS CENTER (O, 360 beds) 33155
Annapolis Road, Wayne, MI Zip 48184; tel. 313/467–4000; Mark
Anthony, Vice President and Administrator

OAKWOOD HOSPITAL BEYER CENTER–YPSILANTI (O, 82 beds) 135 South
Prospect Street, Ypsilanti, MI Zip 48198–5693; tel. 313/484–2200; Richard
Hillbom, Acting Administrator

OAKWOOD HOSPITAL DOWNRIVER CENTER–LINCOLN PARK (O, 49 beds)
25750 West Outer Drive, Lincoln Park, MI Zip 48146–1574;
tel. 313/382–6000; Thomas Kochis, Administrator

OAKWOOD HOSPITAL SEAWAY CENTER (O, 103 beds) 5450 Fort Street,
Trenton, MI Zip 48183; tel. 313/671–3800; Edward Freisinger, Vice
President and Administration

OAKWOOD HOSPITAL AND MEDICAL CENTER–DEARBORN (O, 560 beds)
18101 Oakwood Boulevard, Dearborn, MI Zip 48124, Mailing Address: P.O.
Box 2500, Zip 48123–2500; tel. 313/593–7000; Gerald D. Fitzgerald,
President and Chief Executive Officer

OAKWOOD HOSPITAL–HERITAGE CENTER (O, 243 beds) 10000 Telegraph
Road, Taylor, MI Zip 48180–3349; tel. 313/295–5000; Thomas E. Johnson,
Vice President and Administrator

Owned, leased, sponsored:	6 hospitals	1397 beds
Contract–managed:	0 hospitals	0 beds
Totals:	6 hospitals	1397 beds

★9095: OHIOHEALTH (NP)
3555 Olentangy River Road, 4000, Columbus, OH Zip 43214;
tel. 614/566–5424; William W. Wilkins, President and Chief Executive
Officer

OHIO: BUCYRUS COMMUNITY HOSPITAL (C, 55 beds) 629 North Sandusky
Avenue, Bucyrus, OH Zip 44820–0627, Mailing Address: Box 627, Zip
44820–0627; tel. 419/562–4677; Mark E. Marley, President and Chief
Executive Officer

GALION COMMUNITY HOSPITAL (C, 120 beds) Portland Way South, Galion,
OH Zip 44833–2314; tel. 419/468–4841; Mark E. Marley, Chief Executive
Officer

GRANT/RIVERSIDE METHODIST HOSPITALS–GRANT CAMPUS (O, 460 beds)
111 South Grant Avenue, Columbus, OH Zip 43215–1898;
tel. 614/461–3232; Jay William Eckersley, Chief Executive Officer

GRANT/RIVERSIDE METHODIST HOSPITALS–RIVERSIDE CAMPUS (O, 778
beds) 3535 Olentangy River Road, Columbus, OH Zip 43214–3998;
tel. 614/566–5000; Jay William Eckersley, Chief Executive Officer

HARDIN MEMORIAL HOSPITAL (O, 51 beds) 921 East Franklin Street, Kenton,
OH Zip 43326–2099, Mailing Address: P.O. Box 710, Zip 43326–0710;
tel. 419/673–0761; Don J. Sabol, Administrator

MARION GENERAL HOSPITAL (O, 133 beds) McKinley Park Drive, Marion, OH
Zip 43302–6397; tel. 614/383–8400; Frank V. Swinehart, President and
Chief Executive Officer

MORROW COUNTY HOSPITAL (C, 75 beds) 651 West Marion Road, Mount
Gilead, OH Zip 43338–1096; tel. 419/946–5015; Alan C. Pauley,
Administrator

SOUTHERN OHIO MEDICAL CENTER (O, 281 beds) 1805 27th Street,
Portsmouth, OH Zip 45662–2400; tel. 614/354–5000; Randal M. Arnett,
President and Chief Executive Officer

Owned, leased, sponsored:	5 hospitals	1703 beds
Contract–managed:	3 hospitals	250 beds
Totals:	8 hospitals	1953 beds

**0018: OKLAHOMA STATE DEPARTMENT OF MENTAL
HEALTH AND SUBSTANCE ABUSE SERVICES** (NP)
1000 N.E. Tenth, Oklahoma City, OK Zip 73152, Mailing Address:
P.O. Box 53277, Zip 73152; tel. 405/271–6868; Thomas Peace,
Ph.D., Commissioner

OKLAHOMA: GRIFFIN MEMORIAL HOSPITAL (O, 182 beds) 900 East Main
Street, Norman, OK Zip 73070–0101, Mailing Address: Box 151, Zip
73070; tel. 405/321–4880; William T. Burkett, Superintendent

WESTERN STATE PSYCHIATRIC CENTER (O, 170 beds) Fort Supply, OK
Mailing Address: P.O. Box 1, Zip 73841–0001; tel. 405/766–2311; Steve
Norwood, Director

Owned, leased, sponsored:	2 hospitals	352 beds
Contract–managed:	0 hospitals	0 beds
Totals:	2 hospitals	352 beds

★3355: ORLANDO REGIONAL HEALTHCARE SYSTEM (NP)
1414 Kuhl Avenue, Orlando, FL Zip 32806–2093;
tel. 407/841–5111; J. Gary Strack, Chairman and Chief Executive
Officer

FLORIDA: ORLANDO REGIONAL MEDICAL CENTER (O, 807 beds) 1414 Kuhl
Avenue, Orlando, FL Zip 32806–2093; tel. 407/841–5111; John
Hillenmeyer, President

SOUTH LAKE HOSPITAL (O, 68 beds) 847 Eighth Street, Clermont, FL
Zip 34711; tel. 352/394–4071; P. Shannon Elswick, Administrator and Chief
Executive Officer

SOUTH SEMINOLE HOSPITAL (O, 206 beds) 555 West State Road 434,
Longwood, FL Zip 32750; tel. 407/767–1200; Sue Whelan–Williams, Site
Administrator

ST. CLOUD HOSPITAL, A DIVISION OF ORLANDO REGIONAL HEALTHCARE
SYSTEM (O, 68 beds) 2906 17th Street, Saint Cloud, FL Zip 34769–6099;
tel. 407/892–2135; Jim Norris, Executive Director

Owned, leased, sponsored:	4 hospitals	1149 beds
Contract–managed:	0 hospitals	0 beds
Totals:	4 hospitals	1149 beds

Section B

For explanation of codes following names, see page B2.
★ Indicates Type III membership in the American Hospital Association.

★5335: **OSF HEALTHCARE SYSTEM** (CC)
800 N.E. Glen Oak Avenue, Peoria, IL Zip 61603–3200;
tel. 309/655–2850; Sister Frances Marie Masching, President

ILLINOIS: OSF ST. JOSEPH MEDICAL CENTER (O, 152 beds) 2200 East
Washington Street, Bloomington, IL Zip 61701–4364;
tel. 309/662–3311; Kenneth J. Natzke, Administrator

SAINT ANTHONY MEDICAL CENTER (O, 210 beds) 5666 East State Street,
Rockford, IL Zip 61108–2472; tel. 815/226–2000; David A. Schertz,
Administrator

SAINT FRANCIS MEDICAL CENTER (O, 534 beds) 530 N.E. Glen Oak Avenue,
Peoria, IL Zip 61637; tel. 309/655–2000; Sister M. Canisia, Administrator

SAINT JAMES HOSPITAL (O, 81 beds) 610 East Water Street, Pontiac, IL
Zip 61764; tel. 815/842–2828; David Ochs, Administrator

SAINT JOSEPH HOSPITAL (O, 58 beds) 1005 Julien Street, Belvidere, IL
Zip 61008–9932; tel. 815/544–3411; David A. Schertz, Administrator

ST. MARY MEDICAL CENTER (O, 156 beds) 3333 North Seminary Street,
Galesburg, IL Zip 61401–1299; tel. 309/344–3161; Richard S. Kowalski,
Administrator and Chief Executive Officer

MICHIGAN: ST. FRANCIS HOSPITAL (O, 66 beds) 3401 Ludington Street,
Escanaba, MI Zip 49829; tel. 906/786–3311; Roger M. Burgess,
Administrator

Owned, leased, sponsored:	7 hospitals	1257 beds
Contract–managed:	0 hospitals	0 beds
Totals:	7 hospitals	1257 beds

0110: **OUR LADY OF MERCY HEALTHCARE SYSTEM, INC.**
(CC)
600 East 23rd Street, New York, NY Zip 10466;
tel. 718/920–9500; Gary S. Horan, FACHE, President

NEW YORK: OUR LADY OF MERCY MEDICAL CENTER (O, 508 beds) 600
East 233rd Street, Bronx, NY Zip 10466; tel. 718/920–9000; Gary S.
Horan, FACHE, President and Chief Executive Officer

ST. AGNES HOSPITAL (O, 184 beds) 305 North Street, White Plains, NY
Zip 10605; tel. 914/681–4500; Gary S. Horan, FACHE, President and Chief
Executive Officer

Owned, leased, sponsored:	2 hospitals	692 beds
Contract–managed:	0 hospitals	0 beds
Totals:	2 hospitals	692 beds

0435: **PACIFIC HEALTH CORPORATION** (IO)
249 East Ocean Boulevard, Long Beach, CA Zip 90802;
tel. 310/435–1300; Jens Mueller, Chairman

CALIFORNIA: ANAHEIM GENERAL HOSPITAL (O, 88 beds) 3350 West Ball
Road, Anaheim, CA Zip 92804–9998; tel. 714/827–6700; Timothy L.
Carda, Chief Executive Officer

BELLFLOWER MEDICAL CENTER (O, 145 beds) 9542 East Artesia Boulevard,
Bellflower, CA Zip 90706; tel. 310/925–8355; Stanley Otake, Chief
Executive Officer

BUENA PARK MEDICAL CENTER (O, 58 beds) 5742 Beach Boulevard, Buena
Park, CA Zip 90621; tel. 714/521–4770; Timothy L. Carda, Administrator
and Chief Executive Officer

HAWTHORNE HOSPITAL (O, 73 beds) 13300 South Hawthorne Boulevard,
Hawthorne, CA Zip 90250; tel. 310/679–3321; Marvin Herschberg, Chief
Executive Officer

LOS ANGELES METROPOLITAN MEDICAL CENTER (O, 115 beds) 2231 South
Western Avenue, Los Angeles, CA Zip 90018–1399; tel. 213/737–7372;
Marc A. Furstman, Chief Executive Officer

Owned, leased, sponsored:	5 hospitals	479 beds
Contract–managed:	0 hospitals	0 beds
Totals:	5 hospitals	479 beds

★7555: **PALOMAR POMERADO HEALTH SYSTEM** (NP)
15255 Innovation Drive, Suite 204, San Diego, CA Zip 92128–3410;
tel. 619/675–5100; Victoria M. Penland, Interim President and Chief
Executive Officer

PALOMAR MEDICAL CENTER (O, 395 beds) 555 East Valley Parkway,
Escondido, CA Zip 92025–3084; tel. 619/739–3000; Victoria M. Penland,
Administrator and Chief Operating Officer

POMERADO HOSPITAL (O, 258 beds) 15615 Pomerado Road, Poway, CA
Zip 92064; tel. 619/485–4600; Marvin W. Levenson, M.D., Administrator and
Chief Operating Officer

Owned, leased, sponsored:	2 hospitals	653 beds
Contract–managed:	0 hospitals	0 beds
Totals:	2 hospitals	653 beds

5765: **PARACELSUS HEALTHCARE CORPORATION** (IO)
515 West Greens Road, Suite 800, Houston, TX Zip 77067;
tel. 281/774–5100; Charles R. Miller, President and Chief Operating
Officer

BELLWOOD GENERAL HOSPITAL (O, 65 beds) 10250 East Artesia Boulevard,
Bellflower, CA Zip 90706; tel. 562/866–9028; Joseph Sharp, Administrator

CHICO COMMUNITY HOSPITAL (O, 105 beds) 560 Cohasset Road, Chico, CA
Zip 95926; tel. 916/896–5000; Fredrick W. Hodges, Chief Executive Officer

HOLLYWOOD COMMUNITY HOSPITAL OF HOLLYWOOD (O, 160 beds) 6245
De Longpre Avenue, Los Angeles, CA Zip 90028; tel. 213/462–2271; Steven
Courtier, Chief Executive Officer

LANCASTER COMMUNITY HOSPITAL (O, 123 beds) 43830 North Tenth Street
West, Lancaster, CA Zip 93534; tel. 805/948–4781; Steve Schmidt,
Administrator and Chief Executive Officer

LOS ANGELES COMMUNITY HOSPITAL (O, 186 beds) 4081 East Olympic
Boulevard, Los Angeles, CA Zip 90023; tel. 213/267–0477; Thomas
McClintock, Chief Executive Officer

MONROVIA COMMUNITY HOSPITAL (O, 49 beds) 323 South Heliotrope
Avenue, Monrovia, CA Zip 91016, Mailing Address: Box 707, Zip
91017–0707; tel. 818/359–8341; Steve Courtier, Administrator

ORANGE COUNTY COMMUNITY HOSPITAL OF BUENA PARK (O, 55 beds)
6850 Lincoln Avenue, Buena Park, CA Zip 90620–5703; tel. 562/827–1161;
Joseph Sharp, Acting Administrator

FLORIDA: SANTA ROSA MEDICAL CENTER (O, 129 beds) 1450 Berryhill
Road, Milton, FL Zip 32570, Mailing Address: P.O. Box 648, Zip 32572;
tel. 904/626–7762; Barbara H. Thames, Chief Executive Officer

GEORGIA: FLINT RIVER COMMUNITY HOSPITAL (O, 50 beds) 509 Sumter
Street, Montezuma, GA Zip 31063–0770, Mailing Address: P.O. Box 770,
Zip 31063–0770; tel. 912/472–3100; Michael Clark, Chief Executive
Officer

MISSISSIPPI: SENATOBIA COMMUNITY HOSPITAL (O, 52 beds) 401 Getwell
Drive, Senatobia, MS Zip 38668, Mailing Address: P.O. Box 648, Zip
38668; tel. 601/562–3100; James D. Tesar, Administrator

NORTH DAKOTA: DAKOTA HEARTLAND HEALTH SYSTEM (O, 203 beds)
1720 South Univeristy Drive, Fargo, ND Zip 58103; tel. 701/280–4100;
Bruce A. Baldwin, Interim President and Chief Executive Officer

TENNESSEE: BLEDSOE COUNTY GENERAL HOSPITAL (O, 26 beds) Pikeville,
TN Mailing Address: P.O. Box 699, Zip 37367–0699; tel. 423/447–2112;
Gary Burton, Chief Executive Officer

CUMBERLAND RIVER HOSPITAL NORTH (O, 36 beds) McArthur Street, Celina,
TN Zip 38551, Mailing Address: Box 427, Zip 38551; tel. 615/243–3581;
Patrick J. Gray, Chief Executive Officer

CUMBERLAND RIVER HOSPITAL SOUTH (O, 30 beds) 620 Hospital Drive,
Gainesboro, TN Zip 38562, Mailing Address: Box 36, Zip 38562–0036;
tel. 615/268–0211; Tim Tapp, Administrator

FENTRESS COUNTY GENERAL HOSPITAL (O, 73 beds) Highway 52 West,
Jamestown, TN Zip 38556, Mailing Address: P.O. Box 1500, Zip 38556;
tel. 615/879–8171; Curtis B. Courtney, Administrator

TEXAS: BAYCOAST MEDICAL CENTER (O, 191 beds) 1700 James Bowie
Drive, Baytown, TX Zip 77520, Mailing Address: P.O. Box 1451, Zip
77520; tel. 713/420–6100; Frank T. Beirne, President and Chief
Executive Officer

MEDICAL CENTER OF MESQUITE (O, 176 beds) 1011 North Galloway Avenue, Mesquite, TX Zip 75149; tel. 214/320–7000; Terry J. Fontenot, Administrator

WESTWOOD MEDICAL CENTER (O, 80 beds) 4214 Andrews Highway, Midland, TX Zip 79703; tel. 915/522–2273; Michael S. Potter, President and Chief Executive Officer

UTAH: DAVIS HOSPITAL AND MEDICAL CENTER (O, 126 beds) 1600 West Antelope Drive, Layton, UT Zip 84041–1142; tel. 801/825–9561; Robert Cash, Chief Executive Officer

JORDAN VALLEY HOSPITAL (O, 50 beds) 3580 West 9000 South, West Jordan, UT Zip 84088–8811; tel. 801/561–8888; Jeffrey J. Manley, Chief Executive Officer

PIONEER VALLEY HOSPITAL (O, 127 beds) 3460 South Pioneer Parkway, West Valley City, UT Zip 84120; tel. 801/964–3100; Brian Mottishaw, Chief Executive Officer

SALT LAKE REGIONAL MEDICAL CENTER (O, 200 beds) 1050 East South Temple, Salt Lake City, UT Zip 84102–1599; tel. 801/350–4111; Kay Matsumura, Chief Executive Officer

VIRGINIA: METROPOLITAN HOSPITAL (O, 131 beds) 701 West Grace Street, Richmond, VA Zip 23220; tel. 804/775–4100; Priscilla J. Shuler, Chief Executive Officer

Owned, leased, sponsored:	23 hospitals	2423 beds
Contract–managed:	0 hospitals	0 beds
Totals:	23 hospitals	2423 beds

0335: PARK HEALTHCARE COMPANY (IO)
4015 Travis Drive, Nashville, TN Zip 37211; tel. 615/833–1077; Jerry E. Gilliland, President

KENTUCKY: LINCOLN TRAIL BEHAVIORAL HEALTH SYSTEM (O, 67 beds) 3909 South Wilson Road, Radcliff, KY Zip 40160–9714, Mailing Address: P.O. Box 369, Zip 40159–0369; tel. 502/351–9444; Melvin E. Modderman, Administrator

TEXAS: MEMORIAL HOSPITAL (O, 48 beds) 602 Hurst Street, Center, TX Zip 75935, Mailing Address: Box 1749, Zip 75935–1749; tel. 409/598–2781; Robert V. Deen, Administrator and Chief Executive Officer

Owned, leased, sponsored:	2 hospitals	115 beds
Contract–managed:	0 hospitals	0 beds
Totals:	2 hospitals	115 beds

★1785: PARTNERS HEALTHCARE SYSTEM (NP)
800 Boylston Street, Suite 1150, Boston, MA Zip 02199; tel. 617/278–1000; Samuel O. Thier, M.D., Chief Executive Officer

MASSACHUSETTS: BRIGHAM AND WOMEN'S HOSPITAL (O, 617 beds) 75 Francis Street, Boston, MA Zip 02115–6195; tel. 617/732–5500; Jeffrey Otten, President

MASSACHUSETTS GENERAL HOSPITAL (O, 794 beds) 55 Fruit Street, Boston, MA Zip 02114; tel. 617/726–2000; James J. Mongan, M.D., President and Chief Operating Officer

MCLEAN HOSPITAL (O, 201 beds) 115 Mill Street, Belmont, MA Zip 02178–9106; tel. 617/855–2000; Steven M. Mirin, M.D., President and Psychiatrist in Chief

SALEM HOSPITAL (O, 291 beds) 81 Highland Avenue, Salem, MA Zip 01970; tel. 508/741–1200; Michael J. Geaney Jr., President

SHAUGHNESSY–KAPLAN REHABILITATION HOSPITAL (O, 160 beds) Dove Avenue, Salem, MA Zip 01970; tel. 508/745–9000; Anthony Sciola, President and Chief Executive Officer

SPAULDING REHABILITATION HOSPITAL (O, 284 beds) 125 Nashua Street, Boston, MA Zip 02114; tel. 617/720–6400; Manuel J. Lipson, M.D., President

Owned, leased, sponsored:	6 hospitals	2347 beds
Contract–managed:	0 hospitals	0 beds
Totals:	6 hospitals	2347 beds

★5415: PEACEHEALTH (CC)
15325 S.E. 30th Place, Suite 300, Bellevue, WA Zip 98007; tel. 206/747–1711; Sister Monica F. Heeran, President and Chief Executive Officer

ALASKA: KETCHIKAN GENERAL HOSPITAL (L, 53 beds) 3100 Tongass Avenue, Ketchikan, AK Zip 99901–5746; tel. 907/225–5171; Edward F. Mahn, Chief Executive Officer

OREGON: PEACE HARBOR HOSPITAL (O, 21 beds) 400 Ninth Street, Florence, OR Zip 97439, Mailing Address: P.O. Box 580, Zip 97439; tel. 541/997–8412; James Barnhart, Administrator

SACRED HEART MEDICAL CENTER (O, 412 beds) 1255 Hilyard Street, Eugene, OR Zip 97401, Mailing Address: P.O. Box 10905, Zip 97440; tel. 541/686–7300; Andrew R. McCulloch, Administrator

WASHINGTON: ST. JOHN MEDICAL CENTER (O, 178 beds) 1614 East Kessler Boulevard, Longview, WA Zip 98632, Mailing Address: P.O. Box 3002, Zip 98632–0302; tel. 360/423–1530; Mark E. McGourty, Regional Chief Executive Officer

ST. JOSEPH HOSPITAL (O, 206 beds) 2901 Squalicum Parkway, Bellingham, WA Zip 98225–1898; tel. 360/734–5400; John Hayward, Administrator

Owned, leased, sponsored:	5 hospitals	870 beds
Contract–managed:	0 hospitals	0 beds
Totals:	5 hospitals	870 beds

0091: PIONEER HEALTHCARE (IO)
200 Lake Street, Suite 102, Peabody, MA Zip 01960; tel. 508/536–2777; Bruce A. Shear, President and Chief Executive Officer

MICHIGAN: HARBOR OAKS HOSPITAL (O, 64 beds) 35031 23 Mile Road, New Baltimore, MI Zip 48047; tel. 810/725–5777; Gary J. LaHood, Administrator and Chief Executive Officer

UTAH: HIGHLAND RIDGE HOSPITAL (O, 34 beds) 4578 Highland Drive, Salt Lake City, UT Zip 84117; tel. 801/272–9851; Richard Bell, Administrator

VIRGINIA: MOUNT REGIS CENTER (O, 25 beds) 405 Kimball Avenue, Salem, VA Zip 24153; tel. 703/389–4761; Gail S. Basham, Chief Operating Officer

Owned, leased, sponsored:	3 hospitals	123 beds
Contract–managed:	0 hospitals	0 beds
Totals:	3 hospitals	123 beds

●★0034: PMH HEALTH RESOURCES, INC. (NP)
1201 South Seventh Avenue, Phoenix, AZ Zip 85007–3913, Mailing Address: P.O. Box 21207, Zip 85036–1207; tel. 602/238–3321; Reginald M. Ballantyne III, President

ARIZONA: PMH HEALTH SERVICES NETWORK (O, 183 beds) 1201 South Seventh Avenue, Phoenix, AZ Zip 85007–3995; tel. 602/258–5111; Jeffrey Norman, Chief Executive Officer

Owned, leased, sponsored:	1 hospital	183 beds
Contract–managed:	0 hospitals	0 beds
Totals:	1 hospital	183 beds

★3505: PRESBYTERIAN HEALTHCARE SERVICES (CO)
5901 Harper Drive N.E., Albuquerque, NM Zip 87109, Mailing Address: P.O. Box 26666, Zip 87125–6666; tel. 505/260–6300; James H. Hinton, President and Chief Executive Officer

COLORADO: DELTA COUNTY MEMORIAL HOSPITAL (C, 44 beds) 100 Stafford Lane, Delta, CO Zip 81416–2297, Mailing Address: P.O. Box 10100, Zip 81416–5003; tel. 970/874–7681; Edwin E. Hurysz, Administrator

NEW MEXICO: ARTESIA GENERAL HOSPITAL (C, 38 beds) 702 North 13th Street, Artesia, NM Zip 88210; tel. 505/748–3333; Tony Plantier, Administrator

DR. DAN C. TRIGG MEMORIAL HOSPITAL (L, 37 beds) 301 East Miel De Luna Avenue, Tucumcari, NM Zip 88401, Mailing Address: P.O. Box 608, Zip 88401; tel. 505/461–0141; Dan Noteware, Administrator

---

For explanation of codes following names, see page B2.
★ Indicates Type III membership in the American Hospital Association.
● Single hospital health care system

ESPANOLA HOSPITAL (O, 80 beds) 1010 Spruce Street, Espanola, NM Zip 87532; tel. 505/753–7111; Marcella A. Romero, Administrator

LINCOLN COUNTY MEDICAL CENTER (L, 38 beds) 211 Sudderth Drive, Ruidoso, NM Zip 88345, Mailing Address: P.O. Drawer 3C/D, Hollywood Station, Zip 88345; tel. 505/257–7381; Valerie Miller, Administrator

PLAINS REGIONAL MEDICAL CENTER (O, 84 beds) 2100 North Thomas Street, Clovis, NM Zip 88101, Mailing Address: P.O. Box 1688, Zip 88101–1688; tel. 505/769–2141; Dennis E. Headlee, Administrator

PRESBYTERIAN HOSPITAL (O, 424 beds) 1100 Central Avenue S.E., Albuquerque, NM Zip 87106, Mailing Address: P.O. Box 26666, Zip 87125–6666; tel. 505/841–1234; William Fitzpatrick, M.D., Senior Vice President and Chief Operating Officer

PRESBYTERIAN KASEMAN HOSPITAL (O, 120 beds) 8300 Constitution Avenue N.E., Albuquerque, NM Zip 87110, Mailing Address: P.O. Box 26666, Zip 87125–6666; tel. 505/291–2000; Jim Purdy, Administrative Director

SOCORRO GENERAL HOSPITAL (O, 30 beds) 1202 Highway 60 West, Socorro, NM Zip 87801, Mailing Address: P.O. Box 1009, Zip 87801–1009; tel. 505/835–1140; Jeff Dye, Administrator

Owned, leased, sponsored:	7 hospitals	813 beds
Contract–managed:	2 hospitals	82 beds
Totals:	9 hospitals	895 beds

★1130: **PRESBYTERIAN HEALTHCARE SYSTEM** (NP)
8220 Walnut Hill Lane, Suite 700, Dallas, TX Zip 75231; tel. 214/345–8500; Douglas D. Hawthorne, President and Chief Executive Officer

TEXAS: PRESBYTERIAN HOSPITAL OF DALLAS (O, 637 beds) 8200 Walnut Hill Lane, Dallas, TX Zip 75231–4402; tel. 214/345–6789; Mark H. Merrill, Executive Director

PRESBYTERIAN HOSPITAL OF KAUFMAN (O, 68 beds) 850 Highway 243 West, Kaufman, TX Zip 75142–9998, Mailing Address: Box 310, Zip 75142; tel. 214/932–7200; Michael J. McBride, CHE, Executive Director

PRESBYTERIAN HOSPITAL OF PLANO (O, 91 beds) 6200 West Parker Road, Plano, TX Zip 75093–7914; tel. 972/608–8000; Philip M. Wentworth, FACHE, Executive Director

PRESBYTERIAN HOSPITAL OF WINNSBORO (O, 50 beds) 719 West Coke Road, Winnsboro, TX Zip 75494–3098, Mailing Address: P.O. Box 628, Zip 75494–0628; tel. 903/342–5227; Jerry Hopper, FACHE, Executive Director

Owned, leased, sponsored:	4 hospitals	846 beds
Contract–managed:	0 hospitals	0 beds
Totals:	4 hospitals	846 beds

★5255: **PRESENTATION HEALTH SYSTEM** (CC)
610 West 23rd Street, Yankton, SD Zip 57078, Mailing Address: P.O. Box 38, Zip 57078; tel. 605/357–7050; John T. Porter, President and Chief Executive Officer

IOWA: HEGG MEMORIAL HEALTH CENTER (C, 123 beds) 1202 21st Avenue, Rock Valley, IA Zip 51247–1497; tel. 712/476–5305; Daniel L. Drees, Administrator and Chief Executive Officer

HOLY FAMILY HEALTH SERVICES (C, 36 beds) 826 North Eighth Street, Estherville, IA Zip 51334–1598; tel. 712/362–2631; Thomas Nordwick, President and Chief Executive Officer

SIOUX CENTER COMMUNITY HOSPITAL AND HEALTH CENTER (C, 90 beds) 605 South Main Avenue, Sioux Center, IA Zip 51250; tel. 712/722–1271; Marla Toering, Administrator

MINNESOTA: DIVINE PROVIDENCE HEALTH CENTER (C, 79 beds) 312 East George Street, Ivanhoe, MN Zip 56142–0136, Mailing Address: P.O. Box G, Zip 56142–0136; tel. 507/694–1414; James C. Rossow, Administrator

PIPESTONE COUNTY MEDICAL CENTER (C, 76 beds) 911 Fifth Avenue S.W., Pipestone, MN Zip 56164, Mailing Address: P.O. Box 370, Zip 56164; tel. 507/825–5811; Carl P. Vaagenes, Administrator

TYLER HEALTHCARE CENTER (C, 63 beds) 240 Willow Street, Tyler, MN Zip 56178–0280; tel. 507/247–5521; James Rotert, Administrator

SOUTH DAKOTA: EUREKA COMMUNITY HOSPITAL (C, 10 beds) 410 Ninth Street, Eureka, SD Zip 57437–0517; tel. 605/284–2661; Robert A. Dockter, Administrator

FLANDREAU MUNICIPAL HOSPITAL (C, 18 beds) 214 North Prairie Avenue, Flandreau, SD Zip 57028–1243; tel. 605/997–2433; Paul Bergman, Administrator

HAND COUNTY MEMORIAL HOSPITAL (C, 23 beds) 300 West Fifth Street, Miller, SD Zip 57362; tel. 605/853–2421; Clarence A. Lee, Administrator

MARSHALL COUNTY MEMORIAL HOSPITAL (C, 38 beds) 413 Ninth Street, Britton, SD Zip 57430–0230, Mailing Address: Box 230, Zip 57430–0230; tel. 605/448–2253; Stephanie Lulewicz, Administrator

MCKENNAN HOSPITAL (O, 521 beds) 800 East 21st Street, Sioux Falls, SD Zip 57105, Mailing Address: P.O. Box 5045, Zip 57117–5045; tel. 605/322–8000; Fredrick Slunecka, President and Chief Executive Officer

PLATTE COMMUNITY MEMORIAL HOSPITAL (C, 63 beds) 609 East Seventh, Platte, SD Zip 57369, Mailing Address: P.O. Box 200, Zip 57369–0200; tel. 605/337–3364; Mark Burket, Chief Executive Officer

PRAIRIE LAKES HOSPITAL AND CARE CENTER (C, 122 beds) 400 Tenth Avenue N.W., Watertown, SD Zip 57201, Mailing Address: P.O. Box 1210, Zip 57201–1210; tel. 605/882–7000; Edmond L. Weiland, President and Chief Executive Officer

QUEEN OF PEACE HOSPITAL (O, 183 beds) 525 North Foster, Mitchell, SD Zip 57301–2999; tel. 605/995–2000; Ronald L. Jacobson, President and Chief Executive Officer

SACRED HEART HEALTH SERVICES (C, 257 beds) 501 Summit, Yankton, SD Zip 57078–3899; tel. 605/668–8000; Dennis A. Sokol, President and Chief Executive Officer

ST. BENEDICT HEALTH CENTER (C, 105 beds) Glynn Drive, Parkston, SD Zip 57366, Mailing Address: P.O. Box B, Zip 57366; tel. 605/928–3311; Gale Walker, Administrator

ST. LUKE'S MIDLAND REGIONAL MEDICAL CENTER (O, 313 beds) 305 South State Street, Aberdeen, SD Zip 57402–4450; tel. 605/622–5000; Dale J. Stein, President and Chief Executive Officer

Owned, leased, sponsored:	3 hospitals	1017 beds
Contract–managed:	14 hospitals	1103 beds
Totals:	17 hospitals	2120 beds

0108: **PRINCIPAL HOSPITAL GROUP** (IO)
109 Westpark Drive, Suite 180, Brentwood, TN Zip 37026; tel. 615/370–1377; Marty Rash, President and Chief Executive Officer

CALIFORNIA: OJAI VALLEY COMMUNITY HOSPITAL (O, 116 beds) 1306 Maricopa Highway, Ojai, CA Zip 93023–3180; tel. 805/646–1401; William E. Price, Interim Chief Executive Officer

COLORADO: COLORADO PLAINS MEDICAL CENTER (O, 40 beds) 1000 Lincoln Street, Fort Morgan, CO Zip 80701; tel. 970/867–3391; Keith Mesmer, Administrator and Chief Executive Officer

TEXAS: PARKVIEW REGIONAL HOSPITAL (O, 28 beds) 312 East Glendale Street, Mexia, TX Zip 76667–3608; tel. 817/562–5332; Karl R. Stinson, Administrator

WISCONSIN: DIVINE SAVIOR HOSPITAL AND NURSING HOME (O, 160 beds) 1015 West Pleasant Street, Portage, WI Zip 53901–9987, Mailing Address: P.O. Box 387, Zip 53901; tel. 608/742–4131; Michael Decker, President and Chief Executive Officer

Owned, leased, sponsored:	4 hospitals	344 beds
Contract–managed:	0 hospitals	0 beds
Totals:	4 hospitals	344 beds

★0995: **PROMINA NORTHWEST HEALTH SYSTEM** (NP)
1791 Mulkey Road, Suite 102, Austell, GA Zip 30001–1124; tel. 770/732–5501; Thomas E. Hill, Chief Executive Officer

GEORGIA: KENNESTONE HOSPITAL (O, 439 beds) 677 Church Street, Marietta, GA Zip 30060; tel. 770/793–5000; Thomas E. Hill, Chief Executive Officer

For explanation of codes following names, see page B2.
★ Indicates Type III membership in the American Hospital Association.

PROMINA COBB HOSPITAL (O, 311 beds) 3950 Austell Road, Austell, GA Zip 30001–1121; tel. 770/732–4000; Betty Whisenant, Site Manager

PROMINA DOUGLAS HOSPITAL (O, 98 beds) 8954 Hospital Drive, Douglasville, GA Zip 30134–2282; tel. 770/949–1500; Tom Hill, Chief Executive Officer

PROMINA PAULDING MEMORIAL MEDICAL CENTER (O, 208 beds) 600 West Memorial Drive, Dallas, GA Zip 30132–1335; tel. 770/445–4411; T. Mark Haney, Administrator

PROMINA WINDY HILL HOSPITAL (O, 100 beds) 2540 Windy Hill Road, Marietta, GA Zip 30067; tel. 770/644–1000; T. Mark Haney, Administrator

Owned, leased, sponsored:	5 hospitals	1156 beds
Contract–managed:	0 hospitals	0 beds
Totals:	5 hospitals	1156 beds

★5265: PROVIDENCE SERVICES (CC)

9 East Ninth Avenue, Spokane, WA Zip 99202; tel. 509/742–7337; Richard J. Umbdenstock, President and Chief Executive Officer

MONTANA: BENEFIS HEALTH CARE (S, 357 beds) 500 15th Avenue South, Great Falls, MT Zip 59403; tel. 406/727–3333; Lloyd V. Smith, President and Chief Executive Officer

ST. JOSEPH HOSPITAL (S, 22 beds) Skyline Drive and 14th Avenue, Polson, MT Zip 59860, Mailing Address: P.O. Box 1010, Zip 59860–1010; tel. 406/883–5377; John W. Glueckert, President

ST. PATRICK HOSPITAL (S, 191 beds) 500 West Broadway, Missoula, MT Zip 59802–4096, Mailing Address: Box 4587, Zip 59806–4587; tel. 406/543–7271; Lawrence L. White Jr., President

WASHINGTON: DEER PARK HEALTH CENTER AND HOSPITAL (S, 26 beds) East 1015 D Street, Deer Park, WA Zip 99006, Mailing Address: P.O. Box 742, Zip 99006; tel. 509/276–5061; Cathy Simchuk, Chief Operating Officer

HOLY FAMILY HOSPITAL (S, 190 beds) North 5633 Lidgerwood Avenue, Spokane, WA Zip 99220; tel. 509/482–0111; Ronald J. Schurra, Chief Executive Officer

MOUNT CARMEL HOSPITAL (S, 32 beds) 982 East Columbia Street, Colville, WA Zip 99114–0351, Mailing Address: Box 351, Zip 99114–0351; tel. 509/684–2561; Gloria Cooper, Chief Executive Officer

SACRED HEART MEDICAL CENTER (S, 607 beds) West 101 Eighth Avenue, Spokane, WA Zip 99220, Mailing Address: P.O. Box 2555, Zip 99220–2555; tel. 509/455–3040; Ryland P. Davis, President

ST. JOSEPH'S HOSPITAL (S, 65 beds) 500 East Webster Street, Chewelah, WA Zip 99109, Mailing Address: P.O. Box 197, Zip 99109; tel. 509/935–8211; Gary V. Peck, Chief Executive Officer

ST. MARY MEDICAL CENTER (S, 134 beds) 401 West Poplar Street, Walla Walla, WA Zip 99362, Mailing Address: Box 1477, Zip 99362–0312; tel. 509/525–3320; John A. Isely, President

Owned, leased, sponsored:	9 hospitals	1624 beds
Contract–managed:	0 hospitals	0 beds
Totals:	9 hospitals	1624 beds

0011: PUERTO RICO DEPARTMENT OF HEALTH (NP)

Building A – Medical Center, San Juan, PR Zip 00936, Mailing Address: Call Box 70184, Zip 00936; tel. 809/274–7676; Carmen Feliciano De Melecio, M.D., Secretary of Health

PUERTO RICO: AGUADILLA GENERAL HOSPITAL (O, 110 beds) Carr Aguadilla San Juan, Aguadilla, PR Zip 00605, Mailing Address: P.O. Box 4036, Zip 00605; tel. 787/891–3000; William Rodriguez Castro, Executive Director

ARECIBO REGIONAL HOSPITAL (O, 183 beds) San Luis Avenue, Arecibo, PR Zip 00612; tel. 809/878–7272; Jose L. Mirauda, M.D., Executive Director

DR. JOSE RAMOS LEBRON HOSPITAL (O, 180 beds) General Valero Avenue, #194, Fajardo, PR Zip 00738, Mailing Address: P.O. Box 1283, Zip 00738–1283; tel. 809/863–0505; Victor R. Marrero, Executive Administrator

HOSPITAL UNIVERSITARIO DR. RAMON RUIZ ARNAU (O, 372 beds) Avenue Laurel, Santa Juanita, Bayamon, PR Zip 00956; tel. 809/787–5151; Iris J. Vazquez Rosario, Executive Director

PONCE REGIONAL HOSPITAL (O, 407 beds) Barrio Machuelo, Ponce, PR Zip 00731; tel. 809/844–2080; Julio Andino, Executive Director

STATE PSYCHIATRIC HOSPITAL (O, 425 beds) San Juan, PR Mailing Address: Call Box 2100, Caparra Heights Station, Zip 00922–2100; tel. 787/766–4646; Guadalupe Alvarez, Administrator

UNIVERSITY HOSPITAL (O, 297 beds) Puerto Rico Medical Center, Rio Piedras Station, San Juan, PR Zip 00935; tel. 809/754–3654; Roberto Hernandez, Administrator

Owned, leased, sponsored:	7 hospitals	1974 beds
Contract–managed:	0 hospitals	0 beds
Totals:	7 hospitals	1974 beds

★0040: QUEEN'S HEALTH SYSTEMS (NP)

1099 Alakea Street, Suite 1100, Honolulu, HI Zip 96813; tel. 808/532–6100; Richard L. Griffith, President and Chief Executive Officer

HAWAII: MOLOKAI GENERAL HOSPITAL (O, 30 beds) Kaunakakai, HI Mailing Address: P.O. Box 408, Zip 96748–0408; tel. 808/553–5331; Calvin M. Ichinose, Administrator

QUEEN'S MEDICAL CENTER (O, 496 beds) 1301 Punchbowl Street, Honolulu, HI Zip 96813; tel. 808/538–9011; Arthur A. Ushijima, President and Chief Executive Officer

Owned, leased, sponsored:	2 hospitals	526 beds
Contract–managed:	0 hospitals	0 beds
Totals:	2 hospitals	526 beds

★0002: QUORUM HEALTH GROUP/QUORUM HEALTH RESOURCES, INC. (IO)

103 Continental Place, Brentwood, TN Zip 37027; tel. 615/371–7979; James E. Dalton Jr., President and Chief Executive Officer

ALABAMA: FLOWERS HOSPITAL (O, 215 beds) 4370 West Main Street, Dothan, AL Zip 36301, Mailing Address: Box 6907, Zip 36302–6907; tel. 334/793–5000; Keith Granger, President and Chief Executive Officer

GADSDEN REGIONAL MEDICAL CENTER (O, 257 beds) 1007 Goodyear Avenue, Gadsden, AL Zip 35999; tel. 205/494–4000; William Russell Spray, Chief Executive Officer

JACKSONVILLE HOSPITAL (O, 56 beds) 1701 Pelham Road South, Jacksonville, AL Zip 36265, Mailing Address: P.O. Box 999, Zip 36265; tel. 205/435–4970; Richard L. McConahy, Chief Executive Officer

MEDICAL CENTER ENTERPRISE (O, 113 beds) 400 North Edwards Street, Enterprise, AL Zip 36330–9981; tel. 334/347–0584; John L. Robertson, Chief Executive Officer

MONROE COUNTY HOSPITAL (C, 59 beds) 1901 South Alabama Avenue, Monroeville, AL Zip 36460, Mailing Address: P.O. Box 886, Zip 36461–0886; tel. 334/575–3111; Joe Zager, Chief Executive Officer

WIREGRASS HOSPITAL (C, 151 beds) 1200 West Maple Avenue, Geneva, AL Zip 36340; tel. 334/684–3655; H. Randolph Smith, Administrator

ALASKA: BARTLETT REGIONAL HOSPITAL (C, 64 beds) 3260 Hospital Drive, Juneau, AK Zip 99801; tel. 907/586–2611; Robert F. Valliant, Administrator

ARIZONA: MARICOPA MEDICAL CENTER (C, 481 beds) 2601 East Roosevelt Street, Phoenix, AZ Zip 85008, Mailing Address: P.O. Box 5099, Zip 85010; tel. 602/267–5011; Frank D. Alvarez, Chief Executive Officer

PHOENIX GENERAL HOSPITAL AND MEDICAL CENTER (C, 97 beds) 19829 North 27th Avenue, Phoenix, AZ Zip 85027–4002; tel. 602/879–6100; H. Douglas Garner, Chief Executive Officer

ARKANSAS: CHICOT COUNTY MEMORIAL HOSPITAL (C, 35 beds) 2729 Highway 65 and 82 South, Lake Village, AR Zip 71653–0000, Mailing Address: Box 512, Zip 71653–0441; tel. 501/265–5351; Robert R. Reddish, Administrator and Chief Executive Officer

DELTA MEMORIAL HOSPITAL (C, 35 beds) 300 East Pickens Street, Dumas, AR Zip 71639, Mailing Address: Box 887, Zip 71639–0887; tel. 501/382–4303; Rodney McPherson, Administrator

For explanation of codes following names, see page B2.
★ Indicates Type III membership in the American Hospital Association.

Section B

HELENA REGIONAL MEDICAL CENTER (C, 125 beds) 155 Newman Drive, Helena, AR Zip 72342, Mailing Address: Box 788, Zip 72342–0788; tel. 501/338–5800; Steve Reeder, Chief Executive Officer

HOWARD MEMORIAL HOSPITAL (C, 50 beds) 800 West Leslie Street, Nashville, AR Zip 71852–0381, Mailing Address: Box 381, Zip 71852–0381; tel. 501/845–4400; Lynn Crowell, Chief Executive Officer

MENA MEDICAL CENTER (C, 42 beds) 311 North Morrow Street, Mena, AR Zip 71953; tel. 501/394–6100; Albert Pilkington III, Administrator and Chief Executive Officer

REBSAMEN REGIONAL MEDICAL CENTER (C, 113 beds) 1400 West Braden Street, Jacksonville, AR Zip 72076; tel. 501/985–7000; Thomas R. Siemers, Chief Executive Officer

SALINE MEMORIAL HOSPITAL (C, 141 beds) 1 Medical Park Drive, Benton, AR Zip 72015; tel. 501/776–6000; Roger D. Feldt, FACHE, President and Chief Executive Officer

SILOAM SPRING MEMORIAL HOSPITAL (C, 52 beds) 205 East Jefferson Street, Siloam Springs, AR Zip 72761; tel. 501/524–4141; Donald E. Patterson, Administrator

SOUTHWEST HOSPITAL (C, 125 beds) 11401 Interstate 30, Little Rock, AR Zip 72209; tel. 501/455–7100; Timothy E. Hill, President and Chief Executive Officer

CALIFORNIA: SANTA PAULA MEMORIAL HOSPITAL (C, 54 beds) 825 North Tenth Street, Santa Paula, CA Zip 93060–0270, Mailing Address: P.O. Box 270, Zip 93060–0270; tel. 805/525–7171; William M. Greene, FACHE, President

COLORADO: GRAND RIVER HOSPITAL DISTRICT (C, 75 beds) 701 East Fifth Street, Rifle, CO Zip 81650–2970, Mailing Address: P.O. Box 912, Zip 81650–0912; tel. 970/625–1510; Edwin A. Gast, Administrator

HEART OF THE ROCKIES REGIONAL MEDICAL CENTER (C, 38 beds) 448 East First Street, Salida, CO Zip 81201–0429, Mailing Address: P.O. Box 429, Zip 81201–0429; tel. 719/539–6661; Howard D. Turner, Administrator and Chief Executive Officer

MEMORIAL HOSPITAL (C, 27 beds) 785 Russell Street, Craig, CO Zip 81625–9906; tel. 970/824–9411; M. Randell Phelps, Administrator

MONTROSE MEMORIAL HOSPITAL (C, 60 beds) 800 South Third Street, Montrose, CO Zip 81401–4291; tel. 970/249–2211; Tyler Erickson, Administrator

MOUNT SAN RAFAEL HOSPITAL (C, 31 beds) 410 Benedicta Avenue, Trinidad, CO Zip 81082–2093; tel. 719/846–9213; James P. D'Agostino, Chief Executive Officer

PARKVIEW EPISCOPAL MEDICAL CENTER (C, 259 beds) 400 West 16th Street, Pueblo, CO Zip 81003; tel. 719/584–4000; C. W. Smith, President

PIONEERS HOSPITAL OF RIO BLANCO COUNTY (C, 41 beds) 345 Cleveland Street, Meeker, CO Zip 81641–0000; tel. 970/878–5047; Jim Murphy, Administrator

PROWERS MEDICAL CENTER (C, 40 beds) 401 Kendall Drive, Lamar, CO Zip 81052–3993; tel. 719/336–4343; Earl J. Steinhoff, Chief Executive Officer

SOUTHWEST MEMORIAL HOSPITAL (C, 56 beds) 1311 North Mildred Road, Cortez, CO Zip 81321; tel. 970/565–6666; Stephen R. Selzer, Administrator

VALLEY VIEW HOSPITAL (C, 61 beds) 1906 Blake Avenue, Glenwood Springs, CO Zip 81601, Mailing Address: Box 1970, Zip 81602; tel. 970/945–6535; Norman L. McBride, Chief Executive Officer

FLORIDA: BASCOM PALMER EYE INSTITUTE–ANNE BATES LEACH EYE HOSPITAL (C, 35 beds) 900 N.W. 17th Street, Miami, FL Zip 33136–1199, Mailing Address: Box 016880, Zip 33101–6880; tel. 305/326–6000; David Bixler, Administrator

BERT FISH MEDICAL CENTER (C, 82 beds) 401 Palmetto Street, New Smyrna Beach, FL Zip 32168; tel. 904/424–5000; James R. Foster, President and Chief Executive Officer

BROOKSVILLE REGIONAL HOSPITAL (C, 91 beds) 55 Ponce De Leon Boulevard, Brooksville, FL Zip 34601–0037, Mailing Address: Box 37, Zip 34605–0037; tel. 352/796–5111; Robert Foreman, Associate Administrator

DESOTO MEMORIAL HOSPITAL (C, 62 beds) 900 North Robert Avenue, Arcadia, FL Zip 34265, Mailing Address: P.O. Box 2180, Zip 34265–2180; tel. 941/494–3535; Gary M. Moore, President and Chief Executive Officer

GLADES GENERAL HOSPITAL (C, 47 beds) 1201 South Main Street, Belle Glade, FL Zip 33430; tel. 561/996–6571; Michael G. Layfield, Chief Executive Officer

HENDRY REGIONAL MEDICAL CENTER (C, 45 beds) 500 West Sugarland Highway, Clewiston, FL Zip 33440; tel. 941/983–9121; J. Rudy Reinhardt, Administrator

JACKSON HOSPITAL (C, 84 beds) 4250 Hospital Drive, Marianna, FL Zip 32446, Mailing Address: P.O. Box 1608, Zip 32447–1608; tel. 904/526–2200; Richard L. Wooten, Administrator

JUPITER MEDICAL CENTER (C, 276 beds) 1210 South Old Dixie Highway, Jupiter, FL Zip 33458; tel. 407/747–2234; Donald A. Mayer, Chief Executive Officer

LEESBURG REGIONAL MEDICAL CENTER (C, 414 beds) 600 East Dixie Avenue, Leesburg, FL Zip 34748; tel. 352/323–5000; Joe D. DePew, President and Chief Executive Officer

SPRING HILL REGIONAL HOSPITAL (C, 75 beds) 10461 Quality Drive, Spring Hill, FL Zip 34609; tel. 904/688–3053; Sonia I. Gonzalez, R.N., Chief Operating Officer

SUN COAST HOSPITAL (C, 241 beds) 2025 Indian Rocks Road, Largo, FL Zip 34644, Mailing Address: Box 2025, Zip 34649–2025; tel. 813/581–9474; Jeffrey A. Collins, Chief Executive Officer

UNIVERSITY OF MIAMI HOSPITAL AND CLINICS (C, 40 beds) 1475 N.W. 12th Avenue, Miami, FL Zip 33136–1002; tel. 305/243–6418; John Rossfeld, Administrator

GEORGIA: CAMDEN MEDICAL CENTER (C, 40 beds) 2000 Dan Proctor Drive, Saint Marys, GA Zip 31558–0805, Mailing Address: Box 805, Zip 31558–0805; tel. 912/576–4200; Warren Manley, Administrator

ELBERT MEMORIAL HOSPITAL (C, 52 beds) 4 Medical Drive, Elberton, GA Zip 30635–1897; tel. 706/283–3151; Tim Merritt, Administrator

EMANUEL COUNTY HOSPITAL (C, 119 beds) 117 Kite Road, Swainsboro, GA Zip 30401, Mailing Address: P.O. Box 879, Zip 30401; tel. 912/237–9911; Richard W. Clarke, Chief Executive Officer

HABERSHAM COUNTY MEDICAL CENTER (C, 140 beds) Highway 441, Demorest, GA Zip 30535, Mailing Address: Box 37, Zip 30535; tel. 706/754–2161; C. Richard Dwozan, President

HANCOCK MEMORIAL HOSPITAL (C, 35 beds) 453 Boland Street, Sparta, GA Zip 31087, Mailing Address: P.O. Box 490, Zip 31087; tel. 706/444–7006; Daniel D. Holtz, FACHE, Administrator and Chief Executive Officer

MACON NORTHSIDE HOSPITAL (O, 103 beds) 400 Charter Boulevard, Macon, GA Zip 31210, Mailing Address: P.O. Box 4627, Zip 31208; tel. 912/757–8200; Richard Gaston, Administrator

MCDUFFIE COUNTY HOSPITAL (C, 47 beds) 521 Hill Street S.W., Thomson, GA Zip 30824; tel. 706/595–1411; Douglas C. Keir, Chief Executive Officer

MEMORIAL MEDICAL CENTER (C, 373 beds) 4700 Waters Avenue, Savannah, GA Zip 31404, Mailing Address: Box 23089, Zip 31403–3089; tel. 912/350–8000; Robert A. Colvin, President and Chief Executive Officer

MIDDLE GEORGIA HOSPITAL (O, 119 beds) 888 Pine Street, Macon, GA Zip 31201, Mailing Address: Box 6278, Zip 31208–6278; tel. 912/751–1111; William W. Fox III, Chief Executive Officer

OCONEE REGIONAL MEDICAL CENTER (C, 145 beds) 821 North Cobb Street, Milledgeville, GA Zip 31061, Mailing Address: Box 690, Zip 31061; tel. 912/454–3500; Brian L. Riddle, Chief Executive Officer

RIDGECREST HOSPITAL (C, 45 beds) 393 Ridgecrest Circle, Clayton, GA Zip 30525; tel. 706/782–4297; Gerald E. Knepp, Chief Executive Officer

SOUTHEAST GEORGIA REGIONAL MEDICAL CENTER (C, 337 beds) 3100 Kemble Avenue, Brunswick, GA Zip 31520, Mailing Address: Box 1518, Zip 31521; tel. 912/264–7000; E. Berton Whitaker, President and Chief Executive Officer

TANNER MEDICAL CENTER (C, 183 beds) 705 Dixie Street, Carrollton, GA Zip 30117–3818; tel. 770/836–9666; Loy M. Howard, Chief Executive Officer

TANNER MEDICAL CENTER–VILLA RICA (C, 45 beds) 601 Dallas Road, Villa Rica, GA Zip 30180, Mailing Address: Box 638, Zip 30180; tel. 770/459–7100; Larry N. Steed, Administrator

UPSON REGIONAL MEDICAL CENTER (C, 115 beds) 801 West Gordon Street, Thomaston, GA Zip 30286–2831, Mailing Address: Box 1059, Zip 30286; tel. 706/647–8111; Samuel S. Gregory, Administrator

For explanation of codes following names, see page B2.
★ Indicates Type III membership in the American Hospital Association.

Section B

WALTON MEDICAL CENTER (C, 115 beds) 330 Alcovy Street, Monroe, GA Zip 30655, Mailing Address: Box 1346, Zip 30655; tel. 770/267–8461; Edgar L. Belcher, Administrator

WAYNE MEMORIAL HOSPITAL (C, 110 beds) 865 South First Street, Jesup, GA Zip 31598, Mailing Address: Box 408, Zip 31598; tel. 912/427–6811; Charles R. Morgan, Administrator

WILLS MEMORIAL HOSPITAL (C, 50 beds) 120 Gordon Street, Washington, GA Zip 30673, Mailing Address: Box 370, Zip 30673–0370; tel. 706/678–2151; Vincent DiFranco, Chief Executive Officer

WOODRIDGE HOSPITAL (C, 32 beds) 394 Ridgecrest Circle, Clayton, GA Zip 30525; tel. 706/782–3100; Gerald E. Knepp, Chief Executive Officer

IDAHO: BINGHAM MEMORIAL HOSPITAL (C, 115 beds) 98 Poplar Street, Blackfoot, ID Zip 83221–1799; tel. 208/785–4100; Robert M. Peterson, Administrator

GRITMAN MEDICAL CENTER (C, 35 beds) 710 South Washington Street, Moscow, ID Zip 83843; tel. 208/882–4511; Daniel R. Smigelski, Chief Executive Officer

ILLINOIS: CARMI TOWNSHIP HOSPITAL (C, 126 beds) 400 Plum Street, Carmi, IL Zip 62821–1799; tel. 618/382–4171; Joe E. Gamble, Chief Executive Officer

COMMUNITY MEMORIAL HOSPITAL (C, 57 beds) 400 Caldwell Street, Staunton, IL Zip 62088–1499; tel. 618/635–2200; Patrick B. Heise, Chief Executive Officer

CRAWFORD MEMORIAL HOSPITAL (C, 102 beds) 1000 North Allen Street, Robinson, IL Zip 62454, Mailing Address: P.O. Box 151, Zip 62454; tel. 618/544–3131; William E. Schirmer, FACHE, Interim Chief Executive Officer

GIBSON COMMUNITY HOSPITAL (C, 82 beds) 1120 North Melvin Street, Gibson City, IL Zip 60936, Mailing Address: P.O. Box 429, Zip 60936–0429; tel. 217/784–4251; Craig A. Jesiolowski, Chief Executive Officer

ILLINI COMMUNITY HOSPITAL (C, 45 beds) 640 West Washington Street, Pittsfield, IL Zip 62363; tel. 217/285–2113; Jete Edmisson, President and Chief Executive Officer

MEMORIAL HOSPITAL (C, 59 beds) South Adams Street, Carthage, IL Zip 62321, Mailing Address: P.O. Box 160, Zip 62321; tel. 217/357–3131; Keith E. Heuser, Chief Executive Officer

MEMORIAL HOSPITAL (C, 50 beds) 1900 State Street, Chester, IL Zip 62233–0609, Mailing Address: Box 609, Zip 62233; tel. 618/826–4581; Eric Freeburg, Administrator

SANDWICH COMMUNITY HOSPITAL (C, 50 beds) 11 East Pleasant Avenue, Sandwich, IL Zip 60548–0901; tel. 815/786–8484; Roland R. Carlson, Administrator

THOMAS H. BOYD MEMORIAL HOSPITAL (C, 60 beds) 800 School Street, Carrollton, IL Zip 62016–1498; tel. 217/942–6946; Deborah Campbell, Administrator

INDIANA: DAVIESS COUNTY HOSPITAL (C, 85 beds) 1314 Grand Avenue, Washington, IN Zip 47501–2198, Mailing Address: P.O. Box 760, Zip 47501–0760; tel. 812/254–2760; Marc Chircop, Chief Executive Officer

LUTHERAN HOSPITAL OF INDIANA (O, 342 beds) 7950 West Jefferson Boulevard, Fort Wayne, IN Zip 46804–1677; tel. 219/435–7001; William L. Anderson, Chief Executive Officer

MARY SHERMAN HOSPITAL (C, 53 beds) 320 North Section Street, Sullivan, IN Zip 47882, Mailing Address: P.O. Box 10, Zip 47882–0010; tel. 812/268–4311; Thomas J. Hudgins, Administrator

IOWA: BOONE COUNTY HOSPITAL (C, 57 beds) 1015 Union Street, Boone, IA Zip 50036–4898; tel. 515/432–3140; Joseph S. Smith, Chief Executive Officer

DES MOINES GENERAL HOSPITAL (C, 112 beds) 603 East 12th Street, Des Moines, IA Zip 50309–5515; tel. 515/263–4200; Roy W. Wright, Chief Executive Officer

FORT MADISON COMMUNITY HOSPITAL (C, 50 beds) Highway 61 West, Fort Madison, IA Zip 52627–0174, Mailing Address: Highway 61 West, Box 174, Zip 52627–0174; tel. 319/372–6530; C. James Platt, Administrator

KNOXVILLE AREA COMMUNITY HOSPITAL (C, 52 beds) 1002 South Lincoln Street, Knoxville, IA Zip 50138–3121; tel. 515/842–2151; Daryl Mackender, Chief Executive Officer

WASHINGTON COUNTY HOSPITAL (C, 83 beds) 400 East Polk Street, Washington, IA Zip 52353, Mailing Address: P.O. Box 909, Zip 52353; tel. 319/653–5481; Ronald D. Davis, Chief Executive Officer

KANSAS: BOB WILSON MEMORIAL GRANT COUNTY HOSPITAL (C, 39 beds) 415 North Main Street, Ulysses, KS Zip 67880; tel. 316/356–1266; Bruce K. Birchell, Administrator

COFFEYVILLE REGIONAL MEDICAL CENTER (C, 123 beds) 1400 West Fourth, Coffeyville, KS Zip 67337–3306; tel. 316/251–1200; Gerald Joseph Marquette Jr., Administrator

NEOSHO MEMORIAL REGIONAL MEDICAL CENTER (C, 60 beds) 629 South Plummer, Chanute, KS Zip 66720; tel. 316/431–4000; Murray L. Brown, Administrator

NEWMAN MEMORIAL COUNTY HOSPITAL (C, 110 beds) 1201 West 12th Avenue, Emporia, KS Zip 66801–2597; tel. 316/343–6800; Terry R. Lambert, Chief Executive Officer

WILSON COUNTY HOSPITAL (C, 38 beds) 205 Mill Street, Neodesha, KS Zip 66757, Mailing Address: Box 360, Zip 66757; tel. 316/325–2611; Deanna Pittman, Administrator

KENTUCKY: CRITTENDEN COUNTY HOSPITAL (C, 67 beds) Highway 60 South, Marion, KY Zip 42064–0386, Mailing Address: Box 386, Zip 42064; tel. 502/965–5281; Rick Napper, Chief Executive Officer

CUMBERLAND COUNTY HOSPITAL (C, 31 beds) Highway 90 West, Burkesville, KY Zip 42717–0280, Mailing Address: P.O. Box 280, Zip 42717–0280; tel. 502/864–2511; Mark Thompson, Chief Executive Officer

FLEMING COUNTY HOSPITAL (C, 52 beds) 920 Elizaville Avenue, Flemingsburg, KY Zip 41041, Mailing Address: Box 388, Zip 41041–0388; tel. 606/849–5000; Bobby B. Emmons, Administrator

FRANKLIN–SIMPSON MEMORIAL HOSPITAL (C, 36 beds) Brookhaven Road, Franklin, KY Zip 42135–2929, Mailing Address: P.O. Box 2929, Zip 42135–2929; tel. 502/586–3253; William P. Macri, Administrator

JENNIE STUART MEDICAL CENTER (C, 139 beds) 320 West 18th Street, Hopkinsville, KY Zip 42240–6315; tel. 502/887–0100; Lewis T. Peeples, Chief Executive Officer

MARSHALL COUNTY HOSPITAL (C, 80 beds) 503 George McClain Drive, Benton, KY Zip 42025, Mailing Address: P.O. Box 630, Zip 42025; tel. 502/527–4800; David G. Fuqua, R.N., Chief Executive Officer

MONROE COUNTY MEDICAL CENTER (C, 49 beds) 529 Capp Harlan Road, Tompkinsville, KY Zip 42167; tel. 502/487–9231; Carolyn E. Riley, Chief Executive Officer

MUHLENBERG COMMUNITY HOSPITAL (C, 135 beds) 440 Hopkinsville Street, Greenville, KY Zip 42345, Mailing Address: P.O. Box 387, Zip 42345; tel. 502/338–8000; Charles D. Lovell Jr., Chief Executive Officer

OHIO COUNTY HOSPITAL (C, 54 beds) 1211 Main Street, Hartford, KY Zip 42347; tel. 502/298–7411; Blaine Pieper, Administrator

LOUISIANA: BOGALUSA COMMUNITY MEDICAL CENTER (C, 102 beds) 433 Plaza Street, Bogalusa, LA Zip 70429–0940; tel. 504/732–7122; Terry G. Whittington, Chief Executive Officer and Administrator

FRANKLIN FOUNDATION HOSPITAL (C, 60 beds) 1501 Hospital Avenue, Franklin, LA Zip 70538, Mailing Address: Box 577, Zip 70538–0577; tel. 318/828–0760; A. Dale Morgan, Administrator

LAKEWOOD MEDICAL CENTER (C, 122 beds) 1125 Marguerite Street, Morgan City, LA Zip 70380, Mailing Address: Drawer 2308, Zip 70381; tel. 504/384–2200; Joyce Grove Hein, Chief Executive Officer

LANE MEMORIAL HOSPITAL (C, 136 beds) 6300 Main Street, Zachary, LA Zip 70791–9990; tel. 504/658–4000; Charlie L. Massey, Administrator

NORTH OAKS MEDICAL CENTER (C, 245 beds) 15790 Medical Center Drive, Hammond, LA Zip 70403, Mailing Address: Box 2668, Zip 70404; tel. 504/345–2700; James E. Cathey Jr., Chief Executive Officer

OPELOUSAS GENERAL HOSPITAL (C, 126 beds) 520 Prudhomme Lane, Opelousas, LA Zip 70570, Mailing Address: Box 1208, Zip 70571–1208; tel. 318/948–3011; Patrick Brian Carrier, Administrator

THIBODAUX REGIONAL MEDICAL CENTER (C, 130 beds) 602 North Acadia Road, Thibodaux, LA Zip 70301, Mailing Address: Box 1118, Zip 70302–1118; tel. 504/447–5500; Greg K. Stock, Chief Executive Officer

MAINE: CALAIS REGIONAL HOSPITAL (C, 57 beds) 50 Franklin Street, Calais, ME Zip 04619–1398; tel. 207/454–7521; Ray H. Davis Jr., Chief Executive Officer

For explanation of codes following names, see page B2.
★ Indicates Type III membership in the American Hospital Association.

CARY MEDICAL CENTER (C, 59 beds) 37 Van Buren Road, Caribou, ME Zip 04736–2599; tel. 207/498–3111; Kris Doody–Chabre, Interim Executive Director

DOWN EAST COMMUNITY HOSPITAL (C, 38 beds) Upper Court Street, Machias, ME Zip 04654, Mailing Address: Rural Route 1, Box 11, Zip 04654; tel. 207/255–3356; Richard Hanley, Chief Executive Officer

HOULTON REGIONAL HOSPITAL (C, 69 beds) 20 Hartford Street, Houlton, ME Zip 04730–9998; tel. 207/532–9471; Thomas J. Moakler, Administrator and Chief Executive Officer

INLAND HOSPITAL (C, 44 beds) Kennedy Memorial Drive, Waterville, ME Zip 04901; tel. 207/861–3000; Wilfred J. Addison, Administrator

MAINE COAST MEMORIAL HOSPITAL (C, 48 beds) 72 Union Street, Ellsworth, ME Zip 04605–1599; tel. 207/667–5311; Paul Raymond Barrette, President and Chief Executive Officer

MAYO REGIONAL HOSPITAL (C, 46 beds) 75 West Main Street, Dover–Foxcroft, ME Zip 04426; tel. 207/564–8401; George Avery, Interim Chief Executive Officer

MILLINOCKET REGIONAL HOSPITAL (C, 20 beds) 200 Somerset Street, Millinocket, ME Zip 04462; tel. 207/723–5161; Craig A. Kantos, Chief Executive Officer

PENOBSCOT VALLEY HOSPITAL (C, 42 beds) Transalpine Road, Lincoln, ME Zip 04457–0368, Mailing Address: P.O. Box 368, Zip 04457–0368; tel. 207/794–3321; Ronald D. Victory, Administrator

MARYLAND: ATLANTIC GENERAL HOSPITAL (C, 62 beds) 9733 Healthway Drive, Berlin, MD Zip 21811–1151; tel. 410/641–1100; Donald E. Annis, Chief Executive Officer

MASSACHUSETTS: HALE HOSPITAL (C, 113 beds) 140 Lincoln Avenue, Haverhill, MA Zip 01830; tel. 508/374–2000; Jeffrey Doran, Chief Executive Officer

HUBBARD REGIONAL HOSPITAL (C, 34 beds) 340 Thompson Road, Webster, MA Zip 01570–0608; tel. 508/943–2600; Gerald J. Barbini, Administrator and Chief Executive Officer

JORDAN HOSPITAL (C, 123 beds) 275 Sandwich Street, Plymouth, MA Zip 02360–2196; tel. 508/746–2001; Alan D. Knight, President and Chief Executive Officer

MASSACHUSETTS RESPIRATORY HOSPITAL (C, 110 beds) 2001 Washington Street, Braintree, MA Zip 02184; tel. 617/848–2600; Edward F. Kittredge, Chief Executive Officer

QUINCY HOSPITAL (C, 254 beds) 114 Whitwell Street, Quincy, MA Zip 02169–1899; tel. 617/773–6100; Ralph DiPisa, Chief Executive Officer

MICHIGAN: ALLEGAN GENERAL HOSPITAL (C, 63 beds) 555 Linn Street, Allegan, MI Zip 49010–1594; tel. 616/673–8424; James Klun, President

COMMUNITY HEALTH CENTER OF BRANCH COUNTY (C, 96 beds) 274 East Chicago Street, Coldwater, MI Zip 49036–2088; tel. 517/279–5489; Douglas L. Rahn, Chief Executive Officer

COMMUNITY HOSPITAL (C, 54 beds) Medical Park Drive, Watervliet, MI Zip 49098–0158, Mailing Address: Box 158, Zip 49098; tel. 616/463–3111; Dennis Turney, Chief Executive Officer

LAKEVIEW COMMUNITY HOSPITAL (C, 168 beds) 408 Hazen Street, Paw Paw, MI Zip 49079, Mailing Address: Box 209, Zip 49079–0209; tel. 616/657–3141; Sue E. Johnson–Phillippe, Chief Executive Officer

MARLETTE COMMUNITY HOSPITAL (C, 91 beds) 2770 Main Street, Marlette, MI Zip 48453–0307, Mailing Address: P.O. Box 307, Zip 48453–0307; tel. 517/635–4000; David S. McEwen, Chief Executive Officer

MECOSTA COUNTY GENERAL HOSPITAL (C, 74 beds) 405 Winter Avenue, Big Rapids, MI Zip 49307–2099; tel. 616/796–8691; Thomas E. Daugherty, Chief Executive Officer

STURGIS HOSPITAL (C, 67 beds) 916 Myrtle, Sturgis, MI Zip 49091–2001; tel. 616/659–4400; David James, Chief Executive Officer

THREE RIVERS AREA HOSPITAL (C, 60 beds) 1111 West Broadway, Three Rivers, MI Zip 49093–9362; tel. 616/278–1145; Bradley Solberg, President and Chief Executive Officer

MINNESOTA: FALLS MEMORIAL HOSPITAL (C, 35 beds) 1400 Highway 71, International Falls, MN Zip 56649–2189; tel. 218/283–4481; James F. Hanko, Administrator and Chief Executive Officer

VIRGINIA REGIONAL MEDICAL CENTER (C, 199 beds) 901 Ninth Street North, Virginia, MN Zip 55792–2398; tel. 218/741–3340; Kyle Hopstad, Administrator

MISSISSIPPI: BOLIVAR COUNTY HOSPITAL (C, 142 beds) Highway 8 East, Cleveland, MS Zip 38732, Mailing Address: P.O. Box 1380, Zip 38732; tel. 601/846–0061; Robert L. Hawley Jr., Chief Executive Officer

CROSBY MEMORIAL HOSPITAL (C, 61 beds) 801 Goodyear Boulevard, Picayune, MS Zip 39466, Mailing Address: Box 909, Zip 39466; tel. 601/798–4711; Calvin Green, Administrator

DELTA REGIONAL MEDICAL CENTER (C, 159 beds) 1400 East Union Street, Greenville, MS Zip 38703–3246, Mailing Address: Box 5247, Zip 38704–5247; tel. 601/378–3783; George Repa, Chief Executive Officer

FIELD MEMORIAL COMMUNITY HOSPITAL (C, 66 beds) 270 West Main Street, Centreville, MS Zip 39631, Mailing Address: Box 639, Zip 39631–0639; tel. 601/645–5221; Brock A. Slabach, Administrator

H. C. WATKINS MEMORIAL HOSPITAL (C, 43 beds) 605 South Archusa Avenue, Quitman, MS Zip 39355–2398; tel. 601/776–6925; Thomas G. Bartlett, President and Chief Executive Officer

HANCOCK MEDICAL CENTER (C, 66 beds) 149 Drinkwater Boulevard, Bay St. Louis, MS Zip 39520, Mailing Address: P.O. Box 2790, Zip 39521; tel. 601/467–9081; Thomas B. Symonds, Chief Executive Officer

KING'S DAUGHTERS HOSPITAL (C, 102 beds) Highway 51 North, Brookhaven, MS Zip 39601, Mailing Address: P.O. Box 948, Zip 39601; tel. 601/833–6011; Wallace Cooper, Chief Executive Officer

MAGNOLIA REGIONAL HEALTH CENTER (C, 157 beds) 611 Alcorn Drive, Corinth, MS Zip 38834; tel. 601/293–1000; Rohn J. Butterfield, Chief Executive Officer

NATCHEZ REGIONAL MEDICAL CENTER (C, 121 beds) Seargent S Prentiss Drive, Natchez, MS Zip 39120, Mailing Address: Box 1488, Zip 39121–1488; tel. 601/443–2100; David M. Snyder, Executive Director and Chief Executive Officer

NESHOBA COUNTY GENERAL HOSPITAL (C, 192 beds) 1001 Holland Avenue, Philadelphia, MS Zip 39350, Mailing Address: P.O. Box 648, Zip 39350; tel. 601/663–1200; Lawrence Graeber, Administrator

PARKVIEW REGIONAL MEDICAL CENTER (O, 197 beds) 100 McAuley Drive, Vicksburg, MS Zip 39180–2897, Mailing Address: P.O. Box 590, Zip 39181–0590; tel. 601/631–2131; Charles Mitchener Jr., Chief Operating Officer and Administrator

UNIVERSITY HOSPITALS AND CLINICS, UNIVERSITY OF MISSISSIPPI MEDICAL CENTER (C, 524 beds) 2500 North State Street, Jackson, MS Zip 39216–4505; tel. 601/984–4100; Frederick Woodrell, Associate Vice Chancellor and Director

MISSOURI: NEVADA REGIONAL MEDICAL CENTER (C, 97 beds) 800 South Ash Street, Nevada, MO Zip 64772; tel. 417/667–3355; Michael L. Mullins, President

MONTANA: CENTRAL MONTANA MEDICAL CENTER (C, 124 beds) 408 Wendell Avenue, Lewistown, MT Zip 59457, Mailing Address: P.O. Box 580, Zip 59457; tel. 406/538–7711; David M. Faulkner, Chief Executive Officer and Administrator

COMMUNITY HOSPITAL OF ANACONDA (C, 101 beds) 401 West Pennsylvania Street, Anaconda, MT Zip 59711; tel. 406/563–5261; Sam J. Allen, Administrator

NORTH VALLEY HOSPITAL (C, 99 beds) 6575 Highway 93 South, Whitefish, MT Zip 59937; tel. 406/863–2501; Kenneth E. S. Platou, Chief Executive Officer

NEBRASKA: GREAT PLAINS REGIONAL MEDICAL CENTER (C, 99 beds) 601 West Leota Street, North Platte, NE Zip 69101, Mailing Address: P.O. Box 1167, Zip 69103; tel. 308/534–9310; Lucinda A. Bradley, President

MIDLANDS COMMUNITY HOSPITAL (O, 160 beds) 11111 South 84th Street, Papillion, NE Zip 68046; tel. 402/593–3000; Diana Smalley, Chief Executive Officer

PHELPS MEMORIAL HEALTH CENTER (C, 55 beds) 1220 Miller Street, Holdrege, NE Zip 68949, Mailing Address: P.O. Box 828, Zip 68949–0828; tel. 308/995–2211; Jerome Seigfried Jr., Chief Executive Officer

NEVADA: DESERT SPRINGS HOSPITAL (O, 225 beds) 2075 East Flamingo Road, Las Vegas, NV Zip 89119, Mailing Address: P.O. Box 19204, Zip 89132; tel. 702/733–8800; Thomas L. Koenig, Chief Executive Officer

For explanation of codes following names, see page B2.
★ Indicates Type III membership in the American Hospital Association.

NYE REGIONAL MEDICAL CENTER (C, 45 beds) 825 South Main, Tonopah, NV Zip 89049, Mailing Address: Box 391, Zip 89049; tel. 702/482–6233; Roger Mayers, Interim Administrator

NEW HAMPSHIRE: LITTLETON REGIONAL HOSPITAL (C, 49 beds) 262 Cottage Street, Littleton, NH Zip 03561; tel. 603/444–7731; Robert S. Pearson, Administrator

MONADNOCK COMMUNITY HOSPITAL (C, 62 beds) 452 Old Street Road, Peterborough, NH Zip 03458; tel. 603/924–7191; Frank A. Niro, Chief Executive Officer

NEW MEXICO: CIBOLA GENERAL HOSPITAL (C, 22 beds) 1212 Bonita Avenue, Grants, NM Zip 87020; tel. 505/287–4446; Polly Pine, Administrator

GERALD CHAMPION MEMORIAL HOSPITAL (C, 74 beds) 1209 Ninth Street, Alamogordo, NM Zip 88310–0597, Mailing Address: P.O. Box 597, Zip 88311–0597; tel. 505/439–2100; Carl W. Mantey, Administrator

GILA REGIONAL MEDICAL CENTER (C, 68 beds) 1313 East 32nd Street, Silver City, NM Zip 88061; tel. 505/538–4000; Alfredo Ontiveros, Administrator

HOLY CROSS HOSPITAL (C, 42 beds) 630 Paseo De Pueblo Sur, Taos, NM Zip 87571, Mailing Address: P.O. Box DD, Zip 87571; tel. 505/758–8883; Rita Campbell, Chief Executive Officer

NEW YORK: AURELIA OSBORN FOX MEMORIAL HOSPITAL (C, 238 beds) 1 Norton Avenue, Oneonta, NY Zip 13820–2697; tel. 607/432–2000; John R. Remillard, President

ELLIS HOSPITAL (C, 434 beds) 1101 Nott Street, Schenectady, NY Zip 12308–2487; tel. 518/382–4124; G. B. Serrill, President and Chief Executive Officer

NORTH CAROLINA: ALEXANDER COMMUNITY HOSPITAL (C, 36 beds) 326 Third Street S.W., Taylorsville, NC Zip 28681–3096; tel. 704/632–4282; Joe W. Pollard Jr., Administrator

ALLEGHANY COUNTY MEMORIAL HOSPITAL (C, 46 beds) 233 Doctor's Street, Sparta, NC Zip 28675–0009, Mailing Address: P.O. Box 9, Zip 28675–0009; tel. 910/372–5511; James Yarborough, Chief Executive Officer

ANGEL MEDICAL CENTER (C, 59 beds) Riverview and White Oak Streets, Franklin, NC Zip 28734, Mailing Address: P.O. Box 1209, Zip 28734–1209; tel. 704/524–8411; Michael E. Zuliani, Chief Executive Officer

ASHE MEMORIAL HOSPITAL (C, 115 beds) Highway 221 South–Box 8, Jefferson, NC Zip 28640–0008; tel. 910/246–7101; R. D. Williams, Administrator

CHATHAM HOSPITAL (C, 42 beds) West Third Street and Ivy Avenue, Siler City, NC Zip 27344–2343, Mailing Address: P.O. Box 649, Zip 27344; tel. 919/663–2113; Ted G. Chapin, Chief Executive Officer

COLUMBUS COUNTY HOSPITAL (C, 117 beds) 500 Jefferson Street, Whiteville, NC Zip 28472–9987; tel. 910/642–8011; William S. Clark, Chief Executive Officer

GOOD HOPE HOSPITAL (C, 72 beds) 410 Denim Drive, Erwin, NC Zip 28339–0668, Mailing Address: P.O. Box 668, Zip 28339–0668; tel. 910/897–6151; David T. Boucher, Chief Executive Officer

GRANVILLE MEDICAL CENTER (C, 146 beds) 1010 College Street, Oxford, NC Zip 27565–2507, Mailing Address: Box 947, Zip 27565–0947; tel. 919/690–3000; Andrew Mannich, Administrator

HUGH CHATHAM MEMORIAL HOSPITAL (C, 160 beds) Parkwood Drive, Elkin, NC Zip 28621–0560, Mailing Address: P.O. Box 560, Zip 28621–0560; tel. 910/527–7000; Richard D. Osmus, Chief Executive Officer

JOHNSTON MEMORIAL HOSPITAL (C, 127 beds) 509 North Bright Leaf Boulevard, Smithfield, NC Zip 27577–1376, Mailing Address: P.O. Box 1376, Zip 27577–1376; tel. 919/934–8171; Leland E. Farnell, President

MOREHEAD MEMORIAL HOSPITAL (C, 236 beds) 117 East King's Highway, Eden, NC Zip 27288–5299; tel. 910/623–9711; Robert Enders, President

NORTHERN HOSPITAL OF SURRY COUNTY (C, 115 beds) 830 Rockford Street, Mount Airy, NC Zip 27030, Mailing Address: Box 1101, Zip 27030–1101; tel. 910/719–7000; William B. James, Chief Executive Officer

PENDER MEMORIAL HOSPITAL (C, 86 beds) 507 Freemont Street, Burgaw, NC Zip 28425; tel. 910/259–5451; James L. Jarrett, Chief Executive Officer

PERSON COUNTY MEMORIAL HOSPITAL (C, 93 beds) 615 Ridge Road, Roxboro, NC Zip 27573–4630; tel. 910/503–4800; H. James Graham, Administrator

RUTHERFORD HOSPITAL (C, 293 beds) 308 South Ridgecrest Avenue, Rutherfordton, NC Zip 28139–3097; tel. 704/286–5000; Robert D. Jones, President

WASHINGTON COUNTY HOSPITAL (C, 49 beds) 1 Medical Plaza, Plymouth, NC Zip 27962; tel. 919/793–4135; Lawrence H. McAvoy, Administrator

OHIO: BARBERTON CITIZENS HOSPITAL (O, 272 beds) 155 Fifth Street N.E., Barberton, OH Zip 44203; tel. 330/745–1611; Mike A. Bernatovicz, Chief Executive Officer

DEFIANCE HOSPITAL (C, 96 beds) 1206 East Second Street, Defiance, OH Zip 43512–2495; tel. 419/783–6955; Richard C. Sommer, Administrator

DOCTORS HOSPITAL OF STARK COUNTY (O, 142 beds) 400 Austin Avenue N.W., Massillon, OH Zip 44646–3554; tel. 216/837–7200; Thomas E. Cecconi, Chief Executive Officer

FAYETTE COUNTY MEMORIAL HOSPITAL (C, 48 beds) 1430 Columbus Avenue, Washington Court House, OH Zip 43160–1791; tel. 614/335–1210; Francis G. Albarano, Administrator

GREENFIELD AREA MEDICAL CENTER (C, 36 beds) 545 South Street, Greenfield, OH Zip 45123–1400; tel. 513/981–2116; Mark E. Marchetti, Chief Executive Officer

KNOX COMMUNITY HOSPITAL (C, 117 beds) 1330 Coshocton Road, Mount Vernon, OH Zip 43050–1495; tel. 614/393–9000; Robert G. Polahar, Chief Executive Officer

MEMORIAL HOSPITAL (C, 132 beds) 715 South Taft Avenue, Fremont, OH Zip 43420–3200; tel. 419/332–7321; John A. Gorman, Chief Executive Officer

PARK MEDICAL CENTER (O, 145 beds) 1492 East Broad Street, Columbus, OH Zip 43205–1546; tel. 614/251–3000; Cornelius Serle, Chief Executive Officer

PAULDING COUNTY HOSPITAL (C, 51 beds) 11558 State Road 111, Paulding, OH Zip 45879–9220; tel. 419/399–4080; Joseph M. Dorko, Chief Executive Officer

SELBY GENERAL HOSPITAL (C, 44 beds) 1106 Colegate Drive, Marietta, OH Zip 45750–1323; tel. 614/373–0582; James J. Cliborne Jr., Chief Executive Officer

WOOSTER COMMUNITY HOSPITAL (C, 90 beds) 1761 Beall Avenue, Wooster, OH Zip 44691–2342; tel. 330/263–8100; William E. Sheron, Chief Executive Officer

OKLAHOMA: ATOKA MEMORIAL HOSPITAL (C, 30 beds) 1501 South Virginia Avenue, Atoka, OK Zip 74525; tel. 405/889–3333; Bruce A. Bennett, Administrator and Chief Executive Officer

CUSHING REGIONAL HOSPITAL (C, 75 beds) 1027 East Cherry, Cushing, OK Zip 74023, Mailing Address: Box 1409, Zip 74023–1409; tel. 918/225–2915; Ron Cackler, President and Chief Executive Officer

HENRYETTA MEDICAL CENTER (C, 28 beds) Dewey Bartlett and Main Streets, Henryetta, OK Zip 74437, Mailing Address: P.O. Box 1269, Zip 74437–1269; tel. 918/652–4463; James P. Bailey, Administrator and Chief Executive Officer

HOLDENVILLE GENERAL HOSPITAL (C, 27 beds) 100 Crestview Drive, Holdenville, OK Zip 74848–9700; tel. 405/379–6631; Joseph J. Mitchell, Chief Executive Officer and Administrator

KINGFISHER REGIONAL HOSPITAL (C, 25 beds) 500 South Ninth Street, Kingfisher, OK Zip 73750, Mailing Address: Box 59, Zip 73750–0059; tel. 405/375–3141; Steven G. Daniel, Administrator

LOGAN HOSPITAL AND MEDICAL CENTER (C, 32 beds) Highway 33 West at Academy Road, Guthrie, OK Zip 73044, Mailing Address: P.O. Box 1017, Zip 73044; tel. 405/282–6700; James R. Caton, Chief Executive Officer

MCCURTAIN MEMORIAL HOSPITAL (C, 89 beds) 1301 Lincoln, Idabel, OK Zip 74745; tel. 405/286–7623; Ronald Campbell, Administrator

PERRY MEMORIAL HOSPITAL (C, 28 beds) 501 14th Street, Perry, OK Zip 73077–5099; tel. 405/336–3541; Judith K. Feuquay, Chief Executive Officer

PURCELL MUNICIPAL HOSPITAL (C, 22 beds) 1500 North Green Avenue, Purcell, OK Zip 73080, Mailing Address: P.O. Box 511, Zip 73080–0511; tel. 405/527–6524; Joe Duerr, Administrator

For explanation of codes following names, see page B2.
★ Indicates Type III membership in the American Hospital Association.

© 1997 AHA Guide   Networks, Health Care Systems and Alliances   **B127**

SAYRE MEMORIAL HOSPITAL (C, 46 beds) 501 East Washington Street, Sayre, OK Zip 73662, Mailing Address: Box 680, Zip 73662; tel. 405/928–5541; Larry Anderson, Administrator

SEMINOLE MUNICIPAL HOSPITAL (C, 39 beds) 606 West Evans Street, Seminole, OK Zip 74868, Mailing Address: P.O. Box 2130, Zip 74818–2130; tel. 405/382–0600; Stephen R. Schoaps, Chief Executive Officer

SHARE MEDICAL CENTER (C, 120 beds) 800 Share Drive, Alva, OK Zip 73717, Mailing Address: P.O. Box 727, Zip 73717–0727; tel. 405/327–2800; Barbara Oestmann, Chief Executive Officer

TAHLEQUAH CITY HOSPITAL (C, 63 beds) 1400 East Downing Street, Tahlequah, OK Zip 74464, Mailing Address: Box 1008, Zip 74465–1008; tel. 918/456–0641; L. Gene Matthews, Chief Executive Officer

WATONGA MUNICIPAL HOSPITAL (C, 24 beds) 500 North Nash Boulevard, Watonga, OK Zip 73772–0370, Mailing Address: Box 370, Zip 73772–0370; tel. 405/623–7211; Terry Buckner, Administrator

WOODWARD HOSPITAL AND HEALTH CENTER (C, 68 beds) 900 17th Street, Woodward, OK Zip 73801; tel. 405/256–5511; Warren K. Spellman, Administrator

PENNSYLVANIA: BERWICK HOSPITAL CENTER (C, 409 beds) 701 East 16th Street, Berwick, PA Zip 18603–2397; tel. 717/759–5000; Thomas R. Sphatt, President and Chief Executive Officer

BROWNSVILLE GENERAL HOSPITAL (C, 116 beds) 125 Simpson Road, Brownsville, PA Zip 15417; tel. 412/785–7200; Richard D. Constantine, Chief Executive Officer

CARLISLE HOSPITAL (C, 183 beds) 246 Parker Street, Carlisle, PA Zip 17013–0310; tel. 717/249–1212; Michael J. Halstead, President and Chief Executive Officer

CLARION HOSPITAL (C, 88 beds) One Hospital Drive, Clarion, PA Zip 16214; tel. 814/226–9500; John J. Shepard, President and Chief Executive Officer

CORRY MEMORIAL HOSPITAL (C, 55 beds) 612 West Smith Street, Corry, PA Zip 16407–1196; tel. 814/664–4641; Joseph T. Hodges, President

J. C. BLAIR MEMORIAL HOSPITAL (C, 104 beds) Warm Springs Avenue, Huntingdon, PA Zip 16652; tel. 814/643–2290; Richard E. D'Alberto, Chief Executive Officer

JERSEY SHORE HOSPITAL (C, 64 beds) 1020 Thompson Street, Jersey Shore, PA Zip 17740–0689; tel. 717/398–0100; Louis A. Ditzel Jr., President and Chief Executive Officer

LOCK HAVEN HOSPITAL (C, 195 beds) 24 Cree Drive, Lock Haven, PA Zip 17745; tel. 717/893–5000; Gary R. Rhoads, President and Chief Executive Officer

MEMORIAL HOSPITAL (C, 99 beds) One Hospital Drive, Towanda, PA Zip 18848–9767; tel. 717/265–2191; Gary A. Baker, President

METRO HEALTH CENTER (C, 112 beds) 252 West 11th Street, Erie, PA Zip 16501; tel. 814/870–3400; J. B. Frith, Chief Executive Officer

MINER'S MEMORIAL MEDICAL CENTER (C, 110 beds) 360 West Ruddle, Coaldale, PA Zip 18218–0067, Mailing Address: P.O. Box 67, Zip 18218–0067; tel. 717/645–2131; Michael R. Miller, President and Chief Executive Officer

MINERS HOSPITAL NORTHERN CAMBRIA (C, 40 beds) 2205 Crawford Avenue, Spangler, PA Zip 15775; tel. 814/948–7171; Roger P. Winn, Chief Executive Officer

OHIO VALLEY GENERAL HOSPITAL (C, 102 beds) 25 Heckel Road, McKees Rocks, PA Zip 15136–1694; tel. 412/777–6161; William Provenzano, President

POTTSVILLE HOSPITAL AND WARNE CLINIC (C, 196 beds) 420 South Jackson Street, Pottsville, PA Zip 17901–3692; tel. 717/621–5000; Donald R. Gintzig, President and Chief Executive Officer

TYRONE HOSPITAL (C, 59 beds) One Hospital Drive, Tyrone, PA Zip 16686–1898; tel. 814/684–1255; Philip J. Stoner, Chief Executive Officer

SOUTH CAROLINA: ABBEVILLE COUNTY MEMORIAL HOSPITAL (C, 48 beds) Highway 72, Abbeville, SC Zip 29620–0887, Mailing Address: P.O. Box 887, Zip 29620; tel. 864/459–5011; Bruce P. Bailey, Administrator

CAROLINAS HOSPITAL SYSTEM (O, 316 beds) 121 East Cedar Street, Florence, SC Zip 29501, Mailing Address: P.O. Box 100550, Zip 29501–0549; tel. 803/661–3000; J. Michael Cowling, Chief Executive Officer

CAROLINAS HOSPITAL SYSTEM–KINGSTREE (O, 47 beds) 500 Nelson Boulevard, Kingstree, SC Zip 29556, Mailing Address: P.O. Drawer 568, Zip 29556–0568; tel. 803/354–9661; Richard L. Gamber, Administrator

CAROLINAS HOSPITAL SYSTEM–LAKE CITY (O, 40 beds) U.S. Highway 52 North, Lake City, SC Zip 29560–1029, Mailing Address: P.O. Box 1029, Zip 29560–1029; tel. 803/394–2036; Richard L. Gamber, Administrator

GEORGETOWN MEMORIAL HOSPITAL (C, 131 beds) 606 Black River Road, Georgetown, SC Zip 29440, Mailing Address: Drawer 1718, Zip 29442–1718; tel. 803/527–7000; Paul D. Gatens Sr., Administrator

LAURENS COUNTY HEALTHCARE SYSTEM (C, 216 beds) Highway 76 West, Clinton, SC Zip 29325, Mailing Address: P.O. Box 976, Zip 29325–0976; tel. 864/833–9100; Michael A. Kozar, Chief Executive Officer

MARY BLACK MEMORIAL HOSPITAL (O, 197 beds) 1700 Skylyn Drive, Spartanburg, SC Zip 29307, Mailing Address: Box 3217, Zip 29304–3217; tel. 864/573–3000; Ronald J. Vigus, Chief Executive Officer

NEWBERRY COUNTY MEMORIAL HOSPITAL (C, 75 beds) 2669 Kinard Street, Newberry, SC Zip 29108–0497, Mailing Address: P.O. Box 497, Zip 29108–0497; tel. 803/276–7570; Lynn W. Beasley, President and Chief Executive Officer

REGIONAL MEDICAL CENTER OF ORANGEBURG AND CALHOUN COUNTIES (C, 295 beds) 3000 St. Matthews Road, Orangeburg, SC Zip 29118–1470; tel. 803/533–2200; Thomas C. Dandridge, President

TUOMEY REGIONAL MEDICAL CENTER (C, 206 beds) 129 North Washington Street, Sumter, SC Zip 29150–4983; tel. 803/778–9000; Jay Cox, President and Chief Executive Officer

WALLACE THOMSON HOSPITAL (C, 107 beds) 322 West South Street, Union, SC Zip 29379–2857, Mailing Address: Box 789, Zip 29379; tel. 864/429–2600; Harrell L. Connelly, Chief Executive Officer

SOUTH DAKOTA: HURON REGIONAL MEDICAL CENTER (C, 55 beds) 172 Fourth Street S.E., Huron, SD Zip 57350–2590; tel. 605/353–6200; John L. Single, Chief Executive Officer

TENNESSEE: CITY OF MILAN HOSPITAL (C, 62 beds) 4039 South Highland, Milan, TN Zip 38358; tel. 901/686–1591; Mark D. Le Neave, Chief Executive Officer

LINCOLN REGIONAL HOSPITAL (C, 63 beds) 700 West Maple Street, Fayetteville, TN Zip 37334; tel. 615/438–1111; Gary G. Kendrick, Chief Executive Officer

MACON COUNTY GENERAL HOSPITAL (C, 43 beds) 204 Medical Drive, Lafayette, TN Zip 37083, Mailing Address: P.O. Box 378, Zip 37083; tel. 615/666–2147; Dennis A. Wolford, FACHE, Administrator

RHEA MEDICAL CENTER (C, 125 beds) 7900 Rhea County Highway, Dayton, TN Zip 37321; tel. 423/775–1121; Kennedy L. Croom Jr., Administrator and Chief Executive Officer

WELLMONT HEALTH SYSTEM–BRISTOL (C, 339 beds) 1 Medical Park Boulevard, Bristol, TN Zip 37620; tel. 423/844–4200; Randall M. Olson, Administrator

WELLMONT HEALTH SYSTEM–HOLSTON VALLEY (C, 384 beds) West Ravine Street, Kingsport, TN Zip 37662–0224, Mailing Address: Box 238, Zip 37662–0224; tel. 423/224–5001; Louis H. Bremer, President and Chief Executive Officer

TEXAS: ABILENE REGIONAL MEDICAL CENTER (O, 160 beds) 6250 Highway 83–84 at Antilley Road, Abilene, TX Zip 79606; tel. 915/695–9900; Woody Gilliland, Chief Executive Officer

BRAZOSPORT MEMORIAL HOSPITAL (C, 156 beds) 100 Medical Drive, Lake Jackson, TX Zip 77566–9983; tel. 409/297–4411; Wesley W. Oswald, Chief Executive Officer

CAMPBELL HEALTH SYSTEM (C, 78 beds) 713 East Anderson Street, Weatherford, TX Zip 76086–9971; tel. 817/596–8751; John B. Millstead, Chief Executive Officer

DALLAS–FORT WORTH MEDICAL CENTER (C, 162 beds) 2709 Hospital Boulevard, Grand Prairie, TX Zip 75051–1083; tel. 972/641–5000; Robert A. Ficken, Chief Executive Officer and Chief Financial Officer

DOCTORS HOSPITAL (C, 72 beds) 5500 39th Street, Groves, TX Zip 77619–9805; tel. 409/962–5733; John Isbell, Chief Executive Officer

FORT DUNCAN MEDICAL CENTER (C, 71 beds) 350 South Adams Street, Eagle Pass, TX Zip 78852; tel. 210/757–7501; Don Spaulding, Administrator and Chief Executive Officer

For explanation of codes following names, see page B2.
★ Indicates Type III membership in the American Hospital Association.

© 1997 AHA Guide

HENDERSON MEMORIAL HOSPITAL (C, 96 beds) 300 Wilson Street, Henderson, TX Zip 75652; tel. 903/657–7541; George T. Roberts Jr., Chief Executive Officer

HIGHLAND LAKES MEDICAL CENTER (C, 42 beds) Highway 281 South, Burnet, TX Zip 78611, Mailing Address: P.O. Box 840, Zip 78611; tel. 512/756–6000; James R. Giffin, Interim Administrator

HUNTSVILLE MEMORIAL HOSPITAL (C, 130 beds) 3000 I–45, Huntsville, TX Zip 77340, Mailing Address: P.O. Box 4001, Zip 77342–4001; tel. 409/291–3411; Ralph E. Beaty, Administrator

MISSION HOSPITAL (C, 110 beds) 900 South Bryan Road, Mission, TX Zip 78572; tel. 210/580–9000; Paul H. Ballard, Chief Executive Officer

TITUS REGIONAL MEDICAL CENTER (C, 165 beds) 2001 North Jefferson, Mount Pleasant, TX Zip 75455; tel. 903/577–6000; Steven K. Jacobson, Chief Executive Officer

VERMONT: NORTHEASTERN VERMONT REGIONAL HOSPITAL (C, 64 beds) Hospital Drive, Saint Johnsbury, VT Zip 05819–9962, Mailing Address: P.O. Box 905, Zip 05819–9962; tel. 802/748–8141; Paul R. Bengtson, Chief Executive Officer

NORTHWESTERN MEDICAL CENTER (C, 70 beds) Fairfield Street, Saint Albans, VT Zip 05478–1004, Mailing Address: Box 1370, Zip 05478; tel. 802/524–5911; Peter A. Hofstetter, Chief Executive Officer

VIRGINIA: BUCHANAN GENERAL HOSPITAL (C, 99 beds) Grundy, VA Mailing Address: Route 5, Box 20, Zip 24614–9611; tel. 540/935–1000; John West, Administrator

GREENSVILLE MEMORIAL HOSPITAL (C, 130 beds) 214 Weaver Avenue, Emporia, VA Zip 23847–1482; tel. 804/348–2000; Rosemary C. Check, Chief Executive Officer

HALIFAX REGIONAL HOSPITAL (C, 157 beds) 2204 Wilborn Avenue, South Boston, VA Zip 24592; tel. 804/575–3100; Chris A. Lumsden, Administrator

MEMORIAL HOSPITAL OF MARTINSVILLE AND HENRY COUNTY (C, 152 beds) 320 Hospital Drive, Martinsville, VA Zip 24112–1981, Mailing Address: Box 4788, Zip 24115–4788; tel. 540/666–7200; Joseph Roach, Executive Director

RICHMOND EYE AND EAR HOSPITAL (C, 32 beds) 1001 East Marshall Street, Richmond, VA Zip 23219; tel. 804/775–4500; William E. Holmes, Chief Executive Officer

SOUTHSIDE REGIONAL MEDICAL CENTER (C, 287 beds) 801 South Adams Street, Petersburg, VA Zip 23803–5133; tel. 804/862–5000; David S. Dunham, President

WASHINGTON: KADLEC MEDICAL CENTER (C, 125 beds) 888 Swift Boulevard, Richland, WA Zip 99352–9974; tel. 509/946–4611; Marcel Loh, President and Chief Executive Officer

WEST VIRGINIA: CITY HOSPITAL (C, 163 beds) Dry Run Road, Martinsburg, WV Zip 25401, Mailing Address: P.O. Box 1418, Zip 25402–1418; tel. 304/264–1000; Peter L. Mulford, Administrator

FAIRMONT GENERAL HOSPITAL (C, 249 beds) 1325 Locust Avenue, Fairmont, WV Zip 26554–1435; tel. 304/367–7100; Richard W. Graham, FACHE, President

PRESTON MEMORIAL HOSPITAL (C, 60 beds) 300 South Price Street, Kingwood, WV Zip 26537–1495; tel. 304/329–1400; Raymond E. Wood, President and Chief Executive Officer

WISCONSIN: APPLE RIVER HOSPITAL (C, 10 beds) 230 Deronda Street, Amery, WI Zip 54001–1407; tel. 715/268–7151; Michael Karuschak Jr., Administrator

OCONTO MEMORIAL HOSPITAL (C, 17 beds) 405 First Street, Oconto, WI Zip 54153; tel. 414/834–8800; Steve Dewoody, Chief Executive Officer

RIVERSIDE MEDICAL CENTER (C, 40 beds) 800 Riverside Drive, Waupaca, WI Zip 54981–1999; tel. 715/258–1000; Jan V. Carrell, Chief Executive Officer

WYOMING: CAMPBELL COUNTY MEMORIAL HOSPITAL (C, 119 beds) 501 South Burma Avenue, Gillette, WY Zip 82716, Mailing Address: Box 3011, Zip 82717; tel. 307/682–8811; David Crow, Chief Executive Officer

WEST PARK HOSPITAL (C, 171 beds) 707 Sheridan Avenue, Cody, WY Zip 82414; tel. 307/527–7501; Gary Bishop, Administrator

Owned, leased, sponsored:	18 hospitals	3106 beds
Contract–managed:	239 hospitals	24492 beds
Totals:	257 hospitals	27598 beds

0405: RAMSAY HEALTH CARE, INC. (IO)
1 Alhambra Plaza, Suite 750, Coral Gobles, FL Zip 33134; tel. 305/569–6993; Bert Cibran, President and Chief Operating Officer

ALABAMA: HILL CREST BEHAVIORAL HEALTH SERVICES (O, 100 beds) 6869 Fifth Avenue South, Birmingham, AL Zip 35212; tel. 205/833–9000; Steve McCabe, Chief Executive Officer

ARIZONA: DESERT VISTA BEHAVIORAL HEALTH SERVICES (L, 119 beds) 570 West Brown Road, Mesa, AZ Zip 85201; tel. 602/962–3900; Allen S. Nohre, Chief Executive Officer

FLORIDA: GULF COAST TREATMENT CENTER (O, 79 beds) 1015 Mar–Walt Drive, Fort Walton Beach, FL Zip 32547; tel. 904/863–4160; Raul D. Ruelas, M.D., Administrator

LOUISIANA: BAYOU OAKS HOSPITAL (L, 86 beds) 8134 Main Street, Houma, LA Zip 70360, Mailing Address: P.O. Box 4374, Zip 70361–4374; tel. 504/876–2020; George H. Perry, Ph.D., Chief Executive Officer

GREENBRIER HOSPITAL (O, 66 beds) 201 Greenbrier Boulevard, Covington, LA Zip 70433; tel. 504/893–2970; Pam McCullough Broughton, Chief Executive Officer

MICHIGAN: HAVENWYCK HOSPITAL (O, 120 beds) 1525 University Drive, Auburn Hills, MI Zip 48326–2675; tel. 810/373–9200; Robert A. Kercorian, Chief Executive Officer

MISSOURI: HEARTLAND BEHAVIORAL HEALTH SERVICES (O, 60 beds) 1500 West Ashland Street, Nevada, MO Zip 64772; tel. 417/667–2666; Eugene Hastings, Chief Executive Officer

NORTH CAROLINA: BRYNN MARR BEHAVIORAL HEALTHCARE SYSTEM (O, 76 beds) 192 Village Drive, Jacksonville, NC Zip 28546; tel. 910/577–1400; Dale Armstrong, Chief Executive Officer

OKLAHOMA: MEADOWLAKE BEHAVIORAL HEALTH SYSTEM (O, 50 beds) 2216 South Van Buren, Enid, OK Zip 73703, Mailing Address: P.O. Box 5409, Zip 73702; tel. 405/234–2220; Dave Lamerton, Chief Executive Officer

SOUTH CAROLINA: COASTAL CAROLINA HOSPITAL (O, 27 beds) 152 Waccamaw Medical Park Drive, Conway, SC Zip 29526; tel. 803/347–7156; Dale Armstrong, Chief Executive Officer

TEXAS: HAVEN HOSPITAL (O, 27 beds) 800 Kirnwood Drive, De Soto, TX Zip 75115–2092; tel. 972/709–3700; Sheila C. Kelly, R.N., MS, Chief Executive Officer

MISSION VISTA BEHAVIORAL HEALTH SYSTEM (L, 30 beds) 14747 Jones Maltsberger, San Antonio, TX Zip 78247–3713; tel. 210/490–0000; James M. Hunt, Chief Executive Officer

UTAH: BENCHMARK BEHAVIORAL HEALTH SYSTEMS (O, 68 beds) 592 West 1350 South, Woods Cross, UT Zip 84087–1665; tel. 801/299–5300; Richard O. Hurt, Ph.D., Chief Executive Officer

WEST VIRGINIA: CHESTNUT RIDGE HOSPITAL (O, 70 beds) 930 Chestnut Ridge Road, Morgantown, WV Zip 26505; tel. 304/293–4000; Lawrence J. Drake, Chief Executive Officer

Owned, leased, sponsored:	14 hospitals	978 beds
Contract–managed:	0 hospitals	0 beds
Totals:	14 hospitals	978 beds

4810: RIVERSIDE HEALTH SYSTEM (NP)
606 Denbigh Boulevard, Suite 601, Newport News, VA Zip 23608; tel. 757/875–7500; Nelson L. St. Clair, President

VIRGINIA: LAKE TAYLOR HOSPITAL (C, 304 beds) 1309 Kempsville Road, Norfolk, VA Zip 23502–2286; tel. 757/461–5001; David B. Tate Jr., President and Chief Executive Officer

RIVERSIDE REGIONAL MEDICAL CENTER (O, 576 beds) 500 J. Clyde Morris Boulevard, Newport News, VA Zip 23601–1976; tel. 757/594–2000; Gerald R. Brink, President and Chief Executive Officer

For explanation of codes following names, see page B2.
★ Indicates Type III membership in the American Hospital Association.

RIVERSIDE TAPPAHANNOCK HOSPITAL (O, 100 beds) Tappahannock, VA Mailing Address: Route 2, Box 612, Zip 22560; tel. 804/443–3311; Elizabeth J. Martin, Vice President and Administrator

RIVERSIDE WALTER REED HOSPITAL (O, 71 beds) Gloucester, VA Mailing Address: Route 17, Box 1130, Zip 23061–1130; tel. 804/693–8800; Grady W. Philips III, Vice President and Administrator

Owned, leased, sponsored:	3 hospitals	747 beds
Contract–managed:	1 hospital	304 beds
Totals:	4 hospitals	1051 beds

★0109: RURAL HEALTH MANAGEMENT CORPORATION (NP)
549 North 400 East, Nephi, UT Zip 84648; tel. 801/623–4924; Mark R. Stoddard, President

UTAH: ALLEN MEMORIAL HOSPITAL (L, 31 beds) 719 West 400 North Street, Moab, UT Zip 84532, Mailing Address: Box 998, Zip 84532; tel. 801/259–7191; Charles A. Davis, Administrator

CENTRAL VALLEY MEDICAL CENTER (L, 20 beds) 549 North 400 East, Nephi, UT Zip 84648; tel. 801/623–1242; Mark R. Stoddard, President

GUNNISON VALLEY HOSPITAL (C, 21 beds) 64 East 100 North, Gunnison, UT Zip 84634, Mailing Address: P.O. Box 759, Zip 84634; tel. 801/528–7246; Greg Rosenvall, Administrator

MILFORD VALLEY MEMORIAL HOSPITAL (C, 34 beds) 451 North Main Street, Milford, UT Zip 84751–0640, Mailing Address: Box 640, Zip 84751–0640; tel. 801/387–2411; John E. Gledhill, Administrator

TOOELE VALLEY REGIONAL MEDICAL CENTER (C, 122 beds) 211 South 100 East, Tooele, UT Zip 84074–2794; tel. 801/882–1697; Mark F. Dalley, Chief Executive Officer

Owned, leased, sponsored:	2 hospitals	51 beds
Contract–managed:	3 hospitals	177 beds
Totals:	5 hospitals	228 beds

★3855: RUSH–PRESBYTERIAN–ST. LUKE'S MEDICAL CENTER (NP)
1653 West Congress Parkway, Chicago, IL Zip 60612–3864; tel. 312/942–5000; Leo M. Henikoff, President

ILLINOIS: COPLEY MEMORIAL HOSPITAL (O, 140 beds) 2000 Ogden Avenue, Aurora, IL Zip 60504–4206; tel. 630/978–6200; D. Chet McKee, President

RUSH NORTH SHORE MEDICAL CENTER (O, 229 beds) 9600 Gross Point Road, Skokie, IL Zip 60076–1257; tel. 847/677–9600; John S. Frigo, President

RUSH–PRESBYTERIAN–ST. LUKE'S MEDICAL CENTER (O, 783 beds) 1653 West Congress Parkway, Chicago, IL Zip 60612–3833; tel. 312/942–5000; Leo M. Henikoff, President and Chief Executive Officer

Owned, leased, sponsored:	3 hospitals	1152 beds
Contract–managed:	0 hospitals	0 beds
Totals:	3 hospitals	1152 beds

0118: SAINT BARNABAS HEALTH CARE SYSTEM (NP)
94 Old Short Hills Road, Livingston, NJ Zip 07039; tel. 201/533–5000; Ronald Del Mauro, Chairman and Chief Executive Officer

NEW JERSEY: COMMUNITY KIMBALL HEALTH CARE SYSTEM (O, 510 beds) 99 Highway 37 West, Toms River, NJ Zip 08755–6423; tel. 908/240–8000; Kevin R. Burchill, Executive Director

IRVINGTON GENERAL HOSPITAL (O, 157 beds) 832 Chancellor Avenue, Irvington, NJ Zip 07111–0709; tel. 201/399–6000; Thomas A. Biga, Executive Director

KIMBALL MEDICAL CENTER (O, 292 beds) 600 River Avenue, Lakewood, NJ Zip 08701–5281; tel. 908/363–1900; Joanne Carrocino, Executive Director

MONMOUTH MEDICAL CENTER (O, 435 beds) 300 Second Avenue, Long Branch, NJ Zip 07740–6303; tel. 908/222–5200; Cynthia N. Sparer, Executive Director and Chief Operating Officer

NEWARK BETH ISRAEL MEDICAL CENTER (O, 451 beds) 201 Lyons Avenue, Newark, NJ 07112–2027; tel. 201/926–7000; Ronald W. Weitz, Executive Director

SAINT BARNABAS MEDICAL CENTER (O, 615 beds) 94 Old Short Hills Road, Livingston, NJ Zip 07039; tel. 201/533–5000; Ronald Del Mauro, Chairman and Chief Executive Officer

UNION HOSPITAL (O, 148 beds) 1000 Galloping Hill Road, Union, NJ Zip 07083–1652; tel. 908/687–1900; Kathryn W. Coyne, Executive Director and Chief Operating Officer

WAYNE GENERAL HOSPITAL (O, 146 beds) 224 Hamburg Turnpike, Wayne, NJ Zip 07470–2100; tel. 201/942–6900; Kenneth H. Kozloff, Executive Director

WEST HUDSON HOSPITAL (O, 217 beds) 206 Bergen Avenue, Kearny, NJ Zip 07032; tel. 201/955–7051; Carmen Bruce Alecci, Executive Director

Owned, leased, sponsored:	9 hospitals	2971 beds
Contract–managed:	0 hospitals	0 beds
Totals:	9 hospitals	2971 beds

0120: SAINT LUKE'S SHAWNEE MISSION HEALTH SYSTEM (NP)
10920 Elm Avenue, Kansas City, MO Zip 64134; tel. 816/932–3377; G. Richard Hastings, President and Chief Executive Officer

KANSAS: ANDERSON COUNTY HOSPITAL (O, 66 beds) 421 South Maple, Garnett, KS Zip 66032, Mailing Address: Box 309, Zip 66032; tel. 913/448–3131; James K. Johnson, Administrator

SHAWNEE MISSION MEDICAL CENTER (O, 333 beds) 9100 West 74th Street, Shawnee Mission, KS Zip 66204–4019, Mailing Address: Box 2923, Zip 66201–1323; tel. 913/676–2000; William G. Robertson, Senior Executive Officer

MISSOURI: CRITTENTON (O, 28 beds) 10918 Elm Avenue, Kansas City, MO Zip 64134–4199; tel. 816/765–6600; Robert D. Gray, Ed.D., Chief Executive Officer

SAINT LUKE'S HOSPITAL (O, 508 beds) 4400 Wornall Road, Kansas City, MO Zip 64111; tel. 816/932–2000; James M. Brophy, Senior Executive Officer

SAINT LUKE'S NORTHLAND HOSPITAL (O, 55 beds) 5830 N.W. Barry Road, Kansas City, MO Zip 64154–9988; tel. 816/891–6000; James M. Brophy, FACHE, Senior Executive Officer

WRIGHT MEMORIAL HOSPITAL (O, 48 beds) 701 East First Street, Trenton, MO Zip 64683–0648, Mailing Address: P.O. Box 628, Zip 64683–0628; tel. 816/359–5621; Johnnye L. Dennis, Chief Executive Officer

Owned, leased, sponsored:	6 hospitals	1038 beds
Contract–managed:	0 hospitals	0 beds
Totals:	6 hospitals	1038 beds

★2535: SAMARITAN HEALTH SYSTEM (NP)
1441 North 12th Street, Phoenix, AZ Zip 85006–2666; tel. 602/495–4000; James C. Crews, President and Chief Executive Officer

ARIZONA: DESERT SAMARITAN MEDICAL CENTER (O, 511 beds) 1400 South Dobson Road, Mesa, AZ Zip 85202–9879; tel. 602/835–3000; Bruce E. Pearson, Vice President and Chief Executive Officer

GOOD SAMARITAN REGIONAL MEDICAL CENTER (O, 714 beds) 1111 East McDowell Road, Phoenix, AZ Zip 85006, Mailing Address: Box 2989, Zip 85062; tel. 602/239–2000; Steven L. Seiler, Senior Vice President and Chief Executive Officer

HAVASU SAMARITAN REGIONAL HOSPITAL (O, 118 beds) 101 Civic Center Lane, Lake Havasu City, AZ Zip 86403; tel. 520/855–8185; Kevin P. Poorten, Vice President and Chief Executive Officer

MARYVALE SAMARITAN MEDICAL CENTER (O, 213 beds) 5102 West Campbell Avenue, Phoenix, AZ Zip 85031; tel. 602/848–5101; Robert H. Curry, Senior Vice President and Chief Executive Officer

PAGE HOSPITAL (C, 25 beds) North Navajo Drive and Vista Avenue, Page, AZ Zip 86040, Mailing Address: P.O. Box 1447, Zip 86040; tel. 520/645–2424; Preston M. Simmons, Administrator

---

For explanation of codes following names, see page B2.
★ Indicates Type III membership in the American Hospital Association.

Section B

SAMARITAN BEHAVIORAL HEALTH CENTER–SCOTTSDALE (O, 60 beds) 7575 East Earll Drive, Scottsdale, AZ Zip 85251–6998; tel. 602/941–7500; Robert F. Meyer, M.D., Chief Executive Officer

SAMARITAN–WENDY PAINE O'BRIEN TREATMENT CENTER (O, 23 beds) 5055 North 34th Street, Phoenix, AZ Zip 85018; tel. 602/955–6200; Mike Todd, Chief Executive Officer

THUNDERBIRD SAMARITAN MEDICAL CENTER (O, 227 beds) 5555 West Thunderbird Road, Glendale, AZ Zip 85306; tel. 602/588–5555; Robert H. Curry, Senior Vice President and Chief Executive Officer

CALIFORNIA: COLUMBIA SAN CLEMENTE HOSPITAL AND MEDICAL CENTER (O, 86 beds) 654 Camino De Los Mares, San Clemente, CA Zip 92673; tel. 714/496–1122; Tony Struthers, Chief Executive Officer

Owned, leased, sponsored:	8 hospitals	1952 beds
Contract–managed:	1 hospital	25 beds
Totals:	9 hospitals	1977 beds

★0037: SCOTTSDALE MEMORIAL HEALTH SYSTEMS, INC. (NP)
3621 Wells Fargo Avenue, Scottsdale, AZ Zip 85251; tel. 602/481–4324; Max Poll, President and Chief Executive Officer

ARIZONA: SCOTTSDALE MEMORIAL HOSPITAL–NORTH (O, 242 beds) 9003 East Shea Boulevard, Scottsdale, AZ Zip 85260; tel. 602/860–3000; Thomas J. Sadvary, FACHE, Senior Vice President and Administrator

SCOTTSDALE MEMORIAL HOSPITAL–OSBORN (O, 258 beds) 7400 East Osborn Road, Scottsdale, AZ Zip 85251; tel. 602/481–4000; David R. Carpenter, FACHE, Senior Vice President and Administrator

Owned, leased, sponsored:	2 hospitals	500 beds
Contract–managed:	0 hospitals	0 beds
Totals:	2 hospitals	500 beds

★1505: SCRIPPS HEALTH (NP)
4275 Campus Point Court, San Diego, CA Zip 92121, Mailing Address: P.O. Box 28, La Jolla, Zip 92038; tel. 619/678–7470; Martin B. Buser, Executive Vice President Health Services

CALIFORNIA: GREEN HOSPITAL OF SCRIPPS CLINIC (O, 165 beds) 10666 North Torrey Pines Road, La Jolla, CA Zip 92037–1093; tel. 619/455–9100; Glenn W. Chong, Senior Vice President and Administrator

SCRIPPS HOSPITAL–EAST COUNTY (O, 105 beds) 1688 East Main Street, El Cajon, CA Zip 92021; tel. 619/593–5600; Robin B. Brown, Vice President and Administrator

SCRIPPS MEMORIAL HOSPITAL–CHULA VISTA (O, 159 beds) 435 H Street, Chula Vista, CA Zip 91912–1537, Mailing Address: Box 1537, Zip 91910–1537; tel. 619/691–7000; Thomas A. Gammiere, Vice President and Administrator

SCRIPPS MEMORIAL HOSPITAL–ENCINITAS (O, 145 beds) 354 Santa Fe Drive, Encinitas, CA Zip 92024, Mailing Address: P.O. Box 817, Zip 92023; tel. 619/753–6501; Gerald E. Bracht, Vice President and Administrator

SCRIPPS MEMORIAL HOSPITAL–LA JOLLA (O, 431 beds) 9888 Genesee Avenue, La Jolla, CA Zip 92037–1276, Mailing Address: Box 28, Zip 92038–0028; tel. 619/626–4123; Glenn W. Chong, Senior Vice President and Administrator

SCRIPPS MERCY MEDICAL CENTER (O, 417 beds) 4077 Fifth Avenue, San Diego, CA Zip 92103–2180; tel. 619/260–7101; Nancy Wilson, Senior Vice President and Regional Administrator

Owned, leased, sponsored:	6 hospitals	1422 beds
Contract–managed:	0 hospitals	0 beds
Totals:	6 hospitals	1422 beds

★2565: SENTARA HEALTH SYSTEM (NP)
6015 Poplar Hall Drive, Norfolk, VA Zip 23502; tel. 757/455–7000; David L. Bernd, President and Chief Executive Officer

VIRGINIA: SENTARA BAYSIDE HOSPITAL (O, 141 beds) 800 Independence Boulevard, Virginia Beach, VA Zip 23455–6076; tel. 757/363–6100; Virginia Bogue, Site Administrator

SENTARA HAMPTON GENERAL HOSPITAL (O, 242 beds) 3120 Victoria Boulevard, Hampton, VA Zip 23661, Mailing Address: Drawer 640, Zip 23669; tel. 804/727–7000; Les A. Donahue, President and Chief Executive Officer

SENTARA LEIGH HOSPITAL (O, 220 beds) 830 Kempsville Road, Norfolk, VA Zip 23502; tel. 757/466–6000; Darleen S. Anderson, R.N., MSN, Site Administrator

SENTARA NORFOLK GENERAL HOSPITAL (O, 598 beds) 600 Gresham Drive, Norfolk, VA Zip 23507–1999; tel. 804/668–3000; Roger M. Eitelman, Site Administrator

WILLIAMSBURG COMMUNITY HOSPITAL (C, 100 beds) 301 Monticello Avenue, Williamsburg, VA Zip 23187–8700, Mailing Address: Box 8700, Zip 23187–8700; tel. 757/259–6000; Les A. Donahue, President and Chief Executive Officer

Owned, leased, sponsored:	4 hospitals	1201 beds
Contract–managed:	1 hospital	100 beds
Totals:	5 hospitals	1301 beds

★4025: SERVANTCOR (CC)
1475 Harvard Drive, Kankakee, IL Zip 60901–9465; tel. 815/937–2034; Joseph S. Feth, President

ILLINOIS: CENTRAL COMMUNITY HOSPITAL (C, 33 beds) 335 East Fifth Avenue, Clifton, IL Zip 60927, Mailing Address: Box 68, Zip 60927; tel. 815/694–2392; Steve Wilder, President and Chief Executive Officer

COVENANT MEDICAL CENTER (O, 268 beds) 1400 West Park Street, Urbana, IL Zip 61801; tel. 217/337–2000; Joseph W. Beard, President and Chief Executive Officer

ST. MARY'S HOSPITAL (O, 209 beds) 500 West Court Street, Kankakee, IL Zip 60901; tel. 815/937–2400; Allan C. Sonduck, President and Chief Executive Officer

Owned, leased, sponsored:	2 hospitals	477 beds
Contract–managed:	1 hospital	33 beds
Totals:	3 hospitals	510 beds

0111: SHANDS HEALTH SYSTEM, UNIVERSITY OF FLORIDA HEALTH SCIENCE CENTER (NP)
1600 S.W. Archer Road, Gainesville, FL Zip 32610–0326; tel. 352/395–0421; J. Richard Gaintner, M.D., Chief Executive Officer

FLORIDA: SHANDS AT AGH (O, 269 beds) 801 S.W. Second Avenue, Gainesville, FL Zip 32601; tel. 352/372–4321; Robert B. Williams, Administrator

SHANDS AT LAKE SHORE (O, 128 beds) 560 East Franklin Street, Lake City, FL Zip 32055, Mailing Address: Box 1989, Zip 32056–1989; tel. 904/755–3200; Linda A. McKnew, R.N., Chief Operating Officer

SHANDS AT LIVE OAK (O, 16 beds) 1100 S.W. 11th Avenue, Live Oak, FL Zip 32060, Mailing Address: P.O. Drawer X, Zip 32060; tel. 904/362–1413; Rhonda Sherrod, Administrator

SHANDS AT STARKE (O, 23 beds) 922 East Call Street, Starke, FL Zip 32091, Mailing Address: P.O. Box 1210, Zip 32091–1210; tel. 904/964–6000; Jeannie Baker, Chief Operating Officer

SHANDS AT THE UNIVERSITY OF FLORIDA (O, 564 beds) 1600 S.W. Archer Road, Gainesville, FL Zip 32610–0326, Mailing Address: P.O. Box 100326, Zip 32610–0326; tel. 352/395–0111; J. Richard Gaintner, M.D., Chief Executive Officer

UPREACH REHABILITATION HOSPITAL (O, 40 beds) 8900 N.W. 39th Avenue, Gainesville, FL Zip 32606–5625; tel. 352/338–0091; Cynthia M. Toth, Administrator

Owned, leased, sponsored:	6 hospitals	1040 beds
Contract–managed:	0 hospitals	0 beds
Totals:	6 hospitals	1040 beds

2065: SHARP HEALTHCARE (NP)
3131 Berger Avenue, Suite 100, San Diego, CA Zip 92123; tel. 619/541–4000

For explanation of codes following names, see page B2.
★ Indicates Type III membership in the American Hospital Association.

CALIFORNIA: GROSSMONT HOSPITAL (C, 377 beds) 5555 Grossmont Center Drive, La Mesa, CA Zip 91942, Mailing Address: Box 158, Zip 91944–0158; tel. 619/465–0711; Michele T. Tarbet, R.N., Chief Executive Officer

SHARP CABRILLO HOSPITAL (O, 227 beds) 3475 Kenyon Street, San Diego, CA Zip 92110–5067; tel. 619/221–3400; Randi Larsson, Senior Vice President and Administrator

SHARP CHULA VISTA MEDICAL CENTER (O, 306 beds) 751 Medical Center Court, Chula Vista, CA Zip 91911, Mailing Address: Box 1297, Zip 91912; tel. 619/482–5800; Britt Berrett, Chief Executive Officer

SHARP CORONADO HOSPITAL (C, 195 beds) 250 Prospect Place, Coronado, CA Zip 92118; tel. 619/522–3600; Marcia K. Hall, Chief Executive Officer

SHARP HEALTHCARE MURRIETA (O, 91 beds) 25500 Medical Center Drive, Murrieta, CA Zip 92562–5966; tel. 909/696–6000; Juanice Lovett, Chief Executive Officer

SHARP MEMORIAL HOSPITAL (O, 488 beds) 7901 Frost Street, San Diego, CA Zip 92123–2788; tel. 619/541–3400; Dan Gross, Chief Executive Officer

Owned, leased, sponsored:	4 hospitals	1112 beds
Contract–managed:	2 hospitals	572 beds
Totals:	6 hospitals	1684 beds

★4125: SHRINERS HOSPITALS FOR CHILDREN (NP)
2900 Rocky Point Drive, Tampa, FL Zip 33607–1435, Mailing Address: Box 31356, Zip 33631–3356; tel. 813/281–0300; Joseph E. Melchiorre Jr., CHE, Executive Administrator

SHRINERS HOSPITALS FOR CHILDREN, LOS ANGELES (O, 50 beds) 3160 Geneva Street, Los Angeles, CA Zip 90020–1199; tel. 213/388–3151; Paul D. Hargis, Administrator

SHRINERS HOSPITALS FOR CHILDREN, SAN FRANCISCO (O, 48 beds) 1701 19th Avenue, San Francisco, CA Zip 94122–4599; tel. 415/665–1100; Margaret Bryan–Williams, Administrator

FLORIDA: SHRINERS HOSPITALS FOR CHILDREN, TAMPA (O, 60 beds) 12502 North Pine Drive, Tampa, FL Zip 33612–9499; tel. 813/972–2250; John Holtz, Administrator

HAWAII: SHRINERS HOSPITALS FOR CHILDREN, HONOLULU (O, 40 beds) 1310 Punahou Street, Honolulu, HI Zip 96826–1099; tel. 808/941–4466; James B. Brasel, Administrator

ILLINOIS: SHRINERS HOSPITALS FOR CHILDREN–CHICAGO (O, 60 beds) 2211 North Oak Park Avenue, Chicago, IL Zip 60607–3392; tel. 773/622–5400; A. James Spang, Administrator

KENTUCKY: SHRINERS HOSPITALS FOR CHILDREN–LEXINGTON UNIT (O, 50 beds) 1900 Richmond Road, Lexington, KY Zip 40502; tel. 606/266–2101; Tony Lewgood, Administrator

LOUISIANA: SHRINERS HOSPITALS FOR CHILDREN, SHREVEPORT (O, 45 beds) 3100 Samford Avenue, Shreveport, LA Zip 71103; tel. 318/222–5704; Thomas R. Schneider, Administrator

MASSACHUSETTS: SHRINERS HOSPITALS FOR CHILDREN, BURNS INSTITUTE BOSTON UNIT (O, 30 beds) 51 Blossom Street, Boston, MA Zip 02114–2699; tel. 617/722–3000; Robert F. Bories Jr., FACHE, Administrator

SHRINERS HOSPITALS FOR CHILDREN, SPRINGFIELD (O, 40 beds) 516 Carew Street, Springfield, MA Zip 01104–2396; tel. 413/787–2000; Mark L. Niederpruem, Administrator

MINNESOTA: SHRINERS HOSPITALS FOR CHILDREN, TWIN CITIES UNIT (O, 40 beds) 2025 East River Road, Minneapolis, MN Zip 55414–3696; tel. 612/335–5300; Laurence E. Johnson, Administrator

MISSOURI: SHRINERS HOSPITALS FOR CHILDREN, ST. LOUIS (O, 76 beds) 2001 South Lindbergh Boulevard, Saint Louis, MO Zip 63131–3597; tel. 314/432–3600; Carolyn P. Golden, Administrator

OHIO: SHRINERS HOSPITALS FOR CHILDREN, CINCINNATI BURNS INSTITUTE (O, 30 beds) 3229 Burnet Avenue, Cincinnati, OH Zip 45229–3095; tel. 513/872–6000; Ronald R. Hitzler, Administrator

OREGON: SHRINERS HOSPITALS FOR CHILDREN, PORTLAND (O, 25 beds) 3101 S.W. Sam Jackson Park Road, Portland, OR Zip 97201; tel. 503/241–5090; Nancy Jones, Administrator

PENNSYLVANIA: SHRINERS HOSPITALS FOR CHILDREN, ERIE UNIT (O, 30 beds) 1645 West 8th Street, Erie, PA Zip 16505; tel. 814/875–8700; Richard W. Brzuz, Administrator

SHRINERS HOSPITALS FOR CHILDREN, PHILADELPHIA UNIT (O, 80 beds) 8400 Roosevelt Boulevard, Philadelphia, PA Zip 19152–1299; tel. 215/332–4500; Sharon J. Rajnic, Administrator

SOUTH CAROLINA: SHRINERS HOSPITALS FOR CHILDREN, GREENVILLE (O, 60 beds) 950 West Faris Road, Greenville, SC Zip 29605–4277; tel. 864/271–3444; Gary F. Fraley, Administrator

TEXAS: SHRINERS HOSPITALS FOR CHILDREN, GALVESTON BURNS INSTITUTE (O, 30 beds) 815 Market Street, Galveston, TX Zip 77550–2725; tel. 409/770–6600; John A. Swartwout, Administrator

SHRINERS HOSPITALS FOR CHILDREN, HOUSTON (O, 40 beds) 6977 Main Street, Houston, TX Zip 77030; tel. 713/797–1616; Steven B. Reiter, Administrator

UTAH: SHRINERS HOSPITALS FOR CHILDREN–INTERMOUNTAIN (O, 40 beds) Fairfax Road and Virginia Street, Salt Lake City, UT Zip 84103–4399; tel. 801/536–3500; Douglas P. Schweikhart, Administrator

WASHINGTON: SHRINERS HOSPITALS FOR CHILDREN–SPOKANE (O, 30 beds) 911 West Fifth Avenue, Spokane, WA Zip 99204–2901, Mailing Address: P.O. Box 2472, Zip 99210–2472; tel. 509/455–7844; Charles R. Young, Administrator

Owned, leased, sponsored:	20 hospitals	904 beds
Contract–managed:	0 hospitals	0 beds
Totals:	20 hospitals	904 beds

0067: SINGING RIVER HOSPITAL SYSTEM (NP)
2809 Denny Avenue, Pascagoula, MS Zip 39581; tel. 601/938–5062; Robert L. Lingle, Executive Director

MISSISSIPPI: OCEAN SPRINGS HOSPITAL (O, 95 beds) 3109 Bienville Boulevard, Ocean Springs, MS Zip 39564; tel. 601/872–1111; Dwight Rimes, Administrator

SINGING RIVER HOSPITAL (O, 314 beds) 2809 Denny Avenue, Pascagoula, MS Zip 39581; tel. 601/938–5000; James S. Kaigler, FACHE, Administrator

Owned, leased, sponsored:	2 hospitals	409 beds
Contract–managed:	0 hospitals	0 beds
Totals:	2 hospitals	409 beds

0078: SIOUX VALLEY HEALTH SYSTEM (NP)
1100 South Euclid Avenue, Sioux Falls, SD Zip 57105–0496; tel. 605/333–1000; Kelby K. Krabbenhoff, President

IOWA: MERRILL PIONEER COMMUNITY HOSPITAL (L, 30 beds) 801 South Greene Street, Rock Rapids, IA Zip 51246–1998; tel. 712/472–2591; Gordon Smith, Administrator

NORTHWEST IOWA HEALTH CENTER (L, 95 beds) 118 North Seventh Avenue, Sheldon, IA Zip 51201; tel. 712/324–5041; Charles R. Miller, Chief Executive Officer

MINNESOTA: ARNOLD MEMORIAL HEALTH CARE CENTER (C, 50 beds) 601 Louisiana Avenue, Adrian, MN Zip 56110–0279, Mailing Address: Box 279, Zip 56110–0279; tel. 507/483–2668; Gerald E. Carl, Administrator

CANBY COMMUNITY HEALTH SERVICES (L, 99 beds) 112 St. Olaf Avenue South, Canby, MN Zip 56220–1433; tel. 507/223–7277; Robert J. Salmon, Chief Executive Officer

JACKSON MEDICAL CENTER (C, 41 beds) 1430 North Highway, Jackson, MN Zip 56143–1098; tel. 507/847–2420; Charlotte Heitkamp, Chief Executive Officer

LUVERNE COMMUNITY HOSPITAL (C, 38 beds) 305 East Luverne Street, Luverne, MN Zip 56156–2519, Mailing Address: P.O. Box 1019, Zip 56156; tel. 507/283–2321; Gerald E. Carl, Administrator

MURRAY COUNTY MEMORIAL HOSPITAL (C, 30 beds) 2042 Juniper Avenue, Slayton, MN Zip 56172; tel. 507/836–6111; Jerry Bobeldyk, Administrator

TRACY MUNICIPAL HOSPITAL (C, 28 beds) 251 Fifth Street East, Tracy, MN Zip 56175–1536; tel. 507/629–3200; Thomas J. Quinlivan, Administrator

---

For explanation of codes following names, see page B2.
★ Indicates Type III membership in the American Hospital Association.

WESTBROOK HEALTH CENTER (C, 8 beds) 920 Bell Avenue, Westbrook, MN Zip 56183, Mailing Address: P.O. Box 188, Zip 56183–0188; tel. 507/274–6121; Judy Lichty, Administrator

WINDOM AREA HOSPITAL (C, 17 beds) Highways 60 and 71 North, Windom, MN Zip 56101, Mailing Address: P.O. Box 339, Zip 56101; tel. 507/831–2400; J. Stephen Pautler, CHE, Administrator

WORTHINGTON REGIONAL HOSPITAL (C, 83 beds) 1018 Sixth Avenue, Worthington, MN Zip 56187, Mailing Address: P.O. Box 997, Zip 56187; tel. 507/372–2941; Melvin J. Platt, Administrator

SOUTH DAKOTA: CANTON–INWOOD MEMORIAL HOSPITAL (L, 25 beds) 440 North Hiawatha Drive, Canton, SD Zip 57013–9404, Mailing Address: Rural Route 3, Box 7, Zip 57013; tel. 605/987–2621; John Devick, Chief Executive Officer

DAKOTA MEDICAL CENTER (L, 95 beds) 20 South Plum Street, Vermillion, SD Zip 57069; tel. 605/624–2611; Larry W. Veitz, Chief Executive Officer

DEUEL COUNTY MEMORIAL HOSPITAL (O, 20 beds) 701 Third Avenue South, Clear Lake, SD Zip 57226–1037, Mailing Address: P.O. Box 1037, Zip 57226–1037; tel. 605/874–2141; Robert J. Salmon, Interim Administrator

LAKE AREA HOSPITAL (C, 26 beds) North First Street, Webster, SD Zip 57274, Mailing Address: P.O. Box 489, Zip 57274–0489; tel. 605/345–3336; Donald J. Finn, Administrator

MID DAKOTA HOSPITAL (L, 54 beds) 300 South Byron Boulevard, Chamberlain, SD Zip 57325; tel. 605/734–5511; Mick Penticoff, Administrator

PIONEER MEMORIAL HOSPITAL (C, 77 beds) 315 North Washington Street, Viborg, SD Zip 57070, Mailing Address: P.O. Box 368, Zip 57070–0368; tel. 605/326–5161; Georgia Pokorney, Chief Executive Officer

SIOUX VALLEY HOSPITAL (O, 504 beds) 1100 South Euclid Avenue, Sioux Falls, SD Zip 57105–0496, Mailing Address: P.O. Box 5039, Zip 57117–5039; tel. 605/333–1000; Kelby K. Krabbenhoft, Chief Executive Officer

WINNER REGIONAL HEALTHCARE CENTER (O, 116 beds) 745 East Eighth Street, Winner, SD Zip 57580–2677, Mailing Address: Box 745, Zip 57580–0745; tel. 605/842–2110; Robert Houser, Chief Executive Officer

Owned, leased, sponsored:	9 hospitals	1038 beds
Contract–managed:	10 hospitals	398 beds
Totals:	19 hospitals	1436 beds

5995: SISTERS OF CHARITY CENTER (CC)
Mount St. Vincent on Hudson, New York, NY Zip 10471–1093; tel. 718/549–9200; Sister Elizabeth A. Vermaelen, President

NEW YORK: SAINT VINCENT'S HOSPITAL AND MEDICAL CENTER OF NEW YORK (S, 978 beds) 153 West 11th Street, New York, NY Zip 10011–8397; tel. 212/604–7000; Karl P. Adler, M.D., President and Chief Executive Officer

ST. JOSEPH'S MEDICAL CENTER (S, 394 beds) 127 South Broadway, Yonkers, NY Zip 10701–4080; tel. 914/378–7000; Sister Mary Linehan, President

Owned, leased, sponsored:	2 hospitals	1372 beds
Contract–managed:	0 hospitals	0 beds
Totals:	2 hospitals	1372 beds

★6095: SISTERS OF CHARITY HEALTH CARE SYSTEM CORPORATION (CC)
75 Vanderbilt Avenue, New York, NY Zip 10304–3850; tel. 718/354–5080; John J. DePierro, President and Chief Executive Officer

BAYLEY SETON HOSPITAL (S, 198 beds) 75 Vanderbilt Avenue, Staten Island, NY Zip 10304–3850; tel. 718/354–6000; Dominick M. Stanzione, Chief Operating Officer and Executive Vice President

ST. VINCENT'S MEDICAL CENTER OF RICHMOND (S, 440 beds) 355 Bard Avenue, Staten Island, NY Zip 10310–1699; tel. 718/876–1234; Dominick M. Stanzione, Executive Vice President

Owned, leased, sponsored:	2 hospitals	638 beds
Contract–managed:	0 hospitals	0 beds
Totals:	2 hospitals	638 beds

★5095: SISTERS OF CHARITY OF LEAVENWORTH HEALTH SERVICES CORPORATION (CC)
4200 South Fourth Street, Leavenworth, KS Zip 66048–5054; tel. 913/682–1338; Sister Marie Damian Glatt, President

CALIFORNIA: SAINT JOHN'S HOSPITAL AND HEALTH CENTER (O, 234 beds) 1328 22nd Street, Santa Monica, CA Zip 90404; tel. 310/829–5511; Sister Marie Madeleine Shonka, President

COLORADO: SAINT JOSEPH HOSPITAL (O, 394 beds) 1835 Franklin Street, Denver, CO Zip 80218; tel. 303/837–7111; Sister Marianna Bauder, President and Chief Executive Officer

ST. MARY'S HOSPITAL AND MEDICAL CENTER (O, 273 beds) 2635 North 7th Street, Grand Junction, CO Zip 81501–1628, Mailing Address: P.O. Box 1628, Zip 81502; tel. 970/244–2273; Sister Lynn Casey, President and Chief Executive Officer

KANSAS: PROVIDENCE MEDICAL CENTER (O, 219 beds) 8929 Parallel Parkway, Kansas City, KS Zip 66112–0430; tel. 913/596–4000; Francis V. Creeden Jr., President

SAINT JOHN HOSPITAL (O, 36 beds) 3500 South Fourth Street, Leavenworth, KS Zip 66048–5092; tel. 913/680–6000; Francis V. Creeden Jr., President

ST. FRANCIS HOSPITAL AND MEDICAL CENTER (O, 308 beds) 1700 West Seventh Street, Topeka, KS Zip 66606–1690; tel. 913/295–8000; Sister Loretto Marie Colwell, President

MONTANA: HOLY ROSARY HEALTH CENTER (O, 151 beds) 2600 Wilson, Miles City, MT Zip 59301; tel. 406/233–2600; H. Ray Gibbons, President and Chief Executive Officer

SAINT VINCENT HOSPITAL AND HEALTH CENTER (O, 257 beds) 1233 North 30th Street, Billings, MT Zip 59101, Mailing Address: P.O. Box 35200, Zip 59107–5200; tel. 406/657–7000; Patrick M. Hermanson, President and Senior Executive

ST. JAMES COMMUNITY HOSPITAL (O, 103 beds) 400 South Clark Street, Butte, MT Zip 59701, Mailing Address: P.O. Box 3300, Zip 59702; tel. 406/723–2500; James T. Paquette, Regional Chief Executive Officer

Owned, leased, sponsored:	9 hospitals	1975 beds
Contract–managed:	0 hospitals	0 beds
Totals:	9 hospitals	1975 beds

★3045: SISTERS OF CHARITY OF NAZARETH HEALTH SYSTEM (CC)
135 West Drive, Nazareth, KY Zip 40048, Mailing Address: P.O. Box 171, Zip 40048–0171; tel. 502/349–6250; Mark W. Dundon, President and Chief Executive Officer

ARKANSAS: ST. VINCENT INFIRMARY MEDICAL CENTER (O, 570 beds) Two St. Vincent Circle, Little Rock, AR Zip 72205–5499; tel. 501/660–3000; Diana T. Hueter, President and Chief Executive Officer

KENTUCKY: CARITAS MEDICAL CENTER (O, 177 beds) 1850 Bluegrass Avenue, Louisville, KY Zip 40215–1199; tel. 502/361–6000; Peter J. Bernard, President and Chief Executive Officer

CARITAS PEACE CENTER (O, 156 beds) 2020 Newburg Road, Louisville, KY Zip 40205; tel. 502/451–3330; Peter J. Bernard, President and Chief Executive Officer

FLAGET MEMORIAL HOSPITAL (O, 36 beds) 201 Cathedral Manor, Bardstown, KY Zip 40004–1299; tel. 502/348–3923; Suzanne Reasbeck, President and Chief Executive Officer

MARYMOUNT MEDICAL CENTER (O, 95 beds) 310 East Ninth Street, London, KY Zip 40741–1299; tel. 606/878–6520; Lowell Jones, President

ST. JOSEPH HOSPITAL (O, 324 beds) One St. Joseph Drive, Lexington, KY Zip 40504; tel. 606/278–3436; Thomas J. Murray, President

For explanation of codes following names, see page B2.
★ Indicates Type III membership in the American Hospital Association.

TENNESSEE: MEMORIAL HOSPITAL (O, 296 beds) 2525 De Sales Avenue, Chattanooga, TN Zip 37404–3322; tel. 615/495–2525; L. Clark Taylor Jr., President and Chief Executive Officer

Owned, leased, sponsored:	7 hospitals	1654 beds
Contract–managed:	0 hospitals	0 beds
Totals:	7 hospitals	1654 beds

5125: SISTERS OF CHARITY OF ST. AUGUSTINE HEALTH SYSTEM (CC)

2351 East 22nd Street, Cleveland, OH Zip 44115; tel. 216/696–5560; Sister Mary Ann Andrews, President and Chief Executive Officer

OHIO: COLUMBIA MERCY MEDICAL CENTER (S, 416 beds) 1320 Mercy Drive N.W., Canton, OH Zip 44708–2641; tel. 330/489–1000; Jack W. Topoleski, President and Chief Executive Officer

COLUMBIA ST. VINCENT CHARITY HOSPITAL (S, 266 beds) 2351 East 22nd Street, Cleveland, OH Zip 44115–3111; tel. 216/861–6200; Samuel H. Turner, Chief Executive Officer

ST. JOHN WEST SHORE HOSPITAL (S, 183 beds) 29000 Center Ridge Road, Cleveland, OH Zip 44145–5219; tel. 216/835–8000; Fred M. DeGrandis, President and Chief Executive Officer

SOUTH CAROLINA: COLUMBIA PROVIDENCE HOSPITAL (S, 214 beds) 2435 Forest Drive, Columbia, SC Zip 29204–2098; tel. 803/256–5300; M. John Heydel, President and Chief Executive Officer

Owned, leased, sponsored:	4 hospitals	1079 beds
Contract–managed:	0 hospitals	0 beds
Totals:	4 hospitals	1079 beds

★0605: SISTERS OF CHARITY OF THE INCARNATE WORD HEALTHCARE SYSTEM (CC)

2600 North Loop West, Houston, TX Zip 77092; tel. 713/681–8877; Sister Christina Murphy, President and Chief Executive Officer

ARKANSAS: MAGNOLIA HOSPITAL (C, 65 beds) 101 Hospital Drive, Magnolia, AR Zip 71753–2416, Mailing Address: Box 629, Zip 71753–0629; tel. 501/235–3000; William D. Hedden, Administrator

LOUISIANA: SCHUMPERT MEDICAL CENTER (O, 486 beds) One St. Mary Place, Shreveport, LA Zip 71101, Mailing Address: P.O. Box 21976, Zip 71120–1076; tel. 318/681–4500; Arthur A. Gonzalez, Dr.PH, President and Chief Executive Officer

ST. FRANCES CABRINI HOSPITAL (O, 227 beds) 3330 Masonic Drive, Alexandria, LA Zip 71301; tel. 318/487–1122; Sister Olive Bordelon, Chief Executive Officer

ST. PATRICK HOSPITAL OF LAKE CHARLES (O, 298 beds) 524 South Ryan Street, Lake Charles, LA Zip 70601, Mailing Address: P.O. Box 3401, Zip 70602–3401; tel. 318/436–2511; J. William Hankins, President and Chief Executive Officer

TEXAS: JASPER MEMORIAL HOSPITAL (C, 54 beds) 1275 Marvin Hancock Drive, Jasper, TX Zip 75951; tel. 409/384–5461; George N. Miller Jr., Administrator

ST. ELIZABETH HOSPITAL (O, 480 beds) 2830 Calder Avenue, Beaumont, TX Zip 77702, Mailing Address: P.O. Box 5405, Zip 77726–5405; tel. 409/892–7171; Sister Mary Fatima McCarthy, Administrator

ST. JOHN HOSPITAL (O, 133 beds) 2050 Space Park Drive, Nassau Bay, TX Zip 77058; tel. 281/333–5503; Thomas Permetti, Administrator

ST. JOSEPH HOSPITAL (O, 483 beds) 1919 LaBranch Street, Houston, TX Zip 77002; tel. 713/757–1000; Raymond J. Khoury, Administrator

ST. MARY HOSPITAL (O, 231 beds) 3600 Gates Boulevard, Port Arthur, TX Zip 77642–3601, Mailing Address: P.O. Box 3696, Zip 77643–3696; tel. 409/985–7431; James E. Gardner Jr., Administrator

ST. MICHAEL HEALTH CARE CENTER (O, 80 beds) 2600 St. Michael Drive, Texarkana, TX Zip 75503; tel. 903/614–2009; Don A. Beeler, Chief Executive Officer

Owned, leased, sponsored:	8 hospitals	2418 beds
Contract–managed:	2 hospitals	119 beds
Totals:	10 hospitals	2537 beds

5805: SISTERS OF MARY OF THE PRESENTATION HEALTH CORPORATION (CC)

1102 Page Drive S.W., Fargo, ND Zip 58106–0007, Mailing Address: P.O. Box 10007, Zip 58106–0007; tel. 701/237–9290; Aaron Alton, President

ILLINOIS: ST. MARGARET'S HOSPITAL (O, 127 beds) 600 East First Street, Spring Valley, IL Zip 61362–2034; tel. 815/664–5311; Timothy Muntz, President

IOWA: VAN BUREN COUNTY HOSPITAL (C, 40 beds) Highway 1 North, Keosauqua, IA Zip 52565, Mailing Address: Box 70, Zip 52565; tel. 319/293–3171; Lisa Wagner Schnedler, Administrator

NORTH DAKOTA: PRESENTATION MEDICAL CENTER (O, 102 beds) 213 Second Avenue N.E., Rolla, ND Zip 58367, Mailing Address: P.O. Box 759, Zip 58367–0759; tel. 701/477–3161; Kimber Wraalstad, Chief Executive Officer

ST. ALOISIUS MEDICAL CENTER (O, 165 beds) 325 East Brewster Street, Harvey, ND Zip 58341–1605; tel. 701/324–4651; Ronald J. Volk, President

ST. ANDREW'S HEALTH CENTER (O, 67 beds) 316 Ohmer Street, Bottineau, ND Zip 58318–1018; tel. 701/228–2255; Keith Korman, President

Owned, leased, sponsored:	4 hospitals	461 beds
Contract–managed:	1 hospital	40 beds
Totals:	5 hospitals	501 beds

★5185: SISTERS OF MERCY HEALTH SYSTEM–ST. LOUIS (CC)

2039 North Geyer Road, Saint Louis, MO Zip 63131–3399, Mailing Address: P.O. Box 31902, Zip 63131–1902; tel. 314/965–6100; Sister Mary Roch Rocklage, President and Chief Executive Officer

ARKANSAS: CARROLL REGIONAL MEDICAL CENTER (O, 39 beds) 214 Carter Street, Berryville, AR Zip 72616, Mailing Address: P.O. Box 387, Zip 72616; tel. 501/423–5230; J. Rudy Darling, President and Chief Executive Officer

HARBOR VIEW MERCY HOSPITAL (O, 80 beds) 10301 Mayo Road, Fort Smith, AR Zip 72903, Mailing Address: P.O. Box 17000, Zip 72917–7000; tel. 501/484–5550; Sister Judith Marie Keith, President and Chief Executive Officer

MERCY HOSPITAL OF SCOTT COUNTY (O, 127 beds) Highways 71 and 80, Waldron, AR Zip 72958–9984, Mailing Address: Box 2230, Zip 72958–2230; tel. 501/637–4135; Sister Mary Alvera Simon, Administrator

MERCY HOSPITAL–TURNER MEMORIAL (O, 39 beds) 801 West River, Ozark, AR Zip 72949; tel. 501/667–4138; Sister Mary Werner Keith, Administrator

NORTH LOGAN MERCY HOSPITAL (O, 16 beds) 500 East Academy, Paris, AR Zip 72855–4099; tel. 501/963–6101; Jim L. Maddox, Chief Administrative Officer

ST. EDWARD MERCY MEDICAL CENTER (O, 260 beds) 7301 Rogers Avenue, Fort Smith, AR Zip 72903, Mailing Address: P.O. Box 17000, Zip 72917–7000; tel. 501/484–6000; Sister Judith Marie Keith, President and Chief Executive Officer

ST. JOSEPH'S REGIONAL HEALTH CENTER (O, 274 beds) 300 Werner Street, Hot Springs, AR Zip 71913; tel. 501/622–1000; Randall J. Fale, President and Chief Executive Officer

ST. MARY–ROGERS MEMORIAL HOSPITAL (O, 110 beds) 1200 West Walnut Street, Rogers, AR Zip 72756–3599; tel. 501/636–0200; Michael J. Packnett, President and Chief Executive Officer

ILLINOIS: ST. CLEMENT HEALTH SERVICES (O, 105 beds) One St. Clement Boulevard, Red Bud, IL Zip 62278–1194; tel. 618/282–3831; Michael Thomas McManus, President

KANSAS: MERCY HEALTH SYSTEM OF KANSAS (O, 105 beds) 821 Burke Street, Fort Scott, KS Zip 66701; tel. 316/223–2200; Susan Barrett, President and Chief Executive Officer

For explanation of codes following names, see page B2.
★ Indicates Type III membership in the American Hospital Association.

MERCY HOSPITALS OF KANSAS (O, 58 beds) 800 West Myrtle Street, Independence, KS Zip 67301, Mailing Address: Box 388, Zip 67301–0388; tel. 316/331–2200; Susan Barrett, President and Chief Executive Officer

MISSOURI: ST. ANTHONY'S MEDICAL CENTER (O, 708 beds) 10010 Kennerly Road, Saint Louis, MO Zip 63128; tel. 314/525–1000; David P. Seifert, President

ST. JOHN'S MERCY MEDICAL CENTER (O, 804 beds) 615 South New Ballas Road, Saint Louis, MO Zip 63141–8277; tel. 314/569–6000; Mark Weber, President

ST. JOHN'S REGIONAL HEALTH CENTER (O, 813 beds) 1235 East Cherokee Street, Springfield, MO Zip 65804–2263; tel. 417/885–2000; Allen L. Shockley, President and Chief Executive Officer

ST. LUKE'S HOSPITAL (O, 495 beds) 232 South Woods Mill Road, Chesterfield, MO Zip 63017–3480; tel. 314/434–1500; George Tucker, M.D., President

OKLAHOMA: MERCY HEALTH CENTER (O, 363 beds) 4300 West Memorial Road, Oklahoma City, OK Zip 73120–8362; tel. 405/755–1515; Bruce F. Buchanan, FACHE, President and Chief Executive Officer

MERCY MEMORIAL HEALTH CENTER (O, 193 beds) 1011 14th Street N.W., Ardmore, OK Zip 73401–1889; tel. 405/223–5400; Bobby G. Thompson, President and Chief Executive Officer

ST. MARY'S MERCY HOSPITAL (O, 135 beds) 305 South Fifth Street, Enid, OK Zip 73701–5899, Mailing Address: Box 232, Zip 73702–0232; tel. 405/233–6100; Frank Lopez, President and Chief Executive Officer

TEXAS: MERCY REGIONAL MEDICAL CENTER (O, 320 beds) 1515 Logan Avenue, Laredo, TX Zip 78040, Mailing Address: Drawer 2068, Zip 78044–2068; tel. 210/718–6222; Michael L. Morgan, President and Chief Executive Officer

Owned, leased, sponsored:	19 hospitals	5044 beds
Contract–managed:	0 hospitals	0 beds
Totals:	19 hospitals	5044 beds

6015: SISTERS OF MERCY OF THE AMERICAS–REGIONAL COMMUNITY OF BALTIMORE (CC)
1300 Northern Parkway, Baltimore, MD Zip 21239, Mailing Address: P.O. Box 11448, Zip 21239; tel. 410/435–4400; Sister Margaret Beatty, President

GEORGIA: ST. JOSEPH'S HOSPITAL (O, 305 beds) 11705 Mercy Boulevard, Savannah, GA Zip 31419–1791; tel. 912/927–5404; Paul P. Hinchey, President and Chief Executive Officer

MARYLAND: MERCY MEDICAL CENTER (O, 218 beds) 301 St. Paul Place, Baltimore, MD Zip 21202–2165; tel. 410/332–9000; Sister Helen Amos, President and Chief Executive Officer

Owned, leased, sponsored:	2 hospitals	523 beds
Contract–managed:	0 hospitals	0 beds
Totals:	2 hospitals	523 beds

★5275: SISTERS OF PROVIDENCE HEALTH SYSTEM (CC)
520 Pike Street, Seattle, WA Zip 98101, Mailing Address: P.O. Box 11038, Zip 98111–9038; tel. 206/464–3355; Sister Karin Dufault, Ph.D., Administrator

ALASKA: PROVIDENCE ALASKA MEDICAL CENTER (O, 341 beds) 3200 Providence Drive, Anchorage, AK Zip 99508, Mailing Address: P.O. Box 196604, Zip 99519–6604; tel. 907/562–2211; Douglas A. Bruce, Chief Executive Alaska Service Area

CALIFORNIA: PROVIDENCE HOLY CROSS MEDICAL CENTER (O, 257 beds) 15031 Rinaldi Street, Mission Hills, CA Zip 91345–1285; tel. 818/365–8051; Michael J. Madden, Chief Executive Los Angeles Service Area

PROVIDENCE SAINT JOSEPH MEDICAL CENTER (O, 423 beds) 501 South Buena Vista Street, Burbank, CA Zip 91505–4866; tel. 818/843–5111; Michael J. Madden, Chief Executive Los Angeles Service Area

OREGON: PROVIDENCE MEDFORD MEDICAL CENTER (O, 140 beds) 1111 Crater Lake Avenue, Medford, OR Zip 97504–6241; tel. 541/732–5000; Charles T. Wright, Chief Executive, Southern Oregon Service Area

PROVIDENCE MILWAUKIE HOSPITAL (O, 50 beds) 10150 S.E. 32nd Avenue, Milwaukie, OR Zip 97222–6593; tel. 503/652–8300; Janice Burger, Operations Administrator

PROVIDENCE NEWBERG HOSPITAL (O, 35 beds) 501 Villa Road, Newberg, OR Zip 97132; tel. 503/537–1555; Mark W. Meinert, CHE, Chief Executive, Yamhill Service Area

PROVIDENCE PORTLAND MEDICAL CENTER (O, 420 beds) 4805 N.E. Glisan Street, Portland, OR Zip 97213–2967; tel. 503/215–1111; David T. Underriner, Operations Administrator

PROVIDENCE SEASIDE HOSPITAL (L, 26 beds) 725 South Wahanna Road, Seaside, OR Zip 97138–7735; tel. 503/717–7000; Ronald Swanson, Chief Executive North Coast Service Area

PROVIDENCE ST. VINCENT MEDICAL CENTER (O, 451 beds) 9205 S.W. Barnes Road, Portland, OR Zip 97225–6661; tel. 503/216–1234; Donald Elsom, Operations Administrator

WASHINGTON: MARK REED HOSPITAL (C, 7 beds) 322 South Birch Street, McCleary, WA Zip 98557; tel. 360/495–3244; Jean E. Roberts, Administrator

MORTON GENERAL HOSPITAL (C, 50 beds) 521 Adams Street, Morton, WA Zip 98356, Mailing Address: Drawer C, Zip 98356; tel. 360/496–5112; Mike Lee, Superintendent

PROVIDENCE CENTRALIA HOSPITAL (O, 127 beds) 914 South Scheuber Road, Centralia, WA Zip 98531; tel. 360/736–2803; Maureen Comer, Operations Administrator

PROVIDENCE GENERAL MEDICAL CENTER (O, 290 beds) Pacific and Nassau Streets, Everett, WA Zip 98201, Mailing Address: P.O. Box 1067, Zip 98206–1067; tel. 206/261–2000; Raymond F. Crerand, Interim Chief Executive Northwest Washington Service Area

PROVIDENCE SEATTLE MEDICAL CENTER (O, 334 beds) 500 17th Avenue, Seattle, WA Zip 98122, Mailing Address: P.O. Box 34008, Zip 98124–1008; tel. 206/320–2000; Nancy A. Giunto, Operations Administrator

PROVIDENCE ST. PETER HOSPITAL (O, 327 beds) 413 Lilly Road N.E., Olympia, WA Zip 98506–5166; tel. 360/491–9480; C. Scott Bond, Administrator

PROVIDENCE TOPPENISH HOSPITAL (O, 48 beds) 504 West Fourth Avenue, Toppenish, WA Zip 98948, Mailing Address: P.O. Box 672, Zip 98948–0672; tel. 509/865–3105; Steve Burdick, Administrator

PROVIDENCE YAKIMA MEDICAL CENTER (O, 190 beds) 110 South Ninth Avenue, Yakima, WA Zip 98902–3397; tel. 509/575–5000; Barbara A. Hood, Chief Executive Officer Central Washington Service Area

Owned, leased, sponsored:	15 hospitals	3459 beds
Contract–managed:	2 hospitals	57 beds
Totals:	17 hospitals	3516 beds

•5285: SISTERS OF PROVIDENCE HEALTH SYSTEM (CC)
146 Chestnut Street, Springfield, MA Zip 01103; tel. 413/737–3981; Sister Kathleen Popko, President and Chief Executive Officer

MASSACHUSETTS: MERCY HOSPITAL (O, 262 beds) 271 Carew Street, Springfield, MA Zip 01104, Mailing Address: P.O. Box 9012, Zip 01102–9012; tel. 413/748–9000; Vincent J. McCorkle, President and Chief Executive Officer

Owned, leased, sponsored:	1 hospital	262 beds
Contract–managed:	0 hospitals	0 beds
Totals:	1 hospital	262 beds

★5345: SISTERS OF ST. FRANCIS HEALTH SERVICES, INC. (CC)
1515 Dragoon Trail, Mishawaka, IN Zip 46546–1290, Mailing Address: P.O. Box 1290, Zip 46546–1290; tel. 219/256–3935; Kevin D. Leahy, President and Chief Executive Officer

ILLINOIS: ST. FRANCIS HOSPITAL OF EVANSTON (O, 440 beds) 355 Ridge Avenue, Evanston, IL Zip 60202–3399; tel. 847/316–4000; James C. Gizzi, President and Chief Executive Officer

Section B

For explanation of codes following names, see page B2.
★ Indicates Type III membership in the American Hospital Association.
• Single hospital health care system

ST. JAMES HOSPITAL AND HEALTH CENTERS (O, 332 beds) 1423 Chicago Road, Chicago Heights, IL Zip 60411–9934; tel. 708/756–1000; Peter J. Murphy, President and Chief Executive Officer

INDIANA: SAINT ANTHONY HOSPITAL AND HEALTH CENTERS (O, 190 beds) 301 West Homer Street, Michigan City, IN Zip 46360–4358; tel. 219/879–8511; Bruce E. Rampage, President and Chief Executive Officer

SAINT MARGARET MERCY HEALTHCARE CENTERS (O, 624 beds) 5454 Hohman Avenue, Hammond, IN Zip 46320; tel. 219/933–2074; Eugene C. Diamond, President and Chief Executive Officer

ST. ELIZABETH MEDICAL CENTER (O, 205 beds) 1501 Hartford Street, Lafayette, IN Zip 47904–2126, Mailing Address: Box 7501, Zip 47903–7501; tel. 765/423–6011; Douglas W. Eberle, President and Chief Executive Officer

ST. FRANCIS HOSPITAL AND HEALTH CENTERS (O, 396 beds) 1600 Albany Street, Beech Grove, IN Zip 46107–1593; tel. 317/787–3311; Robert J. Brody, President and Chief Executive Officer

TENNESSEE: ST. JOSEPH HOSPITAL AND HEALTH CENTERS (O, 402 beds) 220 Overton Avenue, Memphis, TN Zip 38105–2789; tel. 901/577–2700; Joan M. Carlson, President and Chief Executive Officer

Owned, leased, sponsored:	7 hospitals	2589 beds
Contract–managed:	0 hospitals	0 beds
Totals:	7 hospitals	2589 beds

★5555:   SISTERS OF ST. JOSEPH HEALTH SYSTEM (CC)
455 East Eisenhower Parkway, Suite 300, Ann Arbor, MI Zip 48108–3324; tel. 313/741–1160; John S. Lore, President and Chief Executive Officer

MICHIGAN: BORGESS MEDICAL CENTER (O, 394 beds) 1521 Gull Road, Kalamazoo, MI Zip 49001–1640; tel. 616/226–7000; R. Timothy Stack, FACHE, President and Chief Executive Officer

GENESYS REGIONAL MEDICAL CENTER (O, 599 beds) One Genesys Parkway, Grand Blanc, MI Zip 48439–1477; tel. 810/606–6600; Young S. Suh, President and Chief Executive Officer

HOLY CROSS HOSPITAL (O, 161 beds) 4777 East Outer Drive, Detroit, MI Zip 48234–0401; tel. 313/369–9100; Michael F. Breen, President

LEE MEMORIAL HOSPITAL (O, 47 beds) 420 West High Street, Dowagiac, MI Zip 49047–1907; tel. 616/782–8681; Fritz Fahrenbacher, Vice President and Regional Hospital Administrator

OAKLAND GENERAL HOSPITAL (O, 166 beds) 27351 Dequindre, Madison Heights, MI Zip 48071; tel. 810/967–7000; Robert Deputat, President

RIVER DISTRICT HOSPITAL (O, 68 beds) 4100 South River Road, East China, MI Zip 48054; tel. 810/329–7111; John E. Knox, President

ST. JOHN HEALTH SYSTEM–SARATOGA CAMPUS (O, 170 beds) 15000 Gratiot Avenue, Detroit, MI Zip 48205–1999; tel. 313/245–1200; Michael F. Breen, President

ST. JOHN HOSPITAL AND MEDICAL CENTER (O, 599 beds) 22101 Moross Road, Detroit, MI Zip 48236–2172; tel. 313/343–4000; Timothy J. Grajewski, President and Chief Executive Officer

ST. JOHN HOSPITAL–MACOMB CENTER (O, 66 beds) 26755 Ballard Road, Harrison Township, MI Zip 48045–2458; tel. 810/465–5501; David Sessions, President

TAWAS ST. JOSEPH HOSPITAL (O, 69 beds) 200 Hemlock Street, Tawas City, MI Zip 48763, Mailing Address: P.O. Box 659, Zip 48764–0659; tel. 517/362–3411; Paul R. Schmidt, President and Chief Executive Officer

Owned, leased, sponsored:	10 hospitals	2339 beds
Contract–managed:	0 hospitals	0 beds
Totals:	10 hospitals	2339 beds

5955:   SISTERS OF THE 3RD FRANCISCAN ORDER (CC)
2500 Grant Boulevard, Syracuse, NY Zip 13208–1713; tel. 315/425–0115; Sister Grace Anne Dillenschneider, General Superior

HAWAII: ST. FRANCIS MEDICAL CENTER (O, 221 beds) 2230 Liliha Street, Honolulu, HI Zip 96817–9979, Mailing Address: P.O. Box 30100, Zip 96820–0100; tel. 808/547–6011; Cynthia Okinaka, Administrator

ST. FRANCIS MEDICAL CENTER–WEST (O, 87 beds) 91–2141 Fort Weaver Road, Ewa Beach, HI Zip 96706; tel. 808/678–7000; Sister Gretchen Gilroy, President and Chief Executive Officer

NEW YORK: ST. ELIZABETH MEDICAL CENTER (O, 201 beds) 2209 Genesee Street, Utica, NY Zip 13501–5999; tel. 315/798–8100; Sister Rose Vincent, President and Chief Executive Officer

ST. JOSEPH'S HOSPITAL HEALTH CENTER (O, 431 beds) 301 Prospect Avenue, Syracuse, NY Zip 13203; tel. 315/448–5111; Theodore M. Pasinski, President

Owned, leased, sponsored:	4 hospitals	940 beds
Contract–managed:	0 hospitals	0 beds
Totals:	4 hospitals	940 beds

5575:   SISTERS OF THE HOLY FAMILY OF NAZARETH–SACRED HEART PROVINCE (CC)
310 North River Road, Des Plaines, IL Zip 60016–1211; tel. 847/298–6760; Sister M. Lucille Madura, Provincial Superior

ILLINOIS: HOLY FAMILY MEDICAL CENTER (O, 183 beds) 100 North River Road, Des Plaines, IL Zip 60016; tel. 847/297–1800; Sister Patricia Ann Koschalke, President and Chief Executive Officer

SAINT MARY OF NAZARETH HOSPITAL CENTER (O, 305 beds) 2233 West Division Street, Chicago, IL Zip 60622–3086; tel. 312/770–2000; Sister Stella Louise, President and Chief Executive Officer

Owned, leased, sponsored:	2 hospitals	488 beds
Contract–managed:	0 hospitals	0 beds
Totals:	2 hospitals	488 beds

★5305:   SISTERS OF THE SORROWFUL MOTHER UNITED STATES HEALTH SYSTEM (CC)
Tulsa, OK Mailing Address: P.O. Box 4753, Zip 74159–0753; tel. 918/742–9988; Sister M. Therese Gottschalk, President

MINNESOTA: ST. ELIZABETH HOSPITAL (O, 183 beds) 1200 Fifth Grand Boulevard West, Wabasha, MN Zip 55981; tel. 612/565–4531; Thomas Crowley, President

NEW JERSEY: NORTHWEST COVENANT MEDICAL CENTER (O, 644 beds) 25 Pocono Road, Denville, NJ Zip 07834–2995; tel. 201/625–6000; Joseph A. Trunfio, President and Chief Executive Officer

OKLAHOMA: ST. JOHN MEDICAL CENTER (O, 589 beds) 1923 South Utica Avenue, Tulsa, OK Zip 74104–5445; tel. 918/744–2345; Sister M. Therese Gottschalk, President

WISCONSIN: FLAMBEAU HOSPITAL (O, 42 beds) 98 Sherry Avenue, Park Falls, WI Zip 54552, Mailing Address: P.O. Box 310, Zip 54552; tel. 715/762–2484; Curtis A. Johnson, Administrator

MERCY MEDICAL CENTER (O, 232 beds) 631 Hazel Street, Oshkosh, WI Zip 54902, Mailing Address: P.O. Box 1100, Zip 54902–1100; tel. 414/236–2000; Otto L. Cox, President and Chief Executive Officer

SACRED HEART–ST. MARY'S HOSPITALS (O, 51 beds) 1044 Kabel Avenue, Rhinelander, WI Zip 54501–3998, Mailing Address: P.O. Box 20, Zip 54501; tel. 715/369–6600; Kevin J. O'Donnell, President and Chief Executive Officer

SAINT JOSEPH'S HOSPITAL (O, 524 beds) 611 St. Joseph Avenue, Marshfield, WI Zip 54449–1898; tel. 715/387–1713; Michael A. Schmidt, President and Chief Executive Officer

SAINT MICHAEL'S HOSPITAL (O, 104 beds) 900 Illinois Avenue, Stevens Point, WI Zip 54481; tel. 715/346–5000; Jeffrey L. Martin, President and Chief Executive Officer

VICTORY MEDICAL CENTER (O, 127 beds) 230 East Fourth Avenue, Stanley, WI Zip 54768; tel. 715/644–5571; Cynthia Eichman, Chief Executive Officer and Administrator

Owned, leased, sponsored:	9 hospitals	2496 beds
Contract–managed:	0 hospitals	0 beds
Totals:	9 hospitals	2496 beds

For explanation of codes following names, see page B2.
★ Indicates Type III membership in the American Hospital Association.

★0106: SOUTHERN CALIFORNIA HEALTHCARE SYSTEM (NP)
1300 East Green Street, Pasadena, CA Zip 91106; Frederick C. Meyer, President and Chief Executive Officer

CALIFORNIA: BEVERLY HOSPITAL (O, 120 beds) 309 West Beverly Boulevard, Montebello, CA Zip 90640; tel. 213/726–1222; Matthew S. Gerlach, Chief Executive Officer and Administrator

HUNTINGTON EAST VALLEY HOSPITAL (O, 128 beds) 150 West Alosta Avenue, Glendora, CA Zip 91740–4398; tel. 818/335–0231; James W. Maki, Chief Executive Officer

HUNTINGTON MEMORIAL HOSPITAL (O, 472 beds) 100 West California Boulevard, Pasadena, CA Zip 91105, Mailing Address: P.O. Box 7013, Zip 91109–7013; tel. 818/397–5000; Stephen A. Ralph, President and Chief Executive Officer

METHODIST HOSPITAL OF SOUTHERN CALIFORNIA (O, 304 beds) 300 West Huntington Drive, Arcadia, CA Zip 91007, Mailing Address: P.O. Box 60016, Zip 91066–6016; tel. 818/445–4441; Dennis M. Lee, President

VERDUGO HILLS HOSPITAL (O, 134 beds) 1812 Verdugo Boulevard, Glendale, CA Zip 91208, Mailing Address: P.O. Box 1431, Zip 91209–1431; tel. 818/790–7100; Bernard Glossy, President

Owned, leased, sponsored:	5 hospitals	1158 beds
Contract–managed:	0 hospitals	0 beds
Totals:	5 hospitals	1158 beds

★4175: SOUTHERN ILLINOIS HOSPITAL SERVICES (NP)
608 East College Street, Carbondale, IL Zip 62901, Mailing Address: P.O. Box 3988, Zip 62902–3988; tel. 618/457–5200; John J. Buckley Jr., President

ILLINOIS: FERRELL HOSPITAL (O, 51 beds) 1201 Pine Street, Eldorado, IL Zip 62930; tel. 618/273–3361; E. T. Seely, Acting Administrator and Chief Financial Officer

FRANKLIN HOSPITAL AND SKILLED NURSING CARE UNIT (L, 117 beds) 201 Bailey Lane, Benton, IL Zip 62812; tel. 618/439–3161; Ron Slaviero, Administrator

HERRIN HOSPITAL (O, 84 beds) 201 South 14th Street, Herrin, IL Zip 62948; tel. 618/942–2171; Virgil Hannig, Administrator

MEMORIAL HOSPITAL OF CARBONDALE (O, 132 beds) 405 West Jackson Street, Carbondale, IL Zip 62902, Mailing Address: P.O. Box 10000, Zip 62902–9000; tel. 618/549–0721; George Maroney, Administrator

ST. JOSEPH MEMORIAL HOSPITAL (O, 59 beds) 2 South Hospital Drive, Murphysboro, IL Zip 62966; tel. 618/684–3156; Betty Gaffney, Administrator

UNITED MINE WORKERS OF AMERICA UNION HOSPITAL (O, 32 beds) 507 West St. Louis Street, West Frankfort, IL Zip 62896–1999; tel. 618/932–2155; Ronald Slaviero, Administrator

Owned, leased, sponsored:	6 hospitals	475 beds
Contract–managed:	0 hospitals	0 beds
Totals:	6 hospitals	475 beds

★4195: SPARTANBURG REGIONAL HEALTHCARE SYSTEM (NP)
101 East Wood Street, Spartanburg, SC Zip 29303–3016; tel. 864/560–6000; Joseph Michael Oddis, President

SOUTH CAROLINA: B.J. WORKMAN MEMORIAL HOSPITAL (O, 32 beds) 751 East Georgia Street, Woodruff, SC Zip 29388, Mailing Address: P.O. Box 699, Zip 29388–0699; tel. 864/476–8122; G. Curtis Walker, R.N., Administrator

SPARTANBURG REGIONAL MEDICAL CENTER (O, 471 beds) 101 East Wood Street, Spartanburg, SC Zip 29303–3016; tel. 864/560–6000; Joseph Michael Oddis, President

Owned, leased, sponsored:	2 hospitals	503 beds
Contract–managed:	0 hospitals	0 beds
Totals:	2 hospitals	503 beds

★5455: SSM HEALTH CARE SYSTEM (CC)
477 North Lindbergh Boulevard, Saint Louis, MO Zip 63141–7813; tel. 314/994–7800; Sister Mary Jean Ryan, President and Chief Executive Officer

GEORGIA: ST. FRANCIS HOSPITAL (C, 281 beds) 2122 Manchester Expressway, Columbus, GA Zip 31904–6878, Mailing Address: Box 7000, Zip 31908–7000; tel. 706/596–4000; Michael E. Garrigan, President and Chief Executive Officer

ILLINOIS: GOOD SAMARITAN REGIONAL HEALTH CENTER (O, 152 beds) 605 North 12th Street, Mount Vernon, IL Zip 62864; tel. 618/242–4600; Leo F. Childers Jr., FACHE, President

ST. FRANCIS HOSPITAL AND HEALTH CENTER (O, 258 beds) 12935 South Gregory Street, Blue Island, IL Zip 60406–2470; tel. 708/597–2000; Jay E. Kreuzer, President

WASHINGTON COUNTY HOSPITAL (C, 53 beds) 705 South Grand Street, Nashville, IL Zip 62263–1532; tel. 618/327–8236; Michael P. Ellermann, President

MISSOURI: ARCADIA VALLEY HOSPITAL (O, 50 beds) Highway 21, Pilot Knob, MO Zip 63663, Mailing Address: P.O. Box 548, Zip 63663–0548; tel. 573/546–3924; H. Clark Duncan, Administrator

CARDINAL GLENNON CHILDREN'S HOSPITAL (O, 172 beds) 1465 South Grand Boulevard, Saint Louis, MO Zip 63104–1095; tel. 314/577–5600; Douglas A. Ries, President

DEPAUL HEALTH CENTER (O, 371 beds) 12303 DePaul Drive, Saint Louis, MO Zip 63044–2588; tel. 314/344–6000; Robert G. Porter, President

PIKE COUNTY MEMORIAL HOSPITAL (C, 25 beds) 2305 West Georgia Street, Louisiana, MO Zip 63353–0020; tel. 573/754–5531; Thomas E. Lefebvre, President

SSM REHABILITATION INSTITUTE (O, 78 beds) 6420 Clayton Road, Suite 600, Saint Louis, MO Zip 63117; tel. 314/768–5300; Melinda Clark, President

ST. FRANCIS HOSPITAL AND HEALTH SERVICES (O, 55 beds) 2016 South Main Street, Maryville, MO Zip 64468–2693; tel. 816/562–2600; Michael Baumgartner, President

ST. JOSEPH HEALTH CENTER (O, 316 beds) 300 First Capitol Drive, Saint Charles, MO Zip 63301–2835; tel. 314/947–5000; Kurt Weinmeister, President

ST. JOSEPH HOSPITAL (O, 250 beds) 525 Couch Avenue, Saint Louis, MO Zip 63122–5594; tel. 314/966–1500; Carla S. Baum, President

ST. JOSEPH HOSPITAL WEST (O, 100 beds) 100 Medical Plaza, Lake Saint Louis, MO Zip 63367–1395; tel. 314/625–5200; Kurt Weinmeister, President

ST. MARY'S HEALTH CENTER (O, 440 beds) 6420 Clayton Road, Saint Louis, MO Zip 63117–1811; tel. 314/768–8000; Michael E. Zilm, President

ST. MARYS HEALTH CENTER (O, 151 beds) 100 St. Marys Medical Plaza, Jefferson City, MO Zip 65101; tel. 573/761–7000; John S. Dubis, President

OKLAHOMA: BONE AND JOINT HOSPITAL (O, 89 beds) 1111 North Dewey Avenue, Oklahoma City, OK Zip 73103–2615; tel. 405/552–9100; James A. Hyde, Administrator

HILLCREST HEALTH CENTER (O, 181 beds) 2129 S.W. 59th Street, Oklahoma City, OK Zip 73119–7001; tel. 405/685–6671; Ray Brazier, President

ST. ANTHONY HOSPITAL (O, 445 beds) 1000 North Lee Street, Oklahoma City, OK Zip 73102, Mailing Address: Box 205, Zip 73101–0205; tel. 405/272–7000; Steven L. Hunter, President

SOUTH CAROLINA: SAINT EUGENE COMMUNITY HOSPITAL (O, 87 beds) 301 East Jackson Street, Dillon, SC Zip 29536–2509, Mailing Address: P.O. Box 1327, Zip 29536–1327; tel. 803/774–4111; Ronald W. Webb, President

WISCONSIN: ST. CLARE HOSPITAL AND HEALTH SERVICES (O, 76 beds) 707 14th Street, Baraboo, WI Zip 53913–1597; tel. 608/356–5561; David B. Jordahl, FACHE, President

Section B

For explanation of codes following names, see page B2.
★ Indicates Type III membership in the American Hospital Association.

ST. MARYS HOSPITAL MEDICAL CENTER (O, 319 beds) 707 South Mills Street, Madison, WI Zip 53715–0450; tel. 608/251–6100; Gerald W. Lefert, President

Owned, leased, sponsored:	18 hospitals	3590 beds
Contract–managed:	3 hospitals	359 beds
Totals:	21 hospitals	3949 beds

★2255: ST. FRANCIS HEALTH SYSTEM (NP)
4401 Penn Avenue, Pittsburgh, PA Zip 15224–1334; tel. 412/622–4214; Sister M. Rosita Wellinger, President and Chief Executive Officer

PENNSYLVANIA: ST. FRANCIS CENTRAL HOSPITAL (O, 143 beds) 1200 Centre Avenue, Pittsburgh, PA Zip 15219–3594; tel. 412/562–3000; Robin Z. Mohr, Chief Executive Officer

ST. FRANCIS HOSPITAL OF NEW CASTLE (O, 193 beds) 1000 South Mercer Street, New Castle, PA Zip 16101–4673; tel. 412/658–3511; Sister Donna Zwigart, Chief Executive Officer

ST. FRANCIS MEDICAL CENTER (O, 885 beds) 400 45th Street, Pittsburgh, PA Zip 15201–1198; tel. 412/622–4343; Sister Florence Brandt, Chief Executive Officer

Owned, leased, sponsored:	3 hospitals	1221 beds
Contract–managed:	0 hospitals	0 beds
Totals:	3 hospitals	1221 beds

★5425: ST. JOSEPH HEALTH SYSTEM (CC)
440 South Batavia Street, Orange, CA Zip 92868–3995, Mailing Address: P.O. Box 14132, Zip 92613–1532; tel. 714/997–7690; Richard Statuto, Chief Executive Officer

CALIFORNIA: MISSION HOSPITAL REGIONAL MEDICAL CENTER (O, 208 beds) 27700 Medical Center Road, Mission Viejo, CA Zip 92691; tel. 714/364–1400; Peter F. Bastone, President and Chief Executive Officer

PETALUMA VALLEY HOSPITAL (C, 84 beds) 400 North McDowell Boulevard, Petaluma, CA Zip 94954–2339; tel. 707/778–1111; Neil Martin, President and Chief Executive Officer

QUEEN OF THE VALLEY HOSPITAL (O, 176 beds) 1000 Trancas Street, Napa, CA Zip 94558, Mailing Address: Box 2340, Zip 94558; tel. 707/252–4411; Howard Levant, President and Chief Executive Officer

REDWOOD MEMORIAL HOSPITAL (O, 35 beds) 3300 Renner Drive, Fortuna, CA Zip 95540; tel. 707/725–3361; Paul J. Chodkowski, President and Chief Executive Officer

SAINT JOSEPH HOSPITAL (O, 62 beds) 2700 Dolbeer Street, Eureka, CA Zip 95501; tel. 707/445–8121; Paul J. Chodkowski, President and Chief Executive Officer

SANTA ROSA MEMORIAL HOSPITAL (O, 225 beds) 1165 Montgomery Drive, Santa Rosa, CA Zip 95405, Mailing Address: Box 522, Zip 95402; tel. 707/546–3210; Robert H. Fish, President and Chief Executive Officer

ST. MARY REGIONAL MEDICAL CENTER (O, 137 beds) 18300 Highway 18, Apple Valley, CA Zip 92307–0725, Mailing Address: Box 7025, Zip 92307–0725; tel. 619/242–2311; Catherine M. Pelley, President and Chief Executive Officer

ST. JOSEPH HOSPITAL (O, 367 beds) 1100 West Stewart Drive, Orange, CA Zip 92668, Mailing Address: P.O. Box 5600, Zip 92613–5600; tel. 714/633–9111; Larry K. Ainsworth, President and Chief Executive Officer

ST. JUDE MEDICAL CENTER (O, 347 beds) 101 East Valencia Mesa Drive, Fullerton, CA Zip 92635; tel. 714/992–3000; Robert J. Fraschetti, President and Chief Executive Officer

TEXAS: CROSBYTON CLINIC HOSPITAL (C, 35 beds) 710 West Main Street, Crosbyton, TX Zip 79322; tel. 806/675–2382; Michael Johnson, Administrator and Chief Executive Officer

D. M. COGDELL MEMORIAL HOSPITAL (C, 65 beds) 1700 Cogdell Boulevard, Snyder, TX Zip 79549–6198; tel. 915/573–6374; Jeff Reecer, Chief Executive Officer

ST. MARY OF THE PLAINS HOSPITAL (O, 410 beds) 4000 24th Street, Lubbock, TX Zip 79410; tel. 806/796–6000; Charley O. Trimble, President and Chief Executive Officer

SWISHER MEMORIAL HOSPITAL DISTRICT (C, 25 beds) 539 Southeast Second, Tulia, TX Zip 79088, Mailing Address: P.O. Box 808, Zip 79088; tel. 806/995–3581; Tony Staynings, Chief Executive Officer

YOAKUM COUNTY HOSPITAL (C, 24 beds) 412 Mustang Avenue, Denver City, TX Zip 79323, Mailing Address: P.O. Drawer 1130, Zip 79323; tel. 806/592–5484; Edward Rodgers, Chief Executive Officer

Owned, leased, sponsored:	9 hospitals	1967 beds
Contract–managed:	5 hospitals	233 beds
Totals:	14 hospitals	2200 beds

5845: ST. LUKE'S HEALTH SYSTEM, INC. (NP)
2720 Stone Park Boulevard, Sioux City, IA Zip 51104–2000; tel. 712/279–3500; John D. Daniels, President and Chief Executive Officer

IOWA: FLOYD VALLEY HOSPITAL (C, 44 beds) Highway 3 East, Le Mars, IA Zip 51031, Mailing Address: P.O. Box 10, Zip 51031; tel. 712/546–7871; G. Frank LaBonte, FACHE, Chief Executive Officer

ORANGE CITY MUNICIPAL HOSPITAL (C, 113 beds) 400 Central Avenue N.W., Orange City, IA Zip 51041–1398; tel. 712/737–4984; Martin W. Guthmiller, Administrator

Owned, leased, sponsored:	0 hospitals	0 beds
Contract–managed:	2 hospitals	157 beds
Totals:	2 hospitals	157 beds

3555: STATE OF HAWAII, DEPARTMENT OF HEALTH (NP)
1250 Punchbowl Street, Honolulu, HI Zip 96813; tel. 808/586–4416; Bertrand Kobayashi, Deputy Director

HAWAII: HILO MEDICAL CENTER (O, 274 beds) 1190 Waianuenue Avenue, Hilo, HI Zip 96720–2095; tel. 808/974–4743; William Carnett, D.O., Acting Administrator

HONOKAA HOSPITAL (O, 50 beds) Honokaa, HI Mailing Address: P.O. Box 237, Zip 96727–0237; tel. 808/775–7211; Romel de la Cruz, Administrator

KAU HOSPITAL (O, 21 beds) Pahala, HI Mailing Address: P.O. Box 40, Zip 96777; tel. 808/928–8331; Dawn S. Pung, Administrator

KAUAI VETERANS MEMORIAL HOSPITAL (O, 49 beds) Waimea Canyon Road, Waimea, HI Zip 96796, Mailing Address: P.O. Box 337, Zip 96796–0337; tel. 808/338–9431; Orianna A. Skomoroch, Administrator

KOHALA HOSPITAL (O, 26 beds) Kohala, HI Mailing Address: P.O. Box 10, Kapaau, Zip 96755–0010; tel. 808/889–6211; Manuel Anduha, Administrator

KONA COMMUNITY HOSPITAL (O, 75 beds) Kealakekua, HI Mailing Address: P.O. Box 69, Zip 96750–0069; tel. 808/322–4429; David W. Patton, Chief Executive Officer

KULA HOSPITAL (O, 105 beds) 204 Kula Highway, Kula, HI Zip 96790–9499; tel. 808/878–1221; Michael P. Gagne, Administrator

LANAI COMMUNITY HOSPITAL (O, 14 beds) 628 Seventh Street, Lanai City, HI Zip 96763–0797, Mailing Address: P.O. Box 797, Zip 96763–0797; tel. 808/565–6411; Herbert K. Yim, Administrator

LEAHI HOSPITAL (O, 192 beds) 3675 Kilauea Avenue, Honolulu, HI Zip 96816; tel. 808/733–8000; Fred D. Horwitz, Administrator

MAUI MEMORIAL HOSPITAL (O, 180 beds) 221 Mahalani Street, Wailuku, HI Zip 96793–2581; tel. 808/244–9056; Alan G. Lee, Administrator

SAMUEL MAHELONA MEMORIAL HOSPITAL (O, 82 beds) 4800 Kawaihau Road, Kapaa, HI Zip 96746–1998; tel. 808/822–4961; Neva M. Olson, Administrator

Owned, leased, sponsored:	11 hospitals	1068 beds
Contract–managed:	0 hospitals	0 beds
Totals:	11 hospitals	1068 beds

0044: STERLING HEALTHCARE CORPORATION (IO)
1500 114th Avenue S.E., Suite 100, Bellevue, WA Zip 98004; tel. 206/453–5445; David Jacobsen, President

INDIANA: KOALA BEHAVIORAL HEALTH–COLUMBUS CAMPUS (O, 60 beds) 2223 Poshard Drive, Columbus, IN Zip 47203; tel. 812/376–1711; Thomas N. Theroult, Administrator

For explanation of codes following names, see page B2.
★ Indicates Type III membership in the American Hospital Association.

KOALA HOSPITAL AND COUNSELING CENTER (O, 80 beds) 1800 North Oak Road, Plymouth, IN Zip 46563; tel. 219/936–3784; Wayne T. Miller, Administrator

OKLAHOMA: OAK CREST HOSPITAL AND COUNSELING CENTER (O, 50 beds) 1601 Gordon Cooper Drive, Shawnee, OK Zip 74801; tel. 405/275–9610; Eugene Suksi, Administrator

WILLOW CREST HOSPITAL (O, 50 beds) 130 A Street S.W., Miami, OK Zip 74354; tel. 918/542–1836; Cornelia Willis, Administrator and Chief Executive Officer

OREGON: PACIFIC GATEWAY HOSPITAL AND COUNSELING CENTER (O, 66 beds) 1345 S.E. Harney, Portland, OR Zip 97202; tel. 503/234–5353; W. Michael Johnson, Executive Director

Owned, leased, sponsored:	5 hospitals	306 beds
Contract–managed:	0 hospitals	0 beds
Totals:	5 hospitals	306 beds

0805: STORMONT–VAIL HEALTHCARE (NP)
1500 Southwest Tenth Street, Topeka, KS Zip 66604–1353; tel. 913/354–6121; Maynard F. Oliverius, President and Chief Executive Officer

KANSAS: DECHAIRO HOSPITAL (O, 13 beds) First and North Streets, Westmoreland, KS Zip 66549; tel. 913/457–3311; Paula Lauer, Administrator

STORMONT–VAIL HEALTHCARE (O, 313 beds) 1500 S.W. Tenth Street, Topeka, KS Zip 66604–1353; tel. 913/354–6000; Maynard F. Oliverius, President and Chief Executive Officer

WAMEGO CITY HOSPITAL (C, 26 beds) 711 Genn Drive, Wamego, KS Zip 66547; tel. 913/456–2295; Lisa J. Freeborn, Administrator

Owned, leased, sponsored:	2 hospitals	326 beds
Contract–managed:	1 hospital	26 beds
Totals:	3 hospitals	352 beds

★0030: SUN HEALTH CORPORATION (NP)
13180 North 103rd Drive, Sun City, AZ Zip 85351, Mailing Address: P.O. Box 1278, Zip 85372–1278; tel. 602/876–5301; Leland W. Peterson, President and Chief Executive Officer

ARIZONA: DEL E. WEBB MEMORIAL HOSPITAL (O, 181 beds) 14502 West Meeker Boulevard, Sun City West, AZ Zip 85375, Mailing Address: P.O. Box 5169, Zip 85375; tel. 602/214–4000; Thomas C. Dickson, Executive Vice President and Chief Operating Officer

WALTER O. BOSWELL MEMORIAL HOSPITAL (O, 297 beds) 10401 West Thunderbird Boulevard, Sun City, AZ Zip 85351, Mailing Address: Box 1690, Zip 85372; tel. 602/977–7211; George Perez, Executive Vice President and Chief Operating Officer

Owned, leased, sponsored:	2 hospitals	478 beds
Contract–managed:	0 hospitals	0 beds
Totals:	2 hospitals	478 beds

★8795: SUTTER HEALTH (NP)
2800 L Street, Sacramento, CA Zip 95816, Mailing Address: P.O. Box 160727, Zip 95816; tel. 916/733–8800; Van R. Johnson, President and Chief Executive Officer

CALIFORNIA: ALTA BATES MEDICAL CENTER–ASHBY CAMPUS (O, 453 beds) 2450 Ashby Avenue, Berkeley, CA Zip 94705; tel. 510/204–4444; Albert Lawrence Greene, President and Chief Executive Officer

CALIFORNIA PACIFIC MEDICAL CENTER (O, 520 beds) Clay at Buchanan Street, San Francisco, CA Zip 94115, Mailing Address: P.O. Box 7999, Zip 94120; tel. 415/563–4321; Martin Brotman, M.D., President and Chief Executive Officer

COMMUNITY HOSPITAL (O, 128 beds) 3325 Chanate Road, Santa Rosa, CA Zip 95404; tel. 707/576–4000; Cliff Coates, Chief Executive Officer

MARIN GENERAL HOSPITAL (O, 108 beds) 250 Bon Air Road, Greenbrae, CA Zip 94904, Mailing Address: Box 8010, San Rafael, Zip 94912–8010; tel. 415/925–7000; Henry J. Buhrmann, President and Chief Executive Officer

MEMORIAL HOSPITALS ASSOCIATION (O, 373 beds) Modesto, CA Mailing Address: P.O. Box 942, Zip 95353; tel. 209/526–4500; David P. Benn, President and Chief Executive Officer

MILLS–PENINSULA HEALTH SERVICES (O, 414 beds) 1783 El Camino Real, Burlingame, CA Zip 94010–3205; tel. 415/696–5400; Robert W. Merwin, Chief Executive Officer

NOVATO COMMUNITY HOSPITAL (O, 30 beds) 1625 Hill Road, Novato, CA Zip 94947, Mailing Address: P.O. Box 1108, Zip 94948; tel. 415/897–3111; Anne Hosfeld, Chief Administrative Officer

SUTTER AMADOR HOSPITAL (O, 85 beds) 810 Court Street, Jackson, CA Zip 95642–2379; tel. 209/223–7500; Scott Stenberg, Chief Executive Officer

SUTTER AUBURN FAITH HOSPITAL (O, 105 beds) 11815 Education Street, Auburn, CA Zip 95604, Mailing Address: Box 8992, Zip 95604–8992; tel. 916/888–4518; Joel E. Grey, Chief Executive Officer

SUTTER CENTER FOR PSYCHIATRY (O, 69 beds) 7700 Folsom Boulevard, Sacramento, CA Zip 95826–2608; tel. 916/386–3000; Diane Gail Stewart, Administrator

SUTTER COAST HOSPITAL (O, 47 beds) 800 East Washington Boulevard, Crescent City, CA Zip 95531; tel. 707/464–8511; John E. Menaugh, Chief Executive Officer

SUTTER COMMUNITY HOSPITALS (O, 499 beds) 5151 F Street, Sacramento, CA Zip 95819–3295; tel. 916/454–3333; Lou Lazatin, Chief Executive Officer

SUTTER DAVIS HOSPITAL (O, 48 beds) 2000 Sutter Place, Davis, CA Zip 95616, Mailing Address: P.O. Box 1617, Zip 95617; tel. 916/756–6440; Lawrence A. Maas, Administrator

SUTTER DELTA MEDICAL CENTER (O, 111 beds) 3901 Lone Tree Way, Antioch, CA Zip 94509; tel. 510/779–7200; Linda Horn, Administrator

SUTTER LAKESIDE HOSPITAL (O, 54 beds) 5176 Hill Road East, Lakeport, CA Zip 95453–6111; tel. 707/262–5001; Paul J. Hensler, Chief Executive Officer

SUTTER MERCED MEDICAL CENTER (O, 158 beds) 301 East 13th Street, Merced, CA Zip 95340–6211, Mailing Address: Box 231, Zip 95341–0231; tel. 209/385–7000; Brian S. Bentley, Administrator

SUTTER ROSEVILLE MEDICAL CENTER (O, 183 beds) One Medical Plaza, Roseville, CA Zip 95661–3477; tel. 916/781–1000; Joel E. Grey, Chief Executive Officer

SUTTER SOLANO MEDICAL CENTER (O, 63 beds) 300 Hospital Drive, Vallejo, CA Zip 94589–2517, Mailing Address: P.O. Box 3189, Zip 94589; tel. 707/554–4444; Patrick R. Brady, Administrator

TRACY COMMUNITY MEMORIAL HOSPITAL (O, 63 beds) 1420 North Tracy Boulevard, Tracy, CA Zip 95376–3497; tel. 209/835–1500; Larry L. Meyer, Vice President and Administrator

HAWAII: KAHI MOHALA (O, 88 beds) 91–2301 Fort Weaver Road, Ewa Beach, HI Zip 96706; tel. 808/671–8511; Margi Drue, Administrator

Owned, leased, sponsored:	20 hospitals	3599 beds
Contract–managed:	0 hospitals	0 beds
Totals:	20 hospitals	3599 beds

0039: TARRANT COUNTY HOSPITAL DISTRICT (NP)
1500 South Main Street, Fort Worth, TX Zip 76104; tel. 817/927–1230; Anthony J. Alcini, President and Chief Executive Officer

TEXAS: TARRANT COUNTY HOSPITAL DISTRICT (O, 359 beds) 1500 South Main Street, Fort Worth, TX Zip 76104–4941; tel. 817/921–3431; Anthony J. Alcini, President and Chief Executive Officer

For explanation of codes following names, see page B2.
★ Indicates Type III membership in the American Hospital Association.

TRINITY SPRINGS PAVILION–EAST (O, 34 beds) 1500 South Main Street, Fort Worth, TX Zip 76104–4917; tel. 817/927–3636; Robert N. Bourassa, Executive Director

Owned, leased, sponsored:	2 hospitals	393 beds
Contract–managed:	0 hospitals	0 beds
Totals:	2 hospitals	393 beds

0063: TENET HEALTHCARE CORPORATION (IO)

3820 State Street, Santa Barbara, CA Zip 93105, Mailing Address: P.O. Box 31907, Zip 93130; tel. 805/563–7000; Jeffrey Barbakow, Chairman and Chief Executive Officer

ALABAMA: BROOKWOOD MEDICAL CENTER (O, 515 beds) 2010 Brookwood Medical Center Drive, Birmingham, AL Zip 35209; tel. 205/877–1000; Gregory H. Burfitt, President and Chief Executive Officer

LLOYD NOLAND HOSPITAL AND HEALTH SYSTEM (O, 222 beds) 701 Lloyd Noland Parkway, Fairfield, AL Zip 35064–2699; tel. 205/783–5106; Gary M. Glasscock, Administrator

ARIZONA: COMMUNITY HOSPITAL MEDICAL CENTER (O, 59 beds) 6501 North 19th Avenue, Phoenix, AZ Zip 85015; tel. 602/249–3434; Randall Hempling, Chief Executive Officer

MESA GENERAL HOSPITAL MEDICAL CENTER (L, 125 beds) 515 North Mesa Drive, Mesa, AZ Zip 85201; tel. 602/969–9111

ST. LUKE'S MEDICAL CENTER (L, 296 beds) 1800 East Van Buren Street, Phoenix, AZ Zip 85006–3742; tel. 602/251–8100; Mary Starmann–Harrison, FACHE, Chief Executive Officer

TEMPE ST. LUKE'S HOSPITAL (L, 110 beds) 1500 South Mill Avenue, Tempe, AZ Zip 85281–6699; tel. 602/784–5501; Thomas A. Salerno, Chief Executive Officer

TUCSON GENERAL HOSPITAL (O, 80 beds) 3838 North Campbell Avenue, Tucson, AZ Zip 85719; tel. 520/318–6300; William C. Behnke Jr., Chief Executive Officer

ARKANSAS: CENTRAL ARKANSAS HOSPITAL (O, 173 beds) 1200 South Main, Searcy, AR Zip 72143; tel. 501/278–3131; David C. Laffoon, Executive Director

METHODIST HOSPITAL OF JONESBORO (O, 104 beds) 3024 Stadium Boulevard, Jonesboro, AR Zip 72401; tel. 501/972–7000; Philip H. Walkley Jr., Chief Executive Officer

NATIONAL PARK MEDICAL CENTER (O, 166 beds) 1910 Malvern Avenue, Hot Springs, AR Zip 71901; tel. 501/321–1000; Jerry D. Mabry, Executive Director

SAINT MARY'S REGIONAL MEDICAL CENTER (O, 152 beds) 1808 West Main Street, Russellville, AR Zip 72801; tel. 501/968–2841; Mike McCoy, Chief Executive Officer

CALIFORNIA: ALVARADO HOSPITAL MEDICAL CENTER (O, 144 beds) 6655 Alvarado Road, San Diego, CA Zip 92120–5298; tel. 619/229–3100; Barry G. Weinbaum, Chief Executive Officer

BROOKSIDE HOSPITAL (O, 286 beds) 2000 Vale Road, San Pablo, CA Zip 94806; tel. 510/235–7000; Michael P. Lawson, President and Chief Executive Officer

BROTMAN MEDICAL CENTER (O, 240 beds) 3828 Delmas Terrace, Culver City, CA Zip 90231–2459, Mailing Address: Box 2459, Zip 90231–2459; tel. 310/836–7000; John V. Fenton, Chief Executive Officer

CENTINELA HOSPITAL MEDICAL CENTER (O, 375 beds) 555 East Hardy Street, Inglewood, CA Zip 90301–4073, Mailing Address: Box 720, Zip 90307–0720; tel. 310/673–4660; John Smithhisler, CHE, Chief Executive Officer

CENTURY CITY HOSPITAL (L, 135 beds) 2070 Century Park East, Los Angeles, CA Zip 90067; tel. 310/553–6211; John R. Nickens III, Chief Executive Officer

CHAPMAN MEDICAL CENTER (L, 135 beds) 2601 East Chapman Avenue, Orange, CA Zip 92869; tel. 714/633–0011; Maxine T. Cooper, Chief Executive Officer

COASTAL COMMUNITIES HOSPITAL (O, 177 beds) 2701 South Bristol Street, Santa Ana, CA Zip 92704–9911, Mailing Address: P.O. Box 5240, Zip 92704–0240; tel. 714/754–5454; Mark Meyers, Chief Executive Officer

COMMUNITY HOSPITAL OF HUNTINGTON PARK (L, 226 beds) 2623 East Slauson Avenue, Huntington Park, CA Zip 90255; tel. 213/583–1931; Charles Martinez, Ph.D., Chief Executive Officer

COMMUNITY HOSPITAL OF LOS GATOS (L, 209 beds) 815 Pollard Road, Los Gatos, CA Zip 95030; tel. 408/378–6131; Truman L. Gates, Chief Executive Officer

DOCTORS HOSPITAL OF MANTECA (O, 73 beds) 1205 East North Street, Manteca, CA Zip 95336, Mailing Address: Box 191, Zip 95336; tel. 209/823–3111; Patrick W. Rufferty, Chief Executive Officer

DOCTORS HOSPITAL OF PINOLE (L, 137 beds) 2151 Appian Way, Pinole, CA Zip 94564; tel. 510/724–5000; Gary Sloan, Chief Executive Officer

DOCTORS MEDICAL CENTER (O, 289 beds) 1441 Florida Avenue, Modesto, CA Zip 95350–4418, Mailing Address: P.O. Box 4138, Zip 95352–4138; tel. 209/578–1211; Chris DiCicco, Chief Executive Officer

ENCINO–TARZANA REGIONAL MEDICAL CENTER (L, 382 beds) 18321 Clark Street, Tarzana, CA Zip 91356; tel. 818/881–0800; Arnold R. Schaffer, Chief Executive Officer

FOUNTAIN VALLEY REGIONAL HOSPITAL AND MEDICAL CENTER (O, 413 beds) 17100 Euclid at Warner, Fountain Valley, CA Zip 92708; tel. 714/966–7200; Richard E. Butler, Chief Executive Officer

FRENCH HOSPITAL MEDICAL CENTER (O, 124 beds) 1911 Johnson Avenue, San Luis Obispo, CA Zip 93401; tel. 805/543–5353; William L. Gilbert, Chief Executive Officer

GARDEN GROVE HOSPITAL AND MEDICAL CENTER (O, 167 beds) 12601 Garden Grove Boulevard, Garden Grove, CA Zip 92843–1959; tel. 714/741–2700; Timothy Smith, President and Chief Executive Officer

GARFIELD MEDICAL CENTER (O, 207 beds) 525 North Garfield Avenue, Monterey Park, CA Zip 91754; tel. 818/573–2222; Philip A. Cohen, Chief Executive Officer

GREATER EL MONTE COMMUNITY HOSPITAL (O, 113 beds) 1701 South Santa Anita Avenue, South El Monte, CA Zip 91733–9918; tel. 818/579–7777; Elizabeth A. Primeaux, Chief Executive Officer

HARBOR VIEW MEDICAL CENTER (O, 146 beds) 120 Elm Street, San Diego, CA Zip 92101; tel. 619/232–4331; Steve Hall, Chief Executive Officer

IRVINE MEDICAL CENTER (L, 153 beds) 16200 Sand Canyon Avenue, Irvine, CA Zip 92618–3714; tel. 714/753–2000; Richard H. Robinson, Chief Executive Officer

JOHN F. KENNEDY MEMORIAL HOSPITAL (O, 130 beds) 47–111 Monroe Street, Indio, CA Zip 92201, Mailing Address: P.O. Drawer LLLL, Zip 92202–2558; tel. 619/347–6191; Michael A. Rembis, Chief Executive Officer

LAKEWOOD REGIONAL MEDICAL CENTER (O, 148 beds) 3700 East South Street, Lakewood, CA Zip 90712; tel. 310/531–2550; Gustavo A. Valdespino, Chief Executive Officer

LOS ALAMITOS MEDICAL CENTER (O, 173 beds) 3751 Katella Avenue, Los Alamitos, CA Zip 90720; tel. 310/598–1311; Gustavo A. Valdespino, Chief Executive Officer

MIDWAY HOSPITAL MEDICAL CENTER (O, 291 beds) 5925 San Vicente Boulevard, Los Angeles, CA Zip 90019; tel. 213/938–3161; John V. Fenton, Chief Executive Officer

MONTEREY PARK HOSPITAL (O, 95 beds) 900 South Atlantic Boulevard, Monterey Park, CA Zip 91754; tel. 818/570–9000; Dan F. Ausman, Chief Executive Officer

NORTH HOLLYWOOD MEDICAL CENTER (O, 150 beds) 12629 Riverside Drive, North Hollywood, CA Zip 91607–3495; tel. 818/980–9200; Dale Surowitz, President and Chief Executive Officer

PLACENTIA–LINDA HOSPITAL (O, 114 beds) 1301 Rose Drive, Placentia, CA Zip 92870; tel. 714/993–2000; Maxine T. Cooper, Chief Executive Officer

REDDING MEDICAL CENTER (O, 162 beds) 1100 Butte Street, Redding, CA Zip 96001–0853, Mailing Address: Box 496072, Zip 96049–6072; tel. 916/244–5454; Jeff Koury, Chief Executive Officer

SAN DIMAS COMMUNITY HOSPITAL (O, 93 beds) 1350 West Covina Boulevard, San Dimas, CA Zip 91773–0308; tel. 909/599–6811; Larry Peterson, Chief Executive Officer

SAN RAMON REGIONAL MEDICAL CENTER (O, 103 beds) 6001 Norris Canyon Road, San Ramon, CA Zip 94583; tel. 510/275–9200; Philip P. Gustafson, Chief Executive Officer

For explanation of codes following names, see page B2.
★ Indicates Type III membership in the American Hospital Association.

SANTA ANA HOSPITAL MEDICAL CENTER (O, 90 beds) 1901 North Fairview Street, Santa Ana, CA Zip 92706; tel. 714/554–1653; Michael H. Sussman, Acting Chief Executive Officer

SIERRA VISTA REGIONAL MEDICAL CENTER (O, 117 beds) 1010 Murray Street, San Luis Obispo, CA Zip 93405, Mailing Address: Box 1367, Zip 93406–1367; tel. 805/546–7600; Harold E. Chilton, Chief Executive Officer

SOUTH BAY MEDICAL CENTER (L, 149 beds) 514 North Prospect Avenue, Redondo Beach, CA Zip 90277; tel. 310/376–9474; Jerald R. Happel, Executive Director

ST. LUKE MEDICAL CENTER (O, 120 beds) 2632 East Washington Boulevard, Pasadena, CA Zip 91107–1994; tel. 818/797–1141; Mark Uffer, Chief Executive Officer

SUBURBAN MEDICAL CENTER (L, 130 beds) 16453 South Colorado Avenue, Paramount, CA Zip 90723; tel. 310/531–3110; Michael D. Kerr, Chief Executive Officer

TWIN CITIES COMMUNITY HOSPITAL (O, 84 beds) 1100 Las Tablas Road, Templeton, CA Zip 93465; tel. 805/434–3500; Harold E. Chilton, Chief Executive Officer

VALLEY COMMUNITY HOSPITAL (L, 70 beds) 505 East Plaza Drive, Santa Maria, CA Zip 93454–9943; tel. 805/925–0935; William C. Rasmussen, Chief Executive Officer

WESTERN MEDICAL CENTER HOSPITAL ANAHEIM (O, 171 beds) 1025 South Anaheim Boulevard, Anaheim, CA Zip 92805; tel. 714/533–6220; Doug Norris, Chief Operating Officer

WESTERN MEDICAL CENTER–SANTA ANA (O, 288 beds) 1001 North Tustin Avenue, Santa Ana, CA Zip 92705–3502; tel. 714/835–3555; Richard E. Butler, Chief Executive Officer

WHITTIER HOSPITAL MEDICAL CENTER (O, 159 beds) 15151 Janine Drive, Whittier, CA Zip 90605; tel. 562/907–1541; Sandra M. Chester, Chief Executive Officer

WOODRUFF COMMUNITY HOSPITAL (O, 96 beds) 3800 Woodruff Avenue, Long Beach, CA Zip 90808; tel. 310/421–8241; Robert Glass, Executive Director

FLORIDA: CORAL GABLES HOSPITAL (O, 205 beds) 3100 Douglas Road, Coral Gables, FL Zip 33134–6990; tel. 305/445–8461; Martha Garcia, Chief Executive Officer

DELRAY COMMUNITY HOSPITAL (O, 211 beds) 5352 Linton Boulevard, Delray Beach, FL Zip 33484; tel. 407/498–4440; Mitchell S. Feldman, Chief Executive Officer

FLORIDA MEDICAL CENTER HOSPITAL (O, 459 beds) 5000 West Oakland Park Boulevard, Fort Lauderdale, FL Zip 33313–1585; tel. 305/735–6000; Denny De Narvaez, Chief Executive Officer

FLORIDA MEDICAL CENTER SOUTH (O, 127 beds) 6701 West Sunrise Boulevard, Plantation, FL Zip 33313; tel. 954/581–7800; Denny DeNaruaez, Chief Executive Officer

HIALEAH HOSPITAL (O, 411 beds) 651 East 25th Street, Hialeah, FL Zip 33013–3878; tel. 305/693–6100; Clifford J. Bauer, Chief Executive Officer

HOLLYWOOD MEDICAL CENTER (O, 238 beds) 3600 Washington Street, Hollywood, FL Zip 33021; tel. 954/966–4500; Holly Lerner, Chief Executive Officer

MEMORIAL HOSPITAL OF TAMPA (O, 174 beds) 2901 Swann Avenue, Tampa, FL Zip 33609–4057; tel. 813/873–6400; Stephen Mahan, Chief Executive Officer

NORTH BAY MEDICAL CENTER (O, 122 beds) 6600 Madison Street, New Port Richey, FL Zip 34652; tel. 813/842–8468; Dennis A. Taylor, Administrator

NORTH RIDGE MEDICAL CENTER (O, 391 beds) 5757 North Dixie Highway, Fort Lauderdale, FL Zip 33334; tel. 305/776–6000; Emil P. Miller, Chief Executive Officer

NORTH SHORE MEDICAL CENTER (O, 286 beds) 1100 N.W. 95th Street, Miami, FL Zip 33150–2098; tel. 305/835–6000; Steven M. Klein, President and Chief Executive Officer

PALM BEACH GARDENS MEDICAL CENTER (L, 204 beds) 3360 Burns Road, Palm Beach Gardens, FL Zip 33410–4304; tel. 407/622–1411

PALMETTO GENERAL HOSPITAL (O, 360 beds) 2001 West 68th Street, Hialeah, FL Zip 33016; tel. 305/823–5000; John C. Johnson, Chief Executive Officer

PALMS OF PASADENA HOSPITAL (O, 267 beds) 1501 Pasadena Avenue South, Saint Petersburg, FL Zip 33707; tel. 813/381–1000; John D. Bartlett, Chief Executive Officer

PARKWAY REGIONAL MEDICAL CENTER (O, 392 beds) 160 N.W. 170th Street, North Miami Beach, FL Zip 33169; tel. 305/654–5050; Stephen M. Patz, Chief Executive Officer

SEVEN RIVERS COMMUNITY HOSPITAL (O, 128 beds) 6201 North Suncoast Boulevard, Crystal River, FL Zip 34428; tel. 904/795–6560; Michael L. Collins, Chief Executive Officer

TOWN AND COUNTRY HOSPITAL (O, 148 beds) 6001 Webb Road, Tampa, FL Zip 33615–3291; tel. 813/885–6666; Stephen Mahan, Chief Executive Officer

WEST BOCA MEDICAL CENTER (O, 150 beds) 21644 State Road 7, Boca Raton, FL Zip 33428–1899; tel. 407/488–8000; Richard Gold, Chief Executive Officer

GEORGIA: NORTH FULTON REGIONAL HOSPITAL (L, 168 beds) 3000 Hospital Boulevard, Roswell, GA Zip 30076–9930; tel. 404/751–2500; Frederick R. Bailey, Chief Executive Officer

SPALDING REGIONAL HOSPITAL (O, 160 beds) 601 South Eighth Street, Griffin, GA Zip 30224, Mailing Address: P.O. Drawer V, Zip 30224–1168; tel. 770/228–2721; Phil Shaw, Executive Director

INDIANA: CULVER UNION HOSPITAL (O, 98 beds) 1710 Lafayette Road, Crawfordsville, IN Zip 47933; tel. 765/362–2800; Gregory D. Starnes, Chief Executive Officer

WINONA MEMORIAL HOSPITAL (O, 159 beds) 3232 North Meridian Street, Indianapolis, IN Zip 46208–4693; tel. 317/924–3392; Keith R. King, Chief Executive Officer

IOWA: DAVENPORT MEDICAL CENTER (O, 106 beds) 1111 West Kimberly Road, Davenport, IA Zip 52806; tel. 319/391–2020; Richard A. Seidler, Chief Executive Officer

LOUISIANA: DOCTORS HOSPITAL OF JEFFERSON (L, 114 beds) 4320 Houma Boulevard, Metairie, LA Zip 70006–2973; tel. 504/456–5800; Gerald L. Parton, Chief Executive Officer

KENNER REGIONAL MEDICAL CENTER (O, 213 beds) 180 West Esplanade Avenue, Kenner, LA Zip 70065; tel. 504/468–8600; Steven J. Greene, Chief Executive Officer

MEADOWCREST HOSPITAL (O, 181 beds) 2500 Belle Chase Highway, Gretna, LA Zip 70056; tel. 504/392–3131; Jaime A. Wesolowski, Chief Executive Officer

MEMORIAL MEDICAL CENTER (O, 522 beds) 2700 Napoleon Avenue, New Orleans, LA Zip 70115; tel. 504/899–9311; Randall L. Hoover, Chief Executive Officer

MINDEN MEDICAL CENTER (O, 121 beds) 1 Medical Plaza, Minden, LA Zip 71055; tel. 318/377–2321; George E. French III, Chief Executive Officer

NORTHSHORE REGIONAL MEDICAL CENTER (L, 147 beds) 100 Medical Center Drive, Slidell, LA Zip 70461–8572; tel. 504/649–7070; Charles F. Miller, Chief Executive Officer

ST. CHARLES GENERAL HOSPITAL (O, 137 beds) 3700 St. Charles Avenue, New Orleans, LA Zip 70115; tel. 504/899–7441; Lynn C. Orfgen, Chief Executive Officer

MASSACHUSETTS: SAINT VINCENT HOSPITAL (O, 369 beds) 25 Winthrop Street, Worcester, MA Zip 01604–4593; tel. 508/798–1234; Robert E. Maher Jr., President and Chief Executive Officer

MISSISSIPPI: GULF COAST MEDICAL CENTER (O, 189 beds) 180–A Debuys Road, Biloxi, MS Zip 39531–4405, Mailing Address: Box 4518, Zip 39531–4518; tel. 601/388–6711; Gary L. Stokes, Chief Executive Officer

MISSOURI: COLUMBIA REGIONAL HOSPITAL (O, 265 beds) 404 Keene Street, Columbia, MO Zip 65201–6698; tel. 573/875–9000; Thomas G. Neff, Chief Executive Officer

LUCY LEE HOSPITAL (L, 185 beds) 2620 North Westwood Boulevard, Poplar Bluff, MO Zip 63901–2341, Mailing Address: P.O. Box 88, Zip 63901–2341; tel. 573/785–7721; David L. Archer, Chief Executive Officer

LUTHERAN MEDICAL CENTER (O, 232 beds) 2639 Miami Street, Saint Louis, MO Zip 63118–3999; tel. 314/772–1456; Cliff Yeager, Chief Executive Officer

For explanation of codes following names, see page B2.
★ Indicates Type III membership in the American Hospital Association.

TWIN RIVERS REGIONAL MEDICAL CENTER (O, 119 beds) 1301 First Street, Kennett, MO Zip 63857; tel. 573/888–4522; Carol Hanes, Chief Executive Officer

NEBRASKA: ST. JOSEPH HOSPITAL (O, 284 beds) 601 North 30th Street, Omaha, NE Zip 68131–2197; tel. 402/449–5021; Matthew A. Kurs, President and Chief Executive Officer

NEVADA: LAKE MEAD HOSPITAL MEDICAL CENTER (O, 140 beds) 1409 East Lake Mead Boulevard, North Las Vegas, NV Zip 89030; tel. 702/649–7711; Ernest Libman, Administrator and Chief Executive Officer

NORTH CAROLINA: CENTRAL CAROLINA HOSPITAL (O, 137 beds) 1135 Carthage Street, Sanford, NC Zip 27330; tel. 919/774–2100; L. Glenn Davis, Executive Director

FRYE REGIONAL MEDICAL CENTER (L, 355 beds) 420 North Center Street, Hickory, NC Zip 28601; tel. 704/322–6070; Dennis Phillips, Chief Executive Officer

OREGON: EASTMORELAND HOSPITAL (O, 77 beds) 2900 S.E. Steele Street, Portland, OR Zip 97202; tel. 503/234–0411; Ken Giles, Administrator

WOODLAND PARK HOSPITAL (O, 123 beds) 10300 N.E. Hancock, Portland, OR Zip 97220; tel. 503/257–5500; Jack Dusenbery, Chief Executive Officer

SOUTH CAROLINA: EAST COOPER REGIONAL MEDICAL CENTER (O, 100 beds) 1200 Johnnie Dodds Boulevard, Mount Pleasant, SC Zip 29464; tel. 803/881–0100; John Holland, President

HILTON HEAD MEDICAL CENTER AND CLINICS (O, 68 beds) Hilton Head Island, SC Mailing Address: P.O. Box 21117, Zip 29925–1117; tel. 803/681–6122; Dennis Ray Bruns, President and Chief Executive Officer

PIEDMONT HEALTHCARE SYSTEM (O, 276 beds) 222 Herlong Avenue, Rock Hill, SC Zip 29732; tel. 803/329–1234; Paul A. Walker, President

TENNESSEE: HARTON REGIONAL MEDICAL CENTER (O, 137 beds) 1801 North Jackson Street, Tullahoma, TN Zip 37388, Mailing Address: P.O. Box 460, Zip 37388; tel. 615/393–3000; Brian T. Flynn, Administrator and Chief Executive Officer

MEDICAL CENTER OF MANCHESTER (L, 49 beds) 481 Interstate Drive, Manchester, TN Zip 37355, Mailing Address: P.O. Box 1409, Zip 37355; tel. 615/728–6354; Sherry Collier, Chief Nursing Officer and Chief Operating Officer

SAINT FRANCIS HOSPITAL (O, 559 beds) 5959 Park Avenue, Memphis, TN Zip 38119–5198, Mailing Address: P.O. Box 171808, Zip 38187–1808; tel. 901/765–1000; Charles R. Slaton, President and Chief Executive Officer

UNIVERSITY MEDICAL CENTER (O, 225 beds) 1411 Baddour Parkway, Lebanon, TN Zip 37087; tel. 615/444–8262; Nanette Todd, R.N., Acting Administrator

TEXAS: BROWNSVILLE MEDICAL CENTER (O, 196 beds) 1040 West Jefferson Street, Brownsville, TX Zip 78520–5829, Mailing Address: Box 3590, Zip 78523–3590; tel. 210/544–1400; Robert Collete, Chief Executive Officer

DOCTORS HOSPITAL OF DALLAS (O, 197 beds) 9440 Poppy Drive, Dallas, TX Zip 75218; tel. 214/324–6100; Robert S. Freymuller, Chief Executive Officer

GARLAND COMMUNITY HOSPITAL (O, 113 beds) 2696 West Walnut Street, Garland, TX Zip 75042; tel. 214/276–7116; K. Dwayne Ray, Administrator and Chief Executive Officer

HOUSTON NORTHWEST MEDICAL CENTER (O, 370 beds) 710 FM 1960 West, Houston, TX Zip 77090–3496; tel. 281/440–1000; J. O. Lewis, Chief Executive Officer

LAKE POINTE MEDICAL CENTER (O, 92 beds) 6800 Scenic Drive, Rowlett, TX Zip 75088–1550, Mailing Address: P.O. Box 1550, Zip 75030–1500; tel. 972/412–2273; Kenneth R. Teel, Administrator

MID–JEFFERSON HOSPITAL (O, 138 beds) Highway 365 and 27th Street, Nederland, TX Zip 77627, Mailing Address: P.O. Box 1917, Zip 77627–1917; tel. 409/727–2321; Wilson J. Weber, Chief Executive Officer

NACOGDOCHES MEDICAL CENTER (O, 113 beds) 4920 N.E. Stallings, Nacogdoches, TX Zip 75961, Mailing Address: Box 631604, Zip 75963–1604; tel. 409/568–3380; Bryant H. Krenek Jr., Director

ODESSA REGIONAL HOSPITAL (O, 100 beds) 520 East Sixth Street, Odessa, TX Zip 79761, Mailing Address: Box 4859, Zip 79760; tel. 915/334–8200; Lex A. Guinn, Chief Executive Officer

PARK PLACE MEDICAL CENTER (O, 219 beds) 3050 39th Street, Port Arthur, TX Zip 77642, Mailing Address: Box 1648, Zip 77641; tel. 409/983–4951; Bob McCurry, Interim Chief Executive Officer

PARK PLAZA HOSPITAL (O, 370 beds) 1313 Hermann Drive, Houston, TX Zip 77004; tel. 713/527–5000; Judith Novak, President and Chief Executive Officer

PROVIDENCE MEMORIAL HOSPITAL (O, 348 beds) 2001 North Oregon Street, El Paso, TX Zip 79902; tel. 915/577–6011; L. Marcus Fry Jr., Chief Executive Officer

RHD MEMORIAL MEDICAL CENTER (L, 117 beds) Seven Medical Parkway, Dallas, TX Zip 75234, Mailing Address: P.O. Box 819094, Zip 75381–9094; tel. 214/247–1000; Thomas E. Casaday, President

SHARPSTOWN GENERAL HOSPITAL (O, 121 beds) 6700 Bellaire at Tarnef, Houston, TX Zip 77074–4999, Mailing Address: P.O. Box 740389, Zip 77274–0389; tel. 713/774–7611; Glenn Robinson, Chief Executive Officer

SIERRA MEDICAL CENTER (O, 365 beds) 1625 Medical Center Drive, El Paso, TX Zip 79902–5044; tel. 915/747–4000; L. Marcus Fry Jr., Chief Executive Officer

SOUTH PARK HOSPITAL (O, 101 beds) 6610 Quaker Avenue, Lubbock, TX Zip 79413–5938; tel. 806/791–8000; D. Clinton Matthews, Chief Executive Officer

SOUTHWEST GENERAL HOSPITAL (O, 223 beds) 7400 Barlite Boulevard, San Antonio, TX Zip 78224–1399; tel. 210/921–2000; Keith Swinney, Chief Executive Officer

TRINITY MEDICAL CENTER (L, 149 beds) 4343 North Josey Lane, Carrollton, TX Zip 75010; tel. 214/492–1010; Thomas E. Casaday, President

TRINITY VALLEY MEDICAL CENTER (O, 150 beds) 2900 South Loop 256, Palestine, TX Zip 75801; tel. 903/731–1000; Larry C. Bozeman, Chief Executive Officer

TWELVE OAKS HOSPITAL (O, 199 beds) 4200 Portsmouth Street, Houston, TX Zip 77027; tel. 713/623–2500; Steve Altmiller, Chief Executive Officer

WASHINGTON: PUGET SOUND HOSPITAL (O, 146 beds) 215 South 36th Street, Tacoma, WA Zip 98408, Mailing Address: P.O. Box 11412, Zip 98411–0412; tel. 206/474–0561; Bruce Brandler, Administrator

WEST VIRGINIA: PLATEAU MEDICAL CENTER (O, 79 beds) 430 Main Street, Oak Hill, WV Zip 25901; tel. 304/469–8600

WYOMING: LANDER VALLEY MEDICAL CENTER (O, 102 beds) 1320 Bishop Randall Drive, Lander, WY Zip 82520; tel. 307/332–4420; Andrew Gramlich, Chief Executive Officer

Owned, leased, sponsored:	122 hospitals	23362 beds
Contract–managed:	0 hospitals	0 beds
Totals:	122 hospitals	23362 beds

0020: TEXAS DEPARTMENT OF HEALTH (NP)
1100 West 49th Street, Austin, TX Zip 78756; tel. 512/458–7111; Patti J. Patterson, Commissioner

TEXAS: SOUTH TEXAS HOSPITAL (O, 85 beds) 1301 Rangerville Road, Harlingen, TX Zip 78552–7609, Mailing Address: P.O. Box 592, Zip 78551–0592; tel. 210/423–3420; James N. Elkins, FACHE, Director

TEXAS CENTER FOR INFECTIOUS DISEASE (O, 109 beds) 2303 S.E. Military Drive, San Antonio, TX Zip 78223–3597; tel. 210/534–8857; James N. Elkins, FACHE, Director

Owned, leased, sponsored:	2 hospitals	194 beds
Contract–managed:	0 hospitals	0 beds
Totals:	2 hospitals	194 beds

0093: TRANSITIONAL HOSPITALS CORPORATION (IO)
5110 West Sahara Avenue, Las Vegas, NV Zip 89102; tel. 702/257–4000; Richard L. Conte, Chief Executive Officer and Chairman of the Board

CALIFORNIA: THC–ORANGE COUNTY (O, 48 beds) 875 Brea Boulevard, Brea, CA Zip 92821; tel. 714/529–6842; Donna Hoover, Chief Executive Officer

For explanation of codes following names, see page B2.
★ Indicates Type III membership in the American Hospital Association.

FLORIDA: TRANSITIONAL HOSPITAL OF TAMPA (O, 102 beds) 4801 North Howard Avenue, Tampa, FL Zip 33603; tel. 813/874–7575; Robert N. Helms Jr., Divisional Vice President, Operations

ILLINOIS: TRANSITIONAL HOSPITAL OF CHICAGO (O, 81 beds) 4058 West Melrose Street, Chicago, IL Zip 60641; tel. 773/736–7000; Darryl L. Duncan, Chief Executive Officer

LOUISIANA: THC–NEW ORLEANS (O, 78 beds) 3601 Coliseum Street, New Orleans, LA Zip 70115; tel. 504/899–1555; John R. Watkins, Chief Executive Officer

MASSACHUSETTS: THC–BOSTON (O, 59 beds) 15 King Street, Peabody, MA Zip 01960; tel. 508/531–2900; Della Underwood, Chief Executive Officer

MINNESOTA: TRANSITIONAL HOSPITAL CORPORATION OF MINNEAPOLIS (O, 111 beds) 4101 Golden Valley Road, Golden Valley, MN Zip 55422; tel. 612/588–2750; Patrick A. Auman, Ph.D., Chief Executive Officer

NEVADA: THC–LAS VEGAS HOSPITAL (O, 52 beds) 5100 West Sahara Avenue, Las Vegas, NV Zip 89102; tel. 702/871–1418; Dale A. Kirby, Chief Executive Officer

NEW MEXICO: THC–ALBUQUERQUE (O, 61 beds) 700 High Street N.E., Albuquerque, NM Zip 87102; tel. 505/242–4444; Jean Koester, Chief Executive Officer

TEXAS: THC–ARLINGTON (O, 75 beds) 1000 North Cooper, Arlington, TX Zip 76011; tel. 817/543–0200; Darryl S. Dubroca, Administrator

THC–FORT WORTH (O, 80 beds) 7800 Oakmont Boulevard, Fort Worth, TX Zip 76132; tel. 817/346–0094; Barbara Schmidt, Chief Executive Officer

WASHINGTON: THC–SEATTLE HOSPITAL (O, 30 beds) 10560 Fifth Avenue N.E., Seattle, WA Zip 98125–0977; tel. 206/364–2050; Deborah L. Abrams, Chief Executive Officer

WISCONSIN: THC–MILWAUKEE (O, 34 beds) 5017 South 110th Street, Greenfield, WI Zip 53228; tel. 414/427–8282; Lee Jaeger, Chief Executive Officer

Owned, leased, sponsored:	12 hospitals	811 beds
Contract–managed:	0 hospitals	0 beds
Totals:	12 hospitals	811 beds

★9255: TRUMAN MEDICAL CENTER (NP)
2301 Holmes Street, Kansas City, MO Zip 64108–2677; tel. 816/556–3153; E. Ratcliffe Anderson Jr., M.D., Executive Director

MISSOURI: TRUMAN MEDICAL CENTER–EAST (C, 302 beds) 7900 Lee's Summit Road, Kansas City, MO Zip 64139–1241; tel. 816/373–4415; Ross P. Marine, Administrator and Chief Executive Officer

TRUMAN MEDICAL CENTER–WEST (C, 229 beds) 2301 Holmes Street, Kansas City, MO Zip 64108; tel. 816/556–3000; Rosa L. Miller, R.N., Administrator

Owned, leased, sponsored:	0 hospitals	0 beds
Contract–managed:	2 hospitals	531 beds
Totals:	2 hospitals	531 beds

9195: U. S. PUBLIC HEALTH SERVICE INDIAN HEALTH SERVICE (FG)
2275 Research Boulevard, Rockville, MD Zip 20850; tel. 202/619–0257; Michael Trujillo, M.D., M.P.H., Director

ALASKA: KANAKANAK HOSPITAL (O, 16 beds) Dillingham, AK Mailing Address: P.O. Box 130, Zip 99576; tel. 907/842–5201; Darrel C. Richardson, Chief Operating Officer

MANIILAQ HEALTH CENTER (O, 17 beds) Kotzebue, AK Zip 99752–0043; tel. 907/442–3321; Jan Harris, Vice President

NORTON SOUND REGIONAL HOSPITAL (O, 34 beds) Bering Street, Nome, AK Zip 99762, Mailing Address: Box 966, Zip 99762; tel. 907/443–3311; Charles Fagerstrom, Vice President

SAMUEL SIMMONDS MEMORIAL HOSPITAL (O, 15 beds) Barrow, AK Zip 99723; tel. 907/852–4611; John Morrow, Administrator

SEARHC MT. EDGECUMBE HOSPITAL (O, 72 beds) 222 Tongass Drive, Sitka, AK Zip 99835–9416; tel. 907/966–2411; Arthur C. Willman, Vice President Operations

U. S. PUBLIC HEALTH SERVICE ALASKA NATIVE MEDICAL CENTER (O, 140 beds) 255 Gambell Street, Anchorage, AK Zip 99501, Mailing Address: P.O. Box 107741, Zip 99510; tel. 907/279–6661; Richard Mandsager, M.D., Director

YUKON–KUSKOKWIM DELTA REGIONAL HOSPITAL (O, 50 beds) P.O. Box 528, Bethel, AK Zip 99559–3000; tel. 907/543–6300; Edwin L. Hansen, Vice President

ARIZONA: CHINLE COMPREHENSIVE HEALTH CARE FACILITY (O, 60 beds) Highway 191, Chinle, AZ Zip 86503, Mailing Address: P.O. Drawer PH, Zip 86503; tel. 520/674–5281; Ronald Tso, Chief Executive Officer

HUHUKAM MEMORIAL HOSPITAL (O, 10 beds) Seed Farm Road, Sacaton, AZ Zip 85247–0038, Mailing Address: P.O. Box 38, Zip 85247; tel. 602/562–3321; Viola L. Johnson, Chief Executive Officer

TUBA CITY INDIAN MEDICAL CENTER (O, 69 beds) Main Street, Tuba City, AZ Zip 86045–6211, Mailing Address: P.O. Box 600, Zip 86045–6211; tel. 520/283–2827; Susie John, M.D., Chief Executive Officer

U. S. PUBLIC HEALTH SERVICE FORT DEFIANCE INDIAN HEALTH SERVICE HOSPITAL (O, 49 beds) Fort Defiance, AZ Mailing Address: P.O. Box 649, Zip 86504; tel. 520/729–3223; Franklin Freeland, Ed.D., Chief Executive Officer

U. S. PUBLIC HEALTH SERVICE INDIAN HOSPITAL (O, 18 beds) Parker, AZ Mailing Address: Route 1, Box 12, Zip 85344; tel. 520/669–2137; Gary Davis, Service Unit Director

U. S. PUBLIC HEALTH SERVICE INDIAN HOSPITAL (O, 34 beds) Sells, AZ Mailing Address: P.O. Box 548, Zip 85634; tel. 520/383–7251; Darrell Rumley, Service Unit Director

U. S. PUBLIC HEALTH SERVICE INDIAN HOSPITAL (O, 28 beds) San Carlos, AZ Mailing Address: P.O. Box 208, Zip 85550; tel. 520/562–3382; Viola L. Johnson, Service Unit Director

U. S. PUBLIC HEALTH SERVICE INDIAN HOSPITAL (O, 45 beds) State Route 73, Box 860, Whiteriver, AZ Zip 85941–0860; tel. 520/338–4911; Carla Alchesay–Nachu, Service Unit Director

U. S. PUBLIC HEALTH SERVICE PHOENIX INDIAN MEDICAL CENTER (O, 137 beds) 4212 North 16th Street, Phoenix, AZ Zip 85016–5389; tel. 602/263–1200; Anna Albert, Chief Executive Officer

U. S. PUBLIC HEALTH SERVICES INDIAN HOSPITAL (O, 17 beds) Keams Canyon, AZ Mailing Address: P.O. Box 98, Zip 86034; tel. 520/738–2211; Taylor Satala, Service Unit Director

CALIFORNIA: U. S. PUBLIC HEALTH SERVICE INDIAN HOSPITAL (O, 17 beds) Winterhaven, CA Mailing Address: P.O. Box 1368, Yuma, AZZip 85366–8368; tel. 619/572–0217; Hortense Miguel, R.N., Acting Service Unit Director

MARYLAND: WARREN G. MAGNUSON CLINICAL CENTER, NATIONAL INSTITUTES OF HEALTH (O, 330 beds) 9000 Rockville Pike, Bethesda, MD Zip 20892–1504; tel. 301/496–4114; John I. Gallin, M.D., Director

MINNESOTA: U. S. PUBLIC HEALTH SERVICE INDIAN HOSPITAL (O, 13 beds) 7th Street and Grant Utley Avenue N.W., Cass Lake, MN Zip 56633; tel. 218/335–2293; Luella Brown, Service Unit Director

U.S. PUBLIC HEALTH SERVICE INDIAN HOSPITAL (O, 23 beds) Redlake, MN Zip 56671; tel. 218/679–3912; Essimae Stevens, Service Unit Director

MISSISSIPPI: CHOCTAW HEALTH CENTER (O, 35 beds) Highway 16 West, Philadelphia, MS Zip 39350, Mailing Address: Route 7, Box R–50, Zip 39350; tel. 601/656–2211; Jim Wallace, Executive Director

MONTANA: U. S. PUBLIC HEALTH SERVICE BLACKFEET COMMUNITY HOSPITAL (O, 25 beds) Browning, MT Mailing Address: P.O. Box 760, Zip 59417–0760; tel. 406/338–6100; Mary Ellen LaFromboise, Service Unit Director

U. S. PUBLIC HEALTH SERVICE INDIAN HOSPITAL (O, 24 beds) Crow Agency, MT Mailing Address: Box 9, Zip 59022; tel. 406/638–2626; Tennyson Doney, Service Unit Director

U. S. PUBLIC HEALTH SERVICE INDIAN HOSPITAL (O, 12 beds) Rural Route 1, Box 67, Harlem, MT Zip 59526; tel. 406/353–2651; Charles D. Plumage, Director

NEBRASKA: U. S. PUBLIC HEALTH SERVICE INDIAN HOSPITAL (O, 30 beds) Winnebago, NE Zip 68071; tel. 402/878–2231; Shirley A. Poor Thunder, Service Unit Director

NEVADA: U. S. PUBLIC HEALTH SERVICE OWYHEE COMMUNITY HEALTH FACILITY (O, 15 beds) Owyhee, NV Mailing Address: P.O. Box 130, Zip 89832–0130; tel. 702/757–2415; Kay C. Jewett, Administrative Officer

For explanation of codes following names, see page B2.
★ Indicates Type III membership in the American Hospital Association.

NEW MEXICO: ACOMA–CANONCITO–LAGUNA HOSPITAL (O, 15 beds) San Fidel, NM Mailing Address: P.O. Box 130, Zip 87049; tel. 505/552–6634; Richard L. Zephier, Ph.D., Service Unit Director

GALLUP INDIAN MEDICAL CENTER (O, 99 beds) 516 East Nizhoni Boulevard, Gallup, NM Zip 87301–1334, Mailing Address: Box 1337, Zip 87305; tel. 505/722–1000; Timothy G. Fleming, M.D., Chief Executive Officer

NORTHERN NAVAJO MEDICAL CENTER (O, 59 beds) Shiprock, NM Mailing Address: Box 160, Zip 87420; tel. 505/368–6001; Dee Hutchison, Chief Executive Officer

PHS SANTA FE INDIAN HOSPITAL (O, 39 beds) 1700 Cerrillos Road, Santa Fe, NM Zip 87505; tel. 505/988–9821; Lawrence A. Jordan, Director

PUBLIC HEALTH SERVICE INDIAN HOSPITAL (O, 28 beds) 801 Vassar Drive N.E., Albuquerque, NM Zip 87106–2799; tel. 505/256–4000; Raymond L. Rodgers, Administrator

U. S. PUBLIC HEALTH SERVICE INDIAN HOSPITAL (O, 32 beds) Crownpoint, NM Mailing Address: Box 358, Zip 87313–0358; tel. 505/786–5291; Anita Muneta, Chief Executive Officer

U. S. PUBLIC HEALTH SERVICE INDIAN HOSPITAL (O, 13 beds) Mescalero, NM Mailing Address: Box 210, Zip 88340–0210; tel. 505/671–4441; Joe Wahnee Jr., Service Unit Director

U. S. PUBLIC HEALTH SERVICE INDIAN HOSPITAL (O, 29 beds) Zuni, NM Mailing Address: P.O. Box 467, Zip 87327; tel. 505/782–4431; Jean Othole, Service Unit Director

NORTH CAROLINA: U. S. PUBLIC HEALTH SERVICE INDIAN HOSPITAL (O, 30 beds) Hospital Road, Cherokee, NC Zip 28719; tel. 704/497–9163; Janet Belcourt, Administrator

NORTH DAKOTA: U. S. PUBLIC HEALTH SERVICE INDIAN HOSPITAL (O, 42 beds) Belcourt, ND Mailing Address: P.O. Box 160, Zip 58316–0130; tel. 701/477–6111; Ray Grandbois, M.P.H., Service Unit Director

U. S. PUBLIC HEALTH SERVICE INDIAN HOSPITAL (O, 14 beds) Fort Yates, ND Mailing Address: P.O. Box J, Zip 58538; tel. 701/854–3831; Terry Pourier, Service Unit Director

OKLAHOMA: CARL ALBERT INDIAN HEALTH FACILITY (O, 53 beds) 1001 North Country Club Road, Ada, OK Zip 74820–2847; tel. 405/436–3980; Kenneth R. Ross, Administrator

CHOCTAW NATION INDIAN HOSPITAL (O, 44 beds) Route 2, Box 1725, Talihina, OK Zip 74571; tel. 918/567–2211; Rosemary Hooser, Acting Administrator

CREEK NATION COMMUNITY HOSPITAL (O, 34 beds) 309 North 14th Street, Okemah, OK Zip 74859; tel. 918/623–1424; Philip Barnoski, Chief Executive Officer

U. S. PUBLIC HEALTH SERVICE COMPREHENSIVE INDIAN HEALTH FACILITY (O, 50 beds) 101 South Moore Avenue, Claremore, OK Zip 74017–5091; tel. 918/342–6434; John Daugherty Jr., Service Unit Director

U. S. PUBLIC HEALTH SERVICE INDIAN HOSPITAL (O, 11 beds) Clinton, OK Mailing Address: P.O. Box 279, Zip 73601; tel. 405/323–2884; Thedis V. Mitchell, Director

U. S. PUBLIC HEALTH SERVICE INDIAN HOSPITAL (O, 44 beds) 1515 Lawrie Tatum Road, Lawton, OK Zip 73507; tel. 405/353–0350; George F. Howell, Service Unit Director

WILLIAM W. HASTINGS INDIAN HOSPITAL (O, 60 beds) 100 South Bliss Avenue, Tahlequah, OK Zip 74464–3399; tel. 918/458–3100; Hickory Starr Jr., Administrator

SOUTH DAKOTA: INDIAN HEALTH SERVICE–SIOUX SAN HOSPITAL (O, 32 beds) 3200 Canyon Lake Drive, Rapid City, SD Zip 57702; tel. 605/355–2280; James Cournoyer, Director

U. S. PUBLIC HEALTH SERVICE INDIAN HOSPITAL (O, 27 beds) Eagle Butte, SD Mailing Address: P.O. Box 1012, Zip 57625–1012; tel. 605/964–3001; Orville Night Pipe, Service Unit Director

U. S. PUBLIC HEALTH SERVICE INDIAN HOSPITAL (O, 46 beds) Pine Ridge, SD Zip 57770–1201; tel. 605/867–5131; Vern F. Donnell, Service Unit Director

U. S. PUBLIC HEALTH SERVICE INDIAN HOSPITAL (O, 35 beds) Rosebud, SD Zip 57570; tel. 605/747–2231; Gayla J. Twiss, Service Unit Director

U. S. PUBLIC HEALTH SERVICE INDIAN HOSPITAL (O, 18 beds) Chestnut Street, Sisseton, SD Zip 57262, Mailing Address: P.O. Box 189, Zip 57262; tel. 605/698–7606; Richard Huff, Administrator

Owned, leased, sponsored:	50 hospitals	2189 beds
Contract–managed:	0 hospitals	0 beds
Totals:	50 hospitals	2189 beds

★2315: UNIHEALTH (NP)
3400 Riverside Drive, Burbank, CA Zip 91505; tel. 818/238–6000; David R. Carpenter, FACHE, President and Chairman of the Board

CALIFORNIA: CALIFORNIA HOSPITAL MEDICAL CENTER (O, 309 beds) 1401 South Grand Avenue, Los Angeles, CA Zip 90015; tel. 213/748–2411; Melinda D. Beswick, President and Chief Executive Officer

GLENDALE MEMORIAL HOSPITAL AND HEALTH CENTER (O, 273 beds) 1420 South Central Avenue, Glendale, CA Zip 91204–2594; tel. 818/502–1900; Roger E. Seaver, President and Chief Executive Officer

LA PALMA INTERCOMMUNITY HOSPITAL (O, 139 beds) 7901 Walker Street, La Palma, CA Zip 90623–5850, Mailing Address: P.O. Box 5850, Buena Park, Zip 90622; tel. 714/670–7400; Stephen E. Dixon, President and Chief Executive Officer

LONG BEACH COMMUNITY MEDICAL CENTER (O, 290 beds) 1720 Termino Avenue, Long Beach, CA Zip 90804; tel. 310/498–1000; Makoto Nakayama, Interim President and Chief Executive Officer

MARTIN LUTHER HOSPITAL–ANAHEIM (O, 205 beds) 1830 West Romneya Drive, Anaheim, CA Zip 92801–1854; tel. 714/491–5200; Stephen E. Dixon, President and Chief Executive Officer

NORTHRIDGE HOSPITAL MEDICAL CENTER–ROSCOE BOULEVARD CAMPUS (O, 368 beds) 18300 Roscoe Boulevard, Northridge, CA Zip 91328; tel. 818/885–8500; Roger E. Seaver, President and Chief Executive Officer

NORTHRIDGE HOSPITAL AND MEDICAL CENTER, SHERMAN WAY CAMPUS (O, 195 beds) 14500 Sherman Circle, Van Nuys, CA Zip 91405; tel. 818/997–0101; Richard D. Lyons, President and Chief Administrative Officer

SAN GABRIEL VALLEY MEDICAL CENTER (O, 271 beds) 218 South Santa Anita Street, San Gabriel, CA Zip 91776, Mailing Address: P.O. Box 1507, Zip 91778–1507; tel. 818/289–5454; Makoto Nakayama, President and Chief Executive Officer

Owned, leased, sponsored:	8 hospitals	2050 beds
Contract–managed:	0 hospitals	0 beds
Totals:	8 hospitals	2050 beds

★2445: UNITED HEALTH GROUP (NP)
Five Innovation Court, Appleton, WI Zip 54914, Mailing Address: P.O. Box 8025, Zip 54913–8025; tel. 414/730–0330; James Edward Raney, President and Chief Executive Officer

WISCONSIN: APPLETON MEDICAL CENTER (O, 146 beds) 1818 North Meade Street, Appleton, WI Zip 54911; tel. 414/731–4101; Paul E. Macek, Senior Vice President

THEDA CLARK MEDICAL CENTER (O, 216 beds) 130 Second Street, Neenah, WI Zip 54956, Mailing Address: P.O. Box 2021, Zip 54957–2021; tel. 414/729–3100; Paul E. Macek, Senior Vice President

Owned, leased, sponsored:	2 hospitals	362 beds
Contract–managed:	0 hospitals	0 beds
Totals:	2 hospitals	362 beds

1765: UNITED HOSPITAL CORPORATION (IO)
6189 East Shelby Drive, Memphis, TN Zip 38115; tel. 901/794–8440; James C. Henson, President

ALABAMA: FLORALA MEMORIAL HOSPITAL (O, 23 beds) 515 East Fifth Avenue, Florala, AL Zip 36442–0189, Mailing Address: P.O. Box 189, Zip 36442–0189; tel. 334/858–3287; Blair W. Henson, Administrator

ARKANSAS: VAN BUREN COUNTY MEMORIAL HOSPITAL (C, 144 beds) Highway 65 South, Clinton, AR Zip 72031, Mailing Address: Box 206, Zip 72031; tel. 501/745–2401; Alan Finley, Administrator

For explanation of codes following names, see page B2.
★ Indicates Type III membership in the American Hospital Association.

Owned, leased, sponsored:	1 hospital	23 beds
Contract–managed:	1 hospital	144 beds
Totals:	2 hospitals	167 beds

9605: UNITED MEDICAL CORPORATION (IO)
603 Main Street, Windermere, FL Zip 34786, Mailing Address: P.O. Box 1100, Zip 34786–1100; tel. 407/876–2200; Donald R. Dizney, Chairman

KENTUCKY: TEN BROECK HOSPITAL (O, 94 beds) 8521 Old LaGrange Road, Louisville, KY Zip 40242; tel. 502/426–6380; Pat Hammer, Chief Executive Officer

LOUISIANA: ST. CLAUDE MEDICAL CENTER (O, 136 beds) 3419 St. Claude Avenue, New Orleans, LA Zip 70117; tel. 504/948–8200; Joseph R. Tucker, President

PUERTO RICO: DOCTORS GUBERN'S HOSPITAL (O, 51 beds) 110 Antonio R. Barcelo, Fajardo, PR Zip 00738, Mailing Address: Box 846, Zip 00738; tel. 809/863–0924; Roberto Acevedo, Administrator

HOSPITAL PAVIA (O, 183 beds) 1462 Asia Street, San Juan, PR Zip 00909, Mailing Address: Box 11137, Santurce Station, Zip 00910; tel. 809/727–6060; Jose Luis Suarez Fonseca, Executive Director

HOSPITAL PEREA (O, 82 beds) 15 Basora Street, Mayaguez, PR Zip 00681, Mailing Address: Box 170, Zip 00681; tel. 809/834–0101; Jaime F. Maestre, Executive Director

SAN JORGE CHILDREN'S HOSPITAL (O, 85 beds) 258 San Jorge Avenue, San Juan, PR Zip 00912; tel. 809/727–1000; Domingo Cruz Vivaldi, Administrator

Owned, leased, sponsored:	6 hospitals	631 beds
Contract–managed:	0 hospitals	0 beds
Totals:	6 hospitals	631 beds

9555: UNIVERSAL HEALTH SERVICES, INC. (IO)
367 South Gulph Road, King of Prussia, PA Zip 19406; tel. 610/768–3300; Alan B. Miller, President and Chief Executive Officer

ARKANSAS: BRIDGEWAY (L, 70 beds) 21 Bridgeway Road, North Little Rock, AR Zip 72113; tel. 501/771–1500; Barry Pipkin, Chief Executive Officer

CALIFORNIA: DEL AMO HOSPITAL (O, 166 beds) 23700 Camino Del Sol, Torrance, CA Zip 90505; tel. 310/530–1151; E. Daniel Thomas, Administrator and Chief Executive Officer

INLAND VALLEY REGIONAL MEDICAL CENTER (L, 80 beds) 36485 Inland Valley Drive, Wildomar, CA Zip 92595; tel. 909/677–1111; B. Ann Kuss, Chief Executive Officer and Managing Director

FLORIDA: MANATEE MEMORIAL HOSPITAL (O, 512 beds) 206 Second Street East, Bradenton, FL Zip 34208; tel. 941/745–7373; Michael Marquez, Chief Executive Officer

WELLINGTON REGIONAL MEDICAL CENTER (L, 93 beds) 10101 Forest Hill Boulevard, West Palm Beach, FL Zip 33414; tel. 561/798–8500; Gregory E. Boyer, Chief Executive Officer

GEORGIA: TURNING POINT HOSPITAL (O, 59 beds) 319 East By–Pass, Moultrie, GA Zip 31776, Mailing Address: P.O. Box 1177, Zip 31768; tel. 912/985–4815; Ben Marion, Chief Executive Officer

ILLINOIS: THE PAVILION (O, 38 beds) 809 West Church Street, Champaign, IL Zip 61820; tel. 217/373–1700; Nina W. Eisner, Chief Executive Officer

LOUISIANA: CHALMETTE MEDICAL CENTERS (L, 196 beds) 9001 Patricia Street, Chalmette, LA Zip 70043; tel. 504/277–8011; Larry M. Graham, Chief Executive Officer

DOCTORS' HOSPITAL OF SHREVEPORT (L, 118 beds) 1130 Louisiana Avenue, Shreveport, LA Zip 71101, Mailing Address: Box 1526, Zip 71165; tel. 318/227–1211; Charles E. Boyd, Administrator

RIVER OAKS HOSPITAL (O, 94 beds) 1525 River Oaks Road West, New Orleans, LA Zip 70123; tel. 504/734–1740; Daryl Sue White, R.N., Managing Director

RIVER PARISHES HOSPITAL (O, 60 beds) 500 Rue De Sante, Laplace, LA Zip 70068; tel. 504/652–7000; John Lloyd Hummer, Chief Executive Officer and Managing Director

MASSACHUSETTS: ARBOUR HOSPITAL (O, 118 beds) 49 Robinwood Avenue, Boston, MA Zip 02130, Mailing Address: P.O. Box 9, Zip 02130; tel. 617/522–4400; Roy A. Ettlinger, Chief Executive Officer

FULLER MEMORIAL HOSPITAL (O, 46 beds) 200 May Street, South Attleboro, MA Zip 02703–5599; tel. 508/761–8500; Landon Kite, President

H. R. I. HOSPITAL (O, 51 beds) 227 Babcock Street, Brookline, MA Zip 02146; tel. 617/731–3200; Roy A. Ettlinger, Chief Executive Officer

MICHIGAN: FOREST VIEW HOSPITAL (O, 62 beds) 1055 Medical Park Drive S.E., Grand Rapids, MI Zip 49546; tel. 616/942–9610; John F. Kuhn, Chief Executive Officer

MISSOURI: TWO RIVERS PSYCHIATRIC HOSPITAL (O, 80 beds) 5121 Raytown Road, Kansas City, MO Zip 64133–2141; tel. 816/356–5688; Craig Nuckles, Administrator

NEVADA: NORTHERN NEVADA MEDICAL CENTER (O, 110 beds) 2375 East Prater Way, Sparks, NV Zip 89434–9645; tel. 702/331–7000; James R. Pagels, Chief Executive Officer and Managing Director

VALLEY HOSPITAL MEDICAL CENTER (O, 365 beds) 620 Shadow Lane, Las Vegas, NV Zip 89106; tel. 702/388–4000; Roger Collins, Chief Executive Officer and Managing Director

PENNSYLVANIA: CLARION PSYCHIATRIC CENTER (O, 52 beds) 2 Hospital Drive, Clarion, PA Zip 16214, Mailing Address: Rural Delivery 3, Box 188, Zip 16214; tel. 814/226–9545; Michael R. Keefer, CHE, Chief Executive Officer

HORSHAM CLINIC (O, 138 beds) 722 East Butler Pike, Ambler, PA Zip 19002; tel. 215/643–7800; David A. Baron, D.O., Medical Director

KEYSTONE CENTER (O, 76 beds) 2001 Providence Avenue, Chester, PA Zip 19013–5504; tel. 610/876–9000; Jimmy Patton, Chief Executive Officer and Managing Director

MEADOWS PSYCHIATRIC CENTER (O, 101 beds) Centre Hall, PA Mailing Address: Rural Delivery 1, Box 259, Zip 16828; tel. 814/364–2161; Joseph Barszczewski, Chief Executive Officer

SOUTH CAROLINA: AIKEN REGIONAL MEDICAL CENTER (O, 233 beds) 202 University Parkway, Aiken, SC Zip 29801–2757, Mailing Address: P.O. Box 1117, Zip 29802–1117; tel. 803/641–5000; Richard H. Satcher, Chief Executive Officer

TEXAS: EDINBURG HOSPITAL (O, 94 beds) 333 West Freddy Gonzalez Drive, Edinburg, TX Zip 78539–6199; tel. 210/383–6211; Leon J. Belila, Administrator

GLEN OAKS HOSPITAL (O, 54 beds) 301 East Division, Greenville, TX Zip 75401; tel. 903/454–6000; Thomas E. Rourke, Administrator

MCALLEN MEDICAL CENTER (L, 472 beds) 301 West Expressway 83, McAllen, TX Zip 78503; tel. 210/632–4000; John L. Mims, Executive Director

MERIDELL ACHIEVEMENT CENTER (L, 78 beds) Austin, TX Mailing Address: P.O. Box 87, Liberty Hill, Zip 78642; tel. 800/366–8656; Scott McAvoy, Managing Director

NORTHWEST TEXAS HEALTHCARE SYSTEM (O, 332 beds) 1501 South Coulter Avenue, Amarillo, TX Zip 79106–1790, Mailing Address: P.O. Box 1110, Zip 79175–1110; tel. 806/354–1000; Michael A. Callahan, Chief Executive Officer

RIVER CREST HOSPITAL (O, 80 beds) 1636 Hunters Glen Road, San Angelo, TX Zip 76901–5016; tel. 915/949–5722; Larry Grimes, Managing Director

TIMBERLAWN MENTAL HEALTH SYSTEM (O, 124 beds) 4600 Samuell Boulevard, Dallas, TX Zip 75228, Mailing Address: Box 151489, Zip 75315–1489; tel. 214/381–7181; Debra S. Lowrance, R.N., Chief Executive Officer and Managing Director

VICTORIA REGIONAL MEDICAL CENTER (O, 108 beds) 101 Medical Drive, Victoria, TX Zip 77904; tel. 512/573–6100; J. Michael Mastej, Chief Executive Officer and Managing Director

WASHINGTON: AUBURN GENERAL HOSPITAL (O, 100 beds) 202 North Division, Plaza One, Auburn, WA Zip 98001; tel. 206/833–7711; Michael M. Gherardini, Managing Director

Owned, leased, sponsored:	32 hospitals	4360 beds
Contract–managed:	0 hospitals	0 beds
Totals:	32 hospitals	4360 beds

For explanation of codes following names, see page B2.
★ Indicates Type III membership in the American Hospital Association.

0112: UNIVERSITY HOSPITALS HEALTH SYSTEM (NP)

11100 Euclid Avenue, Cleveland, OH Zip 44106; tel. 216/844–1000; Farah M. Walters, President and Chief Executive Officer

OHIO: UHHS GEAUGA REGIONAL HOSPITAL (O, 121 beds) 13207 Ravenna Road, Chardon, OH Zip 44024; tel. 216/269–6000; Richard J. Frenchie, President and Chief Executive Officer

UHHS–MEMORIAL HOSPITAL OF GENEVA (O, 14 beds) 870 West Main Street, Geneva, OH Zip 44041–1295; tel. 216/466–1141; Gerard D. Klein, Chief Executive Officer

UNIVERSITY HOSPITALS HEALTH SYSTEM BEDFORD MEDICAL CENTER (O, 110 beds) 44 Blaine Avenue, Bedford, OH Zip 44146–2799; tel. 216/439–2000; Arlene A. Rak, R.N., President

UNIVERSITY HOSPITALS OF CLEVELAND (O, 725 beds) 11100 Euclid Avenue, Cleveland, OH Zip 44106–2602; tel. 216/844–1000; Farah M. Walters, President and Chief Executive Officer

Owned, leased, sponsored:	4 hospitals	970 beds
Contract–managed:	0 hospitals	0 beds
Totals:	4 hospitals	970 beds

6405: UNIVERSITY OF CALIFORNIA–SYSTEMWIDE ADMINISTRATION (NP)

300 Lakeside Drive, 18th Floor, Oakland, CA Zip 94612–3550; tel. 510/987–9701; Cornelius L. Hopper, M.D., Vice President Health Affairs

CALIFORNIA: SANTA MONICA–UCLA MEDICAL CENTER (O, 221 beds) 1250 16th Street, Santa Monica, CA Zip 90404–1200; tel. 310/319–4000; William D. Parente, Director and Chief Executive Officer

UNIVERSITY OF CALIFORNIA LOS ANGELES MEDICAL CENTER (L, 610 beds) 10833 Le Conte Avenue, Los Angeles, CA Zip 90095–1730; tel. 310/825–9111; Michael Karpf, M.D., Vice Provost Hospital System and Director Medical Center

UNIVERSITY OF CALIFORNIA LOS ANGELES NEUROPSYCHIATRIC HOSPITAL (O, 117 beds) 760 Westwood Plaza, Los Angeles, CA Zip 90024–1759; tel. 310/825–9548; G. Michael Arnold, Interim Director

UNIVERSITY OF CALIFORNIA SAN DIEGO MEDICAL CENTER (O, 412 beds) 200 West Arbor Drive, San Diego, CA Zip 92103–8970; tel. 619/543–6222; David B. Coats, President

UNIVERSITY OF CALIFORNIA SAN FRANCISCO MEDICAL CENTER (O, 663 beds) 500 Parnassus, San Francisco, CA Zip 94143–0296; tel. 415/476–1000; William B. Kerr, Director

UNIVERSITY OF CALIFORNIA, DAVIS MEDICAL CENTER (O, 448 beds) 2315 Stockton Boulevard, Sacramento, CA Zip 95817–2282; tel. 916/734–2011; Frank J. Loge, Director

UNIVERSITY OF CALIFORNIA, IRVINE MEDICAL CENTER (O, 383 beds) 101 The City Drive, Orange, CA Zip 92668–3298; tel. 714/456–7890; Mark R. Laret, Executive Director

Owned, leased, sponsored:	7 hospitals	2854 beds
Contract–managed:	0 hospitals	0 beds
Totals:	7 hospitals	2854 beds

0021: UNIVERSITY OF NEW MEXICO (NP)

915 Camino De Salud, Albuquerque, NM Zip 87131; tel. 505/272–5849; Jane E. Henney, M.D., Vice President Health Sciences

NEW MEXICO: CARRIE TINGLEY HOSPITAL (O, 18 beds) 1127 University Boulevard N.E., Albuquerque, NM Zip 87102–1715; tel. 505/272–5200; Kurt Sams, Interim Administrator

UNIVERSITY HOSPITAL (O, 267 beds) 2211 Lomas Boulevard N.E., Albuquerque, NM Zip 87106; tel. 505/272–2121; Stephen McKernan, Chief Executive Officer

UNIVERSITY OF NEW MEXICO CHILDREN'S PSYCHIATRIC HOSPITAL (O, 53 beds) 1001 Yale Boulevard N.E., Albuquerque, NM Zip 87131; tel. 505/272–2945; Christina B. Gunn, Chief Executive Officer

UNIVERSITY OF NEW MEXICO MENTAL HEALTH CENTER (O, 60 beds) 2600 Marble N.E., Albuquerque, NM Zip 87131–2600; tel. 505/272–2870; Christina B. Gunn, Chief Executive Officer

Owned, leased, sponsored:	4 hospitals	398 beds
Contract–managed:	0 hospitals	0 beds
Totals:	4 hospitals	398 beds

0057: UNIVERSITY OF SOUTH ALABAMA HOSPITALS (NP)

2451 Fillingim Street, Mobile, AL Zip 36617–2293; tel. 205/471–7110; Stephen H. Simmons, Senior Administrator

ALABAMA: USA DOCTORS HOSPITAL (O, 131 beds) 1700 Center Street, Mobile, AL Zip 36604–3391; tel. 334/415–1000; Thomas J. Gibson, Administrator

UNIVERSITY OF SOUTH ALABAMA KNOLLWOOD PARK HOSPITAL (O, 150 beds) 5600 Girby Road, Mobile, AL Zip 36693–3398; tel. 334/660–5120; Stanley K. Hammack, Administrator

UNIVERSITY OF SOUTH ALABAMA MEDICAL CENTER (O, 316 beds) 2451 Fillingim Street, Mobile, AL Zip 36617; tel. 334/471–7000; Stephen H. Simmons, Administrator

Owned, leased, sponsored:	3 hospitals	597 beds
Contract–managed:	0 hospitals	0 beds
Totals:	3 hospitals	597 beds

0033: UNIVERSITY OF TEXAS SYSTEM (NP)

601 Colorado Street, Austin, TX Zip 78701–2982; tel. 512/499–4224; Charles B. Mullins, Executive Vice Chancellor

TEXAS: HARRIS COUNTY PSYCHIATRIC CENTER (O, 250 beds) 2800 South MacGregor, Houston, TX Zip 77021, Mailing Address: P.O. Box 20249, Zip 77225–0249; tel. 713/741–5000; Robert W. Guynn, M.D., Executive Director

UNIVERSITY OF TEXAS HEALTH CENTER AT TYLER (O, 117 beds) Gladewater Highway, Tyler, TX Zip 75708, Mailing Address: Box 2003, Zip 75710–2003; tel. 903/877–3451; George A. Hurst, M.D., Director

UNIVERSITY OF TEXAS M. D. ANDERSON CANCER CENTER (O, 417 beds) 1515 Holcombe Boulevard, Box 506, Houston, TX Zip 77030–4096; tel. 713/461–0529; David J. Bachrach, Professor, Health Services Management

UNIVERSITY OF TEXAS MEDICAL BRANCH HOSPITALS (O, 858 beds) 301 University Boulevard, Galveston, TX Zip 77555–0138; tel. 409/772–1011; James F. Arens, M.D., Chief Executive Officer

Owned, leased, sponsored:	4 hospitals	1642 beds
Contract–managed:	0 hospitals	0 beds
Totals:	4 hospitals	1642 beds

★0038: UPPER CHESAPEAKE HEALTH SYSTEM (NP)

1916 Belair Road, Fallston, MD Zip 21047; tel. 410/893–0322; Lyle Ernest Sheldon, President and Chief Executive Officer

MARYLAND: FALLSTON GENERAL HOSPITAL (O, 115 beds) 200 Milton Avenue, Fallston, MD Zip 21047–2777; tel. 410/877–3700; Lyle Ernest Sheldon, Executive Vice President and Chief Operating Officer

HARFORD MEMORIAL HOSPITAL (O, 168 beds) 501 South Union Avenue, Havre De Grace, MD Zip 21078–3493; tel. 410/939–2400; Lyle Ernest Sheldon, President and Chief Executive Officer

Owned, leased, sponsored:	2 hospitals	283 beds
Contract–managed:	0 hospitals	0 beds
Totals:	2 hospitals	283 beds

★1965: UPPER VALLEY MEDICAL CENTERS (NP)

3130 North Dixie Highway, Troy, OH Zip 45373; tel. 937/332–7921; David J. Meckstroth, President and Chief Executive Officer

OHIO: DETTMER HOSPITAL (O, 49 beds) 3130 North Dixie Highway, Troy, OH Zip 45373–1039; tel. 937/332–7500; Keith Achor, Assistant Administrator

For explanation of codes following names, see page B2.
★ Indicates Type III membership in the American Hospital Association.

PIQUA MEMORIAL MEDICAL CENTER (O, 85 beds) 624 Park Avenue, Piqua, OH Zip 45356–2098; tel. 513/778–6500; Eva L. Fine, R.N., MS, Assistant Administrator

STOUDER MEMORIAL HOSPITAL (O, 131 beds) 920 Summit Avenue, Troy, OH Zip 45373; tel. 937/332–8500; Patricia Meyer, Assistant Administrator

Owned, leased, sponsored:	3 hospitals	265 beds
Contract–managed:	0 hospitals	0 beds
Totals:	3 hospitals	265 beds

0043: VALLEY HEALTH SYSTEM (NP)
1117 East Devonshire Avenue, Hemet, CA Zip 92543; tel. 909/652–2811; Geoffrey Lang, Chief Executive Officer

CALIFORNIA: HEMET VALLEY MEDICAL CENTER (O, 285 beds) 1117 East Devonshire Avenue, Hemet, CA Zip 92543; tel. 909/652–2811; John Ruffner, Administrator

MENIFEE VALLEY MEDICAL CENTER (O, 84 beds) 28400 McCall Boulevard, Sun City, CA Zip 92585–9537; tel. 909/679–8888; Susan Ballard, Administrator

MORENO VALLEY COMMUNITY HOSPITAL (O, 66 beds) 27300 Iris Avenue, Moreno Valley, CA Zip 92555; tel. 909/243–0811; Janice Ziomek, Administrator

Owned, leased, sponsored:	3 hospitals	435 beds
Contract–managed:	0 hospitals	0 beds
Totals:	3 hospitals	435 beds

0097: VALLEYCARE HEALTH SYSTEM (NP)
5575 West Las Positas Boulevard, 300, Pleasanton, CA Zip 94588

VALLEY MEMORIAL HOSPITAL (O, 110 beds) 1111 East Stanley Boulevard, Livermore, CA Zip 94550; tel. 510/447–7000; Richard E. Herington, President and Chief Executive Officer

VALLEYCARE MEDICAL CENTER (O, 68 beds) 5555 West Los Positas Boulevard, Pleasanton, CA Zip 94588; tel. 510/847–3000

Owned, leased, sponsored:	2 hospitals	178 beds
Contract–managed:	0 hospitals	0 beds
Totals:	2 hospitals	178 beds

0081: VALUEMARK HEALTHCARE SYSTEMS, INC. (IO)
300 Galleria Parkway, Suite 650, Atlanta, GA Zip 30339; tel. 770/933–5500; James T. McAfee Jr., Chairman, President and Chief Executive Officer

VALUEMARK PINE GROVE BEHAVIORAL HEALTHCARE SYSTEM (O, 62 beds) 7011 Shoup Avenue, Canoga Park, CA Zip 91307; tel. 818/348–0500; Diane Sharpe, Chief Executive Officer

FLORIDA: VALUEMARK BEHAVIORAL HEALTHCARE OF FLORIDA (O, 52 beds) 6601 Central Florida Parkway, Orlando, FL Zip 32821; tel. 407/345–5000; Marni Berger, Chief Executive Officer

GEORGIA: VALUEMARK–BRAWNER BEHAVIORAL HEALTHACARE SYSTEM–NORTH (O, 108 beds) 3180 Atlanta Street S.E., Smyrna, GA Zip 30080; tel. 404/436–0081; John J. Cascone, Chief Executive Officer

MISSOURI: VALUEMARK BEHAVIORAL HEALTHCARE SYSTEM OF KANSAS CITY (O, 72 beds) 4800 N.W. 88th Street, Kansas City, MO Zip 64154; tel. 816/436–3900; David C. Nissen, Chief Executive Officer

VIRGINIA: VALUEMARK WEST END BEHAVIORAL HEALTHCARE SYSTEM (O, 84 beds) 12800 West Creek Parkway, Richmond, VA Zip 23238; tel. 804/784–2200; Jonathan A. Garber, Chief Executive Officer

Owned, leased, sponsored:	5 hospitals	378 beds
Contract–managed:	0 hospitals	0 beds
Totals:	5 hospitals	378 beds

0026: VENCOR, INCORPORATED (IO)
400 West Market Street, Suite 3300, Louisville, KY Zip 40202–3360; tel. 502/596–7300; W. Bruce Lunsford, Board Chairman, President and Chief Executive Officer

ARIZONA: VENCOR HOSPITAL–PHOENIX (O, 58 beds) 40 East Indianola, Phoenix, AZ Zip 85012; tel. 602/280–7000; John L. Harrington Jr., FACHE, Administrator

CALIFORNIA: VENCOR HOSPITAL–LOS ANGELES (O, 81 beds) 5525 West Slauson Avenue, Los Angeles, CA Zip 90056; tel. 310/642–0325; Billie Anne Schoppman, R.N., Administrator

VENCOR HOSPITAL–ONTARIO (O, 100 beds) 550 North Monterey, Ontario, CA Zip 91764; tel. 909/391–0333; Virgis Narbutas, Administrator

VENCOR HOSPITAL–SACRAMENTO (O, 32 beds) 223 Fargo Way, Folsom, CA Zip 95630; tel. 916/351–9151; Meredith Taylor, Administrator

VENCOR HOSPITAL–SAN DIEGO (O, 70 beds) 1940 El Cajon Boulevard, San Diego, CA Zip 92104; tel. 619/543–4500; Michael D. Cress, Administrator

VENCOR HOSPITAL–SAN LEANDRO (O, 42 beds) 2800 Benedict Drive, San Leandro, CA Zip 94577; tel. 510/357–8300; Wayne M. Lingenfelter, Ed.D., Administrator and Chief Executive Officer

FLORIDA: VENCOR HOSPITAL–CORAL GABLES (O, 53 beds) 5190 S.W. Eighth Street, Coral Gables, FL Zip 33134; tel. 305/445–1364; Theodore Welding, Chief Executive Officer

VENCOR HOSPITAL–FORT LAUDERDALE (O, 64 beds) 1516 East Las Olas Boulevard, Fort Lauderdale, FL Zip 33301–2399; tel. 954/764–8900; Lewis A. Ransdell, Administrator

VENCOR HOSPITAL–ST PETERSBURG (O, 60 beds) 3030 Sixth Street South, Saint Petersburg, FL Zip 33705; tel. 813/894–8719; Pamela M. Riter, R.N., Administrator

VENCOR HOSPITAL–TAMPA (O, 73 beds) 4555 South Manhattan Avenue, Tampa, FL Zip 33611; tel. 813/839–6341; Theresa Hunkins, Administrator

VENCOR–NORTH FLORIDA (O, 48 beds) 801 Oak Street, Green Cove Springs, FL Zip 32043; tel. 904/284–9230; Tim Simpson, Administrator

GEORGIA: VENCOR HOSPITAL–ATLANTA (O, 66 beds) 705 Juniper Street N.E., Atlanta, GA Zip 30365; tel. 404/873–2871; Skip Wright, Administrator

ILLINOIS: VENCOR HOSPITAL–CHICAGO NORTH (O, 111 beds) 2544 West Montrose Avenue, Chicago, IL Zip 60618; tel. 773/267–2622; Steven A. Matarelli, Administrator

VENCOR HOSPITAL–SYCAMORE (O, 50 beds) 225 Edward Street, Sycamore, IL Zip 60178; tel. 815/895–2144; Donald Van Voorhis, Administrator

INDIANA: VENCOR HOSPITAL–LAGRANGE (O, 57 beds) 207 North Townline Road, LaGrange, IN Zip 46761; tel. 219/463–2143; Joe Murrell, Administrator

KENTUCKY: VENCOR HOSPITAL–LOUISVILLE (O, 156 beds) 1313 St. Anthony Place, Louisville, KY Zip 40204; tel. 502/627–1102; James H. Wesp, Administrator

MICHIGAN: VENCOR HOSPITAL–DETROIT (O, 112 beds) 26400 West Outer Drive, Lincoln Park, MI Zip 48146; tel. 313/594–6000; Judith A. Curtiss, Administrator

MISSOURI: VENCOR HOSPITAL–KANSAS CITY (O, 100 beds) 8701 Troost Avenue, Kansas City, MO Zip 64131; tel. 816/995–2000; Suzanne R. Wilsey, Administrator

NORTH CAROLINA: VENCOR HOSPITAL–GREENSBORO (O, 124 beds) 2401 Southside Boulevard, Greensboro, NC Zip 27406; tel. 910/271–2800; James R. Vroom, Chief Executive Officer

PENNSYLVANIA: VENCOR HOSPITAL–PHILADELPHIA (O, 52 beds) 6129 Palmetto Street, Philadelphia, PA Zip 19111; tel. 215/722–8555; Debra Condon, Administrator

VENCOR HOSPITAL–PITTSBURGH (O, 63 beds) 7777 Steubenville Pike, Oakdale, PA Zip 15071; tel. 412/494–5500; Patricia B. Speak, Administrator

TENNESSEE: VENCOR HOSPITAL–CHATTANOOGA (O, 43 beds) 709 Walnut Street, Chattanooga, TN Zip 37402; tel. 423/266–7721; Steven E. McGraw, Administrator

TEXAS: VENCOR HOSPITAL–DALLAS (O, 55 beds) 1600 Abrams Road, Dallas, TX Zip 75214–4499; tel. 214/818–2400; Dorothy J. Elford, Administrator

VENCOR HOSPITAL–FORT WORTH SOUTH (O, 94 beds) 1802 Highway 157 North, Mansfield, TX Zip 76063–9555; tel. 817/473–6101

VENCOR HOSPITAL–HOUSTON (O, 94 beds) 6441 Main Street, Houston, TX Zip 77030; tel. 713/790–0500; Darrell L. Pile, Administrator

For explanation of codes following names, see page B2.
★ Indicates Type III membership in the American Hospital Association.

VIRGINIA: VENCOR HOSPITAL–ARLINGTON (O, 206 beds) 601 South Carlin Springs Road, Arlington, VA Zip 22204–1096; tel. 703/671–1200; Joseph A. Stuber, Administrator

WISCONSIN: VENCOR HOSPITAL–MILWAUKEE (O, 60 beds) 5700 West Layton Avenue, Milwaukee, WI Zip 53202; tel. 414/325–5900; E. Kay Gray, Interim Administrator

Owned, leased, sponsored:	27 hospitals	2124 beds
Contract–managed:	0 hospitals	0 beds
Totals:	27 hospitals	2124 beds

0114: VENDELL HERALTHCARE, INC. (IO)
3401 West End Avenue, Suite 500, Nashville, TN Zip 37203–0376; tel. 615/383–0376; H. Neil Campbell, Chief Executive Officer

ARKANSAS: RIVENDELL PSYCHIATRIC CENTER (O, 77 beds) 100 Rivendell Drive, Benton, AR Zip 72015; tel. 501/794–1255; Mark E. Schneider, Chief Executive Officer

MICHIGAN: RIVENDELL OF MICHIGAN (O, 63 beds) 101 West Townsend Road, Saint Johns, MI Zip 48879; tel. 517/224–1177; Michael Talmo, Chief Executive Officer

TEXAS: GULF PINES BEHAVIORAL HEALTH SERVICES (O, 140 beds) 205 Hollow Tree Lane, Houston, TX Zip 77090; tel. 713/537–0700; Lawrence Story, Chief Executive Officer and Administrator

RED RIVER HOSPITAL (O, 50 beds) 1505 Eighth Street, Wichita Falls, TX Zip 76301–3106; tel. 817/322–3171; Ricky Powell, Administrator

Owned, leased, sponsored:	4 hospitals	330 beds
Contract–managed:	0 hospitals	0 beds
Totals:	4 hospitals	330 beds

★5435: VIA CHRISTI HEALTH SYSTEM (CC)
929 North St. Francis, Wichita, KS Zip 67214; tel. 316/268–5000; LeRoy E. Rheault, President and Chief Executive Officer

CALIFORNIA: ST. ROSE HOSPITAL (C, 175 beds) 27200 Calaroga Avenue, Hayward, CA Zip 94545–4383; tel. 510/264–4000; Michael P. Mahoney, President and Chief Executive Officer

KANSAS: MERCY HEALTH CENTER OF MANHATTAN (O, 178 beds) Manhattan, KS Mailing Address: 1823 College Avenue, Zip 66502; E. Michael Nunamaker, President and Chief Executive Officer

MOUNT CARMEL MEDICAL CENTER (O, 119 beds) Centennial and Rouse Streets, Pittsburg, KS Zip 66762–6686; tel. 316/231–6100; John Daniel Lingor, President and Chief Executive Officer

VIA CHRISTI REGIONAL MEDICAL CENTER (O, 1098 beds) 929 North St. Francis Street, Wichita, KS Zip 67214–3882; tel. 316/268–5000; Randall G. Nyp, President and Chief Executive Officer

OKLAHOMA: ST. JOSEPH REGIONAL MEDICAL CENTER OF NORTHERN OKLAHOMA (O, 88 beds) 14th Street and Hartford Avenue, Ponca City, OK Zip 74601–2035, Mailing Address: Box 1270, Zip 74602–1270; tel. 405/765–3321; Garry L. England, President and Chief Executive Officer

Owned, leased, sponsored:	4 hospitals	1483 beds
Contract–managed:	1 hospital	175 beds
Totals:	5 hospitals	1658 beds

0012: VIRGINIA DEPARTMENT OF MENTAL HEALTH (NP)
109 Governor Street, Richmond, VA Zip 23219, Mailing Address: P.O. Box 1797, Zip 23218; tel. 804/786–3921; Timothy A. Kelly, Ph.D., Commissioner

VIRGINIA: CENTRAL VIRGINIA TRAINING CENTER (O, 1112 beds) 210 East Colony Road, Madison Heights, VA Zip 24572, Mailing Address: P.O. Box 1098, Lynchburg, Zip 24505; tel. 804/947–6326; S. J. Butkus, Ph.D., Director

DE JARNETTE CENTER (O, 60 beds) 1355 Richmond Road, Staunton, VA Zip 24401–1091, Mailing Address: Box 2309, Zip 24402–2309; tel. 540/332–2100; Andrea C. Newsome, FACHE, Director

EASTERN STATE HOSPITAL (O, 727 beds) Williamsburg, VA Mailing Address: P.O. Box 8791, Zip 23187–8791; tel. 804/253–5161; John M. Favret, Director

NORTHERN VIRGINIA MENTAL HEALTH INSTITUTE (O, 62 beds) 3302 Gallows Road, Falls Church, VA Zip 22042–3398; tel. 703/207–7111; Antoni Sulikowski, Facility Director

PIEDMONT GERIATRIC HOSPITAL (O, 210 beds) Highway 460/360, Burkeville, VA Zip 23922–9999; tel. 804/767–4401; Willard R. Pierce Jr., Director

SOUTHERN VIRGINIA MENTAL HEALTH INSTITUTE (O, 96 beds) 382 Taylor Drive, Danville, VA Zip 24541–4023; tel. 804/799–6220; Constance N. Fletcher, Ph.D., Director

SOUTHWESTERN VIRGINIA MENTAL HEALTH INSTITUTE (O, 266 beds) 502 East Main Street, Marion, VA Zip 24354; tel. 540/783–1200; Gerald E. Deans, Director

WESTERN STATE HOSPITAL (O, 488 beds) 1301 Richmond Avenue, Staunton, VA Zip 24401, Mailing Address: Box 2500, Zip 24402–2500; tel. 540/332–8000; Lynwood F. Harding, Director

Owned, leased, sponsored:	8 hospitals	3021 beds
Contract–managed:	0 hospitals	0 beds
Totals:	8 hospitals	3021 beds

★6725: WEST JERSEY HEALTH SYSTEM (NP)
1000 Atlantic Avenue, Camden, NJ Zip 08104; tel. 609/342–4604; Richard P. Miller, President and Chief Executive Officer

NEW JERSEY: WEST JERSEY HOSPITAL–BERLIN (O, 79 beds) 100 Townsend Avenue, Berlin, NJ Zip 08009; tel. 609/768–6006; Ellen Guarnieri, Acting Executive Director

WEST JERSEY HOSPITAL–CAMDEN (O, 117 beds) 1000 Atlantic Avenue, Camden, NJ Zip 08104–1595; tel. 609/342–4000; Frederick M. Carey, Executive Director

WEST JERSEY HOSPITAL–MARLTON (O, 167 beds) Route 73 and Brick Road, Marlton, NJ Zip 08053; tel. 609/596–3500; Leroy J. Rosenberg, Executive Director

WEST JERSEY HOSPITAL–VOORHEES (O, 253 beds) 101 Carnie Boulevard, Voorhees, NJ Zip 08043–1597; tel. 609/772–5000; Joan T. Meyers, R.N., Executive Director

Owned, leased, sponsored:	4 hospitals	616 beds
Contract–managed:	0 hospitals	0 beds
Totals:	4 hospitals	616 beds

★0004: WEST TENNESSEE HEALTHCARE, INC. (NP)
708 West Forest Avenue, Jackson, TN Zip 38301; tel. 901/425–5000; James T. Moss, President

TENNESSEE: BOLIVAR GENERAL HOSPITAL (O, 47 beds) 650 Nuckolls Road, Bolivar, TN Zip 38008; tel. 901/658–3100; George L. Austin, Chief Executive Officer

CAMDEN GENERAL HOSPITAL (O, 40 beds) 175 Hospital Drive, Camden, TN Zip 38320; tel. 901/584–6135; Alfred P. Taylor, Administrator and Chief Executive Officer

GIBSON GENERAL HOSPITAL (O, 41 beds) 200 Hosptial Drive, Trenton, TN Zip 38382, Mailing Address: Box 488, Zip 38382; tel. 901/855–2551; Kelly R. Yenawine, Administrator

HUMBOLDT GENERAL HOSPITAL (O, 51 beds) 3525 Chere Carol Road, Humboldt, TN Zip 38343–3699; tel. 901/784–0301; Karen Utley, Administrator

JACKSON–MADISON COUNTY GENERAL HOSPITAL (O, 567 beds) 708 West Forest Avenue, Jackson, TN Zip 38301–3855; tel. 901/425–5000; James T. Moss, President

PATHWAYS OF TENNESSEE (O, 57 beds) 238 Summar Drive, Jackson, TN Zip 38301; tel. 901/935–8200; James T. Moss, President and Chief Executive Officer

Owned, leased, sponsored:	6 hospitals	803 beds
Contract–managed:	0 hospitals	0 beds
Totals:	6 hospitals	803 beds

For explanation of codes following names, see page B2.
★ Indicates Type III membership in the American Hospital Association.

© 1997 AHA Guide

0119: WEST VIRGINIA UNITED HEALTH SYSTEM (NP)
Morgantown, WV Mailing Address: P.O. Box 8010, Zip 26506–8010; tel. 304/598–6000; Bernard G. Westfall, President

WEST VIRGINIA: UNITED HOSPITAL CENTER (O, 309 beds) Route 19 South, Clarksburg, WV Zip 26301, Mailing Address: P.O. Box 1680, Zip 26302–1680; tel. 304/624–2121; Bruce C. Carter, President

WEST VIRGINIA UNIVERSITY HOSPITALS (O, 334 beds) Medical Center Drive, Morgantown, WV Zip 26506–4749; tel. 304/598–4000; Bruce McClymonds, President and Chief Executive Officer

Owned, leased, sponsored:	2 hospitals	643 beds
Contract–managed:	0 hospitals	0 beds
Totals:	2 hospitals	643 beds

★6745: WHEATON FRANCISCAN SERVICES, INC. (CC)
26W171 Roosevelt Road, Wheaton, IL Zip 60189–0667, Mailing Address: P.O. Box 667, Zip 60189–0667; tel. 708/462–9271; Wilfred F. Loebig Jr., President and Chief Executive Officer

ILLINOIS: MARIANJOY REHABILITATION HOSPITAL AND CLINICS (O, 107 beds) 26 West 171 Roosevelt Road, Wheaton, IL Zip 60187, Mailing Address: P.O. Box 795, Zip 60189–0795; tel. 630/462–4000; Bruce A. Schurman, President

OAK PARK HOSPITAL (O, 176 beds) 520 South Maple Avenue, Oak Park, IL Zip 60304–1097; tel. 708/383–9300; Leonard J. Muller, President

IOWA: COVENANT MEDICAL CENTER (O, 293 beds) 3421 West Ninth Street, Waterloo, IA Zip 50702–5499; tel. 319/272–8000; Raymond F. Burfeind, President

MERCY HOSPITAL OF FRANCISCAN SISTERS (O, 64 beds) 201 Eighth Avenue S.E., Oelwein, IA Zip 50662; tel. 319/283–6000; Richard Schrupp, President and Chief Executive Officer

WISCONSIN: ELMBROOK MEMORIAL HOSPITAL (O, 136 beds) 19333 West North Avenue, Brookfield, WI Zip 53045–4198; tel. 414/785–2000; Kimry A. Johnsrud, President

SAINT MARY'S MEDICAL CENTER (O, 226 beds) 3801 Spring Street, Racine, WI Zip 53405; tel. 414/636–4011; Edward P. Demeulenaere, President and Chief Executive Officer

ST. ELIZABETH HOSPITAL (O, 155 beds) 1506 South Oneida Street, Appleton, WI Zip 54915–1397; tel. 414/738–2000; Otto L. Cox, President and Chief Executive Officer

ST. FRANCIS HOSPITAL (S, 265 beds) 3237 South 16th Street, Milwaukee, WI Zip 53215–4592; tel. 414/647–5000; Gregory A. Banaszynski, President

ST. JOSEPH'S HOSPITAL (O, 484 beds) 5000 West Chambers Street, Milwaukee, WI Zip 53210–9988; tel. 414/447–2000; Jon L. Wachs, President

ST. LUKE'S MEMORIAL HOSPITAL (C, 183 beds) 1320 Wisconsin Avenue, Racine, WI Zip 53403–1987; tel. 414/636–2011; Edward P. Demeulenaere, President and Chief Executive Officer

ST. MICHAEL HOSPITAL (O, 152 beds) 2400 West Villard Avenue, Milwaukee, WI Zip 53209; tel. 414/527–8000; Jeffrey K. Jenkins, President

Owned, leased, sponsored:	10 hospitals	2058 beds
Contract–managed:	1 hospital	183 beds
Totals:	11 hospitals	2241 beds

★9575: WILLIAM BEAUMONT HOSPITAL CORPORATION (NP)
3601 West Thirteen Mile Road, Royal Oak, MI Zip 48073–6769; tel. 810/551–5000; Ted D. Wasson, President and Chief Executive Officer

MICHIGAN: WILLIAM BEAUMONT HOSPITAL–ROYAL OAK (O, 856 beds) 3601 West Thirteen Mile Road, Royal Oak, MI Zip 48073–6769; tel. 810/551–5000; John D. Labriola, Vice President and Director

WILLIAM BEAUMONT HOSPITAL–TROY (O, 189 beds) 44201 Dequindre Road, Troy, MI Zip 48098–1198; tel. 810/828–5100; Eugene F. Michalski, Vice President and Hospital Director

Owned, leased, sponsored:	2 hospitals	1045 beds
Contract–managed:	0 hospitals	0 beds
Totals:	2 hospitals	1045 beds

••★0068: YORK HEALTH SYSTEM (NP)
1001 South George Street, York, PA Zip 17405; tel. 717/851–2121; Bruce M. Bartels, President

PENNSYLVANIA: YORK HOSPITAL (O, 435 beds) 1001 South George Street, York, PA Zip 17405–3676; tel. 717/851–2345; Bruce M. Bartels, President

Owned, leased, sponsored:	1 hospital	435 beds
Contract–managed:	0 hospitals	0 beds
Totals:	1 hospital	435 beds

For explanation of codes following names, see page B2.
★ Indicates Type III membership in the American Hospital Association.
• Single hospital health care system

© 1997 AHA Guide · · · Networks, Health Care Systems and Alliances **B149**

Geographically

United States

ALABAMA

Birmingham: 0345 ★ BAPTIST HEALTH SYSTEM 3500 Blue Lake Drive, Suite 100, Zip 35243, Mailing Address: P.O. Box 830605, Zip 35283–0605; tel. 205/715–5319; Dennis A. Hall, President, p. B68

2455 BRADFORD HEALTH SERVICES 2101 Magnolia Avenue South, Suite 518, Zip 35205; tel. 205/251–7753; Jerry W. Crowder, President and Chief Executive Officer, p. B72

0100 ★ EASTERN HEALTH SYSTEM, INC. 48 Medical Park East Drive, 450, Zip 35235; tel. 205/838–3999; Robert C. Chapman, FACHE, President and Chief Executive Officer, p. B96

0023 HEALTHSOUTH CORPORATION One Healthsouth Parkway, Zip 35243; tel. 205/967–7116; Anthony J. Tanner, Executive Vice President, p. B102

0089 INNOVATIVE HEALTHCARE SYSTEMS, INC. 1900 International Park Drive, Suite 220, Zip 35243; tel. 205/967–3455; Kerry Teel, President and Chief Executive Officer, p. B105

Brewton: 1255 ESCAMBIA COUNTY HEALTH CARE AUTHORITY 1301 Belleville Avenue, Zip 36426; tel. 334/368–2500; Phillip L. Parker, Administrator, p. B96

Guntersville: 1975 MARSHALL COUNTY HEALTH CARE AUTHORITY 8000 Alabama Highway 69, Zip 35976; tel. 205/753–8000; L. C. Couch, Board Chairman, p. B112

Huntsville: 0117 HUNTSVILLE HOSPITAL SYSTEM 101 Silvey Road, Zip 35801; tel. 205/517–8020; Edward D. Boston, Chief Executive Officer, p. B105

Mobile: 2025 INFIRMARY HEALTH SYSTEM, INC. 3 Mobile Infirmary Circle, Zip 36607; tel. 334/431–5500; E. Chandler Bramlett Jr., President and Chief Executive Officer, p. B105

0057 UNIVERSITY OF SOUTH ALABAMA HOSPITALS 2451 Fillingim Street, Zip 36617–2293; tel. 205/471–7110; Stephen H. Simmons, Senior Administrator, p. B146

Tuscaloosa: 1825 ★ DCH HEALTHCARE AUTHORITY 809 University Boulevard East, Zip 35401; tel. 205/759–7111; Bryan Kindred, Chief Executive Officer, p. B89

ARIZONA

Phoenix: 8810 ★ BAPTIST HOSPITALS AND HEALTH SYSTEMS, INC. 2224 West Northern Avenue, Suite D–300, Zip 85021; tel. 602/864–1184; Gerald L. Wissink, President and Chief Executive Officer, p. B68

0034 ★ PMH HEALTH RESOURCES, INC. 1201 South Seventh Avenue, Zip 85007–3913, Mailing Address: P.O. Box 21207, Zip 85036–1207; tel. 602/238–3321; Reginald M. Ballantyne III, President, p. B121

2535 ★ SAMARITAN HEALTH SYSTEM 1441 North 12th Street, Zip 85006–2666; tel. 602/495–4000; James C. Crews, President and Chief Executive Officer, p. B130

Scottsdale: 0037 ★ SCOTTSDALE MEMORIAL HEALTH SYSTEMS, INC. 3621 Wells Fargo Avenue, Zip 85251; tel. 602/481–4324; Max Poll, President and Chief Executive Officer, p. B131

Sun City: 0030 ★ SUN HEALTH CORPORATION 13180 North 103rd Drive, Zip 85351, Mailing Address: P.O. Box 1278, Zip 85372–1278; tel. 602/876–5301; Leland W. Peterson, President and Chief Executive Officer, p. B139

ARKANSAS

Little Rock: 0355 ★ BAPTIST HEALTH 9601 Interstate 630, Exit 7, Zip 72205–7299; tel. 501/202–2000; Russell D. Harrington Jr., President, p. B67

CALIFORNIA

Burbank: 2315 ★ UNIHEALTH 3400 Riverside Drive, Zip 91505; tel. 818/238–6000; David R. Carpenter, FACHE, President and Chairman of the Board, p. B144

Covina: 0101 CITRUS VALLEY HEALTH PARTNERS 210 West San Bernardino Road, Zip 91723; tel. 818/938–7577; Peter E. Makowski, President and Chief Executive Officer, p. B78

Fairfield: 2075 ★ NORTHBAY HEALTHCARE SYSTEM 1200 B Gale Wilson Boulevard, Zip 94533–3587; tel. 707/429–3600; Gary J. Passama, President and Chief Executive Officer, p. B119

Fresno: 1085 COMMUNITY HOSPITALS OF CENTRAL CALIFORNIA Fresno and R Streets, Zip 93721, Mailing Address: P.O. Box 1232, Zip 93721; tel. 209/442–6000; Philip Hinton, Chief Executive Officer, p. B87

Hemet: 0043 VALLEY HEALTH SYSTEM 1117 East Devonshire Avenue, Zip 92543; tel. 909/652–2811; Geoffrey Lang, Chief Executive Officer, p. B147

Huntington Beach: 0076 COLLEGE HEALTH ENTERPRISES 7711 Center Avenue, Suite 300, Zip 92647; tel. 714/891–5000; Elliot A. Sainer, President and Chief Executive Officer, p. B78

Loma Linda: 2175 ADVENTIST HEALTH SYSTEM–LOMA LINDA 11161 Anderson Street, Zip 92350; tel. 909/824–4540; B. Lyn Behrens, President, p. B64

Long Beach: 0084 MEMORIAL HEALTH SERVICES 2801 Atlantic Avenue, Zip 90801, Mailing Address: P.O. Box 1428, Zip 90801–1428; tel. 562/933–2000; Thomas J. Collins, President and Chief Executive Officer, p. B113

0435 PACIFIC HEALTH CORPORATION 249 East Ocean Boulevard, Zip 90802; tel. 310/435–1300; Jens Mueller, Chairman, p. B120

Los Angeles: 5755 LOS ANGELES COUNTY–DEPARTMENT OF HEALTH SERVICES 313 North Figueroa Street, Room 912, Zip 90012; tel. 213/240–8101; Mark Finucane, Director Health, p. B109

Oakland: 2105 ★ KAISER FOUNDATION HOSPITALS One Kaiser Plaza, Zip 94612–3600; tel. 510/271–5910; David M. Lawrence, M.D., Chairman and Chief Executive Officer, p. B107

6405 UNIVERSITY OF CALIFORNIA–SYSTEMWIDE ADMINISTRATION 300 Lakeside Drive, 18th Floor, Zip 94612–3550; tel. 510/987–9701; Cornelius L. Hopper, M.D., Vice President Health Affairs, p. B146

Orange: 5425 ★ ST. JOSEPH HEALTH SYSTEM 440 South Batavia Street, Zip 92868–3995, Mailing Address: P.O. Box 14132, Zip 92613–1532; tel. 714/997–7690; Richard Statuto, Chief Executive Officer, p. B138

Pasadena: 0106 ★ SOUTHERN CALIFORNIA HEALTHCARE SYSTEM 1300 East Green Street, Zip 91106; Frederick C. Meyer, President and Chief Executive Officer, p. B137

Pleasanton: 0097 VALLEYCARE HEALTH SYSTEM 5575 West Las Positas Boulevard, 300, Zip 94588, p. B147

Roseville: 0235 ★ ADVENTIST HEALTH 2100 Douglas Boulevard, Zip 95661–3898, Mailing Address: P.O. Box 619002, Zip 95661–9002; tel. 916/781–2000; Frank F. Dupper, President, p. B63

Sacramento: 8795 ★ SUTTER HEALTH 2800 L Street, Zip 95816, Mailing Address: P.O. Box 160727, Zip 95816; tel. 916/733–8800; Van R. Johnson, President and Chief Executive Officer, p. B139

San Diego: 7555 ★ PALOMAR POMERADO HEALTH SYSTEM 15255 Innovation Drive, Suite 204, Zip 92128–3410; tel. 619/675–5100; Victoria M. Penland, Interim President and Chief Executive Officer, p. B120

1505 ★ SCRIPPS HEALTH 4275 Campus Point Court, Zip 92121, Mailing Address: P.O. Box 28, La Jolla, Zip 92038; tel. 619/678–7470; Martin B. Buser, Executive Vice President Health Services, p. B131

2065 SHARP HEALTHCARE 3131 Berger Avenue, Suite 100, Zip 92123; tel. 619/541–4000, p. B131

San Francisco: 5205 ★ CATHOLIC HEALTHCARE WEST 1700 Montgomery Street, Suite 300, Zip 94111–9603; tel. 415/438–5500; Richard J. Kramer, President and Chief Executive Officer, p. B77

San Leandro: 0225 ALAMEDA COUNTY HEALTH CARE SERVICES AGENCY 1850 Fairway Drive, Zip 94577; tel. 510/618–3452; David J. Kears, Director, p. B64

Santa Barbara: 0103 COTTAGE HEALTH SYSTEM Pueblo at Bath Streets, Zip 93102, Mailing Address: P.O. Box 689, Zip 93102; tel. 805/682–7111; James L. Ash, President and Chief Executive Officer, p. B87

0063 TENET HEALTHCARE CORPORATION 3820 State Street, Zip 93105, Mailing Address: P.O. Box 31907, Zip 93130; tel. 805/563–7000; Jeffrey Barbakow, Chairman and Chief Executive Officer, p. B140

Yuba City: 2115 FREMONT–RIDEOUT HEALTH GROUP 989 Plumas Street, Zip 95991; tel. 916/751–4010; Thomas P. Hayes, Chief Executive Officer, p. B98

COLORADO

Denver: 0092 ★ CATHOLIC HEALTH INITIATIVES 1999 Broadway, Suite 2605, Zip 80202; tel. 303/298–9100; Patricia A. Cahill, Chief Executive Officer, p. B75

5395 MARYCREST HEALTH SYSTEM 2861 West 52nd Avenue, Zip 80221–1259; tel. 303/458–8611; Dale G. Budde, President, p. B112

CONNECTICUT

Hartford: 0014 CONNECTICUT STATE DEPARTMENT OF MENTAL HEALTH 90 Washington Street, Zip 06106; tel. 203/566–3650; Albert J. Solnit, M.D., Commissioner, p. B87

DELAWARE

Dover: 0107 ★ BAYHEALTH MEDICAL CENTER 640 South State Street, Zip 19901; Dennis E. Klima, President and Chief Executive Officer, p. B69

DISTRICT OF COLUMBIA

Washington: 9655 DEPARTMENT OF NAVY Zip 20066, p. B89

9495 DEPARTMENT OF THE AIR FORCE Zip 20333; tel. 202/767–5066; Major General Charles H. Roadman II, Deputy Surgeon General, p. B89

9295 DEPARTMENT OF VETERANS AFFAIRS 810 Vermont Avenue N.W., Zip 20420; tel. 202/273–5781; Kenneth W. Kizer, M.D., M.P.H., Under Secretary for Health, p. B91

2015 ★ GREATER SOUTHEAST HEALTHCARE SYSTEM 1310 Southern Avenue S.E., Zip 20032; tel. 202/574–6926; Dalton A. Tong, CPA, FACHE, President and Chief Executive Officer, p. B99

6615 ★ MEDLANTIC HEALTHCARE GROUP 100 Irving Street N.W., Zip 20010–2975; tel. 202/877–6006; John P. McDaniel, Chief Executive Officer, p. B113

FLORIDA

Clearwater: 0071 ACCORD HEALTH CARE CORPORATION 3696 Ulmerton Road, Zip 34622; tel. 813/573–1755; Stephen H. Noble, President, p. B63

Coral Gobles: 0405 RAMSAY HEALTH CARE, INC. 1 Alhambra Plaza, Suite 750, Zip 33134; tel. 305/569–6993; Bert Cibran, President and Chief Operating Officer, p. B129

Fort Lauderdale: 3115 ★ NORTH BROWARD HOSPITAL DISTRICT 303 S.E. 17th Street, Zip 33316–2510; tel. 305/355–5100; G. Wil Trower, President and Chief Executive Officer, p. B118

Gainesville: 0111 SHANDS HEALTH SYSTEM, UNIVERSITY OF FLORIDA HEALTH SCIENCE CENTER 1600 S.W. Archer Road, Zip 32610–0326; tel. 352/395–0421; J. Richard Gaintner, M.D., Chief Executive Officer, p. B131

Hollywood: 0083 ★ MEMORIAL HEALTHCARE SYSTEM 3501 Johnson Street, Zip 33021; tel. 954/985–5805; Frank V. Sacco, FACHE, Chief Executive Officer, p. B114

Jacksonville: 2715 METHODIST HEALTH SYSTEM 580 West Eighth Street, Zip 32209–6553; tel. 904/798–8000; Marcus E. Drewa, President, p. B116

Naples: 1775 HEALTH MANAGEMENT ASSOCIATES 5811 Pelican Bay Boulevard, Suite 500, Zip 33963–2710; tel. 941/598–3175; William J. Schoen, President, p. B100

Orlando: 3355 ★ ORLANDO REGIONAL HEALTHCARE SYSTEM 1414 Kuhl Avenue, Zip 32806–2093; tel. 407/841–5111; J. Gary Strack, Chairman and Chief Executive Officer, p. B119

Ormond Beach: 2615 ★ MEMORIAL HEALTH SYSTEMS 875 Sterthaus Avenue, Zip 32174–5197; tel. 904/676–6114; Richard A. Lind, President and Chief Executive Officer, p. B113

Palm Harbor: 1335 MEASE HEALTH CARE 135 Annwood Road, Zip 34648; tel. 813/733–1111; Philip K. Beauchamp, FACHE, President and Chief Executive Officer, p. B113

Pensacola: 0185 BAPTIST HEALTH CARE CORPORATION 1717 North E Street, Suite 320, Zip 32501–6335; tel. 904/469–2337; James F. Vickery, President, p. B67

Tampa: 1385 ★ ALLEGANY HEALTH SYSTEM 6200 Courtney Campbell Causeway, Zip 33607–1458; tel. 813/281–9098; Sister Marie Celeste Sullivan, President and Chief Executive Officer, p. B64

4125 ★ SHRINERS HOSPITALS FOR CHILDREN 2900 Rocky Point Drive, Zip 33607–1435, Mailing Address: Box 31356, Zip 33631–3356; tel. 813/281–0300; Joseph E. Melchiorre Jr., CHE, Executive Administrator, p. B132

Windermere: 9605 UNITED MEDICAL CORPORATION 603 Main Street, Zip 34786, Mailing Address: P.O. Box 1100, Zip 34786–1100; tel. 407/876–2200; Donald R. Dizney, Chairman, p. B145

Winter Park: 4165 ★ ADVENTIST HEALTH SYSTEM SUNBELT HEALTH CARE CORPORATION 111 North Orlando Avenue, Zip 32789–3675; tel. 407/975–1417; Mardian J. Blair, President, p. B63

GEORGIA

Adel: 2335 MEMORIAL HEALTH SERVICES 706 North Parrish Avenue, Zip 31620, Mailing Address: Box 677, Zip 31620; tel. 912/896–2251; Wade E. Keck, Chief Executive Officer, p. B113

Atlanta: 0073 BOWDON CORPORATE OFFICES 4250 Perimeter Park South, Suite 102, Zip 30341; tel. 770/452–1221; Bill E. Ehrhardt, Executive Director, p. B72

0695 MAGELLAN HEALTH SERVICES 3414 Peachtree Road N.E., Suite 1400, Zip 30326; tel. 404/841–9200; E. Mac Crawford, President, Chief Executive Officer and Chairman, p. B110

0081 VALUEMARK HEALTHCARE SYSTEMS, INC. 300 Galleria Parkway, Suite 650, Zip 30339; tel. 770/933–5500; James T. McAfee Jr., Chairman, President and Chief Executive Officer, p. B147

Austell: 0995 ★ PROMINA NORTHWEST HEALTH SYSTEM 1791 Mulkey Road, Suite 102, Zip 30001–1124; tel. 770/732–5501; Thomas E. Hill, Chief Executive Officer, p. B122

Macon: 1585 HEALTHCARE MANAGEMENT GROUP, INC. 776 Baconsfield Drive, Suite 209, Zip 31211–0101; tel. 912/743–5606; Earl Bonds Jr., Chief Executive Officer, p. B102

Thomasville: 0104 ARCHBOLD MEDICAL CENTER 910 South Broad Street, Zip 31792; tel. 912/228–2739; Ken B. Beverly, President and Chief Executive Officer, p. B67

HAWAII

Honolulu: 0040 ★ QUEEN'S HEALTH SYSTEMS 1099 Alakea Street, Suite 1100, Zip 96813; tel. 808/532–6100; Richard L. Griffith, President and Chief Executive Officer, p. B123

3555 STATE OF HAWAII, DEPARTMENT OF HEALTH 1250 Punchbowl Street, Zip 96813; tel. 808/586–4416; Bertrand Kobayashi, Deputy Director, p. B138

ILLINOIS

Arlington Heights: 0113 CANCER TREATMENT CENTERS OF AMERICA 3455 West Salt Creek Lane, Zip 60005–1080; tel. 847/342–7400; Robert Mayo, President and Chief Executive Officer, p. B73

Carbondale: 4175 ★ SOUTHERN ILLINOIS HOSPITAL SERVICES 608 East College Street, Zip 62901, Mailing Address: P.O. Box 3988, Zip 62902–3988; tel. 618/457–5200; John J. Buckley Jr., President, p. B137

Chicago: 0079 ★ CATHOLIC HEALTH PARTNERS 2913 North Commonwealth, Zip 60657; tel. 773/665–3170; Sister Theresa Peck, President and Chief Executive Officer, p. B76

0016 COOK COUNTY BUREAU OF HEALTH SERVICES 1835 West Harrison Street, Zip 60612; tel. 312/633–8533; Ruth M. Rothstein, Chief, p. B87

0058 ★ LOUIS A WEISS MEMORIAL HOSPITAL/UNIVERSITY OF CHICAGO HOSPITALS 4646 North Marine Drive, Zip 60640; tel. 773/878–8700; Gregory A. Cierlik, President and Chief Executive Officer, p. B109

3855 ★ RUSH–PRESBYTERIAN–ST. LUKE'S MEDICAL CENTER 1653 West Congress Parkway, Zip 60612–3864; tel. 312/942–5000; Leo M. Henikoff, President, p. B130

Des Plaines: 5575 SISTERS OF THE HOLY FAMILY OF NAZARETH–SACRED HEART PROVINCE 310 North River Road, Zip 60016–1211; tel. 847/298–6760; Sister M. Lucille Madura, Provincial Superior, p. B136

Elk Grove Village: 0065 ALEXIAN BROTHERS HEALTH SYSTEM, INC. 600 Alexian Way, Zip 60007–3395; tel. 847/640–7550; Brother Felix Bettendorf, President, p. B64

Evergreen Park: 2295 LITTLE COMPANY OF MARY SISTERS HEALTHCARE SYSTEM 9350 South California Avenue, Zip 60805; tel. 708/229–5491; Sister Carol Pacini, Provincialate Superior, p. B109

Frankfort: 1415 ★ FRANCISCAN SISTERS HEALTH CARE CORPORATION 9223 West St. Francis Road, Zip 60423–8334; tel. 815/469–4888; Gerald P. Pearson, President, p. B98

Kankakee: 4025 ★ SERVANTCOR 1475 Harvard Drive, Zip 60901–9465; tel. 815/937–2034; Joseph S. Feth, President, p. B131

Naperville: 5215 MERCY–CHICAGO REGION HEALTHCARE SYSTEM 55 Shuman Boulevard, Suite 150, Zip 60563–8469; tel. 708/778–2164; Sister Catherine C. Gallagher, President, p. B115

Oakbrook: 0064 ★ ADVOCATE HEALTH CARE 2025 Windsor Drive, Zip 60521–0222; tel. 708/990–5003; Richard R. Risk, President and Chief Executive Officer, p. B64

Peoria: 5335 ★ OSF HEALTHCARE SYSTEM 800 N.E. Glen Oak Avenue, Zip 61603–3200; tel. 309/655–2850; Sister Frances Marie Masching, President, p. B120

Springfield: 5355 ★ HOSPITAL SISTERS HEALTH SYSTEM Mailing Address: P.O. Box 19431, Zip 62794–9431; tel. 217/523–4747; Sister Jomary Trstensky, President, p. B105

0086 ★ MEMORIAL HEALTH SYSTEM 800 North Rutledge Street, Zip 62781–0001; tel. 217/788–3000; Robert T. Clarke, President and Chief Executive Officer, p. B113

Wheaton: 6745 ★ WHEATON FRANCISCAN SERVICES, INC. 26W171 Roosevelt Road, Zip 60189–0667, Mailing Address: P.O. Box 667, Zip 60189–0667; tel. 708/462–9271; Wilfred F. Loebig Jr., President and Chief Executive Officer, p. B149

INDIANA

Hobart: 0135 ★ ANCILLA SYSTEMS INC. 1000 South Lake Park Avenue, Zip 46342; tel. 219/947–8500; William D. Harkins, President and Chief Executive Officer, p. B66

Kendallville: 0098 ★ CONTINUUM 111 Cedar Street, Zip 46755, Mailing Address: P.O. Box 249, Zip 46755; tel. 219/347–6344; John Berhow, President, p. B87

Mishawaka: 5345 ★ SISTERS OF ST. FRANCIS HEALTH SERVICES, INC. 1515 Dragoon Trail, Zip 46546–1290, Mailing Address: P.O. Box 1290, Zip 46546–1290; tel. 219/256–3935; Kevin D. Leahy, President and Chief Executive Officer, p. B135

South Bend: 5585 ★ HOLY CROSS HEALTH SYSTEM CORPORATION 3606 East Jefferson Boulevard, Zip 46615–3097; tel. 219/233–8558; Sister Patricia Vandenberg, President and Chief Executive Officer, p. B104

IOWA

Des Moines: 0061 ★ IOWA HEALTH SYSTEM 1200 Pleasant Street, Zip 50309–1453; tel. 515/241–6212; Samuel T. Wallace, President, p. B106

Sioux City: 5845 ST. LUKE'S HEALTH SYSTEM, INC. 2720 Stone Park Boulevard, Zip 51104–2000; tel. 712/279–3500; John D. Daniels, President and Chief Executive Officer, p. B138

KANSAS

Leavenworth: 5095 ★ SISTERS OF CHARITY OF LEAVENWORTH HEALTH SERVICES CORPORATION 4200 South Fourth Street, Zip 66048–5054; tel. 913/682–1338; Sister Marie Damian Glatt, President, p. B133

Phillipsburg: 1535 ★ GREAT PLAINS HEALTH ALLIANCE, INC. 625 Third, Zip 67661, Mailing Address: P.O. Box 366, Zip 67661–0366; tel. 913/543–2111; Roger S. John, President and Chief Executive Officer, p. B99

Topeka: 0805 STORMONT–VAIL HEALTHCARE 1500 Southwest Tenth Street, Zip 66604–1353; tel. 913/354–6121; Maynard F. Oliverius, President and Chief Executive Officer, p. B139

Wichita: 5435 ★ VIA CHRISTI HEALTH SYSTEM 929 North St. Francis, Zip 67214; tel. 316/268–5000; LeRoy E. Rheault, President and Chief Executive Officer, p. B148

KENTUCKY

Lexington: 0145 APPALACHIAN REGIONAL HEALTHCARE 1220 Harrodsburg Road, Zip 40504, Mailing Address: Box 8086, Zip 40533–8086; tel. 606/226–2440; Forrest Calico, M.D., President, p. B66

Louisville: 2285 ★ ALLIANT HEALTH SYSTEM 234 East Gray Street, Suite 225, Zip 40202, Mailing Address: P.O. Box 35070, Zip 40232–5070; tel. 502/629–8025; Stephen A. Williams, President, p. B65

0315 ★ BAPTIST HEALTHCARE SYSTEM 4007 Kresge Way, Zip 40207–4677; tel. 502/896–5000; Tommy J. Smith, President and Chief Executive Officer, p. B68

0052 ★ JEWISH HOSPITAL HEALTHCARE SERVICES 217 East Chestnut Street, Zip 40202; tel. 502/587–4011; Henry C. Wagner, President, p. B107

0026 VENCOR, INCORPORATED 400 West Market Street, Suite 3300, Zip 40202–3360; tel. 502/596–7300; W. Bruce Lunsford, Board Chairman, President and Chief Executive Officer, p. B147

Nazareth: 3045 ★ SISTERS OF CHARITY OF NAZARETH HEALTH SYSTEM 135 West Drive, Zip 40048, Mailing Address: P.O. Box 171, Zip 40048–0171; tel. 502/349–6250; Mark W. Dundon, President and Chief Executive Officer, p. B133

LOUISIANA

Baton Rouge: 1475 ★ FRANCISCAN MISSIONARIES OF OUR LADY HEALTH SYSTEM, INC. 4200 Essen Lane, Zip 70809; tel. 504/923–2701; John J. Finan Jr., President and Chief Executive Officer, p. B97

0775 ★ GENERAL HEALTH SYSTEM 3849 North Boulevard, Suite 200, Zip 70806; tel. 504/387–7810; Thomas H. Sawyer, President and Chief Executive Officer, p. B98

0715 LOUISIANA HEALTH CARE AUTHORITY 8550 United Plaza Boulevard, 4th Floor, Zip 70809; tel. 504/922–0488; Cary Doughtery, Acting Chief Executive Officer, p. B109

New Orleans: 0047 LOUISIANA STATE HOSPITALS 210 State Street, Zip 70118; tel. 504/897–3400; M. E. Teague, Chief Executive Officer, p. B109

MAINE

Bangor: 0555 ★ EASTERN MAINE HEALTHCARE 489 State Street, Zip 04401, Mailing Address: P.O. Box 404, Zip 04402–0404; tel. 207/973–7051; Norman A. Ledwin, President, p. B96

MARYLAND

Baltimore: 1015 ★ JOHNS HOPKINS HEALTH SYSTEM 600 North Wolfe Street, Zip 21287–1193; tel. 410/955–9540; Ronald R. Peterson, President, p. B107

6015 SISTERS OF MERCY OF THE AMERICAS–REGIONAL COMMUNITY OF BALTIMORE 1300 Northern Parkway, Zip 21239, Mailing Address: P.O. Box 11448, Zip 21239; tel. 410/435–4400; Sister Margaret Beatty, President, p. B135

Fallston: 0038 ★ UPPER CHESAPEAKE HEALTH SYSTEM 1916 Belair Road, Zip 21047; tel. 410/893–0322; Lyle Ernest Sheldon, President and Chief Executive Officer, p. B146

Landover: 0029 ★ DIMENSIONS HEALTH CORPORATION 9200 Basil Court, Zip 20785; tel. 301/925–7000; Winfield M. Kelly Jr., President and Chief Executive Officer, p. B95

Lutherville: 2355 ★ HELIX HEALTH 2330 West Joppa Road, Suite 301, Zip 21093; tel. 410/847–6700; James A. Oakey, President and Chief Executive Officer, p. B104

Marriottsville: 5085 ★ BON SECOURS HEALTH SYSTEM, INC. 1505 Marriottsville Road, Zip 21104–1399; tel. 410/442–5511; Christopher M. Carney, President and Chief Executive Officer, p. B71

Rockville: 9195 U. S. PUBLIC HEALTH SERVICE INDIAN HEALTH SERVICE 2275 Research Boulevard, Zip 20850; tel. 202/619–0257; Michael Trujillo, M.D., M.P.H., Director, p. B143

MASSACHUSETTS

Boston: 0096 ★ CAREGROUP 375 Longwood Avenue, Zip 02215; tel. 617/667–2222; Mitchell T. Rabkin, Chief Executive Officer, p. B74

1125 ★ CARITAS CHRISTI HEALTH CARE SYSTEM 736 Cambridge Street, Zip 02135; tel. 617/789–2500; Michael F. Collins, M.D., President, p. B74

0013 MASSACHUSETTS DEPARTMENT OF MENTAL HEALTH 25 Staniford Street, Zip 02114; tel. 617/727–5600; Marylou Sudders, Commissioner, p. B112

1785 ★ PARTNERS HEALTHCARE SYSTEM 800 Boylston Street, Suite 1150, Zip 02199; tel. 617/278–1000; Samuel O. Thier, M.D., Chief Executive Officer, p. B121

Lexington: 5885 ★ COVENANT HEALTH SYSTEMS, INC. 420 Bedford Street, Zip 02173–1502; tel. 617/862–1634; David R. Lincoln, President and Chief Executive Officer, p. B88

Norwood: 3175 NEPONSET VALLEY HEALTH SYSTEM 800 Washington Street, Zip 02062–3487; tel. 617/769–4000; Yolanda Landrau, R.N., Ed.D., President and Chief Executive Officer, p. B117

Peabody: 0091 PIONEER HEALTHCARE 200 Lake Street, Suite 102, Zip 01960; tel. 508/536–2777; Bruce A. Shear, President and Chief Executive Officer, p. B121

Pittsfield: 2435 ★ BERKSHIRE HEALTH SYSTEMS, INC. 725 North Street, Zip 01201; tel. 413/447–2743; David E. Phelps, President and Chief Executive Officer, p. B70

Springfield: 1095 ★ BAYSTATE HEALTH SYSTEMS, INC. 759 Chestnut Street, Zip 01199–0001; tel. 413/784–0000; Michael J. Daly, President, p. B69

5285 SISTERS OF PROVIDENCE HEALTH SYSTEM 146 Chestnut Street, Zip 01103; tel. 413/737–3981; Sister Kathleen Popko, President and Chief Executive Officer, p. B135

Wellesley Hills: 0215 COMMUNITY CARE SYSTEMS, INC. 15 Walnut Street, Zip 02181–0001; tel. 617/431–3000; Frederick J. Thacher, Chairman, p. B86

MICHIGAN

Ann Arbor: 5555 ★ SISTERS OF ST. JOSEPH HEALTH SYSTEM 455 East Eisenhower Parkway, Suite 300, Zip 48108–3324; tel. 313/741–1160; John S. Lore, President and Chief Executive Officer, p. B136

Dearborn: 1165 ★ OAKWOOD HEALTHCARE SYSTEM 18101 Oakwood Boulevard, Zip 48124, Mailing Address: P.O. Box 2500, Zip 48123–2500; tel. 313/593–7000; Gerald D. Fitzgerald, President, p. B119

Detroit: 2145 ★ DETROIT MEDICAL CENTER 4201 St. Antoine Boulevard, Zip 48201–2194; tel. 313/745–5192; David J. Campbell, President and Chief Executive Officer, p. B94

9505 ★ HENRY FORD HEALTH SYSTEM One Ford Place, Zip 48202; tel. 313/876–8715; Gail L. Warden, President and Chief Executive Officer, p. B104

Farmington Hills: 5165 ★ MERCY HEALTH SERVICES 34605 Twelve Mile Road, Zip 48331–3221; tel. 810/489–6000; Judith Pelham, President and Chief Executive Officer, p. B114

Kalamazoo: 0595 ★ BRONSON HEALTHCARE GROUP, INC. One Healthcare Plaza, Zip 49007–5345; tel. 616/341–6000; Frank J. Sardone, President and Chief Executive Officer, p. B73

Midland: 0001 ★ MIDMICHIGAN REGIONAL HEALTH SYSTEM 4005 Orchard Drive, Zip 48670; tel. 517/839–3000; Terence F. Moore, President, p. B116

Port Huron: 0053 ★ BLUE WATER HEALTH SERVICES CORPORATION 1221 Pine Grove Avenue, Zip 48060; tel. 810/989–3717; Donald C. Fletcher, President and Chief Executive Officer, p. B71

Royal Oak: 9575 ★ WILLIAM BEAUMONT HOSPITAL CORPORATION 3601 West Thirteen Mile Road, Zip 48073–6769; tel. 810/551–5000; Ted D. Wasson, President and Chief Executive Officer, p. B149

Saint Joseph: 0056 ★ LAKELAND REGIONAL HEALTH SYSTEM, INC. 1234 Napier Avenue, Zip 49085–2158; tel. 616/983–8300; Joseph A. Wasserman, President and Chief Executive Officer, p. B108

Southfield: 2055 MICHIGAN HEALTH CARE CORPORATION 23100 Providence Drive, Suite 300, Zip 48075; tel. 810/304–3400; Charles E. Housley, FACHE, President and Chief Executive Officer, p. B116

Traverse City: 1465 ★ MUNSON HEALTHCARE 1105 Sixth Street, Zip 49684–2386; tel. 616/935–6502; John M. Rockwood Jr., President, p. B117

Warren: 0042 ★ DETROIT–MACOMB HOSPITAL CORPORATION 12000 East Twelve Mile Road, Zip 48093; tel. 810/573–5914; Timothy J. Ryan, JD, President and Chief Executive Officer, p. B95

MINNESOTA

Duluth: 0515 BENEDICTINE HEALTH SYSTEM 503 East Third Street, Zip 55805–1964; tel. 218/720–2370; Sister Kathleen Hofer, Chair Person and Chief Executive Officer, p. B70

Minneapolis: 0041 ★ ALLINA HEALTH SYSTEM 5601 Smetana Drive, Zip 55440, Mailing Address: P.O. Box 9310, Zip 55440–9310; tel. 612/992–2000; Gordon M. Sprenger, Executive Officer, p. B65

1325 ★ FAIRVIEW HOSPITAL AND HEALTHCARE SERVICES 2450 Riverside Avenue, Zip 55454–1400; tel. 612/672–6300; Richard A. Norling, President and Chief Executive Officer, p. B97

Rochester: 1875 ★ MAYO FOUNDATION 200 S.W. First Street, Zip 55905; tel. 507/284–2511; Robert R. Waller, M.D., President and Chief Executive Officer, p. B112

Saint Louis Park: 1985 HEALTHSYSTEM MINNESOTA 6500 Excelsior Boulevard, Zip 55426–4702; tel. 612/932–6300, p. B103

Saint Paul: 2185 ★ HEALTHEAST 559 Capitol Boulevard, 6–South, Zip 55103–0000; tel. 612/232–2300; Timothy H. Hanson, President and Chief Executive Officer, p. B102

MISSISSIPPI

Batesville: 1275 FIRST HEALTH, INC. 107 Public Square, Zip 38606; tel. 601/563–7676; Sandra Skinner, Chief Executive Officer, p. B97

Jackson: 0017 MISSISSIPPI STATE DEPARTMENT OF MENTAL HEALTH 1101 Robert E Lee Building, Zip 39201–1101; tel. 601/359–1288; Roger McMurtry, Chief Mental Health Bureau, p. B117

Pascagoula: 0067 SINGING RIVER HOSPITAL SYSTEM 2809 Denny Avenue, Zip 39581; tel. 601/938–5062; Robert L. Lingle, Executive Director, p. B132

Tupelo: 0032 NORTH MISSISSIPPI HEALTH SERVICES, INC. 830 South Gloster Street, Zip 38801; tel. 601/841–3136; Jeffrey B. Barber, Dr.PH, President and Chief Executive Officer, p. B118

MISSOURI

Kansas City: 8815 ★ HEALTH MIDWEST 2304 East Meyer Boulevard, Suite A–20, Zip 64132–4104; tel. 816/276–9181; Richard W. Brown, President and Chief Executive Officer, p. B101

0120 SAINT LUKE'S SHAWNEE MISSION HEALTH SYSTEM 10920 Elm Avenue, Zip 64134; tel. 816/932–3377; G. Richard Hastings, President and Chief Executive Officer, p. B130

9255 ★ TRUMAN MEDICAL CENTER 2301 Holmes Street, Zip 64108–2677; tel. 816/556–3153; E. Ratcliffe Anderson Jr., M.D., Executive Director, p. B143

Saint Louis: 0051 ★ BJC HEALTH SYSTEM 4444 Forest Park Avenue, Zip 63108–2259; tel. 314/286–2030; Fred L. Brown, President and Chief Executive Officer, p. B71

5945 ★ CARONDELET HEALTH SYSTEM 13801 Riverport Drive, Suite 300, Zip 63043–4810; tel. 314/770–0333; Gary Christiansen, President and Chief Executive Officer, p. B75

1855 ★ DAUGHTERS OF CHARITY NATIONAL HEALTH SYSTEM 4600 Edmundson Road, Zip 63134, Mailing Address: P.O. Box 45998, Zip 63145–5998; tel. 314/253–6700; Donald A. Brennan, President and Chief Executive Officer, p. B88

5185 ★ SISTERS OF MERCY HEALTH SYSTEM–ST. LOUIS 2039 North Geyer Road, Zip 63131–3399, Mailing Address: P.O. Box 31902, Zip 63131–1902; tel. 314/965–6100; Sister Mary Roch Rocklage, President and Chief Executive Officer, p. B134

5455 ★ SSM HEALTH CARE SYSTEM 477 North Lindbergh Boulevard, Zip 63141–7813; tel. 314/994–7800; Sister Mary Jean Ryan, President and Chief Executive Officer, p. B137

NEBRASKA

Norfolk: 2855 MISSIONARY BENEDICTINE SISTERS AMERICAN PROVINCE 300 North 18th Street, Zip 68701; tel. 402/371–3438; Sister M. Agnes Salber, Prioress, p. B116

NEVADA

Las Vegas: 0093 TRANSITIONAL HOSPITALS CORPORATION 5110 West Sahara Avenue, Zip 89102; tel. 702/257–4000; Richard L. Conte, Chief Executive Officer and Chairman of the Board, p. B142

NEW JERSEY

Camden: 6725 ★ WEST JERSEY HEALTH SYSTEM 1000 Atlantic Avenue, Zip 08104; tel. 609/342–4604; Richard P. Miller, President and Chief Executive Officer, p. B148

Edison: 8855 ★ JFK HEALTH SYSTEMS, INC. 80 James Street, 2nd Floor, Zip 08820–3998; tel. 908/632–1500; John P. McGee, President and Chief Executive Officer, p. B107

Livingston: 0118 SAINT BARNABAS HEALTH CARE SYSTEM 94 Old Short Hills Road, Zip 07039; tel. 201/533–5000; Ronald Del Mauro, Chairman and Chief Executive Officer, p. B130

Newark: 6545 CATHEDRAL HEALTHCARE SYSTEM, INC. 219 Chestnut Street, Zip 07105–1558; tel. 201/690–3600; Frank L. Fumai, President and Chief Executive Officer, p. B75

Trenton: 0010 DIVISION OF MENTAL HEALTH SERVICES, DEPARTMENT OF HUMAN SERVICES, STATE OF NEW JERSEY Capital Center, CN 727, Zip 08625–0727; tel. 609/777–0702; Alan G. Kaufman, Director, p. B95

NEW MEXICO

Albuquerque: 3505 ★ PRESBYTERIAN HEALTHCARE SERVICES 5901 Harper Drive N.E., Zip 87109, Mailing Address: P.O. Box 26666, Zip 87125–6666; tel. 505/260–6300; James H. Hinton, President and Chief Executive Officer, p. B121

0021 UNIVERSITY OF NEW MEXICO 915 Camino De Salud, Zip 87131; tel. 505/272–5849; Jane E. Henney, M.D., Vice President Health Sciences, p. B146

NEW YORK

Albany: 0009 NEW YORK STATE DEPARTMENT OF MENTAL HEALTH 44 Holland Avenue, Zip 12229; tel. 518/447–9611; Jesse Nixon Jr., Ph.D., Director, p. B118

Manhasset: 0062 ★ NORTH SHORE HEALTH SYSTEM 300 Community Drive, Zip 11030; tel. 516/562–4060; John S. T. Gallagher, President, p. B119

New York: 1485 ★ FRANCISCAN SISTERS OF THE POOR HEALTH SYSTEM, INC. 708 Third Avenue, Suite 200, Zip 10017; tel. 212/818–1987; James H. Flynn Jr., President and Chief Executive Officer, p. B98

3075 NEW YORK CITY HEALTH AND HOSPITALS CORPORATION 125 Worth Street, Room 514, Zip 10013; tel. 212/788–3321; Luis R. Marcos, M.D., President, p. B117

0110 OUR LADY OF MERCY HEALTHCARE SYSTEM, INC. 600 East 23rd Street, Zip 10466; tel. 718/920–9500; Gary S. Horan, FACHE, President, p. B120

5995 SISTERS OF CHARITY CENTER Mount St. Vincent on Hudson, Zip 10471–1093; tel. 718/549–9200; Sister Elizabeth A. Vermaelen, President, p. B133

6095 ★ SISTERS OF CHARITY HEALTH CARE SYSTEM CORPORATION 75 Vanderbilt Avenue, Zip 10304–3850; tel. 718/354–5080; John J. DePierro, President and Chief Executive Officer, p. B133

Rochester: 0046 ★ GREATER ROCHESTER HEALTH SYSTEM, INC. 1040 University Avenue, Zip 14607; tel. 716/756–4280; Roger S. Hunt, President and Chief Executive Officer, p. B99

Syracuse: 5955 SISTERS OF THE 3RD FRANCISCAN ORDER 2500 Grant Boulevard, Zip 13208–1713; tel. 315/425–0115; Sister Grace Anne Dillenschneider, General Superior, p. B136

Uniondale: 0735 ★ EPISCOPAL HEALTH SERVICES INC. 333 Earle Ovington Boulevard, Zip 11553–3645; tel. 516/228–6100; Jack N. Farrington, Ph.D., Executive Vice President, p. B96

NORTH CAROLINA

Charlotte: 0705 CAROLINAS HEALTHCARE SYSTEM 1000 Blythe Boulevard, Zip 28203, Mailing Address: Box 32861, Zip 28232–2861; tel. 704/355–2000; Harry A. Nurkin, Ph.D., President and Chief Executive Officer, p. B74

NORTH DAKOTA

Bismarck: 0545 BENEDICTINE SISTERS OF THE ANNUNCIATION 7520 University Drive, Zip 58504–9653; tel. 701/255–1520; Sister Susan Berger, Prioress, p. B70

Fargo: 2235 ★ LUTHERAN HEALTH SYSTEMS 4310 17th Avenue S.W., Zip 58103, Mailing Address: P.O. Box 6200, Zip 58106–6200; tel. 701/277–7500; Steven R. Orr, Chairman and Chief Executive Officer, p. B110

5805 SISTERS OF MARY OF THE PRESENTATION HEALTH CORPORATION 1102 Page Drive S.W., Zip 58106–0007, Mailing Address: P.O. Box 10007, Zip 58106–0007; tel. 701/237–9290; Aaron Alton, President, p. B134

OHIO

Cincinnati: 0415 ★ BETHESDA HOSPITAL, INC. 619 Oak Street, Zip 45206–1690; tel. 513/569–6141; L. Thomas Wilburn Jr., Chairman, p. B71

0082 ★ HEALTH ALLIANCE OF GREATER CINCINNATI 2060 Reading Road, Suite 400, Zip 45202–1456; tel. 513/632–3700; Jack M. Cook, President and Chief Executive Officer, p. B100

5155 ★ MERCY HEALTH SYSTEM 2335 Grandview Avenue, 4th Floor, Zip 45206–2280; tel. 513/221–2736; Michael D. Connelly, President and Chief Executive Officer, p. B115

Cleveland: 2515 FAIRVIEW HOSPITAL SYSTEM 18101 Lorain Avenue, Zip 44111–5656; tel. 216/476–7000; Kenneth T. Misener, Vice President and Chief Operating Officer, p. B97

5125 SISTERS OF CHARITY OF ST. AUGUSTINE HEALTH SYSTEM 2351 East 22nd Street, Zip 44115; tel. 216/696–5560; Sister Mary Ann Andrews, President and Chief Executive Officer, p. B134

0112 UNIVERSITY HOSPITALS HEALTH SYSTEM 11100 Euclid Avenue, Zip 44106; tel. 216/844–1000; Farah M. Walters, President and Chief Executive Officer, p. B146

Columbus: 1045 DOCTORS HOSPITAL 1087 Dennison Avenue, Zip 43201; tel. 614/297–4000; Richard A. Vincent, President, p. B95

9095 ★ OHIOHEALTH 3555 Olentangy River Road, 4000, Zip 43214; tel. 614/566–5424; William W. Wilkins, President and Chief Executive Officer, p. B119

Mayfield Village: 8835 ★ MERIDIA HEALTH SYSTEM 6700 Beta Drive, Suite 200, Zip 44143; tel. 216/446–8000; Charles B. Miner, President and Chief Executive Officer, p. B115

Sylvania: 5375 ★ FRANCISCAN SERVICES CORPORATION 6832 Convent Boulevard, Zip 43560–2897; tel. 419/882–8373; John W. O'Connell, President, p. B97

Troy: 1965 ★ UPPER VALLEY MEDICAL CENTERS 3130 North Dixie Highway, Zip 45373; tel. 937/332–7921; David J. Meckstroth, President and Chief Executive Officer, p. B146

OKLAHOMA

Oklahoma City: 0305 ★ INTEGRIS HEALTH 3366 Northwest Expressway, Zip 73112; tel. 405/949–6068; Stanley F. Hupfeld, President and Chief Executive Officer, p. B106

0018 OKLAHOMA STATE DEPARTMENT OF MENTAL HEALTH AND SUBSTANCE ABUSE SERVICES 1000 N.E. Tenth, Zip 73152, Mailing Address: P.O. Box 53277, Zip 73152; tel. 405/271–6868; Thomas Peace, Ph.D., Commissioner, p. B119

Tulsa: 0665 CENTURY HEALTHCARE CORPORATION 5555 East 71st Street, Suite 9220, Zip 74136–6540; tel. 918/491–0775; Jerry D. Dillon, President and Chief Executive Officer, p. B78

5305 ★ SISTERS OF THE SORROWFUL MOTHER UNITED STATES HEALTH SYSTEM Mailing Address: P.O. Box 4753, Zip 74159–0753; tel. 918/742–9988; Sister M. Therese Gottschalk, President, p. B136

OREGON

Medford: 0094 ★ ASANTE HEALTH SYSTEM 2650 Siskiyou Boulevard, Suite 200, Zip 97504–8389; tel. 541/608–4100; Jon K. Mitchell, FACHE, President and Chief Executive Officer, p. B67

Portland: 0585 ★ BRIM, INC. 305 N.E. 102nd Avenue, Zip 97220–4199; tel. 503/256–2070; Jim McKinney, President, p. B72

2755 ★ LEGACY HEALTH SYSTEM 1919 N.W. Lovejoy Street, Zip 97209–1503; tel. 503/415–5600; John G. King, President and Chief Executive Officer, p. B108

PENNSYLVANIA

Danville: 5570 GEISINGER HEALTH SYSTEM 100 North Academy Avenue, Zip 17822; tel. 717/271–6211; Frank J. Trembulak, Executive Vice President and Chief Operating Officer, p. B98

Devon: 0845 DEVEREUX FOUNDATION 19 South Waterloo Road, Zip 19333, Mailing Address: Box 400, Zip 19333; tel. 610/964–3000; Ronald P. Burd, President and Chief Exeuctive Officer, p. B95

King of Prussia: 9555 UNIVERSAL HEALTH SERVICES, INC. 367 South Gulph Road, Zip 19406; tel. 610/768–3300; Alan B. Miller, President and Chief Executive Officer, p. B145

Mechanicsburg: 1715 CONTINENTAL MEDICAL SYSTEMS, INC. 600 Wilson Lane, Zip 17055–0715, Mailing Address: P.O. Box 715, Zip 17055–0715; tel. 717/790–8300; Robert Ortenzio, President and Chief Executive Officer, p. B87

Media: 0008 ★ CROZER–KEYSTONE HEALTH SYSTEM 1400 North Providence Road, Suite 4010, Zip 19063–2049; tel. 610/892–8000; John C. McMeekin, President and Chief Executive Officer, p. B88

Philadelphia: 1685 ALBERT EINSTEIN HEALTHCARE NETWORK 5501 Old York Road, Zip 19141–3098; tel. 215/456–7890; Martin Goldsmith, President, p. B64

Pittsburgh: 2305 ★ ALLEGHENY HEALTH, EDUCATION AND RESEARCH FOUNDATION 120 Fifth Avenue, Zip 15222; tel. 412/359–8800; Sherif S. Abdelhak, President and Chief Executive Officer, p. B64

2255 ★ ST. FRANCIS HEALTH SYSTEM 4401 Penn Avenue, Zip 15224–1334; tel. 412/622–4214; Sister M. Rosita Wellinger, President and Chief Executive Officer, p. B138

Radnor: 3595 ★ EASTERN MERCY HEALTH SYSTEM 3 Radnor Corporate Center, Suite 220, Zip 19087; tel. 610/971–9770; Daniel F. Russell, President and Chief Executive Officer, p. B96

7775 ★ JEFFERSON HEALTH SYSTEM 259 Radnor–Chester Road, Suite 290, Zip 19087–5260; tel. 610/293–8200; Douglas S. Peters, President and Chief Executive Officer, p. B107

Sayre: 0675 ★ GUTHRIE HEALTHCARE SYSTEM Guthrie Square, Zip 18840; tel. 717/882–4312; Ralph H. Meyer, President and Chief Executive Officer, p. B100

Wayne: 0455 HOSPITAL GROUP OF AMERICA 1265 Drummers Lane, Suite 107, Zip 19087; tel. 610/687–5151; Mark R. Russell, President and Chief Executive Officer, p. B104

Williamsport: 0066 SUSQUEHANNA HEALTH SYSTEM 1001 Grampian Boulevard, Zip 17703; tel. 717/320–7100; Don A. Crum, President and Chief Executive Officer, p. B146

York: 0068 ★ YORK HEALTH SYSTEM 1001 South George Street, Zip 17405; tel. 717/851–2121; Bruce M. Bartels, President, p. B149

PUERTO RICO

San Juan: 0011 PUERTO RICO DEPARTMENT OF HEALTH Building A – Medical Center, Zip 00936, Mailing Address: Call Box 70184, Zip 00936; tel. 809/274–7676; Carmen Feliciano De Melecio, M.D., Secretary of Health, p. B123

RHODE ISLAND

Providence: 0099 ★ CARE NEW ENGLAND HEALTH SYSTEM 45 Willard Avenue, Zip 02905; tel. 401/453–7900; John J. Hynes, President and Chief Executive Officer, p. B73

0060 ★ LIFESPAN CORPORATION 167 Point Street, Zip 02903; tel. 401/444–6699; William Kreykes, President and Chief Executive Officer, p. B108

SOUTH CAROLINA

Columbia: 4155 ★ BAPTIST HEALTHCARE SYSTEM OF SOUTH CAROLINA Taylor at Marion Street, Zip 29220; tel. 803/771–5010; Charles D. Beaman Jr., President and Chief Executive Officer, p. B68

Greenville: 1555 ★ GREENVILLE HOSPITAL SYSTEM 701 Grove Road, Zip 29605–4211; tel. 864/455–7000; Frank D. Pinckney, President, p. B100

Spartanburg: 4195 ★ SPARTANBURG REGIONAL HEALTHCARE SYSTEM 101 East Wood Street, Zip 29303–3016; tel. 864/560–6000; Joseph Michael Oddis, President, p. B137

SOUTH DAKOTA

Sioux Falls: 0078 SIOUX VALLEY HEALTH SYSTEM 1100 South Euclid Avenue, Zip 57105–0496; tel. 605/333–1000; Kelby K. Krabbenhoff, President, p. B132

Yankton: 5255 ★ PRESENTATION HEALTH SYSTEM 610 West 23rd Street, Zip 57078, Mailing Address: P.O. Box 38, Zip 57078; tel. 605/357–7050; John T. Porter, President and Chief Executive Officer, p. B122

TENNESSEE

Brentwood: 0080 COMMUNITY HEALTH SYSTEMS, INC. 155 Franklin Road, Suite 400, Zip 37027–4600, Mailing Address: P.O. Box 217, Zip 37024–0217; tel. 615/373–9600; Wayne T. Smith, President, p. B86

0108 PRINCIPAL HOSPITAL GROUP 109 Westpark Drive, Suite 180, Zip 37026; tel. 615/370–1377; Marty Rash, President and Chief Executive Officer, p. B122

0002 ★ QUORUM HEALTH GROUP/QUORUM HEALTH RESOURCES, INC. 103 Continental Place, Zip 37027; tel. 615/371–7979; James E. Dalton Jr., President and Chief Executive Officer, p. B123

Chattanooga: 1155 GREENLEAF HEALTH SYSTEMS, INC. One Northgate Park, Zip 37415; tel. 423/870–5110; Dan B. Page, President, p. B99

2795 HEALTHCORP OF TENNESSEE, INC. 735 Broad Street, Zip 37402; tel. 615/267–8406; T. Farrell Hayes, President, p. B102

Franklin: 0074 AMERICAN TRANSITIONAL HOSPITALS, INC. 112 Second Avenue North, Zip 37064; tel. 615/791–7099; T. Jerald Moore, President and Chief Executive Officer, p. B66

Jackson: 0004 ★ WEST TENNESSEE HEALTHCARE, INC. 708 West Forest Avenue, Zip 38301; tel. 901/425–5000; James T. Moss, President, p. B148

Knoxville: 2155 BAPTIST HEALTH SYSTEM OF TENNESSEE 137 Blount Avenue S.E., Zip 37920, Mailing Address: Box 1788, Zip 37901; tel. 615/632–5099; Dale Collins, President and Chief Executive Officer, p. B68

Memphis: 1625 ★ BAPTIST MEMORIAL HEALTH CARE CORPORATION 899 Madison Avenue, Zip 38146; tel. 901/227–2727; Stephen Curtis Reynolds, President and Chief Executive Officer, p. B68

9345 ★ METHODIST HEALTH SYSTEMS, INC. 1211 Union Avenue, Suite 700, Zip 38104; tel. 901/726–2300; Maurice W. Elliott, President, p. B116

1765 UNITED HOSPITAL CORPORATION 6189 East Shelby Drive, Zip 38115; tel. 901/794–8440; James C. Henson, President, p. B144

Nashville: 0069 BEHAVIORAL HEALTHCARE CORPORATION 102 Woodmont Boulevard, Suite 500, Zip 37205; tel. 615/269–3492; Edward A. Stack, President, p. B69

0048 ★ COLUMBIA/HCA HEALTHCARE CORPORATION One Park Plaza, Zip 37203; tel. 615/320–2000; Richard L. Scott, Chairman and Chief Executive Officer, p. B78

0022 METROPOLITAN NASHVILLE GENERAL HOSPITAL 215 Second Avenue North, Zip 37201; tel. 615/862–4000; Tom Deweese, Administrator, p. B116

0116 NETCARE HEALTH SYSTEMS, INC. 424 Church Street, Suite 2100, Zip 37219; tel. 615/742–8500; Michael A. Koban Jr., Chief Executive Officer, p. B117

0335 PARK HEALTHCARE COMPANY 4015 Travis Drive, Zip 37211; tel. 615/833–1077; Jerry E. Gilliland, President, p. B121

0114 VENDELL HERALTHCARE, INC. 3401 West End Avenue, Suite 500, Zip 37203–0376; tel. 615/383–0376; H. Neil Campbell, Chief Executive Officer, p. B148

TEXAS

Austin: 0003 ★ COLUMBIA/ST. DAVID'S MEDICAL CENTER 919 East 32nd Street, Zip 78705, Mailing Address: P.O. Box 4039, Zip 78765; tel. 512/397–4265; Cole C. Eslyn, Chief Executive Officer, p. B85

0395 HEALTHCARE AMERICA, INC. 1407 West Stassney Lane, Zip 78745, Mailing Address: P.O. Box 4008, Zip 78765–4008; tel. 512/464–0200; John P. Harcourt Jr., President and Chief Executive Officer, p. B101

0020 TEXAS DEPARTMENT OF HEALTH 1100 West 49th Street, Zip 78756; tel. 512/458–7111; Patti J. Patterson, Commissioner, p. B142

0033 UNIVERSITY OF TEXAS SYSTEM 601 Colorado Street, Zip 78701–2982; tel. 512/499–4224; Charles B. Mullins, Executive Vice Chancellor, p. B146

Bay City: 2505 MATAGORDA COUNTY HOSPITAL DISTRICT 1115 Avenue G, Zip 77414; tel. 409/245–6383; Wendell H. Baker Jr., Chief Executive Officer, p. B112

Dallas: 0095 ★ BAYLOR HEALTH CARE SYSTEM 3500 Gaston Avenue, Zip 75226; tel. 214/820–0111; Boone Powell Jr., President, p. B69

2735 ★ METHODIST HOSPITALS OF DALLAS 1441 North Beckley, Zip 75203, Mailing Address: P.O. Box 655999, Zip 75265–5999; tel. 214/947–8181; Howard M. Chase, FACHE, President and Chief Executive Officer, p. B116

1130 ★ PRESBYTERIAN HEALTHCARE SYSTEM 8220 Walnut Hill Lane, Suite 700, Zip 75231; tel. 214/345–8500; Douglas D. Hawthorne, President and Chief Executive Officer, p. B122

Fort Worth: 2345 ★ HARRIS METHODIST HEALTH SYSTEM 6000 Western Place, Suite 200, Zip 76107; tel. 817/570–8900; Ronald L. Smith, President, p. B100

0039 TARRANT COUNTY HOSPITAL DISTRICT 1500 South Main Street, Zip 76104; tel. 817/927–1230; Anthony J. Alcini, President and Chief Executive Officer, p. B139

Houston: 0077 CAMBRIDGE INTERNATIONAL, INC, 7505 Fannin, Suite 680, Zip 77225; tel. 713/790–1153; Timothy Sharma, M.D., President, p. B73

2645 ★ MEMORIAL HEALTHCARE SYSTEM 7737 S.W. Freeway, Suite 200, Zip 77074–1800; tel. 713/776–6992; Dan S. Wilford, President, p. B114

7235 ★ METHODIST HEALTH CARE SYSTEM 6565 Fannin Street, D–200, Zip 77030; tel. 713/790–2221; Larry L. Mathis, FACHE, President and Chief Executive Officer, p. B115

5765 PARACELSUS HEALTHCARE CORPORATION 515 West Greens Road, Suite 800, Zip 77067; tel. 281/774–5100; Charles R. Miller, President and Chief Operating Officer, p. B120

0605 ★ SISTERS OF CHARITY OF THE INCARNATE WORD HEALTHCARE SYSTEM 2600 North Loop West, Zip 77092; tel. 713/681–8877; Sister Christina Murphy, President and Chief Executive Officer, p. B134

Lubbock: 0036 ★ LUBBOCK METHODIST HOSPITAL SYSTEM 3615 19th Street, Zip 79410–1201; tel. 806/792–1011; James P. Houser, President and Chief Executive Officer, p. B109

San Antonio: 0265 BAPTIST HEALTH SYSTEM 660 North Main Street, Suite 300, Zip 78205–1222; tel. 210/302–3000; Fred R. Mills, President and Chief Executive Officer, p. B67

5565 ★ INCARNATE WORD HEALTH SERVICES 9311 San Pedro, Suite 1250, Zip 78216–4469; tel. 210/524–4100; Joseph Blasko Jr., President and Chief Executive Officer, p. B105

Tyler: 1895 EAST TEXAS MEDICAL CENTER REGIONAL HEALTHCARE SYSTEM 1000 South Beckham Street, Zip 75701–1996, Mailing Address: P.O. Drawer 6400, Zip 75711–6400; tel. 903/535–6211; Elmer G. Ellis, President and Chief Executive Officer, p. B95

UTAH

Nephi: 0109 ★ RURAL HEALTH MANAGEMENT CORPORATION 549 North 400 East, Zip 84648; tel. 801/623–4924; Mark R. Stoddard, President, p. B130

Salt Lake City: 1815 ★ INTERMOUNTAIN HEALTH CARE, INC. 36 South State Street, 22nd Floor, Zip 84111; tel. 801/442–2000; Scott S. Parker, President, p. B106

VIRGINIA

Falls Church: 9395 DEPARTMENT OF THE ARMY, OFFICE OF THE SURGEON GENERAL 5109 Leesburg Pike, Zip 22041; tel. 703/681–3114; Major Beverly Pritchett, Executive Officer, p. B90

Lynchburg: 2265 ★ CENTRA HEALTH, INC. 1920 Atherholt Road, Zip 24501–1104; tel. 804/947–4700; George W. Dawson, President, p. B77

Newport News: 4810 RIVERSIDE HEALTH SYSTEM 606 Denbigh Boulevard, Suite 601, Zip 23608; tel. 757/875–7500; Nelson L. St. Clair, President, p. B129

Norfolk: 2635 FIRST HOSPITAL CORPORATION 240 Corporate Boulevard, Zip 23502; tel. 757/459–5100; Ronald I. Dozoretz, M.D., Chairman, p. B97

Section B Index

2565 ★ SENTARA HEALTH SYSTEM 6015 Poplar Hall Drive, Zip 23502; tel. 757/455–7000; David L. Bernd, President and Chief Executive Officer, p. B131

Richmond: 0012 VIRGINIA DEPARTMENT OF MENTAL HEALTH 109 Governor Street, Zip 23219, Mailing Address: P.O. Box 1797, Zip 23218; tel. 804/786–3921; Timothy A. Kelly, Ph.D., Commissioner, p. B148

Roanoke: 0070 ★ CARILION HEALTH SYSTEM 1212 Third Street S.W., Zip 24016, Mailing Address: P.O. Box 13727, Zip 24036–3727; tel. 540/981–7000; Thomas L. Robertson, President and Chief Executive Officer, p. B74

Springfield: 1305 ★ INOVA HEALTH SYSTEM 8001 Braddock Road, Zip 22151–2150; tel. 703/321–4213; J. Knox Singleton, President, p. B105

WASHINGTON

Bellevue: 5415 ★ PEACEHEALTH 15325 S.E. 30th Place, Suite 300, Zip 98007; tel. 206/747–1711; Sister Monica F. Heeran, President and Chief Executive Officer, p. B121

0044 STERLING HEALTHCARE CORPORATION 1500 114th Avenue S.E., Suite 100, Zip 98004; tel. 206/453–5445; David Jacobsen, President, p. B138

Seattle: 9995 ★ GROUP HEALTH COOPERATIVE OF PUGET SOUND 521 Wall Street, Zip 98121–1536; tel. 206/326–3000; Phil Nudelman, Ph.D., President and Chief Executive Officer, p. B100

5275 ★ SISTERS OF PROVIDENCE HEALTH SYSTEM 520 Pike Street, Zip 98101, Mailing Address: P.O. Box 11038, Zip 98111–9038; tel. 206/464–3355; Sister Karin Dufault, Ph.D., Administrator, p. B135

Spokane: 0945 EMPIRE HEALTH SERVICES West 800 Fifth Avenue, Zip 99204, Mailing Address: P.O. Box 248, Zip 99210–0248; tel. 509/458–7960; Thomas M. White, President, p. B96

5265 ★ PROVIDENCE SERVICES 9 East Ninth Avenue, Zip 99202; tel. 509/742–7337; Richard J. Umbdenstock, President and Chief Executive Officer, p. B123

Tacoma: 6555 MULTICARE HEALTH SYSTEM 315 Martin Luther King Jr. Way, Zip 98405, Mailing Address: P.O. Box 5299, Zip 98405–0299; tel. 206/552–1000; William B. Connoley, President, p. B117

WEST VIRGINIA

Charleston: 0955 ★ CAMCARE, INC. 501 Morris Street, Zip 25301, Mailing Address: P.O. Box 1547, Zip 25326; tel. 304/348–5432; Phillip H. Goodwin, President, p. B73

Morgantown: 0119 WEST VIRGINIA UNITED HEALTH SYSTEM Mailing Address: P.O. Box 8010, Zip 26506–8010; tel. 304/598–6000; Bernard G. Westfall, President, p. B149

WISCONSIN

Appleton: 2445 ★ UNITED HEALTH GROUP Five Innovation Court, Zip 54914, Mailing Address: P.O. Box 8025, Zip 54913–8025; tel. 414/730–0330; James Edward Raney, President and Chief Executive Officer, p. B144

Fond Du Lac: 5695 CONGREGATION OF ST. AGNES 475 Gillett Street, Zip 54935–4598; tel. 414/923–0804; Rosann Geiser, Corporate Director, p. B87

La Crosse: 9650 ★ FRANCISCAN SKEMP HEALTHCARE 700 West Avenue South, Zip 54601; tel. 608/791–9710; Brian C. Campion, M.D., President and Chief Executive Officer, p. B98

Manitowoc: 1455 ★ FRANCISCAN SISTERS OF CHRISTIAN CHARITY HEALTHCARE MINISTRY, INC 2409 South Alverno Road, Zip 54220–9320; tel. 920/684–7071; Sister Laura J. Wolf, President, p. B98

Milwaukee: 2215 ★ AURORA HEALTH CARE 3000 West Montana, Zip 53215–3268, Mailing Address: P.O. Box 343910, Zip 53234–3910; tel. 414/647–3000; G. Edwin Howe, President, p. B67

0027 ★ HORIZON HEALTHCARE, INC. 2300 North Mayfair Road, Suite 550, Zip 53226–1508; tel. 414/257–3888; Sister Renee Rose, President and Chief Executive Officer, p. B104

Alliances

ALLIANCE OF INDEPENDENT ACADEMIC MEDICAL CENTERS
435 N Michigan Ave, Ste 2700, Chicago, IL Zip 60611; tel. 312/923–9770; Ms Nancie Noie, Managing Director

ARIZONA
Phoenix
Member
  Good Samaritan Regional Medical Center
  Maricopa Medical Center
  St. Joseph's Hospital and Medical Center

CALIFORNIA
Long Beach
Member
  Long Beach Memorial Medical Center

Los Angeles
Member
  Cedars–Sinai Medical Center

Oakland
Member
  Kaiser Foundation Hospital

CONNECTICUT
Hartford
Member
  Saint Francis Hospital and Medical Center

DELAWARE
Wilmington
Member
  Medical Center of Delaware

DISTRICT OF COLUMBIA
Washington
Member
  Washington Hospital Center

FLORIDA
Miami Beach
Member
  Mount Sinai Medical Center

Orlando
Member
  Orlando Regional Medical Center

ILLINOIS
Berwyn
Member
  MacNeal Hospital

Chicago
Member
  Columbia Michael Reese Hospital and Medical Center
Shareholder
  Illinois Masonic Medical Center

Park Ridge
Member
  Lutheran General Hospital

INDIANA
Indianapolis
  St. Vincent Hospitals and Health Services
Member
  Methodist Hospital of Indiana

LOUISIANA
New Orleans
Member
  Ochsner Foundation Hospital

MAINE
Portland
Member
  Maine Medical Center

MARYLAND
Lutherville
Member
  Helix Health

MASSACHUSETTS
Springfield
Member
  Baystate Medical Center

MICHIGAN
Detroit
Member
  Henry Ford Health System

Royal Oak
Member
  William Beaumont Hospital–Royal Oak

MISSOURI
Kansas City
Member
  Saint Luke's Hospital

Saint Louis
  St. John's Mercy Medical Center

NEW JERSEY
Livingston
Member
  Saint Barnabas Medical Center

Long Branch
Member
  Monmouth Medical Center

Paterson
Member
  St. Joseph's Hospital and Medical Center

NEW YORK
Bronx
Member
  Bronx–Lebanon Hospital Center

Brooklyn
Member
  Maimonides Medical Center

Buffalo
Member
  Millard Fillmore Health System

Jamaica
Member
  Catholic Medical Center of Brooklyn and Queens

Mineola
Member
  Winthrop–University Hospital

New Hyde Park
Member
  Long Island Jewish Medical Center

New York
Member
  Beth Israel Medical Center
  St. Luke's–Roosevelt Hospital Center

NORTH CAROLINA
Charlotte
Member
  Carolinas Medical Center

OHIO
Akron
Member
  Akron General Medical Center
  Summa Health System

Cleveland
Member
  Cleveland Clinic Hospital

Columbus
Member
  Grant/Riverside Methodist Hospitals–Riverside Campus
  Mount Carmel Health System

OKLAHOMA
Tulsa
Member
  Hillcrest Healthcare System

PENNSYLVANIA
Philadelphia
Member
  Albert Einstein Medical Center

Pittsburgh
Member
  Mercy Hospital of Pittsburgh
  Shadyside Hospital
  Western Pennsylvania Hospital

SOUTH CAROLINA
Columbia
Member
  Richland Memorial Hospital

Greenville
Member
  Greenville Hospital System

TEXAS
Dallas
Member
  Baylor University Medical Center

WASHINGTON
Seattle
Member
  Virginia Mason Medical Center

ASSOCIATION OF INDEPENDENT HOSPITALS
8300 Troost, Kansas City, MO Zip 64131; tel. 816/276–7580; Mr Jeff Tindle, President and Chief Executive Officer

ILLINOIS
Mount Vernon
Member
  Good Samaritan Regional Health Center

Woodstock
Member
  Memorial Medical Center

KANSAS
Columbus
Member
  Maude Norton Memorial City Hospital

Council Grove
Member
  Morris County Hospital

Garnett
Member
  Anderson County Hospital

Girard
Member
  Crawford County Hospital District One

Holton
Member
  Holton Community Hospital

Iola
Member
  Allen County Hospital

Junction City
Member
  Geary Community Hospital

Kansas City
Member
  Providence Medical Center
  University of Kansas Hospital

Lawrence
Member
  Lawrence Memorial Hospital

Leavenworth
Member
  Saint John Hospital

Manhattan
Member
  Mercy Health Center of Manhattan

Marysville
Member
  Community Memorial Hospital

Section B

Olathe
Member
Olathe Medical Center

Onaga
Member
Community Hospital Onaga

Ottawa
Member
Ransom Memorial Hospital

Overland Park
Member
Menorah Medical Center

Paola
Member
Miami County Medical Center

Pittsburg
Member
Mount Carmel Medical Center

Seneca
Member
Nemaha Valley Community Hospital

Topeka
Member
C. F. Menninger Memorial Hospital
St. Francis Hospital and Medical Center

Winchester
Member
Jefferson County Memorial Hospital

MISSOURI
Albany
Member
Gentry County Memorial Hospital

Belton
Member
Research Belton Hospital

Bethany
Member
Harrison County Community Hospital

Boonville
Member
Cooper County Memorial Hospital

Brookfield
Member
General John J. Pershing Memorial Hospital

Carrollton
Member
Carroll County Memorial Hospital

Carthage
Member
McCune–Brooks Hospital

Chillicothe
Member
Hedrick Medical Center

Clinton
Member
Golden Valley Memorial Hospital

Columbia
Member
University Hospitals and Clinics

Excelsior Springs
Member
Excelsior Springs Medical Center

Fairfax
Member
Community Hospital Association

Farmington
Member
Mineral Area Regional Medical Center

Hannibal
Member
Hannibal Regional Hospital

Harrisonville
Member
Cass Medical Center

Hermann
Member
Hermann Area District Hospital

Independence
Member
Medical Center of Independence

Jefferson City
Member
Capital Region Medical Center–Southwest

Joplin
Member
St. John's Regional Medical Center

Kansas City
Member
Baptist Medical Center
Park Lane Medical Center
Research Medical Center
Trinity Lutheran Hospital

Lees Summit
Member
Lee's Summit Hospital

Lexington
Member
Lafayette Regional Health Center

Macon
Member
Samaritan Memorial Hospital

Mexico
Member
Audrain Medical Center

Moberly
Member
Moberly Regional Medical Center

Nevada
Member
Nevada Regional Medical Center

North Kansas City
Member
North Kansas City Hospital

Richmond
Member
Ray County Memorial Hospital

Saint Joseph
Member
Heartland Regional Medical Center

Saint Louis
Member
DePaul Health Center
Saint Louis University Hospital

Warrensburg
Member
Western Missouri Medical Center

CHILD HEALTH CORPORATION OF AMERICA
6803 West 64th Street, Ste 208, Shawnee Mission, KS Zip 66202; tel. 913/262–1436; Mr Don C Black, President and Chief Executive Officer

ALABAMA
Birmingham
Member
Children's Hospital of Alabama

ARKANSAS
Little Rock
Member
Arkansas Children's Hospital

CALIFORNIA
Fresno
Member
Valley Children's Hospital

Los Angeles
Member
Childrens Hospital of Los Angeles

Oakland
Member
Children's Hospital Oakland

Orange
Member
Children's Hospital of Orange County

Palo Alto
Member
Lucile Salter Packard Children's Hospital at Stanford

San Diego
Member
Children's Hospital and Health Center

COLORADO
Denver
Member
Children's Hospital

DISTRICT OF COLUMBIA
Washington
Member
Children's National Medical Center

FLORIDA
Miami
Member
Miami Children's Hospital

Saint Petersburg
Member
All Children's Hospital

GEORGIA
Atlanta
Member
Egleston Children's Hospital at Emory University

ILLINOIS
Chicago
Member
Children's Memorial Hospital

LOUISIANA
New Orleans
Member
Children's Hospital

MASSACHUSETTS
Boston
Member
Children's Hospital

MICHIGAN
Detroit
Member
Children's Hospital of Michigan

MINNESOTA
Minneapolis
Member
Children's Health Care, Minneapolis

MISSOURI
Kansas City
Member
Children's Mercy Hospital

Saint Louis
Member
St. Louis Children's Hospital

NEBRASKA
Omaha
Member
Children's Hospital

NEW YORK
Buffalo
Member
Children's Hospital

OHIO
Akron
Member
Children's Hospital Medical Center of Akron

Cincinnati
Member
Children's Hospital Medical Center

Columbus
Member
Children's Hospital

Dayton
Member
Children's Medical Center

PENNSYLVANIA
Philadelphia
Member
Children's Hospital of Philadelphia

Pittsburgh
Member
  Children's Hospital of Pittsburgh

TENNESSEE

Memphis
Member
  Le Bonheur Children's Medical Center

TEXAS

Corpus Christi
Member
  Driscoll Children's Hospital

Dallas
Member
  Children's Medical Center of Dallas

Fort Worth
Member
  Cook Children's Medical Center

Houston
Member
  Texas Children's Hospital

VIRGINIA

Norfolk
Member
  Children's Hospital of the King's Daughters

WASHINGTON

Seattle
Member
  Children's Hospital and Medical Center

WISCONSIN

Milwaukee
Member
  Children's Hospital of Wisconsin

CONSOLIDATED CATHOLIC HEALTH CARE
  1301 W 22nd Street, Suite 202, Oak Brook, IL Zip 60521-2011; tel. 708/990-2242; Mr Roger N Butler, Executive Director

CALIFORNIA

Orange
Member
  St. Joseph Health System

COLORADO

Denver
Member
  Catholic Health Initiatives

FLORIDA

Tampa
Member
  Allegany Health System

ILLINOIS

Frankfort
Member
  Franciscan Sisters Health Care Corporation

Kankakee
Member
  ServantCor

INDIANA

Mishawaka
Member
  Sisters of St. Francis Health Services, Inc.

South Bend
Member
  Holy Cross Health System Corporation

KANSAS

Leavenworth
Member
  Sisters of Charity of Leavenworth Health Services Corporation

Wichita
Member
  Via Christi Health System

MASSACHUSETTS

Springfield
Member
  Sisters of Providence Health System

MICHIGAN

Ann Arbor
Member
  Sisters of St. Joseph Health System

MISSOURI

Saint Louis
Member
  Carondelet Health System

NEW YORK

New York
Member
  Franciscan Sisters of the Poor Health System, Inc.

OHIO

Cincinnati
Member
  Mercy Health System

Sylvania
Member
  Franciscan Services Corporation

HOSPITAL NETWORK, INC.
  One Healthcare Plaza, Kalamazoo, MI Zip 49007; tel. 616/341-8888; Mr Richard Fluke, President and Chief Executive Officer

MICHIGAN

Allegan
Member
  Allegan General Hospital

Hastings
Member
  Pennock Hospital

Kalamazoo
Member
  Bronson Healthcare Group, Inc.
  Bronson Methodist Hospital

Marshall
Member
  Oaklawn Hospital

Sturgis
Member
  Sturgis Hospital

Vicksburg
Member
  Bronson Vicksburg Hospital

INTERHEALTH
  2550 University Ave W, Ste 233, Saint Paul, MN Zip 55114; tel. 612/646-5574; Mr Benjamin Aune, President and Chief Executive Officer

ALABAMA

Birmingham
Member
  Baptist Health System

ILLINOIS

Normal
Member
  BroMenn Healthcare

Oakbrook
Member
  Advocate Health Care

Rock Island
Member
  Trinity Medical Center–West Campus

LOUISIANA

New Orleans
Member
  Southern Baptist Health System

MICHIGAN

Bay City
Member
  Bay Health Systems

MINNESOTA

Duluth
Member
  Benedictine Health System

Saint Paul
Member
  HealthEast

MISSISSIPPI

Jackson
Member
  Mississippi Baptist Medical Center

MISSOURI

Saint Louis
Member
  Deaconess Incarnate Word Health System

OHIO

Cleveland
Member
  Fairview Hospital System

Columbus
Member
  OhioHealth

Kettering
Member
  Kettering Medical Center

TEXAS

Houston
Member
  Memorial Healthcare System

MERIDIAN HEALTH SYSTEM
  1945 State Highway 33, Neptune, NJ Zip 07753; tel. 908/776-4215; Mr John K Lloyd, Chief Executive Officer

NEW JERSEY

New Brunswick
Member
  University Health System of New Jersey

PREMIER, INC.
  3 Westbrook Corporate Center, 9th Floor, Westchester, IL Zip 60154-5735; tel. 708/409-4100; Mr Alan Weinstein, President

ALABAMA

Daphne
Member
  Mercy Medical

Dothan
Member
  Southeast Alabama Medical Center

Florala
Member
  Florala Memorial Hospital

Opelika
Member
  East Alabama Medical Center

Valley
Member
  George H. Lanier Memorial Hospital and Health Services

ALASKA

Fairbanks
Member
  Fairbanks Memorial Hospital

Homer
Member
  South Peninsula Hospital

Ketchikan
Member
  Ketchikan General Hospital

Kodiak
Member
  Providence Kodiak Island Hospital and Medical Center

Palmer
Member
  Valley Hospital

Sitka
Member
  Searhc MT. Edgecumbe Hospital
  Sitka Community Hospital

Section B

Soldotna
Member
　Central Peninsula General Hospital

Valdez
Member
　Valdez Community Hospital

ARIZONA

Ganado
Member
　Sage Memorial Hospital

Mesa
Member
　Mesa Lutheran Hospital
　Valley Lutheran Hospital

ARKANSAS

Batesville
Shareholder
　White River Medical Center

Berryville
Shareholder
　Carroll Regional Medical Center

Crossett
Shareholder
　Ashley Memorial Hospital

Danville
Shareholder
　Chambers Memorial Hospital

Dardanelle
Shareholder
　Dardanelle Hospital

De Witt
Shareholder
　DeWitt City Hospital

El Dorado
Shareholder
　Medical Center of South Arkansas

Eureka Springs
Shareholder
　Eureka Springs Hospital

Gravette
Shareholder
　Gravette Medical Center Hospital

Harrison
Shareholder
　North Arkansas Medical Center

Hot Springs National Park
Shareholder
　Levi Hospital

Little Rock
Shareholder
　Arkansas Children's Hospital
　St. Vincent Infirmary Medical Center

Magnolia
Shareholder
　Magnolia Hospital

McGehee
Shareholder
　McGehee–Desha County Hospital

Monticello
Shareholder
　Drew Memorial Hospital

Morrilton
Shareholder
　Conway County Hospital

Mountain Home
Shareholder
　Baxter County Regional Hospital

Paragould
Shareholder
　Arkansas Methodist Hospital

Pine Bluff
Shareholder
　Jefferson Regional Medical Center

Springdale
Shareholder
　Northwest Medical Center

Warren
Shareholder
　Bradley County Memorial Hospital

West Memphis
Shareholder
　Crittenden Memorial Hospital

CALIFORNIA

Anaheim
Member
　Martin Luther Hospital–Anaheim

Apple Valley
Member
　St. Mary Regional Medical Center

Bakersfield
Member
　Kern Medical Center
　San Joaquin Community Hospital

Burbank
Member
　UniHealth

Chula Vista
Member
　Sharp Chula Vista Medical Center

Clearlake
Member
　Redbud Community Hospital

Corona
Member
　Corona Regional Medical Center

Coronado
Member
　Sharp Coronado Hospital

Deer Park
Member
　St. Helena Hospital

Delano
Member
　Delano Regional Medical Center

Escondido
Member
　Palomar Medical Center

Eureka
Member
　Saint Joseph Hospital

Fortuna
Member
　Redwood Memorial Hospital

Fullerton
Member
　St. Jude Medical Center

Glendale
Member
　Glendale Adventist Medical Center
　Glendale Memorial Hospital and Health Center

Hanford
Member
　Hanford Community Medical Center

La Mesa
Member
　Grossmont Hospital

La Palma
Member
　La Palma Intercommunity Hospital

Long Beach
Member
　Long Beach Community Medical Center

Los Angeles
Member
　California Hospital Medical Center
　White Memorial Medical Center

Mission Viejo
Member
　Mission Hospital Regional Medical Center

Murrieta
Member
　Sharp Healthcare Murrieta

Napa
Member
　Queen of the Valley Hospital

National City
Member
　Paradise Valley Hospital

Northridge
Member
　Northridge Hospital Medical Center–Roscoe Boulevard
　　Campus

Oakland
Member
　Summit Medical Center

Orange
Member
　St. Joseph Health System
　St. Joseph Hospital

Paradise
Member
　Feather River Hospital

Poway
Member
　Pomerado Hospital

Rancho Mirage
Member
　Eisenhower Memorial Hospital and Betty Ford Center
　　at Eisenhower

Roseville
Member
　Adventist Health

San Diego
Member
　Palomar Pomerado Health System
　Sharp Cabrillo Hospital
　Sharp Healthcare
　Sharp Memorial Hospital

San Gabriel
Member
　San Gabriel Valley Medical Center

San Jose
Member
　Alexian Brothers Hospital

Santa Rosa
Member
　Santa Rosa Memorial Hospital

Simi Valley
Member
　Simi Valley Hospital and Health Care Services

Sonora
Member
　Sonora Community Hospital

Ukiah
Member
　Ukiah Valley Medical Center

Van Nuys
Member
　Northridge Hospital and Medical Center, Sherman
　　Way Campus

Willits
Member
　Frank R. Howard Memorial Hospital

COLORADO

Brush
Member
　East Morgan County Hospital

Delta
Member
　Delta County Memorial Hospital

Durango
Member
　Mercy Medical Center

Greeley
Member
　North Colorado Medical Center

Loveland
Member
　McKee Medical Center

Sterling
Member
　Sterling Regional Medcenter

CONNECTICUT

Hartford
Member
　Saint Francis Hospital and Medical Center

New Haven
Member
 Hospital of Saint Raphael

Stafford Springs
Member
 Johnson Memorial Hospital

DELAWARE

Dover
Member
 Kent General Hospital

Lewes
Member
 Beebe Medical Center

Wilmington
Member
 Medical Center of Delaware

DISTRICT OF COLUMBIA

Washington
Member
 Columbia Hospital for Women Medical Center
 George Washington University Hospital
 Sibley Memorial Hospital

FLORIDA

Altamonte Springs
Member
 Florida Hospital–Altamonte

Apopka
Member
 Florida Hospital–Apopka

Avon Park
Member
 Florida Hospital–Walker

Bunnell
Member
 Memorial Hospital–Flagler

Cape Coral
Member
 Cape Coral Hospital

Coral Springs
Member
 Coral Springs Medical Center

DeLand
Member
 Memorial Hospital–West Volusia

Dunedin
Member
 Mease Hospital Dunedin

Eustis
Member
 Florida Hospital Waterman

Fernandina Beach
Member
 Baptist Medical Center–Nassau

Fort Lauderdale
Member
 Broward General Medical Center
 Cleveland Clinic Hospital
 Imperial Point Medical Center
 North Broward Hospital District

Gainesville
Member
 AvMed–Santa Fe
 Shands at AGH
 Shands at the University of Florida

Hollywood
Member
 Memorial Regional Hospital

Homestead
Member
 Homestead Hospital

Jacksonville
Member
 St. Vincent's Medical Center

Jacksonville Beach
Member
 Baptist Medical Center–Beaches

Kissimmee
Member
 Florida Hospital Kissimmee

Lake City
Member
 Shands at Lake Shore

Lake Wales
Member
 Lake Wales Medical Centers

Largo
Member
 Sun Coast Hospital

Naples
Member
 Naples Community Hospital

Orlando
Member
 Florida Hospital

Ormond Beach
Member
 Memorial Health Systems
 Memorial Hospital–Ormond Beach

Pembroke Pines
Member
 Memorial Hospital Pembroke
 Memorial Hospital West

Pensacola
Member
 Sacred Heart Hospital of Pensacola

Pinellas Park
Member
 Pinellas Community Hospital

Plant City
Member
 South Florida Baptist Hospital

Pompano Beach
Member
 North Broward Medical Center

Port Charlotte
Member
 Bon Secours–St. Joseph Hospital

Rockledge
Member
 Wuesthoff Hospital

Safety Harbor
Member
 Mease Countryside Hospital

Saint Petersburg
Member
 St. Anthony's Hospital

Sarasota
Member
 Sarasota Memorial Hospital

Starke
Member
 Shands at Starke

Tampa
Member
 St. Joseph's Hospital

Tarpon Springs
Member
 Helen Ellis Memorial Hospital

Tavernier
Member
 Mariners Hospital

Titusville
Member
 Parrish Medical Center

Venice
Member
 Bon Secours–Venice Hospital

Vero Beach
Member
 Indian River Memorial Hospital

West Palm Beach
Member
 St. Mary's Hospital

Winter Haven
Member
 Winter Haven Hospital

Winter Park
Member
 Adventist Health System Sunbelt Health Care
  Corporation

Zephyrhills
Member
 East Pasco Medical Center

GEORGIA

Athens
Member
 St. Mary's Health Care System

Atlanta
Member
 Crawford Long Hospital of Emory University
 Georgia Baptist Health Care System
 Saint Joseph's Hospital of Atlanta

Augusta
Member
 Walton Rehabilitation Hospital

Blairsville
Member
 Union General Hospital

Calhoun
Member
 Gordon Hospital

Columbus
Member
 St. Francis Hospital

Cumming
Member
 Baptist North Hospital

Fort Oglethorpe
Member
 Hutcheson Medical Center

Glenwood
Member
 Wheeler County Hospital

Hiawassee
Member
 Chatuge Regional Hospital and Nursing Home

La Grange
Member
 West Georgia Health System

Riverdale
Member
 Southern Regional Medical Center

Savannah
Member
 Memorial Medical Center
 St. Joseph's Hospital

Smyrna
Member
 Emory–Adventist Hospital

Tifton
Member
 Tift General Hospital

HAWAII

Honolulu
Member
 Kuakini Medical Center

Kailua
Member
 Castle Medical Center

IDAHO

Nampa
Member
 Mercy Medical Center Extended Care Facility

ILLINOIS

Aurora
Member
 Mercy Center for Health Care Services

Barrington
Member
 Good Shepherd Hospital

Blue Island
Member
 St. Francis Hospital and Health Center

Section B

Alliances

Canton
Member
  Graham Hospital

Chicago
Member
  Bethany Hospital
  Mercy Hospital and Medical Center
  Mount Sinai Hospital Medical Center of Chicago
  Our Lady of the Resurrection Medical Center
  Ravenswood Hospital Medical Center
  Resurrection Medical Center
  St. Elizabeth's Hospital
  Thorek Hospital and Medical Center
  Trinity Hospital

Downers Grove
Member
  Good Samaritan Hospital

East St Louis
Member
  St. Mary's Hospital

Elk Grove Village
Member
  Alexian Brothers Medical Center

Fairfield
Member
  Fairfield Memorial Hospital

Galesburg
Member
  Galesburg Cottage Hospital

Geneseo
Member
  Hammond–Henry Hospital

Geneva
Member
  Delnor–Community Hospital

Hazel Crest
Member
  South Suburban Hospital

Hoopeston
Member
  Hoopeston Community Memorial Hospital

Melrose Park
Member
  Gottlieb Memorial Hospital

Metropolis
Member
  Massac Memorial Hospital

Morrison
Member
  Morrison Community Hospital

Mount Carmel
Member
  Wabash General Hospital District

Mount Vernon
Member
  Good Samaritan Regional Health Center

Naperville
Member
  Mercy–Chicago Region Healthcare System

Nashville
Member
  Washington County Hospital

Oak Lawn
Member
  Christ Hospital and Medical Center

Oak Park
Member
  West Suburban Hospital Medical Center

Oakbrook
Member
  Advocate Health Care

Ottawa
Member
  Community Hospital of Ottawa

Paris
Member
  Paris Community Hospital

Park Ridge
Member
  Lutheran General Hospital

Peoria
Member
  Methodist Health Services Corporation
  Methodist Medical Center of Illinois

Urbana
Member
  Carle Foundation Hospital

Winfield
Member
  Central DuPage Hospital

INDIANA

Bluffton
Member
  Caylor–Nickel Medical Center

Brazil
Member
  Clay County Hospital

Bremen
Member
  Community Hospital of Bremen

Charlestown
Member
  Medical Center of Southern Indiana

Crown Point
Member
  St. Anthony Medical Center

East Chicago
Member
  St. Catherine Hospital

Evansville
Member
  Welborn Memorial Baptist Hospital

Fort Wayne
Member
  St. Joseph Medical Center of Fort Wayne

Gary
Member
  Methodist Hospitals
  Northlake Campus

Greensburg
Member
  Decatur County Memorial Hospital

Hartford City
Member
  Blackford County Hospital

Hobart
Member
  St. Mary Medical Center

Jeffersonville
Member
  Clark Memorial Hospital

Mishawaka
Member
  St. Joseph Community Hospital

North Vernon
Member
  Jennings Community Hospital

Portland
Member
  Jay County Hospital

Princeton
Member
  Gibson General Hospital

Rushville
Member
  Rush Memorial Hospital

Salem
Member
  Washington County Memorial Hospital

Scottsburg
Member
  Scott Memorial Hospital

South Bend
Member
  St. Mary Community Hospital

Tell City
Member
  Perry County Memorial Hospital

Wabash
Member
  Wabash County Hospital

Williamsport
Member
  St. Vincent Williamsport Hospital

Winchester
Member
  Randolph County Hospital

IOWA

Algona
Member
  Kossuth Regional Health Center

Ames
Member
  Mary Greeley Medical Center

Belmond
Member
  Belmond Community Hospital

Britt
Member
  Hancock County Memorial Hospital

Cedar Rapids
Member
  Mercy Medical Center
  St. Luke's Hospital

Centerville
Member
  St. Joseph's Mercy Hospital

Clinton
Member
  Samaritan Health System

Corning
Member
  Alegent Health Mercy Hospital

Council Bluffs
Member
  Alegent Health Mercy Hospital

Cresco
Member
  Howard County Hospital

Des Moines
Member
  Iowa Health System
  Iowa Lutheran Hospital
  Iowa Methodist Medical Center

Dubuque
Member
  Mercy Health Center

Dyersville
Member
  Mercy Health Center–St. Mary's Unit

Eldora
Member
  Eldora Regional Medical Center

Elkader
Member
  Central Community Hospital

Emmetsburg
Member
  Palo Alto County Hospital

Hampton
Member
  Franklin General Hospital

Hawarden
Member
  Hawarden Community Hospital

Iowa City
Member
  Mercy Hospital

Marengo
Member
  Marengo Memorial Hospital

Marshalltown
Member
  Marshalltown Medical and Surgical Center

Mason City
Member
  North Iowa Mercy Health Center

Missouri Valley
Member
  Alegent Health Community Memorial Hospital

New Hampton
Member
  Saint Joseph Community Hospital

Oelwein
Member
  Mercy Hospital of Franciscan Sisters

Osage
Member
  Mitchell County Regional Health Center

Osceola
Member
  Clarke County Hospital

Oskaloosa
Member
  Mahaska County Hospital

Primghar
Member
  Baum Harmon Memorial Hospital

Rock Valley
Member
  Hegg Memorial Health Center

Shenandoah
Member
  Shenandoah Memorial Hospital

Sioux City
Member
  Marian Health Center

Spencer
Member
  Spencer Municipal Hospital

Storm Lake
Member
  Buena Vista County Hospital

Waterloo
Member
  Allen Memorial Hospital

KANSAS
Iola
Member
  Allen County Hospital

Marion
Member
  St. Luke Hospital

Neodesha
Member
  Wilson County Hospital

Oberlin
Member
  Decatur County Hospital

KENTUCKY
Bardstown
Member
  Flaget Memorial Hospital

Berea
Member
  Berea Hospital

Bowling Green
Member
  The Medical Center at Bowling Green

Campbellsville
Member
  Taylor County Hospital

Carrollton
Member
  Carroll County Memorial Hospital

Corbin
Member
  Baptist Regional Medical Center

Elizabethtown
Member
  Hardin Memorial Hospital

Glasgow
Member
  T. J. Samson Community Hospital

Greensburg
Member
  Jane Todd Crawford Memorial Hospital

Hardinsburg
Member
  Breckinridge Memorial Hospital

Harrodsburg
Member
  The James B. Haggin Memorial Hospital

Henderson
Member
  Community Methodist Hospital

Horse Cave
Member
  Caverna Memorial Hospital

Irvine
Member
  Marcum and Wallace Memorial Hospital

La Grange
Member
  Tri County Baptist Hospital

Lancaster
Member
  Garrard County Memorial Hospital

Leitchfield
Member
  Twin Lakes Regional Medical Center

Lexington
Member
  Central Baptist Hospital
  Lexington Hospital
  St. Joseph Hospital

London
Member
  Marymount Medical Center

Louisville
  Charter louisville Behavioral Health System
Member
  Alliant Health System
  Alliant Hospitals
  Baptist Healthcare System
  Baptist Hospital East
  Caritas Medical Center
  Caritas Peace Center
  Jewish Hospital
  Jewish Hospital Healthcare Services
  Kosair Children's Hospital
  Norton Hospital
  University of Louisville Hospital

Madisonville
Member
  Regional Medical Center of Hopkins County

Manchester
Member
  Memorial Hospital

Morganfield
Member
  Union County Methodist Hospital

Mount Sterling
Member
  Mary Chiles Hospital Extended Care Facility

Mount Vernon
Member
  Rockcastle Hospital

Murray
Member
  Murray–Calloway County Hospital

Nazareth
Member
  Sisters of Charity of Nazareth Health System

Owensboro
Member
  Owensboro Mercy Health System

Paducah
Member
  Lourdes Hospital
  Western Baptist Hospital

Pikeville
Member
  Pikeville United Methodist Hospital of Kentucky

Princeton
Member
  Caldwell County Hospital

Richmond
Member
  Pattie A. Clay Hospital

Russell Springs
Member
  Russell County Hospital

Scottsville
Member
  Medical Center at Scottsville

Shelbyville
Member
  Jewish Hospital–Shelbyville

Stanford
Member
  Fort Logan Hospital

Versailles
Member
  Woodford Hospital

Winchester
Member
  Clark Regional Medical Center

LOUISIANA
Baton Rouge
Member
  Baton Rouge General Health Center
  Baton Rouge General Medical Center
  General Health System
  Woman's Hospital

Bossier City
Member
  Bossier Medical Center

Cut Off
Member
  Lady of the Sea General Hospital

Farmerville
Member
  Union General Hospital

Homer
Member
  Homer Memorial Hospital

Houma
Member
  Terrebonne General Medical Center

Jena
Member
  La Salle General Hospital

Lafayette
Member
  Lafayette General Medical Center

Mansfield
Member
  De Soto Regional Health System

Marrero
Member
  West Jefferson Medical Center

New Orleans
Member
  Touro Infirmary

Raceland
Member
  St. Anne General Hospital

Shreveport
Member
  Schumpert Medical Center

Sterlington
Member
  Sterlington Hospital

West Monroe
Member
  Glenwood Regional Medical Center

MAINE
Blue Hill
Member
  Blue Hill Memorial Hospital

Brunswick
Member
Parkview Hospital

Lewiston
Member
St. Mary's Regional Medical Center

Portland
Member
Mercy Hospital Portland

South Portland
Member
Jackson Brook Institute

MARYLAND

Annapolis
Member
Anne Arundel Medical Center

Baltimore
Member
Bon Secours Hospital
Children's Hospital and Center for Reconstructive Surgery
Church Hospital Corporation
Franklin Square Hospital Center
Good Samaritan Hospital of Maryland
Harbor Hospital Center
Mercy Medical Center
Mt. Washington Pediatric Hospital
Sinai Hospital of Baltimore
Union Memorial Hospital

Bethesda
Member
Suburban Hospital

Cambridge
Member
Dorchester General Hospital

Columbia
Member
Howard County General Hospital

Cumberland
Member
Memorial Hospital and Medical Center of Cumberland

Elkton
Member
Union Hospital

Frederick
Member
Frederick Memorial Hospital

Hagerstown
Member
Washington County Hospital Association

Lanham
Member
Doctors Community Hospital

Lutherville
Member
Helix Health

Marriottsville
Member
Bon Secours Health System, Inc.

Olney
Member
Montgomery General Hospital

Randallstown
Member
Northwest Hospital Center

Rockville
Member
Shady Grove Adventist Hospital

Salisbury
Member
Peninsula Regional Medical Center

Takoma Park
Member
Washington Adventist Hospital

Westminster
Member
Carroll County General Hospital

MASSACHUSETTS

Andover
Member
Yankee Alliance

Attleboro
Member
Sturdy Memorial Hospital

Ayer
Member
Deaconess–Nashoba Hospital

Boston
Member
New England Baptist Hospital

Brockton
Member
Brockton Hospital

Cambridge
Member
Youville Lifecare

Framingham
Member
Columbia MetroWest Medical Center

Gardner
Member
Heywood Hospital

Great Barrington
Member
Fairview Hospital

Greenfield
Member
Franklin Medical Center

Lowell
Member
Saints Memorial Medical Center

Needham
Member
Deaconess–Glover Hospital Corporation

Palmer
Member
Wing Memorial Hospital and Medical Centers

Pittsfield
Member
Berkshire Medical Center

Salem
Member
Salem Hospital

Springfield
Member
Baystate Health Systems, Inc.
Baystate Medical Center

Stoneham
Member
Boston Regional Medical Center

Ware
Member
Mary Lane Hospital

Winchester
Member
Winchester Hospital

Worcester
Member
Memorial Health Care

MICHIGAN

Alma
Member
Gratiot Community Hospital

Ann Arbor
Member
St. Joseph Mercy Health System

Battle Creek
Member
Battle Creek Health System

Cadillac
Member
Mercy Health Services–North

Clinton Township
Member
St. Joseph's Mercy Hospitals and Health Services

Commerce Township
Member
Huron Valley Hospital

Deckerville
Member
Deckerville Community Hospital

Detroit
Member
Detroit Medical Center
Detroit Receiving Hospital and University Health Center
Detroit Riverview Hospital
Grace Hospital
Harper Hospital
Henry Ford Health System
Henry Ford Hospital
Hutzel Hospital
Mercy Hospital
Sinai Hospital
St. John Health System–Saratoga Campus

Farmington Hills
Member
Botsford General Hospital
Mercy Health Services

Flint
Member
McLaren Regional Medical Center

Frankfort
Member
Paul Oliver Memorial Hospital

Grand Rapids
Blodgett Memorial Medical Center
Member
Metropolitan Hospital
Saint Mary's Health Services

Grayling
Member
Mercy Health Services North–Grayling

Grosse Pointe
Member
Bon Secours Hospital

Grosse Pointe Farms
Member
Henry Ford Cottage Hospital of Grosse Pointe

Howell
Member
McPherson Hospital

Jackson
Member
W. A. Foote Memorial Hospital

Kalamazoo
Member
Borgess Medical Center

Lansing
Member
Sparrow Health System
St. Lawrence Hospital and Healthcare Services

Lapeer
Member
Lapeer Regional Hospital

Madison Heights
Member
Madison Community Hospital
Oakland General Hospital

Marshall
Member
Oaklawn Hospital

Monroe
Member
Mercy Memorial Hospital

Mount Clemens
Member
Mount Clemens General Hospital

Muskegon
Member
Mercy General Health Partners–Oak Avenue Campus
Mercy General Health Partners–Sherman Boulevard Campus

Northport
Member
Leelanau Memorial Health Center

Pontiac
Member
Pontiac Osteopathic Hospital
St. Joseph Mercy Oakland

Port Huron
Member
Mercy Hospital

Saint Johns
Member
Clinton Memorial Hospital

Saline
Member
Saline Community Hospital

Southfield
Member
Straith Hospital for Special Surgery

Traverse City
Member
Munson Medical Center

Trenton
Member
Riverside Osteopathic Hospital

Warren
Member
Bi–County Community Hospital
Macomb Hospital Center

Wyandotte
Member
Henry Ford Wyandotte Hospital

MINNESOTA

Adrian
Member
Arnold Memorial Health Care Center

Aitkin
Member
Riverwood Health Care Center

Albany
Member
Albany Area Hospital and Medical Center

Albert Lea
Member
Naeve Hospital

Alexandria
Member
Douglas County Hospital

Austin
Member
Austin Medical Center

Baudette
Member
Lakewood Health Center

Brainerd
Member
St. Joseph's Medical Center

Breckenridge
Member
St. Francis Medical Center

Burnsville
Member
Fairview Ridges Hospital

Chisago City
Member
Chisago Health Services

Cloquet
Member
Community Memorial Hospital and Convalescent and Nursing Care Section

Cook
Member
Cook Hospital and Convalescent Nursing Care Unit

Crosby
Member
Cuyuna Regional Medical Center

Detroit Lakes
Member
St. Mary's Regional Health Center

Duluth
Member
Miller Dwan Medical Center

Ely
Member
Ely–Bloomenson Community Hospital

Fairmont
Member
Fairmont Community Hospital

Forest Lake
Member
District Memorial Hospital

Hastings
Member
Regina Medical Center

Hibbing
Member
University Medical Center–Mesabi

Litchfield
Member
Meeker County Memorial Hospital

Little Falls
Member
St. Gabriel's Hospital

Luverne
Member
Luverne Community Hospital

Madison
Member
Lac Qui Parle Hospital of Madison

Minneapolis
Member
Fairview Hospital and Healthcare Services
Fairview Southdale Hospital

Monticello
Member
Monticello Big Lake Hospital

Moose Lake
Member
Mercy Hospital and Health Care Center

Mora
Member
Kanabec Hospital

New Prague
Member
Queen of Peace Hospital

Northfield
Member
Northfield Hospital

Ortonville
Member
Ortonville Area Health Services

Park Rapids
Member
St Joseph's Area Health Services

Pipestone
Member
Pipestone County Medical Center

Princeton
Member
Fairview Northland Regional Hospital

Red Wing
Member
St. John's Regional Health Center

Robbinsdale
Member
North Memorial Health Care

Rochester
Member
Olmsted Medical Center

Rush City
Member
Rush City Hospital

Saint Louis Park
Member
HealthSystem Minnesota

Sandstone
Member
Pine Medical Center

Sauk Centre
Member
St. Michael's Hospital

Staples
Member
Greater Staples Hospital and Care Center

Thief River Falls
Member
Northwest Medical Center

Tyler
Member
Tyler Healthcare Center

Wadena
Member
Tri–County Hospital

Warren
Member
North Valley Health Center

Westbrook
Member
Westbrook Health Center

Winona
Member
Community Memorial Hospital and Convalescent and Rehabilitation Unit

MISSISSIPPI

Amory
Member
Gilmore Memorial Hospital

Bay Springs
Member
Jasper General Hospital

Brandon
Member
Rankin Medical Center

Columbia
Member
Methodist Hospital of Marion County

Greenville
Member
King's Daughters Hospital

Grenada
Member
Grenada Lake Medical Center

Hattiesburg
Member
Methodist Hospital of Hattiesburg

Jackson
Member
Methodist Medical Center
Mississippi Baptist Medical Center

Laurel
Member
South Central Regional Medical Center

Lexington
Member
Methodist Hospital of Middle Mississippi

Louisville
Member
Winston Medical Center

Magee
Member
Magee General Hospital

Meridian
Member
Rush Foundation Hospital

Union
Member
Laird Hospital

Yazoo City
Member
King's Daughters Hospital

MISSOURI

Albany
Member
Gentry County Memorial Hospital

Belton
Member
Research Belton Hospital

Carrollton
Member
Carroll County Memorial Hospital

Farmington
Member
Mineral Area Regional Medical Center

Harrisonville
Member
Cass Medical Center

Independence
Member
Medical Center of Independence

Jefferson City
Member
St. Marys Health Center

Joplin
Member
St. John's Regional Medical Center

Kansas City
Member
Baptist Medical Center
Health Midwest
Park Lane Medical Center
Research Medical Center
Trinity Lutheran Hospital

Lake Saint Louis
Member
St. Joseph Hospital West

Lees Summit
Member
Lee's Summit Hospital

Lexington
Member
Lafayette Regional Health Center

Louisiana
Member
Pike County Memorial Hospital

Maryville
Member
St. Francis Hospital and Health Services

Mexico
Member
Audrain Medical Center

Pilot Knob
Member
Arcadia Valley Hospital

Saint Charles
Member
St. Joseph Health Center

Saint Louis
Member
Cardinal Glennon Children's Hospital
DePaul Health Center
SSM Health Care System
St. Joseph Hospital
St. Mary's Health Center

MONTANA
Bozeman
Member
Bozeman Deaconess Hospital

Great Falls
Member
Benefis Health Care–West Campus

Miles City
Member
Holy Rosary Health Center

Missoula
Member
St. Patrick Hospital

Polson
Member
St. Joseph Hospital

Sidney
Member
Sidney Health Center

NEBRASKA
Ainsworth
Member
Brown County Hospital

Albion
Member
Boone County Health Center

Alliance
Member
Box Butte General Hospital

Atkinson
Member
West Holt Memorial Hospital

Auburn
Member
Nemaha County Hospital

Aurora
Member
Memorial Hospital

Bassett
Member
Rock County Hospital

Central City
Member
Litzenberg Memorial County Hospital

Chadron
Member
Chadron Community Hospital

Cozad
Member
Cozad Community Hospital

Crawford
Member
Legend Buttes Health Services

Creighton
Member
Creighton Area Health Services

Fairbury
Member
Jefferson Community Health Center

Fremont
Member
Fremont Area Medical Center

Friend
Member
Warren Memorial Hospital

Geneva
Member
Fillmore County Hospital

Genoa
Member
Genoa Community Hospital

Gordon
Member
Gordon Memorial Hospital District

Gothenburg
Member
Gothenburg Memorial Hospital

Hebron
Member
Thayer County Health Services

Henderson
Member
Henderson Health Care Services

Humboldt
Member
Community Memorial Hospital

Imperial
Member
Chase County Community Hospital

Lincoln
Member
Lincoln General Hospital

Lynch
Member
Niobrara Valley Hospital

Oakland
Member
Oakland Memorial Hospital

Ogallala
Member
Ogallala Community Hospital

Omaha
Member
Alegent Health Bergan Mercy Medical Center
Alegent Health Immanuel Medical Center
Bishop Clarkson Memorial Hospital
Boys Town National Research Hospital

Ord
Member
Valley County Hospital

Osceola
Member
Annie Jeffrey Memorial County Health Center

Oshkosh
Member
Garden County Hospital

Pawnee City
Member
Pawnee County Memorial Hospital

Pender
Member
Pender Community Hospital

Red Cloud
Member
Webster County Community Hospital

Saint Paul
Member
Howard County Community Hospital

Sargent
Member
Sargent District Hospital

Schuyler
Member
Alegent Health–Memorial Hospital

Seward
Member
Memorial Health Care Systems

Superior
Member
Brodstone Memorial Hospital

Syracuse
Member
Community Memorial Hospital

Tecumseh
Member
Johnson County Hospital

Valentine
Member
Cherry County Hospital

Wahoo
Member
Saunders County Health Service

Wayne
Member
Providence Medical Center

West Point
Member
St. Francis Memorial Hospital

NEVADA
Fallon
Member
Churchill Community Hosptial

Lovelock
Member
Pershing General Hospital

NEW HAMPSHIRE
Manchester
Member
Catholic Medical Center
Elliot Hospital

Nashua
Member
St. Joseph Healthcare

NEW JERSEY
East Orange
Member
East Orange General Hospital

Edison
Member
JFK Health Systems, Inc.
JFK Medical Center

Englewood
Member
Englewood Hospital and Medical Center

Freehold
Member
Centrastate Medical Center

Holmdel
Member
Bayshore Community Hospital

Irvington
Member
Irvington General Hospital

Long Branch
Member
Monmouth Medical Center

Newark
Member
Newark Beth Israel Medical Center

Passaic
Member
Beth Israel Hospital

Paterson
Member
Barnert Hospital

Salem
Member
Memorial Hospital of Salem County

NEW MEXICO

Albuquerque
Member
Presbyterian Healthcare Services
Presbyterian Hospital
Presbyterian Kaseman Hospital

Artesia
Member
Artesia General Hospital

Clayton
Member
Union County General Hospital

Clovis
Member
Plains Regional Medical Center

Espanola
Member
Espanola Hospital

Los Alamos
Member
Los Alamos Medical Center

Ruidoso
Member
Lincoln County Medical Center

Socorro
Member
Socorro General Hospital

Truth or Consequences
Member
Sierra Vista Hospital

Tucumcari
Member
Dr. Dan C. Trigg Memorial Hospital

NEW YORK
Member
St. John's Queens Hospital

Albany
Member
Albany Medical Center
St. Peter's Hospital

Batavia
Member
St. Jerome Hospital

Bath
Member
Ira Davenport Memorial Hospital

Brockport
Member
Lakeside Memorial Hospital

Bronx
Member
Montefiore Medical Center

Brooklyn
Member
Kings Highway Hospital Center
Long Island College Hospital
Maimonides Medical Center
St. Mary's Hospital

Buffalo
Member
Mercy Hospital
Millard Fillmore Health System
Sheehan Memorial Hospital

Cambridge
Member
Mary McClellan Hospital

Canandaigua
Member
F. F. Thompson Health System

Clifton Springs
Member
Clifton Springs Hospital and Clinic

Corning
Member
Corning Hospital

Dansville
Member
Nicholas H. Noyes Memorial Hospital

Dobbs Ferry
Member
Community Hospital at Dobbs Ferry

Elmira
Member
Arnot Ogden Medical Center
St. Joseph's Hospital

Flushing
Member
St. Joseph's Hospital

Glens Falls
Member
Glens Falls Hospital

Hornell
Member
St. James Mercy Hospital

Irving
Member
Lake Shore Hospital

Jamaica
Member
Catholic Medical Center of Brooklyn and Queens

Kenmore
Member
Kenmore Mercy Hospital

Medina
Member
Medina Memorial Hospital

Mineola
Member
Winthrop–University Hospital

Montour Falls
Member
Schuyler Hospital

New Hyde Park
Member
Long Island Jewish Medical Center

New York
Member
Beth Israel Medical Center
Mount Sinai Medical Center

Newark
Member
Newark–Wayne Community Hospital

Newfane
Member
Inter–Community Memorial Hospital

Penn Yan
Member
Soldiers and Sailors Memorial Hospital of Yates County

Port Jefferson
Member
St. Charles Hospital and Rehabilitation Center

Port Jervis
Member
Mercy Community Hospital

Poughkeepsie
Member
Saint Francis Hospital
Vassar Brothers Hospital

Rochester
Member
Genesee Hospital
Rochester General Hospital
Strong Memorial Hospital of the University of Rochester

Sleepy Hollow
Member
Phelps Memorial Hospital Center

Smithtown
Member
St. John's Episcopal Hospital–Smithtown

Sodus
Member
Myers Community Hospital

Staten Island
Member
Doctors' Hospital of Staten Island
Staten Island University Hospital

Uniondale
Member
Episcopal Health Services Inc.

Warsaw
Member
Wyoming County Community Hospital

NORTH CAROLINA

Albemarle
Member
Stanly Memorial Hospital

Asheboro
Member
Randolph Hospital

Asheville
Member
Memorial Mission Medical Center
St. Joseph's Hospital
Thoms Rehabilitation Hospital

Banner Elk
Member
Charles A. Cannon Jr. Memorial Hospital

Blowing Rock
Member
Blowing Rock Hospital

Boiling Springs
Member
Crawley Memorial Hospital

Boone
Member
Watauga Medical Center

Brevard
Member
Transylvania Community Hospital

Burgaw
Member
Pender Memorial Hospital

Burlington
Member
Alamance Regional Medical Center

Charlotte
Member
Mercy Hospital
Presbyterian Hospital
Presbyterian Specialty Hospital
Presbyterian–Orthopaedic Hospital

Clinton
Member
Sampson Regional Medical Center

Clyde
Member
Haywood Regional Medical Center

Columbus
Member
St. Luke's Hospital

Concord
Member
Cabarrus Memorial Hospital

Crossnore
Member
Sloop Memorial Hospital

Danbury
Member
Stokes–Reynolds Memorial Hospital

Durham
Member
Durham Regional Hospital

Edenton
Member
Chowan Hospital

Elizabethtown
Member
Bladen County Hospital

Fayetteville
Member
Cape Fear Valley Health System

Gastonia
Member
Gaston Memorial Hospital

Goldsboro
Member
Wayne Memorial Hospital

Henderson
Member
Maria Parham Hospital

Hendersonville
Member
Margaret R. Pardee Memorial Hospital

Hickory
Member
Catawba Memorial Hospital

Jacksonville
Member
Onslow Memorial Hospital

Kenansville
Member
Duplin General Hospital

Kinston
Member
Lenoir Memorial Hospital

Laurinburg
Member
Scotland Memorial Hospital

Lenoir
Member
Caldwell Memorial Hospital

Lexington
Member
Lexington Memorial Hospital

Lincolnton
Member
Lincoln Medical Center

Lumberton
Member
North Carolina Cancer Institute
Southeastern Regional Medical Center

Marion
Member
McDowell Hospital

Morganton
Member
Grace Hospital

New Bern
Member
Craven Regional Medical Authority

North Wilkesboro
Member
Wilkes Regional Medical Center

Pinehurst
Member
Moore Regional Hospital

Roanoke Rapids
Member
Halifax Memorial Hospital

Sealevel
Member
Sea Level Hospital Extended Care Facility

Shelby
Member
Cleveland Regional Medical Center

Statesville
Member
Iredell Memorial Hospital

Supply
Member
Columbia Brunswick Hospital

Sylva
Member
Harris Regional Hospital

Troy
Member
Montgomery Memorial Hospital

Wadesboro
Member
Anson County Hospital and Skilled Nursing Facilities

Williamston
Member
Martin General Hospital

Wilmington
Member
New Hanover Regional Medical Center

Wilson
Member
Wilson Memorial Hospital

Winston–Salem
Member
North Carolina Baptist Hospital

Yadkinville
Member
Hoots Memorial Hospital

NORTH DAKOTA

Cavalier
Member
Pembina County Memorial Hospital and Wedgewood Manor

Dickinson
Member
St. Joseph's Hospital and Health Center

Fargo
Member
Dakota Heartland Health System
Lutheran Health Systems

Lisbon
Member
Lisbon Medical Center

Minot
Member
UniMed Medical Center

OHIO

Akron
Member
Summa Health System

Barberton
Member
Barberton Citizens Hospital

Batavia
Member
Clermont Mercy Hospital

Bellevue
Member
Bellevue Hospital

Bowling Green
Member
Wood County Hospital

Cincinnati
Member
Bethesda Hospital, Inc.
Bethesda North Hospital
Bethesda Oak Hospital
Jewish Health Systems, Inc.
Jewish Hospital

Cleveland
Member
Cleveland Clinic Hospital
Meridia Hillcrest Hospital
Meridia Huron Hospital
Mount Sinai Medical Center

Euclid
Member
Meridia Euclid Hospital

Gallipolis
Member
Holzer Medical Center

Garfield Heights
Member
Marymount Hospital

Green Springs
Member
St. Francis Health Care Centre

Hamilton
Member
Mercy Hospital

Kettering
Member
Kettering Medical Center

Lima
Member
St. Rita's Medical Center

Mayfield Village
Member
Meridia Health System

Norwalk
Member
Fisher–Titus Medical Center

Oregon
Member
St. Charles Hospital

Sandusky
Member
Providence Hospital

Springfield
Member
Mercy Medical Center

Tiffin
Member
Mercy Hospital

Toledo
Member
St. Vincent Mercy Medical Center

Urbana
Member
Mercy Memorial Hospital

Warren
Member
St. Joseph Health Center

Warrensville Heights
Member
Meridia South Pointe Hospital

Wauseon
Member
Fulton County Health Center

Willard
Member
Mercy Hospital–Willard

Willoughby
Member
Laurelwood Hospital

Youngstown
Member
St. Elizabeth Health Center

OKLAHOMA

Beaver
Member
Beaver County Memorial Hospital

Boise City
Member
Cimarron Memorial Hospital

Clinton
Member
Clinton Regional Hospital

Cordell
Member
  Cordell Memorial Hospital

El Reno
Member
  Park View Hospital

Frederick
Member
  Memorial Hospital

Hobart
Member
  Elkview General Hospital

Kingfisher
Member
  Kingfisher Regional Hospital

Lawton
Member
  Comanche County Memorial Hospital

Mangum
Member
  Mangum City Hospital

Marietta
Member
  Love County Health Center

Okeene
Member
  Okeene Municipal Hospital

Oklahoma City
Member
  Bone and Joint Hospital
  Hillcrest Health Center
  St. Anthony Hospital

Watonga
Member
  Watonga Municipal Hospital

OREGON

Bend
Member
  St. Charles Medical Center

Burns
Member
  Harney District Hospital

Cottage Grove
Member
  Cottage Grove Healthcare Community

Dallas
Member
  Valley Community Hospital

Eugene
Member
  Sacred Heart Medical Center

Florence
Member
  Peace Harbor Hospital

Gold Beach
Member
  Curry General Hospital

Gresham
Member
  Legacy Mount Hood Medical Center

Heppner
Member
  Pioneer Memorial Hospital

Hood River
Member
  Hood River Memorial Hospital

John Day
Member
  Blue Mountain Hospital

Lakeview
Member
  Lake District Hospital

Lebanon
Member
  Lebanon Community Hospital

Lincoln City
Member
  North Lincoln Hospital

Newport
Member
  Pacific Communities Hospital

Ontario
Member
  Holy Rosary Medical Center

Portland
Member
  Adventist Medical Center
  Legacy Good Samaritan Hospital and Medical Center
  Legacy Health System

Prineville
Member
  Pioneer Memorial Hospital

Redmond
Member
  Central Oregon District Hospital

Roseburg
Member
  Mercy Medical Center

Salem
Member
  Salem Hospital

Springfield
Member
  McKenzie–Willamette Hospital

Stayton
Member
  Santiam Memorial Hospital

Tillamook
Member
  Tillamook County General Hospital

Tualatin
Member
  Legacy Meridian Park Hospital

PENNSYLVANIA

Abington
Member
  Abington Memorial Hospital

Allentown
Member
  Allentown Osteopathic Medical Center

Bala Cynwyd
Member
  Mercy Health System of Southeastern Pennsylvania

Bethlehem
Member
  St. Luke's Hospital

Bryn Mawr
Member
  Bryn Mawr Hospital
  Bryn Mawr Hospital

Danville
Member
  Geisinger Medical Center

Doylestown
Member
  Doylestown Hospital

Easton
Member
  Easton Hospital

Erie
Member
  Millcreek Community Hospital
  Saint Vincent Health Center

Greenville
Member
  Horizon Hospital System

Harrisburg
Member
  PinnacleHealth System
  PinnacleHealth at Polyclinic Hospital

Havertown
Member
  Mercy Community Hospital

Hazleton
Member
  Hazleton–St. Joseph Medical Center

Jeannette
Member
  Jeannette District Memorial Hospital

Langhorne
Member
  Delaware Valley Medical Center

Meadville
Member
  Meadville Medical Center

Monroeville
Member
  Forbes Regional Hospital

Nanticoke
Member
  Mercy Special Care Hospital

Palmerton
Member
  Palmerton Hospital

Paoli
Member
  Paoli Memorial Hospital

Philadelphia
Member
  Albert Einstein Healthcare Network
  Albert Einstein Medical Center
  Belmont Center for Comprehensive Treatment
  Germantown Hospital and Medical Center
  Neumann Medical Center
  Northeastern Hospital of Philadelphia

Pittsburgh
Member
  Forbes Metropolitan Hospital
  Mercy Hospital of Pittsburgh
  Mercy Providence Hospital
  Suburban General Hospital
  Western Pennsylvania Hospital

Quakertown
Member
  St. Luke's Quakertown Hospital

Radnor
Member
  Jefferson Health System

Ridley Park
Member
  Taylor Hospital

Scranton
Member
  Mercy Hospital of Scranton

Titusville
Member
  Titusville Area Hospital

Union City
Member
  Union City Memorial Hospital

Warren
Member
  Warren General Hospital

Wilkes–Barre
Member
  Geisinger Wyoming Valley Medical Center
  Mercy Hospital of Wilkes–Barre

Wynnewood
Member
  Lankenau Hospital

PUERTO RICO

Mayaguez
Member
  Bella Vista Hospital

Ponce
Member
  Hospital De Damas

RHODE ISLAND

Providence
Member
  Roger Williams Medical Center

SOUTH CAROLINA

Anderson
Member
  Anderson Area Medical Center

Camden
Member
Kershaw County Medical Center

Charleston
Member
Bon Secours–St. Francis Xavier Hospital
Roper Hospital
Roper Hospital North

Columbia
Member
Richland Memorial Hospital

Conway
Member
Conway Hospital

Dillon
Member
Saint Eugene Community Hospital

Edgefield
Member
Edgefield County Hospital

Florence
Member
McLeod Regional Medical Center

Greenville
Member
Greenville Hospital System
Greenville Memorial Hospital
Shriners Hospitals for Children, Greenville

Greenwood
Member
Self Memorial Hospital

Greer
Member
Allen Bennett Hospital

Pickens
Member
Cannon Memorial Hospital

Simpsonville
Member
Hillcrest Hospital

Spartanburg
Member
Spartanburg Regional Medical Center

West Columbia
Member
Lexington Medical Center

Winnsboro
Member
Fairfield Memorial Hospital

Woodruff
Member
B.J. Workman Memorial Hospital

SOUTH DAKOTA
Aberdeen
Member
St. Luke's Midland Regional Medical Center

Armour
Member
Douglas County Memorial Hospital

Belle Fourche
Member
Belle Fourche Health Care Center

Clear Lake
Member
Deuel County Memorial Hospital

Custer
Member
Custer Community Hospital

Deadwood
Member
Northern Hills General Hospital

Dell Rapids
Member
Dell Rapids Community Hospital

Eureka
Member
Eureka Community Hospital

Faulkton
Member
Faulk County Memorial Hospital

Flandreau
Member
Flandreau Municipal Hospital

Gettysburg
Member
Gettysburg Medical Center

Gregory
Member
Gregory Community Hospital

Hot Springs
Member
Southern Hills General Hospital

Hoven
Member
Holy Infant Hospital

Lemmon
Member
Five Counties Hospital

Martin
Member
Bennett County Community Hospital

Milbank
Member
St. Bernard's Providence Hospital

Miller
Member
Hand County Memorial Hospital

Mitchell
Member
Queen of Peace Hospital

Pierre
Member
St. Mary's Hospital

Platte
Member
Platte Community Memorial Hospital

Rapid City
Member
Rapid City Regional Hospital

Redfield
Member
Community Memorial Hospital

Sioux Falls
Member
McKennan Hospital

Spearfish
Member
Lookout Memorial Hospital

Sturgis
Member
Sturgis Community Health Care Center

Wagner
Member
Wagner Community Memorial Hospital

Watertown
Member
Prairie Lakes Hospital and Care Center

Webster
Member
Lake Area Hospital

Yankton
Member
Presentation Health System
Sacred Heart Health Services

TENNESSEE
Chattanooga
Member
Memorial Hospital
North Park Hospital
Siskin Hospital for Physical Rehabilitation

Cleveland
Member
Bradley Memorial Hospital

Copperhill
Member
Copper Basin Medical Center

Crossville
Member
Cumberland Medical Center

Dyersburg
Member
Methodist Hospital of Dyersburg

Erwin
Member
Unicoi County Memorial Hospital

Etowah
Member
Woods Memorial Hospital District

Gallatin
Member
Sumner Regional Medical Center

Greeneville
Member
Takoma Adventist Hospital

Jefferson City
Member
Jefferson Memorial Hospital

Jellico
Member
Jellico Community Hospital

Johnson City
Member
Johnson City Medical Center Hospital

Knoxville
Member
Baptist Hospital of East Tennessee
St. Mary's Health System

La Follette
Member
La Follette Medical Center

Lexington
Member
Methodist Hospital of Lexington

Madison
Member
Tennessee Christian Medical Center

Maryville
Member
Blount Memorial Hospital

McKenzie
Member
Methodist Hospital of McKenzie

Memphis
Member
Methodist Health Systems, Inc.
Methodist Hospitals of Memphis

Morristown
Member
Morristown–Hamblen Hospital

Nashville
Member
Vanderbilt University Hospital

Rockwood
Member
Baptist Urgent Care

Rogersville
Member
Hawkins County Memorial Hospital

Somerville
Member
Methodist Hospital of Fayette

Tazewell
Member
Claiborne County Hospital

TEXAS
Abilene
Member
Hendrick Health System

Albany
Member
Shackelford County Hospital District

Alpine
Member
Big Bend Regional Medical Center

Arlington
Member
Huguley Willow Creek Hospital

Aspermont
Member
Stonewall Memorial Hospital

Austin
Member
Specialty Hospital of Austin

Azle
Member
Harris Methodist Northwest

Baytown
Member
San Jacinto Methodist Hospital

Bedford
Member
Harris Methodist–HEB

Beeville
Member
Spohn Bee County Hospital

Bellville
Member
Bellville General Hospital

Big Lake
Member
Reagan Memorial Hospital

Bowie
Member
Bowie Memorial Hospital

Brady
Member
Heart of Texas Memorial Hospital

Breckenridge
Member
Stephens Memorial Hospital

Brenham
Member
Trinity Community Medical Center of Brenham

Bryan
Member
St. Joseph Regional Health Center

Burleson
Member
Huguley Memorial Medical Center

Caldwell
Member
Burleson St. Joseph Health Center

Canadian
Member
Hemphill County Hospital

Canyon
Member
Palo Duro Hospital

Carrizo Springs
Member
Dimmit County Memorial Hospital

Childress
Member
Childress Regional Medical Center

Chillicothe
Member
Chillicothe Hospital District

Clarksville
Member
East Texas Medical Center–Clarksville

Cleburne
Member
Walls Regional Hospital

Clifton
Member
Goodall–Witcher Hospital

Coleman
Member
Coleman County Medical Center

Colorado City
Member
Mitchell County Hospital

Columbus
Member
Columbus Community Hospital

Comanche
Member
Comanche Community Hospital

Commerce
Member
Presbyterian Hospital of Commerce

Crane
Member
Crane Memorial Hospital

Crosbyton
Member
Crosbyton Clinic Hospital

Dalhart
Member
Coon Memorial Hospital and Home

Dallas
Member
Charlton Methodist Hospital
Methodist Hospitals of Dallas
Methodist Medical Center
Presbyterian Healthcare System
Presbyterian Hospital of Dallas
St. Paul Medical Center

De Leon
Member
De Leon Hospital

Decatur
Member
Decatur Community Hospital

Del Rio
Member
Val Verde Memorial Hospital

Denison
Member
Texoma Medical Center Restorative Care Hospital

Denver City
Member
Yoakum County Hospital

Dimmitt
Member
Plains Memorial Hospital

Eagle Lake
Member
Rice Medical Center

Eastland
Member
Eastland Memorial Hospital

Eden
Member
Concho County Hospital

Edna
Member
Jackson County Hospital

El Campo
Member
El Campo Memorial Hospital

El Paso
Member
R. E. Thomason General Hospital

Eldorado
Member
Schleicher County Medical Center

Electra
Member
Electra Memorial Hospital

Fairfield
Member
Fairfield Memorial Hospital

Fort Stockton
Member
Pecos County Memorial Hospital

Fort Worth
Member
Harris Methodist Fort Worth
Harris Methodist Health System
Harris Methodist Southwest
Osteopathic Medical Center of Texas

Fredericksburg
Member
Hill Country Memorial Hospital

Friona
Member
Parmer County Community Hospital

Galveston
Member
University of Texas Medical Branch Hospitals

Gatesville
Member
Coryell Memorial Hospital

Georgetown
Member
Georgetown Hospital

Gonzales
Member
Memorial Hospital

Graham
Member
Graham General Hospital

Greenville
Member
Hunt Memorial Hospital District

Hale Center
Member
Hi–Plains Hospital

Hallettsville
Member
Lavaca Medical Center

Hamilton
Member
Hamilton General Hospital

Hamlin
Member
Hamlin Memorial Hospital

Haskell
Member
Haskell Memorial Hospital

Hemphill
Member
Sabine County Hospital

Henrietta
Member
Clay County Memorial Hospital

Hondo
Member
Medina Community Hospital

Houston
Member
Diagnostic Center Hospital
Methodist Health Care System
St. Luke's Episcopal Hospital
The Institute for Rehabilitation and Research
The Methodist Hospital
University of Texas M. D. Anderson Cancer Center

Iraan
Member
Pecos County General Hospital

Jacksboro
Member
Faith Community Hospital

Junction
Member
Kimble Hospital

Kaufman
Member
Presbyterian Hospital of Kaufman

Kenedy
Member
Otto Kaiser Memorial Hospital

Kermit
Member
Memoria! Hospital

Killeen
Member
Metroplex Hospital

Knox City
Member
Knox County Hospital

La Grange
Member
  Fayette Memorial Hospital

Lamesa
Member
  Medical Arts Hospital

Livingston
Member
  Memorial Medical Center–Livingston

Llano
Member
  Llano Memorial Hospital

Lubbock
Member
  St. Mary of the Plains Hospital
  University Medical Center

Lufkin
Member
  Memorial Medical Center of East Texas

Luling
Member
  Edgar B. Davis Memorial Hospital

Madisonville
Member
  St. Francis Health Center

Marlin
Member
  Falls Community Hospital and Clinic

McCamey
Member
  McCamey Hospital

Memphis
Member
  Hall County Hospital

Mexia
Member
  Parkview Regional Hospital

Midland
Member
  Westwood Medical Center

Mineral Wells
Member
  Palo Pinto General Hospital

Monahans
Member
  Ward Memorial Hospital

Morton
Member
  Cochran Memorial Hospital

Muenster
Member
  Muenster Memorial Hospital

Muleshoe
Member
  Muleshoe Area Medical Center

Nacogdoches
Member
  Nacogdoches Memorial Hospital

Nocona
Member
  Nocona General Hospital

Odessa
Member
  Medical Center Hospital

Olney
Member
  Hamilton Hospital

Palestine
Member
  Memorial Mother Frances Hospital

Paris
Member
  McCuistion Regional Medical Center

Pearsall
Member
  Frio Hospital

Perryton
Member
  Ochiltree General Hospital

Plano
Member
  Presbyterian Hospital of Plano

Quanah
Member
  Hardeman County Memorial Hospital

Rankin
Member
  Rankin Hospital District

Refugio
Member
  Refugio County Memorial Hospital

Rio Grande City
Member
  Starr County Memorial Hospital

Rockdale
Member
  Richards Memorial Hospital

Rotan
Member
  Fisher County Hospital District

San Marcos
Member
  Central Texas Medical Center

Seminole
Member
  Memorial Hospital

Seymour
Member
  Seymour Hospital

Shamrock
Member
  Shamrock General Hospital

Snyder
Member
  D. M. Cogdell Memorial Hospital

Sonora
Member
  Lillian M. Hudspeth Memorial Hospital

Spearman
Member
  Hansford Hospital

Stamford
Member
  Stamford Memorial Hospital

Stanton
Member
  Martin County Hospital District

Stephenville
Member
  Harris Methodist–Erath County

Sulphur Springs
Member
  Hopkins County Memorial Hospital

Sweetwater
Member
  Rolling Plains Memorial Hospital

Tahoka
Member
  Lynn County Hospital District

Taylor
Member
  Johns Community Hospital

Temple
Member
  Olin E. Teague Veterans' Center
  Scott and White Memorial Hospital

Throckmorton
Member
  Throckmorton County Memorial Hospital

Trinity
Member
  Trinity Memorial Hospital

Tulia
Member
  Swisher Memorial Hospital District

Van Horn
Member
  Culberson Hospital District

Weimar
Member
  Colorado–Fayette Medical Center

Wellington
Member
  Collingsworth General Hospital

Weslaco
Member
  Knapp Medical Center

West
Member
  West Community Hospital

Wheeler
Member
  Parkview Hospital

Whitney
Member
  Lake Whitney Medical Center

Winnsboro
Member
  Presbyterian Hospital of Winnsboro

Winters
Member
  North Runnels Hospital

Woodville
Member
  Tyler County Hospital

UTAH

Monticello
Member
  San Juan Hospital

VERMONT

Burlington
Member
  Fletcher Allen Health Care

VIRGINIA

Abingdon
Member
  Johnston Memorial Hospital

Alexandria
Member
  Inova Mount Vernon Hospital

Bedford
Member
  Carilion Bedford Memorial Hospital

Big Stone Gap
Member
  Lonesome Pine Hospital

Chesapeake
Member
  Chesapeake General Hospital

Culpeper
Member
  Culpeper Memorial Hospital

Danville
Member
  Danville Regional Medical Center

Dunn Loring
Member
  Iliff Nursing Home

Fairfax
Member
  Inova Fair Oaks Hospital

Falls Church
Member
  Inova Fairfax Hospital

Farmville
Member
  Southside Community Hospital

Front Royal
Member
  Warren Memorial Hospital

Galax
Member
  Twin County Regional Hospital

Gloucester
Member
  Riverside Walter Reed Hospital

Leesburg
Member
 Loudoun Hospital Center

Lexington
Member
 Stonewall Jackson Hospital

Luray
Member
 Page Memorial Hospital

Manassas
Member
 Prince William Hospital

Marion
Member
 Smyth County Community Hospital

Nassawadox
Member
 Northampton–Accomack Memorial Hospital

Newport News
Member
 Riverside Health System
 Riverside Regional Medical Center
 Riverside Rehabilitation Institute

Norfolk
Member
 Bon Secours–DePaul Medical Center
 Lake Taylor Hospital

Norton
Member
 Norton Community Hospital

Pearisburg
Member
 Carilion Giles Memorial Hospital

Portsmouth
Member
 Bon Secours–Maryview Medical Center
 Portsmouth General Hospital

Radford
Member
 Carilion Radford Community Hospital

Richmond
Member
 Bon Secours–Richmond Community Hospital
 Bon Secours–Stuart Circle
 Richmond Memorial Hospital
 St. Mary's Hospital

Roanoke
Member
 Carilion Health System
 Carilion Roanoke Community Hospital
 Carilion Roanoke Memorial Hospital
 Gill Memorial Eye, Ear, Nose and Throat Hospital

Rocky Mount
Member
 Carilion Franklin Memorial Hospital

South Hill
Member
 Community Memorial Healthcenter

Springfield
Member
 Inova Health System

Stuart
Member
 R. J. Reynolds–Patrick County Memorial Hospital

Suffolk
Member
 Louise Obici Memorial Hospital

Virginia Beach
Member
 Tidewater Health Care, Inc.
 Virginia Beach General Hospital

Warrenton
Member
 Fauquier Hospital

Woodbridge
Member
 Potomac Hospital

Woodstock
Member
 Shenandoah Memorial Hospital

Wytheville
Member
 Wythe County Community Hospital

WASHINGTON
Aberdeen
Member
 Grays Harbor Community Hospital

Arlington
Member
 Cascade Valley Hospital, North Snohomish County Health System

Bellevue
Member
 Overlake Hospital Medical Center
 PeaceHealth

Bellingham
Member
 St. Joseph Hospital

Brewster
Member
 Okanogan–Douglas County Hospital

Burien
Member
 Highline Community Hospital

Chelan
Member
 Lake Chelan Community Hospital

Chewelah
Member
 St. Joseph's Hospital

Clarkston
Member
 Tri–State Memorial Hospital

Colfax
Member
 Whitman Hospital and Medical Center

Colville
Member
 Mount Carmel Hospital

Coupeville
Member
 Whidbey General Hospital

Davenport
Member
 Lincoln Hospital

Edmonds
Member
 Stevens Healthcare

Ephrata
Member
 Columbia Basin Hospital

Fort Steilacoom
Member
 Western State Hospital

Goldendale
Member
 Klickitat Valley Hospital

Grand Coulee
Member
 Coulee Community Hospital

Kirkland
Member
 Evergreen Hospital Medical Center

Longview
Member
 St. John Medical Center

Medical Lake
Member
 Eastern State Hospital

Moses Lake
Member
 Samaritan Healthcare

Newport
Member
 Newport Community Hospital

Odessa
Member
 Odessa Memorial Hospital

Omak
Member
 Mid–Valley Hospital

Othello
Member
 Othello Community Hospital

Prosser
Member
 Prosser Memorial Hospital

Pullman
Member
 Pullman Memorial Hospital

Puyallup
Member
 Good Samaritan Community Healthcare

Quincy
Member
 Quincy Valley Medical Center

Redmond
Member
 The Eastside Hospital

Renton
Member
 Valley Medical Center

Republic
Member
 Ferry County Memorial Hospital

Richland
Member
 Kadlec Medical Center

Ritzville
Member
 East Adams Rural Hospital

Seattle
Member
 Group Health Cooperative of Puget Sound
 Northwest Hospital
 Swedish Health Services

Shelton
Member
 Mason General Hospital

Snoqualmie
Member
 Snoqualmie Valley Hospital

Spokane
Member
 Deaconess Medical Center–Spokane
 Holy Family Hospital
 Providence Services
 Sacred Heart Medical Center
 Shriners Hospitals for Children–Spokane
 Valley Hospital and Medical Center

Sunnyside
Member
 Sunnyside Community Hospital

Tonasket
Member
 North Valley Hospital

Vancouver
Member
 Southwest Washington Medical Center

Walla Walla
Member
 St. Mary Medical Center
 Walla Walla General Hospital

Wenatchee
Member
 Central Washington Hospital

White Salmon
Member
 Skyline Hospital

WEST VIRGINIA
Berkeley Springs
Member
 Morgan County War Memorial Hospital

Bluefield
Member
 Bluefield Regional Medical Center

Alliances

Buckhannon
Member
St. Joseph's Hospital

Clarksburg
Member
United Hospital Center

Elkins
Member
Davis Memorial Hospital

Huntington
Member
St. Mary's Hospital

Keyser
Member
Potomac Valley Hospital

Kingwood
Member
Preston Memorial Hospital

Morgantown
Member
Monongalia General Hospital

Parkersburg
Member
Camden–Clark Memorial Hospital

Petersburg
Member
Grant Memorial Hospital

Point Pleasant
Member
Pleasant Valley Hospital

Ranson
Member
Jefferson Memorial Hospital

Romney
Member
Hampshire Memorial Hospital

Sistersville
Member
Sistersville General Hospital

South Charleston
Member
Thomas Memorial Hospital

Summersville
Member
Summersville Memorial Hospital

Weirton
Member
Weirton Medical Center

Weston
Member
Stonewall Jackson Memorial Hospital

WISCONSIN
Baldwin
Member
Baldwin Hospital

Baraboo
Member
St. Clare Hospital and Health Services

Barron
Member
Barron Memorial Medical Center and Skilled Nursing Facility

Berlin
Member
Community Health Network

Burlington
Member
Memorial Hospital Corporation of Burlington

Cumberland
Member
Cumberland Memorial Hospital

Elkhorn
Member
Lakeland Medical Center

Green Bay
Member
Bellin Hospital

Hartford
Member
Hartford Memorial Hospital

Madison
Member
St. Marys Hospital Medical Center

Marinette
Member
Bay Area Medical Center

Milwaukee
Member
Aurora Health Care
Sinai Samaritan Medical Center

Monroe
Member
The Monroe Clinic

Plymouth
Member
Valley View Medical Center

Sheboygan
Member
Sheboygan Memorial Medical Center

Two Rivers
Member
Two Rivers Community Hospital and Hamilton Memorial Home

Wauwatosa
Member
Milwaukee Psychiatric Hospital

West Allis
Member
West Allis Memorial Hospital

Woodruff
Member
Howard Young Medical Center

WYOMING
Buffalo
Member
Johnson County Memorial Hospital

Lusk
Member
Niobrara County Hospital District

Newcastle
Member
Weston County Memorial Hospital

Sundance
Member
Crook County Medical Services District

Wheatland
Member
Platte County Memorial Hospital Nursing Home

Worland
Member
Washakie Memorial Hospital

SYNERNET, INC.
222 St John Street, Portland, ME Zip 04102; tel. 207/775–6081; Mr Paul I Davis, III, President

MAINE
Bangor
Member
St. Joseph Hospital

Bar Harbor
Member
Mount Desert Island Hospital

Bath
Member
Mid Coast Hospital

Belfast
Member
Waldo County General Hospital

Biddeford
Member
Southern Maine Medical Center

Blue Hill
Member
Blue Hill Memorial Hospital

Bridgton
Member
Northern Cumberland Memorial Hospital

Damariscotta
Member
Miles Memorial Hospital

Farmington
Member
Franklin Memorial Hospital

Fort Kent
Member
Northern Maine Medical Center

Lewiston
Member
St. Mary's Regional Medical Center

Norway
Member
Stephens Memorial Hospital

Pittsfield
Member
Sebasticook Valley Hospital

Portland
Member
Brighton Campus of Maine Medical Center
Mercy Hospital Portland

Rockport
Member
Penobscot Bay Medical Center

Rumford
Member
Rumford Community Hospital

Sanford
Member
Henrietta D. Goodall Hospital

Skowhegan
Member
Redington–Fairview General Hospital

Waterville
Member
Inland Hospital

Westbrook
Member
Westbrook Community Hospital

York
Member
York Hospital

UNIVERSITY HEALTH SYSTEM OF NEW JERSEY
317 George Street, New Brunswick, NJ Zip 08901; tel. 908/235–7000; Dr Thomas E Terrill, Ph.D., President

NEW JERSEY
Atlantic City
Member
Atlantic City Medical Center

Camden
Member
Our Lady of Lourdes Medical Center
The Cooper Health System

Cherry Hill
Member
Kennedy Memorial Hospitals–University Medical Center

Florham Park
Member
Atlantic Health System

Hackensack
Member
Hackensack University Medical Center

Hamilton
Member
Robert Wood Johnson University Hospital at Hamilton

New Brunswick
Member
Robert Wood Johnson University Hospital

Newark
Member
Saint Michael's Medical Center
University of Medicine and Dentistry of New
Jersey–University Hospital

Paramus
Member
Bergen Pines County Hospital

Phillipsburg
Member
Warren Hospital

Somerville
Member
Somerset Medical Center

Trenton
Member
Helene Fuld Medical Center

West Orange
Member
Kessler Institute for Rehabilitation

UNIVERSITY HEALTHSYSTEM CONSORTIUM, INC.
2001 Spring Road, Suite 700, Oak Brook,
IL Zip 60521; tel. 708/954–1700; Mr
Robert J Baker, President and Chief
Executive Officer

ALABAMA
Birmingham
Member
University of Alabama Hospital

Mobile
Member
University of South Alabama Medical Center

ARIZONA
Tucson
Member
University Medical Center

ARKANSAS
Little Rock
Member
University Hospital of Arkansas

CALIFORNIA
Los Angeles
Member
University of California Los Angeles Medical Center

Orange
Member
University of California, Irvine Medical Center

Sacramento
Member
University of California, Davis Medical Center

San Diego
Member
University of California San Diego Medical Center

San Francisco
Member
San Francisco General Hospital Medical Center
University of California San Francisco Medical Center

Stanford
Member
Stanford University Hospital

COLORADO
Denver
Member
University of Colorado Hospital

CONNECTICUT
Farmington
Member
University of Connecticut Health Center, John
Dempsey Hospital

New Haven
Member
Yale–New Haven Hospital

DISTRICT OF COLUMBIA
Washington
Member
Georgetown University Hospital
Howard University Hospital

FLORIDA
Gainesville
Member
Shands at the University of Florida

GEORGIA
Atlanta
Member
Crawford Long Hospital of Emory University
Emory University Hospital

Augusta
Member
Medical College of Georgia Hospital and Clinics

ILLINOIS
Chicago
Member
University of Chicago Hospitals
University of Illinois at Chicago Medical Center

Maywood
Member
Loyola University Medical Center

INDIANA
Indianapolis
Member
Indiana University Medical Center

IOWA
Iowa City
Member
University of Iowa Hospitals and Clinics

KANSAS
Kansas City
Member
University of Kansas Hospital

KENTUCKY
Lexington
Member
University of Kentucky Hospital

LOUISIANA
Shreveport
Member
LSU Medical Center–University Hospital

MARYLAND
Baltimore
Member
University of Maryland Medical System

MASSACHUSETTS
Boston
Member
Brigham and Women's Hospital
Massachusetts General Hospital

Worcester
Member
University of Massachusetts Medical Center

MICHIGAN
Ann Arbor
Member
University of Michigan Hospitals

MISSOURI
Saint Louis
Member
Saint Louis University Hospital

NEBRASKA
Omaha
Member
University of Nebraska Medical Center

NEW JERSEY
New Brunswick
Member
Robert Wood Johnson University Hospital

Newark
Member
University of Medicine and Dentistry of New
Jersey–University Hospital

NEW YORK
Albany
Member
Albany Medical Center

Brooklyn
Member
University Hospital of Brooklyn–State University of
New York Health Science Center at Brooklyn

New York
Member
New York University Medical Center
Presbyterian Hospital in the City of New York

Stony Brook
Member
University Hospital

Syracuse
Member
University Hospital–SUNY Health Science Center at
Syracuse

NORTH CAROLINA
Chapel Hill
Member
University of North Carolina Hospitals

Greenville
Member
Pitt County Memorial Hospital–University Medical
Center of Eastern Carolina–Pitt County

Winston–Salem
Member
North Carolina Baptist Hospital

OHIO
Cincinnati
Member
Univerisity Hospital

Cleveland
Member
University Hospitals of Cleveland

Columbus
Member
Ohio State University Medical Center

Toledo
Member
Medical College Hospitals

OKLAHOMA
Oklahoma City
Member
The University Hospitals

OREGON
Portland
Member
University Hospital

PENNSYLVANIA
Hershey
Member
Penn State University Hospital–Milton S. Hershey
Medical Center

Philadelphia
Thomas Jefferson University Hospital
Member
Allegheny University Hospitals, Hahnemann
Hospital of the University of Pennsylvania

Pittsburgh
Member
University of Pittsburgh Medical Center
University of Pittsburgh Medical Center, St. Margaret

SOUTH CAROLINA
Charleston
Member
MUSC Medical Center of Medical University of South
Carolina

TENNESSEE
Knoxville
Member
University of Tennessee Memorial Hospital

Memphis
Member
University of Tennessee Bowld Hospital

Nashville
Member
Vanderbilt University Hospital

TEXAS
Dallas
Member
Zale Lipshy University Hospital

Section B

Galveston
Member
   University of Texas Medical Branch Hospitals

Houston
Member
   Hermann Hospital

UTAH

Salt Lake City
Member
   University of Utah Hospitals and Clinics

VIRGINIA

Charlottesville
Member
   University of Virginia Medical Center

Richmond
Member
   Medical College of Virginia Hospitals, Virginia
      Commonwealth University

WASHINGTON

Seattle
Member
   Harborview Medical Center
   University of Washington Medical Center

WEST VIRGINIA

Morgantown
Member
   West Virginia University Hospitals

WISCONSIN

Madison
Member
   University of Wisconsin Hospital and Clinics

Milwaukee
Member
   Froedtert Memorial Lutheran Hospital

VHA, INC.

   220 East Las Colinas Boulevard, Irving,
   TX Zip 75039–5500; tel. 214/830–0000;
   Mr C Thomas Smith, President and Chief
   Executive Officer

ALABAMA

Anniston
Partner
   Northeast Alabama Regional Medical Center

Athens
Partner
   Athens–Limestone Hospital

Birmingham
Shareholder
   Baptist Health System

Cullman
Partner
   Cullman Regional Medical Center

Decatur
Partner
   Decatur General Hospital

Florence
Partner
   Eliza Coffee Memorial Hospital

Guntersville
Partner
   Marshall County Health Care Authority

Jackson
Partner
   Vaughn Jackson Medical Center

Mobile
Shareholder
   Infirmary Health System, Inc.

Montgomery
Shareholder
   Baptist Medical Center

Scottsboro
Partner
   Jackson County Hospital

Tuscaloosa
Partner
   DCH Healthcare Authority

ARIZONA

Phoenix
Shareholder
   Samaritan Health System

Tucson
Shareholder
   Health Partners of Southern Arizona

ARKANSAS

Fayetteville
Partner
   Washington Regional Medical Center

Fort Smith
Shareholder
   Sparks Regional Medical Center

Jonesboro
Partner
   St. Bernards Regional Medical Center

Little Rock
Shareholder
   Baptist Health

CALIFORNIA

Anaheim
Partner
   Anaheim Memorial Hospital

Bakersfield
Partner
   Bakersfield Memorial Hospital

Covina
Partner
   Citrus Valley Health Partners

Fresno
Shareholder
   Community Hospitals of Central California

La Jolla
Shareholder
   Scripps Memorial Hospital–La Jolla

Lancaster
Partner
   Antelope Valley Hospital

Long Beach
Shareholder
   Memorial Health Services

Los Angeles
Shareholder
   Cedars–Sinai Medical Center

Modesto
Partner
   Memorial Hospitals Association

Newport Beach
Shareholder
   Hoag Memorial Hospital Presbyterian

Pasadena
Partner
   Southern California Healthcare Systems

Pomona
Partner
   Pomona Valley Hospital Medical Center

Riverside
Partner
   Riverside Community Hospital

Sacramento
Shareholder
   Sutter Health

San Francisco
Shareholder
   California Pacific Medical Center

Santa Barbara
Partner
   Santa Barbara Cottage Hospital

Stockton
Partner
   St. Joseph's Regional Health System

Torrance
Partner
   Torrance Memorial Medical Center

Turlock
Partner
   Emanuel Medical Center

Valencia
Partner
   Santa Clarita Health Care Association

Van Nuys
Partner
   Valley Presbyterian Hospital

Walnut Creek
Partner
   John Muir Medical Center

Whittier
Partner
   Presbyterian Intercommunity Hospital

COLORADO

Alamosa
Partner
   San Luis Valley Regional Medical Center

Aspen
Partner
   Aspen Valley Hospital District

Boulder
Partner
   Boulder Community Hospital

Colorado Springs
Partner
   Memorial Hospital

Englewood
Shareholder
   HealthONE Healthcare System

Fort Collins
Partner
   Poudre Valley Hospital

Grand Junction
Partner
   Community Hospital

La Junta
Partner
   Arkansas Valley Regional Medical Center

Longmont
Partner
   Longmont United Hospital

Steamboat Springs
Partner
   Routt Memorial Hospital

Vail
Shareholder
   Vail Valley Medical Center

Wheat Ridge
Shareholder
   Lutheran Medical Center

CONNECTICUT

Danbury
Partner
   Danbury Hospital

Greenwich
Partner
   Greenwich Hospital

Hartford
Shareholder
   Hartford Hospital

Meriden
Partner
   Veterans Memorial Medical Center

Middletown
Partner
   Middlesex Hospital

Stamford
Partner
   Stamford Hospital

Torrington
Partner
   Charlotte Hungerford Hospital

DELAWARE

Milford
Partner
   Bayhealth Medical Center, Milford Memorial Campus

DISTRICT OF COLUMBIA

Washington
Shareholder
   Medlantic Healthcare Group

FLORIDA

Boca Raton
Partner
Boca Raton Community Hospital

Boynton Beach
Partner
Bethesda Memorial Hospital

Fort Myers
Partner
Lee Memorial Health System

Inverness
Partner
Citrus Memorial Hospital

Jacksonville
Partner
Methodist Medical Center
St. Luke's Hospital

Lakeland
Shareholder
Lakeland Regional Medical Center

Melbourne
Shareholder
Holmes Regional Medical Center

Miami
Partner
South Miami Hospital

Ocala
Partner
Munroe Regional Medical Center

Orlando
Shareholder
Orlando Regional Healthcare System

Panama City
Partner
Bay Medical Center

Pensacola
Shareholder
Baptist Health Care Corporation

Saint Petersburg
Partner
Bayfront Medical Center

Stuart
Partner
Martin Memorial Health System

Tallahassee
Shareholder
Tallahassee Memorial Regional Medical Center

Tampa
Partner
University Community Hospital

West Palm Beach
Partner
Good Samaritan Medical Center

GEORGIA

Albany
Partner
Phoebe Putney Memorial Hospital

Athens
Partner
Athens Regional Medical Center

Atlanta
Partner
Northside Hospital
Shareholder
Piedmont Hospital

Columbus
Partner
Columbus Regional Health Care System, Inc

Dalton
Partner
Hamilton Medical Center

Decatur
Partner
DeKalb Medical Center

East Point
Partner
South Fulton Medical Center

Gainesville
Partner
Northeast Georgia Health Services

Lawrenceville
Partner
Promina Gwinnett Hospital System

Macon
Partner
Medical Center of Central Georgia

Marietta
Partner
Kennestone Hospital

Riverdale
Partner
Southern Regional Medical Center

Rome
Partner
Floyd Medical Center

Royston
Partner
Cobb Memorial Hospital

Savannah
Partner
Candler Hospital

Thomasville
Partner
John D. Archbold Memorial Hospital

Valdosta
Partner
South Georgia Medical Center

HAWAII

Honolulu
Shareholder
Queen's Medical Center

IDAHO

Boise
Shareholder
St. Luke's Regional Medical Center

Coeur D'Alene
Partner
Kootenai Medical Center

Pocatello
Partner
Bannock Regional Medical Center

Twin Falls
Partner
Magic Valley Regional Medical Center

ILLINOIS

Berwyn
Partner
MacNeal Hospital

Carbondale
Partner
Southern Illinois Hospital Services

Chicago
Shareholder
Northwestern Memorial Hospital
Rush–Presbyterian–St. Luke's Medical Center

De Kalb
Partner
Kishwaukee Community Hospital

Decatur
Shareholder
Decatur Memorial Hospital

Dixon
Partner
Katherine Shaw Bethea Hospital

Elgin
Partner
Sherman Hospital

Elmhurst
Partner
Elmhurst Memorial Hospital

Evanston
Shareholder
Evanston Hospital

Evergreen Park
Partner
Little Company of Mary Hospital and Health Care Centers

Freeport
Partner
Freeport Memorial Hospital

Harvey
Shareholder
Ingalls Health System
Ingalls Memorial Hospital

Highland Park
Partner
Highland Park Hospital

Jacksonville
Partner
Passavant Area Hospital

Joliet
Partner
Silver Cross Hospital

Kankakee
Partner
Riverside Healthcare

Macomb
Partner
McDonough District Hospital

Maryville
Partner
Anderson Hospital

Mattoon
Partner
Sarah Bush Lincoln Health System

Normal
Partner
BroMenn Healthcare

Oakbrook
Shareholder
Advocate Health Care

Quincy
Partner
Blessing Hospital

Rock Island
Partner
Trinity Medical Center–West Campus

Rockford
Partner
Rockford Memorial Hospital

Springfield
Shareholder
Memorial Medical Center
Memorial Medical Center System

INDIANA

Anderson
Partner
Community Hospital of Anderson and Madison County

Bloomington
Partner
Bloomington Hospital

Columbus
Partner
Columbus Regional Hospital

Danville
Partner
Hendricks Community Hospital

Elkhart
Partner
Elkhart General Hospital

Evansville
Shareholder
Deaconess Hospital

Fort Wayne
Partner
Parkview Memorial Hospital

Indianapolis
Partner
Indiana University Medical Center
Shareholder
Community Hospitals Indianapolis
Methodist Hospital of Indiana

Alliances

La Porte
Partner
La Porte Hospital

Madison
Partner
King's Daughters' Hospital

Marion
Partner
Marion General Hospital

Muncie
Shareholder
Ball Memorial Hospital

New Albany
Partner
Floyd Memorial Hospital and Health Services

Noblesville
Partner
Riverview Hospital

Richmond
Partner
Reid Hospital and Health Care Services

South Bend
Shareholder
Memorial Health System, Inc.

Terre Haute
Partner
Union Hospital

Valparaiso
Partner
Porter Memorial Hospital

Vincennes
Partner
Good Samaritan Hospital

IOWA
Atlantic
Shareholder
Cass County Memorial Hospital

Council Bluffs
Shareholder
Jennie Edmundson Memorial Hospital

Keokuk
Shareholder
Keokuk Area Hospital

Red Oak
Shareholder
Montgomery County Memorial Hospital

Sioux City
Shareholder
St. Luke's Regional Medical Center

KANSAS
Atchison
Shareholder
Atchison Hospital

Colby
Shareholder
Citizens Medical Center

Hays
Shareholder
Hays Medical Center

Hutchinson
Shareholder
Hutchinson Hospital Corporation

Kansas City
Shareholder
Bethany Medical Center

Liberal
Shareholder
Southwest Medical Center

Phillipsburg
Shareholder
Great Plains Health Alliance, Inc.

Pratt
Shareholder
Pratt Regional Medical Center

Shawnee Mission
Shareholder
Shawnee Mission Medical Center

Topeka
Partner
St. Francis Hospital and Medical Center
Shareholder
Stormont–Vail HealthCare

KENTUCKY
Fort Thomas
Partner
St. Luke Hospital East

Madisonville
Partner
Regional Medical Center of Hopkins County

Owensboro
Partner
Owensboro–Daviess County Hospital

LOUISIANA
Baton Rouge
Member
Our Lady of the Lake Regional Medical Center
Partner
Woman's Hospital

Crowley
Partner
American Legion Hospital

De Ridder
Partner
Beauregard Memorial Hospital

Lafayette
Partner
Our Lady of Lourdes Regional Medical Center

Lake Charles
Partner
Lake Charles Memorial Hospital

Monroe
Partner
St. Francis Medical Center

New Orleans
Partner
Pendleton Memorial Methodist Hospital
Shareholder
Ochsner Foundation Hospital

Ruston
Partner
Lincoln General Hospital

Shreveport
Shareholder
Willis–Knighton Medical Center

MAINE
Augusta
Shareholder
Kennebec Valley Medical Center

Biddeford
Shareholder
Southern Maine Medical Center

Lewiston
Shareholder
Central Maine Medical Center

Portland
Shareholder
Maine Medical Center

Waterville
Shareholder
Mid–Maine Medical Center

MARYLAND
Easton
Partner
Memorial Hospital at Easton Maryland

Fallston
Partner
Upper Chesapeake Health System

MASSACHUSETTS
Beverly
Partner
Beverly Hospital

Boston
Partner
Massachusetts Eye and Ear Infirmary
Shareholder
New England Medical Center
Partners HealthCare System

Cambridge
Partner
Mount Auburn Hospital

Concord
Partner
Emerson Hospital

Fall River
Member
Southcoast Hospitals Group

Hyannis
Partner
Cape Cod Hospital

Lawrence
Owner
Lawrence General Hospital

Leominster
Partner
Health Alliance Hospitals

Lowell
Partner
Lowell General Hospital

Medford
Partner
Lawrence Memorial Hospital of Medford

Melrose
Partner
Melrose–Wakefield Hospital

Newton
Partner
Newell Home Health Service

South Weymouth
Partner
South Shore Health & Education Corporation

Southbridge
Partner
Harrington Memorial Hospital

Worcester
Partner
Saint Vincent Hospital

MICHIGAN
Bay City
Partner
Bay Medical Center

Dearborn
Member
Oakwood Healthcare System

Detroit
Partner
St. John Hospital and Medical Center

Flint
Partner
Genesys Health System

Grand Rapids
Shareholder
Butterworth Hospital

Holland
Partner
Holland Community Hospital

Kalamazoo
Partner
Bronson Healthcare Group, Inc.

Lansing
Partner
Michigan Capital Healthcare

Monroe
Partner
Mercy Memorial Hospital

Petoskey
Partner
Healthshare Group

Port Huron
Partner
Blue Water Health Services Corporation

Royal Oak
Shareholder
William Beaumont Hospital–Royal Oak

Saginaw
Partner
Saginaw General Hospital

Saint Joseph
Partner
  Lakeland Regional Health System, Inc.

MINNESOTA
Bemidji
Partner
  North Country Regional Hospital

Duluth
Partner
  St. Luke's Hospital

Fergus Falls
Partner
  Lake Region Hospital Corporation

Mankato
Partner
  Immanuel St. Joseph's–Mayo Health System

Minneapolis
Shareholder
  Allina Health System

Saint Cloud
Partner
  St. Cloud Hospital

Saint Paul
Shareholder
  HealthEast

Waconia
Partner
  Ridgeview Medical Center

Willmar
Partner
  Rice Memorial Hospital

MISSISSIPPI
Greenwood
Partner
  Greenwood Leflore Hospital

Gulfport
Partner
  Memorial Hospital at Gulfport

Hattiesburg
Partner
  Forrest General Hospital

Jackson
Partner
  St. Dominic–Jackson Memorial Hospital

McComb
Partner
  Southwest Mississippi Regional Medical Center

Meridian
Partner
  Jeff Anderson Regional Medical Center

Pascagoula
Partner
  Singing River Hospital System

Tupelo
Shareholder
  North Mississippi Health Services, Inc.

MISSOURI
Bolivar
Partner
  Citizens Memorial Hospital

Branson
Partner
  Skaggs Community Health Center

Cameron
Partner
  Cameron Community Hospital

Cape Girardeau
Partner
  Saint Francis Medical Center
  Southeast Missouri Hospital

Carthage
Partner
  McCune–Brooks Hospital

Joplin
Partner
  Freeman Hospital West

Kansas City
Shareholder
  Saint Luke's Hospital

Liberty
Partner
  Liberty Hospital

Saint Louis
Shareholder
  BJC Health System

Springfield
Shareholder
  Cox Health Systems

West Plains
Partner
  Ozarks Medical Center

MONTANA
Billings
Partner
  Deaconess Medical Center

Great Falls
Partner
  Benefis Health Care–East Campus

Helena
Partner
  St. Peter's Community Hospital

NEBRASKA
Aurora
Partner
  Memorial Hospital

Beatrice
Partner
  Beatrice Community Hospital and Health Center

Columbus
Partner
  Columbus Community Hospital

Hastings
Partner
  Mary Lanning Memorial Hospital

Lincoln
Partner
  Bryan Memorial Hospital

Omaha
Partner
  Children's Hospital
Shareholder
  Nebraska Methodist Hospital

Scottsbluff
Partner
  Regional West Medical Center

NEW HAMPSHIRE
Concord
Partner
  Capital Region Family Health Center

Dover
Partner
  Wentworth–Douglass Hospital

Keene
Partner
  Cheshire Medical Center

Nashua
Partner
  Southern New Hampshire Regional Medical Center

Rochester
Partner
  Frisbie Memorial Hospital

NEW JERSEY
Belleville
Shareholder
  Clara Maass Health System

Camden
Partner
  Our Lady of Lourdes Medical Center

Elizabeth
Partner
  Elizabeth General Medical Center

Flemington
Partner
  Hunterdon Medical Center

Hackettstown
Partner
  Hackettstown Community Hospital

Hammonton
Partner
  William B. Kessler Memorial Hospital

Jersey City
Partner
  Christ Hospital

Mount Holly
Shareholder
  Memorial Hospital of Burlington County

Newton
Partner
  Newton Memorial Hospital

Phillipsburg
Partner
  Warren Hospital

Plainfield
Partner
  Muhlenberg Regional Medical Center

Pompton Plains
Partner
  Chilton Memorial Hospital

Rahway
Partner
  Rahway Hospital

Somers Point
Partner
  Shore Memorial Hospital

Toms River
Shareholder
  Community Kimball Health Care System

Trenton
Partner
  Mercer Medical Center

Woodbury
Partner
  Underwood–Memorial Hospital

NEW MEXICO
Albuquerque
Partner
  University Hospital

Farmington
Partner
  San Juan Regional Medical Center

Gallup
Partner
  Rehoboth McKinley Christian Hospital

Las Cruces
Partner
  Memorial Medical Center

Roswell
Partner
  Eastern New Mexico Medical Center

NEW YORK
Binghamton
Shareholder
  United Health Services Hospitals–Binghamton

Brooklyn
Partner
  Brooklyn Hospital Center

Cobleskill
Partner
  Bassett Hospital of Schoharie County

Geneva
Partner
  Geneva General Hospital

Ithaca
Partner
  Cayuga Medical Center at Ithaca

Jamestown
Partner
  Woman's Christian Association Hospital

Manhasset
Partner
  North Shore Health System

Mount Kisco
Partner
  Northern Westchester Hospital Center

New Rochelle
Partner
  Sound Shore Medical Center of Westchester

New York
Partner
  Lenox Hill Hospital
  New York University Medical Center
  St. Luke's–Roosevelt Hospital Center
Shareholder
  Presbyterian Hospital in the City of New York
  Society of the New York Hospital

North Tonawanda
Partner
  De Graff Memorial Hospital

Plattsburgh
Partner
  Champlain Valley Physicians Hospital Medical Center

Rochester
Partner
  Highland Hospital of Rochester
  Park Ridge Health System

Rockville Centre
Partner
  Mercy Medical Center

Southampton
Partner
  Southampton Hospital

Suffern
Partner
  Good Samaritan Hospital

Syracuse
Partner
  Crouse Hospital

Troy
Partner
  Samaritan Hospital

Utica
Partner
  Mohawk Valley Psychiatric Center

White Plains
Partner
  White Plains Hospital Center

Yonkers
Partner
  St. John's Riverside Hospital

NORTH CAROLINA
Charlotte
Shareholder
  Carolinas HealthCare System

Greensboro
Partner
  Wesley Long Community Hospital

Raleigh
Partner
  Wake Medical Center

Rocky Mount
Partner
  Nash Health Care Systems

Thomasville
Partner
  Community General Hospital of Thomasville

Winston–Salem
Shareholder
  Carolina Medicorp, Inc.

NORTH DAKOTA
Bismarck
Partner
  MedCenter One

Fargo
Shareholder
  MeritCare Health System

Grand Forks
Partner
  United Health Services

Jamestown
Partner
  Jamestown Hospital

Minot
Partner
  Trinity Medical Center

OHIO
Akron
Shareholder
  Akron General Medical Center

Ashtabula
Partner
  Ashtabula County Medical Center

Cincinnati
Partner
  Bethesda Corporate Health Services
Shareholder
  Christ Hospital

Columbus
Shareholder
  OhioHealth

Dover
Partner
  Union Hospital

Elyria
Partner
  EMH Regional Medical Center

Fremont
Partner
  Memorial Hospital

Garfield Heights
Partner
  Marymount Hospital

Hamilton
Partner
  Fort Hamilton–Hughes Memorial Hospital

Lima
Partner
  Lima Memorial Hospital

Mansfield
Partner
  Mansfield Hospital

Maumee
Partner
  St. Luke's Hospital

Middletown
Partner
  Middletown Regional Hospital

Painesville
Partner
  Lake Hospital System

Springfield
Partner
  Community Hospital

Toledo
Shareholder
  The Toledo Hospital

Troy
Partner
  Upper Valley Medical Centers

Warren
Partner
  Trumbull Memorial Hospital

Xenia
Partner
  Greene Memorial Hospital

OKLAHOMA
Ada
Partner
  Valley View Regional Hospital

Altus
Partner
  Jackson County Memorial Hospital

Ardmore
Partner
  Mercy Memorial Health Center

Chickasha
Partner
  Grady Memorial Hospital

Duncan
Partner
  Duncan Regional Hospital

McAlester
Partner
  McAlester Regional Health Center

Midwest City
Partner
  Midwest City Regional Medical Center

Muskogee
Partner
  Muskogee Regional Medical Center

Norman
Partner
  Norman Regional Hospital

Oklahoma City
Partner
  Deaconess Hospital
Shareholder
  Oklahoma Health System

Poteau
Partner
  Eastern Oklahoma Medical Center

Stillwater
Partner
  Stillwater Medical Center

Tulsa
Shareholder
  Hillcrest Healthcare System

PENNSYLVANIA
Allentown
Shareholder
  Lehigh Valley Hospital

Altoona
Partner
  Altoona Hospital

Beaver
Partner
  The Medical Center

Bristol
Partner
  Lower Bucks Hospital

Butler
Partner
  Butler Health System

Erie
Shareholder
  Hamot Health Systems

Johnstown
Partner
  Conemaugh Valley Memorial Hospital

Kingston
Partner
  Wyoming Valley Health Care System

Lancaster
Partner
  Lancaster General Hospital

Latrobe
Partner
  Latrobe Area Hospital

Media
Shareholder
  Crozer–Keystone Health System

Natrona Heights
Partner
  Allegheny Valley Hospital

Norristown
Partner
  Montgomery Hospital

Philadelphia
Partner
  Chestnut Hill Hospital
  Episcopal Hospital
  Frankford Hospital of the City of Philadelphia
  Jeanes Health System
Shareholder
  Pennsylvania Hospital

Pittsburgh
Partner
  Shadyside Hospital
  St. Clair Memorial Hospital
  University of Pittsburgh Medical Center, St. Margaret
Shareholder
  Allegheny Health, Education and Research Foundation

Pottstown
Partner
  Pottstown Memorial Medical Center

Reading
Partner
  Reading Hospital and Medical Center

Sayre
Shareholder
  Guthrie Healthcare System

Scranton
Partner
  Community Medical Center

Sellersville
Partner
  Grand View Hospital

Sewickley
Partner
  Sewickley Valley Hospital, (A Division of Valley Medical
    Facilities)

Uniontown
Partner
  Uniontown Hospital

Washington
Partner
  Washington Hospital

West Chester
Partner
  Chester County Hospital

Williamsport
Partner
  Susquehanna Health System

York
Partner
  York Health System

RHODE ISLAND
Providence
Shareholder
  Rhode Island Hospital

SOUTH CAROLINA
Columbia
Shareholder
  Baptist Healthcare System of South Carolina

SOUTH DAKOTA
Sioux Falls
Shareholder
  Sioux Valley Hospital

TENNESSEE
Jackson
Shareholder
  West Tennessee Healthcare, Inc.

Knoxville
Shareholder
  Fort Sanders Alliance

Memphis
Shareholder
  Baptist Memorial Hospital

Nashville
Shareholder
  Baptist Hospital

Oak Ridge
Partner
  Methodist Medical Center of Oak Ridge

TEXAS
Amarillo
Partner
  Baptist–St. Anthony Health System

Arlington
Partner
  Arlington Memorial Hospital

Austin
Partner
  Columbia St. David's Hospital

Beaumont
Partner
  Baptist Hospital of Southeast Texas

Dallas
Shareholder
  Baylor Health Care System

El Paso
Partner
  Providence Memorial Hospital

Fort Worth
Shareholder
  All Saints Episcopal Hospital of Fort Worth

Grapevine
Partner
  Baylor Medical Center at Grapevine

Harlingen
Partner
  Valley Baptist Medical Center

Houston
Shareholder
  Memorial Hospital Southwest

Irving
Partner
  Irving Healthcare System

Lubbock
Shareholder
  Lubbock Methodist Hospital System

Marshall
Partner
  Marshall Regional Medical Center

Midland
Partner
  Memorial Hospital and Medical Center

San Antonio
Partner
  Baptist Health System

Sherman
Partner
  Wilson N. Jones Regional Health System

Temple
Partner
  King's Daughters Hospital

Texarkana
Partner
  Wadley Regional Medical Center

Waco
Partner
  Hillcrest Baptist Medical Center

Wichita Falls
Partner
  Wichita General Hospital

VERMONT
Barre
Partner
  Central Vermont Medical Center

Burlington
Shareholder
  Fletcher Allen Health Care

Rutland
Partner
  Rutland Regional Medical Center

VIRGINIA
Alexandria
Partner
  Alexandria Hospital

Arlington
Partner
  Arlington Hospital

Charlottesville
Partner
  Martha Jefferson Hospital

Franklin
Partner
  Southampton Memorial Hospital

Fredericksburg
Partner
  MWH Medicorp

Harrisonburg
Partner
  Rockingham Memorial Hospital

Lynchburg
Partner
  Centra Health, Inc.

Norfolk
Shareholder
  Sentara Health System

Richmond
Partner
  Children's Hospital

Warrenton
Partner
  Fauquier Hospital

WEST VIRGINIA
Charleston
Shareholder
  Camcare, Inc.

Glen Dale
Partner
  Reynolds Memorial Hospital

Huntington
Partner
  Cabell Huntington Hospital

Morgantown
Partner
  West Virginia University Hospitals

Parkersburg
Owner
  St. Joseph's Hospital

Princeton
Partner
  Princeton Community Hospital

Wheeling
Partner
  Wheeling Hospital

WISCONSIN
Beaver Dam
Partner
  Beaver Dam Community Hospitals

Eau Claire
Partner
  Luther Hospital

Green Bay
Partner
  Bellin Hospital

Kenosha
Partner
  Kenosha Hospital and Medical Center

La Crosse
Shareholder
  Lutheran Hospital–La Crosse

Madison
Shareholder
  Meriter Hospital

Menomonee Falls
Partner
  Community Memorial Hospital

Milwaukee
Partner
  Columbia Hospital
  Froedtert Memorial Lutheran Hospital
  Horizon Healthcare, Inc.

Rice Lake
Partner
  Lakeview Medical Center

Watertown
Partner
  Watertown Memorial Hospital

Waukesha
Partner
  Waukesha Health System, Inc.

West Bend
Owner
  St. Joseph's Community Hospital of West Bend

WYOMING
Casper
Partner
  Wyoming Medical Center

Cheyenne
Partner
  United Medical Center

Laramie
Partner
  Ivinson Memorial Hospital

Sheridan
Partner
  Memorial Hospital of Sheridan County

VANTAGE HEALTH GROUP
  265 Conneaut Lake Road, Meadville, PA
  Zip 16335; tel. 814/337–0000; Mr David
  C Petno, Vice President Business
  Development

COLORADO
Denver
Member
  Catholic Health Initiatives

ILLINOIS
Kankakee
Member
  ServantCor

OHIO
Cincinnati
Member
  Mercy Health System

PENNSYLVANIA
Erie
Member
  Millcreek Community Hospital
  Saint Vincent Health Center

Franklin
Member
  Northwest Medical Center

Greenville
Member
  Horizon Hospital System

Meadville
Member
  Meadville Medical Center

Titusville
Member
  Titusville Area Hospital

Warren
Member
  Warren General Hospital

YANKEE ALLIANCE
  300 Brickstone Square, 5th Floor,
  Andover, MA Zip 01810–1429;
  tel. 508/475–2000; Mr R Paul O'Neill,
  President

CONNECTICUT
New Haven
Member
  Hospital of Saint Raphael

MAINE
Blue Hill
Affiliate
  Blue Hill Memorial Hospital

Lewiston
Member
  St. Mary's Regional Medical Center

MASSACHUSETTS
Attleboro
Affiliate
  Sturdy Memorial Hospital

Boston
Member
  Boston Medical Center

Fall River
Member
  Southcoast Hospitals Group

Great Barrington
Member
  Fairview Hospital

Lexington
Member
  Covenant Health Systems, Inc.

Lowell
Member
  Saints Memorial Medical Center

Needham
Affiliate
  Deaconess–Glover Hospital Corporation

Pittsfield
Member
  Berkshire Health Systems, Inc.
  Berkshire Medical Center

Waltham
Member
  Maristhill Nursing Home

Winchester
Member
  Winchester Hospital

NEW HAMPSHIRE
Manchester
Affiliate
  Catholic Medical Center
  Elliot Hospital

Nashua
Member
  St. Joseph Healthcare

NEW YORK
Albany
Member
  Albany Medical Center

Glens Falls
Member
  Glens Falls Hospital

Plattsburgh
Affiliate
  Champlain Valley Physicians Hospital Medical Center

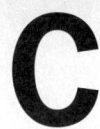

C

**Health Organizations,
Agencies, and Providers**

†List supplied by the Joint Commission on
Accreditation of Healthcare Organizations

For more information on membership contact:
Manager, Department of Membership
American Hospital Association
One North Franklin
Chicago, Illinois 60606-3401

Section C

Description of Lists

This section was compiled to provide a directory of information useful to the health care field.

National and International Organizations

The national and international lists include many types of voluntary organizations concerned with matters of interest to the health care field. The organizational information includes address, telephone number, FAX number, and the contact person. For organizations that maintain permanent offices, office addresses and telephone numbers are given. For organizations not maintaining offices, the addresses and telephone numbers given are those of their corresponding secretaries. The information was obtained directly from the organizations.

National Organizations are listed alphabetically by their full names. International Organizations are grouped alphabetically by country.

Also included is the Healthfinder listings. The Healthfinder is composed of two listing types: toll–free numbers for health information and federal health information centers and clearinghouses. Organizations are listed alphabetically by topic area.

We present this list simply as a convenient directory. Inclusion or omission of any organization's name indicates neither approval nor disapproval by Healthcare InfoSource, Inc., a subsidiary of the American Hospital Association.

United States Government Agencies

National agencies concerned with health–related matters are listed by the major department of government under which the different functions fall.

State and Local Organizations and Agencies

The lists of organizations in states, associated areas, and provinces include Blue Cross–Blue Shield plans, health systems agencies, hospital associations and councils, hospital licensure agencies, medical and nursing licensure agencies, peer review organizations, state health planning and development agencies, and statewide health coordinating councils.

There are many active local organizations that do not fall within these categories. Contact the hospital association of the state or province for information about such additional groups. The hospital association and councils listed have offices with full-time executives.

The selected state and provincial government agencies include those within state departments of health and welfare, and other agencies, such as comprehensive health planning, crippled children's services, maternal and child health, mental health, and vocational rehabilitation.

Health Care Providers

Lists of JCAHO Accredited Freestanding Long–Term Care Organizations, Health Maintenance Organizations, Freestanding Ambulatory Surgery Centers, Freestanding Hospices, JCAHO Accredited Freestanding Substance Abuse Organizations, JCAHO Accredited Freestanding Mental Health Care Organizations are provided in this section. The lists were developed from information supplied by the providers themselves.

As with the lists of National and International Organizations, these lists are provided simply as a convenient directory. Inclusion or omission of any organization's name indicates neither approval nor disapproval by Healthcare InfoSource, Inc.

National Organizations

A

ADARA: Professionals Networking for Excellence in Service Delivery, with Individuals Who are Deaf or Hard of Hearing, P.O. Box 251554, Little Rock, AR 72225; tel. 501/868–8850; FAX. 501/868–8812; Steve Larew, President

AVSC International, 79 Madison Avenue, Seventh Floor, New York, NY 10016; tel. 212/561–8065; Bob Geisler, Director, Information Services

Academy for Implants and Transplants, P.O. Box 223, Springfield, VA 22150; tel. 703/451–0001; FAX. 703/451–0004; Anthony J. Viscido, D.D.S., Secretary–Treasurer

Academy of Dentistry for Persons with Disabilities, 211 East Chicago Avenue, Suite 948, Chicago, IL 60611; tel. 312/440–2660; FAX. 312/440–2824; John S. Rutkauskas, M.S., D.D.S., Executive Director

Academy of General Dentistry, 211 East Chicago Avenue, Suite 1200, Chicago, IL 60611–2670; tel. 312/440–4300; FAX. 312/440–0559; Harold E. Donnell, Jr., Executive Director

Academy of Oral Dynamics, 5950 Elmer Derr Road, Frederick, MD 21703; tel. 301/473–9719; Joseph P. Skellchock, D.D.S., Treasurer

Academy of Organizational and Occupational Psychiatry, 6728 Old McLean Village Drive, McLean, VA 22101; tel. 703/556–9222; George K. Degnon, Executive Director

Accreditation Association for Ambulatory Health Care, 9933 Lawler Avenue, Skokie, IL 60077–3708; tel. 847/676–9610; FAX. 847/676–9628; Christopher A. Damon, Executive Director

Aerospace Medical Association, 320 South Henry Street, Alexandria, VA 22314–3579; tel. 703/739–2240; FAX. 703/739–9652; Russell B. Rayman, M.D., Executive Director

Alexander Graham Bell Association for the Deaf, Inc., 3417 Volta Place, N.W., Washington, DC 20007; tel. 202/337–5220; Donna McCord Dickman, Ph.D., Executive Director

Allergy Associates, 133 East 58th Street, Suite 502, New York, NY 10022; tel. 212/355–1005; FAX. 212/355–1019; Joseph D'Amore, M.D.

Alliance for Healthcare Strategy and Marketing, 11 South LaSalle, Suite 2300, Chicago, IL 60603; tel. 312/704–9700; FAX. 312/704–9709; Carla Windhorst, President

Alzheimer's Association, (Alzheimer's Disease and Related Disorders Association, Inc.), 919 North Michigan Avenue, Suite 1000, Chicago, IL 60611; tel. 312/335–8700; FAX. 312/335–1110; Thomas Kirk, Vice President, Patient, Family and Education Services

Ambulatory Pediatric Association, 6728 Old McLean Village Drive, McLean, VA 22101; tel. 703/556–9222; FAX. 703/556–8729; Marge Degnon, Executive Secretary

America's Blood Centers, 725 15th Street, N.W., Suite 700, Washington, DC 20005–2109; tel. 202/393–5725; FAX. 202/393–1282; Jim MacPherson, Executive Director

American Academy for Cerebral Palsy and Developmental Medicine, 6300 North River Road, Suite 727, Rosemont, IL 60018–4226; tel. 847/698–1635; FAX. 847/823–0536; Sheril King, Executive Director

American Academy of Allergy, Asthma and Immunology, 611 East Wells Street, Milwaukee, WI 53202; tel. 414/272–6071; FAX. 414/272–6070; Rick Iber, Executive Vice President

American Academy of Child and Adolescent Psychiatry, 3615 Wisconsin Avenue, N.W., Washington, DC 20016; tel. 202/966–7300; FAX. 202/966–2891; Virginia Q. Anthony, Executive Director

American Academy of Dental Electrosurgery, Planetarium Station, P.O. Box 374, New York, NY 10024; tel. 212/595–1925; Maurice J. Oringer, D.D.S., Executive Secretary

American Academy of Dental Practice Administration, 1063 Whippoorwill Lane, Palatine, IL 60067; tel. 847/934–4404; Kathleen Uebel, Executive Director

American Academy of Dermatology, P.O. Box 4014, Schaumburg, IL 60168–4014; tel. 847/330–0230; FAX. 847/330–0050; Bradford W. Claxton, Executive Director

American Academy of Environmental Medicine, 4510 West 89th Street, Suite 110, Prairie Village, KS 66207–2282; tel. 913/642–6062; FAX. 913/341–6912; Matt Tidwell, Executive Director

American Academy of Facial Plastic and Reconstructive Surgery, Inc., 1110 Vermont Avenue, N.W., Suite 220, Washington, DC 20005; tel. 202/842–4500; FAX. 202/371–1514; Stephen C. Duffy, Executive Vice President

American Academy of Family Physicians, 8880 Ward Parkway, Kansas City, MO 64114; tel. 816/333–9700; FAX. 816/822–0580; Robert Graham, M.D., Executive Vice President

American Academy of Healthcare Attorneys (AHA), One North Franklin, Chicago, IL 60606–3491; tel. 312/422–3700; FAX. 312/422–4574; Marietta B. Gaden, Executive Director

American Academy of Implant Dentistry, 6900 Grove Road, Thorofare, NJ 08086; tel. 609/848–7027; FAX. 609/853–5991; Christine Malin, Executive Secretary

American Academy of Insurance Medicine, 2211 Congress Street, Portland, ME 04122; tel. 207/770–6454; FAX. 207/770–6772; Paul R. Bell, M.D., Secretary

American Academy of Medical Administrators, 30555 Southfield Road, Suite 150, Southfield, MI 48076–7747; tel. 810/540–4310; FAX. 810/645–0590; Thomas R. O'Donovan, Ph.D., FAAMA, President

American Academy of Neurology, 2221 University Avenue, S.E., Suite 335, Minneapolis, MN 55414; tel. 612/623–8115; FAX. 612/623–2491; Jan W. Kolehmainen, Executive Director

American Academy of Ophthalmology, 655 Beach Street, P.O. Box 7424, San Francisco, CA 94120; tel. 415/561–8500; FAX. 415/561–8533; H. Dunbar Hoskins, Jr., M.D., Executive Vice President

American Academy of Optometry, 6110 Executive Boulevard, Suite 506, Rockville, MD 20852; tel. 301/984–1441; FAX. 301/984–4737; Lois Schoenbrun, Executive Director

American Academy of Oral Medicine, 631 South 29th Street, Arlington, VA 22202; tel. 703/684–6649; FAX. 703/684–2008; Ronald S. Brown, D.D.S., M.S., Secretary

American Academy of Orthopaedic Surgeons, 6300 North River Road, Rosemont, IL 60018–4262; tel. 847/823–7186; FAX. 847/823–8125; William W. Tipton, Jr., M.D., Executive Vice President

American Academy of Otolaryngic Allergy, 8455 Colesville Road, Suite 745, Silver Spring, MD 20910; tel. 301/588–1800; FAX. 301/588–2454; Donald J. Clark, Executive Director

American Academy of Otolaryngology–Head and Neck Surgery, Inc., One Prince Street, Alexandria, VA 22314; tel. 703/836–4444; FAX. 703/683–5100; Michael D. Maves, M.D., M.B.A., Executive Vice President

American Academy of Pain Management, 13947 Mono Way, Suite A, Sonora, CA 95370–2807; tel. 209/533–9744; FAX. 209/533–9750; Richard S. Weiner, Ph.D., Executive Director

American Academy of Pediatric Dentistry, 211 East Chicago Avenue, Suite 700, Chicago, IL 60611; tel. 312/337–2169; FAX. 312/337–6329; Dr. John A. Bogert, Executive Director

American Academy of Pediatrics, 141 Northwest Point Boulevard, P.O. Box 927, Elk Grove Village, IL 60009–0927; tel. 847/228–5005; FAX. 847/228–5097; Joe M. Sanders, Jr., M.D., Executive Director

American Academy of Physical Medicine and Rehabilitation, One IBM Plaza, Suite 2500, Chicago, IL 60611–3604; tel. 312/464–9700; FAX. 312/464–0227; Ronald A. Henrichs, CAE, Executive Director

American Academy of Physician Assistants, 950 North Washington Street, Alexandria, VA 22314; tel. 703/836–2272; FAX. 703/684–1924; Stephen C. Crane, Ph.D., M.P.H., Executive Vice President

American Academy of Physiologic Dentistry, 567 South Washington Street, Naperville, IL 60540; tel. 630/355–2625; Dr. William Kopperud, Secretary

American Academy of Psychoanalysis, 47 East 19th Street, Sixth Floor, New York, NY 10003; tel. 212/475–7980; FAX. 212/475–8101; James J. D. Tendean–Luce, Executive Director

American Academy of Restorative Dentistry, 1235 Lake Plaza Drive, Suite 251, Colorado Springs, CO 80906; tel. 719/576–8840; Donald H. Downs, D.D.S., Secretary–Treasurer

American Aging Association, 2129 Providence Avenue, Chester, PA 19013–5506; tel. 610/874–7550; FAX. 610/876–7715; Arthur K. Balin, M.D., Ph.D., Executive Director

American Alliance for Health, Physical Education, Recreation, and Dance, 1900 Association Drive, Reston, VA 22091; tel. 703/476–3400; FAX. 703/476–9527; Michael G. Davis, Executive Vice President

American Ambulance Association, 3800 Auburn Boulevard, Suite C, Sacramento, CA 95821; tel. 916/483–3827; FAX. 916/482–5473; David A. Nevins, Executive Vice President

American Art Therapy Association, 1202 Allanson Road, Mundelein, IL 60060; tel. 847/949–6064; FAX. 847/566–4580; Edward J. Stygar, Jr., Executive Director

American Assembly for Men in Nursing, 437 Twin Bay Drive, Pensacola, FL 32534–1350; tel. 904/474–0144; FAX. 904/484–8762; Robert T. Rupp, Executive Director

American Association for Adult and Continuing Education, 1200 19th Street, N.W., Suite 300, Washington, DC 20036; tel. 202/429–5131; FAX. 202/223–4579; Dr. Drew Allbritten, Executive Director

American Association for Clinical Chemistry, Inc., 2101 L Street, N.W., Suite 202, Washington, DC 20037; tel. 202/857–0717; FAX. 202/887–5093; Richard Flaherty, Executive Vice President

American Association for Dental Research, 1619 Duke Street, Alexandria, VA 22314–3406; tel. 703/548–0066; FAX. 703/548–1883; John J. Clarkson, BDS, Ph.D., Executive Director

American Association for Laboratory Animal Science, 70 Timber Creek Drive, Cordova, TN 38018; tel. 901/754–8620; FAX. 901/753–0046; Michael R. Sondag, Executive Director

American Association for Respiratory Care, 11030 Ables Lane, Dallas, TX 75229; tel. 214/243–2272; FAX. 214/484–2720; Sam P. Giordano, Executive Director

American Association for the Advancement of Science, 1200 New York Avenue, N.W., Washington, DC 20005; tel. 202/326–6400; FAX. 202/842–1603; Richard S. Nicholson, Executive Officer

American Association for the Study of Headache, 875 Kings Highway, Suite 200, Woodbury, NJ 08096; tel. 609/845–0322; FAX. 609/384–5811; Linda McGillicuddy, Executive Director

American Association for the Surgery of Trauma, Harborview Medical Center, AAST/Department of Surgery, 325 Ninth Avenue, Box 359796, Seattle, WA 98104–2499; tel. 206/731–3299; FAX. 206/731–8582; Ronald V. Maier, M.D., Secretary–Treasurer

American Association of Ambulatory Surgery Centers, 401 North Michigan Avenue, Chicago, IL 60611–4267; tel. 800/237–3768; FAX. 312/527–6636; Thomas E. Stautzenbach, Executive Director

American Association of Anatomists, Department of Anatomy, Tulane Medical School, 1430 Tulane Avenue, New Orleans, LA 70112; FAX. 504/584-1687; Robert Yates, Secretary-Treasurer

American Association of Bioanalysts, 818 Olive Street, Suite 918, St. Louis, MO 63101-1598; tel. 314/241-1445; FAX. 314/241-1449; Mark S. Birenbaum, Ph.D., Administrator

American Association of Certified Orthoptists, 501 Hill Street, Waycross, GA 31501; tel. 912/285-2020; FAX. 912/285-8112; Jill Clark, President

American Association of Colleges of Nursing, One Dupont Circle, N.W., Suite 530, Washington, DC 20036; tel. 202/463-6930; FAX. 202/785-8320; Geraldine Bednash, Ph.D., RN, FAAN, Executive Director

American Association of Colleges of Pharmacy, 1426 Prince Street, Alexandria, VA 22314-2841; tel. 703/739-2330; FAX. 703/836-8982; Richard P. Penna, Pharm.D., Executive Vice President

American Association of Colleges of Podiatric Medicine, 1350 Piccard Drive, Suite 322, Rockville, MD 20850-4307; tel. 301/990-7400; FAX. 301/990-2807; Anthony J. McNevin, CAE, President

American Association of Critical-Care Nurses, 101 Columbia, Aliso Viejo, CA 92656-1491; tel. 714/362-2000; FAX. 714/362-2020; Sarah J. Sanford, RN, M.A., CNAA, FAAN, Chief Executive Officer

American Association of Dental Consultants, Inc., P.O. Box 3345, Lawrence, KS 66046; tel. 913/749-2727; FAX. 913/749-1140; Alan M. Helerstein, D.D.S., Secretary-Treasurer

American Association of Dental Schools, 1625 Massachusetts Avenue, N.W., Washington, DC 20036; tel. 202/667-9433; FAX. 202/667-0642; Preston A. Littleton, Jr., D.D.S., Ph.D., Executive Director

American Association of Endodontists, 211 East Chicago Avenue, Suite 1100, Chicago, IL 60611; tel. 312/266-7255; FAX. 312/266-9867; Irma S. Kudo, Executive Director

American Association of Fund-Raising Counsel, Inc., 25 West 43rd Street, New York, NY 10036; tel. 212/354-5799; FAX. 212/768-1795; Ann Kaplan, Research Director

American Association of Health Plans, (AAHP), 1129 20th Street, N.W., Suite 600, Washington, DC 20036-3421; tel. 202/778-3200; FAX. 202/778-8486; Charles W. Stellar, Executive Vice President

American Association of Healthcare Consultants, 11208 Waples Mill Road, Suite 109, Fairfax, VA 22030; tel. 800/362-4674; FAX. 703/691-2247; Vaughan A. Smith, President

American Association of Homes and Services for the Aging, 901 E Street, N.W., Suite 500, Washington, DC 20004-2037; tel. 202/783-2242; FAX. 202/783-2255; Sheldon L. Goldberg, President

American Association of Hospital Dentists, Inc., 211 East Chicago Avenue, Suite 948, Chicago, IL 60611; tel. 312/440-2661; FAX. 312/440-2824; John S. Rutkauskas, M.S., D.D.S., Executive Director

American Association of Kidney Patients, 100 South Ashley Drive, Suite 280, Tampa, FL 33602; tel. 800/749-2257; FAX. 813/223-0001; Kris Robinson, Executive Director

American Association of Medical Assistants, 20 North Wacker Drive, Suite 1575, Chicago, IL 60606-2903; tel. 312/899-1500; FAX. 312/899-1259; Donald A. Balasa, J.D., M.B.A., Executive Director, Legal Counsel

American Association of Neuroscience Nurses, 224 North DesPlaines, Suite 601, Chicago, IL 60661; tel. 312/993-0043; FAX. 312/993-0362; John F. Settich, Executive Director

American Association of Nurse Anesthetists, 222 South Prospect Avenue, Park Ridge, IL 60068-4001; tel. 847/692-7050, ext. 302; FAX. 847/692-7084; John F. Garde, CRNA, M.S., FAAN, Executive Director

American Association of Nutritional Consultants, 880 Canarios Court, Suite 210, Chula Vista, CA 91910; tel. 619/482-8533; FAX. 619/482-0938; Lenda Summerfield, Administrator

American Association of Occupational Health Nurses, Inc., 50 Lenox Pointe, Atlanta, GA 30324; tel. 404/262-1162; FAX. 404/262-1165; Ann R. Cox, CAE, Executive Director

American Association of Oral and Maxillofacial Surgeons, 9700 West Bryn Mawr Avenue, Rosemont, IL 60018-5701; tel. 847/678-6200; FAX. 847/678-6286; Barbara N. Moles, Executive Director

American Association of Orthodontists, 401 North Lindbergh Boulevard, St. Louis, MO 63141-7816; tel. 314/993-1700; FAX. 314/997-1745; Ronald S. Moen, Executive Director

American Association of Pastoral Counselors, 9504A Lee Highway, Fairfax, VA 22031-2303; tel. 703/385-6967; FAX. 703/352-7725; C. Roy Woodruff, Ph.D., Executive Director

American Association of Physicists in Medicine, One Physics Ellipse, College Park, MD 20740-3846; tel. 301/209-3350; FAX. 301/209-0862; Salvatore Trofi, Jr., Executive Director

American Association of Plastic Surgeons, 2317 Seminole Road, Atlantic Beach, FL 32233; tel. 904/359-3759; FAX. 904/359-3789; Francis A. Harris, Executive Secretary

American Association of Poison Control Centers, 3201 New Mexico Avenue, N.W., Suite 310, Washington, DC 20016; tel. 202/362-7217; Rose Ann Soloway, RN

American Association of Preferred Provider Organizations, 601 13th Street, N.W., 370 South, Washington, DC 20005; tel. 202/347-7600; FAX. 202/347-7601; Gordon Wheeler, President, Chief Operating Officer

American Association of Psychiatric Technicians, Inc., A.A.P.T., 336 Johnson Road, Michigan City, IN 46360; tel. 219/879-2911; FAX. 219/879-1887; George Blake, Ph.D., Director, President

American Association of Public Health Dentistry, A.A.P.H.D. National Office, 10619 Jousting Lane, Richmond, VA 23235-3838; tel. 804/272-8344; FAX. 804/272-0802; Robert Collins, D.M.D., M.P.H., President

American Association of Public Health Physicians, Department of Preventive Medicine and Public Health, 1600 Canal Street, Room 801, New Orleans, LA 70112; tel. 504/568-6935; FAX. 504/568-6905; Joel L. Nitzkin, M.D., President

American Association on Mental Retardation, 444 North Capitol Street, N.W., Suite 846, Washington, DC 20001-1512; tel. 202/387-1968; FAX. 202/387-2193; M. Doreen Croser, Executive Director

American Baptist Homes and Hospitals Association, P.O. Box 851, Valley Forge, PA 19482-0851; tel. 215/768-2254; FAX. 215/768-2470; Milton E. Owens, Jr., Executive Director

American Board of Allergy and Immunology, A Conjoint Board of the American Board of Internal Medicine and the American Board of Pediatrics, University City Science Center, 3624 Market Street, Philadelphia, PA 19104; tel. 215/349-9466; FAX. 215/222-8669; John W. Yunginger, M.D., Executive Secretary

American Board of Anesthesiology, 4101 Lake Boone Trail, Suite 510, Raleigh, NC 27607-7506; tel. 919/881-2570; FAX. 919/881-2575; D. David Glass, M.D., Secretary-Treasurer

American Board of Cardiovascular Perfusion, 207 North 25th Avenue, Hattiesburg, MS 39401; tel. 601/582-3309; Beth A. Richmond, Ph.D., Mark G. Richmond, Ed.D., Co-Executive Directors

American Board of Colon and Rectal Surgery, 20600 Eureka Road, Suite 713, Taylor, MI 48180; tel. 313/282-9400; FAX. 313/282-9402; Herand Abcarian, M.D., Executive Director

American Board of Dermatology, Inc., Henry Ford Hospital, One Ford Place, Detroit, MI 48202-3450; tel. 313/874-1088; FAX. 313/872-3221; Harry J. Hurley, M.D., Executive Director

American Board of Emergency Medicine, 3000 Coolidge Road, East Lansing, MI 48823; tel. 517/332-4800; FAX. 517/332-2234; Benson S. Munger, Ph.D., Executive Director

American Board of Family Practice, Inc., 2228 Young Drive, Lexington, KY 40505; tel. 606/269-5626; FAX. 606/266-9699; Paul R. Young, M.D., Executive Director

American Board of Internal Medicine, 3624 Market Street, Philadelphia, PA 19104; tel. 215/243-1500; FAX. 215/382-4702; Harry R. Kimball, M.D., President

American Board of Medical Management, 4890 West Kennedy Boulevard, Suite 200, Tampa, FL 33609-2575; tel. 813/287-2815; FAX. 813/287-8993; Roger S. Schenke, Executive Vice President

American Board of Medical Specialties, 1007 Church Street, Suite 404, Evanston, IL 60201-5913; tel. 847/491-9091; FAX. 847/328-3596; J. Lee Dockery, M.D., Executive Vice President

American Board of Neurological Surgery, 6550 Fannin Street, Suite 2139, Houston, TX 77030; tel. 713/790-6015; Mary Louise Sanderson, Administrator

American Board of Nuclear Medicine, 900 Veteran Avenue, Los Angeles, CA 90024; tel. 310/825-6787; FAX. 310/825-9433; Joseph F. Ross, M.D., President

American Board of Ophthalmology, 111 Presidential Boulevard, Suite 241, Bala Cynwyd, PA 19004; tel. 610/664-1175; Denis M. O'Day, M.D., Executive Director

American Board of Oral and Maxillofacial Surgery, 625 North Michigan Avenue, Suite 1820, Chicago, IL 60611; tel. 312/642-0070; FAX. 312/642-8584; Cheryl E. Mounts, Executive Secretary

American Board of Orthopedic Surgery, Inc., 400 Silver Cedar Court, Chapel Hill, NC 27514; tel. 919/929-7103; FAX. 919/942-8988; G. Paul De Rosa, M.D., Executive Director

American Board of Otolaryngology, 5615 Kirby Drive, Suite 936, Houston, TX 77005-2452; tel. 713/528-6200; FAX. 713/528-1171; Robert W. Cantrell, M.D., Executive Vice President

American Board of Pathology, One Urban Centre, 4830 West Kennedy Boulevard, P.O. Box 25915, Tampa, FL 33622-5915; tel. 813/286-2444; FAX. 813/289-5279; William H. Hartmann, M.D., Executive Vice President

American Board of Pediatric Dentistry, 1193 Woodgate Drive, Carmel, IN 46033-9232; tel. 317/573-0877; FAX. 317/846-7235; James R. Roche, D.D.S., Executive Secretary-Treasurer

American Board of Pediatrics, Inc., 111 Silver Cedar Court, Chapel Hill, NC 27514; tel. 919/929-0461; FAX. 919/929-9255; James A. Stockman III, M.D., President

American Board of Physical Medicine and Rehabilitation, Norwest Center, Suite 674, 21 First Street, S.W., Rochester, MN 55902; tel. 507/282-1776; FAX. 507/282-9242; Mark R. Raymond, Ph.D., Executive Director

American Board of Podiatric Orthopedics and Primary Podiatric Medicine, 401 North Michigan Avenue, Suite 2400, P.O. Box 39, Chicago, IL 60611-4267; tel. 312/321-5139; FAX. 312/881-1815; Jeffrey P. Knezovich, Executive Director

American Board of Podiatric Surgery, 1601 Dolores Street, San Francisco, CA 94110-4906; tel. 415/826-3200; FAX. 415/826-4640; James A. Lamb, Executive Director

American Board of Preventive Medicine, Inc., 9950 West Lawrence Avenue, Suite 106, Schiller Park, IL 60176; tel. 847/671-1750; FAX. 847/671-1751; Alice R. Ring, M.D., M.P.H., Executive Director

American Board of Prosthodontics, P.O. Box 8437, Atlanta, GA 31106; tel. 404/876-2625; FAX. 404/872-8804; William D. Culpepper, D.D.S., M.S.D., Executive Director

American Board of Psychiatry and Neurology, Inc., 500 Lake Cook Road, Suite 335, Deerfield, IL 60015; tel. 847/945-7900; FAX. 847/945-1146; Stephen C. Scheiber, M.D., Executive Vice President

American Board of Quality Assurance and Utilization Review Physicians, 4890 West Kennedy Boulevard, Suite 260, Tampa, FL 33609; tel. 813/286-4411; FAX. 813/286-4387; Gene Hartsell, Chief Operating Officer

American Board of Radiology, Inc., 5255 East Williams Circle, Suite 6800, Tucson, AZ 85711; tel. 520/790-2900; FAX. 520/790-3200; M. Paul Capp, M.D., Executive Director

American Board of Surgery, Inc., 1617 John F. Kennedy Boulevard, Suite 860, Philadelphia, PA 19103; tel. 215/568-4000; FAX. 215/563-5718; Wallace P. Ritchie, Jr., M.D., Executive Director

American Board of Thoracic Surgery, One Rotary Center, Suite 803, Evanston, IL 60201; tel. 847/475-1520; FAX. 847/475-6240; Richard J. Cleveland, M.D., Secretary-Treasurer

American Board of Urology, 31700 Telegraph Road, Suite 150, Bingham Farms, MI 48025; tel. 810/646-9720; FAX. 810/644-0039; Stuart S. Howards, M.D., Executive Secretary

American Broncho-Esophagological Association, Vanderbilt University Medical Center, Department of Otolaryngology, S-2100 MCN, Nashville, TN 37232-2559; tel. 615/322-7267; FAX. 615/343-7604; James A. Duncavage, M.D., Secretary

American Burn Association, Department of Surgery, University of Utah, 50 North Medical Drive, Salt Lake City, UT 84132; tel. 800/548-2876; FAX. 801/585-2435; Jeffrey R. Saffle, M.D., Secretary

American Cancer Society, 1599 Clifton Road, N.E., Atlanta, GA 30329; tel. 404/320-3333; Gerald P. Murphy, M.D., Senior Vice President, Medical Affairs

American Center for the Alexander Technique, Inc., 129 West 67th Street, New York, NY 10023; tel. 212/799-0468; Kathryn Miranda, Executive Director

American Chiropractic Association, 1701 Clarendon Boulevard, Arlington, VA 22209; tel. 703/276-8800; FAX. 703/243-2593; Garrett F. Cuaco, Executive Vice President

American Cleft Palate-Craniofacial Association, 1218 Grandview Avenue, Pittsburgh, PA 15211; tel. 412/481-1376; FAX. 412/481-0847; Nancy C. Smythe, Executive Director

American Clinical Neurophysiology Society, (formerly the American Electroencephalographic Society), One Regency Drive, P.O. Box 30, Bloomfield, CT 06002; tel. 203/243-3977; FAX. 203/286-0787; Jacquelyn T. Coleman, Executive Director

American College Health Association, P.O. Box 28937, Baltimore, MD 21240-8937; tel. 410/859-1500; FAX. 410/859-1510; Charles H. Hartman, Ed.D, CAE, Executive Director

American College of Allergy, Asthma and Immunology, 85 West Algonquin Road, Suite 550, Arlington Heights, IL 60005; tel. 847/427-1200; FAX. 847/427-1294; James R. Slawny, Executive Director

American College of Apothecaries, P.O. Box 341266, Bartlett, TN 38184; tel. 901/383-8119; FAX. 901/383-8882; D. C. Huffman, Jr., Ph.D., Executive Vice President

American College of Cardiology, 9111 Old Georgetown Road, Bethesda, MD 20814; tel. 301/897-2622; FAX. 301/897-9745; Penny S. Mills, Associate Executive Vice President

American College of Cardiovascular Administrators, 30555 Southfield Road, Suite 150, Southfield, MI 48076-7747; tel. 810/540-4598; FAX. 810/645-0590; Michael Flaherty, FAAMA, FACCA

American College of Chest Physicians, 3300 Dundee Road, Northbrook, IL 60062-2348; tel. 847/498-1400; FAX. 847/498-5460; Alvin Lever, Executive Vice President

American College of Dentists, 839 Quince Orchard Boulevard, Suite J, Gaithersburg, MD 20878-1603; tel. 301/977-3223; FAX. 301/977-3330; Sherry Keramidas, Ph.D., CAE

American College of Emergency Physicians, P.O. Box 619911, Dallas, TX 75261-9911; tel. 972/550-0911; FAX. 972/580-2816; Colin C. Rorrie, Jr., Ph.D., CAE, Executive Director

American College of Foot and Ankle Orthopedics and Medicine (ACFAOM), 4603 Highway 95 South, P.O. Box 39, Cocolalla, ID 83813-0039; tel. 208/683-3900; FAX. 208/683-3700; Judith A. Baerg, Executive Director

American College of Foot and Ankle Surgeons, 515 Busse Highway, Park Ridge, IL 60068; tel. 847/292-2237; FAX. 847/292-2022; Teri Gargano Barabash, Director, Communications

American College of Health Care Administrators, 325 South Patrick Street, Alexandria, VA 22314; tel. 703/549-5822; FAX. 703/739-7901; Richard L. Thorpe, CAE, Executive Vice President

American College of Healthcare Executives, One North Franklin, Suite 1700, Chicago, IL 60606-3491; tel. 312/424-2800; FAX. 312/424-0023; Thomas C. Dolan, Ph.D., FACHE, CAE, President/Chief Executive Officer

American College of Healthcare Information Administrators, 30555 Southfield Road, Suite 150, Southfield, MI 48076-7747; tel. 810/540-4310; FAX. 810/645-0590; Robert J. Berger, Ph.D., President

American College of Legal Medicine, 611 East Wells Street, Milwaukee, WI 53202; tel. 800/433-9137; FAX. 414/276-3349; Janet Haynes, Director, Administration

American College of MOHS Micrographic Surgery and Cutaneous Oncology, 930 North Meacham, Schaumburg, IL 60173-4965; tel. 847/330-9830, ext. 379; FAX. 847/330-0050; Christina Achziger, Executive Director

American College of Managed Care Administrators, 30555 Southfield Road, Suite 150, Southfield, MI 48076-7747; tel. 810/540-4310; FAX. 810/645-0590; Eugene Migilaccio, Dr.P.H., Chairman

American College of Medical Staff Development, 3150 Holcomb Bridge Road, Suite 205, Norcross, GA 30071; tel. 800/897-9494; FAX. 404/417-2176; Susan Woodbury, Executive Director

American College of Nurse-Midwives, 818 Connecticut Avenue, N.W., Suite 900, Washington, DC 20006; tel. 202/728-9860; FAX. 202/728-9897; Deanne Williams, Director, Professional Services

American College of Obstetricians and Gynecologists, 409 12th Street, S.W., Washington, DC 20024-2188; tel. 202/638-5577; FAX. 202/484-5107; Ralph W. Hale, M.D., Executive Director

American College of Occupational and Environmental Medicine, (Includes ACOEM Research and Education Fund, and Occupational Physicians Scholarship Fund OPSF), 55 West Seegers, Arlington Heights, IL 60005; tel. 847/228-6850, ext. 11; FAX. 847/228-1856; Donald L. Hoops, Ph.D., Executive Vice President

American College of Oncology Administrators, 30555 Southfield Road, Suite 150, Southfield, MI 48076-7747; tel. 810/540-4310; FAX. 810/645-0590; Jeanne M. Walter, RN, M.S., OCN, President

American College of Osteopathic Pediatricians, 5301 Wisconsin Avenue, NW, Suite 630, Washington, DC 20015; tel. 202/362-3229; FAX. 202/537-1362; David Kushner, Executive Director

American College of Physician Executives, 4890 West Kennedy Boulevard, Suite 200, Tampa, FL 33609-2575; tel. 813/287-2000; FAX. 813/287-8993; Roger S. Schenke, Executive Vice President

American College of Physicians, Independence Mall West, Sixth Street at Race, Philadelphia, PA 19106; tel. 215/351-2800; FAX. 215/351-2829; Walter J. McDonald, M.D., FACP, Executive Vice President

American College of Preventive Medicine, 1660 L Street, N.W., Washington, DC 20036; tel. 202/466-2044; FAX. 202/466-2662; Hazel K. Keimowitz, M.A., Executive Director

American College of Radiology, 1891 Preston White Drive, Reston, VA 20191-4397; tel. 703/648-8900; FAX. 703/648-9176; John J. Curry, Executive Director

American College of Rheumatology, 60 Executive Park South, Suite 150, Atlanta, GA 30329; tel. 404/633-3777; FAX. 404/633-1870; Lynn Bonfiglio, Director, Membership

American College of Sports Medicine, P.O. Box 1440, Indianapolis, IN 46206-1440; tel. 317/637-9200; FAX. 317/634-7817, ext. 100; James R. Whitehead, Executive Vice President

American College of Surgeons, 55 East Erie Street, Chicago, IL 60611; tel. 312/664-4050, ext. 201; FAX. 312/440-7014; Paul A. Ebert, M.D., Director

American Congress of Rehabilitation Medicine, 4700 West Lake Avenue, Glenview, IL 60025; tel. 847/375-4725; FAX. 847/375-4777; Diane Burgher, Executive Director

American Council on Pharmaceutical Education, Inc., 311 West Superior Street, Suite 512, Chicago, IL 60610; tel. 312/664-3575; FAX. 312/664-4652; Daniel A. Nona, Ph.D., Executive Director

American Dental Assistants Association, 203 North LaSalle, Suite 1320, Chicago, IL 60601; tel. 312/541-1550, ext. 204; FAX. 312/541-1496; Lawrence H. Sepin, Executive Director

American Dental Association, 211 East Chicago Avenue, Chicago, IL 60611; tel. 312/440-2500; FAX. 312/440-7494; John S. Zapp, D.D.S., Executive Director

American Dental Society of Anesthesiology, Inc., 211 East Chicago Avenue, Suite 780, Chicago, IL 60611; tel. 312/664-8270; FAX. 312/642-9713; Christopher LoFrisco, D.M.D., Executive Director

American Diabetes Association, Inc., 1660 Duke Street, Alexandria, VA 22314; tel. 703/549-1500; FAX. 703/836-7439; John H. Graham IV, Chief Executive Officer

American Dietetic Association, 216 West Jackson Boulevard, Suite 800, Chicago, IL 60606-6995; tel. 312/899-0040, ext. 4889; FAX. 312/899-1758; Beverly Bajus, Association Management Group

American Federation for Medical Research, 1200 19th Street, N.W., Suite 300, Washington, DC 20036-2422; tel. 202/429-5161; FAX. 202/223-4579; Susan Eisenberg, Executive Director

American Foundation for Aging Research, North Carolina State University, Biochemistry Department, P.O. Box 7622, Raleigh, NC 27695-7622; tel. 919/515-5679; FAX. 919/515-2047; Paul F. Agris, President

American Foundation for Aids Research, 733 Third Avenue, 12th Floor, New York, NY 10017; tel. 212/682-7440; Mathilde Krim, Ph.D., Founding Co-Chair

American Foundation for the Blind, Inc., 11 Penn Plaza, Suite 300, New York, NY 10001; tel. 212/502-7600; Liz Greco, Vice President, Communications

American Fracture Association, 2406 East Washington Street, Bloomington, IL 61704; tel. 309/663-6272; Sarah Olson, Executive Secretary

American Geriatrics Society, 770 Lexington Avenue, Suite 300, New York, NY 10021; tel. 212/308-1414; FAX. 212/832-8646; Linda Hiddemen Barondess, Executive Vice President

American Group Practice Association, Inc., 1422 Duke Street, Alexandria, VA 22314-3430; tel. 703/838-0033; FAX. 703/548-1890; Donald W. Fisher, Ph.D., Executive Vice President and Chief Executive Offi

American Group Psychotherapy Association, Inc., 25 East 21st Street, Sixth Floor, New York, NY 10010; tel. 212/477-2677; FAX. 212/979-6627; Marsha S. Block, CAE, Chief Executive Officer

American Guild of Patient Account Management, 1200 19th Street, N.W., Suite 300, Washington, DC 20036; tel. 202/857-1179; FAX. 202/223-4579; Dennis E. Smeage, Executive Director

American Health Care Association, 1201 L Street, N.W., Washington, DC 20005; tel. 202/842-4444; FAX. 202/842-3860; Paul R. Willging, Ph.D., Executive Vice President

American Health Foundation, One Dana Road, Valhalla, NY 10595; tel. 914/789-7122; FAX. 914/592-6317; Ernst L. Wynder, M.D., President

American Health Information Management Association, 919 North Michigan Avenue, Suite 1400, Chicago, IL 60611; tel. 312/787-2672, ext. 210; FAX. 312/787-9793; Linda Kloss, R.R.A., Executive Director

American Health Planning Association, 7245 Arlington Boulevard, Suite 300, Falls Church, VA 22042; tel. 202/371-1515; FAX. 703/573-1276; Dean Montgomery

American Healthcare Radiology Administrators, P.O. Box 334, Sudbury, MA 01776; tel. 508/443-7591; FAX. 508/443-8046; Teresa Cryan, Office Administrator

American Heart Association, Inc., Office of Scientific Affairs, 7320 Greenville Avenue, Dallas, TX 75231; tel. 214/706–1446; Mary Jane Jesse, M.D., Senior Vice President

American Hospital Association, One North Franklin, Chicago, IL 60606–3491; tel. 312/422–3000, Office of the President: 325 Seventh Street, N.W., Washington, DC 20004; tel. 202/638–1100; FAX. 202/626–2345; Richard J. Davidson, President

American Hospital Association, National Grassroots/Political Project Director, 3405 22nd Street, Boulder, CO 80304; tel. 800/999–1462; FAX. 303/442–7158; Mary Lynne Shickich, National Grassroots/Political Project Director

American Hospital Association, Mid–Atlantic Legislative Office, 325 Seventh Street, N.W., Washington, DC 20004; tel. 800/555–7218; FAX. 202/626–2254; Stephanie Nelson, Regional Legislative Director

American Hospital Association, Midwest Regional Legislative Office, 5721 Odana Road, Madison, WI 53719; tel. 800/999–1438; FAX. 608/288–0976; Dave Hewett, Regional Legislative Director

American Hospital Association, Northeast Regional Legislative Office, Five New England Executive Park, Burlington, MA 01803–5006; tel. 800/999–1561; FAX. 617/273–3708; Jack Barry, Regional Legislative Director

American Hospital Association, Southern Regional Legislative Office, 1675 Terrell Mill Road, Suite 250, Marietta, GA 30067; tel. 800/999–1560; FAX. 770/933–8230; Paul D. Bolster, Regional Legislative Director

American Hospital Association, Washington Office, 325 Seventh Street, N.W., Suite 700, Washington, DC 20004; tel. 202/638–1100; FAX. 202/626–2345; Richard Pollack, Executive Vice President, Federal Relations

American Hospital Association, Western Regional Legislative Office, 5412 Idylwild Trail, Suite 108, Boulder, CO 80301; tel. 303/516–9709; FAX. 303/516–9710; Marcia Desmond, Regional Legislative Director

American Institute of Architects, Committee on Architecture for Health, 1735 New York Avenue, N.W., Washington, DC 20006; tel. 202/626–7366; FAX. 206/626–7518; Todd S. Phillips, Ph.D., Director

American Juvenile Arthritis Organization, a Council of the Arthritis Foundation, 1330 West Peachtree Street, Atlanta, GA 30309; tel. 404/872–7100, ext. 6271; FAX. 404/872–9559; Janet S. Austin, Ph.D., Vice President

American Laryngological Association, 300 Longwood Avenue, Fegan 9, Boston, MA 02115; tel. 617/335–6417; FAX. 617/355–8041; G. B. Healy, M.D., Secretary

American Laryngological, Rhinological, and Otological Society, Inc., (The Triological Society), 10 South Broadway, Suite 1401, St. Louis, MO 63102–1741; tel. 314/621–6550; FAX. 314/621–6688; Daniel Henroid, Sr., Executive Director

American Library Association, 50 East Huron Street, Chicago, IL 60611; tel. 312/280–3205; FAX. 312/944–3897; Elizabeth Martinez, Executive Director

American Lung Association, 1740 Broadway, New York, NY 10019–4374; tel. 212/315–8700; FAX. 212/265–5642; John R. Garrison, Managing Director

American Lung Association of Ohio, Dayton Office, 7560 McEwen Road, Dayton, OH 45459; tel. 513/291–0451; FAX. 513/291–0453; Roberta M. Taylor, Director

American Medical Association, 515 North State Street, Chicago, IL 60610; tel. 312/464–5000; FAX. 312/464–4184; P. John Seward, M.D., Executive Vice President

American Medical Association Alliance, 515 North State Street, Chicago, IL 60610; tel. 312/464–4470; FAX. 312/464–5020; Hazel J. Lewis, Executive Director

American Medical Student Association/Foundation, 1902 Association Drive, Reston, VA 22091; tel. 703/620–6600; FAX. 703/620–5873; Paul R. Wright, Executive Director

American Medical Technologists, 710 Higgins Road, Park Ridge, IL 60068; tel. 847/823–5169; FAX. 847/823–0458; Gerard P. Boe, Ph.D., Executive Director

American Medical Women's Association, Inc., 800 North Fairfax Street, Suite 400, Alexandria, VA 22314; tel. 703/838–0500; FAX. 703/549–3864; Eileen McGrath, J.D., CAE, Executive Director

American Medical Writers Association, 9650 Rockville Pike, Bethesda, MD 20814–3998; tel. 301/493–0003; FAX. 301/493–6384; Lillian Sablack, Executive Director

American National Standards Institute, 11 West 42nd Street, New York, NY 10036; tel. 212/642–4900; FAX. 212/398–0023; Sergio Mazza, President

American Nephrology Nurses' Association, East Holly Avenue, P.O. Box 56, Pitman, NJ 08071; tel. 609/256–2320; FAX. 609/589–7463; Ron P. Brady, Executive Director

American Neurological Association, 5841 Cedar Lake Road, Suite 108, Minneapolis, MN 55416; tel. 612/545–6284; FAX. 612/545–6073; Linda Wilkerson, Executive Director

American Nurses' Association, 600 Maryland Avenue, S.W., Suite 100 W, Washington, DC 20024–2571; tel. 202/651–7012; FAX. 202/651–7006; Geri Marullo, M.S.N., RN, Executive Director

American Occupational Therapy Association, Inc., 4720 Montgomery Lane, P.O. Box 31220, Bethesda, MD 20824–1220; tel. 301/652–2682, ext. 2101; FAX. 301/652–7711; Jeanette Bair, M.B.A., O.T.R., F.A.O.T.A.

American Ophthalmological Society, Duke University Eye Center, Box 3802, Durham, NC 27710–3802; tel. 919/684–5365; FAX. 919/684–2230; W. Banks Anderson, Jr., M.D., Secretary–Treasurer

American Optometric Association, 243 North Lindbergh Boulevard, St. Louis, MO 63141; tel. 314/991–4100, ext. 252; FAX. 314/991–4101; Jeffrey G. Mays, Executive Director

American Organization of Nurse Executives (AONE), One North Franklin, 34th Floor, Chicago, IL 60606; tel. 312/422–2800; FAX. 312/422–4503; Marjorie Beyers, RN, Ph.D., FAAN

American Orthopsychiatric Association, 330 Seventh Avenue, 18th Floor, New York, NY 10001; tel. 212/564–5930; FAX. 212/564–6180; Gale Siegel, M.S.W., Executive Director

American Orthoptic Council, 3914 Nakoma Road, Madison, WI 53711; tel. 608/233–5383; FAX. 608/263–7694; Leslie France, Administrator

American Osteopathic Academy of Addiction Medicine, 5301 Wisconsin Avenue, N.W., Suite 630, Washington, DC 20015; tel. 202/966–7732; FAX. 202/537–1362; David Kushner, Executive Director

American Osteopathic Association, 142 East Ontario Street, Chicago, IL 60611; tel. 312/280–5800; FAX. 312/280–3860; Ann M. Wittner, Director, Department of Administration

American Osteopathic Healthcare Association, 5301 Wisconsin Avenue, N.W., Suite 630, Washington, DC 20015; tel. 202/686–1700; FAX. 202/686–7615; David Kushner, President and Chief Executive Officer

American Otological Society, Inc., Loyola University Medical Center, 2160 South First Avenue, Building 105, Number 1870, Maywood, IL 60153; tel. 708/216–8526; FAX. 708/216–4834; Gregory J. Matz, M.D., Secretary–Treasurer

American Parkinson Disease Association, Inc., 1250 Hylan Boulevard, Suite 4B, Staten Island, NY 10305; tel. 800/223–2732; FAX. 718/981–4399; G. Maestrone, D.V.M., Scientific and Medical Affairs Director

American Pediatric Society, Inc., 141 Northwest Point Boulevard, P.O. Box 675, Elk Grove Village, IL 60009–0675; tel. 847/427–0205; FAX. 847/427–1305; Kathy Cannon, Associate Executive Director

American Pharmaceutical Association, 2215 Constitution Avenue, N.W., Washington, DC 20037; tel. 202/628–4410; FAX. 202/783–2351; John A. Gans, Pharm.D., Executive Vice President

American Physical Therapy Association, 1111 North Fairfax Street, Alexandria, VA 22314; tel. 703/684–2782; FAX. 703/684–7343; Francis J. Mallon, Esq., Chief Executive Officer

American Physiological Society, 9650 Rockville Pike, Bethesda, MD 20814–3991; tel. 301/530–7118; FAX. 301/571–8305; Martin Frank, Ph.D., Executive Director

American Podiatric Medical Association, 9312 Old Georgetown Road, Bethesda, MD 20814–1698; tel. 301/571–9200; FAX. 301/530–2752; Frank J. Malouff, Executive Director

American Psychiatric Association, 1400 K Street, N.W., Washington, DC 20005; tel. 202/682–6000; FAX. 202/682–6114; Melvin Sabshin, M.D., Medical Director

American Psychoanalytic Association, 309 East 49th Street, New York, NY 10017; tel. 212/752–0450; FAX. 212/593–0571; Ellen B. Fertig, Administrative Director

American Psychological Association, 750 First Street, N.E., Washington, DC 20002–4242; tel. 202/336–5500; FAX. 202/336–6069; Russ Newman, Ph.D., J.D., Executive Director, Professional Practice

American Psychosomatic Society, 6728 Old McLean Village Drive, McLean, VA 22101; tel. 703/556–9222; George K. Degnon, Executive Director

American Public Health Association, 1015 15th Street, N.W., Washington, DC 20005; tel. 202/789–5600; FAX. 202/789–5681; Fernando M. Trevino, Ph.D., M.P.H., Executive Director

American Public Welfare Association, 810 First Street, N.E., Suite 500, Washington, DC 20002; tel. 202/682–0100; FAX. 202/289–6555; Sidney Johnson III, Executive Director

American Red Cross, National Headquarters, 8111 Gatehouse Road, Falls Church, VA 22042; tel. 703/206–7764; FAX. 703/206–7765; Susan M. Livingstone, Vice President, Health and Safety Services

American Registry of Medical Assistants, 69 Southwick Road, Suite A, Westfield, MA 01085–4729; tel. 413/562–7336; Annette H. Heyman, R.M.A., Director

American Registry of Radiologic Technologists, 1255 Northland Drive, St. Paul, MN 55120; tel. 612/687–0048; Jerry B. Reid, Ph.D., Executive Director

American Rhinologic Society, Department of Otolaryngology, LSU Medical Center, 1501 Kings Highway, Shreveport, LA 71130; tel. 318/675–6262; FAX. 318/675–6260; Fred J. Stucker, M.D., Secretary

American Roentgen Ray Society, 1891 Preston White Drive, Reston, VA 22091; tel. 703/648–8992; FAX. 703/264–8863; Paul R. Fullagar, Executive Director

American School Health Association, 7263 S.R. 43, P.O. Box 708, Kent, OH 44240–0708; tel. 330/678–1601; FAX. 330/678–4526; Thomas M. Reed, Acting Executive Director

American Society for Adolescent Psychiatry, 4340 East West Highway, Suite 401, Bethesda, MD 20814; tel. 301/718–6502; FAX. 301/656–0989; Ann T. Loew, Ed.M.

American Society for Biochemistry and Molecular Biology, Inc., 9650 Rockville Pike, Bethesda, MD 20814–3996; tel. 301/530–7145; FAX. 301/571–1824; Charles C. Hancock, Executive Officer

American Society for Clinical Laboratory Science, 7910 Woodmont Avenue, Suite 530, Bethesda, MD 20814; tel. 301/657–2768; FAX. 301/657–2909; Elissa Passiment, Executive Director

American Society for Clinical Pharmacology and Therapeutics, 1718 Gallagher Road, Norristown, PA 19401–2800; tel. 610/825–3838; FAX. 610/834–8652; Elaine Galasso, Executive Director

American Society for Cytotechnology, 920 Paverstone Drive, Suite D, Raleigh, NC 27615; tel. 919/848–9911; FAX. 919/848–9853; Sue Brenzel, Executive Assistant, Office Manager

American Society for Head and Neck Surgery, c/o Dr. Jonas Johnson, Eye and Ear Institute, 203 Lothrop Street, Suite 250, Pittsburgh, PA 15213; tel. 410/955–7400; Charles W. Cummings, M.D., Secretary

American Society for Healthcare Central Service Professionals (AHA), One North Franklin, 30th Floor, Chicago, IL 60606; tel. 312/422–3570; FAX. 312/422–4573; J. D. Meacham, Director, Continuing Education

American Society for Healthcare Education and Training (AHA), One North Franklin, Chicago, IL 60606; tel. 312/422–3720; FAX. 312/422–4579; Linda H. Brooks, Executive Director

American Society for Healthcare Engineering (AHA), One North Franklin, Chicago, IL 60606; tel. 312/422–3800; FAX. 312/422–4571; Joseph Martori, Executive Director

American Society for Healthcare Food Service Administrators (AHA), One North Franklin, Chicago, IL 60606; tel. 312/422–3870; FAX. 312/422–4581; Patricia Burton, Executive Director

American Society for Healthcare Human Resources Administration (AHA), One North Franklin, 31st Floor, Chicago, IL 60606; tel. 312/422–3720; FAX. 312/422–4579; Linda H. Brooks, Executive Director

American Society for Healthcare Materials Management (AHA), One North Franklin, Chicago, IL 60606–3491; tel. 312/422–3840; FAX. 312/422–4573; Shelly Johnson, Executive Director

American Society for Healthcare Risk Management (AHA), One North Franklin, Chicago, IL 60606; tel. 312/422–3980; FAX. 312/422–4580; Christy Kessler, Executive Director

American Society for Investigative Pathology, 9650 Rockville Pike, Bethesda, MD 20814–3993; tel. 301/530–7130; FAX. 301/571–1879; Frances A. Pitlick, Ph.D., Executive Officer

American Society for Laser Medicine and Surgery, Inc., 2404 Stewart Square, Wausau, WI 54401; tel. 715/845–9283; FAX. 715/848–2493; Richard O. Gregory, M.D.

American Society for Microbiology, 1325 Massachusetts Avenue, N.W., Washington, DC 20005; tel. 202/924–9265; FAX. 202/942–9333; Michael I. Goldberg, Ph.D., Executive Director

American Society for Pharmacology and Experimental Therapeutics, Inc., 9650 Rockville Pike, Bethesda, MD 20814–3995; tel. 301/530–7060; FAX. 301/530–7061; Kay A. Croker, Executive Officer

American Society for Psychoprophylaxis in Obstetrics, Inc. (ASPO/LAMAZE), 1200 19th Street, N.W., Suite 300, Washington, DC 20036; tel. 202/857–1128; FAX. 202/223–4579; Linda L. Harmon, Executive Director

American Society for Public Administration, 1120 G Street, N.W., Suite 700, Washington, DC 20005; tel. 202/393–7878; FAX. 202/638–4952; Mary Hamilton, Executive Director

American Society for Reproductive Medicine, (formerly The American Fertility Society), 1209 Montgomery Highway, Birmingham, AL 35216–2809; tel. 205/978–5000; FAX. 205/978–5005; Robert D. Visscher, M.D., Executive Director

American Society for Therapeutic Radiology and Oncology, 1891 Preston White Drive, Reston, VA 22091; tel. 800/962–7876; FAX. 703/476–8167; Gregg Robinson, Chief Operating Officer

American Society for the Advancement of Anesthesia in Dentistry, Six East Union Avenue, P.O. Box 551, Bound Brook, NJ 08805; tel. 201/469–9050; David Crystal, D.D.S., Executive Secretary

American Society of Anesthesiologists, 520 North Northwest Highway, Park Ridge, IL 60068; tel. 847/825–5586; FAX. 847/825–1692; Glenn W. Johnson, Executive Director

American Society of Cardiovascular Professionals, Society for Cardiovascular Management ASCP/SCM, 120 Falcon Drive, Suite Three, Fredericksburg, VA 22408; tel. 540/891–0079; FAX. 540/898–2393; Peggy McElgunn, Executive Director

American Society of Clinical Oncology, 435 North Michigan Avenue, Suite 1717, Chicago, IL 60611–4067; tel. 312/644–0828; FAX. 312/644–8557; Robert E. Becker, J.D., CAE, Executive Director

American Society of Clinical Pathologists., (Includes Board of Registry), 2100 West Harrison Street, Chicago, IL 60612–3798; tel. 312/738–1336; FAX. 312/738–9798; Robert C. Rock, M.D., Senior Vice President

American Society of Colon and Rectal Surgeons, 85 West Algonquin Road, Suite 550, Arlington Heights, IL 60005; tel. 847/290–9184; FAX. 847/290–9203; Richard Billingham, M.D., Secretary

American Society of Consultant Pharmacists, 1321 Duke Street, Alexandria, VA 22314–3563; tel. 703/739–1300; FAX. 703/739–1321; R. Timothy Webster, Executive Director

American Society of Contemporary Medicine and Surgery, 4711 Golf Road, Suite 408, Skokie, IL 60076; tel. 800/621–4002; FAX. 847/568–1527; Randall T. Bellows, M.D., Director

American Society of Contemporary Ophthalmology, 4711 Golf Road, Suite 408, Skokie, IL 60076; tel. 800/621–4002; FAX. 847/568–1527; Randall T. Bellows, M.D., Director

American Society of Cytopathology, 400 West Ninth Street, Suite 201, Wilmington, DE 19801; tel. 302/429–8802; FAX. 302/429–8807; Petrina M. Smith, RN, M.B.A., Executive Secretary

American Society of Dentistry for Children, John Hancock Center, 875 North Michigan Avenue, Suite 4040, Chicago, IL 60611; tel. 312/943–1244; FAX. 312/943–5341; Dr. Peter Fos, Interim Executive Director

American Society of Directors of Volunteer Services (AHA), One North Franklin, Chicago, IL 60606; tel. 312/422–3938; FAX. 312/422–4575; Nancy A. Brown, Executive Director

American Society of Electroneurodiagnostic Technologists, Inc., 204 West Seventh Street, Carroll, IA 51401–2317; tel. 712/792–2978; FAX. 712/792–6962; M. Fran Pedelty, Executive Director

American Society of Extra–Corporeal Technology, Inc., 11480 Sunset Hills Road, Suite 210E, Reston, VA 20190–5208; tel. 703/435–8556; FAX. 703/435–0056; George M. Cate, Executive Director

American Society of Group Psychodrama and Psychotherapy, 6728 Old McLean Village Drive, McLean, VA 22101; tel. 703/556–9222; George K. Degnon, Executive Director

American Society of Health–System Pharmacists, 7272 Wisconsin Avenue, Bethesda, MD 20814; tel. 301/657–3000; FAX. 301/652–8278; Joseph A. Oddis, Executive Vice President

American Society of Internal Medicine, 2011 Pennsylvania Avenue, N.W., Suite 800, Washington, DC 20006–1808; tel. 202/835–2746; FAX. 202/835–0443; Alan R. Nelson, M.D., Executive Vice President

American Society of Law, Medicine & Ethics, 765 Commonwealth Avenue, 16th Floor, Boston, MA 02215; tel. 617/262–4990; FAX. 617/437–7596; Michael Vasko, M.A., Managing Director

American Society of Maxillofacial Surgeons, 444 East Algonquin Road, Arlington Heights, IL 60005; tel. 847/228–8375; FAX. 847/228–6509; Gina Cappellania, Administrative Coordinator

American Society of Neuroimaging, 5841 Cedar Lake Road, Suite 108, Minneapolis, MN 55416; tel. 612/545–6204; FAX. 612/545–6073; Linda Wilkerson, Executive Director

American Society of Plastic and Reconstructive Surgeons, 444 East Algonquin Road, Arlington Heights, IL 60005; tel. 847/228–9900; FAX. 847/228–9131; Dave Fellers, CAE, Executive Director

American Society of Radiologic Technologists, 15000 Central Avenue, S.E., Albuquerque, NM 87123–3917; tel. 505/298–4500; FAX. 505/298–5063; Joan L. Parsons, Executive Vice President, Operations

American Speech–Language–Hearing Association, Consumer Division, 10801 Rockville Pike, Rockville, MD 20852; tel. 800/638–8255; FAX. 301/571–0457; Frederick T. Spahr, Ph.D., Executive Director

American Surgical Association, 13 Elm Street, Manchester, MA 01944; tel. 508/526–8330; FAX. 508/526–4018; John L. Cameron, M.D., Secretary

American Thoracic Society, 1740 Broadway, New York, NY 10019–4374; tel. 212/315–8700, ext. 778; FAX. 212/315–6498; Marilyn Hansen, Executive Director

American Thyroid Association, Inc., Montefiore Medical Center, 111 East 210th Street, Room 311, Bronx, NY 10467; tel. 718/882–6047; FAX. 718/882–6085; Martin I. Surks, M.D., Secretary

American Trauma Society, 8903 Presidential Parkway, Suite 512, Upper Marlboro, MD 20772–2656; tel. 800/556–7890; FAX. 301/420–0617; Harry Teter, Executive Director

American Urological Association, Inc., 1120 North Charles Street, Baltimore, MD 21201; tel. 410/223–4300; FAX. 410/223–4370; G. James Gallagher, Executive Director

Arthritis Foundation, 1330 West Peachtree Street, Atlanta, GA 30309; tel. 404/872–7100, ext. 6200; FAX. 404/872–0457; Don L. Riggin, President, Chief Executive Officer

Association for Applied Psychophysiology and Biofeedback, 10200 West 44th Avenue, Suite 304, Wheat Ridge, CO 80033; tel. 303/422–8436; FAX. 303/422–8894; Francine Butler, Ph.D.

Association for Clinical Pastoral Education, Inc., 1549 Clairmont Road, Suite 103, Decatur, GA 30033; tel. 404/320–1472; FAX. 404/320–0849; Russell H. Davis, Executive Director

Association for Healthcare Philanthropy, 313 Park Avenue, Suite 400, Falls Church, VA 22046; tel. 703/532–6243; FAX. 703/532–7170; Dr. William C. McGinly, CAE, President, Chief Executive Officer

Association for Hospital Medical Education, 1200 19th Street, N.W., Suite 300, Washington, DC 20036–2401; tel. 202/857–1196; FAX. 202/223–4579; Dennis Smeage, Executive Director

Association for Professionals in Infection Control and Epidemiology, Inc., 1016 16th Street, Sixth Floor, Washington, DC 20036; tel. 202/296–2742; FAX. 202/296–5645; Christopher E. Laxton, Executive Director

Association for Quality HealthCare, Inc., P.O. Box 670, Columbus, GA 31902; tel. 404/571–2122; FAX. 404/571–2650; L. B. Skip Teaster, Executive Director

Association for Volunteer Administration, 10565 Lee Highway, Suite 104, Fairfax, VA 22030; tel. 703/352–6222; FAX. 703/352–6767; Joan Shephard, Executive Director

Association for the Advancement of Automotive Medicine, 2340 DesPlaines Avenue, Suite 106, Des Plaines, IL 60018; tel. 847/390–8927; Elaine Petrucelli, Executive Director

Association for the Advancement of Medical Instrumentation, 3330 Washington Boulevard, Suite 400, Arlington, VA 22201–4598; tel. 703/525–4890; FAX. 703/276–0793; Michael J. Miller, J.D., President

Association for the Care of Children's Health (ACCH), 7910 Woodmont Avenue, Suite 300, Bethesda, MD 20814; tel. 301/654–6549; FAX. 301/986–4553; Heather Bennett McCabe, Ph.D., Executive Director

Association of American Medical Colleges, 2450 N Street, N.W., Washington, DC 20037–1127; tel. 202/828–0400; FAX. 202/828–1125; Jordan J. Cohen, M.D., President

Association of American Physicians, Krannert Institute of Cardiology, Indiana University School of Medicine, 1111 West 10th Street, Indianapolis, IN 46202–4800; tel. 317/630–7712; FAX. 317/274–9697; David R. Hathaway, M.D., Secretary

Association of American Physicians and Surgeons, Inc., 1601 North Tucson Boulevard, Suite Nine, Tucson, AZ 85716; tel. 520/327–4885; FAX. 520/325–4230; Jane M. Orient, M.D., Executive Director

Association of Birth Defect Children, 827 Irma Avenue, Orlando, FL 32803; tel. 407/245–7035; FAX. 407/245–7087; Betty Mekdeci, Executive Director

Association of Community Cancer Centers, 11600 Nebel Street, Suite 201, Rockville, MD 20852; tel. 301/984–9496; FAX. 301/770–1949; Lee E. Mortenson, DPA, Executive Director

Section C

Association of Mental Health Administrators, 60 Revere Drive, Suite 500, Northbrook, IL 60062; tel. 847/480–9626; FAX. 847/480–9282; Alison C. Brown, Executive Director

Association of Mental Health Clergy, Inc., 1701 East Woodfield Road, Suite 311, Schaumburg, IL 60173–5191; tel. 847/240–1014; FAX. 847/240–1015; David E. Carl, President

Association of Military Surgeons of the U.S., 9320 Old Georgetown Road, Bethesda, MD 20814; tel. 301/897–8800; FAX. 301/530–5446; Lt. General Max B. Bralliar, USAF MC Ret., Executive Director

Association of Operating Room Nurses, Inc., 2170 South Parker Road, Suite 300, Denver, CO 80231–5711; tel. 303/755–6300; FAX. 303/750–2927; Lola M. Fehr, RN, M.S., CAE, FAAN, Executive Director

Association of Osteopathic Directors and Medical Educators, 5301 Wisconsin Avenue, N.W., Suite 630, Washington, DC 20015; tel. 202/537–1021; FAX. 202/537–1362; David Kushner, Executive Director

Association of Schools of Allied Health Professions, 1730 M Street, N.W., Suite 500, Washington, DC 20036; tel. 202/293–4848; FAX. 202/293–4852; Thomas W. Elwood, Dr.P.h., Executive Director

Association of Schools of Public Health, Inc., 1660 L Street, N.W., Suite 204, Washington, DC 20036; tel. 202/296–1099; FAX. 202/296–1252; Michael K. Gemmell, CAE, Executive Director

Association of Specialized and Cooperative Library Agencies, 50 East Huron Street, Chicago, IL 60611; tel. 312/280–4399; FAX. 312/944–8085; Cathleen Bourdon, ASCLA, Executive Director

Association of State and Territorial Health Officials, 415 Second Street, N.E., Suite 200, Washington, DC 20002; tel. 202/546–5400; FAX. 202/544–9349; Cheryl A. Beversdorf, RN, M.H.S., CAE, Executive Vice President

Association of Surgical Technologists, Inc., 7108–C South Alton Way, Englewood, CO 80112–2106; tel. 303/694–9130; FAX. 303/694–9169; William J. Teutsch, Executive Director

Association of University Anesthesiologists, 2033 Sixth Avenue, Suite 804, Seattle, WA 98121–2586; tel. 206/441–6020; FAX. 206/441–8262; Shirley Bishop

Association of University Programs in Health Administration, 1911 North Fort Myer Drive, Suite 503, Arlington, VA 22209; tel. 703/524–5500; FAX. 703/525–4791; Henry A. Fernandez, J.D., President, Chief Executive Officer

Asthma Foundation of Southern Arizona, P.O. Box 30069, Tucson, AZ 85751–0069; tel. 602/323–6046; FAX. 602/324–1137; Lynn Krust, Executive Director

Asthma and Allergy Foundation of America, 1125 15th Street, N.W., Suite 502, Washington, DC 20005; tel. 202/466–7643; FAX. 202/466–8940; Mary E. Worstell, M.P.H., Executive Director

B

BCS Financial Corporation, 676 North St. Clair, Chicago, IL 60611; tel. 312/951–7700; FAX. 312/951–7777; Edward J. Baran, Chairman, Chief Executive Officer

Bereavement Services/RTS, Gundersen Lutheran Medical Center, 1910 South Avenue, La Crosse, WI 54601; tel. 800/362–9567, ext. 4747; FAX. 608/791–5137; Fran Rybarik, Director

Biological Photographic Association, Inc., 1819 Peachtree Road, N.E., Suite 620, Atlanta, GA 30309; tel. 404/351–6300; FAX. 404/351–3348; William Just, Executive Director

Biological Stain Commission, Inc., University of Rochester, Department Pathology, Box 626, Rochester, NY 14642–0001; tel. 716/275–6335; FAX. 716/273–1027; David P. Penney, Ph.D., Treasurer

Blinded Veterans Association, 477 H Street, N.W., Washington, DC 20001; tel. 800/669–7079; FAX. 202/371–8258; Ronald L. Miller, Ph.D., Executive Director

Blue Cross and Blue Shield Association, 676 North St. Clair Street, Chicago, IL 60611; tel. 312/440–6000; FAX. 312/440–6609; Patrick G. Hays, President, Chief Executive Officer

C

Catholic Health Association of the United States, 4455 Woodson Road, St. Louis, MO 63134–3797; tel. 314/427–2500; FAX. 314/427–0029; John E. Curley, Jr., President, Chief Executive Officer

Center for Health Administration Studies, University of Chicago, 969 East 60th Street, Chicago, IL 60637; tel. 773/702–7104; FAX. 773/702–7222; Edward F. Lawlor, Ph.D., Director

Central Neuropsychiatric Association, 128 East Milltown Road, Wooster, OH 44691; tel. 330/345–6555; FAX. 330/345–6648; Dennis O. Helmuth, M.D., Secretary–Treasurer

Central Society for Clinical Research, Inc., 1228 West Nelson Street, Chicago, IL 60657; tel. 312/871–1618; Morton F. Arnsdorf, M.D., Secretary–Treasurer

Central Surgical Association, Northwestern University Medical School, Department of Surgery, 250 East Superior Street, Suite 201, Chicago, IL 60611–2950; tel. 312/908–8060; FAX. 312/908–7404; David L. Nahrwold, M.D., Secretary

Children's Rights Council (CRC), a/k/a National Council for Children's Rights, 220 Eye Street, N.E., Suite 140, Washington, DC 20002; tel. 202/547–6227; FAX. 202/546–4272; David L. Levy, Esq., President

Christian Record Services, Inc., 4444 South 52nd Street, Lincoln, NE 68516; tel. 402/488–0981; FAX. 402/488–7582; Rikki Stenbakken, Assistant to the President

College of American Pathologists, 325 Waukegan Road, Northfield, IL 60093–2750; tel. 847/832–7000; FAX. 847/832–8151; Lee VanBremen, Ph.D., Executive Vice President

College of Osteopathic Healthcare Executives, 5301 Wisconsin Avenue, N.W., Suite 630, Washington, DC 20015; tel. 202/686–1700; FAX. 202/686–7615; David Kushner, President

Commission on Accreditation of Rehabilitation Facilities, 4891 East Grant Road, Tucson, AZ 85712; tel. 520/325–1044; FAX. 520/318–1129; Donald E. Galvin, Ph.D., President, Chief Executive Officer

Commission on Recognition of Postsecondary Accreditation, Inc., One Dupont Circle, N.W., Suite 305, Washington, DC 20036; tel. 202/452–1433; FAX. 202/331–9571; Dorothy Fenwick, Ph.D., Executive Director

Committee of Interns and Residents, 386 Park Avenue, S., New York, NY 10016; tel. 212/725–5500; FAX. 212/779–2413; John Ronches, Executive Director

Cooley's Anemia Foundation, Inc., 129–09 26th Avenue, Suite 203, Flushing, NY 11354; tel. 800/522–7222; FAX. 718/321–3340; Gina Cioffi, Esq. National Executive Director

Corporate Angel Network, Inc., CAN (Arranges Free Air Transportation for Cancer Patients), Westchester County Airport, Building One, White Plains, NY 10604; tel. 914/328–1313; FAX. 914/328–3938; Laura Adler, Administrator

Council of Jewish Federations, Inc., 730 Broadway, New York, NY 10003; tel. 212/475–5000; FAX. 212/529–5842; Martin S. Kraar, Executive Vice President

Council of Medical Specialty Societies, 51 Sherwood Terrace, Suite Y, Lake Bluff, IL 60044; tel. 847/295–3456; FAX. 847/295–3759; Rebecca R. Gschwend, M.A., M.B.A., Executive Vice President

Council of State Administrators of Vocational Rehabilitation, P.O. Box 3776, Washington, DC 20007; tel. 202/638–4634; Jack G. Duncan, General Counsel, Rehabilitation Policy

Council on Education for Public Health, 1015 Fifteenth Street, N.W., Washington, DC 20005; tel. 202/789–1050; FAX. 202/789–1895; Patricia P. Evans, Executive Director

Council on Social Work Education, 1600 Duke Street, Alexandria, VA 22314; tel. 703/683–8080; FAX. 703/683–8099; Donald W. Beless, Ph.D., Executive Director

Crohn's and Colitis Foundation of America, Inc., 386 Park Avenue, S., 17th Floor, New York, NY 10016–8804; tel. 800/932–2423; FAX. 212/779–4098; Dr. Stephen E. Torkelsen, President, Chief Executive Officer

Cystic Fibrosis Foundation, 6931 Arlington Road, Bethesda, MD 20814; tel. 301/951–4422; FAX. 301/951–6378; Robert J. Beall, Ph.D., President/Chief Executive Officer

D

Damien Dutton Society for Leprosy Aid, Inc., 616 Bedford Avenue, Bellmore, NY 11710; tel. 516/221–5829; FAX. 516/221–5909; Howard E. Crouch, President

Delta Dental Plans Association, 211 East Chicago Avenue, Suite 800, Chicago, IL 60611; tel. 312/337–4707; FAX. 312/337–7991; James Bonk, President

Dermatology Foundation, 1560 Sherman Avenue, Evanston, IL 60201–4802; tel. 847/328–2256; FAX. 847/328–0509; Sandra Rahn Goldman, Executive Director

Dietary Managers Association, One Pierce Place, Suite 1220W, Itasca, IL 60143; tel. 630/775–9200; FAX. 630/775–9250; William St. John, President

Dysautonomia Foundation, Inc., 20 East 46th Street, Suite 302, New York, NY 10017; tel. 212/949–6644; FAX. 212/682–7625; Lenore F. Roseman, Executive Director

E

ECRI, 5200 Butler Pike, Plymouth Meeting, PA 19462; tel. 610/825–6000, ext. 140; FAX. 610/834–1275; Joel J. Nobel, M.D., President

Eastern Orthopaedic Association, Inc., Pier Five North, Suite 5D, Seven North Columbus Boulevard, Philadelphia, PA 19106–1486; tel. 215/351–4110; FAX. 215/351–1825; Elizabeth F. Capella, Executive Director

Educational Commission for Foreign Medical Graduates, 3624 Market Street, Philadelphia, PA 19104–2685; tel. 215/386–5900; FAX. 215/387–9963; Nancy E. Gary, M.D., President, Chief Executive Officer

Ehlers–Danlos National Foundation, P.O. Box 13157, Richmond, VA 23225; tel. 804/320–8192; FAX. 804/320–8192; Susan L. Stephenson, Vice President, Patient Advocate

Emergency Nurses Association, 216 Higgins Road, Park Ridge, IL 60068–5736; tel. 847/698–9400; FAX. 847/698–9406; H. Stephen Lieber, CAE, Executive Director

Environmental Management Association, 4350 Dipaolo Center, Suite C, Glenview, IL 60025; tel. 847/699–6362; FAX. 847/699–6369; Carl Wangman, President

Epilepsy Foundation, 1800 Sialas, Rocky Hill, CT 06067; tel. 860/721–9226; Linda Wallace

Epilepsy Foundation of America, 4351 Garden City Drive, Landover, MD 20785–2267; tel. 301/459–3700; FAX. 301/577–2684; Paulette V. Maehara, Chief Executive Officer

F

Family Service America, Inc., 11700 West Lake Park Drive, Milwaukee, WI 53224; tel. 414/359–1040; FAX. 414/359–1074; Peter B. Goldberg, President, Chief Executive Officer

Federation of American Health Systems, 1111 19th Street, N.W., Suite 402, Washington, DC 20036; tel. 202/833–3090; FAX. 202/861–0063; Ken Murphy, Assistant Vice President, Communications

Federation of State Medical Boards of the United States, Inc., 400 Fuller Wiser Road, Suite 300, Euless, TX 76039–3855; tel. 817/868–4000; FAX. 817/868–4099; James R. Winn, M.D., Executive Vice President

Financial Accounting Standards Board, 401 Merritt 7, P.O. Box 5116, Norwalk, CT 06856–5116; tel. 203/847–0700, ext. 250; FAX. 203/849–9714; Timothy S. Lucas, Director, Research, Technical Activities

Foundation for Chiropractic Education and Research, 1701 Clarendon Boulevard, Arlington, VA 22209; tel. 703/276–7445; FAX. 703/276–8178; Stephen R. Seaten, CAE, Executive Director

Foundation for Osteopathic Health Services, 5301 Wisconsin Avenue, N.W., Suite 630, Washington, DC 20015; tel. 202/686–1700; FAX. 202/686–7615; David Kushner, President

G

Gerontological Society of America, 1275 K Street, N.W., Suite 350, Washington, DC 20005; tel. 202/842–1275; FAX. 202/842–1150; Carol A. Schutz, Executive Director

Great Plains Health Alliance, Inc., 625 Third Street, Box 366, Phillipsburg, KS 67661; tel. 913/543–2111; FAX. 913/543–5098; Roger S. John, President, Chief Executive Officer

Greater Flint Area Hospital Assembly, 702 South Ballenger Highway, Flint, MI 48532–3803; tel. 810/766–8898; FAX. 810/766–6422; Marlene Soderstrom, Executive Director

Guide Dog Users, Inc., 57 Grandview Avenue, Watertown, MA 02172; tel. 617/926–9198; Kim Charlson, Editor

H

HEAR Center, 301 East Del Mar Boulevard, Pasadena, CA 91101; tel. 818/796–2016; FAX. 818/796–2320; Josephine Wilson, Executive Director

Health Industry Distributors Association, 66 Canal Center Plaza, Suite 520, Alexandria, VA 22314; tel. 703/549–4432; FAX. 703/549–6495; Edward Wissing, Chairman

Health Industry Manufacturers Association, 1200 G Street, N.W., Suite 400, Washington, DC 20005; tel. 202/783–8700; FAX. 202/783–8750; Alan H. Magazine, President

Health Insurance Association of America, 1025 Connecticut Avenue, N.W., Suite 1200, Washington, DC 20036–3998; tel. 202/223–7780; FAX. 202/223–7897; Gloria Tibby, Administrative Assistant

Healthcare Financial Management Association, Two Westbrook Corporate Center, Suite 700, Westchester, IL 60154; tel. 708/531–9600; FAX. 708/531–0032; Richard L. Clarke, F.H.F.M.A., President

Healthcare Information and Management Systems Society (HIMSS), 230 East Ohio Street, Suite 600, Chicago, IL 60611–3201; tel. 312/664–4467; FAX. 312/664–6143; John A. Page, Executive Director

Hispanic American Geriatrics Society, One Cutts Road, Durham, NH 03824–3102; tel. 603/868–5757; Eugene E. Tillock, Ed.D., President

Histochemical Society, Inc., Four Barlows Landing Road, Suite Eight, Pocasset, MA 02559; tel. 508/563–1155; FAX. 508/563–1211

Hospital Research and Educational Trust, One North Franklin, Chicago, IL 60606; tel. 312/422–2624; FAX. 312/422–4568; Deborah Bohr, Vice President

Huntington's Disease Society of America, Inc., 140 West 22nd Street, Sixth floor, New York, NY 10011–2420; tel. 212/242–1968; FAX. 212/243–2443; Claudia Archimede, Director, Grants, Administrative Programs

I

Institutes for the Achievement of Human Potential, 8801 Stenton Avenue, Philadelphia, PA 19118; tel. 215/233–2050; FAX. 215/233–3940; Roselise H. Wilkinson, M.D., Medical Director

InterHealth, 2550 University Avenue, W., St. Paul, MN 55114; tel. 612/646–5574; FAX. 612/646–2559; Benjamin Aune, President, Chief Executive Officer

International Childbirth Education Association, Inc., P.O. Box 20048, Minneapolis, MN 55420–0048; tel. 612/854–8660; FAX. 612/854–8772; Doris Olson, Administrator

International College of Surgeons/United States Section, 1516 North Lake Shore Drive, Chicago, IL 60610–1694; tel. 312/787–6274; FAX. 312/787–9289; Susan Zelner, Meeting and Convention Manager

International Council for Health, Physical Education, Recreation, Sport and Dance, 1900 Association Drive, Reston, VA 20191; tel. 703/476–3486; FAX. 703/476–9527; Dr. Dong Ja Yang, Secretary General

International Society for Clinical Laboratory Technology, 818 Olive Street, Suite 918, St. Louis, MO 63101–1598; tel. 314/241–1445; FAX. 314/241–1449; Mark S. Birenbaum, Ph.D., Administrator

Intravenous Nurses Society, Inc., 10 Fawcett Street, Fresh Pond Square, Cambridge, MA 02138; tel. 617/441–3008; FAX. 617/576–5452; Mary Larkin, Chief Executive Officer

J

John Milton Society for the Blind, 475 Riverside Drive, Suite 455, New York, NY 10115; tel. 212/870–3335; FAX. 212/870–3229; Darcy Quigley, Managing Director, Editor–in–Chief

Joint Commission on Accreditation of Healthcare Organizations, One Renaissance Boulevard, Oakbrook Terrace, IL 60181; tel. 630/792–5000; FAX. 630/792–5005; Dennis S. O'Leary, M.D., President

Juvenile Diabetes Foundation International, 432 Park Avenue, S., New York, NY 10016; tel. 212/889–7575; Gloria Pennington, Executive Director

L

Leukemia Society of America, Inc., 600 Third Avenue, New York, NY 10016; tel. 212/573–8484; FAX. 212/856–9686; Marshall Lichtman, M.D., Executive Vice President, Research

Long Term Acute Care Hospital Association of America, 1301 K Street, N.W., Suite 1100 East Tower, Washington, DC 20005–3317; tel. 202/296–4446;

Lupus Foundation of America, Inc., 1300 Piccard Drive, Suite 200, Rockville, MD 20850; tel. 301/670–9292; FAX. 301/670–9486; John Huber, Executive Director

Lutheran Health Systems/Lutheran Hospitals and Homes Society of America, Western Health Network, Box 6200, 4310 17th Avenue, S.W., Fargo, ND 58106–6200; tel. 701/277–7629; FAX. 701/277–7636; Steven R. Orr, Chairman, Chief Executive Officer

M

March of Dimes Birth Defects Foundation, 1275 Mamaroneck Avenue, White Plains, NY 10605; tel. 914/428–7100; FAX. 914/428–8203; Jennifer L. Howse, Ph.D., President

Maternity Center Association, 48 East 92nd Street, New York, NY 10128; tel. 212/369–7300; FAX. 212/369–8747; Maureen P. Corry, M.P.H., General Director

Medic Alert, 2323 Colorado Avenue, Turlock, CA 95382; tel. 800/825–3785; FAX. 209/668–8752; David Roth, News and Information Services Manager

Medical Group Management Association, 104 Inverness Terrace, E., Englewood, CO 80112–5306; tel. 303/799–1111; FAX. 303/643–4427; Thomas L. Adams, CAE, Chief Executive Officer

Medical Library Association, Six North Michigan Avenue, Suite 300, Chicago, IL 60602–4805; tel. 312/419–9094; FAX. 312/419–8950; Carla J. Funk, Executive Director

Medical Staff Recruitment Certification Program, Inc., 3150 Holcomb Road, Suite 205, Norcross, GA 30071; tel. 800/258–4081; FAX. 404/417–2176; Susan Woodbury

Mended Hearts, Inc., 7272 Greenville Avenue, Dallas, TX 75231; tel. 214/706–1442; FAX. 214/987–4334; Darla Bonham, Executive Director

Minnesota Healthcare Conference, 2221 University Avenue, S.E., Suite 425, Minneapolis, MN 55414; tel. 612/331–5571; FAX. 612/331–1001; Peggy Westby, Manager

Muscular Dystrophy Association, 3300 East Sunrise Drive, Tucson, AZ 85718; tel. 602/529–2000; FAX. 602/529–5300; Robert Ross, Senior Vice President and Executive Director

N

NSF International, 3475 Plymouth Road, P.O. Box 130140, Ann Arbor, MI 48113–0140; tel. 313/769–8010, ext. 201; FAX. 313/769–0109; Nina I. McClelland, Ph.D., President, Chief Executive Officer

National Academy of Sciences, National Research Council/Commission on Life Sciences, 2101 Constitution Avenue, N.W., NAS 343, Washington, DC 20418; tel. 202/334–2500; FAX. 202/334–1639; Paul Gilman, Ph.D., Executive Director

Section C

National Accreditation Council for Agencies Serving the Blind and Visually Handicapped, 15 East 40th Street, Suite 1004, New York, NY 10016; tel. 212/683–5068; FAX. 212/683–4475; Ruth Westman, Executive Director

National Accrediting Agency for Clinical Laboratory Sciences, 8410 West Bryn Mawr, Suite 670, Chicago, IL 60631–3402; tel. 773/714–8880; FAX. 773/714–8886; Olive M. Kimball, Executive Director

National Alliance for the Mentally Ill, 2101 Wilson Boulevard, Suite 302, Arlington, VA 22201; tel. 703/524–7600; FAX. 703/524–9094; Laurie Flynn, Executive Director

National Assembly on School Based Health Care, 6728 Old McLean Village Drive, McLean, VA 22101; tel. 703/556–0411; FAX. 703/556–8729; Jenny Mangelli, Account Manager

National Association Medical Staff Services, P.O. Box 23350, Knoxville, TN 37933–1350; tel. 423/531–3571; FAX. 423/531–9939; Robert A. Dengler, CAE, Interim Executive Director

National Association for Home Care, 228 Seventh Street, S.E., Washington, DC 20003; tel. 202/547–7424; FAX. 202/547–3540; Val J. Halamandaris, President

National Association for Medical Equipment Services (NAMES), 625 Slaters Lane, Suite 200, Alexandria, VA 22314–1171; tel. 703/836–6263; FAX. 703/836–6730; Steve Haracznak, Vice President, Communications and Member Relations

National Association for Music Therapy, Inc., 8455 Colesville Road, Suite 1000, Silver Spring, MD 20910; tel. 301/589–3300; FAX. 301/589–5175; Andrea Farbman, Ed.D., Executive Director

National Association for Practical Nurse Education and Service, Inc. (NAPNES), 1400 Spring Street, Suite 310, Silver Spring, MD 20910; tel. 301/588–2491; FAX. 301/588–2839; John H. Word, LPN, Executive Director

National Association of Boards of Pharmacy, 700 Busse Highway, Park Ridge, IL 60068; tel. 847/698–6227; FAX. 847/698–0124; Carmen A. Catizone, R.Ph., M.S., Executive Director, Secretary

National Association of Children's Hospitals and Related Institutions, Inc., 401 Wythe Street, Alexandria, VA 22314; tel. 703/684–1355; FAX. 703/684–1589; Lawrence A. McAndrews, President, Chief Executive Officer

National Association of Dental Assistants, 900 South Washington, Suite G13, Falls Church, VA 22046; tel. 703/237–8616; S. Young, Director

National Association of Dental Laboratories, (Includes National Board for Certification in Dental Laboratory Technology), 555 East Braddock Road, Alexandria, VA 22314–2199; tel. 703/683–5263; FAX. 703/549–4788; Robert W. Stanley, Executive Director

National Association of Health Services Executives, 8630 Fenton Street, Suite 126, Silver Spring, MD 20910; tel. 202/628–3953; FAX. 301/588–0011; Ozzie Jenkins, CMP, Executive Director

National Association of Hospital Hospitality Houses, Inc., 4013 West Jackson Street, Muncie, IN 47304; tel. 800/542–9730; FAX. 317/287–0321; Gerry Beck, Chairperson

National Association of Institutional Laundry Managers, 781 Twin Oaks Avenue, Chula Vista, CA 92010; tel. 619/420–1396; FAX. 619/420–1396; Robert J. Conard, Executive Secretary

National Association of Psychiatric Health Systems, 1317 F Street, N.W., Suite 301, Washington, DC 20004; tel. 202/393–6700, ext. 16; FAX. 202/783–6041; Mark J. Covall, Executive Director

National Association of Social Workers, Inc., 750 First Street, N.E., Suite 700, Washington, DC 20002; tel. 202/408–8600, ext. 233; FAX. 202/336–8311; James P. Brennan, LISW, ACSW, Senior Staff Associate, Health, Mental Health

National Association of State Mental Health Program Directors, 66 Canal Center Plaza, Suite 302, Alexandria, VA 22314; tel. 703/739–9333; FAX. 703/548–9517; Robert W. Glover, Ph.D., Executive Director

National Board for Respiratory Care, 8310 Nieman Road, Lenexa, KS 66214; tel. 913/599–4200; FAX. 913/541–0156; Steven K. Bryant, Executive Director

National Board of Medical Examiners, 3750 Market Street, Philadelphia, PA 19104; tel. 215/590–9500; FAX. 215/590–9755; L. Thompson Bowles, M.D., Ph.D., President

National Children's Eye Care Foundation, P.O. Box 795069, Dallas, TX 75379–5069; tel. 972/407–0404; FAX. 972/407–0616; Suzanne C. Beauchamp, Administrator

National Commission on Certification of Physician Assistants, 2845 Henderson Mill Road, N.E., Atlanta, GA 30341; tel. 404/493–9100; FAX. 404/493–7316; David L. Glazer, Executive Vice President, Managing Director

National Council on Alcoholism and Drug Dependence, Inc., 12 West 21st Street, New York, NY 10010; tel. 212/206–6770; FAX. 212/645–1690; Jeffrey Hon, Director, Public Information

National Council on Radiation Protection and Measurements, 7910 Woodmont Avenue, Suite 800, Bethesda, MD 20814; tel. 301/657–2652; FAX. 301/907–8768; W. Roger Ney, J.D., Executive Director

National Council on the Aging, Inc., 409 Third Street, S.W., Suite 200, Washington, DC 20024; tel. 202/479–1200; FAX. 202/479–0735; James Firman, President

National Dental Association, 5506 Connecticut Avenue, N.W., Suite 24–25, Washington, DC 20015; tel. 202/244–7555; FAX. 202/244–5992; Robert S. Johns, Executive Director

National Depressive and Manic–Depressive Association, 730 North Franklin Street, Suite 501, Chicago, IL 60610; tel. 312/642–0049; FAX. 312/642–7243; Donna DePaul–Kelly, Acting Executive Director

National Easter Seal Society, 230 West Monroe Street, Suite 1800, Chicago, IL 60606–4802; tel. 312/726–6200; FAX. 312/726–1494; James E. Williams, Jr., President

National Environmental Health Association, 720 South Colorado Boulevard, South Tower, Suite 970, Denver, CO 80222; tel. 303/756–9090; FAX. 303/691–9490; Nelson Fabian, Executive Director

National Federation of Catholic Physicians' Guilds, 850 Elm Grove Road, Elm Grove, WI 53122; tel. 414/784–3435; FAX. 414/782–8788; Robert H. Herzog, Executive Director

National Federation of Licensed Practical Nurses, 1418 Aversboro Road, Garner, NC 27529; tel. 919/779–0046; FAX. 919/779–5642; Charlene Barbour, Administrator

National Fire Protection Association, P.O. Box 9101, One Batterymarck Park, Quincy, MA 02269–9101; tel. 617/770–3000; FAX. 617/770–7110; Burton R. Klein, Health Care Fire Protection Engineer

National Gaucher Foundation, 11140 Rockville Pike, Suite 350, Rockville, MD 20852; tel. 301/816–1515; FAX. 301/816–1516; Rhonda Buyers, Executive Director

National Headache Foundation, 428 West St. James Place, Second Floor, Chicago, IL 60614–2750; tel. 800/843–2256; FAX. 773/525–7357; Suzanne Simons, Director, Administration and Development

National Health Council, Inc., 1730 M Street, N.W., Suite 500, Washington, DC 20036; tel. 202/785–3910; FAX. 202/785–5923; Myrl Weinberg, CAE, President

National Health Lawyers Association, 1120 Connecticut Avenue, N.W., Suite 950, Washington, DC 20036; tel. 202/833–1100; FAX. 202/833–1105; Marilou M. King, Esq., Executive Vice President, Chief Executive Officer

National Hemophilia Foundation, 110 Greene Street, Suite 303, New York, NY 10012; tel. 212/219–8180, ext. 3020; FAX. 212/966–9247; Stephen E. Bajard, Executive Director

National Institute for Jewish Hospice, Central Telephone Network, 8723 Alden Drive, Suite S148, Los Angeles, CA 90048; tel. 800/446–4448; Levana Lev, Executive Director

National Kidney Foundation, 30 East 33rd Street, New York, NY 10016; tel. 800/622–9010; FAX. 212/689–9261; John Davis, Executive Director

National League for Nursing, 350 Hudson Street, New York, NY 10014; tel. 212/989–9393; FAX. 212/989–9256; Patricia Moccia, Ph.D., RN, FAAN, Chief Executive Officer

National Medical Association, 1012 10th Street, N.W., Washington, DC 20001; tel. 202/347–1895; FAX. 202/842–3293; Lorraine Cole, Ph.D., Executive Director

National Mental Health Association, 1021 Prince Street, Alexandria, VA 22314–2971; tel. 703/684–7722; FAX. 703/684–5968; Michael M. Faenza, President, Chief Executive Officer

National Multiple Sclerosis Society, 733 Third Avenue, New York, NY 10017; tel. 212/986–3240; FAX. 212/986–7981; Dwayne Howell, Executive Vice President

National Nutrition Consortium, Inc., 24 Third Street, N.E., Suite 200, Washington, DC 20002; tel. 202/547–4819; Betty B. Blouin, Executive Director

National Osteopathic Women Physicians Association, 5301 Wisconsin Avenue, N.W., Suite 630, Washington, DC 20015; tel. 202/686–1700; FAX. 202/537–1362; David Kushner, Executive Director

National Parkinson Foundation, Inc., 1501 Northwest Ninth Avenue, Miami, FL 33136–1494; tel. 305/547–6666; FAX. 305/548–4403; Brian Morton, Controller

National Perinatal Association, 3500 East Fletcher Avenue, Suite 209, Tampa, FL 33613–4712; tel. 813/971–1008; FAX. 813/971–9306; Julie Leachman, Executive Director

National Recreation and Park Association, (Includes National Therapeutic Recreation Society), 2775 South Quincy Street, Suite 300, Arlington, VA 22206; tel. 703/820–4940; FAX. 703/671–6772; R. Dean Tice, Executive Director

National Registry in Clinical Chemistry, 815 15th Street, N.W., Suite 630, Washington, DC 20005; tel. 202/393–7140; FAX. 202/393–4059; Gilbert E. Smith, Ph.D, Executive Director

National Registry of Emergency Medical Technicians, 6610 Busch Boulevard, P.O. Box 29233, Columbus, OH 43229; tel. 614/888–4484; William E. Brown, Jr., Executive Director

National Rehabilitation Association, (Includes Nine National Associations and Sixty Affiliate Chapters), 633 South Washington Street, Alexandria, VA 22314; tel. 703/836–0850; FAX. 703/836–0848; Ann Tourigny Turner, Ph.D., CAE, Executive Director

National Resident Matching Program, 2450 N Street, N.W., Suite 201, Washington, DC 20037–1141; tel. 202/828–0676; FAX. 202/828–1121; Richard R. Randlett, Deputy Executive Director

National Rural Health Association, 1320 19th Street, N.W., Suite 350, Washington, DC 20036; tel. 202/232–6200; FAX. 202/232–1133; Jennifer Rapp, Government Affairs Director

National Safety Council, 1121 Spring Lake Drive, Itasca, IL 60143–3201, P.O. Box 558, Itasca, IL 60143–0558; tel. 630/285–1121; FAX. 630/285–0797; Kimberly D. Spoolstea, Customer Service

National Spinal Cord Injury Association, 545 Concord Avenue, Suite 29, Cambridge, MA 02138; tel. 617/441–8500; FAX. 617/441–3449; Dianne M. Barry, Executive Director

National Student Nurses' Association, Inc., 555 West 57th Street, Suite 1327, New York, NY 10019; tel. 212/581–2211; FAX. 212/581–2368; Diane J. Mancino, Ed.D., RN, CAE, Executive Director

National Tay–Sachs and Allied Diseases Association, 2001 Beacon Street, Brookline, MA 02146; tel. 617/277–4463; FAX. 617/277–0134; Debi Gutter, Executive Director

Neurosurgical Society of America, UCLA Division of Neurosurgery, 10833 Le Conte Avenue, Los Angeles, CA 90024; tel. 310/825–3998; FAX. 310/794–2147; Donald P. Becker, M.D., President

Neurotics Anonymous, 11140 Bainbridge Drive, Little Rock, AR 72212; tel. 501/221–2809; FAX. 501/221–2809; Grover Boydston, Chairman

New England Gerontological Association, One Cutts Road, Durham, NH 03824–3102; tel. 603/868–5757; Eugene E. Tillock, Ed.D., Executive Director

Section C

New England Healthcare Assembly, Inc., 500 Spaulding Turnpike, Suite W–310, Portsmouth, NH 03802–7100; tel. 603/422–6100; FAX. 603/422–6101; James S. Dolph, President

O

Osteogenesis Imperfecta Foundation, Inc., 804 West Diamond Avenue, Suite 210, Gaithersburg, MD 20878; tel. 301/947–0083; FAX. 301/947–0456; Leanna Jackson, Manager

Otosclerosis Study Group, 6465 Yale, Tulsa, OK 74136; Roger E. Wehrs, M.D., Secretary–Treasurer

P

Pan American Health Organization, 525 23rd Street, N.W., Washington, DC 20037; tel. 202/861–3200; Jose M. Paganini, Director HSS

Pathology Practice Association, 1225 Eighth Street, Suite 590, Sacramento, CA 95814; tel. 916/446–2651; J. Michael Allen, Executive Secretary

Physician Executive Management Center, 4014 Gunn Highway, Suite 160, Tampa, FL 33624–4787; tel. 813/963–1800; FAX. 813/264–2207; David R. Kirschman, President

Pilot Dogs, Inc., 625 West Town Street, Columbus, OH 43215; tel. 614/221–6367; FAX. 614/221–1577; J. Jay Gray, Executive Director

Prevent Blindness America, 500 East Remington Road, Schaumburg, IL 60173–4557; tel. 847/843–2020; FAX. 847/843–8458; Richard T. Hellner, President

Public Relations Society of America, 33 Irving Place, New York, NY 10003–2376; tel. 212/995–2230; FAX. 212/995–0757; Ray Gaulke, Chief Operating Officer

R

Radiological Society of North America, Inc., 2021 Spring Road, Suite 600, Oak Brook, IL 60521; tel. 630/571–2670; FAX. 630/571–7837; Delmar J. Stauffer, Executive Director

Recording for the Blind and Dyslexic, 20 Roszel Road, Princeton, NJ 08540; tel. 609/452–0606; FAX. 609/520–7990; Ritchie L. Geisel, President, Chief Executive Officer

Renal Physicians Association, 2011 Pennsylvania Avenue, N.W., Suite 800, Washington, DC 20006–1808; tel. 202/835–0436; FAX. 202/835–0443; Dale Singer, MHA, Executive Director

Robert Wood Johnson Foundation, P.O. Box 2316, Route One and College Road East, Princeton, NJ 08543–2316; tel. 609/452–8701; FAX. 609/987–8845; Edward Robbins, Proposal Manager

S

Shriners Hospitals for Children, P.O. Box 31356, Tampa, FL 33631–3356; tel. 813/281–0300, ext. 8163; FAX. 813/281–8113; Lee M. Woodfin, Executive Secretary

Sickle Cell Disease Foundation of Greater New York, 127 West 127th Street, Suite 421, New York, NY 10027; tel. 212/865–1500; FAX. 212/865–0917; Beryl Murray, Executive Director

Society for Academic Emergency Medicine, 901 North Washington Avenue, Lansing, MI 48906; tel. 517/485–5484; FAX. 517/485–0801; Mary Ann Schropp, Executive Director

Society for Adolescent Medicine, Inc., 1916 Northwest Copper Oaks Circle, Blue Springs, MO 64015; tel. 816/224–8010; FAX. 816/224–8009; Edie Moore, Administrative Director

Society for Health and Human Values, 6728 Old McLean Village Drive, McLean, VA 22101; tel. 703/556–9222; FAX. 703/556–8729; George K. Degnon, Executive Director

Society for Healthcare Consumer Advocacy, One North Franklin, Chicago, IL 60606; tel. 312/422–3999; FAX. 312/422–4580; Richard Koepke, Director

Society for Healthcare Strategy and Market Development, One North Franklin, 31st Floor, Chicago, IL 60606; tel. 312/422–3888; FAX. 312/422–4579; Lauren A. Barnett, Executive Director

Society for Occupational and Environmental Health, 6728 Old McLean Village Drive, McLean, VA 22101; tel. 703/556–9222; FAX. 703/556–8729; Marge Degnon, Executive Director

Society for Pediatric Pathology, 6728 Old McLean Village Drive, McLean, VA 22101; tel. 703/556–9222; FAX. 703/556–8729; Marge Degnon, Executive Director

Society for Social Work Administrators in Health Care, One North Franklin, Chicago, IL 60606–3401; tel. 312/422–3771; FAX. 312/422–4580; Richard Koepke, Executive Director

Society of Critical Care Medicine, 8101 East Kaiser Boulevard, Anaheim, CA 92808–2214; tel. 714/282–6000; FAX. 714/282–6050; Norma J. Shoemaker, M.N., Executive Director

Society of Neurological Surgeons, New England Medical Center, Department of Neurosurgery, 750 Washington Street, P.O. Box 178, Boston, MA 02111; tel. 617/636–5858; William Shucart, M.D., Secretary

Society of Nuclear Medicine, 1850 Samuel Morse Drive, Reston, VA 22090; tel. 703/708–9000; FAX. 703/708–9015; Torry Mark Sansone, Executive Director

Society of University Otolaryngologists–Head and Neck Surgeons, Joint Center for Otolaryngology, Harvard Medical School, 333 Longwood Avenue, Boston, MA 02115; tel. 617/732–7003; FAX. 617/217–1372; Marvin Fried, M.D., Secretary–Treasurer

Southeastern Healthcare Association, 1345 Carmichael Way, P.O. Box 11126, Montgomery, AL 36111–0126; tel. 800/952–0086; FAX. 205/260–0023; Tommy R. McDougal, FACHE, President

T

Technologist Section, Society of Nuclear Medicine, 1850 Samuel Morse Drive, Reston, VA 22090; tel. 703/708–9000, ext. 241; FAX. 703/708–9015; Virginia M. Pappas, Administrator

The American Association of Immunologists, 9650 Rockville Pike, Bethesda, MD 20814; tel. 301/530–7178; FAX. 301/571–1816; M. Michele Hogan, Ph.D., Executive Director

The American Board of Obstetrics and Gynecology, Inc., 2915 Vine Street, Dallas, TX 75204–1069; tel. 214/871–1619; FAX. 214/871–1943; Dr. Norman F. Gant, Executive Director

The American Board of Plastic Surgery, Inc., Seven Penn Center, Suite 400, 1635 Market Street, Philadelphia, PA 19103–2204; tel. 215/587–9322; Kathleen H. Lemly, Administrative Assistant

The American Board of Professional Disability Consultants, 1350 Beverly Road, Suite 115–327, McLean, VA 22101; tel. 703/790–8644; Taras J. Cerkevitch, Ph.D., Director, Operations

The American Orthopaedic Association, 6300 North River Road, Suite 300, Rosemont, IL 60018–4263; tel. 847/318–7330; FAX. 847/318–7339; Hildegard A. Weiler, Executive Director

The Arc, Formerly Association for Retarded Citizens, 500 East Border Street, Suite 300, Arlington, TX 76011; tel. 817/640–0204; FAX. 817/277–3491; Al Abeson, Ed.D., Executive Director

The Association for Research in Vision and Ophthalmology, 9650 Rockville Pike, Suite 1500, Bethesda, MD 20814–3998; tel. 301/571–1844; FAX. 301/571–8311; Joanne G. Angle, Executive Director

The Association of Medical Illustrators, 1819 Peachtree Street, N.E., Suite 712, Atlanta, GA 30309; tel. 404/350–7900; FAX. 404/351–3348; William H. Just, Executive Director

The Association of Women's Health, Obstetric, and Neonatal Nurses, 700 14th Street, N.W., Suite 600, Washington, DC 20005–2019; tel. 202/662–1600, ext. 1608; FAX. 202/737–0575; Gail G. Kincaide, Executive Director

The Duke Endowment, 100 North Tryon Street, Suite 3500, Charlotte, NC 28202; tel. 704/376–0291; FAX. 704/376–9336; Jere W. Witherspoon, Executive Director

The Endocrine Society, 4350 East West Highway, Suite 500, Bethesda, MD 20814–4410; tel. 301/941–0200; FAX. 301/941–0259; Sean Tipton, Director, Public Affairs

The Foundation Fighting Blindness, Executive Plaza I, Suite 800, 11350 McCormick Road, Hunt Valley, MD 21031–1014; tel. 800/683–5555; FAX. 410/771–9470; Robert M. Gray, Chief Executive Officer

The Foundation for Ichthyosis and Related Skin Types, Inc., (F.I.R.S.T.), P.O. Box 20921, Raleigh, NC 27619–0921; tel. 919/782–5728; FAX. 919/781–0679; Nicholas Gattuccio, Executive Director

The Healthcare Forum, 425 Market Street, 16th Floor, San Francisco, CA 94105; tel. 415/356–4300; FAX. 415/356–9300; Kathryn E. Johnson, President, Chief Executive Officer

The Institute for Rehabilitation and Research, Administration, 1333 Moursund, Houston, TX 77030; tel. 713/799–5000; FAX. 713/799–7095; Louisa Adelung, Chief Executive Officer

The Orton Dyslexia Society, Chester Building, Suite 382, 8600 LaSalle Road, Baltimore, MD 21286; tel. 410/296–0232; FAX. 410/321–5069; Susan Brickley, Director, Marketing and Development

The Points of Light Foundation, 1737 H Street, N.W., Washington, DC 20006; tel. 202/223–9186; FAX. 202/223–9256; Virginia Faulkner, Information Representative

The Salvation Army National Corporation, 615 Slaters Lane, P.O. Box 269, Alexandria, VA 22313; tel. 703/684–5500; FAX. 703/684–3478; Commissioner Robert A. Watson, National Commander

The Seeing Eye, Inc., Washington Valley Road, Box 375, Morristown, NJ 07963–0375; tel. 201/539–4425; FAX. 201/539–0922; Kenneth Rosenthal, President

The Southwestern Surgical Congress, 401 North Michigan Avenue, Chicago, IL 60611–4267; tel. 312/527–6667; FAX. 312/321–6869; Thomas E. Stautzenbach, Executive Director

U

United Cerebral Palsy Associations, Inc., 1660 L Street, N.W., Suite 700, Washington, DC 20036; tel. 800/872–5827; Michael Morris, Executive Director

Section C

United Methodist Association of Health and Welfare Ministries, 601 West Riverview Avenue, Dayton, OH 45406–5543; tel. 937/227–9494; FAX. 937/227–9493; Dean W. Pulliam, President, Chief Executive Officer

United Ostomy Association, Inc., 36 Executive Park, Suite 120, Irvine, CA 92714; tel. 800/826–0826; FAX. 714/660–9262; Darlene A. Smith, Executive Director

United Parkinson Foundation, 833 West Washington Boulevard, Chicago, IL 60607; tel. 312/733–1893; FAX. 312/733–1896; Judy Rosner, Executive Director

United States Pharmacopeial Convention, Inc., 12601 Twinbrook Parkway, Rockville, MD 20852; tel. 301/881–0666; FAX. 301/816–8299; Jerome A. Halperin, Executive Vice President

United Way of America, 701 North Fairfax Street, Alexandria, VA 22314–2045; tel. 703/836–7100; FAX. 703/683–7840; William Aramony, President

W

W. K. Kellogg Foundation, One Michigan Avenue East, Battle Creek, MI 49017–4058; tel. 616/968–1611; FAX. 616/968–0413; Robert A. DeVries, Program Director

Western Orthopaedic Association, 2975 Treat Boulevard, Suite D–4, Concord, CA 94518; tel. 510/671–2164; FAX. 510/671–2012; Susan Hanf, Executive Director

Western Surgical Association, Mayo Clinic, 200 First Street, S.W., Rochester, MN 55905; Jon A. VanHeerden, M.D., Secretary

Healthfinder

The healthfinder is composed of two listing types: toll–free numbers for health information and federal health information centers and clearinghouses. Toll–free numbers are denoted with the letter A and federal numbers are denoted with the letter B. Toll–free numbers are listed first, followed by the federal numbers.

This file was released in March 1996. This document is revised annually.

This Federal document is in the public domain, but is distributed subject to two conditions: 1) Any person or organization posting and/or distributing this document in electronic or paper form MUST respect the integrity of the document and post or distribute it ONLY in its entirety, including this paragraph, and without any change whatsoever; and 2) Any person or organization either posting or distributing this document MUST agree to post and/or distribute future editions of the document in the same manner as this edition to ensure that the most current information is made available to those parties who received the earlier version.

At the time of publication, the 1997 healthfinder list was not available. If you would like more information, contact the National Health Information Center at 800/336–4797 or through the internet at nhic–nt:health.org.

TOLL–FREE NUMBERS FOR HEALTH INFORMATION

This Healthfinder lists selected toll–free numbers and describes organizations that provide health–related information. The numbers do not diagnose or recommend treatment for any disease. Some offer recorded information; others provide personalized counseling, referrals, and/or written materials. Unless otherwise stated, numbers can be reached within the continental United States Monday through Friday, and hours of operation are eastern time. Numbers that operate 24 hours a day can be reached 7 days a week unless otherwise noted.

This Healthfinder is one in a series of publications, on a variety of topics, prepared by the National Health Information Center (NHIC). NHIC is a service of the Office of Disease Prevention and Health Promotion, Public Health Service, U.S. Department of Health and Human Services. The information contained on the following pages in no way should be construed as an endorsement, real or implied, by the U.S. Department of Health and Human Services.

ADOPTION

A–1. Bethany Christian Services
(800)238–4269
Services for women considering adoption as an option. Free counseling. Housing is available. 8 a.m.–12 midnight, every day. (See also B–24)

A–2. National Adoption Center
(800)TO–ADOPT
(215)735–9988
Expands adoption opportunities throughout the United States, particularly for children with special needs. Links all State adoption agencies through a telecommunication network. Addresses adoption and child welfare issues. 9 a.m.–5 p.m.

AGING

Eldercare Locator
(800)677 1116
Provides referrals to local resources nationwide. 9 a.m. 11 p.m. (Eastern)

A–3. National Institute on Aging Information Center
(800)222–2225
(800)222–4225 (TTY)
(301)589–3014 (Fax)
Provides publications on health topics of interest to older adults, to the public, and to doctors, nurses, social activities directors, and health educators. 8:30 a.m.–5 p.m. (See also A–16, A–17, A–18, A–81, B–1)

AIDS/HIV

A–4. AIDS Clinical Trials Information Service
(800)874–2572
(800)243–7012 (TTY/TDD)
(301)217 0023
(301)738 6616 (Fax)
Sponsored by the Centers for Disease Control and Prevention, the Food and Drug Administration, the National Institute of Allergy and Infectious Diseases, and the National Library of Medicine. Provides current information on federally and privately sponsored clinical trials for AIDS patients and others with HIV infection and on the drugs used in those trials. All calls are confidential. Spanish–speaking operators available. 9 a.m.–7 p.m.

A–5. CDC National AIDS Clearinghouse
(800)458–5231
(800)243–7012 (TDD)
(301)217 0023
(301)738–6616 (Fax)
(800)458 5231 (NAC Fax–Back Service)
aidsinfo@cdcnac.aspensys.com (E–Mail)
Sponsored by the Centers for Disease Control and Prevention. A national reference, referral, and distribution service for HIV/AIDS–related information. Answers questions and provides technical assistance; distributes published HIV–related materials including current information on scientific findings, CDC guidelines, and trends in the HIV epidemic; and provides specific information on AIDS–related organizations, educational materials, funding opportunities, and other topics. Services include a 24–hour fax–back service for HIV/AIDS–related information and the Business and Labor Resource Service for resources, technical assistance, publications, and referrals concerning managing AIDS in the workplace. Provides information and publications in English and Spanish. 9 a.m.–7 p.m. (See also B–3)

A–6. CDC National AIDS Hotline
(800)342–2437 (English)
(800)344–7432 (Spanish)
(800)243–7889 (TDD)
Sponsored by the Centers for Disease Control and Prevention. Provides information to the public on prevention and spread of HIV/AIDS. The first toll–free number provides 24–hour service; the second number provides service in Spanish 8 a.m.–2 a.m., everyday except holidays. The third toll–free number is available 10 a.m.–10 p.m., Monday–Friday.

HIV/AIDS Treatment Information Service
(800)HIV 0440
(800)243 7012 (TDD)
(301)217 0023
(301)738 6616 (Fax)
Sponsored by the CDC National AIDS Clearinghouse. Provides timely, accurate treatment information on HIV and AIDS. Answers questions about treatment of HIV disease; distributes copies of federally approved HIV/AIDS treatment guidelines and information; provides services in Spanish and English. 9 a.m. 7 p.m. All calls are confidential.

A–7. National Indian AIDS Hotline
(800)283–2437
(510)444–2051
(510)444–1593 (Fax)
Sponsored by the National Native American AIDS Prevention Center. Provides technical assistance, printed materials and information about AIDS and AIDS prevention in the Native American community. 8:30 a.m.–12 p.m. and 1 p.m.–5 p.m. (Pacific). Leave recorded message after hours.

A–8. Project Inform HIV/AIDS Treatment Hotline
(800)822–7422
(415)558–9051
Provides treatment information and referral for HIV–infected individuals. Information on clinical trials. No diagnosis. 10 a.m.–4 p.m., Monday–Saturday (Pacific).

ALCOHOL ABUSE

See also DRUG ABUSE

A–9. ADCARE Hospital Helpline
(800)ALCOHOL
Provides information and referral for alcohol and other drug concerns. Operates 24 hours.

A–10. Al–Anon Family Group Headquarters
(800)356–9996
Al–Anon and Alateen provide help for families and friends of alcoholics. The headquarters provides literature and refers people who need assistance to local meetings. 9 a.m.–4:30 p.m.

A–11. Alcohol and Drug Helpline
(800)821–4357
(801)272–4357
Sponsored by Pioneer Health Care. Provides referrals to local facilities where adolescents and adults can seek help. Operates 24 hours.

A–12. American Council on Alcoholism
(800)527–5344
(410)889–0297 (Fax)
Offers information and sources for alcoholism treatment to callers concerned about excessive drinking of someone close to them. 9 a.m.–5 p.m.

A–13. National Clearinghouse for Alcohol and Drug Information
(800)729–6686
(301)468–2600
(800)487–4889 (TTY/TDD)
(301)230–2867 (TTY/TDD)
(301)468–6433 (Fax)
Sponsored by the Center for Substance Abuse Prevention, Substance Abuse and Mental Health Services Administration. Gathers and disseminates information on alcohol and other drug–related subjects, including tobacco. Distributes publications. Services include subject searches and provision of statistics and other information. Operates the Regional Alcohol and Drug Awareness Resource Network, a nationwide linkage of alcohol and other drug information centers. Maintains a library open to the public. 8 a.m.–7 p.m.

A–15. National Council on Alcoholism and Drug Dependence, Inc.
(800)622–2255
(212)206–6770
(212)645–1690 (Fax)
Refers to local affiliates for counseling and provides written information on alcoholism and drug dependence. The toll–free number operates 24 hours; the other number is staffed 9 a.m.–5 p.m.

ALLERGY/ASTHMA

See LUNG DISEASE/ASTHMA/ALLERGY

ALZHEIMER'S DISEASE

See also AGING

Section C

A-16. Alzheimer's Association
(800)272-3900
(312)335-8882 (TDD)
(312)335-1110 (Fax)
http://www.alz.org (World Wide Web)
Refers to local chapters and support groups. Offers basic information about Alzheimer's disease and related disorders including research, drug treatments and clinical trials, warning signs of the disease, and caregiving information. Printed materials are available in English and Spanish. Spanish-speaking operators are available. The information and referral line is available 24 hours; operators staff the line 8:30 a.m.-5 p.m. Central, M-F. Leave message after hours.

A-17. Alzheimer's Disease Education and Referral Center
(800)438-4380
(301)495-3334 (Fax)
adear@alzheimers.org (E-mail)
Sponsored by the National Institute on Aging. Provides information and publications on Alzheimer's disease. 8:30 a.m.-5 p.m.

ARTHRITIS

A-18. Arthritis Foundation Information Line
(800)283-7800
Provides information about arthritis and referrals to local chapters. 24 hours. (See also B-7)

Lyme Disease Foundation, Inc.
(800)886 5963
Services include public education; supporting research relating to the condition; guiding and supporting self-help groups; and providing medical referrals. Distributes brochures on Lyme disease and reprints of scientific articles.

AUDIOVISUALS

See LIBRARY SERVICES

AUTISM

See CHILD DEVELOPMENT

BONE MARROW

See CANCER

CANCER

A-19. American Cancer Society Response Line
(800)227-2345 (Voice/TDD/TT)
Provides information and publications about cancer and pain management. Offers support services to cancer patients. Through the One-Day Memorial Response Service, donors can make contributions, during or after hours, in memory of a friend or loved one to help American Cancer Society Programs. 8:30 a.m. 4:30 p.m.

A-20. Cancer Information Service
(800)422-6237
Provides information about cancer and cancer-related resources to patients, the public, and health professionals. Inquiries are handled by trained information specialists. Spanish-speaking staff members are available. Distributes free publications from the National Cancer Institute. Operates 9 a.m.-7 p.m.

A-21. National Marrow Donor Program
(800)MARROW-2
Sponsored by the National Heart, Lung, and Blood Institute and the Department of the Navy. Provides multilingual information on donating marrow and the transplant process. Also provides information on donor centers in the caller's area. Professional staff answer questions from 8 a.m.-6 p.m. (Central); recorded message at all other times. (See also A-117)

Susan G. Komen Breast Cancer Foundation
(800)IM AWARE
Organizes breast health seminars throughout the country and provides education material about breast cancer, mammo-graphy, and breast self-examination.

A-22. Y-Me National Breast Cancer Organization
(800)221-2141
(312)986-8228
Provides breast cancer patients with presurgery counseling, treatment information, peer support, self-help counseling, and patient literature. Also provides information to any and all women concerned about breast health and breast cancer. Y-ME has a matching caller program for men whose partners have been diagnosed with breast cancer. 9 a.m.-5 p.m. (Central). Local number operates 24 hours.

CEREBRAL PALSY

See RARE DISORDERS

CHEMICAL PRODUCTS/PESTICIDES

See also HOUSING

A-23. Chemtrec Non-Emergency Services Hotline
(800)262-8200
Provides nonemergency referrals to companies that manufacture chemicals and to Federal and State agencies for health and safety information and information regarding chemical regulations. 9 a.m.-6 p.m.

A-24. National Pesticide Telecommunications Network
(800)858-7378
Sponsored by the U.S. Environmental Protection Agency and Oregon State University. Provides information about a variety of pesticide-related subjects, including: pesticide product information; information on the recognition and management of pesticide poisonings; toxicology; environmental chemistry; referrals for laboratory analyses, investigation of pesticide incidents, and emergency treatment information; safety information; health and environmental effects; clean-up and disposal procedures. TDD capability. 6:30 a.m.-4:30 p.m. (Pacific); voice mail provided for off-hours calls. (See also B-23)

CHILD ABUSE/MISSING CHILDREN/MENTAL HEALTH

A-25. Boys Town National Hotline
(800)448-3000
(800)448-1833 (TDD)
Provides short-term intervention and counseling and refers callers to local community resources. Counsels on parent-child conflicts, family issues, suicide, pregnancy, runaway youth, physical and sexual abuse, and other issues that impact children and families. Spanish-speaking operators are available. TDD capability. Operates 24 hours.

A-26. Child Find of America, Inc.
(800)426-5678 (I-AM-LOST)
Searches for missing children under age 18 who are victims of parental abduction, stranger abduction, or who have run away. Provides safety prevention information. Operates 24 hours.

(800)292-9688 (A-WAY-OUT)
Provides unique crisis mediation program for parents contemplating abduction of their children, or who have already abducted their children and want to use Child Find Volunteer Family Mediators to resolve their custody dispute. Operates 24 hours.

A-27. CHILDHELP/IOF Foresters National Child Abuse Hotline
(800)4-A-CHILD
(800)2-A-CHILD (TDD)
Provides multilingual crisis intervention and professional counseling on child abuse and domestic violence issues. Gives referrals to local agencies offering counseling and other services related to child abuse, adult survivor issues, and domestic violence. Provides literature on child abuse in English and Spanish. Operates 24 hours.

A-28. Covenant House Nineline
(800)999-9999
Crisis line for youth, teens, and families. Locally based referrals throughout the United States. Help for youth and parents regarding drugs, abuse, homelessness, runaway children, and message relays. Operates 24 hours.

A-31. National Center for Missing and Exploited Children
(800)843-5678
(703)235-3900
(800)826-7653 (TDD)
(703)235-4067 (Fax)
Operates a hotline for reporting missing children and sightings of missing children. Offers assistance and training to law enforcement agents. Takes reports of sexually exploited children. Serves as the National Child Porn TipLine. Provides books and other publications on prevention and issues related to missing and sexually exploited children. Ability to serve callers in over 140 languages. Operates 24 hours.

A-29. National Child Safety Council Childwatch
(800)222-1464
Answers questions and distributes literature on safety, including drug abuse, household dangers, and electricity. Provides safety information to local police departments. Sponsor of the missing kids milk carton program. Operates 24 hours.

A-30. National Clearinghouse on Child Abuse and Neglect Information
(800)394-3366
(703)385-7565
(703)385-3206 (Fax)
nccanch@clark.net (E-mail)
Serves as a national resource for the acquisition and dissemination of child abuse and neglect materials and distributes a free publications catalog upon request. Maintains bibliographic databases of documents, audiovisuals, and national organizations. Services include searches of databases and annotated bibliographies on frequently requested topics. CD-ROM containing Clearinghouse databases is available free to qualified institutions. 8:30 a.m.-5 p.m. (See also B-11, B-12)

A-32. National Resource Center on Child Abuse and Neglect
(800)227-5242
Sponsored by the American Humane Association. Provides general information and statistics about child abuse. 8:30 a.m.-4:30 p.m., Monday Friday (Mountain).

A-33. National Runaway Switchboard
(800)621-4000
(800)621-0394 (TDD)
(312)929-5150 (Fax)
Provides crisis intervention and travel assistance information to runaways. Gives referrals to shelters nationwide. Also relays messages to, or sets up conference calls with, parents at the request of the child. Has access to AT&T Language Line. Operates 24 hours.

A-34. National Youth Crisis Hotline
(800)448-4663
Provides counseling and referrals to local drug treatment centers, shelters, and counseling services. Responds to youth dealing with pregnancy, molestation, suicide, and child abuse. Operates 24 hours.

CHILD DEVELOPMENT

Autism Society of America
(800)3AUTISM
(301)657 0869 (Fax)
Educates parents, professionals, and the public regarding autism; improves the welfare of people with autism; supports research regarding autism; and oversees over 200 local chapters nationwide.

A-36. Human Growth Foundation
(800)451-6434
(703)883-1773
Provides parent education and mutual support, funds research, and promotes public awareness of the physical and emotional problems of short-statured people. Offers brochures on child growth abnormalities. 8:30 a.m.-5 p.m.

Section C

CHILD EDUCATION

A–37. National Association for the Education of Young Children
(800)424–2460
(202)232–8777
(202)328–1846 (Fax)
The National Association for the Education of Young Children is neither a helpline nor hotline. The association publishes books, posters, and brochures for teachers and parents of young children, birth through age 8. Sponsors conferences and public awareness activities concerning quality programs for the education of young children. 9 a.m.–5 p.m.

CLEFT PALATE

See RARE DISORDERS

CYSTIC FIBROSIS

See RARE DISORDERS

DIABETES/DIGESTIVE DISEASES

A–38. American Diabetes Association
(800)232–3472
(703)549–1500
(703)549–6995 (Fax, Customer Service)
(800)ADA ORDER (Fax, Order Fulfillment)
Offers patient assistance in many areas, including general information about diabetes, nutrition, exercise, treatment, and referrals to diabetes medical professionals. For people with diabetes facing discrimination, the association offers referrals from a nationwide attorney's network and information on how to influence public leaders. The association also conducts a variety of patient activities, including educational seminars and workshops, culturally diverse programs, support groups, and youth programs. Spanish–speaking operators available. 8:30 a.m.–5 p.m. (See also B–16)

A–39. Crohn's and Colitis Foundation of America, Inc.
(800)932–2423
(800)343–3637 (Warehouse)
Provides educational materials on Crohn's disease and ulcerative colitis. Refers to local support groups and physicians. 9 a.m.–5 p.m. Recording after hours. Warehouse is open 8 a.m.–5 p.m.

A–40. Juvenile Diabetes Foundation International Hotline
(800)223–1138
(212)785–9500
Answers questions and provides brochures on diabetes. Refers to local chapters, physicians, and clinics. Chapters located worldwide. 9 a.m.–5 p.m.

DISABLING CONDITIONS

See also HEARING AND SPEECH

Americans with Disabilities Act Hotline
(800)514 0301
(800)514 0383 (TTY)
(202)514 6193 (Electronic Bulletin Board)
Sponsored by the U.S. Department of Justice. Provides a 24–hour recording of information on the Americans with Disabilities Act. The recording also allows callers to request publications. ADA Specialists available 10 a.m. 6 p.m. on Monday, Tuesday, Wednesday, and Friday and 1 p.m. 6 p.m. on Thursday.

A–41. Handicapped Media, Inc.
(800)321–8708 (Voice/TDD)
Provides information, referral on services, and advocacy. Operates 8 a.m.–5 p.m. (Mountain).

A–42. Heath Resource Center
(800)544–3284
(202)939–9320
Operates the national clearinghouse on postsecondary education for individuals with disabilities and on learning disabilities. 9 a.m.–5 p.m.

A–43. Job Accommodation Network
(800)ADA–Work (Voice/TDD)
(800)526–7234 (Voice/TDD)
(800)526–2262 (in Canada)
(800)DIAL–JAN (Electronic Bulletin Board)
(304)293–5407 (Fax)

Sponsored by the President's Commission on the Employment of People with Disabilities. Offers ideas for accommodating disabled persons in the workplace and information on the availability of accommodation aids and procedures. Services available in English, Spanish, and French. 8 a.m.–8 p.m., Monday–Thursday; 8 a.m.–5 p.m., Friday.

A–44. Medical Rehabilitation Education Foundation
(800)438–7342
Provides medical rehabilitation information and a referral service for help in locating rehabilitation facilities throughout the country. 8 a.m.–5 p.m.

A–45. National Center for Youth with Disabilities: Adolescent Health Program: University of Minnesota
(800)333–6293
(612)626–2825
(612)626–2134 (Fax)
(612)624–3939 (TDD)
NCYD is an information, policy, and resource center focusing on adolescents with chronic illnesses and disabilities and the issues surrounding their transition to adult life. Offers a number of publications, including a newsletter, Connections, and a series of annotated bibliographies, CYDLINE Reviews. Maintains the National Resource Library, a database containing abstracts of current research literature, information about model programs, training/educational materials, and a list of consultants. 8 a.m.–4:30 p.m. (Central). (See also B–18, B–19)

A–46. National Clearinghouse on Family Support and Children's Mental Health
(800)628–1696
(503)725–4040
(503)725–4165 (Fax)
(503)725–4180 (TDD)
Sponsored by the National Institute on Disability and Rehabilitation Research, U.S. Department of Education, and the Center for Mental Health Services, U.S. Department of Health and Human Services. Provides publications on parent/family support groups, financing, early intervention, various mental disorders, and other topics concerning children's mental health. Also offers a computerized data bank and a State by State resource file. Recording is operated 24 hours.

A–47. National Easter Seal Society
(800)221–6827
(312)726–6200
(312)726–1494 (Fax)
(312)726–4258 (TDD)
Through its 160 affiliates nationwide, provides rehabilitative and other support services to assist children and adults with disabilities to achieve their maximum independence. 8:30 a.m.–5 p.m. (Central).

A–48. National Information Center for Children and Youth with Disabilities
(800)695–0285 (Voice/TT)
(202)884–8200 (Voice/TT)
(202)884–8441 (Fax)
nichcy@capcon.net (Internet)
Sponsored by the U.S. Department of Education. Information and referral service dedicated to disabled children. 9 a.m.–5 p.m. or leave recorded message after hours.

A–49. National Information Clearinghouse for Infants with Disabilities and Life Threatening Conditions
(800)922–9234, ext. 201
Sponsored by the National Center for Child Abuse and Neglect, Administration on Children and Families, U.S. Department of Health and Human Services. Makes referrals to support groups and sources of financial, medical, and educational assistance for families having infants with disabilities (birth to age 3). Spanish–speaking operators available. 9 a.m.–5 p.m.

A–50. National Information System for Vietnam Veterans and their Families
(800)922–9234, ext. 401 (Voice/TDD)
Provides information and referral for Vietnam veterans having children with disabilities or special health care needs. Produces and disseminates fact sheets on health conditions common to Vietnam veterans' children and on advocacy topics. 9 a.m.–5 p.m.

A–51. National Rehabilitation Information Center (NARIC)
(800)346–2742 (Voice/TDD)
(301)588–9284 (Voice/TDD)
(301)587–1967 (Fax)
Sponsored by the National Institute on Disability and Rehabilitation Research. Collects and disseminates the results of federally funded research projects. The collection includes commercially published books, journal articles, and audiovisuals. Spanish–speaking operators available. 8 a.m.–6 p.m. (See also B–49)

Scoliosis Association
(800)800 0669
(407)994 4435 (Fax)
Provides information on scoliosis and related spinal deformities. [new entry 8/16 SM]

DOWN SYNDROME

See RARE DISORDERS

DRINKING WATER SAFETY

A–52. Safe Drinking Water Hotline
(800)426–4791
(202)260–8072 (Fax)
sdwa@epamail.epa.gov (E–mail)
Sponsored by the U.S. Environmental Protection Agency. Provides general and technical information on the Federal drinking water program and referrals to other organizations when appropriate. Does not provide site–specific information on local water quality, bottled water, or home water treatment units. Has the ability to communicate in English, Spanish, French, Lebanese, and Persian. 9 a.m.–5:30 p.m., weekdays, except Federal holidays.

DRUG ABUSE

See also ALCOHOL ABUSE and SUBSTANCE ABUSE

A–53. CSAP Workplace Helpline
(800)843–4971
Sponsored by the Center for Substance Abuse Prevention, Substance Abuse and Mental Health Services Administration. Offers information, publications, and referrals to corporations, businesses, industry, and national organizations on assessing drug abuse within an organization and developing and implementing drug abuse policy and programs. 9 a.m.–8 p.m.

A–54. Housing and Urban Development Drug Information and Strategy Clearinghouse
(800)578–3472
Promotes strategies for eradicating drugs and drug trafficking from public housing. Provides housing officials, residents, and community leaders a source for information and assistance on drug abuse prevention and trafficking control techniques. Maintains a database system consisting of national and community program descriptions, publications, research, and news articles. Provides resource lists. 8 a.m.–5 p.m. (See also B–21)

A–55. "Just Say No" International
(800)258–2766
(510)451–6666
Thirteen thousand clubs. Founded in 1985. Provides materials, technical assistance, and training to help children and teenagers lead healthy, productive, drug–free lives. The New Youth Power program builds on young people's resiliency, drawing on and encouraging the skills and attributes that allow young people to cope with challenges and adversity. Youth Power empowers youth to discover and hone their assets to succeed in all areas of their lives. 7 a.m.–5 p.m. (Pacific).

A–56. National Cocaine Hotline
(800)262–2463
Sponsored by the Phoenix House Foundation. Answers questions on cocaine, alcohol, and other drugs from users, their friends, and families. Provides referrals to drug rehabilitation centers. Operates 24 hours.

Section C

A–57. National Federation TARGET Resource Center
(800)366–6667
(816)464–5400
Sponsored by the National Federation of State High School Associations. Provides education and prevention materials on tobacco, alcohol, and other drugs, including steroids and other performance–enhancing drugs, and on other healthy lifestyle issues surrounding high school athletics and activities. Catalog available. 8 a.m.–4:30 p.m. (Central).

DYSLEXIA

See LEARNING DISORDERS

ENDOMETRIOSIS

See WOMEN

ENVIRONMENT

A–58. Indoor Air Quality Information Clearinghouse
(800)438–4318
Provides information on indoor air quality, including the health effects of passive smoke, formaldehyde, and various indoor air pollutants. 9 a.m.–5 p.m. (See also B–23, B–35)

EPILEPSY

See RARE DISORDERS

ETHICS

A–59. Joseph and Rose Kennedy Institute of Ethics National Reference Center for Bioethics Literature Georgetown University
(800)633–3849
(202)687–3885
(202)687–6770 (Fax)
medethx@guvm.ccf.georgetown.edu (E–mail)
Provides reference assistance and conducts free searches on bioethical topics. Produces a variety of publications, as well as the BIOETHICSLINE database on the MEDLARS information system. 9 a.m.–5 p.m., Monday, Wednesday, Thursday, Friday; 9 a.m.–9 p.m., Tuesday; 10 a.m.–3 p.m., Saturday, except summers and holidays.

FIRE PREVENTION

A–60. National Fire Protection Association
(800)344–3555 (Customer Service)
(617)770–3000
(617)984–7880 (TDD)
(617)770–0200 (Fax)
Develops fire protection codes and standards, fire safety education materials, and provides technical information on fire prevention, firefighting procedures, and the fire loss experience. 8:30 a.m.–5 p.m.

FITNESS

A–61. Aerobics and Fitness Foundation of America
(800)446–2322 (For Professionals)
(800)YOUR–BODY (Consumer Hotline)
Answers questions regarding safe and effective exercise programs and practices. Written health and fitness guidelines also available (shipping and handling charges may apply). 7:30 a.m.–5:30 p.m. (Pacific).

Consumer Fitness Hotline
(800)529 8227
Sponsored by the American Council on Exercise. Provides information on health and fitness, including information on how to start an exercise program. Answers specific questions concerning a variety of fitness topics. 8 a.m. 5 p.m. (Pacific)

A–62. YMCA of the USA
(800)872–9622
(312)977–9063 (Fax)
Provides information about YMCA services and locations of Ys in residential areas. 8 a.m.–5 p.m. (Central).

FOOD SAFETY

A–63. Food Labeling Hotline Meat and Poultry Hotline
(800)535–4555
Sponsored by the U.S. Department of Agriculture. Provides information on safe handling, preparation, and storage of meat, poultry, and eggs. Also provides tips on buying a turkey, holiday food safety, and understanding labels on meat and poultry. 10 a.m.–4 p.m. (See also B–26)

A–64. Seafood Hotline
(800)FDA–4010
(202)205–4314
http://vm.cfsan.fda.gov/list.html (WWW)
Sponsored by the Food and Drug Administration. Provides information on seafood buying, handling, and storage for home consumption. Also provides seafood publications and prerecorded seafood safety messages. Information available on food safety, chemicals and contaminants, food and color additives, biotechnology, food labeling, nutrition, health and disease, and women's health. Messages and publications available in Spanish. Staff are available for assistance 12 p.m.–4 p.m. (Eastern). Automated Hotline operates 24 hours.

FOOT HEALTH

American Podiatric Medical Association, Inc.
(800)FOOTCARE
(301)571–9200
(301)530–2752 (Fax)
Provides a variety of patient education literature on topics including specific foot problems and diseases, sports and fitness activities, and systemic disease manifestations in the foot and ankle. Operates 24 hours.

GENERAL HEALTH

A–65. Agency for Health Care Policy and Research Clearinghouse
(800)358–9295
(301)495–3453
Distributes lay and scientific publications produced by the agency, including clinical practice guidelines on a variety of topics, reports from the National Medical Expenditure Survey, and health care technology assessment reports. 9 a.m.–5 p.m. (See also B–28)

American Osteopathic Association
(800)621 1773
Provides materials on osteopathic medicine and patient education materials. Directories of osteopathic physicians and specialists are also available.

A–66. MedicAlert Foundation
(800)432–5378
(800)344–3226
(209)669–2495 (Fax)
Provides emergency service for people who cannot speak for themselves by means of a unique member number on a Medic-Alert bracelet or necklace. Operates 24 hours.

A–67. National Health Information Center
(800)336–4797
(301)565–4167
(301)984–4256 (Fax)
nhicinfo@health.org (E–Mail)
http://nhic–nt.health.org (World Wide Web)
Helps the public and health professionals locate health information through identification of health information resources, an information and referral system, and publications. Uses a database containing descriptions of health–related organizations to refer inquirers to the most appropriate resources. Does not diagnose medical conditions or give medical advice. Prepares and distributes publications and directories on health promotion and disease prevention topics.

GRIEF

A–68. Grief Recovery Helpline
(800)445–4808
Provides educational services on recovering from loss. 9 a.m.–5 p.m., Monday– Friday (Pacific).

HEADACHE/HEAD INJURY

A–70. Brain Injury Association, Inc.
(800)444–6443 (Family Helpline)
(202)296–6443 (Business office)
(202)296–8850 (Fax)
Formerly the National Head Injury Foundation. Dedicated to improving the quality of life of people with brain injuries and promoting prevention of brain injury. Provides information and resources for people with brain injury, their families, and professionals. Offers educational materials on the impact of brain injury, location of rehabilitative facilities, and availability of community services. 9 a.m.–5 p.m. (Eastern).

A–69. National Headache Foundation
(800)843–2256
(312)907–6278 (Fax)
Disseminates free information on headache causes and treatments, funds research, and sponsors public and professional education programs nationwide. Offers audio and videotapes, brochures, and other helpful materials for purchase. Organized a nationwide network of local support groups. 9 a.m.–5 p.m. (Central) Monday–Friday.

HEARING AND SPEECH

A–71. American Speech–Language–Hearing Association
(800)638–8255
(301)897–5700
Offers information on speech, language, and hearing disabilities. Also provides referrals to speech language pathologists and audiologists certified by the American Speech–Language–Hearing Association. 8:30 a.m.–5 p.m.

A–72. Deafness Research Foundation
(800)535–3323
(212)684–6556 (Voice/TDD)
(212)779–2125 (Fax)
Funds research into causes, treatment, and prevention of hearing loss and other ear disorders. Also offers resource and referral information on ear–related problems. 9 a.m.–5 p.m. (Eastern).

A–73. Dial A Hearing Screening Test
(800)222–3277 (Voice/TDD)
(610)543–2802 (Fax)
Sponsored by Occupational Hearing Services. Answers questions on hearing problems and makes referrals to local numbers for a 2–minute telephone hearing screening test, as well as for ear, nose, and throat specialists. Also makes referrals to organizations that have information on ear–related problems, including broken earing aids. 9 a.m.–5 p.m. (Eastern).

A–74. The Ear Foundation at Baptist Hospital
(800)545–4327
(615)329–7849
(615)329–7935 (Fax)
Committed to integration of hearing and balance impaired people into the mainstream of society through public awareness and medical education. Includes the Meniere's Network and Young EAR's Program. Provides brochure about Meniere's disease and other literature, including newsletters. 8:30 a.m.–4:30 p.m. (Central) or leave recorded message after hours.

A–75. Hear Now
(800)648–4327 (Voice/TDD)
(303)695–7797 (Voice/TDD)
(303)695–7789 (Fax)
Provides hearing aids and cochlear implants for deaf and hard of hearing individuals with limited financial resources. Collects used hearing aids. Applications for assistance available. 8 a.m.–4 p.m. (Mountain).

A–76. Hearing HelpLine
(800)EAR–WELL
(703)642–0580
(703)750–9302 (Fax)
Sponsored by the Better Hearing Institute.
Implements national public information programs on
hearing loss and available medical, surgical, hearing
aid, and rehabilitation assistance for millions with
uncorrected hearing problems. Provides information
on hearing loss and hearing help. 9 a.m.–5 p.m.

A–78. International Hearing Society
(800)521–5247
(810)478–4520 (Fax)
Provides general information on hearing aids and a
listing of local hearing aid specialists. 9 a.m.–5 p.m.

A–77. John Tracy Clinic
(800)522–4582 (Voice/TTY)
(213)749–1651 (Fax)
Provides free diagnostic, habilitative, and
educational services to preschool deaf children and
their families through onsite services and to the
preschool deaf and deaf–blind children through
worldwide correspondence courses in Spanish and
English. 8 a.m.–4 p.m. (Pacific). Leave recorded
message after hours.

National Family Association for Deaf–Blind
(800)255 0411, ext. 275
Provides information and resources; facilitates family
organizations in each state; and develops family/
professional partnerships to benefit people with
deaf–blindness.

**A–79. National Institute on Deafness and Other
Communication Disorders Information
Clearinghouse**
(800)241–1044
(800)241–1055 (TT)
Collects and disseminates information on hearing,
balance, smell, taste, voice, speech, and language
for health professionals, patients, people in industry,
and the public. Maintains a database of references
to brochures, books, articles, fact sheets,
organizations, and educational materials, which is a
subfile on the Combined Health Information
Database (CHID). Develops publications. 8:30
a.m.–5 p.m.

A–80. TRIPOD GRAPEVINE
(800)352–8888 (Voice/TDD in the U.S.)
(800)287–4763 (Voice/TDD in Canada)
(818)972 2090 (Fax)
tripodla@aol (E–Mail)
Offers information on deafness, including raising and
educating a deaf child. Refers callers to parents,
professionals, and other resources in their own
communities nationwide. 8 a.m.–5 p.m. (Pacific) or
leave recorded message after hours.

HEART DISEASE

A–81. American Heart Association
(800)242–8721
Provides English and Spanish publications and
information about heart and blood vessel diseases,
exercise, nutrition, and smoking cessation.
Additional information is available for minority and
senior citizen audiences. Callers are routed to local
AHA offices for additional local information. 9
a.m.–5 p.m.

**National Heart, Lung, and Blood Institute's High
Blood Pressure Program**
(800)575 WELL
Provides a 24–hour recording of information on high
blood pressure and high blood cholesterol in English
and Spanish.

HISTIOCYTOSIS

See RARE DISORDERS

HOMELESSNESS

**A–82. National Resource Center on
Homelessness and Mental Illness**
(800)444–7415
Sponsored by the Center for Mental Health Services,
Substance Abuse and Mental Health Services
Administration. Provides technical assistance and
information about services and housing for the
homeless and mentally ill population. 8 a.m.–5 p.m.

HORMONAL DISORDERS

Thyroid Foundation of America, Inc.
(800)832 8321
Provides health education and support for thyroid
patients and health professionals. Responds to
inquiries on all aspects of thyroid dysfunction.
Provides information on genetically related
autoimmune diseases including vitiligo, diabetes
mellitus, and pernicious anemia.

HOSPITAL/HOSPICE CARE

A–83. Children's Hospice International
(800)242–4453
(703)684–0330
Provides support system and information for health
care professionals, families, and the network of
organizations that offer hospice care to terminally ill
children. Distributes educational materials. 9:30
a.m.–5:30 p.m. [rev 8/14 SM]

A–84. Hill–Burton Hospital Free Care
(800)638–0742
(800)492–0359 (in MD)
Sponsored by the Bureau of Health Resources
Development, Health Resources and Services
Administration. Provides information on hospitals
and other health facilities participating in the
Hill–Burton Hospital Free Care Program. 9:30
a.m.–5:30 p.m. or leave recorded message after
hours.

A–85. Hospice Education Institute "Hospice Link"
(800)331–1620
(860)767–2746 (Fax)
Offers information and advice about hospice and
palliative care, makes referrals to local hospice and
palliative care programs nationwide, and offers
information and advice on grief support programs.
Maintains a current database of hospices and
palliative care units, publishes books and pamphlets,
offers continuing education. No medical advice or
psychological counseling offered, but "sympathetic
listening" is available to patients and families coping
with advanced illness and loss. 9 a.m.–4 p.m.

A–86. Shriners Hospital Referral Line
(800)237–5055
Gives information on free hospital care available to
children under 18 who need orthopedic care or burn
treatment. Sends application forms to requesters
who meet eligibility requirements for treatment
provided by 22 Shriners Hospitals in the United
States, Mexico, and Canada. 8 a.m.–5 p.m.

HOUSING

**See also CHEMICAL PRODUCTS/PESTICIDES,
LEAD**

A–87. Housing and Urban Development User
(800)245–2691
Disseminates publications for U.S. Department of
Housing and Urban Development's Office of Policy
Development and Research. Offers database
searches on housing research. Provides reports on
housing safety, housing for elderly and handicapped
persons, and lead–based paint. 8:30 a.m.–5:15
p.m. (See also B–34)

HUNTINGTON'S DISEASE

See RARE DISORDERS

IMMUNIZATION

CDC Immunization Hotline
(800)232 SHOT
Provides information on childhood immunizations
and specific vaccinations.

IMPOTENCE

A–88. Impotence Information Center
(800)843–4315
(800)543–9632
Provides free information to prospective patients
regarding the causes of and treatments for
impotence. Provides referrals to local physicians.
8:30 a.m.–5 p.m. (Central) or leave recorded
message after hours.

INSURANCE/MEDICARE/MEDICAID

A–90. DHHS Inspector General's Hotline
(800)HHS TIPS
Handles complaints regarding fraud, employee
misconduct, and waste and abuse of U.S.
Department of Health and Human Services' funds,
including medicare, and medicaid. 9 a.m.–8 p.m.

A–91. Medicare Issues Hotline
(800)638–6833
(800)820–1202 (TDD/TTY)
Sponsored by the Health Care Financing
Administration. Gives information on medicare/
medigap insurance and policies, answers general
questions on medicare problems, and sends free
medicare publications. Publications include: Your
Medicare Handbook, The Guide to Health Insurance
for People with Medicare, and publications related to
Mammograms, HMOs, Low Income Beneficiaries,
Hospice Benefits, and Nursing Homes. 8 a.m.–8
p.m.

A–92. National Insurance Consumer Helpline
(800)942–4242
Provides general information and answers questions
regarding life, health, and home and automobile
insurance. Free consumer publications available.
Spanish–speaking operators available. 8 a.m.–8
p.m. (Eastern).

Social Security Administration
(800)772 1213
Provides public information materials about the
Social Security and supplemental security income
(SSI) programs, as well as information on
entitlement to Medicare. Free pamphlets on Social
Security benefits, disability benefits, and
supplemental security income are available.

JUSTICE

**A–93. National Criminal Justice Reference
Service (NCJRS)**
(800)851–3420
(301)738–8895 (Electronic Bulletin Board)
Provides criminal justice research findings and
documents from bureaus within the Office of Justice
Programs, U.S. Department of Justice. The NCJRS
library collection contains more than 130,000
documents and is accessible online. Clearinghouse
resources and activities also can be accessed via
the NCJRS electronic bulletin board. 8:30 a.m.–7
p.m. Leave recorded message after hours.

KIDNEY DISEASE

See UROLOGICAL DISORDERS

LEAD

See also HOUSING

A–94. National Lead Information Hotline
(800)LEAD–FYI (Hotline)
(800)424–LEAD (Clearinghouse)
(800)526–5456 (TDD)
EHC@cais.com (E–mail)
cais.com (Internet gopher)
Hotline supplies a basic information packet to the
public in English or Spanish on lead poisoning and
prevention through a 24–hour automated response
system. Clearinghouse provides technical
information and answers in English or Spanish to
specific lead–related questions for private citizens
and professionals. 8:30 a.m.–5 p.m. (See also
B–34)

LEARNING DISORDERS

See also HANDICAPPING CONDITIONS

**Children and Adults with Attention Deficit
Disorders (CH.A.D.D.)**
(800)233 4050
Provides an information packet on attention deficit
disorders and information on joining CH.A.D.D.

A–95. The Orton Dyslexia Society
(800)222–3123
(410)296–0232
Clearinghouse that provides information on testing;
tutoring; and computers used to aid people with
dyslexia and related disorders and general
information. Operates 24 hours a day.

LIBRARY SERVICES

See also HANDICAPPING CONDITIONS

**A–96. Modern Talking Picture Service, Inc.
Captioned Films/Videos**
(800)237–6213 (Voice/TDD)
(800)538–5636 (Fax)
Provides free loan of captioned films and videos for
deaf and hearing impaired people. 9 a.m.–5 p.m.

Section C

A–99. National Library Service for the Blind and Physically Handicapped
(800)424–8567
(202)707–5100
(202)707–0744 (TDD)
(202)707–0712 (Fax)
A total of over 140 network libraries that work in cooperation with the Library of Congress to provide free library service to anyone who is unable to read standard print because of visual or physical impairment. Provides both audio and braille formats through a network of regional libraries. 8 a.m.–4:30 p.m.

A–100. Recording for the Blind and Dyslexic
(800)221–4792
Serves people who cannot read standard print because of a visual, perceptual or other physical disability. Service includes free lending library of academic textbooks on audio cassette and sale of books on computer diskette and specially adapted tape players and recorders. Provides information on becoming a registered borrower.

LIVER DISEASES

A–101. American Liver Foundation
(800)223–0179
(201)256–2550
Provides information, including fact sheets, and makes physician and support group referrals. Liver disease information brochures and information sheets available upon request. 9 a.m.–5 p.m.

Hepatitis Foundation International
(800)891 0707
(201)857 5044 (Fax)
Educates the public about the prevention, diagnosis and treatment of viral hepatitis. Disseminates a variety of materials on viral hepatitis.

LUNG DISEASE/ASTHMA/ALLERGY

American Lung Association
(800)586 4872
Provides information on such topics as air pollution, smoking, tuberculosis, lung hazards on the job, marijuana, asthma, emphysema, and other lung diseases. Some materials are available in Spanish.

A–102. Asthma and Allergy Foundation of America
(800) 7–ASTHMA (727–8462)
Provides a 24–hour recording for callers to request general information, publications and videotapes.

A–103. Asthma Information Line
(800)822–2762
(414)276–3349 (Fax)
Sponsored by the American Academy of Allergy, Asthma, and Immunology. Provides written materials on asthma and allergies and offers a printed listing of physician referrals. Operates 24 hours.

A–104. Lung Line National Jewish Center for Immuno–logy and Respiratory Medicine
(800)222–5864
(303)355–5864
(800)552–LUNG (LUNG FACTS)
(303)270–2150 (Fax)
http://www.njc.org (Internet)
Answers questions about asthma, emphysema, chronic bronchitis, allergies, juvenile rheumatoid arthritis, smoking, and other respiratory and immune system disorders. Questions answered by registered nurses. 8 a.m.–5 p.m. (Mountain). LUNG FACTS, a companion to LUNG LINE, is a 24–hour, 7–days–a–week automated information service. Using a touch–tone telephone, callers can choose among a selection of recorded topics on lung disease and immunological disorders.

ORAL HEALTH

American Dental Association
(800)947 4746
Distributes educational materials on dental health topics such as dentures, tooth decay, smoking, diet, oral care, and fluoridation.

MATERNAL AND INFANT HEALTH

A–105. La Leche League International
800)LA–LECHE
(708)519–7730
(708)519–0035 (Fax)
Provides breastfeeding information and mother–to–mother support for women who wish to breastfeed. Distributes and sells a wide variety of materials on breastfeeding and parenting. Also organizes training for health professionals and provides a reliable source for current breastfeeding research information through the Center for Breastfeeding Information. Catalogue free of charge upon request. 9 a.m.–5 p.m. (Central).

MEDICARE/MEDICAID

See INSURANCE/MEDICARE/MEDICAID

MENTAL HEALTH

See also CHILD ABUSE/MISSING CHILDREN/ MENTAL HEALTH

American Academy of Child and Adolescent Psychiatry
(800)333 7636
Distributes fact sheets on mental illnesses affecting youngsters.

A–106. Depression Awareness, Recognition, and Treatment (D/ART)
(800)421–4211
Sponsored by the National Institute of Mental Health. Provides a 24 hour recording for callers to request free brochures on clinical depression. Foreign language materials available upon request.

National Alliance for the Mentally Ill
(800)950 6264
Provides information on severe mental illness and its effects on families, support for the rights of patients and families, and help in starting local groups.

A–107. National Clearinghouse on Family Support and Children's Mental Health
(800)628–1696
(503)725–4040
(503)725–4165 (TTD)
(503)725–4180 (Fax)
Sponsored by the National Institute on Disability and Rehabilitation Research, U.S. Department of Education, and the Center for Mental Health Services, U.S. Department of Health and Human Services. Provides publications on parent/family support groups, financing, early intervention, various mental disorders, and other topics concerning children's mental health. Also offers a computerized databank and a State by State resource file. Recording operates 24 hours a day.

A–108. National Foundation for Depressive Illness
(800)248–4344
(212)268–4434 (Fax)
NAFDI@pipeline.com (E–mail)
A 24–hour recorded message describes symptoms of depression and manic depression and gives an address for more information and physician and support group referrals by State.

A–109. National Mental Health Association
(800)969–6642
(703)684–5968 (Fax)
Provides public education, direct services and advocacy for mental health and mental illness concerns in communities across the nation. Distributes information on various mental health topics and provides referrals to other organizations.

National Mental Health Services Clearinghouse
(800)789 2647
Provides referrals to individuals requesting mental health services within their communities. 9 a.m. 5:30 p.m. (Pacific)

National Mental Illness Screening Project
(800)262–4444
National Depression Screening Day (October 5) Site Locator Service Call September 5–October 5 to find a local free depression screening site. After October 5, call for the location of a local health facility that can provide mental health services.

A–110. National Resource Center on Homelessness and Mental Illness
(800)444–7415 [no change 8/16 SM]

See HOMELESSNESS

A–111. Panic Disorder Information Line
(800)64–PANIC
Sponsored by the National Institute of Mental Health. Provides educational materials on panic disorder symptoms, diagnosis, referral, and treatment to health care and mental health professionals and the public. Also disseminates lists of additional resource materials and organizations that can help callers locate a treatment professional. Spanish–speaking operators available. Operates 24 hours a day.

MINORITY HEALTH

A–112. Office of Minority Health Resource Center
(800)444–6472
Responds to consumer and professional inquiries on minority health–related topics by distributing materials, providing referrals, and identifying sources of technical assistance. Spanish– and Asian–speaking operators available. 9 a.m.–5 p.m. (See also B–42)

NUTRITION

A–113. American Dietetic Association's Consumer Nutrition Hotline
(800)366–1655
Provides consumers with direct and immediate access to reliable food and nutrition information. Callers may listen to recorded nutrition messages in English or Spanish, 8 a.m.–8 p.m. (Central). Registered dietitians (RDs) answer food and nutrition questions and provide referrals to RDs in the caller's area 9 a.m.–4 p.m. (Central). TDD available. (See also B–27)

A–114. American Institute for Cancer Research
(800)843–8114
Provides free educational publications about diet, nutrition, and cancer prevention, as well as a Nutrition Hotline staffed by registered dietitians. 9 a.m.–5 p.m.

A–115. National Dairy Council
(800)426–8271
(800)974–6455 (Fax)
(708)803–2077 (Fax)
Develops and provides educational materials on nutrition. 8:30 a.m.–4:30 p.m. (Central).

ORGAN DONATION

See also VISION and UROLOGICAL DISORDERS

A–116. The Living Bank
(800)528–2971
(713)961–0979 (Fax)
The Living Bank is a nonprofit organization established in 1969 to promote organ, tissue, and body donations through public education and registration of donors. Assistance is available in English and Spanish. Operates 24 hours.

A–117. National Marrow Donor Program

(800)MARROW–2

See CANCER

A–118. United Network for Organ Sharing
(800)243–6667
(804)330–8507 (Fax)
http://www.infi.net/shreorg/unos.html (World–Wide Web)
Offers information and referrals for organ donation and transplantation. Answers requests for organ donor cards. Operates 24 hours.

PARALYSIS AND SPINAL CORD INJURY

See also HANDICAPPING CONDITIONS, STROKE

A–119. American Paralysis Association
(800)225–0292
(201)912–9433 (Fax)
Raises money to fund world–wide research to find a cure for paralysis caused by spinal injuries and other central nervous system disorders. Provide information about spinal cord research. 9 a.m.–5 p.m.

A–120. National Rehabilitation Information Center
(800)346–2742 (Voice/TDD)
(301)588–9284 (Voice/TDD)
(301)587–1967 (Fax)
Provides research referrals and information on rehabilitation issues and concerns. Spanish–speaking interpreters available upon request. 8 a.m.–6 p.m.

A–121. National Spinal Cord Injury Association
(800)962–9629 (Members and individuals with spinal cord injuries; no vendors)
(617)441–8500 (Nonmembers, public, professionals)
Provides peer counseling to those with spinal cord injuries through local chapters and organizations. Provides information and referral service. 9 a.m.–5 p.m.

A–122. National Spinal Cord Injury Hotline
(800)526–3456
(410)366–2325 (Fax)
Financially supported by the Paralyzed Veterans of America. Offers information on spinal cord injuries and peer support to those with spinal cord injuries and their families. 24–hour answering service will page for emergency. 9 a.m.–5 p.m.

A–123. National Stroke Association
(800)STROKES
(303)771–1700
(303)771–1887 (TDD)
Provides both written and referral information to individuals, including stroke survivors, families, and health care providers on prevention, treatment, and rehabilitation. 8 a.m.–4:30 p.m., Monday–Thursday; 8 a.m.–4 p.m., Friday (Mountain).

Paralyzed Veterans of America
(800)424 8200
(800)795 4327 (TDD)
An organization for veterans of the armed forces who have experienced spinal cord injury or dysfunction. Advocates for quality health care and civil rights and opportunities for its members. Conducts research and disseminates information addressing spinal cord injury and dysfunction.

PARKINSON'S DISEASE

A–124. American Parkinson's Disease Association
(800)223–2732
(718)981–4399 (Fax)
Operates 51 information and referral centers throughout the United States. Raises funds for Parkinson's disease research and education. Provides information and referrals to patients and families. Multilingual educational literature available. 9 a.m.–5 p.m. (Eastern). Leave recorded message after hours.

A–125. National Parkinson Foundation, Inc.
(800)327–4545
(800)433–7022 (in FL)
(305)548–4403 (Fax)
A worldwide research, clinical, and therapeutic organization. Also provides physician references, support group systems, and educational materials in both English and Spanish. Professional staff answer questions about the disease from 9 a.m.–5 p.m., Monday–Friday; recorded messages at all other times.

PESTICIDES

See CHEMICAL PRODUCTS/PESTICIDES

PHYSICIANS

A–127. American Board of Medical Specialties
(800)776–2378
The ABMS is the umbrella organization for the 24 medical specialty boards authorized and recognized to certify physician specialists in the United States. As a service to the public, a toll–free number is provided to verify board certification of physicians certified by the Member Boards of ABMS from 9 a.m.–6 p.m.

PRACTITIONER REPORTING

A–128. USP Practitioners Reporting Network
(800)4–USP–PRN (487–7776)
(800)23–ERROR (Medication error)
Offers a service for health professionals to report problems with drugs, medical devices, radiopharmaceuticals, animal drugs, and actual or potential medication errors. Recording operates 24 hours a day; staff available 9 a.m.–4:30 p.m., Monday–Friday. Medication error telephone number records information 24 hours a day.

PREGNANCY/MISCARRIAGE

A–129. American Academy of Husband–Coached Childbirth
(800)4–ABIRTH
Provides free listing of teachers of the Bradley Method, including package of information and referral for local classes in natural childbirth. Books and videotapes may be ordered also. 9 a.m. 5 p.m. (Pacific). Leave recorded message after hours.

A–130. ASPO/Lamaze (American Society for Psychoprophylaxis in Obstetrics)
(800)368–4404
(202)857–1128
(202)223–4579 (Fax)
MThompso@SBA.Com (E–mail)
Operates a toll–free telephone service to provide consumers with information about prepared childbirth and how to locate a local ASPO–Certified Childbirth Educator. 9 a.m.–5 p.m. (Eastern).

A–131. International Childbirth Education Association
(800)624–4934 (Book Center orders)
(612)854–8660 (General information)
Provides referrals to local chapters and support groups, membership information, certification, and mail–order service. 7 a.m.–4:30 p.m. (Central).

A–132. Liberty Godparent Home
(800)542–4453
Provides a residential program for unwed mothers. Provides counseling referrals to local and national organizations and distributes brochures on request. An adoption agency is also on site. Operates 24 hours. [rev. 7/25/95 SR unsure re. wording for adoption agency]

RADON

A–133. Radon Hotline
(800)SOS–RADON
(800)526–5456 (TDD)
Operated by the National Safety Council. Provides a 24–hour recording for callers to request a brochure on reducing radon risks in the home and a listing of local contacts. (See also B–23, B–34)

RARE DISORDERS*

*A rare disorder is defined as a disorder that affects less than 1 percent of the population at any given time.

A–134. American Leprosy Missions (Hansen's Disease)
(800)543–3131
(803)271–7040
(803)271–7062 (Fax)
Answers questions and distributes materials on the disease. Also assists in raising funds for people with this disease. 8 a.m.–5 p.m.

A–135. The American Lupus Society
(800)331–1802
(805)339–0467 (Fax)
Provides a 24–hour recording for callers to leave their names and addresses to receive information on services provided.

A–136. American SIDS Institute
(800)232–7437
(800)847–7437 (in GA)
Answers inquiries from families and physicians, distributes literature, and makes referrals to other organizations. 8 a.m. 5 p.m. Leave recorded message after hours.

A–137. Amyotrophic Lateral Sclerosis Association (ALS, Lou Gehrig's Disease)
(800)782–4747
(818)340–2060 (Fax)
Provides names of support groups and locations of clinics and distributes literature. 8 a.m.–5 p.m. (Pacific). Leave recorded message after hours.

A–138. Batten's Disease Support and Research Association
(800)448–4570
Provides a 24 hour recording for callers to request information on Batten's Disease.

The CFIDS Association of America
(800)442 3437
Provides information on chronic Epstein–Barr Virus, myalgic encephalomyelitis, HBLV, and related disorders, such as interstitial cystitis, mitral valve prolapse, and vestibular problems.

A–139. Cleft Palate Foundation
(800)242–5338 (CLEFTLINE)
(412)481–1376
(412)481–0847 (Fax)
Provides information and referral to individuals and families affected by cleft lip, cleft palate, or other craniofacial birth defects. Referrals are made to local cleft palate/craniofacial teams for treatment and to parent/patient support groups. Free information on various aspects of clefting is available; some available in Spanish. CLEFTLINE operates 24 hours. Spanish–speaking operators available 8:30 a.m.–4:30 p.m., Monday–Friday.

A–140. Cooley's Anemia Foundation
(800)522–7222
(718)321–CURE
(718)321–3340 (Fax)
Provides information on patient care, research, fundraising, patient–support groups, and research grants. Makes referrals to local chapters and screening centers. 9 a.m.–5 p.m.

A–141. Cornelia de Lange Syndrome Foundation, Inc.
(800)223–8355
(800)753–2357
(203)693–0159
(203)693–6819 (Fax)
Promotes research and provides a variety of materials for families, friends, and professionals about this syndrome. Services include an international professional network, a newsletter, Family Support Program, and a Scientific Advisory Committee. 9 a.m.–4:30 p.m. (Eastern) Leave recorded message after hours.

A–142. Crohn's and Colitis Foundation of America, Inc.
(800)932–2423
(800)343–3637 (Warehouse) [rev 8/18 SM]
See DIABETES/DIGESTIVE DISEASES

A–143. Cystic Fibrosis Foundation
(800)344–4823
(301)951–6378 (Fax)
Responds to patient and family questions, offers literature, and provides referrals to local clinics. 8:30 a.m.–5:30 p.m.

A–144. Epilepsy Foundation of America
(800)332–1000
(800)213 5821 (Publications)
(301)459–3700
(301)577–2684 or 4941 (Fax)
Provides information on epilepsy and makes referrals to local chapters. Spanish–speaking operators available. 9 a.m.–5 p.m.

Epilepsy Information Service
(800)642 0500
Provides general information on epilepsy. Distributes pamphlets on epilepsy free of charge. 8 a.m. 5 p.m. (Eastern)

Fibromyalgia Network
(800)853 2929
(520)290 5550 (Fax)
Provides information on Fibromyalgia, Chronic Fatigue Syndrome, and Myofascial Pain Syndrome. Maintains state–by–state listings for support group and health professional referrals. 8 a.m. 5 p.m. (Mountain)

A–145. Histiocytosis Association
(800)548–2758
(609)589–6614 (Fax)
Provides patient and family support to those affected with any of the histiocytoses. Quarterly newsletter, information, brochures, networking directory, regional meetings, and funds research. Operates 8:30 a.m.–4 p.m., Monday–Friday. Voice mail at all other times.

Section C

A-146. Huntington's Disease Society of America, Inc.
(800)345-4372
(212)242-1968
(212)243-2443 (Fax)
Provides written and audiovisual materials pertaining to all aspects of Huntington's Disease; information and referral to local support groups, chapter social workers, physicians, nursing homes and a variety of other resources via local representatives; and support for research into the causes, treatment and cure of Huntington's Disease.

A-147. Lupus Foundation of America
(800)558-0121 (English)
(800)558 0231 (Spanish)
(301)670-9292
(301)670 9486 (Fax)
Answers basic questions about the disease and provides health professionals and patients and their families with information and literature. Refers to local affiliates. 9 a.m.-5 p.m. Recording 24 hours a day.

A-148. Meniere's Network
(800)545-4327
(see the Ear Foundation at Baptist Hospital, HEARING AND SPEECH)

Muscular Dystrophy Association
(800)572 1717
(520)529 5300 (Fax)
Provides information on 40 neuromuscular diseases, including the muscular dystrophies, motor neuron diseases, inflammatory myopathies, diseases of the neuromuscular junction, diseases of the peripheral nerve, metabolic diseases of the muscles, myopathies due to endocrine abnormalities, and certain other myopathies.

A-149. Myasthenia Gravis Foundation
(800)541-5454
(312)258-0461 (Fax)
Provides information regarding services for myasthenia patients, and patient and medical literature. Promotes public awareness. Funds research. 8:45 a.m.-4:45 p.m. (Central).

A-150. National Down Syndrome Congress
(800)232-6372
(404)633-2817 (Fax)
ndsc@charitiesusa.com (E-mail)
Responds to questions concerning all aspects of Down syndrome. Refers to local organizations. Information available in Spanish. 9 a.m.-5 p.m. (Eastern). Recording after hours.

A-151. National Down Syndrome Society Hotline
(800)221-4602
(212)460-9330
Sponsors internationally renowned scientific symposia. Advocates on behalf of families and individuals affected by this condition. Provides information and referral services through its toll-free hotline staffed by English and Spanish speakers. Develops educational materials, many of which are distributed free of charge.

A-153. National Lymphedema Network
(800)541-3259
Provides information on the prevention and management of primary and secondary lymphedema to the general public as well as health care professionals. Offers referrals to health care professionals and treatment centers, local support groups, and exercise programs. Provides a quarterly newsletter, resource guide, and information on support groups, conferences, and professional training courses. Leave recorded message.

A-154. National Multiple Sclerosis Society
(800)FIGHT-MS
(212)986-7981 (Fax)
Offers a 24-hour telephone message line. Staff members available to answer questions 11 a.m.-5 p.m., Monday-Thursday.

A-155. National Neurofibromatosis Foundation
(800)323-7938
(212)344-6633
(212)747-0004 (Fax)
Responds to inquiries from health professionals and patients and families. Makes referrals to physicians on clinical advisory board. 9 a.m.-5 p.m.

A-156. National Organization for Rare Disorders
(800)999-6673
(203)746-6518
(203)746-6481 (Fax)
(203)746-6927 (TDD)
A clearinghouse for information on over 3,000 rare diseases, offers networking programs linking patients and family members together, and administers several medication assistance programs for indigent patients. Fees charged for some services. 9 a.m.-5 p.m. (Eastern) Monday-Friday. Leave recorded message after hours.

A-157. National Reye's Syndrome Foundation
(800)233-7393
(419)636-2679
(419)636-3366 (Fax)
Provides awareness materials to the public and medical community, raises funds for research, and offers guidance and counseling to victims. 8 a.m.-5 p.m. Leave recorded message after hours.

A-159. National Sarcoidosis Foundation
(800)223-6429
Provides a 24 hour recording for callers to request information on sarcoidosis.

A-158. National Tuberous Sclerosis Association
(800)225-6872
(301)459-9888
(301)459-0394 (Fax)
ntsa@aol.com (Internet)
Answers questions about the disease and makes parent-to-parent contact referrals. Literature is provided to families and professionals. 8:30 a.m.-5 p.m.

Office of Orphan Products Development Food and Drug Administration
(800)300 7469
Disseminates information on orphan drugs and rare diseases; responds to inquiries from patients, health professionals, and pharmaceutical manufacturers, as well as the general public.

The Paget Foundation for Paget's Disease of Bone and Related Disorders
(800)23-PAGET
(212)229-1582
(212)229-1502 (Fax)
Provides educational literature on Paget's disease of bone, primary hyperparathyroidism and other disorders to patients and the medical community. Gives physician referrals. 9 a.m.-5 p.m. (Eastern).

A-167. Scleroderma Foundation, United
(800)722-HOPE
(408)728-2202
(408)728-3328 (Fax)
outreach@scleroderma.com (E-Mail)
Develops chapter and support groups, distributes printed materials, and provides patient support and information and medical reference lists. 8 a.m.-5 p.m. (Pacific).

A-160. Sickle Cell Disease Association of America, Inc.
(800)421-8453
Offers educational materials, referrals for client services, research support, and public awareness. 8:30 a.m.-5 p.m. (Pacific). Recording after hours and weekends.

A-161. SIDS Alliance
(800)221-SIDS (7437)
(410)653-8226
(410)653-8709 (Fax)
Hotline is available for parents who wish to discuss their concerns with a SIDS counselor, request additional information, and/or be connected to the local SIDS Affiliate for support services in their area. 9 a.m.-5 p.m. (Eastern). Phone line available 24 hours. (See also B-52)

A-162. Spina Bifida Association of America
(800)621-3141
(202)944-3285
(202)944-3295 (Fax)
Provides information to consumers and health professionals and referrals to local chapters. 9 a.m.-5 p.m.

A-163. Spondylitis Association of America (formerly the Ankylosing Spondylitis Association)
(800)777-8189
(818)981-1616
(818)981-9826 (Fax)
Provides information on ankylosing spondylitis, psoriatic arthritis, and Reiter's syndrome. 9 a.m.-5 p.m. (Pacific). Leave recorded message after hours.

A-164. Sturge-Weber Foundation
(800)627-5482
Provides list of publications, long-distance support groups, and referrals for families, friends, and professionals. 9 a.m.-3 p.m., Monday-Friday.

A-165. Tourette Syndrome Association, Inc.
(800)237-0717
(718)224-2999
(718)279-9596 (Fax)
Provides a 24-hour recording for callers to request information and leave name and address. To speak with a staff member, call the local number between 9 a.m.-5 p.m.

A-166. United Cerebral Palsy Association
(800)872-5827
(202)776-0406
(202)776-0414 (Fax)
Provides literature about cerebral palsy and related disorders. Responds to inquiries from people with cerebral palsy and related disorders, their families, and the public. Makes referrals to local affiliates. 8:30 a.m.-5:30 p.m.

REHABILITATION

See DISABLING CONDITIONS, PARALYSIS AND SPINAL CORD INJURY

RETINITIS PIGMENTOSA

See VISION

RURAL

A-168. Rural Information Center Health Service (RICHS)
(800)633-7701
(301)504-5547
(301)504-6856 (TTY/TDD)
(301)504-5181 (Fax)
ric@nalusda.gov (E-mail)
gopher://gopher.nalusda.gov (Internet)
Provides information and referrals to the public and to professionals on rural health issues. Performs brief, complimentary literature searches. 8 a.m.-4:30 p.m. (See also B-50)

SAFETY

See also CHEMICAL PRODUCTS/PESTICIDES

A-169. National Child Safety Council Childwatch
(800)222-1464
(see CHILD ABUSE/MISSING CHILDREN/MENTAL HEALTH)

A-170. National Highway Traffic Safety Administration Auto Safety Hotline
(800)424-9393
(202)366-0123
Provides information and referral on the effectiveness of occupant protection, such as safety belt use, child safety seats, and automobile recalls. Gives referrals to other Government agencies for consumer questions on warranties, service, automobile safety regulations, and reporting safety problems. 8 a.m.-4 p.m. (See also B-32)

A-171. National Institute for Occupational Safety and Health Technical Information Branch
(800)356-4674
Provides information on chemical and physical hazards in the workplace, training courses, publications, and the health hazard evaluation program. 9 a.m.-4 p.m. (See also B-36, B-44, B-48)

National Safety Council
(800)621 7615
Offers a safety training institute, a child safety club, home study courses in safety, and traffic and transportation safety services. Provides materials on all aspects of safety accident prevention, and prevention of occupational illnesses.

Section C

A–172. Office of Navigation Safety and Waterway Services U.S. Coast Guard Customer Infoline
(800)368–5647
(202)267–0780
(800)689–0816 (TDD/TT)
(202)267–6707 (TDD/TT)
Modem #703313591 (Navigation Center Bulletin Board)
http://www.dot.gov/affairs/index.htm (Internet)
Provides information on boating safety, including a kit for consumers, recalls on boating products, makes referrals to other organizations, and other Coast Guard missions. 8 a.m.–4 p.m.

A–173. U.S. Consumer Product Safety Commission Hotline
(800)638–2772
(800)638–8270 (TDD)
info@cpsc.gov (Internet)
Provides 24–hour messages on consumer product safety, including product hazards and product recalls. Covers only products used in and around the home, excluding automobiles, child safety seats, health care products, warranties, foods, drugs, cosmetics, boats, and firearms. (See also B–36, B–48)

SEXUAL EDUCATION

A–174. Planned Parenthood Federation of America, Inc.
(800)669–0156
Provides family planning, reproductive, and sexual health care information.
(800)230–PLAN
Callers will reach the nearest Planned Parenthood center for clinical appointments or education staff. (See also B–24)

SEXUALLY TRANSMITTED DISEASES

A–175. Centers for Disease Control and Prevention National STD Hotline
(800)227–8922
Information regarding all sexually transmitted diseases. Referral to community clinics offering free or low–cost examination and treatment. 8 a.m.–11 p.m. Free written information available.

Herpes Resource Center
(800)230 6039
(800)478 3227 (Canada)
Provides information and support services to persons who suffer from herpes. Sponsors local support groups nationwide, telephone counseling services, information, research and education projects. 9 a.m. 7 p.m.

SPINAL CORD INJURY

See PARALYSIS AND SPINAL CORD INJURY

STROKE

See also PARALYSIS AND SPINAL CORD INJURY

A–176. American Heart Association Stroke Connection
(800)553–6321
(214)696–5211 (Fax)
Maintains a listing of more than 1000 groups across the Nation for referral to stroke survivors, their families, care givers, and interested professionals. Publishes Stroke Connection magazine, a forum for stroke survivors and their families to share information about coping with stroke. Provides information and referral and carries stroke–related books, videotapes, and literature available for purchase. 8:30 a.m.–5 p.m. (Central).

National Institute of Neurological Disorders and Stroke
(800)352 9424
Conducts and supports research on the causes, prevention, diagnosis, and treatment of neurological disorders and stroke. Consumer publications are available on the brain and nervous system and a variety of neurological disorders.

STUTTERING

A–177. National Center for Stuttering
(800)221–2483
Provides treatment for older children (age 7 and above) and adults, training for professionals, and information for parents with young children (below age 7). 9 a.m.–6 p.m.

A–178. Stuttering Foundation of America
(800)992–9392
(901)452–7343
(901)452–3931 (Fax)
stuttersfa@aol.com (E–mail)
Provides materials and makes referrals to speech–language pathologists. 9 a.m.–5 p.m.

SUBSTANCE ABUSE

See also ALCOHOL ABUSE and DRUG ABUSE

National Inhalent Prevention Coalition
(800)269–4237
Provides a free information packet on inhalent abuse. Distributes videotapes and posters on inhalent abuse (a fee is charged for this material when sent to States other than Texas).

SUDDEN INFANT DEATH SYNDROME

See RARE DISORDERS

SURGERY/FACIAL PLASTIC SURGERY

A–179. American Society for Dermatologic Surgery, Inc.
(800)441–2737
Provides information about various dermatologic surgical procedures, as well as referrals to dermatologic surgeons in local areas. 8:30 a.m.–5 p.m. (Central).

A–180. American Society of Plastic and Reconstructive Surgeons, Inc.
(800)635–0635
Provides referrals to board–certified plastic surgeons nationwide and in Canada. 8:30 a.m.–4:30 p.m. (Central). Leave recorded message after hours.

A–181. Facial Plastic Surgery Information Service
(800)332–3223
(202)842–4500
Provides physician referral list and brochures. 24 hours.

TRAUMA

A–182. American Trauma Society (ATS)
(800)556–7890
(301)420–4189
(301)420–0617 (Fax)
Offers information to health professionals and the public; answers questions about trauma prevention and trauma systems. 9 a.m.–5 p.m.

UROLOGICAL DISORDERS

A–183. American Association of Kidney Patients
(800)749–2257
(813)223–0001 (Fax)
Helps renal patients and their families to deal with the physical and emotional impact of kidney disease. Supplies information on renal conditions. 9 a.m.–5 p.m.

A–184. American Foundation for Urologic Disease
(800)242–2383
(410)528–0550 (Fax)
Provides a 24 hour recording for callers seeking patient information on urologic diseases and dysfunctions. (See also B–37)

A–185. American Kidney Fund
(800)638–8299
Offers financial assistance to kidney patients who are unable to pay treatment–related costs. Also provides information on organ donations and kidney–related diseases. 8 a.m.–5 p.m.

Incontinence Information Center
(800)843–4315
(800)543–9632
Provides free information to prospective patients regarding the causes and treatments for incontinence. Provides referrals to local physicians. 8:30 a.m.–5 p.m. (Central) or leave recorded message after hours.

A–186. National Kidney Foundation
(800)622–9010
(212)689–9261 (Fax)
Provides information and referrals to the public and health professionals regarding kidney disorders. 9 a.m.–5 p.m.

A–187. The Simon Foundation for Continence
(800)237–4666 (Patient information)
(708)864–3913
(708)864–9758 (Fax)
Provides information on continence and ordering a quarterly newsletter and other publications. Also has a community–based education program/self–help group and informational videotape. Toll–free number operates 24 hours; second number is staffed 9 a.m.–5 p.m. (Central).

VENEREAL DISEASES

See SEXUALLY TRANSMITTED DISEASES

VISION

See also LIBRARY SERVICES

A–188. American Council of the Blind
(800)424–8666 (Live operators available 3p.m.–5:30 p.m. Eastern)
(202)467–5081 (9 a.m.–5:30 Eastern)
(202)467–5085 (Fax)
(202)331–1058 (Electronic Bulletin Board)
hcraff@ACCESS.DIGEX.NET (E–mail)
Offers information on blindness and referrals to rehabilitation organizations, research centers, and chapters. Publishes resource lists. Leave recorded message after hours.

A–189. Blind Childrens Center
(800)222–3566
(800)222–3567
(213)665–3828 (Fax)
info@blindcntr.org (E–mail)
http://www.blindcntr.org/bcc (World Wide Web)
Nonprofit early intervention program and educational preschool. Family support services. Information and referral line. Educational booklets for parents, educators, and specialists. 7:30 a.m.–5 p.m. (Pacific).

A–199. The Foundation Fighting Blindness
(800)683–5555
(800)683–5551 (TDD)
(410)771—9470 (Fax)
Funds medical research and provides information on retinitis pigmentosa and other inherited retinal degenerations. Scope of information includes current research, genetics, retina donor program, and practical resources available throughout the United States. 8:30 a.m.–5 p.m.

A–190. Guide Dog Foundation for the Blind, Inc.
(800)548–4337
(516)265–2121
(516)361–5192 (Fax)
(516)366–4462 (Electronic Bulletin Board)
School for blind individuals requiring guide dogs. Operates a computer bulletin board system. Operates 24 hours.

A–191. The Lighthouse National Center for Education
(800)334–5497
(212)821–9200
(212)821–9705 (Fax)
(212)821–9713 (TDD)
Provides educational materials and information on vision and child development and age–related vision loss to professionals and consumers. Provides information nationwide on local resources such as low vision centers, support groups, and vision rehabilitation agencies. Some materials in Spanish. 9 a.m.–5 p.m. Leave recorded message after hours.

A–192. Louisiana Center for the Blind
(800)234–4166
(318)251–2891
(318)251–0109 (Fax)
Private, residential training program for legally blind adults and children. 8 a.m.–5 p.m. (Central).

A–193. National Association for Parents of the Visually Impaired
(800)562–6265
(617)972–7444 (Fax)
Provides support and information to parents of visually impaired, blind, deaf–blind, and blind multi–handicapped children. 9 a.m.–5 p.m. (Central).

Section C

A–194. National Eye Care Project Helpline
(800)222–EYES (3937)
Provides medical and surgical eye care to disadvantaged elderly people who can no longer access the ophthalmologists they have visited in the past. 8 a.m.–4 p.m. (Pacific).

A–195. National Eye Research Foundation
(800)621–2258
(708)564–4652
(708)564–0807 (Fax)
Recording provides patient and membership information. Publishes the Green Directory, an international listing of member optometrists for patient referrals. 8:30 a.m.–5 p.m. Leave recorded message after hours.

A–196. The National Eye Research Foundation's Memorial Eye Clinic
(800)621–2258
Provides low–vision care, orthokeratology, and problem contact lens care. 9 a.m. 5 p.m., Monday, Tuesday, Wednesday; 9 a.m.–2 p.m., Friday. Leave recorded message after hours.

National Family Association for Deaf–Blind
(800)255 0411, ext. 275
See HEARING AND SPEECH

A–197. National Federation of the Blind: Job Opportunities for the Blind (JOB)
(800)638–7518
Offers support and factual information to blind individuals seeking jobs, employers, parents, and teachers. Also provides a free sample package and job magazine on cassette. 12:30 p.m.–5 p.m.

A–198. Prevent Blindness Center for Sight
(800)331–2020
Sponsored by Prevent Blindness America. Provides information on a broad range of eye health and safety topics. 8 a.m.–5 p.m. (Central).

VIOLENCE

A–200. Family Violence Prevention Fund
(800)313–1310
Provides information and resources on how to diagnose, treat, and prevent domestic violence. Materials available include a Primary Care Information Packet and an Emergency Department Information Packet, as well as research studies and a variety of other publications. Technical assistance available through a program specialist.

Rape, Abuse, and Incest National Network
(800)656 4673
Connects caller to the nearest counseling center which provides counseling for rape, abuse, and incest victims.

WOMEN

Breast Implant Hotline
(800)532 4440
Sponsored by the Food and Drug Administration. Provides a 24–hour recording of general information on breast implants. Distributes a breast implant information packet.

A–201. Endometriosis Association
(800)992–3636
(414)355 6065 (Fax)
Provides a 24–hour recording for callers to request information and leave name and address.

National Osteoporosis Foundation
(800)464 6700
(202)223 2237 (Fax)
Provides women with information on bone density testing, advice on how to talk to physicians about osteoporosis, and location of bone density testing facilities.

A–202. PMS Access
(800)222–4767
(608)833–7412 (Fax)
Sponsored by Madison Pharmacy Associates, Inc. Provides information, literature, and counseling on premenstrual syndrome (PMS). Gives referrals to physicians and clinics in the caller's area. 9 a.m.–5 p.m. (Central).

A–203. Women's Sports Foundation
(800)227–3988
(516)542–4716 (Fax)
A national, nonprofit, educational organization that promotes and enhances sports and fitness opportunities for all girls and women.

GUIDE TO FEDERAL HEALTH INFORMATION CLEARINGHOUSES

The Federal Government operates many clearinghouses and information centers that focus on specific topics. Their services include distributing publications, providing referrals, and answering inquiries. Many offer toll–free numbers. Unless otherwise stated, numbers can be reached within the continental United States Monday through Friday, during normal business hours, and hours of operation are eastern time. The clearinghouses are listed below by keyword.

B–1. National Institute on AGING Information Center
P.O. Box 8057
Gaithersburg, MD 20898–8057
(800)222–2225 (Voice/TTY)
(301)587–2528
(800)222–4225 (TDD)
(301)589–3014 (Fax)
Provides publications on health topics of interest to older adults, to the public, and to doctors, nurses, social activities directors, and health educators. (See also A–3, A–16, A–17, A–18, A–81)

B–2. U.S. Department of AGRICULTURE Extension Service
See the listing in the Government section of your telephone book for your local extension office. Provides information on health, nutrition, fitness, and family well–being.

B–3. CDC National AIDS Clearinghouse
P.O. Box 6003
Rockville, MD 20849–6003
(800)458–5231
(800)243–7012 (TDD)
(800)874–2572 AIDS Clinical Trials
(800)458–5231 (NAC Fax–Back Service)
(800)448–0440 HIV/AIDS Treatment
(301)217–0023 (International)
(301)738–6616 (Fax)
aidsinfo@cdcnac.aspensys.com (E–Mail)
Sponsored by the Centers for Disease Control and Prevention. A national reference, referral, and distribution service for HIV/AIDS–related information. Answers questions and provides technical assistance; distributes published HIV–related materials including current information on scientific findings, CDC guidelines, and trends in the HIV epidemic; and provides specific information on AIDS–related organizations, educational materials, funding opportunities, and other topics. Services include a 24–hour fax–back service for HIV/AIDS–related information and the Business and Labor Resource Service for resources, technical assistance, publications, and referrals concerning managing AIDS in the workplace. Provides information and publications in English and Spanish. 9 a.m.–7 p.m.

B–4. National Clearinghouse for ALCOHOL and DRUG Information
P.O. Box 2345
Rockville, MD 20847–2345
(800)729–6686
(301)468–2600
(800)487–4889 (TTY/TDD)
(301)230–2867 (TTY/TDD)
(301)468–6433 (Fax)
Sponsored by the Center for Substance Abuse Prevention, Substance Abuse and Mental Health Services Administration. Gathers and disseminates information on alcohol and other drug–related subjects, including tobacco. Distributes publications. Services include subject searches and provision of statistics and other information. Operates the Regional Alcohol and Drug Awareness Resource Network, a nationwide linkage of alcohol and other drug information centers. Maintains a library open to the public. 8 a.m.–7 p.m. (See also A–13, A–53, B–51)

B–5. National Institute of ALLERGY and INFECTIOUS DISEASES
Office of Communications
Building 31, Room 7A50
9000 Rockville Pike
Bethesda, MD 20892
(301)496–5717
Distributes publications to the public and to doctors, nurses, and researchers.

B–6. ALZHEIMER'S DISEASE Education and Referral Center
P.O. Box 8250
Silver Spring, MD 20907–8250
(800)438–4380
(301)495–3311
(301)495–3334 (Fax)
adear@alzheimers.org (E–mail)
Sponsored by the National Institute on Aging. Provides information and publications on Alzheimer's disease to health and service professionals, patients and their families, caregivers, and the public. (See also A–3, A–16, A–17)

B–7. National ARTHRITIS and Musculoskeletal and Skin Diseases Information Clearinghouse
1 AMS Circle
Bethesda, MD 20892–3675
(301)495–4484
(301)587–4352 (Fax)
Identifies educational materials about arthritis and musculoskeletal and skin diseases and serves as an information exchange for individuals and organizations involved in public, professional, and patient education. Conducts subject searches and makes resource referrals. (See also A–3, A–18)

B–8. National AUDIOVISUAL Center
National Technical Information Service
U.S. Department of Commerce
Springfield, VA 22161
(703)487–4650
(703)321–8547 (Fax)
Sells more than 9,000 federally produced audiovisual programs. Provides catalogs at no cost. Several catalogs cover health–related topics, including alcohol and other drug abuse, emergency fire services, industrial safety, and occupational health.

B–9. National Library Service for the BLIND and Physically Handicapped
Library of Congress
1291 Taylor Street NW.
Washington, DC 20542
(800)424–8567
(202)707–5100
(202)707–0744 (TDD)
(202)707–0712 (Fax)
A network of 56 regional and 87 local libraries that work in cooperation with the Library of Congress to provide free library service to anyone who is unable to read standard print due to visual or physical disabilities. Delivers recorded and Braille books and magazines to eligible readers. Specially designed phonographs and cassette players also are loaned. A list of participating local and regional libraries is available.

B–10. CANCER Information Service
Office of Cancer Communications
National Cancer Institute
Building 31, Room 10A16
9000 Rockville Pike
Bethesda, MD 20892
(800)4–CANCER (422–6237)
(301)496–5583
(301)402–2594 (Fax)
Provides information about cancer and cancer–related resources to patients, the public, and health professionals. Inquiries are handled by trained information specialists. Spanish–speaking staff members are available. Distributes free publications from the National Cancer Institute. Operates 9 a.m.–7 p.m. (See also A–19, A–20, A–21, A–22)

B–11. National Clearinghouse on CHILD ABUSE and Neglect Information
P.O. Box 1182
Washington, DC 20013–1182
(800)FYI–3366
(703)385–7565
(703)385–3206 (Fax)
nccanch@clark.net (E–mail)
Serves as a national resource for the acquisition and dissemination of child abuse and neglect materials and distributes a free publications catalog upon request. Maintains bibliographic databases of documents, audiovisuals, and national organizations. Services include searches of databases and annotated bibliographies on frequently requested topics. (See also A–30)

B–12. National Clearinghouse on Family Support and CHILDREN'S MENTAL HEALTH
Portland State University
P.O. Box 751
Portland, OR 97207–0751
(800)628–1696
(503)725–4040
(503)725–4165 (TTD)
(503)725–4180 (Fax)
Sponsored by the National Institute on Disability and Rehabilitation Research, U.S. Department of Education, and the Center for Mental Health Services, U.S. Department of Health and Human Services. Provides publications on parent/family support groups, financing, early intervention, various mental disorders, and other topics concerning children's mental health. Also offers a computerized databank and a State–by– State resource file. Recording operates 24 hours a day. (See also A–107, B–41)

NIH CONSENSUS Program Clearinghouse
P.O. Box 2577
Kensington, MD 20891
(800)644–6627
(301)816–9840 (Electronic Bulletin Board)
(301)816–2494 (Fax)
A service of the Office of Medical Applications of Research (OMAR), National Institutes of Health. Provides up–to–date information on biomedical technologies to all health care providers. Offers a 24–hour voice mail service to order consensus statements produced by non–Federal panels of experts that evaluate scientific information on biomedical technologies. Information Specialists available between 8:30 a.m. and 5 p.m. (Eastern). Consensus statements can also be ordered by mail, fax, and electronic bulletin board.

B–14. CONSUMER INFORMATION Center
Pueblo, CO 81009
(719)948–4000
Distributes Federal agency publications. Publishes quarterly catalog of Federal publications of consumer interest.

B–15. National Institute on DEAFNESS and Other Communication Disorders Information Clearinghouse
1 Communication Avenue
Bethesda, MD 20892–3456
(800)241–1044
(800)241–1055 (TT)
(301)907–8830 (Fax)
Collects and disseminates information on hearing, balance, smell, taste, voice, speech, and language for health professionals, patients, people in industry, and the public. Maintains a database of references to brochures, books, articles, fact sheets, organizations, and educational materials, which is a subfile on CHID. Develops publications, including directories, fact sheets, brochures, information packets, and newsletters.

B–16. National DIABETES Information Clearinghouse
1 Information Way
Bethesda, MD 20892–3560
(301)654–3327
(301)907–8906 (Fax)
NDIC@aerie.com (E–mail)
The National Diabetes Information Clearinghouse (NDIC) is an information and referral service of the National Institute of Diabetes and Digestive and Kidney Diseases, one of the National Institutes of Health. The clearinghouse responds to written inquires, develops and distributes publications about diabetes, and provides referrals to diabetes organizations, including support groups. The NDIC maintains a database of patient and professional education materials, from which literature searches are generated. (See also A–38, A–40)

B–17. National DIGESTIVE DISEASES Information Clearinghouse
2 Information Way
Bethesda, MD 20892–3570
(301)654–3810
(301)907–8906 (Fax)
NDDIC@aerie.com (E–mail)
The National Digestive Diseases Information Clearinghouse (NDDIC) is an information and referral service of the National Institute of Diabetes and Digestive and Kidney Diseases, one of the National Institutes of Health. A central information resource on the prevention and management of digestive diseases, the clearinghouse responds to written inquires, develops and distributes publications about digestive diseases, and provides referrals to digestive disease organizations, including support groups. The NDDIC maintains a database of patient and professional education materials, from which literature searches are generated.

B–18. National Information Center for Children and Youth with DISABILITIES
P.O. Box 1492
Washington, DC 20013–1492
(800)695–0285 (Voice/TT)
(202)884–8200 (Voice/TT)
(202)884–8441 (Fax)
nichcy@capcon.net (E–mail)
Sponsored by the U.S. Department of Education. Assists individuals by providing information on disabilities and disability–related issues, with a special focus on children and youth with disabilities (birth to age 22). Services include responses to questions, referrals, and technical assistance to parents, educators, caregivers, and advocates. Develops and distributes fact sheets on disability and general information on parent support groups and public advocacy. All information and services are provided free of charge. (See also A–45, A–48, A–49)

B–19. Clearinghouse on DISABILITY INFORMATION
Office of Special Education and Rehabilitative Services
U.S. Department of Education
330 C Street SW.
Switzer Building, Room 3132
Washington, DC 20202–2524
(202)205–8241
(202)205–9252 (Fax)
Responds to inquiries on a wide range of topics, especially in the areas of Federal funding, legislation, and programs benefiting people with disabling conditions. Provides referrals. (See also A–45)

B–20. National Center for Chronic DISEASE PREVENTION and Health Promotion (NCCDPHP)
Technical Information Services Branch enters for Disease Control and Prevention
4770 Buford Highway, MS K13
Atlanta, GA 30341–3724
(770)488–5080
(770)488–5969 (Fax)
Provides information and referrals to the public and to professionals. Gathers information on chronic disease prevention and health promotion. Develops the following bibliographic databases focusing on health promotion program information: Health Promotion and Education, Cancer Prevention and Control, Comprehensive School Health with an AIDS school health component, Prenatal Smoking Cessation, and Epilepsy Education and Prevention Activities. Produces bibliographies on topics of interest in chronic disease prevention and health promotion. The NCCDPHP Information Center collections include approximately 400 periodical subscriptions, 4,000 books, and 400 reference books. Visitors may use the collection by appointment. Produces the CDP File CD–ROM, which includes the above databases and the Chronic Disease Prevention Directory, a listing of key contacts in public health.

B–21. Housing and Urban Development DRUG INFORMATION and Strategy Clearinghouse
P.O. Box 6424
Rockville, MD 20850
(800)955–2232
Sponsored by the U.S. Department of Housing and Urban Development. Promotes strategies for eradicating drugs and drug trafficking from public housing. Provides housing officials, residents, and community leaders a source for information and assistance on drug abuse prevention and trafficking control techniques. Maintains an automated database system consisting of national and community program descriptions, publications, research, and news articles. Provides resource lists.

DRUGS and CRIME Data Center and Clearinghouse
1600 Research Boulevard
Rockville, MD 20850
(800)666–3332
A service of the Bureau of Justice Statistics (BJS), Office of Justice Programs, U.S. Department of Justice. Responds to policy makers' need for the most current data about illegal drugs, drug law violations, drug–related crime, drug–using offenders in the criminal justice system, and the impact of drugs on criminal justice administration. The Data Center prepares special reports on drugs and crime; analyzes and evaluates existing drug data; prepares annotated bibliographies of drugs–and–crime reports; and responds to request for drug and crime information. The Clearinghouse disseminates BJS and other Department of Justice publications relating to drugs and crime; distributes information on specific drugs–and–crime topics; maintains a data base of reports, books, and articles on crime; and maintains a reading room where visitors can use the Clearinghouse collection. 8:30 a.m.–5:15 p.m. (Eastern). Leave recorded message after hours.

B–22. ERIC Clearinghouse on Teaching and Teacher EDUCATION
One Dupont Circle NW.
Suite 610
Washington, DC 20036–1186
(202)293–2450
(202)457–8095 (Fax)
Sponsored by the U.S. Department of Education. Acquires, evaluates, abstracts, and indexes literature on the preparation and development of education personnel and on selected aspects of health and physical education, recreation, and dance. Publishes monographs, trends and issues papers, ERIC Digests and ERIC Recent Resources (annotated bibliographies from the ERIC database). Performs computer searches of the ERIC database and sponsors work–shops on searching the ERIC database.

Section C

B–23. U.S. ENVIRONMENTAL PROTECTION Agency Public Information Center
401 M Street S.W., 3404
Washington, DC 20460
(202)260–2080
(202)260–6257 (Fax)
public–access@epamail.epa.gov (E–Mail)
Offers general information about the Agency and nontechnical publications on various environmental topics, such as air quality, pesticides, radon, indoor air, drinking water, water quality, and Superfund. Refers inquiries for technical information to the appropriate regional or program office. The public may visit the PIC Visitor Center between the hours of 10 a.m. and 4 p.m., Monday–Friday, except Federal holidays. (See also A–24, A–58, A–133, B–35)

FEDERAL INFORMATION Center (FIC) Program
(800)688–9889
(800)326–2996 (TDD/TTY)
http://www.gsa.gov/et/fic–firs/fichome.htm (World Wide Web)
Provides information about the Federal Government's agencies, programs, and services. Information specialists use an automated database, printed reference materials, and other resources to provide answers to inquiries or accurate referrals. Callers who speak Spanish will be assisted. A descriptive brochure on the FIC program is available free from Department 584B at the Consumer Information Center (see listing in this publication). 9 a.m. Eastern–5 p.m. Pacific Monday–Friday except Federal holidays.

B–26. FOOD AND DRUG Administration
Office of Consumer Affairs
5600 Fishers Lane, HFE–88
Rockville, MD 20857
(301)443–3170
(301)443–9767 (Fax)
Responds to consumer requests for information and publications on foods, drugs, cosmetics, medical devices, radiation–emitting products, and veterinary products. 1 p.m.–3:30 p.m. (See also A–63, A–64)

B–27. FOOD AND NUTRITION Information Center
National Agricultural Library/FNIC
U.S. Department of Agriculture, ARS
10301 Baltimore Boulevard Room 304
Beltsville, MD 20705–2351
(301)504–5719
(301)504–6409 (Fax)
fnic@nalusda.gov (E–Mail)
Provides information on human nutrition, food service management, and food technology. Acquires and lends books and audiovisual materials. Offers database searching and access through electronic mail. (See also A–113, A–114)

B–28. Agency for HEALTH CARE POLICY and Research Clearinghouse
P.O. Box 8547
Silver Spring, MD 20907–8547
(800)358–9295
(301)495–3453
Distributes lay and scientific publications produced by the agency, including clinical practice guidelines on a variety of topics, reports from the National Medical Expenditure Survey, and health care technology assessment reports. (See also A–65)

B–29. National HEALTH INFORMATION Center
P.O. Box 1133
Washington, DC 20013–1133
(800)336–4797
(301)565–4167
(301)984–4256 (Fax)
nhicinfo@health.org (E–Mail)
http://nhic–nt.health.org (World Wide Web)
Helps the public and health professionals locate health information through identification of health information resources, an information and referral system, and publications. Uses a data–base containing descriptions of health–related organizations to refer inquirers to the most appropriate resources. Does not diagnose medical conditions or give medical advice. Prepares and distributes publications and directories on health promotion and disease prevention topics. (See also A–67)

B–30. National Center for HEALTH STATISTICS
Data Dissemination Branch
6525 Belcrest Road, Room 1064
Hyattsville, MD 20782
(301)436–8500
http://www.cdc.gov/nchshome.htm (World Wide Web)
The Data Dissemination Branch of the National Center for Health Statistics answers requests for catalogs of publications and electronic data products; single copies of publications, such as Advance Data reports; ordering information for publications and electronic products sold through the Government Printing Office and National Technical Information Service; adding addresses to the mailing list for new publications; and specific statistical data collected by the National Center for Health Statistics.

B–31. National HEART, LUNG, AND BLOOD Institute (NHLBI)
Information Center
P.O. Box 30105
Bethesda, MD 20824–0105
(301)251–1222
(301)251–1223 (Fax)
nhlbiic@dgs.dgsys.com (E–Mail)
NHLBI serves as a source of information and materials on risk factors for cardiovascular disease. Services include dissemination of public education materials, programmatic and scientific information for health professionals, and materials on worksite health, as well as responses to information requests. Materials on cardiovascular health are available to consumers and professionals. (See also B–44)

B–32. National HIGHWAY TRAFFIC SAFETY Administration
U.S. Department of Transportation
400 Seventh Street, SW.
Washington, DC 20590
(800)424–9393 (Hotline)
(202)366–0123 (Hotline)
(202)366–5962 (Fax)
Provides information and referral on the effectiveness of occupant protection, such as safety belt use, child safety seats, and automobile recalls. Gives referrals to other Government agencies for consumer questions on warranties, service, automobile safety regulations, and reporting safety problems. Works with private organizations to promote safety programs. Provides technical and financial assistance to state and local governments and awards grants for highway safety.

B–33. The National Resource Center on HOMELESSNESS and Mental Illness
262 Delaware Avenue
Delmar, NY 12054
(800)444–7415
(518)439–7415
(518)439–7612 (Fax)
Collects, synthesizes, and disseminates information on the services, supports, and housing needs of homeless people with serious mental illnesses. Maintains extensive database of published and unpublished materials, prepares customized database searches, holds workshops and national conferences, provides technical assistance. (See also A–82, B–41)

B–34. HOUSING AND URBAN DEVELOPMENT (HUD) User
P.O. Box 6091
Rockville, MD 20850
(800)245–2691
(301)251–5154
(800)483–2209 (TDD)
Disseminates publications for U.S. Department of Housing and Urban Development's Office of Policy Development and Research. Offers database searches on housing research. Provides reports on housing safety, housing for elderly and handicapped persons and lead–based paint. (See also A–87, A–94, A–133)

B–35. INDOOR AIR Quality Information Clearinghouse
P.O. Box 37133
Washington, DC 20013–7133
(800)438–4318
Information specialists provide information, referrals, publications, and database searches on indoor air quality. Information is provided about pollutants and sources, health effects, control methods, commercial building operations and maintenance, standards and guidelines, and Federal and State legislation. (See also A–58, B–23)

B–36. National INJURY Information Clearinghouse
U.S. Consumer Product Safety Commission
4330 East West Highway
Bethesda, MD 20814
(301)504–0424
(301)504–0124 (Fax)
info@cpsc.gov (E–Mail)
Sponsored by the U.S. Consumer Product Safety Commission (CPSC). The clearinghouse collects and disseminates information on the causes and prevention of death, injury, and illness associated with consumer products. Compiles data obtained from accident reports, consumer complaints, death certificates, news clips, and the National Electronic Injury Surveillance System operated by the CPSC. Publications include statistical analyses of data and hazard and accident patterns. (See also A–171, B–48)

B–37. National KIDNEY AND UROLOGIC Diseases Information Clearinghouse
3 Information Way
Bethesda, MD 20892–3580
(301)654–4415
(301)907–8906 (Fax)
NKUDIC@aerie.com
The National Kidney and Urologic Diseases Information Clearinghouse (NKUDIC) is an information and referral service of the National Institute of Diabetes and Digestive and Kidney Diseases, one of the National Institutes of Health. The clearinghouse responds to written inquires, develops and distributes publications about kidney and urologic diseases, and provides referrals to digestive disease organizations, including support groups. The NKUDIC maintains a database of patient and professional education materials, from which literature searches are generated. (See also A–183)

B–38. National LEAD Information Center
1019 19th Street, NW.
Suite 401
Washington, DC 20036–5015
(800)424–LEAD (Clearinghouse)
(800)LEAD–FYI (Hotline)
(800)526–5456 (TDD)
(202)659–1192 (Fax)
EHC@cais.com (E–mail)
cais.com (Gopher)
Sponsored by the National Safety Council. Responds to inquiries regarding lead and lead poisoning. Provides information on lead poisoning and children, lead–based paint, a list of local and State contacts who can help, and other lead–related questions. (See also A–87, A–94)

Section C

B–39. National Center for Education in MATERNAL AND CHILD HEALTH
2000 15th Street, North
Suite 701
Arlington, VA 22201–2617
(703)524–7802
(703)524–9335 (Fax)
ncemch@gumedlib.dml.georgetown.edu (E–mail)
Sponsored by the Maternal and Child Health Bureau, Health Resources and Services Administration. Provides information to health professionals and the public, develops educational and reference materials, and provides technical assistance in program development. Subjects covered are women's health including pregnancy and childbirth; infant, child, and adolescent health; nutrition; children with special health needs; injury and violence prevention; health and safety in day care; and maternal and child health programs and services. Types of materials include professional literature, curricula, patient education materials, audiovisuals, and information about organizations and programs. Appointment preferred for on–site visits. Participates in the following electronic services: the Combined Health Information Database (CHID), National Library of Medicine's DIRLINE, and MCH–NetLink. (See also A–105)

B–40. National MATERNAL AND CHILD HEALTH Clearinghouse
8201 Greensboro Drive
Suite 600
McLean, VA 22102
(703)821–8955, ext. 254 or 265
(703)821–2098 (Fax)
Sponsored by the Maternal and Child Health Bureau, Health Resources and Services Administration. Centralized source of materials and information in the areas of human genetics and maternal and child health. Distributes publications and provides referrals. (See also A–105)

B–41. National Institute of MENTAL HEALTH
Information Resources and Inquiries Branch
5600 Fishers Lane
Room 7C–02
Rockville, MD 20857
(301)443–4513
(301)443–8431 (TDD)
(301)443–0008 (Fax)
(301)443–5158 (MENTAL HEALTH FAX4U Fax Information System)
(800)64–PANIC (PANIC DISORDER Information)
(800)421–4211 (Depression/Awareness, Recognition, and Treatment Information)
Responds to information requests from the public, clinicians, and the scientific community, with a variety of printed materials on such subjects as children's mental disorders, schizophrenia, oppression, bipolar disorder, seasonal affective disorder, anxiety and panic disorders, obsessive–compulsive disorder, eating disorders, learning disabilities, and Alzheimer's disease. Information and publications on the Depression/ Awareness, Recognition, and Treatment Program (D/ART) and on the Panic Disorder Education Program, NIMH–sponsored educational programs on depressive and panic disorders, their symptoms and treatment, are distributed. Single copies of publications are free of charge. A list of NIMH publications, including several in Spanish, is available upon request. (See also A–106)

B–42. Office of MINORITY HEALTH Resource Center
P.O. Box 37337
Washington, DC 20013–7337
(800)444–6472
(301)565–5112 (Fax)
Responds to information requests from health professionals and consumers on minority health issues and locates sources of technical assistance. Provides referrals to relevant organizations and distributes materials. Spanish– and Asian–speaking operators are available. (See also A–112)

B–43. Office of NAVIGATION SAFETY and Waterway Services
U.S. Coast Guard Consumer Affairs and Analysis Branch
2100 Second Street SW.
Washington, DC 20593–0001
(800)368–5647 (Customer InfoLine)
(202)267–0780
(800)689–0816 (TDD/TT)
(202)267–6707 (TDD/TT)
(202)267–4285 (Fax)
Modem #703313591 (Navigation Center Bulletin Board)
http://www.dot.gov/affairs/index.htm (World Wide Web)
Provides safety information to recreational boaters; assists the public in finding boating education classes; answers technical questions; and distributes literature on boating safety, Federal laws, and the prevention of recreational boating casualties.

B–44. Clearinghouse for OCCUPATIONAL SAFETY AND HEALTH INFORMATION
4676 Columbia Parkway
Cincinnati, OH 45226–1998
(800)35–NIOSH
(513)533–8326
(513)533–8573 (Fax)
Provides technical information support for National Institute for Occupational Safety and Health (NIOSH) research programs and disseminates information to others on request. Services include reference and referral, and information about NIOSH studies. Distributes a publications list of NIOSH materials. Maintains automated database covering the field of occupational safety and health. (See also A–171)

B–24. OPA Clearinghouse
P.O. Box 30686
Bethesda, MD 20824–0686
(301)654–6190
(301)907–9655 (Fax)
Sponsored by the Office of Population Affairs. Provides information and distributes publications to health professionals and the public in the areas of family planning, adolescent pregnancy, and adoption. Makes referrals to other information centers in related subject areas. (See also A–1, A–2, A–174)

National ORAL HEALTH Information Clearinghouse
1 NOHIC Way
Bethesda MD 20892–3500
(301)403–7364
(301)907–8830 (Fax)
nidr@aerie.com (E–Mail)
A service of the National Institute of Dental Research (NIDR). Focuses on the oral health concerns of special care patients, including: people with genetic disorders or systemic diseases that compromise oral health, people whose medical treatment causes oral problems, and people with mental or physical disabilities that make good oral hygiene practices and dental care difficult. Develops and distributes information and educational materials on special care topics, maintains a bibliographic database on oral health information and materials, and provides information services with trained staff to respond to specific interests and questions.

OSTEOPOROSIS and Related Bone Diseases
National Resource Center
1150 17th Street NW., Suite 500
Washington, DC 20036
(800)624–BONE
(202)223–0344
(202)466–4315 (TDD)
(202)223–2237 (Fax)
orbdnrc@nof.org (E–Mail)
Sponsored by the National Institute of Arthritis and Musculoskeletal and Skin Diseases. Provides patients, health professionals, and the public with resources and information on metabolic bone diseases such as osteo–porosis, Paget's disease of the bone, osteogenesis imper–fecta, and primary hyperparathyroidism. Specific populations include the elderly, men, women, and adolescents.

B–45. President's Council on PHYSICAL FITNESS and Sports
701 Pennsylvania Avenue NW.
Suite 250
Washington, DC 20004
(202)272–3421
(202)504–2064 (Fax)
Conducts a public service advertising program, prepares educational materials, and works to promote the development of physical fitness leadership, facilities, and programs. Helps schools, clubs, recreation agencies, employers, and Federal agencies design and implement programs. Offers a variety of testing, recognition, and incentive programs for individuals, institutions, and organizations. Materials on exercise and physical fitness for all ages are available.

B–46. POLICY Information Center
Office of the Assistant Secretary for Planning and Evaluation
U.S. Department of Health and Human Services
Hubert H. Humphrey Building
Room 438F
200 Independence Avenue SW.
Washington, DC 20201
(202)690–6445
(202)690–6518 (Fax)
http://www.os.dhhs.gov (World Wide Web)
A centralized repository of evaluations, short–term evaluative research reports and program inspections/audits relevant to the Department's operations, programs, and policies. It also includes relevant reports from the General Accounting Office (GAO), Congressional Budget Office (CBO), Office of Technology Assessment (OTA), and the Institute of Medicine and the National Research Council's Committee on National Statistics, both part of the National Academy of Sciences, Departments of Agriculture, Labor, and Education, as well as from the private sector. Final reports and executive summaries are available for review at the facility, or final reports may be purchased from the National Technical Information Service (NTIS). In addition, the PIC online database of evaluation abstracts are accessible on Internet through HHS HomePage, http://www.os.dhhs.gov or gopher.os.dhhs.gov. The database includes over 6,000 project descriptions of both in–process and completed studies. PIC Highlights, a quarterly publication, features articles of recently completed studies.

B–47. National Clearinghouse for PRIMARY CARE Information
Ticon Courthouse
2070 Chain Bridge Road
Suite 450
Vienna, VA 22182
(703)821–8955, ext. 245
(703)556–4831 (TTY/TDD)
(703)821–2098 (Fax)
Sponsored by the Bureau of Primary Health Care (BPHC), Health Resources and Services Administration. Provides information services to support the planning, development, and delivery of ambulatory health care to urban and rural areas that have shortages of medical personnel and services. A primary role of the clearinghouse is to identify, obtain, and disseminate information to community and migrant health centers. Distributes publications focusing on ambulatory care, financial management, primary health care, and health services administration of special interest to professionals working in primary care centers funded by BPHC. Materials are available on health education, governing boards, financial management, administrative management, and clinical care. Bilingual medical phrase books, a directory of federally funded health centers, and an annotated bibliography are available also.

Section C

B–48. U.S. Consumer PRODUCT SAFETY Commission Hotline

Washington, DC 20207
(800)638–2772
(800)638–8270 (TT)
(301)504–0580
(301)504–0399 (Fax)
Maintains the National Injury Information Clearinghouse, conducts investigations of alleged unsafe/defective products, and establishes product safety standards. Assists consumers in evaluating the comparative safety of products and conducts education programs to increase consumer awareness. Operates the National Electronic Injury Surveillance System, which monitors a statistical sample of hospital emergency rooms for injuries associated with consumer products. Maintains free hotline to provide information about recalls and to receive reports on unsafe products and product–related injuries. Publications describe hazards associated with electrical products and children's toys. Spanish–speaking operator available through the toll–free number listed above. (See also A–171, A–173, B–36)

B–49. National REHABILITATION Information Center

8455 Colesville Road
Suite 935
Silver Spring, MD 20910
(800)346–2742 (Voice/TT)
(301)588–9284 (Voice/TT)
(301)587–1967 (Fax)
The National Rehabilitation Center (NARIC) is a library and information center on disability and rehabilitation. Funded by the National Institute on Disability and Rehabilitation Research, NARIC collects and disseminates the results of federally funded research projects. The collection, which also includes commercially published books, journal articles, and audiovisuals, grows at a rate of about 300 documents per month. (See also A–51)

B–50. RURAL Information Center Health Service (RICHS)

National Agricultural Library
Room 304
10301 Baltimore Boulevard
Beltsville, MD 20705–2351
(800)633–7701
(301)504–5547
(301)504–6856 (TDD)
(301)504–5181 (Fax)
ric@nalusda.gov (E–mail)
gopher://gopher.nalusda.gov (Gopher)
Disseminates information on a variety of rural health issues including health professions, health care financing, special populations and the delivery of health care services. Provides information, referrals, publications, brief complimentary literature searches and access to an electronic bulletin board to professionals and the public. Posts rural health information on the Internet. RICHS is funded by the Federal Office of Rural Health Policy, DHHS and is part of the USDA Rural Information Center, which provides information on rural issues such as economic development, local government viability and community well–being. (See also A–168)

B–51. Office on SMOKING and Health Centers for Disease Control and Prevention

National Center for Chronic Disease Prevention and Health Promotion
Mailstop K–50
4770 Buford Highway, N.E.
Atlanta, GA 30341–3724
(800)CDC–1311
(404)488–5705
(404)488–5939 (Fax)
Develops and distributes the annual Surgeon General's report on smoking and health, coordinates a national public information and education program on tobacco use and health, and coordinates tobacco education and research efforts within the Department of Health and Human Services and throughout both federal and state governments. Maintains the Smoking and Health database, consisting of approximately 60,000 records available on CD–ROM (CDP File) through the Government Printing Office (Superintendent of

Documents, Government Printing Office, Washington, D.C. 20402.) Provides information on smoking cessation, ETS/passive smoking, pregnancy/infants, professional/technical information, and a publications list upon request. Provides specific promotional campaign materials through its toll–free hotline. (See also B–4, B–10, B–23)

B–52. National SUDDEN INFANT DEATH SYNDROME Resource Center

2070 Chan Bridge Road
Vienna, VA 22182
(703)821–8955
(703)821–2098 (Fax)
Sponsored by the Maternal and Child Health Bureau, Health Resources and Services Administration. Provides information and educational materials on sudden infant death syndrome (SIDS), apnea, and other related issues. Responds to information requests from professionals and from the public. Maintains a library of standard reference materials on topics related to SIDS. Maintains and updates mailing lists of State programs, groups, and individuals concerned with SIDS. Also develops fact sheets, catalogs, and bibliographies on areas of special interest to the community. Conducts customized searches of database on SIDS and SIDS–related materials. (See also A–161)

National Clearinghouse for Worker Safety and Health Training for HAZARDOUS MATERIALS, WASTE OPERATIONS, and EMERGENCY RESPONSE

c/o The George Meany Center for Labor Studies
10000 New Hampshire Avenue
Silver Spring, MD 20903
(301)431–5425
(301)434–0371 (Fax)
71112,713@compuserve.com (E–mail)
The Clearinghouse is supported by the Superfund Worker Training Program of the National institute of Environmental Health Sciences (NIEHS) to provide information and support services to NIEHS–funded hazardous materials, waste operations, and emergency response worker training programs. Disseminates related information and materials to the general public.

Section C

International Organizations

ARGENTINA

Argentinan Association of Dermatology, Asociacion Argentina De Dermatologia, Mexico 1720, 1100 Buenos Aires, Argentina; tel. 381–2737; FAX. 381–2737; Dra. Lidia Ester Valle, Chairman

AUSTRALIA

Austrailian Healthcare Association, P.O. Box 54, Deakin West, ACT, 2600, Australia; tel. +61 62851488; FAX. +61 62822395; Tracey Turner, Office Manager

BELGIUM

European Association of Poisons/Centres and Clinical Toxicologists (EAPCCT), City Hospital, Birmingham, B187QH, Belgium; tel. (44) 121 507 4123; FAX. (44) 121 507 5580; Dr. Allister Vale, President

International Federation of Oto–Rhino–Laryngological Societies, 1FOS–MISA–NKO Oosterweldlaan 24, 2610 WKRIJK, Belgium; tel. 3 4433611; Ms. Gadeyne, Administrator, Publication Manager

Verbond der Verzorgingsinstellingen V.Z.W., 1, Guimardstraat, Brussels 1040, Belgium; tel. 2 5118008; FAX. 2 5135269; Mrs. C. Boonen, M.D., General Director

BRAZIL

Fraternidade Crista De Doentes E Deficientes, Cap. Correa Pacheco 134, Americana, SP, 13470, Brazil; tel. 0 194 619754; Celso Zoppi

CANADA

Association des Medecins de langue francaise du Canada, 8355 St. Laurent Boulevard, Montreal, PQ H2P 2Z6, Canada; tel. 514/388–2228; FAX. 514/388–5335; Jacques Lambert, President

Canadian Anaesthetists' Society, One Eglinton Avenue East, Suite 208, Toronto, ON M4P 3A1, Canada; tel. 416/480–0602; FAX. 416/480–0320; Ann Andrews, CAE, Executive Director

Canadian Association of Medical Radiation Technologists, 280 Metcalfe Street, Suite 410, Ottawa, ON K2P 1R7, Canada; tel. 613/234–0012; FAX. 613/234–1097; Earl P. Rooney, Executive Director

Canadian Association of Pathologists, Office of the Secretariat, 774 Echo Drive, Ottawa, ON K1S 5N8, Canada; tel. 613–730–6230; FAX. 613–730–1116; Dr. Rosemary Henderson, Secretary–Treasurer

Canadian Association of Social Workers, 383 Parkdale Avenue, Suite 402, Ottawa, ON K1Y 4R4, Canada; tel. 613/729–6668; FAX. 613/729–9608; Eugenia Repetur Moreno, Executive Director

Canadian Cancer Society, 10 Alcorn Avenue, Suite 200, Toronto, ON M4V 3B1, Canada; tel. 416/961–7223; FAX. 416/961–4189; Dorothy Lamont, Chief Executive Officer

Canadian Cardiovascular Society, 360 Victoria Avenue, Suite 401, Westmount, PQ H3Z 2N4, Canada; tel. 514/482–3407; FAX. 514/482–6574; Linda Theriault, Executive Director

Canadian College of Health Record Administrators, Canadian Health Record Association, 1090 Don Mills Road, Suite 501, Don Mills, ON M3C 3G8, Canada; tel. 416/447–4900; FAX. 416/447–4598; Deborah Del Duca, Executive Director

Canadian Council of the Blind, 396 Cooper Street, Suite 405, Ottawa, ON K2P 2H7, Canada; tel. 613/567–0311; FAX. 613/567–2728; Mary Lee Moran, Executive Director

Canadian Council on Social Development, 441 Maclaren, Fourth Floor, Ottawa, ON K2P 2H3, Canada; tel. 613/236–8977; FAX. 613/236–2750; Nancy Perkins, Communications Coordinator

Canadian Dental Association, 1815 Alta Vista Drive, Ottawa, ON K1G 3Y6, Canada; tel. 613/523–1770; FAX. 613/523–7736; Jardine Neilson, Executive Director

Canadian Healthcare Association/Association Canadienne de soins de sante, 17 York Street, Suite 100, Ottawa, ON K1N 9J6, Canada; tel. 613/241–8005; FAX. 613/241–5055; Joyce Bailey, Acting President

Canadian Medical Engineering Consultants, 594 Bush Street, Belfountain, ON L0N 1B0, Canada; tel. 519/927–3286; FAX. 519/927–9440; A. M. Dolan, President

Canadian Mental Health Association, 2160 Yonge Street, Toronto, ON M4S 2Z3, Canada; tel. 416/484–7750; FAX. 416/484–4617; Edward J. Pennington, General Director

Canadian National Institute for the Blind, 1929 Bayview Avenue, Toronto, ON M4G 3E8, Canada; tel. 416/480–7586; FAX. 416/480–7677; Euclid J. Herie, President, Chief Executive Officer

Canadian Nurses Association, 50 Driveway, Ottawa, ON K2P 1E2, Canada; tel. 613/237–2133; FAX. 613/237–3520; Mary Ellen Jeans, RN, Ph.D., Executive Director

Canadian Orthopaedic Association, 1440 Ste. Catherine Street, W., Suite 421, Montreal, PQ H3G 1R8, Canada; tel. 514/874–9003; FAX. 514/874–0464; Robert F. Martin, M.D., President

Canadian Pharmaceutical Association, 1785 Alta Vista Drive, Ottawa, ON K1G 3Y6, Canada; tel. 613/523–7877; FAX. 613/523–0445; Leroy C. Fevang, Executive Director

Canadian Physiotherapy Association, 890 Yonge Street, 9th Floor, Toronto, ON M4W 3P4, Canada; tel. 416/924–5312; FAX. 416/924–7335; Brenda Myers, Executive Director

Canadian Psychiatric Association, 237 Argyle Street, Suite 200, Ottawa, ON K2P 1B8, Canada; tel. 613/234–2815; FAX. 613/234–9857, ext. 36; Alex Saunders, Chief Executive Officer

Canadian Public Health Association, 1565 Carling Avenue, Suite 400, Ottawa, ON K1Z 8R1, Canada; tel. 613/725–3769; FAX. 613/725–9826; Gerald H. Dafoe, M.H.A., Executive Director

Canadian Rehabilitation Council for the Disabled, 45 Sheppard Avenue, E., Suite 801, Toronto, ON M2N 5W9, Canada; tel. 416/250–7490; FAX. 416/229–1371; Henry Botchford, National Executive Director

Canadian Society of Hospital Pharmacists, 1145 Hunt Club Road, Suite 350, Ottawa, ON K1V OY3, Canada; tel. 613/736–9733; FAX. 613/736–5660; Bill Leslie, Executive Director

Canadian Society of Laboratory Technologists, Box 2830, LCD 1, Hamilton, ON L8N 3N8, Canada; tel. 905/528–8642, ext. 3011; FAX. 905/528–4968; E. Valerie Booth, Executive Director

Catholic Health Association of Canada, 1247 Kilborn Place, Ottawa, ON K1H 6K9, Canada; tel. 613/731–7148; FAX. 613/731–7797; Maryse Blouin, Director, Programs and Communications

College des medecins du Quebec, 2170, boul. Rene–Levesque Ouest, Montreal, PQ H3H 2T8, Canada; tel. 514/933–4441; FAX. 514/993–3112; Joelle Lescop, MD, Secretary General

College of Family Physicians of Canada, 2630 Skymark Avenue, Mississauga, ON L4W 5A4, Canada; tel. 905/629–0900; FAX. 905/629–0893; Dr. Claude A. Renaud, Director, Professional Affairs

College of Physicians and Surgeons of New Brunswick, One Hampton Road, Suite 300, Rothesay, NB E2E 5K8, Canada; tel. 506/849–5050; FAX. 506/849–5069; Ed Schollenberg, M.D., Registrar

National Cancer Institute of Canada, 10 Alcorn Avenue, Suite 200, Toronto, ON M4V 3B1, Canada; tel. 416/961–7223; FAX. 416/961–4189; J. David Beatty, M.D., Executive Director

The Canadian Dietetic Association, 480 University Avenue, Suite 601, Toronto, ON M5G 1V2, Canada; tel. 416/596–0857, ext. 314; FAX. 416/596–0603; Marsha Sharp, Chief Executive Officer

The Canadian Hearing Society, 271 Spadina Road, Toronto, ON M5R 2V3, Canada; tel. 416/964–9595; FAX. 416/964–2066; Gordon Ryall, Executive Director

The Canadian Medical Association, Box 8650, Ottawa, ON K1G 0G8, Canada; tel. 613/731–9331; FAX. 613/731–7314; Leo–Paul Landry, M.D., Secretary General

The Canadian Red Cross Society, National Office, 1800 Alta Vista Drive, Ottawa, ON K1G 4J5, Canada; tel. 613/739–2220; FAX. 613/739–2505; Claude Houde, National Director, Blood Services

The Royal College of Physicians and Surgeons of Canada, 774 Echo Drive, Ottawa, ON K1S 5N8, Canada; tel. 613/730–6201; FAX. 613/730–2410; Mrs. Pierrette Leonard, APR, Head Communications Section

World Federation of Hemophilia, 4616 St. Catherine Street, W., Montreal, PQ H3Z 1S3, Canada; tel. 514/933–7944; FAX. 514/933–8916; The Rev. Prebendary Alan J. Tanner

DENMARK

Amtsradsforeningen, Dampfaergevej 22, Postboks 2593, DK–2100 Copenhagen 0, Denmark; tel. +45 35 29 81 00; FAX. +45 35 29 83 00; Ida Sofie Jensen, Assistant Director

Danish Dental Association, Amaliegade 17, Postboks 143, DK–1004, Copenhagen, Denmark; tel. 45 33157711; FAX. 45 33151637; Karsten Thuen, Chief Executive Director

National Committee for Danish Hospitals, Amtsradsforeningen, Dampfaergevej 22, Postboks 2593, DK–2100 Copenhagen 0, Denmark; tel. +45 35 29 81 00; FAX. +45 35 29 83 00; Ida Sofie Jensen, Assistant Director

ENGLAND

British Medical Association, B.M.A. House Tavistock Square, London, WCH1 9JP, England; tel. 0171/387–4499; FAX. 0171/383–6400; Dr. E. M. Armstrong, B.Sc., FRCP(Glas), FRCGP, Secretary

Institute of Health Services Management (United Kingdom and International), 39 Chalton Street, London, NW1 1JD, England; tel. 071/388–2626; FAX. 071/388–2386; Noel Flannery, Deputy Director

International Hospital Federation, Four Abbots Place, London, NW6 4NP, England; tel. 071–372 7181; FAX. 071/328 7433; Dr. Errol N. Pickering, Director General

King's Fund, 11–13 Cavendish Square, London, W1M OAN, England; tel. 0171/307–2400; FAX. 0171/307–2801; R. J. Maxwell, Chief Executive Officer, Secretary

Nuffield Provincial Hospitals Trust, 59 New Cavendish Street, London W1M 7RD, England; tel. 0171/485–6632; FAX. 0171/485–8215; Max Lehmann, Acting Secretary

FRANCE

World Medical Association, 28 Avenue des Alpes, B.P. 63, 01212 Ferney–Voltaire, Cedex, France; tel. 450 407575; FAX. 450 405937; Dr. Ian Field, Secretary General

GERMANY

Deutsche Krankenhausgesellschaft, (German Hospital Federation), Tersteegenstrasse 9, D40474, Dusseldorf, Germany; tel. 211 454730; FAX. 211 4547361; Jorg Robbers, Director General

International Academy of Cytology, Universitaets–Frauenklinik, Hugstetterstrausse 55, D–79106 Freiburg i. Br., Germany; tel. 761 2703012; FAX. 761 2703112; Manuel Hilgarth, M.D., F.I.A.C.

HUNGARY

Magyar Korhazszovetseg, Furedi utca 9/c. VIII.34., 1144 Hungary, Budapest, Hungary; tel. (36–1) 163–52–73; FAX. (36–1) 163–52–73; Dr. I. Mikola, President

KOREA

Korean Hospital Association, (Mapo Hyun Dai Building), (Mapo–dong, Mapo–gu, Seoul 121–050, Korea; tel. 2 7187521; FAX. 2 7187522; Ho Uk Ha, Ph.D., Vice President

MEXICO

Federacion Latinoamericana de Hospitales, Apartado Postal 107–076, C.P. 06741, Mexico D.F., Mexico; tel. 5 482650; Dr. Guillermo Fajardo, Representative

NETHERLANDS

Federation of Health Care Organizations in the Netherlands, Postbus 9696, NL–3506 GR Utrecht, Netherlands; tel. 30 739911; FAX. 30 739438

PERU

Peruvian Hospital Association, Av. Dos De Mayo 8502 Of. 203, San Isidro, Lima 27, Peru; tel. 14 419546; Arturo Vasi Paez, President

PHILIPPINES

Philippine Hospital Association, 14 Kamias Rd., Quezon City–1102 Metro Ma, Philippines; tel. 2 9227674/75; Thelma Navarrete–Clemente, M.D., M.H.A., President

SOUTH AFRICA

Provincial Administration, Health Services Branch, P.O. Box 517, Bloemfontein 9300, South Africa; tel. 051/4055818; FAX. 051/304958; Dr. J. H. Kotze

SWITZERLAND

Ht Die Spitaler der Schweiz, (Swiss Hospital Association), Rain 32, CH–5001, Aarau, Switzerland; tel. 64 24 12 22; FAX. 64 22 33 35; Mr. Christof Haudenschild, Director

World Health Organization, 20 Avenue Appia, CH–1211 Geneva 27, Switzerland; tel. 22 791 21 11; FAX. 22 791 07 46; Hiroshi Nakajima, M.D., Ph.D., Director–General

UNITED STATES

American College of Gastroenterology, 4900B South 31st Street, Arlington, VA 22206, United States; tel. 703/820–7400; FAX. 703/931–4520; Thomas F. Fise, Executive Director

American Society for Testing and Materials, 100 Barr Harbor Drive, West Conshohocken, PA 19428–2959, United States; tel. 610/832–9672; FAX. 610/832–9666; Kenneth C. Pearson, Vice President

Association for Assessment and Accreditation of Laboratory Animal Care International (AAALACI), 11300 Rockville Pike, Suite 1211, Rockville, MD 20852–3035, United States; tel. 301/231–5353; FAX. 301/231–8282; Dr. John G. Miller, Executive Director

International Academy of Podiatric Medicine (IAPM), 4603 Highway 95 South, P.O. Box 39, Cocolalla, ID 83813–0039, United States; tel. 208/683–3900; FAX. 208/683–3700; Judith A. Baerg, Executive Director

International Aid, Inc., 17011 West Hickory, Spring Lake, MI 49456–9712, United States; tel. 616/846–7490; FAX. 616/846–3842; Warren L. Prelesnik, FACHE, Director, Medical Procurement

International Association for Dental Research, 1619 Duke Street, Alexandria, VA 22314–3406, United States; tel. 703/548–0066; FAX. 703/548–1883; John J. Clarkson, BDS, Ph.D., Executive Director

International Association of Ocular Surgeons, 4711 Golf Road, Suite 408, Skokie, IL 60076, United States; tel. 847/568–1500; FAX. 847/568–1527; Randall T. Bellows, M.D., Director

International Association of Pediatric Laboratory Medicine, 6728 Old McLean Village Drive, McLean, VA 22101, United States; tel. 703/556–9222; George K. Degnon, Executive Director

International Council on Social Welfare/U.S. Committee, 750 First Street, N.E., Washington, DC 20002, United States; tel. 202/336–8274; FAX. 202/336–8311; Toshio Tatara, Chair

International Executive Housekeepers Association, Inc., 1001 Eastwind Drive, Suite 301, Westerville, OH 43081–3361, United States; tel. 800/200–6342; FAX. 614/895–1248; Beth Risinger, Chief Executive Officer, Executive Director

International Tremor Foundation, 833 West Washington Boulevard, Chicago, IL 60607, United States; tel. 312/733–1893

Rehabilitation International, 25 East 21st Street, New York, NY 10010, United States; tel. 212/420–1500; FAX. 212/505–0871; John Stott, President

Sigma Theta Tau International Honor Society of Nursing, 550 West North Street, Indianapolis, IN 46202, United States; tel. 317/634–8171; FAX. 317/634–8188; Nancy A. Dickenson–Hazard, Executive Officer

World Federation of Public Health Associations, c/o APHA, 1015 15th Street, N.W., Washington, DC 20005, United States; tel. 202/789–5696; FAX. 202/789–5681; Diane Kuntz, M.P.H., Executive Secretary

VENEZUELA

Latin American Association for the Study of the Liver (LAASL), P.O. Box 51890, Sabana Grande, Caracas, 1050–A, Venezuela; tel. 58–2–9799380; FAX. 58–2–9799380; Dr. Miguel A. Garassini, President

U. S. GOVERNMENT AGENCIES

Specific addresses have been omitted because of the many changes presently occurring, and scheduled for the future among federal agencies. The telephone numbers given are general public information numbers, unless specifically identified with the officials listed.

The following information is based on data available as of March 1997.

For more information about U.S. government agencies, consult the U.S. Government Manual, *available from the Office of the* Federal Register, *National Archives and Records Service, Washington, DC 20408. A telephone directory of the U.S. Department of Health and Human Services is available from the Superintendent of Documents, Government Printing Office, Washington, DC 20402. Additional assistance may be obtained by contacting the American Hospital Association's Washington office, 325 Seventh Street, N.W., Washington, DC 20004.*

Executive Office of the President
tel. 202/456–1414

Counsel to the President: Charles Ruff; 202/456–2632

Chief of Staff: Erskine Dowles; 202/456–6797

Assistant to the President for Economic Policy: Gene B. Sperling; 202/456–5808

Assistant to the President for Domestic Policy: Bruce Reed; 202/456–2216

Assistant to the President and Director of Public Liaison: Alexis M. Herman; 202/456–2930

COUNCIL OF ECONOMIC ADVISORS
Chairman: Dr. Janet Yellen

OFFICE OF MANAGEMENT AND BUDGET
Director: Franklin D. Raines; 202/395–4840

Department of Agriculture
tel. 202/720–8732

Secretary: Dan Glickman; 202/720–3631

Department of Commerce
tel. 202/482–2000

Secretary: William M. Daley; 202/482–2112
BUREAU OF ECONOMIC ANALYSIS
Director: Steven Landefeld; 202/606–9600
ECONOMIC DEVELOPMENT ADMINISTRATION
Assistant Secretary: Phillip Singerman; 202/482–5067
NATIONAL INSTITUTE OF STANDARDS AND TECHNOLOGY
Director: Arati Prabhakar, Ph.D.; 301/975–2300

Department of Defense
tel. 703/545–6700

Secretary: William S. Cohen; 703/695–5261

Assistant Secretary of Defense (Health Affairs): Dr. Stephen Joseph; 703/697–2111
CIVILIAN HEALTH AND MEDICAL PROGRAMS OF THE UNIFORMED SERVICES (OCHAMPUS) (Denver, CO)
Director: Seileen Mullen; 303/361–1313
UNIFORMED SERVICES UNIVERSITY OF THE HEALTH SCIENCES
President: James A. Zimble; 301/295–3013
DEPARTMENT OF THE AIR FORCE
Surgeon General: Charles H. Roadman II; 202/767–4343
DEPARTMENT OF THE ARMY
Surgeon General: Lt. Gen. Ronald R. Blanck; 703/681–3000
DEPARTMENT OF THE NAVY
Surgeon General of the Navy: V.A.D.M. Harold M. Koenig; 202/762–3701

Department of Education
tel. 202/401–2000

Secretary: Richard W. Riley; 202/401–3000

Department of Health and Human Services
tel. 202/619–0257

Secretary: Donna E. Shalala; 202/690–7000
General Counsel: Harriet Rabb; 202/690–7741
MANAGEMENT AND BUDGET
Assistant Secretary: John J. Callahan, Ph.D.; 202/690–6396
HEALTH
Acting Assistant Secretary: Jo Ivey Boufford; 202/690–7694
ADMINISTRATION FOR CHILDREN AND FAMILIES
Assistant Secretary: Vacant; 202/401–2337
LEGISLATION
Assistant Secretary/Designate: Richard J. Tarplin; 202/690–7627
PLANNING AND EVALUATION
Acting Assistant Secretary: David Garrison; 202/690–7858
PUBLIC AFFAIRS
Assistant Secretary: Melissa Skolfield; 202/690–7850
PUBLIC HEALTH SERVICE
Acting Surgeon General: Audrey F. Manely, M.D., M.P.H.; 301/443–4000
Center for Disease Control, Atlanta 30333
Deputy Director: Dr. Claire V. Broome; 404/639–7000
Food and Drug Administration, Rockville, MD 20857
Commissioner: David Kessler, M.D.; 301/827–2410
Health Resources and Services Administration, Hyattsville, MD 20782
Administrator: Ciro Sumaya, M.D.; 301/443–2216
National Institutes of Health, Bethesda, MD 20892
Director: Harold Varmus, M.D.; 301/496–2433
Substance Abuse and Mental Health Services Administration, Rockville, MD
Administrator: Nelba Chavez, Ph.D.; 301/443–4795
HEALTH CARE FINANCING ADMINISTRATION
Administrator: Bruce C. Vladeck; 202/690–6726
SOCIAL SECURITY ADMINISTRATION: Baltimore, MD 21235
Commissioner: John W. Callahan; 410/965–7700
Regional Commissioners telephone: 800/772–1213
(1) Boston
Manny Vaz
(2) New York
Beatrice M. Disman
(3) Philadelphia
Larry G. Massanari
(4) Atlanta
Gordon M. Sherman
(5) Chicago
Myrtle S. Habersham
(6) Dallas
Horace L. Dickerson
(7) Kansas City
Michael Grochowski
(8) Denver
Horace L. Dickerson
(9) San Francisco
Linda S. McMahon
(10) Seattle
Marty Baer

Department of Housing and Urban Development
tel. 202/708–1112

Secretary: Andrew Cuomo; 202/708–0417

Department of Justice
tel. 202/514–2000

Attorney General: Janet Reno; 202/514–2000

DRUG ENFORCEMENT ADMINISTRATION
Administrator: Thomas A. Constantine; 202/307–8000

Department of Labor
tel. 202/219–5000

Acting Secretary: Cynthia Metzler; 202/219–8271

BUREAU OF LABOR STATISTICS
Commissioner: Katharine G. Abraham; 202/606–7800

EMPLOYMENT AND TRAINING ADMINISTRATION
Acting Assistant Secretary: Ray Uhalde; 202/219–6050

OCCUPATIONAL SAFETY AND HEALTH ADMINISTRATION
Acting Assistant Secretary: Greg Watchman; 202/219–7162

Department of State
tel. 202/647–4000

Secretary: Madeleine Albright; 202/647–6575

AGENCY FOR INTERNATIONAL DEVELOPMENT
Administrator: J. Brian Atwood; 202/647–9620

Independent Agencies

U.S. COMMISSION ON CIVIL RIGHTS
Chairperson: Mary Frances Berry; 202/376–7572

CONSUMER PRODUCT SAFETY COMMISSION
Chairperson: Ann Brown; 301/504–0213

ENVIRONMENTAL PROTECTION AGENCY
Administrator: Carol M. Browner; 202/260–4700

EQUAL EMPLOYMENT OPPORTUNITY COMMISSION
Chairman: Gilbert Casellas; 202/663–4001

FEDERAL EMERGENCY MANAGEMENT AGENCY
Director: James Lee Witt; 202/646–3923

Government-Related Groups *Federally aided corporations and quasi–official agencies, such as American Red Cross, National Academy of Sciences and World Health Organization, are listed with International, National, and Regional Organizations beginning on page C3.*

State and Local Organizations and Agencies

Blue Cross– Blue Shield Plans

The following list of Blue Cross and Blue Shield Plans is based on the Winter 1997 edition of the Directory Blue Cross and Blue Shield Plans, obtained from Blue Cross and Blue Shield Association, 676 North St. Clair, Chicago, IL 60611; tel. 312/440–6000. When addressing mail to a plan, use the post office box number.

United States

ALABAMA: Blue Cross and Blue Shield of Alabama, 450 Riverchase Parkway, E., P.O. Box 995, Birmingham, AL 35298; tel. 205/988–2200; FAX. 205/988–2949; E. Gene Thrasher, President, Chief Executive Officer

ALASKA: Blue Cross of Washington and Alaska, Blue Cross and Blue Shield of Alaska, 7001 220th Street, S.W., Mountlake Terrace, WA 98045–2124, P.O. Box 327, Seattle, WA 98111–0327; tel. 206/670–5900; FAX. 206/670–4900; Betty Woods, President, Chief Executive Officer

ARIZONA: Blue Cross and Blue Shield of Arizona, Inc., 2444 West Las Palmaritas Drive, Phoenix, AZ 85021, P.O. Box 13466, Phoenix, AZ 85002–3466; tel. 602/864–4400; FAX. 602/864–4242; Robert B. Bulla, President, Chief Executive Officer

ARKANSAS: Arkansas Blue Cross and Blue Shield, a Mutual Insurance Company, 601 Gaines Street, Little Rock, AR 72201, P.O. Box 2181, Little Rock, AR 72203; tel. 501/378–2010; FAX. 501/378–2037; Robert L. Shoptaw, President, Chief Executive Officer

CALIFORNIA: Blue Cross of California, CaliforniaCare Health Plans, 21555 Oxnard Street, Woodland Hills, CA 91367, P.O. Box 70000, Van Nuys, CA 91470; tel. 818/703–2345; FAX. 818/703–2848; Leonard D. Schaeffer, Chairman, Chief Executive Officer

Blue Shield of California, California Physicians' Service Corporation, Two North Point, San Francisco, CA 94133, P.O. Box 7168, San Francisco, CA 94120; tel. 415/445–5000; FAX. 415/445–5056; Wayne R. Moon, Chairman

COLORADO: Blue Cross and Blue Shield of Colorado, Rocky Mountain Hospital and Medical Service, 700 Broadway, Denver, CO 80273–0002; tel. 303/831–2131; FAX. 303/830–0887; C. David Kikumoto, President, Chief Executive Officer

CONNECTICUT: Blue Cross and Blue Shield of Connecticut, Inc., 370 Bassett Road, P.O. Box 504, North Haven, CT 06473; tel. 203/239–4911; FAX. 203/239–7742; John F. Croweak, Chairman, Chief Executive Officer

DELAWARE: Blue Cross and Blue Shield of Delaware, Blue Cross and Blue Shield of Delaware, Inc., One Brandywine Gateway, P.O. Box 1991, Wilmington, DE 19899; tel. 302/429–0260; FAX. 302/421–2089; Robert C. Cole, Jr., President, Chief Executive Officer

DISTRICT OF COLUMBIA: Blue Cross and Blue Shield of the National Capital Area, 550 12th Street, S.W., Washington, DC 20065; tel. 202/479–8000; FAX. 202/479–3520; Larry C. Glasscock, President, Chief Executive Officer

FLORIDA: Blue Cross and Blue Shield of Florida, Inc., 532 Riverside Avenue, Jacksonville, FL 32202, P.O. Box 1798, Jacksonville, FL 32231–0014; tel. 904/791–6111; FAX. 904/791–8081; William J. Flaherty, Chairman, Chief Executive Officer

GEORGIA: Blue Cross and Blue Shield of Georgia, Inc., Capital City Plaza, 3350 Peachtree Road, N.E., Atlanta, GA 30326, P.O. Box 4445, Atlanta, GA 30302–4445; tel. 404/842–8000; FAX. 404/842–8010; Richard D. Shirk, President, Chief Executive Officer

HAWAII: Blue Cross and Blue Shield of Hawaii, Hawaii Medical Service Association, 818 Keeaumoku Street, Honolulu, HI 96814, P.O. Box 860, Honolulu, HI 96808–0860; tel. 808/948–5517; FAX. 808/948–5999; Robert P. Hiam, President

IDAHO: Blue Cross of Idaho Health Service, Inc., 1501 Federal Way, Boise, ID 83705, P.O. Box 7408, Boise, ID 83707; tel. 208/345–4550; FAX. 208/331–7311; David L. Barnett, President, Chief Executive Officer

Blue Shield of Idaho, Medical Service Bureau of Idaho, Inc., 1602 21st Avenue, P.O. Box 1106, Lewiston, ID 83501; tel. 208/798–2100; FAX. 208/798–2085; Rich D. Nelson, President, Chief Executive Officer

ILLINOIS: Blue Cross and Blue Shield of Illinois, Health Care Service Corporation, a Mutual Legal Reserve Company, 233 North Michigan Avenue, Chicago, IL 60601, P.O. Box 1364, Chicago, IL 60690; tel. 312/938–7500; FAX. 312/819–1220; Raymond F. McCaskey, President, Chief Executive Officer

INDIANA: Anthem Blue Cross and Blue Shield, Anthem Insurance Companies, Inc., 120 Monument Circle, Indianapolis, IN 46204; tel. 317/488–6489; FAX. 317/488–6477; L. Ben Lytle, President, Chief Executive Officer

IOWA: Blue Cross and Blue Shield of Iowa, IASD Health Services Corp., 636 Grand Avenue, Des Moines, IA 50309; tel. 515/245–4545; FAX. 515/245–5090; John D. Forsyth, President, Chief Executive Officer

KANSAS: Blue Cross and Blue Shield of Kansas, Inc., 1133 Topeka Boulevard, Topeka, KS 66629–0001, P.O. Box 239, Topeka, KS 66601–0239; tel. 800/432–3990; FAX. 913/291–8465; John W. Knack, President, Chief Executive Officer

KENTUCKY: Anthem Blue Cross and Blue Shield, Anthem Insurance Companies, Inc., 9901 Linn Station Road, Louisville, KY 40223; tel. 502/423–2011; FAX. 502/339–5483; James P. Murphy, President, Tri–State Health Operations

LOUISIANA: Blue Cross and Blue Shield of Louisiana, Louisiana Health Service and Indemnity Company, 5525 Reitz Avenue, Baton Rouge, LA 70809–3802, P.O. Box 98029, Baton Rouge, LA 70898–9029; tel. 504/295–2511; FAX. 504/295–2506; P. J. Mills, President, Chief Executive Officer

MAINE: Blue Cross Blue Shield of Maine, Associated Hospital Service of Maine, Two Gannett Drive, South Portland, ME 04106–6911; tel. 207/822–7000; FAX. 207/822–7350; Andrew W. Greene, President, Chief Executive Officer

MARYLAND: Blue Cross and Blue Shield of Maryland, Inc., 10455 Mill Run Circle, P.O. Box 1010, Owings Mills, MD 21117; tel. 800/524–4555; FAX. 410/998–5576; William L. Jews, President, Chief Executive Officer

MASSACHUSETTS: Blue Cross and Blue Shield of Massachusetts, 100 Summer Street, Boston, MA 02110; tel. 617/832–3300; FAX. 617/832–3353; William C. Van Faasen, President, Chief Executive Officer

MICHIGAN: Blue Cross and Blue Shield of Michigan, 600 Lafayette East, Detroit, MI 48226–2998; tel. 313/225–8000; FAX. 313/225–6239; Richard E. Whitmer, President, Chief Executive Officer

MINNESOTA: Blue Cross and Blue Shield of Minnesota, BCBSM, Inc., 3535 Blue Cross Road, St. Paul, MN 55122, P.O. Box 64560, St. Paul, MN 55164; tel. 612/456–5040; FAX. 612/456–1657; Andrew P. Czajkowski, President, Chief Executive Officer

MISSISSIPPI: Blue Cross & Blue Shield of Mississippi, a Mutual Insurance Company, 3545 Lakeland Drive, Jackson, MS 39208–9799, P.O. Box 1043, Jackson, MS 39215–1043; tel. 601/932–3704; FAX. 601/939–7035; Richard J. Hale, President, Chief Executive Officer

MISSOURI: Alliance Blue Cross Blue Shield, 1831 Chestnut Street, St. Louis, MO 63103–2275; tel. 314/923–4444; FAX. 314/923–4809; Roy R. Heimburger, Chairman, Chief Executive Officer

Blue Cross and Blue Shield of Kansas City, 2301 Main, Kansas City, MO 64108, P.O. Box 419169, Kansas City, MO 64141–6169; tel. 816/395–2222; FAX. 816/395–2035; Richard P. Krecker, President, Chief Executive Officer

MONTANA: Blue Cross Blue Shield of Montana, Inc., 560 North Park Avenue, Helena, MT 59601, P.O. Box 4309, Helena, MT 59604–4309; tel. 406/444–8200; FAX. 406/442–6946; Alan F. Cain, President, Chief Executive Officer

NEBRASKA: Blue Cross and Blue Shield of Nebraska, 7261 Mercy Road, P.O. Box 3248 Main P.O. Station, Omaha, NE 68180–0001; tel. 402/390–1800; FAX. 402/392–2141; Richard L. Guffey, Chairman of the Board, Chief Executive Officer

NEVADA: Blue Cross and Blue Shield of Nevada, 5250 South Virginia Street, Reno, NV 89502, P.O. Box 10330, Reno, NV 89520–0330; tel. 702/829–4040; FAX. 702/829–4101; C. David Kikumoto, President, Chief Executive Officer

NEW HAMPSHIRE: Blue Cross and Blue Shield of New Hampshire, New Hampshire–Vermont Health Service, 3000 Goffs Falls Road, Manchester, NH 03111–0001; tel. 603/695–7064; FAX. 603/695–7304; David Jensen, President, Chief Executive Officer

NEW JERSEY: Blue Cross and Blue Shield of New Jersey, Inc., Three Penn Plaza East, P.O. Box 420, Newark, NJ 07105–2200; tel. 201/466–4000; FAX. 201/466–8762; William J. Marino, President, Chief Executive Officer

NEW MEXICO: Blue Cross and Blue Shield of New Mexico, New Mexico Blue Cross and Blue Shield, Inc., 12800 Indian School Road, N.E., Albuquerque, NM 87112, P.O. Box 27630, Albuquerque, NM 87125–7630; tel. 505/291–3500; FAX. 505/237–5324; Norman P. Becker, President, Chief Operating Officer

NEW YORK: Blue Cross and Blue Shield of Central New York, Inc., Excellus Health Plan, Inc., 344 South Warren Street, Syracuse, NY 13202, P.O. Box 4809, Syracuse, NY 13221–4809; tel. 315/448–3902; FAX. 315/448–6763; Albert F. Antonini, President, Chief Executive Officer

Blue Cross and Blue Shield of Western New York, Inc., 1901 Main Street, Buffalo, NY 14208, P.O. Box 80, Buffalo, NY 14240–0080; tel. 716/884–2911; FAX. 716/887–8981; Thomas P. Hartnett, Ph.D., President

Empire Blue Cross and Blue Shield, 622 Third Avenue, New York, NY 10017–6758, P.O. Box 345, New York, NY 10163–0345; tel. 800/261–5962; FAX. 212/983–7615; Michael A. Stocker, M.D., President, Chief Executive Officer

Finger Lakes Blue Cross and Blue Shield, Finger Lakes Medical Insurance Company, Inc., 150 East Main Street, Rochester, NY 14647; tel. 716/454–1700; FAX. 716/238–4400; Howard J. Berman, President, Chief Executive Officer

Utica–Watertown Health Insurance Company, Inc., d/b/a Blue Cross and Blue Shield of Utica–Watertown and HMO Blue, Utica Business Park, 12 Rhoads Drive, Utica, NY 13502–6398; tel. 315/798–4200; FAX. 315/797–5254, ext. 248; Matthew D. Babcock, Acting President

NORTH CAROLINA: Blue Cross and Blue Shield of North Carolina, 5901 Chapel Hill Road, Durham, NC 27707–0718, P.O. Box 2291, Durham, NC 27702; tel. 919/489–7431; FAX. 919/490–0171; Kenneth C. Otis II, President

NORTH DAKOTA: Blue Cross Blue Shield of North Dakota, 4510 13th Avenue, S.W., Fargo, ND 58121–0001; tel. 800/342–4718; FAX. 701/282–1866; Michael B. Unhjem, President, Chief Executive Officer

OHIO: Anthem Blue Cross and Blue Shield, Community Insurance Company, Inc., Anthem Insurance Companies, Inc., 1351 William Howard Taft Road, Cincinnati, OH 45206; tel. 513/977–8811; FAX. 513/977–8812; Dwane R. Houser, Chairman of the Board, Chief Executive Officer
Blue Cross and Blue Shield of Ohio, Blue Cross and Blue Shield Mutual of Ohio, 2060 East Ninth Street, Cleveland, OH 44115–1355; tel. 216/687–7000; FAX. 216/687–6044; John Burry, Jr., Chairman, Chief Executive Officer

OKLAHOMA: Blue Cross and Blue Shield of Oklahoma, (Group Health Service of Oklahoma, Inc.), 1215 South Boulder Avenue, Tulsa, OK 74119–2800, P.O. Box 3283, Tulsa, OK 74102–3283; tel. 918/560–3500; FAX. 918/560–2095; Ronald F. King, Chief Executive Officer

OREGON: Blue Cross and Blue Shield of Oregon, 100 Southwest Market Street, Portland, OR 97201, P.O. Box 1271, Portland, OR 97207; tel. 800/452–7390; FAX. 503/225–5232; Richard L. Woolworth, President, Chief Executive Officer

PENNSYLVANIA: Blue Cross of Northeastern Pennsylvania, Hospital Service Association of Northeastern Pennsylvania, 70 North Main Street, Wilkes Barre, PA 18711; tel. 717/831–3676; FAX. 717/831–3670; Thomas J. Ward, President, Chief Executive Officer
Capital Blue Cross, 2500 Elmerton Avenue, Harrisburg, PA 17177–1032; tel. 717/541–7000; FAX. 717/541–6072; James M. Mead, President, Chief Executive Officer
Highmark Blue Cross Blue Shield, 120 Fifth Avenue, Pittsburgh, PA 15222–3099; tel. 412/255–7000; FAX. 412/255–8158; William M. Lowry, President, Chief Executive Officer
Independence Blue Cross, 1901 Market Street, Philadelphia, PA 19103; tel. 800/358–0050; FAX. 215/241–3824; G. Fred DiBona, Jr., President, Chief Executive Officer
Pennsylvania Blue Shield, Medical Service Association of Pennsylvania, 1800 Center Street, Camp Hill, PA 17011, P.O.Box 890089, Camp Hill, PA 17089–0089; tel. 800/637–3493; FAX. 717/763–3544; Samuel D. Ross, Jr., President, Chief Executive Officer

RHODE ISLAND: Blue Cross and Blue Shield of Rhode Island, 444 Westminster Street, Providence, RI 02903–3279; tel. 401/459–1200; FAX. 401/459–1290; Douglas J. McIntosh, President

SOUTH CAROLINA: Blue Cross and Blue Shield of South Carolina, I–20 East at Alpine Road, Columbia, SC 29219; tel. 803/788–3860; FAX. 803/736–3420; M. Edward Sellers, President, Chief Executive Officer

SOUTH DAKOTA: Blue Cross Blue Shield of South Dakota, South Dakota Health Services Company, 1601 West Madison Street, Sioux Falls, SD 57104; tel. 605/361–5981; FAX. 605/361–5898; F. Joseph DuBray, President, Chief Executive Officer

TENNESSEE: Blue Cross Blue Shield of Tennessee–Memphis, Memphis Hospital Service and Surgical Association, Inc., 85 North Danny Thomas Boulevard, Memphis, TN 38103, P.O. Box 98, Memphis, TN 38101; tel. 901/544–2111; FAX. 901/544–2440; Gene Holcomb, President
Blue Cross and Blue Shield of Tennessee, 801 Pine Street, Chattanooga, TN 37402; tel. 423/755–5600; FAX. 423/755–2178, ext. 5621; Thomas Kinser, Chief Executive Officer

TEXAS: Blue Cross and Blue Shield of Texas, Inc., 901 South Central Expressway, Richardson, TX 75080, P.O. Box 655730, Dallas, TX 75265–5730; tel. 972/766–6900; FAX. 972/766–6060; Rogers K. Coleman, M.D., President, Chief Executive Officer

UTAH: Blue Cross and Blue Shield of Utah, 2455 Parley's Way, P.O. Box 30270, Salt Lake City, UT 84130–0270; tel. 801/481–6198; FAX. 801/481–6994; Jed H. Pitcher, Chairman, President, Chief Executive Officer

VERMONT: Blue Cross and Blue Shield of Vermont, One East Road, Berlin, VT 05602, P.O. Box 186, Montpelier, VT 05601; tel. 802/223–6131; FAX. 802/229–0511; Preston Jordan, President, Chief Executive Officer

VIRGINIA: Trigon Blue Cross Blue Shield, Blue Cross and Blue Shield of Virginia, 2015 Staples Mill Road, Richmond, VA 23230, P.O. Box 27401, Richmond, VA 23279; tel. 804/354–7173; FAX. 804/354–7044; Norwood H. Davis, Jr., Chairman, Chief Executive Officer

WASHINGTON: Blue Cross of Washington and Alaska, Blue Shield in North Central Washington, 7001 220th Street, S.W., Mountlake Terrace, WA 98043–2124, P.O. Box 327, Seattle, WA 98111–0327; tel. 206/670–5900; FAX. 206/670–4900; Betty Woods, President, Chief Executive Officer
King County Medical Blue Shield, 1800 Ninth Avenue, Seattle, WA 98101–1322, P.O. Box 21267, Seattle, WA 98111–3267; tel. 206/464–3600; FAX. 206/389–6778; Dale M. Francis, President, Chief Executive Officer
Medical Service Corporation of Eastern Washington, 3900 East Sprague Avenue, Spokane, WA 99202, P.O. Box 3048, Spokane, WA 99220–3048; tel. 509/536–4500; FAX. 509/536–4770; Betty Woods, Chief Executive Officer
Pierce County Medical Bureau, Inc., 1501 Market Street, Tacoma, WA 98402, P.O. Box 2354, Tacoma, WA 98401–2354; tel. 206/597–6557; FAX. 206/597–7475; Rich Nelson, President
Skagit County Medical Bureau, P.O. Box 699, Mount Vernon, WA 98273; tel. 360/336–9660; FAX. 360/336–2028; Roger B. Mercer, President
Washington Physicians Service Association, 1800 Ninth Avenue, Seattle, WA 98101, P.O. Box 2010, Seattle, WA 98111; tel. 206/389–7520; FAX. 206/389–7521; William Van Hollebeke, Executive Director
Whatcom Medical Bureau, 3000 Northwest Avenue, Bellingham, WA 98225, P.O. Box 9753, Bellingham, WA 98227–9753; tel. 360/734–8000; FAX. 360/734–6676; Michael D. Plenkovich, Acting President

WEST VIRGINIA: Mountain State Blue Cross & Blue Shield, Inc., 700 Market Square, Parkersburg, WV 26101, P.O. Box 1948, Parkersburg, WV 26102; tel. 304/424–7732; FAX. 304/424–7789; Gregory K. Smith, President, Chief Executive Officer

WISCONSIN: Blue Cross and Blue Shield United of Wisconsin, 401 West Michigan Street, Milwaukee, WI 53203, P.O. Box 2025, Milwaukee, WI 53201; tel. 414/224–6100; FAX. 414/226–5488; Thomas R. Hefty, Chairman, Chief Executive Officer

WYOMING: Blue Cross and Blue Shield of Wyoming, 4000 House Avenue, Cheyenne, WY 82001–2266, P.O. Box 2266, Cheyenne, WY 82003–2266; tel. 307/634–1393; FAX. 307/778–8582; C. E. Chapman, President

U. S. Associated Areas

JAMAICA: Blue Cross of Jamaica, 85 Hope Road, Kingston 6, JA, West Indies; tel. 809/927–9821, ext. 224; FAX. 809/927–9817; Henry Lowe, Ph.D., C.D., J.P., President, Chief Executive Officer

PUERTO RICO: La Cruz Azul de Puerto Rico, Blue Cross of Puerto Rico, Carretera Estatal 1, K.M. 17.3–Rio Piedras, PR 00927, P.O. Box 366068, San Juan, PR 00936–6068; tel. 787/272–9898; FAX. 787/272–7867; Jose Julian Alvarez, Executive President
Triple–S, Inc., P.O. Box 363628, San Juan, PR 00936–3628; tel. 809/749–4114; FAX. 809/749–4191; Miguel A. Vazquez–Deynes, President

Canada

ALBERTA: Alberta Blue Cross Plan, 10009–108th Street, Edmonton, AB T5J 3C5, CANADA; tel. 403/428–1100; FAX. 403/498–8532; V. George Ward, President, Chief Executive Officer

BRITISH COLUMBIA: Medical Services Association, 2025 West Broadway, P.O. Box 9300, Vancouver, BC V6B 5M1, CANADA; tel. 604/737–5700; FAX. 604/737–5781; John D. Seney, President, Chief Executive Officer

MANITOBA: Manitoba Blue Cross, United Health Services Corporation, 100A Polo Park Centre, 1485 Portage Avenue, Winnipeg, MB R3G 0W4, P.O. Box 1046, Winnipeg, MB R3C 2X7, CANADA; tel. 204/775–0151; FAX. 204/774–1761; Kerry V. Bittner, President

NEW BRUNSWICK: Blue Cross of Atlantic Canada, 644 Main Street, Moncton, NB E1C 1E2, P.O. Box 220, Moncton, NB E1C 8L3, CANADA; tel. 506/853–1811; FAX. 506/853–4651; Leon R. Furlong, President, Chief Executive Officer

NEWFOUNDLAND: Blue Cross in Ontario, (Moncton Office), 644 Main Street, Moncton, NB E1C 1E2, P.O. Box 220, Moncton, NB E1C 8L3; tel. 506/853–1811; FAX. 506/853–4651; Leon R. Furlong, President, Chief Executive Officer

NOVA SCOTIA: Blue Cross of Atlantic Canada, 644 Main Street, Moncton, NB E1C 1E2, P.O. Box 220, Moncton, NB E1C 8L3; tel. 506/853–1811; FAX. 506/867–4651; L. R. Furlong, President, Chief Executive Officer

ONTARIO: Blue Cross in Ontario, (Ontario Office), 185 The West Mall, Suite 600, P.O. Box 2000, Etobicoke, ON M9C 5P1; tel. 416/626–1688; FAX. 416/626–0997; Andrew Yorke, Chief Operating Officer

QUEBEC: Quebec Blue Cross Quebec Hospital Service Association, 550 Sherbrooke Street, W., Montreal, PQ H3A 1B9, CANADA; tel. 514/286–8472; FAX. 514/286–8475; Claude Ferron, CA, President

SASKATCHEWAN: Group Medical Services, 1992 Hamilton Street, Regina, SK S4P 2C6, CANADA; tel. 306/352–7638; FAX. 306/525–3825; Harold N. Hoffman, President
Saskatchewan Blue Cross, (MSI) Medical Services Incorporated, 516 Second Avenue, N., Saskatoon, SK S7K 2C5, P.O. Box 4030, Saskatoon, SK S7K 3T2, CANADA; tel. 306/244–1192; FAX. 306/664–1945; Terry R. Brash, President, Chief Executive Officer

Section C

Health Systems Agencies

The following is a list of federally funded Health Systems Agencies. The information was obtained from the National Directory of Health Planning Policy and Regulatory Agencies, published by the Missouri Department of Health, Certificate of Need Program. States not listed do not have HSAs. For information about other local agencies and organizations that fulfill similar functions, contact the state or metropolitan hospital associations; see also the list of State Health Planning and Development Agencies in section C.

United States

FLORIDA: Big Bend Health Council, Inc. (District Two), 2629 West 10th Street, Panama City, FL 32401; tel. 904/872–4128; FAX. 904/872–4131; David W. Carter, Executive Director

Broward Regional Health Planning Council (District 10), 915 Middle River Drive, Suite 521, Fort Lauderdale, FL 33304; tel. 305/561–9681; FAX. 305/561–9685; John H. Werner, Executive Director

Health Council of South Florida, Inc., 5757 Blue Lagoon Drive, Suite 170, Miami, FL 33126; tel. 305/263–9020; FAX. 305/262–9905; Sonya Albury, Executive Director

Health Council of West Central Florida (District Six), 9721 Executive Center Drive, N., Suite 114, St. Petersburg, FL 33702–2438; tel. 813/576–7772; FAX. 813/570–3033; Elizabeth Rugg, Director

Health Planning Council of Northeast Florida, Inc., 2236 St. Johns Avenue, Jacksonville, FL 32204; tel. 904/381–6035; FAX. 904/381–6067; Lori A. Billelo, Executive Director

Health Planning Council of Southwest Florida, Inc., 9250 College Parkway, Suite Three, Fort Myers, FL 33919; tel. 941/433–4600; FAX. 941/433–6703; Mary W. Schulthess, Planner, Executive Director

Local Health Council of East Central Florida (District Seven), 1155 South Semoran Boulevard, Suite 1111, Winter Park, FL 32792–5505; tel. 407/671–2005; Steve Windham, Executive Director

North Central Florida Health Planning Council, 11 West University Avenue, Suite Seven, Gainesville, FL 32601; tel. 904/955–2264; FAX. 904/955–3109; Carol J. Gormley, Executive Director

Northwest Florida Health Council, Inc. (District One), 2629 West 10th Street, Panama City, FL 32401; tel. 904/872–4128; FAX. 904/872–4131; David W. Carter, Executive Director

Suncoast Health Council, Inc. (District Five), 9721 Executive Center Drive, N., Suite 114, St. Petersburg, FL 33702–2451; tel. 813/576–7772; FAX. 813/570–3033; Elizabeth Rugg, Executive Director

Treasure Coast Health Council, Inc. (District Nine), 5651 Corporate Way, Suite Four, West Palm Beach, FL 33407–2001; tel. 407/681–6256; FAX. 407/681–6258; Barbara H. Jacobowitz, Executive Director

MARYLAND: Chesapeake Health Planning System, Inc., P.O. Box 773, Cambridge, MD 21613; tel. 410/221–0907; FAX. 410/228–1321

MINNESOTA: Region 1 (Northwest MN) and Region II (Northeast MN), Regional Coordinating Boards, Minnesota Department of Health, P.O. Box 64975, St. Paul, MN 55164–0975; tel. 612/282–5644; FAX. 612/282–5628; Michele Danen

Region III (Central MN) and Region IV (Twin City Metro), Minnesota Department of Health, P.O. Box 64975, St. Paul, MN 55164–0975; tel. 612/282–6330; Kristin Pederson

Region V (Southwest MN) and Region VI (Southeast MN), Minnesota Department of Health, CHS Division, Suite 460, P.O. Box 64975, St. Paul, MN 55164–0975; tel. 612/282–6328; FAX. 612/282–5628; Kay Markling

NEW JERSEY: Essex and Union Advisory Board for Health Planning, Inc., 14 South Orange Avenue, South Orange, NJ 07079; tel. 201/761–6969; FAX. 201/761–7401; Sharon Postel, Executive Director

Fairleigh Dickinson University, Region Two Health Planning Advisory Board, Inc., 1000 River Road, Teaneck, NJ 07666; tel. 201/692–7180; FAX. 201/692–7189; Thomas Pavlak, Ph.D., Executive Director

Health Visions, Inc., 6981 North Park Drive, East Building, Suite 307, Pennsauken, NJ 08109; tel. 609/662–2050; FAX. 609/662–2261; Charles Daly, Vice President, Health Planning

Jersey Coast Health Planning Council, Inc., 515 Route 70, Suite 208, Brick, NJ 08723; tel. 908/262–9047; FAX. 908/262–9049; Eleanor Jaeger, Executive Director

Mid–State Health Advisory Corporation–Rider University, Rider University, 2083 Lawrenceville Road, Lawrenceville, NJ 08648; tel. 609/219–2121; FAX. 609/219–2120; Bernadette West, Executive Director

Region One Health Planning Advisory Board, Five Emery Avenue, Randolph, NJ 07869–1368; tel. 201/361–3390; FAX. 201/361–3864; Robert Schermer, Executive Director

NEW YORK: Central New York Health Systems Agency, Inc., 101 Intrepid Lane, Syracuse, NY 13205; tel. 315/492–8557; FAX. 315/492–8563; Timothy J. Bobo, Executive Director

Finger Lakes Health Systems Agency, 1150 University Avenue, Rochester, NY 14607; tel. 716/461–3520; FAX. 716/461–0997; Martha P. Bond, Acting Executive Director

Health Systems Agency of New York City, 450 Seventh Avenue, 13th Floor, New York, NY 10001; tel. 212/244–8100; FAX. 212/244–8120; Robert D. Gumbs, Executive Director

Health Systems Agency of Northeastern New York, Pine West Plaza, One United Way, Washington Avenue Extension, Albany, NY 12205–5558; tel. 518/452–3300; FAX. 518/452–5943; Bruce R. Stanley, Executive Director

Health Systems Agency of Western New York, 2070 Sheridan Drive, Buffalo, NY 14223; tel. 716/876–7131; FAX. 716/876–4968; Brian G. McBride, Ph.D., Executive Director

Hudson Valley Health Systems Agency, P.O. Box 696, Tuxedo, NY 10987; tel. 914/351–5146; Regina M. Kelly, Executive Director

NY Penn Health Systems Agency, 84 Court Street, Suite 300, Binghamton, NY 13901; tel. 607/772–0336; FAX. 607/772–0158; Denise Murray, Executive Director

Nassau–Suffolk Health Systems Agency, 1537 Old Country Road, Plainview, NY 11803; tel. 516/293–5740; FAX. 516/293–6288; Renee Pekmezaris, Ph.D., Executive Director

OHIO: Health Planning and Resource Development Association of Central Ohio River Valley, 35 East Seventh Street, Suite 311, Cincinnati, OH 45202; tel. 513/621–2434; FAX. 513/621–4307; James F. Sandmann, President

Health Systems Agency, 415 Bulkley Building, 1501 Euclid Avenue, Cleveland, OH 44115; tel. 216/771–6814; FAX. 216/771–2939; Nancy J. Roth, Executive Director

Lake to River Health Care Coalition, 106 Robbins Avenue, Niles, OH 44446; tel. 330/652–8111; FAX. 330/652–0003; Thomas J. Flynn, Executive Director

Miami Valley Health Improvement Council, 7039 Taylorsville Road, Huber Heights, OH 45424–3103; tel. 937/236–5358; FAX. 937/237–9750; Robert P. Thimmes, President, Chief Executive Officer

Northwest Ohio Health Planning, Inc., 635 North Erie Street, Toledo, OH 43624; tel. 419/255–1190; FAX. 419/255–2900; David G. Pollick, Executive Director

Scioto Valley Health Systems Agency (SVHSA), 261 East Livingston Avenue, Columbus, OH 43215–5748; tel. 614/221–1381; FAX. 614/221–7016; Franklin Hirsch, Executive Director

VIRGINIA: Central Virginia Health Planning Agency, Inc., P.O. Box 24287, Richmond, VA 23224; tel. 804/233–6206; FAX. 804/233–8834; Karen L. Cameron, Executive Director

Eastern Virginia Health Systems Agency, Inc., 18 Koger Executive Center, Suite 232, Norfolk, VA 23502; tel. 757/461–4834; FAX. 757/461–3255; Paul M. Boynton, Executive Director

Health Systems Agency of Northern Virginia, 7245 Arlington Boulevard, Suite 300, Falls Church, VA 22042; tel. 703/573–3100, ext. 1500; FAX. 703/573–1276; Dean Montgomery, Executive Director

Northwestern Virginia Health Systems Agency, 1924 Arlington Boulevard, Suite 211, Charlottesville, VA 22903; tel. 804/977–6010; FAX. 804/977–0748; Margaret P. King, Executive Director

Southwest Virginia Health Systems Agency, 3100–A Peters Creek Road, N.W., Roanoke, VA 24019; tel. 540/362–9528; FAX. 540/362–9676; Pamela P. Clark, MPA, Executive Director

The following list of state and metropolitan hospital associations is derived from the American Hospital Association's 1997 Directory of Hospital Associations.

United States

ALABAMA: Alabama Hospital Association, 500 North East Boulevard, Zip 36117, P.O. Box 210759, Montgomery, AL 36121–0759; tel. 334/272–8781; FAX. 334/270–9527; J. Michael Horsley, President, Chief Executive Officer

ALASKA: Alaska State Hospital and Nursing Home Association, 319 Seward Street, Suite 11, Juneau, AK 99801; tel. 907/586–1790; FAX. 907/463–3573; Laraine Derr, President, Chief Executive Officer

ARIZONA: Arizona Hospital and Healthcare Association, 1501 West Fountainhead Parkway, Suite 650, Tempe, AZ 85282; tel. 602/968–1083; FAX. 602/967–2029; John R. Rivers, President, Chief Executive Officer

ARKANSAS: Arkansas Hospital Association, 419 Natural Resources Drive, Little Rock, AR 72205–1539; tel. 501/224–7878; FAX. 501/224–0519; James R. Teeter, President, Chief Executive Officer

CALIFORNIA: California Healthcare Association, 1201 K Street, Suite 800, Sacramento, CA 95814, P.O. Box 1100, Sacramento, CA 95812–1100; tel. 916/443–7401; FAX. 916/552–7596; C. Duane Dauner, President

Healthcare Association of Southern California, 515 South Figueroa Street, Suite 1300, Los Angeles, CA 90071–3322; tel. 213/538–0700; FAX. 213/629–4272; James D. Barber, President, Chief Executive Officer

Hospital Council of Northern and Central California, 7901 Stoneridge Drive, Suite 500, Pleasanton, CA 94588; tel. 510/460–5444, ext. 304; FAX. 510/460–5457; Gregg Schnepple, President, Chief Executive Officer

Hospital Council of San Diego and Imperial Counties, 402 West Broadway, 23rd Floor, San Diego, CA 92101–3542; tel. 619/544–0777; FAX. 619/544–0888; Gary R. Stephany, President, Chief Executive Officer

COLORADO: Colorado Hospital Association, 2140 South Holly Street, Denver, CO 80222–5607; tel. 303/758–1630; FAX. 303/758–0047; Larry Wall, President

CONNECTICUT: The Connecticut Hospital Association, Inc., 110 Barnes Road, P.O. Box 90, Wallingford, CT 06492–0090; tel. 203/294–7200; FAX. 203/284–9318; Dennis P. May, President

DELAWARE: Association of Delaware Hospitals, 1280 South Governors Avenue, Dover, DE 19904–4802; tel. 302/674–2853; FAX. 302/734–2731; Joseph M. Letnaunchyn, President

DISTRICT OF COLUMBIA: District of Columbia Hospital Association, 1250 Eye Street, N.W., Suite 700, Washington, DC 20005–3930; tel. 202/682–1581; FAX. 202/371–8151; Joan H. Lewis, Acting President

FLORIDA: Florida Hospital Association, 307 Park Lake Circle, P.O. Box 531107, Orlando, FL 32853–1107; tel. 407/841–6230; FAX. 407/422–5948; Charles F. Pierce, Jr., President

South Florida Hospital and Healthcare Association, 8181 Miami Lakes Drive, W., Suite 200, Miami Lakes, FL 33016–5817; tel. 305/825–4007; FAX. 305/825–8697; Linda S. Quick, President

The Tampa Bay Hospital Association, Inc., 9455 Koger Boulevard, N., Suite 118, St. Petersburg, FL 33702; tel. 813/579–0252; FAX. 813/579–9494; Willard E. Wisler, FACHE, President

GEORGIA: Georgia Hospital Association, 1675 Terrell Mill Road, Marietta, GA 30067; tel. 770/955–0324; FAX. 770/955–5801; Joseph A. Parker, President

HAWAII: Healthcare Association of Hawaii, 932 Ward Avenue, Suite 430, Honolulu, HI 96814–2126; tel. 808/521–8961; FAX. 808/599–2879; Richard E. Meiers, President, Chief Executive Officer

IDAHO: Idaho Hospital Association, 802 West Bannock Street, Suite 500, Boise, ID 83702–5842, P.O. Box 1278, Boise, ID 83701–1278; tel. 208/338–5100; FAX. 208/338–7800; Steven A. Millard, President

ILLINOIS: Illinois Hospital and HealthSystems Association, Center for Health Affairs, 1151 East Warrenville Road, P.O. Box 3015, Naperville, IL 60566–7015; tel. 630/505–7777; FAX. 630/505–9457; Kenneth C. Robbins, President

Metropolitan Chicago Healthcare Council, 222 South Riverside Plaza, 19th Floor, Chicago, IL 60606; tel. 312/906–6000; FAX. 312/993–0779; Earl C. Bird, President

INDIANA: Indiana Hospital&Health Association, One American Square, P.O. Box 82063, Indianapolis, IN 46282; tel. 317/633–4870; FAX. 317/633–4875; Kenneth G. Stella, President

IOWA: The Association of Iowa Hospitals and Health Systems, 100 East Grand Avenue, Suite 100, Des Moines, IA 50309; tel. 515/288–1955; FAX. 515/283–9366; Stephen F. Brenton, President

KANSAS: Kansas Hospital Association, 215 Southeast Eighth Street, Topeka KS 66603–3906, P.O. Box 2308, Topeka, KS 66601–2308; tel. 913/233–7436; FAX. 913/233–6955; Donald A. Wilson, President

KENTUCKY: KHA, 1302 Clear Spring Trace, P.O. Box 24163, Louisville, KY 40224; tel. 502/426–6220; FAX. 502/426–6226; Michael T. Rust, President, Chief Executive Officer

LOUISIANA: Louisiana Hospital Association, 9521 Brookline Avenue, Baton Rouge, LA 70809, P.O. Box 80720, Baton Rouge, LA 70898–0720; tel. 504/928–0026; FAX. 504/923–1004; Robert D. Merkel, President

Metropolitan Hospital Council of New Orleans, 2450 Severn Avenue, Suite 210, Metairie, LA 70001; tel. 504/837–1171; FAX. 504/837–1174; John J. Finn, Ph.D., President

MAINE: Maine Hospital Association, 150 Capitol Street, Augusta, ME 04330; tel. 207/622–4794; FAX. 207/622–3073; Bruce J. Rueben, President

MARYLAND: Healthcare Council of the National Capital Area, 8201 Corporate Drive, Suite 410, Landover, MD 20785–2229; tel. 301/731–4700; FAX. 301/731–8286; Joseph P. Burns, President, Chief Executive Officer

MHA, 1301 York Road, Suite 800, Lutherville, MD 21093–6087; tel. 410/321–6200; FAX. 410/321–6268; Calvin M. Pierson, President

MASSACHUSETTS: Massachusetts Hospital Association, Five New England Executive Park, Burlington, MA 01803; tel. 617/272–8000; FAX. 617/272–1524, ext. 111; Ronald M. Hollander, President

MICHIGAN: Center for Health Affairs, 3075 Charlevoix Drive, S.E., Grand Rapids, MI 49546; tel. 616/940–3337; FAX. 616/940–0723; Edward A. Rode, President

Greater Flint Area Hospital Assembly, 702 South Ballenger Highway, Flint, MI 48532–3803; tel. 810/766–8898; FAX. 810/766–6422; Marlene Soderstrom, Executive Director

Hospital Council of East Central Michigan, 141 Harrow Lane, Suite 11, Saginaw, MI 48603; tel. 517/792–1725; FAX. 517/792–3099; Randolph K. Flechsig, President

Michigan Health & Hospital Association, 6215 West St. Joseph Highway, Lansing, MI 48917; tel. 517/323–3443; FAX. 517/323–0946; Spencer C. Johnson, President

North Central Council of the Michigan Health & Hospital Association, 114 North Court Street, Gaylord, MI 49735; tel. 517/732–7002; FAX. 517/732–3059; Mary E. Fox, Executive Director

South Central Michigan Hospital Council, 6215 West St. Joseph Highway, Lansing, MI 48917; tel. 517/323–3443; FAX. 517/323–0946; Marlene Soderstrom, President

Southeast Michigan Health and Hospital Council, 24725 West Twelve Mile Road, Suite 104A, Southfield, MI 48034; tel. 810/358–2950; FAX. 810/358–1098; Donald P. Potter, President

Southwestern Michigan Hospital Council, 6215 West St. Joseph Highway, Lansing, MI 48917; tel. 517/323–3443; FAX. 517/323–0946; Clark R. Ballard, President

MINNESOTA: Minnesota Hospital and Healthcare Partnership, 2550 University Avenue, W., Suite 350S, St. Paul, MN 55114–1900; tel. 612/641–1121; FAX. 612/659–1477; Stephen Rogness, President

MISSISSIPPI: Mississippi Hospital Association, 6425 Lakeover Road, Jackson, MS 39213, P.O. Box 16444, Jackson, MS 39236–6444; tel. 601/982–3251; FAX. 601/368–3200; Sam W. Cameron, President, Chief Executive Officer

MISSOURI: Greater Kansas City Health Council, 10401 Holmes Road, Suite 280, Kansas City, MO 64131–3368; tel. 816/941–3800; FAX. 816/941–0818; Sheryl Jacobs, Senior Vice President

Missouri Hospital Association, 4712 Country Club Drive, Jefferson City, MO 65109–4544, P.O. Box 60, Jefferson City, MO 65102–0060; tel. 573/893–3700; FAX. 573/893–2809; Charles L. Bowman, President

MONTANA: Montana Hospital Association, 1720 Ninth Avenue, Helena, MT 59601, P.O. Box 5119, Helena, MT 59604; tel. 406/442–1911; FAX. 406/443–3894; James F. Ahrens, President

NEBRASKA: Nebraska Association of Hospitals and Health Systems, 1640 L Street, Suite D, Lincoln, NE 68508–2509; tel. 402/458–4900; FAX. 402/475–4091; Harlan M. Heald, Ph.D., President

NEVADA: Nevada Association of Hospitals and Health Systems, 4600 Kietzke Lane, Suite A–108, Reno, NV 89502; tel. 702/827–0184; FAX. 702/827–0190; Roy A. Barraclough, Vice President, Chief Executive Officer

NEW HAMPSHIRE: New England Healthcare Assembly, Inc., 500 Spaulding Turnpike, Suite W–310, P.O. Box 7100, Portsmouth, NH 03802–7100; tel. 603/422–6100; FAX. 603/422–6101; James S. Dolph, President

New Hampshire Hospital Association, 125 Airport Road, Concord, NH 03301–7300; tel. 603/225–0900; FAX. 603/225–4346; Michael J. Hill, President

NEW JERSEY: Hospital Alliance of New Jersey, 150 West State Street, Trenton, NJ 08608; tel. 609/989–8200; FAX. 609/989–7768; Suzanne Ianni, Executive Director

New Jersey Healthcare Congress, 760 Alexander Road, CN–1, Princeton, NJ 08543–0001; tel. 609/924–0049; FAX. 609/275–4114; Lisa Heher, Convention Manager

New Jersey Hospital Association, P.O. Box One, 760 Alexander Road, Princeton, NJ 08543–0001; tel. 609/275–4000; FAX. 609/275–4100; Gary S. Carter, President, Chief Executive Officer

NEW MEXICO: New Mexico Hospitals and Health Systems Association, 2121 Osuna Road, N.E., Albuquerque, NM 87113; tel. 505/343–0010; FAX. 505/343–0012; Maureen L. Boshier, Chief Executive Officer, President

NEW YORK: Greater New York Hospital Association, Subsidiaries and Affiliates, 555 West 57th Street, 15th Floor, New York, NY 10019; tel. 212/246–7100, ext. 401; FAX. 212/262–6350; Kenneth E. Raske, President

Healthcare Association of New York State, 74 North Pearl Street, Albany, NY 12207; tel. 518/431–7600; FAX. 518/431–7915; Daniel Sisto, President

Iroquois Healthcare Alliance, 74 North Pearl Street, Albany, NY 12207; tel. 518/431–7900; FAX. 518/431–7976; Gary J. Fitzgerald, President

Nassau–Suffolk Hospital Council, Inc., 888 Veterans Highway, Suite 310, Hauppauge, NY 11788; tel. 516/435–3000; FAX. 516/435–2343; Peter M. Sullivan, Executive Vice President, Chief Executive Officer

Northern Metropolitan Hospital Association, 400 Stony Brook Court, Newburgh, NY 12550; tel. 914/562–7520; FAX. 914/562–0187; Arthur E. Weintraub, President

Rochester Regional Hospital Association, 3445 Winton Place, Rochester, NY 14623; tel. 716/273–8180; FAX. 716/273–8189; Diane Ashley, Acting President. Chief Executive Officer

Western New York Healthcare Association, 1876 Niagara Falls Boulevard, Tonawanda, NY 14150–6499; tel. 716/695–0843; FAX. 716/695–0073, ext. 208; William D. Pike, President

NORTH CAROLINA: NCHA, P.O. Box 80428, Raleigh, NC 27623–0428; tel. 919/677–2400; FAX. 919/677–4200; C. Edward McCauley, President

NORTH DAKOTA: North Dakota Healthcare Association, 1120 College Drive, Suite 214, P.O. Box 7340, Bismarck, ND 58507–7340; tel. 701/224–9732; FAX. 701/224–9529; Arnold R. Thomas, President

OHIO: Akron Regional Hospital Association, 326 Locust Street, Suite 14, Akron, OH 44302–1801; tel. 330/379–8989; FAX. 330/379–8189; Robin Louis, Executive Director

Greater Cincinnati Hospital Council, 2100 Sherman Avenue, Suite 100, Cincinnati, OH 45212–2736; tel. 513/531–0200; FAX. 513/531–0278; Lynn R. Olman, President

Greater Cleveland Hospital Association, 1226 Huron Road at Playhouse, Cleveland, OH 44115; tel. 216/696–6900; FAX. 216/696–1875; C. Wayne Rice, Ph.D., President, Chief Executive Officer

Greater Dayton Area Hospital Association, 32 North Main Street, Suite 1441, Dayton, OH 45402; tel. 937/228–1000; FAX. 937/228–1035; Joseph M. Krella, President

Hospital Council of Northwest Ohio, 5515 Southwyck Boulevard, Suite 203, Toledo, OH 43614; tel. 419/865–1274; FAX. 419/867–4425; W. Scott Fry, President, Chief Executive Officer

OHA, 155 East Broad Street, Columbus, OH 43215; tel. 614/221–7614; FAX. 614/221–4771; James R. Castle, President

OKLAHOMA: Greater Oklahoma City Hospital Council, 4000 Lincoln Boulevard, Oklahoma City, OK 73105; tel. 405/427–9537; FAX. 405/424–4507; Rebecca J. Ellison, Executive Secretary

Oklahoma Hospital Association, 4000 Lincoln Boulevard, Oklahoma City, OK 73105; tel. 405/427–9537; FAX. 405/424–4507; John C. Coffey, President

OREGON: Oregon Association of Hospitals and Health Systems, 4000 Kruse Way Place, Building 2, Suite 100, Lake Oswego, OR 97035–2543; tel. 503/636–2204; FAX. 503/636–8310; Kenneth M. Rutledge, President

PENNSYLVANIA: Hospital Council of Western Pennsylvania, 500 Commonwealth Drive, Warrendale, PA 15086; tel. 412/776–6400; FAX. 412/776–6969; Ian G. Rawson, Ph.D., President

Hospital and Healthsystem Association of Pennsylvania, 4750 Lindle Road, P.O. Box 8600, Harrisburg, PA 17105–8600; tel. 717/564–9200; FAX. 717/561–5334; Carolyn F. Scanlan, President, Chief Executive Officer

The Delaware Valley Healthcare Council, 121 South Broad Street, Philadelphia, PA 19107; tel. 215/735–9695; FAX. 215/790–1267; Andrew B. Wigglesworth, President

RHODE ISLAND: Hospital Association of Rhode Island, Weld Building, Second Floor, 880 Butler Drive, Suite One, Providence, RI 02906; tel. 401/453–8400; FAX. 401/453–8411; Gerald G. McClure, President

SOUTH CAROLINA: South Carolina Hospital Association, 101 Medical Circle, P.O. Box 6009, West Columbia, SC 29171–6009; tel. 803/796–3080; FAX. 803/796–2938; Ken Shull, FACHE, President

SOUTH DAKOTA: South Dakota Association of Healthcare Organizations, 3708 Brooks Place, Suite 1, Sioux Falls, SD 57106; tel. 605/361–2281; FAX. 605/361–5175

TENNESSEE: THA, 500 Interstate Boulevard, S., Nashville, TN 37210–4634; tel. 615/256–8240; FAX. 615/242–4803; Craig A. Becker, President

TEXAS: Dallas–Fort Worth Hospital Council, 250 Decker Court, Irving, TX 75062; tel. 972/719–4900; FAX. 972/719–4009; John C. Gavras, President

Greater Houston Hospital Council, 3333 Eastside, Suite 130, Houston, TX 77098, P.O. Box 66962, Houston, TX 77266–6962; tel. 713/526–9031; FAX. 713/526–1351; Eugene C. Beck, President

Greater San Antonio Hospital Council, 8620 North New Braunfels, Suite 420, San Antonio, TX 78217; tel. 210/820–3500; FAX. 210/820–3888; William Dean Rasco, FACHE, President, Chief Executive Officer

Texas Hospital Association, 6225 U.S. Highway 290, E., P.O. Box 15587, Austin, TX 78761–5587; tel. 512/465–1000; FAX. 512/465–1090; Terry Townsend, FACHE, CAE, President, Chief Executive Officer

UTAH: Utah Association of Healthcare Providers, 2180 South 1300 East, Suite 440, Salt Lake City, UT 84106–2843; tel. 801/486–9915; FAX. 801/486–0882; Richard B. Kinnersley, President

VERMONT: Vermont Association of Hospitals and Health Systems, 148 Main Street, Montpelier, VT 05602; tel. 802/223–3461; FAX. 802/223–0364; Norman E. Wright, President

VIRGINIA: Virginia Hospital & Healthcare Association, 4200 Innslake Drive, Glen Allen, VA 23060, P.O. Box 31394, Richmond, VA 23294; tel. 804/747–8600; FAX. 804/965–0475; Laurens Sartoris, President

WASHINGTON: Washington State Hospital Association, 300 Elliott Avenue, W., Suite 300, Seattle, WA 98119–4118; tel. 206/281–7211; FAX. 206/283–6122; Leo F. Greenawalt, President, Chief Executive Officer

WEST VIRGINIA: West Virginia Hospital Association, The Association for Hospitals and Health Systems, 100 Association Drive, Charleston, WV 25311; tel. 304/344–9744; FAX. 304/344–9745; Steven J. Summer, President

WISCONSIN: Hospital Council of Greater Milwaukee Area, 2300 North Mayfair Road, Suite 360, Milwaukee, WI 53226; tel. 414/258–9610; FAX. 414/258–2103

Wisconsin Health & Hospital Association, 5721 Odana Road, Madison, WI 53719–1289; tel. 608/274–1820; FAX. 608/274–8554; Robert C. Taylor, President, Chief Executive Officer

WYOMING: Wyoming Hospital Association, 2005 Warren Avenue, Cheyenne, WY 82001, P.O. Box 5539, Cheyenne, WY 82003; tel. 307/632–9344; FAX. 307/632–9347; Robert C. Kidd II, President

U. S. Associated Areas

PUERTO RICO: Puerto Rico Hospital Association, Officina 101–103, Villa Nevarez Professional Center, Centro Commercial Villa Nevarez, San Juan, PR 00927; tel. 809/764–0290; FAX. 809/753–9748; Teodoro Muniz, President

Canada

ALBERTA: Provincial Health Authorities of Alberta, 200–44 Capital Boulevard, 10044 108th Street, N.W., Edmonton, AB T5J 3S7; tel. 403/426–8500; FAX. 403/424–4309; E. Michael Higgins, Executive Director

BRITISH COLUMBIA: British Columbia Health Association, 600–1333 West Broadway, Vancouver, BC V6H 4C7; tel. 604/734–2423, ext. 2616; FAX. 604/734–7202; Mary Collins, President

MANITOBA: Manitoba Health Organizations, Inc., 600–360 Broadway, Winnipeg, MB R3C 4G6; tel. 204/942–6591; FAX. 204/956–1373; Hila Willkie, Vice President

NEW BRUNSWICK: New Brunswick Healthcare Association, 861 Woodstock Road, Fredericton, NB E3B 7R7; tel. 506/451–0750; FAX. 506/451–0760; Michel J. Poirier, Executive Director

NEWFOUNDLAND: Newfoundland and Labrador Health Care Association, P.O. Box 8234, Post Station A, 1118 Topsail Raod, Zip A1N 2M3, St. John's, NF A1B 3N4; tel. 709/364–7701; FAX. 709/364–6460; John F. Peddle, Executive Director

NORTHWEST TERRITORY: Northwest Territories Health Care Association, P.O. Box 1709, 206–4817 49th Street, Yellowknife, NT X1A 2P3; tel. 403/873–9253; FAX. 403/873–9254; Sharon Ehaloak, Chairperson

NOVA SCOTIA: Nova Scotia Association of Health Organizations, Bedford Professional Centre, 2 Dartmouth Road, Bedford, NS B4A 2K7; tel. 902/832–8500; FAX. 902/832–8505; Robert A. Cook, President, Chief Executive Officer

ONTARIO: Ontario Hospital Association, 200 Front Street, W., Suite 2800, Toronto, ON M5V 3L1; tel. 416/205–1300; FAX. 416/205–1310; David MacKinnon, President

PRINCE EDWARD ISLAND: Health Association of Prince Edward Island, Inc., 10 Pownal Street, P.O. Box 490, Charlottetown, PE C1A 3V6; tel. 902/368–3901; FAX. 902/368–3231; Carol Gabanna, Executive Director

QUEBEC: The Quebec Hospital Association, 505 boulevard de Maisonneuve, W., Suite 400, Montreal, PQ H3A 3C2; tel. 514/842–4861; FAX. 514/282–4271; Jacques A. Nadeau, Executive Vice President

SASKATCHEWAN: Saskatchewan Association of Health Organizations, 1445 Park Street, Regina, SK S4N 4C5; tel. 306/347–5500; FAX. 306/525–1960; Arliss Wright, President, Chief Executive Officer

Hospital Licensure Agencies

Information for the following list of state hospital licensure agencies was obtained directly from the agencies.

United States

ALABAMA: Division of Licensure and Certification, Alabama Department of Public Health, The RSA Tower, P.O. Box 303017, Montgomery, AL 36130–3017; tel. 334/206–5078; FAX. 334/240–3147; Rick Harris, Director

ALASKA: Health Facilities Licensing and Certification, 4730 Business Park Boulevard, Building H, Suite 18, Anchorage, AK 99503–7137; tel. 907/561–8081; FAX. 907/561–3011; Shelbert Larsen, Administrator

ARIZONA: Arizona Department of Health Services, Office of Health Care Licensure, Medical Facilities Section, 1647 East Morten Avenue, Suite 110, Phoenix, AZ 85020; tel. 602/255–1144; FAX. 602/255–1109; Deon G. Rasmussen, Program Manager

ARKANSAS: Division of Health Facility Services, Arkansas Department of Health, 5800 West 10th Street, Suite 400, Little Rock, AR 72204–9916; tel. 501/661–2201; FAX. 501/661–2468; Valetta M. Buck, Director

CALIFORNIA: Licensing and Certification, Department of Health Services, 1800 Third Street, Suite 210, Zip 95814, P.O. Box 942732, Sacramento, CA 94234–7320; tel. 916/445–2070; FAX. 916/445–6979; Margaret DeBow, Deputy Director

COLORADO: Health Facilities Division, Colorado Department of Public Health and Environment, 4300 Cherry Creek Drive, S., Denver, CO 80222–1530; tel. 303/692–2800; FAX. 303/782–4883; Susan E. Rehak, Deputy Director

CONNECTICUT: Department of Public Health and Addiction Service, Connecticut State Department of Health Services, 150 Washington Street, Hartford, CT 06106; tel. 203/566–1073; FAX. 203/566–1097; Elizabeth M. Burns, RN, M.S., Director

DELAWARE: Office of Health Facilities Licensing and Certification, Department of Health and Social Services, Three Mill Road, Suite 308, Wilmington, DE 19806; tel. 302/577–6666; FAX. 302/577–6672; Ellen T. Reap, Director

DISTRICT OF COLUMBIA: Service Facility Regulation Administration, 614 H Street, N.W., Suite 1003, Washington, DC 20001; tel. 202/727–7190; FAX. 202/727–7780; Geraldine K. Sykes

FLORIDA: Division of Health Quality Assurance, Hospital and Outpatient Services Unit, Agency for Health Care Administration, 2727 Mahan Drive, Tallahassee, FL 32308; tel. 904/487–2717; FAX. 904/487–6240; Daryl Barowicz, Unit Manager

GEORGIA: Health Care Section, Office of Regulatory Services, Department of Human Resources, Two Peachtree Street, N.W., Suite 19.204, Atlanta, GA 30303–3167; tel. 404/657–5550; FAX. 404/657–8934; Susie M. Woods, Director

HAWAII: Hawaii Department of Health, Hospital and Medical Facilities Branch, P.O. Box 3378, Honolulu, HI 96801; tel. 808/586–4080; FAX. 808/586–4747; Helen K. Yoshimi, B.S.N., M.P.H., Chief, HMFB

IDAHO: Bureau of Facility Standards, Department of Health and Welfare, P.O. Box 83720, Boise, ID 83720–0036; tel. 208/334–6626; FAX. 208/332–7204; Sylvia Creswell, Supervisor, Non–Long Term Care

ILLINOIS: Division of Health Care Facilities and Programs, Illinois Department of Public Health, 525 West Jefferson Street, Springfield, IL 62761; tel. 217/782–7412; FAX. 217/782–0382; Catherine Stokes, Chief

INDIANA: Division of Acute Care, Indiana State Department of Health, Two North Meridian Street, Indianapolis, IN 46204; tel. 317/233–7472; FAX. 317/233–7157; John A. Braeckel, Director

IOWA: Division of Health Facilities, Iowa State Department of Inspections and Appeals, Lucas State Office Building, Des Moines, IA 50319; tel. 515/281–4115; FAX. 515/242–5022

KANSAS: Kansas Department of Health and Environment, Bureau of Adult and Child Care, 900 Southwest Jackson, Suite 1001, Topeka, KS 66612–1290; tel. 913/296–1280; FAX. 913/296–1266; George A. Dugger, Medical Facilities Certification Administrator

KENTUCKY: Division of Licensing and Regulation, Cabinet for Health Services, Cabinet for Human Resources Building, 275 East Main Street, Fourth Floor, E., Frankfort, KY 40621; tel. 502/564–2800; FAX. 502/564–6546; Rebecca J. Cecil, R.Ph., Director

LOUISIANA: Health Standards Section, Louisiana Department of Health and Hospitals, P.O. Box 3767, Baton Rouge, LA 70821; tel. 504/342–5782; FAX. 504/342–5292; Lily W. McAlister, RN, Manager

MAINE: Division of Licensing and Certification, Department of Human Services, State House, Station 11, Augusta, ME 04333; tel. 207/624–5443; FAX. 207/624–5378; Louis Dorogi, Director

MARYLAND: Department of Health and Mental Hygiene, Licensing and Certification Administration, 4201 Patterson Avenue, Baltimore, MD 21215; tel. 410/764–4970; FAX. 410/358–0750; James L. Ralls, Assistant Director

MASSACHUSETTS: Division of Health Care Quality, Massachusetts Department of Public Health, 10 West Street, Fifth Floor, Boston, MA 02111; tel. 617/727–5860; FAX. 617/727–1414; Paul I. Dreyer, Ph.D., Director

MICHIGAN: Bureau of Health Systems, Michigan Department of Public Health, 3423 North Logan Street, P.O. Box 30195, Lansing, MI 48909; tel. 517/335–8505; FAX. 517/335–8510; Walter S. Wheeler III, Chief

MINNESOTA: Facility and Provider Compliance Division, Minnesota Department of Health, 393 North Dunlap Street, P.O. Box 64900, St. Paul, MN 55164–0900; tel. 612/643–2100; FAX. 612/643–2593; Linda G. Sutherland, Director

MISSISSIPPI: Division of Health Facilities Licensure and Certification, Mississippi State Department of Health, P.O. Box 1700, Jackson, MS 39215; tel. 601/354–7300; FAX. 601/354–7230; Vanessa Phipps, Director

MISSOURI: Bureau of Hospital Licensing and Certification, Missouri Department of Health, P.O. Box 570, Jefferson City, MO 65102; tel. 314/751–6302; FAX. 314/526–3621; Darrell Hendrickson, Administrator

MONTANA: Division of Quality Assurance, Department of Public Health and Human Services, Cogswell Building, 1400 Broadway, Helena, MT 59620; tel. 406/444–2037; FAX. 406/444–1742; Denzel Davis, Administrator

NEBRASKA: Health Facility Licensure and Inspection Section, Nebraska Department of Health, 301 Centennial Mall, S., P.O. Box 95007, Lincoln, NE 68509–5007; tel. 402/471–2946; FAX. 402/471–0555; Frederick M. Wright, Section Administrator

NEVADA: Bureau of Licensure and Certification, Nevada Health Division, 1550 East College Parkway, Suite 158, Carson City, NV 89706–7921; tel. 702/687–4475; FAX. 702/687–6588; Sharon M. Ezell, Chief

NEW HAMPSHIRE: Bureau of Health Facilities Administration, Office of Program Support, Licensure and Regulation Services, Health and Human Services Building, Six Hazen Drive, Concord, NH 03301; tel. 603/271–4592; FAX. 603/271–4968; Raymond Rusih, Bureau Chief

NEW JERSEY: Certificate of Need and Acute Care Licensing, Health Systems Analysis, CN–360, Trenton, NJ 08625; tel. 609/292–8772; Darcy Saunders, Esq.

NEW MEXICO: Department of Health, Licensing and Certification Bureau, 525 Camino de los Marquez, Suite Two, Santa Fe, NM 87501; tel. 505/827–4200; FAX. 505/827–4222; Sue K. Morris, Bureau Chief

NEW YORK: Bureau of Hospital Services, Office of Health Systems Management, Hedley Park Place, Suite 303, 433 River Street, Troy, NY 12180–2299; tel. 518/402–1003; FAX. 518/402–1010; Frederick J. Heigel, Director

NORTH CAROLINA: Division of Facility Services, Department of Human Resources, 701 Barbour Drive, P.O. Box 29530, Raleigh, NC 27626–0530; tel. 919/733–1610; FAX. 919/733–3207; Steve White, Chief, Licensure and Certification

NORTH DAKOTA: Health Resources Section, State Department of Health, 600 East Boulevard Avenue, Bismarck, ND 58505–0200; tel. 701/328–2352; FAX. 701/328–4727; Fred Gladden, Chief

OHIO: Bureau of Quality Assessment and Improvement, Department of Health, P.O. Box 118, Columbus, OH 43266–0118; tel. 614/466–3325; FAX. 614/644–8661; Louis Pomerantz, Chief, Bureau of Quality Assessment and Improvement

OKLAHOMA: State Department of Health, 1000 Northeast 10th, Oklahoma City, OK 73117; tel. 405/271–4200; FAX. 405/271–3431; Jerry R. Nida, M.D., Commissioner, Health

OREGON: Health Care Licensure and Certification, Oregon Health Division, P.O. Box 14450, Portland, OR 97214–0450; tel. 503/731–4013; FAX. 503/731–4080; Kathleen Smail, Manager

PENNSYLVANIA: Division of Acute and Ambulatory Care Facilities, Bureau of Quality Assurance, Health and Welfare Building, Suite 532, Harrisburg, PA 17120; tel. 717/783–8980; FAX. 717/772–2163; William White, Director

RHODE ISLAND: Rhode Island Department of Health, Division of Facilities Regulation, Three Capitol Hill, Providence, RI 02908–5097; tel. 401/277–2566; FAX. 401/277–3999; Wayne I. Farrington, Chief Division, Facilities Regulation

SOUTH CAROLINA: Department of Health and Environmental Control, Division of Health Licensing, 2600 Bull Street, Columbia, SC 29201; tel. 803/737–7202; FAX. 803/737–7212; Alan Samuels, Director

SOUTH DAKOTA: Office of Health Care Facilities Licensure and Certification, State Department of Health, Anderson Building, 445 East Capitol, Pierre, SD 57501; tel. 605/773–3356; FAX. 605/773–6667; Joan Bachman, Administrator

TENNESSEE: Tennessee Department of Health, Division of Health Care Facilities, 283 Plus Park Boulevard, Nashville, TN 37247–0530; tel. 615/367–6316; Leslie A. Brown, Director

TEXAS: Health Facility Certification Division, Texas Department of Health, 1100 West 49th Street, Austin, TX 78756–3199; tel. 512/834–6650; Nance Stearman, Division Director

UTAH: Utah State Department of Health, Bureau of Health Facility Licensure, Box 142853, Salt Lake City, UT 84114–2853; tel. 801/538–6152; FAX. 801/538–6325; Debra Wynkoop–Green, Director

VERMONT: Health Improvement, Vermont Department of Health, 108 Cherry Street, P.O. Box 70, Burlington, VT 05402; tel. 802/863–7606; FAX. 802/651–1634; Ellen B. Thompson, Planning Chief

VIRGINIA: Office of Health Facilities Regulation, Virginia Department of Health, 3600 Centre, Suite 216, 3600 West Broad Street, Richmond, VA 23230; tel. 804/367–2102; FAX. 804/367–2149; Nancy R. Hofheimer, Director

WASHINGTON: Acute Care and Construction Review Services, Washington Department of Health, Target Plaza, Suite 500, 2725 Harrison Avenue, N.W., P.O. Box 47852, Olympia, WA 98504–7852; tel. 360/705–6612; FAX. 360/705–6654; Byron Plan, Manager

WEST VIRGINIA: Office of Health Facility Licensure and Certification, West Virginia Division of Health, State Capitol Complex, Building Three, Suite 550, Charleston, WV 25305; tel. 304/558–0050; FAX. 304/558–2515; Sandra Daubman, Interim Director

WISCONSIN: Bureau of Quality Assurance, Division of Supportive Living, Department of Health and Family Services, One West Wilson Street, P.O. Box 309, Madison, WI 53701; tel. 608/267–7185; FAX. 608/267–0352; Judy Fryback, Director, Bureau of Quality Assurance

WYOMING: Department of Health, Health Facilities Licensing, Metropolitan Bank Building, Eighth Floor, Cheyenne, WY 82002; tel. 307/777–7123; FAX. 307/777–5970; Charlie Simineo, Program Manager

Medical and Nursing Licensure Agencies

Information for the following list of state medical licensure agencies was obtained from the Federation of State Medical Board and nursing licensure agencies was obtained from the National League for Nursing.

United States

ALABAMA
Alabama Board of Nursing, RSA Plaza, Suite 250, 770 Washington Avenue, Montgomery, AL 36130–3900; tel. 334/242–4060; FAX. 334/242–4360; Judi Crume, Executive Officer
Alabama State Board of Medical Examiners, 848 Washington Avenue, Zip 36104, P.O. Box 946, Montgomery, AL 36101–0946; tel. 334/242–4116; FAX. 334/242–4155; Larry D. Dixon, Executive Director

ALASKA
Alaska Board of Nursing, Division of Occupational Licensing, 3601 C Street, Suite 722, Anchorage, AK 99503; tel. 907/269–8161; FAX. 907/269–8156; Dorothy Fulton, Executive Secretary
Alaska State Medical Board, Division of Occupational Licensing, 3601 C Street, Suite 722, Anchorage, AK 99503; tel. 907/269–8163; FAX. 907/269–8156; Leslie G. Abel, Administrator

ARIZONA
Arizona Board of Osteopathic Examiners in Medicine and Surgery, 141 East Palm Lane, Suite 205, Phoenix, AZ 85004; tel. 602/255–1747; FAX. 602/255–1756; Robert J. Miller, Ph.D., Executive Director
Arizona State Board of Medical Examiners, 1651 East Morton, Suite 210, Phoenix, AZ 85020; tel. 602/255–3751; FAX. 602/255–1848; Mark R. Speicher, Executive Director
Arizona State Board of Nursing, 1651 East Morten, Suite 150, Phoenix, AZ 85020; tel. 602/255–5092; FAX. 602/255–5130; Joey Ridenour, RN, M.N., Executive Director

ARKANSAS
Arkansas State Board of Nursing, University Tower Building, Suite 800, 1123 South University Avenue, Little Rock, AR 72204; tel. 501/686–2700; FAX. 501/686–2714; Faith A. Fields, M.S.N., RN, Executive Director
Arkansas State Medical Board, 2100 Riverfront Drive, Suite 200, Little Rock, AR 72202; tel. 501/296–1802; FAX. 501/296–1805; Peggy P. Cryer, Executive Director

CALIFORNIA
California Board of Registered Nursing, 400 R Street, Suite 4030, Zip 95814, P.O. Box 944210, Sacramento, CA 94244–2100; tel. 916/322–3350; Ruth Ann Terry, RN, M.P.H., Executive Officer
Medical Board of California, 1426 Howe Avenue, Suite 54, Sacramento, CA 95825; tel. 916/263–2344; FAX. 916/263–2487; Neil Fippin, Program Manager
Osteopathic Medical Board of California, 444 North Third Street, Suite A–200, Sacramento, CA 95814; tel. 916/322–4306; FAX. 916/327–6119; Linda J. Bergmann, Executive Director

COLORADO
Colorado State Board of Medical Examiners, 1560 Broadway, Suite 1300, Denver, CO 80202–5140; tel. 303/894–7690; FAX. 303/894–7692; Susan Miller, Program Administrator
Colorado State Board of Nursing, 1560 Broadway, Suite 670, Denver, CO 80202; tel. 303/894–2430; Karen Brumley, Program Administrator

CONNECTICUT
Connecticut Board of Examiners for Nursing, Department of Public Health, 150 Washington Street, Hartford, CT 06106; tel. 860/566–1041; FAX. 860/566–1464; Marie Hilliard, Ph.D., RN, Executive Officer
Connecticut Department of Public Health, 410 Capitol Avenue, MS #12 APP, P.O. Box 340308, Hartford, CT 06134–0308; tel. 860/509–7563; FAX. 860/509–8247; Debra L. Johnson, Health Program Associate

DELAWARE
Delaware Board of Medical Practice, Cannon Building, 861 Silver Lake Boulevard, Suite 203, P.O. Box 1401, Dover, DE 19903; tel. 302/739–4522; FAX. 302/739–2711; Brenda Petty–Ball, Executive Director
Delaware Board of Nursing, Cannon Building, 861 Silver Lake Boulevard, Suite 203, P.O. Box 1401, Dover, DE 19903; tel. 302/739–4522, ext. 216; FAX. 302/739–2711; Iva J. Boardman, RN, M.S.N., Executive Director

DISTRICT OF COLUMBIA
District of Columbia Board of Medicine, 614 H Street, N.W., Room 108, Washington, DC 20001; tel. 202/727–5365; FAX. 202/727–4087; James R. Granger, Jr., Executive Director
District of Columbia Board of Nursing, 614 H Street, N.W., Washington, DC 20001; tel. 202/727–7461; FAX. 202/727–8030; Barbara Hatcher, Chairperson

FLORIDA
Florida Board of Medicine, 1940 North Monroe Street, Northwood Centre, Suite 60, Tallahassee, FL 32399–0750; tel. 904/488–0595; FAX. 904/922–3040; Marm M. Harris, Executive Director
Florida Board of Osteopathic Medicine, 1940 North Monroe Street, Northwood Centre, Suite 60, Tallahassee, FL 32399–0757; tel. 904/922–6725; FAX. 904/921–6184; Melissa Carter
Florida State Board of Nursing, 4080 Woodcock Drive, Suite 202, Jacksonville, FL 32207; tel. 904/858–6940; FAX. 904/858–6964; Marilyn A. Bloss, RNC, M.S.N., Executive Director

GEORGIA
Georgia Board of Nursing, 166 Pryor Street, S.W., Atlanta, GA 30303; tel. 404/656–3943; FAX. 404/657–7489; Shirley A. Camp, Executive Director
Georgia Composite State Board of Medical Examiners, 166 Pryor Street, S.W., Atlanta, GA 30303; tel. 404/656–3913; FAX. 404/656–9723; Andrew Watry, Executive Director

HAWAII
Hawaii Board of Medical Examiners, Department of Commerce and Consumer Affairs, 1010 Richards Street, Zip 96813, P.O. Box 3469, Honolulu, HI 96801; tel. 808/586–2708; Constance Cabral–Makanani, Executive Director
Hawaii Board of Nursing, P.O. Box 3469, Honolulu, HI 96801; tel. 808/586–2695; FAX. 808/586–2689; Kathy Yokouchi, Executive Officer

IDAHO
Idaho State Board of Medicine, State House Mail, 280 North Eighth, Suite 202, P.O. Box 83720, Boise, ID 83720–0058; tel. 208/334–2822; FAX. 203/334–2801; Donald L. Deleski, Executive Director
Idaho State Board of Nursing, 280 North Eighth Street, Suite 210, P.O. Box 83720, Boise, ID 83720–0061; tel. 208/334–3110; FAX. 208/334–3262; Sandra Evans, Executive Director

ILLINOIS
Illinois Department of Professional Regulation, 320 West Washington Street, Springfield, IL 62786; tel. 217/782–0458; FAX. 217/782–7645; Tony Sanders, Public Information Officer
Illinois Department of Professional Regulation, James R. Thompson Center, 100 West Randolph Street, Suite 9–300, Chicago, IL 60601; tel. 312/814–4500; FAX. 312/814–1837; Nikki M. Zollar, Director

INDIANA
Indiana Health Professions Bureau, Medical Licensing Board of Indiana, 402 West Washington, Room 041, Indianapolis, IN 46204; tel. 317/233–4401; FAX. 317/233–4236; Laura Langford, Executive Director

Indiana State Board of Nursing, Health Professions Bureau, 402 West Washington, Suite 041, Indianapolis, IN 46204; tel. 317/233–4405; FAX. 317/233–4236; Gina Voorhies, Board Administrator

IOWA
Iowa Board of Nursing, State Capitol Complex, 1223 East Court Avenue, Des Moines, IA 50319; tel. 515/281–3255; FAX. 515/281–4825; Lorinda K. Inman, RN, M.S.N., Executive Director
Iowa State Board of Medical Examiners, Executive Hills West, 1209 East Court Avenue, Des Moines, IA 50319–0180; tel. 515/281–5171; FAX. 515/242–5908; Ann M. Martino, Ph.D., Executive Director

KANSAS
Kansas State Board of Healing Arts, 235 Southwest Topeka Boulevard, Topeka, KS 66603–3068; tel. 913/296–7413; FAX. 913/296–0852; Lawrence T. Buening, Jr., J.D., Executive Director
Kansas State Board of Nursing, Landon State Office Building, 900 Southwest Jackson, Suite 551–S, Topeka, KS 66612–1230; tel. 913/296–4929; FAX. 913/296–3929; Patsy Johnson, RN, M.N., Executive Administrator

KENTUCKY
Kentucky Board of Medical Licensure, The Hurstbourne Office Park, 310 Whittington Parkway, Suite 1B, Louisville, KY 40222; tel. 502/429–8046; FAX. 502/429–9923; C. William Schmidt, Executive Director
Kentucky Board of Nursing, 312 Whittington Parkway, Suite 300, Louisville, KY 40222; tel. 502/329–7000; FAX. 502/329–7011; Sharon M. Weisenbeck, M.S., RN, Executive Director

LOUISIANA
Louisiana State Board of Medical Examiners, P.O. Box 30250, New Orleans, LA 70190–0250; tel. 504/524–6763; FAX. 504/568–8893; Mrs. Delmar Rorison, Executive Director
Louisiana State Board of Nursing, 912 Pere Marquette Building, New Orleans, LA 70112; tel. 504/568–5464; FAX. 504/568–5467; Barbara L. Morvant, RN, M.N., Executive Director

MAINE
Maine Board of Licensure in Medicine, Two Bangor Street, 137 State House Station, Augusta, ME 04333; tel. 207/287–3601; FAX. 207/287–6590; Randal C. Manning, Executive Director
Maine Board of Osteopathic Licensure, 142 State House Station, Two Bangor Street, Augusta, ME 04333–0142; tel. 207/287–2480; FAX. 207/287–2480; Susan E. Stout, Executive Secretary
Maine State Board of Nursing, 24 Stone Street, 158 State House Station, Augusta, ME 04333; tel. 207/287–1133; FAX. 207/287–1149; Jean C. Caron, RN, Executive Director

MARYLAND
Maryland Board of Nursing, 4140 Patterson Avenue, Baltimore, MD 21215; tel. 410/764–5124; FAX. 410/358–3530; Donna M. Dorsey, RN, M.S., Executive Director
Maryland Board of Physician Quality Assurance, 4201 Patterson Avenue, Third Floor, P.O. Box 2571, Baltimore, MD 21215–0095; tel. 800/492–6836; FAX. 410/764–2478; J. Michael Compton, Executive Director

MASSACHUSETTS
Massachusetts Board of Registration in Medicine, 10 West Street, Third Floor, Boston, MA 02111; tel. 617/727–3086; FAX. 617/451–9568; Alexander F. Fleming, J.D., Executive Director
Massachusetts Board of Registration in Nursing, 100 Cambridge Street, Suite 1519, Boston, MA 02202; tel. 617/727–9961; FAX. 617/727–9961; Theresa M. Bonanno, M.S.N., RN, Executive Director

MICHIGAN

Michigan Board of Medicine, 611 West Ottawa Street, Fourth Floor, Box 30192, Lansing, MI 48909; tel. 517/373–9102; FAX. 517/373–2179; Brenda Rogers, Assistant Licensing Administrator

Michigan Board of Nursing, Department of Consumer and Industry Services, 611 West Ottawa Street, P.O. Box 30018, Lansing, MI 48909; tel. 517/373–9102; FAX. 517/373–2179; Carol S. Johnson, Licensing Administrator

Michigan Board of Osteopathic Medicine and Surgery, 611 West Ottawa Street, Fourth Floor, P.O. Box 30018, Lansing, MI 48909; tel. 517/373–9102; FAX. 517/373–2179; Carol S. Johnson, Licensing Administrator

MINNESOTA

Minnesota Board of Medical Practice, 2829 University Avenue, S.E., Suite 400, Minneapolis, MN 55414–3246; tel. 612/617–2130; FAX. 612/617–2166; Robert A. Leach, Executive Director

Minnesota Board of Nursing, 2829 University Avenue, S.E., Suite 500, Minneapolis, MN 55414–3253; tel. 612/617–2270; FAX. 612/617–2190; Joyce M. Schowalter, Executive Director

MISSISSIPPI

Mississippi Board of Nursing, 239 North Lamar Street, Suite 401, Jackson, MS 39201–1397; tel. 601/359–6170; FAX. 601/359–6185; Marcia M. Rachel, Ph.D., RN, Executive Director

Mississippi State Board of Medical Licensure, 2688–D Insurance Center Drive, Jackson, MS 39216; tel. 601/354–6645; FAX. 601/987–4159; P. Doyle Bradshaw, Executive Officer

MISSOURI

Missouri State Board of Nursing, 3605 Missouri Boulevard, P.O. Box 656, Jefferson City, MO 65102; tel. 573/751–0681; FAX. 573/751–0075; JoAnn Hanley, Executive Assistant

Missouri State Board of Registration for the Healing Arts, 3605 Missouri Boulevard, Zip 65109, P.O. Box Four, Jefferson City, MO 65102; tel. 314/751–0098; FAX. 314/751–3166; Tina M. Steinman, Executive Director

MONTANA

Montana Board of Medical Examiners, 111 North Jackson, P.O. Box 200513, Helena, MT 59620–0513; tel. 406/444–4284; FAX. 406/444–9396; Patricia I. England, J.D., Executive Secretary

Montana State Board of Nursing, 111 North Jackson–4C, P.O. Box 200513, Arcade Building, Helena, MT 59620–0513; tel. 406/444–2071; FAX. 406/444–7759; Dianne Wickham, RN, M.N., Executive Director

NEBRASKA

Nebraska State Board of Examiners in Medicine and Surgery, 301 Centennial Mall, S., P.O. Box 94986, Lincoln, NE 68509–4986; tel. 402/471–2118; FAX. 402/471–3577; Katherine A. Brown, Executive Secretary

NEVADA

Nevada State Board of Medical Examiners, 1105 Terminal Way, Suite 301, Zip 89502, P.O. Box 7238, Reno, NV 89510; tel. 702/688–2559; FAX. 702/688–2321; Larry D. Lessly, Executive Director

Nevada State Board of Nursing, 4335 South Industrial Road, Suite 420, Las Vegas, NV 89103; tel. 702/739–1575; FAX. 702/739–0298; Lonna Burress, Executive Director

Nevada State Board of Osteopathic Medicine, 2950 East Flamingo Road, Suite E–3, Las Vegas, NV 89121; tel. 702/732–2147; FAX. 702/732–2079; Larry J. Tarno, D.O., Executive Director

NEW HAMPSHIRE

New Hampshire Board of Medicine, Two Industrial Park Drive, Concord, NH 03301; tel. 603/271–1203; Karen Lamoureux, Administrator

New Hampshire State Board of Nursing, Six Hazen Drive, Concord, NH 03301; tel. 603/271–2323; FAX. 603/271–6605; Doris G. Nuttelman, RN, Ed.D., Executive Director

NEW JERSEY

New Jersey Board of Nursing, 124 Halsey Street, Newark, NJ 07102, P.O. Box 45010, Newark, NJ 07101; tel. 201/504–6493; FAX. 201/648–3481

New Jersey State Board of Medical Examiners, 140 East Front Street, Second Floor, Trenton, NJ 08608; tel. 609/826–7100; FAX. 609/984–3930; Kevin B. Earle, Executive Director

NEW MEXICO

New Mexico Board of Osteopathic Medical Examiners, 725 St. Michael's Drive, Santa Fe, NM 87501, P.O. Box 25101, Santa Fe, NM 87504; tel. 505/827–7171; FAX. 505/827–7095; Michelle McGinnis, Executive Director

New Mexico State Board of Medical Examiners, 491 Old Santa Fe Trail, Lamy Building, Second Floor, Santa Fe, NM 87501; tel. 505/827–5022; FAX. 505/827–7377; Kristen A. Hedrick, Executive Secretary

State of New Mexico, Board of Nursing, 4206 Louisiana, N.E., Suite A, Albuquerque, NM 87109; tel. 505/841–8340; FAX. 505/841–8347; Nancy L. Twigg, Executive Director

NEW YORK

New York Board for Professional Medical Conduct, State Department of Health, 433 River Street, Suite 303, Troy, NY 12180–2299; tel. 518/402–0855; FAX. 518/402–0866; Anne F. Saile, Director

New York State Board for Nursing, State Education Department, The Cultural Center, Suite 3023, Albany, NY 12230; tel. 518/474–3845; FAX. 518/473–0578; Milene A. Megel, RN, Ph.D., Executive Secretary

New York State Division of Professional Licensing Services, Cultural Education Center, Suite 3021, Empire State Plaza, Albany, NY 12230; tel. 518/474–3817; FAX. 518/473–0578; Robert G. Bentley, Director, Professional Licensing

NORTH CAROLINA

North Carolina Board of Nursing, P.O. Box 2129, Raleigh, NC 27602–2129; tel. 919/782–3211; FAX. 919/781–9461; Carol A. Osman, RN, Ed.D., Executive Director

North Carolina Medical Board, P.O. Box 20007, Raleigh, NC 27619; tel. 919/828–1212; FAX. 919/828–1295; Bryant D. Paris, Jr., Executive Director

NORTH DAKOTA

North Dakota Board of Nursing, 919 South Seventh Street, Suite 504, Bismarck, ND 58504–5881; tel. 701/328–9777; FAX. 701/328–9785; Ida H. Rigley, RN, Executive Director

North Dakota State Board of Medical Examiners, City Center Plaza, Suite 12, 418 East Broadway Avenue, Bismarck, ND 58501; tel. 701/328–6500; FAX. 701/328–6505; Rolf P. Sletten, Executive Secretary–Treasurer

OHIO

Ohio Board of Nursing, 77 South High Street, 17th Floor, Columbus, OH 43266–0316; tel. 614/466–3947; Dorothy Fiorino, RN, Executive Director

State Medical Board of Ohio, 77 South High Street, 17th Floor, Columbus, OH 43266–0315; tel. 614/466–3934; FAX. 614/728–5946; Ray Q. Bumgarner, Executive Director

OKLAHOMA

Oklahoma Board of Nursing, 2915 North Classen Boulevard, Suite 524, Oklahoma City, OK 73106; tel. 405/525–2076; FAX. 405/521–6089; Sulinda Moffett, M.S.N., RN, Executive Director

Oklahoma State Board of Osteopathic Examiners, 4848 North Lincoln Boulevard, Suite 100, Oklahoma City, OK 73105–3321; tel. 405/528–8625; FAX. 405/528–6102; Gary R. Clark, Executive Director

Oklahoma State Board of Medical Licensure and Supervision, 5104 North Francis, Suite C, Oklahoma City, OK 73118, P.O. Box 18256, Oklahoma City, OK 73154–0256; tel. 405/848–2189; FAX. 405/848–8240; Jan Ewing, Deputy Director

OREGON

Oregon Board of Medical Examiners, 620 Crown Plaza, 1500 Southwest First Avenue, Portland, OR 97201–5826; tel. 503/229–5770; FAX. 503/229–6543; Kathleen Haley, J.D., Executive Director

Oregon State Board of Nursing, 800 Northeast Oregon Street, Suite 465, Portland, OR 97232–2162; tel. 503/731–4745; FAX. 503/731–4755; Joan C. Bouchard, Executive Director

PENNSYLVANIA

Pennsylvania State Board of Medicine, 116 Pine Street, Harrisburg, PA 17101, P.O. Box 2649, Harrisburg, PA 17105–2649; tel. 717/783–1400; FAX. 717/787–7769; Cindy L. Warner, Administrative Assistant

Pennsylvania State Board of Nursing, Department of State, P.O. Box 2649, Harrisburg, PA 17105–2649; tel. 717/783–7142; FAX. 717/787–7769; Miriam H. Limo, Executive Secretary

Pennsylvania State Board of Osteopathic Medicine, P.O. Box 2649, Harrisburg, PA 17105–2649; tel. 717/783–4858; Gina Bittner, Administrative Assistant

RHODE ISLAND

Board of Nursing Education and Nurse Registration, Three Capitol Hill, Room 104, Providence, RI 02908–5097; tel. 401/277–2827; FAX. 401/277–1272; Carol Lietar, RN, M.S.N., Director

Rhode Island Board of Medical Licensure and Discipline, Rhode Island Department of Health, Room 205, 3 Capitol Hill, Providence, RI 02908–5097; tel. 401/277–3855; FAX. 401/277–2158; Milton W. Hamolsky, M.D., Chief Administrative Officer

SOUTH CAROLINA

Department of Labor, Licensing and Regulation, State Board of Nursing for South Carolina, P.O. Box 12367, Columbia, SC 29211; tel. 803/731–1648; FAX. 803/731–1647

South Carolina Department of Labor, Licensing and Regulation, Board of Medical Examiners, 3600 Forest Drive, Columbia, SC 29204, P.O. Box 11289, Columbia, SC 29211–1289; tel. 803/737–9300; FAX. 803/737–9314; Henry D. Foster, Jr., J.D., Board Administrator

SOUTH DAKOTA

South Dakota Board of Nursing, 3307 South Lincoln, Sioux Falls, SD 57105; tel. 605/367–5940; FAX. 605/367–5945; Diana Vander Woude, Executive Secretary

South Dakota State Board of Medical and Osteopathic Examiners, 1323 South Minnesota Avenue, Sioux Falls, SD 57105; tel. 605/336–1965; FAX. 605/336–0270; Robert D. Johnson, Executive Secretary

TENNESSEE

Tennessee Board of Nursing, 283 Plus Park Boulevard, Nashville, TN 37217; tel. 615/367–6232; FAX. 615/367–6397; Elizabeth J. Lund, RN, Executive Director

Tennessee State Board of Medical Examiners, First Floor, Cordell Hull Building, 426 Fifth Avenue, N., Nashville, TN 37247–1010; tel. 615/532–4384; FAX. 615/532–5164; Jerry Kosten, Administrator

Tennessee State Board of Osteopathic Examination, First Floor, Cordell Hull Building, 426 Fifth Avenue, N., Nashville, TN 37247–1010; tel. 615/532–5080; FAX. 615/532–5164; Judy Hartman, Administrator

TEXAS

Texas Board of Nurse Examiners, 9101 Burnet Road, Suite 104, Austin, TX 78758; tel. 512/835–4880; Louise Waddill, RN, Ph.D., Executive Director

Texas State Board of Medical Examiners, 333 Guadalupe, Tower Three, Suite 610, Austin, TX 78701, P.O. Box 149134, Austin, TX 78714–9134; tel. 512/305–7008; FAX. 512/305–4700, ext. 8; Bruce A. Levy, M.D., J.D., Executive Director

UTAH

Utah Physicians Licensing Board, Division of Occupational and Professional Licensing, Heber M. Wells Building, Fourth Floor, 160 East 300 South, Salt Lake City, UT 84111, P.O. Box 45805, Salt Lake City, UT 84145–0805; tel. 801/530–6628; FAX. 801/530–6511; Karen Reimherr, Bureau Manager

Utah State Board of Nursing, 160 East 300 South, Box 146741, Salt Lake City, UT 84114–6741; tel. 801/530–6628; FAX. 801/530–6511; Laura Poe, Executive Administrator

VERMONT

Vermont Board of Medical Practice, 109 State Street, Montpelier, VT 05609–1106; tel. 802/828–2673; FAX. 802/828–2853; Barbara Neuman, J.D., Executive Director

Vermont Board of Nursing Licensure and Regulation Division, 109 State Street, Montpelier, VT 05609–1106; tel. 802/828–2396; FAX. 802/828–2484; Anita Ristau, RN, M.S., Executive Director

Vermont Board of Osteopathic Physicians and Surgeons, 109 State Street, Montpelier, VT 05609–1106; tel. 802/828–2373; FAX. 802/828–2496; Peggy Atkins, Staff Assistant

VIRGINIA
Virginia Board of Medicine, 6606 West Broad Street, Fourth Floor, Richmond, VA 23230–1717; tel. 804/662–9908; FAX. 804/662–9943; Warren W. Koontz, Jr., M.D., Executive Director
Virginia Board of Nursing, 6606 West Broad Street, Fourth Floor, Richmond, VA 23230; tel. 804/662–9909; FAX. 804/662–9943; Nancy K. Durrett, RN, Executive Director

WASHINGTON
Washington Quality Medical Assurance Commission, 1300 Southeast Quince Street, P.O Box 47866, Olympia, WA 98504–7866; tel. 360/753–2287; FAX. 360/586–4573; Keith O. Shafer, Executive Director
Washington State Board of Osteopathic Medicine and Surgery, Department of Health, 1300 Southeast Quince Street, P.O. Box 47866, Olympia, WA 98504–7866; tel. 360/586–8438; FAX. 360/586–4573; Arlene Robertson, Program Manager
Washington State Nursing Care Quality Assurance Commission, Department of Health, 1300 Southeast Quince Street, P.O. Box 47864, Olympia, WA 98504–7864; tel. 360/664–4100; FAX. 360/586–5935; Patty L. Hayes, RN, M.N., Executive Director

WEST VIRGINIA
West Virginia Board of Examiners for Registered Professional Nurses, 101 Dee Drive, Charleston, WV 25311–1620; tel. 304/558–3596; FAX. 304/558–3666; Laura S. Rhodes, RN, M.S.N., Executive Secretary
West Virginia Board of Medicine, 101 Dee Drive, Charleston, WV 25311; tel. 304/558–2921; FAX. 304/558–2084; Ronald D. Walton, Executive Director
West Virginia Board of Osteopathy, 334 Penco Road, Weirton, WV 26062; tel. 304/723–4638; FAX. 304/723–2877; Cheryl D. Schreiber, Executive Secretary

WISCONSIN
Division of Health Professions and Services Licensing, 1400 East Washington Avenue, Room 178, P.O. Box 8935, Madison, WI 53708–8935; tel. 608/266–5432; FAX. 608/267–0644; Deanna Zychowski, Administrative Assistant

Wisconsin Medical Examining Board, 1400 East Washington Avenue, Zip 53702, P.O. Box 8935, Madison, WI 53708; tel. 608/266–2811; FAX. 608/267–0644; Patrick D. Braatz, Bureau Director

WYOMING
Wyoming Board of Medicine, The Colony Building, 211 West 19th Street, Second Floor, Cheyenne, WY 82002; tel. 307/778–7053; FAX. 307/778–2069; Carole Shotwell, Executive Secretary
Wyoming State Board of Nursing, 2020 Carey Avenue, Suite 110, Cheyenne, WY 82002; tel. 307/777–7601; FAX. 307/777–3519; Toma A. Nisbet, RN, M.S., Executive Director

U. S. Associated Areas

AMERICAN SAMOA–GUAM
American Samoa Health Services Regulatory Board, LBJ Tropical Medical Center, Pago Pago, AS 96799; tel. 684/633–1222, ext. 206; FAX. 684/633–1869; Marie F. Mao, RN, M.S., Executive Secretary

GUAM
Guam Board of Medical Examiners, 1304 East Sunset Boulevard, Barrigada, GU 96913; tel. 671/475–0251; FAX. 671/477–4733; Chalsea C. Torres, Board Secretary
Guam Board of Nurse Examiners, Department of Public Health and Social Services, 1304 East Sunset Boulevard, Barrigada (Tiyan), Guam 96913, P.O. Box 2816, Agana, GU 96910; tel. 671/475–0251; FAX. 671/477–4733; Teofila P. Cruz, RN, M.S., Administrator

PUERTO RICO
Council on Higher Education of Puerto Rico, UPR Station, P.O. Box 23305, San Juan, PR 00931–3305; tel. 809/758–3356; Madeline Quilichini Paz, Director, Office of Licensing and Accreditation
Puerto Rico Board of Medical Examiners, Kennedy Avenue, ILA Building, Hogar del Obrero Portuario, Piso 8, Puerto Nuevo, Zip 00920, Call Box 13969, San Juan, PR 00908; tel. 787/793–1333; FAX. 787/782–8733; Lorenne E. Montalvo Garcia, Esq., Executive Director

VIRGIN ISLANDS
Virgin Islands Board of Medical Examiners, Virgin Islands Department of Health, 48 Sugar Estate, St. Thomas, VI 00802; tel. 809/774–0117; FAX. 809/777–4001; Lydia T. Scott, Executive Assistant to the Boards
Virgin Islands Board of Nursing Licensure, P.O. Box 4247, St. Thomas, VI 00803; tel. 809/776–7397; FAX. 809/777–4003; Winifred L. Garfield, CRNA, Executive Secretary

Canada

ALBERTA
College of Physicians and Surgeons of Alberta, 9901 108th Street, Edmonton, AB T5K 1G9; tel. 403/423–4764; L. H. le Riche, M.B., CH.B., Registrar

MANITOBA
College of Physicians and Surgeons of Manitoba, 494 St. James Street, Winnipeg, MB R3G 3J4; tel. 204/774–4344; FAX. 204/774–0750; Kenneth R. Brown, M.D., Registrar

NEW BRUNSWICK
College of Physicians and Surgeons of New Brunswick, One Hampton Road, Rothesay, NB E2E 5K8; tel. 506/849–5050; FAX. 506/849–5069

NOVA SCOTIA
College of Physicians and Surgeons of Nova Scotia, Office of the Registrar, 5248 Morris Street, Halifax, NS B3J 1B4; tel. 902/422–5823; FAX. 902/422–5035; Dr. Cameron Little, Registrar

PRINCE EDWARD ISLAND
College of Physicians and Surgeons of Prince Edward Island, 199 Grafton Street, Charlottetown, PE C1A 1L2; tel. 902/566–3861; FAX. 902/566–3861; H. E. Ross, M.D., Registrar

QUEBEC
College des medecins du Quebec, 2170, boul. Rene–Levesque Quest, Montreal, PQ H3H 2T8; tel. 514/933–4441; FAX. 514/933–3112; Joelle Lescop, M.D., Secretary General

SASKATCHEWAN
College of Physicians and Surgeons of Saskatchewan, 211 Fourth Avenue, S., Saskatoon, SK S7K 1N1; tel. 306/244–7355; FAX. 306/244–0090; D. A. Kendel, M.D., Registrar

Section C

Peer Review Organizations

The following list of PROs was obtained from the Office of Medical Review, Division of Program Operation, HCFA. For more information, contact the office at 410/786–8781.

United States

ALABAMA: Alabama Quality Assurance Foundation, One Perimeter Park, S., Suite 200 North, Birmingham, AL 35243–2354; tel. 205/970–1600; FAX. 205/970–1616; H. Terrell Lindsey, President, Chief Executive Officer

ALASKA: PRO–WEST, 10700 Meridian Avenue, N., Suite 100, Seattle, WA 98133–9075; tel. 206/364–9700; FAX. 206/368–2419; John W. Daise, Chief Executive Officer

ARIZONA: Health Services Advisory Group, Inc., 301 East Bethany Home Road, Suite B–157, Phoenix, AZ 85012; tel. 602/264–6382; FAX. 602/241–0757; Lawrence J. Shapiro, M.D., President, Chief Executive Officer

ARKANSAS: Arkansas Foundation for Medical Care, Inc., 809 Garrision Avenue, P.O. Box 2424, Fort Smith, AR 72902; tel. 501/785–2471; FAX. 501/785–3460; Russell G. Brasher, Ph.D., Chief Executive Officer

CALIFORNIA: California Medical Review, Inc., 60 Spear Street, Suite 400, San Francisco, CA 94105; tel. 415/882–5800; FAX. 415/882–5995; Jo Ellen H. Ross, Chief Executive Officer

COLORADO: Colorado Foundation for Medical Care, 2821 South Parker Road, Suite 605, Aurora, CO 80014–2713; tel. 303/695–3300; FAX. 303/695–3350; Arja P. Adair, Jr., Executive Director

CONNECTICUT: Connecticut Peer Review Organization, Inc., 100 Roscommon Drive, Suite 200, Middletown, CT 06457; tel. 860/632–2008; FAX. 860/632–5865; Marcia K. Petrillo, Executive Director

DELAWARE: West Virginia Medical Institute, Inc., 3001 Chesterfield Place, Charleston, WV 25304; tel. 304/346–9864, ext. 269; FAX. 304/346–9863; Harry S. Weeks, Jr., M.D., President

DISTRICT OF COLUMBIA: Delmarva Foundation for Medical Care, Inc., 9240 Centreville Road, Easton, MD 21601; tel. 410/822–0697; FAX. 410/822–1997; Linda E. Clark, RN, Executive Vice President

FLORIDA: Florida Medical Quality Assurance, Inc., 4350 West Cypress Street, Suite 900, Tampa, FL 33607; tel. 813/354–9111; FAX. 813/354–0737; Jennifer Barnett, President, Chief Executive Officer

GEORGIA: Georgia Medical Care Foundation, 57 Executive Park, S., Suite 200, Atlanta, GA 30329; tel. 404/982–0411; FAX. 404/982–7584; Tom W. Williams, Chief Executive Officer

HAWAII: Montana–Wyoming Foundation for Medical Care, 320 South Beretania Street, Honolulu, HI 96814; tel. 808/545–2550; FAX. 808/599–2875; Janice Connors, Executive Director

IDAHO: PRO–WEST, 10700 Meridian Avenue, N., Suite 100, Seattle, WA 98133–9075; tel. 206/364–9700; FAX. 206/368–2419; John W. Daise, Chief Executive Officer

ILLINOIS: Iowa Foundation for Medical Care–Illinois, The Sunderbruch Corporation–Nebraska, 6000 Westown Parkway, Suite 350E, West Des Moines, IA 50266; tel. 515/223–2900; FAX. 515/222–2407; Rebecca Hemann, VP Government Quality Improvement Programs

INDIANA: Health Care Excel, Incorporated, 2901 Ohio Boulevard, P.O. Box 3713, Terre Haute, IN 47803; tel. 812/234–1499; FAX. 812/232–6167; Philip L. Morphew, Chief Executive Officer

IOWA: Iowa Foundation for Medical Care, 6000 Westown Parkway, Suite 350 E, West Des Moines, IA 50266–7771; tel. 515/223–2900; FAX. 515/222–2407; Fred A. Ferree, Executive Vice President

KANSAS: The Kansas Foundation for Medical Care, Inc., 2947 Southwest Wanamaker Drive, Topeka, KS 66614; tel. 913/273–2552, ext. 363; FAX. 913/273–5130; Larry W. Pitman, Chief Executive Officer

KENTUCKY: Health Care Excel, Incorporated, 9502 Williamsburg Plaza, Suite 102, P.O. Box 23540, Louisville, KY 40222; tel. 502/339–7442; FAX. 502/339–8641; Philip L. Morphew, Chief Executive Director

LOUISIANA: Louisiana Health Care Review, Inc., 8591 United Plaza Boulevard, Suite 270, Baton Rouge, LA 70809; tel. 504/926–6353; FAX. 504/923–0957; Leo Stanley, Chief Executive Officer

MAINE: Northeast Health Care Quality Foundation, 15 Old Rollingsford Road, Suite 302, Dover, NH 03820; tel. 603/749–1641; FAX. 603/749–1195; Robert A. Aurilio, Chief Executive Officer

MARYLAND: Delmarva Foundation for Medical Care, Inc., 9240 Centreville Road, Easton, MD 21601; tel. 410/822–0697; FAX. 410/822–7971; Linda E. Clark, M.B.A., RN, Chief Executive Officer

MASSACHUSETTS: Massachusetts Peer Review Organization, Inc., 235 Wyman Street, Waltham, MA 02154–1231; tel. 617/890–0011; FAX. 617/487–0083; Kathleen E. McCarthy, Chief Executive Officer

MICHIGAN: Michigan Peer Review Organization, 40600 Ann Arbor Road, Suite 200, Plymouth, MI 48170–4495; tel. 313/459–0900; FAX. 313/454–7301; Gary Horvat, Chief Executive Officer

MINNESOTA: Stratis Health, 2901 Metro Drive, Suite 400, Bloomington, MN 55425; tel. 612/854–3306; FAX. 612/853–8503; David M. Ziegenhagen, Chief Executive Officer

MISSISSIPPI: Mississippi Foundation for Medical Care, Inc., 735 Riverside Drive, P.O. Box 4665, Jackson, MS 39296–4665; tel. 601/948–8894; FAX. 601/948–8917; James McIlwain, M.D.

MISSOURI: Missouri Patient Care Review Foundation, 505 Hobbs Road, Suite 100, Jefferson City, MO 65109; tel. 573/893–7900; FAX. 573/893–5827; Dan Jaco, Chief Executive Officer

MONTANA: Montana–Wyoming Foundation for Medical Care, 400 North Park Avenue, Second Floor, Helena, MT 59601; tel. 406/443–4020; FAX. 406/443–4585; Robert Henderson, M.D., President

NEBRASKA: Iowa Foundation for Medical Care/The Sunderbruch Corporation/Nebraska, 6000 Westown Parkway, Suite 350E, West Des Moines, IA 50266; tel. 515/223–2900; FAX. 402/474–7410; Fred Ferree, Executive Vice President

NEVADA: HealthInsight, 675 East 2100 South, Suite 270, Salt Lake City, UT 84106–1864; tel. 702/385–9933; FAX. 702/385–4586; Gary D. Lower, M.D., Chairman of the Board

NEW HAMPSHIRE: Northeast Health Care Quality Foundation, 15 Old Rollinsford Road, Suite 302, Dover, NH 03820–2830; tel. 603/749–1641; FAX. 603/749–1195; Robert A. Aurilio, Chief Executive Officer

NEW JERSEY: The Peer Review Organization of New Jersey, Inc., Central Division, Brier Hill Court, Building J, East Brunswick, NJ 08816; tel. 908/238–5570; FAX. 908/238–7766; Martin P. Margolies, Chief Executive Officer

NEW MEXICO: New Mexico Medical Review Association, 707 Broadway, N.E., Suite 200, P.O. Box 27449, Albuquerque, NM 87125–7449; tel. 505/842–6236; FAX. 505/764–0239; Carl L. Boymel, Acting Chief Executive Officer

NEW YORK: IPRO, 1979 Marcus Avenue, First Floor, Lake Success, NY 11042–1002; tel. 516/326–7767, ext. 540; FAX. 516/328–2310; Theodore O. Will, Executive Vice President

NORTH CAROLINA: Medical Review of North Carolina, Inc., 5625 Dillard Drive, Suite 203, Cary, NC 27511–9227; tel. 919/851–2955; FAX. 919/851–8457; Charles Riddick, Executive Director

NORTH DAKOTA: North Dakota Health Care Review Inc., 800 31st Avenue S.W., Minot, ND 58701; tel. 701/852–4231; FAX. 701/838–6009; David Remillard, Chief Executive Officer

OHIO: Peer Review Systems, Inc., 757 Brooksedge Plaza Drive, P.O. Box 6174, Westerville, OH 43086–6174; tel. 614/895–9900; FAX. 614/895–6784; Gregory J. Dykes, Chief Executive Officer

OKLAHOMA: Oklahoma Foundation for Medical Quality, Inc., The Paragon Building, 5801 Broadway Extension, Suite 400, Oklahoma City, OK 73118–7489; tel. 405/840–2891; FAX. 405/840–1343; Jim L. Williams, President, Chief Executive Officer

OREGON: Oregon Medical Professional Review Organization, 1220 Southwest Morrison Street, Suite 200, Portland, OR 97205; tel. 503/279–0100; FAX. 503/279–0190; Robert S. Kinoshita, President

PENNSYLVANIA: Keystone Peer Review Organization, Inc., 777 East Park Drive, P.O. Box 8310, Harrisburg, PA 17105–8310; tel. 717/564 8288; FAX. 717/564–4188; John DiNardi III, Executive Director

RHODE ISLAND: Rhode Island Quality Partners, Inc. (C/O CT PRO), 100 Roscommon Drive, Suite 200, Middletown, CT 06457; tel. 860/632–2008; FAX. 860/632–5865; Marsha K. Petrillo, Executive Director

SOUTH CAROLINA: Carolina Medical Reviews, 101 Executive Center Drive, Suite 123, Columbia, SC 29210; tel. 803/731–8225; FAX. 803/731–8229; Blake Williams, Director of Operations

SOUTH DAKOTA: South Dakota Foundation for Medical Care, 1323 South Minnesota Avenue, Sioux Falls, SD 57105; tel. 605/336–3505; FAX. 605/336–0270; L. Paul Jensen, Chief Executive Officer

TENNESSEE: Mid–South Foundation for Medical Care, Inc., 6401 Poplar Avenue, Suite 400, Memphis, TN 38119; tel. 901/682–0381; FAX. 901/761–3786; Logan Malone, Chief Executive Officer

TEXAS: Texas Medical Foundation, Barton Oaks Plaza Two, Suite 200, 901 Mopac Expressway, S., Austin, TX 78746–5799; tel. 512/329–6610; FAX. 512/327–7159; Phillip K. Dunne, Chief Executive Officer

UTAH: HealthInsight, 675 East 2100 South, Suite 270, Salt Lake City, UT 84106–1864; tel. 801/487–2290; FAX. 801/487–2296; James Q. Cannon, President, Chief Executive Officer

Section C

VERMONT: Northeast Health Care Quality Foundation, 15 Old Rollinsford Road, Suite 302, Dover, NH 03820–2830; tel. 603/749–1641; FAX. 603/749–1195; Robert A. Aurilio, Chief Executive Officer

VIRGINIA: Virginia Health Quality Center, 1604 Santa Rosa Road, Suite 200, Richmond, VA 23229–5008, P.O. Box K–70, Richmond, VA 23288–0070; tel. 804/289–5320; FAX. 804/289–5324; Terrence E. Dwyer, Executive Director

WASHINGTON: PRO–WEST, 10700 Meridian Avenue, N., Suite 100, Seattle, WA 98133–9075; tel. 206/364–9700; FAX. 206/368–2419; John W. Daise, Chief Executive Officer

WEST VIRGINIA: West Virginia Medical Institute, Inc., 3001 Chesterfield Place, Charleston, WV 25304; tel. 304/346–9864, ext. 269; FAX. 304/346–9863; Harry S. Weeks, Jr., M.D., President

WISCONSIN: Meta Star, 2909 Landmark Place, Madison, WI 53713; tel. 608/274–1940; FAX. 608/274–5008; Greg E. Simmons, President, Chief Executive Officer

WYOMING: Montana–Wyoming Foundation for Medical Care, 400 North Park Avenue, Second Floor, Helena, MT 59601; tel. 406/443–4020; FAX. 406/443–4585; Janice Connors, Executive Director

U. S. Associated Areas

PUERTO RICO: Quality Improvement Professional Research Organization, Mercantile Plaza Building, Suite 605, Hato Rey, PR 00918; tel. 809/753–6705; FAX. 809/753–6885; Jose Robles, Executive Director

VIRGIN ISLANDS: Virgin Islands Medical Institute, Inc., 1AD Estate Diamond Ruby, P.O. Box 5989, Sunny Isle, St. Croix, U.S., VI 00823–5989; tel. 809/778–6470; FAX. 809/778–6801; Denyce E. Singleton, Chief Executive Officer

Section C

State Health Planning and Development Agencies

The following is a list of state health planning and development agencies. The information was obtained from the Missouri Department of Health, Certificate of Need Program. For information about other state agencies and organizations that fulfill many of the same functions, contact the state or metropolitan hospital associations.

United States

ALABAMA: State Health Planning Agency, State of Alabama, 100 North Union Street, Suite 870, Montgomery, AL 36104; tel. 334/242–4103; FAX. 334/242–4113; J. Elbert Peters, Executive Director

ALASKA: Facilities and Planning Section, Department of Health and Social Services, P.O. Box 110650, Juneau, AK 99811–0650; tel. 907/465–3015; FAX. 907/465–2499; Larry J. Streuber, Section Chief

ARIZONA: Office of Health Planning, Evaluation and Statistics, 1740 West Adams, Room 301, Phoenix, AZ 85007; tel. 602/542–1216; FAX. 602/542–1244; Merle Lustig, Chief

CALIFORNIA: Office of Statewide Health Planning and Development, 1600 Ninth Street, Suite 440, Sacramento, CA 95814; tel. 916/654–2087; FAX. 916/654–3138; Priscilla Gonzalez–Leiva, RN, Deputy Director, Primary Care Resources

COLORADO: Department of Health, Office of Health, 4300 Cherry Creek Drive, S., Denver, CO 80222–1530; tel. 303/692–2858; FAX. 303/782–4883; Susan Rehak, Deputy Director

CONNECTICUT: Connecticut Department of Public Health and Addiction Services, Office of Policy, Planning and Evaluation, 410 Capitol Avenue, MS# 13PPE, Box 340308, Hartford, CT 06134–0308; tel. 860/509–7123; FAX. 860/509–7160; Donald Iodice, Health Program Associate

DELAWARE: Bureau of Health Planning and Resources Management, Department of Health and Social Services, P.O. Box 637, Dover, DE 19903; tel. 302/739–4776; FAX. 302/739–3008; Robert I. Welch, Director

DISTRICT OF COLUMBIA: Plan Development and Implementation Division, 800 Ninth Street, S.W., Third Floor, Washington, DC 20024; tel. 202/645–5525; FAX. 202/645–0526; Gail Smith, Chief

FLORIDA: Agency for Health Care Administration, Medicaid Program Development, 2727 Mahan Drive, Tallahassee, FL 32308–5403; tel. 904/488–8394; FAX. 904/414–6236; H. Robert Sharpe, Chief

GEORGIA: State Health Planning Agency, Planning and Implementation Division, Four Executive Park Drive, N.E., Suite 2100, Atlanta, GA 30329; tel. 404/679–4821; FAX. 404/679–4914; Karen Butler–Decker, Director, Division of Planning and Implementation

HAWAII: State Health Planning and Development Agency, 335 Merchant Street, Suite 214–E, Honolulu, HI 96813; tel. 808/587–0788; FAX. 808/587–0783; Marilyn A. Matsunaga, Administrator

IDAHO: Center for Vital Statistics and Health Policy, Division of Health, Idaho Department of Health and Welfare, 450 West State Street, First Floor, P.O. Box 83720, Boise, ID 83720–0036; tel. 208/334–5976; FAX. 208/334–0685; Jane Smith, Chief

ILLINOIS: Illinois Department of Public Health, Division of Health Policy, 525 West Jefferson, Springfield, IL 62761; tel. 217/782–6235; FAX. 217/785–6235; Angela Oldfield, M.S.W., L.S.W., Chief

INDIANA: Indiana State Department of Health, Local Liaison Office, Two North Meridian Street, Suite Eight–B, Indianapolis, IN 46204–3003; tel. 317/233–7846; FAX. 317/233–7761; Randall Ritter, M.P.A.

IOWA: Department of Public Health, Division of Substance Abuse and Health Promotion, Lucas State Office Building, Des Moines, IA 50319; tel. 515/281–5914; FAX. 515/281–4958; Ronald Eckoff, Medical Director

KANSAS: Health Care Commission, 900 Southwest Jackson, Ninth Floor, Landon State Office Building, Topeka, KS 66612; tel. 913/296–7488; FAX. 913/296–2664; Steve Ashley

MAINE: Division of Health Planning and State Health Planning, P.O. Box 426, Augusta, ME 04330–0011; tel. 207/624–5424; Stephen LaForge, Director

MARYLAND: Maryland Health Resources Planning Commission, 4201 Patterson Avenue, Baltimore, MD 21215–2299; tel. 410/764–3255; FAX. 410/358–1311; James Stanton, Executive Director

MICHIGAN: Division of Planning and Evaluation, 3423 North Martin Luther King Jr. Boulevard, Lansing, MI 48909; tel. 517/335–9372; FAX. 517/335–8560; Jan Ruff, Chief

MINNESOTA: Division of Community Health Services, Health Systems and Special Populations, Metro Square Building, 121 East Seventh Place, Suite 460, P.O. Box 64975, St. Paul, MN 55164–0975; tel. 612/296–9720; FAX. 612/296–9362; Ryan Church, Director

MISSISSIPPI: Mississippi State Department of Health, Health Planning and Resource Development Division, 2423 North State Street, P.O. Box 1700, Jackson, MS 39215–1700; tel. 601/960–7874; FAX. 601/354–6123; Harold B. Armstrong, Chief

MISSOURI: Missouri Department of Health, Office of Planning, 1738 East Elm Street, P.O. Box 570, Jefferson City, MO 65102; tel. 314/751–6005; FAX. 314/751–6041; Linda Hillemann, Chief

MONTANA: Health Policy and Services Division, Department of Public Health and Human Services, Cogswell Building, P.O. Box 202951, Helena, MT 59620–2951; tel. 406/444–4349; FAX. 406/444–2606; Gary T. Rose, Health Planner

NEBRASKA: Nebraska Health and Human Services, Regulation and Licensure, Performance Accountability Division, P.O. Box 95007, Lincoln, NE 68509; tel. 402/471–2337; Davina Shutzer, Division Director

NEVADA: State Health Division, Bureau of Health Planning and Statistics, 505 East King Street, Suite 102, Carson City, NV 89701–4761; tel. 702/687–4720; FAX. 702/687–6151; Emil DeJan, Chief

NEW HAMPSHIRE: Office of Health Services Planning and Review, Six Hazen Drive, Concord, NH 03301–6527; tel. 603/271–4606; FAX. 603/271–4141; Edmond Duchesne, Administrator, Planning Coordination

NEW JERSEY: Certificate of Need and Acute Care Licensure Program, New Jersey Department of Health, CN 360, John Fitch Plaza, Trenton, NJ 08625–0360; tel. 609/292–8773; FAX. 609/984–3165; Darcy Saunders, Director

NEW MEXICO: New Mexico Health Policy Commission, 435 St. Michael's Drive, Suite A–202, Santa Fe, NM 87505; tel. 505/827–7500; FAX. 505/827–7506; Katherine Ganz, M.D., Director

NEW YORK: New York State Department of Health, Division of Planning, Policy and Resource Development, Corning Tower, Suite 1495, Empire State Plaza, Albany, NY 12237; tel. 518/474–0180; FAX. 518/474–5450; Judith Arnold, Deputy Commissioner

NORTH CAROLINA: State Medical Facilities Planning Section, P.O. Box 29530, Raleigh, NC 27626–0530; tel. 919/733–4130; FAX. 919/715–4413; Robert J. Fitzgerald, Deputy Director, Division of Facility Services

NORTH DAKOTA: Division of Health Information Systems, North Dakota Department of Health, 600 East Boulevard Avenue, Bismarck, ND 58505–0200; tel. 701/328–2894; FAX. 701/328–4727; Fred Larson, Project Review Administrator

OHIO: Ohio Department of Health, Health Systems Planning, Primary Care and Rural Health, 246 North High Street, P.O. Box 118, Columbus, OH 43266–0118; tel. 614/466–3325; FAX. 614/644–8661; Louis Pomerantz, Chief, Health Systems Planning, Primary Care, Rural Health

OKLAHOMA: Oklahoma State Department of Health, Health Promotion and Policy Analysis, 1000 Northeast 10th Street, Oklahoma City, OK 73117–1299; tel. 405/271–1110; FAX. 405/271–1225; Jerry Prilliman, Director Planning

PENNSYLVANIA: Division of Planning and Technical Assistance, Pennsylvania Department of Health, Health and Welfare Building, Suite 1027, P.O. Box 90, Harrisburg, PA 17108; tel. 717/783–1410; FAX. 717/783–3794; Jack W. Means, Jr., Director

RHODE ISLAND: Rhode Island Department of Health, Cannon Building, Three Capitol Hill, Suite 401, Providence, RI 02908; tel. 401/277–2231; FAX. 401/277–6548; William J. Waters, Jr., Ph.D., Deputy Director

SOUTH CAROLINA: DHEC, Division of Planning and Certificate of Need, 2600 Bull Street, Columbia, SC 29201; tel. 803/737–7200; FAX. 803/737–7212, Albert Whiteside, Director

SOUTH DAKOTA: South Dakota Department of Health, Office of Administrative Services, 445 East Capitol Avenue, Pierre, SD 57501–3185; tel. 605/773–3361; FAX. 605/773–5683; Joan Adam, Director, Office of Administrative Services

TENNESSEE: Assessment and Planning, Tennessee Department of Health, Cordell Hull Building, 426 Fifth Avenue, N., Fourth Floor, Nashville, TN 37247–5261; tel. 615/532–2259; FAX. 615/532–7904; Gary Miles, Health Planner

TEXAS: Bureau of State Health Data and Policy Analysis, Texas Department of Health, 1100 West 49th Street, Austin, TX 78756; tel. 512/458–7261; FAX. 512/458–7344; Rick A. Danko, Planning Director

UTAH: Public Health Policy and Planning Committee (PHPPC), Utah Department of Health, Box 142828, Salt Lake City, UT 84114–2828; tel. 801/538–6352; FAX. 801/538–6694; Laverne Snow, Health Policy Consultant

VERMONT: Division of Health Care Administration, Department of Banking Insurance, Securities, and Health Care Administration, 89 Main Street, Drawer 20, Montpelier, VT 05620–3601; tel. 802/828–2900; FAX. 802/828–2949; Stan Lane, Policy Analyst

VIRGINIA: Virginia Department of Health, Division of Certificate of Public Need, 3600 West Broad Street, Suite 216, Richmond, VA 23220; tel. 804/367–2126; FAX. 804/367–2006; Paul E. Parker, Director

WASHINGTON: Washington State Board of Health, 1102 Southeast Quince, P.O. Box 47990, Olympia, WA 98504–7990; tel. 360/586–0399; FAX. 360/586–6033; Sylvia I. Beck, Executive Director

WEST VIRGINIA: West Virginia Health Care Cost Review Authority, 100 Dee Drive, Charleston, WV 25311; tel. 304/558–7000; FAX. 304/558–7001; David W. Forinash

WYOMING: Department of Health, 117 Hathaway Building, Cheyenne, WY 82002; tel. 307/777–7656; FAX. 307/777–7439; Douglas Thiede, Data and Communications Manager

Section C

The following list includes state departments of health and welfare, and their subagencies as well as such independent agencies as those for crippled children's services, maternal and child health, mental health, and vocational rehabilitation. The information was obtained directly from the agencies.

United States

ALABAMA
The Honorable Fob James, Jr., Governor,
334/242-7100
Health
Department of Public Health, 434 Monroe Street, Montgomery, AL 36130-3017; tel. 334/613-5200; FAX. 334/240-3387; Donald E. Williamson, M.D., State Health Officer
Family
Alabama Department of Public Health, Bureau of Family Health Services, The RSA Tower, P.O. Box 303017, Montgomery, AL 36130-3017; tel. 334/206-2940; FAX. 334/206-2950; Thomas M. Miller, M.D., M.P.H., Director
Licensing
Alabama Department of Public Health, Division of Licensure and Certification, The RSA Tower, P.O. Box 303017, Montgomery, AL 36130-3017; tel. 334/206-5078; FAX. 334/240-3147; Rick Harris, Director
Welfare
Department of Human Resources, Gordon Persons Building, 50 Ripley Street, Montgomery, AL 36130; tel. 334/242-1160; FAX. 334/242-0198; Martha S. Nachman, Commissioner
Medical Services
Alabama Medicaid Agency, 501 Dexter Avenue, P.O. Box 5624, Montgomery, AL 36103-5624; tel. 334/242-5600; FAX. 334/242-5097; Gwendolyn H. Williams, Commissioner
Insurance
Department of Insurance, 135 South Union Street, Montgomery, AL 36130; tel. 334/269-3550; FAX. 334/241-4192; Michael DeBellis, Commissioner
Other
Education
State Department of Education, Gordon Persons Building, Suite 5114, P.O. Box 302101, Montgomery, AL 36130-2101; tel. 334/242-9700; FAX. 334/242-9708; Ed Richardson, Superintendent
Mental Health
State Department of Mental Health and Mental Retardation, RSA Union, 100 North Union Street, P.O. Box 301410, Montgomery, AL 36130-1410; tel. 334/242-3107; FAX. 334/242-0684; Virginia A. Rogers, Commissioner
Nursing
Alabama Board of Nursing, RSA Plaza, 770 Washington Avenue, Suite 250, Montgomery, AL 36130; tel. 334/242-4060; FAX. 334/242-4360; Judi Crume, RN, M.S.N., Executive Officer
Rehabilitation
Department of Rehabilitation Services, 2129 East South Boulevard, Montgomery, AL 36116; tel. 800/441-7607; FAX. 334/281-1973; Lamona H. Lucas, Commissioner

ALASKA
The Honorable Tony Knowles, Governor,
907/465-3500
Health
Department of Health and Social Services, 350 Main Street, Room 229, P.O. Box 110601, Juneau, AK 99811-0601; tel. 907/465-3030; FAX. 907/465-3068; Jay A. Livey, Acting Commissioner
Assistance
State of Alaska, Division of Medical Assistance, P.O. 110660, Juneau, AK 99811-0640; tel. 907/465-3355; FAX. 907/465-2204; Bob Labbe, Director
Family
Division of Family and Youth Services, P.O. Box 110630, Juneau, AK 99811; tel. 907/465-3191; FAX. 907/465-3397; L. Diane Worley, Director
Finance
Division of Administrative Services, Department of Health and Social Services, P.O. Box 110650, Juneau, AK 99811-0650; tel. 907/465-3082; FAX. 907/465-2499; Janet E. Clarke, Director

Licensing
Health Facilities Licensing and Certification, 4730 Business Park Boulevard, Suite 18, Building H, Anchorage, AK 99503-7137; tel. 907/561-8081; FAX. 907/561-3011; Shelbert Larsen, Administrator
Medical Assistance
Division of Medical Assistance, P.O. Box 110660, Juneau, AK 99811-0660; tel. 907/465-3355; FAX. 907/465-2204; Kimberly Busch, Director
Mental Health
Division of Mental Health and Developmental Disabilities, P.O. Box 110620, Juneau, AK 99811-0620; tel. 907/465-3370; FAX. 907/465-2668
Substance Abuse
Division of Alcoholism and Drug Abuse, P.O. Box 110607, Juneau, AK 99811-0607; tel. 907/465-2071; FAX. 907/465-2185; Loren A. Jones, Director
Other
State of Alaska, Department of Health and Social Services, 350 Main Street, Room 229, P.O. Box 110601, Juneau, AK 99811-0601; tel. 907/465-3030; FAX. 907/465-3068; Jay A. Livey, Deputy Commissioner
Other
Education
Department of Education, 801 West 10th Street, Suite 200, Juneau, AK 99801-1894; tel. 907/465-8730; FAX. 907/465-3396; Helen Mehrkens, Health Promotion Specialist
Licensing
Department of Commerce and Economic Development, Division of Occupational Licensing, State Medical Board, 3601 C Street, Suite 722, Anchorage, AK 99503; tel. 907/269-8163; FAX. 907/269-8156; Leslie G. Abel, Executive Administrator
Nursing
Alaska Board of Nursing, 3601 C Street, Suite 722, Anchorage, AK 99503; tel. 907/269-8160; FAX. 907/269-8156; Dorothy P. Fulton, RN, M.A., Executive Administrator
Rehabilitation
Division of Vocational Rehabilitation, 801 West 10th Street, Suite 200, Juneau, AK 99801-1894; tel. 907/465-2814; FAX. 907/465-2856; Duane M. French, Director

ARIZONA
The Honorable Fife Symington, Governor,
602/542-4331
Health
Arizona Department of Health Services, 1740 West Adams Street, Suite 407, Phoenix, AZ 85007; tel. 602/542-1025; FAX. 602/542-1062; Jack Dillenberg, D.D.S., M.P.H., Director
Children
Children's Rehabilitative Services, Administrative Offices, 1740 West Adams Street, Suite 200, Phoenix, AZ 85007; tel. 602/542-1860; FAX. 602/542-2589; Susan Burke, Acting Chief
Environment
Arizona Department of Environmental Quality, 3033 North Central Avenue, Phoenix, AZ 85012; tel. 602/207-2300; FAX. 602/207-2218, ext. 2200; Russell F. Rhoades, Director
Family
Community and Family Health Services, 1740 West Adams Street, Suite 307, Phoenix, AZ 85007; tel. 602/542-1223; FAX. 602/542-1265; W. Sundin Applegate, M.D., Acting Bureau Chief
Health
Behavioral Health Services, Arizona Department of Health Services, 2122 East Highland, Suite 100, Phoenix, AZ 85016; tel. 602/381-8999; FAX. 602/553-9140; Rhonda Baldwin, Assistant Director
Licensing
Arizona Department of Health Services, Division of Health and Child Care Review Services, Office of Health Care Licensure, 1647 East Morten, Phoenix, AZ 85020; tel. 602/255-1197; FAX. 602/255-1135; John Zemaitis, Assistant Director

Prevention
Arizona Department of Health Services, Division of Public Health Services, Bureau of Epidemiology and Disease Control Services, 3815 North Black Canyon Highway, Phoenix, AZ 85015; tel. 602/230-5808; FAX. 602/230-5959; Norman J. Petersen, Bureau Chief

Department of Economic Security, Site Code 010A, P.O. Box 6123, Phoenix, AZ 85005; tel. 602/542-5678; FAX. 602/542-5339; Linda J. Blessing, Director
Rehabilitation
Rehabilition Services Administration (930A), 1789 West Jefferson, Second Floor Northwest, Phoenix, AZ 85007; tel. 602/542-3332; FAX. 602/542-3778; Roger J. Hodges, Administrator
Insurance
Department of Insurance, 3030 North Third Street, Suite 1100, Phoenix, AZ 85012; tel. 602/255-5400; FAX. 602/255-5316
Other
Medical Examiners
Arizona Board of Medical Examiners, 1651 East Morten, Suite 210, Phoenix, AZ 85020; tel. 602/255-3751; Mark R. Speicher, Executive Director
Nursing
Arizona State Board of Nursing, 1651 East Morten, Suite 150, Phoenix, AZ 85020; tel. 602/255-5092; FAX. 602/255-5130

ARKANSAS
The Honorable Mike Huckabee, Governor,
501/682-2345
Health
Arkansas Department of Health, 4815 West Markham Street, Slot 39, Little Rock, AR 72205-3867; tel. 501/661-2111; FAX. 501/671-1450; Sandra B. Nichols, M.D., Director
Administration
Bureau of Administrative Support, State Health Building, Little Rock, AR 72205-3867; tel. 501/661-2252; Tom Butler, Director
Community
Arkansas Department of Health, Bureau of Community Health Services, 4815 West Markham Street, Slot 2, Little Rock, AR 72205-3867; tel. 501/661-2167; FAX. 501/661-2601; Jim Mills, Director
Facilities
Division of Health Facility Services, 5800 West 10th Street, Suite 408, Little Rock, AR 72204; tel. 501/661-2201; FAX. 501/661-2165; Valetta M. Buck, Director
Health
Bureau of Public Health Programs, Arkansas Department of Health, 4815 West Markham Street, Slot 41, Little Rock, AR 72205-3867; tel. 501/661-2243; FAX. 501/661-2055; Martha Hiett, Director
Planning
Arkansas Department of Health, Planning and Policy Development, 4815 West Markham, Slot 55, Little Rock, AR 72205; tel. 501/661-2238; FAX. 501/661-2414; Nancy Kirsch, Deputy Director
Resources
Bureau of Health Resources, 4815 West Markham Street, Slot 21, Little Rock, AR 72205-3867; tel. 501/661-2268; FAX. 501/661-2544; Robert L. Robinette, B.S., M.S.E.H., Director
Welfare
Arkansas Department of Human Services, P.O. Box 1437, Little Rock, AR 72203-1437; tel. 501/682-8650; FAX. 501/682-6836; Tom Dalton, Director
Aging
Division of Aging and Adult Services, P.O. Box 1437, Slot 1412, Little Rock, AR 72203-1437; tel. 501/682-2441; FAX. 501/682-8155; Herb Sanderson, Director

Children
Children's Medical Service, Donaghey Plaza South, Seventh and Main Streets, P.O. Box 1437, Slot 526, Little Rock, AR 72203; tel. 501/682–2277; FAX. 501/682–8247; G. A. Buchanan, M.D., Medical Director

Long Term Care
Office of Long–Term Care, Lafayette Building, Sixth and Louisiana Streets, P.O. Box 8059, Slot 400, Little Rock, AR 72203–8059; tel. 501/682–8487; FAX. 501/682–6955; Shirley Gamble, Director

Medical Services
Division of Medical Services, Donaghey Building, Seventh and Main Streets, P.O. Box 1437, Slot 1100, Little Rock, AR 72203; tel. 501/682–8292; FAX. 501/682–1197; Ray Hanley, Director

Mental Health
Division of Mental Health Services, Arkansas State Hospital, 4313 West Markham, Little Rock, AR 72205–4096; tel. 501/686–9000; FAX. 501/686–9182; John Selig, Director

Rehabilitation
Arkansas Rehabilitation Services, 1616 Brookwood, P.O. Box 3781, Little Rock, AR 72203; tel. 501/296–1616; FAX. 501/296–1675; Bobby C. Simpson, Commissioner

Substance Abuse
Bureau of Alcohol & Drug Abuse Prevention, Freeway Medical Center, Suite 907, 5800 West 10th Street, Little Rock, AR 72204; tel. 501/280–4501; FAX. 501/280–4532; Joe M. Hill, Director

Insurance
Arkansas Insurance Department, 1123 South University Avenue, Suite 400, Little Rock, AR 72204; tel. 501/686–2900; FAX. 501/686–2913; Lee Douglass, Commissioner

Other
Nursing
Arkansas State Board of Nursing, University Tower Building, Suite 800, 1123 South University, Little Rock, AR 72204; tel. 501/686–2700; FAX. 501/686–2714; Faith A. Fields, M.S.N., RN, Executive Director

CALIFORNIA
The Honorable Pete Wilson, Governor, 916/445–2864

Health
Department of Health Services, 714 P Street, Suite 1253, Sacramento, CA 95814; tel. 916/657–1425; FAX. 916/657–1156; S. Kimberly Belshe, Director

Welfare
Health and Welfare Agency, Office of the Secretary, 1600 Ninth Street, Suite 460, Sacramento, CA 95814; tel. 916/654–3454; FAX. 916/654–3343

Community
Community Resources Development Section, California Department of Rehabilitation, 830 K Street Mall, Sacramento, CA 95814; tel. 916/323–0390; FAX. 916/322–0503; Sig Brivkalns, Chief

Developmental Disabilities
Department of Developmental Services, 1600 Ninth Street, Suite 240, Sacramento, CA 95814; tel. 916/654–1897; FAX. 916/654–2167; Dennis G. Amundson, Director

Mental Health
Department of Mental Health, 1600 Ninth Street, Room 151, Sacramento, CA 95814; tel. 916/654–2309; FAX. 916/654–3198; Stephen W. Mayberg, Ph.D., Director

Rehabilitation
Department of Rehabilitation, 830 K Street Mall, Sacramento, CA 95814; tel. 916/445–8638

Social Services
Department of Social Services, 744 P Street, MS 17–11, Sacramento, CA 95814; tel. 916/657–2598; FAX. 916/654–6012; Eloise Anderson, Director

Substance Abuse
Department of Alcohol and Drug Programs, 1700 K Street, Sacramento, CA 95814; tel. 916/445–1943; FAX. 916/323–5873; Andrew M. Mecca, Dr.P.H., Director

Other
Nurse Examiners
Board of Vocational Nurse and Psychiatric Technician Examiners, 2535 Capitol Oaks Drive, Suite 205, Sacramento, CA 95833; tel. 916/263–7800; FAX. 916/263–7859; Teresa Bello–Jones, J.D., M.S.N., RN, Executive Officer

Nursing
Board of Registered Nursing, 400 R Street, Suite 4030, P.O. Box 944210, Sacramento, CA 94244–2100; tel. 916/322–3350; Ruth Ann Terry, M.P.H., R.N., Executive Officer

Quality Assurance
Medical Board of California, 1426 Howe Avenue, Suite 54, Sacramento, CA 95825–3236; tel. 916/263–2389; FAX. 916/263–2387; Ron Joseph, Executive Director

Other
Department of Corporations, Health Care Division, 3700 Wilshire Boulevard, Suite 600, Los Angeles, CA 90010–3001; tel. 213/736–2776; Gary G. Hagen, Assistant Commissioner

COLORADO
The Honorable Roy Romer, Governor, 303/866–2471

Health
Colorado Department of Public Health and Environment, 4300 Cherry Creek Drive, S., Denver, CO 80222–1530; tel. 303/692–2000; FAX. 303/782–0095; Patti Shwayder, Acting Executive Director

Facilities
Colorado Department of Public Health and Environment, Health Facilities Division, 4300 Cherry Creek Drive S., Denver, CO 80222–1530; tel. 303/692–2800; FAX. 303/782–4883; Susan E. Rehak, Deputy Director

Family
Family and Community Health Services Division, Colorado Department of Public Health and Environment, 4300 Cherry Creek Drive South, Denver, CO 80222–1530; tel. 303/692–2310; FAX. 303/753–9249; Daniel J. Gossert, ACSW, M.P.H., Director

Substance Abuse
Alcohol and Drug Abuse Division, Colorado Department of Human Services, 4300 Cherry Creek Drive South, Denver, CO 80222; tel. 303/692–2930; FAX. 303/753–9775; Robert Aukerman, Director

Welfare
State Department of Health Care Policy and Financing, 1575 Sherman Street, Fourth Floor, Denver, CO 80203; tel. 303/866–2859; FAX. 303/866–2803; Richard Allen, Manager, Medical Assistance

Aging
Division of Aging and Adult Services, Colorado Department of Human Services, 110 16th Street, Second Floor, Denver, CO 80202; tel. 303/620–4127; FAX. 303/620–4191; Rita A. Barreras, Director

Rehabilitation
State Department of Health Care Policy and Financing, 1575 Sherman Street, 10th Floor, Denver, CO 80203–1714; tel. 303/866–2993; FAX. 303/866–4411; Alan R. Weil, Executive Director

Other
Insurance
Division of Insurance, 1560 Broadway, Suite 850, Denver, CO 80202; tel. 303/894–7499, ext. 311; FAX. 303/894–7455; Jack Ehnes, Commissioner

Medical Examiners
Colorado Board of Medical Examiners, 1560 Broadway, Suite 1300, Denver, CO 80202–5140; tel. 303/894–7690; Susan Miller, Program Administrator

Mental Health
Mental Health Services, 3824 West Princeton Circle, Denver, CO 80236; tel. 303/762–4088; FAX. 303/762–4373; Thomas J. Barrett, Ph.D., Director

Regulatory
Department of Regulatory Agencies, 1560 Broadway, Suite 1550, Denver, CO 80202; tel. 303/894–7855; Joseph A. Garcia, Executive Director

Other
Department of Human Services, 1575 Sherman Street, Eighth Floor, Denver, CO 80203; tel. 303/866–5096; FAX. 303/866–4740; Barbara McDonnell, Executive Director

CONNECTICUT
The Honorable John G. Rowland, Governor, 203/566–4840

Health
Department of Health Services, 150 Washington Street, Hartford, CT 06106; tel. 203/566–2038; Frederick G. Adams, D.D.S., M.P.H., Commissioner

Health
Connecticut Department of Public Health and Addiction Services, Bureau of Health Promotion, 150 Washington Street, Hartford, CT 06106; tel. 203/566–5475; FAX. 203/566–1400; Peter Galbraith, D.M.D., Bureau Chief

Quality
Department of Public Health, 410 Capitol Avenue, Mail Stop 12APP, P.O. Box 340308, Hartford, CT 06134–0308; tel. 860/509–7579; FAX. 860/509–8457; Cinthia Denne, Director

Regulation
Department of Public Health and Addiction Services, Bureau of Health System Regulation, 150 Washington Street, Hartford, CT 06106; tel. 203/566–1174; FAX. 203/566–1097; Stephen A. Harriman, Bureau Chief

Other
Department of Public Health, Division of Health Systems Regulation, 410 Capitol Avenue, Mail Stop 12 HSR, Hartford, CT 06134–0308; tel. 860/509–7407; FAX. 860/509–7539; Cynthia Denne, RN, M.P.A., Director

Welfare
Department of Social Services, 25 Sigourney Street, Hartford, CT 06106; tel. 203/424–5008; Patricia Giardi, Commissioner

Insurance
Department of Insurance, P.O. Box 816, Hartford, CT 06142–0816; tel. 203/297–3800; FAX. 203/566–7410; Allan B. Roby, Jr., Director, Life and Health Division

Other
Aging
Elderly Services Division, Department of Social Services, 25 Sigourney Street, Hartford, CT 06106–5033; tel. 203/424–5274; FAX. 203/424–4966; Christine M. Lewis, Director, Community Services

Education
Department of Education, 165 Capitol Avenue, Hartford, CT 06145; tel. 203/566–5061; FAX. 203/566–8964

Mental Health
State Department of Mental Health and Addiction Services, 90 Washington Street, Hartford, CT 06106; tel. 203/566–3650; FAX. 203/566–6195; Albert J. Solnit, M.D., Commissioner

Nurse Examiners
Connecticut Board of Examiners for Nursing, Department of Public Health, 150 Washington Street, Hartford, CT 06106; tel. 203/566–1041; FAX. 203/566–1464; Marie Hilliard, Ph.D., RN, Executive Officer

Rehabilitation
Department of Social Services, Bureau of Rehabilitation Services, Division of Organizational Support, 10 Griffin Road, N., Windsor, CT 06095; tel. 203/298–2032; FAX. 203/298–9590; John J. Galiette, Chief

DELAWARE
The Honorable Tom Carper, Governor, 302/739–4101

Health
Department of Health and Social Services, 1901 North DuPont Highway, Main Administration Building, New Castle, DE 19720; tel. 302/577–4500; FAX. 302/577–4510

Aging
Division of Services for Aging and Adults with Physical Disabilities, 1901 North DuPont Highway, New Castle, DE 19720; tel. 302/577–4791, ext. 21; FAX. 302/577–4793; Eleanor Cain, Director

Children
Division of Public Health, Community Health Care Access Section, Jesse S. Cooper Building, Federal Street, P.O. Box 637, Dover, DE 19903; tel. 302/739–4785; FAX. 302/739–6617

Section C

Maternal and Child Health, Division of Public Health, P.O. Box 637, Dover, DE 19903; tel. 302/739-3111; FAX. 302/739-6617; Karen DeLeeuw, M.S.W., Director

Health

Bureau of Personal Health Service, Jesse Cooper Building, P.O. Box 637, Dover, DE 19901; tel. 302/739-4768; FAX. 302/739-6617; John A. J. Forest, M.D., Chief

Division of Public Health, P.O. Box 637, Dover, DE 19903; tel. 302/739-4701; FAX. 302/739-6659; Gregg C. Sylvester, M.D., M.P.H., Director, Division of Public Health

Laboratories

Delaware Public Health Laboratory, 30 Sunnyside Road, P.O. Box 1047, Smyrna, DE 19977-1047; tel. 302/653-2870; FAX. 302/653-2877; Christopher K. Zimmerman, M.A., Acting Director

Licensing

Office of Health Facilities Licensing and Certification, Department of Health and Social Services, Three Mill Road, Suite 308, Wilmington, DE 19806; tel. 302/577-6666; FAX. 302/577-6672; Ellen Reap, Director

Medical Assistance

Division of Social Services, P.O. Box 906, New Castle, DE 19720; tel. 302/577-4400; FAX. 302/577-4405; Elaine Archangelo, Director

Medical Services

Emergency Medical Services, Blue Hen Corporate Center, 655 South Bay Road, Suite Four H, Dover, DE 19901; tel. 302/739-4710; FAX. 302/739-2352; Steven Blessing, Executive Assistant

Other

Medicine

Board of Medical Practice of Delaware, Cannon Building, Suite 203, 861 Silver Lake Boulevard, P.O. Box 1401, Dover, DE 19903; tel. 302/739-4522; FAX. 302/739-2711; Brenda Petty-Ball, Executive Director

Nursing

Delaware Board of Nursing, Cannon Building, Suite 203, P.O. Box 1401, Dover, DE 19903; tel. 302/739-4522, ext. 216; FAX. 302/739-2711; Iva J. Boardman, RN, M.S.N., Executive Director

Rehabilitation

Department of Labor, Division of Vocational Rehabilitation, 4425 North Market Street, Wilmington, DE 19802; tel. 302/761-8275; FAX. 302/761-6611; Michelle P. Pointer, Director

Substance Abuse

Delaware State Hospital, Division of Alcoholism, Drug Abuse and Mental Health, 1901 North DuPont Highway, New Castle, DE 19720; tel. 302/577-4000; FAX. 302/577-4359; Charles H. Debnam, Interim Director

DISTRICT OF COLUMBIA
Government Switchboard, 202/727-1000
Health

Department of Human Services, 801 East Building, P.O. Box 54047, Washington, DC 20032; tel. 202/279-6002; FAX. 202/279-6014; Vincent C. Gray, Director

Children

Bureau of Maternal and Child Health Services, Commission of Public Health, DC, 800 Ninth Street, S.W., Washington, DC 20024; tel. 202/645-5653; Lynette Munday, M.D., Administrator

Health

D.C. Commission of Public Health, 800 Ninth Street, S.W., Washington, DC 20024; tel. 202/727-0014; Harvey Sloane, M.D.

Long Term Care

Long-Term Care Administration, 1660 L Street, N.W., 10th Floor, Washington, DC 20036; tel. 202/673-3597; A. Sue Brown, Administrator

Prevention

Preventive Health Services Administration, 800 Ninth Street, S.W., Third Floor, Washington, DC 20024; tel. 202/727-2317; Richard Levinson, M.D.

Rehabilitation

Rehabilitation Services Administration, 800 Ninth Street, S.W., Fourth Floor, Washington, DC 20024; tel. 202/645-5703; FAX. 202/645-0840

Substance Abuse

Alcohol and Drug Abuse Services Administration, 1300 1st Street, N.E., Washington, DC 20002; tel. 202/727-1762, ext. 223; FAX. 202/535-2028

Welfare

Social Services

Commission on Social Services, 609 H Street, N.E., Fifth Floor, Washington, DC 20002; tel. 202/727-5930; FAX. 202/727-5980; Annie J. Goodson, Acting Commissioner of Social Services

Department of Consumer and Regulatory Affairs, 614 H Street, N.W., Suite 1120, Washington, DC 20001; tel. 202/727-7120; FAX. 202/727-7842; Hampton Cross, Director

Facility

Department of Consumer and Regulatory Affairs, Service Facility Regulation Administration, 614 H Street, N.W., Suite 1003, Washington, DC 20001; tel. 202/727-7190; FAX. 202/727-7780; Geraldine K. Sykes, Administrator

Licensing

Occupational and Professional Licensing Administration, Department of Consumer and Regulatory Affairs, 614 H Street, N.W., Suite 903, Washington, DC 20001; tel. 202/727-7480; FAX. 202/727-7662; Winnie R. Huston, Administrator

Mental Health

Commission on Mental Health Services, St. Elizabeth's Campus, 2700 Martin Luther King Jr. Avenue, S.E., A Building, Suite 105, Washington, DC 20032; tel. 202/373-7166; FAX. 202/373-6484; Guido R. Zanni, Ph.D., Commissioner

FLORIDA
The Honorable Lawton Chiles, Governor, 904/488-2272
Health

Health

State Health Office, Secretary's Office, Department of Health, 1317 Winewood Boulevard, Building Six, Room 306, Tallahassee, FL 32399-0700; tel. 904/487-2945; FAX. 904/487-3729; James T. Howell, M.D, M.P.H., State Health Officer, Secretary

Welfare

Department of Health, 1317 Winewood Boulevard, Tallahassee, FL 32399-0700; tel. 904/487-2945; FAX. 904/487-3729; James T. Howell, M.D., M.P.H., Secretary

Aging

Adult Services, 1317 Winewood Boulevard, Building Two, Suite 323-A, Tallahassee, FL 32399-0700; tel. 904/488-8922; Ms. Conchy T. Bretos, Assistant Secretary

Children

Children's Medical Services, 1317 Winewood Boulevard, Tallahassee, FL 32399-0700; tel. 904/487-2690; FAX. 904/488-3813; Eric G. Handler, M.D., M.P.H., Director, CMS

Facilities

Certificate of Need/Budget Review Office, Agency for Health Care Administration, 2727 Mahan Drive, Tallahassee, FL 32308; tel. 904/488-8673; FAX. 904/922-6964; Elizabeth Dudek, Chief

Licensing

Division of Health Quality Assurance, 2727 Mahan Drive, Tallahassee, FL 32308; tel. 904/487-2527; FAX. 904/487-6240; Marshall E. Kelley, Director

Mental Health

Department of Health and Rehabilitative Services, Alcohol, Drug Abuse and Mental Health Program Office, 1317 Winewood Boulevard, Tallahassee, FL 32399-0700; tel. 904/488-8304; FAX. 904/487-2239

Insurance

Department of Insurance, Bureau of Specialty Insurers, 200 East Gaines Street, Tallahassee, FL 32399; tel. 904/488-6766; FAX. 904/488-0313; Al Willis, Chief

Other

Medicine

Florida Board of Medicine, 1940 North Monroe Street, Tallahassee, FL 32399-0750; tel. 904/488-0595; Marm M. Harris, Executive Director

Rehabilitation

Division of Vocational Rehabilitation, 2002 Old St. Augustine Road, Building A, Tallahassee, FL 32399-0696; tel. 904/488-6210; FAX. 904/921-7215; Tamara Allen Bibb, Director

Other

Department of Labor and Employment Security, 2012 Capital Circle, S.E., 303 Hartman Building, Tallahassee, FL 32399-2152; tel. 904/922-7021; FAX. 904/488-8930; Doug Jamerson, Secretary

GEORGIA
The Honorable Zell Miller, Governor, 404/656-1776
Health

Department of Human Resources, 47 Trinity Avenue, S.W., Suite 520 H, Atlanta, GA 30334; tel. 404/656-5680; FAX. 404/651-8669; Tommy C. Olmstead, Commissioner

Health

Division of Public Health, Two Peachtree Street, S.W., Suite 7-300, Atlanta, GA 30303; tel. 404/657-2700; FAX. 404/657-2715; Patrick Meehan, M.D., Director

Laboratories

Diagnostic Services Unit, Health Care Section, Office of Regulatory Services, Two Peachtree Street, N.W., 19th Floor, Room 320, Atlanta, GA 30303-3167; tel. 404/657-5448; FAX. 404/657-8934; Betty J. Logan, Regional Director, Diagnostic Services Unit

Licensing

Child Care Licensing Section, Two Peachtree Street, N.W., 20th Floor, Atlanta, GA 30303; tel. 404/657-5562; FAX. 404/657-8936; Jo Cato, Director

Department of Human Resources, Office of Regulatory Services, Health Care Section, Two Peachtree Street, N.W., Suite 19.204, Atlanta, GA 30303-3167; tel. 404/657-5550; FAX. 404/657-8934; Susie M. Woods, Director

Mental Health

Division of Mental Health, Mental Retardation and Substance Abuse, Two Peachtree Street, Fourth Floor, Atlanta, GA 30303; tel. 404/657-2252; FAX. 404/657-1137; Carl E. Roland, Jr., Director

Radiology

Diagnostic Services Unit, 878 Peachtree Street, N.E., Suite 719, Atlanta, GA 30309-3997; tel. 404/894-4747; FAX. 404/894-2185; Betty Logan, Director

Regulation

Office of Regulatory Services, Georgia Department of Human Resources, Two Peachtree Street, N.W., 21st Floor, Suite 325, Atlanta, GA 30303-3167; tel. 404/657-5700; FAX. 404/657-5708; Martin J. Rotter, Director

Rehabilitation

Division of Rehabilitation Services, Two Peachtree Street, N.W., Suite 23.319, Atlanta, GA 30303-3166; tel. 404/657-3000; FAX. 404/657-3079; Peggy Rosser, Director

Other

Personal Care Home Program, Office of Regulatory Services, Two Peachtree Street, 21st Floor, Atlanta, GA 30303-3167; tel. 404/657-4076; FAX. 404/657-3655; Victoria L. Flynn, Director

Insurance

Georgia Department of Insurance, Two Martin Luther King, Jr. Drive, Seventh Floor, West Tower, Floyd Building, Atlanta, GA 30334; tel. 404/656-2056; FAX. 404/657-7743; John W. Oxendiner, Commissioner, Insurance

Other

Medical Examiners

Composite State Board of Medical Examiners, 166 Pryor Street, S.W., Atlanta, GA 30303; tel. 404/656-3913; FAX. 404/656-9723; Andrew Watry, Executive Director

Nursing

Georgia Board of Nursing, 166 Pryor Street, S.W., Atlanta, GA 30303; tel. 404/656-3943; FAX. 404/657-7489; Shirley A. Camp, Executive Director

Planning

State Health Planning Agency, Four Executive Park Drive, N.E., Suite 2100, Atlanta, GA 30329; tel. 404/679-4821; FAX. 404/679-4914; Pamela S. Stephenson, Esq., Executive Director

HAWAII
The Honorable Benjamin J. Cayetano, Governor, 808/586-0034
Health

Hawaii Department of Health, P.O. Box 3378, Honolulu, HI 96801; tel. 808/586-4410; FAX. 808/586-4444; Lawrence Miike, Director

Section C

Chronic Disease

Communicable Disease Division, P.O. Box 3378, Honolulu, HI 96801; tel. 808/586–4580; FAX. 808/586–4595; Richard L. Vogt, M.D., State Epidemiologist

Dental

Dental Health Division, 1700 Lanakila Avenue, Suite 203, Honolulu, HI 96817–2199; tel. 808/832–5700; FAX. 808/832–5722; Mark H.K. Greer, D.M.D., M.P.H., Chief

Environment

Environmental Health, P.O. Box 3378, Honolulu, HI 96801; Shinji Soneda, Chief

Family

Family Health Services Division, Hawaii State Department of Health, 1250 Punchbowl Street, Room 216, Honolulu, HI 96813; tel. 808/586–4122; FAX. 808/586–9303; Nancy L. Kuntz, M.D, Chief, Family Health Services Division

Licensing

Department of Health/Hospital and Medical Facilities, Licensing and Certification, P.O. Box 3378, Honolulu, HI 96801; tel. 808/586–4080; FAX. 808/586–4747; Helen K. Yoshimi, B.S.N., M.P.H., Chief, H.M.F.B.

Mental Health

Adult Mental Health Division, P.O. Box 3378, Honolulu, HI 96801–9984; tel. 808/586–4686; FAX. 808/586–4745; Sherry Harrison, RN, M.A., Chief

Planning

State Health Planning and Development Agency, 335 Merchant Street, Suite 214 E, Honolulu, HI 96813; tel. 808/587–0788; FAX. 808/587–0783; Patrick J. Boland, Administrator

Substance Abuse

Alcohol and Drug Abuse Division, 1270 Queen Emma Street, Suite 305, Honolulu, HI 96813; tel. 808/586–3961; FAX. 808/586–4016; Elaine Wilson, Chief

Welfare

Medical Services

Department of Human Services, Med–QUEST Division, 820 Mililani Street, Suite 606, Box 339, Honolulu, HI 96813; tel. 808/586–5391; FAX. 808/586–5389; Rueben T. Shimazu, Acting Administrator

Rehabilitation

Vocational Rehabilitation, 1000 Bishop Street, Suite 605, Honolulu, HI 96813; tel. 808/586–5355; FAX. 808/586–5377; Neil Shim, Administrator

Other

Disability

Department of Labor and Industrial Relations, Disability Compensation Division, P.O. Box 3769, Honolulu, HI 96812; tel. 808/586–9151; FAX. 808/586–9219; Gary S. Hamada, Administrator

Medical Examiners

Department of Commerce and Consumer Affairs, Board of Medical Examiners, P.O. Box 3469, Honolulu, HI 96801; tel. 808/586–2708; Constance Cabral–Makanani, Executive Officer

IDAHO
The Honorable Philip E. Batt, Governor, 208/334–2100

Health

Children

Bureau of Clinical and Preventive Services, P.O. Box 83720, Boise, ID 83720–0036; tel. 208/334–5930; FAX. 208/332–7346; Roger Perotto, Chief

Health

Department of Health and Welfare, Division of Health, 450 West State, Fourth Floor, P.O. Box 83720, Boise, ID 83720–0036; tel. 208/334–5945; FAX. 208/334–6581; Richard H. Schultz, Administrator

Laboratories

Bureau of Laboratories, 2220 Old Penitentiary Road, Boise, ID 83712; tel. 208/334–2235; FAX. 208/334–2382; Richard F. Hudson, Ph.D., Chief

Licensing

Bureau of Facility Standards, Department of Health and Welfare, P.O. Box 83720, Boise, ID 83720–0036; tel. 208/334–6626; FAX. 208/332–7204; Sylvia Creswell, Supervisor–Non LTC

Medical Services

Bureau of Emergency Medical Services, P.O. Box 83720, Boise, ID 83720–0036; tel. 208/334–4000; FAX. 208/334–4015; Dia Gainor, Bureau Chief

Statistics

Center for Vital Statistics and Health Policy, 450 West State, First Floor, P.O. Box 83720, Boise, ID 83720–0036; tel. 208/334–5976; FAX. 208/334–0685; Jane S. Smith, State Registrar, Chief

Substance Abuse

Division of Family and Community Services, Bureau of Mental Health and Substance Abuse, P.O. Box 83720, Boise, ID 83720–0036; tel. 208/334–5935; FAX. 208/334–6664; Tina Klamt, Substance Abuse Project Manager

Insurance

Department of Insurance, Division of Examinations, 700 West State Street, Third Floor, P.O. Box 83720, Boise, ID 83720–0043; tel. 208/334–4250; FAX. 208/334–4398; James M. Alcorn, Director

Other

Medicine

Idaho State Board of Medicine, 280 North Eighth Street, Suite 202, P.O. Box 83720, Boise, ID 83720–0058; tel. 208/334–2822; FAX. 208/334–2801; Darleene Thorsted, Executive Director

Nursing

Idaho State Board of Nursing, 280 North Eighth Street, Suite 210, P.O. Box 83720, Boise, ID 83720–0061; tel. 208/334–3110; FAX. 208/334–3262; Sandra Evans, MA.Ed., RN, Executive Director

Rehabilitation

Vocational Rehabilitation, 650 West State, P.O. Box 83720, Len B. Jordan Building, Suite 150, Boise, ID 83720–0096; tel. 208/334–3390; FAX. 208/334–5305; George J. Pelletier, Jr., Administrator

ILLINOIS
The Honorable Jim Edgar, Governor, 217/782–6830

Health

Illinois Department of Public Health, 535 West Jefferson Street, Springfield, IL 62761; tel. 217/782–4977; FAX. 217/782–3987; John R. Lumpkin, M.D. Director

Administration

Office of Finance and Administration, 535 West Jefferson Street, Springfield, IL 62761; tel. 217/785–2033; FAX. 217/782–3987; Gary Robinson, Deputy Director

Facilities

Illinois Department of Public Health, Office of Health Care Regulation, Bureau of Hospitals and Ambulatory Services, 525 West Jefferson Street, Fourth Floor, Springfield, IL 62761; tel. 217/782–7412; FAX. 217/782–0382; Catherine M. Stokes, Assistant Deputy Director

Health

Illinois Department of Public Health, Office of Health Protection, 525 West Jefferson Street, Springfield, IL 62761; tel. 217/782–3984; FAX. 217/524–0802; Dave King, Deputy Director

Laboratories

Illinois Department of Public Health Laboratories, 825 North Rutledge Street, P.O. Box 19435, Springfield, IL 62794–9435; tel. 217/782–6562; FAX. 217/524–7924; David Carpenter, Ph.D., State Laboratory Director

Medical Services

Illinois Department of Public Health, 535 West Jefferson Street, Springfield, IL 62761; tel. 217/785–0245; FAX. 217/524–2491; James R. Nelson, Deputy Director, Community Health

Policy

Office of Epidemiology and Health Systems Development, 525 West Jefferson Street, Springfield, IL 62761; tel. 217/785–2040; FAX. 217/785–4308; Laura B. Landrum, Deputy Director

Regulation

Illinois Department of Public Health, Office of Health Care Regulation, 525 West Jefferson Street, Springfield, IL 62761; tel. 217/782–2913; FAX. 217/524–6292; William A. Bell, Deputy Director

Welfare

Department of Public Aid, 100 South Grand Avenue, E., Springfield, IL 62762; tel. 217/782–1200; FAX. 217/524–7979; Robert W. Wright, Director

Insurance

Department of Insurance, 320 West Washington Street, Fourth Floor, Springfield, IL 62767; tel. 217/782–4515; FAX. 217/782–5020; Mark Boozell, Director

Other

Children

Division of Specialized Care for Children, University of Illinois at Chicago, (Illinois' Title V Program for Children with Special Health Care Needs), 2815 West Washington, Suite 300, Springfield, IL 62794–9481; tel. 217/793–2350; FAX. 217/793–0773; Robert F. Biehl, M.D., Director

Mental Health

Illinois Department of Mental Health and Developmental Disabilities, 401 William G. Stratton Building, Springfield, IL 62765; tel. 217/782–7179; FAX. 217/524–0835; Jess McDonald, Director

Regulatory

Illinois Department of Professional Regulation, James R. Thompson Center, 100 West Randolph, Suite 9–300, Chicago, IL 60601; tel. 312/814–4500; FAX. 312/814–1837; Nikki M. Zollar, Director

Rehabilitation

Department of Rehabilitation Services, 623 East Adams Street, P.O. Box 19509, Springfield, IL 62794–9509; tel. 217/782–2722; FAX. 217/557–0142; Sharon Banks, Field Operations Manager, Home Service Program

INDIANA
The Honorable Frank O'Bannon, Governor, 317/232–4567

Health

Indiana State Department of Health, Two North Meridian Street, Indianapolis, IN 46204; tel. 317/233–7400; FAX. 317/233–7387; Tami Barrett–Coomer

Children

Maternal and Child Health Services, Indiana State Department of Health, Two North Meridian Street, Suite 700, Indianapolis, IN 46204; tel. 317/233–1262; FAX. 317/233–1299; Judith A. Ganser, M.D., M.P.H., Medical Director

Facilities

Division of Long Term Care, Two North Meridian Street, Fourth Floor, Indianapolis, IN 46204; tel. 317/233–6442; FAX. 317/233–7494; Suzanne Hornstein, Director

Other

Indiana State Department of Health, Division of Acute Care, Two North Meridian Street, Indianapolis, IN 46204; tel. 317/233–7472; FAX. 317/233–7157; John A. Braeckel, Director

Welfare

Indiana Family and Social Services Administration, Office of Medicaid Policy and Planning, Indiana Government Center–South, 402 West Washington, Room W 382, Indianapolis, IN 46204–2739; tel. 317/233–4455; FAX. 317/232–7382; Kathleen D. Gifford, Assistant Secretary

Children

Children's Special Health Care Services, Indiana State Department of Health, Two North Meridian Street, Section 7B, Indianapolis, IN 46204; tel. 317/233–5578; FAX. 317/233–5609; Wendy S. Gettelfinger, Acting Director

Insurance

Department of Insurance, 311 West Washington Street, Suite 300, Indianapolis, IN 46204; tel. 317/232–2406; FAX. 317/232–5251; Sally McCarty, Chief Deputy Commissioner

Other

Human Services

Indiana Department of Human Services, 150 West Market, P.O. Box 7083, Indianapolis, IN 46207–7083; tel. 317/232–7000; FAX. 317/232–1240; Jeff Richardson, Commissioner

Licensing

Medical Licensing Board of Indiana, Health Professions Bureau, 402 West Washington, Suite 041, Indianapolis, IN 46204; tel. 317/232–2960; FAX. 317/233–4236

Section C

Mental Health

Indiana Family and Social Services Administration, Division of Mental Health, Indiana Government Center–South, W353, 402 West Washington Street, Indianapolis, IN 46204; tel. 317/232–7800; FAX. 317/233–3472; Patrick Sullivan, Ph.D., Director

Nursing

Indiana State Board of Nursing, Health Professions Bureau, 402 West Washington Street, Room 041, Indianapolis, IN 46204; tel. 317/232–1105; FAX. 317/233–4236; Barbara Powers, Director

IOWA
The Honorable Terry E. Branstad, Governor, 515/281–5211

Health

Department of Public Health, Lucas State Office Building, 1st, 3rd and 4th Floors, Des Moines, IA 50319–0075; tel. 515/281–5605; FAX. 515/281–4958; Christopher G. Atchison, Director

Planning

Center for Health Policy, Iowa Department of Public Health, Lucas State Office Building, Fourth Floor, Des Moines, IA 50319; tel. 515/281–4346; FAX. 515/281–4958; Gerd Clabaugh, Director

Prevention

Division of Health Protection, Iowa Department of Public Health, Lucas State Office Building, First Floor, Des Moines, IA 50319; tel. 515/281–7785; FAX. 515/281–4529; John R. Kelly, Director

Substance Abuse

Division of Substance Abuse and Health Promotion, Iowa Department of Public Health, Lucas State Office Building, 321 East 12th Street, Des Moines, IA 50319–0075; tel. 515/281–3641; FAX. 515/281–4535; Janet Zwick, Director

Governor's Alliance on Substance Abuse, Lucas State Office Building, Des Moines, IA 50319; tel. 515/281–4518; FAX. 515/242–6390; Dale Woolery, Administrator

Welfare

Department of Human Services, Hoover State Office Building, Des Moines, IA 50319; tel. 515/281–5452; FAX. 515/281–4597; Charles M. Palmer, Director

Mental Health

Division of Mental Health/Developmental Disabilities, Hoover State Office Building, Des Moines, IA 50319–0114; tel. 515/281–5874; FAX. 515/281–4597; Division Administrator

Insurance

Division of Insurance, Lucas State Office Building, Sixth Floor, Des Moines, IA 50319; tel. 515/281–5705; FAX. 515/281–3059; Therese M. Vaughan, Commissioner

Other

Aging

Iowa Department of Elder Affairs, 236 Jewett Building, 914 Grand Avenue, Des Moines, IA 50309–2801; tel. 515/281–5187; FAX. 515/281–4036; Betty L. Grandquist, Executive Director

Children

Child Health Specialty Clinics, 247 Hospital School, University of Iowa, Iowa City, IA 52242–1011; tel. 319/356–1469; FAX. 319/356–3715; Richard Nelson, M.D., Director

Facility

Department of Inspection and Appeals, Division of Health Facilities, Lucas State Office Building, Des Moines, IA 50319; tel. 515/281–4115; FAX. 515/242–5022; J. B. Bennett, Administrator

Medical Examiners

Iowa State Board of Medical Examiners, State Capitol Complex, Executive Hills West, Des Moines, IA 50319; tel. 515/281–5171; FAX. 515/242–5908; Ann M. Martino, Ph.D., Executive Director

Nursing

Iowa Board of Nursing, State Capitol Complex, 1223 East Court Avenue, Des Moines, IA 50319; tel. 515/281–3255; FAX. 515/281–4825; Lorinda K. Inman, RN, M.S.N., Executive Director

Rehabilitation

Department of Education, Division of Vocational Rehabilitation Services, 510 East 12th Street, Des Moines, IA 50319; tel. 515/281–4311; Marge Knudsen, Administrator

KANSAS
The Honorable Bill Graves, Governor, 913/296–3232

Health

Kansas Department of Health and Environment, Landon State Office Building, 900 Southwest Jackson, Suite 620, Topeka, KS 66612–1290; tel. 913/296–0461; FAX. 913/368–6368; James J. O'Connell, Secretary, Kansas Health and Environment

Children

Hospital and Medical Programs, Kansas Department of Health and Environment, Bureau of Adult and Child Care Facilities, 900 Southwest Jackson, Suite 1001, Topeka, KS 66612–1290; tel. 913/296–3362; FAX. 913/296–1266; Greg L. Reser, Director, Hospital and Medical Programs

Welfare

State Department of Social and Rehabilitation Services, Docking State Office Building, Suite 628–S, Topeka, KS 66612; tel. 913/296–6750; FAX. 913/296–4813; Robert L. Epps, Commissioner

Medical Services

Adult and Medical Services, Docking State Office Building, 915 Southwest Harrison, Room 628–S, Topeka, KS 66612; tel. 913/296–3981; FAX. 913/296–4813; Ann E. Koci, Commissioner

Mental Health

Mental Health and Development Disabilities, Docking State Office Building, Fifth Floor–N, Topeka, KS 66612; tel. 913/296–3773; FAX. 913/296–6142; Hugh Sage, Ph.D., Commissioner

Rehabilitation

Rehabilitation Services, Biddle Building, 300 Southwest Oakley, First Floor, Topeka, KS 66606; tel. 913/296–3911; FAX. 913/296–0511; Joyce A. Cussimanio, Commissioner

Insurance

Kansas Insurance Department, 420 Southwest Ninth, Topeka, KS 66612; tel. 913/296–3071; FAX. 913/296–2283; Kathleen Sebelius, Commissioner, Insurance

Health

Kansas Insurance Department, Accident and Health Division, 420 Southwest Ninth, Topeka, KS 66612; tel. 913/296–7850; FAX. 913/296–2283; Richard G. Huncker, Supervisor

Other

Nursing

Kansas State Board of Nursing, Landon State Office Building, 900 Southwest Jackson, Suite 551–S, Topeka, KS 66612–1230; tel. 913/296–4929; FAX. 913/296–3929; Patsy Johnson, RN, M.N., Executive Administrator

Other

Kansas State Board of Healing Arts, 235 South Topeka Boulevard, Topeka, KS 66603–3068; tel. 913/296–7413; FAX. 913/296–0852; Lawrence T. Buening, Jr., Executive Director

KENTUCKY
The Honorable Paul E. Patton, Governor, 502/564–2611

Health

Department for Public Health, Cabinet for Health Services, 275 East Main Street, Frankfort, KY 40621; tel. 502/564–3970; FAX. 502/564–6533; Rice C. Leach, M.D., MSHSA, Commissioner

Licensing

Division of Licensing and Regulation, Cabinet for Health Services, C.H.R. Building, Fourth Floor, E., 275 East Main Street, Frankfort, KY 40621; tel. 502/564–2800; FAX. 502/565–6546; Rebecca J. Cecil, R.Ph., Director

Policy

Health Data Branch, 275 East Main Street, Frankfort, KY 40621; tel. 502/564–2757; FAX. 502/564–6533; George Robertson, Manager

Welfare

Department for Social Insurance, 275 East Main Street, Frankfort, KY 40621; tel. 502/564–3703; FAX. 502/564–6907; John L. Clayton, Commissioner

Insurance

Department of Insurance, Life and Health Division, 215 West Main Street, P.O. Box 517, Frankfort, KY 40602; tel. 502/564–6088; FAX. 502/564–6090; Paula Isaacs, Program Manager, Health Care

Other

Children

Commission for Children with Special Health Care Needs, 982 Eastern Parkway, Louisville, KY 40217; tel. 502/595–4459, ext. 267; FAX. 502/595–4673; Denzle L. Hill, Executive Director

Medical Services

Department for Medicaid Services, 275 East Main Street, Frankfort, KY 40621; tel. 502/564–4321; FAX. 502/564–6917; John Morse, Commissioner

Mental Health

Department For Mental Health/Mental Retardation Services, 275 East Main Street, Frankfort, KY 40621; tel. 502/564–4527; FAX. 502/564–5478; Elizabeth Rehm Wachtel, Ph.D., Commissioner

Nursing

Kentucky Board of Nursing, 312 Whittington Parkway, Suite 300, Louisville, KY 40222–5172; tel. 502/329–7000, ext. 226; FAX. 502/329–7011; Sharon M. Weisenbeck, M.S., RN, Executive Director

Rehabilitation

Department of Vocational Rehabilitation, 209 St. Clair Street, Frankfort, KY 40601; tel. 502/564–4440; FAX. 502/564–6745; Sam Srralgio, Commissioner

Other

Commission for Health Economics Control, 275 East Main Street, Frankfort, KY 40621; tel. 502/564–6620; W. R. Hourigan, Ph.D., Chairman

LOUISIANA
The Honorable Mike Foster, Governor, 504/342–7015

Health

Louisiana Department of Health and Hospitals, P.O. Box 629 Bin 2, Baton Rouge, LA 70821; tel. 504/342–9509; FAX. 504/342–9508; Rose V. Forrest, Secretary

Family

Office of Family Support, P.O. Box 94065, Baton Rouge, LA 70804–4065; tel. 504/342–3950; Howard L. Prejean, Assistant Secretary

Finance

Office of The Secretary, P.O. Box 629 Bin 2, Baton Rouge, LA 70821; tel. 504/342–9500; FAX. 504/342–9508; Bobby P. Jindal, Secretary

Health

Louisiana Healthcare Authority, Medical Center of Louisiana at New Orleans, 1532 Tulane Avenue, New Orleans, LA 70140; tel. 504/568–3201; FAX. 504/568–2028; Jonathan Roberts, Dr.P.H., Chief Executive Officer

Licensing

Department of Health and Hospitals, Bureau of Health Services Financing, Health Standards Section, Box 3767, Baton Rouge, LA 70821; tel. 504/342–0138; FAX. 504/342–5292; Lily W. McAlister, RN, Manager, Health Standards Section

Mental Health

Office of Alcohol and Drug Abuse, P.O. Box 2790, Bin 18, Baton Rouge, LA 70821–2790; tel. 504/342–6717; FAX. 504/342–3931; Alton E. Hadley, Assistant Secretary

Other

Health Care Authority, 8550 United Plaza Boulevard, Fourth Floor, Baton Rouge, LA 70809; tel. 504/922–0488; FAX. 504/922–0939; A. Jack Edwards, Assistant Secretary

Office of Community Services, P.O. Box 3318, Baton Rouge, LA 70821; tel. 504/342–2297; FAX. 504/342–2268; Brenda L. Kelley, Assistant Secretary

Insurance

Department of Insurance, P.O. Box 94214, Baton Rouge, LA 70804; tel. 504/342–5900; FAX. 504/342–7401; James H. Brown, Commissioner

Other

Medical Examiners

Louisiana State Board of Medical Examiners, 630 Camp Street, Zip 70130, P.O. Box 30250, New Orleans, LA 70190–0250; tel. 504/524–6763; FAX. 504/568–8893; Paula M. Mensen, Administrative Manager II

Nurse Examiners

Louisiana State Board of Practical Nurse Examiners, 3421 North Causeway Boulevard, Suite 203, Metairie, LA 70002; tel. 504/838–5791; FAX. 504/838–5279; Terry L. De Marcay, RN, Executive Director

Nursing

Louisiana State Board of Nursing, 150 Baronne Street, 912 Pere Marquette Building, New Orleans, LA 70112; tel. 504/568–5464; Barbara L. Movant, RN, M.N.

MAINE
The Honorable Angus S. King, Jr., Governor, 207/287–3531

Health

Maine Department of Human Services, State House, Station 11, Augusta, ME 04333; tel. 207/287–2736; FAX. 207/287–3005; Kevin W. Concannon, Commissioner

Aging

Bureau of Elder and Adult Services, State House, Station 11, Augusta, ME 04333; tel. 207/624–5335; FAX. 207/624–5361; Christine Gianopoulos, Director

Children

Division of Community and Family Health, 151 Capitol Street, 11 State House Station, Augusta, ME 04333; tel. 207/287–3311; FAX. 207/287–5355; Zsolt Koppanyi, M.D., M.P.H.

Health

Bureau of Health, Department of Human Services, 11 State House Station, Augusta, ME 04333; tel. 207/287–3201; FAX. 207/287–4631; Dora Anne Mills, M.D., M.P.H., Director

Licensing

Division of Licensing and Certification, Department of Human Services, 35 Anthony Avenue, Station 11, Augusta, ME 04333; tel. 207/624–5443; FAX. 207/624–5378; Louis Dorogi, Director

Medical Services

Department of Human Services, Bureau of Medical Services, State House, Station 11, Augusta, ME 04333; tel. 207/287–2674; FAX. 207/287–2675; Frances T. Finnegan, Jr., Director

Insurance

Bureau of Insurance, Department of Professional and Financial Regulation, 34 State House Station, Augusta, ME 04333; tel. 207/624–8475; FAX. 207/624–8599; David Stetson, Supervisor, Life and Health Division

Financial

Department of Professional and Financial Regulation, 35 State House Station, Augusta, ME 04333; tel. 207/624–8500; FAX. 207/624–8690; S. Catherine Longley, Commissioner

Other

Medicine

Board of Licensure in Medicine, Two Bangor Street, 137 State House Station, Augusta, ME 04333; tel. 207/287–3601; FAX. 207/287–6590; Randal C. Manning, Executive Director

Mental Health

Department of Mental Health, Mental Retardation and Substance Abuse Services, State House Station 40, Augusta, ME 04333; tel. 207/287–4220; FAX. 207/287–4268; Andrea Blanch, Associate Commissioner, Programs

Mental Retardation

Department of Mental Health, Mental Retardation and Substance Abuse Services, 40 State House Station, Augusta, ME 04333–0040; tel. 207/287–4223; FAX. 207/287–4268; Melodie J. Peet, Commissioner

Nursing

Maine State Board of Nursing, 24 Stone Street, 158 State House Station, Augusta, ME 04333; tel. 207/287–1133; FAX. 207/287–1149; Jean C. Caron, RN, Executive Director

Rehabilitation

Bureau of Rehabilitation Services, 35 Anthony Avenue, Augusta, ME 04333–0150; tel. 207/624–5323; FAX. 207/624–5302; Margaret Brewster, Director

Other

Bureau of Rehabilitation Services, Division of Deafness, 35 Anthony Avenue, Augusta, ME 04333–0150; tel. 207/624–5318; FAX. 207/624–5302; Alice C. Johnson, State Coordinator

Division for the Blind and Visually Impaired, 150 State House Station, Augusta, ME 04333–0150; tel. 207/624–5323; FAX. 207/624–5302; Harold Lewis, Director

MARYLAND

The Honorable Parris N. Glendening, Governor, 410/974–3901

Health

Department of Health and Mental Hygiene, 201 West Preston Street, Baltimore, MD 21201; tel. 410/767–6500; FAX. 410/767–6489; Martin P. Wasserman, M.D., J.D., Secretary

Developmental Disabilities

Developmental Disabilities Administration, 201 West Preston Street., Baltimore, MD 21201; tel. 410/767–5600; FAX. 410/767–5850; Diane K. Ebberts, Director

Environment

Maryland Department of the Environment, Office of Environmental Health Coordination, 2500 Broening Highway, Baltimore, MD 21224; tel. 410/631–3851; FAX. 410/631–4112; Tom Allen, Director

Family

Local and Family Health Administration, 201 West Preston Street, Baltimore, MD 21201; tel. 410/767–5300; FAX. 410/333–7106; Carlessia A. Hussein, Dr.P.H., Director

Health

Local and Family Health Administration, 201 West Preston Street, Baltimore, MD 21201; tel. 410/225–5300; FAX. 410/333–7106; Alan Baker, Interim Director

Laboratories

Laboratories Administration, 201 West Preston Street, Baltimore, MD 21201; tel. 410/767–6100; FAX. 410/333–5403; J. Mehsen Joseph, Ph.D., Director

Licensing

Licensing and Certification Administration, 4201 West Patterson Avenue, Baltimore, MD 21215; tel. 410/764–2750; FAX. 410/764–5969; Carol Benner, Director

Mental Health

Mental Hygiene Administration, 201 West Preston Street, Baltimore, MD 21201; tel. 410/767–6611; FAX. 410/333–5402; Dr. Stuart B. Silver, Director

Planning

Office of Planning and Capital Financing, 201 West Preston Street, Baltimore, MD 21201; tel. 410/767–6816; FAX. 410/333–7525; Elizabeth G. Barnard, Director

Policy

Department of Health and Mental Hygene, 201 West Preston Street, Room 500, Baltimore, MD 21201; tel. 410/767–6500; FAX. 410/767–6489; Martin P. Wasserman, M.D., J.D., Secretary

Substance Abuse

Alcohol and Drug Abuse Administration, 201 West Preston Street, Baltimore, MD 21201; tel. 410/767–6925; FAX. 410/333–7206; Thomas Davis, Director, Alcohol and Drug Abuse Administration

Welfare

Social Services Administration, 311 West Saratoga Street, Fifth Floor, Baltimore, MD 21201; tel. 410/767–7216; FAX. 410/333–0099; Diane Gordy, Executive Director

Insurance

Maryland Insurance Administration, 501 St. Paul Place, Baltimore, MD 21202; tel. 410/333–2521; FAX. 410/333–6650; Dwight K. Bartlett III, Insurance Commissioner

Other

Education

Department of Education, 200 West Baltimore Street, Baltimore, MD 21201–1595; tel. 410/767–0100; FAX. 410/333–6033; Nancy S. Grasmick, State Superintendent of Schools

Medical Examiners

Board of Physician Quality Assurance, 4201 Patterson Avenue, Baltimore, MD 21215; tel. 800/492–6836; FAX. 410/764–2478; J. Michael Compton, Executive Director

Nursing

Maryland Board of Nursing, 4140 Patterson Avenue, Baltimore, MD 21215–2254; tel. 410/764–5124; FAX. 410/358–3530; Donna M. Dorsey, RN, M.S., Executive Director

Rehabilitation

Division of Rehabilitation Services, 2301 Argonne Drive, Baltimore, MD 21218; tel. 410/554–6100; FAX. 410/554–9412; Robert A. Burns, Assistant State Superintendent

MASSACHUSETTS

The Honorable William F. Weld, Governor, 617/727–9173

Health

Massachusetts Department of Public Health, 150 Tremont Street, 10th Floor, Boston, MA 02111; tel. 617/727–2700; FAX. 617/727–2559; David H. Mulligan, Commissioner

Environment

Bureau of Environmental Health Assessment, 250 Washington Street, Seventh Floor, Boston, MA 02108; tel. 617/624–5757; FAX. 617/624–5777; Suzanne K. Condon, Director

Medical Services

Office of Emergency Medical Services, 470 Atlantic Avenue, Second Floor, Boston, MA 02210–2208; tel. 617/753–8300; FAX. 617/753–8350; Louise Goyette, Director

Quality

Division of Health Care Quality, 10 West Street, Fifth Floor, Boston, MA 02111; tel. 617/727–5860, ext. 335; FAX. 617/727–1414; Paul I. Dreyer, Ph.D., Director

Statistics

Bureau of Health Statistics, Research and Evaluation, Massachusetts Department of Public Health, 250 Washington Street, Sixth Floor, Boston, MA 02108–4619; tel. 617/624–5613; FAX. 617/624–5695; Daniel J. Friedman, Ph.D., Assistant Commissioner

Systems

Bureau of Health Quality Management, Massachusetts Department of Public Health, 250 Washington Street, Boston, MA 02108–4619; tel. 617/624–5280; FAX. 617/624–5046; Nancy Ridley, Assistant Commissioner

Welfare

Department of Transitional Assistance, 600 Washington Street, Boston, MA 02111; tel. 617/348–8402; FAX. 617/348–8575; Claire McIntire, Commissioner

Insurance

Division of Insurance, 470 Atlantic Avenue, Boston, MA 02210–2223; tel. 617/521–7301; FAX. 617/521–7770; Linda Ruthardt, Commissioner

Other

Blind

Commission for the Blind, 88 Kingston Street, Boston, MA 02111; tel. 617/727–5550; FAX. 617/727–5960; Charles Crawford, Commissioner

Medicine

Board of Registration in Medicine, Commonwealth of Massachusetts, Ten West Street, Boston, MA 02111; tel. 617/727–3086; FAX. 617/451–9568, ext. 321; Alexander F. Fleming, Executive Director

Mental Health

Massachusetts Department of Mental Health, Central Office, 25 Staniford Street, Boston, MA 02114; tel. 617/727–5500, ext. 448; FAX. 617/727–4350; Marylou Sudders, Commissioner

Nursing

Massachusetts Board of Registration in Nursing, 100 Cambridge Street, Suite 1519, Boston, MA 02202; tel. 617/727–9961; FAX. 617/727–9961; Theresa M. Bonanno, M.S.N., RN, Executive Director

Rehabilitation

Massachusetts Rehabilitation Commission, Fort Point Place, 27–43 Wormwood Street, Boston, MA 02210–1606; tel. 617/727–2172; FAX. 617/727–1354; Elmer C. Bartels, Commissioner

Substance Abuse

Massachusetts Department of Public Health, Bureau of Substance Abuse, 250 Washington Street, Third Floor, Boston, MA 02108–4619; tel. 617/624–5111; FAX. 617/624–5185; Mayra Rodriguez–Howard, Director

MICHIGAN

The Honorable John Engler, Governor, 517/373–3400

Health

Michigan Department of Community Health, Community Public Health Agency, 3423 North Martin Luther King, Jr. Boulevard, P.O. Box 30195, Lansing, MI 48909; tel. 517/335–8024; FAX. 517/335–9476; James K. Haveman, Jr., Director, MDCH

Community

Michigan Department of Community Health, Community Public Health Agency, Division of Planning and Evaluation, 3423 North Martin Luther King, Jr. Boulevard, P.O. Box 30195, Lansing, MI 48906; tel. 517/335–9371; FAX. 517/335–8560; Janice Ruff, Chief

Environment

Division of Environmental Health, Medical Waste Regulatory Program, 3423 North Martin Luther King Jr. Boulevard, Lansing, MI 48909; tel. 517/335–8637; FAX. 517/335–9033

Section C

Facilities

Bureau of Health Systems, 3423 Martin Luther King, Jr. Boulevard, Lansing, MI 48909; tel. 517/335–8505; FAX. 517/335–8510; Walter S. Wheeler III, Chief

Health

Center for Health Promotion and Chronic Disease Prevention, 3423 North Martin Luther King, Jr. Boulevard, P.O. Box 30195, Lansing, MI 48909; tel. 517/335–8368; FAX. 517/335–8593; Jean Chabut, Chief

Laboratories

Michigan Department of Public Health, Laboratory Improvement Section, Division of Health Facility Licensing & Certification, Bureau of Health Systems, 3500 North Martin Luther King, Jr., Boulevard, P.O. Box 30035, Lansing, MI 48909; tel. 517/321–6816; FAX. 517/321–3430; Jeffrey P. Massey, Dr.P.H., Chief

Licensing

Division of Licensing and Certification, 3500 North Logan Street, Lansing, MI 48909; tel. 517/335–8505; Nancy Graham, Supervisor

Medical Services

Division of Managed Care, Michigan Department of Community Health, P.O. Box 30195, Lansing, MI 48909; tel. 517/335–8551; FAX. 517/335–9239; Janet D. Olszewski, Chief

Substance Abuse

Center for Substance Abuse Services, Michigan Department of Community Health, Community Public Health Agency, Community Public Health Agency, 3423 North Martin Luther King, Jr. Boulevard, P.O. Box 30195, Lansing, MI 48909; tel. 517/335–8808; FAX. 517/335–8837; Karen Schrock, Chief

Welfare

Family Independence Agency, 235 South Grand Avenue, P.O. Box 30037, Lansing, MI 48909; tel. 517/373–2035; FAX. 517/373–8471; Mark Murray, Acting Director

Medical Services

Medical Services Administration, 400 South Pine, P.O. Box 30037, Lansing, MI 48909; tel. 517/335–5000; FAX. 517/335–5007; Robert M. Smedes, Chief Executive Officer

Insurance

Department of Consumer and Industry Services, Michigan Insurance Bureau, 611 West Ottawa, Second Floor, P.O. Box 30220, Lansing, MI 48909–7720; tel. 517/373–9273; FAX. 517/335–4978; D. Joseph Olson, Commissioner, Insurance

Other

Aging

Office of Services to the Aging, P.O. Box 30026, Lansing, MI 48909; tel. 517/373–8230; FAX. 517/373–4092; Carol Parr, Acting Director

Education

Department of Education, Box 30008, Lansing, MI 48909; tel. 517/373–7247; FAX. 517/373–1233; Patricia Nichols, Supervisor, Comprehensive Programs

Licensing

Office of Health Services, Department of Consumer and Industry Services, P.O. Box 30018, Lansing, MI 48909; tel. 517/373–8068; FAX. 517/373–2179; Thomas C. Lindsay II, Director

Medical Services

Office of Health Services, Michigan Department of Consumer and Industry Services, Box 30018, Lansing, MI 48909; tel. 517/373–8068; FAX. 517/373–2179; Thomas C. Lindsay II, Director

Medicine

Michigan Board of Medicine, 611 West Ottawa Street, Box 30018, Lansing, MI 48909; tel. 517/373–6873; FAX. 517/373–2179; Mary G. MacDowell, Director, Licensing

Mental Health

Michigan Department of Community Health, Lewis Cass Building, 320 South Walnut, Lansing, MI 48913; tel. 517/373–3500; FAX. 517/335–3090; James K. Haveman, Jr., Director

Nursing

Michigan Board of Nursing, 611 West Ottawa Street, Box 30018, Lansing, MI 48909; tel. 517/335–0918; FAX. 517/373–2179; Doris Foley, Licensing Administrator

Rehabilitation

Bureau of Rehabilitation and Disability Determination, Box 30010, Lansing, MI 48909; tel. 517/373–3390; Ivan L. Cotman, Associate Superintendent

Other

Office of Health and Human Services, Michigan Department of Management and Budget, Lewis Cass Building, Box 30026, Lansing, MI 48909; tel. 517/373–1076; FAX. 517/373–3624; Paul Reinhart, Director

MINNESOTA
The Honorable Arne H. Carlson, Governor, 612/296–3391

Health

Department of Health, 717 Delaware Street S.E., P.O. Box 9441, Minneapolis, MN 55440–9441; tel. 612/623–5712; FAX. 612/623–5794; Anne M. Barry, Commissioner

Administration

Minnesota Department of Health, Division of Finance and Administration, 717 Southeast Delaware Street, P.O. Box 9441, Minneapolis, MN 55440; tel. 612/623–5465; Christine Everson, Director

Children

Minnesota Department of Health, Division of Family Health, 717 Southeast Delaware Street, P.O. Box 9441, Minneapolis, MN 55440; tel. 612/623–5167; FAX. 612/623–5442; Norbert Hirschhorn, M.D., Director

Community

Minnesota Department of Health, Division of Community Health Services, Metro Square Building, Suite 460, 121 East Seventh Place, P.O. Box 64975, St. Paul, MN 55164–0975; tel. 612/296–9720; FAX. 612/296–9362; Ryan Church, Director

Environment

Division of Environmental Health, 121 East Seventh Place, P.O. Box 64975, St. Paul, MN 55164–0975; tel. 612/215–0700; FAX. 612/215–0979; Patricia A. Bloomgren, Director

Laboratories

Public Health Laboratory Division, 717 Southeast Delaware Street, P.O. Box 9441, Minneapolis, MN 55440; tel. 612/623–5331; FAX. 612/623–5514; Pauline Bouchard, J.D., Director

Prevention

Minnesota Department of Health, Division of Disease Prevention and Control, 717 Southeast Delaware Street, P.O. Box 9441, Minneapolis, MN 55440–9441; tel. 612/623–5363; FAX. 612/623–5743; Agnes T. Leitheiser, Director

Resources

Facility and Provider Compliance Division, Minnesota Department of Health, 393 North Dunlap Street, P.O. Box 64900, St. Paul, MN 55164–0900; tel. 612/643–2100; FAX. 612/643–2593; Linda G. Sutherland, Director

Systems

Minnesota Department of Health, Office of Regulatory Reform, 121 East Seventh Place, P.O. Box 64975, St. Paul, MN 55164–0975; tel. 612/282–5627; FAX. 612/282–3839; Nanette M. Schroeder, Director

Other

Licensing and Certification, 393 North Dunlap Street, P.O. Box 64900, St. Paul, MN 55164–0900; tel. 612/643–2130; FAX. 612/643–3534; Carol Hirschfeld, Supervisor Record and Information Unit

Welfare

Minnesota Department of Human Services, 444 Lafayette Road, N., St. Paul, MN 55155–3815; tel. 612/296–6117; FAX. 612/296–6244; David S. Doth, Commissioner

Other

Medical Examiners

Minnesota Board of Medical Practice, 2700 University Avenue, W., Suite 106, St. Paul, MN 55114–1080; tel. 612/642–0538; FAX. 612/642–0393; Robert A. Leach, Executive Director

Nursing

Minnesota Board of Nursing, 2829 University Avenue, S.E., Suite 500, Minneapolis, MN 55414–3253; tel. 612/617–2270; FAX. 612/617–2190; Joyce M. Schowalter, Executive Director

Rehabilitation

Rehabilitation Services Branch, 390 North Robert Street, Fifth Floor, St. Paul, MN 55101; tel. 612/296–1822; FAX. 612/297–5159; Norena A. Hale, Asssistant Commissioner

Other

Department of Commerce, 133 East Seventh Street, St. Paul, MN 55101; tel. 612/296–4026; FAX. 612/296–4328; David B. Gruenes

MISSISSIPPI
The Honorable Kirk Fordice, Governor, 601/359–3150

Health

Department of Health, Felix J. Underwood State Board of Health Building, P.O. Box 1700, Jackson, MS 32915–1700; tel. 601/960–7634; FAX. 601/960–7931; F.E. Thompson, Jr., M.D., M.P.H., State Health Officer

Children

Children's Medical Program, 421 Stadium Circle, P.O. Box 1700, Jackson, MS 39215–1700; tel. 601/987–3965; FAX. 601/987–5560; Mike Gallarno, Director

Environment

Bureau of Environmental Health, Mississippi State Department of Health, Felix J. Underwood State Board of Health Building, P.O. Box 1700, Jackson, MS 32915–1700; tel. 601/960–7680; FAX. 601/354–6794; Ricky Boggan, Director

Health

Bureau of Health Services, Felix J. Underwood State Board of Health Building Annex, P.O. Box 1700, Jackson, MS 32915; tel. 601/960–7472; FAX. 601/960–7480; Michael J. Gandy, Ed.D., Bureau Director, Deputy

Licensing

Division of Health Facilities Licensure and Certification, P.O. Box 1700, Jackson, MS 39215; tel. 601/354–7300; FAX. 601/354–7230; Vanessa Phipps, Director

Medical Services

Mississippi State Department of Health, Felix J. Underwood State Board of Health Building, P.O. Box 1700, Jackson, MS 32915–1700; tel. 601/960–7634; Betty Jane Phillips, Dr.P.H. Deputy State Health Officer

Planning

Health Planning and Resources Development Division, Mississippi State Department of Health, Felix J. Underwood State Board of Health Building, 2423 North State Street, P.O. Box 1700, Jackson, MS 39215–1700; tel. 601/960–7874; FAX. 601/354–6123; Harold B. Armstrong, Chief

Statistics

Public Health Statistics, Felix J. Underwood State Board of Health Building, Box 1700, Jackson, MS 39215–1700; tel. 601/960–7960; FAX. 601/960–7948; Nita C. Gunter, Director

Other

State Epidemiologist, Underwood Annex, P.O Box 1700, Jackson, MS 32915–1700; tel. 601/960–7725; FAX. 601/354–6061; Mary Currier, M.D., M.P.H.

Welfare

Mississippi Department of Human Services, 750 North State Street, Jackson, MS 39202; tel. 601/359–4480; FAX. 601/359–4477; Donald R. Taylor, Executive Director

Other

Mental Health

Department of Mental Health, 1101 Robert E. Lee Building, Jackson, MS 39201; tel. 601/359–1288; FAX. 601/359–6295; Randy Hendrix, Ph.D., Director

Nursing

Mississippi Board of Nursing, 239 North Lamar Street, Suite 401, Jackson, MS 39201–1397; tel. 601/359–6170; FAX. 601/359–6185; Marcia M. Rachel, Ph.D., RN, M.S.N., Executive Director

Rehabilitation

State Department of Rehabilitation Services, P.O. Box 1698, Jackson, MS 39215–1698; tel. 601/853–5100; FAX. 601/853–5205; Pery Winegarden, Interim Director

MISSOURI
The Honorable Mel Carnahan, Governor, 573/751–3222

Health

Department of Health, Box 570, Jefferson City, MO 65102; tel. 314/751–6001; FAX. 314/751–6010; Ronald W. Cates, Interim Director

Licensing

Bureau of Hospital Licensing and Certification, Missouri Department of Health, Box 570, Jefferson City, MO 65102; tel. 314/751–6302; FAX. 314/526–3621; Darrell Hendrickson, Administrator

Resources

Center for Health Information Management and Epidemiology (CHIME), Box 570, Jefferson City, MO 65102; tel. 573/751–6272; FAX. 573/526–4102; Garland H. Land, Director

Insurance

Department of Insurance, P.O. Box 690, Jefferson City, MO 65102; tel. 314/751–4126; FAX. 314/751–1165; Jay Angoff, Director

Health

Life and Health Section, Missouri Department of Insurance, P.O. Box 690, Jefferson City, MO 65102; tel. 573/751–4363; FAX. 573/526–6075; James W. Casey, Supervisor

Other

Children

Division of Maternal, Child and Family Health, 1730 East Elm, Box 570, Jefferson City, MO 65102; tel. 314/526–5520; FAX. 314/526–5348; Gretchen C. Wartmen, Director

Education

Department of Elementary and Secondary Education, 205 Jefferson, P.O. Box 480, Jefferson City, MO 65102; tel. 573/751–4446; FAX. 573/751–1179; Dr. Robert E. Bartman, Commissioner of Education

Mental Health

Department of Mental Health, 1706 East Elm Street, P.O. Box 687, Jefferson City, MO 65102; tel. 573/751–4122; FAX. 573/751–8224; Roy C. Wilson, M.D., Director

Rehabilitation

Vocational Rehabilitation, 3024 West Truman Boulevard, Jefferson City, MO 65109–0525; tel. 314/751–3251; FAX. 314/751–1441; Don L. Gann, Assistant Commissioner

Other

Bureau of Special Health Care Needs, 1730 East Elm, P.O. Box 570, Jefferson City, MO 65102; tel. 314/751–6246; FAX. 314/751–6447; Angela Ford, Interim Bureau Chief

Missouri State Board of Registration for the Healing Arts, 3605 Missouri Boulevard, Zip 65109, P.O. Box 4, Jefferson City, MO 65102; tel. 314/751–0098; FAX. 314/751–3166; Tina Steinman, Executive Director

MONTANA

The Honorable Marc Racicot, Governor, 406/444–3111

Health

Montana Department of Public Health and Human Services, 111 North Sanders, P.O. Box 4210, Helena, MT 59604; tel. 406/444–5622; FAX. 406/444–1970; Laurie Ekanger, Director

Family

Family/Maternal and Child Health Services Bureau, W. F. Cogswell Building, Helena, MT 59620; tel. 406/444–4740; FAX. 406/444–2606; Maxine B. Ferguson, RN, M.N., Chief

Licensing

Quality Assurance Division, Department of Public Health and Human Services, Certification Bureau, Cogswell Building, 1400 Broadway, P.O. Box 202951, Helena, MT 59620–2951; tel. 406/444–2037; FAX. 406/444–3456; Linda Sandman, Chief

Medical Services

Health Policy and Services Division, Montana Department of Public Health and Human Services, 1400 Broadway, P.O. Box 202951, Helena, MT 59620–2951; tel. 406/444–4540; FAX. 406/444–1861; Nancy Ellery, Administrator

Welfare

Department of Public Health and Human Services, 111 North Sanders Street, Box 4210, Helena, MT 59604–4210; tel. 406/444–5622; FAX. 406/444–1970; Laurie Ekanger, Director

Aging

Aging Services, Senior and Long Term Care Division, Department of Public Health and Human Services, 111 Sanders, P.O. Box 4210, Helena, MT 59604; tel. 406/444–7785; FAX. 406/444–7743; Robert E. Bartholomew, Program Manager

Community

Child and Family Services Division, P.O. Box 8005, Helena, MT 59604–8005; tel. 406/444–5902; FAX. 406/444–5956; Hank Hudson, Administrator

Rehabilitation

Division of Disability Services, P.O. Box 4210, Helena, MT 59604; tel. 406/444–2590; FAX. 406/444–3632; Joe A. Mathews, Administrator

Other

Nursing

Department of Commerce, Montana State Board of Nursing, Arcade Building – 4–C, 111 North Jackson, P.O. Box 200513, Helena, MT 59620–0513; tel. 406/444–2071; FAX. 406/444–7759; Joan Bowers, Administrative Assistant

NEBRASKA

The Honorable E. Benjamin Nelson, Governor, 402/471–2244

Health

State Department of Health, 301 Centennial Mall South, Lincoln, NE 68509; tel. 402/471–2133; FAX. 402/471–0383; Mark B. Horton, M.D., M.S.P.H., Director of Health

Children

Section of Family Health, Nebraska Department of Health and Human Services, 301 Centennial Mall South, P.O. Box 95007, Lincoln, NE 68509–9007; tel. 402/471–3980; FAX. 402/471–7049; Paula Eurek, R.D., Section Administrator

Facilities

Nebraska Department of Health, Certificate of Need Program, P.O. Box 95007, Lincoln, NE 68509–5007; tel. 402/471–2105; FAX. 402/471–0180; Charlene Gondring, Program Manager

Health

Nebraska Department of Health, 301 Centennial Mall, S., P.O. Box 95007, Lincoln, NE 68509; tel. 402/471–2781; Sue Medinger, Nutrition Consultant

Licensing

Nebraska Department of Health, Health Facility Licensure and Inspection Section, 301 Centennial Mall, S., P.O. Box 95007, Lincoln, NE 68509–5007; tel. 402/471–2946; FAX. 402/471–0555; Frederick M. Wright, Section Administrator

Policy

Division of Health Policy and Planning, 301 Centennial Mall, S., P.O. Box 95007, Lincoln, NE 68509; tel. 402/471–2337; David Palm, Ph.D., Director

Radiology

Nebraska Department of Health, Division of Radiological Health, 301 Centennial Mall, S., P.O. Box 95007, Lincoln, NE 68509; tel. 402/471–2168; FAX. 402/471–0169; Harold Borchert, Director

Welfare

Nebraska Department of Social Services, 301 Centennial Mall, S., P.O. Box 95026, Lincoln, NE 68509–5026; tel. 402/471–3121; FAX. 401/471–9449; Donald S. Leuenberger, Director

Children

Nebraska Department of Health and Human Services, Special Services for Children and Adults, 301 Centennial Mall, S., P.O. Box 95044, Lincoln, NE 68509; tel. 402/471–9345; FAX. 402/471–9455; Mary Jo Iwan, Administrator

Medical Services

Nebraska Department of Social Services, Medical Services Division, 301 Centennial Mall, S., P.O. Box 95026, Lincoln, NE 68509; tel. 402/471–9147; FAX. 402/471–9092; Robert Seiffert, Administrator

Insurance

Department of Insurance, 941 O Street, Suite 400, Lincoln, NE 68508; tel. 402/471–2201; FAX. 402/471–4610; Robert G. Lange, Director

Other

Rehabilitation

Department of Education, Vocational Rehabilitation, 301 Centennial Mall, S., P.O. Box 94987, Lincoln, NE 68509; tel. 402/471–3644; Frank Lloyd, Director

Other

Professional and Occupational Licensure Division, 301 Centennial Mall, S., Box 94986, Lincoln, NE 68509; tel. 402/471–2115; FAX. 402/471–3577; Helen L. Meeks, Director

NEVADA

The Honorable Bob Miller, Governor, 702/687–5670

Health

Department of Human Resources, Kinkead Building, 505 East King, Suite 600, Carson City, NV 89710; tel. 702/687–4400; FAX. 702/687–4733; Charlotte Crawford, Director

Children

Children With Special Health Care Needs Program, Nevada State Health Division, Kinkead Building, 505 East King, Suite 205, Carson City, NV 89710; tel. 702/687–4885; FAX. 702/687–1383; Gloria Deyhle, MCH Nurse Consultant

Community

Nevada State Health Division, Bureau of Community Health Services, 3656 Research Way, Suite 32, Carson City, NV 89706; tel. 702/687–6944; FAX. 702/687–7693; Mary D. Sassi, Bureau Chief

Health

Nevada Division of Health, Kinkead Building, 505 East King Street, Room 201, Carson City, NV 89701–4761; tel. 702/687–3786; FAX. 702/687–3859; Yvonne Sylva, Administrator

Laboratories

Nevada State Health Laboratory, 1660 North Virginia Street, Reno, NV 89503; tel. 702/688–1335; FAX. 702/688–1460; Arthur F. DiSalvo, M.D., Director

Medical Services

Medicaid, 2527 North Carson Street, Carson City, NV 89710; tel. 702/687–4775; FAX. 702/687–5080; April Townley, Deputy Administrator

Mental Health

Division of Mental Hygiene and Mental Retardation, Kinkead Building, Suite 602, 505 East King Street, Carson City, NV 89701–4761; tel. 702/687–5943; FAX. 702/687–4773; Carlos Brandenburg, Ph.D., Administrator

Regulation

Bureau of Licensure and Certification, Nevada Health Division, 1550 College Parkway, Capitol Complex, Suite 158, Carson City, NV 89706–7921; tel. 702/687–4475; FAX. 702/687–6588; Sharon M. Ezell, Chief

Rehabilitation

Rehabilitation Division, Kinkead Building, 505 East King, Suite 502, Carson City, NV 89710; tel. 702/687–4440; FAX. 702/687–5980; Elizabeth M. Breshears, Administrator

Resources

Bureau of Health Planning and Statistics, Nevada State Health Division, 505 East King Street, Room 102, Carson City, NV 89701–4761; tel. 702/687–4720; FAX. 702/687–6151; Emil DeJan, Chief

Other

Welfare Division, 2527 North Carson Street, Carson City, NV 89710; tel. 702/687–4770; FAX. 702/687–5080; Myla C. Florence, Administrator

Insurance

Department of Business and Industry, Director's Office, 555 East Washington, Suite 4900, Las Vegas, NV 89101; tel. 702/486–2750; FAX. 702/486–2758; Claudia Cormier, Director

Insurance

Division of Insurance, Capitol Complex, 1665 Hot Springs Road, Suite 152, Carson City, NV 89710; tel. 702/687–4270; FAX. 702/687–3937; Alice A. Molasky, Commissioner

Other

Medical Examiners

Nevada State Board of Medical Examiners, 1105 Terminal Way, Suite 301, Zip 89502, P.O. Box 7238, Reno, NV 89510; tel. 702/688–2559; FAX. 702/688–2321; Larry D. Lessly, Executive Director

Nursing

Nevada State Board of Nursing, 2755 East Plumb Lane, Suite 260, Reno, NV 89502; tel. 702/786–2778; FAX. 702/322–6993; Kathy Apple, M.S., RN, Executive Director

NEW HAMPSHIRE

The Honorable Jeanne Shaheen, Governor, 603/271–2121

Health

Department of Health and Human Services, Six Hazen Drive, Concord, NH 03301; tel. 603/271–4334; FAX. 603/271–4232; Kathleen G. Sgambati, Deputy Commissioner

Community

Division of Public Health Services, Office of Family and Community Health, Health and Welfare Building, Six Hazen Drive, Concord, NH 03301; tel. 603/271–4726; FAX. 603/271–4779; Roger Taillefer, Assistant Director

Facilities

Office of Program Support, Licensing and Regulation, Six Hazen Drive, Concord, NH 03301; tel. 603/271–4592; FAX. 603/271–3745; Raymond Rusch, Chief

Health

Department of Health and Human Services, Six Hazen Drive, Concord, NH 03301–6527; tel. 603/271–4372; FAX. 603/271–4727; Charles E. Danielson, M.D., M.P.H., State Medical Director

Mental Health

Office of Community Supports and Long Term Care, State Office Park, S., 105 Pleasant Street, Concord, NH 03301; tel. 603/271–5007; FAX. 603/271–5058; Paul G. Gorman, Ed.D., Director

Prevention

New Hampshire Department of Health and Human Services, Office of Health Management, Six Hazen Drive, Concord, NH 03301; tel. 603/271–4496; FAX. 603/271–4933; Richard DiPentima, Program Chief

Welfare

Department of Health and Human Services, Office of Family Services, Six Hazen Drive, Concord, NH 03301–6521; tel. 603/271–4321; FAX. 603/271–4727; Richard A. Chevrefils, Assistant Commissioner

Health

Department of Health and Human Services, Office of Health Management, Six Hazen Drive, Concord, NH 03301–6527; tel. 603/271–4726; FAX. 603/271–4779; Roger Taillefer, Assistant Director, Family and Community Health

Insurance

Department of Insurance, 169 Manchester Street, Concord, NH 03301; tel. 603/271–2661; FAX. 603/271–1406; Sylvio L. Dupuis, O.D., Commissioner

Other

Examination Division, 169 Manchester Street, Concord, NH 03301; tel. 603/271–2241; FAX. 603/271–1406; Thomas S. Burke, Director

Other

Education

State Department of Education, 101 Pleasant Street, State Office Park, S., Concord, NH 03301; tel. 603/271–3494; FAX. 603/271–1953; Elizabeth M. Twomey, Commissioner

Environment

Department of Environmental Services, Six Hazen Drive, Concord, NH 03301; tel. 603/271–3503; FAX. 603/271–2867; Robert W. Varney, Commissioner

Medicine

New Hampshire Board of Medicine, Board of Medicine, Two Industrial Park Drive, Suite Eight, Concord, NH 03301; tel. 603/271–1203; FAX. 603/271–6702; Karen Lamoureux, Administrator

Nursing

New Hampshire Board of Nursing, Six Hazen Drive, Concord, NH 03301–6527; tel. 603/271–2323; Doris G. Nuttelman, RN, Ed.D., Executive Director

Rehabilitation

Vocational Rehabilitation Division, 78 Regional Drive, Concord, NH 03301; tel. 603/271–3471; Bruce A. Archambault, Director

NEW JERSEY
The Honorable Christine T. Whitman, Governor, 609/292–6000

Health

New Jersey Department of Health and Senior Services, Office of the Commissioner, CN–360, Trenton, NJ 08625–0360; tel. 609/292–7837; FAX. 609/984–5474; Len Fishman, State Commissioner of Health and Senior Services

Children

Maternal and Child Health Planning and Regional Services, 50 East State Street, CN 364, Trenton, NJ 08625–0364; tel. 609/292–5656; FAX. 609/292–3580; Roberta B. McDonough, RN, M.A., Director

Facilities

Health Facilities Construction Service, CN–367, 300 Whitehead Road, Trenton, NJ 08625; tel. 609/588–7731; FAX. 609/588–7823; Kenneth A. Hess, Director

Office of the Commissioner, CN–360, Trenton, NJ 08625; tel. 609/292–7874; FAX. 609/984–5474; Susan C. Reinhard, RN, Ph.D., Deputy Commissioner Senior Services

Family

Division of Family Health Services, 50 East State Street, CN–364, Trenton, NJ 08625; tel. 609/292–4043; FAX. 609/292–9599; Jean R. Marshall, M.S.N., RN., FAAN, Assistant Commissioner

Licensing

Division of Health Care Systems Analysis, Certificate of Need and Acute Care Licensing, CN–360, Trenton, NJ 08625; tel. 609/292–8773; Darcy Saunders, Director

Planning

Division of Health Care Systems Analysis, CN–360, Trenton, NJ 08625; tel. 609/292–8772; FAX. 609/984–3165; Maria Morgan, Assistant Commissioner

Systems

Office of Managed Care, New Jersey State Department of Health, CN–367, Trenton, NJ 08625; tel. 609/588–2510; FAX. 609/588–7823; Edwin V. Kelleher, Chief

Welfare

Division of Family Development, CN–716, Hamilton Township, NJ 08625; tel. 609/588–2000; FAX. 609/588–3369; Karen D. Highsmith, Director

Other

Medical Examiners

State Board of Medical Examiners, 140 East Front Street, Second Floor, Trenton, NJ 08608; tel. 609/826–7100; FAX. 609/984–3930; Kevin B. Earle, Executive Director

Nursing

New Jersey Board of Nursing, P.O. Box 45010, Newark, NJ 07101; tel. 201/504–6430; FAX. 201/648–3481; Harriet L. Johnson, Assistant Executive Director

Other

Department of Law and Public Safety, CN080, Trenton, NJ 08625; tel. 609/292–4925; FAX. 609/292–3508; Peter Verniero, Attorney General

Division of Consumer Affairs, 124 Halsey Street, P.O. Box 45027, Newark, NJ 07101; tel. 201/504–6534; FAX. 201/648–3538; Mark S. Herr, Director

NEW MEXICO
The Honorable Gary E. Johnson, Governor, 505/827–3000

Health

Department of Health, 1190 St. Francis Drive, Santa Fe, NM 87502; tel. 505/827–2613; FAX. 505/827–2530; J. Alex Valdez, Secretary

Health

Public Health Division, Department of Health, P.O. Box 26110, Santa Fe, NM 87502–6110; tel. 505/827–2389; FAX. 505/827–2329; Pat Cleaveland, Director

Other

Federal Program Certification Section, 525 Camino de los Marquez, Suite Two, Santa Fe, NM 87501; tel. 505/827–4200; FAX. 505/827–4200; Matthew M. Gervase, Bureau Chief

Welfare

Human Services Department, P.O. Box 2348, Santa Fe, NM 87504–2348; tel. 505/827–7750; FAX. 505/827–6286; Duke Rodriguez, Secretary

Social Services

Social Services Division, P.O. Box 2348, Santa Fe, NM 87504–2348; tel. 505/827–4439; Jack Callaghan, Ph.D., Director

Other

Income Support Division, P.O. Box 2348, Santa Fe, NM 87504–2348; tel. 505/827–7252; FAX. 505/827–7203

Insurance

New Mexico Department of Insurance, P.O. Drawer 1269, Santa Fe, NM 87504–1269; tel. 505/827–4601; FAX. 505/827–4734; Helen Hordes, Manager, Life and Health Forms Division

Other

State Corporation Commission, P.O. Drawer 1269, Santa Fe, NM 87504; tel. 505/827–4529; Eric P. Serna, Chairman

Other

Education

State Department of Education, Education Building, 300 Don Gaspar, Santa Fe, NM 87501–2786; tel. 505/827–6516; FAX. 505/827–6696; Alan D. Morgan, State Superintendent of Public Instruction

Medical Examiners

New Mexico Board of Medical Examiners, 491 Old Santa Fe Trail, Lamy Building, Second Floor, Santa Fe, NM 87501; tel. 505/827–5022; FAX. 505/827–7377; Kristen A. Hedrick, Executive Secretary

Nursing

State of New Mexico, Board of Nursing, 4206 Louisiana, N.E., Suite A, Albuquerque, NM 87109; tel. 505/841–8340; FAX. 505/841–8340; Nancy Twigg, Executive Director

Rehabilitation

Division of Vocational Rehabilitation, 435 St. Michaels Drive, Building D, Santa Fe, NM 87505; tel. 505/827–3511; FAX. 505/827–3746; Terry Brigance, Director

NEW YORK
The Honorable George E. Pataki, Governor, 518/474–7516

Health

State Department of Health, Tower Building, Empire State Plaza, Albany, NY 12237; tel. 518/474–2011; FAX. 518/474–5450; Barbara A. DeBuono, M.D., M.P.H., Commissioner

Health

Bureau of Home Health Care Services, New York State Department of Health, Tower Building, Room 1970, Empire State Plaza, Albany, NY 12237; tel. 518/474–2006; FAX. 518/474–2031; Dr. Nancy Barhydt, Director

New York State Department of Health, Tower Building, Empire State Plaza, Room 1482, Albany, NY 12237; tel. 518/474–6462; FAX. 518/473–3824

Laboratories

Wadsworth Center for Laboratories and Research, Clinical Lab Evaluation, P.O. Box 509, Empire State Plaza, Albany, NY 12201–0509; tel. 518/474–7592; Dr. Herbert W. Dickerman, M.D., Ph.D., Director

Systems

New York State Department of Health, Office of Managed Care, Bureau of Managed Care Certification and Surveillance, 1911 Corning Tower Building, Empire State Plaza, Albany, NY 12237; tel. 518/473–4842; FAX. 518/473–3583; Gary Riviello, Director

Office of Health Systems Management, Tower Building, Empire State Plaza, Room 1441, Albany, NY 12237–0701; tel. 518/474–7028; Raymond Sweeney, Director

Other

Bureau of Project Management, New York State Department of Health, Tower Building, Empire State Plaza, Albany, NY 12237; tel. 518/473–7915; FAX. 518/474–3209; Robert J. Stackrow, Director

Welfare

New York State Department of Social Services, 40 North Pearl Street, Albany, NY 12243; tel. 518/474–9003; FAX. 518/474–9004; Brian J. Wing, Acting Commissioner

Other

Education

New York State Education Department, Main Education Building, Room 111, 89 Washington Avenue, Albany, NY 12234; tel. 518/474–5844; FAX. 518/473–4909

Medicine

New York State Board for Medicine, Cultural Education Center, Albany, NY 12230; tel. 518/474–3841; FAX. 518/473–6995; Thomas J. Monahan, Executive Secretary

Mental Health

New York State Office of Mental Health, 44 Holland Avenue, Albany, NY 12229; tel. 518/474–4403; FAX. 518/474–2149; James L. Stone, M.S.W., Commissioner

Mental Retardation

Office of Mental Retardation and Developmental Disabilities, 44 Holland Avenue, Albany, NY 12229; tel. 518/473–1997; FAX. 518/473–1271; Thomas A. Maul, Commissioner

Nursing

State Board for Nursing, New York State Education Department, Cultural Education Center, Room 3023, Albany, NY 12230; tel. 518/474–3843; FAX. 518/473–0578; Milene A. Sower, Ph.D., RN, Executive Secretary

Rehabilitation

New York State Education Department, Vocational and Educational Services for Individuals with Disabilities, One Commerce Plaza, Suite 1606, Albany, NY 12234; tel. 518/474–2714; Lawrence C. Gloeckler, Deputy Commissioner

Substance Abuse

New York State Office of Alcoholism and Substance Abuse Services, 1450 Western Avenue, Albany, NY 12203; tel. 518/457–2061; FAX. 518/457–5474; Marguerite T. Saunders, Commissioner

NORTH CAROLINA
The Honorable James B. Hunt, Jr., Governor, 919/733–4240

Health

Department of Human Resources, 101 Blair Drive, Raleigh, NC 27603; tel. 919/733–4534; FAX. 919/715–4645; C. Robin Britt, Sr., Secretary

Facilities

Department of Human Resources, Division of Facility Services, 701 Barbour Drive, Raleigh, NC 27603; tel. 919/733–2342; FAX. 919/733–2757; Lynda D. McDaniel, Director

Health

Department of Environment, Health and Natural Resources, P.O. Box 27687, Raleigh, NC 27611–7687; tel. 919/715–4126; FAX. 919/715–3060; Ronald H. Levine, M.D., M.P.H., State Health Director

Mental Health

Division of Mental Health, Developmental Disabilities and Substance Abuse Services, 325 North Salisbury Street, Raleigh, NC 27603; tel. 919/733–7011; FAX. 919/733–9455; Michael S. Pedneau, Director

Rehabilitation

Division of Vocational Rehabilitation Services, 805 Ruggles Drive, P.O. Box 26053, Raleigh, NC 27611; tel. 919/733–3364; FAX. 919/733–7968; Bob H.. Philbeck, Director

Welfare

Medical Assistance

Division of Medical Assistance, 1985 Umstead Drive, P.O. Box 29529, Raleigh, NC 27626–0529; tel. 919/733–2060; FAX. 919/733–6608

Insurance

Department of Insurance, P.O. Box 26387, Raleigh, NC 27611; tel. 919/733–7343; FAX. 919/733–6495; James E. Long, Commissioner

Other

Medical Examiners

North Carolina Medical Board, P.O. Box 20007, Raleigh, NC 27619; tel. 919/828–1212; FAX. 919/828–1295; Bryant D. Paris, Jr., Executive Director

Nursing

North Carolina Board of Nursing, P.O. Box 2129, Raleigh, NC 27602; tel. 919/782–3211; FAX. 919/781–9461; Carol A. Osman, RN, Ed.D., Executive Director

NORTH DAKOTA
The Honorable Edward T. Schafer, Governor, 701/328–2200

Health

State Department of Health, 600 East Boulevard Avenue, Bismarck, ND 58505–0200; tel. 701/328–2372; FAX. 701/328–4727; Londa Rodahl, Administrative Assistant

Children

Division of Maternal and Child Health, North Dakota State Department of Health and Consolidated Laboratories, State Capitol, 600 East Boulevard Avenue, Bismarck, ND 58505–0200; tel. 701/328–2493; FAX. 701/328–1412; Sandra Anseth, Director

Facilities

Division of Health Facilities, North Dakota Department of Health, 600 East Boulevard Avenue, Bismarck, ND 58505–0200; tel. 701/328–2352; FAX. 701/328–4727; Fred Gladden, Director

Resources

Health Resources Section, North Dakota Department of Health, 600 East Boulevard Avenue, Bismarck, ND 58505–0200; tel. 701/328–2352; FAX. 701/328–4727; Fred Gladden, Chief

Welfare

Children

Children's Special Health Services (Formerly Crippled Children's Services), Department of Human Services, State Capitol, 600 East Boulevard Avenue, Bismarck, ND 58505–0269; tel. 701/328–2436; FAX. 701/328–2359; Robert W. Nelson, Director

Developmental Disabilities

Developmental Disabilities Unit, Disability Services Division, Department of Human Services, 600 South Second Street, Suite One A, Bismarck, ND 58504–5729; tel. 701/328–8930; FAX. 701/328–8969; Gene Hysjulien, Director

Medical Services

Medical Services Division, North Dakota Department of Human Services, 600 East Boulevard Avenue, Bismarck, ND 58505–0261; tel. 701/328–2321; FAX. 701/328–1544; David J. Zentner, Director

Mental Retardation

Mental Health Services, Department of Human Services, Judicial Wing, Third Floor, 600 East Boulevard Avenue, Bismarck, ND 58505–0271; tel. 701/224–2766; FAX. 701/224–2359; Samih Ismir, Director

Rehabilitation

Office of Vocational Rehabilitation, Department of Human Services, 400 East Broadway Avenue, Suite 303, Bismarck, ND 58501–4038; tel. 701/328–3999; FAX. 701/328–3976; Gene Hysjulien, Director

Substance Abuse

Division of Alcoholism and Drug Abuse, 1839 East Capitol Avenue, Professional Building, Bismarck, ND 58501–2152; tel. 701/328–9769; FAX. 701/328–9770; Karen Larson, Acting Director

Other

Office of Economic Assistance, North Dakota Department of Human Services, 600 East Boulevard Avenue, Bismarck, ND 58505–0250; tel. 701/328–4060; FAX. 701/328–1545; Wayne J. Anderson, Deputy Director

Program and Policy, State Capitol, 600 East Boulevard Avenue, Bismarck, ND 58505–0265; tel. 701/224–4217; FAX. 701/224–2359; Lori Wightman, Deputy Director

Insurance

Department of Insurance, State Capitol, 600 East Boulevard, Bismarck, ND 58505–0320; tel. 701/328–2440; FAX. 701/328–4880; Glenn Pomeroy, Commissioner

Other

Medical Examiners

North Dakota State Board of Medical Examiners, City Center Plaza, 418 East Broadway Avenue, Suite 12, Bismarck, ND 58501; tel. 701/328–6500; FAX. 701/328–6505; Rolf P. Sletten, Executive Secretary, Treasurer

Nurse Examiners

North Dakota Board of Nursing, 919 South Seventh Street, Suite 504, Bismarck, ND 58504–5881; tel. 701/224–2974; FAX. 701/224–4614; Ida H. Rigley, RN, Executive Director

Other

Facility Management Division, Office of Management and Budget, 600 East Boulevard, State Capitol, Bismarck, ND 58505; tel. 701/328–2471; Greg Larson, Director, Facility Management

OHIO
The Honorable George V. Voinovich, Governor, 614/466–3555

Health

Ohio Department of Health, 246 North High Street, Columbus, OH 43266–0588; tel. 614/466–2253; FAX. 614/644–0085; Peter Somani, M.D., Ph.D., Director

Children

Division of Family and Community Health Services, 246 North High Street, P.O. Box 118, Columbus, OH 43266–0118; tel. 614/466–3263; FAX. 614/728–3616; Kathryn K. Peppe, RN, M.S., Chief

Licensing

Division of Quality Assurance, Ohio Department of Health, 246 North High Street, Columbus, OH 43266–0588; tel. 614/466–8739; FAX. 614/644–0208; Rebecca S. Maust, Chief

Nursing

Ohio Department of Health, Bureau of Local Services, 246 North High Street, Columbus, OH 43266–0118; tel. 614/466–5190; FAX. 614/466–4556; John Wanchick, M.P.A., R.S., Chief

Resources

Ohio Department of Health, Bureau of Quality Assessment and Improvement, 246 North High Street, P.O. Box 118, Columbus, OH 43266–0118; tel. 614/466–3325; FAX. 614/644–8661; Louis Pomerantz, Chief, Bureau of Quality Assessment and Improvement

Substance Abuse

Ohio Department of Alcohol and Drug Addiction Services, Two Nationwide Plaza, 280 North High Street, 12th Floor, Columbus, OH 43215–2537; tel. 614/466–3445; FAX. 614/752–8645; Luceille Fleming, Director

Welfare

Ohio Department of Human Services, 30 East Broad Street, 32nd Floor, Columbus, OH 43266–0423; tel. 614/466–6282; FAX. 614/466–1504; Arnold R. Tompkins, Director

Medical Assistance

Bureau of Medical Assistance, 30 East Broad Street, 31st Floor, Columbus, OH 43266–0423; tel. 614/466–2365; John J. Nichols, Chief

Medical Services

Ohio Department of Human Services, Office of Medicaid, 30 East Broad Street, 31st Floor, Columbus, OH 43266–0423; tel. 614/644–0140; FAX. 614/752–3986; Kathryn Glynn, Deputy Director

Insurance

Department of Insurance, 2100 Stella Court, Columbus, OH 43215–1067; tel. 614/644–2658; FAX. 614/728–0069; Harold T. Duryee, Director

Other

Managed Care Division, 2100 Stella Court, Columbus, OH 43215–1067; tel. 614/644–2661; FAX. 614/644–3741; Teresa Reedus, Senior Contract Analyst

Other

Disability

Bureau of Disability Determination, P.O. Box 359001, Columbus, OH 43235–9001; tel. 614/438–1500; FAX. 614/438–1504; Linda Krauss, Director

Medicine

State Medical Board of Ohio, 77 South High Street, 17th floor, Columbus, OH 43266–0315; tel. 614/466–3934; FAX. 614/728–5946; Ray Q. Bumgarner, Executive Director

Mental Health

Department of Mental Health, 30 East Broad Street, Eighth Floor, Columbus, OH 43266–0414; tel. 614/466–2596; FAX. 614/752–9453; Michael F. Hogan, Ph.D. Director

Mental Retardation

Department of Mental Retardation and Developmental Disabilities, 30 East Broad Street, Suite 1280, Columbus, OH 43266–0415; tel. 614/466–5214; FAX. 614/644–5013; Jerome C. Manuel, Director

Nursing

Ohio Board of Nursing, 77 South High Street, 17th Floor, Columbus, OH 43266–0316; tel. 614/466–3947; Dorothy Fiorino, RN, M.S., Executive Director

Rehabilitation

Ohio Rehabilitation Services Commission, Bureau of Vocational Rehabilitation, 400 East Campus View Boulevard (SW3), Columbus, OH 43235–4604; tel. 614/438–1250; FAX. 614/438–1257; June K. Gutterman, Ed.D., Director

Other

Ohio Rehabilitatioin Services Commission,, Bureau of Services for the Visually Impaired, 400 East Campus View Boulevard, Columbus, OH 43235–4604; tel. 614/438–1255; FAX. 614/438–1257; William A. Casto II, Director

OKLAHOMA
The Honorable Frank Keating, Governor, 405/521–2342

Oklahoma State Board of Medical Licensure and Supervision, P.O. Box 18256, Oklahoma City, OK 73154–0256; tel. 405/848–6841; FAX. 405/848–8240; Jan Ewing, Deputy Director

State Department of Health, 1000 Northeast 10th, Oklahoma City, OK 73117–1299; tel. 405/271–4200; FAX. 405/271–3431; Jerry R. Nida, M.D., Commissioner of Health

Children

Child Health and Guidance Service, 1000 Northeast 10th Street, Oklahoma City, OK 73117–1299; tel. 405/271–4477; FAX. 405/271–1011; Edd D. Rhoades, M.D., M.P.H., Chief

Maternal and Infant Health Service, 1000 Northeast 10th Street, Oklahoma City, OK 73117–1299; tel. 405/271–4476; FAX. 405/271–6199; Shari Kinney, RN, M.S., Acting Assistant Chief

Dental

State Department of Health, Dental Services, 1000 Northeast 10th Street, Oklahoma City, OK 73117–1299; tel. 405/271–5502; FAX. 405/271–6199; Michael L. Morgan, D.D.S., Chief

Facilities

Special Health Services, 1000 Northeast 10th, Oklahoma City, OK 73117; tel. 405/271–6576; FAX. 405/271–1308; Gary Glover, Chief, Medical Facilities

Health

State Department of Health, Special Health Services, 1000 Northeast 10th, Oklahoma City, OK 73117–1299; tel. 405/271–4200; FAX. 405/271–3431; Brent E. VanMeter, Deputy Commissioner

Laboratories

Public Health Laboratory Services, 1000 Northeast 10th, Oklahoma City, OK 73117–1299; tel. 405/271–5070; FAX. 405/271–4850; Garry McKee, Ph.D., Chief

Nursing

State Department of Health, Nursing Service, 1000 Northeast 10th, Oklahoma City, OK 73117–1299; tel. 405/271–5183; FAX. 405/271–1897; Toni Frioux, M.S., RN, C.N.S.

Welfare

Oklahoma Health Care Authority, 4545 North Lincoln, Suite 124, Oklahoma City, OK 73105; tel. 405/530–3439; FAX. 405/530–3471; Garth L. Splinter, M.D., M.B.A., Chief Executive Officer

Aging

Aging Services Division, 312 Northeast 28th, Oklahoma City, OK 73105; tel. 405/521–2327; FAX. 405/521–2086; Roy R. Keen, Division Administrator

Children

Oklahoma Health Care Authority, Special Health Care Outreach and Development, 4545 North Lincoln Boulevard, Suite 124, Oklahoma City, OK 73105; tel. 405/530–3400; FAX. 405/530–3470; Peggy Davis, Supervisor, Special Health Care Outreach and Development

Medical Services

Oklahoma Health Care Authority, 4545 North Lincoln Boulevard, Suite 124, Oklahoma City, OK 73105; tel. 405/530–3439; FAX. 405/530–3472; Mike Fogarty, State Medical Director

Rehabilitation

Rehabilitation Services, 3535 Northwest 58th Street, Suite 500, Oklahoma City, OK 73112–4815; tel. 405/951–3400; FAX. 405/951–3529; Linda Parker, Director

Other

Mental Health

Department of Mental Health and Substance Abuse Services, P.O. Box 53277, Oklahoma City, OK 73152; tel. 405/522–3877; FAX. 405/522–3650; Sharron D. Boehler, Commissioner

Nursing

Oklahoma Board of Nursing, 2915 North Classen Boulevard, Suite 524, Oklahoma City, OK 73106; tel. 405/525–2076; FAX. 405/521–6089; Sulinda Moffett, RN, Executive Director

OREGON
The Honorable John A. Kitzhaber, Governor, 503/378–3111

Health

Oregon Health Division, 800 Oregon Street, Suite 925, Portland, OR 97232; tel. 503/731–4000; FAX. 503/731–4078; Elinor Hall, M.P.H., Administrator

Facilities

Oregon Health Division, Health Care Licensure and Certification, P.O. Box 14450, Portland, OR 97214–0450; tel. 503/731–4013; FAX. 503/731–4080; Kathleen Smail, Manager

Laboratories

Oregon State Public Health Laboratory, P.O. Box 275, Portland, OR 97207–0275; tel. 503/229–5882; FAX. 503/229–5682; Michael R. Skeels, Ph.D., M.P.H.

Welfare

Family

Adult and Family Services Division, 500 Summer Street, N.E., Salem, OR 97310–1013; tel. 503/945–5601; Sandie Hoback, Administrator

Insurance

Department of Consumer and Business Services, 350 Winter Street, N.E., Salem, OR 97310; tel. 503/378–4100; FAX. 503/378–6444; Kerry Barnett

Other

Children

Child Development and Rehabilitation Center, Oregon Health Sciences University, Box 574, Portland, OR 97207; tel. 503/494–8362; FAX. 503/494–6868; Clifford J. Sells, M.D., Director

Mental Health

Mental Health and Developmental Disability Services Division, 2575 Bittern Street, N.E., Salem, OR 97310; tel. 503/945–9449; FAX. 503/378–3796; Barry S. Kast, M.S.W., Administrator

Nursing

Oregon State Board of Nursing, 800 Northeast Oregon Street, Suite 465, Portland, OR 97232–2162; tel. 503/731–4745; FAX. 503/731–4755; Joan C. Bouchard, RN, M.N., Executive Director

Rehabilitation

Vocational Rehabilitation Division, Human Resources Building, 500 Summer Street N.E., Salem, OR 97310–1018; tel. 503/945–5880; FAX. 503/378–3318; Mr. Joil A. Southwell, Administrator

Substance Abuse

Office of Alcohol and Drug Abuse Programs, 500 Summer Street, N.E., Salem, OR 97310–1016; tel. 503/945–5763; FAX. 503/378–8467

PENNSYLVANIA
The Honorable Tom Ridge, Governor, 717/787–2500

Health

Pennsylvania Department of Health, Health and Welfare Building, Suite 802, Harrisburg, PA 17120; tel. 717/787–6436; FAX. 717/787–0191; Daniel F. Hoffmann, Secretary–Designate

Administration

Pennsylvania Department of Health, Health and Welfare Building, Suite 806, Harrisburg, PA 17120; tel. 717/783–8770; FAX. 717/772–6959

Community

Bureau of Primary Care Resources and Systems Development, 709 Health and Welfare Building, Harrisburg, PA 17120; tel. 717/772–5298; Joseph B. May, Director

Health

Pennsylvania Department of Health, Division of Primary Care and Home Health, 132 Kline Plaza, Suite A, Harrisburg, PA 17104; tel. 717/783–1379; FAX. 717/787–3188; Robert Bastian, Director

Pennsylvania Department of Health, Public Health Programs, 801 Health and Welfare Building, Harrisburg, PA 17120; tel. 717/783–8804; FAX. 717/783–3794; Jeannie D. Peterson, M.P.A., Deputy Secretary

Laboratories

Department of Health, Bureau of Laboratories, P.O. Box 500, Exton, PA 19341–0500; tel. 610/363–8500; FAX. 610/436–3346; Dr. Bruce Kleger, Director

Planning

Pennsylvania Department of Health, Quality Assurance, Health and Welfare Building, Room 805, P.O. Box 90, Harrisburg, PA 17108; tel. 717/783–1078; FAX. 717/772–6959; Raphael Molly, Deputy Secretary

Quality

Bureau of Quality Assurance, Health and Welfare Building, Room 930, Harrisburg, PA 17120; tel. 717/787–8015; FAX. 717/787–1491; Andrew Major, Director

Substance Abuse

Drug and Alcohol Programs, Health and Welfare Building, Lionville, PA 19353; tel. 717/783–8200; FAX. 717/787–6285; Eugene Boyle, Director

Other

Division of Acute and Ambulatory Care Facilities, Health and Welfare Building, Room 532, Harrisburg, PA 17120; tel. 717/783–8980; William White, Director

Welfare

Pennsylvania Department of Public Welfare, Health and Welfare Building, Harrisburg, PA 17120; tel. 717/787–1870; FAX. 717/787–4639; Darlene C. Collins, M.Ed., M.P.H., Deputy Secretary

Family

Office of Children, Youth, and Families, Department of Public Welfare, P.O. Box 2675, Harrisburg, PA 17105–2675; tel. 717/787–4756; FAX. 717/787–0414; Jo Ann R. Lawer, Deputy Secretary

Medical Assistance

Office of Medical Assistance, Health and Welfare Building, Harrisburg, PA 17120; tel. 717/787–1870; FAX. 717/787–4639; Robert S. Zimmerman, Acting Deputy Secretary

Mental Health

Mental Health, Health and Welfare Building, Room 502, P.O. Box 2675, Harrisburg, PA 17120; tel. 717/787–6443; FAX. 717/787–5394; Charles G. Curie, Deputy Secretary, Mental Health

Other

Office of Income Maintenance, Health and Welfare Building, Room 432, Harrisburg, PA 17120, P.O. Box 2675, Harrisburg, PA 17105; tel. 717/783–3063; FAX. 717/787–6765; Sherri Z. Heller, Deputy Secretary

Insurance

Department of Insurance, 1326 Strawberry Square, Harrisburg, PA 17120; tel. 717/783–0442; FAX. 717/772–1969; Linda S. Kaiser, Insurance Commissioner

Business Regulation

Pennsylvania Insurance Department, Office of Rate and Policy Regulation, 1311 Strawberry Square, Harrisburg, PA 17120; tel. 717/783–5079; FAX. 717/787–8555; Gregory Martino, Deputy Insurance Commissioner

Other

Laboratories

Division of Laboratory Improvement, Bureau of Laboratories, P.O. Box 500, Exton, PA 19341–0500; tel. 610/363–8500; FAX. 610/436–3346; Joseph W. Gasiewski, Director

Medicine

State Board of Medicine, P.O. Box 2649, Harrisburg, PA 17105 2649; tel. 717/783 1400; FAX. 717/787–7769; Cindy L. Warner, Administrative Assistant

Nursing

Pennsylvania State Board of Nursing, Department of State, P.O. Box 2649, Harrisburg, PA 17105–2649; tel. 717/783–7142; FAX. 717/783–0822; Miriam H. Limo, Executive Secretary

Rehabilitation

Office of Vocational Rehabilitation, Labor and Industry Building, Room 1300, Seventh and Forster Streets, Harrisburg, PA 17120; tel. 717/787–5244; FAX. 717/783–5221; Gil Selders, Executive Director

RHODE ISLAND
The Honorable Lincoln Almond, Governor, 401/277–2080

Health

Department of Health, Three Capitol Hill, Providence, RI 02908–5097; tel. 401/277–2231; FAX. 401/277–6548; Barbara A. DeBuono, M.D., M.P.H., Director, Health

Facilities

Rhode Island Department of Health, Division of Facilities Regulation, Three Capitol Hill, Providence, RI 02908–5097; tel. 401/277–2566; FAX. 401/277–3999; Wayne I. Farrington, Chief

Family

Rhode Island Department of Health, Division of Family Health, Three Capitol Hill, Room 302, Providence, RI 02908–5097; tel. 401/277–1185, ext. 142; FAX. 401/277–1442; William H. Hollinshead, M.D., M.P.H., Medical Director

Section C

Mental Health

Rhode Island Department of Mental Health, Retardation and Hospitals, Aime J. Forand Building, 600 New London Avenue, Cranston, RI 02920; tel. 401/464-3201; FAX. 401/464-3204; A. Kathryn Power, Director

Policy

Rhode Island Department of Health, Three Capitol Hill, Providence, RI 02908-5097; tel. 401/277-2231; FAX. 401/277-6548; William J. Waters, Jr., Ph.D., Deputy Director

Regulation

Division of Professional Regulation, Three Capitol Hill, Suite 104, Providence, RI 02908-5097; tel. 401/277-2827; FAX. 401/277-1272; Russell J. Spaight, Administrator

Systems

Rhode Island Department of Health, Office of Health Systems Development, Three Capitol Hill, Providence, RI 02908-5097; tel. 401/277-2788; FAX. 401/273-4350; John X. Donahue, Chief

Insurance

Division of Insurance, 233 Richmond Street, Suite 233, Providence, RI 02903-4233; tel. 401/277-2223; FAX. 401/751-4887; Charles P. Kwolek, Jr, CPA, Associate Director, Superintendent of Insurance

Business Regulation

Department of Business Regulation, 233 Richmond Street, Suite 237, Providence, RI 02903-4237; tel. 401/277-2246; FAX. 401/277-6098; Barry G. Hittner, Director

Other

Human Services

Department of Human Services, 600 New London Avenue, Cranston, RI 02920; tel. 401/464-3575; FAX. 401/464-2174; John Young, Associate Director, Division of Medical Services

Rehabilitation

Office of Rehabilitation Services, 40 Fountain Street, Providence, RI 02903; tel. 401/421-7005, ext. 301; FAX. 401/421-9259; Raymond A. Carroll, Acting Administrator

Other

Division of Medical Services, 600 New London Avenue, Cranston, RI 02920; tel. 401/464-5274; John Young, Associate Director

SOUTH CAROLINA

The Honorable David M. Beasley, Governor, 803/734-9818

Health

Department of Health and Environmental Control, 2600 Bull Street, Columbia, SC 29201; tel. 803/734-4880; FAX. 803/734-4620; Douglas E. Bryant, Commissioner

Children

Bureau of Maternal and Child Health, South Carolina Department of Health and Environmental Control, Robert Mills Complex, P.O. Box 101106, Columbia, SC 29211; tel. 803/737-4190; FAX. 803/734-4442; Marie Meglen, M.S., C.N.M., Bureau Director

Environment

Bureau of Environmental Health, 2600 Bull Street, Columbia, SC 29201; tel. 803/935-7945; FAX. 803/935-7825; Jack H. Vaughan, Jr., Chief

Laboratories

Bureau of Laboratories, P.O. Box 2202, Columbia, SC 29202; tel. 803/935-7045; FAX. 803/935-7357; Sarah J. Robinson, Acting Chief

Licensing

Department of Health and Environmental Control, Division of Health Licensing, 2600 Bull Street, Columbia, SC 29201; tel. 803/737-7202; FAX. 803/737-7212; Alan Samuels, Director

Long Term Care

South Carolina Department of Health and Environmental Control, Bureau of Home Health Services and Long Term Care, 2600 Bull Street, Columbia, SC 29201; tel. 803/737-3955; FAX. 803/734-3352; Michael Byrd, Chief

Prevention

Bureau of Preventive Health Services, South Carolina Department of Health and Environmental Control, 2600 Bull Street, Columbia, SC 29201; tel. 803/737-4040; FAX. 803/737-4036; G. Larry Sandifer, M.P.H., Acting Bureau Chief

Substance Abuse

Bureau of Drug Control, South Carolina Department of Health and Environmental Control, 2600 Bull Street, Columbia, SC 29201; tel. 803/935-7817; FAX. 803/935-7820; Wilbur L. Harling, Director

Welfare

South Carolina Department of Social Services, P.O. Box 1520, Columbia, SC 29202; tel. 803/734-5760; FAX. 803/734-5597; James T. Clark, State Director

Other

Aging

South Carolina Governor's Office, Division on Aging, 202 Arbor Lake Drive, Suite 301, Columbia, SC 29223; tel. 803/737-7500; FAX. 803/737-7501; Constance C. Rinehart, M.S.W., Director

Blind

South Carolina Commission for the Blind, 1430 Confederate Avenue, Columbia, SC 29201; tel. 803/734-7522; FAX. 803/734-7885; Donald Gist, Commissioner

Medical Examiners

South Carolina Department of Labor, Licensing and Regulation, Board of Medical Examiners, 3600 Forest Drive, Columbia, SC 29204, P.O. Box 11289, Columbia, SC 29211-1289; tel. 803/737-9300; FAX. 803/737-9314; Henry D. Foster, Jr., Board Administrator

Mental Health

State Department of Mental Health, 2414 Bull Street, P.O. Box 485, Columbia, SC 29202; tel. 803/734-7780; FAX. 803/734-7879

Mental Retardation

South Carolina Department of Disabilities and Special Needs, 3440 Harden Street Extension, P.O. Box 4706, Columbia, SC 29240; tel. 803/737-6444; FAX. 803/737-6323; Philip S. Massey, Ph.D, State Director

Nursing

Department of Labor, Licensing and Regulation, State Board of Nursing for South Carolina, 220 Executive Center Drive, Suite 220, Columbia, SC 29210; tel. 803/731-1648; FAX. 803/731-1647; Renatta S. Loquist, RN, Executive Director

Rehabilitation

Vocational Rehabilitation Department, 1410 Boston Avenue, P.O. Box 15, West Columbia, SC 29171-0015; tel. 803/896-6500; P. Charles LaRosa, Jr., Commissioner

Services

Department of Health and Human Services, 1801 Main Street, P.O. Box 8206, Columbia, SC 29202-8206; tel. 803/253-6100; FAX. 803/253-4137; Gwen Power, Interim Director

Substance Abuse

South Carolina Department of Alcohol and Other Drug Abuse Services, 3700 Forest Drive, Suite 300, Columbia, SC 29204; tel. 803/734-9520; FAX. 803/734-9663; Beverly G. Hamilton, Director

SOUTH DAKOTA

The Honorable William J. Janklow, Governor, 605/773-3212

Health

Department of Health, 445 East Capitol, Pierre, SD 57501-3185; tel. 605/773-3361; FAX. 605/773-5683; Doneen B. Hollingsworth, Secretary of Health

Health

Division of Health Systems Development and Regulation, South Dakota Department of Health, Anderson Building, 445 East Capitol, Pierre, SD 57501; tel. 605/773-3364; FAX. 605/773-5904; Kevin Forsch, Division Director

Licensing

Office of Health Care Facilities Licensure and Certification, State Department of Health, Anderson Building, 445 East Capitol, Pierre, SD 57501; tel. 605/773-3356; FAX. 605/773-6667; Joan Bachman, Administrator

Medical Services

Division of Health, Medical and Laboratory Services, 615 East Fourth Street, Pierre, SD 57501; tel. 605/773-3737; FAX. 605/773-5509; John N. Jones, Director

Policy

Office of Administrative Services, South Dakota Department of Health, 445 East Capitol Avenue, Pierre, SD 57501-3185; tel. 605/773-3693; FAX. 605/773-5683; Joan Adam, Director

Substance Abuse

Division of Alcohol and Drug Abuse, 3800 East Highway 34, Hillsview Plaza, c/o 500 East Capitol, Pierre, SD 57501; tel. 605/773-3123; FAX. 605/773-5483; Gilbert Sudbeck, Director

Welfare

Developmental Disabilities

Division of Developmental Disabilities, Hillsview Plaza, E. Highway 34, c/o 500 East Capitol, Pierre, SD 57501-5070; tel. 605/773-3438; FAX. 605/773-5483; Betty Oldenkamp, Director

Medical Services

Office of Medical Services, 700 Governor's Drive, Pierre, SD 57501-2291; tel. 605/773-3495; FAX. 605/773-4855; David Christensen, Administrator

Social Services

Department of Social Services, 700 Governor's Drive, Pierre, SD 57501-2291; tel. 605/773-3165; FAX. 605/773-4855; James W. Ellenbecker, Secretary

Other

Medical Examiners

State Board of Medical and Osteopathic Examiners, 1323 South Minnesota Avenue, Sioux Falls, SD 57105; tel. 605/336-1965; FAX. 605/336-0270; Robert D. Johnson, Executive Secretary

Rehabilitation

Department of Human Services, East Highway 34, Hillsview Plaza, c/o 500 East Capitol, Pierre, SD 57501; tel. 605/773-5990; FAX. 605/773-5483; William Podhradsky, Secretary

TENNESSEE

The Honorable Don Sundquist, Governor, 615/741-2001

Health

Department of Health, Cordell Hull Building, 426 Fifth Avenue, N., Third Floor, Nashville, TN 37247-0101; tel. 615/741-3111; FAX. 615/741-2491; Fredia Wadley, Commissioner

Administration

Bureau of Administrative Services, Tennessee Department of Health, Cordell Hull Building, Third Floor, Nashville, TN 37247-0301; tel. 615/741-3824; FAX. 615/741-2491; Robert G. Maxwell, Director

Environment

Bureau of Environment, L & C Tower–21st Floor, 401 Church Street, Nashville, TN 37243-1530; tel. 615/532-0220; FAX. 615/532-0120; Wayne K. Scharber, Deputy Commissioner

Facilities

Department of Health, Bureau of Manpower and Facilities, Cordell Hull Building, 426 Fifth Avenue, N., First Floor, Nashville, TN 37247-0501; tel. 615/741-8402; FAX. 615/741-5542; Sherryl L. Midgett, Assistant Commissioner

Division of Health Care Facilities, Cordell Hull Building, 426 Fifth Avenue, N., Nashville, TN 37247-0508; tel. 615/741-7221; FAX. 615/741-7051; Marie Fitzgerald, Director

Health

Tennessee Department of Health, Commissioner's Office, Cordell Hull Building, 426 Fifth Avenue, N., Third Floor, Nashville, TN 37247-0101; tel. 615/741-3111; FAX. 615/741-2491

Laboratories

Tennessee Medical Laboratory Board, Cordell Hull Building, 426 Fifth Avenue, N., First Floor, Nashville, TN 37247-1010; tel. 615/532-5080; FAX. 615/532-5164; Lynda England, Facility Licensure

Licensing

Board for Licensing Health Care Facilities, Cordell Hull Building, 426 Fifth Avenue, N., Nashville, TN 37247-0530; tel. 615/741-7351; FAX. 615/741-7051; Melanie Hill, Director

Medical Services

Medicaid/TennCare, 729 Church Street, Nashville, TN 37247-6501; tel. 615/741-0213; FAX. 615/741-0882; Theresa Clarke, Assistant Commissioner

Welfare

Tennessee Department of Human Services, 400 Deaderick Street, Nashville, TN 37248; tel. 615/741-3241; FAX. 615/741-4165; Robert A. Grunow, Commissioner

Family

Family Assistance, 400 Deaderick Street, Nashville, TN 37248-0070; tel. 615/313-4712; FAX. 615/741-4165; Michael O'Hara, Assistant Commissioner

Section C

Rehabilitation
Division of Rehabilitation Services, Citizens Plaza State Office Building, 15th Floor, 400 Deaderick Street, Nashville, TN 37248–0060; tel. 615/313–4714; FAX. 615/741–4165; Jack Van Hooser, Assistant Commissioner

Tennessee Rehabilitation Center, 460 Ninth Avenue, Smyrna, TN 37167; tel. 615/741–4921; FAX. 615/355–1373; Joseph J. DiDomenico, Superintendent

Social Services
Department of Children's Services, Program Operations which includes Departmental Services, Regional Services and Resource Management, Cordell Hull Building, 436 Sixth Avenue, N., Seventh Floor, Nashville, TN 37243–1290; tel. 615/532–1102; FAX. 615/532–6495; Cathy Rogers Smith, Assistant Commissioner, Department Children's Services

Other
Aging
Tennessee Commission on Aging, 500 Deaderick Street, Ninth Floor, Nashville, TN 37243–0860; tel. 615/741–2056; FAX. 615/741–3309; Emily Wiseman, Director

Medical Examiners
Tennessee Board of Medical Examiners, Cordell Hull Building, 426 Fifth Avenue, N., First Floor, Nashville, TN 37247–1010; tel. 615/532–4384; Jerry Kosten, Administrator

Mental Health
Tennessee Department of Mental Health and Mental Retardation, 710 James Robertson Parkway, Nashville, TN 37243–0675; tel. 615/532–6500; FAX. 615/532–6514; Ben Dishman, Acting Commissioner

Nursing
Tennessee Board of Nursing, 283 Plus Park Boulevard, Nashville, TN 37217; tel. 615/367–6232; FAX. 615/367–6397; Elizabeth J. Lund, RN, Executive Director

Substance Abuse
Bureau of Alcohol and Drug Abuse Services, Cordell Hull, 426 Fifth Avenue, N., Third Floor, Nashville, TN 37247–4401; tel. 615/741–1921; FAX. 615/532–2419; Stephanie W. Perry, M.D., Assistant Commissioner

TEXAS
The Honorable George W. Bush, Governor, 512/463–2000
Health
Texas Department of Health, 1100 West 49th Street, Austin, TX 78756; tel. 512/458–7111, ext. 7375; Patti J. Patterson, M.D., Commissioner

Children
Bureau of Children's Health, (Texas Department of Health), 1100 West 49th Street, Austin, TX 78756; tel. 512/458–7700; FAX. 512/458–7203; Jack Baum, D.D.S., Chief

Texas Department of Health, Centers for Minority Health Initiatives and Cultural Competency, 1100 West 49th Street, Suite M543, Austin, TX 78756; tel. 512/458–7555, ext. 3005; FAX. 512/458–7713; John E. Evans, Executive Director

Data Analysis
Texas Department of Health, Bureau of State Health Data and Policy Analysis, 1100 West 49th Street, Austin, TX 78756; tel. 512/458–7261; FAX. 512/458–7344; Dora McDonald, Bureau Chief

Licensing
Bureau of Licensing and Certification, Texas Department of Health, 1100 West 49th Street, Austin, TX 78756–3199; tel. 512/834–6645; FAX. 512/834–6653; Maurice B. Shaw, Chief

Health Facility Compliance Division, 1100 West 49th Street, Austin, TX 78756; tel. 512/834–6650; FAX. 512/834–6653; Nance Stearman, RN, M.S.N., Director

Welfare
Texas Department of Health, 1100 West 49th Street, Austin, TX 78756–3167; tel. 512/338–6501; FAX. 512/338–6945; Randy P. Washington, Associate Commissioner, Health Care Financing

Insurance
Texas Department of Insurance, P.O. Box 149104, Mail Code 106–1A, Austin, TX 78714–9104; tel. 512/322–3401; FAX. 512/322–3552; Tyrette Hamilton, Deputy Commissioner, Life/Health Group

Other
Mental Health
Texas Department of Mental Health and Mental Retardation, 909 West 45th Street, P.O. Box 12668, Capitol Station, Austin, TX 78711–2668; tel. 512/454–3761; FAX. 512/206–4560; Tex Killion, Deputy Medical Director for Administration

Nurse Examiners
Board of Nurse Examiners for the State of Texas, P.O. Box 140466, Austin, TX 78714; tel. 512/305–7400; FAX. 512/305–7401; Katherine A. Thomas, M.N., RN, Executive Director

Board of Vocational Nurse Examiners, William P. Hobby Building, 333 Guadalupe Street, Suite 3–400, Austin, TX 78701; tel. 512/305–8100, ext. 205; FAX. 512/305–8101; Marjorie Bronk, Executive Director

UTAH
The Honorable Michael O. Leavitt, Governor, 801/538–1500
Health
Utah Department of Health, 288 North 1460 West, Salt Lake City, UT 84116; tel. 801/538–6111; FAX. 801/538–6306; Rod L. Betit, Executive Director

Environment
Department of Environmental Quality, 288 North, 1460 West, Salt Lake City, UT 84116; tel. 801/538–6121; FAX. 801/538–6016; Kenneth Alkema, Executive Director

Family
Community and Family Health Services Division, P.O. Box 144100, Salt Lake City, UT 84114–4100; tel. 801/538–6901; FAX. 801/538–6510; George Delavou, M.D., M.P.H., Director

Finance
Division of Health Care Financing (Utah Medicaid), P.O. Box 142901, Salt Lake City, UT 84114–2901; tel. 801/538–6406; FAX. 801/538–6099; Michael J. Deily, Director

Health
Utah Department of Health, Bureau of Primary Care and Rural Health Systems, Box 142856, Salt Lake City, UT 84114–2856; tel. 801/538–6113; FAX. 801/538–6387; Robert W. Sherwood, Jr., Bureau Director

Laboratories
Utah Department of Health, Division of Epidemiology and Laboratory Services, 46 North Medical Drive, Salt Lake City, UT 84113; tel. 801/584–8400; FAX. 801/584–8486; Charles D. Brokopp, Dr.P.H., Director

Licensing
Utah Department of Health, Bureau of Health Facility Licensure, Box 142853, Salt Lake City, UT 84114–2853; tel. 801/538–6152; FAX. 801/538–6325; Debra Wynkoop–Green, Director

Medical Examiner
Office of The Medical Examiners, State of Utah, 48 North Medical Drive, Salt Lake City, UT 84113; tel. 801/584–8410; FAX. 801/584–8435; Todd C. Grey, M.D., Director

Insurance
Insurance Department, State Office Building, Suite 3110, Salt Lake City, UT 84114; tel. 801/538–3800; FAX. 801/538–3829; Robert E. Wilcox, Commissioner

Other
Aging
Division of Aging and Adult Services, 120 North 200 West, Room 401, Salt Lake City, UT 84103; tel. 801/538–3910; FAX. 801/538–4395; Helen Goddard, Director

Children
Youth Corrections, P.O. Box 45500, Salt Lake City, UT 84145–0500; tel. 801/538–4330; FAX. 801/538–4334; Gary K. Dalton, Director

Education
State Office of Education, 250 East 500 South, Salt Lake City, UT 84111; tel. 801/538–7500; FAX. 801/538–7521; Scott W. Bean, Superintendent

Family
Division of Child and Family Services, P.O. Box 45500, Salt Lake City, UT 84145–0500; tel. 801/538–4100; FAX. 801/538–3993; Mary T. Noonan, Director

Licensing
Division of Occupational and Professional Licensing, Heber M. Wells Building, 160 East 300 South, Box 146741, Salt Lake City, UT 84114–6741; tel. 801/530–6628; FAX. 801/530–6511; J. Craig Jackson, Director

Mental Health
Mental Health, P.O. Box 45500, Salt Lake City, UT 84145–0500; tel. 801/538–4270; Paul Thorpe, Director

Rehabilitation
Utah State Office of Rehabilitation, 250 East 500 South, Salt Lake City, UT 84111; tel. 801/538–7530; FAX. 801/538–7522; Blaine Petersen, Ed.D., Executive Director

Services
Department of Human Services, 120 North 200 West, P.O. Box 45500, Salt Lake City, UT 84145–0500; tel. 801/538–4001; FAX. 801/538–4016; Robin Arnold–Williams, Director

Division of Services for People With Disabilities, 120 North 200 West, Suite 201, Salt Lake City, UT 84103; tel. 801/538–4200; FAX. 801/538–4279; Sue Geary, Ph.D., Director

Substance Abuse
Division of Substance Abuse, 120 North 200 West, Room 201, Salt Lake City, UT 84145; tel. 801/538–3939; FAX. 801/538–4696; F. Leon PoVey, Director

VERMONT
The Honorable Howard Dean, M.D., Governor, 802/828–3333
Health
Vermont Department of Health, 108 Cherry Street, P.O. Box 70, Burlington, VT 05402; tel. 802/863–7280; FAX. 802/863–7425; Jan K. Carney, M.D., M.P.H., Commissioner

Environment
Environmental Health Division, 108 Cherry Street, P.O. Box 70, Burlington, VT 05402; tel. 802/863–7220; FAX. 802/863–7425; Robert O'Grady, Director

Laboratories
Vermont Department of Health Laboratory, 195 Colchester Avenue, P.O. Box 1125, Burlington, VT 05402–1125; tel. 802/863–7335; FAX. 802/863–7632; Burton W. Wilcke, Jr., Ph.D., Laboratory Director

Licensing
Licensing and Protection, Ladd Hall, 103 South Main Street, Waterbury, VT 05671–2306; tel. 802/241–2345; FAX. 802/241–2358; Laine Lucenti, Director

Medical Services
Vermont Department of Health, Division of Community Public Health, P.O. Box 70, Burlington, VT 05402; tel. 802/863–7347; FAX. 802/863–7229; Patricia Berry, Director

Regulation
Vermont Department of Aging and Disabilities, Division of Licensing and Protection, Ladd Hall, 103 South Main Street, Waterbury, VT 05671–2306; tel. 802/241–2345; FAX. 802/241–2358; Robert Aiken, Director

Statistics
Vermont Department of Health, Division of Health Surveillance, Public Health Statistics, 108 Cherry Street, P.O. Box 70, Burlington, VT 05402–0070; tel. 802/863–7300; FAX. 802/865–7701; Margaret Brozicevic, Acting Director

Other
Vermont Department of Health Epidemiology and Disease Prevention, 108 Cherry Street, P.O. Box 70, Burlington, VT 05402; tel. 802/863–7240; FAX. 802/865–7701; Peter Galbraith, Epidemiologist

Welfare
Agency of Human Services, 103 South Main Street, Waterbury, VT 05676; tel. 802/241–2220; FAX. 802/244–8103; Cornelius Hogan, Secretary

Department of Social Welfare, 103 South Main Street, Waterbury, VT 05671–1201; tel. 802/241–2853; FAX. 802/241–2830; M. Jane Kitchel, Commissioner

Medical Services
Office of Vermont Health Access/Medicaid, 103 South Main Street, Waterbury, VT 05671–1201; tel. 802/241–2880; FAX. 802/241–2974; Paul Wallace–Brodeur, Acting Director

Section C

Mental Health

Department of Developmental and Mental Health Services, Weeks Building, 103 South Main Street, Waterbury, VT 05671–1601; tel. 802/241–2610; FAX. 802/241–1129; Rodney E. Copeland, Ph.D., Commissioner

Rehabilitation

Department of Social and Rehabilitation Services, 103 South Main Street, Waterbury, VT 05671–2401; tel. 802/241–2100; FAX. 802/241–2980; William M. Young, Commissioner

Vocational Rehabilitation Division, 103 South Main Street, Osgood Building, Waterbury, VT 05671–2303; tel. 802/241–2186; FAX. 802/241–3359; Diane P. Dalmasse, Director

Substance Abuse

Office of Alcohol and Drug Abuse Programs, 108 Cherry Street, Burlington, VT 05401; tel. 802/651–1550; FAX. 802/651–1573; Thomas E. Perras, Director

Insurance

Department of Banking, Insurance, Securities and Health Care Administation, 89 Main Street, Drawer 20, Montpelier, VT 05620–3101; tel. 802/828–3301; FAX. 802/828–3306; Elizabeth R. Costle, Commissioner

Other

Nursing

Vermont State Board of Nursing, 109 State Street, Montpelier, VT 05609–1106; tel. 802/828–2396; FAX. 802/828–2484; Anita Ristau, RN, M.S., Executive Director

VIRGINIA
The Honorable George Allen, Governor,
804/786–2211

Health

State Department of Health, Main Street Station, P.O. Box 2448, Richmond, VA 23218; tel. 804/786–3561; FAX. 804/786–4616; Randolph L. Mordon, M.D., M.P.H., Commissioner

Children

Division of Children's Specialty Services, Virginia Department of Health, P.O. Box 2448, Room 135, Richmond, VA 23218; tel. 804/786–3691; FAX. 804/225–3307; Nancy R. Bullock, RN, M.P.H., Director

Division of Women's and Infants' Health, 1500 East Main Street, Suite 135, P.O. Box 2448, Richmond, VA 23218–2448; tel. 804/786–5916; FAX. 804/371–6032; Carolyn L. Beverly, M.D., M.P.H., Director

Licensing

Office of Health Facilities Regulation, Virginia Department of Health, 3600 Centre, Suite 216, 3600 West Broad Street, Richmond, VA 23230; tel. 804/367–2102; FAX. 804/367–2149; Nancy R. Hofheimer, Director

Welfare

Virginia Department of Social Services, 730 East Broad Street, Richmond, VA 23219–1949; tel. 804/692–1900; FAX. 804/692–1849; Carol A. Brunty, Commissioner

Insurance

State Corporation Commission–Bureau of Insurance, P.O. Box 1157, Richmond, VA 23218; tel. 804/371–9869; FAX. 804/371–9511; Douglas C. Stolte, Deputy Insurance Commissioner

Business Regulation

State Corporation Commission Bureau of Insurance, Company Licensing and Regulatory Compliance Section, P.O. Box 1157, Richmond, VA 23209; tel. 904/371–9636; FAX. 904/371–9396; Andy Delbridge, Supervisor

Insurance

Bureau of Insurance, Virginia State Corporation Commission, P.O. Box 1157, Richmond, VA 23218; tel. 804/371–9691; FAX. 804/371–9944; Life and Health Consumer Services Section

Other

Aging

Department for the Aging, 700 East Franklin Street, 10th Floor, 700 Centre, Richmond, VA 23219–2327; tel. 804/225–2271; FAX. 804/371–8381; Thelma Bland, Commissioner

Medical Assistance

Department of Medical Assistance Services, 600 East Broad Street, Suite 1300, Richmond, VA 23219; tel. 804/786–8099; FAX. 804/371–4981; Joseph M. Teefey, Director

Medicine

Virginia State Board of Medicine, 6606 West Board Street, Fourth Floor, Richmond, VA 23230–1717; tel. 804/662–9908; FAX. 804/662–9943; Warren W. Koontz, Jr., M.D., Executive Director

Mental Health

Department of Mental Health, Mental Retardation and Substance Abuse Services, P.O. Box 1797, Richmond, VA 23214; tel. 804/786–3921; FAX. 804/371–6638; Timothy A. Kelly, Ph.D., Commissioner

Rehabilitation

Department of Rehabilitative Services, 8004 Franklin Farms Drive, Richmond, VA 23288; tel. 804/662–7000; FAX. 804/662–9532; John Vaughan, Commissioner

WASHINGTON
The Honorable Gary Locke, Governor,
360/753–6780

Health

State Department of Social and Health Services, P.O. Box 45080, Olympia, WA 98504–5080; tel. 206/753–1777; FAX. 206/586–5874; Jane Beyer, Assistant Secretary, Medical Assistance, Administration

Facilities

Office of Field Services, Department of Health, Target Plaza, 2725 Harrison Avenue, N.W., Suite 500, P.O. Box 47852, Olympia, WA 98504–7852; tel. 206/705–6622; FAX. 206/705–6654; Fern Bettridge, Program Manager

Health

Department of Health, Facilities and Services Licensing, P.O. Box 47852, Olympia, WA 98504–7852; tel. 206/705–6652; FAX. 206/705–6654; Kathy Stout, Director

Department of Health, Office of Emergency Medical and Trauma Prevention, P.O. Box 47853, Olympia, WA 98504–7853; tel. 360/705–6700; FAX. 360/705–6706; Janet Griffith, Director

Medical Assistance

Medical Assistance Administration, P.O. Box 45080, Olympia, WA 98504–5080; tel. 360/902–7807; FAX. 360/902–7855; Jane Beyer, Assistant Secretary

Policy

Medical Assistance Administration, P.O. Box 45500, Olympia, WA 98504–5500; tel. 360/753–5839; FAX. 360/586–7448; Eric Houghton, M.D., Acting Medical Director

Rehabilitation

Division of Vocational Rehabilitation, P.O. Box 45340, Olympia, WA 98504–5340; tel. 206/438–8000; FAX. 206/438–8007; Jeanne Munro, Director

Substance Abuse

Division of Alcohol and Substance Abuse, P.O. Box 45330, Mail Stop 5330, Olympia, WA 98504–5330; tel. 206/438–8200; FAX. 206/438–8078; Ken Stark, Director

Other

Washington State Department of Health, P.O. Box 47812, Mail Stop 7812, Olympia, WA 98504–7812; tel. 206/705–6060; FAX. 206/705–6043; Dan Rubin, Director, Special Projects Office

Insurance

Office of the Insurance Commissioner, Insurance Building, P.O. Box 40255, Olympia, WA 98504–0255; tel. 206/753–7300; FAX. 206/586–3535; Deborah Senn, Insurance Commissioner

Other

Licensing

Health Systems Quality Assurance, Department of Health, 1112 Quince, Mail Stop 7850, Olympia, WA 98504–7850; tel. 360/753–2241; FAX. 360/664–0398; Sherman Cox, Assistant Secretary

Nursing

Washington State Nursing Care Quality Assurance Commission, 1300 Southeast Quince Street, P.O. Box 47864, Olympia, WA 98504–7864; tel. 206/664–4100; FAX. 206/586–5935; Patty L. Hayes, RN, M.N., Interim Executive Director

WEST VIRGINIA
The Honorable Cecil Underwood, Governor,
304/558–2000

Health

Bureau for Public Health, Building Three, Room 518, State Capitol Complex, Charleston, WV 25305; tel. 304/558–2971; FAX. 304/558–1035; Henry G. Taylor, M.D., M.P.H., Commissioner

Community

Office of Community and Rural Health Services, Bureau for Public Health, 1411 Virginia Street, E., Charleston, WV 25301–3013; tel. 304/558–0580; FAX. 304/558–1437

Environment

Office of Environmental Health Services, Morrison Building, 815 Quarrier Street, Suite 418, Charleston, WV 25301–2616; tel. 304/558–2981; FAX. 304/558–0691; Joseph P. Schock, M.P.H., P.E., Director

Licensing

Office of Health Facility Licensure and Certification, West Virginia Division of Health, Capitol Complex, 1900 Kanawha Boulevard, E., Building Three, Suite 550, Charleston, WV 25305; tel. 304/558–0050; FAX. 304/558–2515; Sandra Daubman, Interim Director

Medical Examiner

Office of Chief Medical Examiner, State of West Virginia, 701 Jefferson Road, South Charleston, WV 25309; tel. 304/558–3920; FAX. 304/558–7886; Irvin Sopher, M.D., Chief Medical Examiner

Substance Abuse

Division on Alcoholism and Drug Abuse, Capitol Complex, Building Six, Room B–738, Charleston, WV 25305; tel. 304/558–2276; FAX. 304/558–1008; Jack C. Clohan, Jr., Director

Other

West Virginia Department of Health and Human Resources, Division of Primary Care and Recruitment, 1411 Virginia Street, E., Charleston, WV 25301; tel. 304/558–4007; FAX. 304/558–1437; Charles W. Dawkins, Director

Welfare

Department of Health and Human Resources, Capitol Complex, Building Three, Room 206, Charleston, WV 25305; tel. 304/558–0684; FAX. 304/558–1130; Gretchen O. Lewis, Secretary

Children

Children with Special Health Care Needs, 1116 Quarrier Street, Charleston, WV 25301; tel. 304/558–3071; FAX. 304/558–2866; Patricia Kent, Administrative Director

Other

Division of Medical Care, Department of Human Services, 1900 Washington Street, E., Charleston, WV 25305; tel. 304/348–8990; Helen Condry, Director

Insurance

Insurance Commissioners Office, P.O. Box 50540, Charleston, WV 25305–0540; tel. 304/558–3354; FAX. 304/558–0412; Hanley C. Clark, Commissioner

Financial

Insurance Commissioner's Office, 1124 Smith Street, Charleston, WV 25301; tel. 304/558–2100; FAX. 304/558–0412; Jeffrey W. VanGilder, Director, Chief Examiner

Other

Education

West Virginia Department of Education, Division of Technical and Adult Education, State Capitol, 1900 Kanawha Boulevard, E., Charleston, WV 25305; tel. 304/558–2346; FAX. 304/558–0048; Adam Sponaugle, Assistant State Superintendent

Medicine

West Virginia Board of Medicine, 101 Dee Drive, Charleston, WV 25311; tel. 304/558–2921; FAX. 304/558–2084; Ronald D. Walton, Executive Director

Nurse Examiners

West Virginia Board of Examiners for Registered Professional Nurses, 101 Dee Drive, Charleston, WV 25311–1620; tel. 304/558–3596; FAX. 304/558–3666; Laura S. Rhodes, M.S.N., RN, Executive Secretary

Rehabilitation

Division of Rehabilitation Services, P.O. Box 50890, State Capitol Complex, Charleston, WV 25305–0890; tel. 304/766–4601; FAX. 304/766–4671; William C. Dearien, Director

WISCONSIN
The Honorable Tommy G. Thompson, Governor,
608/266–1212

Section C

Health

Department of Health and Social Services, P.O. Box 7850, Madison, WI 53707; tel. 608/266-9622; FAX. 608/266-7882; Joe Green, Secretary

Environment

Bureau of Public Health, P.O. Box 309, Madison, WI 53701; tel. 608/266-1704; FAX. 608/267-4853

Finance

Bureau of Health Care Financing (Wisconsin Medicaid), One West Wilson Street, Suite 250, P.O. Box 309, Madison, WI 53701-0309; tel. 608/266-2522; FAX. 608/266-1096; Peggy L. Bartels, Director

Health

Bureau of Health Services, P.O. Box 7925, Madison, WI 53707-7925; tel. 608/267-1720; FAX. 608/267-1751; Sharon Zunker, Director

State Division of Health, One West Wilson Street, Room 218, P.O. Box 309, Madison, WI 53701-0309; tel. 608/266-1511; FAX. 608/267-2832; John D. Chapin, Interim Administrator

Policy

Bureau of Health Management and Analysis, Division of Health, P.O. Box 309, Madison, WI 53701; tel. 608/266-7384; FAX. 608/267-2832

Prevention

Bureau of Public Health, 1414 East Washington Avenue, Room 233, Madison, WI 53703-3044; tel. 608/266-1251; FAX. 608/264-6078; Kenneth Baldwin, Director

Quality

Bureau of Quality Assurance, Division of Supportive Living, Department of Health and Family Services, P.O. Box 309, Madison, WI 53701; tel. 608/267-7185; FAX. 608/267-0352; Judy Fryback, Director, Bureau of Quality Assurance

Rehabilitation

Division of Vocational Rehabilitation, Box 7852, Madison, WI 53707-7852; tel. 608/243-5600; FAX. 608/243-5680; Judy Norman-Nunnery, Administrator

Statistics

Center for Health Statistics, P.O. Box 309, Madison, WI 53701-0309; tel. 608/266-1334; FAX. 608/261-6380; R. D. Nashold, Ph.D., Director

Insurance

Office of the Commissioner of Insurance, 121 East Wilson Street, P.O. Box 7873, Madison, WI 53707-7873; tel. 608/266-3585; FAX. 608/266-9935

Other

Children

Division for Learning Support: Equity and Advocacy, 125 South Webster Street, P.O. Box 7841, Madison, WI 53707-7841; tel. 608/266-8960; FAX. 608/267-3746; Nancy F. Holloway, Student Services, Prevention and Wellness

Medical Examiners

Wisconsin Medical Examining Board, 1400 East Washington Avenue, P.O. Box 8935, Madison, WI 53708; tel. 608/266-2811; FAX. 608/267-0644; Patrick D. Braatz, Bureau Director

Professions

Department of Regulation and Licensing, 1400 East Washington Avenue, Room 173, P.O. Box 8935, Madison, WI 53708-8935; tel. 608/266-8609; FAX. 608/267-0644; Grace Schwingel, Secretary

Regulatory

State of Wisconsin, Department of Regulation and Licensing, 1400 East Washington Avenue, Suite 173, P.O. Box 8935, Madison, WI 53708-8935; tel. 608/266-8609; FAX. 608/267-0644; Marlene A. Cummings, Secretary

Other

State Department of Public Instruction, 125 South Webster Street, P.O. Box 7841, Madison, WI 53707-7841; tel. 608/266-1771; FAX. 608/267-1052; John T. Benson, State Superintendent

WYOMING

The Honorable Jim Geringer, Governor, 307/777-7434

Health

Department of Health, 117 Hathaway Building, Cheyenne, WY 82002; tel. 307/777-7656; FAX. 307/777-7439

Children

Childrens Health Service, Department of Health, Hathaway Building, Fourth Floor, Cheyenne, WY 82002; tel. 307/777-7941; FAX. 307/777-5402; Cathy Parish, Program Manager

Facilities

Health Facilities Licensing, Department of Health, Metropolitan Bank Building, Eighth Floor, Cheyenne, WY 82002; tel. 307/777-7123; FAX. 307/777-5970; Charlie Simineo, Program Manager

Medical Assistance

Division of Health Care Financing, 6101 Yellowstone Road, Room 259B, Cheyenne, WY 82002; tel. 307/777-7531; FAX. 307/777-6964; Cheryl McVay, Administrator

Medical Services

Department of Health, 117 Hathaway Building, Cheyenne, WY 82002; tel. 307/777-7656; FAX. 307/777-7439

Prevention

Preventive Medicine, Hathaway Building, 2300 Capitol Avenue, Cheyenne, WY 82002; tel. 307/777-6004; FAX. 307/777-5402

Welfare

Department of Family Services, Hathaway Building, Third Floor, Cheyenne, WY 82002-0490; tel. 307/777-7561; FAX. 307/777-7747; Shirley R. Carson, Director

Other

Aging

Wyoming Divison on Aging, Hathaway Building, Suite 139, Cheyenne, WY 82002-0480; tel. 800/442-2766; FAX. 307/777-5340; Deborah Fleming, Administrator

Community

Division of Behavioral Health, 447 Hathaway Building, Cheyenne, WY 82002-0480; tel. 307/777-7094; FAX. 307/777-5580

Medical Examiners

Wyoming Board of Medicine, The Colony Building, Second Floor, 211 West 19th Street, Cheyenne, WY 82002; tel. 307/778-7053; FAX. 307/778-2069; Carole Shotwell, Executive Secretary

Nursing

Wyoming State Board of Nursing, 2020 Carey Avenue, Suite 110, Cheyenne, WY 82002; tel. 307/777-7601; FAX. 307/777-3519; Toma A. Nisbet, RN, M.S., Executive Director

Rehabilitation

Division of Vocational Rehabilitation, Herschler Building, Room 1128, Cheyenne, WY 82002; tel. 307/777-7385; FAX. 307/777-5939; Gary W. Child, Administrator

U. S. Associated Areas

GUAM

The Honorable Carl T. C. Gutierrez, Governor, 011 671/472-8931

Health

Department of Public Health and Social Services, Box 2816, Agana, GU 96910; tel. 671/735-7102; FAX. 671/734-5910; Dennis G. Rodriguez, Director

Planning

Guam Health Planning and Development Agency, P.O. Box 2950, Agana, GU 96910; tel. 671/477-3920; FAX. 671/477-3956; Helen B. Ripple, Director

Welfare

Division of Public Welfare, Box 2816, Agana, GU 96910; tel. 671/735-7274; FAX. 671/734-7015; John W. Leon-Guerrero, Chief Human Services Administrator

Other

Rehabilitation

Department of Vocational Rehabilitation, Government of Guam, 122 Harmon Plaza, Suite B201, Harmon Industrial Park, GU 96911; tel. 671/646-9468; FAX. 671/649-7672; Albert San Agustin, Acting Director

PUERTO RICO

The Honorable Pedro Rossello, Governor, 787/721-7000

Health

Puerto Rico Department of Health, Building A-Medical Center, Call Box 70184, San Juan, PR 00936; tel. 809/766-1616; FAX. 809/766-2240; Carmen A. Feliciano-De-Melecio, Secretary, Health

Administration

Administration, Building A-Medical Center, Call Box 70184, San Juan, PR 00936; tel. 809/765-1616; FAX. 809/250-6547; Icelia Medina Medina, Assistant Secretary for Administration

Dental

Dental Health, Building A-Medical Center, Call Box 70184, San Juan, PR 00936; tel. 809/751-4750; FAX. 809/765-5675; Wanda Urbiztondo, D.M.D., Oral Health Coordinator

Environment

Environmental Health, Department of Health, Building A, Psiq Hospital, Box 70184, San Juan, PR 00936-0184; tel. 787/274-7798; FAX. 787/758-6285; Hernan Horta, Assistant Secretary, Environmental Health

Mental Health

Mental Health and Anti-Addiction Services Administration, P.O. Box 21414, San Juan, PR 00928-1414; tel. 809/764-3670; FAX. 809/765-5895; Astrid Oyola, Administrator

Prevention

Department of Health, Secretaryship for Preventive Medicine and Family Health, Building E-Medical Center, Call Box 70184, San Juan, PR 00936; tel. 809/765-0482; FAX. 809/765-5675; Dr. Raul G. Castellanos Bran, Director, Division of Family Health

Other

Legal Services, Building A-Medical Center, Call Box 70184, San Juan, PR 00936; tel. 809/766-1616; FAX. 809/766-2240; Ricardo L. Torres-Munoz, Esquire Director

Welfare

Department of Family, Call Box 11398, San Juan, PR 00910; tel. 809/721-4624; FAX. 809/723-1223; Carmen L. Rodriguez de Rivera, Secretary

Other

Rehabilitation

Vocational Rehabilitation Program, Department of Social Services, Apartado 191118, San Juan, PR 00919-1118; tel. 809/725-1792; FAX. 809/721-6286; Sr. Francisco Vallejo, Assistant Secretary

VIRGIN ISLANDS

The Honorable Roy L. Schneider, M.D., Governor, 809/774-0001

Health

Virgin Islands Department of Health, St. Thomas Hospital, 48 Sugar Estate, St. Thomas, VI 00802; tel. 809/774-0117; FAX. 809/777-4001; Ralph A. de Chabert, M.D., Acting Commissioner

Children

Division of Maternal and Child Health Services, Virgin Islands Department of Health, Nisky Center Suite 210, St. Thomas, VI 00801; tel. 809/776-3580; FAX. 809/774-8633; Dr. Mavis Matthew, Director

Environment

Division of Environmental Health, Old Hospital Complex, Charlotte Amalie, St. Thomas, VI 00802; tel. 809/774-9000, ext. 4644; FAX. 809/776-7899; Laura A. Hassell, Director

Medical Services

Division of Hospitals and Medical Services, Roy Lester Schneider Hospital, 9048 Sugar Estate, St. Thomas, VI 00802; tel. 809/776-3687; FAX. 809/777-8421; Evelyn McLaughlin, Acting Chief Executive Officer

Mental Health

Division of Mental Health, Alcoholism, and Drug Dependency Services, Oswald Harris Court, Street C, St. Thomas, VI 00801; tel. 809/774-4888; FAX. 809/774-4701

Prevention

Prevention, Health, Promotion and Protection, Department of Health, Charles Harwood Hospital, 3500 Richmond Christiansted, St. Croix, VI 00820-4300; tel. 809/773-1311; FAX. 809/772-5895; Olaf G. Hendricks, M.D., Assistant Commissioner

Other

Department of Health, Division of Financial Services, Knud Hansen Complex, St. Thomas, VI 00802; tel. 809/774-3171; FAX. 809/777-5120; Alphonse J. Stalliard, Deputy Commissioner

Welfare
Virgin Islands Department of Human Services,
Knud Hansen Complex, Building A, 1303 Hospital
Ground, St. Thomas, VI 00802; tel.
809/774–1166; FAX. 809/774–3466; Catherine L.
Mills, Commissioner

Other
Rehabilitation
Disabilities and Rehabilitation Services,
Department of Human Services, Knud Hansen
Complex–Building A, 1303 Hospital Ground, St.
Thomas, VI 00802; tel. 809/774–0930; FAX.
809/774–3466; Sedonie Halbert, Administrator

Canada

ALBERTA
Health
Department of Family and Social Services, 109
Street and 97 Avenue, 104 Legislature Building,
Edmonton, AB T5K 2B6; tel. 403/427–2606; FAX.
403/427–0954; The Honorable Mike Cardinal

BRITISH COLUMBIA
Health
Ministry of Health, Parliament Building, Room 306,
Victoria, BC V8V 1X4; tel. 604/387–5394; FAX.
604/387–3696; The Honorable Joy K. MacPhail

MANITOBA
Health
Department of Health, 302 Legislative Building,
Winnipeg, MB R3C 0V8; tel. 204/945–3731; FAX.
204/945–0441; The Honorable Darren Praznik,
Minister

Other
Community
Department of Manitoba Family Services, 450
Broadway, Room 357, Legislative Building,
Winnipeg, MB R3C 0V8; tel. 204/945–4173; FAX.
204/945–5149; The Honorable Bonnie Mitchelson,
Minister

NEW BRUNSWICK
Health
Department of Health and Community Services,
Box 5100, Fredericton, NB E3B 5G8; tel.
506/453–2581; FAX. 506/453–5243; The
Honorable Russell H. T. King, M.D.

NEWFOUNDLAND
Health
Department of Health, Confederation Building, P.O.
Box 8700, St. John's, NF A1B 4J6; tel.
709/729–3124; FAX. 709/729–0121; The
Honorable Lloyd Matthews, Minister, Health

NOVA SCOTIA
Health
Department of Health, P.O. Box 488, Halifax, NS
B3J 2R8; tel. 902/424–4310; FAX.
902/424–0559; The Honorable Ronald D. Stewart,
M.D.

PRINCE EDWARD ISLAND
Health
Department of Health and Social Services,
Sullivan Building, Second Floor, P.O. Box 2000,
Charlottetown, PE C1A 7N8; tel. 902/368–4930;
FAX. 902/368–4969; The Honorable Walter A.
McEwen, Q.C./Minister

QUEBEC
Health
Ministry of Health and Social Services, Ministere
de la Sante et des Services Sociaux, 1075 Chemin
Ste–Foy, 15e Etage, Quebec, PQ G1S 2M1; tel.
418/643–3160; FAX. 418/644–4534; Jean
Rochon, Minister

SASKATCHEWAN
Health
Department of Health, 3475 Albert Street, Third
Floor, Regina, SK S4S 6X6; tel. 306/787–3168;
FAX. 306/787–8677; The Honorable Eric Cline,
Minister

Section C

Health Care Providers

Health Maintenance Organizations

The following is a list of Health Maintenance Organizations developed with the assistance of state government agencies and the individual facilities listed. The list is current as of January 1, 1997.

We present this list simply as a convenient directory. Inclusion or omission of any organization indicates neither approval nor disapproval by Healthcare InfoSource, Inc., a subsidiary of the American Hospital Association.

United States

ALABAMA

Apex Healthcare of Alabama, Inc., 104 Inverness Center Parkway, Suite 230, Birmingham, AL 35243; tel. 334/279–5000; Rea Jabour, Executive Director

Complete Health, Inc., 2160 Highland Avenue, Birmingham, AL 35205; tel. 205/933–7661; FAX. 205/933–0083; William W. Featheringill, President, Chief Executive Officer

Complete Health/United Health Care South, 2160 Highland Avenue, Birmingham, AL 35205; tel. 205/933–7661; Blair R. Sullentrop, President

Foundation Health, 2100 Southbridge Parkway, Suite 675, Birmingham, AL 35209; tel. 205/803–4400; Drew Wood

Health Advantage Plans, Inc., 140 Riverchase Parkway, E., Birmingham, AL 35244; tel. 205/982–8402; FAX. 205/982–8411; Pam Nichols, Executive Vice President, Chief Executive Officer

Health Maintenance Group of Birmingham, 495 Wynn Drive, Huntsville, AL 35805; tel. 205/729–9100; FAX. 205/726–9117; Adina Bishop, Director

Health Options, Inc., 532 Riverside Avenue, Jacksonville, FL 32203; tel. 904/791–6086; Harvey Matoren, President

Health Partners of Alabama, Inc., 600 Beacon Parkway, W., Suite 500, Birmingham, AL 35209; tel. 205/942–5787; FAX. 205/945–9450; Carole Zimbrolt, Vice President, Chief Operating Officer

Healthcare USA–Alabama, Inc., 1855 Data Drive, Suite 250, Birmingham, AL 35244; tel. 205/988–9400; Christopher T. Fey, President

Humana Health Plan of Alabama, Inc., 303 Williams Avenue, S.W., Suite 121, Huntsville, AL 35801; tel. 205/532–2000; FAX. 205/532–2025; Rene Moret, Executive Director

PCA Health Plans of Alabama, Inc., 104 Inverness Parkway W., Suite 280, Birmingham, AL 35242; tel. 205/991–6000; Bill Whitaker, President, Chief Operating Officer

Prime Health, 1400 South University Boulevard, Suite A, Mobile, AL 36609; tel. 334/342–0022; FAX. 334/342–6428; Becky S. Holliman, Executive Director

Primehealth of Alabama, Inc., 1400 South University Boulevard, Suite M, Mobile, AL 36609; tel. 334/342–0022; Becky S. Holliman, President

Principal Health Care of Florida, Inc., 1200 Riverplace Boulevard, Suite 500, Jacksonville, FL 32207–1802; tel. 904/390–0935, ext. 200; FAX. 904/390–0950; James F. H. Henry, Regional Vice President

Viva Health, Inc., 1401 South 21st Street, Birmingham, AL 35205; tel. 205/939–1718; John Davis, Interim President

ARIZONA

Aetna Health Plan of Arizona, Inc., 7878 North 16th Street, Suite 210, Phoenix, AZ 85020; tel. 602/395–8800; FAX. 602/395–8813; James W. Jones, Acting Vice President, Market Manager

CIGNA HealthCare of Arizona, Inc., 11001 North Black Canyon Highway, Suite 400, Phoenix, AZ 85029; tel. 602/942–4462; FAX. 602/371–2625; Clyde Wright, M.D., President, General Manager

FHP Inc., 410 North 44th Street, P.O. Box 52078, Phoenix, AZ 85072–2078; tel. 602/244–8200; FAX. 602/681–7680; Clifford Klima, President, Arizona Region

First Health of Arizona, Inc., 10448 West Coggins Drive, Sun City, AZ 85351; tel. 602/933–1344; FAX. 602/977–8808; Glenn D. Jones, Administrative Director

HMO Arizona, 2444 West Las Palmaritas, P.O. Box 13466, Phoenix, AZ 85002–3466; tel. 602/864–4250; FAX. 602/864–4035; Deborah Marshall, Director

HealthPartners Health Plans, Inc., (formerly Partners Health Plan of Arizona, Inc.), 333 East Wetmore, Tucson, AZ 85705; tel. 520/696–8020; Jeannie M. Byrne, Administrative Secretary

Humana Health Plan, Inc., Anchor Centre III, 2231 East Camelback Road, Suite 208, Phoenix, AZ 85016; tel. 602/381–4300; FAX. 602/381–4381; Elizabeth Kelly, Associate Executive Director

Intergroup Prepaid Health Plan of Arizona, Inc., 1010 North Finance Center Drive, Suite 100, Tucson, AZ 85710; tel. 602/290–7350; FAX. 602/290–7389; Edward J. Munno, Jr., President, Chief Operating Officer

Premier Healthcare, Inc., d/b/a Premier Healthcare of Arizona, 100 East Clarendon, Suite 400, Phoenix, AZ 85013; tel. 602/248–0404; FAX. 602/248–7771; David K. Stewart, Vice President, Marketing, Sales

United Healthcare of Arizona, Inc., (formerly MetraHealth Care Plan of Arizona, Inc.), 3020 East Camelback, Suite 100, Phoenix, AZ 85016; tel. 602/553–1300; FAX. 602/553–1331; Kathleen Garast, President, Chief Executive Officer

University Physicians Health Maintenance Organization, Inc., 575 East River Road, Tucson, AZ 85704–5822; tel. 520/795–3500

ARKANSAS

American Dental Providers, Inc., 614 Center Street, P.O. Box 34045, Little Rock, AR 72203–4045; tel. 501/376–0544; FAX. 501/371–3820; Robert E. Iriana

American Health Care Providers, Inc., 142 Town Center Road, Matteson, IL 60443–2254; tel. 708/503–5000; FAX. 708/503–5001; Asif Sayeed, President

DentiCare of Arkansas, Inc., Regional Administration Office, 7112 South Mingo, Suite 108, Tulsa, OK 74133; tel. 918/254–9055; FAX. 918/254–9076; John K. Wright, Secretary

HMO Partners, Inc., d/b/a HEALTH ADVANTAGE, 26 Corporate Hill Drive, P.O. Box 8069, Little Rock, AR 72203–8069; tel. 501/954–5250; FAX. 501/954–5481; Jack L. Blackshear, M.D., FACP, Chief Medical Officer

Healthsource Arkansas, Inc., 333 Executive Court, Little Rock, AR 72205–4548; tel. 501/227–7222; Donald T. Jack

Healthwise of Arkansas, Ltd., Three Financial Centre, 900 South Shackleford, Suite 400, Little Rock, AR 72211; tel. 501/228–9473; FAX. 501/221–0974; Caralee Pruitt

Mercy Health Plans of Missouri, Inc., 12935 North Outer 40 Drive, St. Louis, MO 63141–8636; tel. 314/214–8100; FAX. 314/214–8101; Thomas L. Kelly, President

Prudential Health Care Plan Inc., d/b/a Prucare of Arkansas, 1701 Centerview Drive, Suite 101, Little Rock, AR 72211; tel. 501/224–8977; Norine Yukon

QCA Health Plan, Inc., 10800 Financial Centre Parkway, Suite 540, Little Rock, AR 72211; tel. 501/954–9595; FAX. 501/228–0135; James M. Stewart, President, Chief Executive Officer

United HealthCare of Arkansas, Inc., 415 North McKinley Street, Plaza West Building, Suite 820, Little Rock, AR 72205; tel. 501/664–7700; FAX. 501/664–7768; V. Rob Herndon III

CALIFORNIA

Access Dental Plan, Inc., 555 University Avenue, Suite 182, Sacramento, CA 95825; tel. 916/922–5000, ext. 310; FAX. 916/646–9000; Reza Abbaszaden, D.D.S., Chief Executive Officer

Advanced Dental Systems, Inc., 3162 Newberry Drive, San Jose, CA 95118; tel. 800/448–1942; FAX. 408/448–5418; Dr. Roy Ingram, President

Aetna Dental Care of California, Inc., 201 North Civic Drive, Suite 300, Walnut Creek, CA 94596; tel. 510/977–7865; FAX. 510/746–6560; Bryan J. Geremia, Chief Executive Officer

Aetna Health Plans of California, 201 North Civic Drive, Suite 300, Walnut Creek, CA 94596; tel. 909/386–3145; FAX. 909/386–3330; Michael Dobbs, Market Vice President

Almeda Alliance for Health, 1850 Fairway Drive, San Leandro, CA 94577; tel. 510/895–4500; FAX. 510/483–6038; David J. Kears, President, Chief Executive Officer

Alternative Dental Care of California, Inc., 21700 Oxnard Street, Suite 500, Woodland Hills, CA 91367; tel. 818/710–9400, ext. 421; FAX. 818/704–9817; Sargis Khaziran, Chief Finance Officer

American Chiropractic Network Health Plan, Inc., 8989 Rio San Diego Drive, Suite 250, San Diego, CA 92108; tel. 619/297–8100; FAX. 619/297–8189; George DeVries, President

American Healthguard Corporation, Centaguard Dental Plan, 21031 Ventura Boulevard, Suite 506, Woodland Hills, CA 91364–1836; tel. 818/884–7645; David Kutner, M.D., President

Ameritas Managed Dental Plan, 151 Kalmus Drive, Suite B–250, Costa Mesa, CA 92626; tel. 714/437–5966; FAX. 714/437–5967; Karin Truxillo, President

Baycare Health Plan, 101 Skyport Drive, Suite B, San Jose, CA 95110; tel. 408/441–9340; Tracy K. Herta, D.D.S., President

Blue Cross of California/Wellpoint Health Network Inc./, CaliforniaCare Health Plans, 21555 Oxnard Street, Woodland Hills, CA 91367; tel. 818/703–2497; Brian J. Donnelly, Senior Vice President

CIGNA Dental Health of California, Inc., 5990 Sepulveda Boulevard, Suite 500, Van Nuys, CA 91411; tel. 818/756–2900; FAX. 818/756–2997; Claire Marie Burchill, President, Chief Executive Officer

CMG Behavioral Health of California, Inc., 865 South Figueroa Street, Suite 1450, Los Angeles, CA 90017; tel. 213/312–9400; FAX. 213/312–9413; Michael L. Jospe, Ph.D., Executive Director

California Benefits Dental Plan, 4911 Warner Avenue, Suite 208, Huntington Beach, CA 92649; tel. 714/840–2852; FAX. 714/840–3213; Robert F. Gosin, D.D.S., President

California Dental Health Plan, 14471 Chambers Road, 92680, P.O. Box 899, Tustin, CA 92681–0899; tel. 714/731–4751; FAX. 714/731–2049; James R. Lindsey, President

California Pacific Medical Group, d/b/a Brown and Toland Medical Group, 1388 Sutter Street, Suite 400, P.O. Box 640469, San Francisco, CA 94109; tel. 415/776–5140; Michael Abel, M.D., President

California Physicians' Service, Blue Shield of California, Two NorthPoint, San Francisco, CA 94133; tel. 415/445–5195; FAX. 415/445–5343; Patricia Ernsberger, Associate General Counsel

Care 1st Health Plan, 6255 Sunset Boulevard, Suite 1700, Los Angeles, CA 90028; tel. 213/957–4310; Bill Gil, President, Chief Executive Officer

CareAmerica, 6300 Canoga Avenue, Woodland Hills, CA 91367; tel. 818/228–2207; FAX. 818/228–5117; Robert P. White, President, Chief Executive Officer

Chinese Community Health Plan, 170 Columbus Avenue, Suite 210, San Francisco, CA 94133; tel. 415/397–3190; FAX. 415/397–6140; Thomas M. Harlan, Chief Executive Officer

Chrioserve, Inc., 3833 Atlantic Avenue, Long Beach, CA 90808; tel. 310/595–8164; Rodney Shelley, President, Chief Executive Officer

Cohen Medical Corporation, d/b/a Tower Health Service, 200 Ocean Gate, Sixth Floor, Long Beach, CA 90802; tel. 310/435–2676; Robert Cohen, M.D., Vice President

Community Dental Services, Smilecare, 18101 Von Karman Avenue, Irvine, CA 92715; tel. 714/756–1111; M. E. Hardin, President, Chief Executive Officer

Community Health Group, 740 Bay Boulevard, Chula Vista, CA 91910; tel. 619/422–0422; FAX. 619/422–5930; Gabriel Arce, Chief Executive Officer

ConsumerHealth, Inc., d/b/a Newport Dental Plan, 1401 Dove Street, Suite 290, Newport Beach, CA 92660; tel. 714/752–8522, ext. 220; FAX. 714/833–9172; Stephen R. Casey, President

Continental Dental Plan, 300 Corporate Pointe, Suite 385, Culver City, CA 90230; tel. 310/216–1154; James M. Hubbard, President

Contra Costa Health Plan, 595 Center Avenue, Suite 100, Martinez, CA 94553; tel. 510/313–6000; FAX. 510/313–6002; Milton Camhi, Executive Director

County of Los Angeles, Department of Health Services, d/b/a Community Health Plan, 3l3 North Figueroa Street, Los Angeles, CA 90012; tel. 213/974–8136; Westley Sholes, Deputy Director, Administrative Services

County of Ventura, Ventura County Health Care Plan, 133 West Santa Clara Street, Ventura, CA 93001; tel. 805/648–9562; FAX. 805/648–9593; Patricia S. Neumann, Insurance Administrator

Dedicated Dental Systems, Inc., 3990 Ming Avenue, Bakersfield, CA 93309; tel. 805/397–5513; FAX. 805/397–2888; Robert J. Newman, Vice President

Delta Dental Plan of California, 100 First Street, San Francisco, CA 94105; tel. 415/972–8312; Carl W. Ludwig, Director, Northern California Sales

Dental Benefit Providers of California, Inc., 1999 Harrison Street, Suite 2750, Oakland, CA 94612; tel. 510/832–2655; FAX. 510/832–2405; Carolyn Suminski, Operating Officer

Dental Health Services, 3833 Atlantic Avenue, Long Beach, CA 90807–3505; tel. 310/595–6000; FAX. 310/424–0150; Godfrey Pernell, D.D.S., President, Chief Executive Officer

Denticare of California, Inc., 28202 Cabot Road, Suite 600, Zip 92677, P.O. Box 30019, Laguna Niguel, CA 92607–0019; tel. 714/365–8010, ext. 215; FAX. 714/347–7612; Robert E. Wergin, President

Dr. Leventhal's Vision Care Centers of America, 3680 Rosecrans Street, Zip 92110, P.O. Box 87808, San Diego, CA 92138; tel. 619/223–5656; FAX. 619/223–2318; Debra Brant, Chief Operating Officer

Eyecare Service Plan, Inc., 9090 Burton Way, Beverly Hills, CA 90211; tel. 310/271–0145; FAX. 310/271–0784; Matthew Rips, Vice President

Eyexam 2000 of California, Inc., 700 El Real Camino, Menlo Park, CA 94025; tel. 415/329–9966; FAX. 415/572–9313; Evyn L. Shomer, Corporate Counsel

FHP, Inc., 18000 Studebaker Road, Suite 750, Cerritos, CA 90701; tel. 213/809–5399; FAX. 714/968–7159; Stuart Byer, Associate Vice President, Consumer, Government Affairs

For Eyes Vision Plan, Inc., 2104 Shattuck Avenue, Berkeley, CA 94704; tel. 510/843–0787; Robert Schoen, President

Foundation Health, a California Health Plan, 3400 Data Drive, Rancho Cordova, CA 95670; tel. 916/631–5299; FAX. 916/631–5294; Marshall Bentley, Vice President, Counsel

Foundation Health Psychcare Services, Inc., 125 East Sir Francis Drake Boulevard, Suite 300, Larkspur, CA 94939–1860; tel. 510/655–0535; Cathy Clement, Administrator

Foundation Health Vision Services, Vision Plans, 28202 Cabot Road, Suite 600, Laguna Niguel, CA 92677; tel. 714/365–7775, ext. 215; FAX. 714/347–1466; Robert E. Wergin, President

Golden West Dental and Vision Plan, 888 West Ventura Boulevard, Camarillo, CA 93010; tel. 805/987–8941, ext. 138; Karl H. Lehmann, President

Great American Health Plan, 2525 Camino Del Rio, S., Suite 350, San Diego, CA 92108; tel. 619/574–6600; Riley McWilliams, Chief Executive Officer

Greater California Dental Plan, Smilesaver, Signature Dental Plan, 22144 Clarendon Street, First Floor, P.O. Box 4281, Woodland Hills, CA 91365–4281; tel. 818/348–1500; FAX. 818/348–2942; Mark Johnson, President

Greater Pacific HMO, Inc., 2005 North Garey Avenue, Pomona, CA 91767; tel. 909/596–4835; FAX. 909/593–2185; Lee Reynolds, President

HMO California, 4675 MacArthur Court, Suite 1400, Newport Beach, CA 92660; tel. 800/795–8755; FAX. 714/756–5550; Robin Friend, Chief Executive Officer

Health Benefits, Inc., H.B.I. Prepaid Dental Plans, 4557 Quail Lakes Drive, Stockton, CA 95207; tel. 800/331–0903; FAX. 209/478–2918; Sherri E. Crowl, Vice President

Health Net, 21600 Oxnard Street, Woodland Hills, CA 91367, P.O. Box 9103, Van Nuys, CA 91409–9103; tel. 818/719–6800; FAX. 818/719–5450; Arthur Southam, M.D., Chief Executive Officer

Health Plan of the Redwoods, 3033 Cleveland Avenue, Santa Rosa, CA 95403; tel. 707/525–4231; FAX. 707/547–4101; William D. Hughes, Chief Executive Officer

Health and Human Resource Center, 7798 Starling Drive, San Diego, CA 92123; tel. 619/571–1698; FAX. 619/571–1868; Stephen H. Heidel, M.D., President, Chief Executive Officer

Healthdent of California, Inc., 2848 Arden Way, Suite 100, Sacramento, CA 95825; tel. 916/486–0749; FAX. 916/486–3642; Edward L. Cruchley, D.D.S., President

Holman Professional Counseling Centers, 21050 Van Owen Street, Canoga Park, CA 91303; tel. 818/704–1444, ext. 235; FAX. 818/704–9339; Ron Holman, Ph.D., President

Human Affairs International of California, 300 North Continental Boulevard, Suite 200, El Segundo, CA 90245; tel. 310/414–0066; FAX. 310/414–9282; Jonathan Wormhoudt, Ph.D., Chief Executive Officer

Ideal Dental Health Plan, 1720 South San Gabriel Boulevard, Suite 102, San Gabriel, CA 91776; tel. 818/288–2203; Richard Sun, D.D.S., President

Inland Empire Health Plan, 1250 East Cooley Drive, Colton, CA 92324; tel. 909/430–2700; FAX. 909/430–2703; Richard Bruno, Chief Executive Officer

Inter Valley Health Plan, 300 South Park Avenue, Suite 300, Pomona, CA 91766; tel. 909/623–6333; FAX. 909/622–2907; Mark C. Covington, President, Chief Executive Officer

Kaiser Foundation Health Plan, Inc., 2770 Ordway Building, One Kaiser Plaza, Oakland, CA 94612; tel. 510/271–2680; FAX. 510/271–5917; H. Paul Brandes, Assistant Secretary, Senior Counsel

Kern Health Systems, 1600 Norris Road, Bakersfield, CA 93380; tel. 805/391–4000; FAX. 805/391–4097; Carol L. Sorrell, RN, Chief Executive Officer

Key Health Plan, Inc., 5959 South Mooney Boulevard, Visalia, CA 93277–9329; tel. 209/730–4175; Dean K. Ward, Chief Executive Officer

Laurel Dental Plan, Inc., 5451 Laurel Canyon Boulevard, Suite 209, North Hollywood, CA 91607; tel. 818/980–0929; FAX. 818/980–4668; Dr. Victor Sands, President

Lifeguard, Inc., 1851 McCarthy Boulevard, Milpitas, CA 95035; tel. 408/943–9400; FAX. 408/383–4259; Mark G. Hyde, President, Chief Executive Officer

MAXICARE, 1149 South Broadway Street, Los Angeles, CA 90015; tel. 213/765–2000, ext. 2101; FAX. 213/765–2694; Peter J. Ratican, Chairman, President, Chief Executive Officer

MCC Behavioral Care of California, Inc., 801 North Brand Boulevard, Suite 1150, Glendale, CA 91203; tel. 818/551–2200; Bernhild E. Quintero, Vice President

Managed Dental Care of California, 6200 Canoga Avenue, Suite 100, Woodland Hills, CA 91367; tel. 800/273–3330; FAX. 818/347–7302; Michael Gould, President, Chief Executive Officer

Managed Health Network, Inc., 5100 West Goldleaf Circle, Suite 300, Los Angeles, CA 90056; tel. 213/299–0999; FAX. 213/298–2765; Alethea Caldwell, President

Merit Behavioral Care of California, Inc., 400 Oyster Point Boulevard, Suite 306, South San Francisco, CA 94080; tel. 415/742–0980; FAX. 415/742–0988; Douglas Studebaker, President

Molina Medical Centers, One Golden Shore, Long Beach, CA 90802; tel. 310/435–3666; John Molina, J.D., Vice President

Monarch Plan, Inc., 201 North Salsipuedes, Suite 206, Santa Barbara, CA 93103–3256; tel. 805/963–0566; FAX. 805/564–4167; Peter J. Leeson, D.O., Chief Executive Officer

National Health Plans, 1005 West Orangeburg Avenue, Suite B, Modesto, CA 95350–4163; tel. 209/527–3350; FAX. 209/527–6773; Clive Riddle, Senior Vice President, Chief Executive Officer

Omni Healthcare, 2450 Venture Oaks Way, Suite 300, Sacramento, CA 95833–3292; tel. 916/921–4000; FAX. 916/921–4100; Robert E. Edmonson, President, Chief Executive Officer

One Health Plan of California, Inc., 1740 Technology Drive, Suite 530, San Jose, CA 95110; tel. 408/437–4100; FAX. 408/437–0253; Fred Riggall, President

Oral Health Services, Inc., Mida Dental Plan, 21700 Oxnard Street, Suite 500, Woodland Hills, CA 91367; tel. 818/710–9400, ext. 421; FAX. 818/710–9400; Sargis Khaziran, Chief Financial Officer

PacifiCare Behavioral Health of California, 23046 Avenida de la Carlota, Suite 700, Laguna Hills, CA 92653; tel. 714/859–7971; Heidi Prescott, National Sales Manager

PacifiCare of California, Secure Horizons, 5701 Katella Avenue, Zip 90630–5019, P.O. Box 6006, Cypress, CA 90630–6006; tel. 714/952–1121; FAX. 714/236–7887; Jon Wampler, President

Pacific Union Dental, Inc., 2200 Powell Street, Suite 805, Emeryville, CA 94608; tel. 510/547–8227; FAX. 510/547–7305; Carl Legreca, Vice President, Marketing

Pearle Vision Care, Inc., 12625 High Bluff Drive, Suite 108, San Diego, CA 92130; tel. 800/843–6706; FAX. 619/793–4090; Nan Johnson, President

Pioneer Provider Network, Inc., 5000 Airport Plaza Drive, Long Beach, CA 90815; tel. 310/627–6019; David Maggenti, Chief Operating Officer

Preferred Health Plan, Inc., Personal Dental Services, 4034 Park Boulevard, San Diego, CA 92103; tel. 619/297–6670; FAX. 619/297–0317; Philip G. Menna, D.D.S., President

Preventive Dental Systems, Inc., 2000 L Street, Sacramento, CA 95814; tel. 916/448–2994; FAX. 916/448–2997; Carolyn Brodt, Executive Director

Priority Health Services, Central Valley Health Plan, Inc., P.O. Box 25790, Fresno, CA 93729–5790; tel. 209/446–6810; FAX. 209/435–7693; John M. Cronin, President, Chief Executive Officer

Private Medical–Care, Inc., PMI, 12898 Towne Center Drive, Cerritos, CA 90701; tel. 310/924–8311; FAX. 310/924–8039; Robert B. Elliott, President

Prudential Health Care Plan of California, Inc., 5800 Canoga Avenue, Woodland Hills, CA 91367; tel. 818/712–5705; FAX. 818/992–2474; Jeff Kamil, President

Ross–Loos Health Plan of California, Inc., d/b/a CIGNA HealthCare of California, 505 North Brand Boulevard, P.O. Box 2125, Glendale, CA 91203; tel. 818/500–6726; FAX. 818/500–6831; Leslie A. Margolin, Chief Counsel

SCAN Health Plan, 3780 Kilroy Airport Way, Suite 600, P.O. Box 22616, Zip 90801–5616, Long Beach, CA 90806–2460; tel. 310/989–5100; FAX. 310/989–5200; Sam L. Ervin, President, Chief Executive Officer

Safeguard Health Plans, 505 North Euclid Street, P.O. Box 3210, Anaheim, CA 92803–3210; tel. 714/778–1005; FAX. 714/778–4383; Ronald I. Brendzel, Senior Vice President

San Francisco Health Plan, 568 Howard Street, Fifth Floor, San Francisco, CA 94105; tel. 415/547–7800; FAX. 415/547–7824; Shahnaz Nikpay, Ph.D., Chief Executive Officer

San Joaquin County Health Commission, d/b/a The Health Plan of San Joaquin, 1550 West Fremont Street, Stockton, CA 95203–2643; tel. 209/939–3500; FAX. 209/939–3535; Leona M. Butler, Chief Executive Officer

San Joaquin Valley Dental Plan, Inc., 2000 Fresno Street, Suite 201, Fresno, CA 93721; tel. 209/442–1111; Debra Ann Dominquez, Vice President, Operations

Santa Clara Valley Medical Center, Valley Health Plan, 750 South Bascom Avenue, San Jose, CA 95l28; tel. 408/885–5704; FAX. 408/885–4050; Roger Wells, Executive Director

Sharp Health Plan, 9325 Sky Park Court, Suite 300, San Diego, CA 92123; tel. 619/637–6530; FAX. 619/637–6504; Kathlyn Mead, President, Chief Executive Officer

UDC Dental California, Inc., (formerly The Dental Advantage/National Dental Health), 3111 Camino Del Rio North, Suite 1000, San Diego, CA 92108; tel. 800/288–9992; FAX. 619/283–9437; Keith C. Macumber, Senior Vice President, Western Regional Manager

United Behavioral Health, 425 Market Street, 27th Floor, San Francisco, CA 94105–2426; tel. 415/547–5273; FAX. 415/547–5512; Caryl Rosner, Assistant Vice President, Client Services, Marketing

United Healthcare of California, Inc., d/b/a MetraHealth Care Plan, UHC Healthcare, 4500 East Pacific Coast Highway, Suite 120, Long Beach, CA 90804–6441; tel. 310/498–5106; FAX. 310/498–5137; George S. Goldstein, Ph.D., Chief Executive Officer

Universal Care, 1600 East Hill Street, Signal Hill, CA 90806; tel. 310/424–6200, ext. 4003; FAX. 310/427–4634; Howard E. Davis, President, Chief Executive Officer

Value Behavioral Health of California, Inc., (formerly American Psychmanagement of California, Inc.), 340 Golden Shore, Long Beach, CA 90802; tel. 310/590–9004; FAX. 310/951–6130; Annie–Claude Sanchis, Regional Vice President

Value Healthplan of California, Inc., 5251 Viewridge Court, San Diego, CA 92123; tel. 619/278–2273; Lory Wallach, Vice President, Chief Operating Officer

Vision Plan of America, 8111 Beverly Boulevard, Suite 306, Los Angeles, CA 90048; tel. 213/658–6113; FAX. 213/658–8611; Dr. Stuart Needleman

Vision Service Plan, 3333 Quality Drive, Rancho Cordova, CA 95670; tel. 800/852–7600; Al Schubert, Vice President, Managed Care

Visioncare of California, d/b/a Sterling Visioncare, 6540 Lusk Boulevard, Suite 234, San Diego, CA 92121; tel. 619/458–9983; Martin J. Shomank, President

Vista Behavioral Health Plans, 2355 Northside Drive, Third Floor, San Diego, CA 92108; tel. 619/521–4440; FAX. 619/497–5244; Keith Dixon, Ph.D., President, Chief Executive Officer

Viva Health Plan, d/b/a BPS HMO, 17 Cupania Circle, Monterey Park, CA 91754; tel. 213/724–8770; FAX. 213/890–5845; Mitchell Zevin, President

Watts Health Foundation, Inc., United Health Plan, 10300 Compton Avenue, Los Angeles, CA 90002; tel. 310/412–3591; FAX. 310/412–4198; Clyde W. Oden, M.P.H., O.D., President, Chief Executive Officer

Wellpoint Dental Plan, 21555 Oxnard Street, Woodland Hills, CA 91367; tel. 818/703–2412; Thomas C. Geiser, Senior Vice President, General Counsel

Wellpoint Health Networks, Inc., 21555 Oxnard Street, Woodland Hills, CA 91367; tel. 818/703–2412; FAX. 818/703–4406; Thomas Geiser, Executive Vice President, General Counsel

Wellpoint Pharmacy Plan, 27001 Agoura Road, Suite 325, Calabasas Hills, CA 91301–5339; tel. 818/878–2675; FAX. 818/880–4981; Richard C. Bleil, General Manager

Western Dental Services, Inc., Western Dental Plan, 300 Plaza Alicante, Suite 800, Garden Grove, CA 92640; tel. 714/938–1600; FAX. 714/938–1611; Robert C. Schur, President

COLORADO

Antero Healthplans, 600 Grant Street, Suite 900, Denver, CO 80203; tel. 303/830–3150; FAX. 303/830–2392; Charlie Stark, President, Chief Executive Officer

CIGNA HealthCare of Colorado, Inc., 3900 East Mexico Avenue, Suite 1100, Denver, CO 80210–3946; tel. 303/782–1500; FAX. 303/782–1577; Dennis Mouras, General Manager

Colorado Access, 501 South Cherry Street, Suite 700, Denver, CO 80222; tel. 303/333–0900; Judith M. Fenhart, Health Plan Director

Community Health Plan of the Rockies, Inc., 400 South Colorado Boulevard, Suite 300, Denver, CO 80222; tel. 303/355–3220; Laura Barribo, Human Resources

FHP of Colorado, Inc., 6455 South Yosemite Street, Englewood, CO 80111; tel. 303/220–5800; FAX. 303/714–3999; James J. Swayze, Vice President, Sales and Marketing

Foundation Health, a Colorado Health Plan, Inc., P.O. Box 958, Pueblo, CO 81002; tel. 719/583–7500

Frontier Community Health Plans, Inc., 6312 South Fiddler's Green Circle, Suite 260–N, Englewood, CO 80111; tel. 303/771–7200; FAX. 303/771–0366; Dr. Thomas J. Hazy

HMO Colorado, Inc., 700 Broadway, Suite 612, Denver, CO 80203; tel. 303/831–2131

HMO Health Plans, Inc., d/b/a San Luis Valley HMO, Inc., 95 West First Avenue, Monte Vista, CO 81144; tel. 719/852–4055; FAX. 719/852–3481; Douglas Johnson, Executive Director, Chief Executive Officer

HSI Health Plans, Inc., P.O. Box 1668, Fort Collins, CO 80522; tel. 970/482–8403; FAX. 970/482–8911; Karen Morgan, Vice President, Group and Member Services

Health Network of Colorado Springs, Inc., 555 East Pikes Peaks Avenue, Suite 108, Colorado Springs, CO 80903; tel. 719/365–5025; FAX. 719/365–5004; Ron Burnside, Chief Executive Officer

Humana Health Plan, Inc., P.O. Box 740036, Louisville, KY 40201–7436; tel. 502/580–5804; Craig Drablos, Executive Director

Kaiser Foundation Health Plan, Rocky Mountain Division, 10350 East Dakota Avenue, Denver, CO 80231–1314; tel. 303/344–7200; FAX. 303/344–7290; Kathryn A. Paul, President

One Health Plan of Colorado, Inc., 8505 East Orchard Road, Englewood, CO 80111; tel. 303/804–6800

Prudential Health Care Plan, Inc., d/b/a Prudential HealthCare HMO, 4643 South Ulster Street, Suite 1000, Denver, CO 80237; tel. 303/796–6161; FAX. 303/796–6183; Denise Saabye, Communication Manager

Qual–Med Plans for Health of Colorado, Inc., P.O. Box 1986, Pueblo, CO 81002–1986; tel. 719/542–0500; FAX. 719/542–4921; Malik Hasan, M.D., Chairman, President

Rocky Mountain Health Maintenance Organization, d/b/a Rocky Mountain HMO, P.O. Box 10600, Grand Junction, CO 81502–5500; tel. 303/244–7760; FAX. 303/244–7880; Michael J. Weber, Executive Director

Sloans Lake Health Plan, Inc., 1355 South Colorado Boulevard, Suite 902, Denver, CO 80222; tel. 303/691–2200

Unicare, 1840 West Mountain View Avenue, Suite Four, Longmont, CO 80501; tel. 303/678–4035; FAX. 303/678–5588; Rick Spears, Chief Executive Officer

United Healthcare of Colorado, Inc., 6251 Greenwood Plaza Boulevard, Englewood, CO 80111; tel. 303/694–9336

CONNECTICUT

Aetna Health Plans of Southern New England, 80 Lamberton Road, Conveyor LB2B, Windsor, CT 06095; tel. 203/298–4000; Craig W. Gage, M.D., Vice President, Health Services Management

Blue Care Health Plan, 370 Bassett Road, North Haven, CT 06473; tel. 203/239–8483; FAX. 203/234–8573; Robert Scalettar, M.D., M.P.H., Vice President, Medical Policy

CIGNA HealthCare of Connecticut, Inc., 900 Cottage Grove Road, A–118, Hartford, CT 06152–1118; tel. 860/769–2300; FAX. 860/769–2399; Donald S. Grossman, M.D., Medical Director

ConnectiCare, Inc., 30 Batterson Park Road, Farmington, CT 06032–3006; tel. 203/674–5700; FAX. 203/674–5728; Marcel Gamache, President, Chief Executive Officer

Healthsource Connecticut, Inc., 40 Stanford Drive, Farmington, CT 06032; tel. 860/674–9922; FAX. 860/674–9924; Steven T. Burnett, Chief Executive Officer

Kaiser Foundation Health Plan, 76 Batterson Park Road, P.O. Box 4011, Farmington, CT 06034–4011; tel. 203/678–6178; FAX. 203/678–6160; Pat Parkerton, Area Operations Manager

M.D. Health Plan, Six Devine Street, North Haven, CT 06473; tel. 800/772–5869; FAX. 203/407–2899; Barbara G. Bradow, President

MedSpan, Inc., 55 Farmington Avenue, Hartford, CT 06105; tel. 860/541–6789; Kevin W. Kelly, President, Chief Executive Officer

NYLCare Health Plans of Connecticut, Inc., Four Armstrong Road, Shelton, CT 06484; tel. 203/944–1900; Theresa Atwood, Regional Vice President

Oxford Health Plans, 800 Connecticut Avenue, Norwalk, CT 06854; tel. 800/444–6222; Julie Summers, Marketing Associate

Physicians Health Services, Inc., 120 Hawley Lane, Trumbull, CT 06611–5343; tel. 800/848–4747, ext. 5642; FAX. 203/381–7665; Sharon Williams, Director, Marketing Administration

Prudential Health Care of Connecticut, Inc., 101 Merritt Seven, Norwalk, CT 06851; tel. 203/849–1800; FAX. 203/849–8387; Lewis E. Devendorf, Executive Director

Suburban Health Plan, Inc., 680 Bridgeport Avenue, Shelton, CT 06484; tel. 203/926–8882; FAX. 203/925–1202; Tim Pusch, Manager, Sales, Marketing

U.S. Healthcare, Inc., 1000 Middle Street, Middletown, CT 06457; tel. 860/636–8300; Leonard Abramson, President

Wellcare of Connecticut, Inc., 1781 Highland Avenue, Cheshire, CT 06410; tel. 203/250–9355; FAX. 203/699–8593; G. William Strein, President

Yale Preferred Health, Inc., 23 Maiden Lane, North Haven, CT 06473; tel. 203/239–7444; FAX. 203/239–5308; Sylvia B. Kelly, Operations Director

DELAWARE

Aetna Health/U.S. Healthcare, Rockwood Office Park, 501 Carr Road, Third Floor, Wilmington, DE 19809; tel. 800/231–8430; Cynthia Mazer, Manager

Amerihealth HMO, Inc., 919 North Market Street, Suite 1200, Wilmington, DE 19801–3021; Alfred F. Meyer, Executive Director

CIGNA HealthCare of Pennsylvania, New Jersey and Delaware, One Beaver Valley Road, Suite CHP, Wilmington, DE 19803; tel. 302/477–3000, ext. 3725; FAX. 302/477–3707; Norman Scott, M.D., Medical Director

CareLink, Georgetown Professional Park, Route 113 North, Suite 109, Georgetown, DE 19947; tel. 302/856–3100; FAX. 302/856–3999; Craig Gieseman, Vice President, Managed Care Services

Delmarva Health Plan, Inc., 106 Marlboro Road, Easton, MD 21601; tel. 410/822–7223; Richard Moore, Chief Executive Officer

HMO of Delaware, Inc., The Health Care Center at Christiana, 200 Hygeia Drive, P.O. Box 6008, Newark, DE 19714; tel. 302/421–2518; FAX. 302/421–2577; Paul C. King, Chief Operating Officer

Healthcare Delaware, Inc., Seventh and Clayton Streets, P.O. Box 7498, Wilmington, DE 19803; tel. 302/652–8038, ext. 4799; FAX. 215/358–5238; James J. Thomas III, Senior Vice President

Optimum Choice Inc./MDIPA, Inc./Alliance PPO, Inc., Four Taft Court, Rockville, MD 20850; tel. 301/762–8205, ext. 3994; Gloria Stem, Human Resource, Senior Director

Principal Health Care of Delaware, Inc., 2751 Centerville Road, Suite 400, Wilmington, DE 19808; tel. 302/955–6100; FAX. 302/633–4044; Robert J. White, Executive Director

Total Health, Inc., One Brandywine Gateway, P.O. Box 8792, Wilmington, DE 19899; tel. 302/421–3034; FAX. 302/421–2577; Robert C. Cole, Jr., President

U.S. Healthcare, Inc., 980 Jolly Road, P.O. Box 1109, Blue Bell, PA 19422; tel. 215/628–4800; Leonard Abramson, President

DISTRICT OF COLUMBIA

Aetna Health Plans of the Mid–Atlantic, Inc., 7799 Leesburgh Pike South, Suite 1100, Falls Church, VA 22045; tel. 703/903–7100; Russ Dickhart, Executive Director

CIGNA HealthCare Mid–Atlantic, Inc., 9700 Patuxent Woods Drive, Columbia, MD 21046; tel. 410/720–5800; Linda Hacker

CapitalCare, Inc., 550 12th Street, S.W., Washington, DC 20065–0001; tel. 202/479–3678; FAX. 202/479–3660; M. Bruce Edwards, President

D.C. Chartered Health Plan, Inc., 820 First Street, N.E., Suite LL100, Washington, DC 20002–4205; tel. 202/408–4710; Robert L. Bowles, Jr., DBA, Chairman, President and Chief Executive Officer

George Washington University Health Plan, Inc., 4550 Montgomery Avenue, Suite 800, Bethesda, MD 20814; tel. 301/941–2000, ext. 2100; FAX. 301/941–2005; Dr. John E. Ott, Executive Director, Chief Executive Officer

HealthPlus, Inc., NYLCare Health Plans of the Mid–Atlantic, Inc., 7601 Ora Glen Drive, Suite 200, Greenbelt, MD 20770–3641; tel. 301/441–1600, ext. 3308; FAX. 301/489–5282; Jeff D. Emerson, President, Chief Executive Officer

Humana Group Health Association, Inc., 430l Connecticut Avenue, N.W., Washington, DC 20008; tel. 202/364–2000; FAX. 202/364–7418; Robert Pfotenhauer, President, Chief Executive Officer

Kaiser Foundation Health Plan of the Mid–Atlantic States, 2101 East Jefferson Street, Box 6611, Rockville, MD 20849–6611; tel. 301/468–6000; FAX. 301/816–7465; Robert A. Essink, Acting President

M.D. Individual Practive Association, Inc., Four Taft Court, Rockville, MD 20850; tel. 800/544–2853; Susan Goff, President

Optimum Choice, MAMSI, Four Taft Court, Rockville, MD 20850; tel. 301/294–5100; FAX. 301/309–1709; George Jochum, President

Physicians Health Plan, Inc./Physicians Care, d/b/a Health Keepers, 2111 Wilson Boulevard, Suite 11510, Arlington, VA 22201; tel. 703/525–0602; Wyndahm Kidd

Prudential Health Care Plan, 2800 North Charles Street, Baltimore, MD 21218; tel. 410/554–7222

United Mine Workers of America, 4455 Connecticut Avenue, N.W., Washington, DC 20008; tel. 202/895–3960; Robert Condra

FLORIDA

Aetna Health Plans of Florida, Inc., 4890 West Kennedy, Suite 545, Tampa, FL 33630–3123; tel. 813/287–7820; FAX. 813/282–0893; James R. Gilmour, Administrator

American Medical Healthcare, 1900 Summit Tower Boulevard, Suite 700, Orlando, FL 32810; tel. 407/660–1611; FAX. 407/660–0203; Sandra K. Johnson, President, Chief Executive Officer

Anthem Health Plan of Florida, Inc., 10199 Southside Boulevard, Suite 301, Jacksonville, FL 32256; tel. 904/363–7601; FAX. 904/363–7627; Ann F. Dehgan, Senior Vice President, Chief Operating Officer

AvMed Health Plan, P.O. Box 749, Gainesville, FL 32606–0749; tel. 904/372–8400; FAX. 904/372–5155; Edward C. Peddie, President, Chief Executive Officer

Beacon Health Plans, Inc., 2511 Ponce de Leon Boulevard, Coral Gables, FL 33134; tel. 305/460–2000; Emilio Nunez

CIGNA HealthCare of Florida, Inc., 5404 Cypress Center Drive, P.O. Box 24203, Tampa, FL 33623; tel. 813/281–1000; FAX. 813/282–0356; Betty Kimmel, President, General Manager

Capital Group Health Services of Florida, Inc., 2140 Centerville Place, P.O. Box 13267, Tallahassee, FL 32317; tel. 904/386–3161; FAX. 904/385–3193; John Hogan, Administrator

Champion Healthcare, 7406 Fullerton Street, Suite 200, Jacksonville, FL 32256; tel. 904/519–0900; FAX. 904/519–0838; Richard C. Powell, President, Chief Executive Officer

Community Health Care Systems, Inc., 1414 Kuhl Avenue, Orlando, FL 32806; tel. 407/481–7100

Florida Health Care Plan, Inc., 1340 Ridgewood Avenue, Holly Hill, FL 32117; tel. 904/676–7193; FAX. 904/676–7196; Edward F. Simpson, Jr., President, Chief Executive Officer

Florida Ist Health Plan, Inc., 3425 Lake Alfred Road, P.O. Box 9126, Winter Haven, FL 33883–9126; tel. 813/293–0785, ext. 5125; FAX. 813/297–9095; John J. Torti, President

Foundation Health, a Florida Health Plan, Inc., 7950 Northwest 53rd Street, Miami, FL 33166; tel. 305/591–3311; Gary Lewison, Executive Director

Foundation Health, a South Florida Health Plan, Inc., 7950 Northwest 53rd Street, Miami, FL 33166; tel. 305/591–3311

HIP Health Plan of Florida, Inc., 200 South Park Road, Hollywood, FL 333021; tel. 954/962–3008, ext. 4100; FAX. 954/985–4379; Steven M. Cohen, President, Chief Executive Officer

Health First HMO, Inc., 8247 Devereux Drive, Suite 103, Melbourne, FL 32940–7955; tel. 407/953–5600; FAX. 407/752–1129; Jerry Seme, President, Chief Executive Officer

Health Options, Inc., 532 Riverside Avenue, P.O. Box 60729, Jacksonville, FL 32236–0729; tel. 904/791–6105; FAX. 904/791–8082; William E. Flaherty, President

Healthcare USA, Inc., 8705 Perimeter Park Boulevard, Suite Three, Jacksonville, FL 32216; tel. 904/565–2950; FAX. 904/646–9238; Christopher Fey, President, Chief Executive Officer

Healthplan Southeast, Inc., 3520 Thomasville Road, Suite 200, Tallahassee, FL 32308; tel. 904/668–3000; FAX. 904/668–3133; Deborah L. Redd, President, Managed Care Division

Healthplans of America, Inc., 405 Douglas Avenue, Altaonte Springs, FL 32714; tel. 407/786–3551

Humana Medical Plan, Inc., 3400 Lakeside Drive, Miramar, FL 33027; tel. 305/626–5619; FAX. 305/626–5297; Joe Berding, Vice President, South Florida Market Operations

Neighborhood Health Partnership, Inc., 7600 Corporate Center Drive, Miami, FL 33126; tel. 800/354–0222; FAX. 305/715–2660; Ruben King–Shaw, Chief Operating Officer

PCA Health Plans of Florida, Inc., 6101 Blue Lagoon Drive, Suite 300, Miami, FL 33126; tel. 305/267–6633; FAX. 305/265–5393; Bert Cibran, President

PacifiCare of Florida, Inc., One Alhambra Plaza, Suite 1000, Coral Gables, FL 33134; tel. 800/887–6888; FAX. 305/447–6625; C. Daniel Koon, Vice President, Operations

Physicians Healthcare Plans, Inc., One Harbour Place, 777 South Harbor Island Boulevard, Tampa, FL 33602; tel. 813/229–5300; FAX. 813/229–5301; Miguel B. Fernandez, Chief Executive Officer

Preferred Choice, HMO of Florida Health Choice, Inc., 5300 West Atlantic Avenue, Delray Beach, FL 33484; tel. 561/496–0505; FAX. 561/496–0513; W. Brent Casey, President, Chief Executive Officer

Preferred Medical Plan, Inc., 6090 Bird Road, Miami, FL 33155; tel. 305/669–1501; FAX. 305/669–4121; Sylvia Urlich, President

Principal Health Care of Florida, Inc., 1200 Riverplace Boulevard, Jacksonville, FL 32207; tel. 904/390–0935, ext. 200; FAX. 904/390–0948; James F. H. Henry, Regional Director

Prudential Health Care Plan, Inc., d/b/a PruCare, 2301 Lucien Way, Suite 230, Maitland, FL 32751–7086; tel. 404/933–6700; FAX. 404/933–6885; David A. George, Administrator

Riscorp Health Plan, Inc., 1390 Main Street, Zip 34236, P.O. Box 1598, Sarasota, FL 34230–1598; tel. 800/226–9899; FAX. 813/954–4611; Barbara Corbett, Administrator

St. Augustine Health Care, Inc., 3550 Buschwood Park Drive, Tampa, FL 33618; tel. 813/935–2896

Sunrise Healthcare Plan, Inc., 900 West Cypress Creek Road, Suite 740, Suite 740, Fort Lauderdale, FL 33309; tel. 954/492–4243; FAX. 954/267–9673; Sheila D. Williams, Executive Administrator

The Public Health Trust of Dade County, 1500 Northwest 12th Avenue, JMT, Suite West 1001, Miami, FL 33136; tel. 305/585–7120; FAX. 305/545–5212; Jose R. Paredes, Executive Director

Ultramedix Health Care Systems, Inc., 3450 West Buschwood Park Drive, Suite 245, Tampa, FL 33618; tel. 813/933–6200; FAX. 813/930–2949; John S. Zaleskie, Chief Executive Officer

United Healthcare Plans of Florida, Inc., 75 Valencia Avenue, Coral Gables, FL 33134; tel. 800/543–3145; FAX. 305/447–3292; Luis E. Lamela, Administrator

Vantage Health Plan, Inc., 4250 Lakeside Drive, Jacksonville, FL 32210; tel. 904/387–4451

Well Care HMO, Inc., 11016 North Dale Mabry, Suite 301, Tampa, FL 33618; tel. 813/963–6128; FAX. 813/960–1623; Pradip C. Patel, Administrator

GEORGIA

AETNA Health Plans of Georgia, Inc., 3500 Piedmont Road, Suite 300, Atlanta, GA 30305; tel. 404/814–4300; FAX. 404/814–4294; Teresa L. Kline, President

American Medical Plans of Georgia, Inc., 1355 Peachtree Street, N.E., Suite 1500, Atlanta, GA 30309; tel. 404/347–8005; Tom Stockdale, Executive Director

CIGNA Healthcare of Georgia, Inc., 1349 West Peachtree Street, N.E., Suite 1300, Atlanta, GA 30309; tel. 404/881–9779; FAX. 404/898–4701; J.C. Ranelli,, General Manager

Complete Health of Georgia, Inc., 2970 Clairmont Road, N.E., Atlanta, GA 30329; tel. 404/698–8600; Gail Smallridge, Executive Director

FamilyPlus Health Plans of Georgia, Inc., Two Decatur Town Center, 125 Clairemont Road, Suite 360, Decatur, GA 30030; tel. 404/315–3851; FAX. 404/248–3858; Brenda A. Williams, Vice President Legislative Public Affairs

HMO Georgia, Inc., 3350 Peachtree Road, N.E., P.O. Box 3417, Atlanta, GA 30326; tel. 404/842–8422; FAX. 404/842–8451; John Harris, President

Healthsource Georgia, Inc., 7130 Hodgson Memorial Drive, Suite 4000, Savannah, GA 31406; tel. 912/351–2140; FAX. 912/351–2416; James L. Boone, Executive Director

Healthsource Georgia, Inc., 400 Interstate North Parkway, Suite 200, Atlanta, GA 30339; tel. 404/858–1900; Steve Parham, Executive Director

Humana Employers Health Plan of Georgia, Inc., 115 Perimeter Center Place, N.E., Suite 540, Atlanta, GA 30346; tel. 770/399–5916; Mr. Rene P. Moret, Executive Director

Kaiser Foundation Health Plan of Georgia, Inc., 3495 Piedmont Road, N.E., Building Nine, Atlanta, GA 30305–1736; tel. 404/364–7000; Herman Weil, Associate Regional Manager

Master Health Plan, Inc., 3652 J. Dewey Gray Circle, Augusta, GA 30909; tel. 706/863–5955; Libby Young, Executive Director

Metrahealth Care Plan of Georgia, Inc., 1130 Northchase Parkway, Suite 250, Marietta, GA 30067; tel. 404/980–0740; Thomas David, Administrator

PCA Health Plans of Georgia, Inc., Two Midtown Plaza, 1349 West Peachtree Street, N.E., Suite 1000, Atlanta, GA 30309; tel. 404/815–7160; Rodney Spencer, Acting President

Principal Health Care of Georgia, Inc., 400 North Creek, Suite 300, Atlanta, GA 30327; tel. 404/231–9911; Ken Bryant, Executive Director

Prudential Health Care Plan of Georgia, Inc., Prudential Health Care, 2839 Paces Ferry Road, Suite 1000, Atlanta, GA 30339; tel. 770/955–8010; FAX. 770/433–0616; Harvey Ludlam, President

U.S. Healthcare of Georgia, Inc., 115 Perimeter Center Place, Suite 777, South Terraces, Atlanta, GA 30346; tel. 770/481–0100; FAX. 770/481–0800; J. Scott Murphy, Senior Vice President

United Healthcare of Georgia, Inc., 2970 Clairmont Road, Atlanta, GA 30329; tel. 404/364–8800; FAX. 404/364–8818; A. Kelly Atkinson, Executive Director

HAWAII

HMO Hawaii (HMSA), 818 Keeaumoko Street, P.O. Box 860, Honolulu, HI 96808; tel. 808/948–5408; FAX. 808/948–5999; Robert C. Nickel, Vice President

Health Plan Hawaii (HMSA), 818 Keeaumoku Street, P.O. Box 860, Honolulu, HI 96814; tel. 808/948–5408; FAX. 808/948–5063; Robert C. Nickel, Vice President

Health Plan Partners, d/b/a Kapi'olani HealthHawai'i, 677 Ala Moana Boulevard, Suite 602, Honolulu, HI 96813; tel. 808/522–5107; FAX. 808/522–6137; Kevin Somerfield, Vice President, Managed Care Systems

Island Care (HMO), Queen's Hawaii Care (HMO), Two Waterfront Plaza, Suite 200, 500 Ala Moana Boulevard, Honolulu, HI 96813; tel. 808/532–4114; FAX. 808/532–7996; Nate Nygaard, Vice President, Director, Tricare

Kaiser Foundation Health Plan, Inc., 711 Kapiolani Boulevard, Honolulu, HI 96813; tel. 808/834–5333; FAX. 808/529–5495; Cora M. Tellez, Vice President, Regional Manager

Pacific Health Care, 1946 Young Street, Suite 450, Honolulu, HI 96826; tel. 808/973–3000; FAX. 808/949–3259; John Kim, M.D., President, Medical Director

Straub Plan, 888 South King Street, Honolulu, HI 96813; tel. 808/522–4540; FAX. 808/522–4544; Karen Lennox, Executive Director

IDAHO

Group Health Northwest, West 5615 Sunset Highway, Spokane, WA 99204; tel. 509/838–9100; FAX. 509/458–0368; Henry S. Berman, M.D., President, Chief Executive Officer

HealthSense, 1602 21st Avenue, Lewiston, ID 83501; tel. 208/746–2671; FAX. 208/746–1030; Carolyn Steinbrecher–Loera, Manager, Managed Care Programs

Healthplus, P.O. Box 2113, Seattle, WA 98111–2113; tel. 206/670–4700; FAX. 206/670–4505; Gary Meade, President, Chief Executive Officer

IHC Health Plans, Inc., 36 South State Street, 15th Floor, Salt Lake City, UT 84111; tel. 801/442–5000; Sid Paulson, Chief Operating Officer

Primary Health Network, Inc., 800 Park Boulevard, Suite 760, Boise, ID 83712; tel. 208/344–1811; FAX. 208/344–4262; Elden Mitchell, President, Chief Executive Officer

QualMed Washington Health Plan, Inc., West 508 Sixth Avenue, Suite 700, P.O. Box 2470, Spokane, WA 99210–2470; tel. 509/459–6690, ext. 469; FAX. 509/459–9299; Nicolette Crowley, Provider Services Manager

ILLINOIS

Aetna Health Plans of Illinois, 100 North Riverside Plaza, 20th Floor, Chicago, IL 60606; tel. 312/441–3000, ext. 3231; FAX. 312/441–3000, ext. 3215; Kevin F. Hickey, President

Aetna Health Plans of Illinois, Inc., d/b/a Aetna Health Plans of the Midwest, 100 North Riverside Plaza, Chicago, IL 60606; tel. 312/441–3000

Americaid Illinois, Inc., 4425 Corporation Lane, Suite 100, Virginia Beach, VA 23462; tel. 804/490–6900

American Health Care Providers, Inc., 142 Towncenter Road, Matteson, IL 60443; tel. 708/503–5000; Roger Carlson, Director, Operations

BCI HMO, Inc., 233 North Michigan Avenue, Zip 60601–5655, P.O. Box A3694, Chicago, IL 60690; tel. 312/938–7491; Eileen Holderbaum, Executive Director

Benchmark Health Insurance Company, 1313 East State Street, Rockford, IL 61104–2227; tel. 815/966–2085; FAX. 815/966–2089; Michael J. Gallagher

CIGNA HealthCare of Illinois, Inc., 1700 East Higgins Road, Suite 600, Des Plaines, IL 60018; tel. 847/699–5600; FAX. 847/699–5675; Bert B. Wagener, General Manager

Cigna HealthCare of St. Louis, Inc., 8182 Maryland Avenue, Suite 900, St. Louis, MO 63105; tel. 314/726–7860; FAX. 314/726–7819; Eric Schultz, Executive Director

Community Health Plan of Sarah Bush Lincoln, 1000 Health Center Drive, P.O. Box 372, Mattoon, IL 61938–0372; tel. 217/258–2572; Eugene A. Leblond, FACHE, President and Chief Executive Officer

Compass Health Care Plans, 310 South Michigan Avenue, Chicago, IL 60604; tel. 312/294–0200; FAX. 312/294–5826; Aldo Giacchino, Chief Executive Officer

Dreyer Health Plans, 1877 West Downer Place, Aurora, IL 60506; tel. 630/859–1100, ext. 5501; FAX. 630/906–5100; Richard A. Lutz, President

Exclusive Healthcare, Inc., Mutual of Omaha Plaza, Omaha, NE 68175; tel. 402/342–7600; David Creamer, Senior Managed Care Development Specialist

FHP of Illinois, Inc., One Lincoln Centre, Suite 700, Oakbrook Terrace, IL 60181–4260; tel. 630/916–8400; FAX. 630/916–4275; Paula C. Mazvrkiewicz, Director, Marketing, Public Relations

Gencare Health Systems, Inc., P.O. Box 419079, St. Louis, MO 63141–9079; tel. 314/434–6114

Group Health Plan, 940 Westport Plaza, Suite 300, St. Louis, MO 63146; tel. 314/453–1700; FAX. 314/453–1958; Richard H. Jones, President, Chief Executive Officer

HMO Illinois a product of Health Care Services Corporation, 233 North Michigan Avenue, Chicago, IL 60601–5655; tel. 312/938–6359; Don Pebworth, J.D., Director

HMO Missouri (Blue Choice), 1831 Chestnut Street, P.O. Box 66828, St. Louis, MO 63166–6828; tel. 314/923–8623; FAX. 314/923–8958; Ken Evelyn, President, Chief Operating Officer

Harmony Health Plan of Illinois, Inc., 125 South Wacker Drive, Suite 2900, Chicago, IL 60606; tel. 312/630–2025; Keri Rosenbloom, Operations

Health Alliance Medical Plans, Inc., d/b/a Health Alliance HMO, 102 East Main, Suite 200, P.O. Box 6003, Urbana, IL 61801; tel. 217/337–8010; FAX. 217/337–8093; John W. Pollard, M.D., Chief Executive Officer Interim

Health Alliance Midwest, Inc., P.O. Box 6003, Urbana, IL 61801; tel. 217/337–8000

Health Direct Insurance, Inc., 1011 East Touhy Avenue, Suite 500, Des Plaines, IL 60018–2808; tel. 847/391–9600; Kerry Finnegan, Vice President, Sales, Marketing

Healthlink HMO, Inc., 777 Craig Road, St. Louis, MO 63141; tel. 314/569–7200

Heritage National Healthplan of Tennessee, Inc., 1515 Fifth Avenue, Suite 200, Moline, IL 61265; tel. 309/765–1200; G. Michael Hammes, President

Heritage National Healthplan, Inc., 1515 Fifth Avenue, Suite 200, Moline, IL 61265–1368; tel. 309/765–1200; FAX. 309/765–1322; G. Michael Hammes, President

Humana Health Chicago, Inc., P.O. Box 740036, Louisville, KY 40201–7436; tel. 312/441–9111; Barry Averill, Vice President

Humana Health Plan, Inc., P.O. Box 740036, Louisville, KY 40201–7436; tel. 502/580–5804; Craig Drablos, Executive Director

Illinois Masonic Community Health Plan, 836 West Wellington, Chicago, IL 60657; tel. 312/975–1600; Bruce C. Campbell, President

John Deere Family Healthplan, Inc., 1515 Fifth Avenue, Suite 600, Moline, IL 61265–1368; tel. 309/765–1287; James K. Thomson, Operations

Maxicare Health Plans of the Midwest, Inc., 111 East Wacker Drive, Suite 1500, Chicago, IL 60601; tel. 312/616–4700; FAX. 312/616–4998; Mark Hanrahan, Vice President, General Manager

Medical Associates Health Plan, Inc., 700 Locust Street, Suite 230, Dubuque, IA 52001–6800; tel. 319/556–8070; FAX. 319/556–5134; Lawrence E. Cremer, Executive Director

Medical Center Health Plan, d/b/a Partners HMO, One City Place Drive, Suite 670, St. Louis, MO 63141; tel. 314/567–6660; Dalbert E. Snoberger, Chief Executive Officer

Mercy Care Corporation, 2600 South Michigan Avenue, Chicago, IL 60616–2477; tel. 312/567–5649; FAX. 312/567–2786; Ramesh Joshi, Director

Mercy Health Plans of Missouri, Inc., 12935 North Outer 40 Drive, St. Louis, MO 63141–8636; tel. 314/214–8100; FAX. 314/214–8101; Thomas L. Kelly, President

NYLCare Health Plans of the Midwest, Inc., 1111 West 22nd Street, Suite 800, Oak Brook, IL 60521; tel. 630/368–1800; FAX. 630/368–1802; William P. Donahue, President

OSF Health Plans, Inc., 300 S.W. Jefferson Street, Peoria, IL 61602–1413; tel. 309/677–8200; FAX. 309/677–8330; Richard H. Bohn, President, Chief Executive Officer

One Health Plan of Illinois, Inc., 6250 River Road, Suite 3030, Rosemont, IL 60018; tel. 847/518–0490; FAX. 847/685–3844

Personal Care Insurance of Illinois, Inc., 510 Devonshire Drive, Champaign, IL 61820; tel. 217/366–1226; FAX. 217/366–5571; Raymond E. DeWitte, Chairman

Principal Health Care of Illinois, Inc., One Lincoln Center, Suite 1040, Oakbrook Terrace, IL 60181–4267; tel. 630/916–6622; FAX. 630/916–9595, ext. 200; Lee Green, Executive Director

Principal Health Care of St. Louis, Inc., 12312 Olive Boulevard, Suite 150, St. Louis, MO 63141; tel. 314/434–6990; FAX. 314/434–7540; Barbara C. Buenemann, Executive Director

Rockford Health Plans, 3401 North Perryville Road, Rockford, IL 61114; tel. 815/654–3600; FAX. 815/654–5186; D. Michael Elliott, President

Rush Prudential Health Plans, 233 South Wacker Drive, Suite 3900, Chicago, IL 60606; tel. 312/234–7000; FAX. 312/234–0050; Barbara B. Hill, President, Chief Executive Officer

UIHMO, Inc., 2023 West Ogden Avenue, Suite 205, M/C 692, Chicago, IL 60612–3741; tel. 312/996–3553; FAX. 312/413–7872; Diane S. Eng, Vice President, University Programs

Union Health Service, 1634 West Polk, Chicago, IL 60612; tel. 312/829–4224; FAX. 312/829–8241; Helen M. Hrynkiw, Executive Director

United HealthCare of Illinois, Inc., d/b/a Chicago HMO, Ltd., One South Wacker Drive, P.O. Box 909714, Chicago, IL 60609–9714; tel. 312/424–4460; FAX. 312/424–4448; Marshall Rozzi, President, Chief Executive Officer

Unity HMO, of Illinois, Inc., 150 South Wacker Drive, Suite 2100, Chicago, IL 60606; tel. 312/251–0955; FAX. 312/251–0294; Norris A. Stevenson, Chief Operating Officer

INDIANA

Aetna Health Plans of Ohio, Inc., 3690 Orange Place, Suite 200, Cleveland, OH 44122; tel. 203/636–9279

Alternative Dental Care of Indiana, Inc., One Penmark, Suite 200, 11595 Meridian Street, Carmel, IN 46032; tel. 800/237–7727; David P. McSweeney, President

Alternative Health Delivery Systems, Inc., 1901 Campus Place, Louisville, KY 40299; tel. 502/261–2176; FAX. 502/261–2255; Carol H. Muldoon, Vice President, Chief Operating Officer

American Health Care Providers, Inc., 4801 Southwick Drive, Matteson, IL 60443; tel. 708/503–5000; Asif Sayeed, President

Anthem Health Plan, d/b/a Key Health Plan, 120 Monument Circle, Indianapolis, IN 46204; tel. 317/488–6000; FAX. 317/290–5695; Dijuana Lewis, Vice President, Health Care Management

Arnett HMO, Inc., 3768 Rome Drive, Lafayette, IN 47905; tel. 317/448–8200; FAX. 317/448–8660; James A. Brunnemer, Executive Director

BCI HMO, Inc., (formerly HMO Illinois, Inc.), 233 North Michigan Avenue, Chicago, IL 60601; tel. 312/938–6347; FAX. 312/819–1220; Simeon Martin Hickman, President

Benefit Directions, Inc., 3901 West 86th Street, Suite 230, Indianapolis, IN 46268; tel. 317/872–2202

CIGNA Healthplan of Illinois, Inc., 1700 Higgins, Suite 600, Des Plaines, IL 60018; tel. 708/699–5600; FAX. 708/699–5675; John W. Rohfritch, Senior Vice President

ChoiceCare Health Plans, Inc., 655 Eden Park Drive, Cincinnati, OH 45202; tel. 513/784–5200; FAX. 513/784–5300; Daniel A. Gregorie, M.D., Chief Executive Office

CompDent Corporation, 1930 Bishop Lane, 16th Floor, Louisville, KY 40218; tel. 800/456–5500, ext. 201; FAX. 502/456–2772; Allan Brockway Morris, President, Chief Executive Officer

Coordinated Care Corporation Indiana, Inc., d/b/a Managed Health Services, 8688 Broadway, Merrillville, IN 46410; tel. 219/756–7134

Delta Dental Plan of Indiana, Inc., 5875 Castle Creek Parkway, North Drive, Indianapolis, IN 46250; tel. 317/842–4022

Dental Care Plus, Inc., 4500 Lake Forest Drive, Suite 512, Cincinnati, OH 45242; tel. 513/554–1100; FAX. 513/554–3187; Dennis K. Coleman, President, Chief Executive Officer

FHP of Illinois, 747 East 22nd Street, Suite 100, Lombard, IL 60148; tel. 708/916–8400

Family Health Plan of Indiana, Inc., 3510 Park Place West, Mishawaka, IN 46545; tel. 219/271–8901; FAX. 219/271–8911; Larry L. Donaldson, Chief Executive Officer

First Commonwealth, Inc., 444 North Wells, Suite 600, Chicago, IL 60610; tel. 312/644–1800, ext. 8638; FAX. 312/644–1822; Mark R. Lundberg, Vice President, Sales

HMO Kentucky, Inc., 9901 Linn Station Road, Louisville, KY 40223; tel. 502/423–2282; FAX. 502/423–6979; G. Douglas Sutherland, President

HMPK, Inc., P.O. Box 740036, Louisville, KY 40201–7436; tel. 502/580–5804; Craig Drablos, Executive Director

HPlan, Inc., 101 East Main Street, 12th Floor, Louisville, KY 40204; tel. 800/245–4446; FAX. 502/580–5044

Health Resources, Inc., 314 Southeast Riverside Drive, P.O. Box 3607, Evansville, IN 47735–3607; tel. 812/424–l444; FAX. 812/424–2096; Edward L. Fritz, D.D.S., President

Healthpoint, LLC, 8900 Keystone Crossing, Suite 500, Indianapolis, IN 46240; tel. 317/574–8181; FAX. 317/574–8182; L. Denise Smith, Administrative Assistant

Healthsource Indiana Managed Care Plan, Inc., 225 South East Street, Suite 240, Indianapolis, IN 46206; tel. 800/933–3466; FAX. 317/687–8500; David H. Smith, Chief Executive Officer

Humana Health Plan, Inc., 500 West Main Street, Louisville, KY 40202; tel. 502/580–1860; FAX. 502/580–3127; Greg Donaldson, Director, Corporate Communications

Humana HealthChicago, Inc., 500 West Main Street, P.O. Box 1438, Louisville, KY 40201–1438; tel. 502/580–1000; Norman J. Beles, President

Indiana Vision Services, Inc., 115 West Washington Street, Suite 1370, Indianapolis, IN 46204; tel. 317/687–1066

M Plan, Inc., 8802 North Meridian Street, Suite 100, Indianapolis, IN 46260; tel. 317/571–5300; FAX. 317/571–5306; Alex Slabosky, President

MIDA Dental Plans, Inc., 2000 Town Center, Suite 2200, Southfield, MI 48075; tel. 810/353–6410; Walter Knysz, Jr., D.D.S., President

Maxicare Health Plans of the Midwest, Maxicare Illinois, 111 East Wacker Dr., Suite 1500, Chicago, IL 60601; tel. 312/616–4700

Maxicare Indiana, Inc., 9480 Priority Way, West Drive, Indianapolis, IN 46240–3899; tel. 317/844–5775; FAX. 317/574–0713; Vicki F. Perry, Vice President, General Manager

Metrahealth Care Plan of Illinois, Inc., 1900 East Golf Road, Suite 501, Schaumburg, IL 60173; tel. 708/619–2222

Metrahealth Care Plan of Kentucky, Inc., Northmark Business Center III, 4501 Erskin, Suite 100, Cincinnati, OH 45242–4713; tel. 513/745–9700; Charles Stark, President

National Foot Care Program, Inc., Pinewood Plaza, 22255 Greenfield, Suite 550, Southfield, MI 48075; tel. 313/559–2579

Partners National Health Plans of Indiana, Inc., One Michiana Square, 100 East Wayne, Suite 502, South Bend, IN 46601; tel. 219/233–4899; FAX. 219/234–7484; Richard C. Born, Senior Vice President Finance, Operations

Physicians Health Network, Inc., One Riverfront Place, Suite 400, P.O. Box 3357, Evansville, IN 47732; tel. 812/465–6000; FAX. 812/465–6014; Kevin M. Clancy, Chairman, President, Chief Executive Officer

Physicians Health Plan of Northern Indiana, Inc., 8101 West Jefferson Boulevard, Fort Wayne, IN 46804; tel. 219/432–6690; FAX. 219/432–0493; John P. Smith, M.D., President

Physicians Health Plan of Northern Indiana, Inc., 8101 West Jefferson Boulevard, Fort Wayne, IN 46804–4163; tel. 800/982–6257; FAX. 219/432–0493

Principal Health Care of Indiana, Inc., One North Pennsylvania, Suite 1100, Indianapolis, IN 46204; tel. 317/263–0920; FAX. 317/972–8249; Douglas Stratton, Executive Director

Prudential Health Care Plan, Inc., PruCare, 24 Greenway Plaza, Suite 500, Houston, TX 77046; tel. 201/716–8174

Riverside Dental Care of Indiana, Inc., 1100 Dennison Avenue, Columbus, OH 43201; tel. 614/297–4870; Richard A. Mitchell, President

Rush Prudential HMO, Inc., 233 South Wacker Drive, Suite 3900, Chicago, IL 60606; tel. 312/234–7000; FAX. 312/234–8555; Carmeline Esposito, Public Relations Manager

Sagamore Health Network, Inc., 11555 North Meridian, Suite 400, Carmel, IN 46032; tel. 317/573–2904; FAX. 317/580–8488; Malinda Hinkle, Vice President, Marketing

Southeastern Indiana Health Organization, Inc. (SIHO), 432 Washington Street, P.O. Box 1787, Columbus, IN 47202–1787; tel. 812/378–7000; FAX. 812/378–7048; Roy H. Flaherty, President, Chief Executive Officer

SpecialMed of Indiana, Inc., 120 Monument Circle, Indianapolis, IN 46204–4903; tel. 317/488–6128; Mike Hostetter, M.D., President

The Dental Concern, Ltd., 222 North LaSalle Street, Suite 2140, Chicago, IL 60601; tel. 312/201–1260; Polly Reese, D.D.S., Dental Director

United Dental Care of Indiana, Inc., 50 South Meridian, Suite 700, Indianapolis, IN 46204–3542; tel. 800/262–5388

Universal Health Services, Inc., 403 West 14th Street, Chicago Heights, IL 60411–2498; tel. 708/755–2462; Ralph R. Crescenzo, President

Welborn Clinic/Welborn HMO, Welborn Health Options, 421 Chestnut Street, Evansville, IN 47713; tel. 812/425–3939; David Christeson, M.D., Medical Director

IOWA

Care Choices HMO, 600 Fourth Street, Terra Centre, Suite 401, Sioux City, IA 51101; tel. 712/252–2344; FAX. 712/233–3684; Karen Pederson, Executive Director

Exclusive Healthcare, Mutual of Omaha Plaza, Omaha, NE 68175; tel. 402/978–2700; FAX. 402/978–2999; Dick L. Easley, President

HMO Nebraska, Inc., 10040 Regency Circle, Suite 300, Omaha, NE 68114; tel. 402/392–2800; Richard L. Guffey, President

Health Alliance Midwest, Inc., 102 East Main Street, Suite 200, P.O. Box 6003, Urbana, IL 61801; tel. 217/337–8000; Robert C. Parker, M.D., President

Heritage National Healthplan, 1515 Fifth Avenue, Suite 200, Moline, IL 61265–1368; tel. 309/765–1200; G. Michael Hammes, President

John Deere Family Health Plan, 1515 Fifth Avenue, Suite 200, Moline, IL 61265–1368; tel. 309/765–1600; G. Michael Hammes, President

Medical Associates Health Plan, Inc., 700 Locust Street, Dubuque, IA 52001–6800; tel. 319/556–8070; FAX. 319/556–5134; Lawrence Cremer, Chief Executive Officer

Principal Health Care of Iowa, Inc., 4600 Westown Parkway, Suite 301, West Des Moines, IA 50266–1099; tel. 515/225–1234; FAX. 515/223–0097; Louis Garcia, Executive Director

Principal Health Care of Nebraska, Inc., 10810 Farnam Drive, Suite 425, Omaha, NE 68154; tel. 402/333–1720; FAX. 402/333–1116; Louis B. Garcia, Executive Director

United HealthCare of Midlands, Inc., 2717 North 118th Circle, Omaha, NE 68164; tel. 402/445–5600; FAX. 402/445–5572; John Michael Braasch, President

KANSAS

BMA Selectcare, Inc., One Penn Valley Park, Zip 64108, P.O. Box 419458, Kansas City, MO 64141; tel. 816/753–8000, ext. 5309; FAX. 816/751–5571; John R. Barton, President

Blue–Care, Inc., 2301 Main, Zip 64108–2428, P.O. Box 413163, Kansas City, MO 64141–6163; tel. 816/395–2222; Richard P. Krecker, President

CIGNA HealthCare of Ohio, Inc., 3700 Corporate Drive, Suite 200, Business Campus N.E. # Five, Columbus, OH 43231; tel. 614/823–7500; FAX. 614/823–7519; James D. Massie, General Manager

Community Health Plan, 5301 Faraon, St. Joseph, MO 64506; tel. 402/978–2425; Joan Copeland, President

Exclusive Healthcare, Inc., 7300 College Boulevard, Suite 208, Overland Park, KS 66210; tel. 913/451–1777; FAX. 913/451–7742; Kim Daniels, Executive Director

FirstGuard Health Plan, Inc., 3801 Blue Parkway, Kansas City, MO 64130; tel. 816/922–7645; Mark Bryant

GenCare Health Systems, Inc., 969 Executive Parkway, Suite 100, P.O. Box 27379, St. Louis, MO 63141–6301; tel. 314/434–6114; FAX. 314/434–6328; Tom Zorumski, President, Chief Executive Officer

HMO Kansas, Inc., 1133 Topeka Boulevard, P.O. Box 110, Topeka, KS 66601–0110; tel. 913/291–8600; John W. Knack, Jr., President

HealthNet, Inc., Two Pershing Square, 2300 Main Street, Suite 700, Kansas City, MO 64108; tel. 816/221–8400; FAX. 816/221–7709; Andrew Dahl, Sc.D., Chief Executive Officer

Healthcare America Plans, Inc., 453 South Webb Road, Wichita, KS 67207–1309; tel. 316/262–7400; FAX. 316/262–1395; Garland L. Bugg, President

Horizon Health Plan, Inc., 623 Southwest 10th Avenue, Suite 300, Topeka, KS 66612–1627; tel. 913/235–0402; Bruce M. Gosser, President

Humana Health Plan, Inc., 10450 Holmes, Suite 330, Kansas City, MO 64131–1471; tel. 816/941–8900; FAX. 816/941–8630; David Fields, Executive Director

Humana Kansas City, Inc., 10405 Holmes, Second Floor, Kansas City, MO 64131–3471; tel. 816/941–8900; Gregory H. Wolf, President

Kaiser Foundation Health Plan of Kansas City, Inc., 10561 Barkley, Suite 200, Overland Park, KS 66212–1886; tel. 913/967–4600; FAX. 913/642–0209; Kathryn Paul, President, Regional Manager

Lawrence Community Health Plan, Inc., 1112 West Sixth, Suite 210, Lawrence, KS 66044; tel. 913/832–6850; FAX. 913/832–6875; Michael J. Herbert, Chief Operating Officer

MetraHealth Care Plan of Kansas City, Inc., (a wholly owned subsidiary of United HealthCare of the Midwest, Inc.), 9300 West 110th Street, Suite 350A, Overland Park, KS 66210; tel. 913/451–5656; FAX. 913/451–0492; Robert S. Bonney, Vice President

Preferred Plus of Kansas, Inc., 345 Riverview, Suite 103, P.O. Box 49288, Wichita, KS 67203; tel. 316/268–0390; Marlon Dauner, President

Premier Health, Inc., d/b/a Premier Blue, 1133 Topeka Avenue, Topeka, KS 66629–0001; tel. 913/291–7000; John W. Knack, Jr., President

Principal Health Care of Kansas City, Inc., 1001 East 101st Terrace, Suite 230, Kansas City, MO 64131; tel. 816/941–3030; FAX. 816/941–8516; Kenneth J. Linde, President

Prudential Health Care Plan, Inc., 4600 Madison Avenue, Suite 300, Kansas City, MO 64112; tel. 816/756–5588; FAX. 816/756–5667; David W. Dingley, Executive Director

Total Health Care, 2301 Main Street, 64108–2428, P.O. Box 413613, Kansas City, MO 64141–6163; tel. 816/395–2222; Richard P. Krecker, President

TriSource HealthCare, Inc., d/b/a Blue Advantage, 2301 Main Street, P.O. Box 419130, Kansas City, MO 64141–6130; tel. 816/395–3636; FAX. 816/395–3811; Larry K. Chastain, President, Chief Executive Officer

Trucare, Inc., 2301 Holmes, Kansas City, MO 64108; tel. 816/556–3186; Joseph Cecil, President

KENTUCKY

Advantage Care, Inc., 700 Bob–O–Link Drive, Suite 200, Lexington, KY 40504–3758; tel. 606/276–0306; FAX. 606/276–2839; Jeffrey P. Johnson, Chief Executive Officer

Aetna Health Plans, 3690 Orange Place, Suite 200, Cleveland, OH 44122; tel. 216/486–8979; David K. Ellwanger, Administrator

Alternative Health Delivery Systems, 1901 Campus Place, Blankenbaker Crossing, Louisville, KY 40299; tel. 502/261–2100; Cheryl Kutchinski, Vice President, Operations

American Health Network of Kentucky, Inc., 300 West Main, Suite 100, Louisville, KY 40202; tel. 502/681–0960; Denise Schifano, Regional Director, Operations

Anthem Blue Cross Blue Shield, 9901 Linn Station Road, Louisville, KY 40223; tel. 502/423–2277; FAX. 502/423–2729; Robert McIntire, Vice President

Anthem Blue Cross and Blue Shield, 9901 Linn Station Road, Louisville, KY 40223; tel. 502/423–2373; FAX. 502/423–6974; George L. Walker, Chief Operating Officer

Bluegrass Family Health, Inc., 651 Perimeter Drive, Suite Two B, Lexington, KY 40517; tel. 606/269–4475; Katherine Schaefer

CHA Health, 3220 Nicholasville Road, Suite 11, Zip 40503, P.O. Box 23468, Lexington, KY 40523–3468; tel. 606/257–8074; Ronald K. Davy, Chief Executive Officer

ChoiceCare, 655 Eden Park Drive, Cincinnati, OH 45202; tel. 513/784–5200; FAX. 513/784–5300; Daniel Gregorie, M.D., President, Chief Executive Officer

FHP Health Care, 11260 Chester Road, Suite 800, Cincinnati, OH 45246; tel. 513/772–7325; John Davren

HMPK, 101 East Main Street, Louisville, KY 40202; tel. 502/580–5005; FAX. 502/580–5044; Betty Chowning, Executive Director

HPLAN, Inc., P.O. Box 740023, Louisville, KY 40201; tel. 502/580–5804; Craig Drablos, Executive Director

Healthsource Kentucky, Inc., 100 Mallard Creek Road, Suite 300, Louisville, KY 40207; tel. 502/899–7500; Paul E. Stamp, Interim Executive Director

Healthwise of Kentucky, Ltd., 2409 Harodsburg Road, Lexington, KY 40504; tel. 606/296–6100; FAX. 606/255–9134; Harold Bischoff, Executive Director

Heritage National Healthplan, Inc., 909 River Drive, Moline, IL 61265; tel. 309/765–7660; Douglas R. Niska, Director

Humana Health Plan, Inc., 101 East Main Street, Louisville, KY 40202; tel. 502/580–5005; FAX. 502/580–5018; Craig A. Drablos, Executive Director

MetraHealth Care Plan of Kentucky, 4501 Erskine Road, Suite 150, Cincinnati, OH 45242; tel. 502/339–8481; Charles Stark, Administrator

Owensboro Community Health Plan, 2211 Mayfair Avenue, Suite 205, Owensboro, KY 42301; tel. 502/686–6368; Ronald T. Derstadt, Executive Director

Prudential HealthCare, 312 Elm Street, Suite 1400, Cincinnati, OH 45202; tel. 513/784–7500; FAX. 513/784–7020; Kim Bellard, Executive Director

LOUISIANA

Advantage Health Plan, Inc., 829 St. Charles Avenue, New Orleans, LA 70130; tel. 504/568–9009; FAX. 504/568–0301; Jane Cooper, President, Chief Executive Officer

Aetna Health Plans of Louisiana, Inc., 3900 North Causeway Boulevard, Suite 410, Metairie, LA 70002–7283; tel. 504/830–5600; FAX. 504/837–6571; Michael L. Rogers, President

Apex Healthcare of Louisiana, Inc., 639 Loyola Avenue, Suite 1725, New Orleans, LA 70113; tel. 504/585–0508; Warwick D. Syphers

CIGNA HealthCare of Louisiana, Inc., 4354 South Sherwood Forest Boulevard, Suite 240, Baton Rouge, LA 70816; tel. 504/295–2800; FAX. 504/295–2888; Nancy T. Horstmann, Executive Director

CIGNA HealthCare of North Louisiana, Inc., 4354 South Sherwood Forest Boulevard, Suite 240, Baton Rouge, LA 70816; tel. 504/295–2800; FAX. 504/295–2888; Nancy T. Horstmann, Executive Director

Capitol Health Network, Inc., 4700 Wichers Drive, Suite 300, Marrero, LA 70072; tel. 504/347–4515; John Sudderth, Chief Executive Officer

Community Health Network of Louisiana, 2431 South Acadian Thruway, Suite 350, P.O. Box 80159, Baton Rouge, LA 70898–0159; tel. 504/237–2106; FAX. 504/237–2222; Glen J. Golemi, President, Chief Executive Officer

Foundation Health, Louisiana Health Plan, Inc., 5353 Essen Lane, Suite 450, Baton Rouge, LA 70809; tel. 504/763–5300; Joseph Klinger

Futurecare Health Plans of Louisiana, Inc., 3029 South Sherwood Forest Boulevard, Suite 300, Baton Rouge, LA 70816; tel. 800/764–5201; David P. Giles

Gulf South Health Plans, Inc., 5615 Corporate Boulevard, Suite Three, P.O. Box 80339, Baton Rouge, LA 70898–0339; tel. 504/237–1700; FAX. 504/237–1939; Jack W. Walker, President

HMO of Louisiana, Inc., P.O. Box 98029, Baton Rouge, LA 70898–8024; tel. 504/295–2383; FAX. 504/295–2491; Michael A. Hayes, Executive Director

Section C

Health Plus of Louisiana, Inc., 2600 Greenwood Road, Shreveport, LA 71103; tel. 318/632–4590; FAX. 318/632–4463; Peter J. Babin, President

Humana Health Plan of Louisiana, Inc., 500 West Main Street, P.O. Box 740036, Louisville, KY 40201–7436; tel. 502/580–1000; James E. Murray, Vice President, Finance

Life Net Health Plans HMO, Inc., 9100 Bluebonnet Centre Boulevard, Suite 200, Baton Rouge, LA 70809; tel. 504/295–7000; Robert Jackson

Maxicare Louisiana, Inc., 3850 North Causeway Boulevard, Suite 990, Metairie, LA 70002; tel. 504/836–2022; FAX. 504/835–0493; Alan M. Preston, Vice President, General Manager

Medfirst Health Plans of Louisiana, Inc., 3500 North Causeway Boulevard, Suite 520, Metairie, LA 70002; tel. 504/837–4000; FAX. 504/831–1107; Carol A. Solomon, President

MetraHealth Corporation, 3900 North Causeway Boulevard, Suite 860, Metairie, LA 70002; tel. 504/832–7655; FAX. 504/836–5506; Susan Sharkey, Vice President, Executive Director

NYLCare Health Plans of Louisiana, Inc., 2014 West Pinhook Road, Suite 200, Lafayette, LA 70508; tel. 800/825–0568; FAX. 318/237–1703; Burley J. Pellerin II, Director, Operations

Ochsner Health Plan, Inc. (HMO), One Galleria Boulevard, Suite 1224, Metairie, LA 70001; tel. 504/836–6600; FAX. 504/836–6566; R. Lyle Luman, President, Chief Executive Officer

OmniCare Health Plan of Louisiana, Inc., 400 Poydras Street, Suite 2400, New Orleans, LA 70130; tel. 504/523–9751; FAX. 504/523–2638; Joan G. Savoy, Director, Operations

Principal Health Care of Louisiana, 3421 North Causeway Boulevard, Suite 600, Metairie, LA 70002; tel. 504/834–0840; FAX. 504/834–2694; Erin R. Glynn, Executive Director

SMA HMO, Inc., 111 Veteran's Memorial Boulevard, Heritage Plaza, Suite 500, Metairie, LA 70005; tel. 504/837–7374; FAX. 504/837–7366; Barbara B. Louviere, President

Sunbelt Health Plan of Louisiana, Inc., 3434 South Causeway Boulevard, Suite 901, Metairie, LA 70001; tel. 504/922–9142; John F. Ales

Vantage Health Plan, Inc., 909 North 18th Street, Suite 201, Monroe, LA 71201; tel. 318/323–2269; Angela Olden, Executive Director

MAINE

AssureCare of Maine, Inc., 2367 Congress Street, Portland, ME 04102; tel. 800/600–5905; Courtney Hudson, Vice President

Blue Cross and Blue Shield of Maine, Two Gannett Drive, South Portland, ME 04106; tel. 800/527–7706; Nancy Hutchings, Director, Customer Service

Harvard Community Health Plan, Inc., 10 Brookline Place West, Brookline, MA 02146; tel. 617/421–6400; Laura Peabody, Assistant General Counsel

Health Plans, Inc., 202 US Route One, P.O. Box 165, Falmouth, ME 04105; tel. 207/781–9890; FAX. 207/828–2408; Jeffrey W. Kirby, Controller

Healthsource Maine, Inc., Two Stonewood Drive, P.O. Box 447, Freeport, ME 04032–0447; tel. 207/865–5000, ext. 5201; FAX. 207/865–5632; Richard White, Chief Executive Officer

Healthsource New Hampshire, Donovan Street Extension, P.O. Box 2041, Concord, NH 03302; tel. 603/225–5077; FAX. 603/225–7621; Susan Berry, Director, Marketing

NYLCare of Maine Health Plans, Inc., One Monument Square, Portland, ME 04102; tel. 207/791–7916; Charlotte Pease, Manager

Tufts Health Plan of New England, Inc., 333 Wyman Street, Waltham, MA 02254–9112; tel. 617/466–9055; Theresa Gallinaro, Manager

MARYLAND

Aetna Health Plans of the Mid–Atlantic, Inc., 7600 A Leesburg Pike, Falls Church, VA 22043; tel. 703/903–7100; Jon Glaudemans, Vice President, Health Services

CIGNA Healthplan of the MidAtlantic, Inc., 9700 Patuxent Woods Drive, Columbia, MD 21046; tel. 410/720–5800; FAX. 410/720–5860

Capital Care, Inc., 550 12th Street, S.W., Washington, DC 20065; tel. 202/479–3678; FAX. 202/479–3660; M. Bruce Edwards, President

Chesapeake Health Plan, Inc., Executive Office, 814 Light Street, Baltimore, MD 21230; tel. 410/539–8622; FAX. 410/752–0271; Leon Kaplan, President, Chief Executive Officer

Columbia Medical Plan, Inc., Two Knoll North Drive, Columbia, MD 21045; tel. 410/997–8500; FAX. 410/964–4563; Marilyn M. Levinson, Director, Patient Services

Delmarva Health Care Plan, 106 Marlboro Road, P.O. Box 2410, Easton, MD 21601; tel. 410/822–7223; FAX. 410/822–8152; Richard Moore, President

Free State Health Plan, Inc., 100 South Charles Street, Tower II, Baltimore, MD 21201; tel. 410/528–7000

George Washington University Health Plan, Inc., 4550 Montgomery Avenue, Suite 800, Bethesda, MD 20814; tel. 301/941–2000; FAX. 301/941–2005; Lawrence E. Berman, Director, Government Relations and Legal Affairs

Healthcare Corporation of Mid–Atlantic, 100 South Charles Street, Baltimore, MD 21201; tel. 301/828–7000; David D. Wolf, Chief Executive Officer

Healthcare Corporation of the Potomac, Inc., Care First–Free State Potomac, Equitable Bank Center's Tower–II, 100 South Charles Street, Baltimore, MD 21201; tel. 410/528–7025; FAX. 410/528–7013; David Wolf, President

Humana Group Health Association, Inc., 4301 Connecticut Avenue, N.W., Washington, DC 20008; tel. 202/364–2000; FAX. 202/364–7418; Robert P. Pfotenhauer, President, Chief Executive Officer

Kaiser Foundation Health Plan of the Mid–Atlantic States, Inc., 2101 East Jefferson Street, Rockville, MD 20852; tel. 301/816–6420; FAX. 301/816–7478; Cleve Killingsworth, President

MD Individual Practice Association, MDIPA/Optimum, Four Taft Court, Rockville, MD 20850; tel. 301/762–8205; FAX. 301/762–2479; Steve B. Griffin, President

NYL Care Health Plans of the Mid–Atlantic, Inc., 7601 Ora Glen Drive, Suite 200, Greenbelt, MD 20770; tel. 301/982–0098, ext. 3308; FAX. 301/489–5282; Jeff D. Emerson, President, Chief Executive Officer

Optimum Choice, Inc., Four Taft Court, Rockville, MD 20850; tel. 301/762–8205

PHN–HMO, Inc., 5700 Executive Drive, Suite 104, Baltimore, MD 21228–1798; tel. 410/747–9060; FAX. 410/788–7543; L. David Taylor, President, Chief Executive Officer

Physicians Health Plan, Inc., 2111 Wilson Boulevard, Suite 1150, Arlington, VA 22201; tel. 703/525–0602; FAX. 703/243–3066; Suellen Rainey, Executive Director

Primehealth Corporation, 9602 C Martin Luther King Jr. Highway, Lanham, MD 20706; Edward L. Mosley, Jr., President

Principal Health Care Plan of the Mid–Atlantic, Inc., 1801 Rockville Pike, Suite 110, Rockville, MD 20852; tel. 301/881–4903; FAX. 301/881–9808; Julia Campion, Executive Director

Principal Health Care of Delaware, Inc., One Corporate Commons, 100 West Commons Boulevard, Suite 300, New Castle, DE 19720; tel. 302/322–4700

Prudential Health Care Plan, Inc., Seton Court, 2800 North Charles Street, Baltimore, MD 21218; tel. 410/554–7000; FAX. 410/554–7070

Total Health Care, Inc., 2305 North Charles Street, Baltimore, MD 21218; tel. 410/383–8300; FAX. 410/554–9012; Edwin R. Golden, President

U.S. Healthcare, 980 Jolly Road, Blue Bell, PA 19422; tel. 215/628–4800; FAX. 215/283–6858

MASSACHUSETTS

CIGNA HealthCare of Massachusetts, Inc., 20 Speen Street, Third Floor, Framingham, MA 01701; tel. 508/935–2100

Central Massachusetts Health Care, Mechanics Tower, 100 Front Street, Suite 300, Worcester, MA 01608; tel. 508/798–8667; FAX. 508/798–4197, ext. 4201; Brian D. Wells, Chief Executive Officer

Community Health Plan, One CHP Plaza, Latham, NY 12110–1080; tel. 800/638–0668; Fred H. Hooven, Regional Administrator

ConnectiCare of Massachusetts, Inc., P.O. Box 522, Farmington, CT 06032–0522; tel. 800/474–1466

Coordinated Health Partners, Inc., d/b/a Blue Chip/Coordinated Health Partners, Inc., 30 Chestnut Street, Providence, RI 02903; tel. 401/459–5500; James E. Bobbitt, Chief Operating Officer

Fallon Community Health Plan, One Chestnut Place, 10 Chestnut Street, Worcester, MA 01608; tel. 508/799–2100; FAX. 508/831–0921; Gary J. Zelch, Executive Director

HMO Blue, 100 Summer Street, Boston, MA 02110; tel. 617/832–7797; FAX. 617/832–7973; Maureen Coneys, Executive Director

Harvard Community Health Plan, 10 Brookline Place West, Brookline, MA 02146; tel. 617/731–8240; FAX. 617/730–4695; Manuel M. Ferris, President, Chief Executive Officer

Harvard Pilgrim Health Care, 10 Brookline Place West, Brookline, MA 02146; tel. 617/745–1000; FAX. 617/982–9668; Allan Greenberg, Chief Executive Officer

Harvard Pilgrim Health Care of New England, One Hoppin Street, Providence, RI 02903–4199; tel. 401/331–3000; FAX. 401/331–0496; Stephen Schoenbaum, M.D., Medical Director

Health New England, One Monarch Place, Springfield, MA 01144; tel. 413/787–4000; FAX. 413/734–3356; Phil M. Pin, Interim President

Healthsource New Hampshire, 54 Regional Drive, P.O. Box 2041, Concord, NH 03302–2041; tel. 603/225–5077; FAX. 603/229–2983; Donna K. Lencki, Chief Executive Officer

Kaiser Foundation Health Plan, 170 University Drive, P.O. Box 862, Amherst, MA 01002; tel. 413/256–0151, ext. 5162; FAX. 413/549–1601; Linda Todaro, Massachusetts Area Administrator

Neighborhood Health Plan, 253 Summer Street, Boston, MA 02210; tel. 617/772–5500; FAX. 617/772–5513; James Hooley, Chief Executive Officer

Prudential HealthCare of New England, 10 New England Business Center, Suite 200, P.O. Box 1827, Andover, MA 01810; tel. 508/681–4723; FAX. 508/659–4198; Larry L. Hsu, M.D., Executive Director

Tufts Health Plan, 333 Wyman Street, P.O. Box 9112, Waltham, MA 02254–9112; tel. 617/466–9400; FAX. 617/466–9430; Harris A. Berman, M.D., President, Chief Executive Officer

Tufts Health Plan of New England, Inc., 333 Wyman Street, P.O. Box 9112, Walthma, MA 02254–9112; tel. 800/442–0422

U.S. Healthcare, Inc., Three Burlington Woods Drive, Burlington, MA 01803; tel. 617/273–5600; Robert Roy, M.D., Medical Director

United Health Plans of NE, Inc., 475 Kilvert Street, Warwick, RI 02886–1392; tel. 800/447–1245; FAX. 401/732–7208; Robert K. Winston, Director, Corporate Communications

MICHIGAN

Apex Healthcare, Inc., 104 Inverness Center Parkway, Suite 320, Birmingham, AL 35242; tel. 205/991–3233

Blue Care Network of East Michigan, 4200 Fashion Square Boulevard, Saginaw, MI 48603; tel. 517/249–3200; FAX. 517/249–3730; Arnold C. DuFort, President, Chief Executive Officer

Blue Care Network of Southeast Michigan, 25925 Telegraph, P.O. Box 5043, Southfield, MI 48086–5043; tel. 313/354–7450; FAX. 313/799–6970; David H. Smith, President, Chief Executive Officer

Blue Care Network–Great Lakes, 1769 South Garfield Avenue, Suite B, Traverse City, MI 49684; tel. 616/941–6000, ext. 6030; FAX. 616/941–6012; Sharon Carlin, Regional Director

Blue Care Network–Great Lakes, 3624 South Westnedge, Kalamazoo, MI 49008; tel. 616/388–9500; FAX. 616/388–5156; Marcia Lallaman, Regional Manager

Blue Care Network–Great Lakes, 611 Cascade West Parkway, S.E., Grand Rapids, MI 49546; tel. 616/957–5057; FAX. 616/956–5866; Sharon Carlin, President, Chief Executive Officer

Blue Care Network–Great Lakes, 3375 Merriam Avenue, Muskegon Heights, MI 49444–3173; tel. 616/739–6600; FAX. 616/739–6670; Barbara Carlson, Regional Manager

Blue Care Network–Health Central, 1403 South Creyts Road, Lansing, MI 48917; tel. 517/322–8000; FAX. 517/322–8015; Arnold C. DuFort, President, Chief Executive Officer

Care Choices HMO, Mercy Health Plans, 34605 Twelve Mile Road, Farmington Hills, MI 48331; tel. 313/489–6203; FAX. 810/489–6278; Robert J. Flanagan, Ph.D., President, Chief Executive Officer

Care Choices–Brighton, 7990 West Grand River, Brighton, MI 48116; tel. 810/229–6866; FAX. 810/229–6811; Louise Zackmann

Care Choices–Eastern Michigan, South East Region–Michigan, 2000 Hogback Road, Suite 15, Ann Arbor, MI 48105; tel. 313/971–7667; FAX. 313/971–7455; Dennis Angellis, M.D., Medical Director, South East Region

Care Choices–Grand Rapids, 1500 East Beltline S.E., Suite 300, Grand Rapids, MI 49506; tel. 616/285–3801; FAX. 616/285–3810; Janie Begeman, Site Manager

Care Choices–Lansing, 2111 University Park, Suite 100, Okemos, MI 48864; tel. 517/349–2111; FAX. 517/349–6449; Jeffrey Ash, Executive Director

Care Choices–Muskegon, 950 West Norton Avenue, Suite 500, Muskegon, MI 49441; tel. 616/737–0307; FAX. 616/733–6352; Molly McCarthy, Site Director

Family Health Plan of Michigan, 901 North Macomb, Monroe, MI 48162–3048; tel. 313/457–5370; FAX. 313/457–5506; Robert Campbell, Executive Vice President

Grand Valley Health Plan, 829 Forest Hill Avenue, S.E., Grand Rapids, MI 49546; tel. 616/949–2410; FAX. 616/949–4978; Roland Palmer, President

Great Lakes Health Plan, Inc., 17117 West Nine Mile Road, Suite 1600, Southfield, MI 48075; tel. 810/559–5656; FAX. 810/559–4640; Donald A. Zinner, President

Health Alliance Plan, 2850 West Grand Boulevard, Detroit, MI 48202; tel. 313/874–8310; FAX. 313/874–8301; Joseph E. Schmitt, Chief Financial Officer

HealthPlus of Michigan, 2050 South Linden Road, P.O. Box 1700, Flint, MI 48501–1700; tel. 810/230–2000; FAX. 810/230–2208; Paul A. Fuhs, Ph.D., President, Chief Executive Officer

HealthPlus of Michigan–Saginaw, 5560 Gratiot Avenue, Saginaw, MI 48603; tel. 517/797–4000; FAX. 517/799–6471; Bruce Hill, Regional Vice President

M–Care, 2301 Commonwealth Boulevard, Ann Arbor, MI 48105–1573; tel. 313/747–8700; FAX. 313/747–7152; Peter W. Roberts, President

NorthMed HMO, 109 East Front Street, Suite 204, Traverse City, MI 49684; tel. 616/935–0500; FAX. 616/935–0505; Walter J. Hooper III, President

OmniCare Health Plan, 1155 Brewery Park, Suite 250, Detroit, MI 48207–2602; tel. 313/259–4000, ext. 4570; FAX. 313/393–7944; Ronald R. Dobbins, President, Chief Executive Officer

PHP–Kalamazoo, 106 Farmers Alley, P.O. Box 50271, Kalamazoo, MI 49005; tel. 616/349–6692; FAX. 616/349–1476; Michael Koehler, Executive Director

Parmount Care of Michigan, Inc., 1339 North Telegraph Road, Monroe, MI 48162; tel. 313/241–5604; FAX. 313/241–5998; Robert J. Kolodgy, Vice President, Finance

Physicians Health Plan, P.O. Box 30377, Lansing, MI 48909–7877; tel. 517/349–2101; FAX. 517/347–9460; John G. Ruther, President, Chief Executive Officer

Physicians Health Plan–Jackson, 209 East Washington Avenue, Suite 315 E, Jackson, MI 49201; tel. 517/782–7154; FAX. 517/782–4512; Susan K. Sharkey, Chief Executive Officer

Physicians Health Plan–Muskegon, Terrace Plaza, 250 Morris Avenue, Suite 550, Muskegon, MI 49440–1143; tel. 616/728–3900; FAX. 616/728–5189; Ronald Franzese, Chief Executive Officer

Priority Health, 1231 East Beltline, Suite 300, Grand Rapids, MI 49505; tel. 616/942–0954; FAX. 616/942–0145; Vic Turvey, President, Chief Executive Officer

Priority Health Managed Benefits, Inc., 1231 East Beltline, N.E., Grand Rapids, MI 49503; tel. 800/942–0954; FAX. 616/942–5651; Kimberly K. Horn, Chief Executive Officer

SelectCare HMO, Inc., 2401 West Big Beaver Road, Suite 700, Troy, MI 48084; tel. 810/637–5300, ext. 5571; FAX. 810/637–6710; Roman T. Kulich, President, Chief Executive Officer

The Wellness Plan, Comprehensive Health Services, Inc., 6500 John C. Lodge, Detroit, MI 48202; tel. 313/875–6960; FAX. 313/875–7416; Sharon P. Matthews, Regional Administrator

The Wellness Plan, 1060 West Norton Avenue, Suite Four B, Muskegon, MI 49442; tel. 616/780–4722; FAX. 616/780–3557; Evangeline Zimmerman, Health Systems Manager

The Wellness Plan, One East First Street, Genesse Tower, Suite 1620, Flint, MI 48502; tel. 810/767–7400; FAX. 810/767–6338; Sharon P. Matthews, Regional Administrator

The Wellness Plan, 320 North Washington Square, Lansing, MI 48933; tel. 517/484–1400; FAX. 517/484–8801; Mary Anne Sesti, Health Systems Manager

Total Health Care, Inc., 1600 Fisher Building, Detroit, MI 48202; tel. 313/871–7800; FAX. 313/871–0196; Kenneth G. Rimmer, Executive Director

MINNESOTA

Blue Plus, P.O. Box 64179, St. Paul, MN 55164; tel. 612/456–8438; FAX. 612/456–6768; Mark Banks, M.D., President, Chief Executive Officer

First Plan HMO, 1010 Fourth Street, Two Harbors, MN 55616; tel. 218/834–7210; John Bjorum, Executive Director

HealthPartners, 8100–34th Avenue South, P.O. Box 1309, Minneapolis, MN 55440–1309; tel. 612/883–5382; FAX. 612/883–5120; George Halvorson, President, Chief Executive Director

HealthPartners, 8100–34th Avenue South, P.O. Box 1309, Minneapolis, MN 55440–1309; tel. 612/883–7000; George Halvorson, President, Chief Executive Officer

Mayo Health Plan, 21 First Street S.W., Suite 401, Rochester, MN 55902; tel. 507/284–5811; FAX. 507/284–0528; Shirley A. Weis, Executive Director

Medica Choice, 5601 Smetana Drive, Minneapolis, MN 55440–7001; tel. 612/992–5450; James Ehlen, M.D., Chief Executive Officer

Medica Health Plans, 5601 Smetana Drive, P.O. Box 9310, Minneapolis, MN 55440–9310; tel. 612/992–3952; FAX. 612/992–3998; David Strand, President

Metropolitan Health Plan, 822 South Third Street, Suite 140, Minneapolis, MN 55415; tel. 612/347–2340; FAX. 612/904–4214; John Bluford, Executive Director

Northern Plains Health Plan, 1000 South Columbia Road, Grand Forks, ND 58201; tel. 800/675–2467; FAX. 701/780–1683; Tim Sayler, Executive Director

UCARE Minnesota, 2550 University Avenue, W., Suite 201 S, St. Paul, MN 55114; tel. 612/647–2630; FAX. 612/603–0650; Nancy Feldman, Chief Executive Officer

MISSISSIPPI

AmeriCan Medical Plans of Mississippi, Inc., 633 North State Street, Suite 211, Jackson, MS 39202; tel. 601/968–9000; FAX. 601/968–9800; Rissa P. Richardson, Director, Provider Relations

Apex Healthcare of Mississippi, Inc., 405 Briarwood Drive, Suite 104A, Jackson, MS 39206; tel. 601/991–0505

Canton Management Group, Inc., 3330 South Liberty Street, Suite 300, Canton, MS 39046; tel. 601/859–4450

Cigna Healthcare of Tennessee, Inc., 6555 Quince Road, Suite 215, Memphis, TN 38119; tel. 901/755–7411; David O. Hollis, M.D., Medical Director

Family Healthcare Plus, 118 Service Drive, Suite 10, Brandon, MS 39042; tel. 601/825–7280

HMO of Mississippi, Inc., 3545 Lakeland Drive, Jackson, MS 39208; tel. 601/932–3704; Thomas C. Fenter, M.D., Executive Director

Health Link, Inc., 830 South Gloster Street, Tupelo, MS 38801; tel. 800/453–7536; FAX. 800/453–0648; Pamela J. Hansen, Director

Integrity Health Plan of Mississippi, Inc., 6360 I–55 North, Suite 460, Jackson, MS 39211; tel. 601/977–0010; FAX. 601/977–0019; Robert S. Parenteau, Director, Marketing

Mississippi Managed Care Network, Inc., 713 South Pear Orchard Road, Suite B–102, Ridgeland, MS 39157; tel. 601/977–9834; FAX. 601/977–9553; Jesse Buie, President

Phoenix Healthcare of Mississippi, Inc., 795 Woodlands Parkway, Suite 200, Ridgeland, MS 39157; tel. 601/956–2706; FAX. 601/957–0847; Stephen G. Braden, Executive Director

PrimeHealth of Alabama, Inc., 1400 University Boulevard, South, Mobile, AL 36609; tel. 334/342–0022

Prudential Health Care Plan, Inc., One Prudential Circle, Sugar Land, TX 77478–3833; tel. 713/276–3940

South East Managed Care Organization, Inc., (SEMCOs Magnolia Health Plan), 713 South Pear Orchard Road, Suite 404, Ridgeland, MS 39157; tel. 601/977–7557, ext. 9001; Elizabeth M. Mitchell, President, Chief Executive Officer

United HealthCare of Mississippi, Inc., 713 South Pear Orchard Road, Suite 205, Ridgeland, MS 39157; tel. 601/956–8030; FAX. 601/957–1306; Charles C. Pitts, Chief Executive Officer

MISSOURI

Alliance for Community Health, Inc., d/b/a Community Care Plus, 5615 Pershing, Suite 29, St. Louis, MO 63112; tel. 314/454–0055, ext. 234; FAX. 314/454–9595; James D. Sweat, Chief Executive Officer

AmeriCan Medical Plans of Missouri, Inc., 4741 Central Avenue, Suite 358, Kansas City, MO 64112; tel. 816/561–2883

BMA Selectcare, Inc., One Penn Valley Park, P.O. Box 419458, Kansas City, MO 64141; tel. 816/751–5336; FAX. 816/751–5571; Sara L. Adams, Vice President

CIGNA HealthCare of Kansas/Missouri, 7400 West 110th Street, Suite 600, Overland Park, KS 66210; tel. 913/339–4700; FAX. 913/451–0974; Cynthia Finter, President, General Manager

CIGNA HealthCare of St. Louis, Inc., 8182 Maryland Avenue, Suite 900, St. Louis, MO 63105–3721; tel. 314/726–7860; FAX. 314/726–7819; Jim Young, General Manager, President

Childrens Mercy Family Plan, 2401 Gilham Road, Kansas City, MO 64108

Childrens Mercy Hospital/Truman Medical Center Family Health Partners, Inc., d/b/a Family Health Partners, 2301 Holmes Road, Kansas City, MO 64108; tel. 816/234–3000

Community Health Plan, 801 Faraon, St. Joseph, MO 64501; tel. 816/271–1247; FAX. 816/271–1248; Joan E. Copeland, Executive Vice President, Chief Operating Officer

Exclusive Healthcare, Inc., Mutual of Omaha Plaza, Omaha, NE 68175; tel. 402/978–2869; FAX. 402/978–2999; Kurt Irlbeck, Administrative Services Coordinator

FirstGuard Health Plan, Inc., 3801 Blue Parkway, Kansas City, MO 64130; tel. 816/922–7250; FAX. 816/922–7251; Joy Haug, Executive Director, Chief Operating Officer

Gencare Health Systems, Inc., d/b/a Sanus Health Plan, Inc., P.O.Box 27379, St. Louis, MO 63141–6301; tel. 800/627–0687, ext. 3307; FAX. 314/469–9854; Thomas Zorumski, Chief Executive Officer

Good Health HMO, Inc., d/b/a Blue–Care, Inc., One Pershing Square, 2301 Main Street, Kansas City, MO 64108; tel. 816/395–3636; FAX. 816/395–3811; Larry K. Chastain, President, Chief Operating Officer

Group Health Plan, Inc., 940 West Port Plaza, Suite 300, St. Louis, MO 63146; tel. 314/453–1700; FAX. 314/453–0375; Richard H. Jones, President, Chief Executive Officer

HMO Missouri, Inc., d/b/a BlueChoice, 4444 Forest Park, St. Louis, MO 63108–2292; tel. 314/658–4444; FAX. 314/289–6239; Seymour Kaplan, President, Chief Executive Officer

HealthCare American Plans, Inc., P.O. Box 780467, Wichita, KS 67278–0467

HealthFirst Health Management Organization, 1102 West 32nd Street, Joplin, MO 64804–3599

HealthLink HMO, Inc., d/b/a HealthLink HMO, 777 Craig Road, Suite 110, Creve Coeur, MO 63141; tel. 314/569–7200; FAX. 314/569–3268; Dennis McCart, Executive Director

HealthNet, Inc., 2300 Main Street, Suite 700, Kansas City, MO 64108–2415; tel. 816/221–8400; FAX. 816/221–7709; Beth Johnson, Executive Assistant

Healthcare USA of Missouri LLC, 100 South Fourth Street, Suite 1100, St. Louis, MO 63102; tel. 800/213–7792; FAX. 314/241–8010; Davina Lane, President, Chief Executive Officer

Humana Health Plan, Inc., 11861 Westline Industrial Boulevard, Maryland Heights, MO 63146; tel. 314/993–3593

Humana Kansas City, Inc., 10450 Holmes Road, Kansas City, MO 64131–3471; tel. 816/941–8900; FAX. 816/941–3910; David W. Fields, Executive Director

Kaiser Foundation Health Plan of Kansas City, Inc., 10561 Barkley, Suite 200, Overland Park, KS 66212–1886; tel. 913/967–4600; Robert Biblo, Regional Manager

Medical Center Health Plan, d/b/a Partners HMO, One City Place Drive, Suite 670, St. Louis, MO 63141; tel. 314/567–6660; FAX. 314/567–3627; Del Snoberger, Executive Director

Mercy Health Plans of Missouri, Inc., d/b/a Premier Health Plans, 12935 North Outer Forty Drive, Suite 200, St. Louis, MO 63141–8636; tel. 314/214–8100; FAX. 314/214–8101; Thomas L. Kelly, President

MetraHealth Care Plan of Kansas City, Inc., (a wholly owned subsidiary of United HealthCare of the Midwest, Inc.), 9300 West 110th Street, Suite 350A, Building 55, Overland Park, KS 66210; tel. 913/451–5656; Robert S. Bonney, Vice President

Missouri Advantage LLC, P.O. Box 699, 113 East Broadway, Bolivar, MO 65613; tel. 417/777–6000; FAX. 417/777–4603; Kevin G. McRoberts, Executive Director

Physicians Health Plan of Greater St. Louis, Inc., 77 West Port Plaza, Suite 500, St. Louis, MO 63146; tel. 314/275–7000; FAX. 314/542–1155; Thomas Zorumski, President, Chief Executive Officer

Physicians Health Plan of Midwest, Inc., 77 Westport Plaza, Suite 500, St. Louis, MO 63146; tel. 314/275–7000; FAX. 314/542–1155

Principal Health Care Plan of St. Louis, Inc., 12312 Olive Boulevard, Suite 150, St. Louis, MO 63141; tel. 314/434–6990; FAX. 314/434–7540; Barbara C. Buenemann, Executive Director

Principal Health Care of Kansas City, Inc., 1001 East 101st Terrace, Suite 300, Kansas City, MO 64131; tel. 816/941–3030; FAX. 816/941–8516; Jan Stallmeyer, Executive Director

Prudential Health Care Plan, Inc., 12312 Olive Boulevard, Suite 500, St. Louis, MO 63141; tel. 314/567–1100; Gary C. Hawkins, Executive Director

TriSource HealthCare, Inc., d/b/a Blue Advantage HMO, 2400 Pershing, Suite 310, Kansas City, MO 64108; tel. 816/395–2016; FAX. 816/395–3325; Tom Bowser, Chief Operating Officer, HMO Programs

Truman Medical Center, Inc., 2301 Holmes Street, Kansas City, MO 64108; tel. 816/556–3094; James J. Mongan, M.D., Executive Director

MONTANA

Glacier Community Health Plan, 1297 Burns Way, Suite Three, Kalispell, MT 59901; tel. 406/758–6900; FAX. 406/758–6907; Patsy Stinger, Administrative Assistant

HMO Montana, 404 Fuller Avenue, Helena, MT 59604; tel. 406/447–8753; Carol Wood, Manager

Yellowstone Community Health Plan, 1222 North 27th Street, Suite 201, Billings, MT 59101; tel. 406/238–6868; FAX. 406/238–6898; Jennifer A. Parise, Director, Marketing

NEBRASKA

Care Choices HMO, 34605 Twelve Mile Road, Farmington Hills, MI 48331; tel. 810/489–6200

Exclusive Healthcare, Inc., Mutual of Omaha Plaza, Omaha, NE 68175; tel. 402/978–2700; Dick L. Easley, President

HMO Nebraska, Inc., P.O. Box 241739, Omaha, NE 68124–5739; tel. 402/392–2800; FAX. 402/392–2761; Maxine E. Crossley, Executive Vice President, Chief Operating Officer

Humana Health Plan, Inc., 101 East Main Street, Louisville, KY 40202; tel. 502/580–5005

Mutual of Omaha Health Plans of Lincoln, Inc., 220 South 17th Street, Lincoln, NE 68508; tel. 402/475–7000; FAX. 402/475–6005; Steve Burnham, Chief Operating Officer

Principal Health Care of Nebraska, Inc., 330 North 117th Street, Omaha, NE 68154–2595; tel. 402/333–1720; FAX. 402/333–1116; Ken Klaasmeyer, Executive Director

United Health Care of Midlands, Inc., d/b/a Share Health Plan of Nebraska, Inc., 2717 North 118 Circle, Omaha, NE 68164; tel. 402/445–5000; Sara Hemenway, Marketing Communications Manager

NEVADA

Amil International of Nevada, 1050 East Flamingo Road, Suite E–120, Las Vegas, NV 89119; tel. 702/693–5250; FAX. 702/693–5399; Jeff Allen, Director, Provider Relations Director

Exclusive Healthcare, Inc., Mutual of Omaha Plaza, Omaha, NE 68175

FHP Health Care, Inc., 2300 West Sahara, Suite 700, Box 14, Las Vegas, NV 89102; tel. 702/222–4641; FAX. 702/222–4705; R. Lyle Luman, President, Nevada Region

HMO Colorado, Inc., d/b/a HMO Nevada, 6900 Westcliff Drive, Suite 600, Las Vegas, NV 89128; tel. 702/228–2583; Norman P. Becker, CLU, Regional Vice President

Health Plan of Nevada, Inc., 2720 North Tenaya Way, Mailing Address: P.O. Box 15645, Las Vegas, NV 89114–5645; tel. 702/242–7300; Jon Bunker, President

Hometown Health Plan, Inc., 400 South Wells Avenue, Reno, NV 89502; tel. 702/325–3000; FAX. 702/325–3220; Ed Holme, Executive Director

Humana Health Plan, Inc., 3107 South Maryland Parkway, Las Vegas, NV 89109; tel. 702/737–7211; FAX. 702/791–5826; Craig A. Drablos, General Manager

John Alden Nevadaplus Health Plan, 7300 Corporate Center Drive, Miami, FL 33126

Med One Health Plan, 2085 East Sahara Avenue, Las Vegas, NV 89104; tel. 702/650–4000; FAX. 702/650–4030; Joy McClenahan, Vice President, Administration

Nevadacare, Inc., 85 Washington Street, Reno, NV 89503

Silmo Healthcare Services, Inc., 6655 West Sahara Avenue, Las Vegas, NV 89102–0846

St. Mary's HealthFirst, 5290 Neil Road, Reno, NV 89502; tel. 702/829–6000; FAX. 702/829–6010; Lin Howland, Executive Director

NEW HAMPSHIRE

HMO Blue, c/o Blue Cross Blue Shield of New Hampshire, 3000 Goffs Falls Road, Manchester, NH 03111–0001; tel. 800/621–3724

Harvard Community Health Plan of New England, Inc., 10 Brookline Place, W., Brookline, MA 02146; tel. 617/731–8250

Healthsource New Hampshire, Inc., Donovan Street Extension, P.O. Box 2041, Concord, NH 03302–2041; tel. 603/225–5077; FAX. 603/225–7621; Sally Crawford, Chief Executive Officer

Matthew Thornton Health Plan, 43 Constitution Drive, Bedford, NH 03110–6020; tel. 603/695–1100; FAX. 603/695–1157; Everett Page, President

Oxford Health Plans, 10 Tara Boulevard, Nashua, NH 03062; tel. 603/891–7000; FAX. 603/891–7015; Craig Tobin, Regional Chief Executive Officer

Tufts Associated Health Maintenance Organization, Inc., 333 Wyman Street, P.O. Box 9112, Waltham, MA 02254–9112; tel. 617/466–9400

U.S. Healthcare New Hampshire, Inc., U.S. Healthcare Massachusetts, Inc., Three Burlington Woods Drive, Burlington, MA 01803; tel. 617/273–5600; FAX. 617/238–8999; James J. Broderick, General Manager

NEW JERSEY

Aetna Health Plans of New Jersey, 8000 Midlantic Drive, Suite 100 North, Mount Laurel, NJ 08054; tel. 609/866–7880; Dennis Allen, Medical Director

AltantiCare Health Plans, 6727 Delilah Road, Egg Harbor Township, NJ 08234; tel. 609/272–6330; FAX. 609/407–7770; Patricia Koelling, Chief Operating Officer

Americaid, Inc., 550 Broad Street, 11th Floor, Newark, NJ 07102; tel. 201/242–8840; Gerry McNair, Chief Executive Officer

American Preferred Provider Plan, Inc., 810 Broad Street, Newark, NJ 07102; tel. 201/799–0900; FAX. 201/799–0911; Harold E. Smith, President, Chief Executive Officer

Amerihealth HMO, Inc., 8000 Midlantic Drive, Suite 333, Mount Laurel, NJ 08054; tel. 609/778–6500; FAX. 609/778–6550; Leo Carey, Chief Executive Director

CIGNA Health Plan of Southern New Jersey, CIGNA HealthCare of PA, NJ & DE, One Beaver Valley Road, Suite CHP, Wilmington, DE 19803; tel. 302/477–3700; FAX. 302/477–3707; Norman Scott, M.D.

CIGNA of Northern New Jersey, Inc., Three Stewart Court, Denville, NJ 07834–1028; tel. 201/262–7700; FAX. 201/262–9135; Diane Foy–Noa, Vice President, General Manager

Chubbhealth, Inc., 380 Madison Avenue, 20th Floor, New York, NY 10017; tel. 212/880–5455; Keith Collins, M.D., President

Community Healthcare Plan, 309 Market Street, Camden, NJ 08102; tel. 609/541–7526; FAX. 609/635–9328; Mark R. Bryant, President

First Option Health Plan, The Galleria, Two Bridge Avenue, Building Six, Second Floor, Red Bank, NJ 07701–1106; tel. 908/842–5000; Donald Parisi, Senior Vice President, Secretary, General Counsel

Garden State Health Plan, CN–712, Trenton, NJ 08625–0712; tel. 800/525–0047; FAX. 609/588–4643; Beverly Blacher, EIDG, Chief Executive Officer

HIP Health Plan of New Jersey, One HIP Plaza, North Brunswick, NJ 08902; tel. 908/937–7600; FAX. 908/937–7870; Victoria A. Wicks, President, Chief Executive Officer

HMO Blue, Three Penn Plaza East, Newark, NJ 07105–2000; tel. 201/466–8120; FAX. 201/466–6745; Donna M. Celestini, Acting President, Chief Operating Officer

HMO New Jersey, U.S. HealthCare, 55 Lane Road, Fairfield, NJ 07004; tel. 201/575–5600; Andrew Schuyler, M.D., Medical Director

Harmony Health Plan, 200 Executive Drive, Suite 230, West Orange, NJ 07052; tel. 201/669–2900; FAX. 201/669–4666; Stephan N. Yelenik, President, Chief Executive Officer

Liberty Health Plan, 115 Christopher Columbus Drive, Jersey City, NJ 07302; tel. 201/946–6800; FAX. 201/946–1740; Donald L. Picuri, Senior Vice President, Chief Operating Officer

Managed Health Care Systems of New Jersey, Inc., One Gateway Center, Newark, NJ 07102; tel. 201/645–0800; Tony Welters, Chief Executive Officer

MetraHealth Care Plan of New Jersey, 485 B. Route One, Suite 150, Iselin, NJ 08830; tel. 908/602–6500; FAX. 908/602–6519; William Lamoreaux, Director

Metrahealth Care Plan of Upstate New York, Two Penn Plaza, Suite 700, New York, NY 10121; tel. 212/216–6591; James T. Kerr, Chief Executive Officer

NYLCare Health Plans of New Jersey, Inc., 530 East Swedesford Road, Suite 201, Wayne, PA 19087; tel. 610/971–0404; FAX. 610/971–0159; Peter Linder, Executive Director

Oxford Health Plans, Inc., 800 Connecticut Avenue, Norwalk, CT 06854; tel. 800/889–7546; Stephen Wiggins, Chief Executive Officer

Physician Health Services of New Jersey, Inc., Mack Centre IV, South 61 Paramus Road, Paramus, NJ 07652; tel. 201/291–9300; Ronald L. Hjelm, Executive Director

Physician Healthcare Plan of New Jersey, 1009 Lenox Drive, Building Four East, Lawrenceville, NJ 08648; tel. 609/896–1233; FAX. 609/896–3041; Joseph D. Billotti, M.D., Chairman

PruCare of New Jersey, (Northern Division), 200 Wood Avenue, S., Iselin, NJ 08830; tel. 908/632–7333; FAX. 908/494–8207; Paul Conlin, Vice President, Group Operations

QualMed Plans for Health, Inc., 1835 Market Street, Ninth Floor, Philadelphia, PA 19103; tel. 215/209–6704; FAX. 215/209–6708, ext. 6701; Kenneth B. Allen, Director, Legal Services

University Health Plans, Inc., 60 Park Place, 15th Floor, Newark, NJ 07102; tel. 201/623–8700; FAX. 201/623–3635; Steven Marcus, Chief Executive Officer

NEW MEXICO

Cimarron HMO, 2801 East Missouri, Suite 15, Las Cruces, NM 88011; tel. 505/521–1234; FAX. 505/521–1262; Garrey Carruthers, President, Chief Executive Officer

FHP of New Mexico, Inc., 4300 San Mateo, N.E., Albuquerque, NM 87110; tel. 505/881–7900; FAX. 505/883–0102; John Tallent, President

HMO New Mexico, 12800 Indian School Road, N.E., Zip 87112, P.O. Box 11968, Albuquerque, NM 87192; tel. 505/271–4441; FAX. 505/237–5324; Blair Christensen, President

Lovelace, Inc., P.O. Box 27107, Albuquerque, NM 87125–7107; tel. 505/262–7363; Derick Pasternak, M.D., President

Presbyterian Health Plan, 7500 Jefferson, N.E., Building Two, Albuquerque, NM 87109; tel. 505/823–0700; FAX. 505/823–0718; Robert L. Simmons, President

Qual–Med, Inc.–New Mexico Health Plan, 6100 Uptown Boulevard, N.E., Suite 400, Albuquerque, NM 87110; tel. 505/889–8800; FAX. 505/889–8819; Michael J. Mayer, President

NEW YORK

Aetna Health Plans of New York, Inc., 2700 Westchester Avenue, Purchase, NY 10577; tel. 914/251–0600; FAX. 914/251–0260; Paula Adderson, President

Better Health Plan, Inc., 120 Pineview Drive, Amherst, NY 14228; tel. 518/482–1200; Daniel Tillotson, Chief Executive Officer

Blue Cross and Blue Shield of Western New York, Community Blue, 1901 Main Street, P.O. Box 159, Buffalo, NY 14240–0159; tel. 716/887–8874; FAX. 716/887–7911; Nora K. McGuire, Executive Director

Bronx Health Plan, One Fordham Plaza, Bronx, NY 10458; tel. 718/733–4747; Maura Bluestone, Chief Executive Officer

CIGNA HealthCare of New York, Inc., 195 Broadway, Eighth Floor, New York, NY 10007; tel. 212/618–4200; FAX. 212/618–4258; Tom Garvey, Assistant Vice President, Network Management

Capital Area Community Health Plan, Inc., 1201 Troy–Schenectady Road, Latham, NY 12110; tel. 518/783–1864, ext. 4216; FAX. 518/783–0234; John Baackes, President, Chief Executive Officer

Capital District Physicians' Health Plan, 17 Columbia Circle, Albany, NY 12203; tel. 518/862–3700; FAX. 518/452–0003; Diane E. Bergman, President

CarePlus, 350 Fifth Avenue, Suite 5119, New York, NY 10118; tel. 212/563–5570; Robert Porper, M.D., Chief Executive Officer

Catholic Health Services of Brooklyn/Queens, 26 Court Street, Brooklyn, NY 11242; tel. 718/935–1164; Father Patrick Frawley, Chief Executive Officer

CenterCare, Inc., 555 West 57th Street, 18th Floor, New York, NY 10019–2925; tel. 212/293–9200; FAX. 212/293–9298; Paul Accardi, Executive Vice President

ChubbHealth, Inc., 380 Madison Avenue, 20th Floor, New York, NY 10017; tel. 212/880–5400; FAX. 212/880–5454; Keith Collins, M.D., President, Chief Executive Officer

Community Choice Health Plan of Westchester, Inc., 35 East Grassy Sprain Road, Suite 300, Yonkers, NY 10710; tel. 914/337–6908; FAX. 914/337–6919; Kristen M. Johnson, Chief Executive Officer

Community Premier Plus, Inc., 161 Fort Washington Avenue, Suite AP1220, New York, NY 10032; tel. 212/305–7040; FAX. 212/305–3301; Harris Lampert, M.D., President, Medical Director

Compre–Care, Inc., Two Broad Street Plaza, P.O. Box 222, Glens Falls, NY 12801; tel. 518/798–3555; John Rugge, M.D., Chief Executive Officer

Elderplan, Inc., 6323 Seventh Avenue, Brooklyn, NY 11220; tel. 718/921–7990; FAX. 718/921–7962; Eli S. Feldman, Executive Vice President, Chief Executive Officer

Empire Blue Cross and Blue Shield Healthnet/Blue Choice, Three Park Avenue, New York, NY 10016; tel. 212/251–2623; FAX. 212/779–7876; Victor Botnick, Vice President, Managed Care

Empire Health Choice, Inc., 622 Third Avenue, New York, NY 10017–6758; tel. 800/453–0113; Michael Stocker, M.D., Chief Executive Officer

Finger Lakes Blue Cross/Blue Shield, Blue Choice, 150 East Main Street, Rochester, NY 14647; tel. 716/454–1700; FAX. 716/238–4526; Richard D. Dent, M.D., Senior Vice President, Managed Care

GENESIS Healthplan, Inc., One Executive Boulevard, Second Floor, Yonkers, NY 10701; tel. 914/476–6000; Ms. M. A. Chagnon, President

HMO–CNY, Inc., 344 South Warren Street, P.O. Box 4809, Syracuse, NY 13221; tel. 315/448–4931; FAX. 315/448–6802; Ralph Carelli, Jr., Senior Vice President

HUM HealthCare Systems, Inc., d/b/a Partner's Health Plans, Two Broad Street Plaza, P.O. Box 140, Glens Falls, NY 12801; tel. 518/745–0903; FAX. 518/745–1099; Richard Sanford, Chief Executive Officer

Health Care Plan, Inc., 900 Guaranty Building, Buffalo, NY 14202; tel. 716/847–1480; FAX. 716/847–1817; Arthur R. Goshin, M.D., Plan President, Chief Executive Officer

Health Insurance Plan of Greater New York (HIP), Seven West 34th Street, New York, NY l000l; tel. 212/630–5110; FAX. 212/630–5078; Anthony Watson, President

Health Services Medical Corporation of Central New York, Inc., a/k/a Prepaid Health Plan (PHP) in Syracuse, NY, PHP/SDMN in Utica, NY, 8278 Willett Parkway, Baldwinsville, NY 13027; tel. 315/638–2133; FAX. 315/638–0985; Frederick F. Yanni, Jr., President, Chief Executive Officer

HealthFirst PHSP, Inc., 25 Broadway, Ninth Floor, New York, NY 10004; tel. 212/801–6000; FAX. 212/801–1799; Paul Dickstein, Chief Executive Officer

HealthPlus, Inc., 5800 Third Avenue, Brooklyn, NY 11220; tel. 718/745–0030; Thomas Early, Chief Executive Officer

Healthsource HMO of New York, Inc., P.O. Box 1498, Syracuse, NY 132011498; tel. 315/449–1100; FAX. 315/449–2200; Ron Harms, Chief Executive Officer

Independent Health Association, Inc., 511 Farber Lakes Drive, Buffalo, NY 14221; tel. 716/631–3001; FAX. 716/635–3838; Frank Colantuono, President, Chief Executive Officer

Institute for Urban Family Health, Inc., d/b/a ABC Health Plan, 16 East 16th Street, New York, NY 10003; tel. 212/633–0800; FAX. 212/691–4610; Neil Calman, M.D., Chief Executive Officer

Kaiser Foundation Health Plan of New York, 210 Westchester Avenue, White Plains, NY l0604; tel. 914/682–6401; FAX. 914/682–6403; Maura Carley, New York Area Operations Manager

MD:LI, 275 Broad Hollow Road, Melville, NY 11747; tel. 516/454–1900; Richard Ridoccia, Chief Executive Officer

MVP Health Plan, Inc., 111 Liberty Street, Schenectady, NY 12305; tel. 518/370–4793; FAX. 518/370–0852; David W. Oliker, President, Chief Executive Officer

MagnaHealth, 100 Garden City Plaza, Garden City, NY 11530; tel. 516/294–0700; Anthony Bacchi, Chief Executive Officer

Managed Health, Inc., 162 EAB Plaza, Uniondale, NY 11556–0162; tel. 516/683–1010; FAX. 516/683–1034; James Molbihill, M.D., President

Managed Healthcare Systems of New York, Inc., Seven Hanover Square, Fifth Floor, New York, NY 10004; tel. 212/509–5999; FAX. 212/509–2151; Karen Clark, Chief Executive Officer

MetraHealth Care Plan of Upstate NY, Inc., 5015 CampusWood Drive, Suite 303, East Syracuse, NY 13057; tel. 315/433–5851; David Barker, Chief Executive Officer

Metroplus Health Plan, 11 West 42nd Street, Second Floor, New York, NY 10036; tel. 212/597–8600; FAX. 212/597–8666; Denice F. Davis, J.D., Executive Director

Mohawk Valley Physicians Health Plan, 111 Liberty Street, Schenectady, NY 12305; tel. 518/370–4793; David Oliker, Chief Executive Officer

NYLCare Health Plans of New York, Inc., 75–20 Astoria Boulevard, Jackson Heights, NY 11370; tel. 718/899–5200; Arthur J. Drechsler, Executive Director

Neighborhood Health Providers, 630 Third Avenue, New York, NY 10017; tel. 212/808–4775; Steven Bory, Chief Executive Officer

New York Hospital Community Health Plan, 333 East 38th Street, New York, NY 10016; tel. 212/297–5547; FAX. 212/297–5923; Rosaire McDonald, Chief Executive Officer

North American HealthCare, Inc., 300 Corporate Parkway, Amherst, NY 14226; tel. 716/446–5500; Ronald Zoeller, Chief Executive Officer

North Medical Community Health Plan, Inc., 5112 West Taft Road, Suite R, Liverpool, NY 13088; tel. 315/452–2500; James Butler, Chief Executive Officer

OLM/Soundview, 190 East 162nd Street, Bronx, NY 10451; tel. 718/681–5070; FAX. 718/681–5281; John Connors, Chief Executive Officer

Oxford Health Plans of New York, 521 Fifth Avenue, 15th Floor, New York, NY 10175; tel. 212/599–2266; FAX. 212/599–3552; Stephen F. Wiggins, Chief Executive Officer

Physicians Health Services of New York, Inc., Crosswest Office Center, 399 Knollwood Road, Suite 212, White Plains, NY 10603; tel. 914/682–8006; FAX. 914/682–5692; Ronald L. Hjelm, Executive Director

PruCare of New York, Tri–State Health Care Management, The Office Center at Monticello, 400 Rella Boulevard, Suffern, NY 10901; tel. 914/368–4497

Rochester Area HMO, Inc., d/b/a Preferred Care, 259 Monroe Avenue, Suite A, Rochester, NY 14607; tel. 716/325–3920; FAX. 716/325–3122; John Urban, President

SCHC Total Care, Inc., 819 South Salina Street, Syracuse, NY 13202; tel. 315/476–7921; Rueben Cowart, D.D.S., Chief Executive Officer

St. Barnabas Community Health Plan, 183rd Street and Third Avenue, Bronx, NY 10457; tel. 718/960–6232; Steven Anderman, Chief Executive Officer

Suffolk County Department of Health Services, 225 Rabro Drive, E., Happauge, NY 11788–4290; tel. 516/342–0063; Mary Hibberd, M.D., Chief Executive Officer

U.S. Healthcare, Inc., Nassau Omni West, 333 Earle Ovington Boulevard, Suite 502, Uniondale, NY 11553; tel. 516/794–6565; Michael A. Stocker, M.D., President

United HealthCare Plan of NY, Inc., United HealthCare Plan of NJ, Two Penn Plaza, Suite 700, New York, NY 10121; tel. 212/216–6401; FAX. 212/216–6595; R. Channing Wheeler, Chief Executive Officer

Utica–Watertown Health Insurance Co., Inc., The Utica Business Park, 12 Rhoads Drive, Utica, NY 13502; tel. 315/798–4358; FAX. 315/797–4298; Thomas Flannery, M.D.

Vytra Healthcare, Corporate Center, 395 North Service Road, Melville, NY 11747–3127; tel. 516/694–4000; FAX. 516/694–5780; David S. Reynolds, Ph.D., President

WellCare of New York, Inc., P.O. Box 4059, Park West/Hurley Avenue Ext., Kingston, NY 12402; tel. 914/334–7185; FAX. 914/338–0566; Robert Goff, Chief Executive Officer

Westchester Prepaid Health Services Plan, Inc., d/b/a HealthSource, 303 South Broadway, Suite 321, Tarrytown, NY 10591; tel. 914/631–1611; FAX. 914/631–1615; Georganne Chapin, Chief Executive Officer

NORTH CAROLINA

Aetna Health Plans of the Carolinas, Inc., 201 South College Street, Suite 1010, Charlotte, NC 28244; tel. 704/353–7176; FAX. 704/353–7180; Amy Williams, General Manager

American Dental Plan of North Carolina, Inc., 130 Edinburgh South, Suite 107, Cary, NC 27511; tel. 919/380–9267; FAX. 919/380–1729; John Arnold

Association of Eye Care Centers Total Vision Health Plan, Inc., P.O. Box 7185, 110 Zebulon Court, Rocky Mount, NC 27804; tel. 919/937–6650; FAX. 919/451–2182; Samuel B. Petteway, Jr., President

Atlantic Health Plan, Inc., 7415 Pineville–Matthews Road, Suite 200, Charlotte, NC 28226; tel. 704/544–1075; Lance Hunsinger

Blue Cross Blue Shield of North Carolina, P.O. Box 2291, Durham, NC 27702; tel. 919/489–7431; FAX. 919/419–1082; Ken Otis II, President

CIGNA Dental Health of North Carolina, Inc., 600 East Las Colinas, Suite 1000, Irving, TX 75039; tel. 800/237–2904; David O. Cannady, President

CIGNA Health Plan of North Carolina, Inc., 7400 Carmel Executive Park, Charlotte, NC 28235; tel. 800/235–5707; FAX. 704/544–4375; Debbie Walters, Manager

Carolina Summit Healthcare, Inc., Four North Blount Street, Raleigh, NC 27601; tel. 919/571–4691; William Bull

Community Choice of North Carolina, Inc., 100 North Green Street, Greensboro, NC 27401; tel. 910/691–3001; Randolph Ferguson

Doctors Health Plan of North Carolina, Inc., 2828 Croasdaile Drive, P.O. Box 15309, Durham, NC 27704; tel. 919/383–4175, ext. 6124; FAX. 919/383–3286; Richard A. Felice, President

Health Maintenance Organization of North Carolina, Inc., P.O. Box 2291, Durham, NC 27702; tel. 919/489–7431; FAX. 919/419–1338; Earl Ridout, Senior Director

Healthsource North Carolina, Inc., 701 Corporate Center Drive, Raleigh, NC 27607; tel. 919/854–7000, ext. 7700; FAX. 919/854–7102; Robert J. Greczyn, Jr., President, Chief Executive Officer

Kaiser Foundation Health Plan of North Carolina, 3120 Highwoods Boulevard, Suite 300, Raleigh, NC 27604–1038; tel. 919/981–6000; FAX. 919/878–5835; Ted Carpenter, Vice President, Regional Manager

Maxicare North Carolina, Inc., 5550 77 Center Drive, Suite 380, Charlotte, NC 28217–0700; tel. 704/525–0880, ext. 6451; FAX. 704/529–0382; Richard T. Hedlund, Vice President, General Manager

Optimum Choice of the Carolinas, Inc., Crabtree Center, 4600 Marriott Drive, Suite 300, Raleigh, NC 27612; tel. 919/881–8481; George T. Jochum

PARTNERS National Health Plans of North Carolina, Inc., P.O. Box 24907, Winston–Salem, NC 27114–4907; tel. 910/760–4822; FAX. 910/659–2950; John W. Jones, President

Personal Care Plan of North Carolina, Inc., Blue Cross and Blue Shield of North Carolina Personal Care Plan, P.O. Box 30004, Durham, NC 27702; tel. 919/490–4003; FAX. 919/419–1338; Don W. Bradley, M.D., Executive Director

Principal Health Care of the Carolinas, Inc., 1801 Rockville Pike, Suite 601, Rockville, MD 20852; tel. 301/881–1033; Kenneth J. Linde, President

Prudential Health Care Plan, Inc., 2701 Coltsgate Road, Suite 300, Charlotte, NC 28211; tel. 704/365–6070; FAX. 704/365–9959; Jim Ebitt, Vice President

QualChoice of North Carolina, Inc., 2000 West First Street, Suite 210, Winston–Salem, NC 27104; tel. 919/716–0907; FAX. 910/716–0920; Douglas Cueny, President

Spectera Dental Services, Inc., (formerly United Dental Services), 2811 Lord Baltimore Drive, Baltimore, MD 21244–2644; tel. 410/265–6033; Oscar B. Camp, President

The Wellness Plan of North Carolina, Inc., 4601 Park Road, Suite 550, Charlotte, NC 28209–3239; tel. 704/679–3700; FAX. 704/679–3706; Timothy O'Brien, Chief Executive Officer

U. S. Healthcare of the Carolinas, Inc., 205 Regency Executive Park, Suite 410, Charlotte, NC 28217; tel. 704/672–2700; Amy N. Williams, General Manager

United Health Care of North Carolina, Northwestern Plaza, 2307 West Cone Boulevard, Greensboro, NC 27408; tel. 910/282–0900; FAX. 910/545–5099; Frank R. Mascia, President, Chief Executive Officer

Wellpath Select, Inc., 6320 Quadrangle Drive, Suite 180, Chapel Hill, NC 27514; tel. 919/493–1210; Anna Lore

NORTH DAKOTA

Heart of America HMO, 802 South Main, Rugby, ND 58368; tel. 701/776-5848; FAX. 701/776-5425; Mary Ann Jaeger, Executive Director

Northern Plains Health Plan, 1000 South Columbia Road, Grand Forks, ND 58201; tel. 701/780-1600; Raymond Kuntz

OHIO

Aetna Health Plans of Ohio, Inc., 3690 Orange Place, Suite 200, Cleveland, OH 44122-4438; tel. 216/464-2722; FAX. 216/464-2723; David K. Ellwanger, Executive Director

Aultcare HMO, 2600 Sixth Street, S.W., Canton, OH 44710; tel. 216/438-6360; Rick L. Haines, Vice President, Managed Care

Bethesda Managed Care, Inc., 619 Oak Street, Cincinnati, OH 45206; tel. 513/569-6490; FAX. 513/569-6233; Robert Smith, M.D., Medical Director

Butler Health Plan, 111 Buckeye Street, Suite 107, Hamilton, OH 45011; tel. 800/872-9093; FAX. 513/863-6437; Pamela A. Poland, Executive Director

ChoiceCare, 655 Eden Park Drive, Suite 400, Cincinnati, OH 45202; tel. 513/784-5200; FAX. 513/784-5300; Daniel A. Gregorie, M.D., Chief Executive Officer

Cigna Healthcare of Ohio, Inc., 3700 Corporate Drive, Suite 200, Business Campus, N.E., Columbus, OH 43231-4963; tel. 614/823-7500; FAX. 614/823-7775; James Massie, General Manager

Community Health Plan of Ohio, 1915 Tamarack Road, Newark, OH 43055-3699; tel. 614/348-4901; FAX. 614/348-4909; Robert R. Kamps, M.D., President, Chief Executive Officer

Day-Med Health Maintenance Plan, 9797 Springboro Pike, Suite 200, Miamisburg, OH 45342; tel. 937/847-5646, ext. 120; FAX. 513/847-5620; Jeanette Prear, President, Chief Executive Officer

Dayton Area Health Plan, One Dayton Centre, One South Main Street, Suite 440, Dayton, OH 45402-9794; tel. 513/224-3300; FAX. 513/224-2272, ext. 2200; Pamela B. Morris, President, Chief Executive Officer

Emerald HMO, Inc., Diamond Building, 1100 Superior Avenue, 16th Floor, Cleveland, OH 44114-2591; tel. 216/241-4133; FAX. 216/241-4158; Randolph C. Hoffman, President

FHP of Ohio, Inc., Spectrum Office Tower, 11260 Chester Road, Suite 800, Cincinnati, OH 45246-9928; tel. 513/772-9191; FAX. 513/772-1466; John Davren, M.D., Plan Director

Family Health Plan, Inc., 1001 Madison Avenue, Toledo, OH 43264-1916; tel. 419/241-6501; FAX. 419/241-5441; Robert Campbell, Executive Vice President

Genesis Health Plan of Ohio, Inc., Two Summit Park Drive, Suite 340, Cleveland, OH 44131; tel. 216/642-3344; FAX. 216/642-3345; Karl Rajani, President

HMO Health Ohio, 2060 East Ninth Street, Cleveland, OH 44115-1353; tel. 216/687-7730; FAX. 216/687-6585; Gerry P. Long, Director, ADS Products

Health Guard, d/b/a Advantage Health Plan, 3000 Guernsey Street, Bellaire, OH 43906-1598; tel. 614/676-4623; Daniel Splain, President

Health Maintenance Plan, 4665 Cornell Road, Suite 351, Cincinnati, OH 45241; tel. 513/247-6688; FAX. 513/247-6789; Bradford A. Buxton, Executive Director

Health Power HMO, Inc., 560 East Town Street, Columbus, OH 43215-0346; tel. 614/461-9900; FAX. 614/461-0960; Thomas Beaty, Jr., President

HealthFirst, 372 East Center Street, Marion, OH 43302-3831; tel. 614/387-6355; FAX. 614/387-0665; N. Robert Jones, President, Chief Executive Officer

HealthPledge, a product of U.S. Health HMO, 300 East Wilson Bridge Road, Suite 200, Worthington, OH 43085-2339; tel. 614/566-0111; FAX. 614/566-0403; Colleen M. Tincher, Director, Operations

Healthassurance HMO, 2601 Market Place, Harrisburg, PA 17110-9339; tel. 412/577-4340; FAX. 412/497-5880; Deborah Zuroski, Senior Compliance Analyst

Healthsource Ohio, 225 South East Street, Suite 240, Indianapolis, IN 46202; tel. 317/685-8300; FAX. 317/686-0148; David Smith, Chief Executive Officer

HomeTown Hospital Health Plan, 100 Lillian Gish Boulevard, Suite 301, Massillon, OH 44647; tel. 216/837-6880; FAX. 216/837-6869; William C. Epling, Vice President, Chief Operating Officer

Humana Health Plan of Ohio, Inc., 8044 Montgomery Road, Suite 460, Cincinnati, OH 45236; tel. 513/792-0511; FAX. 513/792-0520; Bill Wakefield, Executive Director

InHealth, Inc., 200 East Campus View Boulevard, Worthington, OH 43235; tel. 614/888-2223; Jeralyn Green, President

John Alden Health Systems, Inc., 5500 Glendon Court, Dublin, OH 43017; tel. 614/798-2930; William F. Sterling, Vice President, Senior Associate Counsel

Kaiser Permanente, North Point Tower, 1001 Lakeside Avenue, Suite 1200, Cleveland, OH 44114-1153; tel. 216/621-5600, ext. 5296; FAX. 216/623-8776; Jeffrey Werner, Vice President, Marketing

Medical Value Plan, 405 Madison Avenue, P.O. Box 2147, Toledo, OH 43603-2147; tel. 419/244-2900; FAX. 419/252-8251; Hal A. White, M.D., Medical Director

Mutual of Omaha Health Plans of Ohio, Inc., Rockside Square I, 6155 Rockside Road, Suite 201, Independence, OH 44131; tel. 216/524-3555; FAX. 216/524-5035; Susan Mego, Executive Director

Paramount Health Care, 1715 Indian Wood Circle, Suite 200, P.O. Box 928, Toledo, OH 43697-0928; tel. 419/891-2500; FAX. 419/891-2530; John C. Randolph, President

Personal Physician Care, Inc., Sterling Building, 1255 Euclid Avenue, Suite 500, Cleveland, OH 44115-1807; tel. 216/687-0015; FAX. 216/687-9484; Wilton A. Savage, Executive Director

Prudential Health Care Plan, Inc., PruCare of Central Ohio, 485 Metro Place S., Suite 450, Dublin, OH 43017; tel. 614/761-0002; FAX. 614/761-1757; Budd Fisher, Director, Group Operations

QualChoice Health Plan, 6000 Parkland Boulevard, Cleveland, OH 44124; tel. 216/460-4010; FAX. 216/460-4000; Ray S. Herschman, Chief Financial Officer

SummaCare, Inc., 400 West Market Street, P.O. Box 3620, Akron, OH 44309-3620; tel. 330/996-8410; FAX. 330/996-8415; Martin P. Hauser, President

Super Blue HMO, 2060 East Ninth Street, Cleveland, OH 44115; tel. 216/687-7730; FAX. 216/687-6585; Gerry Long, Director, ADS Products

The Health Plan, 52160 National Road, East, St. Clairsville, OH 43950-9365; tel. 614/695-3585; Philip D. Wright, President, Chief Operating Officer

Total Health Care Plan, Inc., 12800 Shaker Boulevard, Cleveland, OH 44120; tel. 216/991-3000, ext. 2221; FAX. 222/991-3011; James G. Turner, President, Chief Executive Officer

USHC, 375 Carriage Lane, Canfield, OH 44406; tel. 215/283-6656; FAX. 215/654-6078; Jean Moriarity

United Healthcare of Ohio, Inc., 3650 Olentangy River Road, Columbus, OH 43216-1138; tel. 614/442-7106; Shirley Reynolds, Director Product Administration

OKLAHOMA

CIGNA HealthCare of Oklahoma, Inc., Cigna Center, 5100 North Brookline, Ninth Floor, Oklahoma City, OK 73112; tel. 405/943-7711; FAX. 405/946-9568; Cynthia A. Finter, General Manager

Comanche County Hospital Authority, d/b/a Prime Advantage Health Plan, 4411 West Gore Boulevard, Suite B4, Lawton, OK 73505; tel. 405/357-6684; FAX. 405/357-9064; Tanya Case, Director

Community Care HMO, Inc., 4720 South Harvard, Suite 202, Tulsa, OK 74135; tel. 918/749-1171; FAX. 918/749-7970; David J. Pynn, President

Foundation Health, An Oklahoma Health Plan, Inc., 5810 East Skelly Drive, Suite 1100, Tulsa, OK 74135; tel. 918/621-5900; Richard McCutchen, Senior Vice President, Executive Officer

GHS Health Maintenance Organization, Inc., d/b/a BlueLincs HMO, 1400 South Boston, Tulsa, OK 74119-3630; tel. 918/592-9414; FAX. 918/592-0611; Robert D. Pearcy, Group Vice President

Healthcare Oklahoma, Inc., 3030 Northwest Expressway, Suite 140, Oklahoma City, OK 73112-4481; tel. 405/951-4700; FAX. 405/951-4701; Jon H. Friesen, President, Chief Executive Officer

PROklahoma Care, Inc., 5005 North Lincoln, P.O. Box 25127, Oklahoma City, OK 73126; tel. 405/521-8253; Joe Crosthwait, M.D., Vice President, Medical Director

PacifiCare of Oklahoma, 7666 East 61st Street, Tulsa, OK 74133-1112; tel. 918/459-1100; FAX. 918/459-1451; Chris Whitty, Vice President, General Manager

Prudential Health Care Plan, Inc., d/b/a Prudential Health Care HMO, 7912 East 31st Court, Tulsa, OK 74145; tel. 918/624-4600; FAX. 918/627-9759; Ann Paul, Executive Director

Prudential HealthCare Plan, Inc., 4005 Northwest Expressway, Suite 300, Oklahoma City, OK 73116; tel. 405/879-1780; James K. McNaughton, Executive Director

OREGON

HMO Oregon, Inc., P.O. Box 12625, Salem, OR 97309; tel. 503/364-4868; FAX. 503/588-4350; Roger B. Lyman, President

Health Maintenance of Oregon, Inc., P.O. Box 139, Portland, OR 97207-0139; tel. 503/274-0755; FAX. 501/223-5993; Richard Woolworth, President, Chief Executive Officer

Health Masters of Oregon, 201 High Street, S.E., Salem, OR 97301; tel. 503/779-9468; FAX. 503/779-3238; Jud Holtey, Chief Operating Officer, Southern Regional Office, BCBSO

HealthGuard Services, Inc., d/b/a SelectCare, 600 Country Club Road, Zip 97401, P.O. Box 10106, Eugene, OR 97440; tel. 541/686-3948; FAX. 541/984-4030; Larry Abramson, President

Kaiser Foundation Health Plan of the Northwest, 500 Northeast Multnomah Street, Suite 100, Portland, OR 97232-2099; tel. 503/813-2800; Michael H. Katcher, President

Liberty Health Plan, Inc., 825 Northeast Multnomah Street, Suite 1600, Portland, OR 97232; tel. 503/234-5345; FAX. 503/234-5381; Kristen A. Fassenfelt, Vice President

PACC, P.O. Box 286, Clackamas, OR 97015-0286; tel. 503/659-4212; FAX. 503/794-3409; Martin A. Preizler, President, Chief Executive Officer

Pacificare of Oregon, Inc., Five Centerpointe Drive, Suite 600, Lake Oswego, OR 97035-8650; tel. 503/620-9324; FAX. 503/603-7377; Mary O. McWilliams, President

Providence Health Plans, 1235 Northeast 47th Avenue, Suite 220, Portland, OR 97213; tel. 503/215-2981; FAX. 503/215-7655; Jack Friedman, Executive Director

QualMed Oregon Health Plan, Inc., 4800 Southwest Macadam, Suite 400, Portland, OR 97201; tel. 503/222-5217; FAX. 503/796-6366; Chris du Laney, Executive Director

PENNSYLVANIA

Aetna Health Plans of Central and Eastern Pennsylvania, Inc., 955 Chesterbrook Boulevard, Suite 200, Wayne, PA 19087; tel. 610/644-3800; FAX. 610/251-6441; Anthony Buividas, Chief Executive Officer

Alliance Health Network, 1700 Peach Street, Suite 244, Erie, PA 16501; tel. 814/878-1700; FAX. 814/452-4358; James R. Smith, President, Chief Executive Officer

Best Health Care of Western Pennsylvania, Towne Centre Offices, P.O. Box 8440, Pittsburgh, PA 15218-0440; tel. 800/699-3527

Central Medical Health Plan, d/b/a Advantage Health, 121 Seventh Avenue, Suite 500, Pittsburgh, PA 15222-3408; tel. 412/391-9300, ext. 509; FAX. 412/391-0457; Elizabeth Stolkowski, Executive Vice President, Chief Operating Officer

Cigna Health Plan of Pennsylvania, Inc., One Beaver Valley Road, Suite CHP, Wilmington, DE 19803; tel. 302/477-3700

Geisinger Health Plan, Geisinger Office Building, 100 North Academy Avenue, Danville, PA 17822-3020; tel. 717/271-8760; FAX. 717/271-5268; Howard G. Hughes, M.D., Senior Vice President Health Plans

HIP of Pennsylvania, d/b/a HIP Health Plan, Six Neshaminy Interplex, Suite 600, Trevose, PA 19053; tel. 215/633-7780

HMO of Northeastern Pennsylvania, d/b/a First Priority Health, 70 North Main Street, Wilkes-Barre, PA 18711; tel. 717/829-6044; FAX. 717/830-6319; Denise S. Cesare, Executive Vice President, Chief Operating Officer

Health Partners of Philadelphia, 4700 Wissachickon Avenue, Suite 118, Philadelphia, PA 19144-4283; tel. 215/849-9606

HealthAmerica of Pennsylvania, Inc., Five Gateway Center, Pittsburgh, PA 15222; tel. 412/553–7300; FAX. 412/553–7384; Mike Blackwood, Chief Executive Officer

HealthGuard of Lancaster, Inc., 280 Granite Run Drive, Suite 105, Lancaster, PA 17601–6810; tel. 717/560–9049; FAX. 717/581–4580; James R. Godfrey, President

Healthcare Management Alternatives, Inc., 5070 Parkside Avenue, Suite 6200, Philadelphia, PA 19131; tel. 215/473–7511; FAX. 215/473–0446; Dr. Denise Ross, Chief Executive Officer

Healthcentral, Inc., 2605 Interstate Drive, Suite 140, Harrisburg, PA 17110; tel. 717/540–0033; Martin R. Miracle, President, Chief Executive Officer

Keystone Health Plan Central, Inc., 300 Corporate Center Drive, P.O. Box 898812, Camp Hill, PA 17089–8812; tel. 717/763–3458; FAX. 717/975–6895; Joseph M. Pfister, President, Chief Executive Officer

Keystone Health Plan East, Inc., 1901 Market Street, Philadelphia, PA I9101–7516; tel. 215/241–2001; John Daddis, Executive Vice President, Chief Operating Officer

Keystone Health Plan West, Inc., Fifth Avenue Place, 120 Fifth Avenue, Suite 3116, Pittsburgh, PA 15222; tel. 412/255–7245; FAX. 412/255–7583; Kenneth R. Melani, M.D., President

Medigroup HMO, Inc., 1700 Market Street, Suite 1050, Philadelphia, PA 19103; tel. 215/575–0530

Optimum Choice, Inc. of Pennsylvania, 1755 Oregon Pike, First Floor, Lancaster, PA 17601; tel. 800/474–6647; FAX. 717/569–7820; J. Steve DuFresne, President

Oxford Health Plans, The Curtis Center, 601 Walnut Street, Suite 900E, Philadelphia, PA 19106; tel. 215/625–8800; FAX. 215/625–5601; Michael C. Gaffney, Chief Executive Officer

Philcare Health Systems, Inc., 2005 Market Street, Commerce Square, Philadelphia, PA 215/564–4050

Prudential Health Care Plan, Inc., Prudential HealthCare, 220 Gibraltar Road, Suite 200, P.O. Box 901, Horsham, PA 19044–0901; tel. 215/672–1944; FAX. 215/442–2946; Brian J. Keane, Senior Director, Network Management, Operations

QualMed Plans for Health of Pennsylvania, Inc., 1835 Market Street, Ninth Floor, Philadelphia, PA 19103; tel. 215/209–6300; FAX. 215/209–6561; Diane C. Chiponis, Chief Financial Officer

Qualmed Plans for Health, Inc., (formerly Greater Atlantic Health Service, Inc.), 3550 Market Street, Philadelphia, PA 19104; tel. 215/823–8600; Ernest Monfiletto, President, Chief Executive Officer

Three Rivers Health Plans, Inc., 300 Oxford Drive, Monroeville, PA 15146; tel. 412/858–4000; FAX. 412/858–4060; Warren Carmichael, Chairman, Chief Executive Officer

United States Health Care Systems, Inc., d/b/a The Health Maintenance Organization of Pennsylvania, 980 Jolly Road, P.O. Box 1109, Blue Bell, PA 19422; tel. 215/628–4800; Leonard Abramson, President

RHODE ISLAND
Blue Cross & Blue Shield of Rhode Island, 444 Westminster Street, Providence, RI 02903; tel. 401/459–1000; Douglas J. McIntosh, President

Coordinated Health Partners, Inc., 30 Chestnut Street, Providence, RI 02903; tel. 401/274–6644; FAX. 401/453–5586; Paula Nordhoff, Executive Vice President

Delta Dental of Rhode Island, 50 Park Row West, Providence, RI 02903–1143; tel. 401/453–0800; Colin MacGillvary

Harvard Pilgrim Health Care of New England, One Hoppin Street, Providence, RI 02903; tel. 401/331–3000; FAX. 401/331–0496; Stephen Schoenbaum, M.D., Medical Director

Neighborhood Health Plan of Rhode Island, Inc., 32 Branch Avenue, Providence, RI 02904; tel. 401/459–6000; Chris Schneider

Pilgrim Health Care, 10 Accord Executive Drive, P.O. Box 200, Norwell, MA 02061; tel. 617/871–3950; FAX. 617/982–9668; Allan Greenberg, Executive Vice President

U. S. Healthcare, Inc., 980 Jolly Road, P.O. Box 1109, Blue Bell, PA 19422; tel. 215/283–6656; Timothy Nolan, President

United Health Plans of New England, Inc., 475 Kilvert Street, Suite 310, Warwick, RI 02886–1392; tel. 401/737–6900; FAX. 401/737–6957; Max Powell, Chief Executive Officer

SOUTH CAROLINA
Aetna Health Plans of the Carolinas, Inc., 1010 Charlotte Plaza, Suite 1010, Charlotte, NC 28244; tel. 704/353–7201

American Medical Plans of South Carolina, Inc., 246 Stoneridge Drive, Suite 101, Columbia, SC 29210; tel. 803/748–7395; FAX. 803/748–9597; George A. Schneider, Chief Executive Officer

Carolina Care Health Plan, Inc., 111 Stonemark Lane, Suite 202, Columbia, SC 29210; tel. 800/641–5584; FAX. 813/265–6213; Laurie Burrell, Chief Operating Officer

Companion HealthCare Corporation, I–20 at Alpine Road, Columbia, SC 29219–2401; tel. 803/786–8466; FAX. 803/699–2374; Harvey L. Galloway, Executive Vice President, Chief Operating Officer

Doctors Health Plan, Inc., 2828 Croasdaile Drive, Durham, NC 27705; tel. 919/383–4173; FAX. 919/383–4175; Richard Allan Felice, President

Health First, Inc., 255 Enterprise Boulevard, Suite 200, Greenville, SC 29615; tel. 864/455–4098; FAX. 864/455–1120; R. Wesley Champion, Chief Financial Officer

Healthsource South Carolina, Inc., 215 East Bay Street, Suite 401, Charleston, SC 29401; tel. 803/723–5520; FAX. 803/723–7715; Michael V. Clark, President, Chief Executive Officer

Heritage National Healthplan, Inc., 1515 Fifth Avenue, Suite 200, Moline, IL 61265–1368; tel. 309/765–1200; G. Michael Hammes, President

Kaiser Foundation Health Plan of North Carolina, 3120 Highwoods Boulevard, Raleigh, NC 27604; tel. 704/551–1986; William Dewey Brown, Jr.

Maxicare North Carolina, Inc., 5550 77 Center Drive, Suite 380, Charlotte, NC 28210; tel. 704/525–0880; FAX. 704/529–0382; Richard T. Hedlund, Vice President, General Manager

Optimum Choice of the Carolinas, Inc., 4600 Marriott Drive, Suite 300, Raleigh, NC 27612; tel. 800/373–5879; Jim Bendel, Sales Manager

Partners National Health Plans of NC, Inc., 2085 Frontis Plaza Boulevard, Winston–Salem, NC 27103; tel. 910/760–4822; FAX. 910/760–6218; Cosby M. Davis, III, Chief Financial Officer

Physicians Health Plan of South Carolina, Inc., 110 Centerview Drive, Suite 301, Columbia, SC 29210–8438; tel. 803/750–7400, ext. 4; FAX. 803/750–7474; William E. Martin, Chief Executive Officer

Preferred Health Systems, Inc., I–20 at Alpine Road, Columbus, SC 29219; tel. 803/788–0222; FAX. 803/736–2851; Gail Bragg, Senior Director

Principal Health Care of the Carolinas, Inc., One Coliseum Center, 2300 Yorkmont Road, Suite 710, Charlotte, NC 28217; tel. 704/357–1421; FAX. 704/357–3164; Chuck Trinchitella, Executive Director

Provident Health Care Plan, Inc. of South Carolina, 201 Brookfield Parkway, Suite 100, Greenville, SC 29607; tel. 803/987–3100; James D. Kollefrath

Select Health of South Carolina, Inc., 7410 Northside Drive, Suite 208, North Charleston, SC 29420; tel. 803/569–1759; FAX. 803/569–0702; Michael Jernigan, President, Chief Executive Officer

U. S. Healthcare of the Carolinas, Inc., 205 Regency Executive Park Drive, Charlotte, NC 28217; tel. 800/278–0122; Vaughn Delk

WellPath Select, Inc., 6330 Quadrangle Drive, Suite 500, Chapel Hill, NC 27514; tel. 919/493–1210; FAX. 919/419–3872; Anna M. Lore, President, Chief Executive Officer

SOUTH DAKOTA
Mutual of Omaha of South Dakota and Community Health Plus HMO, Inc., 4009 West 49th Street, Suite 301, Sioux Falls, SD 57106; tel. 605/361–9591; FAX. 605/361–9593; William P. Jetter, Executive Director

South Dakota State Medical Holding Company, Inc., d/b/a Dakota Care, 1323 South Minnesota Avenue, Sioux Falls, SD 57105; tel. 605/334–4000; FAX. 605/336–0270; Robert D. Johnson, Chief Executive Officer

TENNESSEE
Aetna Health Plans of Tennessee, 1801 West End Avenue, Suite 500, Nashville, TN 37203; tel. 615/322–1600; FAX. 615/322–1217; David R. Field, President

American Medical Security Health Plan, Inc., 22 North Front Street, Suite 960, Memphis, TN 38103; tel. 901/523–2672; Eric B. Taylor, President

CIGNA HealthCare of Tennessee, Inc., Palmer Plaza, Suite 800, 1801 West End Avenue, Nashville, TN 37203; tel. 615/340–3059; FAX. 615/340–3590; Sherri A. Silvas, Administrative Assistant

Community Health Plan of Chattanooga, Inc., d/b/a Wellport Health Plan, Franklin Building, Suite 101, Chattanooga, TN 37411; tel. 423/490–1120; Brian E. Dalbey, President

Erlanger Health Plan Trust, 979 East Third Street, Chattanooga, TN 37403; tel. 423/778–8255; John Barnes, President

Health 123, Inc., 706 Church Street, Suite 500, Nashville, TN 37203; tel. 615/782–7811; FAX. 615/782–7812; Thomas J. Nagle, President, Chief Executive Officer

HealthNet HMO, Inc., 44 Vantage Way, Suite 300, Nashville, TN 37228; tel. 800/881–9466; Gary Brukardt, President

HealthWise of Tennessee, Inc., 404 BNA Drive, Suite 204, Nashville, TN 37217; tel. 615/366–6010; FAX. 615/367–5008; Len Cantrell, Chief Executive Officer

Healthsource Tennessee, Inc., 5409 Maryland Way, Suite 300, Brentwood, TN 37027; tel. 615/373–6995; FAX. 615/370–9396; Steve White, Chief Executive Officer

Humana Health Plan, Inc., P.O. Box 740036, Louisville, KY 40201–7436; tel. 502/580–5804; Craig Drablos, Executive Director

Mid–South Health Plan, Inc., 889 Ridge Lake Boulevard, Suite 111, Memphis, TN 38120; tel. 901/766–7500; William C. Stewart, Jr., Chief Executive Director, Medical Director

PHP Health Plans, Inc., 1420 Centrepoint Boulevard, Knoxville, TN 37932; tel. 423/470–7470; Jerry M. Marsh, CPA, Director, Finance

Phoenix Healthcare of Tennessee, Inc., 3401 West End Avenue, Suite 470, Nashville, TN 37203; tel. 615/298–3666, ext. 260; FAX. 615/297–2036; Samuel H. Howard, Chairman

Provident Health Care Plan, Inc. of Tennessee, Two Northgate Park, Chattanooga, TN 37415

Prudential Health Care Plan, Inc., 227 French Landing Drive, Suite 200, Nashville, TN 37228

Southern Health Plan, Inc., 600 Jefferson, Memphis, TN 38105; tel. 901/544–2336; FAX. 901/544–2220; Bill Graham, Executive Director

Tennessee Health Care Network, Inc., P.O. Box 1407, Chattanooga, TN 37401–1407; tel. 423/755–2033; FAX. 615/755–5630; Robert M. Fox, President

Vanderbilt Health Plans, Inc., 706 Church Street Building, Suite 500, Nashville, TN 37203; tel. 615/343–2670; FAX. 615/343–2823; Randal B. Farr, Executive Vice President

TEXAS
AECC Total Vision Health Plan of Texas, Inc., 3010 LBJ Freeway, Suite 240, Dallas, TX 75234; tel. 800/268–8847; Samuel Petteway, Jr., President

Aetna Dental Care of Texas, Inc., 2350 Lakeside Boulevard, Suite 740, Richardson, TX 75082; tel. 214/470–7990; Jackie Eveslage, Chief Operating Officer

Aetna Health Plans of North Texas, Inc., 2350 Lakeside Boulevard, Suite 500, Richardson, TX 75082; tel. 214/470–7878; John Coyle, President

Aetna Health Plans of Texas, Inc., 2900 North Loop West, Suite 200, Houston, TX 77092; tel. 713/683–7500; FAX. 713/683–5819; Joseph T. Blanford III, General Manager

Alpha Dental Programs, Inc., d/b/a Delta Care, 1431 Greenway Drive, Suite 230, Irving, TX 75038; tel. 972/580–1616; FAX. 972/580–1333; Lee Schneider, Vice President, Marketing, Western Region

Alternative Dental Care of Texas, Inc., 2023 South Gessner K–3, Houston, TX 77063; tel. 713/781–6607; Thomas Anthony Dzuryachko, President

Americaid Texas, Inc., d/b/a Americaid Community Care, 617 Seventh Avenue, Second Floor, Fort Worth, TX 76104; tel. 817/870–1281; James Donovan, Jr., President

Anthem Health Plan of Texas, Inc., 5055 Keller Springs Road, Dallas, TX 75243; tel. 972/732–2000; FAX. 972/732–2043; Joseph W. Hrbek, President

Block Vision of Texas, Inc., 4445 Alpha Road, Suite 100, Dallas, TX 75244; tel. 800/914–9795; FAX. 972/991–4704; Andrew Alcorn, President

CIGNA Dental Health of Texas, Inc., d/b/a CIGNA Dental Health, 600 East Las Colinas Boulevard, Suite 1000, Irving, TX 75039; tel. 800/367–1037; Brent Martin, D.D.S., M.B.A., Chief Executive Officer, Regional Vice Pres.

CIGNA HealthCare of North Texas, Inc., 600 East Las Colinas Boulevard, Suite II00, Irving, TX 75039; tel. 214/401–5200; FAX. 214/401–5209; Vernon W. Walters, M.D., Vice President, Medical Director

Certus Healthcare, L.L.C., 1300 North 10th Street, Suite 450, McAllen, TX 78501; tel. 210/630–1956, ext. 106; FAX. 210/630–1957; David Rodriguez, President

Community First Health Plans, Inc., P.O. Box 7548, San Antonio, TX 78207–0548; tel. 210/227–2347; FAX. 210/244–3014; Charles L. Knight, President, Chief Executive Officer
Comprehensive Heatlh Services of Texas, Inc., 100 Northeast Loop 410, Suite 675, San Antonio, TX 78217; tel. 210/321–4050; Thomas C. Jackson, Chief Executive Officer
Dental Benefits, Inc., d/b/a Bluecare Dental HMO, 12170 Abrams Road, Dallas, TX 75243; tel. 972/766–5185; Doyle C. Williams, President
Denticare, Inc., 14141 Southwest Freeway, Suite 1300, Sugar Land, TX 77478–9990; tel. 713/242–1099; FAX. 713/242–1007; Henry New, President
Dorsey Dental Plans of America, Inc., 1177 West Loop South, Suite 725, Houston, TX 77027; tel. 713/621–6050; Michael P. Stern, President, Chief Executive Officer
ECCA Managed Vision Care, Inc., 11103 West Avenue, San Antonio, TX 78213–1392; tel. 800/340–0129; FAX. 210/524–6587; Melissa Kazen, Director
Exclusive Healthcare, Inc., 12790 Merit Drive, Suite 714, Dallas, TX 75251; tel. 214/450–4500; Robert Robidou, Plan Manager
FHP of New Mexico, d/b/a FHP of El Paso, 4300 San Mateo Boulevard, N.E., Albuquerque, NM 87110; tel. 505/881–7900; FAX. 505/875–3305; Mark Zobel, Regional Compliance Officer
FHP of Texas, Inc., 12 Greenway Plaza, Suite 500, Houston, TX 77046–1201; tel. 800/455–4156; FAX. 713/621–9647; Patrick Stewart, President
First American Dental Benefits, Inc., 14800 Landmark Boulevard, Suite 700, Dallas, TX 75240; tel. 214/661–5848; Jim Davenport, President, Acting Chief Executive Officer
Foundation Health, a Texas Health Plan, Inc., 9101 Barnet Road, Suite 104, Austin, TX 78758; tel. 512/873–6100; Penny Zagroba, Operations Manager
HMO Texas, L.C., P.O. Box 42416, Houston, TX 77242–2416; tel. 713/952–6868; FAX. 713/974–1650; John Micale, President
Harris Health Plan, Inc., d/b/a Harris Methodist Health Plan, 611 Ryan Plaza Drive, Suite 900, Arlington, TX 76011–4009; tel. 817/462–7000; Donna A. Goldin, Chief Operating Officer
Harris Methodist Texas Health Plan, Inc., d/b/a Harris Methodist Health Plan, 611 Ryan Plaza Drive, Suite 900, Arlington, TX 76011–4009; tel. 817/462–7000; FAX. 817/462–7235; Tom Keenan, Chief Operating Officer
Healthcare Partner HMO, 821 ESE, Loop 323, Two American Center, Zip 75701, P.O. Box 130187, Zip 75713, Tyler, TX 75701; tel. 903/581–2600; Tom Slack, Chief Executive Officer
Healthplan of Texas, Inc., 534 South Beckham, Tyler, TX 75701; tel. 903/531–4730; Edwin McClusky, M.D., Chief Executive Officer
Healthsource North Texas, Inc., 1612 Summit Avenue, Suite 300, Fort Worth, TX 76102; tel. 817/336–1044; FAX. 817/332–2330; David Mier, Manager, Provider Relations
Healthsource Texas, Inc., 1122 Colorado, Suite 205, Austin, TX 78701; tel. 512/494–1090; Terry Steven Shilling, President, Chief Executive Officer
Humana Health Plan of Texas, Inc., d/b/a Humana Health Plan of San Antonio, 8431 Fredericksburg Road, Suite 570, San Antonio, TX 78229; tel. 210/617–1000; FAX. 210/617–1704; Michael A. Seltzer, Director, Texas Operations
Humana Health Plan of Texas, Inc., d/b/a Humana Health Plan of Dallas, 8431 Fredericksburg Road, San Antonio, TX 78229; tel. 512/617–1000; Brenda Luckett, Executive Director
Kaiser Foundation Health Plan of Texas, 12720 Hillcrest Road, Suite 600, Dallas, TX 75230; tel. 214/458–5000; FAX. 214/233–5281; Sharon Flaherty, President
Memorial Sisters of Charity HMO, LLC, 9494 Southwest Freeway, Suite 300, Houston, TX 77074; tel. 713/430–1400; FAX. 713/778–2375; Brigid Pace, President, Chief Executive Officer
Mercy Health Plans of Missouri, Inc., 1919 Cedar Street, Larado, TX 78740; tel. 210/718–8764; Ernesto Seguna, Vice President
MethodistCare, 6500 Fannin, Suite 902, Houston, TX 77030; tel. 713/793–7052; FAX. 713/793–7064; James Henderson, President, Chief Executive Officer
Mid–Con Health Plans, L.C., d/b/a HMO Blue, SouthWest Texas, 500 Chestnut Street, Suite 1699, Abilene, TX 79602; tel. 915/738–3518; FAX. 915/738–3519; Harold Rubin, President
NYLCare Dental Plan of the Southwest, Inc., 4500 Fuller Drive, Irving, TX 75038; tel. 972/650–5500; FAX. 972/650–5707; Steve Yerxa, Chief Executive Officer, Executive Director
NYLCare Health Plan of the Southwest, 4500 Fuller Drive, Irving, TX 75038; tel. 972/650–5500; FAX. 972/650–5703; Steve Yerxa
NYLCare Health Plans of the Gulf Coast, 2425 West Loop South, Suite 1000, Houston, TX 77027; tel. 713/624–5000; FAX. 713/963–9417; Thomas S. Lucksinger, President, Chief Executive Officer
One Health Plan of Texas, Inc., 10000 North Central Expressway, Suite 900, Lock Box 46, Dallas, TX 75231; tel. 800/866–3136; Jim White, President
Orthopedic Healthcare of Texas, Inc., 729 Bedford–Euless Road, W., Suite 100, Hurst, TX 76053; tel. 817/282–6905; Edward William Smith, D.O., President
PCA Health Plans of Texas, Inc., 8303 MoPac, Suite 450, Austin, TX 78759; tel. 512/338–6100; FAX. 512/338–6137; Donald Gessler, M.D., President, Chief Executive Officer
Pacificare of Texas, Inc., 1420 West Mockingbird Lane, Suite 800, Dallas, TX 75247; tel. 214/631–5312; FAX. 214/640–1658; Patrick Feyen, President
Parkland Community Health Plan, Inc., 5201 Harry Hines Boulevard, Dallas, TX 75235; tel. 214/590–2800; Ron J. Anderson, President
Parliament Dental Plans, Inc., 2909 Hillcroft, Suite 515, Houston, TX 77057; tel. 713/784–6262; FAX. 713/784–0488; Paul H. Michael, President
Physicians Care HMO, Inc., 5959 Harry Hines Boulevard, Suite 620, Dallas, TX 75235; tel. 214/915–1300; FAX. 214/905–9369; Amanullah Khan, President
Principal Health Care of Texas, Inc., 555 North Caracahua, Suite 500, Corpus Christi, TX 78478; tel. 512/887–0101; Diana Tchida, Executive Director
Prudential Dental Maintenance Organization, Inc., Stop 206, One Prudential Circle, Sugar Land, TX 77478–3833; tel. 281/494–6000; FAX. 281/276–3752; Royce Rosemond, Executive Director
Prudential Health Care Plan, Inc. of Houston, Stop 300–D, One Prudential Circle, Sugar Land, TX 77478; tel. 713/276–3850; FAX. 713/276–8254; Dennis Edmonds, Executive Director
Rio Grande HMO, Inc., d/b/a HMO Blue, 4150 Pinnacle, Suite 203, El Paso, TX 79902; tel. 800/831–0576; Anne McDow, Vice President, Operations
Safeguard Health Plans, Inc., 7502 Greenville Avenue, Suite 210, Dallas, TX 75231; tel. 214/265–7041; FAX. 214/265–7702; David Branstetter, Executive Director
Scott & White Health Plan, 2401 South 31st Street, Temple, TX 76508; tel. 817/742–3030; FAX. 817/742–3011; Deny Radefeld, Executive Director
Seton Health Plan, Inc., 1201 West 38th Street, Austin, TX 78705; tel. 800/749–7404; FAX. 512/323–1952; John H. Evler III, President, Chief Operating Officer
Sha, L.L.C., d/b/a Firstcare, 12940 Research, Austin, TX 78750; tel. 800/431–7737; Dale Bowerman, President and Chief Executive Officer
Spectera Dental, Inc., (formerly United Healthcare Dental, Inc.), 1445 North Loop West, Suite 1000, Houston, TX 77008; tel. 713/861–3231; Arlene Sheldon, Executive Director
Superior Healthplan, L.P., 701 Brazos Street, Suite 500, Austin, TX 78701; tel. 512/320–9155; Jose Comacho, Executive Director
Texas Children's Health Plan, Inc., 1919 South Braeswood Boulevard, P.O. Box 301011, Houston, TX 77230–1011; tel. 713/770–2600; FAX. 713/770–2686; Christopher Born, President
Unicare of Texas Health Plans, Inc., (formerly Affiliated Health Plans, Inc.), 11200 Westheimer, Suite 700, Houston, TX 77042; tel. 713/782–4555; Sam John Nicholson II, President
United Dental Care of Texas, Inc., 14755 Preston Road, Suite 300, Dallas, TX 75240; tel. 214/458–7474; James B. Kingston, President
United Healthcare of Texas, Inc., (formerly Metrahealth Care Plan of Texas, Inc.), Arboretum Plaza Building Two, Suite 600, 9442 Capital of Texas Highway N., Austin, TX 78759; tel. 800/424–6480; FAX. 512/338–6812; Karen England, Director, Network Operations
United Healthcare of Texas, Inc., Dallas/Fort Worth Division, 4835 LBJ Freeway, Suite 1100, Dallas, TX 75244; tel. 214/866–6000; FAX. 214/866–6018; Richard Cook, Chief Executive Officer
Vista Health Plan, Inc., (formerly The Wellness Health Plan of Texas, Inc.), 7801 North IH–35, Austin, TX 78753; tel. 512/433–1000; Paul Tovar, President
West Texas Health Plans, d/b/a HMO Blue, West Texas, Sentry Plaza II, 5225 South Loop 289, Suite 117, Lubbock, TX 79424; tel. 806/798–6367; Michael A. Huesman, President

UTAH

American Family Care of Utah, Inc., 3098 South Highland Drive, Suite 335, Salt Lake City, UT 84106; tel. 801/486–1664; Jose Fernandez, President
Benchoice, Inc., 310 East 4500 South, Suite 550, Murray, UT 84157–0906; tel. 801/262–2999; Talmage Pond, President
CIGNA Health Plan of Utah, Inc., 5295 South 320 West, Suite 280, Salt Lake City, UT 84107; tel. 801/265–2777, ext. 7501; FAX. 801/261–5349; Robert Immitt, President
Delta Care Dental Plan, Inc., 257 East 200 South, Suite 375, Salt Lake City, UT 84111; tel. 801/575–5168
Educators Health Care, 852 East Arrowhead Lane, Murray, UT 84107–5298; tel. 801/262–7476; FAX. 801/269–9734; Andy I. Galano, Ph.D., President
Employees Choice Health Option, 35 West Broadway, Salt Lake City, UT 84101; tel. 801/355–1234; Larry Bridge, President
FHP of Utah, Inc., 35 West Broadway, Salt Lake City, UT 84101; tel. 801/355–1234, ext. 3500; FAX. 801/531–9003; Larry Bridge, President
HealthWise, 2455 Parley's Way, P.O. Box 30270, Salt Lake City, UT 84130–0270; tel. 801/481–6184; FAX. 801/481–6994; Jed H. Pitcher, Chairman
Humana Health Plan of Utah, Inc., 500 West Main Street, 20th Floor, Louisville, KY 40201; tel. 502/580–1000
IHC Care, Inc., 36 South State Street, 15th Floor, Salt Lake City, UT 84111; tel. 801/442–5000; FAX. 801/538–5003; Sid Paulson, Chief Operating Officer
IHC Group, Inc., 36 South State Street, 15th Floor, Salt Lake City, UT 84111; tel. 801/442–5000; Sid Paulson, Chief Operating Officer
IHC Health Plans, Inc., 36 South State Street, 15th Floor, Salt Lake City, UT 84111; tel. 801/442–5000; Sid Paulson, Chief Operating Officer
Intergroup Healthcare Corporation of Utah, 127 South 500 East, Suite 410, Salt Lake City, UT 84102; tel. 801/532–7665; FAX. 801/297–4585; Elden Mitchell, President
Opticare of Utah, 159 1/2 South Main Street, Salt Lake City, UT 84111; tel. 801/363–0950; Stephen H. Schubach, President
Safeguard Health Plans, Inc., P.O. Box 3210, Anaheim, CA 92803–3210; tel. 714/778–1005; Steven J. Baileys, D.D.S., President
U. S. Dental Plan, Inc., 4001 South 700 East, Suite 300, Salt Lake City, UT 84107; tel. 801/263–8884; Christopher A. Jehle, President
United HealthCare of Utah, 7910 South 3500 East, Salt Lake City, UT 84121; tel. 801/942–6200; FAX. 801/944–0940; Colin Gardner, Chief Executive Officer
Utah Community Health Plan, 36 South State Street, Suite 1020, Salt Lake City, UT 84111–1418; tel. 801/442–3780; FAX. 801/442–3791; William K. Willson, Executive Director

VERMONT

Capital District Physicians Health Plan, 17 Columbia Circle, Albany, NY 12203; tel. 518/862–3923; FAX. 518/452–3767; Ellen M. Pierce, Director, Accounting
Community Health Plan (CHP), 1201 Troy–Schenectady Road, Latham, NY 12110; tel. 518/783–1864; FAX. 518/783–0234; John Baackes, President, Chief Executive Officer
Harvard Community Health Plan, 10 Brookline Place West, Brookline, MA 02146; tel. 617/731–8240
MVP Health Plan, 111 Liberty Street, P.O. Box 2207, Schenectady, NY 12301–2207; tel. 518/370–4793; David W. Oliker, President
Matthew Thornton Health Plan, 43 Constitution Drive, Bedford, NH 03110–6020; tel. 603/695–1100; FAX. 603/695–1157; Everett Page, President

VIRGINIA

Aetna Health Plans of the Mid–Atlantic, Inc., 7799 Leesburg Pike, Suite 1100 South, Falls Church, VA 22043; tel. 703/903–7100; FAX. 703/903–0316; Russell R. Dickhart, President, Executive Director

CIGNA HealthCare of Virginia, Inc., 4050 Innslake Drive, Glen Allen, VA 23060; tel. 804/273–1100; John E. Sharp, Vice President, Executive Director

CIGNA Healthplan Mid–Atlantic, Inc., 9700 Patuxent Woods Drive, Columbia, MD 21046; tel. 301/720–5800; Timothy P. Fitzgerald, President

CapitalCare, Inc., Tysons International Plaza, 550 12th Street, S.W., Suite 2, Washington, DC 20065–0001; tel. 703/761–5400; FAX. 703/761–5576; David L. Ward, President, Chief Executive Officer

Chesapeake Health Plan, Inc., 814 Light Street, Baltimore, MD 21230; tel. 410/539–8622

George Washington University Health Plan, Inc., 4550 Montgomery Avenue, Suite 800, Bethesda, MD 20814; tel. 301/941–2000; FAX. 301/941–2005; Dr. Kenneth A. Tannenbaum, Chief Executive Officer

Group Health Association, Inc., 4301 Connecticut Avenue, N.W., Washington, DC 20008; tel. 202/364–7523

HMO Virginia, Inc., Health Keepers, 2220 Edward Holland Drive, Richmond, VA 23230; tel. 804/354–7961; FAX. 804/354–3554; Sam Weidman, Vice President, Finance

Health First, Inc., 621 Lynnhaven Parkway, Suite 450, Virginia Beach, VA 23452–7330; tel. 804/431–5298; Russell F. Mohawk, President

HealthKeepers, Inc., 2220 Edward Holland Drive, P.O. Box 26623, Richmond, VA 23230; tel. 804/354–7961; FAX. 804/354–3554; Sam Weidman, Vice President, Finance

Heritage National Healthplan, Inc., 1515 Fifth Avenue, Suite 200, Moline, IL 61265–1358; tel. 309/765–1203

Humana Group Health Plan, Inc., 4301 Connecticut Avenue, N.W., Washington, DC 20008; tel. 202/364–2000; FAX. 202/364–7418; Ted W. LaBedz

Kaiser Foundation Health Plan of the Mid–Atlantic States, Inc., 2101 East Jefferson Street, Rockville, MD 20852; tel. 301/816–2424; FAX. 301/816–7478; Alan J. Silverstone, President

MD–Individual Practice Association, Inc., Four Taft Court, Rockville, MD 20850; tel. 301/294–5100; FAX. 301/309–1709; Susan Goff, President

NYLCare Health Plans of Mid–Atlantic, Inc., 7601 Ora Glen Drive, Suite 200, Greenbelt, MD 20770; tel. 301/982–0098, ext. 3308; FAX. 301/489–5282; Jeff D. Emerson, President, Chief Executive Officer

National Capital Health Plan, Inc., 5850 Versar Center, Suite 420, Springfield, VA 22151; tel. 703/914–5650

Optimum Choice, Inc., Four Taft Court, Rockville, MD 20850; tel. 301/738–7920; FAX. 301/309–3782; George T. Jochum, President, Chief Executive Officer

Partners National Health Plans of NC, Inc., 2000 Frontis Plaza Boulevard, P.O. Box 24907, Winton–Salem, NC 27114–4907; tel. 910/760–4822

Peninsula Health Care, Inc., 606 Denbigh Boulevard, Suite 500, Newport News, VA 23608; tel. 757/875–5760; FAX. 757/875–5785; C. Burke King, President

Physicians Health Plan, Inc., Health Keepers, 2220 Edward Holland Drive, Richmond, VA 23230; tel. 804/354–7961; FAX. 804/354–3554; Sam Weidman, Vice President, Finance

Principal Health Care, Inc., 1801 Rockville Pike, Suite 601, Rockville, MD 20852; tel. 301/881–1033, ext. 2211; FAX. 301/881–5403; Kenneth J. Linde, President

Priority Health Plan, Inc., 621 Lynnhaven Parkway, Suite 450, Virginia Beach, VA 23452–7330; tel. 804/463–4600; Russell F. Mohawk, President

Prudential Health Care Plan, Inc., d/b/a PruCare and Prudential Health Care Plan of the Mid–Atlantic, 1000 Boulders Parkway, Richmond, VA 23225; tel. 804/323–0900; William Patrick Link, President

QualChoice of VA Health Plan, Inc., 1807 Seminole Trail, Suite 201, Charlottesville, VA 22901; tel. 804/975–1212; FAX. 804/975–1414; Jay V. Garriss, President, Chief Executive Officer

Sentara Health Management, 4417 Corporation Lane, Virginia Beach, VA 23462; tel. 804/552–7400; FAX. 804/552–7396; Michael M. Dudley, President

Sentara Health Plans, Inc., d/b/a Sentara Health Plan, 4417 Corporation Lane, Virginia Beach, VA 23462; tel. 804/552–7100; FAX. 804/552–7396; John E. McNamara III, President

Southern Health Services, 9881 Mayland Drive, P.O. Box 85603, Richmond, VA 23285–5603; tel. 804/747–3700; FAX. 804/747–8723; James L. Gore, President

U. S. Healthcare, Inc., 980 Jolly Road, P.O. Box 1109, Blue Bell, PA 19422; tel. 215/628–4800

United Optical, d/b/a Spectera, Inc., 2811 Lord Baltimore Drive, Baltimore, MD 21244; tel. 410/265–6033; FAX. 410/594–9862; Dave Hall, Vice President, Marketing

VA Chartered Health Plan, Inc., 4701 Cox Road, Glen Allen, VA 23060; tel. 804/967–0747; Sheila Blackman, Chief Operating Officer

WASHINGTON

Good Health Plan of Washington, Century Square, 1501 Fourth Avenue, Suite 500, Seattle, WA 98101; tel. 206/622–6111; FAX. 206/346–0969; Lee Hooks, Executive Director

Group Health Cooperative of Puget Sound, Administration and Conference Center, 521 Wall Street, Seattle, WA 98121–1535; tel. 206/448–6460; FAX. 206/448–6080; Phil Nudelman, Ph.D., President, Chief Executive Officer

Group Health Northwest, 5615 West Sunset Highway, Spokane, WA 99204; tel. 509/838–9100; FAX. 509/838–3823; Henry S. Berman, M.D., President, Chief Executive Officer

HMO Washington, 1800 Ninth Avenue, P.O. Box 2088, Seattle, WA 98111–2088; tel. 206/389–6721; FAX. 206/389–6719; Bryan Heinrich, Executive Director

Health Maintenance of Oregon, Inc., 1800 First Avenue, Suite 505, P.O. Box 139, Portland, OR 97201; tel. 503/274–0755; FAX. 503/225–5431; Eric Bush

HealthFirst Partners, Inc., 601 Union Street, Suite 700, Seattle, WA 98101; tel. 206/667–8070; FAX. 206/667–8060; Eileen Duncan

HealthGuard Services, Inc., d/b/a SelectCare, 600 Country Club Road, P.O. Box 10106, Eugene, OR 97401–2240; tel. 541/485–1850; FAX. 503/686–2504; David L. Slade, President

HealthPlus, P.O. Box 2113, Seattle, WA 98111–2113; tel. 206/670–4700; FAX. 206/670–4766; Gary L. Meade, President, Chief Executive Officer

Humana Health Plan of Washington, Inc., P.O. Box 1438, Louisville, KY 40201–1438; tel. 502/580–3620; FAX. 502/580–3942; Sandra Lewis, Director, Government Compliance

Kaiser Foundation Health Plan of the Northwest, 500 Northeast Multnomah, Suite 100, Portland, OR 97232–2099; tel. 503/813–2800; FAX. 503/813–2283; Denise L. Honzel, Vice President

PACC, d/b/a PACC Health Plans of Washington, 12901 Southeast 97th Avenue, P.O. Box 286, Clackamas, OR 97015–0286; tel. 503/659–4212; FAX. 503/786–5319; Ron Morgan

PacifiCare of Oregon, Inc., Five Centerpointe Drive, Suite 600, Lake Oswego, OR 97035; tel. 503/620–9324; Patrick Feyen, President

PacificCare of Washington, 600 University Street, Suite 700, Seattle, WA 98101; tel. 206/326–4645; FAX. 206/442–5399; Brad Bowlus, President, Chief Executive Officer

QualMed Washington Health Plan, Inc, d/b/a Qual–Med Health Plan, 2331 130th Avenue, N.E., Suite 200, Zip 98009, P.O. Box 3387, Bellevue, WA 98009–3387; tel. 206/869–3500; FAX. 206/869–3568; C.F. du Laney, President

Sisters of Providence, Good Health Plan of Oregon, Inc., 1235 Northeast 47th Avenue, Suite 220, Portland, OR 97213; tel. 503/249–2981; Jack Friedman, Executive Director

Unified Physicians of Washington, Inc., 33301 Ninth Avenue, S., Suite 200, Federal Way, WA 98003–6394; tel. 206/815–1888; FAX. 206/815–0486; Dodie Wine, Associate Director, Communications

Virginia Mason Health Plan, Inc., Metropolitan Park West, 1100 Olive Way, Suite 1580, Seattle, WA 98101–1828; tel. 206/223–8844; FAX. 206/223–7506; John Clarke, Director, Operations

WEST VIRGINIA

Anthem Health Plan of West Virginia, Inc., d/b/a PrimeONE, 602 Virginia Street, East, Charleston, WV 25301; tel. 304/353–8728; FAX. 304/353–8732; A. Paul Holdren, President, Chief Executive Officer

Carelink Health Plans, 141 Summers Square, P.O. Box 1711, Charleston, WV 25326–1711; tel. 304/348–2901; FAX. 304/348–2948; Alan L. Mytty, President

Coventry Health Plan of West Virginia, Inc., (Health Assurance HMO), 887 National Road, Wheeling, WV 26003; tel. 304/234–5100; FAX. 304/234–5119; Marilyn White, Manager

Health Guard, Inc., d/b/a Advantage Health Plan, Inc., 300 Guernsey Street, Bellaire, OH 43906; tel. 614/676–4623; Dan Splain

Optimum Choice, 3025 Hamaker Court, Suite 301, Fairfax, VA 22031; tel. 703/207–6570; Susan Hrubes, Senior Director

The Health Plan of the Upper Ohio Valley, 52160 National Road, E., St. Clairsville, OH 43950; tel. 614/695–3585; Philip D. Wright, President

WISCONSIN

Atrium Health Plan, Inc., 2215 Vine Street, Suite E, Hudson, WI 54016–5802; tel. 800/535–4041; FAX. 715/386–8326; Michael L. Christensen, Director of Operations

Compcare Health Services Insurance Corp., 401 West Michigan Street, P.O. Box 2947, Milwaukee, WI 53201–2025; tel. 414/226–6171; FAX. 414/226–6229; Jeffrey J. Nohl, President, Chief Operating Officer

Dean Health Plan, Inc., P.O. Box 56099, Madison, WI 53705–9399; tel. 608/836–1400; FAX. 608/836–9620; John A. Turcott, President, Chief Executive Officer

Emphesys Wisconsin Insurance Company, 1100 Employers Boulevard, DePere, WI 54115; tel. 800/558–4444; Mark R. Minsloff, Executive Director

Family Health Plan Cooperative, 11524 West Theo Trecker Way, Milwaukee, WI 53214–7260; tel. 414/256–0006; FAX. 414/256–5681; Conrad Sobczak, Executive Director

Genesis Health Plan Insurance Corporation, P.O. Box 20007, Greenfield, WI 53220–0007; tel. 414/425–3323; FAX. 414/425–3034; Karl Rajani, Chief Executive Officer

Greater La Crosse Health Plans, Inc., 1285 Rudy Street, Onalaska, WI 54650; tel. 608/782–2638; FAX. 608/781–8862; Steven M. Kunes, Plan Administrator

Group Health Cooperative of Eau Claire, P.O. Box 3217, Eau Claire, WI 54702–3217; tel. 715/836–8552; FAX. 715/836–7683; Claire W. Johnson, General Manager

Group Health Cooperative of South Central Wisconsin, 8202 Excelsior Drive, P.O. Box 44971, Madison, WI 53744–4971; tel. 608/251–4156; FAX. 608/257–3842; Lawrence Zanoni, Executive Director

Gundersen Lutheran Health Plan, Inc., 1836 South Avenue, LaCrosse, WI 54601; tel. 608/798–8020; FAX. 608/791–8042; Jeff Treasure, Chief Executive Officer

Humana Wisconsin Health Organization Insurance Corporation, 111 West Pleasant Street, P.O.Box 12359, Milwaukee, WI 53212–0359; tel. 414/223–3300; FAX. 414/223–7777; William L. Carr, Executive Director

Managed Health Services, 10607 West Oklahoma Avenue, Milwaukee, WI 53227; tel. 414/328–5005; FAX. 414/321–9724; Michael F. Neidorff, President, Chief Executive Officer

Maxicare Health Insurance Company, 790 North Milwaukee Street, Milwaukee, WI 53202; tel. 414/271–6371; John F. Southworth, Administrator

Medica Health Plans of Wisconsin, Inc., 5901 Smetana Drive, P.O. Box 9310, Minneapolis, MN 55440–9310; tel. 612/992–2000

Medical Associates Clinic Health Plan of Wisconsin, 700 Locust Street, Suite 230, Dubuque, IA 52001–6800; tel. 319/556–8070; FAX. 319/556–5134; Ross A. Madden, Chairman of the Board, Director

MercyCare Health Plan, Inc., One Parker Place, Suite 750, Janesville, WI 53545; tel. 608/752–3431; FAX. 608/752–3751; Don Schreiner, Senior Vice President

Network Health Plan of Wisconsin, Inc., 1165 Appleton Road, P.O. Box 120, Menasha, WI 54952–0120; tel. 414/727–0100; FAX. 414/727–5634; Michael D. Wolff, President, Chief Executive Officer

North Central Health Protection Plan, 2000 Westwood Drive, Zip 54401, P.O. Box 969, Wausau, WI 54402–0969; tel. 715/847–8866; Larry A. Baker, Administrator

Physicians Plus Insurance Corporation, 340 West Washington Avenue, P.O. Box 2078, Madison, WI 53703; tel. 608/282–8900; FAX. 608/282–8944; Thomas R. Sobocinski, President, Chief Executive Officer

PrimeCare Health Plan, Inc., 10701 West Research Drive, Milwaukee, WI 53226–0649; tel. 414/443–4000; FAX. 414/443–4750; James Schultz, Administrator

Security Health Plan of Wisconsin, Inc., 1000 North Oak Avenue, Marshfield, WI 54449; tel. 715/387–5534; FAX. 715/387–5240; Richard A. Leer, President

United Health of Wisconsin Insurance Company, Inc., P.O. Box 507, Appleton, WI 54912–0507; tel. 414/735–6440; FAX. 414/731–7232; Jay Fulkerson, Chief Executive Officer

Unity Health Plans Insurance Corp., 840 Carolina Street, Sauk City, WI 53583; tel. 800/362–3308; FAX. 608/643–2564; Mary Traver, Interim President

Valley Health Plan, 2270 East Ridge Center, P.O. Box 3128, Eau Claire, WI 54702–3128; tel. 715/832–3235; FAX. 715/836–1298; Kathyrn R. Teeters, Director

WYOMING

IHC Health Plans, Inc., 36 South State Street, Salt Lake City, UT 84111; tel. 801/442–5000; FAX. 801/442–5003; Martin Byrnes, Compliance Supervisor

WINhealth Partners, 2600 East 18th Street, Cheyenne, WY 82001; tel. 307/633–7051; FAX. 307/633–7053; Beth Wasson, Executive Director

U. S. Associated Areas

GUAM

F.H.P., Inc., P.O. Box 6578, Tamunig, GU 96911; tel. 671/646–5824; FAX. 671/646–6923; Edward English, Associate Regional Vice President

Guam Memorial Health Plan, 142 West Seaton Boulevard, Agana, GU 96910; tel. 671/472–4647; FAX. 671/477–1784; James W. Gillan, Chief Operating Officer

PUERTO RICO

First Medical Comprehensive Health Care, Inc., (Antes Plan Comprensivo de Salud, Inc.), Apartado 40954, Estacion Minillas, Santurce, PR 00940; tel. 809/723–6016; FAX. 809/723–6014; J. A. Soler, President

Golden Cross HMO Health Plan Corporation, Antes HMO Medical System Corporation, Apartado 1727, Estacion Viejo San Juan, San Juan, PR 00902; tel. 809/721–0427; FAX. 809/724–7249; Maria J. Gonzalez

Medical One, Inc., (Antes Plan Medico Doctor Gubern, Inc.), Miramar Plaza, Ave. Ponce de Leon 954, Suite 102A, Santurce, PR 00907; tel. 809/289–6969; Montserrat G. de Garcia, Chief Executive Officer

Mennonite General Hospital, Inc., Calle Jose C. Vazquez, Apartado 1379, Aibonito, PR 00705; tel. 809/735–8001; FAX. 809/735–8073; Domingo Torres Zayas, Chief Executive Officer

PCA Health Plans, 383 F. D. Roosevelt Avenue, San Juan, PR 00918–2131; tel. 809/282–7900; FAX. 809/793–1450; Jose A. Cuevas, President, Chief Executive Officer

Plan Medico U.T.I. de Puerto Rico, Inc., Apartado 23316–Estacion U.P.R., Rio Piedras, PR 00924; tel. 809/758–1500; FAX. 809/758–3210; David Munoz, President

Plan de Salud Hospital de la Concepcion, Inc., Calle Luna 41, Apartado 285, San German, PR 00683; tel. 809/892–1860; Ivonne Montaluo, Executive Director

Plan de Salud U.I.A., Inc., Calle Mayaguez #49, San Juan, PR 00917; tel. 787/763–4004; FAX. 787/763–7095; Jose E. Sanchez, Consultant

Plan de Salud de la Federacion de Maestros, de Puerto Rico, Inc., P.O. Box 71336, San Juan, PR 00936–8436; tel. 787/758–5610; FAX. 787/281–7392; Eugenio Aponte, Executive Director

Ryder Health Plan, Inc., Call Box 859, Humacao, PR 00792; tel. 809/852–0846; FAX. 809/850–4863; Juan L. De Le Rosa, Director

Servi Medical, Inc., Avenida Munoz Rivera 402, Parada 31, Hato Rey, PR 00917; tel. 809/758–5555; FAX. 809/250–1425; Lexie Gomez

Servicios de Salud Bella Vista, Bella Vista Gardens Numero 43, Carr. 349–Cerro Las Mesas, Mayaguez, PR 00680; tel. 787/833–8070; FAX. 787/832–5400; Victor Prosper–Rios, President

United Healthcare Plans of Puerto Rico, Inc., (Antes Group Sales and Service of Puerto Rico, Inc.), Rexco Office Park, Apartado 364864, San Juan, PR 00936–4864; tel. 809/782–7005; FAX. 809/782–5269; Luis A. Salgado Munoz, Executive Vice President

State Government Agencies for HMO's

United States

ALABAMA: Department of Insurance, 135 South Union Street, Montgomery, AL 36130; tel. 334/269–3550; FAX. 334/241–4192; Michael DeBellis, Commissioner of Insurance

ALASKA: Alaska Division of Insurance, P.O. Box 110805, Juneau, AK 99811–0805; tel. 907/465–2596; FAX. 907/465–3422; Marianne K. Burke, Director

ARIZONA: Department of Insurance, 2910 North 44th Street, Suite 210, Phoenix, AZ 85018; tel. 602/912–8443; FAX. 602/912–8453; Mary Butterfield, Assistant Director, Life and Health Division

ARKANSAS: Arkansas Insurance Department, 1200 West Third Street, Little Rock, AR 72201–1904; tel. 501/371–2600; FAX. 501/371–2618; Mike Pickens, Insurance Commissioner

CALIFORNIA: Department of Corporations, Health Care Service Plan Division, 3700 Wilshire Boulevard, Los Angeles, CA 90010; tel. 213/736–2776; Gary G. Hagen, Assistant Commissioner, Health Care Division

COLORADO: Department of Regulatory Agencies, Colorado Division of Insurance, 1560 Broadway, Suite 850, Denver, CO 80202; tel. 303/894–7499; FAX. 303/894–7455, ext. 322; Nancy Litwinski, Assistant Commissioner of Financial Regulation

CONNECTICUT: Department of Insurance, P.O. Box 816, Hartford, CT 06142–0816; tel. 203/297–3800; FAX. 203/566–7410; Mary Ellen Breault, Director, Life and Health Division

DELAWARE: Department of Health and Social Services, Office of Health Facilities Licensure and Certification, Three Mill Road, Suite 308, Wilmington, DE 19806; tel. 302/577–6666; FAX. 302/577–6672; Ellen T. Reap, Director

DISTRICT OF COLUMBIA: District of Columbia Department of Insurance, 441 Fourth Street, N.W., Suite 850 North, Washington, DC 20001; tel. 202/727–8000, ext. 3031; FAX. 202/727–8055; Herman Hunter, Chief Consumer Services Division

FLORIDA: Florida Department of Insurance, Bureau of Life and Health Insurer Solvency and Market Conduct, 200 East Gaines, Larson Building, Tallahassee, FL 32399–0327; tel. 904/922–3153, ext. 2471; FAX. 904/413–9019; Tom Warring, HMO Financial Examiner/Analyst Supervisor

GEORGIA: Department of Insurance, 716 West Tower, Floyd Building, Two Martin Luther King Jr. Drive, Atlanta, GA 30334; tel. 404/656–5826; FAX. 404/657–7743; John Oxendine, Commissioner

HAWAII: State of Hawaii Department of Labor and Industrial Relations, Disability Compensation Division, P.O. Box 3769, Honolulu, HI 96812; tel. 808/586–9151; Gary S. Hamada, Administrator

IDAHO: Department of Insurance, 700 West State Street, Third Floor, P.O. Box 83720, Boise, ID 83720–0043; tel. 208/334–4250; FAX. 208/334–4398; Joan Krosch, Health Insurance Coordinator

ILLINOIS: Department of Insurance, 320 West Washington Street, Fourth Floor, Springfield, IL 62767–0001; tel. 217/782–6369; FAX. 217/782–5020; David E. Grant, Health Care Coordinator

INDIANA: Department of Insurance, 311 West Washington Street, Suite 300, Indianapolis, IN 46204; tel. 317/232–2408; FAX. 317/232–5251; Shelly Hitch, Supervising Life and Health Auditor, HMO Coordinator

IOWA: Iowa Department of Commerce, Division of Insurance, Lucas State Office Building, Sixth Floor, Des Moines, IA 50319; tel. 515/281–5705; FAX. 515/281–3059; Therese M. Vaughan, Commissioner

KANSAS: Kansas Insurance Department, 420 Southwest Ninth Street, Topeka, KS 66612; tel. 913/296–3071; FAX. 913/296–2283; Kathleen Sebelius, Commissioner

KENTUCKY: Department of Insurance, Life and Health Division, 215 West Main Street, P.O. Box 517, Frankfort, KY 40602; tel. 502/564–6088; FAX. 502/564–6090; Janie Miller, Director

LOUISIANA: Department of Insurance, P.O. Box 94214, Baton Rouge, LA 70804; tel. 504/342–5900; FAX. 504/342–3078; James H. Brown, Commissioner

MAINE: Department of Professional and Financial Regulation, Bureau of Insurance, 34 State House Station, Augusta, ME 04333; tel. 207/624–8416; FAX. 207/624–8599; Michael F. McGonigle, Senior Insurance Analyst

MARYLAND: Department of Health and Mental Hygiene, Insurance Division, 201 West Preston Street, Baltimore, MD 21201–2399; tel. 410/225–6860; Martin P. Wasserman, M.D., J.D., Secretary

MASSACHUSETTS: Division of Insurance, 470 Atlantic Avenue, Boston, MA 02210–2223; tel. 617/521–7301; FAX. 617/521–7770; Linda Ruthardt, Commissioner

MICHIGAN: Department of Public Health, Bureau of Health Systems, Division of Managed Care, 3423 North Logan/Martin Luther King Boulevard, P.O. Box 30195, Lansing, MI 48909; tel. 517/335–8551; FAX. 517/335–8582; Janet Olszewski, Chief, Managed Care Division

MINNESOTA: Department of Health, Health Systems Development Division, 121 East Seventh Place, Suite 450, P.O. Box 64975, St. Paul, MN 55164–0975; tel. 612/282–5600; Nanette M. Schroeder, Director

MISSISSIPPI: Mississippi Department of Insurance, P.O. Box 79, Jackson, MS 39205; tel. 601/359–3577; FAX. 601/359–2474; George W. Neville, Special Assistant Attorney General

MISSOURI: Department of Insurance, Division of Company Regulation Life and Health Section, P.O. Box 690, Jefferson City, MO 65102; tel. 573/751–4363; FAX. 573/526–6075; James W. Casey, Supervisor

MONTANA: Montana State Auditor, Insurance Department, Insurance Examinations Division, Mitchell Building, Room 270, 126 North Sanders, P.O. Box 4009, Helena, MT 59604–4009; tel. 406/444–2040; FAX. 406/444–3497; James Borchardt, Chief Examiner, Montana Insurance Department

NEBRASKA: Department of Insurance, 941 O Street, Suite 400, Lincoln, NE 68508; tel. 402/471–2201; FAX. 402/471–4610; Robert G. Lange, Director

NEVADA: Nevada Division of Insurance, Capitol Complex, 1665 Hot Springs Road, Suite 152, Carson City, NV 89710; tel. 702/687–4270; FAX. 702/687–3937; Alice A. Molasky, Esq., Commissioner

NEW HAMPSHIRE: Department of Health and Human Services, Office of Medical Services, Hazen Drive, Concord, NH 03301–6521; tel. 603/271–4365; FAX. 603/271–4376; Diane Kemp, Program Specialist

NEW JERSEY: Department of Health, Division of Health Facilities, Evaluation, Licensing and Resource Development, Alternative Health Systems, CN–367, Trenton, NJ 08625; tel. 609/588–2510; FAX. 609/588–7823; Edwin V. Kelleher, Chief

NEW MEXICO: State Corporation Commission, Department of Insurance, P.O. Drawer 1269, Santa Fe, NM 87504; tel. 505/827–4601; FAX. 505/827–4734; Helen S. Hordes, Manager, Life and Health Forms Division

NEW YORK: Department of Health, Office of Health Systems Management, Empire State Plaza, Corning Tower Building, Albany, NY 12237; tel. 518/474–5515

NORTH CAROLINA: Department of Insurance, Financial Evaluation Division, P.O. Box 26387, Raleigh, NC 27611; tel. 919/733–5633; L. W. Cannady, Financial Analyst

NORTH DAKOTA: North Dakota Department of Insurance, State Capitol, 600 East Boulevard, Bismarck, ND 58505–0320; tel. 701/328–2440; FAX. 701/328–4880; Glenn Pomeroy, Commissioner

OHIO: Department of Insurance, Managed Care Division, 2100 Stella Court, Columbus, OH 43215–1067; tel. 614/644–3313; FAX. 614/644–3741; Kip May, Assistant Director

OKLAHOMA: Oklahoma State Department of Health, 1000 Northeast 10th Street, Oklahoma City, OK 73117–1299; tel. 405/271–6868; FAX. 405/271–3442; Lajuana Wire, Senior Health Planner

OREGON: Department of Consumer and Business Services, Insurance Division, 440 Labor and Industries Building, Salem, OR 97310; tel. 503/378–4271, ext. 640; FAX. 503/378–4351

PENNSYLVANIA: Pennsylvania Insurance Department, Company Licensing Division, 1345 Strawberry Square, Harrisburg, PA 17120; tel. 717/787–2735; FAX. 717/787–8557; Steven Harman, Chief

RHODE ISLAND: Department of Business Regulation, Division of Insurance, 233 Richmond Street, Suite 233, Providence, RI 02903–4233; tel. 401/277–2223; FAX. 401/751–4887; Alfonso E. Mastrostefano, Associate Director, Superintendent, Insurance

SOUTH CAROLINA: Solvency Licensing and Taxation Services, South Carolina Department of Insurance, 1612 Marion Street, Columbia, SC 29201; tel. 803/737–6221; Timothy W. Campbell, Chief Financial Analyst

SOUTH DAKOTA: Health Policy and External Affairs, South Dakota Department of Health, 445 East Capitol Avenue, Pierre, SD 57501–3185; tel. 605/773–3361; FAX. 605/773–5683; Terrance L. Dosch, Division Director

TENNESSEE: Department of Commerce and Insurance, 500 James Robertson Parkway, Nashville, TN 37243–1135; tel. 615/741–6796; Kathy Fussell, Chief Financial Executive, Insurance Examiner

TEXAS: Texas Department of Insurance, Mail Code 106–3A, P.O. Box 149104, Austin, TX 78714–9104; tel. 512/322–4266; FAX. 512/322–3552; Leah Rummel, Deputy Commissioner, HMO/URA

UTAH: Utah Insurance Department, 3110 State Office Building, Salt Lake City, UT 84114; tel. 801/538–3800; FAX. 801/538–3829

VERMONT: Department of Banking, Insurance and Securities, 89 Main Street, Drawer 20, Montpelier, VT 05620–3101; tel. 802/828–2900; FAX. 802/828–3306; Theresa Alberghini, Deputy Commissioner

Section C

VIRGINIA: State Corporation Commission, Bureau of Insurance, P.O. Box 1157, Richmond, VA 23219; tel. 804/371–9637; FAX. 804/371–9511; Laura Lee Viergever, Senior Insurance Examiner

WASHINGTON: Office of the Insurance Commissioner, Insurance Building, P.O. Box 40255, Olympia, WA 98504–0255; tel. 360/664–8002; FAX. 360/586–3535; Paula M. Strain, Manager, Health Care Contract

WEST VIRGINIA: Insurance Commissioner's Office, Financial Conditions Division, 1124 Smith Street, Charleston, WV 25301; tel. 304/558–2100; FAX. 304/558–0412; Jeffrey W. Van Gilder, Director, Chief Examiner

WISCONSIN: Office of the Commissioner of Insurance, P.O. Box 7873, Madison, WI 53707–7873; tel. 608/266–3585; FAX. 608/266–9935; Josephine W. Musser, Commissioner

WYOMING: Department of Insurance, Herschler Building, Third Floor East, 122 West 25th Street, Cheyenne, WY 82002; tel. 307/777–6807; FAX. 307/777–5895; Lloyd Wilder, Insurance Standards Consultant

U. S. Associated Areas

GUAM: Department of Public Health and Social Services, Government of Guam, P.O. Box 2816, Agana, GU 96932; tel. 671/735–7102; FAX. 671/734–5910; Dennis G. Rodriguez, Director

PUERTO RICO: Aurea Lopez, Chief Examiner, Office of the Commissioner of Insurance, P.O. Box 8330, Fernandez Juncos Station, Santurce, PR 00910–8330; tel. 809/722–8686, ext. 2212; FAX. 809/722–4400; Aurea Lopez, Chief Examiner

Freestanding Ambulatory Surgery Centers

The following list of freestanding ambulatory surgery centers was developed with the assistance of state government agencies and the individual facilities listed. It is current as of January 1, 1997.

The AHA Guide contains two types of ambulatory surgery center listings; those that are hospital based and those that are freestanding. Hospital based ambulatory surgery centers are listed in section A of the AHA Guide and are identified by Facility Code F44. Please refer to that section for information on the over 5,000 hospital based ambulatory surgery centers.

Those freestanding ambulatory surgery centers accredited by the Joint Commission on Accreditation of Healthcare Organizations (JCAHO) are identified by a hollow square (□). These surgery centers have been found to be in substantial compliance with the Joint Commission standards for ambulatory health care facilities, as found in the Ambulatory Health Care Standards Manual.

We present this list simply as a convenient directory. Inclusion or omission of any organization's name indicates neither approval nor disapproval by Healthcare InfoSource, Inc., a subsidiary of the American Hospital Association.

United States

ALABAMA

American Surgery Centers of Alabama, d/b/a American Surgery Center, 2802 Ross Clark Circle, S.W., Dothan, AL 36301; tel. 334/793-3411; FAX. 334/712-0227; Carlotta McCallister, Administrator

Baptist Surgery Center, 2035 East South Boulevard, Montgomery, AL 36111-0000; tel. 334/286-3180; FAX. 334/286-3381; Faye Wimberly, RN, Administrator

Birmingham Outpatient Surgery Center, Ltd., d/b/a Columbia Outpatient CareCenter, 2720 University Boulevard, Birmingham, AL 35233; tel. 205/933-0050; FAX. 205/933-8212; Jackie Harrison, RN, Administrator

Columbia Montgomery Surgical Center, 855 East South Boulevard, Montgomery, AL 36116; tel. 334/284-9600; FAX. 334/284-4233; Susan N. Lamar, Administrator

Columbia Surgicare of Mobile, 2890 Dauphin Street, Mobile, AL 36606; tel. 334/473-2020; FAX. 334/478-6737; Sandy Bunch, Administrator

Dauphin West Surgery Center, 3701 Dauphin Street, Mobile, AL 36608; tel. 334/341-3405; FAX. 334/341-3404; James L. Spires, Executive Director

□ **Decatur Ambulatory Surgery Center,** 2828 Highway 31, S., Decatur, AL 35603; tel. 205/340-1212; FAX. 205/340-0252; Andrew Hetrick, Administrator

□ **Dothan Surgery Center,** 1450 Ross Clark Circle, S.E., Dothan, AL 36301; tel. 334/793-3442; FAX. 334/793-3318; Donna Bernstrom, Facility Administrator

□ **Florence Surgery Center,** 103 Helton Court, Florence, AL 35630; tel. 205/760-0672; FAX. 205/766-4547; Levonne Rhodes, CPA, Administrator

□ **Gadsden Surgery Center,** 418 South Fifth Street, Gadsden, AL 35901; tel. 205/543-1253; FAX. 205/543-1260; Lisa LeQuire, RN, B.S.N., Administrator

□ **Health South Mobile Surgery Center,** 1721 Springhill Avenue, Mobile, AL 36604; tel. 334/438-3614; Julie Saucier, RN, B.S.N., Facility Administrator

Huntsville Endoscopy Center, Inc., 119 Longwood Drive, Huntsville, AL 35801; tel. 205/533-6488; FAX. 205/533-6495; Michael W. Brown, M.D.

Medplex Outpatient Medical Centers, Inc., 4511 Southlake Parkway, Birmingham, AL 32544; tel. 205/985-4398; FAX. 205/985-4486; Dawn Ousley, RN, Administrator

□ **Outpatient Services East, Inc.,** 52 Medical Park Drive, E., Suite 401, Birmingham, AL 35235; tel. 205/838-3888, ext. 211; FAX. 205/838-3875; James E. Stidham, Chief Executive Officer, President

The Kirklin Clinic Ambulatory Surgical Center, 2000 Sixth Avenue, S., Birmingham, AL 35233; tel. 205/801-8000; Steven C. Schultz, Executive Vice President

The Surgery Center of Huntsville, 721 Madison Street, Huntsville, AL 35801; tel. 205/533-4888; FAX. 205/532-9510; Bobbye H. Riggs, Chief Executive Officer

Tuscaloosa Endoscopy Center, 100 Rice Mine Road, N.E., Suite E, Tuscaloosa, AL 35406; tel. 205/345-0010; FAX. 205/752-1175; A. B. Reddy, M.D., Medical Director

Tuscaloosa Surgical Center, 1400 McFarland Boulevard, N., Tuscaloosa, AL 35406; tel. 205/345-5500; J. Russell Peake, Administrator

ALASKA

Alaska Surgery Center, 4001 Laurel Street, Anchorage, AK 99508; tel. 907/563-3327, ext. 226; FAX. 907/562-7042; Louise M. Bjornstad, Executive Director

Alaska Women's Health Services, Inc., 4115 Lake Otis Drive, Anchorage, AK 99508; tel. 907/563-7228; FAX. 907/563-6278; Lisa Weston, Administrator

Geneva Woods Surgical Center, 3730 Rhone Circle, Suite 100, Anchorage, AK 99508; tel. 907/562-4764; FAX. 907/561-8519; J. David Williams, M.D.

Susitna Surgery Center, 950 East Bogard Road, Wasilla, AK 99645, P.O. Box 1687, Palmer, AK 99645; tel. 907/746-8625; Patsy Crofford, RN, Chief Clinical Officer

ARIZONA

A.I.M.S. Outpatient Surgery, 3636 Stockton Hill Road, Kingman, AZ 86401; tel. 602/757-3636; FAX. 602/757-7224; Bill Margita

Adobe Plastic Surgery, 2585 North Wyatt Drive, Tucson, AZ 85712; tel. 602/322-5295; FAX. 602/325-7763; Lucricia Banks, Administrative Assistant

Aesthetic Reconstructive Associates, P.C., 4222 East Camelback, Suite H-150, Phoenix, AZ 85018; tel. 602/952-8100; FAX. 602/952-9519; Martin L. Johnson, M.D.

Ambulatory Surgicenter, Inc., 1940 East Southern Avenue, Tempe, AZ 85282; tel. 602/820-7101; FAX. 602/820-9291; H. William Reese, D.P.M., Medical Director

Arizona Diagnostic and Surgical Center, 545 North Mesa Drive, Mesa, AZ 85201; tel. 602/461-4407; FAX. 602/461-4401; Lynnette King, RN, Administrator

Arizona Foot Institute, P.C., 1901 West Glendale Avenue, Phoenix, AZ 85021; tel. 602/246-0816; FAX. 602/433-2257; Barry Kaplan

Arizona Medical Clinic, Ltd., 13640 North Plaza Del Rio Boulevard, Peoria, AZ 85381; tel. 602/876-3800; Jan Kaplan, Director, Operations

Arizona Surgical Arts, Inc., 1245 North Wilmot Road, Tucson, AZ 85712; tel. 520/296-7550; Marilyn C. Mazeika, Administrator

Barnet Dulaney Eye Center, 9425 West Bell Road, Sun City, AZ 85351; tel. 602/974-1000; FAX. 602/933-5462; David D. Dulaney, Executive Director

Barnet Dulaney Eye Center, 13760 North 93rd Avenue, Peoria, AZ 85381; tel. 602/977-4291; Ronald W. Barnet, M.D.

Barnet Dulaney Eye Center, 1375 West 16th Street, Yuma, AZ 85364; tel. 602/955-1000; Imelda Kelly, Administrator

Barnet Dulaney Eye Center–Phoenix, 3333 East Camelback Road, Suite 122, Phoenix, AZ 85018; tel. 602/955-1000; FAX. 602/957-9202; Ronald W. Barnet, M.D.

Barnet Eye Center–Mesa, 6335 East Main Street, Mesa, AZ 85205; tel. 602/981-1000; FAX. 602/981-0467; Carolyn Miller, Administrator

Boswell Eye Institute, 10541 West Thunderbird Boulevard, Sun City, AZ 85351; tel. 602/933-3402; FAX. 602/972-5014; Jan Zellmann, Administrator

CIGNA Healthplan of Arizona, Outpatient Surgery, 755 East McDowell Road, Phoenix, AZ 85006; tel. 602/371-2500; Clifton Worsham, M.D., Administrator

Carriker Eye Center, 6425 North 16th Street, Phoenix, AZ 85016; tel. 602/274-1703; FAX. 602/274-3216; Richard G. Carriker, M.D.

Casa Blanca Clinic I.P.L.L.C., 4001 East Baseline Road, Gilbert, AZ 85234; tel. 602/926-6200; FAX. 602/926-6202; Stanley W. Decker, Executive Director

Cataract Surgery Clinic, 215 South Power Road, Suite 112, Mesa, AZ 85206; tel. 602/981-1345; Robert P. Gervais, M.D., Administrator

Cochise Eye and Laser, PC, 2445 East Wilcox Drive, Sierra Vista, AZ 85635; tel. 520/458-8131; FAX. 520/458-0422; Douglas R. Knolles, Administrator

Cottonwood Day Surgery Center, Inc., 55 South Sixth Street, P.O. Box 400, Cottonwood, AZ 86326; tel. 602/634-2444; Linda Davis, Administrator

Desert Mountain Surgicenter, Ltd., 7776 Pointe Parkway West, Suite 135, Phoenix, AZ 85044; tel. 602/431-8500; FAX. 602/431-1677; David M. Creech, M.D.

Desert Samaritan Surgicenter, 1500 South Dobson Road, Suite 101, Mesa, AZ 85202; tel. 602/835-3590; FAX. 602/890-4675; Brenda Hollander, Administrator

Dooley Outpatient Surgery Center, 151 Riviera Drive, Lake Havasu City, AZ 86403; tel. 602/855-9477; FAX. 602/855-2983; William J. Dooley, Jr., M.D., Medical Director

East Valley Surgical Associates, Ltd., 6424 East Broadway Road, Suite 102, Mesa, AZ 85206; tel. 602/833-2216; Manuel J. Chee

FH–Arizona Surgery Centers, Inc., 750 North Alvernon Way, Tucson, AZ 85711; tel. 602/322-8440; FAX. 602/322-2653; Vicki Gagnier, RN, Manager

Fifty–Ninth Avenue Surgical Facility, Ltd., 8608 North 59th Avenue, Glendale, AZ 85302; tel. 602/934-0272; FAX. 602/930-1891; Mark Gorman, Administrator

Fishkind and Bakewell Eye Care and Surgery Center, 5599 North Oracle Road, Tucson, AZ 85704; tel. 602/293-6740; FAX. 602/293-6771; Kathleen A. Brown, Surgery Center Supervisor

Flagstaff Outpatient Surgery Center, 77 West Forest Avenue, Suite 306, Flagstaff, AZ 86001; tel. 520/773-2597; FAX. 520/773-2327; Jackie Mosier, RN, Administrator

Footcare Surgi Center, 10249 West Thunderbird, Suite 100, Sun City, AZ 85351; tel. 602/979-4466; FAX. 602/933-8354; Gary N. Friedlander, D.P.M.

Footcare Surgi Center of Northern Arizona, 10 West Columbus Avenue, Flagstaff, AZ 86001; tel. 602/774-4191; Dr. Edward L. Wiebe

Gary Hall Eye Surgery Institute, 2501 North 32nd Street, Phoenix, AZ 85008; tel. 602/957-6799; FAX. 602/957-0172; Gary W. Hall, M.D., President

Glendale Surgicenter, 5757 West Thunderbird Road, Suite E-150, Glendale, AZ 85306; tel. 602/843-1900; FAX. 602/843-5607; Douglas G. Merrill, M.D., Medical Director

Section C

Good Samaritan Surgicenter, 1111 B East McDowell Road, Phoenix, AZ 85006; tel. 602/239-2776; FAX. 602/239-5352; Brenda Hollander, Administrator

Greenbaum Outpatient Surgery and Recovery Care Center, 3624 Wells Fargo Avenue, Scottsdale, AZ 85251; tel. 602/481-4958; Craig Stout, Administrator

Grimm Eye Clinic and Cataract Institute, P.C., 1502 North Tucson Boulevard, Tucson, AZ 85716; tel. 602/326-4321; Stephen F. Grimm, M.D.; Eleanor M. Grimm, M.D.

Havasu Arthritis and Sports Medicine Institute, 1840 Mesquite Avenue, Suite G, Lake Havasu, AZ 86403; tel. 602/453-2663; Marc H. Zimmerman, M.D., Administrator

Havasu Foot and Ankle Surgi-Center, 90 Riviera Drive, Lake Havasu, AZ 86403; tel. 520/855-7800; FAX. 520/855-5392; Robert Novack, D.P.M., Director

HealthSouth Surgery Center of Tucson, 310 North Wilmot Road, Suite 309, Tucson, AZ 85711; tel. 520/296-7080; FAX. 520/886-6518; Aaron Chatterson, Administrator

Lear Surgery Clinic-Scottsdale, 7351 East Osborn Road, Suite 104, Scottsdale, AZ 85251-6452; tel. 602/990-9400; FAX. 602/990-2664; David E. Marine, Executive Director

Lear Surgery Clinic-Sun City, 10615 West Thunderbird, Suite A-100, Sun City, AZ 85351; tel. 602/974-9375; FAX. 602/977-2598; David E. Marine, Executive Director

Mayo Clinic Scottsdale Ambulatory Surgery Center, 13400 East Shea Boulevard, Scottsdale, AZ 85259; tel. 602/301-8188; FAX. 602/301-8367; Karen A. Biel, Administrator

McCready Eye Surgery Center, 310 North Wilmot Road, Suite 106, Tucson, AZ 85711; tel. 520/885-6783; FAX. 520/885-5366; Joseph L. McCready, M.D., Administrator

Medivision of Tucson, Inc./Columbia HCA, 5632 East Fifth Street, Tucson, AZ 85711; tel. 602/790-8888; FAX. 602/790-1427; Clara Dupnik

Metro Ambulatory Surgery, Inc., a/k/a Metro Recovery Care Center, 3131 West Peoria Avenue, Phoenix, AZ 85029; tel. 602/375-1083; FAX. 602/789-6833; Jody M. Jones, RN, Chief Executive Officer

Mohave Surgery Center, Inc., 1919 Florence Avenue, Kingman, AZ 86401; tel. 520/753-5454; FAX. 520/753-7790, ext. 11; Frank Brown, Administrator

Moon Valley Surgery Center, Inc., 14045 North Seventh Street, Suite Two, Phoenix, AZ 85022; tel. 602/942-3966; Andrew E. Lowy

Nogales Medical Clinic Outpatient Surgery, 480 North Morley Avenue, Nogales, AZ 85621; tel. 520/287-2726; Imogene A. Bell, Administrator

Osborn Ambulatory Surgical Center, 3330 North Second Street, Suite 300, Phoenix, AZ 85012; tel. 602/265-0113; FAX. 602/277-8580; Donna Klamm, RN, Administrator

Outpatient Surgical Care, Ltd., 1530 West Glendale, Suite 105, Phoenix, AZ 85021; tel. 602/995-3395; FAX. 602/995-1853; James Kennedy, M.D., Medical Director

Outpatient Surgical Center, 456 North Mesa Drive, Mesa, AZ 85201; tel. 602/464-8000; FAX. 602/969-7107; Maddie Dauernheim, Administrator

Phoenix Center for Outpatient Surgery, 1950 West Heatherbrae Drive, Suite Seven, Phoenix, AZ 85015; tel. 602/230-0437; Eric Reints, Administrator

Porter, Michael, D.P.M., 3620 East Campbell, Suite B, Phoenix, AZ 85018; tel. 602/954-6224; Michael Porter

Prescott Outpatient Surgery Center, Inc., 815 Ainsworth Drive, Prescott, AZ 86301; tel. 602/778-9770; Gail Reidhead, Administrative Director

Prescott Urocenter, Ltd., 811 Ainsworth, Suite 101, Prescott, AZ 86301; tel. 520/771-5282; FAX. 520/771-5283; Gregory Oldani

Romania Eye Care, P.C., 2820 North Glassford Hill Road, Suite 106, Prescott Valley, AZ 86314; tel. 520/775-5606; FAX. 520/772-4999; Linda Talerico, Administrator

Safford Surgi-Care, 825 20th Avenue, Safford, AZ 85546; tel. 602/428-6930; FAX. 602/428-7272; James Holder, O.D.

Santa Cruz Ambulatory Surgical Center, 699 West Ajo Way, Tucson, AZ 85713; tel. 602/746-1711; Richard Edward Quint, Administrator

Scottsdale Eye Surgery Center, P.C., 3320 North Miller Road, Scottsdale, AZ 85251; tel. 602/949-1208; FAX. 602/994-3316; Karen Borowiak, Administrator

Southwestern Eye Center-Casa Grande, 1919 North Trekell Road, Casa Grande, AZ 85222; tel. 520/426-9224; FAX. 520/426-1554; Lothaire Bluth, Administrator

Southwestern Eye Center-Yuma, 2179 West 24th Street, Yuma, AZ 85364; tel. 520/726-4120; FAX. 520/341-0315; Lance K. Wozniak, M.D.

Southwestern Eye Surgi Center-Falcon Field, 4760 Falcon Drive, Mesa, AZ 85205; tel. 602/985-7400; Karen Buck, Administrator

Southwestern Eye Surgicenter-Dobson Ranch, 2150 South Dobson Road, Mesa, AZ 85202; tel. 602/839-1717; FAX. 602/839-2862; Pat Bray, RN, CRNO, Director, Surgical and Medical Services

Southwestern Eye Surgicenter-Flagstaff, 1355 North Beaver, Suite 140, Flagstaff, AZ 86001; tel. 520/773-1184; FAX. 520/773-1815; Suzi Jensen, Surgical Services

Southwestern Eye Surgicenter-Nogales, 1815 North Mastick Way, Nogales, AZ 85621; tel. 520/281-0160; Pat Bray, Administrator

Sun City Endoscopy Center, Inc., 13203 North 103rd Avenue, Suite C 3, Sun City, AZ 85351; tel. 602/972-2116; John E. Phelps, M.D., Medical Director

Sun City Surgical Center, 13260 North 94th Drive, Suite 300, Peoria, AZ 85381; tel. 602/277-0619; FAX. 602/933-5787; H. William Reese, D.P.M., Director

Surgi-Care, 5115 North Central Avenue, Suite B, Phoenix, AZ 85012; tel. 602/264-1818; FAX. 602/264-2172; Ellison F. Herro, M.D., Administrator

Surgi-Tech Centers, 3271 North Civic Center Plaza, Suite Three, Scottsdale, AZ 85251; tel. 602/994-5978; FAX. 602/990-9397; Richard Jacoby, D.P.M., President

SurgiCenter, 1040 East McDowell Road, Phoenix, AZ 85006; tel. 602/258-1521; FAX. 602/340-0889; Sharon Shafer, RN, Administrator

Surgical Eye Center of Arizona, Inc., 5133 North Central Avenue, Suite 100, Phoenix, AZ 85012; tel. 602/277-7997; Robert Lorenzen, Administrator

Surginet of Arizona, Ltd., 7725 North 43rd Avenue, Suite 510, Phoenix, AZ 85051; tel. 602/931-9400; FAX. 602/930-9884; Steve McLaughlin, Administrator

Swagel Wootton Eye Center, 220 South 63rd Street, Mesa, AZ 85206; tel. 602/641-3937; FAX. 602/924-5096; S. Joyce Graham

T.A.S.I. Surgery Center, 5585 North Oracle Road, Suite B, Tucson, AZ 85704; tel. 602/293-4730; John A. Pierce, M.D., Medical Director

Tempe Surgical Center, Inc., 2000 East Southern Avenue, Suite 106, Tempe, AZ 85282; tel. 602/838-9313; Richard F. Pavese, M.D.

Thunderbird Samaritan Surgicenter, 5555 B West Thunderbird Road, Glendale, AZ 85306-4622; tel. 602/588-5475; FAX. 602/588-5472; Diane Elmore, RN, Administrator

Valley Outpatient Surgery Center, 160 West University Drive, Mesa, AZ 85201; tel. 602/835-7373; FAX. 602/969-7981; Craig R. Cassidy, D.O., President

Warner Medical Park Outpatient Surgery, Inc., 604 West Warner Road, Building A, Chandler, AZ 85224; tel. 602/899-2571; FAX. 602/899-4263; Robert Thunberg, Managing Director

White Mountain Ambulatory Surgery Center, 2650 East Show Low Lake Road, Suite Two, Show Low, AZ 85901; tel. 602/537-4240; William J. Waldo

Yuma Outpatient Surgery Center, L.P., 2475 Avenue A, Suite B, Yuma, AZ 85364; tel. 520/726-6910; FAX. 520/726-7423; Cairne-Lee Larson, RN, Facility Manager

ARKANSAS

Ambulatory Surgical Center, Inc., d/b/a Fort Smith Surgi-Center, 7306A Rogers Avenue, Fort Smith, AR 72903; tel. 501/452-7333; Reem Zofari, Administrator

Arkansas Endoscopy Center, P.A., 9501 Lile Drive, Suite 100, Little Rock, AR 72205; tel. 501/224-9100; FAX. 501/224-0420; Ronald D. Hardin, M.D.

☐ **Arkansas Otolaryngology Ambulatory Surgery Center,** 1200 Medical Towers Building, 9601 Lile Drive, Little Rock, AR 72205; tel. 501/227-5050; Joseph R. Phillips, RN, Administrator

Arkansas Surgery Center, 10 Hospital Circle, Batesville, AR 72501; tel. 501/793-4040; Fredric J. Sloan, M.D., Administrator

Arkansas Surgery Center of Fayetteville, 3873 North Parkview Drive, Suite One, Fayetteville, AR 72703; tel. 501/582-3200; FAX. 501/582-1338; Russ Greene, Administrator

Arkansas Surgery and Endoscopy Center, L.L.C., 4800 Hazel Street, Pine Bluff, AR 71603; tel. 501/536-4800; Mazahir Husain, Administrator

BEC Surgery Center, One Mercy Lane, Suite 201, P.O. Box 6409, Hot Springs, AR 71902; tel. 501/623-0755; Terry D. Brown

Boozman-Hof Eye Surgery and Laser Center, 3737 West Walnut Street, P.O. Box 1353, Rogers, AR 72757-1353; tel. 501/636-7506; Michael D. Malone, Administrator

Cooper Clinic Ambulatory Surgery Center, 6801 Rogers Avenue, P.O. Box 3528, Fort Smith, AR 72903; tel. 501/452-2077; FAX. 501/484-4611; Jerry Stewart, M.D., Administrator

Dempsey-McKee, Inc., d/b/a McKee Outpatient Surgery Center, 601 East Matthews, Jonesboro, AR 72401; tel. 501/935-6396; FAX. 501/935-4063; Terry V. DePriest, Administrator

Doctors Surgery Center, 303 West Polk Street, Suite B, West Memphis, AR 72301; tel. 501/732-2100; Doris Davis, Administrator

Gastroenterology and Surgery Center Of Arkansas, P.A., 8908 Kanis Road, Little Rock, AR 72205; tel. 501/227-7688; FAX. 501/225-2930; Alonzo D. Williams, M.D., Medical Director

H. Lewis Pearson Eye Institute, 3211 Surger Hill Road, Texarkana, AR 71854-9265; tel. 501/772-4440; FAX. 501/772-7190; F. Douglas Kesner, Administrator

Holt-Krock Clinic, 1500 Dodson Avenue, Fort Smith, AR 72901; tel. 501/788-4000; Harold H. Mings, M.D., Chief Executive Officer

Hot Springs Outpatient Surgery, 100 Ridgeway Boulevard, Suite Seven, Hot Springs, AR 71901; tel. 501/624-4464; FAX. 501/624-4602; Edwin L. Harper, M.D., Administrator

James Trice, M.D., P.A., d/b/a Digestive Disease Center, 7005 South Hazel Street, Pine Bluff, AR 71603; tel. 501/536-3070; Louis Triace, Administrator

Little Rock Diagnostic Clinic ASC, 10001 Lile Drive, Little Rock, AR 72205; tel. 501/227-8000, ext. 845; Roger J. St. Onge, Administrator

Little Rock Pain Clinic, Two Lile Court, Suite 100, Little Rock, AR 72205; tel. 501/224-7246; FAX. 501/224-7644; Virginia Johnson, Administrator

☐ **Little Rock Surgery Center,** 8820 Knoedl Court, Little Rock, AR 72205; tel. 501/224-6767; FAX. 501/224-8203; Pamela J. Hooper, Administrator

Lowery Medical/Surgical Eye Center, P.A., 105 Central Avenue, Searcy, AR 72143; tel. 501/268-7154; FAX. 501/268-9071; Benjamin R. Lowery, M.D., Administrator

North Hills Gastroenterology Endoscopy Center, Inc., 3344 North Futrall Drive, Fayetteville, AR 72703; tel. 501/582-7280; William C. Martin, M.D.

Northeast Arkansas Surgery Center, Inc., 505 East Matthews, Jonesboro, AR 72401; tel. 501/972-1723; FAX. 501/972-5941; Carol D. Crawford, Administrator

Ozark Eye Center, 360 Highway Five North, Mountain Home, AR 72653; tel. 501/425-2277; Rick Galkoski, Administrator

Physicians Day Surgery Center, 3805 West 28th, Pine Bluff, AR 71603; tel. 501/536-4100; FAX. 501/536-3100; Joan Fletcher, Administrator

Russellville Surgery Center, L.L.C., 2205 West Main Street, P.O. Box 2654, Russellville, AR 72801; tel. 501/890-2654; FAX. 501/890-5101; James Kennedy, Administrator

South Arkansas Surgery Center, 4310 South Mulberry, Pine Bluff, AR 71603; tel. 501/535-5719; Tammy L. Studdard, Administrator

☐ **The Center for Day Surgery,** 4200 Jenny Lind, Suite A, Fort Smith, AR 72901; tel. 501/648-9496; Monte Wilson, Administrator

The Endoscopy Center of Hot Springs, 151 McGowan Court, Hot Springs, AR 71913; tel. 501/623-4101; FAX. 501/623-0103; Rebecca Bates, Administrator

The Gastro-Intestinal Center, 405 North University, Little Rock, AR 72205; tel. 501/663-1074; James G. Dunlap, Administrator

The Physicians Surgery Center of Arkansas, Inc., d/b/a Physicians Surgery Center, 1024 North University Avenue, Little Rock, AR 72207; tel. 501/663-0158; FAX. 501/663-4652; Martha Plant, Administrator

CALIFORNIA

Advanced Surgery Center, 5771 North Fresno Street, Suite 101, Fresno, CA 93710; tel. 209/448–9900; David B. Singh, Administrator

Aesthetic Facial Surgery Center of Menlo Park, 2200 Sand Hill Road, Suite 130, Menlo Park, CA 94025; tel. 415/854–6444; Dr. Harry Mittelman

Aestheticare Outpatient Surgery Center, 30260 Rancho Viejo Road, San Juan Capistrano, CA 92675; tel. 714/661–1700; FAX. 714/661–4913; Ronald E. Moser, M.D.

Alvarado Family Surgery Center, 215 West Madison Avenue, El Cajon, CA 92020; tel. 619/593–2110; Noreen K. Valentine, R.N., Administrator

Ambulatory Surgical Center of Chico, 1950 East 20th Street, Suite 102, Chico, CA 95928; tel. 916/343–1674; Robert G. Basinger, D.P.M.

Ambulatory Surgical Center of Southern California, 880 South Atlantic Boulevard, Monterey Park, CA 91754; tel. 213/483–9080; Marco Sprintis, M.D.

Ambulatory Surgical Center of the Zeiter Eye, 117 North San Joaquin Street, Stockton, CA 95202; tel. 209/466–5566; FAX. 209/466–0535; Donna M. Tschirky

Ambulatory Surgical Center, Inc., 14400 Bear Valley Road, Victorville, CA 92392; tel. 916/951–5162; FAX. 818/368–2290; Garey L. Weber, D.P.M., Administrator

Ambulatory Surgical Centers, Inc., 18952 Mac Arthur Boulevard, Suite 102, Irvine, CA 92612; tel. 714/833–3406; FAX. 818/368–2290; Garey L. Weber, D.P.M., Administrator

Anaheim Surgical Center, 1324 South Euclid Street, Anaheim, CA 92802; tel. 714/533–9880; FAX. 714/533–1802; Debra Berntsen, RN, Charge Nurse

Antelope Valley Surgery Center, 44301 North Lorimer Avenue, Lancaster, CA 93534; tel. 805/940–1112; FAX. 805/940–6856; Yolanda Gomez

Apple Valley Surgery Center, 18122 Outer Highway 18, Apple Valley, CA; tel. 619/946–1170; FAX. 619/946–2646; Virginia Budington, Administrator

Arlington Podiatry Surgery Center, 7310 Magnolia Avenue, Riverside, CA 92504; tel. 909/354–8787; FAX. 909/354–0350; James A. De Silva, Administrator

Aspen Outpatient Center, 2750 North Sycamore Drive, Simi Valley, CA 93065; tel. 805/583–5923; FAX. 805/583–0952; Jay Evans, Administrator

Associates Outpatient Surgery Center, 2128 Eureka Way, Redding, CA 96001; tel. 916/246–9737; FAX. 916/246–4052; Reed Lockwood, M.D., Administrator

Atherton Plastic Surgery Center, 3351 El Camino Real, Suite 201, Atherton, CA 94027; tel. 415/363–0300; FAX. 415/363–0302; David Apfelberg

Auburn Surgery Center, 3123 Professional Drive, Suite 100, Auburn, CA 95603; tel. 916/888–8899; FAX. 916/888–1464; Charles Smith, Administrator

Bakersfield Endoscopy Center, 1902 B Street, Bakersfield, CA 93301; tel. 805/327–4455; Ramesh Gupta, M.D., Medical Director

Bakersfield Surgery Center, 2120 19th Street, Bakersfield, CA 93301; tel. 805/323–2020; FAX. 805/323–6552; Kathleen Allman, Administrator

Beverly Hills Ambulatory Surgery Center, Inc., 9201 Sunset Boulevard, Suite 405, Los Angeles, CA 90069; tel. 310/887–1730; Sandra Cericola, Administrator

Beverly Hills Outpatient Surgery Center, 250 North Robertson Boulevard, Suite 104, Los Angeles, CA 90211; tel. 310/273–9255; FAX. 310/273–6167; Peter Golden, M.D., Medical Director

Beverly Surgical Center, 105 West Beverly Boulevard, Montebello, CA 90640–4375; tel. 213/728–5400; FAX. 213/887–0058; James G. Ovieda, Administrator

Blackhawk Surgery Center, Inc., 4165 Blackhawk Plaza Circle, Suite 195, Danville, CA 94506; tel. 510/736–7881; Molly Healy, Administrator

Bolsa Out–Patient Surgery Center, 10362 Bolsa Avenue, Westminster, CA 92683; tel. 714/531–2091; D. L. Pham, M.D., Medical Director

Bonaventure Surgery Center, 221 North Jackson Avenue, San Jose, CA 95116; tel. 408/729–2848; FAX. 408/729–2880; Virginia Field, RN, M.B.A., Director

Brawley Endoscopy and Surgery Center, 205 West Legion Road, Brawley, CA 92227; tel. 619/351–3655; FAX. 619/351–3675; Mahomed Suliman, M.D., Administrator

Brockton Surgical Center, 5905 Brockton Avenue, Suite B, Riverside, CA 92506; tel. 909/686–5373; FAX. 909/778–9064; Michael N. Durrant, D.P.M., M.P.H.

Bruce A. Kaplan, M.D., 39000 Bob Hope Drive, Wright Building, Suite 209, Rancho Mirage, CA 92270; tel. 619/346–5603; FAX. 619/346–5604; Jessie Schumaker

California Eye Clinic, 3747 Sunset Lane, Suite A, Antioch, CA 94509; tel. 510/754–2300; Jean Kemp, Administrator

Camden Surgery Center of Beverly Hills, 414 North. Camden Drive, Suite 800, Beverly Hills, CA 90210; tel. 310/859–3991; FAX. 310/859–7126; Yasmin Sibulo, Administrator

Capistrano Surgicenter, Inc., 30280 Rancho Viejo Road, San Juan Capistrano, CA 92675; tel. 714/248–5757; FAX. 714/248–9339; Jeffrey A. Klein, President

Cedars–Sinai, Saint John's, Daniel Freeman SurgiCenter, 9675 Brighton Way, Suite 100, Beverly Hills, CA 90210; tel. 310/205–6080; FAX. 310/205–6090; Diane Tharp, Program Coordinator

Center for Ambulatory Medicine and Surgery, 111 East Noble Avenue, Visalia, CA 93277; tel. 209/739–8383; FAX. 209/739–7929; James J. Shea, M.D., Administrator

Central Coast Surgery Center, 1941 Johnson Avenue, Suite 103, San Luis Obispo, CA 93406; tel. 805/546–9999; FAX. 804/546–8904; Helen Swanagon, Nurse Administrator

Channel Islands Surgicenter, 2300 Wankel Way, Oxnard, CA 93030; tel. 805/485–1908; FAX. 805/485–5767; Mary K. Fish, Administrator

Children's Surgery Center, 744 Fifty–Second Street, Oakland, CA 94609; tel. 510/428–3133; FAX. 510/450–5606; Terry Hawes, Administrator

Columbia Arcadia Outpatient Surgery, Inc., 614 West Duarte Road, Arcadia, CA 91006; tel. 818/445–4714; Sandy Lazare, Administrator

Columbia Los Gatos Surgical Center, 15195 National Avenue, Los Gatos, CA 95032; tel. 408/356–0454; FAX. 408/358–3924; Martha Ponce, Administrator

Columbia North Coast Surgery Center, 3903 Waring Road, Oceanside, CA 92056; tel. 619/940–0997; FAX. 619/940–0407; Donna Danley, Administrator

Columbia Saddleback Valley Outpatient Surgery, 24302 Paseo De Valencia, Laguna Hills, CA 92653; tel. 714/472–0244; FAX. 714/472–0380; Brian FitzGerald, Administrator

Columbia Sereno Surgery Center, 14601 South Bascom Avenue, Suite 100, Los Gatos, CA 95032–2043; tel. 408/358–2727; FAX. 408/358–2950; Martha Ponce, Administrator

Columbia Southwest Surgical Clinic, Inc., 4201 Torrance Boulevard, Suite 240, Torrance, CA 90503; tel. 310/540–7803; FAX. 310/316–3903; Otto Munchow, M.D., Director

Columbia Surgicenter of South Bay, 23500 Madison Street, Torrance, CA 90505; tel. 310/539–5120; Debra Saxton

Columbia West Hills Surgical Center, 7240 Medical Center Drive, West Hills, CA 91307; tel. 818/226–6170; Carol Valeri, R.N., Administrator

Columbia/Woodward Park Surgicenter, 7055 North Fresno Street, Suite 100, Fresno, CA 93720; tel. 209/449–9977; FAX. 209/449–9350; Lori Ruffner, RN, Administrator

Community Surgery Centre, 17190 Bernado Center Drive, Suite 100, San Diego, CA 92128; tel. 619/675–3270; FAX. 619/675–3260; Regina S. Boore, B.S.N., M.S.

Corona Del Mar Plastic Surgery, 1101 Bayside Drive, Suite 100, Corona Del Mar, CA 92625; tel. 714/644–5000; W. Graham Wood, M.D.

Crown Valley Surgicenter, 26921 Crown Valley Parkway, Suite 110, Mission Viejo, CA 92691; tel. 714/348–7252; FAX. 714/348–7246; Maurice Chammas, M.D., Administrator

Cypress Outpatient Surgical Center, Inc., 1665 Dominican Way, Suite 120, Santa Cruz, CA 95065; tel. 408/476–6943; FAX. 408/476–1473; Sandra Warren, Administrator

Cypress Surgery Center, 842 South Akers Road, Visalia, CA 93277; tel. 209/740–4094; FAX. 209/740–4100; Jack K. Waller

Del Rey Surgery Center, 4640 Admiralty Way, Suite 1020, Marina Del Rey, CA 90292; tel. 310/305–7570; Lee Estes, Administrator

Digestive Disease Center, 24411 Health Center Drive, Suite 450, Laguna Hills, CA 92653; tel. 714/586–9386; FAX. 714/586–0864; Crisynda Buss, RN

Doctors Surgery Center of Whittier, 8135 South Painter Avenue, Suite 103, Whittier, CA 90602; tel. 310/945–8961; FAX. 310/698–3578; Veronica Coughenour, RN

Doctors Surgical Center, Inc., 9461 Grindlay Street, Suite 102, Cypress, CA 90630; tel. 714/995–3001; R. Wayne Ives, Administrator

Doctors' Surgery Center, 1441 Liberty Street, Suite 104, Redding, CA 96001; tel. 916/244–6300; FAX. 916/246–2051; Charles Kassis, Administrator

Downey Surgery Center, 8555 East Florence Avenue, Downey, CA 90240; tel. 310/923–9784; Marisol Magana, Administrator

E. N. T. Facial Surgery Center, 1351 East Spruce, Fresno, CA 93720; tel. 209/432–3724; FAX. 209/432–8579; JoAnn LoForti, RN, Division of Nursing

East Bay Medical Surgical Center, 20998 Redwood Road, Castro Valley, CA 94546; tel. 510/538–2828; FAX. 510/538–2508; Yoshitsugu Teramoto, M.D., Administrator

El Camino Surgery Center, 2480 Grant Road, Mountain View, CA 94040–4300; tel. 415/961–1200; FAX. 415/960–7041; Nancy Kessler

El Mirador Surgical Center, 1180 North Indian Canyon Drive, Palm Springs, CA 92263; tel. 619/416–4600; Marilyn M. Perkins, Nurse Administrator

Endoscopy Center of Chula Vista, 681 Third Avenue, Suite B, Chula Vista, CA 91910; tel. 619/425–2150; Robert Penner, M.D., Administrator

Endoscopy Center of Southern California, 2336 Santa Monica Boulevard, Suite 204, Santa Monica, CA 90404; tel. 310/453–4477; FAX. 310/453–4811; Parviz D. Afshani

Endoscopy Center of the Central Coast, 77 Casa Street, Suite 106, San Luis Obispo, CA 93405; tel. 805/541–1021; FAX. 805/541–3142; Judy Grossi, Clinical Director

☐ **Escondido Surgery Center,** 343 East Second Avenue, Escondido, CA 92025; tel. 619/480–6606; FAX. 619/480–6671; Marvin W. Levenson, M.D., Managing Medical Director

Eye Center of Northern California Surgicenter, 6500 Fairmount Avenue, Suite Two, El Cerrito, CA 94530; tel. 510/525–2600; FAX. 510/524–1887; William Ellis

Eye Life Institute, 6283 Clark Road, Suite Seven, Paradise, CA 95969; tel. 916/877–2020; FAX. 916/877–4641; Almary Hivale, RN, Administrator

Eye Surgery Center of Southern California, Inc./Med. Group, 2023 West Vista Way, Suite E, Vista, CA 92083; tel. 619/941–8152; FAX. 619/726–4822; Regg V. Antle, M.D., Medical Director

Eye Surgery Center of the Desert, 39700 Bob Hope Drive, Suite 111, Rancho Mirage, CA 92270; tel. 619/340–3937; FAX. 619/340–1940; Albert T. Milauskas, Administrator

Feather River Surgery Center, 370 Del Norte Avenue, Yuba City, CA 95991; tel. 916/751–4800; FAX. 916/751–4884; Elizabeth LaBouyer, RN, CNOR, Perioperative Coordinator

Fig Garden Surgi–Med Center, 1332 West Herndon Avenue, Suite 102, Fresno, CA 93711–0431; tel. 209/439–3100

Foothill Ambulatory Surgery Center, 1030 East Foothill Boulevard, Suite 101B, Upland, CA 91786; tel. 909/981–5859; FAX. 909/981–8293; Montra M. Kanok, M.D.

Fort Sutter Surgery Center, 2801 K Street, Suite 525, Sacramento, CA 95816; tel. 916/733–5017; FAX. 916/733–8738; Bill Davis, Administrator

Fountain Valley Outpatient Surgical Center, 11160 Warner Avenue, Suite 421, Fountain Valley, CA 92708; tel. 714/751–5621; Eugene Elliott, M.D.

Four Thirty–Six North Bedford Surgicenter, Inc., 436 North Bedford, Suite 101, Beverly Hills, CA 90210; tel. 310/278–0188; FAX. 310/278–1791; Robert Kotler, M.D.

Fritch Eye Care Medical Center, 2525 Eye Street, Suite A and B, Bakersfield, CA 93301; tel. 805/327–8511; FAX. 805/327–9809; Charles D. Fritch, M.D.

Frost Street Outpatient Surgical Center, Inc., 8008 Frost Street, Suite 200, San Diego, CA 92123; tel. 619/576–8320; FAX. 619/576–8568; Jacqueline McWilliams

GastroDiagnostics, A Medical Group, 1140 West La Veta, Suite 550, Orange, CA 92868; tel. 714/835–5100; FAX. 714/835–5567; Stephanie Quinn, Administrator

Section C

Glendale Eye Surgery Center, 607 North Central, Suite 103, Glendale, CA 91203; tel. 818/956–1010; FAX. 818/543–6083; James M. McCaffery, M.D.

Glenwood Surgical Center, L.P., 8945 Magnolia Avenue, Suite 200, Riverside, CA 92503; tel. 909/688–7270; Calvin Nash

Golden Empire Surgical Center, 1519 Graces Highway, Suite 103, Delano, CA 93215; tel. 805/721–7900; Lucy Lara

Golden Triangle Surgicenter, 25405 Hancock Avenue, Suite 103, Murrieta, CA 92562; tel. 909/698–4670; FAX. 909/698–4675; Ella Stockstill, Administrator

Golden West Pain Therapy Center, 25405 Hancock Avenue, Suite 110, Murrieta, CA 92562–5964; tel. 909/698–4710; FAX. 909/698–4715; Richard Harris, Administrator

Greater Long Beach Endoscopy Center, 2880 Atlantic Avenue, Suite 180, Long Beach, CA 90806; tel. 310/426–2606; FAX. 310/426–5866; Andrea Campbell, Business Office Manager

Greater Sacramento Surgery Center, 2288 Auburn Boulevard, Suite 201, Sacramento, CA 95821; tel. 916/929–7229; FAX. 916/929–2590; Susan Brunone, MHS, Administrator

Grossmont Plaza Surgery Center, 5525 Grossmont Center Drive, La Mesa, CA 91942; tel. 619/644–4561; Lois Hoke, Administrator

Grossmont Surgery Center, 8881 Fletcher Parkway, Suite 100, La Mesa, CA 91942; tel. 619/698–0930; FAX. 619/698–3093; Mary Ribulotta, Administrator

Halcyon Laser and Surgery Center, Inc., 303 South Halcyon Road, Arroyo Grande, CA 93420; tel. 805/489–8254; Sanja Batista, Administrator

Harbor–UCLA Medical Foundation, Inc., Ambulatory Surgery Center, 21840 South Normandie Avenue, Suite 700, Torrance, CA 90502; tel. 310/222–5189; Lee Scher, R.N., Administrator

☐ **HealthSouth Center for Surgery of Encinitas,** 477 North El Camino Real, Suite C–100, Encinitas, CA 92024; tel. 619/942–8800; FAX. 619/942–0106; John Cashman, Co–Administrator

HealthSouth Forest Surgery Center, 2110 Forest Avenue, San Jose, CA 95128; tel. 408/297–3432; FAX. 408/298–3338; Helen Maloney, RN, Administrator

☐ **HealthSouth South Bay Ambulatory Surgical Center,** 251 Landis Street, Chula Vista, CA 91910; tel. 619/585–1020; FAX. 619/585–0247; Arthur E. Casey, Administrator

HealthSouth Surgery Center of San Luis Obispo, 1304–C Ella Street, San Luis Obispo, CA 93401; tel. 805/544–7874; FAX. 805/544–6057; Linda M. Harris, RN, M.S.N., Administrator

HealthSouth Surgery Center–J Street, 3810 J Street, Sacramento, CA 95816; tel. 916/929–9431; FAX. 916/929–0132; Charlene Nakayama, Administrator

HealthSouth Surgery Center–Scripps, 75 Scripps Drive, Sacramento, CA 95825; tel. 916/929–9431; FAX. 916/929–0132; Charlene Nakayama, Administrator

HealthSouth Surgery Center–Solano, 991 Nut Tree Road, Suite 100, Vacaville, CA 95687; tel. 707/447–5400; FAX. 707/447–2356; Bill Davis, Administrator

Heart Institute of the Desert, 39–600 Bob Hope Drive, Rancho Mirage, CA 92270; tel. 619/324–3278; Jack J. Sternlieb, Administrator

Hemet Cataract Surgery Clinic, 162 North Santa Fe, Hemet, CA 92343; tel. 714/929–3200; Stephen K. Schaller, M.D., Administrator

Hemet Endoscopy Center, 2390 East Florida Avenue, Suite 101, Hemet, CA 92544; tel. 909/652–2252; FAX. 909/925–9252; Milan S. Chakrabarty, M.D.

Hemet Healthcare Surgicenter, 301 North San Jacinto Avenue, Hemet, CA 92543; tel. 909/765–1717; FAX. 909/765–1716; Kali Chaudhuri, M.D.

Henry Tahl, M.D., 790 East Latham, Hemet, CA 92343; tel. 714/658–3224

Hesperia Podiatry Surgery Center, 14661 Main Street, Hesperia, CA 92345; tel. 619/244–0222; FAX. 619/244–1242; William S. Beal

Hi–Desert Surgery Center, 18002 Outer Highway 18, Apple Valley, CA 92307; tel. 619/242–5505; FAX. 619/242–3502; Venkat R. Vangala, M.D.

High Desert Endoscopy, 18523 Corwin Road, Suite H2, Apple Valley, CA 92307; tel. 619/242–3000; FAX. 619/262–1802; Raman S. Poola, M.D., Administrator

Hospitality Surgery Center, 275 West Hospitality Lane, Suite 106, San Bernardino, CA 92408; tel. 909/885–0180; Milton A. Miller, M.D., Administrator

Huntington Outpatient Surgery Center, 797 South Fair Oaks Avenue, Pasadena, CA 91105; tel. 818/397–3173; FAX. 818/397–8003; Sandra Bidlack, Administrator

Imperial Valley Surgery Center, 608 G Street, Brawley, CA 92227; tel. 619/344–IIOl; FAX. 619/344–4985; Vida C. Baron, M.D., Administrator

Inland Endoscopy Center, Inc., d/b/a Mountain View Surgery Center, 10408 Industrial Circle, Redlands, CA 92374; tel. 909/796–0363; FAX. 909/796–0614; Khushal Stanisai

Inland Eye Surgicenter, 361 North San Jacinto, Hemet, CA 92543; tel. 909/652–4343; R. Michael Duffin, M.D., Medical Director

Inland Surgery Center, 1620 Laurel Avenue, Redlands, CA 92373; tel. 909/793–4701; FAX. 909/792–6397; Rodger Slininger, Facility Administrator

Irvine Multi–Specialty Surgical Care, 4900 Barranca Parkway, Suite 104, Irvine, CA 92604–8603; tel. 714/726–0677; FAX. 714/726–0678; Carol R. Stevenson, RN, Administrator

John Muir/Mt. Diablo HealthCare System, Inc., d/b/a Diablo Valley Surgery Center, 2222 East Street, Suite 200, Concord, CA 94520; tel. 510/671–2222; FAX. 510/671–2672; Virginia Goodrich, Administrator

Kaiser Ambulatory Surgical Center, 2025 Morse Avenue, Sacramento, CA 95825; tel. 916/973–7675; FAX. 916/973–7786; Richard R. Stading, RN, Team Facilitator

Kaiser Ambulatory Surgical Center, 10725 International Drive, Rancho Cordova, CA 95670; tel. 916/973–7675; FAX. 916/631–2013; Angela Hardiman, RN, M.S., Manager

Kaiser Permanente Medical Facility–Stockton, 7373 West Lane, Stockton, CA 95210; tel. 209/476–3300; Jose R. Rivera, Administrator

Klaus Kuehn, M.D., Inc.–Eye Center, 1900 North Waterman Avenue, San Bernardino, CA 92404; tel. 909/882–3728; FAX. 909/881–2078; Klaus Kuehn, M.D., Director

La Jolla Gastroenterology Medical Group, Inc., Endoscopy Center, 9850 Genesee Avenue, Suite 980, La Jolla, CA 92037; tel. 619/453–5200; FAX. 619/453–5753; Otto T. Nebel, M.D., Medical Director

La Veta Surgical Center, 725 West La Veta, Suite 270, Orange, CA 92668; tel. 714/744–0900; Joyce Hall, Administrator

Laser Surgery Center, LTD., 2021 Ygnacio Valley Road, Building H–102, Walnut Creek, CA 94598; tel. 510/944–9400; FAX. 510/947–2160; Lori Fried, Administrator

Laser and Skin Surgery Center of La Jolla, 9850 Genesee Avenue, Suite 480, La Jolla, CA 92037; tel. 619/558–2424; Nancy Fritzenkotter

Lassen Surgery Center, 103 Fair Drive, P.O. Box 1150, Susanville, CA 96130; tel. 916/257–7773; FAX. 916/257–2939; Deborah L. Sutton, Medical Staff Secretary

Lodi Outpatient Surgical Center, 521 South Ham Lane, Suite F, Lodi, CA 95242; tel. 209/333–0905; FAX. 209/333–0219; Marklin E. Brown, Administrator

Loma Linda Foot and Ankle Center, Ambulatory Surgical Center, 11332 Mountain View Avenue, Suite A, Loma Linda, CA 92354; tel. 909/796–3707; FAX. 909/796–3709; Sheldon Collis, D.P.M., Administrator

Los Robles Surgicenter, 2190 Lynn Road, Suite 100, Thousand Oaks, CA 91360; tel. 805/497–3737; FAX. 805/373–8878; Le Anne Schai, Administrative Director

M/S Surgery Center, 3510 Martin Luther King Boulevard, Lynwood, CA 90262; tel. 310/635–7550; FAX. 310/603–8749; John H. Shammas, M.D., Medical Director

Madera Ambulatory Endoscopy Center, 1015 West Yosemite Avenue, Suite 101, Madera, CA 93637; tel. 209/673–4000; FAX. 209/673–1430; Naeem M. Akhtar, M.D.

Madison Park Surgery and Laser Center, 3445 Pacific Coast Highway, Suite 250, Torrance, CA 90505; tel. 310/530–2900; FAX. 310/891–0367; Lawrence Saks, M.D., Administrator

Magnolia Outpatient Surgery Center, 14571 Magnolia Street, Suite 107, Westminster, CA 92683; tel. 714/898–6448; FAX. 714/893–1681; Cynthia Begg, Administrator

Magnolia Plastic Surgery Center, 10694 Magnolia Avenue, Riverside, CA 92505; tel. 909/358–1445; FAX. 909/688–2803; Alexander Carli

Marin Opthalmic Ambulatory Surgi Clinic, 901 E Street, Suite 270, San Rafael, CA 94901; tel. 415/454–2112; FAX. 415/454–6542; Audrey M. DeMars, Administrator

Mariners Bay Surgical Medical Center, 318 South Lincoln Boulevard, Suite 100, Venice, CA 90291; tel. 310/314–2191; FAX. 310/392–8020; Gregory Panos II, Administrator

Martel Eye Surgical Center, 11216 Trinity River, Suite G, Rancho Cordova, CA 95670; tel. 916/635–6161; FAX. 916/635–5145; Joseph Martel, M.D.

McHenry Surgery Center, 1524 McHenry Street, Suite 240, Modesto, CA 95350; tel. 209/576–2900; FAX. 209/575–5815; Syd Fuentes, RN, Director

Medical Arts Ambulatory Surgery Center, 205 South West Street, Suite B, Visalia, CA 93291; tel. 209/625–9601; FAX. 209/625–3124; Thomas F. Mitts, M.D., Administrator

Medical Plaza Orthopedic Surgery Center, 1301 20th Street, Suite 140, Santa Monica, CA 90404; tel. 310/315–0333; FAX. 310/315–0341; Carolyn A. Hankinson, RN, Director, Nursing

Merced Ambulatory Endoscopy Center, 750 West Olive Avenue, Suite 107A, Merced, CA 95348; tel. 209/384–3116; Monika Grasley, Administrator

Mercy Surgical and Diagnostic Center, 3303 North M Street, Merced, CA 95348; tel. 209/384–3533; FAX. 209/383–5047; Lynda Pitts, Administrator

Mirage Center Outpatient Surgery, 39–935 Vista Del Sol, P.O. Box 6000, Rancho Mirage, CA 92270; tel. 619/779–9951; Dr. Peter Scheer

Mission Ambulatory Surgicenter, Ltd., 26730 Crown Valley Parkway, First Floor, Mission Viejo, CA 92691; tel. 714/364–2201; FAX. 714/364–5372; Thomas H. Catlett, Administrator

Mission Valley Surgery Centre, 39263 Mission Boulevard, Fremont, CA 94539; tel. 510/796–4500; FAX. 510/796–4573; Sarb S. Hundal, M.D.

Mittleman/King Reconstructive Surgery, 2200 Sandhill Road, Suite 130, Menlo Park, CA 94025; tel. 415/854–2000; Victoria King, Administrator

Modesto Surgery Center, Inc., 400 East Orangeburg Avenue, Suite One, Modesto, CA 95350; tel. 209/526–3000; Dr. Greg Teslue, Administrator

Monterey Bay Endoscopy Center, 833 Cass Street, Suite B, Monterey, CA 93940; tel. 408/375–3598; FAX. 408/375–1478; James Farrow, Administrator

Monterey Peninsula Surgery Center, Inc., 966 Cass Street, Suite 210, Monterey, CA 93940; tel. 408/372–2169; FAX. 408/372–6323; William McAfee, M.D., Chairman

Moreno Valley Ambulatory Surgery Center, 24384 Sunnymead Boulevard, Moreno Valley, CA 92388; tel. 714/247–8080; FAX. 714/247–9381; John E. Bohn, Administrator

Napa Surgery Center, 3444 Valle Verde Drive, Napa, CA 94558; tel. 707/252–9660; Eric Grigsby, M.D., Medical Director

Newport Beach Orange Coast Endoscopy Center, 1525 Superior Avenue, Suite 114, Newport Beach, CA 92663; tel. 714/646–6999; FAX. 714/646–9699; Donald Abrahm

☐ **Newport Beach Surgery Center,** 361 Hospital Road, Suite 124, Newport Beach, CA 92663; tel. 714/631–0988, ext. 3002; FAX. 714/631–2036; Eric Reints, Administrator

Newport Surgery Institute, 360 San Miguel Drive, Suite 406, Newport Beach, CA 92660; tel. 714/759–0995; Linda Shelman, Office Manager

North Anaheim Surgicenter, 1154 North Euclid, Anaheim, CA 92801; tel. 714/635–6272; FAX. 714/635–0943; Monica Briton, Administrator

North County Outpatient Surgery Center, 1101 Las Tablas Road, P.O. Box 147, Templeton, CA 93465; tel. 805/434–l333; FAX. 805/434–3171; Carolyn Lash, RN, Surgery Center Manager

Northern California Kidney Stone Center, 15195 National Avenue, Suite 204, Los Gatos, CA 95032; tel. 408/358–2111; FAX. 408/356–2359; John Kersten Kraft, Medical Director

Northern California Plastic Surgery Medical Group, 2650 Edith Avenue, Redding, CA 96001; tel. 916/241–2028

Northridge Maxillofacial Surgery Center, 18546 Roscoe Boulevard, Suite 120, Northridge, CA 91324; tel. 818/349–8851; Robert G. Hale, D.D.S., Administrator

Section C

Northridge Surgery Center, 8327 Reseda Boulevard, Northridge, CA 91324; tel. 818/993-3131; FAX. 818/993-3347; Robert Vassey, Administrator

Optima Ophthalmic Medical Associates, Inc., 1237 B Street, Hayward, CA 94541-2977; tel. 510/886-3937; FAX. 510/886-4465; Nora J. McQuinn, Administrative Director

Orange County Institute of Gastroenterology and Endoscopy, 26732 Crown Valley Parkway, Suite 241, Mission Viejo, CA 92691; tel. 714/364-2611; FAX. 714/364-0226; Ahmad M. Shaban, M.D., Medical Director

Orange County Litho Center, Inc., 12555 Garden Grove Boulevard, Suite 200, Garden Grove, CA 92843; tel. 714/530-6000; Guy A. Biagiotti, M.D.

Orange Surgical Services, 302 West La Veta Avenue, Suite 100, Orange, CA 92866; tel. 714/771-3432; FAX. 714/741-7606; Elizabeth E. Grant, RN, M.S.

Out-Patient Surgery Center, 17752 Beach Boulevard, Huntington Beach, CA 92647; tel. 714/842-1426; FAX. 714/847-1503; Madelyn Tinkler, Administrator

Outpatient Care Surgery Center South, 5225 Kearny Villa Way, Suite 110, San Diego, CA 92123; tel. 619/278-1611; FAX. 619/278-5853; Ronald Gertsch, M.D.

PFC Surgicenter, 3445 Pacific Court Highway, Suite 110, Torrance, CA 90505; tel. 213/539-9100; Rifaat Salem, M.D., Ph.D.

Pacific Dental Surgery Center, 820 34th Street, Suite 201, Bakersfield, CA 93301; tel. 805/327-7878; Charles Nicholson III, Administrator

Pacific Eye Institute, 555 North 13th Avenue, Upland, CA 91786; tel. 909/982-8846; FAX. 909/949-3967; Robert Fabricant, M.D., FACS, Medical Director

Pacific Hills Surgery Center, Inc., 24022 Calle De La Plata, Suite 180, Laguna Hills, CA 92653; tel. 714/951-9470; FAX. 714/951-9478; Norman D. Peterson, M.D., Medical Director

Pacific Surgicenter, Inc., 1301 20th Street, Suite 470, Santa Monica, CA 90404; tel. 310/315-0222; FAX. 310/828-8852; Jocelyne Rosenthal, RN, Administrator

Palm Desert Ambulatory Surgery Center, 73-345 Highway 111, Palm Desert, CA 92260; tel. 619/346-4780; FAX. 619/340-4650; S. C. Shah, M.D., Administrator

Paul L. Archambeau, M.D., Inc., Ambulatory Surgery Center, 380 Tesconi Court, Santa Rosa, CA 95401; tel. 707/544-3375; FAX. 707/544-0808; Paul L. Archambeau, M.D., Administrator

Petaluma Surgicenter, 1400 Professional Drive, Suite 102, Petaluma, CA 94954; tel. 707/769-8481; FAX. 707/769-0751; Ronald M. La Vigna, D.P.M.

Physician's Surgery Center, 901 Campus Drive, Suite 102, Daly City, CA 94015; tel. 415/991-2000; FAX. 415/755-8638; Kathleen O'Riordan

Physicians Plaza Surgical Center, 6000 Physicians Boulevard, Bakersfield, CA 93301; tel. 805/322-4744, ext. 26; FAX. 805/322-2938; Michael G. Clark, Administrator

Physicians Resource Group, d/b/a Barr Eye Surgery Center, 1805 North California Street, Stockton, CA 95204; tel. 209/948-3241; FAX. 209/948-9321; Susan Ford, Administrator

Plastic Surgery Center, 1515 El Camino Real, Palo Alto, CA 94304; tel. 415/322-2723; FAX. 415/322-3260; Julia Solinger, Administrator

Plastic and Reconstructive Surgery Center, 1387 Santa Rita Road, Pleasanton, CA 94566; tel. 510/462-3700; FAX. 510/462-4681; Ronald Iverson, Administrator

Plaza Surgical Center, Inc., 168 North Brent Street, Suite 403B, Ventura, CA 93003; tel. 805/643-5438; FAX. 805/643-1625; Dale P. Armstrong, M.D.

Podiatric Surgery Center, 255 North Gilbert, Suite B, Hemet, CA 92543; tel. 909/925-2186; FAX. 909/925-4947; Robert Drake, D.P.M., Administrator

Point Loma Surgical Center, 3434 Midway Drive, Suite 1006, San Diego, CA 92110; tel. 619/223-0910; David M. Kupfer, M.D., Medical Director

Porterville Surgical Center, 577 West Putnam Avenue, Porterville, CA 93257; tel. 209/788-6400; Lucy Lara, Administrator

Premier Endoscopy Center of the Desert, 1100 North Palm Canyon Drive, Suite 209, Palm Springs, CA 92262; tel. 619/776-7580; Phillip R. Roy, Administrator

Premier Surgery of Palm Desert, 73-180 El Paseo, Palm Desert, CA 92660; tel. 619/776-7580; Phillip R. Roy

Premiere Surgery Center, Inc., 700 West El Norte Parkway, Escondido, CA 92026; tel. 619/738-7830; FAX. 619/738-7841; R. K. Massengill, M.D., Medical Director

Providence Ambulatory Surgical Center, 1310 West Stewart Drive, Suite 310, Orange, CA 92668; tel. 714/771-6363; FAX. 714/771-0754; Harrell E. Robinson, M.D., President

Providence Holy Cross Surgery Center, 11550 Indian Hills Road, Suite 160, Mission Hills, CA 91345; tel. 818/898-1061; FAX. 818/898-3866; Laura Moore, Administrator

Pueblo Nuevo Aesthetic and Reconstructive Surgery, 1334 Nelson Avenue, Modesto, CA 95350; tel. 209/524-9904; FAX. 209/524-4101; Diane Payne, Administrator

Redlands Dental Surgery Center, 1180 Nevada Street, Suite 100, Redlands, CA 92374; tel. 909/335-0474; Russell O. Seheult, D.D.S.

Richburg Valley Eye Institute Ambulatory Surgical Center, 1680 East Herndon Avenue, Fresno, CA 93710-1234; tel. 209/432-4200; FAX. 209/432-0147; Frederick Richburg, M.D., Administrator

Riverside Community Surgi-Center, 3980 14th Street, Riverside, CA 92501; tel. 909/787-0580; FAX. 909/787-8201; Pat Finley, Administrator

Riverside Eye, Ear, Nose and Throat Institute Surgery Center, 4500 Brockton Avenue, Suite 105, Riverside, CA 92501; tel. 714/788-2788; FAX. 909/788-4374; B. G. Smith, M.D., Medical Director

Riverside Medical Clinic Surgery Center, 7160 Brockton Avenue, Riverside, CA 92506; tel. 714/782-3801; FAX. 909/782-3861; Jan Gough, RN, Office Manager

Rose Eye Cataract Surgical Center, 3325 North Broadway, Los Angeles, CA 90031; tel. 213/221-6121; Michael R. Rose, Administrator

Ross Valley Medical Group, 1350 So Eliseo Drive, Greenbrae, CA 94904; tel. 415/461-1350; Edward J. Boland, Administrator

Sacramento Eye Surgicenter, 3150 J Street, Sacramento, CA 95816; tel. 916/446-2020; Jill Quinn, RN

Sacramento Midtown Endoscopy Center, 3941 J Street, Suite 460, Sacramento, CA 95819; tel. 916/733-6940; FAX. 916/733-6934; Tommy Poirier, M.D.

Saddleback Eye Center, 23161 Moulton Parkway, Laguna Hills, CA 92653; tel. 714/951-4641; FAX. 714/951-4601; Linda Riley, Administrator

Salinas Surgery Center, 955-A Blanco Circle, Salinas, CA 93901; tel. 408/753-5800; FAX. 408/753-5808; Christine Gallagher, Administrator

Samaritan Pain Management Center, 2520 Samaritan Drive, San Jose, CA 95124; tel. 408/356-2731; FAX. 408/356-6366; Ilka E. McAlister, Administrator

San Buenaventura Surgery Center, A Partnership, 3525 Loma Vista Road, Ventura, CA 93003; tel. 805/641-6434; FAX. 805/641-6437; M. P. Bacon, Medical Director

San Diego Endoscopy Center, A Partnership, 4033 Third Avenue, Suite 106, San Diego, CA 92103; tel. 619/291-6064; FAX. 619/291-3078; John D. Goodman, M.D.

San Diego Outpatient Surgical Center, 770 Washington Street, Suite 101, San Diego, CA 92103; tel. 619/299-9530; FAX. 619/296-5386; Carla G. Ramirez, Administrator

San Francisco Surgi Center, 1635 Divisidero Street, Suite 200, San Francisco, CA 94115; tel. 415/346-1218; FAX. 415/346-1819; Peggy Wellman, Administrator

San Gabriel Valley Surgical Center, 1250 South Sunset Avenue, Suite 100, West Covina, CA 91790; tel. 818/960-6623; FAX. 818/962-4341; Susan Raub, Administrator

San Jose Eye Ambulatory Surgicenter, Inc., 4585 Stevens Creek Boulevard, Suite 500, Santa Clara, CA 95051; tel. 408/247-2706; FAX. 408/296-2020; Lolita Ancheta, Clinical Coordinator

San Leandro Surgery Center, 15035 East 14th Street, San Leandro, CA 94578; tel. 510/276-2800; FAX. 510/276-2890; Sheila L. Cook, Executive Director

Sani Eye Surgery Center, 1315 Las Tablas Road, Templeton, CA 93465; tel. 805/434-2533; FAX. 805/434-3037

Santa Cruz Surgery Center, 3003 Paul Sweet Road, Santa Cruz, CA 95065; tel. 408/462-5512; FAX. 408/462-2451; Donald S. Harner, M.D.

Santa Monica Surgery and Laser Center, 2001 Santa Monica Boulevard, Suite 1288W, Santa Monica, CA 90404; tel. 310/829-2005; FAX. 310/453-9201; Cindy Schlaak, RN, Administrator

Scoffield Foot Care Center, 3796 North Fresno Street, Suite 103, Fresno, CA 93726; tel. 209/228-1475; Mark H. Scoffield, Administrator

Sebastopol Ambulatory Surgery Center, 6880 Palm Avenue, Sebastopol, CA 95472; tel. 707/823-7628; FAX. 707/823-1521; Edward J. Boland, Administrator

Sequoia Endoscopy Center, 2900 Whipple Avenue, Suite 100, Redwood City, CA 94062; tel. 415/363-5200; FAX. 415/369-4609; Stuart Weisman, Administrator

Shepard Eye Center Medical Group, 1414 East Main Street, Santa Maria, CA 93454-4806; tel. 805/925-2637; FAX. 809/928-2067; Dennis D. Shepard, M.D.

Sierra Plastic Surgery Center, 6153 North Thesta, Fresno, CA 93710; tel. 209/432-5156; FAX. 209/432-2247; Terry A. Gillian, M.D., Medical Director

Sierra Vista Medical Pavilion Ambulatory Surgery, 77 Casa Street, Suite 203, San Luis Obispo, CA 93405; tel. 805/544-6471; James W. Thornton, M.D., Administrator

Simi Health Center, 1350 Los Angeles Avenue, Simi Valley, CA 93065; tel. 805/522-3782; FAX. 805/522-1283; Lorna Holland, Administrator

Solis Surgical Arts Center, 4940 Van Nuys Boulevard, Suite 105, Sherman Oaks, CA 91403; tel. 818/787-1144; Dr. H. William Gottschalk, Administrator

Sonora Eye Surgery Center, 940 Sylva Lane, Suite G, Sonora, CA 95370; tel. 209/532-2020; FAX. 209/532-1687; Pamela Donaldson

South Area Procedure Center, 8120 Timberlake Way, Suite 103, Sacramento, CA 95823; tel. 916/854-4400; Debra Quast, Administrator

South Bay Endoscopy Center, 256 Landis Avenue, Suite 100, Chula Vista, CA 91910; tel. 619/420-6864; FAX. 619/420-0477; Janet Lemon, Director

South Coast Eye Institute, A Medical Clinic, 3420 Bristol Street, Suite 701, Costa Mesa, CA 92626; tel. 714/957-0272; FAX. 714/641-2020; Michael R. Rose, M.D., Medical Director

Southern California Surgery Center, 7305 Pacific Boulevard, Huntington Park, CA 90255; tel. 213/584-8222; Amgad A. Awad, Administrator

Southland Endoscopy Center, 949 East Calhoun Place, Suite B, Hemet, CA 92543; tel. 909/929-1177; FAX. 909/765-9111; Sreenivasa R. Nakka, M.D., F.A.C.P.

Southwest Surgical Center, 201 New Stine Road, Suite 130, Bakersfield, CA 93309; tel. 805/396-8900; FAX. 805/397-2929; Mark Miller, M.D., Administrator

St. Joseph Surgery and Laser Center, Inc., 436 South Glassell Street, Orange, CA 92666; tel. 714/633-9566; FAX. 714/633-1593

Stanislaus Surgery Center, 1421 Oakdale Road, Modesto, CA 95355; tel. 209/572-2700; Michael Lipomi, Administrator

Stevenson Surgery Center, 2675 Stevenson Boulevard, Fremont, CA 94538; tel. 510/793-4987; FAX. 510/745-0136; Margaret Holmes, Director, Nursing

Stockton Eye Surgery Center, 36 West Yokuts Avenue, Stockton, CA 95207; tel. 209/473-2940; FAX. 209/474-1181

Surgecenter of Palo Alto, 400 Forest Avenue, Palo Alto, CA 94301; tel. 415/324-1832; FAX. 415/324-2282; Rose Parkes, Chief Executive Officer

Surgery Center of Corona, 1124 South Main Street, Suite 102, Corona, CA 91720; tel. 909/737-9091; FAX. 909/737-9093; Teri Ransbury, Administrator

Surgery Center of Northern California, 950 Butte Street, Redding, CA 96001; tel. 916/241-4044; FAX. 916/241-1408; Keveta Andersen, RN, Director

Surgery Center of San Bernardino, 2150 North Sierra Way, San Bernardino, CA 92405; tel. 909/881-2595; FAX. 909/881-1146; Patricia Bishop, RN, Administrator

Surgery Center of Santa Monica, 2121 Wilshire Boulevard, Santa Monica, CA 90403; tel. 310/260-5577; Carolyn G. Catton

Surgery Centers of the Desert, 1180 North Palm Canyon, Palm Springs, CA 92262; tel. 619/320-7600; FAX. 619/320-1694; Rosemary Coombs, Executive Director

Surgery Centers of the Desert, 39700 Bob Hope Drive, Suite 301, Rancho Mirage, CA 92270; tel. 619/346-7696; FAX. 619/776-1069; Marilee Kyler, Administrator

Surgical Eye Care Center, 655 Laguna Drive, Carlsbad, CA 92008; tel. 619/729-7101; Ellen Powers, Administrator

Surgitek Outpatient Center, Inc., 460 North Greenfield Avenue, Suite Eight, Hanford, CA 93230; tel. 209/582-0238; Wiley Elick, Owner, Administrator

Sutter Alhambra Surgery Center, 1201 Alhambra Boulevard, Sacramento, CA 95816; tel. 916/733-8222; FAX. 916/733-8224; Bill Davis, Administrator

Sutter North Procedure Center, 550 B Street, Yuba City, CA 95991; tel. 916/749-3650; Brenda Nakayama, Manager

Sutter Street Surgery Center, 450 Sutter Street, San Francisco, CA 94108; tel. 415/981-1666; Jack K. Waller, Administrator

The Beverly Hills Center for Special Surgery, 1125 South Beverly Drive, Suite 505, Los Angeles, CA 90035; tel. 310/277-6780; Alina Pnini, Administrator

The Center for Endoscopy, 3921 Waring Road, Suite B, Oceanside, CA 92056; tel. 619/940-6300; FAX. 619/940-8074; Barbara Bockover, RN, Administrator

☐ **The Centre for Plastic Surgery,** 401 East Highland Avenue, Suite 352, San Bernardino, CA 92404; tel. 909/883-8686; FAX. 909/881-6537; Dennis K. Anderson, Administrator

The Darr Eye Clinic Surgical Medical Group, Inc., 44139 Monterey Avenue, Suite A, Palm Desert, CA 92260; tel. 619/773-3099; FAX. 619/341-6863; Joseph L. Darr, M.D., Administrator

The Endoscopy Center, 870 Shasta Street, Suite 100, Yuba City, CA 95991; tel. 916/671-3636; FAX. 916/671-4099; Floyd V. Burton, M.D.

The Endoscopy Center of the South Bay, 23560 Madison Street, Suite 109, Torrance, CA 90505; tel. 310/325-6331; FAX. 310/325-6335; Norman M. Panitch, M.D.

The Eye Surgery Center (Colton), 1900 East Washington, Colton, CA 92324; tel. 909/825-8002; FAX. 909/422-8930; Sally Chalk, RN, Operating Room Manager

The Eye Surgery Center of Northern California, 5959 Greenback Lane, Citrus Heights, CA 95621; tel. 916/723-7400; Shari Sloan, Administrator

The Eye Surgery Center of Riverside, Inc., 8990 Garfield, Suite One, Riverside, CA 92503; tel. 909/785-5421; FAX. 909/785-0130

The Montebello Surgery Center, 229 East Beverly Boulevard, Montebello, CA 90640; tel. 213/728-7998; Clifton M. Baker, Administrator

The Palos Verdes Ambulatory Surgery Medical Center, 3400 West Lomita Boulevard, Suite 307A, Torrance, CA 90505; tel. 310/517-8689; FAX. 310/517-9916; Christine Petti, M.D., Administrator

The Plastic Surgery Center Medical Group, Inc., 95 Scripps Drive, Sacramento, CA 95825; tel. 916/929-1833; FAX. 916/929-6730; Mark L. Ross, Administrator

The Sinskey Eye Institute, 2232 Santa Monica Boulevard, Santa Monica, CA 90411; tel. 310/453-8911; FAX. 310/453-2519; Sherry Bennett, Administrator

The Specialists Surgery Center, 2450 Martin Road, Fairfield, CA 94533; tel. 707/422-2325; FAX. 707/429-6088; Ronald D. Fike, Jr.

The Surgery Center, 1111 Sonoma Avenue, Santa Rosa, CA 95405; tel. 707/578-4100; Ken Alban, Administrator

The Surgery Center, 6840 Sepulveda Boulevard, Van Nuys, CA 91405-4401; tel. 818/785-6840; FAX. 818/785-3931; Gail Morales, RN, Nurse Manager

The Surgery Center, A HealthSouth Surgery Center, 3875 Telegraph Avenue, Oakland, CA 94609; tel. 510/547-2244; Peggy S. Wellman, Director, Operations

The Valley Endoscopy Center, 18425 Burbank Boulevard, Suite 525, Tarzana, CA 91356; tel. 818/708-6050; FAX. 818/708-6009; Betty Asato, RN, Clinical Director

Third Street Surgery Center, 420 East Third Street, Suite 604, Los Angeles, CA 90013; tel. 213/680-1551

Thousand Oaks Endoscopy Center, 227 West Janss Road, Suite 240, Thousand Oaks, CA 91360; tel. 805/371-0455; FAX. 805/371-0455; Hector Caballero, M.D., Administrator

Time Surgical Facility, 720 North Tustin Avenue, Suite 202, Santa Ana, CA 92705; tel. 714/972-1811; Denise Reale, Administrator

Torrance Surgicenter, 22410 Hawthorne Boulevard, Suite Three, Torrance, CA 90505; tel. 310/373-2238; FAX. 310/373-8238; Lindon KenKawahara, M.D., Medical Director

Tri-Valley Surgery Center, 4487 Stoneridge Drive, Pleasanton, CA 94588; tel. 510/484-3100; FAX. 510/484-3113; Karen Stevens, RN, CNOR, Administrator

Truxtun Surgery Center, Inc., 4260 Truxtun Avenue, Suite 120, Bakersfield, CA 93309; tel. 805/327-3636; Velma Reed, Administrator

Twin Cities Surgicenter, Inc., 812 Fourth Street, Suite A, Marysville, CA 95901; tel. 916/741-3937; FAX. 916/743-0427; Bonnie Archuleta, Administrator

☐ **UTC Surgicenter,** 8929 University Center Lane, Suite 103, San Diego, CA 92122; tel. 619/554-0220; FAX. 619/554-0458; Dawn Ainsworth, RN, Administrator

University Surgi-Center Medical Group, 23961 Calle De La Magdalena, Suite 430, Laguna Hills, CA 92653; tel. 714/830-5500; Bernard Berry, M.D., Administrator

Upland Outpatient Surgical Center, Inc., 1330 San Bernardino Road, Upland, CA 91786; tel. 909/981-8755; FAX. 909/981-9462; Roger E. Murken, M.D., President

Valencia Outpatient Surgical Center, L.P., d/b/a Valencia Surgical Center, 24355 Lyons Avenue, Suite 120, Santa Clarita, CA 91321; tel. 805/255-6644; FAX. 805/255-6717; Nina Turner, Administrative Director

Valley Surgical Center, 5555 West Las Positas Boulevard, Pleasanton, CA 94566; tel. 510/734-3360; FAX. 510/734-3358; Beth Combs, RN, Director, Nursing

Ventura Out-Patient Surgery, Inc., 3555 Loma Vista Road, Suite 204, Ventura, CA 93003; tel. 805/653-5460; FAX. 805/653-1470; Brian D. Brantner, M.D.

Victorville Ambulatory Surgery Center, 15030 Seventh Street, Victorville, CA 92392; tel. 619/241-2273; FAX. 619/245-6798; John D. Amar, M.D., Medical Director

Vision Care Surgery Center, 1045 S Street, Fresno, CA 93721; tel. 209/486-2000; Lynn Horton, Executive Director

Walnut Creek Ambulatory Surgery Center, 112 La Casa Via, Suite 300, Walnut Creek, CA 94598; tel. 510/933-0290; Catherine Nichol, Administrator

Wardlow Surgery Center, 200 West Wardlow Road, Long Beach, CA 90806; tel. 310/424-3574; FAX. 310/490-0329; Marisol Magana, Administrator

Washington Outpatient Surgery Center, 2299 Mowry Avenue, First Floor, Fremont, CA 94538; tel. 510/791-5374; FAX. 510/790-8916; Gerald G. Pousho, M.D.

West Olympic Surgery Center and Laser Institute, 11570 West Olympic Boulevard, Los Angeles, CA 90064; tel. 310/479-4211; FAX. 310/473-6069; Chris Klimaszewski, Operating Room Supervisor

West Valley Surgery Center, 3803 South Bascom Avenue, Suite 106, Campbell, CA 95008; tel. 408/559-4886; FAX. 408/559-4908; Annette Wunderlich, RN, Administrator

Westlake Eye Surgery Center, 2900 Townsgate Road, Suite 201, Westlake Village, CA 91361; tel. 805/496-6789; FAX. 805/494-8392; Don Hirschman, M.H.A., Administrator

Westwood Surgery Center, 11819 Wilshire Boulevard, Suite 214, Los Angeles, CA 90025; tel. 310/575-1616; FAX. 310/575-1622; Thomas Cloud, M.D., Administrator

Women's Health Care and Cosmetic Surgical Center, 15306 Devonshire Street, Mission Hills, CA 91311; tel. 818/893-4044; Martha P. Nazemi, Administrator

Woodland Surgery Center, 1321 Cottonwood Street, Woodland, CA 95695; tel. 916/662-9112; FAX. 916/668-5783; Donna Fields, Manager

COLORADO

Ambulatory Surgery, Ltd., 320 East Fontanero, Colorado Springs, CO 80907; tel. 719/634-8878; Dana Alexander, Vice President, Clinical Operations

Aurora Outpatient Surgery, 2900 South Peoria Street, Suite D, Aurora, CO 80014; tel. 303/752-2496; FAX. 303/752-2577; L. F. Peede, Jr., M.D., Administrator

Aurora Surgery Center, Ltd., 13701 Mississippi Avenue, Suite 200, Aurora, CO 80012; tel. 303/363-8646; FAX. 303/363-8689; Beverly Kirchner, RN, Administrator

Avista Surgery Center, 2525 Fourth Street, Lower Level, Boulder, CO 80304; tel. 303/443-3672; John Sackett, Administrator

Boulder Medical Center, P.C., 2750 Broadway, Boulder, CO 80304; tel. 303/440-3000; Bradford B. McKane

Centennial Healthcare Plaza, a Division of Healthone/Columbia, 14200 East Arapahoe Road, Englewood, CO 80112; tel. 303/699-3000; FAX. 303/699-3182; Ginger McNally, Administrator

Center for Reproductive Surgery, 799 East Hampden Avenue, Suite 300, Englewood, CO 80110; tel. 303/788-8309; FAX. 303/788-8310; Dr. William Schoolcraft, Administrator

Cherry Creek Eye Surgery Center, (Rose Medical Center), 4999 East Kentucky Avenue, Denver, CO 80222; tel. 303/692-0903; Jeffrey Dorsey, Administrator

Colorado Outpatient Eye Surgical Center, 2480 South Downing, Suite G-20, Denver, CO 80210; tel. 303/777-3882; FAX. 300/778-0738; Thomas P. Larkin, M.D.

Colorado Springs Eye Surgery Center, 2920 North Cascade Avenue, Colorado Springs, CO 80907; tel. 719/636-5054; FAX. 719/520-3576; Paul Angotti, Administrator

Colorado Springs Health Partners Ambulatory Surgery Unit, 209 South Nevada Avenue, Colorado Springs, CO 80903; tel. 719/475-7700; FAX. 719/475-1241; Bruce B. Minear, Executive Vice President

Columbia Centrum Surgical Center, 8200 East Belleview, Suite 300, East Tower, Englewood, CO 80111; tel. 303/290-0600; FAX. 303/290-6359; Jane Klinglesmith, Administrator

DTC Eye Surgery Center, 8400 East Prentice Avenue, Suite 1200, Englewood, CO 80111; tel. 303/793-3000; Jon Dishler, M.D., President

Denver Eye Surgery Center, Inc., 13772 Denver West Parkway, Building 55, Golden, CO 80401; tel. 303/273-8770; Larry W. Kreider, M.D., Administrator

Denver Midtown Surgery Center, 1919 East 18th Avenue, Denver, CO 80206; tel. 303/322-3993; Connie Holtz, Administrator

Denver West Surgery Center, 13952 Denver West Parkway, Building 53, Suite 100, Golden, CO 80401; tel. 303/271-1112; FAX. 303/271-1117; Annette Kancilia, Facility Manager

ENT Surgicenter, Inc., 1032 Luke, Fort Collins, CO 80524; tel. 970/484-8686; FAX. 970/484-1064; Debbie Brown, Manager

Eye Surgery Center of Colorado, 8403 Bryant Street, Westminster, CO 80030; tel. 303/426-4810; FAX. 303/426-8708; William G. Self, Jr., M.D., Administrator

HealthSouth Surgery Center of Colorado Springs, 1615 Medical Center Point, Colorado Springs, CO 80907; tel. 719/635-7740; FAX. 719/635-7750; B. J. Schott, Administrator

HealthSouth Surgery Center of Fort Collins, 1100 East Prospect Road, Fort Collins, CO 80525; tel. 970/493-7200; FAX. 970/493-2380; Karen Cox, Administrator

Kaiser Permanente Ambulatory Surgery Center, 2045 Franklin Street, Denver, CO 80205; tel. 303/764-4444; Rosemarie Polemi, Director

Lakewood Surgical Center, 2201 Wadsworth Boulevard, Lakewood, CO 80215; tel. 303/234-0445; FAX. 303/232-7182; Kenneth R. Richardson, Medical Director

Littleton Day Surgery Center, 8381 South Park Lane, Littleton, CO 80120; tel. 303/795-2244; FAX. 303/795-5965; Keith A. Chambers, Administrator

North Denver Surgical Center, Ltd., 10001 North Washington, Thornton, CO 80229; tel. 303/252-0083; FAX. 303/252-9095; Charlotte Santoro, Administrator

Orthopaedic Center of the Rockies Ambulatory Surgery Center, 2500 East Prospect Road, Fort Collins, CO 80525; tel. 303/493-0112; FAX. 303/493-0521; Scott M. Thomas, Executive Director

Provenant Medical Center at Summit Surgical Services, Highway Nine at School Road, P.O. Box 4460, Frisco, CO 80443; tel. 303/668-1458; FAX. 970/668-1703; Carol Turrin, Administrator

Pueblo Ambulatory Surgery Center, 25 Montebello Road, Pueblo, CO 81001; tel. 719/544-1600; FAX. 719/544-2599; Marlene Keithley

Section C

Rocky Mountain Surgery Center, LTD., 2405 Broadway, Boulder, CO 80304–4108; tel. 303/449–2020; FAX. 303/440–6893; James R. Schubert, Executive Director

South Denver Endoscopy Center, Inc., 499 East Hampden Avenue, Suite 430, Englewood, CO 80110; tel. 303/788–8888; Dr. Pete Baker, Administrator

Southern Colorado Center for Endoscopy and Surgery, 2002 Lake Avenue, Pueblo, CO 81004; tel. 719/560–7111; FAX. 719/564–0122; D. Alan Taylor, Executive Director

Spring Creek Surgery Center, Spring Creek Medical Park, 2001 South Shields Street, Building H, Suite 100, Fort Collins, CO 80526; tel. 970/221–9363; FAX. 970/221–9636; Natalie Coubrough, Facility Administrator

Springs Pain Research and Surgery Facility, 1625 Medical Center Point, Suite 240, Colorado Springs, CO 80907; tel. 719/577–9063; FAX. 719/577–9124; Charles Ripp, Administrator

Sterling Eye Surgical Center, 1410 South Seventh Avenue, Sterling, CO 80751; tel. 303/522–1833; FAX. 970/522–3677; Inez C. Plank, General Manager

Surgicenter of the San Luis Valley Medical, P.C., 2115 Stuart, Alamosa, CO 81101; tel. 719/589–8010; FAX. 719/589–8112; Lauriann Blakeman, RN, Supervisor

Western Rockies Surgery Center, Inc., 1000 Wellington Avenue, Grand Junction, CO 81501; tel. 970/243–9000; FAX. 970/245–4936; Marilyn M. Smith, RN, Surgery Center Administrator

CONNECTICUT

Bridgeport Surgical Center, 4920 Main Street, Bridgeport, CT 06606; tel. 203/374–1515; FAX. 203/374–4702; Anthony German, Administrative Director

Connecticut Foot Surgery Center, 318 New Haven Avenue, Milford, CT 06460; tel. 203/882–0065; Martin Pressman, D.P.M., Administrator

☐ **Connecticut Surgical Center,** 81 Gillett Street, Hartford, CT 06105; tel. 203/247–5555; FAX. 203/249–5860; Margaret Rubino, President

Danbury Surgical Center, 73 Sandpit Road, Suite 101, Danbury, CT 06810; tel. 203/743–2400; Bernard A. Kershner, President

Hartford Surgical Center, 100 Retreat Avenue, Hartford, CT 06106; tel. 860/549–7970; FAX. 860/247–4121; Christine M. Quallen, Administrative Director

Johnson Surgery Center, 148 Hazard Avenue, P.O. Box 909, Enfield, CT 06083; tel. 860/763–7650; FAX. 860/763–7675; Anthony T. Valente, Vice President, Chief Operating Officer

Middlesex Surgical Center, 530 Saybrook Road, Middletown, CT 06457; tel. 203/343–0400; FAX. 203/343–0396; Louise DeChesser, RN, CNOR, M.S.

Naugatuck Valley Surgical Center, Ltd., 160 Robbins Street, Waterbury, CT 06708; tel. 203/755–6663; FAX. 203/756–9645; Bernard A. Kershner, President

Stamford Surgical Center, 1290 Summer Street, Stamford, CT 06905; tel. 203/961–1345; FAX. 213/324–1470; Charles Tienken, Administrative Director

Waterbury Outpatient Surgical Center, 87 Grandview Avenue, Waterbury, CT 06708; tel. 203/574–2020; Nancy Noll, Administrator

Woman's Surgical Center, 40 Temple Street, New Haven, CT 06510; tel. 203/624–3080; Bruce I. Fisher, Administrator

Yale–New Haven Ambulatory Services Corporation, d/b/a Temple Surgical Center, 60 Temple Street, New Haven, CT 06510; tel. 203/624–6008; Alvin D. Greenberg, M.D., Administrator

DELAWARE

Bayview Endoscopy Center, Inc., 1539 Savannah Road, Lewes, DE 19958; tel. 302/644–0455; FAX. 302/645–9325; Harry J. Anagnostakos, D.O., President

Central Delaware Endoscopy Unit, 644 South Queen Street, Suite 105, Dover, DE 19904; tel. 302/672–1617; William M. Kaplan, M.D., Medical Director

☐ **Central Delaware Surgery Center,** 100 Scull Terrace, Dover, DE 19901; tel. 302/735–8290; Paul Fransisco, Administrator

Endoscopy Center of Delaware, Inc., 1090 Old Churchman's Road, Newark, DE 19713; tel. 302/892–2710; FAX. 302/892–2715; Jean–Marie M. Taylor, Administrator

Glasgow Medical Center, L.L.C., 2400 Summit Bridge Road, Newark, DE 19702–4777; tel. 302/536–8350; Arthur C. Kretz IV, General Manager

Limestone Medical Center, Inc., 1941 Limestone Road, Wilmington, DE 19808; tel. 302/992–9259; FAX. 302/992–9248; Thomas Mulhern, Chief Financial Officer

DISTRICT OF COLUMBIA

Capitol Women's Center, 1339 22nd Street, N.W., Washington, DC 20037; tel. 202/338–2772; Kelly Turner–Minor, Administrator

Hillcrest Northwest, 7603 Georgia Avenue, N.W., Washington, DC 20012; tel. 202/829–5620; FAX. 202/882–8387; Alice Harper, Administrator

Hillcrest Women's Surgi–Center, 3233 Pennsylvania Avenue, S.E., Washington, DC 20020; tel. 202/584–6500; Ms. Caridad V. Wright, Administrator

Medlantic Center for Ambulatory Surgery, Inc., 1145 19th Street, N.W., Suite 850, Washington, DC 20036; tel. 202/223–9040; FAX. 202/223–9047; Marcia F. Zensinger, President

New Summit Medical Center II, Inc., 1630 Euclid Street, N.W., Suite 130, Washington, DC 20037; tel. 202/337–7200; Johnette Anderson, RNC, Administrator

Planned Parenthood of Metropolitan Washington, D.C., Schumacher Center, 1108 16th Street, N.W., Washington, DC 20036; tel. 202/483–3999; FAX. 202/347–0281; Claudia Allers, Center Manager

Premier Ambulatory Center, 6323 Georgia Avenue, N.W., Washington, DC 20011; tel. 202/291–0036; Gwen S. Robinson–Terry, Chief Operating Officer

The Endoscopy Center of Washington, DC, L.P., 2021 K Street, N.W., Suite T–115, Washington, DC 20006; tel. 202/775–8692; FAX. 202/296–9122; Phyllis J. Krchma, Administrator

Washington Surgi–Clinic, 1018 22nd Street, N.W., Washington, DC 20037; tel. 202/659–9403; FAX. 202/467–0056; Maria Barrera, Administrator

FLORIDA

Aker–Kasten Cataract and Laser Institute, 1445 Northwest Boca Raton Boulevard, Boca Raton, FL 33432; tel. 407/338–7722, ext. 238; FAX. 407/338–7785; Kim Harrington, Administrator

Alpha Ambulatory Surgery, Inc., 2160 Capital Circle, N.E., Tallahassee, FL 32308; tel. 904/385–0033; FAX. 904/422–0201; Gloria Jeter, Office Manager

Ambulatory Ankle and Foot Center of Florida, 1509 South Orange Avenue, P.O. Box 536951, Orlando, FL 32853; tel. 407/895–2432; Craig C. Maguire, D.P.M.

☐ **Ambulatory Surgery Center of Brevard,** 719 East New Haven Avenue, Melbourne, FL 32901; tel. 407/726–4106; Dwight Miller, General Manager

Ambulatory Surgery Center of Naples, 1351 Pine Street, Naples, FL 33942; tel. 941/793–0664; FAX. 941/793–4318; L. Christian Mogelvang, M.D., Medical Director

☐ **Ambulatory Surgery Center/Bradenton,** 5817 21st Avenue, W., Bradenton, FL 34209; tel. 813/794–0379; J. Leikensohn, M.D. Medical Director

☐ **Ambulatory Surgical Care,** 1045 North Courtenay Parkway, Merritt Island, FL 32953; tel. 407/452–4448; FAX. 407/452–5404; John L. Stellner, MHA, Administrative Director

Ambulatory Surgical Center of Central Florida, Inc., 801 North Stone Street, DeLand, FL 32720; tel. 904/734–4431; FAX. 904/738–1045; Albert C. Neumann, M.D., Medical Director

Ambulatory Surgical Center of Lake County, Inc., 803 East Dixie Avenue, Leesburg, FL 32748; tel. 904/787–6656; FAX. 904/787–9008; Patricia R. Hux, RN, Business Manager

Ambulatory Surgical Centre, 8700 North Kendall Drive, Suite 100, Miami, FL 33176; tel. 305/595–9511; FAX. 305/271–0383; Gail Tauriello, Administrator

Ambulatory Surgical Facility of South Florida, LTD–East, 4470 Sheridan Street, Hollywood, FL 33021; tel. 305/962–3210; FAX. 305/962–3466; Ross S. Ackerman, Executive Director, Administrator

American Surgery Center of Tallahassee, 3411 Capital Medical Boulevard, P.O. Box 13675, Tallahassee, FL 32317–3675; tel. 904/878–4830; FAX. 904/656–1692; Brenda J. Fletcher, Surgical Coordinator

American Surgery Centers of Coral Gables, Inc., 1097 Le Jeune Road, Miami, FL 33134

Atlantic Surgery Center, 541 Health Boulevard, Daytona Beach, FL 32114; tel. 904/239–0021

Atlantic Surgery Center, A HealthSouth Facility, 1707 South 25th Street, Fort Pierce, FL 34947; tel. 561/464–8900; FAX. 561/879–4416; Roni Brockington, Business Office Coordinator

Atlantic Surgical Center, 150 Southwest 12th Avenue, Suite 450, Pompano Beach, FL 33069; tel. 305/941–3369; Ruben Paradela, Chief Executive Officer

Ayers Surgery Center, 720 Southwest Second Avenue, Suite 101, Gainesville, FL 32601; tel. 904/338–7100; FAX. 904/338–7102; Barbara Hyder, RN, Nurse Manager

Barkley Surgicenter, 63 Barkley Circle, Suite 104, Fort Myers, FL 33907; tel. 813/275–8452; Kerri Gantt, Administrative Director

Bay Med Surgery, 1936 Jenks Avenue, Panama City, FL 32405; tel. 904/763–6700; FAX. 904/763–5779; Riyad Albibi, M.D., Director

Bayfront Medical Plaza Same Day Surgery, 603 Seventh Street South, St. Petersburg, FL 33701; tel. 813/553–7906; FAX. 813/553–7992; Gail A. Cook, RN, Assistant Nurse Manager

Beraja Clinics Laser and Surgery Center, 2550 Douglas Road, Suite 301, Coral Gables, FL 33134

Bethesda Health City Same Day Surgery, 10301 Hagen Ranch Road, Boynton Beach, FL 33437; tel. 561/374–5400; FAX. 561/374–5405; Constance Hillman, Clinical Coordinator

Boca Raton Outpatient Surgery and Laser Center, 501 Glades Road, Boca Raton, FL 33432; tel. 561/362–4400; FAX. 561/362–4440; Karen Raiano, Administrator

Bon Secours–Venice HealthPark, 1283 Jacaranda Boulevard, Venice, FL 34292; tel. 941/497–5660; FAX. 941/492–3942; Kermit Knight, Administrator

Bonita Bay Surgery Center, 26711 Tamiami Trail South, Bonita Springs, FL 33923

Brevard Surgery Center, 665 Apollo Boulevard, Melbourne, FL 32901; tel. 407/984–0300; FAX. 407/984–0032; Narda Cotman, Surgical Director

Cape Coral Endoscopy and Surgery Center, 1413 Viscaya Parkway, Cape Coral, FL 33990; tel. 941/772–0404; Nancy Rhodes, Administrator

☐ **Cape Surgery Center,** 1941 Waldemere Street, Sarasota, FL 34239–3555; tel. 941/917–1900; FAX. 941/917–2356; Sharon Tolhurst, RN, M.B.A., Director

Capital Eye Surgery Center, 2535 Capital Medical Boulevard, Tallahassee, FL 32308; tel. 904/942–3937; FAX. 904/942–6279

Center for Advanced Eye Surgery, L.P., 3920 Bee Ridge Road Building, Suite C, Sarasota, FL 34233; tel. 941/925–0000; FAX. 941/927–2726; E. Helen Smith, RN, Nurse Manager

Central Florida Eye Institute, 3133 Southwest 32nd Avenue, Ocala, FL 34474; tel. 904/237–8400; Thomas L. Croley, M.D.

Clearwater Endoscopy Center, 401 Corbett Street, Suite 220, Clearwater, FL 34616; tel. 813/443–0100; Roberta Hayer, RN, Clinical Director

Cleveland Clinic Florida, 3000 West Cypress Creek Road, Fort Lauderdale, FL 33309

Columbia Ambulatory Surgery Center, 4500 East Fletcher Avenue, Tampa, FL 33613; tel. 813/977–8550; FAX. 813/977–7941; Carole Cornell, Administrator

☐ **Columbia Belleair Surgery Center,** 1130 Ponce de Leon Boulevard, Clearwater, FL 34616; tel. 813/581–4800; FAX. 813/585–0319; Margie Maddock, Administrator

☐ **Columbia Brandon Surgery Center,** 711 South Parsons, Brandon, FL 33511; tel. 813/654–7771, ext. 29; FAX. 813/654–3347; Charlene Harrell, RN, Administrator

Columbia Cape Coral Surgery Center, 2721 Del Prado Boulevard, S., Suite 100, Cape Coral, FL 33904; tel. 941/458–9000; Barry Kandell, Administrator

Columbia Center for Special Surgery, 4650 Fourth Street, N., St. Petersburg, FL 33703; tel. 813/527–1919; FAX. 813/527–0714; Paula Russo, RN, CNOR, Administrator

Columbia Central Florida SurgiCenter, 814 Griffin Road and 900 Griffin Road, Lakeland, FL 33805; tel. 941/686–1010; FAX. 941/686–1711; Jan Townsend, Administrator

Columbia Countryside Surgery Center, 3291 North McMullen Booth Road, Clearwater, FL 34621; tel. 813/725–5800; FAX. 813/797–4002; Sandra McFarland, Administrator

Section C

Columbia DeLand Surgery Center, 651 West Plymouth Avenue, Deland, FL 32720; tel. 904/738–6811; FAX. 904/822–4316; Reid Anderson, Administrator

Columbia Florida Surgery Center, 180 Boston Avenue, Altamonte Springs, FL 32701; tel. 407/830–0573; FAX. 407/830–4373; Paige L. Adams, Administrator

☐ **Columbia Gulf Coast Surgery Center,** 411 Second Street, E., Bradenton, FL 34208; tel. 941/746–1121; FAX. 941/746–7816; Carlene Bailey, RN, Administrator

Columbia Kissimmee Surgery Center, 2275 North Central Avenue, Kissimmee, FL 34741; tel. 407/870–0573; FAX. 407/870–1859; Lou Warmijak, Administrator

☐ **Columbia New Port Richey Surgery Center,** 5415 Gulf Drive, New Port Richey, FL 34652; tel. 813/848–0446; FAX. 813/842–3166; Sandra McFarland, RN, Administrator

☐ **Columbia North County Surgicenter,** 4000 Burns Road, Palm Beach Gardens, FL 33410; tel. 407/626–6446; Theresa Vasquez, Business Manager

Columbia Outpatient Surgical Services, Ltd., 301 Northwest 82nd Avenue, Plantation, FL 33324; tel. 954/424–1766; FAX. 954/424–1966; Debbie Haga–Cofu, Controller

☐ **Columbia Parkside Surgery Center,** 2731 Park Street, Jacksonville, FL 32205; tel. 904/389–1077; FAX. 904/389–9959; Chris Edmond, Administrator

Columbia Plaza Surgery Center, 3901 Beach Boulevard South, Jacksonville, FL 32216; tel. 904/448–1948; Debbie Overton–Raines, Administrator

☐ **Columbia Surgery Center Merritt Island,** 270 North Sykes Creek Parkway, Merritt Island, FL 32953; tel. 407/459–0015; Cynthia Johnson, Administrator

Columbia Surgery Center at Coral Springs, 967 University Drive, Coral Springs, FL 33071; tel. 954/975–4166; FAX. 954/344–7054

Columbia Surgery Center at St. Andrews, Inc., 1350 East Venice Avenue, Venice, FL 34292; tel. 941/488–2030; FAX. 941/484–2010; Judy Miller, Business Office Manager

Columbia Surgery Center of Stuart, 2096 Southeast Ocean Boulevard, Stuart, FL 34996; tel. 561/223–0174; FAX. 561/223–0946; Jill Logan, Administrator

Coral View Surgery Center, 8390 West Flager, Suite 216, Miami, FL 33144; tel. 305/226–5574; Victor Suarez, M.D., President

Cordova Ambulatory Surgical Center, 545 Brent Lane, Pensacola, FL 32503; tel. 904/477–5437; Cynthia Blake, Assistant Administrator

Cortez Foot Surgery Center, PA, 1800 Cortez Road, W., Suite B, Bradenton, FL 34207; tel. 941/758–4608, ext. 27; FAX. 941/755–2901; Margaret Provencher, Administrator

Day Surgery, Inc., 1715 Southeast Tiffany Avenue, Port St. Lucie, FL 34952; tel. 407/335–7005; Mary Holobaugh, RN, Administrator

Dermatologic and Cosmetic Surgery Center, 2668 Swamp Cabbage Court, Fort Myers, FL 33901; tel. 813/275–7546; FAX. 813/275–5074; Charles Eby, M.D.

Diagnostic Clinic Center for Outpatient Surgery, 1401 West Bay Drive, Largo, FL 34640; tel. 813/581–8767; FAX. 813/584–1938; Robert R. Dippong, Administrator, Chief Executive Officer

Doctors Surgery Center, 921 North Main Street, Kissimmee, FL 34744; tel. 407/933–7800

East Lake Outpatient Center, 3890 Tampa Road, Palm Harbor, FL 34684

Endoscopy Associates of Citrus, 6412 West Gulf to Lake Highway, Crystal River, FL 34429

Endoscopy Center of Ocala, Inc., 1160 Southeast 18th Place, Ocala, FL 34471; tel. 352/732–8679, ext. 203; FAX. 352/732–2440; Linda L. Brooks, RN, Nurse Manager

Endoscopy Center of Sarasota, 1435 Osprey Avenue, Suite 100, Sarasota, FL 34239; tel. 941/366–4475; FAX. 941/366–4390; Susan M. Brongel, RN, Administrator

Eye Care and Surgery Center of Ft. Lauderdale, 2540 Northeast Ninth Street, Ft. Lauderdale, FL 33304; tel. 305/561–3533; FAX. 305/565–9706; Michael Goldstone, Administrator

Eye Surgery Facility, P.A., 2808 West Martin Luther King Boulevard, Tampa, FL 33607; tel. 813/876–1331; FAX. 813/872–0647; Phyllis S. Chisholm, RN, M.A., Executive Director

Eye Surgery and Laser Center, 4120 Del Prado Boulevard, Cape Coral, FL 33904; tel. 813/542–2020; FAX. 813/542–0704; Louise Bennett, RN, Administrator

Eye Surgery and Laser Center of Mid–Florida, Inc., 409 Avenue K, S.E., Winter Haven, FL 33880; tel. 941/294–3504, ext. 303; FAX. 941/294–8305; Sue Koha, ASC Supervisor

Eye Surgicenter, 2521 Northwest 41st Street, Gainesville, FL 32606; tel. 904/377–7733; William A. Newsome, M.D.

Faculty Clinic, Inc., 653 West Eighth Street, Jacksonville, FL 32209; tel. 904/350–6708

Family Medical Center, 100 Commercial Drive, Keystone Heights, FL 32656; tel. 352/473–6595; FAX. 352/473–6597; Sue Russell, Office Manager

Florida Eye Clinic Ambulatory Surgical Center, 160 Boston Avenue, Altamonte Springs, FL 32701; tel. 407/834–7776; FAX. 407/831–8607; Genevieve Parm, Chief Executive Officer

Florida Eye Institute Surgicenter, Inc., 2750 Indian River Boulevard, Vero Beach, FL 32960; tel. 407/569–9500; FAX. 407/569–9507; Mary Lynne Schlitt, Administrator

Florida Medical Clinic Special Procedures Center, 38135 Market Square, Zephyrhills, FL 33540

Forest Oaks Ambulatory Surgical Center, Inc., 7320 Forest Oaks Boulevard, Spring Hill, FL 34606; tel. 904/683–5666; Thomas D. Stelnicki, D.P.M.

Foundation for Advanced Eye Care, 3737 Pine Island Road, Sunrise, FL 33351; tel. 305/572–5888; FAX. 305/572–5994; Andrea B. Lettman, Administrator

Gaskins Eye Care and Surgery Center, 2335 Ninth Street, N., Suite 304, Naples, FL 34103; tel. 941/263–7750; FAX. 941/263–1754; Cindy Gaskins, RN, M.S.N., R.M.

☐ **Gulf Coast Endoscopy Center, Inc.,** 665 Del Prado Boulevard, Cape Coral, FL 33990; tel. 813/772–3800; FAX. 813/772–5073; Mrs. Lee Caruso, Administrator

Gulfshore Endoscopy Center, 1064 Goodletter Road, Naples, FL 33940

Harborside Surgery Center, 610 East Olympia Avenue, Punta Gorda, FL 33950

HealthSouth Central Florida Outpatient Surgery Center, 11140 West Colonial Drive, Suite Three, Ocoee, FL 34761; tel. 407/656–2700; FAX. 407/877–9432; Antonio Caos, M.D., Medical Director

HealthSouth Citrus Surgery Center, 110 North Lecanto Highway, Lecanto, FL 34461; tel. 352/527–1825; FAX. 352/527–1827; Douglas Vybiral, Facility Administrator

HealthSouth Collier Surgery Center, 800 Goodlette Road, N., Suite 120, Naples, FL 33940; tel. 813/262–5757; FAX. 813/262–6073; Donna Rae Malone, Administrator

☐ **HealthSouth Emerald Coast Surgery Center,** 995 Northwest Mar Walt Drive, Fort Walton Beach, FL 32547; tel. 904/863–7887; FAX. 904/863–4955; Teresa French, Facility Administrator

HealthSouth Indian River Surgery Center, 1200 37th Street, Vero Beach, FL 32960; tel. 407/770–5600; FAX. 407/770–1793; Regina Ludicke, Clinical Administrator

HealthSouth Melbourne Surgery Center, 624 East Hibiscus Boulevard, Suite 101, Melbourne, FL 32901; tel. 407/729–9493; FAX. 407/768–6043; Robert C. Miner, Administrator

HealthSouth Oakwater Surgical Center, 3885 Oakwater Circle, Suite B, Orlando, FL 32806; tel. 407/438–9533; FAX. 407/438–9542; Doug Oakley, Business Office Manager

HealthSouth Orlando Center for Outpatient Surgery, 1405 South Orange Avenue, Suite 400, Orlando, FL 32806; tel. 407/426–8331; FAX. 407/425–9582

Hialeah Ambulatory Care Center, 445 East 25th Street, Hialeah, FL 33176; tel. 305/691–4450; FAX. 305/693–0823; Jose Kone, Administrative Director

Highlands Surgery Center, 7200 South George Boulevard, Sebring, FL 33872; tel. 941/471–6336; FAX. 941/471–6654; Mary Roger, Administrator

Institute for Plastic and Reconstructive Surgery, 820 Arthur Godfrey Road, Third Floor, Miami Beach, FL 33140; tel. 305/673–6164; FAX. 305/534–9759; Lawrence B. Robbins, M.D.

Jacksonville Surgery Center, 4253 Salisbury Road, Jacksonville, FL 32216; tel. 904/281–0021; FAX. 904/281–0988; Katherine Anderson, RN, B.S.N., Center Director

Johnson Eye Institute Surgery Center, Inc., 5923 Seventh Street, Zephyrhills, FL 33539; tel. 813/788–7656; FAX. 813/788–6011; Jane Dempsey, RN, Surgery Services Coordinator

Kimmel Outpatient Surgical Center, 903 45th Street, West Palm Beach, FL 33407; tel. 407/845–8343; FAX. 407/840–8970; Pamela V. Burgering, Administrator

Lake Surgery and Endoscopy Center, 8100 CR 44A, Leesburg, FL 34788

Lazenby Eye Care Center, 1109 U.S. Highway 19, Suite B, Holiday, FL 34691; tel. 813/934–5705; Laverne Peyton, Administrator

Lee County Center for Foot and Ankle Surgery, Inc., 12734 Kenwood Lane, Suite 44, Fort Myers, FL 33907; tel. 941/936–2454; FAX. 941/936–1974; Steve Ostendorf, D.P.M.

Leesburg Regional Day Surgery Center, 601 East Dixie Avenue, Plaza 501, Leesburg, FL 34748; tel. 904/365–0700; FAX. 904/365–0758; Renae Vaughn, RN, B.S.N., CNOR, Clinical Director

Lowrey Eye Clinic, 1840 North Highland Avenue, Clearwater, FL 34615–1915; tel. 813/442–4147; FAX. 813/446–9297; Miquel E. Mulet, Jr., M.D.

Manatee Endoscopy Center, Inc., 6010 Pointe West Boulevard, Bradenton, FL 34209; tel. 813/792–4239

Martin Memorial SurgiCenter, 509 Riverside Drive, Suite 100, Stuart, FL 34994; tel. 407/223–5920; FAX. 407/288–1821

Martin Memorial Surgicenter at St. Lucie West, 1095 Northwest St. Lucie West Boulevard, Port St. Lucie, FL 34986; tel. 561/223–5945, ext. 6678; FAX. 561/223–6862; Charles S. Immordino, RN, Director, Clinical Operations

Mayo Clinic Jacksonville Ambulatory Surgery Center for G.I., 4500 San Pablo Road, Jacksonville, FL 32224; tel. 904/223–2000; Evelyn Leddy, ASC for GI Coordinator

Mayo Outpatient Surgery Center, 4500 San Pablo Road, Jacksonville, FL 32224

Mease Countryside Ambulatory Care Center, 1880 Mease Drive, Safety Harbor, FL 34695; tel. 813/726–2873; FAX 813/791–4317; William G. Harger, Administrator

Medical Development Corporation of Pasco County, 7315 Hudson Avenue, Hudson, FL 34667; tel. 813/868–9563, ext. 251; FAX. 813/869–6918; Dawn M. Ernst, Director, Nursing

Medical Partners Surgery Center, 4545 Emerson Expressway, Jacksonville, FL 32207; tel. 904/399–2600; Kim Chitty, Director

Medivision of Northern Palm Beach County, 2889 10th Avenue, N., Suite 201, Lake Worth, FL 33461; tel. 407/969–0139; FAX. 407/642–1167; Denise Brower, Administrator

Medivision of Orange County, 116 West Sturtevant Street, Orlando, FL 32806; tel. 407/423–4090; Margie Brill, Administrator

Miami Eye Center, 619 Northwest 12th Avenue, Miami, FL 33136; tel. 305/326–0260; FAX. 305/326–1907; Edward C. Gelber, M.D., F.A.C.S.

Mid Florida Surgery Center, 17564 West Highway 441, Mt. Dora, FL 32757; tel. 904/735–4100; FAX. 904/735–2444; Patsy Lentz, RN, Administrative Director

Montgomery Eye Center, 700 Neapolitan Way, Naples, FL 33940; tel. 813/261–8383; FAX. 813/261–8443; Mary Lee Montgomery, Administrator

Mullis Eye Institute, Inc., 1600 Jenks Avenue, Panama City, FL 32405; tel. 904/763–6666; FAX. 904/763–6665; O. Lee Mullis, M.D., Administrator

☐ **Naples Day Surgery,** 790 Fourth Avenue, N., Naples, FL 33940; tel. 813/263–3863; FAX. 813/263–7429; Sara May McCallum, Executive Director

Naples Day Surgery North, 11161 Health Park Boulevard, Naples, FL 34110; tel. 813/598–3111; FAX. 813/598–1707; Sara May McCallum, Executive Director

New Smyrna Beach Ambulatory Care Center, Inc., 612 Palmetto Street, New Smyrna Beach, FL 32168; tel. 904/423–5500

Newgate Surgery Center, Inc., 5200 Tamiami Trail, Suite 202, Naples, FL 34103; tel. 941/263–6766; FAX. 941/263–3320; Dr. R. Crane

North Florida Eye Clinic Surgicenter, 590 Dundas Drive, Jacksonville, FL 32218; tel. 904/751–3600; FAX. 904/757–8922; Mary Miller, RN, Director Surgical Services

North Florida Surgery Center, 4600 North Davis, Pensacola, FL 32503; tel. 904/494–0048; FAX. 904/494–0065; D. M. Whitehead, Administrator, Chief Executive Officer

North Florida Surgery Center, 2745 South First Street, Lake City, FL 32025; tel. 904/758–8937; Angela Kohlhepp, Administrator

North Florida Surgical Pavilion, 6705 Northwest 10th Place, Gainesville, FL 32605; tel. 352/333–4555; FAX. 352/333–4569; Becky Hite, Administrative Director

North Ridge Surgery Center, 4650 North Dixie Highway, Fort Lauderdale, FL 33334; tel. 305/772–7995

Northwest Florida Gastroenterology Center, Inc., 202 Doctors Drive, Panama City, FL 32405; tel. 904/769–7599; FAX. 904/769–7389

Northwest Florida Surgery Center, 767 Airport Road, Panama City, FL 32405; tel. 904/747–0400; FAX. 904/913–9744; Ron Samuelian, Chief Executive Officer

Oak Hill Ambulatory Surgery and Endoscopy Center, 11377 Cortez Boulevard, Spring Hill, FL 34613; tel. 904/597–3060; FAX. 904/597–3077

Orange Park Surgery Center, 2050 Professional Center Drive, Orange Park, FL 32073; tel. 904/272–2550; FAX. 904/272–7911; Michele K. Cook, RN, Administrator, Nursing Director

Orlando Surgery Center, LTD., 2000 North Orange Avenue, Orlando, FL 32804; tel. 407/894–5808; FAX. 407/894–7802; Pat Churchwell, Administrator

Ormond Eye Surgi Center, 26 North Beach Street, Suite A, Ormond Beach, FL 32174; tel. 904/673–3344; FAX. 904/672–1854; Karen S. LaMotte, RN, Assistant Administrator

Pal–Med Same Day Surgery, 6950 West 20th Avenue, Hialeah, FL 33016; tel. 305/821–0079, ext. 321; FAX. 305/558–7494; Mario Machado, RN, Director

Palm Beach Endoscopy Center, 2015 North Flagler Drive, West Palm Beach, FL 33407; tel. 407/659–6543; FAX. 407/659–3533

Palm Beach Eye Clinic, 130 Butler Street, West Palm Beach, FL 33407; tel. 407/832–6113; FAX. 407/833–3003; Andre J. Golino, M.D.

Palm Beach Lakes Surgery Center, 2047 Palm Beach Lakes Boulevard, West Palm Beach, FL 33409; tel. 561/684–1375; FAX. 561/683–0332; Marjorie F. Konigsberg, Administrator

Parikh Volusia Ambulatory Surgery Center, 598 Sterthaus Avenue, Ormond Beach, FL 32174; tel. 904/673–2262; FAX. 904/677–3808; Robin Hess, Administrator

☐ **Physician's Surgical Care Center,** 2056 Aloma Avenue, Winter Park, FL 32792; tel. 407/647–5100; FAX. 407/647–1966

Physicians Ambulatory Surgery Center, 300 Clyde Morris Boulevard, Suite B, Ormond Beach, FL 32174; tel. 904/672–1080; FAX. 904/672–8628

☐ **Physicians Surgery Center, Ltd.,** 4035 Evans Avenue, Fort Myers, FL 33901; tel. 941/939–7375; FAX. 941/275–5248; Caryl A. Serbin, RN, Administrator

Pinebrook Surgery Center, 14540 Cortez Boulevard, Brooksville, FL 34613; tel. 904/596–1130, ext. 7260; FAX. 904/596–1063

Premier Medical Group, P.A., Surgical Center of Florida, 1799 Woolbright Road, Boynton Beach, FL 33426; tel. 407/737–5500; FAX. 407/737–7055; Lily Lee, Administrator

Premier Surgery Center of Zephyrhills, 37834 Medical Arts Court, Zephyrhills, FL 33541; tel. 813/782–8778; FAX. 813/782–2811; Debra Fortenberry, RN, Director, Nursing

Presidential Surgicenter, Inc., 1501 Presidential Way, Suite Nine, West Palm Beach, FL 33401; tel. 407/689–7255; FAX. 407/683–7342; Steve S. Spector, M.D.

Rand Surgical Pavillion Corp., Five West Sample Road, Pompano Beach, FL 33064; tel. 800/782–1711; FAX. 954/782–7490; Deborah Rand, Administrator

Reed Centre for Ambulatory Urological Surgery, 1111 Kane Concourse, Suite 311, Bay Harbor, FL 33154; tel. 305/865–2000

Riverside Park Surgicenter, 2001 College Street, Jacksonville, FL 32204; tel. 904/355–9800; Janice Carter, RN, Director, Nursing

☐ **Same–Day Surgicenter of Orlando, Ltd.,** 88 West Kaley Street, Orlando, FL 32806; tel. 407/423–0573; Barbara Starr, Administrator

Samuel Wells Surgicenter, Inc., 3599 University Boulevard, S., Suite 604, Jacksonville, FL 32216; tel. 904/399–0905; FAX. 904/346–0757; Faye T. Evans, Administrator

San Pablo Surgery Center, 14444 Beach Boulevard, Suite 50, Jacksonville, FL 32250; tel. 904/223–7800; FAX. 904/223–0081; Kim Chitty, Director

Santa Lucia Surgical Center Inc., 2441 Southwest 37th Avenue, Miami, FL 33145; tel. 305/442–0066; FAX. 305/445–6896

☐ **Sarasota Surgery Center,** 983 South Beneva Road, Sarasota, FL 34232; tel. 813/365–5355; FAX. 813/953–7080; Margo Post, Administrator

Seven Springs Surgery Center, Inc., 2024 Seven Springs Boulevard, New Port Richey, FL 34655; tel. 813/376–7000; Barbara Perich, Administrator

Southwest Florida Endoscopy Center, 5050 Mason Corbin Court, Ft. Myers, FL 33907; tel. 813/275–6678; FAX. 813/275–1785; Nancy Rhodes, Administrator

Southwest Florida Institute of Ambulatory Surgery, 3700 Central Avenue, Suite Two, Ft. Myers, FL 33901; tel. 941/275–0665; Susan Hanzevack, Executive Director

St. Augustine Endoscopy Center, 212 South Park Circle, E., St. Augustine, FL 32086; tel. 904/824–6108; Michael D. Schiff, M.D., President

St. John's Surgery Center, Inc., Conference Drive, Southpointe Commercial Park, Fort Myers, FL 33919; tel. 941/481–8833; FAX. 941/481–7898

St. Joseph's Same Day Surgery Center, 3003 West Martin Luther King Boulevard, Tampa, FL 33607; tel. 813/870–4711; FAX. 813/870–4907; Paula McGuiness, Executive Director

St. Lucy's Outpatient Surgery Center, 21275 Olean Boulevard, Port Charlotte, FL 33952; tel. 813/625–1325; FAX. 813/625–6482; Anthony Limoncelli, M.D.

St. Luke's Surgical Center, 43309 U.S. Highway 19, N., P.O. Box 5000, Tarpon Springs, FL 34688–5000; tel. 813/938–2020; FAX. 813/938–5606; Glenn S. Wolfson, M.D., Medical Director

St. Petersburg Medical Clinic P.A., Ambulatory Surgery Center, 1099 Fifth Avenue, N., St. Petersburg, FL 33705–1419; tel. 813/821–1221, ext. 8740; FAX. 813/892–8770; Iverson Pace, RN, Facility Manager, Director of Nursing, SPMC

☐ **St. Petersburg Surgery Center,** 539 Pasadena Avenue, S., St. Petersburg, FL 33707; tel. 813/345–8337; FAX. 813/347–4675; Patty Grover, Administrator

Suburban Medical Ambulatory Surgical Center, 17615 Southwest 97th Avenue, Miami, FL 33157; tel. 305/255–3950; FAX. 305/233–2503; Jules G. Minkes, D.O., Administrator

Suncoast Endoscopy Center, 601 Seventh Street, S., St. Petersburg, FL 33701; tel. 813/824–7116; FAX. 813/824–7177; Denise Epstein, RN, Director, Nursing

Suncoast Eye Center, Eye Surgery Institute, 14003 Lakeshore Boulevard, Hudson, FL 34667; tel. 813/868–9442; FAX. 813/862–6210; Lawrence A. Seigel, M.D., P.A., Medical Director

Suncoast Skin Surgery Clinic, 4519 U.S. Highway 19, New Port Richey, FL 34652; tel. 813/849–8922; FAX. 813/841–7553; Bethany Carvallo, Administrator

Suncoast Surgery Center of Hernando, Inc., 5060 Commercial Way, Spring Hill, FL 34606; tel. 904/596–3696; FAX. 904/596–2707; Bethany Carvallo, Administrator

Sunrise Surgical Center, 110 Yorktowne Drive, Daytona Beach, FL 32119; tel. 904/788–6696

Surgery Center of Jupiter, Inc., 102 Coastal Way, Jupiter, FL 33477; tel. 407/747–1111; FAX. 407/747–4151; Jane MacDonald, Administrator

Surgery Center of North Florida, Inc., 6520 Northwest Ninth Boulevard, Gainsville, FL 32615; tel. 352/331–7987; FAX. 352/331–2787; Joy Ingram, Administrator

Surgery Center of Ocala, 3241 Southwest 34th Avenue, Ocala, FL 34474; tel. 352/237–5906; FAX. 352/237–5785; Verla Heffrin, Administrator

Surgical Center of Central Florida, 3601 South Highlands Avenue, Sebring, FL 33870; tel. 813/382–7500; FAX. 813/385–7332; Sharon Keiber, RN, Administrator

Surgical Licensed Ward, 110 West Underwood Street, Suite B, Orlando, FL 32806; tel. 407/648–9151; FAX. 407/426–7017; Cheryl Modica, RN, Administrator

Surgical Park Center, Ltd., 9100 Southwest 87th Avenue, Miami, FL 33176; tel. 305/271–9100; FAX. 305/270–8527; Deborah O'Connor, Administrator

Surgicare Center, 4101 Evans Avenue, Ft. Myers, FL 33901; tel. 813/939–3456; FAX. 813/939–1164; Robin Fox, Administrative Coordinator

Surgicare Center of Venice, 950 Cooper Street, Venice, FL 34285; tel. 813/485–4868; FAX. 813/484–4084; Cherie Mooney, Administrator

Tallahassee Endoscopy Center, 2400 Miccosukee Road, Tallahassee, FL 32308; tel. 904/877–2105; FAX. 904/942–1761; Noel Withers, Administrator

☐ **Tallahassee Outpatient Surgery Center, Inc.,** 3334 Capital Medical Boulevard, Suite 500, Tallahassee, FL 32308; tel. 904/877–4688; FAX. 904/877–0368; Martin Shipman, Administrator

☐ **Tallahassee Single Day Surgery,** 1661 Phillips Road, Tallahassee, FL 32308; tel. 904/878–5165; FAX. 904/942–9711; Susan Kizirian, Executive Director

Tampa Bay Surgery Center, Inc., 11811 North Dale Mabry, Tampa, FL 33618; tel. 813/961–8500; FAX. 813/968–6818; Jay L. Rosen, M.D., Executive Director

Tampa Eye Surgery Center, 4302 North Gomez, Tampa, FL 33607; tel. 813/870–6330; FAX. 813/871–3956; Margie Brill, Administrator

☐ **Tampa Outpatient Surgical Facility,** 5013 North Armenia Avenue, Tampa, FL 33603; tel. 813/875–0562; FAX. 813/875–1983; Dianne Pugh, Facility Administrator

The Aesthetic Plastic Surgery Center, 135 San Marco Drive, Venice, FL 34285; tel. 941/484–6836; Claudell Crowe, Administrative Director

☐ **The Center for Digestive Health,** 12700 Creekside Lane, Suite 202, P.O. Box 60157, Fort Myers, FL 33919; tel. 941/489–4454; FAX. 941/489–2114

The Endoscopy Center of Naples, 150 Tamiami Trail, N., Suite One, Naples, FL 34102; tel. 941/262–6665; Marjorie Rogers, Office Manager

The Endoscopy Center of Pensacola, Inc., 4810 North Davis Highway, Pensacola, FL 32503; tel. 904/474–8988; FAX. 904/478–9903; Alice Cartee, Administrator

The Endoscopy Center, Inc., 5101 Southwest Eighth Street, Miami, FL 33134

The Eye Associates Surgery Center, 6002 Pointe West Boulevard, Bradenton, FL 34209; tel. 941/792–2020; FAX. 941/792–2832; Linda Colson, RN, Director

The Gastrointestinal Center of Hialeah, 135 West 49th Street, Hialeah, FL 33012; tel. 305/825–0500; FAX. 305/826–6910; Darlene Boytell, M.S.N, ARNP

The Ocala Eye Surgery Center, 3330 Southwest 33rd Street, Ocala, FL 34474; tel. Carol Hiatt, RN, Nurse Administrator

The Sheridan Surgery Center, 95 Bulldog Boulevard, Melbourne, FL 32901; tel. 407/952–9800; FAX. 407/952–7889; Patrice Curtis, RN, Clinical Director

The Treasure Coast Cosmetic Surgery Center, 1901 Port St. Lucie Boulevard, Port St. Lucie, FL 34952; tel. 407/335–3954; Donato A. Viggiano, M.D.

Total Surgery Center, 130 Tamiami Trail, Suite 210, Naples, FL 33940; tel. 941/434–4118; FAX. 941/434–6343; Elizabeth Ross, Administrator

Treasure Coast Center for Surgery, 1411 East Ocean Boulevard, Stuart, FL 34996; tel. 561/286–8028; FAX. 561/283–6628; Andrea Scoville, Business Office Manager

Trinity Outpatient Center, 2101 Trinity Oaks Boulevard, New Port Richey, FL 34655; tel. 813/372–4000; FAX. 813/372–4082; Nancy Burden, Director

United Surgical Center, 2589 North State Road Seven, Lauderhill, FL 33313

☐ **University Surgical Center, Inc.,** 7251 University Boulevard, Suite 100, Winter Park, FL 32792; tel. 407/677–0066; FAX. 407/677–4199; Laura Hofma, RRA, Director, Operations

☐ **Urological Ambulatory Surgery Center, Inc.,** 1812 North Mills Avenue, Orlando, FL 32803; tel. 407/897–5499; FAX. 407/894–8746; Susan A. Wuerz, Administrator

Urology Center of Florida, Inc., 3201 Southwest 34th Street, Ocala, FL 34474; tel. 904/237–8100; FAX. 904/237–5684; Christopher S. Hill, Administrator

Urology Health Center, 5652 Meadow Lane, New Port Richey, FL 34652; tel. 813/842–9561; FAX. 813/848–7270; Greg Toney, Administrator

Venture Ambulatory Surgery Center, 16853 Northeast Second Avenue, Suite 400, North Miami Beach, FL 33162; tel. 305/652–2999; FAX. 305/652–8156; Claire D. Maze, RN, B.S.N., Clinical Director

Vero Eye Center, 70 Royal Palm Boulevard, Vero Beach, FL 32960; tel. 407/569–6600

Volusia Endoscopy & Surgery Center, Inc., 550 Memorial Circle, Suite G, Ormond Beach, FL 32174; tel. 904/672–0017; FAX. 904/676–0506

☐ **Winter Park Ambulatory Surgical Center,** 1000 South Orlando Avenue, Winter Park, FL 32789; tel. 407/629–1500; FAX. 407/629–1741; Linda Dingman, Administrator

GEORGIA

Advanced Aesthetics Plastic Surgery Center, 499 Arrowhead Boulevard, Jonesboro, GA 30236; tel. 770/603–6000; FAX. 770/603–7064; Paul D. Feldman, President

☐ **Advanced Surgery Center of Georgia,** 220 Hospital Road, Canton, GA 30114; tel. 770/479–2202; FAX. 770/479–6666; Debbie Moore, Administrator

Aesthetica, P.C., 975 Johnson Ferry Road, Suite 500, Atlanta, GA 30342; tel. 404/256–1311; FAX. 404/705–2774; G. Marshall Franklin, Jr., Administrator

Affinity Outpatient Services, 712 East 18 Street, Tifton, GA 31794; tel. 912/382–3814; Barry L. Cutts, Administrator

Albany Ambulatory Surgery Center, 531 Seventh Avenue, Albany, GA 31701; tel. 912/883–3535; FAX. 912/888–1079; J. Kenneth Durham, Medical Director

Ambulatory Foot and Leg Surgical Center, 1652 Mulkey Road, Austell, GA 30001; tel. 404/941–3633; Alan Shaw, D.P.M., Chief Executive Officer

Ambulatory Laser and Surgery Center, 425 Forest Parkway, Suite 103, Forest Park, GA 30050; tel. 404/363–1087; FAX. 404/363–9951; Dr. Paul A. Colon, Administrator

Ambulatory Surgical Facility of Brunswick, Eight Tower Medical Park, 3215 Shrine Road, Brunswick, GA 31520; tel. 912/264–4882; Jimmy L. Dixon, Administrator

Athens Plastic Surgery Clinic, 2325 Prince Avenue, Athens, GA 30606; tel. 706/546–0280; FAX. 404/548–0258; James C. Moore, M.D., Administrator

Atlanta Aesthetic Surgery Center, Inc., 4200 Northside Parkway, Building Eight, Atlanta, GA 30327; tel. 404/233–3833; Debbie Clotfelter, Administrator

☐ **Atlanta Endoscopy Center, LTD,** 2665 North Decatur Road, Suite 545, Decatur, GA 30033; tel. 404/297–5000; FAX. 404/296–9890; Ronda L. Knapp, RN, Clinical Coordinator

Atlanta Eye Surgery Center, P.C., 3200 Downwood Circle, Suite 200, Atlanta, GA 30327; tel. 404/355–8721; Robert J. Allen, Administrator

Atlanta Outpatient Peachtree Dunwoody Center, 5505 Peachtree–Dunwoody Road, Suite 150, Atlanta, GA 30342; tel. 404/847–0893; FAX. 404/843–8664; Janie Ellison, Administrator

Atlanta Outpatient Surgery Center, 993 Johnson Ferry Road, Suite 300, Atlanta, GA 30342; tel. 404/252–3074; FAX. 404/843–2089; Marjane Ellison, Administrator

Atlanta Surgi–Center, Inc., 1113 Spring Street, Atlanta, GA 30309; tel. 404/892–8608; FAX. 404/892–8143; Elizabeth Petzelt, Administrator

Atlanta Women's Medical Center, Inc., 235 West Wieuca Road, Atlanta, GA 30342; tel. 404/257–0057; FAX. 404/257–1245; Ann Garzia, Administrator

Center for Plastic Surgery, Inc., 365 East Paces Ferry Road, Atlanta, GA 30305; tel. 404/814–0868; Dr. Vincent Zubowicz, Medical Director

Center for Reconstructive Surgery, 5335 Old National Highway, College Park, GA 30349; tel. 404/768–3668; FAX. 404/763–2929; Gregory Alvarez, D.P.M.

Clayton Outpatient Surgical Center, Inc., 6911 Tara Boulevard, Jonesboro, GA 30236; tel. 770/477–9535; FAX. 770/471–7826; Yvonne Guettler, Operating Room Supervisor

Cobb Foot and Leg Surgery Center, 792 Church Street, Suite Two, Marietta, GA 30060; tel. 404/422–9864; FAX. 404/984–0303; Glya Lewis, Administrator

☐ **Coliseum Same Day Surgery,** 310 Hospital Drive, P.O. Box 6154, Macon, GA 31208; tel. 912/742–1403; FAX. 912/742–1671; Michael Boggs, Chief Executive Officer, Executive Director

Columbia Augusta Surgical Center, 915 Russell Street, Augusta, GA 30904; tel. 706/738–4925; FAX. 706/738–7224; Beryl Barrett, RN, Administrator

Columbia County Medical Plaza–Surgery, 635 Washington West, Evans, GA 30809; tel. 706/868–1050; Jeff Simless, Assistant Vice President, Finance

Columbus Women's Health Organization, Inc., 3850 Rosemont Drive, Columbus, GA 31901; tel. 404/323–8363

☐ **DeKalb Gastroenterology Associates,** 2675 North Decatur Road, Suite 506, Decatur, GA 30033; tel. 404/299–1679; FAX. 404/501–7558; Peter Leff, M.D.

Decatur Urological Clinic–Ambulatory Surgery Center, Inc., 428 Winn Court, Decatur, GA 30030; tel. 404/292–3727; FAX. 404/294–9674; Diane Moore, RN, M.B.A., Administrator

Dennis Surgery Center, Inc., 3193 Howell Mill Road, Suite 215, Atlanta, GA 30327; tel. 404/355–1312; Valerie Garrett, Administrator

Dunwoody Outpatient Surgicenter, Inc., 4553 North Shallowford Road, Suite 60–C, Atlanta, GA 30338; tel. 770/457–6303; FAX. 770/457–2823; Hank D. Fender, Administrator

Endoscopy Center of Southeast Georgia, Inc., 200 Maple Drive, Vidalia, GA 30474; tel. 912/537–9851; Dixie Calhoun, RN, Administrator

Feminist Women's Health Center, 580 14th Street, N.W., Atlanta, GA 30318; tel. 404/874–7551; FAX. 404/875–7644; Nancy Boothe, Executive Director

Friedrich Surgical Center, 2916 Glynn Avenue, Brunswick, GA 31530

☐ **G.I. Endoscopy Center,** 6555 Professional Place, Suite B, Riverdale, GA 30274; tel. 404/996–8830; FAX. 404/991–1596; Aruna Jaya Prakash, Administrator

Gastrointestinal Endoscopy of Gwinnett, 600 Professional Drive, Suite 130, Lawrenceville, GA 30245; tel. 770/995–7989; FAX. 770/339–8646; Elizabeth Bonner, Office Manager

Georgia Lithotripsy Center, 120 Trinity Place, Athens, GA 30607; tel. 404/543–2718; David C. Allen, M.D., Administrator

Gwinnet Endoscopy Center, 575 Professional Drive, Suite 150, Lawrenceville, GA 30245; tel. 770/822–5560; FAX. 770/822–4989; Kerry H. King, M.D., President

HealthSouth Surgery Center of Gwinnett, 2131 Fountain Drive, Snellville, GA 30278; tel. 770/979–8200; FAX. 770/979–1327; Dianne Barrow, RN, Administrator

☐ **Healthsouth Surgery Center of Atlanta,** 1140 Hammond Drive, Building F, Suite 6100, Atlanta, GA 30328; tel. 770/551–9944; FAX. 770/551–8826; Nichole Busch, Administrator

☐ **Hollis Eye Surgery Center, Inc.,** 7351 Old Moon Road, Columbus, GA 31909; tel. 706/323–8127; Kenneth Hopkins, Administrator

Marietta Surgical Center, Ambulatory Surgery Division, Columbia Healthcare Corporation, 796 Church Street, Marietta, GA 30060; tel. 770/422–1579; FAX. 770/422–1057; Charlotte Bellantoni, Administrator

Medical Eye Associates, Inc., 1429 Oglethorpe Street, Macon, GA 31201; tel. 912/743–7061; FAX. 912/743–6296; Susan Branand, Office Manager

☐ **Midtown Urology Surgical Center,** 128 North Avenue, N.E., Suite 100, Atlanta, GA 30308; tel. 404/881–0966; FAX. 404/874–5902; Jenelle E. Foote, M.D., Administrator

☐ **North Atlanta Endoscopy Center, L.P.,** 5555 Peachtree–Dunwoody Road, Suite G–70, Atlanta, GA 30342; tel. 404/843–0500; FAX. 404/843–0675; Laura Dixon, Clinical Supervisor

North Atlanta Head and Neck Surgery Center, 980 Johnson Ferry Road, Northside Doctors Building, Suite 110, Atlanta, GA 30342; tel. 404/256–5428; Ramon S. Franco, M.D.

North Fulton Diagnostic Gastrointestinal, 2500 Hospital Boulevard, Suite 480, Roswell, GA 30076; tel. 770/475–3085; David A. Atefi, M.D.

North Georgia Endoscopy Center, Inc., 320 Hospital Road, Canton, GA 30114; tel. 770/479–5535; FAX. 770/479–8821; Florene Brookshire, Administrator

North Georgia Outpatient Surgery Center, 795 Red Bud Road, Calhoun, GA 30701; tel. 706/629–1852; Herbert E. Kosmahl, President

North Oak Ambulatory Surgical Center, 2718 North Oak Street, Valdosta, GA 31602; tel. 912/242–3668; FAX. 912/242–9905; A. R. Pitts, Jr., D.P.M.

Northeast Georgia Plastic Surgery Center, 1296 Sims Street, Gainesville, GA 30501; tel. 404/534–1856; FAX. 404/531–0355; Sam Richwine, Medical Director

Northlake Ambulatory Surgical Center, 2193 Northlake Parkway, Building 12, Suite 114, Tucker, GA 30084–4193; tel. 404/938–4860; Winfield Butlin, Administrator

Northlake Endoscopy Center, 1459 Montreal Road, Suite 204, Tucker, GA 30084; tel. 770/939–4721; FAX. 770/939–1187; Gayle Carter, Administrator

Northlake–Tucker Ambulatory Surgery Center, 1491 Montreal Road, Tucker, GA 30084; tel. 404/934–1984; FAX. 404/493–4900; Doris Boye–Mintz

Northside Foot and Ankle Outpatient Surgical Center, 3415 Holcomb Bridge Road, Norcross, GA 30091; tel. 770/449–1122; FAX. 770/242–8709; Steven T. Arminio, Administrator

Northside Hospital Outpatient Surgical Center, 3400–A State Bridge Road, Suite 240, Alpharetta, GA 30202; tel. 404/667–4060; Sidney Kirscher, Administrator

Northside Surgery Center, Inc., 5505 Peachtree–Dunwoody Road, Suite 115, Atlanta, GA 30358–2091; tel. 404/843–1008; Irving Miller, Administrator

Northside Women's Clinic, Inc., 3543 Chamblee–Dunwoody Road, Atlanta, GA 30341; tel. 404/455–4210; FAX. 404/451–9529; James W. Gay, M.D., Administrator

Outpatient Center for Foot Surgery, 730 South Eighth Street, Griffin, GA 30224; tel. 770/228–6644; FAX. 770/228–5769; Janice Parker, Administrator

Paces Plastic Surgery Center, Inc., 3200 Downwood Circle, Suite 640, Atlanta, GA 30327; tel. 404/351–0051; FAX. 404/351–0632; Dawn Faille, Operating Room Supervisor

Parkwood Ambulatory Surgical Center, 2605 Parkwood Drive, Brunswick, GA 31520; tel. 912/265–4766; FAX. 912/267–9857; Betty Bauer, RN

Piedmont Surgery Center, 4660 Riverside Park Boulevard, Macon, GA 31210; tel. 912/471–6300; Stephen N. Barnes, M.D.

Planned Parenthood of East Central Georgia, 1289 Broad Street, Augusta, GA 30911; tel. 706/724–5557; FAX. 706/724–5293; Karen Gates, Clinic Manager

Podiatric Surgi Center, 215 Clairemont Avenue, Decatur, GA 30030; tel. 404/373–2529; FAX. 404/370–1688; Jerald N. Kramer, President

Pulliam Ambulatory Surgical Center, 4167 Hospital Drive, Covington, GA 30209, P.O. Box 469, Covington, GA 30210; tel. 404/786–1234; M.M. Pulliam, P.C., Medical Director

Resurgens Surgical Center, 5671 Peachtree Dunwoody Road, Suite 800, Atlanta, GA 30342; tel. 404/847–9999; Kay F. Elliott, RN

Roswell Ambulatory Surgery Center, 1240 Upper Hembree Road, Roswell, GA 30076; tel. 404/663–8011

Savannah Medical Clinic, 120 East 34th Street, Savannah, GA 31401; tel. 912/236–1603; FAX. 912/236–1605; William Knorr, M.D., Administrator

Savannah Outpatient Foot Surgery Center, 310 Eisenhower Drive, Suite Seven, Savannah, GA 31406; tel. 912/355–6503; Dr. Kalman Baruch, President

Savannah Plastic Surgicenter, 4750 Waters Avenue, Suite 505, Savannah, GA 31404; tel. 912/351–5050; Dr. E. D. Deloach

Southeastern Fertility Institute Surgical Associates, 5505 Peachtree Dunwood Road, Suite 400, Atlanta, GA 30342; tel. 404/250–6859; FAX. 404/256–1528; Melissa Weider, Nursing Director

Statesboro Ambulatory Surgery Center, 95 Bel–Air Drive, Statesboro, GA 30458; tel. 912/489–6519; FAX. 912/764–7882; Marie E. Autry, Office Manager

Surgery Center of Rome, 16 John Maddox Drive, Rome, GA 30161; tel. 404/234–0315; Jan Routledge, Director

The Cosmetic and Plastic Surgicenter of South Atlanta, 6524 Professional Place, Riverdale, GA 30274; tel. 770/991–1733; FAX. 770/997–7204; Nabil Elsahy, M.D.

The Emory Clinic Ambulatory Surgery Center, 1365 Clifton Road, N.E., Atlanta, GA 30322; tel. 404/778–5000; W. Mike Mason, Administrator

The Foot Surgery Center, 2520 Windy Hill Road, Suite 105, Marietta, GA 30067; tel. 770/952–0868; L. Susan Rothstein, Administrator

The Rome Endoscopy Center, Inc., 11 John Maddox Drive, Rome, GA 30165; tel. 706/295–3992; FAX. 706/290–5384; Stephen M. Patton, Administrator

HAWAII

Aloha Eye Clinic and Surgical Center Ltd., 239 East Wakea Avenue, Kahului, HI 96732; tel. 808/877–3984; FAX. 808/871–6498; Russell T. Stodd, M.D., Administrator

Cataract and Retina Center of Hawaii, 1712 Liliha Street, Suite 400, Honolulu, HI 96817; Worldster Lee, M.D., Administrator

Hawaiian Eye Surgicenter, 606 Kilani Avenue, Wahiawa, HI 96786; tel. 808/621–8448; FAX. 808/621–2082; John M. Corboy, M.D., Surgeon, Director

Kaiser Honolulu Clinic, 1010 Pensacola Street, Honolulu, HI 96814; tel. 808/593–2950; Jonathan Gans, Administrator

Kaiser Wailuku Clinic, 80 Mahalani Street, Wailuku, HI 96793; tel. 808/243–6000; FAX. 808/243–6009; Mary Hew, Clinics Manager

Surgical Suites at Thomas Square, 1100 Ward Avenue, Suite 1001, Honolulu, HI 96814; tel. 808/521–2305; FAX. 808/599–4818; Gerald D. Faulkner, M.D., President

Surgicare of Hawaii, Inc., 550 South Beretania Street, Honolulu, HI 96813; tel. 808/528–2511; FAX. 808/526–0651; Eileen M. Peyton, Facility Manager

The Endoscopy Center, 134 Pu'uhou Way, Hilo, HI 96720; tel. 808/969–3979; FAX. 808/935–7657; Jody Montell, Administrator

IDAHO

Boise Center for Foot Surgery, 1400 West Bannock, Boise, ID 83702; tel. 208/345–1871; FAX. 208/368–9707; Marshall D. Ogden, D.P.M., Medical Director

Boise Gastroenterology Associates, P.A., Idaho Endoscopy Center, 5680 West Gage, Boise, ID 83706; tel. 208/378–2894; Samuel S. Gibson, M.D., President

Coeur D'Alene Foot and Ankle Surgery Center, 101 Ironwood Drive, Suite 131, Coeur D'Alene, ID 83814; tel. 208/666–0814; Stephen A. Isham, D.P.M., Chairman, Board of Directors

Coeur d'Alene Surgery Center, 2121 Ironwood Center Drive, Coeur d'Alene, ID 83814; tel. 208/765–9059; FAX. 208/664–9998; Peter C. Jones, M.D., President

Emerald Surgical Center, 811 North Liberty, Boise, ID 83704; tel. 208/323–4522; FAX. 208/376–5258; Stanley B. Leis, D.P.M., Medical Director

Idaho Ambucare Center, Inc., 211 West Iowa, Nampa, ID 83686; tel. 208/467–4222; FAX. 208/466–0328; Gary Botimer, Administrator

Idaho Eye Surgicenter, 2025 West 17th Street, Idaho Falls, ID 83404; tel. 208/524–2025; FAX. 208/529–1924; Kenneth W. Turley, M.D., Medical Director

Idaho Falls Surgical Center, 1945 East 17th Street, Idaho Falls, ID 83404; tel. 208/529–1945; James A. Haney, M.D., Medical Director

Idaho Foot Surgery Center, 782 South Woodruff, Idaho Falls, ID 83401; tel. 208/529–8393; FAX. 208/529–8078; Bruce G. Tolman, D.P.M., Facility Director

Jefferson Day Surgery Center, 220 West Jefferson, Boise, ID 83702; tel. 208/343–3802; William Stano, President

Lake City Surgery Center, 2201 Ironwood Place, Suite B, Coeur d'Alene, ID 83814; tel. 208/667–9362; FAX. 208/765–1310; Rachel Muthersbaugh, Director

North Idaho Cataract and Laser Center, Inc., 1814 Lincoln Way, Coeur d'Alene, ID 83814; tel. 208/667–2531; Marilyn Miller, Administrator

North Idaho Day Surgery and Laser Center, Inc., 2205 North Ironwood Place, Coeur d'Alene, ID 83814; tel. 208/664–0543; FAX. 208/765–2867; Michael P. Christensen, M.D., President

Pacific Cataract and Laser Institute, 250 Bobwhite Court, Suite 100, Boise, ID 83706–3983; tel. 208/385–7576; Debbie Eldredge, Vice President, Chief Operating Officer

Rock Creek Endoscopy Center, 284 Martin Street, Suite Two, Twin Falls, ID 83301; tel. 208/734–1266; FAX. 208/736–0390; Arlene Hansen, Administrator

South Idaho Surgery Center, 191 Addison Avenue, Twin Falls, ID 83301; tel. 208/734–5993; David A. Blackmer, D.P.M., Administrator

Surgicare Center of Idaho, L.C., 360 East Mallard Drive, Suite 125, Boise, ID 83706; tel. 208/336–8700; W. Andrew Lyle, M.D., Medical Director

The Surgery Center, 115 Falls Avenue, W., P.O. Box 1864, Twin Falls, ID 83303–1864; tel. 208/733–1662; FAX. 208/734–3632; Larry Maxwell, M.D., Administrator

ILLINOIS

☐ **25 East Same Day Surgery,** 25 East Washington, Chicago, IL 60602; tel. 312/726–3329; FAX. 312/726–3823; Tom Mallon, Administrator

A.C.T. Medical Center, 5714 West Division Street, Chicago, IL 60651; tel. 312/921–4300; Anthony Centrachio

A.C.U. Health Center, LTD., 736 York Road, Hinsdale, IL 60521; tel. 630/794–0645

Able Health Center, Ltd., 1640 Arlington Heights Road, Suite 110, Arlington Heights, IL 60004; tel. 847/255–7400

☐ **Access Health Center, Ltd.,** 1700 75th Street, Downers Grove, IL 60516; tel. 630/964–0000; FAX. 630/964–0047; Lisa Shyne, Administrative Director

Albany Medical Surgical Center, 5086 North Elston, Chicago, IL 60630; tel. 312/725–0200; FAX. 312/725–6152; Diana Lammon, Administrator

Alton Surgical and Imaging Center L.L.C., 4325 Alby, P.O. Box 3195, Alton, IL 62002; tel. 618/474–8000, ext. 8052; FAX. 618/474–8054; Bruce T. Vest, Jr., M.D., Director, Surgery

AmSurg/Columbia HCA, 330 North Madison Street, Joliet, IL 60435; tel. 815/744–3000; FAX. 815/744–7916; Anne M. Cole, Administrator

Ambulatory Surgicenter of Downers Grove, Ltd., 4333 Main Street, Downers Grove, IL 60515; tel. 630/322–9451; FAX. 630/322–9455; Amos E. Madanes, M.D., Administrator

American Women's Medical Center, 2744 North Western, Chicago, IL 60647; tel. 773/772–7726; FAX. 773/772–3696; Jan Barton, M.D., Administrator

Arlington Health Center, Ltd., 1640 Arlington Heights Road, Suite 210, Arlington Heights, IL 60004; tel. 847/255–7474

Bel–Clair Ambulatory Surgical Treatment Center, 325 West Lincoln, Belleville, IL 62220; tel. 618/235–2299; FAX. 618/235–2556; Linda Soteropoulos, Assistant Administrator

Bio Enterprises, Ltd., P.O. Box 56069, Chicago, IL 60656–0069; tel. 312/266–1235; Laura Palomino

CMP Surgicenter, 3412 West Fullerton Avenue, Chicago, IL 60647; tel. 773/235–8000; FAX. 773/235–7018; Carlos G. Baldoceda, M.D., Medical Director

Carbondale Clinic Ambulatory Surgical Treatment Center, 2601 West Main Street, Carbondale, IL 62901; tel. 618/549–5361, ext. 218; FAX. 618/549–5128; William R. Hamilton, M.D., Chief Executive Officer, Medical Director

Carle Surgicenter, 1702 South Mattis Avenue, Champaign, IL 61821; tel. 217/326–2030; Julie Root, RN, Administrator

Center for Reconstructive Surgery, 6309 West 95th Street, Oak Lawn, IL 60453; tel. 708/499–3355; FAX. 708/423–2305; James D. Schlenker, M.D., Administrator

Chang's Medical Arts Surgicenter, Apple Tree Health Care, 2809 North Center Street, Maryville, IL 62062; tel. 618/288–1882; FAX. 618/288–3575; Donna Evans, RN

Children's Outpatient Services at Westchester, 2301 Enterprise Drive, Westchester, IL 60154; tel. 630/947–4000; FAX. 630/947–4044; Jill Keats, Director Satellite Services

Columbia Surgery Center of Southern Illinois, 806 North Treas, Marion, IL 62959; tel. 618/993–2113; FAX. 618/993–2041; Linda Bickers, RN, Administrator

Columbia Surgicare–North Michigan Avenue, L.P., 60 East Delaware, 15th Floor, Chicago, IL 60611; tel. 312/440–5100; FAX. 312/440–5114; Barbara Villa, Administrator

Columbia–Northwest Surgicare, 1100 West Central Road, Arlington Heights, IL 60005; tel. 847/259–3080; FAX. 847/259–3190; Barbara Cerwin, RN, Administrator

Community Health and Emergency Services, R.R. 1, Box 11, P.O. Box 233, Cairo, IL 62914; tel. 618/734–4400, ext. 303; FAX. 618/734–2884; Frederick L. Bernstein, Executive Director

☐ **Concord Medical Center,** 17 West Grand, Chicago, IL 60610; tel. 312/467–6555; FAX. 312/467–9683; Faramarz Farahati, Managing Director

Concord West Medical Center, Ltd., 530 North Cass Avenue, Westmont, IL 60559; tel. 630/963–2500; Faramarz Farahati, Managing Director

Day SurgiCenters, Inc., 18 South Michigan Avenue, Suite 700, Chicago, IL 60603; tel. 312/726–2000; FAX. 312/726–3921; Andy Andrikos, Regional Vice President

Day Surgicenters, Inc., One South 224 Summit Avenue, Suite 201, Oakbrook Terrace, IL 60181; tel. 630/916–7008; Andrew Andrikos, Administrator

☐ **Dimensions Medical Center, Ltd.,** 1455 East Golf Road, Suite 108, Des Plaines, IL 60016; tel. 847/390–9300; FAX. 847/390–0035; Alan Snider, Executive Director

Doctors Surgicenter, Ltd., 1045 Martin Luther King Jr. Drive, Centralia, IL 62801; tel. 618/532–3110; FAX. 618/532–7226; Charles K. Fischer, M.D., Medical Director

Dreyer Ambulatory Surgery Center, 1221 North Highland Avenue, Aurora, IL 60506; tel. 630/264–8400; James Shear

Eastland Medical Plaza SurgiCenter, 1505 Eastland Drive, Bloomington, IL 61701; tel. 309/662–2500, ext. 1284; FAX. 309/662–7143; Anna Lee Fenger, B.S.N., M.A., Administrator

Edwardsville Ambulatory Surgical Center, LLC, 12, Ginger Creek Parkway, Glen Carbon, IL 62034; tel. 618/656–8200; FAX. 618/656–8204; Maxine Johnson, Interim Administrator

☐ **Effingham Ambulatory Surgical Treatment Center, LTD.,** 904 West Temple Street, Effingham, IL 62401; tel. 217/342–1234; FAX. 217/342–1230; Leanne Fish, RN, CNOR, Administrator

☐ **Foot and Ankle Surgical Center, Ltd.,** 1455 Golf Road, Suite 134, Des Plaines, IL 60016; tel. 847/390–7666; Michelle Gormish, Administrator

Golf Surgical Center, 8901 Golf Road, Des Plaines, IL 60016; tel. 847/299–2273; FAX. 847/299–2297; Bernard Abrams, M.D., Administrator

☐ **Hauser–Ross Surgicenter, Inc.,** 2240 Gateway Drive, Sycamore, IL 60115; tel. 815/756–8571; FAX. 815/756–1226; Karen Rouse, RN, Surgicenter Manager

HealthSouth Surgery Center of Hawthorn, 1900 Hollister Drive, Libertyville, IL 60048; tel. 847/367–8100; FAX. 847/367–8335; Jane Collins, Administrator

☐ **Hinsdale Surgical Center, Inc.,** 908 North Elm Street, Suite 401, Hinsdale, IL 60521; tel. 630/325–5035; FAX. 630/325–5134; Judith L. McCammon, M.S., RN, Administrator

Hope Clinic for Women, Ltd., 1602 21st Street, Granite City, IL 62040; tel. 618/451–5722; Sally Burgess–Griffin, Director

Horizons Ambulatory Surgery Center, 630 Locust Street, Carthage, IL 62321; tel. 217/357–2173; James E. Coeur, M.D., Administrator

Hugar Surgery Center, 1614 North Harlem Avenue, Elmwood Park, IL 60707; tel. 708/452–6102; FAX. 708/452–1614; Frank A. Salvino, FACHA, Administrator

Illinois Eye Surgeons Cataract Surgery, 3990 North Illinois Street, Belleville, IL 62221; tel. 618/277–1130; Cathy Vieluf, Administrator

☐ **Ingalls Same Day Surgery,** 6701 West 159th Street, Tinley Park, IL 60477; tel. 708/429–0222; FAX. 708/429–0293; Barbara A. Bertucci, RN, Director

Lakeshore Physicians and Surgery Center, 7200 North Western Avenue, Chicago, IL 60645; tel. 312/743–6700; FAX. 312/761–9226; Phyllis J. Allen, Administrator

☐ **Magna Surgical Center,** 9831 South Western Avenue, Chicago, IL 60643; tel. 312/445–9696; FAX. 312/445–9590; Nader Bozorgi, M.D., Medical Director

Midwest Ambulatory Surgicenter, 7340 West College Drive, Palos Heights, IL 60463; tel. 708/361–3233; FAX. 708/361–4876; Thomas A. Evans, Administrator

☐ **Midwest Center for Day Surgery,** 3811 Highland Avenue, Downers Grove, IL 60515; tel. 630/852–9300; FAX. 630/852–7773; Ronald P. Ladniak, Administrator

Midwest Eye Center, S.C., 1700 East West Road, Calumet City, IL 60409; tel. 708/891–3330; FAX. 708/891–0904; Jill Stevenson, Administrator

☐ **Naperville Surgical Centre,** 1263 Rickert Drive, Naperville, IL 60540; tel. 630/305–3300; FAX. 630/305–3301; Ronald P. Ladniak

Natioinal Health Care Services of Peoria, Inc., 7501 N. University Road, Suite 200, Peoria, IL 61614; tel. 309/691–9073; Margaret A. Vanduyn

North Shore Endoscopy Center, 101 South Waukegan Road, Suite 980, Lake Bluff, IL 60044; tel. 847/604–8700; FAX. 847/604–8711; Everett P. Kirch, M.D., Administrator

North Shore Outpatient Surgicenter, L.P., 815 Howard Street, Evanston, IL 60202; tel. 847/869–8500; FAX. 847/869–0028; Edward Atkins, M.D., Medical Director

Northern Illinois Surgery Center, 1620 Sauk Road, Dixon, IL 61021; tel. 815/288–7722; Gail Larkin, Director

Northern Illinois Women's Center, Ltd., 1400 Broadway Street, Suite 201, Rockford, IL 61104; tel. 815/963–4101; FAX. 815/963–6122; Richard Ragsdale

Northwest Community Day Surgery Center, 675 West Kirchoff Road, Arlington Heights, IL 60005; tel. 847/506–4361; FAX. 847/577–4001; Judith Knupp, RN, Clinical Director

Notre Dame Hills Surgical Center, 28 North 64th Street, Belleville, IL 62223; tel. 618/398–5705; FAX. 618/398–5764; Kathleen Claunch, RN, Administrator

Nova Med Eye Surgery Center of Maryville, L.L.C., 12 Maryville Professional Center, Maryville, IL 62062; tel. 618/288–7483; Melinda Smith, RN, Administrator

NovaMed Eye Surgery Center River Forest, 7427 Lake Street, River Forest, IL 60305; tel. 708/771–3334; FAX. 708/771–0841; John G. Yeatman, Administrator

NovaMed Eye Surgery Center–Northshore, 3034 West Peterson Avenue, Chicago, IL 60659; tel. 312/973–7432; FAX. 312/973–1119; Susan Vaughn, Administrator

☐ **Oak Brook Surgical Centre, Inc.,** 2425 West 22nd Street, Oak Brook, IL 60521; tel. 630/990–2212; FAX. 630/990–3130; Dr. K. Jafari, President, Medical Director

☐ **Oak Park Eye Center, S.C.,** 7055–61 West North Avenue, Oak Park, IL 60302; tel. 708/848–1182; FAX. 708/848–5033; James L. McCarthy, M.D., Administrator

One Day Surgery Center, 4211 North Cicero Avenue, Chicago, IL 60641–1699; tel. 773/794–1000, ext. 228; FAX. 773/794–9738; Christopher Lloyd, Administrator

Orthopedic Institute of Illinois Ambulatory Surgery Center, 303 North Kumpf Boulevard, Peoria, IL 61605; tel. 309/676–5559; FAX. 309/676–5045; Donna Adair, Administrator

Paulina Surgi–Center, Inc., 7616 North Paulina, Chicago, IL 60626; tel. 312/761–0500; Sheldon Schecter, Administrator

Peoria Ambulatory Surgery Center, 4909 North Glen Park Place, Peoria, IL 61514; tel. 309/691–9069; FAX. 309/691–9286

Peoria Day Surgery Center, 7309 North Knoxville, Peoria, IL 61614; tel. 309/692–9210; FAX. 309/692–9055; Wanda Spacht, RN, CNOR, Nursing Administrator

Physicians' Surgical Center, Ltd., 311 West Lincoln, Suite 300, Belleville, IL 62220; tel. 618/233–7077; FAX. 618/234–5650; Cindy Chapman, RN, Administrator

Planned Parenthood of East Central Illinois, 302 East Stoughton Street, Champaign, IL 61820; tel. 217/359–8022; FAX. 217/359–2683; Karen Cody Carlson, President

Poplar Creek Surgical Center, 1800 McDonough Road, Hoffman Estates, IL 60192; tel. 847/742–7272; FAX. 847/697–3210; JoAnn Uteg, Administrative Director

Quad City Ambulatory Surgery Center, 520 Valley View Drive, Moline, IL 61265; tel. 309/762–1952; FAX. 309/762–3642; Vicki Sullivan, RN, CNOR, Director, Surgical Services

Quad City Endoscopy, 2525 24th Street, Rock Island, IL 61201; tel. 309/788–5624; FAX. 309/788–5668; Najwa Bayrakdar, Administrator

☐ **Regional Surgicenter, Ltd.,** 545 Valley View Drive, Moline, IL 61265; tel. 309/762–5560; FAX. 309/762–7351; Patt Hunter, Administrator

Resurrection Health Care Surgery Center, 3101 North Harlem Avenue, Chicago, IL 60634; tel. 773/282–9700, ext. 304; FAX. 312/745–5522; Sandra Ankebrant, Executive Director

River North Same Day Surgery, One East Erie, Suite 115, Chicago, IL 60611; tel. 312/649–3939; FAX. 312/649–5747; Patricia Wamsley, Administrator

Rockford Ambulatory Surgery Center, 1016 Featherstone Drive, Rockford, IL 61107; tel. 815/226–3300; FAX. 815/226–9990; Dr. Steven Gunderson, Administrator

☐ **Rockford Endoscopy Center,** 401 Roxbury Road, Rockford, IL 61107; tel. 815/397–7340; FAX. 815/397–7388; Nancy Norman, Administrator

South Shore Surgicenter, Inc., 8300 South Brandon Avenue, Chicago, IL 60617; tel. 312/721–6000; FAX. 312/721–9861; Lucy Morales, RN, Administrator

Spiritus Dei Eye Surgery Center, 7600 West College Drive, Palos Heights, IL 60463; tel. 708/361–0010; Peggy A. Toth, Administrator

Springfield Clinic Ambulatory Surgical Treatment Center, Inc., 1025 South Seventh Street, Springfield, IL 62794–9248; tel. 217/528–7541; Michael Maynard

Suburban Otolaryngology SurgiCenter, 3340 South Oak Park Avenue, Berwyn, IL 60402; tel. 708/749–3070; FAX. 708/749–3410; Edward A. Razim, M.D., Administrator

Surgicare Center, Inc., 333 Dixie Highway, Chicago Heights, IL 60411; tel. 708/754–4890; FAX. 708/756–1149; Paul Katz, Administrator

Surgicore, Inc., 10547 South Ewing Avenue, Chicago, IL 60617; tel. 773/221–1690; William Wood, Medical Director

The Center for Orthopedic Medicine, LLC, 2502–B East Empire, Bloomington, IL 61704; tel. 309/662–6120; FAX. 309/663–8972; Tracy J. Silver, RN, Administrator

The Center for Surgery, 475 East Diehl Road, Naperville, IL 60563–1253; tel. 630/505–7733; FAX. 630/505–0656; Eric Myers

Valley Ambulatory Surgery Center, 2210 Dean Street, St. Charles, IL 60175; tel. 630/584–9800; FAX. 630/584–9805; Mark Mayo, Facility Director

☐ **Watertower Surgicenter Corp.,** 845 North Michigan Avenue, Suite 994–W, Chicago, IL 60611; tel. 312/944–2929; FAX. 312/944–7769; John M. Sevcik, President, Chief Executive Officer

Women's Aid Clinic, 4751 West Touhy Avenue, Lincolnwood, IL 60646; tel. 847/676–2428; Iris Schneider

INDIANA

☐ **Akin Medical Center,** 2019 State Street, New Albany, IN 47150–4963; tel. 812/945–3557; FAX. 812/949–3469; Karyn Cureton, RN, Director, Surgery

Calumet Surgery Center, 7847 Calumet Avenue, Munster, IN 46321–1296; tel. 219/836–5102; FAX. 219/836–4493; Gloria J. Portney, RN, Chief Administrative Officer

Central Indiana Surgery Center, 9002 North Meridian, Lower Level, Indianapolis, IN 46260; tel. 317/846–9906; FAX. 317/846–9949; William E. Whitson, M.D., Medical Director

Columbia Physiciancare Outpatient Surgery Center, L.L.P., 7460 North Shadeland, Indianapolis, IN 46250; tel. 317/577–7450; FAX. 317/577–7462; Maureen Chernoff, RN, Administrator

Columbus Surgery Center, 940 North Marr Road, Suite B, Columbus, IN 47201; tel. 812/372–1370; Colleen M. Norta, Executive Director

Digestive Health Center, 1120 AAA Way, Suite A, Carmel, IN 46032–3210; tel. 317/848–5494; FAX. 317/575–0392; Ellen Hairston, Administrative Assistant

Dupont Ambulatory Surgery Center, 2510 East Dupont Road, Suite 130, Fort Wayne, IN 46825; tel. 219/489–8785; FAX. 219/489–2148; Rick C. Trego, Administrator

☐ **Evansville Surgery Center,** 1212 Lincoln Avenue, Evansville, IN 47714–1076; tel. 812/428–0810; FAX. 812/421–6070; Cathy Head, RN, Facility Manager

Foot and Ankle Surgery Center, Inc., 1950 West 86th Street, Suite 105, Indianapolis, IN 46260; tel. 317/334–0232; FAX. 317/334–0268; Eva Stemler, RN, B.S.N., Director

Fort Wayne Cardiology Outpatient Catheterization Laboratory, 1819 Carew Street, Fort Wayne, IN 46805; tel. 219/481–4866; FAX. 219/481–4808; Douglas W. Martin, Director, Clinical Operations

Fort Wayne Ophthalmic Surgical Center, 321 East Wayne Street, Ft. Wayne, IN 46802–2713; tel. 219/422–5976; FAX. 219/424–4511; J. Rex Parent, M.D., Chief Executive Officer

Fort Wayne Orthopaedics LLC Surgicenter, 7601 West Jefferson Boulevard, P.O. Box 2526, Fort Wayne, IN 46801–2526; tel. 219/436–8383; FAX. 219/436–8477; Ronald W. Cousino, Jr., Administrator

Gastrointestinal Endoscopy Center, 801 St. Mary's Drive, Suite 110, West, Evansville, IN 47714; tel. 812/477–6103; FAX. 812/477–4897; Christine Wittman, Administrator

Grand Park Surgical Center, 1479 East 84th Place, Merrillville, IN 46410; tel. 219/738–2828; FAX. 219/756–3349; Chris Macarthy, Administrator

Grossnickle Eye Surgery Center, Inc., 2251 DuBois Drive, Warsaw, IN 46580–3292; tel. 219/269–3777; FAX. 219/269–9828; Shirley Rhodes, RN, Administrative Director

IMA Endoscopy Surgicenter, P.C., 8895 Broadway, Merrillville, IN 46410; tel. 219/738–2081; FAX. 219/736–4658; Sandra K. Shaw, Administrator

Illiana Surgery Center, 701 Superior Avenue, Munster, IN 46321; tel. 219/924–1300; FAX. 219/922–4856; Virgil Villaflor, Executive Director

Indiana Eye Clinic, 30 North Emerson Avenue, Greenwood, IN 46143–9760; tel. 317/881–3937; FAX. 317/887–4008; Mr. B. H. Draffen, Executive Director

Indiana Surgery Center, 8040 Clearvista Parkway, Indianapolis, IN 46256–1695; tel. 317/841–2000; FAX. 317/841–2005; Amy Glover, Administrator

Indiana Surgery Center, South Campus, 1550 East County Line Road, Suite 100, Indianapolis, IN 46227; tel. 317/887–7600; FAX. 317/887–7687; Peggy Davidson, Administrator

Indianapolis Endoscopy Center, 7353 East 21st Street, Indianapolis, IN 46219; tel. 317/353–2232; FAX. 317/353–2522; David Hollander, M.D.

Lafayette Ambulatory Surgery Center, 3733 Rome Drive, Box 6477, Lafayette, IN 47903–6477; tel. 317/449–5272; FAX. 317/477–8723; Dale T. Krynak, Executive Director

MHC Surgical Center Associates, Inc., d/b/a Broadwest Surgical Center, 315 West 89th Avenue, Merrillville, IN 46410–2904; tel. 219/757–5275; FAX. 219/757–5290; Lisa M. Goranovich, Administrator

Medivision, 1305 Wall Street, Suite 101, Jeffersonville, IN 47130–3898; tel. 812/288–9674; FAX. 812/283–6955; Marsha Parker, Administrator

Meridian Endoscopy Center, 1801 North Senate, Suite 400, Indianapolis, IN 46202; tel. 317/929–5660; FAX. 317/929–2346; John C. Kohne, M.D., Executive Director

Meridian Plastic Surgery Center, 170 West 106th Street, Indianapolis, IN 46290–1004; tel. 317/575–0110; FAX. 317/846–5719; Sally Gentner, Director

Midwest Surgery Centers, Inc., 650 Surgery Center Drive, Terre Haute, IN 47802; tel. 812/232–8325; FAX. 812/234–8385; Joanne Floyd, M.D., Administrator

Muncie Ambulatory Surgicenter, LLC, 200 North Tillotson Avenue, Muncie, IN 47304–3988; tel. 317/286–8888; FAX. 317/747–7962; L. Marshall Roch, M.D., Medical Director

Munster Same Day Surgery Center, 761 Forty Fifth Avenue, Suite 116, Munster, IN 46321; tel. 219/924–3090; FAX. 219/924–2160; Thomas Mallon, Partner

Nasser Smith and Pinkerton Cardiac Cath Lab, 8333 Naab Road, Suite 400, Indianapolis, IN 46260; tel. 317/338–6094; FAX. 317/338–6066; Rodger P. Pinto, Ph.D., Administrator

North Indianapolis Surgery Center, 8651 North Township Line Road, Indianapolis, IN 46260–1578; tel. 317/876–2090; FAX. 317/876–2097; Dean E. Lehmkuhler, Facility Administrator

North Meridian Surgery Center, 10601 North Meridian, Indianapolis, IN 46290; tel. 317/574–5400; FAX. 317/575–2713; Julie Hammersley, Director

Northeast Indiana Endoscopy Center, 7900 West Jefferson Boulevard, Fort Wayne, IN 46804; tel. 219/436–6213; FAX. 219/432–6388; Michael T. Isenberg, M.D., Director

Northside Cardiac Cath Lab, 8333 Naab Road, Suite 180, Indianapolis, IN 46260; tel. 317/338–9001; FAX. 317/338–9045; Mary Ellen Boyd, Administrator

NovaMed Eyecare Management, L.L.C., d/b/a NovaMed Eye Surgery Center–Hammond, 6836 Hohman Avenue, Hammond, IN 46324; tel. 219/937–5063; FAX. 219/937–5068; Renee Peters, Administrator

NovaMed Eyecare Management, L.L.C., 8514 Broadway, Merrillville, IN 46410; tel. 219/756–5010; Eldi E. Deschamps, M.D., Executive Director

Outpatient Surgery Center of Indiana, Inc., 711 Gardner Drive, Marion, IN 46952; tel. 317/664–2000; FAX. 317/668–6797; Sheryl Miller, RN, Director

Premier Ambulatory Surgery of Fort Wayne, 1333 Maycrest Drive, Fort Wayne, IN 46805–5478; tel. 219/423–3339; FAX. 219/423–6344; Mary Schafer, Administrator

Richmond Surgery Center, 1900 Chester Boulevard, Richmond, IN 47374; tel. 317/966–1776; FAX. 317/962–1191; Debra Day, Director

Sagamore Surgical Services, Inc., 2320 Concord Road, Suite B, Lafayette, IN 47905; tel. 317/474–7838; FAX. 317/474–7853; Carol Blanar, Administrator

South Bend Clinic Surgicenter, 211 North Eddy Street, P.O. Box 4061, South Bend, IN 46634–4061; tel. 219/237–9366; FAX. 219/237–9329; Teresa Roberts, Executive Director

Southern Indiana Surgery Center, 2800 Rex Grossman Boulevard, Bloomington, IN 47403; tel. 812/333–8969; FAX. 812/335–2309; Miriam Malone, RN, B.S.N., Executive Director

Surgery Center Plus, 7430 North Shadeland Avenue, Suite 100, Indianapolis, IN 46250–2025; tel. 317/841–8005; FAX. 317/577–7538; James Hansen, Administrator

Surgery Center of Eye Specialists, 1901 North Meridian Street, Indianapolis, IN 46202; tel. 317/925–2200; FAX. 317/921–6614; Dan Bradford, Administrator

Surgery One, 5052 North Clinton, Fort Wayne, IN 46825–5822; tel. 219/482–5194; FAX. 219/482–5686; William H. Couch, Jr., M.D., Executive Officer

Surgical Care Center, Inc., 8103 Clearvista Parkway, Indianapolis, IN 46256–4600; tel. 317/842–5173; FAX. 317/576–9644; Larry Gardner, Executive Director

Surgical Center of New Albany, 2201 Green Valley Road, New Albany, IN 47150–4648; tel. 812/949–1223; FAX. 812/945–4765; Tamara E. Hay, RN, Administrator

Talley Cataract and Laser Institute, Inc., 220 East Virginia, Evansville, IN 47711; tel. 812/435–1600; FAX. 812/435–1603; Patricia S. Fisher, Facility Manager

The Ambulatory Care Center, 1125 Professional Boulevard, Evansville, IN 47714; tel. 812/475–1000; FAX. 812/475–1001; Diana McDaniel, Clinical Administrator

The Center for Specialty Surgery of Fort Wayne, Inc., 2730 East State Boulevard, Fort Wayne, IN 46805–4731; tel. 219/483–2540; FAX. 219/483–3097, ext. 2; Andrea Kelley, RN, Director, Nursing

The Endoscopy Center, 8051 South Emerson, Suite 150, Indianapolis, IN 46237; tel. 317/865–2950; FAX. 317/865–2952; Janet Miller, Director, Nurses

The Heart Group Outpatient Cath Lab, 415 West Columbia Street, Evansville, IN 47710; tel. 812/464–9133; FAX. 812/426–6023; Lisa Attebery, Director, Ancillary Services

The Indiana Hand Surgery Center, 8501 Harcourt Road, P.O. Box 80434, Indianapolis, IN 46280–0434; tel. 317/471–4388; FAX. 317/471–4382; Mark S. Fritz, Chief Executive Officer

Unity Surgery Center, 1011 West Second Street, Bloomington, IN 47403–2216; tel. 812/334–1213, ext. 250; FAX. 812/333–5039; Dawana Page, RN, CNOR, Director, Surgical Services

Valparaiso Physican and Surgery Center, 1700 Pointe Drive, Valparaiso, IN 46383; tel. 219/531–5000; FAX. 219/531–5010; Lilly Veljovic, RN, Manager

☐ **Zollman Surgery Center, Inc.,** 7439 Woodland Drive, Indianapolis, IN 46268; tel. 317/328–1100; FAX. 317/328–6948; Susan Matouk, RN, B.S.M., Clinical Administrator

IOWA

Iowa Endoscopy Center, 2600 Grand Avenue, Suite 418, Des Moines, IA 50312; tel. 515/288–3342; Gloria Dayton, Administrator

Iowa Eye Institute, 1721 West 18th Street, Spencer, IA 51301; tel. 712/262–8878; FAX. 712/262–8807; Dennis D. Gordy, M.D., Administrator

Jones Eye Clinic, 4405 Hamilton Boulevard, Sioux City, IA 51104; tel. 712/239–3937; Charles E. Jones, M.D., Medical Director

Land–Barowsky Ambulatory Surgery Center, Center for Sight, Iowa/Illinois, 931 13th Avenue, N., P.O. Box 608, Clinton, IA 52733–0608; tel. 319/242–3937; FAX. 319/242–3845; Renelda Ebensberger, Supervisor

Mississippi Valley Surgery Center, L.C., 3400 Dexter Court, Suite 200, Davenport, IA 52807; tel. 319/344–6600; FAX. 319/344–6699

Surgery Center of Des Moines, 1301 Penn Avenue, Suite 100, Des Moines, IA 50312; tel. 515/266–3140; FAX. 515/266–3073; Kathleen Supplee, RN, Administrator

Tower Surgical Center, 3200 Grand Avenue, Des Moines, IA 50312; tel. 515/271–1735; FAX. 515/271–1726; L. Duane Murray, Administrator

Uro Surgery Center, 3319 Spring Street, Suite 202–A, Davenport, IA 52807; tel. 319/359–1641; FAX. 319/359–9492; Paul Rohlf, M.D., Administrator

KANSAS

College Park Family Care Center, 11725 West 112th Street, Overland Park, KS 66210–2761; tel. 913/469–5579; Chuck Chambers, Administrator

Columbia Mt. Oread Surgery Centre, 3500 Clinton Parkway Place, Lawrence, KS 66047–1985; tel. 913/843–9300; FAX. 913/843–9301; Nancy Sturgeon, Administrator

Columbia Surgicenter of Johnson County, 8800 Ballentine Street, Overland Park, KS 66214–1985; tel. 913/894–4050; FAX. 913/894–0384; Nancy E. Sturgeon, Administrator

Comprehensive Health for Women, 4401 West 109th Street, Overland Park, KS 66211–1303; tel. 913/345–1400; Sheila Kostas, Director, Human Resources

Cotton–O'Neil Clinic Endoscopy Center, 823 Southwest Mulvane Street, Suite 375, Topeka, KS 66606–1679; tel. 913/354–0538; FAX. 913/368–0735; Irene Hasenbank, RN, Administrator

Emporia Ambulatory Surgery Center, 2528 West 15th Avenue, Emporia, KS 66801–6102; tel. 316/343–2233; J. E. Bosiljevac, M.D., Administrator

Endoscopic Services, P.A., 1431 South Bluffview Street, Suite 215, Wichita, KS 67218–3000; tel. 316/687–0234; FAX. 316/687–0360; Jace Hyder, M.D.

☐ **Endoscopy and Surgery Center of Topeka, L.P.,** 2200 Southwest Sixth Avenue, Suite 103, Topeka, KS 66606–1707; tel. 913/354–1254; FAX. 913/354–1255; Ashraf M. Sufi, M.D., Medical Director

EyeSurg of Kansas City, 5520 College Boulevard, Overland Park, KS 66211–1600; tel. 913/491–3757; FAX. 913/469–6686; Phillip Hoopes, M.D., Medical Administrator

Great Plains Clinic, 201 East Seventh, Hays, KS 67601; tel. 913/628–8251; William Norris, Administrator

Hutchinson Clinic Ambulatory Surgery Center, 2101 North Waldron, Hutchinson, KS 67502; tel. 316/669–2500; Murray Holcomb, Administrator

Kansas Ambulatory Surgery Center, 7015 East Central Street, Wichita, KS 67206–1940; tel. 316/684–9300; FAX. 316/652–7618; Robert G. Clark, M.D., Medical Director

Laser Center, 1518A East Iron Avenue, Salina, KS 67401–3236; tel. 913/825–6016; Brian E. Conner, M.D., Administrator

Laser Center–Russell, 222 South Kansas, Suite A, Russell, KS 67665–3029; tel. 913/825–6016; Brian Conner, Administrator

Microsurgery, Inc., 920 Southwest Washburn Avenue, Topeka, KS 66606–1527; tel. 913/233–3939; Adrienne V. Prokop, Administrator

Newman–Young Clinic–A.S.C., 710 West Eighth Street, Fort Scott, KS 66701–2404; tel. 316/223–3100; FAX. 316/223–5390; Thomas W. Smith, Administrator

Newton Surgery Centre, 215 South Pine Street, Newton, KS 67114–3761; tel. 316/283–4400; Sondra L. Leatherman, Administrator

Ochsner Eye Medical/Associated Eye Surgical Center, 1100 North Topeka Street, Wichita, KS 67214–2810; tel. 316/263–6273; FAX. 316/263–5568; Bruce B. Ochsner, Medical Director

South Pointe Surgery Center, 151 West 151st Street, Suite 200, Olathe, KS 66061–5351; tel. 913/782–3631; FAX. 913/782–2606; Katherine Thon, RN, Administrator

Surgery Center of Kansas, Inc., 1507 West 21st Street, Wichita, KS 67203–2449; tel. 316/838–8388; FAX. 316/838–2999; Karen Gabbert, RN, B.S.N., Administrator

☐ **Surgicare of Wichita, Inc.,** 810 North Lorraine, Wichita, KS 67214–4841; tel. 316/685–2207; FAX. 316/685–2861; Carolyn J. Exley, Administrator

Team Vision Surgery Center East, 6100 East Central Street, Suite Six, Wichita, KS 67208–4237; tel. 316/684–8013; Linda S. Buettner, Vice President

Team Vision Surgery Center West, 834 North Socora, Suite One, Wichita, KS 67212–3238; tel. 316/681–2020; Linda Buettner, Administrator

The Center for Same Day Surgery, 818 North Emporia Street, Suite 108, Wichita, KS 67214–3725; tel. 316/262–7263; FAX. 316/262–6253; Michele LeGate, RN, B.S., Administrator

The Headache and Pain Center, 11111 Nall Avenue, Suite 222, Leawood, KS 66211–1625; tel. 913/491–3999; FAX. 913/491–6453; Steven D. Waldman, Administrator

The Wichita Clinic DaySurgery, 3311 East Murdock Street, Wichita, KS 67208–3054; tel. 316/689–9349; James A. Greer, Jr., Administrator

Topeka Single Day Surgery, 823 Southwest Mulvane Street, Suite 101, Topeka, KS 66606–1679; tel. 913/354–8737; FAX. 913/354–1440; Linda Daniel, Executive Director

KENTUCKY

☐ **Ambulatory Surgery Center,** 2831 Lone Oak Road, Paducah, KY 42003; tel. 502/554–8373; FAX. 502/554–8987; Laxmaiah Manchikanti, M.D.

Caritas Surgical Center, 4414 Churchman Avenue, Louisville, KY 40215; tel. 502/366–9525; Danny Cain

Center For Surgical Care, 7575 U.S. 42, Florence, KY 41042; tel. 606/283–9100; FAX. 606/283–6046; Thomas Mayer, M.D., Medical Director

Columbia Owensboro Surgery Center, 1100 Walnut Street, Suite 13, Owensboro, KY 42301; tel. 502/683–2751; FAX. 502/926–1618; Donna R. Norton, Administrator

Dupont Surgery Center, 4004 Dupont Circle, Louisville, KY 40207; tel. 502/896–6428; FAX. 502/895–6787; Vicki Lococo, Nurse Manager

E.M.W. Women's Surgical Center, 138 West Market Street, Louisville, KY 40202; tel. 502/589–2124; FAX. 502/589–1588; Dona F. Wells, Administrator

East Bernstadt Outpatient Surgery Center, 2737 North U.S. Highway 25, East Bernstadt, KY 40729; tel. 606/843–6100; Darby Radmanedsh, Administrator

HEALTHSOUTH Surge Center of Louisville, 4005 DuPont Circle, Louisville, KY 40207; tel. 502/897–7401; FAX. 502/897–5652; Sheila S. Boros, Administrator

Lexington Clinic, 1221 South Broadway, Lexington, KY 40504; tel. 606/258–4000; FAX. 606/258–4795; Thomas Holets, Executive Director

Lexington Surgery Center, 1725 Harrodsburg Road, Lexington, KY 40504; tel. 606/276–2525; FAX. 606/277–6497; Bemedji Asher, Administrator

Louisville Surgery Center, 614 East Chestnut Street, Louisville, KY 40202; tel. 502/589–9488; FAX. 502/589–9928; Jane E. Burbank, Administrator

McPeak Center For Eye Care, 1507 Bravo Boulevard, Glasgow, KY 42141; tel. 502/651–2181; FAX. 502/651–2183; Nancy McPeak, Administrator

Medical Heights Surgery Center, 2374 Nicholasville Road, Lexington, KY 40503; tel. 606/278–1460; FAX. 606/278–0115; John Johnson, Facility Director

Outpatient Care Center at Jewish Hospital, 225 Abraham Flexner Way, Louisville, KY 40202; tel. 502/587–4709; FAX. 502/587–4323; Kim Tharp–Barrie, Administrator

Pikeville United Methodist Hospital of Kentucky, Inc., 911 South By-Pass Road, Pikeville, KY 41501; tel. 606/437–3500; FAX. 606/432–9479; Martha O'Regan Chill, Administrator, Chief Executive Officer

Somerset Surgery Center, 353 Bogle Street, Suite 101, Somerset, KY 42501; tel. 606/679–9322; FAX. 606/678–2666; Kathy Turner, Administrator

Stone Road Surgery Center, 280 Pasadena Drive, Lexington, KY 40503; tel. 606/278–1316; FAX. 606/276–3847; Ballard Wright, President

☐ **Surgical Center of Elizabethtown,** 708 Westport Road, Elizabethtown, KY 42701; tel. 502/737–5200; FAX. 502/765–5362; Suzanne Broadwater, Administrator

The Eye Surgery Center of Paducah, 100 Medical Center Drive, P.O. Box 8269, Paducah, KY 42002–8269; tel. 502/442–1024; FAX. 502/442–1001; Kelly Harris, RN, Administrator

Tri–State Digestive Disorder Center Ambulatory Surgery Center, 196 Barnwood Drive, Edgewood, KY 41017; tel. 606/341–3575; Stephen W. Hiltz, M.D.

Section C

LOUISIANA

Acadiana Endoscopy Center, 113 St. Louis Street, Lafayette, LA 70506; tel. 318/269–1126; FAX. 318/269–0553; Stephen M. Person, M.D., Administrator

☐ **Acadiana Surgery Center, Inc.,** 1100 Andre Street, Suite 300, New Iberia, LA 70560; tel. 318/364–9680; FAX. 318/364–9689

Alexandria Laser and Surgery Center, 4100 Parliment Drive, Alexandria, LA 71303; tel. 318/487–8342, ext. 318; FAX. 318/487–9942; M. L. Revelett, Administrator

Ambulatory Eye Surgery Center of Louisiana, 3900 Veterans Boulevard, Suite 100, Metairie, LA 70002; tel. 504/455–1550; FAX. 504/455–2011; Mark Brown, Administrator

Baton Rouge Ambulatory Surgicare Services, 5328 Didesse Drive, Baton Rouge, LA 70808; tel. 504/766–1718; FAX. 504/767–3034; Laura B. Cronin, Administrator

Broussard Surgery Institute, 1250 Pecanland Road, Suite E–1, Monroe, LA 71203; tel. 318/387–2015; FAX. 318/387–2097; Gerald Broussard, M.D., Administrator

Browne–McHardy Outpatient Surgery Center, 4315 Houma Boulevard, Metairie, LA 70006–2981; tel. 504/889–5218; FAX. 504/889–5224; Robert L. Goldstein, Chief Administrative Officer

Central Louisiana Ambulatory Surgical Center, 720 Madison Street, P.O. Box 8646, Alexandria, LA 71301; tel. 318/443–3511; Louise Barker, RN, Administrator

Colonnade Surgery, 555 South Ryan Street, Lake Charles, LA 70601; tel. 318/439–6226; FAX. 312/436–6223; Pam Ragusa, Administrator

Columbia Greater New Orleans Surgery Center, 3434 Houma Boulevard, Metairie, LA 70006; tel. 504/888–7100; Claire G. Manuel, RN, Administrator

Columbia Surgicare of Lake Charles, 214 South Ryan Street, Lake Charles, LA 70601; tel. 318/436–6941; FAX. 318/439–3384; Debbie Boudreaux, Administrator

Eye Care and Surgery Center, 10423 Old Hammond Highway, Baton Rouge, LA 70816; tel. 504/923–0960; FAX. 504/923–2419; M. Brian Roper

Foot Surgery Center of Shreveport, 9308 Mansfield Road, Suite 300, Shreveport, LA 71118; tel. 318/686–9622; Arnold M. Castellano, Administrator

Gamble Ambulatory Surgery Center, 2601 Line Avenue, Suite B, Shreveport, LA 71104; tel. 318/424–3291; Michael Drews, D.P.M., Administrator

Green Clinic Surgery Center, 1200 South Farmerville Street, Ruston, LA 71270; tel. 318/255–3690; FAX. 318/251–6116; Glenn Scott, Executive Director

Hedgewood Surgical Center, 2427 St. Charles Avenue, New Orleans, LA 70130; tel. 504/895–7642; FAX. 504/895–0728; Sally Carpenter, RN

Houma Outpatient Surgery Center, Ltd., 3800 Houma Boulevard, Suite 250, Metairie, LA 70006; tel. 504/456–1515; Jay Weil III, President, Chief Executive Officer

Houma Surgi Center, Inc., 1020 School Street, Houma, LA 70360; tel. 504/868–4320; FAX. 504/868–3617; Robert M. Alexander, M.D., Administrator

LSU Eye Surgery Center, 2020 Gravier Street, Suite B, New Orleans, LA 70112; tel. 504/568–6700; W. L. Blackwell, Chief Executive Officer

LaHaye Center for Advanced Care, 201 Rue Iberville, Lafayette, LA 70508; tel. 318/235–2149; Darryl Wagley

LaHaye Eye and Ambulatory Surgical Center, 100 Harry Guilbeau Road, Opelousas, LA 70570; tel. 318/942–2024; FAX. 318/948–8869; Dana Cockran, Administrator

Lake Forest Surgical Center, 10545 Lake Forest Boulevard, New Orleans, LA 70127; tel. 504/244–3000; FAX. 504/246–2600; Nina Ory, RN, Facility Manager

Lakeview Surgery and Diagnostic Center, Inc., 800 Heavens Drive, Mandeville, LA 70471; tel. 504/845–7100; FAX. 504/845–7596; Glenda P. Escudero–Dobson, Administrator

Laser and Surgery Center of Acadiana, 514 St. Landry Street, Lafayette, LA 70506; tel. 318/234–2020; FAX. 318/234–8230; Barbara L. Azar, Administrator

Laser and Surgery Center of the South, 1101 Audubon Avenue, Suite S–Four, Thibodaux, LA 70301; tel. 504/447–7258; FAX. 504/448–1521; M. L. Revelett, Administrator

Louisiana Endoscopy Center, Inc., 8150 Jefferson Highway, Baton Rouge, LA 70809; tel. 504/927–0970; FAX. 504/927–0988; Lorrie Rogerson, Administrator

Louisville Plaza Surgery Center, 3101 Kilpatrick Boulevard, Suite B, Monroe, LA 71201; tel. 318/322–5916; FAX. 318/322–5916; Frank Wilderman, D.P.M., Administrator

MGA GI Diagnostic and Therapeutic Center, 1111 Medical Center Boulevard, Suite 310, Marrero, LA 70072; tel. 504/349–6401; FAX. 504/349–6444; Thomas D. McCaffery, Jr., President

MGA GI Diagnostic and Therapeutic Center, 2633 Napolean Avenue, Suite 707, New Orleans, LA 70115; tel. 504/349–6401; FAX. 504/349–6444; Thomas D. McCaffery, Jr., Administrator

Magnolia Surgical Facility, 3939 Houma Boulevard, Suite 216, Metairie, LA 70006; tel. 504/455–7771; FAX. 504/885–5063; Hamid Massiha, M.D., Administrator

Marrero SurgiCenter, Inc., 4511 Westbank Expressway, Suite B, Marrero, LA 70072; tel. 504/340–1993; John Schiro, M.D., Administrator

Ochsner Clinic–Center for Cosmetic Surgery, 1514 Jefferson Highway, Fifth Floor, New Orleans, LA 70121; tel. 504/842–3950; FAX. 504/842–5003; Rachel Franz, RN, B.S.N., Manager

Omega Ambulatory Surgical Institute, One Galleria Boulevard, Suite 810, Metairie, LA 70001; tel. 504/832–4200; Rene Rosenson, Administrator

Outpatient Eye Surgery Center, 4324 Veterans Boulevard, Metairie, LA 70006; tel. 504/455–4046; FAX. 504/455–9890; Cheryl Crouse, RN, Administrator

Outpatient Surgery Center for Sight, 550 Connell's Park Lane, Baton Rouge, LA 70809; tel. 504/924–2020; Alan DeCorte, Administrator

Physicians Surgery Center, 106 Corporate Drive, Houma, LA 70360; tel. 504/853–1390; FAX. 504/853–1470; Connie K. Martin, Administrator

Prytania Surgery, Inc., 3525 Prytania Street, New Orleans, LA 70115; tel. 504/897–8880; Jay Weil III, Administrator

Saints Streets ASC Endoscopy Center, Inc., 201 St. Patrick Street, Suite 202, Lafayette, LA 70506; tel. 318/232–6697; FAX. 318/233–8065; Stephen G. Abshire, M.D., Administrator

Shreveport Endoscopy Center, A.M.C., 3217 Mabel Street, P.O. Box 37045, Shreveport, LA 71133–7045; tel. 318/631–0072; FAX. 318/631–9688; Linda Sibley, Administrator

Shreveport Surgery Center, 745 Olive Street, Suite 100, Shreveport, LA 71104; tel. 318/227–1163; FAX. 318/227–0413; Mary Jones, Administrator

St. Charles Avenue Surgical Facility, Inc., 3600 St. Charles Avenue, New Orleans, LA 70115; tel. 504/897–2237; George W. Hoffman, Administrator

St. Francis P and S Surgery Center, 312 Grammont Street, P.O. Box 3187, Monroe, LA 71201–3187; tel. 318/388–4040; FAX. 318/388–4099; Keith Kelley, Administrator

Surgery Center, Inc., 1101 South College Road, Suite 100, Lafayette, LA 70503; tel. 318/233–8603; FAX. 318/234–0341; Russell J. Arceneaux, Administrator

☐ **Surgi–Center of Baton Rouge,** 5222 Brittany Drive, Baton Rouge, LA 70809; tel. 504/767–5636; FAX. 504/769–9107; Celeste M. Wiggins, Administrator

Surginet of Louisiana, LTD, 101 La Rue France, Suite 400, Lafayette, LA 70508; tel. 318/269–9828; FAX. 318/269–9823; August J. Rantz III, Administrator

Surgiunit, Inc., 4204 Teuton Street, Metairie, LA 70006; tel. 504/888–3836; Gustavo A. Colon, M.D., Administrator

The Endoscopy Center of Monroe, 316 South Sixth Street, Monroe, LA 71201; tel. 318/325–2649; FAX. 318/325–0717; Andy W. Waldo, Administrator

The Endoscopy Clinic of Lake Charles Medical and Surgical Clinic, 501 South Ryan, Lake Charles, LA 70601; tel. 318/433–8400; Robert Oates, Administrator

The Outpatient Surgery Center of Baton Rouge, 505 East Airport Drive, Baton Rouge, LA 70806; tel. 504/925–2031; FAX. 504/924–2809; Lorraine Caraway, Administrator

The Plastic Surgery Center, Inc., 4224 Houma Boulevard, Suite 430, Metairie, LA 70006; tel. 504/456–5150; FAX. 504/456–5055; James B. Johnson, M.D., Administrator

The Surgery Suite, 103 Medical Center Drive, Slidell, LA 70461; tel. 504/646–4466; FAX. 504/646–4485; Allison F. Maestri, RN, Administrator

Urology Specialty and Surgery Center, 234 South Ryan Street, Lake Charles, LA 70601; tel. 318/433–5282; FAX. 318/433–1159; Charles Enright, Administrator

West Monroe Endoscopy Center, 102 Thomas Road, Suite 506, West Monroe, LA 71291; tel. 318/388–8878; Fred W. Ortmann III, Administrator

Westbank Medical Clinic Surgical Facility, Inc., 4700 Wichers Drive, Suite 200, Marrero, LA 70072; Robert L. Sudderth, Administrator

Young Eye Surgery Center, Inc., 204 North Magdalen Square, Abbeville, LA 70510; tel. 318/893–4452; FAX. 318/893–7870; Virginia Y. Hebert, Administrator

MAINE

Acadia Medical Arts Ambulatory Surgical Suite, 404 State Street, Bangor, ME 04401; tel. 207/990–0928; Jordan J. Shubert, M.D., President

Aroostook County Regional Ophthalmology Center, 148 Academy Street, Presque Isle, ME 04769; tel. 207/764–0376; FAX. 207/764–7612; Craig W. Young, M.D., Director

Eye Care and Surgery Center of Maine, P.A., 53 Sewall Street, Portland, ME 04102; tel. 207/773–6336; FAX. 207/773–7034; William S. Holt, M.D., President

Maine Cataract and Eye Center, 386 Bridgton Road, Route 302, Westbrook, ME 04092; tel. 207/797–9214; FAX. 207/797–8236; Elliot Schweid, D.O., Director

Maine Eye Center, P.A., 15 Lowell Street, Portland, ME 04102; tel. 207/774–8277; FAX. 207/871–1415; Frank Read, M.D., Director

Northern Maine Ambulatory Endoscopy Center, 11 Martin Street, P.O. Box 748, Presque Isle, ME 04769–0151; tel. 207/764–2482; FAX. 207/764–1569; Shelley Kenney, RN, Nurse Manager

Orthopaedic Surgery Center, 33 Sewall Street, Portland, ME 04102; tel. 207/828–2130; FAX 207/828–2190; Linda M. Ruterbories, Medical Director

Portland Endoscopy Center, 131 Chadwick Street, Portland, ME 04102–3266; tel. 207/773–7964; FAX. 207/773–9073; Michael Roy, M.D., President

Western Avenue Day Surgery Center, a/k/a Plastic and Hand Surgical Associates, P.A., 244 Western Avenue, South Portland, ME 04106; tel. 207/775–3446; FAX. 207/879–1646; Jean J. Labelle, M.D., President

MARYLAND

Albert Shoumer, D.P.M., Dundalk Professional Center, 40 South Dundalk Avenue, Dundalk, MD 21222; tel. 410/282–6434; FAX. 410/284–4636; Darleen Grupp, Office Manager

Albert Shoumer, D.P.M., 1645 Liberty Road, Eldersburg, MD 21784; tel. 310/795–2889

Amber Meadows Ambulatory Care Center, Inc., 198 Thomas Johnson Drive, Suite Three, Frederick, MD 21702; tel. 301/695–9669; FAX. 301/695–0346

Amber Ridge Operating Room Center, 1475 Taney Avenue, Suite 101, Frederick, MD 21702; tel. 301/694–5656; FAX. 301/846–4117; Lorin F. Busselberg, M.D., Director

Ambulatory Foot Surgery Center of Burtonsville, Inc., 15300 Spencerville Court, Suite 101, Burtonsville, MD 20866; tel. 301/421–4286; Dr. Kressin, President

Ambulatory Plastic Surgery–Robert Conrad, M.D., 9715 Medical Center Drive, Rockville, MD 20850; tel. 301/948–5670; FAX. 301/948–5598; Linda Quesenberry, Assistant Office Manager

American Podiatric Surgery, 10236 River Road, Potomac, MD 20854; tel. 301/983–9873; FAX. 301/299–3985; Amy Meehan, Administrator

Annapolis Plastic Surgery Center, 1300 Ritchie Highway, Arnold, MD 21012; tel. 410/544–0707; FAX. 410/544–0724; Jack Frost, M.D., President

Anne Arundel Gastroenterology Endoscopy Center, 703 Giddings Avenue, Suite M, Annapolis, MD 21401; tel. 410/224–2116; Cheryl L. Smith, Office Manager

Armiger, William G., M.D., P.A., d/b/a Chesapeake Plastic Surgery Associates, 1421 South Caton Avenue, Suite 203, Baltimore, MD 21227; tel. 410/646–3226; FAX. 410/644–2134; Sandra Pappas, Administrator

☐ **Arundel Ambulatory Center for Endoscopy,** 621 Ridgley Avenue, Suite 101, Annapolis, MD 21401; tel. 410/224–3636; FAX. 410/224–6971; Jeff Hazel, Practice Administrator

Ashok K. Narang, M.D., P.A., Two North Avenue, Suite 102, Belair, MD 21014; tel. 410/877–7595

Baltimore Ambulatory Center for Endoscopy, 19 Fontana Lane, Suite 104, Baltimore, MD 21237; tel. 410/574–7776; FAX. 410/574–9038; Dr. V. Sivan, Medical Director

Baltimore County Out–Patient Plastic Surgery Center, 1205 York Road, Suite 36, Lutherville, MD 21093; tel. 410/828–9570; FAX. 410/583–9120; Bernard McGibbon, M.D.

Baltimore Podiatry Group, 5205 East Drive, Suite I, Arbutus, MD 21227; tel. 410/247–5333; FAX. 410/242–5449; Neil Scheffler, D.P.M., President

Baltimore Washington Eye Center, 200 Hospital Drive, Suite 600, Glen Burnie, MD 21061; tel. 410/761–1267; FAX. 410/761–4386; Phillip L. Harrington, Administrator

Bayside Foot and Ankle Center, 8023 Ritchie Highway, Pasadena, MD 21122; tel. 410/761–4190; Sheila Freeze, Office Manager

Beitler, Samuel D., D.P.M. Ambulatory Surgery Center, 795 Aquahart Road, Suite 125, Glen Burnie, MD 21061; tel. 410/768–0702; Samuel D. Beitler, D.P.M.

Benson Surgery Center, Inc., 3421 Benson Avenue, Baltimore, MD 21227; tel. 410/644–3311; FAX. 410/247–9446; Ann Rogowski, Assistant Administrator

Bethesda Ambulatory Surgical Center, 8000 Old Georgetown Road, Bethesda, MD 20814; tel. 301/652–2248; FAX. 301/654–1150; John Lydon, D.P.M., Administrator

Bowie Health Center, 15001 Health Center Drive, Bowie, MD 20716; tel. 301/262–5511; FAX. 301/464–3572

Breschi, Sclama and Hoofnagle (Drs.), 6830 Hospital Drive, Suite 204, Baltimore, MD 21237; tel. 410/391–6131; FAX. 410/391–6144; Anthony O. Sclama, M.D., President

Carroll Medicine, d/b/a Steven Shaffer, M.D., 211 Hanover Pike, Hampstead, MD 21074; tel. 410/239–7073

Center for Eye Surgery P.C., 5550 Friendship Boulevard, Suite 270, Chevy Chase, MD 20815; tel. 301/215–7347; FAX. 301/215–7345; Leila Cabrera–Reid, RN, Administrator

Center for Plastic Surgery, 5550 Friendship Boulevard, Suite 130, Chevy Chase, MD 20815; tel. 301/652–7700; Jean, Administrator

Chesapeake Ambulatory Surgery Center, 8028 Governor Ritchie Highway, Suite 100, Pasadena, MD 21122; tel. 410/768–5800; FAX. 410/768–5806; Ira J. Gottlieb, D.P.M., Owner, Administrator

Clinical Associates, 515 Fairmont Avenue, Suite 500, Towson, MD 21286; tel. 410/494–1335

Columbia Surgery Center, Inc., 1105 Little Patuxent Parkway, Columbia, MD 21044; tel. 410/730–6673; Paul Valvoe, Administrator

De Leonibus and Palmer, L.L.C., A.S.C., MedSurg Foot Center, 2086 Generals Highway, Suite 101, Annapolis, MD 21401; tel. 410/266–7666; FAX. 410/266–7703

Digestive Disease Consultant of Frederick, 915 Toll House Avenue, Suite 201, Frederick, MD 21701; tel. 301/662–7822; James A. Frizzell, M.D.

Dr. Gary Lieberman, P.A., A.S.C., d/b/a Four Corners Ambulatory Surgical Center, 10101 Lorain Avenue, Silver Spring, MD 20901; tel. 301/681–8400

Dr. Michael K. Schwartz, D.D.S., P.A., 723 South Charles Street, Baltimore, MD 21230; tel. 410/727–4886

Dr. W. Alan Hopson, P.A., 560 Riverside Drive, Suite A–101, Salisbury, MD 21801; tel. 410/749–0121; FAX. 410/749–6807; Pat Timmons, Office Manager

Drs. Abelson and Cameron, P.A., ASC, 1212 York Road, Suite A201, Lutherville, MD 21093; tel. 410/337–7755; FAX. 410/337–7922; Laurie Kolmer, Office Manager

Drs. Smith and Schwartz, D.D.S., P.A., 10 Warren Road, Suite 330, Cockeysville, MD 21030; tel. 410/666–5225; FAX. 410/666–7220; Mary Thompson, Office Manager

Dulaney Eye Institute, 901 Dulaney Valley Road, Towson, MD 21204; tel. 410/583–1000; Andrea Hyatt, Administrator

Dundalk Ambulatory Surgery Center, 1123 Merritt Boulevard, Baltimore, MD 21222; tel. 410/282–6666

Easton Foot Center, 8579 Commerce Drive, Suite 100A, Easton, MD 21061; tel. 410/822–0645

Endocenter of Baltimore, 7211 Park Heights Avenue, Baltimore, MD 21208; tel. 410/764–6107; FAX. 410/358–4167

Eye Surgery Center at Greenspring Station of Ophthalmology Associates, L.L.C., 10755 Falls Road, Suite 110B, Lutherville, MD 21093; tel. 410/583–2810; FAX. 410/583–2807; Shalini Pahuja, Operations Manager

Eye Surgical Center Associates of Baltimore, 1122 Kenilworth Drive, Suite 18, Towson, MD 21204; tel. 410/321–4400; FAX. 410/321–4909; Terry Lewis, Administrator

Facial Plastic Surgicenter, Ltd., 21 Crossroads Drive, Suite 310, Owings Mills, MD 21117; tel. 410/356–1100; Ira D. Papel, M.D., President

Family Foot Health Specialists, P.C., 339 East Antietam Street, Hagerstown, MD 21740; tel. 301/797–7272; Judy Cline, Office Manager

Flaum, Martin/Rockville Podiatry Center, 50 West Edmonston Drive, Suite 306, Rockville, MD 20852; tel. 301/340–8666; Martin C. Flaum, Owner

Foot Care Associates Ambulatory Care Center at Hamilton Foot Care, 5508 Harford Road, Baltimore, MD 21214; tel. 410/426–5508

Foot Care Associates Ambulatory Care Center at Joppa Foot Care, 2316 East Joppa Road, Baltimore, MD 21234; tel. 410/882–5100

Foot and Ankle Surgical Center, 2415 Musgrove Road, Suite 103, Silver Spring, MD 20904; tel. 301/384–6500

Footer, Ronald, D.P.M., P.A., 16220 Frederick Avenue, Suite 200, Gaithersburg, MD 20877; tel. 301/948–2995; FAX. 301/948–6056; Maryrose Hanks, Office Manager

Frederick Surgical Center, 915 Toll House Avenue, Suite 103, Frederick, MD 21701; tel. 301/694–3400; FAX. 301/694–3620; Barbara Smith, Administrator

Gastrointestinal Diagnostic Center, 4660 Wilkens Avenue, Suite 302, Baltimore, MD 21229; tel. 410/242–3636; FAX. 410/242–4404; Mary c. Harrison, Business Manager

Gaurdino and Glubo, P.A., 4660 Wilkens Avenue, Baltimore, MD 21229; tel. 410/242–7066; FAX. 410/242–4126; Eileen Giardina, RN

Gehris, Heroy and Associates of Lutherville, 1212 York Road, Suite 201B, Lutherville, MD 21093; tel. 410/821–6130; James H. Heroy III, Administrator

Gynemed Surgi–Center, 17 Fontana Lane, Suite 201, Baltimore, MD 21237; tel. 410/686–8220; FAX. 410/391–0943; David O'Neil, M.D.

☐ **HEALTHSOUTH Central Maryland Surgery,** 1500 Joh Avenue, Baltimore, MD 21227; tel. 410/536–0012; FAX. 410/536–0016; Thelma Hoerl, RN, Facility Manager

☐ **Johns Hopkins Plastic Surgery Associates,** JHOC 8, 601 North Caroline Street, Baltimore, MD 21287; tel. 410/955–6897; FAX. 410/614–1296

Kaiser–Permanente–Kensington, 10810 Connecticut Avenue, Kensington, MD 20895; tel. 301/929–7100; FAX. 301/929–7433; Kathleen Owens, RN, M.S.N., Director, Surgical Services

Kenneth Margolis, M.D., P.A., Ambulatory Endoscopy Surgical Center, 9101 Franklin Square Drive, Suite 213, Baltimore, MD 21237; tel. 410/687–0202; FAX. 410/687–0985; Jo Ann Smith, Office Manager

Klatsky Plastic Surgery Facility, 122 Slade Avenue, Pikesville, MD 21208; tel. 410/484–0400; FAX. 410/484–2993; Stanley A. Klatsky, M.D., Director

Lake Forest Ambulatory Surgical Center, 702 Russell Avenue, Gaithersburg, MD 20877; tel. 301/948–3668; FAX. 301/926–7787

Laser Surgery Center, 484A Ritchie Highway, Severna Park, MD 21146; tel. 410/544–4600; Stan Karloff, Office Manager

Laurel Foot and Ankle Center, 14440 Cherry Lane Court, Suite 104, Laurel, MD 20707; tel. 301/953–3668; Dr. Frank Smith, Administrator

Maclean, Kishel, Applestein, M.D., A.S.C., 11085 Little Patuxent Parkway, Columbia, MD 21044; tel. 410/997–1930

Maple Springs Ambulatory Surgery Center, 10810 Darnstown Road, Suite 101, Gaithersburg, MD 20878; tel. 301/762–3338; FAX. 301/762–1585

Maryland Digestive Disease Center, 7350 Van Ducen Road, Suite 230, Laurel, MD 20707; tel. 301/498–5500

Maryland Ear, Nose and Throat Group, P.A., 2112 Bell Air Road, Suite Three, Fallston, MD 21047; tel. 410/879–7049; Barbara Huckeba, Corporate Secretary

☐ **Maryland Endoscopy Center, L.L.C.,** 100 West Road, Suite 115, Towson, MD 21204; tel. 410/494–0144; FAX. 410/494–0147; Gretchen Caron, RN, Administrator

Maryland Kidney Stone Center, 6115 Falls Road, Baltimore, MD 21209; tel. 410/377–2622; FAX. 410/377–4410; Walter Weinstein, General Manager

Maryland Outpatient Foot Surgery Center, Dennis M. Weber D.P.M., 4701 Randolph Road, Suite 115, Rockville, MD 20852; tel. 301/770–5741; FAX. 301/468–1093; Dennis M. Weber, D.P.M., Director

McCone, Jonathan, Jr., M.D., 6196 Oxon Hill Road, Suite 640, Oxon Hill, MD 20745; tel. 301/567–2400

Metropolitan Ambulatory Urologic Institute Inc., 7753 Belle Point Drive, Greenbelt, MD 20770; tel. 301/474–5583; FAX. 301/513–5087; Amy Boone, Manager

Michetti, Michael, Dr. of District Heights, 6400 Marlboro Pike, District Heights, MD 20747; tel. 301/736–6900

Mid Shore Surgical Eye Center, 8420 Ocean Gateway, Suite One, Easton, MD 21601; tel. 410/822–0424; FAX. 410/822–2283; Adrienne Welch, RN

Mid–Atlantic Surgery Center, 1120 Professional Court, Hagerstown, MD 21740; tel. 301/739–7900

Montgomery Endoscopy Center, Montgomery Gastroenterology P.A., 12012 Veirs Mill Road, Wheaton, MD 20906; tel. 301/942–3550; FAX. 301/933–3621; Howard Goldberg, M.D., A.S.C Director

☐ **Montgomery Surgical Center,** 46 West Gude Drive, Rockville, MD 20850; tel. 301/424–6901; FAX. 301/294–7847; Jeannie M. Lohmeyer, RN, CNOR, Administrative Director

Moulsdale, Murphy, Siegelbaum and Lerner, 7505 Osler Drive, Suite 508, Towson, MD 21204; tel. 410/296–0166; FAX. 410/828–7275

Neil J. Napora, D.P.M., 7809 Wise Avenue, Baltimore, MD 21222; tel. 410/285–0310; FAX. 410/288–1569; Neil J. Napora, D.P.M.

North Arundel Plastic Surgery Specialists, 203 Hospital Drive, Suite 308, Glen Burnie, MD 21061; tel. 410/841–5355; FAX. 410/766–7145; Ajia S. Layman, Administrator

Parris–Castro Eye Association, Six North Boulton Street, Bel Air, MD 21014; tel. 410/836–7010; Michael Grasham, Administrator

Peninsula Obstetrics and Gynecology, 314 West Carroll Street, Salisbury, MD 21801; tel. 410/546–3125; FAX. 410/546–3128

Peninsula Surgery Center, P.A., 145 East Carroll Street, Salisbury, MD 21801; tel. 410/548–1108; FAX. 410/546–8338; Joseph G. Walters, PA–C Administrative Director

Plastic Surgery Specialists, 2448 Holly Avenue, Suite 400, Annapolis, MD 21401; tel. 410/841–5355; FAX. 410/841–6589; Ajia S. Layman, Administrator

Plastic and Aesthetic, Surgical Center of Maryland, Orchard Square, 1212 York Road, Suite B101, Lutherville, MD 21093; tel. 410/337–2551; FAX. 410/321–1550; Oscar M. Ramirez, M.D., Medical Director

Plaza Podiatry, 6568 Reisterstown Road, Suite 501, Baltimore, MD 21215; tel. 410/764–7044; Brian Kashan, Administrator

Podiatry Associates of Hagerstown, A.S.C., 12821 Oak Hill Avenue, Hagerstown, MD 21742; tel. 301/739–1575; FAX. 301/739–1578; Crystal Shockey, Office Manager

Podiatry Associates, P.A., 9712 Bel Air Road, Baltimore, MD 21236; tel. 410/574–6060; FAX. 410/256–2727; Stanley Book

Podiatry Associates, P.A., One North Main Street, Bel Air, MD 21014; tel. 410/879–1212; FAX. 410/893–1081

Podiatry Associates, P.A., 10840 Little Patuxent Parkway, Columbia, MD 21044; tel. 410/730–0970; FAX. 410/730–0161; Dr. Cappello, Podiatrist

Podiatry Associates, P.A., 6569 North Charles Street, Suite 702, Towson, MD 21204; tel. 410/828–5420; Nancy L. Patterson, Billing Manager

Podiatry Associates, P.A., 9101 Franklin Square Drive, Baltimore, MD 21237; tel. 410/574–3900; FAX. 410/574–3902; Vincent J. Martorana, D.P.M.

Podiatry Group, P.A. of Annapolis, 139 Old Solomons Island Road, Suite C, Annapolis, MD 21401; tel. 410/224–4448; FAX. 410/841–5200; Kate Pearson, Administrator

Podiatry Group, P.A. of Laurel, Ambulatory Surgery Center, 1433 Laurel–Bowie Road, Suite 205, Laurel, MD 20708; tel. 301/725–5650; Bruce A. Wenzel, Administrator

☐ **Prince George's Ambulatory Care Center/Endoscopy Suites, Inc.,** 6001 Landover Road, Suite One, Cheverly, MD 20785; tel. 301/773–1111; Jeannette Figueroa, Administrator

Prince George's Multi–Specialty Surgery Centre, Inc., 8700 Central Avenue, Suite 106, Landover, MD 20785; tel. 301/808–9298; FAX. 301/499–1266; Banner E. Williams, Administrator

Professional Village Surgical Center, 356 Mill Street, Hagerstown, MD 21740; tel. 301/791–1800

Queen Anne Plastic, L.L.C., 2110 Red Apple Plaza, Chester, MD 2161; tel. 410/643–7207; FAX. 410/643–6945

Queen Anne Podiatry Center, 2108 DiDonato Drive, Chester, MD 21619; tel. 410/643–7207; FAX. 410/643–9274; Grace LeSage, Administrator

Rafiq Patel, M.D., Ambulatory Surgery Center, 1952 Pulaski Highway, Edgewood, MD 21040; tel. 410/679–5800

River Reach Outpatient Surgery Center, 790 Governor Ritchie Highway, Suite E–35, Severna Park, MD 21146; tel. 410/544–2487

Rivertowne Surgery Center, 6196 Oxon Hill Road, Suite 650, Oxon Hill, MD 20745; tel. 301/839–7499; FAX. 301/839–8726; Beth Smith, Manager

Robinwood Surgery, 11110 Medical Campus Road, Hagerstown, MD 21742; tel. 301/714–4300; FAX. 301/714–4324; Niki Showe, Office Supervisor

Roger J. Oldham, M.D., Ambulatory Surgery Center, 10215 Fernwood Road, Suite 412, Bethesda, MD 20817; tel. 301/530–6100; Nancy Aprill, RN

Rotunda Ambulatory Surgery Center, 711 West 40th Street, Suite 410, Baltimore, MD 21211; tel. 410/889–4885

Sagoskin and Levy, M.D., 9707 Medical Center Drive, Suite 230, Rockville, MD 20850; tel. 301/340–1188; Arthur Sagoskin, M.D., Administrator

Saint Mary's Ambulatory Foot Surgery Center, Route 235 and Chancellors Run Road, Suite 15, California, MD 20619; tel. 301/862–3338; Douglas H. Hallgren, D.P.M., Administrator

Siegel and Langer (Drs.), P.A., Ambulatory Surgery Center, 1001 Pine Heights Avenue, Suite 104, Baltimore, MD 21229; tel. 410/644–0929; Narang Ashok, Administrator

Silver Spring Ambulatory Surgical Center, Inc., 1104 Spring Street, Suite T110, Silver Spring, MD 20910; tel. 301/589–7664; FAX. 301/589–3410; Todd A. Nitkin, D.P.M., President

Silverman, David H., M.D., 6490 Landover Road, Suite D, Cleverly, MD 20785; tel. 301/322–5885

Smith and Harne, M.D., P.A., 2007 Rock Spring Road, Forest Hill, MD 21050; tel. 410/879–4879; FAX. 410/893–4763; Louise Pollard, Office Manager

Smith, Schwartz and Hyatt, D.D.S., P.A. of Owings Mills, 25 Crossroads Drive, Owings Mills, MD 21117; tel. 410/363–7780; Michael K. Schwartz, D.D.S., Administrator

Spector, Adam, D.P.M., Ambulatory Surgery Center, 1111 Spring Street, Silver Spring, MD 20910; tel. 301/589–8886; FAX. 301/589–8889; Adam Spector, D.P.M., Administrator

St. Agnes Surgery Center of Ellicott City, 2850 North Ridge Road, Ellicott City, MD 21043; tel. 410/461–1600; FAX. 410/750–7615

Suburban Endoscopy Center, L.L.C., 10215 Fernwood Road, Suite 206, Bethesda, MD 20817; tel. 301/530–2000

Sugar, Mark, D.P.M., A.S.C., 6505 Belcrest Road, Suite One, Hyattsville, MD 20782; tel. 301/699–5900; FAX. 301/699–9297; Mark H. Sugar, D.P.M.

Suhayl Kalash, Ambulatory Surgery Center, 3455 Wilkens Avenue, Suite 203, Baltimore, MD 21229; tel. 410/646–0330; Bridget Vracar, Accounts Coordinator

SurgiCenter of Baltimore, Formerly Health Specialists, P.A., 23 Crossroads Drive, Suite 100, Owings Mills, MD 21117; tel. 410/356–0300; FAX. 410/356–7507, ext. 101; Jerry W. Henderson, Executive Director, Chief Operating Officer

Surgical Center of Greater Annapolis, Inc., 83 Church Road, Arnold, MD 21012; tel. 410/757–5018; FAX. 410/757–0632; LoRain Potter, RN, Administrator

The Ambulatory Urosurgical Center, 401 East Jefferson Street, Suite 105, Rockville, MD 20850; tel. 301/309–8219; FAX. 301/309–9370; Jacqueline Hillman, RN, B.S.N., M.S., Director, Nursing

The Endoscopy Center, 7402 York Road, Suite 101, Towson, MD 21204; tel. 410/494–0156; FAX. 410/828–1706; Dianne M. Johnson, General Manager

Total Foot Care Surgery Center, Inc., 7525 Greenway Center Drive, Suite 112, Greenbelt, MD 20770; tel. 301/345–4087; FAX. 301/345–0482; Dale Scoville, Office Manager

Towson Ambulatory Surgical Center, 912 A Tower Avenue, Towson, MD 21204; tel. 410/583–8637; FAX. 410/583–8691

Tri County Endoscopy, Shanti Medical Center, P.O. Box 664, Leonardstown, MD 20650; tel. 301/475–5579; Dr. A. Shah

Tri County Endoscopy, Charlotte Hall, Route Five, Charlotte Hall, MD 20622; tel. 301/884–7322; Dr. Shah

Tri County Endoscopy, Calvert Medical Office Building, Suite 303, 110 Hospital Road, Prince Frederick, MD 20678; tel. 410/535–4333; Dr. A. Shah

United Foot Care Center, 420 South Crain Highway, Glen Burnie, MD 21061; tel. 410/766–7500; Steven Brownstein, Administrator

Urology Center, 120 Sister Pierre Drive, Towson, MD 21204; tel. 410/494–1396; Dr. Schonwald, Administrator

Urology Center at Charles North, 1104 Kenilworth Avenue, Suite 300, Towson, MD 21204; tel. 410/823–1565

Urology Center at Glen Burnie, 203 Hospital Drive, Glen Burnie, MD 21162; tel. 410/582–4002; Robert B. Goldstein, M.D., Administrator

Urology Center at Security, 7000 Security Boulevard, Baltimore, MD 21207; tel. 410/281–1892; Mary Hall, Administrator

Urology Center at White Marsh, 8114 Sandpiper Court, Suite 215, Baltimore, MD 21236; tel. 410/931–3229; Michael J. McCormick, Administrator

Vahos Aesthetic Plastic Surgery Institute, 1001 Pine Heights Avenue, Suite 100, Baltimore, MD 21229; tel. 410/644–4877; FAX. 410/525–1346; Mario Vahos, M.D., Director

Waldorf Endoscopy Center Inc., 11340 Pembrooke Square, Suite 202, Waldorf, MD 20603; tel. 301/645–7220; FAX. 301/843–5184; Mary Lou Champney, Office Manager

Washington Surgi Center, 6228 Oxon Hill Road, Oxon Hill, MD 20745; tel. 301/839–0770; FAX. 301/839–1350

Western Maryland Eye Surgical Center, 1003 West Seventh Street, Suite 400, Frederick, MD 21701; tel. 301/662–3721; FAX. 301/698–8164

MASSACHUSETTS

Advanced Pain Management Center, Three Woodland Road, Suite 206, Stoneham, MA 02180; tel. 617/662–2243; FAX. 617/662–4878

Andover Surgical Day Care Clinic, 138 Haverhill Street, Andover, MA 01810; tel. 508/475–2880; FAX. 508/475–9562; Edward G. George, Administrator

☐ **Boston Center for Ambulatory Surgery, Inc.,** 170 Commonwealth Avenue, Boston, MA 02116; tel. 617/267–0701; FAX. 617/236–8704

Boston Eye Surgery & Laser Center, P.C., 50 Staniford Street, Boston, MA 02114; tel. 617/723–2015; FAX. 617/723–7787; Sheila M. Harney, Business Manager

Cataract and Laser Center West, P.C., 171 Interstate Drive, West Springfield, MA 01089; tel. 413/732–2333; FAX. 413/732–3514; John Dunne, Administrator

Cataract and Laser Center, Inc., 333 Elm Street, Dedham, MA 02026; tel. 617/326–3800; John Dunne, Administrator

Cosmetic Surgery Center, 68 Camp Street, Hyannis, MA 02601; tel. 508/775–7026; FAX. 508/778–6327; Laura Norkatis, Office Manager

Eye Institute of the Merrimack Valley, 280 Haverhill Street, Lawrence, MA 01840; tel. 508/685–5366

Goddard Medical Association Outpatient Surgery, One Pearl Street, Caputo Building First Floor, Brockton, MA 02401; tel. 508/586–3600

☐ **Greater New Bedford Surgicare, Inc.,** 540 Hawthorne Street, North Dartmouth, MA 02747; tel. 508/997–1271; FAX. 508/992–7701; George A. Picord, Administrator

HealthSouth Maple Surgery Center, 298 Carew Street, Springfield, MA 01104; tel. 413/739–9668; FAX. 413/781–3652; Kathleen S. Loomis, RN, Facility Administrator

McGowan Eye Care Center, 297 Union Avenue, Framingham, MA 01701; tel. 800/873–4590; FAX. 508/872–0038; Bernard L. McGowan, M.D., Director

New England Eye Surgery Center, 696 Main Street, Weymouth, MA 02190; tel. 617/331–3820; FAX. 617/331–1076; Kenneth Camerota

New England Surgicare, One Brookline Place, Suite 201, Brookline, MA 02146; tel. 617/730–9650; Gratia S. Chase, RN, Administrator

Plymouth Laser and Surgical Center, 40 Industrial Park Road, Plymouth, MA 02360; tel. 508/746–8600; FAX. 508/747–0824; Kathleen Murphy, Administrator

☐ **Same Day SurgiClinic,** 272 Stanley Street, Fall River, MA 02720; tel. 508/672–2290; FAX. 508/679–3766; John Harries, M.D., Chief Executive Officer

☐ **Surgery Center of Waltham,** 40 Second Avenue, Suite 200, Waltham, MA 02154

The Eye Center, 15 Florence Street, Route 128, Danvers, MA 01923; tel. 508/774–2040; FAX. 508/750–4463

☐ **University Eye Associates, Inc.,** 90 New State Highway, Raynham, MA 02767; tel. 508/822–8839; FAX. 508/880–3616; Judith A. Orsie, RN, Nurse Manager

Worcester Surgical Center, Inc., 300 Grove Street, Worcester, MA 01650; tel. 508/754–0700; FAX. 508/831–9989; Andy H. Poritz, M.D., Professional Services Director

MICHIGAN

Balian Eye Center, 432 West University Drive, Rochester, MI 48307; tel. 313/651–6122; John V. Balian, M.D.

Birth Control Center, Inc., 2783 Fourteen Mile Road, Sterling Height, MI 48310; tel. 810/939–4000; Armen Vartanian, Administrator

Blodgett Memorial Medical Center, 1000 East Paris S.E., Suite 100, Grand Rapids, MI 49506; Lori Streeter, Office Manager

Borgess at Woodbridge Hills Outpatient Surgery, 7901 Angling Road, Portage, MI 49024; tel. 616/324–8406; FAX. 616/324–8476; Renee Langeland, Administrator

Bronson Outpatient Surgery–Crosstown Center, 150 East Crosstown Parkway, Suite One, Kalamazoo, MI 49007; tel. 616/341–6166; Frank Sardone, Administrator

Castleman Eye Center, 14050 Dix–Toledo Road, Southgate, MI 48195; tel. 313/283–0500; FAX. 313/283–2720

Centre for Plastic Surgery, 426 Michigan Street, N.E., Suite 300, Grand Rapids, MI 49503; tel. 616/454–1256; FAX. 616/454–0308; Daniel Reeder, Administrator

Community Surgical Center, 30671 Stephenson Highway, Madison Heights, MI 48071; tel. 810/588–8000; FAX. 810/588–9140; C. J. Yanos, Administrator

Detroit Medical Center Surgery Center, 27207 Lahser Road, Suite 100, Southfield, MI 48034; tel. 810/357–0880; FAX. 810/357–1738; Patrick Voight, Administrative Manager

☐ **East Michigan Eye Surgery Center,** 701 South Ballenger, Flint, MI 48532; tel. 810/238–3603; FAX. 810/767–5194; Judith A. Kirby, RN, Administrative Director

Eastside Endoscopy Center, 28963 Little Mack, Suite 103, St. Clair Shores, MI 48081; tel. 810/447–5110; FAX. 810/774–6091; Beth Miller, Administrator

Feminine Health Care Clinic of Flint, 2032 South Saginaw Street, Flint, MI 48503; tel. 800/323–6205; FAX. 313/232–8071; Dawn LoRec, Director

☐ **Glascco Ambulatory Surgery Center,** 1707 West Lake Lansing Road, Lansing, MI 48912; tel. 517/267–0033; FAX. 517/267–0430; Jane Beshore, Administrator

Hemmorrhoid Clinics of America, 22000 Greenfield Road, Oak Park, MI 48237; tel. 810/967–4140; FAX. 810/967–0745; Max Ali, M.D., President

Henry Ford Hospital Fairlane Center, 19401 Hubbard Drive, Dearborn, MI 48126; tel. 313/593–8100; Jay Zerwekh, Administrator

Henry Ford Medical Center–Lakeside Ambulatory Surgery, 14500 Hall Road, Sterling Heights, MI 48313; tel. 810/247–2680; FAX. 810/247–2682; Paul Szilagyi, Administrator

Henry Ford Medical Center–West Bloomfield, Ambulatory Surgery Center, 6777 West Maple Road, West Bloomfield, MI 48033; tel. 810/663–4100; FAX. 810/661–6494; Linda Messina, Administrator

Holland Eye Clinic, 999 South Washington, Holland, MI 49423; tel. 616/396–2316; FAX. 616/396–0085; Kristine Curtis, Assistant Administrator

Hutzel Health Center, 4050 East 12 Mile Road, Warren, MI 48092; tel. 810/573–3140

Section C

☐ **John Michael Garrett, P.C.,** 1301 Carpenter Avenue, Iron Mountain, MI 49801; tel. 906/774-1404; FAX. 906/774-8132; Cathy Hartwig, RN, Supervisor

M.D. Surgicenter, 375 Barclay Circle, Rochester Hills, MI 48307; tel. 810/852-3636; FAX. 810/852-3631; Robert Swartz, Administrator

Metropolitan Eye Center, 21711 Greater Mack, St. Clair Shores, MI 48080; tel. 313/774-6820; FAX. 313/777-2214; Richard C. Mertz, Jr., M.D., Director

Michigan Center for Outpatient Ocular Surgery, 33080 Utica Road, P.O. Box 26010, Fraser, MI 48026; tel. 810/296-7250; FAX. 810/296-0276; Norbert P. Czajkowski, M.D., Director

Midwest Health Center, 5050 Schaefer Avenue, Dearborn, MI 48126; tel. 313/581-2600, ext. 286; FAX. 313/581-6013; Mark B. Saffer, M.D., President, Chief Executive Officer

☐ **Oakland Surgi Center,** 2820 Crooks Road, Rochester Hills, MI 48309; tel. 810/852-7484; Ravindranath Kambhampati, M.D., Administrator

Oakwood Healthcare Center–Dearborn, 10151 Michigan Avenue, Dearborn, MI 48126; tel. 313/436-2430; FAX. 313/436-2411; Dan West, Regional Director, Ambulatory Services

Park Eye and Surgicenter, 5014 Villa Linde Parkway, Flint, MI 48532

Planned Parenthood League, Inc., 25932 Dequindre, Warren, MI 48091; tel. 810/758-2100; FAX. 810/758-2104; Carrie Haneckow, Administrator

Planned Parenthood of Mid–Michigan, 3100 Professional Drive, P.O. Box 3673, Ann Arbor, MI 48106-3673; tel. 313/973-0710, ext. 131; FAX. 313/973-0595; Cindy Bourland, Clinic Manager

Planned Parenthood of South Central Michigan, 4201 West Michigan Avenue, Kalamazoo, MI 49006-5833; tel. 616/372-1205; FAX. 616/372-1279; Louise D. Safron, Executive Director

Port Huron Eye Surgery Center, 1131 Erie Street, Port Huron, MI 48060; tel. 810/984-2681; FAX. 810/984-1024; Richard Engle, Administrator

Providence Hospital Ambulatory Surgery Center, 47601 Grand River, Novi, MI 48374; tel. 810/380-4170; Brian Connolly, Administrator

Providence Surgical Center, 29877 Telegraph Road, Suite 200, Southfield, MI 48034

Reconstructive Surgery Center, 125 West Walnut, Kalamazoo, MI 49007; tel. 616/343-1381; Frank J. Newman, M.D., Medical Director

Saginaw General North, 5400 Mackinaw, Saginaw, MI 48603; tel. 517/797-5000

Sinai Surgery Center, 28500 Orchard Lake Road, Farmington Hills, MI 48334; tel. 810/851-9215; FAX. 810/851-2077; Michael K. Rosenberg, M.D., Medical Director

Somerset Troy Surgical Center, 1565 West Big Beaver Road, Building F, Troy, MI 48084; tel. 810/643-7775; FAX. 810/643-0999; Reza S. Mohajer, M.D., Administrator

St. John Surgery Center, 21000 12 Mile Road, St. Clair Shore, MI 48081; tel. 810/447-5015; FAX. 810/447-5012; Cheri Dendy, Administrator

St. Mary's Ambulatory Care Center, 4599 Towne Centre, Saginaw, MI 48604; tel. 517/797-3000; FAX. 517/797-3010; Donna Juhala, Director

Superior Endoscopy Center/U P Digestive Disease Associates, P.C., 1414 West Fair Avenue, Suite 135, Marquette, MI 49855; tel. 906/226-6025; Jeffrey P. Shaffer, Administrator

Surgery Center of Michigan, 44650 Delco Boulevard, Sterling Height, MI 48313; tel. 810/254-3391; Jay Novetsky, Administrator

Surgical Care Center of Michigan, 750 East Beltline, N.E., Grand Rapids, MI 49505; tel. 616/940-3600; FAX. 616/954-0216; Kris Kilgore, RN, B.S.N, Administrative Director

Troy Bloomfield Surgery Center, 2515 North Woodward Avenue, Bloomfield Hill, MI 48304; tel. 810/332-3332; Joseph Posch, Administrator

University of Michigan Surgery Center, 19900 Haggerty Road, Livonia, MI 48152; tel. 313/462-1888; FAX. 313/462-1944; Pamela Cittan, Administrator

Upper Peninsula Surgery Center, 1414 West Fair Avenue, Suite 232, Marquette, MI 49855; tel. 906/225-7547; FAX. 906/225-7548; Sally J. Achatz, R.N., Administrator

Waterford Ambulatory Surgi–Center, 1305 North Oakland Boulevard, Waterford, MI 48327; tel. 810/666-5519; FAX. 810/666-5550; Sandra K. Parrott, General Manager

MINNESOTA

Centennial Lakes Same Day Surgery Center, 7373 France Avenue, S., Suite 404, Edina, MN 55435; tel. 612/921-0100; FAX. 612/921-0999; Kathleen L. Whatley, Administrator

Children's Health Care–West, 6050 Clearwater Drive, Minnetonka, MN 55343; tel. 612/930-8600; FAX. 612/930-8650; Jane Price, Director

Columbia St. Cloud Surgical Center, 1526 Northway Drive, St. Cloud, MN 56303; tel. 320/251-8385; FAX. 320/251-1267; Jeanette I. Stack, Administrator

Dakota Clinic, Ltd., 125 East Frazee Street, Detroit Lakes, MN 56501; tel. 218/847-3181; FAX. 218/847-2795; Linda L. Walz, Division Manager

First Eye Care Center, Inc., 9117 Lyndale Avenue, S., Bloomington, MN 55420; tel. 612/884-7568; FAX. 612/884-2656; Barbara McGovern, Administrator

Healtheast Maplewood Surgery Center, 1655 Beam Avenue, Maplewood, MN 55109; tel. 612/232-7780; FAX. 612/232-7786; Sandra Todd, Director

Healtheast St. Paul Endoscopy Center, 17 West Exchange Street, Suite 215, St. Paul, MN 55102; tel. 612/224-9677; FAX. 612/223-5683; Glenda Tims, RN, Clinical Manager

Landmark Surgical Center, 17 West Exchange Street, Suite 307, St. Paul, MN 55102; tel. 612/223-7400; FAX. 612/223-5903; Peg Olin, Administrator

Midwest Surgicenter, d/b/a Midwest Eye and Ear Institute, 393 North Dunlap Street, Suite 900, St. Paul, MN 55104; tel. 612/642-9199; FAX. 612/645-3346; H. Joseph Drannen, Administrator

Park Nicollet Clinic Health System Minnesota, 3800 Park Nicollet Boulevard, St. Louis Park, MN 55416; tel. 612/993-1953; FAX. 612/993-9250; Kathy Beckman, RN, Manager

WestHealth, Inc., 2855 Campus Drive, Plymouth, MN 55441; tel. 612/577-7120, ext. 7123; FAX. 612/577-7130; Paula Witke, Administrator

Willmar Surgery Center, 1320 South First Street, P.O. Box 773, Willmar, MN 56201; tel. 612/235-6506; Keith Zempel, Manager

MISSISSIPPI

Ambu–Care Outpatient Surgery Center, 6204 North State Street, Jackson, MS 39213; tel. 601/956-3251; FAX. 601/957-8456; Frank McCune, M.D., Administrator

Better Living Clinic Endoscopy Center, 3000 Halls Ferry Road, Vicksburg, MS 39180; tel. 601/638-9800; Linda Antoine, Administrative Assistant

Biloxi Outpatient Surgery and Endoscopy Center, Inc., 111 Lameuse Street, Suite 104, Biloxi, MS 39530; tel. 601/374-2130; FAX. 601/374-0938; Michael T. Gossman, Administrator

Columbia Mississippi Surgical Center, 1421 North State Street, Jackson, MS 39202; tel. 601/353-8000; Virginia Brown, Administrator

ENT and Facial Plastic Surgery, 107 Millsaps Drive, P.O. Box 17829, Hattiesburg, MS 39402; tel. 601/268-5131; FAX. 601/268-5138; Pam Carter, Office Manager

Gastroenterology Clinic of Laurel, P.A., 1020 Adams Street, Laurel, MS 39440; tel. 601/649-0633

Gulf South Outpatient Center, 1206 31st Avenue, P.O. Box 1778, Gulfport, MS 39501; tel. 601/864-0008; FAX. 601/863-1747; Jason V. Smith, M.D., President

Gulfport Outpatient Surgical Center, 1240 Broad Avenue, Gulfport, MS 39501; tel. 601/868-1120; William Peaks, Administrator

Lowery A. Woodall Outpatient Surgery Facility, 105 South 28th Avenue, Hattiesburg, MS 39401; tel. 601/288-1072; FAX. 601/288-3111; Marshall H. Tucker, FACHE, Administrator

North Mississippi Surgery Center, 500 West Eason Boulevard, Tupelo, MS 38801; tel. 601/841-4700; FAX. 601/841-3101; Beth Taylor, RN, Director

Southern Eye Center of Excellence, 1420 South 28th Avenue, Hattiesburg, MS 39402; tel. 601/264-3937; Lynn McMahan, M.D., Medical Director

Southwest Mississippi Ambulatory Surgery Center, 215 Marion Avenue, McComb, MS 39648; tel. 601/249-1477; FAX. 601/249-1375; Norman M. Price, Administrator

Surgicare of Jackson, 766 Lakeland Drive, Jackson, MS 39216; tel. 601/362-8700; FAX. 601/362-6439; Sheila Grillis, RN, Administrator

MISSOURI

Arnold Eye Surgery Center, Inc., 1265 East Primrose, Springfield, MO 65804; tel. 417/886-3937; FAX. 417/886-1285; Stephen C. Sheppard, Administrator

Associated Plastic Surgeons Ambulatory Surgical Center, 6420 Prospect, Suite 115, Kansas City, MO 64132; tel. 816/333-5524; Joni Reist, RN

BarnesCare, 401 Pine Street, St. Louis, MO 63102; tel. 314/331-3000; FAX. 314/331-3012; Gary Payne, Vice President, BJC Corporate Health

CMMP Surgical Center, 1705 Christy Drive, Jefferson City, MO 65101; tel. 573/635-7022; FAX. 573/635-7029; Angela R. Sumner–Hahn, Business Director

Cape Girardeau Outpatient Surgery Center, 1429 Mount Auburn Road, Cape Girardeau, MO 63701; tel. 573/334-5895; FAX. 573/335-2392; Katherine Bloodworth, RN, Administrator

Cataract Surgery Center of St. Louis, Inc., 900 North Highway 67 (Lindbergh), Florissant, MO 63031; tel. 314/838-0321; FAX. 314/838-4682; Karen E. Wilson, RN, Nurse Manager

Cataract Surgery Center of Young Eye Clinic, Inc., 3201 Ashland Avenue, St. Joseph, MO 64506; tel. 816/279-0079; FAX. 816/364-1100; Judy Watowa, RN, B.S.N., Administrator

Cataract and Glaucoma Outpatient Surgicenter, 7220 Watson Road, St. Louis, MO 63119; tel. 314/352-5515; Stanley C. Becker, M.D.

Center for Eye Surgery, 6650 Troost, Suite 305, Kansas City, MO 64131; tel. 816/276-7757; FAX. 816/926-2231; Connie B. Watson, Administrator

Creekwood Surgery Center, 211 Northeast 54th Street, Suite 100, Kansas City, MO 64118; tel. 816/455-4214; FAX. 816/455-4216; Carol Ohmes, Administrator

Creve Coeur Surgery Center, 633 Emerson, Creve Coeur, MO 63141; tel. 314/872-7100; Judy Henderson, Nursing Administrator

Doctors' Park Surgery, Inc., 30 Doctors' Park, Cape Girardeau, MO 63701; tel. 314/334-9606; FAX. 314/334-9608; Ronald G. Wittmer, President

ENT/Urology Surgical Care, Inc., 5301 Faraon Street, St. Joseph, MO 64506; tel. 816/364-2772; Sidney G. Christiansen, M.D.

Eye Surgery Center–The Cliffs, 4801 Cliff Avenue, Suite 100, Independence, MO 64055; tel. 816/478-4400; FAX. 816/478-8240; Patricia Thomas, RN, Director, Nursing

G.I. Diagnostics, Inc., 4321 Washington, Suite 5700, Kansas City, MO 64111; tel. 816/561-2000; FAX. 816/931-7559; Craig B. Reeves, Administrator

HealthSouth Surgery Center of West County, 1130 Town and Country Commons, Chesterfield, MO 63017; tel. 314/394-0698; FAX. 314/394-7493; Sherry Mohr, Administrator

Hunkeler Eye Surgery Center, Inc., 4321 Washington, Suite 6000, Kansas City, MO 64111; tel. 816/753-6511; FAX. 816/931-9498; Deborah M. Highfill, R.N.

Kansas City Surgicenter, Ltd., 1800 East Meyer Boulevard, Kansas City, MO 64132; tel. 816/523-0100; FAX. 816/523-6241; Barbara Klein, RN, Administrator

Laser Surgery Center North, 7700 South Florissant Road, St. Louis, MO 63122; tel. 314/261-2020; FAX. 314/821-4080; Irvin C. Hoffman, Administrator

Laser Surgery Center West, 1028 South Kirkwood, St. Louis, MO 63122; tel. 314/984-0080; FAX. 314/821-4080; Irvin C. Hoffman, Administrator

Midwest Eye Institute, 5139 Mattis Road, St. Louis, MO 63128; tel. 314/849-8400; Anwar Shah, M.D.

Missouri Surgery Center, Inc., 300 South Mount Auburn Road, Suite 200, Cape Girardeau, MO 63701; tel. 314/339-7575; FAX. 314/339-7887; Steve Telford, Administrator

North County Surgery Center, One Village Square, Hazelwood, MO 63042; tel. 314/895-4001; FAX. 314/895-1791; Connie Moore, Administrator

Outpatient Surgery Center, 450 North New Ballas Road, Suite 103, St. Louis, MO 63141; tel. 314/991-0776; FAX. 314/991-3076; Karen Barrow, Administrator

Regional Surgery Center, P.C., 1531 West 32nd Street, Suite 107, Joplin, MO 64804; tel. 417/781-9595; FAX. 417/781-9814; Cynthia Shofner, Administrator

South County Outpatient Surgery Center, 13303 Tesson Ferry Road, St. Louis, MO 63128; tel. 314/842-3200; Stephen L. Partridge, Administrator

St. Charles County Surgery Center, Inc., 4203 South Cloverleaf Drive, St. Peters, MO 63376; tel. 314/928–0087; FAX. 314/928–1242; Sandi Baber, Administrator

Surgery Center of Springfield, L.P., 1350 East Woodhurst Drive, Springfield, MO 65804; tel. 417/887–5243; FAX. 417/887–6507; Celine Snyder, RN, Administrator

☐ **Surgi–Care Center of Independence,** 2311 Redwood Avenue, Independence, MO 64057; tel. 816/373–7995; FAX. 816/373–8580; Dolores Sabia, Administrator

The Ambulatory Head and Neck Surgical Center, 1965 South Fremont, Suite 1940, Springfield, MO 65804; tel. 417/887–5750; FAX. 417/887–6612; Charles R. Taylor, Administrator

☐ **The Endoscopy Center,** 3800 South Whitney, Independence, MO 64055; tel. 816/478–6868; John A. Woltjen, M.D.

The Endoscopy Center II, 5330 North Oak Trafficway, Suite 100, Kansas City, MO 64118; tel. 816/836–1616; Jean Thompson, Public Relations, Marketing

The Surgery Center, 802 North Riverside Road, St. Joseph, MO 64507; tel. 816/364–5030; FAX. 816/364–5810; Nancy Moore, RN

The Tobin Eye Institute, 3902 Sherman Avenue, St. Joseph, MO 64506; tel. 816/279–1363; FAX. 816/233–8936; Linda S. Wildhagen, Administrator

Tri County Surgery Center, 1111 East Sixth Street, Washington, MO 63090; tel. 314/239–1766; FAX. 314/239–2964; Sharry Mohr, RN, Administrator

MONTANA

Billings Cataract and Laser Surgicenter, 1221 North 26th Street, Billings, MT 59101; tel. 406/252–5681

Eye Microsurgery Center, Inc., 1232 North 30th Street, Billings, MT 59101; tel. 406/256–9006; Nancy Oliphant, Office Manager

Flathead Outpatient Surgical Center, 66 Claremont Street, Kalispell, MT 59901; tel. 406/752–8484; FAX. 406/756–8008; Victoria L. Johnson, RN, Facility Manager

Great Falls Eye Surgery Center, Inc., 1717 Fourth Street South, Great Falls, MT 59405; tel. 406/727–9920; FAX. 406/727–9904

Montana Surgical Center, Inc., 840 South Montana, Butte, MT 59701; tel. 406/782–2391; Charles Harris, Manager

Northern Rockies Surgicenter, Inc., 1020 North 27th Street, Suite 100, Billings, MT 59101; tel. 406/248–7186; FAX. 406/248–6889; Sharon McLeod, RN, OR Supervisor

Rocky Mountain Eye Surgery Center, 700 West Kent, Missoula, MT 59801; tel. 406/543–8179; Darlene Timmerhoff, Administrator

Same Day Surgery Center, Inc., 300 North Willson, Bozeman, MT 59715; tel. 406/586–1956; Ann Guenther, Supervisor

The Eye Surgicenter, 2475 Village Lane, Billings, MT 59102; tel. 406/252–6608; FAX. 406/252–6600; Sara Coleman, Supervisor

NEBRASKA

Aesthetic Surgical Images, P.C., 8900 West Dodge Road, Omaha, NE 68114; tel. 402/390–0100; FAX. 402/390–2711; Carl H. Dahl, M.D.

Anis Eye Institute, P.C., d/b/a The Nebraska Eye Surgical Center, 1500 South 48th Street, Suite 612, Lincoln, NE 68506; tel. 402/483–4448; FAX. 402/483–4750; Dr. Aziz Y. Anis

Bergan Mercy Surgical Center, 11704 West Center Road, Omaha, NE 68124; tel. 402/333–3111; Richard A. Hachten III

Clarkson Hospital Outpatient Surgery, 4353 Dodge Street, Omaha, NE 68131; tel. 402/442–2000; D. Max Francis

Clarkson West Medical Center–Outpatient Surgery, 14505 West Center Road, Omaha, NE 68144; tel. 402/334–1243; Cindy Alloway, Director

Jones Eye Clinic, 825 North 90th Street, Omaha, NE 68114; tel. 402/397–2010

Lincoln Surgery Center, 1710 South 70th, Lincoln, NE 68506; tel. 402/483–1550; FAX. 402/483–0476; Larry W. Wood, M.D., Administrator

Omaha Surgical Center, 8051 West Center Road, Omaha, NE 68124; tel. 402/391–3333; James Quinn, M.D., Administrator

The Omaha Eye Institute Surgery Center, 11606 Nicholas Street, Omaha, NE 68154; tel. 402/493–2020; FAX. 402/493–8987; Dr. Robert S. Vandervort, Administrator

The Urology Center, P.C., 111 South 90th Street, Omaha, NE 68114; tel. 402/397–9800; Laura Forehead

Tobin Eye Institute, 4151 E Street, Omaha, NE 68107; tel. 402/731–1363; Dr. Robert Livingston, Administrator

NEVADA

Aesthetic Associates Day Surgery Center, 1580 East Desert Inn Road, Las Vegas, NV 89109; tel. 702/735–6755; FAX. 702/733–8221; Charles A. Vinnik, M.D., Administrator

☐ **Carson Ambulatory Surgery Center, Inc.,** 1299 Mountain Street, Carson City, NV 89703; tel. 702/883–1700; FAX. 702/883–8905; Joan P. Lapham, RN, Executive Director

☐ **Center for Outpatient Surgery,** 343 Elm Street, Suite 100, Reno, NV 89503; tel. 702/789–6500; FAX. 702/789–6535; Christine Balascoe, Executive Director

Columbia Reno Medical Plaza, 2005 Silverada Boulevard, Suite 100, Reno, NV 89512; tel. 702/359–0212; FAX. 702/359–0645; Sandra Walker–Wright, Director, Operations

Columbia Sunrise Flamingo Surgery Center, 2565 East Flamingo Road, Las Vegas, NV 89121; tel. 702/697–7900; FAX. 702/697–5383; Carolyn C. Weaver, Administrator

Columbia Sunrise Surgical Center–Sahara, 2401 Paseo Del Prado, Las Vegas, NV 89102; tel. 702/362–7874; FAX. 702/362–3567; Stephanie Finkelstein, Administrator

Desert Surgery Center, 1569 East Flamingo Road, Suite B, Las Vegas, NV 89119; tel. 792/735–5177; FAX. 702/735–3140; Roseanne Davis, RN, Director, Nursing

Diagnostic Imaging of South Nevada, ASC, 1661 East Flamingo Road, Las Vegas, NV 89119; tel. 702/791–0380; Judith L. Atwell, Administrator

Digestive Disease Center, 2136 East Desert Inn Road, Suite B, Las Vegas, NV 89109; tel. 702/734–0075; Osama Haikal, M.D., Administrator

Digestive Health Center, 5250 Kietzke Lane, Reno, NV 89511; tel. 702/829–7600; FAX. 702/829–3757; Kenneth A. Griggs, Jr., Administrator

Endoscopic Institute of Nevada, 3777 Pecos–McLeod, Suite 102, Las Vegas, NV 89121; tel. 702/433–5686; Vicki A. Montijo, Administrator

Endoscopy Center of Nevada, LTD, 700 Shadow Lane, Suite 165B, Las Vegas, NV 89106; tel. 702/382–8101; Dipak K. Desai, Administrator

Eye Surgery Center of Nevada, 3839 North Carson Street, Carson City, NV 89706; tel. 702/882–3950; FAX. 708/882–1726; Michael J. Fischer, M.D., Administrator

Foot Surgery Center of Northern Nevada, 1300 East Plumb Lane, Suite A, Reno, NV 89502; tel. 702/829–8066; FAX. 702/829–8069; Dr. Frank M. Davis, Jr., Administrator

Ford Center for Foot Surgery, 2321 Pyramid Way, Sparks, NV 89431; tel. 702/331–1919; FAX. 702/331–2008; Dr. L. Bruce Ford, Administrator

Gastrointestinal Diagnostic Clinic, 3196 South Maryland Parkway, Suite 207, Las Vegas, NV 89109; tel. 702/369–3400; Luis Tupac, Administrator

Goldring Surgical Center, 2020 Goldring, Suite 300, Las Vegas, NV 89106; tel. 817/922–9042; Texas Gustavson, Administrator

Institute for Pain Surgery, 630 South Rancho Drive, Suite A, Las Vegas, NV 89106; tel. 702/870–1111; FAX. 702/870–7121; Mona Dever, Administrator

La Tourette Surgical Center, 2300 South Rancho Drive, Suite 216, Las Vegas, NV 89102; tel. 702/386–6979; FAX. 702/386–8700; Gary J. La Tourette, Administrator

Las Vegas Surgicare, Ltd., 870 South Rancho Drive, Las Vegas, NV 89106; tel. 702/870–2090; FAX. 702/870–5468; Stephanie Finkelstein, Administrator

NMC–Red Rock Surgical Center, 5701 West Charleston Boulevard, Suite 102, Las Vegas, NV 89102; tel. 702/870–3443; FAX. 702/258–8238; Diane McNamee, Administrator

Nevada Institute of Ambulatory Surgery, 2316 West Charleston, Suite 120, Las Vegas, NV 89102; tel. 702/878–5668; FAX. 702/878–0265; Lois M. Webb, RN, Administrator

Nevada Surgery Center, 4187 Pecos Road, Las Vegas, NV 89121; tel. 702/458–3179; Lyndell Kewley, Administrator

Northern Nevada Plastic Surgery Associates, 932 Ryland Street, Reno, NV 89502; tel. 702/322–3446; FAX. 702/322–4529; Kathleen Richards, Office Manager

Reno Endoscopy Center, Inc., 753 Ryland Street, Reno, NV 89502; tel. 702/329–1009; FAX. 702/329–4992; Lew Fisher, RN

Reno Outpatient Surgery Center, LTD., 350 West Sixth Street, Reno, NV 89502; tel. 702/334–4888; Sandra Walker–Wright, Administrator

SMA Surgery Center, 2450 West Charleston, Las Vegas, NV 89106; tel. 702/877–8660; FAX. 702/877–5180; Steve Evans, M.D., Medical Director

Sahara–Lindell Surgery Center, 2575 Lindell Road, Las Vegas, NV 89102; tel. 702/362–3937; FAX. 702/362–7935; Elizabeth Sayers, Administrator

Shepherd Eye Surgicenter, 3575 Pecos McLeod, Las Vegas, NV 89121; tel. 702/731–2088; FAX. 702/734–7836; John R. Shepherd, M.D., Medical Director

Sierra Center for Foot Surgery, 1801 North Carson, Suite B, Carson City, NV 89701; tel. 702/885–1790; FAX. 702/882–6844; Beverlee J. Gillette, RN, B.S.N. CNOR, OCN, Administrator

☐ **Valley View Surgery Center,** 1330 Valley View Boulevard, Las Vegas, NV 89102; tel. 702/870–7101; FAX. 702/870–7118; Dale A. Kirby

NEW HAMPSHIRE

Bedford Ambulatory Surgical Center, 11 Washington Place, Bedford, NH 03110; tel. 603/622–3670; FAX. 603/626–9750; Linda Dwyer, RN, B.S.N., Director

Day Surgery, 590 Court Street, Keene, NH 03431; tel. 603/357–3411; Michael Chelstowski, Director

Dunning Street Ambulatory Care Center, Seven Dunning Street, Claremont, NH 03743; tel. 603/543–3501; Jyl Bradley, Administrator

Elliot One Day Surgery Center, 445 Cypress Street, Manchester, NH 03103; tel. 603/627–4889; FAX. 603/626–4300; Donna Quinn, RN, B.S.N., M.B.A., Director

Nashua Eye Surgery Center, Inc., Five Coliseum Avenue, Nashua, NH 03063; tel. 603/882–9800; FAX. 603/882–0556; Paul O'Leary, Administrator

New Hampshire Eye Surgicenter, 19 Riverway Place, Bedford Commons, Building One, Bedford, NH 03110; tel. 603/627–9540; FAX. 603/668–7952; Paul Pender, M.D.

Northeast Pain Consultation and Management PC, 255 State Route 16, Somersworth, NH 03878; tel. 603/692–3166; FAX. 603/692–3168; Michael J. O'Connell, M.D., M.H.A., Director

Nutfield Surgicenter, Inc., 44 Birch Street, Suite 304, Derry, NH 03038; tel. 603/432–8104; Dr. Keith D. Jorgensen, Director

Orthopeadic Surgery Center, 264 Pleasant Street, Concord, NH 03301; tel. 603/228–7211; FAX. 603/228–7192; Elaine Lambert, Director

Salem Surgery Center, 32 Stiles Road, Salem, NH 03079; tel. 603/898–3610; FAX. 603/890–3313; Dale Spracklin, O.R., Administrator

Seacoast Outpatient Surgical Center, 200 Route 108, Somersworth, NH 03878; tel. 603/749–4327; FAX. 603/749–5379; David M. Laplante, Executive Director

The Clinic Surgery Center, 253 Pleasant Street, Concord, NH 03301; tel. 603/226–2200; Kevin Appleton, Administrator

NEW JERSEY

A Center for Advanced Surgery, Three Winslow Place, Paramus, NJ 07652; tel. 201/843–9390; FAX. 201/843–0591; Marc L. Reichman, Director of Administration

Affiliated Ambulatory Surgery PA, 182 South Street, Suite One, Morristown, NJ 07960; tel. 201/267–0300; FAX. 201/984–2670; Sylvia Wexler, Administrator

Allan H. Schoenfeld, M.D., PA, 501 Lakehurst Road, Toms River, NJ 08753

Arthur W. Perry, MD, FACS Plastic Surgery Center, 3055 Route 27, Franklin Park, NJ 08823; tel. 908/422–9600; FAX. 908/422–9606; Arthur W. Perry, Director

Associated Surgeon of Northern New Jersey, 25 Rockwood Place, Englewood, NJ 07631; tel. 201/567–3999; FAX. 201/567–9288

Atlantic Eye Physicians, P.A., d/b/a Monmouth Opthalmic Associates, P.A., 279 Third Avenue, Suite 204, Long Branch, NJ 07740; tel. 908/222–7373; FAX. 908/229–1556; Daniel B. Goldberg, M.D., President

Atrium Surgery Center, Inc., 195 Route 46, Suite 202, Mine Hill, NJ 07803; tel. 201/989–5185; FAX. 201/328–4097; Jennifer Rand, RN, CNOR, President

Bergen Gastroenterology, 466 Old Hook Road, Suite One, Emerson, NJ 07630; tel. 201/967–8221; FAX. 201/967–0340; Robert Ein, M.D., President

☐ **Bergen Surgical Center,** One West Ridgewood Avenue, Paramus, NJ 07652; tel. 201/444–7666; Ralph Perricelli, Administrator

Burlington County Internal Medicine, 651 John F Kennedy Way, Willingboro, NJ 08046

Campus Eye Group, 1700 Whitehorse Hamilton Square Road, Suite A, Hamilton Square, NJ 08690

Cataract Surgery and Laser Center, Inc., 19 21 Fair Lawn Avenue, Fair Lawn, NJ 07410

Cataract and Laser Institute, PA, 101 Prospect Street, Suite 102, Lakewood, NJ 08701; tel. 908/367–0699; FAX. 908/367–0937

Center for Special Surgery, 104 Lincoln Avenue, Hawthorne, NJ 07506; tel. 201/427–6800; FAX. 201/427–9602; John Tauber, Business Administrator

Clifton Surgery Center, 1117 Route 46 East Suite 303, Clifton, NJ 07013; tel. 201/779–7210; FAX. 201/779–7387; Ramon Silen, M.D., President, Medical Director

Drs. Scherl Scherl Chessler and Zingler, P.A., 1555 Center Avenue, Fort Lee, NJ 07024; tel. 201/945–6564; FAX. 201/461–9038; Dorothy Hoffmann–Freeman, Office Manger

Eichler Surgeye Center, 50 Newark Avenue, Belleville, NJ 07109; tel. 201/751–6060; FAX. 201/450–1464; Eileen Beltramba, Administrator

Endo–Surgi Center, 1201 Morris Avenue, Union, NJ 07083; tel. 908/686–0066; Sharon DeMato, Administrator

Endo/Surgical Center of New Jersey, 925 Clifton Avenue, Clifton, NJ 07013; tel. 201/777–3938; FAX. 201/777–6738; Pauline Perrino, RN, CGRN, Director of Nursing

Englewood Endoscopic Associates, 420 Grand Avenue, Englewood, NJ 07631

Enrico Monti and Murphy, PA, 715 Broadway, Second Floor, Paterson, NJ 07514

Essex Eye Surgery and Laser Center, 1460 Broad Street, Bloomfield, NJ 07003; tel. 201/338–5566; FAX. 201/338–0753

Eye Physician of Sussex County Surgical Center, 183 High Street, Newton, NJ 07860; tel. 201/383–6345; FAX. 201/383–0032; Patricia Fowler, RN

Eye Surgery Princeton, 419 North Harrison Street, Princeton, NJ 08540; tel. 609/921–9437; FAX. 609/921–0277; Richard H. Wong, M.D., Medical Director

Freehold Ent, d/b/a Face to Face, Patriots Park, 222 Schanck Road, Freehold, NJ 07728; tel. 908/431–1666; FAX. 908/431–1665

Garden State Ambulatory Surgical Center, One Plaza Drive, Suite 20–21, Toms River, NJ 08757; tel. 908/341–7010; FAX. 908/341–5066; Moshe Rothkopf, M.D., FACS

Garden State Surgi–Center, 550 Newark Avenue, Jersey City, NJ 07306; tel. 201/795–0646; FAX. 201/795–0744; Gary P. Pard, Executive Director

Gastroenterology Diag Northern New Jersey, 205 Browertown Road, West Paterson, NJ 07424; Barbara Wattenberg, Administrative Director

Hackensack Surgery Center, 321 Essex Street, Hackensack, NJ 07601

Hand Surgery and Rehabilitation Center of New Jersey, P.A., 5000 Sagemore Drive, Suite 103, Marlton, NJ 08053; tel. 609/983–4263; FAX. 609/983–9362

☐ **HealthSouth Surgical Center of South Jersey,** 130 Gaither Drive, Suite 160, Mount Laurel, NJ 08054; tel. 609/722–7000; FAX. 609/722–8962; Eleanor O. Peschko, Administrator

Horizon Laser and Eye Surgery Center, 9701 Ventnor Avenue, Suite 301, Margate City, NJ 08402; tel. 609/822–7171; FAX. 609/822–3211; Suzanne D. Bruno, Administrator

Hunterdon Center for Surgery, 121 Highway 31, Flemington, NJ 08822; tel. 908/806–7017; David I. Rosen, M.D., Medical Director

James Street Surgical Suite, 261 James Street, Morristown, NJ 07960

☐ **Mediplex Surgery Center,** 98 James Street, Suite 108, Edison, NJ 08820–3998; tel. 908/632–1600; FAX. 908/632–1678; Ruth Mosher, Administrator

Metropolitan Surgical Association, 40 Eagle Street, Englewood, NJ 07631

Mid Atlantic Eye Center, 70 East Front Street, Red Bank, NJ 07701; tel. 908/741–0858; FAX. 908/219–0180; Walter J. Kahn, M.D.

Middlesex Same Day Surgical Center, 561 Cranbury Road, East Brunswick, NJ 08816; tel. 908/390–4300; FAX. 908/390–4405; Evelyn Tornquist, Office Manager

Monmouth Surgi Center, Inc., 370 State Highway 35, Middletown, NJ 07748

Newark Mini–Surgi Site, Inc., 145 Roseville Avenue, Newark, NJ 07107; tel. 201/485–3300; FAX. 201/485–2404; Monica Chomsky

North Jersey Center for Surgery, 39 Newton Sparta Road, Newton, NJ 07860; tel. 201/383–0153; FAX. 201/383–3201; Bruno J. Casatelli, D.P.M., Administrator

North Jersey Women's Medical Center, Inc., 6000 Kennedy Boulevard, West New York, NJ 07093; tel. 201/869–9293; Saul Luchs, M.D.

Northern New Jersey Eye Institute, 71 Second Street, South Orange, NJ 07079; tel. 201/763–2203; FAX. 201/762–9449; Shirley Vitale, Medical, Business Director

Northwest Jersey Ambulatory Surgery Center, 350 Sparta Avenue, Sparta, NJ 07871; tel. 201/729–8580; FAX. 201/729–8185; Sharon L. Marquardt, RN, Operating Room Coordinator

Ocean County Eye Associates, P.C., 18 Mule Road, Toms River, NJ 08755

☐ **Ocean Surgical Pavilion, Inc.,** 1907 Highway 35, Suite Nine, Oakhurst, NJ 07755; tel. 908/517–8885; FAX. 908/517–8589; Marie T. Scoles, RN, Administrator

Ophthalmic Physicians of Monmouth, 733 North Beers Street, Holmdel, NJ 07733; tel. 908/739–0707; FAX. 908/739–6722; Beverly Savlov, Office Manager

Pavonia Surgery Center, Inc., 600 Pavonia Avenue, Fourth Floor, Jersey City, NJ 07306; tel. 201/216–1700; FAX. 201/216–1800; William H. Constad, M.D., President

Princeton Ambulatory Surgery Center, Inc., 281 Witherspoon Street, Third Floor, Princeton, NJ 08542; tel. 609/497–4380; FAX. 609/497–4986; Dennis Doody, President

Princeton Orthopedic Association, 727 State Road, Princeton, NJ 08540; tel. 609/924–8131; William G. Hyncik, Jr., Executive Director

Retina Consultants Surgery Center, 39 Sycamore Avenue, Little Silver, NJ 07739

☐ **Ridgedale Surgery Center,** 14 Ridgedale Avenue, Suite 120, Cedar Knolls, NJ 07927; tel. 201/605–5151; FAX. 201/605–1208; Enza Guagenti, Administrator

Ridgewood Ambulatory Surgery Center, 1200 Ridgewood Avenue, Ridgewood, NJ 07450; tel. 201/444–4499; FAX. 201/612–8114

Roseland Surgery Center, 556 Eagle Rock Avenue, Roseland, NJ 07068; tel. 201/226–1717; FAX. 201/403–9034; Joseph Brandspiegel, Executive Director

Saddle Brook Surgicenter, Inc., 289 Market Street, Saddle Brook, NJ 07663; tel. 201/843–4444; FAX. 201/368–2817

Seashore Surgery Center, 1907 New Road, Northfield, NJ 08225; tel. 609/646–2323; FAX. 609/645–9780; Michael J. Lahoud, Administrator

☐ **Shore Surgicenter, Inc.,** 142 Route 35, Eatontown, NJ 07724; tel. 908/542–9666; FAX. 908/542–9393; Simone Bendary, Manager

Somerset Eye Institute, P.C., 562 Easton Avenue, Somerset, NJ 08873

Somerset Surgical Center, P.A., 1081 Route 22 West, Bridgewater, NJ 08807

South Jersey Endoscopy Center, 17 West Red Bank Avenue, Suite 302, Woodbury, NJ 08096; tel. 609/848–4464; FAX. 609/848–8706; Sue Lampman, Billing Manager

South Jersey Surgicenter, 2835 South Delsea Drive, Vineland, NJ 08360; tel. 609/696–0020; FAX. 609/794–9799; James Yondura, RN, Administrator

Springfield Eye Surgery Laser Center, 105 Morris Avenue, Springfield, NJ 07081; tel. 201/376–3113; FAX. 201/376–1378; Dr. Christine Zolli

St. Barnabas Outpatient Centers, Same Day Surgery Center, 101 Old Short Hills Road, West Orange, NJ 07052; tel. 201/325–6565; FAX. 201/325–6551; Veronica Rose, RN, Acting Administrative Director

Summit Eye Group T/A Suburban Eye Institute, 369 Springfield Avenue, Berkeley Heights, NJ 07922; tel. 908/464–4600; FAX. 908/464–4737; Patricia K. Ketcham, RN, Administrator

Summit Surgical and Endoscopy Center, 110 Carnie Boulevard, Voorhees, NJ 08043; tel. 609/770–5813; FAX. 609/751–8960; Maureen Miller, Executive Director

Surgery Center of Cherry Hill, 408 Route 70 East, Cherry Hill, NJ 08034; tel. 609/354–1600; FAX. 609/429–7555; Yvonne M. Bley, Director of Nursing

Surgicare Surgical Associates, PC, 15 01 Broadway, Route 4 West, Suite One and Three, Fairlawn, NJ 07410; tel. 201/791–6585; John H. Haffar, M.D., Medical Director

Surgicare of Central Jersey, Inc., 40 Stirling Road, Watchung, NJ 07060; tel. 908/769–8000; FAX. 908/668–3139; Jacqueline Jerko, Executive Director

Teaneck Gastroenterology and Endoscopy Center, 1086 Teaneck Road, Suite Three B, Teaneck, NJ 07666; tel. 201/837–9636; FAX. 201/837–9544

The Endoscopy Center of Red Bank, 365 Broad Street, Red Bank, NJ 07701; tel. 908/842–4294; FAX. 908/842–3854; Elizabeth Boyle, Provider Relations

The Endoscopy Center of South Jersey, 2791 South Delsea Drive, South Vineland, NJ 08360; tel. 609/691–1400; FAX. 609/691–7117; Richard Wagar, Assistant Director

The Eye Care Center, 500 West Main Street, Freehold, NJ 07728; tel. 908/462–8707; FAX. 908/462–1296; Dale A. Ingram, Administrator

The Hernia Center, 222 Schanck Road, Suite 100, Freehold, NJ 07728; tel. 908/462–2999; FAX. 908/462–7760; Jackie Porter, RN

The New Jersey Eye Center, 21 West Main Street, Bergenfield, NJ 07621; tel. 201/384–7333; FAX. 201/385–3881; Joyce Katzman, Administrator

The Peck Center Incorporated, 1200 Route 46, Clifton, NJ 07013; tel. 201/471–3906; FAX. 201/471–7048; George C. Peck, Jr., M.D.

The Surgical Center at South Jersey Eye Physicians, P.A., 509 South Lenola Road, Building 11, Moorestown, NJ 08057; tel. 609/727–9333; FAX. 609/727–0064; Janet Daniels, RN, ASC Nurse Manager

Trocki Plastic Surgery Center, PA, 635 Tilton Road, Northfield, NJ 08225

United Hospital Community Health Center, 194 Clinton Avenue, Newark, NJ 07108; tel. 201/242–2300; Delores Henderson

NEW MEXICO

Alamogordo Eye Clinic and Surgical Center, 1124 10th Street, Alamogordo, NM 88310; tel. 505/434–1200; FAX. 505/437–3947; Donald J. Ham, Administrator

Eastern New Mexico Eye Clinic, 1820 West 21st Street, Clovis, NM 88101; tel. 505/762–2207; Dik S. Cheung, M.D.

HealthSouth Albuquerque Surgery Center, 1720 Wyoming Boulevard, N.E., Albuquerque, NM 87112; tel. 505/292–9200; FAX. 505/292–1398; Sharon Prudhomme, Administrator

Lazaro Eye Surgical Center, 1131 Mall Drive, Las Cruces, NM 88011; tel. 505/522–7676; Corine B. Lazaro, M.D., Administrator

Northside Presbyterian, P.O. Box 26666, 5901 Harper Drive, NE, Albuquerque, NM 87125; tel. 505/823–8500; FAX. 505/823–8088; Robert Garcia, Administrator

Presbyterian Family Healthcare, 4100 High Resort Boulevard, Rio Rancho, NM 87124; tel. 505/823–8804; Andrew Scianimanico, Administrator

☐ **The Endoscopy Center of Santa Fe,** 1650 Hospital Drive, Suite 900, Santa Fe, NM 87505; tel. 505/988–3373; FAX. 505/984–1858; Jim Howlett, Administrator

Valley Eye Surgery Center, 110 North Coronado Avenue, Espanola, NM 87532; tel. 505/753–7391; FAX. 505/753–2749; Dr. Gary Puro

NEW YORK

Ambulatory Surgery Center of Brooklyn, 313 43rd Street, Brooklyn, NY 11232; tel. 718/369–1900; FAX. 718/965–4157; Michael M. Levi, M.D., Ph.D., Governing Authority

Ambulatory Surgery Center of Greater New York, Inc., 1101 Pelham Parkway, N., Bronx, NY 10469; tel. 718/515–3500; FAX. 718/655–1795, ext. 3204; Joanne McLaughlin, Administrator

Brook Plaza Ambulatory Surgical Center, 1901 Utica Avenue, Brooklyn, NY 11234; tel. 718/968–8700; Sharron Resnick, Office Manager

Brooklyn Eye Surgery Center, 1301–1311 Avenue J, Brooklyn, NY 11230; tel. 718/645–0600; FAX. 718/692–4456; Rosalind A. Kochman, Administrator

Buffalo Ambulatory Services, Inc., 3095 Harlem Road, Cheektowaga, NY 14225; tel. 716/896–7234

Central New York Eye Center, 22 Green Street, Poughkeepsie, NY 12601; tel. 914/471–3720; Maureen Lashway

Day-Op Center of Long Island, Inc., 110 Willis Avenue, Mineola, NY 11501; tel. 516/294-0030; FAX. 516/294-0228; Robin Fishman, Executive Director

Fifth Avenue Surgery Center, 1049 Fifth Avenue, New York, NY 10028; tel. 212/772-6667; Francois Simon, Vice President

Harrison Center Outpatient Surgery, Inc., 550 Harrison Street, Suite 230, Syracuse, NY 13202; tel. 315/472-4424; FAX. 315/475-8056; Margaret M. Alteri, Administrator, Chief Executive Officer

Hurley Avenue Surgical Center, Inc., 40 Hurley Avenue, Kingston, NY 12401; tel. 914/338-4777; FAX. 914/339-7339; Steven L. Kelley, Administrator

Lattimore Community Surgicenter, 125 Lattimore Road, Rochester, NY 14620; tel. 716/473-9000; FAX. 716/473-9018; John J. Goehle, CPA, Administrator

Long Island Eye Surgery Center, 601 Suffolk Avenue, Brentwood, NY 11717; tel. 516/231-4455

☐ **Long Island Surgi-Center,** 1895 Walt Whitman Road, Melville, NY 11747; tel. 516/293-9700; FAX. 516/293-1018; Howard Leemon, D.D.S.

Mackool Eye Institute, 31-27 41st Street, Astoria, NY 11103; tel. 718/728-3400; Jeanne Mackool, Administrator

☐ **Millard Fillmore Ambulatory Surgery Center,** 215 Klein Road, Williamsville, NY 14221; tel. 716/689-2300; FAX. 716/689-2385; Gary Schultz, Fiscal Officer

Nassau Center for Ambulatory Surgery, Inc., 400 Endo Boulevard, Garden City, NY 11530; tel. 516/832-8504; FAX. 516/832-1085; Miriam DeJesus, RN, Operating Room Supervisor

New York Institute for Same Day Surgery, Inc., 99 Dutch Hill Plaza, Orangeburg, NY 10962; tel. 914/359-9000; FAX. 914/359-1495; Richard Sherman, CPA, Director of Finance and Business Development

North Shore Surgi Center, Inc., 989 Jericho Turnpike, Smithtown, NY 11787; tel. 516/864-7100; FAX. 516/864-7129; Gerald Mazzola, Administrator

Our Lady of Victory Surgery Center, 6300 Powers Road, Orchard Park, NY 14127; tel. 716/667-3222; FAX. 716/667-3120; Dana M. Mata, Administrative Director

Queens Surgi-Center, 83-40 Woodhaven Boulevard, Glendale, NY 11385; tel. 718/849-8700; FAX. 718/849-6523; Stanley H. Kornhauser, Ph.D., Chief Operating Officer

Queens Surgical Community Center, 46-04 31st Avenue, Long Island City, NY 11103; tel. 718/545-5050; FAX. 718/721-8709; Mr. Misk, Partner

Same Day Surgery of Latham, Inc., Seven Century Hill Drive, Latham, NY 12110; tel. 518/785-5741; FAX. 518/785-5741; Bruce Woods, Administrator

Westfall Surgery Center, LLP, 919 Westfall Road, Rochester, NY 14618; tel. 716/256-1330; FAX. 716/256-3823; Gary J. Scott, Administrative Director

NORTH CAROLINA

☐ **Asheboro Endoscopy Center,** 700 Sunset Avenue, P.O. Box 4830, Asheboro, NC 27203; tel. 910/626-4328; FAX. 910/625-9941; Trudy Hogan, RN, Clinical Director

Asheville Hand Ambulatory Surgery Center, 34 Granby Street, P.O. Box 1980, Asheville, NC 28802; tel. 704/258-0847; FAX. 704/258-0374; E. Brown Crosby, M.D., Executive Officer

☐ **Blue Ridge Day Surgery Center,** 2308 Wesvill Court, Raleigh, NC 27607; tel. 919/781-4311; FAX. 919/781-0625; Susan S. Swift, Facility Manager

Carteret Surgery Center, 3714 Guardian Avenue, Morehead City, NC 28557; tel. 919/247-2101; Frances Meyer, Administrator

☐ **Chapel Hill Surgical Center,** 109 Conner Drive, Suite 1201, Chapel Hill, NC 27514; tel. 919/968-0611; FAX. 919/967-8637; Gary S. Berger, M.D., President

☐ **Charlotte Surgery and Laser Center,** 2825 Randolph Road, Charlotte, NC 28211; tel. 704/377-1647; FAX. 704/358-8267; Margaret Slattery, Manager

Christenbury Ambulatory Surgical Center, 449 North Wendover Road Park Place, Charlotte, NC 28211; tel. 704/332-9365; Terry Coman

☐ **Cleveland Ambulatory Services,** 1100 North Lafayette Street, Shelby, NC 28150; tel. 704/482-1331; Thomas D. Bailey, M.D., Medical Director

Columbia Medivision Inc., 2200 East Seventh Street, Charlotte, NC 28204; tel. 704/334-4317; FAX. 704/377-1830; Dian H. Matthews, Administrator

Durham Ambulatory Surgical Center, 120 Carver Street, P.O. Box 15727, Durham, NC 27704; tel. 919/477-9677; FAX. 919/479-6755; Joseph T. Jordan, Director

Eye Surgery Center of Shelby, 1622 East Marion Street, Shelby, NC 28150; tel. 704/482-0696; FAX. 704/482-7707; Dennis Lee, Business Manager

Eye Surgery and Laser Clinic, 500 Lake Concord Road, N.E., Concord, NC 28025; tel. 704/782-1127; FAX. 704/782-1207; J. W. Wheatley, Co-Chief Administrator

Fayetteville Ambulatory Surgery Center, 1781 Metromedical Drive, Fayetteville, NC 28304; tel. 910/323-1647; FAX. 910/323-4142; John T. Henley, Jr., M.D., Director

FemCare, 62 Orange Street, Asheville, NC 28801; tel. 704/255-8400; Philip J. Kittner, M.D., Executive Director

Gaston Ambulatory Surgery, 2511 Court Drive, Gastonia, NC 28054; tel. 704/834-2086; FAX. 704/834-2085; Elizabeth Kohli, Director

Goldsboro Endoscopy Center, Inc., 2705 Medical Office Place, Goldsboro, NC 27534; tel. 919/580-9111; FAX. 919/580-0988; Venkata C. Motaparthy, M.D., Chief Executive Officer

☐ **Greensboro Center for Digestive Diseases,** 520 North Elam Avenue, P.O. Box 10829, Greensboro, NC 27403; tel. 910/547-1718; FAX. 910/547-1711; Paul Green, Clinical Operations Director

Greensboro Specialty Surgical Center, 522 North Elam Avenue, Greensboro, NC 27403; tel. 910/294-1833; FAX. 910/294-8831; Lee Youngblood, Administrator

☐ **Hawthorne Surgical Center,** 1999 South Hawthorne Road, Winston-Salem, NC 27103; tel. 910/718-6800; FAX. 910/718-6847; Teresa L. Carter, Facility Director

High Point Endoscopy Center, Inc., 624 Quaker Lane, Suite C-106, High Point, NC 27262; tel. 910/885-1400; Lester E. Hurrelbrink

High Point Surgery Center, 600 Lindsay Street, P.O. Box 2476, High Point, NC 27261; tel. 910/884-6068; FAX. 910/888-6111; Joan Gayle, Administrator

Iredell Head, Neck and Ear Ambulatory Surgery Center, Inc., 707 Bryant Street, Statesville, NC 28677; tel. 704/873-5224; FAX. 704/873-5984; Scott Seagle, Administrator

Iredell Surgical Center, 1720 Davie Avenue, Statesville, NC 28677; tel. 704/871-0081; Jeannie Naylor, Administrator

Lexington Ambulatory Surgery, Inc., Seven Medical Park Drive, Lexington, NC 27292; tel. 704/243-2431; FAX. 704/243-2359; Lloyd D. Lohr, President

MediVision of Hickory, Outpatient Surgery Center, 27 13th Avenue, N.E., Hickory, NC 28601; tel. 704/328-1493; FAX. 704/322-6097; Marie Hudson, Administrator

MediVision, Inc., 3312 Battleground Avenue, Greensboro, NC 27410; tel. 919/282-8330; Jeanne Justice, Administrator

MediVision, Inc., 2170 Midland Road, Southern Pines, NC 28387; tel. 910/295-1221; FAX. 910/295-0512; Joy Powers, Business Office Manager

New Bern Outpatient Surgery Center, 801 College Court, P.O. Box 12446, New Bern, NC 28561; tel. 919/633-2000; FAX. 919/633-0096; Lila Cotten, Business Manager

Piedmont Gastroenterology Center, Inc., 1901 South Hawthorne Road, Suite 308, Winston-Salem, NC 27103; tel. 910/760-4340; FAX. 919/765-2869; Charles H. Hauser, Administrator

Plastic Surgery Center of North Carolina, Inc., 2901 Maplewood Avenue, Winston-Salem, NC 27103; tel. 910/768-6210; FAX. 910/768-6236; Ronald C. Stewart, M.D., Chief of Staff

Quandrangle Endoscopy Center, 620 South Memorial Drive, Greenville, NC 27834; tel. 919/757-3636; Mark Dellasega

RMS Surgery Center, 5200 North Croatan Highway, Kitty Hawk, NC 27949; tel. 919/261-9009; FAX. 919/261-4329; Cindy Nilson, RN, Clinical Manager

☐ **Raleigh Endoscopy Center,** 3320 Wake Forest Road, Raleigh, NC 27609; tel. 919/878-1151; Robert N. Harper, Jr., Medical Director

Raleigh Plastic Surgery Center, Inc., 1112 Dresser Court, Raleigh, NC 27609; tel. 919/872-2616; FAX. 919/872-2771; Arlene Roessler, Administrator

Raleigh Women's Health Organization, Inc., 3613 Haworth Drive, Raleigh, NC 27609; tel. 919/783-0444; FAX. 919/781-8432; Susan Hill, Vice President

SameDay Surgery Center at Presbyterian, 1800 East Fourth Street, P.O. Box 34425, Charlotte, NC 28234; tel. 704/384-4200; Anne McKelvey, Vice President, CNO

Southern Eye Associates, P.A., Ophthalmic Surgery Center, 2801 Blue Ridge Road, Suite 200, Raleigh, NC 27607; tel. 919/571-0081; Gloria Johnson, Executive Director

Surgery Center of Morganton Eye Physicians, P.A., 335 East Parker Road, Morganton, NC 28655; tel. 704/433-6225; L. A. Raynor, M.D., Medical Director

☐ **SurgiCenter of Wilson,** 209 Richards Street, Wilson, NC 27893; tel. 919/237-5649; FAX. 919/237-4977; Phyllis Renfrow, President

Surgical Center of Greensboro, Inc., 1211 Virginia Street, P.O. Box 29347, Greensboro, NC 27429; tel. 919/272-0012; FAX. 919/272-4063; Donald E. Linder, M.D., Medical Director

☐ **Surgicenter Services of Pitt, Inc.,** 102 Bethesda Drive, Greenville, NC 27834; tel. 919/816-7700; FAX. 919/816-7733; Anna Letchworth, RN, B.S.N., President

The Endoscopy Center, 191 Biltmore Avenue, Asheville, NC 28801; tel. 704/254-0881; Michael Grier, M.D.

The Surgery Center, 166 Memorial Court, Jacksonville, NC 28546; tel. 910/353-9565; FAX. 919/353-5497; Takey Crist, M.D., President

WHA Medical Center, PLLC, 1202 Medical Center Drive, Wilmington, NC 28401; tel. 910/341-3433; Diane A. Atkinson, Executive Director

☐ **Wilmington SurgCare, Inc.,** 1801 South 17th Street, Wilmington, NC 28401; tel. 910/763-4555; FAX. 910/763-9044; Catherine Peterman, President, Chief Executive Officer

Wilson OB-GYN, 2500 Horton Boulevard, Zip 27893, P.O. Box 7639, Wilson, NC 27895; tel. 919/206-1000; FAX. 919/237-0704; Debbie Baker, LPN

Woman Care and Carolina Birth Center, 712 North Elm Street, High Point, NC 27262; tel. 910/889-3646; Robert C. Crawford, M.D., Chief Executive Officer

NORTH DAKOTA

Centennial Medical Center, 1500 24th Avenue, S.W., Minot, ND 58702; tel. 701/852-0777; John C. Tescher, Controller

Dakota Day Surgery, 1717 South University Drive, P.O. Box 6014, Fargo, ND 58103; tel. 701/280-4700; FAX. 701/280-4703; Lynn R. Wold, Business Manager

Day Surgery-Wahpeton, 275 South 11th Street, Wahpeton, ND 58075; tel. 701/642-2000; FAX. 701/671-4153; Keith Robberstad, Administrator

Grand Forks Clinic Ltd., ASC, 1000 South Columbia Road, Grand Forks, ND 58201; tel. 701/780-6000; Wayne K. Larson, Associate Administrator

Great Plains Clinic Surgery Center, 33 Ninth Street, W., Dickinson, ND 58601; tel. 701/225-6017; FAX. 701/225-5018; Brian Rahman, Administrator

Medical Arts, ASC, Inc., 400 East Burdick Expressway, Minot, ND 58702; tel. 701/857-7000; Phil Gorby, Administrator

Western Dakota Medical Group, 1102 Main, Williston, ND 58801; tel. 701/572-7711; FAX. 701/572-2283; Jeff Neuberger, Administrator

OHIO

Advanced Cosmetic and Laser Surgery Center, Inc., 2200 Philadelphia Drive, Suite 651, Dayton, OH 45406; tel. 513/278-0809

Amend Center for Eye Surgery, 5939 Colerain Avenue, Cincinnati, OH 45239; tel. 513/923-3900; FAX. 513/923-3012

☐ **Aultman Center for One Day Surgery,** 4715 Whipple Avenue, N.W., Canton, OH 44718; tel. 216/492-3050; Eric Draime, Administrator

☐ **Austintown Ambulatory Healthcare Center,** 45 North Canfield-Niles Road, Youngstown, OH 44515; tel. 216/792-2722; FAX. 216/793-4883; James M. Conti, President, Chief Executive Officer

Big Run Surgery Center, 950 Georgesville Road, Columbus, OH 43228; tel. 614/234-2144

Bloomberg Eye Center, 1651 West Main Street, Newark, OH 43055; tel. 614/522-3937; FAX. 614/522-6766; John E. Reid, Executive Director

☐ **Carnegie Surgery Center,** 10681 Carnegie Avenue, Cleveland, OH 44106; tel. 216/231–5566; FAX. 216/231–1441; K. L. Rosacco, RN, CNOR, Nurse Administrator

Central Ohio Eye Surgery Center, 210 Sharon Road, Suite B, Circleville, OH 43113; tel. 614/477–7200; FAX. 614/477–8349; Debbie Neal, RN, B.S.N.

Cincinnati Eye Institute and Outpatient Eye Surgery Center, 10494 Montgomery Road, Cincinnati, OH 45242; tel. 513/984–5133; FAX. 513/984–4240; Doris Holton, Administrator

Cincinnati Foot Clinic, Inc., 9600 Colerain Avenue, Suite 400, Cincinnati, OH 45239; tel. 513/385–6946; Robert Hayman, M.D., President

☐ **Columbia The Surgery Center,** 19250 East Bagley Road, Middleburg Heights, OH 44130; tel. 216/826–3240; FAX. 216/826–3250

☐ **Columbus Eye Surgery Center,** 5965 East Broad Street, Suite 460, Columbus, OH 43213; tel. 614/751–4080; FAX. 614/751–4092; Terri Gatton, RN, CNOR, Director Surgery

Consultants in Gastroenterology, Inc., 29001 Cedar Road, Suite 110, Lyndhurst, OH 44124; tel. 216/461–2550; FAX. 216/461–5319; Gloria Bradshaw, Office Manager

☐ **Crystal Clinic Surgery Center,** 3975 Embassy Parkway, Akron, OH 44313; tel. 216/668–4085; Katherine L. McNeal, RN, Administrator

Dayton Ear, Nose and Throat Surgeons, Inc., 7076 Corporate Way, Centerville, OH 45459; tel. 937/434–0555; FAX. 937/434–7413; K. Jean Christian, Administrator

Digestivecare Endoscopy Unit, 75 Sylvania Drive, Beavercreek, OH 45440; tel. 513/325–5065; FAX. 513/325–5060; Patty Mannix, RN, CGRN Endoscopy Coordinator

Endoscopy Center West, 3654 Werk Road, Cincinnati, OH 45248; tel. 513/451–6001; FAX. 513/451–7310

Endoscopy Center of Dayton LTD, 4200 Indian Ripple Road, Beaver Creek, OH 45440; tel. 937/427–1680; FAX. 937/427–9496; Christy L. McBride, Office Manager

Eye Care Center of Cincinnati, 5300 Cornell Road, Cincinnati, OH 45242; tel. 513/489–6161; FAX. 513/489–6442; Amy D. Riegler, Coordinator

Eye Institute of Northwestern Ohio, Inc., 5555 Airport Highway, Suite 110, Toledo, OH 43615; tel. 419/865–3866; FAX. 419/865–3451; Carol R. Kollarits, M.D., President

Eye Surgery Center of Wooster, 3519 Friendsville Road, Wooster, OH 44691; tel. 330/345–6371; FAX. 330/345–8029; Michelle Morrison, Director

Facial Surgery Center, 1130 Congress Avenue, Glendale, OH 45246; tel. 513/772–2442; FAX. 513/772–2844; Joseph J. Moravec, M.D., Medical Director

Firas Atassi, M.D. Outpatient Surgery Center, 34500 Center Ridge Road, North Ridgeville, OH 33039; tel. 216/327–2414

Gastroenterology Associates of Cleveland, 6801 Mayfield Road, Suite 142, Mayfield Heights, OH 44124; tel. 216/461–8800; James Andrassy, Administrator

Gastroenterology Associates, Inc., 4665 Belpar Street, NW, P.O. Box 36329, Canton, OH 44735; tel. 216/493–1480; FAX. 216/493–6805

Gastroenterology Specialists, Inc., 2732 Fulton Drive, N.W., Canton, OH 44718; tel. 330/455–5011; FAX. 330/588–7127; Melissa Smith, RN, C.G.C.

Halpin–Poweleit Eye Surgery Center, (Division of Tri–State Eye Care), 8044 Montgomery Road, Suite 155, Cincinnati, OH 45236; tel. 513/791–3937; FAX. 513/791–1473

Heritage Surgical Associates of Cincinnati, d/b/a Healthsouth Surgery Center of Cincinnati, 2925 Vernon Place, Suite 101, Cincinnati, OH 45219; tel. 513/872–4541; FAX. 513/872–4558; Patti Murphy, RN, Director

Innova Surgery Center East, d/b/a Eastside Surgical Center, 3755 Orange Place, Beachwood, OH 44122; tel. 216/464–7300; FAX. 216/464–3050; Nancy Halkerston, RN, Director Clinical Services

☐ **Kahn and Diehl Center for Progressive Eye Care,** 2740 Navarre Avenue, Oregon, OH 43616; tel. 419/697–3658; FAX. 419/697–2149; Karen R. Hess, RN, C.O.T., O.R. Supervisor

Kunesh Eye Surgery Center, 2601 Far Hills Avenue, Dayton, OH 45419–1665; tel. 937/298–1093; FAX. 937/298–6344; Lucy Helmers, Administrator

Mercy Ambulatory Surgery Center, 2990 Mack Road, Fairfield, OH 45014; tel. 513/874–6440; FAX. 513/874–6005; Patricia Ann Clark, RN, M.S., Administrator

Mid–Ohio Outpatient Surgery Center, 245 Taylor Station Road, Columbus, OH 43213; tel. 614/861–0448; FAX. 614/861–7717; Dr. Grace Z. Kim, Director

MidWest Eye Center, 119 West Kemper Road, Cincinnati, OH 45246; tel. 513/671–6112; FAX. 513/671–6386; Lorrie Walters, Business Office Supervisor

North Coast Endoscopy, Inc., 9500 Mentor Avenue, Suite 380, Mentor, OH 44060; tel. 216/352–9400; FAX. 216/352–9407; Ahmad Ascha, M.D.

Northshore Endoscopy Center, 850 Columbia Road, Suite 201, Westlake, OH 44145; tel. 216/808–1212

Northwest Ohio Urologic, A.S.C., P.O. Box 351837, Toledo, OH 43635–6254; tel. 419/535–1837; FAX. 419/535–6254; Carl V. Dreyer, M.D., President

Ohio Eye Associates Eye Surgery Center, 466 South Trimble Road, Mansfield, OH 44906; tel. 419/756–8000; FAX. 419/756–7100; John L. Marquardt, M.D.

Ohio Gastroenterology Group, Inc., Endoscopy Center, 777 West State Street, Suite 402, Columbus, OH 43222; tel. 614/221–8368; FAX. 614/341–2408; Jean Yarletts, RN, B.S.N.

Parkside Women's Center, Inc., 1011 Boardman–Canfield Road, Boardman, OH 44512; tel. 216/758–0975; FAX. 216/758–8453

☐ **Parkway Urology Center, Inc.,** 3500 Executive Parkway, Toledo, OH 43606; tel. 419/531–8349; FAX. 419/534–5337; Gregor K. Emmert, Sr., M.D., Chief Executive Officer

☐ **Ram Bandi M.D. A.S.C.,** 1037 North Main Street, Suite B, Akron, OH 44310; tel. 330/923–0094; FAX. 330/923–0193; Ann Marie Faber, RN

Restorative Vision Center, 4452 Eastgate Boulevard, Suite 305, Cincinnati, OH 45245; tel. 513/752–5700; FAX. 513/752–5716; Holly Schwab, RN, Surgery Manager

Richfield Surgery Center, Inc., 3030 Streetsboro Road, Richfield, OH 44286; tel. 216/659–4790; FAX. 216/659–3355; Carol A. Westfall, Vice President

☐ **Rockside Surgery Center,** 6701 Rockside Road, Suite 101, Independence, OH 44131; tel. 216/520–3030; FAX. 216/520–3068; Elizabeth A. Bus, Administrator

Ross Park Surgical Services, One Ross Park, Steubenville, OH 43952; tel. 614/282–4790; Kathy Lemasters, RN, Manager

☐ **Sandusky Surgeons, Inc.,** 1221 Hayes Avenue, Sandusky, OH 44870; tel. 419/625–1374; Donald Lenhart, M.D., President

Sidney Foot and Ankle Surgical Center, 1000 Michigan, Sidney, OH 45365; tel. 513/492–1211; FAX. 513/492–6557; Micki Heater, Administrative Director

South Dayton Urological Associates, Inc., 10 Southmoor Circle, N.W., Kettering, OH 45429; tel. 513/294–1489; FAX. 513/294–7999; Donald Bailey, Practice Administrator

Stoneridge Endoscopy Center, 3900 Stoneridge Lane, Dublin, OH 43017; tel. 614/889–5001, ext. 1236; FAX. 614/889–5913; Cheryl Miller, Clinic Manager

☐ **Surgery Alliance Ltd.,** 975 Sawburg Avenue, Alliance, OH 44601; tel. 216/821–7997; Hazel Thomas, Administrator

☐ **Surgery Center At Southwoods,** 7525 California Avenue, Youngstown, OH 44513; tel. 330/758–1954

Surgery Center West, 850 Columbia Road, Westlake, OH 44145; tel. 216/808–4000; FAX. 216/808–4010; Michelle Padden, RN, Administrator

Surgiplex, 950 Clague Road, Westlake, OH 44145; tel. 216/333–1020; FAX. 216/333–3278

Taylor Station Surgery Center, 275 Taylor Station Road, Columbus, OH 43213; tel. 614/751–4466; FAX. 614/751–4475; Bridget A. Huston, Manager

☐ **The Endoscopy Center,** 3439 Granite Circle, Toledo, OH 43617; tel. 419/843–7993; FAX. 419/841–7789; Myung S. Lee, RN, Nurse Manager

☐ **The LCA Center for Surgery,** 7840 Montgomery Road, Cincinnati, OH 45236; tel. 513/792–9099; FAX. 513/792–5634; Rene Fischer, President, Chief Executive Officer

The Surgical Center of East Liverpool, 16480 St. Clair Avenue, P.O. Box 2640, East Liverpool, OH 43920; tel. 216/386–9000; FAX. 216/386–1255; Robin Menchen, Chief Executive Officer

The Zeeba Clinic, A Meridia Outpatient and Laser Surgery Center, 29017 Cedar Road, Lyndhurst, OH 44124; tel. 216/461–7774; FAX. 216/461–5401; Sharon Luke, RN, B.S.N., Clinical Manager

☐ **Tippecanoe Endoscopy, Inc.,** 1210 Boardman Canfield Road, Youngstown, OH 44512; tel. 330/726–0132; FAX. 330/726–0571; Mary Amorn, RN, Administrator

Toledo Clinic, Inc., 4235 Secor Road, Toledo, OH 43623; tel. 419/473–3561; FAX. 419/472–0838; David J. Sobczak, Senior Vice President, Chief Financial Officer

Toledo Community Lithotripter Center, 3158 West Central Avenue, Toledo, OH 43606; tel. 419/531–3538

Toledo Plastic Surgeons Center, 2865 North Reynolds Road, Toledo, OH 43615; tel. 419/534–3330; FAX. 419/534–5716; Charles E. Jaeger, General Manager, Chief Executive Officer

Wedgewood Surgery Center, 10330 Sawmill Parkway, Powell, OH 43065; tel. 614/234–0500; FAX. 614/234–0540; Kim Heimlich, RN, Nurse Manager

Western Reserve Surgery Center, LP, 1930 State Route 59, Kent, OH 44240; tel. 216/677–3292; FAX. 330/677–3624; Laurie Simon, Office Manager

Wilson Eye Clinic Surgicenter, 300 West National Road, Vandalia, OH 45377; tel. 513/890–8992

☐ **Wright Surgery Center,** 1611 South Green Road, Suite 124, South Euclid, OH 44121; tel. 216/382–1868; Barbara McCann, Director of Marketing and Communications

OKLAHOMA

A.M. Surgery, Inc., d/b/a Lawton Physician's Surgery Center, 3617 West Gore Boulevard, Suite D, Lawton, OK 73505; tel. 405/357–1900; FAX. 405/357–1775; Roxanne H. Gibson, Administrator

Ambulatory Surgery Associates, 6160 South Yale Avenue, Tulsa, OK 74136; tel. 918/495–2625; FAX. 918/495–2601; Jaquelyn S. Moore, RN, Director

Center for Plastic Surgery, P.C., 1826 East 15th Street, Tulsa, OK 74104; tel. 918/749–7177; Mark L. Mathers, D.O., Administrator

Central Oklahoma Ambulatory Surgical Center, Inc., 3301 Northwest 63rd Street, Oklahoma City, OK 73116; tel. 405/842–9732; FAX. 405/842–9771; Paul Silverstein, M.D., Administrator

Columbia Oklahoma Surgicare, 13313 North Meridian, Suite B, Oklahoma City, OK 73120; tel. 405/755–6240; FAX. 405/752–1819; Lindie Slater, Administrator

Columbia Surgicare of Tulsa, 4415 South Harvard Avenue, Suite 100, Tulsa, OK 74135; tel. 918/742–2502; FAX. 918/745–9750; Dirk Foxworthy, Administrator

Columbia Surgicare–Midtown, 1000 North Lincoln, Suite 150, Oklahoma City, OK 73104; tel. 405/232–8696; FAX. 405/232–6002; Connie M. Belding, RN, Administrator

☐ **Digestive Disease Specialists, Inc.,** 3366 Northwest Expressway, Suite 400, P.O. Box 99521, Oklahoma City, OK 73199; tel. 405/943–2001; FAX. 405/947–1966; Larry A. Bookman, M.D.

Eastern Oklahoma Surgery Center, L. L. C., 5020 East 68th Street, Tulsa, OK 74136; tel. 918/492–1539, ext. 138; FAX. 918/494–8683; Bobbie Huff, RN, Director

Grisham Eye Surgery Center, P.O. Box 1437, Bartlesville, OK 74005; tel. 918/333–1990, ext. 119; Dennis McKinley

☐ **Heritage Eye Surgicenter of Oklahoma,** Heritage Building, 6922 South Western, Suite 104, Oklahoma City, OK 73139; tel. 405/636–1508; Edward D. Glinski, D.O., Administrator

Medical Plaza Endoscopy Unit, 1125 North Porter, Suite 304, Norman, OK 73071; tel. 405/360–2799; FAX. 405/447–0321; Philip C. Bird, M.D.

Oklahoma Ambulatory Surgery Center, 6908–B East Reno, Midwest City, OK 73110; tel. 405/737–6900; FAX. 405/732–0885; A.C. Vyas, M.D., Administrator

Oklahoma City Clinic, 701 Northwest 10th Street, Oklahoma City, OK 73104; tel. 405/280–5700; FAX. 405/280–5200; Mike Klein, Executive Director

Section C

☐ **Orthopedic Associates Ambulatory Surgery Center, Inc.,** 3301 Northwest 50th Street, P.O. Box 57027, Oklahoma City, OK 73157–7027; tel. 405/947–5610; FAX. 405/947–1341; Thomas H. Flesher, President

Outpatient Surgical Center of Ponca City, 400 Fairview, Ponca City, OK 74601; tel. 405/762–0695; FAX. 405/765–9406; Peggy Maples, RN, Executive Director

Physicians Surgical Center, 805 East Robinson, Norman, OK 73071–6610; tel. 405/364–9789; FAX. 405/366–8081; Ruth Beller, RN, Director

Southern Oklahoma Surgical Center, Inc., 2412 North Commerce, Ardmore, OK 73401; tel. 405/226–5000; Ann Willis, RN, Administrator

Southern Plains Ambulatory Surgery Center, 2222 Iowa Avenue, P.O. Box 1069, Chickasha, OK 73023; tel. 405/224–8111; FAX. 405/222–9557; H. Wayne Delony, Executive Director

☐ **Southwest Orthopedic Ambulatory Surgery Center, Inc.,** 8125 South Walker Avenue, Oklahoma City, OK 73139; tel. 405/631–1014; Anthony L. Cruse, D.O., President

Surgery Center of Edmond, 1700 South State Street, Edmon, OK 73013; tel. 405/330–1003; FAX. 405/330–1087; Timothy A. Gee, Administrator

Surgery Center of Enid, Inc., 1133 West Willow Road, Enid, OK 73703, P.O. Box 5069, Enid, OK 73702; tel. 405/233–6680; Tina C. Brooks, Administrator

Surgery Center of Midwest City, 8121 National Avenue, Suite 108, Midwest City, OK 73110; tel. 405/732–7905; FAX. 405/732–3561; Jackie Reed, Administrator

Surgery Center of Oklahoma, 815 Northwest 12th Street, Oklahoma City, OK 73106; tel. 405/235–4525; Olivia Dick, RN, Administrator

Surgery Center of South Oklahoma City, 100 Southeast 59th Street, Oklahoma City, OK 73109; tel. 405/634–9300; FAX. 405/634–8300; Larry Smith, Administrator

The Cataract Center of Lawton, 4214 Southwest Lee Boulevard, Lawton, OK 73505; tel. 405/353–5860; Stephen W. Gilkeson, Executive Administrator

Three Rivers Surgery Center, 3800 West Okmulgee, Muskogee, OK 74401; tel. 918/682–9899; FAX. 918/687–0786; Doug Blessen, Chief Executive Officer

Tower Day Surgery, 1044 Southwest 44th Street, Suite 100, Oklahoma City, OK 73109; tel. 405/636–1701; FAX. 405/636–4314; Marie Smith, RN, Director

Triad Eye Medical Clinic and Cataract Institute, 6140 South Memorial, Tulsa, OK 74133; tel. 918/252–2020; FAX. 918/252–7466; Marc L. Abel, D.O., Medical Director

Wilson Surgery Center, 5404 West Lee Boulevard, Lawton, OK 73505; tel. 405/357–2020; Gary Wilson, M.D., Administrator

OREGON

Aesthetic Breast Care Center, 10201 Southeast Main, Suite 20, Portland, OR 97216; tel. 503/253–3458; FAX. 503/253–0856; Mary K. Barnhart, M.D., Administrator

Center for Cosmetic and Plastic Surgery, 1353 East McAndrews Road, Medford, OR 97504; tel. 503/770–6776; FAX. 503/770–5791; Robert M. Jensen, M.D., Administrator

Eye Surgery Center, 2925 Siskiyou Boulevard, Medford, OR 97504; tel. 541/779–2020; FAX. 541/770–6838; Loren R. Barrus, M.D., Administrator

Futures Outpatient Surgical Center, Inc., 1849 Northwest Kearney, Suite 302, Portland, OR 97209; tel. 503/224–0723; FAX. 503/224–0722; Bryce E. Potter, M.D.

GI Endoscopy Center, 2560 N.W. Medical Park Drive, Roseburg, OR 97470; tel. 541/673–2046; FAX. 541/673–0454; Ruth E. Harpole, RN, Administrator

Lawrence W. O'Dell, d/b/a Northwest Eye Center, 9975 Southwest Nimbus Avenue, Beaverton, OR 97005; tel. 503/646–7644; Jim Heath, Administrator

Lovejoy Surgicenter, Inc., 933 Northwest 25th Avenue, Portland, OR 97210; tel. 503/221–1870; FAX. 503/221–1488; Allene M. Klass, Administrator

Medford Clinic, P.C., 555 Black Oak Drive, Medford, OR 97504; tel. 541/734–3434; FAX. 541/734–3598; Jon D. Ness, Chief Executive Officer

Medford Plastic Surgeons, 1690 East McAndrews Road, Medford, OR 97504; tel. 541/779–5655; FAX. 541/770–6943; R. Kenneth Pons, M.D., Administrator

North Bend Medical Center, Inc., 1900 Woodland Drive, Coos Bay, OR 97420; tel. 503/267–5151, ext. 298; FAX. 503/269–0797; Sally Kay, RN, Day Surgery Manager

Northbank Surgical Center, 700 Bellevue Street, S., Suite 300, Salem, OR 97301; tel. 503/364–3704; Peggy Seidler, Administrator

Northwest Eye Center, 1700 Valley River Drive, Eugene, OR 97401; tel. 503/343–3900; FAX. 503/343–3913; Jim Health, Administrator

Oregon Cataract and Laser Institute, 2700 Southeast 14th Avenue, Albany, OR 97321; tel. 503/928–1666; Darrell Genstler, M.D., Administrator

Oregon Eye Surgery Center, Inc., 1550 Oak Street, Eugene, OR 97401; tel. 503/683–8771; William E. Spangler, M.D., Medical Director

Roseburg Surgicenter, 631 West Stanton, Roseburg, OR 97470; tel. 503/440–6311; FAX. 503/440–6394; William I Calhoun, M.D., Executive Officer

The Gastroenterology Endoscopy Center, Inc., 6464 Southwest Borland Road, Suite D–4, Tualatin, OR 97062; tel. 503/692–4537; FAX. 503/691–2324; Gale R. Dupek, M.B.A., Administrator

The Oregon Clinic Gastroenterology Division Gresham Office, 24900 Southeast Stark, Suite 205, Gresham, OR 97030; tel. 503/661–2000; FAX. 503/661–2001; Jeffrey S. Albaugh, M.D., Administrator

The Portland Clinic Surgical Center, 800 Southwest 13th Avenue, Portland, OR 97205; tel. 503/221–0161; FAX. 503/274–1697; J. Michael Schwab, Administrator

Tigard Surgery Center, 13240 Southwest Pacific Highway, Suite 200, Tigard, OR 97223; tel. 503/639–6571; FAX. 503/624–6037; Ivan L. Bakos, M.D., Administrator

Willamette Valley Eye SurgiCenter, 2001 Commercial Street, S.E., Salem, OR 97302; tel. 503/363–1500; FAX. 503/588–2028; Gordon Miller, M.D., Administrator

PENNSYLVANIA

☐ **Abington Surgical Center,** 2701 Blair Mill Road, Suite 35, Willow Grove, PA 19090; tel. 215/443–8505; FAX. 215/957–0565; Deborah S. Kitz, Ph.D., Executive Director

Aesthetic and Reconstructive Surgery, 816 Belvedere Street, Carlisle, PA 17013

Aestique Ambulatory Surgical Center, One Aesthetic Way, Greensburg, PA 15601; tel. 412/832–7555; FAX. 412/832–7568; Theordore A. Lazzaro, M.D., Medical Director

Apple Hill Surgical Center, 25 Monument Road, Suite 270, York, PA 17403; tel. 717/741–8250; FAX. 717/741–8254; Gwendolyn J. Grothouse, RN, Administrative Director

Delaware Valley Laser Surgery Institute, Two Bala Plaza, PI 33, Bala Cynwd, PA 19004; tel. 215/668–2847; FAX. 215/668–1509; Herbert J. Nevyas, M.D., Medical Director

Dermatologic Surgical Center, P.C., 6415 Bustleton Avenue, Philadelphia, PA 19149

Dermatologic SurgiCenter, 1200 Locust Street, Philadelphia, PA 19107; tel. 215/546–3666; FAX. 215/546–6060; Anthony V. Benedetto, D.O., FACP, Medical Director

Dermatologic SurgiCenter, 2221 Garrett Road, Drexel Hill, PA 19026; tel. 610/623–5885; FAX. 610/623–7276; Anthony V. Benedetto, D.O. Medical Director

Digestive Disease Institute, 897 Poplar Church Road, Camp Hill, PA 17011; tel. 717/763–1239; FAX. 717/763–9854; Iris Garman, Administrator

Eye Clinic Ambulatory Surgical Center, Inc., 601 Wyoming Avenue, Kingston, PA 18704; tel. 717/288–7405; Mark Kelly, Administrator

Fairgrounds Surgical Center, 400 North 17th Street, Suite 300, Allentown, PA 18104; tel. 610/821–2020; FAX. 610/821–2016; Darlene G. Hinkle, Administrative Director

Fort Washington Surgery Center, 467 Pennsylvania Avenue, Fort Washington, PA 19034; tel. 215/628–4300; FAX. 215/628–4253; Elizabeth Brennan, Administrator

Grandview Surgery & Laser Center, 205 Grandview Avenue, Camp Hill, PA 17011; tel. 717/731–5444; FAX. 717/731–0415; Sherry L. Rhodes, RN, Administrative Director

Hanover Surgicenter, 3130 Grandview Road, Building B, Hanover, PA 17331; tel. 717/633–1600; FAX. 717/633–6556; Melvin L. Brooks, Jr., CRNA, Administrator

☐ **HealthSouth Scranton Surgery and Laser Center,** 425 Adams Street, Scranton, PA 18510; tel. 717/348–1114; FAX. 717/347–4351; Nancy A. Nealon, RN, B.S.N., Administrative Director

☐ **HealthSouth Surgery Center of Lancaster,** 217 Harrisburg Avenue, Suite 103, Lancaster, PA 17603; tel. 717/295–2500; FAX. 717/295–4898; Debra K. Sanders, RN, Administrative Director

☐ **Healthsouth Mt. Pleasant Surgery Center,** 200 Bessemer Road, Mt. Pleasant, PA 15666; tel. 412/547–5432; FAX. 412/547–2435; Brian Kowleczny, Administrative Director

☐ **Jefferson Surgery Center,** Coal Valley Road, P.O. Box 18420, Pittsburgh, PA 15236; tel. 412/469–6060; FAX. 412/469–7322; Sheran Sullivan, Manager

John A. Zitelli, M.D., P.C., Ambulatory Surgery Facility, 5200 Centre Avenue, Suite 303, Pittsburgh, PA 15232; tel. 412/681–9400; FAX. 412/681–5240; John A. Zitelli, M.D.

Kremer Laser Eye Center, 200 Mall Boulevard, King of Prussia, PA 19406; tel. 610/337–1580; FAX. 610/337–1815; Tara Hopewell, RN

Lebanon Outpatient Surgical Center, L.P., 830 Tuck Street, Lebanon, PA 17042; tel. 717/228–1620; FAX. 717/228–1642; Anita Gingrich Fuhrman, Manager

Lowry SurgiCenter, 1115 Lowry Avenue, Jeannette, PA 15644; tel. 412/527–2885; FAX. 412/527–6885; K. Diddle, M.D., Medical Director

Mt. Lebanon Surgical Center, Professional Office Building, 1050 Bower Hill Road, Suite 102, Pittsburgh, PA 15243; tel. 412/563–6808; FAX. 412/563–6857; Patricia Strosnider, Director, Nursing

N.E.I. Ambulatory Surgery, Inc., 204 Mifflin Avenue, Scranton, PA 18503; tel. 717/342–3145, ext. 2400; FAX. 717/342–3136

North Shore Surgi–Center, Two Allegheny Center, Suite 530, Pittsburgh, PA 15212–5493; tel. 412/231–0200; FAX. 412/231–0613; Jack Demos, M.D., FACS

☐ **Northwood Surgery Center,** 3729 Easton–Nazareth Highway, Easton, PA 18045; tel. 610/559–7110; FAX. 610/559–7317; Pankesh Kadam, Administrator

Ophthalmology Laser and Surgery Center, Inc., 92 Tuscarora Street, Harrisburg, PA 17104; tel. 717/233–2020; FAX. 717/232–3294; Jeanne Megella, RN, Director, Nursing

☐ **Paoli Surgery Center,** One Industrial Boulevard, Paoli, PA 19301; tel. 610/408–0822; FAX. 610/408–9933; Marcia L. Collymore, Facility Manager

Pennsylvania Eye Surgery Center, 4100 Linglestown Road, Harrisburg, PA 17112; tel. 717/657–2020; FAX. 717/657–2071; Sandra Benner, RN, Director, Surgical Services

Pocono Ambulatory Surgery Center, One Veterans Place, Stroudsburg, PA 18360; tel. 717/421–4978; Mary P. Hayden RN, B.S., A.S.C. Coordinator

Ridgeway Esper Medical Center Ambulatory Surgical Center, 5050 West Ridge Road, Erie, PA 16506–1298; tel. 814/833–8800; FAX. 814/833–2079; Deborah Hartmann, RN, Director, Nursing

Sewickley Surgical Center at Edgeworth Commons, 301 Ohio River Boulevard, Edgeworth, Suite 100, Sewickley, PA 15143; tel. 412/741–5866; FAX. 412/741–5884; Carol Figas, RN, CNOR, Supervisor

Shadyside Surgi–Center, Inc., 5727 Centre Avenue, Pittsburgh, PA 15206; tel. 412/363–6626; FAX. 412/363–7008; Susan M. Katch, RN, Director

☐ **Southwestern Ambulatory Surgery Center,** 500 Lewis Run Road, Pittsburgh, PA 15236; tel. 412/469–6964; FAX. 412/469–6948; Pamela Wrobleski, CRNA, M.P.M., Director

Southwestern Pennsylvania Eye Surgery Center, 750 East Beau Street, Washington, PA 15301; tel. 412/228–7477; FAX. 412/228–8117; Karen A. Dynice, Clinical Director

☐ **Specialists Health Care Clinic of Monroeville,** 125 Daugherty Drive, Monroeville, PA 15146–2749; tel. 412/374–9385, ext. 224; FAX. 412/374–9490; Carol Fiske, CMSC, Administrative Assistant, Medical Staff Manager

St. Francis Surgery Center North, One St. Francis Way, Cranberry Township, PA 16066; tel. 412/772–5360; FAX. 412/772–4644; Gerry Matt, RN, M.Ed., Director

Surgery Center of Bucks County, 401 North York Road, Warminster, PA 18974; tel. 215/443–3022; FAX. 215/443–5859; JoAnn Quinn, Director, Nursing

☐ **Surgical Center of York,** 1750 Fifth Avenue, P.O. Box 290, York, PA 17405; tel. 717/843–7613; Thomas R. Harlow, Administrative Director

Surgical Eye Institute of Western Pennsylvania, 618 Monongahela Avenue, Glassport, PA 15045; tel. 412/664–7874; FAX. 412/673–5720; Shirley A. Smith, RN

The Surgery Center of Chester County, 460 Creamery Way, Oaklands Corporate Center, Exton, PA 19341–2500; tel. 610/594–8900; FAX. 215/594–8907; Stephen P. Barainyak, Executive Director

The SurgiCenter at Ligonier, 221 West Main Street, Ligonier, PA 15658; tel. 412/238–9573; FAX. 412/238–4709; Kim Kenney–Ciarimboli, Supervisor

West Shore Endoscopy Center, 423 North 21st Street, Camp Hill, PA 17011; tel. 717/975–2430; Marilee Ball, RN, Director

Wills Eye Surgery Center of the Northeast, 1815 Cottman Avenue, Philadelphia, PA 19111; tel. 215/722–2505; FAX. 215/742–6386; Lawrence S. Schaffzin, M.D., Medical Director

☐ **Wyoming Valley Surgery Center,** 1130 Highway 315, Wilkes-Barre, PA 18702; tel. 717/821–2830; FAX. 717/825–7962; David N. Culp, Chief Executive Officer

RHODE ISLAND

Bayside Endoscopy Center, 120 Dudley Street, Suite 103, Providence, RI 02905; tel. 401/274–1810; FAX. 401/273–9689; Nicholas Califano, M.D., Administrator

Blackstone Valley Surgicare, Inc., 333 School Street, Pawtucket, RI 02860; tel. 401/728–3800; FAX. 401/723–2440; Ann Dugan, Administrator

Koch Eye Surgi Center, Inc., 566 Tollgate Road, Warwick, RI 02886; tel. 401/738–4800; FAX. 401/738–8153; Paul S. Koch, M.D., Administrator

Ocean State Endoscopy, 100 Highland Avenue, Providence, RI 02906; tel. 401/421–6306; Joel Spellun, M.D.

Planned Parenthood of Rhode Island, 111 Point Street, Providence, RI 02903; tel. 401/421–9620; FAX. 401/621–6250; Miriam Inocencio, President, Chief Executive Officer

Wayland Square Surgicare, 17 Seekonk Street, Providence, RI 02906; tel. 401/453–3311; FAX. 401/351–1280; Ann Dugan, Administrator

Women's Medical Center, 1725 Broad Street, Cranston, RI 02905; tel. 401/467–9111; FAX. 401/461–1390; Carol Belding, Administrator

SOUTH CAROLINA

Ambulatory Eye Surgery and Laser Center, Inc., 9297 Medical Plaza Drive, Charleston, SC 29406; tel. 803/572–2888; Margaret A. Thompson

Bay Microsurgical Unit, Inc., 400 Marina Drive, P.O. Drawer L, Georgetown, SC 29442; tel. 803/546–8421; FAX. 803/546–1173; Rebecca Lammonds, Administrator, Director, Nursing

Bearwood Ambulatory Surgery Center, 3031 Highway 81, N., Anderson, SC 29621; tel. 864/226–0837; FAX. 864/226–8367; Patricia P. Smith, Administrator

Bishopville Ambulatory Surgical Center, 800 West Church Street, Bishopville, SC 29010; tel. 803/484–6976; Carolyn Sellers, Administrator

Carolina Eye Ambulatory Surgery Center, 210 University Parkway, Suite 1500 B, Aiken, SC 29801; tel. 803/649–3953; FAX. 803/641–3801; Stephen K. VanDerVliet, M.D.

Carolina Regional Surgery Center, Ltd., 900 Medical Circle, Myrtle Beach, SC 29572; tel. 803/449–7885; FAX. 803/497–5137; Mary Garvey, RN, Administrator

Carolina Surgical Center, 198 South Herlong Avenue, Rock Hill, SC 29732; tel. 803/327–4664; Jackie Ridley, Administrator

Charleston Plastic Surgery Center, Inc., 159 Rutledge Avenue, Charleston, SC 29403; tel. 803/722–1985; FAX. 803/722–4840; Anna Lambert, Office Manager

Columbia Ambulatory Plastic Surgery Center, Inc., 338 Harbison Boulevard, Columbia, SC 29212; tel. 803/732–6655; FAX. 803/732–6644; Vickie H. Ott, Administrator

Columbia Eye Surgery Center, Inc., 1920 Pickens Street, P.O. Box 1754, Columbia, SC 29202; tel. 803/254–7732; FAX. 803/748–7199; Kenneth W. Gibbons, Administrator

Columbia Gastrointestinal Endoscopy Center, 2739 Laurel Street, Suite One–B, Columbia, SC 29240; tel. 803/254–9588; FAX. 803/252–0052; Frederick F. DuRant III, Administrator

Cross Creek Surgery Center of Greenville Hospital System, Nine Doctors Drive, Crosscreek Medical Park, Greenville, SC 29605; tel. 803/455–8400; Greg Rusnak, Administrator

Greenville Endoscopy Center, Inc., 317 St. Francis Drive, Suite 150, Greenville, SC 29601; tel. 803/232–7338; Rebecca K. Swoyer, Administrator

☐ **HealthSouth Surgery Center of Charleston,** 2690 Lake Park Drive, North Charleston, SC 29406; tel. 803/764–0992; FAX. 803/764–3187; Donna Padgette, RN, M.S.N., Facility Manager

☐ **Healthsouth Surgery Center of Greenville,** Five Memorial Medical Court, Greenville, SC 29605; tel. 864/295–3067; FAX. 864/295–3096; Vickie Waters, Facility Manager

Outpatient Surgery Center of Lexington Medical Center in Irmo, 7035 Saint Andrews Road, Columbia, SC 29212; tel. 803/749–0924; Barbara Willm, Administrator

Pee Dee Ambulatory Surgery Center, 602 Cheves, P.O. Box F–17, Florence, SC 29506; tel. 803/669–3822; Joseph J. McEvoy, Administrator

Roper West Ashley Surgery Center, 18 Farmfield Avenue, Charleston, SC 29407; tel. 803/763–3763; FAX. 803/763–3881; Maria I. Sample, Administrator

Same Day Surgery East, 10 Enterprise Boulevard, Suite 104, Greenville, SC 29615; tel. 803/458–7141; FAX. 803/676–9116; Mary Jane Knottek, RN, B.S.N., CNOR, Clinical Nurse Manager

Spartanburg Urology Surgicenter, Inc., 391 Serpentine Drive, Suite 330, Spartanburg, SC 29303; tel. 864/585–2002; FAX. 864/585–3300; Anita Womick, RN, OR Director

The Greenwood Endoscopy Center, 103 Liner Drive, Greenwood, SC 29646; tel. 803/227–3838; FAX. 803/227–6116; A. A. Ramage, M.D., Administrator

The Microsurgery Center, Inc., 1655 East Greenville Street, P.O. Box 1886, Anderson, SC 29622–1886; tel. 864/225–1933; FAX. 864/225–9035; Ann Geier, Director, Clinical Services

Trident Surgery Center, 9313 Medical Plaze Drive, Suite 102, Charleston, SC 29406; tel. 803/797–8992; FAX. 803/797–4094; Leah J. Dawson, Administrator

SOUTH DAKOTA

Aberdeen Surgical Center, 1200 South Main, Box 1150, Aberdeen, SD 57401–1150; tel. 605/225–2466; Scott H. Berry, M.D., Administrator

Black Hills Regional Eye Surgery Center, 2800 Third Street, Rapid City, SD 57701–7394; tel. 605/341–4100; FAX. 605/341–0278; Richard B. Hanafin, Executive Director

Jones Eye Clinic, 3801 South Elmwood Avenue, Sioux Falls, SD 57105–6565; tel. 605/336–3142; FAX. 605/334–0737; Charles E. Jones, M.D.

Mallard Pointe Surgical Center, 1201 Mickelson Drive, Watertown, SD 57201–7100; tel. 605/882–4743; FAX. 605/882–6064; James Arlt, Operations Director

Medical Associates Surgi Center, 772 East Dakota, Pierre, SD 57501–3399; tel. 605/224–5901; Michael Pfeifer, Administrator

Sioux Falls Surgical Center, 910 East 20th Street, Sioux Falls, SD 57105–1012; tel. 605/334–6730; Donald A. Schellpfeffer, M.D., Ph.D., Medical Director

Spearfish Surgery Center, Inc., 1316 10th Street, Spearfish, SD 57783–1530; tel. 605/642–3113; FAX. 605/642–3117; Linda Redding, Administrator

SurgiClinic, 1010 Ninth Street, Rapid City, SD 57701–3599; tel. 605/348–7607; FAX. 605/342–1359; Ray G. Burnett, M.D., Medical Director

Women's Health Clinic, 909 South Miller, Mitchell, SD 57301; tel. 605/995–5560; Donna Gerlach, RN, Clinic Director

Yankton Medical Clinic P.C., 1104 West Eighth Street, Yankton, SD 57078–3306; tel. 605/665–7841; FAX. 605/665–0546; Don P. Lake, Administrator

TENNESSEE

Appalachian Ambulatory Surgical Center, Medical Arts Building, 106 Rogosin Drive, Elizabethton, TN 37643; tel. 615/543–5888

Arrowsmith Eye Surgery Center, Parkview Tower, Suite 900, 210 25th Avenue, N., Nashville, TN 37203; tel. 615/327–2244; FAX. 615/321–3175; Cyndi Hamill, RN, Operating Room Supervisor

Atrium Memorial Surgical Center, 1949 Gunbarrel Road, Suite 290, Chattanooga, TN 37421; tel. 615/495–3550; FAX. 615/495–3580; Sandy Proctor, Administrator

Baptist Physicians Pavilion Surgery Center, 360 Wallace Road, Nashville, TN 37211; tel. 615/781–9020; FAX. 615/781–9944; Sandra Holshouser, Administrator

Bristol Surgery Center, 350 Blountville Highway, Suite 108, Bristol, TN 37620; tel. 423/844–6120; FAX. 423/844–6126; David Paul Gross, Administrator

Cataract Surgery Center, 5406 Knight Arnold Road, Memphis, TN 38115; tel. 901/360–8081; FAX. 901/368–3822

☐ **Centennial Surgery Center,** 340 23rd Avenue, N., Nashville, TN 37203; tel. 615/327–1123; FAX. 615/327–0261; Cynthia S. Duvall, RN, B.S., Administrator

☐ **Chattanooga Surgery Center,** 400 North Holtzclaw Avenue, Chattanooga, TN 37404; tel. 615/698–6871; Becky Myers, Administrator

Clarksville Encoscopy Center, 132 Hillcrest Drive, Clarksville, TN 37043; tel. 615/552–0180; FAX. 615/572–0915

Cleveland Surgery Center, L.P., 137 25th Street, N.E., Cleveland, TN 37311; tel. 423/472–7874; R. Scott Peterson, Executive Director

Columbia Endoscopy Center, Inc., 1510 1/2 Hatcher Lane, Columbia, TN 38401; tel. 615/381–7818; FAX. 615/381–5625; Dianne Roberts, RN, Head Nurse

Columbia Outpatient Surgery, Inc., 1405 Hatcher Lane, Columbia, TN 38401; tel. 615/381–3700; Deborah Woodard, Administrator

Columbia Sullins Surgery Center, 2761 Sullins Street, Knoxville, TN 37919; tel. 423/522–2949; FAX. 423/637–3259; Tina Shelby–Kahl, Assistant Administrator

D D C Surgery Center, Nine Physicians Drive, Jackson, TN 38305; tel. 901/661–0086; Regina Phelps, Billing Manager

Digestive Disease Endoscopy Center, 2021 Church Street, Suite 303, Nashville, TN 37203; tel. 615/340–4625; FAX. 615/340–4628

East Memphis Surgery Center, 80 Humphreys Center Drive, Suite 101, Memphis, TN 38120; tel. 901/747–3233; FAX. 901/747–3230

☐ **Endoscopy Center of Kingsport,** 2204 Pavilion Drive, Kingsport, TN 37660; tel. 423/392–6100; FAX. 423/392–6159; Barbara Light, Office Manager

Endoscopy Center of Northeast Tennessee, 310 State of Franklin Road, Suite 202, Johnson City, TN 37604; tel. 615/929–7111

Eye Surgery Center of East Tennessee, 1124 Weisgarber Road, Suite 110, Knoxville, TN 37909; tel. 423/588–1037, ext. 108; FAX. 423/909–9104; Donna Chambless, RN

Fort Sanders West Outpatient Surgery Center, Ltd., 210 Fort Sanders West Boulevard, Knoxville, TN 37922; tel. 615/531–5222; FAX. 615/531–5043; Leslie Irwin, Administrator

Franklin Surgery Center at MedCore, 2105 Edward Curd Lane, Franklin, TN 37067; tel. 615/794–7320

G. Baker Hubbard Ambulatory Surgery Center, 616 West Forest Avenue, Jackson, TN 38301; tel. 901/422–0330

☐ **G. I. Diagnostic and Therapeutic Center,** 1068 Cresthaven Road, Suite 300, Memphis, TN 38119; tel. 901/682–6700; FAX. 901/683–3046; Randolph M. McCloy, M.D., Medical Director

Germantown Ambulatory Surgical Center, Inc., 7499 Old Poplar Pike, Germantown, TN 38138; tel. 901/755–6465; FAX. 901/757–5543; Carol Harper, Facility Manager

Health South Surgery Center of Clarksville, 121 Hillcrest Drive, Clarksville, TN 37043; tel. 615/552–9992

☐ **HealthSouth Nashville Surgery Center,** 1717 Patterson Street, Nashville, TN 37203; tel. 615/329–1888; FAX. 615/329–0179; Patricia Middleton, Facility Manager

HealthSouth Surgery Center of Chattanooga, 924 Spring Creek Road, Chattanooga, TN 37412; tel. 423/899–1600; FAX. 423/899–2171; Melissa Powers, Administrator

Kingsport Bronchoscopy Center, Inc., 135 West Ravine Road, Suite Eight–A, Kingsport, TN 37660; tel. 615/247–5197; FAX. 615/247–5254; Shirley Hawkins, Administrator

Section C

Kingsport Endoscopy Corporation, 135 West Ravine Street, Suite 7A, Kingsport, TN 37660; tel. 423/246-6777; Bettye Reed, Administrator

Knoxville Center for Reproductive Health, 1547 West Clinch Avenue, Knoxville, TN 37916; tel. 423/637-3861; Bernadette McNabb, Executive Director

☐ **Knoxville Surgery Center,** 9300 Park West Boulevard, Knoxville, TN 37923; tel. 615/691-2725; FAX. 615/691-3090; Ranae Thompson, RN, Facility Administrator

LeBonheur East Surgery Center, L.P., 786 Estate Place, Memphis, TN 38120; tel. 901/681-4100; FAX. 901/681-4140; Diane Swain, Director

Lebanon Surgery Center, Inc., 1414 Baddour Parkway, P.O. Box 549, Lebanon, TN 37088; tel. 615/444-8944; Sheena Sloan, Administrator

Maternity Center of East Tennessee, 1925-B Ailor Avenue, Knoxville, TN 37921; tel. 615/524-4422

Medical Center Endoscopy Group, 930 Madison, Suite 870, Memphis, TN 38103; tel. 901/578-2538; FAX. 901/578-2572; John W. Flowers, Business Manager

Memphis Area Medical Center for Women, 29 South Bellevue Boulevard, Memphis, TN 38104; tel. 901/722-8050

Memphis Center for Reproductive Health, 1462 Poplar Avenue, Memphis, TN 38104; tel. 901/274-3550

Memphis Eye and Cataract Ambulatory Surgery Center, 6485 Poplar Avenue, Memphis, TN 38119; tel. 901/767-3937

Memphis Gastroenterology Group, 80 Humphrey's Blvd., Suite 220, Memphis, TN 38120; tel. 901/747-3630; FAX. 901/747-4039; Sylvia Hawkins, RN, Nurse Manager

Memphis Planned Parenthood, Inc., 1407 Union Avenue, Third Floor, Memphis, TN 38104; tel. 901/725-1717

Memphis Regional Gamma Knife Center, 1265 Union Avenue, Memphis, TN 38104; tel. 901/726-6444

☐ **Memphis Surgery Center,** 1044 Cresthaven Road, Memphis, TN 38119; tel. 901/682-1516; FAX. 901/682-1545; Barbara Hopper, RN, B.S., CNOR, Facility Manager

Mid-State Endoscopy Center, 2010 Church Street, Suite 420, Nashville, TN 37203; tel. 615/329-2141; FAX. 615/321-0522; Allan H. Bailey, M.D., Medical Director

Nashville Endoscopy Center, 300 20th N., Eighth Floor, Nashville, TN 37203; tel. 615/284-1335; FAX. 615/284-1316; Margaret Sullivan, RN

Nashville Gastrointestinal Endoscopy Center, 4230 Harding Road, Suite 309, Nashville, TN 37205; tel. 615/383-0165; FAX. 615/292-4657; Ron E. Pruitt, M.D.

Ophthalmic Ambulatory Surgery Center, P.C., 342 22nd Street, Nashville, TN 37203; tel. 615/327-2001; FAX. 615/327-2069; Alec Dryden, Administrator

Oral Facial Surgery Center, 322 22nd Avenue, N., Nashville, TN 37203; tel. 615/321-6160; FAX. 615/327-9612; Kelly Ingle, Administrator

PRISM Aesthetic Surgery Center, 80 Humphreys Center, Suite 310, Memphis, TN 38120; tel. 901/747-0446; FAX. 901/747-4406; Judy Sharp, Director, PRISM ASC

Physicians Surgery Center, 207 Stonebridge, Jackson, TN 38305; tel. 901/661-6340; FAX. 901/661-6363; Judy Haskins, RN, Manager

Planned Parenthood Association of Nashville, 412 D.B. Todd Boulevard, Nashville, TN 37203; tel. 615/321-7216

Ridge Lake Ambulatory Surgery Center, 825 Ridge Lake Boulevard, Memphis, TN 38119; tel. 901/685-0777

☐ **Rivergate Surgery Center,** 647 Myatt Drive, Madison, TN 37115; tel. 615/868-8942; FAX. 615/860-3820; Brenda Cruse, Director

Shea Clinic, 6133 Poplar Pike, Memphis, TN 38119; tel. 901/761-9720; FAX. 901/683-8440

Southern Endoscopy Center, 397 Wallace Road, Suite 407, Nashville, TN 37211; tel. 615/832-5530; FAX. 615/832-5713; Robert W. Herring, Jr., M.D., Medical Director

St. Thomas Medical Group Endoscopy Center, 4230 Harding Road, Suite 400, Nashville, TN 37205; tel. 615/297-2700

Surgical Services, P.C., 604 South Main Street, Sweetwater, TN 37874; tel. 423/337-4508; FAX. 423/337-4588

Surgicenter Of Murfreesboro Medical Clinic, P.A., 1004 North Highland Avenue, Murfreesboro, TN 37130; tel. 615/893-4480, ext. 351; FAX. 615/895-6212

Tennessee Endoscopy Center, 1706 East Lamar Alexander Parkway, Maryville, TN 37804; tel. 615/983-0073; FAX. 615/984-1731; Craig Jarvis, M.D., Administrator

The Cookeville Surgery Center, 100 West Fourth Street, Suite 100, Cookeville, TN 38501; tel. 615/528-6115; FAX. 615/526-2962; Diana Welch, RN, Administrator

☐ **The Endoscopy Center,** 801 Weisgarber Road, Suite 100, Knoxville, TN 37909, P.O. Box 59002, Knoxville, TN 37950-9002; tel. 615/588-5121; Gayle Mahan, Office Manager

The Endoscopy Center of Centennial, L.P., 2400 Patterson Street, Suite 515, Nashville, TN 37203; tel. 615/327-2111; FAX. 615/327-9292; Dawn Lynn Gray, RN, B.S., Endoscopy Administrator

The Eye Surgery Center Oak Ridge, 90 Vermont Avenue, Oak Ridge, TN 37830; tel. 423/482-8894; Sally Jones

The Pain Clinic and Rehabilitation Center, 55 Humphreys Center Drive, Suite 200, Memphis, TN 38120; tel. 901/747-0040; FAX. 901/747-3424; Lori Parris, RN, Administrator

Tullahoma Outpatient Surgery Center, 1918 North Jackson, Tullahoma, TN 37388; tel. 615/455-2006

Urology Surgery Center, Inc., 2011 Church Street, Sixth Floor, Nashville, TN 37203; tel. 615/329-7700; Robert B. Barnett, M.D., Medical Director

Van Dyke Ambulatory Surgery Center, 1024 Kelley Drive, Paris, TN 38242; tel. 901/642-5003; FAX. 901/642-8756; John T. VanDyck III, M.D., Owner

Volunteer Medical Clinic, 313 Concord Street, Knoxville, TN 37919; tel. 423/522-5173; FAX. 423/522-9907

Wesberry Surgery Center, 2900 South Perkins Road, Memphis, TN 38118-3237; tel. 901/362-3100; FAX. 901/362-3372; Jess Wesberry, Jr., M.D., President

Wesley Ophthalmic Plastic Surgery Center, 250 25th Avenue North, Suite 213, Nashville, TN 37203; tel. 615/329-3624

Women's Wellness and Maternity Center, Inc., 3459 Highway 68, Madisonville, TN 37354; tel. 423/442-6624; FAX. 423/442-5746; Betti Wilson, Administrator

TEXAS

AHCA-Mainland Outpatient Surgery Center, 3810 Hughes Court, Dickinson, TX 77539; tel. 713/337-7001; FAX. 713/337-7091; Terry R. Williams, Administrator

Abilene Cataract and Refractive Surgery Center, 2120 Antilley Road, Abilene, TX 79606; tel. 915/695-2020; FAX. 915/695-2326; Robert W. Cameron, M.D., Medical Director

☐ **Abilene Endoscopy Center,** 1249 Ambler Avenue, Abilene, TX 79601; tel. 915/695-2020; Royce Harrell

Amarillo Cataract and Eye Surgery Center, Inc., 7310 Fleming Avenue, Amarillo, TX 79106; tel. 806/354-8891; FAX. 806/354-2591; Carol A. Pearson, Director

Ambulatory Urological Surgery Center, Inc., 1149 Ambler, Abilene, TX 79601; tel. 915/676-3557; FAX. 915/673-2143; Angela X. Young, RN, Manager

American Cataract Centers of South Texas, LTD, 7810 Louis Pasteur, Suite 101, San Antonio, TX 78229; tel. 210/692-0218; Britt F. Mitchell, C.O.T., Director, Operations

Bailey Square Surgical Center, Ltd., 1111 West 34th Street, Austin, TX 78705; tel. 512/454-6753; FAX. 512/454-4314; Katherine S. Wilson, RN, M.H.A., Administrator

Barbara Jean Bartlett Memorial Surgery Center, 4200 Andrews Highway, Midland, TX 79707; tel. 915/520-5888; Sylvan Bartlett, M.D., Administrator

Bay Area Endoscopy Center, 444 FM 1959, Houston, TX 77034; tel. 281/481-9400; FAX. 281/481-9490; N. S. Bala, Medical Director

Bay Area Surgery, 7101 South Padre Island Drive, Corpus Christi, TX 78412; tel. 512/985-3500; FAX. 512/985-3754; Gene Hybner, Administrator

Bay Area Surgicare Center, Inc., 502 Medical Center Boulevard, P.O. Box 57767, Webster, TX 77598; tel. 713/332-2433; FAX. 713/332-0619; Mary P. Colombo, Administrator

Baylor SurgiCare, 3920 Worth Street, Dallas, TX 75246; tel. 214/820-2581; FAX. 214/820-7484; Patty Crabb, Administrative Director

Bellaire Surgicare, Inc., 6699 Chimney Rock, Suite 200, Houston, TX 77081; tel. 713/665-1406; FAX. 713/665-8262; Sheila M. Liccketto, Administrator

Brazosport Eye Institute, 103 Parking Way, P.O. Box 369, Lake Jackson, TX 77566; tel. 409/297-2961; FAX. 409/297-2395; Frank J. Grady, M.D., Ph.D., FACS, Director

Brownsville Surgicare, 1024 Los Ebanos Boulevard, Brownsville, TX 78520; tel. 210/548-0101; FAX. 210/541-3752; Norberto J. Sanchez, Administrator

Central Texas Day Surgery Center, L.P., 1817 Southwest Dodgen, Loop, Temple, TX 76502; tel. 817/773-7785; FAX. 817/773-9333; Debby Meyer, Director

Coastal Bend Ambulatory Surgical Center, 900 Morgan, Corpus Christi, TX 78404; tel. 512/888-4288; FAX. 512/888-4786; Barbara VandenBout

Columbia Endoscopy Center of Dallas, 6390 LBJ Freeway, Suite 200, Dallas, TX 75240; tel. 972/934-3691; Jeane Suggs, Administrator

Columbia North Texas Surgi-Center, 917 Midwestern Parkway, E., Wichita Falls, TX 76302; tel. 817/767-7273; FAX. 817/723-9059; Barbara Dawson, Administrator

☐ **Columbia Physicians Daysurgery Center,** 3930 Crutcher Street, Dallas, TX 75246; tel. 214/827-0760; FAX. 214/827-0944; Vickie Roberts, RN, Administrator

Columbia Surgery Center at Park Central, 12200 Park Central Drive, Third Floor, Dallas, TX 75251; tel. 972/661-0505; FAX. 972/661-0505; Molly Paulose, Administrator

Columbia Surgery Center of Las Colinas, 4255 North Macarthur Boulevard, Irving, TX 75038; tel. 214/257-0144; FAX. 214/258-0436; Bill Beaman, Administrator

Columbia Surgery Center of Sherman, 3400 North Calais Drive, Sherman, TX 75090; tel. 903/813-3377; FAX. 903/870-7617; Brian Roland, Business Office Manager

Columbia Surgical Center, 2800 East 29th Street, Bryan, TX 77802, P.O. Box 2700, Bryan, TX 77805; tel. 409/776-4300; FAX. 409/774-7149; Joan Dougan, Interim Chief Operating Officer

Columbia Surgical Center of Southeast Texas, 3127 College Street, Beaumont, TX 77701; tel. 409/835-2607; Jim Hoeks, Administrator

Columbia Surgicare Outpatient Center of Victoria, 1903 East Sabine, Victoria, TX 77901; tel. 512/576-4105; FAX. 512/576-9830; Margaret Coleman, RN, Administrator

Columbia West Houston Surgicare, 970 Campbell Road, Houston, TX 77024-2804; tel. 713/461-3547; FAX. 713/722-8921; Penny A. Menge, RN, M.S.N., Administrator

Columbia/Waco Medical Group Surgery Center, 2911 Herring, Waco, TX 76708; tel. 817/755-4430; FAX. 817/755-4590; Kay H. O'Leary, RN, Administrator

Crystal Outpatient Surgery Center, Inc., 215 Oak Drive, S., Suite J, Lake Jackson, TX 77566; tel. 409/299-6118; FAX. 409/299-1007; R. Scott Yarish, M.D., Administrator

Cy-Fair Surgery Center, 11250 Fallbrook Drive, Houston, TX 77065; tel. 713/955-7194; FAX. 713/890-0895; Scott Washko, Administrator

Dallas Day Surgery Center, Inc., 411 North Washington, Suite 5400, Dallas, TX 75246; tel. 214/821-8613; Henry S. Byrd, President

Dallas Eye Surgicenter, Inc., 720 South Cedar Ridge Road, Duncanville, TX 75137; tel. 214/296-6634; William Hamilton, Administrator

Dallas Opthalmology Center, Inc., 2811 Lemmon Avenue E., Suite 102, Dallas, TX 75204; tel. 214/520-7600; FAX. 214/528-6522; Jean Vining, RN, Administrator

Dallas Surgi Center, 8230 Walnut Hill Lane, Suite 808, Dallas, TX 75231; tel. 214/696-8828; FAX. 214/696-1444

DeHaven Surgical Center, Inc., 1424 East Front Street, Tyler, TX 75702; tel. 903/595-4168; FAX. 903/595-6821; Barbara Shamburger, RN, Administrator

☐ **Diagnostic Clinic of San Antonio Ambulatory Surgical Center,** 4647 Medical Drive, P.O. Box 29249, San Antonio, TX 78224-3100; tel. 210/692-3382; FAX. 512/692-3397; Nancy Nixon, RN, ASC Supervisor

Doctors Surgery Center, Inc., 5300 North Street, Nacogdoches, TX 75961; tel. 409/569-8278; Robert P. Lehmann, M.D., Director

Duncanville Surgery Center, (an affiliate of ASC Network Corporation), 1018 East Wheatland Road, Duncanville, TX 75116; tel. 214/296-6912; Michael Kincaid, Vice President

East El Paso Surgery Center, 7835 Corral Drive, El Paso, TX 79915; tel. 915/595–3353; FAX. 915/595–6796; Ruth Robertson, Administrator

East Side Surgery Center, Inc., 10918 East Freeway, Houston, TX 77029; tel. 713/451–4299; FAX. 713/451–4383; Clifford E. Kirby, Administrator

☐ **East Texas Eye Associates Surgery Center,** 1306 Frank Avenue, Lufkin, TX 75901; tel. 409/634–8381; Jo Ann O'Neill, C.O.T., Administrator

El Paso Institute of Eye Surgery, Inc., 1717 North Brown Street, Building Three, El Paso, TX 79902; tel. 915/544–0526; FAX. 915/544–2877; Esthern A. Calderon, Administrator

Elm Place Ambulatory Surgical Center, 2217 South Danville Drive, Abilene, TX 79605; tel. 915/695–0600; FAX. 915/695–3908; Susan King, RN, Director

Eye Surgery Center, 2001 Ed Carey Drive, Suite Three, Harlingen, TX 78550; tel. 210/423–2100; Michael Laney, C.O.M.T., Administrator

Facial Plastic and Cosmetic Surgical Center, 6300 Humana Plaza, Suite 475, Abilene, TX 79606; tel. 915/695–3630; FAX. 915/695–3633; Howard A. Tobin, M.D., FACS, Medical Director

Forest Park Surgery Pavilion, 5920 Forest Park Road, Suite 700, Dallas, TX 75235; tel. 214/350–2400; FAX. 214/352–3853; Mark Turner, Administrator

Fort Worth Endoscopy Center, 1201 Summit Avenue, Suite 400, Fort Worth, TX 76102; tel. 817/332–6500; Donna Drerup, RN, M.S.N., Administrator

Garland Surgery Center L.P., 777 Walter Reed Boulevard, Suite 105, Garland, TX 75042; tel. 214/494–2400; FAX. 214/494–3873; Dan Nicholson, President

☐ **Gastroenterology Consultants Outpatient Surgical Center,** 8214 Wurzbach, San Antonio, TX 78229; tel. 210/614–1234; FAX. 210/614–7749; Bonnie Draude, B.S.N., RN, C.G.R.N., Clinical Manager

Gastrointestinal Endoscopy Center Number Two, LTD, 1600 Coit Road, Suite 401A, Plano, TX 75075; tel. 214/867–0019; Brian Cooley, M.D., Administrator

Gonzaba Surgical Center, 720 Pleasanton Road, San Antonio, TX 78214; tel. 210/921–3826; FAX. 210/921–3825; William Gonzaba, M.D., Chief Executive Officer

☐ **Gramercy Outpatient Surgery Center, LTD,** 2727 Gramercy, Houston, TX 77025; tel. 713/660–6900; FAX. 713/660–0704; Elaine Hand, RN, CNOR, Clinical Director

HEALTHSOUTH Surgery Center of Beaumont, 3050 Liberty, Beaumont, TX 77702; tel. 409/835–3535; FAX. 409/835–6005; Tammie Clodfelter, Administrator

☐ **HEALTHSOUTH Surgery Center of Conroe,** 233 Interstate 45 N., P.O. Box 3091, Conroe, TX 77304; tel. 409/760–3443; FAX. 409/760–1322; Kathy Schutz, RN, B.S.N., Facility Administrator

☐ **HEALTHSOUTH Surgery Center of Dallas,** 7150 Greenville Avenue, Suite 200, Dallas, TX 75231; tel. 214/891–0466; FAX. 214/739–4702; Vicki V. Schultz, RN, Administrator

HealthSouth Surgery Center of Southwest Houston, 8111 Southwest Freeway, Houston, TX 77074; tel. 713/988–7600; FAX. 713/988–4070; Karen Whigham, Administrator

☐ **Healthsouth Arlington Day Surgery,** 918 North Davis Street, Arlington, TX 76012; tel. 817/860–9933; FAX. 817/860–2314; Diane Wood, RN, Administrator

☐ **Healthsouth Outpatient Surgery Center,** 7515 South Main Street, Suite 800, Houston, TX 77030; tel. 713/796–9666; FAX. 713/796–9660; Joan M. Culberson, RN, Administrator

Heart of Texas Outpatient Cataract Center, 100 South Park Drive, Brownwood, TX 76801; tel. 915/643–3561; FAX. 915/646–0670; Larry Smith, CRNA, Administrator

Heritage Surgery Center, 1501 Redbud, McKinney, TX 75069; tel. 214/548–0771; FAX. 214/562–2300; Rudolf Churner, M.D., Administrator

Houston Eye Clinic Partnership, 1200 Binz, Suite 1000, Houston, TX 77004; tel. 713/526–1600; FAX. 713/529–5254; Darcy Falbey, Director, Nursing

Howerton Eye and Laser Surgical Center, 2610 I.H. 35 South, Austin, TX 78704–5703; tel. 512/443–9715; FAX. 512/443–9845; Ernest E. Howerton, M.D., Administrator

☐ **Key Whitman Surgery Center,** 2801 Lemmon Avenue, Suite 400, Dallas, TX 75204; tel. 214/754–0000; FAX. 214/754–0079; Jeffrey Whitman, M.D.

Knolle Ocular Surgery Center, 4126 Southwest Freeway, Suite 108, Houston, TX 77027; tel. 713/621–3920; FAX. 713/621–7217; Guy E. Knolle, Jr., M.D., Administrator

Lipsky Sight Center, 1060 Hercules, Houston, TX 77058; tel. 713/488–7213; Ed Bercier, Administrator

☐ **Longview Ambulatory Surgical Center,** 703 East Marshall Avenue, Suite 2000, Longview, TX 75601–5563; tel. 903/236–2111; FAX. 903/236–2479; Jerry D. Adair, President, Chief Executive Officer

Lubbock Surgi Center, LLP, 3610 34th Street, Suite D, Lubbock, TX 79410; tel. 806/793–0255; Robert M. Brodkin, D.P.M., Administrator

Lufkin Endoscopy Center, 317 Gaslight Boulevard, Lufkin, TX 75901; tel. 409/634–3713; FAX. 409/634–8136; Bhagvan R. Malladi, M.D., Administrator

☐ **MSCH Health Center,** 1211 Highway Six, Suite One, Sugarland, TX 77478; tel. 713/242–7200; John Araiza, Administrator

Maddox Outpatient Eye Surgery Center, 1755 Curie Drive, El Paso, TX 79902; tel. 915/544–9597; FAX. 915/533–3460; Robert M. Maddox, M.D., Administrator

Mann Cataract Surgery Center, 18850 South Memorial Boulevard, Humble, TX 77338; tel. 713/446–9164; Elpidio Fahel, Administrator

Medical City Dallas Ambulatory Surgery Center, 7777 Forest Lane, Suite C–150, Dallas, TX 75230; tel. 214/661–7000; FAX. 214/788–6181; Michael D. Pugh, President, Chief Executive Officer

Medical Mall Surgery Center, Inc., 1665 Antilley Road, Suite 170, Abilene, TX 79606; tel. 915/692–6694; FAX. 915/691–1568; Melissa Boyd, RN

Methodist Ambulatory Surgery Center–Central San Antonio, 1008 Brooklyn Avenue, San Antonio, TX 78215–1600; tel. 210/225–0496; FAX. 210/225–8462; Carl J. Collazo, Administrator

Methodist Malone and Hogan–Texas Surgery, 1501 West 11th Place, Suite A, Big Spring, TX 79720–4199; tel. 915/267–1623; FAX. 915/267–1137; Penny Phillips, Administrator

Metroplex Ambulatory Surgical Center, 2717 Osler Drive, Suite 102, Grand Prairie, TX 75051; tel. 214/647–6272; FAX. 214/660–1822; Glenda Daniels, RN, Director

☐ **Metroplex Surgicare,** 1600 Central Drive, Suite 180, Bedford, TX 76022; tel. 817/571–1999; FAX. 817/571–1220; Julie Walker, Administrator

Mid–Cities Surgi–Center, 2012 Plaza Drive, Bedford, TX 76021; tel. 817/283–5994; Melany Pierson

Mid–Town Surgical Center, Inc., 2105 Jackson Street, Suite 200, Houston, TX 77003; tel. 713/659–3050; FAX. 713/659–3037; Glory Gee, Administrator

North Carrier Surgicenter, 517 North Carrier Parkway, Suite A, Grand Prairie, TX 75050–5494; tel. 214/264–0533; FAX. 214/262–5974; Abraham F. Syrquin, M.D., Medical Director

North Dallas Surgicare, 375 Municipal Drive, Suite 214, Richardson, TX 75080; tel. 214/918–9400; FAX. 214/918–9749; Bill MacKnight, Administrator

Northeast Surgery Center, 18929 Highway 59, Humble, TX 77338; tel. 713/446–4053; Harold Taylor

Northeast Texas Surgical Center, 1801 Galleria Oaks Drive, Texarkana, TX 75503; tel. 903/792–2108; FAX. 903/792–0606; Ruby Bearden, Business Manager

Northwest Ambulatory Surgery Center, 2833 Babcock Road, San Antonio, TX 78229; tel. 210/705–5100; FAX. 210/705–5025; Jim Brown, Administrator

Outpatient Surgical Center, 2507 Medical Row, Suite 101, Grand Prairie, TX 75051; tel. 214/647–8520; Jack Gray, Administrator

Outpatient Surgisite, 401–A East Pinecrest Drive, Marshall, TX 75670; tel. 903/938–3110; Carol C. Hall

Piney Point Ambulatory Surgery Center, 2500 Fondren, Suite 350, Houston, TX 77063; tel. 713/782–8279; FAX. 713/782–3139

Plano Ambulatory Surgery Associates, L.P., d/b/a Columbia Surgery Center of Plano, 1620 Coit Road, Plano, TX 75075–7799; tel. 972/519–1100; Dolores Holland

Plastic and Reconstructive Surgery Centre of the SW, 461 Westpark Way, Euless, TX 76040; tel. 817/540–1755; Catherine Lugger, Director

Plaza Day Surgery, 909 Ninth Avenue, Fort Worth, TX 76104–3986; tel. 817/336–6060; Nancy Kilekas, RN, B.S., CNOR, Administrator

Port Arthur Day Surgery Center, 3449 Gates Boulevard, Port Arthur, TX 77642; tel. 409/983–6144; Vicki Clark, Administrative Director

Premier Ambulatory Surgery of Austin, 4207 James Casey, Suite 203, Austin, TX 78745; tel. 512/440–7894; FAX. 512/440–1932; Patricia Philbin, Executive Director

Regional Eye Surgery Center, 107 West 30th Street, Pampa, TX 79065; tel. 806/665–0051; FAX. 806/665–0640; George R. Walters, M.D., President

☐ **Rio Grande Surgery Center,** 1809 South Cynthia, McAllen, TX 78503; tel. 512/618–4402; FAX. 210/618–4174; Janet R. West, Director

San Antonio Digestive Disease Endoscopy Center, 1804 Northeast Loop 410, Suite 101, San Antonio, TX 78217; tel. 210/828–8400; FAX. 210/828–8648

San Antonio Eye Surgicenter, 800 McCullough, San Antonio, TX 78215; tel. 210/226–6169; FAX. 210/226–6383; Carol Harris, Administrator

San Antonio Gastroenterology Endoscopy Center, 520 Euclid Avenue, San Antonio, TX 78212; tel. 210/271–0606; FAX. 210/271–0180; Ernesto Guerra, M.D.

☐ **San Antonio Surgery Center, Inc.,** 5290 Medical Drive, San Antonio, TX 78229; tel. 210/614–0187; FAX. 210/692–7757; Ann Finney, RN, Facility Administrator

Santa Rose Diagnostic and Surgical Center, 315 North San Saba, San Antonio, TX 78207; tel. 210/704–4000; FAX. 210/704–4014; Julie Meador, Clinical Manager

South Plains Endoscopy Center, 3610 24th Street, Lubbock, TX 79410; tel. 806/797–1015; Pat S. Wheeler, Administrator

South Texas Eye Surgicenter, Inc., 4406 North Laurent, Victoria, TX 77901; tel. 800/352–5928; Robert T. McMahon, M.D., Chief Executive Officer

South Texas Outpatient Surgical Center, Inc., 4025 East Southcross Boulevard, Building Three, Suite 15, San Antonio, TX 78222; tel. 210/333–0633; FAX. 210/333–0671; Michael P. Lewis, Administrator

South West Surgery Center, 1717 Precinct Line Road, Suite 101, Hurst, TX 76054; tel. 817/498–0525; FAX. 817/656–1490; Kim Gustin, Office Manager

Southwest Endoscopy Center, 11803 South Freeway, Suite 115, Fort Worth, TX 76115; tel. 817/293–9292; FAX. 817/551–0616; Pamela Payne, RN

St. Mary Surgicenter, Ltd., 2301 Quaker Avenue, Lubbock, TX 79410; tel. 806/793–8801; David S. Weil, Executive Director

SurgEyeCare, Inc., 5421 La Sierra Drive, Dallas, TX 75231; tel. 214/361–1443; FAX. 214/691–3299; Sandra J. Yankee, Administrator

☐ **Surgery Center Southwest,** 8230 Walnut Hill Lane, Suite 102, Dallas, TX 75231; tel. 214/345–4076; FAX. 214/345–4055; Tom Blair, Director, PHS

☐ **Surgery Center of Fort Worth,** 2001 West Rosedale, Fort Worth, TX 76104; tel. 817/877–4777; Debra Delain, RN, Administrator

Surgi–Care Center of Midland, Inc., 3001 West Illinois, Suite Five–A, Midland, TX 79701; tel. 915/697–1067; FAX. 915/697–8802; Michelle Edelbrock, RN, B.S.N., Director

SurgiSystems, Inc., 427 West 20th Street, Houston, TX 77008; tel. 713/868–3641; FAX. 713/865–5460; Jo McBeth, RN

Surgical Center of El Paso, 1815 North Stanton, El Paso, TX 79902; tel. 915/533–8412; FAX. 915/542–0367; Thomas Reynolds, Managing Director

Surgical and Diagnostic Center, Inc., 729 Bedford Euless Road West 100, Hurst, TX 76053; tel. 817/282–6905; FAX. 817/285–8114; Edward William Smith, D.O., Medical Director

☐ **Surgicare of Travis Centre, Inc.,** 6655 Travis, Suite 200, Houston, TX 77030; tel. 713/526–5100; Carol Simons, Administrator

Surgicare, Ltd., 3534 Vista, Pasadena, TX 77504; tel. 713/947–0330; Evelyn Grimes, Administrator

Surgicenter of San Antonio, L.P., 7902 Ewing Halsell Drive, San Antonio, TX 78229; tel. 210/614–7372; FAX. 210/614–7362; Russell Furth, Executive Director

Texarkana Surgery Center, 5404 Summerhill Road, Texarkana, TX 75503; tel. 903/792–7151; Karen Stephens, Director

Section C

Texas Ambulatory Surgical Center, Inc., 2505 North Shepherd, Houston, TX 77008; tel. 713/880–3940; FAX. 713/880–1923; Kwang S. Park, Administrator

Texas Institute of Surgery, 12700 North Featherwood Drive, Suite 100, Houston, TX 77034; tel. 713/481–9303; FAX. 713/481–4263; Glenn Rodriguez, Administrator

Texoma Outpatient Surgery Center, Inc., 1712 Eleventh Street, Wichita Falls, TX 76301; tel. 817/723–1274; Tracy Youngblood, Administrator

The Birth Center of Southeast Texas, Inc., 2400 Highway 96 S., Lumberton, TX 77656; tel. 409/755–0252; Dennis D. Riston, M.D., Administrator

The Cataract Center of East Texas, P.A., 802 Turtle Creek Drive, Tyler, TX 75701; tel. 903/595–4333; FAX. 903/535–9845; Connie Bryan, RN

The Center for Sight, P.A., Two Medical Center Boulevard, Lufkin, TX 75904–3175; tel. 409/634–8434; FAX. 409/639–2581; Richard J. Ruckman, M.D.

The Endoscopy Center of Southeast Texas, 950 North 11th Street, Beaumont, TX 77702; tel. 409/833–5555; FAX. 409/833–9911; Royce D. Harrell

The Eye Surgery Center of the Rio Grande Valley, 1402 East Sixth Street, Weslaco, TX 78596; tel. 210/968–6155; FAX. 210/968–8291; Linda Funston, Administrator

The Ocular Surgery Center, Inc., 1100 North Main Avenue, San Antonio, TX 78212; tel. 210/222–2154; FAX. 512/222–0706; Jane Wilson, Administrator

The Surgery Center of Mesquite, 2690 North Galloway Avenue, Mesquite, TX 75150; tel. 972/279–8100; FAX. 972/279–3300; Jeffrey S. Houston, Administrator

☐ **The Surgery Center of Texas,** 155 East Loop 338, Suite 500, Odessa, TX 79762; tel. 915/367–3906; FAX. 915/367–3895; Ann Wilson, Interim Administrator

The Surgery Center of the Woodlands, 1441 Woodstead Court, Suite 100, The Woodlands, TX 77380; tel. 281/363–0058; FAX. 281/363–0450; Kathy Budd, Administrator

Thorstenson Eye Clinic Surgery Center, 3302 Northeast Stallings Drive, Nacogdoches, TX 75963–2020; tel. 409/564–2411; FAX. 409/564–1280; Lyle S. Thorstenson, M.D., FACS, Administrator

University Surgery Center, Inc., 311 University Drive, Fort Worth, TX 76107; tel. 817/877–1002; FAX. 817/877–1006; Lori Schooler, Administrator

Urological Surgery Center of Fort Worth, 418 South Henderson, Fort Worth, TX 76104; tel. 817/338–4637; Charles Bamberger, M.D.

Valley Endoscopy Center, LLP, 3101 South Sunshine Strip, Harlingen, TX 78550; tel. 210/421–2324; FAX. 210/428–2561; Noel B. Searle, MD

Valley Eye Surgery Center, 1515 North Ed Carey Drive, Harlingen, TX 78550; tel. 210/423–2773; FAX. 210/423–5618; Michael D. Laney, Administrator

☐ **Valley View Surgery Center,** 5744 LBJ Freeway, Suite 200, Dallas, TX 75240; tel. 972/490–4333; FAX. 972/490–3408; Ronald W. Disney, Chief Executive Officer

Vista Healthcare, Inc., 4301 Vista, Pasadena, TX 77504; tel. 713/947–0891; FAX. 713/947–1377; Chiu M. Chan, Administrator

WestPark Surgery Center, 130 South Central Expressway, McKinney, TX 75070; tel. 214/542–9382; FAX. 214/548–5303; Debbie Taylor

Westside Surgery Center, Ltd., 16100 Cairnway, Houston, TX 77084; tel. 713/550–5556; FAX. 713/550–7888; Harold F. Taylor, President, Chief Executive Officer

Wilson Surgicenter, 4315 28th Street, Lubbock, TX 79410; tel. 806/792–2104; Bill W. Wilson, M.D., Chief Executive Officer

UTAH

Central Utah Surgical Center, 1067 North 500 West, Provo, UT 84604; tel. 801/374–0354; FAX. 801/374–2615; Jane Sowards, Administrator

Institute of Facial and Cosmetic Surgery, 5929 Fashion Boulevard, Murray, UT 84107; tel. 801/261–3637; FAX. 801/261–4096; Pam J. Groves, Facility Manager

Intermountain Surgical Center, 359 Eighth Avenue, Salt Lake City, UT 84103; tel. 801/321–3200; FAX. 801/321–3035; Joan W. Lelis, Ambulatory Director

McKay–Dee Surgical Center, 3903 Harrison Boulevard, Suite 100, Ogden, UT 84403; tel. 801/625–2809; FAX. 801/629–5938; Suzanne Richins, Administrator

Provo Surgical Center, 585 North 500 West, Provo, UT 84601; tel. 801/375–0983; Brent K. Ashby, Administrator

Salt Lake Endoscopy Center, 24 South 1100 East, Salt Lake City, UT 84102; tel. 801/355–2987; FAX. 801/531–9704; Clifford G. Harmon, M.D., Administrator

☐ **Salt Lake Surgical Center,** 617 East 3900 South, Salt Lake City, UT 84107; tel. 801/261–3141; FAX. 801/268–2599; Jay T. Lighthall, Administrator

St. George Surgical Center, 676 South Bluff Street, St. George, UT 84770; tel. 801/673–8080; FAX. 801/673–0096; Terrill Dick, Administrator

☐ **St. Mark's Outpatient Surgery Center,** 1250 East 3900 South, Suite 100, Salt Lake City, UT 84124; tel. 801/262–0358; FAX. 801/262–0901; Marjorie Kimes, Administrator

The SurgiCare Center of Utah, 755 East 3900 South, Salt Lake City, UT 84107; tel. 801/266–2283, ext. 706; FAX. 801/268–6151; LuAnn Woodall, LPN

Wasatch Endoscopy, 1220 East 3900 South, Suite 1B, Salt Lake City, UT 84124; tel. 801/281–3657; Marjorie Kimes, R.N., Administrator

Wasatch Surgery Center, 555 South Foothill Boulevard, Salt Lake City, UT 84112; tel. 801/585–3088; FAX. 801/581–8962; Patricia Carroll, Administrator, Manager

Western Surgery Center, Inc., 850 East 1200 North, Logan, UT 84341; tel. 801/797–3670; FAX. 801/797–3848; Steven V. Hodson, Administrator

VERMONT

David S. Chase, M.D., Ambulatory Surgical Center, 183 St. Paul Street, Burlington, VT 05401; tel. 802/864–0381; David S. Chase, M.D., Administrator

VIRGINIA

Ambulatory Surgery Center, 844 Kempsville Road, Norfolk, VA 23502; tel. 804/466–6900; FAX. 804/461–6796; Darleen S. Anderson, Site Administrator

Cataract and Refractive Surgery Center, 2010 Bremo Road, Suite 128, Richmond, VA 23226; tel. 804/285–0680; FAX. 804/282–6365; Jeffry A. Staples, Administrator

Columbia Fairfax Surgical Center, 10730 Main Street, Fairfax, VA 22030; tel. 703/691–0670; Sharon B. Johnson, Chief Executive Officer

CountrySide Ambulatory Surgery Center, Four Pidgeon Hill Drive, Sterling, VA 20165; tel. 703/444–6060; FAX. 703/444–2278; Deborah F. Arminio, RN, Director

Fredericksburg Ambulatory Surgery Center, Inc., 2216 Princess Anne Street, Fredericksburg, VA 22401; tel. 540/899–3403; FAX. 540/899–6893; Jeane Bullock, Administrator

Kaiser Permanente Falls Church Medical Center Ambulatory Surgery Center, 201 North Washington Street, Falls Church, VA 22046; tel. 703/237–4046; FAX. 703/536–1400; Debbie Bland, Director, Surgical Services

Lakeview Medical Center, Inc., 2000 Meade Parkway, Suffolk, VA 23424; tel. 804/539–0251; FAX. 804/934–2620; Michael B. Stout, Administrator

Lewis–Gale Clinic, Inc., Same Day Surgery, 1802 Braeburn Drive, Salem, VA 24153; tel. 703/772–3673; FAX. 703/989–0879; Lyndell B. Brooks, President

Piedmont Day Surgery Center, Inc., 1040 Main Street, P.O. Box 1360, Danville, VA 24543–1360; tel. 804/792–1433, ext. 258; FAX. 804/797–1398; Aaron Lieberman, Chief Operating Officer

Retreat Regional Medical Center, 7016 Lee Park Road, Mechanicsville, VA 23111; tel. 804/730–9000; FAX. 804/730–1460; Timothy E. Wildt, Administrator

Riverside Surgery Center–Warwick, 12420 Warwick Boulevard, Building Three, Suite C, Newport News, VA 23606; tel. 804/594–2796; FAX. 804/594–3911; M. Caroline Martin, Executive Vice President

Sentara Care Plex, 3000 Coliseum Drive, Hampton, VA 23666; tel. 804/827–2000; FAX. 804/827–6748; Jeri Eastridge, Director

Surgi Center of Central Virginia, Inc., 223 Willow Street, Fredericksburg, VA 22405; tel. 703/371–5349; FAX. 703/373–1745; Janet P. O'Keefe, Facility Administrator

Surgi–Center of Winchester, Inc., 1860 Amherst Street, P.O. Box 2660, Winchester, VA 22604; tel. 703/722–8934; FAX. 703/722–8936; H. Emerson Poling, M.D., Administrator

Tuckahoe Surgery Center, Inc., 8919 Three Chopt Road, Richmond, VA 23229; tel. 804/285–4763; FAX. 804/288–2850; Charles A. Stark, CHE, Administrator

Urosurgical Center of Richmond, 5224 Monument Avenue, Richmond, VA 23226; tel. 804/288–4137; FAX. 804/288–3529; Terry W. Coffey, Administrator

Urosurgical Center of Richmond–North, 8228 Meadowbridge Road, Mechanicsville, VA 23111; tel. 804/730–5023; FAX. 804/746–4015; Terry W. Coffey, Administrator

Urosurgical Center of Richmond–South, 7001 Jahnke Road, Richmond, VA 23225; tel. 804/560–4483; FAX. 804/272–1178; Terry W. Coffey, Administrator

Virginia Ambulatory Surgery Center, 337–15th Street, S.W., Charlottesville, VA 22903; tel. 804/295–4800; FAX. 804/977–0544; Gerry Dobrasz, Administrator

Virginia Beach Ambulatory Surgery Center, 1700 Will–o–Wisp Drive, Virginia Beach, VA 23454; tel. 804/496–6400; FAX. 804/496–3137; Brian Murray, M.D., Administrator

Virginia Eye Institute/Eye Surgeons of Richmond, Inc., 400 Westhampton Station, Richmond, VA 23226; tel. 804/282–3931; FAX. 804/287–4256; Kenneth J. Newell, Administrator

Virginia Heart Institute, LTD., 205 North Hamilton Street, Richmond, VA 23221; tel. 804/359–9265; Charles L. Baird, Jr., M.D., Director

Woodburn Surgery Center, 3289 Woodburn Road, Suite 100, Annandale, VA 22003; tel. 703/207–7520; Jolene Tornabeni, Senior Vice President, Administrator

WASHINGTON

AEsteem Outpatient Surgery Center, 1200 North Northgate Way, Seattle, WA 98133–8916; tel. 206/522–0200; FAX. 206/522–7019; Peter R. N. Chatard, Jr., M.D., Medical Director

Aesthetic Eye Associates, P.S., 1810 116th Avenue, N.E., Suite B, Bellevue, WA 98004; tel. 206/462–0400; FAX. 206/454–1085; Janet Jordan, Business Manager

Bel–Red Ambulatory Surgical Facility, 1370 116th Avenue, N.E., Suite 209, Bellevue, WA 98004; tel. 206/455–7225; FAX. 206/455–0045

Bellingham Surgery Center, 2980 Squalicum Parkway, Bellingham, WA 98225; tel. 206/671–6933; Richard Brumenschenkel, Managing Agent

Boyd Davis Eye Center, 1051 116th Avenue, N.E., Bellevue, WA 98004; tel. 206/454–2018; Herschell H. Boyd, M.D.

Cascade Ambulatory Surgery Center, 407 Northeast 87th Street, Vancouver, WA 98664; tel. 360/253–9201; Joseph R. McFarland, M.D.

Cascade Regional Eye Surgery Center, 16404 Smokey Point Boulevard, Suite 111, Arlington, WA 98223; tel. 206/653–4000; FAX. 206/658–1266; Smokey Simons, Director

Central Washington Cataract Surgery, 1450 North 16th Avenue, Building J, Yakima, WA 98902; tel. 509/457–5000; FAX. 509/457–6498; Paul Almeida, CRNA

Central Washington Surgicare, 307 South 12th Avenue, Suite Nine, Yakima, WA 98902; tel. 509/248–4900; FAX. 509/248–0609

Covington Day Surgery Center, 17700 Southeast 272nd Street, Kent, WA 98042; tel. 206/639–8302; FAX. 206/639–8301; Victoria Fitzpatrick, B.S.N., Director

Dietrich Von Feldmann, M.D., Inc., 16259 Sylvester S.W., Suite 401, Seattle, WA 98166; tel. 206/244–5335; FAX. 206/244–4147; Dietrich Von Feldmann, M.D.

Ear, Nose, Throat and Plastic Surgery, 101 Second Street, N.E., Auburn, WA 98002; tel. 206/833–6241; FAX. 206/833–4113; William Portuese, M.D., Medical Director

Eastside Podiatry Ambulatory Surgery Center, 15617 Bel–Red Road, Bellevue, WA 98008; tel. 206/881–5592; G. Curda, D.P.M.

Edmonds Surgery Center, 21229 84th Avenue W., Edmonds, WA 98026; tel. 206/775–1505; FAX. 206/775–9078; Mark A. Kuzel, D.P.M.

Everett Surgical Center, Inc., 3025 Rucker Avenue, Everett, WA 98201; tel. 206/339–2464; FAX. 206/252–4700; Rita Sweeney, RNFA, CNOR, Administrator

Evergreen Endoscopy Center, 13030 121st Way, N.E., Suite 101, Kirkland, WA 98034; tel. 206/899–4500; Lynn Bookkeeper

Evergreen Eye Surgery Center, 34719 Sixth Avenue South, Federal Way, WA 98003; tel. 206/874–3969; Richard A. Boudreau, Administrator

Evergreen Surgical Center, 12034 Northeast 130th Lane, Kirkland, WA 98034; tel. 206/821–3131; Ronald E. Abrams, M.D.

☐ **Good Samaritan Surgery Center,** 1322 Third Street S.E., Suite 100, Puyallup, WA 98372; tel. 206/840–2200; FAX. 206/840–2352; Roger D. Robinett, M.D., Medical Director

Health South, Green River Surgical Center, 126 Auburn Avenue, Suite 200, Auburn, WA 98002; tel. 206/735–0500; FAX. 206/939–8526; Gail A. Okon, Facility Manager

Hernia Treatment Center, NW, 205 Lilly Road, NE, Suite D, Olympia, WA 98506; tel. 360/491–8667; Robert Kugel, M.D., Director

Inland Empire Endoscopy Center, South 820 McClellan, Suite 314, Spokane, WA 99204; tel. 509/747–0143; J. D. Fitterer, M.D.

Inland Eye Center, South 842 Cowley, Spokane, WA 99202; tel. 509/624–5300; FAX. 509/747–1348; Michael H. Cunningham, M.D., President

Kruger Clinic Day Surgery, 21600 Highway 99, Suite 150, Edmonds, WA 98026; tel. 206/774–2636

Laboratory for Reproductive Health, 1370 116th Avenue, N.E., Suite 100, Bellevue, WA 98004; tel. 206/462–6100

Lomas Surgery Center, 17800 Talbot Road, S., Renton, WA 98055; tel. 425/255–0986; FAX. 425/271–5703; Inese A. Lomas, Administrator

Madrona Medical Group, ASC, 4370 Cordata Parkway, Bellingham, WA 98226; tel. 360/676–1712

McIntyre Eye Surgical Center, 1920 116th Avenue, N.E., Bellevue, WA 98004; tel. 206/454–3937; FAX. 206/646–5914; David McIntyre, M.D., FACS

Mid–Columbia Surgical Suite, Inc., 471 Williams Boulevard, Suite Four, Richland, WA 99352; tel. 509/943–1134; Robert C. Luckey, M.D., Medical Director

Minor & James Medical, PLLC, 515 Minor Avenue, Suite 200, Seattle, WA 98104; tel. 206/386–9500; FAX. 206/386–9605; Sylvia Croy, RN, ASC Coordinator

Monroe Foot Care Associates Ambulatory Surgery Center, 14692 179th Avenue, S.E., Suite 300, Monroe, WA 98272; tel. 206/794–1266; Dr. Brunsman, Medical Director

Moses Lake Surgery Center, 840 East Hill Avenue, Moses Lake, WA 98837; tel. 509/765–0216; John Rodriguez, ASC Manager

NW Aesthetic Surgery Center, 550 16th Avenue, Suite 404, Seattle, WA 98122; tel. 206/328–2250; Mary Ann Beberman, Administrator

NW Center for Corrective Jaw Surgery, 550 16th Avenue, Seattle, WA 98122; tel. 206/324–6570; FAX. 206/324–9936; Carolyn Conroy, Office Administrator

North Cascade ENT Facial Plastic Surgery, 20302 77th Avenue, N.E., Arlington, WA 98223; tel. 360/435–6300; FAX. 360/435–8381; Alex O'Dell

North Cascade ENT and Facial Plastic Surgery, 111 South 13th Street, Mount Vernon, WA 98273; tel. 206/336–2178

North Kitsap Ambulatory Surgical Center, 20696 Bond Road, N.E., Poulsbo, WA 98370; tel. 360/779–6527; FAX. 360/697–2743; Susan Chu, RN

Northwest Center for Plastic and Reconstructive Surgery, 16259 Sylvester Road, S.W., Suite 302, Seattle, WA 98166; tel. 206/241–5400; FAX. 206/241–8591; Sindi Miller, Office Manager

Northwest Eye Surgery, P.C., N1120 Pines Road, Spokane, WA 99206; tel. 509/927–0700

Northwest Gastroenterology, d/b/a Northwest Endoscopy, 2930 Squalicum, Suite 202, Bellingham, WA 98225; tel. 360/733–3231; FAX. 360/734–8748; Kathy Bruns, Manager

Northwest Nasal Sinus Center, 10330 Meridan Avenue, N., Suite 240, Seattle, WA 98133; tel. 206/525–2525; FAX. 206/525–0346

Northwest Surgery Center, 1920 100th Street, S.E., Everett, WA 98208; tel. 206/316–3700; Chris Vance, President

Northwest Surgery Center, Inc., West 123 Francis, Spokane, WA 99205; tel. 509/483–9363; FAX. 509/483–0355; Douglas P. Romney

Northwest Surgical Center, 3120 Squalicum Parkway, Bellingham, WA 98225; tel. 360/647–0557; FAX. 360/733–2892; Marianne Karuza, A.R.T.

Olympic Ambulatory Surgery Center, Inc., 2601 Cherry Avenue, Suite 115, Bremerton, WA 98310; tel. 206/479–5990; FAX. 360/377–5731; Audrey E. Harris, RN

Olympic Plastic Surgery Suite, 2600 Cherry Avenue, Suite 201, Bremerton, WA 98310; tel. 206/479–4370

Pacific Cataract and Laser Institute, 2517 Northeast Kresky, Chehalis, WA 98532; tel. 206/748–8632; Debbie Eldredge, Vice President, Chief Operating Officer

Pacific Cataract and Laser Institute, 10500 Northeast Eighth Street, Suite 1650, Bellevue, WA 98004–4332; tel. 206/462–7664; FAX. 206/462–6429; Maynard Pohl, O.D., Clinical Director

Pacific Cataract and Laser Institute, 8200 West Grandridge, Kennewick, WA 99336

Pacific Medical Center, 1200 12th Avenue, S., Seventh Floor, Seattle, WA 98144; tel. 206/326–4000, ext. 2469; Carolyn Bodeen, RN, Clinic Director

Pacific NW Facial Plastic Ambulatory Surgery Center, 600 Broadway, Suite 280, Seattle, WA 98122; tel. 206/386–3550; FAX. 206/386–3553

Parkway Surgical Center, 2940 Squalicum Parkway, Suite 204, Bellingham, WA 98225; tel. 206/676–8350; FAX. 206/676–8351; Orville Vandergriend, M.D., Administrator

Physicians Eye Surgical Center, 3930 Hoyt Avenue, Everett, WA 98201; tel. 206/259–2020; Carol Schoenfelder, Administrator

Plastic Surgery Center, 1017 South 40th Avenue, Yakima, WA 98904; tel. 509/966–6000; FAX. 509/966–6565; Julie Marquis, RN, Quality Assurance Manager

Plastic Surgicenter of Olympia, 400 Lilly Road, N.E., Building Four, Olympia, WA 98506; tel. 360/456–4400; FAX. 360/491–7619; Wayne L. Dickason, M.D.

Plastic and Reconstructive Surgeons, 17930 Talbot Road, S., Renton, WA 98055; tel. 206/228–3187; Mack D. Richey, M.D.

Professional Surgical Specialists, 1609 Meridian South, Puyallup, WA 98371; tel. 206/841–1331

Redmond Foot Care Associates, ASC, 16146 Cleveland Street, Redmond, WA 98052; tel. 206/885–7004

Rockwood Clinic, d/b/a Gastrointestinal Endoscopy Unit, Sacred Heart Building, West 105 Eighth Avenue, Suite 7050, Spokane, WA 99204; tel. 509/838–2531; FAX. 509/459–1527; Stephen Burgert, M.D., Administrator

Rockwood Clinic, PS, East 400 Fifth Avenue, Spokane, WA 99202; tel. 509/838–2531; FAX. 509/455–5315; William R. Poppy, Chief Executive Officer, Administrator

Seattle Endoscopy Center, 11027 Meridian Avenue, N., Suite 100, Seattle, WA 98133; tel. 206/363–8502; FAX. 206/365–3456; Patty Carroll, CGRN, Manager

Seattle Eye Plastic Surgery Center, 1229 Madison Street, Suite 1190, Seattle, WA 98104; tel. 206/621–0800; FAX. 206/621–7023; R. Toby Sutcliffe, M.D.

Seattle Hand Surgery Group, P.C., 600 Broadway, Suite 440, Seattle, WA 98122; tel. 206/292–6252; FAX. 206/292–7893; Suzann H. Demianew, Administrator

Seattle Head and Neck Office Surgery, 515 Minor Avenue, Suite 130, Seattle, WA 98104; tel. 206/682–6103; Adrienne C. Peach, RN, Director

Seattle Microsurgical Eyecare Center, 5300 17th Avenue, N.W., Seattle, WA 98107; tel. 206/783–3929; Jack C. Bunn, M.D., Medical Director

Seattle Plastic Surgery Center, 600 Broadway, Suite 320, Seattle, WA 98122; tel. 206/324–1120; FAX. 206/720–0800; Wendy Discher, Manager

Seattle Surgery Center, Columbus Pavilion, 900 Terry Avenue, Fourth Floor, Seattle, WA 98104–1240; tel. 206/382–1021; FAX. 206/382–1026; Naya Kehayes, M.P.H., Administrator

Sequim Same Day Surgery, 777 North Fifth Avenue, Sequim, WA 98382; tel. 360/681–0358; Tammy Paolini, Surgical Technician

South Hill Ambulatory Surgical Center, South 3028 Grand Boulevard, Spokane, WA 99203; tel. 509/747–0279; FAX. 509/747–3220

Southwest Washington Ambulatory Surgery Center, Inc., 416 Northeast 87th Avenue, Vancouver, WA 98664; tel. 206/696–4000; FAX. 206/696–4287

Southwest Washington Ambulatory Surgery Center, Inc., 102 West Fourth Plain Boulevard, Vancouver, WA 98666; tel. 206/696–4400; Kim Fehly

Spokane Digestive Disease Center, 105 West Eighth Avenue, Suite 6010, Spokane, WA 99204–2318; tel. 509/838–5950; FAX. 509/838–5961; Margie Troske–Johnson, RN, B.S.N., Director

Spokane Eye Surgery Center, West 208 Fifth Street, Spokane, WA 99204; tel. 509/456–8150; FAX. 509/455–9887; Donald Ellingsen, M.D.

Spokane Foot and Ankle Surgery Center, 9405 East Sprague Avenue, Spokane, WA 99206; tel. 509/922–3199; Rita Kinney, RN

Spokane Surgery Center, North 1120 Pines Road, Spokane, WA 99206; tel. 509/924–3235; Stewart P. Brim, D.P.M.

St. Mark's Micro Surgical Center, Inc., 502 South M Street, Tacoma, WA 98405; tel. 206/627–8266; Roy Baker, Chief Executive Officer

Stanley M. Jackson, M.D., Plastic and Reconstructive Surgery, 105 27th Avenue, S.E., Puyallup, WA 98374; tel. 206/848–8110; FAX. 206/845–3561; Karen Smith, RN

TLC Northwest Eye, Inc., 10330 Meridian Avenue N., Suite 370, Seattle, WA 98133–9451; tel. 206/528–6000, ext. 114; FAX. 206/528–0014; Wendy R. Williams, Marketing Director

Tacoma Ambulatory Surgery Center, 1112 Sixth Avenue, Suite 100, Tacoma, WA 98405; tel. 206/272–3916, ext. 324; FAX. 206/627–1713; Joan Hoover, Administrator

Tacoma Endoscopy Center, 1112 Sixth Avenue, Suite 200, Tacoma, WA 98405; tel. 206/272–8664; FAX. 206/627–7880; Richard Baerg, M.D., Medical Director

Tacoma Speciality ASU, 209 Martin Luther King Jr. Way, Tacoma, WA 98405; tel. 206/596–3590; Linda Bradley, Manager

The Eastside Endoscopy Center, P.L.L.C., 1700 116th Avenue, N.E., Suite 100, Bellevue, WA 98004–3049; tel. 206/451–7335; FAX. 206/451–7335; Bunny McCormack, RN, Director, Nursing

The Plastic SurgiCentre, Inc., 535 South Pine Street, Spokane, WA 99202; tel. 509/623–2160; FAX. 509/623–1135; Pamala Silvers, RN, Manager

The Polyclinic, Inc., 1145 Broadway, Seattle, WA 98122; tel. 206/329–1760; Lloyd David, Chief Executive Officer

Trenton J. Spolar, 505 Northeast 87th Avenue, Suite 203, Vancouver, WA 98664; tel. 206/254–8596

Valley Outpatient Surgery Center, North 1414 Houk Road, Suite 204, Spokane, WA 99216; tel. 509/922–0362; FAX. 509/927–8316; Dr. Douglas Norquist, President

Valley Surgi Centre, Five South 14th Avenue, Yakima, WA 98902; tel. 509/248–6813; FAX. 509/457–9691

Virginia Mason Clinic South, 33501 First Way South, Federal Way, WA 98003; tel. 206/874–1635; Steve Alley

Virginia Mason–Issaquah, 100 Northeast Gilman Boulevard, Issaquah, WA 98027; tel. 206/557–8000; Bobbie Eatmon, Manager

Washington Orthopaedic Center, Inc., PS, 1900 Cooks Hill Road, Centralia, WA 98531; tel. 360/736–2889, ext. 400; JoAnn Wilkey, Director

Wenatchee Surgical Center, 600 Orondo Avenue, Wenatchee, WA 98807; tel. 509/662–8956; Shirley DeWitz, RN, Manager

Wenatchee Valley Clinic/Cascade Surgery Center, 820 North Chelan, Wenatchee, WA 98801; tel. 509/663–8711; FAX. 509/665–2309; Dr. Don Paugh, Chief, Cascade Surgery Center

Westlake Surgical Center, 509 Olive Way, Third Floor, Seattle, WA 98101; tel. 206/623–4755; Maria T. Burrows, Administrative Assistant

Whidbey SurgiCare, 31775–SR 20, Suite A Two, Oak Harbor, WA 98277–2334; tel. 360/679–3117; FAX. 360/679–3118

Whitehorse Surgical Center, 875 Wesley Street, Suite 160, Arlington, WA 98223; tel. 360/435–6969; FAX. 360/435–1068

WEST VIRGINIA

Anwar Eye Center, 1500 Lafayette Avenue, Moundsville, WV 26041; tel. 304/845–0908; M. F. Anwar, M.D.

☐ **Cabell Huntington Surgery Center,** 1201 Hal Greer Boulevard, Huntington, WV 25701; tel. 304/523–1885; FAX. 304/523–8942; John Stone, Facility Administrator

Section C

Cook Eye Surgery Center, 1300 Third Avenue, Huntington, WV 25701; tel. 304/522-1802; FAX. 304/529-6752; David W. Cook, M.D., President

Jerry N. Black, M.D., Surgical Suite, 10 Amalia Drive, Buckhannon, WV 26201; tel. 304/472-2100; Jerry N. Black, M.D., Medical Director

Kanawha Valley Surgi-Center, 4803 MacCorkle Avenue, S.E., Charleston, WV 25304; tel. 304/925-6390; Gorli Harish, M.D., Medical Director

Lee's Surgi-Center, 415 Morris Street, Suite 200, Charleston, WV 25301; tel. 304/342-1113; FAX. 304/346-2271; Hans Lee, M.D., President

SurgiCare, 3200 MacCorkle Avenue, S.E., Charleston, WV 25304; tel. 304/348-9556; Robert L. Savage, President

West Virginia Surgery Center, Inc., 425 Greenway Avenue, South Charleston, WV 25309; tel. 304/768-7310; FAX. 304/768-8211; Nancy Jo Vinson, Administrator

WISCONSIN

Aurora Health Center, 10400 75th Street, Kenosha, WI 53142; tel. 414/697-6901; FAX. 414/697-3022; Carol Ragalie, Administrator

Bay Lake Surgery Outpatient Surgery Center, Inc., 1843 Michigan Street, P.O. Box 678, Sturgeon Bay, WI 54235; tel. 414/746-1070; FAX. 414/746-1072; Michael Herlache, Administrator

Baycare Surgery Center, 2253 West Mason, P.O. Box 33227, Green Bay, WI 54303-0102; tel. 414/592-9100; FAX. 414/497-6830; Jeff Mason, Administrator

Center for Digestive Health, 2901 West Kinnickinnic River Parkway, Suite 560, Milwaukee, WI 53215; tel. 414/649-3522; FAX. 414/649-5454; Robert Chang, Administrator

Davis Duehr Day Surgery, 1025 Regent Street, Madison, WI 53715; tel. 608/282-2050; Rodney Sturm, M.D., President

Dean St. Mary's Surgery Center, 800 South Brooks Street, Madison, WI 53715; tel. 608/259-3510; FAX. 608/255-1272; Patricia Klitzman, Director

Eau Claire Surgery Center, 950 West Clairemont Avenue, Eau Claire, WI 54701; tel. 715/839-9339; FAX. 715/839-9033; Kathryn Hentz, RN, Facility Manager

Green Bay Surgical Center, Ltd., 704 South Webster Avenue, Green Bay, WI 54301; tel. 414/432-7433; FAX. 414/432-6313; Herbert F. Sandmire, M.D., Medical Director, Administrator

HealthSouth Surgery Center of Wausau, 2809 Westhill Drive, Wausau, WI 54401; tel. 715/842-4490; FAX. 715/842-4645; Kathy Eisenschink, RN, Facility Administrator

Kenosha Surgical Center, Inc., 3505 30th Avenue, Kenosha, WI 53142; tel. 414/656-8638; FAX. 414/656-8631; David Bittner, Business Manager

LaSalle Surgery Center, 1550 Midway Place, Menasha, WI 54952; tel. 414/727-8200; FAX. 414/727-8203; Laura Ruys, Manager

Marshfield Clinic Ambulatory Surgery Center, 1000 North Oak Avenue, Marshfield, WI 54449; tel. 715/387-5315; FAX. 715/387-5240; Robert J. DeVita, Executive Director

Menomonee Falls Ambulatory Surgery Center, W180 N8045 Town Hall Road, Menomonee Falls, WI 53051; tel. 414/250-0950; FAX. 414/250-0955; Robert W. Scheller Jr, CPA, Business Director

Mercy Walworth, ASC, N2950 State Road 67, Lake Geneva, WI 53147; tel. 414/245-0535; Cynthia Job, Administrator

Meriter Ambulatory Surgery Center, 20 South Park Street, Madison, WI 53715; tel. 608/267-6479; FAX. 608/267-6370; Robert L. Coats, President, Chief Operating Officer

North Shore Surgical Center, 7007 North Range Line Road, Milwaukee, WI 53209; tel. 414/352-3341; FAX. 414/352-3218; Robert Lonergan, Executive Director

Northlake Surgery Center, 2110 Medical Drive, Box 636, Menomonee, WI 54751; tel. 715/235-8884; Douglas Carson

Northwest Surgery Center, 2300 North Mayfair Road, Wauwatosa, WI 53226; tel. 414/257-3322; Nancy Jones, Administrator

Oshkosh Surgery Center, 1925 Surgery Center Drive, Oshkosh, WI 54901; tel. 414/233-1233; FAX. 414/233-2101; Jean Cox, Administrator

Riverview Surgery Center, 616 North Washington Street, Janesville, WI 53545; tel. 608/758-7300; FAX. 608/758-1050; Cheryl A. Wilson, Director

Surgery Center of Wisconsin, 10401 West Lincoln Avenue, Suite 201, West Allis, WI 53227; tel. 414/321-7850; Penny Leinbeck, Administrator

Surgicenter of Greater Milwaukee, 3223 South 103rd Street, Milwaukee, WI 53227; tel. 414/328-5800; Raymond E. Grundman, General Manager

Surgicenter of Racine, Ltd., 5802 Washington Avenue, Racine, WI 53406; tel. 414/886-9100; Dennis J. Kontra, Administrator

Wauwatosa Surgery Center, d/b/a HealthSouth Surgery Center of Wauwatosa, 10900 West Potter Road, Wauwatosa, WI 53226-3424; tel. 414/774-9227; FAX. 414/774-0957; Carol Leitinger, RN, B.S.N., CNOR, Administrator

WYOMING

Casper Endoscopy Center, 167 South Conwell, Suite Seven, Casper, WY 82601; tel. 307/262-3896; Robert A. Schlidt, M.D., Administrator

Gem City Bone and Joint Surgery Center, 1909 Vista Drive, Laramie, WY 82070; tel. 307/745-8851; Trent Kaufman, Executive Director

Wyoming Endoscopy Center, 1200 East 20th Street, Cheyenne, WY 82001; tel. 307/635-5439; John W. Beckman

Wyoming Outpatient Services, 5050 Powderhouse Road, Cheyenne, WY 82009; tel. 307/634-1311; FAX. 307/638-6820; Peter Perakos, M.D., Director

Yellowstone Surgery Center, Ltd., 5201 Yellowstone Road, Cheyenne, WY 82009; tel. 307/635-7070; FAX. 307/632-9920; Linnea McNair, RN, B.S.N., Director

---

U. S. Associated Areas

PUERTO RICO

ASC Centro Inst de Gastroenterologia y Endoscopia Las Americas, Suite 206, Hato Rey, PR 00919; tel. 787/764-8787

ASC Espanola Clinic, Box 490, La Quinta, Mayaguez, PR 00681; tel. 787/832-2094

ASC Hato Rey Comm., 435 Ponce de Leon Avenue, Hato Rey, PR 00919; tel. 787/754-0909; FAX. 787/753-1625

ASC Mimiya, P.O. Box 41245, 303 De Diego Avenue, Santurce, PR 00940; tel. 809/721-2590

Arecibo Medical Center, Carr. 2 Km 80.1, Call Box AMC, Arecibo, PR 00613; tel. 809/878-3185

Cirugia Ambulatoria y Centro de Diagnostico y Tratamiento de San Sebastian, Box 486, San Sebastian, PR 00755; tel. 809/896-1850

Clinica de Cirugia Ambulatoria de Puerto Rico, Box 3748, Marina Station, Mayaguez, PR 00681; tel. 787/833-4400; Roberto Ruiz, Asencio, Administrator

Clinica del Turabo, P.O. Box 1900, Caguas, PR 00626; tel. 787/746-8899; FAX. 787/258-1776; Loda A. M. Negron, M.H.S.A.

Instituto Cirugia, Plastica del Oeste, 165 Este Mendez Virgo Street, Mayaguez, PR 00680; tel. 787/833-3248; FAX. 787/831-4400; Mrs. Leonor M. Jaume, Executive Director

Instituto Quirurgico De Un Dia - Dr. Pila, P.O. Box 1910, Ponce, PR 00733; tel. 809/844-5600

Instituto de Ojos y Piel, Carr Three, KM 12.3, Carolina, PR 00985; tel. 809/769-2477

Las Americas Ambulatory Surgical Center, P.O. Box 194236, San Juan, PR 00919-4236; tel. 787/756-8418; FAX. 787/250-8597; Carmen Martin, MHSA, Administrator

OJOS, Inc., Calle Hipodromo, Esquina Las Palmas, Pda. 20, Santurce, PR 00908; tel. 787/721-8330; FAX. 787/722-3222; Maria Delos A. Tirado, Administrator

San Juan Health Centre, 150 De Diego Avenue, Esquina Baldorioty, San Juan, PR 00911; tel. 809/725-0202

Sothern SurgiCenter, Edificio Parra, Ofic. 201, Ponce By Pass, Ponce, PR 00731; tel. 787/841-0303; FAX. 787/841-0387; Roberta Rentas

State Government Agencies for FASC's

United States

ALABAMA
Alabama Department of Public Health, Division of Licensure and Certification, 434 Monroe Street, Montgomery, AL 36130–1701; tel. 334/240–3503; FAX. 334/240–3147; L. O'Neal Green, Director

ALASKA
Health Facilities Licensing and Certification, 4730 Business Park Boulevard, Suite 18, Anchorage, AK 99503–7137; tel. 907/561–8081; FAX. 907/561–3011; Shelbert Larsen, Administrator

ARIZONA
Arizona Department of Health Services, Health and Child Care Review Services, 1647 East Morten, Suite 220, Phoenix, AZ 85020; tel. 602/255–1221; FAX. 602/255–1108; John Zemaitis, Assistant Director

ARKANSAS
Department of Health, Division of Health Facility Services, 5800 West 10th Street, Suite 400, Little Rock, AR 72204–9916; tel. 501/661–2201; FAX. 501/661–2165; Valetta Buck, Director

CALIFORNIA
Department of Health Services, Licensing and Certification Division, 1800 Third Street, Suite 210, P.O. Box 942732, Sacramento, CA 94234–7320; tel. 916/445–2070; FAX. 916/445–6979; Michael Rodrian, Branch Manager

COLORADO
Department of Health, Division of Health Facilities, 4210 East 11th Avenue, Denver, CO 80220; tel. 303/331–6600; FAX. 303/331–6559; Diane Carter, Deputy, Director

CONNECTICUT
Department of Health and Addiction Services, Hospital and Medical Care Division, 150 Washington Street, Hartford, CT 06106; tel. 203/566–1073; FAX. 203/566–1097; Elizabeth M. Burns, RN, M.S., Director

DELAWARE
Department of Health and Social Services, Licensing and Certification, Office of Health Facilities, 3000 Newport Gap Pike, Wilmington, DE 19808; tel. 302/995–6674; FAX. 302/995–8332; Ellen T. Reap, Director

DISTRICT OF COLUMBIA
Department of Consumer and Regulatory Affairs, Service Facility Regulation Administration, 614 H Street, N.W., Suite 1003, Washington, DC 20001; tel. 202/727–7190; FAX. 202/727–7780; Geraldine K. Sykes

FLORIDA
Division of Health Quality Assurance, Agency for Health Care Administration, Fort Knox Executive Office Center, 2727 Mahan Drive, Suite 214, Tallahassee, FL 32308–5407; tel. 904/487–2527; FAX. 904/487–6240; Gloria Crawford–Henderson, Director

GEORGIA
Health Care Section, Office of Regulatory Services, Department of Human Resources, Two Peachtree Street, N.W., Suite 19.204, Atlanta, GA 30303–3167; tel. 404/657–5550; FAX. 404/657–8934; Susie M. Woods, Director

HAWAII
Hawaii Department of Health, Hospital and Medical Facilities Branch, P.O. Box 3378, Honolulu, HI 96801; tel. 808/586–4080; FAX. 808/586–4747; Helen K. Yoshimi, B.S.N., M.P.H., Chief, HMFB

IDAHO
Bureau of Facility Standards, Department of Health and Welfare, P.O. Box 83720, Boise, ID 83720–0036; tel. 208/334–6626; FAX. 208/332–7204; Sylvia Creswell, Supervisor–Non Long Term Care

ILLINOIS
Department of Public Health, Division of Health Care Facilities and Programs, 525 West Jefferson Street, Springfield, IL 62761; tel. 217/782–7412; FAX. 217/782–0382; Michelle Gentry–Wiseman, Chief

INDIANA
Indiana State Department of Health, Division of Acute Care, Two North Meridian Street, Indianapolis, IN 46204; tel. 317/233–7472; FAX. 317/233–7157; John A. Braeckel, Director

IOWA
Department of Inspection and Appeals, Division of Health Facilities, Lucas State Office Building, Des Moines, IA 50319; tel. 515/281–4115; FAX. 515/242–5022; J. Bennett, Administrator

KANSAS
Kansas Department of Health and Environment, Bureau of Adult and Child Care, 900 Southwest Jackson, Suite 1001, Topeka, KS 66612–1290; tel. 913/296–1280; FAX. 913/296–1266; George A. Dugger, Medical Facilities Certification Administrator

KENTUCKY
Cabinet for Health Services, Division of Licensing and Regulation, C.H.R. Building, 275 East Main Street, 4th Floor East, Frankfort, KY 40621; tel. 502/564–2800; FAX. 502/564–6546; Rebecca J. Cecil, Director

LOUISIANA
Department of Health and Hospitals, Bureau of Health Services Financing–Health Standards Section, P.O. Box 3767, Baton Rouge, LA 70821; tel. 504/342–0138; FAX. 504/342–5292; Lily W. McAlister, RN, Manager

MAINE
Division of Licensing and Certification, Department of Human Services, 35 Anthony Avenue, Station 11, Augusta, ME 04333; tel. 207/624–5443; FAX. 207/624–5378; Louis Dorogi, Director

MARYLAND
Department of Health and Mental Hygiene, Office of Licensing and Certification, 4201 Patterson Avenue, Baltimore, MD 21215; tel. 410/764–4980; FAX. 410/764–5969

MASSACHUSETTS
Department of Public Health, Division of Health Care Quality, 80 Boylston Street, Suite 1100, Boston, MA 02116; tel. 617/727–5860; Irene McManus, Director

MICHIGAN
Department of Public Health, Division of Licensing and Certification, 3500 North Logan, Lansing, MI 48909; tel. 517/335–8505; Pauline DeRose

MINNESOTA
Department of Health, Facility and Provider Compliance Division, Licensing and Certification Section, 393 North Dunlap Street, P.O. Box 64900, St. Paul, MN 55164–0900; tel. 612/643–2130; FAX. 612/643–3534; Carol Hirschfeld, Supervisor, Records and Information Unit

MISSISSIPPI
Department of Health, Division of Health Facilities Licensure and Certification, P.O. Box 1700, Jackson, MS 39215; tel. 601/354–7300; FAX. 601/354–7230; Vanessa Phipps, Director

MISSOURI
Missouri Department of Health, Bureau of Hospital Licensing and Certification, P.O. Box 570, Jefferson City, MO 65102; tel. 573/751–6302; FAX. 573/526–3621; Darrell Hendrickson, Administrator

MONTANA
Health Facilities Division, Department of Health and Environmental Sciences, Cogswell Building, Helena, MT 59620; tel. 406/444–2037; FAX. 406/444–1742; Denzel C. Davis, Division Administrator

NEBRASKA
Health Facility Licensure and Inspection Section, Nebraska Department of Health, 301 Centennial Mall, S., P.O. Box 95007, Lincoln, NE 68509–5007; tel. 402/471–2946; FAX. 402/471–0555; Frederick M. Wright, Section Administrator

NEVADA
Bureau of Licensure & Certification, Nevada Health Divison, 505 East King Street, Suite 202, Carson City, NV 89710; tel. 702/687–4475; FAX. 702/687–5751; Sharon M. Ezell, Chief

NEW HAMPSHIRE
Office of Program Support, Licensing and Regulation, Six Hazen Drive, Concord, NH 03301; tel. 603/271–4592; FAX. 603/271–3745

NEW JERSEY
Division of Health Systems Analysis, Certificate of Need and Acute Licensing, CN–360, Trenton, NJ 08625; tel. 609/292–5960; FAX. 609/588–7823; Darcy Saunders, Esq., Director

NEW MEXICO
Department of Health and Environment, Health Facility Licensing and Certification Bureau, 525 Camino de los Marquez, Suite Two, Santa Fe, NM 87501; tel. 505/727–4200; FAX. 505/827–4222; Sue K. Morris, Chief, Licensing and Certification Bureau

NEW YORK
Health Education Services, P.O. Box 7126, Albany, NY 12224; tel. 518/439–7286; FAX. 518/439–7286

NORTH CAROLINA
Department of Human Resources, Division of Facility Services, 701 Barbour Drive, P.O. Box 29530, Raleigh, NC 27626–0530; tel. 919/733–1610; FAX. 919/733–3207; Steve White, Chief, Licensure and Certification

NORTH DAKOTA
North Dakota Department of Health, Health Resources Section, 600 East Boulevard Avenue, Bismarck, ND 58505–0200; tel. 701/328–2352; FAX. 701/328–4727; Fred Gladden, Chief

OHIO
Division of Quality Assurance, Ohio Department of Health, 246 North High Street, Columbus, OH 43266–0588; tel. 614/466–7857; FAX. 614/644–0208; Rebecca Maust, Chief

OKLAHOMA
Department of Health, Special Health Services, 1000 Northeast 10th Street, P.O. Box 53551, Oklahoma City, OK 73152; tel. 405/271–6576; FAX. 405/271–3442; Gary Glover, Chief, Medical Facilities

OREGON
  Health Care Licensure and Certification, Oregon Health Division, 800 Northeast Oregon Street, Suite 640, # 21, Portland, OR 97232; tel. 503/731–4013; FAX. 503/731–4080; Kathleen Smail, Manager

PENNSYLVANIA
  Bureau of Quality Assurance, Division of Acute and Ambulatory Care Facilities, Health and Welfare Building, Suite 532, Harrisburg, PA 17120; tel. 717/783–8980; FAX. 717/772–2163; William White, Director

RHODE ISLAND
  Rhode Island Department of Health, Division of Facilities Regulation, Three Capitol Hill, Providence, RI 02908–5097; tel. 401/277–2566; FAX. 401/277–3999; Wayne I. Farrington, Chief

SOUTH CAROLINA
  Department of Health and Environmental Control, Division of Health Licensing, 2600 Bull Street, Columbia, SC 29201; tel. 803/737–7202; FAX. 803/737–7212; Alan Samuels, Director

SOUTH DAKOTA
  Department of Health, Office of Health Care Facilities, Licensure and Certification, 445 East Capitol, Pierre, SD 57501; tel. 605/773–3356; Joan Bachman, Administrator

TENNESSEE
  Department of Health, Division of Health Care Facilities, Cordell Hull Building, First Floor, 426 Fifth Avenue, N., Nashville, TN 37247–0508; tel. 615/741–7221; Marie Fitzgerald, Director

TEXAS
  Department of Health, Health Facility Licensure and Certification Division, 8407 Wall Street, Zip 78754, 1100 West 49th Street, Austin, TX 78756; tel. 512/834–6650; FAX. 512/834–6653; Nance Stearman, RN, M.S.N., Director

UTAH
  Utah Department of Health, Bureau of Health Facility Licensure, P.O. Box 16990, Salt Lake City, UT 84116–0990; tel. 801/538–6152; FAX. 801/538–6325; Debra Wynkoop–Green, Director

VERMONT
  Department of Aging and Disability, 103 South Main Street, Waterbury, VT 05676; tel. 802/241–2345

VIRGINIA
  Virginia Department of Health, Office of Health Facilities Regulation, 3600 Centre, Suite 216, 3600 West Broad Street, Richmond, VA 23230; tel. 804/367–2102; FAX. 804/367–2149; Nancy R. Hofheimer, Director

WASHINGTON
  Washington Department of Health, Facilities and Services Licensing, Target Plaza, Suite 500, 2725 Harrison Avenue N.W., P.O. Box 47852, Olympia, WA 98504–7852; tel. 360/705–6780; FAX. 360/705–6654; Byron R. Plan, Manager

WEST VIRGINIA
  Office of Health Facility Licensure and Certification, West Virginia Division of Health, 1900 Kanawha Boulevard, E., Charleston, WV 25305; tel. 304/558–0050; FAX. 304/588–2515; Jeannie Miller, Program Administrator

WISCONSIN
  Bureau of Quality Assurance, Division of Supportive Living, Department of Health and Family Services, P.O. Box 309, Madison, WI 53701; tel. 608/267–7185; FAX. 608/267–0352; Judy Fryback, Director, Bureau of Quality Assurance

WYOMING
  Wyoming Department of Health, Health Facilities Licensing, Metropolitan Bank Building, Eighth Floor, Cheyenne, WY 82001; tel. 307/777–7123; FAX. 307/777–5970; Charlie Simineo, Program Manager

U. S. Associated Areas

PUERTO RICO
  Department of Health, P. O. Box 70184, San Juan, PR 00936; tel. 809/766–1616; FAX. 809/766–2240; Carmen Feliciano de Melecio, M.D., Secretary of Health

Section C

Freestanding Hospices

The following list of freestanding hospices was developed with the assistance of state government agencies and the individual facilities listed. The list is current as of January 1, 1997. For a complete list of hospital based hospice programs please refer to Section A. In Section A, hospice programs are identified by Facility Code F33.

We present this list simply as a convenient directory. Inclusion or omission of any organization's name indicates neither approval nor disapproval by Healthcare InfoSource, Inc., a subsidiary of the American Hospital Association.

United States

ALABAMA

Alacare Hospice, 1945 Hoover Court, Birmingham, AL 35226; tel. 205/823–7081, ext. 8605; FAX. 205/956–8021; Jackie Lawrence, Director, Hospice, Palliative Care

BHS Hospice–Walker, Medical Arts Tower, Suite 215, Jasper, AL 35502; tel. 205/387–4514; FAX. 205/387–4888; Frances Glenn, Director

Baptist Hospice, 2055 Normandie Drive, Suite 214, Montgomery, AL 36111; tel. 334/286–3321; Mark Johnson

Birmingham Area Hospice, 1400 Sixth Avenue, S., P.O. Box 2648, Birmingham, AL 35233; tel. 205/930–1330; FAX. 205/930–1390; Flora Y. Blackledge, Director

Chattahoochee Hospice, Inc., 604 Cusseta Road, Valley, AL 36854; tel. 334/756–8043; FAX. 334/756–8059; Judy Guin, RN, Administrator

Columbia Community Hospice, Six East Court Square, Andalusia, AL 36420; tel. 334/222–2172; Charlotte Parker

Community Hospice of Baldwin County, 1113B North McKenzie Street, Foley, AL 36535; tel. 334/943–5015; Matthew Bowdoin, Administrator

Health Services East, Inc., Hospice Care, 7916 Second Avenue, S., Birmingham, AL 35206; tel. 205/838–5730; FAX. 205/838–5757; Jeff Johnson, Director, Home Care Services

Hospice Care, Division of St. Clair Care, A Hospice, Inc., 17 Lake Plaza, P.O. Box 544, Pell City, AL 35125; tel. 205/884–1111; FAX. 205/884–1114; Nancy Odom, Director

Hospice of Blount County, Inc., 204 Washington Avenue, E., Oneonta, AL 35121; tel. 205/274–0549; FAX. 205/274–0550; Debbie Hyde

Hospice of Cullman County, Inc., 402 Fourth Avenue, N.E., P.O. Box 1227, Cullman, AL 35055; tel. 205/739–5185; Jackie H. Cook

Hospice of EAMC, 459 North Dean Road, Auburn, AL 36830; tel. 334/826–1899; Nancy A. Penaskovic

Hospice of East Alabama, Inc., 825 Keith Avenue, Anniston, AL 36207; tel. 205/236–5334; FAX. 205/231–4558; Jeannie Stanko, RN, M.S.N., Executive Director

Hospice of Huntsville, Inc., 806 Governors Drive, Suite 202, Huntsville, AL 35801; tel. 205/536–1889; FAX. 205/536–9541; Jim Higgins, Executive Director

Hospice of Limestone County, 405 South Marion Street, P.O. Box 626, Athens, AL 35612; tel. 205/232–5017; FAX. 205/230–0085; Patricia P. Jackson, Administrator

Hospice of Marshall County, 8787 U.S. Highway 431, Albertville, AL 35950; tel. 205/891–7724; FAX. 205/891–7754; Rhonda Floyd, RN, B.S.N., OCN, CRNH, Executive Director

Hospice of Montgomery, 1111 Holloway Park, Montgomery, AL 36117; tel. 334/279–6677; FAX. 334/277–2223; Clare W. Lacey, Executive Director

Hospice of Northeast Alabama, a Member of the Baptist Health System, 112 College Street, P.O. Box 981, Scottsboro, AL 35768; tel. 205/574–4622; FAX. 205/259–3772; Virginia Stone, Director

Hospice of Northwest Alabama, 40 First Avenue East, P.O. Box 1216, Winfield, AL 35594; tel. 205/487–8140; FAX. 205/487–8740; Linda Martin Sewell, Executive Director

Hospice of West Alabama, 1800 McFarland Boulevard, N., Suite 310, Tuscaloosa, AL 35406; tel. 205/345–0067; FAX. 205/345–9806; Julie Sittason, Executive Director

Hospice of the Shoals, Inc., 1106 Bradshaw Drive, P.O. Box 307, Florence, AL 35630–0000; tel. 205/767–6699; FAX. 205/767–3116; Blake Edwards, Executive Director

Hospice of the Valley, Inc., 216 Johnston Street, S.E., P.O. Box 2745, Decatur, AL 35602; tel. 205/350–5585; FAX. 205/350–5567; Carolyn Dobson, Executive Director

Huntsville Hospice Cares, Inc., 509 Madison Street, Huntsville, AL 35801–4206; tel. 205/534–1095; FAX. 205/534–1096; Florence M. Helman, Executive Director

Huntsville Hospice Cares, Inc., 2225 Drake Avenue, S.W., Suite 14, Huntsville, AL 35805; tel. 205/880–9898; FAX. 205/880–2929

Mercy Medical Hospice–Mobile, 3712 Dauphin Street, Mobile, AL 36608–5917; tel. 334/344–7126; FAX. 334/304–3012; Cheryl Robinson, Medical Program Manager

Providence Hospice of Seton Home Health Services, 6051 Airport Boulevard, Building B, Suite Two, Mobile, AL 36608; tel. 334/344–2234; FAX. 334/344–4642; Katherine Bradshaw, Director

Saad's Hospice Services, Inc., 3725 Airport Boulevard, Suite 180, Mobile, AL 36608; tel. 334/343–9600; FAX. 334/380–3328; Barbara S. Fulgham

Southern Hospice Care, Inc., 2663 Valleydale Road, Suite 334, Birmingham, AL 35244; tel. 205/408–2933; Michael J. Pardy

St. Vincent's Hospice, 2112 11th Avenue, S., Suite 335, Birmingham, AL 35205; tel. 205/252–9727; Sue Cacioppo

Tombigbee Hospice, Inc., 1448 22nd Avenue, Tuscaloosa, AL 35401; tel. 205/366–9681; FAX. 205/652–5212; Bobby T. Williams, Ph.D., M.B.A., Chief Executive Officer

Tombigbee Hospice, Inc., 2608 Eighth Street, Tuscaloosa, AL 35401; tel. 205/345–2696; Dr. Bobby T. Williams

Tombigbee Inpatient Hospice, 1406 East Pushmataha Street, Butler, AL 36904; tel. 334/459–5506; Bobby T. Williams, Ph.D., Administrator

Wiregrass Hospice, Inc., Post Office Drawer 2127, Dothan, AL 36301; tel. 334/794–9101; FAX. 334/794–0009; Ray L. Shrout, Administrator

Wiregrass Hospice, Inc., 557 Colony Square, Suite Five and Six, Glover Avenue, Enterprise, AL 36330; tel. 334/347–3353; FAX. 334/347–7349; Donna Mosholder, RN, PCC

ALASKA

Alaska Home Health Care Agency, Inc., 1200 Airport Heights, Suite 170, Anchorage, AK 99508; tel. 907/272–0018; FAX. 907/272–0014; Lawrence Smith, Title Company President

Hospice of Anchorage, 3305 Arctic Road, Suite 105, Anchorage, AK 99503; tel. 907/561–5322; FAX. 907/561–0334; Paula McCarron

Hospice of Mat–Su, 950 East Bogard Road, Suite 133, Wasilla, AK 99654; tel. 907/352–2845; FAX. 907/352–2844; Donna J. Harding, Director

ARIZONA

Community Hospice, 4330 North Campbell Avenue, Suite 256, Tucson, AZ 85718; tel. 520/544–2273; FAX. 520/577–8862; Bonnie Lindstrom

Community Hospice, 340 East Palm Lane, Suite 150, Phoenix, AZ 85004; tel. 602/252–2273; FAX. 602/254–6166; Dan Johnson, Interim Executive Director

Dignita Home Hospice, 202 East Earll Drive, Suite 478, Phoenix, AZ 85012; tel. 602/279–0677; FAX. 602/279–1085; Gary Polsky

FHP Hospice, 540 West Iron, Suite 110, Mesa, AZ 85210; tel. 602/244–8200; Donna O'Brien

Hospice Family Care, 3443 East Fort Lowell Road, Tucson, AZ 85716; tel. 520/323–3288; FAX. 520/323–6557; Dan Johnson

Hospice Family Care Inpatient Unit, 5037 East Broadway Road, Mesa, AZ 85206; tel. 602/807–2655; FAX. 602/807–2660; Donna Jazz

Hospice Family Care Inpatient Unit–Santa Rita, 150 North La Canada Drive, Green Valley, AZ 85614; tel. 520/648–3099; Nancy Smith

Hospice Family Care Inpatient Unit–Sonora, 1920 West Rudasill, Tucson, AZ 85704; tel. 602/797–3442; Nancy Smith

Hospice Family Care, Inc., 7330 North 16th Street, Suite A100, Phoenix, AZ 85020; tel. 602/331–9200; FAX. 602/331–9222; Vicki Moscow, Regional Public Relations Coordinator

Hospice Family Care, Inc., 10240 West Bell Road, Suite E, Sun City, AZ 85351; tel. 602/876–9100; Vicki Mascaro, Regional Public Relations Coordinator

Hospice Family Care, Inc., 1125 East Southern Avenue, Suite 202, Mesa, AZ 85204; tel. 602/926–6089; Don Johnson

Hospice Family Care, Inc. Green Valley Program, 210 West Continental Road, Suite 134, Green Valley, AZ 85614; tel. 520/648–6166; FAX. 520/648–6165; Karen Hoefle

Hospice Family Care–Greenfield Inpatient Unit, 13617 North 55th Avenue, Glendale, AZ 85304; tel. 602/547–9939; Mike Reimann

Hospice of Arizona, 7600 North 15th Street, Suite 165, Phoenix, AZ 85020; tel. 602/678–1313; FAX. 602/678–5220; Jerene Maierle

Hospice of Havasu, 1685 Mesquite Avenue, Suite I, Lake Havasu City, AZ 86403; tel. 520/453–2111; FAX. 520/453–3003; Nancy Iannone, Administrator

Hospice of Yuma, 1824 South Eighth Avenue, Yuma, AZ 85364; tel. 602/343–2222; FAX. 602/343–0688; Phyllis K. Swanson, Executive Director

Hospice of the Valley, 1510 East Flower Street, Phoenix, AZ 85014; tel. 602/530–6900; FAX. 602/530–6901; Susan Goldwater, Executive Director

Hospice of the Valley Gardiner Hospice Home, 1522 West Myrtle Avenue, Phoenix, AZ 85021; tel. 602/995–9323; Susan Goldwater, Executive Director

In Home Health Hospice, 4600 South Mill Avenue, Suite 170, Tempe, AZ 85282; tel. 602/839–5686; FAX. 602/839–3872; Walter Bendick, Director

Jacob C. Fruchthendler Jewish Community Hospice, 5100 East Grant Road, P.O. Box 13090, Tucson, AZ 85732–3090; tel. 602/881–5300; FAX. 602/322–3620; Jo Turnbull, RN, B.S.

LHS Home and Community Care–Hospice, 325 East Elliot Road, Suite 27, Chandler, AZ 85225; tel. 602/497–5535; FAX. 602/497–8250; Jennifer P. Huppenthal, Executive Director

Mt. Graham Community Hospital–Hospice Services, 1600 20th Avenue, Building E, Safford, AZ 85546; tel. 520/348–4045; FAX. 520/428–3868; Carol Bradford, Clinical Coordinator

Northern Arizona/Cottonwood, 203 South Candy Lane, Suite Two–B, Cottonwood, AZ 86326; tel. 520/634–2251; Renate Atkins

Northland Hospice, 702 North Beaver, P.O. Box 997, Flagstaff, AZ 86001; tel. 520/779–1227; FAX. 520/779–5884; Marilyn J. Pate, Executive Director

Olsten Kimberly Qualitycare Hospice, 711 East Missouri, Suite 140, Phoenix, AZ 85014; tel. 602/279–9898; FAX. 602/279–2019

RTA Hospice, 107 East Frontier, Payson, AZ 85541; tel. 602/472–6340, ext. 12; FAX. 602/472–6464; Vicki Dietz, RN, B.S.N., Executive Director

RTA Hospice, Inc., 177 West Cottonwood Lane, Suite 10, Casa Grande, AZ 85222; tel. 520/421–7143; FAX. 520/421–7315; Hope A. Hood, Patient Care Administrator

Samaritan Hospice, 2222 South Dobson Road, Suite 401, Mesa, AZ 85202; tel. 602/835–0711; FAX. 602/730–6078; Sandra Rose Simmons

Special Care Hospice, 1514 C Gold Rush Road, Suite 236, Bullhead City, AZ 86442; tel. 602/758–3800; FAX. 602/758–4403; Jayne Knox, Director

Sun Health Hospice, 13101 North 103rd Avenue, Sun City, AZ 85351; tel. 602/974–7819; FAX. 602/974–7894; Marlene Stolz, Acting Director

Vista Hospice Care, Inc., 6991 East Camelback Road, Suite C–250, Scottsdale, AZ 85251; tel. 602/945–2200; Roseanne Berry

ARKANSAS

Area Agency of Aging Hospice of West Central Arkansas, 103 West Parkway Drive, Suite Two A, Russellville, AR 72801; tel. 501/967–9300; Oren Yates, Program Administrator

Area Agency on Aging Hospice of Western Arkansas, 524 Garrison Avenue, P.O. Box 1724, Fort Smith, AR 72902; tel. 501/783–4500; FAX. 501/783–0029; Jim Medley, Executive Director

Area Agency on Aging of Southeast Arkansas Hospice Two, 529 West Trotter, P.O. Box 722, Monticello, AR 71655; tel. 501/367–9873; Betty Bradshaw, Administrator

Area Agency on Aging of Southeast Arkansas, Inc. Hospice, 709 East Eighth Avenue, P.O. Box 8569, Pine Bluff, AR 71611; tel. 501/534–3268; Betty Bradshaw, President, Chief Executive Officer

Area Agency on Aging of Western Arkansas, Inc., Mena Hospice, 600 Seventh Street, Mena, AR 71953; tel. 501/394–5458; FAX. 501/394–7675; Mary Keith, RNC, Vice President

Area Agency on Aging of Western Arkansas, Inc., d/b/a Visiting Nurses Agency of Western Arkansas, Inc., 389 School Street, Winslow, AR 72959; tel. 501/634–3812; Jim Medley, Executive Director

Area Three Hospice, Faulkner County Health Unit, 811 North Creek Drive, P.O. Box 1726, Conway, AR 72032; tel. 501/450–4941; FAX. 501/450–4946; John Selig, Administrator

Ark La Tex Visiting Nurses, Inc., d/b/a Ark La Tex Home Health and Hospice Care, 421 Hickory Street, Texarkana, AR 71854; tel. 501/772–0958; Debbie Turner, Director of Nursing

Arkansas Department of Health Hospice 10, 40 Allen Chapel Road, P.O. Box 4267, Batesville, AR 72503; tel. 501/251–2848; FAX. 501/251–3449; Susan Coleman, Hospice Specialist

Arkansas Department of Health Hospice Five, Miller County Health Unit, 1007 Jefferson Avenue, Texarkana, AR 75502; tel. 501/773–2108; John Selig, Administrator

Arkansas Department of Health Hospice Four, 301 East McNeil, Benton, AR 72015; tel. 501/776–1606; FAX. 501/776–5654; John Selig, Administrator

Arkansas Department of Health Hospice Nine West, Monroe County Health Unit, 306 West King Drive, Brinkley, AR 72021; tel. 501/734–1461; FAX. 501/734–1024; John Selig, Administrator

Arkansas Department of Health Hospice Six, Area Six Office, Highway 167 South, P.O. Drawer E, Hampton, AR 71744; tel. 501/798–3113; John Selig, Administrator

Arkansas Department of Health–Hospice Area Nine, Crittenden County Health Unit, 901 North Seventh, West Memphis, AR 72301; tel. 501/735–4334; FAX. 501/735–1393; John Selig, Administrator

Baptist Health, d/b/a Baptist Hospice, 11900 Colonel Glenn Road, Suite 2300, Little Rock, AR 72210; tel. 501/223–7494; FAX. 501/223–7443; Becky Pryor, Administrator

Baptist Memorial Regional Home Health Care, d/b/a Arkansas Home Health and Hospice, 824 North Washington, P.O. Box 90, Forrest City, AR 72335; tel. 501/633–6184; Gary Hughes, Administrator

Baptist Memorial Regional Home Health Care, Inc., d/b/a Arkansas Home Health and Hospice–West Memphis, 310 Mid–Continent Building, Suite 400, P.O. Box 2013, West Memphis, AR 72303; tel. 501/735–0363; FAX. 501/735–7156; Gary Hughes, Administrator

Best Care Hospice Services, 4425 Jefferson, Suite 115, Texarkana, AR 75502; tel. 501/773–4671; Patricia Stevens, Administrator

CareNetwork, Inc., d/b/a CareNetwork Hospice of Rogers, 1227 West Walnut, Rogers, AR 72756; tel. 501/636–1700; Barry Solomon, Administrator

CareNetwork, Inc., d/b/a CareNetwork of Hot Springs Hospice, 2212 Malvern, Suite 3, Hot Springs, AR 71901; tel. 501/623–5656; Cheryl Drake, Director, Hospice Services

CareNetwork, Inc., d/b/a CareNetwork Hospice of Little Rock, 9712 West Markham, Little Rock, AR 72205; tel. 501/223–3333; FAX. 501/228–0252; Barry Solomon, Administrator

CareNetwork, Inc., d/b/a CareNetwork Hospice of Fort Smith, Central Mall, Suite 600, Fort Smith, AR 72903; tel. 501/484–7273; Barny Solomon, Administrator

Central Arkansas Area Agency on Aging, d/b/a Hospice of Central Arkansas, 706 West Fourth Street, P.O. Box 5988, North Little Rock, AR 72119; tel. 501/372–5300, ext. 223; FAX. 501/688–7443; Beth Landon, Director

County Medical Services of Arkansas, Inc., d/b/a Eastern Ozarks Home Health and Hospice, Route Two, Box 79, Hardy, AR 72542; tel. 501/856–3241; Norman Steinig, Administrator

Hospice Care for Southeast Arkansas, Inc., d/b/a Hospice Care Services, 2214 South Blake, Pine Bluff, AR 71603; tel. 501/534–4847; Bud Millenbaugh

Hospice Home Care, Inc., Prospect Building, 1501 North University Avenue, Suite 340, Little Rock, AR 72207; tel. 501/666–9697; FAX. 501/666–4616; Cecilia Troppoli, Administrator

Hospice of Cherokee Village, Inc., 13 Minentonka, P.O. Box 986, Cherokee Village, AR 72525; tel. 501/257–3108; Sally Lindemood, Administrator

Hospice of Preferred Choice, Inc., d/b/a Fort Smith Community Hospice, 1115 South Waldron, Suite 108, Fort Smith, AR 72903; tel. 501/478–3200; Jim Petrus, Administrator

Hospice of St. Michael Health Care Center, 300 East Fifth Street, Texarkana, AR 75502; tel. 501/779–2720; Steven F. Wright, Administrator

Hospice of Texarkana, 122 East Broad Street, Suite 207, P.O. Box 2341, Texarkana, AR 75502; tel. 501/773–1899; Cynthia L. Marsh, Administrator

Jonesboro Health Services, L.L.C., d/b/a Methodist Hospital of Jonesboro Hospice, Forrest City, 815 North Washington, P.O. Box 1388, Forrest City, AR 72335; tel. 501/633–8977; Phillip H. Walkley Jr., FACHE, Chief Executive Officer

Leo N. Levi National Arthritis Hospital Hospice, 300 Prospect Avenue, Hot Springs AR 71901, P.O. Box 850, Hot Springs, AR 71902; tel. 501/624–1281, ext. 416; FAX. 501/622–3500; Patrick G. McCabe, Jr., Administrator

Northwest Health System, Inc., Circle of Life Hospice, 205 Northwest A Street, P.O. Box 1169, Bentonville, AR 72712; tel. 501/273–3658; FAX. 501/273–9080; Gail Hubbell, Hospice Manager

Share Foundation, d/b/a Community Hospice, 516 West Faulkner, El Dorado, AR 71730; tel. 501/862–0337; FAX. 501/862–0727; Linda D. Stringfellow, Administrator

Texarkana Memorial Hospital, Inc., d/b/a Wadley Care Source Hospice, 718 East Fifth Street, Texarkana, AR 71854; tel. 903/798–7660; FAX. 903/798–7667; Hugh R. Hallgren, President, Chief Executive Officer

Visiting Nurses Agency of Western Arkansas, Inc., 207 College Avenue, Clarksville, AR 72830; tel. 501/754–8280; Lois Phillips, RNC, Regional Nursing Supervisor

Washington Regional Medical Center Hospice, 4209 Frontage Road, Fayetteville, AR 72703; tel. 501/442–1000; Patrick D. Flynn, Administrator

CALIFORNIA

AIDS Hospice Foundation, 1300 Scott Boulevard, Los Angeles, CA 90026; tel. 213/482–2500; FAX. 213/962–8513; Tay Aston, Cesar Mier, Admissions Officers

All Nations Hospice, Inc., 3325 Wilshire Boulevard, Los Angeles, CA 90010; tel. 213/738–9741; Ugochi Obuge, Chief Executive Officer

Allied Home Health and Hospice, 1916 Orange Tree Lane, Suite 450–E, Redlands, CA 92374; tel. 909/798–8006; Ruth R. Jackson

Alternative Health Care Inc., Home Health and Hospice, 21601 Devonshire Street, Suite 215, Chatsworth, CA 91311; tel. 818/998–0525; FAX. 818/998–2529; John Teige

American Home Health Hospice, 1800 East McFadden Avenue, Suite 100, Santa Ana, CA 92705; tel. 714/550–0800; FAX. 714/550–0521; Marylyn A. Hagerty, Chief Executive Officer

American Home Health Hospice, 245 East Main Street, Suite 118, Alhambra, CA 91801; tel. 818/457–9825; Kim Loan To

Assisted Home Hospice, 16909 Parthenia Street, Suite 201, North Hills, CA 91343; tel. 818/894–8117; FAX. 818/894–8707; Sherry Netherland, M.A., Executive Director, Hospice

Avalon Home Health Services, Inc., 9608 Van Nuys Boulevard, Suite 209, Panorama, CA 91046; tel. 818/830–5898; Anatoly Smolyansky

Care One Health Center, 1252 Turley Street, Riverside, CA 92501; tel. 909/780–5455; Viola Delphine Donton

Carl Bean House, 2146 West Adams Boulevard, Los Angeles, CA 90018; tel. 213/766–2326; FAX. 213/730–8244; Roland Palencia, Executive Director

Casa Encino, 4600 Woodley Avenue, Encino, CA 91316; tel. 818/905–8625; Ronald Morgan

Children's Homecare–Hospice, 9550 Chesapeake Drive, Suite 201, San Diego, CA 92123; tel. 619/495–4941; James Rodisch, Director

Community Home Care Services/Hospice, 1925 East Dakota, Suite 208, Fresno, CA 93726; tel. 209/221–5615; FAX. 209/221–5798; Jami L. de Santigo, Service Integrator

Community Hospice Care–Orange County, 333 South Anita Drive, Suite 950, Orange, CA 92668; tel. 714/921–2273

Community Hospice of the Bay Area, d/b/a Hospice by the Bay, 1540 Market Street, Suite 350, San Francisco, CA 94102–6035; tel. 415/626–5900; FAX. 415/626–7800; Constance L. Borden, Executive Director

Community Hospice, Inc., 601 McHenry Avenue, Modesto, CA 95350; tel. 209/577–0615; FAX. 209/577–0738; Harold A. Peterson III, Executive Director

Community Hospice–San Diego, 8880 Rio San Diego Drive, Suite 950, San Diego, CA 92108; tel. 619/280–2273; Catherine Estherfeld, RN

Companion Hospice, 12072 Trask Avenue, Suite 100, Garden Grove, CA 92643; tel. 714/741–0953; FAX. 714/534–0998; Michael Uranga, Administrator

Compassionate Care Hospice of San Francisco, L.P., 785 Market Street, Suite 850, San Francisco, CA 94103; tel. 415/979–0925; Victoria A. Condon

Coordinated Hospice, 13800 Arizona Street, Suite 202, Westminster, CA 92683; tel. 714/898–7106; FAX. 714/898–0407; Kay Donald, Hospice Manager

Covina Health Care Center, 5109 North Greer, Covina, CA 91724; tel. 818/339–9460; Rajinder Kutty

Crossroads Home Health Care and Hospice, Inc., 320 Judah Street, Suite Seven, San Francisco, CA 94122; tel. 415/682–2111; Virginia A. Kahn

Elizabeth Hospice, l845 East Valley Parkway, Escondido, CA 92027; tel. 619/737–2050; FAX. 619/737–2088; Laura Miller, Executive Director

Fremont–Rideout Home Health Valley Hospice, 16911 Willow Glen Road, Brownsville, CA 95919; tel. 916/692–1410; Cindy White, RN, Supervisor, Patient Care Coordinator

Garden Grove Hospice, 12882 Shackelford Lane, Garden Grove, CA 92841; tel. 714/638–9470; Rosa Valdivia

Gran Care Hospice, 19682 Hesperian Boulevard, Suite 200, Hayward, CA 94541; tel. 510/887–1622; Virginia Bartow

Group One, 14520 Hesby Street, Sherman Oaks, CA 91403; tel. 818/906–7825; FAX. 818/906–7151; Elizabeth Dean

Group One Health, Inc.–Erwin, 13634 Erwin Street, Van Nuys, CA 91401; tel. 818/906–7825; Elizabeth Dean

Harmony Hospice, 888 Prospect Street, Suite 201, LaJolla, CA 92037; tel. 619/456–9703; Robert Cohn, Administrator

Helping Hands–Hospice, 1310 South Imperial Avenue, El Centro, CA 92243; tel. 619/352–7100; FAX. 619/352–7448; Suzi Jacobson, Executive Director

Hinds Hospice Services, 1616 West Shaw Avenue, Suite B–Six, Fresno, CA 93711; tel. 209/226–5683; FAX. 209/226–1028; Nancy Hinds, Administrator, Director of Nursing

Hoffman Hospice of the Valley, Inc., 3550 Q Street, Suite 204, Bakersfield, CA 93301; tel. 805/833–3900; M. Earl Ward, Director

Home Health Plus, 2005 De La Cruz Boulevard, Suite 221, Santa Clara, CA 95050; tel. 408/986–1801; Anne Mason

Home Health Plus, 2511 Garden Road, Suite B–200, Monterey, CA 93940; tel. 408/373–8442; Anne Mason

Home Health Plus, 1200 Concord Avenue, Suite 150, Concord, CA 94520; tel. 510/674–8610; Marie Wisniewski, Hospice Supervisor

Home Health Plus, 2334 Merced Street, San Leandro, CA 94577; tel. 510/357–5852; Anne Mason

Home Health Plus, 411 Borel Avenue, San Mateo, CA 94402; tel. 510/357–5852; Michelle V. Gillmore

Home Health Plus–Hospice, 3558 Round Barn Boulevard, Suite 212, Santa Rosa, CA 95403; tel. 707/523–0111; Suzanne Chevalier

Home Health Plus/Hospice, 1770 Iowa Avenue, Suite 500, Riverside, CA 92507; tel. 909/369–8054; Judith K. Kafantaris

Home Health/Hospice of San Luis Obispo, 285 South Street, Suite J, P.O. Box 1489, San Luis Obispo, CA 93406; tel. 805/781–4141; FAX. 805/781–1236; Michele S. Groff, Administrator

Hope Hospice, 6500 Dublin Boulevard, Suite 100, Dublin, CA 94568–3151; tel. 510/829–8770; FAX. 510/829–0868; Joanne Howard, Executive Director

Horizon Hospice, 12709 Poway Road, Suite E–Two, Poway, CA 92064; tel. 619/748–3030; Thomas Dusmu–Johnson

Hospice Care of California, 377 East Chapman Avenue, Suite 280, Placentia, CA 92670; tel. 714/577–9656; FAX. 714/577–9679; Ann Hablitzel, Executive Director

Hospice Care of California, 1340 East Alosta, Suite 200–J, Glendora, CA 91740; tel. 818/335–1399; Ann Hablitzel

Hospice Cheer, 4032 Wilshire Boulevard, Suite 305, Los Angeles, CA 90010; tel. 213/383–9905; FAX. 213/383–9908; Bonnie Farwell, RN, B.S.N.

Hospice Family Care, Inc., 17291 Irvine Boulevard, Suite 412, Tustin, CA 92680; tel. 714/730–1114; FAX. 714/730–9236; Sandy Dunn, General Manager

Hospice Preferred Choice, Inc., d/b/a HPC–Concord, 1470 Enea Circle, Suite 1710, Concord, CA 94520; tel. 510/798–1014; Victoria Condon, Executive Director

Hospice Services of California, 11266 Washington Place, Culver City, CA 90230; tel. 310/636–8484; FAX. 310/636–8480; Fred Jackson, Executive Director

Hospice Services of Lake County, 1717 South Main Street, Lakeport, CA 95453; tel. 707/263–6222; FAX. 707/263–6045; Michael Brooks

Hospice Services of Santa Barbara, a Division of the Santa Barbara Visiting Nurse Association, 222 East Canon Perdido, Santa Barbara, CA 93101; tel. 805/963–6794; Carol Brainerd, RN, M.N., Vice President, Professional Services

Hospice by the Sea, 312 South Cedros Street, Suite 205, Solana Beach, CA 92075; tel. 619/794–0195; FAX. 619/794–0147; Kathie Jackson, Administrator

Hospice of Amador, 839 North Highway 49/88, Suite F, P.O. Box 595, Jackson, CA 95642; tel. 209/223–5500; FAX. 209/223–4964; Hazel Joyce, Executive Director

Hospice of Contra Costa, 2051 Harrison Street, Concord, CA 94520; tel. 510/609–1830; FAX. 510/609–1841; Cindy Siljestrom, Executive Director

Hospice of Emanuel, 2101 Geer Road, Suite 120, Turlock, CA 95382; tel. 209/667–4663; Renette Bronken

Hospice of Humboldt, Inc., 2010 Myrtle Avenue, Eureka, CA 95501; tel. 707/445–8443; FAX. 707/445–2209; Jacqueline Berry, Executive Director

Hospice of Madera County, 115 North P Street, P.O. Box 1325, Madera, CA 93639; tel. 209/674–0407; Nancy Hinds, Administrator

Hospice of Marin, 150 Nellen Avenue, Corte Madera, CA 94925; tel. 415/927–2273; FAX. 415/927–2284; Mary Tavema, President

Hospice of Merced, 149 16th Street, Suite A, P.O. Box 763, Merced, CA 95341; tel. 209/383–3123; FAX. 209/383–5308; Nancy Hinds, RN, Administrator

Hospice of Napa Valley, Five Financial Plaza, Suite 201, Napa, CA 94558; tel. 707/258–9080; FAX. 707/258–9088; Judy Garrison, Executive Director

Hospice of Saddleback Valley, 24022 Calle De La Plata, Suite 200, Laguna Hills, CA 92653; tel. 714/458–8551; Ann Buchanan, Administrator

Hospice of San Joaquin, 2609 East Hammer Lane, Stockton, CA 95210; tel. 209/957–3888; FAX. 209/957–3986; Barbara Tognoli, Administrator

Hospice of Tulare County, Inc., 332 North Johnson, Visalia, CA 93291; tel. 209/733–0642; FAX. 209/733–0658; Debbie Westfall

Hospice of the Canyon, 5045 Parkway Calabasas, Calabasas, CA 91302; tel. 818/591–1459; FAX. 815/591–1486; David Bernstein, D.D.S., Executive Director

Hospice of the Central Coast/Adobe Home Health, 100 Barnet Segal Lane, Monterey, CA 93940; tel. 408/648–7744; FAX. 408/648–7746; Patricia Cincone

Hospice of the East San Gabriel Valley, d/b/a Home Care Advantage, 820 North Phillips Avenue, West Covina, CA 91791; tel. 818/859–2263; FAX. 818/859–2272

Hospice of the North Coast, 4002 Vista Way, Oceanside, CA 92056; tel. 619/724–8411; John P. Lauri, President, Chief Executive Officer

Hospice of the Sierra, 20100 Cedar Road North, Sonora, CA 95370; tel. 209/532–7166; Judy Villalobos, Administrator

Hospice of the Valley, 1150 South Bascom Avenue, Suite Seven A, San Jose, CA 95128; tel. 408/947–1233; FAX. 408/288–4172; Barbara Noggle

Hospital Home Health Care–Hospice, 2601 Airport Drive, Suite 110, Torrance, CA 90505; tel. 310/530–3800; FAX. 310/534–1754; Kaye Daniels, President

Inland Valley Hospice, 7710 Limonite Avenue, Suite E, Riverside, CA 92509; tel. 909/360–5848; Katherine L. Allen

Kern Hospice, 4300 Stine Road, Suite 720, Bakersfield, CA 93313; tel. 805/327–1012; David Christen, Vice President, General Manager

Lifecare Hospice, 1588 West 48th Street, Los Angeles, CA 90062; tel. 213/734–3945; James A. Miller

Livingston Memorial VNA and Hospice, 1996 Eastman Avenue, Suite 101, Ventura, CA 93003; tel. 805/642–0239; FAX. 805/642–2320; Deborah Roberts, RN, B.S.N., Ph.D., President, Chief Executive Officer

Madrone Hospice, Inc., 107 South Broadway, P.O. Box 1193, Yreka, CA 96097; tel. 916/842–3160; FAX. 916/842–4025; Audrey Flower, Executive Director

Marian Hospital Homecare and Hospice, 1300 East Cypress, Suite G, Santa Maria, CA 93454; tel. 805/922–9609; FAX. 805/349–9229; Marie Whitford, Vice President, Alternate Care Services

Matched Caregivers Home Health and Hospice, 211 Town and Country Village, Palo Alto, CA 94301; tel. 415/321–2273; FAX. 415/321–2352; Darrell Owens, M.S., CRNH, Vice President

Memorial Hospice Program, 3711 Long Beach Boulevard, Suite 621, Long Beach, CA 90807; tel. 213/595–2000

Metropolitan Hospice, 4904 Crenshaw Boulevard, Los Angeles, CA 90043; tel. 213/293–6163; FAX. 213/296–3913; Kathleen I. Jones, RN, B.S., Director

Midpeninsula HomeCare and Hospice, 201 San Antonio Circle, Suite 135, Mountain View, CA 94040; tel. 415/949–3029; FAX. 415/949–4317; John D. Hart, Executive Director

Mission Hospice, Inc. of San Mateo County, 1515 Trousdale Drive, Suite 109, Burlingame, CA 94010; tel. 415/692–3080; Carol L. Gray, RN, Administrator

Mountain Home Health Services, Inc., 35680 Wish–i–ah Road, Auberry, CA 93602; tel. 209/855–2200; FAX. 209/855–2284; Lori M. Harshman

My Father's House–Hospice, 2429 Leeward Circle, Westlake Village, CA 91361; tel. 805/495–7368; FAX. 805/495–6466; May Isobel Oxx

Nations Healthcare, Inc.–Hospice, 9823 Pacific Heights Boulevard, Suite N, San Diego, CA 92121; tel. 619/546–3834; FAX. 619/546–0701; David Golman, Administrator

Orangegrove Hospice, 12332 Garden Grove Boulevard, Garden Grove, CA 92843; tel. 714/534–1041; FAX. 714/534–7921; Maria Aguilar, Director, Hospice Services

Pacific Home Health Group, 106 East Manchester, Inglewood, CA 90301; tel. 310/677–4574; Evadne Wright

Pacific Home Health and Hospice, 1168 Park Avenue, San Jose, CA 95126–2913; tel. 408/971–4151; Lemuel F. Ignacio, M.S.W., Administrator

Pathways to Care, Hospice, 1650 Iowa Avenue, Suite 220, Riverside, CA 92507; tel. 909/320–7070; FAX. 909/320–7060; Ed Gardner, President

Quality Continuum Hospice, 5505 Garden Grove Boulevard, Westminster, CA 92683; tel. 800/797–2686; FAX. 714/379–7910; Janet Horn, Administrator

Ramona Care Center Hospice, 11900 Ramona Boulevard, El Monte, CA 91732; tel. 818/442–5721

San Diego Hospice Corporation, 4311 Third Avenue, San Diego, CA 92103; tel. 619/688–1600; FAX. 619/688–9665; Jan Cetti, President, Chief Executive Officer

San Pedro Peninsula Home Care/Hospice, 1386 B West Seventh Street, San Pedro, CA 90732; tel. 310/548–4106; FAX. 310/514–5328; Susan Nowinski, M.S.N., Executive Director

Self–Help HomeCare and Hospice, 407 Sansome Street, Suite 300, San Francisco, CA 94111; tel. 415/982–9171; FAX. 415/398–5903; Nellie Kwan, RN

Spectrum Health Services, Home Health and Hospice, 2421 Mendocino Avenue, Suite 150, Santa Rosa, CA 95403; tel. 707/528–4663, ext. 365; FAX. 707/528–2301; Charmaine Noon, RN, Intake/Referral and Triage

St. Ambrose Hospice Care, 15022 Pacific Street, Suite #A, Midway City, CA 92655; tel. 714/379–6738; FAX. 714/379–6740; Mike Peiton, Director, Operations

St. Joseph Health System Home Care Services–Hospice, 1845 West Orangewood Avenue, Suite 100 A, Orange, CA 92868; tel. 714/712–9559; FAX. 714/712–9529; June van den Noort, Hospice Director

St. Joseph Medical Center Home Hospice, 2101 West Alameda Avenue, Burbank, CA 91506; tel. 818/843–5111, ext. 7051; Roosevelt Travis, Jr., Manager, Home Hospice

Tender Loving Care Home Hospice, 2139 Tapo Street, Suite 205, Simi Valley, CA 93063; tel. 805/520–3166; FAX. 805/520–3167; Shelley Hurt, Administrator

Tendercare Hospice and Home Health, 10882 Kyle Street, Suite A, Los Alamitos, CA 90720; tel. 310/596–5033; Susan Falkner

The Miller Project, 970 North Van Ness, Fresno, CA 93728; tel. 209/264–0061

Tri–Med Hospice, 534 West Manchester Boulevard, Inglewood, CA 90301; tel. 310/419–4836; Margaret R. Lanam

VNA Home Health Systems–Hospice, 1337 Braden Court, Orange, CA 92668; tel. 714/288–4500; Mavis Scott, Director of Hospice

VNA and Home Hospice, 1110 North Dutton Avenue, Santa Rosa, CA 95401–4606; tel. 707/542–5045; FAX. 707/542–6731; Rebecca LaLonde, Regional Director

Verdugo Hills VNA Hospice in the Home, 1101 East Broadway, Suite 201, Glendale, CA 91205–1386; tel. 818/956–1860; FAX. 818/956–1881; Marie Reynolds, RN, Executive Director

Visiting Nurse Association Los Angeles, Inc., 2461 208th Street, Torrance, CA 90501; tel. 310/782–8886; FAX. 310/782–9172; Judy Regotti, PHN

Visiting Nurse Association and Hospice of Northern California, 1900 Powell Street, Suite 300, Emeryville, CA 94608; tel. 510/450–8596; FAX. 510/450–8532; Pat Sussman, Director

Visiting Nurse Association and Hospice of Pomona/San Bernardino, Inc., 150 West First Street, P.O. Box 908, Claremont, CA 91711; tel. 714/624–3574; FAX. 714/624–8904; Karen H. Green, President

Visiting Nurse Association of Long Beach–Hospice, 3295 Pacific Avenue, Long Beach, CA 90807; tel. 310/426–8856; FAX. 310/988–9474; Jean Lawrence, Director, Agency Operations

Visiting Nurse Association of Los Angeles and Yvette Luque Hospice, 520 South Lafayette Park Place, Suite 500, Los Angeles, CA 90057; tel. 213/386–7200; FAX. 213/386–4227; June Simmons, Chief Executive Officer

Visiting Nurse Service Hospice, Serving Santa Barbara County and San Luis Obispo County, 521 East Chapel Street, P.O. Box 1029, Santa Maria, CA 93454; tel. 805/925–8694; FAX. 805/925–1387; John W. Puryear, Executive Director

West Healthcare Hospice Services, 180 Otay Lakes Road, Suite 100, Bonita, CA 91902; tel. 619/472–7500; FAX. 619/472–1534; Suzanne L. Purdy

Wilcare Hospice and Home Health, 2001 Gateway Place, Suite 150, San Jose, CA 95110; tel. 408/467–0777; FAX. 408/467–0770; Sandra K. Rohlfing, Administrator

COLORADO

Angel of Shavano Hospice, 543 East First Street, Salida, CO 81201; tel. 719/539–7638; FAX. 719/539–3699; Claudia Dixon

Arkansas Valley Hospice, 118 West Fourth Street, Box 1067, LaJunta, CO 81050; tel. 719/384–8827; FAX. 719/384–2045; Erma J. Isaac, Executive Director

Baca County Hospice, 373 East 10th Avenue, Springfield, CO 81073; tel. 719/523–4851; FAX. 719/523–4763; Shirley Close, RN

Boulder County Hospice, Inc., 2825 Marine Street, Boulder, CO 80303; tel. 303/449–7740; FAX. 303/449–6961; Constance Holden, Director

Section C

Bristlecone Home Care and Hospice, Inc., 416 Main Street, Suite Six, P.O. Box 1327, Frisco, CO 80443; tel. 970/668–5604; FAX. 970/668–3189; Rebecca Greene, RN, Patient Care Coordinator, Administrator

Caring Unlimited Hospice Services, Inc., 4491 Bent Bros Boulevard, Colorado City, CO 81019; tel. 719/676–3637; FAX. 719/676–3695; Karen Clouse, RN

Colorado Palliative Care Hospice, 1425 Senter Street, Burlington, CO 80807; tel. 719/346–7700; FAX. 719/346–7754; Nancy Hendricks

Colorado Palliative Care Hospice, 559 East Pikes Peak, #300, Colorado Springs, CO 80903; tel. 719/447–1511; Mary Hahns, RN

Colorado Palliative Care Hospice, 6795 East Tennessee, Suite 250, Denver, CO 80224; tel. 303/355–5890; Art Holtz, Chief Operating Officer

Community Hospice/Roaring Fork Valley, P.O. Box 5016, Aspen, CO 81612; tel. 303/925–4885; FAX. 303/963–4566; Lou Cunningham, RN, B.S.N., Executive Director

Grand Valley Hospice, Inc., d/b/a Hospice of the Grand Valley, 2754 Compass Drive, Suite 377, Grand Junction, CO 81506; tel. 970/241–2212; FAX. 970/257–2400; Christy Whitney, Executive Director

Hospice Del Valle, Inc., 231 State Avenue, P.O. Box 1554, Alamosa, CO 81101; tel. 719/589–9019; FAX. 719/589–5094; Jan Bezuidenhout, Executive Director

Hospice Services of Northwest Colorado, 135 Sixth Street, P.O. Box 775816, Steamboat Springs, CO 80477; tel. 970/879–9218; FAX. 970/870–1326; Janet Fritz, Executive Director

Hospice of Larimer County, 7604 Colland Drive, Fort Collins, CO 80525; tel. 970/663–3500; FAX. 970/663–1180; Brian Hoag, Executive Director

Hospice of Metro Denver, Inc., 425 South Cherry Street, Suite 700, Denver, CO 80222–1234; tel. 303/321–2828; FAX. 303/321–7171; Jacob S. Blass, President, Chief Executive Officer

Hospice of Montezuma, Inc., 44 North Ash, Cortez, CO 81321; tel. 970/565–4400; FAX. 970/565–9543; Claudia Poynter, Administrator

Hospice of Northern Colorado, 2726 11th Street Road, Greeley, CO 80631; tel. 970/352–8487; FAX. 970/352–6685; Jane M. Schnell, RN, Executive Director

Hospice of Peace, 1601 A Lowell Boulevard, Denver, CO 80204–1545; tel. 303/575–8393; FAX. 303/575–8390; Ann Luke, Supervisor

Hospice of St. John, 1320 Everett Court, Lakewood, CO 80215; tel. 303/232–7900; FAX. 303/232–3614; Kathy Cure, Administrator

Hospice of the Comforter, 3715 Parkmoor Village Drive, Suite 108, Colorado Springs, CO 80917; tel. 719/573–4166, FAX. 719/573–4164; Ronald Coffin, Ph.D., M.B.A., Executive Director

Hospice of the Gunnison Valley, 1500 West Tomichi Avenue, Gunnison, CO 81230; tel. 970/641–0704; FAX. 970/641–5593; Robert Patterson, Administrator

Hospice of the Rockies, 826 1/2 Grand Avenue, P.O. Box 1025, Glenwood Springs, CO 81602; tel. 970/928–8796; FAX. 970/945–8661; Rachael Windh, M.S.W., Administrator

Integra Hospice/Home Health, 1401 17th Street, Suite 700, Denver, CO 80202; tel. 303/293–2273; FAX. 303/293–2262; Edward Lowe, Regional Director

Lamar Area Hospice Association, Inc., 1001 South Main, P.O. Box 843, Lamar, CO 81052; tel. 719/336–2100; Linda Earl, Executive Director

Lutheran Homecare and Hospice, 3964 Youngfield, Wheat Ridge, CO 80033; tel. 303/467–4700; FAX. 303/424–5260; Marge Bassett, Manager

Mount Evans Hospice, 3721 Evergreen Parkway, P.O. Box 2770, Evergreen, CO 80439; tel. 303/674–6400; Louisa B. Walthers, Executive Director

Pikes Peak Hospice, Inc., 3630 Sinton Road, Suite 302, Colorado Springs, CO 80907; tel. 719/633–3400; FAX. 719/633–1150; Martha Barton, RN, Chief Executive Officer

Porter Care Hospice, 2465 South Downing Street, Suite 202, Denver, CO 80210; tel. 303/871–0835; FAX. 303/778–5859; Terri Walter, Director

Prospect Home Care Hospice, Inc., 321 West Henrietta Avenue, Suite E, P.O. Box 6278, Woodland Park, CO 80866; tel. 719/687–0549; FAX. 719/687–8558; Joleen Bailey, Executive Director

Sangre de Cristo Hospice, 704 Elmhurst Place, Pueblo, CO 81004; tel. 719/542–0032; FAX. 719/542–1413; Joni Fair, President, Chief Executive Officer

Vail Valley Home Health, and Maintenance Hospice, 100 West Beaver Creek Boulevard, #222, Avon, CO 81620; tel. 970/845–9155; Ray McMahan

Visiting Nurse Association Hospice at Home, 3801 East Florida, Suite 800, Denver, CO 80210; tel. 303/757–6363, ext. 413; FAX. 303/782–2573; Linda Gaetani, Director

CONNECTICUT

Bristol Hospital Home Care Agency, Seven North Washington Street, Plainville, CT 06062; tel. 860/585–4752; FAX. 860/747–6719; Mary C. Smith, RN, Administrator

East Hartford Visiting Nurse Association, Inc., 60 Hartland Street, East Hartford, CT 06108–3213; tel. 860/528–2273; FAX. 860/920–6777; Karen Stone, RN, President

Foothills Visiting Nurse & Home Care, Inc., 32 Union Street, Winsted, CT 06098; tel. 860/379–8561; FAX. 860/738–7479; Jeannette Jakubiak, RN, Administrator

Home and Community Health Services, Inc., The Nirenberg Medical Center, 140 Hazard Avenue, P.O. Box 1199, Enfield, CT 06083; tel. 860/763–7600; FAX. 860/763–7613; Kathryn D. Roby, RN, B.S.N., Administrator

Hospice Care, Inc., 461 Atlantic Street, Stamford, CT 06902; tel. 203/324–2592; Janice Casey, RN

Hospice at Home, a program of Visiting Nurse Services of Connecticut, Inc., 765 Fairfield Avenue, Bridgeport, CT 06606; tel. 203/366–3821, ext. 310; FAX. 203/334–0543; Lois Ravage – Mass, RN, M.S.N, Director, Hospice

Hospice of Eastern Connecticut, a Program at Visiting Nurse and Community Health of Eastern Connecticut, Inc., 34 Ledgebrook Drive, P.O. Box 716, Mansfield Center, CT 06250; tel. 860/456–7288; FAX. 860/456–4267; Susan Lund, Hospice Director

Hospice of Northeastern Connecticut, 13 Railroad Street, P.O. Box 203, Pomfret Center, CT 06259; tel. 860/928–0422; FAX. 860/928–4545

Hospice of Southeastern Connecticut, Inc., 179 Gallivan Lane, P.O. Box 902, Uncasville, CT 06382–0902; tel. 860/848–5699; FAX. 860/848–6898

McLean Community and Home Services, 75 Great Pond Road, Simsbury, CT 06070; tel. 860/658–3950; FAX. 860/408–1319; Nancy E. Ryan, RN, Administrator

Mid–Fairfield Hospice, Inc., 112 Main Street, Norwalk, CT 06851; tel. 203/847–7646; FAX. 203/847–8394; Carol Yoder, RN, M.S.N., Administrator, Supervisor

Middlesex Visiting Nurse and Home Health Services, Inc., 51 Broad Street, Middletown, CT 06457; tel. 860/704–5600; Janine Fay, Administrator

New Milford Visiting Nurse Association, Inc., 68 Park Lane Road, New Milford, CT 06776; tel. 860/354–2216; FAX. 860/350–2852; Andrea Wilson, B.S., M.P.A., Executive Director

Project Care, Inc., Home and Hospice Services, 51 Depot Street, Suite 203, Watertown, CT 06795; tel. 860/274–9239; FAX. 860/945–3625; Joel Schlank, Administrator

Regional Hospice of Western Connecticut, Inc., 30 West Street, Danbury, CT 06810; tel. 203/797–1685; Patricia Coyle, RN, Administrator, Supervisor

Salisbury Public Health Nursing Association, Inc., 30 Salmon Kill Road, Salisbury, CT 06068; tel. 203/435–0816; Marilyn Joseph, RN, Administrator, Supervisor

Southington Visiting Nurse Association, Inc., 80 Meriden Avenue, Southington, CT 06489; tel. 203/621–0157; Mary Jane Corn, RN, Administrator

The Connecticut Hospice, Inc., 61 Burban Drive, Branford, CT 06405; tel. 203/481–6231; FAX. 203/483–9539; Rosemary J. Hurzeler, President, Chief Executive Officer

The Greater Bristol VNA, Inc., 10 Maltby Street, P.O. Box 2826, Bristol, CT 06011–2826; tel. 860/583–1644; FAX. 860/584–2100; Anita Baldwin, Hospice Coordinator

United Home Care, Inc., United Home Hospice, 1931 Black Rock Turnpike, Fairfield, CT 06430; tel. 203/330–9198; Karen Speer, RN, B.S.N., Hospice Administrator

VNA Health at Home, Inc., 27 Princeton Road, Watertown, CT 06795; tel. 860/274–7531; FAX. 860/274–8492; W. Rennard Wieland, President

VNA Hospice, Inc., 103 Woodland Street, Hartford, CT 06105; tel. 860/525–7001; FAX. 860/278–0581; Judith Milewsky Bigler, Executive Director

VNA Valley Care, Inc., Eight Old Mill Lane, Simsbury, CT 06070–1932; tel. 860/651–3539; FAX. 860/651–5082; Incy Severance, RN, M.P.A., Executive Director

Visiting Nurse Association and Hospice, of Pioneer Valley, Inc., 701 Enfield Street, Enfield, CT 06082; tel. 203/253–5316; Kimberly A. Barbaro, RN, M.B.A., Administrator

Visiting Nurse Association of Central Connecticut, Inc., 205 West Main Street, P.O. Box 1327, New Britain, CT 06050; tel. 860/224–7131; FAX. 860/224–8303; Mary Jane Corn, B.S.N., R.N., President, Chief Executive Officer

Visiting Nurse and Community Care, Inc., Eight Keynote Drive, Vernon, CT 06066; tel. 860/872–9163; FAX. 860/872–3030; Rafael Sciullo, Administrator

Visiting Nurse and Home Care Northwest, Inc., Four Old Middle Street, P.O. Box 266, Goshen, CT 06756; tel. 860/491–3740; FAX. 860/491–8635; Pamela Duchaine, Hospice Coordinator

Visiting Nurse and Home Care of Manchester, Inc., 545 North Main Street, Manchester, CT 06040; tel. 860/647–1481; FAX. 860/643–4942; Mary Lavery, Hospice Supervisor

DELAWARE

Compassionate Care Hospice of Delaware, 256 Chapman Road, Suite 201–A, Newark, DE 19702; tel. 302/454–7002; FAX. 302/454–7003; Cathy Stauffer Kimble, M.P.H., Regional Director

Delaware Hospice, 100 Clayton Building, 3515 Silverside Road, Wilmington, DE 19810; tel. 302/478–5707; FAX. 302/479–2586; Susan D. Lloyd, RN, M.S.N., Executive Director

Delaware Hospice, Inc.–Georgetown, 600 Dupont Highway, Suite 107, Georgetown Professional Park, Georgetown, DE 19947; tel. 302/856–7717; Susan D. Lloyd, RN, M.S.N., Executive Director

Delaware Hospice–Central Division, Lotus Plaza, 911 South Dupont Highway, Dover, DE 19901; tel. 302/678–4444; FAX. 302/678–4451; Judi Tulak, RN, M.S., Program Coordinator

First State Hospice, 5165 West Woodmill Drive, Suite 12, Wilmington, DE 19808; tel. 302/995–2273; FAX. 302/995–2280; Terry L. Hastings, RN, Executive Director

Hospice of the Delaware Valley, 527 Plymouth Road, Suite 417, Plymouth Meeting, PA 19462; tel. 610/941–6700; Marsha Cook, Administrator

DISTRICT OF COLUMBIA

American Home Health Care/Hospice, 6856 Eastern Avenue, N.W., Washington, DC 20012; tel. 202/541–0810; Hakim Abdullah Alkalim

Americare InHome Nursing, 5203 Leesburg Pike, Suite 705, Falls Church, VA 22041; tel. 703/931–9002; FAX. 703/826–0076; Mary L. Tatum

Health Cap Medical Service, 3332 Georgia Avenue, N.W., Washington, DC 20010; tel. 202/882–0112; Terrance Monkou

Home Health Partners NCA, 1234 Massachusetts Avenue, N.W., Washington, DC 20005; tel. 202/638–2382; Margaret Terry

Hospice Care of the District of Columbia, 1325 Massachusetts Avenue, N.W., Suite 606, Washington, DC 20005–4171; tel. 202/347–1700; FAX. 202/347–4285; Darla Schueth, Executive Director

Hospice of Washington, 3720 Upton Street, N.W., Washington, DC 20016; tel. 202/966–3720; FAX. 202/895–0177; Mary Ann Griffin, Vice President Hospice

Housecall Hospice, 801 Pennsylvania Avenue, S.E., Washington, DC 20003; tel. 202/546–6764; Karlene Conrad, Regional Manager

Inova Health Care–District of Columbia Branch, 1331 Pennsylvania Avenue, N.W., S–500, Washington, DC 20005; tel. 202/638–5828; Regina Silver

Interim HealthCare Inc., 8401 Colesville Road, Silver Spring, MD 20910; tel. 301/587–3136; FAX. 301/587–3478; Arlene Berger, RN, B.S.N., Executive Director

Jewish Social Service Home Health Association, 6123 Montrose Road, Rockville, MD 20852; tel. 301/881–3700; Laura Freiden

Optimum Home Health Care, 1050 17th Street, N.W., Washington, DC 20036; tel. 202/496–1289; FAX. 202/296–2854; Patricia Austin

Personal Touch, 4400 Jenifer Street, N.W., Washington, DC 20015; tel. 202/537–7200; Mary Ellen Conway

Section C

Potomac Home Health Care, 6001 Montrose Road, Rockville, MD 20852; tel. 301/896–6999; Lauren Simpson, Chief Executive Officer

Urgent Home Health Care, 1535 P Street, N.W., Washington, DC 20005; tel. 202/483–3355; Pauline NGO Bapack

Visiting Nurses Association, 5151 Wisconsin Avenue, N.W., Washington, DC 20016; tel. 202/686–2862; Susan Walker, Hospice Director

FLORIDA

Big Bend Hospice, Inc., 1723 Mahan Center Boulevard, Tallahassee, FL 32308–5428; tel. 904/878–5310; FAX. 904/309–1638; Elaine C. Bartelt, M.S., Executive Director

Bon Secours Hospice, 21234 Olean Boulevard, Suite Four, Port Charlotte, FL 33952; tel. 813/764–8204; FAX. 813/764–6494; Jackie Homes, Team Manager

Brevard Hospice, 14 Suntree Place, Melbourne, FL 32940; tel. 407/253–2222; FAX. 407/253–2238; Cynthia P. Harris Panning, RN, B.B.A., Executive Director

Catholic Hospice, Inc., 14100 Palmetto Frontage Road, Suite 370, Miami, FL 33016; tel. 305/822–2380; FAX. 305/824–0665; Janet L. Jones, President, Chief Executive Officer

Good Shepherd Hospice of Mid–Florida, Inc., 247 South Commerce Avenue, Sebring, FL 33870; tel. 941/471–3700; FAX. 941/471–9452; Ruth Angus, RN, Director Highlands/Hardee

Good Shepherd Hospice of Mid–Florida/Winter Haven, Inc., 105 Arneson Avenue, Auburndale, FL 33823; tel. 813/297–1880; FAX. 813/965–5601; Mary Ellen Poe, Administrator

Hernando–Pasco Hospice, Inc., 12107 Majestic Boulevard, Hudson, FL 34667; tel. 813/863–7971; FAX. 813/868–9261; Rodney Taylor, Executive Director

Holmes Regional Hospice, Inc., 1900 Dairy Road, West Melbourne, FL 32904; tel. 407/952–0494; FAX. 407/952–0382; Roberta Van Dusen, Director

Hope Hospice of Lee County, Inc., 9470 Health Park Circle, Ft. Myers, FL 33908; tel. 941/482–4673; FAX. 941/482–2488; Samira K. Beckwith, President, Chief Executive Officer

Hospice Care of Broward County, Inc., 309 Southeast 18th Street, Ft. Lauderdale, FL 33316; tel. 954/467–7423; FAX. 954/524–6067; Susan G. Telli, Executive Director

Hospice Care of South Florida, 7270 Northwest 12th Street, Penthouse Six, Miami, FL 33126; tel. 305/591–1606; FAX. 305/591–1618; Rose Marie R. Marty, Executive Director

Hospice by the Sea, Inc., 1531 West Palmetto Park Road, Boca Raton, FL 33486–3395; tel. 561/395–5031; FAX. 561/393–7137; Trudi Webb, Executive Director

Hospice of Citrus County, Inc., 3350 West Audubon Park Path, Lecanto, FL 34461–8450; tel. 904/527–2020; FAX. 904/527–0386; William J. Murphy, Executive Director

Hospice of Hillsborough, Inc., 3010 West Azeele Street, Tampa, FL 33609–3139; tel. 813/877–2200; FAX. 813/872–7037; Anne E. Thal, President, Chief Executive Director

Hospice of Lake and Sumter, Inc., 12300 Lane Park Road, Taveres, FL 32778–9660; tel. 904/343–1341; FAX. 904/343–6115; Rebecca A. McDonald, Chief Executive Officer

Hospice of Marion County, Inc., 3231 Southwest 34th Avenue, Ocala, FL 34474, P.O. Box 4860, Ocala, FL 34478–4860; tel. 352/873–7434; FAX. 352/873–7435; Alice J. Privett, Chief Executive Director

Hospice of Naples, Inc., 1095 Whippoorwill Lane, Naples, FL 34105; tel. 941/261–4404; FAX. 941/261–3278; Diane S. Cox, Executive Director

Hospice of Northeast Florida, Inc., 4266 Sunbeam Road, The Earl Hadlow Center for Caring, Jacksonville, FL 32257; tel. 904/268–5200; FAX. 904/268–9674; Susan Ponder–Stansel, President, Chief Executive Officer

Hospice of Northwest Florida, Inc., 2001 North Palafox Street, Pensacola, FL 32501; tel. 904/433–2155; FAX. 904/433–7212; Dale O. Knee, President, Chief Executive Officer

Hospice of Okeechobee, Inc., 411 Southeast Fourth Street, Okeechobee, FL 34973; tel. 813/467–2321; FAX. 813/467–8330; Pat Ballengee, Executive Director

Hospice of Palm Beach County, Inc., 5300 East Avenue, West Palm Beach, FL 33407; tel. 561/848–5200; FAX. 561/863–2955; Deborah S. Dailey, M.B.A., President, Chief Executive Officer

Hospice of Pasco, Inc., 6224–6230 Lafayette Street, New Port Richey, FL 34652–2626; tel. 813/845–5707; Michael Wilson, Executive Director

Hospice of Southwest Florida, Inc., 6055 Rand Boulevard, Sarasota, FL 34238; tel. 941/923–5822; FAX. 941/921–7431; Bonnie Harvey, President, Chief Executive Officer

Hospice of St. Francis, Inc., 6770 South U.S. Highway 1, P.O. Box 5563, Titusville, FL 32783–5563; tel. 407/269–4240; FAX. 407/269–5428; Cheryl M. Parker, Executive Director

Hospice of Treasure Coast, Inc., 805 Virginia Avenue, P.O. Box 1748, Ft. Pierce, FL 34982–1748; tel. 407/465–0504; FAX. 407/465–6309; Sharon A. Rivers, President, Chief Executive Officer

Hospice of Volusia and Flagler, 3800 Woodbriar Trail, Port Orange, FL 32119; tel. 904/322–4701; FAX. 904/322–4702; Debbie Harley, Director

Hospice of the Comforter, 595 Montgomery Road, Altamonte Springs, FL 32714; tel. 407/682–0808; FAX. 407/682–5787; Robert G. Wilson, President, Director

Hospice of the Florida Keys, 1319 William Street, Key West, FL 33040; tel. 305/294–8812; FAX. 305/292–9466; Liz Kern, Chief Executive Officer

Hospice of the Florida Suncoast, Inc., 300 East Bay Drive, Largo, FL 33770; tel. 813/586–4432; FAX. 813/581–5846; Mary Labyak, M.S.S.W., L.C.S.W., President

Hospice of the Gold Coast H.H.S., 911 East Atlantic Boulevard, Suite 200, Pompano Beach, FL 33060; tel. 305/785–2990; FAX. 305/785–2993; Lynda Friedman, Administrator

The Hospice of Martin & St. Lucie, Inc., 2030 Southeast Ocean Boulevard, Stuart, FL 34996; tel. 561/287–7860; FAX. 561/287–7982; Mary C. Knox, Executive Director

The Hospice of North Central Florida, 3615 Southwest 13th Street, Gainesville, FL 32608; tel. 352/378–2121; FAX. 352/378–4111; Patrice Moore, Administrator

VITAS Healthcare Corporation of Central Florida, Inc., 2500 Maitland Center Parkway, Suite 300, Maitland, FL 32751; tel. 407/875–0028; FAX. 407/875–2074; Brenda K. Horne, General Manager

VNA Hospice of Indian River County, 1111 36th Street, Vero Beach, FL 32960; tel. 407/567–5551; FAX. 407/567–9308; Sharon L. Kennedy, President, Chief Executive Officer

Vitas Healthcare Corporation of Florida, 3323 West Commercial Boulevard, Suite 200, Ft. Lauderdale, FL 33309; tel. 305/486–4085; FAX. 305/777–5328; Deirdre Lawe, Regional Vice President

Vitas Healthcare Corporation of Florida, 3700 Executive Way, Miramar, FL 33025; tel. 954/437–5433; FAX. 954/704–2797; Barbara Gray, General Manager

GEORGIA

Albany Community Hospice, 416 Fifth Avenue, P.O. Box 1828, Albany, GA 31703; tel. 912/889–7050; FAX. 912/889–7447; Patty Woodall, Executive Director

Atlanta Hospice International L.L.C., 236 Forsyth Street, Suite 405, Atlanta, GA 30303; tel. 404/681–1212; Renee M. Folsom

Avondale Hospice Services, Inc., 3500 Kensington Road, Decatur, GA 30032; tel. 404/299–6111; Rachel Waldemar

Blue–Gray Community Hospice, Perry House Road, P.O. Box 1349, Fitzgerald, GA 31750–1447; tel. 912/424–7152; Lenora Kirby, RN, Executive Director

Central Hospice Care, 1150 Hammond Drive, Suite B–2100, Atlanta, GA 30328; tel. 404/391–9531; FAX. 404/391–9732; Sharon Compton, Administrator

Columbus Hospice, Inc., 3228 University Avenue, Suite 101, Columbus, GA 31907; tel. 706/569–7992; FAX. 706/569–8560; Mike Smajd, Executive Director

Community Hospice Care, 206 Hospital Circle, Rome, GA 30162; tel. 706/295–9731; Joy Jones, Director

Elysium House, 6490 West Fayetteville Road, Riverdale, GA 30274; tel. 404/997–0889; FAX. 404/997–8559; Kimberly K. Partain, Director

Georgia Baptist Hospice, 100 10th Street, N.E., Suite 800, Atlanta, GA 30309–4007; tel. 770/265–1144; FAX. 770/265–1414; Mary Jo Wilson, RN, Director

Georgia Mountain Hospice, Inc., 1452 East Church Street, P.O. Box 881, Jasper, GA 30143; tel. 706/692–3125; FAX. 706/692–4300; Lynn Corliss, Executive Director

Hamilton Medical Center–Hospice, P.O. Box 1168, 1103 Memorial Drive, Dalton, GA 30720–1168; tel. 404/226–2848; Johnnie Bradley, Vice President

Hand In Hand Hospice, 2150 Limestone Parkway, Gainesville, GA 30501; tel. 404/536–0497; FAX. 404/536–0157; Ellen Patterson, Director

Haven House at Midtown, Inc., 250 14th Street, Atlanta, GA 30309; tel. 404/874–8313; FAX. 404/875–4363; Clyde W. Johnson, Jr., President, Chief Executive Officer

Hospice Atlanta, 1244 Park Vista Drive, Atlanta, GA 30319; tel. 404/869–3000; FAX. 404/869–3099; Pat Szucs, Vice President

Hospice Care of Carroll County, Inc., 906 South Park Street, Carrollton, GA 30117; tel. 770/214–2355; FAX. 770/214–8301; Margaret Davis, Director

Hospice Care, Inc., 1310 13th Avenue, Suite 200, P.O. Box 9401, Columbus, GA 31901; tel. 706/660–8899; FAX. 706/660–8899; Mr. Adeleye Tokes, Ph.D., Administrator

Hospice Satilla of Memorial Hospital, Inc., 1906 Tebeau Street, Waycross, GA 31501; tel. 912/287–2664; FAX. 912/283–0200; Rai B. Duane, Director

Hospice Savannah, Inc., 1352 Eisenhower Drive, Zip 31406, P.O. Box 13190, Savannah, GA 31416; tel. 912/355–2289; FAX. 912/355–2376; Judith B. Brunger, Executive Director

Hospice of Americus and Sumter County, 119 Brannan Street, P.O. Box 1434, Americus, GA 31709; tel. 912/928–4000; FAX. 912/928–1322; Anne F. Speer, Executive Director

Hospice of Baldwin, Inc., 811 North Cobb Street, Milledgeville, GA 31061; tel. 912/453–8572; FAX. 912/453–8432; Bob Karlinski,

Hospice of Central Georgia, 3312 Northside Drive, Building D, Suite 100, Macon, GA 31201; tel. 912/477–0335; FAX. 912/477–0690; Gary Thomas, Director

Hospice of Chattanooga, Inc., 165 Hamm Road, Chattanooga, TN 37405; tel. 615/267–6828; Viston Taylor III, Executive Director

Hospice of Georgia, Inc., 3450 New High Shoals Road, P.O. Box 10, High Shoals, GA 30645; tel. 706/769–5341; FAX. 706/769–5944; Magda D. Bennett, President

Hospice of Houston Co., Inc., 2066 Watson Boulevard, P.O. Box 1023, Warner Robins, GA 31099; tel. 912/922–1777; FAX. 912/922–9433; Jackie Connors, Administrator

Hospice of Laurens County, 1103 Bellevue Avenue, P.O. Box 1344, Suite 100, Dublin, GA 31040; tel. 912/272–8333; Kaye Bracewell, Executive Director

Hospice of Northeast Georgia, Inc., Highway 76 West, Parks and Recreation Building, P.O. Box 586, Clayton, GA 30525; tel. 706/782–7505; FAX. 404/782–3343; Irene Perkins, B.S.N., Executive Director

Hospice of South Georgia, 201 Pendleton Drive, Suite 207, Valdosta, GA 31603–1727; tel. 912/249–4100; FAX. 912/249–4102; Frances Rowell, Director

Hospice of Southeast Georgia, Inc., 333 South Ashley Street, P.O. Box 1077, Kingsland, GA 31548; tel. 912/673–7000; Susan Ponder–Stansel, President, Chief Executive Officer

Hospice of Southwest Georgia, 808 Gordon Avenue, Thomasville, GA 31798; tel. 912/227–5520; FAX. 912/227–5526; Patricia Whetsell, Administrator

Hospice of Wilkinson County, Inc., Mission Road, P.O. Box 920, Gordon, GA 31031; tel. 912/628–5655; Edwin Lavender, Administrator

Hospice of the Golden Isles, Inc., 2311 Heron Street, Brunswick, GA 31520; tel. 912/265–4735; Cheryl Johns, RN, Executive Director

HospiceCare, 1424 North Expressway, Suite 114, Griffin, GA 30223; tel. 770/227–1264; FAX. 770/412–0014; Nancy Frederick, RN

House Call Hospice, Inc., Executive Business Park, 6025 Lee Highway, Suite 415, Chattanooga, TN 37421; tel. 615/892–2561; Caroline McBrayer

Metro Hospice, Inc., 2045 Peachtree Road, N.E., Suite 210, Atlanta, GA 30309; tel. 404/355–3134; FAX. 404/352–5193; Shari Silvers, Administrator

Northside Hospice, 5825 Glenridge Drive, Building Four, Atlanta, GA 30328–5544; tel. 404/851–6300; Margot Marcus, Manager

Ogeechee Area Hospice, 209 B South Zetterower Avenue, P.O. Box 531, Statesboro, GA 30459; tel. 912/764–8441; FAX. 912/489–8247; Nancy Bryant, RN

Section C

Olsten Kimberly Quality Care Hospice, 1395 South Marietta Parkway, Suite 222, Marietta, GA 30061; tel. 770/422–5741; FAX. 770/425–3516; Joan Richters, RN, M.N.

Peachtree Hospice, 3600 Dekalb Technology Parkway, Altanta, GA 30340; tel. 404/451–0021; Mary Nixon, Administrator

Portsbridge, Inc., 4598 Barclay Drive, Dunwoody, GA 30350; tel. 770/936–9546, ext. 12; FAX. 770/936–9547; Hugh Henderson, Administrator

Shepherd's Gate Hospice, Inc., P.O. Box 447, Covington, GA 30210–0447; tel. 770/784–9200; FAX. 770/784–7650; John J. McBride, Executive Director

Southwest Christian Hospice, 7225 Lester Road, Union City, GA 30291; tel. 404/969–8354; FAX. 404/969–1940; Mike Sorrow, Executive Director

United Hospice of Calhoun, 1195 Curtis Parkway, Calhoun, GA 30701; tel. 706/602–9546; Jean Coppola, RN

United Hospice of Macon, Inc., 2484 Ingleside Avenue, Building B, Macon, GA 31204; tel. 912/745–9204; FAX. 912/745–9321; Scott Schull

United Hospice, Inc., 3945 Lawrenceville Highway, Lilburn, GA 30247; tel. 800/544–4788; FAX. 770/925–4619; Scott Shull, Vice President

Willow Way Hospice, 6000 Lake Forrest Drive, Suite 400, Atlanta, GA 30328; tel. 404/255–4015; FAX. 404/255–8340; Maxine McCullar

Wiregrass Hospice, Inc., Post Office Drawer 2127, Dothan, AL 36301; tel. 334/794–9101; FAX. 334/794–0009; Ray L. Shrout, Administrator

HAWAII

Hospice Hawaii, 445 Seaside Avenue, Suite 604, Honolulu, HI 96815; tel. 808/924–9255; FAX. 808/922–9161; Stephen A. Kula, President, Chief Professional Officer

Hospice Maui, 400 Mahalani Street, Wailuku, HI 96793; tel. 808/244–5555; Dr. Gregory LaGoy, Executive Director

Hospice of Hilo, 1266 Waianuenue Avenue, Hilo, HI 96720; tel. 808/969–1733; FAX. 808/969–4863; Brenda Ho, Executive Director

Hospice of Kona, Inc., P.O. Box 217, Kailua–Kona, HI 96745; tel. 808/334–0334; FAX. 808/334–0365; Dorothy M. Shepherd, RN, Executive and Clinical Director

Kauai Hospice, 4483 Kuene Street, P.O. Box 3286, Lihue, HI 96766; tel. 808/245–7277; FAX. 808/245–5006; Kathleen Boyle

North Hawaii Hospice, Inc., P.O. Box 1236, Kamuela, HI 96743; tel. 808/885–7547; FAX. 808/885–5592; Nancy Bouvet, Executive Director

St. Francis Hospice, 24 Puiwa Road, Honolulu, HI 96817; tel. 808/595–7566; FAX. 808/595–6996; Michael A. Warren, RN, B.S.N., M.A., Director

IDAHO

Blackfoot Medical Clinic, Home Care & Hospice, Inc., 625 West Pacific, Blackfoot, ID 83221; tel. 208/785–2600; James Marriott, Administrator

Crest Hospice Care, 1009 Highway Two West, Suite E, Sandpoint, ID 83864; tel. 208/265–9200; FAX. 208/265–0622; Lorraine P. Gruner, Administrator

Good Samaritan Community Hospice, 840 East Elva, Idaho Falls, ID 83401; tel. 208/529–8326; FAX. 208/522–7473; Carol Ord, RN, B.S.N., Director

Horizon Hospice, Inc., 1406 East First Street, Suite 107, Meridan, ID 83642; tel. 208/884–5051; FAX. 208/884–5054; Marcella Little, President

Hospice Visions, Inc., 1300 Kimberly Road, Suite 11, Twin Falls, ID 83301; tel. 208/326–4068; Tamala Klinsky, Director

Hospice of Idaho, 812 East Clark, Pocatello, ID 83201; tel. 208/232–0088; FAX. 208/232–7941; Debbie Osborn, Administrator

Hospice of North Idaho, West 280 Prairie Avenue, Coeur d'Alene, ID 83814; tel. 208/772–7994; John Nugent, Administrator

Hospice of the Palouse, P.O. Box 9461, Moscow, ID 83843; tel. 208/882–1228; FAX. 208/883–2239; Norman Bowers, Administrator

Latah Health Home Care & Hospice, 510 West Palouse River Drive, Moscow, ID 83843; tel. 208/882–4802; FAX. 208/882–1819; Irma Laskowski, RNC, Hospice Director

Life's Doors Hospice, Inc., 1111 South Orchard, Suite 400, P.O. Box 5754, Boise, ID 83705; tel. 208/344–6500; FAX. 208/344–6590; Mary L. Langenfeld, Chief Executive Officer

MSTI – Hospice of Boise, 151 East Bannock, Boise, ID 83712; tel. 208/386–2711; Nan Hart, Administrator

Magic Valley Staffing Service, Inc., 200 Second Avenue, N., Twin Falls, ID 83301; tel. 208/734–0600; FAX. 208/733–5980; Debbie Osborn, Administrator

Mercy Hospice, 111 Third Street, S., Nampa, ID 83651; tel. 208/465–5235; Robert A. Fale, Chief Executive Officer

Southeastern District Hospice, 465 Memorial Drive, Pocatello, ID 83201; tel. 208/239–5240; FAX. 208/234–7169; Judy Moyer, Administrator

The Oaks Hospice, 316 West Washington, Boise, ID 83702; tel. 208/343–7755; Shelley Greget, Vice President

XL Hospice, Inc., 1401 North Whitley Drive, Suite 16, Fruitland, ID 83619; tel. 208/452–5911; FAX. 208/452–4090; Leon C. Felder, President

ILLINOIS

Advocate Hospice, 1441 Branding Avenue, Suite 240, Downers Grove, IL 60515; tel. 630/963–6800; FAX. 630/963–6877; Nancy Kitts–Woodworth

Ariston Hospice Service, One Tower Lane, Suite 2620, Oak Brook Terrace, IL 60181; tel. 630/572–6400; Lynn MacMillan, Administrator

Beloit Hospice, Inc., 5512 Elevator Road, Roscoe, IL 61073; tel. 608/365–7421; Virginia Young

Bureau Valley Area Hospice, 530 Park Avenue, E., Princeton, IL 61356; tel. 815/875–2811; Janice Shue, Administrator

CT Willow Hospice, 9730 South Western Avenue, Suite 426, Evergreen, IL 60642; tel. 708/422–8575; Marie E. Vangemert, Director

Cass–Schuyler Area Hospice, 331 South Main Street, Virginia, IL 62691; tel. 217/452–3057; FAX. 217/452–7245; Virginia Hertweck, Administrator

Community Hospices of America Northwest Illinois, 256 South Soangetaha Road, Suite 103, Galesburg, IL 61401–5586; tel. 309/342–3007; FAX. 309/342–6973; Susan Myer, Program Director

DeKalb County Hospice, 615 North First Street, Suite 204, DeKalb, IL 60115; tel. 815/756–3000; Karen Hagen, RN, M.S., Executive Director

Dyna Care Hospice, 4800 North 129th Street, Alsip, IL 60658; tel. 708/389–2700; Marie Van Gemert, Administrator

Family Hospice of Belleville Area, 11B Park Place, Professional Center, Swansea, IL 62226; tel. 618/277–1800; FAX. 618/277–1074; Diane Smith, Administrator

Fox Valley Hospice, 200 Whitfield Drive, P.O. Box 707, Geneva, IL 60134; tel. 630/232–2233; FAX. 630/232–0023; Wilma I. Drummer, Executive Director

Franciscan Hospice of Central Illinois, 107 West Water Street, Pontiac, IL 67764; tel. 815/844–6982; Donna O'Shaughnessy, Administrator

Genesis Hospice Care of VNA, 1705 Second Avenue, Rock Island, IL 61201; tel. 309/794–1626; Sharon Meister, Administrator

Grundy Community Hospice, 1802 North Division Street, Suite 307, Morris, IL 60450; tel. 815/942–8525; Joan Sereno

Harbor Light Hospice, 800 Roosevelt Road, Building C, Suite 206, Glen Ellyn, IL 60137; tel. 800/419–0542; FAX. 630/942–0118; Dorothy M. Stahl, Administrator

Home Health Plus Hospice Program, 2215 Enterprise Drive, Suite 1512, Westchester, IL 60154; tel. 708/531–9339; Mary Schultz, Administrator

Home Health Plus Hospice Program, 333 Salem Place, Suite 165, Fairview Heights, IL 62208; tel. 618/632–0304; Ann Maurutto, Administrator

Horizon Hospice, Inc., 833 West Chicago Avenue, Chicago, IL 60622; tel. 312/733–2233; FAX. 312/733–8931; Kathryn A. Meshenberg, President, Chief Executive Officer

Hospice Alliance, Inc., 3452 North Sheridan Road, Zion, IL 60099; tel. 847/263–1180; Connie Matter, Administrator

Hospice Care, 319 East Madison, Suite Three J, Springfield, IL 62701; tel. 217/789–6506; FAX. 217/525–3739; Janet Thomson

Hospice Care of Illinois, Visiting Nurse Association of Central Illinois, 720 North Bond Street, Springfield, IL 62702; tel. 217/757–7322; Barbara Sullivan, Administrator

Hospice Suburban South, 78 Cherry Street, Park Forest, IL 60466; tel. 708/481–2104; Maureen Rinella, Executive Director

Hospice of Bond County, 503 South Prairie, Greenville, IL 62246; tel. 618/664–1442; Elnora Hamel, Administrator

Hospice of Dubuque, 501 St. Mary's Drive, East Dubuque, IL 61025; tel. 815/747–3622; Barbara Zoeller, Administrator

Hospice of Dupage, Inc., 690 East North Avenue, Carol Stream, IL 60188; tel. 630/690–9000; Wendy Neal, Administrator

Hospice of Kankakee Valley, Inc., 1015 North Fifth Avenue, Suite Five, Kankakee, IL 60901; tel. 815/939–4141; FAX. 815/939–1501; Dorothea MacDonald–Lagesse, Executive Director

Hospice of Lincolnland, 75 Professional Plaza, Mattoon, IL 61938; tel. 217/234–4044; FAX. 217/345–3261; Connie R. Oetinger, President, Chief Executive Officer

Hospice of Northeastern Illinois, Inc., 410 South Hager Avenue, Barrington, IL 60010; tel. 847/381–5599; FAX. 847/381–5713; Jane Bilyeu, Executive Director

Hospice of Northwest Illinois, Inc., 155 West Front Street, P.O. Box 185, Stockton, IL 61085–0185; tel. 815/947–3260; FAX. 815/947–3257; Les Graham, Associate Director

Hospice of Southeastern Illinois, 306 South Fair, Olney, IL 62450; tel. 618/395–2131; Susan G. Batchelor, Administrator

Hospice of Southern Illinois, Inc., 305 South Illinois Street, Belleville, IL 62220; tel. 618/235–1703; FAX. 618/235–2828; Merle L. Aukamp, President, Chief Executive Officer

Hospice of the Calumet Area, Inc., 3224 Ridge Road, Suite 202 and 203, Lansing, IL 60438; tel. 708/895–8332; FAX. 219/922–1947; Penny Karczewski, Admissions Coordinator

Hospice of the Great Lakes, 3130 Commercial Avenue, Northbrook, IL 60062; tel. 847/559–8999; FAX. 847/559–9005; Mary Jo Fox, Administrator

Hospice of the North Shore, A Division of Palliative Care Center of the North Shore, 2821 Central Street, Evanston, IL 60201; tel. 847/467–7423; FAX. 847/866–6023; Dorothy L. Pitner, RN, B.S.N., MM, President

Hospice of the Rock River Valley, 212 Fourth Avenue, P.O. Box 918, Rock Falls, IL 61071; tel. 815/626–9242; FAX. 815/626–7438; Mary Deem, Executive Director

Joliet Area Community Hospice, Inc., 335 West Jefferson Street, Joliet, IL 60435; tel. 815/740–4104; FAX. 815/740–4107; Duane A. Krieger, Executive Director

Lourdes Hospice, 600 Market Street, Metropolis, IL 62960; tel. 618/524–3647; FAX. 618/524–3920; Donna Stewart, Director

Monroe Clinic Hospice, 1301 South Kiwanis Drive, Freeport, IL 61032; tel. 815/235–1406; Carla Stadel, Administrator

Northern Illinois Hospice Association, 4215 Newburg Road, Rockford, IL 61108; tel. 815/398–0500; FAX. 815/398–0588; Judith A. Engblom, Executive Director

Ogle County Hospice Association, 421 Pines Road, P.O. Box 462, Oregon, IL 61061; tel. 815/732–2499; Lorrie Bearrows, RN, Executive Director

Pike County Health Department Hospice Care, 113 East Jefferson Street, Pittsfield, IL 62363; tel. 217/285–4407; FAX. 217/285–4639; Judith Schlieper, Administrator

QLS Community Home Health Based Hospice, 353 South Lewis Lane, Carbondale, IL 62901; tel. 618/529–2262; FAX. 618/457–8599; Monica J. Brahler, Administrator

QV, Inc., 322 South Green Street, Suite 500, Chicago, IL 60607–3599; tel. 312/736–8622; Noreen Hoenig, Administrator

Rainbow Hospice, Inc., 1550 North Northwest Highway, Suite 220, Park Ridge, IL 60068–1427; tel. 847/699–2000; FAX. 847/699–2047; Patricia Ahern, President, Executive Director

Rockford VNA, 4223 East State Street, Rockford, IL 61108; tel. 815/229–1100; FAX. 815/229–2226; Susan Schreier, Administrator

Rush Hospice Partners, 1035 Madison Street, Oak Park, IL 60302; tel. 708/386–9191; FAX. 708/386–9933; Kathleen Nash

Samaritan Care, Inc., 1955 Bernice Road, Suite N, Lansing, IL 60438; tel. 708/418–0100; Linda Mendoza

St. Thomas Hospice, Inc., Seven Salt Creek Lane, Suite 101, Hinsdale, IL 60521; tel. 630/850–3990; FAX. 630/850–3969; JoAnn Shenk, RN, Patient Care Coordinator

Staff Builders Services, Inc., Eight Cottonwood Road, Suite One, Edwardsville, IL 62034; tel. 618/288–8000; FAX. 618/288–8099; Linda Linkes, Administrator

Section C

Tip of Illinois Hospice Program, Four Executive Woods, Swansea, IL 62221; tel. 800/371–3885; FAX. 618/997–0922; Jodell Wheeler, Chief Executive Officer

Unity Hospice, 439 East 31st Street, Suite 213, Chicago, IL 60616; tel. 312/949–1188; FAX. 312/949–0158; Michael Klein, President

VNA Hospice, 3122 North Water Street, Decatur, IL 62526; tel. 217/877–1222; Karen Adell, Administrator

VNA Hospice of Evanston–Glenbrook Hospitals Home Services, 5215 Old Orchard, Suite 700, Skokie, IL 60077; tel. 847/581–1717; FAX. 847/581–1919; Mindy Ferber, Administrator

VNA of Fox Valley Hospice, 1245 Corporate Boulevard, Aurora, IL 60504; tel. 630/978–2532; FAX. 630/978–1129; Janet S. Craft, President, Chief Executive Officer

VNA of Illinois Hospice, 1809 West McCord, Centralia, IL 62801; tel. 618/533–2781; FAX. 618/533–3265; Celeste Krahl, Administrator

VNHA of Western Illinois Pathway Hospice, 500 42nd Street, Rock Island, IL 61201; tel. 309/788–0600; Mary Oelschlaeger, Administrator

Visiting Nurse Association Hospice, 1406 U.S. 45 North, Eldorado, IL 62930; tel. 618/273–9305; FAX. 618/273–2469; Cissy Kraft, Administrator

Vitas Corporation, 100 West 22nd Street, Suite 101, Lombard, IL 60148; tel. 630/495–8484; David Fielding, Administrator

Vitas Corporation, 5215 Old Orchard Road, Suite 800, Skokie, IL 60077; tel. 847/470–9193; Brian D. Wohl, Administrator

Vitas Corporation, 1055 West 175th Street, Suite One, Homewood, IL 60430; tel. 708/957–8777; Jay Koeper, Administrator

Vitas Corporation, 1424 East 53rd Street, Suite 201, Chicago, IL 60615; tel. 312/643–6222; Jay Koeper, Administrator

West Towns Hospice, 6438 West 34th Street, Berwyn, IL 60402; tel. 708/749–7171; FAX. 708/749–7185; Sandra Kubik, Administrator

Woodhaven Hospice and Special Support Services, 800 Hoagland Boulevard, Jacksonville, IL 62650; tel. 217/245–0838; Bette Jackson, Administrator

INDIANA

A Priority Hospice, 761 – 45th Street, Munster, IN 46321; tel. 219/922–8695

Americare Home Health and Hospice Services, 49 East Monroe, Franklin, IN 46131; tel. 317/736–6005

Clarian Hospice, Clarian Health Partners, Inc., 2039 North Capitol Avenue, Indianapolis, IN 46202; tel. 317/927–3800, ext. 134; FAX. 317/927–3815; Cheri McKinney, Program Coordinator

Comprecare Home Health and Hospice, 1607 East Dowling Street, Kendallville, IN 46755–0517; tel. 800/824–5860

Family Hospice of Indiana, LLC, 1710 East 10th L–185, Jeffersonville, IN 47130; tel. 812/284–0455

Harbor Light Hospice, 500 West Lincoln Highway, Suite F, Merrillville, IN 46410; tel. 800/237–4242; FAX. 219/793–9292; Stephanie Mayercik, Director

Heartland Hospice, 1315 Directors Row, Suite 206, Fort Wayne, IN 46808; tel. 219/484–7622; FAX. 219/484–5662; Tim Boon, Administrator

Hoosier Uplands Hospice, 1500 West Main Street, P.O. Box Nine, Mitchell, IN 47446; tel. 812/849–4447; FAX. 812/849–3068; Allen Burris, Director

Hospice Preferred Choice, 9302 North Meridian, Suite 251, Indianapolis, IN 46260; tel. 317/575–8590; FAX. 317/575–8698; James R. Monahan, Executive Director

Hospice of BAM Health Associates, Inc., 9223 Broadway, Suite A, Merrillville, IN 46410; tel. 219/738–5230

Hospice of South Central Indiana, Inc., 2400 East 17th Street, Columbus, IN 47201–5351; tel. 812/376–5813; FAX. 812/376–5929; Sandra Carmichael, Executive Director

Hospice of Southeastern Indiana, 606 Wilson Creek Road, Suite 430, Lawrenceburg, IN 47025; tel. 812/537–8192

Hospice of Southern Indiana, 624 East Market Street, P.O. Box 17, New Albany, IN 47150–4621; tel. 800/895–5633; FAX. 812/945–4733; Paul Elzer, Chief Executive Officer

Hospice of St. Joseph County, Inc., JMS Building, 108 North Main Street, Suite 111–113, South Bend, IN 46601–1625; tel. 219/237–0340; FAX. 219/237–0349; Thomas Burzynski, Executive Director

Hospice of Wabash Valley, 686 Wabash Avenue, Terre Haute, IN 47807; tel. 812/234–2515; FAX. 812/232–2047; Michelle Sly Smith, Hospice Services Director

Hospice of the Calumet Area, Inc., 600 Superior Avenue, Munster, IN 46321–4032; tel. 219/922–2732; FAX. 219/922–1947; Penny Karczewski, Admissions Coordinator

Hospice of the Miami Valley, 706 Eads Parkway, Lawrenceburg, IN 47025; tel. 812/537–5976; Gay Haggard, General Manager

Huntington Hospice, 240 South Jefferson Street, Huntington, IN 46750; tel. 219/356–3000

Jennings Visiting Nurse Association, Inc. Hospice, 945 Veterans Drive, P.O. Box 909, North Vernon, IN 47265; tel. 812/346–8774

Odyssey HealthCare of Central Indiana, Inc., 8765 Guion Road, Indianapolis, IN 46268; tel. 800/307–6021; Courtney McCollum, RN

Saint Joseph at Home Hospice Services, 400 North Main, Kokomo, IN 46903; tel. 317/452–6066; FAX. 317/457–4817; Darcy Herr, RN, Director

Samaritan Care Inc., 1101 East Coolspring Avenue, Michigan City, IN 46360; tel. 219/879–3411

St. Francis Hospice, 438 South Emerson, Greenwood, IN 46143; tel. 317/865–2095; Pamela Franklin, Administrator

The Community Hospice of VNA of NCI, 1354 South B Street, Elwood, IN 46036; tel. 317/552–3393; FAX. 317/552–3994; Karen Jarrett, Hospice Director

VNA Home Care Services Hospice, Inc., 901 South Woodland Avenue, Michigan City, IN 46360–5672; tel. 219/877–2070; FAX. 219/877–2089; Mary Craymer, Chief Executive Officer

VNA Hospice Home Care, and VNA Mary E. Bartz Hospice Center, 501 Marquette Street, Valparaiso, IN 46383–2058; tel. 219/462–5195; FAX. 219/462–6020; Laura Harting, Administrator

VNA Hospice of Southeastern Indiana, 1806 East 10th Street, Jeffersonville, IN 47130; tel. 812/288–2700; FAX. 812/285–8111; Nanci Brill, Hospice Director

Vencare Hospice of Indiana, 2601 Fortune Circle East Drive, Suite 105B, Indianapolis, IN 46241; tel. 317/484–9400; FAX. 317/484–9500; Dianna Pandak, Administrator

Vencor Hospice – Indianapolis, 1700 West 10th Street, Indianapolis, IN 46222; tel. 317/636–4400

Visiting Nurse Association Hospice, 610 East Walnut Street, P.O. Box 3487, Evansville, IN 47734–3487; tel. 800/326–4862; FAX. 812/463–4300; Carole Mattingly, Client Services Supervisor

Visiting Nurse Association of Northwest Indiana, Inc., 201 West 89th Avenue, Merrillville, IN 46410–6283; tel. 219/769–3644; FAX. 219/756–7372; Susan Rehrer, Executive Director

Visiting Nurse Home Health Services, Inc., 2323 Shoshone Court, Lafayette, IN 47905; tel. 317/448–6171; FAX. 317/474–7292; Marguerite Boerger, Executive Director

Visiting Nurse Service Hospice of Central Indiana, 4701 North Keystone Avenue, Indianapolis, IN 46205; tel. 317/722–8200; FAX. 317/722–8223; John L. Pipas, President, Chief Executive Officer

Visiting Nurse Service and Hospice, Inc., 3015 South Wayne Avenue, Fort Wayne, IN 46807; tel. 219/456–9888, ext. 232; FAX. 219/458–3089; Karen Gardner, President

Vitas Healthcare Corporation, 5240 Fountain Drive, Suite E, Crown Point, IN 46307; tel. 219/736–8921; FAX. 219/736–0972; Jay Koeper, General Manager

IOWA

Beacon of Hope Hospice Inc., 3906 Lillie, Suite Six, Davenport, IA 52806; tel. 319/391–6933; FAX. 319/391–5104; Dr. Robin Hall, Executive Director

Bremer–Butler Hospice, 406 West Bremer Avenue, Suites C and D, Waverly, IA 50677; tel. 319/352–1274; FAX. 319/352–9001

Calhoun County HHA/Hospice, 515 Court Street, P.O. Box 71, Rockwell City, IA 50579; tel. 712/297–8323; FAX. 712/297–5309; Tami Kinney, RN, Homecare Director

Cedar Valley Hospice, 2101 Kimball Avenue, Suite 401, Waterloo, IA 50702; tel. 319/292–1450; FAX. 319/292–1256; Cheryl A. Hoerner, Executive Director

Community Hospice of Iowa, 508 East Broadway, Council Bluffs, IA 51503; tel. 712/325–1751; FAX. 712/325–1895; Barbara Coppa, Administrator

Hamilton County PHNS–Hospice Division, 821 Seneca Street, Webster City, IA 50595; tel. 515/832–9565; FAX. 515/832–9554; Jacqueline Butler, Administrator

Homeward Hospice, 1606 South Duff, Suite 400, Ames, IA 50010; tel. 515/239–6730; FAX. 515/233–7556; Pat Fawcett, Director

Hospice of Central Iowa, 3619 1/2 Douglas Avenue, Des Moines, IA 50310; tel. 515/274–3400; FAX. 515/271–1302; William P. Havekost, President, Chief Executive Officer

Hospice of Compassion, 406 Court, P.O. Box 1034, Williamsburg, IA 52361–1034; tel. 319/668–2262; FAX. 319/668–1656; Carole Moore, Executive Director

Hospice of Dubuque, 3448 Hillcrest Road, Dubuque, IA 52002; tel. 319/582–1220; FAX. 319/582–8089; Barbara Zoeller, Director

Hospice of Lee County, Lee County Health Department–Community Nursing, 2218 Avenue H, Fort Madison, IA 52627; tel. 319/372–5225; FAX. 319/372–4374; M. Therese O'Brien, Administrator

Hospice of Mahaska County, 1229 C Avenue, E., Oskaloosa, IA 52577; tel. 515/672–3100; David E. Rutter, Administrator

Hospice of North Iowa, 232 Second Street, S.E., Mason City, IA 50401; tel. 515/423–3508; FAX. 515/423–5250; Ann MacGregor, Administrator

Hospice of Northwest Iowa, 1200 First Avenue East, Spencer, IA 51301; tel. 712/264–6380; FAX. 712/264–6470; Sheryl Thu, Director

Hospice of Siouxland, 500 11th Street, Sioux City, IA 51101; tel. 712/233–1298; FAX. 712/233–1123; Linda Todd, Hospice Director

Hospice of VNA, 242 North Bluff Boulevard, Clinton, IA 52732; tel. 319/242–7165; FAX. 319/242–7197; Denise Schrader, Executive Director

Hospice of Wapello County, 312 East Alta Vista, Ottumwa, IA 52501; tel. 515/682–0684; FAX. 515/684–9209; Cindy Donohue, RN, B.S.N., Director

Humboldt County PHNS and Hospice, Home Care Connection, Courthouse, Dakota City, IA 50529; tel. 515/332–2492; FAX. 515/332–4756; Janna Emick, Administrator

Iowa City Hospice, Inc., 613 Bloomington Street, Iowa City, IA 52245; tel. 319/351–5665; FAX. 319/351–5729; Maggie Elliott, Executive Director

Iowa River Hospice, Inc., 206 West Linn Street, Marshalltown, IA 50158; tel. 515/753–7704; FAX. 515/753–0379; Brent D. Blackwell, Executive Director

Mercy Hospice, 1055 Sixth Avenue, Suite 105, Des Moines, IA 50314; tel. 515/247–8383

Wings of Hope Hospice, Northwest Iowa Home Health Care and Hospice, 160 South Hayes Avenue, Primghar, IA 51245; tel. 712/757–0060; FAX. 712/757–0060; Beverly Van Beek, Executive Director

KANSAS

Central Homecare and Hospice, Inc., 427 S.E. Second, P.O. Box 645, Newton, KS 67114; tel. 316/283–8220; FAX. 316/283–8576; Robert E. Carlton, Executive Director

Community Hospice, 100 West Eighth Street, Onaga, KS 66521; tel. 913/889–7200; FAX. 913/889–4808; Mary Abitz, Director

Community Hospice of Kansas, 1650 South Georgetown, Suite 160, Wichita, KS 67218; tel. 316/686–5999; FAX. 316/686–5634; Karen Everhart, M.Ed., Director

Homecare and Hospice, Inc., 323 Poyntz Avenue, Suite A, Manhattan, KS 66502; tel. 913/537–0688; FAX. 913/537–1309; Pam Oehme, Director, Health Services

Hospice Care in Douglas County, 336 Missouri, Lower Level, Lawrence, KS 66044; tel. 913/749–5006; FAX. 913/843–0757; L. Kay Metzger, Director

Hospice Inc., 313 South Market, P.O. Box 3267, Wichita, KS 67201–3267; tel. 316/265–9441; FAX. 316/265–6066; John G. Carney, President

Hospice Services, Inc., 424 Eighth Street, P.O. Box 116, Phillipsburg, KS 67661; tel. 913/543–2900; FAX. 913/543–5688; Sandy Kuhlman

Hospice of Golden Belt HHS, 3623 Broadway, Great Bend, KS 67530; tel. 316/792–8171; Gayle Edwards

Hospice of Jefferson County, 1212 Walnut, Highway 59, P.O. Box 324, Oskaloosa, KS 66066–0275; tel. 913/863–2447; FAX. 913/863–2652; Marilyn Zieg, RN, Hospice Coordinator

Hospice of NE Kansas Multi–County, 326 East Ninth Street, Holton, KS 66436; tel. 913/364–4921; FAX. 913/364–3001; Patricia Scott, RN

Hospice of Reno County, Inc., Three Compound Drive, Hutchinson, KS 67502; tel. 316/665–2473; FAX. 316/669–5959; Carolyn Carter, RN, M.N., Executive Director

Hospice of Salina, Inc., 333 South Santa Fe, P.O. Box 2238, Salina, KS 67402–2238; tel. 913/825–1717; FAX. 913/825–4949; Kim Fair, Executive Director

Hospice of the Flint Hills, 527 Commercial, Suite 501, P.O. Box 102, Emporia, KS 66801; tel. 316/342–6640; FAX. 316/342–9424; Jay O'Daniel, Interim Director

Hospice of the Heartland, Inc., 400 West Eighth, Suite 207, P.O. Box 21, Beloit, KS 67420; tel. 913/738–9227; FAX. 913/738–9227; Robert Monty, Executive Director

Hospice of the Prairie, Inc., 2010 A First Avenue, P.O. Box 1294, Dodge City, KS 67801–2623; tel. 316/227–7209; FAX. 316/227–7429; Jeannie Reinert–Schuette, Executive Director

Leavenworth County Hospice, 920 Sixth Avenue, Leavenworth, KS 66048; tel. 913/684–1305; Charles L. Rogers

Midland Hospice Care, Inc., 200 Southwest Frazier Circle, Topeka, KS 66606–2800; tel. 913/232–2044; FAX. 913/232–5567; Karren Weichert, Executive Director

Ottawa County Home Health/Hospice Agency, 307 North Concord, Suite 200, Minneapolis, KS 67467; tel. 913/392–2822; June Clark, RN

SCCS Home Health and Hospice, P.A., 1410 North Woodlawn, Suite D, Derby, KS 67037; tel. 316/788–7626; FAX. 316/788–7072; Cheryl Pelaccio, RN, Administrator

South Wind Hospice, Inc., 337 North Pine, P.O. Box 862, Pratt, KS 67124; tel. 316/672–7553; FAX. 316/672–7554; Diane L. Johnson, Director

Southwest Homecare and Hospice, 103 East 11th Street, Liberal, KS 67901; tel. 316/629–2456; FAX. 316/629–2453, ext. 509; Ida Rodkey, Administrator

KENTUCKY

Community Hospice, 1538 Carter Avenue, Ashland, KY 41101; tel. 606/329–1890; FAX. 606/329–0018; Susan Hunt, Administrator

Cumberland Valley District Health Department Hospice, 102 South Court Street, Manchester, KY 40962; tel. 606/287–8437; Dottie Dunsil, RN, Nursing Supervisor

Green River Hospice, P.O. Box 449, Calhoun, KY 42327; tel. 502/273–3486; FAX. 502/273–9794; Jeana Bamberger, Patient Care Coordinator

Heritage Hospice, 337 West Broadway, P.O. Box 1213, Danville, KY 40422; tel. 606/236–2425; FAX. 606/236–6152; Andy Baker, Executive Director

Hospice Association, Inc., 2225 Frederica Street, P.O. Box 1403, Owensboro, KY 42301; tel. 502/926–7565; FAX. 502/926–1223; Linda Domerese, Ph.D., Executive Director

Hospice East, 24 West Lexington Avenue, P.O. Box 115, Winchester, KY 40392; tel. 606/744–9866; FAX. 606/744–1971; Carol Richardson, Director

Hospice of Big Sandy, 236 College Street, Paintsville, KY 41240–1747; tel. 606/789–3841; FAX. 667/789–1527; Claire Arsenault, Executive Director

Hospice of Central Kentucky, 105 Diecks Drive, P.O. Box 2149, Elizabethtown, KY 42701–2444; tel. 502/737–6300; FAX. 502/737–4053; Stephen Connor, Ph.D., Executive Director

Hospice of Hope, One West McDonald Parkway, Maysville, KY 41056; tel. 606/564–4848; FAX. 606/564–7615; Norman McRae, Chief Executive Officer

Hospice of Lake Cumberland, 108 College Street, P.O. Box 651, Somerset, KY 42502; tel. 606/679–4389; FAX. 606/678–0191; Jeanne Travis, Executive Director

Hospice of Louisville, 3532 Ephraim McDowell Drive, Louisville, KY 40205–3224; tel. 502/456–6200; FAX. 502/456–6655; Helen Donaldson, Executive Director

Hospice of Nelson County, 118 East Broadway, Bardstown, KY 40004; tel. 502/348–3660; FAX. 502/349–1292; Sharon Bade, Administrator

Hospice of Pike County, 229 College Street, Pikeville, KY 41501; tel. 606/432–2112; FAX. 606/432–4631; Sharon Branham, President, Chief Executive Officer

Hospice of Southern Kentucky, Inc., 1027 Broadway, Bowling Green, KY 42104; tel. 502/782–3402; FAX. 502/782–3496; Connie Jones, Director of Program Development and Volunteers

Hospice of the Bluegrass, 2312 Alexandria Drive, Lexington, KY 40504; tel. 606/276–5344; FAX. 606/223–0490; Gretchen M. Brown, President, Chief Executive Officer

Hospice of the Kentucky River, Inc., 210 St. George Street, Richmond, KY 40475–2376; tel. 606/624–8820; FAX. 606/624–9230; Gail McGillis, M.S.N., Chief Executive Officer

Jessamine County Hospice, 109 Shannon Parkway, P.O. Box 873, Nicholasville, KY 40356; tel. 606/887–2696; FAX. 606/885–1474; Susan G. Swinford, M.S.W., Executive Director

Lourdes Hospice, 2855 Jackson Street, Paducah, KY 42001; tel. 502/444–2262; FAX. 502/444–2380; Donna Stewart, Administrator

Mountain Community Hospice, P.O. Box 1234, Hazard, KY 41702; tel. 606/439–2111; FAX. 606/439–4198; Amy Asher, RN, Director

Mountain Heritage Hospice, Inc., 163 Belkway, Village Center, Building Two, P.O. Box 189, Harlan, KY 40831–0189; tel. 606/573–6111; FAX. 606/573–7964; Bernice Reynolds, Administrator

Pennyroyal Hospice, Inc., 1821 East Ninth Street, Suite A, Hopkinsville, KY 42240; tel. 502/885–6428; FAX. 502/889–5005; Hanna Sabel, Executive Director

St. Anthony's Hospice, Inc., 2410 South Green Street, P.O. Box 351, Henderson, KY 42420; tel. 502/826–2326; FAX. 502/831–2169; Rebecca S. Curry, Administrator

Tri County Hospice, P.O. Box 395, London, KY 40741; tel. 606/877–3950; Ed Valentine

LOUISIANA

Alternative Care Hospice, P.O. Box 691, Coushatta, LA 71019; tel. 318/932–8855; Faye Ross, Director

Alternative Hospice Care, Inc., 4560 North Boulevard, Suite 103, Baton Rouge, LA 70806; tel. 504/926–1550; Glenn Adams

American Hospice of Louisiana, Inc., 3340 Severn Avenue, Suite 215, Metairie, LA 70002; tel. 504/887–8128; FAX. 504/887–8206; Pat McCue, General Manager

Community Hospice of Bossier Medical Center, 2285 Benton Road, Suite 201D, Bossier City, LA 71111; tel. 318/741–6032; FAX. 318/747–0142; Linda McMillan, Director

Community Hospice of Louisiana, Inc., 5647 Superior Drive, Baton Rouge, LA 70816; tel. 504/293–1948; Frank Reuter, Program Director

Friendship Hospice of New Orleans, Inc., 1406 Esplanade Avenue, New Orleans, LA 70116; tel. 504/522–3183; Valarie Davis, Administrator

Golden Age Hospice, 5627 South Sherwood Forest Boulevard, Baton Rouge, LA 70816; tel. 504/292–2000; Martha C. Sewell

Good Shepherd in Hospice, Inc., 327 North Canal Boulevard, P.O. Box 1223, Thibodaux, LA 70302–1223; tel. 504/448–2200; Barbara Lofton

Hancock Hospice, P.O. Box 329, Tallulah, LA 71282–0329; tel. 318/574–2240; Ronald Hancock

Hospice Home Care of Lake Charles Memorial Hospital, 3050 Aster Street, Lake Charles, LA 70601; tel. 318/494–6444; FAX. 318/494–6451; Carol A. Maikisch, B.S.N., M.B.A., Administrator

Hospice Managed Care, Inc., 1423 Peterman Drive, Alexandria, LA 71301; tel. 318/442–5002; FAX. 318/442–5009; Susan Stephens, Administrator

Hospice of Acadiana, Inc., 125 South Buchanan, P.O. Box 3467, Lafayette, LA 70501; tel. 318/232–1234; FAX. 318/232–1297; Nelson Waguespack, Jr., Executive Director

Hospice of Greater Baton Rouge, 8322 One Calais Avenue, Suite A, Baton Rouge, LA 70809–3412; tel. 504/767–4673; FAX. 504/769–8113; Kathryn Grigsby, Executive Director

Hospice of Greater New Orleans, 3616 South I–10 Service Road, Suite 109, New Orleans, LA 70001; tel. 504/838–8944; FAX. 504/838–9034; Jo–Ann Mueller, Chief Executive Officer

Hospice of Jefferson, 2200 Veterans Highway, Suite 209, Kenner, LA 70062; tel. 504/464–7357; FAX. 504/466–9482; Anne Hedberg, Administrator

Hospice of Louisiana, 2915 Missouri Avenue, Shreveport, LA 71109; tel. 318/632–4697; FAX. 318/632–2382; Peggy Gavin, Hospice Administrative Representative

Hospice of Saint Landry, P.O. Box 488, Palmetto, LA 71358; tel. 318/623–3404; FAX. 318/623–3414; Dorothy Rabalais, RN, Director, Patient Services

Hospice of Shreveport/Bossier, 910 Pierremont, Suite 107, Shreveport, LA 71106; tel. 318/865–7177; Susan P. Stephens

Hospice of South Louisiana, 210 Mystic Boulevard, Houma, LA 70360; tel. 504/851–4273; FAX. 504/872–6543; Dottie Landry, RN, Administration

Hospice of Southwest Louisiana, 1000 South Huntington, Suite C, Sulphur, LA 70663; tel. 318/528–3011; FAX. 318/528–3035; Gail Hale, RN

Hospice of St. Jude, 615 Baronne Street, Suite 300 A, New Orleans, LA 70113; tel. 504/522–7108; Charles C. Harding

Hospice of St. Luke, 237 North Second Street, Eunice, LA 70535; tel. 800/869–2067; Willadean McWhorter, Administrator

Metro Hospice Care, Inc., 714 St. John, Monroe, LA 71201; tel. 318/361–9000; FAX. 318/361–9047; Deeni Shannon, Administrator

North Shore Regional Medical Center Hospice, 104 Smart Place, Slidell, LA 70458; tel. 504/641–7373; FAX. 504/641–4772; Aubrey Price, Director

Peoples Hospice, 1743 Stumpf Boulevard, Gretna, LA 70056; tel. 504/364–1494; FAX. 504/362–1056; Maggie Faucheux, RN, Administrator

Red River Hospice, Inc., 5501 John Eskew Drive, Alexandria, LA 71303; tel. 318/443–5694; E. W. Parker, Administrator

Samaritan Care Hospice of Louisiana, 3000 Knight Street, Suite 3000, Shreveport, LA 71105; tel. 318/869–2722; FAX. 318/869–2744; Toni Camp, Administrator

MAINE

Androscoggin Home Health Services, 15 Strawberry Avenue, P.O. Box 819, Lewiston, ME 04243–0819; tel. 207/777–7740; Richard C. Stephenson, M.D., Medical Director

Community Health And Nursing Services, d/b/a CHANS Hospice Care, 50 Baribeau Drive, Brunswick, ME 04011; tel. 207/729–6782; FAX. 207/725–5640; Jeanne St. Amand, RN, Executive Director

Community Health Services, Inc., 901 Washington Avenue, Suite 104, Portland, ME 04103; tel. 207/775–7231; FAX. 207/775–5520; Robert P. Liversidge, Jr., President, Chief Executive Officer

HealthReach Hospice, Eight Highwood Street, P.O. Box 1568, Waterville, ME 04903–1568; tel. 207/873–1127; FAX. 207/873–2059; Rebecca K. Colwell, Vice President, Home Care

Hospice Volunteers of Kennebec Valley, 150 Dresden Avenue, (First floor, KVMC), Gardiner, ME 04345; tel. 207/626–1779; FAX. 207/626–1798; Barbara Bell, Director

Hospice Volunteers of Waldo County, 118 Northport Avenue, P.O. Box 772, Belfast, ME 04915; tel. 207/338–2268, ext. 119; Michael L. Weaver, RN, Volunteer Coordinator

Hospice Volunteers of Waterville Area, 76 Silver Street, Waterville, ME 04901; tel. 207/873–3615; Susan Hermann–McMorrow, Program Coordinator

Hospice of Aroostook, Route 89 Access Highway, P.O. Box 688, Caribou, ME 04736; tel. 207/498–2578; FAX. 207/493–3111; Saundra Scott–Adams, Executive Director

Hospice of Hancock County, 29 Union Street, P.O. Box 224, Ellsworth, ME 04605; tel. 207/667–2531; FAX. 207/667–9406; Vesta Kowalski, Administrative Director

Hospice of Maine, 693 Rear Congress Street, Portland, ME 04102–3303; tel. 207/774–4417; Martha Wooten, Acting Executive Director

Hospice of Mid Coast Maine, 29 Parkview Circle, Brunswick, ME 04011–0741; tel. 207/729–3602; Gary Araujo, Executive Director

Kno–Wal–Lin Coastal Family Hospice, 170 Pleasant Street, Rockland, ME 04841; tel. 207/594–9561; FAX. 207/594–2527; Kathleen Deupree, RN, Patient Care Coordinator

Miles Home Health Hospice Division, R.R. Two, P.O. Box 4500, Damariscotta, ME 04543–8903; tel. 207/563–4592; FAX. 207/563–8652; Carol Knipping, Executive Director

New Hope Hospice, Inc., Route 46, Eddington, ME 04429; tel. 207/843–7521; Nancy S. Burgess, Director

Pine Tree Hospice, 65 West Main Street, Dover–Foxcroft, ME 04426; tel. 207/564–8401, ext. 346; Theresa Boettner, Program Coordinator

Southern Maine Health and Homecare Services, Route One South, P.O. Box 739, Kennebunk, ME 04043; tel. 207/985–4767; FAX. 207/985–6715; Elaine Brady, Executive Director

Tri–Area Visiting Nurse Association, Inc., 301 High Street, Somersworth, NH 03878–1800; tel. 603/692–2112; FAX. 603/692–9940; Susan Karmeris, President/Chief Executive Officer

Visiting Nurse Association and Hospice, 50 Foden Road, South Portland, ME 04106; tel. 207/780–8624; FAX. 207/756–8676; Delthia Vilasuso, Executive Director

Visiting Nurse Service of Southern Maine, 15 Industrial Park Road, Saco, ME 04072; tel. 207/284–4566; FAX. 207/282–4148; Maryanna Arsenault, Chief Executive Officer

MARYLAND

Bay Area Hospice, Inc., 410 West Lombard Street, Suite 602, Baltimore, MD 21201; tel. 410/328–1160; FAX. 410/328–1165; Karen L. Holland, Director

Bon Secours Home Health/Hospice, 1502 Joh Avenue, Suite 190, Baltimore, MD 21227; tel. 410/837–8500; FAX. 410/536–9739; Vic Ribaudo, Acting Executive Director

Calvert Hospice, 238 Merrimac Court, P.O. Box 838, Prince Frederick, MD 20678; tel. 410/535–0892; FAX. 301/855–1226; Carolyn S. Lewis, Executive Director

Caroline County Home Health/Hospice, 601 North Sixth Street, P.O. Box 10, Denton, MD 21629; tel. 410/479–3500; FAX. 410/479–3425; L. Carol Smith, Administrator

Carroll Hospice, 95 Carroll Street, Westminster, MD 21157; tel. 410/857–1838; Julie Flaherty, Executive Director

Children's Hospice Services, 111 Michigan Avenue, N.W., Washington, DC 20010; tel. 202/884–4663; FAX. 202/884–6950

Coastal Hospice, Inc., 2604 Old Ocean City Road, P.O. Box 1733, Salisbury, MD 21802–1733; tel. 410/742–6044; FAX. 410/548–5669; Marion F. Keenan, President

Dorchester County Home Health Hospice, 751 Woods Road, Cambridge, MD 21613; tel. 410/228–5860; FAX. 410/228–4475; Joyce T. Hyde, RN, M.S., Director

Harford Hospice, Inc., 56 East Bel Air Avenue, Aberdeen, MD 21001–3759; tel. 410/272–2266; FAX. 410/272–8413; Barry E. Yingling, President, Chief Executive Officer

Holy Cross Home Care and Hospice, 9805 Dameron Drive, Silver Spring, MD 20902; tel. 301/754–7740; FAX. 301/754–7743; Margaret Hadley, Assistant Director

Hospice Caring, Inc., Volunteer Hospice, 707 Conservation Lane, Suite 100, Gaithersburg, MD 20878; tel. 301/869–4673; FAX. 301/869–4673; Carol Sheehan, Executive Director

Hospice Services of Howard County, 5537 Twin Knoll Road, Suite 433, Columbia, MD 21045; tel. 410/730–5072; FAX. 410/730–5284; Nancy Weber

Hospice of Baltimore, Gilchrist Center for Hospice Care, 6601 North Charles Street, Baltimore, MD 21204; tel. 410/512–8200; FAX. 410/512–8284; Regina Bodnar, Director, Clinical Services

Hospice of Charles County, 105 La Grange Avenue, P.O. Box 1703, LaPlata, MD 20646; tel. 301/934–1268; FAX. 301/934–6437; Geri Firosz, President

Hospice of Frederick County, 1730 North Market Street, P.O. Box 1799, Frederick, MD 21702; tel. 301/694–6444; FAX. 301/694–9012; Laurel A. Cucchi, Executive Director

Hospice of Garrett County, 2008 Maryland Highway, P.O. Box 271, Mountain Lake Park, MD 21550; tel. 301/334–5151; FAX. 301/334–5800; Brenda Butscher, Executive Director

Hospice of Prince George's County, 96 Harry Truman Drive, Largo, MD 20774; tel. 301/499–0550; FAX. 301/350–7844; Lois Kimber, Director, Nursing Services

Hospice of Queen Anne's, Inc., 206 North Commerce Street, P.O. Box 179, Centreville, MD 21617; tel. 410/758–3043; FAX. 410/758–2838; Mildred H. Barnette, Director

Hospice of St. Mary's, Inc., 100 Courthouse Drive, Leonardtown, MD 20650; tel. 301/475–2023; FAX. 301/475–3497; Dana McGarity, Executive Director

Hospice of Washington County, 101 East Baltimore Street, Hagerstown, MD 21740; tel. 301/791–6360; FAX. 301/791–6579; Robert Rauch, Executive Director

Hospice of the Chesapeake, Inc., 8424 Veterans Highway, Millersville, MD 21108; tel. 410/987–2003; FAX. 410/987–3961; Erwin E. Abrams, President

Jewish Social Service Agency, 22 C Montgomery Village Avenue, Gaithersburg, MD 20879; tel. 301/990–6880; Joanne Nattrass, Director

Joseph Richey Hospice, 828 North Eutaw Street, Baltimore, MD 21201; tel. 410/523–2150; FAX. 410/523–1146; Suzanne Hetzer, RN, Director, Patient Services

Kent Home Health/Hospice, 125 South Lynchburg Street, P.O. Box 359, Chestertown, MD 21620; tel. 410/778–1050; FAX. 410/778–7399; Karen Russum, RN, Director

Mid–Atlantic Hospice Care, 4805 Benson Avenue, Baltimore, MD 21227; tel. 410/247–2900; FAX. 410/247–2581; Darlene Tamburri

Montgomery Hospice Society, 1450 Research Boulevard, Suite 310, Rockville, MD 20850; tel. 301/279–2566; Nancy Taylor, Executive Director

Northern Chesapeake Hospice, Inc., 239 South Bridge Street, Suite Two, Elkton, MD 21921; tel. 410/392–4742; FAX. 410/392–6448; Cathy Stauffer Kimble, Executive Director

Stella Maris Hospice Care Program, 2300 Dulaney Valley Road, Towson, MD 21204; tel. 410/252–4500; FAX. 410/560–9675; Sister Karen McNally, R.S.M., Chief Operating Officer

Talbot County Home Health/Hospice, 100 South Hanson Street, Easton, MD 21601; tel. 410/822–3855; FAX. 410/822–2583; Gloria W. Dill, RN, MS, Nurse Manager

Tri–Home Health Care and Services, 2000 Rock Springs Road, P.O. Box 240, Forest Hills, MD 21050; tel. 410/893–0544; Susan Parks, RN, Hospice Coordinator

VNA Hospice of Maryland L.L.C., 6000 Metro Drive, Suite 101, Baltimore, MD 21215; tel. 410/358–7300; FAX. 410/358–7326; Janet Melancon, RN, Hospice Director

MASSACHUSETTS

Bay State Health Care Center South Shore, 780 Main Street, South Weymouth, MA 02190

Cranberry Area Hospice, Inc., 161 Summer Street, Kingston, MA 02364–1224; tel. 617/585–1881; FAX. 617/585–1898; John A. Brennan, Executive Director

Diversified VNA Hospice, 316 Nichols Road, Fitchburg, MA 01420; tel. 508/342–6013; FAX. 508/343–5629; Noreen Basque, Administrator

Good Samaritan Hospice, Inc., 310 Allston Street, Brighton, MA 02146; tel. 617/566–6242; FAX. 617/566–3055; Leo P. Smith, Executive Director

Hampshire County Hospice, Inc., Seven Denniston Place, P.O. Box 1087, Northampton, MA 01061; tel. 413/586–8288; FAX. 413/584–9615; Joan Keochakian, Executive Director

HealthCare Dimensions, 254 South Street, Waltham, MA 02154–2707; tel. 617/894–1100; FAX. 617/736–0908; Patricia A. Field, Executive Director

Hospice Care of Greater Taunton, One Taunton Green, Taunton, MA 02780; tel. 508/822–1447; Joanne Smith, Vice President, Clinical Services

Hospice Care, Inc., 41 Montvale Avenue, Stoneham, MA 02180; tel. 617/279–4100; FAX. 617/279–4677; Christine Peacock Bauler, Interim Executive Director

Hospice Community Care, 495 Pleasant Street, Winthrop, MA 02152

Hospice Life Care, P.O. Box 10428, Holyoke, MA 01041; tel. 413/533–3923; FAX. 413/536–4513; Patricia Cavanaugh, Director

Hospice Outreach, Inc., 243 Forest Street, Fall River, MA 02721; tel. 508/673–1589; FAX. 508/677–3144; Linda Valley, Executive Director

Hospice of Boston and Hospice of Greater Brockton, 500 Belmont Street, Suite 215, Brockton, MA 02401; tel. 508/583–0383; FAX. 508/583–1193; Ruth Capernaros, Executive Director

Hospice of Cape Cod, Inc., 923 Route 6A, Yarmouthport, MA 02675; tel. 508/362–1103; FAX. 508/362–6885; Marilyn Hannus, RN, Director

Hospice of Central Massachusetts, Inc., 120 Thomas Street, Worcester, MA 01608; tel. 508/756–7176

Hospice of Community Health Services, 423 Main Street, Athol, MA 01331; tel. 508/249–5366

Hospice of Community Nurse Association, 40 Centre Street, P.O. Box 831, Fairhaven, MA 02719; tel. 508/999–3400; FAX. 508/999–6401; Brenda M. Van Laarhoven, RN, Supervisor

Hospice of Community Visiting Nurse Agency, 141 Park Street, Attleboro, MA 02703; tel. 800/220–0110; FAX. 508/226–8939; Kathleen M. Trier, Executive Director

Hospice of Greater Milford, 391 South Main Street, P.O. Box 122, Hopedale, MA 01747; tel. 508/634–8382; FAX. 508/634–8738; Renee Merolli, RN, M.A., Director

Hospice of Northern Berkshire, Inc. at CompCare, 46 Howland Avenue, Adams, MA 01220; tel. 413/743–2960; FAX. 413/743–1515; Camille Richards, Executive Director

Hospice of the Good Shepherd, 2042 Beacon Street, Waban, MA 02168; tel. 617/969–6130; FAX. 617/928–1450; Ellen Rudikoff, Ph.D., Executive Director

Hospice of the North Shore, Inc., 10 Elm Street, Danvers, MA 01923; tel. 508/774–7566; FAX. 508/774–4389; Diane Stringer, Executive Director

Hospice of the South Shore, P.O. Box 334, 100 Bay State Drive, Braintree, MA 02184

HospiceCare of the Berkshires, Inc., 235 East Street, Pittsfield, MA 01201; tel. 413/443–2994; FAX. 413/433–7814; Peter Briguglio, Executive Director

Lighthouse Hospice Association, Inc., 166 Main Street, P.O. Box 448, Wareham, MA 02571–0448; tel. 508/295–8544; FAX. 508/295–0930; Phyllis G. Pheeney, Executive Director

Merrimack Valley Hospice, Inc., One Water Street, Haverhill, MA 01830; tel. 508/470–1615; FAX. 508/470–4690; Raymond Brokill, Director

Neponset Valley Hospice, Inc., Three Edgewater Drive, Norwood, MA 02062; tel. 617/769–8282; FAX. 617/762–0718; Susan DiBona, Hospice Manager

Old Colony Hospice, Inc., 14 Page Terrace, Stoughton, MA 02072; tel. 617/341–4145; FAX. 617/297–7345; Analee Wulfhuhle, Executive Director

Staff Builders Hospice Program, 529 Main Street, Suite 1M07, Boston, MA 02129; tel. 617/242–4872; FAX. 617/241–2880; Victoria Gunfolino, Director

Trinity Hospice of Greater Boston, Inc., 111 Cypress Street, Brookline, MA 02146

VNA Care Choices, Inc., 245 Winter Street, Suite 110, Waltham, MA 02154; tel. 617/890–2931; FAX. 617/890–6627; Patricia O'Brien, M.S., RN, Executive Director, VNA Care Choices, Inc.

VNA of Greater Gardner Hospice, 34 Pearly Lane, Gardner, MA 01440; tel. 508/632–1230; FAX. 508/632–4513; Tina Griffin, Director

Visiting Nurse Association and Hospice of Pioneer Valley, Inc., 50 Maple Street, P.O. Box 9058, Springfield, MA 01102–9058; tel. 413/781–5070; FAX. 413/781–3342; Maureen Skipper, President

Visiting Nurse Association of Greater Lowell Hospice, 336 Central Street, P.O. Box 1965, Lowell, MA 01853–1965; tel. 508/459–9343; FAX. 508/459–0981; Nancy L. Pettinelli, Executive Director

Visiting Nurse Association of Middlesex–East and Affiliated Visiting Nurse Hospice, 12 Beacon Street, Stoneham, MA 02180; tel. 617/438–3770; FAX. 617/438–7994; Jacquelyn Galluzzi, Chief Executive Officer

Wayside Hospice/Parmenter Health Services, 266 Cochituate Road, Wayland, MA 01778; tel. 508/358–3000; FAX. 508/358–3005; Edith L. Murray, Director

Westhills Home Health and Hospice, Inc., 77 Mill Street, Suite 207, Westfield, MA 01085; tel. 413/562–7049; FAX. 413/568–9434; Jacqueline Schmitz, RNC, Hospice Director

MICHIGAN

Allen Hospice–Southfield, 26300 Telegraph Road, Suite 102, Southfield, MI 48034; tel. 810/948–1019; Annette F. Sherry, Executive Director

Andy Scholett Memorial, 12426 State Street, P.O. Box 587, Atlanta, MI 49709–0587; tel. 517/785–3134; FAX. 517/785–2834; Shirley Burnham, Executive Director

Angela Hospice Home Care, Inc. and Care Center, 14100 Newburgh Road, Livonia, MI 48154–5010; tel. 313/464–7810; FAX. 313/464–6930; Clare McAuliffe, Admissions Counselor

Arbor Hospice, Home Care and Care–ousel, 7445 Allen Road, Suite 230, Allen Park, MI 48101; tel. 800/783–5764; FAX. 313/383–0115; Sue Andres, Director, Clinical Services

Arbor Hospice, Home Care, and Care–ousel, 3810 Packard Road, Suite 200, Ann Arbor, MI 48108; tel. 313/677–0500; FAX. 313/677–2014; Mary Lindquist, President

Arcadia Hospice, Inc., 340 East Big Beaver, Suite 200, Troy, MI 48083; tel. 810/740–8778; FAX. 810/740–8726; Pamela Lennig, Director

Baraga County Hospice, Inc., 913 Meador Street, L'Anse, MI 49946; tel. 906/524–5168

Barry Community Hospice, A Division of Good Samaritan Hospice Care, Inc., 450 Meadow Run Drive, Suite 200, P.O. Box 308, Hastings, MI 49058; tel. 616/948–8452; FAX. 616/948–9545; Kay Rowley, Patient Care Coordinator

Barry–Eaton District Health Department – Hospice Program, 528 Beech Street, Charlotte, MI 48813; tel. 517/541–2610; FAX. 517/541–2612; Penny Pierce, RN, Director

Blue Water Hospices, Inc., 1422 Lyon Street, Port Huron, MI 48060; tel. 313/982–8809; FAX. 313/984–1612; Brenda K. Clark, Vice President, Operations

Branch–Hillsdale–St. Joseph District, Health Department Hospice, 809 Marshall Road, Coldwater, MI 49036; tel. 517/279–5961; FAX. 517/278–2923; Helen Jakstas, RN, B.S.N., M.P.H., Director

Branch–Hillside–St. Joseph DHD, 600 South Lakeview, Sturgis, MI 49091; tel. 616/659–4013; Duke Anderson

Cass Branch Hospice Program, 201 M–62 North, Cassopolis, MI 49031; tel. 616/445–2296

Cass County Hospice, Inc., 58253 M52, Cassopolis, MI 49031; tel. 616/782–5078; Jean Maile

Charlevoix County Hospice, 601 Bridge Street, East Jordan, MI 49727; tel. 616/536–2842; FAX. 616/536–7150; Margaret Lasater

Citizens for Hospice, 27 East Chicago Street, Coldwater, MI 49028; tel. 517/278–5903; Sara Semmelroth

Community Home Health and Hospice, G–5095 West Bristol Road, Flint, MI 48507; tel. 313/733–7250; FAX. 313/733–8424; Donna Lloyd, Executive Director

Community Hospice Services, Inc., 32932 Warren Road, Suite 100, Westland, MI 48185; tel. 313/522–4244; FAX. 313/522–2099; Maureen Butrico, Executive Director

Cranbrook Hospice Care, 281 Enterprise Court, Suite 300, Bloomfield, MI 48302–0313; tel. 810/334–6700; FAX. 810/334–7064; Brian Hansen, Director

Dickinson–Iron DHD, 601 Washington Avenue, Stambaugh, MI 49964; tel. 906/265–9913; FAX. 906/265–2950; Linda Piper, RNC, M.P.H.

District Health Department, #3, 220 West Garfield Street, Charleviox, MI 49720; tel. 616/547–6092; FAX. 616/547–1164; Nancy Bottomley, RN, M.S., Director, Adult Health

Downriver Hospice, Inc., 1545 Kingsway Court, Trenton, MI 48183; tel. 313/671–6343

Genesys Hospice, 100 South Dort Highway, Flint, MI 48503; tel. 810/762–3875; FAX. 810/762–0027; LaVerne McCombs, Administrator

Good Samaritan Hospice Care, Inc., 80 North 20th Street, P.O. Box 1695, Battle Creek, MI 49016; tel. 616/965 1391; FAX. 616/965–2833; Jo Cunningham, Executive Director

Grancare Hospice Services, 38935 Ann Arbor Road, Livonia, MI 48150; tel. 313/432–6565; FAX. 313/432–7244; Nancy L. McHugh, Director

Grand Traverse Area Hospice, 1105 Sixth Street, Traverse City, MI 49684; tel. 616/935–6520; FAX. 616/935–7270; Kay Benisek, Manager

Heartland Hospice, 814 Adams, Suite 109, Bay City, MI 48708; tel. 517/892–0355; FAX. 517/892–0896; Christine Satkowiak, RN, Administrator

Heartland Hospice, 700 West Ash Street, Suite Three–A, Mason, MI 48854; Lynn Howes

Heartland Hospice, 6504 28th Street, S.E., Suite T, Grand Rapids, MI 49546; tel. 616/942–7733

Helping Hands Hospice, 545 Apple Tree Drive, Ionia, MI 48846; tel. 616/527–5550; FAX. 616/527–5683; Becky Mason, RN, Administrator

Henry Ford Hospice–West Bloomfield, 6020 West Maple Road, Suite 500, West Bloomfield, MI 48322; tel. 810/539–0660; FAX. 810/539–8868; Laura Zeile, RN, B.S.N., Manager

Home Health Plus Hospice, 26211 Central Park Boulevard, Suite 110, Southfield, MI 48076; tel. 313/357–3650; Sharon Kohlitz, RN, B.S., Director, Operations

Home Hospice, Inc., 315 Ives, Big Rapids, MI 49307; tel. 616/796–7371; FAX. 616/796–4841; Kathy Shefferly, RN, Director

Hospice Care, Inc., 110 South Clay, Sturgis, MI 49091; tel. 616/651–6255

Hospice at Home, Inc., 2626 West John Beers Road, P.O. Box 297, Stevensville, MI 49127; tel. 616/429–7100; FAX. 616/428–3499; Stephen S. Towns, Director

Hospice for Presque Isle County, 658 South Bradley, Rogers City, MI 49779; tel. 517/734–7200; FAX. 517/734–2059; Shirley Haan, Coordinator

Hospice of Bay Area, 1460 West Center Avenue, Essexville, MI 48732; tel. 517/895–4750; FAX. 517/895–4701; Christine Chesny

Hospice of Bay Area, 150 Millwood, Caro, MI 48723; tel. 517/672–2094; Christine Chesny

Hospice of Central Michigan, Inc., 210 North Court Street, Suite B, Mt. Pleasant, MI 48858; tel. 517/773–6137; FAX. 517/773–1072; Deanna L. Heath, Executive Director

Hospice of Chippewa County/Chippewa County Health Department, 125 Arlington Street, Sault Ste. Marie, MI 49783; tel. 906/632–2202; FAX. 906/635–1701; Judy Jones, Supportive Services Director

Hospice of Clinton Memorial and Sparrow, 304 Brush Street, St. Johns, MI 48879; tel. 517/224–5650; FAX. 517/224–1501, ext. 330; Michelle Wiseman, Director

Hospice of Crawford County, P.O. Box Two, Grayling, MI 49738; tel. 517/348–5461

Hospice of Gladwin Area, Inc., 612 North M–18, P.O. Box 557, Gladwin, MI 48624; tel. 517/426–4464; FAX. 517/426–3057; Georgann Schuster, Executive Director

Hospice of Greater Grand Rapids, 1260 Ekhart, N.E., Grand Rapids, MI 49503; tel. 616/454–1426; David G. Zwicky, Program Director

Hospice of Greater Kalamazoo, Inc., 301 West Cedar Street, Kalamazoo, MI 49007–5106; tel. 616/345–0273; FAX. 616/345–8522; Lori Schultz, Director, Client Care

Hospice of Helping Hands, Inc., 801 East Houghton Avenue, P.O. Box 71, West Branch, MI 48661; tel. 517/345–4700; FAX. 517/345–2991; Christopher Lauckner, Director

Hospice of Hillsdale County, 111 South Howell Street, Suite B, Hillsdale, MI 49242; tel. 517/437–5252; FAX. 517/437–5253; Kathryn Aemisegger

Hospice of Holland Home, 2100 Raybrook, S.E., Suite 303, Grand Rapids, MI 49546; tel. 616/235–5100; FAX. 616/235–5111; Karen Bacon Washburn, Director

Hospice of Holland, Inc., 270 Hoover Boulevard, Holland, MI 49423; tel. 616/396–2972; FAX. 616/396–2808; Judith A. Zylman, RN, Executive Director

Hospice of Ionia, 117 North Depot Street, Ionia, MI 48846; tel. 616/527–0681; Bernice Falsetta

Hospice of Jackson, 915 Airport Road, Jackson, MI 49202; tel. 517/783–2648; FAX. 517/783–2674; Michael L. Freytag, M.A., L.P.C., Executive Director

Hospice of Lake County, 735 Third Street, P.O. Box 699, Baldwin, MI 49304; tel. 616/745–6161; FAX. 616/745–7676; Margaret Horner, RN, Program Director

Hospice of Lansing, Inc., 6035 Executive Drive, Suite 103, Lansing, MI 48911; tel. 517/882–4500; FAX. 517/882–3010; Barbara A. Kowalski, M.P.A., Executive Director

Hospice of Lenawee, 415 Mill Road, Adrian, MI 49221; tel. 517/263–2323; FAX. 517/263–1279; Karen Miller, RN, CRNH, Patient Care Coordinator

Hospice of Little Traverse Bay, 416 Connable Avenue, Petoskey, MI 49770; tel. 616/347–9700; FAX. 616/348–4228; Diane Lagerstrom, Executive Director

Hospice of Mason County, Inc., 10 Atkinson Drive, Suite Three, Ludington, MI 49431; tel. 616/845–0321; Glenna Lou Nelson, RN, B.S.N., Interim Executive Director

Hospice of Michigan, Crossroads Building, 16250 Northland Drive, Suite 212, Southfield, MI 48075–5200; tel. 810/559–9209; FAX. 810/559–6489; Carolyn J. Cassin, President, Chief Executive Officer

Hospice of Michigan–Roscommon, 107 South Main, P.O. Box 532, Roscommon, MI 48653; tel. 517/275–8967; FAX. 517/275–6130; Sheila Simpson, Program Director

Hospice of Monroe, 502 West Elm Street, Monroe, MI 48162; tel. 313/457–3220; FAX. 313/457–5060; Teri Turner, RN, M.S., Director

Hospice of Muskegon–Oceana, 1095 Third Street, Suite 209, Muskegon, MI 49441; tel. 616/728–3442; FAX. 616/722–0708; Mary Anne Gorman, Executive Director

Hospice of Muskegon–Oceana, 339B Dewey, Shelby, MI 49455; tel. 616/861–4761; FAX. 616/722–0708

Hospice of Newaygo County, A division of Hospice of Michigan, Inc., 819 West Main Street, Fremont, MI 49412; tel. 616/924–6123; FAX. 616/924–8028; Marie Malone, RN, B.S.N., Hospice Director

Hospice of North Ottawa Community, Inc., 1515 South Despelder, Grand Haven, MI 49417; tel. 616/846–2015; FAX. 616/846–7227; Carolyn K. Howes, Executive Director

Hospice of Northeastern Michigan, Inc., 112 West Chisholm, Alpena, MI 49707; tel. 517/354–5258; Jeraldyne Habermehl, Executive Director

Hospice of Southeast Michigan/Detroit, 2990 West Grand Boulevard, Suite 402, Detroit, MI 48202; tel. 313/874–2000; June William

Hospice of Southeast Michigan/Franklin, 12900 West Chicago Boulevard, Detroit, MI 48228; tel. 313/491–0022; Carolyn Fitzgerald

Hospice of Southeastern Michigan – North Oakland, 530 West Huron, Pontiac, MI 48341; tel. 810/253–2580; FAX. 810/253–2599; Rita Ann Mahon, RN, Director

Hospice of Southeastern Michigan–St. Clair Shores, 22811 Greater Mack Avenue, St. Clair Shore, MI 48080; tel. 313/559–9209; Carolyn Fitzgerald

Hospice of Sturgis, 600 South Lakeview Avenue, Sturgis, MI 49091; Pamela Pope

Hospice of Van Buren County/Greater Kalamazoo, 404 North Hazen Street, Suite L3, Paw Paw, MI 49079; tel. 616/657–7769; FAX. 616/657–7225; Lori Schultz, Director of Client Care

Hospice of Washtenaw, 806 Airport Boulevard, Ann Arbor, MI 48108; tel. 313/741–5777; FAX. 313/741–5757; Stephanie Gilbert, Admissions Coordinator

Hospice of Wexford–Missaukee, A Program of Hospice of Michigan, 932 North Mitchell Street, Cadillac, MI 49601; tel. 616/779–9570; FAX. 616/779–0717; Pat Spragg, RN, Director

Hospice of the North, Inc., 110 South Elm Street, Gaylord, MI 49735; tel. 517/732–3722

Hospice of the Straits/Vital Care, 761 Lafayette, Cheboygan, MI 49721; tel. 616/627–4774; FAX. 616/627–4416; Kimberly L. Sangster, Executive Director

Hospice of the VNA of Southeastern Michigan, 7700 Second Avenue, Detroit, MI 48202; tel. 313/876–8550; FAX. 313/876–8518; Charlene T. Coting, RN

Hospice of the VNA of Southeastern Michigan–East, 26000 Hoover, Warren, MI 48089; tel. 810/756–9000; Charlene T. Cotting, RN

Hospice of the VNA of Southeastern Michigan–Oakland, 26200 Lahser Road, Suite 204, Southfield, MI 48034; tel. 810/354–5250; Charlene T. Cotting, RN

Hospice of the VNA of Southeastern Michigan–West, 8600 Silvery Lane, Dearborn Height, MI 48127; tel. 313/730–8020; Charlene T. Cotting, RN

Hospice's of Henry Ford Health System, 23000 Mack Avenue, Suite 500, St. Clair Shore, MI 48080; tel. 810/774–4141; FAX. 810/774–0515; Sondra Seely, Administrator

Hospice–Partners in Caring, Division of VNA of Saginaw, 500 South Hamilton, Saginaw, MI 48602; tel. 517/799–6020; FAX. 517/799–6062; S. J. Schultz, B.S.N., M.S., President, Chief Executive Officer

Individualized Hospice, 3003 Washtenaw Avenue, Suite Two, Ann Arbor, MI 48104; tel. 313/971–0444; FAX. 313/971–1980; Patricia Love, Clinical Director

International Pediatric Hospice, 2300 Buhl Building, Detroit, MI 48226; tel. 313/965–6100; Paul Manion

Kaleidoscope Kids, 2921 West Grand Boulevard, Detroit, MI 48202; tel. 313/972–1980; Sondra Seely

Karmanos Cancer Institute–Hospice Program, 24601 Northwestern Highway, Southfield, MI 48075; tel. 810/827–1592; FAX. 810/827–0972; Joan McNally, Administrator

Keweenaw Home Nursing and Hospice, 414 Hecla Street, Laurium, MI 49913; tel. 906/337–5700; FAX. 906/337–9929; Diane Tiberg, RN, Director

LMAS DHD Hospice, P.O. Box 398, County Road 428, Newberry, MI 49868; tel. 906/293–5107; FAX. 906/293–5453; Kathleen Nyeste, Hospice Director

LMAS DHD Hospice/St. Ignace, 749 Hombach Street, St. Ignace, MI 49781; tel. 906/643–7700; FAX. 906/643–7719; Judy Misner, Home Health Nursing Supervisor

Section C

Lake Superior Hospice Association, 148 West Washington, Marquette, MI 49855; tel. 906/226–2646; FAX. 906/226–7735; Jill Baker, Executive Director

Lake Superior Hospice Association, 502 North Main Street, L'Anse, MI 49946; tel. 906/524–4477; Jill Baker

MI Home Health Care/Terminal Care, 955 East Commerce Drive, Traverse City, MI 49684; tel. 616/943–8451; FAX. 616/943–4515; Lilo Hoelzel–Seipp

Manistee Area Volunteer Hospice, Inc., P.O. Box 293, Manistee, MI 49660; tel. 616/723–6064; Diane Cameron, President

Marinette–Menominee County Hospice, 3133 Carney Avenue, Marinette, WI 54143; tel. 906/863–6331

McLaren Hospice Service, Inc., 237 Davis Lake Road, Lapeer, MI 48446; tel. 810/667–0042; Terry Morgan, President

Memorial Hospice, 1320 South Carpenter Street, Iron Mountain, MI 48901; tel. 906/774–5589

Mid Michigan VNA Hospice/Clare, 1438 North McEwan, Clare, MI 48617; tel. 800/862–5002; FAX. 517/839–1773; Miriam Markowitz, Director

MidMichigan Visiting Nurses Association and Hospice, 3007 North Saginaw Road, Midland, MI 48640; tel. 517/839–1770; FAX. 517/839–1749; Miriam Markowitz, Hospice Director

Montcalm Area Hospice, 302 1/2 East Main, Stanton, MI 48888; tel. 517/831–5045; Carol Goffnett

North County Hospice, Inc., 301 South Cedar, Kalkaska, MI 49646; tel. 616/258–5286

North Woods Home Nursing and Hospice, 226 South Cedar, P.O. Box 307, Manistique, MI 49854; tel. 906/341–6963; FAX. 906/341–2490; Susan Bjorne, Administrator

Northwest Ohio Hospice Association, 3930 Sunforest Court, Suite 200, Toledo, OH 43624; tel. 419/479–3115; Virginia Clifford

Otsego Area Hospice, a program of Hospice of Michigan, 810 South Otsego, Suite 111, Gaylord, MI 49735; tel. 517/732–2151; FAX. 517/731–2897; Sheila Simpson, Area Director

Samaritan Care, Inc., 24445 Northwestern Highway, Suite 100, Southfield, MI 48075; tel. 800/397–9360; FAX. 810/355–5705; Margaret Karvala, Administrator

South Haven Area Hospice, 05055 Blue Star Highway, P.O. Box 990, South Haven, MI 49090–0990; tel. 616/637–3825; FAX. 616/637–6777; Barbara Reicherts, Executive Director

St. Joseph Huron Home Health and Hospice, Inc., 716 German Street, Suite B, P.O. Box 208, Tawas City, MI 48764; tel. 517/362–4611; FAX. 517/362–8771; Ann Balfour, Administrator

St. Joseph's Hospice/Affiliate of Henry Ford Cottage Hospice, 43411 Garfield Boulevard, Building Two, Suite B, Clinton Township, MI 48038; tel. 810/263–2840; FAX. 810/263–2895; Patti Ciechanovski, CRNH, Manager

United Home Hospice, Inc., 2401 20th Street, Detroit, MI 48216; tel. 313/964–1133; Alice Okwu, Director, Nursing

United Hospice Service, Six Eastgate Plaza, Sandusky, MI 48471; tel. 800/635–7490

Upper Peninsula Home Nursing/Hospice, 1414 West Fair, Suite 44, Marquette, MI 49855; tel. 906/225–4545; FAX. 906/225–4544; Cynthia A. Nyquist, RN, B.S.N., Administrator, Chief Executive Officer

VNA Home Care Services Hospice, Inc., 901 South Woodland Avenue, Michigan City, IN 46360–5672; tel. 219/877–2070; FAX. 219/877–2089; Mary Craymer, Chief Executive Officer

VNA of Southwest Michigan Hospice, County Road #681, Suite D, Hartford, MI 49057; tel. 616/621–3154; Jill Eldred

VNA of Southwest Michigan–Hospice Program, 348 North Burdick Street, Kalamazoo, MI 49007–3843; tel. 616/343–1396; FAX. 616/382–8686; Jill Eldred

Visiting Nurse Hospice, 4801 Willoughby, Suite Seven, Holt, MI 48842; tel. 517/694–8300; FAX. 517/694–4968; Jeanne Zabihaylo, Admissions Coordinator

Visiting Nurse Service of Western Michigan Hospice Program, 1401 Cedar, N.E., Grand Rapids, MI 49503; tel. 616/774–2702; FAX. 616/774–7017; Laurie Sefton, RN, M.S.N., Hospice Program Director

West Bloomfield Hospice, 6777 West Maple Road, West Bloomfield, MI 48322; Sondra Seely

Wings of Hope Hospice, Inc. of Allegan County, 663 North 10th Street, Plainwell, MI 49080; tel. 616/685–1645; FAX. 616/685–2105; Marie Tucker, Executive Director

MINNESOTA

Douglas County PHNS Hospice, 305 Eighth Avenue West, Alexandria, MN 56308; tel. 320/763–6018; FAX. 320/763–4127; Mark Lundin, RN

Fairview Hospice, 2450 26th Avenue South, Minneapolis, MN 55406; tel. 612/728–2380; Mark Enger

Faribault County Area Hospice, 515 South Moore Street, Blue Earth, MN 56013; tel. 507/526–3273, ext. 345; FAX. 507/526–3621; Mavis Hodges, RN

HealthSpan Home Care and Hospice, 2750 Arthur Street, Roseville, MN 55113; tel. 612/635–9173; FAX. 612/635–9074; Karen Harrison, Manager

Homecaring Hospice, 11685 Lake Boulevard North, Chisago City, MN 55013; tel. 612/257–8402; Scott Wordelman, Administrator

Hospice Partners, Inc., 201 North Concord Exchange, Suite 250, South St. Paul, MN 55075–1150; tel. 612/457–5161; FAX. 612/457–5168; Roberta S. Cline, Chief Executive Officer, President

Hospice of Murray County, 2129 Broadway, Slayton, MN 56172; tel. 507/836–8114; Holly Miller, Administrator

Hospice of the Lakes, 8100 34th Avenue, S., P.O. Box 1309, Minneapolis, MN 55440–1309; tel. 612/883–6877; FAX. 612/883–6883; Barry Baines, M.D., Medical Director

Hospice of the Twin Cities Inc., 7100 Northland Circle, Suite 205, Minneapolis, MN 55428; tel. 612/531–2424; FAX. 612/531–2422; Lisa Abicht–Swensen, Administrator

Lakeland Hospice, Inc., 117 East Vasa, P.O. Box 824, Fergus Falls, MN 56538; tel. 218/736–7885; FAX. 218/736–2231; Delores Peterson, Director

Mayo Hospice Program, 200 First Street, S.W., Rochester, MN 55905; tel. 507/284–4002; FAX. 507/284–0161; Margaret Gillard, RN, Program Coodinator

Nobles Community Hospice, 1018 Sixth Avenue, P.O. Box 997, Worthington, MN 56187; tel. 507/372–2941; Melvin J. Platt, Administrator

North Memorial Medical Center Hospice, 3500 France Avenue North, Suite 101, Robbinsdale, MN 55422; tel. 612/520–5770; FAX. 612/520–3920; Elizabeth A. Woll, Manager

Pine to Prairie Hospice Inc., 201 Hillestad Avenue North, Fosston, MN 56542; tel. 218/435–2017; FAX. 218/435–6909; Judy Potvin

Prairie Home Hospice, Inc., 300 South Bruce, Marshall, MN 56258; tel. 507/537–9247; FAX. 507/537–9258; Lynn Yueill, Administrative Director

Red Wing Hospice, 434 West Fourth Street, Suite 200, Red Wing, MN 55066; tel. 612/385–3410; FAX. 612/385–3414; Beth Krehbiel, Director

Shamrock Seasons Hospice, 1242 Whitewater Avenue, St. Charles, MN 55972; tel. 507/932–3949; FAX. 507/932–5125; Doris Oehlke, Director

St. Cloud Hospital Hospice, 48 North 29 Avenue, Suite 15, St. Cloud, MN 56303; tel. 320/259–9375; FAX. 320/240–3266; Kathleen Murphy, Care Center Director

St. Joseph's Home Care and Hospice, 303 Kingwood Street, Brainerd, MN 56401; tel. 218/828–7444; FAX. 218/828–7579; Thomas Prusak, President

St. Marys Medical Center Hospice, 404 East Fourth Street, Duluth, MN 55805; tel. 218/726–4020; FAX. 218/725–7249; Bonnie King, Hospice Nurse Manager

St. Olaf Hospital Home Care and Hospice, 300 Eighth Avenue, N.W., Austin, MN 55912; tel. 507/437–0415; Donald Brezicka, Executive Vice President

Waseca Area Hospice, Inc., 204 Second Street, N.W., P.O. Box 94, Waseca, MN 56093; tel. 507/835–8983; FAX. 507/835–8737; Linda Grant, Director

Winona Area Hospice Services, 825 Mankato Avenue, Suite 111, Winona, MN 55987; tel. 507/457–4461; Roger L. Metz, President

MISSISSIPPI

Appletree Hospice, Inc., 521 Main Street, Suite U–Four, P.O. Box 299, Natchez, MS 39121; tel. 601/446–8000; Linda L. Carlton, Administrator

Baptist Memorial Regional Home Health Care, Inc., Magnolia Health Services and Hospice North, 396 Southcrest Court Five, Southhaven, MS 38671; tel. 601/349–1394; Bill Caldwell, Administrator

Community Hospice of Mississippi, Inc., d/b/a Gulf Coast, 154 Porter Avenue, Biloxi, MS 39530; tel. 601/435–1948; L. Jim Anthis, Ph.D, Administrator

DHS HospiceCare, 862 Goodman Road East, P.O. Box 744, Southaven, MS 38671; tel. 601/349–6711; FAX. 601/349–8826; Linda Crum, Administrator

Delta Area Hospice Care, Ltd., 522 Arnold Avenue, P.O. Box 5915, Greenville, MS 38704–5915; tel. 601/335–7040; FAX. 601/335–7048; Gloria Blakely, Administrator

Friendship Hospice of Natchez, Inc., 133 Jeff Davis Boulevard, Natchez, MS 39120; tel. 601/445–0307; Cynthia Paul, Administrator

Hospice Care, 202 South Washington Avenue, Greenville, MS 38701; tel. 601/335–4298; FAX. 601/335–4292; Emry Oxford, Administrator

Hospice Care Foundation, Inc., P.O. Box 2056, Vicksburg, MS 39181; tel. 800/380–3070; FAX. 601/634–6010; Rachel Y. Goodman, RN, Coordinator

Hospice Care Foundation, Inc., 317–B Highland Avenue, Natchez, MS 39120; tel. 601/442–3070; Janie Calloway, Office Manager

Hospice South, Inc., 112 Lafayette Street, P.O. Box 219, Livingston, AL 35470; tel. 205/652–2451; FAX. 205/652–5212; Bobby T. Williams, Ph.D., Chief Executive Officer

Hospice South, Inc., 1448 22nd Avenue, Tuscaloosa, AL 35401; tel. 205/366–9681; Dr. Bobby T. Williams, Chief Executive Officer

Hospice of Central Mississippi, Inc., 2600 Insurance Center Drive, Suite B–120, Jackson, MS 39216–4911; tel. 601/366–9881; FAX. 601/981–0150; John Fletcher, Executive Director

Hospice of Central Mississippi, Inc., 224 South First Street, Brookhaven, MS 39601; tel. 601/835–1020; FAX. 601/835–1063; Jean Berch, Branch Director

Hospice of Light, 4341 Gautier & Vancleave Road, Suite Four, Gautier, MS 39553; tel. 601/497–2400; FAX. 601/497–9035; Laurie H. Grady, Nurse Coordinator

Hospice of North Mississippi Clarksdale, 130 Desota Avenue, P.O. Box 1490, Clarksdale, MS 38614; tel. 601/624–8144; Jessie Rudd, RN, Patient Care Coordinator

Hospice of North Mississippi Olive Branch, 6920 Oak Forrest Drive, Suite B, Olive Branch, MS 38654; tel. 601/893–8900; FAX. 601/893–8905; Kim M. Ross, RN, Patient Care Coordinator

Hospice of North Mississippi, Inc., 619 East Lee Street, Sardis, MS 38666; tel. 601/487–1827; FAX. 601/487–1060; Renee Wright, Administrator

Hospice–North Mississippi Medical Center, 600 West Main, Tupelo, MS 38801; tel. 601/841–3612; Laura Kelley, Administrator

Magnolia Health Service and Hospice, 2130 Jackson Avenue West, Oxford, MS 38655; tel. 601/234–8553; FAX. 601/236–1459; Susan Eftink, L.M.S.W., Hospice Coordinator

Methodist Alliance Hospice, 930 South White Station Road, Suite 100, Memphis, TN 38117; tel. 901/680–0169; FAX. 901/537–2109; Caby E. Byrne, Administrator

Quality Hospice of Gulf Coast, Inc., P.O. Box 549, Biloxi, MS 39533; tel. 601/374–4434; FAX. 601/436–3679; Patricia Hiers, Administrator

Rush Hospital Hospice, Highway 15, Route Nine, Box 28, Philadelphia, MS 39350; tel. 601/656–8388; Ken Boyette, Patient Care Coordinator, Supervisor

Sta–Home Hospice, 105 North Van Buren, Carthage, MS 39051; tel. 800/898–1159; Claudette Hathcock, Administrator

Sta–Home Hospice, 1620 24th Avenue, Meridan, MS 39305; tel. 601/485–8489; FAX. 601/693–7457; Edwina White, Patient Care Coordinator

Whispering Pines Hospice, 1480 Raymond Road, Jackson, MS 39204; tel. 601/373–2472; Jeanne H. Jones, Consulting Administrator

MISSOURI

American Heartland Hospice, 7555 South Lindbergh Boulevard, St. Louis, MO 63125; tel. 314/894–8189; FAX. 314/894–7334; Susan O'Kane, Administrator

Barnes Jewish Hospice, 9890 Clayton Road, Ladue, MO 63124; tel. 314/993–4600; Ruth Sedano, Administrator

Barr Hospice and Palliative Care, 2701 Rockcreek Parkway, Suite 200, Kansas City, MO 64117; tel. 816/471–2218; FAX. 816/471–2434; Linda Ault, Administrator

Bates County Hospice, 501 North Orange, Butler, MO 64730; tel. 816/679–6108; George Taylor, Administrator

Beacon of Hope Hospice, Inc., 4191 Crescent Drive, Suite A, St. Louis, MO 63129; tel. 314/894–1000; FAX. 314/894–8389; Dawn Counts, Executive Director

Community Hospice of America–Central, 3600 I–70 Drive, S.E., Suite H, Columbia, MO 65201; tel. 314/443–8360; FAX. 314/499–4601; Tom Howard, RN, Patient Care Supervisor

Community Hospice of America–South Central, 101 East Second Street, Mountain Grove, MO 65711; tel. 417/926–4146; FAX. 417/926–6123; Virginia Holtmann, Administrator

Community Hospice of America–Tri Lakes, 1756 Bee Creek Road, Suite G, Branson, MO 65616; tel. 417/335–2004; FAX. 417/335–2012; Janet Gard, Program Director

Comprehealth, Inc., Hospice Services Division, 2001 South Hanley Road, Suite 450, St. Louis, MO 63144; tel. 314/781–2800; FAX. 314/781–4844; Carolynn Ingerson–Hoffman, Interim Administrator

Hands of Hope Hospice, 801 Faraon Street, St. Joseph, MO 64501; tel. 816/271–7190; FAX. 816/271–7191; Jim Pierce, Director

Harrison County Hospice, Highway 136 West, P.O. Box 425, Bethany, MO 64424; tel. 816/425–6324; FAX. 816/425–7642; Nola Martz, RN, B.S.N., Administrator

Hartline Hospice, Inc., Serving Southern Missouri, 3322 South Campbell, Suite T, Springfield, MO 65807; tel. 800/241–3798; FAX. 417/886–0082; Denise Stroud, B.S.N., Patient Care Administrator

HealthCor, Inc., 3215 LeMone Industrial Boulevard, Suite 100, Columbia, MO 65201–8245; tel. 314/449–0206; Rebecca Rastkar, RN, Administrator

Heart of America Hospice, L.C., 9229 Ward Parkway, Suite 350, Kansas City, MO 64114; tel. 816/333–1980; FAX. 816/333–2421; Jacquelin Tuohig, Executive Director

HomeCare of Mid–Missouri Hospice, 102 West Reed Street, Moberly, MO 65270; tel. 816/263–1517; Marsha Ideus Cooper, Administrator

Hospice 2000, Inc., 406 South Fourth, Kirksville, MO 63501; tel. 816/627–9711; FAX. 816/627–7005; Ron McCullough, Administrator

Hospice Care of Mid–America, 3100 Broadway, Suite 300, Kansas City, MO 64111–2415; tel. 816/931–4276; FAX. 816/931–9147; Patricia Walters, Interim Director

Hospice Preferred Choice of Kansas City and Kansas, 1170 West 152 Highway 152, Suite R–Two, Liberty, MO 64068; tel. 816/792–8700; FAX. 816/792–8701; Charlene Jaeger, RN, Executive Director

Hospice of Southwest Missouri, Inc., 3653 South Avenue, Springfield, MO 65807; tel. 417/882–0453; FAX. 417/882–1245; Richard Williams, President, Chief Executive Officer

HospiceCare of Visiting Nurse Association, 531 B South Union, Springfield, MO 65802; tel. 417/866–4374; FAX. 417/866–0233; Suzanne Dollar, Administrator

HospiceCare, Inc., Mineral Area College, North College Center, Park Hills, MO 63601; tel. 573/431–0162; Debra Jones, Administrator

Howard County Home Health and Hospice, 104 East Davis, Fayette, MO 65248; tel. 816/248–1780; FAX. 816/248–3347; Serese M. Wiehardt, Administrator

Kansas City Hospice, 1625 West 92nd Street, Kansas City, MO 64114; tel. 816/363–2600; FAX. 816/523–0068; Elaine McIntosh, President

Kendallwood Hospice, 10015 North Executive Hills Boulevard, Kansas City, MO 64153; tel. 816/891–7766; FAX. 816/891–7748; Charlotte Bruyn, Administrator

Lake Ozark Area Home Health and Hospice, A Department of Pulaski County Health Department, 602 Commercial Street, P.O. Box 498, Crocker, MO 65452; tel. 314/736–2219; FAX. 314/736–5847; Beth Hutton, Administrator

Meramec Hospice, 200 North Main, Rolla, MO 65401; tel. 314/364–2425; FAX. 314/364–1575; Shirley Rutz, Administrator

Missouri River Hospice, 1440 Aaron Court, Jefferson City, MO 65101; tel. 314/635–5643; FAX. 314/635–6552; Marge Borst, Administrator

Pershing Hospice, 225 West Hayden, Marceline, MO 64658; tel. 816/376–2222; FAX. 816/376–2432; Rose Ayers, Director

Pike County Home Health Agency and Hospice, 19 North Main Cross, Bowling Green, MO 63334; tel. 573/324–2111; FAX. 573/324–5517; Lisa Pitzer, RN, Patient Care Coordinator

Providence Hospice Group, Inc., 510 North Main, Sikeston, MO 63801; tel. 314/472–4041; FAX. 314/472–4043; Matthew Brauss, Administrator

Randolph County Health Department, Home Care and Hospice, 425 East Logan, P.O. Box 488, Moberly, MO 65270; tel. 816/263–6643; FAX. 816/263–0333; Mary D. Wolf, M.S.N., RNC, Patient Care Coordinator

Riverways Hospice of Ozarks Medical Center, 114 East Main, West Plains, MO 65775; tel. 417/256–3133; FAX. 417/256–5961; Mary Dyck, Administrator

Samaritan Care Hospice of Missouri, 10910 Kennerly Road, St. Louis, MO 63128; tel. 314/849–3324; FAX. 314/842–9077; Betty Richards, Administrator

St. Clair County Hospice, 101 Hospital Drive, Osceola, MO 64776; tel. 417/646–8157; FAX. 417/646–8159; Candice J. Baker, Administrator

Twin Lakes Hospice, Inc., 304 Main, P.O. Box 211, Warsaw, MO 65355; tel. 816/438–9700; FAX. 816/438–6404; Sandra Spooner, Administrator

VNA of Southeast Missouri Hospice, 100 East Harrison, Kennett, MO 63857; tel. 573/888–5892; FAX. 573/888–0538; Teresa McCulloch, Administrator

Visiting Nurse Association Hospice Care, 1260 Andes Boulevard, St. Louis, MO 63132; tel. 314/993–6800; Susan Pettit, Administrator

Visiting Nurses Association of Central Missouri, 1809 Vandiver Drive, Columbia, MO 65202; tel. 314/474–6000; FAX. 314/474–6400; Ron Barnes, Administrator

MONTANA

Anaconda Pintler Hospice of Community Hospital of Anaconda, 200 Main (Montana Square), P.O. Box 596, Anaconda, MT 59711; tel. 406/563–5422; FAX. 406/563–5427; Alice Cortright, Director

Big Sky Hospice, 3021 Sixth Avenue, N., Suite 205, P.O. Box 1049, Billings, MT 59103–1049; tel. 406/248–7442; FAX. 406/248–2572; Bernice Bjertness, RN, M.N., Director

Highlands Hospice, 2121 Amherst–505 Centennial Avenue, Butte, MT 59701; tel. 406/723–5780; FAX. 406/723–9595; Virginia Mick, Director

Hospice of Powell County, 310 Milwaukee Avenue, P.O. Box 808, Deer Lodge, MT 59722; tel. 406/846–3975; Nora E. Meier, Office Manager

Kootenai Volunteer Hospice, P.O. Box 781, Libby, MT 59923; tel. 406/293–3923; Theresa Schneider, Director

Lake County Home Health Hospice, 830 1/2 Shoreline Drive, Polson, MT 59860

Partners in Home Care Home Health & Hospice, Inc.–Hospice, 500 North Higgins, Suite 201, Missoula, MT 59801; tel. 406/728–8848; Teresa Smith, RN, Patient Care Coordinator

Partners in Home Care, Inc. (Residential Hospice), 10450 West Mullan Road, Missoula, MT 59802; tel. 406/542–1478; FAX. 406/721–0256; Teresa Smith, Clinical Manager

Peace Hospice of Montana, 125 Northwest Bypass H, Great Falls, MT 59404; tel. 406/727–6161; FAX. 406/727–9758; Mary Gray, RNCS, Director

Pondera Hospice, 300 North Virginia, Suite 305, Conrad, MT 59425; tel. 406/278–5566; FAX. 406/278–5569

Stillwater Big Sky Hospice Team, 350 West Pike Avenue, P.O. Box 1109, Columbus, MT 59019; tel. 406/322–5100; FAX. 406/322–5737; Sharon Marten, Chairperson

Westmont Home Health Services Inc Hospice, 2525 Colonial Drive, Helena, MT 59601; tel. 406/443–4140; Lynn Zavalney, RN, M.A., Hospice Coordinator

NEBRASKA

Hospice Care of Nebraska LLC, 1600 South 70th Street, Suite 201, Lincoln, NE 68506; tel. 402/488–1363; FAX. 402/488–5976; Marcia Cederdahl, RN, CRNH, B.S.Ed.

Hospice of Tabitha, 4720 Randolph Street, Lincoln, NE 68510; tel. 402/483–7671; Melody Gagner, Administrator

St. Joe Ville Homecare and Hospice, 2305 South Tenth Street, Omaha, NE 68108–1154; tel. 402/345–3333; FAX. 402/345–3826; Mary Jane Whitsett, Director

Visiting Nurse Association of the Midlands, 10840 Harney Street, Omaha, NE 68154; tel. 402/334–1820; FAX. 402/342–5587; Jim Kelleher, Vice President, Operations

NEVADA

Family Home Hospice, 1701 West Charleston, Suite 150, Zip 89102, P.O. Box 15645, Las Vegas, NV 89114–5645; tel. 702/383–0887; FAX. 702/383–1173; Jerilyn D. Hudgens, Administrator

Hospice of Northern Nevada, 1155 West Fourth Street, Suite 122, Reno, NV 89503; tel. 702/789–3081; FAX. 702/789–3909; Marva Slight, Director

Hospice of Northern Nevada–Carson City, 809 North Plaza, Carson City, NV 89701; tel. 702/884–8900; FAX. 702/884–8909; Elissa DeWolfe, Administrator

Margaret Rose Home Hospice, 1500 East Tropicana Avenue, Las Vegas, NV 89119; tel. 702/626–1966; Jackie Crawley

Nathan Adelson Hospice, 4141 South Swenson Street, Las Vegas, NV 89119; tel. 702/733–0320; FAX. 702/796–3195; Betsy Peirson–Gornet, Chief Executive Officer

PRN Home Hospice, 3022 West Post Road, Las Vegas, NV 89118; tel. 702/361–6801; Marti Norris, Administrator

Proper Care Hospice, 3601 West Sahara, Las Vegas, NV 89102; tel. 702/248–4119; Marlen P. Spagnol, Administrator

Safe Harbor Hospice, Inc., 3910 Pecos McLeod Building, Las Vegas, NV 89121; tel. 702/435–7660; Kristy Thompson, Executive Director

Special Care Hospice, 1514 C Gold Rush Road, Suite 236, Bullhead City, AZ 86442; tel. 520/758–3800; Dianne H. Butler, B.S.N., RNC, Administrator

Vista Care, Inc., 1830 East Sahara Avenue, Suite 102, Las Vegas, NV 89104; tel. 702/734–0307; FAX. 702/734–0310; Diana Hopkins–Weiss, Administrator

Washoe Home Connection, 1000 Ryland, Suite 410, Reno, NV 89502; tel. 702/328–5790; FAX. 702/328–5795; Michael Girard, Administrator

NEW HAMPSHIRE

Community Health and Hospice, Inc., 780 North Main Street, P.O. Box 578, Laconia, NH 03247–0578; tel. 603/524–8444; FAX. 603/524–8217; Alida Millham, Executive Director

Concord Regional VNA–Hospice, 250 Pleasant Street, P.O. Box 1797, Concord, NH 03301; tel. 603/224–4093; FAX. 603/224–4093; Joanne Fadale Wagner, ACSW, Director

Connecticut Valley Home Care Inc., 958 John Stark Highway, Newport, NH 03773; tel. 603/543–0164; Lynn Holland, RN

Elliot Home Care and Hospice, 25 South Maple Street, Manchester, NH 03103; tel. 603/628–4430; FAX. 603/622–4800; Diane LaBossiere, M.S.W.

Heritage Home Health, Inc., 169 Daniel Webster Highway, Suite Seven, Meredith, NH 03253; tel. 603/279–4700; FAX. 603/279–1370; Linda Roberts, Director

Hillsborough Hospice, 400 Mast Road, Goffstown, NH 03045; tel. 603/627–5540; Sandra Kinsey, RN, Hospice Administrator

Home Health and Hospice Care, 22 Prospect Street, Nashua, NH 03060; tel. 603/882–2941; FAX. 603/883–1515; Margaret Gilmour, Chief Executive Officer

Home Healthcare, Hospice and Community Services, Inc., 69L Island Street, P.O. Box 564, Keene, NH 03431; tel. 603/352–2253; FAX. 603/358–3904; Lois Hopkins, Hospice Program Coordinator

Hospice of VNH, 20 South Main Street, White River Junction, VT 05001; tel. 802/295–2604; FAX. 802/295–3163; Marie Kirn, Executive Director

Lake Sunapee Home Care and Hospice, 290 County Road, P.O. Box 2209, New London, NH 03257; tel. 603/526–4077; FAX. 603/526–4272; Barbara Boulton, RN, Hospice Patient Care Coordinator

Merrimack Valley Hospice, Inc., One Union Street, Andover, MA 01810; tel. 508/623–3100; FAX. 508/470–4690; Raymond Brockhill, Administrator

North Country Home Health Agency, 536 Cottage Street, Littleton, NH 03561; tel. 603/444–5317; FAX. 603/444–0980; Mary Ruppert, Director

Optima Health Visiting Nurse Services, VNA Hospice, 1850 Elm Street, Manchester, NH 03104; tel. 603/622–3781; FAX. 603/641–4074; Jane Clough, Director

Pemi–Baker Home Health Agency, 79 Highland Street, Plymouth, NH 03264; tel. 603/536–2232; Margaret Terrasi, Director

Portsmouth Regional Visiting Nurses Association and Hospice, 127 Parrott Avenue, Portsmouth, NH 03801; tel. 603/436–0815; FAX. 603/431–5457; Joan P. Nickell, President

Rochester Visiting Nurse Association, Inc., 89 Charles Street, Rochester, NH 03867; tel. 603/332–1133; FAX. 603/332–9223; Marianne Gagne, Hospice Coordinator

Rochingham VNA and Hospice, 137 Epping Road, Exeter, NH 03833; tel. 603/772–2981; Bonita J. Donovan

Rural District VNA Inc., Charles Street, Farmington, NH 03835; tel. 603/755–2202; FAX. 603/755–3760; Sue Houle

Seacoast Hospice, 10 Hampton Road, Exeter, NH 03833; tel. 603/778–7391; FAX. 603/772–7692; Walter Phinney, Executive Director

Souhegan Nursing Association Inc., 24 North River Road, Milford, NH 03055; tel. 603/673–3460; FAX. 603/673–0159; Lise Coombs, Hospice Coordinator

Squamscott Visiting Nurse and Hospice Care, 89 Old Rochester Road, Dover, NH 03820; tel. 603/742–7921; FAX. 603/742–3835; Mary Jo Sceggell

Tri–Area VNA Hospice, 301 High Street, Somersworth, NH 03878; tel. 603/692–2112; FAX. 603/692–9940; Maxine Lacy, Clinical Services Coordinator

VNA – Hospice of Southern Carroll County and Vicinity, South Main Street, Wolfeboro, NH 03894; tel. 603/569–2729; FAX. 603/569–2409; Carol C. Tubman, RN, CRNH

Visiting Nurse and Hospice Care of Northern Carroll County, Route 16, P.O. Box 432, North Conway, NH 03818; tel. 603/447–6766; FAX. 603/447–6370; Wilma H. Lord, Director

NEW JERSEY

Atlantic City Medical Center Hospice, 1406 Doughty Road, Pleasantville, NJ 08232; tel. 609/272–2424; FAX. 609/272–2414; Diana Ciurczak, Director

Atlantic Home Care and Hospice, 33 Bleeker Street, Millburn, NJ 07041

Barbara E. Cheung Memorial Hospice at Roosevelt Hospital, P.O. Box 151, CN4003 and Parsonage Road, Metuchen, NJ 08840–0151; tel. 908/321–9334; FAX. 908/321–9044; Enory Coughlin, RN, Supervisor

Center for Hope Hospice, Inc., 176 Hussa Street, Linden, NJ 07036; tel. 908/486–0700; FAX. 908/486–2450; Margaret J. Coloney, President

Compassionate Care Hospice, 1373 Broad Street, Suite 304, Clifton, NJ 07013; tel. 201/916–1400; FAX. 201/916–0066; Judith Grey, M.P.H., RNC, Director

Garden State Hospice, 256 Columbia Turnpike, Suite 100 N, Florham Park, NJ 07932; tel. 201/660–9400; FAX. 201/660–1122; Elise Power–Crystal, Chief Executive Officer, Marketing Director

Greater Monmouth VNA Hospice, 111 Union Avenue, Long Branch, NJ 07740; tel. 908/229–0816; FAX. 908/229–0561; Debra Cox, RN, Hospice Supervisor

Holy Redeemer Hospice, 1801 Route Nine North, P.O. Box 280A, Swainton, NJ 08210; tel. 609/465–2082; FAX. 609/465–6185; Arleen Moffitt, ACSW

Home Care Resources Hospice, 615 Hope Road, Building Three, First Floor, Eatontown, NJ 07724; tel. 908/935–1797; FAX. 908/935–0949; Kerri A. Johnston, Hospice Administrator

Hospice Program of Bayonne VNA, 325 Broadway, Bayonne, NJ 07002; tel. 201/339–2500; FAX. 201/339–1255; Barbara Halosz, RN, B.S.N., Coordinator

Hospice at Bergen Community Health Care, 400 Old Hook Road, Westwood, NJ 07675–3131; tel. 201/358–2900; FAX. 201/358–0836; Patricia Hutzelman, RN, Hospice Coordinator

Hospice of Delaware Valley, Inc., 2564 Route 1, Lawrenceville, NJ 08648; tel. 609/695–3461, ext. 2222; FAX. 695/771–8010; Sister Katheleen Manning, RN, M.S.N., ONCSC, Director of Hospice

Hospice of New Jersey, 400 Broadacres Drive, Fourth Floor, Bloomfield, NJ 07003; tel. 201/893–0818; FAX. 201/893–0828; Marcia M. Cook, Administrator

Hospice of VNA of Northern New Jersey, 38 Elm Street, Morristown, NJ 07960

HospiceCare of South Jersey, Inc., 2848 South Delsea Drive, Vineland, NJ 08360; tel. 609/794–1515; FAX. 609/691–7660; Yvonne Crouch, Executive Director

Jerseycare Hospice, 50 Newark Avenue, Suite 101, Belleville, NJ 07109

Karen Ann Quinlan Center of Hope Hospice, 99 Sparta Avenue, Newton, NJ 07860; tel. 201/383–0115; FAX. 201/383–6889; Jackie Petrazzelli, Executive Director

Passaic Valley Hospice, VHS of New Jersey, Inc., 783 Riverview Drive, Totowa, NJ 07511; tel. 201/785–7457; FAX. 201/256–6778; Nancy Jacoby, Associate Director

Samaritan Hospice, 214 West Second Street, Moorestown, NJ 08057; tel. 800/229–8183; FAX. 609/778–0237; Ritamarie A. Frey, President, Chief Executive Officer

Somerset Valley Visiting Nurse Association Hospice, 586 East Main Street, Bridgewater, NJ 08807; tel. 908/725–9355; FAX. 908/725–1033; Anita G. Busch, B.S.N., CRNH, Hospice Manager

The Center for Hospice Care, Inc., Three High Street, Glen Ridge, NJ 07028–2306; tel. 201/429–0300; FAX. 201/429–9274; Lorraine M. Sciara, President, Chief Executive Officer

Trinity Hospice, 150 Ninth Street, Runnemede, NJ 08078; tel. 609/939–9000, ext. 7166; FAX. 609/939–9010; Barbara Billington, Director

Unity Hospice, 17 Academy Street, Newark, NJ 07102; tel. 201/596–9661; FAX. 201/596–9664; Terry M. Copeland, Administrator

VNA of Central Jersey Hospice, 1100 Wayside Road, Asbury Park, NJ 07712; tel. 908/493–2220; FAX. 908/493–4256; Barbara Buczny, Director of Hospice

Valley Hospice, a Division of Valley Home Care, Inc., 505 Goffle Road, Ridgewood, NJ 07450; tel. 201/447–8822; FAX. 201/447–0105; Roberta White, Director

Visiting Nurse Association Somerset Hills Hospice, 12 Olcott Avenue, Bernardsville, NJ 07924; tel. 908/766–0180; FAX. 908/766–2268; Barbara Fox, Hospice Coordinator

Visiting Nurse and Health Services Hospice, 354 Union Avenue, P.O. Box 170, Elizabeth, NJ 07208; tel. 908/352–5694, ext. 302; FAX. 908/352–9216; Shirley Altman, Hospice Administrator

Vitas Health Care Corporation of Penn, Two Executive Campus, Route 70 and Cuthbert Road, Cherry Hill, NJ 08002; tel. 609/661–5600; FAX. 609/661–5650; Emily Fedullo, Director, Operations

West Essex Hospice, 799 Bloomfield Avenue, Verona, NJ 07044; tel. 201/857–7300; FAX. 201/857–3433; Janice Breen, President, Chief Executive Officer

NEW MEXICO

Alamogordo Home Care–Hospice, 505 11th Street, Alamogordo, NM 88310; tel. 800/617–3555; FAX. 505/437–2399; Pat Raub, Administrator

Alternative Home Health Care Hospice, 1118 National Avenue, Las Vegas, NM 87701; tel. 800/296–1538; FAX. 505/425–7682; Maxine E.Gonzales, Administrator

Caring Unlimited Hospice Services, 200 South Third, Raton, NM 87740; tel. 505/445–5113; Jo Ellen Ferguson, Administrator

Carlsbad Hospice, Inc., 1003 West Riverside Drive, P.O. Drawer PP, Carlsbad, NM 88220; tel. 505/885–8257; Nancy Flanagan, Administrator

Esperanza Home Health Care Hospice, Inc., Highway 518 Buena Vista, P.O. Box 270, Mora, NM 87732; tel. 505/387–2215; Josephine P. Garcia

Helping Hand Hospice, 615 South Second, Tucumcari, NM 88401; tel. 505/461–0099; Diana Beck, Administrator

Hospice Services, Inc., 90I East Bender, P.O. Box 249, Hobbs, NM 88241; tel. 800/658–6844; FAX. 505/393–3985; Brenda Chambers

Hospice Services, Inc. – Eddy, 1031 North Thomas, P.O. Box 280, Carlsbad, NM 88220; tel. 505/887–1835; FAX. 505/887–6967; Jan Shields, RN, Branch Manager

Hospice at VNS, 2960 Rodeo Park Drive, W., Santa Fe, NM 87505; tel. 505/984–2571; FAX. 505/984–2571; Janet Rose, Chief Executive Officer

Hospice of Artesia, 702 North 13th, Artesia, NM 88210; tel. 505/748–3333, ext. 604; FAX. 505/746–8918, ext. 424; Beverly Morehead, RN, Director

Los Alamos Visiting Nurse Service Hospice, 901 18th Street, Suite 203, Los Alamos, NM 87544; tel. 505/662–2525; FAX. 505/662–7093; Deborah Simon, Administrator

Mesilla Valley Hospice, Inc., 299 East Montana Avenue, Las Cruces, NM 88005; tel. 505/523–4700; FAX. 505/527–2204; Patti Lyman, RN, Executive Director

Mountain Home Health Hospice, 630 Paseo del Pueblo Sur, Suite 180, Taos, NM 87571; tel. 505/758–4786; Patricia Heinen, Administrator

New Hope Hospice of New Mexico, 4153 Montgomery Boulevard, N.E., Albuquerque, NM 87109; tel. 505/881–7336; Michael Garcia, Administrator

Northwest New Mexico Hospice, 608 Reilly Avenue, P.O. Box 3336, Farmington, NM 87499; tel. 505/327–0301; FAX. 505/325–2477; Lizette Vannest, Program Coordinator

Presbyterian Hospice, 4545 McLeod N.E., Suite G, Albuquerque, NM 87109; tel. 505/888–5656; June Vermillion

Professional Home Health Care, Inc., 1345 Pacheco Street, Santa Fe, NM 87505; tel. 505/982–8581; FAX. 505/982–0457; Debbie Conway

Quality Continuum Hospice, 5608 Zuni, S.E., Albuquerque, NM 87108; tel. 505/256–8360; Kathleen M. Hart, Administrator

Roswell Hospice Home Care, 600 North Richardson, Roswell, NM 88201; tel. 505/623–5887; FAX. 505/624–8566; Nancy Smith, Program Director

Sandia Hospice, 5740 Osuna, N.E., Albuquerque, NM 87109; tel. 505/888–0095; FAX. 505/888–2025; Catherine A. Esterheld, Executive Director

St. Anthony's Hospice, 1008 Douglas Avenue, P.O. Box 1170, Las Vegas, NM 87701; tel. 505/425–3353; Beatrice R. Velasquez, Administrator

Staff Builders Services, Inc., 826 Camino De Monte Rey, P.O. Box 23448, Santa Fe, NM 87502; tel. 505/983–5408; Pamela Brunsell, RN, Administrator

The Hospice Center, 1422 Paseo De Peralta, Santa Fe, NM 87501; tel. 505/988–2211; FAX. 505/986–1833; Barbara Elder Owas, RN, Executive Director

VNS Health Services, Inc., 706 La Joya, N.E., Espanola, NM 87532; tel. 505/753–2284; FAX. 505/756–2179; Beatrice Sceery, Manager, Home Health, Hospice

Victory Home Health Hospice, 624 University, P.O. Box 670, Las Vegas, NM 87701; tel. 505/454–0499; FAX. 505/425–9105; Maria Luisa Padilla, Administrator

NEW YORK

Capital District Hospice, Inc., a/k/a Hospice of Schenectady, Hospice of Saratoga, Hospice of Amsterdam, Hospice of Warren County, 1411 Union Street, Schenectady, NY 12308; tel. 518/377–8846; FAX. 518/377–8868; Philip G. Di Sorbo, Executive Director

Caring Community Hospice of Cortland, 4281 North Homer Avenue, Cortland, NY 13045; tel. 607/753–9105; Mary Beach, Administrator, Patient Care Coordinator

Catskill Area Hospice, Inc., 542 Main Street, Oneonta, NY 13820; tel. 607/432–6773; FAX. 607/432–7741; Lesley Deleski, Executive Director

Christian Nursing Hospice, Inc., d/b/a CNR Hospice, 110 Lake Avenue South, Suite 33, Nesconset, NY 11767; tel. 516/265–5300; FAX. 516/265–5789; Camille Harlow, Executive Director

Comstock Hospice Care Network, 1225 West State Street, Olean, NY 14760; tel. 716/372–2106; FAX. 716/372–4635; Kathleen Mack, Hospice Director

East End Hospice, Inc., 1111 Riverhead Road, P.O. Box 1048, Westhampton Beach, NY 11978; tel. 516/288–8400; FAX. 512/288–8492; Priscilla Ruffin, Executive Director

Herkimer County Hospice, 267 North Main Street, Herkimer, NY 13350; tel. 315/867–1317; FAX. 315/867–1371; Sue Campagna, Administrator

High Peaks Hospice, Inc., P.O. Box 840, Trudeau Road, Saranac Lake, NY 12983; tel. 518/891–0606; FAX. 518/891–0657; Maureen Sayles, Executive Director

Hospicare of Tompkins County, Inc., 172 East King Road, Ithaca, NY 14850; tel. 607/272–0212; FAX. 607/272–0237; Nina K. Miller, Executive Director

Hospice Buffalo, Inc., 225 Como Park Boulevard, Cheektowaga, NY 14227–1480; tel. 716/686–8060; FAX. 716/686–8128; J. Donald Schumacher, Psy.D., President, Chief Executive Officer

Hospice Care Network, 900 Ellison Avenue, Westbury, NY 11590; tel. 516/832–7100; FAX. 516/832–7160; Maureen Hinkleman, Chief Executive Officer

Hospice Care, Inc., 4277 Middlesettlement Road, New Hartford, NY 13413; tel. 315/735–6484; FAX. 315/735–8545; Wes Case, Executive Director

Section C

Hospice Chautauqua County, Inc., Nine Park Street, P.O. Box 503, Sinclairville, NY 14782–0503; tel. 716/962–2010; FAX. 716/962–2020; Susan Schwartz, M.P.A., Executive Director

Hospice Family Care, 550 East Main Street, Batavia, NY 14020; tel. 716/343–7596; FAX. 716/343–7629; Deborah Schafer, Operating Director

Hospice VNSW/WPHC, Inc., d/b/a Hospice of Westchester, 95 South Broadway, White Plains, NY 10601; tel. 914/682–1484; FAX. 914/682–9425; Emily R. Giannattasio, Executive Director

Hospice of Central New York, 1118 B Court Street, P.O. Box 69, Syracuse, NY 13208; tel. 315/476–5552; FAX. 315/476–5559; Peter Moberg–Sarver, President, Chief Executive Officer

Hospice of Chenango County, Inc., 21 Hayes Street, Norwich, NY 13815; tel. 607/334–3556; FAX. 607/334–3688; Laurie Vogel, Executive Director

Hospice of Dutchess County, 70 South Hamilton Street, Poughkeepsie, NY 12601; tel. 914/485–2273; Wayne Herron, Chief Executive Officer

Hospice of Jefferson County, Inc., 425 Washington Street, Watertown, NY 13601; tel. 315/788–7323; FAX. 315/785–9932; Frances Calabrese, Executive Director

Hospice of North Country, 386 Rugar Street, Plattsburgh, NY 12901–2306; tel. 518/561–8465; FAX. 518/561–3182; Sarah Anderson, Executive Director

Hospice of Northern Westchester and Putnam, Inc., an Affiliate of VNA of Hudson Valley, 43 Kensico Drive, Mount Kisco, NY 10549; tel. 914/666–4228; FAX. 914/666–0378; Cornelia Schimert, Director

Hospice of Orange in Hudson Valley, Inc., Hospice of Sullivan County, 70 Dubois Street, Newburgh, NY 12550; tel. 914/561–6111; FAX. 914/561–2179; Daniel Grady, Executive Director

Hospice of Orleans County, 13996 Route 31 West, Albion, NY 14411; tel. 716/589–0809; Mary Ann Fisher, Executive Director

Hospice of Rochester and Hospice of Wayne and Seneca Counties, 49 Stone Street, Rochester, NY 14604; tel. 716/325–1880, ext. 1155; FAX. 716/325–7678; Sue Greer, RN, B.S.N., Vice President, Hospice Services

Hospice of St. Lawrence Valley, Inc., 6439 State Highway 56, P.O. Box 469, Potsdam, NY 13676; tel. 315/265–3105; FAX. 315/265–0323; Brian Gardam, Executive Director

Hospice of the Finger Lakes, 25 William Street, Auburn, NY 13021; tel. 315/255–2733; FAX. 315/252–9080; Theresa Kenny Kline, Executive Director

Jansen Memorial Hospice/Home Nursing Association of Westchester, 69 Main Street, Tuckahoe, NY 10707; tel. 914/961–2818, ext. 307; FAX. 914/961–8654; Lucille D. Winton, Director

Livingston County Hospice, Two Livingston County Campus, Mount Morris, NY 14510; tel. 716/243–7290; FAX. 716/243–7287; Cheryl Pletcher, Administrator

Mercy Hospice, St. Pius X Service Center, 1220 Front Street, Uniondale, NY 11553; tel. 516/485–3060; FAX. 516/485–1007; Sister Dolores Castellano, Executive Director

Mountain Valley Hospice, 73 North Main Street, Gloversville, NY 12078; tel. 518/725–4545; FAX. 518/725–8066; Nancy Dowd, Executive Director

Niagara Hospice, Inc., 4675 Sunset Drive, Lockport, NY 14094; tel. 716/439–4417; FAX. 716/439–6035; Carol E. Gettings, M.S., Executive Director

Ontario–Yates Hospice, 756 Pre–Emption Road, Geneva, NY 14456; tel. 315/781–0071; Bonnie Hollenbeck, Administrator

Oswego County Hospice, Oswego County Health Department, 70 Bunner Street, Oswego, NY 13126; tel. 315/349–8259; FAX. 315/349–8269; Steven D. Rose, Administrator

Pax Christi Hospice, 355 Bard Avenue, Staten Island, NY 10310; tel. 718/876–1022; Patricia Farrington, Executive Director

Southern Tier Hospice, Inc., 244 West Water Street, Elmira, NY 14901; tel. 607/734–1570; FAX. 607/734–1902; Mary Ann Starbuck, Executive Director

The Brooklyn Hospice, 6323 Seventh Avenue, Brooklyn, NY 11220; tel. 718/921–7900; FAX. 718/921–0752; Abby Gordon, Administrator

Tioga County Hospice, 231 Main Street, Owego, NY 13827; tel. 607/687–0682; FAX. 607/684–6041; Janette Swindell, Administrator

United Hospice of Rockland, 18 Thiells–Mount Ivy Road, Pomona, NY 10970; tel. 914/354–5100; FAX. 914/354–2128; Amy Stern, Executive Director

VNS Hospice of Suffolk, 505 Main Street, Northport, NY 11768; tel. 516/261–7200; FAX. 516/261–1985; Virginia Stein, RN, M.S., Director, Patient Services

VNSNY Hospice Care, 1250 Broadway, New York, NY 10001; tel. 212/290–3888; FAX. 212/290–3933; Eileen Hanley, RN, M.B.A., Administrator

Visiting Nurse Hospice, 2180 Empire Boulevard, Webster, NY 14580; tel. 716/787–8315; FAX. 716/787–9726; Dorothy Chilton, Administrator

NORTH CAROLINA

Albemarle Home Care, 103 Charles Street, P.O. Box 189, Hertford, NC 27907; tel. 919/426–5488; Paula Vanhorn, Administrator

Albemarle Home Care, County Office Building, P.O. Box 189, Edenton, NC 27907; tel. 919/482–7001; Angie Layden, Administrator

Albemarle Home Care, Highway 168, P.O. Box 189, Currituck, NC 27907; tel. 919/232–2026; Victoria Rentrop, Administrator

Albemarle Home Care, South 343, Courthouse Complex, P.O. Box 189, Elizabeth City, NC 27907–0189; tel. 800/478–0477; FAX. 919/338–4364; Kay Cherry, Director

Albemarle Home Care and Hospice, 400 South Road Street, P.O. Box 189, Elizabeth City, NC 27907–0189; tel. 919/338–4066; FAX. 919/338–4069; Beth Ehrhardt, M.S.W., Hospice Program Coordinator

Angel Home Health Agency, 268 Highway 19S, Suite Three, P.O. Box 389, Bryson City, NC 28713; tel. 704/488–3877; Sandy Smith, Administrator

Caldwell County Hospice, Inc., 902 Kirkwood Street, N.W., Lenoir, NC 28645; tel. 704/754–0101; FAX. 704/757–3335; Cathy S. Simmons, Executive Director

Cape Fear Valley Home Health and Hospice, 3357 Village Drive, Fayetteville, NC 28304

Cashiers Home Health, Highway 107 South, 59 Hospital Road, Sylva, NC 28779; tel. 704/586–7410

Center of Living Home Health and Hospice, d/b/a Center of Living Healthcare, 416 Vision Drive, Zip 27203, P.O. Box 9, Asheboro, NC 27204–0009; tel. 910/672–9300, ext. 263; FAX. 910/672–0868; Billie Vuncannon, Chief Executive Officer, President

Community Home Care and Hospice, 516 Owen Drive, Fayetteville, NC 28304; tel. 910/323–9816; FAX. 910/484–6724; Brinda L. Williams, Business Office Manager

Comprehensive Home Health Care, 3840 Henderson Drive, Jacksonville, NC 28456; tel. 910/346–4800; Linda Powers, Patient Care Manager

Comprehensive Home Health Care, 819 Jefferson Street, P.O. Box 366, Whiteville, NC 28472; tel. 910/642–5808; FAX. 910/640–1374; Sheila Faulk, Director

Comprehensive Home Health Care, 1120 Ocean Highway W, P.O. Box 200, Supply, NC 28462; tel. 910/754–8133, ext. 212; FAX. 910/754–2096; Crystal Floyd, RN, Director

Comprehensive Home Health Care and Comprehensive Hospice, Inc., 101 South Craig Street, P.O. Drawer 2540, Elizabethtown, NC 28337; tel. 910/862–8538; Sherry Hester, Dirctor, Office Operations

Comprehensive Home Health Care–Hospice, 3311 Burnt Mill Drive, Wilmington, NC 28403; tel. 910/251–8111; FAX. 910/343–1218; Debra Nixion Jones, Patient Case Manager

Comprehensive Home Health Care/Comprehensive Hospice, 1800 Skibo Road, Suite 228, Fayetteville, NC 28303; tel. 910/864–8411; Gwendolynn Harrell, Regional Director

Craven County Home Health–Hospice Agency, 2818 Neuse Boulevard, P.O. Drawer 12610, New Bern, NC 28561; tel. 919/636–4930; FAX. 919/636–5301

Dare Hospice, 8321 Oregon Inlet Road, P.O. Box 2511, Kill Devil Hills, NC 27948; tel. 919/441–6242; Mary A. Burrus, Executive Director

Davie County Health Department, and Home Health, Hospice of Davie County, 210 Hospital Street, P.O. Box 848, Mocksville, NC 27028; tel. 704/634–8770; FAX. 704/634–0335; Dennis E. Harrington, M.P.H. Health Director

Duplin Home Care and Hospice Inc., Duplin Street, Box 887, Kenansville, NC 28349; tel. 910/296–0819; FAX. 910/296–0482; Rhonda Lucus, RN, Hospice Coordinator

Duplin Home Care and Hospice, Inc., 101 East Main Street, Wallace, NC 28466; tel. 919/285–1100, ext. 6637; FAX. 910/285–1172; Glenda Kenan, RN, Home Health Coordinator

Duplin Home Care and Hospice, Inc., 238 Smith Chapel Road, Mount Olive, NC 28365

Edgecombe County HomeCare and Hospice, 2909 North Main Street, Tarboro, NC 27886; tel. 919/641–7558; FAX. 919/641–7004; Jessie Worthington, Hospice Program Director

Four Seasons Hospice, 802 Old Spartanburg Highway, P.O. Box 2395, Hendersonville, NC 28739; tel. 704/692–6178; FAX. 704/692–2365; Barbara W. Stewart, Executive Director

Good Shepherd Home Health and Hospice Agency, Inc., P.O. Box 465, Hayesville, NC 28904; tel. 704/389–6311; Ruth Kraushaar, RN, Hospice Coordinator

Good Shepherd Home Health and Hospice Agency, Inc., Main and May Streets, Hayesville, NC 28904

Good Shepherd Home Health and Hospice Agency, Inc., P.O. Box 465, Hayesville, NC 28904; tel. 704/389–6311; FAX. 704/389–9584; Ruth Onsum, Hospice Coordinator

Home Health Agency of Chapel Hill, Inc., 1101 Weaver Dairy Road, P.O. Box 4126, Chapel Hill, NC 27514; tel. 919/929–7149; Paula Balber, Hospice Coordinator

Home Health and Hospice Care, Inc., 1004 Jenkins Avenue, P.O. Box 190, Maysville, NC 28555; tel. 919/743–2800; Janet Haddow–Green, Administrator

Home Health and Hospice Care, Inc., 1023 Beaman Street, P.O. Box 852, Clinton, NC 28328; tel. 800/695–4442; FAX. 910/592–7392; Richard Stone, Administrator

Home Health and Hospice Care, Inc., d/b/a Kitty Askins Hospice Center, 107 Handley Park Court, Goldsboro, NC 27534; tel. 800/260–4442; FAX. 919/735–8460; Donna Boren, RN

Home Health and Hospice Care, Inc., 2305 Wellington Drive, Suite G, P.O. Box 3673, Wilson, NC 27835–3673; tel. 919/291–4400; Deede Morgan, Hospice Director

Home Health and Hospice Care, Inc., 15 Noble Street, P.O. Box 1524, Smithfield, NC 27577–9300; tel. 919/934–0664; FAX. 919/934–9046; Phil Adams Administrator

Home Health and Hospice Care, Inc., 2419 East Ash Street, Suite Four and Five, Goldsboro, NC 27532; tel. 919/735–1386; FAX. 919/731–4985; Jim Wall, Administrator

Home Health and Hospice Care, Inc., 907A Southeast Second Street, Snow Hill, NC 28580

Home Health and Hospice Care, Inc., 702 BWH Smith Boulevard, Greenville, NC 27834

Home Health and Hospice Care, Inc., 102 North Carolina Highway 55 West, Mount Olive, NC 28365

Home Health and Hospice of Halifax, 1229 Julian R. Allsbrook Road, Roanoke Rapids, NC 27870; tel. 919/308–0700; FAX. 919/537–1872; Sheila Alford, RN, Home Care Director

Home Health and Hospice of Person County, 325 South Morgan Street, Roxboro, NC 27573; tel. 910/597–2542; FAX. 910/597–3367; Joyce Franke, Administrator

Home Technology Health Care–Hospice of Tar Heel, U.S. Highway 11 South and Chapman Road, P.O. Box 1645, Greenville, NC 27835; tel. 919/758–4622; FAX. 919/758–7006; Patti Lotts, Executive Director

HomeHealth and Hospice Care Inc., 744 Airport Road, P.O. Box 1396, Kinston, NC 28503; tel. 919/527–9561; Ann Harrison, Clinical Director

Hometown Hospice, Inc., 2404 South Charles Street, Suite E, Greenville, NC 27835

Hospice Home, 918 Chapel Hill Road, Burlington, NC 27215; tel. 910/513–4460; FAX. 910/513–4471; Judy Bowman, Manager

Hospice at Charlotte, Inc., 1420 East Seventh Street, Charlotte, NC 28204; tel. 704/375–0100; FAX. 704/375–8623; Janet Fortner, President

Hospice at Greensboro, Inc., 2500 Summit Avenue, Greensboro, NC 27405; tel. 910/621–2500; FAX. 910/621–4516; Pamela Barrett, Executive Director

Hospice at Greensboro–Beacon Place, 2502 Summit Avenue, Greensboro, NC 27405

Hospice of Alamance–Caswell, 730 Hermitage Road, P.O. Box 2122, Burlington, NC 27216; tel. 910/538–8040; FAX. 910/538–8049; Peter Barcus, Executive Director

Hospice of Alexander County, Inc., 412 Third Street, S.W., Taylorsville, NC 28681; tel. 704/632-5026; FAX. 704/632-3707; Donna W. AuBuchon, Executive Director

Hospice of Alleghany, P.O. Box 1278, Sparta, NC 28675; tel. 910/373-8018; Wanda Branch, Administrator

Hospice of Ashe, 392 Highway 88 East, P.O. Box 421, Jefferson City, NC 28640; tel. 704/265-3926; FAX. 704/264-2125; Wanda Branch, Administrator

Hospice of Avery County, Inc., 351 West Michelle Street, P.O. Box 1357, Newland, NC 28657; tel. 704/733-0663; FAX. 704/733-0375; Sharon Cole, RN, Patient Care Coordinator

Hospice of Burke County, Inc., P.O. Box 1579, Morganton, NC 28680; tel. 704/879-1601; FAX. 704/879-3500; A. Malanie Price, Executive Director

Hospice of Cabarrus County, Inc., 1060 Diploma Place, S.W., P.O. Box 1235, Concord, NC 28026-1235; tel. 704/788-9434; FAX. 704/788-6013; Shirley McDowell, Executive Director

Hospice of Carteret County, Inc., P.O. Box 1818, Morehead City, NC 28557; tel. 919/247-2808; Ruth Yearick-Jones, Administrator

Hospice of Catawba Valley, Inc., 263 Third Avenue, N.W., Hickory, NC 28601; tel. 704/328-4200; FAX. 704/328-3031; Julie Packer, Interim Executive Director

Hospice of Chatham County, Inc., 200 East Street, P.O. Box 1077, Pittsboro, NC 27312; tel. 919/542-5545; FAX. 919/542-6232; Susan H. Balfour, RN, Executive Director

Hospice of Cleveland County, Inc., 951 Wendover Heights Drive, Shelby, NC 28150; tel. 704/487-4677; FAX. 704/481-8050; Myra McGinnis Hamrick, Executive Director

Hospice of Cumberland County, 711 Executive Place, Suite 207, P.O. Box 53324, Fayetteville, NC 28305; tel. 910/484-1776; FAX. 910/484-6294; Melissa Harris, Hospice Coordinator

Hospice of Davidson County, Inc., 524 South State Street, P.O. Box 1941, Lexington, NC 27293-1941; tel. 910/248-6185; FAX. 910/248-4574; Gary Drake, Executive Director

Hospice of Gaston County, Inc., d/b/a Gaston Hospice, 717 North New Hope Road, P.O. Box 3984, Gastonia, NC 28054; tel. 704/861-8405; FAX. 704/865-0590; Lee Bucci, Executive Director

Hospice of Harnett County, Inc., 111A North Ellis Avenue, Dunn, NC 28334, P.O. Box 373, Erwin, NC 28339; tel. 910/892-1213; FAX. 910/892-1229; Grace E. Tart, Administrator

Hospice of Iredell County, Inc., 2347 Simonton Road, P.O. Box 822, Statesville, NC 28687; tel. 704/873-4719; FAX. 888/464-4673; Ron D. Thompson, Executive Director

Hospice of Iredell County, Inc., 153 North Main Street, Suite One, Mooresville, NC 28115; tel. 704/663-0051; FAX. 704/872-1810; Judy Snowden, Executive Director

Hospice of Lee County, Inc., P.O. Box 1181, Sanford, NC 27331-1181; tel. 919/774-4169; FAX. 919/774-6348; Janet MacLaren Scovil, Executive Director

Hospice of Lincoln County, Inc., 107 North Cedar Street, P.O. Box 1526, Lincolnton, NC 28093-1526; tel. 704/732-6146; FAX. 704/732-9808; Gregory Urban, Executive Director

Hospice of Macon County, Inc., 30 Roller Mill Road, P.O. Box 1594, Franklin, NC 28734; tel. 704/369-6641; Suzanne A. Owens, Executive Director

Hospice of McDowell County, Inc., 116 North Logan Street, P.O. Box 1072, Marion, NC 28752; tel. 704/652-1318; FAX. 704/659-1631

Hospice of Mitchell County, 188 C Highway 226 South, Bakersville, NC 28705; tel. 704/688-4090; FAX. 704/688-3566; Clarice Turner, Executive Director

Hospice of Pamlico County, Inc., 13628 North Carolina Highway 55, Alliance, P.O. Box 959, Bayboro, NC 28515; tel. 919/745-5171; Diane McDaniel, Executive Director

Hospice of Rockingham County, Inc., 2150 North Carolina 65, P.O. Box 281, Wentworth, NC 27375; tel. 910/427-9022; FAX. 919/427-9030; Fran Hughes, Executive Director

Hospice of Rutherford County, Inc., 374 Hudlow Road, P.O. Box 336, Forest City, NC 28043; tel. 704/245-0095; FAX. 704/248-1035; Rita Burch, Executive Director

Hospice of Scotland County, 600 South Main Street, Suite F, P.O. Box 1033, Laurinburg, NC 28353; tel. 910/276-7176; FAX. 910/277-1941; Linda McQueen, RN, Executive Director

Hospice of Stanly County, Inc., 960 North First Street, Albemarle, NC 28001-3350; tel. 704/983-4216; FAX. 704/983-6662; Elvin T. Henry, Executive Director

Hospice of Stokes County, Highway 8 and 89, P.O. Box 10, Danbury, NC 27016; tel. 910/593-5309; FAX. 910/593-5354; Margaret Arey, Executive Director

Hospice of Surry County, Inc., 1326 North Main Street, Mount Airy, NC 27030; tel. 910/789-2922; FAX. 910/789-0856; Laney Johnson, Director

Hospice of Surry County, Inc., 827 North Bridge Street, Elkin, NC 28621; tel. 910/526-2650; FAX. 910/526-2383; Laney Johnson, Executive Director

Hospice of Union County, Inc., 700 West Roosevelt Boulevard, Monroe, NC 28110; tel. 704/292-2100; FAX. 704/292-2190; Charlene C. Broome, Executive Director

Hospice of Wake County, Inc., 4513 Creedmoor Road, Suite 400, Raleigh, NC 27612; tel. 919/782-3959; FAX. 919/782-3598; Karolyn H. Kaye, Executive Director

Hospice of Watauga, 136 Furman Road, Route Five, Box 199, Boone, NC 28607; tel. 704/265-3926; Wanda Branch, Administrator

Hospice of Winston-Salem/Forsyth County, Inc., 1100 South Stratford Road, Building C, Winston-Salem, NC 27103-3212; tel. 910/768-3972; FAX. 910/659-0461; Jo Ann Davis, Chief Executive Officer

Hospice of Yancey County, 314 West Main Street, P.O. Box 471, Burnsville, NC 28714; tel. 704/682-9675; FAX. 704/682-4713; Donna Messenger, Executive Director

Hospice of the Carolina Foothills, Inc., 421 North Trade Street, Tryon, NC 28782; tel. 704/859-2270; FAX. 704/859-2731; Jean H. Eckert, Executive Director

Hospice of the Piedmont/Care Connection, 213 North Lindsay Street, High Point, NC 27262; tel. 910/889-8446; FAX. 910/889-3450; Leslie Kalinowski, President

Lower Cape Fear Care, Inc., 810 Princess Street, Wilmington, NC 28401; tel. 910/762-0200; FAX. 910/762-9146; Eloise Thomas, Executive Director

Lower Cape Fear Hospice, Inc., 121 West Main Street, P.O. Box 636, Whiteville, NC 28472; tel. 919/642-9051; Barbara Godwin, RN, BSN, Patient Care Coordinator

Lower Cape Fear Hospice, Inc., 2507-B North Marine Boulevard, Jacksonville, NC 28546; tel. 919/347-6266; FAX. 910/347-9279; Lori Griffin, Patient Care Coordinator

Lower Cape Fear Hospice, Inc., 112 Pine Street, P.O. Box 1926, Shallotte, NC 28459; tel. 910/754-5356; FAX. 910/754-5351; Jeff Hickey, Director, Operations

Lower Cape Fear Hospice, Inc., 103 North Morehead Street, Elizabethtown, NC 28337

Madison Home Care and Hospice, P.O. Box 909, 170 Carl Eller Road, Mars Hill, NC 28754; tel. 704/689-3491; FAX. 704/689-3496; John H. Estes, Executive Director

Mountain Area Hospice, Inc., 85 Lillicoa Street, P.O. Box 16, Asheville, NC 28802; tel. 704/255-0231; FAX. 704/255-2880; Kit Cosgrove, Associate Director

Northern Hospital Home Care and Hospice, 933 Old Rockford Street, P.O. Box 1605, Mount Airy, NC 27030; tel. 910/719-7434; FAX. 910/719-7435; Mary Alice Culler, Administrator

Onslow Home Health and Hospice, 612 College Street, Jacksonville, NC 28540; tel. 910/577-6660; FAX. 910/577-6636; Shirley P. Moore, RN, Director

Pemberton Hospice, 106 North Main Street, P.O. Box 3069, Pembroke, NC 28372; tel. 910/521-5550; FAX. 910/521-3335

Richmond County Hospice, Inc., 230 South Lawrence Street, Rockingham, NC 28379, P.O. Box 2136, Rockingham, NC 28380; tel. 910/997-4464; FAX. 910/997-4484; Lydia P. Talbert,CRNH, Patient Care Coordinator

Roanoke Home Care, 210 West Liberty Street, Williamston, NC 27892; tel. 919/792-5899; Barbara Owens, Nursing Director

Roanoke Home Care-Hospice, 408 Bridge Street, P.O. Box 238, Columbia, NC 27925; tel. 919/796-2681; FAX. 919/796-0818; Barbara Owens, RN, Director, Nursing

Roanoke Home Care-Hospice, 198 North Carolina Highway 45 North, Plymouth, NC 27962; tel. 800/842-8275; FAX. 919/793-3417; Phyllis McCombs, Referrals and Intake

Roanoke-Chowan Hospice, Inc., 521 Myers Street, P.O. Box 272, Ahoskie, NC 27910; tel. 919/332-3392; FAX. 919/332-5705; Brenda Hoggard, Director

Sandhills Hospice, Inc., Inverness Park, Five Aviemore Drive, P.O. Box 1956, Pinehurst, NC 28374; tel. 910/295-2220; FAX. 910/295-3720; Carole White, RN, Executive Director

St. Joseph of the Pines Home Health Agency, 117 Wortham Street, P.O. Box 974, Wadesboro, NC 28170; tel. 704/694-5992; Kathy Appenzeller, Director, Daily Operations

St. Joseph of the Pines Home Health Agency, 404 North Main Street, Troy, NC 27371; tel. 910/572-4962; FAX. 910/572-5010; Barbara Smith, CRNH Coordinator

St. Joseph of the Pines Home Health Agency, 336 South Main Street, P.O. Box 879, Raeford, NC 28376; tel. 910/875-8198; FAX. 910/875-8862; Ronda Pickler, Administrator

Staff Builders, 112 Broad Street, Oxford, NC 27565

Staff Builders/MedVisit Home Health and Hospice, 1924 Ruin Creek Road, Suite 207, Henderson, NC 27536; tel. 919/492-6046; FAX. 919/492-9967; Dorothy Forrest, Administrator

Staff Builders/MedVisit Home Health and Hospice, Highway 39 North, Route Three, Box 48, Louisburg, NC 27549; tel. 919/496-1900; FAX. 919/496-7052; Sherry Watson, Administrator

Swain County Home Health Agency, Main Street, Robbinsville, NC 28771; tel. 704/479-2110; FAX. 704/479-3848; Betty DeHart, RN

Triangle Hospice at the Meadowlands, 1001 Corporate Drive, Hillsborough, NC 27278; tel. 919/644-0764; FAX. 919/644-0932; Jerome Schiro, RN, M.N., Director

Triangle Hospice, Inc., 1804 Martin Luther King, Jr. Parkway, Suite 112, Durham, NC 27707; tel. 919/490-8480; FAX. 919/493-0242; Lucy Worth, Executive Director

Wendover, 953 Wendover Heights Drive, Shelby, NC 28150; tel. 704/487-7018; FAX. 704/487-7028; Myra McGinnis Hamrick, Executive Director

Wilson Home Care, Inc. d/b/a Hometown Hospice, 1705 South Tarboro Street, P.O. Box 2303, Wilson, NC 27894; tel. 919/237-4333; FAX. 919/237-1125; Gail Brewer, RN, M.P.H., Home Care Manager

Yadkin County Home Health/Hospice Agency, 217 East Willow Street, P.O. Box 457, Yadkinville, NC 27055; tel. 910/679-4207; FAX. 910/679-6358; Jackie Harrell, Nursing Supervisor

NORTH DAKOTA

Hospice of the Red River Valley, 702 28th Avenue, N., Fargo, ND 58102; tel. 701/237-4629; FAX. 701/280-9069; Susan J. Fuglie, Executive Director

Riveredge Hospice of St. Francis, 415 Oak Street, Breckenridge, ND 56520; tel. 218/643-7594; FAX. 218/643-7502; Cindy Splichal, Director

Trinity Hospice, 300 Southwest First Street, Minot, ND 58701; tel. 701/857-5083; Marilyn Bader, Administrator

United Community Hospice, 216 South Broadway, Minot, ND 58701; tel. 701/857-2499; FAX. 701/857-2565; Phil Sisi, Administrator

OHIO

Allen Hospice, 5700 Southwyck Boulevard, Suite 111, Toledo, OH 43614; tel. 419/867-4655; FAX. 419/865-1601; Jane Wilcox, RN, Executive Director

Aultman Hospice Program, 4510 Dressler Road, N.W., Canton, OH 44718; tel. 216/493-3344; FAX. 330/493-8637; Kathy Cummings, RN, Program Coordinator

Bridge Home Health and Hospice, 1900 South Main Street, Findlay, OH 45840; tel. 419/423-5351; FAX. 419/423-8967; Karen Mallett, Vice President, Home Care Services

CHWC-Hospice Care, 909 Snyder Avenue, Montpelier, OH 43543; tel. 419/485-3154

Columbia Mercy Medical Center Hospice, 1445 Harrison Avenue, N.W., Suite 201, Canton, OH 44708; tel. 330/489-6855; FAX. 330/489-6868; Ken Wasiniak, L.I.S.W., Hospice Manager

Community Hospice, 2609 Franklin Boulevard, Cleveland, OH 44113; tel. 216/363-2397; FAX. 216/363-2284; Cheryl Carrino, Patient Care Coordinator

Community Hospice Care, 182 St. Francis Avenue, Rear Suite, Tiffin, OH 44883; tel. 419/447-4040; FAX. 419/447-4657; Rebecca S. Shank, Executive Director

Section C

Crawford County Hospice, 1810 East Mansfield Street, Bucyrus, OH 44820; tel. 419/562–2001; FAX. 419/562–2803; Bert Maglott, RN, Executive Director

Geauga County Visiting Nurse Service and Hospice, 13221 Ravenna Road, Chardon, OH 44024; tel. 216/286–9461; Patricia Huels, RN, Director, Patient Services

Holmes County Hospice, 931 Wooster Road, Millersburg, OH 44654; tel. 330/674–5035; FAX. 330/674–2528; Diana L. Henry, RN, B.S.N., Director

Home Nursing Service and Hospice, 900 Third Street, Marietta, OH 45750; tel. 614/373–8549; FAX. 614/373–3995; Pamela Parr, Director

Hospice Care of Williams Co., Inc., 127 West Butler Street, Bryan, OH 43506; tel. 419/636–8034; FAX. 419/636–8221

Hospice Homecare, 92 Northwoods Boulevard, #A, Columbus, OH 43235; tel. 614/781–1444; FAX. 614/781–1450; Belinda R. Shaw, RN, Clinical Manager

Hospice Service of Licking County, Inc., d/b/a Hospice of Central Ohio, Homecare of Central Ohio, 1435 B West Main Street, Newark, OH 43055; tel. 614/344–0311; FAX. 614/344–6577; Michele McMahon, Executive Director

Hospice and Health Services of Fairfield County, 1111 East Main Street, Lancaster, OH 43130; tel. 614/654–7077; FAX. 614/654–6321; Donna J. Householder, Executive Director

Hospice of Alliance VNA, 2367 West State Street, Alliance, OH 44601; tel. 330/821–7055; Lin Severs, M.S.N., Executive Director

Hospice of Appalachia, 282 East State Street, P.O. Box 768, Athens, OH 45701; tel. 614/592–3493; FAX. 614/594–5591; Carol May, Director

Hospice of Care Corporation, 831 South Street, Chardon, OH 44024; tel. 216/338–6628; FAX. 216/286–7662; Elizabeth A. Petersen, RN, Vice President, Operations

Hospice of Cincinnati, Inc., 2710 Reading Road, Cincinnati, OH 45206; tel. 513/569–5100; Leigh Gerdsen, RN, Director

Hospice of Columbus, 181 South Washington Boulevard, Columbus, OH 43215; tel. 614/645–6471; FAX. 614/645–5895; Larry L. Miracle, Director

Hospice of Coshocton County, Inc., 230 South Fourth, P.O. Box 1284, Coshocton, OH 43812; tel. 614/622–7311; FAX. 614/622–7310; Barbara Brooks–Emmons, Director

Hospice of Darke County, Inc., 122 West Martz Street, Greenville, OH 45331; tel. 937/548–2999; FAX. 937/548–7144; Joy Marchal, Executive Director

Hospice of Dayton, Inc., 324 Wilmington Avenue, Dayton, OH 45420; tel. 513/256–4490; Betty Schmoll, President

Hospice of Guernsey, Inc., 1300 Clark Street, P.O. Box 1537, Cambridge, OH 43725; tel. 614/432–7440; Patricia Howell, RN, Administrator

Hospice of Henry County, 104 East Washington, Suite 302, Napoleon, OH 43545; tel. 419/599–5545; FAX. 419/599–1714

Hospice of Knox County, 302 East High Street, Mount Vernon, OH 43050; tel. 614/397–5188; FAX. 614/397–5189; Linda M. Bales, Interim Executive Director

Hospice of Medina County, 797 North Court Street, Medina, OH 44256; tel. 330/722–4771; FAX. 330/722–5266; Patricia M. Stropko–O'Leary, Executive Director

Hospice of Miami County, Inc., P.O. Box 502, Troy, OH 45373; tel. 937/335–5191; FAX. 937/335–8841; Sidney J. Pinkus, Chief Executive Officer

Hospice of Morrow County, P.O. Box 272, 851 West Marion Road, Mount Gilead, OH 43338; tel. 419/946–9822; FAX. 419/946–9971; Frances Turner, RN, Executive Director

Hospice of North Central Ohio, Inc., 1605 County Road 1095, Ashland, OH 44805; tel. 419/281–7107; FAX. 419/281–8427; Ruth A. Lindsey, Executive Director

Hospice of Northwest Ohio, 30000 East River Road, Perrysburg, OH 43551; tel. 419/661–4001; FAX. 419/661–4015; Virginia Clifford, Executive Director

Hospice of Pickaway County, 702 Pickaway Street, Circleville, OH 43113; tel. 614/474–3525; FAX. 614/474–1832

Hospice of Tuscarawas County, Inc., 201 West Third Street, Dover, OH 44622; tel. 330/343–7605; FAX. 330/343–3542; Janie Jones, Administrator

Hospice of V.N.A., 1195–C Professional Drive, Van Wert, OH 45891; tel. 419/238–9223; FAX. 419/238–9391; Donna Grimm, President, Chief Executive Officer

Hospice of Visiting Nurse Service, 3358 Ridgewood Road, Akron, OH 44333; tel. 800/335–1455; FAX. 216/668–4680; Patricia Waickman, M.S.N., RN, Vice President, Hospice

Hospice of Wayne County, Ohio, 2330 Cleveland Road, Wooster, OH 44691; tel. 330/264–4899; FAX. 330/264–4874; Mary Ellen Walsh, Executive Director

Hospice of Wyandot County, 320 West Maple Street, Suite C, Upper Sandusky, OH 43351; tel. 419/294–5787; FAX. 419/294–4721; Susan Barth, RN, Interim Director

Hospice of the Miami Valley, Inc., 930 Laurel Avenue, Hamilton, OH 45015; tel. 513/863–3433; FAX. 513/867–7444; Rebecca Hight, RN, President, Chief Executive Officer

Hospice of the Valley, Inc., 5190 Market Street, Youngstown, OH 44512; tel. 330/788–1992; FAX. 330/788–1998; Kenneth O. Drees, Executive Director

Hospice of the Western Reserve, 300 East 185th Street, Cleveland, OH 44119; tel. 216/383–2222; FAX. 216/383–3750; David A. Simpson, Executive Director

Hospice, The Caring Way of Defiance County, 197–C Island Park Avenue, Defiance, OH 43512; tel. 419/784–3818; FAX. 419/782–4979; Ruthann Czartoski, Hospice Coordinator

Loving Care Hospice, Inc., 106 West High Street, P.O. Box 445, London, OH 43140; tel. 614/852–7755

M J Nursing Registry, 2534 Victory Parkway, Cincinnati, OH 45206; tel. 513/961–1000; FAX. 513/872–7550; Jan Brown, RN, Assistant Administrator, Home Care

Madison County Home Health Hospice Inc., 212 North Main Street, London, OH 43140; tel. 614/852–3915; FAX. 614/852–5125; Barbara C. Anderson, Executive Director

Mercy Hospice, 7010 Rowan Hill Drive, Cincinnati, OH 45227; tel. 513/271–1440; FAX. 513/271–2405

Mount Carmel Hospice, 1144 Dublin Road, Columbus, OH 43215; tel. 614/234–0200; FAX. 614/234–0201; Mary Ann Gill, Director

NCJW/Montefiore Hospice, One David N. Myers Parkway, Beachwood, OH 44122; tel. 216/360–9080, ext. 338; FAX. 216/360–9697; Jennifer Hooks, Hospice Director

New Life–Choices in LifeCare, 5255 North Abbe Road, Elyria, OH 44035; tel. 216/934–1458; FAX. 216/934–1567; Micki M. Tubbs, President, Chief Executive Officer

Ohio's Integrated Hospice, 2365 Lakeview Drive, Suite B, Beavercreek, OH 45431; tel. 513/427–3074; Patricia B. Kehl, M.A., RN, Administrator

Stein Hospice Services, Inc., 1200 Sycamore Line, Sandusky, OH 44870; tel. 800/625–5269; FAX. 419/625–5761; Rosalie A. Perry, Executive Director

The Hospice of Staff Builders, 6100 Rockside Woods Boulevard, Suite 100, Independence, OH 44131; tel. 216/642–0202; FAX. 216/642–3273; Marion Keathley, Intake Coordinator

The VNA of North Central Ohio Hospice, 188 West Third Street, P.O. Box 1322, Mansfield, OH 44901–1322; tel. 419/524–4663; FAX. 419/524–4862

Tri County Hospice, Inc., One Park Centre, Suite 209, Wadsworth, OH 44281; tel. 210/336–6595

Tricare Hospice, 701 Park Road, Bellefontaine, OH 43311; tel. 800/886–5936; FAX. 513/593–9783; Jim Hoffman, Director

VNA of Cleveland Hospice, 2500 East 22nd Street, Cleveland, OH 44115; tel. 216/931–1450; FAX. 216/694–6355; Roberta Laurie, Executive Director, Hospice

Valley Hospice, Inc., One Ross Park, Steubenville, OH 43952; tel. 614/283–7487; FAX. 614/283–7507; Karen Nichols, RN, B.S.N., Executive Director

Vencare Hospice, 2055 Reading Road, Suite 240, Cincinnati, OH 45202; tel. 513/241–9209; FAX. 513/241–4012; Rebecca Wright, RN, CRNH, Administrator

Visiting Nurse Hospice and Health Care, 383 West Dussel Drive, Maumee, OH 43537; tel. 419/897–2803; FAX. 419/897–2810; Nancy Host, Executive Director

Vitas Health Care Corporation of Ohio, 4700 Smith Road, Suite M, Cincinnati, OH 45212; tel. 513/531–6317; FAX. 513/531–7551; Gay Haggard, General Manager

OKLAHOMA

Blaine County Hospice, 401 North Clarence Nash, P.O. Box 567, Watonga, OK 73772; tel. 405/623–7414; FAX. 405/623–7412; Lisa Watson, RN

Carter Hospice Care, 1235 Sovereign Row, Suite C–5, Oklahoma City, OK 73108; tel. 405/942–1161; FAX. 405/947–2718; Kathi Egan, RN, Executive Director

Carter Hospice Care, 828 North Porter, Norman, OK 73069; tel. 405/942–1161; Stanley F. Carter, Administrator

Carter Hospice Care, Inc., 9916A East 43rd Street, S., Tulsa, OK 74146; tel. 405/942–1161; FAX. 405/947–2718; Stanley F. Carter, Administrator

Columbia Hospice Oklahoma, 7508 North Broadway Extension, Suite 110, Oklahoma City, OK 73112; tel. 800/243–7776; FAX. 405/848–5135; Sharon Collins, RN, CRNH, Hospice Director

Community Hospice, Inc., 1400 South Broadway, Edmond, OK 73034; tel. 405/359–1948; FAX. 405/359–4913; L. Jim Anthis, Ph.D., President, Chief Executive Officer

Crossroads Hospice of Oklahoma, L.L.C., 10810 East 45th Street, Suite 310, Tulsa, OK 74146; tel. 918/663–3234; FAX. 918/663–3334; G. Perry Farmer, Jr., Executive Director

Eastern Oklahoma Hospice, 1301 Reynolds, Poteau, OK 74953; tel. 918/647–8235; Jody L. Shepherd, RN, Agency Director

Family Hospice of Greater Oklahoma City, 4900 Richmond Square, Suite 203, Oklahoma City, OK 73118; tel. 405/843–4097; FAX. 405/843–5629; Steven L. Edwards, Executive Director

Family Hospice of Tulsa, 7030 South Yale Avenue, Suite 412, Tulsa, OK 74136; tel. 918/488–9477; FAX. 918/488–9506; Robert D. Lane, ARNP, L.C.S.W., Executive Director

Four Square Hospice, 223 Plaza, P.O. Box 827, Madill, OK 73446; tel. 405/795–3384; Norma Howard

Good Shepherd Hospice, 1300 Sovereign Row, Oklahoma City, OK 73108; tel. 405/943–0903; FAX. 405/943–0950; Don Greiner, Executive Director

Hospice Care of Oklahoma, 5901 North Western, Suite 101, Oklahoma City, OK 73118; tel. 405/848–2324; Jean Calder, CRNH

Hospice Circle of Love, 605 South Monroe, Enid, OK 73701; tel. 405/234–2273; FAX. 405/234–1990; Cathy Graber, Director

Hospice of Central Oklahoma, 4549 Northwest 36th Street, Oklahoma City, OK 73122; tel. 405/491–0828; Sharon Holland, President

Hospice of Green Country, Inc., 3010 South Harvard, Suite 110, Tulsa, OK 74114–6136; tel. 918/747–2273; FAX. 918/747–2573; Sue Mosher, M.S., Executive Director

Hospice of Lawton Area, Inc., 1930 Northwest Ferris Avenue, Suite 10, Lawton, OK 73505; tel. 405/248–5885; FAX. 405/355–2446; Lee Young, Executive Director

Hospice of McAlester, First National Center, Suite 112, McAlester, OK 74501; tel. 918/423–3911; FAX. 918/426–6335; Vicki Schaff, Executive Director

Hospice of Oklahoma County, Inc., 4334 Northwest Expressway, Suite 106, Oklahoma City, OK 73116–1515; tel. 405/848–8884; FAX. 405/841–4899; Douglas M. Gibson, Executive Director

Hospice of Ponca City, 1904 North Union, Suite 103, Ponca City, OK 74601; tel. 405/762–9102; FAX. 405/762–9111; Melody Lahann, Director

Hospice of the Heartland, 1002 South College, Tahlequah, OK 74464; tel. 918/458–3011; FAX. 918/458–3067; Deborah Huggins, Administrator

Judith Karman Hospice, Inc., 824 South Main Street, P.O. Box 818, Stillwater, OK 74076; tel. 405/377–8012; FAX. 405/624–9007; Mary Lee Warren, Executive Director

Lawton Community Hospice, Inc., 4645 West Gore Boulevard, Lawton, OK 73505; tel. 405/250–0440; FAX. 405/250–0489; Jerry W. Black, Program Director

Mid–Lakes Hospice Care, 500 East Main Street, P.O. Box 728, Stigler, OK 74462; tel. 918/967–8499; FAX. 918/967–2584; John C. Neal, Administrator

Mission Hospice, Inc., 7301 North Broadway, Suite 225, Oklahoma City, OK 73116; tel. 405/848–3779; FAX. 405/848–8481; Susan Osborne, RN, Administrator

New Hope Hospice of Oklahoma, Inc., 5460 South Garnett, Suite H, Tulsa, OK 74146; tel. 918/622–7744; Tonia Caselman, L.S.W., Executive Director

Norman Community Hospice, 2424 Springer, Suite 105, Norman, OK 73069; tel. 405/360–4884; FAX. 405/360–4913; Debbie Standefer, RN, PCC

Preferred Hospice, 1200 North Walker, Suite 200, Oklahoma City, OK 73103; tel. 405/235–7674; FAX. 405/235–5478; Dean A. Deason, M.D., Director, Operations

Russell–Murray Hospice, Inc., 221 South Bickford, P.O. Box 1423, El Reno, OK 73036; tel. 405/262–3088; FAX. 405/262–3082; Cathie Sales, Administrator

The Hospice, 2023 West Broadway, Muskogee, OK 74401; tel. 918/683–1192; FAX. 918/687–0750; Jamie Bridgewater, Executive Director

Visiting Nurses Agency of Eastern Oklahoma Hospice, 220 South Main Street, Spiro, OK 74959; tel. 918/962–9491; Jim Medley, Chief Executive Officer

Visiting Nurses Agency of Eastern Oklahoma, Inc., Two Eastern Heights Shopping Center, P.O. Box 1647, Muldrow, OK 74948; tel. 918/427–1010; Mary Keith, RNC, Vice President

OREGON

Benton Hospice Service, Inc., 917 Northwest Grant Street, P.O. Box 100, Corvallis, OR 97333; tel. 541/757–9616; FAX. 541/757–1760; Judy List, Executive Director

Curry County Home/Health Hospice, 29984 Ellensburg, P.O. Box 746, Gold Beach, OR 97444; tel. 541/247–7084; FAX. 541/247–2117; Lori Kent, RN

Harney County Home Health/Hospice, 420 North Fairview, Burns, OR 97720; tel. 541/573–8360; FAX. 541/573–8389; Angela Ivey, Director

Hospice of Bend, 1303 Northwest Galveston, Bend, OR 97701; tel. 541/383–3910; FAX. 541/388–4221

Hospice of Redmond and Sisters, P.O. Box 1092, Redmond, OR 97756; tel. 541/548–7483; FAX. 541/548–1507; Ellen Garcia, Executive Director

Hospice of St. Vincent, 9340 Southwest Barnes Road, Suite M, Portland, OR 97225; tel. 503/297–6109; Jerry Hunter

Hospice of the Gorge, Inc., 114 Cascade Street, P.O. Box 36, Hood River, OR 97031; tel. 503/387–6449; FAX. 503/386–6700; Ina Holman, Executive Director

Kaiser Permanente, Home Health/Hospice, 2701 Northwest Vaughn Street, Suite 140, Portland, OR 97210; tel. 503/499–5200; FAX. 503/499–5200; Linda Van Buren, RN, Administrator

Klamath Hospice, Inc., 437 Main Street, Klamath Falls, OR 97601; tel. 541/882–2902; FAX. 541/883–1992; Teresa C. Pastorius

Legacy VNA Hospice, 2701 Northwest Vaughn, Suite 720, P.O. Box 3426, Portland, OR 97208; tel. 503/225–6370; FAX. 503/225–6398; Linda Downey, Director

Lovejoy Hospice, Inc., 132 Northeast B Street, Suite 23, P.O. Box 356, Grants Pass, OR 97526; tel. 503/474–1193; FAX. 503/474–3035; Charlotte Carroll, RN, P.H.N., Executive Director

Lower Umpqua Hospice, 600 Ranch Road, Reedsport, OR 97467; tel. 541/271–2171, ext. 229; FAX. 541/271–1108; Geraldine Simms, RN, Manager

Mid–Willamette Valley Hospice, 1467 13th Street, S.E., Salem, OR 97302; tel. 503/588–3600; FAX. 503/363–3891; Simon B. Paquette, M.S.W., Administrator

Mt. Hood Hospice, 17270 Southeast Bluff Road, P.O. Box 835, Sandy, OR 97055; tel. 503/668–5545; FAX. 503/668–7951; Lindy Blaesing, Executive Director

Pathway Hospice, Inc., 323 West Idaho Avenue, Ontario, OR 97914; tel. 541/889–0847; FAX. 541/889–0849; Betty Cooper, RN

Providence Home Services Hospice, 1235 Northeast 47th, Suite 215, 4805 Northeast Glisan (Mailing Address), Portland, OR 97213; tel. 503/331–4601; FAX. 503/215–4624; Karen Bell, Director

South Coast Hospice, 371 West Anderson, Suite 218, Coos Bay, OR 97420; tel. 503/269–2986; FAX. 503/267–0458; Linda J. Furman, Administrator

Washington County Hospice, Inc., 427 Southeast Eighth Avenue, Hillsboro, OR 97123–4519; tel. 503/648–9565; FAX. 503/648–1282; Christine Larch, Administrator

Willamette Falls Hospice, 1678 Beavercreek Road, Suite K, Oregon City, OR 97045; tel. 503/655–0550; FAX. 503/655–7585; Robert Steed, Administrator

XL Hospice of Lakeview, 100 North D Street, Suite Three, P.O. Box 337, Lakeview, OR 97630; tel. 541/947–5122; FAX. 541/947–2253; Dian Jepson, RN, Patient Care Coordinator

PENNSYLVANIA

Abington Memorial Hospital Home Care and Hospice Program, 2510 Maryland Road, Suite 250, Willow Grove, PA 19090–0520; tel. 215/881–5800; FAX. 215/881–5850; Marilyn D. Harris, Administrator

Albert Gallatin Hospice Program, 20 Highland Park Drive, Suite 203, Uniontown, PA 15401; tel. 412/438–6660; FAX. 412/438–4468; Chris Constantine, RN, Administrator

All Care Hospice, 472 1/2 South Poplar Street, Hazelton, PA 18201; tel. 717/459–2004; Mary Ann Barletta, RN, Administrator

Berks Visiting Nurse Association, Inc., 1170 Berkshire Boulevard, Wyomissing, PA 19610; tel. 610/378–0481; FAX. 610/378–9762; Lucille D. Gough, RN, President, Chief Executive Officer

Brandywine Hospice, 1219 East Lincoln Highway, Coatesville, PA 19320; tel. 610/384–4200; FAX. 610/384–6871; Margaret Zazo, RN, M.S.N., CS

Brookline Home Care & Hospice, 3901 South Atherton Street, State College, PA 16801; tel. 814/238–2121; FAX. 814/466–4806; Diane Good, Administrator

Centre Hospice, A Program of Centre HomeCare, Inc., 221 West High Street, Bellefonte, PA 16823–1385; tel. 814/355–2273; FAX. 814/353–9292; Molly Schwantz, Executive Director

Chandler Hall Hospice, 99 Barclay Street, Newtown, PA 18940; tel. 215/860–4000; FAX. 215/860–3458; Jane W. Fox, Executive Director

Clarion Forest VNA Hospice, R.D. 3, Box 186, Clarion, PA 16214; tel. 814/226–1140; FAX. 814/226–1143; Deborah J. Kelly, Director, Hospice

Cohhcare's Home Hospice Care, 10 Duff Road, Suite 213, Pittsburgh, PA 15235; tel. 412/247–5606; Carole K. Rimer

Columbia–Montour Home Hospice, Locust Court, 599 East Seventh Street, Suite One, Bloomsburg, PA 17815; tel. 717/784–1723; FAX. 717/784–8512; Jane Gittler, Chief Executive Officer

Comfort Care Hospice, 115 South Filbert Street, Mechanicsburg, PA 17055; tel. 800/255–3300; FAX. 717/766–5037; Robyn Schmalz, RN, Director

Community Nurses Professional Health Services/Hospice, 99 Erie Avenue, St. Marys, PA 15857; tel. 814/781–1415; FAX. 814/781–6987; Elizabeth A. Roberts, RN, Executive Director

Community Nursing Hospice, 1425 Scalp Avenue, Johnstown, PA 15904; tel. 814/262–0246; FAX. 814/262–9616; Gayle Petrunak, Patient Care Coordinator

Compassionate Care Hospice, 100 Granite Drive, Suite 200, Media, PA 19063; tel. 610/892–7741; FAX. 610/892–7721; Catherine A. Stevens, Administrator

Compassionate Care of Gwynedd, Inc., 716 Bethlehem Pike, Suite 100, Lower Gwynedd, PA 19002; tel. 215/540–1244; FAX. 215/540–9849; Christine M. Coletta, RNC, B.S.N., CRNH, Program Director

Crozer Hospice, One Medical Center Boulevard, Upland, PA 19013; tel. 610/447–6141; FAX. 215/447–6027; Maryann Dreisbach, RN, Director

Ephrata Community Home Care's Hospice Program, 169 Martin Avenue, Box 1002, Ephrata, PA 17522–1002; tel. 717/738–6599; FAX. 717/738–6343; Susan Auxier, RN, Clinical Supervisor

Family Hospice of Indiana County, a division of the V.N.A. of Indiana County, 119 Professional Center, 1265 Wayne Avenue, Indiana, PA 15701; tel. 412/463–8711; FAX. 412/463–8907; Linda E. Lutz, B.S.N., RN, Director, Special Care Services, Hospice

Family Hospice, Inc., 1910 Cochran Road, Suite 500, Pittsburgh, PA 15220; tel. 412/572–8800; FAX. 412/572–8827; Baylee Gordon, Executive Director

Forbes Hospice–Forbes Health System, 6655 Frankstown Avenue, Pittsburgh, PA 15206; tel. 412/665–3301; FAX. 412/665–3234; Maryanne Fello, RN, Manager

General Care Services, d/b/a Hospice of Warren County, Two Crescent Park, W., P.O. Box 68, Warren, PA 16365; tel. 814/723–2455; FAX. 814/723–1177; Elsa L. Redding, Director

Great Lakes Hospice, 300 State Street, Suite 301–H, Erie, PA 16507; tel. 814/877–6120; Debbie Burbules, Director

Guthrie Hospice, R.R. One, P.O. Box 154, Towanda, PA 18848; tel. 800/598–6155; FAX. 717/265–3570; Jocelyn O'Donnell, Administrator

Healthreach Home Care and Hospice, 409 South Second Street, Harrisburg, PA 17104; tel. 717/231–6363; Janet T. Foreman, RN

Holy Family Home Health and Hospice Care, 900 West Market Street, Owigsburg, PA 17961; tel. 717/366–0990; FAX. 717/366–3735; Arlene L. Mongrain, RN, B.S., Executive Director

Holy Redeemer, Nazarath and St. Home Health Services, 12265 Townsend Road, Philadelphia, PA 19154; tel. 215/671–9200; FAX. 215/671–1950; Jerold S. Cohen, President

Home Hospice Agency of St. Francis, 131 Columbus Innerbelt, New Castle, PA 16101; tel. 412/652–8847; FAX. 412/656–0876; Susan N. Ludu, Executive Director

Home Nursing Agency/VNA Hospice Program, 201 Chestnut Avenue, P.O. Box 352, Altoona, PA 16603–0352; tel. 814/946–5411; FAX. 814/941–2482; Sylvia H. Schraff, RN, Chief Executive Officer

Hospice Care of the VNA, 400 Third Avenue, Suite 100, Kingston, PA 18704; tel. 717/287–4402; FAX. 717/287–4809; Mary Ann Keirans, Administrator

Hospice Community Care, Inc., 385 Wyoming Avenue, Kingston, PA 18704; tel. 717/288–2288; FAX. 717/288–7424; Philip Decker, President

Hospice Preferred Choice, Inc., 2400 Ardmore Boulevard, Suite 302, Pittsburgh, PA 15221; tel. 412/271–2273; FAX. 412/271–3361; Christean Dugan, Administrator

Hospice Program/VNA of Hanover and Spring Grove, 440 North Madison Street, Hanover, PA 17331; tel. 717/637–1227; FAX. 717/637–9772; Sandra L. Wojtkowiak, RN, MSN, Administrator

Hospice Saint John, 665 Carey Avenue, Wilkes–Barre, PA 18702; tel. 717/823–2114; FAX. 717/823–6438; W. David Keating, Administrator

Hospice Services of the VNA of York County, 218 East Market Street, York, PA 17403; tel. 717/846–9900; FAX. 717/846–1933; Marie V. Fraser, President, Chief Executive Officer

Hospice of Central Pennsylvania, 98 South Enola Drive, P.O. Box 266, Enola, PA 17025–0266; tel. 717/732–1000; FAX. 717/732–5348; Karen M. Paris, Chief Executive Officer

Hospice of Community and Home Health Services, 117 North Hanover Street, Carlisle, PA 17013; tel. 717/245–5600; FAX. 717/249–9346; Elizabeth Hain, RN, Administrator

Hospice of Crawford County, Inc., 448 Pine Street, Meadville, PA 16335; tel. 814/333–5403; FAX. 814/333–5407; John E. Brown, Chief Executive Officer

Hospice of Lancaster County, 685 Good Drive, P.O. Box 4125, Lancaster, PA 17604–4125; tel. 717/295–3900; FAX. 717/391–9582; Mary Graner, President, Executive Director

Hospice of North Penn Visiting Nurse Association, 51 Medical Campus Drive, Lansdale, PA 19446; tel. 215/855–8297; FAX. 215/855–1305; Jane Spizzirri, Hospice Coordinator

Hospice of the Delaware Valley, 527 Plymouth Road, Suite 417, Plymouth Meeting, PA 19462; tel. 610/941–6700; FAX. 610/941–6440; Marcia M. Cook, Administrator

Hospice of the VNA of Bethlehem and Vicinity, 1510 Valley Center Parkway, Suite 200, Bethlehem, PA 18017; tel. 215/691–1100; FAX. 610/691–2271; Jean Fiore, RN, Administrator

Hospice of the VNA of Greater Philadelphia, One Winding Way, Philadelphia, PA 19131; tel. 215/581–2046; FAX. 215/473–5047; Beverly Paukstis, Administrator

Hospice–The Bridge, Lewistown Hospital, 1126 West Fourth Street, Lewistown, PA 17044–1909; tel. 717/242–5000; FAX. 717/242–5009; Shirley McNeal, RN, CRNH, Manager

HospiceCare of Pittsburgh, 11 Parkway Center, Suite 275, Pittsburgh, PA 15220; tel. 412/937–8088; FAX. 412/922–9609; Heather Young, RN, Administrator

Section C

In Home Health, Inc., 750 Holiday Drive, Foster Plaza Nine, Suite 110, Pittsburgh, PA 15220; tel. 412/928-2126; Margaret Timm, Director, Operations

Jefferson Hospice–Main Line, Gerhard Building, 130 South Bryn Mawr Avenue, Bryn Mawr, PA 19018; tel. 610/526-3265; Timothy P. Cousounis, Executive Director

Keystone Hospice, 275 Commerce Drive, Suite 314, Fort Washington, PA 19034; tel. 215/628-8592; FAX. 215/628-8491; Gail A. Inoerwies, Director

Lehigh Valley Hospice, 2166 South 12th Street, Allentown, PA 18103; tel. 610/402-7400; FAX. 610/402-7382; William V. Dunstan, Administrator

Lutheran Home Health Care Services/Hospice, 2700 Luther Drive, Chambersburg, PA 17201; tel. 717/264-8178; FAX. 717/264-6347; Diane M. Howell, Executive Director

McKean County VNA Hospice, 20 School Street, P.O. Box 465, Bradford, PA 16701-0465; tel. 814/362-7466; FAX. 814/362-2916; Elizabeth M. Costello, Administrator

Mercy Health Hospice Program, 1500 Lansdowne Avenue, Darby, PA 19023; tel. 610/237-5010; FAX. 610/237-4689; Cathy Franklin

Montgomery Hospital Hospice Program, 25 West Fornance Street, Norristown, PA 19401; tel. 610/272-1080; Elise N. Lamarra, B.S.N.

Neighborhood Visiting Nurse Association, 795 East Marshall Street, West Chester, PA 19380; tel. 610/696-6511; FAX. 610/344-7064; Mahlon R. Fiscel, Chief Executive Officer

North Chester County Community Nursing Service Hospice, 301 Gay Street, Phoenixville, PA 19460; tel. 215/933-1263; Thomasina A. Chamberlain, Administrator

North Penn HH Agency/Hospice Program, 520 Ruah Street, P.O. Box Eight, Blossburg, PA 16912; tel. 717/638-2141, ext. 700; FAX. 717/638-2163; Wilma Hall, Program Director

Northeast Health and Hospice Care, Inc., 38 North Main Street, Pittston, PA 18640; tel. 717/654-0220; FAX. 717/654-0360; Stephan Hannon, Administrator

Odyssey Health Care of Pennsylvania, Park West One, Suite 500, Cliff Mine Road, Pittsburgh, PA 15275; tel. 412/494-0870; Deborah Yakunich

Olsten Kimberly Quality Care Hospice, 4811 Jonestown Road, Suite 235, Harrisburg, PA 17109; tel. 717/541-4466; Susan Gearhart, RN

Olsten Kimberly QualityCare Hospice, 749 Northern Boulevard, Clarks Summit, PA 18411; tel. 800/870-0085; Peggy Durkin, Administrator

Palliative Care Services, Fox Chase Cancer Center, 500 Township Line Road, Cheltenham, PA 19012; tel. 215/728-3011; FAX. 215/728-5270; Susanne Seeber, RN, MSN

Penn Care at Home, 51 North 39th Street, Philadelphia, PA 19104; tel. 215/662-8996; Rita P. Rebman, RN, MSN

Professional Hospice Care, 3605 Vartan Way, Harrisburg, PA 17110; tel. 717/671-3700; FAX. 717/671-3713; Denise K. Harris, M.S.W., Director

Ridgway Community Nurse Service, Inc., Hospice, 20 North Broad Street, P.O. Box 179, Ridgway, PA 15853; tel. 814/773-5705; FAX. 814/776-6246; Catherine M. Grove, RN, Executive Director

SUN Home Hospice, 61 Duke Street, Northumberland, PA 17857; tel. 717/473-8320; FAX. 717/473-3070; Patricia Campbell, Director

Samaritan Care Hospice of Pennsylvania, 6198 Butler Pike, Suite 275, Blue Bell, PA 19422; tel. 215/653-7310; FAX. 215/653-7340; Peggy Bertels

Sivitz Jewish Hospice, 1620 Murry Avenue, Pittsburgh, PA 15217; tel. 412/422-5700; Deborah Shtulman, Executive Director

St. Gregory's Hospice, Inc., 359 Steubenville Pike, Burgettstown, PA 15021; tel. 412/729-3051; FAX. 412/729-3820; Patricia Murphy, RN, M.S.N., Director

Susquehanna Regional Home Health Services and Hospice, 1201 Grampian Boulevard, Suite Three A, Williamsport, PA 17701-1967; tel. 717/323-9891; FAX. 717/323-0716; Pamela B. McCowan, RN, Director, Hospice

Three Rivers Family Hospice, Inc., 3025 Jacks Run Road, White Oak, PA 15131; tel. 412/672-6737; FAX. 412/672-5823; Jan Diehl, RN, M.S.N., Executive Director

Ultimate Home Health and Hospice Care, 212 North Second Street, Girardville, PA 17935; tel. 717/276-1148; Barbara McDonald, Administrator

Unlimited Home Care, Inc., Hospice, P.O. Box 1070, Uniontown, PA 15401; tel. 412/439-1610; FAX. 412/430-6891; Diane Sanner Crossan, Director

Upper Bucks Hospice, a Division of Life Quest Home Care, 2075 Quaker Pointe Drive, Quakertown, PA 18951; tel. 215/529-6100; FAX. 215/529-6253; Beth Gotwals, RN, M.S.N., Hospice Manager

VNA Community Services Hospice, 354 North Prince Street, P.O. Box 4304, Lancaster, PA 17604-4304; tel. 717/397-8251, ext. 1270; FAX. 717/397-8666; Cynthia Theurer, Hospice Director

VNA Health Care Services, 1789 South Braddock Avenue, Pittsburgh, PA 15218; tel. 412/256-6800; Andrew R. Peacock

VNA Hospice, 334 Jefferson Avenue, Scranton, PA 18501; tel. 717/341-6840; Nancy S. Menapace, RN, M.A., Administrator

VNA Hospice Services of Erie County, 1305 Peach Street, Erie, PA 16501; tel. 814/454-2831; Mary Frances Bauman, Administrator

VNA Hospice, Western Pennsylvania, 154 Hindman Road, Butler, PA 16001; tel. 412/282-6806; FAX. 412/282-7517; Liz Powell, RN, M.N., CRNP, Vice President

VNA of Easton Hospice, 3421 Nightingale Drive, Easton, PA 18045; tel. 215/258-7189; Theresa P. Onorata

VNA of Harrisburg, Inc. Hospice, 118 Washington Street, Harrisburg, PA 17104; tel. 717/233-1035; FAX. 717/233-2759; Thomas Tarasewich, Chief Executive Officer

VNA of Pottstown and Vicinity Comprehensive Hospice Program, 1963 East High Street, Pottstown, PA 19464; tel. 610/327-5700; FAX. 610/327-5701; Sandra Levengood, Executive Director

VNA/Hospice of Monroe County, Inc., R.R. Two, P.O. Box 2159A, East Stroudsburg, PA I8360; tel. 7l7/421-5390; FAX. 717/421-7423; Mark Hodgson, Administrator

Visiting Nurse Association of Northumberland County, 101 South Market Street, Shamokin, PA 17872; tel. 800/732-2486; FAX. 717/648-9590; Joseph L. Scopelliti, Jr., Executive Director

Visiting Nurses Association of the Lehigh Valley, Inc., 1710 Union Boulevard, Allentown, PA 18103; tel. 610/434-6134, ext. 177; FAX. 610/821-1982; Patricia Frenduto, President, Chief Executive Officer

Vitas Health Care Corporation, 805 East Germantown Pike, Suite 805, Norristown, PA 19401; tel. 215/275-2370; Emily B. Fedullo, RN, Director, Development

White Rose Hospice, 2870 Eastern Boulevard, York, PA 17402; tel. 717/849-5642; FAX. 717/849-5630; Karen Hook, B.S., Manager

Wissahickon Hospice, 8835 Germantown Avenue, Philadelphia, PA 19118; tel. 215/247-0277; FAX. 215/248-3253; Priscilla D. Kissick, RN, M.N., Executive Director

RHODE ISLAND

Hospice Care of Rhode Island, 169 George Street, Pawtucket, RI 02860-3868; tel. 401/727-7070; FAX. 401/727-7080; David Rehm, Executive Director

Hospice Care of the Visiting Nurse Service of Greater Woonsocket, Marquette Plaza, Woonsocket, RI 02895; tel. 401/769-5670; FAX. 401/762-2966; Elaine D. Bartro, RN, M.P.H., Chief Executive Officer

Hospice of Nursing Placement, 339 Angell Street, P.O. Box 603337, Providence, RI 02906; tel. 401/453-4544; Marcia Bigney, Administrator

Kent County Visiting Nurse Association Hospice, 51 Health Lane, Warwick, RI 02886; tel. 401/737-6050; FAX. 401/738-0247; Nancy Roberts, RN, M.S.N., Chief Executive Director

Northwest Home Care (Hospice), 185 Putnam Pike, P.O. Box 423, Harmony, RI 02829; tel. 401/949-2600; FAX. 401/949-5115; Beverly McGuire, President

VNA of Rhode Island, 157 Waterman Avenue, Providence, RI 02906; tel. 401/444-9400; FAX. 401/444-9430; Sandra L. Hooper, RN, M.B.A., CNAA, Director, Adult Services

VNS Hospice, 14 Woodruff Avenue, Narragansett, RI 02882-3467; tel. 401/788-2000; FAX. 401/788-2064; Lyle Mook, Director, Hospice Services

Valley Hospice–VNS of Pawtucket, Central Falls, Lincoln and Cumberland, 172 Armistice Boulevard, Pawtucket, RI 02860; tel. 401/725-3414; FAX. 401/728-4999; Christopher L. Boys, Chief Executive Officer

Visiting Nurse Health Services Hospice, 1184 East Main Road, P.O. Box 690, Portsmouth, RI 02871; tel. 401/682-2100; FAX. 401/682-2112; Jean Anderson, RN, M.S., Acting Chief Executive Officer

SOUTH CAROLINA

Hitchcock Rehabilitation Center Home Health and Hospice, 721 Richland Avenue, Aiken, SC 29801; tel. 803/643-0001, ext. 226; FAX. 803/649-0490; Gayle Jones, Director, Home Health, Hospice

Hospice Care of Tri-County, 111 Executive Pointe Boulevard, Columbia, SC 29212; tel. 803/750-8690; FAX. 803/750-8695; Edna McClain, RN, M.N., Administrator

Hospice Care of the Low Country, Hospice Care of the Low Country Home Health, 20 Palmetto Parkway, Hilton Head Island, SC 29926; tel. 803/681-7814; FAX. 803/681-7821; Carole B. Klein, Administrator

Hospice Care of the Piedmont, 303 West Alexander Street, Greenwood, SC 29646; tel. 864/227-9393; FAX. 864/227-9377; Nancy B. Corley, Director

Hospice Community Care, (Serving York, Chester, Lancaster, Cherokee, Union and Fairfield Counties), 325 South Oakland Avenue, Rock Hill, SC 29730; tel. 803/329-4663; FAX. 803/329-5935; Janet Dudek, Executive Director

Hospice Health Services, One Carriage Lane, Suite F1, Charleston, SC 29407; tel. 803/852-2177; FAX. 803/769-0148; Sylvia Barnes Green, RN, Executive Director

Hospice of Charleston, Inc., 3896 Leeds Avenue, North Charleston, SC 29405; tel. 803/529-3100; FAX. 803/529-3111; Carol Younker, Executive Director

Hospice of Chesterfield County, Inc., 140 South Page Street, P.O. Box 293, Chesterfield, SC 29709; tel. 803/623-9155; FAX. 803/623-3833; Monnie W. Bittle, Executive Director

Hospice of Colleton County, Inc., 336 Walter Street, Walterboro, SC 29488; tel. 803/549-5948; FAX. 803/549-1451; Alfred S. Givens, Administrator

Hospice of Georgetown County, Inc., 1018 Huger Drive, P.O. Box 1436, Georgetown, SC 29442; tel. 803/546-3410; FAX. 803/527-6964; Brenda Stroup, RN, Executive Director

Hospice of Laurens County, Inc., 16 Peachtree Street, P.O. Box 178, Clinton, SC 29325; tel. 803/833-6287; FAX. 803/833-0556; Martha Ficklin, RN, Executive Director

Hospice of Marlboro County, Inc., P.O. Box 474, Bennettsville, SC 29512; tel. 803/479-5979; FAX. 803/479-3711; Kevin Long, Administrator

Hospice of Polk County, Inc., 423 North Trade Street, Tryon, NC 28782; tel. 803/859-2270; Jean H. Eckert, Administrator

Hospice of the Upstate, Inc., 506 Summit Avenue, Anderson, SC 29621; tel. 803/261-1594; FAX. 803/261-1523; Nancy Garrett-Boyle, Administrator

Interim HealthCare Hospice, 775 Spartan Boulevard, P.O. Box 9199, Greenville, SC 29604; tel. 864/587-6129; Nancy A. Dereng

Island Hospice, 94-C Main Street, Hilton Head Island, SC 29926; tel. 803/681-7035; FAX. 803/681-8506; Pamela D. Walker, Administrator

Lutheran Hospice Ministry, Lowman Home-Bolick Building, P.O. Box 444, White Rock, SC 29177; tel. 803/732-8756; Jean Tilley, Administrator

Mercy Hospice of Horry County, Columbus Plaza, 131 Wesley Street, P.O. Box 1409, Myrtle Beach, SC 29578; tel. 803/347-2282; FAX. 803/236-4306; Connie Fahey, FSM, Executive Director

Saint Francis Hospital Home Care–Hospice Services, 414 Pettigru Street, P.O. Box 9312, Greenville, SC 29601; tel. 864/233-5300; FAX. 864/233-4873; James A. Rogers

United Hospice, Inc., 6300 St. Andrews Road, Columbia, SC 29212; tel. 803/798-6605; FAX. 803/798-3001; Tamra N. West, Administrator

SOUTH DAKOTA

Ellen Stephen Hospice, P.O. Box 1805, Pine Ridge, SD 57770; tel. 605/455-1217; FAX. 605/455-1218; Susan Kay, Administrator

Hospice of the Hills, 1011 11th Street, Rapid City, SD 57701; tel. 605/341-7118; FAX. 605/399-7820; Dorothy Brown, Administrator

Lyon County Hospice, 803 South Greene Street, Rock Rapids, IA 51246; tel. 712/472-3618; FAX. 712/472-3616; Marge Smith, RN

Tekawitha Nursing Home, Sisseton, SD 57262; tel. 605/886-8491; Charleen Thompson, RN

Section C

TENNESSEE

A Plus Hospice, Inc., 116 Wilson Pike Circle, Suite 103, Brentwood, TN 37027; tel. 615/377-6276; FAX. 615/377-6287; Barbara Brown, Director

Advanced Home Care and Hospice, Inc., 507 A Hill Street, Springfield, TN 37172; tel. 615/384-0962

Alive Hospice, Inc., 1718 Patterson Road, Nashville, TN 37203; tel. 615/327-1085; FAX. 615/963-4700; Dick Hamilton, Interim Executive Director

Baptist Community Home Care and Hospice, 139 East Swan Street, Centerville, TN 37033; tel. 615/729-4500; FAX. 615/729-9000

Baptist Homecare Hospice Division, 1988 Rivermont Manor, 433 Sevier Avenue, Knoxville, TN 37901; tel. 615/632-5711

Buckeye Quality HHA, Inc. Hospice, Highway 52W, P.O. Box 697, Jamestown, TN 38556; tel. 615/879-9928; Sandra Hall, RN, Director, Patient Services

Columbia Homecare, 404 F East College, Dickson, TN 37055; tel. 615/441-1365; FAX. 615/446-8109; Susan Brink, RN, Acting Administrator

Columbia Homecare Hospice, 1084 Bradford Hicks Drive, Livingston, TN 38570; tel. 615/823-2050; FAX. 615/823-7982; Denise Elder, RN, Hospice Director

Community Health Services, Inc., 3918 Dickerson Road, Nashville, TN 37207

Comprehensive HHC Hospice Services, Inc., 1720 Church Street, Suite Two, Tazewell, TN 37879; tel. 423/626-0388; FAX. 423/626-0300; Patricia Brooks, Administrator, Coordinator

Country Hospice, 72 Stonebridge, Suite Three, Jackson, TN 38305; tel. 901/661-0800; Andy Gardner, RN, CRNH, Regional Hospice Director

Country Hospice, Highway 45 South, Route Two Box 23A, Selmer, TN 38375; tel. 901/645-6475; Andy Gardner, RN, CRNH, Regional Hospice Director

Country Hospice, 224 Memorial Drive, Paris, TN 38242; tel. 901/644-9200; Andy Gardner, RN, CRNH, Regional Hospice Director

Elk Valley Hospice Services, 303 South Morgan Avenue, Fayetteville, TN 37334; tel. 615/433-7026

Friendship Hospice of Nashville, Inc., 1326 Eighth Avenue, N., Nashville, TN 37203; tel. 615/327-3950; Andre L. Lee, DPA, Chairman of the Board

Home Health Care of East Tennessee, Inc., 1796 Mount Vernon Drive, N.W., Cleveland, TN 37311; tel. 423/479-4581; FAX. 423/479-5422; Annette Green, DOPC

Home-Bound Medical Care, 4355 Highway 58, Suite 101, Chattanooga, TN 37416; tel. 423/855-9128

Home-Bound Medical Care, Inc., 2165 Spicer Cove, Suite One, Memphis, TN 38134; tel. 901/386-5061

Homecare Hospice Services, 115 Vicksburg Avenue, Camden, TN 38320; tel. 901/584-1927; FAX. 901/584-0401

Hospice of Chattanooga, Inc., 165 Hamm Road, Chattanooga, TN 37405; tel. 423/267-6828; FAX. 423/756-4765; Viston Taylor III, Executive Director

Hospice of Cumberland County, Inc., 140 North Maine, Crossville, TN 38555; tel. 615/484-4748; Shirley Freeman, Executive Director

Hospice of Murfreesboro, 417 North University Street, Murfreesboro, TN 37130; tel. 615/896-4663

Hospice of Tennessee, 521 West Main Street, Lebanon, TN 37087; tel. 800/889-4673; FAX. 615/444-2547

Hospice of Tennessee Nursing Services, 900 East Hill Avenue, Suite 270, Knoxville, TN 37915; tel. 423/524-2138

Hospice of Tennessee, Inc., 112 Louise Avenue, Nashville, TN 37203; tel. 800/252-7442; FAX. 615/773-3033; Debbie Baumgart, RN, Regional Director

Hospice of Tennessee, Inc -Franklin, 415 Williamson Square, Franklin, TN 37064

Hospice of West Tennessee, 1804 Highway 45 Bypass, West Tennessee Healthcare, Jackson, TN 38305; tel. 901/664-4220; FAX. 901/664-4231; Shirley Rowe, RN, Director

Housecall Hospice, 117 Center Park Drive, Suite 201, Knoxville, TN 37922; tel. 423/693-2474; FAX. 423/693-4031; Pamela Winch-Matayoshi, Vice President, Palliative Services

Housecall Hospice, 100 Rogosin Drive, Suite B, Elizabethton, TN 37643; tel. 615/547-0852; FAX. 615/543-6449; Rachel Vollman, Hospice Administrator

Housecall Hospice, 6025 Lee Highway, Executive Business Park, Chattanooga, TN 37421; tel. 615/892-2561; Caroline McBrayer

Housecall Hospice, 5350 Poplar Avenue, Suite 118A, Memphis, TN 38119; tel. 901/685-5300; FAX. 901/761-4321; Lynn Thomasson, Hospice Administrator

Housecall Hospice, 3343 Perimeter Hill Drive, Suite 102, Nashville, TN 37211; tel. 615/333-3994

JEM Health Care Inc., 315 10th Avenue, N., Suite 109, Nashville, TN 37207; tel. 615/726-8668; FAX. 615/726-8665; Marilyn McClain, Administrator

Lazarus House Hospice, Inc., 260 West Fifth Street, Cookeville, TN 38501; tel. 615/528-5133; J. Steve Mathias, Executive Director

Methodist Home Care Services, 1716 Parr Avenue, Dyersburg, TN 38024; tel. 901/287-2307; FAX. 901/287-2174

Methodist Hospice and Health Care Services, Inc., d/b/a Methodist Alliance Hospice, 930 South White Station Road, Suite 100, Memphis, TN 38117; tel. 901/680-0169; FAX. 901/537-2109; Caby Byrne, Director

Procare Support Services, Inc., 111 West Main, Jackson, TN 38301; tel. 800/211-7573; FAX. 901/427-1234; Elaine Kirk, Administrator

Robert Ramsey Memorial Hospice, 317 Steam Plant Road, Gallatin, TN 37066

Smoky Mountain Hospice, Inc., 324 West Broadway, Newport, TN 37821

St. Mary's Hospice, 900 Hill Avenue, Suite 120, Knoxville, TN 37915

TLC Hospice, 1200 Mountain Creek Road, Suite 440, Chattanooga, TN 37405; tel. 423/877-0983; FAX. 423/877-4944; Gloria J. Dodds, RN, B.S.N., Administrator

Tennessee Nursing Services of Knoxville, 1530 West Andrew Johnson Highway, Morristown, TN 37816; tel. 615/586-6808

Tennessee Nursing Services of Morristown, Coldwell Bank Building, 415 North Fairmont, Morristown, TN 37816; tel. 423/581-7690; FAX. 423/581-8164; Glena Duffield, Director, Hospice

Tri County Quality Homecare and Hospice, 20 Lee Avenue, Box 308, McKenzie, TN 38201; tel. 901/352-2240; FAX. 901/352-0320; Kay Taylor, RN, Patient Care Coordinator

Trinity Hospice, 1049 Cresthaven Road, Memphis, TN 38119; tel. 901/767-6767; FAX. 901/767-4627; Bradford A. Austin, RN, Hospice Director

University Home Health and Hospice, Inc., 135 Kennedy Drive, Martin, TN 38237; tel. 901/587-2996; FAX. 800/627-3228; Kellie Sims, B.S.W., Hospice Director

Willowbrook Hospice, Inc., 220 Second Avenue South, Franklin, TN 37064; tel. 800/790-8499; June Baldini, RN, Director

TEXAS

AIM Hospice, 703 East Concho, P.O. Box 2300, Rockport, TX 78381-2300; tel. 512/729-0507; FAX. 512/790-0243; Judith Johnson, RN, Ph.D., Administrator

Abacus Home Health Care, Inc., 3626 North Hall Street, Suite 818, Dallas, TX 75219

Absolute Home Care, Inc., 723 North Upper Broadway, Suite 610, Corpus Christi, TX 78401

Advantage Healthcare Services, 800 North Industrial Boulevard, Suite 102, Euless, TX 76039; tel. 817/545-5215; FAX. 817/545-0533; Carla S. Johnston, Administrator

American Home Health and Hospice, 315 South Oak, Pecos, TX 79772

American Hospice, Inc., 1349 Empire Central, Suite 707, Dallas, TX 75247; tel. 214/689-1010; Julie Wallace, Administrator

Ann's Haven/VNA, 216 West Mulberry Street, Denton, TX 76201; tel. 817/566-6550; FAX. 817/383-4000; Karen Pemberton, RN, B.S.N.

Ark-La-Tex Health and Hospice Care, 6500 Summerhill Road, Suite 1-D, Texarkana, TX 75503; tel. 903/792-6430; FAX. 903/792-5537; Doyle Land, Chief Financial Officer

Burton Hospice Care, Inc., 6640 Eastex Freeway, Suite 140, Beaumont, TX 77708; tel. 409/892-7476; FAX. 409/892-7740; Vergie A. Burton, Administrator

Care United Hospice, 801 West Freeway, Suite 500, Grand Prairie, TX 75051

Center for Hospice Care, 1101 Decker Drive, Baytown, TX 77520

Christian Hospice Services, 215 Dalton Drive, Suite B, Desoto, TX 76115

Circle of Hope Hospice of VNA, 2211 East Missouri, Suite 220, El Paso, TX 79923; tel. 915/543-6201; Tom Meagher, Vice President, Hospice

Circle of Life Hospice, 2512 A Grandview, Odesa, TX 79761; tel. 915/367-7771; FAX. 915/367-2932; Jo Cheryl Miller, Administrator

Columbia Hospice Gulf Coast, 1102 North Mechanic, El Campo, TX 77437; tel. 409/543-9487; FAX. 409/543-9426; Ruth Kainer, RN, Director

Community Care Services, Inc., 403 East Blackjack, Dublin, TX 76446; tel. 817/445-4675; Bobbie Nichols, Administrator

Community Hospice of St. Joseph, 1000 Summit, Fort Worth, TX 76102

Community Hospice of Waco, 3215 Pine Avenue, Waco, TX 76708; tel. 817/756-6911; FAX. 817/756-0029; Richard E. Scott, President

Comprehensive Home Health Services, 901 North Galloway Avenue, Suite 101, Mesquite, TX 75149; tel. 972/285-3713; FAX. 972/285-3699; Julie Francis, Director

Country Nurses, Inc. Hospice and Home Care, 608 A North Rockwall Street, Terrell, TX 75160; tel. 972/563-2415; FAX. 972/563-4042; Carla Menasco, RN, B.S.N., Owner, Administrator

Crawford Hospice Services, Inc., 709 West 34th Street, Suite B, Austin, TX 78705; tel. 800/909-5543; FAX. 512/450-1281; Barbara Powell, Administrator

Cross Timbers Hospice, 103 East Frey, Stephenville, TX 76401; tel. 817/968-6142; FAX. 817/965-2388; Jan Hoover, RN, Administrator

Crown of Texas Hospice, 1000 South Jefferson, Amarillo, TX 79101; tel. 806/372-7696; FAX. 806/372-2825; Sharla Roselius, B.S.N., CRNH, RN, President

Crown of Texas Hospice, 100 I-45 North, Suite 240, Box 103, Conroe, TX 77301; tel. 409/788-7707; FAX. 409/788-7708; Marsha J. Irwin, RN, Ph.D., Director

Cypress Basin Hospice, Inc., 1805 North Jefferson, P.O. Box 544, Mount Pleasant, TX 75455; tel. 903/577-1510; FAX. 903/577-9377; Edd C. Hess, Executive Director

DNS Hospice, 2101 Kemp Boulevard, Wichita Falls, TX 76309; tel. 817/723-2771; FAX. 817/322-1754; Helen Dipprey, Chief Operating Officer

Denson Community Hospice, 1100 Gulf Freeway, N., Suite 122, League City, TX 77573; tel. 713/332-4970; FAX. 713/338-1766; Suzanne Denson, Administrator

East Harris County Hospice Services, Inc., Holland Avenue Medical Center, 1313 Holland Avenue, Building B, Houston, TX 77029; tel. 713/450-4500; FAX. 281/450-4006; Ipe Mathai, Executive Director

Family Hospice, 8701 Shoal Creek Boulevard, Suite 104, Austin, TX 78757; tel. 800/444-2405; FAX. 512/453-4165; Annette McDonald, Executive Director

Family Hospice of Dallas, 1140 Empire Central, Suite 235, Dallas, TX 75247; tel. 214/631-7273; FAX. 214/630-4032; Jim Grant, RN, B.S.N., M.S., Executive Director

Family Hospice of Fort Worth, 4040 Fossil Creek Boulevard, Suite 204, Fort Worth, TX 76137; tel. 817/232-3492; FAX. 817/232-3499; Sally Day, RN, B.S.N., Executive Director

Family Hospice of San Antonio, 6800 Park Ten Boulevard, Suite 110 North, San Antonio, TX 78213-4201; tel. 210/738-8141; FAX. 210/738-3507; Rebecca N. McMinn, RN, B.S.N., MBA, Executive Director

Family Hospice, Inc., 819 South Fifth Street, Temple, TX 76504; tel. 800/643-3139; FAX. 817/742-2023; Carrie Carson, Administrator

Family Service, Inc., 1424 Hemphill Street, Fort Worth, TX 76104-4790; tel. 817/927-8884, ext. 311; FAX. 817/926-0701; Oliver W. Gerland, Jr., President

First Community Homecare, 9323 Garland Road, Suite 308, Dallas, TX 75218

Genesis Hospice Care, 6724 South Broadway, Tyler, TX 75703; tel. 903/581-8700; FAX. 903/509-0138; Betty Johnson, RN

Golden Acres Hospice, 2525 Centerville Road, Dallas, TX 75228-2693; tel. 214/327-4503; FAX. 214/320-2683; Robert J. Watson, Director

Harris Hospice, 6000 Western Place, Suite 118, Fort Worth, TX 76107; tel. 817/570-8200; Barbara Hunt, Director

Heart of West Texas Hospice, 1927 Hickory, Colorado City, TX 79512

Heart of the Valley Hospice, 320 North Williams Road, San Benito, TX 78586; tel. 800/333-6131; FAX. 210/399-3553; Rebecca Hernandez, RN, Administrator

Heritage Health Care, 606 Avenue K, Cisco, TX 76437

Home Health Plus, 8122 Datapoint Drive, Suite 200, San Antonio, TX 78229-3264

Home Health Plus, 1900 West Loop South, Suite 150, Houston, TX 77027; tel. 713/622-9050; Mary James, RN

Home Health Plus, 5080 Spectrum Drive, Suite 105 West, Dallas, TX 75248-4641; tel. 800/925-1155; Ruby Marrero, RN

Home Health Services of Dallas, Inc., 2929 Carlisle Street, Suite 375, Dallas, TX 75204-1050

Home Health Specialists, Inc., 813 South Palestine, Athens, TX 75751; tel. 800/801-8126; FAX. 903/657-9513; Linda Johnson, RN, Administrator

Home Hospice, Grayson County Office, 505 West Center Street, P.O. Box 2306, Sherman, TX 75091; tel. 903/868-9315; FAX. 903/893-2772; Marty Barr, Executive Director

Home Hospice, 3053 East University, Odessa, TX 79762; tel. 915/550-4333; FAX. 915/550-2442; Hilton Chancellor, Director

Horizon Hospice Care, Inc., 9535 Forest Lane, Suite 126, Dallas, TX 75243; tel. 972/690-6632; FAX. 972/690-0834; Debbie Hoffpauir, National Director, Hospice Operations

Hospice Austin, 3710 Cedar Street, Suite 299, Austin, TX 78705; tel. 512/458-3261; FAX. 512/467-0767; Marjorie D. Mulanax, Executive Director

Hospice Brazos Valley, Inc., 2729 A East 29th Street, Bryan, TX 77802; tel. 409/776-0793; FAX. 409/774-0041; John Foster, B.S., M.S., CPM, Executive Director

Hospice Family Care, Inc., 1408 19th Street, Lubbock, TX 79401; tel. 806/765-6111; FAX. 806/762-0828; Connie Nutt, Administrator

Hospice Highland Lakes, 2001 South Water Street, Burnet, TX 78611; tel. 512/756-8003; FAX. 512/756-8046; Mary Kay Stephens, RNC, CRNH, Acting Director

Hospice Home Care, 10221 Desert Sands, Suite 108, San Antonio, TX 78216; tel. 210/377-1033; FAX. 210/377-2560; Al Hafer, Business Administrator

Hospice Longview, Inc., 802 Medical Circle, Suite C, Longview, TX 75601; tel. 903/753-7870; Ed Arneson, Executive Director

Hospice New Braunfels, 613 North Walnut, New Braunfels, TX 78130; tel. 210/625-7500; FAX. 210/625-0773; Opal Umpierre, Interim Administrator

Hospice Preferred Choice, 8203 Willow Place South, Suite 530, Houston, TX 77070; tel. 713/469-7990; FAX. 713/894-1294; Diane A. Incognito, Executive Director

Hospice Preferred Choice, 427 West 20th, Suite 603, Houston, TX 77008; tel. 713/864-2626; FAX. 713/864-9476; Diane Incognito, Administrator

Hospice Preferred Choice–DFW, 4425 West Airport Freeway, Suite 450, Irving, TX 75062; tel. 972/256-1881; FAX. 972/257-3740; Serene Smith, Administrator

Hospice Uvalde Area, (a program of Hospice San Antonio), P.O. Box 5280, Uvalde, TX 78802-5280; tel. 210/278-6691; FAX. 210/278-8925; Edwin Sasek, Bereavement Coordinator

Hospice in the Pines, 116 South Raguet, Lufkin, TX 75904; tel. 800/324-8557; FAX. 409/632-1352; Sherri D. Flynt, L.S.W., Social Services

Hospice in the Pines, 1300 South Frazier, Suite 315, Conroe, TX 77301; tel. 888/539-5252; FAX. 409/539-5272; Sheryl Wallace, Executive Director

Hospice of Abilene, Inc., 1682 Hickory, Abilene, TX 79602; tel. 915/677-8516; FAX. 915/675-5031; Lana Cunningham, RN, M.S.N., Clinical Director

Hospice of Cedar Lake, 409 North Third Street, Mabank, TX 75147-8614; tel. 903/887-3772; FAX. 903/887-3700; Karen Gilmore, Director

Hospice of Central Texas, 2007 B Medical Parkway, San Marcos, TX 78666; tel. 512/753-3584; FAX. 512/353-6573; Dawn O'Donnell, RNC, M.A., Administrator

Hospice of East Texas, 3800 Paluxy, Suite 560, Tyler, TX 75703; tel. 903/581-5585; FAX. 903/581-5293; Michael C. Couch, Executive Director

Hospice of El Paso, Inc., 3901 North Mesa, Suite 400, El Paso, TX 79902; tel. 915/532-5699; FAX. 915/532-7822; Charles E. Roark, Ed.D. FACHE

Hospice of Galveston County, Inc., 1708 Amburn Road, Suite C, Texas City, TX 77591; tel. 409/938-0070; FAX. 409/938-1509; Sue Mistretta, Executive Director

Hospice of Lubbock, Inc., 4314 South Loop 289, Zip 79413, P.O. Box 53276, Lubbock, TX 79453; tel. 806/795-2751; FAX. 806/795-8464; Linda McMurry, R.N., B.S.N.

Hospice of Mercy, 500 West Third Avenue, Suite Two, Corsicana, TX 75110; tel. 903/872-4430; FAX. 903/872-4499; Ann Massey, Administrator

Hospice of Midland, Inc., 911 West Texas, Midland, TX 79701; tel. 915/682-2855; FAX. 915/682-2989; Carol Armstrong, Executive Director

Hospice of North Texas, Inc., 1420 Pioneer Road, Suite A, Mesquite, TX 75149; tel. 888/285-8081; FAX. 972/288-0742; Angela Herrin, Director

Hospice of Northeast Texas, 51 North Side Square, Cooper, TX 75432; tel. 903/395-2811; FAX. 903/395-2766; Nicki J. Beeler, Administrator

Hospice of San Angelo, Inc., 36 East Beauregard, Suite 1100, P.O. Box 471, San Angelo, TX 76902; tel. 915/658-6524; David McBride, Executive Director

Hospice of South Texas, 2004 Fagan Circle, Victoria, TX 77901; tel. 512/572-4300; FAX. 512/572-4532; Doug Eaves, Executive Director

Hospice of St. Michael Hospital of Texarkana, 1400 College Drive, Texarkana, TX 75501; tel. 903/794-1206; FAX. 903/735-5390; Tommy McGee, Administrator

Hospice of Texarkana, Inc., 803 Spruce Street, Texarkana, TX 75501; tel. 903/794-4263; FAX. 501/744-1108; Cynthia L. Marsh, Administrator

Hospice of V.N.A., 2905 Sackett, Houston, TX 77098; tel. 713/520-8115; FAX. 713/520-6054; Maggie Kao, Dr.P.H., Chief Executive Officer

Hospice of Wichita Falls, 4909 Johnson Road, Wichita Falls, TX 76310; tel. 817/691-0982; FAX. 817/691-1608; Jan Banta, Executive Director

Hospice of the Big Bend, 611 East Avenue E, Alpine, TX 79830-4817; tel. 915/837-7286; FAX. 915/837-1132; Marvie Burton, RN, Patient Care Coordinator, Executive Director

Hospice of the Big Country, Inc., 3113 Oldham Lane, Abilene, TX 79602; tel. 915/677-1191; FAX. 915/677-1808; Danna L. Clouse, Administrator

Hospice of the Gulf Coast, Inc., 17041 El Camino Real, Suite 102, Houston, TX 77058; tel. 281/282-0116; FAX. 281/282-0122

Hospice of the Heart, 305 North Brazos, Suite 10, P.O. Box 2180, Whitney, TX 76962; tel. 817/694-6009; FAX. 817/694-9926

Hospice of the Panhandle, 800 North Sumner, P.O. Box 2795, 79066-2795, Pampa, TX 79065; tel. 806/665-6677; Sherry McCavit, Executive Director

Hospice of the Plains, Inc., 7109 Olton Road, Plainview, TX 79072; tel. 806/293-5127; FAX. 806/293-5902; Roxey Williams, Executive Director

Hospice of the Southwest, Inc., 3800 East 42nd Street, Suite 500, P.O. Box 14710, Odessa, TX 79768-4710; tel. 915/362-1431; FAX. 915/362-1468; Connie Brinker, Executive Director

Hospice of the Three Rivers, 51 North 11th Street, Beaumont, TX 77702-2224; tel. 800/946-7742; Andi Whitmer, Administrator

Houston Hospice, 8811 Gaylord, Suite 100, Houston, TX 77024; tel. 713/468-2441; FAX. 713/468-0879; Margaret Caddy, RN, Executive Director

Huguley Hospice Care, 11801 South Freeway, Ft. Worth, TX 76115; tel. 817/551-2545; FAX. 817/568-3294; Donna Reddell, RN, Director

La Mariposa Hospice, 2001 North Oregon, El Paso, TX 79902; tel. 915/452-6802; Frances Witt, Director

Lakes Area Hospice, 254 Ethel Street, Jasper, TX 75951; tel. 409/384-5995; FAX. 409/384-9655; Jeanette Coffield, Executive Director

Lion Health Services, Inc., 800 West Airport Freeway, Suite 1100, Irving, TX 75062; tel. 972/445-4105; FAX. 972/445-4104; Susan Cerroni, RN, Director, Patient Services

Lone Star Hospice, 1212 Palm Valley Boulevard, Round Rock, TX 78664; tel. 512/467-7423; FAX. 512/218-9288; Janet A. Baker, Executive Director

Managed Home Health Care, 2211 Calder Avenue, Beaumont, TX 77707; tel. 409/832-4164; FAX. 409/832-4182; Charles Bray, C.E.D.

Nurses Hospice, Inc., 1330 East Eighth, Suite 323, Odessa, TX 79762; tel. 915/550-5066; Patsy Gerron, Administrator

Nurses In Touch Community Hospice, 7410 Blanco Road, Suite 450, San Antonio, TX 78216; tel. 210/979-9771; FAX. 210/979-6644; Mary Helen Tieken, RN, B.S.N., Administrator

Pacesetter Hospice, Inc., 6800 Manhattan, Suite 401, Fort Worth, TX 76120

Personal Touch Hospice of Texas, Inc., 8200 Brookriver Drive, Suite N109, Dallas, TX 75247; tel. 214/638-0357, ext. 305; FAX. 214/905-8687; Roy W. Terry, RN, Director

Rhodes Home Health Care, Inc., 3224 I-30 East, Suite 132, Mesquite, TX 75150; tel. 972/613-9772; Cherie Rhodes Cunigan

Robinson Creek Home Care, Inc., 1000 Westbank Drive, Suite 6B201, Austin, TX 78746; tel. 512/328-7606; Vanessa Nunnelly, Administrator

Rural Hospice, Inc., 501 South Alford, Crane, TX 79731; tel. 888/558-2300; FAX. 915/558-2335; Pam Ross, RN, Director

Samaritan Care Hospice of Texas, 17103 Preston Road, Suite 200, Dallas, TX 75248; tel. 800/669-3695; FAX. 972/407-5021; Martha Schueler, M.S., CRNH, Director Clinical Services

San Juan Home Health and Hospice, 300 North Nebraska Avenue, San Juan, TX 78589; tel. 210/782-0333; FAX. 210/782-0335; Tony Cortez, Director

Spohn Hospice, 600 Elizabeth Street, Corpus Christi, TX 78404; tel. 512/881-3159; FAX. 512/888-7405; Rita Mueller, RN, Director

St. Anthony's Hospice and Life Enrichment Program, 600 North Tyler, Zip 79107, P.O. Box 950, Amarillo, TX 79176-0001; tel. 806/378-6777; FAX. 806/378-5031; Lezlie Roberson, Executive Director

St. Joseph Hospice Houston, 1404 Calhoun Cullen Family Building, Houston, TX 77002; tel. 713/757-7488; FAX. 713/756-5127; Maresa Henry, Associate Director

St. Paul Hospice, 7920 Elmbrook Drive, Suite 116, Dallas, TX 75247; tel. 214/637-7474; Gwendolyn Pipkins, Director

Stephen's Hospice, 925 A North Graham, Stephenville, TX 76401-4216; tel. 817/965-7119; FAX. 817/965-3228; Kim Davis, Administrator

Taras Prime Home Health Care, Inc., 2765 East Trinity Mills, Suite 400, Carrollton, TX 75006

Tender Loving Care Home Health Hospice Agency, 5787 South Hampton Road, Suite 295, Dallas, TX 75232

Texas Health Staffing Services, Inc., 1115 Chihuahua Street, Suite B, Laredo, TX 78040; tel. 210/791-3012; Maria Elena Montemayor, Administrator

Texoma Community Hospice, 3821 Wilbarger Street, Vernon, TX 76384; tel. 800/658-6330; FAX. 817/552-2305; Jean Tucker, Administrator

The Hospice at the Texas Medical Center, 1905 Holcombe Boulevard, Houston, TX 77030; tel. 713/467-7423; FAX. 713/799-9227; Randal A. Condit, Vice President, Operations

The Southeast Texas Hospice, Inc., 912 West Cherry, P.O. Box 2385, Orange, TX 77630; tel. 409/886-0622; FAX. 409/886-0623; Mary McKenna, Administrator

Thee Hospice, Robinson Creek Center, 3100 I-45, Suite 10, Huntsville, TX 77342-6548; tel. 409/291-8439; FAX. 409/295-8582; Mollie Martin, RN, Patient Care Coordinator

Tomlinson Health Services, Hospice Program, 1300 West Mockingbird, Suite 160, Dallas, TX 75247; tel. 214/630-8847; FAX. 817/573-3160; Reba Tomlinson, Chief Executive Officer

Tyler Hospice, 423 South Beckham Avenue, Tyler, TX 75701; tel. 903/592-9703; FAX. 903/593-0639; Sandra L. Bunch, Administrator

Ultimate Hospice Care, 2300 Highway 365, Suite 440, Nederland, TX 77627; tel. 409/722-4993; FAX. 409/721-4930; Lewanna D. Jones, Administrator

Ultra Home Health Care, Inc., 8303 Southwest Freeway, Suite 410, Houston, TX 77074; tel. 713/988-5872; FAX. 713/271-1002; Mr. Tracy Potts, General Manager

VNA and Hospice of South Texas, 8207 Callaghan, Suite 355, San Antonio, TX 78230; tel. 210/377-3882; FAX. 210/349-4896; Frederick W. Hines, President

VNA and Hospice of the Texas Gulf Coast, P.O. Box 1777, Angleton, TX 77516-1777; tel. 409/849-6476; FAX. 409/849-0343; Jenny Carswell, Administrator

Visiting Nurse Association Hospice, 212 Brown Street, Brownwood, TX 76801-2915; tel. 915/646-6500; FAX. 915/646-6412; Mary Suther, President, Chief Executive Officer

Visiting Nurse Association of Texas Hospice, 1440 West Mockingbird Lane, Suite 500, Dallas, TX 75247–4929; tel. 214/689–0000; FAX. 214/689–0010; Shiela Jacobs

Vitas Healthcare Corporation, 5001 LBJ Freeway, Suite 1050, Dallas, TX 75244; tel. 214/661–2004; FAX. 214/661–3474; David C. Gasmire, General Manager

Vitas Healthcare Corporation, 4828 Loop Central Drive, Suite 890, Houston, TX 77081; tel. 713/663–7777; FAX. 713/663–4990, ext. 4912; Diane Incognito, General Manager

Vitas Healthcare Corporation, 801 West Freeway, Suite 620, Grand Prairie, TX 75051; tel. 972/269–4200; Chuck Dowling, Regional Vice President

Vitas Healthcare Corporation, 4241 Piedras Drive East, Suite 111, San Antonio, TX 78228; tel. 210/731–4300; FAX. 210/731–4380; Ruth R. Castillo, Administrator

Vitas Healthcare Corporation, 211 East Parkwood, Suite 211, Friendswood, TX 77546; tel. 713/996–4400; Ruth Castillo, General Manager

Wadley Care Source Hospice, 1001 Main Street, Suite 107, Texarkana, TX 75501; tel. 903/798–7640; FAX. 903/798–7647; Sheri Milam, RN, OCN, Manager

UTAH

CNS Community Hospice, 2970 South Main, Suite 300, Salt Lake City, UT 84115; tel. 801/461–9500; FAX. 801/486–2193; Grant C. Howarth, President, Chief Executive Officer

Castle Country Hospice, 11 West Main Street, Suite 100, Price, UT 84501; tel. 801/637–8070; Paula Miles, Administrator

Creative Health Services, Inc. Hospice Care, 6777 South 1560 East, Salt Lake City, UT 84121; tel. 801/943–8374; FAX. 801/942–2949; Joyce L. Smith, Administrator

Creekside Hospice Care, 1935 East Vine Street, Suite 350, Salt Lake City, UT 84121; tel. 801/272–8617; FAX. 801/277–3790; Maryann Pales, Administrator

Dixie Regional Home Health Hospice, 354 East 400 South, Suite 304, St. George, UT 84770; tel. 801/634–4567; FAX. 801/634–4564; Kathy Andrus, RN, Administrator

East Lake Home Health Hospice/Family Hospice Care, 668 West 980 North, Provo, UT 84601; tel. 801/374–9986; Kory Coleman, Director

Family Hospice Care, 404 East 5600 South, Murray, UT 84107; tel. 801/268–8083; FAX. 801/268–8096; Pat Burns, Director, Home Care Services

Hospice of Cache Valley, 1400 North 500 East, Logan, UT 84341; tel. 801/750–5477; FAX. 801/750–5361; Neil C. Perkes, RN, M.B.A., Administrator

Hospice of Northern Utah, 2404 Washington Boulevard, Suite 304, Ogden, UT 84401; tel. 801/399–5232; FAX. 801/399–2742; Suzanne Phillips, Administrator

IHC Home Health Agency–Hospice of IHC, 2250 South 1300 West, Suite A, Salt Lake City, UT 84119; tel. 801/977–9900; FAX. 801/977–9956; Shauna Einerson, Administrator

Paracelsus Select Hospice, 102 West 500 South, Suite 510, Salt Lake City, UT 84101; tel. 801/288–1900; FAX. 801/288–2939; Gina Coccimiglio, Chief Executive Officer

Rocky Mountain Hospice, 315 East 400 South, Bountiful, UT 84010; tel. 801/299–3990; Carol Holmes

Vista Care of Utah, 4424 South 700 East, Suite 250, Salt Lake City, UT 84107; tel. 801/293–1656; FAX. 801/293–1670; Kim Olsen, Administrator

VERMONT

Addison County Hospice, Inc., P.O. Box 772, Middlebury, VT 05753; tel. 802/388–4111; Catherine Studley, Executive Director

Brattleboro Area Hospice, 31 South Main Street, P.O. Box 1053, Brattleboro, VT 05302–1053; tel. 802/257–0775; Susan Parris, Administrator

Caledonia Home Health Care–Hospice, Sherman Drive, P.O. Box 383, St. Johnsbury, VT 05819; tel. 802/748–8116; FAX. 802/748–4628; Brenda B. Smith, Director, Home Care, Hospice

Central Vermont Home Health and Hospice, Inc., R.R. 3, Box 6694, Barre, VT 05641; tel. 802/223–1878; FAX. 802/223–6835, ext. 249; Diana Peirce, RN, CRNH, Director, Hospice Services

Franklin County Home Health and Hospice, Three Home Health Circle, St. Albans, VT 05478; tel. 802/527–7531; FAX. 802/527–7533; Janet McCarthy, Executive Director

Hospice of Bennington County, Inc., P.O. Box 1231, Bennington, VT 05201; tel. 802/447–0307; Amy Barber–Thomas, Executive Director

Hospice of Champlain Valley, 25 Prim Road, Colchester, VT 05446; tel. 802/860–4410; FAX. 802/860–6149; Barbara Segal, RN, M.S., Program Director

Lamoille Home Health and Hospice, R.R. 3, Box 790, Farr Avenue, Morrisville, VT 05661; tel. 802/888–4651; FAX. 802/888–7822; Linda Taft, Clinical Director

Orleans Essex VNA and Hospice, Inc., Three Lakemont Road, Newport, VT 05855–1550; tel. 802/334–5213, ext. 19; FAX. 802/334–8822, ext. 45; Diana Hamilton, RN, Director, Hospice

Randolph Area Hospice, 36 South Main Street, Randolph, VT 05060; tel. 802/728–6100, ext. 2273

Rutland Area Visiting Nurse Association, Seven Albert Cree Drive, Rutland, VT 05701; tel. 802/775–0568; FAX. 802/775–2304; Sally Tobin, Associate Director, Community Health Programs

Southern Vermont Home Health Agency, Three Holstein Place, Brattleboro, VT 05301; tel. 802/257–4390; FAX. 802/257–2188; Ellen Bristol, M.S.N., CRNH

Springfield Area Hospice, Inc., 366 River Street, Springfield, VT 05156; tel. 802/886–2525; Marisa Bolognese, Volunteer Coordinator

Visiting Nurse Alliance of Vermont and New Hampshire, 20 South Main Street, Old Court House, White River Junction, VT 05001; tel. 802/295–2604; FAX. 802/295–3163; Betsy Davis, Chief Executive Officer

VIRGINIA

At Home Care Hospice, 3386 Holland Road, Suite 102, Virginia Beach, VA 23452; tel. 757/427–0099; FAX. 757/427–0505; Judy Ray, Program Supervisor

Blue Ridge Hospice, Inc., 333 West Cork Street, Winchester, VA 22601; tel. 540/665–5210; FAX. 540/678–0584; Terrie Stevens, Executive Director

Cana Hospice, Route 1, Highway 52 North, P.O. Box Nine, Cana, VA 24317; tel. 800/719–7434; William B. James, Chief Executive Officer

Columbia Hospice and Family Care, 1405 Johnston–Willis Drive, Richmond, VA 23235; tel. 804/330–2300; FAX. 804/330–2280; Robert S. Dendy, Jr., Director

Commonwealth Home Nursing and Hospice, Inc., 990 Main Street, Suite 104, Danville, VA 24541; tel. 804/792–4663; FAX. 804/793–7429; Janet R. Hamilton, Executive Director

Community Hospices of America, Inc., 540 West Main Street, Wytheville, VA 24382; tel. 703/228–5424; FAX. 703/228–9225; Rita C. Cobbs, Program Director

Crater Community Hospice, Inc., 4233 Crossings Boulevard, Prince George, VA 23875; tel. 804/458–4300; FAX. 804/458–9417; Sparky Clark, Executive Director

Edmarc Hospice for Children, 1131 Crawford Parkway, P.O. Box 7188, Portsmouth, VA 23707; tel. 804/397–0432; FAX. 804/397–5827; Julie S. Sligh, Executive Director

Family Care Home Care and Hospice Care, 610 Laurel Street, P.O. Box 592, Culpeper, VA 22701; tel. 540/829–5760; FAX. 540/829–5761; Lee Kirk, President

First Choice Home Services, Inc., 915 Central Avenue, P.O. Box 1146, Harrisonburg, VA 22801; tel. 703/434–3916; Diana Berkshire, Administrator

Gentle Shepherd Hospice, Inc., 4040 Franklin Road, S.W., Roanoke, VA 24014; tel. 540/989–6265; FAX. 540/989–1547; Donald A. Eckenroth III, Administrator

Good Samaritan Hospice, Inc., 3528 Electric Road, Suite A, Roanoke, VA 24018; tel. 540/776–0198; FAX. 540/776–0841; Sue Moore, President

Homedco, Inc., 8210 Cinderked Road, Norton, VA 22079; Elaine Jakubowski, Administrator

Hospice Care of the Eastern Shore, Inc., 20154 Market Street, Onancock, VA 23417; tel. 757/789–5153; Patricia Seekings, RN, CRNH, Director

Hospice Choice, Highway 235, Big Stone Gap, VA 24219; tel. 703/523–7208; Victoria Daniels Smith, Administrator

Hospice Choice, Inc., 444 Orby Cantrell Highway, South, P.O. Box 359, Big Stone Gap, VA 24219; tel. 703/523–7208; FAX. 703/523–1103; Bonnie Elosser, Hospice Director

Hospice of Central Virginia, 5540 Falmouth Street, Suite 307, Richmond, VA 23230; tel. 804/281–0541; FAX. 804/281–0954; Brenda Clarkson, Administrator

Hospice of Northern Virginia, 13168 Centerpointe Way, Suite 201–202, Woodbridge, VA 22193; tel. 703/670–5080; Marjorie Shipley, Regional Vice President

Hospice of Northern Virginia, Inc., 6400 Arlington Boulevard, Suite 1000, Falls Church, VA 22042; tel. 703/534–7070; FAX. 703/538–2163; David J. English, President, Chief Executive Officer

Hospice of Northern Virginia, Inc., 11166 Main Street, Suite 405, Fairfax, VA 22030; tel. 703/352–7115; FAX. 703/591–2376; Jacqueline Wright, Regional Vice President

Hospice of Northern Virginia, Inc., 885 Harrison Street, S.E., Leesburg, VA 22075; tel. 703/777–7866; FAX. 703/771–8904; Elisabeth A. Murphy, NP, CRNH, Regional Vice President

Hospice of the Piedmont, Inc., 1290 Seminole Trail, Charlottesville, VA 22901; tel. 804/975–5500; FAX. 804/975–4040; Victoria Todd, Executive Director

Hospice of the Rapidan, Inc., 1200 Sunset Lane, Suite 2320, Culpeper, VA 22701; tel. 703/825–4840; FAX. 703/825–7752; Patricia Tuffy, Executive Director

House Call Hospice, 603–605 King Street, Fourth Floor, Alexandria, VA 22314; tel. 703/548–2197; Ray Evans, President

Housecall Hospice, Two Main Street, P.O. Box 850, Jonesville, VA 24263; tel. 703/346–1095; Ethel Combs, Administrator

Housecall Hospice, 2167 Apperson Drive, Salem, VA 24153; tel. 540/776–3207; FAX. 540/776–3215; Sara Brown, RN, LCSW, Administrator

Housecall Hospice, Route 8, Box 335, Martinsville, VA 24112; tel. 540/632–9611; Ellen Boone, Administrator

In Home Health, 5040 Corporate Woods Drive, Virginia Beach, VA 23462; tel. 757/490–9323; FAX. 757/490–8711; Rita E. Wool, Director, Operations

In Home Health and Hospice, 542 East Constance Road, Suffolk, VA 23430; tel. 757/934–7935; FAX. 757/934–7940; Rita E. Wool, Director, Operations

Jewish Family Service, 7300 Newport Avenue, P.O. Box 9503, Norfolk, VA 23505; tel. 804/489–3111; Harry Graber, Executive Director

Mary Washington Hospice, 406 Chatham Square Office Park, 312 Butler Road, Falmouth, VA 22405; tel. 540/899–6433; FAX. 540/899–6328; Dianne Tracy, Administrator

Maryview Wellspring Hospice, 485 Rodman Avenue, Portsmouth, VA 23707; tel. 804/398–2338; Marie F. Biggers–Gray, Director

Mountain Regional Hospice, 1533 Ingalls Street, P.O. Box 53, Clifton Forge, VA 24422; tel. 540/863–3333; FAX. 540/863–5353; Glenn Perry, Executive Director

New River Valley Hospice, Inc., 111 West Main Street, Christianborg, VA 24073; tel. 703/381–5001; FAX. 703/381–5008; Bhanu Iyengar, Executive Director

Personal Touch Hospice of Virginia, Inc., 18 Koger Center, Suite 205, Norfolk, VA 23502; tel. 757/459–2523; FAX. 757/459–2615; Dawn Barnes, RNC, B.S.N., Administrator

Rockbridge Area Hospice, Inc., 129 South Randolph Street, P.O. Box 948, Lexington, VA 24450; tel. 540/463–1848; FAX. 540/463–5219; Susan Hogg, Executive Director

Sentara Hospice, Eight Koger Executive Building, Suite 210, Norfolk, VA 23502; tel. 804/628–3602; Dorothy Weeks, Manager

Twin County Hospice, 605 Glendale Road, Galax, VA 24333; tel. 540/236–7935; Patty S. Cooke, Administrator

VNA Community Hospice, 2775 South Quincy Street, Suite 260, Arlington, VA 22206; tel. 703/824–5200; FAX. 703/824–5228; Eileen L. Dohmann, Executive Director

WASHINGTON

Associated Health Services, P.O. Box 5200, Tacoma, WA 98415–0200; tel. 206/552–1825; FAX. 206/552–1838; Beverly Hatter, Director Grief, Loss and Transitional Care

Assured Home Health and Hospice, 1817 South Market Boulevard, Chehalis, WA 98532; tel. 360/748–0151; FAX. 360/748–0518; Wilma Wayson, RN, B.S.N., Director

Central Basin Home Health and Hospice, 410 West Third Avenue, Moses Lake, WA 98837; tel. 509/765–1856; FAX. 509/765–3323; Patti A. Weaver, Administrator

Section C

Community Home Health and Hospice, 1035 11th Avenue, P.O. Box 2067, Longview, WA 98632–8189; tel. 360/425–8510; FAX. 360/425–4667; Lorraine Berndt, Executive Director

Community Hospice of the Northwest, 5610 Kitsap Way, Suite 301, Bremerton, WA 98312; tel. 360/373–5280; FAX. 360/373–5398; Karen Williams, Executive Director

Evergreen Community Home Health and Hospice, 12822 – 124th Lane, N.E., Kirkland, WA 98034; tel. 206/899–1040; FAX. 206/899–1033; Ben Lindekugel, Assistant Administrator

Group Health Cooperative Hospice Program, 83 South King Street, Suite 515, Seattle, WA 98104–2848; tel. 206/882–2022; FAX. 206/881–7147; Barbara Boyd, Administrator, Home and Community Services

Harbors Home Health and Hospice, 201 Seventh Street, Hoquiam, WA 98550; tel. 360/532–5454; DeLila Thorp, Administrator

Highline Home Care Services, 2801 South 128th, Tukwila, WA 98168; tel. 206/439–9095; FAX. 206/433–1031

Home Health Plus Hospice, 13810 Southeast Eastgate Way, Suite 100, Bellevue, WA 98005; tel. 206/644–3027; FAX. 206/644–3286; Carrie Malmberg, RN

Home Health and Hospice of Southeastern Washington, South 106 Mill Street, Colfax, WA 99111; tel. 509/334–6016; FAX. 509/397–4650; Monica Diteman, Chief Executive Officer

Hospice of Kitsap County, 1007 Scott Avenue, Suite D, Bremerton, WA 98310; tel. 360/479–1749; FAX. 360/479–5800; M. Beth Duchaine, Executive Director

Hospice of Snohomish County, 2731 Wetmore Avenue, Suite 520, Everett, WA 98201–3581; tel. 206/261–4800; FAX. 206/258–1097; Mary L. Brueggeman, Executive Director

Hospice of Spokane, West 1325 First Avenue, Suite 200, P.O. Box 2215, Spokane, WA 99210; tel. 509/456–0438; FAX. 509/458–0359; Anne Koepsell, Executive Director

Hospice of the Palouse, 700 South Main Street, P.O. Box 9461, Moscow, ID 83843–0119; tel. 208/882–1228; FAX. 208/883–2239; Norman Bowers, Administrator

Kaiser Permanente Home Health/Hospice, 2701 Northwest Vaughn Street, Suite 140, Portland, OR 97210–5398; tel. 503/499–5200; FAX. 503/499–5213; Linda Van Buren, Administrator

Lower Valley Hospice, 526 South 11th, Sunnyside, WA 98944; tel. 509/837–1676; FAX. 509/837–8622; Vicki Meyer, Executive Director

Okanogan Regional Home Health Care Agency, 217 Second Avenue, S., P.O. Box 1248, Okanogan, WA 98840; tel. 509/422–6721; Bernice Hartzell, Executive Director

Providence Homecare/Hospice of Seattle, 425 Pontius Avenue, N., Suite 300, Seattle, WA 98109; tel. 206/320–4000; FAX. 206/320–3804; Robert Anderson, Administrator, Home Services

Providence SoundHome Care and Hospice, 3706 Griffin Lane, S.E., Olympia, WA 98501; tel. 360/459–8311; FAX. 360/493–4657; Alice G. Armstrong, Chief Executive Officer

Swedish Home Health and Hospice and Infusion, 5701 Sixth Avenue, S., Suite 504, Seattle, WA 98108–2522; tel. 206/386–6602; FAX. 206/386–6613; Betty Jorgensen, Hospice Director

Tri-Cities Chaplaincy/Hospice and Counseling, 2108 West Entiat Avenue, Kennewick, WA 99336; tel. 509/783–7416; FAX. 509/735–7850; Thomas H. Halazon, Executive Director

VNS Hospice, 400 North 34th Street, Suite 202, Seattle, WA 98103–8600; tel. 206/548–2344; FAX. 206/547–6182; Don W. Tarbutton, MHA, Hospice Program Administrator

Walla Walla Community Hospice, P.O. Box 2026, 35 Jade Street, Walla Walla, WA 99362; tel. 509/525–5561; FAX. 509/525–3517; Marlow B. Wootton, Executive Director

Whatcom Hospice, 600 Birchwood Avenue, Bellingham, WA 98225; tel. 360/733–5877; FAX. 360/734–9621; Marsha J. Johnson

WEST VIRGINIA

Albert Gallatin Hospice, 3280 University Avenue, Morgantown, WV 25605; tel. 304/598–0226; Christine Constantine, Administrator

Community Home Care and Hospice, 1209 Warwood Avenue, Wheeling, WV 26003; tel. 304/277–1500; FAX. 304/277–1507; Ruth Prosser, M.S.N., RN, Administrator

Community Hospices of America – The Virginias, RR 2 Box 380, Bluefield, WV 24701; tel. 304/325–7220; FAX. 304/325–9384; Vicki Webb, Program Director

Dignity Hospice, P.O. Box 4455, Chapmanville, WV 25508; tel. 304/855–7104; Regina Bias, RN, M.S.N., OCN, Director

Extend–A–Care Hospice, 103 Guyandotte Avenue, Mullens, WV 25882; tel. 304/294–4732; FAX. 304/294–4735; Violet A. Burdette, Administrator

Greenbrier Valley Hospice, Inc., 540 North Jefferson Street, Box 5, Lewisburg, WV 24901; tel. 304/645–2700; FAX. 304/645–3188; Deb Cashdollar, Executive Director

Hospice Care Corporation, 321 Garden Towers, P.O. Box 229, Kingwood, WV 26537; tel. 304/329–1161; FAX. 304/329–3285; Malene J. Davis, RN, Executive Director

Hospice of Huntington, 1101 Sixth Avenue, P.O. Box 464, Huntington, WV 25709; tel. 304/529–4217; FAX. 304/523–6051; Charlene Farrell, Executive Director

Hospice of Marion County, P.O. Box 1112, Fairmont, WV 26555–1112; tel. 304/366–0700, ext. 8725; FAX. 304/366–9529; Joe Licata, M.S.W., Hospice Director

Hospice of South West Virginia, 105 South Eisenhower Drive, P.O. Box 1472, Beckley, WV 25802; tel. 304/255–6404; FAX. 304/255–6494; Thomas A. Williams, Executive Director

Hospice of the Panhandle, Inc., 2015 Boyd Orchard Court, Martinsburg, WV 25401; tel. 304/264–0406; FAX. 304/264–0409; Margaret Cogswell, RN, Executive Director

Housecalls Home Health and Hospice, Inc., 914 Market Street, Suite 301, Parkersburg, WV 26101; tel. 304/485–1410; FAX. 304/422–7902; Teresa Roby, Director

Journey Hospice, 314 South Wells Street, Sisterville, WV 26175; tel. 304/652–2611; FAX. 304/652–1440; Lynn L. McCormick, Administrator

Kanawha Hospice Care, Inc., 1143 Dunbar Avenue, Dunbar, WV 25064; tel. 304/768–8523; FAX. 304/768–8627; Shirley Hyatt, Director of Patient Services

Lewis County Home Health and Hospice Care, P.O. Box 1750, Weston, WV 26452; tel. 304/269–6432; FAX. 304/269–8220; Nancy Hosey, RN, Patient Care Coordinator

Monongalia County Health Department Hospice, 453 Van Voorhis Road, Morgantown, WV 26505–3408; tel. 304/598–5500; FAX. 304/598–5167; Vicky Kennedy, Hospice Supervisor, Patient Care Coordinator

Morgantown Hospice, 1159 Van Voorhis Road, Suite B, P.O. Box 4222, Morgantown, WV 26505; tel. 304/285–2777; FAX. 304/285–2787; Margaret M. Kearney, Director, Home Health and Hospice

Mountain Hospice, Inc., P.O. Box 661, Philippi, WV 26416; tel. 304/457–2180, ext. 323; FAX. 304/457–2267; Patricia Arnett, Director

People's Hospice, United Hospital Center, P.O. Box 1680, Clarksburg, WV 26302–1680; tel. 304/623–0524; FAX. 304/623–3399; Janice Chapman, Director

St. Gregory's Hospice, Inc., 836 Charles Street, Wellsburg, WV 26070; tel. 800/252–7290; FAX. 304/737–0871; Patricia Murphy, RN, M.S.N., Director

St. Joseph's Hospice, 92 West Main Street, Buckannon, WV 26201; tel. 304/472–6846; Sandra Knotts, Director

Valley Hospice, One Ross Park, Steubenville, OH 43952; tel. 614/264–7161; Karen Nichols, Executive Director

WISCONSIN

All Saints VNA–Hospice/Racine, 4000 Spring Street, P.O. Box 4045, Racine, WI 53404; tel. 414/635–7580; FAX. 414/633–7332; Debra Ostroski, Administrator

Beloit Hospice, Inc., 2958 Prairie Avenue, Beloit, WI 53511; tel. 608/363–7421; FAX. 608/363–7426; Virginia Young, Administrator

Community Home Hospice, 3149 Saemann Avenue, Sheboygan, WI 53081; tel. 414/457–5770; Bobbi Illig

Community Hospice–VNA, 811 Monitor Street, Suite 101, LaCrosse, WI 54603; tel. 608/796–1666; Margaret Mossholder

Crossroads Hospice, 125 Fowler Street, Oconomowoc, WI 53066; tel. 414/569–8711; FAX. 414/569–8744; Barb Lemke, Intake

Dr. Kate–Lakeland Hospice, P.O. Box 770, Woodruff, WI 54568; tel. 715/356–8805; FAX. 715/358–7299; Helen Mozuch, RN, Director, Operations

Fox Cities Community Hospice, 820 Association Drive, Appleton, WI 54914; tel. 414/733–8562; Susan Kostka, Hospice Director

Franciscan Skemp Healthcare Hospice, 212 South 11th Street, LaCrosse, WI 54601; tel. 608/791–9790; FAX. 608/791–9548; Marilyn Viehl, Administrator

Grancare Hospice, N56W 13365 Silver Spring Drive, Menomonee Falls, WI 53051; tel. 414/252–5303; FAX. 414/252–3974; Phyllis Locicero, Administrator

Grant County Hospice, 111 South Jefferson Street, Lancaster, WI 53813; tel. 608/723–6416; FAX. 608/723–6501; Linda S. Adrian, Director, Health Officer

Heartland Hospice, 455 Davis Street, P.O. Box 487, Hammond, WI 54015; tel. 715/796–2223; Mary Troftgruben, Administrator

Hillside Homecare/Hospice, 709 South University Avenue, Beaver Dam, WI 53916; tel. 414/887–4050, ext. 4181; FAX. 414/887–6815; Marla Noordhof, Director

Home Health United Hospice, 520 South Boulevard, P.O. Box 527, Baraboo, WI 53913; tel. 608/356–2288; FAX. 608/356–2290; Thomas H. Brown, President

HomeCaring and Hospice, 11685 Lake Boulevard, N., Chisago City, MN 55013; tel. 612/257–8850; FAX. 612/257–8852; Karen Brohaugh, Manager

Hope Hospice, Inc., 709 McComb Avenue, P.O. Box 237, Rib Lake, WI 54470; tel. 715/427–3532; FAX. 715/427–3537; Barbara Meyer, Director

Horizon Home Care and Hospice, Inc., 8949 Deebrook Trail, Brown Deer, WI 53223; tel. 414/365–8300; FAX. 414/351–8338; Beth Huetting, Hospice Executive Director

Hospice Alliance, Inc., 3410 80th Street, Kenosha, WI 53142; tel. 414/942–1630; Connie Matler, Director, Clinical Services

Hospice Preferred Choice, 3118 South 27th Street, Milwaukee, WI 53215; tel. 414/649–8302; FAX. 414/649–8441; Cathy Ott, Executive Director

Hospice Program of Waupaca County, 811 Harding Street, Waupaca, WI 54981; tel. 715/258–6323; Barbara J. Black

Hospice of Portage County, Inc., 2232 Prais, P.O. Box 1017, Stevens Point, WI 54481–8217; tel. 715/346–5355; FAX. 715/345–1304; Judy N. Mason

Hospice of the Twin Cities, Inc., d/b/a Hospice of the Valley, 7100 Northland Circle, Suite 205, Minneapolis, MN 55428; tel. 800/364–2478; FAX. 612/531–2422; Lisa Abicht Swensen, Administrator

HospiceCare, Inc., 2802 Coho Street, Suite 100, Madison, WI 53713–4521; tel. 608/276–4660; FAX. 608/276–4672; Susan Phillips, Executive Director

Jefferson Home Health and Hospice, 1007 Washington Street, P.O. Box 117, Baraboo, WI 53913; tel. 608/356–7570; FAX. 608/356–2629; William J. Hamilton, Jr., Managing Director

Lafayette County Hospice, 740 East Street, P.O. Box 118, Darlington, WI 53530; tel. 608/776–4895; FAX. 608/776–4885; Kristie Lueck, RN, Coordinator

Lakeview Hospice, 927 West Churchill Street, Stillwater, MN 55082; tel. 612/430–4521; Geri Wagner

Manitowoc County Community Hospice, 1004 Washington Street, Manitowoc, WI 54220; tel. 414/684–7155; FAX. 414/684–8653; Lynn Seidl–Babcock, RN, B.S.N., Administrator

Marquette General Home Health and Hospice, Doctors Park, Suite 105, Escanaba, MI 49829; tel. 906/789–1305; FAX. 906/789–9144; Linda S. Lewandowski, Director, Hospice

Mayo Hospice Program, 200 First Street, S.W., Rochester, MN 55905; tel. 507/284–4002; FAX. 507/284–0161; Ann Bartlett, RN, Coordinator

Milwaukee Hospice Home Care and Residence, 4067 North 92nd Street, Wauwatosa, WI 53222; tel. 414/438–8000; FAX. 414/438–8010; James Ewens, Mary New, Co–Directors

Northwest Wisconsin HomeCare/Hospice, 2321 East Clairemont Parkway, P.O. Box 2060, Eau Claire, WI 54702–2060; tel. 715/831–0100; FAX. 715/831–0108; Jill Hurlburt, RN, B.S.N., Director, Clinical Services

Rainbow Hospice Care, LLC, 147 West Rockwell Street, Jefferson, WI 53549; tel. 414/674–6255; FAX. 414/674–5288; Zelpha Pease, Patient Care Coordinator

Red Wing Hospice, 434 West Fourth, Suite 200, Red Wing, MN 55066; tel. 612/385–3410; FAX. 612/385–3414; Beth Krehbiel, Director

Section C

Regional Hospice, 2101 Beaser Avenue, Ashland, WI 54806; tel. 715/682–8677; FAX. 715/682–6404; Phil Garrison, Executive Director

Rolland Nelson Memorial Home Hospice, 419 Frederick Street, Waukesha, WI 53186; tel. 414/542–0724; FAX. 414/542–0608; Jacalyn Burdick, Program Manager

UPC Health Network–Hospice Services, 3724 West Wisconsin Avenue, Milwaukee, WI 53208; tel. 414/342–9292, ext. 449; FAX. 414/342–8721; Walter Orzechowski, National Director, Hospice Services

Unity Hospice, P.O. Box 22395, Green Bay, WI 54305–2395; tel. 414/433–7470; FAX. 414/437–1934; Donald W. Seibel, Director

V.N.A. Home Care and Hospice, 201 East Bell Street, Neenah, WI 54956; tel. 414/727–5555; FAX. 414/727–5552; Judith Eberhardy, President, Chief Executive Officer

VNA Community Hospice, 11333 West National Avenue, Milwaukee, WI 53227; tel. 414/327–2295; FAX. 414/328–4499; Mary Runge, Chief Operating Officer

Visiting Nurse Association Comfortcare Hospice, 3306 Superior Avenue, Sheboygan, WI 53081; tel. 414/458–4314; FAX. 414/458–1819; Robert W. Walters, Vice President, Regional Operations

Visiting Nurse Health Care Services, 901 Mineral Point Avenue, Janesville, WI 53545; tel. 608/754–2201; FAX. 608/754–1147; Caryn Oleston, Executive Director

Vitas Healthcare, 450 North Sunny Slope Road, Brookfield, WI 53005; tel. 414/821–6500; FAX. 414/821–6533; Jay Koeper, Administrator

WYOMING

Central Wyoming Hospice Program, 319 South Wilson Street, Casper, WY 82601; tel. 307/577–4832; FAX. 307/577–4841; Janace Chapman, RN, Director

Hospice of Laramie, 710 East Garfield, Suite 114, Laramie, WY 82070; tel. 307/745–9254; FAX. 307/742–5967; Connie M. Coca, M.S.W., Director

Hospice of Sweetwater County, 809 Thompson, Rock Springs, WY 82901; tel. 307/362–1990; FAX. 307/352–6769; Pamela L. Jelaca, Executive Director

Hospice of the Tetons, 555 East Broadway, P.O. Box 428, Jackson, WY 83001; tel. 307/739–7465; FAX. 307/739–7645; Wendy Wolff, Director

Little Wind Hospice, 2300 Rose Lane, Riverton, WY 82501; tel. 307/857–3708; FAX. 307/856–4129; Shirley Abrahams, Director

Northeast Wyoming Hospice, 720 West Seventh Street Annex G, Gillette, WY 82716; tel. 307/682–6570; FAX. 307/682–2781; Sally Fletcher, Office Manager

U. S. Associated Areas

PUERTO RICO

Caribbean Hospice, 153 Winston Churchill Avenue, Rio Piedras, PR 00926; tel. 809/764–6565; Adalberto Sandoval

Community Hospice, Inc., Avenue Hipodromo #756, Doctors Medical Building, Santurce, PR 00910; tel. 809/723–4177; FAX. 809/722–4243; Edna Vazquez

Condado Hospice, P.O. Box 5417, Station Hato Rey, PR 00919–5417; tel. 809/758–2325; Manuel de Leon

Condado Hospice, Avenue Laurel Z–U–6, Bayamon, PR 00956; tel. 809/269–0175; Carmen L. Rosa

Divina Presencia Hospice, 52 Se St 1228, Reparto Metropolitano, Rio Piedras, PR 00921; tel. 809/767–5124; Norma Williams, M.D., Medical Director

Emmanuel Hospice Care, Bo Lares Cruce Mijan, Lares, PR 00661; tel. 809/897–7040; Moises Rivera

Font Martelo Hospice, Avenue Munoz Marin, P.O. Box 8924, Humacao, PR 00791; tel. 809/852–3685; Martin Lopez Cosme

Guaynabo Hospice, Nine Jose Julian Acosta Street, Guaynabo, PR 00969; tel. 809/789–7878; Ricardo Larin, President

Hospicio Atencion Medica en el Hogar, Cipres K 1A Turabo, Caguas, PR; tel. 809/743–1121; Sandra Torres

Hospicio Del Oeste, Dr Veve 84, San German, PR 00683; tel. 809/892–1820; Anibal Velez Rodriguez

Hospicio El Nuevo Amanecer, Calle Garcia De La, Noceda 38, Rio Grande, PR 00745; tel. 809/888–8885; Melvin Acosta Roman

Hospicio Fe y Esperanza, P.O. Box 1834, Manati, PR 00674; tel. 809/854–4971; Eduardo Alvarez

Hospicio Font Martelo, Calle Calimano 121 Norte, P.O. box 910, Guayama, PR 00784; tel. 787/866–1925; Ana R. Caraballo

Hospicio La Caridad, Calle Cipres, Villa Turabo, Caguas, PR 00725; tel. 787/286–8745; FAX. 787/746–5750; Glorivette Seneriz

Hospicio La Montana, Road 152 Km 12.4, Cedro Arriba P.O. Box 515, Naranjito, PR 00719; tel. 809/869–5500; Hector A. Rodriguez Ortiz

Hospicio La Paz, Calle Jose Rodriguez, Irizarry 152, Arecibo, PR 00612; tel. 809/879–4733; Luis Monrouzeau

Hospicio Luzamor, P.O. Box 1312, Calle Patron, #11, Morovis, PR 00687; tel. 809/862–0608; Ms. Brunilda Otero Declet, Executive Director

Hospicio Nuestra Sra. de la Guadalupe, P.O. Box 7699, Ponce, PR 00732; tel. 787/259–8210; FAX. 787/259–0206; Lucy Gonzalez, Administrator

Hospicio Santa Rita, La Paz Street, Box 1143, Aguada, PR 00602; tel. 787/868–2945; FAX. 787/868–0010; Licedia Rosado

Hospicio Servicios Suplementarios, Roosevelt Avenue 114, Hato Rey, PR 00919; tel. 809/759–7036; Carmen Martino

Hospicio de Esperanza, Avenue General Valero 267, Fajardo, PR 00738; tel. 809/863–0924; Luis Vazquez

Hospital Sin Paredes, P.O. Box 2015, Hato Rey, PR 00919; tel. 809/767–8959; Luis Serrano

La Piedad Hospice, 626 Escorial Hospice, San Juan, PR 00920; tel. 809/792–2411; Antonio Bisono

La Providencia Hospice, 36 Munoz Street, P.O. Box 10447, Ponce, PR 00731; tel. 787/843–2364; FAX. 787/841–2940; Eyleen Rodriguez Lugo

Monserrate Hospice Care, Inc., P.O. Box 366148, San Juan, PR 00936–6148; tel. 809/754–0449; Luis Class

Programa de Servicios de Adjuntas, Inc., Rius Rivera 18, P.O. Box 993, Adjuntas, PR 00601; tel. 787/829–2953; Abraham Gonzalez

Providencia Hospice, Beleares 354 Puerto, Nuevo, PR 00920; tel. 809/793–7535; Eyleen Rodriguez Lugo

San Francisco Asis Hospice, P.O. Box 877, Aguada, PR 00602; tel. 787/868–2920; FAX. 787/252–0211; Dilia Dajer, Executive Director

Santa Rita Hospice, Inc., Condominio Medical Center Plaza, Box 1143, Aguada, PR 00602; tel. 787/831–7225; Licedia Rosado

Sendero de Luz, Inc., 11 Georgetti Street, P.O. Box 875, Comerio, PR 00782; tel. 787/875–5701; FAX. 787/875–0887; Juan C. Santiago, Executive Director

St. Lukes Hospice, Ponce, Urb. Industrial, Reparada, Edif. A–B, Ponce, PR 00732; tel. 809/843–4185; Annie Grave

Un Toque de Amor Hospice, Marginal A–2 Urb, San Salvador, Manati, PR 00674; tel. 809/884–3326; Jenny Olivo

Vista Bahia Hospice, Barrio Magas, Guayanilla, PR 00656; tel. 809/836–3314; Luisa I. Carrasquillo

State Government Agencies for Freestanding Hospices

United States

ALABAMA
Alabama Department of Public Health, Division of Licensure and Certification, 434 Monroe Street, Montgomery, AL 36130–1701; tel. 334/240–3503; FAX. 334/240–3147; Rick Harris, Director

ALASKA
Division of Medical Assistance, Health Facilities Licensing and Certification Section, 4041 B Street, Suite 101, Anchorage, AK 99503; tel. 907/561–2171; Karen Martz, Superior

ARIZONA
Arizona Department of Health Services, Health Care Facilities, 1647 East Morten, Phoenix, AZ 85020; tel. 602/255–1221; FAX. 602/255–1108; Linda Palmer, Assistant Director

ARKANSAS
Department of Health, Division of Health Facility Services, 5800 West 10th, Suite 400, Little Rock, AR 72204–9916; tel. 501/661–2201; FAX. 501/661–2165; Valetta M. Buck, Director

CALIFORNIA
Department of Health Services, Licensing and Certification Program, 1800 Third Street, Suite 210, P.O. Box 942732, Sacramento, CA 94234–7320; tel. 916/324–8628; FAX. 916/445–6979; Marilyn Pearman, Chief, Policy Section

COLORADO
Colorado Department of Public Health and Environment, Health Facilities Division A–Two, 4300 Cherry Creek Drive, S., Denver, CO 80222–1530; tel. 303/692–2800; FAX. 303/782–4883; Peggy Waldon, RN, Program Administrator

CONNECTICUT
Department of Public Health and Addiction Services, Hospital and Medical Care Division, 150 Washington Street, Hartford, CT 06106; tel. 203/566–1073; FAX. 203/566–1097; Elizabeth M. Burns, RN, M.S., Director

DELAWARE
Department of Health and Social Services, Office of Health Facilities Licensing and Certification, Three Mill Road, Suite 308, Wilmington, DE 19806; tel. 302/577–6666; FAX. 302/577–6672; Ellen T. Reap, Director

DISTRICT OF COLUMBIA
Department of Consumer and Regulatory Affairs, Service Facility Regulation Administration, 614 H Street, N.W., Suite 1003, Washington, DC 20001; tel. 202/727–7190; FAX. 202/727–7780; Geraldine Sykes, Administrator

FLORIDA
Agency for HealthCare Administration, Division of Health Quality Assurance, Long Term Care Unit, Fort Knox Executive Center, 2727 Mahan Drive, Tallahassee, FL 32308–5407; tel. 904/922–8540; FAX. 904/487–6240; Patricia Hall, Unit Manager

GEORGIA
Health Care Section, Office of Regulatory Services, Two Peachtree Street, N.W., Suite 19–204, Atlanta, GA 30303–3167; tel. 404/657–5550; FAX. 404/657–8934; Susie M. Woods, Director

HAWAII
Department of Health, Licensing and Certification, Hospital and Medical Facilities Branch, P.O. Box 3378, Honolulu, HI 96801; tel. 808/586–4080; FAX. 808/586–4747; Helen K. Yoshimi, B.S.N., M.P.H., HMF Branch, Chief

IDAHO
Bureau of Facility Standards, Department of Health and Welfare, P.O. Box 83720, Boise, ID 83720–0036; tel. 208/334–6626; FAX. 208/334–0657; Loyal Perry, Supervisor

ILLINOIS
Department of Public Health, Office of Health Care Regulation, Bureau of Hospitals and Ambulatory Services, 525 West Jefferson Street, Fourth Floor, Springfield, IL 62761; tel. 217/782–7412; FAX. 217/782–0382; Catherine M. Stokes, Assistant Deputy Director

INDIANA
Indiana State Department of Health, Division of Acute Care, Two North Meridian Street, Indianapolis, IN 46204; tel. 317/233–7472; FAX. 317/233–7157; John A. Braeckel, Director

IOWA
Department of Inspection and Appeals, Division of Health Facilities, Lucas State Office Building, Des Moines, IA 50319; tel. 515/281–4115; FAX. 515/242–5022; J.B. Bennett, Administrator

KANSAS
Department of Health and Environment, Bureau of Adult and Child Care, 900 Southwest Jackson, Suite 1001, Topeka, KS 66620–0001; tel. 913/296–1280; FAX. 913/296–1266; George A. Dugger, Medical Facilities Certification Administrator

KENTUCKY
Cabinet for Human Resources, Division of Licensing and Regulation, C.H.R. Building, 275 East Main Street, Fourth Floor, East, Frankfort, KY 40621; tel. 502/564–2800; FAX. 502/564–6546; Rebecca J. Cecil, Director

LOUISIANA
Department of Health and Hospitals, Bureau of Health Services Financing, Health Standards Section Licensing Unit, P.O. Box 3767, Baton Rouge, LA 70821; tel. 504/342–0138; FAX. 504/342–5292; Lily W. McAlister, RN, Manager

MAINE
Division of Licensing and Certification, Department of Human Services, State House, Station 11, Augusta, ME 04333; tel. 207/624–5443; FAX. 207/624–5378; Louis Dorogi, Director

MARYLAND
Department of Health and Mental Hygiene, Office of Licensing and Certification Administration, 4201 Patterson Avenue, Baltimore, MD 21215; tel. 410/764–4980; FAX. 410/358–0750; James Ralls, Assistant Director

MASSACHUSETTS
Massachusetts Department of Public Health, Division of Health Care Quality, 10 West Street, Boston, MA 02111; tel. 617/727–5860; David H. Mulligan, Commissioner

MICHIGAN
Department of Consumer and Industry Services, Division of Licensing and Certification, 3500 North Logan, Lansing, MI 48909; tel. 517/335–8505; Nancy Graham, Superior

MINNESOTA
Department of Health, Facility and Provider Compliance Division, Licensing and Certification Section, 393 North Dunlap Street, P.O. Box 64900, St. Paul, MN 55164–0900; tel. 612/643–2130; FAX. 612/643–3534; Carol Hirschfeld, Supervisor, Records Information Unit

MISSISSIPPI
Department of Health, Division of Health Facilities, Licensure and Certification, P.O. Box 1700, Jackson, MS 39215; tel. 601/354–7300; FAX. 601/354–7230; Vanessa Phipps, Director

MISSOURI
Department of Health, Bureau of Home Health Licensing and Certification, P.O. Box 570, Jefferson City, MO 65102; tel. 573/751–6336; FAX. 573/751–6315; Carol Gourd, RN, Administrator

MONTANA
Department of Public Health and Human Services, Quality Assurance Division, Licensure Bureau, Cogswell Building, 1400 Broadway, P.O. Box 202951, Helena, MT 59620–2951; tel. 406/444–2676; FAX. 406/444–1742; Roy P. Kemp, Chief

NEBRASKA
Nebraska Department of Health, Health Facility Licensure and Inspection Section, 301 Centennial Mall, S., P.O. Box 95007, Lincoln, NE 68509–5007; tel. 402/471–2946; FAX. 402/471–0555; Frederick M. Wright, Section Administrator

NEVADA
Nevada State Health Division, Bureau of Licensure and Certification, 1550 East College Parkway, Suite 158, Carson City, NV 89706–7921; tel. 702/687–4475; FAX. 702/687–6588; Sharon M. Ezell, Chief

NEW HAMPSHIRE
Office of Program Support, Licensing and Regulation, Six Hazen Drive, Concord, NH 03301; tel. 603/271–4592; FAX. 603/271–3745; Raymond Rusin, Bureau Chief

NEW JERSEY
New Jersey Department of Health and Senior Services, Division of Health Care Systems Analysis, Certificate of Need and Acute Care Licensure, Inspections, Compliance and Enforcement, John Fitchway, Market and Warren Streets, CN–360, Trenton, NJ 08625–0360; tel. 609/292–8773; FAX. 609/984–3165; Henry T. Kozek, R.Ph., M.P.A., C.P.M., Program Manager

NEW MEXICO
Department of Health, Health Facility Licensing and Certification Bureau, 525 Camino de los Marquez, Suite Two, Santa Fe, NM 87501; tel. 505/827–4200; FAX. 505/827–4222; Sue K. Morris, Bureau Chief

NEW YORK
Bureau of Home Health Care Services, Department of Health, Frear Building, Two Third Street, Suite 401, Troy, NY 12180–3298; tel. 518/271–2741; FAX. 518/271–2771; Dr. Nancy Barhydt, Director

NORTH CAROLINA
Department of Human Resources, Division of Facility Services, 701 Barbour Drive, Raleigh, NC 27626–0530; tel. 919/733–1610; FAX. 919/733–3207; Steve White, Chief, Licensure and Certification

NORTH DAKOTA
 Department of Health, Health Resources Section, 600 East Boulevard Avenue, Bismarck, ND 58505; tel. 701/328–2352; FAX. 701/328–4727; Fred Gladden, Chief

OHIO
 Division of Quality Assurance, Ohio Department of Health, 246 North High Street, Columbus, OH 43266–0588; tel. 614/466–7857; FAX. 614/644–0208; Rebecca Maust, Chief

OKLAHOMA
 Department of Health, Special Health Services, 1000 Northeast 10th Street, Oklahoma City, OK 73117; tel. 405/271–6576; FAX. 405/271–1308; Gary Glover, Chief, Medical Facilities

OREGON
 Health Care Licensing and Certification, Oregon Health Division, 800 Northeast Oregon Street, # 21, Suite 640, Portland, OR 97232; tel. 503/731–4013; FAX. 503/731–4080; Kathleen Smail, Manager

PENNSYLVANIA
 Department of Health, Division of Primary Care and Home Health, 132 Kline Plaza, Suite A, Harrisburg, PA 17104; tel. 717/783–1379; FAX. 717/787–3188; Robert Bastian, Director

RHODE ISLAND
 Rhode Island Department of Health, Division of Facilities Regulation, Three Capitol Hill, Providence, RI 02908–5097; tel. 401/277–2566; FAX. 401/277–3999; Wayne I. Farrington, Chief

SOUTH CAROLINA
 Department of Health and Environmental Control, Division of Certification, 2600 Bull Street, Columbia, SC 29201; tel. 803/737–7205; FAX. 803/737–7292; Arthur I. Starnes, Division Director

SOUTH DAKOTA
 Department of Health, Office of Health Care Facilities Licensure and Certification, 445 East Capitol, Pierre, SD 57501; tel. 605/773–3356; FAX. 605/773–6667; Joan Bachman, Administrator

TENNESSEE
 Department of Health, Division of Health Care Facilities, 283 Plus Park Boulevard, Nashville, TN 37247–0530; tel. 615/741–7603; FAX. 615/367–6397; Evelyn Foust

TEXAS
 Department of Health, Health Facility Licensure and Certification Division, 8407 Wall Street, Zip 78754, 1100 West 49th Street, Austin, TX 78756; tel. 512/834–6647; FAX. 512/834–6653; Nance Stearman, RN, M.S.N., Director

UTAH
 Utah Department of Health, Bureau of Health Facility Licensure, Box 142853, Salt Lake City, UT 84114–2853; tel. 801/538–6152; FAX. 801/538–6325; Debra Wynkoop–Green, Director

VERMONT
 Hospice Council of Vermont, 52 State Street, Montpelier, VT 05602; tel. 802/229–0579; FAX. 802/229–0579; Virginia L. Fry, Director

VIRGINIA
 Virginia Department of Health, Office of Health Facilities Regulation, 3600 Centre, Suite 216, 3600 West Broad Street, Richmond, VA 23230; tel. 804/367–2102; FAX. 804/367–2149; Nancy R. Hofheimer, Director

WASHINGTON
 Washington Department of Health, Facilities and Services Licensing, Target Plaza, Suite 500, 2725 Harrison Avenue, N.W., P.O. Box 47852, Olympia, WA 98504–7852; tel. 360/705–6611; FAX. 360/705–6654; Fern Bettridge, Manager

WEST VIRGINIA
 Office of Health Facility Licensure and Certification, West Virginia Division of Health, 1900 Kanawha Boulevard, E., Building Three, Suite 550, Charleston, WV 25305; tel. 304/558–0050; FAX. 304/558–2515; Robert P. Brauner, R.Ph., D.P.M., Program Administrator

WISCONSIN
 Bureau of Quality Assurance, Division of Supportive Living, P.O. Box 309, Madison, WI 53701; tel. 608/267–7185; FAX. 608/267–0352; Judy Fryback, Director, Bureau of Quality Assurance

WYOMING
 Department of Health, Office of Health Quality, 2020 Carey Avenue, First Bank Building, Eighth Floor, Cheyenne, WY 82002; tel. 307/777–7123; FAX. 307/777–7127; Gerald E. Bronnenberg, Administrator

U. S. Associated Areas

PUERTO RICO
 Puerto Rico Department of Health, Call Box 70184, San Juan, PR 00936; tel. 787/274–7602; FAX. 787/250–6547; Carmen Feliciano de Melecio, M.D., Secretary of Health

Section C

JCAHO Accredited Freestanding Long–Term Care Organizations

The accredited freestanding long–term care organizations listed have been accredited as of January 1, 1997, by the Joint Commission on Accreditation of Healthcare Organizations by decision of the Accreditation Committee of the Board of Commissioners.

The organizations listed here have been found to be in compliance with the Joint Commission standards for long–term care organizations, as found in the Comprehensive Accreditation Manual for the Long–Term Care Organizations.

Please refer to section A of the AHA Guide for information on hospitals with Long–Term Care services. These hospitals are identified by Facility Code 64. In section A, those hospitals identified by Approval Code 1 are JCAHO accredited.

We present this list simply as a convenient directory. Inclusion or omission of any organization's name indicates neither approval nor disapproval by Healthcare InfoSource, Inc., a subsidiary of the American Hospital Association.

United States

ALABAMA

Canterbury Health Facility, 1720 Knowles Road, Phenix City, AL 36869; tel. 334/291–0485; FAX. 334/297–5816; Laura Saxon, Administrator

Dauphin Health Care Facility, 3717 Dauphin Street, Mobile, AL 36608; tel. 334/343–0909; FAX. 334/344–0953; Sheila McArdle, Chief Executive Officer

Integrated Health Services at Briarcliff, 850 Northwest Ninth Street, Alabaster, AL 35007; tel. 205/663–3859; FAX. 205/663–9791; Andy Clements, Administrator

Integrated Health Services at Hanover, 39 Hanover Circle, Birmingham, AL 35205; tel. 205/933–1828; FAX. 205/933–0900; Vicki Worley, Chief Executive Officer

Northside Health Care, 700 Hutchins Avenue, Gadsen, AL 35901; tel. 205/543–7101; FAX. 205/546–3924; Treieva Ridgeway, Administrator

Tyson Manor Healthcare Facility, 2020 North Country Club Drive, Montgomery, AL 36106; tel. 205/263–1643; FAX. 205/263–1645; Suzanne Sherlock

Westside Health Care Center, 4320 Judith Lane, Huntsville, AL 35805; tel. 205/837–1730; FAX. 205/430–3287; Nanette Collier, Administrator

Windsor House Nursing Home, 441 McAllister Drive, Huntsville, AL 35805; tel. 205/837–8585; FAX. 205/837–2214; Charles Birkett

ARIZONA

Casa Delmar Nursing and Rehabilitation Center, 3333 North Civic Center Plaza, Scottsdale, AZ 85251; tel. 602/994–1333; FAX. 602/990–3895; Patricia A. Phillips

Catalina Care Center, 2611 North Warren, Tucson, AZ 85719; tel. 520/795–9574; FAX. 520/321–4983; James K. Kinsey, Administrator

Coronado Care Center, 11411 North 19th Avenue, Phoenix, AZ 85029; tel. 602/256–7500; FAX. 602/943–7697; Jacqueline Lanter, Administrator

Desert Samaritan Care Center, 2145 West Southern Avenue, Mesa, AZ 85202; tel. 602/890–4800; FAX. 602/890–4829; Steven D. Bakken, Administrator

East Mesa Care Center, 51 South 48th Street, Mesa, AZ 85206; tel. 602/832–8333; FAX. 602/830–2466; W. H. Syckes, Administrator

Good Samaritan Care Center, 901 East Willetta Street, Phoenix, AZ 85006; tel. 602/223–3000; FAX. 602/223–3197; Michael J. Oliver, Administrator

La Mesa Rehabilitation and Care Center, 2470 South Arizona Avenue, Yuma, AZ 85364; tel. 520/344–8541; FAX. 520/344–0823; John E. Bowman, Executive Director

ManorCare Health Services, 3705 North Swan, Tucson, AZ 85718; tel. 520/299–7088; FAX. 520/529–0038; Richard Park, Administrator

Scottsdale Village Square, 2620 North 68th Street, Scottsdale, AZ 85257; tel. 602/946–6571; FAX. 602/946–0082; Colleen Sweet

The Village Green HealthCare Center, 2932 North 14th Street, Phoenix, AZ 85014; tel. 602/264–5274; FAX. 602/277–8455; Gayle Stocking, Executive Director

Villa Campana Healthcare Center, 6651 East Carondelet Drive, Tucson, AZ 85710; tel. 520/296–6100; FAX. 602/721–3601; Robin Gwozdz

CALIFORNIA

Alamitos Belmont Rehabilitation Hospital, 3901 East Fourth Street, Long Beach, CA 90814; tel. 562/434–8421; FAX. 562/433–6732; Alan Anderson, President, Chief Executive Officer

Bayside Nursing and Rehabilitation Center, 1251 South Eliseo Drive, Kentfield, CA 94904; tel. 415/461–1900; FAX. 415/461–2736; Mary Thrower, Administrator

Brittany Healthcare Center, Inc., 3900 Garfield Avenue, Carmichael, CA 95608; tel. 916/481–6455; FAX. 916/481–6489; Diane Hoyt, Administrator

Brookside Skilled Nursing Hospital, 2620 Flores Street, San Mateo, CA 94403; tel. 415/349–2161; FAX. 415/345–3955; Stan Coppel

Burlingame Nursing and Rehabilitation Center, 1100 Trousdale Drive, Burlingame, CA 94010; tel. 415/692–3758; FAX. 415/692–5190; Debby Friedman, Administrator

California Nursing and Rehabilitation Center of Palm Springs, 2299 North Indian Canyon Drive, Palm Springs, CA 92262; tel. 619/325–2937; FAX. 619/322–7250; Linda Jackson, Administrator

California Special Care Center, Inc., 8787 Center Drive, La Mesa, CA 91942; tel. 619/460–4444; FAX. 619/460–6341; Ed Long

Calistoga Nursing and Rehabilitation Center, 1715 Washington Street, Calistoga, CA 94515; tel. 707/942–6253; FAX. 707/942–6288; Dottie Dowswell, Director, Nursing

Canyonwood Nursing and Rehabilitation Center, 2120 Benton Drive, Redding, CA 96003; tel. 916/243–6317; FAX. 916/243–4646; Carole J. Reynolds, Administrator

Care West–Anza Nursing and Rehabilitation Center, 622 South Anza Street, El Cajon, CA 92020; tel. 619/442–0544; FAX. 619/442–6177; John Jimenez

CareWest Gateway Nursing and Rehabilitation Center, 26660 Patrick Avenue, Hayward, CA 94544; tel. 510/782–1845; FAX. 510/782–9913; Helen Jones, Director, Nursing

Carmichael Convalescent Hospital, 8336 Fair Oaks Boulevard, Carmichael, CA 95608; tel. 916/944–3100; FAX. 916/944–4202; Kathy Spake, Administrator

Casa Colina Peninsula Rehabilitation Center, 26303 Western Avenue, Lomita, CA 90717; tel. 310/325–3202; FAX. 310/534–2782; Terry Banta Winkowski, Administrator

Casa Palmera Care Center, 14750 El Camino Real, Del Mar, CA 92014; tel. 619/481–4411; FAX. 619/792–7356; Lee Johnson, Administrator

Chapman Harbor Skilled Nursing Facility, 12232 West Chapman Avenue, Garden Grove, CA 92640; tel. 714/971–5517; FAX. 714/748–7851; Patricia Smith, Administrator

Clear View Sanitarium and Convalescent Center, 15823 South Western Avenue, Gardena, CA 90247–3788; tel. 310/538–2323; FAX. 310/538–3509; W. Lee Towns, President

Country Villa Nursing and Rehabilitation Center, 340 South Alvarado Street, Los Angeles, CA 90057; tel. 213/484–9730; FAX. 213/484–9507; June Silver

Country Villa Sheraton Nursing and Rehabilitation Center, 9655 Sepulveda Boulevard, North Hills, CA 91343; tel. 818/892–8665; FAX. 818/891–1208; Steve Reissman

Country Villa South, 3515 Overland Avenue, Los Angeles, CA 90034; tel. 310/839–5201; FAX. 310/839–4763; Cvia Rosen

Country Villa Westwood Nursing Center, 12121 Santa Monica Boulevard, Los Angeles, CA 90025; tel. 310/826–0821; FAX. 310/826–2768; Jane Corr

Courtyard Care Center, 1625 Denton Avenue, Hayward, CA 94545; tel. 510/782–2133; FAX. 510/783–3659; Nathaniel Fripp

Covina Rehabilitation Center, 261 West Badillo, Covina, CA 91723; tel. 813/967–3874; FAX. 813/332–6532; Michael E. Demchuk, Administrator

Devonshire Care Center, 1350 East Devonshire Avenue, Hemet, CA 92544; tel. 909/925–2571; FAX. 909/929–5469; Jacqueline Arcara

Driftwood Health Care Center, 4109 Emerald Street, Torrance, CA 90503; tel. 310/371–4628; FAX. 310/214–1882; Yasmin Murphy, Director, Case Management, Admissions

El Encanto Healthcare, 555 South El Encanto Road, P.O. Box 3444, La Puente, CA 91745–1090; tel. 818/336–1274; FAX. 818/330–2789; Steve Blackwell

English Oaks Convalescent and Rehabilitation Hospital, 2633 West Rumble Road, Modesto, CA 95350; tel. 209/577–1001, ext. 7601; FAX. 209/577–0366; Terry L. Mundy, Administrator

Evergreen Convalescent Hospital and Rehabilitation Center, 2030 Evergreen Avenue, Modesto, CA 95350; tel. 209/577–1055; FAX. 209/526–6961; Daniel J. Cipponeri, Vice President

Excell Health Care Center, 3025 High Street, Oakland, CA 94619; tel. 510/261–5200; FAX. 510/261–1012

Fairfield Health Care Center, 1255 Travis Boulevard, Fairfield, CA 94533; tel. 707/425–0623; FAX. 707/425–0704; Diane Hinkle, Administrator

Fremont Health Center, 39022 Presidio Way, Fremont, CA 94538; tel. 510/792–3743; FAX. 510/792–1966; Lisa Chestnut, Executive Director

Glendora Rehabilitation Center, 435 East Gladstone, Glendora, CA 91740; tel. 818/963–5955; FAX. 818/963–8683; Gerald R. Hardy, Administrator

Grand Terrace Convalescent Hospital, 12000 Mt. Vernon Avenue, Grand Terrace, CA 92324; tel. 909/825–5221; FAX. 909/783–4811; Ted J. Holt, Administrator

Greenery Rehabilitation Center, 385 Esplanade, Pacifica, CA 94044; tel. 415/993–5576; FAX. 415/359–9388; Janet T. Kempis, Ed.D

Guardian Ygnacio, 1449 Ygnacio Valley Road, Walnut Creek, CA 94598; tel. 510/939–5820; FAX. 510/939–0231; Robert Pierce

Hanford Nursing and Rehabilitation Hospital, 1007 West Lacey Boulevard, Hanford, CA 93230; tel. 209/582–2871; FAX. 209/582–5853; Mark Fisher

Hayward Hills Convalescent Hospital, 1768 B Street, Hayward, CA 94541; tel. 510/538–4424; FAX. 510/538–9221; Terry McGregor

Heritage Paradise, 8777 Skyway Street, Paradise, CA 95969; tel. 916/872–3200; FAX. 916/872–5318; Barbara Wright

Heritage Rehabilitation Center, 21414 South Vermont Avenue, Torrance, CA 90502; tel. 310/320–8714; FAX. 310/320–1809; Doug Nelson, Administrator

Heritage of Stockton, a Convalescent and Rehabilitation Center, 9107 North Davis Road, Stockton, CA 95209; tel. 209/478–6488; FAX. 209/952–1782; Kathleen S. Hill, Administrator

Huntington Beach Convalescent Hospital, 18811 Florida Street, Huntington Beach, CA 92648; tel. 714/847–3515; FAX. 714/847–2852; Carolyn E. Paul, Ph.D., Administrator

Huntington Drive Skilled Nursing Facility, 400 West Huntington Drive, Arcadia, CA 91007; tel. 818/445–2421; FAX. 818/821–5916; Richard Tovar, Executive Director

Huntington Valley Nursing Center, 8382 Newman Avenue, Huntington Valley, CA 92647; tel. 714/842–5551; FAX. 714/848–5359; Tish Gamboni, Director, Nursing

Integrated Health Services at Orange Hills, 5017 East Chapman Avenue, Orange, CA 92669; tel. 714/997–7090; FAX. 714/997–4631; Retha Tyler, Controller for Quality

Integrated Health Services at Park Regency, 1770 West La Habra Boulevard, La Habra, CA 90631; tel. 310/691–8810; FAX. 310/697–8478; Kamran Dideban, Administrator

John Douglas French Center for Alzheimer's Disease, 3951 Katella Avenue, Los Alamitos, CA 90720; tel. 562/493–1555; FAX. 562/596–7526; Ferri Kidane, Executive Director

La Mariposa Nursing and Rehabilitation Center, 1244 Travis Boulevard, Fairfield, CA 94533; tel. 707/422–7750; FAX. 707/422–8102; Lisa Churches, Administrator

La Palma Nursing Center, 1130 West La Palma Avenue, Anaheim, CA 92801; tel. 714/772–7480; FAX. 714/776–1841; Larry Szala, Administrator

Lancaster Health Care Center, 1642 West Avenue J, Lancaster, CA 93534; tel. 805/942–8463; FAX. 805/948–5133; Jeri–Anne I. Shelton, Executive Director

Laurelwood Health Care Center, 13000 Victory Boulevard, North Hollywood, CA 91606; tel. 818/985–5990; FAX. 818/505–1947; Scott Herzig, Executive Director

Magnolia Special Care Center, 635 South Magnolia, El Cajon, CA 92020; tel. 619/442–8826; FAX. 619/442–0288; Harriet Haugen, Administrator

Manor Care Nursing and Rehabilitation Center, 11680 Warneer Avenue, Fountain Valley, CA 92708; tel. 714/241–9800; FAX. 714/966–1654; Christine Davis

ManorCare Health Services, 1150 Tilton Drive, Sunnyvale, CA 94087; tel. 408/735–7200; FAX. 408/736–8619; Jennifer Oldfather, Administrator

Manteca Nursing and Rehabilitation Center, 410 Eastwood Avenue, Manteca, CA 95336; tel. 209/239–1222; FAX. 209/239–9101; Maxine Niel

McClure Convalescent Hospital and Rehabilitation Center, 2910 McClure Street, Oakland, CA 94609; tel. 510/836–3677; FAX. 510/836–1938; Jeremy Grimes, Administrator

Mission Terrace Convalescent Hospital, 623 West Junipero Street, Santa Barbara, CA 93105; tel. 805/682–7443; FAX. 805/682–5311; Evelina Murphy, Administrator

Nursing Inn of Menlo Park, 16 Coleman Place, Menlo Park, CA 94025; tel. 415/326–0802; FAX. 415/326–4145; Asaad Abdelmalek, Administrator

Orinda Rehabilitation and Convalescent Hospital, 11 Altarinda Road, Orinda, CA 94563; tel. 510/254–6500; FAX. 510/254–9063; Charles Speers, Administrator

Pacific Coast Manor, 1935 Wharf Road, Capitola, CA 95010; tel. 408/476–0770; FAX. 408/476–0737; Charles H. Bruffey, Administrator

Pacific Hills Manor, 370 Noble Court, Morgan Hill, CA 95037; tel. 408/779–7346; FAX. 408/779–9435; Laurie Behrend, Administrator

Park Anaheim Healthcare Center, 3435 West Ball Road, Anaheim, CA 92804; tel. 714/827–5880; FAX. 714/874–4015; Rhonda A. Caldwell, Administrator

Park Central Nursing and Rehabilitation Center, 2100 Parkside Drive, Fremont, CA 94536; tel. 510/797–5300; FAX. 510/797–2159; Donna Jeffares

Park Tustin Rehabilitation and Healthcare Center, 2210 East First Street, Santa Ana, CA 92705; tel. 714/547–7091; FAX. 714/547–4516; Mark Schroepfer, Administrator

Parkmont Rehabilitation and Nursing Care Center, 2400 Parkside Drive, Fremont, CA 94536; tel. 510/793–7222; FAX. 510/793–4361; Imogene Ellwanger

Parkview Health Care Center, 27350 Tampa Avenue, Hayward, CA 94544–4429; tel. 510/783–8150; FAX. 810/783–8161; Jeff Lambkin, Executive Director

San Bruno Skilled Nursing Hospital, 890 El Camino Real, San Bruno, CA 94066; tel. 415/583–7768; FAX. 415/583–9710; Nicholas deFina

Scripps Memorial Ocean View Convalescent Hospital, 900 Santa Fe Drive, Encinitas, CA 92024; tel. 619/753–6423; FAX. 619/753–4979; Pamela I. Turner, Administrator

Scripps Memorial Torrey Pines Convalescent Hospital, 2552 Torrey Pines Road, La Jolla, CA 92037; tel. 619/453–5810; FAX. 619/452–4301; Elena M. Gulla, Administrator

Simi Valley Rehabilitation and Nursing Center, 5270 Los Angeles Avenue, Simi Valley, CA 93063; tel. 805/527–6204; FAX. 805/527–2082; Janice Lackey

St. Luke's Subacute Care Hospital and Nursing Centre, 1652 Mono Avenue, San Leandro, CA 94578; tel. 415/357–5351; FAX. 415/278–7912; Belinda Leung, RN, Executive Vice President

Subacute Saratoga Hospital, 18611 Sousa Lane, Saratoga, CA 95070; tel. 408/378–8875; FAX. 408/866–8144; Michael Zarcone, President

Tarzana Rehabilitation Center, 5650 Reseda Boulevard, Tarzana, CA 91356; tel. 818/881–4261; FAX. 818/343–7451; Gene Burleson

Thousand Oaks Health Care Center, 93 West Avenida de los Arboles, Thousand Oaks, CA 91360; tel. 805/492–2444; FAX. 805/493–1643; Michael Gamet, Administrator

Tulare Convalescent Hospital, 680 East Merritt Avenue, Tulare, CA 93274; tel. 209/686–8581; FAX. 209/686–5393; Mark Fisher, Administrator

VA Medical Center, 16111 Plummer Street, Sepulveda, CA 91343; tel. 818/895–9308; FAX. 818/895–9559; Dollie G. Brown, Associate Director

Valley Manor Rehabilitation Care Center, 3806 Clayton Road, Concord, CA 94521; tel. 510/689–2266; FAX. 510/689–0509; Ramona Matthews, Coordinator

Villa Maria Care Center, 425 East Barcellus Avenue, Santa Maria, CA 93454; tel. 805/922–3558; FAX. 805/349–8443; Laurie Smith, Administrator

Village Square Nursing and Rehabilitation Center, 1586 West San Marcos Boulevard, San Marcos, CA 92069; tel. 619/471–2986; FAX. 619/471–5176; Gary Leiderman, Administrator

Western Medical Center Bartlett, 600 East Washington Avenue, Santa Ana, CA 92701; tel. 714/973–1656, ext. 408; FAX. 714/836–4349; Page Van Hoy, Chief Executive Officer

Woodland Nursing Inn, 3721 Mount Diablo Boulevard, Lafayette, CA 94549; tel. 510/284–5544; FAX. 510/284–5673; Daniel Alger

COLORADO

Alpine Living Center, 501 East Thornton Parkway, Denver, CO 80229; tel. 303/452–6101; FAX. 303/452–4330; Bruce Odenthal

Bonell Good Samaritan Center, 708 22nd Street, P.O. Box 1508, Greeley, CO 80632–1508; tel. 303/352–6082; FAX. 303/356–7970; Art Hess, Administrator

Boulder Manor, 4685 East Baseline Road, Boulder, CO 80303; tel. 303/494–0535; FAX. 303/494–0162; Gary W. Walker, Administrator

Cedars Health Care Center, 1599 Ingalls Street, Lakewood, CO 80214; tel. 303/232–3551; FAX. 303/232–8992; Terrance Sharron

Cherrelyn Health Care Center, 5555 South Eldti Street, Littleton, CO 80120; tel. 303/798–8686; FAX. 303/798–0145; Lori Moore

Colorado State Veterans Nursing Home – Walsenburg, 23500 US Highway 160, Walsenburg, CO 81089; tel. 719/738–5133; Sandra Ledbetter, Marketing Director

Integrated Health Services of Colorado Springs, 3625 Parkmoor Village Drive, Colorado Springs, CO 80917; tel. 719/550–0200; FAX. 719/637–0756; Rick Haskell

Kenton Manor Living Center, 850 27th Avenue, Greeley, CO 80631; tel. 303/353–1017; FAX. 303/353–2476; Sieglinde Donohue, Administrator

Manor Care Nursing Center, Medbridge Medical and Physical Rehabilitation Center, 290 South Monaco Parkway, Denver, CO 80224; tel. 303/355–2525; FAX. 303/333–6960; Sandi Novotny, Executive Director

Mariner Health of Greenwood Village, 6005 South Holly Street, Littleton, CO 80121; tel. 303/773–1000; FAX. 303/773–0024; Tracy Scruggs

Spring Creek Health Care Center, 1000 East Stuart, Fort Collins, CO 80525; tel. 970/482–5712; FAX. 970/493–8376; Dennis Ziefel

Terrace Gardens Health Care Center, 2438 East Fountain Boulevard, Colorado Springs, CO 80910; tel. 719/473–8000; FAX. 719/473–7370; Anneliese Hemmings

VA Medical Center Fort Lyon, C Street, Fort Lyon, CO 81038; tel. 719/384–3110; FAX. 719/384–3168; W. David Smith, Director

CONNECTICUT

Abbott Terrace Health Center, 44 Abbott Terrace, Waterbury, CT 06702–1499; tel. 203/755–4870; FAX. 203/755–9016; Diane MacSweeney

Adams House Healthcare, 80 Fern Drive, Torrington, CT 06790; tel. 203/482–7668; FAX. 203/496–7815; Dawn Dempsey, Administrator

Arden House, 850 Mix Avenue, Hamden, CT 06514; tel. 203/282–3500; FAX. 203/287–9534; Harold Moffie

Ashlar of Newtown, Toddy Hill Road, Newtown, CT 06470; tel. 203/426–5847; FAX. 203/270–0695; Thomas Gutner, President

Astoria Park, 725 Park Avenue, Bridgeport, CT 06604; tel. 203/366–3653; FAX. 203/333–6974; Donald Franco

Avery Heights, 705 New Britain Avenue, Hartford, CT 06106; tel. 860/527–9126; FAX. 860/525–2090; Charles Otto

Avon Convalescent Home, Inc., d/b/a Avon Health Center, 652 West Avon Road, Avon, CT 06001; tel. 860/673–2521; FAX. 860/675–1587; Laura L. Nelson, Administrator

Bayview Health Care Center, Inc., 301 Rope Ferry Road, Waterford, CT 06385; tel. 203/444–1175; FAX. 203/437–2173; Susan J. Wilson, Administrator

Beacon Brook Health Center, 89 Weid Drive, Naugatuck, CT 06770; tel. 203/729–9889; FAX. 203/729–9889; Carol Anne Salvietti, Administrator

Beechwood Rehabilitation and Nursing Center, 31 Vauxhall Street, P.O. Box 308, New London, CT 06320; tel. 860/442–4363; FAX. 860/447–3749; Richard C. Brown, Administrator

Bethel Health Care Center, 13 Parklawn Drive, Bethel, CT 06801; tel. 203/830–4180; FAX. 203/830–4185; Roland Butler

Branford Hills Health Care Center, 189 Alps Road, Branford, CT 06405; tel. 203/481–6221; FAX. 203/483–1893; Stephen J. Shelton, Administrator

Brightview of Avon, 220 Scoville Road, Avon, CT 06001; tel. 860/673–3265; FAX. 860/673–4883; Greg Hamley, Administrator

Brittany Farms Health Center, 400 Brittany Farms Road, New Britain, CT 06053; tel. 860/224–3111; FAX. 860/229–0066; Thomas Tolisano

Brook Hollow Health Care Center, 55 Kondracki Lane, Wallingford, CT 06492; tel. 203/265–6771; FAX. 203/284–3883; Pamela R. Miller, Administrator

Brookview Health Care Facility, 130 Loomis Drive, West Hartford, CT 06117; tel. 203/521–8700; FAX. 203/521–7452; Clifton P. Mix, Administrator

Cedar Lane Rehabilitation and Health Care Center, 128 Cedar Avenue, Waterbury, CT 06705; tel. 203/757–9271; FAX. 203/757–2988; Elizabeth J. Schmeizl, Administrator

Cherry Brook Health Care Center, 102 Dyer Avenue, Collinsville, CT 06022; tel. 203/693–7777; FAX. 203/693–7779; David Bordonaro

Cheshire Convalescent Center, 745 Highland Avenue, Cheshire, CT 06410; tel. 203/272–7285; FAX. 203/250–6066; William Thompson, Administrator

Chestelm Health Care, 534 Town Street, P.O. Box 719, Moodus, CT 06469; tel. 203/873–1455; FAX. 203/873–2307; Brenda Epright

Clifton House Rehabilitation Center, 181 Clifton Street, New Haven, CT 06513; tel. 203/467–1666; FAX. 203/469–7213; Earle R. Hollings, Administrator

Colchester Nursing and Rehabilitation Center, 59 Harrington Court, Colchester, CT 06415; tel. 860/537–2339; FAX. 860/537–4747; Moshael Straus

Cook Willow Health Center, 81 Hillside Avenue, Plymouth, CT 06782; tel. 860/283–8208; FAX. 860/283–6667; Susan MacDonald

Crestfield Rehabilitation Center and Fenwood Manor, 565 Vernon Street, Manchester, CT 06040; tel. 203/643–5151; FAX. 203/643–5203; Rolland Castleman

Derby Nursing Center, 210 Chatfield Street, Derby, CT 06418; tel. 203/735–7401; FAX. 203/736–0898; Albert Saunders

Fairview, Starr Hill Road, P.O. Box 7218, Groton, CT 06340; tel. 860/445–7478; FAX. 860/445–9575; Jack Van Verdeghem, Administrator

Forestville Health and Rehabilitation Center, 23 Fair Street, Forestville, CT 06010; tel. 860/589–2923; FAX. 860/589–3148; Linda Bradigo, Administrator

Geer Nursing and Rehabilitation Center, 99 South Canaan Road, P.O. Box 819, Canaan, CT 06018; tel. 203/824–5137; FAX. 203/824–1474; Anthony Nania

Section C

Gladeview Health Care Center, 60 Boston Post Road, Old Saybrook, CT 06475; tel. 203/388–6696; FAX. 203/395–0093; Margaret G. Crescione, Administrator

Glastonbury Health Care Center, 969 Hebron Avenue, 1175 Hebron Avenue, Glastonbury, CT 06033; tel. 203/659–1905; FAX. 203/652–3055; Thomas C. Gaccione, Administrator

Glen Hill Convalescent Center, One Glen Hill Road, Danbury, CT 06811; tel. 203/744–2840; FAX. 203/792–1521; James Malloy, Administrator

Greenery Extended Care Center at Cheshire, 50 Hazel Drive, Cheshire, CT 06410; tel. 203/272–7204; FAX. 203/272–4607; Denis Twigg, Administrator

Greenery Rehabilitation Center at Waterbury, 177 Whitewood Road, Waterbury, CT 06708; tel. 203/757–9491; FAX. 203/575–1714; Charles Chidester, Administrator

Harbor Hill Care Center, Inc., 111 Church Street, Middletown, CT 06457; tel. 860/347–7286; FAX. 860/346–5589; Lewis Abramson, Administrator

Hebrew Home and Hospital, Inc., One Abrahms Boulevard, West Hartford, CT 06117–1525; tel. 203/523–3800; FAX. 203/523–3949; Irving Kronenberg

Heritage Heights Care Center, 22 Hospital Avenue, Danbury, CT 06810; tel. 203/744–3700; FAX. 203/798–8322; Susan Jodoin, Administrator

Hill Crest Health Care Center, Five Richard Brown Drive, Uncasville, CT 06382; tel. 860/848–8466; FAX. 860/848–7456; Judith Hilburger

Honey Hill Care Center, 34 Midrocks Drive, Norwalk, CT 06851; tel. 203/847–9686; FAX. 203/840–1584; Betty Karkut, Administrator

Ingraham Manor, 400 North Main Street, Bristol, CT 06010; tel. 203/584–3400; FAX. 203/589–8686; Linda A. Urbanski, Administrator

Jewish Home for the Elderly of Fairfield County, 175 Jefferson Street, Fairfield, CT 06432; tel. 203/374–9461; FAX. 203/374–8082; Donna Joyce, Vice President

Laurel Woods, 451 North High Street, East Haven, CT 06512; tel. 203/466–6850; FAX. 203/466–6852; Lorraine Franco, Administrator

Laurelwood Rehabilitation and Skilled Nursing Center, 642 Danbury Road, Ridgefield, CT 06877; tel. 203/438–8226; FAX. 203/438–8378; Joanne Maccione, Administrator

Litchfield Woods Health Care Center, 255 Roberts Street, Torrington, CT 06790; tel. 860/489–5801; FAX. 860/489–6102; Gene Heavens, Administrator

Lord Chamberlain Nursing Facility Rehabilitation Center, 7003 Main Street, Stratford, CT 06497; tel. 203/375–5894; FAX. 203/375–1199; Martin Sbriglio, RN, Licensed Administrator, Chief Executive Officer

Maefair Health Care Center, 21 Maefair Court, Trumbull, CT 06611; tel. 203/459–5152; FAX. 203/549–5156; Russell Schwartz, Administrator

Manchester Manor Health Care Center, 385 West Center Street, Manchester, CT 06040; tel. 860/646–0129; FAX. 860/645–0841; Stephen Surprenant, Administrator

Mansfield Center for Nursing and Rehabilitation, 100 Warren Circle, Storrs, CT 06268; tel. 203/487–2300; FAX. 203/487–2312; Kathleen Sutherland

Mariner Health Care at Bride Brook, 23 Liberty Way, Niantic, CT 06357; tel. 860/739–4007; FAX. 860/739–3880; John D. Hooker, Administrator

Mariner Health Care at Pendleton Rehabilitation, Inc., 44 Maritime Drive, Mystic, CT 06355; tel. 203/572–1700; FAX. 203/527–7830; Louise Rief, Director of Nursing

Marlborough Health Care Center, Inc., 85 Stage Harbor Road, P.O. Box 476, Marlborough, CT 06447; tel. 203/295–9531; FAX. 203/295–6232; Thomas Harris, Administrator

McLean Home and Home Care Services, 75 Great Pond Road, Simsbury, CT 06070; tel. 203/658–3700; FAX. 203/651–1247; David R. Bailey

Meadowbrook of Granby, 350 Salmon Brook Street, Granby, CT 06035; tel. 203/653–9888; FAX. 203/653–8938; Samuel Paul

Mediplex Rehabilitation and Skilled Nursing Center of Southern Connecticut, 2028 Bridgeport Avenue, Milford, CT 06460; tel. 203/877–0371; FAX. 203/877–6185; Mary Grabell, Executive Director

Mediplex Rehabilitation and Skilled Nursing Center of Central Connecticut, 261 Summit Street, Plantsville, CT 06479; tel. 203/628–0364; FAX. 203/628–9166; Raymond C. DeBlasio, Administrator

Mediplex of Danbury, 107 Osborne Street, Danbury, CT 06810; tel. 203/792–8102; FAX. 203/731–5306; Donna Deitch, Administrator

Mediplex of Darien Rehabilitation Center, 599 Boston Post Road, Darien, CT 06820; tel. 203/655–7727, ext. 202; FAX. 203/655–6718; Samuel S. Hamilton, Chief Executive Officer

Mediplex of Greater Hartford, 160 Coventry Street, Bloomfield, CT 06002; tel. 203/243–2995; FAX. 203/243–1902; Adrianne Zeoli, Administrator

Mediplex of Milford, 245 Orange Avenue, Milford, CT 06460; tel. 203/876–5123; FAX. 203/876–5129; Donna C. Stango, Administrator

Mediplex of Newington, 240 Church Street, Newington, CT 06111; tel. 203/667–2256; FAX. 203/667–6367; Patricia Salisbury, Administrator

Mediplex of Southbury, 162 South Britain Road, Southbury, CT 06488; tel. 203/264–9600; FAX. 203/264–9603; Ann M. Rogers, Administrator

Mediplex of Westport, One Burr Road, Westport, CT 06880; tel. 203/226–4201; FAX. 203/221–4766; Dorothy H. Feigin, Administrator

Mediplex of Wethersfield, 341 Jordan Lane, Wethersfield, CT 06109; tel. 860/563–0101; FAX. 860/257–6107; J. Kevin Prisco, Administrator

Meriden Nursing and Rehabilitation Center, 845 Paddock Avenue, Meriden, CT 06450; tel. 203/238–2645; FAX. 203/238–7376; Beth Casso, Executive Director

Middlesex Convalescent Center, 100 Randolph Road, Middletown, CT 06457; tel. 860/344–0353; FAX. 860/346–1932; Robert Shepard, Administrator

Milford Health Care Center, Inc., 195 Platt Street, Milford, CT 06460; tel. 203/878–5958; FAX. 203/878–4299; Paul E. Ulatowski, Administrator

Miller Memorial Community, 360 Broad Street, Meriden, CT 06450; tel. 203/237–8815; FAX. 203/630–3714; Sister Ann Noonan, R.S.M., Administrator, Chief Operating Officer

Montowese Health and Rehabilitation Center, Inc., 163 Quinnipiac Avenue, North Haven, CT 06473; tel. 203/624–3303; FAX. 203/787–9243; Judith Andrews, Admissions Director

Noble Horizons, 17 Cobble Road, Salisbury, CT 06068; tel. 860/435–9851; FAX. 860/435–0636; Eileen M. Mulligan, Administrator, Vice President

Plainville Health Care Center, 269 Farmington Avenue, Plainville, CT 06062; tel. 860/747–1637; FAX. 860/747–9757; Terri Golec

Regency House of Wallingford, 181 East Main Street, Wallingford, CT 06492; tel. 203/265–1661; FAX. 203/265–7842; Margaret P. Coburn

Riverside Health and Rehabilitation Center, 745 Main Street, East Hartford, CT 06108; tel. 860/289–2791; FAX. 860/289–7713; Karen Chadderton, Administrator

Rose Haven, Ltd., 33 North Street, P.O. Box 157, Litchfield, CT 06759; tel. 860/567–9475; FAX. 860/567–8132; Elsie Kenney

Saint Regis Health Center, Inc., 1354 Chapel Street, New Haven, CT 06511; tel. 203/867–8300; FAX. 203/867–8370; Sister Anne Virginia

Salmon Brook Nursing and Rehabilitation Center, 72 Salmon Brook Drive, Glastonbury, CT 06033; tel. 203/633–5244; FAX. 203/657–2360; Nancy K. Wright, Executive Director

Shady Knoll Health Center, Inc., 41 Skokorat Street, Seymour, CT 06483; tel. 203/881–2555; FAX. 203/881–0853; Robert Fritz, Administrator

Sharon Health Care Center, 27 Hospital Hill Road, Sharon, CT 06069; tel. 203/364–1002; FAX. 203/364–0237; Sally Erdman, Administrator

Sheriden Woods Health Care Center, 321 Stonecrest Drive, Bristol, CT 06010–5300; tel. 203/583–1827; FAX. 203/589–1976; Dorothy Rossetti

Skyview Nursing and Rehabilitation Center, 35 Marc Drive, Wallingford, CT 06492; tel. 203/265–0981; FAX. 203/284–1759; Robert Guastella, Executive Director

Southington Care Center, 45 Meriden Avenue, Southington, CT 06489; tel. 203/621–9559; FAX. 203/628–9366; Patricia Walden, Executive Director

Southport Manor Convalescent Center, Inc., 930 Mill Hill Terrace, Southport, CT 06490; tel. 203/259–7894; FAX. 203/254–3720; Albert A. Garofalo, Administrator

St. Joseph Living Center, Inc., 14 Club Road, Windham, CT 06280; tel. 860/456–1107; FAX. 860/450–7114; Patricia Hamill, Nursing Home Administrator

Sterling Manor, Inc., 870 Burnside Avenue, East Hartford, CT 06108; tel. 203/289–9571; FAX. 203/289–8348; Thomas Blonski, Administrator

Talmadge Park Health Care, 38 Talmadge Avenue, East Haven, CT 06512; tel. 203/469–2316; FAX. 203/467–5582; Donald Franco

The Center for Optimum Care of Danielson, 111 Westcott Road, Danielson, CT 06239; tel. 203/774–9540; FAX. 203/774–9703; Judy Ann Johnson, Executive Director

The Center for Optimum Care–Sound View, One Care Lane, West Haven, CT 06516; tel. 203/934–7955; FAX. 203/934–1038; Jonathan Sherwin

The Center for Optimum Care–Waterford, 171 Rope Ferry Road, Waterford, CT 06385; tel. 860/443–8357; FAX. 860/447–8351; Peter Madden

The Elim Park Baptist Home, Inc., 140 Cook Hill Road, Cheshire, CT 06410; tel. 203/272–3547; FAX. 203/250–6282; David MacNeill, President

The Kent Specialty Care Center, 46 Maple Street, P.O. Box 340, Kent, CT 06757; tel. 860/927–5368; FAX. 860/927–1594; Peter J. Belval, Administrator

The Madison House, 34 Wildwood Avenue, Madison, CT 06443; tel. 203/245–8008; FAX. 203/245–2107; Kathleen Dess

The Reservoir, One Emily Way, West Hartford, CT 06107; tel. 203/521–7022; FAX. 203/521–7023; Harold Moffie

The Suffield House, One Canal Road, Suffield, CT 06078; tel. 860/668–6111; FAX. 860/668–0061; Harold Moffie

The William and Sally Tandet Center for Continuing Care, 146 West Broad Street, Stamford, CT 06902; tel. 203/964–8500; FAX. 203/356–9925; Daniel Katz

Torrington Extend–A–Care Centre, 225 Wyoming Avenue, Torrington, CT 06790; tel. 203/482–8563; Christine Marek

Valerie Manor, Inc., 1360 Torringford Street, Route 183, Torrington, CT 06790; tel. 203/489–1008; FAX. 203/496–9252; Ann Wallace, Administrator

Vernon Manor Health Care Center, 180 Regan Road, Vernon, CT 06066–2818; tel. 860/871–0385; FAX. 860/871–9098; Kate Shepard, Administrator

Wadsworth Glen Health Care and Rehabilitation Center, 30 Boston Road, Middletown, CT 06457; tel. 860/346–9299; FAX. 860/343–5030; Elaine Madden, Administrator

Waterbury Extended Care Facility, 35 Bunker Hill Road, Watertown, CT 06795; tel. 203/274–5428; FAX. 203/945–3736; Mark Barwise

Watrous Nursing Center, Nine Neck Road, Madison, CT 06443; tel. 203/245–9483; FAX. 203/245–4668; John Sweeney, Administrator

Waveny Care Center, Three Farm Road, New Canaan, CT 06840; tel. 203/966–8725; FAX. 203/966–1641; Jeremy Vickers, Executive Director

Westfield Care and Rehabilitation Center, 65 Westfield Road, Meriden, CT 06450; tel. 203/238–1291; FAX. 203/238–7763; Pam Belcourt, Admissions

Westview Nursing Care and Rehabilitation Center, Inc., 150 Ware Road, P.O. Box 428, Dayville, CT 06241; tel. 860/774–8574; FAX. 860/779–5425; Eileen Panteleakos, Chief Executive Officer, Administrator

Windham Hills Healthcare Center, 595 Valley Street, Willimantic, CT 06226; tel. 203/423–2597; FAX. 203/450–7070; Dawn Dempsey, Administrator

Wintonbury Healthcare Center, 140 Park Avenue, Bloomfield, CT 06002; tel. 860/243–9591; FAX. 860/286–0161; Tracy Haddad

Wolcott View Manor, Inc., 50 Beach Road, P.O. Box 6192, Wolcott, CT 06716; tel. 203/879–8066; FAX. 206/879–8072; Dennis Cleary, RN, Administrator

Woodlake at Tolland, 26 Shenipsit Lake Road, Tolland, CT 06084; tel. 203/872–2999; FAX. 203/872–1848; Martha Dale

DELAWARE

Manor Care Health Services–Pike Creek, 5651 Limestone Road, Wilmington, DE 19808; tel. 302/239–8583; FAX. 302/239–4523; John Fredericks

Methodist Country House, 4830 Kennett Pike, Wilmington, DE 19807; tel. 302/654–5101; FAX. 302/426–8108; William H. James, Jr., Executive Director

DISTRICT OF COLUMBIA

Benjamin King Health Center, U.S. Soldiers' and Airmen's Home, 3700 North Capitol Street, N.W., Washington, DC 20317–0001; tel. 202/722–3323; FAX. 202/722–3570; Paul D. Gleason, M.D., Associate Director, Health Care Services

Center for Aging Health Care Institute, 1380 Southern Avenue, S.E., Washington, DC 20032; tel. 202/279-5880; FAX. 202/574-0192; Vanessa Mattox, Administrator

FLORIDA

Arbors at Bayonet Point/Hudson, 8132 Hudson Avenue, Hudson, FL 34667; tel. 813/863-3100; FAX. 813/862-0941; Stephen Jones, Administrator

Arbors at Brandon, 701 Victoria Street, Brandon, FL 33510; tel. 813/681-4220; FAX. 614/791-2930; Terry L. Hilker, Executive Director

Arbors at Lakeland, 2020 West Lake Parker Drive, Lakeland, FL 33805; tel. 941/682-7580; FAX. 941/683-9564; Janice P. Heidel, RN, NHA

Arbors at Orange Park Nursing and Rehabilitation Center, 1215 Kingsley Avenue, Orange Park, FL 32073; tel. 904/269-8922; FAX. 904/264-2253; Terry Carpenter, Executive Director

Arbors at Orlando Subacute and Rehabilitation Center, 1099 West Town Parkway, Altamonte Springs, FL 32714; tel. 407/865-8000; FAX. 407/865-7288; Mr. Pier Borra

Arbors at Tallahassee Subacute and Rehabilitation Center, 1650 Phillips Road, Tallahassee, FL 32308; tel. 904/942-9868; FAX. 904/942-1074; Joseph M. Jicha, Administrator

Atlantis Center, 6026 Old Congress Road, Lantana, FL 33462; tel. 561/964-4430; FAX. 561/641-9711; Dan E. Dailey, Administrator

Bay Pointe Nursing Pavilion, 4201 31st Street, St. Petersburg,, FL 33712; tel. 813/867-1104; FAX. 813/864-4627; Dianne Roepcke, Director, Nursing

Beverly Health and Rehabilitation Center, 600 Business Parkway, Royal Palm Beach, FL 33411; tel. 407/798-3700; FAX. 407/795-3583; Lisa Ryman-Porelli

Boca Raton Rehabilitation Center, 755 Meadows Road, Boca Raton, FL 33486; tel. 561/391-5200; FAX. 561/391-5487; Linda McClamma, Administrator

Bowman's Health Care Center, 350 South Ridgewood Avenue, Ormond Beach, FL 32174; tel. 904/677-4545; FAX. 904/677-3445; Merle Zinck, Administrator

Brandywyne Health Care Center, 1801 North Lake Mariam Drive, Winter Haven, FL 33884; tel. 813/293-1989; FAX. 813/299-6427; Kathryn Smith

Eagle Crest Rehabilitation and Health Care Center, 2802 Parental Home Road, Jacksonville, FL 32216; tel. 904/721-0088; FAX. 904/774-1654; John Hymans

Golfcrest Nursing Home, 600 North 17th Avenue, Hollywood, FL 33020; tel. 305/927-2531; FAX. 305/927-0425; Fred Balestriero

Golfview Nursing Home, 3636 10th Avenue, N., Saint Petersburg, FL 33712; tel. 813/323-3611; FAX. 813/327-5802; Linda Howard, NHA

Good Samaritan Nursing Home, 3127 57th Avenue, N., Saint Petersburg, FL 33714; tel. 813/527-2171; FAX. 813/522-8929; Lorraine Sedlock

Greynolds Park Manor Rehabilitation Center, 17400 West Dixie Highway, North Miami Beach, FL 33160; tel. 305/944-2361; FAX. 305/949-9464; Martin E. Casper, Executive Director

Harborside Healthcare Tampa Bay Rehabilitation and Nursing Center, 3865 Tampa Road, Oldsmar, FL 34677; tel. 813/855-4661; FAX. 813/854-2129; Michele Forney

Harborside Healthcare-Palm Harbor, 2600 Highlands Boulevard, N., Palm Harbor, FL 34684; tel. 813/785-5671; FAX. 813/787-5486; Sharon Harris, Administrator

Harborside Healthcare-Pinebrook, 1240 Pinebrook Road, Venice, FL 34292; tel. 813/488-6733; FAX. 813/484-7924; Connie Tolley, Administrator

Harborside Healthcare-Sarasota, 4602 Northgate Court, Sarasota, FL 34234; tel. 813/355-2913; FAX. 813/355-4259; Stephen Buillard

Hardee Manor Care Center, 401 Orange Place, Wauchula, FL 33873; tel. 813/773-3231; FAX. 813/773-0959; Mary Love, Administrator

HealthPark Care Center, 16131 Rose Rush Court, Fort Meyers, FL 33908; tel. 813/433-4647; FAX. 813/432-3456; Spring Rosen

Heartland Health Care Center Miami Lakes, 5725 Northwest 186th Street, Hialeah, FL 33015; tel. 305/625-9857; FAX. 305/621-3682; Reid Aaron, FACHE, Administrator

Heartland Health Care Center-Jacksonville, 8495 Normandy Boulevard, Jacksonville, FL 32221; tel. 904/783-3749; FAX. 904/693-9137; Larry Potter, Administrator

Heartland Health Care Center-Sunrise, 9711 West Oakland Park Boulevard, Sunrise, FL 33351; tel. 305/572-4000; FAX. 305/749-4927; Joylin Nation

Heartland Health Care and Rehabilitaiton Center, 5401 Sawyer Road, Sarasota, FL 34233; tel. 941/925-3427; FAX. 941/925-8469; Elizabeth A. Bess, Administrator

Heartland Health Care and Rehabilitation Center, 7225 Boca Del Mar Drive, Boca Raton, FL 33433-5517; tel. 407/362-9644; FAX. 407/362-9641; Jerry Labouene, Chief Executive Officer

Heartland Healthcare Convalescent Center, 3600 Boynton Road, Boynton Beach, FL 33436; tel. 407/736-9992; FAX. 407/369-0019; Martha A. Davis, Mobile Director of Nursing

Heartland Healthcare of Lauderhill, 2599 Northwest 55th Avenue, Fort Lauderdale, FL 33313; tel. 305/485-8873; FAX. 305/484-1951; Mavis Matthews, Administrator

Heartland of Tamarac, 5901 Northwest 79th Avenue, Tamarac, FL 33321; tel. 954/722-7001; FAX. 954/720-5419; Susan Robertson, Administrator

Heartland of Zephyrhills, 38220 Henry Drive, Zephyrhills, FL 33540; tel. 813/788-7114; FAX. 813/788-0758; Joyce Plourde

IHS at Avenel, 7751 West Broward Boulevard, Plantation, FL 33324; tel. 954/473-8040; FAX. 954/473-0897; Rosemary Wedderspoon, Administrator

IHS at Central Park Village, 9311 South Orange Blossom Trail, Orlando, FL 32837; tel. 407/858-0455; FAX. 407/850-2470; Nancy Thompson, Administrator

IHS at Green Briar (Integrated Health Services), 9820 North Kendall Drive, Miami, FL 33176; tel. 305/271-6311; FAX. 305/274-5880; Diane King, Administrator

IHS of Bradenton, 2302 59th Street, W., Bradenton, FL 34209; tel. 941/792-8480; FAX. 941/794-8905; Nina Willingham, NHA

IHS of Florida at Sarasota Pavilion, 2600 Courtland Street, Sarasota, FL 34237; tel. 941/365-2926; FAX. 941/951-2015; Gary Duncanson, Administrator

IHS of Port Charlotte, 4033 Beaver Lane, Port Charlotte, FL 33952; tel. 941/625-3200; FAX. 941/624-2358; Todd B. Mehaffey, Administrator

IHS of Venice North, 437 South Nokomis Avenue, Venice, FL 34285; tel. 941/488-9696; FAX. 941/484-1321; Louis Maltaghati, Administrator

Integrated Health Services, 702 South Kings Avenue, Brandon, FL 33511; tel. 813/651-1818; FAX. 813/654-4252; Jack Lehman

Integrated Health Services at Fort Pierce, 703 South 29th Street, Fort Pierce, FL 34947; tel. 407/466-3322; FAX. 407/466-8057; Max Hauth

Integrated Health Services at Gainesville, 4000 Southwest 20th Avenue, Gainesville, FL 32607; tel. 904/377-1981; FAX. 904/377-7340; Terrye Dubberly

Integrated Health Services of Central Florida at Orlando, 1900 Mercy Drive, Orlando, FL 32808; tel. 407/299-5404; FAX. 407/299-3735; Susan Daube

Integrated Health Services of Florida at Clearwater, 2055 Palmetto Street, Clearwater, FL 34625; tel. 813/461-6613; FAX. 813/422-2839; Ann Dougherty

Integrated Health Services of Florida at Jacksonville, 1650 Fouraker Road, Jacksonville, FL 32221; tel. 904/786-8668; FAX. 904/695-0166; James Lundy

Integrated Health Services of Florida at Lake Worth, 1201 12th Avenue, S., Lake Worth, FL 33460; tel. 407/586-7404; FAX. 407/582-2887; Adela Baldo

Integrated Health Services of Florida at West Palm Beach, 2939 South Haverhill Road, West Palm Beach, FL 33415; tel. 561/641-3130; FAX. 561/641-3167; Victor Field, Administrator

Integrated Health Services of Lakeland at Oakbridge, 3110 Oakbridge Boulevard, E., Lakeland, FL 33803; tel. 941/648-4800; FAX. 941/646-9224; Scott J. Allen, Administrator

Integrated Health Services of Palm Bay, 1515 Port Malabar Boulevard, Palm Bay, FL 32905; tel. 407/723-1235; FAX. 407/724-4292; Gregory Roberts, Administrator

Integrated Health Services of Pinellas Park, 8710 49th Street, N., Pinellas Park, FL 34666; tel. 813/546-4661; FAX. 813/545-8783; Julie Moyer

Integrated Health Services of Sebring, 3011 Kenilworth Boulevard, Sebring, FL 33870; tel. 941/382-2153; FAX. 941/382-2039; Eric Britt

Integrated Health Services of St. Petersburg, 811 Jackson Street, St. Petersburg, FL 33705; tel. 813/896-3651; FAX. 813/821-2453; H. Sandra Hugg, Administrator

Integrated Health Services of Tarpon Springs, 900 Beckett Way, Tarpon Springs, FL 34689; tel. 813/934-0876; FAX. 813/942-6790; Paul Vitale

Integrated Health Services of Vero Beach, 3663 15th Avenue, Vero Beach, FL 32960; tel. 561/567-2552; FAX. 561/567-8929; Ronnie Schuessler, Administrator

Integrated Health Services of Winter Park, 2970 Scarlet Road, Winter Park, FL 32792; tel. 407/671-8030; FAX. 407/671-3746; Todd Werthman, Administrator

Integrated Health Services, Inc., 919 Old Winter Haven Road, Auburndale, FL 33823; tel. 941/967-4125; FAX. 941/551-9407; Nancy Thompson

Leesburg Nursing Center, 715 East Dixie Avenue, Leesburg, FL 34748; tel. 352/728-3020; FAX. 352/728-6071; Robert E. Rice, Administrator

Manor Care Carrollwood, MedBridge Medical and Physical Rehabilitation, 3030 West Bearss Avenue, Tampa, FL 33618; tel. 813/968-8777; FAX. 813/961-5189; Nancy Caras, Administrator

Manor Care Health Services, 870 Patricia Avenue, Dunedin, FL 34968; tel. 813/734-8861; FAX. 813/733-5924; Debra Pattinson, NHA

Manor Care Health Services Nursing and Rehabilitation Center, 6931 West Sunrise Boulevard, Plantation, FL 33313; tel. 305/583-6200; FAX. 305/583-6007; Gilda Anderson, Administrator

Manor Care Nursing Center, 3001 South Congress Avenue, Boynton Beach, FL 33426; tel. 407/737-5600; FAX. 407/731-3049; Alicia Erb

Manor Care Nursing and Rehabilitation Center, 3648 University Boulevard, Jacksonville, FL 32216; tel. 904/733-7440; FAX. 904/731-7219; Clara Corcoran, NHA, Executive Director

ManorCare Health Services of Boca Raton, 375 Northwest 51st Street, Boca Raton, FL 33431; tel. 407/997-8111; FAX. 407/995-0109; Dieudegrace Achille

Mariner Health Care of Orange City, 2810 Enterprise Road, Debary, FL 32713; tel. 407/668-8818; FAX. 407/668-6510; Cathy Holland, NHA

Mariner Health of Palm City, 2505 Southwest Martin Highway, Palm City, FL 34990; tel. 407/288-0060; FAX. 407/288-3218; Tim Kimes

Mariner Health of Port Orange, 5600 Victoria Gardens Boulevard, Daytona Beach, FL 32127; tel. 904/760-7773; FAX. 904/760-8949; Dennis O'Leary

Mediplex Rehabilitation-Bradenton, 5627 Ninth Street, E., Bradenton, FL 34203; tel. 813/753-8941; FAX. 813/753-7576; Raymond Fusco, Chief Executive Officer

Menorah Manor, 255 59th Street, N., Saint Petersburg, FL 33710; tel. 813/345-2775; Marshall Seiden, Chief Executive Officer

Moody Manor, Inc., 7150 Holatee Trail, Fort Lauderdale, FL 33330; tel. 305/434-2016; FAX. 305/434-0561; Leonard J. Hoenig, Medical Director

Mount Sinai St. Francis Nursing and Rehabilitation Center, 201 Northeast 112th Street, Miami, FL 33161; tel. 305/899-4700; FAX. 305/899-4719; Morris Funk, Executive Director

Oakwood Rehabilitation and Health Care Center, 301 South Bay Street, Eustis, FL 32726; tel. 904/357-8105; FAX. 904/589-1182; Susan Chancellor

Palm Garden of Largo, 10500 Starkey Road, Largo, FL 33777; tel. 813/397-8166; FAX. 813/319-3704; David Cross, Administrator

Palm Garden of Pinellas, 200 16th Avenue, S.E., Largo, FL 34641; tel. 813/585-9377; FAX. 813/588-9038; Mary Bladen, Administrator

Palmetto Health Center, 6750 West 22nd Court, Hialeah, FL 33016-3918; tel. 305/823-3119; FAX. 305/825-8255; Diana P. Rodriguez, Administrator

Plantation Bay Rehabilitation Center, 401 Kissimmee Park Road, Saint Cloud, FL 34769; tel. 407/892-7344; FAX. 407/892-5244; Glenn Grissinger

Public Health Trust, Jackson Memorial Medical Center, Human Resources Health Center, 2500 Northwest 22nd Avenue, Miami, FL 33142; tel. 305/585-7137; FAX. 305/585-5355; Sylviane Ward, Vice President

Section C

Rio Pinar, 7950 Lake Underhill Road, Orlando, FL 32822; tel. 407/658–2046; FAX. 407/249–2226; Lou Ann Mathews

River Garden Hebrew Home for the Aged, 11401 Old St. Augustine Road, Jacksonville, FL 32258; tel. 904/260–1818; FAX. 904/260–9733; Martin A. Goetz, Administrator

Southern Pines Nursing Center, 6140 Congress Street, New Port Richey, FL 34653; tel. 813/842–8402; FAX. 813/846–9107; Vern V. Charbonneau, Administrator

St. Catherine Labouré' Manor, Inc., 1750 Stockton Street, Jacksonville, FL 32204; tel. 904/308–4700; FAX. 904/308–2987; Maureen Gartland, CNHA, Vice President, Administrator

Sun Health of the Palm Beaches, 6414 13th Road, S., West Palm Beach, FL 33415; tel. 407/478–9900; FAX. 407/478–5067; Kathryn Saretsky

Surrey Place Center, 110 Southeast Lee Avenue, Live Oak, FL 32060; tel. 904/364–5961; FAX. 904/364–1656; Larry Brincefield

Sutton Place Center, 4405 Lakewood Road, Lake Worth, FL 33461; tel. 561/969–1400; FAX. 561/969–0121; Garland Cline, Administrator

Tierra Pines Center, 7380 Ulmerton Road, Largo, FL 33771; tel. 813/535–9833; FAX. 813/536–4525; Maureen Cunningham

Woodland's Rehabilitation and Health Care Center, 13806 North 46th Street, Tampa, FL 33613; tel. 813/977–4514; Jim Fielding

GEORGIA

American Transitional Care–Northside, 993 East Johnson Ferry Road, Building E, Atlanta, GA 30342; tel. 404/256–5131; FAX. 404/257–1820; Brian Williams, Executive Director

Beverly Health and Rehabilitation Center, 2650 Highway 138, Jonesboro, GA 30236; tel. 404/473–4436; FAX. 404/473–4698; Patricia Osterhout, Executive Director

Brook Run, Facility of the Georgia Department of Human Resource, 4770 North Peachtree Road, Dunwoody, GA 30338; tel. 770/551–7157; FAX. 770/551–7040; Rudy Magnone, Ph.D., Interim Superintendent

Dublinair Health Care and Rehabilitation Center, 300 Industrial Boulevard, Dublin, GA 31021, P.O. Box 1243, Dublin, GA 31040; tel. 912/272–7437; FAX. 912/272–2427; Janice Wiley

Family Life Enrichment Centers, Inc., 3450 New High Shoals Road, High Shoals, GA 30645; tel. 706/769–7738; FAX. 706/769–5944; Magda D. Bennett, Administrator

Georgia War Veterans Nursing Home, 1101 15th Street, Augusta, GA 30901; tel. 706/721–2531; FAX. 706/721–3892; Charles Esposito, Administrator

Integrated Health Services at Briarcliff Haven, Inc., 1000 Briarcliff Road, N.E., Atlanta, GA 30306; tel. 404/875–6456; FAX. 404/874–4606; Stephanie Seay, Administrator

Manor Care Nursing and Rehabilitation Center, 2722 North Decatur Road, Decatur, GA 30033; tel. 404/296–5440; FAX. 404/294–0504; Will Blackwell, Administrator

Mariner Health of Northeast Atlanta, 1500 South Johnson Ferry Road, Atlanta, GA 30319; tel. 404/252–2002; FAX. 404/252–1246; Barbara Barron, MHA, Administrator

Montezuma Health Care Center, 521 Sumter Street, P.O. Box 639, Montezuma, GA 31063; tel. 912/472–8168; FAX. 912/472–8168; Merle Baggett, Administrator

Oak Manor and Pine Manor Nursing Homes, Inc., 2010 Warm Springs Road, P.O. Box 8828, Columbus, GA 31904–8828; tel. 404/324–0387; FAX. 706/324–0927; Caroline L. Nahley, RN, Administrator

Specialty Care of Marietta, 26 Tower Road, Marietta, GA 30060–9109; tel. 770/422–8913; FAX. 770/425–2085; Betsy Hill

Winthrop Manor Nursing Center, 12 Chateau Drive, Rome, GA 30161; tel. 706/235–1422; FAX. 706/236–9247; Bruce Behner

ILLINOIS

Alma Nelson Manor, Inc., 550 South Mulford, Rockford, IL 61108; tel. 815/399–4914; FAX. 815/399–0054; Teresa Wester–Peters, Administrator

Apostolic Christian Restmor, Inc., 935 East Jefferson, Morton, IL 61550; tel. 309/266–7141; FAX. 309/266–7877; James L. Metzger, Executive Director

Ballard, a Healthcare Residence, 9300 Ballard Road, Des Plaines, IL 60016; tel. 847/294–2300; FAX. 847/299–4012; Kristin Joyce, Director, Community Services

Barton W. Stone Christian Home, 873 Grove Street, Jacksonville, IL 62650; tel. 217/479–3400; FAX. 217/243–8553; Marla G. Gregory, Business Manager, Nursing

Bethany Terrace Nursing Centre, 8425 North Waukegan Road, Morton Grove, IL 60053; tel. 847/965–8100; FAX. 847/965–8104; Virginia Barry, Administrator

Carlton at the Lake, Inc., 725 West Montrose Avenue, Chicago, IL 60613; tel. 773/929–1700; FAX. 773/929–3068; Rose Marie Betz, RN

Chateau Village Nursing and Rehabilitation Center, 7050 Madison Street, Willowbrook, IL 60521; tel. 708/323–6380; FAX. 708/323–6416; Nancy Hartman, Administrator

Community Convalescent Center of Naperville, 1136 North Mill Street, Naperville, IL 60563; tel. 630/355–3300; FAX. 630/355–1417; Jill Meyer, Executive Director

Council for Jewish Elderly–Lieberman Geriatric Health Centre, 9700 Gross Point Road, Skokie, IL 60076; tel. 847/674–7210; FAX. 847/674–6366; Barbara Wexler, Administrator

Douglas Healthcare Center, West Route 121, P.O. Box 978, Matoon, IL 61938; tel. 217/234–6401; FAX. 217/258–3300; David Moore, Administrator

DuPage Convalescent Center, 400 North County Farm Road, P.O. Box 708, Wheaton, IL 60189; tel. 630/665–6400; FAX. 630/665–2446; Ronald Reinecke

Fairview Baptist Home, 250 Village Drive, Downers Grove, IL 60516–3099; tel. 630/769–6200; FAX. 630/769–6226; Grace M. Jones, Vice President

Galena Park Home, 5533 North Galena Road, Peoria Heights, IL 61614; tel. 309/682–5428; FAX. 309/682–8478; Jane S. Foster, Administrator

Glenview Terrace Nursing Center, 1511 Greenwood Road, Glenview, IL 60025; tel. 708/729–9090; FAX. 708/729–9135; Mark Hollander

Harmony Nursing and Rehabilitation Center, 3919 West Foster Avenue, Chicago, IL 60625; tel. 312/588–9500; FAX. 312/588–9533; Mark Hollander

Heartland Health Care Center, 833 Sixteen Avenue, Moline, IL 61265; tel. 309/764–6744; FAX. 309/764–8176; Lynn Zuck, Administrator

Heartland Health Care Center of Homewood, 940 Maple Avenue, Homewood, IL 60430; tel. 708/799–0244; FAX. 708/799–1500; John K. Graham, Director, Operation Support

Heartland Health Care Center–Henry, 1650 Indian T Road, P.O. Box 215, Henry, IL 61537; tel. 309/364–3905; FAX. 309/364–3119; Susan Legner

Heartland Health Care Center–Macomb, Eight Doctors Lane, Macomb, IL 61455; tel. 309/833–5555; FAX. 309/833–3749; Ronald Eaker

Heartland of Paxton, 1001 East Pells Street, Paxton, IL 60957; tel. 217/379–4361; FAX. 217/379–3325; Cindy Scharp, Administrator

Hillside Healthcare Center, 1308 Game Farm Road, Yorkville, IL 60560; tel. 708/553–5811; FAX. 708/553–2740; Nancy Tettemer, Administrator

Integrated Health Services at Brentwood, 5400 West 87th Street, Burbank, IL 60459; tel. 708/423–1200; FAX. 708/423–8405; Wm. David Terry, Executive Director

Manor Care Health Services, 6300 West 95th Street, Oak Lawn, IL 60453; tel. 707/599–8800; FAX. 708/599–8820; Brian Gross

Manor Care Health Services, 715 West Central Road, Arlington Heights, IL 60005; tel. 708/392–2020; FAX. 708/392–0174; Katherine Keane

Manor Care Health Services, 9401 South Kostner Avenue, Oak Lawn, IL 60453; tel. 708/423–7882; FAX. 708/423–7947; Susan Lucas

Manor Care Health Services, 2145 East 170th Street, South Holland, IL 60473; tel. 708/895–3255; FAX. 708/895–3315; Gina Weidner

Manor Care Health Services, 600 North Coler, Urbana, IL 61801; tel. 217/367–1191; FAX. 217/367–1194; Dorothy Mikucki

Manor Care Health Services, 600 West Ogden, Hinsdale, IL 60521; tel. 708/325–9630; FAX. 708/325–9648; Jeane Hansen

Manor Health Care Services, 512 East Ogden Avenue, Westmont, IL 60559; tel. 708/323–4400; FAX. 708/323–4583; Patricia Patrick

Oakton Pavilion Healthcare Facility, Inc., 1660 Oakton Place, Des Plaines, IL 60018; tel. 847/299–5588; FAX. 847/298–6017; Jay Lewkowitz, ACSW, Administrator

P.A. Peterson Center for Health, 1311 Parkview Avenue, Rockford, IL 61107; tel. 815/399–8832; FAX. 815/399–8342; Stella L. Schroeder

Park Strathmoor Subacute Hospital, 5668 Strathmoor Drive, Rockford, IL 61107; tel. 815/229–5200; FAX. 815/229–1411; Laura Gruetzmacher, Administrator

Parkway Healthcare Center, 219 East Parkway Drive, Wheaton, IL 60187; tel. 630/668–4635; FAX. 630/668–4649; Beth A. LaPointe, Administrator

Piatt County Nursing Home, 1111 North State Street, Monticello, IL 61856; tel. 217/762–2506; FAX. 217/762–9926; Marilyn E. Benedino, Administrator

Pine Acres Care Center, 1212 South Second Street, DeKalb, IL 60115; tel. 815/758–8151; FAX. 815/758–6832; Rex Pippin

Pinecrest Manor, 414 South Wesley Avenue, Mount Morris, IL 61054; tel. 815/734–4103; FAX. 815/734–7318; Vernon C. Showalter, Administrator

Plymouth Place, Inc., 315 North LaGrange Road, LaGrange Park, IL 60526; tel. 708/354–0340; FAX. 708/482–6847; Gloria E. Bialek, Executive Director

Regency Nursing Centre, 6631 North Milwaukee Avenue, Niles, IL 60714; tel. 847/647–7444; FAX. 847/647–6403; Barbara A. Hecht, Administrator

Rest Haven Central Skilled Nursing Care Residence, 13259 South Central Avenue, Palos Heights, IL 60463; tel. 708/597–1000; FAX. 708/389–9990; Richard Schutt

Rest Haven West Christian Nursing Home, 3450 Saratoga, Downers Grove, IL 60515; tel. 630/969–2900; FAX. 630/969–2148; Jacquelyn Terpstra, Administrator

Resurrection Nursing and Rehabilitation Center, 1001 North Greenwood Avenue, Park Ridge, IL 60068; tel. 847/692–5600; FAX. 847/692–2305; Arthur B. Koenigsberger, Senior Vice President

Sherman West Court, 1950 Larkin Avenue, Elgin, IL 60123; tel. 847/742–7070; FAX. 847/742–7248; Anne Huang, Administrator

St. Matthew Lutheran Home, 1601 North Western Avenue, Park Ridge, IL 60068; tel. 847/825–5531; FAX. 847/318–6659; Rue Anne Harris, Administrator

The Admiral, The Old People's Home of the City of Chicago, 909 West Foster Avenue, Chicago, IL 60640; tel. 312/561–2900; FAX. 312/561–2573; Toby A. Turner

The Anchorage of Bensenville, Lifelink Corporation, 111 East Washington Street, Bensenville, IL 60106; tel. 630/766–5800, ext. 206; FAX. 630/595–5473; Jane M. Muller, Administrator

The Imperial Convalescent and Geriatric Center, 1366 West Fullerton Avenue, Chicago, IL 60614; tel. 312/248–9300; FAX. 312/935–0036; Margaret Carlson, Administrator

INDIANA

American Transitional Care–Brookview, 7145 East 21st Street, Indianapolis, IN 46219; tel. 317/356–0977; FAX. 317/356–2484; Todd Taylor

Americana Healthcare Center of Indianapolis–North, 8350 Naab Road, Indianapolis, IN 46260; tel. 317/872–4051; FAX. 317/879–2314; Robert J. Couch, Administrator

Arbors at Fort Wayne, 2827 Northgate Boulevard, Fort Wayne, IN 46835; tel. 219/492–1400; FAX. 219/486–5725; Carol Simmons, Administrator

Covington Manor Health Care Center, 1600 East Liberty Street, Covington, IN 47932; tel. 317/793–4818; FAX. 317/793–3748; Christopher D. Baldwin, Administrator

Harborside Healthcare of Terre Haute, 1001 East Springhill Drive, Terre Haute, IN 47802; tel. 812/238–2441; FAX. 812/299–4492; Karen Rumple

Holiday Care Center, 1201 West Buena Vista Road, Evansville, IN 47710; tel. 812/429–0700; FAX. 812/429–1849; Don Hester, Administrator

Integrated Health Services of Indianapolis at Cambridge, 8530 Township Line Road, Indianapolis, IN 46260; tel. 317/876–9955; FAX. 317/876–6016; Sara L. Freeman, Executive Director

Lifeline Children's Hospital, 1707 West 86th Street, P.O. Box 40407, Indianapolis, IN 46240–0407; tel. 317/872–0555; FAX. 317/471–0058; David Carter, Executive Director

Manor Care Health Services–Indianapolis South, 8549 South Madson Avenue, Indianapolis, IN 46227; tel. 317/881–9164; FAX. 317/887–4060; Clifford Craddock

Miller's Merry Manor, 1500 Grant Street, Huntington, IN 46750; tel. 219/356–5713; FAX. 219/356–8671; Jack Schaefer, Administrator

Miller's Merry Manor, 200 26th Street, Logansport, IN 46947; tel. 219/722–4006; FAX. 219/753–8753; Gregory Fassett, Administrator

Northwest Manor Health Care Center, 6440 West 34th Street, Indianapolis, IN 46224; tel. 371/293–4930; Jennifer A. Knoll, Administrator

Vermillion Convalescent and Rehabilitation Center, 1705 South Main Street, Clinton, IN 47842; tel. 317/832–3573; FAX. 317/832–3420; Melissa Diane Gum, Administrator

IOWA

Anamosa Care Center, 1209 East Third Street, Anamosa, IA 52205; tel. 319/462–4356; FAX. 319/462–5038; Jeff Wollum, Administrator

Bettendorf Health Care Center, 2730 Crow Creek Road, Bettendorf, IA 52722; tel. 319/332–7463; FAX. 319/332–7464; Susan Morton, Administrator

Danville Care Center, 401 South Birch, Danville, IA 52623; tel. 319/392–4259; Michael W. Hocking, Administrator

Edgewood Convalescent Home, 513 Bell Street, Edgewood, IA 52042; tel. 319/928–6461; FAX. 319/928–6462; Ruth M. Stephens

Elkader Care Center, 116 Reimer Street, Elkader, IA 52043; tel. 319/245–1620; Kris Mitchell, Administrator

Great River Care Center, 1400 West Main, P.O. Box 370, McGregor, IA 52157; tel. 319/873–3527; FAX. 319/873–3723; Raletta W. Thomas, Administrator

Health Care Manor, 703 South Fourth Avenue, New Hampton, IA 50659; tel. 515/394–4153; Michael W. Rissien, Administrator

Iowa Veterans Home, 1301 Summit Street, Marshalltown, IA 50158–5485; tel. 515/752–1501; FAX. 515/753–4278; Jack J. Dack, Commandant

Living Center East, 1220 Fifth Avenue, S.E., Cedar Rapids, IA 52403; tel. 319/366–8701; Thomas Wagg

Living Center West, 1050 Fourth Avenue, S.E., Cedar Rapids, IA 52403; tel. 319/366–8714; FAX. 319/366–8854; Marian Stevenson, NHA

Lone Tree Health Care Center, 501 East Pioneer Road, Lone Tree, IA 52755; tel. 319/629–4255; FAX. 319/629–5300; Roberta Shirkey, Administrator

Mill Valley Care Center, 1201 Park Avenue, Bellevue, IA 52031–1911; tel. 319/872–5521; Glinda L. Manternach, Administrator

Monticello Nursing and Rehabilitation Center, 500 Pinehaven Drive, Monticello, IA 52310; tel. 319/465–5415; FAX. 319/465–3205; Sister Donna Venteicher, Administrator

New London Care Center, 100 Care Circle, New London, IA 52645; tel. 319/367–5753; Michael W. Hocking, Administrator

Ramsey Home, 1611 27th Street, Des Moines, IA 50310; tel. 515/274–3612; FAX. 515/274–6541; Loretta Nelson

State Center Manor, 702 Third Street, N.W., State Center, IA 50247; tel. 515/483–2812; FAX. 515/483–2675; Lance Mehaffey, Administrator

Wheatland Manor, Inc., 515 East Lincolnway, Wheatland, IA 52777; tel. 319/374–1295; FAX. 319/374–1107; Jack L. McIntosh, Administrator

KENTUCKY

American Transitional Care–Hillcreek, 3116 Breckenridge Lane, Louisville, KY 40220; tel. 502/459–9120; FAX. 502/459–6150; Philip Bramer

Christopher East Health Care Center, 4200 Brown's Lane, Louisville, KY 40220; tel. 502/459–8900; FAX. 502/459–5026; Thomas J. Martin, Senior Administrator

Florence Park Care Center, 6975 Burlington Pike, Florence, KY 41042; tel. 606/525–0007; FAX. 606/282–4516; Eileen A. Brennan, Administrator

Hurstbourne Care Center at Stony Brook, 2200 Stony Brook Drive, Louisville, KY 40220; tel. 502/425–3620; FAX. 502/425–3662; Robert Bates

Winchester Centre for Health and Rehabilitation, 200 Glenway Road, Winchester, KY 40391; tel. 606/744–1800; FAX. 606/744–0285; Damie U. Castle, Executive Director

LOUISIANA

Gillis W. Long Hansen's Disease Center, 5445 Point Clair Road, Carville, LA 70721–9607; tel. 504/642–4740; FAX. 504/642–4728; Robert R. Jacobson, M.D., Ph.D., Director

Greenery Neurologic Rehabilitation Center at Slidell, 1400 Lindberg Drive, Slidell, LA 70458; tel. 504/641–4985, ext. 3003; FAX. 504/646–0728; James L. McEwen, Ph.D., Executive Director

Lafon Nursing Home of the Holy Family, 6900 Chef Menteur Highway, New Orleans, LA 70126; tel. 504/246–1100; FAX. 504/241–6672; Sister Ann Elise Sonnier, Chief Executive Officer

MAINE

Brewer Rehab and Living Center, 74 Parkway, S., Brewer, ME 04412; tel. 207/989–7300; FAX. 207/989–4240; Carl F. Hausler, Administrator

Cedar Ridge Center for Health Care and Rehabilitation, Dr. Mann Road, Rural Route 1, Box 1283, Skowhegan, ME 04976; tel. 207/474–9686; FAX. 207/474–8626; Stephen A. Marsden, Administrator

Marshwood Nursing Care Center, Roger Street, Lewistown, ME 04240; tel. 207/784–0108; FAX. 207/784–0752; Paul Schreiber

Oak Grove Nursing Care Center, 27 Cool Street, Waterville, ME 04901; tel. 207/873–0721; FAX. 207/877–2287; Sara Sylvester

Pine Point Nursing Care Center, 67 Pine Point Road, Scarborough, ME 04074; tel. 207/883–2468; FAX. 207/883–3983; Barbara Rentz–Champagne

River Ridge, 33 Cat Mousam Road, Kennebunk, ME 04043; tel. 207/985–3030; FAX. 207/985–6428; Irving Faunce, Executive Director

Sandy River Center for Health Care and Rehabilitation, RFD 4, Box 5121, Farmington, ME 04938; tel. 207/778–6591; FAX. 207/778–4245; Anne Herrick

Springbrook Nursing Care Center, 300 Spring Street, Westbrook, ME 04092; tel. 207/856–1230; FAX. 207/856–1239; Pierre Morneault

Windward Gardens, 105 Mechanic Street, Camden, ME 04843; tel. 207/236–4197; FAX. 207/236–4453; Bill Chase

Woodford Park Center for Health Care and Rehabilitation, 68 Devonshire Street, Portland, ME 04103; tel. 207/772–2893; FAX. 207/772–3230; Ted Purdy, Executive Director

MARYLAND

Carriage Hill Nursing Center, 9101 Second Avenue, Silver Spring, MD 20910; tel. 301/588–5544; FAX. 301/588–0788; Teri Karr, Administrator

Fox Chase Rehabilitation and Nursing Center, 2015 East West Highway, Silver Spring, MD 20910; tel. 301/587–2400; FAX. 301/587–2404; Mary Clinton, Administrator

Horizon Specialty Care Center at Canton Harbor, 1300 South Ellwood Avenue, Baltimore, MD 21224; tel. 410/342–6644; FAX. 410/327–3949; Donna Yorkston, Administrator

Keswick Multi–Care Center, 700 West 40th Street, Baltimore, MD 21211; tel. 410/235–8860, ext. 201; FAX. 410/235–7425; Andrea Braid, Executive Director, Chief Executive Officer

Larkin Chase Nursing and Restorative Center, 15005 Health Center Drive, Bowie, MD 20716; tel. 301/805–6070; FAX. 301/805–9779; Gary Waitt

Manor Care Health Services, 6600 Ridge Road, Baltimore, MD 21237; tel. 410/574–4950; FAX. 410/391–4386; L. Zimmerman

Manor Care Health Services, 11901 Georgia Avenue, Wheaton, MD 20902; tel. 301/942–2500; FAX. 301/949–1152; Barb Feege, NHA

Manor Care Ruxton Center, 7001 North Charles Street, Towson, MD 21204; tel. 410/821–9600; FAX. 410/337–8313; Robert F. Harris, Administrator

Manor Care Towson Nursing and Rehabilitation Center, 509 East Joppa Road, Towson, MD 21285; tel. 410/828–9494; FAX. 410/828–9180; Ann Schiff, Administrator

Manor Care–Largo, 600 Largo Road, Largo, MD 20772; tel. 301/350–5555; FAX. 301/350–2871; Stewart Bainum

Mariner Health at Circle Manor, 10231 Carroll Place, Kensington, MD 20895; tel. 301/949–0230; FAX. 301/949–8244; Melinda Hippchen, NHA

Mariner Health of Kensington, 3000 McComas Avenue, Kensington, MD 20895; tel. 301/933–0060; Deborah Toth

Mariner Health of Silver Spring, 901 Arcola Avenue, Silver Spring, MD 20902; tel. 301/649–2400; FAX. 301/649–2081; Jane Blum

MASSACHUSETTS

Ads Reservoir, Inc., 1841 Trapelo Road, Waltham, MA 02154; tel. 617/890–5000; FAX. 617/290–0535; Paul Brisson, Executive Director

Alden Court Nursing Care and Rehabilitation Center, 389 Alden Road, Fairhaven, MA 02719; tel. 508/991–8600; David Manahan

Apple Valley Nursing and Rehabilitation Center, 400 Groton Road, Ayer, MA 01432; tel. 508/772–1704; FAX. 508/772–1708; Michael Lehrman

Avery Manor, 100 West Street, Needham, MA 02194; tel. 617/433–0202; FAX. 617/433–2777; Diane O'Brien, Administrator

Bay Path at Duxbury Nursing and Rehabilitation Center, 308 Kings Town Way, Duxbury, MA 02332; tel. 617/585–5561; FAX. 617/585–1481; Marianne Welch–Martinez, Administrator

Baypointe Rehabilitation and Skilled Care Center, 50 Christy Place, Brockton, MA 02401; tel. 508/580–6800; FAX. 508/587–6633; Kimberly Tobin Sciacca, Administrator

Beaumont Rehabilitation and Skilled Nursing Center, One Lyman Street, Westborough, MA 01581; tel. 508/366–9933; FAX. 508/898–3931; Michael Murphy, Administrator

Birchwood Care Center, Outpatient Rehab Clinic, 1199 John Fitch Highway, Fitchburg, MA 01420; tel. 508/345–0146; FAX. 508/345–4053; Scott Dickinson

Blaire House of Tewksbury, 10 Erlin Terrace, Tewksbury, MA 01876; tel. 508/851–3121; FAX. 508/640–0981; Frank Romano

Blueberry Hill Healthcare, 75 Brimbal Avenue, Beverly, MA 01915; tel. 508/927–2020; FAX. 508/922–4643; Dan Micherone

Boston Center for Rehabilitative and Subacute Care, 1245 Centre Street, Roslindale, MA 02131; tel. 617/325–5400; FAX. 617/325–3259; Frank Silvia, Executive Director

Bostonian Nursing Care and Rehabilitation Center, 337 Neponset Avenue, Dorchester, MA 02122; tel. 617/265–2350; FAX. 617/265–0577; Wayne Pultman

Braemoor Rehabilitation and Nursing Center, Inc., 34 North Pearl Street, Brockton, MA 02401; tel. 508/586–3696; FAX. 508/584–0470; Michael Roland

Braintree Manor Rehabilitation and Nursing Center, 1102 Washington Street, Braintree, MA 02184; tel. 617/848–3100; FAX. 617/356–7367; Elizabeth Flynn, Administrator

Brandon Woods of Dartmouth, 567 Dartmouth Street, South Dartmouth, MA 02748; tel. 508/997–7787; FAX. 508/997–5598; Frank Romano

Briarwood Healthcare Nursing Center, 150 Lincoln Street, Needham, MA 01292; tel. 617/449–4040; FAX. 617/449–4129; Penny Packard, Director, Nursing Service

Cape Regency Nursing and Rehabilitation Center, 120 South Main Street, Centerville, MA 02632; tel. 508/778–1835; FAX. 508/771–7411; Mary E. Benoit, Administrator

Carlyle Nursing Home, Inc., 342 Winter Street, P.O. Box 2495, Framingham, MA 01701; tel. 508/879–6100; FAX. 508/872–1253; Bruce Bedard

Catholic Memorial Home, 2446 Highland Avenue, Fall River, MA 02720; tel. 508/679–0011; FAX. 508/672–5858; Sister Nina Marie Amaral O. Carm., Administrator

Charlwell House, 305 Walpole Street, Norwood, MA 02062; tel. 617/762–7700; FAX. 617/255–0387; Barbara Iarrobino, Administrator

Chestnut Hill Rehabilitation and Nursing Center, 32 Chestnut Street, East Longmeadow, MA 01028; tel. 413/525–1893; FAX. 413/525–8261; Theresa A. Williams, Director, Nursing

Chetwynde Health and Rehabilitation Center, 1650 Washington Street, West Newton, MA 02165; tel. 617/244–5407; FAX. 617/244–9322; Thomas Sullivan, Executive Director

Clark House Nursing Center at Fox Hill Village, 30 Longwood Drive, Westwood, MA 02090; tel. 617/326–5652; FAX. 617/326–4034; Karen Wilkinson, Administrator

Clifton Rehabilitative Nursing Center, 500 Wilbur Avenue, Somerset, MA 02725; tel. 508/675–7589; FAX. 508/672–7422; Clifton Greenwood

Cohasset Knoll Skilled Nursing and Rehabilitation Facility, One Chief Justice Cushing Highway, Cohasset, MA 02025; tel. 617/383–9060; FAX. 617/383–2327; John Corliss, Administrator

Colonial Nursing and Rehabilitation Center, 125 Broad Street, Weymouth, MA 02188; tel. 617/337-3121; FAX. 617/337-9831; F. Roy Fitzsimmons, Administrator

Colony House Nursing and Rehabilitation Center, 277 Washington Street, Abington, MA 02351; tel. 617/871-0200; FAX. 617/878-0661; Paul Corcoran, Administrator

Coolidge House Nursing Care Center, 30 Webster Street, Brookline, MA 02146; tel. 617/734-2300; FAX. 617/232-1131; Dolores Schermer

Country Estates Nursing and Rehabilitation Center, 1200 Suffield Street, Agawam, MA 01001; tel. 413/789-2200; FAX. 413/789-2269; David D. Kurzman, Executive Director

Country Gardens Skilled Nursing and Rehabilitation Center, 2045 G.A.R. Highway, Swansea, MA 02777; tel. 508/379-9700; FAX. 508/379-0723; Scott Sanborn, Executive Director

Country Manor Rehabilitation and Nursing Center, 180 Low Street, Newburyport, MA 01950; tel. 508/465-5361; FAX. 508/462-5607; Daniel Northrup, Administrator

Cranberry Pointe Rehabilitation and Skilled Care Center, 111 Headwaters Drive, Harwich, MA 02645-1726; tel. 508/430-1717; FAX. 508/432-1809; Patrick J. Sheehan, Administrator

D'Youville Manor, 981 Varnum Avenue, Lowell, MA 01854; tel. 508/454-5681; FAX. 508/453-3561; Steve Johnson, Chief Executive Officer

Deutsches Altenheim, Inc., 2222 Centre Street, West Roxbury, MA 02132; tel. 617/325-1230; FAX. 617/323-7523; Bruce Glass

Devereux House Nursing Home, 39 Lafayette Street, Marblehead, MA 01945-1997; tel. 617/631-6120; FAX. 617/631-6122; Kenneth Bane

Eagle Pond Rehabilitation and Living Center, One Love Lane, P.O. Box 208, South Dennis, MA 02660; tel. 508/385-6034; FAX. 508/385-7064; Scott E. Stone, Executive Director

Eastpointe Rehabilitation and Skilled Care Center, 255 Central Avenue, Chelsea, MA 02150; tel. 617/884-5700; FAX. 617/884-7005; Grace DiFilippo, Director, Nursing

Elihu White Nursing and Rehabilitation Center, 95 Commercial Street, Braintree, MA 02184; tel. 617/848-3678; FAX. 617/356-8559; Kenneth M. Logan, Jr., Administrator

Elizabeth Seton Residence Skilled Nursing and Rehabilitation, 125 Oakland Street, Wellesley Hills, MA 02181; tel. 617/237-2161; FAX. 617/431-2589, ext. 30; Sister Blanche LaRose, Administrator

Elmhurst Nursing Home, 743 Main Street, Melrose, MA 02176; tel. 617/662-7500; FAX. 617/665-2594; William Mathies

Fairlawn Nursing Home, Inc., 370 West Street, Leominster, MA 01453; tel. 508/537-0771; FAX. 508/534-0824; Stephen A. Trudeau, Administrator

Forestview Nursing and Rehabilitation Center, 50 Indian Neck Road, Wareham, MA 02571; tel. 508/295-6264; FAX. 508/294-3484; Edward Turcotte-Shamski

Franklin House Healthcare, 130 Chestnut Street, Franklin, MA 02038; tel. 508/528-4600; FAX. 508/528-7976; James Meola

Franvale Nursing and Rehabilitation Center, 20 Pond Street, Braintree, MA 02184; tel. 617/848-1616; FAX. 617/848-8813; Bruce Shear

Geriatric Authority of Holyoke, 45 Lower Westfield Road, Holyoke, MA 01040; tel. 413/536-8110; FAX. 413/533-7999; Judith Egan

Glen Ridge Nursing Care Center, Hospital Road, Malden, MA 02148; tel. 617/391-0800; FAX. 617/391-9127; Robert Driscoll

Greenery Extended Care Center, 59 Acton Street, Worcester, MA 01604; tel. 508/791-3147; FAX. 508/753-6267; Ivan M. Howard, Administrator

Greenery Extended Care Center at Beverly, 40 Heather Street, Beverly, MA 01915; tel. 508/927-6220; FAX. 508/927-1438; James F. Smith, Administrator

Greenery Extended Care Center at Danvers, A Horizon Healthcare Facility, 56 Liberty Street, Danvers, MA 01923; tel. 508/777-2700; FAX. 508/777-2372; Edward J. Stewart, Administrator

Greenery Extended Care Center at North Andover, 75 Park Street, North Andover, MA 01845; tel. 617/685-3372; FAX. 508/683-2030; David A. Butler, Administrator

Greenery Rehabilitation Center, 99 Chestnut Hill Avenue, Brighton, MA 02135; tel. 617/787-3390; FAX. 617/787-9169; Ivan Howard, Administrator

Greenery Rehabilitation and Skilled Nursing Center at Hyannis, 89 Lewis Bay Road, Hyannis, MA 02601; tel. 508/775-7601; FAX. 508/790-4239; Emmanuel P. Freddura, Executive Director

Greenery Rehabilitation and Skilled Nursing Center at Middleboro, Isaac Street, Middleboro, MA 02346; tel. 508/947-9295; FAX. 508/947-7974; John H. Keeney, Administrator

Hammersmith House Nursing Center, 73 Chestnut Street, Sangus, MA 01906; tel. 617/233-8123; FAX. 617/231-2918; Heidi Paek, Administrator

Hannah Duston Healthcare Center, 126 Monument Street, Haverhill, MA 01830; tel. 508/373-1747; FAX. 508/373-5277; Alfred Arcidi

Harrington House Nursing and Rehabilitation Center, 160 Main Street, Walpole, MA 02081; tel. 508/660-3080; FAX. 508/660-1634; William J. McGinley, Administrator

Heritage Nursing Care Center, 841 Merrimack Street, Lowell, MA 01854; tel. 508/459-0546; FAX. 508/970-0715; W. J. Delaney, Administrator

Hermitage Health and Rehabilitation Center, 383 Mill Street, Worcester, MA 01602; tel. 508/791-8131; FAX. 505/756-5524; Mary L. Davis, Executive Director

Hollingsworth House Nursing Facility, 1120 Washington Street, Braintree, MA 02184; tel. 617/848-4710; FAX. 617/849-6487; Vincent Pattavina

Hollywell, a Flatley Rehabilitation and Nursing Center, 975 North Main Street, Randolph, MA 02368; tel. 617/963-8800; FAX. 617/963-8922; Stephen Esdale

Holy Trinity Nursing and Rehabilitation Center, 300 Barber Avenue, Worcester, MA 01606-2476; tel. 508/852-1000; FAX. 508/854-1622; Karen Laganelli

JML Care Center, Inc., 184 Ter Heun Drive, Falmouth, MA 02540-0250; tel. 508/457-4621; FAX. 508/457-1218; Joyce A. Carroll, Vice President, Nursing

Jewish Nursing Home of Western Massachusetts, Inc., 770 Converse Street, Longmeadow, MA 01106-1786; tel. 413/567-6211; FAX. 413/567-0175; Howard Braverman, President

John Scott House Nursing and Rehabilitation Center, 233 Middle Street, Braintree, MA 02184; tel. 617/843-1860; FAX. 617/843-8834; Thomas D. Nolan, Administrator

Kathleen Daniel, 485 Franklin Street, Framingham, MA 01702; tel. 508/872-8801; FAX. 508/875-1385; Jonathan Shadovitz, Administrator

Kimwell, a Flatley Rehabilitation and Nursing Center, 495 New Boston Road, Fall River, MA 02720; tel. 508/679-0106; FAX. 508/674-1570; Arthur Taylor

Ledgewood Rehabilitation and Skilled Nursing Center, 87 Herrick Street, Beverly, MA 01915; tel. 508/921-1392; FAX. 508/927-8627; Laurie Roberto, Administrator

Liberty Commons of Chatham, 390 Orleans Road, North Chatham, MA 02650; tel. 508/945-4611; FAX. 508/945-2245; William Bogdanovich

Life Care Center of Attleboro, 969 Park Street, Attleboro, MA 02703; tel. 508/222-4182; FAX. 508/226-0457; Kate O'Connor

Life Care Center of Merrimack Valley, 80 Boston Road, North Billerica, MA 01862; tel. 508/667-2166; FAX. 508/670-5625; Antonio Sousa, Executive Director

Life Care Center of West Bridgewater, 765 West Center Street, West Bridgewater, MA 02379; tel. 508/580-4400; FAX. 508/580-2412; Alan Richman

Life Care Center of the North Shore, 111 Birch Street, Lynn, MA 01902; tel. 617/592-9667; FAX. 617/599-6590; Joseph Deveau

Littleton House Nursing Home, 191 Foster Street, Littleton, MA 01460; tel. 508/486-3512; FAX. 508/486-8850; Ellen Levinson

Madonna Manor, Inc., 85 North Washington Street, North Attleboro, MA 02760; tel. 508/699-2740; FAX. 508/699-0481; Susan L. Caldwell, Administrator

Marian Manor, Inc., 33 Summer Street, Taunton, MA 02780; tel. 508/822-4885; FAX. 508/880-3386; Edmund Fitzgerald

Mariner Health Care at Longwood, 53 Parker Hill Road, Boston, MA 02120; tel. 617/278-3700; FAX. 617/277-1530; Patrick J. Stapleton, MHA, Administrator

Mariner Health of Methuen, 480 Jackson Street, Methuen, MA 01844; tel. 508/686-3906; FAX. 508/687-6007; David J. Friedler, M.P.H., Administrator

Mariner Health of Southeastern Massachusetts, 4586 Acushnet Avenue, New Bedford, MA 02745; tel. 508/998-1188; FAX. 508/998-1826; Peter L. Lebrun, Administrator

Mary Ann Morse Nursing and Rehabilitation Center, 45 Union Street, Natick, MA 01760; tel. 508/650-9003; FAX. 508/650-9209; Sarah Porter

Meadow Green Nursing and Rehabilitation Center, 45 Woburn Street, Waltham, MA 02154; tel. 617/899-8600; FAX. 617/899-3124; David L. Bell, Administrator

Meadowbrook Nursing and Rehabilitation Center, One Meadowbrook Way, Canton, MA 02021; tel. 617/961-5600; FAX. 617/961-5688; Mathew Muratore, Executive Director

Meadowview Healthcare Nursing Center, 134 North Street, North Reading, MA 01864; tel. 617/944-1107; FAX. 508/664-5746; John Spears, Administrator

Mediplex Rehabilitation and Skilled Nursing Center of the North Shore, 70 Granite Street, Lynn, MA 01904; tel. 617/581-2400; FAX. 617/581-3080; John A. Holt, Executive Director

Mediplex Rehabilitation and Skilled Nursing Facility of Northampton, 548 Elm Street, Northampton, MA 01060; tel. 413/586-3150; FAX. 413/584-7720; Elizabeth Finney, Director, Admissions

Mediplex Skilled Nursing and Rehabilitation Center of Holyoke, 260 Easthampton Road, Holyoke, MA 01040; tel. 413/538-9733; FAX. 413/538-9919; Kevin F. Henry, Administrator

Mediplex Skilled Nursing and Rehabilitation Center of Lowell, 19 Varnum Street, Lowell, MA 01850; tel. 508/454-5644; FAX. 508/459-6520; James J. Pollard, Jr., Executive Director

Mediplex of Beverly, 265 Essex Street, Beverly, MA 01915; tel. 508/927-3260; FAX. 508/922-8347; John E. Gerety, Jr., Executive Director

Mediplex of Brookline, 99 Park Street, Brookline, MA 02146; tel. 617/731-1050; FAX. 617/731-6516; Brian Freedman, Administrator

Mediplex of East Longmeadow, 135 Benton Drive, East Longmeadow, MA 01028; tel. 413/525-3336; FAX. 413/525-3269; Christopher S. Duncan, Administrator

Mediplex of Lexington, 178 Lowell Street, Lexington, MA 02173; tel. 617/862-7400; FAX. 617/862-9255; Robert Belluche, Administrator

Mediplex of New Bedford, 221 Fitzgerald Drive, New Bedford, MA 02745; tel. 508/996-4600; FAX. 508/995-3709; Susan Martineau

Mediplex of Newton, 2101 Washington Street, Newton, MA 02162; tel. 617/969-4660; FAX. 617/964-4622; Donna Steiermann, Executive Director

Mediplex of Weymouth, 64 Performance Drive, Weymouth, MA 02189; tel. 617/340-9800; FAX. 617/340-1771; Robert Nolan

Milford Meadows Skilled Nursing and Rehabilitation Center, 10 Veteran's Memorial Drive, Milford, MA 01757; tel. 508/473-6414; FAX. 508/473-9974; Peter L. Callagy, Executive Director

Mount St. Vincent Nursing Home, Inc., 35 Holy Family Road, Holyoke, MA 01040; tel. 413/532-3246; FAX. 413/532-0309; Dennis K. McKenna, Administrator

New England Pediatric Care, 78 Boston Road, North Billerica, MA 01862; tel. 508/667-5123; FAX. 508/663-5154; Ellen O'Gorman, Executive Director

Newton and Wellesley Alzheimer Center, 694 Worcester Street, Wellesley, MA 02181; tel. 617/237-6400; FAX. 617/237-2302; Steven Tyer, Administrator

North Hill, 865 Central Avenue, Needham, MA 02192; tel. 617/444-9910; FAX. 617/444-5388; Jesse Lee

Oak Knoll Health Care Center, Nine Arbetter Drive, Framingham, MA 01701; tel. 508/877-3300; FAX. 508/788-0079; Jeffrey Gangi

Our Lady's Haven of Fairhaven, Inc., 71 Center Street, Fairhaven, MA 02719; tel. 508/999-4561; FAX. 508/997-0254; Edmund Fitzgerald

Palm Manor, 40 Parkhurst Road, Chelmsford, MA 01824; tel. 508/256-3151; FAX. 508/250-4942; Wendy LaBate

Parkwell-Flatley Rehabilitation and Nursing Center, 745 Truman Highway, Hyde Park, MA 02136; tel. 617/361-8300; FAX. 617/361-7725; Thomas Flatley

Peabody Glen Nursing Center, 199 Andover Street, Peabody, MA 01960; tel. 508/531-0772; FAX. 508/532-4134; Clyde Tyler, Administrator

Penacook Place, 150 Water Street, Haverhill, MA 01830; tel. 617/374–0707; FAX. 617/521–0495; Julian Rich

Port Rehabilitation and Skilled Nursing Center, 113 Low Street, Newburyport, MA 01950; tel. 508/462–7373; FAX. 508/462–6510; Kathleen Pepe, RNC, Director, Quality Assurance

Prescott House Nursing Home, 140 Prescott Street, North Andover, MA 01845; tel. 508/685–8086; Judith E. Blinn, Executive Director

Randolph Crossings Nursing Center, 49 Thomas Patten Drive, Randolph, MA 02368; tel. 617/961–1160; FAX. 617/963–5744; Mary Elizabeth Weadock, Administrator

Rosewood Nursing and Rehabilitation Center, 22 Johnson Street, Peabody, MA 01960; tel. 508/535–8700; FAX. 508/535–2300; Julian Rich

Sacred Heart Nursing Home, 359 Summer Street, New Bedford, MA 02740–5599; tel. 508/996–6751; FAX. 508/996–6751, ext. 24; Sister Blandine D'Amours, Administrator

Sarah S. Brayton Nursing Care Center, 4901 North Main Street, Fall River, MA 02720; tel. 508/675–1001; FAX. 508/675–1088; Alan Solomont

Seacoast Nursing and Retirement Center, 292 Washington Street, Gloucester, MA 01930; tel. 508/283–0300; FAX. 508/281–6774; George Gougian, Executive Director

Sherrill House, Inc., 135 South Huntington Avenue, Boston, MA 02130; tel. 617/731–2400; FAX. 617/731–8671; Donald M. Powell, Executive Director

Sippican Healthcare Center, 15 Mill Street, Marion, MA 02738; tel. 508/748–3830; FAX. 508/748–3834; Alfred Arcidi

Southpoint Rehabilitation and Skilled Care Center, 100 Amity Street, Fall River, MA 02721; tel. 508/675–2500; FAX. 508/675–8874; Richard Sciacca

Suburban Manor Rehabilitation Nursing Center, One Great Road, Acton, MA 01720; tel. 508/263–9101; FAX. 508/263–3278; Carl H. Anderson, Executive Director

Sunny Acres Nursing Home, Inc., 254 Billerica Road, Chelmsford, MA 01824; tel. 508/256–1616; FAX. 508/256–6229; Shirley Freitas

Sunrise–Mediplex of Boston, 910 Saratoga Street, East Boston, MA 02128; tel. 617/569–1157; FAX. 617/567–2236; Maryann Boyle

Sutton Hill Nursing and Retirement Center, 1801 Turnpike Street, North Andover, MA 01845; tel. 508/688–1212; FAX. 508/794–8265; Katherine Lemay

Sweet Brook, 1561 Cold Spring Road, Williamstown, MA 01267; tel. 413/458–8127; FAX. 413/458–8209; John F. Warren, Chief Operating Officer, Administrator

Taber Street Nursing Home, 19 Taber Street, New Bedford, MA 02740; tel. 508/997–0791; FAX. 508/991–5013; Darrin Johnson, Executive Director

The Center for Optimum Care–Bayview, 26 Sturgis Street, Winthrop, MA 02152; tel. 617/846–2060; FAX. 617/846–3283; Steve Demaranville

The Center for Optimum Care–Wakefield, Bathol Street, Wakefield, MA 01880; tel. 617/245–7600; FAX. 617/245–2238; Judith Gordon

The Center for Optimum Care–Winthrop, 170 Cliff Avenue, Winthrop, MA 02152; tel. 617/846–0500; FAX. 617/539–1306; Karla Fleming

The Ellis Nursing and Rehabilitation Center, 135 Ellis Avenue, Norwood, MA 02062; tel. 617/762–6880; FAX. 617/769–0482; Anthony Franchi

The Highlands, 335 Nichols Road, Fitchburg, MA 01420; tel. 508/343–4411; FAX. 508/343–6464; Kenneth L. Sleeper

The Oaks, 4525 Acushnet Avenue, New Bedford, MA 02745; tel. 508/998–7807; FAX. 508/998–8865; Eileen Hegarty, Executive Director

The Oxford, 689 Main Street, Haverhill, MA 01830; tel. 508/373–1131; FAX. 508/373–3074; John Albert

Town Manor Nursing and Rehabilitation Center, 55 Lowell Street, Lawrence, MA 01840; tel. 508/688–6056; FAX. 508/688–5633; Thomas Dresser, Administrator

Town and Country Nursing Home, 259 Baldwin Street, Lowell, MA 01851; tel. 508/454–5438; FAX. 508/970–3692; Alex Struzziero, Administrator

VFW Parkway Nursing Home, 1190 VFW Parkway, West Roxbury, MA 02132–4219; tel. 617/325–1688; FAX. 617/469–5673; Selma Flash

Wachusett Extended Care Facility, 56 Boyden Road, Holden, MA 01520; tel. 508/829–7383; FAX. 508/829–2620; James Oliver, Administrator

Walden Rehabilitation and Nursing Center, 785 Main Street, Concord, MA 01742; tel. 508/369–6889; FAX. 508/369–8392; Sharon K. Buehrle

West Acres Nursing Home, 804 Pleasant Street, Brockton, MA 02401; tel. 508/583–6000; FAX. 508/580–2468; John Soule

Westford Nursing and Rehabilitation Center, Three Park Drive, Westford, MA 01886; tel. 508/392–1144; FAX. 508/392–0032; Alan Solomont

Westridge Health Care Center, 121 Northboro Road, Marlborough, MA 01752; tel. 508/485–4040; FAX. 508/481–5585; Barbara E. Garbarczyk, Administrator

Willow Manor Health Care and Rehabilitation Center, 30 Princeton Boulevard, Lowell, MA 01851; tel. 508/454–8086; FAX. 508/453–9772; Anne Roth, Executive Director

Willowood Health Care Center, 175 Franklin Street, North Adams, MA 01247; tel. 413/664–4041; FAX. 413/664–8447; Beverly Clark, Administrator

Willowood Healthcare Center, 151 Christian Hill Road, P.O. Box 330, Great Barrington, MA 01230; tel. 413/528–4560; FAX. 413/528–5691; Debbie Richardson, Administrator

Willowood of Williamstown, 25 Adams Road, Williamstown, MA 01267; tel. 413/458–2111; FAX. 413/458–4907; Ronald T. Cerow, Administrator

Wilmington Woods Nursing Care Center, 750 Woburn Street, Wilmington, MA 01887; tel. 508/988–0888; FAX. 508/658–6470; Mark Latham, Administrator

Wingate at Andover Rehabilitative Skilled Nursing, 80 Andover Street, Andover, MA 01810; tel. 508/470–3434; FAX. 508/475–7097; John T. Kain, Administrator

Wingate at Brighton Rehabilitative Skilled Nursing Residence, 100 North Beacon Street, Boston, MA 02134; tel. 617/787–2300; FAX. 617/787–1539; Sister Jacquelyn McCarthy, Administrator

Wingate at Needham, 589 Highland Avenue, Needham, MA 02194; tel. 617/455–9090; FAX. 617/455–9012; Muriel Baum

Wingate at Reading, 1364 Main Street, Reading, MA 01867; tel. 617/942–1210; FAX. 617/942–7251; Catherine M. Congo, Administrator

Wingate at Wilbraham Rehabilitative Skilled Nursing, Nine Maple Street, Wilbraham, MA 01095; tel. 413/596–2411; FAX. 413/599–1738; Duncan Hunter

Woburn Nursing Center, Inc., 18 Frances Street, Woburn, MA 01801; tel. 617/933–8175; FAX. 617/938–8402; Patricia Devereaux, Administrator

Woodbriar of Wilmington, 90 West Street, Wilmington, MA 01887; tel. 508/658–2700; FAX. 508/657–0015; Dennis Sargent, President

Youville Healthcare Center, 1575 Cambridge Street, Cambridge, MA 02138; tel. 617/876–4344; FAX. 617/441–8902; Sister Joan Coyne, Administrator

MICHIGAN

Bay County Medical Care Facility, 564 West Hampton Road, Essexville, MI 48732; tel. 517/892–3591; FAX. 517/892–6991; William R. Mahoney, Administrator

Crestmont Health Care Center, 111 Trealout Drive, Fenton, MI 48430; tel. 810/629–4105; FAX. 810/629–7538; Dane Van Buskirk, Executive Director

Greenery Extended Care Center, 34225 Grand River, Farmington, MI 48335; tel. 313/477–7373; FAX. 810/477–2888; Thomas L. Johnsrud, Administrator

Greenery Health Care Center, 4800 Clintonville Road, Clarkston, MI 48346; tel. 313/674–0903; Maureen L. Hewitt, Executive Director

Greenery Health Care Center at Howell, 3003 West Grand River, Howell, MI 48843; tel. 517/546–4210; FAX. 517/546–7661; Darlena Richman, Administrator

Heartland Health Care Center–Kalamazoo, 3625 West Michigan Avenue, Kalamazoo, MI 49006; tel. 616/375–4550; FAX. 616/375–4687; Dennis Shaffer, FACHE, Administrator

Heartland Health Care Center–University, 28550 Five Mile Road, Livonia, MI 48154; tel. 313/427–8270; FAX. 313/427–2135; Judy Ashton, Administrator

Heartland Health Center–Grand Rapids, 2320 East Baltimore, S.E., Grand Rapids, MI 49546; tel. 616/949–3000; FAX. 616/949–5612; Sue Doherty

Heartland Healthcare Center–Georgian Bloomfield, 2975 North Adams Road, Bloomfield Hills, MI 48034; tel. 810/645–2900; FAX. 810/645–5228; Elizabeth Siebert, Administrator

Integrated Health Services of Michigan at Riverbend, 11941 Belsay Road, Grand Blanc, MI 48439; tel. 313/694–1970; FAX. 810/694–4081; Lee K. Karson, Executive Director, Chief Executive Officer

Isabella County Medical Care Facility, 1222 North Drive, Mount Pleasant, MI 48858; tel. 517/772–2957; FAX. 517/772–3669; Vickie S. Block, Administrator

Martha T. Berry Memorial Medical Care Facility, 43533 Elizabeth Road, Mount Clemens, MI 48043; tel. 810/469–5623; FAX. 810/469–6352; Raymond D. Pietrzak, Administrator

Marvin and Betty Danto Health Care Center, 6800 West Maple, West Bloomfield, MI 48322; tel. 810/788–7113; Robert Possanzo

Mercy Bellbrook, 873 West Avon Road, Rochester Hills, MI 48307; tel. 810/656–3239, ext. 203; FAX. 810/656–8160; Ann L. Eastman, Administrator

Mercy Pavilion of Battle Creek, 80 North 20th Street, Battle Creek, MI 49015; tel. 616/964–5400; FAX. 616/964–5559; Michael Richards, Senior Administrator

North Ottawa Care Center, Inc., 1615 South Despelder, Grand Haven, MI 49417–2633; tel. 616/842–0770; FAX. 616/842–0783; Robert Baldus

Oakland County Medical Care Facility, 1200 North Telegraph Road, Pontiac, MI 48341–0469; tel. 810/858–1415; FAX. 810/858–4026; Shirla F. Kugler, Administrator

Orchard Hills, 532 Orchard Lake Road, Pontiac, MI 48341; tel. 810/338–7151; FAX. 810/338–2563; Marsha Tomas, Administrator

Shore Haven, a Mercy Living Center, 900 South Beacon Boulevard, Grand Haven, MI 49417; tel. 616/846–1850; FAX. 616/846–0971; Nancy J. Ritchie, Administrator

Tendercare–Clare, 600 Southeast Fourth Street, Clare, MI 48617; tel. 517/386–7723; FAX. 517/386–4100; Wilma Shurlow, Administrator

MINNESOTA

Lake Ridge Rehabilitation and Specialty Care Center, 2727 North Victoria, Roseville, MN 55113; tel. 612/483–5431; FAX. 612/486–2461; Todd Carsen, Executive Director

Moorhead Healthcare Center, 2810 North Second Avenue, Moorhead, MN 56560; tel. 218/233–7578; FAX. 218/233–8307; David Erickson

Whitewater Healthcare Center, 525 Bluff Avenue, P.O. Box 8, Saint Charles, MN 55972; tel. 507/932–3283; FAX. 507/932–4756; Michael Maher, Executive Director

MISSISSIPPI

Eupora Health Care Center, 200 Walnut Avenue, P.O. Box 918, Eupora, MS 39744; tel. 601/258–8293; FAX. 601/258–2345; Gerald Gary, Administrator

Lakeland Health Care Center, 3680 Lakeland Lane, Jackson, MS 39216; tel. 601/982–5505; FAX. 601/362–1883; Angela Turner, Executive Director

United States Naval Home, 1800 Beach Drive, Gulfport, MS 39507–1597; tel. 601/897–4003; FAX. 601/897–4013; Michael Fox

MISSOURI

BCC at Lebanon Park Manor, Inc., 514 West Fremont, Lebanon, MO 65536; tel. 417/532–5351; FAX. 417/831–7928; John Foster, Regional President

Harry S. Truman Restorative Center, 5700 Arsenal Street, St. Louis, MO 63139; tel. 314/768–6600, ext. 13; FAX. 314/645–7628; Edward M. Peters, Chief Executive Officer

Integrated Health Services at Alpine North, 4700 Cliff View Drive, Kansas City, MO 64150; tel. 816/741–5105; FAX. 816/746–1301; Karen Leverich, Administrator

Integrated Health Services of St. Louis at Gravois, 10954 Kennerly Road, St. Louis, MO 63128; tel. 314/843–4242; FAX. 314/843–5370; Milissa J. Watkins, Administrator

John Knox Village Care Center, 600 Northwest Pryor Road, Lees Summit, MO 64081; tel. 816/246–4343, ext. 2402; FAX. 816/525–3473; Daniel Rexroth, Vice President, Health Services

ManorCare Health Services, 1200 Graham Road, Florissant, MO 63031; tel. 314/838–6555; FAX. 314/838–4000; Anita Martinez, Administrator

Village North Health Center, 11160 Village North Drive, St. Louis, MO 63136; tel. 314/355–8010; FAX. 314/653–4801; Wes Sperr, Administrator

Village North Manor, 6768 North Highway 67, Florissant, MO 63034; tel. 314/741–9101; FAX. 314/741–4936; Elaine Piper, Administrator

Village North Woods, 9500 Bellefontaine Road, St. Louis, MO 63137; tel. 314/868–1400; FAX. 314/868–0170; Gladys A. Sullivan, Administrator

NEBRASKA

Carl T. Curtis Health Education Center, 100 Main Street, P.O. Box 250, Macy, NE 68039; tel. 402/837–5381; FAX. 402/837–5303; David Beaver

Hartington Nursing Center, 401 West Darlene Street, P.O. Box 107, Hartington, NE 68739; tel. 402/254–3905; FAX. 402/254–3963; Pat Stonacek, Administrator

Lakeview Rehabilitation Nursing Center, 1405 West Highway 34, Grand Island, NE 68801; tel. 308/382–6397; FAX. 308/382–0125; Marilou Luth, Executive Director

The Ambassador Lincoln, 4405 Norman Boulevard, Lincoln, NE 68506; tel. 402/488–2355; FAX. 402/488–2779; Michael Ryan, Director, Operations

NEVADA

Integrated Health Services of Las Vegas, 2170 East Harmon Avenue, Las Vegas, NV 89119; tel. 702/794–0100; FAX. 702/794–0041; Maryanne Smith, Assistant Vice President

NEW HAMPSHIRE

Dover Rehabilitation and Living Center, 307 Plaza Drive, Dover, NH 03820; tel. 603/742–2676, ext. 115; FAX. 603/749–5375; Robert T. Brzycki, Administrator

Good Shepherd Nursing Home, 20 Plantation Dive, Joffrey, NH 03452; tel. 603/532–8762; FAX. 603/532–6057; Judith A. LeBlanc, Administrator

Greenbriar Terrace Healthcare, 55 Harris Road, Nashua, NH 03062; tel. 603/888–1573; FAX. 603/888–5089; Arthur O'Leary, Administrator

Integrated Health Services of Derry, Eight Peabody Road, Derry, NH 03038; tel. 603/434–1566; FAX. 603/434–2299; David Ross, Administrator

Integrated Health Services of New Hampshire at Claremont, RFD 3, Box 47, Hanover Street Extension, Claremont, NH 03743; tel. 603/542–2606; FAX. 603/543–0479; Brian King, Administrator

Integrated Health Services of New Hampshire at Manchester, 191 Hackett Hill Road, Manchester, NH 03102; tel. 603/668–8161; FAX. 603/622–2584; Marcia S. Couitt, Administrator

Mount Carmel Nursing Home, 235 Myrtle Street, Manchester, NH 03104; tel. 603/627–3811; FAX. 603/626–4696; Sister Jacinta Mary Hirner, Administrator

Saint Ann Home, 195 Dover Point Road, Dover, NH 03820; tel. 603/742–2612; FAX. 603/743–3055; Sister Mary Robert Romano, Administrator

St. Francis Home, SNF/ICF, 406 Court Street, Laconia, NH 03246; tel. 603/524–0466; FAX. 603/527–0884; Julieann Fay, Administrator

St. Teresa's Manor, 519 Bridge Street, Manchester, NH 03104; tel. 603/668–2373; FAX. 603/668–0059; Stephen V. Fulchino, Administrator

St. Vincent de Paul Nursing Home, 29 Providence Avenue, Berlin, NH 03570; tel. 603/752–1820; FAX. 603/752–7149; Steven E. Woods, Administrator

NEW JERSEY

Ashbrook Nursing and Rehabilitation Center, 1610 Raritan Road, Scotch Pines, NJ 07076; tel. 908/889–5500; FAX. 908/889–6573; Ronald Delmauro

Barn Hill Convalescent Center, 249 High Street, Route 94 South, Newton, NJ 07860; tel. 201/383–5600; FAX. 201/383–1397; Barbara Rice, Administrator

Cornell Hall, 234 Chestnut Street, Union, NJ 07083; tel. 908/687–7800; FAX. 908/687–1417; Victor Fresolone

Daughters of Miriam Center for the Aged, 155 Hazel Street, Clifton, NJ 07015; tel. 201/772–3700; FAX. 201/772–5044; Steven Schilsky, L.N.H.A., Executive Vice President

Dunroven Health Care Center, 221 County Road, Cresskill, NJ 07656; tel. 201/567–9310; FAX. 201/567–9239; Donald C. DeVries, Executive Director

Franklin Care Center, 3371 Route 27, Franklin Park, NJ 08823; tel. 908/821–8000; FAX. 908/821–9253; Robert J. Kovacs, Administrator

Glenside Nursing Center, 144 Gales Drive, New Providence, NJ 07974; tel. 908/464–8600; FAX. 908/464–6355; Joan Lepore

Green Acres Manor, 1931 Lakewood Road, Route 9, Toms River, NJ 08755; tel. 908/286–2323; FAX. 908/244–9095; Maria Lapid, RN, Administrator

Greenbrook Manor Nursing and Rehabilitation Center, 303 Rock Avenue, Green Brook, NJ 08812–2616; tel. 908/968–5500; FAX. 908/968–7963; Adrienne C. Mayernik, L.N.H.A.

Harborside Healthcare Rehabilitation and Nursing Center–Woods Edge, 875 Route 202/206 North, Bridgewater, NJ 08807; tel. 908/526–8600; FAX. 908/707–0686; James Lindes

Inglemoor Care Center, 311 South Livingston Avenue, Livingston, NJ 07039; tel. 201/994–0221; FAX. 201/992–0696; Daniel Moles

Integrated Health Services of New Jersey at Somerset Valley, 1621 Route 22 West, Bound Brook, NJ 08805; tel. 908/469–2000; FAX. 908/469–8917; Carolyn Allen, Executive Director

JFK Hartwyck at Cedar Brook Nursing Convalescent and Rehabilitation, 1340 Park Avenue, Plainfield, NJ 07060; tel. 908/906–2100; FAX. 908/321–9217; Nanetta Malone, Administrator

King James Care and Rehabilitation Center, 1165 Easton Avenue, Somerset, NJ 08873; tel. 908/246–4100; FAX. 908/246–3926; Allyson Brown, Administrator

Lanfair House Nursing and Rehabilitation Center, 1140 Black Oak Ridge Road, Wayne, NJ 07470; tel. 201/835–7443; Victor Fresolone

Laurelton Village Care Center, 475 Jack Martin Boulevard, Brick, NJ 08724; tel. 908/458–6600; FAX. 908/458–2674; Kathy Bogajevski

Linwood Convalescent Center, New Road and Central Avenue, Linwood, NJ 08221; tel. 609/927–6131; FAX. 609/927–0069; David G. Wolf, CFACHE, President

Manor Care Health Services, 1180 Route 22 West, Mountainside, NJ 07092; tel. 908/654–0020; FAX. 908/654–8661; Melanie J. Lalacoma, Executive Director

ManorCare Health Services, 550 Jessup Road, West Deptford, NJ 08066; tel. 609/848–9551; FAX. 609/848–1817; David Donin, Administrator

Margaret McLaughlin McCarrick Care Center, 15 Dellwood Lane, Somerset, NJ 08873; tel. 908/545–4200; FAX. 908/846–1089; James Caron, Administrator

Meadow View Nursing and Respiratory Care Center, 1328 South Black Horse Pike, Williamstown, NJ 08094; tel. 609/875–0100; FAX. 609/629–4619; Jane Greenberg, Administrator

Mediplex Subacute Center, Two Cooper Plaza, Camden, NJ 08103; tel. 609/342–7600; FAX. 609/541–4059; Mary Beth Schwartz, Executive Director, Administrator

Morris View Nursing Home, 540 West Hanover Avenue, Morris Plains, NJ 07950; tel. 201/285–2820; FAX. 201/285–6062; Joaquin Deniz, Administrator

Neptune ConvaCenter, 101 Walnut Street, Neptune, NJ 07753; tel. 908/774–3550; FAX. 908/775–7534; George Michals, L.N.H.A.

Seacrest Village Nursing Home, 1001 Center Street, P.O. Box 1480, Tuckerton, NJ 08087; tel. 609/296–9292; FAX. 609/296–0508; Brian Holloway

The Manor, 689 West Main Street, Freehold, NJ 07728; tel. 908/431–5200, ext. 11; FAX. 908/409–2446; Mrs. J. Escovar, Administrator

Troy Hills Nursing and Rehabilitation Center, 200 Reynolds Avenue, Parsippany, NJ 07054; tel. 201/887–8080; FAX. 201/386–5906; Anne Marie Gauntlett

Valley Health Care Center, 300 Old Hook Road, Westwood, NJ 07675; tel. 201/664–8888; FAX. 201/664–9577; Chris Asmann–Finch, Administrator

Voorhees Pediatric Facility, 1304 Laurel Oak Road, Voorhees, NJ 08043; tel. 609/346–3300; FAX. 609/435–4223; Carl Underland, Administrator

Woodcrest Center, 800 River Road, New Milford, NJ 07646; tel. 201/967–1700; FAX. 201/967–5423; Nancy A. Bubrick, Administrator

NEW MEXICO

Americare–Las Palomas Nursing and Rehabilitation Center, 8100 Palomas, N.E., Albuquerque, NM 87109; tel. 505/821–4200; FAX. 505/822–0234; Julie Dreike

NEW YORK

Bainbridge Nursing Home, 3518 Bainbridge Avenue, Bronx, NY 10467; tel. 718/655–1991; FAX. 718/655–3903; Isaac Goldbrenner, Administrator

C & C Homecare, Inc., 64 Bethpage Road, Hicksville, NY 11801; tel. 516/433–1030; FAX. 516/433–1260; Stacey L. Granat

CNR Health Care Network, Inc., 520 Prospect Place, Brooklyn, NY 11238; tel. 718/636–1000; FAX. 718/857–4559; Michael Fassler, Executive Vice President

Clove Lakes Health Care and Rehabilitation Center, 25 Fanning Street, Staten Island, NY 10314; tel. 718/289–7900; FAX. 718/761–8701; Eric Kalt, Administrator

Crown Nursing and Rehabilitation Center, 3457 Nostrand Avenue, Brooklyn, NY 11229; tel. 718/615–1100; FAX. 718/769–6901; Sally Gearhart Schnabel

Dumont Masonic Home, 676 Pelham Road, New Rochelle, NY 10805; tel. 914/632–9600; FAX. 914/632–4766; Beth Goldstein, Administrator

East Haven Nursing Home, 2323 Eastchester Road, Bronx, NY 10469; tel. 718/655–2848; FAX. 718/655–2750; Joseph Brachfeld, Administrator

Golden Gate Health Care Center, Inc., 191 Bradley Avenue, Staten Island, NY 10314; tel. 718/698–8800; FAX. 718/698–5536; Alan Chopp, Administrator

Gouverneur Nursing Facility and Certified Home Health Agency, 227 Madison Street, New York, NY 10002; tel. 212/238–8000; FAX. 212/238–8007; Kenneth Gelb, Chief Operating Officer

Grace Plaza of Great Neck, Inc., 15 St. Paul's Place, Great Neck, NY 11021; tel. 516/466–3001; FAX. 516/829–3854; Celia Strow, Administrator

Haven Manor Health Care Center, 1441 Gateway Boulevard, Far Rockaway, NY 11691; tel. 718/471–1500; FAX. 718/868–0030; Aron Cytryn, Administrator

Highgate Manor of Cortland, Inc., 28 Kellogg Road, Cortland, NY 13045; tel. 607/753–9631; FAX. 607/756–2968; Karen Harvatin, Administrator

Highgate, a Center for Health and Rehabilitation, 100 New Turnpike Road, Troy, NY 12182; tel. 518/235–1410; FAX. 518/235–1632; Mark Carden, Administrator

Hilltop Manor of Niskayuna, 1805 Providence Avenue, Niskayuna, NY 12309; tel. 518/374–2212; FAX. 518/374–4330; Chris Alexander, Administrator

M.J.G. Nursing Home Company, Inc., 4915 Tenth Avenue, Brooklyn, NY 11219; tel. 718/851–3710; FAX. 718/972–6120; Eli Feldman, Executive Vice President, Chief Executive Officer

Maplewood Nursing Home, Inc., 100 Daniel Drive, Webster, NY 14580–2983; tel. 716/872–1800; FAX. 716/872–2597; Gregory Chambery, Administrator

Margaret Tietz Center for Nursing Care, 164–11 Chapin Parkway, Jamaica, NY 11432; tel. 718/523–6400, ext. 705; FAX. 718/262–8839; Kenneth M. Brown, President, Chief Executive Officer

Mosolu Parkway Nursing Home, 3356 Perry Avenue, Bronx, NY 10467; tel. 718/655–3568; FAX. 718/515–5713; Issac Schapiro, Administrator

Nassau Extended Care Center, One Greenwich Street, Hempstead, NY 11550; tel. 516/565–4800; FAX. 516/565–4966; Caryl Benjamin

Oakwood Health Care Center, Inc., 200 Bassett Road, Buffalo, NY 14221; tel. 716/689–6681; FAX. 716/689–2547; Carla Chur, Administrator

Palm Gardens Nursing Home, 615 Avenue C, Brooklyn, NY 11218; tel. 718/633–3300; FAX. 718/633–3320; Shoshana Lefkowitz, Administrator

Providence Rest, 3304 Waterbury Avenue, Bronx, NY 10465; tel. 718/931–3000; FAX. 718/863–0185; Sister Seline Mary Flores, C.S.J.B., Administrator

Rosewood Gardens Convalescent Home, Inc., 284 Troy Road, Rensselaer, NY 12144; tel. 518/286–1621; FAX. 518/286–1691; Beverly Benno, Administrator

Saint Cabrini Nursing Home, Inc., 115 Broadway, Dobbs Ferry, NY 10522; tel. 914/693–6800, ext. 500; FAX. 914/693–1731; Robert Gilpatrick, Chief Executive Officer

Sea View Hospital Rehabilitation Center and Home, 460 Brielle Avenue, Staten Island, NY 10314; tel. 718/317–3221; FAX. 718/351–7898; Jane M. Lyons, Executive Director

Shorefront Jewish Geriatric Center, 3015 West 29th Street, Brooklyn, NY 11224; tel. 718/921–8065; FAX. 718/921–1616; Eli Feldman, Executive Vice President, Chief Executive Officer

St. Mary's Hospital for Children, Inc., 29–01 216th Street, Bayside, NY 11360; tel. 718/281–8800, ext. 8850; FAX. 718/279–2141; Stuart C. Kaplan, Executive Vice President

The Center for Extended Care and Rehabilitation, 330 Community Drive, Manhasset, NY 11030; tel. 516/562–4050; FAX. 516/562–4545; John Gallagher

The Nathan Miller Center for Nursing Care, Inc., 220 West Post Road, White Plains, NY 10606; tel. 914/686–8880; FAX. 914/686–8216; Lorraine Goldman, Administrative Director

The Wartburg, Wartburg Place, Mount Vernon, NY 10552; tel. 914/699–0800, ext. 311; FAX. 914/699–2512; Dale Gatz

Throgs Neck Extended Care Facility, 707 Throgs Neck Expressway, Bronx, NY 10465; tel. 718/430–0003; FAX. 718/430–7024; George Stops, Administrator

Victory Lake Nursing Center, 419 North Quaker Lane, Hyde Park, NY 12538; tel. 914/229–9177; FAX. 914/229–9819; Robert C. Farrow, M.P.H., Administrator

Waterview Nursing Care Center, 119–15 27th Avenue, Flushing, NY 11354; tel. 718/461–5000; FAX. 718/321–1984; Larry Slatky, Executive Director

Wayne Nursing Home, 3530 Wayne Avenue, Bronx, NY 10467; tel. 718/655–1700, ext. 541; FAX. 718/515–5650; I. Hartman, Assistant Administrator

Wesley Group, Inc., 630 East Avenue, Rochester, NY 14607–2194; tel. 716/241–2100; FAX. 716/241–2180; Jon R. Zemans, President, Chief Executive Officer

Wingate at Dutchess Rehabilitative Skilled Nursing, Three Summit Court, Fishkill, NY 12524; tel. 914/896–1500; FAX. 914/896–1531, ext. 600; Ross B. Decker, Administrator

NORTH CAROLINA

American Transitional Care–Charlottte, 2616 East Fifth Street, Charlotte, NC 28204; tel. 704/333–5165; FAX. 704/372–6906; Jane Kinard

Beverly Health Care Center, 1000 Western Boulevard, P.O. Box 7008, Tarboro, NC 27886–7008; tel. 919/823–0401; FAX. 919/823–1819; Effie Webb

Brian Center Health and Rehabilitation–Durham, 6000 Fayetteville Road, Durham, NC 27713; tel. 919/544–9021; FAX. 919/544–0345; Carol Drum

Cypress Pointe Rehabilitation and Health Care Centre, 2006 South 16th Street, Wilmington, NC 28401; tel. 910/763–6271; FAX. 910/251–9803; Faye M. Kennedy, Administrator

Horizon Rehabilitation Center, 3100 Erwin Road, Durham, NC 27705; tel. 919/383–1546; FAX. 919/382–0156; Maureen O'Neal, Administrator

Integrated Health Services of Charlotte at Hawthorne, 333 Hawthorne Lane, Charlotte, NC 28204; tel. 704/372–1270; FAX. 704/377–2059; Darryl Ehlers, Administrator

Integrated Health Services of Raleigh at Crabtree Valley, 3830 Blue Ridge Road, Raleigh, NC 27612; tel. 919/781–4900; FAX. 919/571–2583; Paul Vitale, Administrator

North Carolina Special Care Center, 4761 Ward Boulevard, Wilson, NC 27893; tel. 919/399–2112; FAX. 919/399–2138; Mike Moseley, Director

OHIO

Americare Marion Nursing and Rehabilitation Center, 524 James Way, Marion, OH 43302–5890; tel. 614/389–6306; FAX. 614/389–4042; Debra Hart

Arbors East Subacute and Rehabilitation Center, 5500 East Broad Street, Columbus, OH 43213; tel. 614/575–9003; FAX. 614/575–9101; Alexander Bettinger, Administrator

Arbors West, 375 West Main Street, West Jefferson, OH 43162; tel. 614/879–7661; FAX. 614/879–7848; Thomas C. Widney

Arbors at Canton, 2714 13th Street, N.W., Canton, OH 44708; tel. 216/456–2842; FAX. 216/456–5343; Gary L. Van, Administrator

Arbors at Delaware, 2270 Warrensburg Road, Delaware, OH 43015; tel. 614/369–9614; FAX. 614/363–5881; Kelly Darrow, Administrator

Arbors at Marietta, 400 Seventh Street, Marietta, OH 45750; tel. 614/373–3597; FAX. 614/373–3597; Aaron W. Loney, Administrator

Arbors at Milford, 5900 Meadowcreek Drive, Milford, OH 45150; tel. 513/248–1655; FAX. 513/248–0466; Deonne Schenk

Arbors at Toledo Subacute and Rehabilitation Center, 2920 Cherry Street, Toledo, OH 43608; tel. 419/242–7458; FAX. 419/242–6514; Robert Aroesty, Executive Director

Aurora Manor Special Care Centre, 101 Bissell Road, Aurora, OH 44202; tel. 216/562–5000; FAX. 216/562–5181; Scott Bower, Administrator

Broadview Multi–Care Center/Rosepoint Pavilion, 5520 Broadview Road, Parma, OH 44134; tel. 216/749–4010, ext. 2167; FAX. 786/860–; Harold Shachter

Castle Nursing Homes, Inc., Sunset View Unit, 6180 State Road 83, P.O. Box 5001, Millersburg, OH 44654; tel. 330/674–0015; FAX. 330/674–2822; Mick DeWitt, Administrator

Cedarwood Plaza, 12504 Cedar Road, Cleveland Heights, OH 44106; tel. 216/371–3600; FAX. 216/371–3631; Tom Lowenkamp, Administrator

College Park Nursing and Rehabilitation Center, 3201 County Road 16, Coshocton, OH 43812; tel. 614/622–2074; FAX. 614/622–5501; Robert Guilliams

Columbus Rehabilitation and Subacute Institute, 44 South Souder Avenue, Columbus, OH 43222; tel. 614/228–5900, ext. 231; FAX. 614/228–3989; Robert D. Brooks, Executive Director

Community Multicare Center, 908 Symmes Road, Fairfield, OH 45014; tel. 513/868–6500; FAX. 513/844–8579; Anne Dahling, Chief Executive Officer

Continental Manor Nursing and Rehabilitation Center, 820 East Center Street, P.O. Box 157, Blanchester, OH 45107; tel. 937/783–4949; FAX. 937/783–4398; Nancy Hamann, Administrator

Cortland Quality Care Nursing and Rehabilitation Center, 369 North High Street, Cortland, OH 44410; tel. 216/638–4015; FAX. 216/638–4628; Joseph Neelis

Gateway Health Care Center, Three Gateway Drive, Euclid, OH 44119; tel. 216/486–4949; FAX. 216/481–5155; Linda Bliss, Director, Nursing

Greenbriar Quality Care of Boardman, 8064 South Avenue, Boardman, OH 44512; tel. 216/726–3700; FAX. 216/726–2194; Joseph Neelis

Harborside Healthcare–Difiance, 395 Harding Street, Defiance, OH 43512; tel. 419/784–1450; FAX. 419/784–9190; Tim Ross

Harborside Healthcare–Northwestern Ohio, 1104 Wesley Avenue, Bryan, OH 43506; tel. 419/636–5071; FAX. 419/636–3894; Randi Kiphen, Administrator

Harborside Healthcare–Toledo, 28546 Starbright Boulevard, Perrysburg, OH 43551; tel. 419/666–0935; FAX. 419/666–5610; Steven Rankin, Administrator

Heartland of Beavercreek, 1974 North Fairfield Road, Dayton, OH 45432; tel. 937/429–1106; FAX. 937/429–0902; Jim Kyle, Administrator

Heartland of Centerburg, 212 Fairview Avenue, Centerburg, OH 43011; tel. 614/625–5774; FAX. 614/625–7426; Laurie Zinn, Administrator

Heartland of Holly Glen, 4293 Monroe Street, Toledo, OH 43601; tel. 419/474–6021; FAX. 419/475–1946; Myra Knouff

Heartland of Marysville, 755 South Plum Street, Marysville, OH 43040; tel. 937/644–8836; FAX. 937/644–1811; Paul J. LeGrande, Administrator

Heartland of Mentor, 8300 Center Street, Mentor, OH 44060; tel. 216/256–1496; FAX. 216/256–4935; Douglas Mock

Heartland of Perrysburg, 10540 Fremont Pike, Perrysburgh, OH 443551; tel. 419/874–3578; FAX. 419/874–7753; John K. Graham, Director, New Product

Hickory Creek Nursing Center, 3421 Pinnacle Road, Dayton, OH 45418; tel. 513/268–3488; FAX. 513/268–1889; Barbara J. Ater, Administrator

Horizon Village Nursing and Rehabilitation Center, 2473 North Road, Northeast, Warren, OH 44483; tel. 216/372–2251; FAX. 216/372–6478; Albert C. Parton, Administrator

IHS at Waterford Commons Subacute Care and Rehabilitation Center, 955 Garden Lake Parkway, Toledo, OH 43614; tel. 419/382–2200; FAX. 419/381–0188; Mary E. McConnell, Administrator

Manor Care Health Services, 23225 Lorain Road, North Olmsted, OH 44070; tel. 216/779–6900; FAX. 216/779–1859; Shelly Szarek–Skodny, NHA, Administrator

Manor Care Health Services of Willoughby, 37603 Euclid Avenue, Willoughby, OH 44094; tel. 216/951–5551; FAX. 216/951–1914; Kevin Ahmadi, Administrator

Manor Care Health Services–Mayfield Heights, 6757 Mayfield Road, Mayfield Heights, OH 44124; tel. 216/473–0090; FAX. 216/473–1170; Arlene Manross, Administrator

Manor Care Nursing Center–Rocky River, 4102 Rocky River Drive, Cleveland, OH 44135; tel. 216/251–3300; FAX. 216/251–0201; James Kallevig

Manor Care Nursing and Rehabilitation Center, 140 County Line Road, Westerville, OH 43081; tel. 614/882–1511; FAX. 614/882–5318; Sandra Coleman, Administrator

Manor Care Nursing and Rehabilitation Center, 2250 Banning Road, Cincinnati, OH 45239; tel. 513/591–0400; FAX. 513/591–0100; Aileen Baker, Administrator

ManorCare Health Services of Akron, 1211 West Market Street, Akron, OH 44313; tel. 216/867–8530; FAX. 216/867–9159; Jim Kallevig, Administrator

Mayfair Village Subacute and Rehabilitation Center, 3000 Bethel Road, Columbus, OH 43220; tel. 614/889–7532; FAX. 614/889–7532; Cheryl Guyman, Executive Director

Menorah Park Center for the Aging, 27100 Cedar Road, Beachwood, OH 44122–1156; tel. 216/831–6500; FAX. 216/831–5492; Steven Raichilson

Newark Healthcare Centre, 75 McMillen Drive, Newark, OH 43055; tel. 614/344–0357; FAX. 614/344–8615; Amy Cajka, Administrator

Northland Terrace Medical Center for Subacute Care and Rehabilitation, 5700 Karl Road, Columbus, OH 43229; tel. 614/846–5420; FAX. 614/846–3247; Jill Philipp, Provider Relations

Regency Manor Rehabilitation and Subacute Center, 2000 Regency Manor Circle, Columbus, OH 43207; tel. 614/445–8261; FAX. 614/445–8050; Jeffreys Barrett

Secrest/Giffin Long Term Care Facility, 3416 South Columbus Avenue, Sandusky, OH 44870; tel. 419/625–2454, ext. 500; FAX. 419/625–3207; Linda Pegrim, Nursing Home Administrator

St. Augustine Manor, 7801 Detroit Avenue, Cleveland, OH 44102; tel. 216/634–7400; FAX. 216/634–7483; Patrick Gareau, President, Chief Executive Officer

The Franciscan at St. Leonard, 8100 Clyo Road, Dayton, OH 45458; tel. 513/439–7119; FAX. 513/439–7165; Brian Forschner

The Maria–Joseph Center, 4830 Salem Avenue, Dayton, OH 45416–1798; tel. 937/278–2692; FAX. 937/278–9016; Bonnie G. Langdon, President, Chief Executive Officer

The Village at Westerville Nursing Center, 1060 Eastwind Drive, Westerville, OH 43081; tel. 614/895–1038; FAX. 614/895–1094; Pamela M. DeGroodt, Administrator

Walton Manor Health Care Center, 19859 Alexander Road, Walton Hills, OH 44146; tel. 216/439–4433; FAX. 216/439–0691; Patricia Pell, Administrator

West Chester Health Care, 9117 Cincinnati–Columbus Road, West Chester, OH 45069; tel. 513/777–6164; FAX. 513/777–6158; Wilma Willard, President

Willard Quality Care Nursing and Rehabilitation Center, 725 Wessor Avenue, Willard, OH 44890; tel. 419/935–6511; FAX. 419/935–8494; Tracy Head, NHA

Woodridge Retirement Center, 3801 Woodridge Boulevard, Fairfield, OH 45014; tel. 513/874–9933; Michael Snow

OKLAHOMA

Four Seasons Nursing Center, 2425 South Memorial, Tulsa, OK 74129; tel. 918/628–0932; FAX. 918/622–2060; Phillip Howard

Four Seasons Nursing Center of Midwest City, 2900 Parklawn Drive, Midwest City, OK 73110; tel. 405/737–6601; FAX. 405/737–4984; Chiquita Henderson

Georgian Court Nursing Center, 2552 East 21st Street, Tulsa, OK 74114–1788; tel. 918/742–7319; FAX. 918/742–5270; Brian H. Hoyle, Chief Executive Officer

Manor Care Health Services, 5301 North Brookline, Oklahoma City, OK 73112; tel. 405/946–3351; FAX. 405/946–3647; Deborah Burian, Administrator

Saint Simeon's Episcopal Home, Inc., 3701 North Cincinnati, Tulsa, OK 74106; tel. 918/425–3583; FAX. 918/425–6368; Marian Matthews, Executive Director

OREGON

Cascade Terrace Nursing Center, 5601 Southeast 122nd Avenue, Portland, OR 97236; tel. 503/761–3181; FAX. 503/760–6556; Diane Richardson, Administrator

Villa Cascade Care Center, 350 South Eighth Street, Lebanon, OR 97355; tel. 503/259–1221; FAX. 503/451–1349; Alfred H. Jones, Administrator

PENNSYLVANIA

Allegheny Manor, 512 South Paint Boulevard, Shippenville, PA 16254; tel. 814/226–5660; FAX. 814/226–9896; Eric Funk

Section C

American Transitional Care–Oakmont, 26 Ann Street, Oakmont, PA 15139; tel. 412/828–7300; FAX. 412/828–2669; Brad Nowlen, Executive Director

Bishop Nursing Home, Inc., 318 South Orange Street, Media, PA 19063; tel. 215/565–3881; FAX. 610/891–6509; Walter M. Strine, Jr., Chief Executive Officer

Buckingham Valley Rehabilitation and Nursing Center, 820 Durham Road, Route 413, P.O. Box 447, Buckingham, PA 18912; tel. 215/598–7181; Mary Elena Shaw, RN, M.S., NHA, Administrator

Chandler Hall Friends Nursing Home/Hospice Home Health Agency, 99 Barclay Street, Newtown, PA 18940; tel. 215/860–4000; FAX. 215/860–3458; Jane Fox, Executive Director

Chester Care Center, 15th Street and Shaw Terrace, Chester, PA 19013; tel. 215/499–8800; FAX. 610/499–8805; Barbara Quaintance, Administrator

Clara Burke Community, 251 Stenton Avenue, Plymouth Meeting, PA 19462; tel. 610/828–2272; FAX. 610/828–2519; Karen Pulini

Dowden Nursing and Rehabilitation Center, 3503 Rhoads Avenue, Newtown Square, PA 19073; tel. 215/359–0300; FAX. 215/359–1187; Roberta A. Haviland, Administrator

Erie Rehabilitation and Nursing Center, 2686 Peach Street, Erie, PA 16508; tel. 814/453–6641; FAX. 814/453–5546; Donna Stone

Green Acres Rehabilitation and Nursing Center, 1401 Ivy Hill Road, Wyndmoor, PA 19118; tel. 215/233–5605; FAX. 215/836–1050; Allen Segal

Greenery Rehabilitation and Skilled Nursing Center at Meadowlands, 2200 Hill Church–Houston Road, Canonsburg, PA 15317; tel. 412/745–8000, ext. 212; FAX. 412/746–8780; Kathy Carter, Acting Administrator

Hanover Hall Nursing and Rehabilitation Center, 267 Frederick Street, Hanover, PA 17331; tel. 717/637–8937; FAX. 717/633–5700; Christine F. Lorah, NHA, Administrator

Haverford Nursing and Rehabilitation Center, 2050 Old West Chester Pike, Havertown, PA 19083–2798; tel. 610/449–8600; FAX. 610/446–1126

Heartland Health Care Center, 550 South Negley, Pittsburgh, PA 15232; tel. 412/665–2400; FAX. 412/363–6146; Deborah Koch, Administrator

Heatherbank Rehabilitation and Skilled Nursing Center, 745 Chiques Hill Road, Columbia, PA 17512; tel. 717/684–7555; FAX. 717/684–0571; Joanne Loraw, Director, Admissions

Integrated Health Services of Chestnut Hill, 8833 Stenton Avenue, Wyndmoor, PA 19038; tel. 215/836–2100; FAX. 215/233–3551; Karen Pulini

Integrated Health Services of Greater Pittsburgh, 890 Mount Pleasant Road, Greensburg, PA 15601; tel. 412/837–8076; FAX. 412/837–3152; James Anthony Palmer, Administrator

Integrated Health Services of Pennsylvania at Broomall, 50 North Malin Road, Broomall, PA 19008; tel. 610/356–0800; FAX. 610/325–9499; Susan Eccles

Integrated Health Services of Pennsylvania at Plymouth, 900 East Germantown Avenue, Norristown, PA 19401; tel. 610/279–7300; FAX. 610/279–2061; Elaine Addlespurger

Jefferson Manor Health Centers, Rural Route Five, Brookville, PA 15825; tel. 814/849–8026; FAX. 814/849–3889; Diane Endress, Director, Nursing

LAS/St. John Specialty Care Center, 500 Wittenberg Way, P.O. Box 928, Mars, PA 16046; tel. 412/625–1571; FAX. 412/625–0087; Lynn Croushore, Executive Director

Lancashire Hall Nursing and Rehabilitation Center, 2829 Lititz Pike, Lancaster, PA 17601; tel. 717/569–3211; FAX. 717/569–1569; Jeanne Caron

Langhorne Gardens Rehabilitation and Nursing Center, 350 Manor Avenue, Langhorne, PA 19047; tel. 215/757–7667; FAX. 215/750–1426; Deborah Haugh

Laurel Nursing and Rehabilitation Center, 125 Holly Road, Hamburg, PA 19526–6902; tel. 610/562–2284; FAX. 610/562–0775; Denise M. Smith, Director, Nursing

Leader Nursing and Rehabilitation Center, 60 Highland Road, Bethel Park, PA 15102; tel. 412/831–6050; FAX. 412/831–7465; Martin Russell

Leader Nursing and Rehabilitation Center II, 2029 Westgate Drive, Bethlehem, PA 18017; tel. 610/861–0100; FAX. 610/861–4078; Mary Beth Schwartz

Liberty Nursing and Rehabiliation Center, Inter Med Unit, 17th and Allen Streets, Allentown, PA 18104; tel. 610/432–4351; FAX. 610/435–4470; M. J. Specter, N.H.A., Administrator

Main Line Nursing and Rehabilitation Center, 283 East Lancaster Avenue, Malvern, PA 19355; tel. 610/296–4170; FAX. 610/296–7051; John Hadgkiss

Manchester House Nursing and Convalescent Center, 411 Manchester Avenue, Media, PA 19063; tel. 610/565–1800; FAX. 610/891–0471; Donna L. Doyle, RN, NHA, Administrator

Manor Care Health Services, 14 Lincoln Avenue, Yeadon, PA 19050; tel. 610/626–7700; FAX. 610/626–5319; Stewart Bainum

Manor Care Health Services, 3430 Huntingdon Pike, Huntingdon Valley, PA 19006; tel. 215/938–7171; FAX. 215/938–7338; Peter L. Heck, Administrator

Manor Care Health Services, 1848 Greentree Road, Pittsburgh, PA 15220; tel. 412/344–7744; FAX. 412/344–5502; Linda Keith, Executive Director

Manor Care Health Services, 600 West Valley Forge Road, King of Prussia, PA 19406; tel. 610/337–1775; FAX. 610/337–3638; Valerie Palmieri, Administrator

ManorCare Health Services, 425 Buttonwood Street, West Reading, PA 19611; tel. 610/373–5166; FAX. 610/374–7560; Robert McQuillan, NHA

ManorCare Health Services, 1070 Stouffer Avenue, Chambersburg, PA 17201; tel. 717/263–0436; FAX. 717/263–7468; Caroline Lensbower, NHA, Administrator

ManorCare Health Services Nursing and Rehabilitation Center, 1265 South Cedar Crest Boulevard, Allentown, PA 18103; tel. 610/776–7522; FAX. 610/776–0270; Judith Kempf, NHA

Mariner Health at North Hills, 194 Swinderman Road, Wexford, PA 15090; tel. 412/935–3781; FAX. 412/935–0190; Nancy Flenner, Administrator

Mount Lebanon Manor, 350 Gilkeson Road, Pittsburgh, PA 15228; tel. 412/257–4444; FAX. 412/257–8226; Anthony J. Molinaro, Administrator

Presbyterian Medical Center of Oakmont, 1215 Hulton Road, Oakmont, PA 15139; tel. 412/828–5600; FAX. 412/826–6121; Mary Pat Braudis, NHA, Executive Director

Quakertown Nursing and Rehabilitation Center, 1020 South Main Street, Quakertown, PA 18950–1592; tel. 215/536–9300; FAX. 215/536–1970; Theodore Foedisch

Quincy United Methodist Home, 6596 Orphanage Road, P.O. Box 217, Quincy, PA 17247; tel. 717/749–3151; FAX. 717/749–3912; Kathleen R. Hoos, RN, NHA, President

Redstone Highlands Health Care Center, Six Garden Center Drive, Greensburg, PA 15601–1397; tel. 412/832–8400; FAX. 412/836–3710; Judith B. Wohnsiedler, Assistant Administrator

Rest Haven–York, 1050 South George Street, York, PA 17403; tel. 717/843–9866; FAX. 717/846–5894; Nancy A. Underwood, Administrator

Richboro Care Center, 253 Twining Ford Road, Richboro, PA 18954; tel. 215/357–2032; FAX. 215/357–3444; Gale Bupp

Rochester Manor, 174 Virginia Avenue, Rochester, PA 15074; tel. 412/775–6400; FAX. 412/775–4386; Kathryn Kopsack, Administrator

Rose View Manor, Inc., 1201 Rural Avenue, Williamsport, PA 17701; tel. 717/323–4340; FAX. 717/323–0836; Russell Twigg

Saratoga Manor Nursing and Rehabilitation Center, 225 Evergreen Road, Pottstown, PA 19464; tel. 610/323–1800; FAX. 610/323–7914; Russell Twigg

Saunders House, 100 Lancaster Avenue, Wynnewood, PA 19096; tel. 610/658–5100; FAX. 610/658–5101; William Grim

South Mountain Restoration Center, 10058 South Mountain Road, South Mountain, PA 17261; tel. 717/749–3121, ext. 316; FAX. 717/749–3946; Thomas A. Buckus, Administrator

Statesman Health and Rehabilitation Center, 2629 Trenton Road, Levittown, PA 19056; tel. 215/943–7777; FAX. 215/943–1240; Charles Kane

The Fairways at Brookline Village, 1950 Cliffside Drive, State College, PA 16801; tel. 814/238–3139; FAX. 814/235–2074; Clifford Coldren

The Healthcare Campus at Colonial Manor, 970 Colonial Avenue, York, PA 17403; tel. 717/845–2661; FAX. 717/854–0529; George R. Lorah, Administrator

The Presbyterian Medical Center of Washington, 835 South Main Street, Washington, PA 15301; tel. 412/222–4300; FAX. 412/223–5697; Harvey Brown, Jr., Executive Vice President, Chief Executive Officer

Twinbrook Medical Center, 3805 Field Street, Erie, PA 16511; tel. 814/898–5600; FAX. 814/899–9829; Tamara J. Montell, Nursing Home Administrator

Valley Manor Nursing and Rehabilitation Center, 7650 Route 309, Coopersburg, PA 18036; tel. 610/282–1919; FAX. 610/282–2962; Janice Ricchio, NHA

Wallingford Nursing and Rehabilitation Center, 115 South Providence Road, Wallingford, PA 19086; tel. 610/565–3232; FAX. 610/892–0830; Ventura Gutierrez

Western Reserve Health and Rehabilitation Center, 1521 West 54th Street, Erie, PA 16509; tel. 814/864–0671; FAX. 814/864–1424; Linda Jackson, Director, Nursing

Woodhaven Care Center, 2400 McGinley Road, Monroeville, PA 15146; tel. 412/856–4770; FAX. 412/856–6856; Rebecca D. Jobe, Administrator

RHODE ISLAND

Evergreen House Health Center, One Evergreen Drive, East Providence, RI 02914; tel. 401/438–3250; FAX. 410/438–3250; Madeline Ernest

Heatherwood Nursing and Subacute Center, Inc., 398 Bellevue Avenue, Newport, RI 02840; tel. 401/849–6600; FAX. 401/847–0778; Joan Woods

Morgan Health Center, 80 Morgan Avenue, Johnston, RI 02919; tel. 401/944–7800; FAX. 401/944–6037; David Ryan

Oak Hill Nursing and Rehabilitation Center, 544 Pleasant Street, Pawtucket, RI 02860; tel. 401/725–8888; FAX. 401/723–5720; Richard E. Gamache, Administrator

Oakland Grove Health Care Center, 560 Cumberland Hill Road, Woonsocket, RI 02895; tel. 401/769–0800; FAX. 401/766–3661; Susan Laninfa, Administrator

Saint Elizabeth Home, 109 Melrose Street, Providence, RI 02907–1898; tel. 401/941–0200; FAX. 401/941–5231; Steven J. Horowitz, Administrator

Steere House Nursing and Rehabilitation Center, 100 Borden Street, Providence, RI 02903; tel. 401/454–7970; FAX. 401/831–7570; Steven Farrow

SOUTH CAROLINA

C. M. Tucker, Jr./Dowdy Gardner Nursing Care Center, 2200 Harden Street, Columbia, SC 29203–7199; tel. 803/737–5302; FAX. 803/737–5342; Shielda Friendly, Director

Heartland Health Care Center of Charleston, 1800 Eagle Landing Boulevard, Hanahan, SC 29406; tel. 803/553–656; FAX. 803/553–9773; Paul J. Cercone, Administrator

Integrated Health Services of Charleston at Driftwood, 2375 Baker Hospital Boulevard, North Charleston, SC 29405; tel. 803/744–2750; FAX. 803/747–0406; B. C. Davidson, Administrator

Life Care Center of Charleston, 2600 Elms Plantation Boulevard, North Charleston, SC 29418; tel. 803/764–3500; FAX. 803/569–7222; Betty Whittle, Executive Director

Life Care Center of Columbia, 2514 Faraway Drive, Columbia, SC 29223; tel. 803/865–1999; FAX. 803/865–0759; Louis Milite

Manor Care Nursing and Rehabilitation Center, 2416 Sunset Boulevard, West Columbia, SC 29169; tel. 803/796–8024; FAX. 803/796–5485; Colette Pickett

Oakmont East, 601 Sulphur Springs Road, Greenville, SC 29611; tel. 864/246–2721; FAX. 864/246–7563; Deborah Dobson

TENNESSEE

Allen Morgan Health Center, 177 North Highland, Memphis, TN 38111; tel. 901/325–4003; FAX. 901/327–8847; Rebecca D. DeRousse, Administrator

Briarcliff Health Care Center, 100 Elmhurst Drive, Oak Ridge, TN 37803; tel. 615/481–3367; FAX. 615/483–7121; Stan Strauge, Administrator

Laurel Manor Health Care, 902 Buchanan Road, New Tazewell, TN 37825; tel. 615/626–8215; FAX. 615/626–0676; Charles Birkett

Manor House of Dover, 537 Spring Street, Dover, TN 37058–8039; tel. 615/232–6902; FAX. 615/232–4256; Sheila K. McArdle, Regional Vice President

NHC HealthCare, 420 North Univeristy Street, Murfreesboro, TN 37133–2009; tel. 615/893–2602; FAX. 615/890–1224; W. Adams

Woods Memorial Hospital District, Highway 411 and Old Grady Road, P.O. Box 410, Etowah, TN 37331; tel. 615/263–3605; FAX. 615/263–3793; Phil Campbell

TEXAS

Beacon Health, Ltd., 9182 Six Pines Drive, The Woodlands, TX 77380; tel. 281/364–0317; FAX. 281/298–7366; Kathy Roberts

Beechnut Manor Living Center, 12777 Beechnut Street, Houston, TX 77072; tel. 713/879–8040; FAX. 713/879–5616; Kenneth Morgan

Brookhaven Nursing Center, 1855 Cheyenne, Carrollton, TX 75008; tel. 972/394–7141; FAX. 972/492–5534; Stephen Powell, Administrator

Bureau of Prisons–Federal Medical Center, 3150 Horton Road, Fort Worth, TX 76119; tel. 817/535–2111; FAX. 817/535–8937; George Killinger

CASA, a Special Hospital, 1803 Old Spanish Trail, Houston, TX 77054; tel. 713/796–2272; FAX. 713/796–0043; Gretchen Thorp

Hearthstone of Round Rock, 401 Oakwood Boulevard, Round Rock, TX 78681; tel. 512/388–7494; FAX. 512/388–2166; Stacy Adams, Administrator

Heartland Health Care Center, 11406 Rustic Rock Drive, Austin, TX 78750; tel. 512/335–5028; FAX. 512/335–0709; Mary Lou Clem, Administrator

Heartland Health Care Center, 2939 Woodland Park Drive, Houston, TX 77082; tel. 713/870–9100; FAX. 713/558–9700; Terri Humes, Administrator

Heartland Health Care Center–Bedford, 2001 Forst Ridge Drive, Bedford, TX 76021; tel. 817/571–6804; FAX. 817/267–4176; Mack Baldridge, Administrator

Heartland of San Antonio, One Heartland Drive, San Antonio, TX 78247; tel. 210/653–1219; FAX. 210/653–8977; Guy Bowles, Administrator

Hillcrest Manor, 208 Maple, P.O. Box 230, Luling, TX 78648; tel. 210/875–5219; FAX. 210/875–2919; John Berg

IHS Hospital at Houston, 6160 South Loop East, Houston, TX 77087; tel. 713/640–6400; FAX. 713/640–2935; C. Philip Hacker, Executive Director

Integrated Health Services of Dallas at Treemont, 5550 Harvest Hill Road, Dallas, TX 75230; tel. 214/661–1862; FAX. 214/715–5557; Timothy Miller, Administrator

Lampasas Manor, 611 North Broad, P.O. Box 970, Lampasas, TX 76550; tel. 512/556–3588; FAX. 512/556–2507; Sandra Springwater

Manor Care Health Services–Briaridge, 7703 Briaridge Drive, San Antonio, TX 78230; tel. 210/341–6121; FAX. 210/341–1298; Stewart Bainum

Willowbrook Health Care Center, 13631 Ardfield Drive, Houston, TX 77070; tel. 713/955–9572; FAX. 713/955–1597; Sherion Schroeder

Yorktown Manor, 670 West Fourth, Yorktown, TX 78164; tel. 512/564–2275; FAX. 512/564–3593; Janice Tieman, Director, Nursing

UTAH

South Davis Community Hospital, 401 South 400 East, Bountiful, UT 84010; tel. 801/295–2361; FAX. 801/295–1398; Gordon W. Bennet, Administrator

Sunshine Terrace Foundation, Inc., 225 North 200 West, Logan, UT 84321–3805; tel. 801/752–0411, ext. 216; FAX. 801/752–1318

VIRGINIA

Bay Pointe Medical and Rehabilitation Center, 1148 First Colonial Road, Virginia Beach, VA 23454–2499; tel. 757/481–3321; FAX. 757/481–4413; Bruce Busby

Berkshire Health Care Center, 705 Clearview Drive, Vinton, VA 24179; tel. 703/982–6691; FAX. 703/982–6518; Richie Alba, Administrator

Camelot Hall of Lynchburg, 5615 Seminole Avenue, Lynchburg, VA 24502; tel. 804/239–2657; FAX. 804/239–4062; Elizabeth E. Kail, Administrator

Goodwin House West, 3440 South Jefferson Street, Falls Church, VA 22041; tel. 703/578–7230; FAX. 703/578–7228; Fran Casey, Director

Harbour Pointe Medical and Rehabilitation Centre, (a Vencor Facility), 1005 Hampton Boulevard, Norfolk, VA 23507; tel. 757/623–5602; FAX. 757/623–4646; Vickie Archer, Executive Director

Health of Virginia, 2420 Pemberton Road, Richmond, VA 23233–2099; tel. 804/747–9200; FAX. 804/747–1574; Walter W. Regirer, Chief Executive Officer, General Counsel

Iliff Nursing and Rehab Center, 8000 Iliff Drive, Dunn Loring, VA 22027; tel. 703/560–1000; FAX. 703/280–0406; Joan H. Bishop, Administrator

James River Convalescent Center, 540 Aberthaw Avenue, Newport News, VA 23601; tel. 804/595–2273; FAX. 757/595–2271; Nancy Pittman, Administrator, Vice President

Lucy Corr Nursing Home, 6800 Lucy Corr Court, P.O. Drawer 170, Chesterfield, VA 23832; tel. 804/748–1511; FAX. 804/796–6285; Jacob Mast

Manning Convalescent Home, Inc., 175 Hatton Street, Portsmouth, VA 23705; tel. 757/399–1321; FAX. 757/399–4337; T. W. Manning, President

Manor Care Health Services, 550 South Carlin Springs Road, Arlington, VA 22204; tel. 703/379–7200; FAX. 703/578–5788; Mary Jo Sbitani, Administrator

Manor Care Health Services–Fair Oaks Nursing and Rehabilitation Center, 12475 Lee Jackson Memorial Highway, Fairfax, VA 22033; tel. 703/352–7172, ext. 3203; FAX. 703/218–3200; Justin M. Dunie, Administrator

ManorCare Health Services–Stratford, 2125 Hilliard Road, Richmond, VA 23228; tel. 804/266–9666; FAX. 804/266–3599; Vivian Thomas, Administrator

Nansemond Pointe Rehabilitation and Healthcare Centre, 200 West Constance Road, Suffolk, VA 23434; tel. 757/539–8744; FAX. 757/539–6128; Arlene Palmer, Assistant Administrator

Oak Hill Health Care Center, 512 Houston Street, P.O. Box 2565, Staunton, VA 24401; tel. 703/886–2335; FAX. 703/886–7459; Mary Lou DiGrassie, Administrator

Parham Healthcare and Rehabilitation Center, 2400 East Parham Road, Richmond, VA 23228; tel. 804/264–9185; FAX. 804/264–3963; Clifton J. Porter II

Riverside Regional Convalescent Center, 1000 Old Denbigh Boulevard, Newport News, VA 23602; tel. 757/875–2020; FAX. 757/875–2036; Patricia A. Iannetta, Administrator

Williamsburg Health Care and Rehabilitation Center, 1235 Mt. Vernon Avenue, Williamsburg, VA 23185; tel. 804/229–4121; Mark Hamister

Woodbine Rehabilitation and Healthcare Center, 2729 King Street, Alexandria, VA 22302; tel. 703/836–8838; FAX. 703/836–2965; Mary Ann Sleigh, Administrator

Woodmont Health Care Center, 11 Dairy Lane, P.O. Box 419, Fredericksburg, VA 22404–0419; tel. 540/371–9414; FAX. 540/371–4501; Sharon Bartlett

WASHINGTON

Blue Mountain Medical and Rehabilitation Center, 1200 Southeast 12th Street, College Place, WA 99324; tel. 509/529–4080; FAX. 509/529–2173; Gloria Botimer, Chief Executive Officer

Harmony Gardens Care Center, 10010 Des Moines Way, S., Seattle, WA 98168; tel. 206/762–0166; FAX. 206/762–8612; Tom Dhanens, Administrator

Highlands Care Center, 1110 Edmonds Avenue, N.E., Renton, WA 98056; tel. 206/226–6120; FAX. 206/228–8087; Andrew Turner

Integrated Health Services of Seattle, 820 Northwest 95th Street, Seattle, WA 98117; tel. 206/782–0100, ext. 228; FAX. 206/781–1448; Jerry Harvey, Administrator

Laurelwood Care Center, 150–102nd Avenue, S.E., Bellevue, WA 98004; tel. 206/454–6166; FAX. 206/454–7152; Andrew Turner, Chief Executive Officer

Mercer Island Care Center, 7445 Southeast 24th Street, Mercer Island, WA 98040; tel. 206/232–6600; FAX. 206/232–6502; Andrew Turner

Phoenix Rehabilitation Center, 555 16th Avenue, Seattle, WA 98122; tel. 206/324–8200; FAX. 206/324–0780; Skip McDonald, Ph.D., Executive Director

Terrace View Diversified Health Care Center, Inc., 1701–18th Avenue, S., Seattle, WA 98144; tel. 206/329–9586; FAX. 206/325–1750; Maria Joell, Director, Nursing

The Care Center at Kelsey Creek, 2210 132nd Avenue, S.E., Bellevue, WA 98005; tel. 206/957–2400; FAX. 206/957–2425; Betty Mullin

Wedgwood Rehabilitation Center, 9132 Ravenna Avenue, N.E., Seattle, WA 98115; tel. 206/524–6535; FAX. 206/523–1817; Andrew Turner

WEST VIRGINIA

Americare Pine Lodge Nursing and Rehabilitation Center, 405 Stanford Road, Beckley, WV 25801; tel. 304/252–6317; FAX. 304/253–4140; Sherry Johnson

GlenWood Park Retirement Village, Route One, Box 464, Princeton, WV 24740–9244; tel. 304/425–8128; Daniel W. Farley, Ph.D., CNHA, President, Chief Executive Officer

Heartland of Charleston, 3819 Chesterfield Avenue, Charleston, WV 25304; tel. 304/925–4771; FAX. 304/925–1343; Karen Lawson

WISCONSIN

Beaver Dam Care Center, 410 Roedl Court, P.O. Box 617, Beaver Dam, WI 53916; tel. 414/887–7191; FAX. 414/887–2380; Richard Rexrode

Colonial Manor Medical and Rehabilitation Center, 1010 East Wausau Avenue, Wausau, WI 54403–3199; tel. 715/842–2028; FAX. 715/845–5810; Jean Burgener

DePaul Hospital, Inc., 4143 South 13th Street, Milwaukee, WI 53221–1701; tel. 414/281–4400; FAX. 414/325–3172; Kathy Olewinski, Hospital Administrator

Eastview Medical and Rehabilitation Center, 729 Park Street, Antigo, WI 54409; tel. 715/623–2356; FAX. 715/623–2263; Tina A. VerHagen, NHA

Franciscan Villa, 3601 South Chicago Avenue, South Milwaukee, WI 53172; tel. 414/764–4100; FAX. 414/764–0706; Roger L. DeMark, Administrator

Franciscan Woods, 19525 West North Avenue, Brookfield, WI 53045; tel. 414/785–1114; FAX. 414/785–9967; Mary Piette

Greendale Health and Rehabilitation Center, 3129 Michigan Avenue, Sheboygan, WI 53081; tel. 414/458–1155; FAX. 414/458–4869; Suzanne Bruner, Executive Director

Manor Care Health Services, 1335 South Oneida, Appleton, WI 54911; tel. 414/731–6646; FAX. 414/731–5177; Lorie Neumann

Marian Catholic Center, 3333 West Highland Boulevard, Milwaukee, WI 53208; tel. 414/344–8100; FAX. 414/345–4793; Michael Zimmerman

Marian Franciscan Center, 9632 West Appleton Avenue, Milwaukee, WI 53225; tel. 414/461–8850; FAX. 414/461–9570; James Gresham, Regional Vice President, Continuing Care Services Division

Middleton Village Nursing and Rehabilitation Center, 6201 Elmwood Avenue, Middleton, WI 53562; tel. 608/831–8300; FAX. 608/831–4253; Mary Ann Drescher, Administrator

Mount Carmel Health and Rehabilitation Center, 5700 West Layton Avenue, Milwaukee, WI 53220; tel. 414/281–7200; FAX. 414/281–4620; Dennis E. Zoltak, Administrator

Northwest Health Care Center, 7800 West Fond Du Lac Avenue, Milwaukee, WI 53218; tel. 414/464–3950; FAX. 414/464–5110; Candy Gremore, Executive Director

Outagamie County Health Center, 3400 West Brewster Street, Appleton, WI 54914; tel. 414/832–5400; FAX. 414/832–5416; David A. Rothmann, Administrator

Parkview Manor Health and Rehabilitation Center, 2961 St. Anthony Drive, Green Bay, WI 54311; tel. 414/468–0861; FAX. 414/468–8548; Stacie Herzog

The Terrace at St. Francis, 3200 South 20th Street, Milwaukee, WI 53215; tel. 414/389–3200, ext. 3250; FAX. 414/389–3300; Geri Wandrey

Villa Clement and Clement Manor Health Center, 3939 South 92nd Street, Greenfield, WI 53228; tel. 414/321–1800; FAX. 414/546–7333; William H. Lange, President, Chief Executive Officer

Western Village Health and Rehabilitation, 1540 Shawano Avenue, Green Bay, WI 54303; tel. 414/499–5177; FAX. 414/499–6035; Linda Kessenich

Section C

JCAHO Accredited Freestanding Mental Health Care Organizations

The accredited freestanding mental health care organizations listed have been accredited as of January 1, 1997, by the Joint Commission on Accreditation of Healthcare Organizations by decision of the Accreditation Committee of the Board of Commissioners.

The organizations listed here have been found to be in compliance with the Joint Commissions standards for Accreditation Manual for Mental Health, Chemical Dependency, and Mental Retardation/Development Disabilities Services.

Please refer to section A of the AHA Guide for information on hospitals with inpatient and/or outpatient services. These hospitals are identified by Facility Codes F52, F53, F54, F55, F56, F57, F58 and F59. In section A, those hospitals identified by Approval Code 1 are JCAHO accredited.

We present this list simply as a convenient directory. Inclusion or omission of any organization's name indicates neither approval nor disapproval by Healthcare InfoSource, Inc., a subsidiary of the American Hospital Association.

United States

ALABAMA

Bradford Adolescent at Oak Mountain, 2280 Highway, Pelham, AL 35124; tel. 205/664–3460; Eve S. Laxer, Chief Executive Officer

Bradford Health Services at Birmingham Lodge, 1189 Allbritton Road, Warrior, AL 35180; tel. 205/647–1945; Roy M. Ramsey, Executive Director

Bradford at Huntsville, 1600 Browns Ferry Road, Madison, AL 35758; tel. 205/461–7272; Benjamin Y. Lee, Ph.D., Chief Executive Officer

Eufaula Adolescent Center, P.O. Box 1179, Eufaula, AL 36072–1179; tel. 334/687–5741; FAX. 334/687–0693; Carol M. Driggers, Quality Improvement

New Perspectives (Adult), 1000 Fairfax Park, Tuscaloosa, AL 35406; tel. 205/391–4738; FAX. 205/759–4151; Martha Hinkle, Administrator

Noble Army Health Clinic, Building 295, Fort McClellan, AL 36205–5083; tel. 205/848–2151; Col. Robert Reed, Chief Executive Officer

Partial Hospital Institute of America, Inc., 1565 Hillcrest Road, Mobile, AL 36695; tel. 334/607–7610; FAX. 334/607–7621; James S. Harrold, Jr., M.D., Chief Executive Officer

Pathway, Inc., Route 2, Box 352–A, New Brockton, AL 36351; tel. 334/894–6322; Norman G. Hemp, Executive Director

Physicians' Psychiatric Clinic, P.C., 10 Mobile Street, Mobile, AL 36607; tel. 334/450–1200; FAX. 334/450–1207; Maureen Driscoll, M.S., Director, Clinical Services

The Catalyst Center (Adolescent), 1000 Fairfax Park, Tuscaloosa, AL 35406; tel. 205/391–4738; FAX. 205/759–4151; Martha Hinkle, Chief Executive Officer

Thomasville Mental Health Rehabilitation Center, Bashi Road, Thomasville, AL 36784; tel. 334/636–5421, ext. 230; FAX. 334/636–5421, ext. 285; Kimberly S. Ingram, M.S.N., Facility Director

Three Springs Residential Treatment Center, 101 Madison Street, P.O. Box 370, Courtland, AL 35618; tel. 205/637–2199; FAX. 205/637–8911; Gerald Maxwell, M.S., Administrator

ALASKA

Akeela House, Inc., 2805 Bering Street, Suite Four, Anchorage, AK 99503; tel. 907/561–5206; Rosalie Nadeau, Deputy Director

Alaska Children's Services, 4600 Abbott Road, Anchorage, AK 99507; tel. 907/346–2101; FAX. 907/346–2748; James E. Maley, Executive Director

Department of Veterans Affairs Medical and Regional Office Center, 2925 DeBarr Road, Ankorage, AK 99508–2989; tel. 907/257–6774; Mr. Alonzo Poteet, Chief Executive Officer

ARIZONA

ABCS Little Canyon Center, Inc., 3115 West Missouri Avenue, P.O. Box 39239, Phoenix, AZ 85069–9239; tel. 602/943–7760; FAX. 602/943–7864; Bob Garrett, CBSW, Admissions Coordinator

Arizona Children's Home Association, 2700 South Eighth Avenue, Tucson, AZ 85725–7277; tel. 520/622–7611; FAX. 520/624–7042; Fred J. Chaffee, Chief Executive Officer

Calvary Rehabilitation Center, Inc., 720 East Montebello Avenue, Phoenix, AZ 85014; tel. 602/279–1468; FAX. 602/279–3090; Jeffrey Shook, Chief Executive Officer

Chandler Valley Hope, 501 North Washington, Chandler, AZ 85244–1839; tel. 602/899–3335; FAX. 602/899–6697; Julian S. Pickens, Ed.D., Chief Executive Officer

Cottonwood de Tucson, Inc., 4110 West Sweetwater Drive, Tucson, AZ 85745; tel. 520/743–0411; FAX. 520/743–7991; Ronald B. Welch, President, Chief Executive Officer

Desert Hills Center for Youth and Families, 2797 North Introspect Drive, Tucson, AZ 85745; tel. 520/622–5437; FAX. 520/792–6249; Boyd Dover, Chief Executive Officer

Devereux/Arizona, 6436 East Sweetwater Avenue, Scottsdale, AZ 85254; tel. 602/998–2920; FAX. 602/443–1531; Stephen A. Vitali, Executive Director

META Services, 621 West Southern Avenue, Mesa, AZ 85210; tel. 602/649–1111; FAX. 602/649–0149; Eugene Johnson, President, Chief Executive Officer

Mingus Mountain Estate Residential Center, Inc., P.O. Box 848, Dewey, AZ 86327; tel. 602/249–1311; Dr. Pauline H. Don Carlos, Chief Executive Officer

Parc Place, 5116 East Thomas Road, Phoenix, AZ 85018; tel. 602/840–4774, ext. 316; FAX. 602/840–7567; Darcey A. Morrow, M.S.W., Director, Admissions

Prehab of Arizona, Inc., 868 East University, Mesa, AZ 85203; tel. 602/969–4024, ext. 210; FAX. 602/969–0039; Michael T. Hughes, Executive Director

Remuda Ranch Center for Anorexia and Bulimia, Jack Burden Road, Wickenburg, AZ 85358; tel. 602/684–3913; FAX. 602/684–2908; Ward Keller, President

Salvation Army Recovery Center, 2707 East Van Buren, Phoenix, AZ 85008; tel. 602/267–1404; FAX. 602/267–4131; Major John Webb, Chief Executive Officer

Sierra Tucson, Inc., 16500 North Lago Del Oro Parkway, Tucson, AZ 85739; tel. 520/624–4000; FAX. 520/825–3523; Terry A. Stephens, Executive Director

Southeastern Arizona Psychiatric Health Facility, 470 South Ocotillo Avenue, P.O. Box 1296, Benson, AZ 85602; tel. 602/586–9161; FAX. 602/586–7939; Dana J. Dapper, ACSW, Executive Director

The Meadows, 1655 North Tegner, P.O. Box 97, Highway 89/93, Wickenburg, AZ 85358; tel. 800/621–4062; FAX. 602/684–3261; J. P. Mellody, Executive Director

The New Foundation, P.O. Box 3828, Scottsdale, AZ 85271; tel. 602/945–3302; FAX. 602/945–9308; David S. Hedgcock, Executive Director

Touchstone Community, Inc., 4202 East Union Hill Drive, Phoenix, AZ 85024; tel. 602/992–2952; FAX. 602/953–9217; Ida Chiappetta, Director, Admissions

Westbridge Treatment Centers, 1830 East Roosevelt, Phoenix, AZ 85006; tel. 602/254–0884; FAX. 602/258–4033; Michael J. Perry, Chief Executive Officer

Westcenter, 2105 East Allen Road, Tucson, AZ 85719; tel. 520/795–0952; FAX. 520/318–6442; Allan Harrington, Executive Director

ARKANSAS

Centers for Youth and Families, P.O. Box 251970, Little Rock, AR 72225–1970; tel. 501/666–8686; FAX. 501/660–6836; Richard T. Hill, President, Chief Executive Officer

Millcreek of Arkansas, P.O. Box 727, Industrial Park Drive, Highway 79 North, Fordyce, AR 71742; tel. 501/352–8203; FAX. 501/352–5311; Mary Huntley, Interim Administrator

Ozark Guidance Center, Inc., 219 South Thompson Street, P.O. Box 1340, Springdale, AR 72765; tel. 501/751–7052; FAX. 501/751–4346; David L. Williams, Ph.D., President, Chief Executive Officer

Timber Ridge Ranch Neurorehabilitation Center, Inc., 15000 Highway 298, P.O. Box 90, Benton, AR 72015–5009; tel. 501/594–5211; Sharon J. Burleson, Executive Director

Youth Home, Inc., 20400 Colonel Glenn Road, Little Rock, AR 72210–5323; tel. 501/821–5500; FAX. 501/821–5580; Beth Cartwright, ACSW, L.C.S.W. Executive Director

CALIFORNIA

A Touch of Care, 2231 South Carmelina Avenue, Los Angeles, CA 90064; tel. 310/473–6525; FAX. 310/479–1287; Richard B. Cohen, MFCC, Executive Director

Betty Ford Center at Eisenhower, 39000 Bob Hope Drive, Rancho Mirage, CA 92270; tel. 619/773–4100; FAX. 619/773–4141; Michael S. Neatherton, Vice President, Administrator

Broad Horizons of Ramona, Inc., 1236 H Street, P.O. Box 1920, Ramona, CA 92065; tel. 619/789–7060; FAX. 619/789–4062; Ellen Wright, LCSW, Chief Executive Officer

Care Options In Home Treatment Program, 18881 Von Karman, Suite 250, Irvine, CA 92715; tel. 714/740–8040; FAX. 714/442–2196; David F. Ellisor, Chief Executive Officer

Cornerstone of Southern California, 13682 Yorba Street, Tustin, CA 92680; tel. 714/730–5399; FAX. 714/730–3505; Lynda Klinger, Administrator

Creative Care, Inc., 18850 Devonshire Street, Northridge, CA 91324; tel. 818/363–5630; FAX. 818/368–5269; Morteza Khaleghi, Ph.D., Clinical Director

Health Care Children's Campus, 15339 Saticoy Street, Van Nuys, CA 91406; tel. 818/778–6400; Kim Brandi–O'Meara, MAMFCC, Director, Clinical Services

Impact Drug and Alcohol Treatment Center, 1680 North Fair Oaks Avenue, Pasadena, CA 91103; tel. 818/798–0884; James M. Stillwell, Executive Director

Ivy Lea Manor–Parkview, 1379 West Park Western Drive, Suite 310, San Pedro, CA 90732–2217; tel. 310/832–8511; Casey Smart, Administrator

Learning Services – Northern California, 10855 DeBruin Way, Gilroy, CA 95020; tel. 408/848–4379; FAX. 408/848–6509; Randle Mitchell, Chief Executive Officer

Los Angeles Centers for Alcohol and Drug Abuse, 11015 Bloomfield Avenue, Santa Fe Springs, CA 90670; tel. 310/906–2676; FAX. 310/906–2681; John Brown, Chief Executive Officer

Michael's House, The Treatment Center for Men, 430 South Cahuilla Road, Palm Springs, CA 92262; tel. 619/320–5486; FAX. 619/778–6020; Arlene Rosen, President, Chief Executive Officer

Monterey Psychiatric Health Facility, Inc., Five Via Joaquin, Monterey, CA 93940; tel. 408/645–9000; FAX. 408/646–1317; Dr. Thomas Marra, Chief Executive Officer

Oak Grove Institute Foundation, 24275 Jefferson Avenue, Murrieta, CA 92562; tel. 909/677–5599; FAX. 909/698–0461; Elizabeth H. Burnett, Ph.D., Clinical Project Director

Residential Treatment Centers of America, Inc., 1227 East Shepherd Avenue, Fresno, CA 93720; tel. 209/449–2604; Robert F. Norton, Chief Administrative Officer

S. T. E. P. S., 224 East Clara Street, Port Hueneme, CA 93044; tel. 805/488–6424; FAX. 805/488–6717; John J. Megara, M.B.A., Administrator

San Diego Center for Children, 3002 Armstrong Street, San Diego, CA 92111–5798; tel. 619/277–9550, ext. 114; FAX. 619/279–2763; Edwin G. Kofler, M.B.A., Chief Executive Officer

SeaBridge Adolescent Treatment Center, 30371 Morning View Drive, Malibu, CA 90265; tel. 310/457–5802; FAX. 310/457–6093; Martha Zimmerman, Executive Director

Spencer Recovery Centers, Inc., 343 West Foothill Boulevard, Monrovia, CA 91016; tel. 818/358–3662; FAX. 818/357–7405; Cindy Salo Garcia, Chief Operating Officer

Substance Abuse Foundation of Long Beach, Inc., 3125 East Seventh Street, Long Beach, CA 90804; tel. 310/439–7755; Ronald H. Banner, Executive Director

Tarzana Treatment Center, 18646 Oxnard Street, Tarzana, CA 91356; tel. 818/996–1051; FAX. 818/345–3778; Albert Senella, Chief Executive Officer

The Linden Center, 5750 Wilshire Boulevard, Suite 535, Los Angeles, CA 90036; tel. 213/937–3999, ext. 209; FAX. 213/937–6641; David Amitai, Ph.D., Associate Director

Twin Town Treatment Centers, 10741 Los Alamitos Boulevard, Los Alamitos, CA 90720; tel. 310/594–8844; FAX. 310/493–1280; Warren L. Devon, Executive Director

VA Medical Center, 16111 Plummer Street, Sepulveda, CA 91343; tel. 818/895–9466; FAX. 818/895–9559; Dollie Whitehead, Chief Executive Officer

Veterans Affairs Northern California Health Care System, 2300 Contra Costa Boulevard, Suite 440, Pleasant Hill, CA 94523; tel. 510/372–2010; FAX. 510/372–2020; Sheldon Fine, Chief Executive Officer

Vista Del Mar Child and Family Services, 3200 Motor Avenue, Los Angeles, CA 90034; tel. 310/836–1223, ext. 201; FAX. 310/204–1405; Gerald D. Zaslaw, ACSW, Chief Executive Officer

Vista Pacifica, 7989 Linda Vista Road, San Diego, CA 92111; tel. 619/576–1200; FAX. 619/576–8362; Daniel R. Valentine, Administrator

Vista San Diego Center, 3003 Armstrong Street, San Diego, CA 92111; tel. 619/268–3343, ext. 204; FAX. 619/268–8737; Elyce Hoene, M.A., Intake Coordinator

Watts Health Foundation, Inc., 10300 South Compton Avenue, Los Angeles, CA 90002; tel. 213/564–4331; FAX. 213/563–6378; Dr. Clyde Oden, Chief Executive Officer

COLORADO

Adolescent and Family Institute of Colorado, Inc., 10001 West 32nd Avenue, Wheat Ridge, CO 80033; tel. 303/238–1231; FAX. 303/238–0500; Alex M. Panio, Jr., Ph.D., Chief Executive Officer

Aurora Behavioral Health Hospital, 1290 South Potomac Street, Aurora, CO 80012; tel. 303/745–2273; FAX. 303/369–9556; John Thompson, Administrator

Cheyenne Mesa, 1301 South Eighth Street, Colorado Springs, CO 80906; tel. 719/520–1400; FAX. 719/475–1527; Sal Edwards, Chief Executive Officer

Colorado Boys Ranch, 28071 Highway 109, La Junta, CO 81050; tel. 719/384–5981; FAX. 719/384–8119; David Zimmerman, Vice President

Forest Heights Lodge, 4801 Forest Hill Road, Evergreen, CO 80439; tel. 303/674–6681; FAX. 303/674–6805; Russell H. Colburn, M.S.W., LCSW, Executive Director

Harmony Foundation, Inc., 1600 Fish Hatchery Road, P.O. Box 1989, Estes Park, CO 80517; tel. 970/586–4491; Donald R. Hays, J.D., NCACII, CACIII, Director

Learning Services–Rocky Mountain Region, Brain Injury and Stroke Rehabilitation Programs, 7201 West Hampden Avenue, Lakewood, CO 80227; tel. 303/989–6660; FAX. 303/989–2830; Kenneth R. Hosack, Program Director

Parker Valley Hope, 22422 East Main Street, Parker, CO 80134; tel. 303/841–7857; FAX. 303/841–6526; John J. Arnold, Ph.D., Program Director

Pikes Peak Mental Health Center, 220 Ruskin Drive, Colorado Springs, CO 80910; tel. 719/572–6100; FAX. 719/572–6199; Charles J. Vorwaller, President, Chief Executive Officer

CONNECTICUT

Berkshire Woods Chemical Dependence Treatment Center, Fairfield Circle South, P.O. Box 7006, Newtown, CT 06470; tel. 203/426–2531; FAX. 203/426–6285; Sarah Kruel, Chief Executive Officer

Capitol Region Mental Health Center, 500 Vine Street, Hartford, CT 06112; tel. 203/297–0903; FAX. 203/297–0914; Lillian Tamayo, Chief Executive Officer

Cornerstone of Eagle Hill, 32 Alberts Hill Road, Sandy Hook, CT 06482; tel. 203/426–8085; FAX. 203/426–2821; Norman J. Sokolow, President

Greater Bridgeport Community Mental Health Center, 1635 Central Avenue, P.O. Box 5117, Bridgeport, CT 06610; tel. 203/579–6626; FAX. 203/579–6094; James Lehane, Chief Executive Officer

Guenster Rehabilitation Center, Inc., 276 Union Avenue, Bridgeport, CT 06607; tel. 203/384–9301; FAX. 203/336–4395; Thomas Kidder, Clinical Director

High Meadows, 825 Hartford Turnpike, Hamden, CT 06517; tel. 203/281–8300; Ms. Chris Depgen–DeMatteo, RN, Quality Assurance Coordinator

Klingberg Family Centers, Inc., 370 Linwood Street, New Britain, CT 06052; tel. 860/224–9113, ext. 363; FAX. 860/826–1739; Rosemarie A. Burton, President

Reid Treatment Center, Inc., 121 West Avon Road, Avon, CT 06001; tel. 860/673–6115; FAX. 860/675–7433; Mary Ann Reid, Executive Director

Riverview Hospital for Children and Youth, 915 River Road, Middletown, CT 06457–9297; tel. 860/704–4090; FAX. 860/704–4123; Carl H. Sundell, Jr., Superintendent

Rushford Center, Inc., 1250 Silver Street, Middletown, CT 06457; tel. 203/346–0300; Margaret Crafton, Vice President for Clinical Operations

Stonington Institute, Swantown Hill Road, North Stonington, CT 06359; tel. 203/535–1010; Michael J. Angelides, President

The BlueRidge Center, 1095 Blue Hills Avenue, Bloomfield, CT 06002; tel. 860/243–1331; FAX. 860/242–3265; Mary Ellen Doyle, Executive Director

The Center, 4083 Main Street, Bridgeport, CT 06606; tel. 203/365–8400; Susan Dalesandro, Clinical Director

The Children's Center, 1400 Whitney Avenue, Hamden, CT 06517; tel. 203/248–2116; FAX. 203/248–2572; Brian F. Lynch, Chief Executive Officer

The Wellspring Foundation, Inc., 21 Arch Bridge Road, P.O. Box 370, Bethlehem, CT 06751–0370; tel. 203/266–7235; FAX. 203/266–5830; Herbert Hall, M.Ed., Chief Executive Officer

Vitam Center, Inc., 57 West Rocks Road, P.O. Box 730, Norwalk, CT 06852; tel. 203/846–2091; FAX. 203/846–3620; Leonard A. Kenowitz, Ph.D., Executive Director

Wheeler Clinic, Inc., 91 Northwest Drive, Plainville, CT 06062; tel. 203/747–6801; FAX. 203/793–3520; Dennis Keenan, Executive Director

DELAWARE

Brandywine Counseling, Inc., 2713 Lancaster Avenue, Wilmington, DE 19805; tel. 302/656–2348; FAX. 302/656–0746; Sara Taylor Allshouse, Executive Director

Delaware Guidance Services for Children and Youth, Inc., 1213 Delaware Avenue, Wilmington, DE 19806; tel. 302/652–3948; FAX. 302/652–8297; Bruce Kelsey, LCSW, BCD, Executive Director

Lower Kensington Environmental Center, Inc., Recovery Center of Delaware, P.O. Box 546, Delaware City, DE 19706; tel. 302/836–1615; FAX. 302/836–0412; John Moody, Project Director

Sodat–Delaware, Inc., 625 North Orange Street, Wilmington, DE 19801; tel. 302/656–4044; Thomas C. Maloney, Executive Director

DISTRICT OF COLUMBIA

Buena Vista Terrace, 5008 Connecticut Avenue, N.W., Suite 101, Washington, DC 20008; tel. 202/244–0612; Victor B. Smith, President

Devereux Children's Center, 3050 R Street, N.W., Washington, DC 20007; tel. 202/282–1200; FAX. 202/282–1219; Janet Heisse, Director of Management Service

Riverside Hospital, 4460 MacArthur Boulevard, N.W., Washington, DC 20007; tel. 202/333–9355; Dr. Elliot Bovelle, Chief Executive Officer

FLORIDA

45th Street Mental Health Center, Inc., 1041–45th Street, West Palm Beach, FL 33407; tel. 407/844–9741; FAX. 407/844–2373; Terry Allen, Chief Executive Officer

Alternatives in Treatment, Inc., 7601 North Federal Highway, Suite 100B, Boca Raton, FL 33487; tel. 407/998–0866; FAX. 407/241–5042; Jacob Frydman, Executive Director

American Day Treatment Centers of Boca Raton, 2101 Corporate Boulevard, Suite 102, Boca Raton, FL 33431; tel. 407/241–7741; FAX. 407/241–7743; Ralph Levinson, LCSW, Director, Clinical Services

Apalachee Center for Human Services, Inc., 625 East Tennessee Street, Tallahassee, FL 32308; tel. 904/487–2930; FAX. 904/487–0851; Ronald P. Kirkland, Chief Executive Officer

Associated Counseling and Education, Inc., 4563 South Orange Blossom Trail, Orlando, FL 32839; tel. 407/422–7233; FAX. 407/843–9602; Loretta Parrish, Chief Executive Officer

Auburndale Health Care Institute, 602 Melton Avenue, P.O. Box 458, Auburndale, FL 33823; tel. 800/762–3712; FAX. 813/375–4775; JoAnn Summerlin, Chief Executive Officer

Bayview Center for Mental Health, Inc., 12550 Biscayne Boulevard, Suite 919, Miami, FL 33181; tel. 305/892–4646; FAX. 305/893–1224; Robert Ward, Chief Executive Officer

Beachcomber Rehab, Inc., 4493 North Ocean Boulevard, Delray Beach, FL 33483; tel. 407/734–1818; FAX. 408/265–1349; James Bryan, Chief Executive Officer

Camelot Care Centers, Inc., 9180 Oakhurst Road, Largo, FL 34646; tel. 813/593–9000; Stacey Welton, Director

Charter Behavioral Health System at Manatee Palms, 4480 51st Street, W., Bradenton, FL 34210; tel. 941/792–2222; FAX. 941/795–4359; Ray Heckerman, Administrator, Chief Executive Officer

Coastal Recovery Centers, Inc., 3830 Bee Ridge Road, Sarasota, FL 34233; tel. 941/927–8900; FAX. 941/925–3836; James R. Sleeper, President, Chief Executive Officer

Crossroads School, 4650 Southwest 61 Avenue, Fort Lauderdale, FL 33314; tel. 305/584–1100; FAX. 305/584–0150; Aubrey Fein, Administrator

Crossroads–The Recovery Center, 2121 Lisenby Avenue, Panama City, FL 32406; tel. 904/784–0869; Tony Gilchrist, Chief Executive Officer

Daniel Memorial, Inc., 3725 Belfort Road, Jacksonville, FL 32216; tel. 800/737–1677; FAX. 904/448–7700; James D. Clark, Vice President, Programs

David Lawrence Center, Inc., 6075 Golden Gate Parkway, Naples, FL 33999; tel. 813/455–1031; FAX. 813/455–6561; David Schimmel, Executive Director

Disc Village, Inc., Tallahassee/Leon County Human Services Center, 3333 West Pensacola Street, Tallahassee, FL 32304; tel. 904/575–4388; FAX. 904/576–5960; Thomas K. Olk, Executive Director

Eckerd Alternative Treatment Program at E. How–Kee, 197 Culbreath Road, Brooksville, FL 34602; tel. 800/554–4357, ext. 456; Dwight Lord, Director, Admissions

Fairwinds, 1569 South Fort Harrison, Clearwater, FL 34616; tel. 813/449–0300; Mazhar Al–Abed, Chief Executive Officer, Administrator

Green Cross, Inc., 2645 Douglas Road, Suite 601, Miami, FL 33133; tel. 305/443–9990; FAX. 305/443–9498; Dr. Miguel Nunez, Chief Executive Officer

Hanley–Hazelden Center at St. Mary's, 5200 East Avenue, West Palm Beach, FL 33407; tel. 407/848–1666; Jerry Singleton, M.A., Executive Director

High Point, 5960 Southwest 106th Avenue, Cooper City, FL 33328; tel. 954/680–2700; FAX. 954/680–9941; Joseph A. Hartl, Chief Financial Officer

InterPhase Community Mental Health Center, 23123 State Road Seven, Suite A, Boca Raton, FL 33428; tel. 407/487–5400; FAX. 407/852–8872; Daniel L. Carzoli, M.A., CAP, Executive Director

Section C

Jacksonville Therapy Center, 6428 Beach Boulevard, Jacksonville, FL 32216; tel. 904/724–6500; FAX. 904/721–6677; Christopher P. Cheshire, Chief Executive Officer

La Amistad Behavioral Health Services, 1650 Park Avenue North, Maitland, FL 32751; tel. 407/647–0660; FAX. 407/647–3060; Rosemary Cohen, Chief Executive Officer

Lakeside Alternatives, Inc., 434 West Kennedy Boulevard, Orlando, FL 32810; tel. 407/875–3700; FAX. 407/875–5717; Duane Zimmerman, Chief Executive Officer

Leon F. Stewart–Hal S. Marcham Treatment Center, 3875 Tiger Bay Road, Daytona Beach, FL 32124; tel. 904/947–1300; FAX. 904/947–1309; Ernest D. Cantley, President, Chief Executive Officer

LifeStream Behavioral Center and Hospital, 515 West Main Street, P.O. Box 491000, Leesburg, FL 34749–1000; tel. 352/360–6575; FAX. 352/360–6595; Tim Camp, Executive Vice President

Lifeskills of Boca Raton, Inc., 7301A West Palmetto Park Road, Suite 300B, Boca Raton, FL 33433; tel. 561/392–1199; FAX. 561/392–4341; Carol A. Parks, Administrator

Marion Citrus Mental Health Centers, Inc., 717 Southwest Martin Luther King Jr. Avenue, P.O. Box 1330, Ocala, FL 34474; tel. 352/620–7300; FAX. 352/732–1413; Russell Rasco, Chief Executive Officer

Mental Health Care, Inc., 5707 North 22nd Street, Tampa, FL 33610; tel. 813/237–3914; FAX. 813/238–6574; Julian Rice, Executive Director

Mental Health Resource Center, Inc., 11820 Beach Boulevard, Jacksonville, FL 32246; tel. 904/642–9100; FAX. 904/641–6529; Robert A. Sommers, Ph.D., President, Chief Executive Officer

Meridian Behavioral Healthcare, Inc., 4300 Southwest 13th Street, Gainesville, FL 32608; tel. 352/374–5600; FAX. 352/371–9841; Douglas L. Starr, Ph.D., Chief Executive Officer

Montanari Residential Treatment Center, 291 East Second Street, Hialeah, FL 33011–1360; tel. 305/887–7543; FAX. 305/882–1970; Paul Hague, Executive Director

National Recovery Institutes Group, 1000 Northwest 15th Street, Boca Raton, FL 33486; tel. 407/392–8444; FAX. 407/368–0879; Don Russakoff, President, Chief Executive Officer

Northwest Dade Center, Inc., 4175 West 20th Avenue, Hialeah, FL 33012; tel. 305/825–0300; FAX. 305/824–1006; Mario Jardon, LCSW, Chief Executive Officer

Oak Center, 8889 Corporate Square Court, Jacksonville, FL 32216; tel. 904/725–7073; FAX. 904/727–9777; Diana Sourbrine, Administrator

Pathways to Recovery, Inc., 13132 Barwick Road, Delray Beach, FL 33445; tel. 407/496–7532; Allen Bombart, Executive Director

Peace River Center for Personal Development, Inc., 1745 Highway 17, S., Bartow, FL 33830; tel. 941/534–7020; FAX. 941/534–7028; Bert Lacey, Executive Director

Recovery Corner of West Palm Beach, 10800 North Military Trail, Suite 220, Palm Beach Gardens, FL 33410; tel. 407/624–1924; FAX. 407/626–1739; Jay Mills, Executive Director

Renaissance Institute of Palm Beach, Inc., 7000 North Federal Highway, Boca Raton, FL 33487; tel. 561/241–7977; FAX. 561/241–9233; Sid Goodman, M.A., Executive Director

South County Mental Health Center, Inc., 16158 South Military Trail, Delray Beach, FL 33484–6502; tel. 561/637–1000; FAX. 561/495–7975; Joseph S. Speicher, Executive Director

Southern Institute for Treatment and Evaluation, Inc., 660 Linton Boulevard, Suite 112, Delray Beach, FL 33444; tel. 407/278–8411; FAX. 407/278–7774; Michele Michael, Director

Spectrum Programs, Inc., 18441 Northwest Second Avenue, Suite 218, Miami, FL 33169; tel. 305/653–8288, ext. 19; FAX. 305/653–6787; David Freedman, Vice President, Administrative Services

Tampa Bay Academy, 12012 Boyette Road, Riverview, FL 33569; tel. 813/677–6700; FAX. 813/671–3145; Edward C. Hoefle, Executive Director

The Addictions Center for Treatment, 2905 South Federal Highway, Suite C–Eight, Delray Beach, FL 33483; tel. 407/278–0060; FAX. 407/278–0082; Michael Chernak, M.A., M.P.S., M.A.C., Chief Executive Officer

The Inn at Bowling Green Family Recovery Center, 101 North Oak Street, Bowling Green, FL 33834; tel. 800/762–3712; FAX. 813/375–2832; JoAnn Summerlin, Vice President, Administration

The Renfrew Center of Florida, 7700 Renfrew Lane, Coconut Creek, FL 33073; tel. 954/698–9222; FAX. 954/698–9007; Barbara Peterson, Executive Director

The Rose Institute, Inc., 17 Rose Drive, Fort Lauderdale, FL 33316; tel. 954/522–7673; FAX. 954/522–4031; Dr. Richard Maulion, Chief Executive Officer

The Village South, Inc., 3180 Biscayne Boulevard, Miami, FL 33137; tel. 305/573–3784; FAX. 305/576–1348; Matthew Gissen, Chief Executive Officer

The Willough at Naples, 9001 Tamiami Trail, E., Naples, FL 33962; tel. 813/775–4500; FAX. 813/793–0534; Gary D. Centafanti, Executive Director

Transitions Recovery Program, 1928 Northeast 154th Street, North Miami Beach, FL 33162; tel. 305/949–9001; Roselyn McGowan, Administrator

Turning Point of Tampa, Inc., 5439 Beaumont Center Boulevard, Tampa, FL 33634; tel. 813/882–3003; FAX. 813/885–6974; Stephanie Green, Director, Admissions

Twelve Oaks, 2068 Healthcare Avenue, Navarre, FL 32566; tel. 904/939–1200; FAX. 904/939–1257; Candy Henderson, Executive Director

U.S. Life Center of St. Augustine, 1100–3 South Ponce De Leon Boulevard, Saint Augustine, FL 32086; tel. 904/829–5566; FAX. 904/829–0677; James Ferguson, Chief Executive Officer

GEORGIA

Anchor Hospital and the Talbott–Marsh Recovery Campus, 5454 Yorktowne Drive, Atlanta, GA 30349; tel. 770/991–6044; FAX. 770/991–3843; Benjamin H. Underwood, FAAMA, President, Chief Executive Officer

Anxiety Disorders Institute of Atlanta Center, One Dunwoody Park, Suite 112, Atlanta, GA 30338; tel. 404/395–6845; Asaf Aleem, Chief Executive Officer

Bridges Outpatient Center, Inc., 1209 Columbia Drive, Milledgeville, GA 31061; tel. 912/454–1727; FAX. 912/454–1770; James Simmons, Chief Executive Officer

Brightmore Day Hospital, 115 Davis Road, P.O. Box 211849, Martinez, GA 30907–1849; tel. 404/868–1735; FAX. 404/860–6358; R. Adair Blackwood, M.D., Medical Director

Brook Run – Facility of the Georgia Department of Human Resource, 4770 North Peachtree Road, Dunwoody, GA 30338; tel. 770/551–7157; FAX. 770/551–7040; Dr. Rudy Magnone, Chief Executive Officer

CareSouth Homecare Professionals, 1048 Claussen Road, Augusta, GA 30907; tel. 706/738–8856; FAX. 706/736–5007; Jeanette Garrison, Chief Executive Officer

Charter Behavioral Health System of Atlanta at Laurel Heights, 934 Briarcliff Road, N.E., Atlanta, GA 30306; tel. 404/888–7860; FAX. 404/872–5088; Ruth Coody, Director, Clinical Services

Devereux Center In Georgia, 1291 Stanley Road, N.W., Kennesaw, GA 30152–4359; tel. 770/427–0147; FAX. 770/425–1413; Ralph L. Comerford, Executive Director

Learning Services Southeastern Region–Specialists in NeuroRehabilitation, 2400 Highway 29, S., Lawrenceville, GA 30245; tel. 770/962–4828; FAX. 770/995–1253; Heddi Silon, Director, Admissions

Murphy–Harpst–Vashti, Inc., 740 Fletcher Street, Cedartown, GA 30125; tel. 404/748–1500; FAX. 404/749–1094; Robert M. Spaulding II, Admissions Coordinator

Safe Recovery Systems, Inc., 2300 Peachtree Road, Suite 2000, Atlanta, GA 30338; tel. 404/455–7233; FAX. 404/458–1481; Henslee Dutton, Chief Executive Director

Schizophrenia Treatment and Rehabilitation, Inc., 208 Church Street, Decatur, GA 30030; tel. 404/377–9844; FAX. 404/373–5258; Tammie C. Robinson, RN, M.S., C.S., Executive Director

Skyland Trail, 2573 Skyland Trail, N.E., Atlanta, GA 30319; tel. 888/248–4801; FAX. 404/248–8956; Elizabeth Finnerty, Chief Executive Officer

Turning Point Care Center, Inc., 319 Bypass, Moultrie, GA 31776; tel. 912/985–4815; Michael Cornelison, Chief Executive Officer

Willingway Hospital, 311 Jones Mill Road, Statesboro, GA 30458; tel. 912/764–6236; FAX. 912/764–7063; Rodney Battles, Chief Executive Officer

IDAHO

Northview Hospital, 8050 Northview Street, Boise, ID 83704; tel. 208/327–0504; FAX. 208/327–0594; B. Joyce Ellis, Administrator

Walker Center, 1120A Montana Street, Gooding, ID 83330–1858; tel. 208/934–8461; FAX. 208/934–5437; Vayle Mauldin, Program Director

ILLINOIS

Alexian Brothers Lake–Cook Behavioral Health Resources, 999A Leicester, (Mailing address: 3265 North Arlington Heights Road, Suite 307, Arlington Heights, IL 60004), Elk Grove Village, IL 60007; tel. 708/577–1501; FAX. 708/577–0256; Mark Frey, Chief Executive Officer

Allendale Association, Grand Avenue and Offield Road, P.O. Box 1088, Lake Villa, IL 60046; tel. 847/356–2351; FAX. 847/356–2393; Kathryn M. Collins, President

American Day Treatment Centers, 1936 Green Bay Road, Highland Park, IL 60035; tel. 847/480–2625; FAX. 847/480–2624; Carmen Fontanez, Regional Executive Director

Camelot Care Center, Inc., 1502 North Northwest Highway, Palatine, IL 60067; tel. 847/359–5600; FAX. 847/359–2759; Maria Wywialowski, LCSW, Director, Social Services

Chestnut Health Systems, Inc., 1003 Dr. Martin Luther King Jr. Drive, Bloomington, IL 61701; tel. 309/827–6026; Alan R. Sodetz, Clinical Director

DuPage County Health Department/Mental Health Division, 111 North County Farm Road, Wheaton, IL 60187; tel. 708/682–7979; FAX. 708/690–5282; Dr. Gary Noll, Chief Executive Officer

Family Service and Community Mental Health Center/McHenry, 5320 West Elm Street, McHenry, IL 60050; tel. 815/385–6400; FAX. 815/385–8127; Robert Martens, Chief Executive Officer

Gateway Youth Care Foundation, 2200 Lake Victoria Drive, Springfield, IL 62703; tel. 217/529–9266; FAX. 217/529–9151

Great River Recovery Resources, Inc., 428 South 36th Street, Quincy, IL 62301; tel. 217/224–6300; FAX. 217/224–4329; Michael Hutmacher, Chief Executive Officer

Horizons Wellness Center, Inc., 970 South McHenry Avenue, Crystal Lake, IL 60014; tel. 815/477–8881; FAX. 815/477–4886; Linda D. Simko, Clinical Director

Interventions South Wood, 5701 South Wood, Chicago, IL 60636; tel. 312/737–4600; Herb Higgin, Director

Interventions Woodridge, 2221 64th Street, Woodridge, IL 60517; tel. 630/968–6477; FAX. 630/968–5744; Edward Ravine, Director, Clinical Operations

Interventions, City Girls/City Women, 140 North Ashland, Chicago, IL 60607; tel. 312/433–7777; FAX. 312/433–7787; Dr. Peter Bokos, Chief Executive Officer

Interventions–DuPage Adolescent Center, 11 South 250 Route 53, Hinsdale, IL 60521; tel. 630/325–5050; FAX. 630/325–9130; Kathy Hubek, Intake Coordinator

McHenry County Youth Service Bureau, 101 South Jefferson Street, Woodstock, IL 60098; tel. 815/338–7360; FAX. 815/337–5510; Susan H. Krause, Executive Director

New Life Clinic of Wheaton, P.C., 2100 Manchester Road, Suite 1410 and 1510, Wheaton, IL 60187; tel. 708/653–1717; FAX. 708/653–7926; Nancy Brown, Clinic Director

Northwestern University Health Service, 633 Emerson Street, Room 126, Evanston, IL 60208–4000; tel. 847/491–2143; FAX. 847/491–5919; Dr. Margaret Barr, Chief Executive Officer

Rosecrance on Alpine, 1505 North Alpine Road, Rockford, IL 61107; tel. 815/399–5351; FAX. 815/398–2641; Lori Berkes–Nelson, Administrator

Rosecrance on Harrison, 3815 Harrison Avenue, Rockford, IL 61108; tel. 815/391–1000; Philip W. Eaton, President, Chief Executive Officer

Sojourn House, Inc., 565 North Turner Avenue, Freeport, IL 61032; tel. 815/232–5121; FAX. 815/233–4591; Brenda J. Bombard, M.S.W., Executive Director

Southeastern Illinois Counseling Centers, Inc., 504 Micah Drive, P.O. Drawer M, Olney, IL 62450; tel. 618/395–4306; FAX. 618/395–4507; Gary Robertson, Executive Director

The Women's Treatment Center, 140 North Ashland, Chicago, IL 60607; tel. 312/850–0050; FAX. 312/850–9095; Dr. Jewell Oats, Chief Executive Officer

Triangle Center, 120 North 11th Street, Springfield, IL 62703; tel. 217/544-9858; FAX. 217/544-0223; Stephen J. Knox, Executive Director

White Oaks Companies of Illinois, 3400 New Leaf Lane, Peoria, IL 61614; tel. 309/692-6900; FAX. 309/689-3086; Dr. John Gilligan, Chief Executive Officer

INDIANA

Center for Behavioral Health, 645 South Rogers Street, Bloomington, IN 47403; tel. 812/339-1691; FAX. 812/339-8109; Linda Lumsden, Quality Improvement

Community Mental Health Center, Inc., 285 Bielby Road, Lawrenceburg, IN 47025; tel. 812/537-1302; FAX. 812/537-5219; Joseph Stephens, Chief Executive Officer

Comprehensive Mental Health Services, Inc., 240 North Tillotson Avenue, Muncie, IN 47304; tel. 317/288-1928; FAX. 317/741-0310; Suzanne Gresham, Ph.D., Chief Executive Officer

Evansville Psychiatric Children's Center, 3300 East Morgan Avenue, Evansville, IN 47715; tel. 812/477-6436; FAX. 812/474-4248; Thomas C. Andis, Jr., Superintendent

Fairbanks Hospital, Inc., 8102 Clearvista Parkway, Indianapolis, IN 46256-4698; tel. 317/849-8222, ext. 100; FAX. 317/849-1455; Timothy J. Kelly, M.D., Interim Administrator

Four County Counseling Center, 1015 Michigan Avenue, Logansport, IN 46947; tel. 219/722-5151, ext. 281; FAX. 219/722-9523; Laurence Ulrich, Chief Executive Officer

Grant-Blackford Mental Health, Inc., 505 Wabash Avenue, Marion, IN 46952; tel. 317/662-3971; FAX. 317/662-7480; Paul Kuczora, Chief Executive Officer

Hamilton Center, Inc., 620 Eighth Avenue, Terre Haute, IN 47804; tel. 812/231-8323; FAX. 812/231-8400; Galen Goode, Chief Executive Officer

Madison Hospital, 403 East Madison, South Bend, IN 46617; tel. 219/234-0061; FAX. 219/234-0670; John Twardos, Chief Operating Officer

Park Center, Inc., 909 East State Boulevard, Fort Wayne, IN 46805; tel. 219/481-2700; FAX. 219/481-2717; Paul D. Wilson, Chief Executive Officer

Porter-Starke Services, 601 Wall Street, Valparaiso, IN 46383; tel. 219/531-3500; FAX. 219/462-3975; Lee Grogg, Chief Executive Officer

Quinco Behavioral Health Systems, P.O. Box 628, Columbus, IN 47202-0628; tel. 812/379-2341; FAX. 812/376-4875; Robert J. Williams, Ph.D., Chief Executive Officer

Southwestern Indiana Mental Health Center, Inc., 415 Mulberry Street, Evansville, IN 47713; tel. 812/423-7791; FAX. 812/422-7558; John K. Browning, Executive Director

Tara Treatment Center, Inc., 6231 South U.S. Highway 31, R.R. 5, Box 225, Franklin, IN 46131; tel. 812/526-2611; FAX. 812/526-8527; Ann Daugherty-James, Chief Executive Officer

The Center for Mental Health, Inc., 1100 Broadway, P.O. Box 1258, Anderson, IN 46015; tel. 317/649-8161; FAX. 317/641-8238; C. Richard DeHaven, President

The Children's Campus, 1411 Lincoln Way, W., Mishawaka, IN 46544-1690; tel. 219/259-5666, ext. 222; FAX. 219/255-6179; Michael James, Vice President

The Madison Clinic of Saint John's, 2210 Jackson Street, Anderson, IN 46016; tel. 317/644-1414; FAX. 317/646-8462; Kyle DeFur, Vice President, Behavioral Services

Tri-City Comprehensive Community Mental Health Center, 3903 Indianapolis Boulevard, East Chicago, IN 46312; tel. 219/398-7050; FAX. 219/392-6998; Sandy Appleby, Assistant Director, Special Services

Tri-County Center, Inc., 697 Pro-Med Lane, W., Carmel, IN 46032; tel. 317/587-0500; FAX. 317/574-1234; Lesly Davis, Quality Improvement Manager

Wabash Valley Hospital, Inc., 2900 North River Road, West Lafayette, IN 47906; tel. 765/463-2555; FAX. 765/497-3960; R. Craig Lysinger, Chief Executive Officer

IOWA

Boys and Girls Home And Family Service, Inc., 2601 Douglas Street, Sioux City, IA 51104; tel. 712/277-4031; Robert P. Sheehan, Chief Executive Officer

Children and Families of Iowa, 1111 University, Des Moines, IA 50314; tel. 515/288-1981, ext. 346; FAX. 515/288-9109, ext. 402; Dr. Bobbretta M. Brewton, Director, Education, Prevention and Advocacy

Christian Home Association-Children's Square U.S.A., North Sixth Street and Avenue E, P.O. Box 8-C, Council Bluffs, IA 51502-3008; tel. 712/322-3700; FAX. 712/325-0913; Carol D. Wood, ACSW, L.I.S.W., President, Chief Executive Officer

Four Oaks, Inc. Smith Center, 5400 Kirkwood Boulevard, S.W., Cedar Rapids, IA 52404; tel. 319/364-0259; FAX. 319/364-1162; Karen Bruess-Baty, Director, Residential Services

Gerard Treatment Programs, 980 South Iowa Avenue, P.O. Box 1353, Mason City, IA 50401; tel. 515/423-3222; Rita Paxson, Chief Executive Officer

Hillcrest Family Services, 2005 Asbury Road, P.O. Box 1161, Dubuque, IA 52004-1161; tel. 319/583-7357; FAX. 319/583-7026; Barbara Simpson, Clinical Director

Lutheran Social Service of Iowa, 1323 Northwestern, Ames, IA 50010; tel. 515/232-7262; FAX. 515/232-7416; Mary Halbmaier, Office Manager

Orchard Place-Child Guidance, 925 Southwest Porter Avenue, P.O. Box 35425, Des Moines, IA 50315-0304; tel. 515/285-6781, ext. 601; FAX. 515/287-9695; Earl P. Kelly, Chief Executive Officer

Tanager Place, 2309 C Street, S.W., Cedar Rapids, IA 52404; tel. 319/365-9164; FAX. 319/365-6411

KANSAS

22nd Medical Group, 57950 Leavenworth Street, Suite Six E Four, McConnell AFB, KS 67221; tel. 316/652-5000; FAX. 316/652-5014; Col. Scott Garner, Chief Executive Officer

Atchison Valley Hope, 1816 North Second Street, Atchison, KS 66002; tel. 913/367-1618; FAX. 913/367-6224; Dennis Gilhousen, Chief Executive Officer

Columbia Health Systems, Inc., 10114 West 105th Street, Suite 100, Overland Park, KS 66212; tel. 913/492-9875; FAX. 913/492-0187; Robert L. Reed, President

Comprehensive Evaluation and Treatment Unit, CETU-Brigham Building, 300 Southwest Oakley, Topeka, KS 66606; tel. 913/296-2196; FAX. 913/296-2204; James Fairchild, Director

Kaw Valley Center, 4300 Brenner Drive, Kansas City, KS 66104; tel. 913/334-0294; B. Wayne Sims, President, Chief Executive Officer

Norton Valley Hope, 709 West Holme, Norton, KS 67654; tel. 913/877-5101; FAX. 913/877-2322; Dennis R. Gilhousen, President, Chief Executive Officer

S.P.I.R.I.T. Program of United Methodist Youthville, Inc., 900 West Broadway, Newton, KS 67114; tel. 316/283-1950, ext. 305; FAX. 316/283-9540; Karen Baker, Vice President, Programs

The Saint Francis Academy, Incorporated, 509 East Elm Street, Salina, KS 67401; tel. 913/825-0541; FAX. 913/825-2502; Reverend Phillip J. Rapp, President, Chief Executive Officer

KENTUCKY

Bluegrass Regional Mental Health-Mental Retardation Board, 1351 Newton Pike, Lexington, KY 40511; tel. 606/253-1686; David A. Holder, M.S.W., Director, Quality Improvement

Brooklawn, Inc., 2125 Goldsmith Lane, Louisville, KY 40218; tel. 502/451-5177; David A. Graves, President, Chief Executive Officer

Central State Hospital, 10510 LaGrange Road, Louisville, KY 40223; tel. 502/245-4121, ext. 7061; FAX. 502/253-7049; Paula Tamme, CSW, Chief Executive Officer

Christian Church Homes Children's and Family Services, 1151 Perryville Road, P.O. Box 45, Danville, KY 40423-0045; tel. 606/236-5507; FAX. 606/236-7044; Kathy Miles, Chief Executive Officer

Comprehensive Care Centers of Northern Kentucky, Inc., 503 Farrell Drive, Covington, KY 41011; tel. 606/578-3252; FAX. 606/578-3256; Edward G. Muntel, Ph.D., President

Cumberland River Regional Mental Health and Mental Retardation, Inc., American Greeting Road, P.O. Box 568, Corbin, KY 40702; tel. 606/528-7010; Ralph Lipps, Executive Director

Jefferson Alcohol and Drug Abuse Center, 600 South Preston Street, Louisville, KY 40202; tel. 502/583-3951; FAX. 502/581-9234; Diane E. Hague, Director

Pathways, Inc., 3701 Lansdowne Drive, P.O. Box 790, Ashland, KY 41105-0790; tel. 606/329-8588, ext. 142; FAX. 606/329-8195; Lora Reynolds, RNC, Mental Health Director

Presbyterian Child Welfare Agency, One Buckhorn Lane, Buckhorn, KY 41721; tel. 606/398-7245; Charles Baker, President, Chief Executive Officer

RiverValley Behavioral Health, 416 West Third Street, P.O. Box 1637, Zip 42302-1637, Owensboro, KY 42302; tel. 502/684-0696; FAX. 502/683-4696; Gayle DiCesare, Chief Executive Officer

Seven Counties Services, Inc., 101 West Muhammad Ali Boulevard, Louisville, KY 40202-1430; tel. 502/589-8600; Debra Hino, Quality Improvement Officer

Spectrum Care Academy, 4500 Campbellsville Road, Columbia, KY 42728; tel. 502/384-6444; FAX. 502/384-4883; Beverly K. Harvey, Administrator

The Adanta Group-Behavioral Health Srvices, 259 Parkers Mill Road, Somerset, KY 42501; tel. 606/678-2768; FAX. 606/678-5296; Sandra Renfro, Quality Improvement Coordinator

LOUISIANA

Addiction Recovery Resources of New Orleans, 401 Veterans Boulevard, Suite 102, Metairie, LA 70005; tel. 504/828-6700; FAX. 504/831-8949; Julia Clarke, Administrator

Hope Haven Center (Residential Treatment), Includes Hope Haven, Madonna Manor, St. Elizabeth's, 1101 Barataria Boulevard, Marrero, LA 70072; tel. 504/347-5581; FAX. 504/340-2075; Robert J. Guasco, Chief Administrative Officer

LA United Methodist Children and Family Services, Inc., 901 South Vienna Street, P.O. Box 929, Ruston, LA 71273-0929, Ruston, LA 71270; tel. 318/255-5020; FAX. 318/255-5457; Terrel DeVille, Chief Executive Officer

Meadowbrook Residential Treatment Center, 100 Meadowbrook Drive, P.O. Box 725, Zip 71058-0725, Minden, LA 71055; tel. 318/371-9494; FAX. 318/371-9933; Roy Martinez, Chief Executive Officer

New Beginnings Residential Program of Opelousas, 1692 Linwood Loop, Opelousas, LA 70570; tel. 318/942-1171; FAX. 318/948-9101; Kim Signorelli, Chief Executive Officer

Vermilion Hospital for Psychiatric and Addictive Medicine, 2520 North University Avenue, Lafayette, LA 70507; tel. 318/234-5614; FAX. 318/235-0696; Johnny Patout, Administrator

MAINE

Community Health and Counseling Services, 42 Cedar Street, P.O. Box 425, Bangor, ME 04402-0425; tel. 207/947-0366; FAX. 207/990-3581; Joseph H. Pickerling, Jr., Executive Director

Kids Peace National Centers for Kids in Crisis New England, Route 180, P.O. Box 787, Ellsworth, ME 04605; tel. 207/667-0909; FAX. 207/667-6348; John P. Peter, President, Chief Executive Officer

MARYLAND

A. F. Whitsitt Rehabilitation Center, 300 Scheeler Road, P.O. Box 229, Chestertown, MD 21620; tel. 410/778-6404, ext. 38; FAX. 410/778-5431; Terri Dowling, RN, Admissions Coordinator

Allegany County Health Department Addictions Program, Willowbrook Road, Cumberland, MD 21502; tel. 301/777-5680; Rodger D. Simons, Administrator

American Day Treatment Centers of Chevy Chase, LP, Two Wisconsin Circle, Suite 620, Chevy Chase, MD 20815; tel. 301/656-0151; Heidi Brown, Executive Director

Ashley, Inc., 800 Tydings Lane, Havre DeGrace, MD 21078; tel. 410/273-6600; FAX. 410/272-5617, ext. 215; Leonard Angus Dahl, Chief Executive Officer

Baltimore Recovery Center, 16 South Poppleton Street, Baltimore, MD 21201; tel. 410/962-7180; FAX. 410/962-7192; Morris A. Hill, President

Changing Point, 4100 College Avenue, P.O. Box 396, Ellicott City, MD 21041-0396; tel. 410/465-9500; FAX. 410/465-9500, ext. 320; Beatrice Grant, RN, Program Director

Charter Behavioral Health Systems at Hidden Brook, 522 Thomas Run Road, P.O. Box 1607, Bel Air, MD 21014; tel. 410/879-1919; FAX. 410/734-6752; Carol Koffinke, Chief Executive Officer

Chesapeake Treatment Center, P.O. Box 1238, Cambridge, MD 21613; tel. 410/221-0288; FAX. 410/228-9588; Jonathan Sova, Administrator

Crossroads Centers, Two West Madison Street, Baltimore, MD 21201; tel. 410/752–6505; FAX. 410/385–1237; Barbara Q. McKenna, Executive Director

Edgemeade, 13400 Edgemeade Road, Upper Marlboro, MD 20772; tel. 301/888–1330; FAX. 301/579–2342; James Filipczak, Ph.D., Executive Director

Glass Substance Abuse Programs, Inc., 821 North Eutaw Street, Suite 201, 101, Baltimore, MD 21201; tel. 410/225–9185; FAX. 410/225–7964; Herman Jones, President

Good Shepherd Center, 4100 Maple Avenue, Baltimore, MD 21227–4099; tel. 410/247–2770; FAX. 410/247–3242; Sister Mary Rosaria Baxter, M.S., Administrator

Hope House, Marbury Drive, Building 26, Crownsville, MD 21032; tel. 410/923–6700; FAX. 410/923–6213; William H. Rufenacht, Executive Director

Hudson Health Services, 1506 Harting Drive, Salisbury, MD 21802–1096; tel. 410/742–0151; FAX. 410/742–7048; Alfred Grafton, CCDC, Clinical Coordinator

Maryland Treatment Centers, Inc., U. S. Route 15, Emmitsburg, MD 21727; tel. 301/447–2361; FAX. 301/447–6504; Mary A. Roby, President

Melwood Farm Treatment Center, 19715 Zion Road, Olney, MD 20832; tel. 800/368–8313; Sue Krantz, Corporate Director of Quality

New Beginnings at Warwick Manor, 3680 Warwick Road, East New Market, MD 21631; tel. 410/943–8108; Charles J. Hooker, Executive Director

New Life Addiction Counseling Services, Inc., 2528 Mountain Road, Pasadena, MD 21122; tel. 410/255–4475; FAX. 410/255–6277; Thomas S. Porter, Chief Executive Officer

Oakview Treatment Center, 3100 North Ridge Road, Ellicott City, MD 21043; tel. 410/461–9922

Pathways Drug and Alcohol Treatment Center, 2620 Riva Road, Annapolis, MD 21401; tel. 410/573–5400; FAX. 410/573–5401; Marti Potter, Administrative Team Leader

Quarterway Houses, Inc., 730 Ashburton Street, P.O. Box 31419, Baltimore, MD 21216–6119; tel. 410/233–0684; FAX. 410/233–8540; Dr. Joseph Verrett, Chief Executive Officer

Regional Institute for Children and Adolescents–Baltimore, 605 South Chapel Gate Lane, Baltimore, MD 21229; tel. 410/368–7800; FAX. 410/368–7886; Clifford A. Palmer, Chief Executive Officer

Regional Institute for Children and Adolescents/Rockville, 15000 Broschart Road, Rockville, MD 20850–3392; tel. 301/251–6800; FAX. 301/309–9004; John L. Gildner, Chief Executive Officer

Regional Institute for Children and Adolescents/Southern Maryland, 9400 Surratts Road, Cheltenham, MD 20623; tel. 301/372–1800; FAX. 301/372–1906; Brenda Harris, Director, Admissions

Saint Luke Institute, Inc., 8901 New Hampshire Avenue, Silver Spring, MD 20903; tel. 301/445–7970; FAX. 301/422–5400; Reverend Stephen J. Rossetti, Ph.D., President, Chief Executive Officer

Villa Maria, 2300 Dulaney Valley Road, Timonium, MD 21093; tel. 410/252–4700; FAX. 410/252–3040; Mark Greenberg, LCSW, Administrator

Woodbourne Center, Inc., 1301 Woodbourne Avenue, Baltimore, MD 21239; tel. 410/433–1000; FAX. 410/435–4745, ext. 221; Patricia K. Cronin, LCSW, Executive Vice President, Chief Operating Officer

Worcester County Health Department, 6040 Public Landing Road, P.O. Box 249, Snow Hill, MD 21863; tel. 410/632–1100; FAX. 410/632–0906; Deborah Goeller, RN, M.S., Health Officer

MASSACHUSETTS

AdCare Hospital of Worcester, Inc., 107 Lincoln Street, Worcester, MA 01605; tel. 508/799–9000; FAX. 508/753–3733; David W. Hillis, President, Chief Executive Officer

Brighton Center for Children and Families, 77 Warren Street, Building Four, Brighton, MA 02135; tel. 617/789–5547; FAX. 617/787–4494; Richard L. Segal, Program Director

Brockton Multi Service Center, 165 Quincy Street, Brockton, MA 02402; tel. 508/580–0800; FAX. 508/588–2949; John P. Sullivan, Ph.D., Area Director

Cape Cod Alcoholism Intervention and Rehabilitation Unit, Inc., d/b/a Gosnold on Cape Cod, 200 Ter Heun Drive, Box CC, Falmouth, MA 02541; tel. 508/540–6550; FAX. 508/540–6550; Raymond Tamasi, President, Chief Executive Officer

Cape Cod and the Islands, Community Mental Health Center, 259 North Street, Hyannis, MA 02601; tel. 508/775–1199; Richard Dunnells, Center Director, Superintendent

Center for Health and Human Services, Inc., 370 Faunce Corner Road, Mailing Address: P.O. Box 2097, New Bedford, MA 02741, North Dartmouth, MA 02747; tel. 508/995–4853; FAX. 508/995–1868; Warren Davis, Chief Executive Officer

Centerpoint, Tewksbury Hospital, Southgate, 365 East Street, Tewksbury, MA 01876; tel. 508/858–3776; FAX. 508/858–3494; Carolyn Ingalls, Program Director

Charles River Intensive Residential Treatment Program, 60 Hodges Avenue–Goss Three, Taunton, MA 02780–0997; tel. 508/824–7575; FAX. 508/824–7528; Eleni Carr, Program Director

Chauncy Hall Academy, 167 Lyman Street, P.O. Box 732, Westborough, MA 01581; tel. 508/774–0774; FAX. 508/774–8369; Russell Gwilliam, Program Director

Choate Health Systems, Inc., 23 Warren Avenue, Woburn, MA 01801; tel. 617/279–0200, ext. 304; FAX. 617/279–2804; Margaret A. Moran, Vice President, Marketing & Program Development

Dr. Harry C. Solomon Mental Health Center, 391 Varnum Avenue, Lowell, MA 01854; tel. 508/454–8851; FAX. 508/454–7538; Linda Sutter, Chief Executive Officer

Dr. John C. Corrigan Mental Health Center, 49 Hillside Street, Fall River, MA 02720; tel. 508/678–2901; FAX. 508/678–2290; Elaine M. Hill, Superintendent

Dr. Solomon Carter Fuller Mental Health Center, 85 East Newton Street, Boston, MA 02118–2389; tel. 617/266–8800, ext. 436; FAX. 617/421–9190; Dr. Jean Wilkinson, Center Director

Erich Lindermann Mental Health Center, 25 Stanford Street, Boston, MA 02114; tel. 617/727–5500; FAX. 617/727–5500; Carla Saccone, Chief Executive Officer

Fuller Intensive Residential Treatment Program, 85 East Newton Street, Sixth Floor East, Boston, MA 02118; tel. 617/536–1227; FAX. 617/536–1837; Michael Krupa, Chief Executive Officer

High Point, 1233 State Road, Route 3A, Plymouth, MA 02360; tel. 508/224–7701; FAX. 508/224–2845; Daniel Mumbauer, Chief Executive Officer

Intensive Treatment Unit, 3832 Hancock Road, Route 43, (Mailing Address: P.O. Box 4699, Pittsfield, MA 01202–4699), Lanesboro, MA 01237; tel. 413/738–5151; FAX. 413/443–0143; Gerald Burke, Chief Executive Officer

Meadowridge Behavioral Health Center, Residential Psychiatric Care, 664 Stevens Road, Swansea, MA 02777; tel. 800/479–8740; FAX. 508/678–9059; John Lynch, Program Director

Spectrum Health Systems, Inc., 154 Oak Street, P.O. Box 1208, Westboro, MA 01581; tel. 508/898–1570; FAX. 508/898–1578; Roy Ross, Chief Executive Officer

The Grove Adolescent Treatment Center, 320 Riverside Drive, Northampton, MA 01060; tel. 413/586–6210; FAX. 413/586–7852; Victoria Perry, Program Director

The Kolburne School, Inc., Southfield Road, New Marlborough, MA 01230; tel. 413/229–8787; FAX. 413/229–7708; Jeane K. Weinstein, M.A., Executive Director

The May Institute, Inc., 940 Main Street, P.O. Box 899, South Harwich, MA 02661; tel. 508/432–5530; FAX. 508/432–3478; Dr. Walter P. Christian, Chief Executive Officer

The Three Rivers Treatment Program, 94 Mosher Street, Holyoke, MA 01040; tel. 413/536–8833; FAX. 413/536–7907; Carl Cutchins, Chief Executive Officer

The Whitney Academy, Inc., 85 Doctor Braley Road, P.O. Box 619, East Freetown, MA 02717; tel. 508/763–3737; FAX. 508/763–4200; George E. Harmon, Executive Director

University of Massachusetts I.R.T.P., 305 Belmont Street, Seventh Floor, Worcester, MA 01604; tel. 508/856–1455; FAX. 508/856–1435; Aaron Lazare, Chief Executive Officer

Wild Acre Inns, 108 Pleasant Street, Arlington, MA 02174–4813; tel. 617/643–0643, ext. 116; John G. Domaleski, Director, Administration, Finance

MICHIGAN

A.C.T. Specialists, P.C., 20600 Eureka Road, Suite 604, Taylor, MI 48180; tel. 313/285–5000; FAX. 313/285–5863; Karin Chaundy, M.A., Director, Clinical Services

ACAC, Inc., 3949 Sparks Avenue, S.E., Suite 103, Grand Rapids, MI 49546; tel. 616/957–5850; FAX. 616/957–5853; Michael Durco, Chief Executive Officer

AOS, Inc., 1331 Lake Drive, S.E., Grand Rapids, MI 49506; tel. 616/456–8010; FAX. 616/451–0020; Charles Logie, President

Addiction Treatment Services, Inc., 116 East Eighth Street, Traverse City, MI 49684; tel. 616/922–4810; FAX. 616/922–2095; David N. Abeel, M.S.W., Executive Director

Adult/Youth Developmental Services, PC, 23133 Orchard Lake Road, Suite 104, Farmington, MI 48336; tel. 810/477–0107; Dr. George Kates, Chief Executive Officer

Alcohol Information and Counseling Center, 1575 Suncrest Drive, Lapeer, MI 48446; tel. 810/667–0243; FAX. 810/667–9399; Stephen L. Cranfield, Director

Allegan Substance Abuse Agency, Inc., 120 Cutler Street, Allegan, MI 49010; tel. 616/673–8735; FAX. 616/673–1572; Paul Mailloux, Chief Executive Officer

Ann Arbor Consultation Services, 5331 Plymouth Road, Ann Arbor, MI 48105; tel. 313/996–9111; Steven Sheldon, Director

Arborview Hospital, 6902 Chicago Road, Warren, MI 48092; tel. 810/983–3600; FAX. 810/264–6918; Donald Warner, Chief Executive Officer

Auro Medical Center, 1711 South Woodward, Suite 102, Bloomfield Hills, MI 48302; tel. 313/335–1130; FAX. 313/335–4680; Sue Comer, Contact Person

Battle Creek Child Guidance Center, Inc., 155 Garfield Avenue, Battle Creek, MI 49017; tel. 616/968–9280; FAX. 616/966–4123; Charles Dolk, Chief Executive Officer

Boniface Human Services, 25050 West Outer Drive, Suite 201, Lincoln Park, MI 48146; tel. 313/928–8940; FAX. 313/928–5152; Ronald G. Berglund, Executive Director

Brighton Hospital, 12851 East Grand River Avenue, Brighton, MI 48116; tel. 810/227–1211, ext. 235; FAX. 810/227–1869; Deborah Sopo, President, Chief Executive Officer

Catholic Services of Macomb, 235 South Gratiot Avenue, Mount Clemens, MI 48043; tel. 810/468–2616; FAX. 810/468–6234; Thomas J. Reed, President, Chief Executive Officer

Center for Behavior and Medicine, 2004 Hogback Road, Suite 16, Ann Arbor, MI 48105; tel. 313/677–0809; FAX. 313/677–0452; Gerard M. Schmit, M.D., Chief Executive Officer

Center for Personal Growth, P.C., 817 10th Avenue, Port Huron, MI 48060; tel. 810/984–4550; FAX. 810/984–3737; Fredric B. Roberts, Ed.D., Chief Executive Officer

Center of Behavioral Therapy P.C., 24453 Grand River Avenue, Detroit, MI 48219; tel. 313/592–1765; Hollis Evans, Executive Director

Central Michigan Community Mental Health Services, 301 South Crapo, Suite 100, Mount Pleasant, MI 48858; tel. 517/773–6961; FAX. 517/773–1968; George Rouman, Chief Executive Officer

Central Therapeutic Services, Inc., 17600 West Eight Mile Road, Southfield, MI 48075; tel. 313/559–4340; FAX. 313/559–1451; K. G. Thimotheose, Ph.D., President, Chief Executive Officer

Children's Home of Detroit, 900 Cook Road, Grosse Pointe Woods, MI 48236; tel. 313/886–0800; FAX. 313/886–9446; Michael R. Horwitz, Executive Director

Chip Counseling Center, Inc., 14695 Park Avenue, Charlevoix, MI 49720; tel. 616/547–6551; Patrick Q. Nestor, Executive Director

Clinton–Eaton–Ingham Community Mental Health Board, 808–B Southland, Lansing, MI 48910; tel. 517/887–2126; FAX. 517/887–0086; Judith Taylor, Ph.D., Executive Director

Community Care Services, 26184 West Outer Drive, Lincoln Park, MI 48146; tel. 313/389–7525; FAX. 313/389–7515; Mr. Kari Walker, Deputy Director

Community Mental Health Services of St. Joseph County, 210 South Main, Three Rivers, MI 49093; tel. 616/273–2000; FAX. 616/273–9456; Kristine Kirsch, RNC, M.P.A., NMCC, Chief Executive Officer

Community Programs, Inc., 1435 North Oakland Boulevard, Waterford, MI 48327; tel. 810/666-2720; FAX. 810/666-8822; Bernard P. Paige, Esq., Chief Executive Officer

Comprehensive Psychiatric Services, PC, 28800 Orchard Lake Road, Suite 250, Farmington, MI 48334; tel. 810/932-2500; FAX. 810/932-2506; Dr. Alan Rosenbaum, Chief Executive Officer

Comprehensive Services, Inc., 4630 Oakman Boulevard, Detroit, MI 48204-4127; tel. 313/934-8400; Catherine Green, Consultant

Cruz Clinic, 17177 North Laurel Park Drive, Suite 131, Livonia, MI 48152; tel. 313/462-3210; FAX. 313/462-1024; Ida Goutman, Administrator, Program Director

Delta Family Clinic, 2303 East Ameligh Road Bay, Bay City, MI 48706; tel. 517/684-9313; FAX. 517/684-5773; Gary West, Chief Executive Officer

Department of Human Services, Gratiot Clinic, 3506 Gratiot, Detroit, MI 48207; tel. 313/267-6718; Octavius E. Sapp, Assistant Director

Desgranges Psychiatric Center P.C., G-8145 South Saginaw Street, Grand Blanc, MI 48439; tel. 810/694-2730; Louise Desgranges, M.D., Chief Executive Officer

Detroit Central City Community Mental Health, Inc., 10 Peterboro, Detroit, MI 48201; tel. 313/831-3160; FAX. 313/831-2604; George D. Gaines, M.S.W., M.P.H., Executive Director

Dimensions of Life, Inc., 3320 West Saginaw Street, Lansing, MI 48917; tel. 517/886-0340; FAX. 517/886-0505; Alfred K. Doering, Director

Dot Caring Centers, Inc., 3190 Hallmark Court, Saginaw, MI 48603; tel. 517/790-3366; Wendell J. Montney, Ph.D., Executive Director, Behavioral Healthcare

Downriver Guidance Clinic of Wayne County, 13101 Allen Road, Southgate, MI 48195; tel. 313/282-1700; Leroy A. Lott, M.S.W., Chief Executive Officer

Downriver Mental Health Clinic, 20600 Eureka Road, Suite 819, Taylor, MI 48180; tel. 313/285-8282; David S. Monhollen, Administrator

Elrose Health Services, Inc., 1475 East Outer Drive, Detroit, MI 48234; tel. 313/892-4244; FAX. 313/892-1457; Ellsworth E. Jackson, M.A., CSW, Program Director

Fairlane Behavioral Services, 23400 Michigan Avenue, Suite P-24, Dearborn, MI 48124; tel. 313/562-6730; FAX. 313/562-8840; Theresa Reynolds, Adult Services; Millie Shepherd, Child Services

Gateway Services, 333 Turwill Lane, Kalamazoo, MI 49006; tel. 616/382-9827; FAX. 616/342-6440; Thomas E. Lucking, Executive Director

Growth Works, Inc., 271 South Main Street, Plymouth, MI 48170; tel. 313/455-4095; Dale F. Yagiela, Executive Director

Guest House for Women Religious, 1840 West Scripps Road, P.O. Box 420, Lake Orion, MI 48361; tel. 810/391-3100; FAX. 810/391-0210; Richard Frisch, Chief Executive Officer

Hegira Programs, Inc., 8623 North Wayne Road, Suite 200, Westland, MI 48185; tel. 313/458-4601; FAX. 313/458-4611; Edward L. Forry, Chief Executive Officer

Highland Waterford Center, Inc., 4501 Grange Hall Road, Holly, MI 48442; tel. 810/634-0140; FAX. 810/634-3838; Michael J. Filipek, B.A., Executive Director

Huron Valley Consultation Center, 955 West Eisenhower Circle, Suite B, Ann Arbor, MI 48103; tel. 313/662-6300; Janet Ford, Business Manager

Ionia County Community Mental Health Services, 5827 North Orleans, P.O. Box 155, Orleans, MI 48865; tel. 616/761-3135; FAX. 616/761-3992; Richard Visingardi, Chief Executive Officer

Jensen Counseling Centers P.C., 26105 Orchard Lake Road, Suite 301, Farmington Hills, MI 48334; tel. 313/478-4411; Francine Friedman, M.D., Medical Director

Lapeer County Community Mental Health Center, 1570 Suncrest Drive, Lapeer, MI 48446-1154; tel. 810/667-0500; FAX. 810/664-8728; Richard I. Berman, Ph.D., Executive Director

Latino Family Services, Inc., 3815 West Fort, Detroit, MI 48216; tel. 313/841-7380; FAX. 313/841-3730; Cristina Jose-Kampfner, Ph.D., President

LifeLong Center, Inc., 719 Harrison Street, Flint, MI 48502-1613; tel. 810/235-1950; Georgia Herrlich, Chief Executive Officer

LifeWays, 1200 North West Avenue, Jackson, MI 49202; tel. 517/789-1200; FAX. 517/789-1276; Dr. Christina Thompson, Chief Executive Officer

Macomb Child Guidance Clinic, Inc., 7828 22 Mile Road, Utica, MI 48317; tel. 810/254-3737; Mary Vandia, ACSW, Clinic Director

Meridian Professional Psychological Consultants, P.C., 5031 Park Lake Road, East Lansing, MI 48823; tel. 517/332-0811; FAX. 517/332-4452; Thomas S. Gunnings, Ph.D., President, Clinical Director

Metro East Substance Abuse Treatment Corporation, 13929 Harper Avenue, Detroit, MI 48213; tel. 313/371-0055; FAX. 313/371-1409; Leslie B. Carroll, President

Michigan Counseling Services, 1400 East 12 Mile Road, Madison Heights, MI 48071-2651; tel. 810/547-2223; Marylyn Krzeminski, Director, Clinical Services

Monroe County Community Mental Health Authority, 1001 South Raisinville Road, Monroe, MI 48161; tel. 313/243-3371; FAX. 313/243-5564; Sheldon M. Rosen, Executive Director

NPL, Inc., 18641 West Seven Mile Road, Detroit, MI 48219; tel. 313/532-8015; Ken Wolf, Ph.D., Chief Executive Officer

Nardin Park Recovery Center, 9605 Grand River, P.O. Box 04506, Detroit, MI 48204; tel. 313/834-5930; FAX. 313/834-4541; Annie B. Scott, Executive Director

National Council on Alcoholism Lansing Regional Area, 3400 South Cedar, Suite 200, Lansing, MI 48910; tel. 517/887-0851; FAX. 517/887-8121; Nancy L. Siegrist, Executive Director

National Council on Alcoholism and Addictions, 202 East Boulevard, Suite 310, Flint, MI 48503; tel. 810/767-0350; FAX. 810/767-4031; John A. Cnockaert, Ph.D., Executive Director

National Council on Alcoholism and Drug Dependence, 2927 West McNichols, Detroit, MI 48221; tel. 313/341-9891; FAX. 313/341-9776; Benjamin A. Jones, President, Chief Executive Officer

Neighborhood Service Organization, 220 Bagley, Suite 840, Detroit, MI 48226; tel. 313/961-4890; FAX. 313/961-5120; Angela G. Kennedy, Executive Director

New Center Community Mental Health Services, 2051 West Grand Boulevard, Detroit, MI 48208; tel. 313/961-3200; FAX. 313/961-3769; Roberta V. Sanders, Chief Executive Officer

New Era Alternative Treatment Center, 211 Glendale, Suite 513, Highland Park, MI 48203; tel. 313/869-6328, ext. 312; FAX. 313/869-1765; Joseph A. Pitts, Executive Medical Director

New Hope Treatment Center, 3455 Woodward, Second Floor, Detroit, MI 48201; tel. 313/832-6930; FAX. 313/961-8090; Janice Kwiatkowski, Chief Executive Officer

New Perspectives Center, Inc., 1321 South Fayette Street, Saginaw, MI 48602; tel. 517/790-0301; FAX. 517/790-0233; Jimmie D. Westbrook, Executive Director

Northeast Guidance Center, 13340 East Warren, Detroit, MI 48215; tel. 313/824-8000; FAX. 313/824-7779; Cheryl Coleman, Executive Director

Northern Michigan Community Mental Health, One MacDonald Drive, Suite A, Petroskey, MI 49770; tel. 616/347-7890; FAX. 616/347-1241; Alexis Kaczynski, Chief Executive Officer

Northpointe Behavioral Healthcare Systems, 715 Pyle Drive, Kingsford, MI 49802; tel. 906/774-0522; FAX. 906/774-1570; James Gaynor II, Chief Executive Officer

O. Ganesh, M.D., P.C., 28165 Greenfield, Southfield, MI 48076; tel. 313/569-6642; FAX. 810/569-7922; G. Borovsky, M.A., L.L.P., CSW, Administrator

Oakland Psychological Clinic, P.C., 2050 North Woodward Avenue, Suite 110, Bloomfield Hills, MI 48304-2258; tel. 810/594-1200; FAX. 810/594-1306; Barry H. Tigay, Ph.D., President

Orchard Hills Psychiatric Enter, P.C., 40,000 Grand River Avenue, Suite 306, Novi, MI 48375-2137; tel. 810/426-9900; FAX. 810/426-9950; Dr. Hiten Patel, Chief Executive Officer

Orchards Children's Services, Inc., 30215 Southfield Road, Southfield, MI 48076; tel. 810/433-8600; FAX. 810/258-0487; Gerald Levin, Chief Executive Officer

Ottawa County Community Mental Health, 12251 James Street, Holland, MI 49424; tel. 616/393-5600; FAX. 616/393-5687; Dr. Rudolph Lie, Chief Executive Officer

Parkside Mental Health and Clinical Services, 18820 Woodward Avenue, Suite Five, Detroit, MI 48203; tel. 313/893-9771; FAX. 313/368-2605; Victoria Mayberry, Chief Executive Officer

Personal Dynamics Center, 23810 Michigan Avenue, Dearborn, MI 48124; tel. 313/563-4142; FAX. 313/563-2615; Pamela Czuj, Executive Director

Personal Home Care Skilled Services, Inc., 32743 23 Mile Road, New Baltimore, MI 48047; tel. 810/716-1090; FAX. 810/725-0911; Sheila Fullmer, Business Leader

Perspectives of Troy, P.C., 2690 Crooks Road, Suite 300, Troy, MI 48084; tel. 810/244-8644; FAX. 810/244-1330; Timothy Coldiron, ACSW, Ph.D., Chief Executive Officer

Pioneer Counseling Centers, 28511 Orchard Lake Road, Suite A, Farmington Hills, MI 48334; tel. 810/489-1550; Gary J. LaHood, Chief Executive Officer

Program for Alcohol and Substance Treatment, 110 Sanborn, Big Rapids, MI 49307; tel. 616/796-6203; John R. Kelly, Director

Propelled Therapeutic Services, 18820 Woodward Avenue, Detroit, MI 48203; tel. 313/368-2600; FAX. 313/368-2605; Cecelia Wallace, Executive Director, President

Psychological Consultants of Michigan, P.C., 2518 Capital Avenue, S.W., Suite Two, Battle Creek, MI 49015; tel. 616/968-2811; FAX. 616/968-2651; Jeffrey N. Andert, Ph.D., Administrator

Psychotherapy Institute of Mid-Michigan, PC, 5000 Northwind Drive, East Lansing, MI 48823-5032; tel. 517/351-8994; Pamela Vandel, Licensure Coordinator

Redford Counseling Center, 25945 West Seven Mile Road, Redford, MI 48240; tel. 313/535-6560; FAX. 313/535-5266; Jo Ann Sadler, Director, ACSW, BCD

Regional Mental Health Clinic, P.C., 23100 Cherry Hill Road, Suite 10, Dearborn, MI 48124-4144; tel. 313/277-1300; Gena J. D'Alessandro, Ph.D., Chief Executive Officer

River's Bend P.C., 33975 Dequindre, Suite Five, Troy, MI 48083; tel. 810/583-1110; FAX. 810/583-9399; James Keener, Chief Executive Officer

Riverwood Community Mental Health Center, 1485 M-139, P.O. Box 547, Benton Harbor, MI 49023; tel. 616/925-0585; FAX. 616/925-0070; Allen Edlefson, Chief Executive Officer

Rose Hill Center, Inc., 5130 Rose Hill Boulevard, Holly, MI 48442; tel. 810/634-5530; FAX. 810/634-7754; David E. Ballenberger, President, Executive Director

STM Clinic, One Tuscola Street, Suite 302, Saginaw, MI 48607; tel. 517/755-2532; FAX. 517/755-2827; Sara Terry-Moton, Chief Executive Officer

Sacred Heart Rehabilitation Center, Inc., 400 Stoddard Road, Memphis, MI 48041; tel. 810/392-2167; Michael Kelly, Director, Treatment Programs

Saginaw County Mental Health Center, 500 Hancock Street, Saginaw, MI 48602; tel. 517/792-9732; FAX. 517/799-0206; Donald Miller, Chief Executive Officer

Self Help Addiction Rehabilitation, 1852 West Grand Boulevard, Detroit, MI 48208; tel. 313/894-1445; FAX. 313/894-5542; Anne C. Benion, ACSW, Program Services Manager

Star Center, Inc., 13575 Lesure, Detroit, MI 48227; tel. 313/493-4410; FAX. 313/493-4415; Menuel L. Hill, Clinical Director

Substance Abuse Council of St. Joseph County, 222 South Main Street, Three Rivers, MI 49093-1658; tel. 616/279-5187; FAX. 616/273-2083; James Brundirks, M.A., L.L.P., Clinical Director

Suburban West Community Center, 11677 Beech Daly Road, Redford, MI 48239; tel. 313/937-9500; FAX. 313/937-9504; William R. Hart, Clinical Program Director

Summit Pointe, 140 West Michigan Avenue, Battle Creek, MI 49017; tel. 616/966-1460; FAX. 616/966-2844; Ervin Brinker, Chief Executive Officer

Superior Behavioral Health, 200 West Spring Street, Marquette, MI 49855; tel. 906/225-7201; FAX. 906/225-7204; William G. Birch, Ed.D., M.S.W., Chief Executive Officer

Taylor Psychological Clinic, PC, 1172 Robert T. Longway Boulevard, Flint, MI 48503; tel. 810/232-8466; Dr. Maxwell Taylor, Chief Executive Officer

The Center for Human Resources, 1001 Military Street, Port Huron, MI 48060-0541; tel. 313/985-5168; Thomas P. Pope, Executive Director

Section C

The Counseling Center P.C., 1411 South Woodward, Suite 101, Bloomfield Hills, MI 48304; tel. 810/338-2918; FAX. 810/338-1322; Robert L. Bailey, Director

The Guidance Clinic, 2615 Stadium Drive, Kalamazoo, MI 49008; tel. 616/343-1651; FAX. 616/382-7078; Steven L. Smith, Executive Director

The Montcalm Center for Behavioral Health, 611 North State Street, Stanton, MI 48888; tel. 517/831-7520; FAX. 517/831-7578; Robert Brown, Chief Executive Officer

The Salvation Army's Turning Point Programs at Metropolitan Hospital, 1931 Boston, S.E., Grand Rapids, MI 49506; tel. 616/235-1565; FAX. 616/235-1574; Robert E. Byrd, M.A., Director

Thumb Area Behavioral Services Center, 1309 Cleaver Road, P.O. Box 239, Caro, MI 48723; tel. 517/673-7575; FAX. 517/673-7579; Susan H. Clara, Program Director

University Psychiatric Center, 2751 East Jefferson, Suite 200, Detroit, MI 48207; tel. 313/993-3434; FAX. 313/993-3421; G. Robert Miller, Chief Executive Officer

W. D. Lee Center for Life Management, Inc., 11000 West McNichols, Suite 222, Detroit, MI 48221; tel. 313/345-6777; FAX. 313/345-6369; Wendie D. Lee, Director, Chief Executive Officer

West Michigan Community Mental Health System, 920 Diana Street, Ludington, MI 49431; tel. 616/845-6294, ext. 5062; FAX. 616/845-7095; John Sternberg, Director, Clinical Services

MINNESOTA
Anthony Louis Center, 1000 Paul Parkway, Blaine, MN 55434; tel. 612/757-2906; Jon Benson, Chief Executive Officer

Charter Behavioral Health System of Waverly, 109 North Shore Drive, Waverly, MN 55390; tel. 612/658-4811; FAX. 612/658-4128; Clelland Gilchrist, Chief Executive Officer, Director, Clinical Services

Fairview Riverside Woodbury, Extended Care and Halfway House, 1665 Woodbury Drive, Woodbury, MN 55125; tel. 612/436-6623; Richard Peterson, President, Chief Executive Officer

Fountain Lake Treatment Center, Inc., 408 Fountain Street, Albert Lea, MN 56007; tel. 507/377-6411; Garth Barker, Director

Guest House, 4800 48th Street N.E., P.O. Box 954, Rochester, MN 55903; tel. 507/288-4693; FAX. 507/288-1240; William C. Morgan, Treatment Center Director

Hazelden Foundation, 15245 Pleasant Valley Road, Center City, MN 55012; tel. 612/257-4010; FAX. 612/257-1055; Jerry Spicer, President

Mission Care Detox Center, 3409 East Medicine Lake Road, Plymouth, MN 55441; tel. 612/559-1402; FAX. 612/559-2559; Judy Retterath, Program Director

Omegon, Inc., 2000 Hopkins Crossroads, Minnetonka, MN 55343; tel. 612/541-4738; Barbara J. Danielsen, Executive Administrator

Pride Institute, 14400 Martin Drive, Eden Prairie, MN 55344; tel. 800/547-7433; David DuBois, Chief Operating Officer

St. Joseph's Home for Children, 1121 East 46th Street, Minneapolis, MN 55407; tel. 612/827-9366; FAX. 612/827-7954; Lori Squire, Quality Assurance Director

MISSISSIPPI
Cares Center, Inc., 402 Wesley Avenue, Jackson, MS 39202; tel. 601/352-7784; Richard H. Macsherry, Director

Copac, Inc., 3949 Highway 43N, Brandon, MS 39042; tel. 800/446-9727; Jerald Stacy Hughes, Jr., Ph.D., Executive Director

Jackson Recovery Center, 5354 I-55 South Frontage Road, Jackson, MS 39212; tel. 601/372-9788; FAX. 601/372-9505; D. Preston Smith, Jr., President, Chief Executive Officer

Male/Female Receiving Med Psych Services, 3550 Highway 468 West, P.O. Box 157-A, Whitfield, MS 39193; tel. 601/351-8000; FAX. 601/939-0647; James Chastain, Chief Executive Officer

Millcreek, 900 First Avenue, N.E., P.O. Box 1160, Magee, MS 39111; tel. 601/849-4221; FAX. 601/849-7194; Karen L. Lister, Ph.D., Executive Director

Oak Circle Center, P.O. Box 157-A, Whitfield, MS 39193; tel. 601/939-1221; FAX. 601/939-0647; James Chastain, Chief Executive Officer

MISSOURI
Boonville Valley Hope, 1415 Ashley Road, Boonville, MO 65233; tel. 816/882-6547; Dennis Gilhousen, Chief Executive Officer

Boys and Girls Town of Missouri, Route D.D., P.O. Box 189, St. James, MO 65559; tel. 573/265-3251; FAX. 573/265-5370; Richard C. Dunn, ACSW, LCSW, Executive Director

Centrec-Care, Inc., 12401 Olive Street Road, Suite 103, St. Louis, MO 63141; tel. 314/576-9929; FAX. 314/576-1253; Mohammed A. Kabir, M.D., Chief Executive Officer

Child Center of Our Lady, 7900 Natural Bridge Road, St. Louis, MO 63121; tel. 314/383-0200; FAX. 314/383-6334; Milton T. Fujita, M.D., Chief Executive Officer

Comprehensive Mental Health Services, Inc., 10901 Winner Road, Independence, MO 64052; tel. 816/254-3652; FAX. 816/254-9243; William Kyles, Chief Executive Officer

Edgewood Children's Center, 330 North Gore Avenue, Webster Groves, MO 63119; tel. 314/968-2060; FAX. 314/968-8608; Sue Stepleton, Executive Director

Epworth Children and Family Services, Inc., 110 North Elm Avenue, St. Louis, MO 63119; tel. 314/961-5718; FAX. 314/961-3503; Kevin Drollinger, Executive Director

Great Rivers Mental Health Services, 9362 Dielman Industrial Drive, St. Louis, MO 63132; tel. 314/340-6400; Diane McFarland, Director

Industrial Rehabilitation Center, 2701 Rockcreek Parkway, Suite 205, North Kansas City, MO 64117; tel. 816/471-0511; Maurice L. Cummings, Executive Director

Marillac Center, 2826 Main Street, Kansas City, MO 64108; tel. 816/751-4900; FAX. 816/751-4921; R. Michael Bowen, President

Piney Ridge Center, Inc., 1000 Hospital Road, Waynesville, MO 65583; tel. 314/774-5353; FAX. 314/774-2907; Rocky Carroll, Executive Director

Provident Counseling, Inc., 2650 Olive Street, St. Louis, MO 63103; tel. 314/371-6500; FAX. 314/371-6510; Kathleen E. Buescher, President, Chief Executive Officer

Research Mental Health Services, 901 Northeast Independence Avenue, Lees Summit, MO 64086; tel. 816/246-8000; FAX. 816/246-8207; Alan Flory, President

St. Louis Mental Health Center, 1430 Olive Street, Suite 500, St. Louis, MO 63103; tel. 314/877-1776; FAX. 314/877-1709; Bob Kent, Director, Utilization Management

Swope Parkway Health Center, 3801 Blue Parkway, Kansas City, MO 64130; tel. 816/923-5800; FAX. 816/923-9210; Mr. E. Frank Ellis, Chief Executive Officer

The Children's Place, Two East 59th Street, Kansas City, MO 64113; tel. 816/363-1898; FAX. 816/822-7711; Lynn Peck, President, Chief Executive Officer

MONTANA
Intermountain Children's Home, 500 South Lamborn, Helena, MT 59601; tel. 406/442-7920; FAX. 406/442-7949; John Wilkinson, Administrator

Rimrock Foundation, 1231 North 29th Street, Billings, MT 59101; tel. 406/248-3175; FAX. 406/248-3821; David W. Cunningham, M.H.A., Chief Executive Officer

Rocky Mountain Treatment Center, 920 Fourth Avenue North, Great Falls, MT 59401; tel. 406/727-8832; FAX. 406/727-8172; Claree Schulte, Administrator

Yellowstone Treatment Centers, 1732 South 72nd Street, W., Billings, MT 59106; tel. 406/655-2100; FAX. 406/656-0021; JoAnne Rea, Intake/Assessment Clinician

NEBRASKA
Alpha School, 1615 South Sixth Street, Omaha, NE 68108; tel. 402/444-6557; FAX. 402/444-6574; Ray Christensen, Chief Executive Officer

Cedars Youth Services, 770 North Cotner Boulevard, Suite 410, Lincoln, NE 68505; tel. 402/466-6181; FAX. 402/466-6395; James Blue, Chief Executive Officer

Center For The Advancement of Human Development, 503 North Fifth Street, (Mailing Address: 117 South 50th Street, Omaha, NE 68132), Seward, NE 68434; tel. 402/556-6049; FAX. 402/556-0636; William Reay, Chief Executive Officer

Developmental Services of Nebraska, Inc., 5744 Ballard Avenue, (Mailing Address: 5561 South 48th Street, Suite 200, Lincoln, NE 68516), Lincoln, NE 68507; tel. 402/420-2800; FAX. 402/420-2883; Scott LeFevre, Chief Executive Officer

Epworth Village, Inc., 2119 Division, York, NE 68467; tel. 402/362-3353; FAX. 402/362-3248; Kristi Weber, Admissions Coordinator

Lincoln Lancaster County Child Guidance Center, 215 Centennial Mall South, Lincoln, NE 68508; tel. 402/475-7666; FAX. 402/476-9623; Carol Crumpacker, Executive Director

O'Neill Valley Hope, North 10th Street, O'Neill, NE 68763; tel. 402/336-3747; FAX. 402/336-3096; Kaye Chohon, Program Director

Uta Halee Girls Village, 10625 Calhoun Road, P.O. Box 12034, Omaha, NE 68112; tel. 402/453-0803; FAX. 402/453-1247; Denis McCarville, Chief Executive Officer

NEW HAMPSHIRE
Beech Hill Hospital, New Harrisville Road, P.O. Box 254, Dublin, NH 03444; tel. 603/563-8511; FAX. 603/563-8771; Jeffrey A. Baron, Chief Executive Officer

Community Council of Nashua, New Hampshire, Inc., Seven Prospect Street, Nashua, NH 03060-3990; tel. 603/889-6147, ext. 1221; FAX. 603/883-1568; Zlatko Kuftinec, M.D., Executive Director, Chief Medical Officer

Lakeview Neuro Rehab Center, 101 Highwatch Road, Effingham Falls, NH 03814; tel. 603/539-7451; FAX. 603/539-8888; Carolyn Ramsay, Chief Executive Officer

Seaborne Hospital, Inc., Seaborne Drive, Dover, NH 03820; tel. 603/742-9300; Bud Charest, Administrator

Seacoast Mental Health Center, Inc., 1145 Sagamore Avenue, Portsmouth, NH 03801; tel. 603/431-6703; FAX. 603/433-5078; Deborah Lindberg, Quality Assurance and Improvement Coordinator

The Mental Health Center of Greater Manchester, Inc., 401 Cypress Street, Manchester, NH 03103; tel. 603/668-4111; FAX. 603/669-1131; Nicholas Verven, Ph.D., President, Executive Director

NEW JERSEY
American Day Treatment Center, of West Essex Network, Inc., 799 Bloomfield Avenue, Verona, NJ 07044; tel. 201/857-5200; E. Bonnie Lizzio, Director

American Day Treatment Center of West Essex, 799 Bloomfield Avenue, Suite 212, Verona, NJ 07044; tel. 201/857-5200; FAX. 201/857-4920; Barbara A. Hotton, LCSW, Executive Director

Arthur Brisbane Child Treatment Center, Allaire Road, P.O. Box 625, Farmingdale, NJ 07727; tel. 908/938-5061; FAX. 908/751-0813; Raymond Grimaldi, Chief Executive Officer

Cedar Grove Residential Center, 240 Grove Avenue, Cedar Grove, NJ 07009; tel. 201/857-0200; Patrick Lodato, Superintendent

Community Centers for Mental Health, Inc., Two Park Avenue, Dumont, NJ 07628; tel. 201/385-4400; FAX. 201/384-7067; Catherine Small, Chief Executive Officer

Comprehensive Behaviorl Healthcare, Inc., 516 Valley Brook Avenue, Lyndhurst, NJ 07071; tel. 201/935-3322; FAX. 201/460-3698; Peter Scerbo, Chief Executive Officer

Daytop, New Jersey, 80 West Main Street, Mendham, NJ 07945; tel. 201/543-0162; FAX. 201/543-7502; Joseph Hennen, Chief Executive Officer

Discovery, Inc., P.O. Box 177, Marlboro, NJ 07746; tel. 908/946-9444; Henry Crowell, Director, Admissions

Evaluation and Treatment Services, Hopkins Lane, P.O. Box 20, Haddonfield, NJ 08033-0018; tel. 609/429-0010, ext. 259; Lisa Hanway, M.S.N., Senior Director

Ewing Residential Treatment Center, 1610 Stuyvesant Avenue, Trenton, NJ 08618; tel. 609/530-3350; FAX. 609/530-3467; Julius Campbell, Chief Executive Officer

High Focus Centers, Inc., 299 Market Street, Suite 110, Saddle Brook, NJ 07663; tel. 201/291-0055; FAX. 201/291-0888; Peter Balo, Chief Executive Officer

Holley Child Care and Development Center of Youth Consultation Service, 260 Union Street, Hackensack, NJ 07601; tel. 201/343-8803; FAX. 201/343-8563; Richard Mingoia, Associate Executive Director

Honesty House, 1272 Long Hill Road, Stirling, NJ 07980; tel. 908/647-3211; FAX. 908/647-7864; Charles H. Stucky, N.C.A.D.C., Executive Director

JFK Hartwyck at Cedar Brook Nursing, Convalescent and Rehab, 1340 Park Avenue, (Mailing Address: 2048 Oak Tree Road, Edison, NJ 08820), Plainfield, NJ 07060; tel. 908/906-2100; FAX. 908/321-9217; Thomas Lankey, Chief Executive Officer

Lighthouse at Mays Landing, 5034 Atlantic Avenue, Mays Landing, NJ 08330; tel. 609/625–4900; FAX. 609/625–8058; Dr. C. Wm. Brett, Chief Executive Officer

Mid–Bergen Center, Inc., 610 Industrial Avenue, Paramus, NJ 07652; tel. 201/265–8200; FAX. 201/265–3543; Joseph Masciandaro, Chief Executive Officer

Monmouth Chemical Dependency Treatment Center, Inc., 152 Chelsea Avenue, Long Branch, NJ 07740; tel. 908/222–5190; FAX. 908/222–5577; Timothy Harrington, Chief Executive Officer

New Hope Foundation, Inc., Route 520, Marlboro, NJ 07746; tel. 908/946–3030; FAX. 908/946–3507; George J. Mattie, Chief Executive Officer

Ocean Mental Health Services, Inc., 230 Main Street, Toms River, NJ 08753; tel. 908/349–0838; Charles J. Langan, Chief Executive Officer

Patterson Army Health Clinic, Stephenson Road, (Mailing Address: MCXS–QI, Fort Monmouth, NJ 07703–5000), Fort Monmouth, NJ 07703–5607; tel. 908/532–0945; FAX. 908/532–3452; Michele Steinert, Chief, Quality Management

Preferred Behavioral Health of New Jersey, CN 2036–700 Airport Road, Lakewood, NJ 08701; tel. 908/367–4700; FAX. 908/364–2253; William Sette, Chief Executive Officer

Rutgers University Student Health Service, Hurtado Health Center, 11 Bishop Place, New Brunswick, NJ 08903–5069; tel. 908/932–8429; FAX. 908/932–1525; Robert Bierman, Chief Executive Officer

Seabrook House, 133 Polk Lane, P.O. Box 5055, Seabrook, NJ 08302–0655; tel. 800/582–5968; FAX. 609/453–1022; Matt Wolf, Admissions Coordinator

Sunrise House Foundation, Inc., 37 Sunset Inn Road, Lafayette, NJ 07848; tel. 201/383–6300; FAX. 201/383–8458; Beth Anne Nathans, M.S., Chief Executive Officer

U.M.D.N.J–Community Mental Health Center at Piscataway, 671 Hoes Lane, P.O. Box 1392, Piscataway, NJ 08855–1392; tel. 908/235–5900; FAX. 908/235–4594; Gary W. Lamson, Vice President, Chief Executive Officer

Vineland Children's Residential Treatment Center, 2000 Maple Avenue, Vineland, NJ 08360; tel. 609/696–6620; FAX. 609/696–6847; Theodore Allen, Superintendent

West Bergen Mental Healthcare, Inc., 120 Chestnut Street, Ridgewood, NJ 07450–2500; tel. 201/444–3550; FAX. 201/652–1613; Philip Wilson, Chief Executive Officer

Willowglen Academy–New Jersey, Inc., Highway 206, Newton, NJ 07860; tel. 201/579–3700; Jean Mendres, Executive Director

Woodbridge Child Diagnostic and Treatment Center, 15 Paddock Street, Avenel, NJ 07001; tel. 908/499–5050; FAX. 908/815–4874; William Falvo, Chief Executive Officer

NEW MEXICO

Desert Hills Center for Youth and Families, 5310 Sequoia, N.W., Albuquerque, NM 87120; tel. 505/836–7330; FAX. 505/836–7424; Dan Lopez, Chief Executive Officer

Four Corners Regional Adolescent Treatment Center, P.O. Box 567, Shiprock, NM 87420; tel. 505/368–4712; FAX. 505/368–5457; Hoskie Benally, Chief Executive Officer

Innovative Services, 2700 Yale Boulevard, S.E., Albuquerque, NM 87106; tel. 505/242–5466; FAX. 505/242–0099; Christina I. Orona, M.A., QMRP, Chief Executive Officer

NAMASTE, P.O. Box 489, Los Lunas, NM 87031; tel. 505/865–6176; FAX. 505/865–3268; Linda Zimmerman, Executive Director

Pinon Hills Residential Treatment Center, 6930 Weicker Lane, P.O. Box 428, Velarde, NM 87582; tel. 505/852–2704; FAX. 505/852–2022; Jerry Smith, Chief Executive Officer

River's Bend Children's Residential Treatment, 300 East Griggs, Las Cruces, NM 80001; tel. 505/525–2693; FAX. 505/525–2965; Mike Boyce, Chief Executive Officer

Sequoyah Adolescent Treatment Center, 3405 West Pan American Freeway, N.E., Albuquerque, NM 87107; tel. 505/841–4375; FAX. 505/841–4361; W. Henry Gardner, Ph.D., Director

Tender Touch Industries, Inc., 4316 Carlisle Boulevard, N.E., Suite A, Albuquerque, NM 87107; tel. 505/884–6693; FAX. 505/884–4304; Dr. Michael Dismond, Chief Executive Officer

The Adolescent Pointe, 5050 McNutt Street, P.O. Box Six, Santa Teresa, NM 88008; tel. 505/589–0033; FAX. 505/589–2860; Lorenzo Barrios, Chief Executive Officer

The Pointe ARTC for Children, 200 Laura Court, P.O. Box Six, Santa Teresa, NM 88008; tel. 505/589–0033; FAX. 505/589–2860; Scott Pelking, Administrator

NEW YORK

Areba/Casriel Institute, 500 West 57th Street, New York, NY 10019; tel. 212/376–1810; FAX. 212/376–1824; Steven Yohay, Executive Director

Arms Acres, Inc., 75 Seminary Hill Road, Carmel, NY 10512; tel. 914/225–3400; FAX. 914/225–5660; Edward Spauster, Ph.D., Executive Director

Baker Victory Services, 780 Ridge Road, Lackawanna, NY 14218; tel. 716/828–9777; FAX. 716/828–9767; James J. Casion, Chief Executive Officer

Bronx Alcoholism Treatment Center, 1500 Waters Place, Bronx, NY 10461; tel. 718/904–0026, ext. 300; FAX. 718/597–9434; Ronald B. Lonesome, M.D., Director

Charles K. Post Alcoholism Treatment Center, Building One Pilgrim Psychiatric Center, West Brentwood, NY 11717; tel. 516/434–7209; Phillip A. Dawes, Director

Children's Home RTF, Inc., Squirrel Hill Road, P.O. Box 658, Greene, NY 13778; tel. 607/656–9004; FAX. 607/656–9076; Mary Jo Thorn, Program Director

Conifer Park, Inc., 79 Glenridge Road, Glenville, NY 12302; tel. 518/399–6446; John A. Duffy, Executive Officer

Conners Residential Treatment Facility, Inc., 824 Delaware Avenue, Buffalo, NY 14209; tel. 716/884–3802; FAX. 716/884–8689; James D. Lawson, Director

Cornerstone of Medical Arts Center Hospital, 57 West 57th Street, New York, NY 10019; tel. 212/755–0200; FAX. 212/755–0915; Norman J. Sokolow, President

Cortland Medical, Four Skyline Drive, Hawthorne, NY 10532; tel. 914/347–2990; FAX. 914/347–3074; Jeffery Smith, M.D., Chief Executive Officer

Creedmoor Alcoholism Treatment Center, 80–45 Winchester Boulevard, Building 19–D, Queens Village, NY 11427; tel. 718/264–3743; FAX. 718/776–5145; Kay Santiago–Vazquez, Acting Director

Crestwood Children's Center, 2075 Scottsville Road, Rochester, NY 14623–2098; tel. 716/436–4442; FAX. 716/436–0169; Denise M. Groesbeck, OTR, M.P.A., Director, Administration

Dick Van Dyke Alcoholism Treatment Center, P.O. Box 218, Willard, NY 14588–0218; tel. 607/869–9500; FAX. 607/869–5303; James R. Sharp, Ph.D., Assistant Director

Dutchess County Department of Mental Hygiene, 230 North Road, Poughkeepsie, NY 12601; tel. 914/485–9700; FAX. 914/485–2759; Kenneth M. Glatt, Ph.D., Commissioner

Green Chimneys Children's Services, Inc., Putnam Lake Road, Caller Box 719, Brewster, NY 10509; tel. 914/279–2995, ext. 205; FAX. 914/279–2714; Joseph Whalen, Executive Director

Harmony Heights, 57 Sandy Hill Road, Oyster Bay Cove, NY 11771; tel. 516/922–4060; Donald Lafayette, P.D., Quality Assurance Utilization

Hillside Children's Center, 1183 Monroe Avenue, Rochester, NY 14620; tel. 716/256–7500; FAX. 716/256–7510; Dennis M. Richardson, President, Chief Executive Officer

Hope House, Inc., 517 Western Avenue, Albany, NY 12203; tel. 518/482–4673; FAX. 518/482–0873; Mary Ann Finn, Executive Director

Hopevale, Inc., 3780 Howard Road, Hamburg, NY 14075; tel. 716/648–1964; FAX. 716/648–5266; Stanfort J. Perry, Executive Director

J. L. Norris Alcoholism Treatment Center, 1111 Elmwood Avenue, Rochester, NY 14620; tel. 716/461–0410; FAX. 716/461–4545; Thomas E. Nightingale, Director

Jewish Board of Family and Children's Services, Inc., 120 West 57th Street, New York, NY 10019; tel. 212/582–9100, ext. 1750; FAX. 212/956–5676; Alan B. Siskind, Ph.D., Executive Vice President

Julia Dyckman Andrus Memorial, Inc., 1156 North Broadway, Yonkers, NY 10701; tel. 914/965–3700; FAX. 914/965–3883; Dr. Gary Carman, Chief Executive Officer

Kingsboro Alcoholism Treatment Center, 754 Lexington Avenue, Brooklyn, NY 11221; tel. 718/453–6747; JACK. 718/453–7581; Jacqueline Cole, Director

Madonna Heights Services, a Division of St. Christopher/Ottilie, 151 Burrs Lane, P.O. Box 8020, Dix Hills, NY 11746–9020; tel. 516/643–8800; FAX. 516/491–4440; Robert J. McMahon, Executive Director

Manhattan Alcoholism Treatment Center MII, 600 East 125th Street, Ward's Island, New York, NY 10035; tel. 212/369–0703; FAX. 212/369–3507; K. Santiago–Vazquez, RN, Chief Executive Officer

McPike Alcoholism Treatment Center, 1213 Court Street, Utica, NY 13502; tel. 315/797–6800, ext. 4801; FAX. 315/738–4437; Phillip Dranger, Acting Director

Middletown Alcoholism Treatment Center, 141 Monhagen Avenue, Middleton, NY 10940; tel. 914/341–2500; FAX. 914/341–2570; Richard C. Ward, Director

National Recovery Institutes, 455 West 50th Street, New York, NY 10019; tel. 212/262–6000; Roger Cohn, President

Parsons Child and Family Center, 60 Academy Road, Albany, NY 12208; tel. 518/426–2600; FAX. 518/426–2792; John W. Carswell, Executive Director

Psych Services of Long Island, 1600 Stewart Avenue, Suite 202, Westbury, NY 11590; tel. 516/683–1200; Marci Zaslav, Executive Director

Psych Systems of Westchester, 33 West Main Street, Suite 307, Elmsford, NY 10523; tel. 914/345–5676; FAX. 914/345–5610; Richard Santiago, Chief Executive Officer

Research Institute on Addictions, 1021 Main Street, Buffalo, NY 14203; tel. 716/887–2386; FAX. 716/887–2215; Paul R. Stasiewicz, Ph.D., CRC Coordinator, Outpatient Services

Restorative Management Corporation, 15 King Street Third Floor, Middletown, NY 10940; tel. 914/342–5941; FAX. 914/344–2604; Dean Scher, Chief Executive Officer

Rochester Mental Health Center, Hart Building, 490 East Ridge Road, Rochester, NY 14621; tel. 716/544–5220; FAX. 716/544–6694; Connie Aiello, RN, Acting President

Russell E. Blaisdell Alcoholism Treatment Center, R. P. C. Campus, Orangeburg, NY 10962; tel. 914/359–8500; FAX. 914/359–2016; Louis R. Brandes, M.D., Director

Saint Peter's Addiction Recovery Center (SPARC, Inc.), Three Mercy Care Lane, Guiderland, NY 12084; tel. 518/452–6700; FAX. 518/452–6753; Karen A. Giles, Chief Executive Director

Salamanca Hospital District Authority, d/b/a Salamanca Healthcare Complex, 150 Parkway Drive, Salamanca, NY 14779; tel. 716/945–1900; FAX. 716/945–5016; Kenneth Oakley, Administrator

Salvation Army–Wayside Home School For Girls, 1461 Dutch Broadway, Valley Stream, NY 11580; tel. 516/825–1600; FAX. 516/825–1829; Joseph Juliana, Director

Seafield Center, Inc., Seven Seafield Lane, Westhampton Beach, NY 11978; tel. 516/288–1122; John C. Haley, Chief Operating Officer

South Beach Alcoholism Treatment Center, 777 Seaview Avenue, Building One, Second Floor, Staten Island, NY 10305; tel. 718/667–4218; FAX. 718/351–1958; Gerlando A. Verruso, Director

St. Christopher–Ottilie Residential Treatment Facility, 85–70 148th Street, Briarwood, NY 11435; tel. 718/658–4101; FAX. 718/523–2582; James G. Nyreen, Program Director

St. Joseph's Rehabilitation Center, Inc., 99 Glenwood Estates, P.O. Box 470, Saranac Lake, NY 12983–0470; tel. 518/891–3950; FAX. 518/891–3986; Reverend Arthur M. Johnson, Chief Executive Officer

St. Joseph's Villa of Rochester, 3300 Dewey Avenue, Rochester, NY 14616–3795; tel. 716/865–1550; FAX. 716/865–5219; Roger C. Battaglia, President, Chief Executive Officer

St. Lawrence Alcoholism Treatment Center, One Chimney Point Drive, Hamilton Hall, Ogdensburg, NY 13669; tel. 315/393–1180; FAX. 315/393–6160; Phillip Dranger, Director

St. Mary's Children and Family Services, 525 Convent Road, Syosset, NY 11791–3864; tel. 516/921–0808; FAX. 516/921–4542; Liz Giordano, Executive Director

Stutzman Alcoholism Treatment Center, 360 Forest Avenue, Buffalo, NY 14213; tel. 716/882–4900; FAX. 716/882–4426; Steven Schwartz, Director

The Astor Home for Children, 36 Mill Street, P.O. Box 5005, Rhinebeck, NY 12572–5005; tel. 914/876–4081; FAX. 914/876–2020; Sister Rose Logan, D.C., Executive Director

Section C

The August Aichhorn Center for Adolescent Residential Care, Inc., 23 West 106th Street, New York, NY 10025; tel. 212/316–9353; FAX. 212/662–2755; Michael A. Pawel, M.D., Executive Director

The Children's Village, Dobbs Ferry, NY 10522; tel. 914/693–0600, ext. 1201; FAX. 914/674–9208; Nan Dale, Executive Director

The Health Association–MAIN QUEST Treatment Center, 774 West Main Street, Rochester, NY 14620; tel. 716/464–8870; FAX. 716/464–8077; Susan L. Costa, Chief Executive Officer

The House of the Good Shepherd, 1550 Champlin Avenue, Utica, NY 13502; tel. 315/733–0436; FAX. 315/732–0772; William Holicky, Chief Executive Officer

The Long Island Center for Recovery, 320 West Montauk Highway, Hampton Bays, NY 11946; tel. 516/728–3100; Steve Bassis, Chief Executive Officer

The Rhinebeck Lodge for Successful Living, Inpatient Substance Abuse Treatment Program, 500 Milan Hollow Road, Rhinebeck, NY 12572; tel. 800/266–4410; Chandra Singh, Ph.D., Chief Executive Officer

The Saint Francis Academy, Incorporated, Lake Placid (Camelot, The Knight House, Adirondack Experience), 50 Riverside Drive, Lake Placid, NY 12946; tel. 518/523–3605; FAX. 518/523–1470; Reverend Carlos J. Caguiat, FACHE, Vice President, Executive Director

The Villa Outpatient Center, 290 Madison Avenue, Sixth Floor, New York, NY 10017; tel. 212/679–4960; FAX. 212/679–4966; Richard Partridge, Chief Executive Officer

Tully Hill, Route 80, P.O. Box 920, Tully, NY 13159; tel. 315/696–6114; FAX. 315/696–8509; Cathy L. Palm, CPA, M.B.A., Executive Director

Valley View House, Inc., Swiss Hill Road, Kenoza Lake, NY 12750; tel. 800/955–2869; FAX. 914/482–3516; William Coleman, CSW, Chief Executive Officer

Veritas Villa, Inc., R.R. 2, Box 415, Kerhonkson, NY 12446; tel. 914/626–3555; FAX. 914/626–3840; James S. Cusack, President, Owner

Westchester Jewish Community Services, Inc., 141 North Central Avenue, Hartsdale, NY 10530; tel. 914/949–6761; FAX. 914/949–3224; Ronald Gaudia, Chief Executive Officer

NORTH CAROLINA

American Day Treatment Centers Charlotte, 201 Providence Road, Suite 101, Charlotte, NC 28207; tel. 704/370–0800; FAX. 704/370–0001; Sherley Ward, Jr., Executive Director

Amethyst, 1715 Sharon Road, W., Charlotte, NC 28210, P.O. Box 32861, Charlotte, NC 28232–2861; tel. 704/554–8373; FAX. 704/554–8058; Daniel J. Harrison, Assistant Vice President, Administrator

Fellowship Hall, Inc., 5140 Dunstan Road, P.O. Box 13890, Greensboro, NC 27415; tel. 910/621–3381; FAX. 910/621–7513; Rodney Battles, M.B.A., Executive Director

Forsyth–Stokes Mental Health Center, 725 North Highland Avenue, Winston-Salem, NC 27101; tel. 919/725–7777; Roy H. Haberkern, M.D., Medical Director

Robeson Health Care Corporation, 1211 South Walnut Street, Fairmont, NC 28340; tel. 910/628–5200; FAX. 910/628–6205; Jinnie Lowery, Chief Executive Officer

The Alcohol and Drug Abuse Treatment Center, 301 Tabernacle Road, Black Mountain, NC 28711; tel. 704/669–3400; FAX. 704/669–3451; Bill Rafter, Director

The Wilmington Treatment Center, 2520 Troy Drive, Wilmington, NC 28401; tel. 919/762–2727; FAX. 919/762–7923; Charles Sharp, Executive Director

Three Springs of North Carolina, P.O. Box 1370, Pittsboro, NC 27312; tel. 919/542–1104; Peggy Reeder, Administrator

Timber Ridge Treatment Center, 14225 Stokes Ferry Road, Gold Hill, NC 28071; tel. 704/279–1199; FAX. 704/279–7668; Thomas A. R. Hibbert, President, Chief Executive Officer

Unity Regional Youth Treatment Center, P.O. Box C–201, Cherokee, NC 28719; tel. 704/497–3958; Mary Anne Farrell, M.D., Director

Walter B. Jones Alcohol and Drug Abuse Treatment Center, 2577 West Fifth Street, Greenville, NC 27834; tel. 919/830–3426; FAX. 919/830–8585; Phillip A. Mooring, Chief Executive Officer

OHIO

Beech Brook, 3737 Lander Road, Cleveland, OH 44124; tel. 216/831–2255, ext. 309; FAX. 216/831–0638; Mark Groner, Assistant Clinical Director

Bellefaire JCB, 22001 Fairmount Boulevard, Cleveland, OH 44118; tel. 216/932–2800, ext. 335; FAX. 216/932–8520; Allison Weiss, M.S.S.A., L.I.S.W., Intake Coordinator

Blick Clinic, Inc., 640 West Market Street, Akron, OH 44303–1465; tel. 216/762–5425; FAX. 216/762–4019; Dr. Gregory Laforme, Chief Executive Officer

Center for Chemical Addictions Treatment, 830 Ezzard Charles Drive, Cincinnati, OH 45214; tel. 513/381–6672; Sandra L. Kuehn, Executive Director

Central Mental Health/Wellstar, 832 McKinley Avenue, N.W., Canton, OH 44703; tel. 216/455–9407; FAX. 216/453–0007; Richard W. Thompson, Executive Director

Children's Aid Society, 10427 Detroit Avenue, Cleveland, OH 44102; tel. 216/521–6511; FAX. 216/521–6006; Lawrence S. Waldman, Ph.D., Director, Clinical Services

Community Drug Board, Inc., 725 East Market Street, Akron, OH 44305; tel. 330/434–4141; FAX. 330/434–7125; Theodore Paul Ziegler, Chief Executive Officer

Community Support Services, Inc., 150 Cross Street, Akron, OH 44311; tel. 330/253–9388; Alicia Wagner, R.R.A., Quality Improvement

Comprehensive Psychiatry Specialists, 955 Windham Court, Suite Two, Boardman, OH 44512; tel. 330/726–9570; FAX. 330/726–9031; Pradeep Mathur, President

Crisis Intervention Center of Stark County, Inc., 2421 13th Street, N.W., Canton, OH 44708; tel. 216/452–9812; FAX. 216/454–4357; Lori S. Lapp, M.B.A., Executive Director

D and E Counseling Center, 142 Javit Court, Youngstown, OH 44515; tel. 216/793–2487; FAX. 216/793–4559; Gregory Cvetkovic, Chief Executive Officer

Family Recovery Center, 964 North Market Street, Lisbon, OH 44432; tel. 330/424–1468; FAX. 330/424–9844; Eloise V. Traina, Executive Director

Focus Health, 5701 North High Street, Suite Eight, Worthington, OH 43085; tel. 614/885–1944; FAX. 614/885–6665; Jo-Ann Boundy, Director, Operations

Glenbeigh Health Sources, P.O. Box 298, Rock Creek, OH 44084; tel. 216/563–3400; FAX. 216/563–9619; Patricia Weston–Hall, Executive Director

Harbor Behavioral Healthcare, 4334 Secor Road, Toledo, OH 43623–4234; tel. 419/475–4449; FAX. 419/479–3832; Dale E. Shreve, Chief Operating Officer

Health Recovery Services, Inc., 100 Hospital Drive, Suite Two, Athens, OH 45701; tel. 614/592–6720; FAX. 614/592–6728; Kenneth H. Pickering, Executive Director

INTERACT Behavioral Healthcare Services, Inc., a Member of Mount Carmel Health System, Administrative Offices, 1808 East Broad Street, Columbus, OH 43203; tel. 614/251–8242; James M. Shulman, Ph.D., Chief Executive Officer

Interval Brotherhood Home, Alcohol Drug Rehabilitation Center, 3445 South Main Street, Akron, OH 44319; tel. 330/644–4095; FAX. 330/645–2031; Father Samuel R. Ciccolini, Executive Director

Lakeshore Treatment Centers, Inc., 1717 East Perkins Avenue, Sandusky, OH 44870; tel. 419/626–1633; Jack L. Manuel, Chief Operating Officer

Lincoln Center For Prevention and Treatment of Chemical Dependency, 1918 North Main Street, Findlay, OH 45840; tel. 419/423–9242; FAX. 419/423–7854; Nita L. Rider, Executive Director

Mahoning County Chemical Dependency Programs, Inc., 527 North Meridan Road, Youngstown, OH 44509; tel. 330/797–0070; FAX. 330/797–9148; Martin K. Gaudiose, Chief Executive Officer

McKinley Hall, Inc., 1101 East High Street, Springfield, OH 45505; tel. 937/328–5300; FAX. 937/322–4900; Judith O. Hoy, Chief Executive Officer

Mental Health Center of Western Stark County, Inc., 111 Tremont Avenue, S.W., Massillon, OH 44647; tel. 216/833–4132; FAX. 216/833–6548; Lawrence R. Cook, Executive Director

Miami Valley Labor Management, Health Care Delivery Systems, Inc., 136 Heid Avenue, Dayton, OH 45404; tel. 513/236–1367; Thomas Keen, Director

Neil Kennedy Recovery Clinic, 2151 Rush Boulevard, Youngstown, OH 44507; tel. 216/744–1181; FAX. 216/740–2849; Gerald V. Carter, Executive Director

Neo Psych Consultants, 819 McKay Court, Suite 101, Boardman, OH 44512; tel. 216/726–7785; Charles L. Boris, President

New Directions, Inc., 30800 Chagrin Boulevard, Pepper Pike, OH 44124; tel. 216/591–0324; FAX. 216/591–1243; Sally Newman, Intake Coordinator

Nova Behavioral Healthcare, 1207 West State Street, Alliance, OH 44601; tel. 216/821–1995; FAX. 216/821–6080; Carol H. Hales, Chief Executive Officer

Parkside Behavioral Healthcare, Inc., d/b/a Parkside Recovery Services, 349 Olde Ridenour Road, Columbus, OH 43230; tel. 614/471–2552; FAX. 614/471–0167; Christine Gerber, President, Chief Executive Officer

Parmadale Family Services, 6753 State Road, Parma, OH 44134; tel. 216/845–7700; FAX. 216/845–5910; Michael J. Haggerty, Executive Director

Portage Path Community Mental Health Center, 340 South Broadway Street, Akron, OH 44308–8159; tel. 330/253–4118; FAX. 330/376–8002; Shelly Obert, Clinical Services Director

Psycare, Inc., 3530 Belmont Avenue, Suite Seven, Youngstown, OH 44505; tel. 216/759–2310; FAX. 216/759–0018; Douglas Darnall, Ph.D., Chief Executive Officer

Psych Systems of Greater Cincinnati, 11223 Cornell Park Drive, Cincinnati, OH 45242; tel. 513/530–8500; FAX. 513/530–5805

Quest Recovery Services, 1341 Market Avenue, N., Canton, OH 44714; tel. 216/453–8252; FAX. 216/453–6716; Donald C. Davies, Chief Executive Officer

Ravenwood Mental Health Center, 12557 Ravenwood Drive, Chardon, OH 44024; tel. 216/285–3568; FAX. 216/285–4552; David Boyle, Executive Director

Rescue Mental Health Services, 3350 Collingwood Boulevard, Toledo, OH 43610; tel. 419/255–9585; FAX. 419/255–2801; Frank C. Ayers, Executive Director

Serenity Living, Inc., 210 West National Road, P.O. Box 217, Vandalia, OH 45377; tel. 513/898–2788; Joseph J. Trevino, M.D., Chief Executive Officer

Specialty Care Psychiatric Services, 2657 Niles Cortland Road, Warren, OH 44484; tel. 216/652–3533; Donna J. Dyer, M.Ed., President

Springview Developmental Center, 3130 East Main Street, Springfield, OH 45505; tel. 937/325–9263; FAX. 937/325–3593; Dominick S. Dennis, Superintendent

Stepping Stone Recovery Center, 165 East Park Avenue, Niles, OH 44446; tel. 216/544–6355; FAX. 216/652–4781; Pamela Walter, Chief Executive Officer

Substance Abuse Services, Inc., 2012 Madison Avenue, Toledo, OH 43624; tel. 419/243–7274; FAX. 419/243–1505; Carroll Parks, Chief Executive Officer

The Akron Child Guidance Center, Inc., 312 Locust Street, Akron, OH 44302–1878; tel. 330/762–0591; FAX. 330/258–0931; Charles M. Vehlow, Jr., Executive Director

The Buckeye Ranch, 5665 Hoover Road, Grove City, OH 43123; tel. 800/859–5665; FAX. 614/871–6487; Francine Rado, M.S.W., L.I.S.W., Utilization Manager

The Campus, 905 South Sunbury Road, Westerville, OH 43081; tel. 614/895–1000, ext. 13; FAX. 614/895–3010; Robert Stevenson, CCDC III, Intake Coordinator

The Campus Hospital of Cleveland, 18120 Puritas Road, Cleveland, OH 44135; tel. 216/476–0222; FAX. 216/476–2938; Joan Curran, Administrator

The Lake Area Recovery Center, 2801 C Court, Ashtabula, OH 44004; tel. 216/998–0722; FAX. 216/992–1699; Kathleen Kinney, Executive Director

Transitional Living, Inc., 2052 Princeton Road, Hamilton, OH 45011; tel. 513/863–6383; Lila Webb, Administrative Assistant

Tri–State Behavioral Health Center, 3156 Glenmore Avenue, Cincinnati, OH 45211; tel. 513/481–8822; FAX. 513/481–7317; Michael Miller, Chief Executive Officer

Two North Park, Inc., 720 Pine Street, S.E., Warren, OH 44483; tel. 216/399–3677; FAX. 216/394–3815; Ken Lloyd, M.S. Ed., L.S.W., CCDC III, Executive Director

Wellspring Retreat and Resource Center, P.O. Box 67, 32598 Woodyard Road, Albany, OH 45710; tel. 614/698–6277; FAX. 614/698–2053; Dr. Paul Martin, Chief Executive Officer

Wood County Council on Alcoholism and Drug Abuse, Inc., 320 West Gypsy Lane, Bowling Green, OH 43402; tel. 419/352–2551; Randall J. LaFond, Executive Director

OKLAHOMA

Christopher Youth Center, Inc., 2741 East Seventh Street, Tulsa, OK 74104; tel. 918/583–0612; FAX. 918/583–5459; Thomas E. McKee, Ed.D., Director

High Pointe, 6501 Northeast 50th Street, Oklahoma City, OK 73141; tel. 405/424–3383; FAX. 405/424–0729; Charlene Arnett, Chief Executive Officer

Jim Taliaferro Community Mental Health Center, 602 Southwest 38th Street, Lawton, OK 73505–6999; tel. 405/248–5780; FAX. 405/248–3610; Ted Debbs, M.S., Executive Director

Mendros Psychiatric Medical Clinic, 2100 North Broadway, Moore, OK 73160; tel. 405/794–7719; Harry G. Mendros, M.D., Chief Executive Officer

Oklahoma Youth Center, 320 12th Avenue, N.E., Norman, OK 73071–5300; tel. 405/573–3821; FAX. 405/573–3804; Paul Bouffard, Director

Parkside, Inc., 1620 East 12th Street, Tulsa, OK 74120; tel. 918/582–2131; FAX. 918/588–8822; Quentin Henley, Chief Executive Officer

Recovery Plus, 817 South Elm Place, Suite 105, Broken Arrow, OK 74012–2537; tel. 918/258–6900; Karen Doney, Executive Director

Valley Hope Alcohol and Drug Treatment Center, 100 South Jones, P.O. Box 472, Cushing, OK 74023; tel. 918/225–1736; FAX. 918/225–7742; Dennis Gilhousen, Chief Executive Officer

OREGON

Children's Farm House, 4455 Northeast Highway 20, Corvallis, OR 97339–9102; tel. 541/757–1852; FAX. 541/757–1944; Kim Scott, Associate Director

Eastern Oregon Adolescent Multi–Treatment Center, 412 Southeast Dorion, Pendleton, OR 97801; tel. 541/276–0057; FAX. 541/276–1704; Ronald Humiston, Executive Director

Edgefield Children's Center, Inc., 2408 Southwest Halsey Street, Troutdale, OR 97060–1097; tel. 503/665–0157; FAX. 503/666–3066; David Fuks, M.S.W., Executive Director

Kerr Youth and Family Center, 722 Northeast 162nd Avenue, Portland, OR 97230; tel. 503/255–4205; James V. Novell, Administrator

Parry Center for Children, 3415 Southeast Powell Boulevard, Portland, OR 97202; tel. 503/234–9591; FAX. 503/234–4376; Marie Avery, Chief Executive Officer

Pioneer Trail Adolescent Treatment Center, 4101 Northeast Division Street, Gresham, OR 97030; tel. 503/661–0775; FAX. 503/661–4649; Robert E. Marshall, Administrator

RiverBend Youth Center, 15544 South Clackamas River Drive, Oregon City, OR 97045; tel. 503/656–8005; FAX. 503/656–8929; Marcia L. McClocklin, Executive Director

Rosemont Treatment Center and School, 9911 Southeast Mt. Scott Boulevard, Portland, OR 97266; tel. 503/777–8090; FAX. 503/788–1131; Benson Meyers, Chief Executive Officer

Serenity Lane, Inc., 616 East 16th Avenue, Eugene, OR 97401; tel. 541/687–1110; FAX. 541/687–9041; Neil H. McNaughton, Executive Director

Southern Oregon Adolescent Study and Treatment Center, Inc., 210 Tacoma Street, Grants Pass, OR 97526; tel. 503/476–3302; FAX. 503/476–2895; Robert Lieberman, Executive Director

Springbook Northwest, 2001 Crestview Drive, Newberg, OR 97132; tel. 503/537–7000; Greg Skipper, M.D., Medical Director

The Christie School, P.O. Box 368, Marylhurst, OR 97036; tel. 503/635–3416; FAX. 503/697–6932; Daniel A. Mahler, M.S.W., LCSW, Executive Director

PENNSYLVANIA

Abraxas I, Blue Jay Village, Box 59 Forest Road, Marienville, PA 16239; tel. 814/927–6615; FAX. 814/927–8560; James Newsome, Program Director

Alternative Counseling Associates, 438 High Street, Pottstown, PA 19464; tel. 610/970–9060; FAX. 610/970–4280; Charles Beem, Executive Director

American Day Treatment Center of Bryn Mawr, 950 Haverford Road, Suite D, Bryn Mawr, PA 19010; tel. 610/527–7474; FAX. 610/527–7479; Charlotte Yoder, Executive Director

Bowling Green Inn–Brandywine, 1375 Newark Road, Kennett Square, PA 19348; tel. 610/268–3588; FAX. 610/268–2334; Jeffrey J. Kegley, Executive Director

Cedar Manor Drug and Alcohol Treatment Center, 109 Summer Street, P.O. Box 286, Cresson, PA 16630; tel. 814/886–7399; FAX. 814/886–8705; Mary McDermott, Chief Executive Officer

Charter Behavioral Health System at Cove Forge, New Beginnings Road, Williamsburg, PA 16693; tel. 800/873–2131; FAX. 814/832–2882; Jonathan Wolf, Chief Executive Officer

Clear Brook, Inc., 1003 Wyoming Avenue, Forty–Fort, PA 18704; tel. 717/288–6692; Dave Lombard, Chief Executive Officer

Conewago Place, Nye Road, P.O. Box 406, Humelstown, PA 17036; tel. 717/533–0428; Dan Baker, Executive Director

Eagleville Hospital, 100 Eagleville Road, P.O. Box 45, Eagleville, PA 19408; tel. 610/539–6000; FAX. 610/539–9314; Kendria Kurtz, Administrator

Friendship House, 1329 Wyoming Avenue, P.O. Box 3778, Scranton, PA 18505; tel. 717/341–7102; FAX. 717/341–9736; Robert Angeloni, President, Chief Executive Officer

Gateway Rehabilitation Center, Moffett Run Road, Aliquippa, PA 15001; tel. 412/766–8700, ext. 101; FAX. 412/375–8815; Kenneth S. Ramsey, Ph.D., President

Gaudenzia, Inc.–Common Ground, 2835 North Front Street, Harrisburg, PA 17110; tel. 717/238–5553; Gerald McFarland, Program Director

Greenbriar Treatment Center, 800 Manor Drive, Washington, PA 15301; tel. 412/225–9700; FAX. 412/225–9764; Mary Banaszak, Executive Director

Hoffman Homes for Youth, 815 Orphanage Road, Littlestown, PA 17340; tel. 717/359–7148; FAX. 717/359–9536; Frank Deroba, Director

Holy Redeemer Visiting Nurse Association, 12265 Townsend Road, Suite 400, Philadelphia, PA 19154; tel. 215/671–9200; FAX. 215/671–1950; Jerold Cohen, Chief Executive Officer

Keystone Center, 2001 Providence Avenue, Chester, PA 19013–5504; tel. 610/876–9000; FAX. 610/876–5441; Jimmy Patton, Chief Executive Officer

Livengrin Foundation, Inc., 4833 Hulmeville Road, Bensalem, PA 19020–3099; tel. 215/638–5200; FAX. 215/638–2603; Medical Director

Lutheran Youth and Family Services, Beaver Road, P.O. Box 70, Zelienople, PA 16063; tel. 412/452–4453; FAX. 412/452–6576; Charles T. Lockwood, Executive Director

Malvern Institute, 940 King Road, Malvern, PA 19355; tel. 610/647–0330; FAX. 610/647–2572; Valerie Craig, Administrator, Chief Executive Officer

Marworth, Lily Lake Road, Waverly, PA 18471; tel. 717/563–1112; FAX. 717/563–2711; James Dougherty, Senior Vice President

Milestones Community HealthCare, Inc., 1069 Easton Road, Roslyn, PA 19001; tel. 215/884–5566; FAX. 215/885–1746; Dr. Paul Volosov, Chief Executive Officer

Mirmont Treatment Center, 100 Yearsley Mill Road, Lima, PA 19037; tel. 215/565–9232; FAX. 215/565–7497; Thomas F. Crane, Executive Director

New Vitae Partial Hospital and Residential Treatment Center, 5201 St. Joseph Road, Limeport, PA 18060; tel. 610/965–9021; FAX. 610/965–6227; Albert J. Arbogast, Administrator

Northern Southwest Community MH/MR/D & A, Birmingham Center, 21st and Wharton Streets, Suite 321, Pittsburgh, PA 15203; tel. 412/488–4040; Stephanie Murtaugh

Pamm Human Resources Center, Inc., 2400–10 North Front Street, Philadelphia, PA 19133; tel. 215/291–4357; FAX. 215/426–6010; Dr. Melchor Martinez, President, Chief Executive Officer

Penn Foundation, 807 Lawn Avenue, P.O. Box 32, Sellersville, PA 18960; tel. 215/257–6551; FAX. 215/257–9347; Vernon H. Kratz, M.D., President

Renewal Centers, 2705 Old Bethlehem Pike, Quakertown, PA 18951; tel. 215/536–9070; FAX. 215/536–4788; Theresa E. Walsh, Executive Director

Richard J. Caron Foundation, Galen Hall Roads, P.O. Box A, Wernersville, PA 19565; tel. 610/678–2332; FAX. 610/678–5704; Douglas Tieman, Chief Executive Officer

Roxbury, 601 Roxbury Road, P.O. Box L, Shippensburg, PA 17257; tel. 717/532–4217; FAX. 717/532–4003; Claire F. Beckwith, Chief Executive Officer

Salisbury House, Inc., 910 East Emmaus Avenue, Allentown, PA 18103; tel. 610/791–7878; FAX. 610/791–4709; Dr. David Smock, Clinical Director

Serenity Hall, Inc., 414 West Fifth Street, Erie, PA 16507; tel. 814/459–4775; FAX. 814/453–6118; Suzanne C. Mack, Executive Director

St. John Vianney Hospital, 151 Woodbine Road, Downingtown, PA 19335–3080; tel. 610/269–2600; FAX. 610/873–8028; Louis D. Horvath, Administrator

The Bridge, 8400 Pine Road, Philadelphia, PA 19111; tel. 215/342–5000; FAX. 215/342–7709; Star Weiss, Program Director

The Mitchell Clinic, 1259 South Cedar Crest Boulevard, Suite 317, Allentown, PA 18103; tel. 610/435–9257; FAX. 610/435–4633; Dr. John Mitchell, Chief Executive Officer

The Renfrew Center, 475 Spring Lane, Philadelphia, PA 19128; tel. 215/482–5353; FAX. 215/482–7390; Samuel Menaged, Chief Executive Officer

The Terraces, 1170 South State Street, Ephrata, PA 17522; tel. 717/859–4100; FAX. 717/859–2131; Ronald J. Hunsicker, Executive Director

Today, Inc., 1990 North Woodbourne Road, P.O. Box 908, Newtown, PA 18940; tel. 215/968–4713; FAX. 215/968–8742; John E. Howell, Executive Vice President

Twin Lakes Center for Drug and Alcohol Rehabilitation, P.O. Box 909, Somerset, PA 15501–0909; tel. 814/443–3639; FAX. 814/443–2737; Mark Sarneso, Executive Director

White Deer Run, Devitt Camp Road, P.O. Box 97, Allenwood, PA 17810–0097; tel. 717/538–2567; FAX. 717/538–5303; Stephen T. Wicke, Executive Director

Winco Medical Center, 329 East Brown Street, East Stroudsburg, PA 18301; tel. 717/424–6233; FAX. 717/424–6380; Thomas Hudson, Chief Executive Officer

Wordsworth Academy, Pennsylvania Avenue and Camp Hill, Fort Washington, PA 19034; tel. 215/643–5400, ext. 3201; FAX. 215/643–0595; Bernard Cooper, Ph.D., Chief Executive Officer

RHODE ISLAND

Alternatives, 350 Duncan Drive, Providence, RI 02906; tel. 401/453–4742; FAX. 401/274–8086; Dr. Yitzhak Bakal, Chief Executive Officer

CODAC, Inc., 1052 Park Avenue, Cranston, RI 02910; tel. 401/461–5056; FAX. 401/942–3590; Craig Stenning, Chief Executive Officer

Community Counseling Center, 160 Beechwood Avenue, Pawtucket, RI 02860; tel. 401/722–5573, ext. 204; FAX. 401/722–5630; Richard H. Leclerc, President

East Bay Mental Health Center, Inc., Two Old County Road, Barrington, RI 02806; tel. 401/246–1195; FAX. 401/246–1985; John P. Digits, Jr., Chief Executive Officer

Fellowship Health Resources, Inc., 25 Blackstone Valley Place, Lincoln, RI 02865; tel. 401/333–3980; FAX. 401/333–3984; Joseph Dziobek, Chief Executive Officer

Good Hope Center, Inc., P.O. Box 470, East Greenwich, RI 02818; tel. 401/826–2750; Alan Willoughby, Ph.D., Chief Executive Officer

Mental Health Services, Inc., 1516 Alwood Avenue, Johnston, RI 02919–9323; tel. 401/273–8756; FAX. 401/454–0148; Stephen DeRosa, Vice President, Quality Management

South Shore Mental Health Center, Inc., 4705A Old Post Road, P.O. Box 899, Charlestown, RI 02813; tel. 401/364–7705; FAX. 401/364–3310; Richard Antonelli, Chief Executive Officer

The Providence Center for Counseling and Psychiatric Services, 520 Hope Street, Providence, RI 02906; tel. 401/276–4000; FAX. 401/276–4015; Charles Maynard, Chief Executive Officer

SOUTH CAROLINA

Charter Behavioral Health System at Fenwick Hall, 2777 Speissegger Drive, Charleston, SC 29405; tel. 803/559–2461; FAX. 803/745–5196; Anne F. Battin, Acting Chief Executive Officer

New Hope Treatment Centers, Inc., 225 Midland Parkway, Summerville, SC 29485–8104; tel. 803/851–5010; FAX. 803/851–5020; Katherine W. Grego, President, Chief Operating Officer

York Place–Episcopal Church Home for Children, 234 Kings Mountain Street, York, SC 29745; tel. 803/684–8005; FAX. 803/628–1632; Kathryn Peterson, Director, Admissions

Section C

SOUTH DAKOTA

Black Hills Childrens Home, 24100 South Rockerville Road, Rapid City, SD 57701–9277; tel. 605/343–5422; FAX. 605/343–1411; Frederick G. Tully, Clinical Director

Children's Home Society of South Dakota, 801 North Sycamore, P.O. Box 1749, Sioux Falls, SD 57101–1749; tel. 605/334–6004, ext. 146; FAX. 605/335–2776, ext. 146; David P. Loving, Executive Director

Keystone Treatment Center, 1010 East Second Street, Canton, SD 57013; tel. 605/987–2751; FAX. 605/987–2365; Carol A. Regier, RN, CCDC, Executive Director

TENNESSEE

Buffalo Valley, Inc., 501 Park Avenue, S., Hohenwald, TN 38462; tel. 615/796–5427; Jerry T. Risner, Executive Director

Camelot Care Center, Inc., Route 3, Box 267C, 183 Fiddlers Lane, Kingston, TN 37763; tel. 615/376–2296; FAX. 615/376–1850; James E. Spicer, Ph.D., Executive Director

Child and Family Services of Knox County, Inc., 901 East Summit Hill Drive, Knoxville, TN 37915; tel. 423/524–7483; FAX. 423/524–4790; Charles E. Gentry, ACSW, LCSW, Chief Executive Officer

Compass Intervention Center, LLC, 7900 Lowrance Road, Memphis, TN 38125; tel. 901/758–2002; FAX. 901/758–2156; Robin Smith, Director, Clinical Services, Marketing

Cornerstone of Recovery, Inc., 1120 Topside Road, Louisville, TN 37777; tel. 615/970–7747; FAX. 615/681–2266; Dan R. Caldwell, President

Council for Alcohol and Drug Abuse Services, Inc., 207 Spears Avenue, Chattanooga, TN 37405; tel. 615/756–7644; FAX. 615/756–7646; James F. Marcotte, Executive Director

Cumberland Heights Drug and Alcohol Treatment Center, Route 2, 8283 River Road, Nashville, TN 37209; tel. 615/352–1757; FAX. 615/353–4300; James Moore, President, Chief Executive Officer

Daybreak Treatment Center and Specialized School, 2262 Germantown Road, S., Germantown, TN 38138; tel. 901/753–4300; FAX. 901/751–8105; Tina Mills, Chief Executive Officer

FHC Cumberland Hall of Chattanooga, 7351 Standifer Gap Road, Chattanooga, TN 37421; tel. 615/499–9007; FAX. 615/499–9757; Charles Dickens, Administrator

Greene Valley Developmental Center, 4850 East Andrew Johnson Highway, Greeneville, TN 37743; tel. 423/787–6800; Robert G. Erb, Ed.D., Superintendent

Jackson Academy L.L.C., 222 Church Street, Dickson, TN 37055; tel. 615/446–3900; FAX. 615/446–3985; Robert D. Glasner, Psy.D., Chief Executive Officer

New Life Lodge, 999 Girl Scout Road, P.O. Box 430, Burns, TN 37029; tel. 615/446–7034; FAX. 615/446–7987; James Kestner, Chief Executive Officer

Peninsula Village, P.O. Box 100, Louisville, TN 37777; tel. 423/970–1828; FAX. 423/970–1875; Angie Montgomery, Administrative Director

Pine Point Center, Inc., 49 Old Hickory Boulevard, Jackson, TN 38305; tel. 901/664–7196; FAX. 901/661–0640; Britt Whitaker, Executive Director

The Harbours, 804 Youngs Lane, P.O. Box 70158, Nashville, TN 37207; tel. 615/650–0700; FAX. 615/650–0647; Melanie Taylor, Controller, Assistant Administrator

Three Springs Outdoor Therapeutic Program, P.O. Box 297, Centerville, TN 37033; tel. 615/729–5040; FAX. 615/729–9525; David Stephenson, M.S., Director, Referral Development

University of Tennessee Day Treatment Program, 711 Jefferson, Suite 607, Memphis, TN 38105; tel. 901/448–6378; Pamela A. Millsap, Program Director

Youth Villages, 2890 Bekemeyer Drive, Arlington, TN 38002; tel. 901/867–8832; FAX. 901/867–8937; Patrick Lawler, Chief Executive Officer

TEXAS

Alternatives Centre for Behavioral Health, 5001 Alabama Street, El Paso, TX 79930; tel. 915/565–4800; FAX. 915/544–5374; Carol Anderson, Chief Executive Officer

Austin Child Guidance Center, 810 West 45th Street, Austin, TX 78751; tel. 512/451–2242; FAX. 512/454–9204; Donald J. Zappone, Dr.P.H., Executive Director

Canyon Lakes Residential Treatment Center, 2402 Canyon Lake Drive, Lubbock, TX 79415; tel. 806/762–5782; FAX. 806/762–0838; Ray H. Brown, Ph.D., Administrator

Child Study Center, 1300 West Lancaster, Fort Worth, TX 76102; tel. 817/336–8611; FAX. 817/336–2823; Larry D. Eason, Ed.D., Administrator

Columbia Champions' Center for Children and Adolescents, 14320 Walters Road, Houston, TX 77014; tel. 713/537–5050; FAX. 713/537–2726; Cheryl Bautsch, RN, Director, Medical/Nursing Services

Community Residential Centers of San Antonio, 17720 Corporate Woods Drive, San Antonio, TX 78259–3500; tel. 210/494–1060; FAX. 210/490–8672; Patricia McLemore, Administrator

DePelchin Children's Center, 100 Sandman Street, Houston, TX 77007; tel. 713/861–8136; FAX. 713/802–7611; Curtis C. Mooney, Ph.D., Chief Executive Officer

Devereux–Texas Treatment Network, 120 David Wade Drive, Victoria, TX 77902–2666; tel. 512/575–8271; FAX. 512/575–6520; L. Gail Atkinson, Executive Director

Family Opportunity Resources, The F.O.R.G.I.V.E. Program, 6000 Broadway, Suite 106R, Galveston, TX 77551; tel. 409/740–0442; FAX. 409/740–0457; Gordon W. McKee, Administrator

Family Service Center, 4625 Lillian Street, Houston, TX 77007; tel. 713/868–4466; FAX. 713/868–2619; Lloyd Sidwell, Chief Executive Officer

Forest Springs Residential Treatment Center, 1120 Cypress Station Drive, Houston, TX 77090; tel. 713/893–7200; FAX. 713/893–7646; James Muska, Chief Executive Officer

Fort Worth Oak Grove Treatment Center, 6436 Mark Drive, Burleson, TX 76028; tel. 817/483–0989; FAX. 817/561–1309; Elsa Steward, Chief Executive Officer

Glass Treatment Center, Inc., 18838 Memorial, Suite 103, Humble, TX 77338; tel. 713/666–9811; FAX. 713/446–5292; G. Glass, M.D., Medical Director

La Hacienda Treatment Center, FM 1340, Hunt, TX 78024; tel. 512/238–4222; FAX. 512/238–4070; Frank Sadlack, Ph.D., Executive Director

Meridell Achievement Center, Inc., P.O. Box 87, Liberty Hill, TX 78642; tel. 512/515–6650; FAX. 512/515–5873; Scott McAvoy, Chief Executive Officer

New Dimensions Day Treatment, 18333 Egret Bay Boulevard, Suite 560, Houston, TX 77058; tel. 713/333–2284; FAX. 713/333–0221; Valarie Corbett, QA CQI Coordinator

New Spirit, 2411 Fountainview, Suite 175, Houston, TX 77057–4803; tel. 713/975–1580; FAX. 717/975–0228; Thomas A. Blocher, M.D., Chief Executive Officer

New View Partial Hospitalization Centre, Inc., 4310 Dowlen Road, Suite 13, Beaumont, TX 77706; tel. 409/892–0009; Darla Tortorice, Nursing Coordinator

Paul Meier New Life Day Hospital and Outpatient Clinic, 2071 North Collins, Richardson, TX 75080; tel. 972/437–4698; FAX. 972/690–9309; Jacquelyn Jeffrey, Chief Executive Officer

River Oaks Academy, 8120 Westglen, Houston, TX 77063; tel. 713/783–7200; FAX. 713/783–7286; Dr. Sandra Phares, Chief Executive Officer

Saint Joseph's Day Treatment Center, 1201 Corpus Christi, Laredo, TX 78040; tel. 210/718–2273; FAX. 210/726–6357; Dr. Jose Garcia, Chief Executive Officer

Seaview Mental Health Center, P.A., 4529 Weber Road, Corpus Christi, TX 78411; tel. 512/852–3994; FAX. 512/852–6183; Stan Tubbs, Jr., Administrator

Shiloh Treatment Center, Inc., 4227 County Road 89, Manvel, TX 77578; tel. 281/489–1290; FAX. 281/489–0167; Dr. Brenda Gardner, Chief Executive Officer

Shoreline, Inc., 1220 Gregory, P.O. Box 23, Taft, TX 78390; tel. 512/528–3356; FAX. 512/528–3249; Bob O. Nevill, Chief Executive Officer

Summer Sky Treatment Center, 1100 McCart Street, Stephenville, TX 76401; tel. 817/968–2907; FAX. 817/968–4509; Cathern Brooks, Chief Executive Officer

Sundown Ranch, Inc., Route Four, Box 182, Canton, TX 75103; tel. 903/479–3933; FAX. 903/479–3999; Richard Boardman, Chief Executive Officer

The Country Place Adolescent Residential Treatment Center, 7475 Skillman Street, Suite 107D, Dallas, TX 75231; tel. 214/340–1613; FAX. 214/340–1058; Fayteen Marshall, President

The Oaks Treatment Center, Inc., 1407 West Stassney Lane, Austin, TX 78745; tel. 512/464–0400; FAX. 512/464–0444; Mack Wigley, Chief Executive Officer

The Patrician Movement, 222 East Mitchell, San Antonio, TX 78210; tel. 512/532–3126; FAX. 512/534–3779; Patrick Clancey, Administrator

VA Health Care Center, 5001 North Piedras, El Paso, TX 79930–4211; tel. 915/564–7901; FAX. 915/564–7920; Edward Valenzuela, Chief Executive Officer

Waco Center for Youth, 3501 North 19th Street, Waco, TX 76708; tel. 817/756–2171; FAX. 817/745–5119; Thomas Stidvent, M.D., Clinical Director

Westheimer Psychiatric Day Hospital, 5631 Dolores Street, Houston, TX 77057; tel. 713/780–1229; Bernard Levitt, Chief Executive Officer

UTAH

Brightway at St. George, 115 West 1470 South, St. George, UT 84770; tel. 800/345–4828; FAX. 801/673–8420; Paula O. Bell, Managing Director

Highland Ridge Hospital, 4578 Highland Drive, Salt Lake City, UT 84117; tel. 801/272–9851; FAX. 801/272–9857; Robert Boswell, Executive Vice President, Pioneer Healthcare, Inc.

Island View, Inc., 2650 West 2700 South, Syracuse, UT 84075; tel. 801/773–0200; Jared U. Balmer, Executive Director

New Haven, 2096 East 7200 South, (Mailing Address: P.O. Box 50238, Provo, UT 84605–0238), Spanish Fork, UT 84660; tel. 801/794–1218; FAX. 801/794–1223; Mark McGregor, Chief Executive Officer

Provo Canyon School, 4501 North University Avenue, Provo, UT 84604; tel. 801/227–2000; FAX. 801/227–2095; Robert R. Harrison, Chief Executive Officer

Rivendell of Utah, 5899 West Rivendell Drive, West Jordan, UT 84084; tel. 801/561–3377; John T. Young, M.S., Chief Executive Officer

Sorenson's Ranch School, Second East 345 North, Box 440219, Koosharem, UT 84744; tel. 801/638–7318; FAX. 801/638–7582; Burnell D. Sorenson, Owner

The Heritage Center, 5600 North Heritage School Drive, Provo, UT 84604; tel. 801/225–5552; FAX. 801/226–4696; Jerry Spanos, Chief Executive Officer

Youth Care, Inc., 12595 South Minuteman Drive, Draper, UT 84020; tel. 801/572–6989; Polly J. Isaacson, Survey Consultant

VIRGINIA

Altenative Behavioral Services The Pines RTC, 825 Crawford Parkway, Portsmouth, VA 23704; tel. 757/393–0061; FAX. 757/393–9658; Edward Irby, Chief Executive Officer

Barry Robinson Center, 443 Kempsville Road, Norfolk, VA 23502; tel. 757/455–6100; FAX. 757/455–6127; Thomas D. Pittman, M.P.H., Executive Director

CATS–Comprehensive Addiction Treatment Services, 3300 Gallows Road, Falls Church, VA 22042–3300; tel. 703/698–1530; FAX. 703/698–1537; Donald F. Silver, Assistant Vice President, Behavioral Health Services

DeJarnette Center, 1290 Richmond Road, Staunton, VA 24402–2309; tel. 540/332–2100; Donald L. Roe, Ph.D., Program Director

Diamond Healthcare of Williamsburg Place, 5477 Mooretown Road, Williamsburg, VA 23185; tel. 804/565–0106; FAX. 804/565–0620; Thomas J. Brennan, ACSW, Administrator

Graydon Manor, 801 Children's Center Road, S.W., Leesburg, VA 20175–4753; tel. 703/777–3485; FAX. 703/777–4887; Bernard J. Haberlein, Executive Director, Chairman of the Board

Inova Kellar Center, 10396 Democracy Lane, Fairfax, VA 22030–0252; tel. 703/218–8500; Rick Leichtweis, Ph.D., Program Director

Learning Services, 9524 Fairview Avenue, Manassas, VA 22110; tel. 703/335–9771; FAX. 703/330–5277; Randall Mitchell, Chief Executive Officer

Mount Regis Center, 405 Kimball Avenue, Salem, VA 24153; tel. 703/389–4761; Mark S. Cowell, Administrator

The Life Center of Galax, 112 Painter Street, Galax, VA 24333; tel. 800/345–6998; FAX. 703/236–8821; Tina R. Bullins, Executive Director

WASHINGTON

92d Medical Group, 701 Hospital Loop, Fairchild Air Force Base, WA 99011–5300; tel. 509/247–5127; FAX. 509/247–2170; Major Stuart Cowles, Chief Executive Officer

Carondelet Psychiatric Care Center, 1175 Carondelet Drive, Richland, WA 99352; tel. 509/943–9104; Barbara Mead, Quality Assurance Coordinator

Martin Center, 2806 Douglas Avenue, Bellingham, WA 98227–5704; tel. 360/733–5804; J. Ane Berrett, Clinical Director

Pearl Street Center, 815 South Pearl Street, Tacoma, WA 98465; tel. 206/756–5290; FAX. 206/759–7008; Michael Kent Laederich, Ph.D., Director, Children and Family Services

Puyallup Tribal Health Authority, 2209 East 32nd Street, Tacoma, WA 98404; tel. 206/593–0232; FAX. 206/272–6138; Rodney Smith, Chief Executive Officer

Seattle Children's Home, 2142 10th Avenue, W., Seattle, WA 98119; tel. 206/283–3300; FAX. 206/284–7843; R. David Cousineau, Executive Director

Seattle Indian Health Board, 611–12th Avenue S., Suite 200, Seattle, WA 98114; tel. 206/324–9360; FAX. 206/324–8910; Ralph Forquera, Chief Executive Officer

Tamarack Center, Inc., 2901 West Fort George Wright Drive, Spokane, WA 99204; tel. 509/326–8100; FAX. 509/326–9358; Chris Dal Pra, M.C., Assistant Director

WEST VIRGINIA

Elkins Mountain School, 100 Bell Street, Elkins, WV 26241; tel. 304/637–8000; FAX. 304/636–4694; Dr. Eugene Foster, Chief Executive Officer

Olympic Center Preston, Inc., Adolescent Alcohol/Drug Treatment, Route Seven West, P.O. Box 158, Kingwood, WV 26537; tel. 304/329–2400; FAX. 304/329–2405; Arlene Glover, Executive Director

Shawnee Hills, Inc., 603 Morris Square, P.O. Box 3698, Charleston, WV 25336–3698; tel. 304/341–0240; FAX. 304/341–0359; John E. Barnette, Ed.D., President, Chief Executive Officer

Worthington Center, Inc., 3199 Core Road, Suite Two, Parkersburg, WV 26104; tel. 304/485–5185; FAX. 304/485–0051; Dr. Fred Lee, Chief Executive Officer

WISCONSIN

Eau Claire Academy, 550 North Dewey Street, P.O. Box 1168, Eau Claire, WI 54702–1168; tel. 715/834–6681; FAX. 715/834–9954; Marcia R. Van Beek, Executive Director

Lac Courte Oreilles Communtiy Health Center, Route 2, Box 2750, Hayward, WI 54843; tel. 715/634–4795; FAX. 715/634–6107; Don Smith, Chief Executive Officer

Learning Services Mid–Western Region, 1424 North Highpoint Road, Middleton, WI 53562; tel. 608/836–3339; Chauncey J. Hunker, Program Director

Libertas Treatment Center, 1701 Dousman Street, Green Bay, WI 54303; tel. 414/498–8600; Patrick Ryan, Program Director

St. Rose Residence, Inc., 3801 North 88th Street, Milwaukee, WI 53222; tel. 414/466–9450; FAX. 414/466–0730; Kenneth Czaplewski, President

WYOMING

St. Joseph's Children's Home, 1419 South Main, P.O. Box 1117, Torrington, WY 82240; tel. 307/532–4197; FAX. 307/532–8405; Robert Mayor, Chief Executive Officer

Section C

The accredited freestanding substance abuse programs listed have been accredited as of January 1, 1997, by the Joint Commission on Accreditation of Healthcare Organizations by decision of the Accreditation Committee of the Board of Commissioners.

The organizations listed here have been found to be in compliance with the Joint Commission standards for subtance abuse organizations, as found in the Accreditation Manual for Mental Health, Chemical Dependency, and Mental Retardation/Developmental Disabilities Services.

Please refer to section A of the AHA Guide for information on hospitals with inpatient and/or outpatient alcohol and chemical dependency services. These hospitals are identified by Facility Codes F2 and F3. In section A, those hospitals identified by Approval Code 1 are JCAHO accredited.

We present this list simply as a convenient directory. Inclusion or omission of any organization's name indicates neither approval nor disapproval by Healthcare InfoSource, Inc., a subsidiary of the American Hospital Association.

United States

ALABAMA

Bradford Adolescent at Oak Mountain, 2280 Highway 35, Pelham, AL 35124; tel. 205/664–3460; FAX. 205/664–8476; Joseph E. Roche, M.S.W., M.B.A., Chief Executive Officer

Bradford Health Services–Birmingham Lodge, 1189 Allbritton Road, P.O. Box 129, Warrior, AL 35180; tel. 205/647–1945; FAX. 205/647–3626; Roy M. Ramsey, Executive Director

Bradford–Parkside at Huntsville, 1600 Browns Ferry Road, P.O. Box 176, Madison, AL 35758; tel. 205/461–7272; FAX. 205/464–9618; Robert Hinds, Chief Executive Officer

New Perspectives (Adult), 1000 Fairfax Park, Tuscaloosa, AL 35406; tel. 205/391–4738; FAX. 205/759–4151; Martha Hinkle, Administrator

Noble Army Health Clinic, Building 292, Fort McClellan, AL 36205–5083; tel. 205/848–2490; FAX. 205/848–2151; Col. Robert Reed, Chief Executive Officer

The Catalyst Center (Adolescent), 1000 Fairfax Park, Tuscaloosa, AL 35406; tel. 205/391–4738; FAX. 205/759–4151; Martha Hinkle, Chief Executive Officer

ALASKA

Akeela House, Inc., 2805 Bering Street, Suite Four, Anchorage, AK 99503; tel. 907/561–5206; Rosalie Nadeau, Deputy Director

Department of Veterans Affairs Medical and Regional Office Center, 2925 DeBarr Road, Anchorage, AK 99508–2989; tel. 907/257–5460; FAX. 907/257–6774; Alonzo Poteet, Chief Executive Officer

ARIZONA

Calvary Rehabilitation Center, Inc., 720 East Montebello Avenue, Phoenix, AZ 85014; tel. 602/279–1468; FAX. 602/279–3090; Jeffrey Shook, Chief Executive Officer

Chandler Valley Hope, 501 North Washington, Chandler, AZ 85244–1839; tel. 602/899–3335; FAX. 602/899–6697; Julian S. Pickens, Ed.D., Chief Executive Officer

Cottonwood de Tucson, Inc., 4110 Sweetwater Drive, Tucson, AZ 85745; tel. 520/743–0411; FAX. 520/743–7991; Ron Welch, Chief Executive Officer

Desert Hills Center for Youth and Families, 2797 North Introspect Drive, Tucson, AZ 85745; tel. 520/622–5437; FAX. 520/792–6249; Boyd Dover, Chief Executive Officer

Parc Place, 5116 East Thomas Road, Phoenix, AZ 85018; tel. 602/840–4774; FAX. 602/840–7567; Gary Buchik, Program Director

Prehab of Arizona, Inc., 868 East University, Mesa, AZ 85203; tel. 602/969–4024; Michael T. Hughes, Executive Director

Remuda Ranch Center for Anorexia and Bulimia, Jack Burden Road, Wickenburg, AZ 85358; tel. 520/684–3913; Tammy Low, Director, Quality

Salvation Army Recovery Center, 2707 East Van Buren, Phoenix, AZ 85008; tel. 602/267–1404; FAX. 602/267–4131; Major John Webb, Chief Executive Officer

Sierra Tucson, Inc., 16500 North Lago del Oro Parkway, Tucson, AZ 85737; tel. 602/624–4000, ext. 2001; FAX. 602/792–2916; Kenneth J. Whitaker, Executive Director

The Meadows, 1655 North Tegner, P.O. Box 97, Wickenburg, AZ 85358; tel. 602/684–3926; FAX. 602/684–3261; James Mellody, Chief Executive Officer

The New Foundation, 1200 North 77th Street, Scottsdale, AZ 85257; tel. 602/945–3302; FAX. 602/945–9308; David Hedgcock

Westcenter Rehabilitation Facility, Inc., d/b/a Westcenter, 2105 East Allen Road, Tucson, AZ 85719; tel. 520/795–0952; FAX. 602/318–6442; Allan Chip Harrington, Executive Director

CALIFORNIA

Behavioral Care of America, P.O. Box 30018, Laguna Niguel, CA 92607–0018; tel. 714/752–1510; FAX. 714/442–2139; David Ellisor, Director

Betty Ford Center at Eisenhower, 39000 Bob Hope Drive, Rancho Mirage, CA 92270; tel. 619/773–4100; FAX. 619/773–4141; Michael S. Neatherton, Vice President, Administrator

Cornerstone of Southern California, 13682 Yorba Street, Tustin, CA 92780; tel. 714/730–5399; FAX. 714/730–3505; Michael Stone, M.D., Medical Director, President

Impact Drug and Alcohol Treatment Center, 1680 North Fair Oaks Avenue, Pasadena, CA 91103; tel. 818/798–0884; James M. Stillwell, Executive Director

Los Angeles Centers for Alcohol and Drug Abuse, 11015 Bloomfield Avenue, Santa Fe Springs, CA 90670; tel. 310/906–2676; FAX. 310/906–2681; John Brown, Executive Director

Michael's House Treatment Center for Men, 430 South Cahuilla Road, Palm Springs, CA 92262; tel. 619/320–5486; FAX. 619/778–6020; Arlene Rosen, President

Oak Grove Institute Foundation, 24275 Jefferson Avenue, Murrietta, CA 92562; tel. 909/677–5599; Tamara L. Wilson, Program Director

S.T.E.P.S., 224 East Clara Street, Port Hueneme, CA 93044; tel. 805/488–6424; FAX. 805/488–6717; John J. Megara, Administrator

SeaBridge Adolescent Treatment Center, 30371 Morning View Drive, Malibu, CA 90265; tel. 310/457–5802; FAX. 310/457–6093; Martha Zimmerman, Executive Director

Spencer Recovery Centers, Inc., 343 West Foothill Boulevard, Monrovia, CA 91016; tel. 818/358–3662; FAX. 818/357–7405; Chris Spencer, President, Chief Executive Officer

Substance Abuse Foundation of Long Beach, Inc., 3125 East Seventh Street, Long Beach, CA 90804; tel. 310/439–7755; Ronald H. Banner, Executive Director

Tarzana Treatment Center, 18646 Oxnard Street, Tarzana, CA 91356; tel. 818/996–1051; FAX. 818/345–3778; Albert Senella

Twin Town Treatment Centers, 2501 Burbank Boulevard, Suite 212, Burbank, CA 91505; tel. 818/840–0806; FAX. 818/840–0845; Irma Astudillo, CSAC, Program Administrator

VA Medical Center, 16111 Plummer Street, Sepulveda, CA 91343; tel. 818/895–9466; FAX. 818/895–9559; Dollie Whitehead

Veterans Affairs Northern California Health Care System, 2300 Contra Costa Boulevard, Suite 440, Pleasant Hill, CA 94523; tel. 510/372–2010; FAX. 510/372–2020; Sheldon Fine

Vista Pacifica Hospital, 7989 Linda Vista Road, San Diego, CA 92111; tel. 619/576–1200; FAX. 619/576–8362; Daniel R. Valentine, Adminstrator

Watts Health Foundation, Inc., 10300 South Compton Avenue, Los Angeles, CA 90002; tel. 213/564–4331; FAX. 213/563–6378; Clyde Oden

COLORADO

Adolescent and Family Institute of Colorado, Inc., 10001 West 32nd Avenue, Wheat Ridge, CO 80033; tel. 303/238–1231; FAX. 303/238–0500; Alex M. Panio, Jr., Ph.D., Chief Executive Officer

Alpha Drug Abuse Program, 802 Ninth Street #2, 3 and 4, Greeley, CO 80631; tel. 303/346–9546; Robert Warren

Aurora Behavioral Health Hospital, 1290 South Potomac, Aurora, CO 80012; tel. 303/745–2273; FAX. 303/369–9556; Lorry Kenney, Administrator

Cheyenne Mesa, 1301 South Eighth Street, Colorado Springs, CO 80906; tel. 719/520–1400; FAX. 719/475–1527; Letha Mahar, Performance Improvement Director

Harmony Foundation, Inc., 1600 Fish Hatchery Road, P.O. Box 1989, Estes Park, CO 80517; tel. 303/586–4491; FAX. 970/577–0392; Donald R. Hays, J.D., NCACII, CACIII, Director

Parker Valley Hope, 22422 East Main Street, Parker, CO 80134; tel. 303/841–7857; FAX. 303/841–6526; John J. Arnold, Ph.D., Program Director

CONNECTICUT

Cornerstone of Eagle Hill, Inc., 28 Alberts Hill Road, Sandy Hook, CT 06482; tel. 203/426–8085; FAX. 203/426–2821; Norman J. Sokolow, Executive Director

Greater Bridgeport Community Mental Health Center, 1635 Central Avenue, P.O. Box 5117, Bridgeport, CT 06610; tel. 203/579–6626; FAX. 203/579–6094; James Lehane

Guenster Rehabilitation Center, Inc., 276 Union Avenue, Bridgeport, CT 06607; tel. 203/384–9301; FAX. 203/336–4395; Sue Roselle, President

Reid Treatment Center, Inc., 121 West Avon Road, Avon, CT 06001; tel. 860/673–6115; FAX. 860/675–7433; Mary Ann Reid, Executive Director

Rushford Center, Inc., 1250 Silver Street, Middletown, CT 06457; tel. 203/346–0300; FAX. 860/344–8152; Margaret Crafton, Vice President, Clinical Operations

Stonington Institute, Swantown Hill Road, North Stonington, CT 06359; tel. 203/535–1010; FAX. 203/535–4820; William A. Aniskovich, Chief Operating Officer

The BlueRidge Center, 1095 Blue Hills Avenue, Bloomfield, CT 06002; tel. 203/243–1331; FAX. 203/242–3265; Mary Ellen Doyle, Executive Director

The Center, 4083 Main Street, Bridgeport, CT 06606; tel. 203/365–8400; Susan Dalesandro, CISW, CAC, Clinical Director

Vitam Center, Inc., 57 West Rocks Road, P.O. Box 730, Norwalk, CT 06852–0730; tel. 203/846–2091; FAX. 203/846–3620; Leonard A. Kenowitz, Ph.D., Executive Director

Wheeler Clinic, Inc., 91 Northwest Drive, Plainville, CT 06062; tel. 800/793–3588; FAX. 203/793–3520; Dennis Keenan, Executive Director

DELAWARE

Brandywine Counseling, Inc., 2713 Lancaster Avenue, Wilmington, DE 19805; tel. 302/656–2348; FAX. 302/656–0746; Sara Taylor Allshouse, Executive Director

Sodat–Delaware, Inc., 625 North Orange Street, Wilmington, DE 19801; tel. 302/656–4044; Thomas C. Maloney, Executive Director

The Recovery Center of Delaware, Inc., Governor Bacon Health Center, Delaware City, DE 19706; tel. 302/836–1615; Terence McSherry, Executive Director

FLORIDA

Alternatives In Treatment, Inc, 7601 North Federal Highway, Suite 100B, Boca Raton, FL 33487; tel. 407/998–0866; FAX. 407/241–5042; Jacob Frydman, Executive Director

Apalachee Center for Human Services, Inc., 625 East Tennessee Street, Tallahassee, FL 32308; tel. 904/487–2930; Ronald P. Kirkland, Chief Executive Officer

Associated Counseling and Education, Inc., 4563 South Orange Blossom Trail, Orlando, FL 32839; tel. 407/422–7233; FAX. 407/843–9602; Loretta Parrish

Auburndale Health Care Institute, 602 Melton Avenue, P.O. Box 458, Auburndale, FL 33823; tel. 800/762–3712; FAX. 813/375–4775; JoAnn Summerlin

Bayview Center for Mental Health, Inc., 12550 Biscayne Boulevard, Suite 919, Miami, FL 33181; tel. 305/892–4646; FAX. 305/893–1224; Robert Ward

Camelot Care Centers, Inc., 9160 Oakhurst Road, Seminole, FL 33776; tel. 813/596–9960; FAX. 813/593–1784; Lynn Chalache, Chief Operating Officer

Coastal Recovery Centers, Inc., 3830 Bee Ridge Road, Sarasota, FL 34233; tel. 813/927–8900; FAX. 813/925–3836; James R. Sleeper, President, Chief Executive Officer

Crossroads Center, 2121 Lisenby Avenue, Panama City, FL 32406; tel. 800/922–7522; FAX. 904/763–3933; Ernest H. Borders, Chief Executive Officer

DISC Village, Inc., (Tallahassee/Leon County Human Services Center), 3333 West Pensacola Street, Tallahassee, FL 32304; tel. 904/575–4388, ext. 117; FAX. 904/576–5960; Thomas K. Olk, Executive Director

David Lawrence Center, Inc., 6075 Golden Gate Parkway, Naples, FL 33999; tel. 813/455–1031; FAX. 813/455–6561; David Schimmel, Executive Director

Eckerd Alternative Treatment Program at E–How–Kee, 397 Culbreath Road, Brooksville, FL 34602; tel. 904/796–9493; FAX. 904/754–6791; Dwight Lord

Fairwinds Treatment Center, 1569 South Fort Harrison, Clearwater, FL 34616; tel. 800/226–0301; FAX. 813/446–1022; Samuel Teresi, Director, Community Relations

Hanley–Hazelden Center at St. Mary's, 5200 East Avenue, West Palm Beach, FL 33407; tel. 407/848–1666; FAX. 407/848–6333; Jerry Singleton, M.A., Executive Director

High Point, 5960 Southwest 106th Avenue, Cooper City, FL 33328; tel. 954/680–2700; FAX. 954/680–9941; Alan Sherman, Administrator

Jacksonville Therapy Center, 6428 Beach Boulevard, Jacksonville, FL 32216; tel. 904/724–6500; FAX. 904/721–6677; David Cheshire, M.D.

Lakeside Alternatives, Inc., 434 West Kennedy Boulevard, Orlando, FL 32810; tel. 407/875–3700; FAX. 407/875–5717; Duane Zimmerman

Leon F. Stewart–Hal S. Marchman Center, 120 Michigan Avenue, Daytona Beach, FL 32114; tel. 904/255–0447, ext. 298; FAX. 904/238–0877; Dr. Ernest D. Cantley, Executive Director

LifeStream Behavioral Center, 515 West Main Street, P.O. Box 491000, Leesburg, FL 34749–1000; tel. 352/360–6575; FAX. 352/360–6595; Tim Camp, Executive Vice President

Lifeskills of Boca Raton, Inc., 7301A West Palmetto Park Road, Suite 300 B, Boca Raton, FL 33433; tel. 561/392–1199; FAX. 561/392–4341; Carol Parks, Administrator

Marion Citrus Mental Health Centers, Inc., 717 Southwest Martin Luther King Jr. Avenue, P.O. Box 1330, Ocala, FL 34474; tel. 352/620–7300; FAX. 352/732–1413; Russell Rasco

Mental Health Services, Inc. of North Central Florida, 4300 Southwest 13th Street, Gainesville, FL 32608; tel. 904/374–5600; Douglas L. Starr, Chief Executive Officer

National Recovery Institutes Group, Inc., 1000 Northwest 15th Street, Boca Raton, FL 33486; tel. 407/392–8444; Sheldon Russakoff, President, Chief Executive Officer

Northwest Dade Center, Inc., 4175 West 20th Avenue, Hialeah, FL 33012; tel. 305/825–0300; FAX. 305/824–1006; Mario Jardon, LCSW, Chief Executive Officer

Oak Center, 8889 Corporate Square Court, Jacksonville, FL 32216; tel. 904/725–7073; FAX. 904/727–9777; Diana Sourbrine, Administrator

Pathways to Recovery, Inc., 13132 Barwick Road, Delray Beach, FL 33445; tel. 407/496–7532; Allen Bombart, Executive Director

Recovery Corner, 10800 North Military Trail, Suite 220, Palm Beach Gardens, FL 33410; tel. 800/435–3668; FAX. 407/626–1739; Jay C. Mills, Executive Director

Renaissance Institute of Palm Beach, Inc., 7000 North Federal Highway, Boca Raton, FL 33487; tel. 561/241–7977; FAX. 561/241–9233; Sid Goodman, Executive Director

Sandalfoot Community Mental Health Center, 23120 Sandalfoot Square Place Drive, Boca Raton, FL 33428; tel. 561/852–8777; FAX. 561/852–8212; Daniel L. Carzoli, M.A., CAP

South County Mental Health Center, Inc., 16158 South Military Trail, Delray Beach, FL 33484–6502; tel. 561/637–1000; FAX. 561/495–7975; Joseph S. Speicher, Executive Director

Spectrum Programs, Inc., 18441 Northwest Second Avenue, Suite 218, Miami, FL 33169; tel. 305/653–8288, ext. 19; FAX. 305/653–6787; H. Bruce Hayden, President

The Addictions Center for Treatment, 2905 South Federal Highway, Suite C–Eight, Delray Beach, FL 33483; tel. 407/278–0060; FAX. 407/278–0082; Michael Chernak

The Beachcomber, 4493 North Ocean Boulevard, Delray Beach, FL 33483; tel. 561/734–1818; FAX. 561/265–1349; Joseph Bryan, Director

The Inn at Bowling Green, 101 North Oak Street, Bowling Green, FL 33834; tel. 941/375–4373; Joann Summerlin, Vice President, Operations, Administration

The Louis de la Parte/Florida Mental Health Institute, 13301 Bruce B. Downs Boulevard, Tampa, FL 33612–3899; tel. 813/974–1990; FAX. 813/974–4699; David L. Shern, Dean, Ph.D., Professor

The Renfrew Center of Florida, Inc., 7700 Renfrew Lane, Coconut Creek, FL 33073; tel. 954/698–9222; FAX. 954/698–9007; Barbara Peterson, Executive Director

The Rose Institute, Inc., 17 Rose Drive, Fort Lauderdale, FL 33316; tel. 954/522–7673; FAX. 954/522–4031; Richard Maulion

The Southern Institute for Treatment and Evaluation, 660 Linton Boulevard, Suite 112, Delray Beach, FL 33444; tel. 407/278–8411; FAX. 407/278–7774; Diana Burns

The Village South, Inc., 3180 Biscayne Boulevard, Miami, FL 33137; tel. 800/443–3784; FAX. 305/576–1348; Matthew Gissen, Chief Executive Officer

The Willough at Naples, 9001 Tamiami Trail, E., Naples, FL 33962; tel. 941/775–4500; FAX. 941/793–0534; Gary D. Centafanti, Executive Director

Transitions Recovery Program, 1928 Northeast 154th Street, North Miami Beach, FL 33162; tel. 305/949–9001; Roselyn McGowan, Administrator

Turning Point of Tampa, 5439 Beaumont Center Boulevard, Suite 1010, Tampa, FL 33634; tel. 813/882–3003; FAX. 813/885–6974; Michelle Ratcliff, Chief Executive Officer

Twelve Oaks, 2068 Heather Avenue, Navarre, FL 32566; tel. 904/939–1200; FAX. 904/939–1257; Candy Henderson, Administrator

U.S. Life Center of St. Augustine, 1100–3 South Ponce de Leon Boulevard, St. Augustine, FL 32086; tel. 904/829–5566; FAX. 904/829–0677; James Ferguson, President

GEORGIA

Anchor Hospital and The Talbott–Marsh Recovery Campus, 5454 Yorktowne Drive, Atlanta, GA 30349; tel. 770/991–6044, ext. 3201; FAX. 770/991–6044, ext. 298; Benjamin H. Underwood, FAAMA, President, Chief Executive Officer

Bridges Outpatient Center, Inc., 1209 Columbia Drive, Milledgeville, GA 31061; tel. 912/454–1727; FAX. 912/454–1770; James Simmons, Chief Executive Officer

Brightmore Day Hospital, 115 Davis Road, Martinez, GA 30907–7184; tel. 706/868–1735; Joy J. Beaird, Case Manager

Charter Laurel Heights Behavioral Health System, Inc., 934 Briarcliff Road, N.E., Atlanta, GA 30306; tel. 404/888–7860; FAX. 404/872–5088; Jewel Norman

Safe Recovery Systems, Inc., 2300 Peachford Road, Suite 2000, Atlanta, GA 30338; tel. 770/455–7233; FAX. 770/458–1481; Henslee Dutton, Chief Executive Officer

Turning Point Care Center, Inc., 319 Bypass, P.O. Box 1177, Moultrie, GA 31768; tel. 912/985–4815; FAX. 912/890–1614; Ben Marion, Managing Director

Willingway Hospital, 311 Jones Mill Road, Statesboro, GA 30458; tel. 912/764–6236; FAX. 912/764–7063; Jimmy Mooney, Chief Executive Officer

HAWAII

VA Medical and Regional Office Center (VAMROC), 300 Ala Moana Boulevard, P.O. Box 50188, Honolulu, HI 96850; tel. 808/566–1707; FAX. 808/566–1895; Barry Raff, Director

IDAHO

Northview Hospital, 8050 Northview Street, Boise, ID 83704; tel. 208/327–0504; FAX. 208/327–0594; Joyce Ellis, Administrator

Walker Center, 1120–A Montana Street, Gooding, ID 83330–1858; tel. 208/934–8461; FAX. 208/934–5437; Vayle Mauldin, Treatment Coordinator

ILLINOIS

Alexian Brothers Lake Cook Behavioral Health Resources, 901 Biesterfield Road, Suite 400, Elk Grove Village, IL 60007–3392; tel. 847/577–1501; FAX. 847/577–0256; Mark Frey, Chief Executive Officer

Camelot Care Center, Inc., 1502 North Northwest Highway, Palatine, IL 60067; tel. 847/359–5600; FAX. 847/359–2759; Peggy Williams, President, Professional Staff

Chestnut Health Systems, Inc., 1003 Martin Luther King Jr. Drive, Bloomington, IL 61701; tel. 309/827–6026; FAX. 309/827–6496; Alan R. Sodetz, Ph.D., Clinical Director

DuPage County Health Department/Mental Health Division, 111 North County Farm Road, Wheaton, IL 60187; tel. 708/682–7979; FAX. 708/690–5282; Gary Noll

Family Service and Community Mental Health Center/McHenry, 5320 West Elm Street, McHenry, IL 60050; tel. 815/385–6400; FAX. 815/385–8127; Robert Martens

Gateway Youth Care Foundation, 25480 West Cedarcrest Lane, Lake Villa, IL 60046; tel. 847/356–8292; FAX. 847/356–0414; Janet Mason, Director

Great River Recovery Resources, Inc., 428 South 36th Street, Quincy, IL 62301; tel. 217/224–6300; FAX. 217/224–4329; Michael Hutmacher

Interventions South Wood, 5701 South Wood, Chicago, IL 60636; tel. 773/737–4600; FAX. 773/737–5790; Herb Higgin, Director

Interventions Woodridge, 2221 64th Street, Woodridge, IL 60517; tel. 630/968–6477; FAX. 630/968–5744; Edward Ravine, Director of Clinical Operations

Interventions, City Girls/City Women, 140 North Ashland, Chicago, IL 60607; tel. 312/433–7777; FAX. 312/433–7787; Peter Bokos

Interventions–DuPage Adolescent Center, 11 South 250, Route 83, Hinsdale, IL 60521; tel. 708/325–5050; FAX. 630/325–9130; Anthony Kunkemoeller, Director

McHenry County Youth Service Bureau, 101 South Jefferson Street, Woodstock, IL 60098; tel. 815/338–7360; FAX. 815/338–5510; Susan H. Krause, Executive Director

New Life Clinic of Wheaton, P.C., 2100 Manchester Road, Suite 1410 and 1510, Wheaton, IL 60187; tel. 708/653–1717; FAX. 708/653–7926; Nancy Brown, Director

Rosecrance Center, 1505 North Alpine Road, Rockford, IL 61107; tel. 815/399–5351; FAX. 815/398–2641; Philip W. Eaton, President

Rosecrance on Harrison, 3815 Harrison Avenue, Rockford, IL 61108; tel. 815/391–1000; Philip W. Eaton, President, Chief Executive Officer

Sojourn House, Inc., 565 North Turner Avenue, Freeport, IL 61032; tel. 815/232–5121; FAX. 815/233–4591; Brenda J. Bombard, M.S.W., Executive Director

Southeastern Illinois Counseling Centers, Inc., 504 Micah Drive, P.O. Drawer M, Olney, IL 62450; tel. 618/395–4306; FAX. 618/395–4507; Glenn Jackson, Clinical Director

The Women's Treatment Center, 140 North Ashland, Chicago, IL 60607; tel. 312/850–0050; FAX. 312/850–9095; Jewell Oates, Ph.D., Executive Director

Section C

Triangle Center, 120 North 11th Street, Springfield, IL 62703; tel. 217/544–9858; FAX. 217/544–0223; Stephen J. Knox, Executive Director

White Oaks Companies of Illinois, 3400 New Leaf Lane, Peoria, IL 61614; tel. 309/692–6900; FAX. 309/689–3086; Tom Murphy

INDIANA

Center for Behavioral Health, 645 South Rogers Street, Bloomington, IN 47403; tel. 812/339–1691; FAX. 812/339–8109; Linda Lumsden, Quality Improvement

Community Mental Health Center, Inc., 285 Bielby Road, Lawrenceburg, IN 47025; tel. 812/537–1302; FAX. 812/537–5219; Joseph Stephens

Comprehensive Mental Health Services, Inc., 240 North Tillotson, Muncie, IN 47304; tel. 317/288–1928; FAX. 317/741–0310; Suzanne Gresham, Ph.D., Chief Executive Officer

Fairbanks Hospital, Inc., 8102 Clearvista Parkway, Indianapolis, IN 46256; tel. 317/849–8222; FAX. 317/849–1455; Timothy L. Boruff, President, Administrator

Four County Counseling Center, 1015 Michigan Avenue, Logansport, IN 46947; tel. 219/722–5151; FAX. 219/722–9523; Laurence Ulrich

Grant–Blackford Mental Health, Inc., 505 Wabash Avenue, Marion, IN 46952; tel. 317/662–3971; FAX. 317/662–7480; Paul Kuczora

Hamilton Center, Inc., 620 Eighth Avenue, Terre Haute, IN 47804; tel. 812/231–8323; FAX. 812/231–8400; Galen Goode, Chief Executive Officer

Lifespring Mental Health Services, 207 West 13th Street, Jeffersonville, IN 47130; tel. 812/283–4491; John Case, Executive Director

Madison Center and Hospital, 403 East Madison Street, South Bend, IN 46617; tel. 219/234–0061, ext. 1116; FAX. 219/288–5047; Jack Roberts, Executive Director

Madison Clinic, Inc., 2210 Jackson Street, Anderson, IN 46016–4363; tel. 317/644–1414; Gary L. Porter, Chief Executive Officer

Park Center, Inc, 909 East State Boulevard, Fort Wayne, IN 46805; tel. 219/481–2700; FAX. 219/481–2717; Paul Wilson, ACSW, Chief Executive Officer

Porter–Starke Services, 601 Wall Street, Valparaiso, IN 46383; tel. 219/531–3500; FAX. 219/462–3975; Lee Grogg

Quinco Behavioral Health Systems, P.O. Box 628, Columbus, IN 47202–0628; tel. 812/379–2341; Robert J. Williams, Ph.D., Chief Executive Officer

Southwestern Indiana Mental Health Center, Inc., 415 Mulberry Street, Evansville, IN 47713; tel. 812/423–7791; FAX. 812/422–7558; John K. Browning, Executive Director

Tara Treatment Center, Inc., 6231 South US Highway, Franklin, IN 46131; tel. 812/526–2611; FAX. 812/526–8527; Ann Daugherty–James

The Center for Mental Health, Inc., 2020 Brown Street, Anderson, IN 46016; tel. 317/649–8161; FAX. 317/641–8238; Cynthia Goodman, ACSW, Addiction Services Manager

The Children's Campus, 1411 Lincoln Way W., Mishawaka, IN 46544–1690; tel. 219/259–5666; FAX. 219/255–6179; Sylvia Sebert

Tri–City Comprehensive Community Mental Health Center, 3903 Indianapolis Boulevard, East Chicago, IN 46312; tel. 219/398–7050; FAX. 219/392–6998; Sandy Appleby, Assistant Director

Tri–County Center, Inc., 697 Pro–Med Lane, Carmel, IN 46032; tel. 317/587–0500; FAX. 317/574–1234; Larry L. Burch, ACSW, Executive Director

Wabash Valley Hospital, Inc., 2900 North River Road, West Lafayette, IN 47906; tel. 765/463–2555; FAX. 765/497–3960; R. Craig Lysinger

IOWA

Children and Families of Iowa, 1111 University Avenue, Des Moines, IA 50314; tel. 515/288–1981; FAX. 515/288–9109; David Stout, Executive Director

Hillcrest Family Services, 2005 Asbury Road, Dubuque, IA 52001; tel. 319/583–7357; FAX. 319/583–7026; Donald Lewis

KANSAS

22d Medical Group, 57950 Leavenworth, McConnell AFB, KS 67221; tel. 316/652–5000; FAX. 316/652–5014; Colonel Scott Garner

Atchison Valley Hope, 1816 North Second Street, Atchison, KS 66002; tel. 913/367–1618; FAX. 913/367–6224; Dave Ketter, Program Director

Columbia Health Systems, Inc., 10114 West 105th Street, Suite 100, Overland Park, KS 66212; tel. 913/492–9875; FAX. 913/492–0187, ext. 203; Robert L. Reed, President

Kaw Valley Center, 4300 Brenner Drive, Kansas City, KS 66104; tel. 913/334–0294; Anne M. Roberts, Vice President

Norton Valley Hope, 709 West Holme, Norton, KS 67654; tel. 913/877–5101; FAX. 913/877–2322; Dennis Gilhousen, Chief Executive Officer

United Methodist Youthville, Inc., 900 West Broadway, P.O. Box 210, Newton, KS 67114; tel. 316/283–1950; FAX. 316/283–9540; Robert Smith

KENTUCKY

Adanta Group Behavioral Health Services, 259 Parkers Mill Road, Somerset, KY 42501; tel. 606/678–2768; FAX. 606/679–5296; Sandra Renfro, QI Coordinator

Bluegrass Regional Mental Health–Mental Retardation Board, 1351 Newtown Pike, Lexington, KY 40511; tel. 606/253–1686; David Hanna, Director, Quality Assurance

Comprehensive Care Centers of Northern Kentucky, Inc., 722 Scott Boulevard, Covington, KY 41011; tel. 606/431–2225; David Lindemann, M.S.W., Director Substance Abuse Programs

Cumberland River Regional MH/MR Board, Inc., American Greeting Road, Corbin, KY 40701; tel. 606/528–7010; FAX. 606/528–5401; Robert Koehler, Substance Abuse Director

Jefferson Alcohol and Drug Abuse Center, 600 South Preston Street, Louisville, KY 40202; tel. 502/583–3951; FAX. 502/581–9234; Diane E. Hague, Director

Pathways, Inc., 3701 Lansdowne Drive, P.O. Box 790, Ashland, KY 41105–0790; tel. 606/329–8588; FAX. 606/329–8195; Richard Stai

RiverValley Behavioral Health, 416 West Third Street, Owensboro, KY 42301; tel. 502/684–0696; FAX. 502/683–4696; Gayle DiCesare

LOUISIANA

Addiction Recovery Resources of New Orleans, 401 Veterans Boulevard, Suite 102, Metairie, LA 70005; tel. 504/828–6700; FAX. 504/831–8949; Julia Clarke, Administrator

Greenbrier Behavioral Health Care Systems, 201 Greenbrier Boulevard, Covington, LA 70433; tel. 504/893–2970; FAX. 504/867–1150; Marty Dean, Director, Chemical Dependency

Meadowbrook Residential Treatment Center, 101 Meadowbrook Drive, Minden, LA 71055; tel. 318/371–1700; FAX. 318/371–9465; Jeffrey E. Morrow, Administrator

New Beginnings of Opelousas, Inc., 1692 Linwood Loop, Opelousas, LA 70570; tel. 318/942–1171; FAX. 318/948–9101; Kim Signorelli, Administrator

Vermilion Hospital for Psychiatric and Addictive Medicine, 2520 North University Avenue, Lafayette, LA 70507; tel. 318/234–5614; Johnny Patout, Director

MAINE

Community Health and Counseling Services, 42 Cedar Street, P.O. Box 425, Bangor, ME 04402–0425; tel. 207/947–0366; FAX. 207/990–3581; Joseph H. Pickering, Jr., Executive Director

MARYLAND

Allegany County Health Department Addictions Program, Willowbrook Road, Cumberland, MD 21502; tel. 301/777–5680; FAX. 301/777–5674; Rodger D. Simons, Administrator

Ashley, Inc., 800 Tydings Lane, Havre de Grace, MD 21078; tel. 410/273–6600; FAX. 410/272–5617; Leonard Angus Dahl, Chief Executive Officer

Baltimore Recovery Center (Inpatient Center), 16 South Poppleton Street, Baltimore, MD 21201; tel. 410/962–7180; FAX. 410/962–7194; Morris A. Hill, President

Charter at Hidden Brook, 522 Thomas Run Road, P.O. Box 1607, Bel Air, MD 21014; tel. 410/879–1919; Carol Koffinke, Chief Executive Officer

Edgemeade Residential Treatment Center, 13400 Edgemeade Road, Upper Marlboro, MD 20772; tel. 301/888–1330; FAX. 301/579–2342; Dr. James Filipczak

Glass Substance Abuse Program, Inc., 1777 Reisterstown Road, Suite 345, Baltimore, MD 21208; tel. 410/484–2700; FAX. 410/484–1949; Sheldon D. Glass, M.D., President

Hope House, Marbury Drive, Building 26, Crownsville, MD 21032; tel. 410/923–6700; FAX. 410/923–6213; William H. Rufenacht, Executive Director

Hudson Health Services, 1506 Harting Drive, Salisbury, MD 21802–1096; tel. 410/742–0151; FAX. 410/742–7048; Alfred Grafton, Clinical Coordinator

Maryland Treatment Centers, Inc., U.S. Route 15, Emmitsburg, MD 21727; tel. 301/447–2361; Mary A. Roby, Executive Director

Melwood Farm Treatment Center, 19715 Zion Road, P.O. Box 182, Olney, MD 20832; tel. 800/368–8313; Sue Krantz, Director

New Beginnings at Warwick Manor, 3680 Warwick Road, East New Market, MD 21631; tel. 301/943–8108; FAX. 410/943–3976; Larry V. Foxwell, Chief Executive Officer

New Life Addiction Counseling Services, Inc., 2528 Mountain Road, Suite 204, Pasadena, MD 21122; tel. 410/255–4475; FAX. 410/255–6277; Thomas Porter

Oakview Treatment Center, 3100 North Ridge Road, Ellicott City, MD 21043; tel. 301/461–9922; FAX. 301/465–0923; David C. Heebner, Administrator

Pathways Drug and Alcohol Treatment Center, 2620 Riva Road, Annapolis, MD 21401; tel. 410/573–5400; FAX. 410/573–5401; Marti Potter, Administrative Team Leader

Quarterway Houses, Inc., 730 Ashburton Street, P.O. Box 31419, Baltimore, MD 21216; tel. 410/233–0684; FAX. 410/233–8540; John E. Hickey, Ph.D.

Saint Luke Institute, Inc., 2420 Brooks Drive, Suitland, MD 20746; tel. 301/967–3700; FAX. 301/967–3953; Frank L. Valcour, Medical Director

Worcester County Health Department, 6040 Public Landing Road, P.O. Box 249, Snow Hill, MD 21863; tel. 410/632–1100; FAX. 410/632–0906; David A. MacLeod, Addictions Program Director

MASSACHUSETTS

AdCare Hospital of Worcester, Inc., 107 Lincoln Street, Worcester, MA 01605; tel. 508/799–9000; FAX. 508/753–3733; David W. Hillis, President, Chief Executive Officer

Baldpate Hospital, Baldpate Road, Georgetown, MA 01833; tel. 508/352–2131; FAX. 508/352–6755; Subhash C. Mukherjee, Administrator

Cape Cod Alcoholism Intervention and Rehabilitation Unit, Inc., d/b/a Gosnold on Cape Cod, 200 Ter Heun Drive, Box CC, Falmouth, MA 02541; tel. 508/540–6550; FAX. 508/540–6550; Raymond V. Tamasi, President, Chief Executive Officer

Cape Cod and the Islands Community Mental Health Center, 259 North Street, Hyannis, MA 02601; tel. 508/563–2276; FAX. 617/727–1861; Richard Dunnells

Caulfield Center, 23 Warren Avenue, Woburn, MA 01801; tel. 617/933–6700, ext. 328; FAX. 617/933–9119; Gail Hanson–Mayer, RNCS, M.P.H., Chief Operating Officer

Center for Health and Human Services, Inc., 370 Faunce Corner Road, North Dartmouth, MA 02747, P.O. Box 2097, New Bedford, MA 02741; tel. 508/995–4853; FAX. 508/995–1868; Warren Davis

High Point, 1233 State Road, Route 3 A, Plymouth, MA 02360; tel. 508/224–7701; FAX. 508/224–2845; Daniel S. Mumbauer, Chief Executive Officer

Spectrum Health Systems, Inc., 200 East Main Street, Milford, MA 01757–2808; tel. 508/634–1877; FAX. 508/634–1875; Roy Ross, President

MICHIGAN

ACAC, Inc., 3949 Sparks Drive, S.E., Suite 103, Grand Rapids, MI 49546; tel. 616/957–5850; FAX. 616/957–5853; Michael Durco, Program Director

AOS, Inc., (Associated Outpatient Services), 1331 Lake Drive, S.E., Grand Rapids, MI 49506; tel. 616/456–8010; FAX. 616/451–0020; Charles F. Logie, Jr., President

Adult/Youth Developmental Services, P.C., 23133 Orchard Lake Road, Suite 104, Farmington, MI 48336; tel. 810/477–0107; Dr. George Kates

Advanced Counseling Services, P.C., 20600 Eureka Road, Suite 819, Taylor, MI 48180; tel. 313/285–8282; FAX. 313/281–0402; Brian W. Matthews, Administrator

Advanced Counseling Services, P.C., 17199 Laurel Park Drive, Suite 312, Livonia, MI 48152; tel. 313/285–8282; FAX. 313/281–0402; Dr. Arthur Hughett

Alcohol Information and Counseling Center, 1575 Suncrest Drive, Lapeer, MI 48446; tel. 810/667-0243; FAX. 810/667-9399; John Niederhauser

Allegan Behavioral Health Services, Inc., 120 Cutler Street, Allegan, MI 49010; tel. 616/673-8735; FAX. 616/673-1572; Barbara A. Chamberlain, ACSW, CSW, Executive Director

Auro Medical Center, 1711 South Woodward, Suite 102, Bloomfield Hills, MI 48020; tel. 810/335-1130; Yatinder M. Singhal, M.D., Administrator

Boniface Human Services, 25050 West Outer Drive, Suite 201, Lincoln Park, MI 48146; tel. 313/928-8940; FAX. 313/928-5152; Ronald Berglund, Executive Director

Brighton Hospital, 12851 East Grand River Avenue, Brighton, MI 48116; tel. 810/227-1211, ext. 235; FAX. 810/227-1869; Deborah Sopo, President, Chief Executive Officer

Catholic Services of Macomb, 12434 Twelve Mile Road, Suite 201, Warren, MI 48093; tel. 810/558-7551; Linda Stum, Vice President, Client Services

Center for Behavior and Medicine, 2004 Hogback Road, Suite 16, Ann Arbor, MI 48105; tel. 313/677-0809; FAX. 313/677-0452; Gerard M. Schmit, M.D., Chief Executive Officer

Center for Personal Growth, P.C., 817 10th Avenue, Port Huron, MI 48060; tel. 810/984-4550; FAX. 810/984-3737; Fredric B. Roberts, Ed.D., Chief Executive Officer

Center of Behavioral Therapy, P.C., 24453 Grand River Avenue, Detroit, MI 48219; tel. 313/592-1765; FAX. 313/592-1864; Hollis Evans, Executive Director

Central Therapeutic Services, Inc., 17600 West Eight Mile Road, Suite Seven, Southfield, MI 48075; tel. 810/559-4340; FAX. 810/559-1451; K. G. Thimotheose, Ph.D., President, Chief Executive Officer

Charles Allen Ransom Counseling Center, Inc. (CHIP), 14695 Park Avenue, Charlevoix, MI 49720; tel. 616/547-6551; Patrick Q. Nestor, Executive Officer

Clinton-Eaton-Ingham, Community Mental Health Board, 808 Southland, Suite B, Lansing, MI 48910; tel. 517/887-2126; FAX. 517/887-0086; Judith Taylor, Ph.D., Executive Director

Community Care Services, 26184 West Outer Drive, Lincoln Park, MI 48146; tel. 313/389-7525; FAX. 313/389-7515; Kari Walker, Deputy Director

Community Programs, Inc., 1435 North Oakland Boulevard, Waterford, MI 48327; tel. 810/666-2720; FAX. 810/666-8822; Bernard P. Paige, Esq. Chief Executive Officer

Comprehensive Services, Inc., 4630 Oakman Boulevard, Detroit, MI 48204-4127; tel. 313/934-8400; Mary Doss

Cruz Clinic, 17177 North Laurel Park Drive, Livonia, MI 48152; tel. 313/462-3210; Ida Goutman, Administrator

Delta Family Clinic, 2303 East Amelith Road, Bay City, MI 48706; tel. 517/684-9313; FAX. 517/684-5773; Gary West

Detroit Central City, Community Mental Health, Inc., 10 Peterboro, Suite 208, Detroit, MI 48201; tel. 313/831-3160; FAX. 313/831-2604; George Gaines

Dimensions of Life, Inc., 3320 West Saginaw Street, Lansing, MI 48917; tel. 517/886-0340; FAX. 517/886-0505; Alfred K. Doering, Director

Dot Caring Centers, Inc., 3190 Hallmark Court, Saginaw, MI 48603; tel. 517/790-3366; FAX. 517/790-9156; Wendell Montney, Ph.D., Director

Downriver Guidance Clinic of Wayne County, 13101 Allen Road, Suite 200, Southgate, MI 48192; tel. 313/287-1700; FAX. 313/287-1661; Leroy A. Lott, M.S.W., Chief Executive Officer

Elrose Health Services, Inc., 1475 East Outer Drive, Detroit, MI 48234; tel. 313/892-4244; FAX. 313/892-1457; Ellsworth Jackson M.A., CSW, Program Director

Evergreen Counseling Centers, 6902 Chicago Road, Warren, MI 48092; tel. 810/983-3600; FAX. 810/264-6918; Donald Warner

Fairlane Behavioral Services, 23400 Michigan Avenue, Suite P-24, Dearborn, MI 48124; tel. 313/562-6730; FAX. 313/562-8840; Carlos Ruiz, Executive Director

Gateway Services, 333 Turwill Lane, Kalamazoo, MI 49006; tel. 616/382-9827; Thomas E. Lucking, Executive Director

Growth Works, Inc., 271 South Main Street, Plymouth, MI 48170; tel. 313/455-4095; Dale F. Yagiela, Executive Director

Guest House, Inc., Lake Orion Treatment Center, 1840 West Scripps Road, Box 68, Lake Orion, MI 48361; tel. 313/391-3100; Sister Mae Kierans, CSJ, Clinical Services Coordinator

Hegira Programs, Inc., Holiday Park Office Plaza, 8623 North Wayne Road, Second Floor, Suite 200, Westland, MI 48185; tel. 313/458-4601; FAX. 313/458-4611; Edward L. Forry, Chief Executive Officer

Highland Waterford Center, Inc, Holly Gardens, 4501 Grange Hall Road, Holly, MI 48442; tel. 810/634-0140; FAX. 810/634-3838; Michael J. Filipek, Executive Director

Huron Valley Consultation Center, 955 West Eisenhower Circle, Suite B, Ann Arbor, MI 48103; tel. 313/662-6300; Janet Ford, Administrator

Ionia County Community Mental Health Services, 5827 North Orleans, P.O. Box 155, Orleans, MI 48865; tel. 616/761-3135; FAX. 616/761-3992; Richard Visingardi

Jensen Counseling Centers, P.C., 26105 Orchard Lake Road, Suite 301, Farmington Hills, MI 48334; tel. 810/478-4411; FAX. 810/478-5346; Cynthia Sweier

Latino Family Services, Inc., 3815 West Fort, Detroit, MI 48216; tel. 313/841-7380; Pam Lynch, Director, HIV/AIDS

LifeLong Center, Inc., 2712 North Saginaw Street, Oak Business Center, Suite 13 D, Flint, MI 48505; tel. 810/235-1950; FAX. 810/235-2450; Georgia Herrlich

LifeWays, 1200 North West Avenue, Jackson, MI 49202; tel. 517/789-1208; FAX. 517/789-1276; Christina M. Thompson, Chief Executive Officer

Meridian Professional Psychological Consultants, P.C., 5031 Park Lake Road, East Lansing, MI 48823; tel. 517/332-0811; FAX. 517/332-4452; Thomas S. Gunnings, Ph.D., President, Clinical Director

Metro East Substance Abuse Treatment Corporation, Metro East Drug Treatment Corporation, 13929 Harper Avenue, Detroit, MI 48213; tel. 313/371-0055; FAX. 313/371-1409; Leslie B. Carroll, M.S., President

Michigan Counseling Services, 1400 East 12 Mile Road, Madison Heights, MI 48071-2651; tel. 810/547-2223; Marylyn Krzeminski, Clinical Director

Monroe County Community Mental Health Authority, 1001 South Raisinville Road, Monroe, MI 48161; tel. 313/243-7340; FAX. 313/243-5564; James Pacheco, L.L.P., Supervisor

NSD Building Number Five Clinic, 3506 Gratiot, Detroit, MI 48207; tel. 313/267-6718; FAX. 313/267-6110; Rick Talley

Nardin Park Recovery Center, 9605 Grand River, Detroit, MI 48204; tel. 313/834-5930; FAX. 313/834-4541; Annie B. Scott, Director

National Council on Alcoholism Lansing Regional Area, 3400 South Cedar, Suite 200, Lansing, MI 48910; tel. 517/887-0851; FAX. 517/887-8121; Nancy L. Siegrist, Executive Director

National Council on Alcoholism and Addictions, 202 East Boulevard Drive, Suite 310, Flint, MI 48503; tel. 313/767-0350; FAX. 313/767-4031; John A. Cnockaert, Ph.D., Executive Director

National Council on Alcoholism and Drug Dependence, 2927 West McNichols, Detroit, MI 48221; tel. 313/341-9891; FAX. 313/341-9776; Benjamin A. Jones, President, Chief Executive Officer

Neighborhood Service Organization, 220 Bagley, Suite 840, Detroit, MI 48226; tel. 313/961-4890; FAX. 313/961-5120; Angela G. Kennedy, Executive Director

New Center Community Mental Health Services, 2051 West Grand Boulevard, Detroit, MI 48208; tel. 313/961-3200; FAX. 313/961-3769; Roberta Sanders

New Era Alternative Treatment Center, Inc., 211 Glendale, Suite S/B, Highland Park, MI 48203; tel. 313/869-6328; FAX. 313/869-1765; Joseph Pitts, D.O.

New Hope Treatment Center, 3455 Woodward, Second Floor, Detroit, MI 48201; tel. 313/832-6930; FAX. 313/961-8090; Janice Kwiatkowski

New Perspectives Center, Inc., 1321 South Fayette Street, Saginaw, MI 48602; tel. 517/790-0301; FAX. 517/790-2333; Jimmie D. Westbrook, Chief Executive Officer

Northeast Guidance Center, 13340 East Warren, Detroit, MI 48215; tel. 313/824-5641; FAX. 313/824-8000; Cheryl Coleman

Northern Michigan Community Mental Health, One MacDonald Drive, Suite A, Petoskey, MI 49770; tel. 616/347-7890; FAX. 616/347-1241; Alexis Kaczynski

O. Ganesh, M.D., P.C., 28165 Greenfield, Southfield, MI 48076; tel. 810/569-6642; FAX. 810/589-7922; Gerard Borovsky, M.A.

Oakland Psychological Clinic, P.C., 2050 North Woodward, Suite 110, Bloomfield Hills, MI 48304-2258; tel. 810/594-1200; FAX. 810/594-1306; Barry H. Tigay, Ph.D., President

Orchard Hills Psychiatric Center, P.C., 40000 Grand River Avenue, Suite 306, Novi, MI 48375-2137; tel. 810/426-9900; FAX. 810/426-9950; Dr. Hiten C. Patel, Chief Executive Officer

Parkside Mental Health and Clinical Services, Prenobscot Building, 645 Griswold Street, Suite 1808, Detroit, MI 40226; tel. 313/964-4930; FAX. 313/368-2605; Victoria Mayberry, Clinical Psychiatrist

Parkview Counseling Centers, 18641 West Seven Mile Road, Detroit, MI 48219; tel. 313/532-8015, ext. 146; FAX. 313/532-2840; Yvette Woodruff, Chief Executive Officer

Personal Dynamics Center, 23810 Michigan Avenue, Dearborn, MI 48124; tel. 313/563-4142; FAX. 313/563-2615; Pamela Czuj, Executive Director

Perspectives of Troy, P.C., 2690 Crooks Road, Suite 300, Troy, MI 48084; tel. 810/244-8644; FAX. 810/244-1330; Timothy Coldiron, Ph.D., Chief Executive Officer

Pioneer Counseling, 28511 Orchard Lake Road, Suite A, Farmington Hills, MI 48334; tel. 810/489-1550; FAX. 810/489-9767; Gary LaHood, Chief Executive Officer

Program for Alcohol and Substance Treatment, 110 Sanborn Avenue, Big Rapids, MI 49307; tel. 616/796-6203; FAX. 616/796-7430; John R. Kelly, Director

Propelled Therapeutic Services, Inc., 18820 Woodward Avenue, Detroit, MI 48203; tel. 313/368-2600; FAX. 313/368-2605; Cecelia Wallace

Psychological Consultants of Michigan, P.C., 2518 Capital Avenue, S.W., Suite Two, Battle Creek, MI 49015; tel. 616/968-2811; FAX. 616/968-2651; Jeffrey N. Andert, Ph.D. Administrative Director

Psychotherapy Institute of Mid-Michigan, P.C., 5000 Northwind Drive, Suite 226, East Lansing, MI 48823-5032; tel. 517/351-8994; Pamela Vandel, Licensure Coordinator

Redford Counseling Center, 25945 West Seven Mile Road, Redford, MI 48240; tel. 313/535-6560; Jo Ann Sadler, Director

Regional Mental Health Clinic, P.C., 23100 Cherry Hill Road, Suite 10, Dearborn, MI 48124-4144; tel. 313/277-1300; Gena J. D'Alessandro, Ph.D., Chief Executive Officer

River's Bend P.C., 33975 Dequindre, Suite Five, Troy, MI 48083; tel. 810/583-1110; FAX. 810/583-9399; James Keener

STM Clinic, One Tuscola Street, Suite 302, Saginaw, MI 48607; tel. 517/755-2532; FAX. 517/755-2827; Sara Terry-Moton

Sacred Heart Rehabilitation Center, Inc., 400 Stoddard Road, P.O. Box 41038, Memphis, MI 48041; tel. 810/392-2167, ext. 231; FAX. 810/392-2057; Michael Kelly, Director, Treatment Programs

Self Help Addiction Rehabilitation, Parent Facility, 1852 West Grand Boulevard, Detroit, MI 48208; tel. 313/894-1445; FAX. 313/894-5542; Anne C. Benion, Program Services Manager

Star Center, Inc., 13575 Lesure, Detroit, MI 48227; tel. 313/493-4410; Menuel L. Hill, Clinical Director

Sub Area Behavioral Service Center, 1309 Cleaver Road, P.O. Box 365, Caro, MI 48723; tel. 517/673-7575; FAX. 517/673-7579; Susan H. Clara, Program Director

Substance Abuse Council of St. Joseph County, 222 South Main Street, Three Rivers, MI 49093-1658; tel. 616/279-5187; FAX. 616/273-2083; Sally Reames, Administrator

Taylor Psychological Clinic, P.C., 1172 Robert T. Longway Boulevard, Flint, MI 48503; tel. 810/232-8466; Dr. Maxwell Taylor

The Center for Human Resources, 1001 Military Street, Port Huron, MI 48060-5418; tel. 313/985-5168; FAX. 313/985-9011; Thomas P. Pope, Chief Executive Officer

The Counseling Center, P.C., 1411 South Woodward, Suite 101, Bloomfield Hills, MI 48302; tel. 313/338-2988; Robert L. Bailey, Co-Director

Section C

The Kalamazoo Child Guidance Clinic, 2615 Stadium Drive, Kalamazoo, MI 49008; tel. 616/343-1651; Pat Hodskins, Administrative Assistant

The Salvation Army Turning Point Program at Metropolitan Hospital, 1215 East Fulton, Grand Rapids, MI 49503; tel. 616/235-1565; FAX. 616/235-1574; Robert E. Byrd, M.A., Director

VBH-Square Lake Corporation, 10 West Square Lake Road, Suite 300, Bloomfield Hills, MI 48302; tel. 810/338-0250; FAX. 810/338-0175; Andrew Blinder, M.A., L.L.P., Site Director

W. D. Lee Center for Life Management, Inc., 11000 West McNichols Road, Suite 212, Detroit, MI 48221; tel. 313/345-6777; Rose Jackson, Quality Assurance Coordinator

Washtenaw Council On Alcoholism, 2301 Platt Road, Ann Arbor, MI 48104; tel. 313/971-7900; FAX. 313/971-5950; Barry K. Kistner, Executive Director

MINNESOTA

Anthony Louis Center, 1000 Paul Parkway, Blaine, MN 55434; tel. 612/757-2906; FAX. 612/757-2059; Jon Benson, Chief Executive Officer

Charter Behavioral Health System of Waverly, 109 North Shore Drive, Waverly, MN 55390; tel. 612/658-4811; FAX. 612/658-4128; Nina T. Johnson, Director, Treatment

Fountain Lake Treatment Center, Inc., 408 Fountain Street, W., Albert Lea, MN 56007; tel. 507/377-6411; FAX. 507/377-6453; Steve Underdahl, Corporate Administrator

Guest House, Inc., 4800 48th Street, N.E., Rochester, MN 55903; tel. 800/634-4155; FAX. 507/288-1240; William C. Morgan, Director

Hazelden Foundation, 15245 Pleasant Valley Road, Center City, MN 55012; tel. 800/257-7800; FAX. 612/257-1055; Jerry Spicer, MHA, President

Missions, Inc. Programs, 3409 East Medicine Lake Boulevard, Plymouth, MN 55441; tel. 612/559-1883; FAX. 612/559-1195; Patricia Murphy, Executive Director

Omegon, Inc., 2000 Hopkins Crossroads, Minnetonka, MN 55343; tel. 612/541-4738; FAX. 612/541-9546; Barbara J. Danielsen, Executive Administrator

Pride Institute, 14400 Martin Drive, Eden Prairie, MN 55344; tel. 800/547-7433; FAX. 612/934-8764; David Dubois, Chief Operating Officer

MISSISSIPPI

Copac, Inc., 3949 Highway 43 North, Brandon, MS 39042; tel. 800/446-9727; FAX. 601/829-4278; Jerald Stacy Hughes, Jr., Ph.D., Executive Director

Jackson Recovery Center, 5354 I-55 South Frontage Road, Jackson, MS 39212; tel. 800/237-2122; FAX. 601/372-9505; D. Preston Smith, Jr., Executive Director

MISSOURI

Boonville Valley Hope, 1415 Ashley Road, Boonville, MO 65233; tel. 816/882-6547; FAX. 816/882-2391; Juanita L. Krebsbach, Program Director

Boys Town of Missouri, Inc., Route DD, P.O. Box 189, St. James, MO 65559; tel. 573/265-3251; FAX. 573/265-5370; Richard C. Dunn, ACSW, LCSW, Executive Director

Centrec Care, Inc., 12401 Olive Street Road, Suite 103A, St. Louis, MO 63141; tel. 314/576-9929; FAX. 314/576-1253; Mohammed A. Kabir, M.D., Chief Executive Officer

Comprehensive Mental Health Services, Inc., 10901 Winner Road, P.O. Box 520169, Independence, MO 64052; tel. 816/254-3652; FAX. 816/254-9243; William Kyles

Industrial Rehabilitation Center, 2701 Rock Creek Parkway, Suite 205, North Kansas City, MO 64117-7252; tel. 816/471-5013; FAX. 816/471-3808; Maurice L. Cummings, Executive Director

Marillac, 2826 Main Street, Kansas City, MO 64108; tel. 816/751-4900, ext. 4962; FAX. 816/751-4921; Sharon A. McGloin, Associate Director of Clinical Services

Piney Ridge Center, Inc., 1000 Hospital Road, Waynesville, MO 65583; tel. 314/774-5353; FAX. 314/774-2907; Rocky Carroll, Executive Director

Provident Counseling, Inc., 2650 Olive Street, St. Louis, MO 63103; tel. 314/371-6500; FAX. 314/371-6510; Kathleen E. Buescher, President, Chief Executive Officer

Research Mental Health Services, 901 Northeast Independence Avenue, Lee's Summit, MO 64086; tel. 816/246-8000; FAX. 816/246-8207; Melvin D. Fetter, Director, Operations

Swope Parkway Health Center, 3801 Blue Parkway, Kansas City, MO 64130; tel. 816/923-5800; FAX. 816/923-6950; E. Frank Ellis, Chief Executive Officer

MONTANA

Rimrock Foundation, 1231 North 29th Street, Billings, MT 59101; tel. 406/248-3175; FAX. 406/248-3821; David W. Cunningham, MHA, Chief Executive Officer

Rocky Mountain Treatment Center, 920 Fourth Avenue, N., Great Falls, MT 59401; tel. 406/727-8832; FAX. 406/727-8172; Ivan Kuderling, Administrator

NEBRASKA

O'Neill Valley Hope Alcohol and Drug Treatment Center, North 10th Street, P.O. Box 918, O'Neill, NE 68763; tel. 402/336-3747; FAX. 402/336-3096; Kaye Chohon, Program Director

Uta Halee Girls Village, 10625 Calhoun Road, Omaha, NE 68112; tel. 402/453-0803; FAX. 402/453-1247; Denis McCarville, President, Chief Executive Officer

NEW HAMPSHIRE

Beech Hill Hospital, New Harrisville Road, P.O. Box 254, Dublin, NH 03444; tel. 603/563-8511; FAX. 603/563-8771; Barbara R. Duckett, RN, M.S., Chief Executive Officer

Lakeview NeuroRehabilitation Center, Inc., 101 Highwatch Road, Effingham Falls, NH 03814; tel. 603/539-7451; FAX. 603/539-8888; Carolyn Ramsay, Administrator, Chief Executive Officer

Seaborne Hospital, Inc., Seaborne Drive, Dover, NH 03820; tel. 603/742-9300; Bud Charest, Administrator

Seacoast Counseling Associates, Department/Program of Seacoast Mental Health Center, Inc., 58 Washington Street, Portsmouth, NH 03801; tel. 603/431-8883; Deborah Lindberg, Quality Assurance and Improvement Coordinator

The Mental Health Center of Greater Manchester, 401 Cypress Street, Manchester, NH 03103; tel. 603/668-4111, ext. 187; FAX. 603/669-1131; Jane Gulmette, Quality Management Director

NEW JERSEY

Community Centers for Mental Health, Inc., Two Park Avenue, Dumont, NJ 07628; tel. 201/385-4400; FAX. 201/384-7067; Catherine Small

Comprehensive Behavioral Healthcare, Inc., 516 Valley Brook Avenue, Lyndhurst, NJ 07071; tel. 201/935-3322; FAX. 201/460-3698; Peter Scerbo

Daytop, New Jersey, 80 West Main Street, Mendham, NJ 07945; tel. 201/543-0162; FAX. 201/543-7502; Joseph Hennen, Executive Director

Discovery Institute for Addictive Disorders, Inc., P.O. Box 177, Marlboro, NJ 07746; tel. 908/946-9444; FAX. 908/946-0758; Robert C. Denes, Chief Executive Officer

High Focus Centers, Inc., 299 Market Street, Suite 110, Saddle Brook, NJ 07663; tel. 201/291-0055; FAX. 201/291-0888; David Nyman, Ph.D., Director, Program Development

Honesty House, 1272 Long Hill Road, Stirling, NJ 07980; tel. 908/647-3211; FAX. 908/647-7684; Charles H. Stucky, I.C.A.D.C., Executive Director

Lighthouse at Mays Landing, 5034 Atlantic Avenue, Mays Landing, NJ 08330; tel. 609/625-4900; FAX. 609/625-8158; Regina LaVerde, Executive Director

Mid-Bergen Center, Inc., 610 Industrial Avenue, Paramus, NJ 07652; tel. 201/265-8200; FAX. 201/265-3543; Joseph Masciandaro

Monmouth Chemical Dependency Treatment Center, Inc., 152 Chelsea Avenue, Long Branch, NJ 07740; tel. 908/222-5190; FAX. 908/222-5577; Brian J. Rafferty, Executive Director

New Hope Foundation, Inc., Route 520, P.O. Box 66, Marlboro, NJ 07746; tel. 908/946-3030; FAX. 908/946-3507; George J. Mattie, Chief Executive Officer

Patterson Army Health Clinic, Stephenson Road, Attn: MCXS-QI, Fort Monmouth, NJ 07703-5607; tel. 908/532-0945; FAX. 908/532-3452; Michele Steinert, Chief, Quality Management

Rutgers University Student Health Service, Hurtado Health Center, 11 Bishop Place, New Brunswick, NJ 08903; tel. 908/932-8429; FAX. 908/932-1525; Dr. Robert Bierman, Director

Seabrook House, 133 Polk Lane, P.O. Box 5055, Seabrook, NJ 08302; tel. 609/455-7575; FAX. 609/451-7669; Regina Marcacci, Chief Operating Officer

Sunrise House Foundation, Inc., 37 Sunset Inn Road, P.O. Box 600, Lafayette, NJ 07848; tel. 201/383-6300; FAX. 201/383-3940; Beth Anne Nathans, M.S., Chief Executive Officer

UMDNJ-University Behavioral Healthcare, 671 Hoes Lane, P.O. Box 1392, Piscataway, NJ 08855-1392; tel. 908/235-5900; Gary W. Lamson, Vice President, Chief Executive Officer

West Bergen Mental Healthcare, Inc., 120 Chestnut Street, Ridgewood, NJ 07450-2500; tel. 201/444-3550; FAX. 201/652-1613; Philip Wilson

NEW MEXICO

Four Corners Regional Adolescent Treatment Center, NCC Campus, Dorm Unit Two, P.O. Box 567, Shiprock, NM 87420; tel. 505/368-4712; Hoskie Benally, Chief Executive Officer

Tender Touch Industries, Inc., 4316 Carlisle Boulevard, Suite A, Albuquerque, NM 87107; tel. 505/884-6693; FAX. 505/884-4304; Dr. Michael Dismond

The Adolescent Pointe, Residential Treatment Center for Adolescents, 5050 McNutt Street-B, P.O. Box 6-B, Santa Teresa, NM 88008; tel. 505/589-4054; FAX. 505/589-2860; Lorenzo Barrios, L.M.S.W.

NEW YORK

Areba Casriel Institute, Inc. (ACI), 500 West 57th Street, New York, NY 10019; tel. 800/724-4444; FAX. 212/376-1824; Steven Yohay, Executive Director

Arms Acres, Inc., 75 Seminary Hill Road, Carmel, NY 10512; tel. 914/225-3400; FAX. 914/225-5660; Eileen Donohue, RN, MSA, Associate Executive Director

Bronx Alcoholism Treatment Center, 1500 Waters Place, Bronx, NY 10461; tel. 718/904-0026; FAX. 718/597-9434; Ronald B. Lonesome, M.D., Director

Charles K. Post Alcoholism Treatment Center, Building One, PPC Campus, West Brentwood, NY 11717; tel. 516/434-7209; Phillip A. Dawes, Director

Conifer Park, Inc., 79 Glenridge Road, Glenville, NY 12302; tel. 518/399-6446; FAX. 518/399-1361, ext. 240; Mr. Gail Harkness, Executive Officer

Cornerstone of Medical Arts Center Hospital, 57 West 57th Street, New York, NY 10019; tel. 212/755-0200, ext. 3100; FAX. 212/755-0915; Norman J. Sokolow, Chief Executive Officer

Cortland Medical, Four Skyline Drive, Hawthorne, NY 10532; tel. 914/347-2990; FAX. 914/347-3074; Jeffery Smith, M.D., Founding Medical Director

Creedmoor Alcoholism Treatment Center, 80-45 Winchester Boulevard, Queens Village, NY 11427; tel. 718/464-7500; FAX. 718/776-5145; Jose Sarabia, M.D., Medical Director

Dick Van Dyke Alcoholism Treatment Center, P.O. Box 218, Willard, NY 14588; tel. 607/869-4760; FAX. 607/869-4711; Thomas Nightingale, Acting Director

Dutchess County Department of Mental Hygiene, 230 North Road, Poughkeepsie, NY 12601; tel. 914/485-9700; FAX. 914/485-2759; Kenneth M. Glatt, Ph.D., Commissioner

Hope House, Inc., 517 Western Avenue, Albany, NY 12203; tel. 518/482-4673; FAX. 518/482-0873; Mary Ann Finn, Executive Director

Jewish Board of Family and Children's Services, Inc., 120 West 57th Street, New York, NY 10019; tel. 212/582-9100; FAX. 212/956-5676; Alan B. Siskind, Ph.D., Executive Vice President

John L. Norris Alcoholism Treatment Center, 1600 South Avenue, Rochester, NY 14620; tel. 716/461-0410; FAX. 716/461-4545; Thomas E. Nightingale, Director

Kingsboro Alcoholism Treatment Center, 754 Lexington Avenue, Brooklyn, NY 11221; tel. 718/453-3200; FAX. 718/453-4785; Jacqueline Cole, Director

Manhattan Alcoholism Treatment Center and Substance Abuse Services, 600 East 125th Street, New York, NY 10035; tel. 212/369-0500; Vera Ward, Chairperson

McPike Alcoholism Treatment Center, 1213 Court Street, Utica, NY 13502; tel. 315/797-6800, ext. 4801; FAX. 315/738-4437; John F. Crowley, M.S., CAC, Director

Middletown Alcoholism Treatment Center, 141 Monhagen Avenue, Middletown, NY 10940; tel. 914/341-2500; FAX. 914/341-2570; Richard C. Ward, Director

National Expert Care Consultants, Inc., d/b/a National Recovery Institutes, 455 West 50th Street, New York, NY 10019; tel. 212/262-6000; FAX. 212/262-9378; Roger Cohn, Executive Vice President

Research Institute on Addictions, 1021 Main Street, Buffalo, NY 14203; tel. 716/887–2386; FAX. 716/887–2215; Paul R. Stasiewicz, Ph.D., Coordinator of Outpatient Services

Restorative Management Corporation, 15 King Street, Third Floor, Middletown, NY 10940; tel. 914/342–5941; FAX. 914/344–2604; Dean Scher

Rochester Mental Health Center, 490 Ridge Road, E., Rochester, NY 14621; tel. 716/544–5220; FAX. 716/544–6694; Constance Aiello, RN, Acting President

Russell E. Blaisdell Alcoholism Treatment Center, R.P.C. Campus, Orangeburg, NY 10962; tel. 914/359–8500; FAX. 914/359–2016; Louis R. Brandes, M.D., Director

Saint Peter's Addiction Recovery Center (SPARC, Inc.), Three Mercy Care Lane, Guilderland, NY 12084; tel. 518/452–6700; FAX. 518/452–6753; Karen A. Giles, Executive Director

Salamanca Hospital District Authority, d/b/a Salamanca HealthCare Complex, 150 Parkway Drive, Salamanca, NY 14779; tel. 716/945–1900; FAX. 716/945–5016; Kenneth L. Oakley, Ph.D., Administrator

Seafield Center, Inc., Seven Seafield Lane, Westhampton Beach, NY 11978; tel. 516/288–1122; FAX. 516/288–1638; Mark Epley, M.B.A., Executive Director

South Beach Alcoholism Treatment Center, 777 Seaview Avenue, Building A, Second Floor, Staten Island, NY 10305; tel. 718/667–4218; FAX. 718/351–1958; Gerlando A. Verruso, Chief Executive Officer

St. Joseph's Rehabilitation Center, Inc., 99 Glenwood Estates, P.O. Box 470, Saranac Lake, NY 12983–0470; tel. 518/891–3950; FAX. 518/891–3986; Rev. Arthur M. Johnson, President, Chief Executive Officer

St. Joseph's Villa of Rochester, 3300 Dewey Avenue, Rochester, NY 14616–3795; tel. 716/865–1550; FAX. 716/865–5219; M. Judith McKay, President, Chief Executive Officer

St. Lawrence Alcoholism Treatment Center, One Chimney Point Drive, Ogdensburg, NY 13669; tel. 315/393–1180; FAX. 315/393–6160; Phillip Dranger, Director

Stutzman Alcoholism Treatment Center, 360 Forest Avenue, Buffalo, NY 14213; tel. 716/882–4900; FAX. 716/882–4426; Steven Schwartz, Director

The Astor Home for Children, 36 Mill Street, P.O. Box 5005, Rhinebeck, NY 12572–5005; tel. 914/876–4081; FAX. 914/876–2020; Sister Rose Logan, Executive Director

The Health Association–Main Quest Treatment Center, 774 West Main Street, Rochester, NY 14620; tel. 716/464–8870; FAX. 716/464–8077; Susan Costa

The Long Island Center for Recovery, 320 West Montauk Highway, Hampton Bays, NY 11946; tel. 516/728–3100; Steve Bassis

The Rhinebeck Lodge for Successful Living, Inpatient Treatment Program, 500 Milan Hollow Road, Rhinebeck, NY 12572; tel. 914/266–3481; Chandra Singh, Ph.D., Chief Executive Officer

Tully Hill Corporation, P.O. Box 920, Tully, NY 13159; tel. 315/696–6114; FAX. 315/696–8509; Cathy L. Palm, CPA, M.B.A., Executive Director

Valley View House, Inc., Swiss Hill Road, P.O. Box 26, Kenoza Lake, NY 12750; tel. 914/482–3400; FAX. 914/482–3516; William J. Coleman, Chief Executive Officer

Veritas Villa, Inc., RR 2-Box 415, Kerhonkson, NY 12446; tel. 914/626–3555; FAX. 914/626–3840; James Cusack, President

Villa Outpatient Center, 290 Madison Avenue, Sixth Floor, New York, NY 10017; tel. 212/679–4960; FAX. 212/679–4966; Richard Partridge, Executive Director

NORTH CAROLINA

Alcohol and Drug Abuse Treatment Center, 301 Tabernacle Road, Black Mountain, NC 28711; tel. 704/669–3400; FAX. 704/669–3451; William A. Rafter, Director

Amethyst Charlotte, Inc., 1715 Sharon Road, West, Charlotte, NC 28224; tel. 704/554–8373; FAX. 704/554–8058; Daniel J. Harrison, Assistant Vice President, Administrator

Fellowship Hall, Inc., 5140 Dunstan Road, P.O. Box 13890, Greensboro, NC 27415; tel. 910/621–3381; FAX. 910/621–7513; Rodney Battles, M.B.A., Executive Director

Forsyth–Stokes Mental Health Center, 725 North Highland Avenue, Winston–Salem, NC 27101; tel. 919/725–7777; Roy H. Haberkern, M.D., Area Director

Robeson Health Care Corporation, 1211 South Walnut Street, Fairmont, NC 28340; tel. 910/628–5200; FAX. 910/628–6205; Jinnie Lowery

The Wilmington Treatment Center, 2520 Troy Drive, Wilmington, NC 28401; tel. 910/762–2727; FAX. 910/762–7923; Keith G. Lewis, Executive Director

Unity Regional Youth Treatment Center, Highway 441 North, P.O. Box C–201, Cherokee, NC 28719; tel. 704/497–3958; Mary Anne Farrell, M.D., Director

Walter B. Jones Alcohol and Drug Abuse Treatment Center, 2577 West Fifth Street, Greenville, NC 27834; tel. 919/830–3426; Phillip A. Mooring, Director

OHIO

Bellefaire, 22001 Fairmount Boulevard, Cleveland, OH 44118; tel. 216/932–2800; FAX. 216/932–6704; Samuel Kelman

Campus Hospital of Cleveland, 18120 Puritas Avenue, Cleveland, OH 44135; tel. 216/476–0222; FAX. 216/476–2938; Joan Curran, Administrator

Careunit Hospital of Cincinnati, 3156 Glenmore Avenue, Cincinnati, OH 45211; tel. 513/481–8822; FAX. 513/481–7317; Judith Erwin, Director, Quality, Utilization Management

Center for Comprehensive Alcoholism Treatment, Inc., 830 Ezzard Charles Drive, Cincinnati, OH 45214; tel. 513/381–6672; FAX. 513/381–6086; Sandra L. Kuehn, Executive Director

Central Mental Health, 832 McKinley Avenue, N.W., Canton, OH 44703; tel. 216/455–9407; FAX. 216/453–0007; Richard Thompson

Community Drug Board, Inc., 725 East Market Street, Akron, OH 44305; tel. 330/434–4141; FAX. 330/434–7125; Theodore Paul Ziegler, Chief Executive Officer

Community Support Services, Inc., 150 Cross Street, Akron, OH 44311; tel. 330/253–9388; FAX. 330/376–6726; Arthur Wickersham

Crisis Intervention Center of Stark County, Inc., 2421 13th Street, N.W., Canton, OH 44708; tel. 216/452–9812; Lori S. Lapp, Executive Director

Family Recovery Center, 964 North Market Street, Lisbon, OH 44432; tel. 330/424–1468; FAX. 330/424–9844; Eloise V. Traina, Executive Director

Focus Health Care, 5701 North High Street, Suite 8, Worthington, OH 43085–3960; tel. 614/885–1944; FAX. 614/885–6665; Jo-Ann Boundy, Operations Manager

Glenbeigh Health Sources, Route 45, P.O. Box 298, Rock Creek, OH 44084; tel. 216/563–3400; FAX. 216/563–9619; Patricia Weston–Hall, Executive Director

Health Recovery Services, Inc., 28 North College Street, Athens, OH 45701; tel. 614/594–3511; FAX. 614/593–7258; Kenneth H. Pickering, Executive Director

INTERACT Behavioral Healthcare Services, Inc., (a Member of the Mount Carmel Health System), Administrative Offices, 1808 East Broad Street, Columbus, OH 43203; tel. 614/251–8242; James Shulman, D.O., Chief Executive Officer

Interval Brotherhood Home Alcohol–Drug Rehab Center, 3445 South Main Street, Akron, OH 44319; tel. 330/644–4095; Father Samuel R. Ciccolini, Executive Director

Lake Area Recovery Center–Chemical Dependency Treatment, Residential, Outpatient, Adult, and Adolescent, 2801 C Court, Ashtabula, OH 44004; tel. 216/998–0722; FAX. 216/992–2761; Kathleen Kinney, Executive Director

Lakeshore Treatment Centers, Inc., 1717 East Perkins Avenue, Sandusky, OH 44870; tel. 419/626–1633; Jack L. Manuel, Chief Operating Officer

Lincoln Center for Prevention and Treatment of Chemical Dependency, 1918 North Main Street, Findlay, OH 45840; tel. 419/423–9242; FAX. 419/423–7854; Nita L. Rider, Executive Director

Mahoning County Chemical Dependency Programs, Inc., 527 North Meridian Road, Youngstown, OH 44509; tel. 330/797–0070; FAX. 330/797–9148; Martin Gaudiose

McKinley Hall, Inc., 1101 East High Street, Springfield, OH 45505; tel. 937/328–5300; FAX. 937/322–4900; Judith O. Hoy, Chief Executive Officer

Mental Health Center, Inc., 1207 West State Street, Alliance, OH 44601; tel. 330/821–1995; FAX. 330/821–6080; Carol Hales, L.I.S.W.

NEO Psych Consultants, 819 McKay Court, Suite 101, Boardman, OH 44512; tel. 330/726–7785; Charles L. Boris, President

Neil Kennedy Recovery Clinic, 2151 Rush Boulevard, Youngstown, OH 44507; tel. 216/744–1181; FAX. 216/740–2849; Gerald V. Carter, Executive Director

New Directions, Inc., 30800 Chagrin Boulevard, Pepper Pike, OH 44124; tel. 216/591–0324; FAX. 216/591–1243; Michael Matoney, Executive Director

Parkside Behavioral Healthcare, Inc., d/b/a Parkside Recovery Services, 349 Olde Ridenour Road, Columbus, OH 43230; tel. 614/471–2552; FAX. 614/471–0167; Chris Gerber, Ph.D., President, Chief Executive Officer

Parmadale, 6753 State Road, Parma, OH 44134–4459; tel. 216/845–7700; Michael J. Haggerty, Associate Executive Director

PsyCare, Inc., 3530 Belmont Avenue, Suite Seven, Youngstown, OH 44505; tel. 216/759–2310; FAX. 216/759–0018; Douglas Darnall, Ph.D., Chief Executive Officer

Psych Systems of Greater Cincinnati, 11223 Cornell Park Drive, Suite 301, Cincinnati, OH 45242; tel. 513/530–8500; FAX. 513/530–8505; Chris Robinson, Program Director, Addiction Services

Quest Recovery Services, 1341 Market Avenue, N., Canton, OH 44714; tel. 330/453–8252; FAX. 330/453–6716; David Wills, Director Outpatient Services

Ravenwood Mental Health Center, 12557 Ravenwood Drive, Chardon, OH 44024; tel. 216/285–3568; FAX. 216/285–4552; David Boyle, Executive Director

Serenity Living, Inc. and Medical Professional Services, 210 West National Road, P.O. Box 217, Vandalia, OH 45377; tel. 513/898–8979; FAX. 513/898–3258; Justin J. Trevino, M.D., Medical Consultant

Specialty Care Psychiatric Services, Inc., 2657 Niles–Courtland Road, S.E., Warren, OH 44484; tel. 216/652–3533; Donna J. Dyer, M.Ed., L.P.C.C., President

Stepping Stone Recovery Center, 165 East Park Avenue, Niles, OH 44446; tel. 216/544–6355; FAX. 216/652–4781; Pamela Walters

Substance Abuse Services, Inc., 2012 Madison Avenue, Toledo, OH 43624; tel. 419/243–7274; FAX. 419/243–1505; Carroll Parks

The Campus, 905 South Sunbury Road, Westerville, OH 43081; tel. 614/895–1000; FAX. 614/895–3010; Robert J. Stevenson, Ph.B., CCDC, III

Transitional Living, Inc., 2052 Princeton Road, Hamilton, OH 45011; tel. 513/863–6383; Lila Webb, Administrative Assistant

Two North Park, Inc., 720 Pine Street, S.E., Warren, OH 44483; tel. 216/399–3677; FAX. 216/394–3815; Robert M. Kaschak, M.Ed., Executive Director

OKLAHOMA

Cushing Valley Hope, 100 South Jones, Cushing, OK 74023; tel. 800/722–5940; FAX. 918/225–7742; Mary Carder, Ph.D., Program Director

Jim Taliaferro Community Mental Health Center, 602 Southwest 38th Street, Lawton, OK 73505–6999; tel. 405/248–5780; FAX. 405/248–3610; Ted Debbs, Executive Director

Parkside, Inc., 1620 East 12th Street, Tulsa, OK 74120; tel. 918/582–2131; FAX. 918/588–8822; Quentin Henley

OREGON

Pioneer Trail Adolescent Treatment Center, 4101 Northeast Division Street, Gresham, OR 97030; tel. 503/661–0775; FAX. 503/661–4649; Robert E. Marshall, M.Ed., Administrator

Serenity Lane, Inc., 616 East 16th Avenue, Eugene, OR 97401; tel. 541/687–1110; FAX. 541/687–9041; Neil H. McNaughton, Executive Director

Springbrook Northwest, 2001 Crestview Drive, Newberg, OR 97132; tel. 503/537–7000; Carol Peake, Admissions Coordinator

PENNSYLVANIA

Abraxas I, Blue Jay Village, Box 59, Forest Road, Marienville, PA 16239; tel. 814/927–6615; FAX. 814/927–8560; James Newsome, Program Director

Alternative Counseling Associates, 438 High Street, Pottstown, PA 19464; tel. 610/970–9060; FAX. 610/970–4280; James O'Shea

Bowling Green Inn–Brandywine, 1375 Newark Road, Kennett Square, PA 19348; tel. 215/268–3588; FAX. 215/268–2334; Jeffrey J. Keglay, Administrator

Caron Foundation, Galen Hall Road, Box A, Wernersville, PA 19565–0501; tel. 610/678–2332; FAX. 610/678–5704; Douglas Tieman, President, Chief Executive Officer

Cedar Manor Drug and Alcohol Treatment Center, 109 Summer Street, P.O. Box 286, Cresson, PA 16630; tel. 814/886–7399; FAX. 814/886–8705; Mary McDermott

Charter Behavioral Health System at Cove Forge, New Beginnings Road, Williamsburg, PA 16693; tel. 800/873–2131; FAX. 814/832–2882; Jonathan Wolf, Chief Executive Officer

Clear Brook, Inc., 1003 Wyoming Avenue, Forty-Fort, PA 18704; tel. 717/288–6692; Dave Lombard, Chief Executive Officer

Conewago Place, Nye Road, P.O. Box 406, Hummelstown, PA 17036; tel. 717/533–0428; FAX. 717/533–1050; Daniel S. Baker, Executive Director

Eagleville Hospital, 100 Eagleville Road, P.O. Box 45, Norristown, PA 19403–0045; tel. 610/539–6000; FAX. 610/539–6249; Kendria Kurtz

Gateway Rehabilitation Center, Moffett Run Road, Aliquippa, PA 15001; tel. 412/766–8700, ext. 101; FAX. 412/375–8815; Kenneth S. Ramsey Ph.D., President, Chief Executive Officer

Gaudenzia, Inc.–Common Ground, 2835 North Front Street, Harrisburg, PA 17110; tel. 717/238–5553; FAX. 717/232–7362; Jerry McFarland, Program Director

Greenbriar Treatment Center, 800 Manor Drive, Washington, PA 15301; tel. 412/225–9700; FAX. 412/225–9764; Mary Banaszak, Executive Director

Keystone Center, 2001 Providence Road, Chester, PA 19013; tel. 215/876–9000; FAX. 215/876–5441; Daniel A. Kidd, Managing Director

Livengrin Foundation, Inc., 4833 Hulmeville Road, Bensalem, PA 19020–3099; tel. 215/638–5200; FAX. 215/638–2603; Richard M. Pine, M.B.A., President, Chief Executive Officer

Malvern Institute, 940 King Road, Malvern, PA 19355; tel. 610/647–0330; FAX. 610/647–2572; Valerie Craig, Administrator, Chief Executive Officer

Marworth, Lily Lake Road, Waverly, PA 18471; tel. 717/563–1112; FAX. 717/563–2711; James J. Dougherty, Senior Vice President

Milestones Community HealthCare, Inc., 1069 Easton Road, Roslyn, PA 19001; tel. 215/884–5566; FAX. 215/885–1746; Dr. Paul Volosov

Mirmont Treatment Center, 100 Yearsley Mill Road, Lima, PA 19063; tel. 215/565–9232; FAX. 215/565–7497; Thomas F. Crane, Executive Director

Penn Foundation, Inc., 807 Lawn Avenue, P.O. Box 32, Sellersville, PA 18960; tel. 215/257–6551; FAX. 215/257–9347; Bobbi L. Baker, Medical Records Manager

Renewal Centers, 2705 Old Bethlehem Pike, Quakertown, PA 18951; tel. 215/536–9070; FAX. 215/536–4788; Timothy R. Munseh, Program Director

Renfrew Center, Inc., 475 Spring Lane, Philadelphia, PA 19128; tel. 215/482–5353

Roxbury, 601 Roxbury Road, Shippensburg, PA 17257; tel. 717/532–4217; FAX. 717/532–4003; Claire F. Beckwith, Chief Executive Officer

Serenity Hall, Crossroads Program, 414 West Fifth Street, Erie, PA 16507; tel. 814/459–4775; FAX. 814/453–6118; Suzanne C. Mack, Director

The Bridge, 8400 Pine Road, Philadelphia, PA 19111; tel. 215/342–5000; FAX. 215/342–7709; Star Weiss, Program Director

The Terraces, 1170 South State Street, Ephrata, PA 17522; tel. 717/859–4100; FAX. 717/859–2131; Michael W. Beavers, President, Chief Executive Officer

Today, Inc., 1990 North Woodbourne Road, P.O. Box 908, Newtown, PA 18940; tel. 215/968–4713; FAX. 215/968–8742; John E. Howell, M.A., NCAC II, Executive Vice President

Twin Lakes Center for Drug and Alcohol Rehabilitation, P.O. Box 909, Somerset, PA 15501–0909; tel. 814/443–3639; FAX. 814/443–2737; Mark Sarneso, Executive Director

White Deer Run, Inc., Devitt Camp Road, Box 97, Allenwood, PA 17810–0097; tel. 717/538–2567; FAX. 717/538–5303; Stephen Wicke, Executive Director

RHODE ISLAND

CODAC, Inc., 1052 Park Avenue, Cranston, RI 02910; tel. 401/461–5056; FAX. 401/942–3590; Craig Stenning, President

Community Counseling Center, 160 Beechwood Avenue, Pawtucket, RI 02860; tel. 401/722–7855; FAX. 401/722–5630; Betsy Abrams, ACSW, L.S.W., ACDP, Manager

East Bay Mental Health Center, Inc., Two Old County Road, Barrington, RI 02806; tel. 401/246–1195; FAX. 401/246–1985; John P. Digits, Jr., Chief Executive Officer

Good Hope Center, Inc., John Potter Road, East Greenwich, RI 02818; tel. 401/826–2750; Alan Willoughby, Chief Executive Officer

South Shore Mental Health Center, Inc., 4705A Old Post Road, P.O. Box 899, Charlestown, RI 02813; tel. 401/364–7705; FAX. 401/364–3310; Richard Antonelli

The Providence Center for Counseling and Psychiatric Services, 520 Hope Street, Providence, RI 02906; tel. 401/276–4000; FAX. 401/276–4015; Charles Maynard

SOUTH CAROLINA

Charter Fenwick Hall Behavioral Health System, 2777 Speissegger Drive, Charleston, SC 29405; tel. 803/559–2461; FAX. 803/745–5196; Ann Battin, Chief Executive Officer

SOUTH DAKOTA

Keystone Treatment Center, 1010 East Second Street, P.O. Box 159, Canton, SD 57013; tel. 800/992–1921; FAX. 605/987–2365; Carol Regier, Executive Director

TENNESSEE

Camelot Care Center, Inc., 183 Fiddlers Lane, Kingston, TN 37763; tel. 615/376–2296; FAX. 615/376–1850; Dr. James Speiser

Compass Intervention Center, LLC, 7900 Lowrance Road, Memphis, TN 38125; tel. 901/758–2002; FAX. 901/758–2156; Robin Smith, Director of Clinical Services/Marketing

Cornerstone of Recovery, Inc., 1120 Topside Road, Louisville, TN 37777; tel. 615/970–7747; FAX. 615/681–2266; Dan R. Caldwell, President

Council for Alcohol and Drug Abuse Services, Inc., 207 Spears Avenue, Chattanooga, TN 37405; tel. 423/756–7644; FAX. 423/756–7646; James F. Marcotte, Executive Director

Cumberland Heights Foundation, 8283 River Road, Route Two, Nashville, TN 37209; tel. 615/352–1757; FAX. 615/353–4325; James Moore, Executive Director

Jackson Academy, LLC, 222 Church Street, Dickson, TN 37055; tel. 615/446–3900; Robert D. Glasner, Chief Executive Officer

New Life Lodge, 999 Girl Scout Road, P.O. Box 430, Burns, TN 37029; tel. 615/446–7034; FAX. 615/446–2377; Charles E. Anderson

Pine Pointe Center, Inc., 49 Old Hickory Boulevard, Jackson, TN 38305; tel. 901/664–7196; David Johnson, Executive Director

TEXAS

Alternatives Center for Behavioral Health, 5001 Alabama Street, El Paso, TX 79930; tel. 915/565–4800; FAX. 915/565–3163; Carol Anderson

Champions, 14320 Walters Road, Houston, TX 77273–3327; tel. 281/537–5050; FAX. 281/537–2726, ext. 24; Theresa Adams, Director of Intake

Community Residential Centers of San Antonio, 17720 Corporate Woods Drive, San Antonio, TX 78259–3500; tel. 210/494–1060; FAX. 210/490–8672; Patricia McLemore

Family Opportunity Resources, The FORGIVE Program, 6000 Broadway, Suite 106R, Galveston, TX 77551; tel. 409/740–0442; FAX. 409/740–0457; Gordon W. McKee, Administrator

Family Service Center, 4625 Lillian Street, Houston, TX 77007; tel. 713/868–4466; FAX. 713/868–2619; Lloyd Sidwell, Chief Executive Officer

Forest Springs Residential Treatment Center, 1120 Cypress Station Drive, Houston, TX 77090; tel. 713/893–7200; FAX. 713/893–7646; James Muska

Glass Treatment Center, 18838 Memorial South, Suite 103, Humble, TX 77338; tel. 713/666–9811; FAX. 713/446–5292; George S. Glass, M.D., Medical Director

La Hacienda Treatment Center, FM Road 1340, P.O. Box One, Hunt, TX 78024; tel. 210/238–4222; FAX. 210/238–4070; Frank J. Sadlack, Ph.D., C.A.S., Executive Director

New Dimensions Day Treatment, 18333 Egret Bay Boulevard, Suite 560, Houston, TX 77058; tel. 713/333–2284; FAX. 713/333–0221; Valarie Corbett, Quality Assurance, Coordinator

New Spirit, Inc., 2411 Fountainview Drive, Suite 175, Houston, TX 77057–4803; tel. 713/975–1580; FAX. 713/975–0228; Tom Blocher, M.D., President

New View Partial Hospitalization Centre, Inc., 4310 Dowlen Road, Suite 13, Beaumont, TX 77706; tel. 409/892–0009; Darla Tortorice, Nursing Coordinator

River Oaks Academy Day Hospital, 8120 Westglen, Houston, TX 77063; tel. 713/783–7200; FAX. 713/783–7286; Sandra E. Phares, Chief Executive Officer

Saint Joseph's Day Treatment Center, 1201 Corpus Christi, Laredo, TX 78040; tel. 210/718–2273; FAX. 210/726–6357; Jose G. Garcia, M.D., M.P.H., Medical Director

Shoreline, Inc., 1220 Gregory, P.O. Box 23, Taft, TX 78390; tel. 512/528–3356; FAX. 512/528–3249; Bob D. Nevill, Chief Executive Officer

Summer Sky Treatment Center, 1100 McCart Street, Stephenville, TX 76401; tel. 800/588–2907; FAX. 817/968–4509; Cathern Brooks, Chief Executive Officer

Sundown Ranch, Inc., Route Four, Box 182, Canton, TX 75103; tel. 903/479–3933; FAX. 903/479–3999; Richard Boardman, Chief Executive Officer

Synergy Partial Hospital, 5631 Dolores Street, Houston, TX 77057; tel. 713/952–0207; FAX. 713/784–8183; Alfredia J. Reed, Program Administrator

The Country Place Adolescent Residential Treatment Center, 3612 Parker Road, Wylie, TX 75098; tel. 214/442–6002; FAX. 972/442–4804; Michael Hannah, Program Director

The Patrician Movement, 222 East Mitchell Street, San Antonio, TX 78210; tel. 512/532–3126; FAX. 512/534–3779; Patrick Clancey, Administrator

VA Health Care Center, 5001 North Piedras, El Paso, TX 79930–4211; tel. 915/564–7901; FAX. 915/564–7920; Edward Valenzuela

UTAH

Brightway at St. George, 115 West 1470 South, St. George, UT 84770; tel. 800/345–4828; FAX. 801/673–8420; Paula O. Bell, Director

Highland Ridge Hospital, 4578 Highland Drive, Salt Lake City, UT 84117; tel. 801/272–9851; FAX. 801/272–9857; Richard Bell, Chief Operating Officer

New Haven, 2096 East 7200 South, Spanish Fork, UT 84660, P.O. Box 50238, Provo, UT 84605–0238; tel. 801/794–1218; FAX. 801/794–1223; Mark McGregor, Chief Executive Officer

Sorenson's Ranch School, Inc., P.O. Box 440219, Koosharem, UT 84744; tel. 801/638–7318; FAX. 801/638–7582; Burnell D. Sorenson, Owner

Youth Care, Inc., 12595 South Minuteman Drive, Draper, UT 84020; tel. 801/572–6989; Robin Stephens

VIRGINIA

Comprehensive Addiction Treatment Services, 3300 Gallows Road, Falls Church, VA 22046; tel. 703/698–1530; FAX. 703/698–1537; Donald F. Silver, Assistant Vice President, Behavioral Health Services

Inova Kellar Center, 10396 Democracy Lane, Fairfax, VA 22030–0252; tel. 703/281–8500; FAX. 703/359–0463; Richard N. Leichtweis, Ph.D., Program Director

Mount Regis Center, 405 Kimball Avenue, Salem, VA 24153; tel. 540/389–4761; FAX. 540/389–6539; Gail S. Basham, Chief Operating Officer

The Life Center of Galax, 112 Painter Street, Galax, VA 24333; tel. 800/345–6998; FAX. 703/236–8821; Tina Bullins, Executive Director

Williamsburg Place, 5477 Mooretown Road, Williamsburg, VA 23188; tel. 800/582–6066; FAX. 757/565–0620; Thomas J. Brennan, ACSW, Administrator

WASHINGTON

92d Medical Group, 701 Hospital Loop, Fairchild AFB, WA 99011–5300; tel. 509/247–5127; FAX. 509/247–2170; Major Stuart Cowles

Seattle Indian Health Board, 606 12th Avenue, S., Seattle, WA 98114; tel. 206/324–9360; FAX. 206/324–8910; Ralph Forquera, Executive Director

Tamarack Center, 2901 West Ft. George Wright Drive, Spokane, WA 99204; tel. 509/326–8100; Elaine Schoenrock, Director, Nursing

Section C

WEST VIRGINIA

Olympic Center–Preston, (Adolescent Treatment Only–Drug Abuse Only), Route Seven West Manown, P.O. Box 158, Kingwood, WV 26537; tel. 304/329–2400; FAX. 304/329–2405; William W. Perkins, Executive Director

Shawnee Hills, Inc., P.O. Box 3698, Charleston, WV 25336–3698; tel. 304/345–4800; FAX. 304/341–0277; John E. Barnette, Ed.D., President, Chief Executive Officer

Worthington Center, Inc., 3199 Core Road, Suite Two, Parkersburg, WV 26104; tel. 304/485–5185; FAX. 304/485–0051; Dr. Fred Lee

WISCONSIN

DePaul Hospital, Inc., 4143 South 13th Street, Milwaukee, WI 53221–1170; tel. 414/281–4400; FAX. 414/325–3172; Kathleen M. Olewinski, Administrator

Eau Claire Academy Division of Clinicare Corporation, 550 North Dewey Street, P.O. Box 1168, Eau Claire, WI 54702–1168; tel. 715/834–6681; FAX. 715/834–9954; Marcia R. Van Beek, Executive Director

Lac Courte Oreilles Community Health Center, Route Two, Box 2750, Hayward, WI 54843; tel. 715/634–4795; FAX. 715/634–6107; Don Smith

Libertas Treatment Center, 1701 Dousman Street, Green Bay, WI 54303; tel. 414/498–8600; Patrick Ryan, Program Director

Section C

Abbreviations Used in the AHA Guide

AB, Army Base
ACSW, Academy of Certified Social Workers
AEC, Atomic Energy Commission
AFB, Air Force Base
AHA, American Hospital Association
AK, Alaska
AL, Alabama
AODA, Alcohol and Other Drug Abuse
APO, Army Post Office
AR, Arkansas
A.R.T., Accredited Record Technician
A.S.C., Ambulatory Surgical Center
A.T.C., Alcoholism Treatment Center
Ave., Avenue
AZ, Arizona

B.A., Bachelor of Arts
B.B.A., Bachelor of Business Administration
B.C., British Columbia
Blvd., Boulevard
B.S., Bachelor of Science
B.S.Ed., Bachelor of Science in Education
B.S.H.S., Bachelor of Science in Health Studies
B.S.N., Bachelor of Science in Nursing
B.S.W., Bachelor of Science and Social Worker
CA, California; Controller of Accounts

C.A.A.D.A.C., Certified Alcohol and Drug Abuse Counselor
CAC, Certified Alcoholism Counselor
CAE, Certified Association Executive
CAP, College of American Pathologists
CAPA, Certified Ambulatory Post Anesthesia
C.A.S., Certificate of Advanced Study
CCDC, Certified Chemical Dependency Counselor
C.D., Commander of the Order of Distinction
CDR, Commander
CDS, Chemical Dependency Specialist
CFACHE, Certified Fellow American College of Healthcare Executives
CFRE, Certified Fund Raising Executive
C.G., Certified Gastroenterology
CHC, Certified Health Consultant
C.L.D., Clinical Laboratory Director
CLU, Certified Life Underwriter, Chartered Life Underwriter
CMA, Certified Medical Assistant
C.M.H.A., Certified Mental Health Administrator
CNHA, Certified Nursing Home Administrator
CNM, Certified Nurse Midwife
CNOR, Certified Operating Room Nurse
C.N.S., Clinical Nurse Specialist
CO, Colorado; Commanding Officer
COA, Certified Ophthalmic Assistant
COMT, Commandant
C.O.M.T., Certified Ophthalmic Medical Technician
Conv., Conventions
Corp., Corporation; Corporate
C.O.T., Certified Ophthalmic Technician
CPA, Certified Public Accountant
C.P.H.Q., Certified Professional in Health Care Quality
CPM, Certified Public Manager
CRNA, Certified Registered Nurse Anesthetist
CRNH, Certified Registered Nurse Hospice
C.S.J.B, Catholic Saint John the Baptist
CSW, Certified Social Worker
CT, Connecticut
CWO, Chief Warrant Officer

D.B.A., Doctor of Business Administration

DC, District of Columbia
D.D., Doctor of Divinity
D.D.S., Doctor of Dental Surgery
DE, Delaware
Diet, Dietitian; Dietary; Dietetics
D.M.D., Doctor of Dental Medicine
D.MIN., Doctor of Ministry
D.O., Doctor of Osteopathic Medicine and Surgery, Doctor of Osteopathy
DPA, Doctorate Public Administration
D.P.M., Doctor of Podiatric Medicine
Dr., Drive
Dr.Ph., Doctor of Public Health
D.Sc., Doctor of Science
D.S.W., Doctor of Social Welfare
D.V.M., Doctor of Veterinary Medicine

E., East
Ed.D., Doctor of Education
Ed.S., Specialist in Education
ENS, Ensign
Esq., Esquire
Expwy., Expressway
ext., extension

FAAN, Fellow of the American Academy of Nursing
FACATA, Fellow of the American College of Addiction Treatment Administrators
FACHE, Fellow of the American College of Healthcare Executives
FACMGA, Fellow of the American College of Medical Group Administrators
FACP, Fellow of the American College of Physicians
FACS, Fellow of the American College of Surgeons
FAX, Facsimile
FL, Florida
FPO, Fleet Post Office
FRCPSC, Fellow of the Royal College of Physicians and Surgeons of Canada
FT, Full-time

GA, Georgia
Govt., Government; Governmental

HHS, Department of Health and Human Services
HI, Hawaii
HM, Helmsman
HMO, Health Maintenance Organization
Hon., Honorable; Honorary
H.S.A., Health System Administrator
Hts., Heights
Hwy., Highway

IA, Iowa
ID, Idaho
IL, Illinois
IN, Indiana
Inc., Incorporated

J.D., Doctor of Law
J.P., Justice of the Peace
Jr., Junior

KS, Kansas
KY, Kentucky

LA, Louisiana
LCDR, Lieutenant Commander
LCSW, Licensed Certified Social Worker
L.H.D., Doctor of Humanities

L.I.S.W., Licensed Independent Social Worker
LL.D., Doctor of Laws
L.L.P., Limited Licensed Practitioner
L.M.H.C., Licensed Master of Health Care
L.M.S.W., Licensed Master of Social Work
L.N.H.A., Licensed Nursing Home Administrator
L.P.C., Licensed Professional Counselor
LPN, Licensed Practical Nurse
L.P.N., Licensed Practical Nurse
L.S.W., Licensed Social Worker
Lt., Lieutenant
LTC, Lieutenant Colonel
Ltd., Limited
LT.GEN., Lieutenant General
LTJG, Lieutenant (junior grade)

MA, Massachusetts
M.A., Master of Arts
Maj., Major
M.B., Bachelor of Medicine
M.B.A., Masters of Business Administration
MC, Medical Corps; Marine Corps
M.C., Member of Congress
MD, Maryland
M.D., Doctor of Medicine
ME, Maine
M.Ed., Master of Education
MFCC, Marriage/Family/Child Counselor
MHA, Mental Health Association
M.H.S., Masters in Health Science; Masters in Human Service
MI, Michigan
MM, Masters of Management
MN, Minnesota
M.N., Master of Nursing
MO, Missouri
M.P.A., Master of Public Administration; Master Public Affairs
M.P.H., Master of Public Health
M.P.S., Master of Professional Studies; Master of Public Science
MS, Mississippi
M.S., Master of Science
MSC, Medical Service Corps
M.S.D., Doctor of Medical Science
MSHSA, Master of Science Health Service Administration
M.S.N., Master of Science in Nursing
M.S.P.H., Master of Science in Public Health
M.S.S.W., Master of Science in Social Work
M.S.W., Master of Social Work
MT, Montana
Mt., Mount

N., North
NC, North Carolina
N.C.A.D.C., National Certification of Alcohol and Drug Counselors
ND, North Dakota
NE, Nebraska
NH, New Hampshire
NHA, National Hearing Association; Nursing Home Administrator
NJ, New Jersey
NM, New Mexico
NPA, National Perinatal Association
NV, Nevada
NY, New York

OCN, Oncology Certified Nurse
O.D., Doctor of Optometry
O.F.M., Order Franciscan Monks, Order of Friars Minor
OH, Ohio
OK, Oklahoma
OR, Oregon
O.R., Operating Room
O.R.S., Operating Room Supervisor

OSF, Order of St. Francis

PA, Pennsylvania
P.A., Professional Association
P.C., Professional Corporation
Pharm.D., Doctor of Pharmacy
Ph.B., Bachelor of Philosophy
Ph.D., Doctor of Philosophy
PHS, Public Health Service
Pkwy., Parkway
Pl., Place
PR, Puerto Rico
PS, Professional Services
PSRO, Professional Standards Review Organization

RADM, Rear Admiral
RD, Rural Delivery
Rd., Road
R.F.D., Rural Free Delivery
RI, Rhode Island
R.M., Risk Manager
RN, Registered Nurse
RNC, Republican National Committee; Registered Nurse or Board Certified
R.Ph., Registered Pharmacist
RRA, Registered Record Administrator
R.S.M., Religious Sisters of Mercy
Rte., Route

S., South
SC, South Carolina
S.C., Surgery Center
SCAC, Senior Certified Addiction Counselor
Sc.D., Doctor of Science
Sci., Science, Scientific
SD, South Dakota
SHCC, Statewide Health Coordinating Council
Sgt., Sergeant
SNA, Surgical Nursing Assistant
SNF, Skilled Nursing Facility
Sq., Square
Sr., Senior, Sister
St., Saint, Street
Sta., Station
Ste., Saint; Suite

Tel., Telephone
Terr., Terrace
TN, Tennessee
Tpke, Turnpike
Twp., Township
TX, Texas

USA, United States Army
USAF, United States Air Force
USMC, United States Marine Corps
USN, United States Navy
USPHS, United States Public Health Service
UT, Utah

VA, Virginia
VADM, Vice Admiral
VI, Virgin Islands
Vlg., Village
VT, Vermont

W., West
WA, Washington
WI, Wisconsin
WV, West Virginia
WY, Wyoming

Index

Notes

Notes

Notes

Notes

Notes

Notes

Notes

Notes

Notes

Notes

Notes

Notes

Notes